Respiratory Care

Principles and Practice

THIRD EDITION

Dean R. Hess, PhD, RRT, FAARC
Assistant Director of Respiratory Care
Massachusetts General Hospital
Associate Professor of Anesthesia
Harvard Medical School
Editor-in-Chief
RESPIRATORY CARE

Neil R. MacIntyre, MD, FAARC
Professor of Medicine
Medical Director of Respiratory Care Services
Duke University Medical Center

William F. Galvin, MSEd, RRT, CPFT, AE-C, FAARC
Assistant Professor
Frances M. Maguire School of Nursing and Health Professions
Director of Respiratory Care Program
Administrative and Teaching Faculty
TIPS Program
Gwynedd Mercy University

Shelley C. Mishoe, PhD, RRT, FAARC
Dean, College of Health Sciences
Professor, School of Community and Environmental Health
Old Dominion University

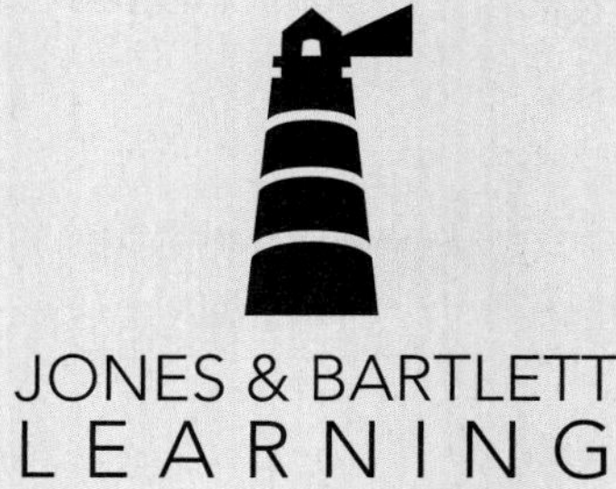

JONES & BARTLETT
LEARNING

World Headquarters
Jones & Bartlett Learning
5 Wall Street
Burlington, MA 01803
978-443-5000
info@jblearning.com
www.jblearning.com

Jones & Bartlett Learning books and products are available through most bookstores and online booksellers. To contact Jones & Bartlett Learning directly, call 800-832-0034, fax 978-443-8000, or visit our website, www.jblearning.com.

Substantial discounts on bulk quantities of Jones & Bartlett Learning publications are available to corporations, professional associations, and other qualified organizations. For details and specific discount information, contact the special sales department at Jones & Bartlett Learning via the above contact information or send an email to specialsales@jblearning.com.

06872-6

Production Credits
Chief Executive Officer: Ty Field
President: James Homer
Chief Product Officer: Eduardo Moura
Executive Publisher: Vernon Anthony
Executive Editor: Rhonda Dearborn
Associate Acquisitions Editor: Kayla Dos Santos
Editorial Assistant: Jamie Dinh
Associate Director of Production: Julie C. Bolduc
Marketing Manager: Grace Richards
VP, Manufacturing and Inventory Control: Therese Connell
Composition: Cenveo Publisher Services
Cover Design: Michael O'Donnell
Rights and Media Manager: Joanna Lundeen
Rights and Media Research Coordinator: Amy Rathburn
Media Development Assistant: Shannon Sheehan
Cover Image: © VikaSuh/ShutterStock, Inc.
Printing and Binding: LSC Communications
Cover Printing: LSC Communications

Library of Congress Cataloging-in-Publication Data
Hess, Dean, author, editor.
Respiratory care : principles and practice / Dean R. Hess, Neil MacIntyre, William F. Galvin, and Shelley C. Mishoe.—Third edition.
p. ; cm.
Preceded by Respiratory care : principles and practice / Dean R. Hess ... [et al.]. 2nd ed. c2012.
Includes bibliographical references and index.
ISBN 978-1-284-05000-4
I. MacIntyre, Neil R., author, editor. II. Galvin, William F., author, editor. III. Mishoe, Shelley C., 1955- , author, editor. IV. Title.
[DNLM: 1. Respiratory Therapy. WF 145]
RC735.I5
616.2'0046—dc23
2014024710

6048

Printed in the United States of America
19 18 10 9 8 7 6 5 4 3

Brief Contents

SECTION IV Applied Sciences for Respiratory Care 1113

SECTION V The Respiratory Care Profession 1299

Contents

Preface

It took 10 years between the first and second editions of *Respiratory Care: Principles and Practice*. The wait is much shorter for this, the *Third Edition*. This edition is, in essence, more of a continuation of a good thing rather than a completely new start. Ten years ago, some might have considered this text dead—but today it is alive and better than ever.

As in the *Second Edition*, patient assessment is covered at the beginning of the text, followed by respiratory therapeutics, respiratory diseases, applied sciences, and, finally, the professional aspects of respiratory care. The new edition offers us a welcome opportunity to build on the successes of the second edition. We have strived to hone this edition to address all of the topics important to contemporary practice in respiratory care. Recognizing the physiologic basis for respiratory care practice, we have added chapters specifically related to physiology; they complement the discussions of physiologic concepts already present in many of the chapters.

Use of extracorporeal membrane oxygenation (ECMO) has expanded considerably in recent years. Consequently, a new chapter dedicated to this topic has been added in the *Third Edition*.

The inclusion of new contributors to this edition has infused this text with new ideas and more thorough and contemporary coverage of many topics. No chapter has remained untouched; indeed, many have been substantially rewritten. This is a brand-new edition of an already solid text—not just the previous edition repackaged with a new cover. Many of the contributors are respiratory therapists, while others are physicians. This diversity underscores the close working relationship between therapists and physicians in everyday respiratory care practice. Many of the contributors are recognized leaders in the field.

All of the successful pedagogical features of the first and second editions of *Respiratory Care: Principles and Practice* have been retained in this edition. These features include the use of clinical practice guidelines, glossary terms, key points, and respiratory recaps. As with previous editions, the text is richly illustrated to enhance the learning experience. We have also added a new feature in this edition: Stop and Think boxes. Our intent in including them is to sharpen students' critical thinking skills. The Stop and Think boxes pose questions that often do not have a clearly right or wrong answer; they should stimulate discussion among students and faculty. The questions are posed, but the answers are intentionally absent.

The respiratory therapist of the 21st century must be a technologist, a physiologist, and a clinician. He or she is expected to be a clinical leader, a role that includes having input into the development of multidisciplinary care plans and implementation of respiratory care protocols. Moreover, contemporary practice is evidence based. Each of these important tenets of modern respiratory care practice is carefully and deliberately incorporated into this text.

The primary audience for this text is respiratory therapy students. We have written this text for students while considering the examination matrix of the National Board for Respiratory Care (NBRC), to ensure that all of the topics on the board exams (and more) are included. Nevertheless, this volume is more than just a text designed to ensure success on the board exams. It includes many topics that go beyond the NBRC exam matrix and that are intended to help students become well-rounded members of the patient care team.

Our goal was to make this text readable and to put the content within reach of students. As part of this effort, we have included boxes, tables, and illustrations to assist learning. We have carefully edited the text for consistency in writing style throughout, but we have not diluted the content. The material may be challenging in some places, but the intent was not to make it difficult. Rather, we seek to help students maximize their contributions when interacting with physicians and other members of the healthcare team. An important aspect of professional interactions is the ability to use the language that others use at the bedside; whether a respiratory therapist, physician, nurse, or other healthcare professional, the language should always be the same.

Although this text is intended primarily for students, it will prove useful for other individuals as a reference text. For the respiratory therapist who graduated from school some time ago, this text will serve as a refresher and update. For readers who are not respiratory therapists, the content should provide insight into respiratory therapy practice and serve as a reference text.

Innumerable persons must be thanked for their contributions to this project. First, I thank my co-editors. They embraced the vision and worked hard to make this text the best that it can be. Second, I thank all of the contributors, who dealt with my prodding to complete their chapters to my own and the publisher's expectations. Finally, I am grateful to the team at Jones & Bartlett Learning, who poured their talents into this project and went out of their way to make this text second to none. The commitment of the Jones & Bartlett team has kept this project alive and moving forward.

It is my hope that the third edition of *Respiratory Care: Principles and Practice* will assist students in mastering the art and science of respiratory care, that it contributes to improvements in the stature of the respiratory care profession, and—most importantly—that it improves the care of patients with respiratory disorders.

Dean R. Hess, PhD, RRT, FAARC

Features

Respiratory Care: Principles and Practice, Third Edition incorporates a number of engaging pedagogical features to aid in the student's understanding and retention of the material. A colorful layout enables ease of comprehension and supports the retention of important concepts. More than 580 full-color photographs and more than 300 tables and equations provide valuable insight into the fundamental aspects of respiratory care practice.

Chapter Outline and Objectives

Each chapter begins with a framework for learning the most important topics by presenting an **Outline** indicating the material to be discussed and **Objectives** that list the chapter's desired learning outcomes.

OUTLINE

Creating a Therapeutic Climate
Components of the Health History
Vital Signs
Techniques of Assessment
Physical Examination of the Lungs and Thorax
Assessment of Other Body Systems

OBJECTIVES

1. Discuss the factors essential in the creation of a therapeutic climate.
2. Explain three considerations of an effective health history.
3. Explain the relevance of cultural diversity in the history-taking process.
4. List the major components of a health history.
5. Identify the four major examination techniques.
6. Define common terms used in assessment of the respiratory system.

Key Terms

Key Terms list the most important new terms covered in the chapter; correlating definitions can be found in the end-of-text glossary.

KEY TERMS

auscultation
barrel chest
Biot respirations
bradypnea
bronchial breath sounds
bronchophony
bronchovesicular
orthopnea
pack years
pallor
palpation
paradoxical respiration
paroxysmal nocturnal dyspnea

Boxed Features

- ***Respiratory Recap*** Provides a review of key study points for core content
- ***Stop and Think*** New feature to this edition, which offers considerations for critical thinking and clinical decision making
- ***Age-Specific Angle*** Covers unique differences that are age specific—pediatric/neonatal focused or geriatric

Respiratory Recap

History of Present Illness

- Onset
- Location
- Duration
- Character
- Associated manifestations
- Relieving factors
- Treatment

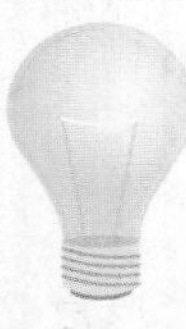

STOP AND THINK

You are seeing a patient for the first time. You are told that the patient has COPD. What information would you collect regarding the patient's health history?

AGE-SPECIFIC ANGLE

Compared with adults, infants and children have higher respiratory rates, higher pulse rates, and lower blood pressures.

Tables

Key information is presented in a clear format for review and reference.

TABLE 1-4
Glasgow Coma Scale

Observation	Score
Eye Opening	
Spontaneous	4
In response to voice	3
In response to pain	2

Equations

Helpful equations provide an example to review and compute clinical calculations.

$$\text{Anion gap} = [Na^+] - ([Cl^-] + [HCO_3^-])$$

Clinical Practice Guidelines

These Guidelines list a review of *Indications, Contraindications, Hazards and Complications,* and *Limitations* according to AARC Clinical Practice Guidelines. The Guidelines are crucial in the evaluation and management of patient care.

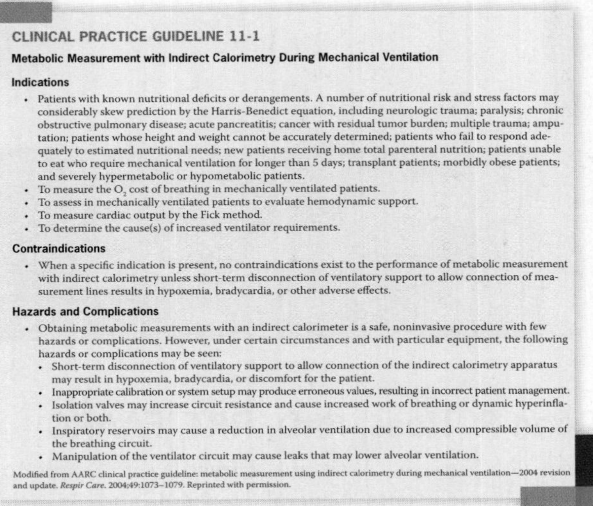

CLINICAL PRACTICE GUIDELINE 11-1

Metabolic Measurement with Indirect Calorimetry During Mechanical Ventilation

Indications

- Patients with known nutritional deficits or derangements. A number of nutritional risk and stress factors may considerably skew prediction by the Harris-Benedict equation, including neurologic trauma; paralysis; chronic obstructive pulmonary disease; acute pancreatitis; cancer with residual tumor burden; multiple trauma; amputation; patients whose height and weight cannot be accurately determined; patients who fail to respond adequately to estimated nutritional needs; new patients receiving home total parenteral nutrition; patients unable to eat who require mechanical ventilation for longer than 5 days; transplant patients; morbidly obese patients; and severely hypermetabolic or hypometabolic patients.
- To measure the O_2 cost of breathing in mechanically ventilated patients.
- To assess in mechanically ventilated patients to evaluate hemodynamic support.
- To measure cardiac output by the Fick method.
- To determine the cause(s) of increased ventilator requirements.

Contraindications

- When a specific indication is present, no contraindications exist to the performance of metabolic measurement with indirect calorimetry unless short-term disconnection of ventilatory support to allow connection of measurement lines results in hypoxemia, bradycardia, or other adverse effects.

Hazards and Complications

- Obtaining metabolic measurements with an indirect calorimeter is a safe, noninvasive procedure with few hazards or complications. However, under certain circumstances and with particular equipment, the following hazards or complications may be seen:
  - Short-term disconnection of ventilatory support to allow connection of the indirect calorimetry apparatus may result in hypoxemia, bradycardia, or discomfort for the patient.
  - Inappropriate calibration or system setup may produce erroneous values, resulting in incorrect patient management.
  - Isolation valves may increase circuit resistance and cause increased work of breathing or dynamic hyperinflation or both.
  - Inspiratory reservoirs may cause a reduction in alveolar ventilation due to increased compressible volume of the breathing circuit.
  - Manipulation of the ventilator circuit may cause leaks that may lower alveolar ventilation.

Modified from AARC clinical practice guideline: metabolic measurement using indirect calorimetry during mechanical ventilation—2004 revision and update. *Respir Care*. 2004;49:1073–1079. Reprinted with permission.

Key Points

A list of bulleted statements appears at the end of each chapter. These **Key Points** recap a summary of the most important points in the chapter.

Key Points

- The health history provides a detailed, chronologic record of the patient.
- The HPI offers a description of the onset of the problem, whether it developed suddenly, and the setting in which it developed.
- The four examination techniques commonly used are inspection, palpation, percussion, and auscultation.
- The use of accessory muscles implies an increased work of breathing.
- The assessment of respiratory expansion helps determine whether the lungs are expanding symmetrically.
- Auscultation of the chest allows assessment of diminished breath sounds, bronchial breath sounds, and adventitious breath sounds, such as crackles, rhonchi, wheezing, stridor, and pleural friction rubs.
- Listening to heart sounds involves notations of the rate and rhythm, extra heart sounds, and murmurs.

About the Editors

Dean R. Hess, PhD, RRT, FAARC

Dean R. Hess is Assistant Director of Respiratory Care, Massachusetts General Hospital, and Associate Professor of Anesthesia, Harvard Medical School. He has more than 40 years of experience in respiratory care, including clinical, research, teaching, and administrative responsibilities. Since 2008, he has been Editor-in-Chief of Respiratory Care, the official science journal of the American Association for Respiratory Care. He is on the Editorial Boards of the *Journal of Aerosol Medicine and Pulmonary Drug Delivery*, and *Simulation in Healthcare*. His research interests include aerosol delivery techniques, adult mechanical ventilation, and critical care monitoring. He is a Fellow of the American Association for Respiratory Care, the American College of Chest Physicians, and the Society of Critical Care Medicine. He has published more than 200 papers and several books. His books have been translated into several foreign languages. He has had a high level of professional activity, including committee appointments with the American Association for Respiratory Care, the American Thoracic Society, the Society of Critical Care Medicine, and two years as President of the National Board for Respiratory Care. He has lectured extensively throughout the United States and around the world. He has received numerous honors including the Forrest M. Bird Lifetime Scientific Achievement Award; American Association for Respiratory Care Life Membership; American College of Chest Physicians Simon Rodbard Memorial Honor Lecture; Jimmy A. Young Medal; Robert H. Miller, RRT, Award; Chadwick Medal; Shubin-Weil Master Clinician/Teaching Award; SCCM Presidential Citation; and the Hector Leon Garza MD Achievement Award. He has received teaching awards from the medicine residents at the Massachusetts General Hospital and the Harvard Pulmonary and Critical Care fellowship program.

Neil R. MacIntyre, MD, FAARC

Neil R. MacIntyre is a native of Southern California but received his medical degree and internal medicine training at Cornell University in New York City. After three years of service as a U.S. Navy flight surgeon at the Naval Aerospace Medical Research Lab in Pensacola, Florida, he returned to California for a pulmonary disease fellowship at the University of California, San Francisco. He was then recruited to the faculty at Duke University where he has spent the remainder of his career. At the present time, he is Professor of Medicine (with tenure), Senior Clinical Advisor of the Pulmonary/Critical Care Division, and Medical Director of Respiratory Care Services. His research interests range from clinical pulmonary physiology to large-scale randomized trials in COPD and acute respiratory failure. Currently he is on the Steering Committee of two large NIH multicenter trials: the Long-Term Oxygen Trial (LOTT), and the COPDgene Network. He was also on the Steering Committee of the NIH Acute Respiratory Distress Syndrome Network (ARDSnet) for its duration. To date he has published more than 200 peer-reviewed articles and reviews, is the editor/co-editor of eight books, and is on the editorial boards of five journals. He is the past president of the American Lung Association of North Carolina, and the National Association of Medical Directors of Respiratory Care, and he is the current Vice-Chair of the American Respiratory Care Foundation. Important honors include Alpha Omega Alpha, the Surgeon General's Award for Aviation Medicine, the Forrest M. Bird Lifetime Scientific Achievement Award, and the Jimmy A. Young Medal from the American Association for Respiratory Care. He is listed in both "Best Doctors in America" and "Who's Who in the World."

William F. Galvin, MSEd, RRT, CPFT, AE-C, FAARC

William F. Galvin is Assistant Professor in the Frances M. Maguire School of Nursing and Health Professions, Program Director for the Respiratory Care Program, and a member of the teaching and administrative faculty for the TIPS (Teacher Improvement Project System) Program at Gwynedd Mercy University (GMU). He has been a respiratory therapist for more than 40 years and has been on faculty at GMU since December 1981;

he first served as Director of Clinical Education for two years before becoming the Director of the Respiratory Care Program in 1983. In addition to his teaching and administrative role at TIPS, he also teaches in the Center for Life Long Learning and in the Bachelor's of Health Science Degree Program. He earned his Bachelor's Degree in Political Science from La Salle College and his Master's Degree in Education (with a concentration in Health) from St. Joseph's University. He is a registered and certified respiratory therapist, certified pulmonary function technologist, and certified asthma educator. He has provided numerous article reviews, abstracts, and contributing chapters for publishing companies such as Springhouse Corporation, Delmar/Cengage Learning, FA Davis, CV Mosby, Williams and Wilkins, W B Saunders/Elsevier, and Jones & Bartlett Learning. He has presented at the local, state, and national levels on topics such as communication skills, wellness, health promotion, disease prevention, patient education, interviewing and assessment skills, programmatic and regional accreditation, outcome assessment, recruitment and retention, test-taking strategies and techniques, and a variety of student survival topics and concepts related to the art of teaching and learning. He has served as a guest presenter for the AARC's Educator Academy, the AARC Asthma Educator Certification Course, the AARC COPD Educator Course, the Adult Critical Care Course, and most recently the AARC Registry Prep Course. He has served on countless professional and college-level boards and committees and is the recipient of numerous awards and honors. In 1996 the AARC distinguished him with the honor of life membership, and in 2005 he was inducted into the AARC Fellowship Program and was the recipient of the Education Section Practitioner of the Year Award. In 2008 he was awarded national honorary life membership in Lambda Beta National Honor Society for Respiratory Care and in 2012 provided the H. Fred Helmholtz Distinguished Education Lecture on the topic of *Excellence in Respiratory Care Education: Creating an Exemplary RC Program*. Bill is an active member of his parish, coaches Little League baseball and high school basketball, and is an avid sports enthusiast. He professes his greatest joy and passion to be in the classroom teaching and learning from his students.

Shelley C. Mishoe, PhD, RRT, FAARC

Shelley C. Mishoe is Dean of the College of Health Sciences at Old Dominion University and a tenured professor in the School of Community and Environmental Health. She has more than 35 years of experience in respiratory care, including teaching, research, and administration. She currently serves on the Board of Directors for the Association of Schools of Allied Health Professions, the Virginia Business Coalition on Health, Physicians for Peace, and Bon Secours Health System. She has held faculty positions at Chang Gung University in Taiwan, Capella University, Medical College of Georgia, and SUNY Upstate Medical University, including roles as director of clinical education and program director in respiratory care. She is an emeritus professor of Respiratory Therapy at Georgia Regents University. She is an inaugural Fellow of the American Association for Respiratory Care, a Fellow of the Association of Schools of Allied Health Professions, and a Fellow of the American Council on Education (ACE) Fellowship Program. Among leadership roles, she was on the Commission on Accreditation for Respiratory Care (CoARC) for 10 years, was the President (2009–2011) and gave the second annual Dr. H. Fred Helmholz Distinguished Education Lecture Series. She served for 15 years on the editorial board for RESPIRATORY CARE and in the AARC House of Delegates in roles as delegate, secretary, and parliamentarian. Other distinctions include the AARC Education Section Practitioner of the Year Award, Delegate of the Year Award from the AARC House of Delegates, and the Forrest M. Bird Literary Award. She has authored or edited numerous books and chapters, original research studies, peer-reviewed articles, case reports, editorials, book reviews, and abstracts, and has published papers on asthma, sleep-disordered breathing, rural health, shared governance, critical thinking, decision making, and problem-based learning. She is a frequent presenter at international, national, regional, and state meetings. She received a PhD in Adult Education from the University of Georgia, a MEd in Education from Augusta State University, and Bachelor of Science and Associate Degrees in Respiratory Therapy from SUNY Upstate Medical University.

Contributing Authors

Allan G. Andrews, MS, RRT
Clinical Specialist in Metabolics
University of Michigan Health System

Sherry Barnhart, RRT-NPS, FAARC
Coordinator of Discharge Planning
Arkansas Children's Hospital

Rhonda Bevis, EdD, RRT
Department of Diagnostic Therapeutic Science
Armstrong Atlantic State University

Rajesh Bhagat, MD
Pulmonary, Critical Care, and Sleep Medicine
University of Mississippi Medical Center

John Boatright, PhD, RRT
Program Director, Associate Professor
Henrietta Schmoll School of Health
Respiratory Care Department
St. Catherine University

Richard D. Branson, MSc, RRT, FAARC
Professor of Surgery
University of Cincinnati

Laura Brenner, MD
Pulmonary & Critical Care Medicine
Massachusetts General Hospital

Melissa K. Brown, BS, RRT-NPS
Neonatal Research Coordinator
Neonatal Research Institute
Sharp Mary Birch Hospital for Women and Newborns

Robert L. Chatburn, MHHS, RRT-NPS, FAARC
Clinical Research Manager, Respiratory Institute
Cleveland Clinic
Adjunct Professor, Department of Medicine
Lerner College of Medicine of Case Western Reserve University

Bashir A. Chaudhary, FAASM, FACCP
Assistant Dean for Clinical Affairs
School of Allied Health Sciences
Director, Sleep Institute of Augusta
Medical College of Georgia

Francis C. Cordova, MD
Associate Professor of Medicine
Division of Pulmonary and Critical Care Medicine
Temple University School of Medicine

Christopher E. Cox, MD, MHA, MPH
Associate Professor of Medicine
Division of Pulmonary, Allergy, and Critical Care
Duke University Medical Center

Gerard J. Criner, MD, FACP, FACCP
Professor of Medicine
Director of Pulmonary and Critical Care Medicine
Temple Lung Center

Rebecca H. Crouch, PT, DPT, MS, CCS, FAACVPR
Clinical Director of Pulmonary Rehabilitation
Duke University Medical Center

John D. Davies, MA, RRT, FAARC
Respiratory Care Services
Duke University Medical Center

William Downey III, MD
Medical Director, Interventional Cardiology
Sanger Heart and Vascular Institute

Crystal L. Dunlevy, EdD, RRT
Clinical Associate Professor, Respiratory Therapy Division
The Ohio State University

Maha Farhat, MD
Pulmonary & Critical Care Medicine
Massachusetts General Hospital

Daniel F. Fisher, MS, RRT
Assistant Director, Respiratory Care Services
Massachusetts General Hospital

Donna D. Gardner, MSHP, RRT
Associate Professor and Department Chair
Department of Respiratory Care
University of Texas Health Science Center at San Antonio

Michael Gentile, MS, RRT, FAARC
Vice-Chair, Institutional Animal Care and Use Committee
Duke University Medical Center

Andrew J. Ghio, MD
Assistant Consulting Professor
Division of Pulmonary and Critical Care Medicine
Department of Medicine
Duke University Medical Center

Lynda T. Goodfellow, EdD, RRT, AE-C, FAARC
Associate Professor and Director
School of Health Professions, College of Health and Human Sciences
Georgia State University

Carl F. Haas, MLS, RRT, FAARC
Educational Coordinator
University of Michigan Health System

Charles William Hargett III, MD
Assistant Professor of Medicine
Division of Pulmonary, Allergy, and Critical Care Medicine
Duke University Medical Center

Jeffrey Haynes, RRT, RPFT
St. Joseph Hospital
Pulmonary Function Laboratory
St. Joseph Hospital

Garry W. Kauffman, MPA, RRT, FAARC
Respiratory Care
Wake Forest Baptist Medical Center

Angela King, BS, RPFT, RRT-NPS
Owner and President
Mobile Medical Maintenance—Clinical Division

Puja Kohli, MD
Pulmonary & Critical Care Medicine
Massachusetts General Hospital

Bryan Kraft, MD
Medical Instructor, Department of Medicine
Division of Pulmonary, Allergy, and Critical Care
Duke University Medical Center

Christopher D. Lyman, PharmD
Department of Pharmacy
Massachusetts General Hospital

Thomas Malinowski, BS, RRT, FAARC
Director, Cardiopulmonary Services
Mary Washington Hospital

Douglas E. Masini, EdD, RPFT, RRT-NPS, AE-C, FAARC
Director, Respiratory Therapy
Armstrong Atlantic State University

Robert McCoy, RRT, FAARC
Managing Director
Valley Inspired Products, Inc.

Christine J. Moore, MEd, RRT-NPS, CPFT
Lecturer and Laboratory Coordinator
Armstrong Atlantic State University

Morgan Mullaney, MD
Medical Instructor, Department of Medicine
Division of Pulmonary, Allergy, and Critical Care
Duke University Medical Center

John Mullarkey, BA, RRT, AE-C
Clinical Manager, Respiratory Care Department
Temple University Hospital

Timothy R. Myers, BS, RRT-NPS
American Association for Respiratory Care

Alexander S. Niven, MD
Director of Medical Education and DIO
Madigan Army Medical Center
Associate Professor of Medicine
Uniformed Services University of the Health Sciences

Catherine O'Malley, RRT
Ann & Robert H. Lurie Children's Hospital of Chicago

Timothy Op't Holt, EdD, RRT, AE-C, FAARC
Professor of Cardiorespiratory Care
University of South Alabama

William C. Pruitt, MBA, RRT, CPFT, AE-C
Director of Clinical Education for the Cardiorespiratory Sciences
University of South Alabama

Craig R. Rackley, MD
Medical Instructor, Department of Medicine
Division of Pulmonary, Allergy, and Critical Care Medicine
Duke University Medical Center

Kyle J. Rehder, MD
Assistant Professor of Pediatrics
Duke Children's Hospital
Duke University Medical Center

Marcos I. Restrepo, MD, MSc
South Texas Veterans Health Care System
The University of Texas Health Sciences Center at San Antonio

Ruben D. Restrepo, MD, RRT, FAARC
Associate Professor, Department of Respiratory Care
The University of Texas Health Sciences Center at San Antonio

Bryce R. H. Robinson, MD
Associate Professor of Surgery
University of Cincinnati

Dario Rodriquez Jr., RRT
Department of Surgery
University of Cincinnati

Bruce K. Rubin, MEngr, MD, MBA, FRCPC
Jessie Ball duPont Professor and Chairman, Department of Pediatrics
Professor of Biomedical Engineering
Children's Hospital of Richmond
Virginia Commonwealth University School of Medicine

Michal Senitko, MD
Medicine, Pulmonary/Critical Care Division
University of Mississippi Medical Center

Georgianna Sergakis, PhD, RRT
Assistant Professor, Clinical Program Director
Respiratory Therapy Division
The Ohio State University

Scott L. Shofer, MD, PhD
Assistant Professor, Division of Pulmonary, Allergy, and Critical Care
Duke University Medical Center

Kathy A. Short, RN, RRT
Director of Respiratory Care
University of North Carolina Hospitals

Mark Simmons, MSed, RRT-NPS, RPFT
Program Director, Respiratory Care
York College of Pennsylvania

Priscilla Simmons, MSN, EdD, APRN, BC
Professor of Nursing
Eastern Mennonite University

Jaspal Singh, MD, MHS, FCCP
Medical Director
Carolinas Medical Center

Mark S. Siobal, BS, RRT, FAARC
Clinical Specialist, Respiratory Care Services
San Francisco General Hospital

Helen M. Sorenson, MS, RRT, FAARC
Associate Professor, Department of Respiratory Care
University of Texas Health Sciences Center

William S. Stigler, MD
Assistant Professor, Pulmonary and Critical Care
University of Alabama at Birmingham

Shawna Strickland, PhD, RRT-NPS, AE-C, FAARC
Associate Executive Director
American Association for Respiratory Care

Arthur Taft, PhD, RRT
Associate Professor, Respiratory Therapy
Georgia Regents University

Amy Treece, MD
Pulmonary Disease, Critical Care and Sleep Medicine/ Lung Center
Greenville Health System

David Turner, MD
Pediatric Critical Care
Duke University Medical Center

Sarah Varekojis, PhD, RRT
Assistant Professor and Director of Clinical Education
Respiratory Therapy Division
The Ohio State University

Ellen Volker, MD, MSPH
Medical Instructor, Department of Medicine
Division of Pulmonary, Allergy, and Critical Care
Duke University Medical Center

Teresa A. Volsko, MHHS, RRT, FAARC
Director of Respiratory Care and Transport
Akron Children's Hospital

Momen M. Wahidi, MD, MBA
Director, Interventional Pulmonology and Bronchoscopy
Associate Professor of Medicine
Duke University Medical Center

Jeffrey J. Ward, MEd, RRT, FAARC
Mayo Clinic Multidisciplinary Medical Simulation Center

Andrew J. Weirauch, BS, RRT
Clinical Specialist
University of Michigan Health System

John Williams, MD
Pulmonary and Critical Care
University of Alabama at Birmingham

Nicholas Wysham, MD
Division of Pulmonary, Allergy, and Critical Care
Duke University Medical Center

Reviewers

Brent Blevins, BSN, RN, RRT
Registered Nurse
Riverpark Hospital

Amy Ceconi, PhD, RRT, RPFT, NPS
Program Director
Bergen Community College

Lea Endress, BS, RRT, RPFT
Respiratory Therapy Instructor
Respiratory Therapy Program
San Joaquin Valley College

David Fry, BS, RRT, CPFT
Director of Clinical Education
Department of Respiratory Care
Temple College

Wesley M. Granger, PhD, RRT
Associate Professor, Program Director
Department of Clinical and Diagnostic Sciences
Respiratory Therapy Program
The University of Alabama at Birmingham

Jennifer Gresham, MA, RRT-NPS
Assistant Professor
Department of Respiratory Care
Midwestern State University

Michael Haines, MPH, RRT-NPS, AE-C
Respiratory Therapy Instructor
San Joaquin Valley College

Suezette Hicks, BA, RRT-CPFT
Director Respiratory Care Program
Black River Technical College

Lisa Johnson, MS, RRT-NPS
Clinical Assistant Professor
Director of Clinical Education
Respiratory Care Program
Stony Brook University

Robert L. Joyner Jr., PhD, RRT, FAARC
Director, Respiratory Therapy Program
Associate Professor and Chair
Department of Health Sciences
Salisbury University

Traci Marin, MPH, RRT
Program Director
Victor Valley College

Cynthia McKinley, RRT
Assistant Professor
Director of Clinical Education, Respiratory Care Program
Lamar Institute of Technology

Larry McMullin, MM, RRT, RPFT
Clinical Coordinator, Assistant Professor
Respiratory Care Program
Ferris State University

Kim J. Morris-Garcia, MEd, RRT, NPS
Associate Master Technical Instructor
Director of Clinical Education
Respiratory Therapy and BAT Programs
University of Texas at Brownsville and Texas Southmost College

Jennifer M. Purdue, MA, RRT-NPS, AE-C, RN
Associate Professor, Program Chair
Department of Respiratory Care
Ivy Tech Community College

Christopher Rowse, MS, RRT, RPFT, RPSGT
Professor
Northern Essex Community College

Georgianna Sergakis, PhD, RRT
Assistant Professor, Clinical Program Director
Respiratory Therapy Division
The Ohio State University

Frank Sinsheimer, RRT, EdD
Professor Emeritus, Respiratory Therapy
Los Angeles Valley College

Stephen G. Smith, MPA, RT, RRT
Chair, New York State Board for Respiratory Therapy
Clinical Assistant Professor
Stony Brook University

Don Steinert, MA, RRT, MT, CLS
Associate Professor
University of the District of Columbia

Chris Trotter, MH, EdS, RRT
Associate Professor, Respiratory Care Coordinator Degree Advancement Program
St Mary's/Marshall University
Staff Therapist
Charleston Area Medical Center

LaVerne Yousey, RRT, MSTE
Professor of Respiratory Care, Emeritus
University of Akron

Rick Zahodnic, PhD, RRT-NPS, RPFT, AE-C
Clinical Coordinator
Respiratory Therapy Program
Macomb Community College

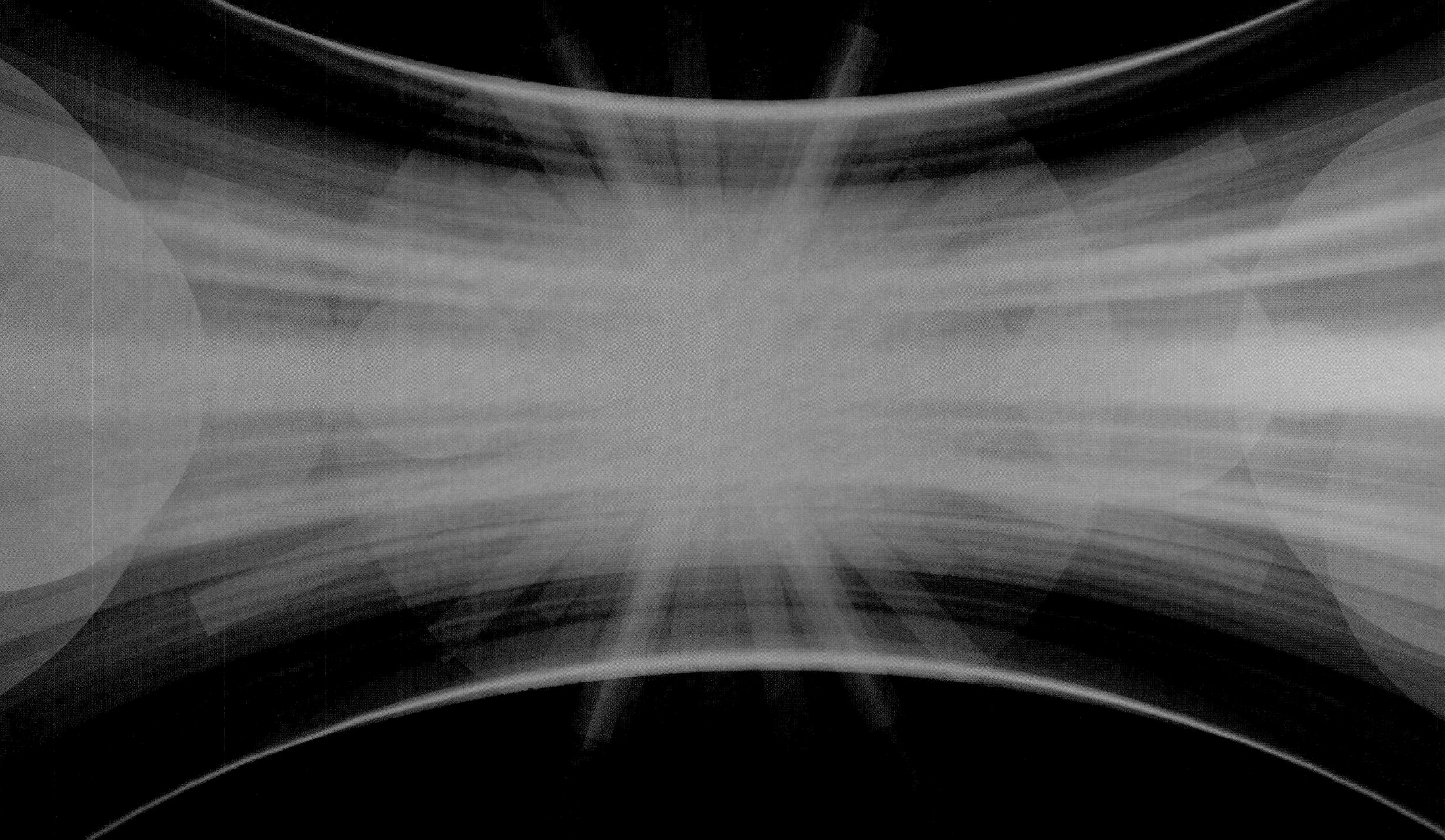

Section I
Respiratory Assessment

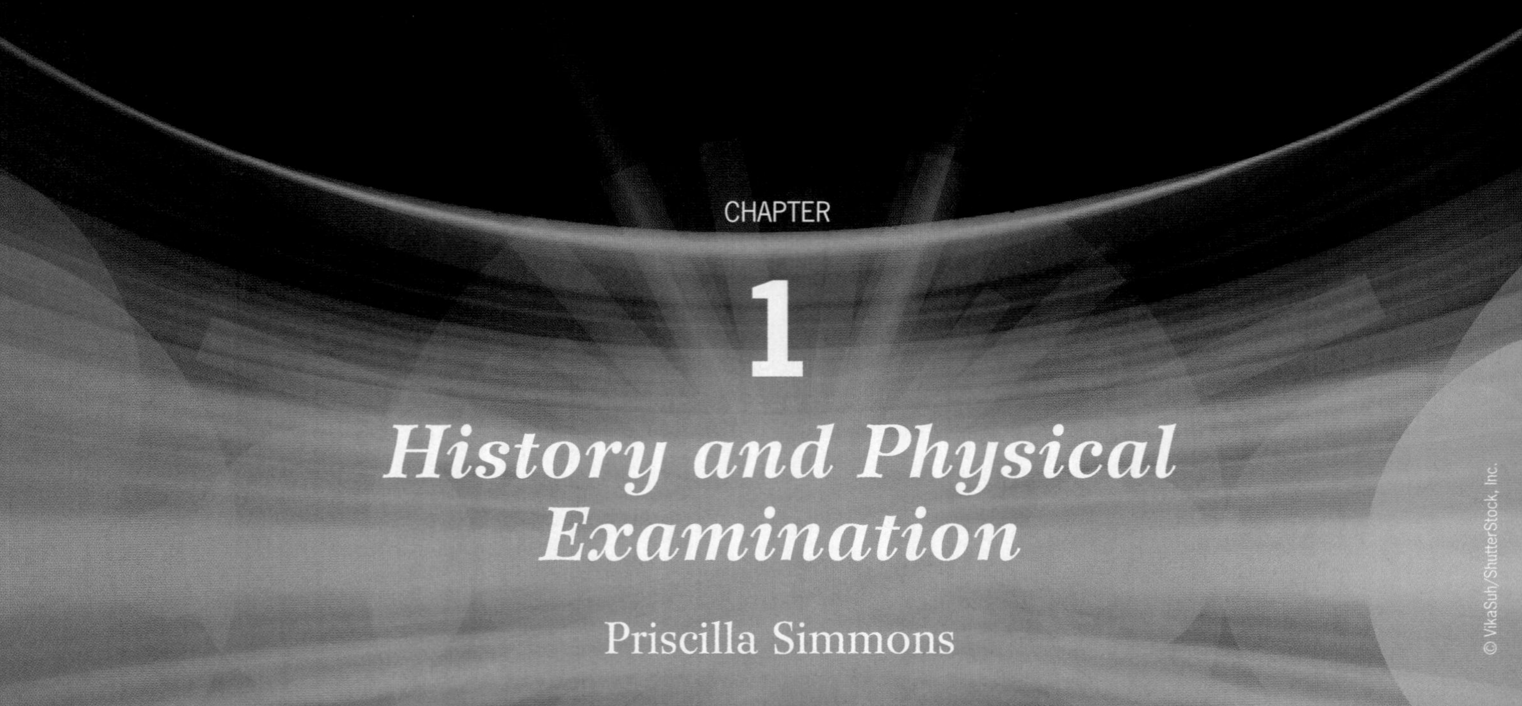

CHAPTER

1

History and Physical Examination

Priscilla Simmons

OUTLINE

OBJECTIVES

1. Discuss the factors essential in the creation of a therapeutic climate.
2. Explain three considerations of an effective health history.
3. Explain the relevance of cultural diversity in the history-taking process.
4. List the major components of a health history.
5. Identify the four major examination techniques.
6. Define common terms used in assessment of the respiratory system.
7. Explain the technique for auscultation of the chest.
8. Define terms associated with normal and abnormal breath sounds.
9. List the signs associated with respiratory distress.
10. Identify common pathologic processes of the respiratory system and pertinent physical findings that extend to other body systems.
11. Identify the significance of various chest landmarks.
12. Explain the significance of sounds heard during cardiac auscultation.
13. Explain the significance of jugular venous distention.
14. Explain common findings associated with an assessment of the neurologic system.

KEY TERMS

auscultation
barrel chest
Biot respirations
bradypnea
bronchial breath sounds
bronchophony
bronchovesicular
Cheyne-Stokes breathing
clubbing
crackles
cyanosis
dyspnea
egophony
flail chest
grunting
hyperpnea
hyperresonant
hyperventilation
inspection
jaundice
Kussmaul respirations
kyphosis
lordosis
murmur
orthopnea
pack years
pallor
palpation
paradoxical respiration
paroxysmal nocturnal dyspnea
pectus carinatum
pectus excavatum
percussion
platypnea
plethora
pleural friction rub
precordium
resonant
rhonchus
scoliosis
stridor
tachypnea
tactile fremitus
tympanic
vesicular breath sounds
wheezes
whispered pectoriloquy

Introduction

This chapter provides a guide to essential assessment techniques used by the respiratory therapist. In the hospital, many members of the healthcare team examine the patient. In the community setting, however, fewer members of the healthcare team assess the patient, thereby warranting a more thorough examination by the respiratory therapist. Whatever the setting, no clinician regularly uses all the available assessment techniques. Some techniques are rarely used. The emphasis of this chapter is on the pathophysiology underlying common respiratory abnormalities and the typical assessment findings associated with them.

Creating a Therapeutic Climate

The patient's perception of the respiratory therapist's competence is of prime importance. When any healthcare provider is perceived as uncaring, the patient may remember that attitude most vividly. Even worse, that poor image may come to characterize all the members of the profession for the patient. To ensure a therapeutic, professional relationship, competence and caring must coexist. A clinician can communicate caring through a gentle demeanor and an unhurried, nonabrupt manner. Maintaining eye contact is essential. Also appropriate is the judicious use of touch, such as patting or squeezing a patient's hand or shoulder. Respiratory therapists should dress appropriately because a professional appearance communicates respect for the patient. A patient's judgment of a healthcare provider often is based on physical appearance. These measures help establish rapport and a climate of professional caring, a goal in every professional relationship.

Components of the Health History

The health history provides a detailed, chronologic health record of the patient's status. For the purpose of developing an individualized plan of care, the health history elicits information about variables affecting the patient's health. The value of the history should not be underestimated because it guides the selection of appropriate physical examination techniques, helps the respiratory therapist develop an accurate index of suspicion, and ultimately leads to appropriate and effective therapeutic intervention. Because obtaining a comprehensive history is time consuming, many healthcare providers assess primarily the body systems of concern. Clearly, the heart and lungs are the systems of primary interest for respiratory therapists.

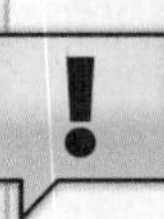

Respiratory Recap

Variables Supporting a Therapeutic Climate

- Caring demeanor
- Competence
- Eye contact
- Judicious use of touch
- Professional image

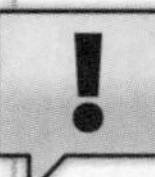

Respiratory Recap

The Health History

- Chief complaint
- History of present illness
- Occupational and environmental history
- Geographic exposure
- Activities of daily living
- Smoking history
- Cough and sputum production
- Family history
- Medical history
- Review of systems

Chief Complaint

The chief complaint (CC) is the problem or concern that prompted the patient to seek healthcare. When documenting the CC in the patient record, the examiner should use the patient's own words in quotation marks.

History of Present Illness

The history of present illness (HPI) is the chronologic, narrative account of the patient's health problem. It should describe in detail information relevant to the CC, including a description of the onset of the problem, the date the symptoms occurred and whether they developed gradually or suddenly, and the setting in which they developed. Also included is a description of the signs and symptoms associated with the problem. The mnemonic *OLD CART* can help the examiner gather information accordingly, as follows:

Onset (when the problem started)
Location of pain, shortness of breath, or other symptoms
Duration of pain, shortness of breath, or other symptoms
Character, quantity, and quality of pain, shortness of breath, or other symptoms
Associated manifestations (the setting in which the pain, shortness of breath, or other symptoms developed)
Relieving factors or factors that diminish or aggravate the pain, shortness of breath, or other symptoms
Treatment (any medications or other remedies that relieve or exacerbate shortness of breath)

Occupational and Environmental History

The examiner should inquire as to whether the patient is employed, retired, or laid off. Are there any current or past hazards at work, such as exposure to asbestos, coal dust, silica, molds, dust, or animals? Is the patient under stress at work? Is the patient satisfied with his or her job?

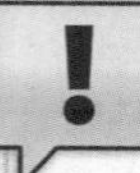

Respiratory Recap

History of Present Illness

- Onset
- Location
- Duration
- Character
- Associated manifestations
- Relieving factors
- Treatment

Geographic Exposure

Has the patient traveled to foreign countries? Has the patient been in military service?

Activities of Daily Living

Has the patient experienced difficulty with or change in the ability to provide self-care?

Smoking History

Does the patient smoke cigarettes, or has the patient done so in the past? How long has the patient smoked cigarettes? This answer is usually expressed in **pack years** and is calculated as follows. A pack a day for 1 year is known as *1 pack year*. Two packs a day for a year is *2 pack years*, and so on. What is the patient's willingness to quit? The examiner should also inquire as to whether the patient smokes a pipe, cigars, or illicit drugs such as marijuana or crack cocaine.

Cough and Sputum Production

The examiner should ask about the presence of cough and sputum. If the patient has a cough, the timing of the cough (for example, in the morning, at night, after eating) and whether sputum is produced should be noted. If sputum is produced, the examiner should determine its amount, consistency, color, and odor, as well as whether the frequency of the cough and the amount of sputum have increased recently.

Family History

Any family history of genetically transmitted disease (for example, cystic fibrosis, alpha-1 antitrypsin deficiency), cancer, heart disease, tuberculosis (TB), or human immunodeficiency virus (HIV) should be noted.

Medical History

Dates of past health problems, hospitalizations, symptoms, and treatment should be noted in the history, as well as whether the problem is ongoing, resolved, or recurrent. Are immunizations current? Does the patient have any food, drug, insect, or environmental allergies?

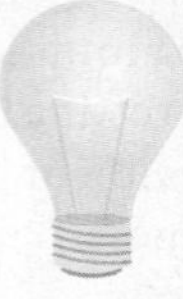

STOP AND THINK

You are seeing a patient for the first time. You are told that the patient has COPD. What information would you collect regarding the patient's health history?

Review of Systems

A review of the systems provides the opportunity for the examiner to methodically question the patient about the health of each body system. It differs from the physical examination in that the data are collected verbally. A thorough review of each system is unnecessary, but the examiner should include a detailed review of the systems affected by the present illness. If the patient answers with a negative response, a denial of that specific complaint should be noted. For example, "Patient denies pain with deep inspiration and coughing."

Vital Signs

Pulse, respirations, and blood pressure are considered *vital signs*. These are commonly measured, along with body temperature, as indicators of the patient's health status. The pulse rate and rhythm can be measured by cardiac auscultation or palpation of any artery, with the radial artery being most commonly used for this purpose. The pulse is counted for a minimum of 15 seconds and then mathematically adjusted to the rate per minute. The normal pulse rate for adults is 60 to 100 beats per minute; the rate is more rapid for infants and children. The respiratory rate is measured by inspection of the movement of the chest for 1 minute. The normal respiratory rate for adults is 12 to 20 breaths per minute; it is more rapid for infants and children.

Blood pressure is measured either with a sphygmomanometer or an indwelling arterial catheter. Normal blood pressure for adults is 120/80 mm Hg. Measurements are lower for infants and children.

Body temperature can be measured via the oral, rectal, or axillary sites using a traditional thermometer. Infrared sensors are also used for the forehead or tympanic sites. Core temperature monitoring is measured in the distal esophagus or pulmonary artery. Normal body temperature is 37° C (98.6° F). The term *fever* refers

AGE-SPECIFIC ANGLE

Compared with adults, infants and children have higher respiratory rates, higher pulse rates, and lower blood pressures.

Respiratory Recap

Respiratory Assessment Techniques

- Inspection
- Palpation
- Percussion
- Auscultation

to a higher-than-normal body temperature (hyperthermia), whereas hypothermia is a temperature lower than normal.

Techniques of Assessment

Inspection

As an examination technique, **inspection** ranges from casual observation to visual scrutiny of the patient.

Palpation

Palpation is the process whereby the examiner uses the hands to feel for body movement, lumps, masses, and skin characteristics. Palpation can be either light or deep.

Percussion

Percussion requires the examiner to place a finger firmly against a body part and strike that finger with a fingertip from the other hand. The technique for the right-handed examiner is as follows:

- Hyperextend the middle finger of the nondominant hand (pleximeter finger).
- Press the distal interphalangeal joint firmly on the surface to be percussed. Avoid contact with any other part of the hand because vibrations may be dampened.
- Hold the forearm of the other arm close to the surface, with the hand turned up at the wrist, and partially flex the middle finger (plexor).
- Strike the pleximeter with the tip of the plexor with a quick, sharp, and relaxed wrist motion and aim at the distal interphalangeal joint (**Figure 1-1**).

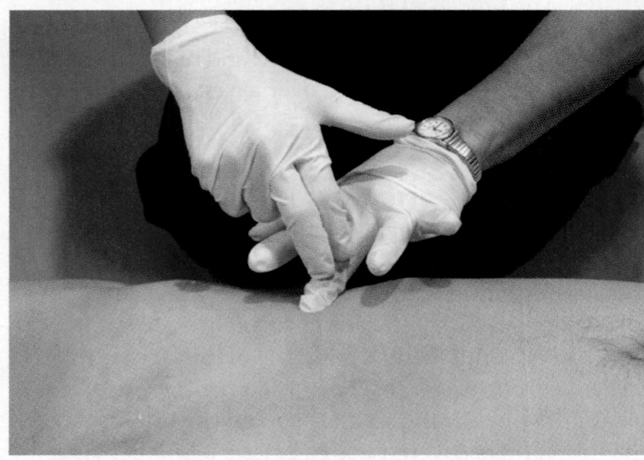

FIGURE 1-1 Percussion technique.

  Withdraw briskly to avoid dampening the vibrations. Use one to two blows at each location.

The resulting sounds can suggest either normal underlying tissue or typical sounds associated with given abnormalities.

Five percussion tones (**Table 1-1**) are commonly recognized: flat, dull, resonant, hyperresonant, and tympanic. A flat percussion note is soft, high pitched, and of short duration. It can be elicited by percussion of the thigh. A dull percussion note is of medium intensity, pitch, and duration. It is heard over the liver or a tumor. A **resonant** note is loud, low in pitch, and of long duration. It may be heard over normal lung tissue. A **hyperresonant** note is very loud, lower in pitch, longer

Respiratory Recap

Percussion Notes

- Flat
- Dull
- Resonant
- Hyperresonant
- Tympanic

TABLE 1-1
Characteristics of Percussion Notes

Type of Tone	Intensity	Pitch	Duration	Quality
Flat	Soft	High	Short	Extremely dull
Dull	Medium	Medium-high	Medium	Thud like
Resonant	Loud	Low	Long	Hollow
Hyperresonant	Very loud	Very low	Longer	Booming
Tympanic	Loud	High	Medium	Drum like

in duration, and commonly heard over an emphysematous lung. A **tympanic** note is loud and drum-like, with a high pitch. It may be heard over a gastric bubble.

Auscultation

After inspection, **auscultation** is the most commonly used physical assessment technique, particularly for assessment of the respiratory system. Auscultation involves listening to body sounds with a stethoscope placed on bare skin. The stethoscope has several important components (**Figure 1-2**). The diaphragm is the larger side of the stethoscope head and is made of rigid plastic. The bell is the smaller cup on the other side of the head and is covered with a plastic or rubber ring. The bell is useful for detection of certain cardiac and vascular sounds. The diaphragm is used more frequently. Note that both adult and pediatric diaphragms and bells exist, with the latter being smaller. Some stethoscopes come with interchangeable parts. The examiner should ensure that the appropriate sizes are being used.

Quality stethoscopes have tubing specifically engineered to conduct sound very well. It is possible to purchase stethoscopes that actually magnify sound. Most stethoscopes, however, simply block out other noise, thereby allowing the examiner to hear body sounds unimpeded. An appropriate tubing length is about 12 inches. Earpieces must fit snugly and comfortably. The earpieces must point toward the nose of the examiner to project sound toward the tympanic membrane of the examiner's ears.

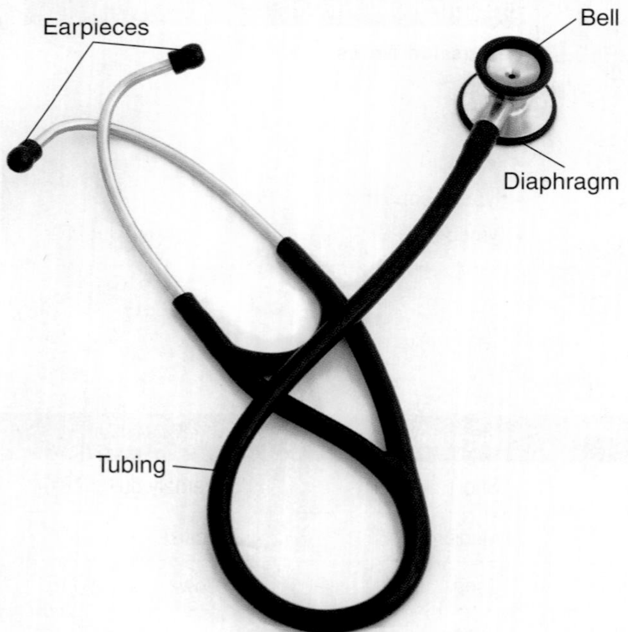

FIGURE 1-2 Stethoscope, illustrating diaphragm and bell.

Physical Examination of the Lungs and Thorax

The astute clinician is thoroughly familiar with human anatomy. An in-depth knowledge of structure and function is vital to the interpretation of assessment findings in terms of underlying pathologic processes. **Figure 1-3** illustrates thoracic landmarks and the surface anatomy of the chest.

Inspection

Observing Respirations

The clinician must be familiar with common respiratory patterns (**Figure 1-4**). **Tachypnea** describes a persistent rate of respiration faster than 20 breaths per minute. It may be present in individuals who are hypoxemic and those who have pain in the thoracic region.

Similarly, if liver enlargement or abdominal distention compromises diaphragmatic movement, tachypnea may result. At times, however, tachypnea is merely a patient response to the realization that respirations are being observed and counted. Tachypnea also occurs in individuals with fever and in those with restrictive ventilatory defects, such as pulmonary fibrosis or pneumonectomy.

Hyperpnea describes breathing that is rapid, deep, and labored. If it results in a lowered P_{CO_2}, **hyperventilation** is the term that applies. **Kussmaul respirations** describe hyperventilation as a compensatory mechanism for metabolic acidosis, most commonly diabetic ketoacidosis. Conversely, **bradypnea** is a rate slower than 12 breaths per minute. It may suggest neurologic impairment or acid–base disturbance but may be a normal finding in physically fit individuals.

Dyspnea is a term that simply means difficult or labored breathing, with the individual feeling short of breath. **Platypnea** refers to an individual's difficulty in breathing unless lying flat. **Orthopnea** indicates that an individual must sit or stand to breathe. Many individuals with chronic lung disease must assume an upright position to breathe well. Such individuals

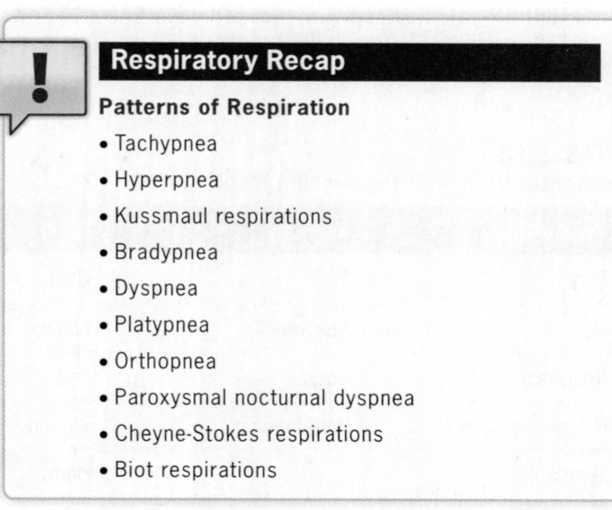
Respiratory Recap

Patterns of Respiration

- Tachypnea
- Hyperpnea
- Kussmaul respirations
- Bradypnea
- Dyspnea
- Platypnea
- Orthopnea
- Paroxysmal nocturnal dyspnea
- Cheyne-Stokes respirations
- Biot respirations

often find it more comfortable to sleep in a chair. **Paroxysmal nocturnal dyspnea** is characterized by sudden shortness of breath that occurs several hours after the individual lies down. It commonly suggests cardiac dysfunction in that the heart is unable to adequately pump a circulatory volume expanded by fluid reabsorbed from the legs, which became edematous during the day.

Cheyne-Stokes breathing is characterized by episodes of slow, shallow breaths, which rapidly increase in depth and rate. This crescendo-decrescendo pattern is followed by periods of apnea. Such breathing may be a normal variant in young children and the elderly. Otherwise, it occurs in individuals with cerebral vascular disease and congestive heart failure.

Biot respirations are symptomatic of elevated intracranial pressure and meningitis. This breathing pattern is characterized by a short burst of uniform, deep respirations, followed by periods of apnea lasting 10 to 30 seconds.

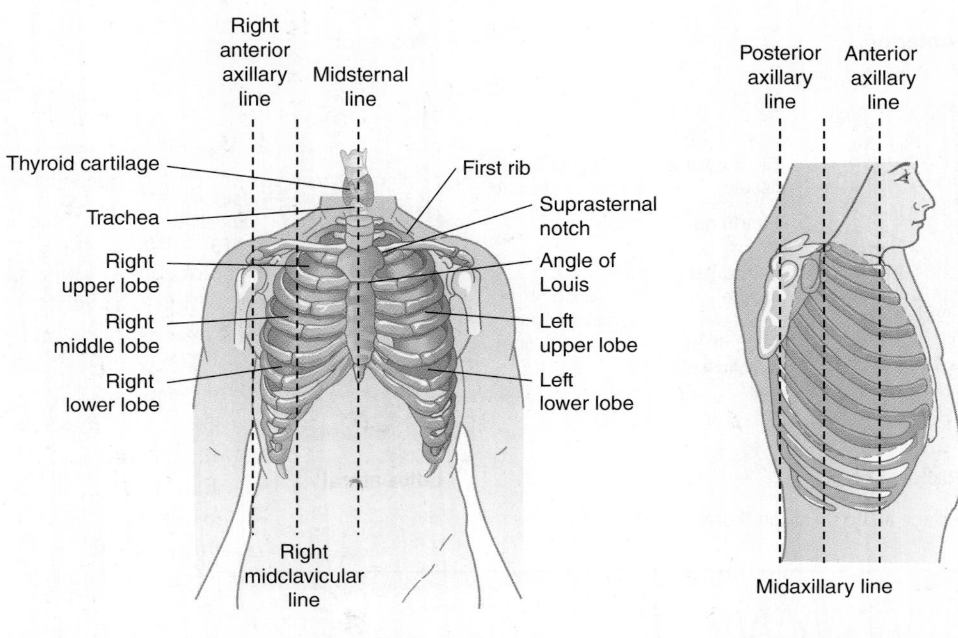

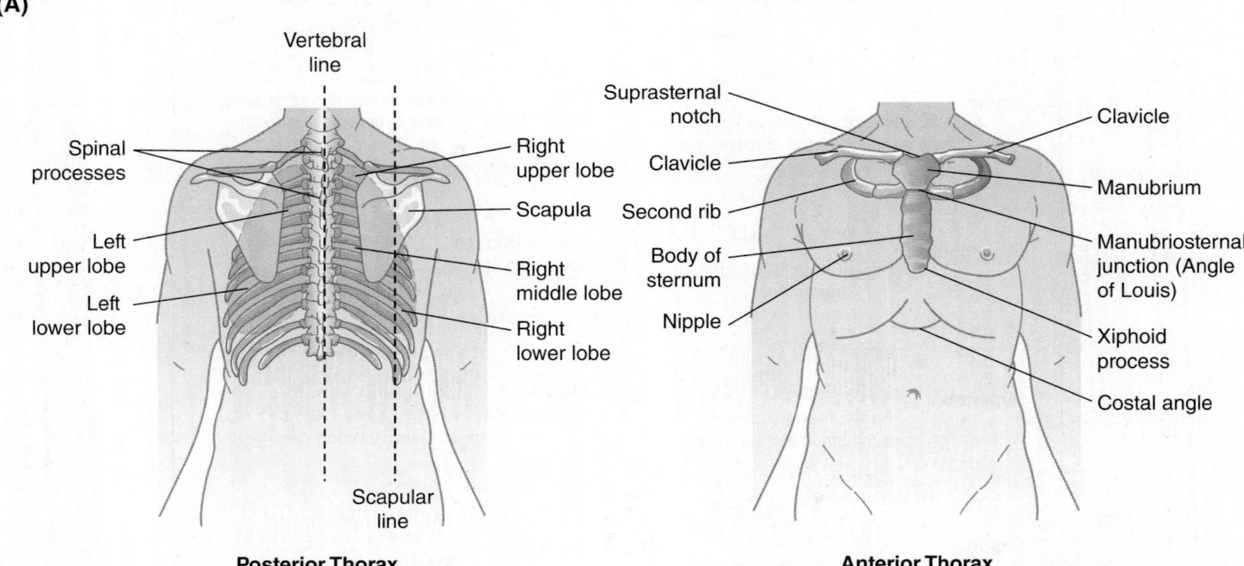

(continues)

FIGURE 1-3 (**A**) Thoracic landmarks. (**B**) Topographic landmarks of the chest.

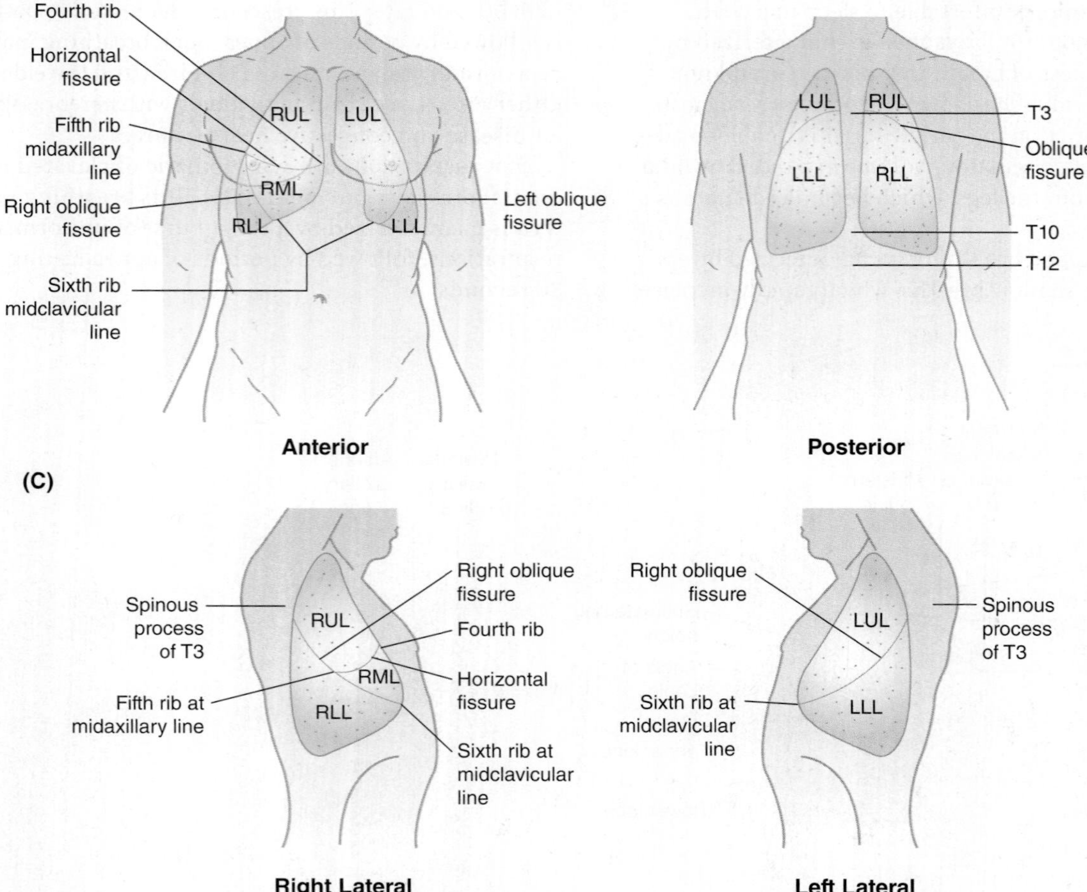

FIGURE 1-3 *(Continued)* (**C**) Surface anatomy of the thorax.

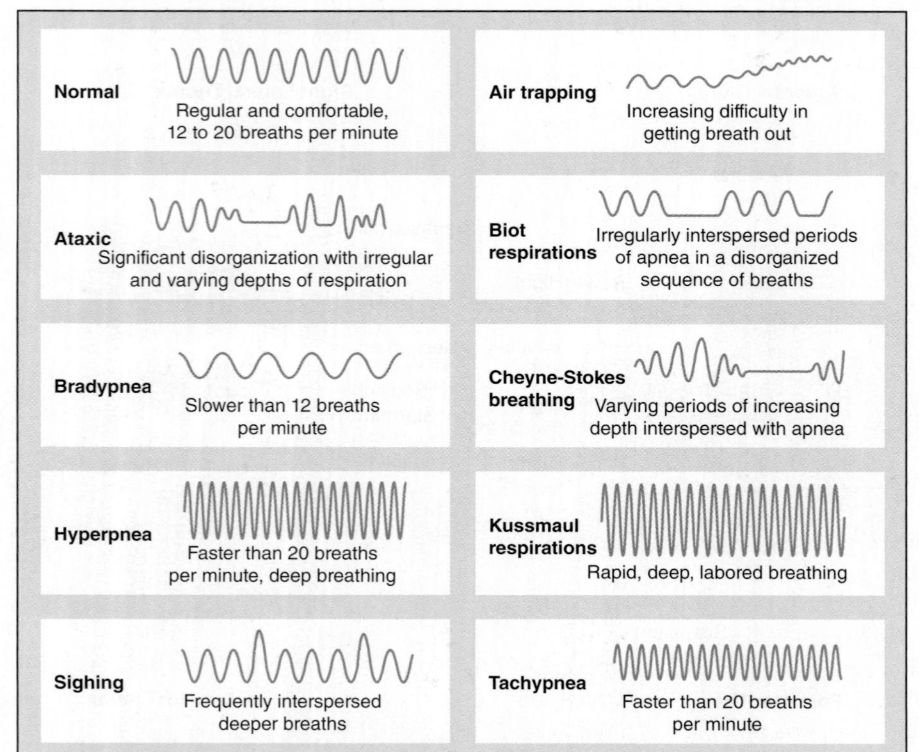

FIGURE 1-4 Patterns of respiration.

Reproduced from *Mosby's Guide to Physical Examination*, Seidel HM, Ball JW, Dains JE, et al., Copyright Elsevier [Mosby] 1999.

Use of Accessory Muscles

Muscles of the back, neck, and abdomen are known as *accessory muscles* of respiration. Although they play a relatively minor role in normal respiration, their function becomes more prominent during exercise or respiratory distress. Use of accessory muscles implies an increased work of breathing or diaphragm weakness.

Retractions suggest a barrier to inspiration, occurring anywhere along the respiratory tract. To overcome this barrier, the respiratory muscles contract more vigorously, resulting in a more negative intrapleural pressure. Retractions resemble a "sucking in" of structures, such as the intercostal spaces, suprasternal space, and subclavian spaces. In such a situation, the examiner documents that the patient "has retractions," "is retracting," or "is using accessory muscles."

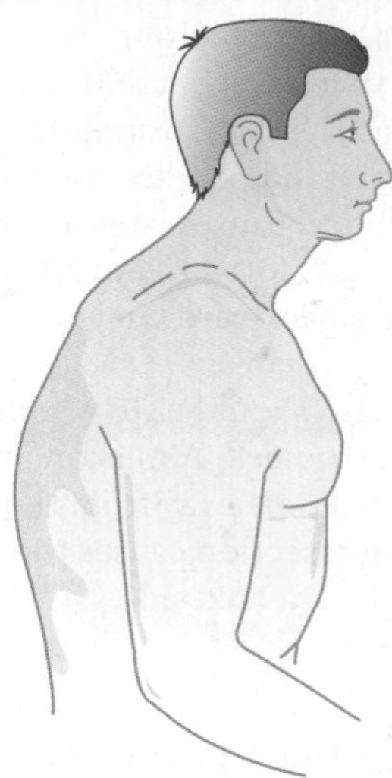

FIGURE 1-5 Barrel chest.

Nasal Flaring and Pursed-Lip Breathing

Individuals in respiratory distress commonly exhibit nasal flaring, presumably in an attempt to decrease the resistance to airflow through the nostrils. Those with emphysema commonly use pursed lips during the expiratory phase to maintain airway patency and better control expiratory flow.

Flail Chest and Paradoxical Respiration

Flail chest is a term describing the appearance of a thorax with multiple rib fractures, causing instability of the chest wall. In this situation the chest wall moves outward on expiration and inward on inspiration. This movement, which is contrary to normal chest movement, is known as **paradoxical respiration**. Flail chest with paradoxical respiration indicates a serious injury and will result in hypoxia if left untreated.

The chest and abdomen also should move in synchrony during the respiratory cycle. Paradoxical inward movement of the abdomen during the inspiratory phase indicates diaphragm weakness or paralysis. Paradoxical inward movement of the chest wall during inspiration indicates paralysis of the chest wall muscles, as may occur with high thoracic spine injury or low cervical spine injury.

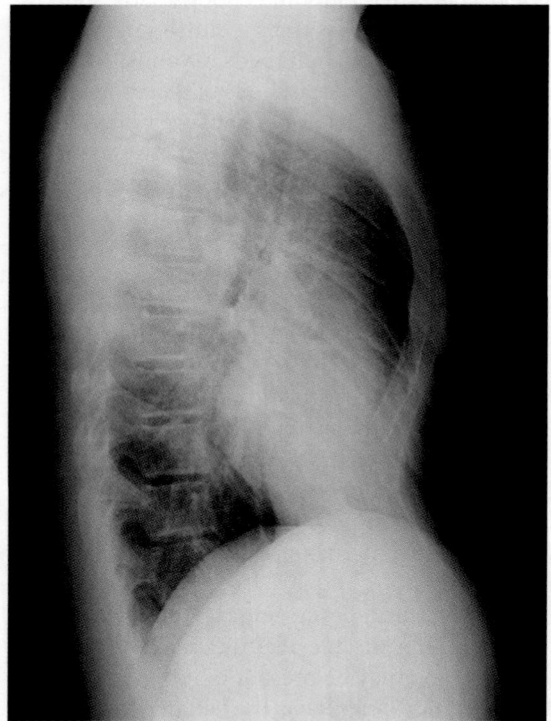

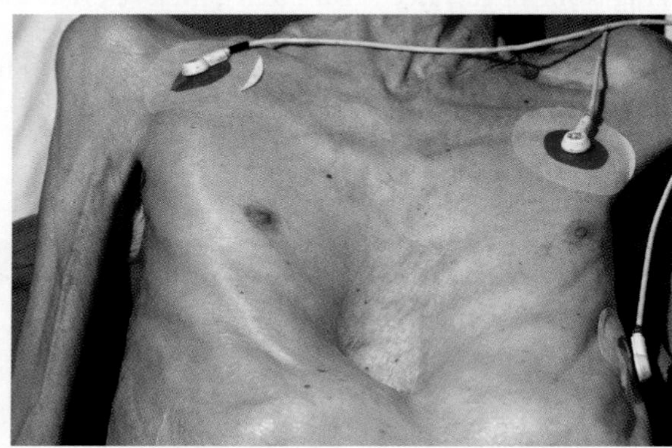

FIGURE 1-6 Pectus excavatum.

Top © Custom Medical Stock Photo; bottom © M. English, MD/Custom Medical Stock Photo.

Shape of the Chest

The examiner should observe the shape of the patient's chest. Abnormalities of the thorax can be significant factors in lung disease. Typically, a patient with emphysema has a **barrel chest** (**Figure 1-5**). The lateral diameter of the chest is normally twice the anteroposterior diameter. With a barrel-shaped chest configuration, the anteroposterior diameter is equal to the lateral diameter. Although obstructive lung disease causes this characteristic change in chest configuration, certain other abnormalities of thoracic shape result in restrictive lung disease. **Pectus excavatum**, or a funnel-shaped sternum, describes a sternum that is depressed and deviated somewhat like a funnel (**Figure 1-6**). Similarly,

pectus carinatum, or a pigeon-breasted sternum, describes a chest that bows out at the sternum, similar to that of a pigeon. These abnormalities in thoracic configuration may result in lung disease as the patient ages. **Scoliosis**, for instance, causes lateral curvature of the spine, **kyphosis** causes forward curvature of the spine, and **lordosis** causes backward curvature of the spine (**Figure 1-7**).

The examiner also should note whether the trachea is midline in the neck. A tension pneumothorax causes tracheal deviation away from the collapsed lung. Atelectasis or lung resection causes the trachea to be deviated toward the affected side.

Skin Color

The color of the patient's skin should be noted. Although several abnormalities in skin color exist, **cyanosis** is of prime significance to the respiratory therapist. When hemoglobin is poorly saturated with oxygen, the skin assumes a bluish hue, which is initially apparent in the nail beds. Cyanosis may be present normally in the nail beds of a person who is vasoconstricted as a result of exposure to cold temperatures. Cyanosis also may be noted in the mucous membranes of the mouth; this site is of particular use in the assessment of individuals with dark skin. Cyanosis also can appear around the mouth (circumoral). In healthy children, circumoral cyanosis is quite common, particularly when they are cold. The significance of cyanosis must be evaluated in light of other clinical findings.

Pallor is the term assigned to describe diminished skin color accompanying anemia. It also may be seen in individuals with severe peripheral vasoconstriction accompanying shock. Detecting pallor is easier in lighter-skinned individuals, but the color of darker skin also appears paler when the individual is severely anemic.

Plethora is a term describing the fullness of blood vessels at the skin surface. Plethora may occur with vasodilation and may be present in individuals who are hypercapnic. **Jaundice** is the yellowish skin color arising from an elevated serum bilirubin level. Any disorder resulting in bile being retained in the liver ultimately causes jaundice. Jaundice is first apparent in the sclera of the eyes.

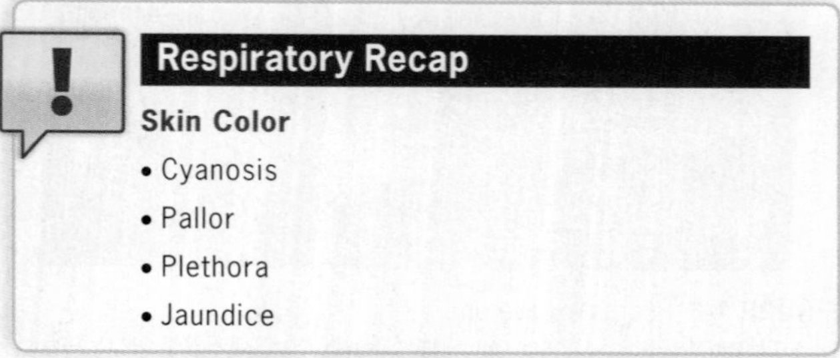

Respiratory Recap

Skin Color

- Cyanosis
- Pallor
- Plethora
- Jaundice

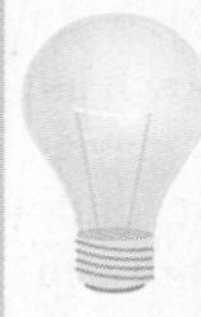

STOP AND THINK

Before initiating a respiratory care plan, you are assessing a patient with a history of COPD. The patient is thought to have pneumonia precipitating an exacerbation. What are your considerations when performing a physical assessment?

Clubbing of Fingers

Clubbed fingers result from enlargement of the distal phalanges and develop as a compensatory mechanism when an individual has chronic hypoxia, such as with congenital heart defects or chronic lung disease. The appearance of **clubbing** is exactly as the term implies: the finger distal to the base of the nail looks like a small club (**Figure 1-8**). Affected fingertips appear full, fleshy, and vascular. Clubbing is associated with lung tumors, bronchiectasis, cystic fibrosis, congenital heart disease, and liver and gastrointestinal disease. It is hereditary in some cases. However, clubbing does *not* occur with chronic obstructive pulmonary disease.

Palpation

Subcutaneous Emphysema

Subcutaneous emphysema is the presence of air in the subcutaneous tissues of the neck, chest, and face. The tissues may be painful and appear swollen. In addition, a crackling or popping sound may be auscultated when a stethoscope is placed over the tissue. An examiner also may detect subcutaneous emphysema by palpating bubbles as the finger pads are rolled over the affected areas.

Respiratory Expansion

The assessment of respiratory expansion is used primarily to determine whether the lungs are expanding symmetrically. Asymmetry of expansion may be present with a pneumothorax, atelectasis, lung resection, or main stem intubation. To perform this examination, the examiner places the thumbs along each costal margin at the back.

The hands then are slid medially to raise loose skin folds between the thumbs. The patient is asked to inhale deeply, and the examiner notes the range and symmetry of respiratory expansion by observing how the skin fold spreads out.

Tactile Fremitus

Tactile fremitus is defined as the palpation of vibrations of the chest wall as a patient speaks. To elicit these vibrations, the examiner presses the bony part of the palm of the hand against the patient's chest wall. For comparison between lungs, both sides are assessed concurrently.

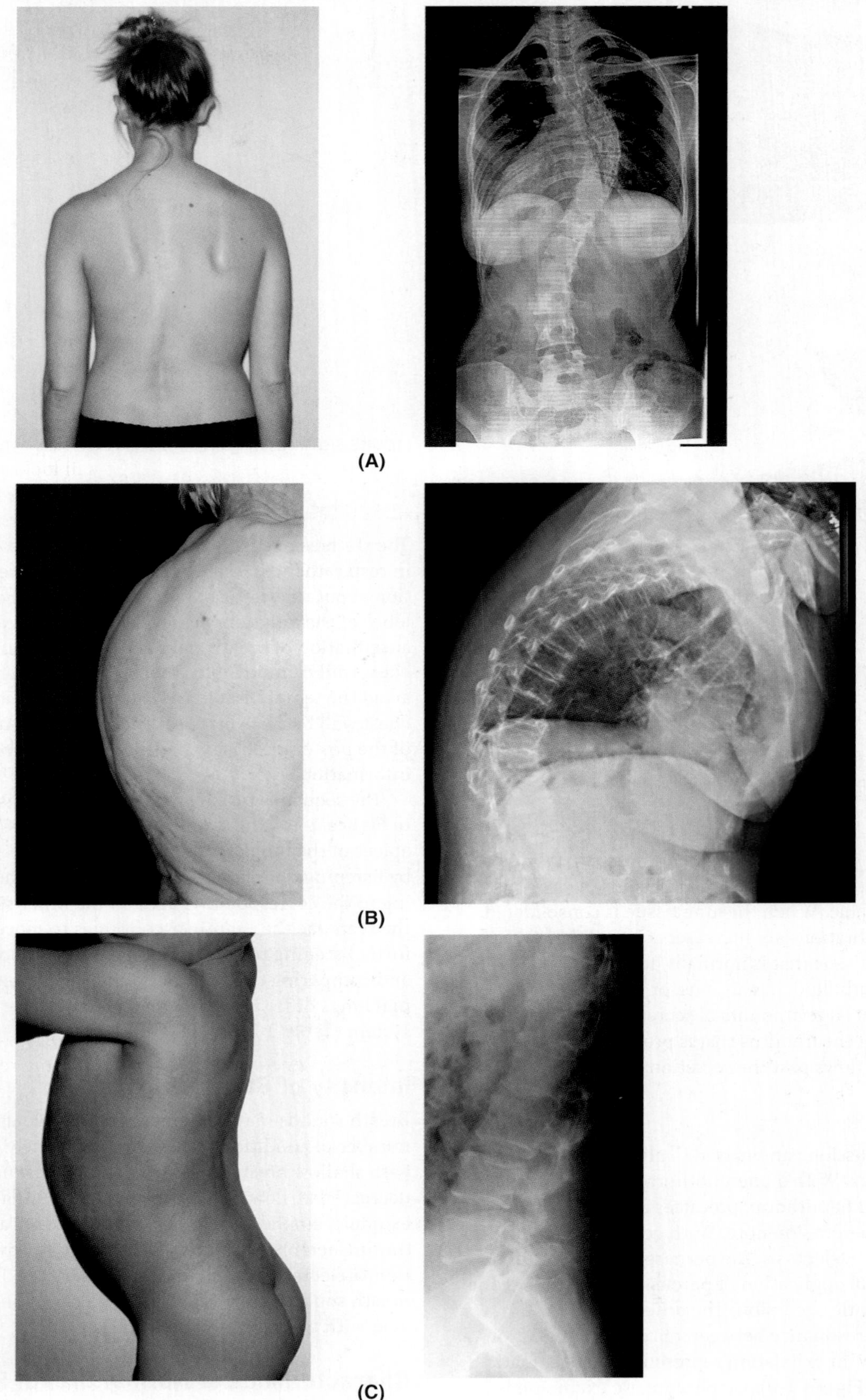

FIGURE 1-7 (**A**) Scoliosis. (**B**) Kyphosis. (**C**) Lordosis.

(**A**) left and right, courtesy of Darci Manley; (**B**) left © Dr. P. Marazzi/SPL/Science Source, right © Apogee/Science Source; (**C**) left © Wellcome Trust Library/Custom Medical Stock Photo, right © medicalpicture/Alamy Images.

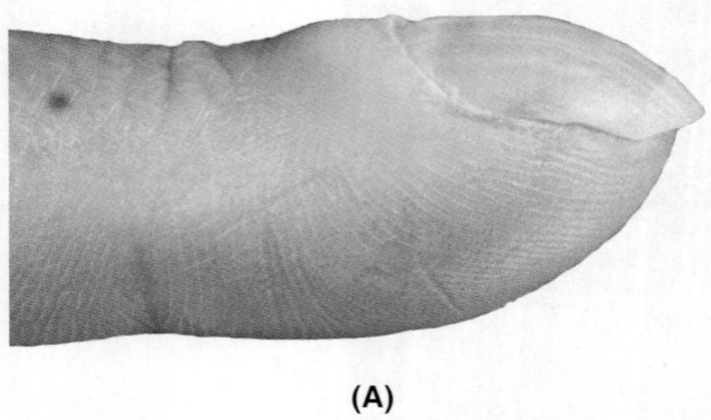

(A)

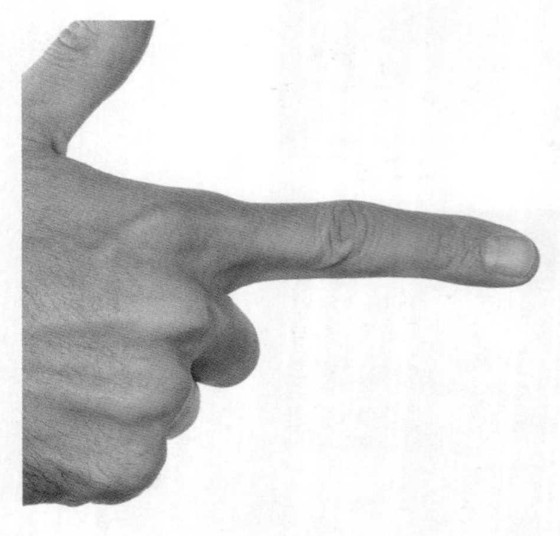

(B)

FIGURE 1-8 (**A**) Clubbing of the finger. (**B**) Normal digit.
(**A**) © Biophoto Associates/Science Source; (**B**) © Jorge Salcedo/ShutterStock, Inc.

The patient is asked to repeat the words *ninety-nine* or *one-one-one*. When the lungs are healthy, vibrations are barely palpable. When the lung tissue is consolidated, however, vibrations are increased. Consolidation occurs when lung tissue that is normally aerated is "made solid" by filling with fluid, mucus, pus, or cellular debris. In the patient with large amounts of secretions in the airways, palpation of the fremitus that is produced may be possible as gas flows past the secretions.

Percussion

Chest percussion can be used to elicit several abnormal findings. With a pneumothorax or emphysema, the affected hemithorax produces a hyperresonant or tympanic percussion note. With consolidation, pleural effusion, or atelectasis, the percussion note is dull or flat. A useful application of percussion is to determine diaphragmatic excursion. The difference in posterior, dependent resonance between maximum inhalation and maximum exhalation represents diaphragmatic excursion (**Figure 1-9**). Diaphragmatic excursion is affected by emphysema, pneumothorax, pleural effusion, atelectasis, consolidation, phrenic nerve injury, and diaphragmatic weakness.

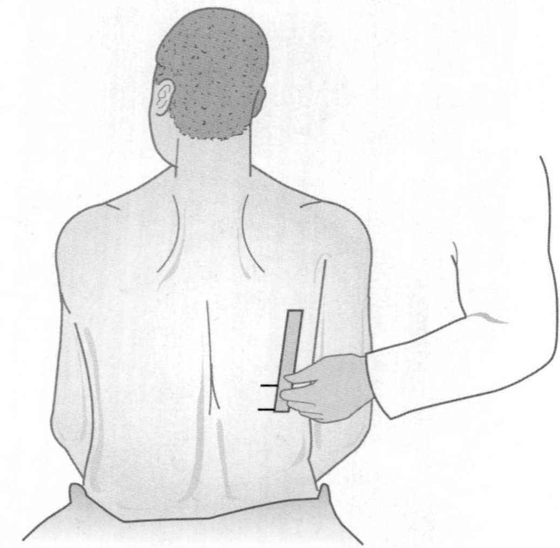

FIGURE 1-9 Measuring diaphragmatic excursion.

Auscultation

The stethoscope is the most frequently used instrument in respiratory assessment and yields valuable information about the status of the lungs. Because the lower lobes of the lungs are posterior in the thorax, complete auscultation of breath sounds through the anterior chest wall is impossible. Therefore, examiners should avoid the temptation to auscultate only the anterior chest wall because of its easy accessibility. Auscultation of the posterior chest wall generally yields more useful information.

The sequence for lung field auscultation is shown in **Figure 1-10**. The examiner first should assess the apices of the lungs as they extend above the scapulae by listening on one side of the thorax and then moving to the corresponding area on the other side. Below the scapulae the examiner continues to move back and forth, listening to corresponding areas on both sides and comparing the sounds. Sounds generated by normal lungs differ according to location in the respiratory system (**Table 1-2**).

Intensity of Breath Sounds

Breath sounds may be reduced in individuals with a number of conditions. They can be diffusely decreased with shallow breathing or with the hyperinflation and decreased airflow that occur with hyperinflation (for example, emphysema or acute asthma). Localized diminished breath sounds occur with airway obstruction, atelectasis, and main stem intubation. Decreased breath sounds at the lung bases are commonly associated with postoperative atelectasis.

Characteristics of Normal Breath Sounds

Bronchial breath sounds are heard over the trachea, at the manubrium anteriorly, and between the scapulae posteriorly. These breath sounds are louder

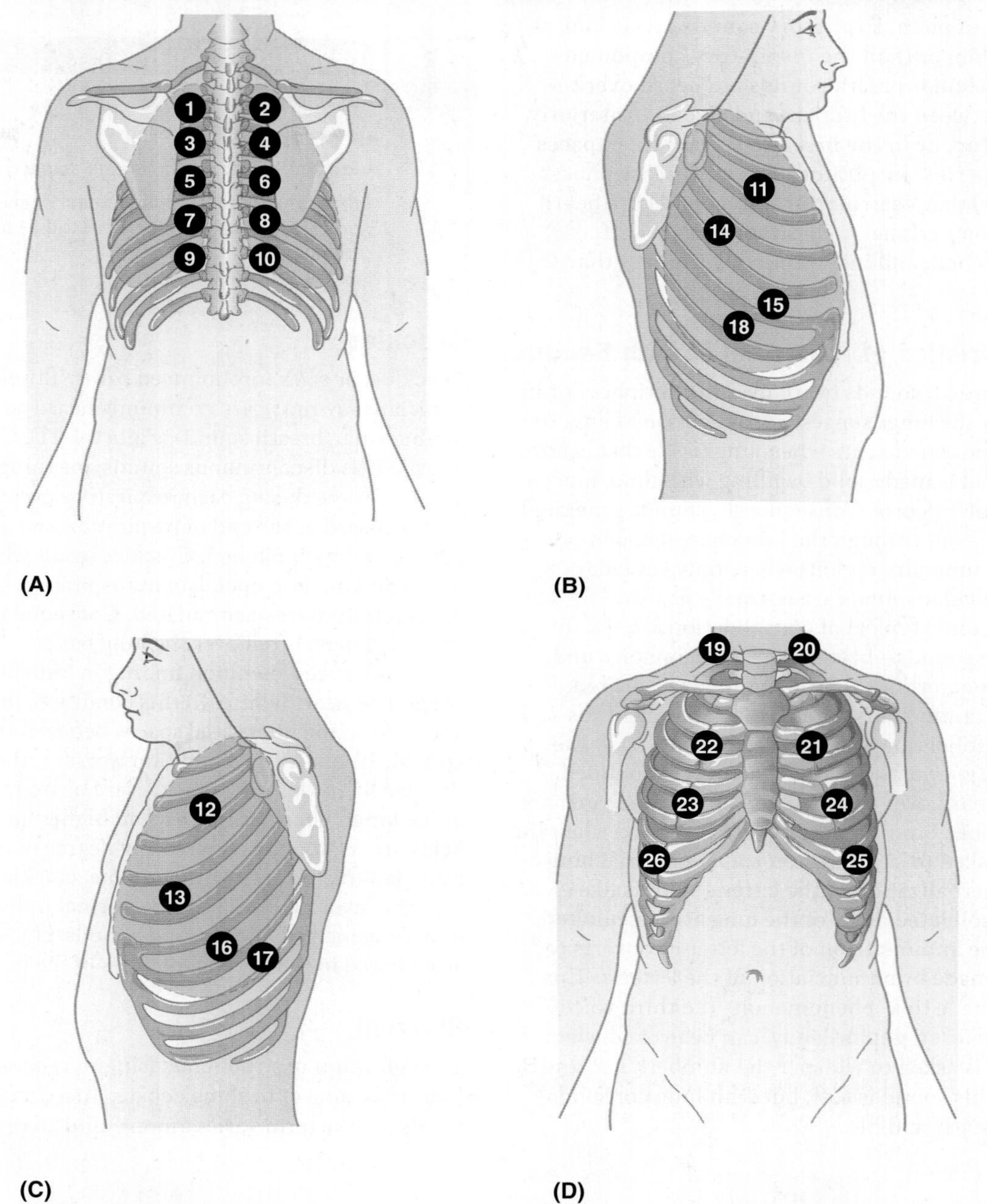

FIGURE 1-10 Suggested sequence for systematic percussion and ausculation of the thorax from the posterior (**A**), right lateral (**B**), left lateral (**C**), and anterior (**D**) views.

TABLE 1-2
Lung Sounds Assessed by Auscultation

Sound	Characteristics
Vesicular	Heard over most lung fields; low pitch; soft and short expirations; accentuated in thin person or child and diminished in overweight or very muscular individuals
Bronchovesicular	Heard over main bronchus area and upper right posterior lung field; medium pitch; expiration equaling inspiration
Bronchial/tracheal (tubular)	Heard only over trachea; high pitch; loud and long expirations, often somewhat longer than inspiration

and higher in pitch. Expiratory sounds are as long as or slightly longer than the inspiratory component. **Bronchovesicular** breath sounds are heard over the junction between the bronchi and alveoli. Anteriorly, the sounds occur in the first and second interspaces between the ribs. Inspiratory and expiratory phases are equally long. **Vesicular breath sounds** are heard over the lung periphery. These sounds are soft and low pitched, and inspiration lasts longer than expiration.

Respiratory Recap

Auscultation

- Intensity of breath sounds
- Presence of bronchial breath sounds
- Presence of adventitious breath sounds: crackles, rhonchi, wheezes, stridor, pleural friction rubs

Characteristics of Abnormal Breath Sounds

Bronchial breath sounds heard over the periphery or in the bases of the lungs suggest consolidation of lung tissue. Consolidation occurs when lung tissue that is normally aerated is made solid by filling with fluid, mucus, pus, or cellular debris. Consequently, sounds generated by air movement through the bronchi resonate more clearly to pulmonary regions where only vesicular or bronchovesicular sounds are normally heard.

Other sounds typical of consolidation are the so-called voice sounds—bronchophony, egophony, and whispered pectoriloquy. **Bronchophony** is elicited when the examiner auscultates over an area of suspected consolidation and asks the patient to say the words *ninety-nine*. Normally, this sound is muffled, but when heard over consolidated lungs, the words are clearly audible. Similarly, **egophony** is elicited when the patient is asked to say the letter *e*. Over normal lung fields, the verbalization of the letter *e* sounds like *e*. When consolidated areas of the lung are auscultated, however, the annunciation of the letter *e* converts to the sound made by annunciation of the letter *a*. This is termed the "e to a" phenomenon. The third voice sound, **whispered pectoriloquy**, can be evoked when the patient is asked to whisper the numbers *1*, *2*, and *3*. Normally this sound is soft, but with lung consolidation, it is clearly audible.

Crackles

Crackles, or rales (pronounced *rawls*, although many clinicians say *rails*), are commonly heard adventitious, or abnormal, breath sounds (**Figure 1-11**). Crackles are classified as discontinuous sounds, meaning that they wax and wane during each respiratory cycle. They are usually heard at the end of inspiration and are fine in quality and high pitched. Crackles result when the terminal airways pop open late in inspiration because fluid or secretions have accumulated. Consequently, crackles are heard most often over the lung bases.

Crackles are a common finding in individuals with congestive heart failure. In this condition, fluid accumulates first in the interstitial spaces between the capillaries and alveoli. As the condition worsens, the fluid fills the alveoli. Initially the crackles are heard in the bases of the lungs. Crackles that ascend higher up the lung fields are related to an increasing degree of congestive heart failure. In cases of pneumonia, crackles are heard over the involved lobe. In some normal individuals who have remained supine for long periods, crackles may be auscultated in the dependent areas of the lung.

Rhonchi

The definition of a **rhonchus** (singular) or *rhonchi* (plural) is subject to some debate. To a certain degree the use of the term varies among clinical practice sites.

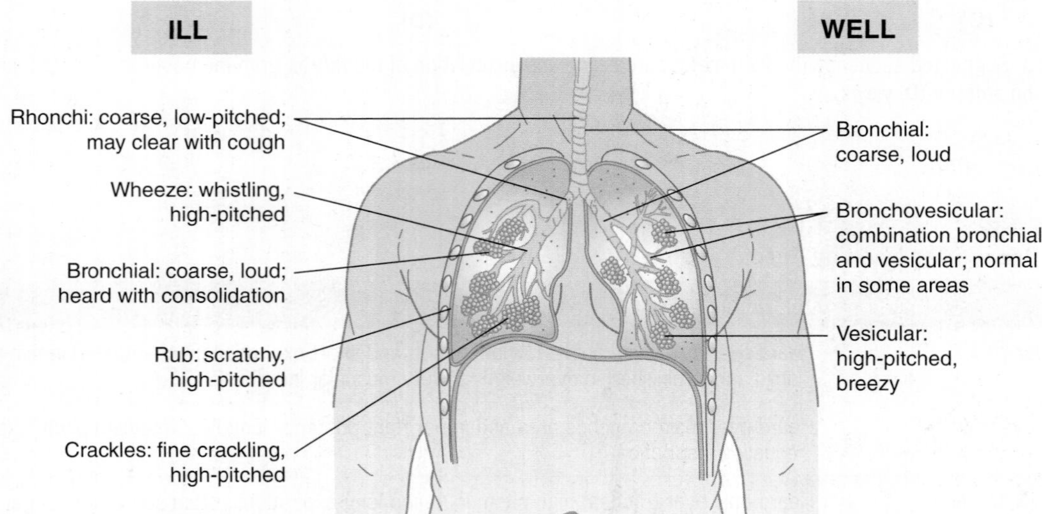

FIGURE 1-11 Breath sounds noted in the ill and well patient.

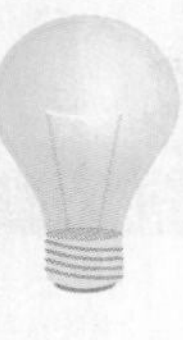

STOP AND THINK

How might the findings during auscultation be different for a patient with COPD, a patient with congestive heart failure, and a patient with both COPD and congestive heart failure?

However, the American Thoracic Society has defined *rhonchi* as being deeper, rumbling sounds that are more pronounced on expiration. These sounds are likely to be continuous. Generally, they are caused by air passing through an airway partially obstructed by thick secretions, spasm of the airways, or presence of a tumor. Higher-pitched or sibilant rhonchi arise in the smaller bronchi, such as in the case of asthma. Lower-pitched, sonorous, or snoring rhonchi are more commonly heard in association with thick secretions in the larger airways. At times the rumbling may be palpable through the chest wall.

Wheezes

Wheezes may be either high or low in pitch. High-pitched wheezes are often called *sibilant* wheezes. They are musical or whistling in nature, caused by air passing through narrowed airways, such as in the bronchospasm of asthma (reactive airway disease). Most often, sibilant wheezes are heard on expiration, although they may be heard throughout the respiratory cycle. Although wheezes are most often associated with asthma, wheezes also can be present in individuals with other conditions, such as congestive heart failure and foreign body aspiration.

Stridor and Grunting

Stridor is a crowing sound commonly caused by inflammation and edema of the larynx and trachea. It may be heard after extubation, when tracheal damage has occurred with resultant edema. Stridor, however, is most commonly associated with croup in children and frequently is accompanied by a barking cough. Usually, stridor is a nocturnal assessment finding probably related to the development of edema in the upper airway while a child is in a dependent position during sleep. Mouth breathing related to nasal congestion often causes a drying and, thus, thickening of secretions that further compounds the stridor. The constellation of findings includes improvement of symptoms with air humidification. Taking the child outside into the cool night air may be an effective intervention. If the child does not improve, however, the stridor must be evaluated further because of the danger of airway obstruction. **Grunting** is a sound heard in newborns with respiratory distress. It occurs when the glottis is closed in an attempt to maintain lung volume.

AGE-SPECIFIC ANGLE

- Stridor is associated with croup in children. Grunting is associated with respiratory distress in the newborn.

Pleural Friction Rubs

A **pleural friction rub** is a continuous grating sound such as is audible when two pieces of leather are rubbed together. Another analogy is that friction rubs sound as though the palms of both hands are sliding against each other. This sound is produced when the visceral and parietal pleurae become inflamed and no longer glide silently against each other during the respiratory cycle. Consequently, the sound is localized and exists only over the area of pleural irritation. Pleural friction rubs may be intermittent.

Pleural friction rubs may accompany a pleural effusion—the accumulation of fluid in the usually empty pleural cavity. Causes of pleural effusion include malignant seeding of metastatic tumors onto the pleural linings. Pleural friction rubs also may be heard in individuals with infectious processes involving the pleural cavity. After thoracic surgery, residual blood in the pleural cavity eventually becomes sludge and may irritate the pleurae, resulting in a friction rub.

Signs of Respiratory Distress

Table 1-3 lists the common physical findings of respiratory diseases.

Assessment of Other Body Systems

The respiratory system interfaces with all other organ systems. Consequently, evaluation of the respiratory system does not occur in an assessment vacuum. The following discussion highlights assessment techniques used to monitor the heart, blood vessels, and brain.

The Heart and Blood Vessels

Location and Significance of Various Chest Landmarks

The chest wall overlying the heart is known as the **precordium**. Each heart valve is auscultated best by placement of the stethoscope in a specific location on the precordium. To do so, the cartilaginous structures—*interspaces*—lying between the ribs must be located, first by identification of the clavicle. Note that the space immediately under the clavicle does not count as an interspace. Next, the first rib should be identified. The cartilage under the first rib is the first interspace. Count the ribs by movement of the fingers down from each rib to the corresponding interspace.

TABLE 1-3
Physical Findings of Respiratory Diseases

Condition	Percussion Note	Fremitus	Breath Sounds	Adventitious Sounds
Normal	Resonant	Normal	Vesicular	None
Left heart failure	Resonant	Normal	Vesicular	Crackles or occasionally wheezes
Pleural effusion	Dull or flat	Decreased	Decreased or absent	None or pleural rub
Consolidation	Dull	Increased	Bronchial	Crackles, rhonchi, or egophony
Bronchitis	Resonant	Normal or decreased	Prolonged exhalation	Wheezes, crackles, or rhonchi
Emphysema	Hyperresonant	Decreased	Decreased or absent	None
Pneumothorax	Hyperresonant	Decreased	Decreased or absent	None
Atelectasis	Dull	Decreased	Decreased or bronchial	None or crackles
Asthma	Resonant or hyperresonant	Normal or decreased	Vesicular	Wheezes
Pulmonary fibrosis	Resonant	Normal	Vesicular	Crackles

The accuracy of the counting process may be verified in the following way. Identify the ridge of bone that is the joint between the manubrium and sternum, known as the *sternal angle* or *angle of Louis*. The interspace to either side immediately below the sternal angle is the second interspace. On the posterior thorax the spinous processes of the vertebrae are useful landmarks. The spinous process of the seventh cervical vertebra (C7) is identified when the patient extends the head and neck forward and down. The most prominent spinous process is C7; directly below that is the first thoracic vertebra (T1). A thorough cardiac auscultation involves systematic movement of the stethoscope over the precordium. A first step taken by the novice examiner is to switch the focus of attention from simply counting each cardiac contraction to a focus on the quality of the sounds created by the valves and any variations in the sounds associated with S_1 and S_2. The examiner should keep the stethoscope in each location for several cardiac cycles.

Bearing in mind that S_1 and S_2 are heard anywhere in the precordium, the examiner begins a thorough examination by focusing on the sounds created by the semilunar valves—the aortic and pulmonic valves. These valves are located at the base of the heart, which is actually the top of the heart where the great vessels exit. Variations associated with alterations of aortic valve function are best assessed in the second interspace to the right of the sternal border, where they are heard best because the valve points in that direction (**Figure 1-12**). The stethoscope then is moved to the second interspace at the left sternal border, the best location for assessment of pulmonic valve function.

All other assessments occur on the left side of the sternum. Tricuspid valve variations are heard best at the fifth interspace at the left sternal border, and the mitral valve is assessed where the fifth interspace intersects the midclavicular line. The mitral valve, or apical area, is not only useful as a landmark for

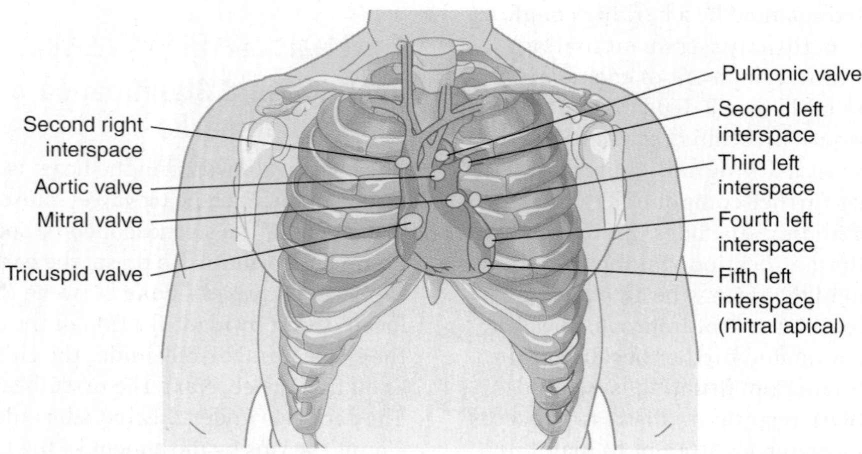

FIGURE 1-12 Areas for auscultation of the heart.

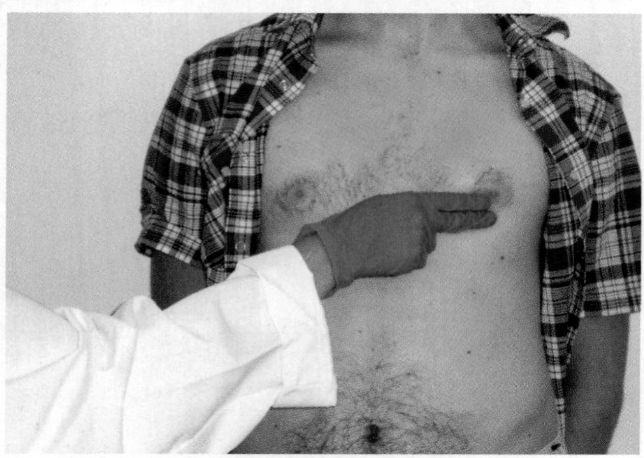

FIGURE 1-13 Palpation of the apical pulse.

auscultation but also provides other useful information. This relatively small left ventricular apex is the area where the left ventricle protrudes from behind the right ventricle, known as the *point of maximal impulse (PMI)*. The left ventricle taps gently against an area of the thoracic wall no more than 2 cm in diameter (**Figure 1-13**). Left ventricular hypertrophy may be the cause of an enlarged PMI.

Cardiac Auscultation

Listening to heart sounds involves notations of rate and rhythm, extra heart sounds, and murmurs. Heart rate and rhythm should be observed first. A regular rhythm with a rate between 60 and 100 beats per minute is ideal; however, certain irregularities represent harmless variants. Conversely, other irregularities may herald serious consequences. Auscultation used to determine rate and rhythm is done with the stethoscope at the apex of the heart, a procedure commonly known as *taking an apical rate*.

S_1 and S_2

Normal heart sounds are classified as S_1 and S_2 (*S* originates simply from the word *sound*). S_1 is the first heart sound and results from closure of the atrioventricular (mitral and tricuspid) valves. S_1 is also described as sounding like *lub*. As the ventricles eject most of their blood, ventricular pressure drops below aortic pressure, resulting in closure of the aortic and pulmonic valves, which in turn produces S_2, or the second heart sound, also known as *dub*.

A normal variant may be auscultated with the stethoscope at the second interspace along the left sternal border. In many individuals, a split S_2 may be heard here during inspiration, a sound that occurs when pulmonic valve closure happens a few milliseconds after closure of the aortic valve. Typically, this action takes place during inspiration, as increasing intrathoracic pressure causes blood to strike the pulmonic valve with greater force.

S_3 and S_4

S_3 and S_4 are extra sounds generated by certain aberrant blood flow mechanisms. These sounds are best heard at the left fifth intercostal space at the midclavicular line, also known as the *mitral*, or *apical, area*. An S_4 immediately precedes the S_1, and the S_3 follows immediately after the S_2. These rhythms are commonly called *gallops* because of their resemblance to the sound of a horse galloping. To auscultate for either an S_3 or an S_4, the bell of a stethoscope is pressed lightly against the skin. Pressing too firmly obliterates the sounds. The S_3 and S_4 are heard best with the patient in a left side-lying position.

An S_3 results from rapid ventricular filling. When ventricular pump failure occurs, an increased amount of residual blood remains in the heart chambers after a contraction. Consequently, the ventricles fill faster during diastole. This pumping of blood into an already partially filled ventricle causes vibrations heard as an S_3. An S_3 occurs immediately after the S_2. It resembles a split S_2 but differs in location and timing. A split S_2 is heard in the pulmonic area and varies with respiratory cycle, whereas the S_3 is heard at the apex.

An S_4 is a sound caused most often by a stiff ventricle, such as may be the case in hypertension or after a myocardial infarction. For an S_4 to be present, an atrial contraction must occur. Consequently, this heart sound is often known as an *atrial gallop*. An S_4 cannot exist in the presence of atrial fibrillation, a condition in which the atria do not contract. The vibrations causing an S_4 are thought to be due to atrial contraction occurring in the presence of a stiffened or *noncompliant* ventricle. The S_4 precedes the S_1.

Murmurs

A simple description of a cardiac **murmur** is an extra sound heard in conjunction with S_1 and S_2. Several mechanisms describe the etiology of murmurs. Murmurs occur when blood regurgitates into the chamber from which it came. Sometimes valvular dysfunction develops as a sequela to rheumatic heart disease after infection with β-hemolytic streptococci. This syndrome results in valves that are distorted in shape and calcified.

Other murmurs arise when a large volume of blood flows through a valve, such as occurs during pregnancy, anemia, or hyperthyroidism. Murmurs also result from blood flowing through a narrowed or stenotic valve. A final category of murmurs arises from congenital defects resulting in blood flow through openings not normally present.

Classification of Murmurs

Murmurs are classified as early, middle, or late systolic—that is, occurring between S_1 and S_2. Others are diastolic, coming between S_2 and the next S_1. The intensity of murmurs is graded from I to VI and is recorded in Roman numerals. A grade I murmur

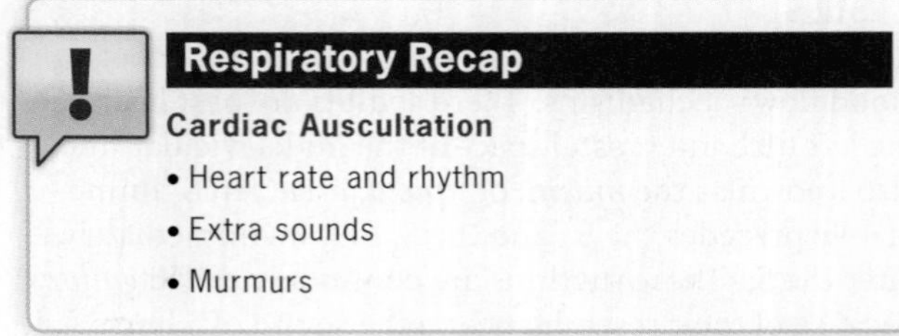

Respiratory Recap

Cardiac Auscultation

- Heart rate and rhythm
- Extra sounds
- Murmurs

is very faint and may not be heard in all positions. Generally, a highly trained ear is required for detection of this sound. Murmurs that are grades II through IV increase progressively in intensity, with a grade V murmur being very loud. A grade VI murmur may be heard without the stethoscope in contact with the chest.

Murmurs differ in quality and are described as blowing, rasping, harsh, coarse, grating, whistling, or musical. In addition, they are classified according to the location at which the sound is loudest. This location corresponds to the area of the precordium where the valve in question is best auscultated, such as the fifth interspace midclavicular line or mitral area.

Murmurs and Infective Endocarditis

Many murmurs are classified as functional, innocent, or physiologic, meaning that they are clinically insignificant. Others are significant in that they suggest a progressive pathologic process that may eventually require surgical intervention. Some murmurs signify a defect that requires prophylaxis against *infective endocarditis*. Formerly known as *subacute bacterial endocarditis*, infective endocarditis develops when bacteria colonize on the heart valves. The immune response causes growth of fibrotic tissue, which consequently results in development of vegetation on valves. Clearly, this interferes with efficient hemodynamics, and a murmur ensues. Another danger exists if the vegetation breaks off and the resulting emboli lodge elsewhere in the body. The bacteria then reproduce in that location. *Prophylaxis against infective endocarditis* is the term given to antibiotic therapy administered before any invasive or surgical procedure, including dental work. Innocent or physiologic murmurs require no such prophylaxis; however, innocence can be determined only by echocardiogram. Diastolic murmurs suggest the need for prophylaxis against infective endocarditis.

Jugular Venous Distention

The inspection component of a cardiac assessment primarily involves observation of the right internal jugular vein, the vessel that reflects pressure changes better than other superficial veins. Oscillations in this vein reflect changing pressures within the right atrium. Similarly, distention of this neck vein suggests a distended right ventricle, which often suggests right ventricular failure. Distended neck veins are normal in an individual in the supine position. Furthermore, neck veins fill temporarily with any activity that raises intrathoracic pressure, such as coughing, conversing, or bearing down (the Valsalva maneuver).

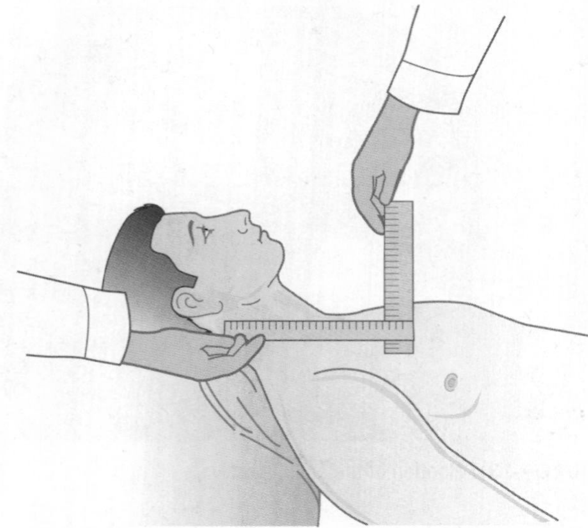

FIGURE 1-14 Technique used to measure jugular venous distention.

To assess for pathologic processes, however, the following technique is used to determine the degree of jugular venous distention. The patient is placed in a supine position, with the head of the bed at a 45-degree angle (**Figure 1-14**). With a centimeter ruler, the vertical distance between the sternal angle and the highest level of jugular vein pulsation then is measured on both sides. Neck veins that fill to a level of 2 cm or less are considered normal. Higher than this level suggests increased right ventricular pressure and is associated with right-sided heart failure.

The Neurologic System

Because of the system's complexity, an assessment of the neurologic system can be daunting. This brief summary focuses on the most common neurologic abnormalities.

Level of Consciousness

When a patient experiences an alteration in the level of consciousness because of trauma or some other hypoxic or metabolic event, the Glasgow Coma Scale (**Table 1-4**) is commonly used. This scale uses a numeric scoring method to document eye-opening response, verbal response, and integrated motor response. Scores range from a low of 3 points, which suggests brain death, to a maximum of 15 points, which indicates full consciousness.

Other indications of neurologic integrity are normality and equality of strength in all extremities. Clearly, any less-than-normal finding suggests impairment and warrants full evaluation. Pupils may be evaluated for size, equality, reaction to light, and

TABLE 1-4
Glasgow Coma Scale

Observation	Score
Eye Opening	
Spontaneous	4
In response to voice	3
In response to pain	2
None	1
Verbal Response	
Oriented response	5
Confused response	4
Inappropriate words	3
Incomprehensible words	2
None	1
Motor Response	
Obeys commands	6
Localizes	5
Withdraws	4
Flexes (decorticate)	3
Extends (decerebrate)	2
None	1

accommodation. Normal reactivity is documented as *PEARLA*, or *pupils equal and reacting to light and accommodation*. Although pupillary assessment is commonly performed, however, abnormalities in size and reaction are a late finding and may indicate significant brain dysfunction.

A decreasing level of consciousness is the first finding to suggest neurologic impairment. Because sleep is itself a decreased level of consciousness, however, it is important to distinguish between normal sleep and a state suggesting a serious pathologic condition—such as is the case in carbon dioxide narcosis or respiratory failure. In critically ill, mechanically ventilated patients, sedation and decreased level of consciousness are often pharmacologically induced. The level

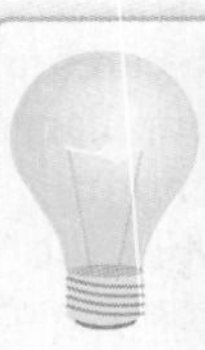

STOP AND THINK

You are assessing a mechanically ventilated patient in the ICU. What considerations are important in the neurologic assessment of the patient?

TABLE 1-5
Ramsay Sedation Scale

Level	Response
1	Anxious, agitated, restless
2	Cooperative, oriented, tranquil
3	Responding to commands only
4	Asleep, brisk response to stimulus
5	Asleep, sluggish response to stimulus
6	Unarousable

of sedation in these patients is often assessed with the Ramsay score (**Table 1-5**) or the Richmond Agitation Sedation Scale (**Table 1-6**). Delirium in the intensive care unit (ICU) is measured with the Confusion Assessment Method for Assessing Delirium in the Intensive Care Unit (CAM-ICU) (**Figure 1-15**).

Posturing

Patients with neurologic injury may demonstrate decerebrate or decorticate posturing (**Figure 1-16**). Decerebrate posturing may result from a painful

TABLE 1-6
Richmond Agitation Sedation Scale (RASS)

Score	Term	Description
+4	Combative	Overtly combative, violent, immediate danger to staff
+3	Very agitated	Pulls or removes tube(s) or catheter(s), aggressive
+2	Agitated	Frequent nonpurposeful movement, fights ventilator
+1	Restless	Anxious, but movements not aggressive or vigorous
0	Alert and calm	
−1	Drowsy	Not fully alert, but has sustained awakening (eye opening/eye contact) to voice (≥10 seconds)
−2	Light sedation	Briefly awakens with eye contact to voice (<10 seconds)
−3	Moderate sedation	Movement or eye opening to voice (but no eye contact)
−4	Deep sedation	No response to voice, but movement or eye opening to physical stimulation
−5	Unarousable	No response to voice or physical stimulation

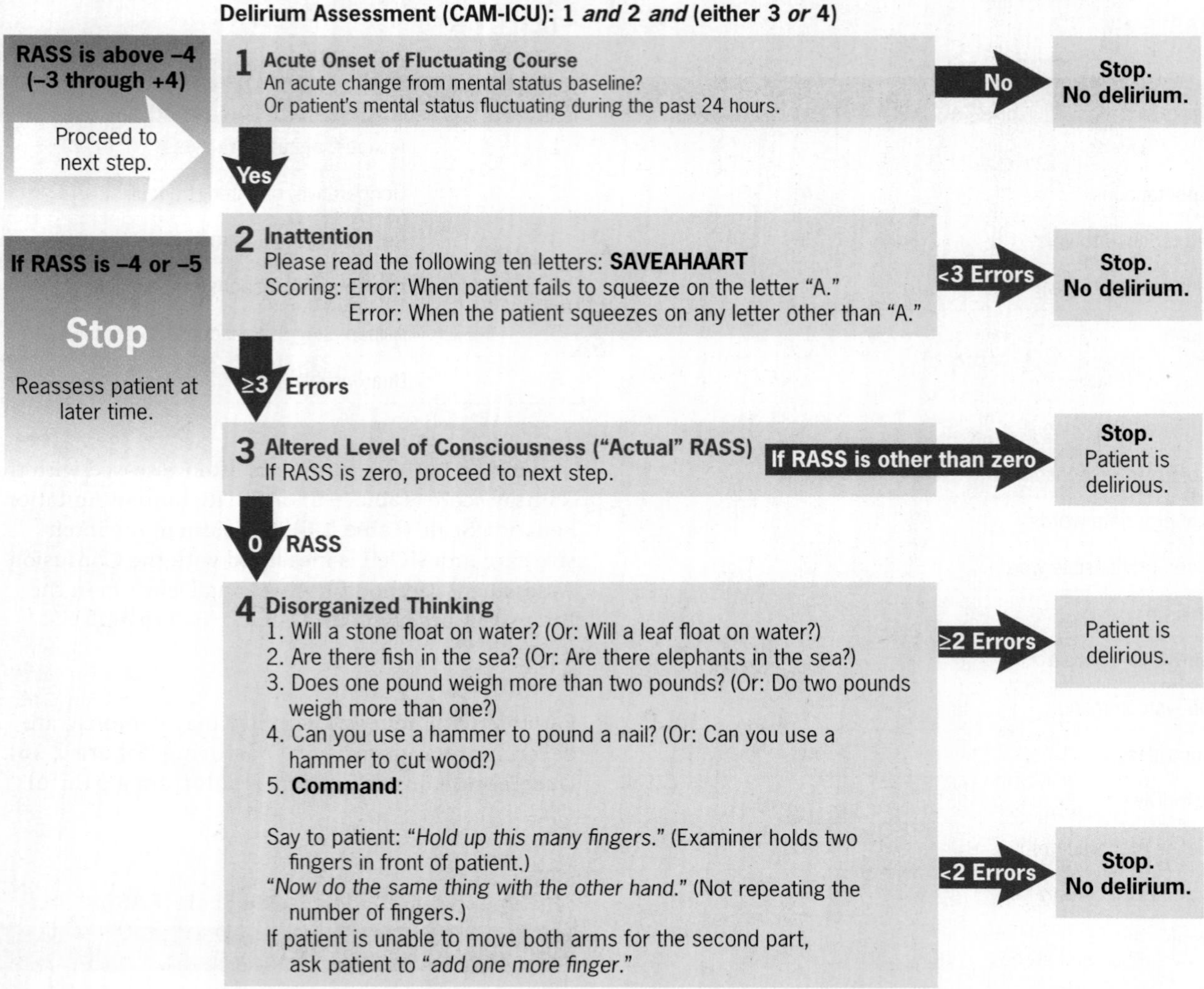

Delirium Assessment (CAM-ICU): 1 *and* 2 *and* (either 3 *or* 4)

RASS is above –4 (–3 through +4)
Proceed to next step.

If RASS is –4 or –5
Stop
Reassess patient at later time.

1 Acute Onset of Fluctuating Course
An acute change from mental status baseline?
Or patient's mental status fluctuating during the past 24 hours.
→ No → **Stop. No delirium.**
↓ Yes

2 Inattention
Please read the following ten letters: **SAVEAHAART**
Scoring: Error: When patient fails to squeeze on the letter "A."
Error: When the patient squeezes on any letter other than "A."
→ <3 Errors → **Stop. No delirium.**
↓ ≥3 **Errors**

3 Altered Level of Consciousness ("Actual" RASS)
If RASS is zero, proceed to next step.
→ **If RASS is other than zero** → **Stop.** Patient is delirious.
↓ 0 **RASS**

4 Disorganized Thinking
1. Will a stone float on water? (Or: Will a leaf float on water?)
2. Are there fish in the sea? (Or: Are there elephants in the sea?)
3. Does one pound weigh more than two pounds? (Or: Do two pounds weigh more than one?)
4. Can you use a hammer to pound a nail? (Or: Can you use a hammer to cut wood?)
5. **Command**:

Say to patient: "*Hold up this many fingers.*" (Examiner holds two fingers in front of patient.)
"*Now do the same thing with the other hand.*" (Not repeating the number of fingers.)
If patient is unable to move both arms for the second part, ask patient to "*add one more finger.*"

→ ≥2 Errors → Patient is delirious.
→ <2 Errors → **Stop. No delirium.**

FIGURE 1-15 Confusion Assessment Method for Assessing Delirium in the Intensive Care Unit (CAM-ICU).

Reproduced from Guenther U, Popp J, Koecher L, et al. Validity and reliability of the CAM-ICU flowsheet to diagnose delirium in surgical ICU patients. *Crit Care.* 2010;25:144–156. Copyright 2010, with permission of Elsevier.

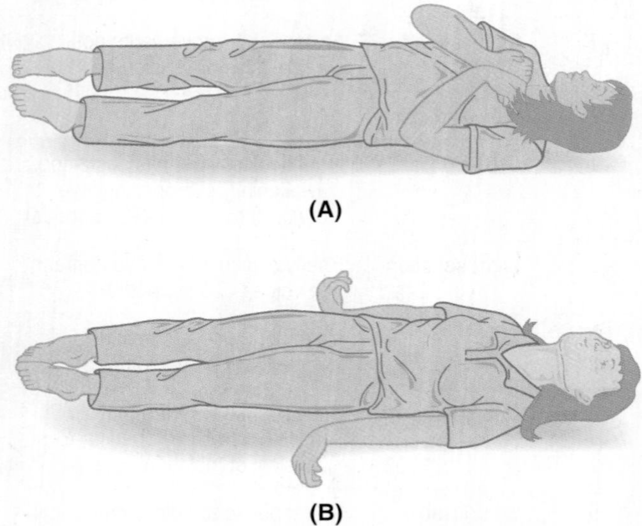

FIGURE 1-16 (**A**) Decorticate posturing. (**B**) Decerebrate posturing.

stimulus of a comatose patient with low-level brain stem compression. The patient responds with extension and internal rotation of the arms and extends the legs. Decorticate posturing results when a painful stimulus is applied to a comatose patient with a lesion in the mesencephalic region of the brain. In response to the stimulus, the patient rigidly flexes the arms at the elbows and wrists. The legs may be flexed as well.

Pupillary Dilation

Pupillary dilation (**Figure 1-17**) can occur with cerebral edema and brain stem compression. Because pupillary dilation is related to compression of the oculomotor nerve, the pupil will be dilated *on the same side* as the causative brain lesion. Either dilation or constriction of the pupils can also be associated with the administration of some medications.

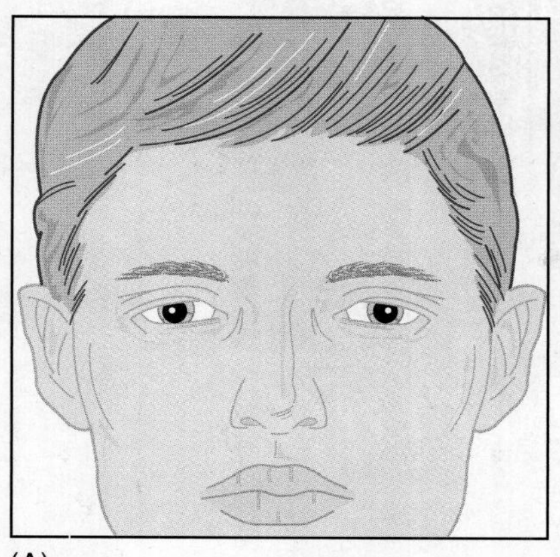
(A)

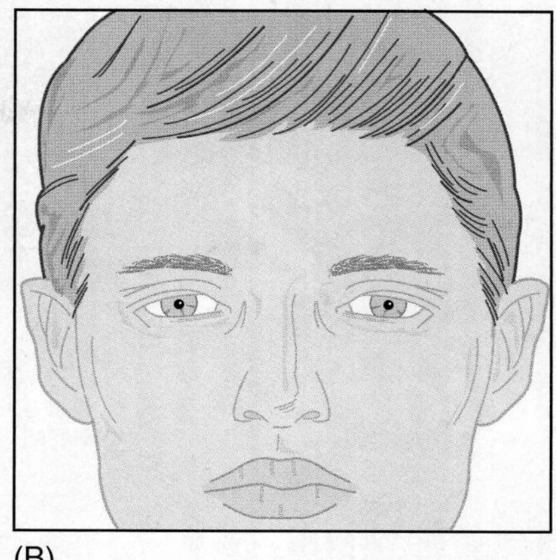
(B)

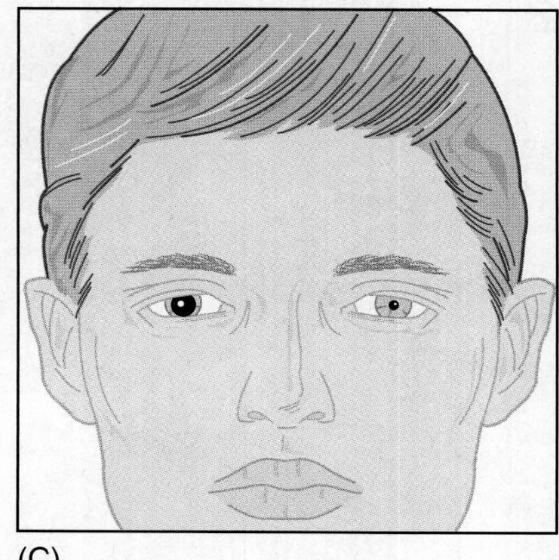
(C)

FIGURE 1-17 (**A**) Dilated pupils. (**B**) Constricted pupils. (**C**) Unequal pupils.

Key Points

- The health history provides a detailed, chronologic record of the patient.
- The HPI offers a description of the onset of the problem, whether it developed suddenly, and the setting in which it developed.
- The four examination techniques commonly used are inspection, palpation, percussion, and auscultation.
- The use of accessory muscles implies an increased work of breathing.
- The assessment of respiratory expansion helps determine whether the lungs are expanding symmetrically.
- Auscultation of the chest allows assessment of diminished breath sounds, bronchial breath sounds, and adventitious breath sounds, such as crackles, rhonchi, wheezing, stridor, and pleural friction rubs.
- Listening to heart sounds involves notations of the rate and rhythm, extra heart sounds, and murmurs.
- The Glasgow Coma Scale is used to assess the level of consciousness.
- The level of sedation in critically ill, mechanically ventilated patients is often assessed with the Ramsay score or the Richmond Agitation Sedation Scale.
- Delirium is measured with the CAM score.

Suggested Reading

Bickley LS. *Bates' Guide to Physical Examination and History Taking.* 11th ed. Philadelphia: JB Lippincott; 2012.

Des Jardins T. *Clinical Manifestation and Assessment of Respiratory Disease.* 6th ed. Philadelphia: Elsevier; 2010.

Jarvis C. *Physical Examination and Health Assessment.* 6th ed. Philadelphia: WB Saunders; 2011.

Mangione S. *Secrets: Heart and Lung Sounds.* 2nd ed. Philadelphia: Elsevier Health Sciences; 2009.

Seidel HM, Flynn JA, Ball JW, Dains JE, Solomon BS *Mosby's Guide to Physical Examination.* 7th ed. St. Louis: Mosby; 2010.

Swartz MH. *Textbook of Physical Diagnosis: History and Examination.* 7th ed. Philadelphia: WB Saunders; 2014.

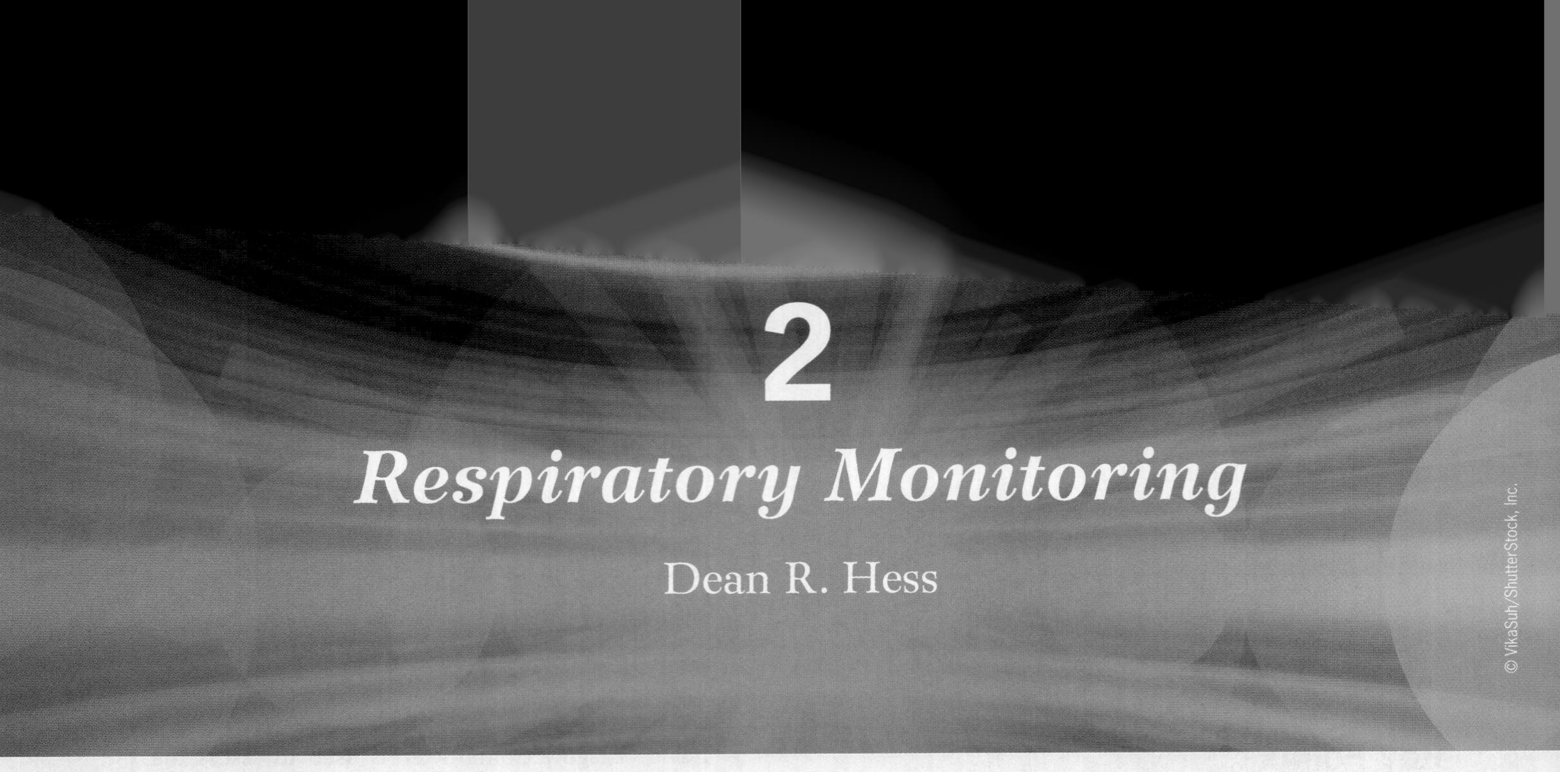

2 Respiratory Monitoring

Dean R. Hess

OUTLINE

Pulse Oximetry
Capnography
Transcutaneous Blood Gas Monitoring
Respiratory Rate and Pattern
Brain Po_2
Near-Infrared Spectroscopy

OBJECTIVES

1. Explain how pulse oximetry estimates arterial oxygen saturation.
2. Discuss the limitations of pulse oximetry.
3. Describe techniques to address errors caused by motion and low perfusion.
4. Explain how the pulse oximeter plethysmographic waveform can be used to assess peripheral perfusion.
5. Describe methods used to measure carbon dioxide in the exhaled gas.
6. Compare sidestream and mainstream capnography.
7. Compare time-based and volume-based capnography.
8. Discuss the physiologic issues related to end-tidal Pco_2 and how they affect the relationship between end-tidal and arterial Pco_2.
9. Explain how volume-based capnography can be used to measure carbon dioxide production and cardiac output.
10. Discuss the principle of operation of transcutaneous blood gas monitors.
11. Discuss the limitations of transcutaneous blood gas monitoring.
12. Describe techniques that can be used to measure respiratory rate.
13. Discuss the use of brain Po_2 monitoring.
14. Describe near-infrared spectroscopy.

KEY TERMS

absorption
acoustic technology
Beer-Lambert law
bradypnea
brain tissue Po_2 ($Pbto_2$)
capnogram
capnography
capnometry
end-tidal Pco_2
fiberoptic plethysmography
impedance pneumography
mass spectrometer
near-infrared spectroscopy (NIRS)
penumbra effect
perfusion index (PI)
piezoelectric plethysmography
plethysmographic variability index (PVI)
pulse oximetry
Raman spectroscopy
respiratory inductance plethysmography (RIP)
spectrophotometry
thermistor
thermocouple
transcutaneous monitoring

Introduction

Monitoring is a continuous, or nearly continuous, evaluation of the physiologic function of a patient in real time to guide management decisions, including when to make therapeutic interventions and assessment of those interventions. Monitoring often is used to ensure patient safety. Monitoring also is used to assess patient response to clinical interventions. In this chapter, respiratory monitoring of oxygenation, ventilation, and respiratory rate is discussed. Also discussed are the newer technologies for monitoring brain Po_2 and tissue oxygenation by near-infrared spectroscopy.

Pulse Oximetry

Pulse oximetry noninvasively estimates the hemoglobin oxygen saturation of arterial blood.[1,2] It is based on **spectrophotometry**, the process by which substances are identified by their **absorption** (also called *extinction*) of specific wavelengths in the electromagnetic spectrum. The various hemoglobin molecules absorb wavelengths between 500 and 1000 nm in the infrared and visible light regions. The **Beer-Lambert law** defines the relationship between the concentration of a substance and the amount of light absorbed:

$$A = L \times C \times \varepsilon$$

where L is the optical path length, C is the concentration of the substance, and ε is the absorption of the particular wavelength used. A separate wavelength is required for each substance to be identified. Most pulse oximeters use two wavelengths, red (660 nm) and infrared (940 nm), at which oxyhemoglobin (HbO_2) and deoxyhemoglobin (Hb) have different absorption characteristics.

Red and infrared light-emitting diodes (LEDs) in the oximeter probe serve as light sources (**Figure 2-1**). Because HbO_2 and Hb differ in light absorption at each wavelength, the amount of red and infrared light transmitted is related to oxygen saturation (**Figure 2-2**). A photodiode positioned on the opposite side of the probe serves as the photodetector. To identify the oxygen saturation of arterial blood only, the device relies on the pulsatile nature of arterial flow. During systole, a new volume of blood enters the arteriolar bed, and light absorption increases. During diastole, absorption decreases to a minimal level (**Figure 2-3**). Measuring pulsatile absorption eliminates the effects of nonpulsatile components such as tissue, bone, and venous blood.

Oxygen saturation (Spo_2) is related to the ratio of minimum and maximum absorption at each wavelength (**Figure 2-4**). A calibration curve is plotted for the pulse-added absorption at the two wavelengths and stored in a software algorithm. Devices vary by manufacturer in the type of LED, photodiode, and

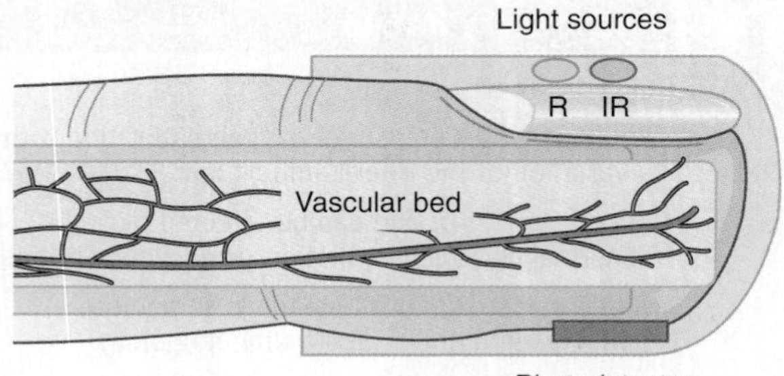

FIGURE 2-1 Pulse oximeter probe fitted over finger, showing position of light sources and detector.

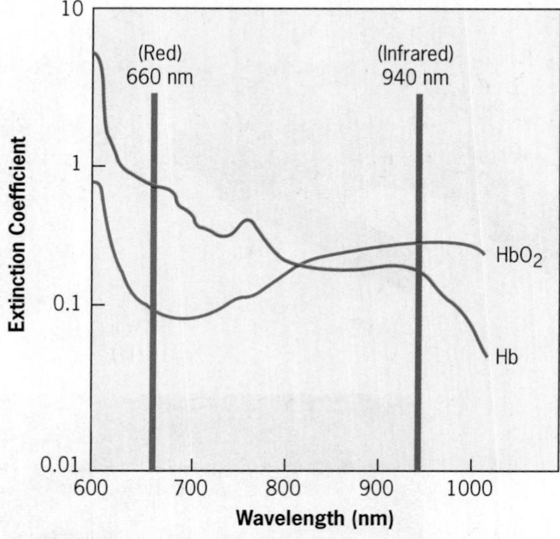

FIGURE 2-2 Absorption spectra for oxyhemoglobin and deoxyhemoglobin for the range of wavelengths relevant to pulse oximetry.

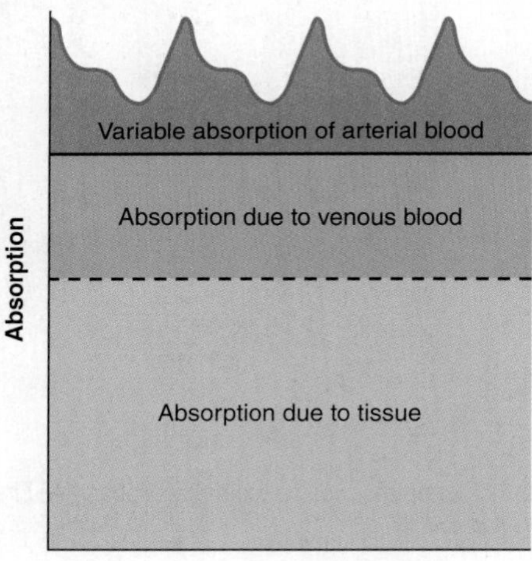

FIGURE 2-3 Dynamic and static light absorption during pulse oximetry.
Used with permission of Philips Respironics.

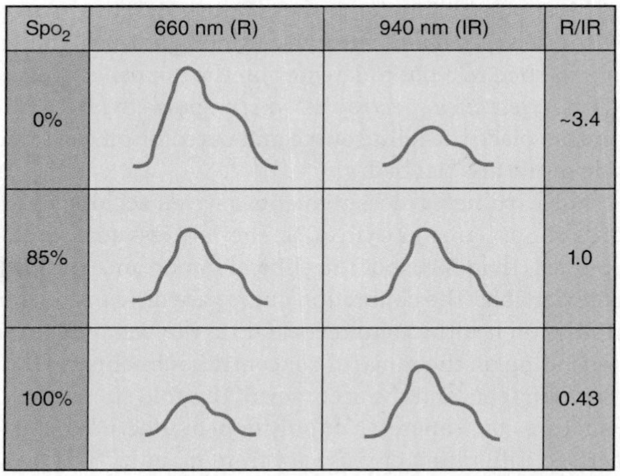

Spo_2	660 nm (R)	940 nm (IR)	R/IR
0%			~3.4
85%			1.0
100%			0.43

FIGURE 2-4 Relationship between red and infrared light absorption for different oxygen saturations.

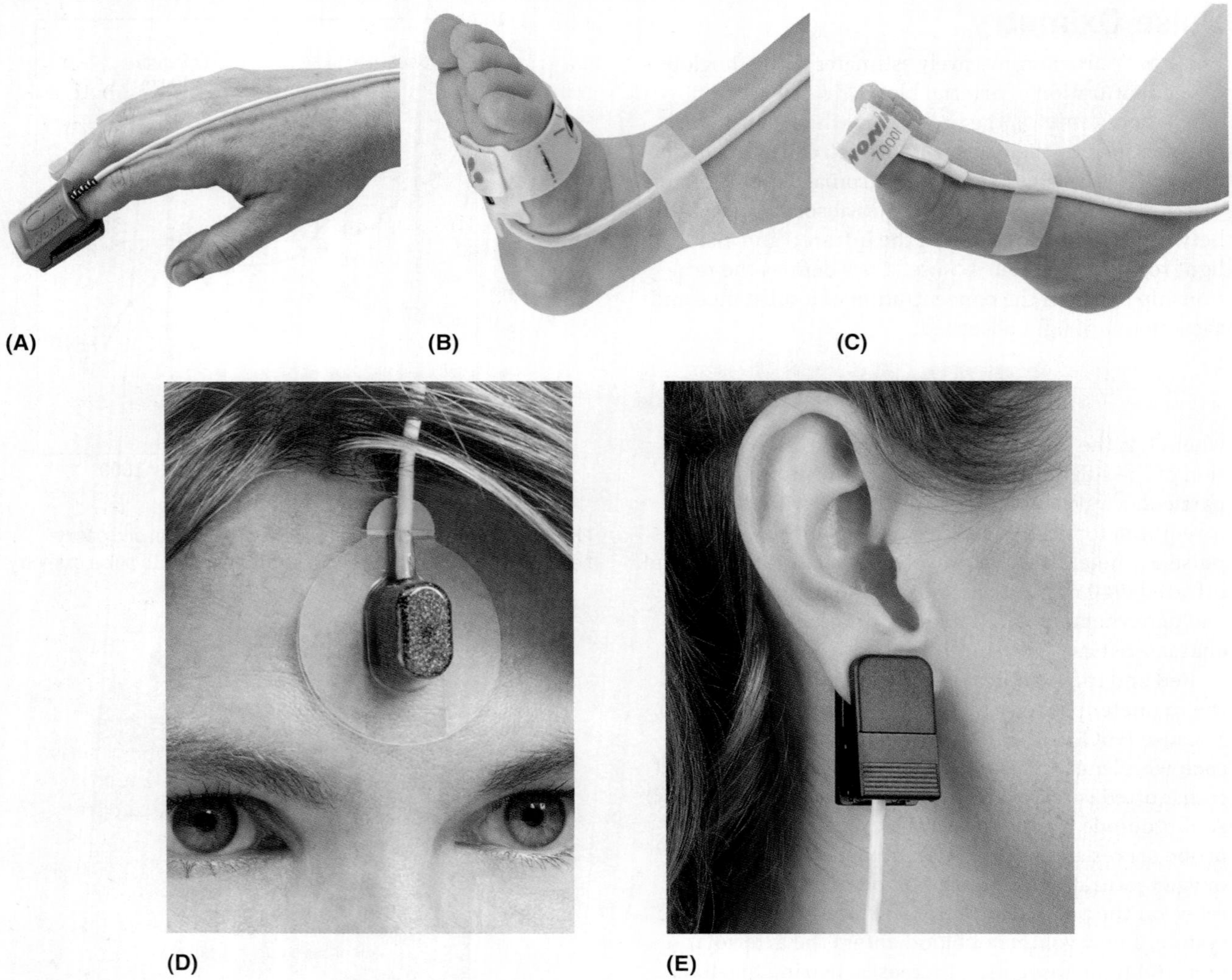

(A) (B) (C)

(D) (E)

FIGURE 2-5 Examples of pulse oximetry probes. (**A**) Finger probe. (**B**) Foot probe. (**C**) Toe probe. (**D**) Forehead probe. (**E**) Ear probe.

microprocessor used. Because the Spo_2 calculation is based on a constantly updated signal ratio, no calibration is required.

Most pulse oximeter probes (**Figure 2-5**) use *transmittance spectrophotometry*, sending light through the arterial bed to a photodetector on the opposite side. With *reflectance spectrophotometry*, pulse oximeter sensors place the light source and detector on the same side of the arterial bed.

Pulse oximeter measurements have an accuracy of ±4% at Spo_2 greater than 80%. They are less accurate at Spo_2 less than 80%, but the clinical importance of this is questionable. The calibration curves are developed from studies on healthy volunteers and vary by manufacturer depending on the range of concentrations achieved by the volunteers and the accuracy of the gold standard, usually a co-oximeter. Not only do manufacturer-derived calibration curves vary from manufacturer to manufacturer but also the output of the LEDs can vary from probe to probe. Ideally, the same pulse oximeter and probe should be used for repeated measurements in the same patient.

To appreciate the implications of the accuracy of pulse oximetry, one must consider the oxyhemoglobin equilibration (or dissociation) curve. If the pulse oximeter displays a Spo_2 of 95%, the true saturation

Respiratory Recap

Pulse Oximetry

- Pulse oximetry measures oxygen saturation with a variation of the Beer-Lambert law.
- Accuracy is ±4% and can be affected by abnormal hemoglobin, motion, and low perfusion.
- Some pulse oximeters measure hemoglobin, carboxyhemoglobin, and methemoglobin.
- Some pulse oximeters display the perfusion index and plethysmogram variability index.

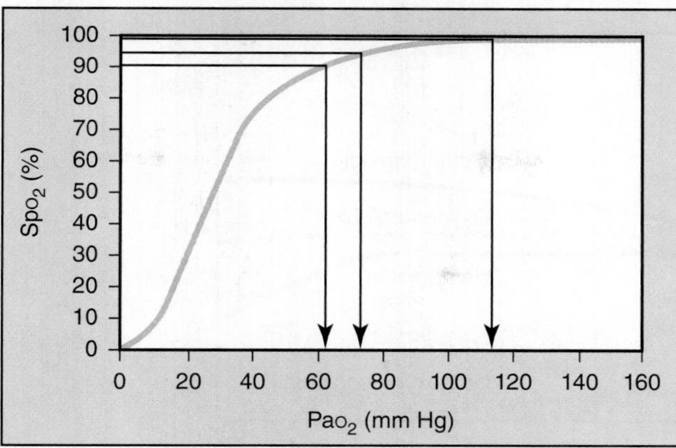

FIGURE 2-6 If the pulse oximeter displays Spo_2 95%, the arterial oxygen saturation could be as low as 91% or as high as 99%. Note that this translates to a wide range of Pao_2.

could be as low as 91% or as high as 99% (**Figure 2-6**). If the true saturation is 91%, the Pao_2 will be about 60 to 70 mm Hg. If the true saturation is 99%, however, the Pao_2 might be very high. A shift of the oxyhemoglobin equilibration curve can change the Spo_2, although no change in Pao_2 has occurred (**Figure 2-7**). For example, a respiratory acidosis will cause the curve to shift to the right, resulting in a decrease in Spo_2 even with no change in Pao_2.

In the intensive care unit (ICU), pulse oximetry is monitored on a continuous basis. Outside the ICU, the availability of portable, battery-powered units has resulted in the common practice of spot-checking hospitalized patients during clinical care or oxygen therapy. Although this practice may enhance appropriate oxygen therapy, allowing weaning or discontinuation of unnecessary prescriptions, it has some potential problems. It provides no direct information about the $Paco_2$ and may not accurately reflect the Pao_2 because of changes in the shape and position of the oxyhemoglobin dissociation curve.

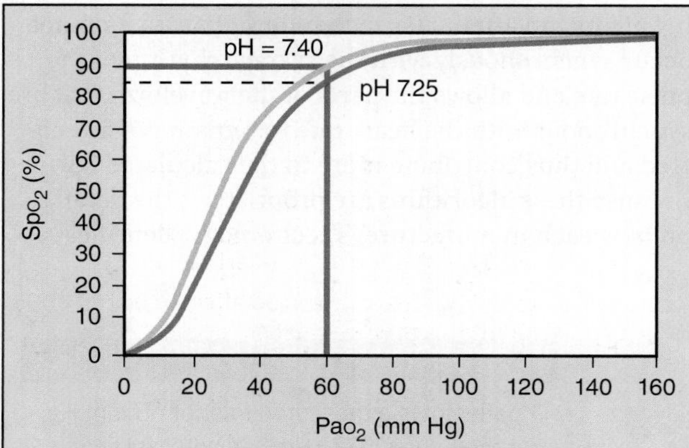

FIGURE 2-7 Note that a shift in the oxyhemoglobin equilibration curve results in a change in Spo_2 without a change in Pao_2.

Limitations

Most pulse oximeters measure only the percentage of HbO_2 relative to the sum of HbO_2 and Hb (functional saturation):

$$Spo_2\ (\%) = HbO_2/(HbO_2 + Hb) \times 100$$

Because of the light absorption characteristics of carboxyhemoglobin (HbCO) relative to HbO_2 (**Figure 2-8A**), the oximeter overestimates HbO_2 saturation by an amount roughly equal to the HbCO level.[3] For methemoglobin (Hbmet), the light absorption for red and infrared light is nearly identical, resulting in a Spo_2 estimate of 85% (**Figure 2-8B**).[3] Thus, Hbmet causes the Spo_2 to be inaccurately low for an arterial oxygen saturation greater than 85% and it causes the Spo_2 to be inaccurately high for an oxygen saturation less than 85%. Fetal hemoglobin and sickle cell anemia[4] do not affect the accuracy of pulse oximetry.

Care must be taken to ensure that the pulse oximeter probe is fitted correctly. If the pulse oximeter probe does not fit correctly, light can be shunted from the LEDs directly to the photodetector. This will cause a falsely low Spo_2 if Sao_2 is greater than 85% and a falsely elevated Spo_2 if Sao_2 is less than 85%. This is called the **penumbra effect**.

The accuracy and performance of pulse oximeters are affected by deeply pigmented skin.[5] Although one study suggests that nail polish may have less effect on the accuracy of pulse oximetry than previously thought, it is prudent to remove nail polish before pulse oximetry is initiated.[6] Intravascular dyes (methylene blue and indocyanine green) also cause an underestimation of Spo_2. Hyperbilirubinemia has no effect on accuracy because the absorption peak for bilirubin (460 nm) is below that used in pulse oximetry. Xenon and fluorescent lighting affect some probes, a problem that can be prevented by shielding.

Pulse oximeters require a pulsating vascular bed. Under conditions of low flow, pulse oximetry becomes unreliable. Under these conditions, an ear probe may be more reliable than a finger probe. Although pulse oximeters are generally reliable over a wide range of hemoglobin levels, they become less accurate and reliable with conditions of severe anemia (hematocrit $<$24 g/dL at low saturations, and hematocrit $<$10% at all saturations). Venous pulses and a large dicrotic notch may affect the accuracy of pulse oximetry.

Pulse oximetry is usually a safe procedure. Tissue injury may result from incorrect probe application or electrical shock and burns from substitution of incompatible probes between instruments.

Approaches to Deal with Errors Caused by Motion and Low Perfusion

Pulse oximetry is accurate when all hemoglobin is either oxyhemoglobin or deoxyhemoglobin, when there are no other absorbers between the LEDs and the

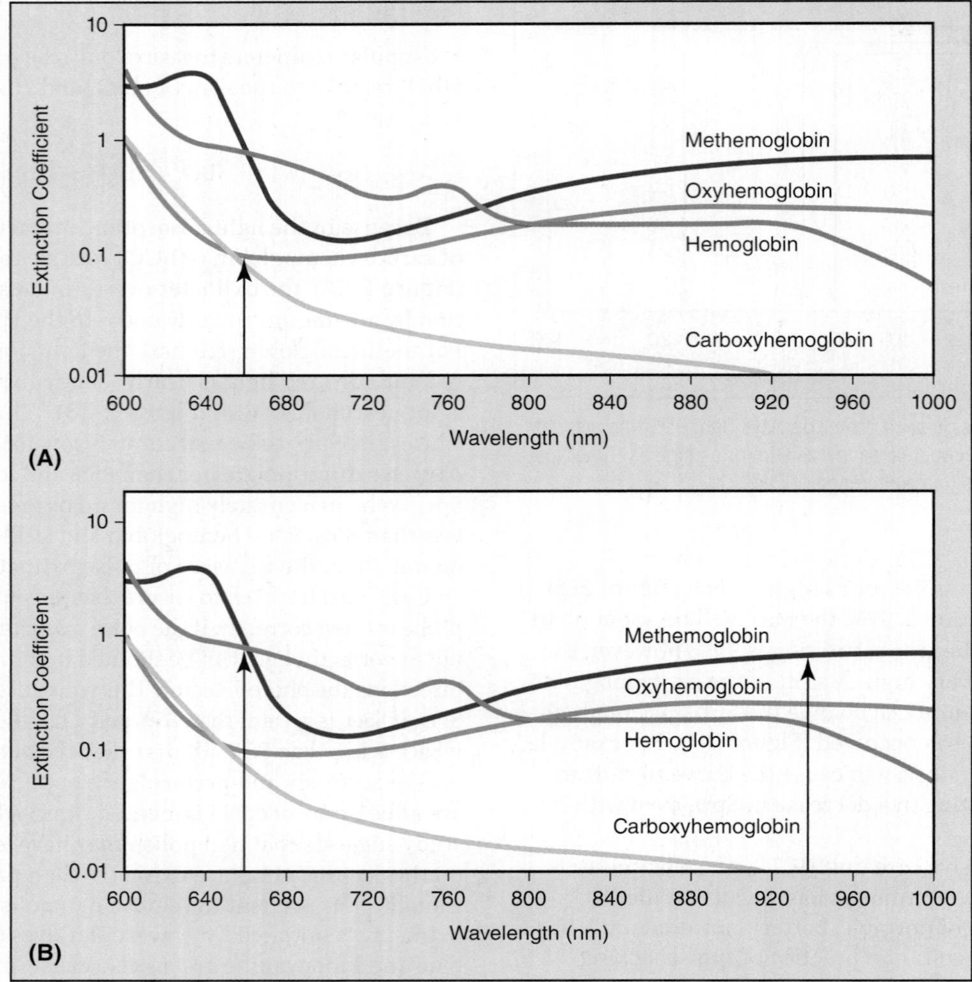

FIGURE 2-8 (**A**) At 660 nm, note that the absorptions for oxyhemoglobin and for carboxyhemoglobin are nearly identical. (**B**) Note that the absorption for methemoglobin is nearly identical at 660 nm and 940 nm.

detector other than those present during the empirical calibration, and when all the blood that pulsates is arterial blood. Motion and low perfusion can induce considerable errors in pulse oximetry accuracy.[7] With low perfusion, there is an increase in the ratio of venous blood to arterial blood at the measuring site. Moreover, lower perfusion is associated with lower pulse amplitude, so the noise of motion has a greater effect when combined with a low signal. Strategies to address issues related to motion and low perfusion include averaging the saturation data over a longer period of time and suspending the reporting of data until clean data are available.

Manufacturers of pulse oximeters have developed motion-resistant technologies and sophisticated algorithms to eliminate motion artifacts from the pulse signal.[8] The discrete saturation transform (DST) uses a reference signal generator, an adaptive filter, and a peak picker, which work in concert to determine the most likely Spo_2 value based on the incoming signals. Signal Extraction Technology (SET) uses DST and parallel signal processing engines to separate the arterial signal from sources of noise to measure Spo_2 and pulse rate accurately. The Fourier artifact-suppression technology (FAST) algorithm identifies the frequency components of the pulse rate and compares those to the frequency components of the incoming signal to select the component that is at the pulse rate for both the red and infrared wavelengths. The variable cardiac gated averaging algorithm attenuates incoming signals that do not occur synchronously with the average rhythm of the pulse rate and allows the parts of the waveform that are synchronous with the heart rate to remain not attenuated and thus contribute more to the calculated Spo_2. Because these algorithms are proprietary, the details on how each manufacturer's technology identifies

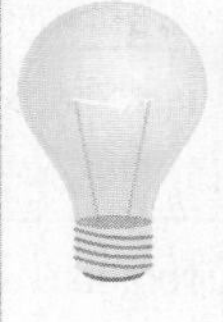

STOP AND THINK

A patient has a measured Pao_2 of 55 mm Hg, but the Spo_2 is 97%. How do you explain this apparent discrepancy?

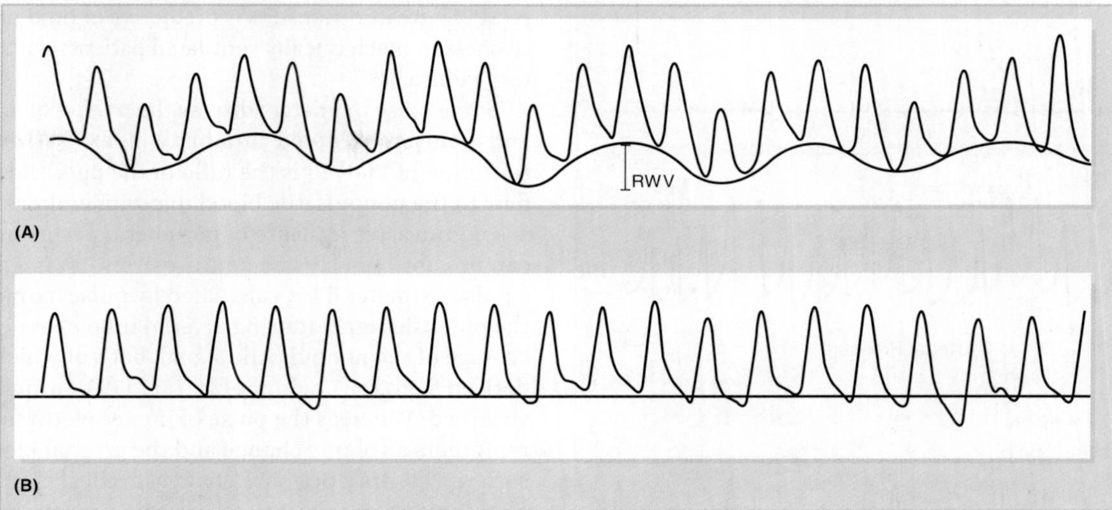

FIGURE 2-9 Pulse oximeter tracings from a 60-year-old woman with an exacerbation of chronic obstructive pulmonary disease who was admitted to the ICU in ventilatory failure. (**A**) The patient's pulse oximetry tracing at the time of admission, revealing the respiratory variability in the pulse oximeter plethysmography tracing. Her measured pulsus paradoxus at this time was 16 mm Hg. (**B**) The patient's pulse oximetry tracing after 12 hours of aggressive therapy. Her pulsus paradoxus at this time was 8 mm Hg. Note the absence of respiratory waveform variation (RWV) in the baseline of the oximeter tracing after the clinical improvement in airflow and the resolution of elevated pulsus paradoxus.

Reproduced from Hartert TV, Wheeler AP, Sheller JR. Use of pulse oximetry to recognize severity of airflow obstruction in obstructive airway disease: correlation with pulsus paradoxus. *Chest.* 1999;115:475–481. Used with permission from the American College of Chest Physicians.

and processes the incoming signals are not available. The clinical performance of new-generation pulse oximeters is better than that of earlier devices, although there is no strong and convincing evidence that the performance of any single new-generation device is superior to that of any of the others.

Pulse Oximetry to Measure Hemoglobin, Carboxyhemoglobin, and Methemoglobin

New pulse oximetry technology uses more than seven wavelengths of light to measure Spo_2 as well as Spco (pulse oximeter estimate of HbCO), SpMet (pulse oximeter estimate of HbMet), and SpHb (pulse oximeter estimate of hemoglobin concentration).[3] There are several limitations of this technology. Because it uses the conventional two-wavelength red and infrared algorithm to determine Spo_2, when there are significant levels of either HbCO or HbMet, the displayed Spo_2 will be subject to the same errors described earlier. However, the presence of a high Spco or SpMet display would alert the user to this error. Another limitation is the crosstalk between the HbMet and HbCO measurement channels. In the presence of significant Hbmet levels, the device will display a falsely elevated Spco but a correct SpMet. In this setting, the device will display an error message indicating that the Spco may not be accurate.

The results of studies evaluating the clinical accuracy of pulse oximetry to detect HbCO suggest caution. The accuracy of Spco is ±6% and, therefore, it should not be used for triage or patient management. An elevated Spco could broaden the diagnosis of CO poisoning in patients without symptoms. But a low Spco in patients suspected of CO poisoning should never rule out CO poisoning and should always be confirmed by blood HbCO.[9–11] Studies evaluating the accuracy of SpHb have reported mixed results.[12,13] Due to this uncertainty, use of SpHb has not been widely adopted.

Use of the Plethysmographic Waveform

Pulse oximetry has non–oxygenation-monitoring applications. The pulse oximetry plethysmographic (POP) waveform may display the effect of pulsus paradoxus, and therefore the severity of air trapping in obstructive airway disease (**Figure 2-9**).[14–18] In patients with obstructive lung disease and elevated pulsus paradoxus, there is an altered pulse oximetry baseline tracing manifested as the respiratory waveform variation. Pulsus paradoxus is significantly correlated with the degree of respiratory waveform variation of the pulse oximetry tracing and the amount of auto-PEEP (positive end-expiratory pressure).

Respiratory variations in POP waveform amplitude during positive pressure ventilation has also been shown to be useful in prediction of fluid responsiveness. POP waveform amplitude during positive pressure ventilation is measured on a beat-to-beat basis as the vertical distance between peak and preceding valley trough in the waveform (**Figure 2-10**). Maximal POP (POP_{max}) and minimal POP (POP_{min}) are determined over the same respiratory cycle. ΔPOP is calculated using the following formula:

$$\Delta POP\ (\%) = 100 \times \frac{POP_{max} - POP_{min}}{(POP_{max} + POP_{min})/2}$$

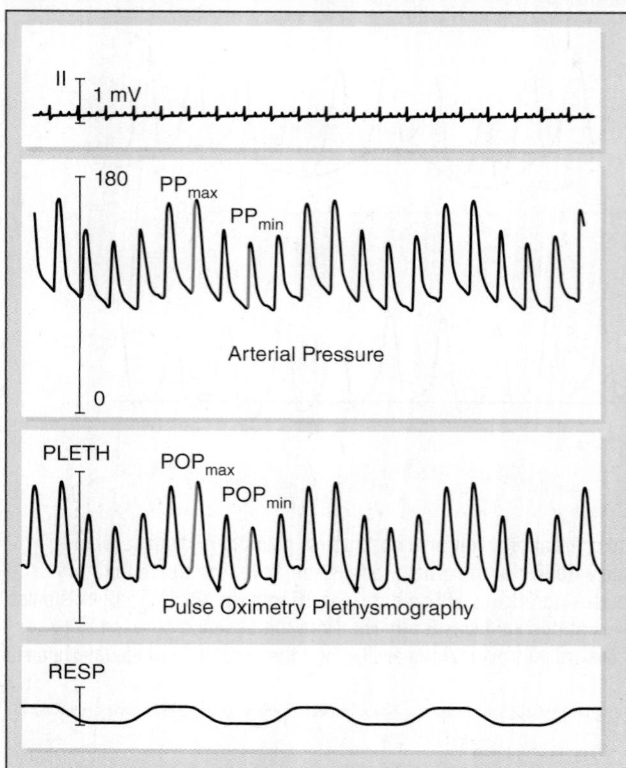

FIGURE 2-10 Comparison of invasive arterial pressure and pulse oximeter plethysmography recordings. Simultaneous recording of electrocardiographic lead (II), systemic arterial pressure (PA), pulse oximetry plethysmography (PLETH), and respiratory signal (RESP) in one illustrative patient. POP, pulse oximetry plethysmographic; PP, pulse pressure.

Reproduced from Cannesson M, Besnard C, Durand PG, et al. Relation between respiratory variations in pulse oximetry plethysmographic waveform amplitude and arterial pulse pressure in ventilated patients. *Crit Care.* 2005;9:R562–R568.

A ΔPOP greater than 15% is predictive of fluid responsiveness in mechanically ventilated patients with circulatory failure.[15,16]

Some pulse oximeters display the **perfusion index (PI)** and **plethysmographic variability index (PVI)** as a reflection of POP. PI is the ratio of the pulsatile blood flow to the nonpulsatile blood in peripheral tissue. It is a noninvasive measure of peripheral perfusion that can be continuously and noninvasively obtained from a pulse oximeter. PI is calculated by pulse oximetry as the pulsatile signal (during arterial inflow) as a percentage of the nonpulsatile signal, both of which are derived from the amount of infrared (940 nm) light absorbed. Whereas the pulse oximeter plethysmogram represents a volume change and the arterial blood pressure represents a pressure change, cyclical shifts in the plethysmogram reflect similar cyclic changes in blood pressure. These changes reflect an intrathoracic pressure relative to the intravascular volume. PVI is a measure of the dynamic changes in the PI that occur during the respiratory cycle:

$$\text{PVI (\%)} = 100 \times (PI_{max} - PI_{min})/PI_{max}$$

Similar to ΔPOP, the greater the PVI, the greater variability there is in the waveform variability over a respiratory cycle.

Capnography

Capnometry and capnography are noninvasive techniques that measure the carbon dioxide levels in expired gas (**CPG 2-1**).[19] **Capnometry** refers to the

CLINICAL PRACTICE GUIDELINE 2-1

Capnometry and Capnography During Mechanical Ventilation

Indications

- To evaluate exhaled CO_2, especially P_{ETCO_2}, which is the maximum partial pressure of CO_2 exhaled during a tidal breath (just before the beginning of inspiration).
- To monitor the severity of pulmonary disease and evaluate the response to therapy, especially therapy intended to improve the ratio of dead space to tidal volume (V_D/V_T).
- As an adjunct to determine that tracheal rather than esophageal intubation has taken place (low or absent cardiac output may negate its use for this indication); colorimetric CO_2 detectors are adequate devices for this purpose.
- To continuously monitor the integrity of the ventilatory circuit, including the artificial airway.
- To evaluate the efficiency of mechanical ventilatory support through determination of the difference between the arterial partial pressure of carbon dioxide (Pa_{CO_2}) and the P_{ETCO_2}, reflecting CO_2 elimination.
- To monitor the adequacy of pulmonary and coronary blood flow; to estimate effective (nonshunted) pulmonary capillary blood flow by a partial rebreathing method; as an adjunctive tool to screen for pulmonary embolism; to monitor the matching of ventilation to perfusion during independent lung ventilation for unilateral pulmonary contusion.

- To monitor inspired CO_2 when CO_2 gas is administered therapeutically.
- To graphically evaluate the ventilator–patient interface; evaluation of the capnogram may be useful in the detection of rebreathing of CO_2, obstructive pulmonary disease, waning neuromuscular blockade (curare cleft), cardiogenic oscillations, esophageal intubation, cardiac arrest, or contamination of the monitor or sampling line with secretions or mucus.
- Measurement of the volume of CO_2 elimination to assess metabolic rate or alveolar ventilation or both.

Contraindications

- There are no absolute contraindications to capnography in mechanically ventilated adults provided the data obtained are evaluated in light of the patient's clinical condition.

Hazards and Complications

- Capnography with a clinically approved device is a safe, noninvasive test associated with few hazards. With mainstream analyzers, use of too large a sampling window may introduce an excessive amount of dead space into the ventilator circuit. Care must be taken to minimize the amount of additional weight placed on the artificial airway by the sampling window or, in the case of a sidestream analyzer, by the sampling line.

Limitations

- The composition of the respiratory gas mixture may affect the capnogram, depending on the measurement technology used; the infrared spectrum of CO_2 has some similarities to the spectra of oxygen and nitrous oxide; the reporting algorithm of some devices (primarily mass spectrometers) assumes that the only gases present in the sample are those that the device is capable of measuring—when a gas that the mass spectrometer cannot detect (such as helium) is present, the reported values of CO_2 are incorrectly elevated in proportion to the concentration of the undetectable gas present.
- The breathing frequency may affect the capnograph. High breathing frequencies may exceed the response capabilities of the capnograph. In addition, a breathing frequency above 10 breaths/min has been shown to affect devices differently.
- The presence of Freon (used as a propellant in metered dose inhalers) in the respiratory gas has been shown to artificially increase the CO_2 reading of mass spectrometers (that is, to show an apparent increase in the CO_2 concentration). A similar effect has not yet been demonstrated with Raman or infrared spectrometers.
- Contamination of the monitor or sampling system by secretions or condensate, use of a sample tube that is too long, a sampling rate that is too high, or obstruction of the sampling chamber can lead to unreliable results.
- Use of filters between the patient airway and the sampling line of the capnograph may lead to lowered P_{ETCO_2} readings.
- Low cardiac output may cause a false-negative result when attempting to verify endotracheal tube position in the trachea. False-positive results have been reported with endotracheal tube position in the pharynx and when antacids or carbonated beverages, or both, are present in the stomach.
- Decreased tidal volume delivery is possible during volume modes, some dual control modes, and time-cycled pressure limited ventilation with low continuous flow rates if the sampling flow rate of a sidestream analyzer is too high, especially in neonates and pediatrics.
- Inaccurate measurement of expired CO_2 may be caused by leaks of gas from the patient/ventilator system preventing collection of expired gases.

Modified from AARC clinical practice guideline: capnometry and capnography during mechanical ventilation—2003 revision and update. *Respir Care.* 2003;48:534–537. Reprinted with permission.

numeric display of CO_2 measurements taken from the airway. When the CO_2 is plotted against time and displayed graphically as a waveform, it is called **capnography**. Most capnometers measure CO_2 by infrared absorption, although mass spectrometry and Raman spectrometry can also be used.

Two airway sampling systems are used in capnometry: *mainstream* sensors and *sidestream* sensors (**Figure 2-11**). There are advantages and disadvantages of each approach (**Table 2-1**). The mainstream capnometer is placed directly into the breathing circuit, usually directly at the airway. Infrared light is passed across the airstream to a photodetector. Improvements in analyzer technology and miniaturization have resulted in the development of low-dead-space, lightweight, and durable mainstream sensors. Because they are positioned on the airway, they may be adversely affected by the accumulation of moisture, secretions, and debris. Mainstream designs are best suited to patients with artificial airways.

The sidestream capnometer uses small-bore tubing to aspirate gas from or adjacent to the airway. The tubing

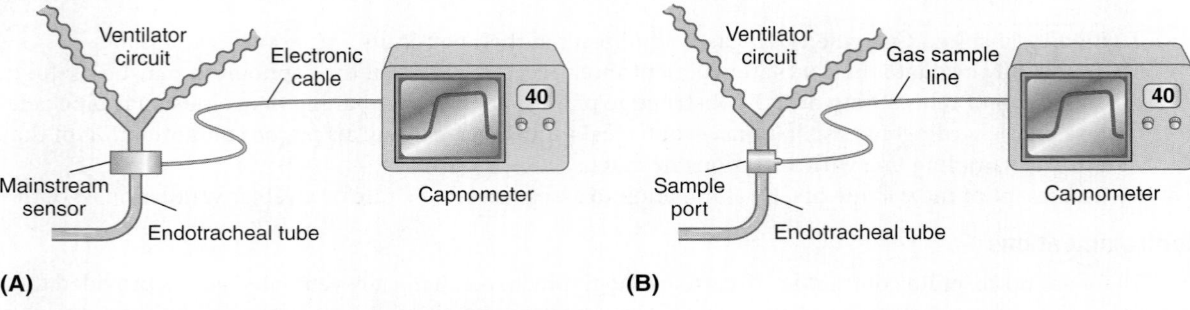

FIGURE 2-11 (**A**) Mainstream capnometry. (**B**) Sidestream capnometry.

aspirates the respiratory gases to a remote measuring chamber for analysis. Moisture and secretions must be removed from the tubing with traps, filters, purging, or reverse flow maneuvers before the sample enters the analysis cell. Some tubing is designed to be water vapor permeable, allowing moisture to escape by diffusion and evaporation. There is always an analysis delay when sidestream monitors are used because of the time required to move the sample from the airway to the sensor. The delay depends on the length of the tubing, its diameter, and the rate at which the gas is aspirated. Sidestream capnometers can be incorporated into nasal cannula designs for nonintubated patients (**Figure 2-12**).

The CO_2 infrared absorption peak (4.26 μm) lies between two peaks for water and very close to a peak for nitrous oxide (**Figure 2-13**). The latter poses an interference problem during the administration of nitrous oxide (N_2O) as an anesthesia gas. Correction factors and filters can be used to address this problem.

TABLE 2-1
Mainstream and Sidestream Capnometers

Advantages	Disadvantages
Mainstream Capnometer	
Sensor at patient airway Fast response (crisp waveform) Short lag time (real-time readings) No sample flow to reduce tidal volume	Secretions and humidity block sensor Sensor heated to prevent condensation Bulky sensor at patient airway Does not measure N_2O Difficult to use with nonintubated patients Cleaning and sterilization of reusable sensor
Sidestream Capnometer	
No bulky sensors or heaters at airway Ability to measure N_2O Disposable sample line Can be used with nonintubated patients	Secretions block sample tubing Water trap required Slow response to CO_2 changes Sample flow may decrease tidal volume

Conventional sidestream infrared analyzers must be calibrated on a regular basis. Room air (zero) and 5% CO_2 are used to perform a two-point calibration. Newer commercially available capnometers allow self-zeroing and calibration features. Until recently, the infrared radiation technique used for capnography was nondispersive blackbody technology. Molecular correlation spectroscopy is also available, which uses a radiation source that emits only CO_2-specific radiation and uses a small sample cell (15 μL) and a low flow rate.

The **mass spectrometer** is used to measure respiratory and anesthetic gases. Multichannel units are available to monitor several patients simultaneously. A mass spectrometer aspirates sample gas into a vacuum chamber, where an electron beam ionizes it. The charged molecules are accelerated through a magnetic field and disperse according to their mass and charge. This dispersion allows them to be separated before they reach a panel of detectors. Because even molecules of similar mass (N_2O and CO_2) ionize to different species (N_2O^+ and CO_2^+), this technique allows accurate measurement of several gases. Mass spectrometers have the advantage of being able to measure all respiratory gases

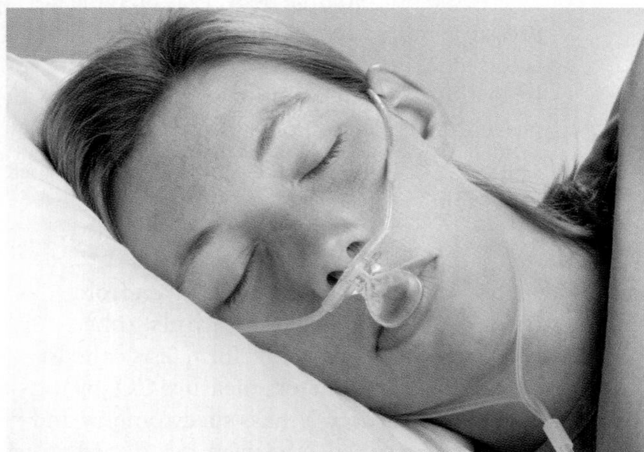

FIGURE 2-12 Nasal cannula designed for CO_2 sampling and oxygen administration (Smart CapnoLine, Oridion). The cannula samples CO_2 from both the nares and the mouth while oxygen is delivered through pinholes directed toward both the nose and mouth.

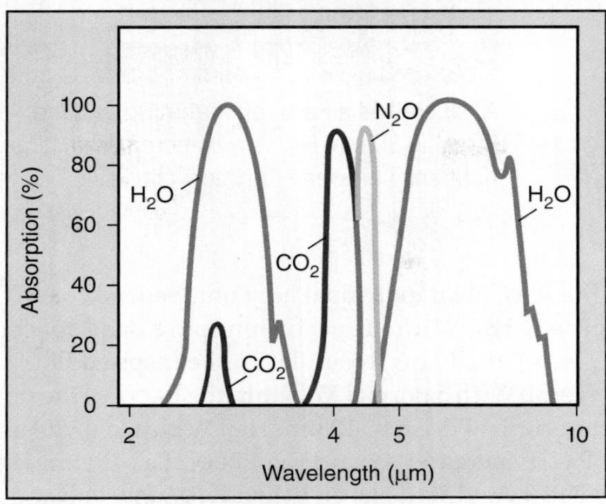

FIGURE 2-13 Carbon dioxide absorption spectra.
Adapted from Decker M, Strohl K. *Pulse Oximetry. Biophysical Measurement Series: Respiration.* SpaceLabs Medical, 1994.

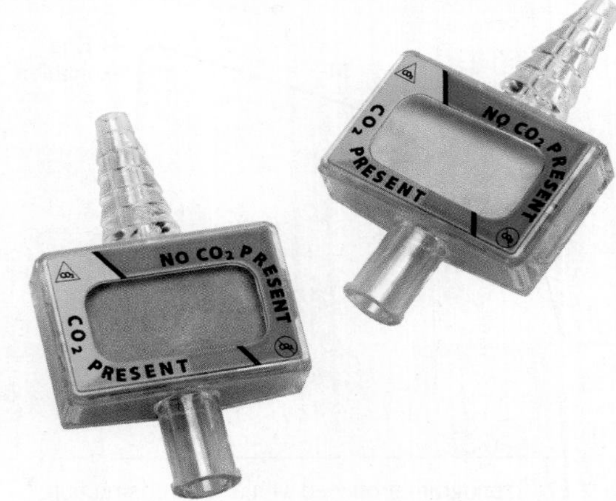

FIGURE 2-15 Colorimetric CO_2 sensor designed to confirm nasogastric tube placement.
Courtesy of Covidien. Used with permission.

breath by breath and are the most accurate analyzers in clinical use. However, they generally are too expensive and cumbersome for use outside the operating room or research settings.

Another method that can be used to measure CO_2 is **Raman spectroscopy.** When ultraviolet or visible light strikes gas molecules, energy is absorbed and reemitted at the same wavelength and direction. A small fraction of the absorbed energy is reemitted at new wavelengths in a phenomenon known as *Raman scattering.* Raman scattering results in reemission at a longer wavelength to produce a red-shifted spectrum. The wavelength shift and amount of scattering can be used to measure the constituents of a gas mixture.

A portable non-electronic single-patient-use device (**Figure 2-14**) is commonly used to produce a color change (colorimetric end-tidal CO_2 detection) in the presence of exhaled CO_2 (i.e., tracheal intubation). The color changes from purple with a low CO_2 concentration to yellow when exposed to a CO_2 concentration of 2.0% to 5.0%. This device is commonly used to confirm the correct position of the endotracheal tube. A color change indicates correct position in the trachea, as opposed to esophageal intubation, in which there is no color change. This technique can also be used to detect accidental tracheal placement of a nasogastric tube (**Figure 2-15**). In this case, a color change indicates incorrect placement of the tube in the trachea.[20]

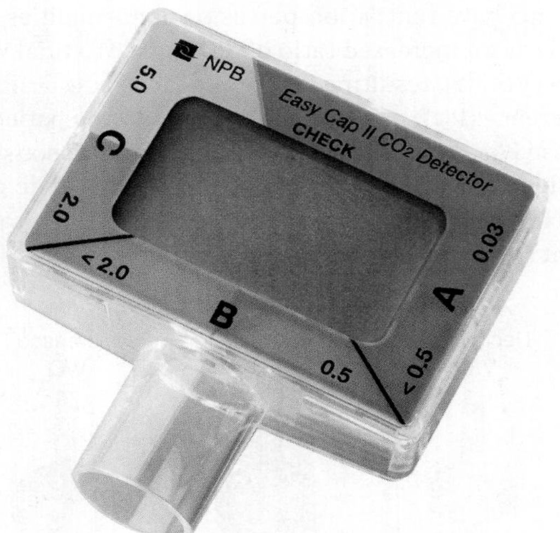

FIGURE 2-14 Colorimetric CO_2 sensor designed to confirm endotracheal intubation. It fits between the endotracheal tube and the manual bag-valve-O_2 device.
Courtesy of Covidien. Used with permission.

Time-Based Capnography

The traditional **capnogram** plots P_{CO_2} on the vertical axis and time on the horizontal axis. During inhalation, P_{CO_2} at the airway equals zero. At the beginning of exhalation, it remains low as the anatomic dead space empties. As the alveolar gas begins to mix with the dead space, CO_2 rises rapidly. A plateau, representing alveolar gas, develops, rising gently, presumably because of CO_2 added to the alveoli from capillary blood during exhalation (**Figure 2-16**). Peak exhaled P_{CO_2} or **end-tidal P_{CO_2}** (P_{ETCO_2}) represents the alveolar P_{CO_2}.

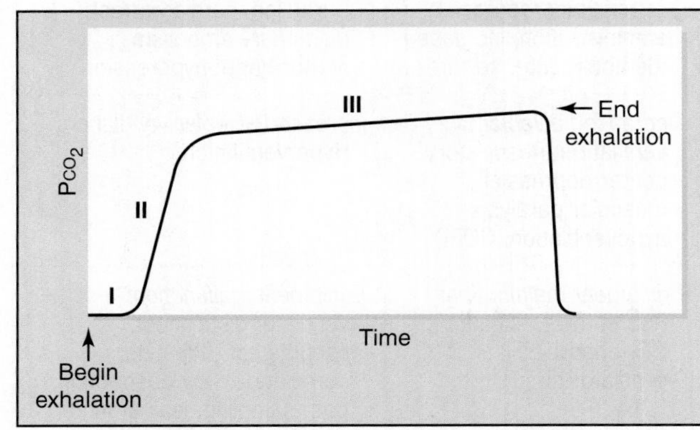

FIGURE 2-16 Time-based capnogram.

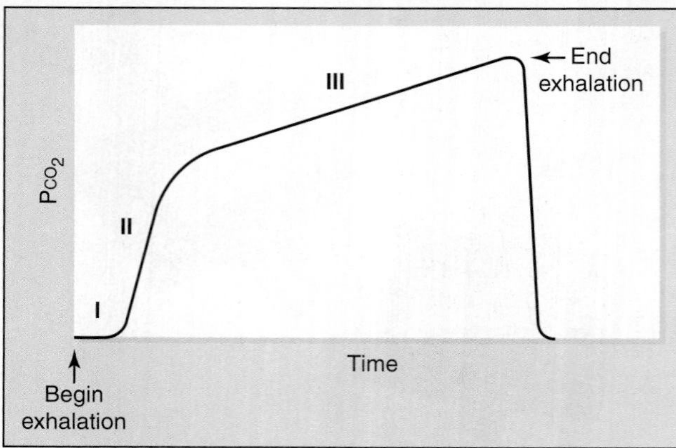

FIGURE 2-17 Capnogram produced with airflow obstruction.

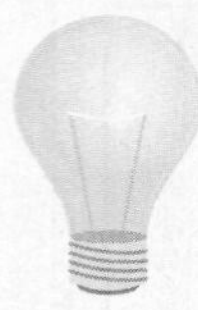

STOP AND THINK

A patient has a Pa_{CO_2} of 55 mm Hg, but the P_{ETCO_2} is 30 mm Hg. Why is there such a large difference between the Pa_{CO_2} and P_{ETCO_2}?

The capnographic waveform can be inspected for specific abnormalities or patterns. In patients with airways obstruction, the slope of the alveolar plateau increases because of inhomogeneous alveolar emptying (**Figure 2-17**). Regions of the lung with delayed emptying caused by increased resistance (long time constants) continue to add CO_2 to expired gas during the latter part of exhalation.

End-Tidal P_{CO_2}

End-tidal P_{CO_2} is determined by the production of CO_2, its subsequent delivery to the lungs by cardiac output, alveolar ventilation, and proper sampling and equipment performance. **Table 2-2** lists causes of an increase or decrease in the P_{ETCO_2}. P_{ETCO_2} is used clinically to ensure that the tracheal tube or mask ventilates the lungs, to estimate the Pa_{CO_2}, to detect changes in pulmonary blood flow or dead space ventilation, and to detect the addition of excess CO_2 to the systemic circulation.

TABLE 2-2
Causes of Increased and Decreased P_{ETCO_2}

Increased P_{ETCO_2}	Decreased P_{ETCO_2}
Increased CO_2 production and delivery to the lungs: Fever, sepsis, bicarbonate administration, increased metabolic rate, seizures	*Decreased CO_2 production and delivery to the lungs*: Hypothermia, low pulmonary perfusion, cardiac arrest, pulmonary embolism, hemorrhage, hypotension
Decreased alveolar ventilation: Respiratory center depression, muscular paralysis, hypoventilation, COPD	*Increased alveolar ventilation*: Hyperventilation
Equipment malfunction: Rebreathing, exhausted CO_2 absorber, leak in ventilator circuit	*Equipment malfunction*: Ventilator disconnect, esophageal intubation, complete airway obstruction, poor sampling, leak around endotracheal tube cuff

The P_{CO_2} of an individual lung unit depends on $\dot{V}/\dot{Q}$ (**Figure 2-18**). Without perfusion (pure dead space; $\dot{V}/\dot{Q} = \infty$), the P_{ACO_2} is similar to the inspired P_{CO_2} (i.e., zero). With a normal $\dot{V}/\dot{Q}$ unit, the P_{ACO_2} is the same as the arterial P_{CO_2} (i.e., 40 mm Hg). With a low $\dot{V}/\dot{Q}$ unit, the P_{ACO_2} increases toward the $P\bar{v}_{CO_2}$ (i.e., 45 mm Hg). The P_{ACO_2}, and thus the end-tidal P_{CO_2}, must always remain between zero and the $P\bar{v}_{CO_2}$. P_{ETCO_2} is normally several mm Hg less than the Pa_{CO_2}. However, the relationship between the Pa_{CO_2} and P_{ETCO_2} will vary depending on the relative contributions of various $\dot{V}/\dot{Q}$ units comprising the lungs.

The presence of CO_2 in exhaled gas usually indicates tracheal intubation. Exhaled CO_2 does not always ensure proper endotracheal tube placement, however, because the tube could be in the main stem bronchus or in the pharynx. Although esophageal intubation generally results in a very low P_{ETCO_2}, falsely elevated readings may occur if the patient ingested antacids or carbonated beverages. The elevated value should diminish with subsequent breaths. Even with proper endotracheal tube placement, the P_{ETCO_2} may remain deceptively low with cardiogenic shock. P_{ETCO_2} is also used to detect tracheal placement of a nasogastric tube. A P_{ETCO_2} near zero suggests that the gastric tube is *not* in the trachea.

Even though P_{ETCO_2} approximates Pa_{CO_2} in normal individuals, capnometry cannot routinely be used as a substitute to measure arterial P_{CO_2}. Most critically ill patients have ventilation-perfusion abnormalities, particularly an increased ratio of dead space to tidal volume (V_D/V_T), resulting in a significant $Pa_{CO_2} - P_{ETCO_2}$ difference ($P[a - ET]CO_2$) (**Table 2-3**).[21] Even patients whose $P(a - ET)CO_2$ is calibrated by simultaneous arterial blood gas and capnometry measurements do not remain stable enough over time to render the measurement a reliable estimate of Pa_{CO_2}.

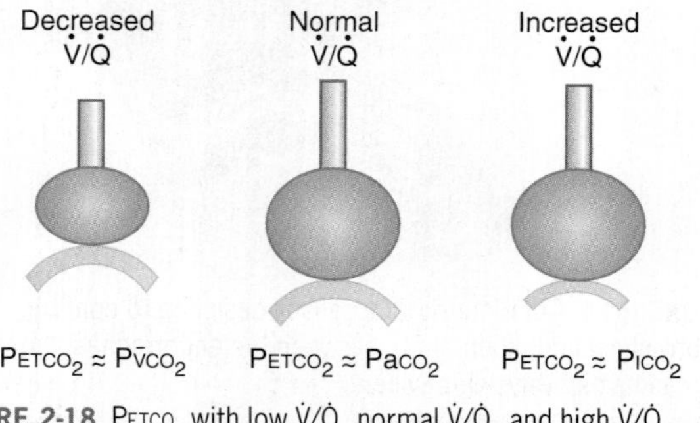

FIGURE 2-18 P_{ETCO_2} with low $\dot{V}/\dot{Q}$, normal $\dot{V}/\dot{Q}$, and high $\dot{V}/\dot{Q}$.

TABLE 2-3
Causes of Increased $P[a - ET]CO_2$

Pulmonary hypoperfusion
Pulmonary embolism
Cardiac arrest
Positive pressure ventilation (especially excessive PEEP)
High-rate, low-tidal-volume ventilation

With no pulmonary blood flow, P_{ETCO_2} equals zero. Because P_{ETCO_2} is partly determined by the amount of blood flow returning to the lungs from the systemic circulation, it has been used to verify the effectiveness of cardiopulmonary resuscitation (CPR). Adequate CPR is associated with increasing P_{ETCO_2} levels. If P_{ETCO_2} does not rise above 10 mm Hg after 20 minutes of pulseless resuscitation, the prognosis is poor. An abrupt increase in P_{ETCO_2} during CPR indicates a return of spontaneous circulation.

Pulmonary embolism is associated with an increased V_D/V_T. The $P(a - ET)CO_2$ is increased with pulmonary embolism. Because many conditions increase V_D/V_T, an increased $P(a - ET)CO_2$ is not specific to pulmonary embolism. However, a normal V_D/V_T suggests that pulmonary embolism is unlikely.

In patients with acute respiratory distress syndrome (ARDS), either too little or too much PEEP increases V_D/V_T and $P(a - ET)CO_2$. If V_D/V_T is excessive, the minute ventilation requirement might indicate that ventilator liberation is unlikely. As noninvasive monitors during the ventilator discontinuation process, capnometric measurements of the respiratory rate and elevated P_{ETCO_2} are unreliable.

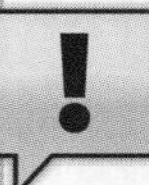

Respiratory Recap

Capnography

- Capnography uses either mainstream or sidestream sampling.
- The CO_2 level is measured by infrared absorption, mass spectrometry, or colorimetric techniques.
- End-tidal P_{CO_2} often is an imprecise reflection of Pa_{CO_2}.
- Capnography is useful in the detection of esophageal intubation.
- End-tidal P_{CO_2} is useful to monitor the effectiveness of cardiopulmonary resuscitation and return of spontaneous circulation.
- Volumetric capnography can be used to measure carbon dioxide production and cardiac output.

Patient safety monitoring during procedural sedation includes pulse rate, blood pressure, respiratory rate, oxygen saturation, ECG, and clinical observation. Noninvasive monitoring of ventilation with capnography is also used in this setting. There are two types of hypoventilation that occur during procedural sedation and analgesia (**Figure 2-19**).[22] An increased P_{ETCO_2} and an increased Pa_{CO_2} characterize bradypneic hypoventilation. Respiratory rate is depressed proportionally greater than tidal volume, resulting in bradypnea, an increase in expiratory time, and an increase in P_{ETCO_2}. Bradypneic hypoventilation is commonly observed with opioids. Hypopneic hypoventilation is

Dead space
Alveolar ventilation
Normal Ventilation
• normal respiratory rate
• normal tidal volume
• normal alveolar ventilation
• normal dead space fraction
• normal Pa_{CO_2}
• normal $P(a - ET)CO_2$
Result
P_{ETCO_2} similar to Pa_{CO_2}
Dead space
Alveolar ventilation
Bradypneic Hypoventilation
• ↓ respiratory rate
• normal tidal volume
• ↓ alveolar ventilation
• normal dead space fraction
• ↑ Pa_{CO_2}
• normal $P(a - ET)CO_2$
Result
↑ P_{ETCO_2}
Dead space
Alveolar ventilation
Hypopneic Hyoventilation
• normal respiratory rate
• ↓ tidal volume
• ↓ alveolar ventilation
• ↑ dead space fraction
• ↑ Pa_{CO_2}
• ↑ $P(a - ET)CO_2$
Result
normal, or ↓ P_{ETCO_2}

FIGURE 2-19 Physiology of hypoventilation states as related to monitoring of end-tidal P_{CO_2}. P_{ETCO_2} = end-tidal P_{CO_2}, Pa_{CO_2} = arterial P_{CO_2}.
Reproduced from Krauss B, Hess DR. Capnography for procedural sedation and analgesia in the emergency department. *Ann Emerg Med.* 2007;50:172–181, with permission from Elsevier.

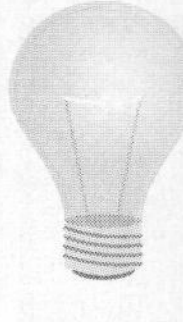

STOP AND THINK

During CPR the P_{ETCO_2} is slowly decreasing from 25 mm Hg to 20 mm Hg to 15 mm Hg. Why is this happening and what is the appropriate response?

characterized by a normal or decreased P_{ETCO_2} with an increased Pa_{CO_2}. This reflects the relationship between tidal volume and airway dead space, in which dead space is constant and tidal volume is decreasing. Because tidal volume is depressed more than respiratory rate, the result is a low tidal volume that leads to an increase in V_D/V_T. The $P(a - ET)CO_2$ increases with the increase in V_D/V_T. Even though Pa_{CO_2} is increasing, P_{ETCO_2} may remain normal or be decreasing. Thus, either an increase or decrease in P_{ETCO_2} might suggest excessive procedural sedation.

Volume-Based Capnography

A normal volume-based capnogram is shown in **Figure 2-20**. It is displayed with the P_{CO_2} on the vertical axis and the volume on the horizontal axis.[23–25] At the beginning of exhalation, the P_{CO_2} remains zero as gas from the anatomic dead space leaves the airway (phase I). The capnogram rises sharply as alveolar gas mixes with dead space gas (phase II). The capnogram then forms a plateau during most of exhalation (phase III). Phase III represents gas flow from the alveoli and therefore is called the *alveolar plateau*. The P_{CO_2} at end-exhalation is the P_{ETCO_2}. Anatomic dead space, alveolar dead space volume, and the volume of exhaled CO_2 ($\dot{V}_{CO_2}$) can be determined from the volume-based capnogram. Volume-based capnography can be measured with stand-alone monitors or with technology incorporated into mechanical ventilators.[26]

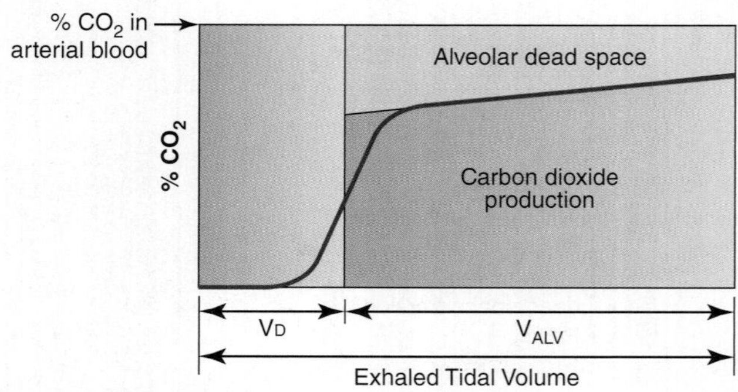

FIGURE 2-20 Components of volume-based capnogram. V_D, anatomic dead space; V_{ALV}, alveolar gas volume.

Reproduced from Longnecker D, Brown D, Newman M, Zapol W. 2008. *Anesthesiology.* McGraw-Hill, New York. (© The McGraw-Hill Companies, Inc.)

Because $\dot{V}_{CO_2}$ is determined by metabolic rate, this can be used to estimate resting energy expenditure (REE):

$$REE = \dot{V}_{CO_2}(L/min) \times 5.52\ kcal/L \times 1440\ min/day$$

Normal $\dot{V}_{CO_2}$ is approximately 200 mL/min (2.8 mL/kg/min).

Using volume-based capnography, it is possible to noninvasively measure cardiac output with the partial CO_2 rebreathing technique (**Figure 2-21**).[27–32] $\dot{V}_{CO_2}$ is calculated on a breath-by-breath basis, and the Fick equation is applied to establish the relationship between $\dot{V}_{CO_2}$ and cardiac output ($\dot{Q}$):

$$\dot{V}_{CO_2} = \dot{Q} \times (C\bar{v}_{CO_2} - Ca_{CO_2})$$

where $C\bar{v}_{CO_2}$ represents the CO_2 content of mixed venous blood and Ca_{CO_2} represents the CO_2 content of arterial blood. CO_2 rebreathing is performed for 35 seconds every 3 minutes. Assuming that $\dot{Q}$ remains constant during the rebreathing procedure yields the following:

$$\Delta\dot{V}_{CO_2} = \dot{Q} \times (\Delta C\bar{v}_{CO_2} - \Delta Ca_{CO_2})$$

where $\Delta\dot{V}_{CO_2}$ is the change in $\dot{V}_{CO_2}$ between normal breathing and rebreathing, $\Delta C\bar{v}_{CO_2}$ is the change in mixed venous carbon dioxide content, and ΔCa_{CO_2} is the change in arterial carbon dioxide content. If $\Delta C\bar{v}_{CO_2}$ remains constant during rebreathing, the following equation is used:

$$\Delta\dot{V}_{CO_2} = \dot{Q} \times (-\Delta C\bar{v}_{CO_2})$$

When end-capillary content (Cc'_{CO_2}) is used in place of Ca_{CO_2}, pulmonary capillary blood flow (PCBF), the blood flow that participates in alveolar gas exchange, is measured rather than $\dot{Q}$, and the following equation is used:

$$\Delta\dot{V}_{CO_2} = PCBF \times (-Cc'_{CO_2})$$

Assuming that $-Cc'_{CO_2}$ is proportional to ΔP_{ETCO_2}, the following equation can be used:

$$PCBF = \Delta\dot{V}_{CO_2}/(S \times \Delta P_{ETCO_2})$$

where ΔP_{ETCO_2} is the change in P_{ETCO_2} between normal breathing and rebreathing, and S is the slope of the carbon dioxide dissociation curve from hemoglobin. Because cardiac output is the sum of PCBF and intrapulmonary shunt flow,

$$\dot{Q} = PCBF/(1 - \dot{Q}_S/\dot{Q}_T)$$

The noninvasive method for estimating $\dot{Q}_S/\dot{Q}_T$ is adapted from Nunn's iso-shunt plots, which are a series of continuous curves indicating the relation between

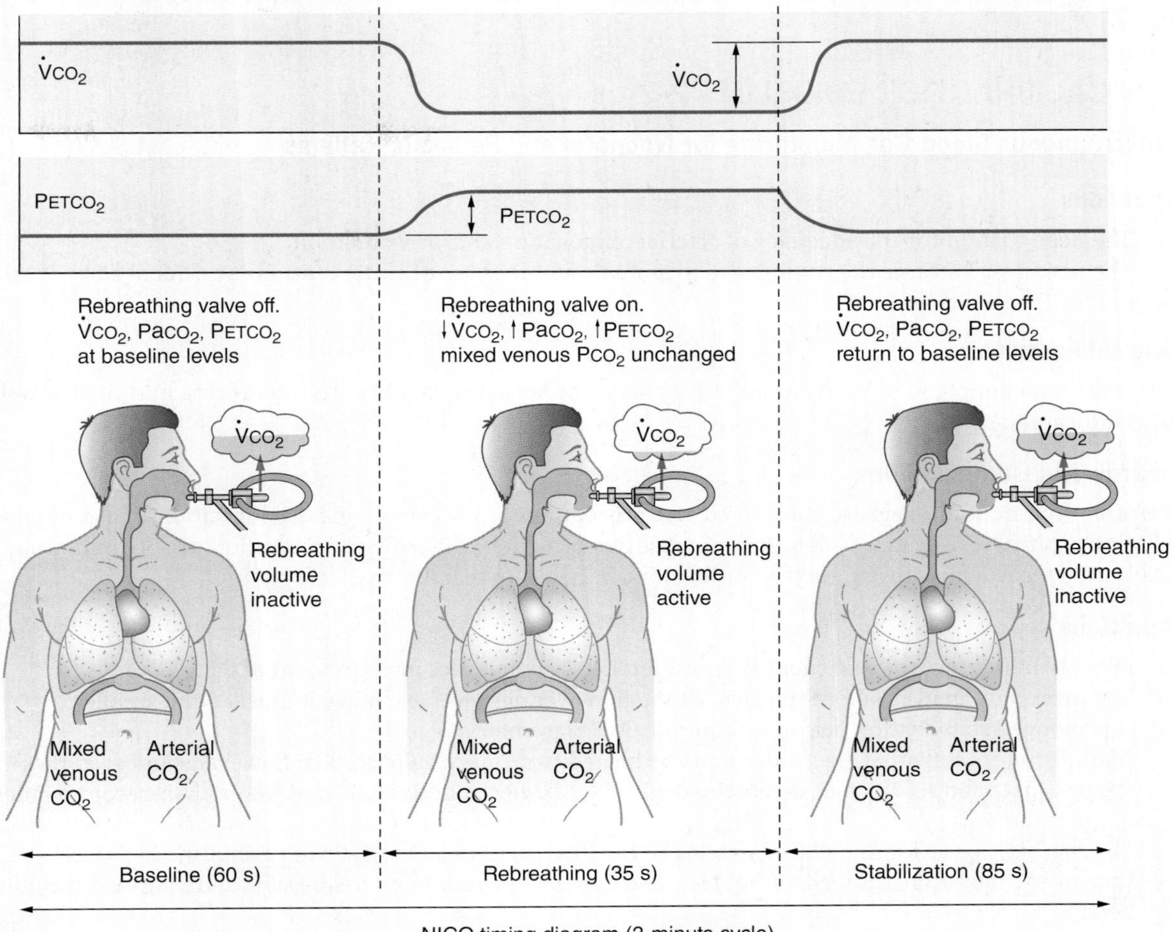

FIGURE 2-21 Rebreathing cycle used to measure cardiac output using the partial CO_2 rebreathing technique.
Modified from Longnecker D, Brown D, Newman M, Zapol W. 2008. *Anesthesiology*. McGraw-Hill, New York. (© The McGraw-Hill Companies, Inc.)

arterial oxygen pressure (Pao_2) and Fio_2 at different levels of right-to-left shunt. Pao_2 is noninvasively estimated using a pulse oximeter.

There are several potential limitations of partial rebreathing for the measurement of cardiac output. In nonparalyzed patients, rebreathing increases the respiratory rate, which reduces the magnitude of the signal and limits the ability to detect changes in P_{ETCO_2} and $\dot{V}co_2$. Noise is increased by respiratory pattern irregularities that produce an unstable P_{ETCO_2} and $\dot{V}co_2$, and these may impair accuracy. Additional cardiac output not calculated due to shunt fraction is estimated from Spo_2 and Fio_2, and these may also introduce errors.

Transcutaneous Blood Gas Monitoring

Transcutaneous monitoring of O_2 and CO_2 ($Ptco_2$ and $Ptcco_2$) uses measurements at the skin surface to provide estimates of Pao_2 and $Paco_2$ (**CPG 2-2**).[33] This type of monitoring has been used with neonates, infants, small children, and patients with peripheral vascular disease. The devices warm the skin to induce hyperemia, and then electrochemically measure oxygen and carbon dioxide partial pressures at the skin surface, providing a noninvasive means of continuously monitoring arterial oxygenation and ventilation. They have been particularly useful in neonates and infants, in whom arterial sampling is technically difficult. Also, because intact circulation is a prerequisite for successful hyperbaric oxygen therapy, candidates with peripheral vascular disease are screened with transcutaneous O_2 monitors. Because $Ptco_2$ is affected by perfusion, it may reflect the quantity of oxygen delivered to the skin under the electrode (the product of cardiac output and arterial oxygen content). $Ptco_2$ has been used in adults to monitor the results of vascular surgery, the intent being to evaluate perfusion rather than Pao_2 per se.

The transcutaneous oxygen electrode uses the polarographic technique. Heating coils surround the

CLINICAL PRACTICE GUIDELINE 2-2

Transcutaneous Blood Gas Monitoring for Neonatal and Pediatric Patients

Indications

- The need to monitor the adequacy of arterial oxygenation and/or ventilation.
- The need to quantitate the response to diagnostic and therapeutic interventions as evidenced by $Ptco_2$ and/or $Ptcco_2$ values.

Contraindications

In patients with poor skin integrity or adhesive allergy, or both, transcutaneous monitoring may be relatively contraindicated.

Hazards and Complications

$Ptco_2$ and $Ptcco_2$ monitoring are considered safe procedures, but because of device limitations, false-negative and false-positive results may lead to inappropriate treatment of the patient. In addition, tissue injury may occur at the measuring site (e.g., erythema, blisters, burns, skin tears).

Limitations

- $Ptco_2$ is an indirect measurement Pao_2 and $Ptcco_2$ is an indirect measurement of $Paco_2$.
- The procedure may be labor intensive, although newer designs have made it quicker and simpler.
- A prolonged stabilization period is required after placement.
- Manufacturers state that electrodes must be heated to produce valid results; however, clinical studies suggest that valid results may be obtained with $Ptcco_2$ electrodes operated at lower-than-recommended temperatures.
- The theoretic basis for mandatory heating of the $Ptco_2$ electrode has not been established.
- Improper calibration, trapped air bubbles, and damaged membranes are possible and may be difficult to detect.
- Hyperoxemia ($Pao_2 > 100$ mm Hg).
- Hypoperfused state (shock, acidosis).
- Improper electrode placement or application.
- Use of vasoactive drugs.
- Nature of the patient's skin and subcutaneous tissue (skinfold thickness, edema).

Modified from AARC clinical practice guideline: transcutaneous blood gas monitoring for neonatal and pediatric patients—2004 revision and update. *Respir Care*. 2004; 49:1069–1072. Reprinted with permission.

anode, and the platinum cathode is centered inside the anode ring. The heating coil induces local hyperemia to arterialize the skin surface. A flat membrane separates the electrode from the skin. Oxygen diffuses from the blood vessels to the skin surface and through the membrane into the electrode.

Respiratory Recap

Transcutaneous Blood Gas Monitors

- Warmed electrodes are placed on the skin to measure $Ptco_2$ and $Ptcco_2$ and estimate Pao_2 and $Paco_2$.
- The electrodes operate on the same principles as blood gas electrodes.
- A miniaturized single sensor combines measurement of pulse oximetry (Spo_2) and $Ptcco_2$.

Transcutaneous carbon dioxide electrodes use a flat glass membrane permeable to CO_2. A pH electrode is positioned behind the membrane in a bicarbonate buffer. Carbon dioxide diffuses from the skin through the membrane and reacts with the buffer to produce a change in [H^+]. Similar to the Pco_2 blood gas electrode, the $Ptcco_2$ electrode detects changes in [H^+] but is calibrated to display Pco_2. Unlike the $Ptco_2$ electrode, a reasonably good correlation with $Paco_2$ can be obtained at a temperature of 37° C (98.6° F). Because $Ptcco_2$ is consistently greater than $Paco_2$, manufacturers incorporate a correction factor so that the $Ptcco_2$ that is displayed approximates the $Paco_2$. Like $Ptco_2$, the proximity with which $Ptcco_2$ approximates $Paco_2$ is the result of a complex set of physiologic events, and thus it is incorrect to believe that $Ptcco_2$ is the $Paco_2$. For example, decreased tissue perfusion causes the $Ptcco_2$ to increase.

A miniaturized single sensor combines the measurement of pulse oximetry (Spo_2) and $Ptcco_2$ (**Figure 2-22**).[34–37] It uses a heated Severinghaus electrode combined with a pulse oximetry sensor and is attached to the earlobe with a clip. The sensor is calibrated using a one-point dry gas calibration with 7% CO_2 when the sensor is placed in its calibration chamber. The sensor is heated to 42° C to induce local vasodilation and enhance skin permeability for CO_2 to improve gas diffusion at the site of measurement. A drop of contact gel is applied in the center of the attachment clip before the sensor is applied. The sensor is removed after 8 hours, recalibrated, and fixed on the other earlobe.

A limitation in the use of transcutaneous blood gas monitoring is the need for a heated electrode. This carries the risk of skin burns and requires that the sensor be rotated among monitoring sites on a regular basis. The reliability of transcutaneous monitoring for accurately estimating arterial blood gases is often questioned, which has led to limited use of this technology.

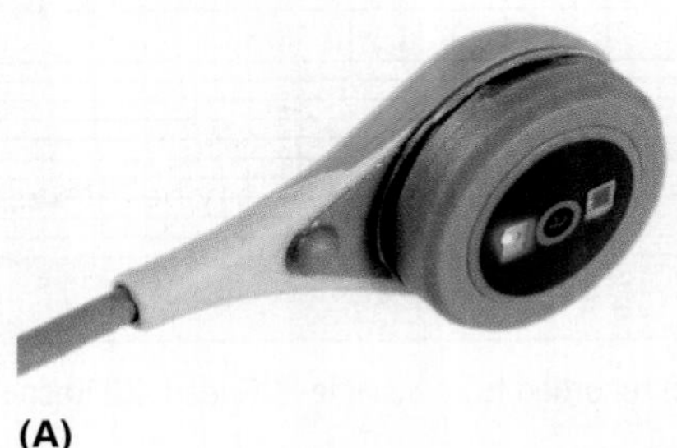

(A)

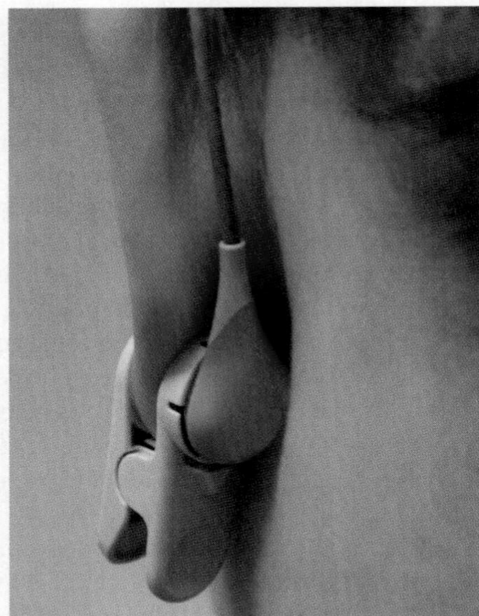

(B)

FIGURE 2-22 A sensor for noninvasive monitoring of transcutaneous carbon dioxide and oxygen saturation.

Courtesy of SenTec AG.

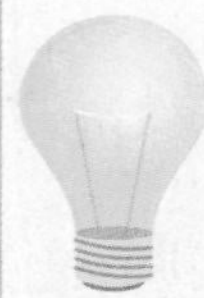

STOP AND THINK

The $Ptcco_2$ suddenly drops to zero. What is the best explanation for this and what is the appropriate clinical response?

Respiratory Rate and Pattern

The respiratory rate is one of the four vital signs. It is a core component of monitoring, because respiratory rate slowing (**bradypnea** or *apnea*) or increasing (*tachypnea*) may warn of clinical deterioration or impending respiratory arrest. In sleep laboratories, sophisticated respiratory rate and pattern monitoring are required during polysomnography. Respiratory (apnea) monitors are also used for infant studies in the home.

The respiratory rate is easily measured at the bedside by counting chest excursions for 30 seconds (and multiplying by 2 to obtain breaths/min) or for 60 seconds. However, this method may be inaccurate, perhaps because clinicians underestimate the importance of this vital sign.

With **impedance pneumography**, the respiratory rate and excursion can be measured by use of two electrodes placed on the chest wall. A high frequency (20 to 100 Hz) and low ampere alternating current (less than 100 μA) is passed between the electrodes on the chest surface (this is, of course, a current too small to be felt by the patient). The strength of the current when it reaches the receiving electrode varies according to the *impedance,* or effective resistance of the tissue between the electrodes. During chest expansion, as the distance between the electrodes increases, impedance increases, causing the current to decrease. The change in current is electronically processed to calculate the respiratory rate (**Figure 2-23**). During normal tidal breathing, the signal can also be calibrated to measure tidal volume. However, volume measurements deteriorate with patient movement or a change in position. Moreover, an obstructive apnea cannot be detected with this method, because the chest wall continues to move despite cessation of airflow. These systems usually are configured as

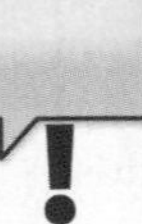

Respiratory Recap

Techniques to Measure the Respiratory Rate

- Counting by inspection at the bedside
- Impedance pneumography
- Respiratory inductance plethysmography
- Fiberoptic plethysmography
- Nasal temperature- and pressure-sensing devices
- Piezoelectric plethysmography
- Acoustic technology
- Capnography

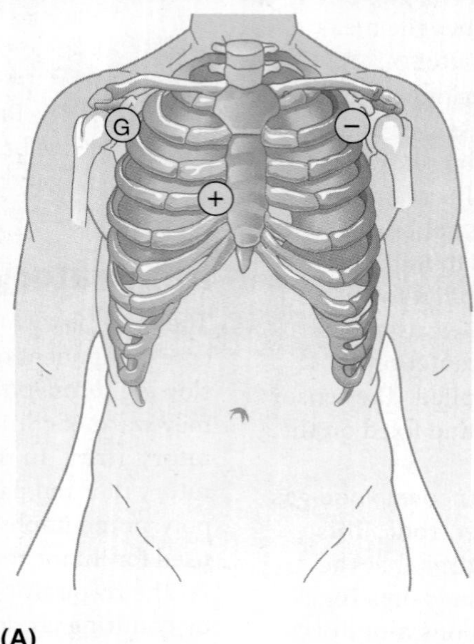

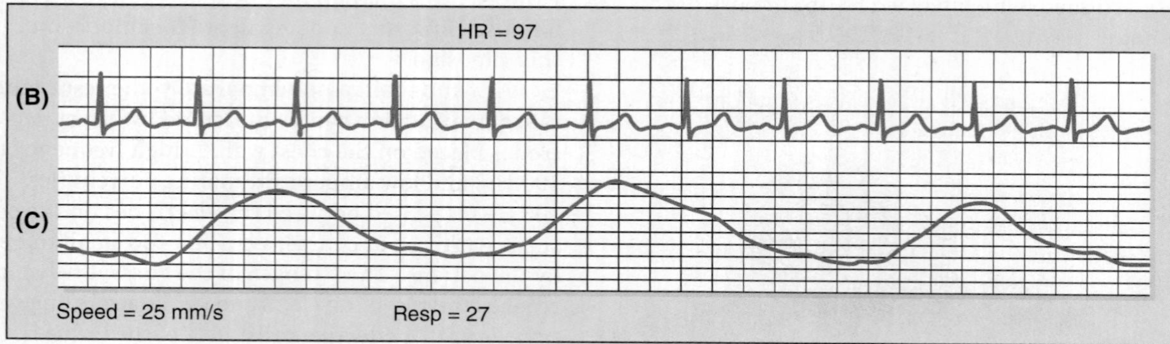

FIGURE 2-23 (**A**) Electrode placement for three-lead array. (**B**) Cardiac rate and rhythm recorded from a single ECG lead. (**C**) Respiratory impedance plethysmography tracing obtained from the same electrode array.

a plug-in module for bedside monitoring of the respiratory rate in the ICU. They use the same electrodes that generally are applied to the patient for cardiac rhythm monitoring. Infant home apnea monitors are based on this technology.

The most accurate method for indirect measurement of tidal volume is **respiratory inductance plethysmography (RIP)**. Inductance sensors use a circuit of coiled wire woven into an elastic band and excited by an AC current. *Inductance* results from alternating electrical currents that create magnetic fields around themselves and the changes in those magnetic fields that alter other electrical currents they encounter. During tidal breathing, the bands stretch and relax. As the belt is displaced during chest expansion, changes in the magnetic fields around the wire coils result in changes in the excitation current. Variations in the excitation current caused by the expansion and contraction of the belt are electronically processed to provide a display of the ventilatory pattern, rate, and change in volume.

When rib cage and abdominal bands are used simultaneously, respiratory motion is described more completely, resulting in tidal volume measurements that correlate well with spirometry (±10%). RIP is stable and comfortable despite patient movement, which makes it suitable for use in sleep laboratories. This noninvasive technique has also been used in the ICU to monitor noninvasive ventilation and to conduct studies of the effect of PEEP on the functional residual capacity. Because it is more expensive than impedance pneumography, its use in the ICU usually is reserved for cases in which noninvasive measurements of tidal volume or changes in functional residual capacity are desired.

A modification of inductance plethysmography, **fiberoptic plethysmography**, uses optical fibers woven into elastic belts. Light is passed through the fibers into a photodetector. When rib cage or abdominal displacements stretch the elastic belt, large changes in light transmission through the fibers result. The change in light transmission is electronically processed to provide data similar to RIP. This technique has the advantage of being free of electrical interference and electrically safe for patients. It also is more sensitive than conventional RIP to small changes in lung volume. Clinical experience with this device is limited.

Temperature and pressure probes can be used to measure the rate and pattern of airflow. Disordered breathing, hypopneas, and apneas are characterized in this way. **Thermistors** and **thermocouples** detect bidirectional airflow at the nose and mouth by sensing the temperature difference between inspired room air and exhaled air that has been warmed to body temperature (**Figure 2-24**). The ability of these devices to detect airflow diminishes if the room air temperature approaches body temperature. Likewise, if the sensor touches skin and rises to body temperature, airflow cannot be detected. Other limitations of thermally based sensors are that they cannot be calibrated in terms of airflow and provide only qualitative information, that moisture condensing on the probe compromises temperature-sensing capabilities, and that loss of signal may occur if the sensor becomes dislodged from the airstream.

To simplify the plethysmography apparatus, the wire coils have been removed from the elastic belts and replaced by a piezoelectric buckle (**piezoelectric plethysmography**). This reduces the cost and allows for belts that can be adjusted to different-size patients. The buckle encloses a sensor, which generates a voltage in response to stretch passed through the ends of the belts. The sensor is not calibrated, however, and provides only a qualitative record of chest or abdominal movement, hence the term *effort belts*. Effort belts based on piezoelectric sensors do not require a battery. As with all belt-type transducers, the quality and interpretability of the respiratory signal are affected if the belt loosens or slips out of the original position.

Most modern mechanical ventilators have integrated airflow transducers designed to monitor and display the respiratory rate. Capnography can also be used to assess respiratory rate. This uses the fact that CO_2 is only present in the exhaled breath. Thus, each decrease in CO_2 to zero represents a respiratory cycle.

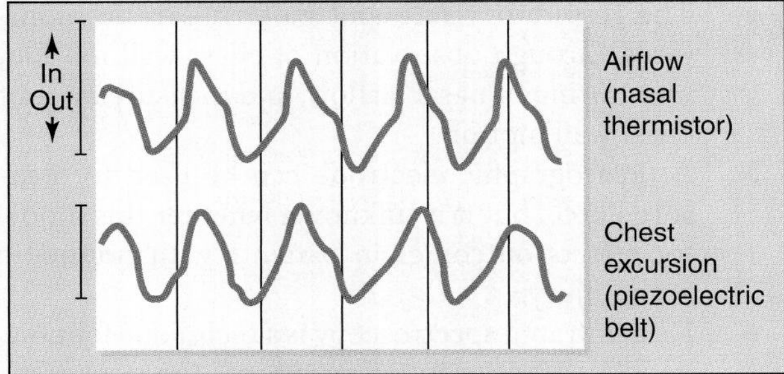

FIGURE 2-24 Airflow and chest and abdominal excursion waveforms are used to monitor respiratory rate and pattern during sleep studies.

Adapted from materials from Pro-Tech Services, Woodinville, WA.

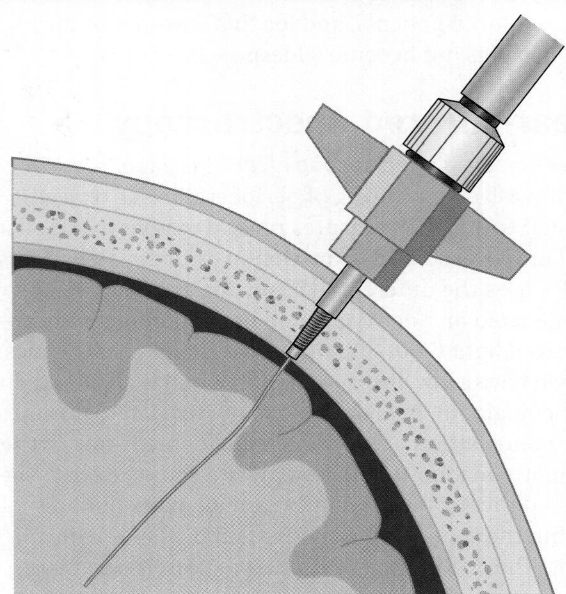

FIGURE 2-25 Coronal section illustrating the placement of the brain tissue oxygenation probe in the brain parenchyma.

Reproduced from Martini RP, Deem S, Treggiari MM. Targeting brain tissue oxygenation in traumatic brain injury. *Respir Care.* 2013;58:162–172.

Acoustic monitoring noninvasively and continuously measures respiration rate using an adhesive sensor with an integrated acoustic transducer applied to the patient's neck. Using acoustic signal processing, the respiratory signal is separated and processed to display continuous respiration rate. This technology is commercially available on the Masimo Rainbow SET Acoustic Monitoring device.

Brain Tissue Po_2

The **brain tissue Po_2 ($Pbto_2$)** measures dissolved oxygen in a small area of brain tissue (**Figure 2-25**).[38] The $Pbto_2$ probe contains polarographic Clark electrodes covered in a semipermeable membrane at the tip of a flexible microcatheter. It is a highly localized measurement, with a sampling area of 7 to 15 mm^2. The probe can be placed through the same burr hole as used with a monitor for intracranial pressure. The location of placement affects the values of $Pbto_2$ measured. Placement into an area of damaged brain, compared to placement into a relatively normal area, will result in data that fail to reflect global dissolved oxygen. Interventions to improve $Pbto_2$ are similar to those used to decrease intracranial pressure. Treatment generally becomes indicated for $Pbto_2$ <20 mm Hg. Periodically, the reliability of measured $Pbto_2$ is assessed by a brief increase in Fio_2 to 1. $Pbto_2$ should rise in tandem with the Pao_2. It is unclear whether targeting strategies to improve $Pbto_2$ result in better outcomes for brain-injured patients, and for this reason monitoring of $Pbto_2$ has not become widespread.

Near-Infrared Spectroscopy

Near-infrared spectroscopy (NIRS) is a technique for noninvasive monitoring of peripheral tissue oxygenation (Sto_2).[39–41] It measures muscle oxygen metabolism and microvascular dysfunction in critically ill patients. NIRS uses the differential absorption properties of oxygenated and deoxygenated hemoglobin. The near-infrared light (700–850 nm) crosses biological tissues, which have a low absorption power, and is absorbed only by hemoglobin, myoglobin, and oxidized cytochrome. The contribution of myoglobin and cytochrome to the light attenuation signal is small and thus the NIRS signal is derived predominantly from hemoglobin present within the volume of tissue crossed by the near-infrared light. The NIRS signal is limited to vessels that have a diameter less than 1 mm (e.g., arterioles, capillaries, and venules).

Commercially available NIRS monitors can provide fractions of oxyhemoglobin and deoxyhemoglobin, used to calculate Sto_2 as well as the total tissue hemoglobin (TTH) and the absolute tissue hemoglobin index (THI), two indicators of blood volume in the region of microvasculature sensed by the probe and expressed in arbitrary units. Light tissue penetration is directly related to the spacing between illumination and detection fibers. At 25 mm spacing, approximately 95% of the detected optical signal is from a depth of 0 to 23 mm. NIRS monitors vary in terms of wavelength selection, number of wavelengths, optode spacing, and algorithms used to calculate data from the absorption data. The NIRS probes in current use measure reflected light and thus the NIRS light source is placed beside the light sensor.

Thenar Sto_2 (**Figure 2-26**) is determined real time at the bedside and may be useful to guide the early resuscitation of critically ill patients, especially in hypodynamic state. However, Sto_2 may be normal in patients with severe sepsis or septic shock, which limits its utilization during resuscitation of septic patients. By inducing an occlusion stress, a variety of dynamic variables can be defined that provide a measure of local metabolic demand and microvascular reactivity. Due to anatomic conditions, both the brachioradial muscle and the muscles of the thenar eminence can be easily subjected to the vascular obstruction test. Alterations in these NIRS-derived dynamic variables are common in patients with severe sepsis and are associated with a poor outcome.

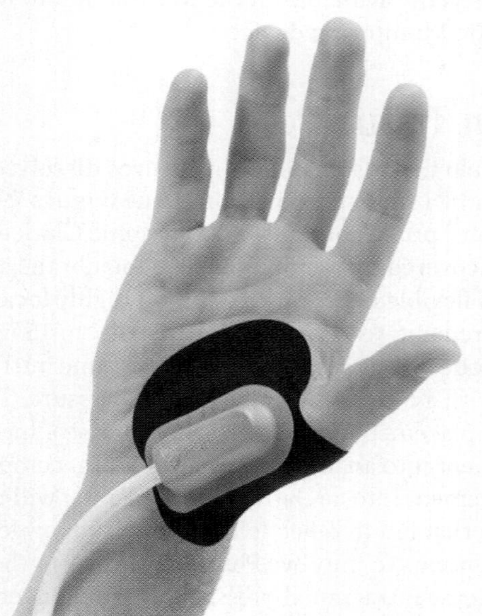

FIGURE 2-26 Near-infrared spectroscopy probe to measure thenar Sto_2.
Courtesy of Hutchinson Technology.

Key Points

- Pulse oximetry measures oxygen saturation by passing two wavelengths of light through a pulsating vascular bed.
- The accuracy of pulse oximetry is ±4%.
- A number of factors can affect the accuracy and performance of pulse oximetry.
- New designs of pulse oximeters measure SpHb, Spco, and SpMet; the clinical utility of these measures is yet to be determined.
- Capnometry measures the concentration of carbon dioxide exhaled from the lungs.
- Capnography can be useful for detection of esophageal intubation, the adequacy of chest compressions, and the return of spontaneous circulation during CPR.
- End-tidal Pco_2 may not be an accurate reflection of $Paco_2$.
- Volumetric capnography can be used to measure carbon dioxide production and cardiac output.
- Transcutaneous Po_2 and Pco_2 are measured with a heated electrode placed on the skin.
- The respiratory rate and pattern can be monitored through observation of chest wall motion, monitoring of nasal airflow, and measurement of chest wall motion.
- A polarographic electrode can be used to measure $Pbto_2$, but it is unknown whether this monitor affects outcomes in patients with traumatic brain injury.
- Near-infrared spectroscopy is a technique for noninvasive monitoring of peripheral tissue oxygenation in various tissues.

References

1. Mannheimer PD. The light–tissue interaction of pulse oximetry. *Anesth Analg.* 2007;105:S10–S17.
2. McMorrow RCN, Mythen MG. Pulse oximetry. *Curr Opin Crit Care.* 2006;12:269–271.
3. Barker SJ, Badal JJ. The measurement of dyshemoglobins and total hemoglobin by pulse oximetry. *Curr Opin Anaesthesiol.* 2008;21:805–810.
4. Kress JP, Pohlman AS, Hall JB. Determinants of hemoglobin saturation in patients with acute sickle chest syndrome. A comparison of arterial blood gases and pulse oximetry. *Chest.* 1999;115:1316–1320.
5. Feiner JR, Severinghaus JW, Bickler PE. Dark skin decreases the accuracy of pulse oximeters at low oxygen saturation: the effects of oximeter probe type and gender. *Anesth Analg.* 2007;105:S18–S23.
6. Yamamoto LG, Yamamoto JA, Yamamoto JB, Yamamoto BE, Yamamoto PP. Nail polish does not significantly affect pulse oximetry measurements in mildly hypoxic subjects. *Respir Care.* 2008;53:1470–1474.
7. Petterson MT, Begnoche VL, Graybeal JM. The effect of motion on pulse oximetry and its clinical significance. *Anesth Analg.* 2007;105:S78–S84.
8. Gehring H, Nornberger C, Matz H, et al. The effects of motion artifact and low perfusion on the performance of a new generation of pulse oximeters in volunteers undergoing hypoxemia. *Respir Care.* 2002;47:48–60.
9. Weaver LK, Churchill SK, Deru K, Cooney D. False positive rate of carbon monoxide saturation by pulse oximetry of emergency department patients. *Respir Care.* 2013;58:232–240.
10. Wilcox SR, Richards JB. Noninvasive carbon monoxide detection: insufficient evidence for broad clinical use. *Respir Care.* 2013;58:376–379.
11. Sebbane M, Claret PG, Mercier G, et al. Emergency department management of suspected carbon monoxide poisoning: role of pulse co-oximetry. *Respir Care.* 2013;58:1514–1620.
12. Rice MJ, Gravenstein N, Morey TE. Noninvasive hemoglobin monitoring: how accurate is enough? *Anesth Analg.* 2013;117:902–907.
13. Frasca D, Dahyot-Fizelier C, Catherine K, et al. Accuracy of a continuous noninvasive hemoglobin monitor in intensive care unit patients. *Crit Care Med.* 2011;39:2277–2282.
14. Bendjelid K. The pulse oximetry plethysmographic curve revisited. *Curr Opin Crit Care.* 2008;14:348–353.
15. Cannesson M, Desebbe O, Rosamel P, et al. Pleth variability index to monitor the respiratory variations in the pulse oximeter plethysmographic waveform amplitude and predict fluid responsiveness in the operating theatre. *Br J Anaesth.* 2008;101:200–206.
16. Desebbe O, Cannesson M. Using ventilation-induced plethysmographic variations to optimize patient fluid status. *Curr Opin Anaesthesiol.* 2008;21:772–778.
17. Shelley KH. Photoplethysmography: beyond the calculation of arterial oxygen saturation and heart rate. *Anesth Analg.* 2007;105(Suppl 6):S31–S36.
18. Hartert TV, Wheeler AP, Sheller JR. Use of pulse oximetry to recognize severity of airflow obstruction in obstructive airway disease: correlation with pulsus paradoxus. *Chest.* 1999;115:475–481.
19. AARC clinical practice guideline: capnometry and capnography during mechanical ventilation—2003 revision and update. *Respir Care.* 2003;48:534–537.
20. Araujo-Preza CE, Melhado ME, Gutierrez FJ, et al. Use of capnometry to verify feeding tube placement. *Crit Care Med.* 2002;30:2255–2259.
21. McSwain SD, Hamel DS, Smith PB, et al. End-tidal and arterial carbon dioxide measurements correlate across all levels of physiologic dead space. *Respir Care.* 2010;55:288–293.
22. Krauss B, Hess DR. Capnography for procedural sedation and analgesia in the emergency department. *Ann Emerg Med.* 2007;50:172–181.
23. Riou Y, Leclerc F, Neve V, et al. Reproducibility of the respiratory dead space measurements in mechanically ventilated children using the CO2SMO monitor. *Intensive Care Med.* 2004;30:1461–1467.
24. Kallet RH, Daniel BM, Garcia O, et al. Accuracy of physiologic dead space measurements in patients with acute respiratory distress syndrome using volumetric capnography: comparison with the metabolic monitor method. *Respir Care.* 2005;50:462–467.
25. Blanch L, Romero PV, Lucangelo U. Volumetric capnography in the mechanically ventilated patient. *Minerva Anesthesiol.* 2006;72:577–585.
26. Siobal MS, Ong H, Valdes J, Tang J. Calculation of physiologic dead space: comparison of ventilator volumetric capnography to measurements by metabolic analyzer and volumetric CO_2 monitor. *Respir Care.* 2013;58:1143–1151.
27. Tachibana K, Imanaka H, Takeuchi M, et al. Noninvasive cardiac output measurement using partial carbon dioxide rebreathing is less accurate at settings of reduced minute ventilation and when spontaneous breathing is present. *Anesthesiology.* 2003;98:830–837.
28. Tachibana K, Imanaka H, Miyano H, et al. Effect of ventilatory settings on accuracy of cardiac output measurement using partial CO_2 rebreathing. *Anesthesiology.* 2002;96:96–102.
29. Yem JS, Tang Y, Turner MJ, et al. Sources of error in noninvasive pulmonary blood flow measurements by partial rebreathing. A computer model study. *Anesthesiology.* 2003;98:881–887.
30. de Abreu MG, Geiger S, Winkler T, et al. Evaluation of a new device for noninvasive measurement of nonshunted pulmonary capillary blood flow in patients with acute lung injury. *Intensive Care Med.* 2002;28:318–323.
31. Odenstedt H, Stenqvist O, Lundin S. Clinical evaluation of a partial CO_2 rebreathing technique for cardiac output monitoring in critically ill patients. *Acta Anaesthesiol Scand.* 2002;46:152–159.
32. de Abreu MG, Winkler T, Pahlitzsch T, et al. Performance of the partial CO_2 rebreathing technique under different hemodynamic and ventilation/perfusion matching conditions. *Crit Care Med.* 2003;31:543–551.
33. AARC clinical practice guideline: transcutaneous blood gas monitoring for neonatal and pediatric patients—2004 revision and update. *Respir Care.* 2004;49:1069–1072.
34. Bernet-Buettiker V, Ugarte MJ, Frey B, et al. Evaluation of a new combined transcutaneous measurement of PCO_2/pulse oximetry oxygen saturation ear sensor in newborn patients. *Pediatrics.* 2005;115:e64–68.
35. Senn O, Clarenbach CF, Kaplan V, et al. Monitoring carbon dioxide tension and arterial oxygen saturation by a single earlobe sensor in patients with critical illness or sleep apnea. *Chest.* 2005;128:1291–1296.
36. Rodriguez P, Lellouche F, Aboab J, et al. Transcutaneous arterial carbon dioxide pressure monitoring in critically ill adult patients. *Intensive Care Med.* 2006;32:309–312.
37. Kocher S, Rohling R, Tschupp A. Performance of a digital PCO_2/SpO_2 ear sensor. *J Clin Monit Comput.* 2004;18:75–79.
38. Martini RP, Deem S, Treggiari MM. Targeting brain tissue oxygenation in traumatic brain injury. *Respir Care.* 2013;58:162–172.
39. Lipcsey M, Woinarski NCZ, Rinaldo Bellomo R. Near infrared spectroscopy (NIRS) of the thenar eminence in anesthesia and intensive care. *Ann Intensive Care.* 2012;2:11.
40. Creteur J. Muscle Sto_2 in critically ill patients. *Curr Opin Crit Care.* 2008;14:361–366.
41. Santora RJ, Moore FA. Monitoring trauma and intensive care unit resuscitation with tissue hemoglobin oxygen saturation. *Critical Care.* 2009;13(Suppl 5):S10.

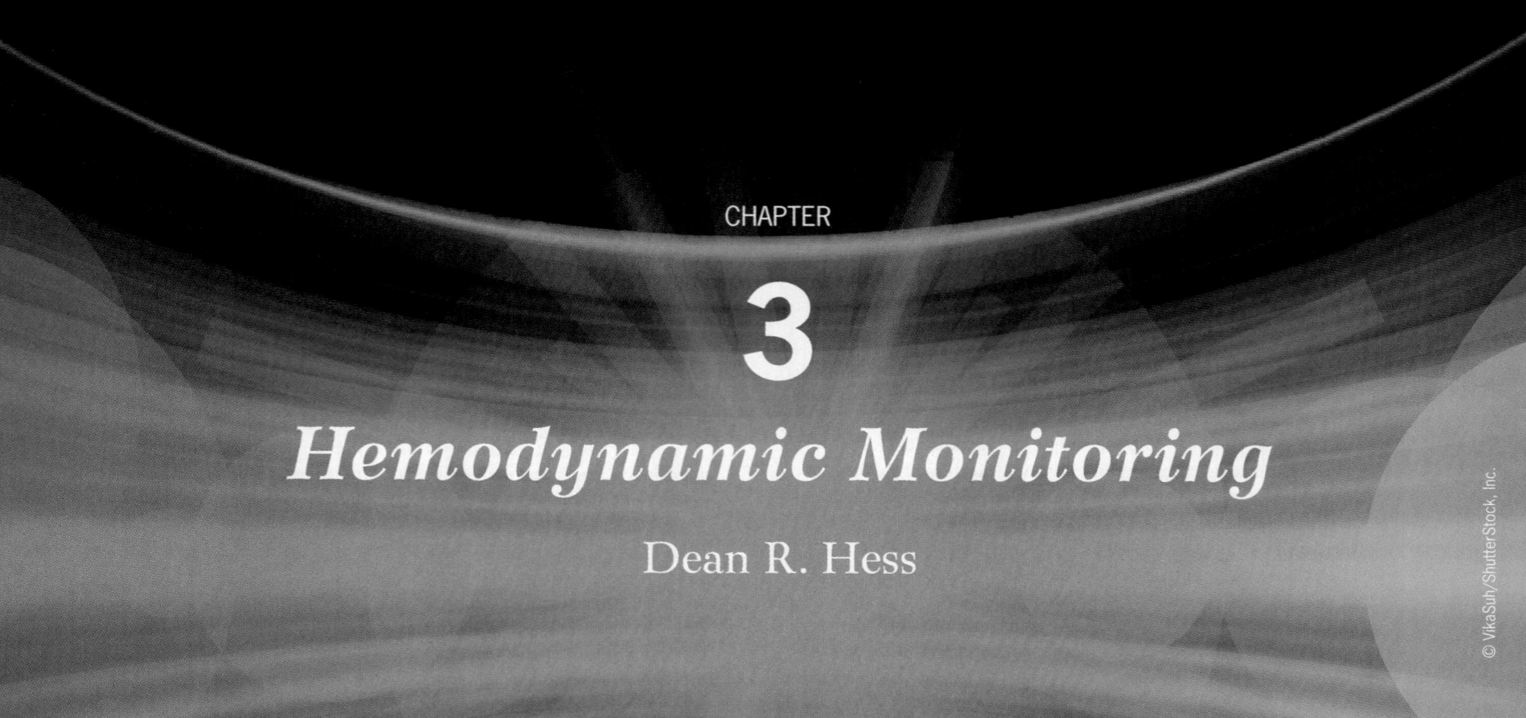

CHAPTER

3
Hemodynamic Monitoring

Dean R. Hess

OUTLINE

OBJECTIVES

1. Discuss the clinical importance of monitoring heart rate and rhythm.
2. Compare noninvasive and invasive techniques used to monitor arterial blood pressure.
3. Describe the clinical significance of systolic pressure variation and pulse pressure variation.
4. Discuss the roles of arterial blood pressure, central venous pressure, and pulmonary artery pressure in hemodynamic monitoring.
5. Describe the pulmonary artery catheter.
6. Identify waveforms from the pulmonary artery catheter.
7. Discuss pitfalls related to measurements of cardiac output.
8. Compare methods used to measure cardiac output.
9. Calculate systemic vascular resistance and pulmonary vascular resistance.

KEY TERMS

arterial blood pressure
a wave
cardiac arrhythmia
central venous pressure (CVP)
diastolic
Fick equation
heart rate
pulmonary artery (PA) catheter
pulmonary artery wedge pressure (PAWP)
pulmonary vascular resistance (PVR)
pulse contour waveform analysis
pulse pressure variation (PPV)
systemic vascular resistance (SVR)
systolic
thermodilution
v wave
Wood units

Introduction

Hemodynamic monitors measure cardiovascular parameters in a continuous or nearly continuous fashion. As shown in **Table 3-1**, there are many different measurable hemodynamic measurements. Some require invasive devices, whereas others can be made by observation. This chapter covers invasive and noninvasive hemodynamic monitors, with particular attention to the role of hemodynamic monitoring of the patient with respiratory disease.

Cardiac Rate and Rhythm

As one of the vital signs, **heart rate** provides a bedside measure of cardiovascular status. With electrocardiographic (ECG) techniques, cardiac rhythms can be displayed at the bedside and/or transmitted to a central monitoring area, where the cardiac rhythms of many patients can be monitored by one individual and, if needed, printed or stored for later review.

The normal adult resting heart rate is 60 to 100 beats/min. It accelerates during exercise and slows during sleep as a result of the direct influence of the autonomic nervous system on the sinus node. During exercise, or with pain or anxiety, the sympathetic nerves act on the sinus node to increase the heart rate. Parasympathetic, or vagal, effects slow the rate. **Cardiac arrhythmias** (excessively fast or slow rates and irregular rhythms) frequently occur during the course of critical illness, especially during cardiopulmonary failure, serious infections, myocardial infarction, and toxic overdose.

Heart rate can be measured at the bedside by counting the peripheral pulse. The radial pulse is most

TABLE 3-1
Normal Ranges for Hemodynamic Measurements

Variable	Units	Normal Range
Systolic blood pressure (SBP)	mm Hg	90–140
Diastolic blood pressure (DBP)	mm Hg	60–90
Mean arterial pressure (MAP)	mm Hg	65–105
Pulmonary artery systolic pressure (PASP)	mm Hg	15–30
Pulmonary artery diastolic pressure (PADP)	mm Hg	4–12
Mean pulmonary artery pressure (MPAP)	mm Hg	9–16
Right ventricular systolic pressure (RVSP)	mm Hg	15–30
Right ventricular end-diastolic pressure (RVEDP)	mm Hg	0–8
Central venous pressure (CVP)	mm Hg	0–8
Pulmonary artery wedge pressure (PAWP)	mm Hg	2–12
Cardiac output (CO)	L/min	Varies with size of patient
Cardiac index (CI)	L/min/m²	2.5–3.5

Reproduced from Nelson LD. The new pulmonary artery catheters: right ventricular ejection fraction and continuous cardiac output. *Crit Care Clin.* 1996;12:795. © 1996, with permission from Elsevier.

commonly used for this purpose. It is counted for 15 to 30 seconds and multiplied to calculate beats per minute. Obtaining an accurate pulse in critically ill patients can be difficult. In hypotensive patients, the only palpable pulses may be over the carotid or femoral arteries. In patients with cardiac arrhythmias, peripheral pulses may vary in intensity because of poor transmission of the irregular beats. In these cases the apical heartbeat should be auscultated at the chest to obtain an accurate measurement.

With ECG electrodes, cardiac electrical activity can be detected at the skin surface and processed to display the heart rate and waveforms. The electrodes are applied to the chest and extremities in standardized arrays, and the electrode array is connected directly to the bedside monitor or ECG machine or is plugged into a radio transmitter that sends the signals to a central telemetry console.

In the intensive care unit (ICU), heart rate and rhythm are displayed on a bedside monitor. These systems accurately measure the heart rate, identify dangerous arrhythmias such as ventricular tachycardia and fibrillation, and recognize episodes of

Respiratory Recap

Cardiac Monitoring

- Bedside ICU monitors measure the heart rate and detect arrhythmias.
- Telemetry is used for cardiac monitoring outside the ICU.

myocardial ischemia. They are equipped with audio and visual alarms that can trigger the printing of a rhythm strip or freeze the monitor screen for immediate review. Patients on hospital telemetry units wear small electronic boxes to transmit the ECG to central monitoring stations. This has allowed early transfer of otherwise stable patients from the ICU to the comfort and convenience of private rooms. The electrodes are connected to a small radio transmitter that encodes the ECG signals into radio frequency waves and transmits them to the receiving unit for display and analysis.

Arterial Blood Pressure

Arterial blood pressure is one of the vital signs. Arterial blood pressure is measured by sphygmomanometry or by an indwelling arterial cannula for continuous pressure measurement and waveform graphics. Blood flow and vascular resistance determine intravascular pressure:

$$\text{Pressure} = \text{Flow} \times \text{Resistance}$$

Flow is determined by cardiac output, and resistance is determined by vascular tone. The arterial waveform consists of peak, or **systolic**, blood pressure corresponding to cardiac contraction; an anacrotic and dicrotic notch; and a nadir, or **diastolic**, blood pressure (**Figure 3-1**). The anacrotic notch is a reflected pressure wave that rebounds from the peripheral vessels. The dicrotic notch represents closure of the aortic valve. In the peripheral vessels a normal increase in elasticity and resistance results in a peaked and narrower waveform. Systolic pressure in the radial artery, therefore, is about 6 mm Hg higher than a simultaneous measurement in the brachial artery. This difference diminishes in patients with inelastic arteries, such as the elderly or those with vascular disease.[1,2]

Noninvasive methods used to measure blood pressure use a blood pressure cuff, which is gradually inflated around an extremity to a pressure above the systolic pressure and then slowly deflated while the artery is auscultated for Korotkoff sounds. Automated noninvasive blood pressure monitors program inflation and deflation of the cuff at selected intervals. Most of these systems are based on oscillometry and use a sensitive transducer to measure not only cuff pressure but also the minute oscillations in the cuff

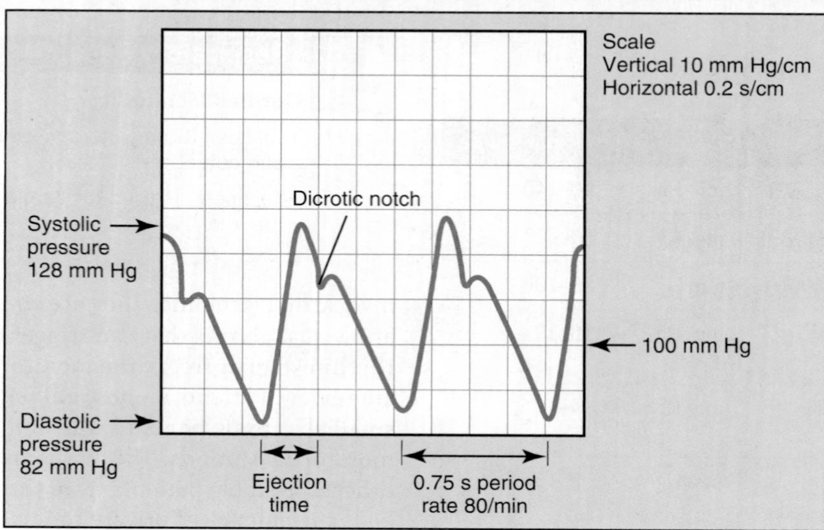

FIGURE 3-1 Arterial blood pressure waveform.

caused by the pulsating vessel. The systolic and diastolic pressures are recognized by changes in oscillation intensity (**Figure 3-2**). These devices are available with programmable blood pressure intervals, memory, display, and print features. Portable units are available for use on hospital wards, and plug-in modules for multifunctional critical care monitors. Manual and automated cuff measurements correlate well with simultaneous intra-arterial values. In adults, however, the first Korotkoff sound generally does not appear until 4 to 15 mm Hg below the intravascular systolic pressure, and the last sound disappears 3 to 6 mm Hg above the intravascular diastolic pressure.[1]

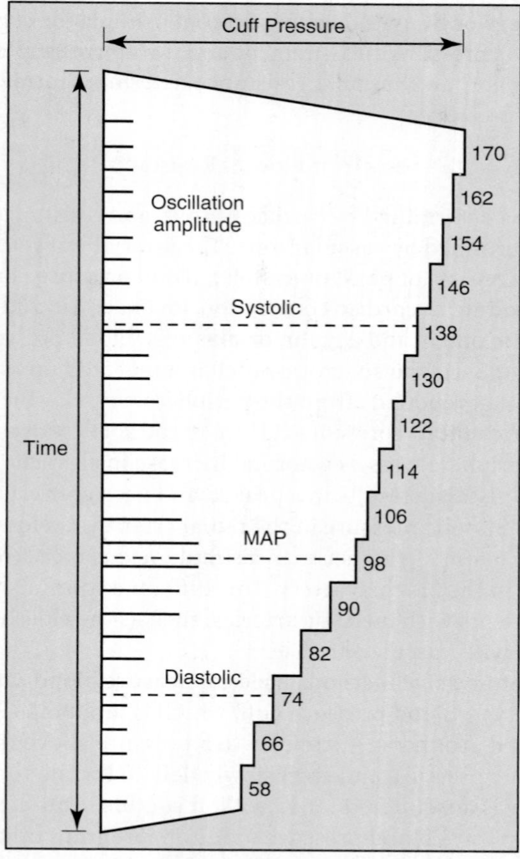

FIGURE 3-2 Noninvasive blood pressure measurements are derived from analysis of oscillation amplitude during a programmed cuff inflation-deflation cycle.

Modified from materials courtesy of Critikon LLC, Tampa, FL. (GE Healthcare Monitoring Solutions).

Noninvasive systems have limitations. Poor-fitting cuffs may lead to measurement errors. Larger cuffs must be used with obese patients, because undersized cuffs can result in an overestimation of arterial pressure. In hypotensive, edematous, or vasoconstricted patients, automated systems may not be able to detect weakly transmitted blood pressure sounds. Programmable noninvasive systems have also been associated with ulnar palsies, skin injury at the site of inflation, and extremity ischemia when used with frequent inflation-deflation cycles.

Intra-arterial monitoring is indicated for critically ill patients with extremes of blood pressure requiring aggressive resuscitation efforts or titration of potent vasoactive agents. Small catheters, usually 18- or 20-gauge, are inserted into the radial, femoral, axillary, dorsalis pedis, or brachial artery based on ease of access and relative frequency of complications. The cannula is connected to a bedside pressure transducer, usually with a stopcock to allow intermittent arterial blood sampling.

Some systematic differences exist between invasive and noninvasive blood pressure measurements. Normally, the intra-arterial systolic pressure is 10% to 20% higher and the diastolic pressure lower in distal extremities because of changes in the elasticity and caliber of the arteries. This effect, known as *distal pulse amplification*, causes a widened pulse pressure without affecting mean arterial pressure. For patients who are rewarming after cardiopulmonary bypass or receiving

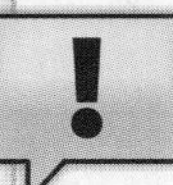

Respiratory Recap

Arterial Blood Pressure

- Automated noninvasive systems are based on oscillometry or photoplethysmography.
- Invasive systems use transducers attached to an intra-arterial catheter.
- Respiratory variation in pulse pressure can be used to assess fluid responsiveness.
- Pulse contour waveform analysis can be used to assess cardiac output.

vasopressors for septic shock, measurements obtained from the radial artery have been shown to underestimate central (femoral artery) pressures. Failure to recognize this phenomenon may lead to the inappropriate use of vasoactive agents.

Intra-arterial monitoring is associated with several complications, including injury to the artery or adjacent nerves, bleeding, ischemia and infection of the extremity, and systemic infection due to catheter-related bloodstream infection. The radial artery is favored for placement of indwelling cannulas because of its accessibility and the presence of vascular collateral circulation to the hand. The ulnar and brachial arteries are avoided, if possible, because of their tenuous and variable collateral blood flow.

Respiratory Variation in Pulse Amplitude

Due to the heart–lung interactions that occur during positive pressure ventilation, the left ventricular stroke volume varies cyclically. It is maximal during inhalation and minimal during exhalation.[3–6] This has been used to assess preload status and predict fluid responsiveness in deeply sedated patients receiving positive pressure ventilation. Using the systolic pressure at end-exhalation as the baseline, the systolic pressure variation is divided into two components: an increase (Δup) and a decrease (Δdown) from baseline (**Figure 3-3**). Volume expansion decreases systolic pressure variation and Δdown. The respiratory changes in systolic pressure result not only from changes in transmural pressure (mainly related to changes in left ventricular stroke volume) but also from changes in extramural pressure (i.e., from changes in pleural pressure). Thus, respiratory changes in systolic pressure may be observed despite lack of variation in left ventricular stroke volume.

Pulse pressure, the difference between the systolic and the diastolic pressure, is proportional to left ventricular stroke volume. Respiratory changes in left ventricular stroke volume are reflected by changes in peripheral pulse pressure during the respiratory cycle. Fluid responsiveness can be assessed by calculating the respiratory **pulse pressure variation (PPV)**:

$$\text{PPV (\%)} = 100 \times (PP_{max} - PP_{min})/PP_{mean}$$

where PP_{max} is the maximal pulse pressure, PP_{min} is the minimal pulse pressure, and PP_{mean} is the average pulse pressure (**Figure 3-4**). PPV greater than 15% allows discrimination between responders and nonresponders to a fluid challenge.[3–6]

Pulse Contour Waveform Analysis

Pulse pressure is determined by stroke volume and vascular tone. Real-time assessment of pulse pressure, **pulse contour waveform analysis**, allows stroke volume to be derived from the arterial pressure waveform.[7,8]

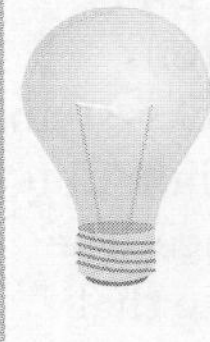

STOP AND THINK

A mechanically ventilated postoperative patient has a blood pressure of 80/50 mm Hg and a significant pulse pressure variation. How would you explain these findings and what would you recommend?

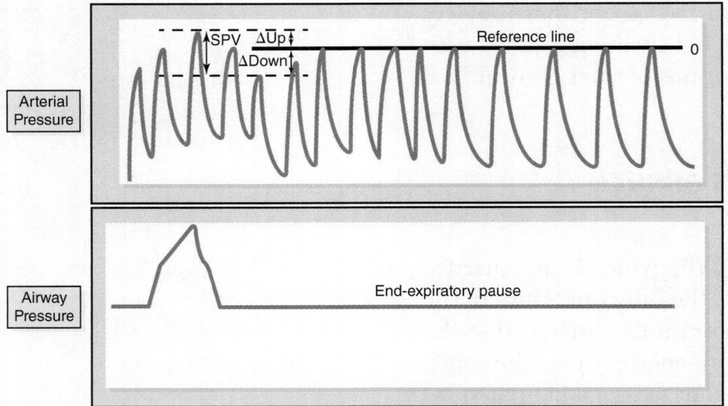

FIGURE 3-3 Systolic pressure variation (SPV) after one positive pressure breath followed by an end-expiratory pause. Reference line permits the measurement of up and down.

Reproduced with kind permission from Springer Science+Business Media: Bendjelid K, Romand J. *Intensive Care Med.*, Fluid responsiveness in mechanically ventilated patients, 2003;29:352–360.

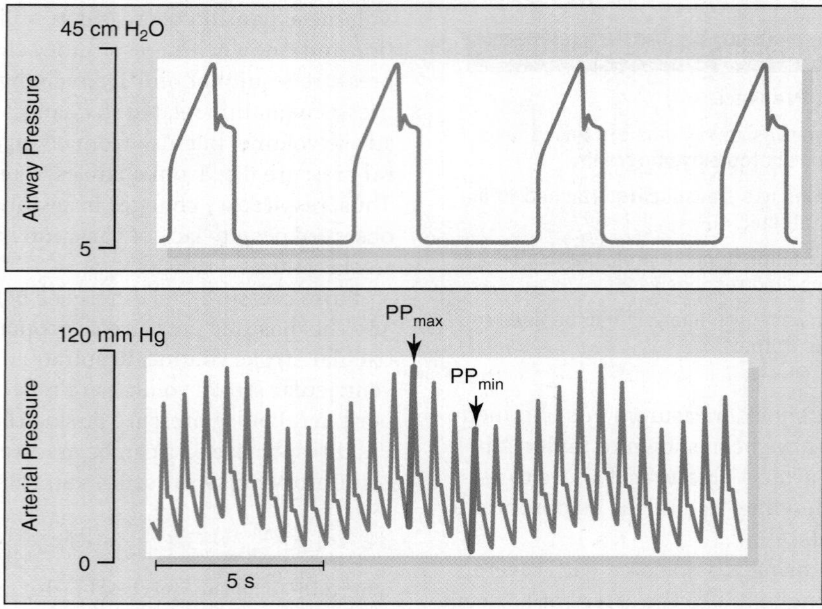

FIGURE 3-4 Respiratory changes in airway and arterial pressures in a mechanically ventilated patient. The pulse pressure (systolic minus diastolic pressure) is maximal (PP_{max}) at the end of the inspiratory period and minimal (PP_{min}) three heartbeats later (i.e., during the expiratory period). The respiratory changes in pulse pressure are calculated as the difference between PP_{max} and PP_{min}, divided by the mean of the two values, and expressed as a percentage.

Reproduced from Michard F, Teboul J. Using heart-lung interactions to assess fluid responsiveness during mechanical ventilation. *Crit Care.* 2000;4:282–289. Reproduced with permission from BioMed Central.

This method uses an arterial catheter to provide a continuous measure of stroke volume and cardiac output. In order to translate pulse pressure into volume, some measure of arterial compliance (vascular tone) is required. There are two calibrated pulse contour waveform analysis devices available. The LiDCO system requires an independent calibration with a lithium dilution technique to account for arterial compliance. The PiCCO system is a pulse contour analysis device that employs transpulmonary **thermodilution**. The Vigileo monitor is a noncalibrated device that uses an arterial pressure transducer to characterize the pulse waveform and that estimates vascular tone using the demographics (age, gender, and body surface area). These devices are commercially available, but their widespread use has been hampered by questions of their clinical accuracy.[9–11]

Central Venous Pressure Monitoring

Central venous pressure (CVP), which is measured in the superior vena cava, is the filling pressure in the right atrium. Single-lumen or multi-lumen catheters are positioned in the superior vena cava via the subclavian (**Figure 3-5**) or internal or external jugular vein to permit CVP monitoring, intravenous access for medication infusions, and venous blood sampling. The femoral vein also is used, especially during emergencies. Femoral catheters positioned in the common iliac vein or inferior vena cava have been shown to provide a reasonable estimate of CVP, at least in the absence of increased abdominal pressure or vena cava injury.

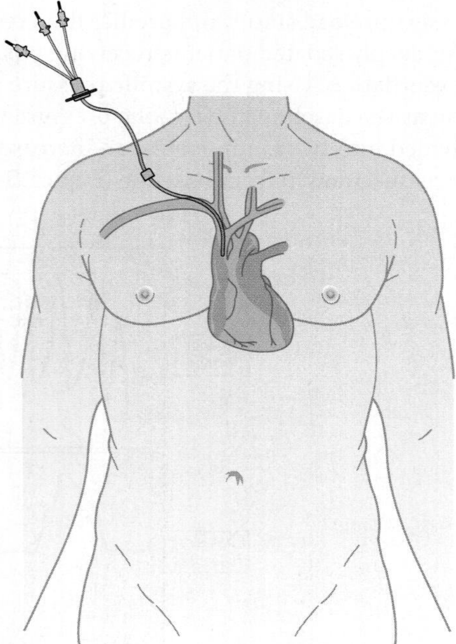

FIGURE 3-5 Placement of triple-lumen central venous catheter.

Adapted from Taylor C, et al. *Fundamentals of Nursing*. 5th ed. Lippincott Williams & Wilkins; 2005.

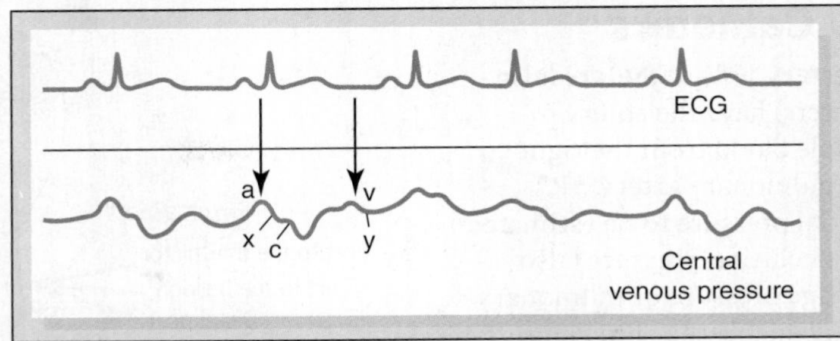

FIGURE 3-6 CVP waveform. The a wave reflects contraction in atrial systole and follows the p wave on the ECG. The x descent reflects the fall in right atrial pressure following atrial systole. The c wave, often small, reflects the closure of the tricuspid valve. The v wave represents ventricular systole, as well as passive atrial diastolic filling, and follows the t wave of the ECG. The y descent reflects the fall in right atrial pressure following opening of the tricuspid valve and the initiation of passive filling of the right ventricle.

When CVP measurements are necessary, the femoral site is usually avoided. In adults, central venous catheters usually measure 7 French (about 2.3 mm) in diameter and 16 to 20 cm in length. They are constructed of biocompatible plastics such as polyethylene, Teflon, and polyurethane. Intravascular catheters are designed with flexibility, a smooth surface, thromboresistance, lack of kink memory, and chemical stability.

In the presence of a competent tricuspid valve, the CVP waveform reflects both venous return to the right atrium (during ventricular systole) and right ventricular end-diastolic pressure. There are normally three positive components and two negative deflections in the right atrial (RA) waveform (**Figure 3-6**). Electrocardiographic correlation is required for correct identification of these events. In the right atrium, there is an 80- to 100-ms delay in the detection of mechanical events from their appearance on the ECG as a result of the length of tubing in the system. Normal right atrial pressures vary from 0 to 7 mm Hg. Elevations in RA pressure are seen in a number of conditions (**Table 3-2**).

A number of cardiac rhythm disturbances can produce characteristic abnormalities in the CVP waveform. Atrial fibrillation is associated with lack of organized atrial activity and therefore loss of the normal **a wave**. Atrial flutter may produce characteristic sawtooth f waves in the CVP tracing (as well as on the ECG) at a rate of 240 to 340 beats per minute. Atrioventricular dissociation (ventricular pacing, complete heart block, ventricular tachycardia) may manifest cannon a waves (or giant a waves) due to the simultaneous contraction of atrium and ventricle while the tricuspid valve is closed.

TABLE 3-2
Conditions Elevating Central Venous Pressure

Volume overload
Impaired right ventricular contractile function
Pulmonary hypertension
Right ventricular infarction
Pulmonic stenosis
Tricuspid valvular disease
Left-to-right shunts

The CVP is particularly useful in volume-depleted states. Low values guide fluid and blood volume replacement in bleeding or hypovolemic patients. However, a normal or elevated CVP correlates poorly with intravascular volume status, especially for patients with heart and lung disease, and cannot be used reliably to guide therapy. Central venous catheters are also used to obtain venous blood samples. A central venous oximetry catheter has the capability for continuous monitoring of central venous oxygen saturation ($Scvo_2$).

Central venous catheterization has well-recognized complications. Mechanical complications related to insertion of the catheter include pneumothorax, bleeding, and injury to nerves, vessels, or the thoracic duct. Fewer complications are seen when the operator is skilled and ultrasound is used to identify the venous anatomy.[12] Malpositioned catheters can cause cardiac arrhythmias, valvular injury, chamber perforation, and cardiac tamponade. Infection can develop at the insertion site, sometimes resulting in bacteremia with prolonged use. Antimicrobial-coated catheters have been developed to reduce the incidence of infectious complications.

Respiratory Recap

Central Venous Pressure

- CVP is measured in the superior vena cava.
- CVP is used to estimate intravascular volume status.
- Central venous catheters can be used to obtain blood samples for laboratory analysis.

Pulmonary Artery Catheters

Flow-directed **pulmonary artery (PA) catheters** (also known as Swan-Ganz catheters) have the ability to measure pressures and sample blood from the right atrium, right ventricle, and pulmonary artery.[12] PA catheters also enable left atrial pressure to be estimated from the pulmonary artery occlusion pressure (also called pulmonary artery wedge pressure or pulmonary capillary wedge pressure) and enable the clinician to measure the cardiac output.

The catheter has a balloon at the tip that is inflated with air, which allows blood flow to direct the catheter through the right ventricle into the pulmonary artery. The right internal jugular vein or the left subclavian vein may be the easiest site to use in difficult access conditions, such as pulmonary hypertension. Fluoroscopic guidance often helps in obtaining accurate catheter placement in patients with marked right atrial or ventricular dilatation, severe tricuspid regurgitation, or left bundle branch block. Fluoroscopy may also be necessary when the cephalic or femoral site is used because of the tortuous vascular pathway to the pulmonary artery. The standard adult thermodilution PA catheter is usually 7 to 7.5 French and approximately 110 cm long, with a balloon capacity of 1.5 mL. Smaller catheters are available for pediatric patients. From the internal jugular or subclavian vein in adults, the catheter generally is positioned at 45 to 60 cm.

Pulmonary artery catheters have three or four ports for pressure measurements, thermodilution injections, and medication infusion (**Figure 3-7**). A proximal port 30 cm from the tip resides in the right atrium–superior vena cava, and a distal port is positioned at the tip in the pulmonary artery. The catheter tip balloon can be inflated intermittently to allow wedging in the distal pulmonary artery. The **pulmonary artery wedge pressure (PAWP)** provides an estimate of left atrial and left ventricular end-diastolic or filling pressure (LVEDP). Each anatomic position produces a characteristic waveform (**Figure 3-8**).

Observation of pressure waveforms permits evaluation of mechanical events within the atria and ventricles and offers important diagnostic information in a wide variety of cardiopulmonary disease states. Consequently, information from the PA catheter can provide diagnostic and therapeutic information (**Table 3-3**). Appropriate use of the PA catheter requires careful data gathering and interpretation.

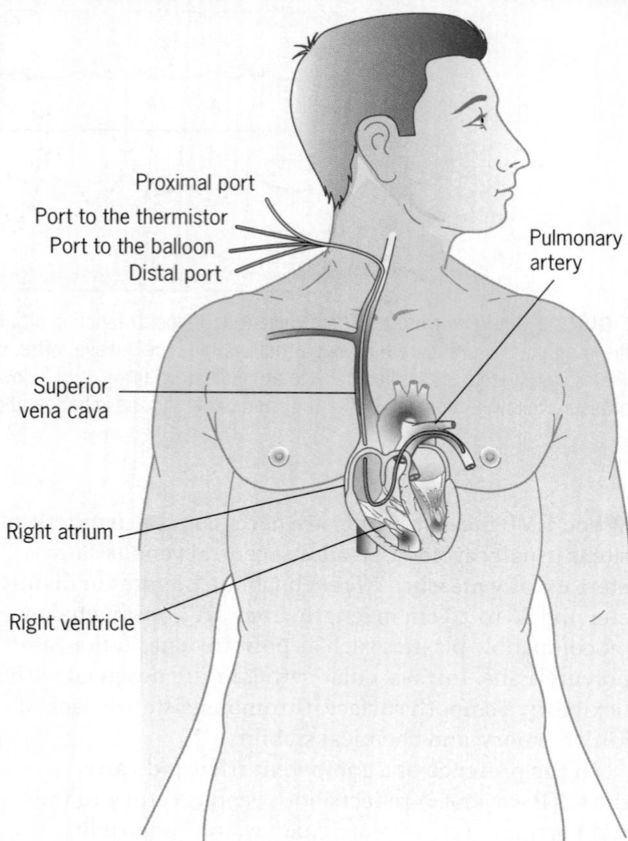

FIGURE 3-7 Monitoring ports on the pulmonary artery catheter.
Adapted from Schulte am Esch J. *Atlas of Anaesthesia*, 3rd ed. Thieme Medical Publishers; 2006.

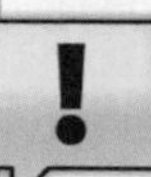

Respiratory Recap

Pulmonary Artery Catheters

- Measures the pulmonary artery pressure and pulmonary artery wedge pressure.
- Thermodilution catheters measure cardiac output.
- Oximetric catheters measure the mixed venous oxygen saturation.
- Samples from pulmonary artery catheters are used to measure mixed venous blood gases.

Catheter Setup

The catheter must be zeroed and referenced for accurate diagnostic information to be obtained. Although zeroing and referencing are done in one step, they represent two separate processes. Opening the system to air establishes atmospheric pressure as zero. Referencing (or leveling) is accomplished by placing the air–fluid interface of the transducer at the level of the right atrium to negate the effects of the weight of the catheter tubing and fluid column.[13] Note that the phlebostatic level changes with differences in the position of the patient.

The pulmonary artery catheter allows simultaneous recording of pressure waveforms from the right atrium and pulmonary artery or pulmonary artery wedge pressure. Pulmonary artery wedge pressure measurements are made by inflating the balloon at the distal tip of the catheter with approximately 1.0

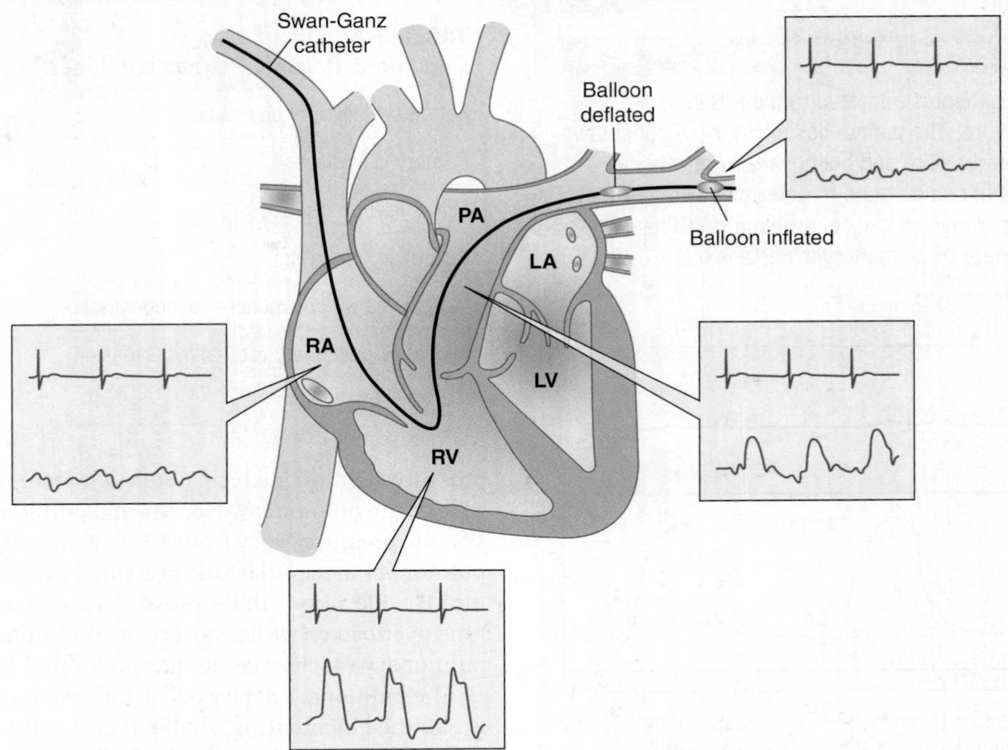

FIGURE 3-8 Waveforms from various sites on the pulmonary artery catheter.
Modified from Longnecker D, Brown D, Newman M, Zapol W. 2008. *Anesthesiology*. McGraw-Hill, New York. © The McGraw-Hill Companies, Inc.

to 1.5 mL of air. Once the balloon is filled, it floats (i.e., is flow directed) until it occludes a segment of the pulmonary artery. The waveform noted following occlusion of the pulmonary artery reflects the transmitted pressure of the left atrium. It does not reflect true left ventricular end-diastolic volume, nor does it reflect capillary hydrostatic pressures or transmural pressures.[14]

TABLE 3-3
Indications for Pulmonary Artery Catheterization

Measure cardiac output
Assess pulmonary hypertension
Assess intravascular volume
Differentiate among shock states (hypovolemic versus heart failure)
Differentiate diffuse pulmonary infiltrates (cardiac versus pulmonary)
Differentiate pericardial constriction, restrictive cardiomyopathy, and tamponade
Assess severity of valvular heart disease
Assess cardiomyopathy
Define intracardiac shunts (e.g., atrial or ventricular septal defects)

Following catheter placement, the dynamic response of the monitoring system should be assessed. Dynamic response is determined by two factors: the resonant frequency and the damping coefficient of the system. Both of these aspects of the monitoring system can be assessed at the bedside using the fast-flush test, performed by briefly opening and closing the valve in the continuous flush device. This produces a square wave displacement on the oscilloscope, followed by ringing and a return to baseline. Stopcocks, excessive tubing lengths, and patient factors (such as tachycardia and high output states) are common causes of under-damping. Air bubbles in the tubing are a common source of overdamping; flushing the system through the stopcock can clear the bubbles.

Pressure Waveforms

CVP measurements are obtained from the proximal port of the PA catheter. Two pressures are typically measured in the right ventricle (RV): the peak right ventricular systolic pressure and the right ventricular end-diastolic pressure. Ventricular diastole is made up of an early rapid filling phase (during which approximately 60% of filling occurs), a slow phase (during which another 25% of filling occurs), and an atrial systolic phase (which produces the a wave in the RV tracing).

If measurement of RV end-diastolic pressure is required (for the diagnosis of cardiac tamponade, cardiac restriction, or pericardial constriction), recordings

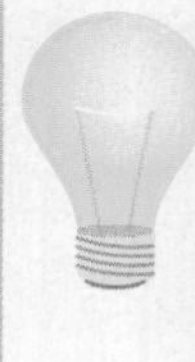

STOP AND THINK

A patient is admitted to the ICU in cardiac failure. The patient has a history of congestive heart failure and pulmonary hypertension. What can be done to determine whether the predominant clinical problem is left heart failure or pulmonary hypertension?

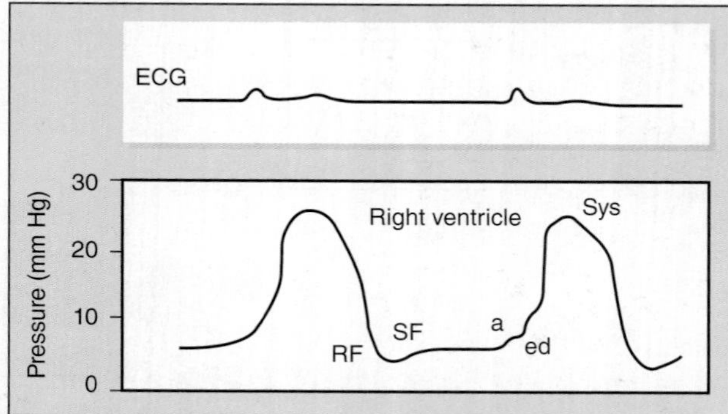

FIGURE 3-9 Right ventricular waveform. RF, rapid filling; SF, slow filling; a, atrial contraction; ed, end-diastole; Sys, systole.
Adapted from Gore JM, et al. *Handbook of Hemodynamic Monitoring*. Little, Brown; 1985.

are made from the distal tip of the catheter during initial catheter insertion. Routine monitoring of RV pressure should be avoided because it is usually not clinically necessary and may induce arrhythmia.

Normal right ventricular systolic pressure varies from 15 to 30 mm Hg, and right ventricular end-diastolic pressure varies from 0 to 8 mm Hg (**Figure 3-9**). An increase in RV systolic pressure is seen in disorders in which there is pulmonary hypertension or in pulmonic valve stenosis. Acute pulmonary embolism can also produce elevations in the RV systolic pressure, although RV systolic pressures rarely exceed 40 to 50 mm Hg in the acute setting. An increase in RV end-diastolic pressure is seen in many forms of cardiomyopathy, as well as in right ventricular ischemia, infarction, and cardiac constriction or tamponade.

The main components of the pulmonary artery (PA) tracing (**Figure 3-10**) are the systolic and diastolic

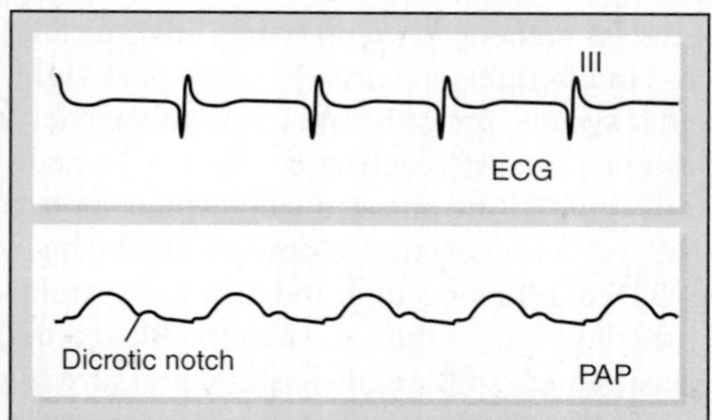

FIGURE 3-10 Pulmonary artery pressure (PAP) waveform.

TABLE 3-4
Conditions Causing Pulmonary Hypertension

Conditions
Left heart failure of any cause
Primary lung disease
Mitral valvular disease
Pulmonary embolism
Hypoxemia with pulmonary vasoconstriction
Idiopathic pulmonary arterial hypertension
Left-to-right shunts

pressures and the dicrotic notch, which represents closure of the pulmonic valve. Normal pulmonary artery systolic pressures vary from 15 to 30 mm Hg, whereas pulmonary artery diastolic pressures vary from 4 to 12 mm Hg. Elevations in PA pressures are seen with volume overload or with a variety of conditions in which pulmonary vascular resistance is elevated (**Table 3-4**).

The pulmonary artery occlusion pressure tracing is obtained by inflating a balloon at the distal tip of the catheter to obstruct forward blood flow through that particular branch of the pulmonary artery. This creates a static column of blood between the catheter tip and the left atrium, allowing the pressure at both ends of the column to equilibrate. The pressure at the distal end of the catheter is then equal to that of the left atrium and is termed the pulmonary artery (or pulmonary capillary) wedge pressure (PAWP). As shown in **Figure 3-11**, the PAWP tracing is similar in general configuration to that seen in the right atrium.

The electrical and mechanical correlation between ECG and PAWP tracings is similar to that seen in the right atrium, but the electromechanical delay is longer because of the time necessary for left atrial mechanical events to be transmitted through the pulmonary vasculature to the distal tip of the catheter. Elevations

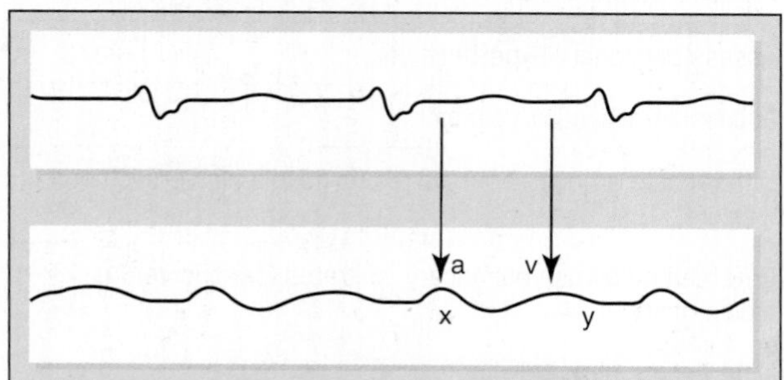

FIGURE 3-11 Pulmonary artery wedge pressure. The a wave reflects contraction in atrial systole, whereas the x descent reflects the fall in left atrial pressure that follows. The c wave, reflecting the closure of the mitral valve, is often not seen. The v wave represents both ventricular systole and passive atrial diastolic filling. The y descent reflects the fall in left atrial pressure following opening of the mitral valve.

TABLE 3-5
Causes of Elevated Pulmonary Artery Wedge Pressure

Left ventricular volume overload
Left ventricular systolic dysfunction
Primary left ventricular diastolic dysfunction
Myocardial ischemia or infarction with decreased left ventricular compliance
Mitral stenosis

in the a wave of the PAWP tracing can be seen with increased resistance to left ventricular filling of any cause (**Table 3-5**). Elevations in the **v wave** of the PAWP tracing represent either mitral regurgitation or an acute volume load to the left atrium. Severe mitral regurgitation is often associated with large v waves in the PAWP tracing, but they are neither sensitive nor specific for this condition. The PAWP generally reflects the left ventricular end-diastolic pressure as long as there is no obstruction to flow between the left atrium and left ventricle. Often the PAWP is used as a surrogate for left ventricular preload (volume status). It is important to note that the PAWP is only a reliable index of left ventricular preload when ventricular compliance is normal or unchanging. Positive pressure ventilation, myocardial ischemia or infarction, cardiac tamponade, and a variety of drugs can profoundly decrease ventricular compliance, thereby interfering with accurate estimation of left ventricular preload via the PAWP.

In patients with pulmonary disease and respiratory failure, the PAWP can exceed the left ventricular end-diastolic pressure secondary to constriction of small veins in hypoxic lung segments, again making the PAWP a poor surrogate for left ventricular preload.

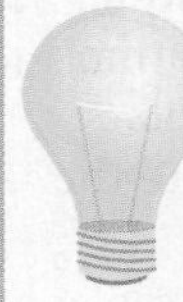

STOP AND THINK

There is a sudden decrease in PAWP with a concomitant increase in CVP. How would you explain this?

Pitfalls in Interpreting Waveforms

The accuracy of the PAWP is dependent on a continuous fluid column between the left atrium and the distal catheter tip. If the pressure in the surrounding alveoli exceeds capillary pressures and compresses the capillaries, the pressure at the catheter tip will reflect alveolar pressure and not left atrial pressure. This concept (**Figure 3-12**) has been used to divide the lungs into three physiologic zones of blood flow, which are based on the relationship between alveolar pressure, mean pulmonary artery pressure, and pulmonary capillary pressure.

The PAWP is an accurate estimate of left atrial pressure only when the pulmonary capillary pressure exceeds the mean alveolar pressure (zone 3). This zone is located in the most dependent portion of the lung, where vascular pressures are the highest (due to gravity). Indicators of non–zone-3 catheter site placement include abnormal position on lateral chest radiographs, marked respiratory variation in the PAWP tracing, and increases in PAWP of more than 50% of the amount of PEEP applied.

During normal spontaneous breathing, alveolar pressure (relative to atmospheric pressure) decreases during inspiration and increases during expiration. Alveolar pressure increases during inhalation and decreases during exhalation with positive pressure ventilation. The changes in alveolar pressure are transmitted to the cardiac structures and are reflected by changes in central venous, pulmonary artery, and PAWP measurements

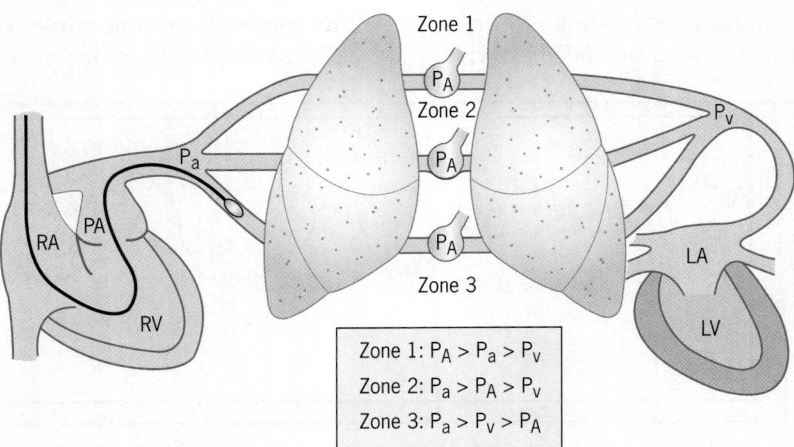

FIGURE 3-12 West zones of the lungs, determined by the relationship between alveolar pressure and pulmonary vascular pressures. RA, right atrium; RV, right ventricle; PA, pulmonary artery; Pa, pulmonary arterial pressure; PA, alveolar pressure; Pv, pulmonary venous pressure; LA, left atrium; LV, left ventricle.

during inspiration and expiration. At end-expiration, pleural and intrathoracic pressures are equal to atmospheric pressures, regardless of the mode of ventilation. The true transmural pressure—and therefore the PAWP—should be measured at end-expiration.

Alveolar pressure will not return to atmospheric pressure at end-expiration in the presence of positive end-expiratory pressure, a change that can affect the measurement of intravascular pressures. PEEP can be applied therapeutically or may result from incomplete expiration of alveolar gas leading to air trapping (auto-PEEP). The effects of either form of PEEP on the PAWP are variable and depend largely on the compliance of the lungs and the chest wall. The effects of PEEP are generally believed not to be important, with notable exceptions. One exception may be in the situation in which the catheter is not in zone 3. By definition, in zone 3 no airway pressure should be transmitted to the vasculature. If the respiratory variation seen in the PAWP tracing exceeds that seen in the pulmonary artery tracing, then the PAWP may be unreliable due to non–zone-3 conditions (**Figure 3-13**).

Even though there may be a small effect of PEEP on intravascular pressure measurements, it is not advisable to eliminate (turn off) PEEP temporarily while pressure measurements are being made, because this may induce hemodynamic instability due to changes in venous return or may cause alveolar de-recruitment with subsequent severe hypoxemia. The effect of PEEP on vascular pressures in the thorax is determined by the relationship between lung compliance and chest wall compliance:[15]

$$\Delta Ppl/\Delta Paw = C_L/(C_L + Ccw)$$

where Ppl is pleural pressure, Paw is airway pressure, C_L is lung compliance, and Ccw is chest wall compliance. A general estimate of the true transmural filling pressures can be made in the presence of PEEP by subtracting one-half of the PEEP from the PAWP if lung and chest wall compliance are normal, 25% of the PEEP if lung compliance is reduced and chest wall compliance is normal, and 75% of the PEEP if chest wall compliance is reduced and lung compliance is normal. The effects of PEEP on PAWP are usually small and rarely affect clinical management.

Cardiac Output Measurement

In addition to providing pressure measurements, the pulmonary artery catheter facilitates measurement of cardiac output via the **Fick equation**:

$$\dot{Q}c = \dot{V}O_2/(CaO_2 - C\bar{v}O_2)$$

where $\dot{Q}c$ is cardiac output, CaO_2 is arterial O_2 content (1.34 × Hb × SaO_2), and $C\bar{v}O_2$ is mixed venous O_2 content (1.34 × Hb × $S\bar{v}O_2$). If arterial blood gases, mixed venous blood gases, and oxygen consumption are measured, cardiac output can be calculated. Mixed venous blood gas samples are obtained from the distal port of the pulmonary artery catheter, and oxygen consumption is measured by indirect calorimetry.

The indicator dilution principle states that when an indicator substance is added to a stream of flowing blood, the flow will be inversely proportional to the mean concentration of the indicator at a downstream site. In the case of a PA catheter, the indicator used is a known volume of saline that is colder than blood. The indicator is injected as a bolus through the proximal port of the pulmonary artery catheter and mixes with blood in the right ventricle. This lowers the temperature of intraventricular blood that flows past the distal temperature sensor. The temperature sensor records the temperature change over time, and the monitor electronically displays a temperature–time curve. The area under this curve is inversely proportional to the flow in the pulmonary artery. This flow should be equal to cardiac output in the absence of intracardiac shunt.

There are several important sources of error in the thermodilution method. Tricuspid regurgitation leads to an attenuated peak and a prolonged washout phase of the temperature–time curve. This is due to cold injectate refluxing into the vena cava, with resultant

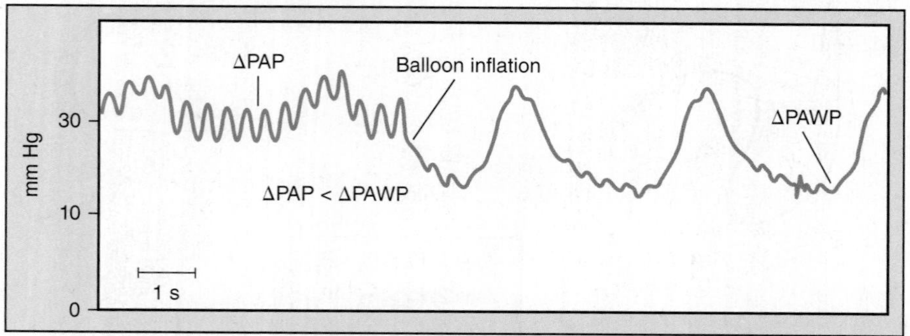

FIGURE 3-13 Pressure trace recorded during positive pressure mechanical ventilation from a pulmonary artery catheter located in West lung zone 1. Pressure swings in the pulmonary artery occlusion pressure (ΔPAWP) reflect changes in airway pressure and are significantly higher than swings in pulmonary artery pressure (ΔPa), which result from changes in pleural pressure.

Modified with permission from Longnecker D, Brown D, Newman M, Zapol W. *Anesthesiology*. New York: McGraw-Hill; 2008. © The McGraw-Hill Companies, Inc.

decreased pulmonary artery cooling (lowered peak) and delayed appearance of injectate that has moved retrograde into the vena cava and is then recirculated (prolonged washout). The net effect is an underestimation of cardiac output. Both right-to-left and left-to-right intracardiac shunts can produce falsely elevated cardiac output measurements by the thermodilution technique. Right-to-left intracardiac shunts produce shunting of cold injectate into the left heart, which reduces pulmonary artery cooling, lowers the peak of the temperature–time curve, and overestimates cardiac output. Left-to-right shunting results in increased right heart volumes and dilution of the injectate, thereby attenuating the height of the temperature–time curve and resulting in an overestimation of cardiac output.

The continuous thermodilution cardiac output catheter is equipped with a 10-cm thermal filament located about 20 cm from the catheter tip. The filament is intermittently warmed to about 44° C. The change in blood temperature is detected at the catheter tip and used to generate a thermodilution curve to determine cardiac output. Although the output is called continuous cardiac output, the measurement is an average cardiac output that is updated every 30 seconds and averaged over 3 to 6 minutes.

Continuous Oximetric Monitoring

Some pulmonary artery catheter designs incorporate continuous oximetric monitoring of pulmonary artery oxygen saturation using fiberoptic reflectance spectrophotometry. These devices employ reflectance spectrophotometry. Light is transmitted through a fiberoptic bundle, reflected from the blood, and the amount of light absorbed by hemoglobin is determined. Oxygen saturation is then determined based on the differential absorption of light by oxyhemoglobin and deoxyhemoglobin. This technology has reasonable correlation with measured mixed venous oxygen saturation determined using co-oximetry but is prone to drift.

The mixed venous oxygen level provides a global indication of the level of tissue oxygenation. Normal $P\bar{v}O_2$ is 35 to 45 mm Hg, and normal $S\bar{v}O_2$ is 65% to 75%. Factors affecting mixed venous oxygen level can be illustrated by the following equation, which is a rearrangement of the Fick equation:

$$S\bar{v}O_2 = SaO_2 - \dot{V}O_2/(\dot{Q}c \times Hb \times 1.34)$$

Note that a decrease in cardiac output results in a decreased $S\bar{v}O_2$. The primary interest in continuous monitoring of $S\bar{v}O_2$ is to detect changes in cardiac output. $P\bar{v}O_2$ and $S\bar{v}O_2$ can be increased with peripheral shunting (e.g., sepsis) and decreased oxygen uptake (e.g., cyanide poisoning).

Other less commonly used applications of pulmonary artery catheters include measurement of right ventricular ejection fraction and extravascular lung water measurements. Pulmonary artery catheters are also available for cardiac pacing.

Vascular Resistance

In addition to calculating cardiac output, the PA catheter facilitates estimation of **systemic vascular resistance (SVR)** and **pulmonary vascular resistance (PVR)**:

$$SVR = (MAP - CVP)/\dot{Q}c$$
$$PVR = (Mean\ PAP - PAWP)/\dot{Q}c$$

Normal SVR is 900 to 1400 dyne $\times$ s $\times$ cm^{-5}, and normal PVR is 150 to 250 dyne $\times$ s $\times$ cm^{-5}. **Wood units** are a simplified system for measuring pulmonary vascular resistance that uses pressure in mm Hg and cardiac output in L/min. To convert to dyne $\times$ s $\times$ cm^{-5}, multiply by 80. These calculations are derived from Ohm's law, which states that resistance in a circuit is equal to the pressure drop across the circuit divided by flow. Vascular resistance is calculated on the basis of both direct and indirect measurements, all with intrinsic sources of error; therefore, of all the hemodynamic information obtained from the pulmonary artery catheter, vascular resistance values are the least accurate and the most sensitive to inaccuracies in data acquisition.

Clinical Use of Hemodynamic Measurements

Hemodynamic monitoring allows differentiation of shock states, determination of intravascular volume status and cardiac performance, and monitoring of interventions such as volume challenges, diuresis, and the infusion of vasoactive agents. Certain cardiopulmonary disorders are associated with characteristic hemodynamic profiles (**Table 3-6**).

Use of PA catheters in the ICU has fallen out of favor in recent years. A randomized controlled trial in patients with acute lung injury reported that PA catheter–guided therapy did not improve survival or organ function and was associated with more complications than CVP-guided therapy.[16] The PA catheter is no longer used commonly for fluid management. Its use is reserved for assessment of left heart failure, pulmonary hypertension, and cardiac output measurement.

Early goal-directed therapy is used in the management of sepsis.[17,18] This protocol (**Figure 3-14**) addresses CVP, arterial blood pressure, and $ScvO_2$ in a systematic manner.

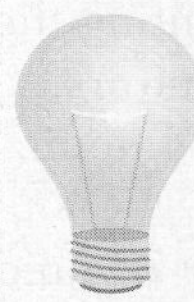

STOP AND THINK

A patient with severe sepsis has a $ScvO_2$ of 55%. What does this indicate and what would be the best clinical approach?

TABLE 3-6
Characteristic Hemodynamic Profiles of Certain Cardiopulmonary Disorders

Condition	CVP/RA	PAP	PAWP	CO	SVR	PVR	BP
Hypovolemic shock	↓	↓	↓	↓	↑	Normal	↓
Cardiogenic shock	↑	↑	↑	↓	↑	Normal	↓
Septic shock	Normal or ↓	Normal or ↓	Normal or ↓	Normal or ↑	↓	Normal or ↓	↓
Pulmonary embolism	↑	↑	Normal or ↓	Normal or ↓	↑	↑	Normal or ↓

CVP/RA, central venous and right atrial pressures; PAP, pulmonary artery pressure; PAWP, pulmonary artery wedge pressure; CO, cardiac output; SVR, systemic vascular resistance; PVR, pulmonary vascular resistance; BP, systemic arterial blood pressure.

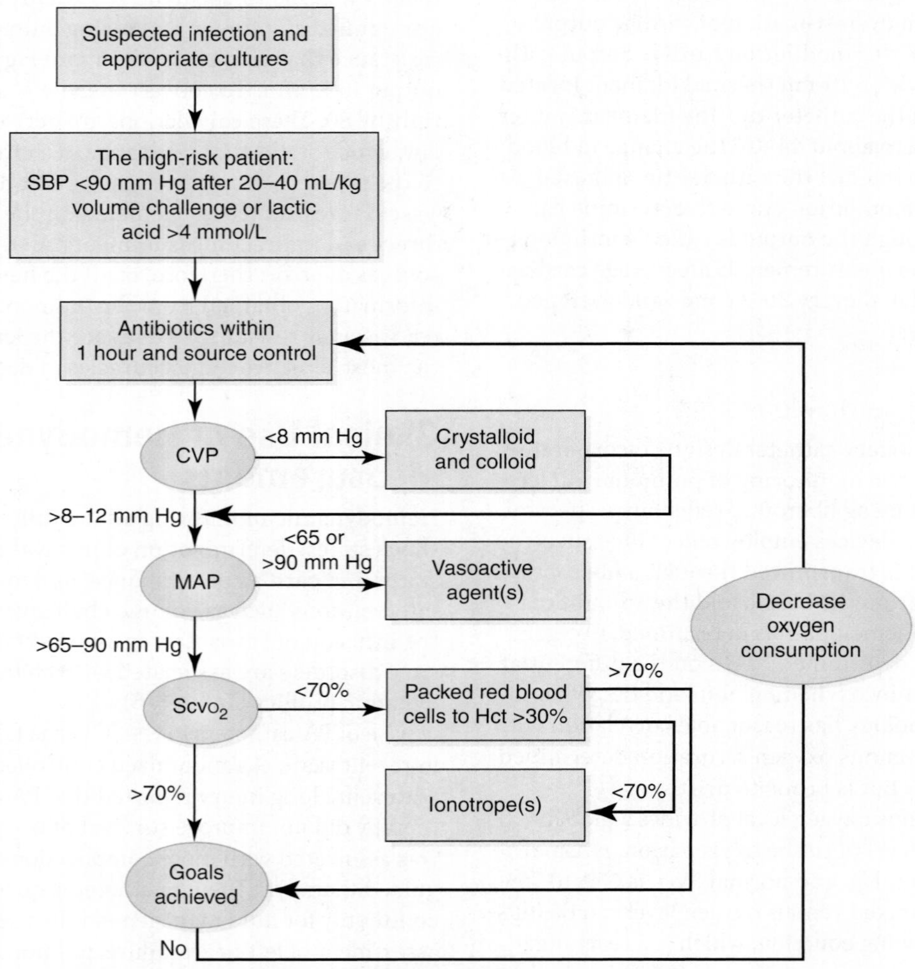

FIGURE 3-14 Algorithm for early management of the septic patient.

Adapted from Rivers EP, et al. Early goal-directed therapy in severe sepsis and septic shock: a contemporary review of the literature. *Curr Opin Anesthesiol.* 2008;21:128–140.

Key Points

- The heart rate can be measured by counting the peripheral pulse or by using bedside monitors.
- Arterial blood pressure can be measured noninvasively or invasively.
- Pulse pressure variation is an indicator of fluid responsiveness.
- Central venous pressure can guide fluid and blood volume replacement.
- The pulmonary artery catheter is used to measure the pulmonary artery pressure, wedge pressure, cardiac output, and mixed venous oxygen saturation.
- Techniques to measure cardiac output include thermodilution, the Fick method, and pulse contour analysis.

References

1. Reeves RA. Does this patient have hypertension? How to measure blood pressure. *JAMA.* 1995;273:1211–1218.
2. Smulyan H, Safar ME. Blood pressure measurement: retrospective and prospective views. *Am J Hypertens.* 2011;24:628–634.
3. Michard F, Teboul JL. Using heart-lung interactions to assess fluid responsiveness during mechanical ventilation. *Crit Care.* 2000;4:282–289.
4. Michard F. Changes in arterial pressure during mechanical ventilation. *Anesthesiology.* 2005;103:419–428.
5. Bendjelid K, Romand JA. Fluid responsiveness in mechanically ventilated patients: a review of indices used in intensive care. *Intensive Care Med.* 2003;29:352–360.
6. Huang CC, Fu JY, Hu HC, et al. Prediction of fluid responsiveness in acute respiratory distress syndrome patients ventilated with low tidal volume and high positive end-expiratory pressure. *Crit Care Med.* 2008;36:2810–2816.
7. Morgan P, Al-Subaie N, Rhodes A. Minimally invasive cardiac output monitoring. *Curr Opin Crit Care.* 2008;14:322–326.
8. de Waal EE, Wappler F, Buhre WF. Cardiac output monitoring. *Curr Opin Anaesthesiol.* 2009;22:71–77.
9. Rajaram SS, Desai NK, Kalra A, et al. Pulmonary artery catheters for adult patients in intensive care. *Cochrane Database Syst Rev.* 2013;2:CD003408.
10. Hadian M, Kim HK, Severyn DA, Pinsky MR. Cross-comparison of cardiac output trending accuracy of LiDCO, PiCCO, FloTrac and pulmonary artery catheters. *Crit Care.* 2010;14:R212.
11. Critchley LA. Pulse contour analysis: is it able to reliably detect changes in cardiac output in the haemodynamically unstable patient? *Crit Care.* 2011;15:106.
12. Summerhill EM, Baram M. Principles of pulmonary artery catheterization in the critically ill. *Lung.* 2005;183:209.
13. Pinsky MR. Pulmonary artery occlusion pressure. *Intensive Care Med.* 2003;29:19–22.
14. Pinsky MR. Clinical significance of pulmonary artery occlusion pressure. *Intensive Care Med.* 2003;29:175–178.
15. Hess DR, Bigatello LM. The chest wall in acute lung injury/acute respiratory distress syndrome. *Curr Opin Crit Care.* 2008;14:94–102.
16. Wheeler AP, Bernard GR, Thompson BT, et al. Pulmonary-artery versus central venous catheter to guide treatment of acute lung injury. *N Engl J Med.* 2006;354:2213–2224.
17. Rivers E, Nguyen B, Havstad S, et al. Early goal-directed therapy in the treatment of severe sepsis and septic shock. *N Engl J Med.* 2001;345:1368–1377.
18. Rivers EP, Coba V, Whitmill M. Early goal-directed therapy in severe sepsis and septic shock: a contemporary review of the literature. *Curr Opin Anaesthesiol.* 2008;21:128–140.

CHAPTER

4

Arterial Blood Gas Sampling, Analysis, and Interpretation

Shelley C. Mishoe

OUTLINE

Blood Gas Analyzers
Blood Gas Sampling
Quality Control and Proficiency Testing
Physiology of Acid–Base Balance
Acid–Base Disorders
Arterial Blood Gas Interpretation

OBJECTIVES

1. Compare methods to measure Po_2, Pco_2, pH, and oxygen saturation.
2. Describe the technique used to obtain blood samples by arterial puncture and by arterial cannulation.
3. Describe preanalytic errors in blood gas analysis.
4. Discuss issues related to temperature correction of blood gases.
5. Describe methods of quality control and proficiency testing of blood gases.
6. Discuss the physiology of acid–base balance.
7. Compare and contrast the use of the anion gap, strong ion difference, and strong ion gap in the assessment of acid–base disorders.
8. Explain why clinical assessment is an essential first step for an acid–base diagnosis.
9. Describe how pH, Pco_2, and HCO_3^- are used to interpret an arterial blood gas as normal, simple, mixed, or compensated acid–base disorder.
10. Describe how the Pao_2 and Sao_2 should be evaluated as normal, hypoxemia, or hyperoxemia.
11. Apply a seven-step process to interpret arterial blood gases.
12. Describe common medical conditions that cause acid–base disorders.

KEY TERMS

acidosis
alkalosis
Allen test
alpha-stat hypothesis
anion
anion gap (AG)
anticoagulant
arterial blood gas (ABG)
bicarbonate buffer system
buffer
cannulation
capillary blood gas
carbonic acid
Clark electrode
Clinical Laboratory Improvement Amendment (CLIA)
Henderson-Hasselbalch equation
hyperoxia
hypoventilation
hypoxemia
hypoxia
metabolic acidosis
metabolic alkalosis
oximeter
oxyhemoglobin
$Paco_2$
Pao_2
pH
point-of-care testing (POCT)
respiratory acidosis
respiratory alkalosis
Sanz electrode
Severinghaus electrode
strong ion difference (SID)
tonometry

Introduction

The analysis of **arterial blood gases (ABGs)** is an important tool in clinical practice. The primary measurements (Po_2, Pco_2, pH, and HCO_3^-) provide important information about oxygenation, ventilation, and acid–base balance. ABGs also guide respiratory and metabolic interventions in critically ill patients. This chapter discusses arterial blood gas sampling, measuring, and interpreting of arterial blood gas data.

Blood Gas Analyzers

Blood gas analyzers use electrodes to measure the partial pressure of oxygen, the partial pressure of carbon dioxide, and the acidity (pH) of the blood. Blood gas analyzers also calculate oxygen saturation (Sao_2) and bicarbonate (HCO_3^-). Some blood gas analyzers incorporate an oximeter to measure Sao_2. ABG analysis evaluates how effectively the lungs are delivering oxygen to the blood and eliminating carbon dioxide. It also indicates how well the lungs and kidneys are interacting to maintain normal blood pH (acid–base balance). Blood gas studies are usually done to assess respiratory disease and other conditions that may affect the lungs. ABGs provide important information to properly manage patients receiving oxygen therapy, anesthesia, mechanical ventilation, and other respiratory therapies.

pH Electrode

The modern pH electrode is sometimes called the **Sanz electrode**. It is based on the linear relationship between the potential differences and pH variations across a pH-sensitive glass membrane. **Figure 4-1** shows the basic design of the modern pH electrode, which consists of two chemical half-cells separated by a pH-sensitive glass membrane. One half-cell has a reference electrode, usually made of mercury-mercurous chloride (calomel), and the other has a measuring electrode, usually composed of silver-silver chloride. The mercury-mercurous chloride of the reference electrode provides a constant reference voltage at a constant temperature. The silver-silver chloride measuring electrode detects the voltage difference across the glass membrane produced by two solutions with different pH levels. The measuring half-cell is embedded within a chamber containing a buffer with a pH of 6.840, which is encased in a constant-temperature water bath. The measuring half-cell is connected to the reference half-cell by a potassium chloride (KCl) contact bridge, which completes the electronic circuit. To prevent contamination, the KCl solution is separated from the unknown blood in the sampling chamber by a membrane.

The pH electrode has a small sampling chamber that can measure blood volume samples as small as 25 μL. The pH electrode incorporates a two-point calibration for accurate measurement of each blood sample. Calibration involves a two-point measure of two buffer solutions. It includes a balance potentiometer set to display 6.840 when the 6.840 buffer solution is placed in the measuring half-cell as well as a slope potentiometer set to display 7.384 when the measuring half-cell is filled with 7.384 buffer solution. Because the potential difference is a linear function of the pH, a two-point calibration, with the pH values of 6.840 and 7.384, is sufficient for accurate blood pH measurement.

Pco_2 Electrode

The principle of Pco_2 measurement is that changes of pH across a semipermeable membrane are proportional to the diffusion of Pco_2 in contact with the membrane. When CO_2 in the blood sample diffuses across the permeable membrane, it undergoes the following reaction:

$$CO_2 + H_2O \rightarrow H_2CO_3 \rightarrow H^+ + HCO_3^-$$

This equation shows that when CO_2 combines with water it produces **carbonic acid**, which results in free hydrogen ion (H^+). The Pco_2 electrode actually

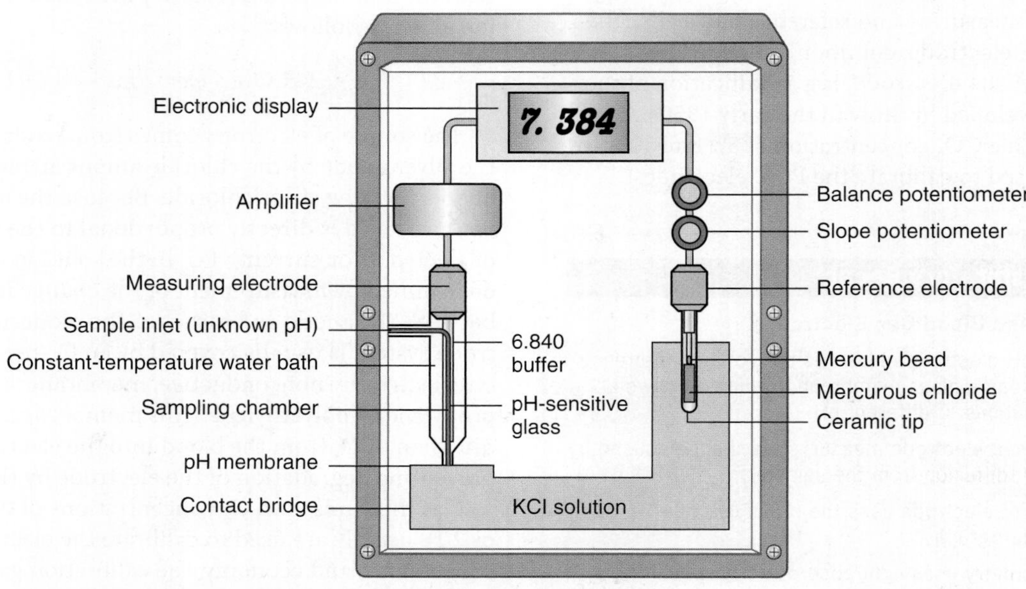

FIGURE 4-1 Schematic illustration of the modern pH electrode.
Adapted from Shapiro BA. *Clinical Application of Blood Gases*. 4th ed. St. Louis: Mosby; 1989.

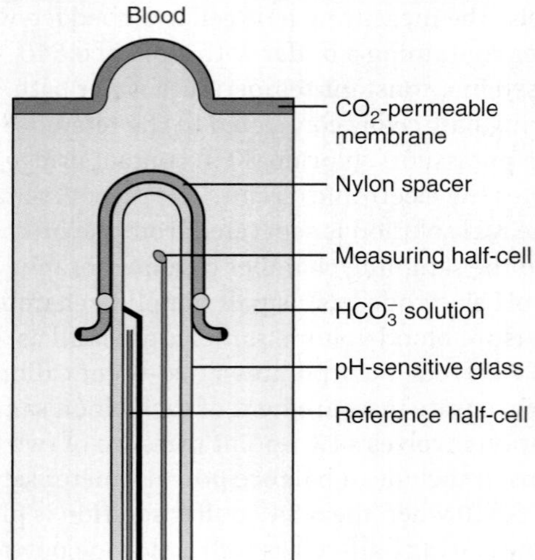

FIGURE 4-2 Schematic illustration of the modern Pco_2 electrode.

measures the acid in the form of the hydrogen ion, produced by CO_2. The basic design of the Pco_2 electrode consists of a CO_2-permeable, but H^+-impermeable, membrane that separates the blood sample from the measuring half-cell (**Figure 4-2**). The measuring half-cell contains a dilute electrolyte solution (sodium bicarbonate and sodium or potassium chloride). Because H^+ concentration is directly proportional to CO_2 in contact with the membrane, pH measured by a pH electrode can be used as an indirect measure of Pco_2.

The design of the Pco_2 electrode is slightly different from the pH electrode in that the pH-sensitive glass electrode is separated from the permeable membrane by nylon mesh or other spacers that allow bicarbonate solution to exist between the glass and membrane. The measuring and reference half-cells are silver-silver chloride. The entire pH electrode is bathed in electrolyte solution, which serves as the electronic bridge between the measuring and reference half-cells. The modern Pco_2 electrode, commonly referred to as the **Severinghaus electrode**, is a modification of the electrode developed by Stow in the early 1950s. Gas mixtures with a CO_2 concentration of 5% and 10% are commonly used to calibrate the Pco_2 electrode.

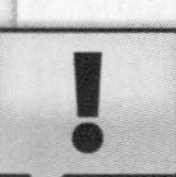

Respiratory Recap

pH and Blood Gas Electrodes

- A pH electrode measures the voltage difference across a glass membrane produced by two solutions of different pH.
- A Pco_2 electrode measures pH change caused by CO_2 diffusion from the sample.
- A Po_2 electrode uses the principles of polarography.
- Oximetry uses light absorption at specific wavelengths.

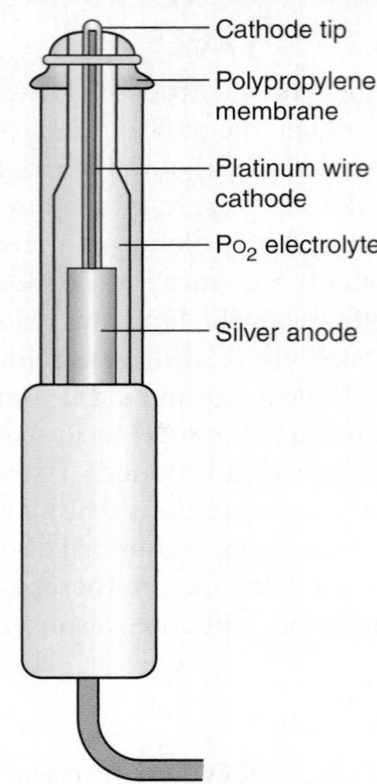

FIGURE 4-3 Schematic illustration of the Po_2 electrode.

Adapted from Shapiro BA. *Clinical Application of Blood Gases*. 4th ed. St. Louis: Mosby; 1989.

Po_2 Electrode

The Po_2 electrode, or **Clark electrode**, measures Po_2 with the principle of polarography. The Clark electrode consists of a platinum cathode and silver anode immersed in a dilute, buffered potassium chloride solution (**Figure 4-3**). The cathode is the negative electrode and the anode is the positive electrode. The electric current produced by the cathode in solution is directly proportional to the availability of O_2 molecules at the cathode tip. When the O_2 molecules come in contact with the platinum cathode, they are reduced to hydroxide **anion**, as follows:

$$O_2 + 2\,H_2O + 4 \text{ electrons} \rightarrow 4\,OH^-$$

The source of electrons comes from oxidation of the silver anode by the chloride anions attracted to the anode, forming silver chloride. Because the amount of O_2 reduced is directly proportional to the number of electrons (or current), Po_2 in the solution can be determined by measurement of the change in current between the anode and cathode. The modern Po_2 electrode system is usually covered by an O_2-permeable, but electrically nonconductive, membrane such as polypropylene or polyethylene. This membrane allows slow diffusion of O_2 from the blood into the electrode while preventing degradation of the electrode by the blood.

Gas mixtures with O_2 concentrations of 0% and 12% or 20% usually are used to calibrate the electrode. For convenience and economy, the calibration gases for the Po_2 and Pco_2 electrodes usually are combined, with one gas composed of 5% CO_2 and 12% or 20% O_2 balanced

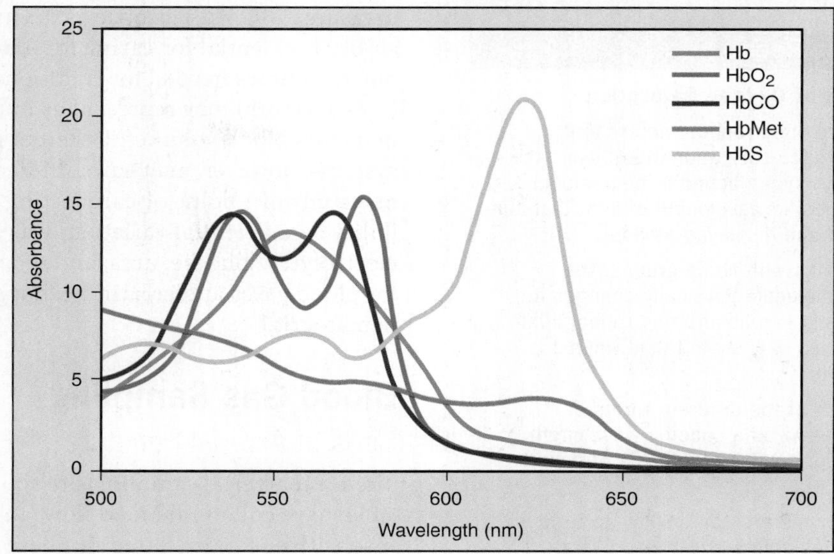

FIGURE 4-4 Absorption spectra for different types of hemoglobin molecules.
Adapted from *Radiometer Medical. Blood Gas, Oximetry, and Electrolyte Systems Reference Manual.* Radiometer Medical; 1996.

with nitrogen and a second gas containing 10% CO_2 and 90% nitrogen. The Po_2 electrode also responds to halothane, resulting in inaccurate Po_2 measurements in blood drawn from patients anesthetized with this drug.

Oximeter

Hemoglobin oxygen content in the blood can be measured by an **oximeter**, which is a spectrophotometer that uses specific wavelengths in the oxyhemoglobin spectrum. As oxygen binds with heme groups, the hemoglobin molecule physically changes its shape, causing it to absorb and reflect light differently when oxygenated than when it is deoxygenated. This phenomenon is responsible for the bright red color of arterial blood that is oxygenated and the bluish-purple color of venous blood that is deoxygenated. Because each of the different forms of hemoglobin absorbs a specific wavelength of light, this principle is the basis of oximeters. The concentration of the molecule in the solution can be determined by the amount of light absorbed by the solution. Based on this principle, the oximeter can display Sao_2 as a percentage of the amount of oxygen bound to hemoglobin (**oxyhemoglobin**) to the total amount of hemoglobin. Modern oximeters measure more than just oxyhemoglobin. The CO-oximeter generates multiple spectra (usually four) that allow distinction among four major hemoglobin species: oxyhemoglobin, deoxyhemoglobin, carboxyhemoglobin, and methemoglobin (**Figure 4-4**).

Point-of-Care Arterial Systems

An ABG can also be measured by a portable analyzer (**Figure 4-5**), which allows testing at the bedside. This is known as **point-of-care testing (POCT)**. These units also offer the ability to measure electrolytes, glucose, and hematocrit. Most use single-use disposable cartridges that contain many of the same devices typically found in traditional laboratory analyzers. The sensors are micro-fabricated thin-film electrodes.

The major advantages of POCT systems are their small sampling volumes and more rapid therapeutic turnaround time of blood gas results, which allows faster and better decision making.[1–3] Some systems can

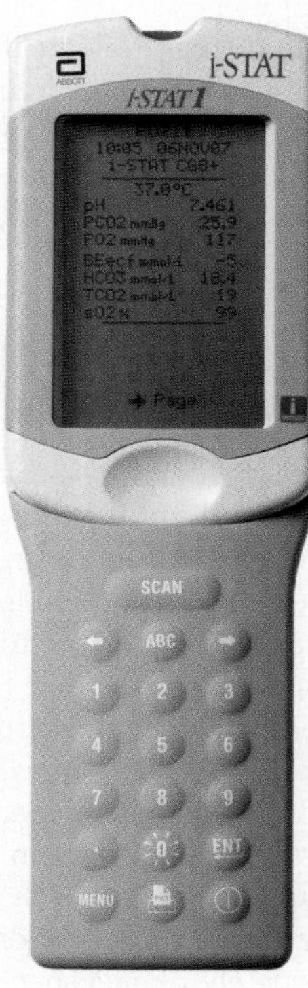

FIGURE 4-5 Point-of-care testing device.
Courtesy of Abbott, Point of Care.

Respiratory Recap

Measurement of Oxygen Saturation

- Oximeters are spectrophotometers that determine oxygen saturation (Sa_{O_2}) using the principle that oxygen bound to hemoglobin absorbs a specific wavelength of light that can be measured and displayed as Sa_{O_2}.
- As oxygen binds with heme groups, the hemoglobin molecule physically changes its shape, causing it to absorb and reflect light differently when oxygenated than when it is deoxygenated.
- Because each of the different forms of hemoglobin absorbs a specific wavelength of light, this principle is the basis of how oximeters work.
- Modern CO-oximeters can display up to four types of hemoglobin showing each as a percentage of the total hemoglobin.
- ABG analyzers report a calculated Sa_{O_2} or incorporate oximetry for direct measurement.

measure ABG with as little as 0.5 mL of blood. This ability is essential for caring for neonates because the blood volumes needed for traditional ABG analyzers (2.7 to 3.0 mL) may represent as much as 10% of the neonate's blood volumes. Different portable blood gas systems, however, may have different accuracies. In one study of a point-of-care testing system, reproducibility (coefficient of variation) was good (<2%) for electrolytes, glucose, urea, and pH; satisfactory (<6.5%) for blood gases and creatinine; but poor (21%) for hematocrit.[4]

Blood Gas Sampling

Sites of Arterial Puncture

The ideal arterial sampling site should be easily accessible, have collateral blood flow, and be relatively insensitive to pain. Based on these criteria, the radial artery is the preferred site for arterial puncture and cannulation for adult patients (**CPG 4-1**). The brachial artery is a good alternative if the radial arteries are unavailable. Femoral artery punctures should be used only if absolutely necessary because the artery

CLINICAL PRACTICE GUIDELINE 4-1

Blood Gas Analysis and Hemoximetry

Indications

- The need to further evaluate the adequacy of a patient's ventilatory (Pa_{CO_2}), acid–base (pH), oxygenation (P_{O_2} and S_{O_2}) status, oxygen-carrying capacity (S_{O_2} and dyshemoglobin saturations), and intrapulmonary shunt
- The need to quantify the response to therapeutic intervention (e.g., supplemental oxygen administration, mechanical ventilation) or diagnostic evaluations (e.g., exercise desaturation)
- The need to assess early goal-directed therapy measuring Scv_{O_2} in patients with sepsis or septic shock and after major surgery
- The need to monitor severity and progression of documented disease processes
- The need to assess inadequacy of circulatory response

Contraindications

- An improperly functioning blood gas analyzer
- A blood gas analyzer that has not had functional status validated
- A specimen that has not been properly anticoagulated
- A specimen containing visible air bubbles
- A specimen that has been stored at room temperature for longer than 30 minutes in a plastic vessel, stored at room temperature for longer than 5 minutes for a shunt study, or stored at room temperature in the presence of an elevated leukocyte or platelet count. In the case of samples that must be kept for longer than 30 minutes, they should be drawn and stored in a glass vessel and chilled to 0–4° C. P_{O_2} in samples drawn from subjects with very high leukocyte counts can decrease rapidly, so immediate cooling and analysis are necessary in this patient population.
- An incomplete requisition that precludes adequate interpretation and documentation of results and for which attempts to obtain additional information has been unsuccessful
- An inadequately labeled specimen lacking the patient's full name and other unique identifier (e.g., medical record number), date, and time of sampling

Hazards and Complications

- Infection of specimen handler from blood carrying the human immunodeficiency virus (HIV), hepatitis C, other bloodborne pathogens
- Inappropriate patient medical treatments based on improperly analyzed blood specimen or from analysis of an unacceptable specimen or from incorrect reporting of results
- In the case of samples received from a contaminated (isolation) room, cross contamination of areas of the hospital or handlers of the sample
- Improperly identified patient

Limitations

- Erroneous results can arise from sample clotting due to improper anticoagulation or improper mixing; sample contamination by air, improper **anticoagulant** and/or improper anticoagulant concentration, saline or other fluids (specimen obtained via an indwelling catheter), inadvertent sampling of venous blood if attempting to obtain an ABG.
- Deterioration or distortion of variables to be measured resulting from delay in sample analysis; inappropriate collection and handling (accurate total hemoglobin concentration).
- Measurement depends on homogeneous mixture of specimen, appropriate anticoagulant concentration and specimen-size ratio, and absence of contamination of specimen by analyzer solutions or calibration gases. The concentration measured may also be dependent on the method incorporated by the specific analyzer; incomplete clearance of analyzer calibration gases and previous waste or flushing solution(s); the presence of hyperlipidemia, methylene blue, and/or hydroxocobalamin, which causes problems with analyzer membranes and may affect CO-oximetry.
- Inappropriate sample size for the type of anticoagulant and/or the sample requirements of the analyzer(s). Attempts should be made to keep sample sizes as small as is technically feasible to limit blood loss, particularly in neonates.
- The presence of dyshemoglobins. Some calculated values may be in error (e.g., calculated Sa_{O_2} may overestimate oxyhemoglobin in the presence of carboxyhemoglobin or methemoglobin, and with changes in 2,3-DPG concentration).
- The presence of excess fetal hemoglobin, as blood gas analyzers assume hemoglobin to be of the adult type (default); therefore, calculated blood gas oxygen saturation values are underestimated in this instance.
- Inappropriate sample site for the analyte being assessed. Arterialized capillary samples and central venous samples may be adequate to assess pH and P_{CO_2}, but not P_{O_2}.
- Hemodynamically stable patients, but may underestimate patient oxygenation.
- Temperature-related errors. The laboratory must have a defined procedure for temperature correction of the measured results. Errors in the measurement of the patient's temperature may cause erroneous temperature-corrected results. If temperature-adjusted results are reported, the report should be clearly labeled as such, and the measured results at 37° C must also be reported. It should be noted that there are no data currently available that can quantify the balance between oxygen delivery and oxygen demand at temperatures other than 37° C. Therefore, temperature correction of blood gas samples is not recommended.
- Hemodilution or altered osmolality when measuring hematocrit using conductometry sensor technology.
- High-speed transport tube systems may produce erroneous P_{O_2} results. Specifically, samples with a P_{O_2} above that of ambient air may be underestimated and those with a P_{O_2} below that of ambient air may be overestimated.
- Results of analysis can be considered valid if analytic procedure conforms to recommended, established guidelines and follows manufacturer's recommendations; results of pH–blood gas analysis fall within the calibration range of the analyzer(s) and quality control product ranges. If a result outside of the usual calibration range is obtained (e.g., P_{O_2} measured as 250 mm Hg, but analyzer calibrated to 140 mm Hg), refer to the manufacturer instructions for the particular machine in use.
- If questionable results are obtained and are consistent with specimen contamination: the labeling of the blood sample container should be rechecked for patient's full name, medical record number or date of birth (patient identifier), date and time of acquisition, and measured F_{IO_2} (or supplemental oxygen liter flow); the residual specimen should be reanalyzed (preferably on a separate analyzer), assuming sufficient sample remains; an additional sample should be obtained if the discrepancy cannot be resolved; results of analysis of discarded samples should be logged with reason for discarding.

(continues)

Clinical Practice Guideline 4-1 *(continued)*

- $Scvo_2$ may not reliably predict (overestimate) $S\bar{v}o_2$ in patients with severe sepsis in early goal-directed therapy.
- Venous blood gas values should be interpreted as interchangeable with ABG *only* in very specific clinical conditions. Available evidence suggests that there is good agreement for pH and HCO_3^- values between arterial and venous blood gas results obtained from a peripheral vein in patients with COPD, but not for Po_2 or Pco_2. Venous blood gas pH and Pco_2 levels have relatively good correlation with ABG values but cannot be substituted for ABG in exacerbation of COPD or in the setting of acute trauma. While a venous blood gas may be used instead of ABG to determine pH, Pco_2, and HCO_3^- in some diseases such as respiratory distress syndrome, neonatal sepsis, renal failure, pneumonia, diabetic ketoacidosis, and status epilepticus, it should not be used as a substitute in other diseases such as neonatal seizure, shock, congestive heart failure, and congenital heart diseases. The presence of a high central venous–arterial Pco_2 gradient helps identify inadequacy of circulatory response as the one present in severe hemorrhagic shock, in poor cardiac output, during cardiopulmonary resuscitation, and after cardiopulmonary bypass.

Recommendations

1. Blood gas analysis and hemoximetry are recommended for evaluating a patient's ventilatory, acid–base, and/or oxygenation status.
2. Blood gas analysis and hemoximetry are suggested for evaluating a patient's response to therapeutic interventions.
3. Blood gas analysis and hemoximetry are recommended for monitoring severity and progression of documented cardiopulmonary disease processes.
4. Hemoximetry is recommended to determine the impact of dyshemoglobins on oxygenation.
5. Capillary blood gas analysis is not recommended to determine oxygenation status.
6. Central venous blood gas analysis and hemoximetry are suggested to determine oxygen consumption in the setting of early goal-directed therapy.
7. For the assessment of oxygenation, a peripheral venous Po_2 is not recommended as a substitute for an arterial Pao_2.
8. It is not recommended to use venous Pco_2 and pH as a substitute for arterial Pco_2 and pH.
9. It is suggested that hemoximetry is used in the detection and evaluation of shunts during diagnostic cardiac catheterization.

Reproduced from Davis MD, Walsh BK, Sittig SE, Restrepo RD. AARC clinical practice guideline. *Respir Care.* 2013;58:1694–1703. Reprinted with permission.

is deep under the skin and the risk of undetected postpuncture bleeding is increased. The limited collateral arterial flow makes the lower limb more susceptible to ischemia if the femoral artery is occluded by clot or hematoma. In addition, the risk of infection is higher because the femoral artery is close to the perineum. The axillary (under the arm) or dorsalis pedis (between the toes) arteries are sometimes used, though not very often.

Most individuals can tolerate a single arterial puncture without local anesthesia. Sometimes a local anesthetic (such as 1% lidocaine) is necessary, especially for arterial cannulation or to decrease the pain and minimize anxiety-induced changes in a patient's blood gas values. Complications associated with arterial puncture include hematoma, arteriospasm, and thrombosis, all of which may result in hand ischemia if perfusion is not restored promptly. Patient reaction to arterial puncture may range from feelings of uneasiness to vasovagal syncope.

Allen Test

Before radial arterial puncture or cannulation is performed, the modified **Allen test** is performed to determine that there is adequate ulnar artery perfusion to the hand (**Figure 4-6**). This test was proposed originally in 1929 by Edgar V. Allen as a noninvasive evaluation of the patency of the arterial supply to the hand of individuals with thromboangiitis obliterans. The test was later modified for use as a test of collateral circulation before arterial cannulation.

To perform the Allen test, the patient makes a fist to force blood from the hand, and pressure is applied to compress the ulnar and radial arteries (Figure 4-6A). The patient then relaxes the hand, and obstructing pressure is removed from the ulnar artery while the radial artery remains compressed (Figure 4-6B). If the ulnar artery is patent, the hand should become flushed within 10 seconds, constituting a normal or positive Allen test. If the Allen test is abnormal, ulnar perfusion to the hand should be assumed to be poor and the

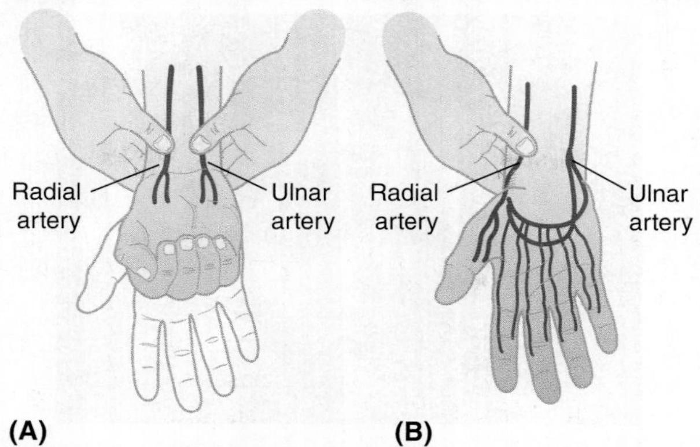

FIGURE 4-6 Allen test. (**A**) The patient is asked to open and close the hand into a fist several times with both radial and ulnar arteries compressed. (**B**) Release the ulnar artery. The entire hand and digits should fill with blood, indicating good collateral flow into the radial artery system.

radial artery in the contralateral wrist or alternative site should be considered for arterial blood sampling. Although not completely accurate, the Allen test remains a simple, useful screening test to assess the adequacy of ulnar collateral perfusion of the hand.

Radial Arterial Puncture

After collateral circulation has been assessed, prepare the patient for puncture of the radial artery (**Figure 4-7**). The radial artery is located via palpation for maximal arterial pulsation (Figure 4-7A). A towel is rolled under the wrist, with the hand hyperextended to bring the radial artery closer to the skin surface (Figure 4-7B). Clean the puncture site with alcohol, iodophor, or other appropriate disinfectant. The arterial puncture can be performed with either a glass syringe lubricated with a minimal amount of liquid heparin or a vented, pre-heparinized (100 to 200 IU), self-filling plastic syringe (Figure 4-7C). If the analysis is delayed, the samples should be drawn and stored in glass.[5] The blood gas syringe should be fitted with a 1-inch 22- or 23-gauge needle.

With the nondominant hand locating the maximal arterial pulsation and the dominant hand holding the syringe needle with the bevel pointing up at a 45-degree angle, puncture the skin and advance the needle. Note that the needle is inserted in the opposite direction of the blood flow, which means that the patient's palm should be facing up with the fingers positioned so that

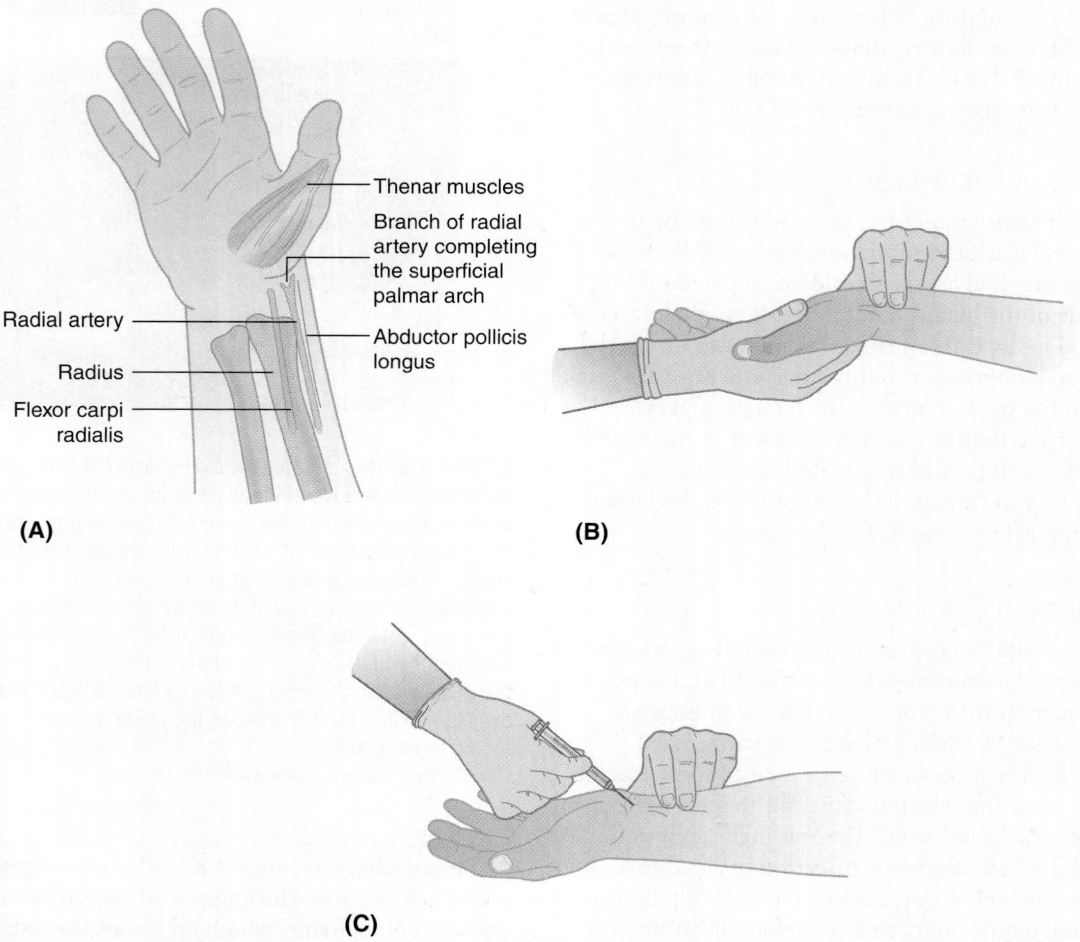

FIGURE 4-7 Radial artery sampling. (A) Anatomic location of radial artery. (**B**) Palpation of radial artery to determine the point of puncture. (**C**) Insertion of needle.

Adapted from Dudley HAF, Eckersely JRT, Paterson-Brown S. *A Guide to Practical Procedures in Medicine and Surgery*. Oxford, UK: Butterworth-Heinemann; 1989.

they point in the same direction as the person's hand inserting the syringe. Because the radial nerve is lateral to the artery, take care not to direct the needle toward the lateral aspect of the wrist. Once the artery is entered, a flash of arterial blood is seen in the needle hub. Collect approximately 2 to 3 mL of arterial blood as the arterial pressure fills the syringe. Usually, aspiration is not necessary, as blood pressure will fill the syringe. If aspiration is necessary, care should be taken to not move the position of the needle during sampling. Apply the needle protective sleeve, remove, and place in the sharp object container. Remove the excess air in the syringe by holding it upright and gently tapping it, allowing any air bubbles present to reach the top of the syringe, from where they can then be expelled. Cap the syringe and send it for analysis.

After the desired blood volume has been obtained, withdraw the needle from the artery and compress the site for at least 5 minutes. This compression decreases the possibility of hematoma formation, compartment syndrome, and ecchymosis, which may interfere with future arterial punctures. Longer compression times may be necessary for patients receiving anticoagulants (e.g., heparin, Coumadin) or those with coagulation defects (e.g., thrombocytopenia, chronic renal failure, disseminated intravascular coagulation). After bleeding has stopped, apply an elastic bandage with moderate pressure.

Punctures of Other Arterial Sites

For brachial artery puncture, the arm should be hyperextended and the hand pronated to best stabilize the artery. The brachial artery should be palpated on the medial side of the biceps tendon, 1 to 2 cm distal to the antecubital fossa. Care must be taken not to direct the puncture medially because this site is the most frequent location of the median nerve. The femoral artery is entered perpendicularly, with the patient in the supine position. The artery is best palpated and fixed just below the inguinal crease. The femoral nerve is lateral and the femoral vein medial to the artery.

Radial Arterial Cannulation

Arterial **cannulation** is performed when frequent arterial blood gas measurements are required and when continuous monitoring of arterial blood pressure is necessary. Usually the radial artery is cannulated (**Figure 4-8**). The arterial catheter is commonly placed through a percutaneous puncture, although a Seldinger technique also can be used. The Seldinger technique is a method of percutaneous insertion of a catheter into a blood vessel or space using a needle to puncture the skin and a guide wire that is threaded through the needle. With this technique, when the needle is withdrawn, the catheter is threaded over the wire and then the wire is withdrawn, leaving the catheter in place.

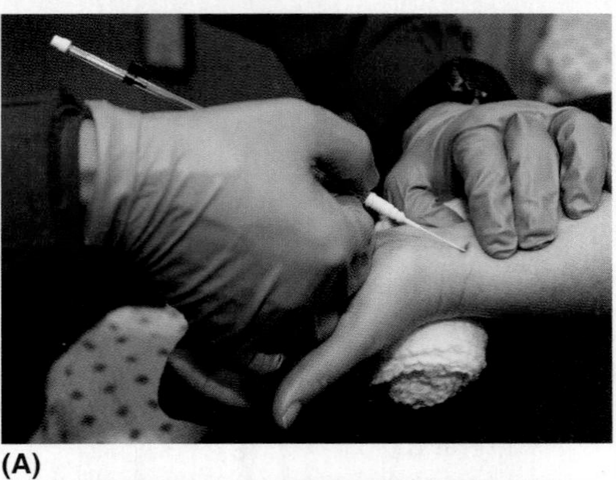

(A)

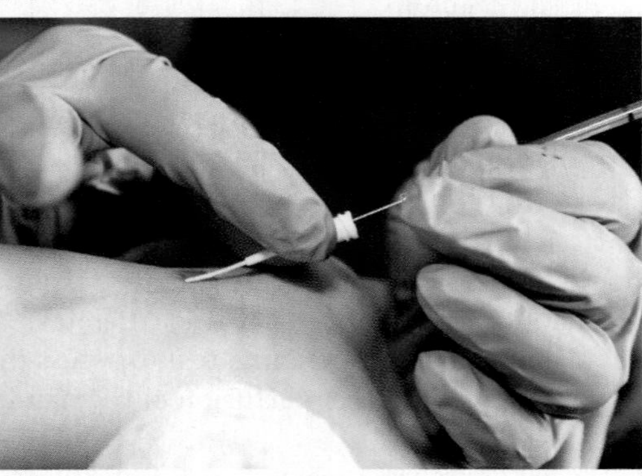

(B)

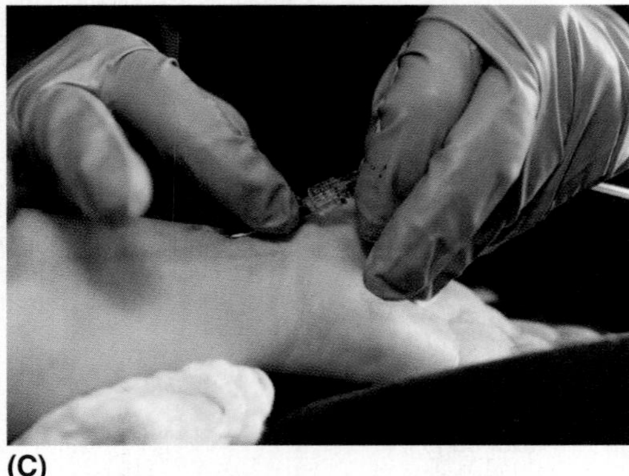

(C)

FIGURE 4-8 The catheter should be inserted using sterile technique. Hyperextend the wrist to bring the artery closer to the surface. Palpate the pulse with two fingers, tracking the course of the vessel. (A) Insert the needle over the radial artery. Advance the needle at an approximately 20 to 40 degree angle until there is a flash of pulsating blood as the needle enters the artery. (B) Immobilize the needle with your free hand and advance the guide wire. Then remove the needle, leaving only the guide wire in the artery. Advance the catheter into the artery over the guide wire. (C) Remove the guide wire and connect the tubing to the catheter.

Before insertion, anesthetize the area of puncture with 2% lidocaine. The anesthetic lidocaine should not contain epinephrine, which increases the risk of arterial spasm. Use a 20-gauge beveled needle with a clear plastic flash chamber. Place a straight stiff Teflon or polyurethane catheter with a hub at its distal end over the needle. After insertion, attach the catheter to a kit consisting of connective tubing, a stopcock for blood gas sampling, a transducer for blood pressure monitoring, and a continuous flush solution to prevent clotting in the catheter. Secure the catheter in place with tape or sutures.

Venous Blood Gases

Blood sampled from a peripheral vein or from the central venous circulation can be measured to provide additional blood gas information. Peripheral venous blood gases reflect the conditions of the tissues from which the venous blood arises. Peripheral venous blood gas values should not be interpreted as interchangeable with ABG for respiratory management. Peripheral venous blood gases might be useful to assess the presence of diabetic ketoacidosis. In the presence of hemodynamic stability, mixed venous or central venous pH and P_{CO_2} might be useful to assess acid–base balance. However, a central venous or mixed venous P_{O_2} should never be assumed to reflect **Pa_{O_2}**. The central venous and mixed venous P_{O_2} reflect tissue P_{O_2}; a low central venous or mixed venous P_{O_2} indicates tissue hypoxia. In the presence of poor blood flow (reduced cardiac output), the central venous and peripheral venous P_{O_2} will be decreased and the P_{CO_2} will be increased. Central venous P_{O_2} is used to assess tissue hypoxia in patients with sepsis. In the presence of peripheral shunting, the central venous and mixed venous P_{O_2} might be elevated.

Capillary Blood Gases

Capillary blood gas samples may be used to estimate pH and P_{CO_2} in infants or other individuals when arterial blood gas analysis is indicated but arterial access is difficult (**CPG 4-2**). Warm the site before the procedure

CLINICAL PRACTICE GUIDELINE 4-2

Capillary Blood Gas Sampling for Neonatal and Pediatric Patients

Indications

- Arterial blood gas analysis is indicated but arterial access is not available.
- Noninvasive monitor readings are abnormal: transcutaneous values, end-tidal CO_2, pulse oximetry.
- Assessment of initiation, administration, or change in therapeutic modalities (i.e., mechanical ventilation) is indicated.
- A change in patient status is detected by history or physical assessment.
- Monitoring the severity and progression of a documented disease process is desirable.

Contraindications

- Capillary punctures should not be performed at or through the following sites: posterior curvature of the heel, as the device may puncture the bone; the heel of a patient who has begun walking and has callus development; the fingers of neonates (to avoid nerve damage); previous puncture sites; inflamed, swollen, or edematous tissues; cyanotic or poorly perfused tissues; localized areas of infection; and peripheral arteries.
- Capillary punctures should not be performed on patients less than 24 hours old, due to poor peripheral perfusion.
- Capillary puncture should not be performed when there is need for direct analysis of oxygenation.
- Capillary puncture should not be performed when there is need for direct analysis of arterial blood.
- Relative contraindications: peripheral vasoconstriction, polycythemia (due to shorter clotting times), hypotension may be a relative contraindication.

Hazards and Complications

- Infection
- Inadvertent puncture or incision and consequent infection in sampler
- Burns
- Hematoma
- Bone calcification
- Nerve damage
- Bruising
- Scarring

(continues)

Clinical Practice Guideline 4-2 *(continued)*

- Puncture of posterior medial aspect of heel may result in tibial artery laceration
- Pain
- Bleeding
- Inappropriate patient management may result from reliance on capillary Po_2 values

Limitations of Method

- Inadequate warming of the site prior to a puncture may result in capillary values that correlate poorly with arterial pH and Pco_2 values.
- Undue squeezing of the puncture site may result in venous and lymphatic contamination of the sample.
- A second puncture may be needed to obtain an adequate amount of blood for analysis.
- Variability in capillary Po_2 values precludes using these samples for assessing oxygenation status.

Modified from AARC clinical practice guideline: capillary blood gases. *Respir Care.* 1994;1180-1183. Reprinted with permission.

to arterialize the blood. Make a puncture or small incision with a lancet into the cutaneous layer of the skin in a highly vascular area. Collect the blood in a heparinized glass capillary tube. Capillary punctures should not be performed through previous puncture sites; through inflamed, edematous, cyanotic, or poorly perfused tissues; through areas of infection; through peripheral arteries; through the posterior curvature of the heel, to avoid injuring bone; or in the fingers of neonates, to avoid nerve damage. Excessive squeezing of the puncture site may result in venous or lymphatic contamination of the sample. Capillary sampling should not be performed on infants younger than 24 hours because of poor peripheral perfusion. Relative contraindications include peripheral vasoconstriction, polycythemia (caused by shorter clotting times), and hypotension.

Capillary blood is handled in a similar way to arterial blood samples; it should be free of contamination by air or blood clots and analyzed in an appropriate time frame. Extreme variability in capillary Po_2 values precludes the use of this technique to assess oxygenation.

Preanalytic Errors

Box 4-1 lists common preanalytic errors. After the arterial blood specimen is obtained, expel any air bubble larger than 5% of the blood sample. Because room air contains a Pco_2 of essentially zero and a Po_2 of approximately 150 mm Hg (at sea level), air bubbles in the blood sample lower the Pco_2 values of the blood sample and cause the Po_2 to approach 150 mm Hg. The syringe must be capped immediately, and the technician in the blood gas laboratory must take great care to ensure that ambient air does not mix with the sample as it is introduced into the blood gas analyzer.

Because sodium heparin has a pH of approximately 7.0, too much heparin may affect the pH measurement. In general, 0.05 to 0.1 mL of heparin per milliliter of blood does not affect the pH value and provides adequate anticoagulation. The volume of the dead space is proportional to the size of the syringe. For example, the dead space of a 5-mL syringe with a needle is about 0.2 mL. Thus, 2 to 4 mL of blood should be obtained so that it contains at least 0.05 mL heparin per 1 mL blood, but no more than 0.1 mL heparin per 1 mL blood. Therefore, flush the syringe with heparin and eject that volume before obtaining arterial blood to keep the volume of heparin in the syringe at a minimum. The commercially available preheparinized syringes have minimized such a contamination problem because they use dry, lyophilized heparin. If electrolyte measurements are performed with the blood sample, use lithium heparin rather than sodium heparin.

Once the arterial blood gas sample is obtained, the syringe should be promptly transported (within 15 minutes at room temperature) to the arterial blood gas laboratory for analysis. Many intensive care units use a vacuum tube transport system to the laboratory, which is ideal for distances of 200 feet or more. A delay could lead to erroneous values because gas diffusion through the plastic syringe wall or between a bubble and blood increases with time, especially when the blood gas tensions differ significantly from those of room air.

BOX 4-1

Common Arterial Blood Gas Preanalytic Errors

Room air contamination of sample
Heparin dilution of sample
Blood clots from inadequate heparin
Hyperventilation during sample collection
Long delay time between sample collection and analysis
Excessive sample metabolism (leukocyte larceny with high WBC count)
Inadequate wait time between change in inspired oxygen or ventilation and collection of blood sample

The diffusion rate is also affected by temperature. If the sample cannot be analyzed immediately, it should be collected in a glass syringe (which decreases diffusion across the barrel of the syringe) and placed in ice (slush or chips) to hasten cooling. Putting the sample in ice slush also slows down oxygen consumption by white blood cells (WBCs), which is approximately 0.1 mL of O_2 from 100 mL blood in 10 minutes at body temperature. This effect is exaggerated if the WBC count is very high (leukocyte larceny). The decrease in Po_2 from the delay is more prominent if the hemoglobin saturation of the arterial blood is high. For example, if the sample is not iced, Po_2 drops to below 250 mm Hg in 1 hour if the original Po_2 is 400 mm Hg. However, if Po_2 is 50 mm Hg, the loss of 0.1 mL O_2 per 100 mL blood makes a very small change in Po_2 because the primary change occurs in the hemoglobin saturation.

Plastic syringes are commonly used for convenience. However, they should not be used if there will be a delay until analysis such that the sample must be placed on ice. The solubility of O_2 and CO_2 in the sample increases when the syringe is cooled, causing more gas to go into solution and thus reducing its partial pressure. Because plastic is relatively permeable to O_2 and CO_2, oxygen diffuses across the plastic into the sample. When the sample is subsequently warmed in the analyzer to 37° C (98.6° F), gas comes out of solution, resulting in a reported Po_2 and Pco_2 greater than what was in the sample drawn from the patient.

Sample Analysis

The blood gas sample should be observed for any air bubble, which must be removed as previously mentioned. Thoroughly mix the blood gas sample before analysis. Although mixing has minimal effect on blood gases and pH, it is necessary if hemoglobin or hematocrit will be measured by a CO-oximeter. Also, remove blood clots from the sample so that the blood gas analyzer does not become clogged. Expelling one or two drops of blood from the syringe tip onto a gauze pad directly before introduction into the analyzer helps ensure that clots are not present and that air bubbles are not introduced.

Blood gas analyzer calibrations are required according to the manufacturer's instructions. Most modern blood gas instruments perform automatic calibration at least every 30 minutes. Calibration reagents are usually standard CO_2 and O_2 gases (for example, 5% CO_2 + 20% O_2 + 75% N_2 and 10% CO_2 + 90% N_2) for Po_2 and Pco_2 sensors, and phosphate buffers (e.g., pH 6.840 and pH 7.384) for pH. The National Institute of Standards and Technology (NIST) provides reference standards for the reagents used for calibration of blood gas analyzers. When a blood gas sample has very high values (for example, a Po_2 value of 600 mm Hg), the operator may need to measure tonometered blood with known values at similar extreme levels to ascertain the instrument's degree of inaccuracy.

Tonometry of Blood

Because of the unique O_2-binding characteristics of hemoglobin and complex viscosity characteristics of normal fresh blood, whole blood must be carefully tonometered so that exact gas tensions can be prepared for analysis by a blood gas instrument. A **tonometry** reference method has been developed and recognized as the internationally accepted standard method. The method requires fresh blood (less than 24 hours old) from asymptomatic donors, which should be nonhemolyzed and without leukocytosis or high blood lipid levels. Gas mixtures, the composition of which has been verified by a mass spectrometer or with a CO_2 and O_2 gas analyzer, can be used to equilibrate the blood. If human blood is not available, bovine hemoglobin solutions (containing both deoxygenated and oxygenated hemoglobin) also can be used. These bovine preparations have been shown to yield data closely resembling those obtained with human blood. These solutions also can be formulated to provide precision data for the pH and electrolytes.

Quality Control and Proficiency Testing

The quality of results is crucial for blood gas analysis. The federal government, through the **Clinical Laboratory Improvement Amendment (CLIA)**, regulates the general aspects of quality control. A properly designed quality control program enables proper function of the blood gas analyzer on a routine basis. Quality control procedures for a blood gas analyzer differ from those of other analyses performed in the clinical laboratory environment because the patient sample is fresh whole blood.

The optimal technique used to establish the extent of inaccuracy and imprecision of an individual blood gas analyzer is the use of whole blood tonometry with samples of fresh, anticoagulated whole blood. However, its hazard potential and labor-intensive process must balance the technical and economic advantages of whole blood tonometry. Alternatives to whole blood tonometry are commercially available prepackaged materials such as aqueous buffer solutions, blood-based

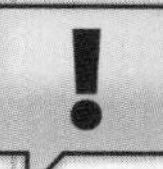

Respiratory Recap

Calibration, Quality Control, and Proficiency Testing

- Calibration adjusts the analyzer to reference standards.
- Quality control analyzes materials of known values for pH, Pco_2, and Po_2.
- Proficiency testing analyzes materials from an external source that have values unknown to the tester.

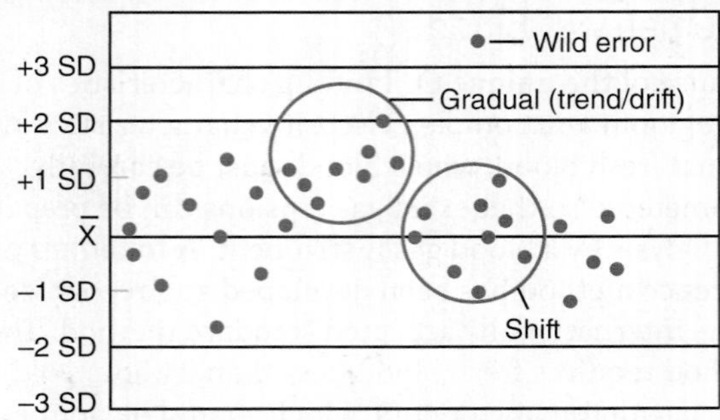

FIGURE 4-9 Three types of analytic errors identified on a Levey-Jennings chart: wild error (outlier), gradual error (trend, drift), and a shift to a new (in this case, lower) mean.

Adapted from Branson RD, Hess DR, Chatburn RL. *Respiratory Care Equipment*. 2nd ed. Lippincott Williams & Wilkins; 1999.

(hemoglobin-containing) materials, and perfluorocarbon-oil emulsions. However, the physical and chemical properties of these controls do not match those of whole blood.

Whichever materials are chosen, the results of the quality control program should be recorded in a manner that allows the operator to easily detect changes in performance of the instrument. This detection is most commonly done with Levey-Jennings charts (**Figure 4-9**). CLIA requires at least two levels of control for pH, Pco_2, and Po_2 on each work shift or every 8 hours of operation. In addition to internal quality control programs, external proficiency testing programs are also used to assess accuracy of measurements. These external proficiency testing programs are available from sources such as the College of American Pathologists (CAP) and the American Thoracic Society (ATS).

Temperature Adjustment

Blood gas analyzers measure and report at normal body temperature of 37° C. Controversy exists whether blood gas values should be adjusted in clinical practice for actual body temperature. The argument for temperature adjustment, also referred to as temperature correction, is that blood gas values measured at 37° C (98.6° F) may not accurately reflect the true oxygenation and acid–base status of the body.[6] Po_2 changes with temperature at 7% per degree Celsius. However, O_2 capacity, O_2 content, and hemoglobin saturation do not. The Po_2 of the arterial blood in a cold extremity thus may be only 40 mm Hg, but the saturation value is 96%. If such a temperature-corrected value of Po_2 is reported, the Po_2 may seem dangerously low to the clinician, whereas in fact the hypothermic patient is adequately oxygenated. The same argument also applies to the acid–base status. Pco_2 and pH change with temperature (4% per degree Celsius for Pco_2; 0.0146 units per degree Celsius for pH), but the bicarbonate and intracellular neutrality do not. Therefore, the pH and Pco_2 values at 37° C (98.6° F) reliably reflect the in vivo acid–base status of the patient. In addition, most acid–base nomograms are valid only at 37° C (98.6° F), and temperature adjustment does not conclusively improve clinical decision making.

Based on these arguments, routine blood gas measurements may be consistently reported at 37° C (98.6° F), without correction for actual body temperature.[7,8] On rare occasions, such as severe hypothermia, the temperature-adjusted arterial (and alveolar) values may be more appropriate, such as for the calculation of the alveolar-arterial O_2 gradient or arterial-alveolar end-tidal CO_2 gradient in patients with abnormal temperatures.[6,8]

The concept of managing pH and $Paco_2$ in which the measurement at 37° C is kept at the normal level, regardless of the patient's body temperature, is called the alpha-stat approach. Nonetheless, it is still unclear whether patients managed by the alpha-stat approach have major differences in outcome compared with those managed by the pH-stat approach. Therefore, the laboratory must have a defined procedure for temperature correction of the measured results. Errors in the measurement of the patient's temperature may cause erroneous temperature-adjusted results. If temperature-adjusted results are reported, the report should be clearly labeled as such, and the measured results at 37° C must also be reported. It should be noted that no data are currently available that can quantify the balance between oxygen delivery and oxygen demand at temperatures other than 37° C and that temperature correction of blood gas samples is not recommended (see CPG 4-2).

Physiology of Acid–Base Balance

Normal physiology generates acids as a by-product of metabolism. These acids are mainly carbonic acid (H_2CO_3), phosphates, and sulfates. H_2CO_3 is also called volatile acid because the lungs eliminate it as carbon dioxide (CO_2). The acids of phosphate and sulfates are also called nonvolatile acids. The kidneys can eliminate only nonvolatile acids. Acid–base balance refers to physiologic mechanisms that regulate the hydrogen ion concentration [H^+] of blood and body fluids within a range compatible with life. The lungs and the kidneys are the primary organs essential in maintaining acid–base balance.

Concept of pH

Sørenson developed the concept of pH in 1909. **pH** is defined as the negative logarithm or exponent (to the base 10) of the [H^+]:

$$pH = -\log [H^+]$$

The pH scale ranges from 0 to 14 pH units. Because pH is the negative logarithm of [H^+], a decrease in pH indicates an increase in [H^+], and vice versa. A logarithm is the power to which a number must be raised in order to get some other number. For example, the base 10 logarithm of 100 is 2, because 10 raised to the power of two is 100:

$$\log 100 = 2$$

This is an example of a base-10 logarithm. It is called a base-10 logarithm because 10 is the number that is raised to a power. The base unit is the number being raised to a power.

The dissociation of pure water molecules (H_2O or HOH) into H^+ and OH^- helps explain this concept. Water dissociates into hydrogen ion and hydroxyl ion.

$$H_2O \leftrightarrow H^+ + OH^-$$

Because water (H_2O) is essentially a constant with very little dissociation, it stays at equilibrium with equal parts of acid and base at 25° C. At equilibrium, pure water contains 10^{-7} mol/L of H^+ and 10^{-7} mol/L of OH^-.

The pH of water, which contains $[H^+]$ of 10^{-7} mol/L (or 100 nmol/L), would be

$$pH = -\log (10^{-7}) = -(-7) = 7$$

When a chemical solution has a pH of 7.0, it is a *neutral solution* (neither acidic nor basic). Water is an example of a neutral solution. A solution with a pH less than 7.0 is called *acidic*; a solution with a pH greater than 7.0 is called *alkaline*. However, remember that the normal pH of the blood is slightly alkaline (7.4), which corresponds to $[H^+]$ of 40 nmol/L. When interpreting arterial blood gases, because blood is slightly alkaline, the normal values of arterial blood (pH of 7.35 to 7.45) are used to describe acidic or alkaline. It is important to remember that the interpretation of an ABG pH is applied differently than it is for chemical solutions.

Buffer Solutions

To understand the concept of pH it is essential to understand how buffers work. A **buffer** is either a weak acid and its conjugate base or a weak base with its conjugate acid. A buffer solution can resist a big change in $[H^+]$, and therefore in pH, when an acid or a base is added. An example of a buffer solution is carbonic acid and its conjugate base, HCO_3^-, or bicarbonate. If we look at the dissociation of carbonic acid, it helps illustrate how buffers work to minimize changes in pH.

The dissociation of carbonic acid is:

$$H_2CO_3 \rightarrow HCO_3^- + H^+$$

If a strong acid, such as hydrochloric acid (HCl), is added to the carbonic acid/sodium bicarbonate ($NaHCO_3$) buffer solution, bicarbonate ions will react with the added H^+ to form more carbonic acid and a neutral salt (NaCl):

$$HCl + NaHCO_3 \rightarrow H_2CO_3 + NaCl$$

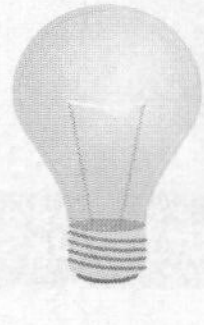

STOP AND THINK

What happens if hydrochloric acid is added to a sodium bicarbonate solution? Explain how this demonstrates the effects of buffers in solution.

The strong acidity of HCl is thus converted to the relatively weak acidity of H_2CO_3, preventing a large drop in pH.

On the other hand, if a strong base, such as sodium hydroxide (NaOH), is added, it will react with the carbonic acid to form sodium bicarbonate ($NaHCO_3$) and water:

$$NaOH + H_2CO_3 \rightarrow NaHCO_3 + H_2O$$

According to this reaction, OH^- from NaOH will react with H^+ to form H_2O; in the process, the strong base, NaOH, is changed to a relatively weak base, $NaHCO_3$, minimizing the large increase in pH that would have otherwise been caused by the addition of NaOH. In an aqueous solution, the sodium bicarbonate readily dissociates into water and bicarbonate (HCO_3^-).

The body has several buffer systems within its extracellular (intravascular and interstitial) and intracellular compartments (**Table 4-1**). The main buffering systems are (1) bicarbonate in plasma, interstitial, and intracellular water and carbonate in bone; (2) intracellular proteins, including hemoglobin in red blood cells; (3) plasma proteins; and (4) intracellular and extracellular phosphates. The extent to which each buffer contributes to the defense of body pH varies with differing kinds of acid–base disturbances. **Table 4-2** shows the individual buffers' contributions to total buffering capacity in whole blood.

Among all the buffering systems, the **bicarbonate buffer system** is the most important because it is present in appreciable quantities in nearly all body fluids and is readily available to stabilize pH. Bicarbonate differs from other body buffers in that the product of

TABLE 4-1
Buffer Systems in Different Body Compartments

Site	Buffer System
Interstitial fluid	Bicarbonate Phosphates Proteins
Blood	Bicarbonate Hemoglobin Plasma proteins Phosphates
Intracellular fluid	Proteins Phosphates Bicarbonate
Bone	Calcium carbonate

TABLE 4-2
Individual Buffer Contributions to Whole Blood Buffering

Buffer Type	Percentage of Total Buffering
Bicarbonate	53
Plasma bicarbonate	35
Erythrocyte bicarbonate	18
Nonbicarbonate	47
Hemoglobin	35
Organic phosphates	3
Inorganic phosphates	2
Plasma proteins	7

Modified from Beachey W. *Respiratory Care Anatomy and Physiology*. 2nd ed. Copyright Elsevier (Mosby) 2007.

its reaction with H^+ is H_2CO_3, an acid that can be converted to CO_2 and eliminated by the lungs as a gas. The reaction between H_2CO_3 and $H_2O + CO_2$ is facilitated by an enzyme called carbonic anhydrase. The carbonic acid is sometimes referred to as volatile acid because it dissociates into a gas that can be exhaled out of the body.

$$H^+ + HCO_3^- \rightarrow H_2CO_3 \rightarrow H_2O + CO_2$$

Henderson-Hasselbalch Equation

In 1909, Lawrence J. Henderson used the law of mass action to express the hydrogen ion equilibrium (**Equation 4-1**). Using the convention in which $[H^+]$ is expressed as pH, Hasselbalch rearranged Henderson's equation and applied it to the carbonic acid buffer system. The **Henderson-Hasselbalch equation** accurately describes the equilibrium relationships among pH, P_{CO_2}, and HCO_3^-. Because the P_{CO_2} of the arterial blood is regulated by alveolar ventilation, it is used to indicate the respiratory component of the acid–base state. $[HCO_3^-]$ is an estimate of the nonrespiratory, or metabolic, component of the acid–base state. Both respiratory and metabolic changes affect HCO_3^-. Therefore, CO_2 and HCO_3^- in the Henderson-Hasselbalch equation are not independently regulated.

The bicarbonate buffer system is influenced by the independent and direct effect of P_{CO_2} on $[HCO_3^-]$. Changes in $[HCO_3^-]$ thus do not indicate metabolic changes alone.

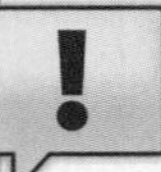

Respiratory Recap

Acids, Bases, and Buffers

- An acid donates a proton in solution.
- A base accepts a proton in solution.
- pH is a measure of hydrogen ion concentration.
- A buffer minimizes the change in pH when a strong acid or strong base is added.

EQUATION 4-1

The Henderson-Hasselbalch Equation

$$pH = pKa + \log\frac{[HCO_3^-]}{[CO_2]}$$

The Henderson equation can be rearranged as follows:

$$[H^+] = 24 \times \frac{P_{CO_2}}{[HCO_3^-]}$$

where $[H^+]$ is in mEq/L, P_{CO_2} is in mm Hg, and $[HCO_3^-]$ is in mmol/L.

Because the pKa of carbonic acid is 6.1 and the solubility constant for CO_2 in plasma is 0.0301, the Henderson-Hasselbalch equation is as follows:

$$pH = 6.1 + \log\frac{[HCO_3^-]}{0.0301 \times P_{CO_2}}$$

This equation suggests the equilibrium that exists between bicarbonate and carbon dioxide, also called a bicarbonate approach to pH. This approach has limitations because changes in HCO_3^- are not due solely to the metabolic component of pH.

Clinical Application of Henderson-Hasselbalch Equation

With the normal pH of 7.4 and **Pa_{CO_2}** of 40 mm Hg, arterial HCO_3^- is calculated using the Henderson-Hasselbalch equation. For clinical application, a modified Henderson-Hasselbalch can be used:

$$\frac{[H^+][HCO_3^-]}{Pa_{CO_2}} = 24$$

The Henderson-Hasselbalch equation is clinically useful to check for inaccuracies due to blood gas analyzer problems, transcription mistakes, or other errors. It is also clinically useful to use the modified Henderson-Hasselbalch equation to anticipate what effect changing one variable will have overall. For example, a clinician could predict how permissive hypercapnia (allowing a high Pa_{CO_2}) would affect the blood pH. By using the patient's most current blood gas showing HCO_3^- of 26 mmol/L, if a pH of at least 7.30 was desired, the level of permissive hypercapnia could be determined using the modified H-H and solving for Pa_{CO_2}:

$$\frac{50 \times 26}{Pa_{CO_2}} = 24$$

TABLE 4-3
Relationship Between pH and [H+]

pH	[H+] (nmol/L)
6.80	158
6.90	126
7.00	100
7.10	79
7.15	71
7.20	63
7.25	56
7.30	50
7.35	45
7.40	40
7.45	35
7.50	32
7.55	28
7.60	25
7.70	20
7.80	16
8.0	10

Modified from Beachey W. *Respiratory Care Anatomy and Physiology*. 2nd ed. Copyright Elsevier (Mosby) 2007.

Using **Table 4-3**, a pH of 7.30 is equivalent to a [H^+] of 50 nmol/L. From this calculation, a $Paco_2$ of 54 mm Hg would drop the pH to 7.30. Therefore, the hypercapnia would be permitted gradually, thereby giving the kidneys a chance to increase bicarbonate to compensate for the higher respiratory acid.

Base Excess

The concept of base excess was introduced by Siggaard-Andersen in the late 1950s. *Base excess* is defined as the amount of strong acid (in mmol/L) that must be added to the blood sample in vitro to return the sample to pH 7.40 after equilibration while maintaining the partial pressure of carbon dioxide at 40 mm Hg. Recall that in vitro means "outside of the body" or removed from the intact physiologic state, while in vivo occurs within living organisms in the normal, intact state. If blood has a pH of 7.40 and a Pco_2 of 40 mm Hg, the base excess will be 0 mmol/L. Siggaard-Andersen developed a nomogram to determine base excess in the clinical setting. This nomogram was later incorporated into blood gas analyzers to allow automatic calculation.

The base excess approach produced the concept of excess [HCO_3^-] in arterial plasma that accounts for changes in the metabolic component of acid–base disorders. However, the concept of base excess did not hold up when applied to whole blood or plasma changes in vivo. First, plasma in vivo is in contiguity with interstitial fluid that has less buffering capacity. The base excess approach deals with this argument by assuming a hemoglobin concentration of 50 g/L, thus reducing the apparent buffer capacity of the blood in vitro. This issue requires standardization of in vitro data to whole blood with a constant hemoglobin concentration. Second, in patients with chronic elevation of $Paco_2$, the base excess approach would have diagnosed a coexisting alkalinizing metabolic process decreasing the acidity. Despite its deficiencies, base excess is still used in some clinical settings because of its simplicity. Normal base excess is ±2 mmol/L and may be reported as part of an ABG analysis.

Assessment of Unmeasured Anions

Bicarbonate-centered approaches to acid–base balance imply that the concentrations of H^+ and HCO_3^- are the main forces regulating acid–base balance. However, unmeasured anions in the plasma have direct impact on arterial blood gas interpretation. As described previously, changes in bicarbonate concentration ([HCO_3^-]) are not solely due to changes in the metabolic or renal component of acid–base (pH) status. Many conditions can result in an increase in unmeasured anion, affecting the pH. Therefore, additional calculations can be used to determine the unmeasured anion to accurately determine an acid–base disorder. Available methods to calculate unmeasured anions are anion gap and strong ion difference, also called strong ion gap.

The **anion gap (AG)** represents the concentration of all the unmeasured anions in the plasma. AG is calculated from the following formula:

$$\text{Anion gap} = [Na^+] - ([Cl^-] + [HCO_3^-])$$

The normal anion gap is 12 ± 4 mmol/L and is mostly caused by negatively charged plasma proteins, sulfate, and phosphate. An increased anion gap represents additional unmeasured anions, which can be endogenous, such as lactate or ketones, or exogenous, such as salicylate. Recall that endogenous means originating from within an organism, tissue, or cell. When excessive acid anions are produced during metabolic **acidosis**, the H^+ produced reacts with bicarbonate anions (buffering),

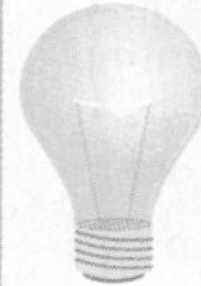

STOP AND THINK

Your patient has a Na^+ of 138 mmol/L, Cl^- of 104 mmol/L, and HCO_3^- of 20 mmol/L. What is the anion gap and what are its implications?

and the CO_2 produced is excreted via the lungs (respiratory compensation). The net effect is a decrease in the concentration of measured anions (i.e., HCO_3^-) and an increase in the concentration of unmeasured anions (the acid anions), so the anion gap increases.

The anion gap is useful clinically to signal the presence of a metabolic acidosis during the interpretation of acid–base disorder, to help differentiate between causes of a metabolic acidosis (high anion gap versus normal anion gap metabolic acidosis), to assist in assessing the biochemical severity of the acidosis, and to follow the response to treatment (e.g., during the treatment of diabetic ketoacidosis). AG can also be lower than normal in myeloma in which immunoglobulin G paraproteins increase. These paraproteins act as weak bases because of the basic amino acids lysine and arginine, which have isoelectric points close to pH = 9.0. They thus have a weak positive charge in the physiologic pH range.

Clinical correlation should be used to interpret AG. For example, lactic acidosis with a lactate level of 5 to 10 mmol/L can be associated with sepsis, but the AG may be within the reference range in as many as 50% of these cases.[9] There are several reasons why this may occur. First, the lactate may not be high enough to push the anion gap out of the reference range. Second, administration of large amounts of intravenous saline solution (NaCl) as in septic shock may increase the levels of chloride and thus decrease AG. Third, in lactic acidosis, plasma lactate may move intracellularly in exchange for chloride via an antiporter. This contributes to an increase in chloride concentration in the plasma, decreasing the AG. Finally, albumin, the major unmeasured anion contributing to the value of the anion gap, may be low in patients with septic shock and lactic acidosis. Because every gram decrease in albumin will decrease the anion gap by 2.5 to 3 mol/L, a high anion gap lactic acidosis may appear as a normal anion gap acidosis in a patient with hypoalbuminemia.

The anion gap (AG) is used routinely in the assessment of metabolic acidosis but can be misleading in patients with hypoalbuminemia and other disorders commonly encountered in intensive care. The AG approach to acid–base analysis relies on assessment of pH, P_{CO_2}, sodium, bicarbonate, and chloride and can lead to underestimation or overestimation of the true electrochemical status of a patient, as it does not include important ions such as lactate, calcium, magnesium, and albumin. Therefore, the strong ion difference, also called the strong ion gap, offers alternative approaches for the assessment of an acid–base disorder in more complicated cases.

The **strong ion difference (SID)**, also called the strong ion gap, is yet another approach to determine unmeasured anions and is considered even more refined than using the anion gap. In the early 1980s, Peter Stewart introduced the strong ion difference approach as an alternative approach to acid–base

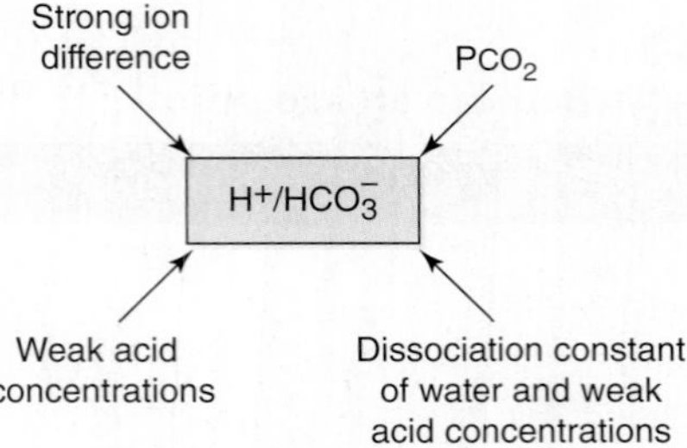

FIGURE 4-10 Important factors in the control of hydrogen and bicarbonate ions using the Stewart approach (strong ion difference).
Modified from Story DA, et al. Bench-to-bedside review. A brief history of clinical acid-base. *Crit Care.* 2004;8:253.

physiology and mass (**Figure 4-10**). This approach is based on the principles of electroneutrality, conversion of mass, and disassociation of electrolytes.

In physiologic fluids the main strong electrolytes are Na^+, K^+, and Cl^-. These strong ions influence $[H^+]$ by the law of electrical neutrality and the dissociation of water, meaning that the net charge must be zero in any system at equilibrium. Thus, in a solution of Na^+, K^+, and Cl^- in water, $[Na^+] + [K^+] + [H^+] - [Cl^-] - [OH^-] = 0$. The effect of strong ions may be lumped into a single term that expresses the net negative or positive charge that they exert. This is the strong ion difference [SID]. In plasma, [SID] is normally calculated as follows:

$$[SID] = [Na^+] + [K^+] - [Cl^-]$$

Strong organic ions, such as lactate or ketones, normally are present in very low concentrations and their effects on [SID] are minimal. In metabolic acidosis, these anions can be present in high concentrations and exert more significant effects on [SID]. Other strong inorganic ions are usually ignored because they are present in low concentrations. Therefore, $[SID] + [H^+] - [OH^-] = 0$, where the independent variable is [SID] and the dependent variables are $[H^+]$ and $[OH^-]$. In normal plasma, $[Na^+]$ is 140 mmol/L, $[K^+]$ is 4 mmol/L, and $[Cl^-]$ is 104 mmol/L. The normal [SID] thus is approximately 40 mmol/L.

Total weak acids (A_{tot}) are all buffers present in a partially dissociated state in the physiologic pH range. Weak acids have dissociation constant (K_a) values between 10^{-4} and 10^{-12}. However, only those with K_a close to 4×10^{-8} (pH = 7.4) are effective buffers. These buffer systems include plasma proteins ($K_a = 3 \times 10^{-7}$), proteins and phosphates in cells ($K_a = 5.5 \times 10^{-7}$), and hemoglobin in red blood cells ($K_a = 2.5 \times 10^{-7}$ for oxyhemoglobin; 6.3×10^{-9} for deoxyhemoglobin). The effectiveness of weak acids as buffers depends not only on the dissociation constant but also on the total concentration $[A_{tot}]$ of the weak, nonvolatile acids, the plasma proteins. $[A_{tot}]$ is the sum of the dissociated (A^-) and undissociated (HA) forms:

$$[A_{tot}] \text{ (mmol/L)} = [HA] + [A^-]$$

In plasma, $[A_{tot}]$ may be estimated via multiplication of the protein content by 0.24. Thus, at a normal total protein of 70 g/L, $[A_{tot}]$ is 0.24 × 70, or 17 mmol/L. This value comprises $[A^-]$ of 15 mmol/L and [HA] of 2 mmol/L at pH = 7.4. Even though plasma proteins behave as weak acids, they are mostly dissociated (15/17 or approximately 90%) at normal arterial pH.

The last independent variable in Stewart's model is P_{CO_2}. The variations in P_{CO_2} and $[H^+]$ alter total CO_2 content, which then governs how the bicarbonate buffer system acts.

Variations in the relative magnitude of the independent variables involved in control of acid–base status produce differing effects in different fluid compartments and tissues. In intracellular fluids, [SID] is large and dominated by a high $[K^+]$. High protein and phosphate concentrations ($[A_{tot}]$) also minimize the effects of reductions in [SID] resulting from falls in $[K^+]$ or accumulation of strong organic ions, such as lactate. In tissues, P_{CO_2} is high and increases by metabolism, but $[HCO_3^-]$ is low. Changes in P_{CO_2} influence $[H^+]$ in tissues much less than in plasma. Control of intracellular $[H^+]$ is achieved through buffering and exchange of strong ions with extracellular fluid, thereby changing [SID], and through diffusion of CO_2 from the cell. In interstitial fluid and other ultrafiltrates of plasma, such as lymph or cerebrospinal fluid, $[H^+]$ is influenced only by changes in [SID] and P_{CO_2} because protein is virtually absent and the weak acid system does not have a role. In plasma, [SID] also tends to regulate the pH, but variations in P_{CO_2} may bring about large and rapid changes in arterial $[H^+]$.

The SID approach appears to provide more explanation than the bicarbonate-centered approaches for many acid–base phenomena seen in the critical care setting.[9–11] This includes explanations for metabolic **alkalosis** associated with decreased plasma albumin concentrations,[12,13] the mechanism of hyperchloremic acidosis,[14] and the role of ammonia in acid–base homeostasis.[10] The SID approach also refines detecting unmeasured ions, or the anion gap. Therefore, it is a methodology for exploring unexplained ions, although the calculations are complex, limiting clinical usefulness.

Respiratory Recap

Anion Gap and Strong Ion Gap

- The anion gap is useful in the interpretation of acid–base disorders.
- Anion gap should be corrected for albumin concentration.
- The Stewart model has three independent variables controlling pH: strong ion difference, the total weak acid concentration, and P_{CO_2}.

Albumin-Corrected Anion Gap

The traditionally defined anion gap does not take into account the large changes in plasma albumin concentration often seen in critically ill patients. Unless a correction factor is used, an increased anion gap may go unrecognized.[11,15] This has led to the concept of albumin-corrected anion gap.[16] Anion gap is reduced by approximately 2.5 mmol/L for every 1 g/dL fall in albumin:

$$\text{Anion gap (corrected)} = \text{Anion gap} + 2.5\,(4.2 - [\text{Albumin}])$$

The SID approach may also provide a better understanding of the various management strategies, including fluid management,[14,17,18] buffer therapy,[19] and renal replacement therapy.[20] Although well supported by clinical evidence, the SID approach is more difficult to use in everyday clinical practice because it is cumbersome to calculate.[21–23]

Regulation of pH

Regulation of pH in the body is described by the alpha-stat hypothesis and the pH-stat hypothesis. The pH-stat hypothesis argues, for ideal body function, the pH should be kept constant despite changes in temperature. This is the same as saying that extracellular fluid (ECF) pH should be kept at 7.4 regardless of the temperature. The alpha-stat hypothesis accommodates changes in temperature as a basis for pH regulation and correction. The alpha-stat hypothesis argues that it is more important to maintain the dissociation constant (K_a) as it varies with temperature rather than maintaining the actual pH. Maintaining the dissociation constant keeps the net charge on all proteins constant despite changes in temperature. This ensures that all proteins, especially enzymes, can function optimally despite temperature changes.

The alpha-stat hypothesis is based on a constant pH gradient between the intracellular and extracellular compartments. The normal pH of arterial blood (7.40) is slightly higher than that of capillary and venous blood (about 7.36). The pH of most remaining ECF (when excluding the arterial blood) is virtually identical to that of capillaries and venous blood because H^+ can permeate across the endothelial barrier. The pH of intracellular fluid (ICF) is lower and ranges from 6.8 to 7.2. Extracellular pH is maintained at 0.6 to 0.8 pH units higher than the prevailing intracellular pH at any given temperature, thereby providing a sink for disposal of the acids produced by intracellular metabolism.

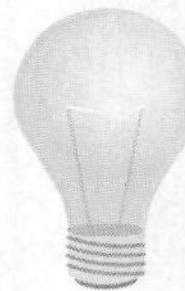

STOP AND THINK

Describe three methods for calculation of unmeasured anions and how to use each to determine an acid–base disorder.

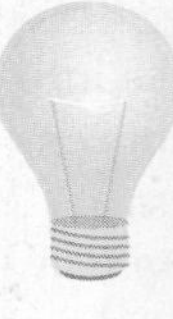

STOP AND THINK

A patient is cooled to 33° C following resuscitation for cardiac arrest. An arterial blood sample that is drawn and analyzed at 37° C is pH 7.40, P_{CO_2} 40 mm Hg, and P_{O_2} 90 mm Hg. The blood gases adjusted to the patient's temperature are pH 7.46, P_{CO_2} 32 mm Hg, and P_{O_2} 68 mm Hg. Would you use the measured blood gases (37° C) or the temperature-adjusted blood gases for ventilator management?

The control mechanism for this constant pH gradient is called the **alpha-stat hypothesis**.

In the body, regulatory mechanisms attempt to keep intracellular pH at or very close to the neutrality of water ($[H^+] = [OH^-]$).[10] The importance of the alpha-stat concept can be illustrated by the following example. During exercise on a cold day, an individual's core temperature is 37° C, and intracellular and blood pH are 6.8 and 7.4, respectively. The intracellular P_{CO_2} is 40 mm Hg. In the exercising muscle, the temperature is 41° C (105.8° F) and P_{CO_2} is 48 mm Hg (due to increased metabolism), but intracellular and blood pH decrease to 6.7 and 7.35, respectively. In the skin, the temperature is cooled to 25° C and intracellular P_{CO_2} is 22 mm Hg, but intracellular and blood pH increase to 7.0 and 7.6, respectively. Thus, despite these striking regional variations in pH and P_{CO_2}, the relative alkalinity, or the net charge of imidazole buffer, between cells and blood is maintained throughout the body.

Erythrocytes and Acid–Base Control

Erythrocytes can buffer sudden changes in ions or P_{CO_2} and help maintain relatively constant conditions in plasma and ECF. Erythrocytes contain hemoglobin, which offers large buffering capacity (by the imidazole group of the histidine residues), which has a pK_a of about 6.8. This is suitable for effective buffering at physiologic pH. Hemoglobin in red blood cells (RBCs) is about six times more important than the plasma proteins as a buffer because it is present in about twice the concentration and contains about three times the number of histidine residues per molecule. These histidine molecules are highly effective buffers. For example, if blood pH changes from 7.5 to 6.5, hemoglobin would buffer 27.5 mmol/L of H^+, and total plasma protein buffering would account for only 4.2 mmol/L of H^+.

When oxygen dissociates from hemoglobin (deoxygenation), $[H^+]$ decreases inside the erythrocyte. As CO_2 enters the erythrocyte, it reacts with water to form carbonic acid. The carbonic anhydrase in the erythrocyte enables the hydration of CO_2 to proceed rapidly. The carbonic acid then ionizes to form H^+ and HCO_3^-. The H^+ offsets the decrease in H^+ during the deoxygenation process. HCO_3^- formed during the process moves out of the cell and Cl^- moves into the cell, a phenomenon called *chloride shift*. CO_2 that enters the erythrocytes also binds at the αNH_2 groups of the β chain of hemoglobin, very rapidly forming carbamates. This reaction is also facilitated by deoxygenation of hemoglobin.

Deoxyhemoglobin is a more effective buffer at physiologic pH than oxyhemoglobin is. Deoxyhemoglobin buffers venous acidity more effectively than oxyhemoglobin does. This phenomenon is called the *isohydric exchange*; that is, the buffer system ($HHbO_2$–HbO_2^-) is converted to another more effective buffer (HHb–Hb^-) exactly at the site where an increased buffering capacity is required. By these mechanisms, erythrocytes can buffer sudden changes in ions or P_{CO_2} and help maintain relatively constant conditions in plasma and ECF. Clinically, RBC transfusion not only increases oxygen delivery by increasing hemoglobin but also provides essential buffer for the management of metabolic acidosis.

The Lungs and Acid–Base Control

The lungs eliminate volatile acid as CO_2 and the kidneys eliminate nonvolatile acid. Oxidative metabolism produces approximately 13,000 to 20,000 mmol/day of volatile acid (H_2CO_3). Because H_2CO_3 is in equilibrium with dissolved CO_2, the lungs can lower blood H_2CO_3 by eliminating CO_2 through ventilation. Through eliminating CO_2 via the exhaled gas, the lungs can produce rapid changes in pH. The Pa_{CO_2} in the alveolar ventilation equation reflects CO_2 elimination:

$$Pa_{CO_2} = 0.863 \times \dot{V}_{CO_2}/\dot{V}_A$$

This equation is useful because neither metabolic rate nor ventilation needs to be measured to assess the adequacy of breathing in relation to metabolic demand. If $\dot{V}_{CO_2}$ and $\dot{V}_A$ are both measured at body temperature and in the same units (e.g., L/min), this equation simplifies to:

$$Pa_{CO_2} = P_b \times \dot{V}_{CO_2}/\dot{V}_A$$

where P_b is barometric pressure at 760 mm Hg (sea level). Examine P_{CO_2} in arterial blood, which represents the balance between metabolic CO_2 production and ventilation. In tissues and venous blood, P_{CO_2} reflects primarily the balance between metabolism and blood flow. The extent to which arterial P_{CO_2} reflects the adequacy of ventilation also depends on carbonic anhydrase activity in allowing rapid equilibration of P_{CO_2} between pulmonary capillary blood and alveolar gas. Drugs that inhibit carbonic anhydrase, such as acetazolamide, thus increase Pa_{CO_2}.

The ventilatory responses to acid–base disorders of nonrespiratory origin are extremely important in the regulation of $[H^+]$ because they change rapidly. The control system for respiratory regulation of acid–base

TABLE 4-4
Control System for Respiratory Regulation of Acid–Base Balance

Control Element	Physiologic or Anatomic Correlate	Comments
Controlled variable	Arterial P_{CO_2}	A change in arterial P_{CO_2} alters arterial pH (as calculated by the Henderson-Hasselbalch equation).
Sensors	Central and peripheral chemoreceptors	Both respond to changes in arterial P_{CO_2} (as well as some other factors).
Central integrator	The respiratory center in the medulla	
Effectors	The respiratory muscles	An increase in minute ventilation increases alveolar ventilation and thus decreases arterial P_{CO_2}. The net result is of negative feedback that tends to restore the P_{CO_2} to the set point.

balance can be considered using the model of a simple servo control system. The components of such a simple model are a controlled variable that is monitored by a sensor, a central integrator that interprets the information from the sensor, and an effector mechanism that can alter the controlled variable (**Table 4-4**). In long-term responses to acid–base disturbances, the response of the central medullary chemoreceptors is the most important factor in the ventilatory set point. The central medullary chemoreceptors respond to the [H^+] in cerebrospinal fluid (CSF).

The Kidneys and Acid–Base Control

The kidneys are responsible for excretion of the fixed acids (nonvolatile acids). These acids amount to about 70 to 100 mmol/day. The kidneys also play an important role in the reabsorption of the filtered bicarbonate. Daily filtered bicarbonate equals the product of the daily glomerular filtration rate (180 L/day) and the plasma bicarbonate concentration (24 mmol/L; i.e., 4320 mmol/day). About 85% to 90% of the filtered bicarbonate is reabsorbed in the proximal tubule, and the intercalated cells of the distal tubule and collecting ducts reabsorb the rest. To understand the kidneys' role in acid–base control, it is helpful to have a basic understanding of renal physiology. You may recall that the kidneys regulate the body's acid–base balance through the proximal tubules, loop of Henle, and the distal tubules.

The proximal tubules are the main site for bicarbonate reabsorption. The mechanisms for bicarbonate reabsorption are shown in **Figure 4-11**. Four major factors regulate bicarbonate reabsorption: luminal [HCO_3^-], luminal flow rate, arterial P_{CO_2}, and angiotensin II (via decrease in cyclic AMP). An increase in any of these four factors causes an increase in bicarbonate reabsorption. Proximal renal tubules also produce ammonium (NH_3) besides reabsorbing bicarbonate. NH_3 is produced from glutamine by the action of the enzyme glutaminase and from glutamate during the conversion to alpha-ketoglutarate. Because the pK_a (dissociation constant) for NH_3 is very high (about 9.2), NH_3 is present entirely in the acid form as ammonium ion, or NH_4^+. The NH_4^+ is not measured as part of the titratable acid. About 75% of the ammonia produced in the proximal tubule is removed from the tubular fluid in the medulla. The amount of ammonium entering the distal tubule therefore is small. A low urine pH greatly increases the ammonium excretion. This ammonium excretion is augmented further if an acidosis is present, helping restore extracellular pH toward normal.

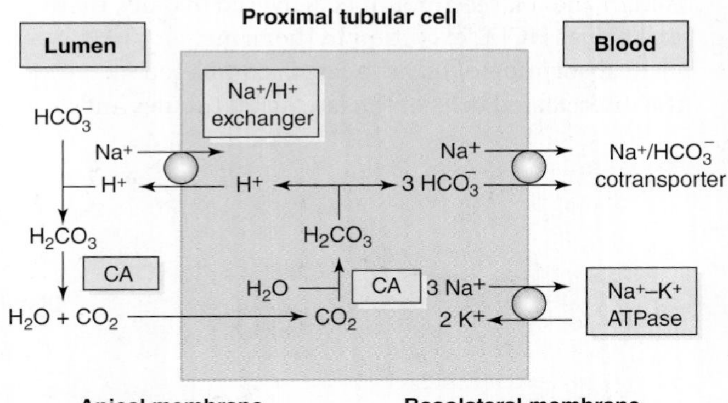

FIGURE 4-11 Schematic representation of the excretion of H^+ in the proximal renal tubules. The Na^+ is reabsorbed in exchange for H^+ via a Na^+–H^+ antiporter. The H^+ reacts with HCO_3 to form H_2O and CO_2 under the influence of brush border carbonic anhydrase (CA). CO_2, which is lipid soluble, then diffuses into the tubular cell. In the cell, CO_2 combines with H_2O to produce HCO_3^-. This process is also facilitated by carbonic anhydrase. The HCO_3^- crosses the basolateral membrane via a Na^+–HCO_3^- cotransporter, which transfers three HCO_3^- for every one Na^+. The basolateral membrane also has an active Na^+–K^+ ATPase (sodium pump), which transports three Na^+ out per two K^+ in. This pump is electrogenic in a direction opposite to that of the Na^+–HCO_3^- cotransporter. The net effect is the reabsorption of one molecule of HCO_3^- and one molecule of Na^+ from the tubular lumen for each molecule of H^+ secreted. This mechanism does not lead to the net excretion of any H^+ from the body because the H^+ is consumed in the reaction with the filtered bicarbonate in the tubular lumen. If the bicarbonate is not reabsorbed, this would be equivalent to an acidifying effect because it would mean that H^+ is accumulating in the cells.

HCO_3^- in the thick ascending limb of the loop of Henle is reabsorbed via mechanisms very similar to those in the proximal tubule. The cells in this part of the tubule also contain carbonic anhydrase. Bicarbonate reabsorption here is stimulated by the presence of luminal furosemide.

Compared with the proximal tubules, the distal renal tubules have a lower capacity for excreting the daily fixed acid load (≈70 mmol/day), although the capacity can increase to as much as 700 mmol/day as needed. The maximal capacity of excreting 700 mmol/day takes about 5 days to reach. The distal tubules can decrease the pH to about 4.5, thus creating a thousand-fold (or 3 pH units) gradient for H^+ across the distal tubular cell. The distal tubules excrete H^+ by reabsorbing the remaining bicarbonate and adding ammonium (NH_4^+) to luminal fluid.

The mechanisms of HCO_3^- reabsorption in the distal tubule are somewhat different from those in the proximal tubule **(Figure 4-12)**. The intercalated cells secrete H^+, involving an H^+–2ATPase (rather than Na^+–H^+ antiporter). HCO_3^- transfer across the basolateral membrane involves a HCO_3^-–Cl^- exchanger (rather than Na^+–HCO_3^- cotransporter). The net effect is the excretion of one H^+ in exchange for one HCO_3^- and one Na^+ to the bloodstream. The distal tubule has only a limited capacity to reabsorb HCO_3^-, so if the filtered HCO_3^- load is high and a large amount is delivered distally, there will be net HCO_3^- excretion in the urine.

Reabsorption of bicarbonate is completed in the intercalated cells of the late distal tubules and collecting ducts. At this site, excess H^+ is actively secreted and combines with phosphate ion and ammonia in the tubules. This process is responsible for reabsorption of the remaining 10% to 15% of the filtered HCO_3^-. This exchange process is achieved by several transporters, including the vacuolar H^+–ATPase (for H^+ secretion across the apical membrane); the Cl^-/HCO_3^- exchanger (for extruding HCO_3^- across the basolateral membrane); and carbonic anhydrase II (for providing both H^+ for luminal secretion and HCO_3^- for basolateral extrusion into the plasma).

As in the proximal tubules, H^+ also combines with ammonium (NH_3) in the distal tubules to form ammonium ion (NH_4^+) in the filtrate. NH_4^+ excretion in severe acidosis can reach 300 mmol/day in humans. H^+ can also be excreted as phosphate, the major component of titratable acids. The amount of phosphate present in the distal tubule, however, does not vary greatly, and changes in phosphate excretion play a minor role in response to an acid load.

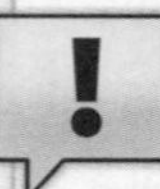

Respiratory Recap

Two Major Functions of the Kidney in Acid–Base Balance

- Excretion of the fixed acids (acid and associated H^+): about 1 mmol/kg/day
- Reabsorption of filtered bicarbonate: 4000 to 5000 mmol/day

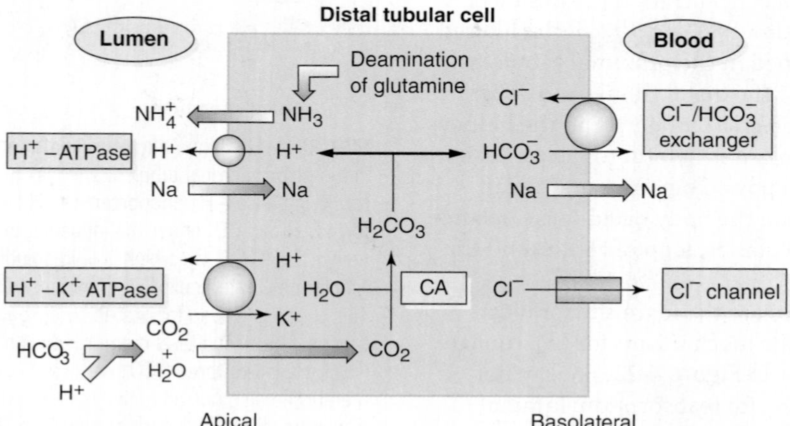

FIGURE 4-12 Schematic representation of the excretion of H^+ in the distal renal tubules. H^+ combines with NH_3 produced by deamination of amino acids to form NH_4^+. This is exchanged for Na^+ that is returned to the bloodstream. H^+ is secreted by the intercalated cells via an H^+–ATPase (rather than a Na^+–H^+ antiporter). Like in the proximal renal cell, HCO_3^- in the distal tubular lumen also combines with H^+ to form H_2O and CO_2. CO_2 then diffuses into the tubular cell, combining with H_2O to produce HCO_3^-. HCO_3^- is transferred across the basolateral membrane via a HCO_3^-–Cl^- exchanger (rather than a Na^+–HCO_3 cotransporter). The net effect is the excretion of one H^+ in exchange for one HCO_3^- and one Na^+ to the bloodstream. The distal tubule has only a limited capacity to reabsorb HCO_3^-, so if the filtered HCO_3^- load is high and a large amount is delivered distally, there will be net HCO_3^- excretion in the urine. CA, carbonic anhydrase.

In summary, the following factors regulate renal bicarbonate reabsorption and acid excretion:

- *Extracellular volume.* When the volume depletion decreases glomerular filtration rate (GFR), the filtered load of bicarbonate is proportionately reduced. The Na^+ retention in response to volume depletion enhances HCO_3^- reabsorption. Conversely, ECF volume expansion results in renal Na^+ excretion and secondary decrease in HCO_3^- reabsorption.
- *Arterial PCO_2.* An increase in arterial PCO_2 (hypercapnia), which increases the production of carbonic acid, increases renal H^+ secretion and HCO_3^- reabsorption. The HCO_3^- retention explains the renal compensation for chronic respiratory acidosis.
- *Potassium and chloride deficiency.* Hypokalemia (low K^+ levels) increases the secretion of H^+ in the renal tubules, resulting in increases in HCO_3^- reabsorption in the kidney. Low chloride increases reabsorption of more HCO_3^- along with Na^+.
- *Phosphate excretion.* Because the amount of phosphate present in the distal tubule does not vary greatly, changes in phosphate excretion play a minor role in response to an acid load.
- *Ammonium.* The kidney responds to an acid load by increasing tubular production and urinary excretion of NH_4^+. Increases in ammonium excretion take several days to reach their maximum. Ammonium excretion increases when urine pH decreases, and this relationship is markedly enhanced with acidosis.
- *Aldosterone and cortisol (hydrocortisone).* Aldosterone at normal levels has no role in renal regulation of acid–base balance. High aldosterone levels (as in hyperaldosteronism) increase Na^+ reabsorption and urinary excretion of H^+ and K^+, resulting in a metabolic alkalosis. Low aldosterone alone, on the other hand, rarely is associated with a metabolic acidosis. Low serum cortisol (as in adrenal insufficiency) can cause a mild metabolic acidosis that has a normal gap.

Acid–Base Disorders

Respiratory Acidosis

There is a low pH and an elevated $PaCO_2$ (hypercapnia) with **respiratory acidosis**. Respiratory acidosis occurs because of alveolar hypoventilation or severe $\dot{V}/\dot{Q}$ mismatch. **Table 4-5** shows common causes of respiratory acidosis. Chronic obstructive pulmonary disease (COPD) is a most common cause of chronic respiratory acidosis. When respiratory acidosis is uncompensated, this implies acute ventilatory failure. Renal compensation for respiratory acidosis begins as soon as $PaCO_2$ rises. Full compensation usually takes days.

TABLE 4-5
Common Causes of Respiratory Acidosis

Associated with Alveolar Hypoventilation
Drugs: anesthetics, sedatives, hypnotics, narcotics
Neuromuscular diseases: poliomyelitis, myasthenia gravis, Guillain-Barré syndrome, amyotrophic lateral sclerosis
Morbid obesity (Pickwickian syndrome)
Severe kyphoscoliosis
Idiopathic (primary alveolar hypoventilation syndrome)
Associated with Severe Ventilation-Perfusion Mismatch
Chronic obstructive pulmonary disease
Advanced diffuse lung parenchymal diseases (such as sarcoidosis or pulmonary fibrosis)

Respiratory Alkalosis

Respiratory alkalosis is associated with reduction in $PaCO_2$ due to hyperventilation. Reduction in $PaCO_2$ reduces H_2CO_3 and thus $[HCO_3^-]$ in plasma. Two compensatory responses minimize the fall in $[H^+]$: (1) retention of Cl^- through a fall in its renal excretion and (2) a small accumulation of lactate resulting from the stimulation of glycolysis in erythrocytes and the liver. Retention of Cl^- characterizes chronic states of hyperventilation, but increases in the concentration of lactate may occur very rapidly. These compensatory changes are associated with increases in $[H^+]$ and a fall in $[HCO_3^-]$. The reductions in $PaCO_2$ and $[H^+]$ in hyperventilation are accompanied by a surprisingly large increase in carbonate (CO_3^{2-}), predisposing to hypocalcemia and tetany. **Table 4-6** lists conditions that lead to respiratory alkalosis. Respiratory alkalosis can also be caused by overly aggressive mechanical ventilation.

Metabolic Acidosis

With **metabolic acidosis**, the pH is decreased with decreased HCO_3^-. Processes that increase the production of nonvolatile acids or lead to an excessive loss of bases from the body can produce metabolic acidosis. Both processes increase $[H^+]$ and decrease pH. Acidosis is a potent stimulus to increase ventilation, and as a consequence PCO_2 falls. The compensatory hyperventilation of metabolic acidosis is characterized by deep and labored breathing with normal or reduced frequency, a breathing pattern referred to as Kussmaul respirations. The initial stimulation of the central chemoreceptors is due to small increases in $[H^+]$

TABLE 4-6
Common Causes of Respiratory Alkalosis

Associated with Normal Lungs
Anxiety
Fever
Drug overdose: salicylates, respiratory stimulants (such as strychnine)
CNS lesions: encephalitis, meningitis, tumor
Pregnancy
Sepsis
Liver cirrhosis
High altitudes
Associated with Ventilation-Perfusion Mismatch
Acute bronchial asthma
Pneumonia
Pulmonary vascular diseases: pulmonary embolism
Early diffuse lung parenchymal diseases (such as sarcoidosis or pulmonary fibrosis)
Pulmonary edema
Iatrogenic
Overly aggressive mechanical ventilation

TABLE 4-7
Common Causes of Metabolic Acidosis

Increased Unmeasured Ions (Increased Gap, Increased Nonvolatile Acids)
Ketoacidosis: diabetic, alcoholic, starvation
Lactic acidosis: hypoxia, circulatory failure, drugs and toxins, enzyme defects
Poisoning: salicylates, ethylene glycol, methanol
Renal failure
Normal Unmeasured Ions (Normal Gap, Loss of Bicarbonate)
Renal tubular acidosis, chronic pyelonephritis, obstructive uropathy
Hypoaldosteronism
Potassium-sparing diuretics (spironolactone)
Diarrhea
Pancreatic or biliary fistulas, ureterosigmoidostomy
Carbonic anhydrase inhibitors: acetazolamide
Excessive intake of ammonium chloride, cationic amino acids

in the CSF. The increase in ventilation causes a fall in arterial P_{CO_2}, which inhibits the ventilatory response. The increase in ventilation in response to metabolic acidosis usually starts within minutes and is usually well advanced at 2 hours of onset, but maximal compensation may take 12 to 24 hours to develop.

The effectiveness of the compensatory hyperventilation also depends on the ventilatory capacity, the efficiency of pulmonary gas exchange, and the ventilatory control mechanisms. Patients with lung diseases and central nervous system diseases may not be able to mount an adequate ventilatory compensation response and thus are prone to more severe acidosis. A number of other factors may also weaken this hyperventilation effect. For example, in diabetic acidosis, severe dehydration may increase [Na^+] and decrease GFR, resulting in increased HCO_3^- reabsorption. The concomitant metabolic alkalosis thus serves to offset some degree of acidosis. In patients with acidosis due to kidney diseases, such as uremia, these adaptive responses may not be available.

Metabolic acidosis is traditionally categorized based on the size of the anion gap into increased anion gap versus normal anion gap acidosis. **Table 4-7** lists common causes of metabolic acidosis.

Metabolic Alkalosis

Metabolic alkalosis is diagnosed by increased pH in association with increased HCO_3^-. Metabolic alkalosis usually occurs when there is a loss of fixed acids or a gain in blood buffer base. Fixed acids can be lost from the renal or gastrointestinal route. In this case, serum Cl^- is usually decreased and metabolic alkalosis can be corrected by replacing intravascular volume with saline (NaCl) (chloride-responsive metabolic alkalosis). Diuresis can cause a contraction alkalosis. High aldosterone and cortisol increase Na^+ reabsorption and urinary excretion of H^+ and K^+. The process increases HCO_3^- reabsorption, resulting in metabolic alkalosis. In these conditions, serum Cl^- is usually unaffected and metabolic alkalosis does not respond to saline replacement (chloride-unresponsive metabolic alkalosis). Ingestion of bicarbonate may also cause metabolic alkalosis, especially when the amount exceeds the bicarbonate-excreting capacity of the kidneys.

Low potassium (hypokalemia) increases H^+ secretion in the renal tubules, resulting in increased reabsorption of HCO_3^-. Severe loss of K^+ may accompany Cl^- in the kidneys, leading to depletion of intracellular [K^+] and a fall in intracellular [H^+]—an intracellular acidosis complicating an extracellular alkalosis. This effect may lead to respiratory muscle weakness, as sometimes seen in periodic paralysis. Correction of metabolic alkalosis requires the correction of hypokalemia in this case. **Table 4-8** lists common causes of metabolic alkalosis.

Arterial Blood Gas Interpretation

ABG interpretation is critical to diagnosing and managing a patient's oxygenation status and acid–base balance. Disorders of acid–base balance can create

TABLE 4-8
Common Causes of Metabolic Alkalosis

Associated with Chloride (Volume) Depletion (Chloride-Responsive)
Vomiting, gastric drainage
Diuretic therapy (contraction alkalosis)
Posthypercapnic alkalosis
Associated with Hyperadrenocorticism (Chloride-Unresponsive)
Cushing syndrome
Primary aldosteronism
Bartter syndrome
Licorice ingestion
Excessive Alkali Intake
Milk-alkali syndrome
Ingestion of sodium bicarbonate
Severe Potassium Depletion

complications in many diseases and the abnormality may become life threatening. Low oxygenation levels in the body (**hypoxia**) or high oxygen levels (**hyperoxia**) also can have harmful effects that can become life threatening. The usefulness of this diagnostic tool is dependent on being able to correctly interpret the results.

A number of variables affect oxygenation, ventilation, and acid–base balance. In most cases, the difficulty stems from trying to make sense of all the measurements at once. By separately considering the values that represent oxygenation and those that indicate acid–base balance, it will not be difficult to make sense of an ABG report to make an interpretation.

Normal Arterial Blood Gas Values

Blood is slightly alkalotic, which affects interpretation of blood pH values (**Table 4-9**). Normal blood pH

TABLE 4-9
Normal Arterial Blood Gases

pH	7.35–7.45
$Paco_2$	35–45 mm Hg
HCO_3^-	22–24 mmol/L
Pao_2	80–100 mm Hg (breathing room air at sea level)
Sao_2	95%–98% (breathing room air at sea level)

ranges from 7.35 to 7.45 and is determined primarily by $Paco_2$ and HCO_3^-. Acids are released as normal waste products of cellular metabolism. Carbonic acid is a volatile acid that is eliminated by the lungs in the form of CO_2. Other acids in the body are fixed acids, which are either excreted by the kidneys or buffered. Acid in the body is in the form of hydrogen ion (H^+) and has an inverse relationship with pH. In other words, high acid (H^+) is reflected as low pH (acidosis).

$$\uparrow H^+ \rightarrow \downarrow pH$$

Abnormalities in the blood pH have a harmful effect on many critical functions of the body, including cardiac contraction, tissue oxygenation, enzyme systems, hormone production, and cellular functions. Normal physiology requires a pH within the normal range. Therefore, the body compensates for acid–base defects to maintain a normal blood pH.

$Paco_2$ is affected by ventilation, which is determined by alveolar ventilation. A normal $Paco_2$ range is 35 to 45 mm Hg. $Paco_2$ is an indicator of the adequacy of ventilation to remove CO_2 from the lungs. High $Paco_2$ indicates alveolar hypoventilation and will cause the arterial pH to go down. $Paco_2$ below normal limits is due to **hypoventilation**, while $Paco_2$ above normal is due to hyperventilation.

$$\uparrow PaCO_2 \rightarrow \downarrow pH$$

HCO_3^- is normally between 22 and 26 mmol/L. Bicarbonate is alkaline and has a direct relationship with the pH because it buffers acid.

$$\uparrow HCO_3^- \rightarrow \uparrow pH$$

The Pao_2 and Sao_2 reflect oxygenation of the arterial blood. Pao_2 is the partial pressure of oxygen in the arterial blood with a normal range of 80 to 100 mm Hg at sea level breathing room air. Sao_2 reflects the hemoglobin saturation of oxygen in arterial blood. Normal Sao_2 is 95% to 98% breathing room air at sea level. To determine acid–base status, pH, $Paco_2$, and HCO_3^- are considered. To determine oxygenation status, Pao_2 and Sao_2 are considered.

Seven-Step Approach to ABG Interpretation

For a consistent approach to ABG interpretation, follow seven steps in consecutive order to first interpret acid–base and then interpret oxygenation. Applying these seven steps in a consistent manner will help make a correct ABG interpretation for most conditions. However, more advanced techniques are sometimes needed when there are multiple conditions requiring complex interventions.

Step 1: Conduct (or review) clinical assessment, including baseline values and overall clinical diagnosis. Clinical assessment, an essential first step, provides insight based on the available clinical information (history, physical examination, and interventions).

When interpreting an ABG, a relevant clinical history of the patient often suggests the etiology of an acid–base disorder. For example, a patient with a history of hypotension, renal failure, and uncontrolled diabetic status or treatment with drugs such as metformin is likely to have metabolic acidosis. A patient with a history of diuretic use, bicarbonate administration, high nasogastric aspirate, and vomiting is likely to have metabolic alkalosis. Respiratory acidosis would occur in COPD, muscular weakness, postoperative cases, and opioid overdose, and respiratory alkalosis is likely to occur in sepsis, hepatic coma, and pregnancy.

Similarly, relevant clinical information can provide insights into the etiology of hypoxemia. For example, acute hypoxemia is a feature of acute respiratory distress syndrome and chronic hypoxemia is associated with COPD.

Step 2: Assess pH. Is it normal, acidic, or alkalotic? Assess the pH and determine if it is normal, acidotic (pH <7.35), or alkalotic (pH >7.45). Note that the pH might be normal, but the acid–base physiology is abnormal because of compensation. This will be assessed in step 4.

Step 3: Assess $Paco_2$. Is it normal, low, or high? Assess the $Paco_2$ and determine if it is normal (35–45 mm Hg), high (>45 mm Hg), or low (<35 mm Hg). High $Paco_2$ indicates respiratory acidosis or compensation for metabolic alkalosis. Low $Paco_2$ indicates respiratory alkalosis or compensation for metabolic acidosis.

Step 4: Assess HCO_3^-. Is it normal (22–26 mmol/L), high (>26 mmol/L), or low (<22 mmol/L)? A bicarbonate <22 mmol/L indicates metabolic acidosis or compensation for respiratory alkalosis; while a bicarbonate >26 mmol/L indicates metabolic alkalosis or compensation for respiratory acidosis.

Step 5: Compare $Paco_2$ and HCO_3^- with pH. Compare the $Paco_2$ and the HCO_3^- with the pH to determine the acid–base disorder. For example, if the pH is low (acidotic), and the $Paco_2$ is high (acidotic) with a normal HCO_3^-, there is a respiratory acid–base disturbance. Therefore, it is a respiratory acidosis. If the pH is low (acidotic) and the HCO_3^- is low (acidotic) with a normal $Paco_2$, the disturbance is metabolic acidosis such as caused by renal failure, diabetic ketoacidosis, or lactic acidosis. Both of these examples are simple acid–base disorders because only one system is contributing to the acid–base disorder and there is no compensation.

If the pH is >7.45, the HCO_3^- is >26 mmol/L, with the $Paco_2$ normal, the acid–base disturbance is a metabolic alkalosis. If the pH is >7.45, the $Paco_2$ is <35 mm Hg, and the HCO_3^- is normal, it is a respiratory alkalosis.

If both the respiratory system and the renal system are contributing to the same acid–base disorder (low or high pH), it is referred to as a mixed or combined disorder. For example, a respiratory and metabolic acidosis occurs when there is high $Paco_2$ and low HCO_3^- creating a low arterial blood pH <7.35. A respiratory and metabolic alkalosis occurs when there is low $Paco_2$ and high HCO_3^- creating a high arterial blood pH of >7.45.

Step 6: Is $Paco_2$ or HCO_3^- in the opposite direction or the same direction as the pH? Look to see if the $Paco_2$ and the pH are moving in the same direction or opposite direction. As explained in the previous step, if both the respiratory system and the renal system move in opposite directions and contribute to more acid, it is a mixed acidosis. If both the respiratory system and the renal system move in the opposite directions and contribute to less acid in the body, it is a mixed alkalosis. However, if the body tries to compensate for acid–base disorders by having the renal and respiratory systems move in the same direction to maintain a normal arterial blood pH, it is a compensated disorder.

Recall from step 1 that the pH can be normal, but the acid–base physiology may be abnormal because the body has compensated for it. Compensation can be seen when both the $Paco_2$ and HCO_3^- rise or fall together to maintain a normal pH. This is because CO_2 is a volatile acid that lowers pH, while HCO_3^- buffers acid and raises pH. Partial compensation occurs when the $Paco_2$ and HCO_3^- rise or fall together, but the pH remains abnormal. This indicates a compensatory mechanism attempted to restore a normal pH. The body will do just enough to compensate to restore blood pH to within normal limits. Knowing this key concept helps to differentiate which system is causing the acid–base disorder and which system is compensating to restore blood pH within normal limits.

Table 4-10 gives a basic overview of how changes in pH, $Paco_2$, and HCO_3^- are used to correctly interpret an acid–base disorder. Note that it is advisable to learn the concepts and apply the steps rather than try to memorize the table. The table is provided to help in grasping the concepts through application of these steps to ABG interpretation. Also note that for the preliminary assessment, the acid–base status is determined before looking at the values for blood oxygenation.

However, determining compensation is challenging because of a nonlinear compensatory response. Additionally, the time lapse between the onset of a primary acid–base disorder and the clinical evaluation may be a problem. Recall it takes time for the body to fully compensate for a primary acid–base disorder. Lung compensation for a metabolic acid–base

TABLE 4-10
Overview of Changes in pH, $Paco_2$, and HCO_3^- for Interpretation of Acid–Base Disorders

Interpretation	pH (acid–base)	$Paco_2$ (respiratory)*	HCO_3^- (metabolic)**
Respiratory Acidosis			
Acute/uncompensated	<7.35	>45	Normal
Partially compensated	<7.35	>45	>26
Compensated	Normal (low range)	>45	>26
Metabolic Acidosis			
Acute/uncompensated	<7.35	Normal	<22
Partially compensated	<7.35	<35	<22
Compensated	Normal (low range)	<35	<22
Respiratory Alkalosis			
Acute/uncompensated	>7.45	<35	Normal
Partially compensated	>7.45	<35	<22
Compensated	Normal (high range)	<35	<22
Metabolic Alkalosis			
Acute/uncompensated	>7.45	Normal	>26
Partially compensated	>7.45	>45	>26
Compensated	Normal (high range)	>45	>26
Respiratory and Metabolic Acidosis			
	<7.35	>45	<22
Respiratory and Metabolic Alkalosis			
	>7.45	<35	>26

*$Paco_2$ in mm Hg; **HCO_3^- in mmol/L

disorder occurs fairly quickly and can take minutes. However, renal compensation for a respiratory acid–base disorder can take as long as 3 to 5 days. Therefore, uncertainty about the onset of a respiratory disorder would complicate the interpretation of renal compensation. Various equations are used to describe the expected degree of compensation. Sample equations are shown in **Box 4-2.** Clinically, the equations for respiratory compensation are most accurate because the relationship is linear and the equations are less accurate for metabolic compensation.

Therefore, the most accurate method is the confidence band technique, shown in **Figure 4-13**. If the expected and actual values match, there is no evidence of a mixed disorder (i.e., changes in $Paco_2$ or HCO_3^- can be fully explained by the compensatory response). Note that maximal compensation does not return the extracellular pH to normal. This is the main reason why pH indicated the primary disorder. The compensatory response for an acid–base disorder should be interpreted in the context of the clinical evaluation of the patient's condition. This clinical assessment should include factors of time, therapies, and the functioning of the pulmonary and renal systems. If the changes in $Paco_2$ or HCO_3^- cannot be adequately explained by the compensatory response, an additional step is needed to determine what kind of second or even third acid–base disorder may be present. This process can be greatly facilitated by reviewing other clues, some of which are summarized in Table 4-10. Once a diagnosis of acid–base disorder is made, additional therapies or tests can be used to determine causes.

Step 7: Are the Pao_2 and Sao_2 normal, low, or high? Only after correctly interpreting the acid–base status using an ABG should the oxygenation status be interpreted. Looking at the arterial oxygenation Pao_2 and Sao_2

BOX 4-2

Expected Compensation for Acid–Base Disturbances*

Renal Compensation for Respiratory Acidosis

Predicted $[HCO_3^-] = 24 + (Paco_2 - 40) \times 0.1$ (acute)
Predicted $[HCO_3^-] = 24 + (Paco_2 - 40) \times 0.35$ (chronic)

Renal Compensation for Respiratory Alkalosis

Predicted $[HCO_3^-] = 24 - (40 - Paco_2) \times 0.2$ (acute)
Predicted $[HCO_3^-] = 24 - (40 - Paco_2) \times 0.5$ (chronic)

Respiratory Compensation for Metabolic Acidosis

Predicted $Paco_2 = 1.5 \times [HCO_3^-] + 8$

Respiratory Compensation for Metabolic Alkalosis

Predicted $Paco_2 = 0.73 \times [HCO_3^-] + 20$

*If the acid–base status exceeds the expected level of compensation, a mixed acid–base disturbance is present.

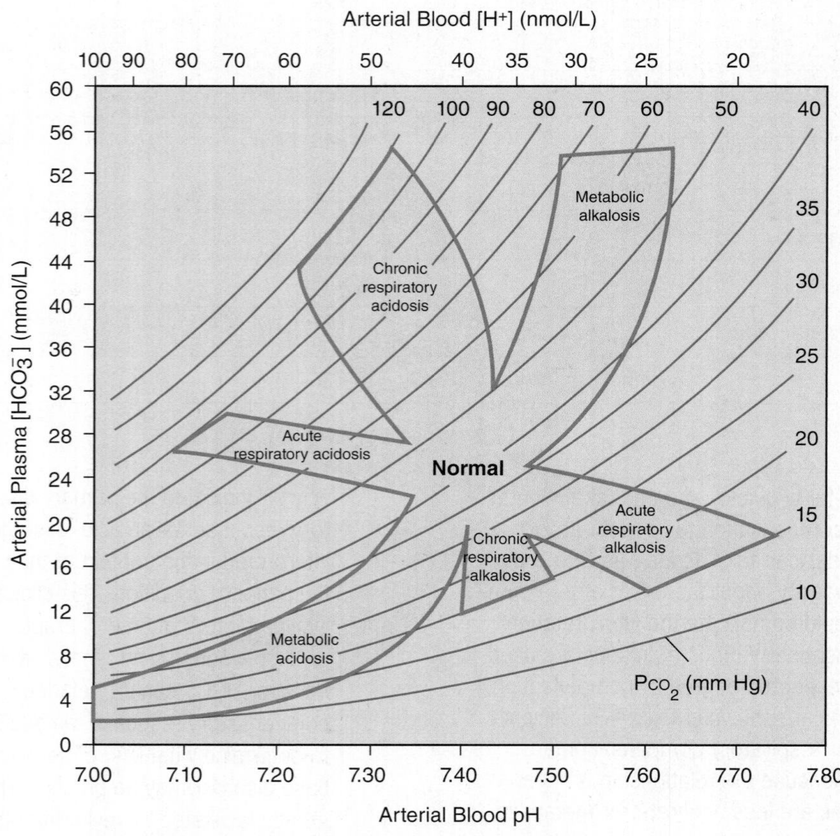

FIGURE 4-13 Davenport diagram for acid–base disorders.

Reproduced from *Fluid & Electrolytes: Physiology & Pathophysiology* by Cogan M.G. (editor). Copyright 1991 by McGraw-Hill Companies, Inc.

provides information about the arterial oxygen supply. Pao_2 = partial pressure of oxygen dissolved in arterial blood, with normal ranges from 80 to 100 mm Hg. Sao_2 = saturation of hemoglobin with normal ranges at 95% or better. Pao_2 and Sao_2 below normal often call for immediate action. Keep in mind that lower oxygen levels are expected at high altitudes, in older people, and in those with COPD.

Pao_2 <40 mm Hg is severe **hypoxemia**. Pao_2 between 40 and 59 mm Hg is moderate hypoxemia.

Pa_{O_2} of 60 mm Hg or greater but less than the predicted normal for age is mild hypoxemia. Pa_{O_2} greater than normal is hyperoxemia. The Pa_{O_2} should be interpreted relative to F_{IO_2} and, if mechanically ventilated, the level of positive end-expiratory pressure (PEEP).

Case Studies

Case 1. Acute Respiratory Acidosis

A 30-year-old unconscious male patient is brought into the emergency room with the following arterial blood gas values breathing room air: pH 7.27, Pa_{CO_2} 56 mm Hg, Pa_{O_2} 70 mm Hg, HCO_3^- 26 mmol/L, $[Na^+]$ 140 mmol/L, $[K^+]$ 4.0 mmol/L, and $[Cl^-]$ 105 mmol/L. The following steps should be performed:

Step 1: Conduct a physical assessment. Physical exam indicates that the patient is unconscious while breathing room air with slow respiratory rate, bradycardia, and hypotension. Body temperature is normal and chest exam is unremarkable.

Step 2: Examine arterial pH. The pH is decreased. Thus, an acidosis is present.

Step 3: Assess the Pa_{CO_2}. The Pa_{CO_2} is increased, indicating hypoventilation.

Step 4: Assess the HCO_3^-. The bicarbonate is in normal range.

Step 5: Compare the Pa_{CO_2} and the HCO_3^- with the pH to determine the acid–base disorder. Determine whether the acidosis is of respiratory or metabolic origin. Because the Pa_{CO_2} is 56 mm Hg and HCO_3^- is normal, this is a respiratory acidosis.

Step 6: Determine if the Pa_{CO_2} and HCO_3^- are moving in the same or the opposite directions. The Pa_{CO_2} is high, but the HCO_3^- is normal. We determine that this is an acute respiratory acidosis with no compensation or secondary acid–base disorder. Because the patient is young and unconscious, with depressed vital signs, it is reasonable to suspect that this patient's acute respiratory acidosis is due to drug overdose with respiratory center depression.

Step 7: Look at the Pa_{O_2} and Sa_{O_2} to determine adequacy of oxygenation. The Sa_{O_2} is not reported, but we would expect a Pa_{O_2} of >90 mm Hg in someone 30 years of age breathing room air. This Pa_{O_2} indicates hypoxemia.

Summarize ABG Interpretation: This is an acute respiratory acidosis with mild hypoxemia. It is not necessary to calculate the anion gap or SID because it is a straightforward case.

Case 2. Partially Compensated Metabolic Acidosis

A 55-year-old woman with a known history of diabetes arrives in the emergency department in a coma having gasping, deep respirations breathing room air. ABG analysis shows pH 7.25, Pa_{CO_2} 20 mm Hg, Pa_{O_2} 90 mm Hg, HCO_3^- 10 mmol/L, $[Na^+]$ 140 mmol/L, $[K^+]$ 4.0 mmol/L, and $[Cl^-]$ 105 mmol/L.

Step 1: Physical exam indicates that the patient is unconscious while breathing room air with rapid respiratory rate, deep breathing, tachycardia, and high blood pressure. Body temperature is normal and chest exam is unremarkable.

Step 2: Examine arterial pH. The pH is decreased. Thus, an acidosis is present.

Step 3: Assess the Pa_{CO_2}. The Pa_{CO_2} is decreased, indicating hyperventilation.

Step 4: Assess the HCO_3^-. The bicarbonate is low.

Step 5: Compare the Pa_{CO_2} and the HCO_3^- with the pH to determine the acid–base disorder. Determine whether the acidosis is of respiratory or metabolic origin. Because the Pa_{CO_2} is low and HCO_3^- is low, this is consistent with metabolic acidosis.

Step 6: Determine if the Pa_{CO_2} and HCO_3^- are moving in the same or the opposite directions. The Pa_{CO_2} is low and HCO_3^- is low. This is an acute metabolic acidosis with partial compensation.

Step 7: Look at the Pa_{O_2} and Sa_{O_2} to determine adequacy of oxygenation. The Sa_{O_2} is not reported, but a Pa_{O_2} of >80 mm Hg is expected in someone 55 years old breathing room air. This ABG indicates a Pa_{O_2} of 90 mm Hg, so there is no hypoxemia.

Additional Step: Because this is a metabolic acidosis and the electrolytes are available, it would be appropriate to calculate the anion gap.

$$\text{Gap} = [Na^+] - ([Cl^-] + [HCO_3^-]) = 140 - (105 + 10) = 25 \text{ mmol/L}$$

This is a high anion gap; normal is 12 ± 4 mmol/L. The anion gap indicates that the metabolic acidosis is due to increase in unmeasured anions.

Summarize ABG Interpretation: This is a partially compensated metabolic acidosis without hypoxemia. The patient history, physical exam, and high anion gap indicate increased unmeasured anions, most likely due to ketoacidosis, consistent with diabetic coma.

Case 3. Partially Compensated Respiratory Acidosis

A 62-year-old man with ARDS is mechanically ventilated. ABG analysis shows pH 7.25, Pa_{CO_2} 70 mm Hg, HCO_3^- 30 mmol/L, Pa_{O_2} 58 mm Hg, and Sa_{O_2} 88%. The F_{IO_2} is 0.8 and the PEEP is set at 12 cm H_2O.

Step 1: Physical exam indicates a comatose patient receiving full respiratory support. Bilateral infiltrates are present on the chest x-ray.

Step 2: Examine arterial pH. The pH is decreased. Thus, acidosis is present.

Step 3: Assess the Pa_{CO_2}. The Pa_{CO_2} is increased, indicating hypoventilation.

Step 4: Assess the HCO_3^-. The bicarbonate is increased.

Step 5: Compare the $Paco_2$ and the HCO_3^- with the pH to determine the acid–base disorder. Because the $Paco_2$ and HCO_3^- are high, the respiratory system is contributing to the acidosis, while the bicarbonate indicates less acid or more base. Given the clinical context, this is likely respiratory acidosis.

Step 6: Determine if the $Paco_2$ and HCO_3^- are moving in the same or the opposite directions. Both the $Paco_2$ and HCO_3^- are elevated. This is most likely a partially compensated respiratory acidosis.

Step 7: Look at the Pao_2 and Sao_2 to determine adequacy of oxygenation. The Sao_2 and Pao_2 are both lower than normal. The Pao_2 is interpreted as moderate hypoxemia.

Summarize ABG Interpretation: This is a partially compensated respiratory acidosis with moderate hypoxemia breathing 80% oxygen.

Key Points

- Arterial blood samples are used to analyze Po_2, Pco_2, pH, and So_2, carboxyhemoglobin, and methemoglobin.
- Common preanalytic errors include sample contamination with air or heparin and a prolonged time between sample procurement and analysis.
- Calibration, quality control, and proficiency testing are used to ensure correct blood gas analyzer function.
- Temperature correction of blood gases is unnecessary.
- The radial artery is the preferred site for arterial puncture because it is easily accessible, it is relatively insensitive to pain, and the hand has collateral circulation.
- Arterial cannulation is performed when frequent arterial blood gas measurements are required.
- Capillary blood gases may be used to estimate pH and Pco_2 in infants or other individuals when arterial blood gas analysis is indicated.
- The Henderson-Hasselbalch equation suggests the equilibrium that exists between bicarbonate and carbon dioxide.
- The modified Henderson-Hasselbalch equation is clinically useful to check for inaccuracies due to blood gas analyzer problems, transcription mistakes, or other errors. It is also useful to anticipate what effect changing one variable will have on overall acid–base balance.
- The lungs regulate nonvolatile acid in the form of CO_2 and the kidneys regulate volatile acids, also called fixed acids, as well as the reabsorption of filtered bicarbonate.
- The anion gap represents the concentration of the unmeasured anions and can be used to determine the general cause of an acid–base disorder.
- The strong ion difference is yet another approach to determine unmeasured anions and is considered even more refined than using the anion gap, though more difficult to calculate.
- The primary acid–base disturbances are respiratory acidosis, respiratory alkalosis, metabolic acidosis, and metabolic alkalosis.
- Combined acid–base disturbances occur when the lungs and kidneys both contribute to either acidosis or alkalosis.
- The lungs can compensate for metabolic acid–base disturbances and the kidneys can compensate for respiratory acid–base disturbances.

References

1. Castro HJ, Oropello JM, Halpern N. Point-of-care testing in the intensive care unit: the intensive care physician's perspective. *Am J Clin Pathol.* 1995;104(4 Suppl 1):S95–S99.
2. Kendall J, Reeves B, Clancy M. Point of care testing: randomised controlled trial of clinical outcome. *BMJ.* 1998;316: 1052–1057.
3. Chen K, Puan RB, Price KJ, Koller CA, Nates JL. The role of point-of-care testing in the early diagnosis of pseudo-hypoxemia in myeloproliferative disorders. *Respir Care.* 2010;55: 777–779.
4. Papadea C, Foster J, Grant S, et al. Evaluation of the i-STAT Portable Clinical Analyzer for point-of-care blood testing in the intensive care unit of a university children's hospital. *Ann Clin Lab Sci.* 2002;32:231–243.
5. Knowles TP, Mullin RA, Hunter JA, Douce FH. Effects of syringe material, sample storage time, and temperature on blood gases and oxygen saturation in arterialized human blood samples. *Respir Care.* 2006;51:732–736.
6. Baher A. Effects of body temperature on blood gases. *Intensive Care Med.* 2005;31:24–27.
7. Rahn H. Body temperature and acid-base regulation. *Pneumonologie.* 1974;151:87–94.
8. Hansen JE. Arterial blood gases. *Clin Chest Med.* 1989;10: 227–237.
9. Dorwart WV, Chalmers L. Comparison of methods for calculating serum osmolality from chemical concentrations, and the prognostic value of such calculations. *Clin Chem.* 1975;21:190–194.
10. Kellum JA. Determinants of blood pH in health and disease. *Crit Care.* 2000;4:6–14.
11. Fencl V, Jabor A, Kazda A, Figge J. Diagnosis of metabolic acid–base disturbances in critically ill patients. *Am J Respir Crit Care Med.* 2000;162:2246–2251.
12. Figge J, Mydosh T, Fencl V. Serum proteins and acid–base equilibria: a follow-up. *J Lab Clin Med.* 1992;120:713–719.
13. Wilkes P. Hypoproteinemia, strong-ion difference, and acid–base status in critically ill patients. *J Appl Physiol.* 1998;84: 1740–1748.
14. Liskaser FJ, Bellomo R, Hayhoe M, et al. Role of pump prime in the etiology and pathogenesis of cardiopulmonary bypass-associated acidosis. *Anesthesiology.* 2000;93:1170–1173.
15. Story DA, Poustie S, Bellomo R. Estimating unmeasured anions in critically ill patients: anion-gap, base-deficit, and strong-ion-gap. *Anaesthesia.* 2002;57:1109–1114.
16. Figge J, Jabor A, Kazda A, Fencl V. Anion gap and hypoalbuminemia. *Crit Care Med.* 1998;26:1807–1810.
17. Scheingraber S, Rehm M, Sehmisch C, Finsterer U. Rapid saline infusion produces hyperchloremic acidosis in patients undergoing gynecologic surgery. *Anesthesiology.* 1999;90:1265–1270.
18. Constable PD. Hyperchloremic acidosis: the classic example of strong ion acidosis. *Anesth Analg.* 2003;96:919–922.

19. Rehm M, Finsterer U. Treating intraoperative hyperchloremic acidosis with sodium bicarbonate or tris-hydroxymethyl aminomethane: a randomized prospective study. *Anesth Analg.* 2003;96:1201–1208.
20. Rocktaschel J, Morimatsu H, Uchino S, et al. Impact of continuous veno-venous hemofiltration on acid–base balance. *Int J Artif Organs.* 2003;26:19–25.
21. Kellum JA. Clinical review: reunification of acid-base physiology. *Crit Care.* 2005;9:500–507.
22. Moviat M, van Haren F, van der Hoeven H. Conventional or physicochemical approach in intensive care unit patients with metabolic acidosis. *Crit Care.* 2003;7:R41–R45.
23. Busse L, Chawla L, Panchamia R, et al. Strong ion gap can be accurately estimated with a simple bedside equation. *Crit Care.* 2013;17(Suppl 2):P444.

CHAPTER

5

Blood Chemistries and Hematology

Michal Senitko, Rajesh Bhagat, Neil R. MacIntyre

OUTLINE

OBJECTIVES

1. Discuss the physiology of normal fluid and electrolyte balance.
2. List causes of abnormal electrolyte levels.
3. Discuss the effects of renal function on serum chemistry.
4. Discuss the role of serum enzymes in assessing liver and cardiac function.
5. Describe laboratory tests used to assess coagulation.
6. Discuss abnormalities of hemoglobin, platelets, and leukocytes.

KEY TERMS

activated partial thromboplastin time (aPTT)
anion gap
anions
bilirubinemia
blood urea nitrogen (BUN)
brain natriuretic peptide (BNP)
cardiac enzymes
cation
C-reactive protein (CRP)
creatinine
diabetic ketoacidosis
extracellular fluid
hematocrit
hemoglobin
hypercalcemia
hyperchloremia
hyperkalemia
hypermagnesemia
hypernatremia
hyperosmolar
hyperphosphatemia
hypocalcemia
hypochloremia
hypokalemia
hypomagnesemia
hyponatremia
hypophosphatemia
intracellular fluid
lactate
leucopenia
leukocytes
leukocytosis
new oral anticoagulants
oncotic pressures
platelets
procalcitonin
proteins
prothrombin time (PT)
pseudohypoxemia
serum electrolytes
troponin
unmeasured anions

Introduction

Circulating blood is composed of water, proteins, electrolytes, and cells. Fluid left after removing the cells from blood is the *plasma*. When both cells and coagulation proteins are removed from blood, the left-over fluid is the *serum*. The water component of blood moves across both tissue barriers and cell membranes, depending on hydrostatic and **oncotic pressures** (osmotic pressure exerted by colloids in a solution; for example, serum proteins in intravascular blood). On the other hand, protein and electrolyte movements into and from blood vessels often depend on complex tissue or cell membrane pumps. Blood cells generally remain within the blood vessels except under conditions of blood vessel injury or inflammation.

Measuring the chemical and cellular properties of blood can yield considerable information about disease states. These measurements are often expressions of concentrations of a substance. Some measurements, however, measure a functional property, such as coagulation activity or osmotic pressure. This chapter covers the common measurements performed on blood samples from patients. For each measurement the discussion includes a review of the physiologic (and pathophysiologic) importance of the blood substance or property, followed by a brief review of commonly used measurement techniques. Diagnoses that should be considered in the event of an abnormal value also are reviewed.

Serum Electrolytes

Body Water

In an average person, approximately 60% of total body weight is water.[1,2] Two-thirds is in the intracellular compartment (i.e., within cells) and one-third is in the extracellular compartment (i.e., interstitium and blood, which make up 75% and 25%, respectively, of this compartment). The compartments are separated by cell membranes that set up active and passive forces regulating water, electrolyte, and solute movement, with resulting electrolyte concentration gradients and oncotic pressures. The most common **serum electrolytes** are the **cations** Na^+, K^+, Ca^{+2}, and Mg^{+2} and the **anions** HCO_3^-, PO_4^-, and SO_4^-.

Extracellular fluid is characterized by higher amounts of Na^+, Cl^-, and HCO_3^-, whereas **intracellular fluid** has higher amounts of K^+, Mg^{+2}, PO_4^-, and SO_4^-. These cations and anions are regulated in the compartments over a narrow normal range. Mechanical, inflammatory, and other pathologic processes frequently affect the integrity of these compartments, with consequent movement of electrolytes, proteins, and water. A change in body or compartment level of one substance often sets off a sequence of compensatory events in the body to maintain fluid homeostasis.

Thus, initial assessment of the overall water volume status is critical in any evaluation of a patient's fluid and electrolyte status. No single test precisely quantifies total body water (TBW) easily in the clinical setting. Instead, clinicians rely on history taking and physical examination. The intent is to decide whether the patient is hypovolemic, euvolemic, or hypervolemic with respect to TBW (**Box 5-1**).

> **BOX 5-1**
>
> **Assessment Tools Used to Evaluate Total Body Water**
>
> Decreased total body water (hypovolemia) is associated with the following:
>
> - *Symptoms*: Thirst, decreased urine output, dizziness on standing up.
> - *Signs*: Thready rapid pulse, low blood pressure, orthostatic hypotension, low skin turgor, sunken eyes, depressed fontanelle in infants, dry, coated tongue; also associated with muscle tremors, rigidity, and even seizures and rarely with hallucinations, delirium, and maniac behavior; development of tachypnea and respiratory arrest before death.
> - *Laboratory data*: Elevated hematocrit (if hypovolemia is not due to blood loss), sodium (hypernatremia), and protein levels. Urine is concentrated, and urine potassium loss (kaliuresis) is seen, associated with decreased serum potassium levels.
>
> Increased total body water (hypervolemia) is associated with the following:
>
> - *Symptoms*: Weight gain, loss of diurnal rhythm of diuresis, pedal edema, dyspnea.
> - *Signs*: Orthopnea, pedal edema, elevated jugular venous pressure, wheezing, ascites.
> - *Laboratory data*: Are not characteristic but may show serum hyponatremia (dilutional) and hypoproteinemia.

Sodium

The sodium cation (Na^+) is the most common electrolyte in extracellular fluid, and the normal serum values range from 135 to 145 mmol/L.[2–9] Na^+ is important for a variety of cell membrane functions and in determinations of serum osmotic pressure. In the hypovolemic patient with normal total body Na^+ content, the relationship between Na^+ and TBW allows for calculation of the free water deficit, as follows:

$$\text{Free water deficit} = \text{TBW} \times \left(1 - \frac{140}{\text{Serum Na}^+}\right)$$

$$\text{Free water deficit} = 0.6 \times \text{Weight (kg)} \times \left(1 - \frac{140}{\text{Serum Na}^+}\right)$$

This formula is useful in calculations of the appropriate amount of free water to be administered in water-deficit states. The relationship between Na^+ and TBW also can be used to predict the change in serum Na^+ after administration of various intravenous fluids, as follows:

$$\text{Free water deficit} = \text{TBW} \times \left(1 - \frac{140}{\text{Serum Na}^+}\right)$$

$$\text{Free water deficit} = 0.6 \times \text{Weight (kg)} \times \left(1 - \frac{140}{\text{Serum Na}^+}\right)$$

$$\text{Change in serum Na}^+ = \frac{(\text{Infusate Na}^+ + \text{Infusate K}^+) - \text{Serum Na}^+}{\text{TBW} + 1}$$

Both low-Na^+ (**hyponatremia**) and high-Na^+ (**hypernatremia**) conditions are evident in a number of disease states and produce important clinical manifestations.

The physiologic effects of Na^+ depend on its concentration in extracellular water.[8] If the serum sample

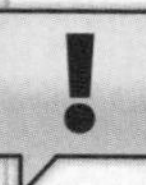

Respiratory Recap

Body Water

- Approximately 60% of total body weight is water.
- Two-thirds of body water is in the intracellular space.
- One-third of body water is in the extracellular space.

has significant amounts of substances that increase the serum volume, but not the water volume, the measured serum Na^+ will appear low even though its water concentration is normal (pseudohyponatremia). Substances that expand serum volume, but not blood volume, include the toxins methanol and ethylene glycol,[9] as well as glucose, mannitol, proteins, and lipids. To assess this instance, osmolality can be measured directly and compared with an estimated value, as follows:

$$\text{Osmolality} = 2\text{Na}^+ + \frac{(\text{BUN mg/dL})}{2.8} + \frac{(\text{Glucose mg/dL})}{18}$$

If the measured osmolality is within 20 of the estimated serum osmolality (that is, no osmolar gap), the Na^+ value reflects the true value and rules out the presence of unmeasured substances.

Decreased serum Na^+ levels are associated with water moving osmotically within cells and creating a significant shift in the relationship between intracellular and extracellular fluid compartments. This shift is associated with weakness, giddiness, lassitude, faintness, muscle cramps, anorexia, nausea, vomiting, confusion, delirium, stupor, and coma. On examination the skin turgor is low, blood pressure may be decreased, and orthostatic hypotension is usually present.

Because the relationship between Na^+ and fluid is so intertwined, a useful practice is to divide the causes of hyponatremia into hypovolemic, euvolemic, and hypervolemic categories, depending on the estimation of TBW by physical examination and the response of the kidney in moving Na^+ into the urine (**Box 5-2**).

A clinically increased Na^+ serum concentration (hypernatremia) is of concern because it suggests dehydration. In contrast, increased total body sodium levels are seen in patients with hypervolemic hyponatremia; however, their serum sodium levels are diluted because of excess water. Hypernatremia is associated with an increased serum osmolality, and its clinical features are classically the same as those associated with water loss. **Box 5-3** lists the causes of hypernatremia.

Laboratory techniques used to estimate sodium concentration include flame atomic emission spectroscopy, ion selective electrode (ISE) potentiometry (direct and indirect), chromogenic ionophore technique, and enzymatic (or enzyme activation) methods. ISE (either direct or indirect) is the most commonly used method. The direct ISE method has the advantage that hyperproteinemic and hyperlipidemic states do not affect accuracy. A potential source of error is protein buildup on membrane surfaces of the measuring electrode.

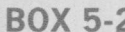

BOX 5-2

Classification of Hyponatremia

Hypovolemic Hyponatremia

Total body sodium deficit higher than TBW deficit
Renal loss (urine sodium >20 mmol/L)
- Diuresis: osmotic or diuretic excess
- Mineralocorticoid deficiency

Extrarenal loss (urine sodium <10 mmol/L)
- Vomiting
- Diarrhea
- Fluid movement into the third space

Euvolemic Hyponatremia

Increased TBW undetectable by clinical evaluation
Syndrome of inappropriate ADH secretion: malignancy (paraneoplastic syndrome), drugs, CNS lesions
Hypothyroidism
Immediate postoperative period (first 24 hours)
Glucocorticoid deficiency

Hypervolemic Hyponatremia

Dilutional: TBW increase greater than total body sodium
Congestive heart failure
Nephrotic syndrome
Cirrhosis
Acute and chronic renal failure

Extracellular space is sometimes grouped into three volumes. The first is plasma volume, the second is interstitial fluid volume, and the third refers to various actual or potential cavities, such as the pleural space, peritoneal space, and gut lumen.

TBW, total body water; ADH, antidiuretic hormone; CNS, central nervous system.

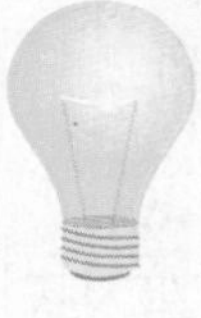

STOP AND THINK

A 60-year-old male smoker with a right upper lobe mass has come for a scheduled outpatient bronchoscopic exam. His pulse is 60/min, blood pressure 120/80 mm Hg. Chest and cardiovascular exam is essentially normal. No pedal edema. His sodium is 130 mmol/L. Remainder of laboratory tests are normal. What is the cause of low sodium?

BOX 5-3

Causes of Hypernatremia

Water Loss More Than Sodium Loss

Osmotic and loop diuretics
Postobstructive nephropathy
Sweating
Diarrhea and fistulas

Pure Water Loss

Diabetes insipidus: central, peripheral, and combination
Excessive sweating: exercise, fever, and hot environment

Increase in Total Body Sodium

Primary hyperaldosteronism
Cushing syndrome
Hypertonic sodium bicarbonate administration in situations such as cardiac arrest

BOX 5-4

Causes of Hypokalemia

Increased loss of potassium
GI losses: vomiting, especially with pyloric obstruction; villous adenoma of colon; diarrhea; non-β islet cell tumor of pancreas
Renal losses: diuretics, such as thiazides and furosemide; renal tubular acidosis I and II; hyperaldosteronism; massive doses of penicillin G, ureteroenterostomy
Intracellular shift of potassium: insulin, testosterone, β_2 agonists, respiratory and metabolic alkalosis, hypokalemic periodic paralysis
Decreased intake: malnutrition, alcoholism, and anorexia nervosa
Miscellaneous: magnesium depletion, Bartter syndrome, Liddle syndrome, licorice abuse

Potassium

Approximately 90% of total body potassium (K^+) is intracellular.[9–12] K^+ homeostasis is regulated by acid–base status, insulin, catecholamines, and aldosterone. Alkalosis and elevated insulin, catecholamine, and aldosterone levels lower serum K^+ through either renal excretion or intracellular potassium shifting. Acidosis and reduced insulin, catecholamine, and aldosterone levels raise serum potassium levels. K^+ is essential for maintenance of the electrical membrane potential; thus, changes in serum K^+ levels affect neuromuscular activity as well as cardiac electrical impulses. Normal serum range is from 3.5 to 5.5 mmol/L.

Serum K^+ levels below normal (**hypokalemia**; **Box 5-4**) affect neuromuscular function, causing muscular weakness, malaise, fatigue, and myalgias. Severe K^+ depletion has been associated with paralysis and rhabdomyolysis. Life-threatening cardiac arrhythmias with electrocardiogram (ECG) changes (U waves, QT prolongation, T wave changes) are commonly associated with severe hypokalemia. Paresthesias, abdominal cramps, and ileus also are common manifestations. Spuriously reduced potassium levels—pseudohypokalemia—may accompany markedly elevated white blood cell (WBC) counts, as in cases of leukemia. Prompt laboratory processing of the sample helps prevent such false-positive results. Hypokalemia may be associated with hypomagnesemia. High doses of inhaled beta-agonist therapy, such as albuterol, can result in hypokalemia.

Serum K^+ levels above normal (**hyperkalemia**; **Box 5-5**) produce hyporeflexia and muscle weakness. Paralysis can occur in cases of severe hyperkalemia, but death due to cardiac arrhythmias usually takes place beforehand. On the ECG, peaked T waves, widened QRS, and eventually sine waves develop before the appearance of actual cardiac arrest. Falsely elevated K^+ levels or pseudohyperkalemia[13] may be seen when the blood sample is hemolyzed or the WBC or platelet count is unusually elevated. Elevated serum potassium levels are frequently encountered in patients with renal disease or failure.

BOX 5-5

Causes of Hyperkalemia

Increased intake or tissue release, especially in the face of compromised renal function: tumor lysis syndrome, rhabdomyolysis, hemolysis, blood transfusion
Drugs: potassium-sparing diuretics, cyclosporin, trimethoprim, ACE inhibitors, heparin, NSAIDs
Renal causes: acute and chronic renal failure, type IV renal tubular acidosis, pseudohypoaldosteronism
Aldosterone deficiency: Addison disease, hereditary adrenal enzyme defects

ACE, angiotensin-converting enzyme; NSAIDs, nonsteroidal anti-inflammatory drugs.

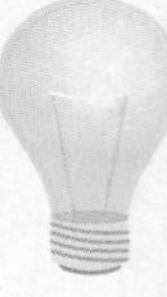

STOP AND THINK

You are asked to provide an albuterol treatment to a patient with acute renal failure. How might this help?

Techniques used to estimate potassium levels include flame atomic emission spectroscopy, ISE (direct and indirect), chromogenic ionophore, and enzymatic (enzyme activation). ISE is the most frequently used technique.

Chloride

Chloride (Cl^-) is the most common anion in the extracellular space.[2–9,13] Changes in serum Cl^- usually follow changes in serum sodium levels. Exceptions are hyperchloremic (elevated serum Cl^-) acidoses and chloride-responsive, hypochloremic (reduced serum Cl^-) alkaloses. Although **hypochloremia** in experimental situations is associated with vasoconstriction and increased reactivity to norepinephrine (especially in cerebral vessels), clinically important isolated chloride changes are almost never seen. Normal Cl^- levels are 98 to 107 mmol/L in the serum and 110 to 250 mmol/L in the urine. Estimation of Cl^- is affected by other halides. Erroneously high values (**hyperchloremia**) may be found with bromide present in the sample. Four laboratory methods are used to estimate Cl^- levels: colorimetric method (mercuric/ferric thiocyanate), coulometric titration, ISE, and enzymatic method. ISE methods are the most commonly used.[14]

Total Serum Carbon Dioxide

Serum contains carbon dioxide in the form of dissolved carbon dioxide (CO_2), carbon dioxide loosely bound to the amine group of plasma proteins, bicarbonate anion (HCO_3^-), carbonate anion (CO_3^{-2}), and carbonic acid. It acts as one of the major buffering systems to control the acid–base milieu of the body. The normal range is 22 to 32 mmol/L. The Henderson-Hasselbalch equation describes the relationship of dissolved CO_2, pH, and HCO_3^-.

Methods used to estimate total serum CO_2 include gas release, pH indicator, carbon dioxide electrodes, enzymatic methods, and calculation from the acid–base estimation. Commonly used methods include the ISE or colorimetric method. Accuracy requires anaerobic handling of the sample. Most autoanalyzers permit immediate analysis of the sample. However, if the sample is left uncapped, the total CO_2 levels can decrease by 6 mmol/L/hour.

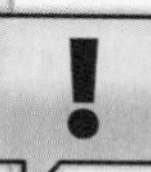

Respiratory Recap

Serum Electrolytes

- Sodium
- Potassium
- Chloride
- Total carbon dioxide
- Unmeasured anions
- Calcium
- Magnesium
- Phosphorus
- Lactate

Unmeasured Anions

Anionic proteins and other substances (**Box 5-6**) also can exist in serum.[15,16] Generally these are not measured in routine serum electrolyte determinations. However, their presence can be suspected by calculation of the **anion gap**, as follows:

$$\text{Anion gap} = ([Na^+] + [K^+]) - ([CO_2] + [Cl^-])$$

If the anion gap exceeds 12 mmol/L, excessive **unmeasured anions** are likely present. Because its concentration is normally low, $[K^+]$ often is omitted from this calculation.

Calcium

Calcium (Ca^{+2}) performs multiple functions in the body.[9,17,18] Besides being a major structural substance in bone, it plays an important role in maintaining cellular conduction in the neuromuscular system. Ca^{+2} is also an important participant or catalyst in several metabolic cascades (e.g., the coagulation pathways). Ca^{+2} is mainly absorbed in the bowel and excreted in the urine. Bones serve as a major calcium reservoir. The important Ca^{+2} level regulators are vitamin D, calcitonin, phosphate, and parathyroid hormone.

BOX 5-6

Unmeasured Anions

Lactate (liver disease, tissue hypoxia)
Ketones (diabetic and alcoholic ketoacidosis)
Salicylates (toxic ingestion)
PO_4^- and SO_4^-
Uremic acidosis
Formate and lactate
Glycolate and oxalate
Ethylene glycol
Free fatty acids
Methyl malonate
Total serum carbon dioxide

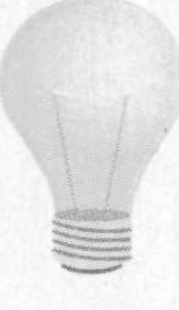

STOP AND THINK

A 72-year-old male with history of hypertension and end-stage renal disease on hemodialysis is admitted to the hospital with pneumonia. You are about to start his albuterol nebulizer treatment. You notice on the bedside cardiac monitor his heart rate is 50/min, T waves are tall, and QRS are wider than what they were with the treatment you gave 4 hours earlier. Which electrolyte abnormality do you need to think about?

In general, vitamin D and parathyroid hormone increase Ca^{+2} levels, whereas calcitonin and phosphate reduce them.

In serum, most Ca^{+2} is bound to albumin. Measured Ca^{+2} levels are thus sensitive to all the factors regulating or affecting serum protein levels (especially albumin). Because unbound (i.e., ionized) calcium is what is metabolically important, measured total serum Ca^{+2} should be corrected for albumin concentration (i.e., a reduction in Ca^{+2} level of 0.8 mg/dL for every gram per deciliter of albumin below normal). Ionized calcium also can be measured directly. In adults, normal total serum Ca^{+2} levels are 8.6 to 10.0 mg/dL (2.15 to 2.50 mmol/L). Normal ionized Ca^{+2} levels are 4.6 to 5.3 mg/dL (1.16 to 1.32 mmol/L).

A low ionized calcium level (**hypocalcemia**) is usually due to either decreased absorption or decreased mobilization of calcium from the bones. Causes include malnutrition, parathyroid hormone activity, vitamin D abnormalities, certain drugs, and renal dysfunction (which produces hyperphosphatemia). Pancreatitis, massive blood transfusions, and tumor lysis syndrome can precipitate Ca^{+2} and thus reduce serum levels. Low Ca^{+2} levels frequently coexist with low magnesium levels, especially in malnourished alcoholics. Alkalosis can disrupt calcium ion balance and cause the symptoms of hypocalcemia. Clinical features of hypocalcemia consist of perioral numbness and tingling progressing to tetany. Physical examination evidence of protein-energy malnutrition, previous parathyroidectomy, pancreatitis, and tumor lysis syndrome should increase the suspicion for reduced Ca^{+2} levels.

Increases in Ca^{+2} levels (**hypercalcemia**) are caused by multiple factors (**Box 5-7**). The clinical features of hypercalcemia include anorexia, vomiting, polyuria, mental confusion, obtundation, and death. The ECG may show a shortened QT interval.

Laboratory tests used to measure serum Ca^{+2} include atomic absorption, cresolphthalein complex formation, arsenazo III dye, and ISE methods to estimate ionic calcium levels. Autoanalyzers frequently use ISE methods. Atomic absorption remains the gold standard, although it is not frequently used for clinical work.

BOX 5-7

Causes of Hypercalcemia

Abnormal Protein Syndromes

Multiple myeloma and paraproteinemias

Increased Parathyroid Hormone or Related Peptides

Malignancy of lung or kidney (paraneoplastic syndrome)

Increased Absorption

Usually vitamin D related (milk alkali syndrome), granulomatous diseases (such as tuberculosis and sarcoidosis), lymphoma

Excessive Renal Phosphate Excretion

Familial syndrome, sarcoidosis

Abnormal Bone Resorption or Formation

Prolonged bed rest, Paget disease

Miscellaneous

Bone metastases, especially from breast and prostate cancers, drugs such as thiazides (rarely)

Magnesium

Magnesium (Mg^{+2}) is the other major cation in the serum (besides Ca^{+2}) that helps maintain membrane potentials at the cellular level.[9,19] Mg^{+2} also is important in maintaining potassium homeostasis through regulation of cell membrane potassium channels. Only 1% to 2% of total body Mg^{+2} is present in the serum, and one-third of this amount is bound to proteins. Mg^{+2} is mainly absorbed in the small bowel (mostly in the initial parts) and is excreted by the kidneys. In adults the normal serum Mg^{+2} range is 1.8 to 3.0 mg/mL (0.7 to 1.1 mmol/L).

Box 5-8 lists causes of low Mg^{+2} levels (**hypomagnesemia**). Low levels often are associated with hypokalemia. Indeed, concurrent hypomagnesemia and hypokalemia makes it difficult to correct the potassium levels until the Mg^{+2} levels are corrected. Hypomagnesemia also is associated with hyponatremia, hypocalcemia, and hypophosphatemia. Low Mg^{+2} levels result in tremulousness, hyperreflexia, ataxia, convulsions, and death in extreme cases.

Hypomagnesemia-induced cardiac dysrhythmias originating in the atria or the ventricles can be

BOX 5-8

Causes of Hypomagnesemia

Absorption Problems

Malnutrition per se or due to alcoholism, diarrhea, intravenous alimentation, intestinal bypass surgery

Psychological problems: bulimia, laxative abuse, or aggressive weight reduction

Others: short bowel syndrome or malignancies, especially in the bowel

Excessive Loss in Urine

Use and abuse of diuretics, postobstructive diuresis, acute tubular necrosis, hypercalcemia, and hereditary renal magnesium wasting

Miscellaneous

Association with hyperaldosteronism, diabetic ketoacidosis, and excessive lactation

Exchange transfusions

Acute intermittent porphyria

BOX 5-9

Causes of Hypophosphatemia

Decreased Absorption

Malnutrition, alcohol abuse, vitamin D deficiency, laxative abuse, and antacid abuse

Intracellular Shift

High-energy states and parenteral nutrition with carbohydrate overload

Increased Excretion

Hyperparathyroidism, diuretics, hyperglycemia, and alcohol abuse

fatal. In patients with rapid polymorphic ventricular tachycardia (torsades de pointes), intravenous magnesium infusion can be life-saving. Hypertension in hypomagnesemic patients can be difficult to control. Hypomagnesemic dysmotility in gastrointestinal muscles is clinically manifested as dysphagia.

High Mg^{+2} levels (**hypermagnesemia**) are uncommon but can be seen in patients suffering from renal failure, especially those undergoing inappropriate dialysis or alimentation regimens. Another cause of hypermagnesemia is abuse of magnesium-based laxatives. In addition, hypermagnesemia is sometimes induced to treat eclampsia. The condition's clinical manifestations include hyporeflexia, muscle weakness, hypotension, bradycardia, coma, and death.

Laboratory methods used to estimate serum levels of Mg^{+2} include colorimetric methods using calmagite, methyl thymol, or chlorophosphonazo III; ISE methods; and atomic absorption, the latter of which remains the gold standard. However, ISE methods are increasingly being used to estimate serum Mg^{+2} levels.

Phosphorus

More than 80% of total body phosphorus is found in bones.[9,20] Phosphate ion (PO_4^-) is a major intracellular anion participating primarily as a cofactor in intracellular metabolic processes. Extracellular phosphate salts function as buffers and play a role in calcium homeostasis. (That is, serum PO_4^- and Ca^{+2} exist in a reciprocal, balanced relationship.) PO_4^- is absorbed through the gastrointestinal tract (vitamin D dependent) and excreted through the kidneys (enhanced by parathyroid hormone). In adults, normal serum PO_4^- levels range between 2.7 and 4.5 mg/dL (0.87 to 1.45 mmol/L).

Low PO_4^- (**hypophosphatemia**) levels are primarily caused by decreased absorption, intracellular shifts, or increased excretion (**Box 5-9**). Severe stress causing glucagon and cortisol release may be responsible for the low serum PO_4^- levels seen in trauma patients. Clinical features of hypophosphatemia include decreased contractility of muscles, causing cardiomyopathy, hyporeflexia, and hypoventilation. If severe, this condition can lead to rhabdomyolysis. Hypophosphatemia also can produce confusion, seizures, and coma. Chronic deficiency can cause osteomalacia.

High PO_4^- levels (**hyperphosphatemia**) are unusual but can be seen in individuals with chronic renal failure, in which the hyperphosphatemia is often overshadowed by other metabolic and electrolyte abnormalities. Other conditions producing hyperphosphatemia include hypoparathyroidism (with low calcium levels also being seen), pseudohypoparathyroidism, and Paget disease of the juvenile, which is characterized by muscle weakness and high alkaline phosphatase levels.

To estimate serum PO_4^- levels, ammonium phosphomolybdate complex levels are read directly by an ultraviolet monitor, or the complex is reduced to molybdenum and its levels estimated.

Lactate

An increase in **lactate** is caused by either increased production as a result of anaerobic metabolism or reduced degradation of lactate as a result of problems in the liver.[21,22] Lactate is most commonly formed in

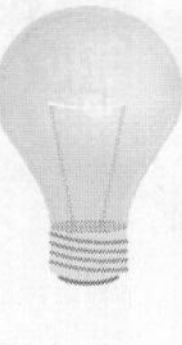

STOP AND THINK

An 85-year-old woman with COPD was admitted last night with abdominal pain. You are called to give her a nebulizer treatment. On arrival you find her lying still, afraid to move, and pale, complaining of abdominal pain. She is breathing 32/minute (was 20/min on admission) and using accessory muscles. On auscultation her lung sounds are normal. You suspect she has metabolic acidosis. What is the likely cause of her increased respiratory rate?

ischemic cells as a consequence of anaerobic glycolysis and the use of pyruvate for generation of adenosine triphosphate (ATP). Thus, it is frequently used to indicate the severity of shock and provides a rough idea of tissue perfusion, oxygen delivery, and oxygen use. For individuals in shock, increased lactate is associated with increased mortality. Increased lactate also is seen in patients with bowel ischemia. A rare cause of increased lactate is high-dose albuterol administration.

An elevated serum lactate level is an important cause of anion gap metabolic acidosis. Lactate has both D and L isomers. Humans normally produce L-lactic acidosis, which most laboratories easily estimate. Theoretically, D-lactate (normally produced by ruminants and bacteria) can be elevated in certain types of individuals (e.g., those with bowel abnormalities). Currently D-lactic acidosis is a research curiosity, with rare cases involving humans. Normal values for lactate in adults are less than 2 mmol/L.

Methods used to estimate lactate levels include chemical oxidation, enzyme reactions, and enzyme electrodes. Other methods use gas chromatography and photometry, but enzyme electrodes have made estimation of serum lactate levels much simpler. Because lactate is unstable, samples should be processed immediately. Lactate increases by 0.4 mmol/L in whole blood kept at room temperature for 30 minutes (0.1 mmol/L on ice).

Serum Chemistries Associated with Renal Function

Good urine production (quantitative as well as qualitative) is a marker of end organ perfusion and renal function. The most important tests are the quantity of urine produced and the characteristics of that urine (i.e., pH, specific gravity, microscopic analysis, and culture).[23] Two other measurements are frequently used to assess renal function, however: the serum blood urea nitrogen (BUN) and creatinine levels.

Blood Urea Nitrogen

Serum **blood urea nitrogen (BUN)** levels indicate the body's ability to clear nitrogenous wastes in the form of urea in the urine. Urea (along with ammonia) is a breakdown product of amino acids; therefore, it can be increased by increases in gastrointestinal protein absorption from either dietary factors or heme in the bowels (i.e., gastrointestinal bleeding). Similarly, urea levels can be decreased with decreases in protein intake or liver impairment. Urea is readily filtered in the glomeruli, but approximately half of it is reabsorbed. It also is broken down into ammonia in the bowel. Levels of BUN thus reflect protein intake and metabolism as well as glomerular and proximal tubule function in the kidney. In the adult, normal BUN values are between 7 and 21 mg/dL.

BUN is estimated from serum urea levels. Almost all the tests used—calorimetric methods, indicator dye, and ISE methods—directly or indirectly estimate the amount of ammonia present in the sample.

Creatinine

Serum **creatinine** levels are a function of skeletal muscle breakdown. Thus, the levels are directly related to the muscle mass of a person. Most creatinine is filtered in the glomeruli, with very little reabsorption. A small amount also is secreted by the tubules into the urine. If the individual's muscle mass is relatively stable, serum creatinine level is a good indicator of glomerular filtration and, hence, renal function. Increased creatinine levels, however, also can occur in conjunction with increased muscle breakdown (e.g., corticosteroids, rhabdomyolysis) or with decreased tubular excretion, such as that seen with use of trimethoprim. Decreased creatinine levels reflect decreased muscle mass, such as those in states of malnutrition or muscle atrophy. In the adult, normal values for creatinine are 0.7 to 1.4 mg/dL.

Serum creatinine level is a relatively insensitive monitor of renal function and may not increase until more than 50% of renal function has deteriorated. With complete renal shutdown, creatinine levels rise approximately 1 mg/dL per day. Creatinine levels also can be used to describe creatinine clearance (the amount of blood per minute cleared of creatinine by the kidney), a more precise measurement of renal function, as follows:

$$\text{Creatinine clearance} = \frac{\text{Urine creatinine concentration} \times \text{24-hour urine volume}}{\text{Plasma creatinine concentration}}$$

A simpler method used to estimate creatinine clearance is as follows:

$$\text{Creatinine clearance} = (140 - \text{Age}) \times \frac{\text{Weight (kg)}}{72} \times \text{Serum creatinine}$$

Normal creatinine clearance is 97 to 137 mL/min (for men) and 88 to 128 mL/min (for women). Creatinine clearance decreases 6.5 mL/min per decade after 40 years of age.

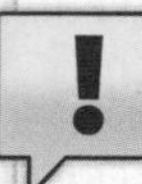

Respiratory Recap

Laboratory Tests Associated with Renal Function

- Urine analysis
- Blood urea nitrogen
- Creatinine

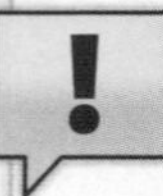

Respiratory Recap

Cardiac Injury Markers

- Cardiac enzymes (CK-MB)
- Troponins T and I
- Brain natriuretic peptide

Estimation of creatinine is done by spectrophotometric analysis of the Jaffe reaction, enzymatic hydrolysis of creatinine, and cation-exchange high-performance liquid chromatography.

Serum Enzyme Activity

Enzymes are chemical substances that facilitate chemical reactions. Most enzymatic reactions occur intracellularly. Nevertheless, a number of these enzymes appear in serum under physiologic conditions. In pathologic conditions, many enzymes appear in serum in increased concentrations because of either cell injury or metabolic abnormalities within the cell.

A number of serum enzymes reflect liver function[24] but also may reflect dysfunction elsewhere. Alanine aminotransferase (ALT) is present in liver cells, and an increased serum level indicates liver cell injury. Aspartate aminotransferase (AST) is present in liver cells but also is present in cardiac, skeletal, kidney, and brain tissue. Serum alkaline phosphatase (ALP) comes from either liver or bone. Elevation of liver ALP indicates intrahepatic or collecting system bile drainage abnormalities (cholestasis). Elevated γ-glutamyltransferase (GGT) serum levels also indicate cholestasis. An AST:ALT ratio greater than 2 suggests alcoholic liver injury.

Lactic dehydrogenase (LDH) enzymes are a family of enzymes in which elevations can reflect liver, bone, cardiac, red blood cell, or pancreatic abnormalities. LDH assays can be fractionated (isoenzymes) to indicate the organ involved if required.

Amylase and lipase are two enzymes that appear elevated as a consequence of pancreatic injury.[25] Both may be elevated in individuals with other gastrointestinal abnormalities as well. Pancreatic disease caused by biliary tract disease usually has accompanying liver-associated abnormalities in the serum.

Cardiac Enzymes and Proteins

Cardiac Enzymes

The term **cardiac enzymes** refers to a group of enzymes that are released from myocardial tissue and appear in the serum as a result of myocardial injury (usually ischemia).[26–28] As the understanding of cardiac ischemia has changed, so has the use of various enzymes to estimate cardiac muscle damage. Nevertheless, cardiac enzyme abnormalities remain a standard used to diagnose cardiac ischemia, in conjunction with history and ECG changes. The initial panel of cardiac enzymes included serum lactate dehydrogenase (LDH), serum glutamic-oxaloacetic transaminase (SGOT), and creatine kinase (CK). The myocardial-specific creatine kinase MB isoform (CK-MB) was used for diagnosing myocardial injury, but recently serum troponin levels have become the standard of care. CK-MB levels begin rising within 4 to 8 hours of myocardial injury, with peak activity by 24 hours. CK-MB levels return to baseline within 2 to 3 days.

Troponins

Serum **troponins** are cardiac regulatory proteins that are involved in the calcium-mediated interaction of actin and myosin in the cardiac muscle. Many centers are now measuring cardiac troponin I or T isoforms for diagnosing myocardial injury. Cardiac troponins begin to rise 2 to 3 hours following an acute myocardial injury, peak by about 14 to 20 hours, and return to baseline within 5 to 10 days. Unfortunately, no uniformity in the measurement of troponins has made the comparison of values from various laboratories difficult. CK, CK-MB, troponin I, and troponin T are estimated by different methods. Rapid assays of these enzymes are very helpful in the quick triaging of patients with suspected acute coronary syndrome. In renal failure and rhabdomyolysis, reduced clearance from the serum or increased production, or both, makes interpretation of the increased serum levels of these proteins difficult. In the future other proteins and enzymes, such as fatty acid-binding protein (FABP) and glycogen phosphorylase isoenzyme (BB), may also prove useful for diagnosing myocardial injury.

Methods used to estimate CK include electrophoresis, ion exchange chromatography, immunoinhibitors, and mass assay (specific for CK-MB). Normal total serum CK is 15 to 130 U/L, and CK-MB is less than 6% of total CK. Potential sources of error are hemolysis, exposure of sample to daylight, and the muscle mass of the patient (either too large or too small). For troponin estimation, enzyme-linked immunosorbent assay (ELISA), immunoenzyme techniques, and rapid immunochromatographic assays are available. The normal range is less than 0.1 ng/mL to 3.1 ng/mL.

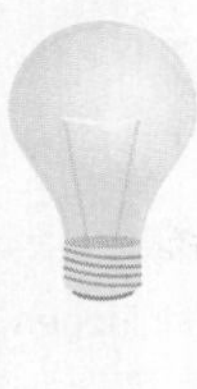

STOP AND THINK

A 68-year-old male is admitted with shortness of breath. Auscultation reveals bilateral basal crackles and pedal edema in both legs. Blood tests show a troponin I of 5.3, BNP of 780, and normal renal function. What is the most likely cause of his shortness of breath?

Brain Natriuretic Peptide

Brain natriuretic peptide (BNP), also known as B-type natriuretic peptide, is a natriuretic hormone similar to atrial natriuretic peptide (ANP). The physiologic actions of BNP include an increase in natriuresis (discharge of sodium through urine) and decrease in systemic vascular resistance and central venous pressure. These actions lead to a decrease in cardiac output and in blood volume. In humans the cardiac ventricles are the major source of BNP.

The N-terminal part of the propeptide of BNP (NT-ProBNP) is an active metabolite of BNP. BNP has a shorter half-life than NT-ProBNP (15–20 min versus 90 min, respectively). Thus, BNP may more closely relate to rapid neurohormonal and hemodynamic changes after acute coronary syndrome. However, elevated NT-ProBNP has a higher circulating concentration, is more stable, and has less biological variability. Nevertheless, elevated serum BNP and NT-ProBNP levels both help to differentiate dyspnea due to heart failure from pulmonary disease. They are elevated in both systolic and diastolic heart failure.

BNP is also useful to guide therapy in and prognostication of heart failure, acute coronary syndrome, and stable angina. BNP levels tend to be higher in people with renal failure and in older people, and lower in obese people and in women. Elevated BNP levels in medical intensive care patients are seen in mild heart failure, values of 600 to 900 pg/mL are seen in moderate heart failure, and values greater than 900 pg/mL are seen in severe heart failure. Recombinant BNP (Nesiritide) is also used for the treatment of acute decompensated congestive heart failure.

BNP and NT-ProBNP are measured by ELISA and chemiluminescent immunometric assay, respectively. Kits are commercially available.

Miscellaneous Serum Chemistries

C-Reactive Protein

C-reactive protein (CRP) was first recognized by its ability to precipitate in the presence of the somatic C polysaccharide of *Pneumococcus*.[29] CRP is a nonspecific marker of acute inflammation produced by the liver and adipocytes. CRP levels are elevated in infections and several long-term diseases, including cancer; rheumatologic diseases such as lupus, rheumatoid arthritis, and giant cell arteritis; inflammatory bowel disease; and osteomyelitis. Recent data suggest that elevation of CRP from baseline within the normal range as well as CRP levels above normal are predictive of risk for myocardial infarction, stroke, peripheral vascular disease, and sudden cardiac death. The availability of high-sensitivity CRP (hs-CRP) measurement techniques has helped to reduce variation and provide reproducible CRP measurements.

CRP values for early risk stratification should be checked in conjunction with serum troponins as soon as possible after a patient presents with acute coronary syndrome to limit the influence of the extent of necrosis. For assessment of long-term risk, CRP values should be assessed at least 4 to 6 weeks after a myocardial infarction to allow for resolution of the acute phase reaction.

Several different ELISA-based assays are available for measuring CRP. All have their own reproducibility as well as characteristics. Ultrasensitive microchip-based systems to measure CRP in other body fluids are currently under investigation.

Bilirubin

Bilirubin is a breakdown product of hemoglobin that is metabolized in the liver.[24] Total serum bilirubin concentration is less than 1.1 mg/dL. Approximately 80% of serum bilirubin is indirect or unconjugated. Elevation of indirect bilirubin levels suggests prehepatic **bilirubinemia** caused by increased bilirubin production (e.g., hemolysis) or decreased liver uptake, as seen in Gilbert syndrome. Parenchymal liver injury and bile collecting system abnormalities (i.e., posthepatic lesions) cause bile stasis (cholestasis) and lead to an increase of conjugated bilirubin.

Proteins

Serum **proteins** include albumin, globulins, and immunoglobulins.[24,30,31] Serum albumin is exclusively synthesized in the liver. Its half-life is approximately 3 weeks, and it can be used as a marker of liver synthetic function. Serum albumin also is a useful marker of nutritional status. Ferritin is an iron-binding protein that also is taken as an index of nutritional status. Serum globulins are mediators of the humoral immune system. Elevations can be seen in individuals with tumors secreting these globulins (e.g., multiple myeloma) and other paraproteinemias. Low values are seen in individuals with congenital immune deficiency states.

Glucose

Glucose metabolism is heavily influenced by a number of nutritional, liver, hormonal, and pancreatic factors.[32] Glucagon and adrenal steroids increase glucose concentrations by promoting liver breakdown of stored glycogen. Insulin is produced by islet cells in the pancreas and is critical for the transfer of glucose into cells. Pancreatic injury or islet cell dysfunction (type 1 diabetes) impairs insulin production and results in serum hyperglycemia. If severe, this condition can produce **diabetic ketoacidosis**. Severe hyperglycemia also can cause a **hyperosmolar** state with coma. In addition, type 2 diabetes (cellular resistance to insulin) can produce hyperglycemia and deranged glucose metabolism. Insulin-secreting tumors or exogenous insulin overdoses produce hypoglycemia. Severe liver injury also can produce hypoglycemia because of a depletion or failure to metabolize liver glycogen; if severe, hypoglycemia can bring about coma and death. Normal fasting glucose is ≤100 mg/dL.

Procalcitonin

Serum **procalcitonin** levels might be a more useful marker for distinguishing bacterial infections from aseptic inflammation than erythrocyte sedimentation rate (ESR) or CRP.[33] Procalcitonin is a precursor protein of the hormone calcitonin and is produced in C cells of the thyroid gland. Procalcitonin is released during infections by microbial toxins or indirectly by humoral factors or the cell-mediated host response. This induction is not as significant in viral or other inflammatory conditions.

Serum procalcitonin levels may be used to guide the need as well as duration of antibiotic therapy. This has the potential to safely reduce the number of antibiotic prescriptions and the duration of antibiotic use in patients. Various studies have reported varying sensitivity and specificity for procalcitonin in diagnosing bacteremia. A meta-analysis reported a sensitivity of 76% and a specificity of 76%. Rapid semiquantitative strip-based and quantitative luminometric immunoassays are being developed to measure serum procalcitonin levels. Higher serum procalcitonin levels indicate a need for a higher level of care and possibly poor outcomes. Soluble triggering receptors expressed on myeloid cells–1 (sTREM-1) also are under investigation as a marker of infections.

Coagulation Tests

The coagulation system (**Figure 5-1**) can be assessed in a number of ways.[34,35] A simple and direct way to evaluate overall coagulation status is the bedside bleeding time. This method is time consuming and difficult to standardize, however. More commonly used techniques are measurements of the prothrombin time, activated partial thromboplastin time, and platelet count.

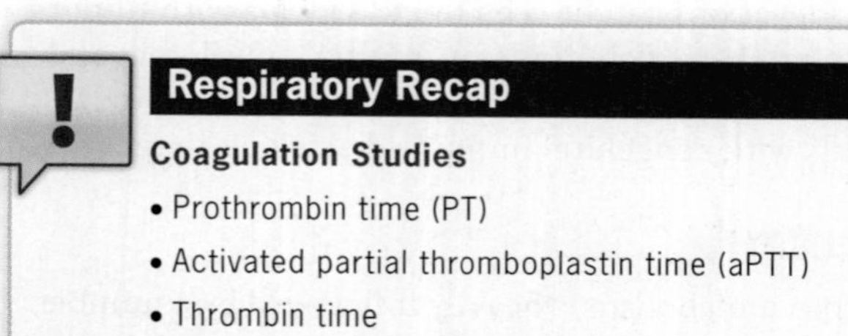

Respiratory Recap

Coagulation Studies

- Prothrombin time (PT)
- Activated partial thromboplastin time (aPTT)
- Thrombin time
- Traditional anticoagulants and newer oral anticoagulants

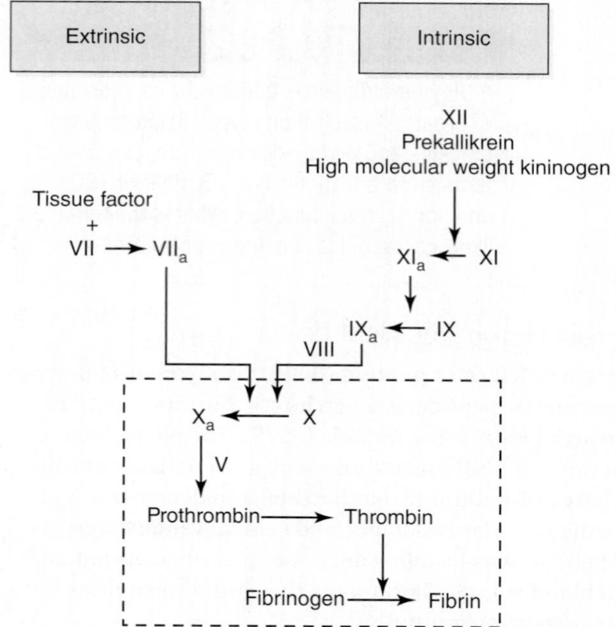

FIGURE 5-1 A simplified version of the role of various clotting factors in the coagulation cascade.

Reproduced from *Cecil Textbook of Medicine*, 21st ed. Goldman L, Bennett JC. Copyright Elsevier [WB Saunders] 2001.

Prothrombin Time

The **prothrombin time (PT)** is used to evaluate the extrinsic pathway, which involves tissue factor, factor VII, and coagulation factors in the common pathway (prothrombin, V, X, and fibrinogen; refer to Figure 5-1). It often is used to monitor adequate anticoagulation in patients on Coumadin (warfarin), which acts on these factors. The result is usually expressed as either a time or ratio of the values with respect to normal pooled sera. To standardize PT monitoring for oral anticoagulation therapy, PT is expressed as an international normalized ratio (INR). The goals of Coumadin therapy are to increase the INR to 2–3. However, in specific conditions, such as mechanical prosthetic heart valves, this ratio must be increased further. The prolonged PT in emergent situations can be reversed with transfusing fresh frozen plasma or in urgent situation with vitamin K. **New oral anticoagulants** like riveroxaban and apixaban can also prolong the PT.

PT can be prolonged in vitamin K deficiency; liver disease; deficiency or inhibition of factors VII, X, II, V, or fibrinogen; and in the presence of antiphospholipid antibodies and sometime heparin treatment, especially after bolus administration of heparin. In the presence of severe, acute liver injury, the PT may rapidly (i.e., within 24 hours) become abnormal. Vitamin K absorption also is impaired in the presence of hepatocellular disease and cholestasis, contributing to the abnormal PT.

Activated Partial Thromboplastin Time

The **activated partial thromboplastin time (aPTT)** is used to assess the intrinsic clotting pathway, especially the early stages involving factors XII, XI, IX, and VIII (refer to Figure 5-1). It often is used to monitor patients on heparin therapy. The goals of heparin therapy are to extend the aPTT to about twice the upper level of normal. In individuals not on anticoagulant therapy, abnormal PT or aPTT values indicate abnormalities in the coagulation system, possibly reflecting liver disorders, hematologic disorders, toxins or drugs, or disseminated intravascular coagulation (DIC) associated with a multiorgan failure syndrome. Further workup might include a number of specific clotting factor assays to identify the exact abnormality. Adding normal clotting factors to the test sample can help determine whether a coagulation abnormality is due to factor deficiency (coagulation normalizing with mix) or a circulating anticoagulant (coagulation not normalizing with mix).

In the clinical setting, prolonged aPTT is frequently seen in patients on intravenous heparin therapy and can be prolonged also with dabigatran. Heparin is an indirect thrombin inhibitor that complexes with antithrombin (AT) and converts it into a rapid inactivator of thrombin, factor Xa, and to a lesser extent factors XIIa, XIa, and IXa. The goal of heparin therapy is to elevate the aPTT to 1.5 times the upper limit of normal range within 24 hours. The goal of maintenance therapy is to maintain the aPTT in the range of 1.5 to 2.5 times the patient's baseline aPTT value. If required, heparin-caused prolonged PTT corrects itself in about 2 hours after stopping IV heparin, or protamine may be used if emergent reversal is indicated. Activated PTT can be prolonged due to a deficiency of, or an inhibitor to, any of the clotting factors except factor VII. Certain lupus anticoagulants can cause aPTT prolongation by interfering with in vitro assembly of the prothrombinase complex. This also causes paradoxical increased risk of venous and arterial thrombus.

Thrombin Time

The thrombin time measures the final step of the clotting pathway, which is the conversion of fibrinogen to fibrin. Thrombin time can be prolonged in the presence of heparin, a direct thrombin inhibitor such as hirudin or argatroban, fibrin degradation products, and hypofibrinogenemia.

The most commonly used anticoagulants are traditional agents such as heparin, low molecular weight heparin (LMWH) and warfarin. Therapeutic levels can be monitored by PTT, antifactor Xa activity and PT respectively. The efficacy of traditional anticoagulants is well established, but they have several limitations, including need for laboratory monitoring, narrow therapeutic window, and need for dose adjustment throughout the course of treatment. Recently approved newer oral anticoagulants (dabigatran, rivaroxabab, apixaban, betrixaban, darexaban) have minimal need for monitoring, but they currently do not have specific antidote for a fast reversal in case of emergencies. We also lack long-term safety data, and their use should be avoided in pregnancy, patients with mechanical valves, and those with severe renal impairment.

Hematology

The complete blood count (CBC) is the most frequently ordered diagnostic test in the hospital. Under the heading of CBC is a long list of indices that vary among laboratories. Automated machines usually directly measure the hemoglobin, WBC count, RBC count, platelet count, differential leukocyte fractions, and RBC distribution list, as well as calculate the hematocrit, mean corpuscular volume, mean corpuscular hemoglobin, mean corpuscular hemoglobin concentration, and differential leukocyte count.

Hemoglobin and Hematocrit

Hemoglobin is an iron-containing globular protein consisting of two pairs of polypeptides.[36,37] Its primary function is the transport of oxygen from the lungs to the tissues. Approximately 1 g of hemoglobin binds with 1.34 mL of oxygen. Normal values for hemoglobin in the adult are 13.5 to 15.5 g/dL (for men) and 12.5 to 14.5 g/dL (for women). The **hematocrit** is the proportion of whole blood that is composed of RBCs (the hemoglobin-carrying cell). Normal hematocrit values in the adult are 42% to 52% (for men) and 37% to 48% (for women). **Box 5-10** lists causes of abnormal hemoglobin and hematocrit levels. High hemoglobin levels are associated with chronic hypoxia and hematologic diseases, such as polycythemia vera. High hemoglobin

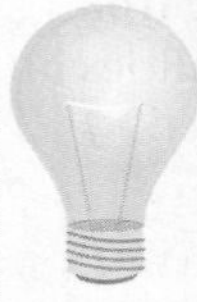

STOP AND THINK

A 25-year-old woman with lupus is admitted for shortness of breath. Her chest x-ray is suggestive of bilateral pneumonia and she is scheduled for bronchoscopy. You notice her hematocrit, which has been 35%, is now 26%, procalcitonin is less than 0.05, and her PTT is prolonged (58 seconds). She is not receiving anticoagulation. What is the reason for her drop in hematocrit and what is the cause of her prolonged PTT?

BOX 5-10

Causes of Low Hemoglobin and Hematocrit Values

Abnormal Hemoglobin

- Iron in the ferric form: methemoglobinemia
- Abnormalities in the polypeptide chain: hemoglobinopathies, such as thalassemias and sickle cell disease

Decreased Hemoglobin Production

- *Bone marrow problems*: aplastic anemia, myelosuppressive drugs, idiosyncratic reaction to drugs, infiltration of bone marrow by other cells
- *Deficiencies*: iron, vitamin B_{12} cofactors, erythropoietin
- *Miscellaneous*: malignancy, chronic diseases, hypothyroidism, hypopituitarism

Increased Loss or Breakdown of RBCs

- Fault in the RBCs: membrane defects, enzymatic deficiencies, hemoglobin disorders
- Acquired causes of hemolysis: drugs, toxins, infections
- Hypersplenism
- Bleeding, alveolar hemorrhage

RBC, red blood cell.

or hematocrit values, or both, also may be seen in individuals with dehydration and hemoconcentration.

Estimation of hemoglobin levels and types of hemoglobin is done by electrophoresis (alkaline or acid), other tests used to estimate abnormal hemoglobin (e.g., solubility test for sickle cell disease), and autoanalyzers.

Platelets

Platelets are blood cells critical to clot formation after vascular injury.[38] They are produced in the bone marrow, with normal blood concentrations ranging from 150,000 to 400,000/μL. **Box 5-11** lists abnormalities in platelet function.

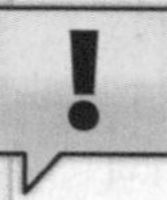

Respiratory Recap

Hematology

- Hemoglobin and hematocrit
- Platelets
- Leukocytes

BOX 5-11

Abnormalities in Platelet Function

Thrombasthenia

- Abnormal platelet function with uremia
- von Willebrand disease
- Drugs

Thrombocytopenia (Decreased Platelet Count)

- *Bone marrow problems*: malignancies, drugs, myelodysplasias
- *Increased breakdown*: structural platelet defects, immune problems (heparin-induced thrombocytopenia)
- Hypersplenism

Thrombocytosis (Increased Platelet Count)

- Essential or idiopathic
- After splenectomy
- Acute blood loss
- Pregnancy

Total and Differential Leukocyte Count

The primary role of **leukocytes** (WBCs) is in fighting infections, and an elevated WBC count (**leukocytosis**) is often a sign of significant infection.[39–41] Leukocytosis, however, also can be associated with elevated glucocorticoids (e.g., stress reaction, steroid administration) and can be seen in a number of cases of hematologic malignancies (**Box 5-12**). A marked elevation in white

BOX 5-12

Causes of Leukocytosis

Physiologic

- Exercise
- Pregnancy
- *Stress:* pain, psychologic, cold exposure, anesthesia, anoxia
- Trauma, hemorrhage
- Menstruation, pregnancy, and labor
- Seizure

Pathologic

- *Infections:* bacterial, fungal, viral, and parasitic
- Leukemoid reaction due to any of the previous causes
- *Leukemias:* uncontrolled malignant proliferation of any of the WBCs in the bone marrow

WBC, white blood cell.

BOX 5-13

Causes of Leukopenia

Overwhelming infection, especially in the very young or very elderly
Drug actions and adverse events
Malignant involvement of the bone marrow
Collagen vascular diseases such as lupus (infrequent cause)
Idiopathic or not-well-understood disease processes, such as myelodysplastic syndromes

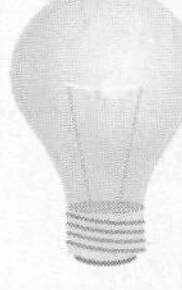

STOP AND THINK

A 60-year-old male with acute myeloid leukemia is feeling short of breath. His white cell count is 150,000/μL. An arterial blood gas is done. His Pao_2 is 50 mm Hg, but the Spo_2 is 96%. How would you explain this discrepancy?

cell count, such as is seen in patients with leukemia, may interfere with the interpretation of arterial blood gas values. A low WBC count (**leukopenia**) is invariably a bad sign in any disease process, especially in infections, in which it often indicates overwhelming infection (**Box 5-13**). The differential percentage of various WBCs in the peripheral smear helps identify the disease process. Once the percentage of different cells is known, the absolute numbers can be calculated from the total WBC counts. Normal WBC counts in adults range from 4000 to 11,000/μL.

Leukocytes are classified into two groups: granulocytes and agranulocytes. The granulocytes (neutrophils, eosinophils, and basophils) have granules in their cell cytoplasm and a multilobed nucleus. They also are called polymorphonuclear leukocytes or polys. The agranulocytes (lymphocytes and monocytes) do not have granules and have nonlobular nuclei. When immature leukocytes are first released from the bone marrow into the peripheral blood, they are called bands or stabs. The normal differentials for leukocyte counts are:

- Bands or stabs: 3–5%
- Neutrophils: 50–70% relative value
- Eosinophils: 1–3% relative value
- Basophils: 0.4–1% relative value
- Lymphocytes: 25–35% relative value
- Monocytes: 4–6% relative value

The differential always adds to 100%.

Years ago, hematology laboratories used visual counting techniques to estimate WBC concentrations. Today, most laboratories have automated instruments that use either resistance changes or flow characteristics to estimate the cell count and size of the cells. To enhance accuracy, RBCs are usually destroyed by chemicals in the blood sample before the WBC counts are performed. Currently, flow-through techniques using electrical resistance (or flow) changes or cytometry alone or in combination with cytochemical techniques are used. The sophistication of the instrument depends on whether it provides a three-, five-, or six-part differential. Ideally, the false-negative rate varies from 2% to 4%, with a false-positive rate of 8% to 15%. Falsely elevated WBC counts may be seen in individuals with undestroyed nucleated RBCs or large or aggregated platelets. Falsely low numbers may be seen in individuals with leukoagglutination; abnormal cells, such as blasts; immature granulocytes; and atypical lymphocytes. Further limitations include an inability to separate mature polymorphonuclear cells from band forms.

In patients with marked leukocytosis, thrombocytosis, and, very rarely, reticulocytosis, hemoglobin oxygen saturation measured by a pulse oximeter (Spo_2) may be substantially higher than Sao_2 or Pao_2 measured by arterial gas analysis. **Pseudohypoxemia**, or factitious hypoxemia, is used to describe this phenomenon. Possible mechanisms for this phenomenon are rapid consumption of the oxygen dissolved in plasma and coating of the sensing electrode by large number of active cells. Various methods of overcoming or minimizing these problems have been reported. Running the sample without delay, drawing the sample in a glass syringe and placing it immediately on ice, or precooling the glass syringes are some of the inexpensive methods. There are more expensive ways that can be used such as adding potassium cyanide or sodium fluoride or using plasma instead of whole blood for arterial blood analysis.

Autoanalyzers for CBC using spectrophotometric methods, electric impedance technique, or light-scattering phenomenon can provide reliable numbers for all the parameters in the majority of samples. Results may be compromised in the presence of hyperlipidemia, cryoproteinemia, agglutination of various cells (e.g., RBCs, WBCs, platelets), and abnormally shaped and sized cells (e.g., schistocytes, sickled cells). Atypical features are usually flagged by the machine and must be assessed by a visual review of the smear.

Laboratory Standards and Quality Control

An enormous amount of clinical information can be derived from examination of blood chemistries and hematology.[42–44] Indiscriminate or routine ordering of these tests should be discouraged, however, because such practices consume resources unnecessarily, cause potential harm from false-positive or false-negative results, and waste patient blood. Indeed, one of the most important causes of ICU anemia is blood drawing.

The clinical relevance and significance of results are a composite product of not only the appropriateness of the test request but also patient sample identification, criteria for sample acceptance, and running of the tests by appropriate standardized methods followed by communication and interpretation of results. Point-of-care testing has made the task even more difficult. All hematology and blood chemistry testing procedures must be standardized to ensure optimal accuracy and precision. To this end, the U.S. federal government in 1988 established published standards under the Clinical Laboratory Improvement Amendment (CLIA). Other organizations, such as the College of American Pathologists (CAP) and the Joint Commission (TJC), also have published certification standards for laboratories. All laboratories must adhere to these standards, not only to ensure quality care but also to ensure appropriate reimbursement.

As testing methodologies are made more portable, so-called point-of-care (POC) devices for measuring electrolytes, glucose, lactate, hemoglobin, and blood gases have become available. In addition to more rapid turnaround times, these devices offer the ability to use smaller samples of blood or even to return the blood to the patient after testing. However, the same quality standards mandated for central laboratories should also be applied to these devices. Recently FDA has requested an addition in labeling for the use of multipatient POC devices under the section of intended use, which reads: "the performance of this system has not been evaluated in the critically ill."

Regardless of the device used, the limitations of various methods must be kept in mind. Interpretation of values requires knowledge of other medical conditions that may affect the numbers. Indeed, an appropriate first step in the assessment of an unexpected abnormality might be to simply repeat the test. Laboratory tests can provide significant information that drives clinical decision making. The clinician assessing the results should fully appreciate both the significance of the results and the potential errors that might exist.

Key Points

- ▶ The most common serum electrolytes are sodium, potassium, calcium, magnesium, chloride, total carbon dioxide, and phosphorus.
- ▶ Two-thirds of body water is intracellular.
- ▶ Sodium is the most common electrolyte in extracellular fluid.
- ▶ Hyponatremia and hypernatremia are associated with a number of disease states.
- ▶ Potassium is found primarily in the intracellular space.
- ▶ Changes in serum potassium concentrations affect neuromuscular activity and cardiac electrical impulses.
- ▶ Changes in serum chloride concentrations usually follow changes in serum sodium concentrations.
- ▶ Unmeasured anions are estimated through calculation of the anion gap.
- ▶ Most calcium is bound to albumin, but only ionized calcium is metabolically important.
- ▶ Magnesium plays an important role in maintaining membrane potential.
- ▶ Phosphorus is a major intracellular anion that participates in many metabolic processes.
- ▶ Increased lactate concentrations are usually due to anaerobic metabolism.
- ▶ Blood urea nitrogen and serum creatinine levels are used to assess renal function.
- ▶ Serum enzyme levels are used to assess liver and cardiac function.
- ▶ Bilirubin is a breakdown product of hemoglobin that is metabolized in the liver.
- ▶ Serum albumin level is a useful marker of nutritional status.
- ▶ Hyperglycemia and hypoglycemia result from derangements in glucose metabolism.
- ▶ Brain natriuretic peptide levels are elevated in patients with congestive heart failure.
- ▶ Elevated serum C-reactive protein levels are a marker for nonspecific inflammation.
- ▶ High-sensitivity CRP is used to monitor patients with coronary artery disease.
- ▶ Serum procalcitonin levels are currently under evaluation to help distinguish inflammation caused by septic bacterial and fungal sources from viral infections and noninfectious conditions.
- ▶ Prolonged prothrombin time and activated partial thromboplastin time are indicative of problems in blood coagulation.
- ▶ Reduced hemoglobin and hematocrit values are seen in anemia.
- ▶ Reduced platelet counts are indicative of problems in clot formation, which can be a problem in patients undergoing bronchoscopic biopsy or arterial blood gas testing.
- ▶ Reduced leukocytes suggest an immunocompromised state. Moderate elevation of leukocyte count is seen in infections or steroid treatment, and a marked elevation in leukemia and leukemoid reactions.

References

1. Gosling P. Salt of the earth or drop in the ocean? A pathophysiological approach to fluid resuscitation. *Emerg Med J.* 2003;20:306–315.
2. Reynolds RM, Padfield PL, Seckl JR. Disorders of sodium balance. *BMJ.* 2006;332:702–705.
3. Schrier RW. Body water homeostasis: clinical disorders of urinary dilution and concentration. *J Am Soc Nephrol.* 2006;17: 1820–1832.

4. Adrogue HJ, Madias NE. Hypernatremia. *N Engl J Med.* 2000;342: 1493–1499.
5. Spital A. Diuretic induced hyponatremia. *Am J Nephrol.* 1999;19: 447–452.
6. Vaidya C, Ho W, Freda BJ. Management of hyponatremia: providing treatment and avoiding harm. *Cleve Clin J Med.* 2010;77:715–726.
7. Arora SK. Hypernatremic disorders in the intensive care unit. *J Intens Care Med.* 2013;28:37–45.
8. Milionis HJ, Liamis GL, Elisaf MS. The hyponatremic patient: a systematic approach to laboratory diagnosis. *CMAJ.* 2002;166: 1056–1062.
9. Kraft MD, Btaiche IF, Sacks GS, Kudsk KA. Treatment of electrolyte disorders in adult patients in the intensive care unit. *Am J Health-Syst Pharm.* 2005;62:1663–1682.
10. McQuade DJ, Dargan PI, Wood DM. Challenges in the diagnosis of ethylene glycol poisoning. *Ann Clin Biochem.* 2014;51(Pt 2): 167–178.
11. Rastergar A, Soleimani M. Hypokalaemia and hyperkalaemia. *Post Grad Med J.* 2001;77:759–764.
12. Elliott MJ, Ronksley PE, Clase CM, Ahmed SB, Hemmelgarn BR. Management of patients with acute hyperkalemia. *CMAJ.* 2010;182:1631–1635.
13. Nikolaos Sevastos N, Theodossiades, G, Archimandritis AJ. Pseudohyperkalemia in serum: a new insight into an old phenomenon. *Clin Med Res.* 2008;6:30–32.
14. Handy JM, Soni N. Physiological effects of hyperchloraemia and acidosis. *Br J Anaesth.* 2008;101:141–150.
15. Kraut JA, Madias NE. Serum anion gap: its uses and limitation in clinical medicine. *Clin J Am Soc Nephrol.* 2007;2:162–174.
16. Ayers P, Warrington L. Diagnosis and treatment of simple acid-base disorders. *Nutr Clin Pract.* 2008;23:122–127.
17. Fong J, Khan A. Hypocalcemia. Updates in diagnosis and management for primary care. *Can Fam Physician.* 2012;58:158–162.
18. Barth JH, Fiddy JB, Payne RB. Adjustment of serum total calcium for albumin concentration: effects of non-linearity and of regression differences between laboratories. *Ann Clin Biochem.* 1996;33:55–58.
19. Kaye P, O'Sullivan I. The role of magnesium in emergency department. *Emerg Med J.* 2002;19:288–291.
20. Schuker JJ, Ward KE. Hyperphosphatemia and binders. *Am J Health Syst Pharm.* 2005;62:2355–2361.
21. Toffaletti J. Elevations in blood lactate: overview of use in critical care. *Scand J Clin Lab Invest.* 1996;56(Suppl 224):107–110.
22. James JH, Luchette FA, McCarter FD, et al. Lactate is an unreliable indicator of tissue hypoxia in injury or sepsis. *Lancet.* 1999;354:505–508.
23. Traynor J, Mactier R, Geddes CC, Fox GJ. How to measure renal function in clinical practice. *BMJ.* 2006;333:733–737.
24. Giannini EG, Testa R, Savarino V. Liver enzyme alteration: a guide for clinicians. *CMAJ.* 2005;172:367–379.
25. Matull WR, Pereira SP, O'Donohue JW. Biochemical markers of acute pancreatitis. *J Clin Pathol.* 2006;59:340–344.
26. Braunwald E, Morrow DA. Unstable angina. Is it time for a requiem? *Circulation.* 2013;127:2452–2457.
27. Apple FS, Wu AHB, Mair J, et al. Future biomarkers for detection of ischemia and risk stratification of acute coronary syndrome. *Clin Chem.* 2005;51:810–824.
28. Clerico A, Fontana M, Zyw L, Passino C, Emdin M. Comparison of the diagnostic accuracy of brain natriuretic peptide (BNP) and the N-terminal part of the propeptide of BNP in chronic and acute heart failure: a systematic review. *Clin Chem.* 2007;53: 813–822.
29. Kao PC, Sheish S-C, Wu T-J. Serum C-reactive protein as a marker for wellness assessment. *Ann Clin Lab Sci.* 2006;36:163–169.
30. Anderson LN, Anderson NG. The human plasma proteome: character and diagnostic prospects. *Mol Cell Proteomics.* 2002;1: 845–867.
31. Anderson LN. The clinical plasma proteome: a survey of clinical assays for proteins in plasma and serum. *Clin Chem.* 2010;56: 177–185.
32. Chiasson J-L, Aris-Jilwan N, Belanger R, et al. Diagnosis and treatment of diabetic ketoacidosis and the hyperglycemic hyperosmolar state. *CMAJ.* 2003;168:859–866.
33. Foushee JA, Hope NH, Grace EE. Applying biomarkers to clinical practice: a guide for utilizing procalcitonin assays. *J Antimicrob Chemother.* 2012;67:2560–2569.
34. Tachil J. Relevance of clotting tests in liver disease. *Postgrad Med J.* 2008;84:177–181.
35. Miyares MA, Davis K. Newer oral anticoagulants: a review of laboratory monitoring options and reversal agents in the hemorrhagic patient. *Am J Health Syst Pharm.* 2012;69:1473–1484.
36. Sihler KC, Napolitano NM. Anemia of inflammation in critically ill patients. *J Intensive Care Med.* 2008;23:295–302.
37. Gulati GL, Hyun BH. The automated CBC: a current perspective. *Hematol Oncol Clin North Am.* 1994;8:593–601.
38. George JN. Platelets. *Lancet.* 2000;355:1531–1539.
39. Dalal BI, Brigden ML. Factitious biochemical measurements resulting from hematologic conditions. *Am J Clin Pathol.* 2009;131: 195–204.
40. George TI. Malignant or benign leukocytosis. *Hematology.* 2012;475–484.
41. Cerny J, Rosemarin AJ. Why does my patient have leukocytosis? *Hematol Oncol Clin North Am.* 2012;26:303–319.
42. Shahangian S, Snyder SR. Laboratory medicine quality indicators. *Am J Clin Pathol.* 2009;131:418–431.
43. Price CP. Regular review: point of care testing. *BMJ.* 2001;322: 1285–1288.
44. Ben ND, Ziath JL. Technology review: discussion of open-source methodologies in laboratory automation. *JALA.* 2009;14:82–89.

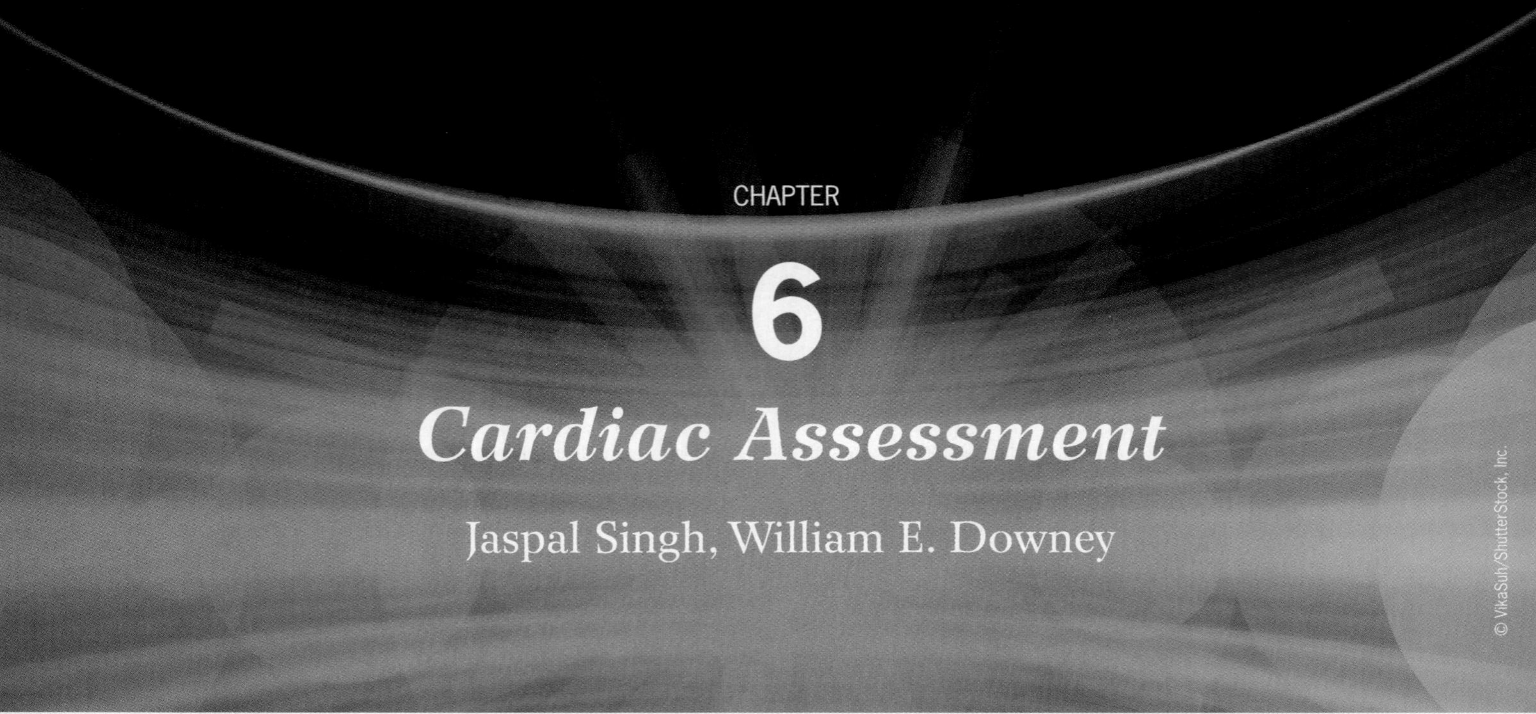

CHAPTER

6
Cardiac Assessment

Jaspal Singh, William E. Downey

OUTLINE

Evaluation of Ventricular Function
Valvular Function
Coronary Artery Disease
Arrhythmias
Refractory Hypoxemia

OBJECTIVES

1. Compare the similarity of symptoms and the interaction between the respiratory and cardiovascular systems.
2. Compare systolic and diastolic dysfunction.
3. Describe tests of cardiac function, their use in clinical practice, and their advantages and disadvantages.
4. Describe tests used to assess left ventricular function and right ventricular function.
5. Describe tests used to evaluate valvular function.
6. Discuss tests to evaluate coronary circulation.
7. Interpret common arrhythmias.
8. Describe intracardiac shunts.
9. Integrate cardiac evaluation into the assessment of the patient with cardiopulmonary disease.

KEY TERMS

afterload
angina
Bubble echocardiogram
cardiac catheterization
cardiac output (c)
cor pulmonale
diastolic dysfunction
echocardiography
ejection fraction (EF)
electrocardiogram (ECG)
ischemia
myocardial perfusion imaging
pulmonary hypertension
radionuclide angiocardiography
stress test
stroke volume
systolic dysfunction
transesophageal echocardiography (TEE)
valvular heart disease
valvular regurgitation
valvular stenosis
ventriculography

Introduction

Diseases of the respiratory and cardiovascular systems interact in pathophysiology, symptoms, treatment, and prognosis. Although primary diseases of either organ system may not involve the other, a significant interaction is more common. This interaction between the respiratory and cardiovascular systems often confounds the diagnosis of the primary problem and complicates its management. Understanding the basics of cardiac function, pathology, and evaluation is important for the respiratory therapist in numerous respects, some of which are described in this chapter.

Evaluation of Ventricular Function

Case 1. Congestive Heart Failure

A 50-year-old man comes to the emergency department with several days of worsening shortness of breath. He has a history of hypertension, diabetes, and high cholesterol. Vital signs show hypertension, hypoxia, and respiratory distress but no fever. On examination he is obese and has an elevated jugular venous pressure (JVP), S_3 gallop, crackles in his lung bases, and prominent bilateral leg swelling. His chest x-ray shows pulmonary edema, and his **electrocardiogram (ECG)** shows no signs of acute myocardial infarction (MI), although there are signs of chronic ischemic heart disease.

This patient may have dyspnea for several reasons, but the clinical clues in this case are derived from the history and physical, with supportive information from the chest x-ray and ECG. All these clues suggest that the patient has acute congestive heart failure (CHF). He has risk factors for heart disease (obese, diabetic, hypertensive, high cholesterol), and the examination demonstrates physical findings of left-sided heart failure (S_3 gallop, crackles in his lung bases) as well as right heart failure (leg edema). The absence of fever helps to exclude an active infectious process such as pneumonia, and additional supportive information is gleaned from the chest x-ray, ECG, and perhaps other laboratory tests. Elevated brain natriuretic peptide (BNP), or B-type natriuretic peptide, levels can be used as a diagnostic tool to evaluate for cardiac dysfunction as a cause of dyspnea and have also been shown to correlate with the presence and severity of cardiac diseases such as CHF.[1] Although an elevated BNP does not give insight into the cause of the dysfunction and its interpretation can be confounded for a number of reasons, it might suggest that cardiac disease is involved in the patient's symptoms. The ECG also points away from an active MI or other diagnosis complicating his picture. At this point, it would be very helpful to understand the patient's cardiac physiology (especially left ventricular function). A transthoracic echocardiogram can be used to evaluate this quickly and noninvasively and would provide the greatest amount of functional and prognostic information.

Left Ventricular Dysfunction

The primary symptom of patients with left ventricular dysfunction is dyspnea, but additional symptoms of CHF such as orthopnea or paroxysmal nocturnal dyspnea may suggest that the primary cause of dyspnea is ventricular dysfunction rather than a pulmonary disorder. The initial diagnostic step used to evaluate patients with symptoms of ventricular dysfunction is to determine whether **systolic dysfunction** (impaired contractility) or **diastolic dysfunction** (impaired filling) is the major pathophysiologic mechanism.

Symptoms of CHF (dyspnea on exertion, orthopnea, paroxysmal nocturnal dyspnea) can also occur with normal systolic function of the left ventricle. Diastolic dysfunction increasingly is recognized as a cause of the symptoms of CHF and may be present with or without systolic dysfunction. Although the history and physical examination are useful for differentiation of cardiac causes from respiratory causes of dyspnea, it may be more difficult to determine whether CHF is due to systolic or diastolic dysfunction without an imaging study of left ventricular function. Moreover, many patients have simultaneous systolic and diastolic heart failure.

Echocardiography uses ultrasonography to examine the heart structures and function. Because of its portability and noninvasiveness (safety), echocardiography often is the primary test used in the assessment of ventricular function. Echocardiography provides information on the **ejection fraction (EF)**, which is the fraction of blood pumped from the ventricle during a single cardiac contraction. The normal left ventricular ejection fraction is more than 0.50. Because the ejection fraction is easily obtained, reproducible, and is an important prognostic factor in critical illness, it is an extremely useful measurement.

In addition to assessing overall function, echocardiography allows more detailed assessment of cardiac structure and function. A regional wall motion abnormality suggests ischemia as the cause of left ventricular systolic dysfunction. In contrast, nonischemic cardiomyopathies usually affect all segments of the myocardium equally (a global process). Moreover, different features of echocardiography (M-mode, Doppler modes) allow more sophisticated assessment of cardiac structure and function.

Cardiac catheterization techniques include other methods used to evaluate ventricular function. **Cardiac output** (c; often expressed in liters per minute) reflects forward blood flow from the heart into the systemic vasculature and provides an overall assessment of cardiovascular function. Cardiac output is often calculated utilizing either the Fick method or thermodilution after placing a catheter into the pulmonary artery. Because numerous assumptions are involved in validating the calculation of cardiac output with both methods, measurements must be interpreted in light of other clinical data.

Other tests evaluating left ventricular function include **radionuclide angiocardiography**, cardiac magnetic resonance imaging (cardiac MRI), and catheter **ventriculography**. Radionuclide tests involve intravenous injection of a radioisotope (most commonly technetium) and the use of a camera to detect the isotope's signal in the left ventricle to allow a reflection of the ejection fraction. Cardiac MRI provides detailed anatomic and functional information, and is now the gold standard for assessment of ventricular function. Its use in critical illness, however, is currently limited by the patient monitoring available during the study and need for breath holding to obtain optimal images. Catheter ventriculography involves injection of radiographic contrast into a cardiac chamber to allow assessment of its size and motion (**Figure 6-1**). This is rarely used solely to assess cardiac function as the same information can be obtained noninvasively. When the patient is undergoing cardiac catheterization for other reasons, this can be a useful adjunctive assessment.

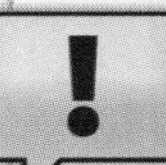

Respiratory Recap

Tests to Assess Left Ventricular Function

- Electrocardiography
- Brain natriuretic peptide elevation
- Radionuclide angiocardiography
- Echocardiography
- Cardiac output
- Left ventriculography by cardiac catheterization
- Cardiac magnetic resonance imaging

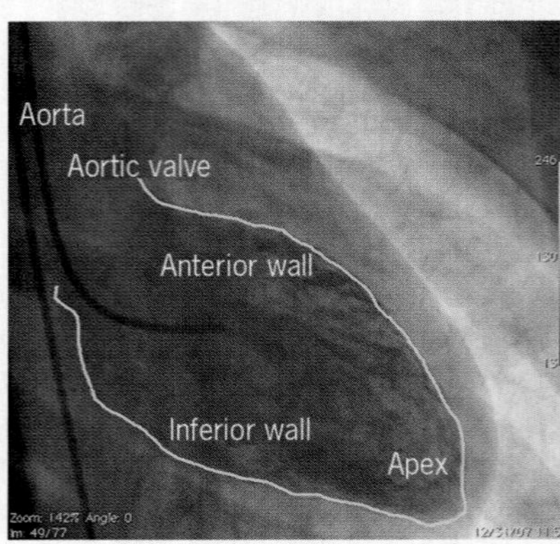

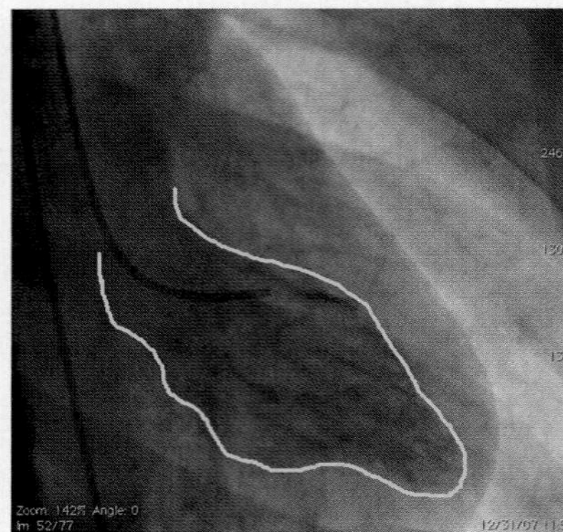

FIGURE 6-1 Left ventriculogram performed during cardiac catheterization, demonstrating (**A**) left ventricular cavity at end-diastole and (**B**) left ventricle at end-systole, with normal contractility of all regions of the myocardium.
Courtesy of Geoffrey A. Rose, MD, FACC, FASE.

Case 2. Right Ventricular Failure

A 53-year-old woman presents with worsening shortness of breath and leg swelling after a long plane ride. She has a history of COPD that was previously well controlled. Vital signs show moderate hypoxemia, tachycardia, and tachypnea. On examination she is obese, has a prominent right ventricular heave, diminished lung sounds throughout, and prominent bilateral leg swelling. Her chest x-ray is clear, and a subsequent ECG **stress test** is unremarkable but was stopped short due to her dyspnea. A computed tomography (CT) scan of the chest with intravenous contrast shows bilateral pulmonary emboli (**Figure 6-2**).

Her clinicians are trying to decide whether to administer thrombolytic therapy, which is more likely to rapidly dissolve the clot than systemic heparin anticoagulation. Thrombolytic therapy is associated with a higher risk of bleeding complications, however. Therefore, it often is reserved for patients with cardiac dysfunction due to the embolism, generally those patients with right ventricular compromise and/or shock.[2] As with assessing left ventricular size and function, echocardiography can be used to evaluate the patient's right ventricle; if a pulmonary embolism is large, it may cause strain on the right heart manifest as dilation and/or hypokinesis of the right ventricle. An echocardiogram demonstrated elevated right ventricular systolic pressures and evidence of strain. Based on this information, the patient received thrombolytic therapy and resolved the clot without further complications.

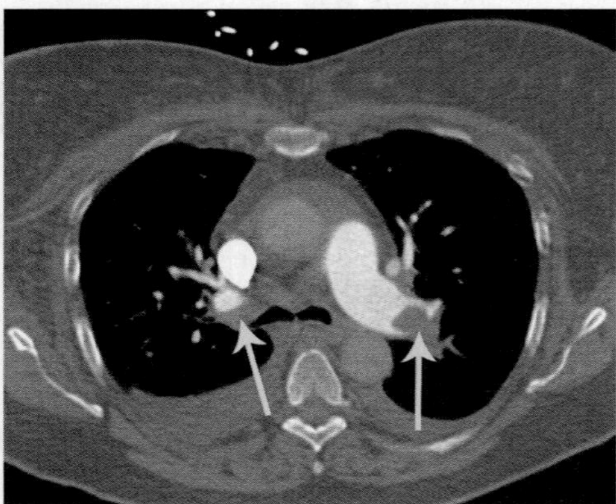

FIGURE 6-2 Bilateral pulmonary emboli.

Right Ventricular Function

Evaluation of pulmonary artery pressures and right ventricular function is important to determine the severity of impact on the heart of pulmonary disease. For example, in patients with severe COPD or severe obstructive sleep apnea, the pulmonary artery pressure may be elevated, resulting in hypertrophy and dilation of the right ventricle, a condition known as **cor pulmonale. Pulmonary hypertension** with chronic respiratory disease (such as COPD) is a poor prognostic finding.[3] Right ventricular dysfunction, or right-sided heart failure, may be suspected in patients with lung disease by the findings of peripheral edema, elevated JVP, hepatomegaly, and ascites.

In the normal situation, the right ventricle is a thin-walled structure that ejects blood into the low resistance of the pulmonary vasculature. Because of its lower muscle mass, it is very sensitive to an acute increase in **afterload** (pulmonary artery pressure), and right ventricular systolic dysfunction may develop. If pulmonary hypertension develops more slowly, the

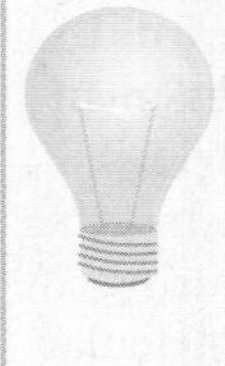

STOP AND THINK

You are providing respiratory care for a patient with COPD and known cardiac disease. What tests might be used to sort out the relative contributions of right-sided and left-sided heart failure?

Respiratory Recap

Tests to Evaluate Right Ventricular Function

- Echocardiography
- Electrocardiogram
- Right heart catheterization (i.e., Swan-Ganz)

right ventricle may adapt by the process of hypertrophy so that the right ventricular ejection fraction remains normal at rest but may decrease during exercise because of an increase in pulmonary artery pressure. A lack of increase in the cardiac output during exercise may result in the symptom of dyspnea. If the pulmonary artery pressure continues to increase over time, further elevation of the right ventricular systolic pressure, and subsequently diastolic pressure, occurs. The elevation in right ventricular diastolic filling pressure results in the signs of right-sided CHF, such as jugular venous distention, lower extremity edema, hepatomegaly, and ascites. Echocardiography provides valuable information about global right ventricular function. In addition to quantitative assessment of right ventricular function and qualitative assessment of right ventricular size and wall thickness, Doppler echocardiography can be used to estimate the pulmonary artery systolic pressure and suggest whether right ventricular dysfunction is caused by pressure overload or volume overload.

Right heart catheterization with the use of a pulmonary artery catheter can be used to assess right heart dysfunction. Right heart catheterization, as mentioned earlier, can also be used as a means to measure cardiac output. Although this is a much more accurate means of measuring right ventricle and pulmonary artery pressures than echocardiogram,[3] it is invasive. As such, it not only exposes the patient to greater risk but also may be difficult to perform when the patient is having acute issues. Because some literature suggests that use of right heart catheterization is associated with poorer clinical outcomes in critically ill patients, its use has fallen out of favor when less invasive means are available.[4]

Valvular Function

Case 3. Valvular Disease

A 26-year-old man comes to the emergency department with 1 day of severe shortness of breath and high fever. He is in respiratory distress, hypoxemic, and unable to provide a history. On examination he is thin, hypotensive, and has a loud, harsh systolic murmur best heard underneath his left nipple. In addition, bilateral crackles are heard on examination. Further inspection shows poor dentition and needle track marks indicating prior intravenous drug use. His chest x-ray shows pulmonary edema, but no discrete infiltrate suggestive of pneumonia. ECG shows only sinus tachycardia. The patient is intubated and placed on mechanical ventilation. Labs show a markedly elevated white blood cell (WBC) count. Blood cultures are drawn, and the patient is started on intravenous antibiotics. He is seen by several specialists who suspect that he has mitral valve endocarditis (a life-threatening infection of the mitral valve).

There are several reasons why this patient might have dyspnea, but the clinical clues in this case are derived from the history and physical, with supportive information from the chest x-ray. These lead one to suspect the patient has endocarditis. The high fever and elevated WBC count are indicative of an acute infectious process. The ensuing hypotension, loud apical murmur, and pulmonary edema are the salient clues to the diagnosis of endocarditis. The chest x-ray and the murmur point away from community-acquired pneumonia as the etiology, whereas the ECG also points away from an active MI and excludes an arrhythmia.

In this case, the valve has been infected and thereby damaged, causing leakage of the valve during each systolic contraction. This leak results in elevated left atrial and, hence, pulmonary venous pressures, causing pulmonary edema and dyspnea. Because a significant proportion of the left ventricular output is then directed backward into the left atrium, hypotension may result from decreased cardiac output. The optimal confirmatory test here is then an echocardiogram, which may be performed via a transthoracic approach (simpler, noninvasive, but lower resolution of the valve) or a transesophageal approach (more invasive but much more sensitive to valvular pathology).

Evaluation of Valvular Function

Acquired or congenital heart disease may affect valvular function. **Figure 6-3** shows the normal valvular anatomy. Hemodynamically, **valvular heart disease** can be differentiated into two types: stenotic lesions resulting in impaired valve opening or regurgitant lesions caused by impaired valve closure. The two types may be present concurrently.

Normally, the valve opens when the pressure in the proximal chamber of the heart exceeds the pressure in the distal chamber. Although the pressure difference (gradient) is responsible for opening the valve and blood flow across the valve, the normal valve gradient is

Respiratory Recap

Types of Valvular Heart Disease

- Stenotic lesions
- Regurgitant lesions

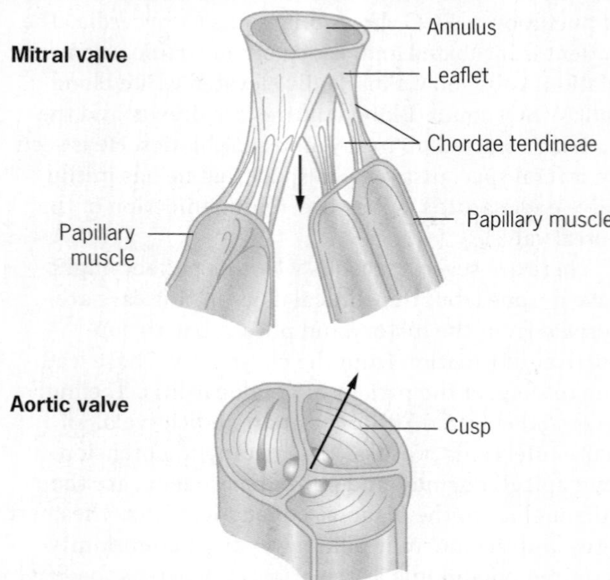

FIGURE 6-3 Normal cardiac valve anatomy.
Reproduced from *Textbook of Medical Physiology*. 8th ed. Guyton AC, Hall JE. Copyright Elsevier [WB Saunders] 1991.

minimal as blood flows between chambers of the heart. When disease causes narrowing of the valve orifice, a greater pressure difference between the chambers of the heart that are separated by the stenotic valve is required to sustain flow. Stenotic valvular lesions thus result in pressure overload of the proximal or upstream heart chamber, eventually resulting in abnormal diastolic function and the symptoms and signs of heart failure.

The severity of valvular stenosis is determined by measurement of the pressure gradient across the valve area. The pressure gradient reflects not only the severity of the stenosis but also the rate of blood flow across the valve. This gradient is then combined mathematically with the measured flow across the valve to calculate the valve area. Valve area measurements have been correlated with severity of disease for left-sided valvular lesions (mitral and aortic stenosis), but the clinical application of valve areas is less clear for the right-sided heart valves; therefore, pressure gradients alone are used to express the severity of stenosis on the right side. Because different chambers have different normal pressures, significant gradients differ from valve to valve. Severe aortic valve stenosis is defined as a mean gradient >40 mm Hg. Severe mitral stenosis is defined as a mean gradient >10 mm Hg. Severe pulmonic stenosis is defined as a peak gradient >64 mm Hg, and tricuspid stenosis, >5 mm Hg.

Valvular regurgitation is caused by abnormal or impaired valve closure. Normally, when pressure in the downstream chamber exceeds pressure in the upstream chamber, the leaflets of the interceding valve close and coapt to prevent regurgitation of blood flow into the proximal chamber. Acquired or congenital valvular disease may result in abnormal valve closure. In such cases a proportion of the ventricular **stroke volume** flows backward rather than contributing to forward blood flow.

With mitral regurgitation a portion of the blood pumped by the left ventricle flows not forward into the aorta but backward into the left atrium, the amount depending on the degree of valvular pathology and relative pressures. The left ventricle therefore needs to increase its workload to meet the forward demands of blood flow as well as account for the additional regurgitant volume going back into the left atrium. This extra work due to chronic severe regurgitation results in volume overload and dilation of the ventricle, and symptoms may develop from the increased pulmonary venous pressure due to the leak itself as well as that due to the resulting systolic dysfunction.

Echocardiography

Echocardiography is the most useful initial test to evaluate valvular function. Two-dimensional echocardiography allows visualization of valve leaflet anatomy and mobility. The appearance of thickened, calcified leaflets with poor mobility suggests **valvular stenosis** (**Figure 6-4**). In addition, with different angles of

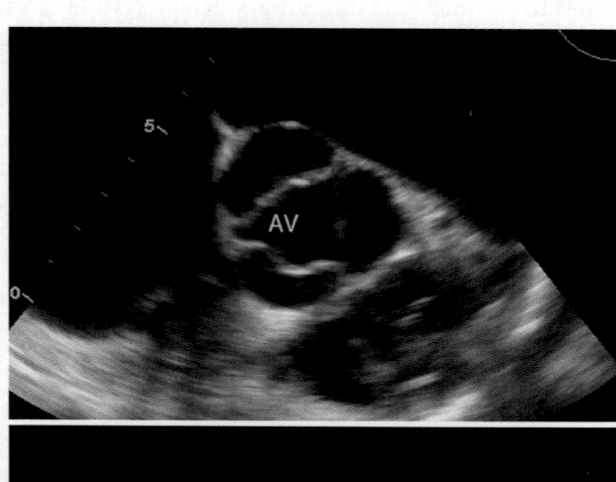

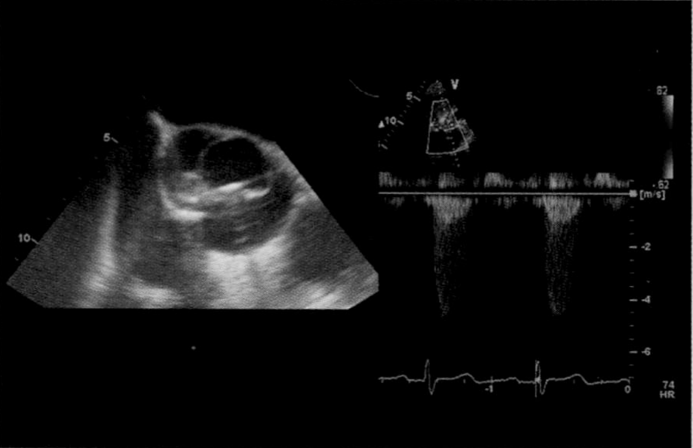

FIGURE 6-4 Two-dimensional echocardiography (short-axis view). (**A**) Normal aortic valve (AV) orifice. (**B**) Calcified, stenotic aortic valve. The continuous wave Doppler analysis across the aortic valve demonstrates a high-velocity jet (>4 meters per second), consistent with severe aortic stenosis.
Courtesy of Geoffrey A. Rose, MD, FACC, FASE.

Respiratory Recap

Tests to Assess Valvular Function

- Electrocardiography
- Radionuclide angiography
- Echocardiography
- Cardiac catheterization

ultrasound transmission, the orifice of the valve can be visualized and measured. Echocardiography is also useful in evaluating the sequelae of valvular stenosis, such as LVH secondary to aortic stenosis or left atrial enlargement secondary to mitral stenosis.

Echocardiography does not measure pressure gradients directly, but Doppler echocardiography allows calculation of the pressure difference across a stenotic valve. Specifically, the modified Bernoulli equation relates flow velocity to pressure gradient ($\Delta P = 4 \times v^2$, where P is measured in mm Hg and v in m/s). Two-dimensional echocardiography is also useful in the assessment of secondary changes of valvular regurgitation, such as increased ventricular size and impaired systolic function, factors that are also used to decide when to intervene. Particularly relevant to the respiratory care provider is the ability of echocardiography to estimate right ventricular systolic pressure, which may reflect the presence of pulmonary hypertension as well as signs of right heart failure.

Transesophageal echocardiography (TEE) is a slightly invasive procedure in which a smaller ultrasound transducer is passed posterior to the heart via the esophagus. This allows closer investigation of valvular heart disease because of the proximity of the transesophageal probe to the heart and the absence of intervening anatomic barriers such as the lungs and ribs.[5] TEE includes all aspects of transthoracic imaging, including two-dimensional, Doppler, and color Doppler techniques, and is useful in assessments of valve morphology and function. It is particularly advantageous in evaluations of both the mitral valve, because of this valve's posterior position (**Figure 6-5**), and prosthetic valves, which may be difficult to visualize by transthoracic echocardiography because of shadowing of the ultrasound beam.

Cardiac Catheterization

Cardiac catheterization is an invasive, accurate means to quantify valvular stenosis and regurgitation. The pressure gradient can be directly assessed with the use of fluid-filled catheters to measure the pressure in the distal and proximal heart chambers across the stenotic valve. The pressure gradient across a stenotic valve is inversely related to the valve area (i.e., the smaller the valve area, the larger the pressure gradient).

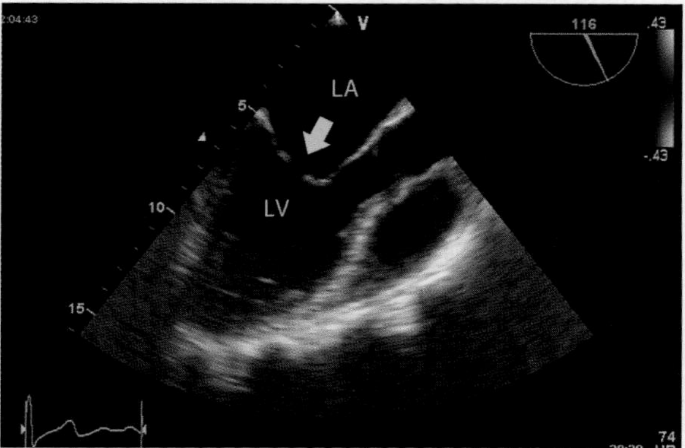

FIGURE 6-5 Transesophageal echocardiography demonstrating significant mitral stenosis. The left atrium (LA) and left ventricle (LV) are depicted, along with the stenotic mitral valve opening (arrow).
Courtesy of Geoffrey A. Rose, MD, FACC, FASE.

Coronary Artery Disease

Case 4. Coronary Artery Disease

A 60-year-old woman comes to the emergency department with several hours of crushing substernal chest pain. Previously this occurred while she was exerting herself and would abate with rest. This time, however, it developed while standing at work. The pain is severe, radiates down her left arm and up to the left side of her face. She also feels sweaty, nauseated, and lightheaded. Her medical history is notable for hypertension, high cholesterol, and a family history of heart disease. Her coworker calls for emergency help, and she is given sublingual nitroglycerin and oxygen, which lessen her pain. An ECG shows ST segment elevation (**Figure 6-6**). She is given aspirin therapy and thereafter transported to the local emergency department. On examination, she is diaphoretic, tachycardic, in mild respiratory distress, and obviously in pain. A chest x-ray is clear. Cardiac troponin is normal.

This patient has classic symptoms of **angina**, which is chest pain due to coronary **ischemia** (lack of oxygen to the heart muscle tissues that are dependent on the blood flow from the blocked vessel). This usually affects the left ventricle, but occasionally may affect the right side of the heart. Before the presentation that brought her to the emergency department, the patient's symptoms would have been classified as stable angina (abates easily with rest), but now her symptoms would be deemed unstable, and in fact she likely has an occluded coronary artery that, if it persists, will result in more extensive cardiac damage. The normal cardiac troponin does not exclude an acute coronary syndrome, as it does not become elevated until approximately 4 hours after the onset of myocardial ischemia.

She therefore undergoes emergent coronary angiography to both definitively assess the coronary arteries and set the stage for emergent coronary revascularization, by means of angioplasty and possibly placing a stent to maintain the patency of the opened artery.

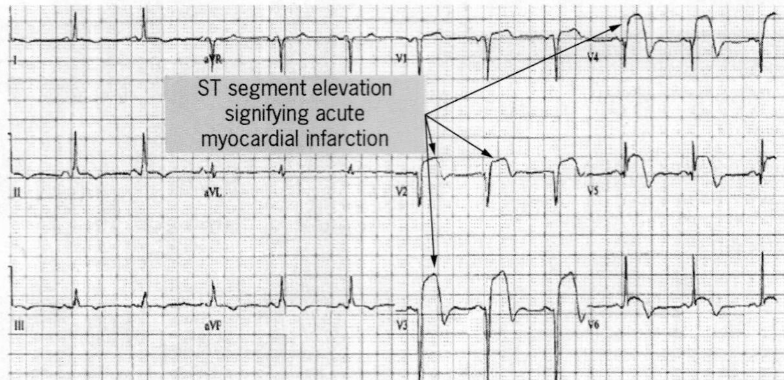

FIGURE 6-6 ECG with ST segment elevation characteristic of cardiac ischemia.

Evaluation of the Coronary Circulation

The most common cause of abnormal coronary circulation is coronary artery disease (CAD) caused by atherosclerosis. Significant CAD primarily affects the left ventricle because of the high metabolic requirement of this chamber. Therefore, left ventricular diastolic dysfunction, systolic dysfunction, and mitral valve dysfunction may occur as a result of limited blood supply to the coronary circulation (i.e., myocardial infarction and/or coronary ischemia). Chest pain and dyspnea are the most common symptoms of CAD.

Coronary artery disease can present as stable angina with symptoms occurring with increased myocardial metabolic demand, such as with exercise. Coronary artery disease can also present as an acute coronary syndrome, typically due to an acute worsening of coronary artery narrowing due to rupture of a cholesterol plaque with superimposed thrombosis. Depending upon the degree of obstruction, the amount of myocardial tissue supplied by the diseased artery, and the extent of collateral supply, acute coronary syndrome may manifest as ST elevation MI (STEMI), myocardial infarction without ST elevations (non-STEMI), or unstable angina. These are differentiated by the presenting ECG (ST elevations or not) and the presence or absence of myocardial necrosis (typically measured via troponin).

Major determinants of myocardial oxygen demand include the myocardial wall tension, contractility, and the heart rate. Furthermore, the response of the heart to ischemia is progressive (the ischemic cascade). As ischemia persists, therefore, additional abnormalities of cardiac function develop. **Figure 6-7** summarizes the ischemic response. When blood flow via a coronary artery is diminished significantly, diastolic dysfunction of the left ventricle is the first demonstrable abnormality of cardiac function. Continued ischemia leads to systolic dysfunction, electrocardiographic changes, and finally, the symptom of angina. Prolonged lack of blood flow results in myocardial infarction. Clinical tests used to evaluate the coronary circulation include the ECG, anatomic assessments, and functional tests. All provide diagnostic and prognostic information, and the rationale for the choice of one test over another is based on the clinical scenario and the information sought.

Specific Tests to Assess Coronary Circulation

Electrocardiogram (ECG)

The ECG is a simple, readily available technique that should be the first test performed in the diagnosis of coronary artery disease.[6] Manifestations of acute ischemia or ongoing infarction on the ECG include T wave inversion, depression of ST segment, and elevation of the ST segment. Completed infarction may be manifest on the ECG as loss of R waves or the development of Q waves. Typically, ischemia is manifest as T wave

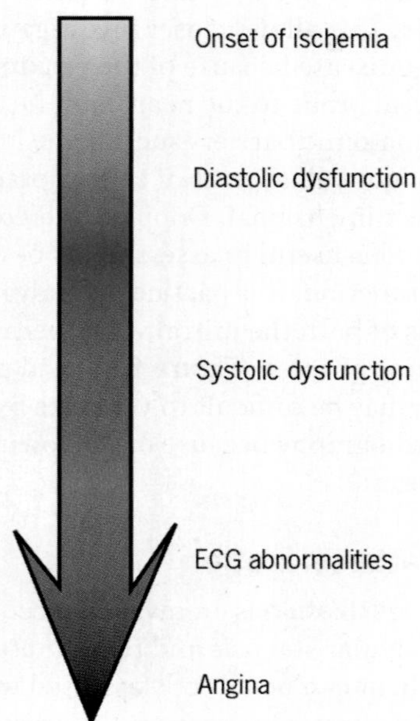

FIGURE 6-7 The ischemic cascade of cardiac dysfunction during coronary artery occlusion.

Adapted from Nesto RW, Kowalchuck GJ. The ischemic cascade: temporal sequence of hemodynamic, electrocardiographic and symptomatic expressions of ischemia. *Am J Cardiol.* 1987;57:23C–27C.

inversion and/or ST depression. ST elevation in the setting of an acute coronary syndrome suggests ongoing infarction of a sizable territory of myocardium. It is important to recognize, however, that myocardial ischemia may occur with minimal or no abnormalities on the ECG. Furthermore, all the ECG changes mentioned may be apparent in conditions other than CAD, such as metabolic abnormalities, LVH, and COPD. For these reasons, such ECG abnormalities must be interpreted in the context of the patient's symptoms, history, and physical examination results.

Anatomic Tests

Anatomic tests provide information on the presence, distribution, and severity of CAD. In some cases the anatomy of CAD provides important prognostic information. For instance, significant stenosis of the left main coronary artery and stenosis involving the proximal segments of all three coronary arteries are known to be associated with a decrease in long-term survival with medical therapy alone, indicating the need to consider revascularization either by percutaneous or surgical means.[7] Most commonly, this information is determined by cardiac catheterization, though cardiac CT angiography is an increasingly viable alternative technique.[8] In general, stenosis of 70% or greater is considered significant (**Figure 6-8**).

Functional Tests

Functional tests assess for impaired blood flow with resultant ischemia or impaired cardiac function. With impaired coronary circulation, the supply of blood to the myocardial tissue may be adequate at rest but insufficient to meet the increased demands of exercise or acute illness. Functional tests assess not the degree of coronary narrowing but the resultant ischemia. Increased myocardial oxygen demand can be induced by exercise or pharmacologically (e.g., with dobutamine). Under these conditions, ECG, perfusion imaging with nuclear agents or MRI, or assessment of resultant dysfunction by echocardiogram can assess ischemia.

Myocardial perfusion imaging involves intravenous injection of a radionuclide agent (such as thallium-201 or technetium-99m), which accumulates in the myocardium in proportion to regional myocardial perfusion. The comparison of perfusion images obtained at rest and with exercise allows determination of whether perfusion is normal both at rest and with exercise, normal at rest but failing to increase with exercise (ischemia), or decreased both at rest and with exercise due to a prior myocardial infarction (**Figure 6-9**). A region of myocardium that is hypoperfused during exercise but that appears normal at rest is called a *reversible perfusion defect.* This abnormality is consistent with the presence of a significant lesion in the coronary artery that limits the increase in myocardial blood flow to that region normally seen during exercise. A region of myocardium that is hypoperfused both during exercise and at rest is called a *fixed perfusion defect* and is consistent with an MI (i.e., the cardiac tissue of the affected area has essentially been replaced by scar tissue, which requires less blood flow than cardiac muscle).

In addition, an individual coronary lesion's physiologic impact can be assessed at cardiac catheterization by measuring the fractional flow reserve (FFR).

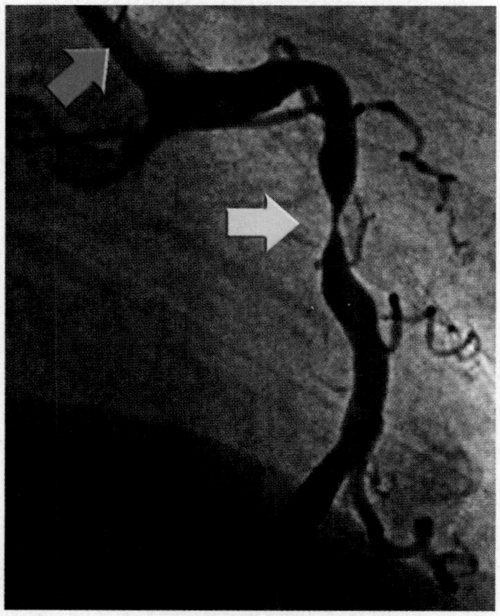

FIGURE 6-8 Right coronary angiogram of a patient with angina and abnormal exercise treadmill test result. The purple arrowhead demonstrates the catheter in the ostium of the right coronary artery. The yellow arrowhead demonstrates a 95% mid–right coronary artery stenosis.

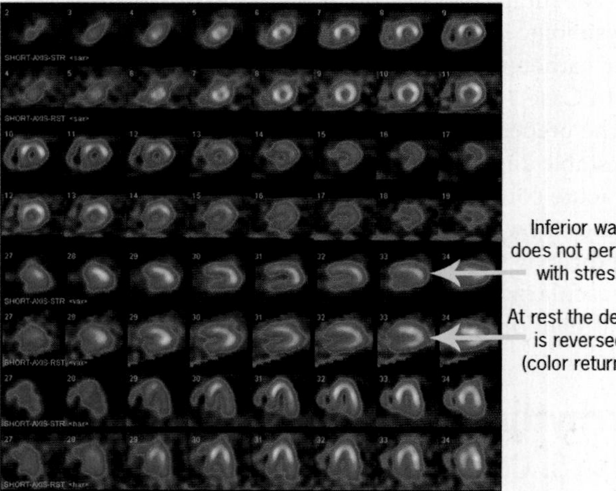
Inferior wall does not perfuse with stress
At rest the defect is reversed (color returns)

FIGURE 6-9 Nuclear cardiology perfusion imaging of the left ventricular myocardium during exercise and rest. The left ventricle is depicted in three different views during exercise and rest. The perfusion images demonstrate hypoperfusion (decreased blood flow) to the inferior wall during exercise (yellow arrows). After the patient rests, the blood flow returns, consistent with myocardial ischemia in that region.

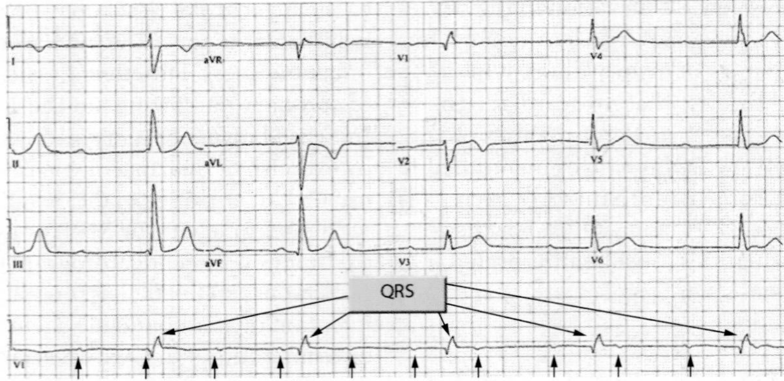

FIGURE 6-10 Complete heart block (third degree).

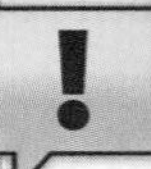

Respiratory Recap

Tests to Assess Coronary Circulation

- Electrocardiogram: ST segment changes
- Exercise stress testing
- Radionuclide angiocardiography
- Echocardiography
- Myocardial perfusion imaging
- Coronary arteriography
- Cardiac CT scanning

The FFR is the ratio of the mean pressure upstream of a lesion compared with that downstream of the lesion under conditions of maximal hyperemia.[9] To measure this, a pressure transducer on a 0.014-inch-diameter coronary guide wire is advanced distal to the lesion and maximal hyperemia is induced by the administration of adenosine or nitroprusside. This technique has the advantage of allowing definitive assessment of the physiologic impact of a given lesion at the time of cardiac catheterization.

In Case 4, a functional test might have been helpful in the preceding weeks to diagnose and target therapy for stable angina, but now, when the patient is having an acute coronary event, revascularization of the culprit lesion will improve outcome. Therefore, proceeding directly to an anatomic test to assess and guide revascularization is appropriate as both diagnostic and treatment options are potentially provided in a single procedure.

Arrhythmias

Case 5. Cardiac Arrhythmia

A 75-year-old woman with a history of CAD develops severe lightheadedness and diaphoresis. On examination, her pulse is 25 beats per minute and blood pressure is 80/45 mm Hg. She is taken to the emergency department where an electrocardiogram (**Figure 6-10**) reveals third-degree block. She is taken immediately for a pacemaker insertion and has a full recovery.

Respiratory therapists commonly encounter cardiac arrhythmias in their patients. Arrhythmias can develop from many medical conditions, both cardiac and noncardiac, as well as from medications or other interventions. Therefore, a basic understanding of the cardiac conduction system is important. In normal function (**Figure 6-11**), the cardiac impulse begins with firing of the sinoatrial (SA) node high in the right atrium with propagation of electrical signal throughout the atria. The ventricles are electrically isolated from the atria with the exception at the atrioventricular (AV) node. The electrical impulse, which begins in the atria, must normally traverse the AV node to allow activation of the ventricles. This electrical impulse is then carried through the right and left bundles to trigger depolarization of the ventricular myocardium.

Dysfunction of this conduction system manifests as arrhythmias. Bradyarrhythmias (slow heart rhythms) may result from slowed or failed firing of the SA node or impaired propagation of the electrical signal at

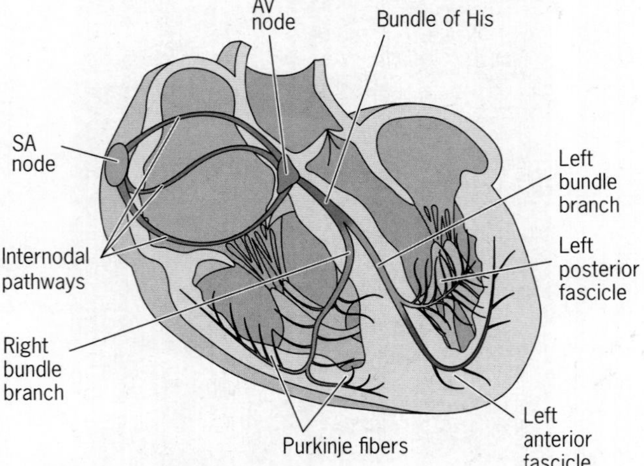

FIGURE 6-11 Electrical activity in the heart. The electrical signal normally starts at the sinus node, which causes the right and left atria to contract. The atrioventricular (AV) node is triggered next. The AV node sends a signal through the His/Purkinje system via the conduction pathways. The conduction pathways then signal the right and left ventricles to contract.

any level. Impaired propagation at the level of the AV node and below is relatively common. AV node dysfunction is commonly a result of medications such as beta blockers or calcium channel blockers and may also be a transient manifestation of increased vagal tone. Impaired propagation in the ventricular conduction system is less likely to be a response to medications or vagal tone. In either case, symptomatic bradycardia arrhythmias can be treated with implantation of a pacemaker. However, asymptomatic bradycardia is common and usually managed conservatively.

Tachyarrhythmias (fast heart rhythms) occur commonly in critically ill patients. The most common tachyarrhythmia is sinus tachycardia, the rapid heart rate induced by increased metabolic stress such as that occurring during exercise or illness. This is not pathologic but an appropriate and necessary physiologic response to stress. Pathologic tachyarrhythmias can be divided into those affecting primarily the atria (supraventricular arrhythmias) versus those affecting the ventricles (ventricular arrhythmias). In general, these are manifest on the ECG as narrow complex and wide complex tachycardia arrhythmias, respectively.

Common supraventricular tachyarrhythmias include atrial flutter, atrial fibrillation, and re-entrant supraventricular tachycardia. Atrial flutter most commonly is a result of a short circuit (reentry) around the tricuspid valve resulting in rapid regular atrial electrical activation (typically 300 beats per minute). This rapid activity bombards the AV node. Usually, the AV node does not transmit all of these electrical signals to the ventricular conduction system, instead allowing only every second or third beat to be conducted; thus atrial flutter with 2:1 or 3:1 block. The resultant ventricular rate is typically 150 or 100 beats per minute. The ECG thus typically manifests multiple P waves at a rate of 300 beats per minute with regular narrow QRS complexes resulting from every second or third of these P waves. The degree of AV block can be increased by medications that slow conduction through the AV node, such as beta blockers and calcium channel blockers.

Atrial fibrillation is a result of disorganized electrical activity within the atria. This disorganized atrial electrical activity results in rapid irregular activation of the AV node, which cannot conduct all of these impulses. The typical ECG manifestation is the absence of P waves and irregular narrow QRS complexes. As in atrial flutter, the ventricular rate can be controlled with medications that slow conduction through the atrioventricular node. Atrial fibrillation, in particular, is commonly paroxysmal and precipitated in times of acute noncardiac illness. Neither atrial flutter nor atrial fibrillation is usually life-threatening when it is the sole problem, but the inappropriate tachycardia can be deleterious to myocardial metabolic demand and cardiac output, thus potentially leading to patient compromise.

In contrast, ventricular tachyarrhythmias are commonly immediately life-threatening. These include ventricular fibrillation and ventricular tachycardia. Ventricular fibrillation is always immediately life-threatening and is treated with emergent electrical defibrillation. Ventricular tachycardia is commonly brief and self-limited. However, sustained ventricular tachycardia is also commonly immediately life-threatening and again treated with emergent electrical cardioversion.

Appendix 6-1 and **Table 6-1** provide a more complete presentation of the different types of cardiac arrhythmias.

ECG in Pulmonary Disease

Characteristic ECG changes may occur with other pulmonary conditions, such as acute pulmonary embolism or obstructive lung disease. If an acute pulmonary embolus results in a significant increase in pulmonary arterial pressure, a number of electrocardiographic features suggestive of acute right ventricular strain may be present: (1) $S_1Q_3T_3$ (development of an S wave in lead I, and Q wave and T wave inversion in lead III); (2) rightward QRS axis shift; (3) transient right bundle branch block; and (4) T wave inversion in the right precordial leads (V_{1-2}). However, these changes are relatively insensitive and transient (as resolution or thrombolysis of the pulmonary embolus occurs).

COPD also may cause characteristic electrocardiographic changes, which are thought to be due to hyperinflation of the lungs and a low position of the diaphragm. As a result, the heart becomes more vertical in the chest and rotates clockwise along its longitudinal axis. Other electrocardiographic abnormalities include right atrial abnormality, right axis deviation, low QRS voltage, T wave abnormalities in the right precordial leads (V_{1-2}), and leftward shift of the transitional zone.

Refractory Hypoxemia

Case 6. Intracardiac Shunt

A 30-year-old woman developed severe streptococcal pneumonia and septic shock for which she was intubated, placed on mechanical ventilation while being treated with antibiotics and supportive care. She initially required vasopressors to maintain her blood pressure. Despite what seemed to be clinical and radiographic stabilization in her condition off vasopressors, oxygenation remained a challenge. On PEEP of 10 cm H_2O and F_{IO_2} of 0.6, her Pa_{O_2} is 50 mm Hg. She had no prior history of cardiac disease and a normal cardiovascular physical exam. Initial echocardiogram did not disclose any cardiac defects and normal right-sided pulmonary pressures were noted. One of the clinicians ordered an echocardiogram with saline bubbles for echo contrast, which demonstrated abnormal flow

TABLE 6-1
Summary of Cardiac Rhythms

	Normal Sinus*	Paroxysmal Supraventricular Tachycardia	Atrial Flutter	Atrial Fibrillation	Ventricular Tachycardia	Ventricular Fibrillation	First-Degree AV Block	Second-Degree AV Block, Type I	Second-Degree AV Block, Type II	Complete AV Block (Type III)
Rate (beats per minute)	60–100	150–250	250–350 atrial; ventricular rate varies	Atrial rate >400; ventricular rate varies	100–250 ventricular	Difficult to discern	Normal	Atrial > ventricular; both usually normal	Atrial >ventricular; both usually normal	Atrial > ventricular; both usually normal
Rhythm	Regular	Regular	Atrial is regular; ventricular can be regular or irregular	Irregular	Regular ventricular	Rapid and chaotic	Regular	Atrial regular; ventricular pauses	Atrial regular; ventricular irregular with pauses	Regular
P waves	Uniform, upright, one before each QRS	May be hard to see	Sawtooth P waves	No P waves identifiable	Usually not discernible	Not discernible	Prolonged, constant PR interval	Progressive widening, then dropped	Some P waves not followed by QRS	No relationship between P and QRS
QRS†	Narrow	Narrow	Narrow	Narrow	Wide	Not discernible	Narrow	Narrow; sometimes dropped	Can be wide	Narrow or wide
Clinical severity‡	Normal	Mild to moderate	Usually mild to moderate	Mild to severe, depending on context	Severe to life threatening	Life threatening	Mild	Mild to moderate, depending on context	Severe to life threatening	Life threatening

*If rate is less than 60, it would be called sinus bradycardia. If rate is greater than 100, it would be sinus tachycardia.

†*Narrow* is defined as less than or equal to 0.12 second and *wide* as greater than 0.12 second.

‡This clinical severity is used as a general guide for clinicians in training, but the actual severity takes into account numerous factors of a patient's illness and the clinical context and thus should be interpreted accordingly.

of bubbles from the right atrium to the left atrium, suggesting an intracardiac shunt. Once the shunt was corrected with the use of a device to close the patent foramen ovale, the patient's hypoxemia resolved and she was extubated without event.

Bubble Echocardiogram

When evaluating patients for persistent hypoxemia, agitated saline may be used as a contrast agent (i.e., echo with bubble study). This method works on the principle that if there is a shunt connecting the right and left heart chambers directly, then bubbles from the venous side of the circulation should travel quickly from the right side of the heart to the left side. Normally, in the absence of any shunt, the pulmonary capillaries filter out the bubbles, so no bubbles appear in the left heart.

When agitated saline is inserted directly into the venous circulation, it can be seen by echocardiogram in the right atrium and right ventricle as a snowstorm appearance (**Figure 6-12**). The air bubbles cause this appearance as air reflects ultrasound waves differently than blood. Normally, the pulmonary capillaries and circulation then filter the air. If there is a cardiac or pulmonary shunt allowing blood to bypass the pulmonary circulation, however, the agitated saline will not only initially show in the right atrium but quickly pass to the left atrium (**Figure 6-13**). In pulmonary shunts, such as in arteriovenous malformations in the lungs, the blood never passes through pulmonary capillaries; therefore, agitated saline may still appear in the left atrium, but it may take several cardiac cycles to do so. **Bubble echocardiogram** may therefore be used as a noninvasive test to detect shunt physiology.

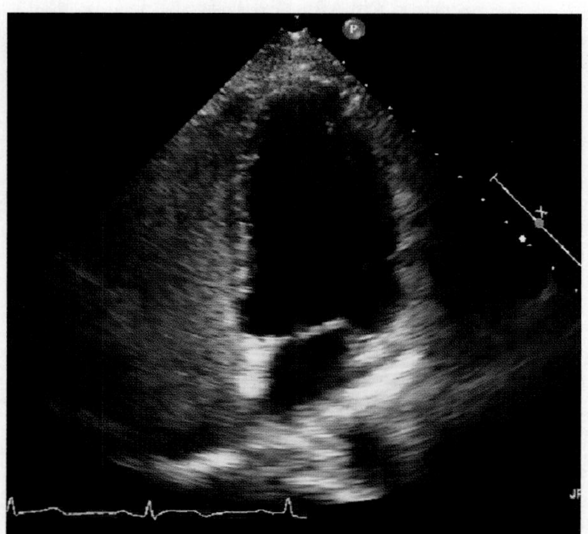

FIGURE 6-12 Normal bubble echocardiogram (no shunt).

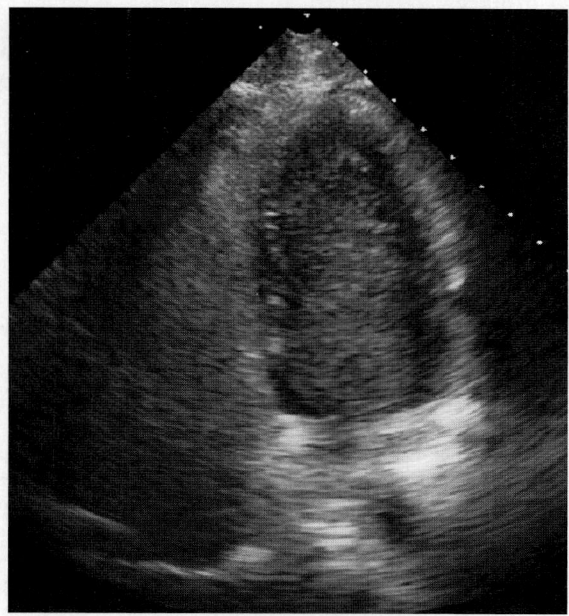

FIGURE 6-13 Bubble echocardiogram with right to left shunt.

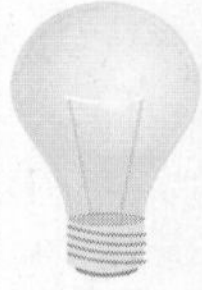

STOP AND THINK

In a mechanically ventilated patient, the Spo_2 decreases from 94% to 86% when the level of positive end-expiratory pressure (PEEP) is increased from 8 cm H_2O to 12 cm H_2O ($Fio_2 = 0.8$). How would you explain this response and what cardiac assessment might be helpful?

Key Points

- Proper cardiac assessment is an important element in the care of patients with symptoms of pulmonary disease or documented pulmonary conditions because of the overlap of symptoms between cardiac and pulmonary disease.
- Clinical assessment involves integrating the history, physical examination, and laboratory studies with other diagnostic studies.
- Clinical tests such as blood tests, electrocardiography, nuclear cardiology, echocardiography, MRI, CT, and cardiac catheterization all have important roles in the diagnosis and prognosis of cardiac conditions, and each test may be used to assess various elements of cardiac function.
- A single test can provide information about several elements of cardiac function, and the advantages and disadvantages of the specific test must be considered in the clinical context of the individual patient.

- Tests of cardiac function may be used not only to help diagnose cardiac disease but also to evaluate the prognosis of patients with these conditions and to guide therapeutic interventions.
- A bubble echocardiogram can be used to assess intracardiac or intrapulmonary shunt.

References

1. Felker GM, Petersen JW, Mark DB. Natriuretic peptides in the diagnosis and management of heart failure. *CMAJ.* 2006;611–617.
2. Guyatt GH, Akl E, Crowder M, et al. Executive summary: *Antithrombotic Therapy and Prevention of Thrombosis*, 9th ed: American College of Chest Physicians evidence-based clinical practice guidelines. *Chest.* 2012;141(Suppl 2):7S–47S.
3. McLaughlin VV, Presberg KW, Doyle RL, et al. Prognosis of pulmonary arterial hypertension. *Chest.* 2004;126(Suppl 1):78S–92S.
4. Shah MR, Hasselblad V, Stevenson LW, et al. Impact of the pulmonary artery catheter in critically ill patients: meta-analysis of randomized clinical trials. *JAMA.* 2005;294:1664–1670.
5. Sheikh KH, de Bruijn NP, Rankin JS, et al. The utility of transesophageal echocardiography and Doppler color flow imaging in patients undergoing cardiac valve surgery. *J Am Coll Cardiol.* 1990;15:363–372.
6. Antman EM, Hand M, Armstrong PW, et al. 2007 focused update of the ACC/AHA 2004 guidelines for the management of patients with ST-elevation myocardial infarction. *J Am Coll Cardiol.* 2008;51:210–247.
7. Wilson PWF, D'Agostino RB, Levy D, et al. Prediction of coronary heart disease using risk factor categories. *Circulation.* 1998;97:1837–1847.
8. Budoff MJ, Achenbach S, Blumenthal RS, et al. Assessment of coronary artery disease by cardiac computed tomography: a scientific statement from the American Heart Association Committee on Cardiovascular Imaging and Intervention, Council on Cardiovascular Radiology and Intervention, and Committee on Cardiac Imaging, Council on Clinical Cardiology. *Circulation.* 2006;114:1761–1791.
9. Watkins S, McGeoch R, Lyne J, et al. Validation of magnetic resonance myocardial perfusion imaging with fractional flow reserve for the detection of significant coronary heart disease. *Circulation.* 2009;120:2163–2165.

APPENDIX 6-1 ECG MONITORING AND DYSRHYTHMIA RECOGNITION

Locations for Chest Electrodes

Lead I

- Positive electrode placed just below the left clavicle
- Negative electrode placed just below the right clavicle
- Provides information about the left lateral wall of the heart

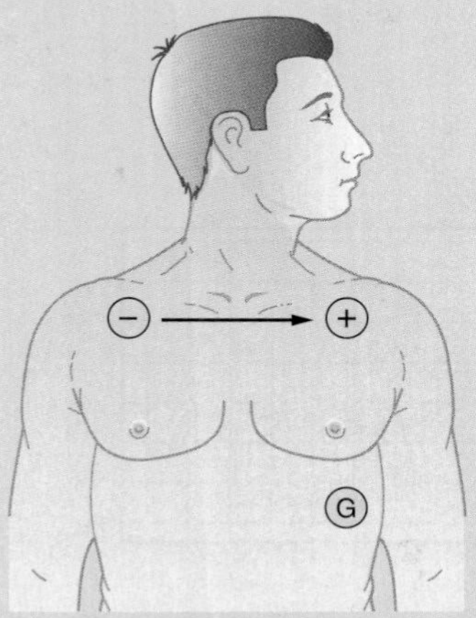

FIGURE 6A-1 Location for chest electrodes: Lead I. G, ground.
Adapted from Aehlert B. *ACLS Quick Review Study Guide*. Mosby; 1994.

Lead II

- Positive electrode just below the left pectoral muscle
- Negative electrode just below the right clavicle
- Provides information about the inferior wall of the heart

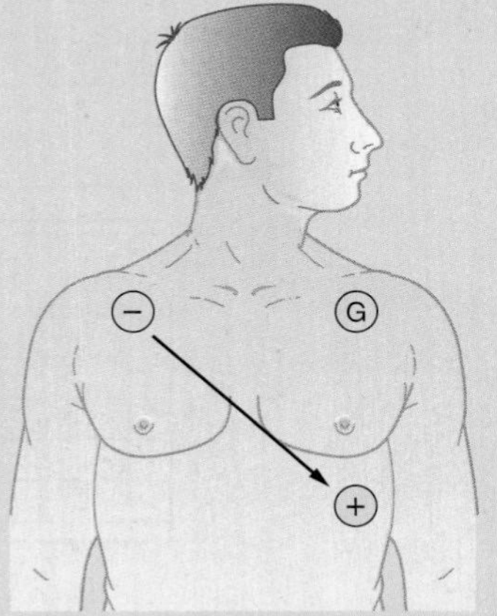

FIGURE 6A-2 Location for chest electrodes: Lead II.
Adapted from Aehlert B. *ACLS Quick Review Study Guide*. Mosby; 1994.

Lead III

- Positive electrode placed just below the left pectoral muscle
- Negative electrode placed just below the left clavicle
- Provides information about the inferior wall of the heart
- P waves seen in this lead usually are of lower amplitude than in leads I and II and are more likely to be biphasic (partly positive and partly negative)

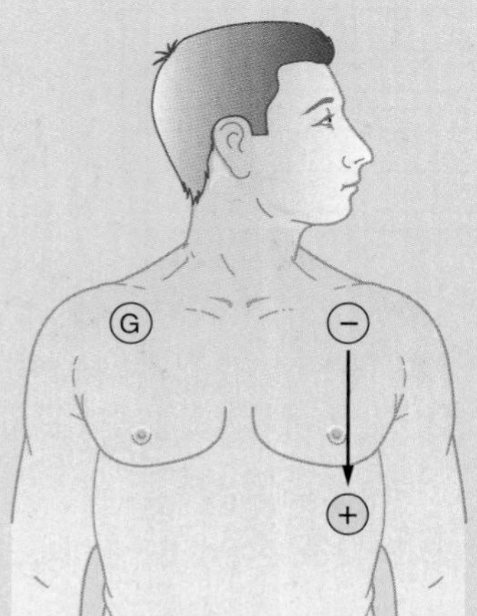

FIGURE 6A-3 Location for chest electrodes: Lead III.
Adapted from Aehlert B. *ACLS Quick Review Study Guide*. Mosby; 1994.

Lead MCL_1 (Modified Chest Lead)

- Negative electrode placed just below the left clavicle
- Positive electrode placed to the right of the sternum at the fourth intercostal space
- Provides information about the anterior wall of the heart
- May prove useful in assessment of the width of the QRS complex to differentiate supraventricular tachycardia (SVT) from ventricular tachycardia (VT)

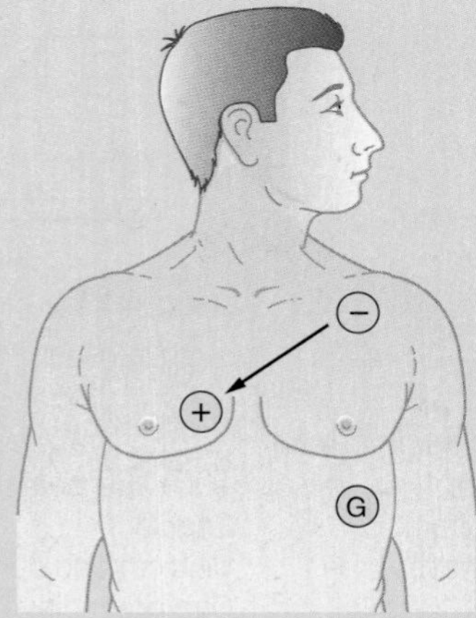

FIGURE 6A-4 Location for chest electrodes: Lead MCL_1.
Adapted from Aehlert B. *ACLS Quick Review Study Guide*. Mosby; 1994.

(*continues*)

Appendix 6-1 *(continued)*

Because the speed of ECG paper is 25 mm/s, the distance between two vertical lines is 1 mm and represents 0.04 second. Thus, the time between two bold vertical lines (five small lines, or 5 mm) represents 0.2 second. The distance between two horizontal lines is also 1 mm. An upward deflection of 10 small lines (or two bold lines) represents 1 mV.

Dysrhythmia Recognition

Normal Sinus Rhythm (NSR)

Rate	60 to 100 beats/min
Rhythm	Regular
P waves	Uniform and upright in appearance One preceding each QRS complex
PR interval	0.12–0.20 s
QRS	<0.10 s

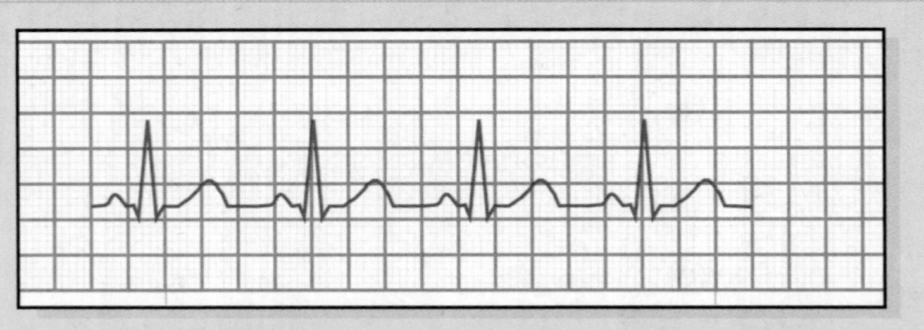

FIGURE 6A-5 Normal sinus rhythm.

Reproduced from *Arrhythmia Recognition: The Art of Interpretation*, courtesy of Tomas B. Garcia, MD.

Sinus Bradycardia

Rate	<60 beats/min
Rhythm	Regular
P waves	Uniform and upright in appearance One preceding each QRS complex
PR interval	0.12–0.20 s
QRS	<0.10 s

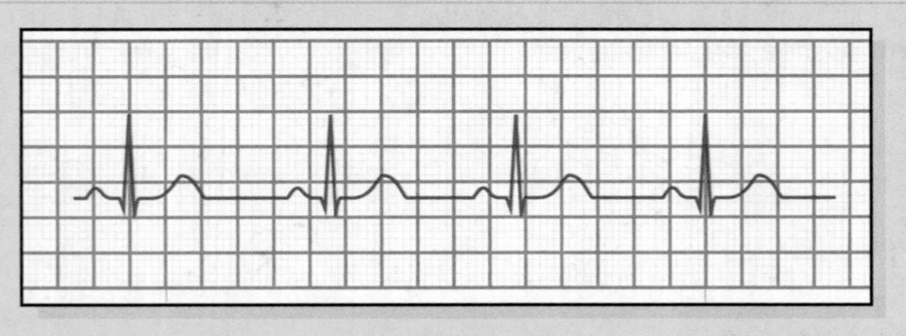

FIGURE 6A-6 Sinus bradycardia.

Reproduced from *Arrhythmia Recognition: The Art of Interpretation*, courtesy of Tomas B. Garcia, MD.

Sinus Tachycardia

Rate	100–160 beats/min
Rhythm	Regular
P waves	Uniform and upright in appearance One preceding each QRS complex
PR interval	0.12–0.20 s
QRS	<0.10 s

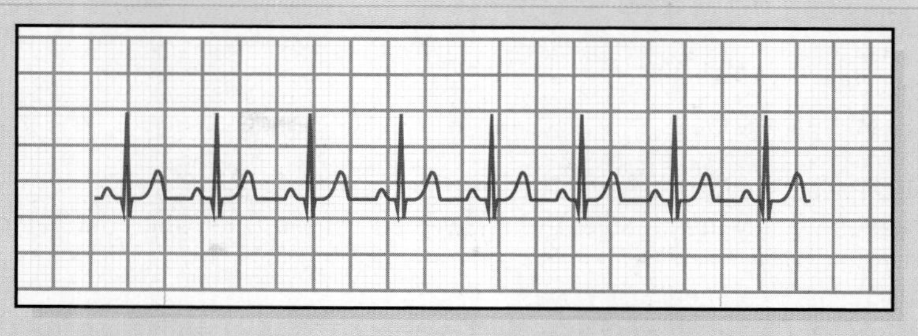

FIGURE 6A-7 Sinus tachycardia.

Reproduced from *Arrhythmia Recognition: The Art of Interpretation*, courtesy of Tomas B. Garcia, MD.

Sinus Arrhythmia

Rate	Usually 60–100 beats/min but may be faster or slower
Rhythm	Irregular
P waves	Uniform and upright in appearance One preceding each QRS complex
PR interval	0.12–0.20 s
QRS	<0.10 s

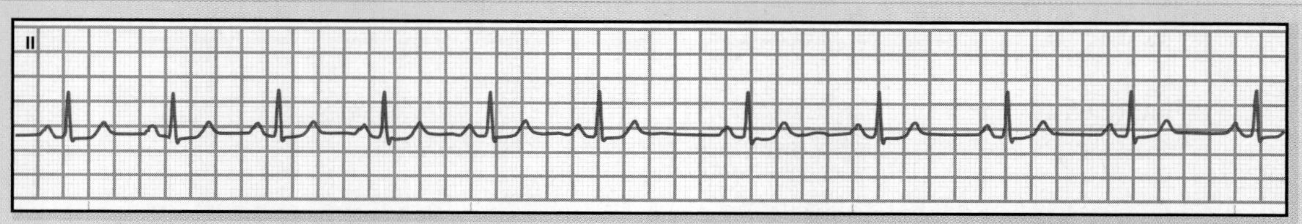

FIGURE 6A-8 Sinus arrhythmia.

Reproduced from *Arrhythmia Recognition: The Art of Interpretation*, courtesy of Tomas B. Garcia, MD.

Premature Atrial Complexes (PACs)

Rate	Usually normal, but depends on underlying rhythm
Rhythm	Irregular because of PACs
P waves	P wave of the early beat differs from sinus P waves Is premature May be flattened or notched May be lost in the preceding T wave
PR interval	Varies from 0.12–0.20 s when the pacemaker site is near the SA node to 0.12 s when the pacemaker site is nearer the AV node
QRS	Usually <0.10 s but may be prolonged

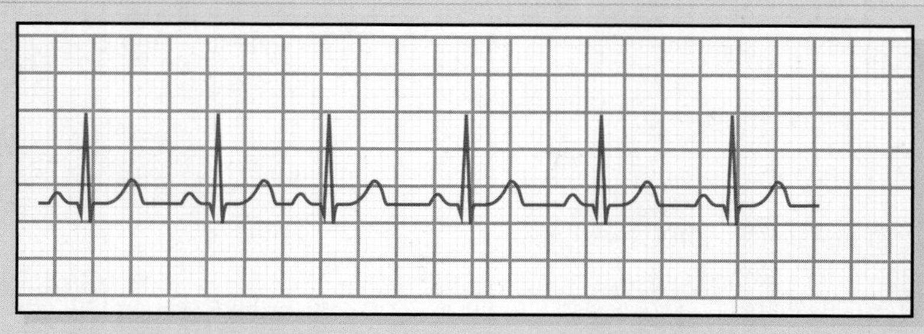

FIGURE 6A-9 Premature atrial complexes.

Reproduced from *Arrhythmia Recognition: The Art of Interpretation*, courtesy of Tomas B. Garcia, MD.

(*continues*)

Appendix 6-1 *(continued)*

Supraventricular Tachycardia

Rate	150–250 beats/min
Rhythm	Regular
P waves	Atrial P waves different from sinus P waves P waves usually identifiable at the lower end of the rate range but seldom identifiable at rates >200 May be lost in preceding T wave
PR interval	Usually not measurable because the P wave is difficult to distinguish from the preceding T wave; if measurable, is 0.12–0.20 s
QRS	<0.10 s

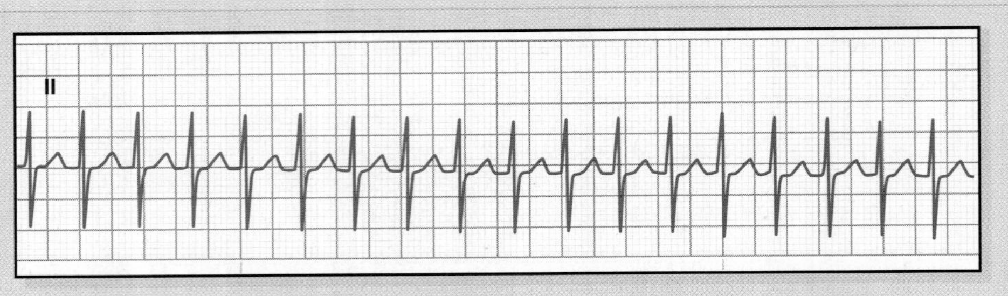

FIGURE 6A-10 Supraventricular tachycardia.

Reproduced from *Arrhythmia Recognition: The Art of Interpretation*, courtesy of Tomas B. Garcia, MD.

Atrial Flutter

Rate	Atrial rate 250–350 beats/min Ventricular rate variable
Rhythm	Atrial rhythm regular Ventricular rhythm usually regular but may be irregular
P waves	Sawtooth flutter waves
PR interval	Not measurable
QRS	Usually <0.10 s but may be widened if flutter waves are buried in the QRS complex

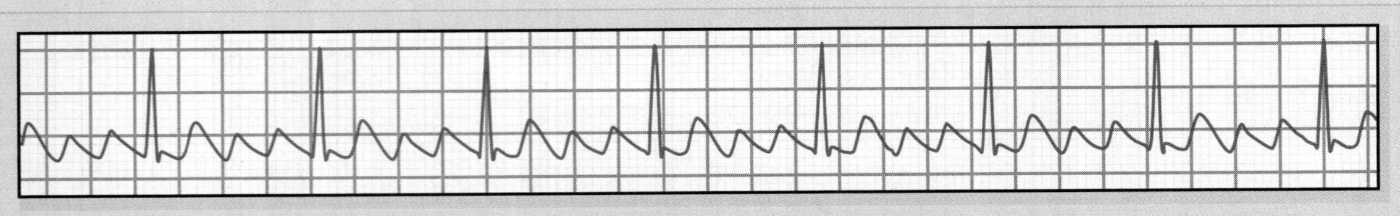

FIGURE 6A-11 Atrial flutter.

Atrial Fibrillation

Rate	Atrial rate usually >400 beats/min Ventricular rate variable
Rhythm	Atrial and ventricular very irregular (regular, bradycardic ventricular rhythm may occur as a result of digitalis toxicity)
P waves	No identifiable P waves Erratic, wavy baseline
PR interval	None
QRS	Usually <0.10 s

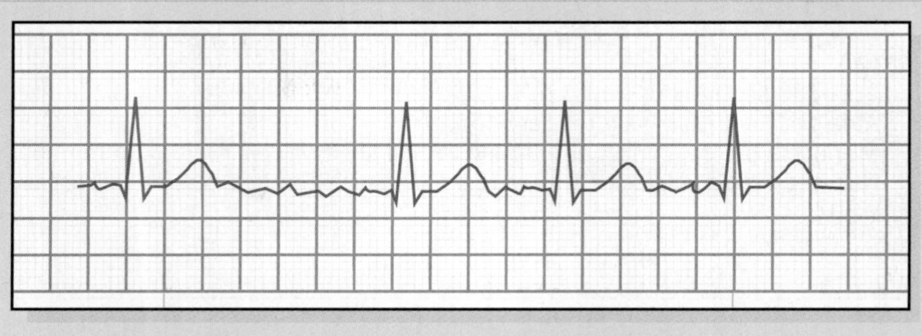

FIGURE 6A-12 Atrial fibrillation.

Reproduced from *Arrhythmia Recognition: The Art of Interpretation*, courtesy of Tomas B. Garcia, MD.

Premature Junctional Complexes (PJCs)

Rate	Atrial and ventricular rates depend on underlying rhythm
Rhythm	Irregular because of premature complex
P waves	May occur before, during, or after the QRS; if seen, will be inverted (retrograde)
PR interval	If the P wave occurs before the QRS, the PR interval will usually be ≤0.12 s
QRS	<0.10 s

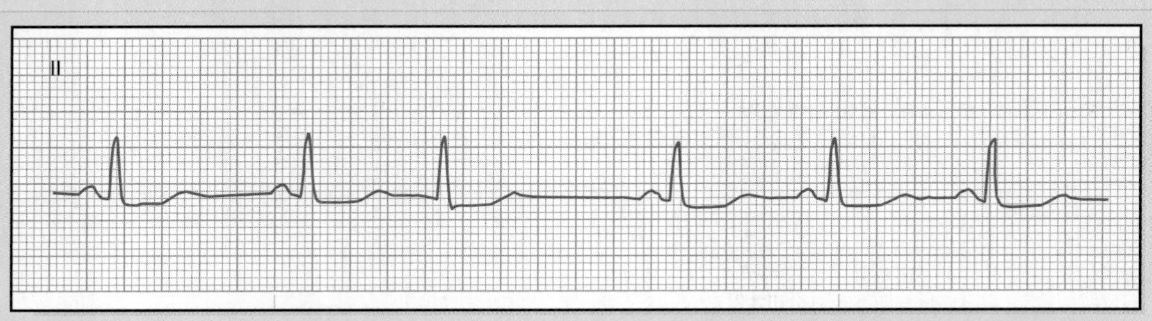

FIGURE 6A-13 Premature junctional complexes.

Reproduced from *Arrhythmia Recognition: The Art of Interpretation*, courtesy of Tomas B. Garcia, MD.

Accelerated Junctional Rhythm

Rate	60–100 beats/min
Rhythm	Atrial and ventricular very regular
P waves	May occur before, during, or after the QRS; if seen, will be inverted (retrograde)
PR interval	Not measurable unless the P wave precedes the QRS; when present, will usually be ≤0.12 s
QRS	<0.10 s

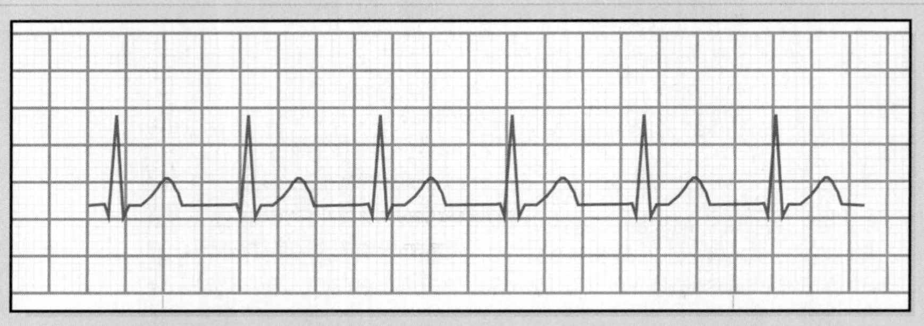

FIGURE 6A-14 Accelerated junctional rhythm.

Reproduced from *Arrhythmia Recognition: The Art of Interpretation*, courtesy of Tomas B. Garcia, MD.

(*continues*)

Appendix 6-1 *(continued)*

Junctional Tachycardia

Rate	100–180 beats/min
Rhythm	Atrial and ventricular very regular
P waves	May occur before, during, or after the QRS; if seen, will be inverted (retrograde)
PR interval	Not measurable unless the P wave precedes the QRS; when present, will usually be ≤0.12 s
QRS	<0.10 s

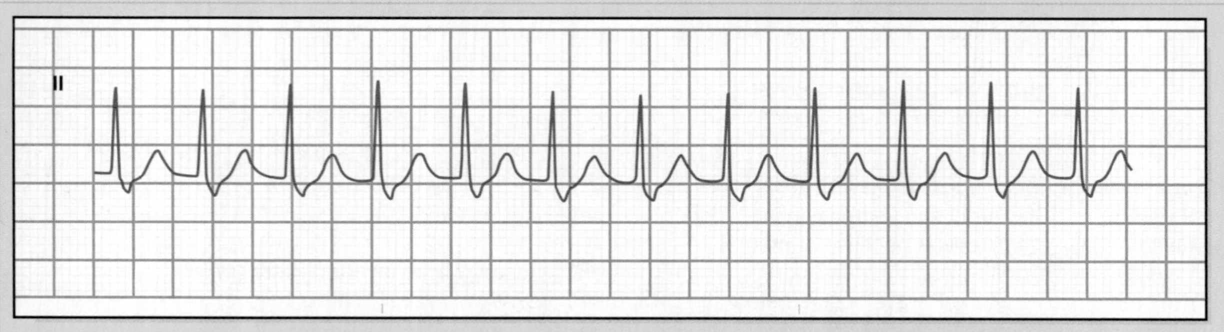

FIGURE 6A-15 Junctional tachycardia.

Reproduced from *Arrhythmia Recognition: The Art of Interpretation*, courtesy of Tomas B. Garcia, MD.

Premature Ventricular Complexes (PVCs)

Rate	Atrial and ventricular rates depend on the underlying rhythm
Rhythm	Irregular because of PVC If the PVC is interpolated (sandwiched between two normal beats), the rhythm will be regular
P waves	No P wave is associated with the PVC
PR interval	None with the PVC because the ectopic originates in the ventricles
QRS	<0.12 s Wide and bizarre T wave frequently in opposite direction of the QRS complex

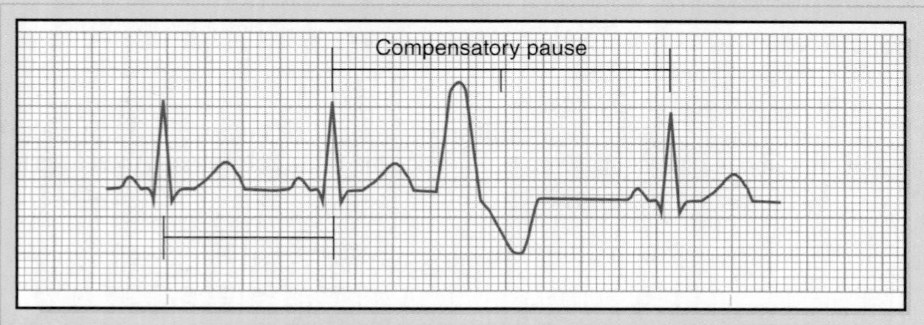

FIGURE 6A-16 Premature ventricular complexes.

Reproduced from *Arrhythmia Recognition: The Art of Interpretation*, courtesy of Tomas B. Garcia, MD.

Ventricular Escape Rhythm (Idioventricular Rhythm [IVR])

Rate	Atrial not discernible; ventricular 20–40 beats/min
Rhythm	Atrial not discernible; ventricular essentially regular
P waves	Absent
PR interval	None
QRS	>0.12 s

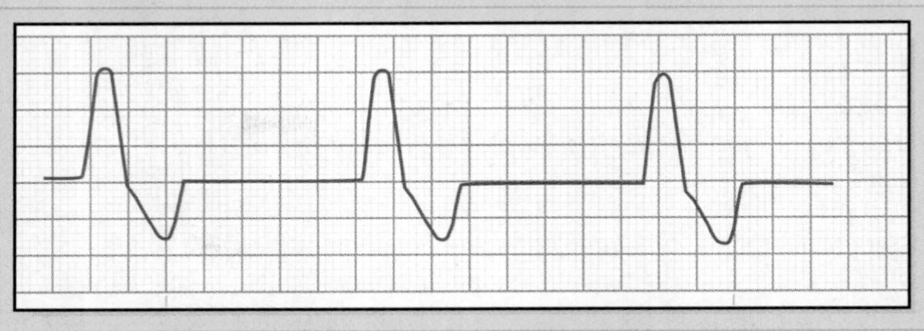

FIGURE 6A-17 Ventricular escape (idioventricular) rhythm.

Reproduced from *Arrhythmia Recognition: The Art of Interpretation*, courtesy of Tomas B. Garcia, MD.

Accelerated Idioventricular Rhythm (AIVR)

Rate	Atrial not discernible; ventricular 40–100 beats/min
Rhythm	Atrial not discernible; ventricular essentially regular
P waves	Absent
PR interval	None
QRS	>0.12 s

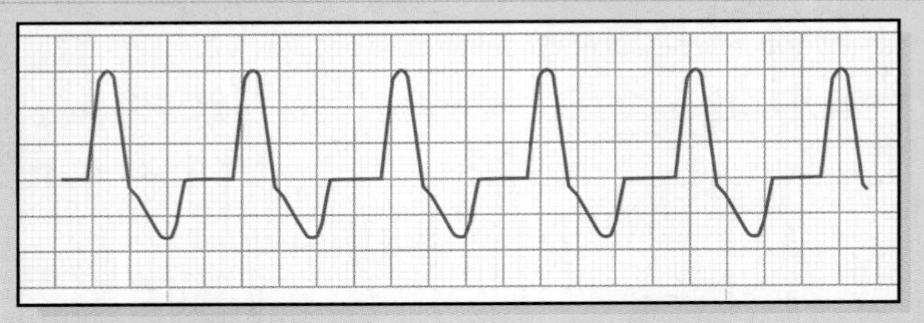

FIGURE 6A-18 Accelerated idioventricular rhythm.

Reproduced from *Arrhythmia Recognition: The Art of Interpretation*, courtesy of Tomas B. Garcia, MD.

Ventricular Tachycardia (Monomorphic VT)

Rate	Atrial not discernible; ventricular 100–250 beats/min
Rhythm	Atrial not discernible; ventricular essentially regular
P waves	May be present or absent; if present, they have no set relationship to the QRS complexes, appearing between the QRSs at a rate different from that of the VT
PR interval	None
QRS	>0.12 s Often difficult to differentiate between the QRS and the T wave

Note: Three or more PVCs occurring sequentially are referred to as a run of VT.

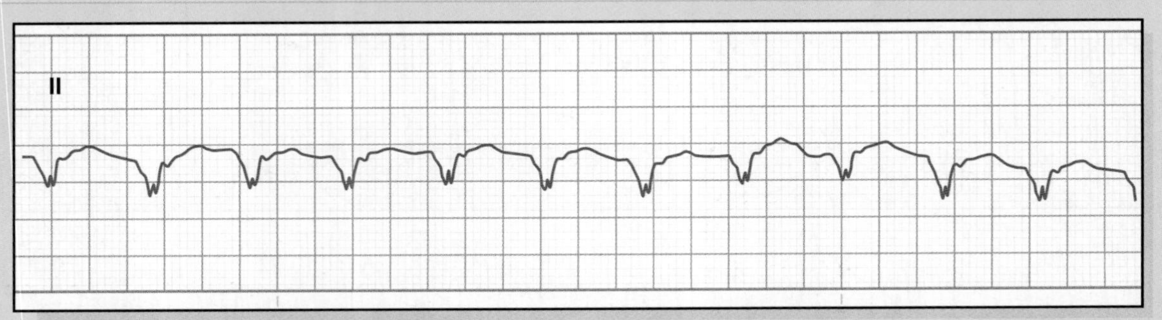

FIGURE 6A-19 Ventricular tachycardia.

Reproduced from *Arrhythmia Recognition: The Art of Interpretation*, courtesy of Tomas B. Garcia, MD.

(continues)

Appendix 6-1 *(continued)*

Torsades de Pointes

Rate	Atrial not discernible; ventricular 150–250 beats/min
Rhythm	Atrial not discernible; ventricular may be regular or irregular
PR interval	None
QRS	>0.12 s
	Gradual alteration in the amplitude and direction of the QRS

Torsades de pointes (French for *twisting of the points*) is a type of polymorphic VT associated with a prolonged QT interval. Symptoms associated with torsades de pointes are related to the decrease in cardiac output, which occurs as a result of the fast ventricular rate. Patients may complain of palpitation or lightheadedness or experience seizures or a syncopal episode. Torsades de pointes is usually initiated by a premature ventricular contraction and may occasionally terminate spontaneously and recur after several seconds or minutes, or it may deteriorate into ventricular fibrillation.

The causes of long QT are many and include the following:

- Drug-induced
  - Cyclic antidepressants (doxepin, imipramine, amitriptyline)
  - Phenothiazines (haloperidol, chlorpromazine, thioridazine)
  - Type I antidysrhythmics (quinidine, procainamide, disopyramide, tocainide, mexiletine)
  - Organophosphate insecticides
- Eating disorders (bulimia, anorexia)
- Electrolyte abnormalities (hypomagnesemia, hypokalemia, hypocalcemia)

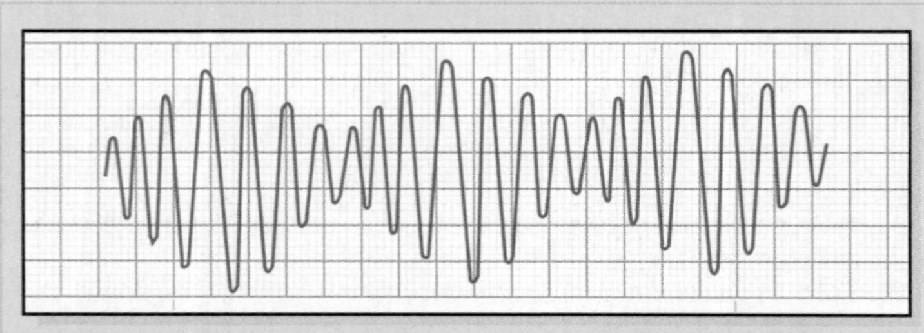

FIGURE 6A-20 Torsades de pointes.

Reproduced from *Arrhythmia Recognition: The Art of Interpretation*, courtesy of Tomas B. Garcia, MD.

Ventricular Fibrillation

Rate	Cannot be determined because waves or complexes are not discernible to measure
Rhythm	Rapid and chaotic with no pattern or regularity
P waves	Not discernible
PR interval	Not discernible
QRS	Not discernible

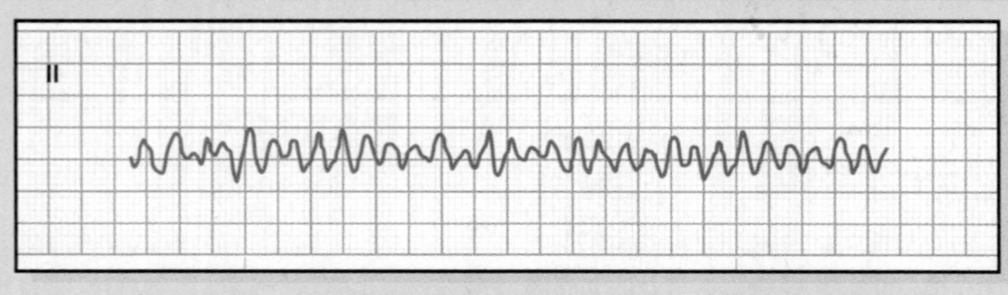

(A)

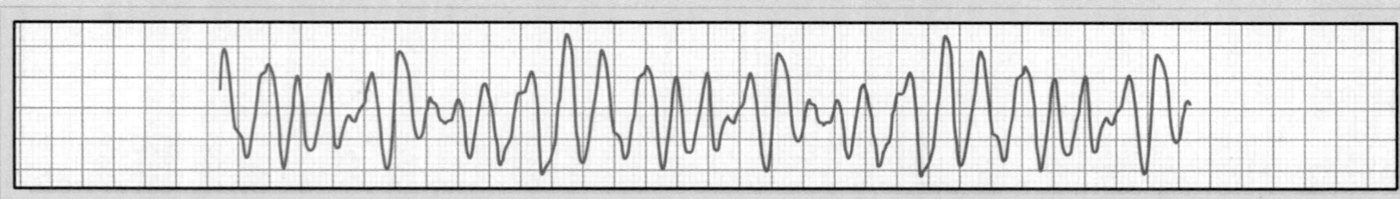

(B)

FIGURE 6A-21 Ventricular fibrillation (**A**) and (**B**).

A reproduced from *Arrhythmia Recognition: The Art of Interpretation*, courtesy of Tomas B. Garcia, MD.

Asystole (Ventricular Asystole, Ventricular Standstill)

Rate	Ventricular usually indiscernible, but may see some atrial activity
Rhythm	Atrial may be discernible; ventricular indiscernible
P waves	Usually not discernible
PR interval	Not measurable
QRS	Absent

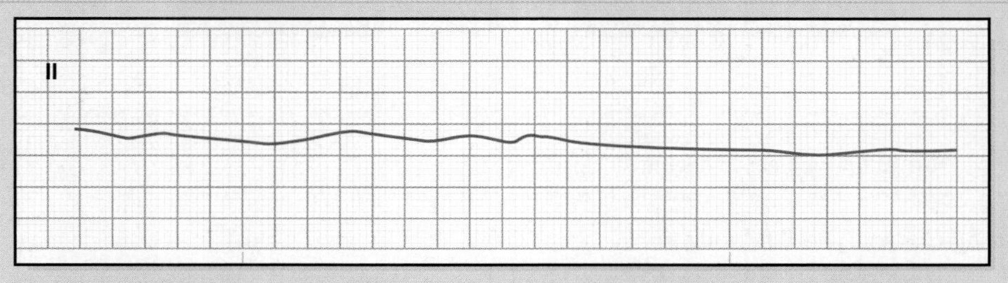

FIGURE 6A-22 Asystole.
Reproduced from *Arrhythmia Recognition: The Art of Interpretation*, courtesy of Tomas B. Garcia, MD.

First-Degree AV Block

Rate	Atrial and ventricular within normal limits and the same
Rhythm	Atrial and ventricular regular
P waves	Normal in size and configuration One P wave for each QRS
PR interval	Prolonged (>0.20 s) but constant
QRS	<0.10 s

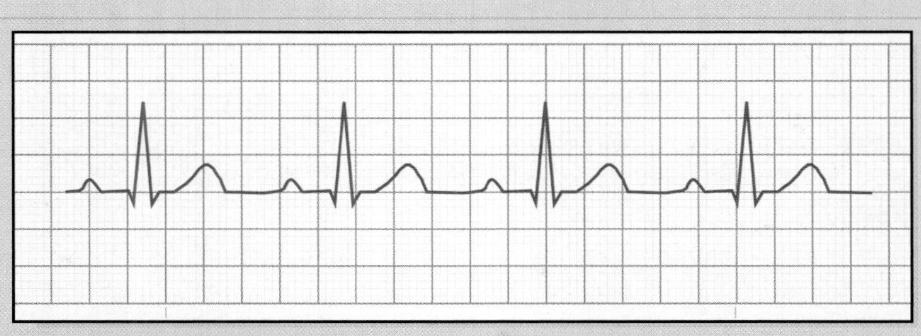

FIGURE 6A-23 Sinus rhythm with first-degree AV block.
Reproduced from *Arrhythmia Recognition: The Art of Interpretation*, courtesy of Tomas B. Garcia, MD.

Second-Degree AV Block, Type I (Wenckebach, Mobitz I)

Rate	Atrial rate > ventricular rate; both are usually within normal limits
Rhythm	Atrial regular (P waves plot through) Ventricular irregular
P waves	Normal in size and configuration Some P waves are not followed by a QRS (more P waves than QRS complexes)
PR interval	Lengthens with each cycle (although lengthening may be slight) until a P wave appears without a QRS
QRS	<0.10 s but is dropped periodically

(*continues*)

Appendix 6-1 *(continued)*

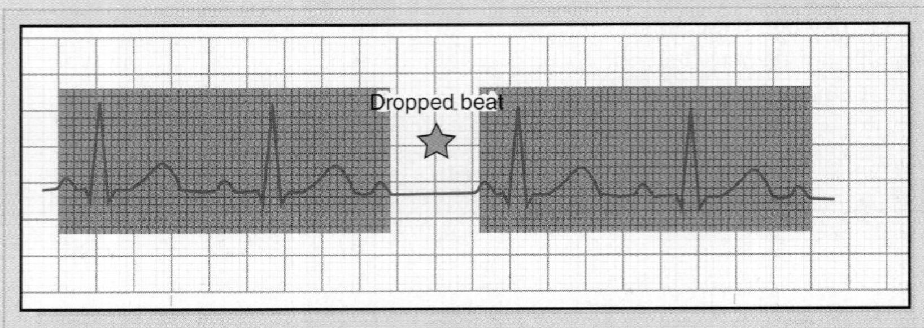

FIGURE 6A-24 Second-degree AV block, type I.

Reproduced from *Arrhythmia Recognition: The Art of Interpretation*, courtesy of Tomas B. Garcia, MD.

Second-Degree AV Block, Type II (Mobitz II)

Rate	Atrial rate > ventricular rate
Rhythm	Atrial regular (P waves plot through) Ventricular irregular
P waves	Normal in size and configuration Some P waves are not followed by a QRS (more P waves than QRS complexes)
PR interval	May be within normal limits or prolonged but is constant for each conducted QRS
QRS	<0.10 s but is dropped periodically

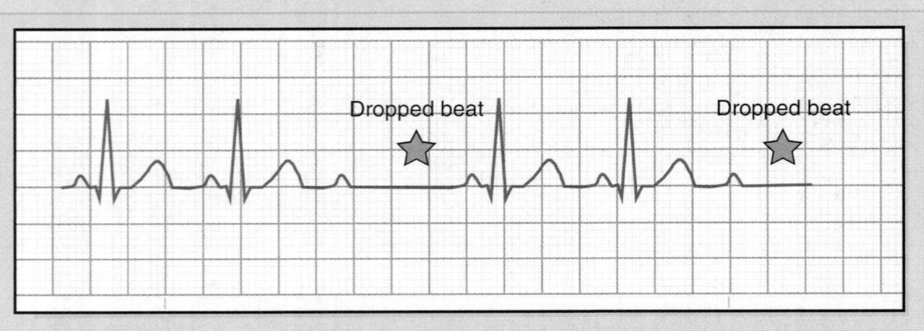

FIGURE 6A-25 Second-degree AV block, type II.

Reproduced from *Arrhythmia Recognition: The Art of Interpretation*, courtesy of Tomas B. Garcia, MD.

Second-Degree AV Block, 2:1 Conduction

Rate	Atrial rate > ventricular rate
Rhythm	Atrial regular (P waves plot through) Ventricular regular
P waves	Normal in size and configuration Every other P wave is followed by a QRS (more P waves than QRS complexes)
PR interval	Constant
QRS	Within normal limits if the block occurs above the bundle of His (probably type I) Wide if the block occurs at or below the bundle of His (probably type II) Absent after every other P wave

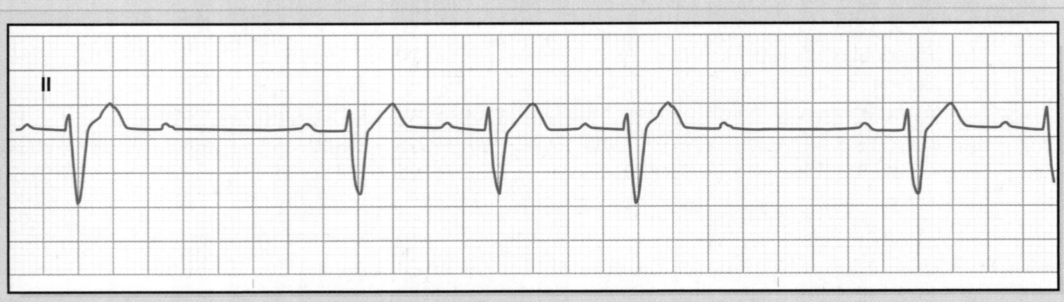

FIGURE 6A-26 Second-degree AV block, 2:1 conduction, probably type I.

Reproduced from *Arrhythmia Recognition: The Art of Interpretation*, courtesy of Tomas B. Garcia, MD.

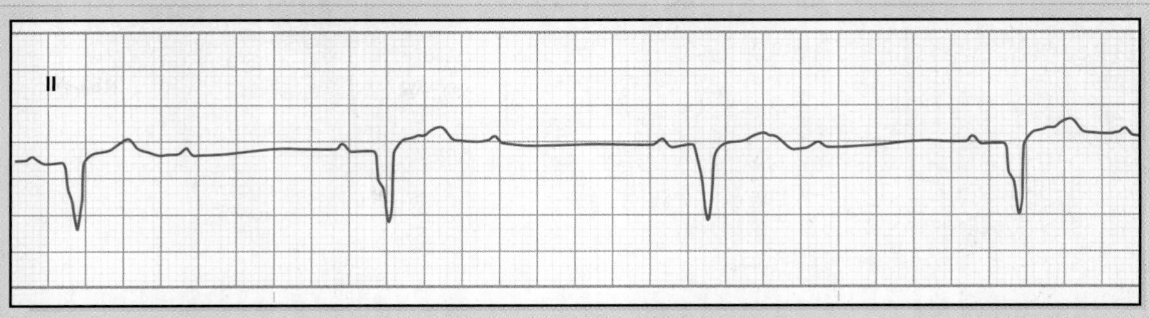

FIGURE 6A-27 Second-degree AV block, 2:1 conduction, probably type II.
Reproduced from *Arrhythmia Recognition: The Art of Interpretation*, courtesy of Tomas B. Garcia, MD.

Complete (Third-Degree) AV Block

Rate	Atrial rate > ventricular rate; ventricular rate determined by the origin of the escape rhythm
Rhythm	Atrial regular (P waves plot through) Ventricular regular
P waves	Normal in size and configuration Some P waves are not followed by a QRS (more P waves than QRS complexes)
PR interval	None—the atria and ventricles beat independently of each other; no relationship between the P waves and QRS complexes
QRS	Narrow or wide depending on the location of the escape pacemaker and the condition of the interventricular conduction system Narrow → junctional pacemaker Wide → ventricular pacemaker

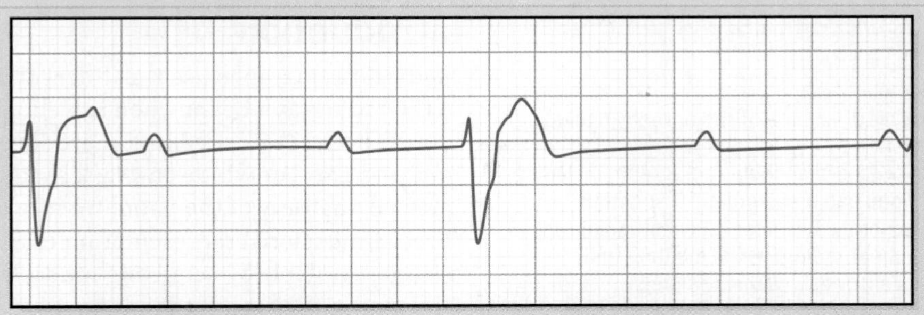

FIGURE 6A-28 Complete (third-degree) AV block.
Reproduced from *Arrhythmia Recognition: The Art of Interpretation*, courtesy of Tomas B. Garcia, MD.

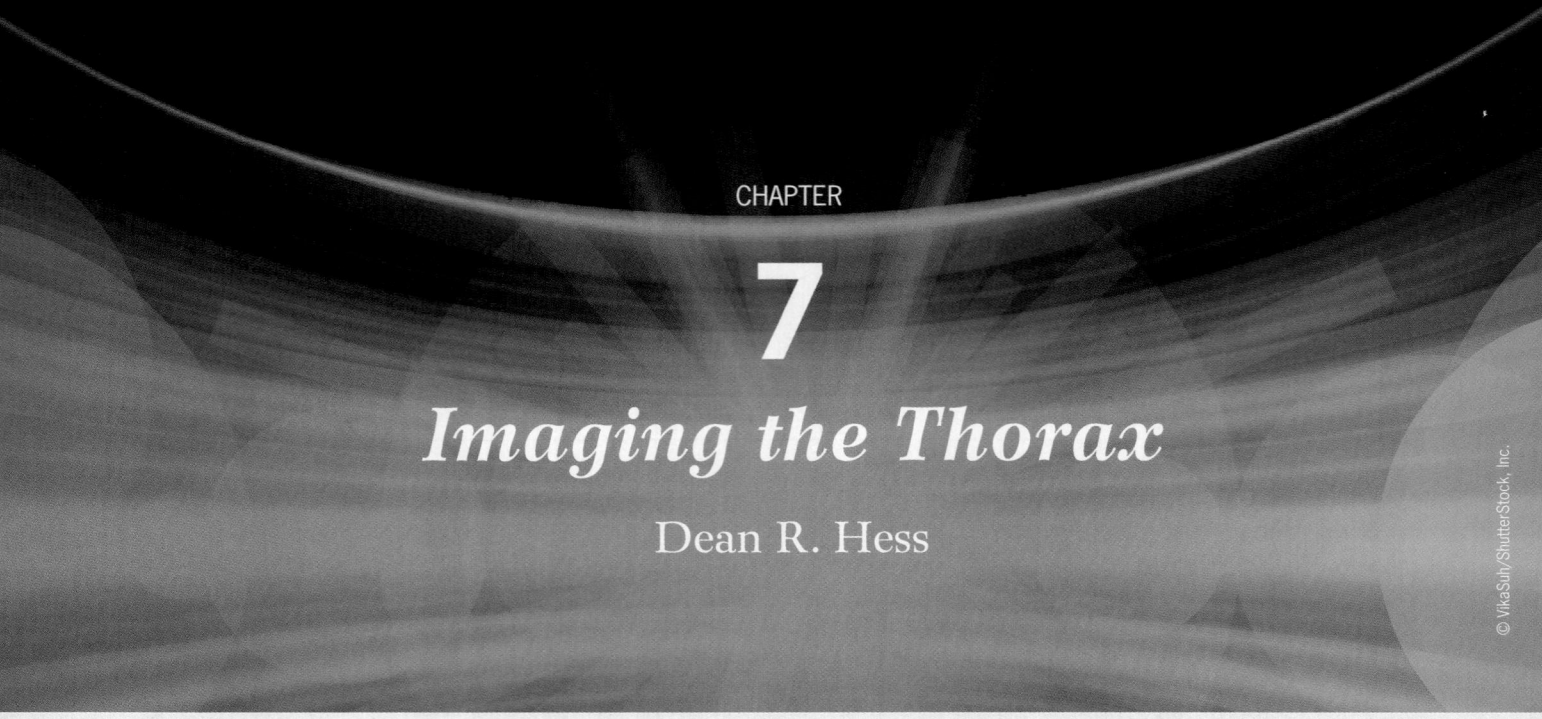

CHAPTER

7

Imaging the Thorax

Dean R. Hess

OUTLINE

OBJECTIVES

1. Describe the underlying principles of radiography, including densities and contrast.
2. Outline the features of a normal chest radiograph, including the different projections and a systematic inspection.
3. Describe the major abnormalities seen on chest radiographs.
4. Explain the use of a chest radiograph in locating and quantifying abnormal air or fluid within the chest.
5. Explain how the chest radiograph is used to verify the proper positioning of monitoring and therapeutic catheters, tubes, and devices.
6. Describe how computed tomography, compared with the chest radiograph, improves diagnostic imaging capabilities.
7. Describe the use of ultrasound, magnetic resonance imaging, and positron emission tomography in imaging studies.
8. Describe the technique of electrical impedance tomography.

KEY TERMS

air bronchogram
anteroposterior (AP) projections
apical lordotic
blunted costophrenic angle
chest radiograph
computed tomography (CT)
deep sulcus sign
electrical impedance tomography (EIT)
ground glass appearance
Hampton hump
honeycomb appearance
Hounsfield units (HU)
Kerley B lines
lateral decubitus
Macklin effect
magnetic resonance imaging (MRI)
mediastinal shift
nodular appearance
opacifications
positron emission tomography (PET)
posteroanterior (PA) projection
radiodensity
radiolucent
radiopaque
silhouette sign
voxels
Westermark sign

Introduction

Medical radiographs use the differential reduction of the radiograph beam when traveling through the human body.[1–9] This reduction produces a superimposed gray- or white-on-black shadow of the internal anatomy of the patient. More recently, a three-dimensional representation of the anatomy has become available by acquiring multiple, angular projections synthesized into tomographic images using **computed tomography (CT)**. CT has revolutionized the use of radiographs in diagnostic imaging even if the traditional radiograph remains the first step in the diagnostic assessment.

Radiographs are produced when electrons interact with matter and convert their kinetic energy into electromagnetic radiation. A **chest radiograph** is produced by x-ray beams (energy) passing through the thorax and exposing a photographic plate or film. Radiographic imaging is based on the anatomy blocking x-ray transmission by varying degrees, which results in an image caused by the degree of exposure of the photographic plate. Before computers and digital imaging, a photographic plate sensitive to x-rays was used to produce radiographic images, and the images were produced directly on film. Digital radiography is replacing film. The major difference between the analog and digital detectors is the digitization of the continuous output signal into discrete spatial sampling locations by an analog-digital converter.

Density and Contrast

The x-ray beam transmitted through the patient will vary in intensity and, when unblocked, completely expose photographic film, converting it from white to black. *Blocking* is the reduction of an x-ray beam, which depends on the penetrating characteristics of the beam and the physical characteristics of the tissue. Blocking of x-rays by intervening tissue is potentially harmful radiation exposure. Therefore, the range of energies used is chosen to optimize the diagnostic information and minimize the radiation absorbed by the patient.

When there is minimal tissue density, such as air or air-filled structures, black areas are produced on the radiograph; these areas are referred to as **radiolucent**. Areas or body tissues that cannot be penetrated by x-rays are **radiopaque** and appear white on the radiograph. Each body tissue or structure has a different **radiodensity**. The four basic radiodensities are:

1. Gas, which appears black or radiolucent; an example is gas in the airways or stomach.
2. Fat, which appears gray or less radiolucent than air; an example is lipid tissue around muscle.
3. Soft tissue (water), which appears gray or less radiolucent than air; examples are heart, blood vessels, and muscles.
4. Bone (or metal), which appears all white or completely radiopaque; examples are bones, calcium deposits, prostheses, and contrast media. Objects placed into the patient, such as endotracheal tubes and vascular catheters, are radiopaque.

Density is determined not only by the composition of an object but also by its thickness. Thus, two objects of different composition can appear to be the same density if they have different thicknesses. Contrast occurs when two objects of different densities are side by side. Radiodense materials are sometimes injected into the body to improve contrast (e.g., arteriograms, bronchograms, barium swallows).

The Normal Chest Radiograph

Technical Factors

Frontal views of the thorax are **posteroanterior (PA)** and **anteroposterior (AP) projections**. In ambulatory patients, PA and lateral projections are commonly obtained

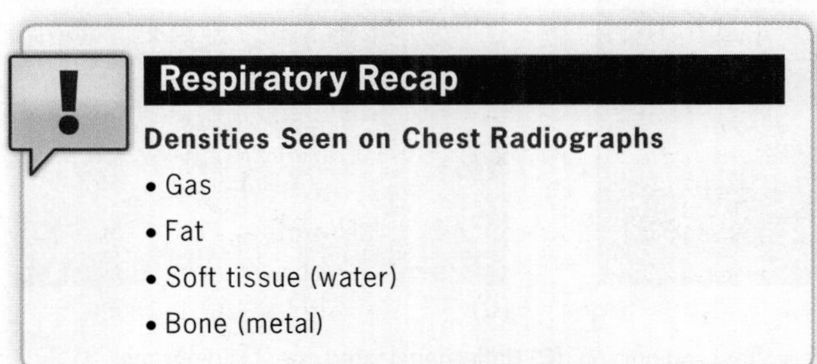

Respiratory Recap

Densities Seen on Chest Radiographs

- Gas
- Fat
- Soft tissue (water)
- Bone (metal)

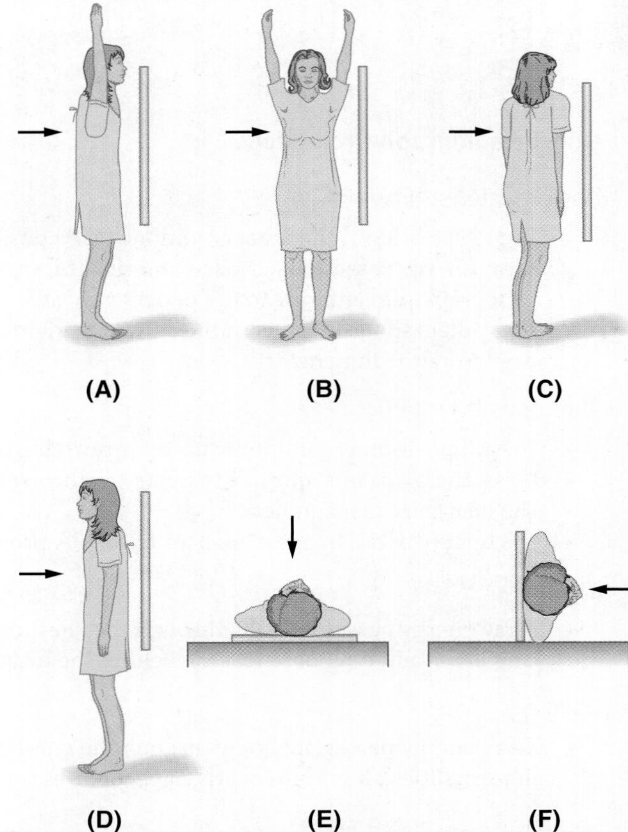

FIGURE 7-1 Various radiographic positions. (**A**) Posteroanterior. (**B**) Lateral. (**C**) Right anterior oblique. (**D**) Anteroposterior. (**E**) Anteroposterior supine. (**F**) Right lateral decubitus.

Adapted from Goodman LR. *Felson's Principles of Chest Roentgenology: A Programmed Text*. 3rd ed. Saunders Elsevier; 2007.

(**Figure 7-1**). Other projections, such as **lateral decubitus** and **apical lordotic**, are used to better visualize the pleural space and the lung apices, respectively (**Box 7-1**). Frontal and lateral radiographs allow the chest to be viewed from two directions (thus, three dimensions) to more easily localize infiltrates and lesions. The lateral view is used to evaluate the mediastinum, the tracheal air column, the inferior vena cava, the retrosternal space, the posterior margin of the heart, the diaphragmatic contour, and the presence of pleural effusions.

For the PA projection, the x-ray beam passes through the chest from the back to the front. For the AP view, the beam passes through the chest from the front to the back. For patients in the intensive care unit (ICU), supine AP views are obtained with a portable x-ray machine. The supine AP view is typically of inferior technical quality. The diaphragm is elevated because of the supine position. Objects that are farther away from the x-ray film are magnified. Thus, the heart appears larger on the AP film.

It is important to assess the technical quality of the chest radiograph. *Penetration* refers to the amount of x-ray exposure. An overpenetrated film will be too black, and an underpenetrated film will appear too white (**Figure 7-2**). With a properly penetrated film,

BOX 7-1

Chest Radiograph Projections

Posteroanterior (PA)

- The PA position is the most commonly used position.
- X-ray energy passes posterior to anterior through the chest of the patient, with the radiograph film anterior to the patient's chest.
- The radiograph is taken with the patient upright, with maximal inspiration, and the scapulae are rotated away from the lung fields.

Anteroposterior (AP)

- The AP position is commonly used for portable radiographs in the critical care unit.
- X-ray energy passes anterior to posterior through the chest of the patient.
- The heart size is magnified.
- The quality of the image is inferior to the PA projection.

Lateral

- X-ray energy passes laterally through the chest of the patient. The lateral position allows visualization of the lung bases and lung parenchyma behind the heart.

Oblique

- X-ray energy passes obliquely through the chest of the patient. The oblique position is used to project abnormalities away from overlying structures.

Lordotic

- The lordotic position provides a better view of the lung apex, lingula, and right middle lobe.

Expiratory

- The expiratory position is used to demonstrate a small pneumothorax or unilateral airway obstruction.

Lateral Decubitus

- The radiograph is taken with the patient in a side-lying position.
- The lateral decubitus position is used to identify the presence of free pleural fluid or to confirm the presence of an air–fluid level in the lung.

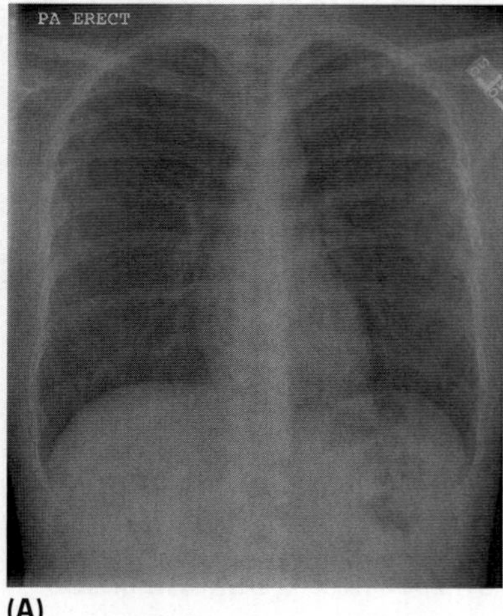

(A)

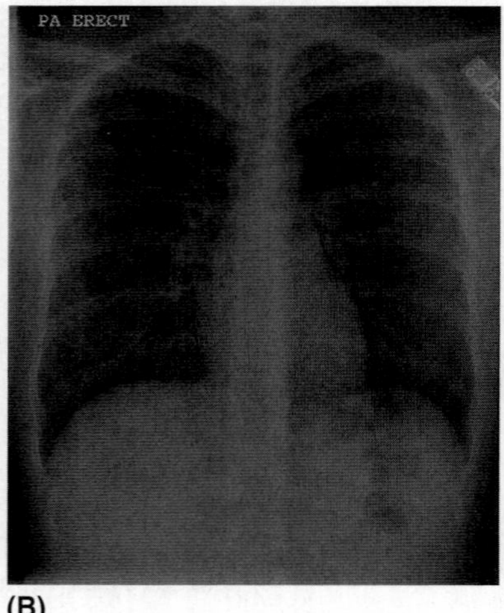

(B)

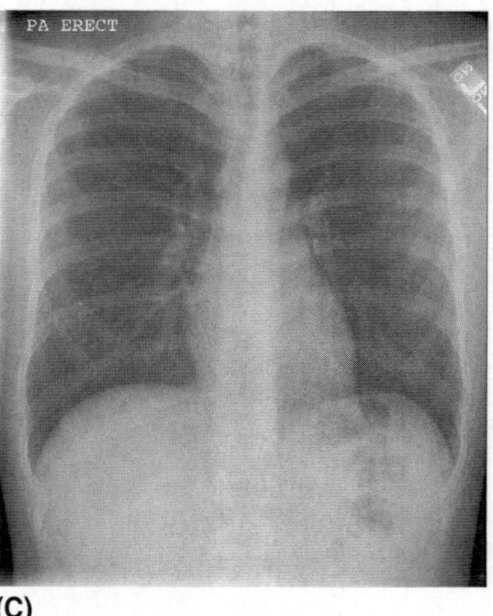

(C)

FIGURE 7-2 (**A**) Correctly penetrated chest radiograph. (**B**) Overpenetrated chest radiograph. (**C**) Underpenetrated chest radiograph.

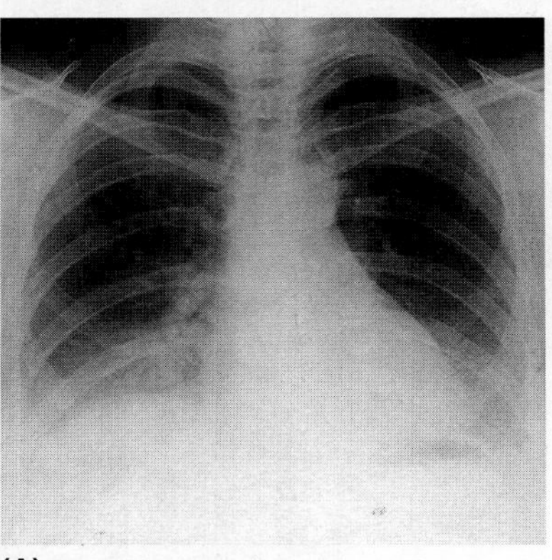

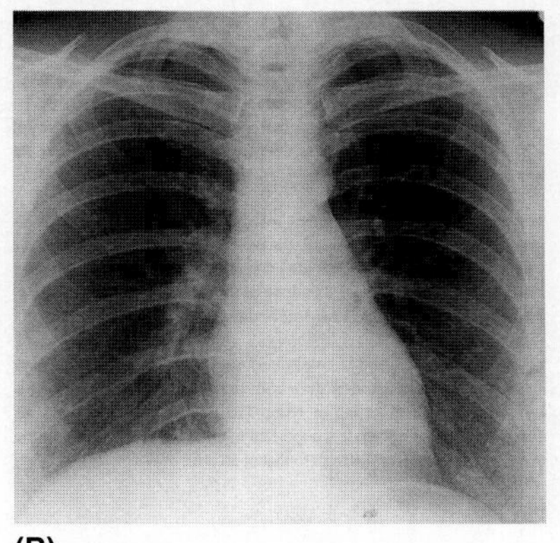

(A) **(B)**

FIGURE 7-3 (**A**) Expiratory film. (**B**) Inspiratory film.
Reproduced from *Chest X-Ray Made Easy*. Corne J, Carroll M, Brown I, Delany D. Copyright Elsevier (Churchill Livingstone), 1997.

the vertebral bodies should be just visible through the cardiac shadow. The patient should be oriented correctly and not rotated to one side or the other. With proper position, the clavicles appear symmetric. The radiograph should be taken at full inspiration. A poor inspiration will make the heart look larger and produce appearance of basilar infiltrates (**Figure 7-3**). The scapulae should be rotated out of position on PA film but will be present on an AP film. The heart should be oriented to the left unless the patient has dextrocardia or situs inversus.

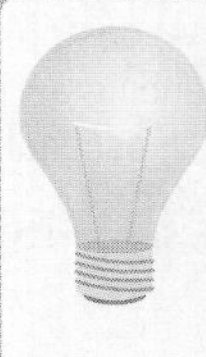

STOP AND THINK

You are examining the chest radiograph of a mechanically ventilated patient in the ICU. What technical aspects would you consider to avoid a misdiagnosis?

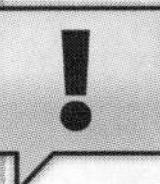

Respiratory Recap

Normal Chest Radiograph

- Right hemidiaphragm higher than the left
- Clear and sharp costophrenic angles
- Left hilum higher than right
- Air tracheogram midline under sternum
- Aortic arch to left of spine
- Heart toward left thorax
- Gastric air bubble on left

Examination of the Chest Radiograph

Examination of the chest radiograph should include systematic inspection of the extrathoracic soft tissues, bony thorax, mediastinal contour, hilar region, pleural surfaces, vascular pattern, and lung fields. The frontal chest radiograph is viewed as though the patient were facing you; in other words, the patient's left is to your right. **Figure 7-4** and **Figure 7-5** show normal chest radiographs.

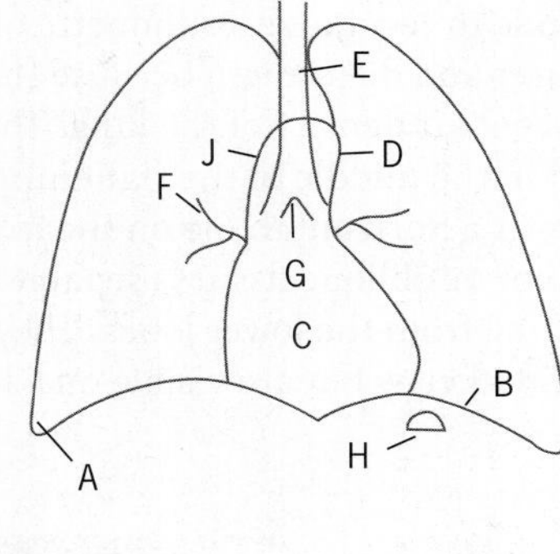

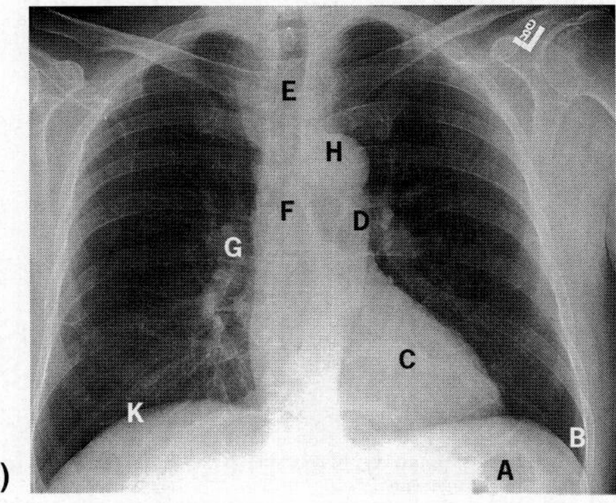

(A) **(B)**

FIGURE 7-4 (**A**) Landmarks on posteroanterior chest radiograph. A, costophrenic angle (sulcus); B, left hemidiaphragm; C, heart; D, aortic arch; E, trachea; F, hilum; G, carina; H, stomach bubble; J, ascending aorta. (**B**) Normal posteroanterior chest radiograph. A, stomach bubble; B, costophrenic angle (sulcus); C, heart; D, descending aorta; E, trachea; F, carina; G, hilum; H, aortic arch; K, right hemidiaphragm.
(**A**) adapted from Goodman LR. *Felson's Principles of Chest Roentgenology: A Programmed Text.* 3rd ed. Saunders Elsevier; 2007; (**B**) reproduced from *Felson's Principles of Chest Roentgenology: A Programmed Text.* 3rd ed. Goodman LR. Copyright Elsevier (Saunders), 2007.

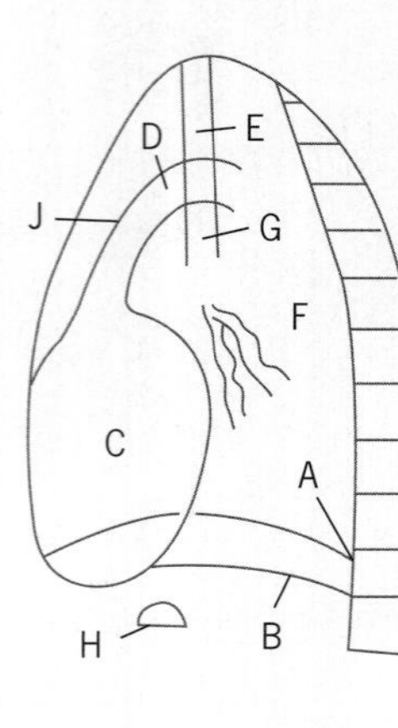

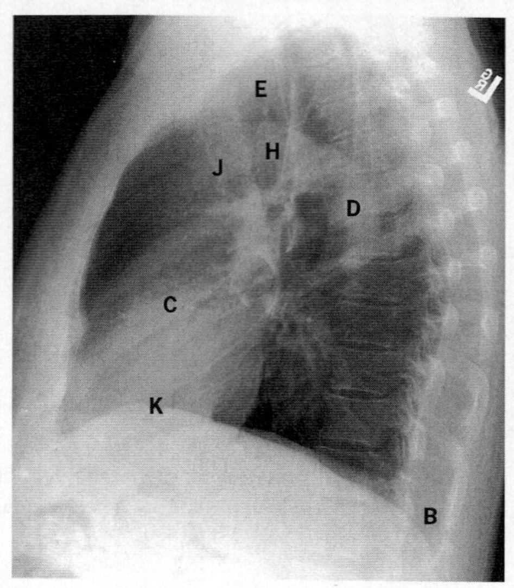

(A) (B)

FIGURE 7-5 (**A**) Landmarks on lateral chest radiograph. A, costophrenic angle (sulcus); B, left hemidiaphragm; C, heart; D, aortic arch; E, trachea; F, hilum; G, carina; H, stomach bubble; J, ascending aorta. (**B**) Normal lateral chest radiograph. B, costophrenic angle (sulcus); C, heart; D, descending aorta; E, trachea; H, aortic arch; J, ascending aorta; K, right hemidiaphragm.

(**A**) adapted from *Felson's Principles of Chest Roentgenology: A Programmed Text.* 3rd ed. Goodman LR. Copyright Elsevier (Saunders), 2007; (**B**) reproduced from *Felson's Principles of Chest Roentgenology: A Programmed Text.* 3rd ed. Goodman LR. Copyright Elsevier (Saunders) 2007.

The trachea appears as a vertically oriented radiolucent structure midway between the clavicles and over the spine. The carina is normally positioned at the level of the sixth posterior rib or T4. Causes of tracheal deviation are chest rotation, tumor, **mediastinal shift**, pneumothorax, or major atelectasis.

Twelve pairs of symmetric ribs should be seen. Each intercostal space is numbered according to the rib above it. Widened intercostal spaces occur in conditions such as chronic obstructive pulmonary disease (COPD), pneumothorax, and pleural effusion. Narrowed intercostal spaces are associated with decreased lung volume (e.g., atelectasis).

The right hemidiaphragm is normally higher than the left because of the liver. The apex of the diaphragm lies at the level of the sixth anterior rib on the PA projection. Flattening of the diaphragm is associated with hyperinflation of the lungs or thorax, as in COPD or pneumothorax. The costal, diaphragmatic, and mediastinal pleura are not visible on plain radiographs. The costophrenic angle should appear sharp. A gastric air bubble is often present under the left hemidiaphragm.

The mediastinum is a narrow, vertically oriented structure between the medial parietal pleural layers of the lung that contains the central cardiovascular structures (heart and major vessels), tracheobronchial structures (trachea and main bronchi), esophagus, lymphatic chain, thoracic duct, and autonomic nerves. The normal heart presents a homogeneous shadow on the chest film without any internal detail. The heart projects toward the left thorax unless the patient has dextrocardia or situs inversus. Detection and identification of heart disease depends mainly on changes in the size and shape of the cardiac silhouette and the great vessels. The cardiothoracic ratio is measured by the horizontal width of the heart divided by the widest width of the thorax and is normally 1:2 or less. The aortic arch is normally to the left of the spine.

The left hilum is slightly higher than the right because the left pulmonary artery is higher than the right. Bronchovascular markings branch out from the hila to the periphery of the lung fields. Hilar elevation is usually present in collapse of the upper lobes of the lung, and hilar depression occurs in collapse of the lower lobes of the lung.

The lung fields are radiolucent because they consist mainly of air and very little tissue or blood. The basis of visualization of a border of a structure depends on its contiguity with another structure of different density. It is possible to recognize a silhouette of the mediastinal structures and diaphragm because they are outlined by adjacent air density of the lung. The minor fissure is located in the middle of the right lung fields, where it appears as a horizontal line on the frontal radiograph. The major or oblique fissures separate the upper lobes of the lung from the lower lobes. They cannot be seen on a frontal view but are visible on a lateral view.

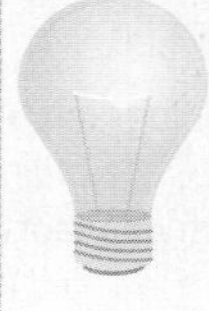

STOP AND THINK

Why might the heart appear on the right side of the chest on a radiograph?

Abnormalities Seen on Chest Radiographs

Abnormalities of the lung fields on chest radiographs include signs and patterns. Two common and important signs are the air bronchogram sign and the silhouette sign. Normally, the airways cannot be visualized on a chest radiograph because there is no contrast between the airway and the surrounding alveoli. If the alveoli become filled with fluid or if they are consolidated or collapsed, an **air bronchogram** will appear; this indicates that the underlying opacity is of pulmonary rather than pleural or mediastinal origin. The **silhouette sign** indicates an obliteration of the borders of the heart, mediastinal structures, or diaphragm by an adjacent opacity of similar density. An intrathoracic lesion that is not anatomically contiguous with one of these structures will not obliterate its border.

Processes involving the medial segment of the right middle lobe obliterate the right heart border. If the lingual is involved, the left heart border is obliterated. Lower lobe processes involving the basilar segments result in obliteration of the border of the diaphragm.

The honeycomb pattern, the nodular pattern, and the ground glass pattern are common patterns seen on the chest radiograph. The **honeycomb appearance** is characterized by the presence of cystic air spaces with thick fibrous walls lined by bronchiolar epithelium. This pattern occurs with idiopathic pulmonary fibrosis, collagen vascular diseases, asbestosis, chronic hypersensitivity pneumonitis, and drug-related fibrosis. A **nodular appearance** refers to multiple round **opacifications** on the chest radiograph. This pattern occurs with sarcoidosis, pneumoconiosis, and metastasis. **Ground glass appearance** is a hazy increased attenuation of the lungs with preservation of bronchial and vascular margins. The ground glass pattern may be associated with air bronchograms. It occurs with pneumonia, pulmonary edema, pulmonary hemorrhage, and pulmonary alveolar proteinosis.

Chronic Obstructive Pulmonary Disease

Several major chest radiograph findings indicate the presence of COPD. The radiograph appears hyperlucent, and bullae may be present. The diaphragms are lowered and flattened. Increased retrosternal airspace is seen on the lateral projection. Two conditions cause the lungs to be more radiolucent: hyperinflation and interstitial destruction. Both of these are present in COPD.

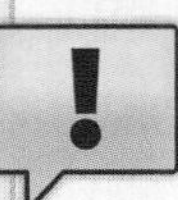

Respiratory Recap

Signs and Patterns on Chest X-Ray

- *Signs:* air bronchogram and silhouette
- *Patterns:* honeycomb, nodular, and ground glass

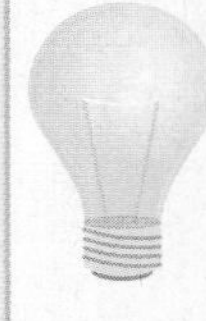

STOP AND THINK

A patient has a right-sided pneumonia. How could you use the chest radiograph to determine whether the infiltrate is in the right lower lobe or right middle lobe?

Pneumonia

Pneumonia can cause a wide variety of abnormalities on the chest radiograph, resulting in segmental or lobar homogeneous opacities or scattered nonsegmental opacities. There may be an extensive and diffuse airspace process. In pneumonia, as opposed to atelectasis, lung volume is preserved and findings persist for days to weeks. Air bronchograms may be present, and there may be associated pleural effusions. The silhouette sign can be used to identify the lobes and segments of the lungs that are involved.

Atelectasis

Direct signs of atelectasis on the chest radiograph include displacement of fissures toward the collapsed lung, increased radiopacity, and air bronchograms (**Figure 7-6** and **Figure 7-7**). Indirect signs of atelectasis include hemidiaphragm elevation, displacement of the mediastinum or hilum, and compensatory overinflation of the remainder of the other lung.

Atelectasis can mimic pneumonia, particularly when other specific signs are absent. Distinguishing atelectasis from pneumonia may be difficult and at times impossible, often requiring corroborative clinical information and follow-up radiographs. If small airways are obstructed, subsegmental opacities result, which often are described as discoid or platelike in appearance. They appear as thin, linear, horizontally or obliquely oriented opacities and frequently are seen in postsurgical patients at the lung bases (**Figure 7-8**). Obstruction of a large airway may result in lobar atelectasis, most commonly involving the left lower lobe or the right lower lobe. Involvement of the left lower lobe is particularly common after cardiac surgery.

Left Heart Failure

With left heart failure (congestive heart failure), the cardiac silhouette is enlarged. With mild failure, interstitial

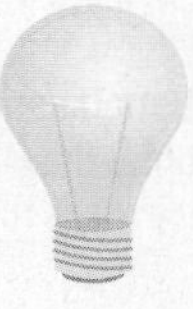

STOP AND THINK

A patient has decreased breath sounds on the left side. How could you use the chest radiograph to determine whether the clinical problem is pneumothorax, atelectasis, pneumonia, or pleural effusion?

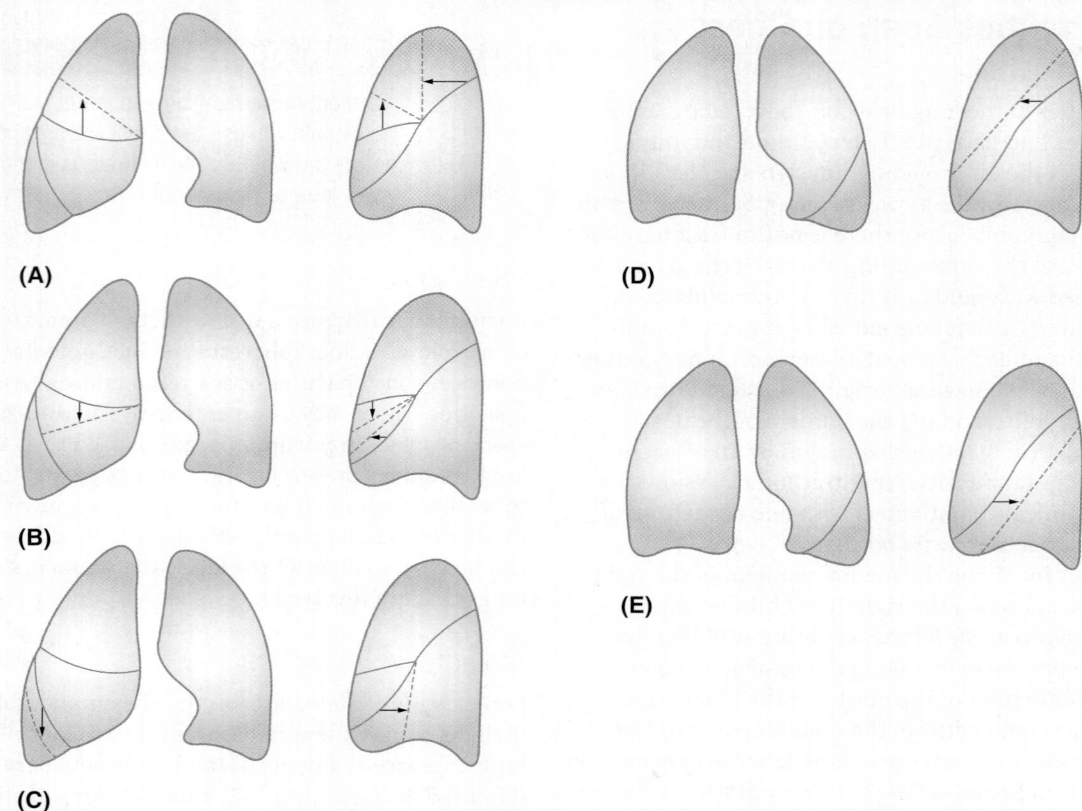

FIGURE 7-6 The best sign of lobar collapse is shift of a fissure. (**A**) Right upper lobe collapse. (**B**) Right middle lobe collapse. (**C**) Right lower lobe collapse. (**D**) Left upper lobe collapse. (**E**) Left lower lobe collapse.

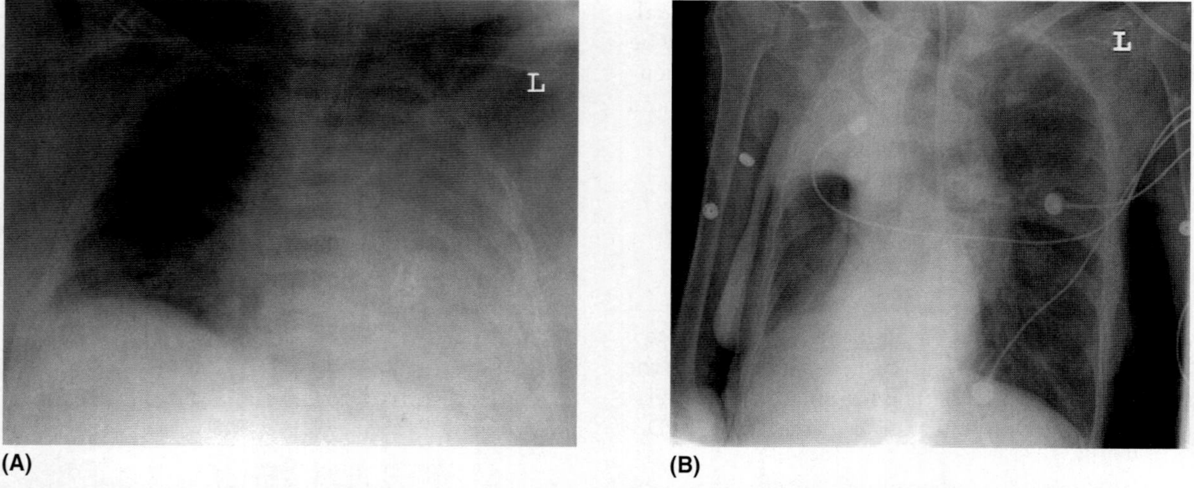

FIGURE 7-7 (**A**) Collapse of left lung. Note tracheal shift, mediastinal shift, and loss of the silhouette of the left hemidiaphragm. (**B**) Right upper lobe collapse. Note upward shift of horizontal fissure and right shift of trachea.

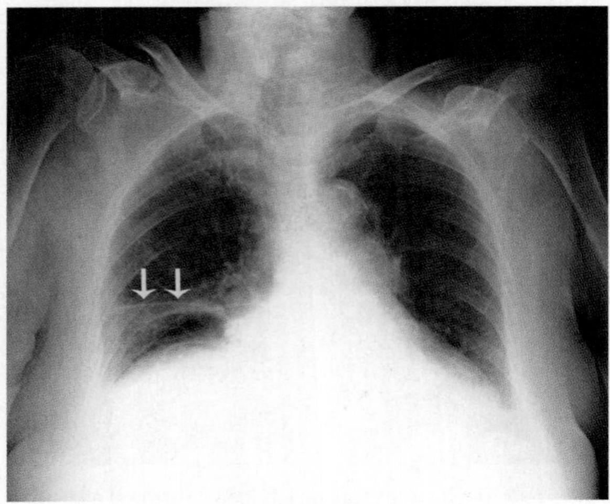

FIGURE 7-8 Platelike atelectasis (arrows).

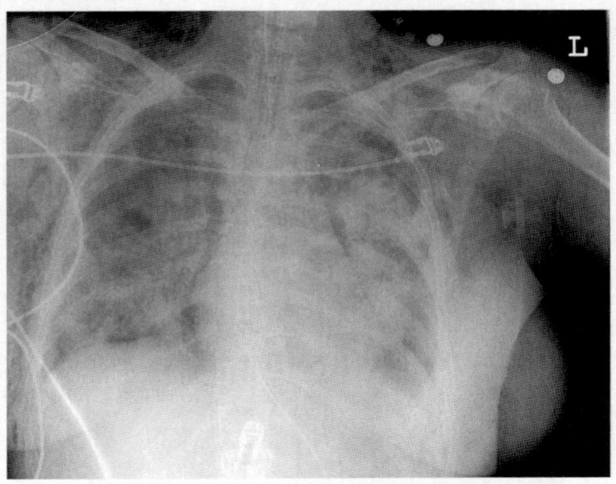

FIGURE 7-9 Pneumomediastinum and subcutaneous emphysema.

edema develops, and the pulmonary vessel margins become less sharp and the peripheral interstitial markings become more prominent. With moderate failure, fluid thickens the interlobular septa, causing short lines to appear perpendicular to the pleural surface. These are called **Kerley B lines** and indicate interstitial edema. Severe failure causes alveolar edema, resulting in opacification (water density) of the lower lung zones. Pleural effusions can also occur with congestive heart failure.

Pneumothorax and Air Leaks

The pathophysiology of extra-alveolar air generally begins with the rupture of distal alveoli into the interstitial space and the subsequent dissection of air into the mediastinum, tissues, and pleural space. Air dissects along bronchovascular bundles, producing the appearance of a pulmonary vessel surrounded by air. Air dissecting into the mediastinum creates vertical linear streaks, which is called the **Macklin effect**. Subcutaneous emphysema results from air leak into the tissues (**Figure 7-9**).

The radiographic diagnosis of pneumothorax is established by identification of the visceral pleural line (**Figure 7-10**). Other radiographic features suggestive of pneumothorax include the absence of vascular markings and increased lucency in the hemithorax. Visualization of the visceral pleura can be enhanced by exposure of the film in expiration. With expiration, the volume of the pneumothorax remains constant, whereas the volume of the hemithorax in which it is contained is reduced.

Pneumothorax is treated by insertion of a chest tube (**Figure 7-11**). A skin fold (**Figure 7-12**) may mimic the visceral pleural line, but whereas the visceral pleural line is a thin line with air on both sides, a skin fold is represented as an interface in which one edge is sharp but gradually fades away.

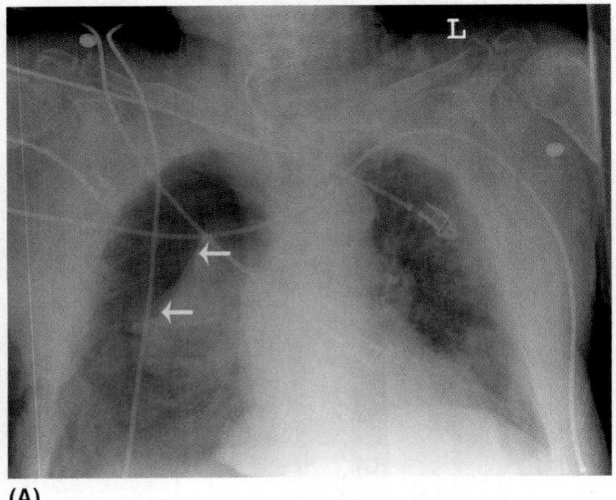

(A)

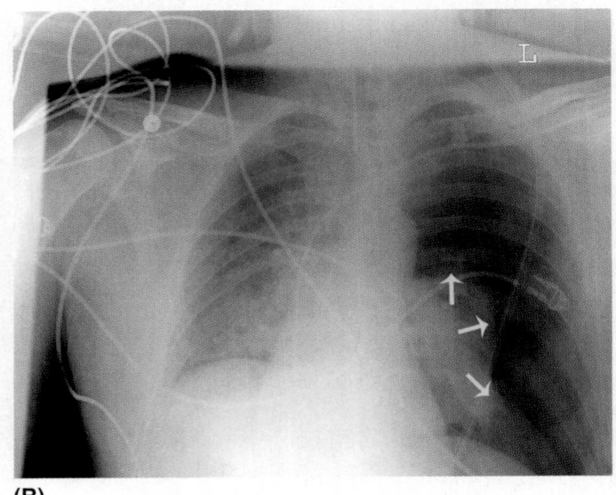

(B)

FIGURE 7-10 (**A**) Right-sided pneumothorax with visceral pleura line. (**B**) Left-sided tension pneumothorax. Note depression of left hemidiaphragm, widened intercostal spaces on left, shift of mediastinum to right, and collapsed left lung.

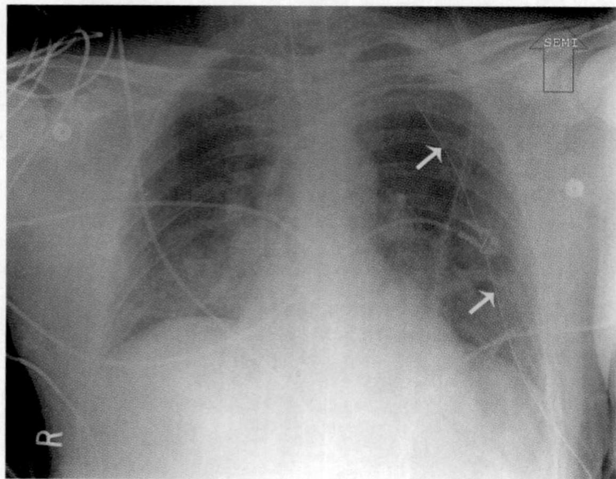

FIGURE 7-11 Note presence of left chest tube (arrows) and reexpansion of the lung after pneumothorax.

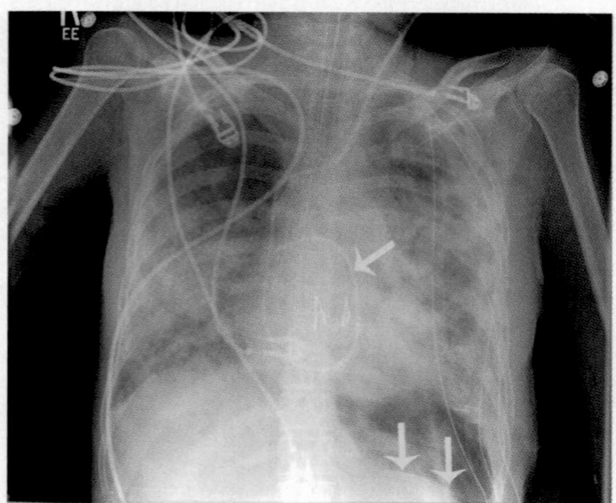

FIGURE 7-13 Deep sulcus sign on left (double arrows) and pulmonary artery catheter (arrow).

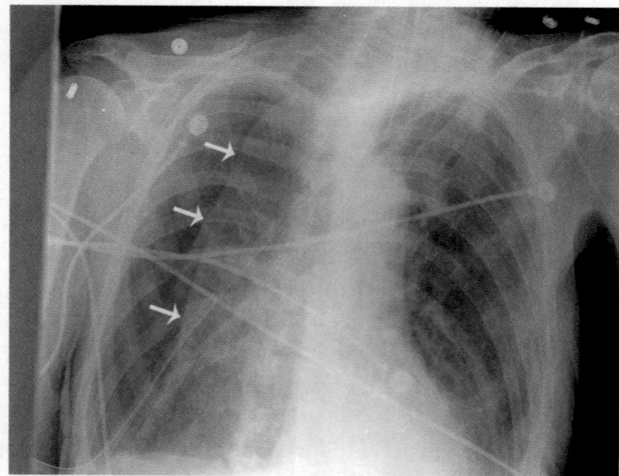

FIGURE 7-12 Skin fold (arrows), which can be confused with a visceral line and pneumothorax.

In the upright position, free air in the pleural space generally collects over the apex of the lung. Most clinicians have been trained to look for air in this location when they suspect a pneumothorax. In patients in the supine position, the highest portion of the thorax is generally the anterior costophrenic sulcus. Free air within the pleural space rises to this position, projecting over the upper abdomen and diaphragm. This results in a distinctive radiographic appearance that is called the **deep sulcus sign** (**Figure 7-13**). If the pneumothorax is on the left side, the apex of the heart and the pericardial fat pad often will be sharply outlined. In addition, the edge of the lung and the visceral pleural line may be identified.

In the supine projection, however, recognition of the deep sulcus sign and increased lucency over the upper abdomen is critical because direct visualization of the visceral pleura in this projection is difficult.

Pleural Effusion

In the supine position, free fluid in the pleural space tends to layer posteriorly. Significant amounts of fluid create a generalized increased opacity over the affected hemithorax. The supine radiograph is relatively insensitive in the detection of pleural fluid and could underestimate its amount. The lateral radiograph is more sensitive than a frontal radiograph to identify a pleural effusion. Decubitus projection allows confirmation of the presence of free fluid in the pleural space (**Figure 7-14**). The presence of pleural effusion should

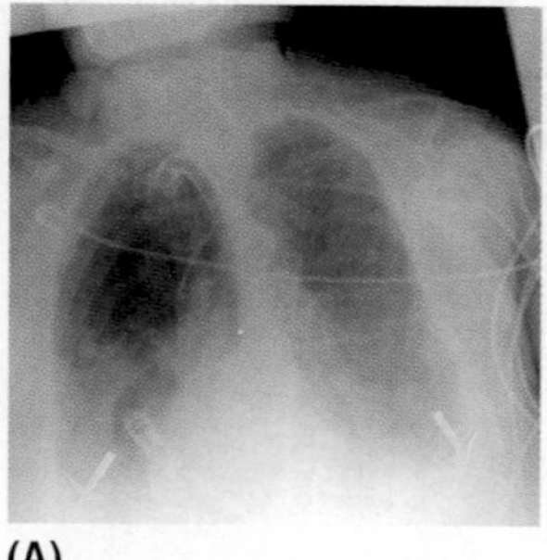

(A)

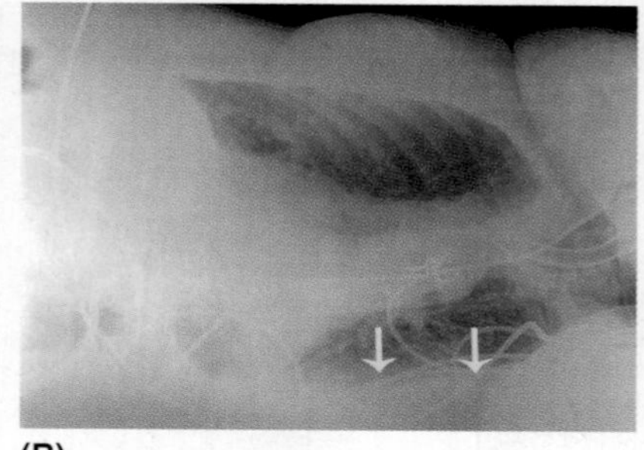

(B)

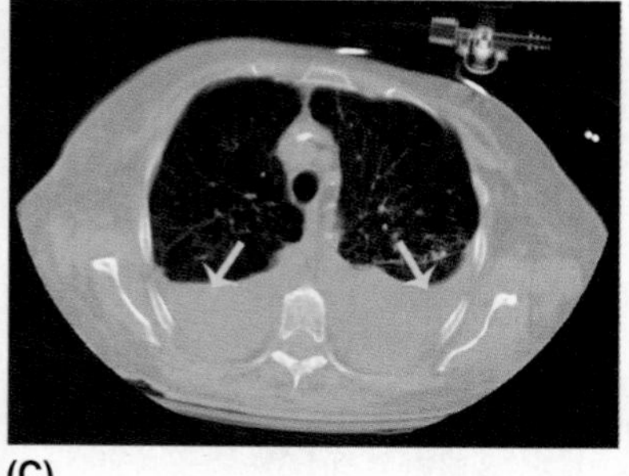

(C)

FIGURE 7-14 (**A**) Anteroposterior projection of patient with bilateral pleural effusions. Note blunted costophrenic angles. (**B**) Lateral decubitus projection. Note layering of the pleural effusion. (**C**) Computed tomographic scan showing large dependent pleural effusions. Lack of air bronchograms suggests this is in the pleural space and not in the lungs.

be suspected with a **blunted costophrenic angle**, which normally appears sharp. Free fluid can track up the pleural space, forming a meniscus, called the *meniscus sign*. There can be an increased homogeneous density on the affected hemithorax and loss of normal silhouette of the hemidiaphragm. There can also be an apparent elevation of the hemidiaphragm, which is actually due to subpulmonic fluid.

Evaluation of Tubes and Catheters

The optimal position of the tip of the endotracheal tube is approximately 4 to 6 cm above the carina with the neck in the neutral position. In the supine position, the correct position of the distal tip of the endotracheal tube should be between the superior clavicular margin and T5. Intubation of a main stem bronchus, usually the right, occurs when endotracheal tube position is too low (**Figure 7-15** and **Figure 7-16**). This results in collapse of the contralateral lung and overinflation of the ipsilateral lung. The tube diameter should be one-half to two-thirds that of the trachea lumen, and the inflated cuff should not cause bulging of the tracheal wall (**Figure 7-17**). Esophageal intubation occasionally occurs and should be considered when significant gastric distension is observed.

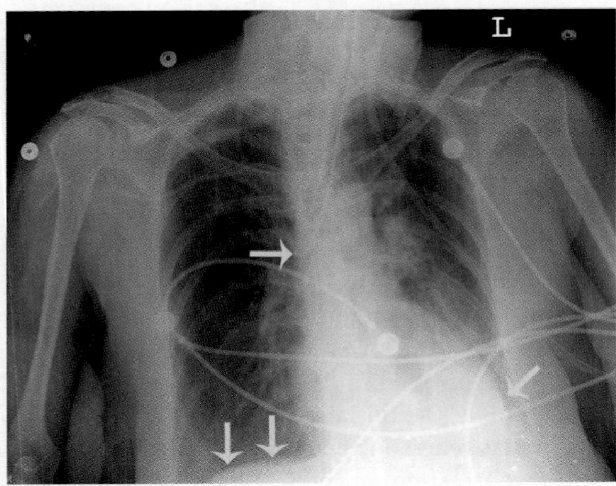

FIGURE 7-15 Right main stem intubation. Also note hyperinflation of right lung and atelectasis on left.

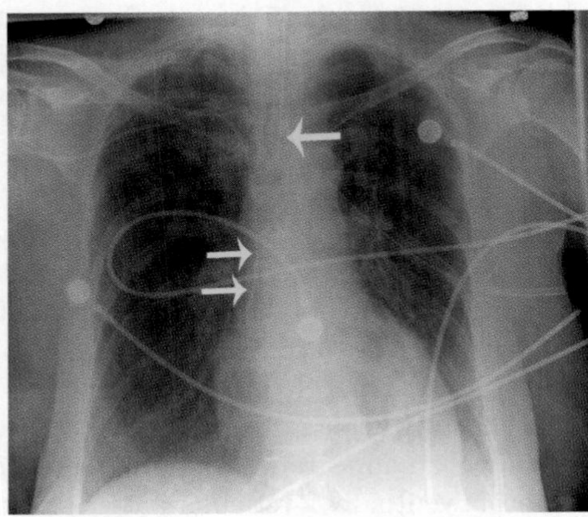

FIGURE 7-16 Endotracheal tube in good position (single arrow). Also note presence of central venous catheter (double arrows).

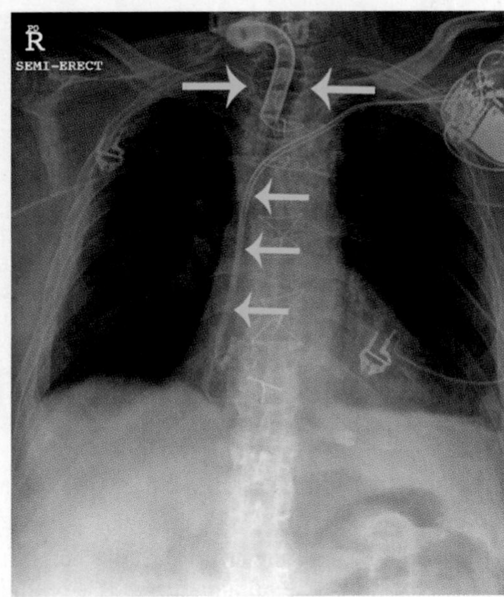

FIGURE 7-17 Tracheal dilation due to overinflation of the cuff of the tracheostomy tube. Also note the presence of a pacemaker. Lowered, flattened diaphragms suggest the presence of chronic obstructive pulmonary disease.

A tracheostomy tube should be midline, and optimal positioning of the tip is one-half to two-thirds of the distance between the stoma and the carina. After insertion of a tracheostomy tube, it is important to be certain that it is in the trachea and not inserted into a false track (**Figure 7-18**).

The tip and the side hole of a feeding tube should be beyond the gastroesophageal junction. Misplacement of the nasogastric tube into the airway may occur (**Figure 7-19**). Radiographic confirmation of feeding tube position is essential before use.

Chest tubes have a radiopaque line that is interrupted by a side hole proximal to the tip, which should be seen medial to the inner margin of the ribs. The side hole should be within the pleural space to ensure proper drainage. Inadvertent insertion of the tube into the soft tissues may be suspected by silhouetting of the

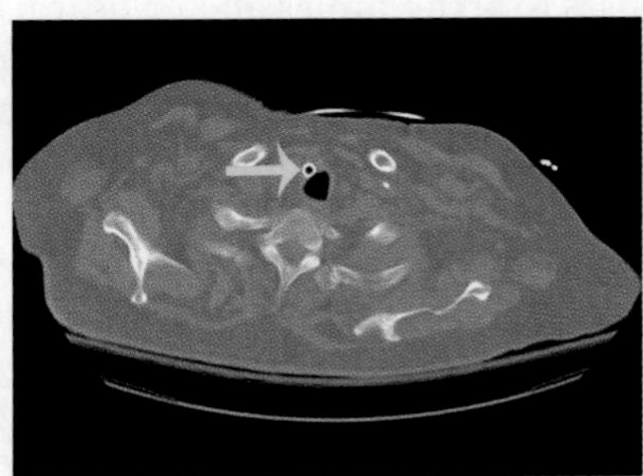

FIGURE 7-18 Computed tomographic scan showing tracheostomy tube in false track.

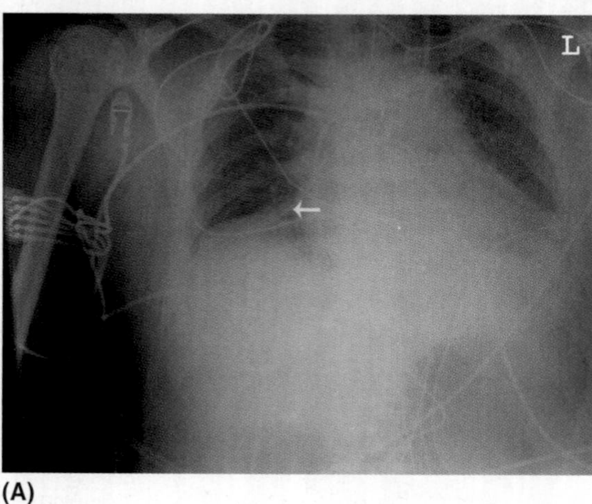

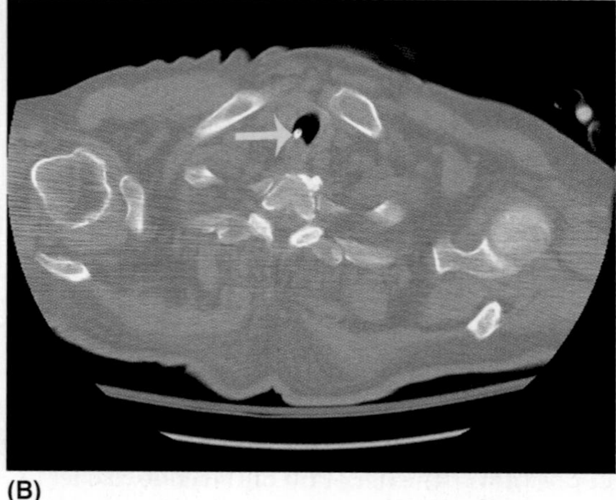

(A) (B)

FIGURE 7-19 (**A**) Gastric tube in right lower lobe bronchus. (**B**) Computed tomographic scan showing gastric tube in trachea.

nonopaque wall of the tube within the adjacent soft tissue density. Normally, the nonopaque wall is rendered visible by surrounding lucent lung. Optimal positioning of the tube depends on whether the air or fluid collection is free or loculated within the pleural space. Intraparenchymal placement may be complicated by a bronchopleural fistula, pulmonary laceration, or hematoma. When a chest tube is inserted into the pulmonary parenchyma, a pulmonary contusion may be seen as opacity near the chest tube. Placement into a fissure is associated with unsatisfactory drainage.

Central venous catheters are inserted peripherally into upper extremity veins or, more commonly, into the subclavian or internal jugular vein. The optimal position of the distal tip of a central venous catheter is the junction of the brachiocephalic vein or superior vena cava, or just proximal to the right atrium in the superior vena cava. Common malpositions of central venous catheters include insertion into the internal mammary and azygous veins, or insertion into the internal jugular vein in the case of a subclavian catheter. A chest radiograph should be used to evaluate the possibility of hemothorax or pneumothorax after line placement.

The optimal position of a pulmonary artery catheter is the right or left pulmonary artery, approximately 5 cm distal to the bifurcation of the main pulmonary artery. Placement of the distal tip into the right ventricle predisposes to arrhythmias and myocardial perforation. Placement too distal in the pulmonary artery may result in pulmonary infarction, hemorrhage, or rupture of the pulmonary artery. The inflated cuff should never be seen on a radiographic study.

An intra-aortic balloon pump catheter is radiolucent, except for the tip, which is radiopaque to permit radiographic localization. The recommended position of the balloon tip is distal to the aortic knob. The carina has been proposed as a practical landmark for positioning of the intra-aortic balloon pump. If the balloon is too high, occlusion of the great vessels may result.

Pulmonary Embolism

Many patients with pulmonary embolism have abnormal chest radiographs. However, the findings are generally nonspecific and may be difficult to appreciate. The most common findings are platelike or discoid atelectasis, peripheral airspace consolidation, and pleural effusion. Other less common abnormalities include enlargement of one or both pulmonary arteries secondary to large emboli, signs of right-sided heart failure, and hemidiaphragm elevation. Decreased vascularity in one lung causing a unilateral increase in radiographic lucency (**Westermark sign**) suggests the presence of a large pulmonary embolus. A wedge-shaped peripheral infiltrate may be seen after a pulmonary embolus that occludes distal vessels in the pulmonary arterial tree (**Hampton hump**). Emboli in the ambulatory patient are more frequent in the lower lobes because of increased blood flow in this region.

Traditionally, the initial investigation of pulmonary embolism has relied on ventilation-perfusion scanning. However, contrast-enhanced spiral CT of the thorax is more sensitive and specific than radionuclide scanning for the detection of pulmonary embolism. Resolution occurs from the periphery, which has been described as the melting of an ice cube. Occasionally, cavitation from an ischemic necrosis or infection occurs during the course of resolution.

Acute Respiratory Distress Syndrome

The chest radiograph in acute respiratory distress syndrome (ARDS) has been traditionally characterized by bilateral diffuse infiltration of the lungs (**Figure 7-20**). The radiographic findings are often progressive, expanding from centrally located, poorly defined opacities to the periphery of the lung fields. The opacified areas often have a fluffy alveolar appearance that progresses to a patchy pattern. Eventually, a reticular pattern develops, and microabscesses with small cavities may become apparent. The CT reveals a gravity-dependent opacity

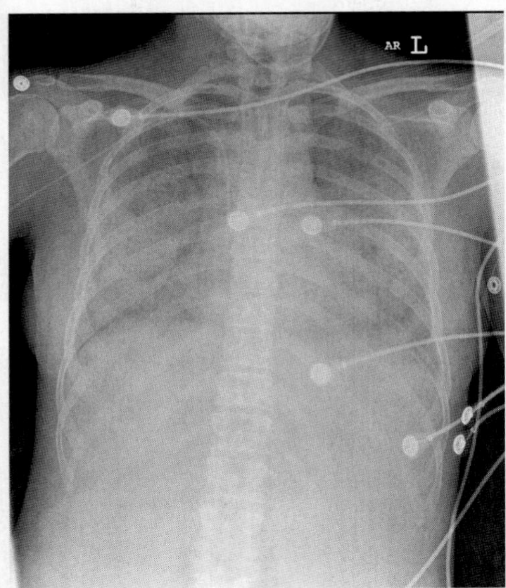

FIGURE 7-20 Anteroposterior projection of patient with severe acute respiratory distress syndrome.

with normal-appearing nondependent regions of the lungs.

Chest Trauma

Chest trauma may be associated with a number of abnormalities on the chest radiograph. These include broken ribs, chest contusion, pneumothorax, and hemothorax.

Cross-Sectional Imaging Techniques

Computed Tomography

The fundamental principle of computed tomography is to acquire multiple views of an object over a range of angular orientations. By this means, additional dimensional data are obtained in comparison with conventional radiographs, in which there is only one view. The CT image is typically called a *slice*, which corresponds to a thickness of the object being scanned. Whereas a digital image is composed of pixels (picture elements), a CT slice image is composed of **voxels** (volume elements). The gray levels in a CT slice correspond to x-ray attenuation, which reflects the proportion of x-rays scattered or absorbed as they pass through each voxel.

Directing x-rays from multiple orientations and measuring their resultant decrease in intensity creates CT images. A specialized algorithm is then used to reconstruct the distribution of x-ray densities in the slice plane. Medical systems generally use **Hounsfield units (HU)**, in which air is given a value of –1000 and water is given a value of 0, causing most soft tissues to have values ranging from –100 to 100 and bone to range from 600 to over 2000. Conventional medical CT exams provide resolution on the order of 1 to 2 mm, whereas high-resolution instruments provide resolution on the order of 100 to 200 micrometers. Ultra-high-resolution instruments provide resolution on the order of a few tens of microns.

Cross-sectional CT images can be viewed in axial, sagittal, coronal, and oblique projections (**Figure 7-21**). New scanners have made it possible to scan the thorax in a single breath hold, thereby eliminating breathing artifact, with advances including high-resolution imaging for the evaluation of interstitial lung disease and a helical technique. Because CT provides exquisite anatomic detail of the thorax, it can be used for a number of different problems (**Figures 7-22** through **7-25**), including soft tissue or bony abnormalities, pleural abnormalities, lung parenchyma and interstitial disease, hilar or mediastinal pathology including the heart and great vessels, pulmonary embolism, and aortic dissection. CT is also useful to guide procedures such as drainage of pleural effusions or to assess the position of drainage catheters. Intravenous contrast, which can be useful for delineating vascular structures, is required in situations such as aortic dissection and the detection of pulmonary embolism. Most CT studies of the thorax do not require IV contrast, however.

A portable chest radiograph may demonstrate a nonspecific area of consolidation. CT can reveal signs of volume loss not otherwise apparent, favoring the diagnosis of atelectasis over pneumonia. Pneumonia on CT is typically space occupying, involving a lobe or part of a lobe and the presence of air bronchograms. Air bronchograms are also seen with atelectasis, noninfectious lung inflammation, and in neoplastic etiologies, including bronchioloalveolar carcinoma and pulmonary lymphoma.

CT is the most accurate examination for detecting and characterizing pleural effusions. Pleural effusion can be difficult to detect on a portable chest radiograph, and its appearance can mimic airspace consolidation. Chest CT in many cases thus may be the only way to accurately assess the size of a pleural effusion. Small pleural effusions can be overlooked easily or be difficult to identify accurately on a supine portable chest radiograph. If an effusion is uncomplicated and free flowing, its appearance will differ with a change in patient position. Pneumothorax is missed frequently when interpreting the portable chest radiograph. CT

Respiratory Recap

Cross-Sectional Imaging Techniques

- Computed tomography
- Ultrasonography
- Magnetic resonance imaging
- Positron emission tomography

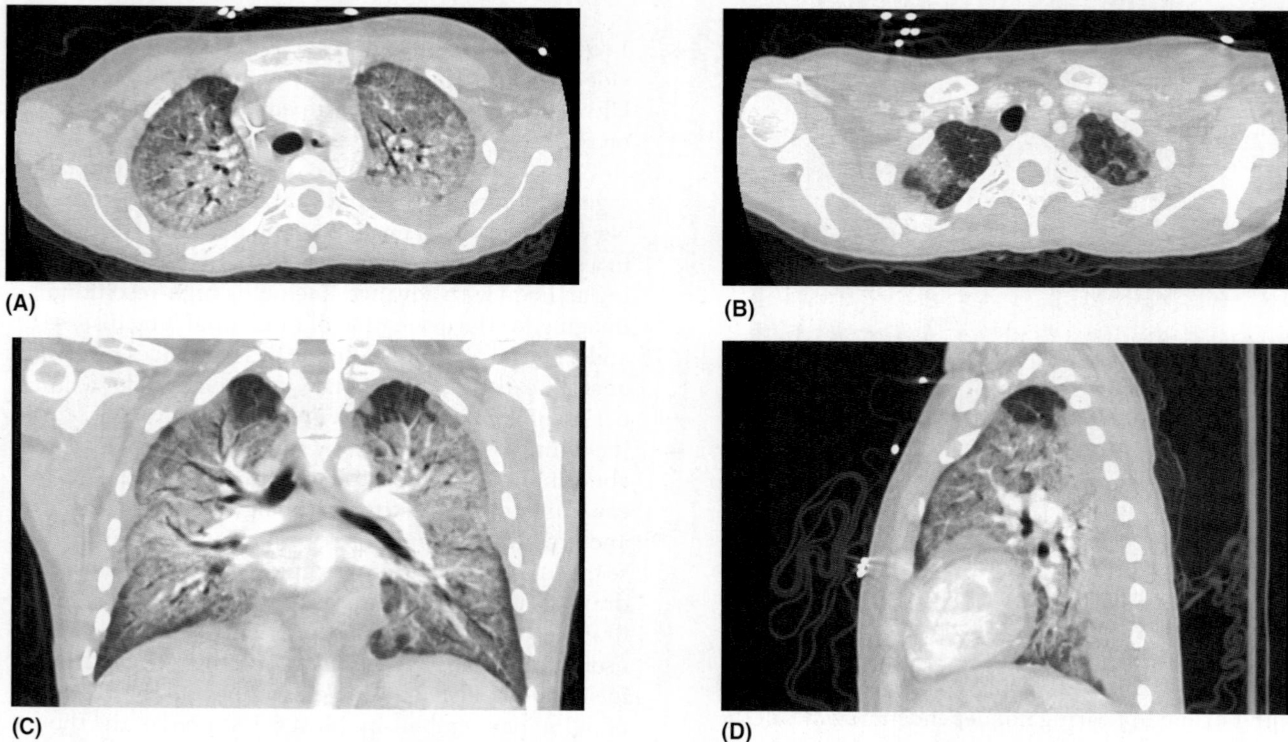

FIGURE 7-21 Computed tomographic scan of patient in Figure 7-20. (**A**) Axial image from mid-lung. (**B**) Axial image from apex. (**C**) Coronal reconstruction. (**D**) Sagittal reconstruction.

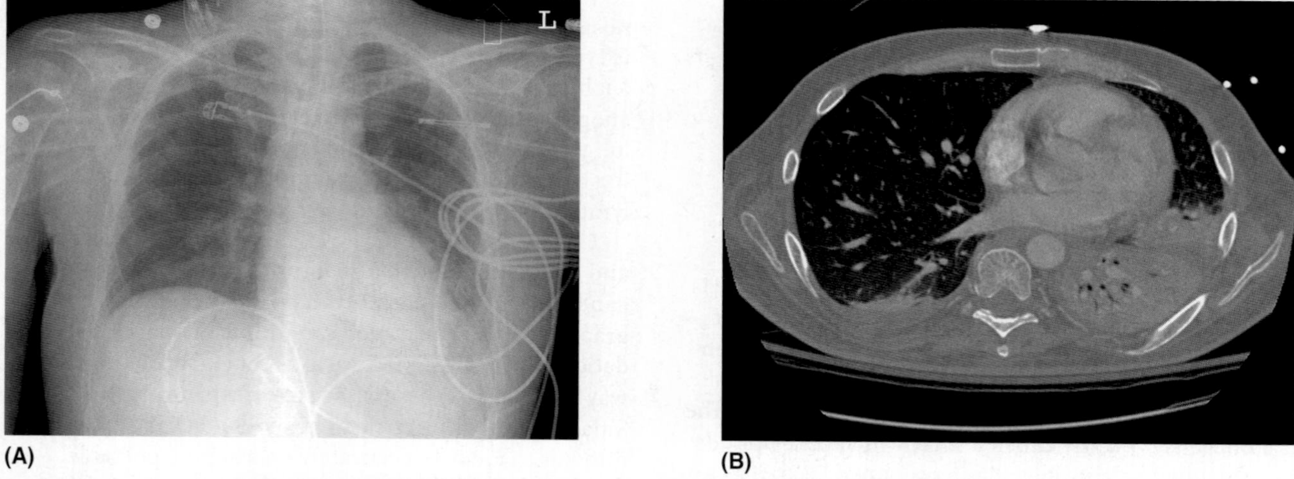

FIGURE 7-22 Left lower lobe pneumonia. (**A**) Note loss of diaphragm border on anteroposterior projection. (**B**) Computed tomography image. Note presence of air bronchograms, indicating that the abnormality is in the lung and not the pleural space.

may be helpful especially for evaluating loculated air collections and the proper location of chest tubes when a pneumothorax persists.

With newer multidetector CT scanners, small emboli to the subsegmental level can be diagnosed confidently. CT pulmonary angiography has reported sensitivities ranging from 53% to 100% and specificities of 83% to 100% when the examination is performed on the newer generation of CT scanners. The clinical validity of using a CT to rule out pulmonary embolism is similar to that reported for conventional pulmonary angiography. A major advantage of CT compared with other diagnostic tests for pulmonary embolism is its ability to diagnose other potential causes of the patient's symptoms.

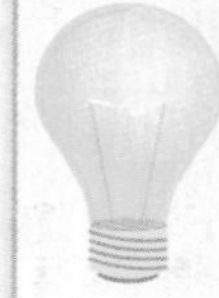

STOP AND THINK

A patient presents in acute respiratory failure. How might a chest CT be helpful?

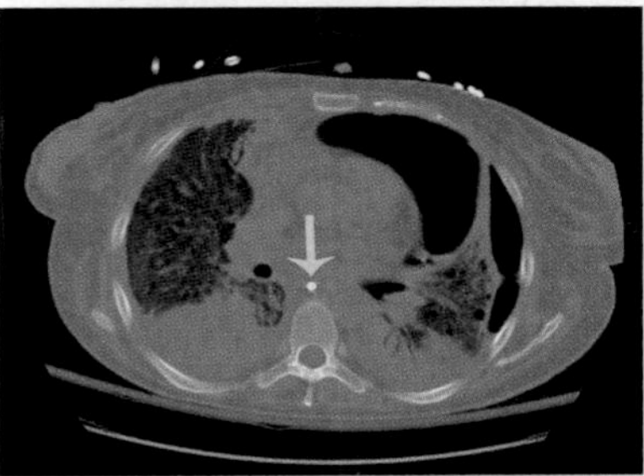

FIGURE 7-23 Computed tomography of the chest of a patient with right pleural effusion and left pneumothorax. Note that the pleural effusion is in the dependent thorax and the pneumothorax is in the nondependent thorax. Also note the air bronchograms in the left lower lobe and the gastric tube in the esophagus (arrow).

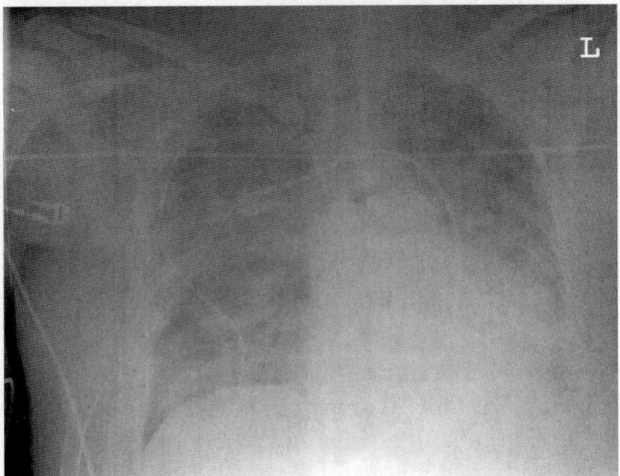

(A)

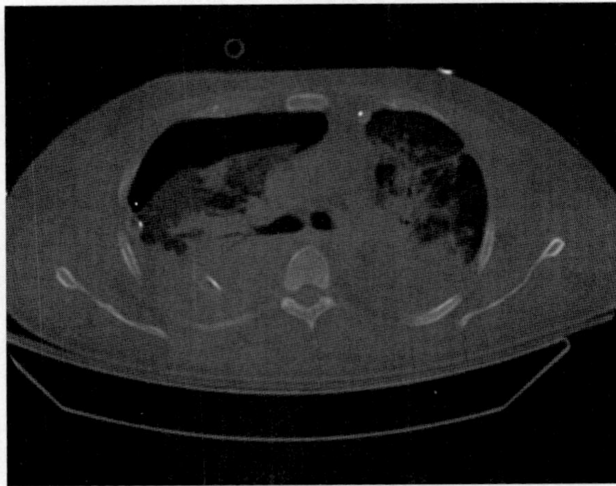

(B)

FIGURE 7-24 (**A**) Anteroposterior projection of patient with bilateral whiteout of the lung fields. (**B**) Computed tomography of the same patient showing large right-sided pneumothorax and dependent consolidation.

Ultrasonography

Ultrasound is increasingly used as a bedside monitor in the ICU.[10–12] Visualization of the lungs is optimized by using a probe with a convex tip placed at the level of an intercostal space. An emission frequency ranging between 4 and 15 MHz is used. High emission frequencies offer an accurate view of the lung periphery and are particularly appropriate for visualizing lung sliding. Low emission frequencies are more appropriate for visualizing the deep lung, particularly pleural effusions and lung consolidations. The diaphragmatic cupola is first identified to avoid confusion because lung consolidation appears similar to those of spleen and liver. Six regions, delineated by anterior and posterior axillary lines, should be examined: upper and lower parts of anterior, lateral and posterior chest wall. Systematic examination of each adjacent intercostal space is used to assess of the extension of ultrasound abnormalities along the cephalocaudal axis. Dorsal lung segments of upper lobes cannot be explored by ultrasound because they lie behind the scapula.

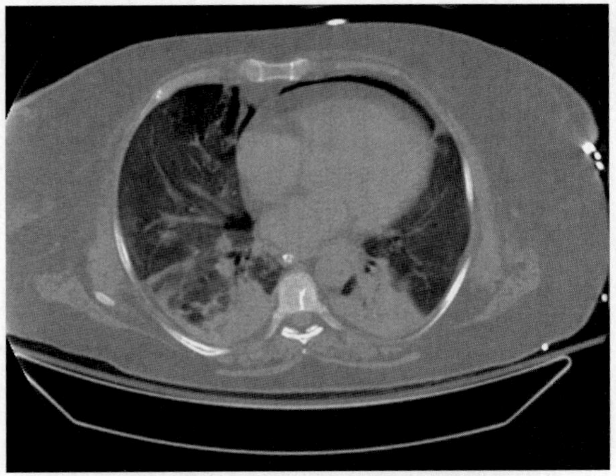

FIGURE 7-25 Computed tomographic scan showing dependent consolidation and pneumopericardium.

Ultrasound waves are not transmitted through anatomic structures that are filled with gas, so normally the lung parenchyma is not visible beyond the pleura. Ultrasound waves are transmitted to deep intrathoracic structures only if lung aeration is absent, as occurs with consolidation, atelectasis, or pleural effusion. Lung ultrasound can be used for detecting and quantifying pleural effusion and lung consolidation. On a longitudinal view, the ribs appear as posterior shadowing and delineate the acoustic window. The pleural line is seen 0.5 cm below the ribs line and appears as a hyperechoic (increased amplitude of waves) and sliding line, moving forward and back with movements of the visceral pleura against the parietal pleura during the respiratory cycle. On time–motion mode, a seashore sign is present, which is characterized by a motionless parietal tissue over the pleural line with a homogeneous granular pattern below. Beyond this pleural line, motionless and regularly spaced horizontal lines are seen, associated with artifacts of repetition. A normal ultrasound pattern is defined by lung sliding associated with horizontal A lines (**Figure 7-26**).

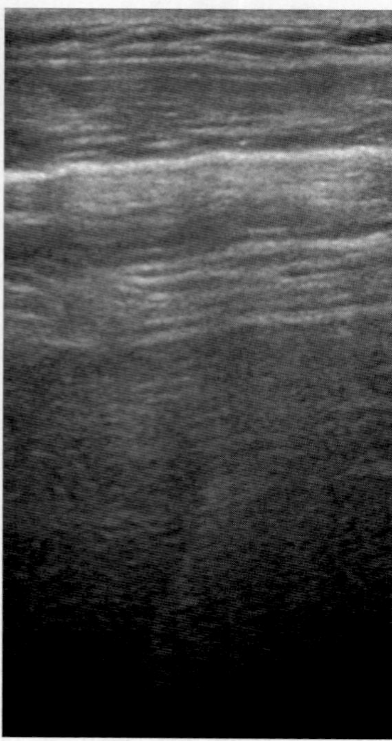

FIGURE 7-26 A lines are artifacts reproducing the pleural line at regular intervals. This is the time required to return the ultrasound beam to the transducer after being reflected one or more times by the pleural line.

Reproduced from Gardelli G, Feletti F, Nanni A, et al. Chest ultrasonography in the ICU. *Respir Care.* 2012;57:773–781.

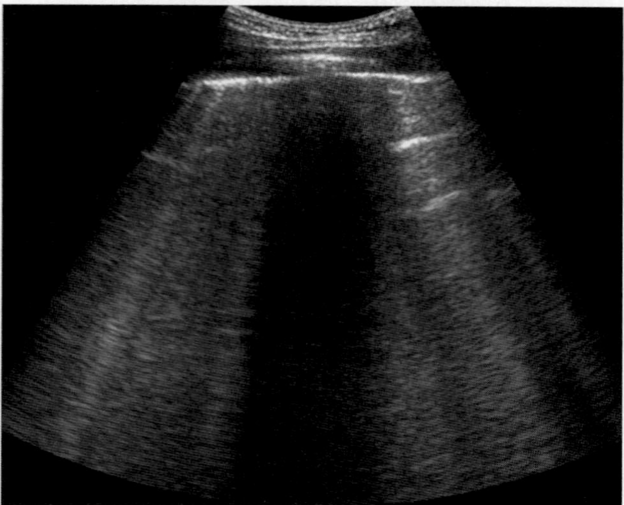

FIGURE 7-27 B lines on thoracic ultrasound.

Reproduced from Gardelli G, Feletti F, Nanni A, et al. Chest ultrasonography in the ICU. *Respir Care.* 2012;57:773–781.

Increased lung tissue creates vertical ultrasound artifacts arising from the pleura. These vertical B lines, called comet tails, extend to the edge of the screen, increase with inspiration, move with the pleural line, and efface A lines (**Figure 7-27**). Multiple B lines are caused by thickened interlobular septa (interstitial edema) when they are 7 mm apart and by ground-glass areas (alveolar edema) when they are 3 mm apart or less. In about a third of healthy humans, a few isolated B lines can be also seen.

Pulmonary ultrasound is used clinically to evaluate pleural effusions and pneumothorax. There is increasingly interest in using ultrasound to evaluate alveolar recruitment during mechanical ventilation in patients with ARDS. With PEEP titration, the recruited areas become hyperreflective, similar to normal lungs, but with many B lines due to interstitial congestion (**Figure 7-28**).

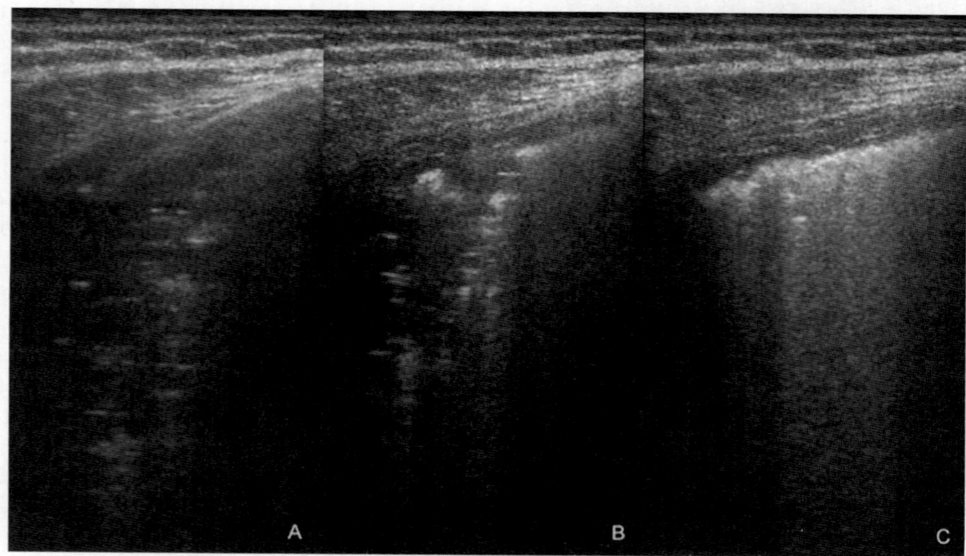

FIGURE 7-28 Evaluation of alveolar recruitment maneuver by ultrasound. (**A**) Consolidated parenchymal area in patient suffering from ARDS. (**B**) The hyperreflectant air aspect reaching the pulmonary consolidation and the progressive reduction of its compactness. (**C**) Recruitment: consolidation is dimensionally reduced and partly replaced by normal air parenchyma, full of B lines, an expression of interstitial thickening.

Reproduced from Gardelli G, Feletti F, Nanni A, et al. Chest ultrasonography in the ICU. *Respir Care.* 2012;57:773–781.

Ultrasound guidance has been demonstrated to facilitate insertion of central venous catheters, especially into the internal jugular vein. A systematic review showed a clear benefit from two-dimensional ultrasound guidance for central venous access compared with the landmark method.[13] This is manifest in a lower technical failure rate (overall and on first attempt), a reduction in complications, and faster access. Ultrasound has also been used for arterial cannulation (**Figure 7-29**).[14,15] The artery is distinguished from nearby veins due to the pulsating nature of the artery or by the use of color Doppler ultrasound. Ultrasound has been used to identify the radial, femoral, axillary, and dorsalis pedis arteries.

Magnetic Resonance Imaging

Magnetic resonance imaging (MRI) takes advantage of nuclear magnetic resonance, in which nuclei with odd numbers of protons and a magnetic moment become aligned when placed in a strong magnetic field. These protons then can be excited to a more energetic state with the addition of a radio-frequency pulse. Once allowed to relax, excited protons emit a resonance signal that reflects the number of protons and their nuclear environment. Different relaxation signals are generated depending on the pulse sequence, that is, the way in which the protons within the nuclei are excited. In the body, the greatest source of odd-number protons, that is, hydrogen nuclei, is used to create a resonance signal. Although some signals have features suggestive of a particular disease process, signal characteristics often are nonspecific.

Once a resonance signal has been generated, the information can be mathematically transformed to produce an image. MRI provides accurate anatomic detail of the thorax. Its current indications include soft tissue and bone marrow pathology, complicated pleural and diaphragmatic diseases, hilar and mediastinal abnormalities (including congenital heart disease, cardiac abnormalities, and vascular pathology), pulmonary embolism, and aortic dissection.

Although MRI often is complementary to CT, it has several advantages. MRI often better serves patients with renal dysfunction because intravenous contrast, which can be nephrotoxic, usually is not required. MRI has several other disadvantages, including limited patient monitoring capabilities and motion artifacts caused by cardiac and respiratory motion, which can obscure the images. MRI is contraindicated in patients with cardiac pacemakers. Despite these limitations, MRI offers information not available from other modalities. In addition, MRI, unlike CT, uses no ionizing radiation.

Positron Emission Tomography

Positron emission tomography (PET) is a recognized tool for the assessment of thoracic pathologic processes, particularly for tumor imaging. Previous PET investigations were performed almost exclusively on the brain, but now some of the same principles have been applied to thoracic abnormalities. Unlike CT and MRI, PET provides physiologic and metabolic information. This test, which focuses on the biochemical properties of cells, has the ability to analyze abnormalities quantitatively. Currently, the positron-emitting agent most commonly used in the thorax is F18-fluorodeoxyglucose (FDG). Metabolically active cells take up and trap this D-glucose analogue. The activity then can be measured and mapped to a specific region within the thorax. More metabolically active tumor cells show increased FDG uptake compared with normal tissues or a benign process.

Indications for PET imaging of the thorax include distinguishing benign and malignant focal pulmonary

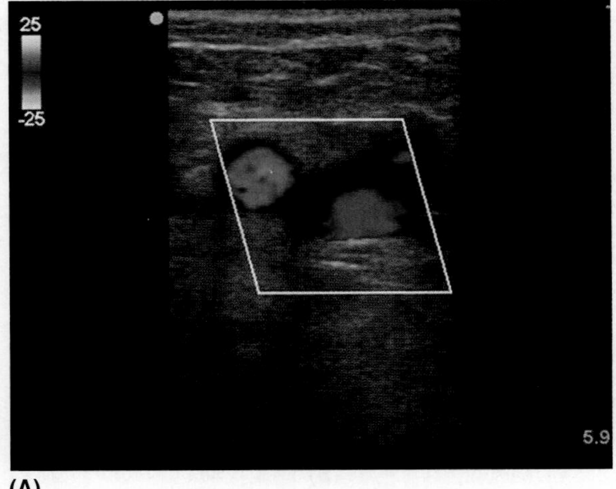

(A)

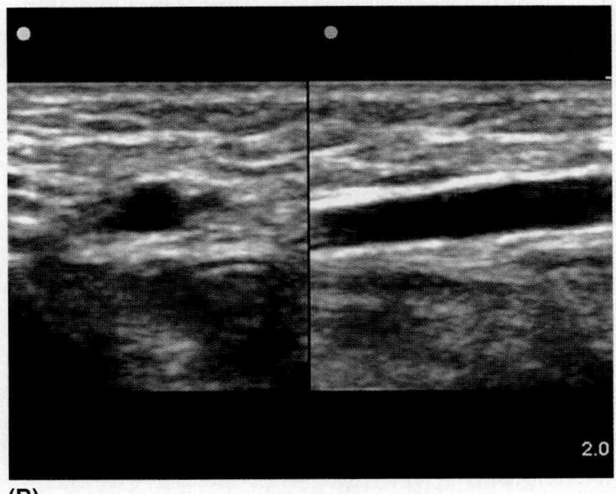

(B)

FIGURE 7-29 (**A**) Femoral artery and vein: color Doppler ultrasound. (**B**) Radial artery in transverse and longitudinal orientations.
Courtesy of Ariel L Shiloh, M.D., Division of Critical Care Medicine, Montefiore Medical Center, The Albert Einstein College of Medicine.

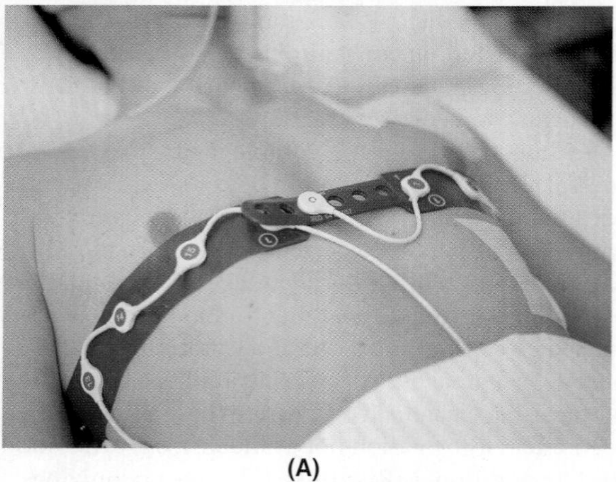

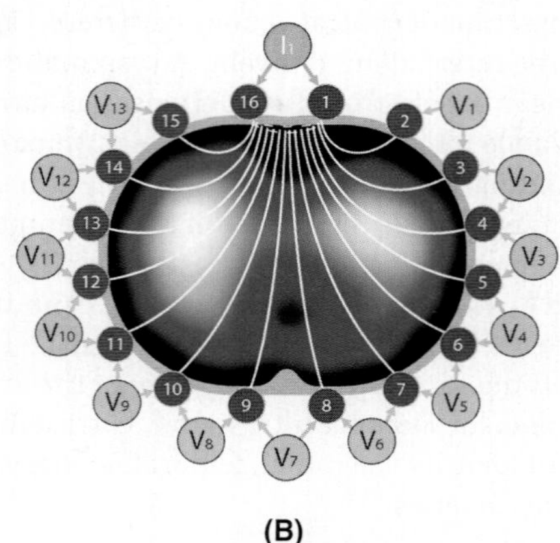

(A) (B)

FIGURE 7-30 Electrical impedance tomography. (**A**) Electrode belt with patient cable connected. (**B**) Current application and voltage measurements around the thorax.

abnormalities, including solitary pulmonary nodules, staging lung cancer, and differentiating fibrosis from tumor in patients treated for lung cancer. PET imaging has a sensitivity of approximately 95% for the detection of cancer in patients who have indeterminate lesions on CT. The specificity of 85% with PET in these lesions is less than the sensitivity because some inflammatory processes, such as granulomatous infection, avidly accumulate FDG. PET is more accurate than CT in determination of the presence or absence of intrathoracic metastatic nodal disease. Intrathoracic and extrathoracic disease can be staged in a single examination with whole-body PET. This allows the detection of occult metastasis. PET is most useful in the management of cancer patients, but its role in critically ill patients is limited.

Electrical Impedance Tomography

Electrical impedance tomography (EIT) is an imaging technique that can be used during mechanical ventilation to detect regional distribution of alveolar ventilation.[16–20] By quantification of local inhomogeneities in lung mechanics, it has the potential to detect recruitment and derecruitment, and the effect of strategies such as titration of positive end-expiratory pressure (PEEP) and tidal volume. EIT is radiation-free, noninvasive, portable, and accessible for bedside monitoring.

EIT data are obtained by application of an alternating current between adjacent electrodes on the skin surface and simultaneous measurements of potential differences between the remaining pairs of 16 to 32 electrodes applied around the thorax (**Figure 7-30**). Current application and voltage measurement are performed in a rotating manner resulting in an update of the image up to 50 times per second. The changes in impedance are explained by the fact that gas is a nonconductor. Tidal inflation decreases the cross-sectional area of the tissue, which results in an increase in impedance inversely proportional to the cross-sectional area. A computer algorithm is used to construct a cross-sectional image of the thorax (**Figure 7-31**).

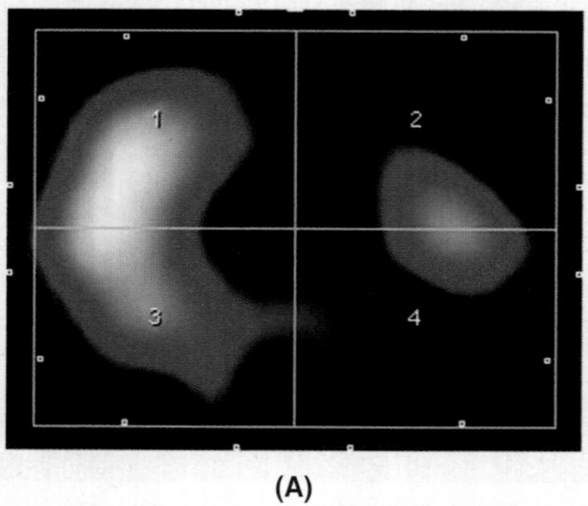

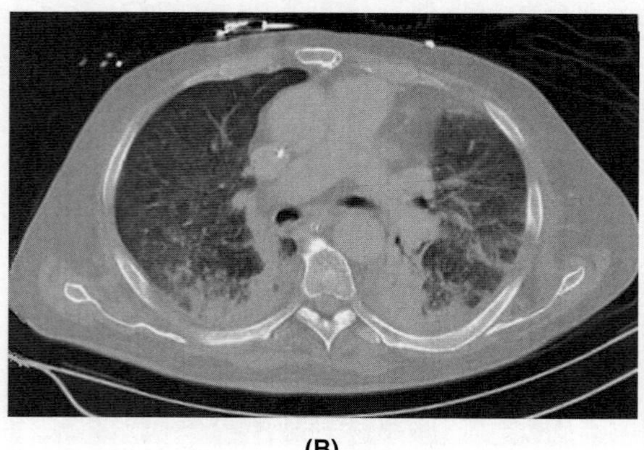

(A) (B)

FIGURE 7-31 Tidal image and corresponding CT image of an ARDS patient.

EIT has yet to receive widespread application. The images generated require training for correct interpretation. Currently, interpretation indices are not available that are simple enough to be used to guide ventilator management.

Key Points

- Structures are seen on the chest radiograph due to density and contrast.
- Positions used for chest radiography include anteroposterior, posteroanterior, lateral decubitus, and apical lordotic.
- The chest radiograph displays anatomic and pathophysiologic features for determining the presence of disorders in the thorax.
- The location and size of abnormal air or fluid pockets within the chest can be evaluated by chest radiography.
- The proper positioning of tubes and catheters is determined by chest radiography.
- The multiple slices of computed tomography provide three-dimensional viewing of the thorax.
- Computed tomography improves the ability to discriminate pneumonia versus atelectasis as well as the location and extent of an effusion or pulmonary emboli.
- Ultrasonography has become useful in vascular cannulation, central venous catheter placements, and bedside assessment of pleural diseases including the presence of air or fluid.
- Magnetic resonance imaging is indicated for detection of soft tissue pathology that includes complicated pleural and diaphragmatic diseases as well as hilar and mediastinal abnormalities.
- Positron emission tomography is indicated for monitoring thoracic pathologic processes, particularly tumor imaging.
- Electrical impedance tomography is an imaging technique that can be used during mechanical ventilation to detect regional distribution of alveolar ventilation.

References

1. Seibert A. X-ray imaging physics for nuclear medicine technologists. Part 1. Basic principles of x-ray production. *J Nucl Med Technol.* 2004;32:139–147.
2. Collins J, Stern EJ. *Chest Radiology: The Essentials.* 2nd ed. Philadelphia: Lippincott Williams & Wilkins; 2008.
3. Godoy MCB, Leitman BS, de Groot PM, et al. (2012). Chest radiography in the ICU: Part 1, Evaluation of airway, enteric, and pleural tubes. *AJR.* 2012;198:563–571.
4. Godoy MCB, Leitman BS, de Groot PM, et al. Chest radiography in the ICU: Part 2, Evaluation of cardiovascular lines and other devices. *AJR.* 2012;198:572–581.
5. Eisenhuber E, Schaefer-Prokop CM, Prosch H, Schima W. Bedside chest radiography. *Respir Care.* 2012;57:427–443.
6. Sheard S, Rao P, Devaraj A. Imaging of acute respiratory distress syndrome. *Respir Care.* 2012;57:607–612.
7. McAdams HP, Samei E, Dobbins J III, et al. Recent advances in chest radiography. *Radiology.* 2008;241:663–683.
8. Hill JR, Horner PE, Primack SL. ICU imaging. *Clin Chest Med.* 2008;29:59–76.
9. Goodman LR. *Felson's Principles of Chest Roentgenology: A Programmed Text.* 3rd ed. Philadelphia: Saunders Elsevier; 2007.
10. Bouhemad B, Zhang M, Lu Q, Rouby JJ. Clinical review: bedside lung ultrasound in critical care practice. *Crit Care.* 2007;11:205.
11. Gardelli G, Feletti F, Nanni A, et al. Chest ultrasonography in the ICU. *Respir Care.* 2012;57:773–781.
12. Arbelot C, Ferrari F, Bouhemad B, Rouby JJ. Lung ultrasound in acute respiratory distress syndrome and acute lung injury. *Curr Opin Crit Care.* 2008;14:70–74.
13. Hind D, Calvert N, McWilliams R, et al. Ultrasonic locating devices for central venous cannulation: meta-analysis. *BMJ.* 2003;327:361.
14. Shiloh AL, Eisen LA. Ultrasound-guided arterial catheterization: a narrative review. *Intensive Care Med.* 2010;36:214–221.
15. Haynes JM, Mitchell H. Ultrasound-guided arterial puncture. *Respir Care.* 2010;55:1754–1756.
16. Bodenstein M, David M, Markstaller K. Principles of electrical impedance tomography and its clinical application. *Crit Care Med.* 2009;37:713–724.
17. Lundin S, Stenqvist O. Electrical impedance tomography: potentials and pitfalls. *Curr Opin Crit Care.* 2012;18:35–41.
18. Muders T, Luepschen H, Putensen C. Impedance tomography as a new monitoring technique. *Curr Opin Crit Care.* 2010;16:269–275.
19. Costa ELV, Lima RG, Amato MBP. Electrical impedance tomography. *Curr Opin Crit Care.* 2009;15:18–24.
20. Putensen C, Wrigge H, Zinserling J. Electrical impedance tomography guided ventilation therapy. *Curr Opin Crit Care.* 2007;13:344–350.

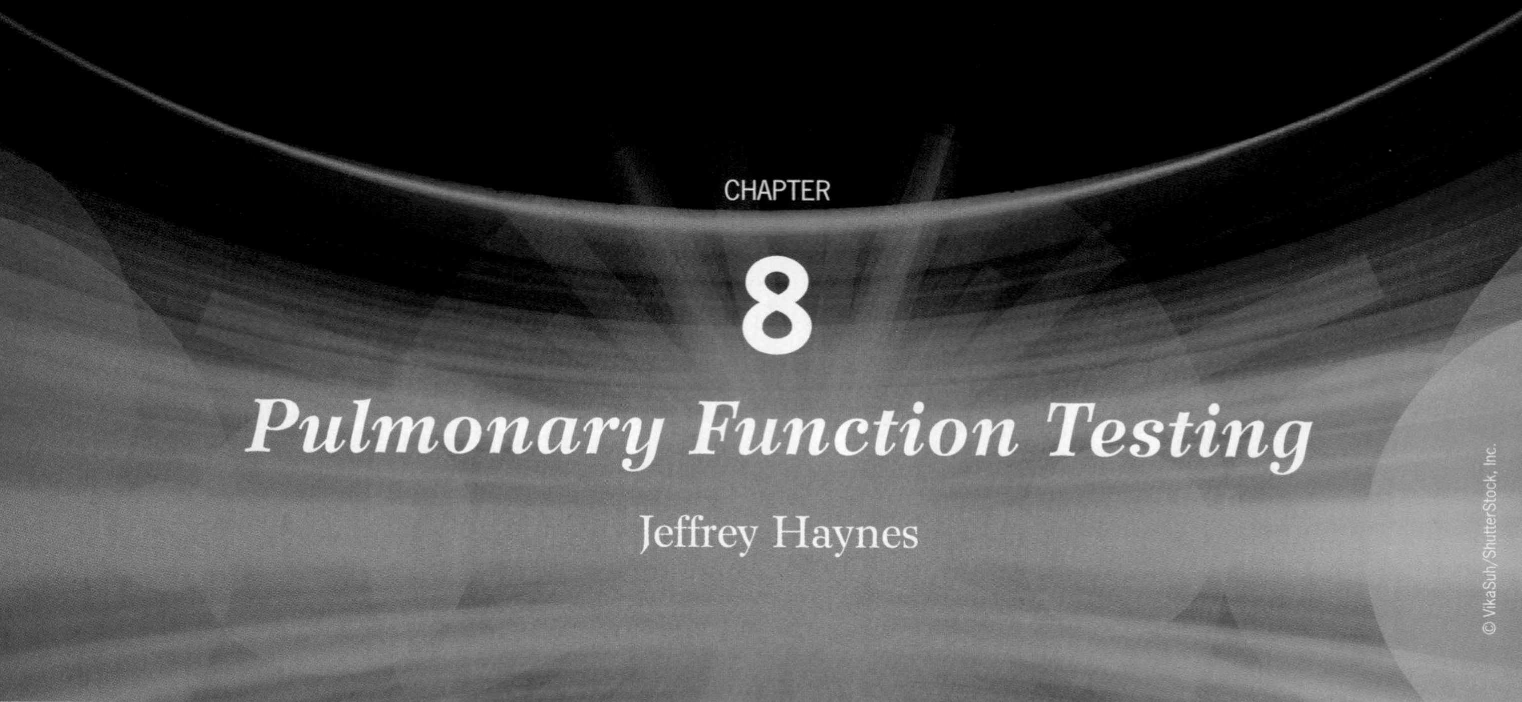

OUTLINE

Goals of Pulmonary Function Testing
Spirometry
Lung Volumes and Capacities
Specialized Pulmonary Function Tests

OBJECTIVES

1. Describe the clinical use of pulmonary function tests.
2. Identify the features of normal and abnormal spirometry tracings.
3. Recognize the common errors seen in spirometry testing.
4. Specify the spirometry values seen in patients with normal lungs, obstructive disease, and restrictive disorders.
5. Explain the importance of spirometry testing before and after administering a bronchodilator.
6. Recognize upper airway obstruction.
7. Define lung volumes and capacities.
8. Compare methods used to measure functional residual capacity.
9. Discuss the American Thoracic Society/European Respiratory Society standards for pulmonary function testing.
10. Explain the importance of diffusing capacity.
11. List the goals of bronchial challenge testing, airways resistance, and tests of respiratory muscle strength.

KEY TERMS

airways resistance
body plethysmography
diffusing capacity
exhaled nitric oxide
forced vital capacity (FVC)
helium dilution
hyperinflation
lung capacity
lung volumes
maximum expiratory pressure
maximum inspiratory pressure
nitrogen washout
obstructive lung disease
pulmonary function tests (PFTs)
restrictive lung disease
single-breath nitrogen washout
spirometer
spirometry
total lung capacity
vital capacity

Introduction

Pulmonary function tests (PFTs) are the primary diagnostic tool for evaluating patients with respiratory symptoms and for guiding the management of such patients' diagnosed lung disease. Unfortunately, many patients are misdiagnosed and improperly treated for lung disease without the guidance of PFTs.

Lord Kelvin famously said: *"When you can measure what you are speaking about, and express it in numbers, you know something about it, when you cannot express it in numbers, your knowledge is of a meager and unsatisfactory kind; it may be the beginning of knowledge, but you have scarcely, in your thoughts advanced to the stage of science."* Lord Kelvin's statement is nowhere more true than in the evaluation of respiratory function. While the evaluation of signs and symptoms is important for formulating a pretest probability of lung disease, these alone are neither sensitive nor specific for diagnosis and have proven to be unreliable in the management of disease states.

The first lung function test, **vital capacity**, was invented in the 1840s to assess lung size (volume) in patients with tuberculosis (TB). An early observation was that patients with TB who had a low vital capacity lived for shorter periods of time compared to those with a higher vital capacity. Since 1950, the most common use of pulmonary function testing has been the assessment of obstructive lung diseases, such as asthma and chronic obstructive pulmonary disease (COPD). Cigarette smokers with lower lung function due to COPD have higher rates of morbidity and mortality.

PFTs have a long, rich history, and the tests performed regularly are relatively well standardized. In 2005 the American Thoracic Society (ATS) and European Respiratory Society (ERS) jointly published guidelines for the most commonly performed PFTs and for the general administration of pulmonary function laboratories.[1–5] PFTs are unique because, unlike most diagnostic tests, PFTs are dependent on the patient and technologist to produce physical actions in accordance with the design of the test. Submaximal efforts and incorrect performance can produce spurious data, which has the potential to misclassify patients. Respiratory therapists performing spirometry and other PFTs must be well trained and be given feedback on the quality of the tests they submit for interpretation.[6–9] The training of personnel conducting the tests should meet minimal criteria as recommended by ATS/ERS guidelines.[1] This chapter describes PFT equipment, patient testing guidelines, and the parameters commonly measured in pulmonary function testing.

Goals of Pulmonary Function Testing

The goal of pulmonary function testing is to classify the patient's lung function as normal or abnormal and, if abnormal, quantify the degree of impairment. While the results of PFTs affect the posttest probability of a disease, PFTs should be regarded as a contributing piece of evidence used in conjunction with other pieces of evidence (risk factors, chest imaging tests) to help make the correct diagnosis. PFTs aid in the detection of restrictive and/or obstructive ventilatory defects, the gas transfer abnormalities that may accompany some lung diseases, and the strength of respiratory muscles. **Restrictive lung diseases** reduce lung volume, whereas **obstructive lung diseases** reduce airflow through the bronchial tree. Obtaining quality data is of the utmost importance during pulmonary function testing. Quality PFT data are dependent on accurate and precise equipment, a competent and motivated technologist, and a capable and cooperative patient.[6,7] Of the three, an incompetent and/or unmotivated technologist is the most common source of poor quality PFT data.

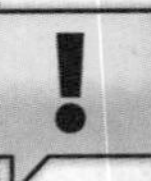

Respiratory Recap

Goals of Pulmonary Function Testing

- Detecting airflow limitation
- Detecting restriction
- Detecting impaired gas transfer abnormalities
- Detecting respiratory muscle weakness

BOX 8-1

Infection Control for Pulmonary Function Testing

Use universal precautions.

For patients with suspected infectious airborne diseases, wear an N95 respirator.

Wear gloves when handling contaminated equipment.

Mouthpieces or flow sensors should be disposable or disinfected between patients.

The use of inline filters does not eliminate the need for regular cleaning and disinfection.

Infection Control

The goal of infection control is to prevent the transmission of infectious organisms from either direct or indirect contact. The guidelines in **Box 8-1** should be applied whenever PFTs are performed.

Spirometry

Spirometry is the most commonly performed PFT. The importance of spirometry has been emphasized by at least three major initiatives to diagnose and treat obstructive lung disease: the National Lung Health Education Program (NLHEP), the Global Initiative for Chronic Obstructive Lung Disease (GOLD), and the Global Initiative for Asthma (GINA). **Box 8-2** lists the most common clinical indications for spirometry.

Equipment

Spirometers can be categorized by their measurement method. In the 1950s, spirometers measured exhaled volume by accumulating exhaled air inside a cylindrical canister. Volume-sensing spirometers, such as water-sealed or dry-rolling seal models, maintain a high accuracy for many years, but are large, difficult to clean, and require leak checks, so they were largely replaced by flow-sensing spirometers in the 1990s. Flow is measured by several methods, including turbines, laminar flow elements (Fleisch pneumotach), Pitot tubes, metal or fiber screens (Lilly or Silverman pneumotach), heated wires, bending vanes, or ultrasonic flow sensors (**Figure 8-1**). Users need to be familiar with conditions that can affect the accuracy of the particular device they are using. Many use single-patient, disposable mouthpieces or filters. The size and cost of spirometers have declined while their ease of use and functionality has improved. **Figure 8-2** shows an example of a modern portable spirometer.

The ATS and ERS have jointly established guidelines for equipment selection and maintenance (**Box 8-3**). Precision and accuracy are key to obtaining reliable test

BOX 8-2

Indications for Spirometry

Diagnostic

- Evaluate symptoms, signs, or abnormal laboratory tests
- Measure effect of disease on pulmonary function
- Screen individuals at risk of having pulmonary disease (e.g., smokers over 40 years of age)
- Assess preoperative risk and/or health status prior to exercise program

Monitoring

- Assess the change in lung function over time or after administration of or change in therapy
- Monitor for adverse reactions to drugs with known pulmonary toxicity
- Assess the potential effects of environmental or occupational exposures

Disability

- Assess impairment or disability from lung disease
- Assess risks as part of insurance evaluation

Public Health

- Epidemiologic surveys
- Derivation of reference equations
- Clinical research

Modified from Miller MR, Hankinson J, Brusasco V, et al. ATS/ERS Task Force: standardisation of spirometry. *Eur Respir J.* 2005;26:319–338. Reproduced with permission of the European Respiratory Society.

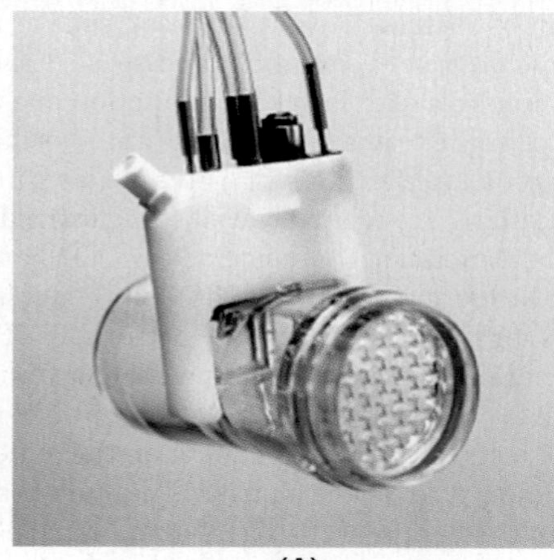

(A)

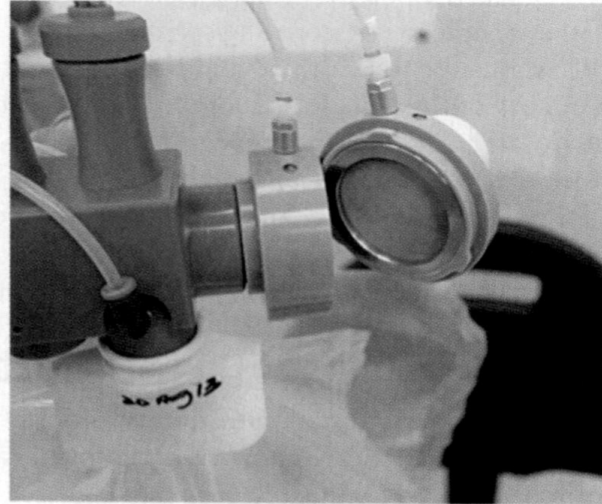

(B)

FIGURE 8-1 Two commonly used pneumotachometers. (A) Pitot tube, pressure is produced within the cross shaped struts in proportion to flow. (**B**) Lilly or Silverman mesh screen pneumotachometer, pressure is measured on each side of the screen, the difference in pressure is proportional to the flow.

data. In addition, equipment must have the capacity, linearity, and output for measuring lung parameters. **Table 8-1** summarizes the ATS/ERS quality control criteria.[2] Once equipment selection has been made, a quality assurance program should be implemented to ensure that minimal ATS/ERS standards are met (**Box 8-4**). The supervising respiratory therapist is responsible for maintaining a log of staff competency, equipment performance, policies and procedures and reporting guidelines. Life-altering medical decisions are made on the basis of PFT data, and it is the responsibility of the respiratory therapist to ensure reliable results.

Pretest Procedures

To determine predicted values, first measure the patient's standing height. Height is the most important factor in determining lung size and is measured in stocking feet. For persons with spinal deformities (e.g., kyphoscoliosis), the arm span measurement from fingertip to fingertip is used to estimate what the patient's height would be without the spinal deformity. Arm span

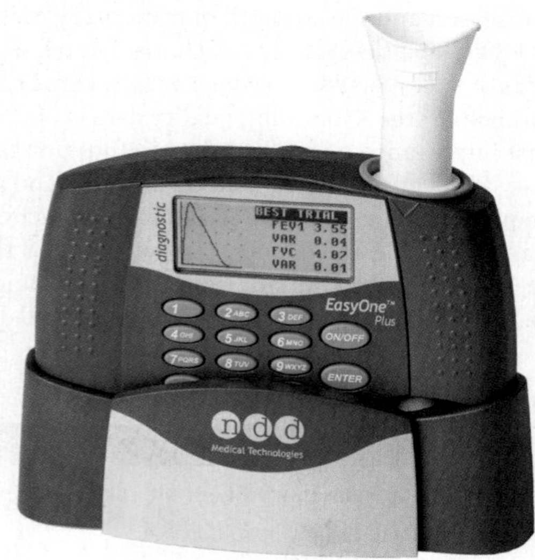

FIGURE 8-2 One of many modern models of portable spirometers. This model measures flow through the disposable white breathing tube using an ultrasonic Doppler technique.

Courtesy of ndd Medical Technologies.

BOX 8-3

Performance Standards for Spirometers

1. Volume accuracy must be within 3% (using a 3-L calibration syringe).
2. FEV_1 and FVC must be corrected to BTPS conditions.
3. A calibration check using a 3-L syringe is required daily.
4. Volumes up to 8 L and flows up to 14 L/s must be measured.
5. Both a volume–time and flow–volume curve must be printed on the report.
6. The highest FEV_1 and the highest FVC should be reported.

FEV_1, forced expiratory volume in 1 second; FVC, forced vital capacity; BTPS, body temperature and pressure saturated.

as a surrogate for standing height can also be used in chair-bound patients. Height reported by patients is unreliable. Other demographics used to predict pulmonary function include age, gender, and race or ethnicity. While weight is entered into pulmonary function systems as a demographic, predicted reference equations using weight should not be used because obese patients will have their pulmonary function overestimated and gaunt individuals will have their pulmonary function underestimated. For a given height and age, healthy males have larger lung volumes than healthy females. Lung function has been shown to differ among races and among regions. For example, the Global Lung Function Initiative 2012 predicted set offers separate equations for patients from northern and southern Asia.[10] For a given height and age, Caucasians and Latinos have larger lungs that African-American and Asian patients. Using Caucasian/Latino predicted equations in African-American and Asian patients may result in the incorrect

TABLE 8-1
Quality Control for Spirometers

Test	Minimum Interval	Action
Volume	Daily	Calibration check with a 3-L syringe
Leak	Daily	3 cm H_2O constant pressure for 1 minute
Volume linearity	Quarterly	1-L increments with a calibrating syringe
Flow linearity	Weekly	Test at least three different flow ranges
Time	Quarterly	Mechanical recorder check with stopwatch
Software	New versions	Log installation date and perform test using known subject

Note: The leak, volume linearity, and time checks only apply to volume-sensing spirometers.

Reproduced from Miller MR, Hankinson J, Brusasco V, et al. ATS/ERS Task Force: standardisation of spirometry. *Eur Respir J.* 2005;26:319–338, Table 3. Reproduced with permission of the European Respiratory Society.

BOX 8-4

Quality Assurance of Spirometry

Volume verification (calibration): at least daily prior to testing, use a calibrated known-volume syringe with a volume of at least 3 liters to ascertain that the spirometer reads a known volume accurately. The known volume should be injected and/or withdrawn at least three times, at flows that vary between 2 and 12 L/s (3-L injection times of approximately 1 second, 6 seconds, and somewhere between 1 and 6 seconds). The tolerance limits for an acceptable calibration are ±3.5% of the known volume. Thus, for a 3-L calibration syringe, the acceptable recovered range is 2.90 to 3.11 L. Practitioners should strive to exceed this guideline whenever possible (i.e., reduce the tolerance limits to less than ±3.5%).

Leak test: volume-displacement spirometers must be evaluated for leaks daily.

Manual: a spirometry procedure manual should be maintained.

Log: a log that documents daily instrument calibration, problems encountered, corrective action required, and system hardware and/or software changes should be maintained.

Calculation verifications: computer software for measurement and computer calculations should be checked against manual calculations. In addition, biologic laboratory standards (i.e., healthy, nonsmoking individuals) can be tested periodically to ensure historic reproducibility, to verify software upgrades, and to evaluate new or replacement spirometers.

Syringe verification: the known-volume syringe should be checked for accuracy at least quarterly using a second known-volume syringe.

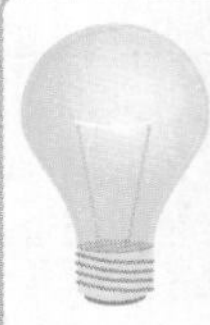

STOP AND THINK

An elderly female with kyphosis arrives for spirometry testing. Her measured height is 58 inches. All of the spirometry data is >120% of predicted. How might her kyphosis contribute to the elevated spirometry data?

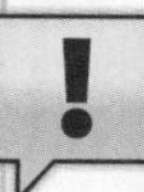

Respiratory Recap

Pretest Procedures

- Calculate reference values using age, height, gender, and race.
- Ascertain the patient's pulmonary history and the number of hours since the patient inhaled a bronchodilator.

diagnosis of lung disease and may falsely disqualify individuals from employment opportunities.

The pulmonary history should include tobacco exposure, current medications, known respiratory disease, cough, allergies, chest surgeries, and occupational exposures. The number of hours since the patient inhaled a bronchodilator should be determined and recorded. The ordering physician may ask the patient to withhold some respiratory medications before spirometry testing (**Table 8-2**).[11] Withholding respiratory medications is more important in patients if a diagnosis has not been determined. In patients with established lung disease, having the patient use the controller medications (e.g., long-acting bronchodilator) on the day of testing may give a better picture of the patient's current disease management. It is imperative for testing personnel to explain each test clearly and concisely and then to demonstrate the correct breathing maneuvers before the patient tries them.

Spirometry Tests

Most spirometers can perform three types of breathing tests: forced vital capacity (FVC), slow vital capacity (SVC), and maximal voluntary ventilation (MVV). Spirometry tests may be performed sitting or standing; however, sitting is recommended to avoid falling due to syncope. Spirometry tests are reported in liters at body temperature and pressure saturated (BTPS), which is the condition of the air in the lungs before it is exhaled and cools toward room temperature. The BTPS calculation is done by the spirometer's computer, which multiplies the measurements by a temperature correction factor (e.g., volume × 1.1 at 20° C). The validity of numeric spirometry results depends largely on the cooperation and effort of the patient. For the results to be valid, the technologist must follow the ATS/ERS guidelines for acceptability and repeatability[2] (**Figure 8-3** and **Box 8-5**).

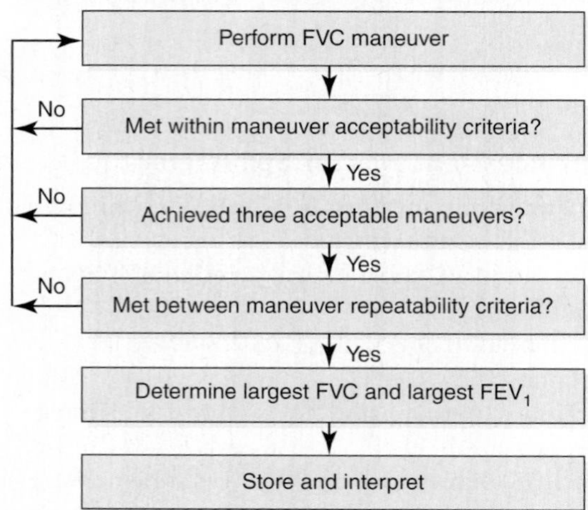

FIGURE 8-3 The American Thoracic Society's acceptability algorithm. FVC, forced vital capacity; FEV_1, forced expiratory volume in 1 second.

Reproduced from Miller MR, Hankinson J, Brusasco V, et al. ATS/ERS Task Force: standardisation of spirometry. *Eur Respir J.* 2005;26:319–338, Figure 3. Reproduced with permission of the European Respiratory Society.

TABLE 8-2
Withholding Medications Before Spirometry (Optional)

Medication	Time to Withhold
Albuterol	4 hours
Long-acting β-agonists	12 hours
Slow-release methylxanthines	24 hours
Ipratropium	4 hours
Tiotropium	24 hours
Inhaled steroids	Maintain dosage

Modified from Ruppel GL. *Manual of Pulmonary Function Testing.* 8th ed. St. Louis: Mosby; 2009:70. Reprinted with permission.

BOX 8-5

American Thoracic Society/European Respiratory Society FVC Quality Goals

Acceptability Criteria

Individual spirometry maneuvers are acceptable if they are free from all of the following conditions:

1. Slow start
2. A cough in the first second
3. Early termination
4. A Valsalva maneuver (glottis closure)
5. A leak
6. An obstructed mouthpiece
7. Evidence of an extra breath

Repeatability Criteria

The difference between the largest and the next largest FVC is 0.150 L or less

The difference between the largest and the next largest FEV_1 is 0.150 L or less

No more than eight maneuvers should be attempted

Adapted from Miller MR, Hankinson J, Brusasco V, et al. ATS/ERS Task Force: standardisation of spirometry. *Eur Respir J.* 2005;26:319–338.

Forced Vital Capacity

The most common PFT is the **forced vital capacity (FVC)** test, in which the patient exhales rapidly into the spirometer for a minimum of 6 seconds (3 seconds for children) and then inhales rapidly to measure the forced inspiratory vital capacity (FIVC). When the FIVC is measured at the end of each FVC maneuver, a flow-volume loop is produced. All FVC tests should be conducted to record a flow-volume loop. The flow-volume loop provides information about test quality and the origin of obstructive defects. Four breathing maneuvers are performed during FVC tests, as shown in **Figure 8-4**. In the first phase, a maximally deep inhalation is taken from the end of a tidal breath. Having the test configured so that several tidal breaths can be taken through the mouthpiece prior to deep inhalation may help to prevent leaks that come from having the patient attempting to coordinate insertion of the mouthpiece after full inhalation. It cannot be understated how important it is to ensure that the patient inhales completely to total lung capacity before exhaling. The second phase lasts for only a split second as the technologist coaches the patient to "blast the air out." It has been traditionally taught that the technologist needs to yell instructions at the patient; however, properly timed key phrases coupled with instructive body language are more important than the loudness of the instructions. A sharp upstroke of flow creating a spike on the flow-volume loop is evidence of adequate force. Rounded or slanted upstrokes should prompt the technologist to reemphasize the importance of blasting the air out. Another effective instruction is to explain that the air should be blasted out with the intensity of a sneeze or like a bullet exiting a gun. If a patient makes humming sounds (generated from adducting the vocal cords) during exhalation instruct the patient to avoid making noises and to blow the air from chest, not from throat.

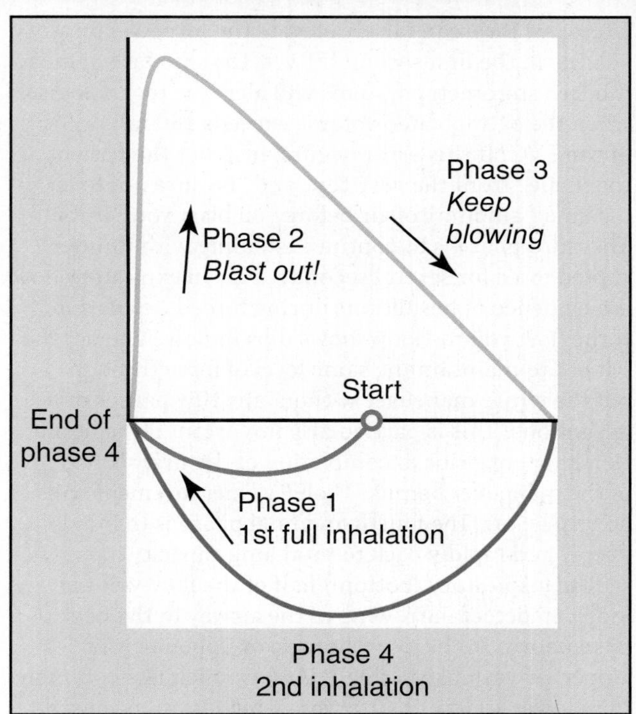

FIGURE 8-4 The forced vital capacity test consists of four breathing maneuvers performed in sequence.

Occasionally patients will inhale to total lung capacity and then let some air escape from their lungs prior to exhaling forcefully. This error is known as excessive back extrapolated volume (BEV; **Figure 8-5**).

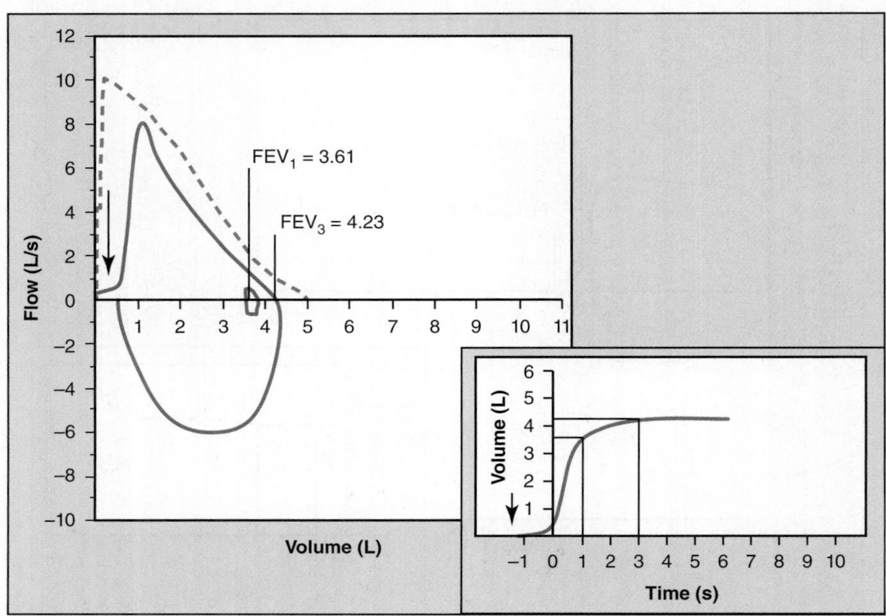

FIGURE 8-5 Excessive back extrapolated volume (BEV). The flow-volume loop shows that approximately 500 mL is allowed to leak from the lungs before forced exhalation begins. The volume-time curve shows that the beginning of the timed measurement (zero on the horizontal axis) begins more than 1 full second after exhalation started.

Excessive BEV can falsely elevate the forced expiratory volume in the first second (FEV_1). The software of most modern spirometry systems will alert the technologist when the extrapolated volume exceeds 150 mL or 5% of the FVC. If this error occurs, instruct the patient to exhale "from the very top" and "be sure not to let out small amounts of air before you blast your air out." The third phase is to continue exhaling with uninterrupted force for several seconds. Dips in expiratory flow are evidence of hesitations during forced exhalation. If the flow-volume loop shows dips in flow, instruct the patient to maintain the same level of force throughout the entire maneuver without any tiny pauses or hesitations. This is particularly important if the hesitation happens prior to completion of the first second of the maneuver because the FEV_1 measurement will be falsely low. The fourth and final phase is to inhale deeply and rapidly back to total lung capacity.

The inspiratory (bottom) half of the flow-volume loop can detect narrowing of the airway in the neck (also known as the extrathoracic or upper airway). Upper airway obstruction (UAO) is much less common than lower airway obstruction, which is often caused by asthma or COPD. If the UAO decreases flow only during forced inhalation, but not forced exhalation, as in vocal cord paralysis, it is categorized as a variable lesion. If the flow is decreased equally during inspiration and expiration, the lesion is considered fixed, as in tracheal stenosis (**Figure 8-6**). Forced inspiratory flows (FIFs) depend greatly on inspiratory effort, which can be influenced by enthusiastic coaching from the technologist. False-positive interpretations of UAO due to submaximal inspiratory efforts are unfortunately very common, so the technologist must strive to obtain maximal inspiratory efforts with repeatable forced inspiratory flows and volumes. The forced expiratory flow at 50% of the FVC to forced inspiratory flow at the FIVC ratio (FEF_{50}/FIF_{50}) can be calculated by most spirometers. The FEF_{50}/FIF_{50} ratio is normally about 1.0 and increases with variable extra-thoracic UAO (**Figure 8-7**). However, the upper limit of the normal range (ULN) for this ratio is poorly established, and may remain normal with fixed UAO, and is normal when both upper and lower airway obstruction exist,

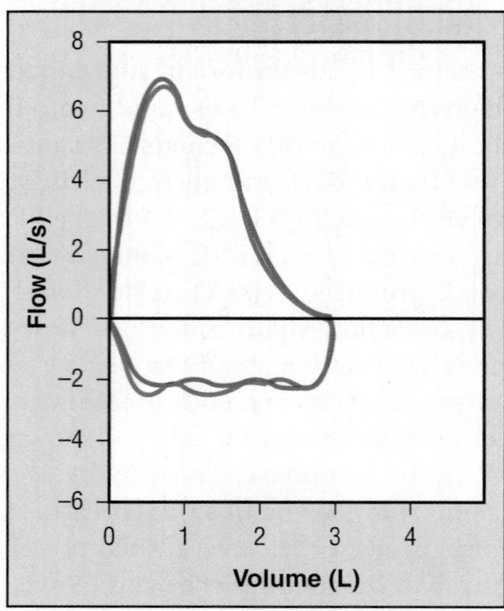

FIGURE 8-7 Consistently low inspiratory flows are compatible with a variable extrathoracic obstruction.

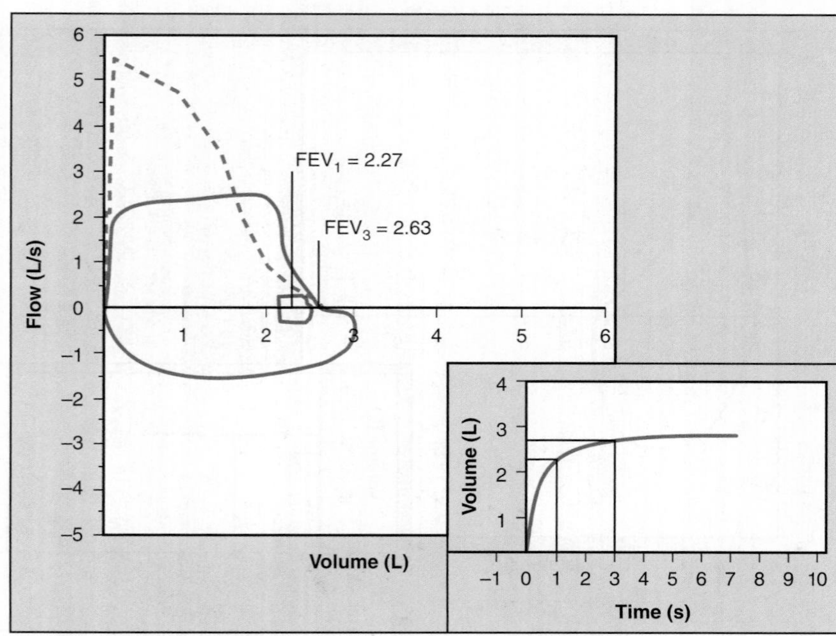

FIGURE 8-6 A flow-volume loop and volume-time curve recorded from a patient with tracheal stenosis. Note that both the expiratory and inspiratory flows are depressed.

such as in patients with asthma who also have vocal cord paralysis. Therefore, the pattern of repeatable flat inspiratory loops is the best method of reliably detecting UAO.

A very important quality indicator is to identify when a patient inhales deeper on the FIVC maneuver than the starting point of the expiratory maneuver. If the FIVC exceeds the FVC, the effort should be discarded and the patient should be instructed to be sure to inhale completely prior to exhalation. The FIVC > FVC error can also be the fault of the technologist if the order to "blast the air out" is premature, before the patient has completed full inhalation (**Figure 8-8**).

The most important values produced from a forced spirometry test are the FVC, FEV_1, and the ratio of FEV_1/FVC. The FVC is the total amount of air that can be rapidly exhaled from total lung capacity for a minimum of 6 seconds; however, most adult patients are coached to exhale for several more seconds. FEV_6 has been introduced as an acceptable replacement for FVC that avoids prolonged expiratory efforts.[12] The FEV_1 is the volume of air that is exhaled after 1 second of the FVC maneuver. Both FVC and FEV_1 can be reduced by obstructive and restrictive ventilator defects. The FEV_1/FVC ratio helps to distinguish between obstructive and restrictive ventilator defects. In the normal adult, this ratio ranges from 0.75 to 0.85; after age 30, this ratio begins to decline (**Figure 8-9**). An obstructive ventilator defect is defined as an FEV_1/FVC ratio below the lower limit of normal (LLN).[5,13–17]

In most cases a normal FEV_1/FVC ratio in the presence of reduced FVC and FEV_1 indicates a restrictive lung disease; however, this pattern can also accompany obstructive lung disease with severe air trapping. The so-called nonspecific pattern is characterized by reduced FVC and FEV_1 coupled with a normal FEV_1/FVC ratio and total lung capacity.[18] The nonspecific pattern is associated with airway hyperresponsiveness. Measurement of the total lung capacity may be necessary to confirm the presence of restrictive lung disease. The peak expiratory flow is the maximum flow rate attained during an FVC maneuver and usually is reported in liters per second. Peak expiratory flow can also be easily measured with disposable, handheld devices; however, these devices report PEF in liters per minute. Although the PEF measurement is very effort dependent, it can be used as an indicator of airway obstruction. For this reason it can be useful in home monitoring of patients with asthma. Home monitoring of PEF or FEV_1 can be used to evaluate the effectiveness of bronchodilator therapy and detect emerging exacerbations of the disease. Other parameters, such as various forced expiratory flow (FEF) measures (e.g., $FEF_{25-75\%}$, FEF_{50}, FEF_{75}) may be depressed in obstructive diseases but do not generally provide clinically important information (**Figure 8-10**).

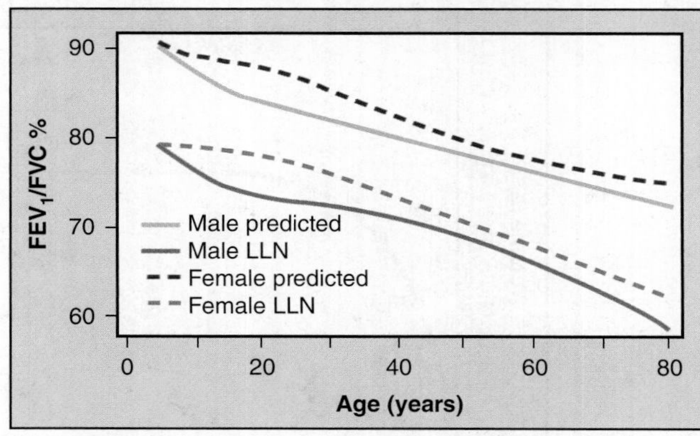

FIGURE 8-9 The lower limit of the normal (LLN) for FEV_1/FVC declines with age; therefore, a fixed LLN should not be used to define airway obstruction.

Adapted from Stanojevic S, et al. Reference ranges for spirometry across all ages: a new approach. *Am J Respir Crit Care Med.* 2008;177(3):253–260. Courtesy of Sanja Stanojevic.

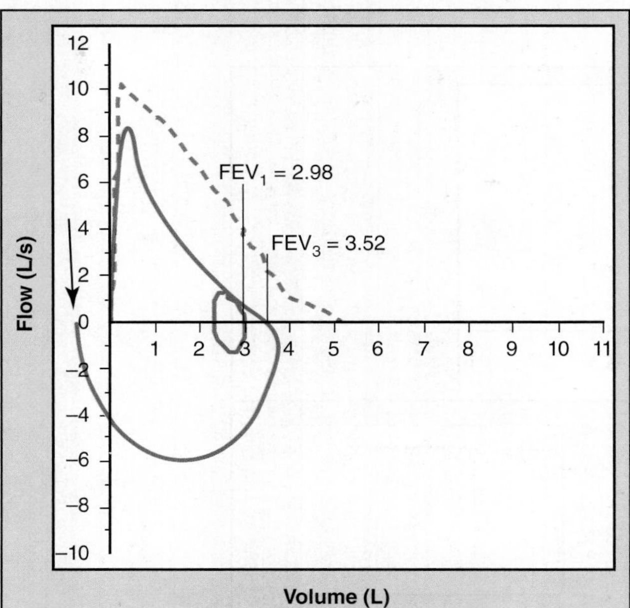

FIGURE 8-8 An example of the inspiratory loop exceeding the starting point of the forced expiratory maneuver (arrow). This indicates that the patient did not fully inhale prior to forced exhalation.

Flow-Volume Loops and Volume-Time Graphs

The examination of flow-volume loops and volume-time graphs are invaluable for both the assessment of test

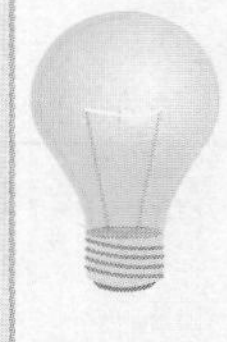

STOP AND THINK

A 20-year-old male has a normal FVC and FEV_1; however, his MVV is 65% of predicted and his FEF_{50}/FIF_{50} is 3.2. What kind of abnormality might be present?

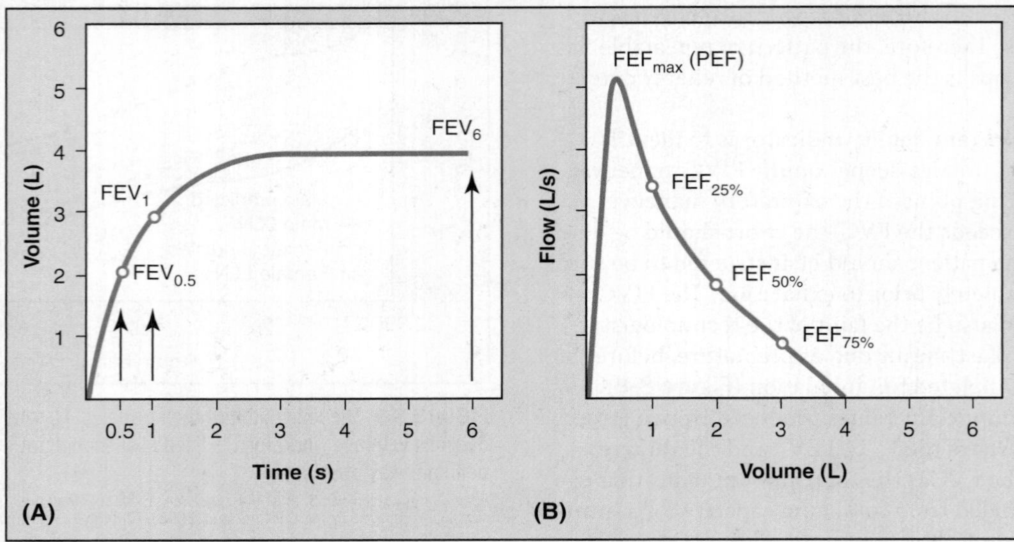

FIGURE 8-10 The volume-time curve (**A**) and the flow-volume curve (**B**). $FEF_{25\%}$, $FEF_{50\%}$, and $FEF_{75\%}$ are the forced expiratory flows after 25%, 50%, and 75% of the forced vital capacity have been exhaled.

quality and the interpretation of the completed test. The flow-volume loop plots the change in breathed volume on the abscissa (horizontal axis) and the flow on the ordinate (vertical axis). The data points above the baseline are from exhalation, while all data points below baseline are generated from inspiration. The volume-time graph plots the change in breathed volume on the ordinate against time in seconds on the abscissa.

The flow-volume loop from a healthy person shows high inspiratory and expiratory flows resembling a sail (**Figure 8-11**). Nonuniform emptying of airways from obstructive airway disease is reflected by a concave downward slope of the flow-volume loop, resembling an ocean wave or the letter "L" in severe cases (dynamic airway collapse) (**Figure 8-12**). The flow-volume loop in patients with restrictive lung disease shows high flows and a rapid emptying of the vital capacity resembling an upside-down ice cream cone (**Figure 8-13**).

The most common causes of airway obstruction are asthma (in patients of any age) and COPD in smokers over age 40 years. If a patient has asthma-like symptoms and demonstrates airway obstruction on spirometry which becomes normal after bronchodilator (post-BD), an asthma diagnosis is likely correct.

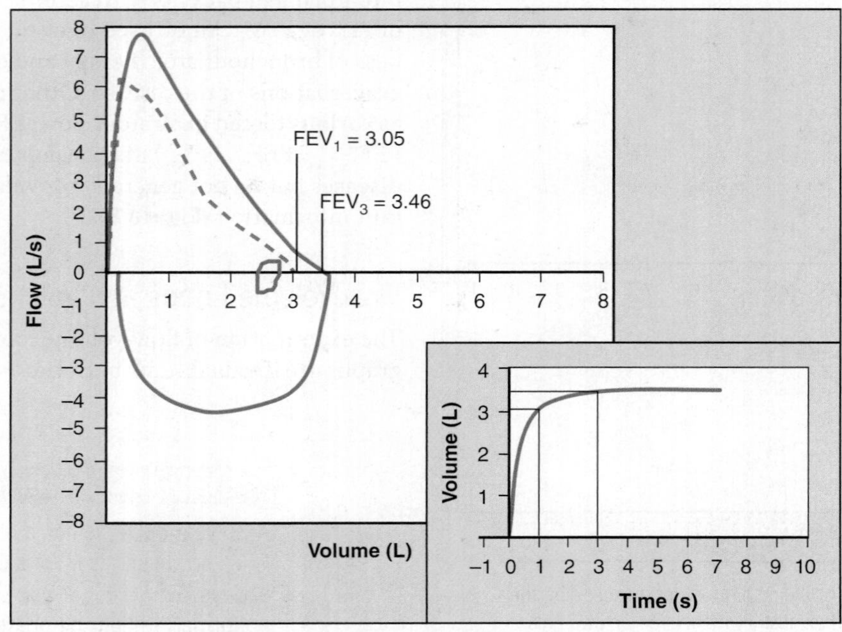

FIGURE 8-11 A flow-volume loop and volume-time curve from a patient with normal pulmonary function.

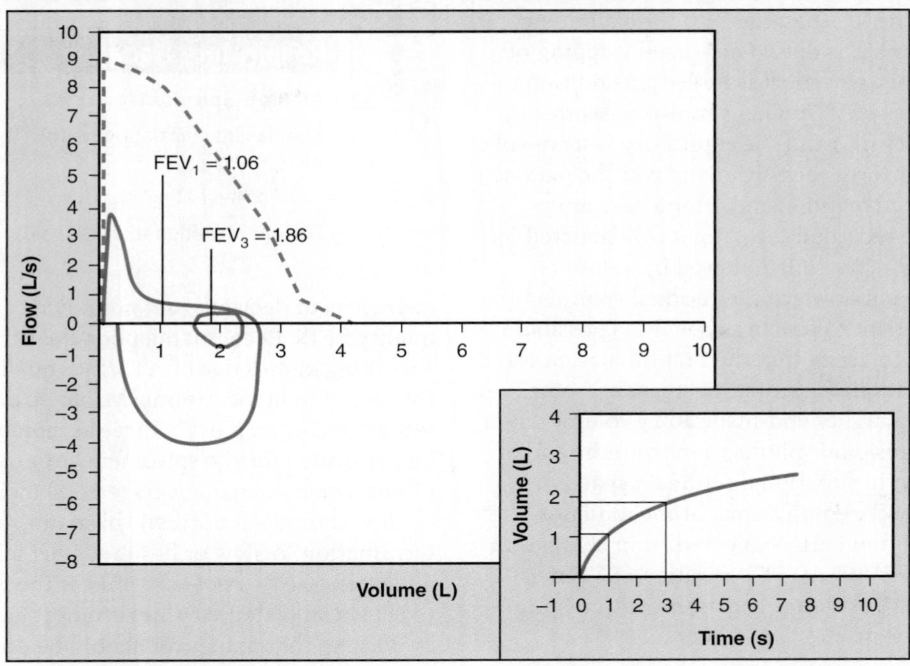

FIGURE 8-12 A flow-volume loop and volume-time curve from a patient with severe emphysema (obstruction).

Respiratory Recap

Spirometry Technique

- The FVC maneuver is the most basic and commonly performed PFT.
- Skilled instruction, coaching, and feedback are needed to avoid errors.
- Technologists must be able to identify technically unacceptable maneuvers.

Pre- and post-BD spirometry can thus be very helpful clinically to confirm asthma. Because asthma is episodic, however, the patient who is currently not experiencing respiratory symptoms may have normal spirometry.

Slow Vital Capacity

Vital capacity measured without a forced effort is called the slow vital capacity (SVC). In many patients with airflow limitation, the SVC provides a larger, more accurate

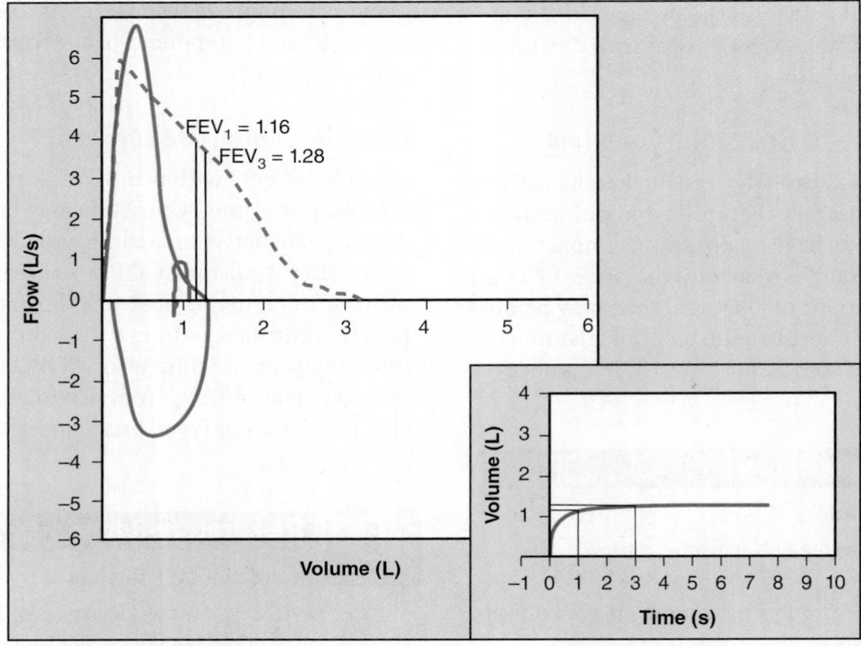

FIGURE 8-13 A flow-volume loop and volume-time curve from a patient with severe pulmonary fibrosis (restriction).

determination of the VC than the FVC. The difference between SVC and FVC is due to increased trapping of air in the lungs when the effort is forced. In addition to the vital capacity, the SVC maneuver also measures the inspiratory capacity (IC) and the expiratory reserve volume (ERV).[2] To perform the SVC maneuver the patient breathes in a relaxed manner, and after a minimum of four breaths are recorded the patient is instructed to inhale as deeply as possible followed by a slow and steady exhalation down to the residual volume. Instructing the patient to inhale as deeply as possible a second time helps to verify that the first inhalation was in fact a full inhalation. For unknown reasons, some patients inhale to a higher end-inspiratory volume when starting from the residual volume than from the end of a tidal volume breath (functional residual capacity).[19] In patients with severe emphysema, bronchodilator responsiveness is often better reflected from changes in SVC and IC than FEV_1.[20] A 15% decrease in SVC measured in the supine position is consistent with respiratory muscle weakness.

Maximum Voluntary Ventilation

The maximum voluntary ventilation (MVV) is the largest volume that a patient can move in and out of his or her lungs during a 12-second interval (expressed in L-min).[2] Patients are instructed to breathe as rapidly and deeply as possible. The recommended breathing frequency during MVV is 90 breaths per minute. Breath volumes should meet or exceed 50% of the patient's best FVC. Two acceptable efforts should be recorded and the variability should not exceed 20%. A low MVV can occur in obstructive, restrictive, or neuromuscular disorders. MVV is performed less frequently than in the past; however, a reduced MVV can present as an isolated defect (in the presence of a normal FVC test) in disorders such a vocal cord dysfunction and tracheal stenosis.

Quality Assurance of Spirometry Testing

Quality assurance of spirometry testing begins with the technologist.[6,7] Respiratory therapists and pulmonary function technologists have an enormous impact on the quality of PFTs.[6–9] Many physicians who order PFTs are unable to recognize poor quality, and thus may be misled by inaccurate PFT results. The technologist must be extremely vigilant so that false-positive diagnoses or treatment decisions are not made based upon poor-quality PFTs. Recognizing poor-quality tests requires a working knowledge of ATS/ERS quality criteria and the ability to identify nonphysiologic data patterns and test errors on graphics.[2] Three acceptable efforts must be performed for the spirometry test to be valid. Types of unacceptable maneuvers (errors) include a delayed or slow start, a suboptimal "blast out" effort, and early termination. A slow or hesitant start leaks volume and alters the start-of-test time. If the volume leaked (back extrapolated volume) is more than 5% of the FVC or 0.150 L, that maneuver should be discarded and repeated. Newer computerized equipment automatically provides an error message so that the therapist can coach the patient appropriately.[6]

Spirometry errors are correctable in 90% of patients, even preschool children and elderly patients, with good demonstrations, enthusiastic coaching, and patience. Most patients are extremely cooperative and provide excellent tests with the proper instruction and coaching. About 10% of patients have difficulties with the maneuvers, however. Many modern spirometry systems include software that alerts the technologist to maneuver errors; but the technologist must also learn how to recognize and correct these errors. Monitoring of technologist performance and providing feedback on ways to improve test quality is a very effective albeit underutilized component of a spirometry quality assurance program.[6,8,9]

Respiratory Recap

FEV_1/FVC Ratio

- A ratio below the LLN indicates airflow obstruction.
- A reduced FVC with a normal ratio is suggestive of restriction.

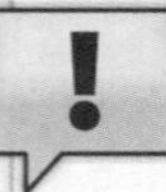

Respiratory Recap

Common Spirometry Errors

- Submaximal inhalation (before the forced exhalation)
- Slow or hesitating start
- Early termination (before 6 seconds in adults)

Bronchodilator Testing

In adult patients with pre-BD airway obstruction, repeating spirometry post-BD may help clinicians to differentiate between asthma and COPD. If post-BD spirometry is normal, COPD is ruled out. If airway obstruction remains post-BD, the patient may have poorly controlled asthma (with considerable airway inflammation and mucus) or COPD. The amount of improvement in FEV_1 from pre-BD to post-BD spirometry is representative of bronchodilator responsiveness,

Respiratory Recap

Bronchodilator Response

- A 12% increase (minimum 200 mL) in FEV_1 or FVC is considered significant.

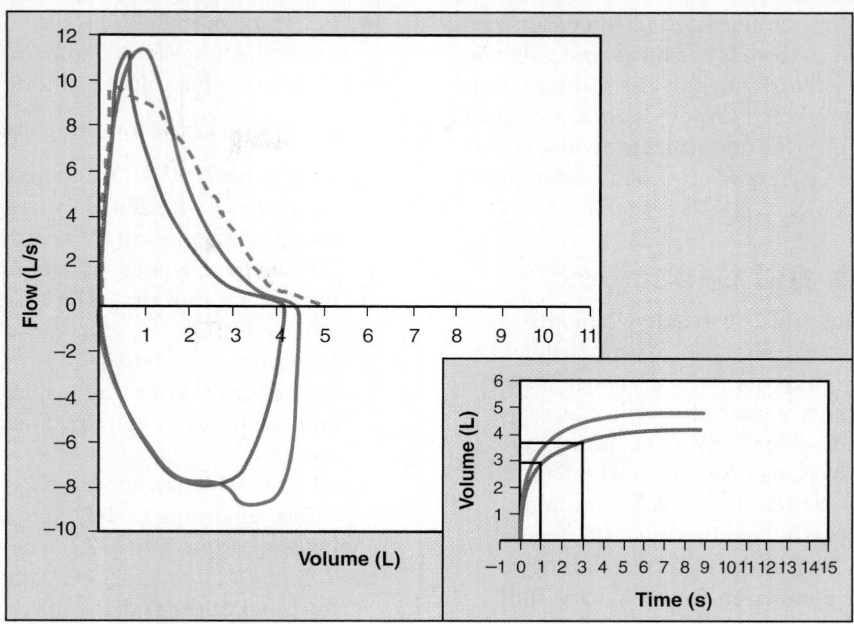

FIGURE 8-14 Prebronchodilator (green) and postbronchodilator (red) flow-volume loops and volume-time curves showing a significant bronchodilator response.

and an increase of 12% (minimum 200 mL) or more is considered significant. Many patients with either asthma or COPD have larger (>20%) changes in post-BD values, however (**Figure 8-14**).

To perform bronchodilator testing, follow good-quality pre-BD spirometry with the administration of albuterol via metered dose inhaler (MDI) with a spacer or small volume nebulizer. A waiting period of 10 to 15 minutes must be observed before repeating spirometry (post-BD). In patients with COPD, a combination of albuterol and a short-acting anticholinergic bronchodilator (ipratropium) may be administered; however, a longer waiting period may be necessary before repeating spirometry (to allow the slower onset of ipratropium to take effect). The technologist should monitor the patient for side effects associated with albuterol (e.g., tremor, nervousness, tachycardia) that may be unpleasant for the patient.

Spirometry Interpretation

The assessment and monitoring of restrictive and obstructive lung diseases always start with spirometry results. A low FEV_1/FVC indicates airway obstruction. A low FVC with a normal FEV_1/FVC suggests spirometric restriction. The percent predicted FEV_1 is usually used to grade the severity of impairment, although the thresholds are arbitrary (**Table 8-3**). Regardless of the type of lung disease causing the impairment, and regardless of the adult patient's age, height, and sex, it is difficult for patients to survive with an FEV_1 below 0.5 L.

Because lung function increases with height and decreases after about age 25 years, even in healthy people, interpretation of PFTs requires comparisons with reference equations derived from population-based samples of healthy people. The threshold between normal and abnormal spirometry results (the lower limit of the normal or LLN) has been traditionally determined by the fifth percentile for each key variable.[5] In other words only 5% of healthy people have values below these fifth percentiles. The LLN should be used to classify data as normal or abnormal. Classifying data based on the "80% of predicted rule" (80% of predicted is the LLN) is statistically invalid and should be abandoned. For example, healthy preschool children and elderly adults have more variability in their normal ranges, so their LLNs can be above or below the 80% of predicted value, respectively.[14] More recently the Lambda Mu Sigma (LMS) method has been applied to spirometry data.[15–17] The LMS method accounts for the skewness of data instead of assuming perfect bell curve distribution (lambda), uses the median of the sample (mu), and incorporates the variance of the data (sigma). This variability

TABLE 8-3
Categorizing the Severity of Impairment Using the FEV_1

FEV_1	Severity
<LLN to 65% predicted	Mild
50% to 65% predicted	Moderate
35% to 50% predicted	Severe
<35% predicted	Very severe

FEV_1, forced expiratory volume in 1 second; LLN, lower limit of the normal range.

may be expressed using standardized residuals (also known as Z scores). A Z score is the measured value minus the predicted value divided by the residual standard deviation. The predicted Z score is zero, a Z score of −1.64 is the LLN (only 5% of normal individuals have a Z score < −1.64), and a Z score of +1.64 is the upper limit of normal (ULN).

Lung Volumes and Capacities

Spirometry testing identifies obstructive lung disease but is only *suggestive* of restrictive impairments. Spirometry is limited in its ability to diagnose restrictive lung disease because a restrictive spirometry pattern (low FVC and normal FEV_1/FVC ratio) can accompany obstructive lung diseases in which the total lung capacity is greater than the LLN. Accordingly, some disorders require the measurement of lung volumes and capacities.[3,21] The classic model of lung volumes and capacities is shown in **Figure 8-15**. A **lung capacity** is two or more **lung volumes**. The four subdivisions that provide the most useful information are the vital capacity, **total lung capacity**, functional residual capacity, and residual volume. A description of the four lung volumes follows:

- *Tidal volume* (V_T) is the volume of gas inhaled or exhaled during normal breathing.
- *Inspiratory reserve volume* (IRV) is the maximum volume of gas that can be inspired from the end of a normal inspiration.
- *Expiratory reserve volume* (ERV) is the maximum volume of gas that can be expired from the end of a resting expiration.
- *Residual volume* (RV) is the volume of gas remaining in the lungs after a maximal expiration. By definition, this volume cannot be exhaled.

A description of the four lung capacities follows:

- *Vital capacity* (VC) is the maximum volume of gas that can be exhaled from the lungs after a maximal inspiration (expiratory vital capacity) or inhaled from a point of maximal exhalation (inspiratory vital capacity). The VC includes the V_T, IRV, and ERV.
- *Inspiratory capacity* (IC) is the maximum volume of gas that can be inspired from the normal end-expiratory position. The IC is the sum of V_T and IRV.
- *Functional residual capacity* (FRC) is the volume of gas remaining in the lungs at the end of a resting expiration. The FRC is the sum of RV and ERV.
- *Total lung capacity* (TLC) is the volume of gas in the lungs at the end of a maximal inspiration and the total volume of air in the lungs seen on most chest radiographs and lung computed tomography (CT) scans.

Measurement of Lung Volumes

Although IC and ERV can be measured with a spirometer during a slow VC maneuver, FRC must be measured separately, using more sophisticated instruments. In PFT labs, the FRC is measured using **nitrogen washout**, **helium dilution**, or **body plethysmography**. Subtracting the ERV from the FRC determines the RV (FRC − ERV = RV). Once the RV is known the TLC can be calculated by simply adding the VC (RV + VC = TLC).

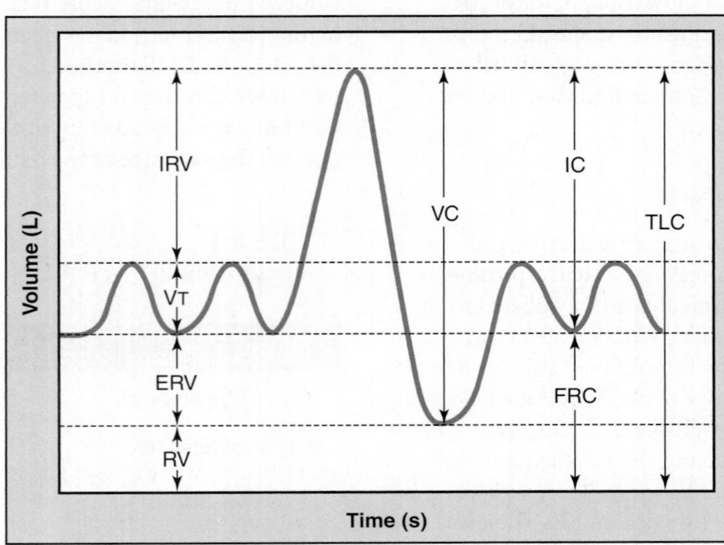

FIGURE 8-15 The volumes and capacities of the lungs. IRV, inspiratory reserve volume; V_T, tidal volume; ERV, expiratory reserve volume; RV, residual volume; VC, vital capacity; IC, inspiratory capacity; FRC, functional residual capacity; TLC, total lung capacity.

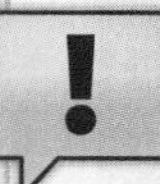

Respiratory Recap

Lung Volumes and Capacities

- *Lung volumes:* tidal volume, inspiratory reserve volume, expiratory reserve volume, residual volume
- *Lung capacities:* vital capacity, inspiratory capacity, functional residual capacity, total lung capacity

Lung volumes can also be determined accurately from lung CT scans; however, this is rarely done due to cost and the need to avoid radiation exposure. **Box 8-6** lists clinical indications for lung volume tests.

Nitrogen Washout Test

The nitrogen washout test calculates the unknown FRC by measuring the volume of nitrogen the patient exhales during several minutes of breathing 100% oxygen. Before starting the test the FRC *volume* is unknown; however, the nitrogen concentration is known to be around 79% when breathing room air. Therefore, by measuring the *volume* of nitrogen gas that is exhaled, the *volume* of FRC can be estimated. So, if the patient has a large FRC, he or she should be expected to exhale a large volume of nitrogen gas, and if the patient has a small FRC, he or she should be expected to exhale a smaller volume of nitrogen gas. To perform a nitrogen washout the subject wears nose clips and breathes through a flanged rubber mouthpiece connected to a pneumotach (to measure exhaled volume), which contains a port from which gas can be sampled to measure the nitrogen concentration. The nitrogen concentration is either measured directly by a nitrogen analyzer or indirectly by measuring the oxygen and carbon dioxide concentrations and subtracting their sum from 100% ($N_2\% + O_2\% + CO_2\% \cong 100\%$). The patient breathes a minimum of four tidal breaths to establish that the exhaled tidal volumes end near FRC, then the patient is switched from breathing room air (79% N_2, 21% O_2) to 100% oxygen. Remember that the nitrogen washout is an attempt to measure the volume of nitrogen in the patient's FRC; by having the patient inhale 100% O_2 (0% N_2) no additional nitrogen volume is added to the patient's lungs. This is called an *open-circuit method* because rebreathing of N_2 cannot be allowed. For this reason it is absolutely critical that no leaks from the mouthpiece, nasal passages, or system exist because nitrogen in the room air will contaminate the sample. An increase in exhaled N_2 during a washout is indicative of a leak. Watch the patient carefully to ensure that he or she does not create leaks by opening the mouth. On rare occasions a ruptured eardrum can introduce a leak large enough to affect the accuracy of this test. If the patient has a ruptured eardrum, a foam earplug can be used to create a seal. As the N_2 washout progresses exhaled tidal volumes are measured (patients are allowed to sigh) until the exhaled nitrogen concentration falls below 1.5% for three consecutive breaths. A nitrogen washout can typically be completed in less than 5 minutes, but the procedure should be terminated after 7 minutes. Once the washout of nitrogen gas is complete the FRC can be calculated from a formula (**Equation 8-1**). This method can underestimate the FRC of patients with airway obstruction because poorly communicating lung regions may not fully wash out their nitrogen volume.

BOX 8-6

Indications for Lung Volume Measurements

In patients with airway obstruction and a low FVC, to determine whether a superimposed restrictive process exists (low TLC)

In patients with a low FVC, but without airway obstruction on spirometry, to determine whether the low FVC is due to a nonspecific abnormality (normal TLC) or a classic restriction of lung volumes (low TLC)

In patients with airway obstruction, to determine the presence and severity of hyperinflation (a high TLC) or to measure the trapped air volume (high RV/TLC)

To correct airway resistance measurements for the lung volume at which airway resistance was measured (usually FRC)

To measure FRC in infants and preschool children who cannot perform spirometry

FVC, forced vital capacity; TLC, total lung capacity; RV, residual volume; FRC, functional residual capacity.

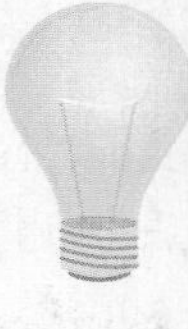

STOP AND THINK

A 15-year-old male is undergoing a nitrogen washout test. After 7 minutes of testing the exhaled nitrogen concentration is 12%. What is the most likely cause of this circumstance?

An increasingly popular test from multiple breath washout testing is the lung clearance index (LCI). The LCI measures the heterogeneity of peripheral airflow that many times cannot be detected by standard spirometry. The patient either performs a standard nitrogen washout or a washout including a small amount of inert gas (e.g., sulfur hexafluoride, helium).[22] LCI is the number of times the FRC needs to be removed (total expired volume/FRC) to reduce the tracer gas or nitrogen concentration in the lungs to 2.5% (often expressed as 1/40) of its initial concentration. More ventilation in relation to the FRC will be required to clear alveolar gas when peripheral airway disease is present. LCI is

EQUATION 8-1

Nitrogen Washout Technique

FRC is calculated from a formula as follows:

$$FRC = \frac{\text{Exhaled } N_2 \text{ volume}}{FeN_2 - FeN_2\text{end}}$$

where

FRC = Unknown functional residual capacity volume

FeN_2 = Fraction of exhaled nitrogen from the FRC at the beginning of the procedure (~ 79%)

Exhaled N_2 volume = The total exhaled nitrogen volume during the washout

FeN_2end = Fraction of nitrogen at the end of the washout

Corrections for nitrogen washed out from tissues are also made based on the patient's body surface area and are subtracted from the exhaled N_2 volume.

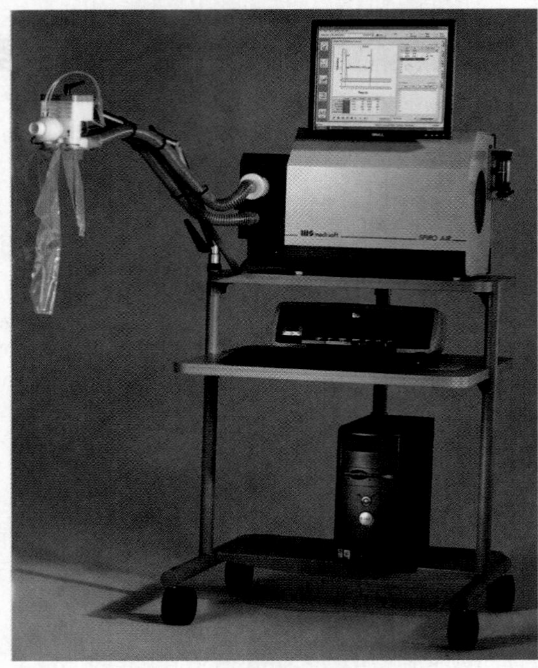

FIGURE 8-16 An instrument used to measure functional residual capacity using the helium dilution technique.
Courtesy of Morgan Scientific, Inc.

proving to be superior to spirometry in the detection of early airway dysfunction in cystic fibrosis.[23]

Helium Dilution Test

As an inert gas, helium can be rebreathed in and out of the lungs without diffusion into the circulatory system. The helium dilution test calculates the unknown FRC by measuring the dilution of helium into the FRC. To perform a helium dilution test the seated patient wears nose clips and breathes through a flanged rubber mouthpiece connected to the spirometer circuit. At the start of the helium dilution test the patient breathes room air for a minimum of four tidal breaths to establish that exhaled tidal volumes end near FRC. The patient is then switched from breathing room air (0% helium) to a volume spirometer system of known volume containing approximately 10% helium (**Figure 8-16** and **Equation 8-2**). This is called a *closed-circuit method* because rebreathing of the helium mixture is necessary. A gas analyzer measures the helium concentration, but the gas doesn't leave the system. Minerals such as sodium or barium hydroxide absorb CO_2 to prevent hypercapnia. The by-product of CO_2 absorption is water vapor, which is then absorbed by desiccant mineral such as calcium sulfate. Failure to remove the water vapor can affect the function of the

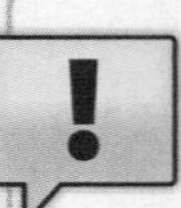

Respiratory Recap

Lung Volume Tests

- Nitrogen washout
- Helium dilution
- Body plethysmography

EQUATION 8-2

Helium Dilution Technique

FRC is calculated from a formula as follows:

$$FRC = \frac{\text{System volume}(F_{He} - F_{He}\text{ end})}{F_{He}\text{ end}}$$

where

FRC = Unknown functional residual capacity volume

System volume = Total spirometer system volume

F_{He} = Fraction of helium in the spirometer system at the beginning of the procedure (~10%)

F_{He} end = Fraction of helium when equilibration between the patient and spirometer system is achieved

gas analyzer. Care must be given to make sure that the gas is passing through mineral chambers in the correct direction. These minerals will change color when they are exhausted, indicating that they should be changed.

As the patient rebreathes through the system, the 10% helium concentration in the spirometer steadily declines from dilution with the patient's FRC (initially 0% helium). The procedure is stopped when the helium concentration in the system (patient and spirometer) reaches equilibration. For example, after several minutes of breathing, the helium concentration steadily declines from 10% and reaches equilibration (plateau) between a normal patient and spirometer at 7%. So if a similar patient has a larger FRC, helium equilibration can be expected to occur at a lower helium concentration (e.g., 6%), and if a similar patient has a smaller FRC, helium equilibration can be expected to occur at a higher helium concentration (e.g., 8%). The larger the patient's FRC volume, the more dilution will occur and vice versa. Moreover, the rate of fall in He concentration (time to equilibrium) is fairly rapid in patients with healthy lungs, but slow in patients with airway obstruction.

As with the nitrogen washout test, it is absolutely critical that no leaks from the mouthpiece, nasal passages, or system exist. On rare occasions a ruptured eardrum can introduce a leak large enough to affect the accuracy of this test. If the patient has a ruptured eardrum, a foam earplug can be used to create a seal. Very rapid declines in helium concentration and failure to reach helium equilibration are indicative of a leak. Any leaks occurring during the procedure will give a falsely high FRC. This method may also underestimate the FRC of patients with airway obstruction because poorly communicating lung regions may not participate in the dilution of helium.

The accuracy of the gas analyzers used for the nitrogen washout or helium dilution tests should be verified at least daily, using a two-point calibration. The first point is zero concentration of the gas, and the second point or span is the concentration of the test gas at the high end of the expected range (e.g., 10% for helium).

Body Plethysmography Test

The measurement of FRC via body plethysmography is performed using a large airtight cabin or body box. The patient sits in the box until the temperature is stable then breathes quietly through a mouthpiece while wearing nose clips and holding their cheeks with their hands (**Figure 8-17**). This method seeks to plot changes in alveolar pressure (mouth pressure) against changes in lung volume (box pressure). Box pressure is representative of lung volume because of a calibration factor. During a body box calibration a small piston repetitively injects and removes small amounts of air in and out of the sealed cabin while measuring the pressure changes associated with the piston action.

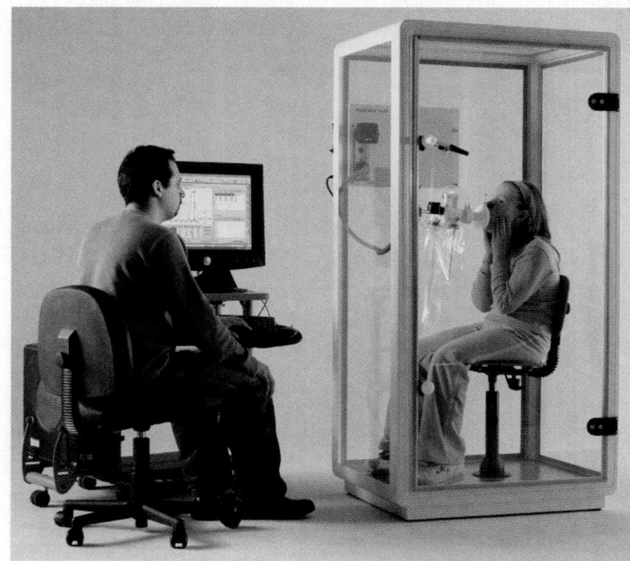

FIGURE 8-17 A body box used to measure static lung volumes and airway resistance. Patients sit on the chair and breathe quietly through the white mouthpiece. Mouth pressure is measured when a shutter in the mouthpiece assembly is closed.
Courtesy of Morgan Scientific, Inc.

Simply stated, if a 50 mL injection of air increases the box pressure by 2 cm H_2O, a 4 cm H_2O increase in box pressure created by a patient's inhalation would represent a 100 mL increase in lung volume. After a minimum of four tidal breaths to establish that the exhaled tidal volumes end near FRC, the patient is instructed to gently pant at a rate of 1 breath per second. Shortly after the panting begins a shutter is closed beyond the mouthpiece, which traps the near-FRC volume (thoracic gas volume or V_{TG}) in the patient's lungs. The patient continues to pant gently, which repeatedly compresses the V_{TG} during exhalation and decompresses the V_{TG} during inhalation. This is the key measurement: gentle inhalation reduces mouth (alveolar) pressure while increasing box pressure (lung volume); gentle exhalation increases mouth (alveolar) pressure while decreasing box pressure (lung volume). The changes in mouth (alveolar) pressure are plotted against the changes in box pressure (lung volume) creating a slope (**Figure 8-18**). A numerical value (tangent) representing the angle of the slope is used to calculate the volume of gas that was just compressed and decompressed. A 45-degree angle has a tangent value of 1 because the rise and the run are equal, whereas a 30-degree angle has a tangent value of 0.58 (rise < run) and a 60-degree angle has a tangent value of 1.7 (rise > run). See **Equation 8-3**.

The V_{TG} calculation is based on Boyle's law, which states that the pressure of a fixed mass of gas is inversely proportional to its volume when temperature is constant. The product of pressure and volume for a fixed mass of gas will always be the same. Compression of a small V_{TG} generates larger proportional changes in pressure compared to comparable compression of a larger V_{TG}.

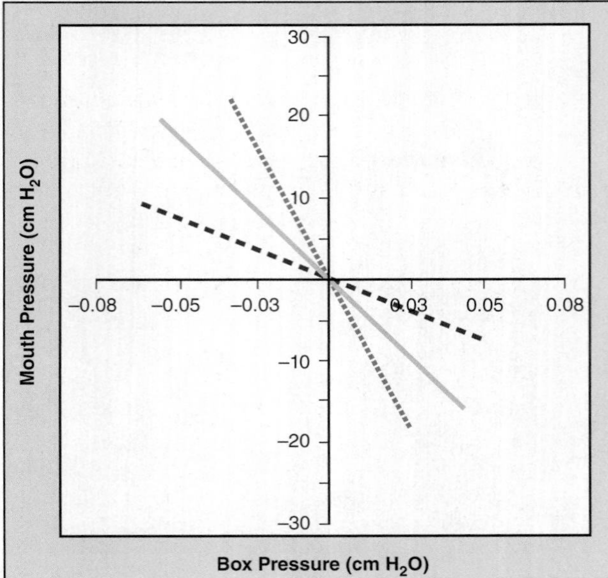

FIGURE 8-18 Thoracic gas volume measurement via body plethysmography. Box pressure (lung volume) is plotted against mouth (alveolar) pressure. The solid line slope represents normal lung volume. If the lung volume increased (e.g., emphysema), the slope would shift to a more horizontal angle (dashed line). If the lung volume decreased (e.g., fibrosis), the slope would shift to a more vertical angle (dotted line).

Accordingly, if the patient has a small FRC due to pulmonary fibrosis, expect to see large changes in mouth (alveolar) pressure when plotted against box pressure (lung volume). This relationship has a more vertical slope (e.g., 60-degree angle, tangent 1.7). If the patient has a large FRC due to emphysema, expect to see small changes in mouth (alveolar) pressure when plotted against box pressure (lung volume). This relationship is represented by a more horizontal slope (e.g., 30-degree angle, tangent 0.58; Figure 8-18).

One advantage of the body box technique is its speed. Several minutes are required to measure FRC once by helium dilution or nitrogen washout where FRC can be determined multiple times within 5 minutes by body plethysmography. Repeating a helium dilution or nitrogen washout test requires a minimum waiting period of 5 and 15 minutes between trials, respectively. In addition, the gas dilution methods measure only communicating gas spaces, whereas body plethysmography measures all gas spaces, regardless of whether they are communicating (e.g., bullae). The difference in the FRC measured by these two techniques is the trapped air volume, which can be significant in patients with airway obstruction.

To ensure instrument accuracy, three signals must be checked daily: mouth pressure, using a manometer; mouth flow and volume, using a 3-L calibration syringe; change in box pressure, using the small piston pump described earlier. Biological controls should be tested on a regular basis (e.g., bimonthly) and recorded in a Levey-Jennings plot. If the biological controls fall outside two standard deviations of the mean, corrective action should be taken. Weekly checks using an isothermal lung are also recommended but aren't widely used due to cost.

EQUATION 8-3

Thoracic Gas Volume (V_{TG}) via Body Plethysmography

V_{TG} is calculated from a formula as follows:

$$V_{TG} = P_B \times \frac{1}{m} \times \frac{\text{Box pressure calibration (mL/cm)}}{\text{Mouth pressure calibration (cm } H_2O\text{/cm)}} \times K$$

where

V_{TG} = unknown thoracic P_B gas volume

P_B = barometric pressure

m = the slope (tangent) of mouth (alveolar) pressure versus box pressure (lung volume)

K = correction factor for the patient's total body volume in the body box

Interpretation of Lung Volumes

Measured static lung volumes and capacities are evaluated in comparison with predicted values. Prediction equations are calculated from height, age, and gender. Lung volumes and capacities should be above the LLN and below the ULN to be considered "normal." When the TLC is below the LLN, a restrictive lung volumes disease may be present, and if the TLC is above the ULN, hyperinflation from obstructive lung disease may be present. A measure of air trapping is an RV/TLC ratio (typically ~25%) above the ULN (**Figure 8-19**). A low ERV is commonly seen in overweight patients. As with spirometry interpretation, classifying data based on the "80% of predicted rule" is statistically invalid and should be abandoned.[14]

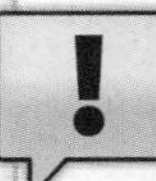

Respiratory Recap

Abnormal Lung Volumes and Capacities

- Reduced lung volumes and capacities generally indicate restrictive disease.
- Elevated residual volume or total lung capacity can indicate air trapping or **hyperinflation**.

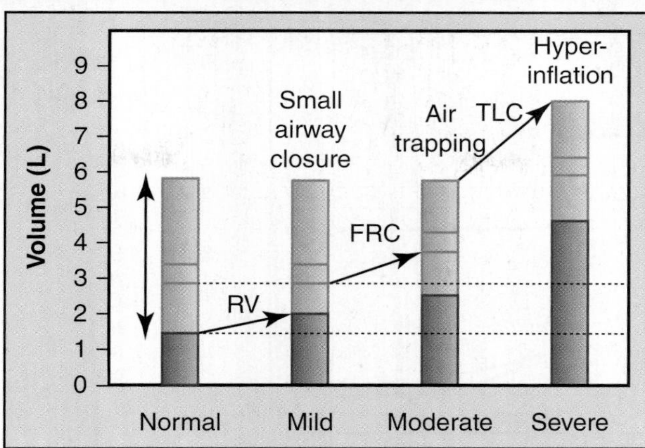

FIGURE 8-19 The effect of increasing airway obstruction on lung volumes. RV, residual volume; FRC, functional residual capacity; TLC, total lung capacity.

Diffusing Capacity

The **diffusing capacity** of the lung for carbon monoxide (DLCO) is a very valuable PFT, with many indications (**Box 8-7**). DLCO is an index of the uptake of gas molecules from the alveoli into the blood at rest.[4,24] This is not only a function of the thickness (resistance) of the alveolar-capillary membrane but also pulmonary perfusion, ventilation/perfusion matching, alveolar volume, and the reaction of CO to hemoglobin. Importantly, the DLCO can be the only abnormal PFT in diseases that are accompanied by normal spirometry and lung volumes (e.g., pulmonary hypertension). DLCO is also predictive of exercise oxygenation desaturation, identifies the presence of toxic medication reactions in the lung (e.g., amiodarone lung toxicity), and provides survival prognosis in many lung diseases.

To perform a DLCO test the seated patient wears nose clips and breathes through a flanged rubber mouthpiece connected to the spirometer circuit. The patient takes several tidal breaths, and then is instructed to exhale to RV. The patient is now instructed to rapidly and fully inhale a gas containing 0.3% carbon monoxide (CO) and an inert tracer gas. The patient passively holds the breath for 10 seconds (8–12) and then rapidly exhales for several seconds. The start and end points of the breath hold time (BHT) have been standardized according to the Jones-Meade method: BHT starts at one-third of the inspiratory time, ends when half of the alveolar sample is collected. The first 750 to 1000 mL of exhaled gas are discarded to prevent dead space (instrument and anatomic) gas from contaminating the alveolar sample (**Figure 8-20**). If the patient's lungs have a normal diffusion capacity, the concentration of CO in the exhaled alveolar sample will be much lower than the CO concentration at the beginning of the breath hold (much of the inhaled CO diffused into the blood and was perfused away). DLCO is expressed as mL/min/mm Hg (SI units are used in European countries). So, DLCO measures the volume (mL) of CO diffused per unit of time (minutes) at a given alveolar-capillary CO pressure gradient (mm Hg).

CO is used to measure the diffusion capacity of the lung because it is soluble in blood, reacts readily with hemoglobin, and is normally present in very small quantities in the blood and alveoli. The inert tracer gas (e.g., helium, methane, neon) is just as important as the CO in a DLCO test. The first function of the tracer gas is to determine the concentration of CO in the alveoli when the breath hold begins. It is known that the initial CO concentration in the PFT system is 0.3%; however, that concentration will decrease once it is diluted by residual volume in the alveoli. To calculate the DLCO, the difference in CO concentration *in the alveoli* from the beginning of the breath hold and the end of the breath hold must be measured. The inert tracer gas concentration will also decrease from dilution by residual volume in the alveoli and, because the tracer gas doesn't enter the blood (insoluble), the extent of that dilution is reflected in the exhaled tracer gas concentration. For example, the initial concentration of helium in a DLCO test gas is 10%. If the helium concentration falls to 7% after being inhaled into the alveoli, it will remain 7% throughout the breath hold and be recorded as 7% in the exhaled alveolar sample. Once the dilution

BOX 8-7

Indications for a DLCO Test

- In a patient with a low FVC or TLC, to differentiate between a chest wall cause of restriction (normal DLCO) and an interstitial lung disease (low DL)
- In a patient with airway obstruction on spirometry, to differentiate between emphysema (low DLCO) versus asthma or simple chronic bronchitis (normal DLCO)
- In a patient with dyspnea but normal spirometry, to detect pulmonary vascular disease (low DLCO) or mild interstitial lung disease (low DLCO)
- To evaluate treatment effects (or disease progression) in patients with interstitial lung diseases
- To evaluate pulmonary involvement in systemic diseases, such as rheumatoid arthritis or systemic lupus erythematosus
- To detect pulmonary side effects from chemotherapy, radiation therapy, or drugs (e.g., amiodarone, bleomycin) known to induce pulmonary dysfunction
- To predict arterial desaturation during exercise in patients with moderate to severe lung disease ($DLCO \leq 50\%$ of predicted increases likelihood of exercise desaturation)

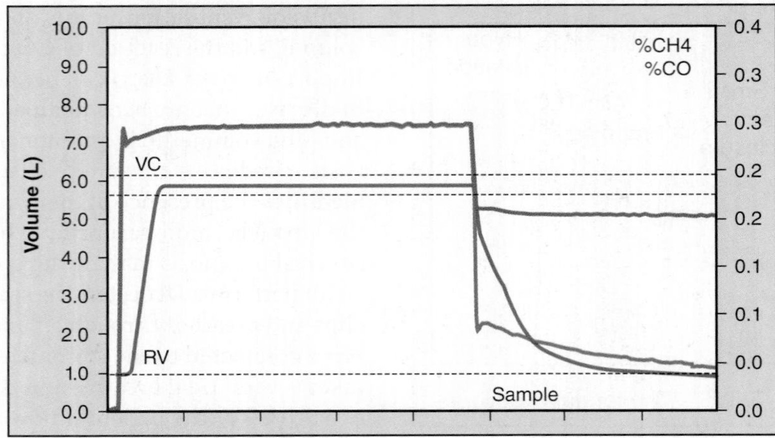

FIGURE 8-20 Graphs produced by a DLCO test. At the lower left corner, the patient begins to inhale the test gas. The red line shows the volume of inspired test gas (V_{in}) of about 6 L. The patient then holds his or her breath for about 10 seconds (the red line plateau), during which some of the carbon monoxide (CO) is absorbed by the red blood cells. The patient then exhales rapidly, and after the anatomic dead space air is discarded (about 1 L), a sample of air from the alveoli is obtained. The concentration of CO (blue line) and the tracer gas (green line) in the sample is measured by two gas analyzers or by gas chromatography.

factor for the tracer gas (3% in this case) is known, that number can be applied to the 0.3% CO concentration to determine what the CO concentration became in the alveoli at the beginning of the breath hold. Again, the difference in alveolar CO concentration at the beginning and end of the breath hold is needed to calculate DLCO. The second function of the tracer gas is to determine the size of the patient's alveolar volume (V_A). This is important because DLCO is the *volume* of CO that diffuses across the lungs for a given time and pressure gradient (mL/min/mm Hg). The larger the V_A, the more diluted the tracer gas concentration will be in the exhaled sample. The measured V_A should be a little smaller than the patient's TLC ($TLC - V_D \cong V_A$) measured by a different method (e.g., body plethysmograph), where V_D is the dead space volume. If the measured V_A is significantly less than the measured TLC, it can be assumed that the DLCO test gas was poorly distributed throughout the lung (e.g., COPD) and this shows a physiologic factor contributing to the patient's abnormal DLCO value. The DLCO can be indexed to the measured V_A, which is called the DLCO/V_A. The DLCO/V_A attempts to adjust the DLCO to the patient's lung size; however, a common misinterpretation of DLCO data is to conclude that a patient's diffusion capacity is normal because the abnormal DLCO value is accompanied by a normal or corrected DLCO/V_A. This conclusion is invalid because the DLCO and the V_A do not rise and fall in an equal or matched manner.[24]

DLCO is commonly low in patients with emphysema due to reduced alveolar surface area, poor $\dot{V}/\dot{Q}$ matching, and reduced pulmonary blood flow. Excessive thickness of the alveolar-capillary membrane and reduced alveolar volume lower DLCO in patients with pulmonary fibrosis. DLCO also is reduced in patients with pulmonary hypertension primarily because of reduced pulmonary blood flow. Anemic patients may have a low DLCO due to the limited hemoglobin volume available to bind with CO. Patients with polycythemia and blood in their airways may have an elevated DLCO. High CO back pressure due to an elevated carboxyhemoglobin (usually caused by recent smoking) can reduce DLCO. DLCO should be corrected for hemoglobin and carboxyhemoglobin whenever possible. Patients should be instructed to avoid smoking for *at least* 1 hour before diffusing capacity tests. Exercise should never be performed before a DLCO test because a higher cardiac output increases pulmonary blood flow and falsely elevates resting DLCO. Patients should remove supplemental O_2 for at least 10 minutes prior to testing if possible because the elevated O_2 pressure will compete with CO for hemoglobin binding.[4]

There are a number of test quality indicators that must be given close attention. First, the patient's inhaled volume must be at least 85% of his or her best vital capacity (ideally SVC). Inhalation of the test gas should be accomplished in no more than 4 seconds. The breath hold time (BHT) should be between 8 and 12 seconds with a target of 10 seconds. The collection of the alveolar sample should be made within 4 seconds. A minimum of two tests must be performed. A minimum of 4 minutes should separate DLCO tests to allow alveolar tracer gas pressures to return to zero. Reproducibility criteria are satisfied if two tests agree within 3 mL/min/mm Hg or 10% of each other. Modern PFT systems have software designed to alert technologists when a test meets (or does not meet) ATS/ERS acceptability and reproducibility criteria.

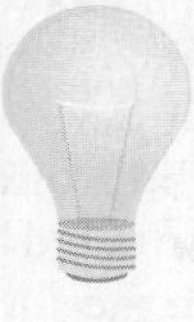

STOP AND THINK

A 50-year-old male with emphysema walks to the restroom after spirometry testing. Upon his return a DLCO measurement is promptly made and the value is 95% of predicted. What may have made this test inaccurate?

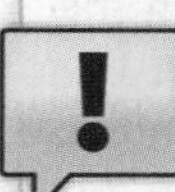

Respiratory Recap

Major Factors Influencing DLCO

- Area and thickness of the alveolar-capillary membrane
- Alveolar volume
- Pulmonary capillary blood volume

Many technical and biologic variables affect the accuracy and reproducibility of the measured DLCO. The accuracy of the DLCO instrumentation is ideally checked using a specialized DLCO simulator; however, very few PFT labs use these devices due to cost. A 3-liter (3-L) calibration syringe can be used to simulate DLCO; with this technique the DLCO should be close to zero. On modern systems, the machine at the beginning of each test does a two-point calibration of the gas analyzers automatically. The accuracy of the flow sensor should be checked every day using a 3-L syringe. The repeatability of DLCO for each machine should be checked at least weekly using a healthy biologic control subject. Biologic control data should be monitored in a Levey-Jennings plot and there should be no drift outside of 2 standard deviations of the mean value for each biologic control subject (**Figure 8-21**).

Interpretation of DLCO

DLCO values are evaluated in comparison with predicted values. Predicted equations are calculated from height, age, and gender. DLCO values should be above the LLN and below the ULN to be considered normal. Altitude has a significant effect on DLCO values (people who live at higher altitudes have higher DLCO values), so choosing a predicted set formulated from a similar altitude as your lab is a good place to start. As with spirometry and lung volume interpretation, classifying data based on the 80% of predicted rule is statistically invalid and should be abandoned.[14]

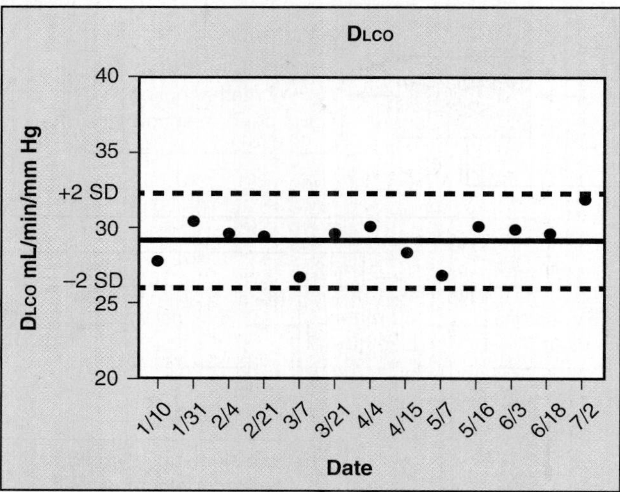

FIGURE 8-21 A Levey-Jennings plot of biological control data from a normal subject. The solid line represents the mean DLCO for the normal subject; the dashed lines represent 2 standard deviations from the mean.

Specialized Pulmonary Function Tests

Several tests of specific aspects of lung function are performed in PFT laboratories. These tests may not be routine in some outpatient testing but can be useful to help further classify the cause, type, or degree of pulmonary disability.

Bronchial Challenge Tests

Asthma is a common lung disease, which causes intermittent attacks with one or more of the following symptoms: wheezing, chest tightness, dyspnea, or coughing. These symptoms can be seen in disorders other than asthma, so PFTs are necessary to make the correct diagnosis. In patients with poorly controlled asthma, baseline spirometry may show airway obstruction and a positive response to bronchodilator compatible with an asthma diagnosis. Most patients with mild asthma spend most of their time with no symptoms and normal spirometry results, however. So unless spirometry testing happens to be scheduled during a symptomatic hour, the test will likely appear within normal limits. Bronchial challenge tests offer a way to provoke airway smooth muscle contraction (bronchospasm) in patients with airway hyper-responsiveness. All airway smooth muscle has the capacity to constrict, but the airway smooth muscle in the asthmatic lung constricts too easily and too much. Airway hyperresponsiveness is a feature of asthma but can also been seen in other disorders, so only patients with a reasonable risk of asthma should be challenged.

Outside of research studies bronchial challenge tests are rarely done when the diagnosis of asthma has already been established. The three most frequently performed bronchial challenge tests are methacholine, mannitol, and exercise challenge tests. Histamine is used in some countries, but more commonly causes uncomfortable systemic side effects, such as flushing or a headache. Less commonly used challenge tests include cold air challenges, eucapnic voluntary hyperventilation of dry gas, and nebulization of hypertonic saline.

Very rarely, specific antigen challenges are done in specialized centers for research studies, or sometimes to confirm occupational asthma due to a single workplace trigger. These patients may require hospitalization for at least 24 hours because of the risk of a delayed response.

Bronchial challenge tests are contraindicated in patients with moderate to severe airway obstruction but are very safe in those with normal baseline spirometry. There are several pretesting instructions for each challenge, which must be followed to obtain accurate results. For example, bronchodilators should not be taken on the day of testing. Exercise is not permitted on the day of testing because if bronchospasm occurs in the pretest exercise, the airways may be in a refractory period and fail to constrict during testing. Patients who arrive with an active or recent chest infection should be rescheduled in 4 to 6 weeks as the infection can increase airway hyperresponsiveness in the asthmatic and cause a false-positive test in the nonasthmatic.

Methacholine Challenge

Methacholine. as a parasympathomimetic, acts directly on bronchial smooth muscle to cause bronchospasm, which typically reverses promptly with bronchodilator administration. Methacholine will cause bronchospasm even in nonasthmatic patients if given in high doses. The methacholine challenge, however, uses small doses of methacholine that are generally large enough to cause bronchospasm in *most* asthmatic patients but are not generally large enough to cause bronchospasm in *most* nonasthmatics patients. The question here, therefore, is not a "yes or no," but rather "how much?"

Two methods of delivering the methacholine have been standardized by the ATS: 2-minute tidal breathing (from a nebulizer) and five-breath dosimeter-actuated nebulizer.[25] The dosimeter delivers gas through the nebulizer for a split second (typically 0.6 second) to control how much methacholine is delivered. The 2-minute tidal breathing method may be more sensitive in mild asthma because the five deep breaths required from the dosimeter method offers protection against bronchospasm.[26]

A methacholine challenge starts with high quality spirometry. If prechallenge spirometry does not show significant airflow obstruction, the patient starts with inhaling very low concentrations of methacholine or a saline diluent. After each step the methacholine is given time to take effect (e.g., 1 minute) and spirometry is repeated. If the FEV_1 remains above 80% of the baseline value, the concentration is increased and the process is repeated (**Figure 8-22**). Higher concentrations of methacholine are administered until the FEV_1 falls more than 20% or the highest concentration of methacholine (e.g., 20 mg/mL) has been given. The patient is then given albuterol to reverse any bronchospasm caused by the methacholine. The results are summarized by the PC_{20} (the provocative concentration of methacholine that caused a 20% fall in the FEV_1) or the PD_{20} (the provocative cumulative dose of methacholine that caused a 20% fall in the FEV_1) (**Figure 8-23**).

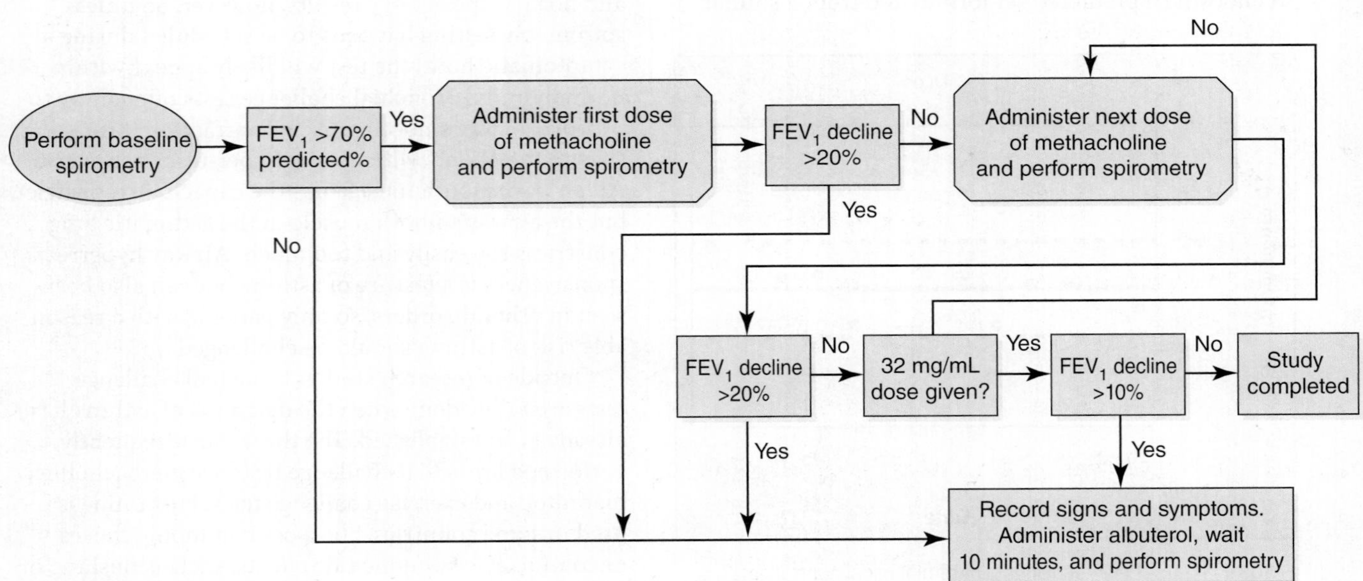

FIGURE 8-22 Algorithm for performance of methacholine challenge testing.
Adapted from Crapo RO, Casaburi R, Coates AL, et al., *Am J Respir Crit Care Med.* 2000;161:309–329.

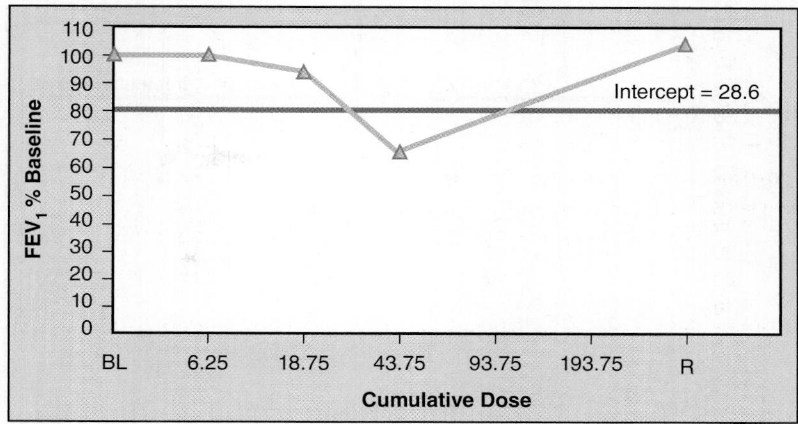

FIGURE 8-23 Methacholine challenge dose response curve. The FEV_1 is plotted against the cumulative methacholine dose (sum of breaths multiplied by methacholine concentration). The patient experienced a 20% decline in FEV_1 (PD_{20}) at a cumulative methacholine dose of 28.6 dose units (provocative dose of methacholine resulting in a 20% decline in FEV_1 [PD_{20}]).

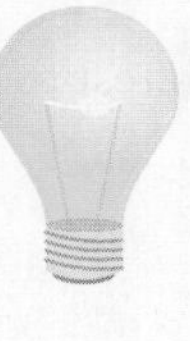

STOP AND THINK

Over the past 3 weeks more patients seem to be reacting to very small doses of methacholine via the five-breath method. What device should you check?

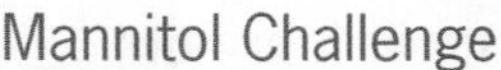

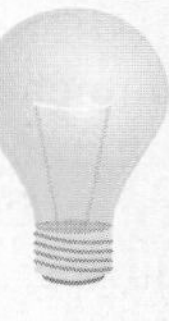

STOP AND THINK

A 23-year-old patient arrives late for a mannitol challenge. She states that she sprinted up the stairs and that she is tardy because she had trouble finding the hospital's bicycle rack. What action should be taken?

Mannitol Challenge

Mannitol challenge is an indirect bronchial challenge. This test is classified as an indirect challenge because unlike methacholine, mannitol doesn't act directly on airway smooth muscle. As an osmotic agent mannitol draws fluid from the surface of the airway. In response fluid is drawn from surrounding cells to replenish the water content of the airway surface. During this process mast cells may degranulate, releasing proinflammatory mediators such as histamine, leukotrienes, and prostaglandins into the airway. These mediators will incite bronchospasm in patients with airway hyperresponsiveness and the FEV_1 will decline.[27]

A mannitol challenge starts with high quality spirometry. If prechallenge spirometry does not show significant airflow obstruction, the patient inhales mannitol powder from an inhaler (**Figure 8-24**). The mannitol challenge has nine dose steps including a 0 mg first step. After each dose a 1-minute waiting period is observed before the patient repeats spirometry.

If the FEV_1 declines by ≥15% from the baseline 0 mg dose or ≥10% between doses, the test is considered positive and the patient is given albuterol to reverse bronchospasm (**Figure 8-25**). It is important to handle the dry powder capsules with metal tweezers because static from exam gloves can reduce the spinning of the capsule within the inhaler. Mannitol is very drying in the upper airway, so a large cup of water should be available for the patient to sip between doses.

Exercise Challenge

Exercise, especially when conducted in cold, dry air, is a common asthma trigger. The mechanism of bronchospasm from exercise is similar to bronchospasm caused by mannitol inhalation: drying of the airway surface leads to mediator release, which incites airway

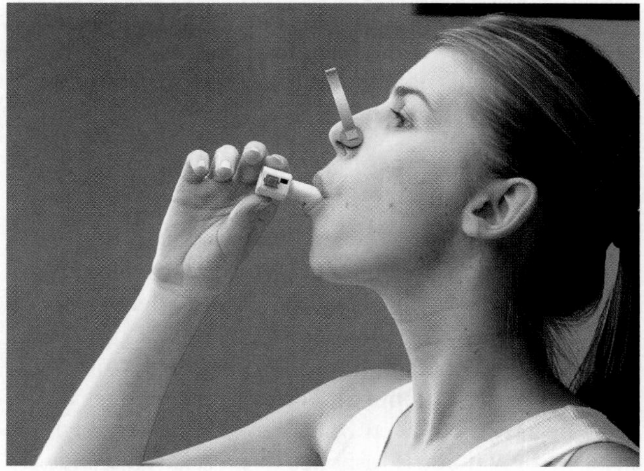

FIGURE 8-24 Inhalation of mannitol from a dry powder inhaler as part of a mannitol challenge test.
Courtesy of Pharmaxis, Inc.

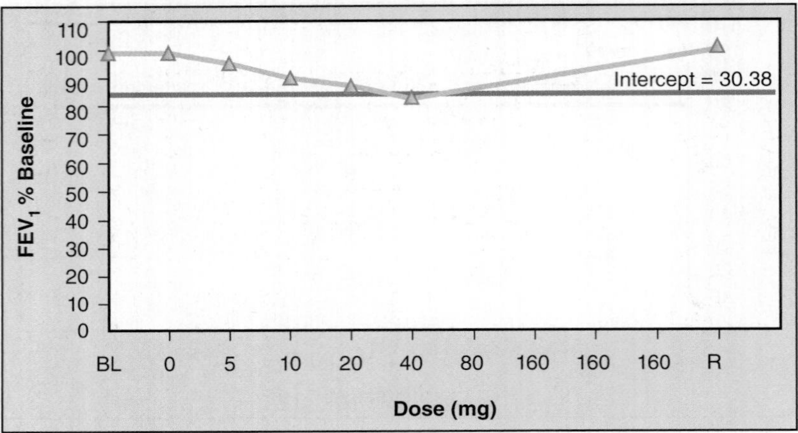

FIGURE 8-25 Mannitol challenge dose response curve. The FEV_1 is plotted against the mannitol dose. The patient experienced a 15% decline in FEV_1 (PC_{15}) at a mannitol concentration of 30.38 mg (provocative concentration of mannitol resulting in a 15% decline in FEV_1 [PC_{15}]).

smooth muscle constriction.[28] However, environmental pollutants such as ozone, trichloramines in swimming pools, and fumes emitted from melted ski wax may also fuel airway inflammation and bronchospasm during exercise.[29]

Exercise challenges are therefore another *indirect* bronchial challenge test. Exercise challenges can be performed on either a treadmill or a bicycle ergometer. Field tests (e.g., Nordic skiing, skating) are sometimes performed on elite athletes, but this is rarely done in a general population. The key to an effective exercise challenge is to produce high minute ventilation with the patient breathing dry gas. Nose clips are recommended to eliminate humidification from the nasal passages if the patient is breathing room air (relative humidity ~50%); however, the most effective strategy is to have the patient exercise while breathing compressed dry air through a valved-breathing circuit. An exercise challenge starts with high quality spirometry. If pre-challenge spirometry does not show significant airflow obstruction, exercise can commence. After approximately 8 minutes of high intensity exercise, the patient is allowed to rest and the FEV_1 is measured every 5 minutes for 30 minutes. A 10% (or 15%) decline in FEV_1 is considered a positive test and the patient is given albuterol to reverse bronchospasm.[25]

Exercise challenge tests have a few disadvantages when compared to methacholine and mannitol challenges. Exercise challenges take longer to perform and may be difficult for patients with orthopedic problems. In addition, the patient must be willing to perform intense exercise; submaximal effort may produce a false-negative test. Even when performed correctly, studies show that the response to exercise challenge has day-to-day variability in some patients. The ATS recommends mannitol challenge as an acceptable alternative to an exercise challenge test; however, methacholine challenge is not a recommended test to diagnose exercise-induced bronchospasm.[28]

What Does a Positive or Negative Challenge Test Mean?

In a perfect world suspicions about the presence of asthma could be ruled-in or ruled-out with near 100% certainty following a bronchial challenge test. Manufacturers of home pregnancy tests boast that their products have more than 99% sensitivity (positive test in pregnant patients) and 99% specificity (negative test in nonpregnant patients). Unfortunately, bronchial challenge tests can't compete with pregnancy tests. In one study, exercise, methacholine, and mannitol challenge tests had sensitivities (positive tests in asthmatics) and specificities (negative tests in nonasthmatics) below 70%. While bronchial challenges are not "yes or no" tests that are correct 100% of time, bronchial challenge tests can play an important role in making the correct diagnosis. When a patient has a "positive" challenge test the probability of asthma increases. The probability of asthma is highest when the patient has a positive response to a small dose of a challenge agent. Likewise, a "negative" challenge test merely reduces the probability of asthma. Asthma is a clinical diagnosis where symptoms, risk factors (e.g., family history, atopy), spirometry, bronchial challenge tests, and ultimately the response to therapy are pooled together to make a case that the patient indeed is asthmatic.

Airways Resistance

A disadvantage of spirometry to measure airway obstruction is that athletic-like breathing maneuvers are necessary. Many preschool children and some elderly adults are unable to perform good-quality spirometry tests. In some patients cough triggered by deep breaths make quality spirometry impossible to obtain. Tests of **airways resistance** require less effort and coordination because they are done during normal breathing or slow panting through a mouthpiece. In addition, obstructions of the upper and large airways may be identified better and quantified by airways resistance than spirometry because FVC and FEV_1 may remain normal.

Airway Resistance via Body Plethysmography

The most common method of measuring airways resistance (Raw) in a PFT lab is using a body box, often done at the same time as the measurement of lung volumes. Resistance is the change in pressure divided by flow. To calculate Raw in a body box, the alveolar pressure is divided by airflow. The airway resistance measurement starts with the patient performing panting (1–1.5 pants per second) through a pneumotach with the mouth shutter open. During this phase inspiratory and expiratory flow is plotted against box pressure. Box pressure is measured because flow and alveolar (mouth) pressure cannot be measured simultaneously. Box pressure will serve as a history of alveolar pressure when panting flow was measured. After capturing several panting flow versus box pressure cycles, the mouth shutter is closed and several closed shutter pants are collected. The closed shutter pants plot alveolar (mouth) pressure against box pressure. This allows the box pressures measured during the open shutter phase (panting flow versus box pressure) to be converted into alveolar pressure values. Alveolar pressures can now be divided by the panting flows to calculate Raw in cm H_2O/L/second.

The other function of measuring box pressure during the Raw procedure is to measure the lung volume when the Raw measurement was made. This is important because Raw is higher at low lung/airway volumes and lower at higher lung/airway volumes. The reciprocal of Raw is conductance (Gaw; 1/Raw = Gaw). Specific conductance (sGaw) is the conductance accounting for the lung volume it was measured at. Therefore, sGaw eliminates the effect of lung volume on the conductance value. For example, a patient with normal airways could have an elevated Raw value if he panted near his RV during the Raw measurement; however, the sGaw would remain normal because sGaw is corrected for lung volume.[30]

Impulse Oscillometry (Forced Oscillation Technique)

Dr. Arthur Dubois is credited with developing both body plethysmograpy and impulse oscillometry (IOS) in the 1950s. Unlike body plethysmography, however, IOS has only recently become widely available for use in PFT labs. The IOS measurement begins with a seated patient breathing through a mouthpiece, wearing nose clips, and holding the cheeks. While the patient breathes quietly, a small speaker generates small flow impulses of various intensities, which are transmitted toward the patient's airways (**Figure 8-26**). The pressure produced by the flow impulses is used to calculate resistance. The most common expression of resistance from IOS testing is R_5, the resistance at a frequency of 5 hertz.[30] IOS can be used to measure resistance and the change in resistance that may accompany bronchodilation or bronchoconstriction (e.g., methacholine challenge). Predicted equations for IOS are not as well established as those for spirometry or sGaw.

IOS is a very attractive test because patients who have difficulty producing quality spirometry data can

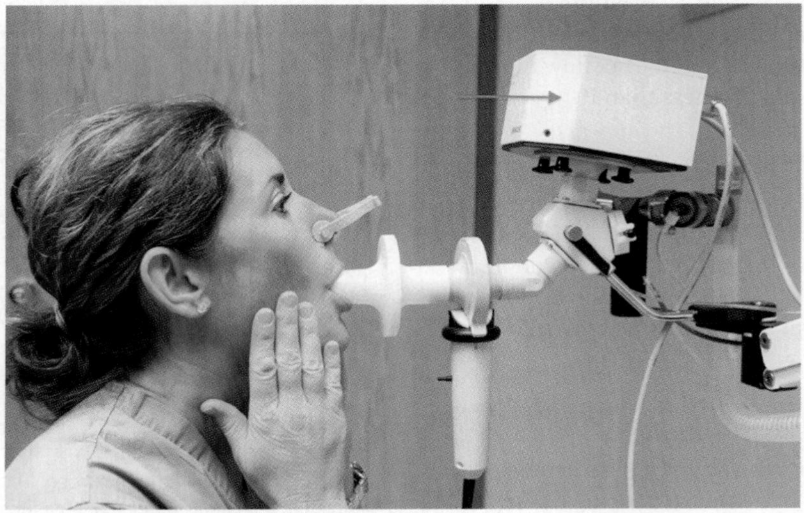

FIGURE 8-26 A respiratory therapist demonstrates impulse oscillometry. A speaker (arrow) sends pulses of flow toward the airway.

Courtesy of Melissa Rowley-Lipman.

often correctly perform IOS. Moreover, many patients cannot perform body plethysmography due to claustrophobia or difficulty performing closed-shutter panting.

Respiratory Muscle Strength

In the past, respiratory therapists often measured the strength of the diaphragm in patients on mechanical ventilation as an index of their ability to tolerate extubation. For example, a **maximum inspiratory pressure** (PI_{max}) of greater than –20 cm H_2O was thought to be highly predictive of extubation readiness. While the usefulness of PI_{max} in making extubation decisions has waned, PI_{max} and **maximum expiratory pressure** (PE_{max}) play an important role in the diagnosis and surveillance of patients with ventilatory insufficiency due to neuromuscular disorders.

The maximum respiratory pressures—PI_{max} and PE_{max}—can be measured by most PFT systems as well as by simple mechanical pressure gauges. Tubing to a pressure gauge connects a mouthpiece. A PI_{max}/PE_{max} system may incorporate a pinhole leak to prevent glottic closure. A flanged rubber mouthpiece and nose clips are used, especially for PE_{max} measurements, to prevent pressure loss from leaks.

To measure PI_{max}, the patient exhales slowly (from FRC toward RV), and then inhales from the mouthpiece as forcefully as possible. The PI_{max} is measured as the highest negative pressure maintained for about 1 second. Up to five PI_{max} maneuvers are performed, with a goal of matching the highest value by less than 10%. The highest value is reported. MEP is measured similarly, but at maximal inhalation (near TLC). Seated and supine SVC measurements are commonly ordered in conjunction with PI_{max}/PE_{max} testing. A 15% decrease in SVC measured in the supine position is consistent with respiratory muscle weakness. Cough peak flow is a test of cough strength in which the patient fully inhales and coughs into a spirometer or hand-held peak flow meter. Low cough peak flows (e.g., <4 L/s) in adults is predictive of respiratory complications associated with the inability to clear secretions. Cough peak flow may be a better judge of cough effectiveness than PE_{max}.

Exhaled Nitric Oxide

Nitric oxide (NO) is a gas molecule, which plays many physiologic roles, most notably the modulation of vascular tone. NO is also produced from eosinophilic inflammation associated with asthma. The fraction of exhaled NO (FENO) can be easily measured in PFT labs, clinics, and physician offices. To perform a FENO measurement, the seated patient inhales to TLC and then without hesitation slowly exhales through a mouthpiece to RV. The patient exhales against an expiratory resistance of +5 cm H_2O to prevent nasal NO (higher than bronchial) from mixing with the pulmonary sample.

The ATS defines FENO levels in the following way: low <25 ppb (parts per billion) adults, <20 ppb children; intermediate: 25–50 ppb adults, 20–35 ppb children; high: >50 ppb adults, >35 ppb children. High FENO may support an asthma diagnosis and low FENO may reduce the likelihood of asthma in some patients. The ATS recommends the use of FENO to *support* the diagnosis of asthma and to determine the likelihood of and the presence of responsiveness to corticosteroid therapy.[31] Limitations to FENO testing include a significant amount of contradictory data in the scientific literature, performance variability among laboratories, and poor correlation with patient symptom scores. The field of exhaled breath condensate (EBC) testing is rapidly growing, measuring of an array of biomarkers such as airway pH.

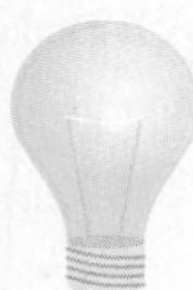

STOP AND THINK

A physician asks you which tests to order for a patient with suspected diaphragm paralysis. What tests would you recommend?

Single Breath Nitrogen Washout (SBN_2)

Ventilation distribution is sometimes measured using the **single-breath nitrogen washout** test. This test involves a maximal inspiration of 100% oxygen followed by a slow exhalation to RV. A one-way valve through a nitrogen analyzer and spirometer directs the slow, complete exhalation. The nitrogen meter continuously records the nitrogen concentration of the expired gas and simultaneously plots the expired nitrogen concentration against expired volume. The normal curve has four portions (**Figure 8-27**).

The slope of phase III and the percent change in nitrogen between 750 mL and 1250 mL of exhaled gas ($\Delta N_{2_{750-1250}}$) are indices of nonuniform ventilation.

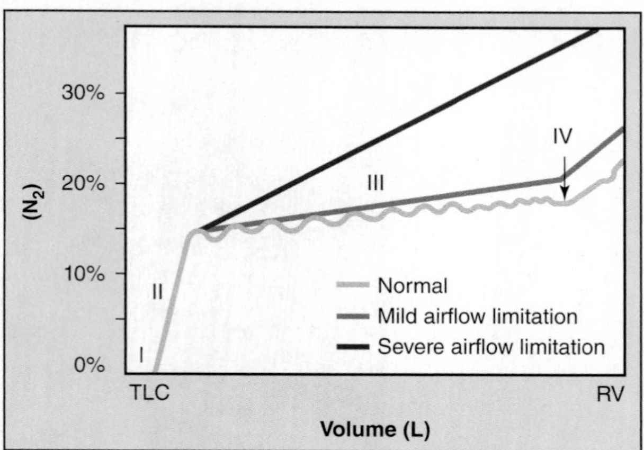

FIGURE 8-27 Single-breath nitrogen test for distribution of ventilation. Phase I is dead space gas, phase II is mixed gas (dead space and alveolar), phase III is alveolar gas, and phase IV is closing volume (arrow). TLC, total lung capacity; RV, residual volume.

The onset of phase IV is considered an indication of the onset of airway closure in the dependent regions. The volume exhaled during phase IV is called the *closing volume*. Relatively uniform gas distribution is identified by a flat phase III. With the onset of obstructive lung disease, closing volume and the slope of phase III are increased. As the distribution of ventilation becomes more heterogeneous, the slope of phase III becomes steeper. In advanced obstructive disease, phase IV becomes lost in the very steep slope of phase III. In obstructive lung disease, the distribution of ventilation worsens because regional differences in airway resistance and airspace compliance affect the rate at which airspace empties and fills.

Exercise Laryngoscopy

Vocal cord dysfunction syndrome (VCD) is a poorly appreciated disorder characterized by abnormal adduction of the vocal cords and/or arytenoid cartilages. The signs and symptoms associated with VCD are similar to asthma: dyspnea; diminished ventilation on auscultation; musical sounds emanating from the respiratory tract. For this reason, many patients with VCD are misdiagnosed with asthma. Complicating matters is the fact that a significant number of patients have overlapping asthma *and* VCD. In many VCD patients PFTs, even the inspiratory portion of the flow/volume loop, appear normal. A common trigger of VCD is exercise; however, because VCD generally only occurs at the peak of exercise, cardiopulmonary exercise tests also can appear normal. Exercise laryngoscopy is a test specifically designed to detect VCD. During an exercise laryngoscopy, an endoscope is situated above the larynx and the laryngeal function is observed while the patient vigorously pedals a cycle ergometer. A scoring system is used to grade the probability of VCD.[32]

Key Points

- To avoid interpretation errors, spirometry requires attentive, vigorous coaching and careful scrutiny of the tracings.
- Spirometry detects airflow limitation due to lung disease, such as asthma or COPD.
- A low FEV_1/FVC indicates airway obstruction.
- A low FEV_1 and FVC with a normal FEV_1/FVC suggests restriction, which can be confirmed by a low TLC.
- A repeatable flat plateau on the inspiratory flow volume curve detects upper airway obstruction.
- DLCO helps in the differential diagnosis when spirometry is abnormal.
- Decreases in lung volumes often indicate restrictive lung disease.
- Increases in residual volume and RV/TLC indicate air trapping, whereas an increase in TLC indicates hyperinflation.
- Specialized pulmonary function tests can be useful to help further classify the cause, type, or degree of respiratory impairment.

References

1. Miller MR, Crapo R, Hankinson J, et al. General considerations for lung function testing. *Eur Respir J.* 2005;26:153–161.
2. Miller MR, Hankinson J, Brusasco V, et al. Standardisation of spirometry. *Eur Respir J.* 2005;26:319–338.
3. Wanger J, Clausen JL, Coates A, et al. Standardisation of the measurement of lung volumes. *Eur Respir J.* 2005;26:511–522.
4. MacIntyre N, Crapo RO, Viegi G, et al. Standardisation of the single-breath determination of carbon monoxide uptake in the lung. *Eur Respir J.* 2005;26:720–735.
5. Pellegrino R, Viegi G, Brusasco V, et al. Interpretative strategies for lung function tests. *Eur Respir J.* 2005;26:948–968.
6. Haynes JM. Quality assurance of the pulmonary function technologist. *Respir Care.* 2012;57:144–152.
7. Blonshine S. Integrating education with diagnostics, patient and technologist. *Respir Care Clin N Am.* 1997;3:139–154.
8. Enright PL, Johnson LR, Connett JE, et al. Spirometry in the lung health study. 1. Methods and quality control. *Am Rev Respir Dis.* 1990;143:1215–1223.
9. Borg BM, Hartley MF, Bailey MJ, Thompson BR. Adherence to acceptability and repeatability criteria for spirometry in complex lung function laboratories. *Respir Care.* 2012;57:2032–2038.
10. Quanjer PH, Stanojevic S, Cole TJ, et al. Multi-ethnic reference values for spirometry for the 3-95-yr age range: the global lung function 2012 equations. *Eur Respir J.* 2012;40:1324–1343.
11. Mottram CD. *Ruppel's Manual of Pulmonary Function Testing.* 10th ed. St. Louis: Mosby; 2012.
12. Swanney MP, Jensen RL, Crichton DA, et al. FEV_6 is an acceptable surrogate for FVC in the spirometric diagnosis of airway obstruction and restriction. *Am J Respir Crit Care Med.* 2000;162: 917–919.
13. Miller A, Enright PL. PFT interpretative strategies: American Thoracic Society/European Thoracic Society 2005 Guideline Gaps. *Respir Care.* 2012;57:127–133.
14. Culver BH. How should the lower limit of normal be defined? *Respir Care.* 2012;57:136–143.
15. Stanojevic S, Wade A, Stocks J, et al. Reference ranges for spirometry across all ages, a new approach. *Am J Respir Crit Care Med.* 2008;177:253–260.
16. Fragoso CA, Gill TM, McAvay G, et al. Use of lambda-mu-sigma-derived Z score for evaluating respiratory impairment in middle-aged persons. *Respir Care.* 2011;56:1771–1777.
17. Fragoso CA, Gill TM, McAvay G, et al. Respiratory impairment in older persons: a novel spirometric approach. *J Investig Med.* 2011;59:1089–1095.
18. Hyatt RE, Cowl CT, Bjoraker JA, Scanlon PD. Conditions associated with an abnormal nonspecific pattern of pulmonary function tests. *Chest.* 2009;135:419–424.
19. Borg BM, Thompson BR. The measurement of lung volumes using body plethysmograpy: a comparison of methodologies. *Respir Care.* 2012;57:1076–1083.
20. O'Donnell DE, Forkert L, Webb KA. Evaluation of bronchodilator responses in patients with "irreversible" emphysema. *Eur Respir J.* 2001;18:914–920.
21. Ruppel GL. What is the clinical value of lung volumes? *Respir Care.* 2012;57:26–35.
22. Horsley A. Lung clearance index in the assessment of airways disease. *Respir Med.* 2009;103:793–799.
23. Kraemer R, Blum A, Schibler A, et al. Ventilation inhomogeneities in relation to standard lung function in patients with cystic fibrosis. *Am J Respir Crit Care Med.* 2005;171:371–378.
24. McCormack MC. Facing the noise: addressing the endemic variability in DLCO testing. *Respir Care.* 2012;57:17–23.

25. Crapo RO, Cassaburi R, Coates AL, et al. Guidelines for methacholine and exercise challenge testing–1999. *Am J Respir Crit Care Med.* 2000;161:309–329.
26. Cockcroft DW, Davis BE. The bronchoprotective effect of inhaling methacholine by using total lung capacity inspirations has a marked influence on the interpretation of the test result. *J Allergy Clin Immunol.* 2006;117:1244–1248.
27. Anderson SD. Indirect challenge tests: airway hyperresponsiveness in asthma: its measurement and clinical significance. *Chest.* 2010;138(Suppl 2):25S–30S.
28. Parsons JP, Hallstrand TS, Mastronarde JG, et al. An official American Thoracic Society clinical practice guideline: exercise-induced bronchoconstriction. *Am J Respir Crit Care Med.* 2013;187:1016–1027.
29. Freberg BI, Olsen R, Thorud S, et al. Chemical exposure among professional ski waxers—characterization of individual work operations. *Ann Occup Hyg.* 2013;57:286–295.
30. Kaminsky DA. What does airway resistance tell us about lung function? *Respir Care.* 2012;57:85–96.
31. Dweik RA, Boggs PB, Erzurum SC, et al. An official ATS clinical practice guideline: interpretation of exhaled nitric oxide levels (FENO) for clinical applications. *Am J Respir Crit Care Med.* 2011;184:602–615.
32. Matt RC, Røksund OD, Halvorsen T, et al. Audiovisual assessment of exercise-induced laryngeal obstruction: reliability and validity of observations. *Eur Arch Otorhinolaryngol.* 2009:266:1929–1936.

CHAPTER

9 Interventional Pulmonary Procedures

Ellen Volker, Amy Treece, Momen M. Wahidi, Scott L. Shofer

OUTLINE

OBJECTIVES

1. Compare flexible fiberoptic bronchoscopy and rigid bronchoscopy.
2. Discuss appropriate patient selection for bronchoscopy.
3. List absolute and relative contraindications for bronchoscopy.
4. Discuss issues related to patient preparation for bronchoscopy.
5. Discuss issues related to sedation for bronchoscopy.
6. Describe the following techniques for flexible fiberoptic bronchoscopy: airway examination, bronchoalveolar lavage, bronchoscopic washing, bronchoscopic brushing, endobronchial biopsy, transbronchial biopsy, and transbronchial needle aspiration.
7. List complications of bronchoscopy.
8. List indications for bronchoscopy.
9. Describe the indications, equipment, and technique for rigid bronchoscopy.
10. Compare the types of stents used for airway stenting.
11. Describe the indications and procedure for thoracentesis.

KEY TERMS

airway stent
brachytherapy
bronchoalveolar lavage (BAL)
bronchoscopic brushing
bronchoscopic washing
bronchoscopy
diagnostic bronchoscopy
endobronchial biopsy
exudative
flexible fiberoptic bronchoscope
hybrid stent
lung-volume reduction
metallic stent
nonprotected bronchial brush
pleural effusion
pleurodesis
procedural sedation
protected bronchial brush
rigid bronchoscope
sclerosing agent
silicone stent
therapeutic bronchoscopy
thoracentesis
transbronchial biopsy
transbronchial needle aspiration (TBNA)
transudative
videobronchoscope

Introduction

Interventional pulmonology is an evolving field within pulmonary medicine that focuses on procedural services provided to patients with airway disorders and pleural diseases. It encompasses three main areas in pulmonary medicine: malignant and nonmalignant airway disorders, pleural diseases, and artificial airways. The topics of diagnostic bronchoscopy, therapeutic bronchoscopy, and pleural interventions are covered in this chapter.

Diagnostic Bronchoscopy

Overview of Bronchoscopy

Bronchoscopy is the most commonly used invasive procedure in pulmonary medicine and can be used to perform both diagnostic and therapeutic procedures (**CPG 9-1**). In the United States alone, approximately 500,000 bronchoscopies are performed each year.[1]

Gustav Killian performed the first bronchoscopy in Germany in 1897 using a laryngoscope and a rigid esophagoscopy tube to remove a foreign body (a piece of pork bone) from the proximal right main stem bronchus. This led to the development of the rigid bronchoscope, consisting of a long, hollow, rigid tube with channels for light and other instruments. In the early 1900s, Chevalier Jackson of Philadelphia further refined the rigid bronchoscope and advocated for its use in clinical practice.

It was not until the late 1960s that the flexible fiberoptic bronchoscope was developed by Shigeto Ikeda in Tokyo, Japan.[2] The development of the flexible bronchoscope significantly simplified the procedure, and it rapidly became widely used by pulmonary physicians, thoracic surgeons, and intensivists with the assistance of a respiratory therapist.

The Flexible Bronchoscope

The **flexible fiberoptic bronchoscope** (**Figure 9-1**) consists of a control unit (or head) and a soft, flexible shaft. The shaft has an external diameter of 3.5 to 6 mm and a tip that can rotate up to 210 degrees. The shaft contains a hollow internal operating channel for suctioning secretions and collecting specimens, and a working channel for administration of solutions (saline, lidocaine) and passage of instruments. The control unit is attached to a light source and can also be fitted with a camera for dynamic or still photography.

There are two types of flexible bronchoscopes: fiberoptic and video chip. The original flexible bronchoscopes were based on fiberoptic technology, with images being transmitted from the instrument's distal objective lens to the proximal eyepiece. The development of video chips led to the creation of the flexible **videobronchoscope**, which works by capturing digital images at the distal tip and transmitting these images via the bronchoscope to a remote television monitor.[3] The videobronchoscope has greatly enhanced the field of bronchoscopy, allowing images to be captured and saved with a camera and aiding in teaching and training purposes with its real-time display. The disadvantages of the flexible videobronchoscope include additional equipment and space requirements.[3]

Flexible Fiberoptic Bronchoscopy

Bronchoscopy is a safe and effective tool for diagnosing and treating a wide variety of pulmonary processes. This safety is dependent on several factors. The bronchoscopist must master the technical skills of manipulating the bronchoscope safely through the airways and have a good understanding of respiratory anatomy. In addition, appropriate patient selection and preparation, careful use of sedatives, and a clear understanding of the indications and expected yields for the various bronchoscopic procedures are critical to making each bronchoscopy a success.

Patient Selection

The ideal patient for fiberoptic bronchoscopy is awake, able to understand and cooperate with the procedure, and free of other conditions that could elevate the risk of the procedure. In particular, major conditions to consider include ischemic or arrhythmic heart disease, bleeding diathesis (coagulopathy, thrombocytopenia, uremia), neurologic disease or head trauma, and respiratory insufficiency. Although bronchoscopy can be performed in patients who fall short of this ideal, the risk of the procedure increases accordingly, and options for more invasive manipulations (biopsies, lengthy procedures, etc.) can be limited. A careful history and physical should be targeted toward ascertaining the presence and severity of any risk factors or comorbidities, documenting previous anesthesia and associated complications, and defining ways in which the timing or nature of the procedure can be modified to minimize risk to the patient.

Preoperative laboratory studies, including platelet count, coagulation studies, blood urea nitrogen level, and creatinine level, are often obtained to assess for bleeding tendencies. Multiple studies examining the utility of preoperative lab work have determined that this is not universally necessary but should be tailored to patients with medical histories suggesting an abnormality. In a retrospective study of 305 bronchoscopies with biopsy, Kozak and Brath identified five clinical risk factors that should prompt further preoperative evaluation: prior anticoagulant therapy, liver disease, family or personal history of bleeding tendencies, active bleeding or recent transfusion requirements, and presence of an unreliable historian.[4]

Box 9-1 lists the absolute and relative contraindications for bronchoscopy and biopsy. Absolute contraindications to bronchoscopy are few and include inability to provide informed consent, status asthmaticus, severe hypoxemia, and unstable cardiovascular conditions. Some of the main factors to consider when selecting a patient for bronchoscopy are discussed next.

Asthma and Bronchospasm

Although bronchoscopy can be safely performed in asthmatic patients, it is associated with a significant drop in FEV_1 and Pao_2 after the procedure. This drop correlates inversely with the concentration of methacholine required to produce a 20% fall in FEV_1 at baseline, but not with the usual measures of asthma

CLINICAL PRACTICE GUIDELINE 9-1

Bronchoscopy Assisting

Indications

- The presence of lesions of unknown etiology on the chest radiograph film or the need to evaluate recurrent pneumonia, persistent atelectasis, or pulmonary infiltrates
- The need to assess patency or mechanical properties of the upper airway
- The need to investigate hemoptysis, persistent unexplained cough, dyspnea, localized wheeze, or stridor
- Suspicious or positive sputum cytology results
- The need to obtain lower respiratory tract secretions, cell washings, and biopsies for cytologic, histologic, and microbiologic evaluation
- The need to determine the location and extent of injury from toxic inhalation or aspiration
- The need to evaluate problems associated with endotracheal or tracheostomy tubes (tracheal damage, airway obstruction, or tube placement)
- The need for aid in performing difficult intubations or percutaneous tracheostomies
- The suspicion that secretions or mucous plugs are responsible for lobar or segmental atelectasis
- The need to remove abnormal endobronchial tissue or foreign material by forceps, basket, or laser
- The need to retrieve a foreign body (although under most circumstances, rigid bronchoscopy is preferred)
- Therapeutic management of endobronchial toilet in ventilator-associated pneumonia
- Achieving selective intubation of a main stem bronchus
- The need to place and/or assess airway stent function
- The need for airway balloon dilation in treatment of tracheobronchial stenosis

Contraindications

Absolute contraindications

- Absence of consent from the patient or his or her representative unless a medical emergency exists and the patient is not competent to give permission
- Absence of an experienced bronchoscopist to perform or closely and directly supervise the procedure
- Lack of adequate facilities and personnel to care for emergencies such as cardiopulmonary arrest, pneumothorax, or bleeding
- Inability to adequately oxygenate the patient during the procedure
- The danger of a serious complication from bronchoscopy is especially high in patients with the disorders listed, and these conditions are usually considered absolute contraindications unless the risk–benefit assessment warrants the procedure:
  - Coagulopathy or bleeding diathesis that cannot be corrected
  - Severe refractory hypoxemia
  - Unstable hemodynamic status, including dysrhythmias

Relative contraindications (or conditions involving increased risk), according to the American Thoracic Society guidelines for fiberoptic bronchoscopy in adults

- Lack of patient cooperation
- Recent (within 6 weeks) myocardial infarction or unstable angina
- Partial tracheal obstruction
- Moderate to severe hypoxemia or any degree of hypercarbia
- Uremia and pulmonary hypertension (possible serious hemorrhage after biopsy)
- Lung abscess (danger of flooding the airway with purulent material)
- Obstruction of the superior vena cava (possibility of bleeding and laryngeal edema)
- Debility and malnutrition
- Disorders requiring laser therapy, biopsy of lesions obstructing large airways, or multiple transbronchial lung biopsies
- Known or suspected pregnancy (safety concern of possible radiation exposure)
- Safety of bronchoscopic procedures in asthmatic patients is a concern, but presence of asthma does not preclude use of these procedures

(continues)

Clinical Practice Guideline 9-1 *(continued)*

- Recent head injury patients susceptible to increased intracranial pressures
- Inability to sedate (including time constraints of oral ingestion of solids or liquids)

Hazards and Complications

- Adverse effects of medication used before and during the bronchoscopic procedure
- Hypoxemia
- Hypercarbia
- Bronchospasm
- Hypotension
- Laryngospasm, bradycardia, or other vagally mediated phenomena
- Mechanical complications such as epistaxis, pneumothorax, and hemoptysis
- Increased airway resistance
- Death
- Infection hazard for healthcare workers or other patients
- Cross-contamination of specimens or bronchoscopes
- Nausea and/or vomiting
- Fever and chills
- Cardiac dysrhythmias

Modified from AARC clinical practice guideline: bronchoscopy assisting—2007 revision and update. *Respir Care.* 2007;52:74–80. Reprinted with permission.

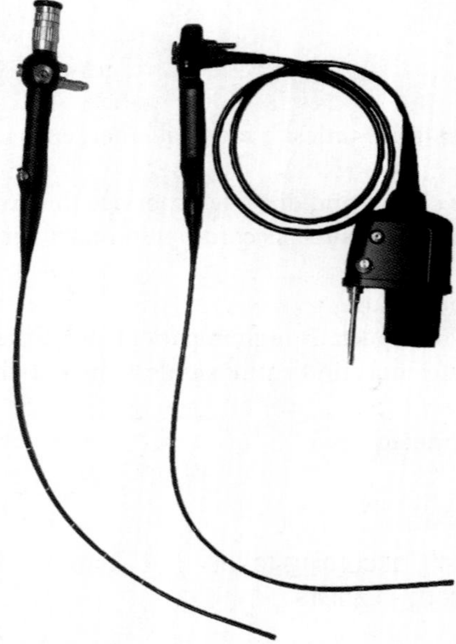

FIGURE 9-1 Flexible fiberoptic (on left) and video chip bronchoscopes.

BOX 9-1

Contraindications to Fiberoptic Bronchoscopy and Transbronchial Biopsy

Absolute

Inability to maintain adequate oxygenation
Operator inexperience
Inadequate facilities
Lack of informed consent
Status asthmaticus

Relative

Active ischemic heart disease
Active cardiac arrhythmia
Refractory hypoxemia
Bleeding diathesis
Uncooperative patient
Active or uncontrolled bronchospasm

severity, such as albuterol use, symptom scoring, and peak flow variation.[5] Bronchoscopy, therefore, should be approached cautiously in the patient with asthma and avoided entirely in the setting of status asthmaticus. In the case of elective bronchoscopy, the procedure should be deferred until bronchospasm is effectively controlled.

Cardiovascular Risk

Fiberoptic bronchoscopy can induce significant hemodynamic changes, including rise in heart rate by 43%, mean arterial pressure by 30%, and cardiac index by 28% when compared with prebronchoscopy controls.[6] Although these changes are well tolerated in a patient with normal cardiovascular function, they can cause significant stress in a patient with underlying heart disease. These hemodynamic changes in combination with episodic oxygen desaturation can lead to an imbalance between myocardial oxygen demand and delivery and precipitate myocardial ischemia, arrhythmias, or both.[7] When possible, patients with active cardiac ischemia or recent myocardial infarction should have their bronchoscopy delayed until their cardiac status is stabilized. The British Thoracic Society's guidelines recommend deferring bronchoscopy a minimum of 6 weeks following myocardial infarction.[8]

Head Trauma and Elevated Intracranial Pressure

Increased intracranial pressure (ICP) has been anecdotally cited as a relative contraindication to bronchoscopy because of concerns that the rise in intrathoracic pressure induced by bronchoscopy-associated cough could abruptly raise ICP and precipitate herniation. A retrospective study found no increase in neurologic complications in patients with space-occupying central nervous system lesions undergoing bronchoscopy, although pretreatment with steroids was recommended to decrease cerebral edema.[9] More recently, a prospective study of 23 patients with intracranial drains in place revealed substantial, though transient, increases in ICP in patients undergoing bronchoscopy, despite adequate levels of sedation, analgesia, and paralysis.[10] No acute deterioration in the patients' clinical status was observed, but, unfortunately, long-term complications or sequelae from these changes remain unknown.[10] Therefore, although fiberoptic bronchoscopy is often necessary in the care of patients after neurologic events, it should be used with caution in this patient population.

Hypoxemia and High Oxygen Requirement

Bronchoscopy carries a higher risk in patients who are hypoxemic at baseline, although determining the cause of hypoxemia is a common indication for bronchoscopy. Unfortunately, hypoxemia is also a complication of bronchoscopy, resulting from sedation-related hypoventilation and ventilation-perfusion mismatch secondary to partial airway occlusion (from the bronchoscope), atelectasis from frequent suctioning, airway bleeding, lavage fluid, and cough.[11] Although there is no absolute amount of supplemental oxygen that is a contraindication for bronchoscopy, caution should be used in patients with high oxygen requirements. Many pulmonologists advocate for elective intubation prior to bronchoscopy in patients with high supplemental oxygen requirements. Severe hypoxemia with Pao_2 less than 65 to 70 mm Hg despite supplemental oxygen therapy is generally considered a contraindication.[12]

Anticoagulant and Antiplatelet Therapy

Use of anticoagulant and antiplatelet agents is common among patients referred for bronchoscopy. Therefore, it is important to carefully review all medications with the patient prior to bronchoscopy and make appropriate recommendations for continuing or holding medications prior to the procedure date.

- *Aspirin.* Aspirin was previously considered a contraindication to bronchoscopy due to its antiplatelet effects and prolongation of bleeding time. However, a large multicenter randomized trial found no difference in bleeding from transbronchial biopsies in the aspirin group compared with the no-aspirin group.[13] Therefore, it is generally accepted that patients can undergo bronchoscopy with transbronchial biopsy without holding aspirin therapy.
- *Clopidogrel.* In contrast to aspirin, clopidogrel significantly increases bleeding risks following transbronchial biopsy. When the effect of clopidogrel on the incidence of bleeding was studied during transbronchial biopsy, significant bleeding rates increased to 89% compared with 3.4% in the control group.[14] In a small number of patients receiving both aspirin and clopidogrel, the incidence of significant bleeding was 100% following transbronchial biopsy.[14] Given the relatively long half-life of clopidogrel, most practices require patients to discontinue clopidogrel a minimum of 5 days prior to undergoing bronchoscopy with transbronchial biopsy.
- *Warfarin and heparin.* No randomized trials exist regarding the use of warfarin in the setting of bronchoscopy. The British Thoracic Society recommends holding warfarin for 3 to 5 days prior to bronchoscopy and/or providing supplemental vitamin K prior to the procedure.[15,16] Laboratory studies should be obtained prior to the procedure to ensure appropriate clearance of anticoagulation effects. Guidelines from the American College of Chest Physicians suggest that an international normalized ratio (INR) of 1.5 is safe for most surgical procedures.[17] In patients who require bridging with therapeutic heparin, consensus statements recommend stopping unfractionated heparin a minimum of 4 to 6 hours prior to the procedure or holding low molecular weight heparin (such as enoxaparin) 24 hours in advance.[17] Heparin and/or warfarin can be resumed 12 to 24 hours after bronchoscopy in the absence of bleeding complications.

Thrombocytopenia

Limited data are available regarding what thresholds for platelets constitute safe levels for bronchoscopy. Transfusion guidelines and expert statements have recommended minimum platelet counts of 20,000 to 50,000/mm^3 for fiberoptic bronchoscopy and greater than 50,000/mm^3 for transbronchial biopsy.[18] When thrombocytopenia is present, an oral route for bronchoscope introduction is preferred to avoid unnecessary epistaxis.

Uremia and Renal Dysfunction

Uremia affects all aspects of platelet function, including secretion, adhesion, and aggregation.[19] No studies specifically examining the effect of uremia on bleeding complications in bronchoscopy currently exist. Some authors have suggested that the use of recombinant arginine vasopressin or desmopressin acetate (DDAVP) may decrease the bleeding time in uremic patients by increasing factor VIII levels and promoting platelet aggregation. The shortening of bleeding time with DDAVP is believed to occur within 1 hour of IV infusion with a dose of 0.3 μg/kg IV and to last up to 6 to 8 hours.[20] The surgical literature reports mixed results in terms of benefit from vasopressin administration in the setting of renal insufficiency. Because of the substantial cost of vasopressin, and in the absence of a large randomized control trial showing clear benefit, its current use remains at the discretion of the physician and the bleeding risks of the individual patient.

Lung transplant recipients have been found to have higher bleeding risks from bronchoscopy independent of traditional risk factors such as coagulation parameters, aspirin use, and renal dysfunction.[21] Many centers are more aggressive about administering vasopressin in lung transplant recipients with coexistent renal insufficiency and have shown this to be beneficial in reducing bleeding complications.[22]

Patient Preparation

Informed Consent

Once the appropriate patient has been selected, informed consent can be obtained. All aspects of the procedure, from the initial application of topical anesthesia to the introduction of the bronchoscope through the nose or mouth, vocal cords, and distal airways, should be explained. The sensations that the patient can anticipate should be described, including the sensation of upper airway closure that is sometimes experienced as topical anesthesia takes effect, pressure in the nose or mouth as the bronchoscope is introduced, and the desire to cough as the bronchoscope is navigated through the airways. Reassurance should be provided about the steps taken to maximize patient comfort throughout the procedure, including the administration of topical anesthesia to alleviate cough and IV sedation as needed.

Procedure Risks and Complications

The risks of bronchoscopy and anesthesia should be specifically reviewed with the patient. The risk of major complications from bronchoscopy, including pneumothorax, pulmonary hemorrhage, infection, and respiratory failure, is 0.6%. When transbronchial biopsy is performed, the risk of serious complications is higher, at 1% to 6%.[23] Minor complications from bronchoscopy include fever, cough, bronchospasm, transient hypoxia, and hemoptysis. Additionally, cardiovascular complications can occur from the stress of the procedure itself, particularly in high-risk patients. Cardiac events can include vasovagal reactions, arrhythmias, myocardial ischemia, angina, and cardiac arrest.[7] The mortality rate from bronchoscopy is approximately 0.01% and has decreased in recent years as monitoring capabilities and technology have improved.[23]

Minimizing Complications

In an effort to minimize aspiration risk, the patient should be kept fasting after midnight prior to a morning procedure. If the procedure is planned for the afternoon, a light liquid breakfast is generally permitted.

Transient hypoxemia has been documented in up to 35% of patients undergoing fiberoptic bronchoscopy but can often be alleviated with the use of supplemental oxygen therapy.[24] Therefore, oxygen supplementation of 2 to 3 L/min is recommended as a preventive measure for all patients undergoing bronchoscopy.[24]

Postprocedure Care and Education

Transient fever has been observed in up to 10% of patients after bronchoscopy and typically resolves within 24 hours. For isolated postprocedure fever, no antibiotic therapy is needed.[25] Additionally, many patients experience a small amount of hemoptysis following bronchoscopy, which gradually subsides over the next 24 hours. Finally, patients receiving procedural sedation should be advised not to drive or operate heavy machinery for 24 hours following the procedure.

Patient Sedation

In one study examining patient perceptions of bronchoscopy, 62% of patients admitted to being anxious and fearful about potential pain, breathing difficulties, and discomfort from the procedure.[26] With careful explanation and reassurance, the physician, nurse, and respiratory therapist can help ease some of these fears. Additionally, use of intravenous sedation can be important in alleviating anxiety, improving patient comfort and cooperation, providing amnestic effects, and facilitating the bronchoscopic procedure.[27] Although bronchoscopy can be performed with topical anesthesia alone, many physicians and patients prefer the judicial use of adjunctive IV sedation.

Procedural sedation is generally used in the outpatient setting, which provides moderate levels of sedation and analgesia with short-acting agents while still maintaining adequate spontaneous ventilation and airway patency. Procedural sedation can only be performed in units where the medical team has had special training, and continuous monitoring and nursing capabilities must be available until the patient has recovered completely.[27]

Many possible sedation regimens are available for bronchoscopy. These regimens can include topical lidocaine for local anesthesia; anticholinergic drugs for reducing secretions and inhibiting vagal tone; codeine for antitussive effects; benzodiazepines for sedation, amnesia, and anxiolysis; and/or opioids for analgesia and cough suppression.[27] **Table 9-1** lists commonly used drugs for fiberoptic bronchoscopy as well as their

TABLE 9-1
Common Pharmacologic Agents Used for Fiberoptic Bronchoscopy

Agent	Dose and Route	Onset	Duration	Effect	Side Effects
Anticholinergic					
Atropine	IM 0.4–1.0 mg	30–60 minutes	Variable	Reduce airway secretions, reduce vagal tone	Tachycardia, tachydysrhythmias, AV dissociation, urinary retention, dry mouth
Local Anesthetics					
Lidocaine	1–10%, topical or inhalation Maximum dose 5–7 mg/kg	5–10 minutes	30–60 minutes	Cough suppression, local anesthesia	Early bronchospasm, dizziness, seizures in high doses; toxic reactions when plasma levels exceed 5 μg/mL
Sedation					
Midazolam	IV 2.5–10.0 mg (0.05–0.075 mg/kg)	1–3 minutes	2 hours	Amnesia, sedation	Respiratory depression
Diazepam	IV 2–7 mg (0.1 mg/kg) PO 5–10 mg	1–3 minutes 15–30 minutes	2–8 hours	Amnesia, sedation	Respiratory depression, thrombophlebitis, pain on injection
Narcotics					
Meperidine	IV/IM 20–75 mg (1 mg/kg)	IV 1–3 minutes, IM 15–30 minutes	2–4 hours	Analgesia	Respiratory depression, nausea
Codeine	IM 20–120 mg	30 minutes	2–4 hours	Cough suppression	Urinary retention
Morphine	IV/IM 2–10 mg (0.1 mg/kg)	IV 5 minutes, IM 15–30 minutes	2–6 hours	Analgesia	Respiratory depression, nausea, itching, bronchospasm, bradycardia, biliary spasm
Fentanyl	IV 50–100 μg (1 μg/kg)	2 minutes	30–60 minutes	Analgesia	Respiratory depression, nausea, chest wall rigidity, bradycardia
Alfentanil	IV 250–1000 μg (10 μg/kg)	1 minute	15–30 minutes	Analgesia	Respiratory depression, nausea, chest wall rigidity
Propofol	IV 50 μg/mg/kg (10–30 mg)	30 seconds	8–10 minutes	Sedation	Respiratory depression, hypotension
Antagonists					
Naloxone	IV 40 μg titrated to effect q 2–3 minutes	1 minute	Dose dependent, lasting 20–60 minutes	Reversal of opioid effect	Tachycardia, hypertension, dysrhythmias
Flumazenil	0.4–1 mg	2 minutes	1 hour	Reversal of benzodiazepine effect	CNS excitation, nausea, residual sedation

AV, atrioventricular; CNS, central nervous system.

Reproduced from Matot I, Kramer MR. Sedation in outpatient bronchoscopy. *Respir Med.* 2000;94:1145–1153, Table 2, with permission from Elsevier.

typical doses, onset, duration of action, therapeutic roles, and side effects. Anticholinergic drugs, such as atropine, were previously considered standard premedications for bronchoscopy given their secretion-drying effects as well as their ability to prevent bradycardia and bronchoconstriction. More recent studies found no increase in bradycardia or excessive secretions when atropine was not used,[28] and many centers have abandoned these agents entirely.

Topical anesthesia is administered immediately prior to the start of the procedure and can be given by a variety of routes. Many agents are available (tetracaine, benzocaine, cocaine, etc.), but lidocaine is the most commonly used because of its wide safety profile and short half-life.[27] An atomizer is often used to spray lidocaine onto the tongue, oropharynx, and pharynx. Lidocaine gel can also be used to lubricate the nose. Alternatively, nebulized lidocaine can be delivered through a face mask to anesthetize the entire airway but takes approximately 20 minutes to administer. Whichever approach is used, careful attention must be given to the total dose of lidocaine delivered before and during the procedure because the serum concentration after topical administration can reach as high as 50% of what would be achieved by IV bolus.[27] The total lidocaine dose should not exceed 5 to 7 mg/kg. This dose should be adjusted downward in patients with significant hepatic or cardiac disease to avoid toxicity or adverse effects.

Entry into the nasopharynx can be facilitated by the application of topical vasoconstrictors such as 4% cocaine or 0.5% phenylephrine, both of which decrease local bleeding and mucosal edema. These can be applied directly into the nose with a cotton-tipped applicator, which can also be used to assess the patency of the nasopharynx and adequacy of topical anesthesia. Once the nasopharynx and/or oropharynx has been adequately anesthetized, additional aliquots (typically 2–3 mL each) of 1% to 2% lidocaine can be applied directly through the bronchoscope during the procedure to the visualized glottis, trachea, carina, and other airways as needed.

In addition to topical agents, IV medications are used both for premedication and sedative effects. Short-acting benzodiazepines, such as midazolam, are commonly used for their amnestic and anxiolytic properties. Although benzodiazepines have few cardiopulmonary effects alone, the risk of respiratory depression is potentiated when used in combination with opioids.[27] Similarly, short-acting opioids, such as fentanyl, can be used for their analgesic effects as well as to decrease the cough reflex and provide modest respiratory depressant effects. When these agents are used, their specific reversal agents (naloxone for narcotics and flumazenil for benzodiazepines) should be readily available.

Propofol is an alternative sedative-hypnotic agent for bronchoscopy given its rapid onset and short duration. It can be used for either procedural sedation or general anesthesia, depending on its dose-dependent sedative effects. Use of propofol often requires a trained anesthesia practitioner, should be reserved for use by experienced administrators, and is not yet approved for procedural sedation in many centers.

Patients should be monitored with telemetry, pulse oximetry, and noninvasive blood pressure measurements throughout the bronchoscopy procedure as well as the recovery period. Additionally, as noted earlier, supplemental oxygen at 2 to 3 L/min should be provided during the procedure to prevent transient hypoxia and weaned appropriately at the conclusion of the procedure. While not yet standard across the country, in 2011 the American Society of Anesthesiologists recommended the adequacy of ventilation should be evaluated by capnography during moderate or deep sedation.[29] Capnography identifies early respiratory compromise, thus reducing frequency of hypoxemia and apnea. Most bronchoscopies are performed on an outpatient basis, and patients are usually safe for discharge within 1 to 2 hours after the procedure. They should be advised not to drive or operate heavy machinery for 24 hours, given the potential for prolonged effects of sedative medications.

Flexible Fiberoptic Bronchoscopy Techniques

Airway Examination

The flexible bronchoscope can be introduced through the nose, mouth, endotracheal tube, or tracheostomy site. The most commonly used approach is transnasal, which is thought to provide more stability (and comfort) by anchoring the scope within the nose and preventing unnecessary fluctuation of the bronchoscope from side to side and interference from the patient's tongue. Either a nasal or oral approach is acceptable, depending on operator preference and patient characteristics. In patients with unfavorable nasal anatomy,

Respiratory Recap

Factors Necessary for Successful Bronchoscopy

- Patient selection
- Patient preparation
- Appropriate sedation

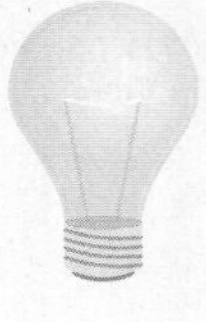

STOP AND THINK

You are about to assist a physician to perform a bronchoscopy. As a respiratory therapist, what would you do to prepare the patient for the procedure?

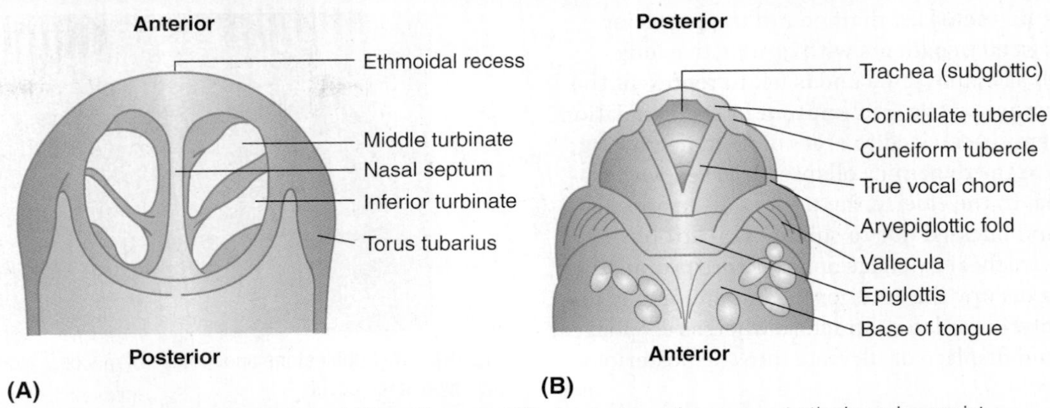

FIGURE 9-2 Normal nasopharyngeal (**A**) and laryngeal (**B**) structures as they appear to the bronchoscopist.

thrombocytopenia, or predilection for sinus infections (e.g., cystic fibrosis), the oral route is often preferred. Many interventional pulmonary procedures require larger bronchoscopes and more equipment, necessitating oral entry. With the oral route, a bite block is used to help anchor the scope and prevent trauma to the bronchoscope from biting. Bronchoscopy via tracheostomy requires a minimum tracheostomy size of 6 mm internal diameter or larger. Similarly, the endotracheal tube must be at least 1.5 mm larger than the bronchoscope (typically 8 mm internal diameter or larger).

The bronchoscope is lubricated with lidocaine gel and introduced under direct visualization into the preanesthetized nare or, alternatively, through a mouthpiece into the posterior hypopharynx. If introducing through a tracheostomy site or endotracheal tube, a medical-grade silicone spray is often necessary for additional lubrication. The nasal and, to a slightly lesser extent, oral approaches allow visualization of the anatomy of the posterior nasopharynx and larynx, including the eustachian tubes, base of the tongue, epiglottis, aryepiglottic folds, and vocal cords (**Figure 9-2**). All approaches allow examination of the trachea, carina, main stem bronchi, and, sequentially, the distal airways to the level of the fourth-order bronchi. A systematic approach to the airway exam is vital for complete evaluation of all upper and lower respiratory tract structures.

The bronchoscopist should pay careful attention to the movement of the vocal cords (**Figure 9-3**) with respiration and phonation to screen for functional as well as structural abnormalities. Paralysis of the left true vocal cord is the most common abnormality seen, which manifests as inability to abduct the left cord. Patients with unilateral vocal cord paralysis are often symptomatic, with laryngospasm or recurrent aspiration.[3] Although sometimes no cause is identified, unilateral vocal cord paralysis, particularly on the left side, can be a sign of malignancy due to compression of the left recurrent laryngeal nerve by a cervical or mediastinal mass (or lymph node) and, in the setting of malignancy, could have important staging implications.[3]

The normal trachea (**Figure 9-4**) has well-defined cartilaginous C-shaped rings along the anterior wall, which serve to maintain airway patency during expiration and cough. The posterior wall consists of a highly organized series of connective tissue and smooth muscle fibers.[3] The shape of the trachea can provide valuable clinical information as well. The scabbard or sabre-sheath trachea, characterized by lateral

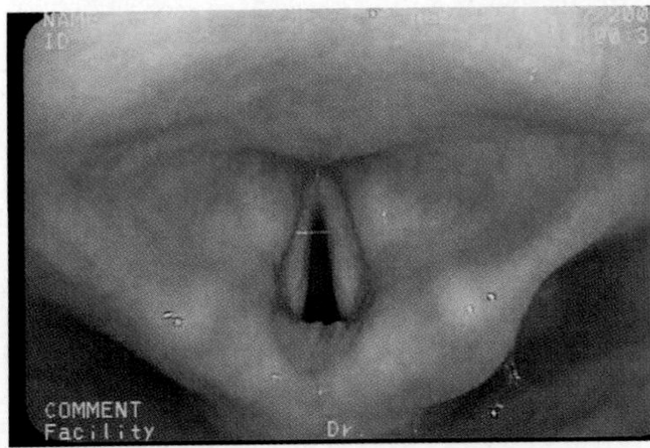

FIGURE 9-3 Normal vocal cord position and appearance.

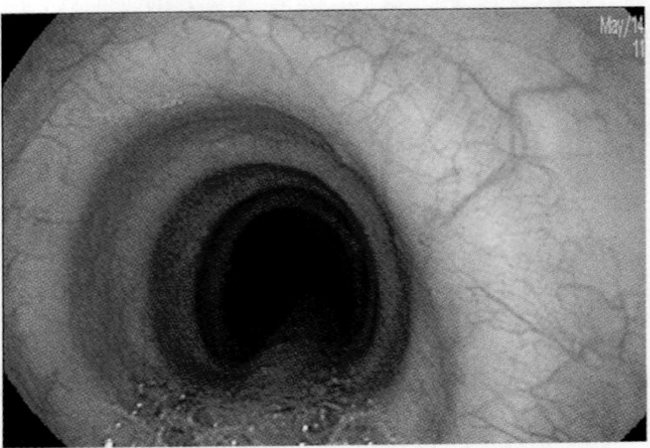

FIGURE 9-4 Normal tracheal anatomy with anterior cartilaginous wall and the posterior membranous wall.

narrowing and increased diameter of the posterior wall, can be seen in patients with obstructive lung disease such as emphysema and is felt to represent the chronic pressure on the trachea from forced exhalation. Tracheal stenosis can lead to areas of fixed narrowing, as opposed to the dynamic collapse observed with tracheomalacia. In the elderly, the trachea often appears elongated and buckled due to submucosal atrophy, making the tracheal cartilage appear more prominent.[30] Masses that occupy the anterior mediastinum may displace the anterior or lateral trachea, whereas esophageal tumors would displace or ulcerate into the posterior trachea.

The site where the trachea divides into the right and left main stem bronchi is termed the *carina*. The normal carina is a sharply angled structure with a smooth mucosal covering (**Figure 9-5**). When the lymph nodes in the subcarinal space become enlarged as a result of infection, inflammation, or malignancy, the carina may develop a splayed or deformed appearance (**Figure 9-6**).

The appearance of the respiratory mucosa can also provide diagnostic clues. For example, an inflamed hypopharynx may represent severe gastroesophageal reflux disease. A characteristic cobblestone appearance is often noted of endobronchial mucosa in sarcoidosis (**Figure 9-7**), and diffuse edema and inflammation are typically seen in chronic bronchitis. In contrast, a focal area of inflamed, friable, or irregular mucosa may represent the presence of submucosal tumor invasion (**Figure 9-8**).

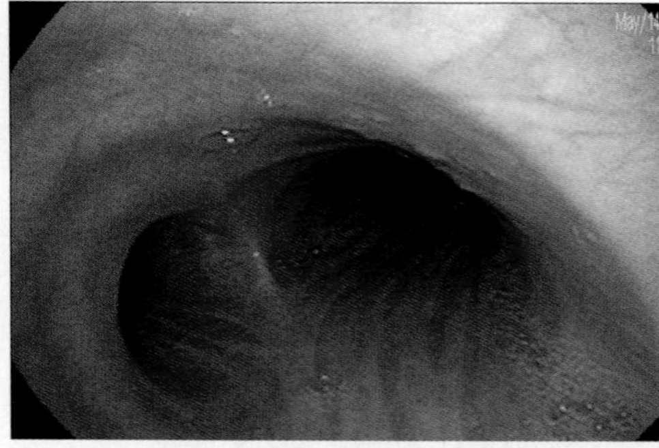

FIGURE 9-5 Normal-appearing main carina with sharply defined bifurcation.

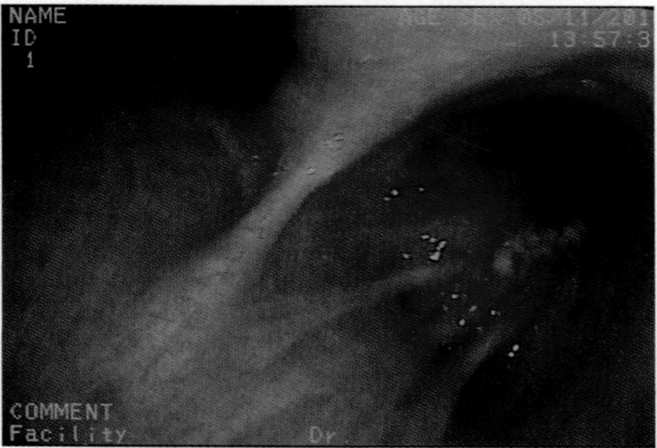

FIGURE 9-6 Tumor infiltrating the proximal right mainstem bronchus.

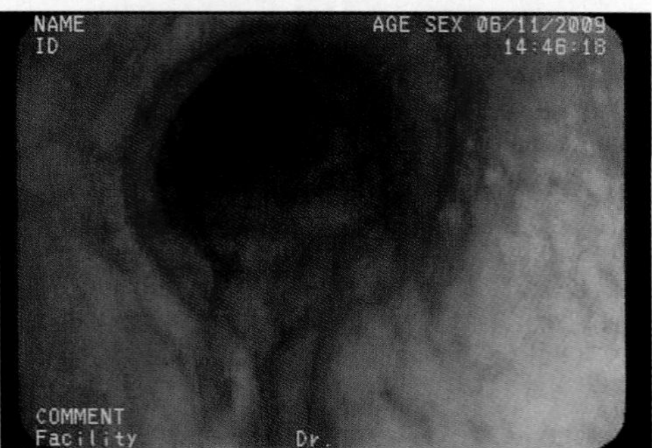

FIGURE 9-7 Cobblestone appearance of mucosa, a characteristic finding in sarcoidosis.

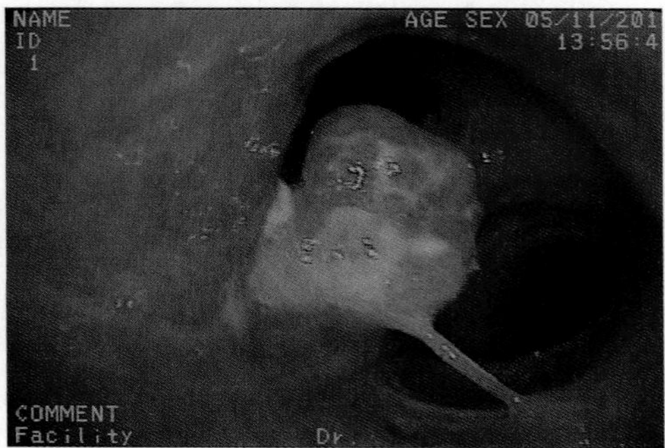

FIGURE 9-8 Endobronchial squamous cell carcinoma arising from the left upper lobe.

After examination of the trachea and carina, the right and left bronchial trees are examined to the subsegmental level. Knowledge of normal endobronchial anatomy and nomenclature is essential for a complete and thorough exam. Each bronchial division is examined to the subsegmental level, with notation made of anatomic variant, mucosal abnormality, presence of endobronchial tumor or secretions, patency of bronchial lumens, and evidence of extrinsic compression. A complete airway exam should almost always precede any other diagnostic maneuvers.

Bronchoalveolar Lavage

Bronchoalveolar lavage (BAL) is the method traditionally used to sample the cellular and microbiologic components of the alveolar space. Although it has been used as a research tool to establish the cellular and biochemical features of several pulmonary diseases such as sarcoidosis, asthma, and interstitial lung disease, its primary use in daily clinical practice is for cytologic and microbiologic sampling. Additionally, BAL can be a tool for pulmonary toilet in rare diseases such as pulmonary alveolar proteinosis by helping to remove the abnormal surfactant material that accumulates with this disease.

Radiographic imaging is frequently used to determine the location for sample collection with the highest yield. The yield of bronchial lavage is generally better from nondependent areas such as anterior segments, the right middle lobe, or lingula. When a specific radiographic abnormality is present, the bronchoscope is directed to the closest correlating subsegmental bronchial lumen for lavage. However, in the presence of diffuse radiographic infiltrates, the right middle lobe or lingula is generally preferred due to the ease of intubation and occlusion so as to maximize return of lavage fluid.

When obtaining a BAL sample, the bronchoscope is advanced as far as possible into a third- or fourth-order bronchus to create a wedge or seal. Room-temperature sterile buffered saline is then introduced, allowed to wash out over the lung, and then retrieved by suction for analysis. The suction pressure is typically maintained below 120 cm H_2O to prevent premature collapse of the bronchus.[3] Some clinicians believe that having the patient hold a large breath also improves the volume of the BAL return.

Lavage amounts and techniques vary among bronchoscopists. The amount of normal saline used for diagnostic BAL should be limited to no more than 200 mL, even though most patients require less than 100 mL for adequate return. Usually, approximately 60% of instilled fluid will be collected on lavage.[3] The most common lavage techniques include manual suction, gravity drainage, and mechanical suction at a moderate negative pressure. Additionally, multiple aliquots can be sequentially introduced before aspiration; alternatively, lavage fluid can be suctioned back after each 20- to 60-mL instillation. Some argue that serial lavage with manual suction produces a greater yield, although few data exist comparing the different bronchoscopic techniques.

If concern for diffuse alveolar hemorrhage (DAH) exists, serial lavage can be helpful for diagnosis because the return will become increasingly bloody as more alveolar fluid is sampled. This technique avoids false positives from scope trauma, in which fluid may initially appear hemorrhagic but will clear with additional aliquots of lavage fluid. Alternatively, DAH should be considered if BAL fluid exhibits more than 20% hemosiderin-laden macrophages on Prussian blue staining.[31]

Complications from bronchoalveolar lavage include hypoxemia and, rarely, bleeding. The incidence of bleeding from BAL in thrombocytopenic patients has been shown to be minimal.[32] Pneumothorax is an extremely rare complication of BAL and has been reported in the literature exclusively in intubated patients.

Bronchoscopic Washing

Bronchoscopic washing is similar to a lavage but is designed to sample the airway rather than the alveolar space. It is commonly used to obtain a cytologic specimen from an endobronchial mass, abnormal mucosa, or an obstructed orifice. When possible, bronchoscopic washing should be used in conjunction with other diagnostic methods such as bronchoscopic brushing or endobronchial biopsy. The timing of the wash, in respect to other procedures, is somewhat controversial. Some bronchoscopists advocate washing a lesion before any other manipulations to avoid contamination of the specimen with blood. Prior to biopsy, washing can also help to assess bleeding risk by evaluating how easily the lesion bleeds with suction alone. Others believe that the best yield for bronchoscopic washing is after biopsy or brushing, believing that more malignant cells may be recovered after the brush or biopsy disrupts the tumor surface. Additionally, bronchoscopic washings can be used when collection of fluid from BAL is inadequate or large amounts of secretions are present in the airway. In this setting, microbiology results can be difficult to interpret because of contamination from upper airway flora.

Similar to BAL, the suction apparatus is fitted with a collection trap reserved for the wash sample alone. The bronchoscope is then placed in close proximity to the lesion while 5- to 10-mL aliquots of sterile buffered saline are introduced and then suctioned back into the collection trap. The sample is then sent to cytology and/or microbiology for processing.

Bronchoscopic Brushing

Two types of brushes are available for **bronchoscopic brushing**. A standard **nonprotected bronchial brush** is used to collect cytologic samples of abnormalities in the proximal airways under direct visualization as well as peripheral lesions under fluoroscopic guidance. A catheter with a brush at its distal end (**Figure 9-9**) is introduced through the working channel of the bronchoscope. This brush may be open or enclosed within an open-ended sheath, which can be advanced and retracted by the assistant at the bronchoscopist's request. Because the sheath is open ended, the brush is not protected from upper airway contamination (within the bronchoscope) but is protected from losing samples when it is withdrawn from the bronchoscope at the conclusion of the procedure.

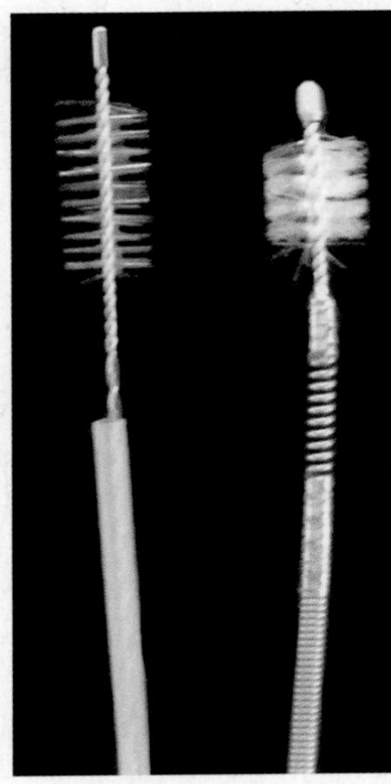

FIGURE 9-9 Instruments used for bronchoscopy. Brushes.

Alternatively, a **protected bronchial brush** is available to collect microbiologic samples (for suspected infection) to ensure that the bacteria collected represent lower-tract pathogens and not upper airway contaminants. The protected specimen brush (PSB) is enclosed within two telescoping catheters, the outer of which is occluded at its tip by a biodegradable plug. This outer catheter protects the catheter tip from contamination as it is advanced through the bronchoscope and the proximal airways.[33] The protected brush is also designed with denser bristles and a more flexible head to maximize secretion recovery. When the area of interest is reached, the plug is dislodged, the inner catheter advanced, and the brush directed into the distal airway through the inner catheter. After the specimen is obtained, the brush is withdrawn into the inner catheter first, followed by the outer catheter, and then withdrawn from the bronchoscope. The outer catheter is cleaned with 70% alcohol and then cut off distal to the inner catheter in sterile fashion. The inner catheter is then advanced, cleaned with alcohol, and cut distal to the brush. Finally, the brush is advanced, cut off, and placed in sterile saline for processing.

With both brushes, the technique for sampling the airway itself is identical. For proximal lesions that are directly visualized, the brush is advanced through the tip of the bronchoscope, placed adjacent to the site of interest, and vigorously advanced back and forth in short strokes. This movement disrupts the mucosa and enables dislodged cells and tissue to become caught within the bristles. The brush is then withdrawn into its sheath and removed from the bronchoscope. For more peripheral lesions, the bronchoscope is advanced to the nearest segmental lumen and then the brush is advanced under fluoroscopic guidance to reach the lesion of interest.

The brush can be processed several ways, depending on the diagnostic goals. For cytologic analysis, including staining for special infections (such as acid-fast bacilli, fungi, *Pneumocystis carinii* pneumonia, or viral inclusions), the contents of the brush can be smeared directly onto glass slides that are then fixed by immediate immersion into 95% alcohol or application of a fixative spray. Alternatively, the entire brush can be placed in a sterile saline solution, vigorously agitated to dislodge its contents, and sent to a laboratory for culture.

Because of the vigorous brushing technique required to obtain samples, brushing does carry a slightly higher risk of bleeding than BAL or bronchial washing. This is particularly true if friable mucosa is being evaluated. In rare instances, pneumothorax can occur, particularly if very peripheral lesions are being sampled.

Endobronchial Biopsy

Endobronchial biopsy is the method used to sample abnormalities directly visualized within the airway, including visible tumors (**Figure 9-10**) or mucosal irregularities. A variety of tools are available, including cupped-tip forceps with a cutting edge, alligator forceps with a toothed jaw, and needle forceps with a sharp prong positioned between the jaws that can be used to help position the forceps over the area of interest.[2] Forceps with a central needle are particularly useful in obtaining biopsies from flat endobronchial lesions in the trachea or main stem bronchi, or when significant flexion of the bronchoscope is required.[2] Generally, the choice of forceps depends on operator preference.

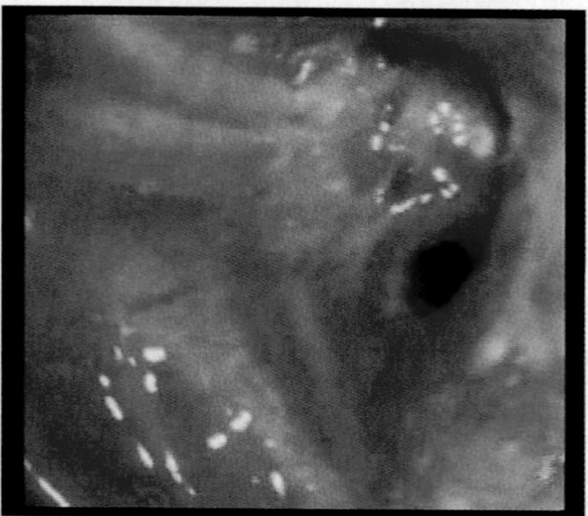

FIGURE 9-10 Endobronchial obstruction.

When the biopsy area has been identified, the forceps (**Figure 9-11**) are advanced through the working channel of the bronchoscope in the closed position. Once the forceps have been completely visualized within the airway lumen, the jaws can be opened and positioned directly over the lesion of interest. The bronchoscopist will then direct the assistant to close the jaws of the forceps, and the closed forceps and sample are removed together through the working channel of the bronchoscope. The sample is then dislodged from the forceps and placed in the appropriate medium for processing (formalin for histology, sterile saline for microbiologic culture). Multiple biopsy samples (three

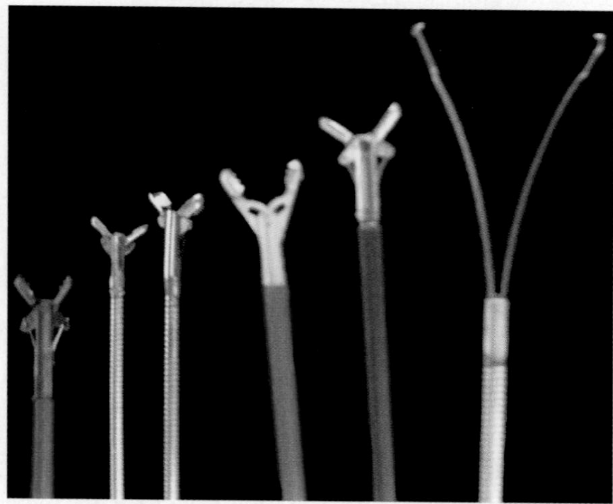

FIGURE 9-11 Instruments used for bronchoscopy. Biopsy forceps.

to six) should be obtained to maximize yield, particularly in the setting of an exophytic endobronchial mass, due to the common presence of surface necrosis and inflammation, which may otherwise preclude an actual pathologic diagnosis.[34] The major complication of endobronchial biopsy is bleeding.

Transbronchial Biopsy

Transbronchial biopsy (TBB) is used to collect small samples of lung tissue for histopathologic review. Careful study of a prebronchoscopy computed tomography (CT) scan is useful in determining the best pulmonary segment to access for biopsy. In diffuse pulmonary diseases, use of fluoroscopy is not necessary, although the risk of significant pneumothorax may be reduced. In focal disease that is visible on chest x-ray, use of fluoroscopy during the procedure may significantly increase the diagnostic yield of the study.

More recent diagnostic tools for peripheral pulmonary lesions include radial endobronchoscopic ultrasound (R-EBUS) and electromagnetic navigation. A R-EBUS probe provides a 360-degree ultrasonographic image of structures surrounding an airway via a transducer housed at the end of the probe introduced through the working channel and advanced to the desired location, providing confirmation of the location for sampling a peripheral nodule. A meta-analysis found the pooled sensitivity and specificity for R-EBUS detecting lung cancer in a peripheral lesion to be 73% and 100%, respectively.[35] Electromagnetic navigation allows use of a high-resolution CT scan of the chest to guide an endobronchial probe to a nodule of interest to permit histologic sampling. Preliminary data suggest yields of 67% for lesions smaller than 2 cm in diameter, far superior to yields with fluoroscopically guided techniques.[36] Addition of a radial endobronchial ultrasound probe in combination with the electromagnetic system enhances yield to 88%.[37] As promising as these new techniques are, further data are needed to establish their efficacy before they are widely accepted into general pulmonary practice.

After a careful airway examination, the pulmonary segment of interest is intubated with the tip of the bronchoscope, and the pulmonary forceps are passed through the working channel of the bronchoscope. As the forceps are visualized entering the pulmonary subsegment, the fluoroscopy unit should be activated to visualize the forceps as they enter the distal segments of the lung. To take a biopsy of peripheral portions of the lung, the forceps should be gently advanced in the closed position until resistance is encountered. If fluoroscopy is used, the forceps may not appear to move very far within the lung if the direction of motion is within the plane of imaging due to the two-dimensional nature of fluoroscopic imaging. If the fluoroscopy unit is equipped with a C-arm, the camera head may be rotated out of plane from the forceps to detect movement in the anterior-posterior direction relative to the patient. Next, the forceps are withdrawn approximately 1 cm, and the command is given to open the forceps' jaws. The forceps are then advanced close to the area where resistance was encountered, and the forceps jaws are closed. With the fluoroscopy unit still activated, the forceps are retracted with firm, continuous pressure to allow the biopsy specimen to be removed from the surrounding lung parenchyma. The lung parenchyma should be watched on the fluoroscopy monitor for retraction during the collection of the biopsy sample. If there is excessive resistance or extensive retraction of the lung parenchyma during sampling, the forceps should be opened to release the lung tissue, and the biopsy procedure should be restarted. Once a sample is obtained, the forceps are removed from the working channel of the bronchoscope and the biopsy is placed in formalin.

Two schools of thought exist as to how best to manage the airway after a biopsy sample is collected. One school advocates use of the wedge technique, in which the tip of the bronchoscope is lodged firmly (wedge position) in the airway subsegment that was sampled to monitor for bleeding. It is thought that leaving the bronchoscope wedged permits control of potential bleeding by continuous suctioning to remove extravasated blood, thereby preventing soiling of the remainder of the lung. Continuous suctioning also allows the operator to assess the quantity of bleeding present, and collapsing the distal airways (with suction) produces a tamponade effect. When bleeding has slowed, the tip of the bronchoscope may be slowly withdrawn from the wedge position to allow observations of the bleeding segment and, if necessary, to facilitate repeating the wedge maneuver if the bleeding continues to be significant. The disadvantage of the wedge maneuver is that the bronchoscopist is not able either to visualize the airways due to blood obscuring the optics of the bronchoscope or to assess the effectiveness of the wedge in isolating the bleeding subsegment.

In the alternative strategy, the tip of the bronchoscope is withdrawn from the subsegment of interest so that the bronchoscopist can watch for welling up of blood from the distal lung. Blood is suctioned with a back-and-forth motion to clear the airway and maintain vision. This suctioning permits a more global assessment of the extent of bleeding and potential seepage of blood into the other portions of the lung. There are currently no data to support the superiority of either approach. One practice is to have novice bronchoscopists maintain a wedge after each biopsy and use the observational technique after they have acquired more experience with the bronchoscope.

Several studies have examined how best to enhance biopsy yield in terms of number of samples to be collected and characteristics of the collected specimens. Most studies report a range of 4 to 10 pieces of tissue to optimize sampling sensitivity.[38–40] The British Thoracic Society's guidelines on flexible bronchoscopy recommend 4 to 6 samples in patients with diffuse lung disease and 7 to 8 in patients with focal lung disease.[8] Our practice is to obtain a minimum of 6 tissue pieces of a minimum size of 1 to 2 mm in the long axis for patients with either focal or diffuse lung disease.

Several studies have examined the optimal size of biopsy forceps for performing TBB. No clear difference has been established regarding size of tissue samples or diagnostic sensitivity between large and small forceps, although one study using large, alligator-type forceps showed lower yields compared with large or small forceps. The lower yield was attributed to difficulty in passing the larger forceps past the various subcarinae of the small airways.[41,42] A third study examined the size and quality of tissue samples obtained using a small round-cup, medium oval-cup, or large round-cup forceps. Tissue sample sizes were equal using the medium or large forceps, and larger in size than those obtained with the small forceps. The quality of samples was greater using the oval forceps, revealing less crush artifact and more intact basement membrane on pathologic analysis.[43]

An additional study examined the ability of physicians to predict the quality of TBB at the time of bronchoscopy. The authors found no significance of floating of the tissue sample in formalin (suggesting alveolated tissue) and no ability of the physicians to predict the quality of the sample at the time the specimen was obtained. The authors did find that alligator forceps obtained larger samples when compared with cup-type forceps of a similar size (3 mm), although the samples were graded for size using a technician's observation as the assessment tool (as opposed to the microscopic measurement used in the other studies described earlier).[44] Our practice is to use medium-sized oval-cup forceps for all of our TBBs because they do not entirely occlude the working channel of the bronchoscope while the forceps are extended, thereby permitting continued use of the working channel for suctioning. Larger forceps show no clear advantage in biopsy quality but do preclude effective suctioning while they are deployed.

Following bronchoscopy with TBB, patients should be observed in a recovery unit, similar to other patients receiving procedural sedation. Given the increased risk of hemorrhage with TBB, outpatients should continue to hold their anticoagulant or antiplatelet agents until the morning after the procedure. Inpatients may resume anticoagulants such as heparin or enoxaparin 12 hours after the procedure.

Transbronchial Needle Aspiration

Transbronchial needle aspiration (TBNA) is a simple and safe procedure that can provide useful diagnostic information in benign and malignant conditions. It is used to evaluate mediastinal and hilar lymphadenopathy, exophytic endobronchial disease, and submucosal disease as well as extrinsic compression of the proximal airways.[45]

For endobronchial disease, the ability of TBNA to bypass surface necrosis and sample viable tumor from deeper within the mass can significantly increase bronchoscopic yield. The sensitivity of TBNA in exophytic mass lesions has been reported to be from 65% to 92% alone, and one study noted an increase in yield from 65% to 96% when TBNA was combined with other conventional methods.[34]

Successful TBNA in lymph node evaluation can provide important diagnostic as well as staging information. Until recently, surgical procedures, including mediastinoscopy, thoracotomy, and video-assisted thoracoscopy, have been the preferred methods for sampling hilar and mediastinal lymphadenopathy. In contrast to bronchoscopy, surgery is more invasive, carries higher risk, and requires general anesthesia. Recent advances in TBNA techniques, including rapid on-site cytologic evaluation, the use of 19-gauge needles for performing core biopsies, and the availability of endobronchial ultrasound (EBUS) guidance, have significantly increased the diagnostic yield of this procedure.[43] Several studies have now documented reduced need for surgical procedures with the use of TBNA, both with and without EBUS guidance.[46,47]

The sensitivity of TBNA for mediastinal lymphadenopathy varies from 15% to 85% and depends largely on lymph node location, size, operator experience, needle type, and number of aspirates obtained.[48] TBNA has a higher yield in malignancy (compared with benign conditions), as well as in small cell lung cancer (SCLC) compared with non–small-cell lung cancer (NSCLC). Other predictors of positive aspirates include increased lymph node size, subcarinal or right tracheobronchial position, visible mucosal abnormalities, and exophytic endobronchial lesions.[49]

Herth et al. reported an overall diagnostic yield of 80% using EBUS-guided TBNA, compared with 71% with conventional TBNA techniques. Although results were similar at the subcarinal location, the diagnostic yield significantly increased (from 58% to 84%) with EBUS guidance in all other stations.[50] EBUS-guided TBNA is now being used with increasing frequency to not only diagnose but also simultaneously stage lung cancer. Mediastinoscopy, previously considered the gold standard to stage the mediastinum, is an invasive surgical procedure requiring general anesthesia, with its associated costs, surgical morbidities, and usually postoperative admission.[51] Furthermore, mediastinoscopy cannot reach the posterior and hilar lymph node stations accessible to EBUS, limiting complete staging evaluation. When compared to mediastinoscopy, EBUS-TBNA has increased sensitivity, specificity, negative predictive value, and positive predictive value.[52–55] Currently, the availability of EBUS guidance is limited to select centers because of its additional training requirements and equipment needs.

The diagnostic yield of TBNA can be enhanced by the on-site assessment of bronchoscopy specimens by cytopathologists. In one study, the diagnostic yield for malignancy was increased from 50% to 81% with the addition of rapid on-site cytologic evaluation (ROSE).[56] Additionally, ROSE can allow additional biopsy passes to be deferred without any loss in diagnostic yield, likely reducing procedural complications and overall costs.[57]

There is no clear consensus regarding the number of biopsy passes needed to establish a diagnosis. Diacon et al.[49] reported diagnosis with the first, second, third, and fourth needle pass at 64%, 87%, 95%, and 98%, respectively, and ultimately concluded that three passes is adequate when only tissue diagnosis is needed or when TBNA is combined with other modalities. For isolated lymph node aspiration in the setting of cancer staging, a minimum of four to five biopsies should be obtained. Similarly, Chin et al. demonstrated a plateau effect in diagnostic yield by the seventh biopsy, with all positive results obtained in seven or fewer biopsies.[58]

TBNA should be obtained before other procedures, such as endobronchial or transbronchial biopsies or brushings, to prevent contamination of the area causing false-positive results. The aspiration needle is available in 19-, 20-, 21-, and 22-gauge sizes and is used to obtain cytologic specimens.[59] The apparatus (**Figure 9-12**) consists of a long, flexible plastic catheter or sheath with a needle retracted within the tubing and controlled by a metal spring.

When the site of interest is located, the sheathed needle can be passed through the working channel of the bronchoscope. Once the tip of the sheath is visualized within the bronchial lumen, the needle can be exposed and subsequently inserted into the intercartilaginous space adjacent to the lymph node targeted for aspiration.[3] Caution must be used to avoid deployment of the needle within the bronchoscope because this can cause

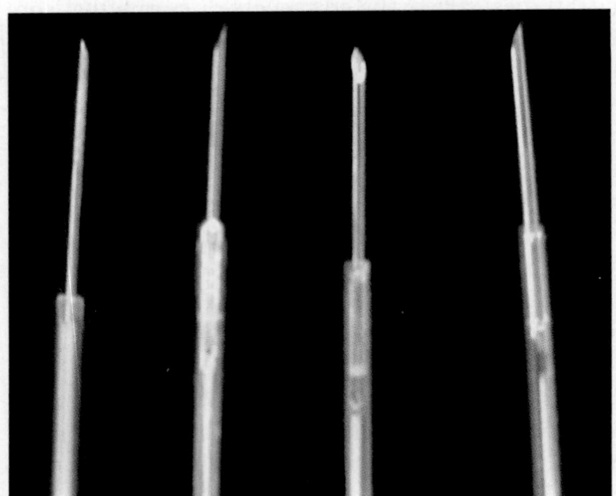

FIGURE 9-12 Instruments used for bronchoscopy. Needles.

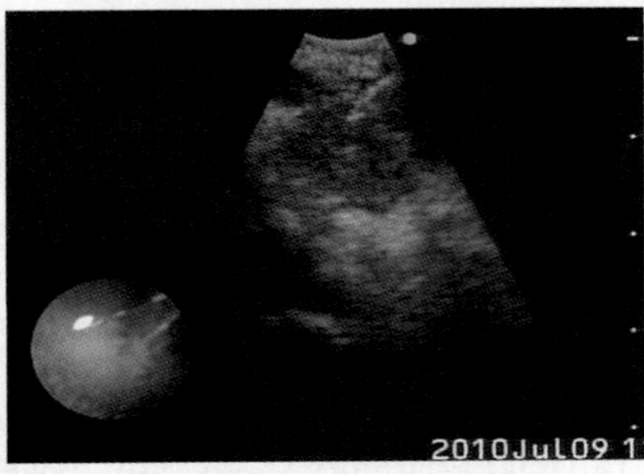

FIGURE 9-13 Ultrasonographic view of transbronchial needle aspiration of a paratracheal lymph node. The visible light image of the needle catheter against the airway wall is shown on the inset.

significant damage to the bronchoscope itself. Once the needle has been completely inserted into the tissue (**Figure 9-13**), an assistant applies suction at the proximal end of the catheter. Typically, a 20- to 60-mL syringe is attached to the proximal end of the bronchoscope, and the plunger is withdrawn to create negative suction.

If no resistance is felt when the syringe plunger is withdrawn, the needle is not adequately fixed in tissue and should be repositioned under direct visualization. Alternatively, aspiration of blood with negative pressure indicates inadvertent cannulation of a blood vessel and should result in removal of the needle, retraction of the needle in the sheath under direct endoscopic guidance, and observation of the site. Notably, vessel puncture during TBNA procedures rarely results in significant bleeding, because of the small gauge of the needles used. If blood is obtained on aspiration, the catheter should be withdrawn from the bronchoscope and flushed before subsequent aspiration attempts because the presence of blood may obscure further cytologic diagnosis. If no blood is aspirated, then suction should be maintained for 1 to 2 minutes as the needle is gently advanced back and forth to maximize recovery of cells.[3] After the sample is obtained, the needle is removed from the aspiration site, retracted into the catheter under direct visualization, and then withdrawn from the bronchoscope. The sample is recovered by flushing the catheter/needle apparatus with saline. Cytologic sampling by TBNA has inherent limitations. False-positive results can be obtained if malignant cells from the tracheobronchial tree contaminate the tip of the bronchoscope, particularly if the primary malignancy is close in proximity to the biopsy site, or other maneuvers, including airway exam, are conducted prior to TBNA. Additionally, site contamination (and false positives) can occur from secretions that have migrated into the proximal airways with coughing. False-negative results can also occur as a result of the small sample size and the blind nature of the technique.

The bleeding at the site of needle puncture is usually negligible. Hemomediastinum, pneumothorax, pneumomediastinum, and bacteremia have been reported in sporadic cases.[3]

Complications of Bronchoscopy

Pneumothorax

Pneumothorax occurs in 1% to 6% of patients undergoing TBB.[23,60] Symptoms include chest pain, hemoptysis, and shortness of breath after the procedure. The need for chest radiography after TBB is controversial. In a single study examining the incidence of pneumothorax after TBB, pneumothorax was identified in 10 of 259 non–lung transplant patients, 7 of whom developed symptoms suggestive of pneumothorax. The 3 patients who were asymptomatic had small pneumothoraces that did not require additional intervention, whereas 4 of 7 symptomatic patients had large pneumothoraces that required chest tube insertion. Severity of symptoms coincided with the size of the pneumothorax. The authors concluded that routine radiography is not necessary after TBB in patients who are able to describe symptoms after biopsy.[60] The use of fluoroscopy during TBB has not been shown to reduce risk of pneumothorax,[8] although a survey of 328 chest physicians in the United Kingdom showed a significantly lower incidence of reported pneumothorax requiring chest tube drainage in the past year for those who routinely used fluoroscopy.[61] No significant difference in the number of pneumothoraces was noted between the two groups (0.86% vs. 1.15%).

Bleeding Complications

Significant hemorrhage, defined as more than 50 mL of blood, is observed in 2% to 9% of patients undergoing TBB. No randomized studies have been published on the optimal management of hemorrhage related to TBB, although recognized experts have proposed several recommendations. Zavala first described the wedge technique in 1976, whereby the tip of the bronchoscope is placed within the subsegment that is being biopsied. The forceps used for the biopsy are passed through the working channel of the bronchoscope and extended into the subsegment, and the biopsy obtained. Afterward, the forceps are removed and the bronchoscope is left in position to isolate the subsegment and prevent the seepage of blood into the remainder of the bronchial tree. Blood is suctioned for a recommended period of 5 minutes to permit clotting, and the bronchoscope is cautiously withdrawn from the subsegment so that it can be observed for further bleeding.[12] As noted previously, no data exist to suggest that the wedge technique decreases significant bleeding or related complications.

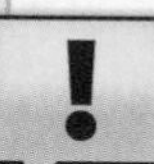

Respiratory Recap

Fiberoptic Bronchoscopy Techniques

- Airway examination
- Bronchoalveolar lavage
- Bronchoscopic washing
- Bronchial brushing
- Endobronchial biopsy
- Transbronchial lung biopsy
- Transbronchial needle aspiration

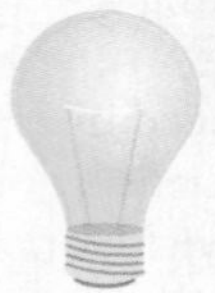

STOP AND THINK

You are caring for a patient who just had a bronchoscopic procedure. For what complications should you be aware?

Additional therapeutic modalities that have been suggested include the use of iced saline administered via the working channel of the bronchoscope placed in the wedge position. Our practice is to give a 20-mL bolus of iced saline and withhold suctioning for several minutes to allow the cold fluid to induce local vasoconstriction. If the first bolus is unsuccessful, the fluid is suctioned and a second bolus is administered, repeating the observation period for several minutes. If this process is unsuccessful in controlling bleeding, 20 mL of 1:20,000 epinephrine is administered, and the patient is placed with the hemorrhaging lung down to prevent soiling of the uninvolved lung.[8] Using these measures, the majority of hemorrhages related to TBB will be controlled. Occasionally, the bleeding may be severe enough to require placement of an endobronchial blocker.

Indications for Bronchoscopy

Acute Lung Collapse, Atelectasis, and Secretion Management

The use of bronchoscopy for acute atelectasis, lobar collapse, and clearance of retained secretions is common, particularly in the intensive care unit (ICU), although there has been very little research dedicated to the safety and utility of bronchoscopy in this clinical setting. Studies have reported success rates ranging from 19% to 89%.[62] When compared with bronchoscopy for subsegmental atelectasis or retained secretions alone, bronchoscopy for lobar collapse seems to be more beneficial, likely due to the presence of large central plugs that are easily accessible by the bronchoscope. Some studies indicate that the adjunctive use of bronchoalveolar lavage may be helpful in clearing more distal mucous plugs. Notably, the presence of an air bronchogram, suggesting a more distal obstruction, is considered a predictor of delayed resolution of the collapse, independent of the treatment interventions used.[63]

Practice opinions vary regarding when to use bronchoscopy instead of conservative therapy alone. In one study comparing bronchoscopy followed by chest physiotherapy with chest physiotherapy alone for acute atelectasis, Marini et al. observed no difference in improvement between the two groups.[63] Many other new tools are available for conservative management of secretions and atelectasis in addition to chest physiotherapy, including kinetic beds, mucolytic agents, percussion vests, and mechanical vibration therapy with handheld devices such as flutter valves.[62] The efficacy of most of these tools has not been formally compared with bronchoscopy. In general, conservative management should be tried first, particularly in patients with modest oxygen requirements who are able to cooperate with therapy. For selected patients in whom conservative management has failed, as well as those with rapidly progressive respiratory failure or distorted airway anatomy, bronchoscopy may have a role.

Hemoptysis

The role of bronchoscopy in the patient with hemoptysis remains controversial. Unfortunately, many of the studies designed to clarify bronchoscopy's role in this setting have been small cohort studies, with results that vary dramatically depending on geographic location, time of publication, and diagnostic studies available.[64] It, therefore, has been difficult to develop consensus recommendations for management of hemoptysis, and practice patterns vary widely.

Indications for bronchoscopy in hemoptysis include identifying the cause of bleeding, localizing the bleeding source, and evaluating for endobronchial malignancy. In massive or persistent hemoptysis, localizing the bleeding source can be helpful in planning surgical intervention or vascular embolization procedures. The most common reason for bronchoscopy in the setting of hemoptysis is for diagnosis of suspected malignancy.

The yield of bronchoscopy for diagnosing malignancy is highest when the chest radiograph is abnormal.[65] Approximately 5% to 6% of patients presenting with hemoptysis and a normal chest radiograph are found to have an endobronchial malignancy.[66] Hemoptysis can be the only clue to localized and potentially resectable disease. Screening airway exams for hemoptysis are widely performed, particularly in patients with other risk factors for malignancy.[67] The factors associated with the highest yield for lung cancer on bronchoscopy include significant smoking history (>40 pack years), male sex, and age greater than 40 years.[67] Other factors, including severity of bleeding, persistent hemoptysis for more than 1 week, and prior episodes of hemoptysis, have not been shown to correlate directly with risk of malignancy.[68]

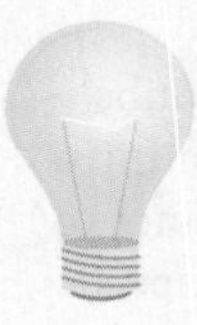

STOP AND THINK

You are caring for a patient who is having difficulty with airway clearance. What therapies would you recommend ahead of bronchoscopy?

Bronchoscopy can also be useful in massive or life-threatening hemoptysis. In this setting, bronchoscopy is used primarily to assist efforts to maintain ventilation. Rigid bronchoscopy is often preferred because of its superior suctioning and ventilation capabilities.[69] Rigid bronchoscopy does require general anesthesia and access to an operating room, however, which can limit its utility in emergency settings. Flexible bronchoscopy is more readily available, but limited in its ability to rapidly suction blood and prevent obstruction of visibility from blood. When flexible bronchoscopy is used, endotracheal intubation should be performed first to secure the airway, facilitate selective intubation to protect the nonbleeding lung, and allow for repeated reintroduction of the bronchoscope should vision become obscured by blood. Bronchoscopy can then be used to direct endobronchial blockade maneuvers to isolate bleeding from other areas of the lung, as well as to guide the endotracheal tube into the main stem bronchus for protective ventilation strategies.[69]

Cough

Chronic cough is a common problem that can be very bothersome for patients. Asthma, postnasal drip/allergic rhinitis, and gastroesophageal reflux disease remain the most common etiologies for chronic cough. Diagnostic workup often includes pulmonary function testing, methacholine challenge, chest radiograph, empiric reflux treatment, 24-hour pH probe (to assess for silent reflux), allergy evaluation, and/or sinus CT, depending on patient history. Prior studies suggest that a diagnosis will be achieved in close to 100% of chronic cough patients when worked up systematically by a set algorithm or protocol screening for common conditions.[70] If cough persists despite aggressive workup and empiric treatment, bronchoscopy should be considered.

The largest study of bronchoscopy in refractory cough consisted of 82 patients referred from a dedicated specialty cough clinic. In this study, 11% of subjects received a diagnosis based on bronchoscopic findings. These diagnoses included tracheal or upper airway abnormalities and tracheal malformations such as tracheobronchopathia osteochondroplastica, stenosis, and broncholithiasis.[70] Ultimately, the authors agreed that bronchoscopy does have a role in chronic cough evaluation but should be reserved for patients who elude diagnosis despite extensive workup.

Suspected Malignancy

Bronchoscopy has a variety of roles in the evaluation of suspected malignancy. An airway exam can be used to evaluate for the presence of endobronchial tumor, particularly when the possibility of obstruction is suggested on the radiograph by volume loss, hyperinflation, or recurrent or unresolving pneumonitis. Similarly, the presence of a localized wheeze, hemoptysis, or chronic cough can be due to endobronchial disease. In these settings, bronchoscopy is often used to evaluate for malignancy, even in the absence of a clear mass on chest radiograph. A careful airway exam will also include evaluation for oropharyngeal or nasopharyngeal lesions and vocal cord paralysis, which can be a sign of recurrent laryngeal nerve entrapment by bulky mediastinal disease.

Bronchoscopy is commonly used to evaluate specific lesions noted on chest radiograph or computed tomography. The diagnostic yield for suspected malignancy is highly dependent on the location of the tumor as well as the sampling technique used. The sensitivity of bronchoscopy for evaluating central lesions has been documented to be as high as 71%, compared with 49% for more peripheral lesions.[71] Adequate sampling of peripheral nodules is more difficult and relies on the ability to visualize the lesion fluoroscopically during the procedure as well as on accessibility from a nearby bronchus.[72] Overall, the diagnostic yield of bronchoscopy for detection of proven malignancy has been reported to be as high as 75% and up to 92% in macroscopically visible endobronchial lesions.[73]

For endobronchial disease, the highest sensitivity is seen with endobronchial biopsy (74%), followed by brushing for cytology (59%), and washing (49%). When all modalities are combined, sensitivity can reach as high as 88%.[71] In contrast, for peripheral lesions, brushing demonstrated the highest sensitivity (52%), followed by transbronchial biopsy (46%) and BAL/washing (43%), with a combined sensitivity of 69% when all modalities were used.[71] The diagnostic yield was significantly less for peripheral lesions smaller than 2 cm in diameter (33%) compared with larger lesions (62%).[71]

Although less commonly used, transbronchial needle aspiration can also be helpful in evaluating endobronchial disease due to the prevalence of submucosal involvement. Even in visible endobronchial tumor, endobronchial biopsy results can be nondiagnostic due to the presence of surface necrosis and inflammation.[34] The ability of TBNA to bypass surface necrosis and sample viable tumor from deeper within the mass can increase the diagnostic yield of the bronchoscopy. The sensitivity of TBNA in exophytic mass lesions has been reported to be from 65% to 92% alone, and one study noted an increase in yield from 65% to 96% when added to other conventional methods.[34]

In addition to discreet masses, bronchoscopy can be helpful in evaluating mediastinal and hilar lymphadenopathy in both undiagnosed and known malignancy. Many lymph nodes, particularly in subcarinal and hilar regions, are easily accessible by bronchoscopy because of their location just beyond the tracheal or bronchial wall. The ability to sample lymph nodes has greatly enhanced the role of bronchoscopy in cancer staging, and it is now possible to provide patients with diagnosis and staging information from a single procedure. The benefits of TBNA and EBUS to diagnose and stage lung cancer are described above under transbronchial needle aspiration.

Infection

Bronchoscopy is used in infection to help define the causative microbiological organism. It can also be helpful to rule out infection in the setting of other lung processes. Initially, bronchoscopy had little to offer as a diagnostic tool for pulmonary infection because of contamination of the instrument during passage through the upper airways. The development of protected catheters and quantitative cultures has significantly increased the utility of bronchoscopy in this setting.[74] Nonetheless, the yield of bronchoscopy in the diagnosis of pneumonia remains directly related to the immune status of the host, the index of suspicion for associated endobronchial disease based on radiographic findings, and the specific techniques used to obtain and process the sample. Although it has been shown to be very helpful in immunocompromised patients, its indication in the immunocompetent host is less clear.

The role of bronchoscopy in community-acquired pneumonia (CAP), particularly in the immunocompetent host, remains uncertain. According to most guidelines, testing for microbial diagnosis in outpatients with CAP is optional because these patients almost always respond to empiric antibiotics (such as a macrolide or fluoroquinolone), and isolation of an organism might not lead to changes in management. Testing for microbial diagnosis is always recommended in patients who require hospitalization, have comorbid conditions, or have risk factors for more resistant pathogens.

In a study of 262 patients hospitalized with CAP, a microbial diagnosis was achieved in only 60% of cases, using routine measures such as blood and sputum cultures, urine serologic detection for *Legionella* and pneumococcal antigens, and selective bronchoscopy.[75] Bronchoscopy was reserved for patients who did not expectorate sputum within 24 hours or patients with treatment failure 72 hours after antibiotic administration. In these cases, bronchoscopy provided microbial diagnosis in 49% of patients who did not expectorate sputum within 24 hours and 52% of patients presenting with treatment failure 72 hours after antibiotic administration. Bronchoscopy provided an additional diagnosis, not detected by other methods, in 25% of patients. These results were validated by Ortqvist et al., who reported obtaining a diagnosis with fiberoptic bronchoscopy in 54% of patients with antibiotic treatment failure.[74]

Therefore, although bronchoscopy should not be routinely used for microbial diagnosis in community-acquired pneumonia, it offers a reasonable adjunct to other forms of testing and can be helpful in hospitalized patients not responding to treatment, particularly those who are severely ill, are immunocompromised, or require ICU care. Additionally, it is useful for patients who are unable to produce sputum samples and any patients with treatment failure, especially if suspicion of anatomic obstruction is considered. Interestingly, the presence of prior or ongoing antibiotic therapy did not appear to influence the bronchoscopic yield, because microbial diagnosis was obtained in 54% of patients with treatment failure.

Pulmonary infections account for significant morbidity and mortality in immunocompromised patients. It is important, therefore, to quickly identify the cause of lung infiltrates in these patients and institute specific treatment. Unfortunately, many infectious and noninfectious diseases can present with similar clinical and radiologic features in immunocompromised patients. The etiology of immunosuppression (HIV, malignancy, drug induced, rheumatologic) should also be considered when constructing a differential diagnosis. In general, common infections in immunocompromised patients include bacterial pneumonia, cytomegalovirus, *Legionella*, aspergillosis, *Pneumocystis carinii* (PCP), and tuberculosis. Other possibilities for pulmonary infiltrates in these patients can include diffuse alveolar hemorrhage, nonspecific interstitial pneumonitis (NSIP), drug-induced pneumonitis, radiation pneumonitis, congestive heart failure, and diffuse alveolar damage or acute respiratory distress syndrome (ARDS).[76] Flexible bronchoscopy was more likely to provide definitive diagnosis when infiltrate was due to infection (81%) than to a noninfectious etiology (56%).

In one study of 104 immunocompromised patients with pulmonary infiltrates, fiberoptic bronchoscopy was the primary source of diagnosis in 78% of patients; notably, all but one of these patients was receiving antibiotics at the time of bronchoscopy.[76] Additionally, similar to bronchoscopy for suspected malignancy, when multiple diagnostic modalities (BAL, brushing, biopsy, etc.) are used together, the overall diagnostic yield is enhanced. Notably, the yield of BAL for fungal infections, compared with bacterial infections, is reduced (47%), and multiple studies have advocated the importance of obtaining multiple sputum samples in addition to BAL to optimize the diagnostic yield for fungal infections.[31,77,78] In immunosuppressed patients, bronchoalveolar lavage samples should always be sent for cytologic evaluation (in addition to culture) because the diagnosis can often be made based on features such as viral inclusion bodies or fungal forms on special stains for various infectious organisms.[79] In addition, cytology may be available sooner than information from cultures, which can take days to weeks for growth and identification, depending on the organism in question.

Suspected Foreign Body Aspiration

Foreign body aspiration is a common (and serious) problem in children but can occur in any age group. Tracheobronchial foreign body aspiration can result in severe airway compromise and death, as well as more long-term complications such as bronchiectasis and/or recurrent or persistent pneumonia. Foreign body aspiration is often suspected by history alone, although the classic diagnostic triad includes the sudden onset of paroxysmal coughing, wheezing, and diminished breath sounds on one side.[80] The chest radiograph can also provide valuable information. In a study of 140 patients with foreign body aspiration, radiographic findings included visualization of a radiopaque foreign body (34%), hyperinflation (18%), atelectasis (12%), and lung infiltrate/consolidation (11%). Normal radiographs were seen in 34% of subjects.[77] Although suspected foreign body aspiration is a definite indication for bronchoscopy, it is also important to remember that the absence of appropriate history or lack of visualization of a radiopaque object on chest radiograph does not exclude this diagnosis, particularly because many aspirated objects, especially food, are radiolucent.

Successful foreign body extraction requires an experienced bronchoscopy team because unexpected complications often arise. When foreign body aspiration is suspected on clinical or radiographic grounds, either flexible or rigid bronchoscopy can be performed. Flexible bronchoscopy allows visualization of more distal airways and does not require general anesthesia. Objects can be extracted by forceps retrieval or use of a basket extraction device through the working channel of the scope. The bronchoscopist must be careful to avoid dislodging the object because it could lead to acute airway obstruction if not securely retrieved. In contrast, rigid bronchoscopy is sometimes preferred because of the wider range of extraction devices available, ability to ventilate the patient throughout the procedure, better visualization (in the large airways), and ability to provide rapid suctioning in the event of substantial bleeding. The rigid bronchoscope remains the instrument of choice for foreign body aspiration in the pediatric population.[76,78] More complicated cases may necessitate intubation or tracheotomy to maintain adequate ventilation and assist in extraction of large objects.

Although many opinions exist, most research suggests that early bronchoscopy is associated with a lower risk of complication. Delayed bronchoscopy can be complicated by the formation of granulation tissue around the foreign material, leading to less visibility and increased risk of bleeding with extraction.[81,82]

Interstitial Lung Disease

The diagnosis of interstitial lung disease often requires a tissue sample for pathology evaluation. Bronchoscopy with transbronchial biopsy is often considered. The yield of transbronchial lung biopsies in patients with interstitial lung disease depends heavily on the diagnosis in question. For example, a diagnosis of sarcoidosis may be easily obtained by transbronchial biopsy, in contrast to other forms of idiopathic interstitial lung disease, which require surgical biopsy for adequate diagnostic material.

Given the high rate of pulmonary involvement in patients with sarcoidosis, bronchoscopy is the diagnostic procedure of choice, with yields as high as 90% in some studies.[38] Transbronchial biopsy has a high yield in other interstitial lung diseases, such as Langerhans cell histiocytosis, pulmonary alveolar proteinosis, lipoid pneumonia, eosinophilic pneumonia, and drug-induced pneumonitis.[83] These diseases all have characteristic appearances under the microscope, and if the affected lung is adequately sampled, transbronchial biopsy can be reliable.[83] In contrast, the diagnosis of other lung diseases, such as various forms of interstitial fibrosis, requires that a larger surgical biopsy be obtained.

Lung Transplant

Lung transplantation is a well-recognized treatment for end-stage pulmonary disease. Flexible bronchoscopy with bronchoalveolar lavage and/or transbronchial biopsy has proven to be a valuable tool for evaluating lung allograft complications. These complications can include infection, rejection (acute or chronic), and airway compromise. Transbronchial biopsy remains the gold standard for determining the presence or absence of acute pulmonary allograft rejection in lung transplant patients.[84] The role of surveillance bronchoscopy, in the absence of clinical worsening, remains controversial and varies between institutions. Many transplant centers endorse routine surveillance bronchoscopy with the hope that early detection and treatment of clinically silent episodes of acute rejection or infection may lead to reduced rates of chronic rejection or bronchiolitis obliterans syndrome (BOS). The impact of surveillance bronchoscopy on overall survival remains unknown.[85]

In lung transplant patients, bronchoscopy also allows for visualization of the airway anastomosis and management of mechanical complications, such as airway stenosis, with interventional techniques such as stent placement, balloon dilatation, and laser therapy.[86]

Respiratory Recap

Diagnostic Indications for Bronchoscopy

- Lung collapse/atelectasis
- Hemoptysis
- Cough
- Suspected malignancy
- Infection
- Foreign body aspiration
- Interstitial lung disease
- Lung transplant
- Trauma

Trauma

Blunt trauma to the chest can be associated with tracheal and bronchial injuries that are life threatening. Although tracheal rupture remains uncommon, its incidence has increased in recent years due to an increasing number of motor vehicle accidents as well as improved paramedic services, which enable patients with major chest trauma to survive transportation to a hospital.[87] Injuries to the tracheobronchial tree are found at autopsy in 3% to 11% of motor vehicle accident victims.[88] Tracheal injury can also occur as an iatrogenic complication of orotracheal intubation. Despite a lack of clear clinical symptoms, the need for early diagnosis and surgical repair is imperative.

Although most trauma patients do receive chest CT imaging, tracheal trauma is not always seen radiographically. In a retrospective analysis of 10 patients with tracheal rupture at a university trauma center, the diagnosis was definitively made by CT in only 1 case, with the remaining 9 diagnosed at bronchoscopy.[87] In many of these cases, indirect clues were seen radiographically, including pneumomediastinum, pneumothorax, hemothorax, persistent atelectasis, and lung contusion. In addition to radiographic signs, the presence of mediastinal or cervical emphysema on clinical exam, unexplained hemoptysis, or continuous air leak through a chest tube following blunt trauma is also suggestive of tracheobronchial injury and should be considered an urgent indication for bronchoscopy.[87] Bronchoscopy remains the gold standard for diagnosing tracheobronchial injuries following blunt trauma and should be obtained early in all patients with suspected tracheal injury to avoid the significant morbidity and mortality associated with untreated or unrecognized airway injuries.

Therapeutic Bronchoscopy

Therapeutic bronchoscopy is most commonly employed to treat patients with central airway obstruction due to benign or malignant etiology. Although the incidence of central airway obstruction is unknown, it is a commonly encountered clinical problem present in 20% to 30% of patients with primary lung cancer and 7% to 18% of patients following lung transplantation.[89,90] Additional common causes of central airway obstruction include tracheal stenosis, either posttracheostomy or idiopathic, tracheomalacia, and foreign body aspiration (**Box 9-2**).[85] Although many of the techniques that are described in this section are amenable to use with the flexible bronchoscope, rigid bronchoscopy provides definitive control of the airway, permitting the use of general anesthesia to maximize patient comfort (**Box 9-3**).[91] In addition, the rigid bronchoscope becomes a conduit for

BOX 9-2

Causes of Central Airway Obstruction

Malignant Causes

- Primary endoluminal carcinoma
- Metastatic carcinoma to the airway
- Laryngeal carcinoma
- Esophageal carcinoma
- Mediastinal tumors
- Lymphoma

Nonmalignant Causes

- Sarcoidosis
- Infectious
  - Tuberculosis
  - Histoplasmosis
  - Human papillomavirus
- Vascular
- Relapsing polychondritis
- Granulation tissue formation
  - Wegener granulomatosis
  - Foreign bodies
  - Airway stents
  - Surgical anastomosis
  - Amyloid
  - Hamartomas
  - Tracheomalacia

use of a variety of tools and suction devices to perform minimally invasive airway surgery. The bronchoscope itself can become a therapeutic tool useful for dilation of airway stenoses and coring out of airway tumor, providing rapid relief of central airway obstruction.[91]

BOX 9-3

Indications for Rigid Bronchoscopy

- Massive hemoptysis
- Foreign body removal
- Dilation of airway stenosis
- Airway stent placement
- Resection of central airway tumor

Rigid Bronchoscopy

The **rigid bronchoscope** was the only method of bronchoscopy available from the advent of bronchoscopy in 1897 by Gustav Killian until the introduction of the flexible fiberoptic scope in 1967 by Ikeda. After the introduction of flexible bronchoscopy, use of the rigid bronchoscope declined by pulmonologists in North America. Its distinct advantages in controlling the airway while facilitating the passage of a wide variety of tools for minimally invasive airway surgery have been rediscovered by the pulmonary community, resulting in an increased interest in training and application of the technique.[92]

Indications

Rigid bronchoscopy can be used for any bronchoscopic indication; however, the additional requirements of general anesthesia generally result in most centers limiting its use to therapeutic indications such as relief of central airway obstruction and foreign body removal, and for investigation of massive hemoptysis. Patient selection for rigid bronchoscopy is similar to that for flexible bronchoscopy. Patients should be able to tolerate general anesthesia, and not have an excessive oxygen requirement. Relative contraindications are similar to those described for **diagnostic bronchoscopy**, including uncontrolled coagulopathy and high O_2 requirement, with the addition of limitation in cervical neck extension due to the need to hyperextend the neck during bronchoscope insertion; an absolute contraindication is inability to provide informed consent.

Equipment

The rigid bronchoscope is essentially a stainless steel tube with a beveled tip at the distal end (**Figure 9-14**), while the proximal end usually contains a series of ports for ventilation, passage of suction catheters, grasping tools, a telescope, or a flexible bronchoscope. Fenestrated caps may be placed over the ports to permit

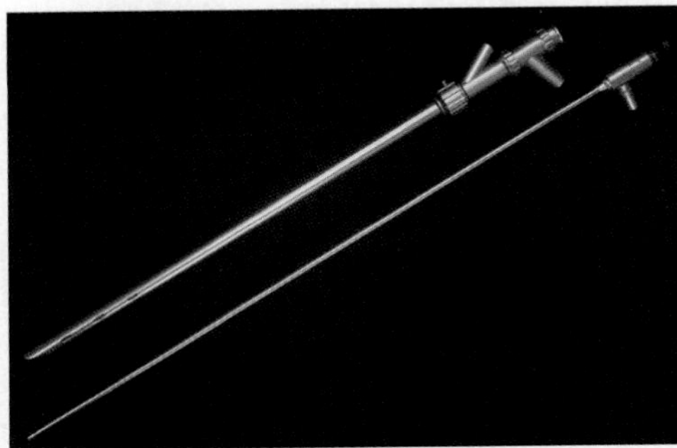

FIGURE 9-14 Rigid bronchoscope with articulated head and multiple ports for passage of a variety of tools or for connection to a closed ventilation system when the appropriate silicone caps are attached to the ports. Below is a telescope unit that may be used to visualize the airway directly or that may be fitted with a video camera for inspection of the airway using a video monitor.

closed ventilation during the procedure. Adult bronchoscopes are generally 9 to 13 mm in diameter and 40 cm long, whereas tracheoscopes are of similar diameter but are only 25 cm in length. Fenestrations are present in the sidewall at the distal end of the bronchoscope to allow for continued ventilation of the opposite lung if the scope is passed down one of the main stem bronchi during the procedure.

Insertion

Prior to bronchoscope insertion, the patient must be adequately sedated with general anesthesia. Many centers choose to administer a muscle relaxant as well, although this is not absolutely required. The patient's neck is hyperextended, and with the fingers of the left hand, the upper lip and teeth are covered with the operator's thumb, the index finger is inserted into the patient's mouth to displace the tongue toward the left side of the patient's mouth, and the middle finger is used to cover the patient's lower lip and teeth to prevent injury to these structures. The bronchoscope is held in the right hand with the barrel of the scope resting between the thumb and first finger, with the bevel of the distal end of the scope facing down. The tip of the scope is inserted into the patient's mouth against the base of the tongue. The tongue is visualized via the telescope inserted through the bronchoscope, and the scope is advanced along the base of the tongue until the epiglottis is visualized. The bevel of the scope is advanced under the epiglottis, and the tip of the scope is rotated upward using the thumb located over the patient's upper mandible as a fulcrum to lift the epiglottis and bring the vocal cords into view. The scope is then rotated 90 degrees to allow the beveled tip to slide between the cords. Rotation is continued an additional 90 degrees as the bronchoscope enters the trachea to run the bevel against the posterior wall of the trachea to prevent injury to the membranous tracheal wall.[91]

Anesthesia and Ventilation

Because of the irritating nature of the rigid intubation, virtually all centers perform rigid bronchoscopy under general anesthesia. If the bronchoscope is capped appropriately, inhalational anesthesia may be used to maintain the patient's sedation; however, most centers in the United States use a total intravenous anesthetic approach in combination with either spontaneous assisted ventilation or jet ventilation using a Sander's jet ventilator.[93] Some centers provide jet ventilation via an automated system, which allows the anesthesiologist to be freed from managing the Sander's jet.[94,95] Limited data exist comparing outcomes between ventilation strategies; however, there is some evidence to suggest that spontaneous assisted ventilation may reduce rates of reintubation following rigid bronchoscopy.[93] This result may be partially explained by the need for use of muscle relaxants with jet ventilation.

Therapeutic Procedures

Central airway obstruction may result from benign or malignant conditions. Benign conditions include tracheal stenosis secondary to endotracheal intubation or following tracheostomy, tracheomalacia from disorders such as relapsing polychondritis, stenosis at anastomotic sites following lung transplantation, and secondary to human papillomavirus infections of the airway. Virtually any type of malignancy can involve the airways, but the most common types are lung cancer, breast cancer, and renal cell carcinoma. Airway obstruction may take one of three forms: extrinsic compression, endobronchial obstruction (**Figure 9-15**), and mixed types.[96] Identification of the type of obstruction is important because it helps the physician determine the best course of treatment for relief of central airway obstruction and whether a procedure is likely to be effective.

A variety of therapeutic procedures are available to relieve airway obstruction due to malignancy or benign airway stenosis (**Table 9-2**). Rapid relief of airway obstruction may be obtained using heat therapy such as endobronchial laser or electrocautery. Laser (light amplification of stimulated emission of radiation) was first described for use in the airway in 1976 and is used in many centers as the primary tool for rapid resection of central airway tumors.[96,97] The most commonly used

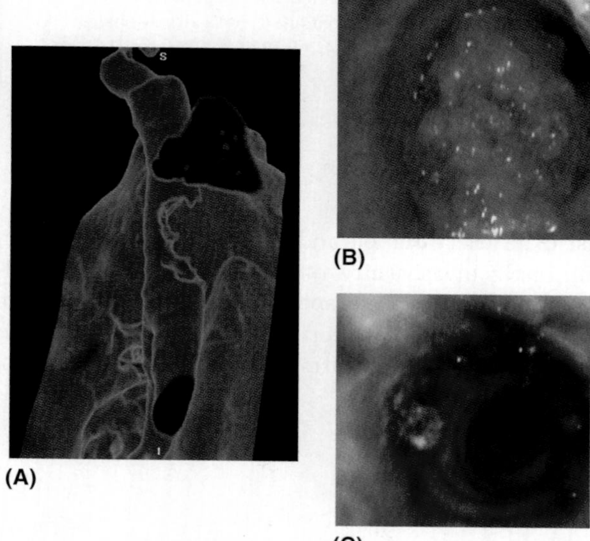

FIGURE 9-15 Intrinsic airway obstruction due to human papillomavirus (HPV) in a patient with HIV infection. (**A**) CT reconstruction of the trachea showing near complete obstruction by the mass of HPV-induced granulation tissue. (**B**) Bronchoscopic view of airway obstruction showing characteristic cluster-of-grapes appearance of HPV disease. (**C**) Trachea after removal of the mass using a combination of argon plasma coagulation and mechanical debridement. Note areas of superficial thermal injury on the tracheal mucosa due to argon plasma coagulation use.

TABLE 9-2
Currently Available Bronchoscopic Ablative Therapies

Modality	Mechanism	Effect	Advantages	Disadvantages
Nd:YAG	Thermal energy produced by laser light	Coagulation and vaporization of tissue	Excellent debulking	Expensive; cumbersome setup
Electrocautery	Thermal energy produced by an electrical current	Coagulation of tissue, but more superficial than laser	Excellent safety profile; multiple instrument designs; inexpensive	Contact mode requiring frequent cleaning of probe
Argon plasma coagulation	Thermal energy produced by the interaction between argon gas and an electrical current	Superficial coagulation of tissue	No undesired deep tissue effects	Ineffective for in-depth tissue coagulation or debulking
Photodynamic therapy	Injection of a photosensitizer followed by the destruction of presensitized tumor cells through illumination with nonthermal laser	Delayed destruction of tissue (24–48 hours)	Relatively long-lasting effects	Expensive; need for multiple bronchoscopies; skin photosensitivity lasting up to 6 weeks
Brachytherapy	Direct delivery of radiation therapy into the airway	Delayed and in-depth destruction of tissue	Long-lasting effect; synergistic with external beam radiation	Higher incidence of complications, particularly hemorrhage
Cryotherapy	Destruction of tissue by alternating cycles of freezing to extreme cold temperatures and thawing	Delayed destruction of tissue (1–2 weeks)	Useful for retrieval of foreign objects and removal of large mucous plugs or clots	Not suitable for debulking in acute airway obstruction; need for multiple bronchoscopies

Adapted from Wahidi M, Herth F, Ernst A. State of the art interventional pulmonology. *Chest*. 2007;131:261–274.

laser is the Nd:YAG device, which causes photocoagulation rather than vaporization of tumor tissue. This allows for devitalization of tumor tissue followed by removal with forceps to open the airway. When using heat therapy in the airway, care must be taken that the inspired FIO_2 is reduced to 40% or less to avoid ignition of flammable components in the airway. Using this technique, 70% of central airway obstructions are relieved.[96]

Similar effect can be obtained using a pulsed electrical field and an electrocautery probe extended through the rigid or flexible bronchoscope. In this case the tissue is devitalized using direct contact, permitting excellent control of tissue destruction. The electrocautery is fired in short bursts, with frequent observation of the underlying tissue injury to avoid unwanted extension of the coagulation effect. Similar to laser therapy, devitalized tissue may then be removed with the use of grasping forceps with a minimum of bleeding.[89,92] There have been no direct comparisons of laser therapy and electrocautery for the relief of central airway obstruction; however, reported efficacy has been similar with both techniques. Electrocautery has an advantage in that it requires less investment in equipment and does not require the use of special eye protection or the avoidance of reflective surfaces during its use.[98]

An additional technique that uses heat therapy is argon plasma coagulation (APC). This technique employs argon gas to form a plasma that when exposed to high voltage conducts electricity to underlying tissue, resulting in a superficial coagulation effect. APC is a noncontact technique in that the electrical energy is carried by the gas to the underlying tissue, and so this technique may be used to deliver energy around corners and in difficult-to-reach locations in the airway. The effect of APC is more superficial than either laser or electrocautery, causing coagulation to a depth of 2 to 3 mm within the airway.[99,100] This limited penetration provides the ability to spray the coagulating effect within the airway, making APC a useful tool for control of airway bleeding and devitalization of granulation tissue. The superficial coagulation effect also makes APC extremely safe, resulting in lower rates of complications such as airway perforation and massive hemorrhage,[101] although there are theoretical concerns about the development of gas embolism with higher flow rates and longer pulse duration with the use of APC.[102]

Treatment of airway stenosis following tracheostomy or lung transplantation may be performed using inflatable balloons or rigid dilators to disrupt the fibrous connective tissue that forms at the site of the prior airway injury.[102] Often, a combination of techniques, such as use of an electrocautery knife to cut the membranous region of a stenosis followed by dilation with an inflatable balloon and removal of granulation tissue with forceps, is required to achieve the desired result. Finally, the rigid bronchoscope itself can be used as a therapeutic instrument to core out central airway tumors after adequate desiccation and coagulation have been performed using laser therapy or electrocautery.[96]

In addition to the rapidly acting procedures described earlier, there are several therapies that provide delayed effect in debulking airway malignancies. Cryotherapy is a safe and effective method that uses nitrous oxide gas to cool the tip of a metal probe placed through the working channel of the flexible bronchoscope. Once the gas flow is activated, the tip of the catheter rapidly cools to induce freezing of tissues at the point of contact and a small margin of surrounding tissue. The tissue thaws and the cycle may be repeated. The freeze–thawing of tissues results in delayed necrosis and sloughing of the treated area over the next several days.[103] This technique has been shown to be effective in debulking tumors and improving central airway obstruction. Cryotherapy is also useful for removal of foreign bodies.[104] The tip of the probe is placed on the foreign body, and the gas flow is activated, resulting in the foreign body being frozen to the catheter tip. The foreign body is then removed from the patient by removing the flexible bronchoscope with the catheter still in the working channel without turning off the gas flow.

Additional delayed-efficacy treatments include photodynamic therapy, which employs a systemically administered photosensitizing agent prior to the procedure that is preferentially concentrated by tumor cells. Photophrin is currently the only sensitizing agent licensed for use in the United States. When stimulated by light of 630 nm via an argon/dye or diode laser applied through a light guide, oxygen radicals are produced in tissues that have concentrated the previously administered medication, resulting in tissue necrosis.[105] Often necrosis is so exuberant that a repeat procedure in needed 24 to 48 hours after light administration to debride necrotic tumor that can cause airway obstruction. Efficacy is good in patients with central airway tumors, where up to 70% report improvement in symptoms of dyspnea.[103] Primary complications include severe sunburn due to the photosensitizing effect of the medication, which may last as long as 6 weeks, and bleeding due to the destruction of vascular tumors.[106]

Finally, **brachytherapy** is a palliative technique that employs locally delivered radionuclide for treatment of endobronchial tumor resulting in central airway obstruction. The advantages of this approach are the delivery of high-dose radiation directly to the tumor tissue with limited penetration to surrounding tissue due to the rapid drop-off of radiation dose with distance from the source, the ability to modify the area of treatment to conform to the shape of the tumor, and the ability to precisely target the tissue of interest.[106] The radionuclide most commonly used is iridium-192 delivered in an encapsulated form via a polyethylene catheter inserted via the working channel of the flexible bronchoscope. The catheter is placed adjacent to the area to be treated, and the bronchoscope is removed. The catheter is then secured at the nose or mouth, and the position is confirmed using fluoroscopy. The iridium source is then after-loaded into the catheter and dwells for a period of time until the desired dose is delivered, generally 7 Gy for high-dose applications; the catheter and source are then removed from the patient. Efficacy for symptom palliation ranges from 65% to 95%.[107–109] A Cochrane review compared the efficacy of external beam radiation therapy and high-dose endobronchial therapy and showed no difference between the two treatments.[110] Complications are rare, although fatal hemoptysis is reported in 2% to 11% of treated patients.[109]

Choice of therapeutic approach is based on a variety of variables, including the patient's degree of dyspnea, the location of the tumor, whether the tumor is primarily endobronchial or the airway obstruction is secondary to extrinsic compression, available equipment, and the level of local experience with the various techniques. Generally speaking, the rapid effect of heat-based therapies may have a less durable effect in the absence of additional treatment such as airway stenting, palliative radiation, or chemotherapy. Treatments such as photodynamic therapy or brachytherapy may delay the recurrence of tumor, and thus may result in a longer-lasting tumor reduction. Currently, there are no data available comparing the efficacy of techniques. There is no demonstrated increase in life expectancy with use of any of the treatments described here; however, substantial data exist that suggest efficacy for providing symptomatic relief.

Airway Stenting

Modern airway stenting began as a modification of the Montgomery T-tube, with silicone stents popularized by Dumon in the late 1980s.[111] Shortly afterward, the

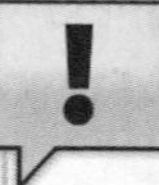

Respiratory Recap

Airway Stents

- Self-expandable metal stents, silicone stents, and hybrid metal-silicone stents are available.
- Rigid bronchoscopy is required for silicone stent placement.
- Stents are generally effective in improving airway patency.
- Common complications include stent migration and occlusion by secretions.

self-expandable metal stent was developed and became widely used because of its ease of deployment without the need for rigid bronchoscopy as is required for silicone stent placement.[112] More recently, hybrid metal-silicone stents have been developed, which share some of the advantages and disadvantages of each type of **airway stent**.

Silicone Stents

Silicone stents are composed of silicone sleeves fitted with external studs to retard stent migration in the airway. The stent wall is relatively thick at 2 mm, and therefore significant portions of the airway lumen may be occupied in smaller (<10 mm outer diameter) stents. Stents are sized from 10 mm to 20 mm in outer diameter and come in lengths ranging from 2 to 8 cm. In addition, Y-shaped stents are available for placement at the main carina with limbs of the Y extending proximally into the trachea and distally into each of the main stem bronchi. The limbs of the Y are not symmetrically angled, but instead are more acute for the left main stem bronchus take-off to accommodate the positioning of the two main stem bronchi.

Rigid bronchoscopy is required for silicone stent placement. During deployment, the stent is rolled along the long axis and placed into a steel delivery tube sized the same length as the rigid bronchoscope. The bronchoscope is advanced to the midpoint of the desired airway obstruction, and the deployment tube is inserted into the bronchoscope. The stent is then pushed forward using a pushrod placed down the deployment tube, followed by removal of both the pushrod and deployment tube (**Figure 9-16**). The rigid scope is then withdrawn while holding the incompletely expanded stent in place until the proximal end is free from the bronchoscope. Generally, the stent will fully expand but occasionally may need to be opened using a dilation balloon. If the stent has been positioned distal to the area of narrowing, it may be dragged proximally using large forceps; however, stents that have been placed too proximally cannot be advanced and must be removed and reinserted (**Figure 9-17**).

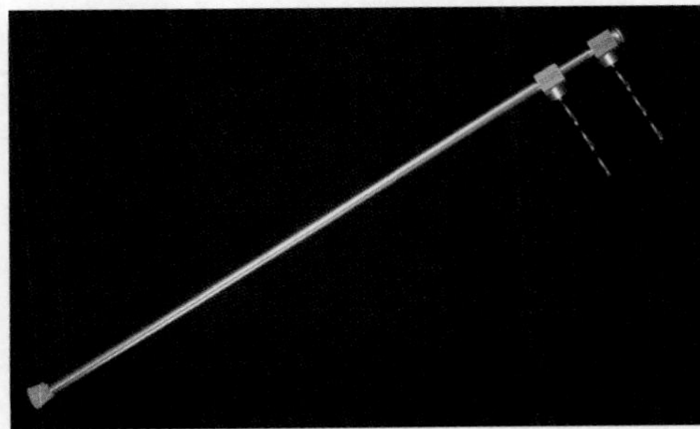

FIGURE 9-16 Silicone stent deployment system. A stent is pictured in partial deployment to illustrate the manner in which the stent is folded to be fitted into the deployment tube.

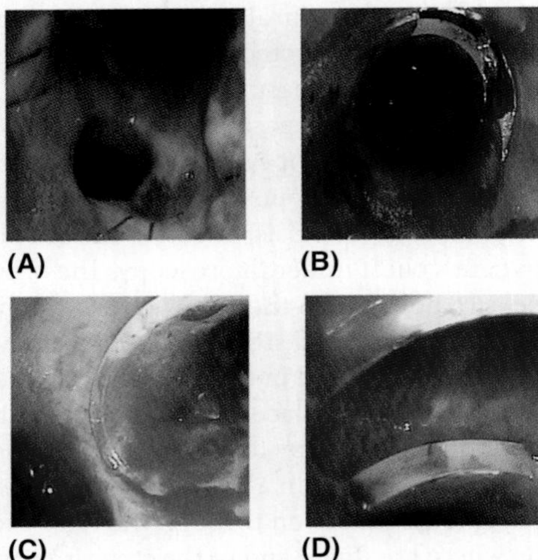

FIGURE 9-17 Lung transplant anastomosis dehiscence treated with a silicone stent. (**A**) Anastomosis dehiscence showing fistula in communication with the patient's mediastinum. (**B**) Proximal view of the silicone stent seen from the distal trachea. (**C**) Axial view of the stent that extends from the right main stem to the distal bronchus intermedius. Note complete occlusion of the underlying fistula, minimizing continued passage of secretions into the mediastinum. (**D**) View of window cut in the stent for ventilation of the right upper lobe.

Self-Expanding Metal Stents

Self-expanding **metallic stents** were introduced in the mid-1990s as an alternative to silicone stents. The majority of these stents are constructed of nitinol, an alloy composed of nickel and titanium. This metal has the properties of being flexible while retaining excellent shape memory, and so the stent can be compressed onto a factory-packaged deployment rod and then will expand to its initial diameter after it is deployed. These stents are less likely to migrate than silicone stents,[113] because they rapidly embed into the surrounding mucosa. They are also less likely to become occluded with secretions, because the open meshwork of the stent allows normal ciliary function of the underlying mucosa to move secretions into the upper airway. Lumen occlusion with granulation tissue can be a significant problem with metallic stents. In addition, once metallic stents are placed, they are rapidly incorporated into the airway wall, making removal very difficult.[114] Over time, stress fractures often develop in the stents, resulting in loose wires, which may migrate through the airway wall and cause injury to the surrounding lung and mediastinal structures. Because of these complications, the American College of Chest Physicians and the Food and Drug Administration have issued warnings against the use of metallic airway stents for benign airway diseases.[115]

An advantage of metal stents over silicone stents is their ability to be placed without the need for rigid bronchoscopy, but rather using a flexible bronchoscope and fluoroscopic guidance. To achieve this, the patient is examined using procedural sedation with a flexible bronchoscope. The obstructed airway of interest is identified, the lesion is measured using the bronchoscope, and a guide wire is passed through the working channel of the bronchoscope across the area of stenosis. Next, the bronchoscope is positioned at the distal and proximal ends of the stenosis, and markers are placed on the patient's chest under fluoroscopy. The bronchoscope is removed with the guide wire left in place. The self-expandable metal stent is then passed over the guide wire, positioned in the airway using fluoroscopy and the previously placed surface markers, and deployed under fluoroscopy to ensure accurate positioning. Metallic stents can also be placed using flexible bronchoscopic visualization through the rigid bronchoscope where the distal end of the stent is monitored during placement to ensure correct positioning.

Hybrid Stents

Hybrid silicone and nitinol stents have been developed that share some of the characteristics of silicone and metallic stents. These **hybrid stents** are constructed of a polyurethane or silicone sleeve with supporting nitinol struts. They share many of the advantages of metal stents in that they are self-expanding and so may be deployed across a tight stenosis and act to open the lesion via the radial force exerted by the wire mesh. The silicone sleeve prevents tumor ingrowth through the stent and also prevents the stent from granulating into the airway wall. This enhances patency as well as allows for removal of the stent at a later time if needed.

One disadvantage of the hybrid stents has recently been recognized and is related to the open nature of the nitinol struts. These struts may fold inward on themselves during vigorous coughing or breathing. Generally they will re-expand to their original dimensions, but occasionally they remain collapsed. Case reports exist describing severe shortness of breath associated with collapsed hybrid tracheal stents, requiring urgent removal, although recent reconfiguring of these devices seems to have decreased the incidence of this complication.[116]

Efficacy and Complications of Stent Placement

Stents are generally effective in improving airway patency and are associated with increases in FEV_1.[117,118] There are no randomized trials evaluating stent efficacy, survival benefit, or head-to-head comparisons of efficacy between types of stent. In addition, optimal placement of airway stents may be more complicated than previously perceived. Miyazawa et al. examined flow-limiting segments of malignant airway stenosis in 64 patients using ultrathin bronchoscopy, flow volume loops, and three-dimensional CT reconstruction before and after central airway stenting. They found that the flow-limiting segment migrated distally in 15% of patients after stent placement, requiring additional airway stent deployment to optimize respiratory function.[119]

Potential complications specific to each type of stent are mentioned above.[120–124] Significant complications are common and are as high as 50% in some series. Common complications include stent migration and occlusion by secretions, occasionally with significant airway obstruction requiring emergent procedures to clear the impacted secretions.

Pleural Disease

Pleural effusions are a commonly encountered medical problem in both inpatient and outpatient medicine. Although no good data are available regarding the incidence of pleural effusions, it is estimated that over one million new effusions are diagnosed annually in the United States.[125] Pleural effusions may be caused by a variety of medical conditions (**Box 9-4**). The most common causes are related to congestive heart failure, malignancy, pneumonia, and pulmonary embolism, however.[125] The first step in determining the etiology of the newly recognized pleural effusion is to perform **thoracentesis**.

Indications for Thoracentesis

Thoracentesis is a safe procedure that may be performed at the bedside and is the first step in the diagnosis of a newly recognized pleural effusion. Indications include diagnosis of a new pleural effusion of unknown etiology and relief of dyspnea in a patient with a large pleural effusion resulting in significant loss of lung

BOX 9-4

Causes of Pleural Effusions

Transudative

- Congestive heart failure
- Cirrhosis of the liver
- Renal failure
- Urinothorax

Exudative

- Malignancy
- Pneumonia
- Pulmonary embolism
- After thoracic surgery
- Tuberculosis
- Chyle
- Connective tissue diseases (e.g., rheumatoid arthritis, systemic lupus erythematosus)

Respiratory Recap

Thoracentesis

- The most common causes of pleural effusions are related to congestive heart failure, malignancy, pneumonia, and pulmonary embolism.
- Indications for thoracentesis include diagnosis of a new pleural effusion of unknown etiology and relief of dyspnea in a patient with a large pleural effusion.
- Removal of 1500 mL of fluid at a time is safe.
- Pleural fluid with pH < 7.20 and glucose < 60 mg/dL may indicate a complicated parapneumonic effusion.
- Light's criteria are used to discriminate between exudative and transudative pleural fluid.
- Pleurodesis is the traditional approach to recurrent pleural effusions.

volume due to the occupation of the hemithorax with fluid.[126] Contraindications are few and include inability to provide informed consent, uncorrected coagulopathy, and operator inexperience.

Thoracentesis Procedure

It is generally considered safe to perform a blind thoracentesis if the fluid layers to a depth of 1 cm on ipsilateral decubitus radiographs of the chest. Using percussion of the chest, the fluid level is identified by listening for loss of the resonant note as the examiner continues to firmly tap the chest wall of both hemithoraces moving from the cephalad to caudal position along the patient's back in the mid-scapular line. The first rib below the area where dullness is first encountered should be identified by palpation and a site marked at the superior aspect of the rib. To avoid injury to the neurovascular bundle that runs below each rib, the finder needle should be inserted at the middle of the rib body, below the marked site.

After the area is cleaned with an appropriate antiseptic such as chlorhexidine or Betadine, a fenestrated sterile drape is applied to the patient's back and a wheal of 1% lidocaine is raised using a 21- or 22-gauge needle and syringe at the needle insertion site. The tissues between the skin and rib are infiltrated with lidocaine until the rib body is contacted with the tip of the finder needle. The finder needle is then angled in the cephalad direction and walked over the top of the rib until it is able to pass into the intercostal space. While maintaining negative pressure on the syringe plunger, the needle is advanced into the pleural space. Often, the patient will flinch as the parietal pleura is contacted by the needle tip. Once the needle has passed through the pleural lining, fluid will be seen to fill the syringe. The needle should not be advanced at this point, but rather retracted 1 to 2 mm and lidocaine administered at this position to provide adequate analgesia to proceed with a sampling needle.

Once the fluid has been located, a clean 20-gauge needle and syringe should be inserted as just described to collect diagnostic pleural fluid samples. Approximately 100 mL should be collected to provide sufficient fluid for all necessary laboratory testing. If a large-volume therapeutic thoracentesis is to be performed, a 4-cm, 18-gauge angiocatheter may be inserted and connected to a three-way stopcock to withdraw fluid. Several convenient, commercially available kits for performing therapeutic thoracentesis have been produced that contain all of the necessary materials, including antiseptic, lidocaine, and long flexible catheters with one-way valves to prevent the entrainment of air into the thoracic cavity during drainage of pleural fluid.

Although no good data exist, it is generally thought that removal of 1500 mL of fluid at a time is safe to avoid the rare, but potentially fatal, complication of re-expansion pulmonary edema.[127,128] Fluid removal should be stopped if the patient develops intractable cough or sensation of chest discomfort during the procedure. To remove the catheter, the patient is asked to hum to produce positive intrathoracic pressure while the catheter is quickly removed. For an uncomplicated thoracentesis, it is not necessary to perform a postprocedure chest x-ray, although in any case in which air was aspirated, intractable cough was present, or chest pain occurred that persists after the procedure is completed, an x-ray should be performed to evaluate for procedural complications.

In obese patients whose body habitus does not permit accurate physical exam, or in patients with small or loculated pleural effusions, thoracic ultrasonography may be useful in localizing pleural fluid for thoracentesis.[129] Several studies suggest that ultrasound-guided thoracentesis is associated with lower complication rates than blind thoracentesis.[130–132] To perform ultrasound-guided thoracentesis, the patient should be placed in the seated position similar to the procedure for blind thoracentesis. The hemithorax of interest is examined, and the diaphragm with subdiaphragmatic structures (liver on the right and spleen on the left), visceral and parietal pleura, and pleural fluid are identified. A site is marked just superior to a rib where there is a clear path on ultrasound from the chest wall to underlying pleural fluid. Once the site is marked, the area is reexamined with the ultrasound probe to confirm the correct location, and the thoracentesis is performed as previously described. Ultrasound-guided thoracentesis should be performed in a single sitting. Use of ultrasound marking followed by performance of thoracentesis at a later time, such as when the patient returns to his or her room from the radiology suite, has not been shown to decrease procedural complications, because the patient is unlikely to be in the same position for both the imaging and thoracentesis.[133] Thoracic ultrasonographic images can be difficult for the novice operator to interpret, and thus ultrasound-guided thoracentesis should only be performed by an adequately trained operator.

Interpretation of Results

The primary purpose of performing diagnostic thoracentesis is to categorize pleural fluid as either **transudative**, suggesting benign, noninflammatory causes, or **exudative**, suggesting a malignant, infectious, or inflammatory etiology. Light's criteria were introduced in 1972 to discriminate between exudative and transudative pleural fluid and are composed of the measurement of pleural fluid and serum protein and lactate dehydrogenase (LDH).[134] A fluid is deemed exudative if the ratio of pleural fluid to serum protein is 0.5 or greater or if the ratio of pleural fluid to serum LDH is 0.6 or greater. Either criterion is adequate to classify the pleural fluid. Alternatively, if the pleural fluid LDH is greater than two-thirds the upper limit of the normal local laboratory values, the fluid is considered to be an exudate.[135]

Additional studies may also be performed on the pleural fluid to establish particular diagnoses. Pleural fluid with pH less than 7.20 and glucose less than 60 mg/dL may indicate a complicated parapneumonic effusion, an indication for chest tube insertion to complete drainage of the pleural space.[136,137]

Pleural fluid cytology has a 70% sensitivity for diagnosis of a malignant pleural effusion,[138] whereas pleural fluid adenosine deaminase levels may be helpful when there is a high suspicion of a tuberculous effusion.[126] Should the cause of an exudative effusion not be determined after initial fluid analysis, medical pleuroscopy or surgical thoracoscopy may be indicated for direct visualization and biopsy of the pleura (**Figure 9-18**). Up to 15% of effusions may elude a definitive diagnosis.[126]

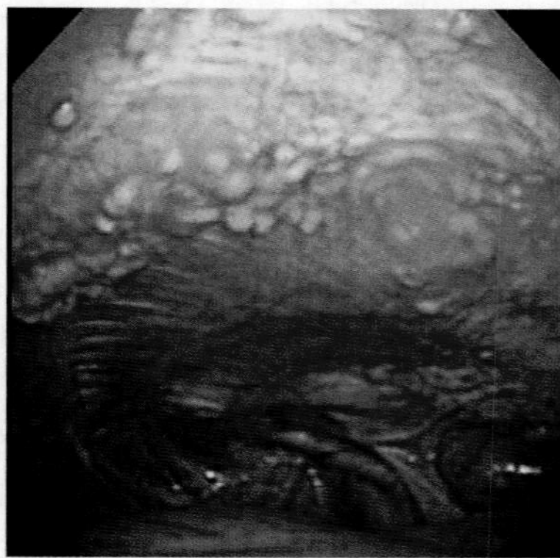

FIGURE 9-18 Thoracoscopic view of parietal pleura showing malignant nodules lining the interior aspect of the chest cavity. These were metastatic breast cancer.

Management of Recurrent Pleural Effusions

Many pleural effusions are self-limited and resolve with treatment of the underlying etiology of the effusion; however, some effusions may be recurrent and result in significant dyspnea and limitation of functional status for the affected patient. Malignant effusions in particular result in substantial morbidity for the patient and often require palliative intervention to alleviate the dyspnea that results from the fluid.

The traditional approach to recurrent pleural effusions is to provide **pleurodesis**, either with mechanical abrasion during a thoracotomy or thoracoscopic surgery or by administering a **sclerosing agent** via tube thoracostomy. Many sclerosing agents have been evaluated, including tetracycline or doxycycline, bleomycin, and talc. Talc is currently considered to be the most efficacious agent available, with 30-day success rates of 80% for control of the recurrent effusion as compared with a 60% success rate at 30 days for doxycycline or bleomycin.[139–141] There is some controversy as to what is the best form in which to administer the talc, either as a slurry suspended in normal saline, or aerosolized as a talc poudrage during medical thoracoscopy or video-assisted thoracoscopy (**Figure 9-19**). The largest study available suggests a small increase in efficacy when talc is delivered as a poudrage in patients with effusions due to metastatic lung, renal, or breast cancer.[139] Although pleurodesis is generally effective, it requires an inpatient stay and usually several days of chest tube drainage following the administration of the sclerosing agent to allow for drainage of pleural fluid as the pleurodesis takes place.

An alternative to pleurodesis is the placement of a tunneled pleural catheter, which allows patients to manage their effusion in the outpatient setting. The catheter is a 15.5 French silicone tube fitted with a polyester cuff that is tunneled beneath the skin of the chest wall and into the pleural space (**Figure 9-20**). The catheter is fitted at the distal end with a one-way valve that is accessed using a specially designed catheter attached to a vacuum bottle for drainage at home. The tunneled catheter permits outpatient management of recurrent pleural effusions with simple insertion done in a radiology or endoscopy suite. Complications are primarily

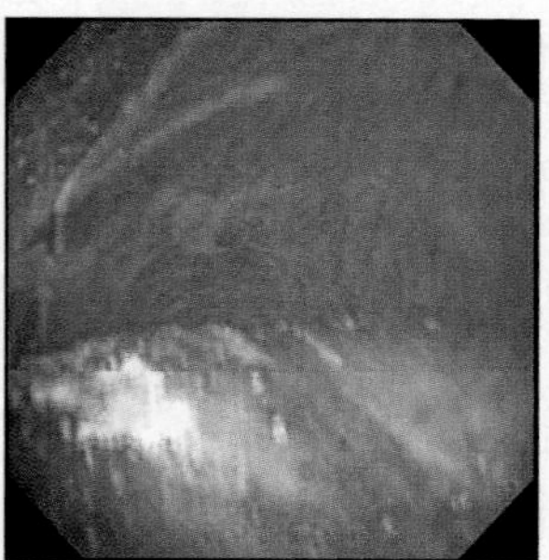

FIGURE 9-19 Thoracoscopic view of a talc poudrage pleurodesis. Note the characteristic snowstorm appearance of the insufflated talc sclerosant.

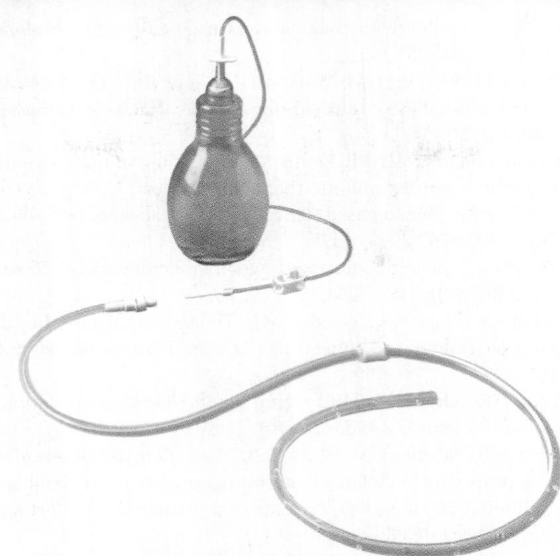

FIGURE 9-20 Pleurx tunneled pleural catheter system with attached drainage bottle. The catheter is tunneled below the skin and inserted into the chest cavity for repeated drainage of pleural fluid. The catheter has a polyester cuff that induces granulation tissue at the skin insertion site, reducing infectious risk with long-term use of the device.

Reproduced with permission from CareFusion.

related to inability to adequately drain a loculated fluid collection, and infection rates are low, between 2% and 8%.[142,143] The catheter may be left in place as long as the effusion continues to recur. A large systematic review examining tunneled pleural catheters for malignant effusion including 1370 patients found symptomatic improvement in 95.6% of patients, spontaneous pleurodesis in 45.6% of patients, allowing for catheter removal in 47.1% of patients.[144] Hybrid techniques for treatment of malignant pleural effusion are also emerging. Reddy and colleagues performed medical pleuroscopy with talc poudrage, together with insertion and subsequent drainage with a tunneled pleural catheter (after removal of surgical chest tube 24 hours after pleuroscopy). Ninety-two percent of patients achieved successful pleurodesis and the tunneled pleural catheter was removed at a mean of 16.7 days after placement.[145]

Future Directions

Interventional pulmonology is a rapidly advancing, technologically driven field of medicine. One current area of intense interest is endoluminal **lung-volume reduction** for treatment of advanced emphysema using one-way endobronchial valves. The valves are inserted bronchoscopically into subsegmental airways with the goal of allowing air to escape via the one-way valve but not reenter the area of emphysema, producing an effective collapse of the abnormal area of lung. This is thought to permit the surrounding lung parenchyma to expand, resulting in improved ventilation-perfusion matching as well as permitting the diaphragm to assume a more normal position in the chest, improving muscle mechanics. Studies to date show good safety and tolerance profiles, but significant changes in physiologic parameters are lacking.[146–149] Other techniques designed to alleviate hyperinflation due to emphysema currently under investigation include biologic lung-volume reduction that uses a fibrin glue-like substance to occlude target airways, and nitinol coils to compress diseased tissue and tether open small airways.

Diagnostic and therapeutic bronchoscopies are useful tools in appropriately trained hands for the management of patients with complex pulmonary disease. Although invasive, procedures may be safely performed when proper precautions are taken to prevent and avoid complications. Given the degree of interest in new technology associated with bronchoscopic techniques, a growing role for the interventional pulmonologist is likely in the coming years.

Key Points

- Bronchoscopy is the most commonly used invasive procedure in pulmonary medicine and can be used to perform both diagnostic and therapeutic procedures.
- The flexible fiberoptic bronchoscope consists of a control unit (or head) and a soft, flexible shaft.
- Bronchoscopy is a safe and effective tool for diagnosing and treating a wide variety of pulmonary processes.
- Factors necessary for a successful bronchoscopy include proper patient selection, patient preparation, and appropriate anesthesia.
- The ideal patient for fiberoptic bronchoscopy is awake, able to understand and cooperate with the procedure, and free of other conditions that could elevate the risk of the procedure.
- Although bronchoscopy can be performed with topical anesthesia alone, many physicians and patients prefer the judicial use of adjunctive IV sedation.
- Common bronchoscopy techniques include airway examination, bronchoalveolar lavage, bronchoscopic washing, bronchial brushing, endobronchial biopsy, transbronchial lung biopsy, and transbronchial needle aspiration.
- Indications for bronchoscopy include atelectasis, hemoptysis, cough, suspected malignancy, infection, foreign body aspiration, interstitial lung disease, lung transplant, and trauma.
- Rigid bronchoscopy can be used for any bronchoscopic indication; however, the additional requirements of general anesthesia generally result in most centers limiting its use to therapeutic indications such as relief of central airway obstruction

and foreign body removal, and for investigation of massive hemoptysis.

- Modern airway stenting uses self-expandable metal stents, silicone stents, and hybrid metal-silicone stents.
- Pleural effusions may be caused by a variety of medical conditions.
- Indications for thoracentesis include diagnosis of a new pleural effusion of unknown etiology and relief of dyspnea in a patient with a large pleural effusion resulting in significant loss of lung volume due to the occupation of the hemithorax with fluid.
- Pleural fluid is deemed exudative if the ratio of pleural fluid to serum protein is 0.5 or greater or if the ratio of pleural fluid to serum LDH is 0.6 or greater.
- The traditional approach to recurrent pleural effusions is to provide pleurodesis, either with mechanical abrasion during a thoracotomy or thoracoscopic surgery or by administering a sclerosing agent via tube thoracostomy.

References

1. Ernst A, Silvestri GA, Johnstone D. Interventional pulmonary procedures: guidelines from the American College of Chest Physicians. *Chest.* 2003;123:1693–1717.
2. Murray JF. *Textbook of Respiratory Medicine.* 3rd ed. Philadelphia: Saunders; 2000.
3. Murray JF, Nadel JA. *Murray and Nadel's Textbook of Respiratory Medicine.* 4th ed. Philadelphia: Elsevier Saunders; 2005.
4. Kozak EA, Brath LK. Do "screening" coagulation tests predict bleeding in patients undergoing fiberoptic bronchoscopy with biopsy? *Chest.* 1994;106:703–705.
5. Djukanovic R, Wilson JW, Lai CK, Holgate ST, Howarth PH. The safety aspects of fiberoptic bronchoscopy, bronchoalveolar lavage, and endobronchial biopsy in asthma. *Am Rev Respir Dis.* 1991;143:772–777.
6. Lundgren R, Haggmark S, Reiz S. Hemodynamic effects of flexible fiberoptic bronchoscopy performed under topical anesthesia. *Chest.* 1982;82:295–299.
7. Matot I, Kramer MR, Glantz L, Drenger B, Cotev S. Myocardial ischemia in sedated patients undergoing fiberoptic bronchoscopy. *Chest.* 1997;112:1454–1458.
8. British Thoracic Society guidelines on diagnostic flexible bronchoscopy. *Thorax.* 2001;56:1–21.
9. Bajwa MK, Henein S, Kamholz SL. Fiberoptic bronchoscopy in the presence of space-occupying intracranial lesions. *Chest.* 1993;104:101–103.
10. Kerwin AJ, Croce MA, Timmons SD, et al. Effects of fiberoptic bronchoscopy on intracranial pressure in patients with brain injury: a prospective clinical study. *J Trauma.* 2000;48:878–882; discussion 882–883.
11. Wahidi MM, Rocha AT, Hollingsworth JW, et al. Contraindications and safety of transbronchial lung biopsy via flexible bronchoscopy. A survey of pulmonologists and review of the literature. *Respiration.* 2005;72:285–295.
12. Zavala DC. Pulmonary hemorrhage in fiberoptic transbronchial biopsy. *Chest.* 1976;70:584–588.
13. Herth FJ, Becker HD, Ernst A. Aspirin does not increase bleeding complications after transbronchial biopsy. *Chest.* 2002;122:1461–1464.
14. Ernst A, Eberhardt R, Wahidi M, Becker HD, Herth FJ. Effect of routine clopidogrel use on bleeding complications after transbronchial biopsy in humans. *Chest.* 2006;129:734–737.
15. Guidelines on oral anticoagulation: third edition. *Br J Haematol.* 1998;101:374–387.
16. Baglin TP, Keeling DM, Watson HG. Guidelines on oral anticoagulation (warfarin): third edition—2005 update. *Br J Haematol.* 2006;132:277–285.
17. Douketis JD, Berger PB, Dunn AS, et al. The perioperative management of antithrombotic therapy: American College of Chest Physicians evidence-based clinical practice guidelines (8th edition). *Chest.* 2008;133:299S–339S.
18. Rebulla P. Platelet transfusion trigger in difficult patients. *Transfus Clin Biol.* 2001;8:249–254.
19. Sohal AS, Gangji AS, Crowther MA, Treleaven D. Uremic bleeding: pathophysiology and clinical risk factors. *Thromb Res.* 2006;118: 417–422.
20. Lohr JW, Schwab SJ. Minimizing hemorrhagic complications in dialysis patients. *J Am Soc Nephrol.* 1991;2:961–975.
21. Diette GB, Wiener CM, White P Jr. The higher risk of bleeding in lung transplant recipients from bronchoscopy is independent of traditional bleeding risks: results of a prospective cohort study. *Chest.* 1999;115:397–402.
22. Dransfield MT, Garver RI, Weill D. Standardized guidelines for surveillance bronchoscopy reduce complications in lung transplant recipients. *J Heart Lung Transplant.* 2004;23:110–114.
23. Pue CA, Pacht ER. Complications of fiberoptic bronchoscopy at a university hospital. *Chest.* 1995;107:430–432.
24. Milman N, Faurschou P, Grode G, Jorgensen A. Pulse oximetry during fibreoptic bronchoscopy in local anaesthesia: frequency of hypoxaemia and effect of oxygen supplementation. *Respiration.* 1994;61:342–347.
25. Witte MC, Opal SM, Gilbert JG, et al. Incidence of fever and bacteremia following transbronchial needle aspiration. *Chest.* 1986;89:85–87.
26. Poi PJ, Chuah SY, Srinivas P, Liam CK. Common fears of patients undergoing bronchoscopy. *Eur Respir J.* 1998;11:1147–1149.
27. Matot I, Kramer MR. Sedation in outpatient bronchoscopy. *Respir Med.* 2000;94:1145–1153.
28. Williams T, Brooks T, Ward C. The role of atropine premedication in fiberoptic bronchoscopy using intravenous midazolam sedation. *Chest.* 1998;113:1394–1398.
29. American Society of Anesthesiologists. *Standards for Basic Anesthetic Monitoring.* Accessed July 2, 2014, from http://www.asahq.org/for-members/~/media/For%20Members/documents/Standards%20Guidelines%20Stmts/Basic%20Anesthetic%20Monitoring%202011.ashx
30. Adam A, Dixon AK, Grainger RG, Allison DJ. *Grainger and Allison's Diagnostic Radiology: A Textbook of Medical Imaging.* Philadelphia: Churchill Livingstone/Elsevier; 2008.
31. Peikert T, Rana S, Edell ES. Safety, diagnostic yield, and therapeutic implications of flexible bronchoscopy in patients with febrile neutropenia and pulmonary infiltrates. *Mayo Clin Proc.* 2005;80:1414–1420.
32. Weiss SM, Hert RC, Gianola FJ, Clark JG, Crawford SW. Complications of fiberoptic bronchoscopy in thrombocytopenic patients. *Chest.* 1993;104:1025–1028.
33. Baughman RP. Protected-specimen brush technique in the diagnosis of ventilator-associated pneumonia. *Chest.* 2000;117:203S–206S.
34. Dasgupta A, Jain P, Minai OA, et al. Utility of transbronchial needle aspiration in the diagnosis of endobronchial lesions. *Chest.* 1999;115:1237–1241.
35. Steinfort D, Khor Y, Manser R, Irving L. Radial probe endobronchial ultrasound for the diagnosis of peripheral lung cancer: systematic review and meta-analysis. *Eur Respir J.* 2011;37:902–910.
36. Eberhardt R, Anantham D, Herth F, et al. Electromagnetic navigation diagnostic bronchoscopy in peripheral lung lesions. *Chest.* 2007;131:1800–1805.
37. Eberhart R, Anantham D, Ernst A, et al. Multimodality bronchoscopic diagnosis of peripheral lung lesions. *Am J Respir Crit Care Med.* 2007;176:36–41.

38. Gilman MJ, Wang KP. Transbronchial lung biopsy in sarcoidosis. An approach to determine the optimal number of biopsies. *Am Rev Respir Dis.* 1980;122:721–724.
39. Popovich J Jr, Kvale PA, Eichenhorn MS, et al. Diagnostic accuracy of multiple biopsies from flexible fiberoptic bronchoscopy. A comparison of central versus peripheral carcinoma. *Am Rev Respir Dis.* 1982;125:521–523.
40. Scott JP, Fradet G, Smyth RL, et al. Prospective study of transbronchial biopsies in the management of heart-lung and single lung transplant patients. *J Heart Lung Transplant.* 1991;10:626–636; discussion 636–637.
41. Loube DI, Johnson JE, Wiener D, et al. The effect of forceps size on the adequacy of specimens obtained by transbronchial biopsy. *Am Rev Respir Dis.* 1993;148:1411–1413.
42. Smith LS, Seaquist M, Schillaci RF. Comparison of forceps used for transbronchial lung biopsy. Bigger may not be better. *Chest.* 1985;87:574–576.
43. Aleva RM, Kraan J, Smith M, et al. Techniques in human airway inflammation: quantity and morphology of bronchial biopsy specimens taken by forceps of three sizes. *Chest.* 1998;113:182–185.
44. Curley FJ, Johal JS, Burke ME, Fraire AE. Transbronchial lung biopsy: can specimen quality be predicted at the time of biopsy? *Chest.* 1998;113:1037–1041.
45. Le Jeune I, Baldwin D. Measuring the success of transbronchial needle aspiration in everyday clinical practice. *Respir Med.* 2007;101:670–675.
46. Patel NM, Pohlman A, Husain A, et al. Conventional transbronchial needle aspiration decreases the rate of surgical sampling of intrathoracic lymphadenopathy. *Chest.* 2007;131:773–778.
47. Larsen SS, Vilmann P, Krasnik M, et al. Endoscopic ultrasound guided biopsy performed routinely in lung cancer staging spares futile thoracotomies: preliminary results from a randomised clinical trial. *Lung Cancer.* 2005;49:377–385.
48. Kennedy MP, Jimenez CA, Bruzzi JF, et al. Endobronchial ultrasound-guided transbronchial needle aspiration in the diagnosis of lymphoma. *Thorax.* 2008;63:360–365.
49. Diacon AH, Schuurmans MM, Theron J, et al. Transbronchial needle aspirates: how many passes per target site? *Eur Respir J.* 2007;29:112–116.
50. Herth F, Becker HD, Ernst A. Conventional vs endobronchial ultrasound-guided transbronchial needle aspiration: a randomized trial. *Chest.* 2004;125:322–325.
51. Herth F, Eberhardt R. Kransik M, Ernst A. Endobronchial ultrasound-guided transbronchial needle aspiration of lymph nodes in the radiologically and positron emission tomography-normal mediastinum in patients with lung cancer. *Chest.* 2008;133:887–891.
52. Ernst A, Anantham D, Eberhardt R, Krasnik M, Herth FJ. Diagnosis of mediastinal adenopathy-real-time endobronchial ultrasound guided needle aspiration versus mediastinoscopy. *J Thorac Oncol.* 2008;3:577–582.
53. Annema JT, van Meerbeeck JP, Rintoul RC, et al. Mediastinoscopy vs endosonography for mediastinal nodal staging of lung cancer: a randomized trial. *JAMA.* 2010;304:2245–2252.
54. Yasufuku K, Pierre A, Darling G, et al. A prospective controlled trial of endobronchial ultrasound-guided transbronchial needle aspiration compared with mediastinoscopy for mediastinal lymph node staging of lung cancer. *J Thorac Cardiovasc Surg.* 2011;142:1393–1400.
55. Dong X, Qui X, Qian L, Jia J. Endobronchial ultrasound-guided transbronchial needle aspiration in the mediastinal staging of non-small cell lung cancer: a meta-analysis. *Ann Thorac Surg.* 2013;96:1502–1507.
56. Diette GB, White P Jr, Terry P, et al. Utility of on-site cytopathology assessment for bronchoscopic evaluation of lung masses and adenopathy. *Chest.* 2000;117:1186–1190.
57. Baram D, Garcia RB, Richman PS. Impact of rapid on-site cytologic evaluation during transbronchial needle aspiration. *Chest.* 2005;128:869–875.
58. Chin R Jr, McCain TW, Lucia MA, et al. Transbronchial needle aspiration in diagnosing and staging lung cancer: how many aspirates are needed? *Am J Respir Crit Care Med.* 2002;166:377–381.
59. Prakash UB. Advances in bronchoscopic procedures. *Chest.* 1999;116:1403–1408.
60. Izbicki G, Shitrit D, Yarmolovsky A, et al. Is routine chest radiography after transbronchial biopsy necessary? A prospective study of 350 cases. *Chest.* 2006;129:1561–1564.
61. Smyth CM, Stead RJ. Survey of flexible fibreoptic bronchoscopy in the United Kingdom. *Eur Respir J.* 2002;19:458–463.
62. Kreider ME, Lipson DA. Bronchoscopy for atelectasis in the ICU: a case report and review of the literature. *Chest.* 2003;124:344–350.
63. Marini JJ, Pierson DJ, Hudson LD. Acute lobar atelectasis: a prospective comparison of fiberoptic bronchoscopy and respiratory therapy. *Am Rev Respir Dis.* 1979;119:971–978.
64. Hirshberg B, Biran I, Glazer M, Kramer MR. Hemoptysis: etiology, evaluation, and outcome in a tertiary referral hospital. *Chest.* 1997;112:440–444.
65. Weaver LJ, Solliday N, Cugell DW. Selection of patients with hemoptysis for fiberoptic bronchoscopy. *Chest.* 1979;76:7–10.
66. Colice GL. Detecting lung cancer as a cause of hemoptysis in patients with a normal chest radiograph: bronchoscopy vs CT. *Chest.* 1997;111:877–884.
67. Thirumaran M, Sundar R, Sutcliffe I, Currie D. Is investigation of patients with haemoptysis and normal chest radiograph justified? *Thorax.* 2009;64:854–856.
68. Poe RH, Israel RH, Marin MG, et al. Utility of fiberoptic bronchoscopy in patients with hemoptysis and a nonlocalizing chest roentgenogram. *Chest.* 1988;93:70–75.
69. Karmy-Jones R, Cuschieri J, Vallieres E. Role of bronchoscopy in massive hemoptysis. *Chest Surg Clin N Am.* 2001;11:873–906.
70. Decalmer S, Woodcock A, Greaves M, Howe M, Smith J. Airway abnormalities at flexible bronchoscopy in patients with chronic cough. *Eur Respir J.* 2007;30:1138–1142.
71. Schreiber G, McCrory DC. Performance characteristics of different modalities for diagnosis of suspected lung cancer: summary of published evidence. *Chest.* 2003;123:115S–128S.
72. Tan BB, Flaherty KR, Kazerooni EA, Iannettoni MD. The solitary pulmonary nodule. *Chest.* 2003;123:89S–96S.
73. Joos L, Patuto N, Chhajed PN, Tamm M. Diagnostic yield of flexible bronchoscopy in current clinical practice. *Swiss Med Wkly.* 2006;136:155–159.
74. Ortqvist A, Kalin M, Lejdeborn L, Lundberg B. Diagnostic fiberoptic bronchoscopy and protected brush culture in patients with community-acquired pneumonia. *Chest.* 1990;97:576–582.
75. van der Eerden MM, Vlaspolder F, de Graaff CS, et al. Value of intensive diagnostic microbiological investigation in low- and high-risk patients with community-acquired pneumonia. *Eur J Clin Microbiol Infect Dis.* 2005;24:241–249.
76. Jain P, Sandur S, Meli Y, et al. Role of flexible bronchoscopy in immunocompromised patients with lung infiltrates. *Chest.* 2004;125:712–722.
77. Horvath JA, Dummer S. The use of respiratory-tract cultures in the diagnosis of invasive pulmonary aspergillosis. *Am J Med.* 1996;100:171–178.
78. Yu VL, Muder RR, Poorsattar A. Significance of isolation of *Aspergillus* from the respiratory tract in diagnosis of invasive pulmonary aspergillosis. Results from a three-year prospective study. *Am J Med.* 1986;81:249–254.
79. Woods GL, Walker DH. Detection of infection or infectious agents by use of cytologic and histologic stains. *Clin Microbiol Rev.* 1996;9:382–404.
80. Eren S, Balci AE, Dikici B, Doblan M, Eren MN. Foreign body aspiration in children: experience of 1160 cases. *Ann Trop Paediatr.* 2003;23:31–37.
81. Soysal O, Kuzucu A, Ulutas H. Tracheobronchial foreign body aspiration: a continuing challenge. *Otolaryngol Head Neck Surg.* 2006;135:223–226.

82. Daines CL, Wood RE, Boesch RP. Foreign body aspiration: an important etiology of respiratory symptoms in children. *J Allergy Clin Immunol.* 2008;121:1297–1298.
83. Leslie KO, Gruden JF, Parish JM, Scholand MB. Transbronchial biopsy interpretation in the patient with diffuse parenchymal lung disease. *Arch Pathol Lab Med.* 2007;131:407–423.
84. Glanville AR. The role of bronchoscopic surveillance monitoring in the care of lung transplant recipients. *Semin Respir Crit Care Med.* 2006;27:480–491.
85. McWilliams TJ, Williams TJ, Whitford HM, Snell GI. Surveillance bronchoscopy in lung transplant recipients: risk versus benefit. *J Heart Lung Transplant.* 2008;27:1203–1209.
86. Chhajed PN, Tamm M, Glanville AR. Role of flexible bronchoscopy in lung transplantation. *Semin Respir Crit Care Med.* 2004;25: 413–423.
87. Kunisch-Hoppe M, Hoppe M, Rauber K, Popella C, Rau WS. Tracheal rupture caused by blunt chest trauma: radiological and clinical features. *Eur Radiol.* 2000;10:480–483.
88. Dennie CJ, Coblentz CL. The trachea: pathologic conditions and trauma. *Can Assoc Radiol J.* 1993;44:157–167.
89. Ernst A, Feller-Kopman D, Becker H, Mehta A. Central airway obstruction. *Am J Respir Crit Care.* 2004;169:1278–1297.
90. Santacruz J, Mehta A. Airway complications and management after lung transplantation. *Proc Am Thorac Soc.* 2009;6:79–93.
91. Beamis J. Modern use of rigid bronchoscopy. In: Bollinger CT, Mathur PN, eds. *Interventional Bronchoscopy.* Basel, Switzerland: S. Karger; 2000.
92. Wahidi M, Herth F, Ernst A. State of the art interventional pulmonology. *Chest.* 2007;131:261–274.
93. Perrin G, Colt HG, Martin C, et al. Safety of interventional rigid bronchoscopy using intravenous anesthesia and spontaneous assisted ventilation. A prospective study. *Chest.* 1992;102: 1526–1530.
94. Conacher ID. Anaesthesia and tracheobronchial stenting for central airway obstruction in adults. *Br J Anaesthesia.* 2003;90: 367–374.
95. Godden DJ, Willey RF, Fergusson RJ, et al. Rigid bronchoscopy under intravenous general anesthesia with oxygen Venturi ventilation. *Thorax.* 1987;37:532–534.
96. Bollinger CT, Sutedja TG, Strausz J, Freitag L. Therapeutic bronchoscopy with immediate effect: laser, electrocautery, argon plasma coagulation and stents. *Eur Respir J.* 2006;27:1258–1271.
97. Laforet EG, Berger RL, Vaughan CW. Carcinoma obstructing the trachea. Treatment by laser resection. *N Engl J Med.* 1976;294: 941.
98. Wahidi M, Unroe M, Adlakha N, et al. The use of electrocautery as the primary ablation modality for malignant and benign airway obstruction. *J Thorac Oncol.* 2011;6:1516–1520.
99. Keller CA, Hinerman R, Singh A, Alvarez F. The use of endoscopic argon plasma coagulation in airway complications after solid organ transplantation. *Chest.* 2001;119:1968–1975.
100. Morice R, Ece T, Ece F, Keus L. Endobronchial argon plasma coagulation for treatment of hemoptysis and neoplastic airway obstruction. *Chest.* 2001;119:781–787.
101. Feller-Kopman D, Lukanich JM, Shapira G, et al. Gas flow during bronchoscopic ablation therapy causes gas emboli to the heart: a comparative animal study. *Chest.* 2008;33:892–896.
102. Vergnon J, Huber R, Moghissi K. Place of cryotherapy, brachytherapy and photodynamic therapy in therapeutic bronchoscopy of lung cancers. *Eur Respir J.* 2006;28:200–218.
103. Ferretti G, Jouvan FB, Thony F, Pison C, Coulomb M. Benign noninflammatory bronchial stenosis: treatment with balloon dilation. *Radiology.* 1995;196:831–834.
104. Reddy A, Govert J, Sporn T, Wahidi M. Broncholith removal using cryotherapy during flexible bronchoscopy. *Chest.* 2007;132: 1661–1663.
105. Mang T. Lasers and light sources for PDT: past, present, and future. *Photodiag Photodyn Ther.* 2004;1:43–48.
106. Lee P, Kupeli E, Mehta A. Therapeutic bronchoscopy in lung cancer. *Clin Chest Med.* 2002;23:241–256.
107. Spratling L, Speiser BL. Endoscopic brachytherapy. *Chest Surg Clin N Am.* 1996;6:293–304.
108. Huber RM, Fischer R, Hautmann H, et al. Palliative endobronchial brachytherapy for central lung tumors: a prospective randomized comparison of two fractionation schedules. *Chest.* 1995;107: 463–470.
109. Ozkok S, Karakoyun-Celik O, Goksel T, et al. High dose rate endobronchial brachytherapy in the management of lung cancer: response and toxicity evaluation in 158 patients. *Lung Cancer.* 2008;62:326–333.
110. Cardona Zorrilla AF, Reveiz L, Ospina EG, Yepes A. Palliative endobronchial brachytherapy for non-small cell lung cancer. *Cochrane Database System Rev.* 2008;2:CD004284.
111. Dumon JF. A dedicated tracheobronchial stent. *Chest.* 1990;97: 328–332.
112. Freitag L. Tracheobronchial stents. In: Bollinger CT, Mathur PN, eds. *Interventional Bronchoscopy.* Basel, Switzerland: S. Karger; 2000:171–186.
113. Chan A, Juarez MM, Allen RP, Albertson TE. Do airway metallic stents for benign lesions confer too costly a benefit? *BMC Pulm Med.* 2008;8:7–15.
114. Lunn W, Feller-Kopman D, Wahidi M, et al. Endoscopic removal of metallic airway stents. *Chest.* 2005;127:2106–2112.
115. Lund W, Force S. Airway stenting for patients with benign airway disease and the Food and Drug Administration advisory: a call for restraint. *Chest.* 2007;132:1107–1108.
116. Trisolini R, Paioli D, Fornario V, et al. Collapse of a new type of self-expanding metallic tracheal stent. *Monaldi Arch Chest Dis.* 2006;65:56–58.
117. Dumon JF, Cavaliere S, Diaz-Jimenez JP, et al. Seven-year experience with the Dumon prosthesis. *J Bronchol.* 1996;2:6–10.
118. Vergnon JM, Costes F, Bayon MC, Emonot A. Efficacy of tracheal and bronchial stent placement on respiratory functional tests. *Chest.* 1995;107:741–746.
119. Miyazawa T, Miyazu Y, Iwamoto Y, et al. Stenting at the flow-limiting segment in tracheobronchial stenosis due to lung cancer. *Am J Respir Crit Care Med.* 2004;169:1096–1102.
120. Wood DE, Liu YH, Vallieres E, Karmy-Jones R, Mulligan MS. Airway stenting for malignant and benign tracheobronchial stenosis. *Ann Thorac Surg.* 2003;76:167–172.
121. Saad CP, Murthy S, Krizmanich G, Mehta AC. Self-expandable metallic airway stents and flexible bronchoscopy: long-term outcomes analysis. *Chest.* 2003;124:1993–1999.
122. Dasgupta A, Dolmatch BL, Abi-Saleh WJ, Mathur PN, Mehta AC. Self-expandable metallic airway stent insertion employing flexible bronchoscopy: preliminary results. *Chest.* 1998;114:106–109.
123. Bollinger CT, Probst R, Tschopp K, Soler M, Perruchoud AP. Silicone stents in the management of inoperable tracheobronchial stenosis: indications and limitations. *Chest.* 1993;104: 1653–1659.
124. Lemaire A, Burfeind WR, Toloza E, et al. Outcomes of tracheobronchial stents in patients with malignant airway disease. *Ann Thorac Surg.* 2005;80:434–438.
125. Light RW. *Pleural Diseases.* 4th ed. Philadelphia: Lippincott Williams & Wilkins; 2001.
126. Light RW. Pleural effusion. *N Engl J Med.* 2002;346:1971–1977.
127. Feller-Kopman D, Walkey A, Berkowitz D, Ernst A. The relationship of pleural pressure to symptom development during therapeutic thoracentesis. *Chest.* 2006;129:1556–1560.
128. Feller-Kopman D, Parker MJ, Schwartzstein RM. Assessment of pleural pressure in the evaluation of pleural effusions. *Chest.* 2009;135:201–209.
129. Feller-Kopman D. Ultrasound-guided thoracentesis. *Chest.* 2006;129:1709–1714.
130. Seneff MG, Corwin RW, Gold LH, Irwin RS. Complications associated with thoracentesis. *Chest.* 1986;90:97–100.

131. Mayo PH, Goltz HR, Tafreshi M, Doelken P. Safety of ultrasound-guided thoracentesis in patients receiving mechanical ventilation. *Chest.* 2004;125:1059–1062.
132. Jones PW, Moyers JP, Rogers JT, et al. Ultrasound-guided thoracentesis: is it a safer method? *Chest.* 2003;123:418–423.
133. Raptopoulos V, Davis LM, Lee G, et al. Factors affecting the development of pneumothorax associated with thoracentesis. *Am J Roentgenol.* 1991;156:917–920.
134. Light RW, Macgregor MI, Luchsinger PC, Ball WC Jr. Pleural effusions: the diagnostic separation of transudates and exudates. *Ann Intern Med.* 1972;77:507–513.
135. Burgess LJ, Maritz FJ, Taljaard JJF. Comparative analysis of the biochemical parameters used to distinguish between pleural transudates and exudates. *Chest.* 1995;107:1604–1609.
136. Colice GL, Curtis A, Deslauriers J, et al. Medical and surgical treatment of parapneumonic effusions. *Chest.* 2000;118:1158–1171.
137. Maskell NA, Butland RJA. BTS guidelines for the investigation of a unilateral pleural effusion in adults. *Thorax.* 2003;58: ii8–ii17.
138. Prakash UBS, Reiman HM. Comparison of needle biopsy with cytologic analysis for the evaluation of pleural effusion: analysis of 414 cases. *Mayo Clin Proc.* 1985;60:158–164.
139. Dresler CM, Olak J, Herndon JE, et al. Phase III intergroup study of talc poudrage vs talc slurry sclerosis for malignant pleural effusion. *Chest.* 2005;127;909–915.
140. Diacon AH, Wyser C, Bolliger CT, et al. Prospective randomized comparison of thoracoscopic talc poudrage under local anesthesia versus bleomycin instillation for pleurodesis in malignant pleural effusions. *Am J Respir Crit Care Med.* 2000;162:1445–1449.
141. Seaton KG, Patz EF, Goodman PC. Palliative treatment of malignant pleural effusions: value of small-bore catheter thoracostomy and doxycycline sclerotherapy. *AJR.* 1995;164:589–591.
142. Putnam JB, Light RW, Rodriquez RM, et al. A randomized comparison of indwelling pleural catheter and doxycycline pleurodesis in the management of malignant pleural effusions. *Cancer.* 1999;86:1992–1999.
143. Tremblay A, Michaud G. Single-center experience with 250 tunnelled pleural catheter insertions for malignant pleural effusion. *Chest.* 2006;129:362–368.
144. VanMeter M, McKee K, Kohlew R. Efficacy and safety of tunneled pleural catheters in adults with malignant pleural effusions: a systematic review. *J Gen Intern Med.* 2011;26:70–76.
145. Reddy C, Ernst A, Lamb C, et al. Rapid pleurodesis for malignant pleural effusions. *Chest.* 2011;139:1419–1423.
146. Wood ED, McKenna RJ, Yusen RD, et al. A multicenter trial of an intrabronchial valve for treatment of severe emphysema. *J Thorac Cardiovasc Surg.* 2007;133:65–73.
147. Ingenito EP, Wood DE, Utz JP. Bronchoscopic lung volume reduction in severe emphysema. *Proc Am Thorac Soc.* 2008;5: 454–460.
148. Criner GJ, Pinto-Plata V, Strange C, et al. Biologic lung volume reduction in advanced upper lobe emphysema. *Am J Respir Crit Care Med.* 2009;179:791–798.
149. Slebos DJ, Klooster K, Ernst A, et al. Bronchoscopic lung volume reduction coil treatment of patients with severe heterogeneous emphysema. *Chest.* 2012;142:574–582.

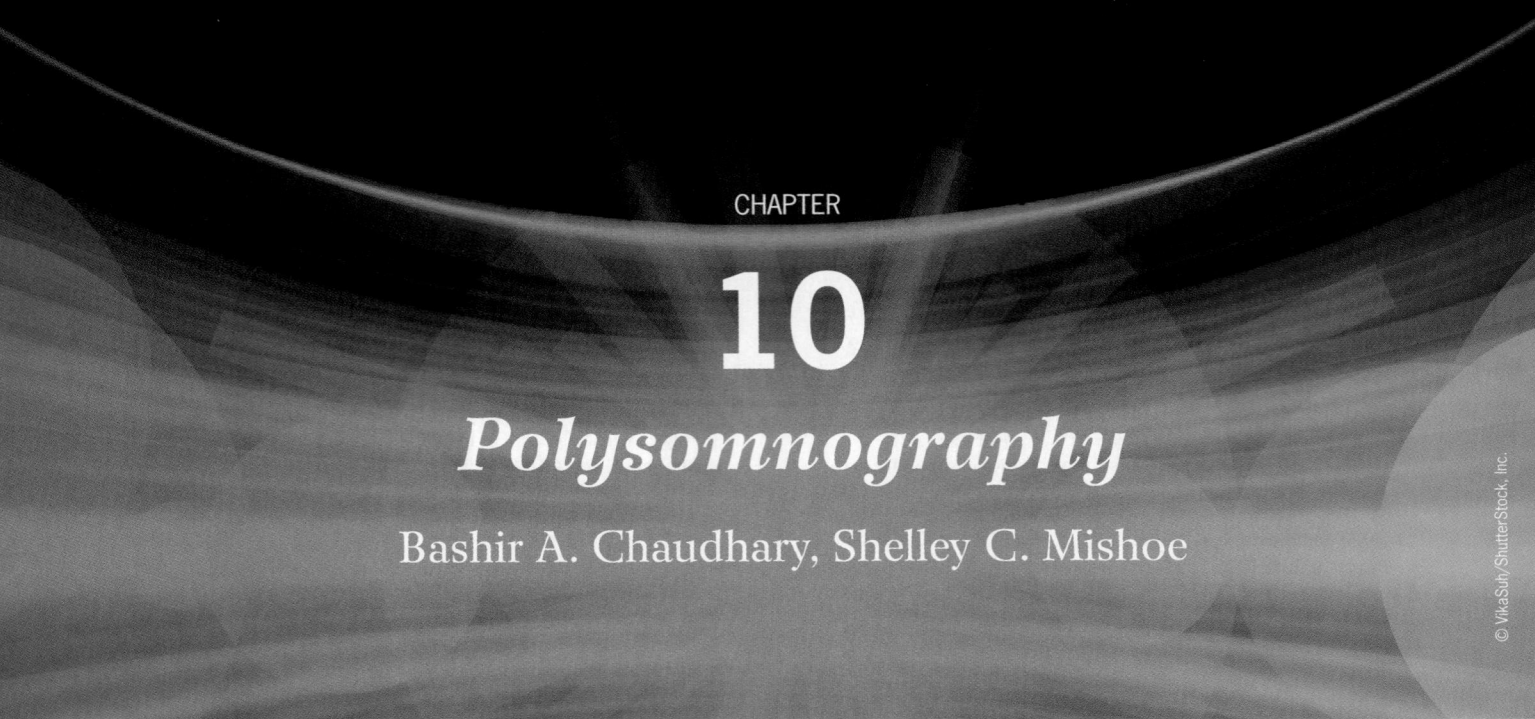

CHAPTER

10

Polysomnography

Bashir A. Chaudhary, Shelley C. Mishoe

OUTLINE

Normal Sleep and Sleep Stages
Polysomnography Components
Scoring Criteria
Polysomnography Report

OBJECTIVES

1. Discuss the 10-20 system of electrode placement for electroencephalography (EEG).
2. Describe how amplifiers, gain, and sensitivity are applied in polysomnography.
3. Describe low-cut, high-cut, and notch filters.
4. Explain the basics of electrooculography and electromyography.
5. Identify common EEG rhythms.
6. Explain the scoring of sleep stages.
7. Apply the rules of disordered breathing.
8. Explain the scoring of leg movements.
9. Discuss the concepts and identification of arousals during sleep.
10. Describe the preparation of a polysomnography report.

KEY TERMS

amplifiers
apnea
arousals
arousal index
delta wave
EEG rhythms
electroencephalogram (EEG)
electromyogram (EMG)
electrooculogram (EOG)
hypopnea
international 10-20 system
K complexes
nonrapid eye movement (NREM) sleep
oximetry
periodic limb movements (PLMs) of sleep
polysomnogram
rapid eye movement (REM) sleep
respiratory effort–related arousal
sleep efficiency
sleep latency
sleep spindles
sleep stages

Introduction

About one-third of our lives is spent sleeping. Although there is considerable variation, most young adults sleep about 7.5 hours during the weeknights and 8.5 hours during the weekends. During sleep, major changes to the organ systems of the body occur, the most important of which are in the neurologic and respiratory systems. Sleep decreases the direct neurologic control of ventilation and ventilatory muscle tone. Changes also occur to neurochemical reflexes that maintain respiration, so there is a reduced drive to breathe and airway resistance increases during normal sleep. Acute and chronic diseases can compound these normal changes, leading to apnea, hypopnea, and sleep-disordered breathing. This chapter focuses on the study of sleep.

Normal Sleep and Sleep Stages

Normal sleep consists of two states: **nonrapid eye movement (NREM) sleep** and **rapid eye movement (REM) sleep**. These sleep states alternate during the night. A combination of NREM and REM sleep makes one sleep cycle. Typically, there are three to five sleep cycles during one night of sleep, and the average duration of a sleep cycle is about 100 ± 10 minutes (mean ± standard deviation). The first sleep cycle is usually the shortest (85 ± 15 minutes). Each sleep cycle starts with NREM sleep, which lasts about 90 minutes before REM sleep begins. NREM sleep has been subdivided into three **sleep stages**: stages N1, N2, and N3 (**Table 10-1**). Stages N1 and N2 represent superficial sleep, whereas stage N3 sleep represents deep sleep.

TABLE 10-1
Sleep Stages in Young Adults

Sleep Stage	Time Spent
NREM Sleep	75–80%
Stage N1	2–5%
Stage N2	45–55%
Stage N3	15–20%
REM or R Sleep	20–25%

Respiratory Recap

Physiologic Changes During Sleep

- Alterations in neurochemical reflexes
- Increased airway resistance
- Reductions in airway space, drive to breathe, upper airway muscle tone, ventilatory muscle tone, ventilation (rate and depth of breathing)

The first sleep cycle starts with sleep stage N1, which lasts only 1 to 7 minutes. During this stage of sleep, the person wakes up easily and may not even realize that he or she was asleep. Stage N2 sleep lasts for 10 to 30 minutes, followed by 25 to 45 minutes of stage N3 sleep. Usually the stage N3 sleep changes back to stage N2 sleep for 5 to 10 minutes before the start of stage R (REM) sleep. The duration of stage R sleep in the first sleep cycle is usually less than 5 minutes. During the subsequent sleep cycles stage N3 sleep decreases in duration, and it is usually absent in the last sleep cycle. On the other hand, stage R increases in duration in the subsequent sleep cycles. The change to and from stage R sleep is through stage N2 sleep. Distribution of sleep stages in a given night can be affected by many factors, including age, the amount of sleep during the previous nights, medications, and the presence of sleep-related medical disorders.[1]

During the first year of life, the onset of sleep frequently is with stage R sleep instead of NREM sleep, and the sleep cycles are about 60 minutes long. The amount of stage N3 sleep is at maximum during the first decade of life and decreases significantly (by about 40%) in the second decade (**Figure 10-1**). The duration of stage N3 sleep decreases progressively with aging and is frequently absent after age 60, particularly in men. The percentage of REM sleep usually does not change much with age.

Sleep deprivation significantly changes the sleep stage pattern. Stage N3 sleep and stage R sleep are increased in duration, as if the body were trying to recover these components of sleep lost during the earlier nights. Stage N3 sleep is usually recovered the first night, and stage R sleep during the subsequent nights. Chronic sleep deprivation or disturbance of sleep and irregular sleep

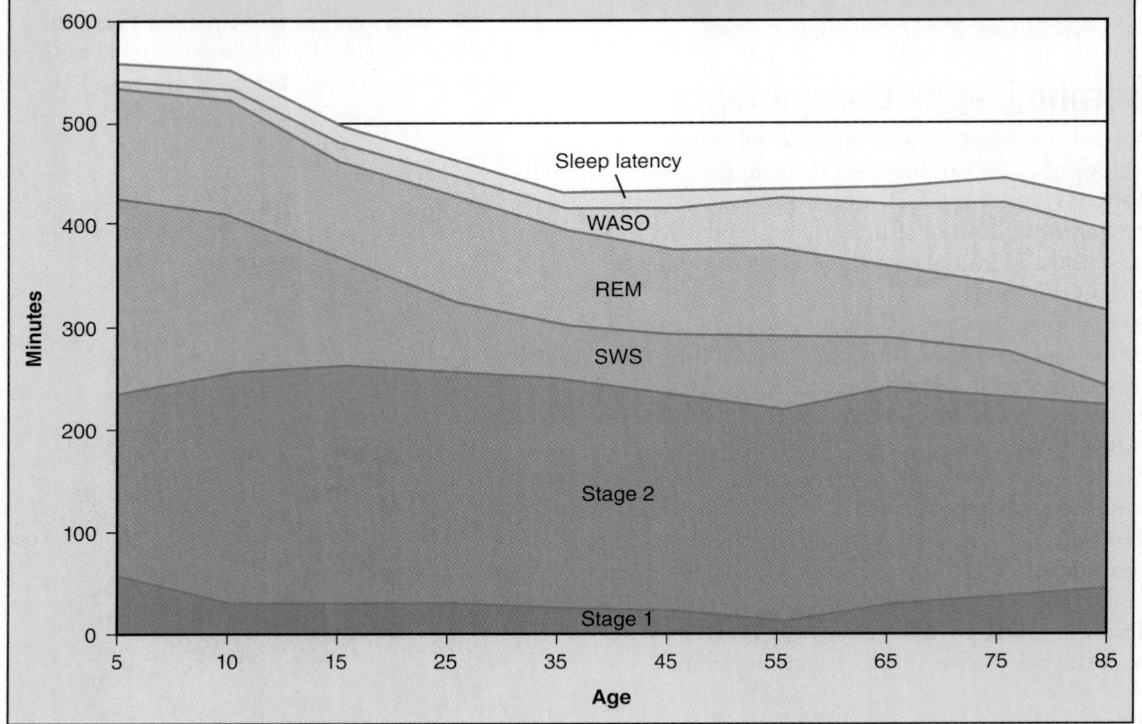

FIGURE 10-1 Age-related sleep stage changes.

Reproduced from Ohayon MM, et al. Metaanalysis of quantitative sleep parameters from childhood to old age in healthy individuals: developing normative sleep values across the human lifespan. *Sleep*. 2004;27:1255–1273. Reprinted with permission of American Academy of Sleep Medicine; permission conveyed through Copyright Clearance Center, Inc.

AGE-SPECIFIC ANGLE

During the first year of life, the onset of sleep is frequently with stage R sleep and sleep cycles are about 60 minutes. The duration of stage N3 sleep decreases progressively with aging and is frequently absent after age 60. The percentage of REM sleep usually does not change much with age.

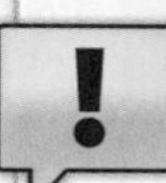

Respiratory Recap

Sleep Stages

- Stage W (wakefulness)
- Stage N1 (old NREM 1)
- Stage N2 (old NREM 2)
- Stage N3 (old NREM 3 and 4)
- Stage R (old REM)

schedule can cause earlier onset of stage R sleep. Most antidepressants, particularly tricyclics, suppress stage R sleep. Benzodiazepines prolong the duration of sleep, but the amount of stage N3 sleep is actually decreased. Withdrawal of the medications suppressing stage N3 or R sleep results in rebound of these stages.

Any medical illness that disturbs sleep, causing arousal, can reduce the amount of stage N3 and stage R sleep. In severe sleep apnea these two stages are frequently reduced. Continuous positive airway pressure (CPAP) therapy is associated with rebound. Narcolepsy is characterized by early onset of stage R sleep.

Polysomnography Components

A typical **polysomnogram** (Current Procedural Terminology code 95810) includes recording of **electroencephalogram (EEG)**, **electrooculogram (EOG)**, **electromyogram (EMG)** of chin muscles, oronasal airflow, chest and abdominal movements, leg movements, snoring, and **oximetry**.[2]

Rechtschaffen and Kales (R&K) developed a manual in 1968 that had been used since that time as the standardized system for sleep stages.[3] In 2007, the American Academy of Sleep Medicine (AASM), previously called the American Sleep Disorders Association, published a new manual, which made significant changes in sleep stages.[4] This manual also added rules about arousals, cardiac rhythm, muscle movements, and sleep-related breathing problems. The AASM rules became the new standard for performing and interpreting polysomnograms in 2008. Following is a discussion of some of the basic aspects of polysomnography.

Electroencephalography

Brain electrical activity is recorded through surface electrodes placed on the skull in accordance with an

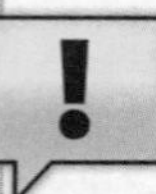

Respiratory Recap

Components of Polysomnography

- Electroencephalogram (EEG)
- Electrooculogram (EOG)
- Electromyogram (EMG) of chin muscles
- Oronasal airflow
- Chest and abdominal movements
- Leg movements
- Snoring
- Oximetry

internationally accepted method. These electrical signals pass from the electrodes and through amplifiers, where they are modified before being recorded on paper (analog) or digital recorders.

International 10-20 System

The **international 10-20 system** was developed in 1958 to standardize the placement of electrodes for EEG recording.[5] The system is termed *10-20* because electrodes are placed either at 10% or 20% of the total distance between two skull landmarks (**Figure 10-2**). The use of percentages instead of absolute distances allows for variation in head sizes. Based on specific anatomic correlates, this system of electrode placement allows for comparison of electrical activity from different areas of the brain and serial comparison of follow-up EEGs in a single patient. Also, it is consistent from one patient to another.

The four landmarks used are the nasion (the indentation between the forehead and the nose), the inion

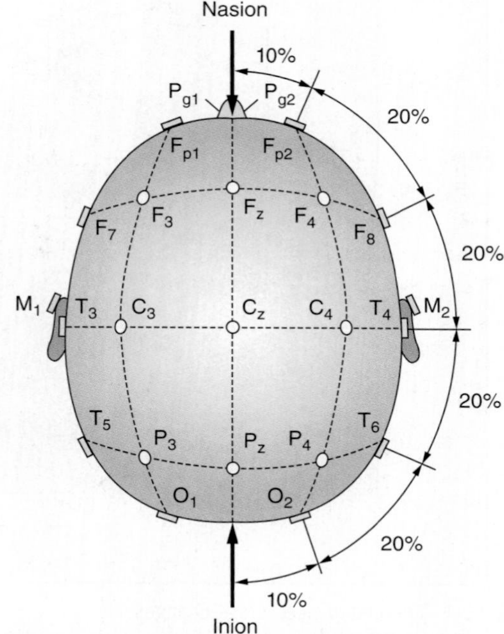

FIGURE 10-2 Electrode placement in the international 10-20 system.

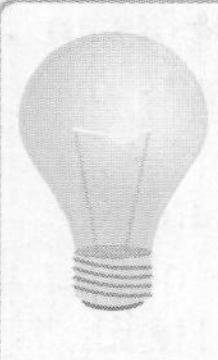

STOP AND THINK

Why should respiratory therapists understand how sleep varies with age? How should this information be considered when interpreting a sleep study?

(the ridge at the back of the skull), and two preauricular points (indentations just in front of the tragus cartilage). The nomenclature gives each electrode a site pertaining to a certain area of the brain (F, frontal; P, parietal; T, temporal; C, central; O, occipital; A, auricular), with the exception of the z electrode, which refers to the midline or zero line. Appended numbers refer to the right (even numbers) and the left (odd numbers) side of the brain. The numbers also define the electrode location in relation to the midline. The smaller the number, the closer the electrode position is to the midline.

The three measurements made to locate the electrode sites are the nasion to inion, right and left preauricular points, and the circumference of the head at the level of Fpz (which is at 10% of the distance from the nasion) and Oz (which is at 10% of the distance from the inion). Frontal (F3 and F4) electrodes are located on the sides of Fz, which is at 30% of the distance from the nasion. Cz is located at the top of the head, at the crossing of the nasion-to-inion line and the line between the two preauricular points. The C3 and C4 electrodes are located on the line between the two auricular points at 20% of the distance from the Cz point or at 30% of the distance from the preauricular points. The O1 and O2 electrodes are separated by 10% of the circumference measurement. These electrodes are at the sides of the Oz electrode at 5% of the circumference measurement.

EEG is recorded using either referential or bipolar deviations. A referential deviation is used when the exploring electrode is compared with a relatively inactive reference site such as the mastoid. A bipolar derivation is used when the two exploring electrodes are compared with each other.

According to Rechtschaffen and Kales, the standard scoring channel for sleep stages was the central channel (C3/A2 or C4/A1).[3] Usually both of these channels were used to minimize the possibility of electrode displacement during the recording. Sleep spindles, K complexes, vertex waves, and delta waves are clearly recorded from these channels. Slow waves and K complexes are maximally expressed in the frontal region, spindles in the central region, and alpha rhythm in the occipital region. Occipital channels are helpful in defining sleep onset.

The AASM has recommended that EEG derivations be increased to three (**Table 10-2**). The major change is the addition of frontal electrodes (F) to better diagnose K complexes and delta waves. With three backup EEG derivations, the total number becomes six. The location of EEG electrodes has been modified, and the recommended derivations are F4-M1, C4-M1, and O2-M1. The backup derivations are F3-M2, C3-M2, and O1-M2. The alternative derivations are Fz-Cz, Cz-Oz, and C4-M1, with backup derivations of Fpz-C3, C3-O1, and C3-M2.

TABLE 10-2
Standard Montage for Monitoring of Sleep States

Parameter	Derivation
EEG	F4-M1 C4-M1 O2-M1
EOG	E1-M2 E2-M2
EMG	One electrode above the inferior edge of mandible Two electrodes below the inferior edge of mandible

Amplifiers

The amplitudes (voltage) of the EEG signals recorded at the scalp are too small. Therefore, **amplifiers** are needed to increase the signal to make them suitable for interpretation. Modern amplifiers also have calibration devices and filters to reduce unwanted EEG frequencies. Amplifiers are able to receive large inputs (volts). Sometimes, amplifiers are arbitrarily referred to as *preamplifiers* if they receive small inputs (microvolts [μV] and millivolts [mV]).

An amplifier multiplies an input signal with a constant, which is usually in the range of 2 to 1000. This amplification factor is referred to as *gain*. The gain can also be expressed as V_{out}/V_{in}. Differential alternating-current (AC) amplifiers used for EEG monitoring receive voltage input from two sources (grid 1 and grid 2, or G1 and G2); the difference between the two voltages is passed through. For example, if the input at G1 is −70 μV and the input at G2 is −10 μV, the difference (i.e., 60 μV) will be amplified and passed further. Signals common to both inputs—for example, the noise from a 60-Hz line current—are called *in phase* or *common mode* and are not passed further. The ability of an amplifier to enlarge the difference in voltage and to reject the voltage common to both inputs is expressed as the *common-mode rejection ratio*.

The ability of a recording system to respond (i.e., pen deflection) to a given input signal is a function of its sensitivity. *Sensitivity* describes the amount of voltage needed to produce a fixed amount of pen deflection and is usually expressed in microvolts per centimeter. The usual sensitivity setting for sleep stages in adults is 50 μV/cm. That is, in order to have a pen deflection of 1 cm, an input of 50 μV is needed. If the amount of pen deflection needs to be increased, then the number of microvolts needed to produce 1 cm of pen deflection has to be decreased. This will give a lower numeric value for sensitivity (e.g., 25 μV/cm). Similarly, if the amplitude of the EEG waves is too high, as is often the case in children, this amplitude may have to be decreased by increasing the number of microvolts needed to produce 1 cm of pen deflection. This change (e.g., 75 μV/cm) will give a higher number for sensitivity even though the amplitude for pen deflection is being decreased. Because the electrocardiographic (ECG) signal is very strong compared with the EEG signal, the sensitivity of the ECG signal has to be very high. The typical sensitivity setting for the ECG signal is 1 to 10 millivolts per centimeter (mV/cm). The mV/cm value is 1000 times more than the μV/cm value.

The relationship of sensitivity, voltage, and pen deflection is similar to the relationship of voltage, current, and resistance in Ohm's law (Voltage = Current × Resistance). In the EEG, sensitivity represents resistance, and pen deflection represents current. If the resistance (sensitivity) goes up, then the current (pen deflection) will decrease, provided there is no change in voltage.

Amplifiers not only increase the size of the input signal but also are able to filter out undesirable signals. The three main types of filters used are high-frequency filters, low-frequency filters, and notch filters. High-frequency filters (HFFs) are used to attenuate frequencies higher than the desired frequency (e.g., muscle activity–related artifacts). These filters are also called *low-pass filters*. Most frequencies of interest in EEG range from 0.16 to 100 Hz. The HFF for EEG is set at 35 Hz. Higher EEG frequencies are seen in patients with seizures. The upper frequency of spike discharge (with a 20-ms base) is 50 Hz. Spikes by definition have a base of 20 to 70 ms, with a frequency of 14 to 50 Hz. In such cases the HFF may be set at a higher frequency (e.g., at 70 Hz). A filter does not have a static or single level of attenuation. The HFF usually attenuates the designated frequency by 80%, and this percentage increases progressively for frequencies higher than the designated frequency of the HFF.

Low-frequency filters (LFFs) are used to attenuate undesirable frequencies in the lower frequency range. These filters are also called *high-pass filters*. These filters attenuate the signal at the designated frequency by 20%. For example, a standard LFF set at 0.3 Hz will attenuate a 0.3-Hz signal of 100 μV to 80 μV. EEG frequencies lower than the designated frequency of the LFF are progressively attenuated more. The *time constant* is another form of expressing filtration of low frequencies. The time constant is defined as the time it takes for a square wave signal to drop to 37% of the original baseline. Frequently, time constant and LFF are used interchangeably, although the numeric values are not the same. A time constant of 1 s represents an LFF of 0.1, and a time constant of 0.3 s represents an LFF of 0.5.

Notch filters are designed to sharply attenuate a narrow-frequency bandwidth within the range of 50 to 60 Hz. Notch filters are also known as 60-Hz filters. These filters are used to eliminate the noise from electric power lines. Routine use of notch filters is not appropriate because they can mask frequencies that may be of interest in seizure monitoring. This filter can also hide high electrode impedance and poor signal transmission. In EMG channels, the notch filter may excessively attenuate the muscle tone, leading to misinterpretation of the sleep stage.

Electrical interference can be minimized if the power cords are kept away from the circuit. Low impedance of the electrodes also helps in minimizing the electric line noise. By convention, EEG signals using differential amplifiers are displayed such that negative waveforms cause an upward deflection and positive waveforms cause a downward deflection.

Electrooculography

Using the R&K manual system, eye movements were recorded from electrodes placed near the outer canthus of each eye.[3] The right outer canthus electrode (ROC) was attached about 1 cm above and out from the outer canthus of the right eye. The left outer canthus electrode (LOC) was attached about 1 cm below and out from the outer canthus of the left eye. These electrodes were usually referred to the same auricular electrode (e.g., ROC/A1 and LOC/A1).

The AASM manual modified the placement of EOG electrodes. Because the highest amplitude of EOG signals is obtained when the electrodes are placed above and below the eyes at the level of the outer canthi, the lateral part of the electrodes' placement has been eliminated. The nomenclature has changed: E1 and E2 represent the left and right eye electrodes, and M1 and M2 represent the left and the right mastoid electrodes. The recommended EOG derivations are E1-M2 and E2-M2. The location of eye electrodes has also changed. E1 is placed 1 cm below the left outer canthus. The E2 electrode is placed 1 cm above the right outer canthus. This new arrangement provides higher-amplitude signals for the eye movements.

Eye movements occur in all directions. Generally only about 10% of eye movements are horizontal, whereas 30% are vertical and 60% are oblique. If it is important to evaluate the direction of eye movements, then an alternative derivation may be helpful. The alternative EOG electrodes are E1-Fpz and E2-Fpz. The alternative E1 electrode is placed 1 cm below and 1 cm lateral to the outer canthus of the left eye. Similarly, the alternative E2 electrode is placed 1 cm below and 1 cm lateral to the outer canthus of the right eye.

Placement of electrodes just above one eye and just below the opposite eye produces out-of-phase deflections for conjugate eye movements. This is helpful in distinguishing artifacts coming to the ROC and LOC from other channels. Delta waves are frequently seen in these channels but can be distinguished by being in the same direction (i.e., in phase).

The small electropotential difference that normally exists between the front and the back of the eye is responsible for the eye movements recorded during polysomnography. The eyeball is like a dipole in which the cornea is positive and the retina is negative. When the eyes move to one side, the electrode placed on the same side as the eye movement will record a positive deflection (downward), while the other electrode will record a negative deflection (upward) because the other eye is going away from that electrode.

Eye movements can be divided into slow eye movements (SEMs) and rapid eye movements (REMs). There are no well-defined criteria to distinguish SEMs from REMs. The frequency of SEMs is usually less than 0.5 Hz (i.e., more than 2 s in duration) and the duration of the entire waveform of REMs is less than 1 s. The main feature that helps in distinguishing these two types of eye movements is that the duration of initial deflection of REMs is less than 500 ms, whereas the initial deflection of SEMs is greater than 500 ms.

The main reason for recording eye movements is to establish the presence of REM sleep. REM sleep cannot be diagnosed without the presence of REMs. The frequency of REMs per hour of REM sleep is designated as *REM density* and is a reflection of REM sleep intensity. The presence of SEMs usually means that sleep stage 1 either has begun or is about to begin. Hence, it is helpful in defining the onset of sleep.

Electromyography

In routine polysomnography, EMG is recorded from chin muscles and anterior tibialis muscles. The AASM manual has recommended placing three electrodes for recording chin EMG. One electrode should be placed 1 cm above the inferior edge of the mandible. The second electrode should be placed 2 cm below the inferior edge of the mandible and 2 cm to the right of the midline. The third electrode should be placed 2 cm below the inferior edge of the mandible and 2 cm to the left of the midline. The EMG is recorded bipolar, and a combination of any two electrodes can be used. The third electrode serves as the backup electrode and is particularly helpful for studies extending to the daytime, when there is a greater likelihood of electrodes coming off during eating and talking.

The limb electrodes are attached about 2 to 4 cm apart over the anterior tibialis muscle on both legs. Additional electrodes are attached in certain situations. EMG from the masseter muscle is helpful in the evaluation of bruxism. In patients suspected of having **periodic limb movements (PLMs) of sleep**, electrodes also may be attached to the upper limbs because PLMs of sleep occur in all four limbs.

Chin-muscle EMG is recorded mainly to distinguish REM sleep from NREM sleep. Reduction of muscle tone is one of the requirements for diagnosing REM sleep. PLMs of sleep are diagnosed from limb EMG channels. Because intercostal muscle activity ceases during REM sleep, sometimes an intercostal EMG is used to determine respiratory effort. The normal EMG frequency is between 20 and 200 Hz and generally is greater than 40 Hz. The use of a 60-Hz filter can substantially reduce the amplitude of the EMG signal. Conversely, reduction in muscle tone may be difficult to detect in the presence of significant 60-Hz artifact.

Respiratory Measurement

Respiratory effort can be measured in many ways, including esophageal pressure monitoring, flow monitoring by pneumotachometer, flow monitoring by thermistor and thermocouple, nasal pressure monitoring, intercostal EMG monitoring, and inductive plethysmography. As yet there is no consensus as to which method of monitoring is the best method for polysomnography.

Thermistors and thermocouples detect airflow indirectly and semiquantitatively by sensing the temperature change during breathing. The sensors sense the temperature difference between the cooler inspiration and warmer expiration. The change in temperature of the sensor is associated with a change in resistance. A thermistor measures this as a change in resistance, and a thermocouple as a change in electromotive force. These sensors are well tolerated by patients. The correlation between the temperature change and the flow is relatively poor. Although apneas are detected reliably, hypopneas are usually underestimated.

A pneumotachometer, placed in tightly fitted masks, measures total oronasal airflow by detecting changes in pressure between inspiration and expiration. In central sleep apnea, respiratory effort, and hence pressure change, is absent. Monitoring of airflow by this method requires a tightly fitting mask, which can cause discomfort and disruption of sleep. Because of these problems, a mask pneumotachometer has not become popular for clinical studies.

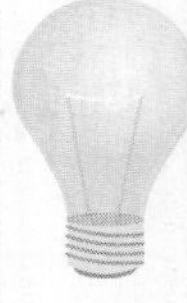

STOP AND THINK

What are the key components of polysomnography for a complete sleep study? Articulate the key information provided by each component and why it is essential for assessment of sleep-disordered breathing.

Nasal pressure can be measured through nasal cannulas placed inside the nares and connected to pressure transducers. Airflow is estimated by measuring nasal airway pressure, which decreases during inspiration and increases during expiration. The flattened contour of inspiratory flow is suggestive of upper airway resistance. Nasal pressure monitoring is more sensitive but less specific than thermistors. Because this technique underestimates the degree of airflow reduction in patients with nasal obstruction, it is not recommended in patients who are mouth breathers. Newer cannulas have been introduced that can detect both nasal and oral airflow. One advantage of nasal cannulas is the detection of inspiratory flow limitation, which is missed by thermistors.

Respiratory inductive plethysmography measures the volume changes in the chest and abdomen during a breathing cycle. The sum of these measurements provides an estimate of tidal volume. Asynchronous breathing can be detected with this method. Asynchronous breathing is paradoxical chest wall and abdominal movements associated with disordered breathing, which means that the chest and abdomen move in opposite directions, rather than together. While this method does not allow for an accurate distinction between apneas and hypopneas in the absence of an airflow measurement, it has been suggested for identification of upper airway resistance syndrome by looking at the ratio of the peak inspiratory flow to mean flow. The loops generated by this technique may also be useful for titration of continuous positive airway pressure.

The AASM manual[4] has recommendations for the detection of sleep-related breathing events. The type of sensor to detect absence of airflow for identification of an apnea is an oronasal thermal sensor, and the one to detect airflow for identification of hypopneas is a nasal air pressure transducer. The sensor used to detect respiratory effort is either esophageal manometry or inductive plethysmography. Flattening of the nasal air pressure waveform leading to an arousal from sleep can also be used for detection of respiratory effort–related arousal.

Scoring Criteria

The main categories of scoring during polysomnography include sleep stages, respiratory events, leg movements, and arousals. Many other parameters, such as oximetry, ECG, snoring, CPAP titration, and effect of posture, also are evaluated.

Sleep Stages

Depending on the frequency (i.e., cycles per second), EEG waves are divided into **EEG rhythms** such as beta, alpha, theta, and delta rhythms (**Table 10-3**).

The sleep state is divided into NREM sleep and REM sleep. NREM sleep was once further subdivided into four stages, with stage 1 being the most superficial and stage 4 the deepest. The AASM manual recommends that NREM stages be named stages N1, N2, N3, the latter of which represents the combined stages 3 and 4 of the R&K manual.[4,6] Sleep stages are scored in 30-s segments (epochs) based on EEG, EOG, and EMG.

Stage W (wakefulness) is characterized by low-amplitude, mixed-frequency EEG (**Figure 10-3**). When the eyes are closed, the alpha rhythm becomes prominent and then diminishes at sleep onset (**Figure 10-4**). Eye movements are present and muscle tone is high. Stage W is scored when more than 50% of the epochs have an alpha rhythm over the occipital region. In those subjects who do not have a discernible alpha rhythm, stage W can be scored if any of the following three items are present: eye blinks with a frequency of 0.5 to 2 Hz, reading eye movements, or irregular conjugate

TABLE 10-3
EEG Rhythms

Rhythm	Frequency (cycles/second)
Beta	>14
Alpha	8–13
Theta	4–7
Delta	<4

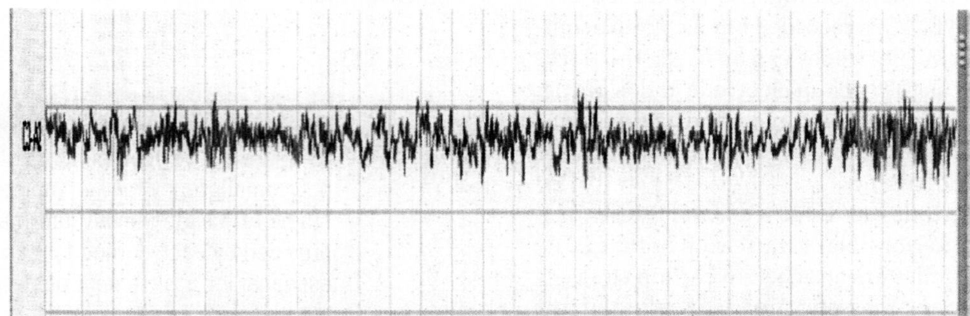

FIGURE 10-3 Thirty-second epoch of low-voltage, mixed-frequency EEG (mostly alpha) of stage W.

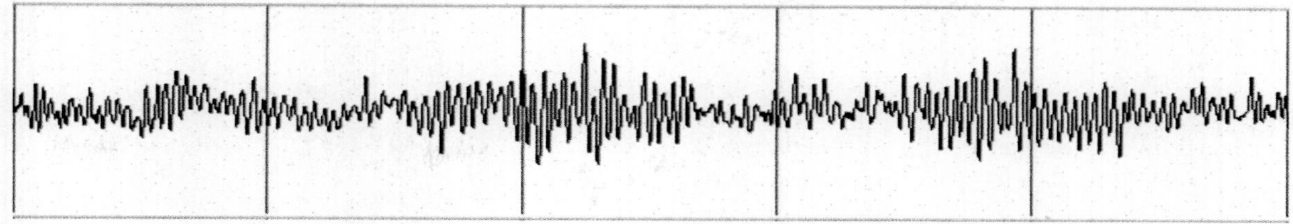

FIGURE 10-4 Ten-second epoch of stage W with eyes closed showing alpha frequency EEG.

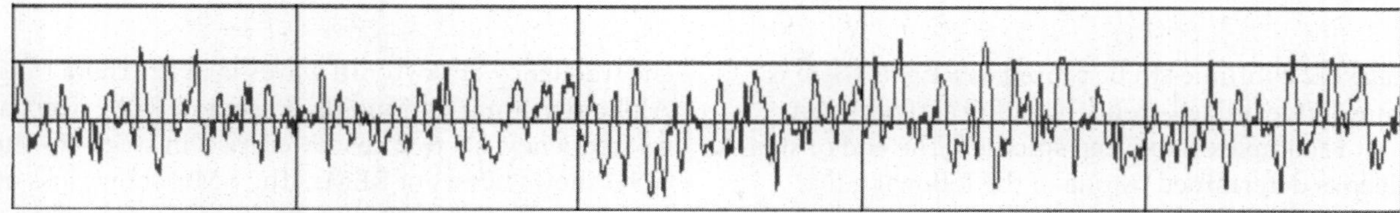

FIGURE 10-5 Ten-second epoch of stage N1 sleep showing predominantly theta frequency EEG.

eye movements associated with normal or high chin muscle tone.

Stage N1 sleep is characterized by a change from alpha activity to theta activity (**Figure 10-5**). SEMs are usually present at sleep onset. Muscle tone usually diminishes at sleep onset compared with stage W. Ten percent to 20% of the population do not have a discernible alpha rhythm. In these subjects, N1 sleep can be scored by the presence of any of the following three items: theta activity with slowing of background frequencies greater than 1 Hz from those of stage W, vertex sharp waves, or slow eye movements.

Sleep onset was previously defined by the presence of sleep for at least three consecutive epochs of stage 1 sleep. The AASM manual has recommended that sleep onset be defined from the start of the first epoch scored as any stage other than stage W.

Stage N2 sleep is characterized by the continuation of the same low-amplitude, mixed-frequency EEG of stage 1 sleep and the appearance of two markers: sleep spindles and K complexes (**Figure 10-6**). **Sleep spindles** have a frequency of 12 to 14 cps (11–16 Hz) and duration of 0.5 to 1.5 s. Incipient (mini, baby) spindles are less than 0.5 s in duration and are seen in stage 1 sleep that precedes stage 2 sleep. Sleep spindles occur with a frequency of 3 to 8 spindles per minute in normal adults. **K complexes** have a sharp upward (negative) deflection followed by a downward (positive) component and are at least 0.5 s in duration. Amplitude is not a criterion for defining a K complex. The usual frequency of K complexes during stage 2 sleep is about 1 to 3 per minute. K complexes occur either spontaneously or are associated with arousals (K arousals). According to the AASM manual, only K complexes unassociated with arousal signal the presence of stage N2 sleep. The presence of K complexes associated with arousal signals the change from stage N2 sleep to stage N1 sleep. The muscle tone is lower than in stage W, and eye movements are uncommon.

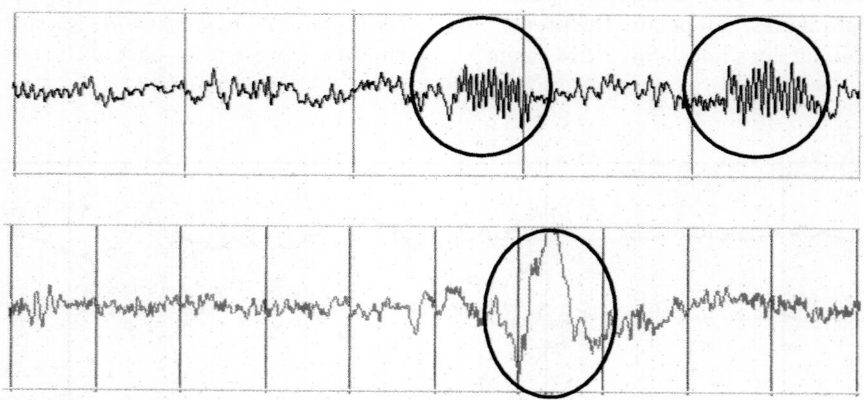

FIGURE 10-6 Ten-second epochs of stage N2 sleep showing sleep spindles in the upper tracing and a K complex in the lower tracing.

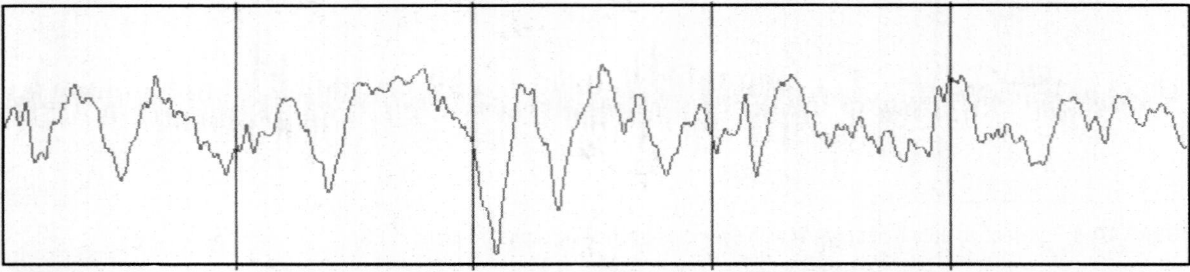

FIGURE 10-7 Ten-second epoch of stage N3 sleep showing high-amplitude, low-frequency delta waves.

Stage N2 continues to be scored as long as there is low-amplitude, mixed-frequency EEG activity even without K complexes or sleep spindles. The end of stage N2 sleep is determined by one of the following five events: (1) transition to stage W, (2) transition to stage N1 because of an arousal, (3) transition to stage N1 because of major body movement followed by slow eye movements, (4) transition to stage N3, or (5) transition to stage R.

Sleep stages 3 and 4 have been called delta sleep and are characterized by the presence of high-voltage (≥75 μV) waves with slow frequency (≤2 cps or slower) (**Figure 10-7**). A **delta wave** should be at least 0.5 s in duration. Stage 3 sleep is defined by the presence of delta waves that occupy at least 20% of an epoch. Stage 4 sleep was scored if delta waves covered at least 50% of an epoch. In the AASM manual system, stages 3 and 4 are combined into stage N3. Stage N3 is scored when 20% or more of an epoch consists of slow wave activity. Occasional sleep spindles may be present in stage N3 sleep. K complexes may be present but are difficult to distinguish from delta waves. Muscle tone is usually still high, but it can be low enough that it resembles the muscle tone of REM sleep. Eye movements are usually absent, but delta waves are frequently seen in eye channels because of the high voltage of delta waves.

REM sleep (stage R) has three cardinal features: low-amplitude, mixed-frequency EEG; bursts of REMs; and loss of muscle tone (**Figure 10-8**). The background EEG is similar to that seen in stage N1 or stage N2 sleep. During this stage, a notched morphology EEG pattern, referred to as *sawtooth waves*, can occur. The presence of this pattern alone does not define REM sleep; the frequency of sawtooth waves is in the theta range. Alpha rhythm is commonly present in REM sleep, and its frequency is 1 to 2 cps lower than in stage W. The EOG shows bursts of REMs. The EMG shows loss of muscle tone. There are occasional muscle twitches. REM sleep is divided into phasic and tonic components based on the presence or absence of eye movements and muscle twitches.

Once stage R sleep has been established, the stage is extended both forward and backward, even in the absence of REMs, until there is evidence of another stage of sleep, as long as there is no change in EMG and EEG. Because stage R can be extended in both directions, we often describe this "REM rule" as "REM rules."

The end of stage R sleep is determined by any of the following: (1) transition to stage W, (2) transition to stage N1 because of increase in muscle tone, (3) transition to stage N1 because of arousal followed by slow eye movements, (4) transition to stage N1 because of major body movement followed by slow eye movements, (5) transition to stage N2, or (6) transition to stage N3 sleep.

Major Body Movements

Movements occur frequently during sleep and obscure EEG and EOG recordings. It becomes difficult to ascertain whether the patient is awake or asleep. If movement occurred for 15 seconds or more, the epoch was scored as "Movement Time" according to the R&K manual.[3] The AASM manual has recommended the term *major body movements* for such artifacts.[4] If alpha rhythm is present for part of the epoch (even less than

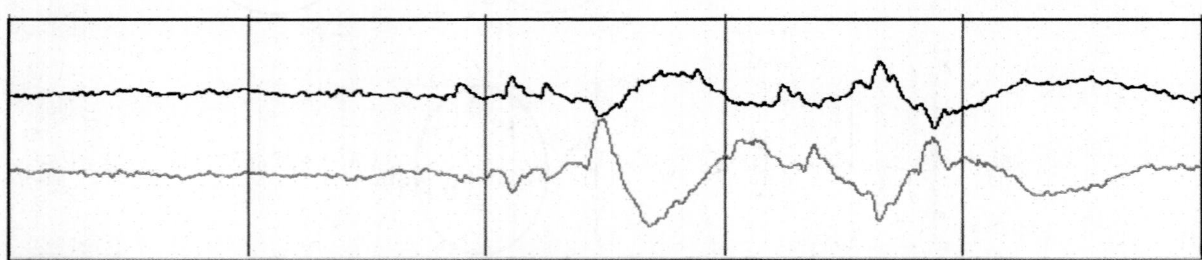

FIGURE 10-8 Ten-second epoch stage R sleep showing eye movements in EOG channels.

15 s in duration), it should be scored as stage W. If stage W either precedes or follows the epoch with major body movement, then it should also be scored as stage W. In other cases the epoch should be scored as the epoch that follows.

Sleep-Disordered Breathing

Sleep-disordered breathing includes apneas, hypopneas, and respiratory effort–related arousals.[7,8] There has been a great deal of controversy about the definition of these events, with the most recent recommendations for detection and scoring coming from the AASM manual.[4,9] **Apnea** is defined as cessation of airflow for more than 10 s. The reduction in airflow should be 90% or more of baseline. At least 90% of the event's duration should meet the amplitude reduction criteria for apnea. Baseline is defined as the mean amplitude of stable breathing and oxygenation in the preceding 2 minutes or the mean amplitude of the three largest breaths in the preceding 2 minutes.

Apnea is classified as *obstructive* if it is associated with continued or increased inspiratory effort throughout the entire period of absent airflow; it is classified as *central* if it is associated with absent inspiratory effort throughout the entire period of absent airflow. Apnea is classified as *mixed* if it is associated with absent inspiratory effort in the initial portion of the event, followed by resumption of inspiratory effort in the second portion of the event.

Hypopnea is defined as a 30% or more decrease (compared with baseline) in airflow or thoracoabdominal movements lasting at least 10 s associated with 4% or more oxygen desaturation. At least 90% of the event's duration should meet the amplitude reduction criteria for hypopneas. Hypopnea can also be scored by an alternative method that requires airflow reduction by 50% and associated oxygen desaturation of 3%.

A **respiratory effort–related arousal** event is defined as a sequence of breaths lasting 10 s characterized by increasing respiratory effort or flattening of the nasal pressure waveform leading to an arousal from sleep when the sequence of breaths does not meet the criteria for an apnea or hypopnea. Esophageal pressure measurement is the preferred method of assessing change in respiratory effort, although nasal pressure and inductive plethysmography can be used.

Respiratory Recap

Sleep Disordered Breathing

- *Apnea*: Reduction of airflow by ≥90% of baseline for ≥10 seconds
- *Obstructive apnea*: Apnea with continued respiratory effort
- *Central apnea*: Apnea with absent respiratory effort
- *Mixed apnea*: Apnea with initial absence and then resumption of respiratory effort
- *Hypopnea*: Reduction of airflow by ≥30% for ≥10 seconds and O_2 desaturation by ≥4%

Arousals

Cortical **arousals** (i.e., those seen on EEG) indicate sleep disruption and are important in defining upper airway resistance syndrome and in determining the clinical impact of nocturnal myoclonic episodes. Arousals were a part of the criteria used to define hypopneas; however, the recommendations of the Centers for Medicare and Medicaid Services do not include arousals as part of the definition of hypopneas.

Arousal is defined as an abrupt shift in EEG frequency that may include theta waves, alpha waves, or frequencies higher than 16 Hz, but not spindles (**Figure 10-9**).[4] Because this change in EEG activity lasts less than 15 s, it does not change the sleep stage. The epoch is scored as awake stage if the change in EEG activity lasts 15 s or more.

The AASM suggests the following rules for scoring of arousals:[4,10]

1. There should be at least 10 s of continuous sleep prior to an arousal.
2. There should be 10 s of continuous sleep prior to a second arousal.
3. An arousal should be at least 3 s long.
4. Arousal in NREM sleep can be scored without EMG elevation.
5. Arousals in REM sleep must have concurrent elevation of chin EMG.
6. Arousals should not be scored based on submental EMG alone.

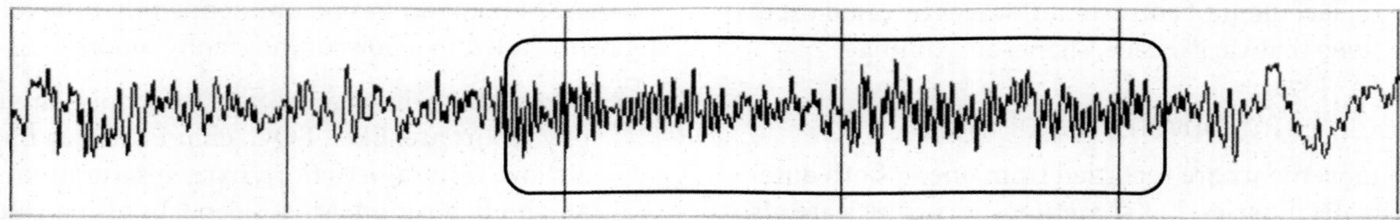

FIGURE 10-9 Ten-second epoch showing an EEG arousal in stage N1 sleep.

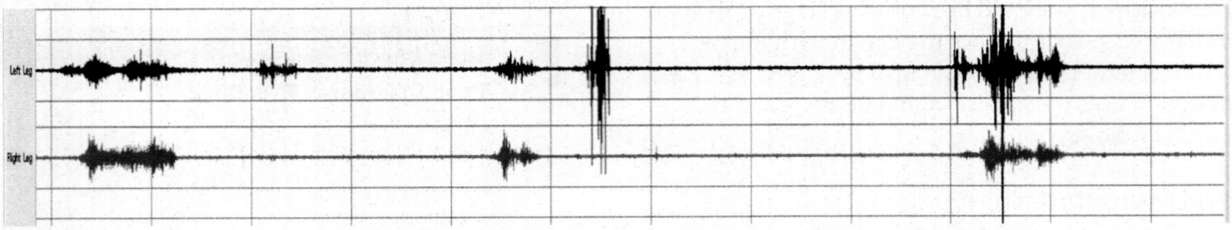

FIGURE 10-10 Two-minute epoch showing leg movements in two EMG channels.

7. Artifacts, K complexes, and delta waves are not arousals unless there is a change in EEG.
8. Pen-deflection artifacts are not arousals unless there is a change in EEG.
9. Nonconcurrent, but contiguous, EEG and EMG changes that last less than 3 s individually but more than 3 s together are not arousals.
10. Alpha sleep is not arousal.
11. Transition from one sleep stage to another sleep stage is not arousal.

Some authors use a different duration criterion (e.g., 1.5 s) for defining an arousal. Arousals are also seen during normal sleep, and there is no consensus at the present time about the normal frequency of arousals. An **arousal index** (number of arousals per hour of sleep) of less than 10 is generally considered within the normal range. Arousal indices of more than 20 (or 25) may be abnormal.

Cardiac Rules

The AASM manual recommends the following rules for scoring of cardiac events:[4,11]

1. Sinus tachycardia is scored if the heart rate is greater than 90 beats/min.
2. Bradycardia is scored if the heart rate is less than 40 beats/min.
3. Asystole is scored if the cardiac pause is greater than 3 seconds.
4. Wide complex tachycardia is scored if the rhythm lasts for a minimum of three consecutive beats at a rate of greater than 100 beats/min and QRS duration of 120 ms or more.
5. Narrow complex tachycardia is scored for a rhythm lasting for a minimum of three consecutive beats at a rate of greater than 100 beats/min and QRS duration of less than 120 ms.
6. Atrial fibrillation is scored if there is an intermittently irregular ventricular rhythm associated with replacement of consistent P waves by rapid oscillations that vary in size, shape, and timing.

Periodic Limb Movements of Sleep

Limb movements are recorded from one or both anterior tibialis muscles, but sometimes recordings are also made from upper extremities. A limb movement is a burst of muscle activity with a mean duration of 1.5 to 2.5 s (**Figure 10-10**).

The AASM manual has recommended the following rules for a significant leg movement (LM) event:[4,12]

1. The minimum duration of an LM is 0.5 s.
2. The maximum duration of an LM event is 10 s.
3. The minimum amplitude of an LM is an 8-μV increase in EMG voltage above resting EMG.

Limb movements are called *periodic* when they occur in a stereotypic manner at intervals of 20 to 40 s. Random aperiodic limb movements are not counted. The AASM has recommended the following rules for defining a periodic limb movement (PLM) series:

1. The minimum number of consecutive LM events needed is four.
2. The minimum period length between LMs is 5 s.
3. The maximum period length between LMs is 90 s.
4. Leg movements on two different legs separated by less than 5 s between movement onsets are counted as a single leg movement.

The total number of limb movements divided by the number of hours of sleep is called the *PLM index*. Limb movements with arousals are counted separately, and the PLM with arousal index is calculated.

Leg movements occurring within 0.5 s of beginning or termination of apneas or hypopneas are not considered a part of periodic limb movements of sleep. On the other hand, leg movements associated with arousals may be a marker of upper airway resistance syndrome. Leg movements without arousals are very common in patients taking antidepressants.

Muscle twitches with duration shorter than 150 ms are called *fragmentary myoclonus*. Excessive fragmentary myoclonus (EFM) is diagnosed if at least 5 potentials per minute are present.

Polysomnography Report

The AASM manual[4] has recommended that the following be included in a polysomnography report:

- *Parameters*. Nine parameters for a polysomnography report are: EEG, EOG, chin EMG, leg EMG, airflow, respiratory effort, oxygen saturation, ECG, and body position. Most sleep labs also include the monitoring of snoring.

- *Sleep scoring data.* Ten respiratory events of data for sleep scoring are light-out time, light-on time, total sleep time, total recording time, **sleep latency**, stage R latency, wake after sleep onset (WASO), percent **sleep efficiency**, time in each sleep stage in minutes, and percentage of total sleep time in each stage.
- *Arousal events.* Total number of arousals and the arousal index (i.e., arousals per hour of sleep).
- *Respiratory events.* Eleven recommended respiratory events are number of obstructive apneas, mixed apneas, central apneas, hypopneas, total apneas and hypopneas, apnea index, hypopnea index, apnea-hypopnea index, mean oxygen saturation, minimum oxygen saturation, and the presence or absence of Cheyne-Stokes breathing. In addition, five optional respiratory events are total respiratory effort–related arousals, respiratory effort–related arousal index, total number of oxygen desaturation episodes (3% or 4%), oxygen desaturation index, and the occurrence or absence of hypoventilation.
- *Cardiac events.* Three cardiac events are the average heart rate during sleep, highest heart rates during sleep, and total recording. In addition the presence or absence of bradycardia, tachycardia, asystole, narrow complex tachycardia, wide complex tachycardia, atrial fibrillation, or any other arrhythmia should be noted.
- *Movement events.* Four recommended movement events are number of periodic limb movements of sleep, number of periodic limb movements with arousals, PLM index, and PLM arousal index.
- *Summary statements.* Four summary events are the findings related to sleep diagnoses, EEG abnormalities, ECG abnormalities, and behavioral observations. Inclusion of sleep hypnogram is an option.

Key Points

- Normal sleep consists of two states: nonrapid eye movement (NREM) sleep and rapid eye movement (REM) sleep.
- NREM and REM sleep states alternate during the night.
- The amount and type of sleep are affected by many variables, such as age, posture, circadian cycle, diseases, alcohol, and medications.
- Polysomnography is used to determine sleep stages and various sleep disorders.
- A typical polysomnogram includes recordings of electroencephalogram (EEG), electrooculogram (EOG), electromyogram (EMG) of chin muscles, oronasal airflow, chest and abdominal movements, leg movements, snoring, and oximetry.
- The main categories of scoring during polysomnography include sleep stages, respiratory events, leg movements, and arousals.
- Many other parameters, such as oximetry, ECG, snoring, continuous positive airway pressure titration, and the effects of posture, are also evaluated.
- The American Academy of Sleep Medicine (AASM) rules became the new standard for the performance and interpretation of polysomnograms in 2008.
- Knowing the basics of polysomnography is important for comprehension of sleep-disordered breathing and common sleep disorders.

References

1. Ohayon MM, Carskadon MA, Guilleminault C, Vitiello MV. Metaanalysis of quantitative sleep parameters from childhood to old age in healthy individuals: developing normative sleep values across the human lifespan. *Sleep*. 2004;27:1255–1273.
2. Carskadon MA, Rechtschaffen A. Monitoring and staging of human sleep. In: Kryger M, Roth T, Dement W, eds. *Principles and Practice of Sleep Medicine*. 4th ed. Philadelphia: WB Saunders; 2005:1359–1377.
3. Rechtschaffen A, Kales A, eds. *A Manual of Standardized Terminology: Techniques and Scoring System for Sleep Stages of Human Subjects*. Los Angeles: UCLA Brain Information Service/Brain Research Institute; 1968.
4. Berry RB, Brooks R, Garnaldo CE, et al. *The AASM Manual for Scoring of Sleep and Associated Events: Rules, Terminology and Technical Specification*, Version 2.0. Darien, IL: American Academy of Sleep Medicine; 2012. Available at http://www.aasmnet.org. Accessed October 1, 2013.
5. Jasper H. The ten-twenty electrode system of the International Federation. *EEG Clin Neurophysiol*. 1958;10:371–375.
6. Silber MH, Ancoli-Israel S, Bonnet MH, et al. The visual scoring of sleep in adults. *J Clin Sleep Med*. 2007;3:121–131.
7. Meoli AL, Casey KR, Clark RW, et al. Hypopnea in sleep-disordered breathing in adults. *Sleep*. 2001;24:469–470.
8. Sleep-related breathing disorders in adults: recommendations for syndrome definition and measurement techniques in clinical research. The report of an American Academy of Sleep Medicine Task Force. *Sleep*. 1999;22:667–689.
9. Redline S, Bhudiraja R, Kapur V, et al. Reliability and validity of respiratory event measurement and scoring. *J Clin Sleep Med*. 2007;3:169–200.
10. EEG arousals: scoring rules and examples. A preliminary report from the Sleep Disorders Atlas Task Force of the American Sleep Disorders Association. *Sleep*. 1992;15:173–184.
11. Caples SM, Rosen CL, Shen WK, et al. The scoring of cardiac events during sleep. *J Clin Sleep Med*. 2007;3:147–154.
12. Walters AS, Lavigne G, Hening W, et al. The scoring of movements in sleep. *J Clin Sleep Med*. 2007;3:155–167.

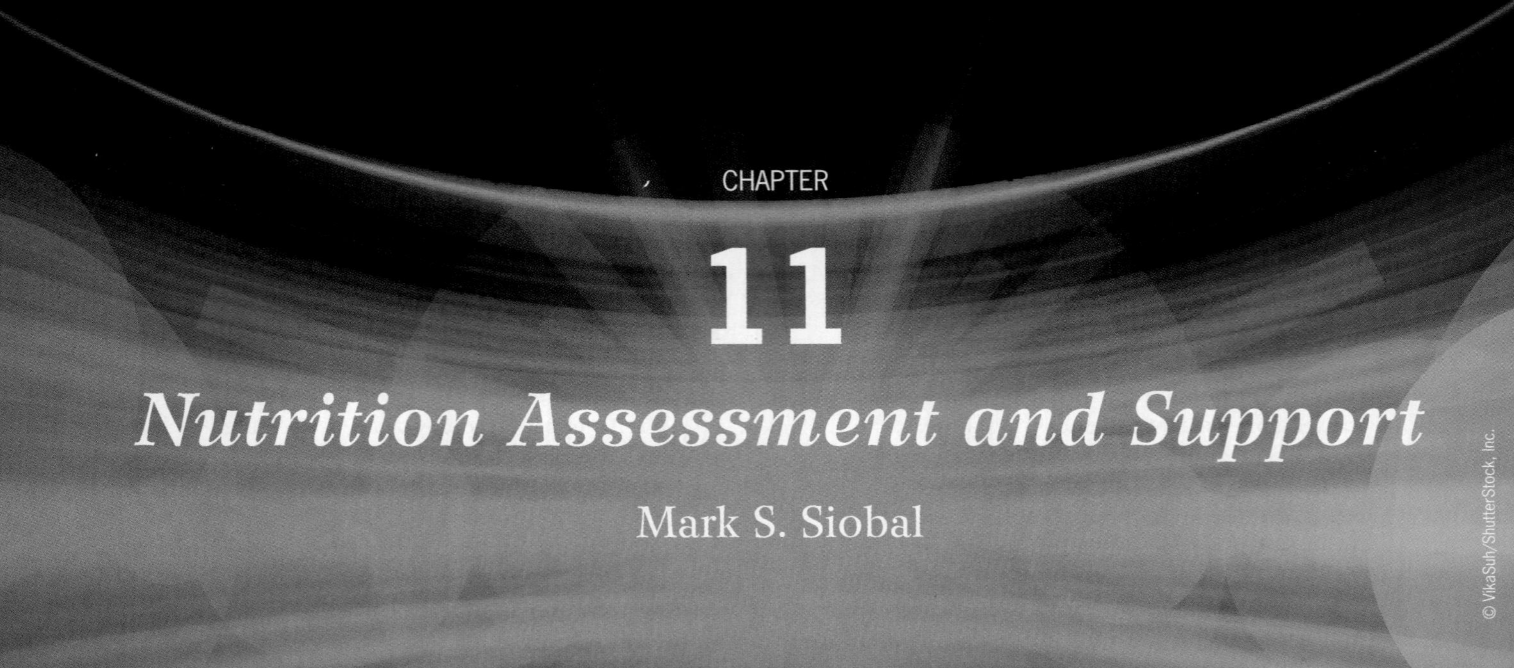

OUTLINE

Effects of Nutrition on Respiratory Function and Critical Illness
Nutrition Assessment
Calculation and Measurement of Energy Requirements
Nutritional Support Guidelines

OBJECTIVES

1. Discuss the effects of nutritional status on the respiratory system.
2. Discuss the effects of nutritional status during critical illness.
3. Explain the principles of nutrition assessment.
4. Compare methods used to estimate nutrient needs.
5. Compare approaches to nutritional support for patients with acute and chronic lung disease.
6. Discuss the role of indirect calorimetry in nutrition assessment.
7. Describe alternative methods to indirect calorimetry.
8. Describe nutrition therapies for acute and chronic lung disease.

KEY TERMS

anthropometry
basal metabolic rate (BMR)
cell-mediated immunity
diet-induced thermogenesis
enteral nutrition
indirect calorimetry
metabolic cart
nitrogen balance
parenteral nutrition
protein-calorie malnutrition (PCM)
refeeding syndrome
respiratory quotient
resting energy expenditure (REE)
stress response to critical illness

Introduction

Nutrition is defined as a series of processes by which an organism uses food for energy, growth, and replacing tissues. Assessment of nutritional status is an important part of the overall assessment of a patient. The human body requires an adequate supply of energy, protein, vitamins, and minerals to maintain an optimal state of health and normal physiology. Without these life-sustaining nutrients, organ system functions become compromised. The respiratory system is no exception.

During periods of prolonged semistarvation and hypercatabolism, the diaphragm and other respiratory muscle groups are not spared, but rather may be broken down for use as a fuel source.[1] Malnutrition is common in critically ill patients.[2,3] Malnutrition and unmet nutritional requirements can lead to prolonged duration of mechanical ventilation, increased length of hospital stay, increased morbidity and mortality, and higher healthcare costs. Caloric overfeeding, on the other hand, may also adversely affect lung function by increasing ventilatory demand and carbon dioxide production ($\dot{V}O_2$).[4]

Critically ill patients with respiratory failure require specialized nutritional support to prevent muscle wasting while avoiding complications associated with nutritional care. Lack of proper nutrition can affect respiratory muscle strength and endurance and impact the immune system response. A careful assessment of the nutritional status of individuals with pulmonary disease and critical illness is essential.[1,3,5]

Effects of Nutrition on Respiratory Function and Critical Illness

Minute Ventilation

The waste products of metabolism are CO_2 and nonvolatile acids. The kidney removes approximately 2% of the waste products that are in the form of nonvolatile acids. The lungs remove 98% of the waste products in the form of CO_2. Metabolic rate determines the amount of carbon dioxide produced and excreted by the process of ventilation. The amount of CO_2 produced by metabolizing nutrients is specific to the amount and type of nutrient being metabolized.[6]

Diet-induced thermogenesis is an increase in metabolic rate of 10% to 15% that occurs after eating as a result of the energy cost of digesting and storing nutrients. Starvation reduces the metabolic rate and results in the use of endogenous fat stores for energy. The reduction in metabolic rate and the metabolism of fat both reduce carbon dioxide production, resulting in lower ventilatory needs.[7] Overfeeding of carbohydrates will result in the production of stored fats (lipogenesis). This process produces an excessive amount of CO_2, resulting in higher ventilatory needs. Amino acids in proteins may increase respiratory drive, which in turn will also increase ventilatory needs. In a patient with limited ventilator reserves, overfeeding may lead to respiratory failure or prolonged mechanical ventilation.[8]

Muscle Weakness

When the body is faced with an energy deficit, it turns to its reserves of glycogen, fat, and protein for the release of fuel. Initially protein is spared, because the body mobilizes and oxidizes fat to serve as the principal fuel source in starvation. If the deficit continues and undernutrition is prolonged, however, catabolism of muscle tissue occurs. In a stressed, critically ill patient, this muscle breakdown occurs within days as a result of the body's hypermetabolic stress response to injury.[5] This circumstance has important implications for an individual with respiratory disease, because the diaphragm, intercostal muscles, and other accessory muscles make up part of the body's skeletal muscle pool and can be catabolized in time of need. Patients whose body weight is below their ideal weight have less diaphragmatic muscle than individuals at healthier weights.[9]

Although **protein-calorie malnutrition (PCM)** affects all types of muscle fibers, it impairs fast twitch fibers most profoundly, resulting in diminished contractile strength. This effect is seen clinically as a decline in maximum inspiratory and expiratory pressures, vital capacity, and voluntary ventilation.[10] Malnutrition also contributes to muscle weakness by depleting the body of phosphorus, which is essential for the production of adenosine triphosphate and 2,3-diphosphoglycerate, without which oxygen release to tissues is limited. This results in impairment of the expiratory muscles' contractility and endurance. Magnesium deficiency also has been associated with muscle weakness and may hinder attempts at weaning from mechanical ventilation. Hypophosphatemia and hypomagnesemia may be caused by gastrointestinal losses, the use of antacids and diuretics, severe malabsorption conditions, and refeeding syndrome. With aggressive repletion of these minerals, diaphragmatic strength and contractility improve.[11,12]

Surfactant Production

Severe starvation causes loss of pulmonary surfactant, which is essential for maintaining alveolar stability and reducing the work of breathing. The size, number, and internal surface area of the alveoli are reduced. Lung lipid content also declines because of multiple factors associated with malnutrition, including alterations in elastin metabolism and a decrease in lipogenesis. PCM has also been shown to reduce the number and size of the lamellar bodies of the granular alveolar pneumocytes, which are the storage sites for surfactant.[13]

Obesity

Mass loading of the chest wall in obesity causes restriction of lung volumes. The most common finding is a decreased expiratory reserve volume, but in extreme obesity vital capacity may also be reduced. The decrease of functional residual capacity may create ventilation-perfusion mismatch, which could cause hypoxemia. The work of breathing may be increased, which increases metabolic rate and carbon dioxide production and may lead to carbon dioxide retention. Weight loss in obese patients can improve lung function, presumably by reducing the work of breathing. Obesity also contributes to problems such as obstructive sleep apnea and obesity hypoventilation syndrome.[14,15]

Immune Function

The primary component of the immune system adversely affected by PCM is **cell-mediated immunity**. Secretory immunoglobulin A (IgA) antibody response, neutrophilic bactericidal capacity, and the complement system also are adversely affected. Protein deficiency triggers a reduction in T4 helper cells and T8 cytotoxic cells and through these T cells impairs B cell activity as well. With the reduction in IgA secretion, the lungs may be more susceptible to bacterial colonization and infection.[16,17]

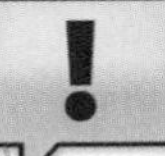

Respiratory Recap

Effects of Poor Nutrition on Respiratory Function

- Muscle weakness
- Impaired immune function
- Impaired surfactant production
- Hypoalbuminemia
- Overnutrition and obesity

Hypoalbuminemia

In a critically ill or malnourished patient, the serum albumin and prealbumin levels are likely to be low. In critical illness this is a consequence of the body's metabolic response to injury, inflammatory damage, or sepsis because the synthesis of albumin is deferred to allow for the manufacture of other acute-phase proteins such as fibrinogen, haptoglobin, and ceruloplasmin. Albumin is essential for the maintenance of plasma colloid oncotic pressure, which controls the movement of fluid from the interstitial space into the capillaries or intracellular space. When the serum albumin concentration is low, interstitial lung fluid increases, which may compromise lung function by increasing the risk of pulmonary edema.[18]

Stress Response to Critical Illness

The **stress response to critical illness** causes wide fluctuation in metabolic rate. The hypercatabolic phase can last for 7 to 10 days and is manifested by an increase in oxygen demands, cardiac output, and $\dot{V}CO_2$. Caloric needs may be increased by up to 100% during this phase.[19] The goal of nutritional treatment is to provide ongoing monitoring and support with high protein feedings while avoiding overfeeding and underfeeding.[5,20]

Refeeding Syndrome

Refeeding syndrome describes the metabolic and clinical disturbances that occur after the reinstitution of nutrition to patients who are malnourished or starved. Severe electrolyte imbalance, vitamin deficiency, and hyperglycemia development during refeeding can result in serious cardiovascular and pulmonary complications. Confusion, coma, seizures, cardiac arrhythmias, congestive heart failure, pulmonary edema, respiratory failure, diaphragm and intercostal muscle weakness, decreased tissue oxygen delivery, and increased $\dot{V}CO_2$ can prolong mechanical ventilation and make weaning from ventilatory support more difficult.[12,21,22]

Acute and Chronic Inflammation

Inflammation is a normal mechanism of defense against infection and injury. Conversely, the inflammatory response can be damaging if mediators of inflammation are not regulated appropriately. There is an increasing understanding that malnutrition and the presence of varying degrees of acute or chronic inflammation play a key role in the pathophysiology of disease or injury.[23] Critical illness causes severe acute systemic inflammation to develop. Mild to moderate degrees of inflammation are associated with chronic conditions (**Table 11-1**).[24]

TABLE 11-1
Example of Conditions Associated with Acute and Chronic Inflammation

Acute Inflammatory Conditions	Chronic Inflammatory Conditions
Major sepsis and infection Acute respiratory distress syndrome Systemic inflammatory response syndrome Major abdominal surgery Multiple trauma Severe burns Traumatic brain injury	Cardiovascular disease Congestive heart failure Organ failure Chronic obstructive pulmonary disease Cystic fibrosis Inflammatory bowel disease Chronic pancreatitis Rheumatoid arthritis Cancer Diabetes mellitus Metabolic syndrome Neuromuscular disease Pressure ulcers Obesity

Traditional markers of malnutrition, serum albumin and prealbumin, are reduced during the presence of inflammation and become ineffective as markers for nutritional assessment. High serum levels of C-reactive protein in the presence of low albumin and prealbumin is an indication of an inflammatory process. During inflammatory states nutritional intervention alone can be ineffective in preventing muscle protein loss.[18]

Obesity is associated with a state of low-grade chronic inflammation. Adipose tissue releases inflammatory mediators and proinflammatory signaling molecules and is thought to be a factor in the development of metabolic disturbances such as metabolic syndrome and type 2 diabetes. The presence of insulin resistance and hyperglycemia during critical illness is believed to be an indicator of acute inflammation.[25]

The presence of inflammation can have significant implications for nutritional support and care. Nutritional supplementation with dietary components such as omega-3 fatty acids, antioxidants, flavonoids, prebiotics, and probiotics have the potential to modulate the predisposition, development, and resolution of inflammatory conditions and may have an increasing role in medical therapy.[1]

Nutrition Assessment

The components of a nutrition evaluation are the patient history, a physical examination, anthropometric measurements, biochemical tests, and indicators of immune system function.[20] Information from the patient's history should help determine the individual's

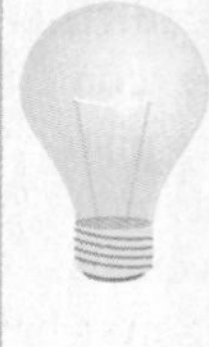

STOP AND THINK

You are caring for a mechanically ventilated patient with septic ARDS. In what ways might you consider nutritional status related to ventilator management and eventual liberation from the ventilator?

TABLE 11-2
Objective Parameters of Malnutrition

Parameter	Malnutrition		
	Mild	Moderate	Severe
Ideal body weight	80–90%	70–79%	<70%
Usual weight	90–95%	80–89%	<80%
Triceps skinfold thickness	40th–50th percentile	30th–39th percentile	<30th percentile
Serum albumin	2.8–3.4 g/dL	2.1–2.7 g/dL	<2.1 g/dL
Serum transferrin	150–200 mg/dL	100–149 mg/dL	<100 mg/dL
Serum prealbumin	12–17 mg/dL	7–11 mg/dL	<7 mg/dL

baseline nutritional state and should reveal signs of nutrition compromise such as weight loss, anorexia, dysphagia, early satiety, nausea, or vomiting.

Anthropometry is the study of human body measurements and components. It includes measurement of height, weight, body mass index, midarm muscle circumference, skinfold thicknesses, and skeletal breadths. An individual's weight as a percentage of usual weight and calculation of the percentage of weight loss over time are particularly important indices of nutritional risk and the extent of illness. A weight loss of 10% or more of the usual body weight over a 6-month period or a body weight below 80% of ideal is considered a sign of significant nutritional risk and indicates a need for aggressive nutritional intervention.[26–32]

Biochemical assessment of nutritional status should accompany the physical and historical assessments. Along with other objective tests (**Table 11-2**), laboratory measurements help reflect the status of a subject's protein stores and therefore the degree of nutritional risk. The serum albumin, transferrin, and transthyretin (prealbumin) levels, along with the retinol-binding protein level, are commonly used to assess the visceral protein stores (**Table 11-3**).[18,33,34] Studies of **nitrogen balance**, which involve a 24-hour urine collection and calculation of the difference between nitrogen intake and excretion, can help determine protein requirements and assess changes in visceral protein stores over time. Interpretation of these values as indicators of nutritional status is difficult, however, because serum concentrations of proteins are affected by many factors, such as acute illness, infection, inflammation, stress, sepsis, hepatic disease, renal disease, malignancy, and hydration status.[34]

TABLE 11-3
Biochemical Measurements of Nutritional Status and Inflammation

Marker	Normal Range
Albumin	3.5–5 g/dL
Transferrin	200–400 mg/dL
Prealbumin	18–50 mg/dL
Retinol-binding protein	3–8 mg/dL
C-reactive protein	0–1.0 mg/dL

The ideal protein for use as a marker of nutritional status has a short half-life, a relatively small body pool, and a rapid rate of synthesis and remains unaffected by a disease or its severity. Albumin, transferrin, and transthyretin all have been used in attempts to fit this role.[34]

Albumin, a protein synthesized by the liver, is required for the transport of molecules, maintenance of the vascular system, and prevention of edema. Its body pool is large, and most of this protein (60%) is present in the extravascular space. The 40% found in the intravascular compartment functions primarily to maintain the plasma colloid oncotic pressure. Because of its abundance in the body and its long half-life (18 to 21 days), albumin does not respond quickly to acute changes in nutritional status. It more often reflects the severity of disease and the metabolic response to injury or infection and therefore can be used as an important prognostic indicator; low albumin levels have been associated with morbidity and mortality and with longer hospitalization.[34]

Transferrin is a ß-globulin synthesized by the liver, which functions as a transport protein for iron. Its biologic half-life is 8 to 10 days, and its body pool is small. It thus may be a more sensitive indicator of protein status than the serum albumin level, although its levels also may be affected by disease and should be interpreted with caution. Transferrin levels may be low with liver disease, after surgery or trauma, or with infection, even

Respiratory Recap

Components of Nutrition Assessment

- Anthropometric measurements
- Biochemical assessments

in patients with good nutritional status. Its serum levels may be elevated in individuals with iron deficiency anemia, acute hepatitis, dehydration, or acute blood loss.[34]

Transthyretin (thyroxine-binding prealbumin) is a carrier protein that aids in the transport of thyroxine and retinol-binding protein. It has a small body pool and a short half-life of 2 to 3 days. Transthyretin is not affected by iron deficiency, but decreased levels may be seen with zinc deficiency and with inflammation, hepatitis, or cirrhosis. Increased levels are seen in patients with renal disease, presumably because of a decrease in protein breakdown by the kidneys. Even so, changes and trends in the serum level of this protein can be monitored and used to assess acute changes in protein status and response to nutritional support.[34]

Immune function measurements also can be used as objective markers of nutritional status. The measurements most commonly evaluate cell-mediated immunity, the immune system component most affected by malnutrition. A reduced total lymphocyte count, lack of delayed cutaneous hypersensitivity to antigens, and abnormal lymphocyte stimulation assay results all may reveal poor immune function. At least one study has shown that nutrition therapy for malnourished individuals with chronic obstructive pulmonary disease (COPD) resulted in improvements in these markers.[16,17]

Calculation and Measurement of Energy Requirements

Equations Versus Measurements

Inadequate energy and protein nutrition may compromise the ability to heal and thrive. Overfeeding of calories may impair bodily functions and lead to respiratory compromise in subjects with limited ventilatory reserve. Energy requirements may be estimated by prediction equations or measured by calorimetry.[35] The use of prediction equations is the most common method to estimate **resting energy expenditure (REE)**. The equations (**Equation 11-1**) work well to predict REE in healthy nonobese subjects, but they work less well in obese or critically ill patients.[36]

EQUATION 11-1

Equations Used to Estimate Energy Expenditure

Harris-Benedict Equation

$$\text{BMR (men)} = 66 + (13.7 \times W) + (5.0 \times H) - (6.8 \times A)$$

$$\text{BMR (women)} = 655 + (9.6 \times W) + (1.7 \times H) - (4.7 \times A)$$

where:
BMR = Basal metabolic rate
W = Weight (kg)
H = Height (cm)
A = Age (years)

Ireton-Jones Formula

$$\text{EEE (obese person)} = [(606 \times G) + (9 \times W) - (12 \times A)] + (400 \times V) + 1444$$

where:
EEE = Estimated energy expenditure
G = Gender (male = 1; female = 0)
W = Actual body weight (kg)
A = Age (years)
V = Ventilator (present = 1; absent = 0)

$$\text{EEE (ventilated person)} = 1925 - (10 \times A) + (5 \times W) + (281 \times G) + (292 \times T) + (851 \times B)$$

where:
EEE = Estimated energy expenditure
A = Age (years)
W = Weight (kg)
G = Gender (male = 1; female = 0)
T = Trauma (present = 1; absent = 2)
B = Burn (present = 1; absent = 0)

The original work of Harris and Benedict (see Equation 11-1) in 1919 first described the amount of energy required to maintain the most basic bodily functions in normal subjects.[35] This amount of energy, expressed as kilocalories (kcal) per day, is known as the **basal metabolic rate (BMR).** The BMR has a fixed relationship with gender, weight in kilograms, height in centimeters, and age in years. The BMR does not take into account stress factors due to illness. For this reason the term *resting energy expenditure* is used in the clinical setting. Critically ill patients may not be at their BMR due to the stress of the disease process. This makes predictions based on BMR invalid for some critically ill patients. In obese subjects, adipose tissue does not contribute to the BMR. For this reason, an ideal body weight or adjusted body weight is usually substituted for actual weight in the equation, which diminishes the ability to predict energy expenditure.[36] The Ireton-Jones formula (refer to Equation 11-1) is a commonly used equation and adjusts for obesity and mechanical ventilation. Energy needs also may be estimated with calories per kilogram of body weight (usually 25 to 35 kcal/kg) if other data are unavailable. Prediction equations may fail to predict REE in a significant number of obese subjects[36] or critically ill patients.[35]

Calorimetry

During direct measurement of energy expenditure (direct calorimetry), an individual is placed in a sealed, thermally insulated chamber. The heat liberated from the individual is determined by measurement of the temperature change in water circulated through the walls of the chamber. The energy produced during metabolism is equal to the heat generated when the organism is at rest. Direct calorimetry is impractical in the clinical setting and is rarely performed even in research studies.[37–41]

Indirect Calorimetry

For clinical purposes, the most common technique to measure energy requirements is **indirect calorimetry,**[20,42,43] which is based on the measurement of inspired and expired gases using a metabolic analyzer. The amounts of oxygen consumed ($\dot{V}O_2$) and carbon dioxide produced ($\dot{V}CO_2$) are equal to the energy produced and at rest equal the metabolic rate.[44,45]

Open-circuit calorimetry measures $\dot{V}O_2$ and $\dot{V}CO_2$. The simplest example of this approach is the Douglas bag technique. In this configuration oxygen and carbon dioxide concentrations are measured in samples of inspired and expired gases. These concentrations can be precisely determined by mass spectrometry or, more routinely, by infrared carbon dioxide and paramagnetic or zirconium oxide oxygen analyzers. Accurate measurement of exhaled or inhaled minute volume is also required, usually by a precision pneumotachometer.[45]

Indirect calorimetry can be performed in mechanically ventilated and spontaneously breathing patients (**CPG 11-1**; **Figure 11-1**, **Figure 11-2**, and **Figure 11-3**). Devices designed for spontaneous breathing use various methods, including a ventilated canopy, masks, and mouthpieces with nose clips. The devices are commonly called **metabolic carts.** $\dot{V}O_2$ is determined by subtraction of the volume of expired oxygen from the volume of inspired oxygen. Mixed exhaled gas analysis is a simple, accurate method of indirect calorimetry in relatively healthy individuals breathing room air. The accuracy of this technique, however, requires precise knowledge of the inspired oxygen fraction (F_{IO_2}). With mechanical ventilation, the F_{IO_2} may vary during the breath or between breaths. Commercial devices currently measure the peak F_{IO_2} to determine F_{IO_2}. This is not a problem with interbreath variation, but these devices cannot measure intrabreath variation. Small errors in the measurement of F_{IO_2} cause large errors in $\dot{V}O_2$, and this error is magnified as the F_{IO_2} rises. For these reasons, this method of indirect calorimetry generally is limited to patients who are spontaneously breathing in room air and to those who are mechanically ventilated with an F_{IO_2} below 0.6.[43,45,46]

When gas exchange measurements are performed for nutritional assessment, every effort must be made to ensure that the measurement conditions are at steady state. Generally, the patient should be resting and recumbent during the measurement period. If the patient is mechanically ventilated, appropriate adjustments should be made to duplicate the patient's usual F_{IO_2}, minute ventilation, and airway pressure. If the patient is breathing spontaneously, measurements should be taken only after the patient has adjusted to breathing through the interface. After steady-state conditions have been confirmed, gas exchange measurements should be averaged over a period of at least 15 minutes. The patient's body temperature and other vital signs should be noted at the time of measurement as a reference for future studies.[45]

After a measurement has been completed, a quality assessment should be performed. The **respiratory quotient** ($R = \dot{V}O_2/\dot{V}CO_2$) should be in the physiologic range (0.67–1.3)[47,48] and be consistent with the patient's condition and nutritional status. The collection time should be sufficient to ensure at least

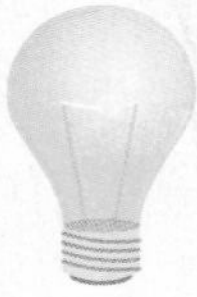

STOP AND THINK

The dietician asks for your help in the nutritional assessment of a mechanically ventilated patient. What information can you provide from the perspective of a respiratory therapist?

CLINICAL PRACTICE GUIDELINE 11-1

Metabolic Measurement with Indirect Calorimetry During Mechanical Ventilation

Indications

- Patients with known nutritional deficits or derangements. A number of nutritional risk and stress factors may considerably skew prediction by the Harris-Benedict equation, including neurologic trauma; paralysis; chronic obstructive pulmonary disease; acute pancreatitis; cancer with residual tumor burden; multiple trauma; amputation; patients whose height and weight cannot be accurately determined; patients who fail to respond adequately to estimated nutritional needs; new patients receiving home total parenteral nutrition; patients unable to eat who require mechanical ventilation for longer than 5 days; transplant patients; morbidly obese patients; and severely hypermetabolic or hypometabolic patients.
- To measure the O_2 cost of breathing in mechanically ventilated patients.
- To assess in mechanically ventilated patients to evaluate hemodynamic support.
- To measure cardiac output by the Fick method.
- To determine the cause(s) of increased ventilator requirements.

Contraindications

- When a specific indication is present, no contraindications exist to the performance of metabolic measurement with indirect calorimetry unless short-term disconnection of ventilatory support to allow connection of measurement lines results in hypoxemia, bradycardia, or other adverse effects.

Hazards and Complications

- Obtaining metabolic measurements with an indirect calorimeter is a safe, noninvasive procedure with few hazards or complications. However, under certain circumstances and with particular equipment, the following hazards or complications may be seen:
  - Short-term disconnection of ventilatory support to allow connection of the indirect calorimetry apparatus may result in hypoxemia, bradycardia, or discomfort for the patient.
  - Inappropriate calibration or system setup may produce erroneous values, resulting in incorrect patient management.
  - Isolation valves may increase circuit resistance and cause increased work of breathing or dynamic hyperinflation or both.
  - Inspiratory reservoirs may cause a reduction in alveolar ventilation due to increased compressible volume of the breathing circuit.
  - Manipulation of the ventilator circuit may cause leaks that may lower alveolar ventilation.

Modified from AARC clinical practice guideline: metabolic measurement using indirect calorimetry during mechanical ventilation—2004 revision and update. *Respir Care.* 2004;49:1073–1079. Reprinted with permission.

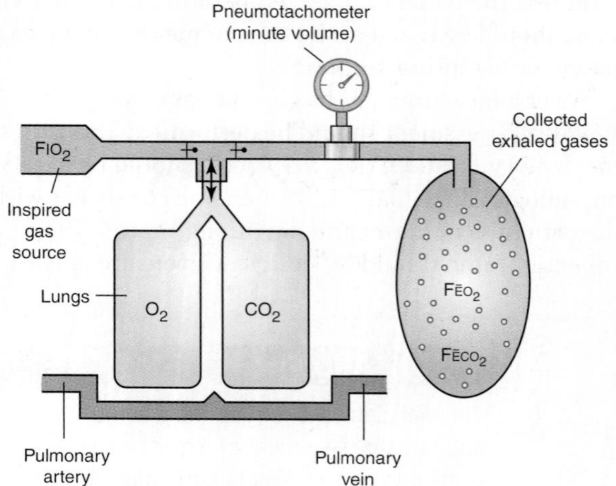

FIGURE 11-1 Diagram illustrating measurement of $\dot{V}O_2$ and $\dot{V}CO_2$ by indirect calorimetry.

Reproduced from *Comprehensive Respiratory Care.* Dantzker DR, MacIntyre NR, Bakow ED, eds. Copyright Elsevier (WB Saunders) 1995.

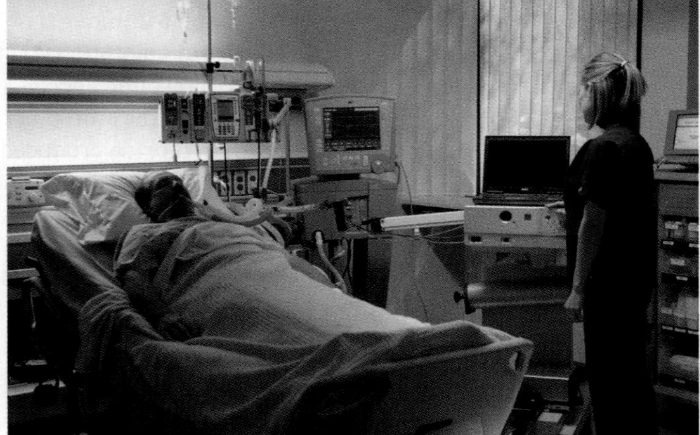

FIGURE 11-2 Use of a metabolic cart (indirect calorimetry) in a mechanically ventilated patient.

Reproduced with permission from CareFusion.

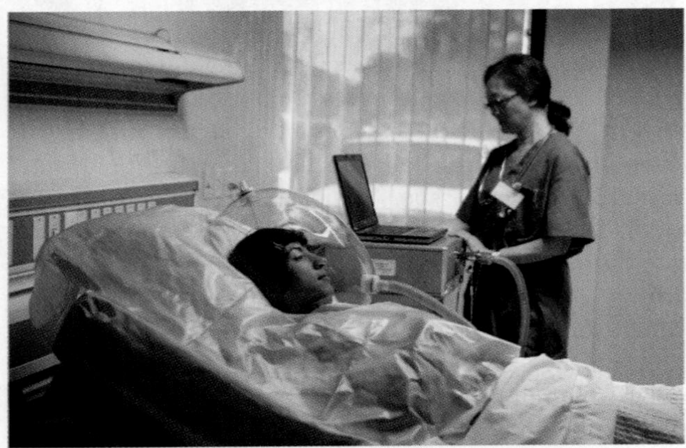

FIGURE 11-3 Use of a metabolic cart (indirect calorimetry) in a spontaneously breathing patient using a hood.
Reproduced with permission from CareFusion.

a 5-min period with the variability of the $\dot{V}CO_2$ and $\dot{V}O_2$ measurements less than 5%.[7] If these conditions have not been met, technical errors such as calibration mistakes, non–steady-state conditions, or tubing leaks may have occurred during the measurement period. After these factors have been corrected, the gas exchange measurement should be repeated. After the results of a gas exchange measurement have been confirmed, the corresponding energy expenditure can be calculated.[45,49]

Through measurement of $\dot{V}O_2$, $\dot{V}CO_2$, and urinary nitrogen excretion (in grams), the Weir equation can be used to determine the REE. Determination of the REE without the measurement of nitrogen excretion is acceptable because it results in an error of 2% or less. The abbreviated Weir equation therefore is used in clinical practice:

$$\text{REE (kcal/day)} = [(3.9 \times \dot{V}O_2) + (1.1 \times \dot{V}CO_2)] \times 1.44$$

where the factor 1.44 calculates kcal requirements for 24 hours.[45]

Modified Weir Equation Method

Modification of the abbreviated Weir equation to calculated REE could be used. By substituting a derived value for either $\dot{V}CO_2$ or $\dot{V}O_2$ adjusted for a normal R of 0.85, the REE based on $\dot{V}CO_2$ (REE-CO_2) or $\dot{V}O_2$ (REE-O_2) can be calculated.[50] Because $\dot{V}CO_2$ is technically easier to measure, is increasingly more available, and can be determined at any F_{IO_2}, use of the REE-CO_2 calculation may be preferable where:

$$\text{REE-}CO_2 = (3.9 \times [\dot{V}CO_2/0.85]) + (1.1 \times \dot{V}CO_2) \times 1.44$$

When the actual R is equal to 0.85, the REE-CO_2 equation calculates a REE value equal to the value derived by the standard Weir equation. When the actual R varies within the normal physiologic range, the REE-CO_2 calculation estimates REE with an accuracy of ±10% compared to the actual REE.[50]

Caloric Equivalent Method

A caloric equivalent has been derived for each class of foodstuffs (substrates). The caloric equivalent of a given energy substrate is the amount of heat (in kilocalories) liberated when the substrate is burned in 1 L of oxygen. Similarly, each class of foodstuffs has a unique respiratory quotient (**Table 11-4**).[51–53]

The caloric equivalence of carbon dioxide and oxygen can be used to calculate an estimate of REE. Critically ill patients have an average R of approximately 0.90, and because $\dot{V}CO_2$ is easier to measure, the CO_2 caloric equivalent factor of 5.52 kcal/L can be used where:

$$\text{REE-}CO_2\text{-Equivalent} = 5.52 \times \dot{V}CO_2 \times 1.44$$

The REE-CO_2-Equivalent calculation has been compared to the Harris-Benedict equation and the standard abbreviated Weir equation. The Harris-Benedict equation underestimated the measured REE, but there was no statistically significant difference between the Weir and REE-CO_2-Equivalent calculations.[51]

TABLE 11-4
Energy and Respiratory Values of Energy Substrates

		Caloric Equivalent (kcal/L)		
Energy Substrate	**Caloric Value (kcal/g)**	**O_2**	**CO_2**	**Respiratory Quotient**
Carbohydrate	4.1	5.05	5.05	1.0
Mixed	—	4.83	5.52	0.90
Protein	4.1	4.46	5.57	0.80
Fat	9.3	4.74	6.67	0.71
Alcohol	7.1	4.86	7.25	0.67

Use of a metabolic analyzer and the standard abbreviated Weir equation for indirect calorimetry is a superior method for determining REE especially when R approaches the physiologic limits of 0.67 and 1.3.[47] When metabolic analyzers are not available or the FIO_2 is greater than 0.60, however, REE measurements based on $\dot{V}CO_2$ are a reasonable alternative. The accuracy of these alternative methods are within acceptable limits needed for clinical monitoring of nutritional support.[50,51]

Fick Method

REE can be determined from $\dot{V}O_2$ alone with the use of an estimated respiratory quotient of 0.8 (to generate a value for $\dot{V}CO_2$) if $\dot{V}CO_2$ is not available. The Fick equation also may be used to determine $\dot{V}O_2$ and the corresponding energy expenditure (**Equation 11-2**).[45,54,55] This technique requires the presence of a pulmonary artery catheter. The range of error for this calculation is significant when the individual errors of thermodilution, cardiac output, blood gas determinations, hemoglobin measurement, and estimation of the oxygen-carrying capacity of hemoglobin are added. For these reasons, the Fick method to calculate $\dot{V}O_2$ and energy expenditure should be regarded as only an approximation of the metabolic rate.[55,56] Because pulmonary artery catheters are used less frequently, use of the Fick method for energy expenditure is usually not practical.

Protein Requirements

In both acute and chronic disease, focusing nutritional support efforts on the maintenance of protein stores is important. With prolonged inadequate nutrient intake, endogenous protein catabolism occurs, with most of the loss from muscle tissue. As mentioned previously, this includes the respiratory muscles, and weakness and fatigue are likely to result, causing increased difficulty breathing. Providing patients with an adequate supply of nutrients for nitrogen building and endogenous protein sparing is, therefore, important.[57] It is suggested that 25 to 35 nonprotein calories per kilogram of body weight be provided to allow for metabolic utilization of 1 g of protein. For most patients, in the absence of renal or liver disease, 1.0 to 2.0 g of dietary protein per kilogram of body weight is recommended.[20,58] Based on the assessment of the protein catabolism, however, protein intake may need to be increased as high as 1.5 to 2.5 g/kg/day.[57] Visceral protein stores are difficult to monitor, but attempts should be made to evaluate the adequacy of a feeding regimen, the response to nutrition therapy, and changes in protein status. Common tools include measurement of transferrin and prealbumin (transthyretin) and 24-hour urine collections to calculate urinary urea nitrogen (UUN).[34]

The UUN, or calculation of nitrogen balance, requires an accurate 24-hour urine collection and can be helpful in the assessment of a patient's response to

EQUATION 11-2

Calculation of Oxygen Consumption with the Fick Equation

$$\dot{V}O_2 = \dot{Q}c \times C(a-\bar{v})O_2$$

where:

$\dot{V}O_2$ = Oxygen consumption
$\dot{Q}c$ = Cardiac output
$C(a-\bar{v})O_2$ = Difference between arterial and mixed venous oxygen content

To perform this calculation, an indwelling pulmonary artery catheter is required to determine the $\dot{Q}c$ (by thermodilution) and obtain a mixed venous blood sample (which must be obtained from the distal port of the catheter positioned in the pulmonary artery). An arterial blood sample also must be obtained. Blood gas analysis is performed on both samples, and the $C(a-\bar{v})O_2$ is then calculated, as follows:

$$C(a-\bar{v})O_2 = [(SaO_2 - S\bar{v}O_2) \times Hb \times 1.34] + [0.003 \times (PaO_2 - P\bar{v}O_2)]$$

where:

$C(a-\bar{v})O_2$ = Difference between arterial and mixed venous oxygen content
SaO_2 = Oxygen saturation of arterial blood
$S\bar{v}O_2$ = Oxygen saturation of venous blood
Hb = Hemoglobin
PaO_2 = Partial pressure of arterial oxygen
$P\bar{v}O_2$ = Partial pressure of oxygen in mixed venous blood

nutrition therapy. The goal of nutritional support is to achieve positive nitrogen balance, which occurs when protein in the diet provides nitrogen in excess of its loss. Nitrogen balance is calculated as follows:

$$\text{Nitrogen balance (g)} = \left[\frac{\text{24-hour protein intake (g)}}{6.25}\right] - [\text{24-hour urinary urea nitrogen (g)} + 4\text{ g}]$$

The 4 g added to the UUN value is an estimate of insensible nitrogen loss (e.g., from the feces, skin, and hair).[34]

A negative nitrogen balance indicates protein catabolism, whereas a positive nitrogen balance reflects an anabolic state. The clinician should aim for a positive nitrogen balance of approximately 1 to 4 g a day. In certain diseases and conditions, however, this measurement may be misleading and is most likely to present the clinician with unreliable results that may not accurately reflect the patient's nutritional state. It also should be kept in mind that in critically ill patients with infection, sepsis, or inflammatory disease and in those receiving steroid therapy, a positive nitrogen balance may not be achieved even with aggressive nutritional support. Because of inaccurate 24-hour urine collections, the presence of renal or liver dysfunction, significant immeasurable insensible losses of protein from burns and large wounds, high-output gastrointestinal fistulas and ostomies, and the presence of inflammatory conditions, nitrogen balance calculations are often negative and may not be an accurate reflection of nutrition status. It might result in increased risk of overfeeding.[34]

Nutritional Support Guidelines

The primary goal of nutrition therapy in patients with respiratory disease is to improve respiratory function through the prevention or minimization of the loss of muscle mass. Other goals are to prevent infection, enhance the immune system, increase exercise tolerance, and improve the patient's quality of life.

Nutrition Delivery

The preferred and most convenient method of nutrient delivery is the oral route. It may be difficult, however, for many individuals with severe respiratory disease to consume enough to maintain their weight and meet their increased nutrient needs. This may occur for several reasons, such as dyspnea on food preparation and consumption, early satiety, gastroesophageal reflux, bloating caused by air swallowing, nausea, and vomiting. Much of the gastrointestinal discomfort can be caused or exacerbated by medications commonly prescribed to treat respiratory symptoms and infection, including bronchodilators, anticholinergics, corticosteroids, antibiotics, and mucolytics. The reflux many patients experience may also be attributed to the effects of lung hyperinflation on the position of the stomach or an increase in abdominal pressure associated with coughing.[34]

If oral intake is inadequate to meet daily energy needs despite the use of high-calorie, high-protein supplements and snacks, enteral delivery of nutrients by means of a feeding tube should be considered. This should also be the method of choice to feed patients requiring ventilatory support.[59]

Enteral nutrition should always be considered when a patient has a functioning gastrointestinal (GI) tract.[20,59] The benefits of enteral nutrient delivery are well documented. Nutrients absorbed via the portal system with delivery to the liver may allow for better absorption and result in enhanced immune competence. The presence of nutrients in the gut prevents intestinal atrophy and maintains the absorptive capacity of the GI mucosa by directly nourishing the enterocytes, supporting epithelial cell repair and replication. Enteral nutrition also helps preserve normal gut flora and gastric pH, which may guard against bacterial overgrowth in the small intestine. Finally, nutrients, especially fats and proteins, stimulate feeding-dependent neuroendocrine activity, which results in the secretion of immunoglobulins. These substances, particularly secretory IgA, are important in the prevention of bacterial translocation and gut sepsis. Although enteral nutrition is not entirely devoid of risk, if administered carefully and sensibly, it is safer than parenteral nutrition and considerably less expensive.[20,59]

The route of delivery varies and may depend on the ease and availability of enteral access; the patient's risk of aspiration, tolerance to feedings, and clinical condition; and the length of time feeding is likely to be needed.[20] Nasogastric or orogastric tubes often are used because they are easy to place at the bedside and are also needed for medication administration. They are considered short-term feeding tubes (less than 3 to 4 weeks) and may be contraindicated in patients who have severe reflux or delayed gastric emptying or gastroparesis, or who are otherwise at high risk of aspiration. In these latter cases a feeding tube placed past the stomach (postpyloric) into the small intestine should be considered. These tubes are also indicated for short-term tube feeding and allow for uninterrupted duodenal or jejunal feeding in patients with gastric dysmotility and large gastric residual volumes, which would otherwise prevent the administration of adequate nutrition support. In this case, the feeding would be infused via the small-bowel (enteric) tube, and a larger gastric tube could be used to decompress the stomach and allow for the drainage of gastric secretions. Presumably the more distal to the stomach the feeding is delivered, the less likely aspiration related to the feeding is to occur. The optimal postpyloric tube

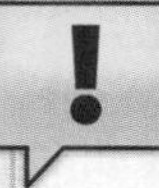

Respiratory Recap

Routes of Nutrition Delivery

- Oral
- Enteral
- Parenteral

placement thus is past the ligament of Treitz, or in the fourth portion of the duodenum.[5]

A Dobhoff tube is a small-bore, flexible, nasogastric feeding tube that typically has an inside diameter of 4 mm. It is smaller and more flexible than other NG tubes, and, therefore, is usually more comfortable for the patient. The tube is inserted by use of a guide wire (stylet), which is removed after the tube's correct placement has been confirmed. A Dobhoff tube typically has a weighted end that helps guide it through the digestive system. Peristalsis helps to move the weight through the esophagus into the stomach or beyond.

If long-term feeding is anticipated, tubes can be placed through the skin into the stomach or small intestine by surgical, endoscopic, radiologic, or laparoscopic techniques. The percutaneous endoscopic gastrostomy (PEG) tube is placed endoscopically. The patient is sedated, and an endoscope is passed through the mouth and esophagus into the stomach. The position of the endoscope can be visualized on the outside of the patient's abdomen because it contains a powerful light source. A needle is inserted through the abdomen and visualized within the stomach by the endoscope, and a suture passed through the needle is grasped by the endoscope and pulled up through the esophagus. The suture is then tied to the end of the PEG tube and pulled back down through the esophagus and stomach and out through the abdominal wall. The insertion takes about 20 minutes. The tube is kept within the stomach either by a balloon or by a retention dome. Gastric tubes are suitable for long-term use and can be replaced without an additional endoscopic procedure. The PEG tube is useful when there is difficulty with swallowing because of neurologic or anatomic disorders and to avoid the risk of aspiration pneumonia. These tubes generally are more comfortable than the nasogastric, orogastric, or enteric tubes.[60]

Many enteral formulas are available (**Table 11-5**), and selection of the most cost-effective, beneficial product presents a great challenge to the clinical nutrition specialist. General-purpose formulas are quite cost effective, palatable, and well tolerated by most patients, except those individuals with malabsorption syndromes or other special conditions. These formulas generally provide 1 calorie per mL and are approximately 50% carbohydrate, 30% fat, and 15% to 20% protein.[61–63]

Many specialized enteral nutrition formulas have been developed for patients with specific conditions, such as diabetes mellitus, hepatic disease, renal disease, and pulmonary disease.[20] The composition of these formulas is different from that of more general formulas, and they tend to be higher in price. The formula designed for patients with pulmonary disease is based on the theory that through the provision of fewer calories from carbohydrate and more from fat, total carbon

TABLE 11-5
Composition of Select Enteral Formulas

Formula	Kcal/mL	Carbohydrate (g/mL)	Protein (g/mL)	Fat (g/mL)
Ensure Plus*	1.5	200	55	53
Boost High Protein†	1.06	140	61	23
Boost Plus	1.5	190	61	57
Isocal†	1.06	138	34	44
Isocal HN†	1.06	123	44	46
TraumaCal†	1.5	162	82	68
Deliver 2.0†	2.0	200	75	102
TwoCal HN†	2.0	217	84	91
Pulmocare*	1.5	106	63	93
Oxepa*	1.5	106	63	93
Respalor†	1.5	148	76	71

* Ross Products Division, Abbott Laboratories, Columbus, OH.

† Mead-Johnson Nutritionals, Evansville, IN.

dioxide production will be decreased, reducing carbon dioxide retention. These formulas contain a higher percentage of calories from fat, or 40% to 55% of total calories. The carbohydrate sources typically contribute less than 40% of total calories. The caloric density typically is 1.5 kcal/mL, which reduces the amount of overall volume necessary to provide full nutritional support. This may be beneficial for patients at risk for the development of fluid overload and pulmonary edema. Studies that have shown positive outcomes with these specialty formulas have been criticized for their small sample sizes, and frequently reports of carbohydrate overfeeding have been based on studies with patients receiving excessive calorie loads (approximately 50 kcal/kg) via parenteral nutrition. If overall calories are not excessive, carbon dioxide production is more affected by total calories than by the percentage of carbohydrate calories. Use of higher-priced specialized formulas for pulmonary patients therefore is controversial.[61,62]

Intravenous delivery of substrate may be necessary when the GI tract is not functioning or if stimulation of the gastrointestinal or pancreatic systems would worsen the patient's condition.[64] **Parenteral nutrition**, which bypasses the GI system, may be indicated for nutritional support in patients with severe pancreatitis, gastrointestinal fistulas, short bowel syndrome, prolonged ileus, and some cancers. It should not be initiated if the expected duration of support is less than 7 days. Placement of a central or peripheral venous catheter is required for the infusion of nutrients into the bloodstream; central venous access usually is preferred. Complications involved in the placement of a central venous catheter include pneumothorax, arterial puncture, catheter malposition, catheter embolization, site infection, air embolus, thoracic duct injury, mediastinal injury, and cardiac injury. The most common complication of percutaneously placed subclavian catheters is pneumothorax, with an incidence rate of 1% to 4%. Pericardial tamponade, a lethal complication, has a mortality rate of 65% to 90%. Furthermore, the infusion of nutrients into the central circulation leaves the GI tract unstimulated, which can lead to gut atrophy, mucosal compromise, and a weakening of the gut barrier, which may increase the risk of bacterial contamination.[20,65]

Nutritional Support in Mechanically Ventilated Patients

The importance of nutrition in the hospital setting cannot be overstated. This is particularly important in critical illness, which is associated with a catabolic stress state in which patients commonly demonstrate a systemic inflammatory response. Nutritional support in critically ill patients has three objectives: to preserve lean body mass, to maintain immune function, and to avert metabolic complications. Important aspects of nutritional support in critically ill patients include early enteral nutrition, appropriate macronutrient and micronutrient delivery, and meticulous glycemic control.[1,3] Early nutritional support using the enteral route is a proactive therapeutic strategy that may reduce disease severity, diminish complications, decrease length of stay in the intensive care unit, and favorably affect patient outcome.[20,59]

A nutritional product rich in antioxidants and supplemented with omega-3 fatty acids such as eicosapentaenoic acid and gamma-linoleic acid can modulate pro-inflammatory properties in patients with acute respiratory distress syndrome (ARDS) and septic shock, resulting in improved oxygenation.[64,66–68] Recent results of a study performed by the ARDS Network, however, did not find that omega-3 and antioxidant supplementation had any benefit in terms of important patient outcomes.[69,70] Glycemic control is important in critically ill patients, and some have advocated for intensive insulin therapy to maintain blood glucose levels at or below 110 mg/dL. Current evidence does not support tight glucose control in terms of improved patient outcomes, however. Tight glucose control is associated with a higher risk of hypoglycemia. Current recommendations are for maintaining blood glucose between the range of 140–180 mg/dL and treating a blood glucose value of <70 mg/dL as hypoglycemia during nutritional support.[71–74]

The following best practice recommendations are adapted from guidelines of the Society of Critical Care Medicine, the American Society of Parenteral and Enteral Nutrition, the Academy of Nutrition and Dietetics, the Canadian Clinical Practice Guideline for Nutritional Support, and the European Society for Clinical Nutrition and Metabolism.[75–80] Nutritional support should be initiated within the first 24 to 48 hours following intubation. Primary goals of nutritional therapy are to:

- Preserve lean muscle mass
- Optimize outcome by ongoing assessment and modification to the nutritional care plan
- Prevent complications such as refeeding syndrome by continuous monitoring
- Prevent protein-energy malnutrition
- Provide adequate total calories
- Prevent accumulation of a caloric deficit
- Achieve goal of >50% of target calories within the first week

Respiratory Recap

Nutritional Support in Critically Ill Patients

- Early enteral nutrition
- Macronutrient and micronutrient delivery
- Glycemic control

In critically ill patients, neither the presence nor the absence of bowel sounds or evidence of passage of flatus and stool is required for the initiation of enteral feeding. Indirect calorimetry should be used when available. Predictive equations should be verified by indirect calorimetry during critical illness. Enteral nutrition practice recommendations are to:

- Feed preferentially via the enteral route
- Initiate enteral nutrition within the first 24 to 48 hours
- Avoid interruptions of enteral nutrition for procedures to prevent underfeeding
- Reduce aspiration risk by head of bed elevation
- Accept gastric residual volumes up to 500 mL in the absence of clear signs of intolerance
- Use motility agents to reduce gastric residual volumes and improve tolerance
- Use postpyloric feeding tube placement when feasible

Parenteral nutrition practice recommendations are to:

- Use parenteral nutrition only when the enteral route is not feasible
- Use parenteral nutrition based on the patient's risk assessment for malnutrition
- Initiate parenteral nutrition early in the presence of moderate and severe malnutrition
- Delay parenteral nutrition up to 7 days if the risks of malnutrition are low
- Convert to EN as soon as tolerated
- Consider trophic (trickle feeding) and permissive underfeeding in obese patients

If unable to meet energy requirements after 7 to 10 days by the enteral route alone, consider initiating supplemental parenteral nutrition. Initiating supplemental parenteral nutrition before this time in the patient receiving enteral nutrition does not improve outcome and may be detrimental. Fluid-restricted calorically dense formulations should be considered for patients with acute respiratory failure. Following are recommendations for use of immunonutrition and pharmaconutrients:

- Omega-3 fatty acids in patients with ARDS may be beneficial
- Increase omega-3 to omega-6 fatty acids ratio
- Arginine, glutamine, nucleotides, antioxidants, and probiotics may be beneficial
- Arginine should be avoided in patients with severe sepsis

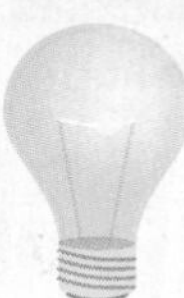

STOP AND THINK

You are working in a pulmonary rehabilitation clinic. What tips related to nutritional support might you provide for a patient with COPD?

BOX 11-1

Nutritional Guidelines for Patients with Chronic Respiratory Disease

Choose high-calorie, nutrient-dense foods.

Plan for small frequent meals or snacks rather than fewer large ones.

Drink liquids between meals, not with them.

Add fats to foods to increase calories, and add dry milk powder to boost the protein content.

Set alarm clocks as reminders to eat, and keep your favorite foods visible.

Avoid gas-forming foods (e.g., cabbage, onions, beans) that may cause bloating and indigestion.

Use home-delivered meal services, frozen foods, and convenience foods to decrease food preparation time.

Supplement your food intake with medical nutritional products (e.g., Ensure, Boost) if you are unable to consume an adequate diet.

Review your medications and consult your physician about adjusting the dosage or type, if possible, of those that have an adverse effect on your food intake.

Nutritional Support in Chronic Respiratory Disease

The goals of nutrition therapy in acute respiratory disease are the same as for patients with chronic disease. Maintaining nutritional status with an adequate energy, protein, vitamin, and mineral intake is essential. For individuals participating in pulmonary rehabilitation programs, poor nutrition may adversely affect their state of health and well-being in several ways. It decreases exercise tolerance, hinders the body's ability to regenerate healthy muscle tissue, increases susceptibility to infection, and ultimately may prevent successful progression through the program. These individuals need practical, simple guidelines to optimize their nutrient intake, such as those listed in **Box 11-1**.

Key Points

- ▶ Respiratory function is affected by nutritional status, which also can affect muscle function, immunity, fluid balance, and surfactant production, in addition to other systems.
- ▶ Caloric overfeeding should be avoided in patients requiring mechanical ventilation because it may result in hypercapnia and a prolonged ventilatory period.

- Indirect calorimetry using a metabolic analyzer is the most accurate method to determine energy expenditure in hospitalized patients with critical illness.
- Alternative methods for estimating energy expenditure should be considered when a metabolic analyzer is not available.
- Enteral delivery of nutrients is preferred to parenteral nutrition because it carries fewer risks of infection, may have a protective effect on the gastrointestinal mucosa, and is less costly.
- The objectives of nutritional support in critically ill patients are to preserve lean body mass, to maintain immune function, and to avert metabolic complications.
- A complete nutrition assessment and support process should be included in the plan of care for patients with acute or chronic lung disease.

References

1. Mueller CM, Merritt RJ, McClave S. *The ASPEN Adult Nutrition Support Core Curriculum*, 2nd ed. Rockville, MD: American Society for Parenteral and Enteral Nutrition; 2012.
2. Coats KG, Morgan SL, Bartolucci AA, Weinsier RL. Hospital-associated malnutrition: a reevaluation 12 years later. *J Am Diet Assoc*. 1993;93:27–33.
3. Grover A, Khashu M, Mukherjee A, Kairamkonda V. Iatrogenic malnutrition in neonatal intensive care units: Urgent need to modify practice. *J Parenter Enteral Nutr*. 2008;32:140–144.
4. Barker LA, Gout BS, Crowe TC. Hospital malnutrition: prevalence, identification and impact on patients and the healthcare system. *Int J Environ Res Public Health*. 2011;8:514–527.
5. Baudouin SV, Evans TW. Nutritional support in critical care. *Clin Chest Med*. 2003;24:633–644.
6. Talpers SS, Romberger DJ, Bunce SB, Pingleton SK. Nutritionally associated increased carbon dioxide production. Excess total calories vs high proportion of carbohydrate calories. *Chest*. 1992;102:551–555.
7. McClave SA, Snider HL. Use of indirect calorimetry in clinical nutrition. *Nutr Clin Pract*. 1992;7:207–221.
8. McClave SA. The consequences of overfeeding and underfeeding. *J Resp Care Pract*. 1997;10:57–58, 62–64.
9. Murciano D, Rigaud D, Pingleton S, et al. Diaphragmatic function in severely malnourished patients with anorexia nervosa. Effects of renutrition. *Am J Respir Crit Care Med*. 1994;150:1569–1574.
10. Birmingham CL, Tan AO. Respiratory muscle weakness and anorexia nervosa. *Int J Eat Disord*. 2003;33:230–233.
11. Marinella MA. The refeeding syndrome and hypophosphatemia. *Nutr Rev*. 2003;61:320–323.
12. Kraft MD, Btaiche IF, Sacks GS. Review of the refeeding syndrome. *Nutr Clin Pract*. 2005;20:625–633.
13. Dias CM, Pássaro CP, Cagido VR, et al. Effects of undernutrition on respiratory mechanics and lung parenchyma remodeling. *J Appl Physiol*. 2004;97:1888–1896.
14. Mokhlesi B. Obesity hypoventilation syndrome: a state-of-the-art review. *Respir Care*. 2010;55:1347–1362.
15. Kapur VK. Obstructive sleep apnea: diagnosis, epidemiology, and economics. *Respir Care*. 2010;55:1155–1167.
16. Krawinkel MB. Interaction of nutrition and infections globally: an overview. *Ann Nutr Metab*. 2012;61(Suppl 1):39–45.
17. Chandra RK, Kumari S. Nutrition and immunity: an overview. *J Nutr*. 1994;124(Suppl 8):1433S–1435S.
18. Don BR, Kaysen G. Serum albumin: relationship to inflammation and nutrition. *Semin Dial*. 2004;17:432–437.
19. Long CL, Schaffel N, Geiger JW, et al. Metabolic response to injury and illness: estimation of energy and protein needs from indirect calorimetry and nitrogen balance. *J Parenter Enteral Nutr*. 1979;3:452–456.
20. Elamin EM, Camporesi E. Evidence-based nutritional support in the intensive care unit. *Int Anesthesiol Clin*. 2009;47:121–138.
21. Mehanna HM, Moledina J, Travis J. Refeeding syndrome: what it is, and how to prevent it and treat it. *BMJ*. 2008;336:1495–1498.
22. Boateng AA, Sriram K, Meguid MM, Crook M. Refeeding syndrome: treatment considerations based on collective analysis of literature case reports. *Nutrition*. 2010;26:156–167.
23. Jensen GL, Wheeler D. A new approach to defining and diagnosing malnutrition in adult critical illness. *Curr Opin Crit Care*. 2012;18:206–211.
24. Jensen GL. Inflammation as the key interface of the medical and nutrition universes: a provocative examination of the future of clinical nutrition and medicine. *J Parenter Enteral Nutr*. 2006;30: 453–463.
25. Stienstra R, Tack CJ, Kanneganti TD, et al. The inflammasome puts obesity in the danger zone. *Cell Metab*. 2012;15:10–18.
26. Jensen GL, Hsiao PY, Wheeler D. Adult nutrition assessment tutorial. *J Parenter Enteral Nutr*. 2012;36:267–274.
27. World Health Organization. *Report of a WHO Consultation on Obesity. Obesity: Preventing and Managing the Global Epidemic*. Geneva: World Health Organization; 1998.
28. Lee RD, Neiman DC. *Nutritional Assessment*, 4th ed. Boston: McGraw-Hill; 2007.
29. Soler-Cataluna JJ, Snachez-Sanchez L, Martinez-Garcia MA, et al. Mid-arm muscle area is a better predictor of mortality than body mass index in COPD. *Chest*. 2005;128:2108–2115.
30. Janssen I, Katzmarzyk PT, Ross R. Waist circumference and not body mass index explains obesity related health risk. *Am J Clin Nutr*. 2004;79:379–384.
31. Snijder MB, van Dam RM, Visser M, Seidell JC. What aspects of body fat are particularly hazardous and how do we measure them? *Int J Epidemiol*. 2006;35:83–92.
32. Ness-Abramof R, Apovian CM. Waist circumference measurement in clinical practice. *Nutr Clin Pract*. 2008;23:397–404.
33. Forse RA, Shizgal HM. Serum albumin and nutritional status. *JPEN J Parenter Enteral Nutr*. 1980;4:450–454.
34. Mahan LK, Escott-Stump S, eds. *Krauses's Food, Nutrition and Diet Therapy*, 11th ed. Philadelphia: Saunders; 2004.
35. da Rocha EE, Alves VG, Silva MH, et al. Can measured resting energy expenditure be estimated by formulae in daily clinical nutrition practice? *Curr Opin Clin Nutr Metab Care*. 2005;8: 319–328.
36. Elamin EM. Nutritional care of the obese intensive care unit patient. *Curr Opin Crit Care*. 2005;11:300–303.
37. Atwater WO, Rosa EB. Description of neo respiration calorimeter and experiments on the conservation of energy in the human body. US Department Agriculture, *Off Exp Sta Bull*. 63, 1899.
38. Atwater WO, Benedict FG. *A Respiration Calorimeter with Appliances for the Direct Determination of Oxygen*. Washington, DC: Carnegie Institute of Washington; Publication 42, 1905.
39. Harris JA, Benedict FG. A biometric study of human basal metabolism. *Proc Natl Acad Sci USA*. 1919;4:370–373.
40. Benedict FG, Carpenter TM. *Metabolism and Energy Transformations of Healthy Man During Rest*. Washington, DC: Carnegie Institution of Washington; 1910.
41. Benedict FG, Tompkins EH. Respiratory exchange, with a description of a respiration apparatus for clinical use. *Boston Med Surg J*. 1916;174:857–864.
42. Lev S, Cohen J, Singer P. Indirect calorimetry measurements in the ventilated critically ill patient: facts and controversies—the heat is on. *Crit Care Clin*. 2010;26:e1–9.
43. Branson RD, Wooley JA, Rodriguez J, Tajchman S. *Indirect Calorimetry in the Ventilated Patient. Critical Decisions*. Burlington, VT: Saxe Healthcare Communications; 2001.

44. Aliprandi G, Bissolotti L, Turla D, et al. The use of REE determination in a clinical setting applied to respiratory disease. *Acta Diabetol.* 2001;38:27–30.
45. Haugen HA, Chan LN, Li F. Indirect calorimetry: a practical guide for clinicians. *Nutr Clin Pract.* 2007;22:377–388.
46. Ultman JS, Bursztein S. Analysis of error in the determination of respiratory gas exchange at varying FIO_2. *J Appl Physiol.* 1981;50:210–216.
47. Branson RD, Johannigman JA. The measurement of energy expenditure. *Nutr Clin Pract.* 2004;19:622–636.
48. McClave SA, Lowen CC, Kleber MJ, et al. Clinical use of the respiratory quotient obtained from indirect calorimetry. *J Parenter Enteral Nutr.* 2003;27:21–26.
49. Wooley JA, Sax HC. Indirect calorimetry: applications to practice. *Nutr Clin Pract.* 2003;18:434–439.
50. Siobal MS, Hammoudeh H, Snow M. Accuracy of resting energy expenditure calculated by a modification of the abbreviated Weir equation in mechanically ventilated adult ICU patients. *Respir Care.* 2012;57:1721.
51. Hess D, Daugherty A, Large E, Agarwal NN. A comparison of four methods of determining caloric requirements of mechanically ventilated trauma patients. *Respir Care.* 1986;31:1197–1205.
52. McCamish MA, Dean RE, Ouellette TR. Assessing energy requirements of patients on respirators. *J Parenter Enteral Nutr.* 1981;5:513–516.
53. Wilmore DW. *The Metabolic Management of the Critically Ill.* New York: Plenum Medical Book Company; 1977.
54. AARC clinical practice guideline: metabolic measurement using indirect calorimetry during mechanical ventilation—2004 revision and update. *Respir Care.* 2004;49:1073–1079.
55. Flancbaum L, Choban PS, Sambucco S, et al. Comparison of indirect calorimetry, the Fick method, and prediction equations in estimating the energy requirements of critically ill patients. *Am J Clin Nutr.* 1999;69:461–466.
56. Malone AM. Methods of assessing energy expenditure in the ICU. *Nutr Clin Pract.* 2002;17:21–28.
57. Whitney EN, Rolfes SR. *Understanding Nutrition.* 13th ed. Belmont, CA: Wadsworth; 2012.
58. Skikora SA, Benotti PN. Nutritional support of the mechanically ventilated patient. *Respir Care Clin North Am.* 1997;3:69–90.
59. de Aguilar-Nascimento JE, Kudsk KA. Early nutritional therapy: the role of enteral and parenteral routes. *Curr Opin Clin Nutr Metab Care.* 2008;11:255–260.
60. Bankhead R, Boullata J, Brantley S, et al. Enteral nutrition practice recommendations. *JPEN J Parenter Enteral Nutr.* 2009;33:122–167.
61. Malone A. Enteral formula selection: a review of selected product categories. *Pract Gastroenterol.* 2005;29:77–74.
62. Cohen DA, Byham-Gray L, Denmark RM. Impact of two pulmonary enteral formulations on nutritional indices and outcomes. *J Hum Nutr Diet.* 2013;26:286–293.
63. Chen Y, Peterson SJ. Enteral nutrition formulas: which formula is right for your adult patient? *Nutr Clin Pract.* 2009;24:344–355.
64. McClave SA, Martindale RG, Vanek VW, et al. Guidelines for the Provision and Assessment of Nutrition Support Therapy in the Adult Critically Ill Patient: Society of Critical Care Medicine (SCCM) and American Society for Parenteral and Enteral Nutrition. *J Parenter Enteral Nutr.* 2009;33:277–316.
65. Griffiths RD, Bongers T. Nutrition support for patients in the intensive care unit. *Postgrad Med J.* 2005;81:629–636.
66. Gadek JE, DeMichele SJ, Karlstad MD, et al. Effect of enteral feeding with eicosapentaenoic acid, gamma-linolenic acid, and antioxidants in patients with acute respiratory distress syndrome. *Crit Care Med.* 1999;27:1409–1420.
67. Singer P, Theilla M, Fisher H, et al. Benefit of an enteral diet enriched with eicosapentaenoic acid and gamma-linolenic acid in ventilated patients with acute lung injury. *Crit Care Med.* 2006;34:1033–1038.
68. Pontes-Arruda A, Aragao AM, Albuquerque JD. Effects of enteral feeding with eicosapentaenoic acid, gamma-linolenic acid, and antioxidants in mechanically ventilated patients with severe sepsis and septic shock. *Crit Care Med.* 2006;34:2325–2333.
69. Rice TW, Wheeler AP, Thompson BT, et al. Enteral omega-3 fatty acid, gamma-linolenic acid, and antioxidant supplementation in acute lung injury. *JAMA.* 2011;306:1574–1581.
70. Cook DJ, Heyland DK. Pharmaconutrition in acute lung injury. *JAMA.* 2011;306:1599–1600.
71. McMahon MM, Nystrom E, Braunschweig C, et al. ASPEN clinical guidelines: nutrition support of adult patients with hyperglycemia. *J Parenter Enteral Nutr.* 2013;37:23–36.
72. Jacobi J, Bircher N, Krinsley J, et al. Guidelines for the use of an insulin infusion for the management of hyperglycemia in critically ill patients. *Crit Care Med.* 2012;40:3251–3276.
73. Mechanick JI, Scurlock C. Glycemic control and nutritional strategies in the cardiothoracic surgical intensive care unit—2010: state of the art. *Semin Thorac Cardiovasc Surg.* 2010;22:230–235.
74. Reeds D. Near-normal glycemia for critically ill patients receiving nutrition support: fact or folly. *Curr Opin Gastroenterol.* 2010;26:152–155.
75. Heyland DK, Dhaliwal R, Drover JW, et al. Canadian clinical practice guidelines for nutrition support in mechanically ventilated, critically ill adult patients. *J Parenter Enteral Nutr* 2003;27:355–373.
76. American Dietetic Association Evidence Library. Critical Illness. Academy of Nutrition and Dietetics. Updated 2012. Available at: https://andevidencelibrary.com/topic.cfm?cat=4800
77. Dhaliwal R, Cahill N, Lemieux M, Heyland DK. The Canadian critical care nutrition guidelines in 2013: an update on current recommendations and implementation strategies. *Nutr Clin Pract.* 2014;29:29–43.
78. Canadian clinical practice guidelines for nutrition support in mechanically ventilated, critically ill adult patients. American Dietetic Association Evidence Library. Critical Illness. Academy of Nutrition and Dietetics. Updated 2011. Available at: http://andevidencelibrary.com/topic.cfm?cat=4063
79. Kreymann KG, Berger MM, Deutz NE, et al. ESPEN Guidelines on Enteral Nutrition: Intensive Care. *Clin Nutr.* 2006;25:210–223.
80. Singer P, Berger MM, Van den Berghe G, et al. ESPEN Guidelines on Parenteral Nutrition: Intensive Care. *Clin Nutr.* 2009;28:387–400.

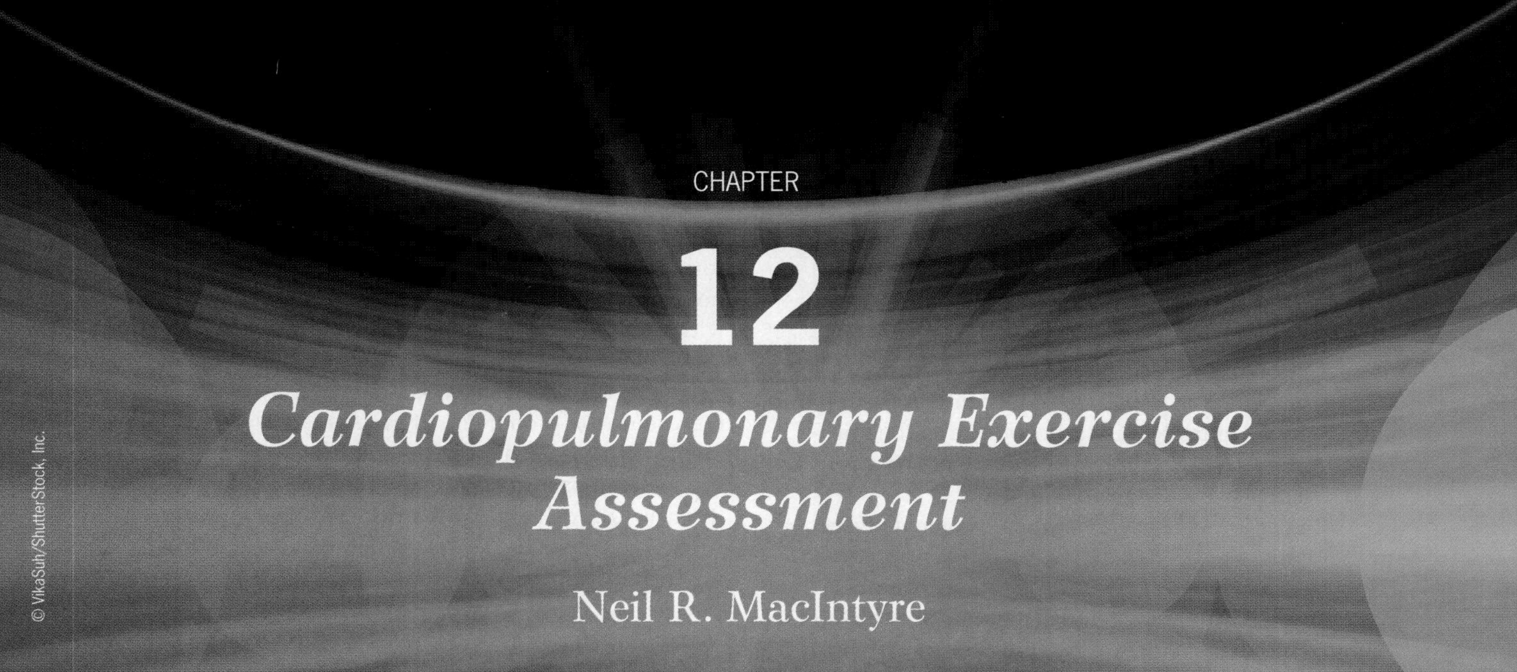

OUTLINE

OBJECTIVES

1. Describe the normal physiologic responses of the respiratory, cardiac, skeletal muscle, and peripheral and pulmonary vascular systems to exercise.
2. Describe the various approaches to exercise assessment and the primary measurements obtained during exercise testing.
3. Describe interpretation strategies for exercise testing.
4. Discuss the indications for exercise testing.
5. Discuss safety issues related to exercise testing.
6. Compare cardiopulmonary exercise testing and timed walk tests.

KEY TERMS

carbon dioxide production ($\dot{V}CO_2$)
cardiopulmonary exercise testing (CPET)
lactate
lactate threshold
metabolic equivalent (MET)
oxygen consumption ($\dot{V}O_2$)
oxygen delivery (DO_2)
oxygen extraction
oxygen pulse
respiratory exchange ratio
timed walk test
ventilatory equivalent
work rate

Introduction

Assessing cardiopulmonary function under exercise conditions can provide considerable insight into a patient's ability to function, tolerate surgical stress, and rehabilitate.[1–4] These assessments can also help clarify pathophysiology (e.g., cardiac versus pulmonary diseases), focus diagnostic processes, and predict disease trajectory. Exercise responses can be assessed in a variety of ways. These range from simple procedures such as measuring heart rate and dyspnea while walking up a set of stairs to complex assessments using invasive instrumentation of the heart and lungs (e.g., pulmonary artery catheters). In this chapter, the normal cardiopulmonary response to exercise is first described. Common approaches to cardiopulmonary exercise testing used and timed walk tests are then discussed as well as interpretation strategies for exercise testing.

Normal Cardiopulmonary Response to Exercise

With increasing muscle activity (e.g., exercise), cellular metabolism increases and the cardiopulmonary system must provide the necessary oxygen and nutrients to fuel this activity.[1–6] The system must also help clear the by-products of metabolism, including carbon dioxide and other substances (e.g., lactate). To accomplish this, both the lungs and the heart have the capability to increase ventilation and cardiac output, respectively, severalfold over resting values.

Oxygen Consumption and Carbon Dioxide Production

Exercise is often quantified by measuring **oxygen consumption ($\dot{V}O_2$)**. $\dot{V}O_2$ at rest is approximately 3.5 mL/kg/min. With slow walking, $\dot{V}O_2$ is 8 to 10 mL/kg/min, which is the minimal requirement to perform simple daily activity. At maximal exertion,

$\dot{V}O_2$ increases to 30 mL/kg/min in a sedentary 70-year-old and to more than 80 mL/kg/min in a young, elite athlete.[1–5] The maximum $\dot{V}O_2$ ($\dot{V}O_2max$) depends on genetics, level of conditioning, and presence of disease.[3] At low to moderate levels of exercise, cellular metabolism is largely aerobic (i.e., O_2 reacts with nutrients to produce energy, H_2O, and CO_2). Under these conditions, increases in $\dot{V}O_2$ and **carbon dioxide production ($\dot{V}CO_2$)** parallel each other as a function of the **respiratory exchange ratio** or respiratory quotient (R). R-values depend on the relative contributions of fat versus carbohydrate as the mitochondrial nutrient–carbohydrate nutrients have R of 1, fat nutrients have R closer to 0.7.[5]

At higher levels of exercise when oxygen delivery to the tissues begins to plateau, oxygen extraction from capillary blood increases to maintain aerobic metabolism. Ultimately, cellular metabolism converts to nonaerobic mechanisms that produce metabolic acids (e.g., **lactate**). This point in exercise has often been called the *anaerobic threshold*, but a better term is the **lactate threshold**, reflecting the fact that lactate buildup is multifactorial and includes hormonal and regional blood flow effects as well as anaerobic metabolism.[1–7] Lactate is buffered by bicarbonate, which then results in $\dot{V}CO_2$ rising faster than VO_2, thus increasing the measured R to as high as 1.1. This change in R is a commonly used indicator for the lactate threshold and normally occurs at 50% to 65% of peak exercise. Bicarbonate buffering capacity may be exceeded at higher levels of exertion. The resulting acidemic stimulus to the medullary receptor and carotid bodies produces levels of exercise ventilation disproportionate to the level of $\dot{V}CO_2$. This relative hyperventilation results in decreased $PaCO_2$ at higher levels of exertion.

Ventilatory Responses

As oxygen demand and $\dot{V}CO_2$ increase, the lungs increase minute ventilation ($\dot{V}E$) to meet these demands according to the relationship between alveolar ventilation ($\dot{V}A$) and $\dot{V}CO_2$ and partial pressure of arterial carbon dioxide ($PaCO_2$):

$$\dot{V}A = (0.863 \times \dot{V}CO_2)/PaCO_2$$

$\dot{V}E$ increases initially as an increase in tidal volume, up to 55% of the vital capacity with a relatively stable end-expiratory lung volume.[1–8] Thereafter, $\dot{V}E$ increases are largely driven by breathing frequency. Measurements of $\dot{V}E$ often are referenced to the maximal ventilatory capacity of the subject, a value commonly represented by the maximum voluntary ventilation (MVV), in L/min, from a maximal effort over 12 to 15 seconds. In referencing $\dot{V}E$ to MVV ($\dot{V}E$/MVV%), a ventilatory reserve can be defined. The normal range for this ratio at maximal exercise is 70% to 80%, indicating that 20% to 30% of the maximal ventilatory capacity remains unused at this level of exercise. This reserve reflects the fact that in normal subjects, cardiovascular factors reach limits at maximal exercise before ventilatory factors do. It is important to recognize that this notion of ventilatory reserve assumes that the resting MVV is indeed reflective of the maximal ventilatory capacity during exercise, an assumption that may not be valid if respiratory system mechanics change with exercise (e.g., bronchospasm, air trapping, edema formation, muscle fatigue).

The ratio of dead space to tidal volume (VD/VT) represents the proportion of each breath that is not involved in gas exchange. This represents both the anatomic dead space (airways) and physiologic dead space (high $\dot{V}/\dot{Q}$). Although absolute dead space may rise slightly during exercise, it is generally less than the rise in VT, and thus the VD/VT ratio should fall with exercise. VD/VT is less than 0.35 at rest and should decrease with increasing exercise.

Gas Exchange Responses to Exercise

Despite severalfold increases in ventilation and cardiac output ($\dot{Q}c$) with exercise, the $\dot{V}/\dot{Q}$ is remarkably stable.[1–7] As a consequence, the alveolar–arterial oxygen gradient remains stable or only increases slightly with exercise. The PaO_2 thus is maintained in the normal range throughout exercise in normal subjects. Interestingly, at extremely high $\dot{Q}c$ in elite athletes, the exposure time of red blood cells to alveolar gas in the pulmonary capillaries (transit time) can become so brief that alveolocapillary O_2 transfer can be short and mild hypoxemia can develop.

Cardiovascular Responses to Exercise

The cardiac response to exercise is an increase in $\dot{Q}c$.[1–8] In normal subjects, up to a fivefold increase in $\dot{Q}c$ can occur, and trained athletes can increase this further. Importantly, it is the limit on $\dot{Q}c$ that ultimately limits exercise capabilities in normal subjects. The increase in $\dot{Q}c$ involves an increase in stroke volume during the initial phase of exercise. At higher levels of exercise, however, the entire increase in $\dot{Q}c$ is related to increases in heart rate. Of note is that the heart rate is higher for any given power output with exercise that uses smaller muscle mass. Heart rate during arm exercise therefore is greater than during bicycle exercise, which is greater than during treadmill exercise for any given power output.

Oxygen Delivery

The integrated effect of increases in the output of the cardiopulmonary system is often expressed as **oxygen delivery (DO_2)**, which is determined by $\dot{Q}c$ and arterial oxygen content (CaO_2). At rest in normal subjects, CaO_2 is 200 mL/L of blood and $\dot{Q}c$ is approximately 5 L/min. DO_2 thus is 1000 mL/min at rest and can increase severalfold with exercise.[1–7] CaO_2 is determined not only by alveolocapillary gas transport properties but also by the ability of the blood to carry oxygen. This is heavily dependent on the hemoglobin concentration and its oxygen-binding properties (expressed as the oxyhemoglobin dissociation curve). In the lungs, the higher pH and lower temperature of the alveolar spaces shift this oxyhemoglobin dissociation curve to the left to increase oxygen loading. The lower pH and increased temperature of exercising muscle result in shifts of the oxyhemoglobin dissociation curve to the right to facilitate the unloading of oxygen into the contracting muscle.

Oxygen Extraction

Similar to $\dot{V}/\dot{Q}$ matching in the lungs, the peripheral circulation responds to exercise with an increase in blood flow to active skeletal muscle to ensure that oxygen delivery is matched to oxygen demand.[1–7] Peripheral vascular resistance decreases with exercise, but systolic blood pressure rises because of disproportionate increases in $\dot{Q}c$. The oxygen delivered to the tissues (muscles) must be extracted (i.e., delivered to muscle mitochondria) to provide energy for muscle contraction. **Oxygen extraction** is quantified by the extraction ratio:

$$\text{Extraction ratio} = \dot{V}O_2/DO_2 = (CaO_2 - C\bar{v}O_2)/CaO_2$$

In normal subjects at rest, the extraction ratio is 25%, but this can increase to over 50% at maximal exercise. Oxygen extraction can be further increased with endurance training through increases in muscle mitochondrial density, capillary density, and metabolic enzymes. Oxygen extraction can be decreased in a variety of pathologic states that impair cellular metabolism and oxygen utilization (e.g., congenital mitochondrial disorders).

Incremental Exercise Testing

Exercise stresses the cardiopulmonary system, and thus assessing physiologic responses can give valuable information on cardiopulmonary function.[1–11] The most comprehensive way to assess this is **cardiopulmonary exercise testing (CPET)** using incremental or ramped exercise to a symptom-limited maximum. Both bicycles and treadmills have been used for this purpose, with the increment or ramped increases designed to get 8 to 12 minutes of data before symptoms terminate the test. A practical approach uses bicycle exercise ramped at 12.5-watt increases per minute for poorly conditioned subjects and at 25-watt increases per minute for better conditioned subjects. The optimal duration, however, may be disease specific. For example, in patients with chronic obstructive pulmonary disease (COPD), a 5- to 9-minute duration may produce a higher maximal workload.

Symptom-Limited Work Rate

A useful way to quantify exercise capacity is to measure the maximal work performed (watts). The relationship between $\dot{V}O_2$ and **work rate** ($\Delta\dot{V}O_2/\Delta$watts) reflects the change in the internal metabolic demand of exercise for a given change in external load and thus remains relatively constant under most circumstances (approximately 10 mL/min/watt during bicycle exercise).[9–11] Values less than 8.8 mL/min/watt may be associated with significant impairments in oxygen delivery or use, such as severe cardiac disease or myopathy. Sudden drops in this value during an exercise study may indicate cardiac ischemia. If it is consistently less than 10 in all patients tested in a laboratory, the calibration of the ergometer should be questioned.

Symptoms at Maximal Exercise

Subjects stop exercising because they achieve intolerable symptoms. The sense of effort at maximal exercise thus is a useful parameter to collect. The modified Borg ratings for dyspnea and perceived leg effort (**Figure 12-1**) offer a validated technique to assess symptoms during exertion.[12]

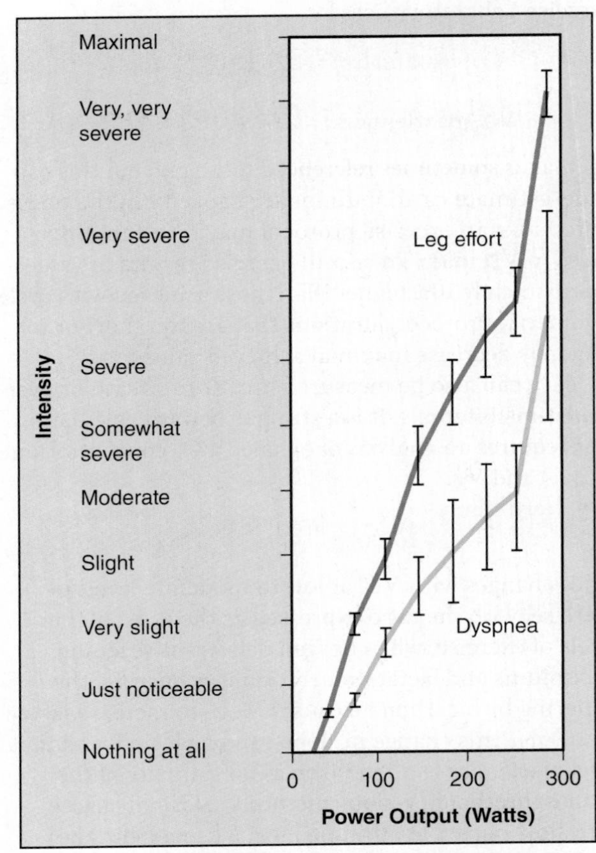

FIGURE 12-1 Exertion scale for perceived effort and sense of dyspnea during incremental exercise testing in normal subjects.

Reproduced from Kearon MC, Summers E, Jones NL, et al. Effort and dyspnea during work of varying intensity and duration. *Eur Respir J.* 1991;4:917–925. Reproduced with permission of the European Respiratory Society.

Oxygen Consumption and Carbon Dioxide Production

$\dot{V}O_2$ is calculated breath-to-breath or averaged over short periods of time. When the inspired gas is room air, it is a straightforward calculation using the measured mixed exhaled O_2 concentration ($F\bar{E}O_2$) and the minute ventilation:

$$\dot{V}O_2 = (0.21 - F\bar{E}O_2) \times \dot{V}E$$

Analysis of inhaled O_2 concentration must be included if the patient requires supplemental O_2. A simple way to express $\dot{V}O_2$ is a **metabolic equivalent (MET)**. One MET approximates the resting $\dot{V}O_2$ (3.5 mL/kg), and exercise increases in $\dot{V}O_2$ can be reported in METs.

$\dot{V}O_2$ is usually the most important parameter used to quantify exercise tolerance, and many other variables derived during exercise testing are often plotted as a function of $\dot{V}O_2$ to measure the appropriateness of their responses throughout exertion. At maximal exertion, this function is called $\dot{V}O_2$max and represents an individual's cardiopulmonary fitness and level of conditioning. $\dot{V}O_2$max is reported as a percentage of predicted normal values and a normal $\dot{V}O_2$max percentage is often taken as greater than 80%. Numerous $\dot{V}O_2$max prediction equations exist.[6,9,11,13] The Duke University Exercise Laboratory uses:[14]

$$\dot{V}O_2\,\max(\text{males}) = 4.2 - (0.032 \times \text{Age})$$

$$\dot{V}O_2\,\max(\text{females}) = 2.6 - (0.014 \times \text{Age})$$

$\dot{V}O_2$max is sometimes referenced to weight, but this can underestimate cardiopulmonary capacity in the obese. Differences in exercise protocol may result in differences in $\dot{V}O_2$max. Treadmill exercise results in values approximately 10% higher than those achieved with cycle ergometry. Protocol durations that are too short or too long may decrease maximal achieved values.

$\dot{V}CO_2$ can also be measured breath-to-breath or over short time intervals. It is a straightforward calculation that requires an analysis of exhaled CO_2 concentration ($F\bar{E}CO_2$) and $\dot{V}E$:

$$\dot{V}CO_2 = F\bar{E}CO_2 \times \dot{V}E$$

$\dot{V}CO_2$ changes with $\dot{V}O_2$ at low to moderate levels of exercise, with the ratio expressed as the R. At higher levels of exercise, when oxygen delivery is reaching maximums and lactate generation is occurring, the buffering by bicarbonate causes $\dot{V}CO_2$ to increase faster than $\dot{V}O_2$. This change in slope can be plotted, and that level of exercise is often taken as an estimate of the lactate threshold (V-slope method).[4] Normal lactate threshold occurs at 50% to 65% of $\dot{V}O_2$max, but the confidence limits extend as low as 40% in groups of individuals without known disease. Lactate threshold can be protocol dependent and varies with rate of incremental work increases and type of exercise, with cycle ergometry resulting in values approximately 10% lower than those seen with treadmill exercise.

The **ventilatory equivalents** for both CO_2 and O_2 are commonly reported during exercise ($\dot{V}E/\dot{V}CO_2$ and $\dot{V}E/\dot{V}O_2$, respectively).[4–11] $\dot{V}E/\dot{V}CO_2$ has been used as an indirect estimate of dead space in the absence of arterial blood gas or end tidal measurements to calculate V_D/V_T. Normal values for $\dot{V}E/\dot{V}CO_2$ and $\dot{V}E/\dot{V}O_2$ at the lactate threshold are less than 34 and 31, respectively. Increases in the $\dot{V}E/\dot{V}CO_2$ and $\dot{V}E/\dot{V}O_2$ can be associated with psychogenic hyperventilation, malingering, metabolic acidosis, or other causes of increased ventilatory drive.

Plots of $\dot{V}E/\dot{V}CO_2$ and $\dot{V}E/\dot{V}O_2$ as a function of $\dot{V}O_2$ are alternative approaches commonly used in the detection of the lactate threshold. Both values initially fall and then plateau at moderate levels of exertion. In cases of early lactic acidosis, during which time bicarbonate buffering results in increasing $\dot{V}CO_2$, but not in acidemia (the isocapnic buffering period), the $\dot{V}E/\dot{V}O_2$ rises while the $\dot{V}E/\dot{V}CO_2$ remains constant. With increasing acidemia, $\dot{V}E/\dot{V}CO_2$ increases. In respiratory conditions such as COPD, increased tissue stores of CO_2 associated with hypoventilation may make the noninvasive determination of lactate threshold impossible.[4]

Exercise Ventilation

Exercise ventilation ($\dot{V}E$) is largely driven by pH and P_{CO_2} (and thus $\dot{V}CO_2$). $\dot{V}E$ can be measured breath-to-breath or over discrete intervals. In normal subjects, the maximal ventilatory capacity of the lung is generally much larger than the ventilation requirements at maximal exercise. There thus exists a substantial ventilatory reserve in normal subjects at maximal exercise (i.e., $\dot{V}E$/MVV is less than 70% to 80% at maximal exercise).

An additional ventilation assessment is the end-expiratory lung volume (EELV).[15–17] EELV should remain relatively stable during increases in exercise ventilation. An increase in EELV suggests air trapping. Changes in EELV can be estimated by changes in inspiratory capacity (IC). Multiple IC maneuvers can be performed throughout exertion, and EELV then is calculated as the difference between total lung capacity and IC.

Arterial Blood Gas Measurements

Arterial blood gas values can be analyzed at different levels of exercise either from an indwelling arterial catheter or intermittent sampling. Because $\dot{V}/\dot{Q}$ matching is well maintained even at exercise with maximal $\dot{Q}c$, Pa_{O_2} does not change significantly during exercise in healthy individuals. Both resting and exercise $P(A - a)O_2$ increase with age, however.[18] Pa_{CO_2} and pH are generally well maintained through low and moderate exercise by appropriate increases in the minute ventilation. Above the lactate threshold, however, accelerated increases in ventilation will lower Pa_{CO_2} in order to preserve the pH.[1–7] Because ventilatory capacity is not the limiting step to exercise in normal subjects, this ability to protect the pH is well maintained until the very highest levels of exercise.

Surrogates for arterial blood gas assessments are pulse oximetry and either end-tidal or transcutaneous CO_2 analyzers. Pulse oximeters need to have visual displays of the pulse waveform to ensure accurate measurements are made under exercise conditions where superficial skin perfusion may be reduced. Similar concerns exist for transcutaneous CO_2 measurements. In healthy individuals, the end-tidal P_{CO_2} (P_{ETCO_2}) can be used to estimate Pa_{CO_2}. Even with healthy lungs, however, small differences exist between the Pa_{CO_2} and the P_{ETCO_2}. In diseased lungs with increases in physiologic dead space, the P_{ETCO_2} may differ considerably from Pa_{CO_2}.

Ratio of Dead Space to Tidal Volume

In addition to calculating $\dot{V}_{CO_2}$, exhaled CO_2 (both mixed exhaled [$P\bar{E}_{CO_2}$] and P_{ETCO_2}) can be used either alone or with a measurement of Pa_{CO_2} to calculate V_D/V_T:

$$V_D/V_T = (Pa_{CO_2} - P\bar{E}_{CO_2})/Pa_{CO_2}$$

$$V_D/V_T = (P_{ETCO_2} - P\bar{E}_{CO_2})/P_{ETCO_2}$$

One weakness with the use of V_D/V_T is that it is influenced by the ventilatory pattern. Because of the 150 to 200 mL of anatomic dead space, respiratory patterns with shallow V_T have a greater proportion of dead space independent of parenchymal gas exchange characteristics. Importantly, in the computation of the dead space and the V_D/V_T, subtraction of the dead space of the measuring device used to perform the gas analysis is necessary.

Cardiovascular Assessment

Cardiac assessment during CPET in most pulmonary laboratories consists of heart rate (HR), blood pressure (BP), and cardiac rhythm.[9–11] $\dot{Q}_C$ increases with exercise are initially stroke volume increases followed by heart rate increases until maximal exercise.[1–7] Because of this, heart rate approaches the predicted maximum of 220 minus age (predicted HRmax) as maximal exercise is approached in normal subjects. A heart rate less than 80% to 90% of predicted at maximal exercise should raise the suspicion of noncardiovascular limitations to exertion (e.g., ventilatory/gas exchange limitation, submaximal effort). On the other hand, identification of significant metabolic acidosis in the presence of a large heart rate reserve may indicate chronotropic insufficiency (as with β-blocker, calcium-channel blocker, or conduction system abnormalities or heart transplantation). It also may reflect large-extremity ischemia if associated with symptoms of claudication, however. Importantly, heart rate recovery after maximal exercise is becoming increasingly recognized as an important indicator of cardiac function. If heart rate has not decreased more than 12 to 13 beats/min after 1 min of recovery, cardiac disease should be suspected.[10]

Heart rate is often plotted as a function of $\dot{V}_{O_2}$ to assess the appropriateness of its response ($\dot{V}_{O_2}$/HR or **oxygen pulse**).[9–11] Normally the O_2 pulse rises linearly with exercise to values approaching predicted $\dot{V}_{O_2}$max/predicted HRmax. Reductions in the O_2 pulse are associated with abnormal stroke volume because heart rate must increase to maintain $\dot{Q}_C$ for a given $\dot{V}_{O_2}$. Hemoglobin, Sa_{O_2}, and peripheral muscle function independently affect the body's ability to increase $\dot{V}_{O_2}$, however, and may result in decreased O_2 pulse independent of stroke volume.

In most pulmonary laboratories, the electrocardiogram (ECG) is routinely measured throughout exercise. A two lead rhythm strip can detect dysrhythmias and a full 12 lead ECG can also be used to detect ischemic events. Blood pressure measurements are also commonly done periodically throughout exercise. Normally, diastolic pressure changes little while systolic pressure rises roughly 10 mm Hg/MET with a maximum of 210 mm Hg in men and 190 mm Hg in women.[10]

In some laboratories, measurements of $\dot{Q}_C$ are made.[10,19] The gold standard for $\dot{Q}_C$ assessment is the direct Fick method, which requires placement of a pulmonary artery catheter. Mixed venous blood is sampled from the pulmonary artery catheter, arterial blood is sampled, and $\dot{V}_{O_2}$ measurements are made from expired gas. Arterial and venous oxygen content (Ca_{O_2} and $C\bar{v}_{O_2}$) are then calculated and $\dot{Q}_C$ is calculated from the Fick equation:

$$\dot{Q}_C = \dot{V}_{O_2}/(Ca_{O_2} - C\bar{v}_{O_2})$$

This technique is reliable during submaximal steady-state exercise, but its use is limited because of its invasive nature and inaccuracy in non-steady-state exercise. Pulmonary artery catheter measurements can also include right and left heart pressures during exercise.

Acetylene and other inert soluble gas rebreathing or single-breath methods can also be used to assess $\dot{Q}_C$ based on the assumption that the rate of disappearance of such gases is directly proportional to the flow of blood through the lungs.[20] The technique is accurate and simple to perform at maximal exercise in healthy individuals but can be inaccurate in persons with ventilation abnormalities caused by lung disease. Of note is that CO uptake (diffusing capacity of the lungs for CO; D_{LCO}) can also be calculated during exercise using similar gas analyzers. D_{LCO} normally increases 25% to 30% with exercise, reflecting capillary recruitment from the increased $\dot{Q}_C$.[20]

Although not routinely used in pulmonary laboratories, echocardiography is becoming increasingly common in many cardiac laboratories.[10,11] This technology can be very useful in detecting beat-to-beat changes in $\dot{Q}c$ (Doppler echocardiography) as well as in assessing both right and left ventricular function under exercise conditions. Interestingly, these laboratories often simulate exercise with drugs such as dobutamine to stimulate HR.

Interpreting the Results of Incremental Cardiopulmonary Exercise Testing

A common approach to interpreting the results of symptom-limited CPET first describes the level of impairment, often using maximal $\dot{V}O_2$ as a percentage of predicted. The exercise-limiting factors can then be defined as ventilatory limitations, gas exchange limitations, or cardiovascular limitations (**Table 12-1**).[4,21–23]

The first question that then should be answered is whether an individual has a normal exercise capacity. A $\dot{V}O_2$max of greater than 80% of predicted indicates a normal physiologic capacity to perform metabolic work. In obese or otherwise inefficient individuals, significant discrepancies may exist between their physiologic capacity to perform work ($\dot{V}O_2$max) and the actual work performed on their environment, or power output, which may be abnormally decreased. Furthermore, in obese individuals $\dot{V}O_2$max adjusted for weight (mL/min/kg) may be decreased into the mild (<25 mL/min/kg) or even severe (<15 mL/min/kg) disability range in the setting of normal $\dot{V}O_2$max% predicted, which is calculated based on height or lean body mass.

TABLE 12-1
A General Scheme for Interpretation of Common CPET Responses

Step one: Exercise capability	$\dot{V}O_2$max < 80% predicted indicates reduced exercise capacity
Step two: Cardiovascular limitations	HRmax and O_2 pulse both > 80% predicted is normal HRmax > 80% predicted, O_2 pulse < 80% predicted suggests cardiac disease or deconditioning HRmax < 80% predicted suggests cardiac limitations not present, HR response limited (drugs, pacer), or poor effort Dysrhythmias, systolic BP decrease or increase above 190 mm Hg (women) or 210 mm Hg (men), diastolic BP increase more than 10–15 mm Hg, ischemic ECG tracings suggest cardiac disease
Step three: Ventilatory limitations	$\dot{V}E$/MVV > 80% or $PaCO_2$ rising indicates ventilatory limits present MVV reduced during exercise from exercise bronchospasm (>15–20% fall in FEV_1) or air trapping (reduced inspiratory capacity)
Step four: Gas exchange limitations	PaO_2 (or SpO_2) falling to 55–79 mm Hg (88–89%) is abnormal, PaO_2 (or SpO_2) falling to < 55 mm Hg (SpO_2 < 88%) is exercise limiting V_D/V_T above 0.35 or rises with exercise indicates inability to match perfusion to exercise ventilation (vascular disease)

Cardiovascular limitation to exercise occurs when the cardiac and peripheral vascular components of the Fick equation are maximized.[1–7] Further increases in $\dot{V}O_2$ thus cannot occur, resulting in unbearable symptoms that lead to exercise termination. The most common indicator is a heart rate greater than 80% to 90% of predicted maximum. In addition, a decrease in base excess or a lactate increase of more than 3 mmol/L can indicate cardiovascular limitation. Healthy individuals exhibit a cardiovascular limitation at normal maximal exercise. Reaching this limit at a normal maximal $\dot{V}O_2$ therefore does not imply abnormalities in the cardiovascular system. The differential diagnosis for isolated abnormalities in the cardiovascular response includes any condition that affects the delivery or use of oxygen, including severe deconditioning, left or right heart systolic or diastolic dysfunction, anemia, hemoglobinopathy, carboxyhemoglobin, myopathy, or peripheral shunt.

Ventilatory limitation occurs when an individual approaches the mechanical limits of the respiratory system, resulting in intolerable dyspnea that leads to exercise termination.[1–8] $\dot{V}O_2$ thus cannot increase further despite significant reserves in the cardiovascular system. Indicators of ventilatory limitation include a $\dot{V}E$max/MVV ratio of greater than 0.70 to 0.80, a rising $PaCO_2$, or a developing respiratory acidosis.

Individuals demonstrating ventilatory limitation nearly all have abnormalities in ventilatory mechanics and thus MVV. Exceptions include the elite athlete, who has trained the cardiovascular system to challenge the limits of the capacity for the ventilatory system and the individual with increased ventilatory drive, as may occur in cases of severe acute or chronic metabolic acidosis. Importantly, because MVV is conventionally measured at rest, acute reductions in MVV because of bronchospasm or because of development of air trapping may be unappreciated as a cause of ventilatory limitations. Thus, intraexercise measurements of inspiratory capacity and postexercise spirometry should be performed in these subjects.[8,16]

Gas exchange limitations (i.e., hypoxemia) leading to intolerable dyspnea are commonly considered a separate category of exercise limitation. Parameters indicating an abnormal gas exchange response include increased V_D/V_T, abnormally widened $P(A - a)O_2$, a decrease in PaO_2 or SpO_2, elevated $\dot{V}E/\dot{V}O_2$ at the lactate threshold, and increased $P(a - ET)CO_2$. Common criteria defining a gas exchange limit to exercise are a Pa_{O_2} less than 55 to 60 mm Hg or an Sp_{O_2} less than 88% to 89%.[21] The finding of abnormalities in gas exchange supports the presence of, and quantifies the magnitude of, overt or occult parenchymal lung disease or airways disease. Note that the impairment in oxygen delivery associated with hypoxemia and the elevation in $\dot{V}_E$ associated with dead space abnormalities may contribute to premature cardiovascular and ventilatory limitations.

Combined limitation occurs when cardiovascular, gas exchange, and/or ventilatory parameters approach physiologic limits together. In such cases, symptoms from each process likely contribute to exercise termination.[21] Combined abnormalities involving cardiovascular, gas exchange, and ventilatory parameters may be characteristic of disease processes, such as primary pulmonary vascular disease. In other cases the response pattern helps subcategorize disease. For example, although COPD is primarily associated with significant deficits in gas exchange, abnormalities in the cardiovascular parameters may indicate the presence of secondary pulmonary hypertension, myopathy, deconditioning, or left ventricular abnormalities. Whereas patients with idiopathic pulmonary fibrosis have qualitatively similar findings, the disease process is characterized by more profound arterial desaturation and rapid respiratory rates, which often exceed 60 breaths/min at maximal exertion. More subtle abnormalities in gas exchange can be observed in subjects with cardiomyopathy, in whom abnormalities in cardiovascular response are prominent.

A submaximal response occurs when exercise is symptom terminated but cardiovascular, gas exchange, and ventilatory system parameters have not approached their physiologic limits. This finding may be a valid measure of exercise capacity if symptoms arise from peripheral muscle weakness, intolerable dyspnea, or musculoskeletal pain, but the values are less meaningful if exercise is terminated due to a lack of effort, dry mouth, or sore buttocks.

Importantly, abnormalities in the various cardiovascular and ventilatory/gas exchange parameters can occur without these abnormalities actually limiting maximal exercise. For example, a low MVV may still be more than enough to provide $\dot{V}_E$ for an exercise test limited by cardiovascular factors. Similarly, a Pa_{O_2} reduction of 87 to 69 mm Hg with exercise is an abnormal response but would not be the exercise-limiting factor in a subject with other limitations.

> **Respiratory Recap**
>
> **Interpretative Strategies for CPET**
>
> - Is the subject's maximal exercise capacity abnormal?
> - What is the major limiting factor to maximal exertion: cardiac, ventilatory, gas exchange, or combined?
> - Are non-exercise-limiting abnormalities present in the cardiovascular and ventilatory gas exchange response?

Timed Walk Tests

Timed walk tests are of two types: the six minute walk test (6MWT) and the shuttle walk test.[24] The 6MWT allows patients to pace themselves and thus focuses primarily on functional performance.[24–27] In contrast, the shuttle walk tests ramp up the walking speed in an attempt to replicate CPET performance.[24]

6MWT are generally easy to perform. Patients usually prefer them to other forms of exercise testing because the exercise is familiar to them and the tests allow patients to set their own pace (including rests) and adaptive maneuvers (e.g., pursed-lip breathing). Patients are encouraged to go as far as they can over a 6-minute period of time. Importantly, a practice walk may result in a very slight (25–27 m) increase in the subsequent walk test.[24] Walking course configuration can impact results and the recent ATS-ERS Guidelines[24] recommend a 30-m course along a flat surface (not a treadmill). The clinician performing the test should offer standard encouragement phrases but should otherwise not interfere with the patient walk. 6MWT often detect exercise hypoxemia that is not observed during a CPET. If the patient has known or suspected exercise hypoxemia, O_2 thus should be supplied at a constant flow known to keep $Sp_{O_2} > 88\%$. This may require a separate O_2 titration assessment prior to the 6MWT.[24] During the walk, supplemental O_2 should be supplied from a portable tank that the patient can pull (not carry). The ATS-ERS Guidelines recommend monitoring both HR and Sp_{O_2} during the walk.[24] This can be done by the clinician following behind the patient with a pulse oximeter or, in the future, using devices with wireless capabilities. **Box 12-1** gives a suggested protocol similar to that used for the National Emphysema Treatment Trial.[28]

At the end of the walk, distance is recorded and usually referenced to a predicted value. Numerous prediction equations exist;[24] the ones used in the Duke University laboratory are:[29]

$$6MWD\ (males) = (7.57 \times Height\ cm) - (5.02 \times Age) - (1.76 \times Weight\ kg) - 309\ m$$

$$6MWD\ (females) = (2.11 \times Height\ cm) - (5.78 \times Age) - (2.29 \times Weight\ kg) + 667\ m$$

Both the nadir and end walk Sp_{O_2} should also be recorded. Some argue for the Sp_{O_2} area over either distance or time. Heart rate is also important to report and notations should be made if there are reasons the HR response might be blunted (i.e., drugs or pacemakers). Heart rate recovery is the change in heart rate during

BOX 12-1

Six-Minute Walk Test Procedures

Walk Course

- Course should be 30 m long, unobstructed, flat, and indoors.
- If testing site is moved, configuration should remain constant.

Patient Preparation

- Prewalk bronchodilator should be administered at least 15 minutes in advance.
- The need for oxygen supplementation should be determined prior to the walk and kept constant (a separate oxygen titration assessment may be required prior to walk).
- The test should take place 2 hours after the last meal.
- The patient should sit at rest at least 10 minutes before the test.
- The patient should wear comfortable clothes and shoes.

Procedure

- Instruct the patient to cover as much ground as possible.
- Allow the patient to slow down or rest as needed (included in the 6 minutes).
- Ask the patient not to talk.
- If oxygen is used, it should be on wheels and not carried.
- Provide the patient with encouragement and the time remaining at each 1-minute mark.
- At the end of 6 minutes, ask the patient to stop. Then perform the following:
    - Record the distance traveled.
    - Record dyspnea (Borg scale).
    - Record the patient's heart rate, blood pressure, and Spo_2.

Information from the National Emphysema Treatment Trial Research Group. A randomized trial comparing lung-volume-reduction surgery with medical therapy for severe emphysema. *N Engl J Med.* 2003;348:2059–2073.

the first minute after exercise stopped and can also be useful to record after a 6MWT. If the HR has not reduced 12 to 13 beats/min over this first minute, cardiac disease should be suspected. The modified Borg scale for dyspnea and perceived exertion is commonly used to assess subjective response to the walk.

Walk test distance has a fair correlation with maximal exercise tolerance but a very strong correlation with an individual's ability to perform activities of daily living and quality of life.[24] Indeed, this latter correlation makes the 6MWT attractive in the evaluation of novel therapies such as vasodilator response or lung volume reduction surgery. 6MWT distance has also been correlated with important outcomes such as mortality, often in conjunction with integrated indices such as the BODE score (Body mass index, Obstructed airways, Dyspnea, and Exercise [6MWT]).[30]

The minimum important change in distance (MID) in the 6MWT following an intervention that correlates with real functional improvement has been studied extensively.[24] The ATS-ERS Guidelines suggest that 30 m be considered the MID for the 6MWT, at least in COPD patients.[24]

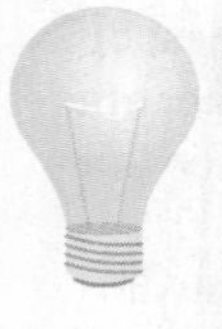

STOP AND THINK

You are seeing a patient with COPD as part of your pulmonary rehabilitation program. How might the six-minute walk distance help in your assessment of the patient?

Shuttle walk tests have been studied less than the 6MWT and are of two types: the incremental shuttle walk test (ISWT) and the endurance shuttle walk test (ESWT).[24] The ISWT uses a 10-m track and a metronome that gradually increases the walking pace until patients cannot keep up. The ultimate walk distance is recorded along with HR, Spo_2, and symptoms similar to the 6MWT. As noted above, the ISWT results tend to mimic CPET results but with less requirement for complex equipment. The ESWT is an endurance test that records the distance a patient can walk at a set percentage (usually 75–85%) of the maximal ISWT walking pace. Because of the standardization of the walk track and the metronome pacer, variability with the shuttle walk tests is less than in the 6MWT.[24]

Indications for Cardiopulmonary Exercise Testing

When routine history, physical, and basic pulmonary function and blood tests fail to determine the cause of dyspnea, exercise testing, especially the CPET, can help document impairment and distinguish abnormal cardiopulmonary physiologic responses from inorganic causes associated with anxiety or even malingering.[9,21,22] A normal study can serve to reassure the individual and avoid expensive and invasive testing. An abnormal study may direct the workup toward more invasive testing, such as right or left heart catheterization, pulmonary angiography, lung biopsy, or muscle biopsy or may indicate specific therapy, such as exercise training or specific medication use.[9–11,31,32] Because of the wide variation of normal values, serial tests in the case of persistent or progressive symptoms may be necessary to document progression of an abnormal physiologic response. CPET can help determine the relative contributions of cardiovascular and ventilatory abnormalities to exercise impairment in individuals with known disease. Such determinations can direct therapy toward the appropriate organ system.

CPET has shown promise for research and clinical use in the assessment of physiologic and functional change associated with an intervention. For example, CPET has been used to document the effects of immunosuppressive therapy in those with idiopathic pulmonary fibrosis,[33] lung transplantation in those with COPD,[34] prostacyclin therapy in individuals with primary pulmonary hypertension,[35] and the effects of lung volume reduction surgery.[36,37] More recently, timed walk tests (especially the 6MWT) have been used to assess functional responses to a number of these interventions.

Measurements of $\dot{V}o_2max$ are predictive of survival in individuals with cystic fibrosis and congestive heart failure.[38] In COPD, exercise tolerance and exercise hypoxemia have also been shown to predict mortality. For example, in COPD patients a Vo_2max below 10 mL/min/kg was associated with a 5-year mortality of 62%, and a $Pao_2/\dot{V}o_2$ slope of less than −80 mm Hg/L/min was associated with a 5-year mortality of 80%.[39] Moreover, incorporating 6MWT into an integrated index including dyspnea, body mass index, and FEV_1 (the BODE index) is an easy technique that allows for accurate mortality predictions in COPD.[30]

$\dot{V}o_2$ measurements have been used to assess preoperative risk before both cardiac and noncardiac surgery.[40–44] The rationale for its use is that CPET mimics the hypermetabolism and tachycardia of the perioperative state and represents an objective evolution of the stair-climbing techniques traditionally used by surgeons. Other investigators have demonstrated low morbidity rates in patients with a good response to CPET who were otherwise considered high risks for thoracotomy by use of traditional criteria.[45] **Table 12-2** presents risk stratification based on the $\dot{V}o_2$ and extent of the operation. In elderly patients undergoing abdominal surgery, cutoff values for $\dot{V}o_2max$ of 11 mL/kg/min have been shown to accurately identify patients with significantly higher mortality rates.[45]

In a large, randomized, controlled trial of lung volume reduction surgery (LVRS) in severe emphysema, low exercise tolerance was a key marker of patients likely to benefit from the surgery (i.e., less than 25 watts for females and 40 watts for males).[28] On the other hand, very low exercise tolerance (as reflected in 6-minute walk distances of less than 200 m) predicted high postoperative mortality from LVRS.[36,37]

Resting pulmonary function measurements clearly do not adequately predict functional status in disability assessments. One standard commonly used to determine disability is to compare Vo_2 measurements in the laboratory to published energy requirements for different jobs.[46] The average energy requirement on the job should not exceed 40% to 50% of an individual's maximal work capacity.

CPET or timed walk tests before pulmonary rehabilitation are recommended to define safety and determine exercise prescription.[47,48] These exercise assessments permit supervised observation of cases of potential ischemia, arrhythmia, hypotension, and hemoglobin oxygen desaturation. Although optimum exercise intensity is not well defined in respiratory patients, individuals who do not reach the lactate threshold are known to be able to train at a higher percentage of maximal exercise tolerance than those who reach the lactate threshold.[49] Although some argue that beneficial effects

TABLE 12-2
Risk Stratification Based on Type of Procedure and Maximum Oxygen Consumption

	$\dot{V}o_2max$ (mL/kg/min)			
Procedure	**<10**	**10 to 15**	**15 to 20**	**>20**
Pneumonectomy	High risk	High risk	Moderate risk	Low risk
Lobectomy	High risk	Moderate risk	Low risk	Low risk
VATS/wedge	Moderate risk	Low risk	Low risk	Low risk

High risk: avoid surgery; moderate risk: consider alternatives; low risk: proceed with surgery. Vo_2max, maximum oxygen consumption; VATS/wedge, video-assisted thoracic surgery/wedge resection.

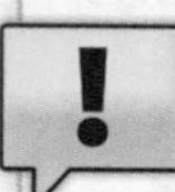

Respiratory Recap

Indications for CPET

- Unexplained or disproportionate dyspnea
- Assessment of the impact of an intervention
- Determination of prognosis
- Disability assessment
- Determination of a pulmonary rehabilitation prescription

of pulmonary rehabilitation can be gained with lower-intensity work, evidence suggests that higher-work-intensity training results in greater reductions in lactic acidosis and ventilation requirements.[49]

Assessment for exercise-induced asthma can be performed as an add-on to CPET or as a separate diagnostic maneuver. If performed as an add-on to routine CPET, spirometry measurements are made before and then every 5 minutes for 30 minutes after a maximal exercise maneuver.[23,50] A decrease in FEV_1 of greater than 15% to 20% is considered diagnostic. If the testing is performed as a stand-alone procedure, the work rate is incremented until the subject achieves an exercise heart rate of 80% of the maximum predicted value and continues at this pace for 6 to 10 minutes. Spirometry is again performed.

The European Respiratory Society published an evidence-based report on the use of exercise testing in clinical practice.[9] **Figure 12-2** summarizes the relationship of various specific CPET measurements and outcomes found in the report. **Table 12-3** and **Table 12-4** summarize the society's recommendations and evidence grades for cardiopulmonary exercise testing and timed walk tests, respectively.

Safety Issues

CPET is generally a very safe procedure if patients are carefully screened for unstable medical conditions (especially cardiac, orthopedic, and neuromuscular issues).[51]

	COPD	ILD	PVD	CF	CHF
$\dot{V}O_2$, peak	+	+	+	+	+
Lactate threshold					+
$\dot{V}E$–$\dot{V}CO_2$ slope and $\dot{V}E$–$\dot{V}CO_2$ at lactate threshold		+			++
Arterial desaturation		++	+	+	
6-minute walk test distance	+		+		+

+, sensitive; ++, more sensitive.

COPD, chronic obstructive pulmonary disease; ILD, interstitial lung disease; PVD, pulmonary vascular disorders; CF, cystic fibrosis; CHF, chronic heart failure; $\dot{V}O_2$, peak, peak oxygen uptake; $\dot{V}E$–$\dot{V}CO_2$, ventilatory equivalent for carbon dioxide.

FIGURE 12-2 Exercise indices that have been shown to predict the prognosis of patients with chronic cardiopulmonary diseases.

Reproduced from Palange P, Ward SA, Carlsen KH, et al. Recommendations on the use of exercise testing in clinical practice. *Eur Respir J.* 2007;29:185–209. Reproduced with permission of the European Respiratory Society.

TABLE 12-3
Indications for CPET in Clinical Practice, with Strength of Evidence Supporting the Recommendation

Indication	Recommendation Grade
Detection of exercise-induced bronchoconstriction	A
Detection of exercise-induced arterial oxygen desaturation	B
Functional evaluation of subjects with unexplained dyspnea and/or exercise intolerance and normal resting lung and heart function	D
To recognize specific disease exercise response patterns that may help in the differential diagnosis of ventilatory versus circulatory causes of exercise limitation	C
Functional and prognostic evaluation of patients with COPD	B, C
Functional and prognostic evaluation of patients with ILD	B, B
Functional and prognostic evaluation of patients with CF	C, C
Functional and prognostic evaluation of patients with PPH	B, B
Functional and prognostic evaluation of patients with CHF	B, B
Evaluation of interventions:	
Maximal incremental test	C
High-intensity constant-work-rate endurance tests	B
Prescription of exercise training	B

With the use of this grading system, A is relatively rare and B is usually considered the best achievable grade. COPD, chronic obstructive pulmonary disease; ILD, interstitial lung disease; CF, cystic fibrosis; PPH, primary pulmonary hypertension; CHF, congestive heart failure.

Reproduced from Palange P, Ward SA, Carlsen KH, et al. Recommendations on the use of exercise testing in clinical practice. *Eur Respir J.* 2007;29: 185–209. Reproduced with permission of the European Respiratory Society.

Indeed, in one report of 5060 CPETs in cardiac patients, only 8 serious cardiac events occurred.[51] Similarly, complications from 6MWT are also quite rare with one report documenting only 6 of 741 patients had to stop the test due to symptoms.[24] Appropriate resuscitation equipment and personnel trained in its use are critical to have immediately available, however. After a maximal exercise maneuver, the patient must continue to pedal with unloaded or low resistance on the bicycle to maintain venous return. This action is especially important for patients with primary or secondary pulmonary hypertension who have a poorly compliant right ventricle and are particularly prone to postexercise hypotension and syncope. **Box 12-2** lists criteria for exercise termination.

TABLE 12-4
Indications for Six-Minute Walk Test in Clinical Practice, with Strength of Evidence Supporting the Recommendation (A through C)

Indication	Recommendation Grade
Diagnosis of exercise-induced arterial desaturation	B
Functional evaluation of patients with COPD, ILD, PPH, and CHF	B
Prognostic evaluation of patients with CF	B
Functional evaluation of patients with CF	C
Prognostic evaluation of patients with COPD or CHF prior to surgery (LVRS, transplantation)	C
Evaluation of the benefits of therapeutic interventions (oxygen supplementation, rehabilitation, surgery)	B

With the use of this grading system, A is relatively rare and B is usually considered the best achievable grade. COPD, chronic obstructive pulmonary disease; ILD, interstitial lung disease; PPH, primary pulmonary hypertension; CHF, congestive heart failure; CF, cystic fibrosis; LVRS, lung volume reduction surgery.

Reproduced from Palange P, Ward SA, Carlsen KH, et al. Recommendations on the use of exercise testing in clinical practice. *Eur Respir J.* 2007;29:185–209. Reproduced with permission of the European Respiratory Society.

BOX 12-2

Criteria for Exercise Test Termination

- Chest pain suggestive of angina
- Evolving mental confusion or lack of coordination
- Evolving lightheadedness
- ECG evidence of ischemia or serious arrhythmia or conduction system abnormality (evolving complex ventricular ectopy, sustained SVT, new LBBB, second- or third-degree heart block)
- Blood pressure: systolic > 250 mm Hg; diastolic > 120 mm Hg
- Fall in systolic blood pressure > 20 mm Hg
- Chronotropic insufficiency in absence of β-blockers
- Spo_2 < 80%
- Inability to sustain cadence on bicycle above 40 rpm
- Subject's request to stop despite encouragement because of symptoms of dyspnea, leg or global fatigue, or otherwise

ECG, electrocardiogram; SVT, supraventricular tachycardia; LBBB, left bundle branch block; Spo_2, oxygen saturation measured by pulse oximetry.

Key Points

- ▶ The normal physiologic response to exercise includes increases in cardiac output and ventilation along with alterations in peripheral circulation, hemoglobin oxygen affinity, and cellular metabolism.
- ▶ CPET stresses the cardiopulmonary system and allows better assessment of the limits of this system.
- ▶ Important indications for exercise testing include diagnosis of unexplained dyspnea, determination of prognosis and risk, and evaluation of responses that follow interventions such as pulmonary rehabilitation.
- ▶ A global interpretive strategy involves definition of the physiologic systems responsible for exercise limitation and subsequent determination of the abnormal responses within these systems.
- ▶ Timed walk tests focus primarily on functional performance.

References

1. Arena R, Kathy E, Sietsema K. Cardiopulmonary exercise testing in the clinical evaluation of patients with heart and lung disease. *Circulation.* 2011;123:668–680.
2. Roca J, Whipp BJ, Agusti AGN, et al. Clinical exercise testing with reference to lung diseases; indications, standardization and interpretation strategies. *Eur Respir J.* 1997;10:2662–2689.
3. Gajulapalli RD, Aneja A, Rovner A. Cardiac stress testing for the diagnosis and management of coronary artery disease. *South Med J.* 2012;105:93–100.
4. Wasserman K, Hansen J, Sue D, et al. *Principles of Exercise Testing and Interpretation.* Philadelphia: Lea & Febiger; 1994.

5. Passmore R, Durnin JY. Human energy expenditure. *Physiol Rev.* 1955;35:801–840.
6. Jones N, Killian, KJ. Mechanisms of disease; exercise limitation in health and disease. *N Engl J Med.* 2000;343:632–641.
7. Martinez F, Stanopoulos I, Acero R, et al. Graded, comprehensive, cardiopulmonary exercise testing in the evaluation of dyspnea unexplained by routine evaluation. *Chest.* 1994;105:168–174.
8. Johnson B, Saupe K, Dempsey J. Mechanical constraints on exercise hyperpnea in endurance athletes. *J Appl Physiol.* 1992;73: 874–886.
9. Palange P, Ward SA, Carlsen KH, et al. Recommendations on the use of exercise testing in clinical practice. *E Respir J.* 2007;29: 185–209.
10. Guazzi M, Adams V, Conraads V, et al. Clinical recommendations for cardiopulmonary exercise testing data assessment in specific patient populations. *Circulation.* 2012;126:2261–2274.
11. Balady G, Arena R, Sietsema K, et al. Clinician's guide to cardiopulmonary exercise testing in adults: a scientific statement from the American Heart Association. *Circulation.* 2010;122:191–225.
12. Kearon MC, Summers E, Jones NL, et al. Effort and dyspnea during work of varying intensity and duration. *Eur Respir J.* 1991;4: 917–925.
13. Hansen J, Sue D, Wasserman K. Predicted values for clinical exercise testing. *Am Rev Respir Dis.* 1984;129(Suppl):S49–S55.
14. Jones NL. *Clinical Exercise Testing.* 4th ed. Philadelphia: W.B. Saunders; 1997.
15. Benzo RP, Paramesh S, Patel SA, et al. Optimal protocol selection for cardiopulmonary exercise testing in severe COPD. *Chest.* 2007;132:1500–1505.
16. Babb T, Viggiano R, Hurley B, et al. Effect of mild-to-moderate airflow limitation on exercise capacity. *J Appl Physiol.* 1991;70: 223–230.
17. O'Donnell DE, Webb KA. Exertional breathlessness in patients with chronic airflow limitation; the role of lung hyperinflation. *Am Rev Respir Dis.* 1993;148:1351–1357.
18. Johnson BD, Badr MS, Dempsey JA. Impact of the aging pulmonary system on the response to exercise. *Clin Chest Med.* 1994;15: 229–246.
19. Maron B, Cockrill B, Waxman A, Systom DM. The invasive cardiopulmonary exercise test. *Circulation.* 2013;127:1157–1164.
20. Huang YC, Helms MJ, MacIntyre NR. Normal values for single exhalation diffusing capacity and pulmonary capillary blood flow in sitting, supine positions and during mild exercise. *Chest.* 1994;105:501–508.
21. Weisman I, Zeballos R. An integrated approach to the interpretation of cardiopulmonary exercise testing. *Clin Chest Med.* 1994;15:421–445.
22. Wasserman K. Diagnosing cardiovascular and lung pathophysiology from exercise gas exchange. *Chest.* 1997;112:1091–1101.
23. American Thoracic Society. Guidelines for methacholine and exercise challenge testing—1999. *Am J Respir Crit Care Med.* 2000;161:309–329.
24. Holland A. for the ATS-ERS Evidence Based Task Force. Field walking tests: a systematic review and evidence based guidelines. *Eur Resp J.* 2014 Chapr; in press.
25. Guyatt GW, Sullivan MJ, Thompson PJ, et al. The 6 minute walk: a new measure of exercise capacity in patients with chronic heart failure. *CMAJ.* 1985;132:919–923.
26. Sciurba F, Criner G, Lee SM, et al. Six minute walk distance in COPD. *Am J Respir Crit Care Med.* 2003;167:1522–1527.
27. Solway S, Brooks D, Lacasse Y, Thomas S. A qualitative systematic overview of the measurement properties of functional walk tests used in the cardiorespiratory domain. *Chest.* 2001;119: 256–270.
28. National Emphysema Treatment Trial Research Group. A randomized trial comparing lung-volume-reduction surgery with medical therapy for severe emphysema. *N Engl J Med.* 2003;348:2059–2073.
29. Enright PL, Sherrill DL. Reference equations for the 6 minute walk in healthy adults. *Am J Respir Crit Care Med.* 1998;158: 1384–1387.
30. Martinez FJ, Han MK, Adin-Cristian A, et al. Longitudinal change in the BODE index predicts mortality in severe emphysema. *Am J Respir Crit Care Med.* 2008;178:491–499.
31. Mezzani A, Hamm L, Jones A, et al. Aerobic exercise intensity assessment and prescription in cardiac rehabilitation. *J Cardiopulm Rehab Prevent.* 2012;32:327–350.
32. Zainuldin R, Mackey M, Alison J. Prescription of walking exercise intensity from the incremental shuttle walk test in people with chronic obstructive pulmonary disease. *Am J Phys Med Rehabil.* 2012;91:592–600.
33. Watters L, Schwarz M, Cherniack R, et al. Idiopathic pulmonary fibrosis: pretreatment bronchoalveolar lavage cellular constituents and their relationships with lung histopathology and clinical response to therapy. *Am Rev Respir Dis.* 1987;135:696–704.
34. Kawut SM, O'Shea MK, Bartels MN, et al. Exercise testing determines survival in patients with diffuse parenchymal lung disease evaluated for lung transplantation. *Respir Med.* 2005;99:1431–1439.
35. Oudiz RJ. The role of exercise testing in the management of pulmonary arterial hypertension. *Semin Respir Crit Care Med.* 2005;26:379–384.
36. Sciurba FC. Early and long-term functional outcomes following lung volume reduction surgery. *Clin Chest Med.* 1997;18: 259–276.
37. Szekely S, Oldberg DA, Wright C, et al. Preoperative predictors of operative morbidity and mortality in COPD patients undergoing bilateral LVRS. *Chest.* 1997;111:550–558.
38. Nixon P, Orenstein D, Kelsey S, et al. The prognostic value of exercise testing in patients with cystic fibrosis. *N Engl J Med.* 1992;327:1785–1788.
39. Hiraga T, Maekuar R, Okuda Y, et al. Prognostic predictors for survival in patients with COPD using cardiopulmonary exercise testing. *Clin Physiol Funct Imaging.* 2003;23:324–331.
40. Mancini D, Eisen H, Kussmaul W, et al. Value of peak exercise oxygen consumption for optimal timing of cardiac transplantation in ambulatory patients with heart failure. *Circulation.* 1991;83: 778–786.
41. Lorio A, Magrì D, Paolillo S, et al. Rationale for cardiopulmonary exercise test in the assessment of surgical risk. *J Cardiovasc Med.* 2013;14:254–261.
42. Benzo R, Kelley GA, Recchi L. Complications of lung resection and exercise capacity: a meta analysis. *Respir Med.* 2007;101: 1790–1797.
43. Morice RC, Peters EJ, Ryan MB, et al. Exercise testing in the evaluation of patients at high risk for complications from lung resection. *Chest.* 1992;101:356–361.
44. Bolliger C, Jordan P, Soler M, et al. Exercise capacity as a predictor of postoperative complication in lung resection candidates. *Am J Respir Crit Care Med.* 1995;151:1472–1480.
45. Older P, Smith R, Courtney P, et al. Preoperative evaluation of cardiac failure and ischemia in elderly patients by cardiopulmonary exercise testing. *Chest.* 1993;104:663–664.
46. Cotes J, Zejda J, King B. Lung function impairment as a guide to exercise limitation in work-related lung disorders. *Am Rev Respir Dis.* 1988;137:1089–1093.
47. Ries AL, Bauldoff GS, Carlin BW, et al. Pulmonary rehabilitation: joint ACCP/AACVPR evidence-based clinical practice guidelines. *Chest.* 2007;131(Suppl 5):4S–42S.
48. Punzal PA, Ries AL, Kaplan RM, et al. Maximum intensity exercise training in patients with chronic obstructive pulmonary disease. *Chest.* 1991;100:618–623.
49. Casaburi R, Patessio A, Ioli F, et al. Reductions in exercise lactic acidosis and ventilation as a result of exercise training in patients with obstructive lung disease. *Am Rev Respir Dis.* 1991;143: 9–18.
50. Cypcar D, Lemanske RF. Asthma and exercise. *Clin Chest Med.* 1994;15:351–368.
51. Skalski J, Allison T, Miller T. The safety of cardiopulmonary exercise testing in a population with high-risk cardiovascular diseases. *Circulation.* 2012;126:2465–2472.

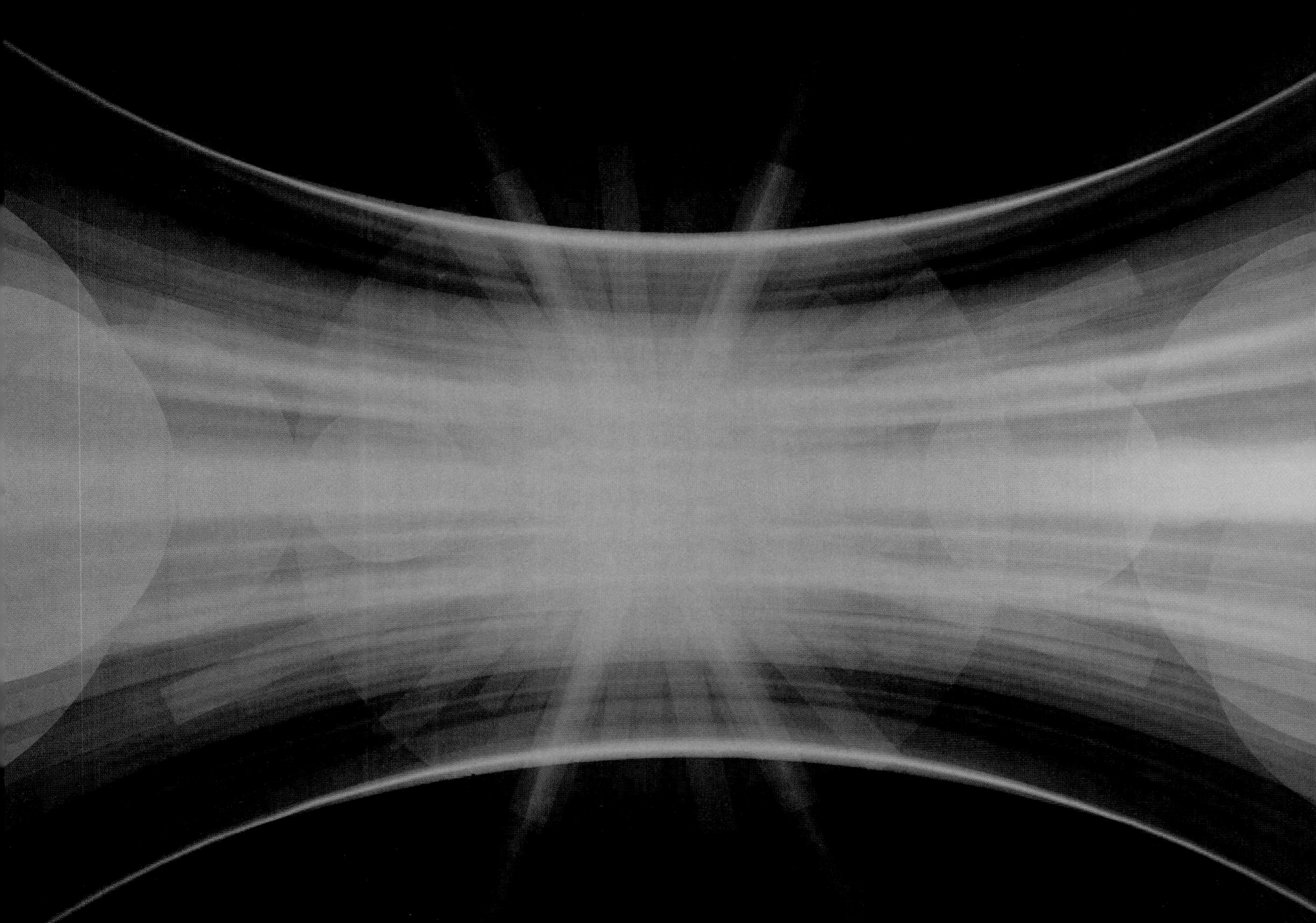

Section II
Respiratory Therapeutics

CHAPTER

13

Therapeutic Gases: Manufacture, Storage, and Delivery

John Boatright, Jeffrey J. Ward

OUTLINE

OBJECTIVES

1. Describe the manufacture, storage, distribution, and regulation (to working outlet pressure/flows) of medical therapeutic gases.
2. Describe the physical properties, chemical symbols, and uses of air, oxygen, carbon dioxide, helium, nitric oxide, and nitrogen.
3. Describe the processes for production of various medical gases.
4. Compare and contrast gaseous and liquid storage methods.
5. Describe the production, safety features, types, and uses of medical gas cylinders.
6. Discuss the established safety systems for the various equipment connections to ensure delivery of a specific gas, such as oxygen.
7. Calculate the duration of flow from a gas cylinder.
8. Describe the design, use, and troubleshooting of various bulk gas supply systems.

KEY TERMS

American Standard Safety System (ASSS)
carbogen
carbon dioxide
Compressed Gas Association (CGA)
Department of Transportation (DOT)
Diameter Index Safety System (DISS)
Food and Drug Administration (FDA)
fractional distillation of liquefied air
heliox
helium
hydrostatic testing
medical gas cylinders
nitric oxide
nitrogen
Pin Index Safety System (PISS)

Introduction

Many therapeutic and diagnostic procedures routinely used in respiratory therapy or by multidisciplinary teams involve one or more medical gases.[1] Consequently, the respiratory therapist frequently serves as the resource for expertise in gas properties, handling, and equipment use. This would also include how to troubleshoot equipment malfunction to ensure the safe delivery of medical gases as needed by patients. This chapter provides descriptions of the physical and chemical characteristics of commonly used therapeutic gases, followed by information about their manufacture, storage, and distribution and the regulation of these gases typically used in acute care hospitals.

Chemical and Physical Properties of Therapeutic Gases

Table 13-1 summarizes the physical properties of the therapeutic gases discussed in this chapter, as well as of nitrogen, which is provided for comparison. The following sections describe these various properties in more detail.

Flammability

All medical gases can be classified either as nonflammable or as flammable or inflammable (terms that are used interchangeably). Nonflammable gases do not burn; examples include nitrogen, oxygen (O_2), helium, air, and carbon dioxide (CO_2). In fact, some nonflammable gases (such as nitrogen and CO_2) are used to extinguish fire because they displace the O_2 that is necessary for combustion to occur. In contrast, a flammable or inflammable gas is one that can ignite, burn, and potentially explode. Cyclopropane and natural gas, not currently used for medical purposes, are examples of flammable gases. O_2, although not explosive or combustible, must be present for combustion to occur, and thus O_2 and air support combustion, meaning that their presence aids and accelerates combustion.

Life Support

O_2 and air are life supportive because the presence of appropriate quantities of these gases supports the metabolic production of energy in the carbon-based organisms found on Earth. Gases that do not support life do not contain substances that are essential for the production of energy but are also included in this discussion because they have physiologic effects and therapeutic potential for humans.

Atmospheric Concentration (by Volume)

Atmospheric concentrations are given in percentage values (%), which represent the relative quantities of gas, as they are present in the earth's atmosphere. Most clinical discussions of gas quantities use this unit of measure.

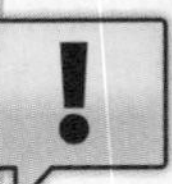

Respiratory Recap

Gas Flammability

- Nonflammable gases do not burn, but some support combustion.
- The terms *flammable* and *inflammable* are used interchangeably.
- Inflammable gases burn and are rarely used for medical purposes.
- O_2 is a nonflammable gas; it does not burn and will not explode.
- O_2 supports combustion, making burning brighter, hotter, and faster.

Atmospheric Pressure

The total pressure of gas in Earth's atmosphere is an expression of absolute quantity rather than a relative value, as in concentration amounts. Atmospheric total pressure, or barometric pressure (P_B), is a convenient expression of gas quantity; in other words, it is an expression about how many molecules of gas are present in the atmosphere.

Standard temperature and pressure of dry gas (STPD) is a designation that the physical conditions for a gas are a temperature of 0° C, at a pressure of 760 mm Hg, without any humidity (dry gas). The term *dry* describes a condition that would rarely be experienced on Earth—that is, an atmospheric condition without any humidity—because even the most dry, cold Earth environments have some amount of water molecules in the ambient gas atmosphere. Water as humidity is not a gas but a vapor; they are not the same but coexist. Water vapor does exert a pressure effect (P_{H2O}) as part of the total barometric pressure.

Ambient temperature and pressure dry (ATPD) means that the physical conditions for a given gas are at ambient temperature and the P_B of the moment without any humidity (dry gas). *Ambient* refers to the actual atmospheric temperature and pressure conditions experienced around an observer, such as in your classroom or hospital. In situations where no specific ATPD is specified, the default total is assumed to be the ambient pressure at sea level (760 mm Hg).

The atmospheric partial pressure column in Table 13-1 represents the partial pressure of each gas in mm Hg under ATPS (ambient temperature and pressure saturated) conditions with the total atmospheric pressure of 760 mm Hg. In contrast to gas concentrations, respiratory therapists use the partial pressure of gases because it is a more precise clinical expression of the absolute amount of a constituent gas present in an environment (e.g., P_{IO_2}).

Viscosity

The viscosity, density, and specific gravity of gases have relevance under special clinical or environmental conditions, such as treatment of patients with extreme airflow obstruction or under highly hyperbaric conditions. In fluid mechanics, which apply to the behavior of liquids and gases, viscosity is best described as the thickness of a substance. Viscosity affects the resistance or friction of a substance to flow. The viscosity of water is thin, whereas the viscosity of oil or honey is thick. The SI unit used for viscosity in Table 13-1 is pascal-second (Pa-s).

Density

Density is a measure of how close the molecules of a substance are to each other. It is most easily defined

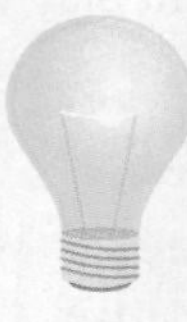

STOP AND THINK

A patient is receiving O_2 via a nasal cannula. Can you explain why the 100% O_2 delivered by the nasal cannula tends to cling to the patient's face, torso, and clothing?

as the mass per unit of volume, and the formula used to determine it is Mass/Volume (m/V). With regard to gases, mass is the molecular weight (grams), and the standard molar volume at ATPD is 22.4 L. The unit of measure for density in Table 13-1 is kilograms per cubic meter (kg/m^3).

Relative Density

The relative density (specific gravity) of a liquid is a relative measurement that compares the density of a fluid with the density of water (at 4° C, 760 mm Hg). For the relative density of a gas, the density of a gas at 4° C and 760 mm Hg is compared with the density of air. A relative density of 1 indicates that the density of the gas is identical to the density of air (for a gas).

Boiling Point

The boiling point of a substance is the temperature at which it changes from a liquid to a gas (at 760 mm Hg). The change of state between a liquid and a gas is known as evaporation or vaporization. The freezing point is the temperature where a substance changes state from a liquid to a solid, and the process of a change of state from a solid directly to a gas is called sublimation. Dry ice, the solid form of CO_2, sublimates directly from a solid to a gas.

Critical Temperature

Critical temperature (T_C) is the temperature at which a substance no longer can be characterized as either a liquid or a gas, nor can it be forced into a liquid state by applying pressure, although with enough pressure it can be changed into a solid. Gases can be more easily converted to liquids at certain temperatures, because as a gas's temperature increases, it becomes more difficult to change it from a gas to a liquid. For example, the T_C of O_2 is –118.6° C. Above this temperature, O_2 cannot become a liquid no matter how much pressure is applied.

TABLE 13-1
Physical Properties of Commonly Used Therapeutic Gases

Gas	Symbol	Molecular Weight	Atmospheric Concentration (% by volume)	Atmospheric Partial Pressure (mm Hg)	Viscosity (× 10^{-6} Pa-s)	Density (kg/m^3)	Relative Density	Boiling Point (°C)
Air	Air	28.975	—	—	182.7	1.2	—	–194.3
Nitrogen	N_2	28.013	78.084	593.44	—	1.153	0.967	–195.9
Oxygen	O_2	31.99	20.946	158	201.8	1.326	1.105	–182.9
Carbon dioxide	CO_2	44.01	0.0335	0.25	148.0	1.833	1.522	–29.0
Helium	He	4.003	0.00052	—	194.1	0.166	0.138	–268.9
Nitric oxide	NO	30.006	0	—	—	1.245	1.040	–151.8

Critical Pressure

The critical pressure (P_C) is the pressure (1 = one Earth atmosphere) required at a critical temperature to change a gas to a liquid. For example, O_2 will become a liquid if 49.7 atmospheres of pressure are applied to −118.6° C gas. It should be noted that H_2O is considered an anomalous substance because water's critical temperature and pressure do not correspond to the typical change of state model. In a solid state, water is a crystalline form (ice), which is in fact less dense than the liquid form of water (which is why ice floats in a glass of water).

Triple Point

The triple point of a substance is the pressure and temperature at which the substance can exist in the three phases of matter in equilibrium. That is, the substance can exist in a liquid, gas, or solid, especially with a small shift in pressure or temperature in any direction. When the temperature is −219° C and the pressure is 0.22 psia (pounds per square inch, absolute), O_2 can exist as a liquid, gas, or solid. Note that at this very cold temperature, the pressure condition is nearly a total vacuum (0 psia).

Solubility in Water

Solubility is the physical property of a substance to dissolve in a solvent—in this case, water. Water solubility is relevant to the respiratory therapist in understanding gas transport physiology. For example, the solubility of O_2 is much less than the solubility of CO_2, which affects differences in the rate of solution and dissolution in plasma, and the migration of the two gases through the alveolar capillary membrane and the cell wall.

Physical State in Cylinder

The physical state of some gases, as contained in a cylinder, may be as a liquid (e.g., CO_2) or as a gas (e.g., O_2). This occurs because some gases assume a liquid state at the pressures required to store them in a cylinder. For example, the degree of compression that is required to store CO_2 in a cylinder causes it to change states from a gas to a liquid. When the cylinder valve is opened and the pressure in the cylinder drops a little (below critical pressure), the liquid at the surface evaporates and returns to the gaseous state. When the liquid in the cylinder has completely evaporated, the cylinder pressure will begin to drop and will reach zero when the cylinder is empty. Because the pressure drop

TABLE 13-1 (*Continued*)
Physical Properties of Commonly Used Therapeutic Gases

Critical Temperature (° C)	Critical Pressure (psia)	Triple Point	Solubility in H_2O	Color	Odor	Taste	Life Support	Flammability	Physical State in Cylinder
−140.7	547	—	0.292	Colorless	Odorless	Tasteless	Supports life	Nonflammable/ supports combustion	Gas
−146.9	493	−210° C @ 1.81 psia	0.023	Colorless	Odorless	Tasteless	Does not support life	Nonflammable	Liquid or gas
−18.6	731.4	−218.8° C @ 60.4 psia	0.049	Colorless	Odorless	Tasteless	Supports life	Nonflammable/ supports combustion	Gas
31.1	1076.6	−56.6° C @ 60.4 psia	0.900	Colorless	Odorless/ pungent	Tasteless/ slightly acidic	Does not support life	Nonflammable	Liquid and gas
−297.9	33	—	0.009	Colorless	Odorless	Tasteless	Does not support life	Nonflammable	Gas
−92.9	949.4	—	0.073	Colorless	Slightly metallic	Tasteless	Does not support life	Nonflammable	Gas

All values are at ATPD (21.1° C, 760 mm Hg, and dry) unless otherwise noted.

Adapted from Langenderfer R, Branson R. Compressed gases: manufacture, storage, and piping systems. In: Branson R, Hess D, Chatburn R, eds. *Respiratory Care Equipment.*
2nd ed. Philadelphia: Lippincott Williams & Wilkins; 1999.

in a CO_2 cylinder begins very near the point at which the cylinder is empty, cylinder weight is monitored to determine the remaining amount of liquid CO_2.

Air

At normal atmospheric conditions, air is an odorless, colorless, transparent, tasteless mixture of gases and water vapor that is nonflammable and supports combustion. Air is composed of about 78% nitrogen and 21% O_2 by volume. The remaining 1% consists of extremely small amounts of chemically inert trace and rare gases, such as argon, neon, helium, krypton, and xenon (**Figure 13-1**). The largest component of air is nitrogen, which is not directly involved in metabolic reactions and is thus considered inert. Nonetheless, nitrogen gas is important in maintaining the inflation of gas-filled body cavities such as alveoli, sinus cavities, and the middle ear.

Compressed air may also be referred to in medical settings as *room air* or *ambient air*. **Table 13-2** shows the relative quantities of the various gases that compose our atmosphere (in both volume percent and fraction).[2] The composition of the major components in dry air is relatively constant. For clinical purposes, gas quantities are commonly referred to as percentages (of concentrations by volume). Fraction of inhaled gas (FI*x*) is commonly required in certain physiologic calculations.

TABLE 13-2
Composition of Room Air

Gas	Concentration by Volume (%)	Fraction
Nitrogen	78.083	0.78083
Oxygen	20.946	0.20946
Argon	0.934	0.00934
Carbon dioxide	0.033	0.00033
Neon	0.001818	—
Helium	0.000524	—
Methane	0.00016	—
Krypton	0.000114	—
Hydrogen	0.00005	—
Nitrous oxide	0.00003	—

Therapeutic Uses

Compressed air has two primary uses in respiratory therapy: (1) to dilute 100% O_2 to provide 22% to 99% mixtures, and (2) as a driving gas for breathing devices when used on patients who do not require O_2 supplementation.

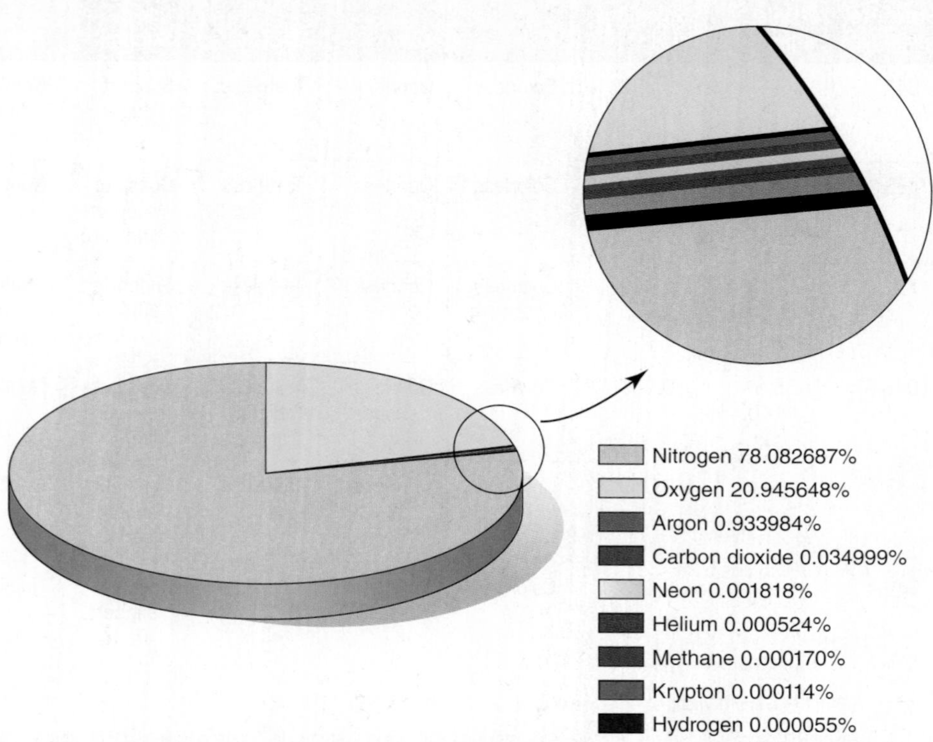

FIGURE 13-1 Constituents of the atmosphere. Values represent percent concentration in the earth's atmosphere.
Information from *Encyclopedia of Earth*. Atmospheric composition. Available at http://www.eoearth.org/article/atmospheric_composition.

Manufacture

Compressed air can be manufactured by a precise mixing of nitrogen and O_2. More commonly, however, atmospheric air is filtered, compressed, and stored in cylinders or directly delivered through a central piping system. The **Compressed Gas Association (CGA)** specifies grades of gaseous air. Medical-grade compressed air (CGA grade J) contains 19.5% to 23.5% O_2, no water vapor, and minimal amounts of hydrocarbons and other impurities. Aside from its medical applications, compressed air is the breathing gas that is supplied in many self-contained breathing devices used in industry, scuba diving, aerospace technology and firefighting.

Cylinders

Compressed air is supplied in cylinders that are color-coded yellow. Compressed air cylinders are similar in composition and size to O_2 cylinders. Regulators (for both compressed air and O_2 cylinders) reduce the high cylinder pressure (greater than 200 lb/in^2 gauge [psig]) to working pressure (50 psig), the pressure needed to adequately operate clinical equipment such as flow meters and other respiratory therapy equipment. The size and shape of the regulator cylinder connections are specifically designed to prevent the inadvertent application of an O_2 regulator. The design for these connections is designated the **American Standard Safety System (ASSS)** and has been established by agreement among the various manufacturers of gas cylinders. Further reductions of working pressure for more refined control of flow or pressure are standardized specifically for compressed air via the Diameter Index Safety System (DISS) of connections or brand-specific quick-connects.

Piped Air Systems

Piped compressed air is commonly provided in hospital medical gas systems for use in areas such as the operating room and intensive care units. Many mechanical ventilators and O_2–air blenders require separate sources of both medical air and O_2. Large compressors provide the supply of compressed air for these piped distribution systems. Various designs of these large compressors are available, but the piston type is most common. A pressure-sensitive switch senses changes in the line pressure and turns the compressor on and off to maintain line pressures of 50 psig. Normally a holding reservoir is added to the system to provide a ready supply and prevent the compressor from running all the time. In large institutions, it is common to have two compressors that alternate operation, prolonging compressor life.

Portable Compressors

Smaller, portable air compressors are available for hospital or home use. Because the air source of these systems is the hospital's ambient air, high humidity and dust may foul the mechanism of these compressors and contaminate the delivered air. It is therefore important that portable compressed air systems incorporate condensers and filters to remove water and dust. Water trap drains must also be maintained to prevent wet air from fouling flow meters and ventilators. Inline desiccant dryers or filters may also be needed, especially during humid months.

Oxygen

Physical Characteristics

The specific individual who should be credited with the scientific discovery of O_2 has been a matter of dispute. For many years, English theologian-scientist and politician Joseph Priestley was credited with first publishing findings on "dephlogisticated air" in 1774. Yet Swedish apothecary Carl Scheele, who co-published Priestley's findings, appears to have been the first to have chemically generated what he termed "fire air." Neither scientist, however, developed a clear, complete comprehension of O_2; that distinction belongs to France's Antoine Lavoisier, who named the gas *oxygen*, meaning "acid generator."

The atomic weight of oxygen (O) is 16 g/mole, and its gram molecular weight (O_2) is 32 g/mole. There is some difference in the proportion of atomic and molecular O_2 with changes in altitude. At about 20 km, photodissociation produces atomic oxygen, which is accompanied by an increase in ozone (O_3); these reach their maximum concentrations at 30 km (0.003%) and 90 km

Respiratory Recap

Properties of Oxygen

- O_2 is a colorless, transparent, odorless, tasteless, nonflammable gas, only slightly heavier than air at STP.
- Only 10.2 mL of O_2 dissolves in 1 L of water at STP.
- Gaseous O_2 can be liquefied when its temperature is lowered to −297.3° F (−182.9° C).
- Liquid O_2 has a pale-blue color and is 1.1 times heavier than water.
- O_2 stays in the liquid state as long as its temperature remains below the boiling point.
- O_2 forms when two oxygen atoms combine by sharing two electrons in their outer orbital shell.
- F_{IO_2} in air is 0.2095 and remains constant with changes in altitude up to 60 miles (96.5 km) above sea level.
- P_{O_2} varies depending on the P_B.

(7%), respectively. Radiation strips off an electron from atomic oxygen, producing the ionized species O^+ and O^{++}. The ionic forms are quite reactive, however, occurring only at high altitudes, and oxygen most commonly exists in molecular form.

The element oxygen exists in molecular form in the atmosphere and, in combination with other elements, is present in a large number of compounds. Molecular O_2 is formed when two oxygen atoms combine by sharing two electrons in their outer orbital shell. This unique molecular bonding characteristic gives O_2 a paramagnetic property—that of being attracted to a magnet—that can be used to determine O_2 concentration in a gas mixture.

At standard temperature and pressure (STP), O_2 is a colorless, transparent, odorless, tasteless gas, only slightly heavier than air, with a density of 1.326 kg/m^3 and a specific gravity of 1.051 at STPD. O_2 is not very soluble in water. At STP, 10.2 mL of O_2 dissolves in 1 L of fresh water (7.8 mL in 1 L of seawater), which nonetheless is enough to sustain all aquatic life.

About half of Earth's crust by weight is oxygen, and gaseous O_2 makes up 20.95%, or 0.2095, by volume of the atmosphere. Although the F_{IO_2} does not normally change, the partial pressure of O_2 inspiratory gas (P_{IO_2}) will vary considerably. The fraction of O_2 in air normally remains constant at 0.2095 to an altitude of 60 miles (96.5 km) above sea level. The P_{IO_2}, however, varies with changes in barometric pressure (P_B), which decreases at higher or lower altitudes compared with sea level. At 1 atmosphere (P_B = 760 mm Hg), the P_{IO_2} is 159 mm Hg. The P_{IO_2} for any P_B can be calculated with the following formula:

$$P_{IO_2} = P_B \times F_{IO_2}$$

where P_{IO_2} is the partial pressure of O_2 in inspiratory gas, P_B is the barometric pressure, and F_{IO_2} is the fraction of O_2 in the inspiratory gas.

The above equation is a demonstration of an application of Dalton's law, which quantifies the O_2 portion of the total atmospheric gas pressure, that is, its partial pressure (P_{IO_2}). For example, on Mount Everest the P_B is about 220 mm Hg, whereas the P_{IO_2} is only 47 mm Hg, which is the sea level equivalent of 6% O_2 (F_{IO_2} is 0.062 under normobaric conditions). These changes in P_{IO_2} account for the need for some mountain climbers to use supplemental O_2 and for pressurizing aircraft during high-altitude flights. This also relates to and explains in part why scuba divers need to stage their return to the surface in order to normalize their bodies to the normobaric P_B. **Table 13-3** illustrates several examples of the effect of altitude on P_{IO_2}.

Below sea level, 1 atm (760 mm Hg) is added for each 33 ft (10 m) of seawater. (*Note*: Freshwater has a slightly lower density than saltwater and, therefore, the pressure increases 1 atm in each 34 feet of depth.) Because the density of water is so much greater than that of atmospheric air, the pressure increases experienced by a diver are dramatically more rapid than the pressure decreases experienced by the climber at altitude. For a diver 66 feet below sea level (or for a patient in a hyperbaric chamber at 3 atm), the total gas pressure thus is 2280 mm Hg, the P_{IO_2} is 478 mm Hg, and the equivalent sea level F_{IO_2} is 0.63 (**Table 13-4**).

TABLE 13-3
Effects of Altitude on Barometric Pressure and Partial Pressure of Inspired Oxygen

Altitude (Feet)	Atmospheres (atm)	P_B (mm Hg)	P_{IO_2} (mm Hg)
Sea level	1.0	760	159
5,000	0.83	630	132
10,000	0.69	523	109
20,000	0.46	349	73
30,000	0.30	226	47

P_B, barometric pressure; P_{IO_2}, partial pressure of inspired oxygen.

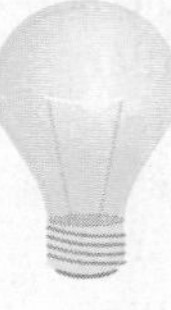

STOP AND THINK

A patient in a hyperbaric chamber is exposed to 3 atm and provided 100% O_2 by tight-fitting mask. What is the P_{O_2} in the patient's trachea?

Support of Combustion

O_2 is a nonflammable gas; that is, it is not capable of being ignited. O_2 vigorously accelerates and supports combustion. The higher the partial pressure of O_2,

TABLE 13-4
Effects of Depth on Barometric Pressure and Partial Pressure of Inspiratory Oxygen

Depth (Feet of Seawater)	Atmospheres (atm)	P_B (mm Hg)	P_{IO_2} (mm Hg)
Sea level (0)	1	760	159
33	2	1520	318
66	3	2280	478
99	4	3040	637
132	5	3800	796

the hotter, faster, and brighter is the burning. Burning (combustion) commonly occurs in air at 21% O_2. A burning match exposed to a 42% O_2 atmosphere (which contains twice the quantity of O_2 as room air) will burn twice as hot, bright, and fast as with 21% O_2. In concentrations greater than 21%, therefore, O_2 not only supports combustion but also accelerates the burning process. In the presence of high concentrations of O_2, certain combustible items, especially petroleum-based products (e.g., oil, grease, petroleum jelly, clothing), can easily and violently ignite with great force from a spark, friction, pressure, or impact.

Manufacture and Distribution

Photosynthesis

All green land and aquatic plants produce O_2 through photosynthesis—a process in which chlorophyll-containing plant cells in the presence of sunlight convert CO_2 and water into glucose and release O_2 as a by-product into the atmosphere, produce O_2 naturally. This process of biologic photosynthesis is the main source and regulator of O_2 levels in the atmosphere. Chlorophyll is the chemical agent necessary for this transformation. A normal human must consume 2 to 5 lb of O_2 a day (4.5 to 11.2 kg) to convert carbohydrates, fats, and proteins into heat, energy, and CO_2. As a result of photosynthesis by green land and aquatic plants, the CO_2 produced by animals and the burning of fossil fuels is converted to O_2. The formula for photosynthesis is as follows:

$$6\,CO_2 + 6\,H_2O + \text{Sunlight} + \text{Chlorophyll} \rightarrow C_6H_{12}O_6 + 6\,O_2$$

Isolating Metallic Oxides

The laboratory or commercial manufacture of O_2 can be accomplished using one of the four following methods: (1) heating and isolating metallic oxides, (2) electrolysis, (3) fractional distillation of liquefied air, and (4) filtration by membrane or molecular sieve. Scheele and Priestley, the scientists who first discovered and described O_2, generated O_2 by heating metallic oxides of mercury, silver, or barium. This method is not commonly used to mass manufacture O_2.

Electrolysis of Water

An electric current passed through water causes the water to separate into its component parts—hydrogen and O_2—with hydrogen bubbling off at the cathode in a 2:1 ratio to the O_2 at the anode. This process, the electrolysis of water, is impractical for the commercial production of O_2.

Fractional Distillation of Liquefied Air

The two major components of air—O_2 and nitrogen—can be produced in bulk, commercial quantities by a process first described in 1907 by Karl von Linde. This process, the **fractional distillation of liquefied air**, relies on the Joule-Kelvin principle, which states that when gases under pressure are released into a vacuum, the gas molecules tend to lose their kinetic energy. In a vacuum, the reduction in kinetic energy causes a decrease in temperature and a reduction in the cohesive forces between the molecules, leading to liquefaction.

Air liquefaction plants are large, complex industrial sites that somewhat resemble a small oil refinery. The actual fractional distillation process consists of multiple stages and steps (**Figure 13-2**). The process begins with atmospheric air being drawn through filters and scrubbers to remove airborne contaminants, and then it is compressed and cooled in several stages to 2000 psig and –50° F. Along the way, water vapor in the air freezes and is removed. The air then is cooled further to –265° F at a pressure of 200 psig, and then allowed to expand to 90 psig in a separator, where partial liquefaction takes place. The liquefied air from the separator is pumped to the top of the fractional distillation column. As it flows down the column, the nitrogen boils off and can be captured and stored in a gaseous or liquid state. O_2 collects at the bottom of the column in liquid form. This liquid O_2 still contains a number of trace gas contaminants, primarily argon and krypton, and is further distilled to recover the argon. Distillation continues with careful control of temperature and pressure until the remaining liquid exceeds 99.0% O_2, the standard of purity required by the United States Pharmacopoeia/National Formulary (USP/NF) for medical-grade O_2.

Molecular Filtration

Another method used to produce O_2 is molecular filtration.[3] This process is used widely in respiratory home

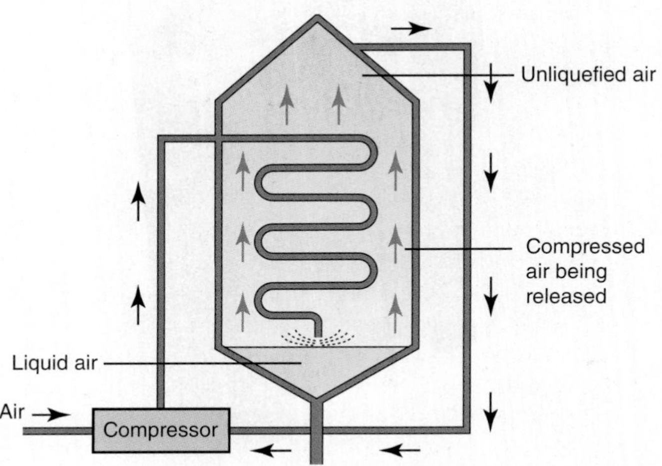

FIGURE 13-2 The process of fractional distillation. Because the boiling points of N_2 and O_2 are different, the two gases can be separated on the basis of the temperature of the distillation chamber.

care with O_2 concentrator devices. *Molecular filtration* is a generic term that refers to the filtering out of gas molecules other than O_2 through various methods. A common method for O_2 production by molecular filtration is the molecular sieve or pressure swing absorbent method (**Figure 13-3**). In this method, a vacuum draws room air into cylinders packed with crystallized zeolite, a silicate with ion exchange properties. The air is compressed (to 100 to 300 psig), and environmental nitrogen is filtered out, that is, temporarily absorbed by the zeolite. Switching to a depressurization phase, which causes the crystals to release the nitrogen as gas, reverses the process.

The final concentration of O_2, as well as the flow setting exiting the sieve, varies among manufacturers. Most concentrators deliver O_2 in the 1 to 5 L/min range at between 0.95 and 0.98 but fall to 0.92 to 0.95 when run at higher flows. This decrease in O_2 concentration is caused by the increasing concentration of argon gas.

An alternative type of commercial device for O_2 production is the membrane O_2 concentrator. Membrane O_2 concentrators use a set of plastic polymer membranes through which room air is filtered. A pump provides the pressure gradient across the membrane cells, and O_2 and water vapor, which are more permeable than nitrogen, move through the membranes to be collected. These concentrators are less commercially popular because they produce only 30% to 40% O_2 and are not currently being manufactured.

All O_2 concentrators require routine mechanical maintenance and should be periodically checked (with an O_2 analyzer and calibrated flow-measuring device) to verify proper flow setting and O_2 concentration.

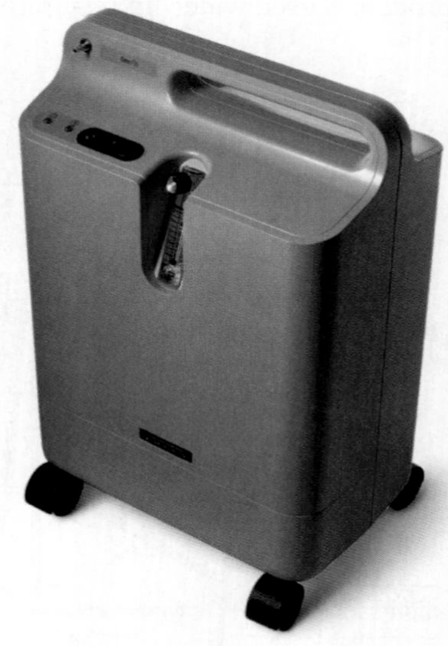

FIGURE 13-3 Molecular sieve. Oxygen concentrators concentrate oxygen from ambient air by filtering out nitrogen.

Used with permission of Philips Respironics.

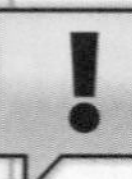

Respiratory Recap

Ways to Produce Oxygen

- Photosynthesis
- Electrolysis of water
- Fractional distillation of air
- Molecular filtration

Distribution

The normal physical state of O_2 is as a gas. As a gas, O_2 can be stored in cylinders and may easily be distributed by flexible and rigid piping systems. Because liquid O_2 can be stored in much larger volumes more efficiently, most hospitals and many patients have liquid O_2 (LOX) storage systems designed to contain O_2 in the liquid state. These systems are designed to maintain the storage tanks at the pressure and temperature required to maintain O_2 in the liquid state: 716 psig and –118° C. The process of returning the liquid O_2 to gaseous O_2 (which is more easily distributed and therapeutically usable) involves heating the liquid O_2 and subsequent evaporation. To accomplish this heat gain, large liquid O_2 storage and distribution systems use evaporator coils in which external ambient heat is absorbed to raise the temperature of the liquid O_2 above its boiling point (which is still very cold). The heat absorption from the atmosphere needed to accomplish the evaporation of liquid O_2 and its conversion to a gas results in ice formation on the evaporative coils of the storage system.

Carbon Dioxide

Physical Characteristics

Carbon dioxide (CO_2) is a colorless, transparent, odorless to pungent, and tasteless or slightly acid-tasting gas with a specific gravity of 1.522, making it heavier than air. It is nonflammable and does not support combustion or animal life. Carbonic acid (H_2CO_3), which forms when CO_2 dissolves in water, is corrosive to metals. Under normal atmospheric conditions, the atmospheric concentration of CO_2 gas is very low, 0.03% (F_{CO_2} of 0.0003). CO_2 in an unrefined form is released by the combustion of wood, coal, coke, natural gas, or oil and by lime kilns, the fermentation process, volcanoes, and natural springs. Animals exhale CO_2 as a by-product of metabolism:

$$O_2 + \text{Glucose} \rightarrow \text{ATP} + H_2O + CO_2$$

Humans exhale 5% CO_2 ($F_{E CO_2}$ 0.05), which, along with exhaled H_2O, constitutes the vast majority of the hydrocarbon by-product resulting from energy production by the mitochondria. Adenosine triphosphate (ATP) is the energy molecule produced by the mitochondria.

Because CO_2 is a by-product of animal metabolism and the burning of carbonaceous fuels, the atmospheric concentration of CO_2 is increasing. The increase of atmospheric CO_2 (along with increases in methane gas concentrations) has resulted in an abnormal retention of planetary heat (the greenhouse effect) and is implicated in global warming.

Therapeutic Uses

Pure, or 100%, CO_2 is not used therapeutically. Small amounts of CO_2 gas have been added to breathing gas for control-ventilated patients to increase $Paco_2$ and correct respiratory alkalosis. This application has served as an alternative to the addition of mechanical dead space to ventilator breathing circuits. Because CO_2 does not support life, CO_2 must be mixed with O_2 to create **carbogen** if it is to be administered via inhalation. The usual available carbogen mixtures are 90% O_2 to 10% CO_2 or 95% O_2 to 5% CO_2. There are significant differences in the density, specific gravity, and viscosity of CO_2 when compared with O_2 or air (refer to Table 13-2). Accurate metering of gas through tubes and orifices must accommodate this factor.

Carbogen has historically been used to treat hiccups (singultus), atelectasis, retinal revascularization after reattachment, anxiety-related hyperventilation, and cerebrovascular conditions. In fact, breathing elevated CO_2 by inspiring and expiring into a paper bag is still a common treatment for anxiety-related hyperventilation. The theorized mechanism of action in this treatment is that increasing the CO_2 concentration of inspiratory gas through rebreathing the patient's own exhaled CO_2 will correct the hypocarbia (low $Paco_2$) that accompanies hyperventilation. Although this technique can no doubt be an effective distraction from the events that induced the patient's anxiety-related hyperventilation, whether the suggested mechanism of action is at all related to increasing the CO_2 in breathing gas—that is, whether the inspiratory CO_2 level is in fact increased by the technique—requires further study. When carbogen is used therapeutically, it is used for short treatment intervals of about 10 minutes, during which the patient must be carefully monitored.

The current Occupational Safety and Health Act (OSHA) standard for the maximal allowable concentration is 0.5% for 8 hours of continuous exposure, or 3% CO_2 over a 10-minute period. Today, CO_2 mixtures are used primarily in medicine for the calibration of capnographs, blood gas analyzers, and other laboratory and diagnostic equipment. CO_2 is also used to insufflate the abdomen during laproscopic surgery. CO_2 is used because it is absorbed and removed by the respiratory system. It is also nonflammable, which is important because electrosurgical devices are commonly used in laparoscopic procedures.

Nonmedical uses of CO_2 include carbonated beverage bottling, food preservation, refrigeration, and fire extinguishing. Solid CO_2 (dry ice) exists at temperatures below its triple point of 69° F (21° C) and at a pressure above 60 psig. At temperatures below its triple point, dry ice will sublimate into a gas without passing through a liquid phase. CO_2 also has a low thermal conductivity, which allows dry ice to remain relatively stable.

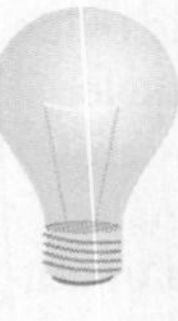

STOP AND THINK

A fire occurs in a small kitchen where a patient's family was using a hot plate to warm food. A CO_2 fire extinguisher was available. What characteristics of that gas would promote its use?

Manufacture and Distribution

The manufacture of CO_2 for medical purposes involves refining atmospheric CO_2. This refinement process removes carbon monoxide, hydrogen sulfide, nitric acid, water, and other pollutants and impurities. For medical purposes, the purity of CO_2 gas must be at least 99.5%. Three forms of CO_2 are available: cylinders at ambient temperatures, liquid at subambient temperatures, and solid CO_2 (dry ice). Cylinders of CO_2 commonly contain both liquid and gas if the temperature is below 31° C with pressures above 60 psig. This possibility requires that cylinders be weighed to determine the quantity of liquid CO_2 in the cylinder. This phenomenon does not occur with medical mixtures of 95%-to-5% and 90%-to-10% O_2–CO_2. **Figure 13-4** illustrates a cylinder containing both liquid and gas CO_2.

Helium

Physical Characteristics

Helium (He) is a rare gas naturally occurring in the atmosphere in extremely small amounts (0.000524% by volume). It is colorless, transparent, odorless, tasteless, and nonflammable; it does not support combustion or life. Helium is the second-lightest element (hydrogen being lighter), with an extremely low density (0.165 kg/m^3) and specific gravity (0.138), slightly more than one-eighth that of air. It is a rare gas in the sense that it is not generally present in the atmosphere (less than 5 parts per million [ppm]) and is chemically and physiologically nonreactive (inert).

Therapeutic Uses

Because helium is an inert, non-life-supporting gas, it must be mixed with at least 20% O_2. Helium and O_2 mixtures are often referred to as **heliox**. In higher concentrations helium (>50%), it is used medically for its low-density and ability to reduce turbulence within natural or artificial airways for palliative treatment

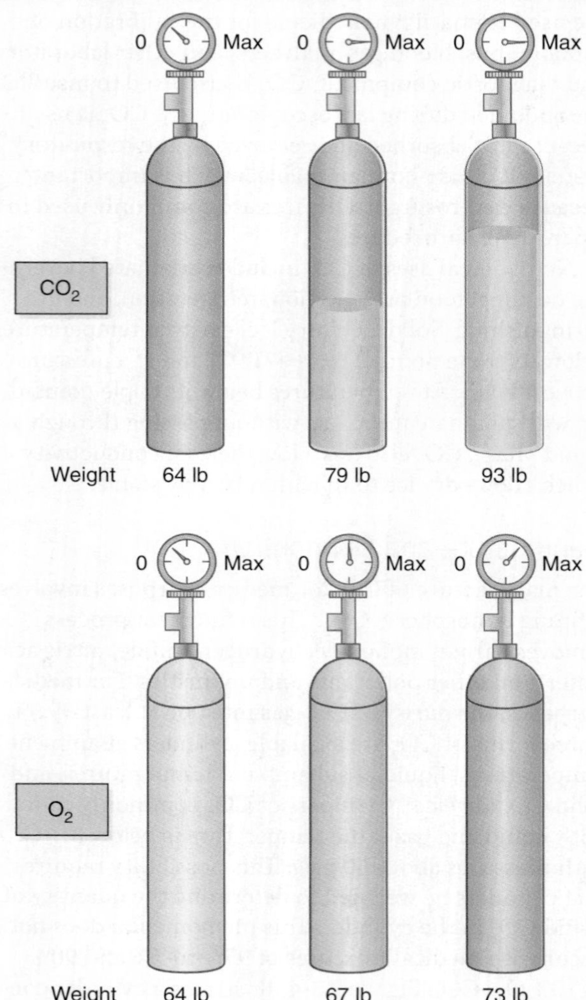

FIGURE 13-4 A cylinder containing liquid and gas carbon dioxide (top) compared to a cylinder containing oxygen (bottom). In gases that assume the liquid state under typical cylinder pressure conditions, gas quantity and flow duration evaluation will require accounting for the amount of liquefied gas that remains in the cylinder.

Modified from Dorsch JA, Dorsch SE. *Understanding Anesthesia Equipment*. 3rd ed. Lippincott Williams & Wilkins; 1994. Reprinted with permission.

of large airway obstructions (such as encountered in asthma, chronic obstructive pulmonary disease, croup, and bronchiolar cancer), because it decreases the work of breathing. Clinical applications may be via mask or via mechanical ventilation.

Heliox is also used in place of normal compressed nitrogen and O_2 mixtures (N_2/O_2) for extreme hyperbaric conditions, such as in commercial and scientific deep-water operations. The use of heliox rather than N_2/O_2 decreases the risk of nitrogen narcosis and the low density of heliox lowers the work of breathing. Low concentrations (<5%) of helium are also used in pulmonary function laboratories as a test gas in lung volume and diffusing testing. Commercially, helium is also used as a nuclear reactor coolant, in cryogenic research, as a shield in arc welding, in silicon and germanium crystal-growing atmospheres, in lighter-than-air aircraft, and for breathing mixtures in deep-water diving.

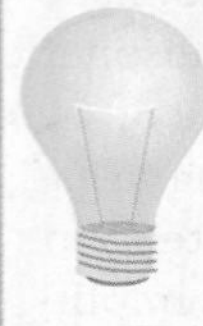

STOP AND THINK

In deep-water diving conditions such as are encountered in commercial, scientific, or military applications, heliox is used as a breathing gas, instead of nitrogen/oxygen mixtures. Why is this done?

Manufacture and Distribution

Helium is not manufactured. On Earth, natural gas containing up to 2% helium is found in the southern United States, Canada, Algeria, and Qatar. The fixed quantity of helium available on Earth has been identified as a future critical shortage. Helium is vital in some medical applications, for example, in MRI equipment it is used to cool the electromagnets.[4] Helium also is produced by fusion reaction from hydrogen in nuclear weapons and in stars. In medical settings, helium gas is supplied in compressed gas cylinders containing 100% helium or various concentrations blended with at least 20% O_2.

Nitric Oxide

Physical Characteristics

Nitric oxide (NO) is a colorless, tasteless gas with a slight metallic odor. This nonflammable and non-life-supporting gas supports combustion, is toxic, and is found in the atmosphere in extremely small amounts (10 to 100 parts per billion) as an air pollutant byproduct of combustion. Nitric oxide, also known as nitrogen monoxide, is an unstable free radical that was originally regarded as an environmental pollutant (e.g., in smog and cigarette smoke) and an impurity of nitrous oxide manufacture. The NO molecule is highly diffusible and lipid soluble. The half-life of NO ranges from 3 to 50 seconds because of its conversion to nitrates and nitrites and the high affinity of hemoglobin for NO.

Therapeutic Uses

In 1987 NO was found to normally biosynthesize in vascular endothelial cells. It is an important signaling messenger molecule, a mediator of physiologic functions, including vasodilation, neurotransmission, long-term memory, and immunologic defense. Nitric oxide plays an important role in vascular smooth muscle relaxation, inhibition of platelet aggregation, neurotransmission, and immune regulation. Abnormally low NO levels in humans have been implicated in atherosclerosis, hypertension, diabetes, erectile dysfunction, and immune deficiency diseases. Exhaled NO (eNO) is a marker of airway inflammation associated with asthma and is gaining importance as a diagnostic adjunct in asthma care.

The inhalation of nitric oxide (iNO) in low concentrations (5 to 80 ppm) causes selective pulmonary vascular dilation, which has led to the use of nitric oxide to treat persistent pulmonary hypertension of the newborn (PPHN), meconium aspiration, bronchopulmonary dysplasia, refractory hypoxemia, and hypertension-associated congenital heart disease in infants. In conjunction with ventilatory support and other appropriate agents, iNO is indicated for the treatment of term and near-term neonates with hypoxic respiratory failure associated with clinical or echocardiographic evidence of pulmonary hypertension, where it improves oxygenation and reduces the need for extracorporeal membrane oxygenation. This gas has also been used for treatment of acute respiratory distress syndrome in adult patients, primarily as a method to improve oxygenation. At the present time, however, the use of iNO as a therapeutic practice in patients other than term neonates with hypoxic respiratory failure remains controversial. To date there have been no large-scale clinical research trials to determine the safety of long-term use of iNO.

Manufacture and Distribution

Nitric oxide is produced in the reaction of sulfur dioxide with nitric acid and through the oxidation of ammonia at temperatures above 500° C in the presence of platinum as a catalyst. Nitric oxide is also produced as a by-product of the anesthetic gas nitrous oxide (N_2O). Medical NO is supplied in concentrations of 100 to 2200 ppm diluted by nitrogen (N_2) for a purity of 99.0%. The usual concentration is 800 ppm, which is further reduced before delivery to the patient. Nitric oxide is supplied in specially cleaned, high-pressure aluminum cylinders. In a cylinder, NO will remain in stable form and not convert to nitrogen dioxide for approximately 18 months.

Nitrogen

Physical Characteristics

Nitrogen (N_2) is the major component of the atmosphere, 78% by volume. Nitrogen gas is responsible for the blue color of the sky on Earth.

Therapeutic Uses

To inflate the abdomen for some minimally invasive procedures and, because it does not support combustion, 100% N_2 is used to power pneumatic instruments in the operating room. N_2 also is used to provide the zero-point reference in some O_2 analyzers, is used as a diagnostic gas in pulmonary function testing, and is applied in a subatmospheric pressure dressing (SPD) to treat aerobic wound infections such as are sometimes encountered with burns, frostbite, or diabetes. There are also reports of the use of inhaled administration of subatmospheric or subambient O_2 concentrations (created by adding N_2 to gaseous air or O_2) to temporarily increase pulmonary vascular resistance and thus reduce pulmonary blood flow in congenital heart defects such as hypoplastic left heart syndrome.

Manufacture and Distribution

Nitrogen gas is produced in large quantities (along with O_2) during fractional distillation of liquefied air. In medical settings, it is usually supplied as compressed gas in cylinders.

Storage and Distribution of Medical Gases

Since the 1890s, steel cylinders have been used to store compressed O_2 and other gases. They continue to be frequently used in medical care today despite the widespread use of piped gas supply systems. Properly handled, they are quite safe, and small cylinders offer portability for patient transport or ambulation. Medical gases can be stored and transported in the gaseous state or as liquefied gas in various-sized cylinders and cryogenic bulk containers. Available high-pressure **medical gas cylinders** range from small, lightweight units containing a few ft^3 of gas to large cylinders of several hundred ft^3 (**Figure 13-5**).

Medical Gas Cylinders

Federal regulation of the construction of cylinders used to transport compressed gas began in 1948 under the jurisdiction of the U.S. Interstate Commerce Commission (ICC) and in 1968 was transferred to the U.S. **Department of Transportation (DOT)**. In Canada, cylinder standards are set by Transport Canada. DOT regulations specify that high-pressure medical gas cylinders be made with seamless construction from high-quality steel, chromium-molybdenum alloy, or aluminum. Today, numerous federal, state, and local statutes as well as industry standards and guidelines regulate the storage, transport, distribution, and use of medical gases. **Table 13-5** summarizes these government agencies and private organizations and their areas of responsibilities and expertise.

Steel cylinders are produced by one of two methods. One involves the pressing of soft steel into a tubular form and using heat to shape and seal the bottom and form the shoulder and neck at the outlet end. Hot steel also can be spun to form a seamless cylinder. Aluminum cylinders are produced by extrusion with an alloy often containing a blend of magnesium and silicon. Aluminum cylinders are as much as 40% lighter than those constructed of steel. Another type of construction available for cylinders, the composite

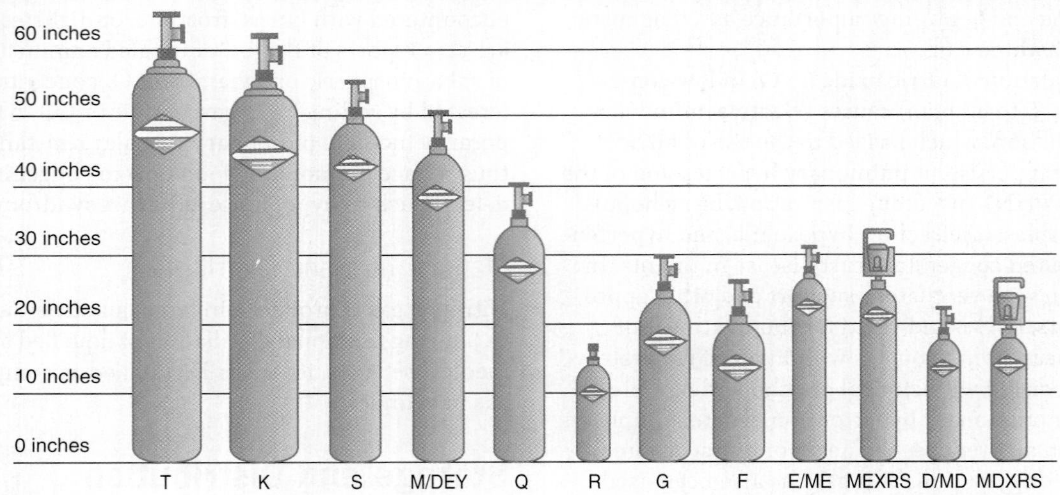

FIGURE 13-5 Cylinder sizes. Cylinders are available in many sizes for a variety of applications (not all sizes are pictured here).

TABLE 13-5
Regulatory and Standards Organizations in the Manufacture, Storage, and Distribution of Medical Gases

ANSI—American National Standards Institute: a private, not-for-profit organization that coordinates U.S. private-sector voluntary standards development
ASME—American Society of Mechanical Engineers: an organization that issues design, mechanical, and structural standards for items such as components of central piping systems
ASTM—American Society for Testing and Materials: a not-for-profit organization that aids in the development and publication of voluntary consensus standards for medical devices and many consumer products
CGA—Compressed Gas Association: a trade organization that has developed numerous safety standards involving cylinders, fittings, and connections
CSA—Canadian Standards Association: an independent Canadian organization that recommends standards for the safety, quality, and performance of equipment
DOT—(U.S.) Department of Transportation: the federal body that regulates cylinder manufacture and testing and the transport of hazardous materials, including compressed gases and cryogenic liquids
EPA—(U.S.) Environmental Protection Agency: the government agency that establishes standards and administers regulations concerning potential and actual environmental hazards
FDA—(U.S.) Food and Drug Administration: an agency of the Department of Health and Human Services (HHS) that enforces regulations and standards concerning the purity of medical gases and their manufacture, packaging, and labeling
HHS—(U.S.) Department of Health and Human Services: the principal government agency dealing with health and social services, with the following subsets: FDA, Centers for Disease Control and Prevention (CDC), National Institutes of Health (NIH), and Centers for Medicare and Medicaid Services (CMS)
ICC—(U.S.) Interstate Commerce Commission: a government bureau that before 1967 set and administered the regulations currently the domain of the DOT
ISO—International Organization for Standardization: a worldwide agency that coordinates and establishes technologic standards in manufacturing and safety
NFPA—(U.S.) National Fire Protection Association: a private independent agency that recommends standards related to fire and safety, which are routinely adopted as regulations by state and local government building and safety codes
NIOSH—(U.S.) National Institute for Occupational Safety and Health: a part of the CDC responsible for conducting research
OSHA—(U.S.) Occupational Safety and Health Administration: an agency of the Department of Labor that establishes and enforces standards of safety in the workplace
TC—Transport Canada: Canadian government agency that administers regulations concerning the manufacture and testing of compressed gas cylinders and their distribution
USP/NF—United States Pharmacopoeia/National Formulary: a not-for-profit private organization founded to develop officially recognized quality standards for drugs, including medical gases
Z-79: a committee of ANSI that establishes standards for oxygen and respiratory and anesthesia equipment and devices

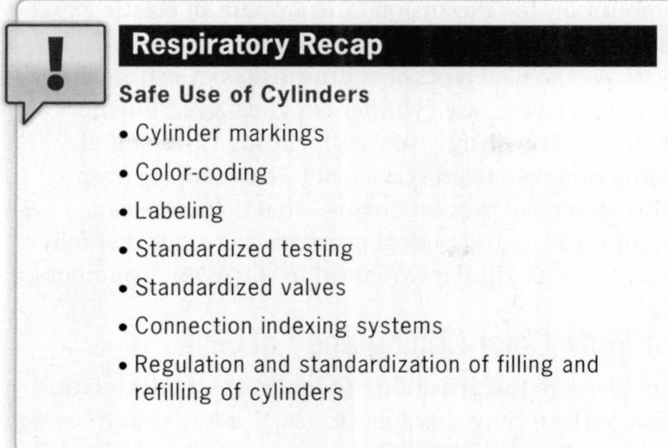

Respiratory Recap

Safe Use of Cylinders

- Cylinder markings
- Color-coding
- Labeling
- Standardized testing
- Standardized valves
- Connection indexing systems
- Regulation and standardization of filling and refilling of cylinders

cylinder, is up to 70% lighter than steel. Composite cylinders are manufactured by overwrapping a thin-walled aluminum cylinder with multiple layers of carbon, fiberglass, or Kevlar fibers in an epoxy resin wrap. Steel and aluminum cylinders have flat bottoms, whereas composite cylinder bottoms are rounded. Composite cylinders are available only in small sizes, up to 22 ft^3 of gas (623 liters), whereas steel and aluminum cylinders are available in a wide range of sizes, as described in **Table 13-6**.

Cylinder Markings

Figure 13-6 shows the typical DOT-required markings found permanently struck into the shoulder of all cylinders. In Canada, the mark TC is used. The DOT specifications to which cylinders are manufactured are DOT 3A, seamless carbon-steel; DOT 3AA, seamless heat-treated, tempered alloy-steel; or DOT 3AL, seamless cylinders made from specified aluminum alloys. The service pressure in psig immediately follows the DOT specification marking and is 2015 for most medical gas cylinders. Cylinders may be filled to 10% more than the service pressure, most being filled to 2200 psig. Also

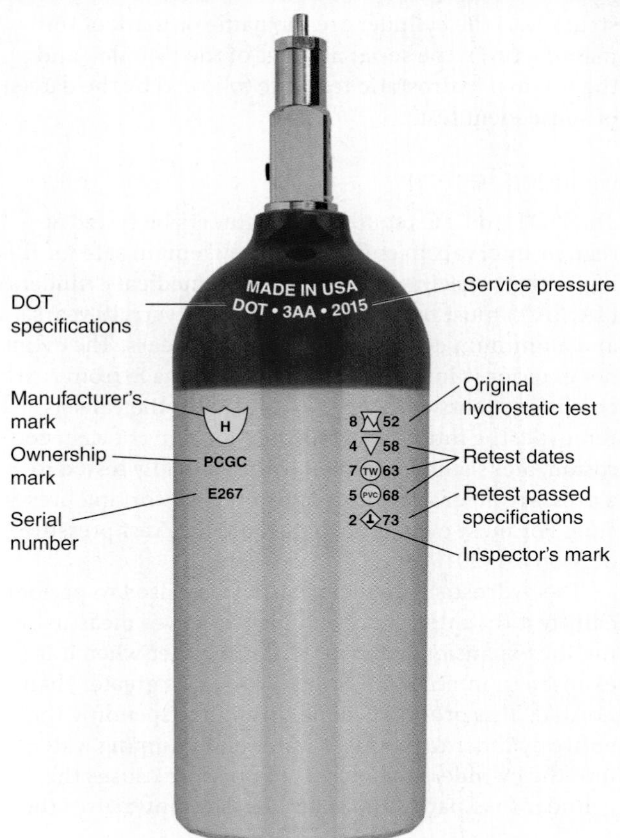

FIGURE 13-6 Typical cylinder markings.

TABLE 13-6
Physical Characteristics of Common-Sized Aluminum and Steel Cylinders

	Aluminum						Steel					
	B or M6	ML6	C or M9	D	E	N or M60	M or MM	D	E	M	H or K	T
Service pressure (psig)	2216	2015	2015	2015	2015	2216	2216	2015	2015	2015	2265	2400
Height without valve (inches)	11.6	7.7	10.9	16.5	25.6	23	35.75	16.75	25.75	43	51	55
Diameter (inches)	3.2	4.4	4.4	4.4	4.4	7.25	8	4.2	4.2	7	9	9.25
Weight empty (without valve, lb)	2.2	2.9	3.7	5.3	7.9	21.7	38.6	7.9	11.3	58	117	139
Capacity (oxygen, ft^3)	6	6	9	15	24	61.4	122	15	24	110	250	300
Capacity (oxygen, L)	170	170	255	425	680	1738.0	3455	425	680	33,113	7075	8490

struck into the cylinder are the name or mark of the manufacturer, the serial number of the cylinder, and the original hydrostatic test date followed by the date(s) of subsequent tests.

Cylinder Testing

The DOT and TC require that cylinders be tested at regular intervals to ensure that they remain safe for filling to their specified pressures. Steel medical cylinders (3A, 3AA) must be tested at least once every 10 years, and aluminum cylinders (3AL) every 5 years. The cylinder exterior is inspected for signs of damage from rust, corrosion, dents, or deep scarring. After the valve is removed, the interior is inspected for signs of rust, corrosion, and scaling and then hydrostatically tested to a pressure at least five-thirds its normal working pressure. For most cylinders, that would be a test pressure of 3358 psi (2015 × 5⁄3).

The hydrostatic challenge procedure used to periodically test the integrity of cylinders involves measuring the expansion behavior of the cylinder when it is exposed to internal pressures two-thirds greater than normal. This process is done through suspending the entire cylinder in a tank of water and pumping water into the cylinder. The increased pressure causes the cylinder to expand. The water displaced measures the amount of this expansion. The amount of elastic expansion is directly related to the thickness of the cylinder wall. As the wall thickness diminishes over time due to normal wear, the cylinder expands more during **hydrostatic testing**, eventually failing the test and being removed from service before becoming unsafe. This challenge process ensures that cylinders can accommodate the typical pressure increases that may occur when cylinders are used in warm environments.

Cylinder Color-Coding and Labeling

To decrease the possibility of inadvertent administration of the wrong therapeutic gas, a safety system using color-coding, labels, and connection devices is used. A standard color-coding system for medical gas cylinders was suggested by the CGA and adopted by the U.S. Department of Commerce on the recommendation of the Bureau of Standards. **Table 13-7** shows this system and a slightly different color-coding scheme used internationally. In addition to the color code, each medical gas cylinder must feature a label meeting the specifications of the U.S. **Food and Drug Administration (FDA)** that indicates the gas contained, that the gas meets U.S. Pharmacopeia (USP) specifications, relevant warnings and dangers, and that a prescription is necessary for dispensing.

TABLE 13-7
Color Codes and Purity of Medical Gases

Gas	Chemical		Color Code	
	Symbol	Purity* (%)	U.S.	International
Oxygen	O_2	99.0	Green	White
Air	—	99.0	Yellow	Black and white
Nitrogen	N_2	99.0	Black	Black
Nitrogen/oxygen†	N_2/O_2	99.0	Black and green	Pink
Carbon dioxide	CO_2	99.0	Gray	Gray
Carbon dioxide/oxygen (carbogen)†	CO_2/O_2	99.0	Gray and green	Gray and white
Helium	He	99.0	Brown	Brown
Helium/oxygen (heliox)†	He/O_2	99.0	Brown and green	Brown and white
Nitrous oxide	N_2O	97.0	Blue	Blue
Nitric oxide/nitrogen†	NO/N_2	99.0	Teal and black	Teal and black
Cyclopropane‡	C_2H_6	99.0	Orange	Orange
Ethylene‡	C_2H_4	99.0	Red	Red

* U.S. Pharmacopoeia/National Formulary standards.

† Labels should always be checked for the percentage of each gas.

‡ Flammable anesthetic gas (rarely used).

Cylinder Valves

Many of the safety systems involved in gas storage systems involve the manufacturer's use of the cylinder valve. Most high-pressure medical gas cylinders use a direct-acting valve, shown in **Figure 13-7**, in which turning the handle moves the stem up or down, thereby raising or lowering the seat and allowing gas to flow from the cylinder or stopping the gas flow. Small cylinders (sizes A through E) use a four-sided rectangular post valve, whereas larger cylinders feature a faucet-like valve with a threaded outlet.

Because the pressure in a closed cylinder is directly related to the temperature (Gay-Lussac's law), all cylinder valves have pressure-relief safety devices that allow for the controlled release of excessive pressure from the cylinder if it is exposed to high temperatures, thus preventing an explosive rupture. If a cylinder is exposed to fire or heat that raises its internal pressure to 1.5 times its normal filled pressure, a safety valve opens and vents the gas. This response prevents the cylinder wall from exploding. Some valves use a frangible (breakable) disk or fusible (meltable) metal plug or a combination. Wood's metal, an alloy of bismuth, lead, cadmium, and tin, is commonly used for the fusible plug material and will yield when the temperature reaches 208° F (97.8° C) to 220° F (104° C). Copper is used as a frangible disk material. **Figure 13-8** illustrates examples of cylinder valve pressure-relief safety devices.

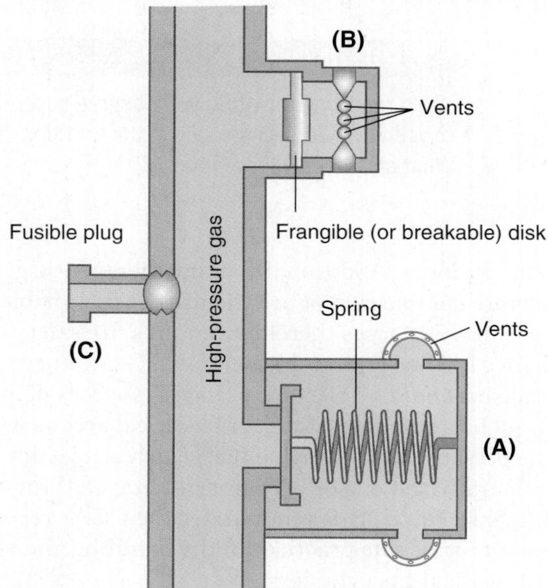

FIGURE 13-8 Cylinder pressure-relief systems. (**A**) Spring-loaded device. When gas pressure exceeds the spring tension, the spring is compressed to the top, allowing gas to escape through the vents. When gas pressure is reduced to normal, the spring tension recluses the valve. (**B**) Frangible disk. When gas pressure exceeds safe limits, the disk ruptures, allowing all of the contents of the cylinder to escape into the atmosphere through the vents. (**C**) Fusible plug. If the temperature inside or outside the cylinder exceeds safe limits, the plug melts, allowing all of the gas in the cylinder to safely escape.

Adapted from Branson RD, Hess DR, Chatburn RL. *Respiratory Care Equipment*. 2nd ed. Lippincott Williams & Wilkins; 1999.

Safe Storage and Handling of Cylinders

Most medical gas cylinders of any size are filled to the same high pressure—2200 to 2500 psig. This pressure involves a formidable force of more than a ton pushing against every square inch of the inside of the cylinder. Because cylinders are shaped awkwardly and steel cylinders are quite heavy, they may fall or be dropped. Therefore, respiratory therapists should practice pressure awareness and lifting precautions whenever handling gas cylinders. Cylinder rupture may result in metal shrapnel or a spinning or rapidly

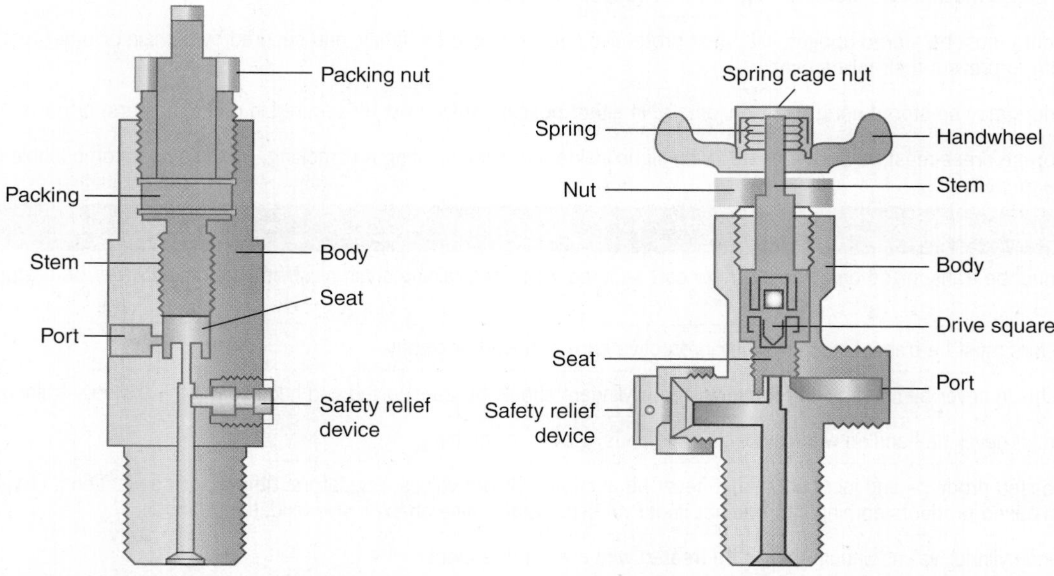

FIGURE 13-7 Direct-acting cylinder valve. When closed, the stem and seat are screwed together by the handwheel. To open the valve, the stem is screwed away from the seat using the handwheel.

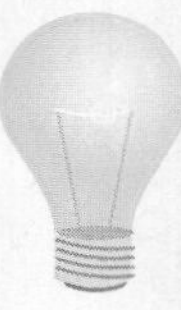

STOP AND THINK

While reporting for work, you observe several oxygen cylinders lying loose in the corridor. What should be your response?

moving cylinder. Additionally, many therapeutic gases accelerate combustion or are themselves flammable; the use of these gases therefore requires fire safety vigilance by the respiratory therapist. Respiratory therapists should be alert for potential sources of ignition, such as smoking, static, or electrical arcs as well as the presence of flammable fuels (such as plastics, petroleum-based oils or jelly, or synthetic clothing and bed linens). **Table 13-8** summarizes the CGA's recommendations for safe practices in the handling and storing of medical gas cylinders.

The Joint Commission has also provided compliance and safety tips for freestanding medical gas cylinders. As much as 300 ft^3 of O_2 can be stored in cylinders in the means of egress (out in the open, the path available for a person to leave a space; e.g., hallways, nursing stations, etc.). This means, for example, that up to 12 E cylinders can be in an alcove in a means of egress without being protected in a cabinet or room. The volume calculation does not include opened or used cylinders, nor does it include cylinders currently in use. The Joint Commission provides two examples of acceptable storage in the means of egress. An operating suite is lined with 15 gurneys, each with an E cylinder attached. A rack of 12 E cylinders sits in an alcove open to the same corridor. This totals 15 cylinders in use, which are not used in volume calculation, and 12 cylinders in storage. Another acceptable example is a clean utility room with two racks holding 12 full E cylinders and a third rack with 12 empty or partially full cylinders. In an alcove outside the room, another storage rack holds 12 E cylinders. This totals 36 E cylinders in the smoke compartment (a space within a building enclosed by smoke barriers on all sides, including the top and bottom), with 12 stored in a means of egress. The Joint Commission regulations also state that full cylinders

TABLE 13-8
Guidelines for Safe Cylinder Storage and Handling

Storage
Cylinder storage must be in compliance with NFPA standards and all local, state, and federal regulations.
Cylinders must be stored in a cool, dry, fire-resistant enclosure that has good ventilation to prevent accumulation of gas if leaks occur.
Cylinder storage areas must be protected from the elements to prevent exposure to rain, snow, ice, and temperatures above 125° F.
Cylinder storage areas must be locked and secured from access and tampering by all unauthorized persons and should not be located near flammable or combustible substances.
Segregated locations for full and empty cylinders within the cylinder storage area must be clearly labeled to prevent their commingling.
Flammable gases must not be stored with gases that support combustion.
Large cylinders must be stored upright, with their protective caps screwed on tightly, and secured by a chain or other restraint mechanism to prevent their falling over.
Small cylinders may be stored upright or horizontally. In either position, they must be secured in racks, holders, or carts.
Cylinder storage areas must be clearly posted with signs inside and out indicating no smoking, open flames, combustible materials, oil or grease, etc.
Transport and Handling
Cylinders must be transported on an appropriate cart secured with a restraining chain or strap. They must never be dragged, rolled, or slid.
Large cylinders must be transported with their protective caps screwed on tightly.
A cylinder should never be lifted by its protective cap. Cylinders should be transported and handled only by properly trained personnel.
Cylinders must never be handled with oily or greasy hands, gloves, or clothing.
Petroleum-based products and lubricants must never be used on cylinder valves, regulators, fittings, or connections. Oxygen and petroleum-based products coming into contact under pressure may cause an explosive oxidation reaction.
Cylinders and cylinder valves should always be treated with care and respect.

in racks must be segregated from those that have been opened or used.

Regulators

Gas-powered respiratory therapy equipment in the United States is designed and calibrated to operate with an inlet gas pressure of 50 psig, which is referred to as the *working pressure.* Central piping systems incorporate pressure-reducing valves that regulate and maintain the pressure at the station (room) outlets at 50 psig. Ventilators, blenders, and flow meters can be connected directly to the station outlets without further need for pressure control.

When cylinders of gas are used, the pressure in a full cylinder may be 2200 to 2500 psig and must be reduced to the standard and safe working pressure of 50 psig through attachment of a high-pressure-reducing valve called a *regulator* to the cylinder outlet.

High-pressure regulators can be direct acting or indirect acting; configured in single or multiple stages; and preset or adjustable. For most respiratory therapy applications, the single-stage regulator is adequate. **Figure 13-9** illustrates the basic components and operating functions of a direct acting, single-stage, preset high-pressure-reducing regulator. Regulators are attached to cylinders with a leak-proof connection using either pin or threaded fittings. The high-pressure source of gas enters at the inlet, usually passing through a fine-sintered brass filter to remove any debris. A pressure gauge is positioned at the inlet to indicate the pressure in the cylinder, which is directly related to the volume of gas in the cylinder. A flexible diaphragm divides the body of the regulator into two chambers: a high-pressure chamber and a chamber open to ambient pressure. A spring is attached to the ambient-pressure side of the diaphragm. A valve stem is attached to the high-pressure side of the diaphragm, and its end is positioned in the high-pressure inlet. In the regulator, the very high pressure from the cylinder is exerted on a very small area of the valve stem, which is balanced by the much larger area of the diaphragm. The tension of the spring exerts a preset pressure on the diaphragm and moves the valve stem to hold the high-pressure inlet open.

When the gas outlet is open, the high-pressure inlet remains open and a balance is maintained between the flow through the outlet and the pressure at the high-pressure inlet. This balance between the force of the spring upward on the diaphragm and the gas pressure above the diaphragm maintains a near-constant outlet pressure, usually preset at 50 psig. When the outlet is closed, pressure increases in the chamber above the diaphragm until it exceeds that of the spring, causing the diaphragm to move downward, pulling the valve stem down and closing the high-pressure inlet. A pressure relief (pop-off) valve is part of the high-pressure chamber. If a malfunction occurs, allowing excessive pressure to develop, this safety valve will open and vent the pressure, preventing a rupture of the diaphragm or regulator body. Modern regulator design has added a second spring, allowing regulators to become more compact because the size of the diaphragm can be reduced.

For applications in which more precise control of pressure and flow are necessary, a multistage regulator is used by connecting two or more single-stage regulators in a series (**Figure 13-10**). The first stage reduces

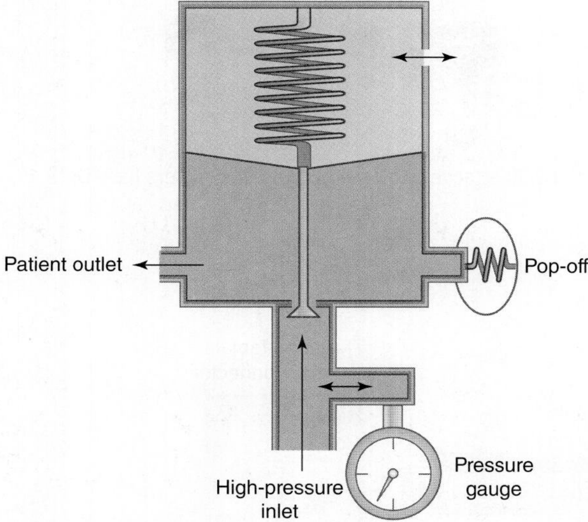

FIGURE 13-9 Single-stage regulator. These regulators are commonly used in clinical settings to regulate gas pressures.

Reproduced from *Egan's Fundamentals of Respiratory Care*, 7th ed. Scanlan CL, Wilkins RL, Stoller JK. Copyright Elsevier (Mosby) 1999.

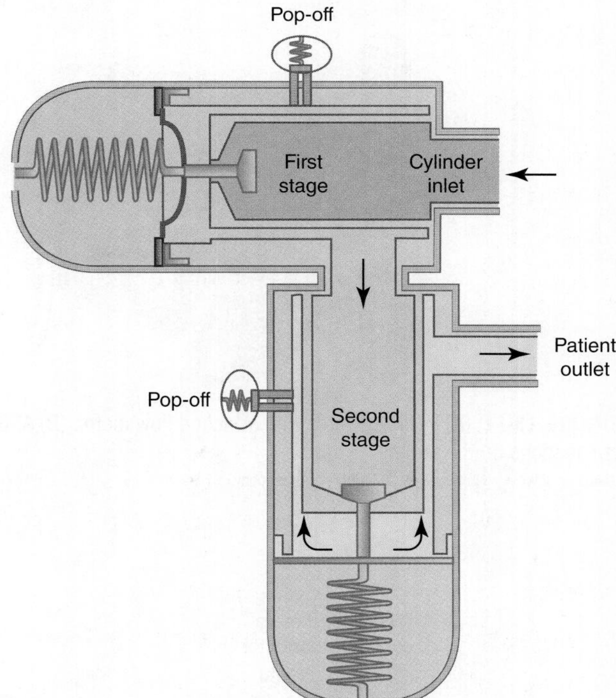

FIGURE 13-10 Multiple-stage regulator. These regulators are more complex than single-stage regulators and thus more expensive. Multiple-stage regulators may be needed for situations in which very consistent gas pressures are necessary.

Modified from Cairo JM, Pilbeam SP. *Mosby's Respiratory Care Equipment*. 6th ed. Mosby; 1999. Reprinted with permission.

the high pressure from the cylinder to a preset intermediate pressure of 500 to 700 psig. The next stage (or stages) further reduces the pressure until the 50-psig outlet pressure is reached. Each stage of a multistage regulator must have a safety pressure-relief valve. The gradual reduction of pressure in two or more stages allows for better pressure control and a smoother flow than can be attained in a single stage. These qualities may be important when precise instrumentation is being used, such as in research and diagnostic applications. Multistage regulators are larger, heavier, and more expensive than the more common single-stage units.

Safety-Indexed Connection Systems

The outlets of cylinder valves are manufactured so that only the regulator or connector specific for that gas or mixture can be attached. Three indexed safety systems are available for medical gases: the American Standard Compressed Gas Cylinder Outlet and Inlet Connections, usually referred to as the American Standard Safety System (ASSS); the Pin Index Safety System (PISS); and the Diameter Index Safety System (DISS). **Figure 13-11** compares these three safety systems.

American Standard Safety System

The threaded outlets of the faucet-like valves found on large cylinders (larger than E) conform to the American Standard Safety System. This system uses a combination of the following factors specific for each gas or gas combination:

- Diameter of the outlet (in thousandths of an inch)
- Number of threads per inch
- Right-handed or left-handed threads
- External or internal threads
- The shape of the mating nipple on the corresponding regulator

The large high-pressure O_2 cylinder (G, H, T or K) has an outlet that meets the specification of 0.903-14-RH-Ext; that is, its outlet diameter is 0.903 inch with 14 threads to the inch, the connections will screw on clockwise, and the threads are external. This configuration is referred to as CGA 540 by the CGA. **Figure 13-12** illustrates selected ASSS valve outlets and connections.

Pin Index Safety System

High-pressure medical gas cylinders, size E and smaller, use another indexing system known as the

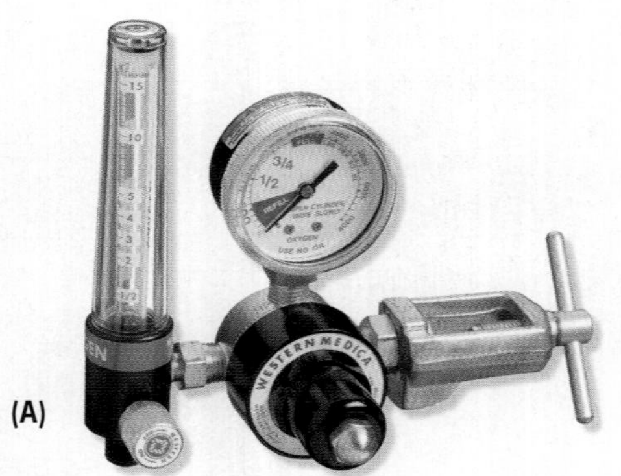

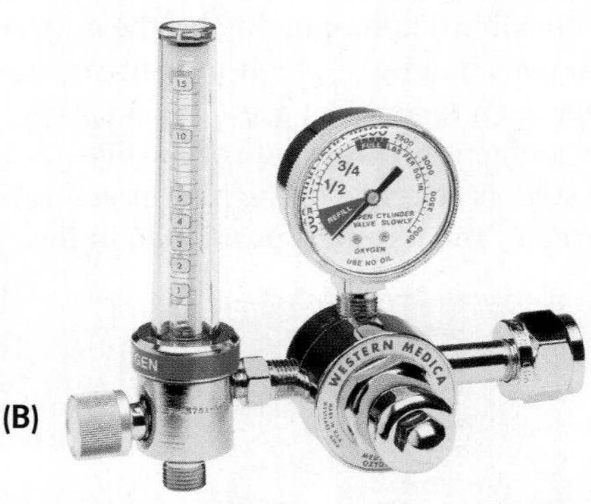

FIGURE 13-11 (**A**) PISS regulator with attached flow meter. (**B**) ASSS regulator with attached flow meter. Both flow meters have DISS connections on the outlets.

Courtesy of Western Enterprises, a Scott Fetzer company.

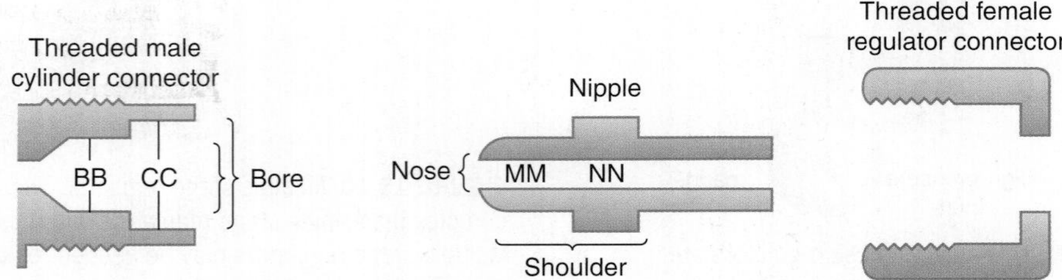

FIGURE 13-12 Cross-sectional diagram of ASSS valve outlet components.

Modified from Dorsch JA, Dorsch SE. *Understanding Anesthesia Equipment*. 3rd ed. Lippincott Williams & Wilkins; 1994.

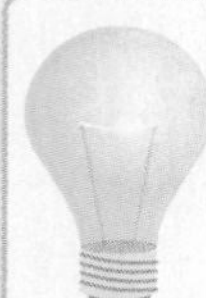

STOP AND THINK

You find an E-cylinder O_2 regulator with both pins removed. What would you do?

Pin Index Safety System (PISS). This system uses a metallic yoke attached to the regulator which surrounds the valve post. The yoke has a specific combination of pins which fit into corresponding holes in the valve post just below the gas outlet. The pin and hole combinations are gas specific to prevent inadvertent connection of regulators to incorrect gases. Any regulator or device intended to connect to the valve has pins that correspond to those holes, allowing for a proper connection. The pin index for O_2 is 2–5, also referred to as CGA 870. **Figure 13-13** shows the connection of a pin-indexed regulator to the post valve. **Figure 13-14** illustrates the pin-indexed positions for some common therapeutic gases.

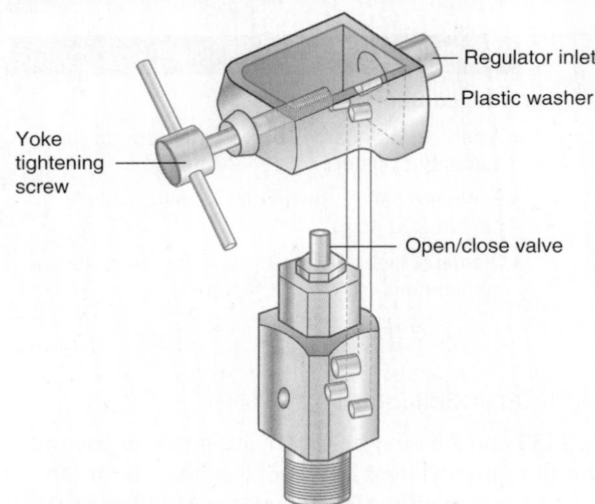

FIGURE 13-13 PISS valve outlet.

Modified from Barnes TA, ed. *Core Textbook of Respiratory Care Practice.* 2nd ed. Mosby; 1994.

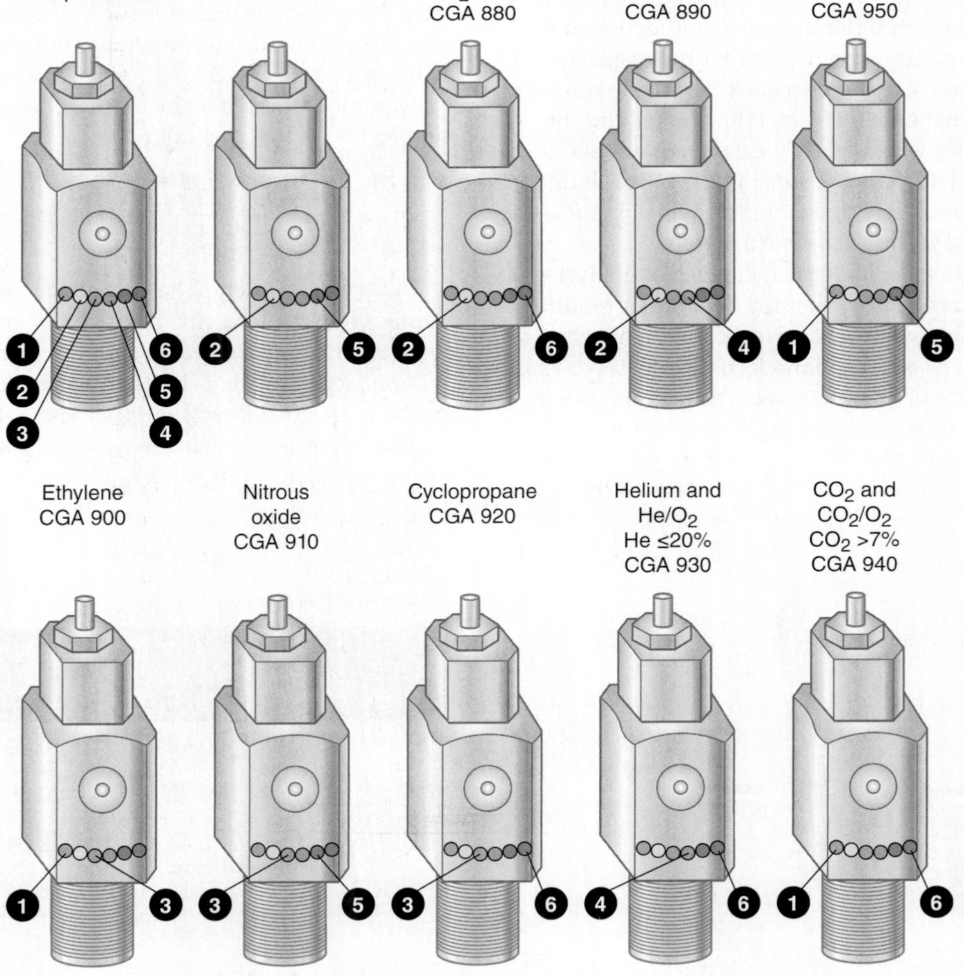

FIGURE 13-14 PISS pin positions for various therapeutic, laboratory and anesthetic gas mixtures.

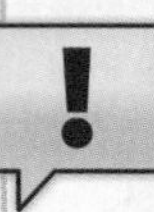

Respiratory Recap

Indexed Safety Systems

- American Standard Safety System for large-capacity cylinders (above 200 psig)
- Pin Index Safety System for small cylinders (above 200 psig)
- Diameter Index Safety System for low-pressure connections (below 200 psig)

Diameter Index Safety System

The PISS and ASSS systems are designed for use on high-pressure cylinders. In contrast, the **Diameter Index Safety System (DISS)** was designed by the CGA for low-pressure (0–200 psig) connections and fittings. The DISS utilizes specific diameter-threaded male outlets that mate with a corresponding female nut and nipple. Different diameters, thread pitch, and nipple configurations are assigned to various gases and gas mixtures. The common O_2 DISS connection (CGA 1240) has a diameter of 9⁄16 of an inch and 18 threads to the inch, often indicated as 9⁄16 2 18. This number will be found at the outlet of an O_2 flow meter, the inlet to a bubble humidifier, and the threaded connection at the end of an O_2 hose. It is important that the respiratory therapist recognize that this means that the relatively low gas flows that emerge from a flow meter and the threaded 50-psig working gas pressure connections have the same DISS connection. **Figure 13-15** illustrates the DISS safety systems for both flow meter outlets and 50-psig working-pressure outlets.

One factor that reduces the incidence of inadvertent connection of respiratory therapy equipment requiring relatively low flows (such as a nasal cannula) directly to working-pressure outlets in modern clinical settings is the common use of quick-connect connectors rather than threaded DISS connections.

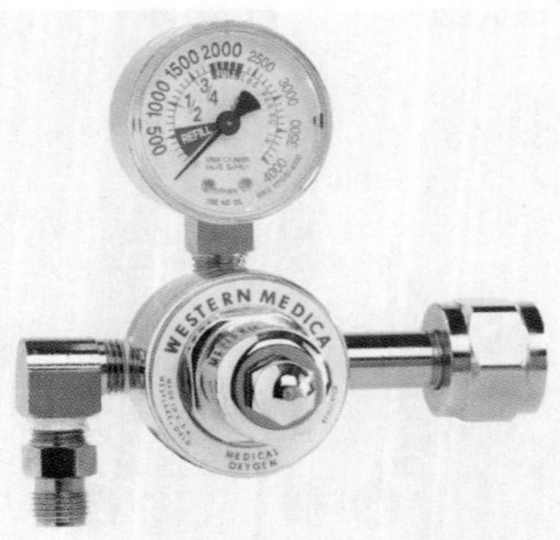

FIGURE 13-15 ASSS regulator with DISS outlet.
Courtesy of Western Enterprises, a Scott Fetzer company.

Calculating Duration of Flow from a Gas Cylinder

Providers of gas therapy cannot expect that a bulk gas distribution system will always be available, and cylinders must be used in transport, during bulk system repair or failure, and whenever wall outlets are inaccessible. In such cases, it is important to calculate how long the contents of any size cylinder will last at a specified flow.

Calculating the remaining volume of cylinder gas or duration at a specific flow requires data in both English and metric units, because cylinders are commonly sized by ft^3, whereas gas is administered in liters per minute (L/min). The calculation requires two steps. First, a conversion factor is determined that reveals how many liters will be released for each psig drop in pressure (L/psig). This will vary based on liters of gas contained in different size cylinders. The second step uses the pressure remaining in the cylinder to determine the gas volume (L). By dividing cylinder content (L) by flow (L/min), the duration of cylinder time (min) can be determined.

Step one of the calculation can be eliminated as commonly used conversion factors have been calculated for specific cylinder sizes. Any cylinder's conversion factor can be determined by converting cubic feet to liters (factor is 28.3 L/ft^3). As an example, the following equation illustrates the calculation of the conversion factor for an E cylinder:

$$\frac{22\ \text{ft}^3 \times 28.3\ \text{L/ft}^3}{2200\ \text{psig}} = 0.28\ \text{L/psig}$$

Table 13-9 presents the conversion factors for a number of cylinder sizes. To calculate duration of flow, multiply the pressure in the cylinder (psig) by the conversion factor for the cylinder, and divide that product by the prescribed flow (L/min). It also is important to realize the serious consequences of allowing a cylinder to run completely out when in clinical use. For this

TABLE 13-9
Cylinder Conversion Factors

	Conversion Factors		
Cylinder Size	**O_2, Air, O_2/N_2**	**O_2/CO_2**	**He/O_2**
D	0.16	0.20	0.14
E	0.28	0.35	0.23
G	2.41	2.94	1.93
H or K	3.14	3.84	2.50
T	3.54		

O_2, oxygen; N_2, nitrogen; CO_2, carbon dioxide; He, helium.

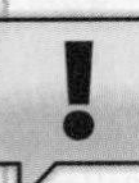

Respiratory Recap

Determining Duration of Flow

- Such calculations are necessary to determine how long an O_2 supply will last when a patient is transported.
- For compressed gas cylinders, duration of flow is calculated by use of the actual pressure in the cylinder, the conversion factor for the size of the cylinder, and the O_2 flow.
- For cylinders containing liquefied gas, the weight of the cylinder is used to infer the amount remaining because the gauge shows a constant pressure.

reason, most respiratory therapists consider cylinders with 500 psig to be effectively empty. Below is an example using a simplified equation based on already knowing the specific conversion factor.

How long before a full E-size cylinder will need to be changed if the cylinder contains 2200 psig and is delivering a flow of 4 L/min? (Assume that it will be changed when it drops to 500 psig.)

$$\text{Time remaining (min)} = \frac{(2200 - 500 \text{ psig}) \times 0.28 \text{ L/psig}}{4 \text{ L/min}}$$
$$= 425 \text{ minutes}$$
$$\frac{(425 \text{ minutes})}{60 \text{ min/hr}} = 7.083 \text{ hrs}$$
or 7 hours and 5 minutes

Calculating the duration of large-volume cylinders may also be necessary. For example, a respiratory therapist is asked to manage a mechanical ventilator in an ICU which has lost its piped gas supply of oxygen. The ventilator is using 10 L/min and connected to a K cylinder with a gauge pressure of 1,600 psig. How long will the cylinder last? The therapist will use the K cylinder conversion factor of 3.14 L/psig and plans to replace the cylinder when its contents reach 500 psig.

$$\text{Time remaining (min)} = \frac{(1{,}600 - 500 \text{ psig}) \times 3.14 \text{ L/psig}}{10 \text{ L/min}}$$
$$= 345.4 \text{ minutes}$$
or 5.42 hours
or 5 hours and 25 minutes

It also is important to note that cylinders of pure CO_2 and nitrous oxide contain a mixture of liquid and gas and that the cylinder pressures will remain constant until the last bit of liquid has evaporated. A pressure gauge on a cylinder containing liquefied gas shows a constant pressure—the vapor pressure of that gas. This pressure bears no relationship to the contents until all the liquid gas has been vaporized, when the pressure will begin to drop. Cylinders containing these gases therefore must be weighed to determine their remaining contents. The contents are directly related to the weight of the contents minus the weight of the cylinder. For example, if the weight of the liquid in the full cylinder is 30 pounds, it follows that when the weight decreases by 15 pounds, half of the contents would have been used.

Central Medical Gas Distribution

Medical gases are available to medical consumers in portable high-pressure gas cylinders, bulk (liquid) cylinders, and fixed liquid systems that feed pipelines for gas supply. Containers of liquefied gases such as O_2 are portable, containing a few liters or gallons to several hundred gallons in a delivery vehicle or several thousand gallons in a tanker truck or railway car. Bulk liquid O_2 storage vessels, such as those found at most hospitals, contain from 500 to 10,000 gallons. O_2 and other medical gases from bulk storage containers are distributed where needed through a piping system throughout the hospital.

Most hospitals and many other healthcare facilities, such as skilled nursing homes, rehabilitation centers, and outpatient surgical or diagnostic clinics, commonly feature piped medical gas distribution systems for O_2, air, and vacuum. Depending on usage, systems for nitrous oxide and occasionally for nitrogen and other gases may also be centrally distributed from a bulk source. Central O_2, air, and vacuum piping systems have made these commodities as common as water faucets and available at every bedside and other locations throughout most healthcare facilities.

Because of the potential hazards medical gases pose to the general public during transportation and to handlers and patients in healthcare settings, a number of agencies have become involved, each providing extremely detailed information, specifications, regulations, and safety procedures.

Systems for Gas Storage and Distribution

Acute care facilities use an enormous amount of O_2 daily. As an example, 50 patients using O_2 at 2 L/min require a total of 144,000 liters of O_2 gas in 24 hours, the equivalent of 21 H cylinders a day, or 625 a month. A large, active facility may require many times more. To satisfy this demand, a bulk liquid O_2 storage system is generally used.

Containers for the bulk supply of liquid O_2 are referred to as *stand tanks, vessels,* or *dewars* (named for Scottish chemist and physicist Sir James Dewar, its inventor). These containers are available in sizes ranging from as small as 500 gallons to 6000 gallons or more. Because 1 gallon of liquid O_2 is equal to 3.785 liters of liquid O_2, and 1 liter of liquid converts to 861 liters of gaseous O_2, a 500-gallon stand tank can deliver 1.6 million liters of gas, and a 6000-gallon vessel can deliver 19.5 million liters. Refilling a liquid bulk supply tank is much more cost effective than physically handling and exchanging the equivalent amount of gas stored in cylinders. (For example, a full H or K cylinder only contains 7075 L of O_2.)

Liquid O_2 stand tanks are refilled by tanker trucks as needed. Alarm systems often are designed to directly communicate the need for a refill to the distributor. All liquid storage containers, from small portable units for individual patient use to the largest stand tanks, are similarly designed and constructed, as shown in **Figure 13-16**. The liquid O_2 is held in an inner stainless steel vessel surrounded by an outer exterior shell similar to cold/hot beverage thermos bottles. Between the inner vessel and the outer shell is an insulation-filled space in which a vacuum is drawn. The inner reservoir contains O_2 both as a liquid and as a gas.

The liquid O_2 is converted to the gaseous state (evaporated) by the vaporizer coil system. So much heat is necessary for this vaporization process that the coils are extremely cold and are frequently coated with ice as a result of moisture in the ambient air condensing and freezing on them. As it is used, gaseous O_2 flows out through the pressure regulation system to the hospital or to the user device. The pressure of the gas is regulated to enter the facility at 50 to 55 psig. If the liquid in the vessel warms up too much and some boils off as gas, thereby increasing the gas pressure, the pressure-relief valve will open, allowing a controlled release of pressure. This release of gas causes the remaining gas in the vessel to expand and, according to Gay-Lussac's law, lowers the temperature in the vessel and helps maintain the liquid between its boiling point and critical pressure so that most of the contents remain in the liquid state.

The National Fire Protection Association (NFPA) issues standards concerning the placement, construction, and maintenance of bulk vessels and piping systems that have been widely adopted by local and state regulatory authorities.[5]

Liquid Oxygen Systems for Home and Transport

Miniature versions of hospital bulk liquid systems are often used in homes, alternate medical sites and patient transport when large-volume supply is needed. Both small stationary and portable vessels are commercially available and resemble a thermos bottle.

To estimate the remaining gas capacity, the contents must be weighed; some units have built-in scales to allow a spot determination.

The key data for calculation includes the following:

- Conversion of gas from liquid: 860/1 (860 liters of gaseous oxygen will vaporize from 1 liter of liquid oxygen)
- Conversion of liquid oxygen weight to gaseous liters: 2.5 lbs/1 L or (1.1 kg/1 L)

Step 1: determine total content of gaseous liters in liquid vessel, L = (liquid weight [lbs] × 860)/2.5 lbs/L

Step 2: determine the duration of contents remaining (time) = Liters of gas/flow (L/min)

For example, a respiratory therapist added 2 lbs to a portable liquid reservoir for patient transport. How long will that supply last if the patient requires oxygen flow of 2 L/min?

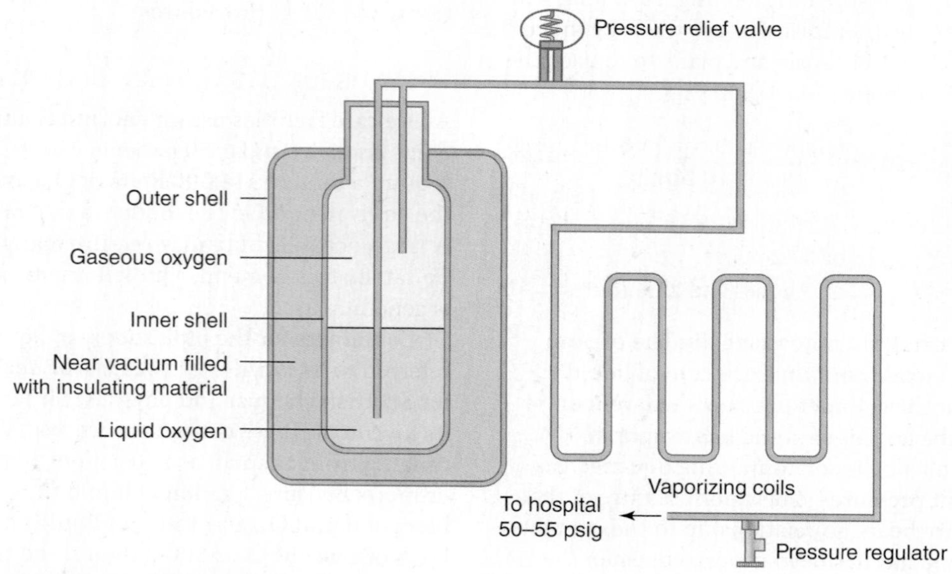

FIGURE 13-16 Bulk liquid O_2 storage.

Adapted from Branson RD, Hess DR, Chatburn RL. *Respiratory Care Equipment*, 2nd ed. Lippincott Williams & Wilkins.; 1999.

Step 1. Liters of gas content

(2 lbs × 860)/(2.5 lbs/L) = 688 L

Step 2: Duration of contents

688 L/(2 L/min) = 344 minutes

344 minutes/(60 min/hr) = 5.73 hours
or 5 hours and 43 minutes

Incidents involving bulk O_2 systems are not rare. A lack of preventive maintenance or miscommunication between respiratory care and facilities management departments can lead the O_2 system to abruptly stop, which is a major emergency. O_2 loss in the operating room or critical care unit must be quickly corrected with easily available backup cylinder gas. Without predetermined emergency protocols in place, the response will usually be slow and disorganized. Analysis of catastrophic loss of the O_2 supply in hospitals has implicated the following causes:

- False alarms caused by calibration drift of pressure sensors
- Excessive depletion of the reserve supply because of pressure imbalance between the main and reserve supply
- Failure of the vacuum seal on the reserve supply
- Inappropriate manipulation of supply valves
- Leakage around valves and ruptured piping
- Failure of monitoring personnel to notify appropriate service personnel
- Occlusion of pressure sensors with foreign substance

Other potentially serious problems include the following:

- Filling bulk cylinders with the wrong gas
- Misconnection of pipelines following remodeling
- Damage from high winds, tornadoes, earthquakes, and fires

Because of the potential for catastrophic failure of O_2 supply systems and the serious injury that would occur under such circumstances, hospitals and clinics should have procedures in place for response to such a failure. Procedures should minimally include standards for maintaining adequate numbers of backup cylinders as well as a rapid distribution plan for operating rooms and critical care areas. It has also been suggested that institutions should regularly provide practice opportunities for such a possibility. For extreme catastrophic failures of the bulk storage facility, an emergency connection to the distribution system is also provided so that a liquid O_2 delivery truck can be directly connected into the distribution system to provide a temporary gas supply.[6–10]

The NFPA requires that the reserve supply be equal to a 1-day average supply.[4] A reserve supply in a second liquid bulk reservoir may be used. Besides acting as a backup, this second reservoir also continuously adds a small amount of gas as normal vaporization occurs. Check valves (one-way valves) prevent any leaks in either system from inadvertently draining the other. Facilities with less volume demand may need only a reserve bank of large gas cylinders (as discussed in the following section concerning alternating supply systems). Alarms that alert personnel to problems in a bulk system traditionally signal the following:

- Low liquid level in either primary or reserve systems
- Reserve in use following a switchover when the main supply falls to 85 psig
- Main supply line pressure variations exceeding ±20%

O_2 piping systems may be supplied from the central source of liquid O_2 or combination of liquid and gas or from cylinders of gaseous O_2. The volume of gas used and the costs of supply dictate the choice of the supply source. Three central bulk supply systems are used: alternating supply systems with or without a reserve emergency supply, and continuous supply systems.

Alternating Supply Systems

Alternating supply systems are used in smaller facilities to supply O_2 or specialty gases such as nitrous oxide and nitrogen (**Figure 13-17**). Figure 13-17A shows the arrangement of an alternating supply system without a reserve supply. It consists of two banks of cylinders, each of which contains anywhere from 2 to as many as 20 cylinders, usually size H or the larger T. A flexible pigtail pipe containing a one-way check valve that allows flow from the cylinder only to a high-pressure header and a pressure regulator connects each cylinder. The combination of the header with its pigtails, valves, and regulator is often referred to as a *manifold*.

Gas flows from one bank of cylinders, the supply bank, through its manifold valve and regulator, where the pressure is reduced to 100 to 200 psig, and then to the main-line pressure regulator, where it is further reduced to 50 to 55 psig and proceeds through the main shut-off valve and into the piping system. Flow continues until the pressure in the supply bank approaches 100 to 200 psig, which activates the changeover switch, automatically opening the valve from the second bank of cylinders, which now becomes the supply bank, and closing the valve from the first bank. The switchover process also activates an alarm, usually located in a manned location, such as the security, maintenance, or central telephone operator area, to alert the responsible party that one bank is empty and needs to be refilled or replaced.

Figure 13-17B shows an alternating supply system with an emergency reserve supply. This system is similar to that in the previous description but adds a third gas supply as an emergency reserve in case either the

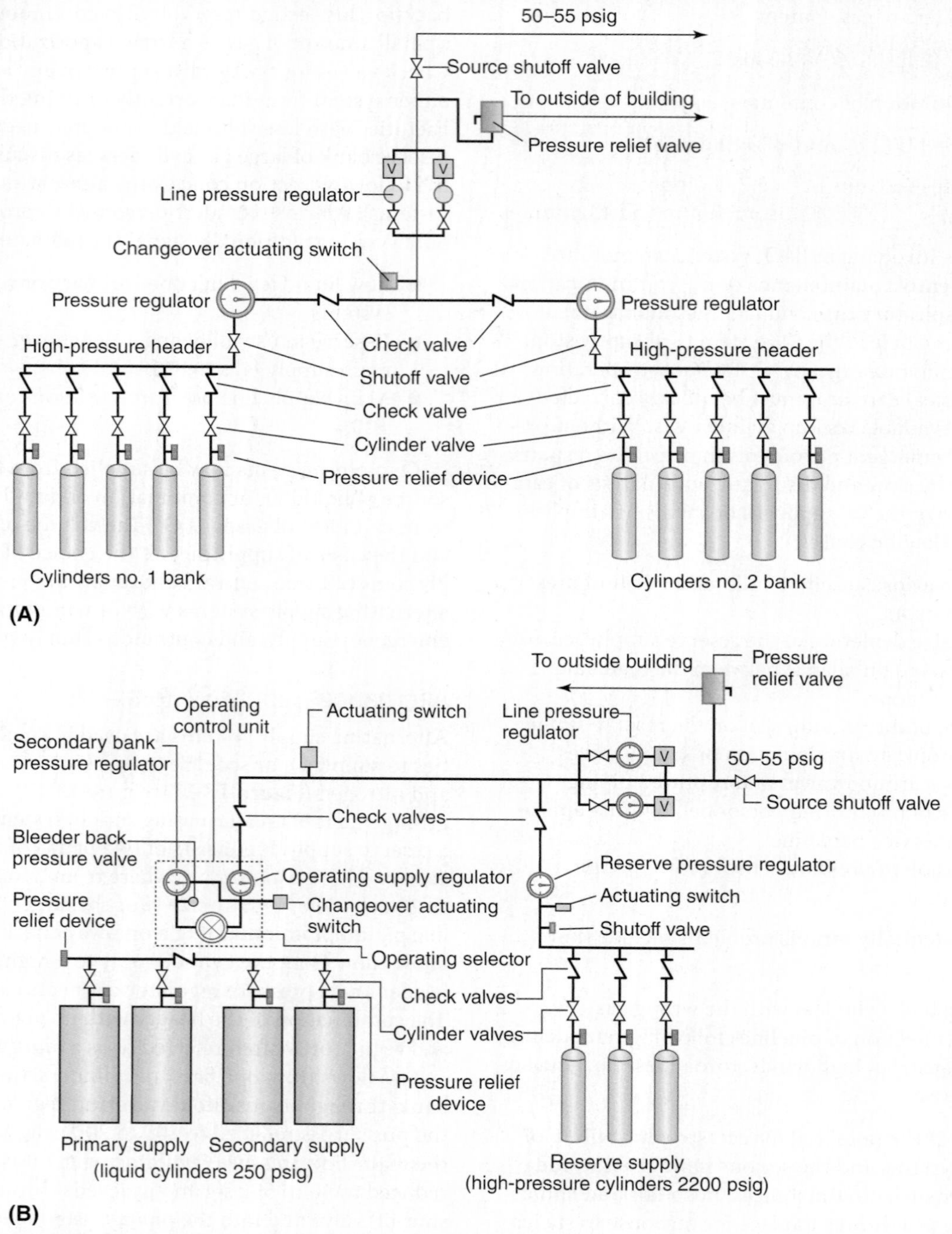

FIGURE 13-17 (**A**) Alternating supply system without a reserve supply. (**B**) Alternating primary and secondary LOX supply system with an emergency reserve supply (high pressure gas cylinders).

primary or the secondary supply or both fail. The system depicted shows liquid vessels being used as the primary and secondary sources of the O_2 supply. Banks of cylinders of gaseous O_2 also can be used.

Gas Piping Systems

Gases stored in bulk quantities are distributed throughout the facility via a system of pipes, valves, and outlets, as shown in **Figure 13-18**. The entire system must meet the standards of the NFPA for construction, installation, testing, and maintenance. The pipe must be type K or L seamless copper tubing specially cleaned to remove all traces of oxidizable material. Engineering studies determine the size (diameter) of pipe required to maintain 50 psig and maximum flows throughout the system. In most cases the pipe decreases in diameter size the farther it is from the main supply. Each pipe must be clearly labeled at regular intervals to indicate

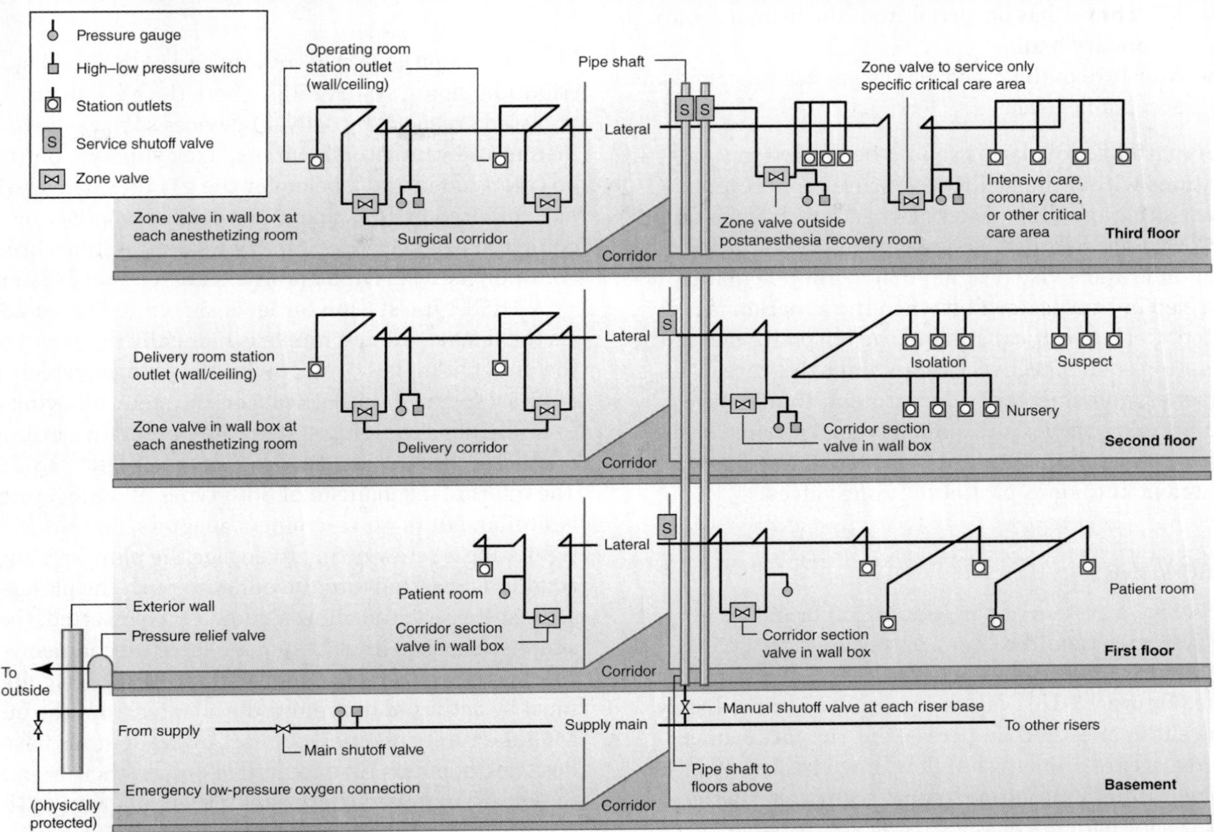

FIGURE 13-18 Gas distribution system in an acute care facility.

the gas contained. All joints and fittings are sweat-soldered with silver solder.[5]

Before any outlets are attached or added to the piping system, the system is blown clean with oil-free dry air or nitrogen to dislodge and eliminate debris such as solder, flux, and metallic filings. When construction is completed, the entire system is pressurized to a minimum of 150 psig with oil-free dry air or nitrogen. Every fitting, connection, valve, and outlet is individually inspected for leaks, and the system then must hold that pressure for at least 24 hours. This cleaning and testing procedure is conducted on each of the piping systems, including those for O_2, air, nitrous oxide, and any others. Before any piping system can be put into use, the test gas must be purged and the gas supply for that system attached. Every outlet must then be tested to ensure that it functions properly, that flow and pressure meet specifications, and that the correct gas is present.

Valves

A primary supply shutoff valve must exist at the point at which the main distribution pipe leaves the bulk supply and, when the bulk supply is located outside the building, at the point at which the main supply pipe enters the facility. From the main line, pipes extend laterally and usually further branch into zones serving groups of patient rooms or other service areas. Risers proceed vertically from the main line to service upper floors.

A shutoff valve must be located at the beginning of each lateral branch and at the base of each riser. Additionally, zone valves are placed in strategic locations so as to isolate specific areas in case of fire or during maintenance or construction. Zone valves are frequently grouped so that several gases may be controlled from the same box, as shown in Figure 13-18. In addition to groups of patient rooms, zone valves would be located to control gas flow to nurseries, each intensive care unit, the emergency department, recovery rooms, and other necessary areas. Each anesthetizing location (operating rooms or special procedures rooms, for example) must have its own dedicated shutoff valve. All shutoff valves must be easily accessible, clearly marked to indicate the area being controlled, and protected from tampering.

Gauges and Alarms

Each gas distribution system must have an automated continuous-monitoring and alarm system to alert personnel to such changes in the system as the following:

- The normal operating pressure has increased or decreased.
- The liquid O_2 supply has reached a low level.

- Switchover has occurred from the primary to the secondary bank.
- Moisture in the piped air system has exceeded an acceptable level.

A master set of alarms should be located in two locations within the facility to ensure rapid response to any situation. The master alarms must be located in areas that are manned 24 hours a day and have both an audible and a visual signal that cannot be manually canceled but turns itself off when the situation is corrected. Certain critical areas of the hospital, such as the operating rooms, recovery room, intensive care units, nurseries, and emergency department, should have line-pressure gauges and audible/visual alarms for high and low system pressure. Area alarms are frequently located next to or as part of the zone valves.

Zone Valves

For safety, a system of partitioning off branches of the system is required. Zone valves are strategically installed to allow isolation of outlets in a certain area or zone (**Figure 13-18**). Valves are required immediately adjacent to anesthetizing areas, life-support rooms, or intensive care units to shut flow down in case of a leak, repair, or fire. Practitioners must secure alternative gas sources for patients before closing a zone valve.

Station Outlets

The station outlet is the working end of the gas distribution piping system. It is where the gas can be accessed and used by delivery devices such as flow meters and ventilators. Outlets, like cylinders, must be color-coded and labeled for the gas they deliver and have indexed fittings that allow connection only to compatible delivery devices. Two safety systems are in common use: the DISS and the quick-connect system.

A DISS-type station outlet is shown in **Figure 13-19**. As the female nut and nipple is manually tightened onto the outlet, it makes contact with the plunger, which moves it forward until it seats on the stem, allowing gas to flow from the piping system. Representative examples of quick-connect adapters are shown in **Figure 13-20**. The internal mechanism of both types of outlet systems is similar, but in quick-connect adapters, instead of tightening a screw fitting to engage the plunger, a male adapter is inserted into the outlet to push the plunger against the seat and allow airflow. Once inserted, the adapter is locked in place and a release mechanism, such as the pressing of a button or twisting of a collar, must be activated to remove the adapter from the outlet. Manufacturers of quick-connect outlet stations have designed adapters that are usable only in their brand of outlet. All manufacturers design their adapters so that only an adapter made for O_2 can fit into an O_2 outlet and

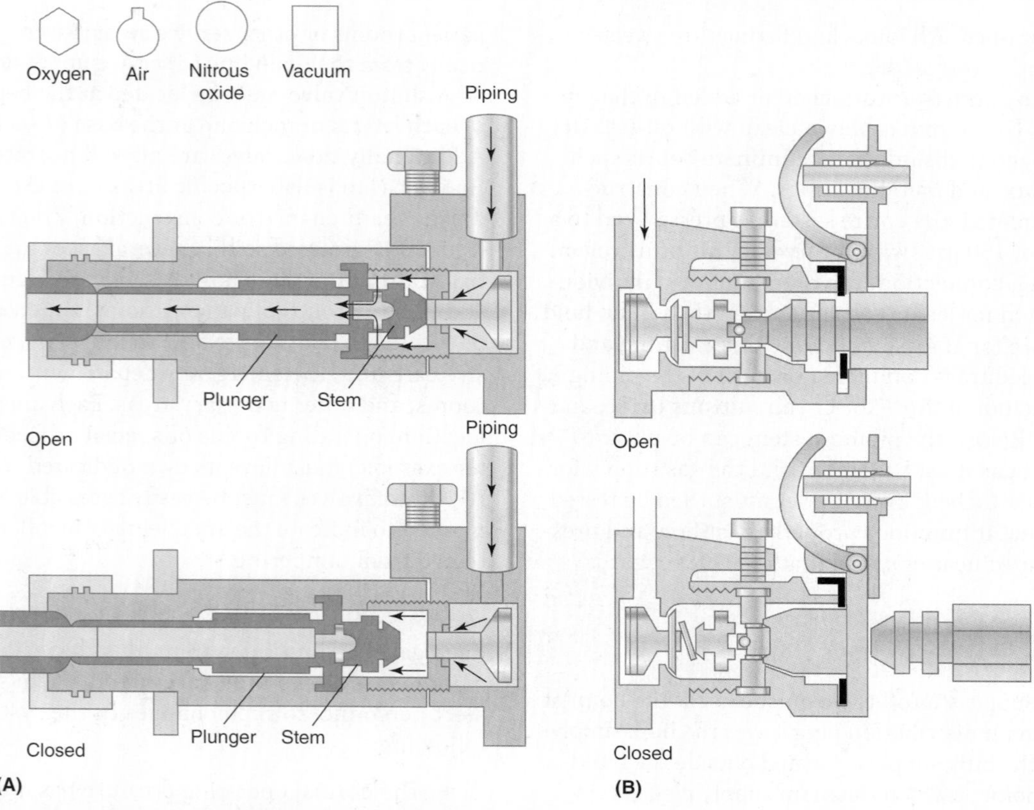

FIGURE 13-19 (**A**) DISS and (**B**) quick-connect station outlets.

Modified from Cairo JM, Pilbeam SP. *Mosby's Respiratory Care Equipment*, 6th ed. Mosby; 1999. Reprinted with permission.

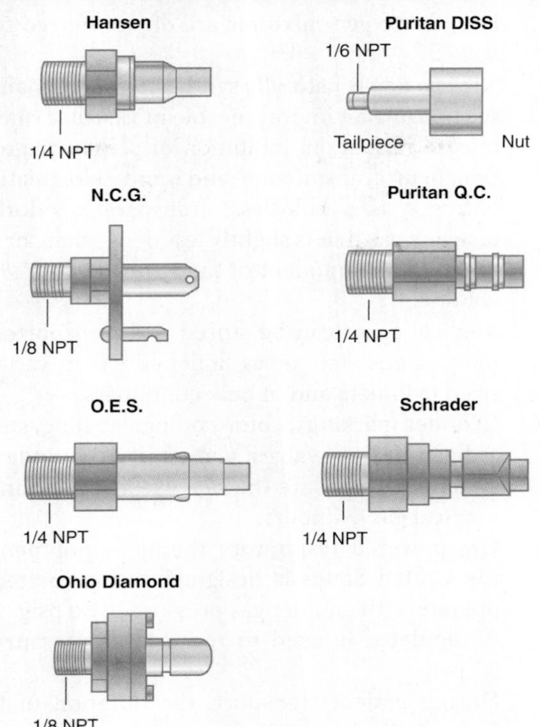

FIGURE 13-20 Quick-connects. Wall outlets only open when a quick-connect is fully locked in place.

Modified from Cairo JM, Pilbeam SP. *Mosby's Respiratory Care Equipment*, 6th ed. Mosby; 1999. Reprinted with permission.

would be physically incompatible with an air, nitrous oxide, or vacuum outlet.

Central Compressed Medical Air Distribution

Compressed medical-grade air is commonly used as the source gas to aerosolize medications, activate large-volume nebulizers, and mix with O_2 in ventilators and blenders to provide a specific FIO_2. The central air distribution system is similar to the O_2 system in the layout of the piping, valves, alarms, and station outlets. The source of the compressed air may be banks of cylinders, but this scenario would be practical only in the case of a very small facility or a facility with a minimal need for compressed air.

In most cases the bulk of the air comes from dual central compressors, as shown in **Figure 13-21**. The compressors can operate together or alternate, but in either case each must be able to supply the full demands of the facility for compressed air when the other needs maintenance. For medical use, the compressors must deliver oil-free air. The compressors used for central systems are usually of the piston or centrifugal/rotary type. Piston compressors use carbon or Teflon rings to create the seal against the cylinder

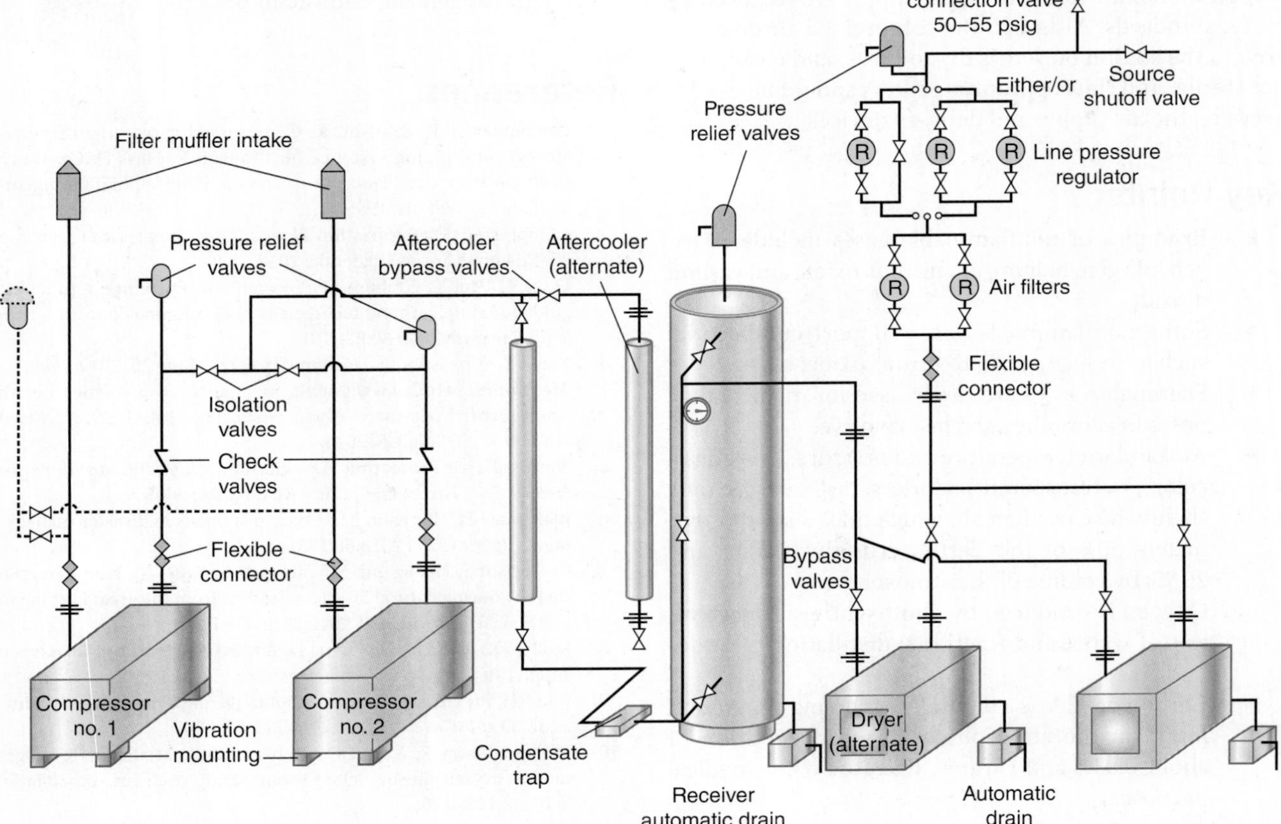

FIGURE 13-21 Bulk air supply compressor system. Dual compressors ensure that the supply of compressed air will be maintained. Note the engineering required to manage the considerable amount of water produced in compressing ambient air.

Modified from Cairo JM, Pilbeam SP. *Mosby's Respiratory Care Equipment*, 6th ed. Mosby; 1999. Reprinted with permission.

wall and eliminate the need for an oil lubricant. High-pressure rotary compressors use a liquid sealant, usually water, between the impeller blades and the housing, again eliminating the need for oil lubrication.

To meet NFPA standards, the air being drawn into the compressor must come from an intake located outside the building, above the roof, and in a location where the air is free from particulates, odors, engine exhaust, and vacuum system discharges. The air is filtered, compressed, and passed through an aftercooler, where cooling causes water vapor to condense and be removed. The air then is stored in a large tank called a reservoir or receiver. Air is stored in the receiver tank at a pressure higher than the 50 to 55 psig required in the facility's piping system, allowing the air to flow in a steady stream from the line pressure regulator. In addition, the compressor turns off when a sufficient supply of air is stored in the reservoir, thus minimizing wear, and additional water vapor condenses in the tank and is eliminated.

After leaving the reservoir, the air passes through a dryer to remove any remaining water vapor. Removal of water vapor, water droplets, and humidity from the compressed air supply is important to prevent microbial growth (e.g., bacteria, fungi, molds) within the piping system. Water in the air supply causes serious damage to ventilators, blenders, and other devices. Alarm systems to monitor dew point (humidity) and carbon monoxide in the main air supply are required by NFPA standards. Although the compressed air delivered to the station outlets is dry, oil free, and clean, it is not sterile, and thus appropriate filters should be used between the air supply and delivery devices.

Key Points

- Examples of nonflammable gases include nitrogen, oxygen, helium, air, nitrous oxide, and carbon dioxide.
- Some nonflammable gases support combustion, such as oxygen, air, and nitrous oxide.
- Flammable gases are rarely used for medical purposes because they can be explosive.
- At standard temperature and pressure, oxygen is a colorless, transparent, odorless, tasteless gas, only slightly heavier than air, which makes up approximately 50% of the Earth's crust by weight and 20.9% by volume of the atmosphere.
- Oxygen is produced by photosynthesis, electrolysis of water, and fractional distillation of liquefied air.
- Carbon dioxide is a naturally occurring compound found in the atmosphere in a concentration of about 0.03% and is rarely used today for medical purposes.
- Helium/oxygen mixtures are often referred to as *heliox*.
- Nitric oxide is naturally synthesized in human tissue, playing an important role in vascular smooth muscle relaxation, inhibition of platelet aggregation, neurotransmission, and immune regulation.
- Nitrogen is a colorless, transparent, odorless, tasteless gas that is slightly less dense than air and the major component of the atmosphere, 78% by volume.
- Medical gases can be stored and transported in the gaseous state or as liquefied gas in various-sized cylinders and in bulk containers.
- Cylinder markings, color-coding, labeling, standardized testing, valves, and connection indexing systems help ensure the safe use and handling of medical gas cylinders.
- Gas-powered respiratory therapy equipment in the United States is designed and calibrated to operate with an inlet gas pressure of 50 psig.
- A regulator is used to reduce gas pressure to 50 psig.
- During patient transport, the duration of flow for a medical gas cylinder must be calculated to determine how many cylinders are needed.
- Most hospitals and many other healthcare facilities have piped medical gas distribution systems for oxygen, air, and vacuum.

References

1. Langenderfer R, Branson R. Compressed gases: manufacture, storage, and piping systems. In: Branson R, Hess D, Chatburn R. *Respiratory Care Equipment*. 2nd ed. Philadelphia: Lippincott Williams & Wilkins; 1999.
2. Compressed Gas Association. *Handbook of Compressed Gases*. 5th ed. Boston: Kluwer Academic; 2013.
3. Duke T, Peel D, Graham SH Oxygen concentrators: a practical guide for clinicians and technicians in developing countries. *Ann Trop Paediatr.* 2010;30:87–101.
4. Magil B. Why is there a Helium Shortage? June 25, 2012. *Popular Mechanics*. http://www.popularmechanics.com/science/health/med-tech/why-is-there-a-helium-shortage-10031229. Accessed January 7, 2013, July 8, 2014.
5. National Fire Protection Association. *NFPA 99: Standard for Health Care Facilities*. Quincy, MA: NFPA; 2005.
6. Blakeman TC, Branson RD. Oxygen supplies in disaster management. *Respir Care.* 2013;58:173–183.
7. Kobayashi S, Hanagama M, Yamanda S, Yanai M. Home oxygen therapy during natural disasters: lessons from the great East Japan earthquake. *Eur Respir J.* 2012;39:1047–1048.
8. Stoller JK, Stefanak M, Orens D, Burkhart J. The hospital oxygen supply: an "O2K" problem. *Respir Care.* 2000;45:300–305.
9. Ritz RH, Previtera J. Oxygen supplies during a mass casualty situation. *Respir Care.* 2008;53:215–225.
10. Weller J, Merry A, Warman G, Robinson B. Anaesthetists' management of oxygen pipeline failure: room for improvement. *Anaesthesia.* 2007;62:122–126.

CHAPTER

14

Therapeutic Gases: Management and Administration

John Boatright, Jeffrey J. Ward

OUTLINE

The Rationale for Supplemental Oxygen
Indications for Oxygen Therapy
Limitations of Supplemental Oxygen
Complications and Hazards of Oxygen Therapy
Dosage Regulation and Administration Devices
Oxygen Administration Devices
Monitoring the Physiologic Effects of Oxygen
Clinical Application of Oxygen Therapy
Helium–Oxygen Therapy
Carbon Dioxide Therapy
Nitric Oxide Therapy

OBJECTIVES

1. Identify indications for supplemental oxygen therapy based on patient history, clinical findings, and physiologic indices.
2. Recognize complications for supplemental oxygen therapy and methods to prevent or minimize untoward effects.
3. Discuss the effect of downstream resistance on the accuracy of flow control devices.
4. Identify clinical circumstances in which low-flow/variable performance oxygen appliances are not meeting patient's needs and require change to high-flow/fixed performance systems.
5. Identify variables that affect the delivered oxygen concentration with low-flow oxygen delivery devices.
6. Describe the use of gaseous oxygen analysis, arterial blood gas measurements, and pulse oximetry monitoring for oxygen therapy.
7. Develop a logical approach to the therapeutic application of medical gases, including equipment selection, dosage regulation, patient interface, and therapy outcome monitoring.
8. Describe clinical applications for the rational use of heliox and nitric oxide.

KEY TERMS

air-entrainment mask
air–oxygen blender
air-to-oxygen mix ratio
Bourdon gauge flow meter
carbogen
carboxyhemoglobin
diffusion defect
flow restrictor
heliox
high-flow nasal cannula
high-flow/fixed-performance device
hyperbaric oxygen (HBO) therapy
hypercarbia
hypoxemia
hypoxemic drive
hypoxia
low-flow/variable-performance device
nasal oxygen cannula
nitric oxide (NO)
nitrogen washout atelectasis
nonrebreathing mask
oxygen analyzer
oxygen hood
oxygen-induced hypoventilation
oxygen tent
oxygen toxicity
partial rebreathing mask
retinopathy of prematurity (ROP)
shunt
simple oxygen mask
Thorpe tube flow meter
ventilation-perfusion ($\dot{V}/\dot{Q}$) mismatch

Introduction

This chapter presents information relevant to the therapeutic application of gases typically used in respiratory care. Not discussed are anesthetic gases, gases used for diagnostic purposes, or invasive oxygenation using extracorporeal membrane (ECMO) techniques. The primary focus of the chapter is the use of oxygen (O_2) to treat hypoxemia, but other gases are also discussed, including helium–oxygen mixtures (heliox), inhaled nitric oxide (iNO), and carbon dioxide–oxygen mixtures (carbogen).

The Rationale for Supplemental Oxygen

Supplemental O_2 is indicated when **hypoxemia** is suspected by history or physical examination or is documented by laboratory data (**CPG 14-1**). The short-term application of high concentrations of O_2 is relatively free of complications, and withholding O_2 can have grave consequences. Tachycardia, cardiac dysrhythmias, dyspnea, tachypnea, use of accessory muscles, increased difficulty breathing, mental confusion, and disorientation may indicate the need for oxygen therapy. In adults, children, and infants (older than 1 month) at rest breathing room air, a PaO_2 below 60 mm Hg or SpO_2 below 90% indicates the need for O_2 therapy. In neonates, a PaO_2 below 50 mm Hg, SpO_2 below 88%, or capillary PO_2 below 40 mm Hg indicates the need for O_2 therapy. In the non–critically ill patient, the medical history and previous laboratory findings are key data.

Hypoxemia can be caused by low ambient barometric pressure or subambient FIO_2, hypoventilation, **ventilation-perfusion ($\dot{V}/\dot{Q}$) mismatch, shunt**, or **diffusion defect**. Hypoxemia caused by all but hypoventilation results in a widened $P(A–a)O_2$. Only with hypoxemia due to low atmospheric PIO_2 (e.g., altitude) or hypoventilation is the $P(A–a)O_2$ normal. Further differentiation requires either testing after 100% oxygen breathing (for quantifying abnormal shunt) or carbon monoxide diffusion testing (for quantifying diffusion defect).

The physiologic mechanism by which increased inspiratory O_2 concentration (expressed either as a percentage of O_2 [O_2%] in the total atmosphere or as a fraction [FIO_2]) increases the PaO_2 is by an increase in the inspired partial pressure of oxygen (PIO_2), resulting in the increased partial pressure of O_2 in ventilated alveolar units (PAO_2). The increased PAO_2 results in an increase in PaO_2 and oxygen saturation of hemoglobin.

O_2 therapy is supportive and does not correct the underlying pulmonary pathology that resulted in hypoxemia. The cause of the hypoxemia must be addressed. For example, if the clinical problem is atelectasis (alveolar collapse), recruitment of collapsed alveoli is the definitive care, even if O_2 therapy is temporarily needed to prevent vital organ injury related to the hypoxemia and the resultant tissue **hypoxia** caused by the maldistribution of ventilation.

CLINICAL PRACTICE GUIDELINE 14-1

Oxygen Therapy in the Acute Care Hospital

Indications

- Documented hypoxemia, defined as a decreased PaO_2 in the blood below normal range (PaO_2 of less than 60 mm Hg or SpO_2 below 90% in subjects breathing room air or with PaO_2 and/or SpO_2 below the desirable range for the specific clinical situation)
- An acute care situation in which hypoxemia is suspected; substantiation of hypoxemia is required within an appropriate period of time following initiation of therapy
- Severe trauma
- Acute myocardial infarction
- Short-term therapy or surgical intervention (e.g., postanesthesia recovery, hip surgery)

Contraindications

- No specific contraindications to oxygen therapy exist when indications are judged to be present.

Precautions and Possible Complications

- With $PaO_2 < 60$ mm Hg, ventilatory depression may occur in spontaneously breathing patients with elevated $PaCO_2$.
- With $FIO_2 > 0.5$, absorption atelectasis, oxygen toxicity, and/or depression of ciliary and/or leukocytic function may occur.
- Supplemental oxygen should be administered with caution to patients suffering from paraquat poisoning and to patients who have received or are undergoing bleomycin drug therapy.
- During laser bronchoscopy, minimal levels of supplemental oxygen should be used to avoid intratracheal ignition.
- Fire hazard is increased in the presence of increased oxygen concentrations.
- Bacterial contamination associated with certain nebulization and humidification systems is a possible hazard.

Modified from AARC clinical practice guideline: oxygen therapy for adults in the acute care facility—2002 revision and update. *Respir Care.* 2002;47:717–720. Reprinted with permission.

Respiratory Recap

Oxygen Therapy

- O_2 therapy should be considered for hypoxemic conditions.
- Short-term use of high O_2 concentrations is relatively free of serious complications.
- Hypoxemia can be caused by low ambient O_2, partial pressure (e.g., altitude) or pulmonary conditions caused by hypoventilation, $\dot{V}/\dot{Q}$ mismatch, right-to-left shunt, or diffusion defect.
- O_2 therapy tends to increase the Pa_{O_2} best in conditions causing hypoventilation, $\dot{V}/\dot{Q}$ mismatch, and diffusion defect; it is least effective when right-to-left shunt predominates.
- The cause of hypoxemia should be corrected; O_2 therapy is a supportive therapy.

The net improvement in Pa_{O_2} with supplemental O_2 is variable. Previously normal subjects with carboxyhemoglobinemia who are given 100% O_2 can achieve a Pa_{O_2} of more than 500 mm Hg very rapidly. At the opposite extreme, patients with a very high shunt will have only a small increase in Pa_{O_2} breathing 100% O_2. With hypoventilation, an increase in F_{IO_2} increases Pa_{O_2} sufficiently to compensate for the effect of the increased Pa_{CO_2} on Pa_{O_2} until the primary hypoventilation can be corrected. Under normal barometric conditions, patients cannot tolerate the arterial hypoxemia that will result from Pa_{CO_2} levels of over 90 mm Hg without O_2-enriched atmospheres due to the level of displaced Pa_{O_2} (**Figure 14-1**). Oxygen therapy also has a very limited role in correcting tissue hypoxia in patients with significant anemia for which transfusion is the corrective treatment.

Indications for Oxygen Therapy

Patients with hypoxemia due to $\dot{V}/\dot{Q}$ mismatch or diffusion defect require O_2 therapy until more definitive therapies take effect. Hypoxemia is caused by $\dot{V}/\dot{Q}$ mismatch in asthma and chronic obstructive pulmonary disease (COPD), with or without hypercapnia. Continuous long-term O_2 therapy in COPD is life prolonging, but evidence for the use of O_2 during exercise training in COPD is limited.[1–3] Patients with interstitial pulmonary fibrosis may also require supplemental oxygen if the diffusion defect is significant. O_2 does improve nocturnal hemoglobin O_2 saturation in patients with obstructive sleep apnea (OSA), but it may also increase duration of apnea-hypopnea events.[2,4]

The perioperative state predisposes patients to the need for supplemental O_2 (**Table 14-1**). General anesthesia commonly causes a decrease in Pa_{O_2} secondary to increased $\dot{V}/\dot{Q}$ mismatch (hypoventilation) and

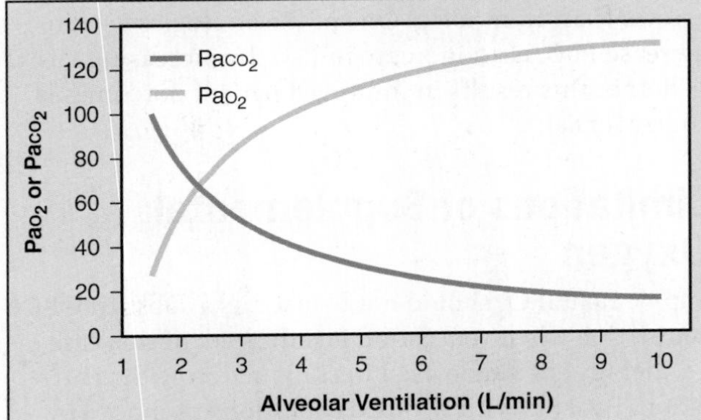

FIGURE 14-1 Relationship between alveolar ventilation, Pa_{O_2}, and Pa_{CO_2}. Note that a reduction in alveolar ventilation causes Pa_{CO_2} to increase and Pa_{O_2} to decrease.

TABLE 14-1
Summary of Conditions Commonly Requiring Treatment with Oxygen

Condition Causing Hypoxemia	General Approach
Perioperative	Treat with O_2 to maintain adequate Sp_{O_2} or Pa_{O_2}.
Chronic obstructive pulmonary disease	Use care to identify patients with chronic hypercarbia because CO_2 retention may occur with O_2 administration. Patients who are chronically hypoxemic may tolerate a lower Pa_{O_2}.
Acute respiratory distress syndrome	Treat with O_2, PEEP, and prone positioning to maintain adequate Pa_{O_2}.
Cardiopulmonary resuscitation	Use of 100% O_2 is standard practice with mask-bag-valve ventilation.
Myocardial infarction or acute coronary syndrome	Use of supplemental oxygen has been standard practice for initial therapy for MI or ACS if $Sa_{O_2} < 94\%$ or clinical signs of heart failure. Recent research has demonstrated detrimental effects of 100% oxygen during and in early recovery following CPR. Clear evidence for reoxygenation strategies are not available at this time.
Cardiogenic pulmonary edema	Treat with O_2 and positive pressure (e.g., CPAP or PEEP) to maintain adequate Sp_{O_2} or Pa_{O_2}.
Cor pulmonale	Treat with O_2 to maintain adequate Sp_{O_2} or Pa_{O_2}.
Carbon monoxide poisoning	Treat with high-concentration O_2. Sp_{O_2} or Pa_{O_2} may not be reflective of the degree of disruption in O_2 transport caused by carboxyhemoglobin. Consider hyperbaric oxygen treatment.
Absorption of air in body cavities	Unusual indication for O_2 therapy, such as pneumocephalus, subcutaneous emphysema, or small pneumothorax.

decreased functional residual capacity (atelectasis).[5] The effects are greatest with thoracic and abdominal surgery, elderly or obese patients, and preexisting pulmonary disease. Hypoxemia usually responds to intraoperative or postoperative supplemental oxygen. Postoperative alveolar recruitment techniques are used to prevent or reverse the underlying ventilatory pathology. General anesthetics can also reduce the respiratory center's responsiveness to hypoxemia. Postoperative O_2 administration has been used to decrease the risk of surgical site infection, but evidence for effectiveness is limited.[6]

Acute respiratory distress syndrome (ARDS) is a common pulmonary disorder with high mortality in the critical care unit; approximately one-third of patients diagnosed with ARDS die. ARDS is characterized by hypoxemia that is difficult to correct with supplemental oxygen. ARDS patients often require a high F_{IO_2} and mechanical ventilation with positive end-expiratory pressure (PEEP). Prone position may be required for severe cases.[7]

Although based on a different etiology (prematurity), RDS (neonatal respiratory distress syndrome, formerly known as hyaline membrane disease, infant or idiopathic respiratory distress syndrome) also results in pulmonary atelectasis, causing increased work of breathing and hypoxemia. Supplemental oxygen is used to improve Pa_{O_2} in the setting of pulmonary (and/or intracardiac) right-to-left shunting and $\dot{V}/\dot{Q}$ mismatch; adjuncts of continuous positive airway pressure (CPAP) or PEEP with mechanical ventilation are added as indicated.

During cardiopulmonary resuscitation (CPR) in adults, as much O_2 as possible should be provided.[8,9] Typically, manual mask-valve-bag resuscitation devices are designed to deliver 100% O_2 when connected to O_2 supply during typical CPR conditions. Respiratory therapists should ensure that adequate O_2 is provided during CPR. To minimize the possibility of retinopathy of prematurity, it is advisable that premature infants requiring frequent or repeated resuscitative efforts be ventilated using concentrations of O_2 that have been previously determined to meet the patient's oxygenation needs.[10]

Although there is a lack of high level evidence to suggest that it alters mortality in uncomplicated care of patients after a myocardial infarction (MI), it is rational to use supplemental oxygen to avoid hypoxemia and decrease the incidence of dysrhythmias. Tissue hypoxia and lactic acidemia often occur after MI as the result of reduced cardiac output rather than hypoxemia. Cardiogenic pulmonary edema commonly requires the use of high-concentration O_2 therapy to sustain the patient while diuretics and vasoactive drugs reduce the effects of the left ventricular failure. If present, tissue hypoxia is commonly the result of reduced cardiac output and hypoxemia from $\dot{V}/\dot{Q}$ mismatching, right-to-left shunting, and diffusion defect in the lung. O_2 therapy is indicated in such cases and commonly used in conjunction with CPAP or ventilation with PEEP to combine that additional alveolar recruitment effect.

Cor pulmonale is a common manifestation of chronic hypoxemia. Low P_{AO_2} induces hypoxic pulmonary vasoconstriction. O_2 administration can reverse the arteriolar constriction unless the vascular changes have become fixed or destructive vascular disease has occurred. One of the goals of long-term O_2 therapy is to reverse or prevent cor pulmonale.

In carbon monoxide poisoning, **carboxyhemoglobin** reduces the hemoglobin O_2 saturation. The treatment of choice for carbon monoxide poisoning is 100% O_2, sometimes in conjunction with hyperbaric conditions, to achieve the highest Pa_{O_2} possible. The use of 100% O_2 is considered an essential therapy in the treatment of carbon monoxide poisoning. In addition to maximizing the quantity of O_2 dissolved in serum, the high Pa_{O_2} resulting from breathing 100% O_2 causes a rapid dissociation of carbon monoxide from hemoglobin. High O_2 concentrations are also used in severe acquired methemoglobinemia until treatment with methylene blue.

High concentrations of O_2 have been used to treat patients who have collection of air in body cavities or tissues. Such conditions include pneumothorax, pneumomediastinum, subcutaneous emphysema, pneumocephalus, and distended bowel.[11,12] When pure O_2 is breathed, nitrogen is displaced from the lungs and the blood. The elimination of nitrogen results in diffusion of nitrogen from the trapped gas into the bloodstream, thus reducing the volume of trapped gas. This phenomenon can be undesirable in the case of a middle ear with a blocked eustachian tube or paranasal sinuses with blocked ostia. Pulmonary atelectasis is also more likely to occur during high-concentration oxygen breathing.

Recently, brain tissue P_{O_2} (Pb_{O_2}) monitoring has been introduced to guide management of patients with severe traumatic brain injury.[13] An electrode that is inserted with intracranial pressure monitoring[14,15] measures brain tissue oxygen. The target Pb_{O_2} is greater than 15 mm Hg. One of the strategies used to increase Pb_{O_2} is an increase in Pa_{O_2} by increasing F_{IO_2}. Whether this results in improved patient outcomes is controversial.

Limitations of Supplemental Oxygen

Supplemental O_2 should not be used as a substitute for ventilation when ventilation is indicated; in this case, O_2 therapy should be used in conjunction with ventilation. Patients with hypoxic conditions produced by acute anemia (Hb < 10 g/dL) can be temporarily supported by high-concentration supplemental O_2, but only a small portion of resting O_2 needs can be met with supplemental O_2. Patients with hypoxia produced by low cardiac output or low tissue perfusion may also be placed on O_2 therapy, but again only a small portion of resting oxygen needs can be met with supplemental O_2. The goal of oxygen therapy in these situations is to maximize the blood's O_2 content. Once hemoglobin is 100% saturated, however, further increases in Pa_{O_2} have a marginal effect on O_2 content and oxygen delivery. Patients with large cardiac or pulmonary right-to-left shunts will have a disappointing response to oxygen therapy because increasing the P_{AO_2} in the areas of good $\dot{V}/\dot{Q}$ matching cannot supersaturate hemoglobin with O_2 to overcompensate for poorly saturated blood from areas with shunting.

Complications and Hazards of Oxygen Therapy

Supplemental O_2 is a relatively benign drug. Far more patients die from hypoxia than suffer complications from (ambient or nonhyperbaric) oxygen therapy. Respiratory therapists must take precautions to minimize untoward effects of O_2 therapy, however. **Table 14-2** summarizes possible complications caused by supplemental O_2 and how to prevent them.

Oxygen Toxicity

Pulmonary **oxygen toxicity** refers to cellular injury of lung parenchyma and airway epithelium.[15] When intracellular P_{O_2} is elevated, cytotoxic free radicals are generated in excessive amounts. The free radicals include superoxide anions (O_2^-), singlet oxygen molecules, hydroxyl radicals (OH^-), and partially reduced oxygen metabolites such as hydrogen peroxide (H_2O_2). Some free radical production occurs as a normal aspect of cellular metabolism; intracellular enzymes such as superoxide dismutase and catalase eliminate most toxic products. Nonenzymatic antioxidants include vitamin A, ascorbate, cysteine carotene, tocopherol, and hemoglobin.

Toxic effects depend on the concentration, length of exposure to O_2, and underlying lung condition. Because cellular levels cannot be directly measured, dosage relationships can only be presumed. To date, no exact threshold O_2 concentration has been established at which toxicity occurs. Onset and severity are more severe in hyperbaric O_2 therapy and may include neuropathologic effects such as vertigo and nausea followed by altered behavior, clumsiness, and convulsions.

Clinical manifestations of high-concentration O_2 breathing include symptoms of mild to severe substernal pain, dyspnea, fatigue, and paresthesias. There is tracheobronchitis, and ciliated airway cells have depressed activity within 6 hours of 100% O_2 exposure. Clinical signs of gas exchange abnormalities can occur within 24 to 48 hours at an F_{IO_2} of 1.0. They include hypoxemia caused by right-to-left shunting from atelectasis, decreased lung compliance, and infiltrates on chest radiograph that reflect the cellular pathology. Inflammatory changes, edema, and fibrosis occur with exposure longer than 72 to 96 hours. Pulmonary

TABLE 14-2
Summary of Complications and Hazards of Oxygen Therapy

Complication or Hazard	Patients Affected	Etiology	Prevention
O_2 toxicity	All ages, patients on 50% or higher O_2	Additional free radicals of O_2 in increased O_2 atmospheres	Use minimal O_2 to maintain normal Sp_{O_2} and/or Pa_{O_2}.
Nitrogen washout atelectasis	All ages, patients receiving 90% to 100% O_2	Sedentary breathing, obstruction, absorption of Pa_{O_2} by blood	Alveolar recruitment; deep breathing; ambulate if possible; avoid 100% O_2.
Oxygen-induced hypoventilation	Patients with chronic hypercarbia	Haldane effect, $\dot{V}/\dot{Q}$ change, or ventilatory drive suppression	Limit O_2 to minimum necessary to correct hypoxemia (Sp_{O_2} 88% to 92%).
Retinopathy of prematurity	Premature infants	Retinal vasoconstriction in the presence of Pa_{O_2} > 80 mm Hg	Maintain Pa_{O_2} of premature infants between 50 and 80 mm Hg.
Closure of the ductus arteriosis	Infants with congenital heart defects that require ductal blood flow	High Pa_{O_2} triggers closure of the ductus	Maintain modest Pa_{O_2}.
Support of combustion	All patients	O_2 accelerates combustion	Maintain fire-safe environment: no sparks, open flames, or smoking. Use no oil or other petroleum products with O_2 therapy. Avoid the use of flammable clothing and plastics.

O_2 toxicity is considered a comorbid condition with ARDS, because the clinical manifestations of O_2 toxicity are identical to the clinical manifestations of ARDS.

Multiple factors affect O_2 tolerance, including hormones, catecholamine levels, vitamin E levels, and drugs such as paraquat. Bleomycin therapy may accelerate the onset of O_2 toxicity, but this claim remains controversial because of the difficulty of human research.[16]

In practice, high-concentration O_2 should not be withheld from critically ill patients or for transport. An F_{IO_2} less than 0.5 for 2 to 7 days does not result in significant lung impairment. Extended exposure to an F_{IO_2} above 0.6 should be avoided if possible. A goal of respiratory therapists is to use the minimum O_2 concentration required to achieve adequate tissue oxygenation. Mechanical ventilation with PEEP should be considered when high F_{IO_2} is required.

Nitrogen Washout Atelectasis

Absorption atelectasis can occur with high-concentration O_2 breathing, secondary to washout of nitrogen from the lungs (**nitrogen washout atelectasis**). During room air breathing, the partial pressure of nitrogen in the lungs is approximately 570 mm Hg. When F_{IO_2} is increased, nitrogen molecules are displaced with O_2 molecules in the alveoli. When airway obstruction or reduction in ventilation occurs, hemoglobin in the pulmonary circulation extracts O_2 from the alveolus. Alveolar collapse occurs when a critically low volume is reached and hypoxemia results from increased physiologic shunting.

Oxygen-Induced Hypoventilation

To understand **oxygen-induced hypoventilation**, it is necessary to review both neurologic control of breathing and pulmonary vascular changes related to oxygen. Under normoxic conditions, the control of ventilation is managed by the CO_2 drive (carbic ventilatory drive). Chemoreceptors in the central nervous system respond to the hydrogen ion concentration ($[H^+]$) of the cerebral spinal fluid (CSF). The $[H^+]$ in the CSF is determined primarily by the Pa_{CO_2}. That is, when the Pa_{CO_2} increases, so does the $[H^+]$ of the CSF. Receptors on the surface of the brain stem sense changes in $[H^+]$ of the CSF and respond by changing the level of ventilation to maintain a normal Pa_{CO_2}. These central chemoreceptors are very sensitive to small changes in H^+ and will maintain the Pa_{CO_2} very closely.

A second, more primitive chemo-ventilatory drive is the **hypoxemic drive** (also called *hypoxic drive*). The peripheral chemoreceptors, which are located in the chest and neck (in the aortic arch and the carotid bodies), respond when the Pa_{O_2} falls below about 60 mm Hg. Whenever the Pa_{O_2} decreases below the hypoxemic threshold of 60 mm Hg, increased ventilation is stimulated. For example, when a person climbing a mountain reaches an altitude where P_{IO_2} causes a Pa_{O_2} of less than 60 mm Hg (at approximately 12,000 to 15,000 ft), the climber will experience an increased ventilatory rate and tidal volume. The hypoxemic drive and the carbic drive act independently of each other, but the hypoxemic drive will override the carbic drive.

O_2-induced hypoventilation may occur in some patients who have adapted to long-term **hypercarbia** (elevated baseline Pa_{CO_2}).[16–21] Examples of diagnoses associated with chronic hypercarbia are end-stage COPD or cystic fibrosis, severe neuromuscular failure, and obesity hypoventilation syndrome. In these patients, the carbic drive is no longer appropriately responsive to Pa_{CO_2} levels, and the hypoxemic drive becomes the primary ventilatory drive. These patients require hypoxemia to stimulate their ventilation ($Pa_{O_2} \approx 60–65$ mm Hg and $Sa_{O_2} \approx 92\%$). Administration of supplemental oxygen to return the Pa_{O_2} to normal or above normal levels may suppress the hypoxemic ventilatory drive, and ventilation may diminish. As a result of the oxygen-induced hypoventilation, the Pa_{CO_2} increases and the patient becomes more hypoxemic.

The role of hypoxemic drive suppression to completely explain oxygen-induced hypoventilation has been challenged.[16–21] Studies have shown that the hypoxemic drive is only marginally affected when oxygen is administered. It has been suggested that: (1) worsening $\dot{V}/\dot{Q}$ mismatching results in increased dead space; (2) abolition of the normal hypoxic vasoconstriction allows blood to flow to poorly ventilated lung zones; and (3) O_2 influences the ability of hemoglobin to bind CO_2 (the Haldane effect). Regardless of the mechanism, clinicians must be alert to the possibility of an increase in Pa_{CO_2} when administering supplemental O_2 to patients with chronic hypercapnia. Oxygen should be titrated to produce a Pa_{O_2} of 50 to 60 mm Hg with a Sp_{O_2} in the 88% to 92% level. Oxygen must never be withheld or withdrawn in the face of high or rising Pa_{CO_2}. If oxygen-induced hypercapnia results in a severely elevated Pa_{CO_2}, mechanical ventilation is indicated.

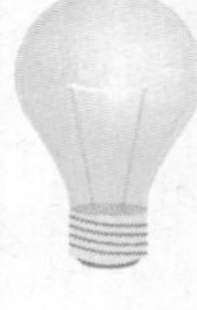

STOP AND THINK

A patient with severe COPD has a Pa_{CO_2} of 90 mm Hg and a pH of 7.35. He is using O_2 at 2 L/min by cannula and has a Sp_{O_2} of 91%. Why is it important that you tell the patient to never increase the O_2 flow?

Retinopathy of Prematurity

Retinopathy of prematurity (ROP) is an insult to the developing retinal vasculature from an elevated $Pa{O_2}$. It was first described in 1942 and termed *retrolental fibroplasia* (RLF). In ROP, oxygen radicals attack the incompletely developed retinal tissue, resulting in vasoconstriction, which can progress to complete obliteration and retinal detachment. It was initially thought that supplemental oxygen was the culprit in ROP. Elevated $Pa{O_2}$ in retinal vessel walls is only one of several predisposing factors that can result in visual defects, however, which can progress to total blindness. Low birth weight, sepsis, gestational age, apnea, acidemia/hypercarbia, oxygen levels, and length of exposure all interact as multiple causes. ROP is also seen in low-birth-weight babies who did not receive supplemental oxygen. Occurrence of blindness varies from 1% to 3% in all live births and from 40% to 70% in infants weighing less than 1 kg. The incidence is inversely proportional to birth weight and highest in neonates weighing less than 1 kg.

In the 1940s and 1950s, the incidence of ROP reached epidemic proportions because oxygen was used without monitoring. Arbitrary guidelines limiting oxygen concentration to 0.4 resulted in increased infant mortality and cerebral palsy. Perinatal oxygen-related complications were reduced with the development of arterial blood gas measurements and pulse oximetry monitoring. Dietary supplementation with vitamin E can also ameliorate the effect and reduce the incidence of ROP through the vitamin's antioxidant action. The $FI{O_2}$ of critically ill infants should be analyzed, and $Pa{O_2}$ and $Sp{O_2}$ monitored both by periodic blood gases and continuous pulse oximetry. In spite of extensive research, the clinically appropriate range for oxygen saturation in preterm infants is unknown. Initial studies suggested that a $Sa{O_2}$ target of 85–89% versus 91–95% may reduce incidence of ROP. More recent research, however, has identified a $Sa{O_2}$ target where <90% was associated with increased risk of death in extremely premature infants. It appears that the extent of prematurity, the duration of oxygen use, as well as the $Pa{O_2}$ are all factors in developing ROP.[22]

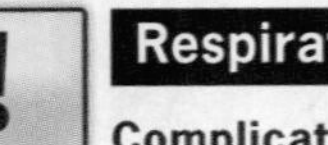

Respiratory Recap

Complications of Oxygen Therapy

- Oxygen toxicity is damage to lung tissue caused by breathing high concentrations of O_2.
- A patient's need for O_2 must override concerns about O_2 toxicity.
- Nitrogen washout atelectasis can occur with high concentrations of O_2.
- O_2-induced hypoventilation may occur in patients who rely on their hypoxemic drive.
- ROP occurs only in infants.
- Some infants with congenital heart defects need a low $Pa{O_2}$ to maintain an open ductus.
- O_2 is not explosive, but it increases the combustibility of other flammable materials.

Closure of the Ductus Arteriosis

Prior to the birth transition (in utero), while the fetal lungs develop, the placenta provides oxygen to the fetus. During this time it is important that the quantity of blood flow into the pulmonary capillary bed be limited. Therefore, fetal circulation has a blood flow bypass (shunt) to redirect blood directly from the right heart into the left heart and aorta. This right-to-left shunting is accomplished via blood flow through the foramen ovale (between the two fetal atria) and the ductus arteriosis (between the pulmonary artery and the aorta). At the time of birth, both the foramen ovale and ductus effectively close. The foramen ovale flow ceases because the pressures in the atria equalize; the ductus arteriosis must be actively closed by smooth muscle contraction.

The biochemical signal that initiates and stimulates ductus closure during the birth event is the dramatic, sudden increase in $Pa{O_2}$ that the infant experiences after beginning breathing. Neonates that experience postpartum hypoxemia are known to open the ductus (patent ductus arteriosis), which considerably exacerbates hypoxemia due to the return to the previously necessary fetal shunt. It is also notable that neonates with congenital heart defects (CHDs) often depend on patency of the ductus arteriosus for either pulmonary or systemic blood flow. Those with pulmonary atresia form the majority of cases, but cases also include those with coarctation of the aorta, tricuspid atresia, and aortic arch interruption. Newborns with these CHDs will experience profound hypoxia or circulatory collapse if the ductus closes. Increasing $P{O_2}$ is the chief trigger of ductal smooth muscle contraction, and thus a modest $Pa{O_2}$ is also indicated as a palliative measure or until corrective surgery is performed. Prostaglandin E_1 has been identified as an important drug for minimizing closure of ductus for these newborns.[23]

Support of Combustion

Fire hazard is a concern when dealing with normobaric oxygen and a major hazard in hyperbaric applications. While it should be emphasized that O_2 is not combustible, flammable, or inflammable, O_2 does support more intense combustion of fuels in proportion to its concentration. Ignition can result in a flash flame via fine surface fibers of fabric or body hair. Combustible materials (e.g., cigarettes), sparking friction toys, and electric razors should be avoided in enclosures or close to open sources of O_2. O_2 administration is a fire risk during laser bronchoscopy.

Dosage Regulation and Administration Devices

Once the gas pressure has been reduced to the safe working pressure of 50 psig (by a cylinder/pressure regulator system or as supplied by a bedside gas distribution station connector), a device to provide more refined control of flow is usually needed. For example, when O_2 or gas mixtures are administered directly to the patient via mask, aerosol, or nasal cannula, a method for metering the flow is necessary. On the other hand, some equipment (such as blenders and ventilators) meter flow internally and do not need an external flow meter device. The respiratory therapist must understand this difference. Flow control devices can be categorized as follows:

- *Flow restrictor:* A preset, fixed flow controller.
- *Bourdon gauge flow meter:* An adjustable flow controller, with adjustable inlet pressure from a fixed outlet orifice.
- *Thorpe tube flow meter:* An adjustable flow controller, with preset inlet pressure from an adjustable outlet orifice.

Flow Restrictor

The most basic flow meter is commercially known as a **flow restrictor**. It is a carefully machined orifice attached to a 50-psig gas source. There are no adjustments and no gauges. A flow restrictor (**Figure 14-2**) has a specific-size orifice that allows a specific flow of gas to pass, provided the inlet pressure is a constant 50 psig. Flow restrictors are uncomplicated, require no maintenance (because they have no moving parts), can be used in any position, and do not allow accidental changes in flow. When a flow change is necessary, however, the single-flow flow restrictor must be removed and replaced by another with an orifice delivering the appropriate flow.

This need can be met by the use of an adjustable flow restrictor that allows the selection of one of a number of orifices, depending on the flow required. Adjustable multiorifice flow meters in combination with an indirect single-stage, preset regulator are commonly used on small cylinders in home care or patient transport because of their compact and lightweight configuration. Other applications include emergency resuscitation packs, in which compact, lightweight devices require relatively high flows to a bag-valve-mask device. Because there is no way to indicate the actual flow, flow restrictors should be periodically checked with a calibration flow meter.

The outlet flow on a flow restrictor can be calculated using the following equation:

$$\dot{V} = (P_1 - P_2)/R$$

where $\dot{V}$ is the flow per unit of time (L/min), P_1 is the inlet pressure (50 psig), P_2 is the outlet pressure (atmospheric), and R is the resistance to gas flow through the orifice. Any change to the $P_1 - P_2$ relationship alters the accuracy of the output flow, which occurs if the inlet pressure varies from 50 psig or if increased resistance is present downstream from the orifice outlet, creating backpressure.

Bourdon Gauge Flow Meters

Like the flow restrictor, the **Bourdon gauge flow meter** has a fixed outlet orifice, but the pressure regulator is adjustable, which facilitates the adjustment of flow output by varying the pressure supply. The change in pressure is displayed on the Bourdon gauge face, which has been calibrated (labeled) in L/min, corresponding to the predictable flows at the variable inlet pressures. The Bourdon gauge is positioned between the pressure source and the fixed orifice. The gas pressure is transmitted to the gauge through a hollow tube. As the pressure increases, the closed distal end of the curved hollow tube is straightened (**Figure 14-3**).

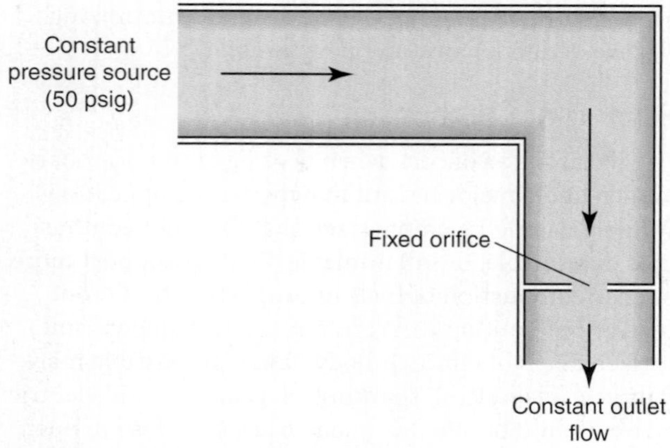

FIGURE 14-2 Fixed orifice flow restrictor.

Reproduced from *Egan's Fundamentals of Respiratory Care*, Seventh Edition. Scanlan CL, Wilkins RL, Stoller JK. Copyright Elsevier (Mosby) 1999.

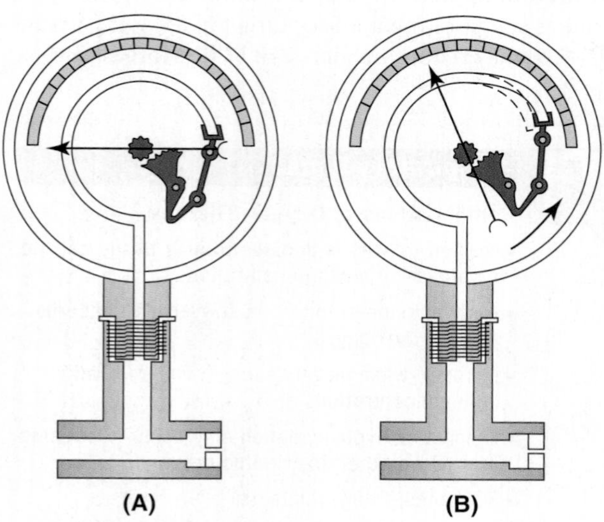

FIGURE 14-3 Bourdon flow gauge, showing the hollow pressure tube and gearing mechanism in an unpressurized state (**A**) and a pressurized state (**B**). An increase in pressure causes straightening of the tube and movement of the indicator needle.

Modified from Ward JJ. Equipment for mixed gas and oxygen therapy. In: Barnes TA, ed. *Core Textbook of Respiratory Care Practice*, 2nd ed. Mosby; 1994.

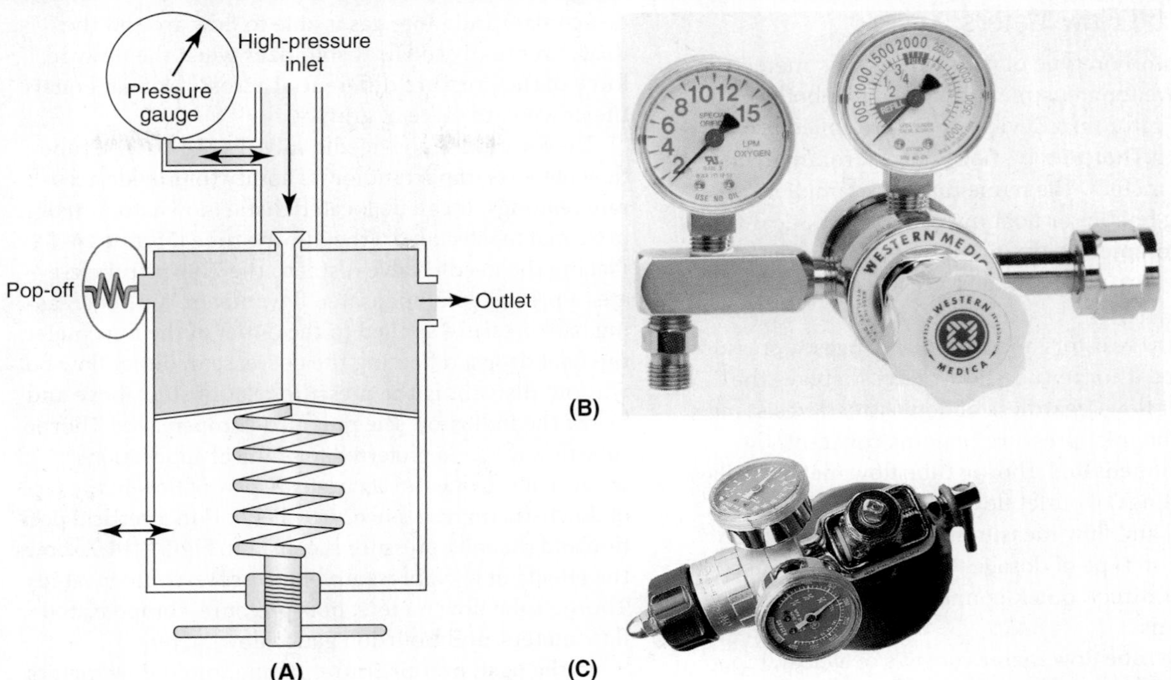

FIGURE 14-4 (**A**) Adjustable, direct-acting, single-stage, high-pressure-reducing regulator. (**B**) A single-stage, adjustable American Standard Safety System (ASSS) regulator with two Bourdon gauges. The gauge to the right, closest to the connection to the gas source, is calibrated in pounds per square inch (psi), indicating the contents of the cylinder. The Bourdon gauge closest to the outlet is calibrated in liters per minute (L/min). Flow is set by turning the knob, increasing or decreasing the regulator pressure and thus the outlet flow through the fixed orifice. (**C**) Pin indexed (PISS) Bourdon gauge flow meter on an oxygen cylinder.

(**A**) reproduced from *Egan's Fundamentals of Respiratory Care*, Seventh Edition. Scanlan CL, Wilkins RL, Stoller JK. Copyright Elsevier (Mosby) 1999; (**B**) courtesy of Western Enterprises, a Scott Fetzer company.

It is linked to a gear system and an indicator needle pointing to the calculated output flow for that pressure. Clinical devices frequently have two gauges: one that indicates cylinder pressure, and one that indicates the flow output (**Figure 14-4**). The gauge closest to the cylinder indicates the pressure contents of the cylinder.

With Bourdon gauge flow meters, the flow meter will deliver accurate flow rates if the outlet flow is unrestricted. When resistance is added downstream of the fixed outlet orifice, however, such as the addition of a long length of tubing and respiratory equipment, the outlet pressure (P_2) rises and the actual outlet flow is decreased (**Figure 14-5**). In fact, if the Bourdon gauge outlet were completely obstructed, the gauge would continue to show flow when none would be present. Because pneumatic nebulizers present a large downstream resistance to the flow meter, they should not be used with a Bourdon gauge if accurate indication of flow rate is necessary.

Bourdon gauges are commonly used on medical gas cylinders for transport and when a mask or nasal cannula is used. These compact flow meters are handy because flow can be changed (in contrast to flow restrictors) and they can be read correctly without being held in a vertical (gravity-dependent position).

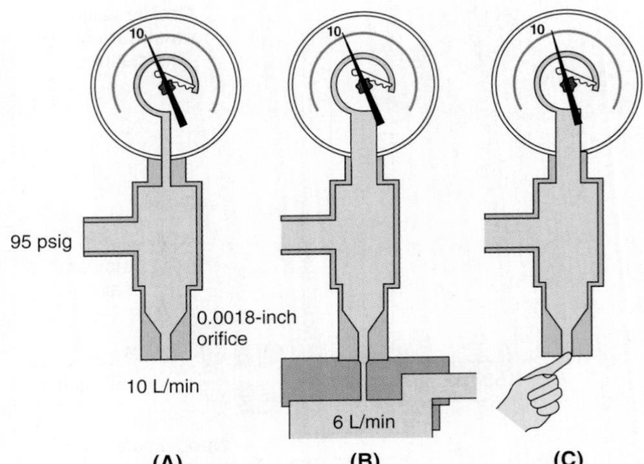

FIGURE 14-5 Bourdon gauge illustrating (**A**) that with a constant inlet pressure and a known fixed outlet orifice size, a predictable outlet flow is achieved and is indicated on the gauge face. Adding resistance downstream of the fixed outlet orifice (**B**) causes flow to be diminished, yet the gauge reading remains unchanged because it measures the pressure prior to the resistance. If the outlet orifice is completely obstructed (**C**), allowing no flow, the gauge continues to read a flow even though there is none because it continues to read preobstruction pressure.

Thorpe Tube Flow Meters

The most common type of medical gas flow meter has a needle valve for adjustment of flow and a hollow tube with an indicator float device. These are called pressure-compensated **Thorpe tube flow meters**, rotameters, or simply flow meters. The name *rotameter* implies use of a rotating bobbin or float instead of a spherical-type indicator. Rotameters are often used to administer anesthetic gases, which require greater accuracy in flow indication.

Unlike flow resistors and Bourdon gauges, a pressure-compensated Thorpe tube flow meter displays the actual outlet flow regardless of downstream resistance. As long as the inlet pressure remains constant, the pressure-compensated Thorpe tube flow meter displays correct readings of outlet flow. For this reason, these flow control and flow measurement devices are the most common type of dosage regulation device used in hospitals for direct, quick-connect application to piped outlet stations.

A Thorpe tube flow meter consists of a clear, tapered glass tube with a diameter that is larger at the top than at the bottom. The tube has graduated markings calibrated to indicate flow (usually liters or milliliters per minute). A float in the glass tube indicates the gas flow and a needle valve controls the flow. When the needle valve is opened, gas flows from the pressure source. Gas entering the bottom of the Thorpe tube creates a pressure differential significant enough to lift the float. As the float rises in the tapered tube, the diameter of the tube increases (equivalent to an increase in the outlet orifice size) and more gas is able to flow around the float. Eventually the float stabilizes when the upward force of the pressure differential across the float equals the downward force of gravity.

The location of the needle valve in the Thorpe tube flow meter is important for its ability to provide accurate readings. It can be located distal (downstream) or proximal (upstream) to the Thorpe tube (**Figure 14-6**). Placing the needle valve distal to the Thorpe tube creates a pressure-compensated flow meter. With increasing backpressure applied to the outlet of the flow meter, the float drops, reflecting the decrease in outlet flow but without disturbing the pressure relationship above and below the indicator. The pressure-compensated Thorpe tube flow meter is preferred for clinical applications because it provides an accurate display of flow in the face of downstream resistance, provided it is in a vertical position and the inlet pressure is constant. **Figure 14-7** shows the effects of back pressure on pressure-compensated Thorpe tube flow meters, non-pressure-compensated flow meters, and Bourdon gauge flow meters.

In the past, non-pressure-compensated flow meters were commonly used for medical applications. They are still used for laboratory or industrial applications. The non-pressure-compensated version of the Thorpe tube flow meter has the needle valve located proximal to the Thorpe tube. When a flow-restricting device is attached to a non-pressure-compensated Thorpe tube flow meter, increasing the downstream resistance, the pressure relationship above and below the ball is distorted within the Thorpe tube, which forces the float downward and provides a reading lower than the actual flow.

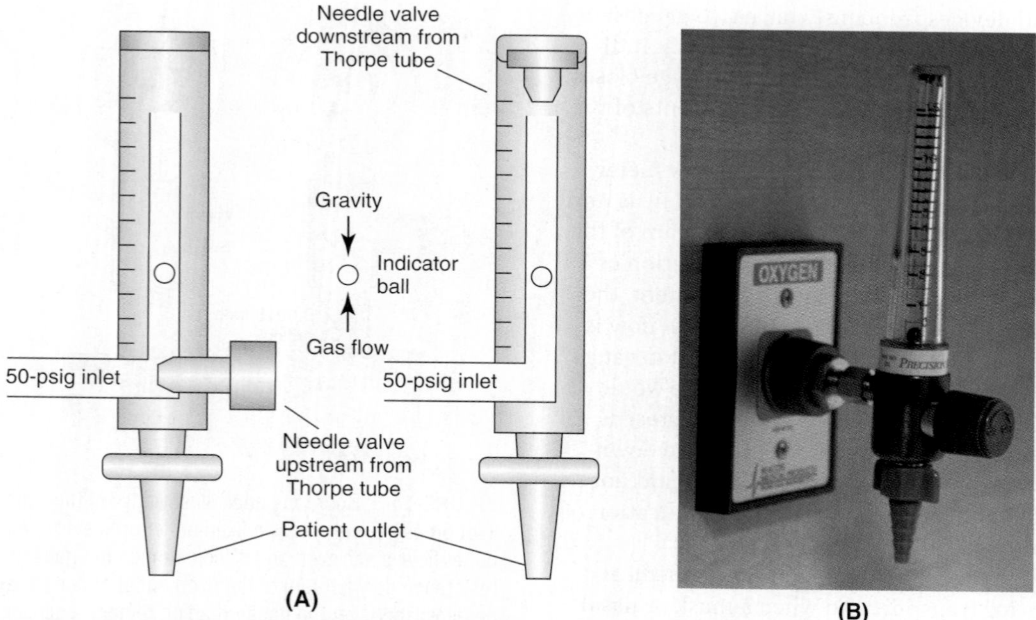

FIGURE 14-6 (**A**) Non-pressure compensated Thorpe tube flow meter (left) in which the needle valve is placed before the Thorpe tube and diagram of a flow meter (right) with the needle valve placement after the Thorpe tube (back-pressure-compensated). (**B**) Commercially available Thorpe tube flow meter.

(**A**) modified from Cairo JM, Pilbeam SP. *Mosby's Respiratory Care Equipment*, 6th ed. Mosby; 1999; (**B**) © Jones & Bartlett Learning. Courtesy of MIEMSS.

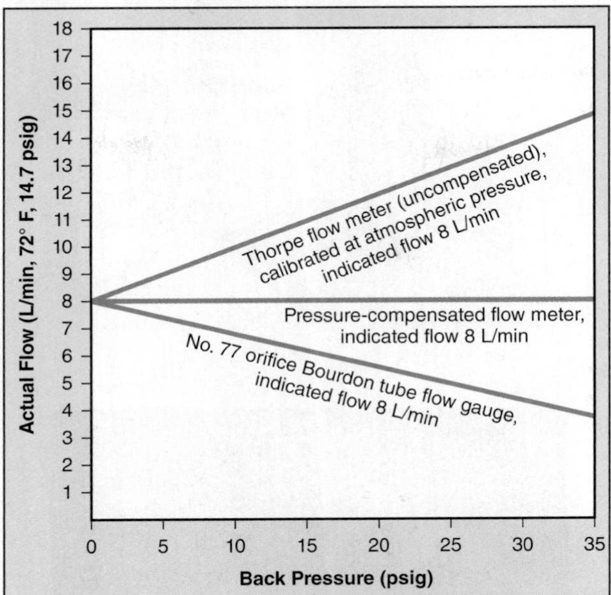

FIGURE 14-7 Comparison of the accuracy of pressure-compensated and noncompensated Thorpe tube flow meters and a Bourdon gauge when faced with increasing levels of downstream back pressure. The pressure-compensated Thorpe tube's indicated flow is the actual flow regardless of back pressure. With a noncompensated Thorpe tube, actual flow is higher than the indicated flow at increasing downstream pressure. With the Bourdon gauge, indicated flow is progressively higher than actual flow as back pressure increases.

Modified from McPherson SP, Spearman CB. *Respiratory Therapy Equipment*. 5th ed. Mosby; 1995.

Determining whether a Thorpe tube flow meter is pressure compensated can be done when the needle valve is closed and the flow meter subsequently pressurized as the cylinder valve is opened or is connected to a station outlet. If the Thorpe tube flow meter is pressure compensated, the float will rise to the top of the tube and then fall back as gas rushes in and fills the tube to the needle valve.

Most Thorpe tube flow meters commonly used in respiratory therapy use a ball as the float, although the float may assume various shapes and configurations. Sighting the float at eye level is important to avoid inaccuracy due to parallax. A ball float is read through the center of the ball, whereas rotameter floats are read at the top surface. The majority of clinical flow meters are scaled from 0 to 16 L/min. The need for more accurate reading of low flows for infants and oxygen-sensitive adult patients has fostered development of 0- to 1-L/min or 0- to 5-L/min flow meters. Most Thorpe-type flow meters also have a flush setting beyond the calibrated range. Although there is no industry standard, most flow meters provide greater than 60 L/min on the flush setting. High-flow oxygen delivery systems (requiring calibrated flow measurements) have prompted manufacturers to develop 0- to 75-L/min Thorpe tubes.

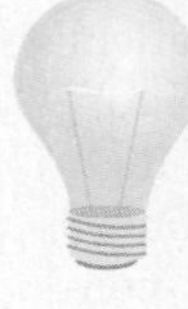

STOP AND THINK

A patient is receiving O_2 by nasal cannula at 4 L/min. She needs to be transported to magnetic resonance imaging (MRI). The E-cylinder must be attached horizontal to the hospital bed. What would be your considerations when selecting a cylinder and flow meter?

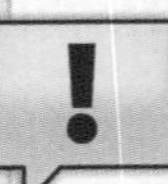

Respiratory Recap

Flow Meters

- Flow restrictors are preset, fixed flow meters.
- Pressure-compensated Thorpe flow meters indicate actual flow unless the source gas pressure varies from 50 psig or the float tube is not set in the vertical position.
- Bourdon gauges, although less accurate, are used whenever a patient application requires that the regulator not be vertical.

Oxygen Administration Devices

O_2 therapy systems generally are categorized as either **low-flow/variable-performance** or **high-flow/fixed-performance devices**. Variable-performance devices (commonly referred to as low-flow devices) provide variable and approximate FIO_2, whereas fixed-performance devices (commonly referred to as high-flow devices) are designed to provide a fixed and known FIO_2.

The descriptive names most commonly employed (low flow and high flow) can be confusing to the respiratory therapy student. The distinguishing characteristic of the two devices is whether the device in question provides a premixed, precise, and known FIO_2 (fixed performance) or whether the FIO_2 received by the patient will be a function of the patient's breathing pattern and volume in combination with supplemental 1.0 FIO_2 gas administered by the device (variable performance).

For example, a patient using a nasal cannula (which is a low-flow device) receives a flow of 100% O_2 at 0 to 6 L/min. The flow of gas coming from the nasal cannula is continuous across both inspiration and expiration, but during inspiration the patient will inhale an inspiratory volume composed of some of the 100% O_2 and some air present in the room (0.21 FIO_2). The FIO_2 that enters the trachea and is eventually delivered to the alveoli thus varies from patient to patient, and in fact from breath to breath, depending on the tidal volume and respiratory rate and pattern. This means that low-flow devices provide variable performance in the sense that the delivered FIO_2 cannot be accurately known.

On the other hand, high-flow devices are designed to produce flow outputs that meet or exceed the patient's full inspiratory flow demand and are more likely to maintain a fixed FIO_2. As with low-flow devices, high-flow devices provide gas continuously (throughout inspiration and expiration) but at the desired O_2 concentration (FIO_2). The major difference between high-flow and low-flow devices is that the high-flow device provides such a high flow of premixed gas that the patient is not likely to inhale any room air. Examples of high-flow devices include air-entrainment devices such as masks and large-volume nebulizers.

Low-Flow (Variable-Performance) Devices

The primary distinguishing feature of low-flow O_2 administration devices is that the patient experiences a variable FIO_2 as changed through variations in minute ventilation (especially changes in tidal volume, inspiratory flow, and respiratory rate). This is because the device delivers 100% O_2 to the patient's upper airway, which is mixed during inspiration with variable amounts of inhaled room air to produce the final delivered FIO_2. Examples of low-flow O_2 administration devices are the nasal cannula, simple mask, partial rebreathing mask, nonrebreathing mask, and transtracheal O_2 catheter.

Low-Flow Nasal Cannula (LFNC)

The **nasal oxygen cannula** (**Figure 14-8**) is the most widely used device for administering low-flow O_2 to infants, children, and adults in the hospital and the home. The LFNC is easily applied and well tolerated by most patients when used with flows up to 6 L/min. The nasal cannula consists of a delivery tube that ends in two short prongs, each about one-half inch long and made of soft, pliable plastic. Cannula prongs are available in a variety of styles, sizes for adults and infants, curved or straight, tapered or nontapered. The nasal prongs are held in place either with an elastic band around the head or by loops of the delivery tubing over the ears, which are then held in place with an adjustable slide placed under the chin.

When oxygen is delivered by LFNC to adults, the expected delivery may be an FIO_2 of 0.22 to 0.24 at 1 L/min and up to about 0.40 at 5 to 6 L/min. Actual FIO_2 levels achieved with a nasal cannula at specific oxygen flows have been debated for many years. A wide range of FIO_2 levels are delivered to the trachea because of the variability of this device.[24–30] Although the standard cannula is usually used at flows of 1 to 6 L/min, flow can be increased to 10 to 15 L/min, which can achieve tracheal concentrations of 0.4 to 0.5. That level of flow is uncomfortable and should be considered only for short-term use.

Figure 14-9 provides a graphic representation of the factors that affect the FIO_2 by nasal cannula.[35] One area

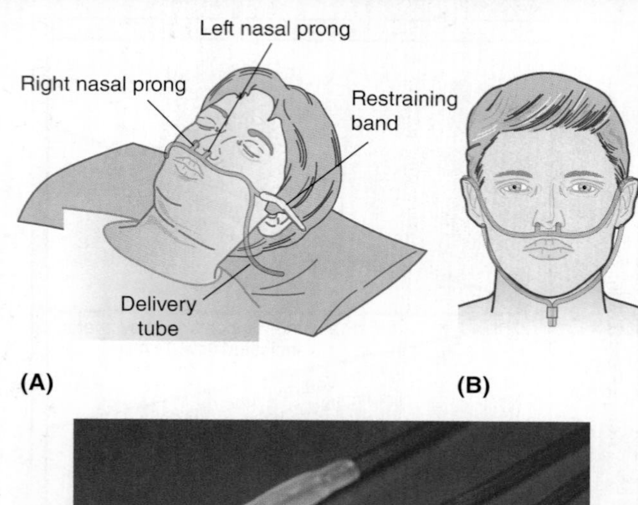

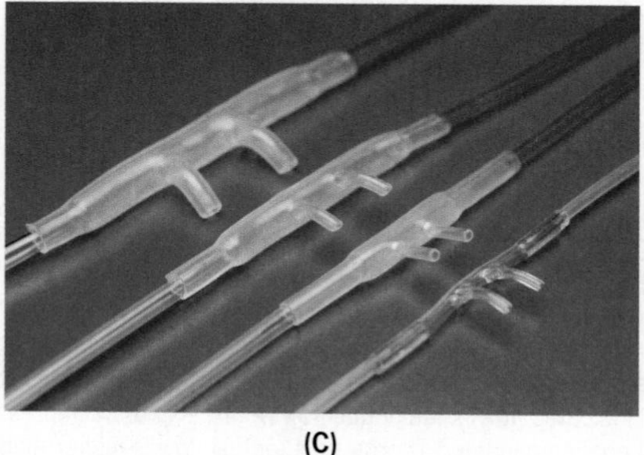

FIGURE 14-8 (**A**) Nasal cannula with elastic strap. (**B**) Over-the-ear style nasal cannula. (**C**) Various styles of nasal prongs.

(**A**) and (**B**) adapted from Scanlan CL, et al. *Egan's Fundamentals of Respiratory Care*. 7th ed. Mosby; 1999; (**C**) courtesy of Teleflex Incorporated. Unauthorized use prohibited.

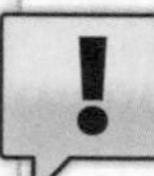

Respiratory Recap

Low-Flow Oxygen Delivery Devices

- FIO_2 is the actual dose of O_2 administered.
- Low-flow devices provide only a portion of the patient's tidal volume.
- FIO_2 of low-flow devices will vary depending on patient breathing patterns as well as the oxygen flow delivered.
- Low-flow devices are titrated with pulse oximetry or arterial blood gases to achieve acceptable SpO_2 and/or PaO_2.
- The low-flow nasal cannula consists of nasal prongs delivering 1 to 6 L/min in adults, which provide 0.24–0.40 FIO_2 when breathing patterns are normal.
- With a high-flow nasal cannula, larger bore nasal prongs are fitted to nearly fill the naris, and warmed, humidified O_2 is delivered at flows up to 40 L/min.
- The partial rebreathing mask uses low-flow oxygen yet can achieve higher concentrations with an attached unvalved reservoir bag (0.40–0.70 FIO_2).
- The nonrebreathing mask uses low-flow oxygen yet can achieve higher concentrations with an attached valved reservoir bag (0.60–0.90 FIO_2).

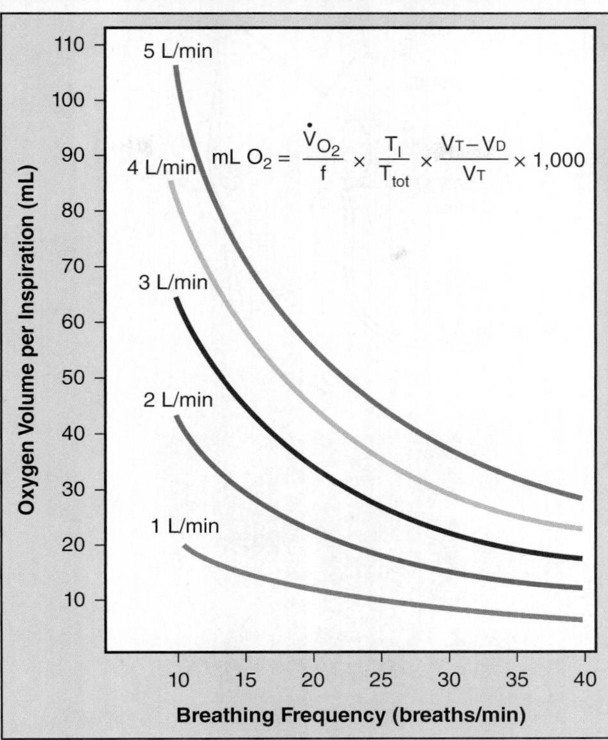

FIGURE 14-9 Factors that affect the volume of oxygen inspired by nasal cannula.

Reproduced from Shigeoka JW, Bonekat HW. The current status of oxygen-conserving devices (editorial). *Respir Care*. 1985;30:833–836.

of confusion is the effect of mouth breathing with nasal cannula. Although mouth breathing might lower the FIO_2, the nasal cannula is an effective O_2 delivery device even when the patient inspired through the mouth because O_2 still flows through the nose into the pharynx.

Physical examination findings and SpO_2 measurements are the most important clinical assessments with the LFNC. A bedside estimate may be useful when initiating therapy for patients with normal breathing conditions and flows up to 5 L/min, however. The delivered FIO_2 will increase approximately 0.025 (2.5%) per each 1 L/min above ambient oxygen level (**Equation 14-1**).

When the LFNC is applied to the patient, clinicians should confirm actual flow from the distal prongs by feeling for gas flow. Absent or inappropriately low flow should prompt the operator to troubleshoot the gas source, flow meter, or whether the cannula or connecting tubing may be kinked. A leak at the humidifier bottle seal (if used) is also possible.

O_2 flow to a LFNC should initially be titrated to each patient using vital signs and pulse oximetry. At a minimum, the respiratory therapist should record set O_2 flow, respiratory rate and SpO_2 in the patient's record. When adult patients' respiratory rates approach or exceed 20 breaths/min, FIO_2 will likely be well below textbook guidelines or calculated bedside estimates. Further titration of flow to the LFNC is ultimately guided by a combination of patient exam findings and SpO_2 or arterial

EQUATION 14-1

Estimation of FIO_2 with Adult Low-Flow Nasal Cannula

Estimated FIO_2 = (Flow × 0.025) + 0.21 ± 0.005
or Estimated % O_2 = (Flow × 2.5) + 21% ± 0.5%

Example: If cannula flow = 2 L/min, estimated FIO_2 = (2 L/min × 0.025) + 0.21 = 0.5 + 0.21= 0.26, with a range of 0.25 to 0.265, or estimated % O_2 = 26%

Example: If cannula flow = 5 L/min, estimated FIO_2 = (5 L/min × 0.025) + 0.21 = 0.125 + 0.21= 0.33, with a range of 0.32 to 0.335, or estimated % O_2 = 33%

blood gas values. The most practical application of an estimated FIO_2 is to determine the approximate FIO_2 for patients whose pulmonary conditions have worsened in order to establish an FIO_2 starting point to selecting higher FIO_2 and/or high-flow O_2 therapy systems. As a comfort compromise, some clinicians combine a LFNC with additional flow from an oxygen mask to provide a higher FIO_2 by additional nonnasal O_2 flow.

A frequent patient complaint while using a LFNC is drying of the nasal mucosa. This problem has been partially addressed by use of bubble humidifiers.[31,32] Because these devices are unheated, they are inefficient, and some hospitals do not routinely use them. Patients may also experience discomfort due to pressure of tubing or elastic when in long-term contact with the face or ears. Gauze padding can be added to protect pressure points on the ears and/or cheekbones. Commercially available foam ear protectors are also available for this purpose (**Figure 14-10**).

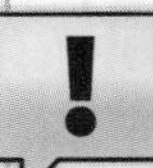

Respiratory Recap

Low-Flow Nasal Cannula

- Factors affecting the inhaled volume of oxygen: flow, concentration of O_2 from flow meter, volume inspired, respiratory rate, total respiratory time or cycle time, inspiratory time, inspiratory flow, inspiratory flow pattern
- Factors that might cause air dilution of inspired oxygen: open-mouth or closed-mouth breathing, diameter of cannula compared to lumen of nares, volume of anatomic airways acting as a reservoir and dead space
- Secondary variables that might alter CPAP effect with high flows: total gas flow, resistance characteristics of airways, sealing characteristics of cannula in patient's nares

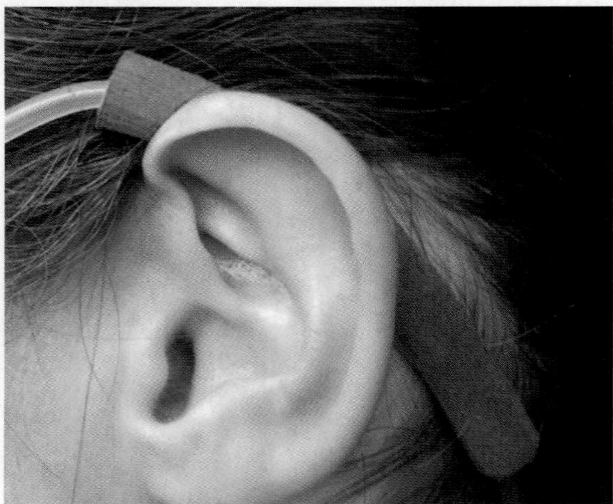

FIGURE 14-10 Ear pads to decrease pressure sores with use of nasal cannula.
Courtesy of Westmed, Inc.

Low-flow nasal cannulas are available in sizes appropriate for infants, toddlers, and children. Because of these patients' small tidal volumes and rapid respiratory frequencies, the O_2 flow to infants and children should be precisely controlled by use of flow meters with an appropriate scale (0 to 1 or 2 L/min in increments of 0.25 or 0.0625 L/min). A flow of 0.25 L/min by nasal cannula to an infant can achieve an F_{IO_2} of 0.35, and more than 0.60 at 1 L/min is possible. Because even minor alterations in flow can result in drastic F_{IO_2} changes, O_2/air blenders have been used to independently set both flow and F_{IO_2} to the cannula to allow greater control. When flows to infants approach or exceed 2 L/min a CPAP-like effect may occur.[33]

Simple Mask

The **simple or nonreservoir oxygen mask** is used when a higher F_{IO_2} is needed than can be attained with a nasal cannula or when a cannula is not appropriate because of nasal obstruction, such as in emergency situations and during and after minor surgical procedures. The simple oronasal mask is a disposable plastic product available in infant, child, and adult sizes, with a length of small-diameter oxygen supply tubing connected to the base of the mask. The masks fit over the bridge of the nose and often are held in place with a malleable aluminum strip, which helps minimize leakage toward the eyes. They cover the nose and mouth down to below the lower lip or to under the chin and are held in place by an elastic band around the head. There is no sealing device (similar to resuscitation masks) and exhaled air leaves via side holes and between the mask and face; inboard inhalation of room air also can occur (**Figure 14-11**).

The simple O_2 mask increases the inspired oxygen concentration by acting as an oxygen reservoir, adding a volume in an adult mask of 100 to 200 mL, which is inhaled at the beginning of inspiration. The patient also inhales room air through a series of small holes in the mask. The amount of oxygen enrichment of the inspired air depends on mask volume, pattern of ventilation, and the oxygen flow to the mask. It is difficult to predict the delivered F_{IO_2} at specific flows. During normal breathing, it is reasonable to expect a range from 0.3 to 0.6 with flows of 5 to 10 L/min, respectively. Oxygen levels can be higher with small tidal volumes or slow breathing rates. With higher flows and normal breathing patterns, F_{IO_2} may approach 0.4 to 0.8.

Because the mask accumulates CO_2 during exhalation, the oxygen flow rate must be sufficient to wash out the mask and prevent rebreathing.[34] A general recommendation is that a minimum flow of 5 L/min should be used to avoid accumulation of exhaled CO_2. The simple mask is a low-flow, variable-performance oxygen delivery system capable of providing an F_{IO_2} of from 0.3

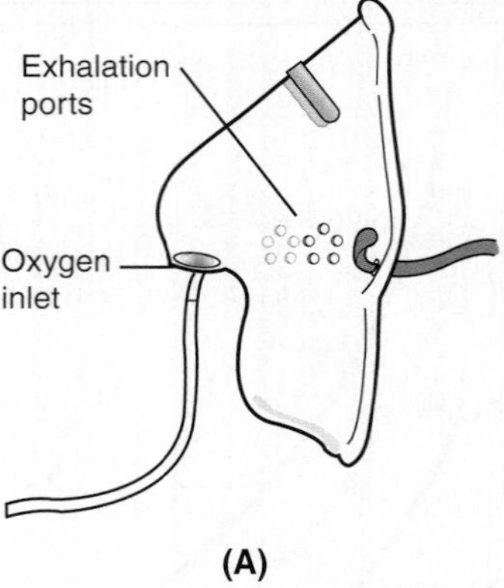

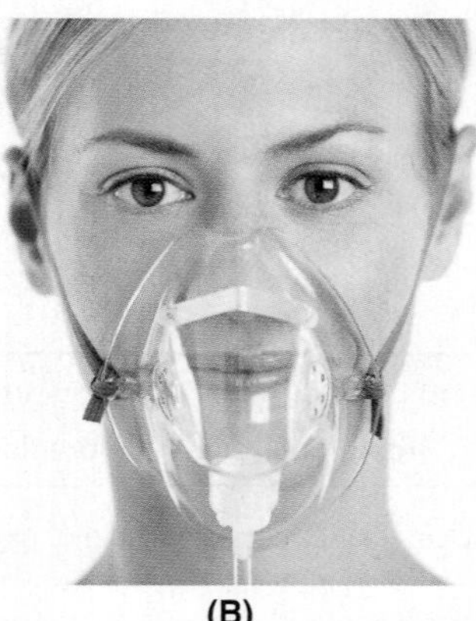

FIGURE 14-11 (**A**) Components of a simple O_2 mask. (**B**) Simple O_2 mask on patient.
(**A**) modified from Scanlan CL, et al. *Egan's Fundamentals of Respiratory Care.* 7th ed. Mosby; 1999; (**B**) © corbis/age fotostock.

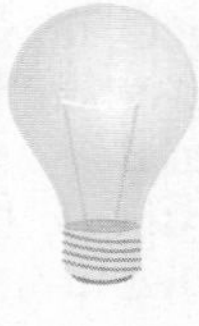

STOP AND THINK

You are asked to assess a patient with COPD. When you arrive at the bedside, you note that he is receiving O_2 at 2 L/min by simple mask. His Sp_{O_2} is 90%. What would be your response?

to 0.6 at flows of 5 to 10 L/min, depending on the size of the mask and the patient's respiratory pattern.

All oronasal masks present the same problems, which include claustrophobic feelings for some patients, speech muffling, and difficulty with eating and drinking. Additionally, any mask administration device increases the possibility of aspirating regurgitated stomach contents.

Partial Rebreathing Mask

The **partial rebreathing mask (Figure 14-12)** combines the simple mask with the addition of an attached nonvalved 300- to 600-mL reservoir bag. The partial rebreathing mask is somewhat misnamed because although there is some insignificant rebreathing of exhaled gas, the mask's actual indication is primarily for administering relatively high O_2 concentrations to severely hypoxemic patients. The oxygen supply tube is positioned between the mask and the reservoir bag. The oxygen flow is set at a rate sufficient to keep the bag at least partially inflated throughout inspiration. This flow varies depending on the patient's respiratory pattern but is usually between 8 and 15 L/min, which produces an F_{IO_2} in the range of 0.4 to 0.7, depending on the patient's respiratory pattern.

When the patient exhales, the exhaled gas exits the mask through the vents on the sides, because fresh 100% O_2 from the supply tubing continues to inflate the reservoir. When the patient then takes the next breath, the inspiratory gas is composed of a mixture of 100% O_2 from the O_2 source, the 100% O_2 that filled the reservoir during exhalation, and some room air inhaled through the mask ports.

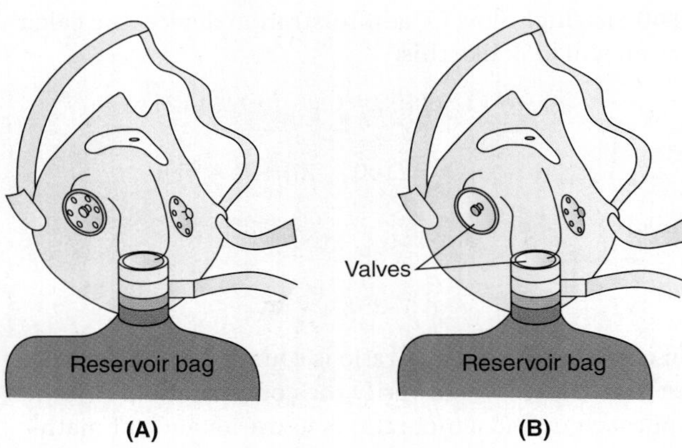

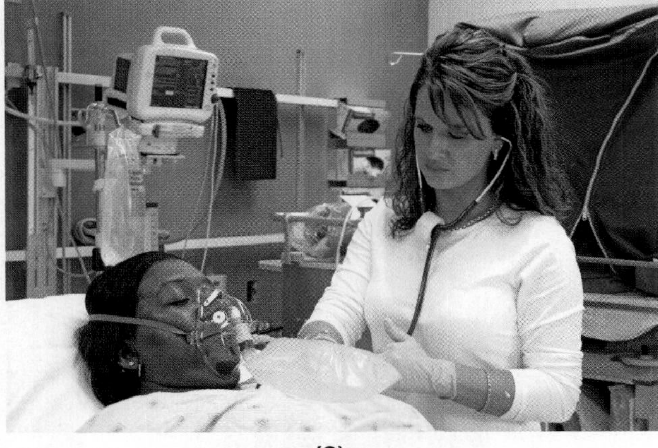

FIGURE 14-12 **(A)** Partial rebreathing mask. **(B)** Nonrebreathing mask. **(C)** Commercially available nonrebreathing mask.

(A) and **(B)** are modified from Scanlan CL, et al. *Egan's Fundamentals of Respiratory Care.* 7th ed. Mosby; 1999; **(C)** © Andrew Gentry/Shutterstock, Inc.

Nonrebreathing Mask

The **nonrebreathing mask (NRB)** uses the same basic system as the partial rebreathing mask but incorporates valves both between the bag and mask and on at least one of the exhalation side ports. O_2 is directed into the mask and into the reservoir bag by small-bore tubing. A one-way valve prevents exhaled gas from entering the reservoir; the entire exhaled volume exits the mask through the mask ports and between face and mask. During exhalation, the reservoir bag can refill with O_2. At the beginning of inspiration, the mask exhalation port valves close, minimizing room air from being drawn in, and the reservoir valve opens, allowing the patient to inhale 300 to 500 mL of O_2 from the reservoir in addition to the oxygen flow. If the system were perfect, delivery of 100% oxygen would be possible. These inexpensive disposable masks cannot provide an airtight fit on the face, however, and their valves are simple rubber or vinyl disks that do not provide a perfect seal. But at flows of 10 to 15 L/min, an F_{IO_2} of 0.6 to 0.8 is achievable during normal breathing conditions. As with the partial rebreathing mask, the O_2 flow must be set at a rate high enough to prevent the bag from emptying more than half. A NRB is indicated for patients who require a high F_{IO_2} but tend to have a relatively normal respiratory pattern. Such patients may include victims of trauma, MI, or carbon monoxide exposure.

Because there is a risk of suffocation if the mask valves stick or the O_2 supply fails, some safety system must be provided to allow room air to enter and prevent suffocation. Some manufacturers provide spring-loaded antisuffocation valves at the neck of the reservoir bag. The spring-loaded antisuffocation valve opens if the pressure in the mask becomes subatmospheric, as happens when the O_2 supply fails. Other manufacturers provide the nonrebreathing mask with a valve on only one side of the mask.

High-Flow (Fixed-Performance) Devices

Precise delivery of F_{IO_2} is required to supply therapeutic levels of O_2 and avoid complications. Several methods exist for control of F_{IO_2} and delivery of adequate flow to meet inspiratory demands. High-flow O_2 administration devices blend 100% O_2 and room air (21% O_2) to produce a gas with the desired F_{IO_2} and provide a flow of the gas high enough to prevent the patient from

Respiratory Recap

High-Flow Oxygen Delivery Devices

- High-flow, fixed-performance O_2 administration devices deliver a predictable FIO_2.
- Mix ratios can be calculated or memorized.
- FIO_2 and flow affect delivered FIO_2 and, in some devices, can be controlled independently.
- FIO_2 is reduced if patient inspiratory flow exceeds the device's total flow output.
- Flow minimum is 3 to 4 times the minute ventilation.
- Minimum total flow for infants is 4 to 6 L/min, and for adults it is 40 L/min.
- Large-volume nebulizers use an air-entrainment mechanism for FIO_2 mixing.
- Air-entrainment masks deliver a precise low FIO_2 but have limited flow for $FIO_2 > 0.4$.
- High-flow generators are engineered to maintain accurate FIO_2 at high levels of flow.
- Dual flow meters can be used to accurately mix O_2 and air and also adjust flows.
- Air–oxygen blenders require 50-psig sources of both air and O_2.

diluting the FIO_2 with room air. High-flow O_2 delivery devices accomplish this by exceeding any tidal volume, respiratory frequency, or inspiratory flow that the patient might produce. Adult patients with gasping inspirations with flows >40 to 60 L/min and/or sustained respiratory rates >20 breaths/min are potential candidates for high-flow delivery systems.

Although high-flow O_2 administration devices potentially offer a constant FIO_2, this may not occur in all clinical situations. The respiratory therapist, thus, must understand the performance characteristics, design, and engineering constraints of each device. For example, if the patient's inspiratory flow exceeds the flow from the device, the patient will dilute the FIO_2 by breathing in additional room air. If this is not recognized, clinicians might be misled into falsely thinking that the patient is receiving a specific concentration of O_2.

Proportioning 100% O_2 and 21% O_2 (room air) to produce a specific FIO_2 is very much like making any solution, except that the solvent and the solute each contain some amount of O_2. For example, if the respiratory therapist wishes to provide a 40% mixture of O_2, each liter of 100% O_2 must be diluted with approximately 3 liters of 21% room air. Because of quality differences between devices and discrepancies in the calibration of flow meters, it is clinically important to verify any O_2 concentration from any high-flow O_2 administration device with an O_2 analyzer.

Air-to-oxygen mix ratios are highly predictable and can be mathematically modeled using relatively simple processes. One strategy used by some respiratory therapists is to memorize key mix ratios for common FIO_2 levels (**Table 14-3**). Another strategy is to use a variant of the volume-concentration formula:

TABLE 14-3
Air-to-Oxygen Mix Ratios for Various FIO_2 Levels

FIO_2	Mix Ratio (Air:O_2 Ratio)
0.24	25:1
0.28	10:1
0.30	8:1
0.35	5:1
0.40	3:1
0.50	1.7:1
0.60	1:1
0.70	0.6:1
0.80	0.3:1

$$V_1 \times C_1 = V_2 \times C_2$$

For example, if one wishes to find the mix ratio for a 0.40 FIO_2 high-flow O_2 administration device, the calculation will look like this:

$$\text{Air-to-}O_2 = (100 - O_2\%)/(O_2\% - 21){:}1$$

$$\text{Air-to-}O_2 = (100 - 40)/(40 - 21){:}1$$

$$\text{Air-to-}O_2 = (60/19){:}1$$

$$\text{Air-to-}O_2 = 3{:}1$$

In clinical use, this mix ratio is rounded to 3:1, because an O_2 analyzer would verify the concentration. Another approach to find a mix ratio is to use an ancient mathematical shortcut, which is known as the *alligation alternate* (sometimes referred to as the magic box). **Figure 14-13** illustrates this approach.

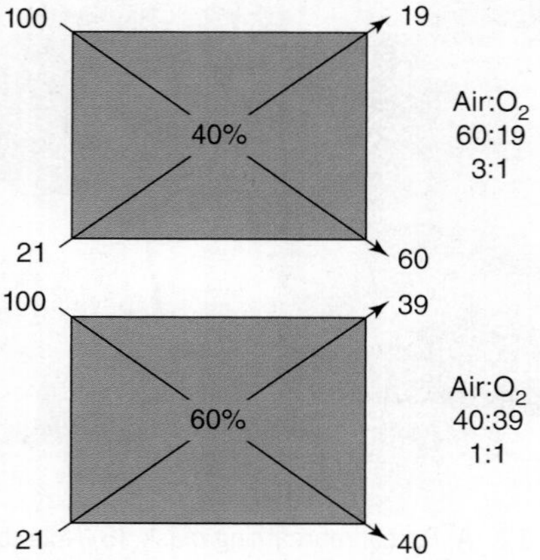

FIGURE 14-13 Magic box to determine oxygen-to-air ratio when mixing O_2 and air. Examples are shown for 40% and 60% O_2.

TABLE 14-4
Flows of Oxygen, Air, and Total Flow for a 40% O_2 Mixing Device

L/min of Oxygen	L/min of Air	Total Flow in L/min
1	3	4
2	6	8
3	9	12
4	12	16
10	30	40

Once the mix ratio is determined, the total gas flow must be determined. A total flow of 40 L/min is sufficient to meet or exceed the inspiratory demands of almost all adult patients. To obtain the desired F_{IO_2} in sufficient quantities, one can calculate various increasing 100% O_2 flows, proportionally increasing the air flow to maintain the desired F_{IO_2}. Note the increasing sum, as demonstrated in **Table 14-4**. Note that to reach an acceptable total flow of 40 L/min, the O_2 flow will need to be set at least 10 L/min for an F_{IO_2} of 0.40.

It is important to note that the 40-L/min minimum flow guideline is based on the assumption that the patient's minute ventilation will not exceed 10 L/min and that the I:E ratio will be 1:3. The therapist should realize that some patients have a higher minute ventilation and may, therefore, require more total gas flow to be certain that the F_{IO_2} delivery is as desired. A general rule is that more gas flow is better from an F_{IO_2} delivery standpoint. A higher gas flow produces more noise, can be annoying, and may deplete the gas source, however.

High-Flow Nasal Cannula

The **high-flow nasal cannula** (HFNC) has gained favor as a more comfortable alternative to mask-delivered O_2 therapy in adults and nasal CPAP for newborns (**Figure 14-14**).[34,35] HFNC devices have advantages (over LFNCs) as they are designed to provide higher delivered flow, which may meet or exceed the patient's inspiratory demand. They are also capable of providing an adjustable range of F_{IO_2} (0.21–1.0) independently of flow meter settings. This flexibility has allowed them to successfully treat patients with moderate levels of hypoxemic respiratory failure. This may be considered an alternative delivery interface for adult patients whose hypoxemia or dyspnea is not relieved following LFNC, nonrebreathing mask, or air-entrainment mask with F_{IO_2} >0.4. There is increased comfort and patient acceptance of HFNC compared with mask therapy. Moreover, eating, drinking, and speaking are not compromised. In neonates, the HFNC has been advocated for prophylaxis or treatment of RDS and as postextubation therapy.

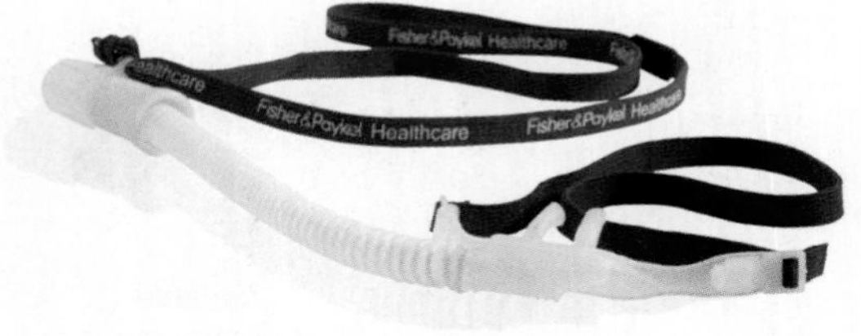

(A)

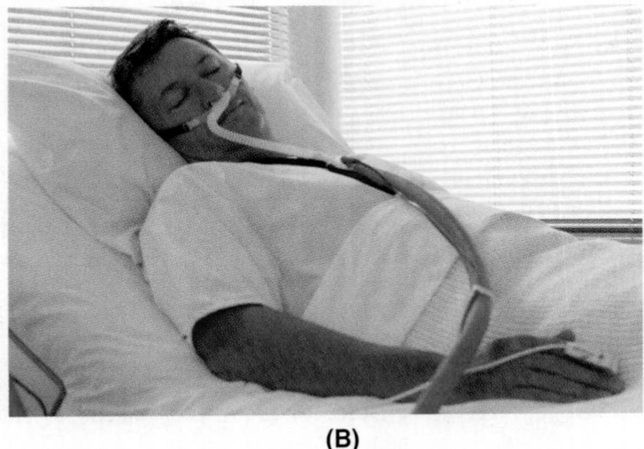

(B)

FIGURE 14-14 High-flow nasal cannula.
Courtesy of Fisher & Paykel Healthcare.

The HFNC uses larger delivery prongs intended to entirely fill each naris, with flows up to 50 L/min used for adults, 20 to 30 L/min for children, and 2 to 8 L/min for neonates. Humidification via high-efficiency heated humidifiers is used for this therapy to ameliorate the mucosal drying effects of such high gas flow. HFNC flow results in variable amounts of increased upper airway positive pressure, and thus some of the therapeutic effects of HFNC relate to the CPAP effect that occurs. The approximate level of CPAP is in the 3 to 5 cm H_2O range, but this effect can be lost when the mouth is opened. Unlike designated CPAP systems with oronasal masks or tight-fitting nasal prongs, the exact level of HFNC distending pressure cannot be specifically set or measured. The HFNC might also flush the upper airway dead space of CO_2 and in that way decrease the minute ventilation requirement.

Large-Volume Air-Entrainment Nebulizers

Large-volume, high-output, all-purpose nebulizers with either cool or heated aerosols have been used in respiratory therapy for many years to provide bland mist therapy with some control of the F_{IO_2} (**Figure 14-15**). With these devices, the clinician can adjust F_{IO_2} by manipulating the size of the orifice, which limits air dilution of gas flow from the driving-gas flow meter (usually O_2). An adjustable collar below the flow meter connection allows F_{IO_2} settings to be controlled from approximately 0.3 to 1.0 (when used with O_2). To increase F_{IO_2},

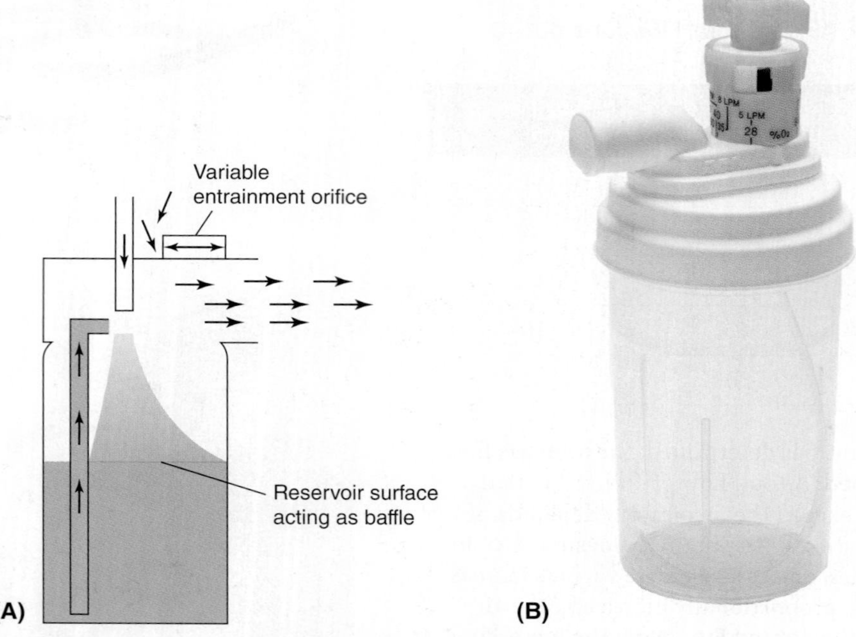

FIGURE 14-15 (**A**) Large-volume air entrainment nebulizer. (**B**) Commercially available large-volume nebulizer.

(**A**) modified from Cohen N, Fink J. Humidity and aerosols. In: Eubanks DH, Bone RC, eds. *Principles and Applications of Cardiorespiratory Care Equipment.* Mosby; 1994; (**B**) courtesy of Teleflex Incorporated. Unauthorized use prohibited.

the collar is set to a small orifice, which limits entrained as well as the total flow delivered to the system. At the 100% O_2 setting, the entrainment orifice is closed, and thus the only flow delivered is from the flow meter itself (typically 15 L/min). The opposite occurs at the low end of F_{IO_2}: as more room air is entrained total flow output increases. At the 35% O_2 setting with 15 L/min oxygen flow, the total output flow approaches 90 L/min. The large-volume air entrainment nebulizer should only be considered a high-flow device when set at $F_{IO_2} \leq 0.4$. Most commercial units have a driving-gas inlet orifice diameter that limits flow to 12 to 15 L/min (at 50 psig). When the O_2 input flow is 15 L/min, the total flows at F_{IO_2} 0.6, 0.7, and 1.0 are 30, 25, and 15 L/min, respectively.

The limited inlet flows may prevent the air-entrainment system flows from meeting the flow demand of tachypneic patients, who often are also hypoxemic and need the high F_{IO_2} settings. Another concern is that with aerosol droplet deposition, water can collect in dependent portions of corrugated delivery tubing. This damming effect can increase resistance to gas flow, which causes back pressure to build within the nebulizing chamber and limit air entrainment. Gas flow can also be blocked completely and gas flows exit via the entrainment port.

Respiratory therapists should be alert to patients who, when using an entrainment aerosol system, increase inspiratory flow demand level as a result of clinical deterioration. In such circumstances, an alternate system should be considered that ensures the required F_{IO_2} with higher flow capability. One approach is to use two nebulizers in tandem (**Figure 14-16**). Another approach is to use of a gas injector nebulizer (GIN), in which an additional flow is added downstream from the nebulizer output (**Figure 14-17**). Yet another option is substitution of specially designed high-flow air-entrainment nebulizers in which manufacturers use larger diameter gas inlet orifices to facilitate higher flows at a higher F_{IO_2}.

Nebulizer systems can direct gas flow to the patient's face or artificial airways with a variety of appliances. The aerosol mask, tracheostomy collar, face tent, and T piece or Briggs adapter (**Figure 14-18**) is attached to the large-volume nebulizer by large-bore 22-mm corrugated tubing. Each of these interfaces provides an open system that freely vents inspiratory and expiratory gases around the patient's face or out the mask hole openings, or the distal port of a Briggs adapter. The open-ended system also can allow considerable secondary dilution of the F_{IO_2}. Because these nebulizers produce an aerosol, respiratory therapists can use that as a visual clue to whether total gas flow is matching patient's inspiratory flow demand. Additional flow may be required if during inspiration the aerosol exiting the interface disappears. Providing adequate flow is especially important if a patient's oxygenation status is poor or deteriorating, as these patients frequently dramatically increase inspiratory flow and minute ventilation.

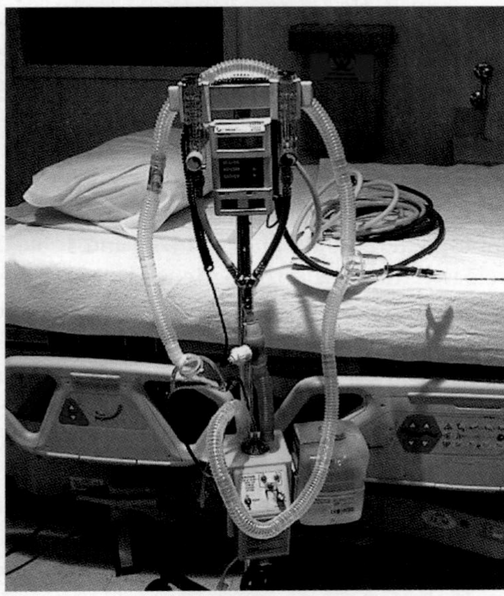

FIGURE 14-16 High-flow oxygen delivery system using flowmeters (for manually mixing air and O_2), an O_2 analyzer, tracheostomy mask and humidifer.

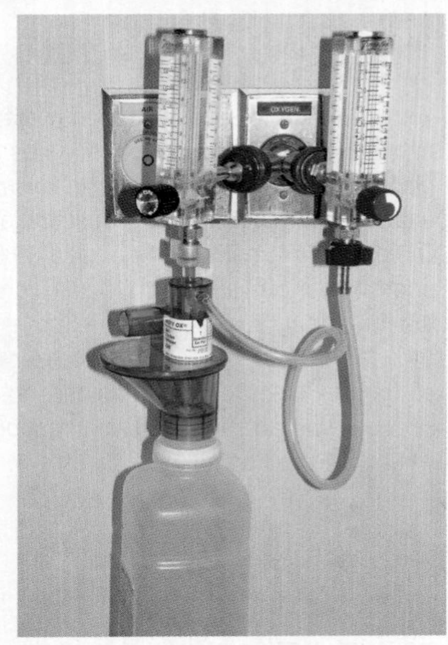

FIGURE 14-17 Injection nebulizer, in which additional flow is injected at the outlet of the nebulizer.

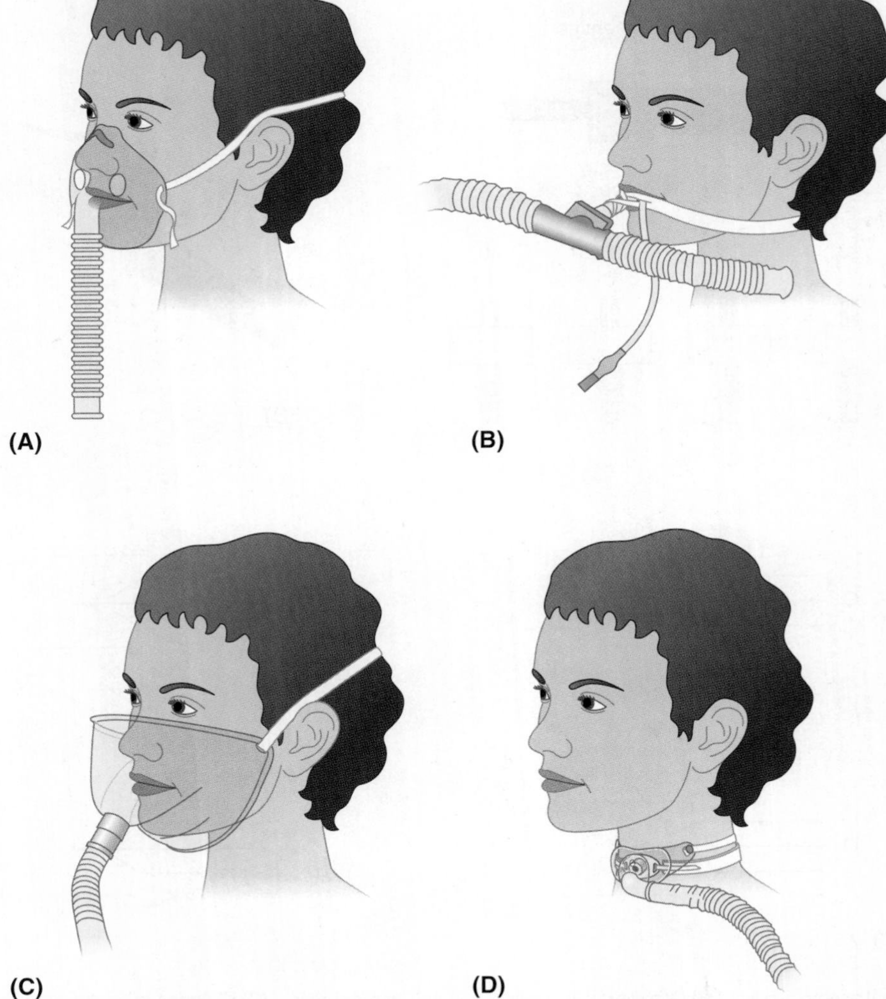

FIGURE 14-18 (**A**) Aerosol mask. (**B**) T-piece and reservoir. (**C**) Face tent. (**D**) Tracheostomy mask.

Adapted from Fink JR, Hunt GE. *Clinical Practice of Respiratory Care*. Lippincott Williams & Wilkins; 1999.

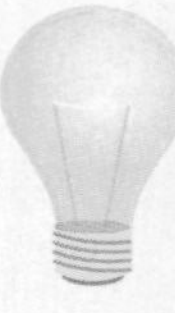

STOP AND THINK

You are asked to assess a recently extubated patient. Following extubation, she was placed on a face mask with large-volume air-entrainment nebulizer at 40% dilution and an O_2 flow of 14 L/min. The Spo_2 was 88% just prior to your arrival. The physician increased the Fio_2 setting to 60%, and the Spo_2 is now 84%. When you increase the nebulizer dilution setting to 80%, the Spo_2 decreases to 82%. How can you explain this clinical response and what would you do next?

Air-Entrainment Masks

An **air-entrainment mask** consists of a single-patient-use, disposable mask, a jet nozzle, and entrainment ports. 100% O_2 is delivered through the jet nozzle, which increases its velocity. This gas at high velocity entrains (or slipstreams) ambient air into the mask because of the viscous shearing forces between the gas traveling through the nozzle and the stagnant ambient air. The Fio_2 depends on the nozzle size and the size of the entrainment ports. Commercially available systems use interchangeable jets, adjustable entrainment ports, or a combination of these (**Figure 14-19** and **Table 14-5**). Fio_2 levels will increase if the patient's hands or bed sheets obstruct the entrainment ports. The patient should be encouraged to keep the mask on the face constantly. A limitation of this device is that patients often do not keep the mask on their face while speaking, eating, or drinking. This potentially can result in hypoxemia unless an alternative device such as LFNC or HFNC is substituted. Air-entrainment masks are a reasonable choice for patients whose hypoxemia cannot be controlled on lower-Fio_2 devices such as the cannula (because of changes in breathing pattern). Patients who hypoventilate with a moderate Fio_2 are candidates for the air-entrainment mask.

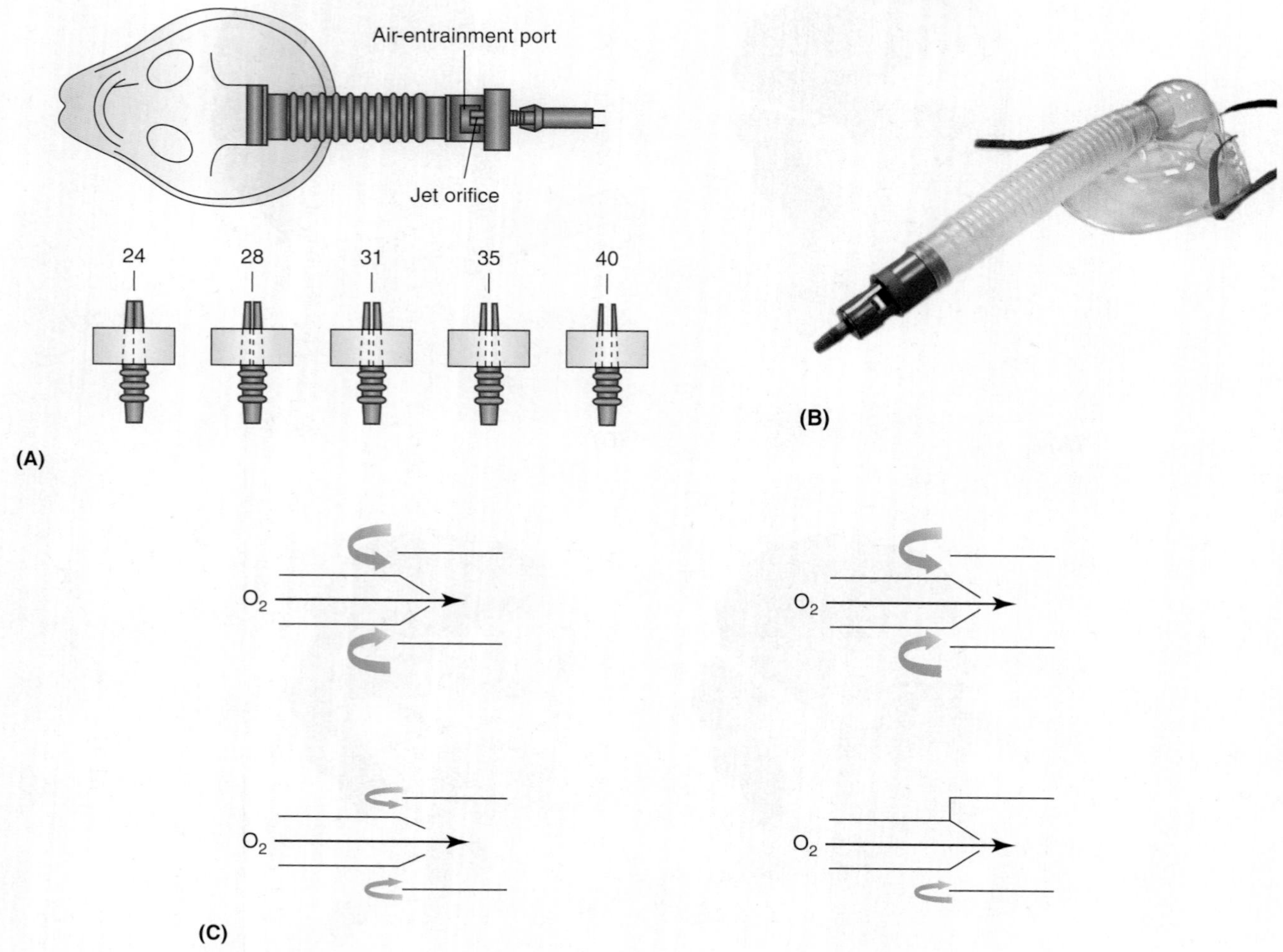

FIGURE 14-19 (**A**) Air-entrainment mask. (**B**) Commercially available air-entrainment mask. (**C**) Changes in air entrainment by changing jet size or changing size of the entrainment port.

(**A**) adapted from Kacmarek RM. Methods of oxygen delivery in the hospital. *Prob Respir Care.* 1990;3:536–574. Reprinted with permission.

TABLE 14-5
FIO_2, Minimum Flow Requirements, Outputs, and Entrainment Ratios for an Air-Entrainment Mask

FIO_2 Setting	Minimum O_2 Flow (L/min)	Entrainment Ratio (Air:O_2)	Total Flow (L/min)
0.24	4	25:1	104
0.28	4	10:1	44
0.31	6	7:1	48
0.35	8	5:1	48
0.40	8	3:1	32
0.50	12	1.7:1	32
0.60	12	1:1	24
0.70	12	0.6:1	19

Information from Branson RD. The nuts and bolts of increasing arterial oxygenation: devices and techniques. *Respir Care.* 1993;38:672–686.

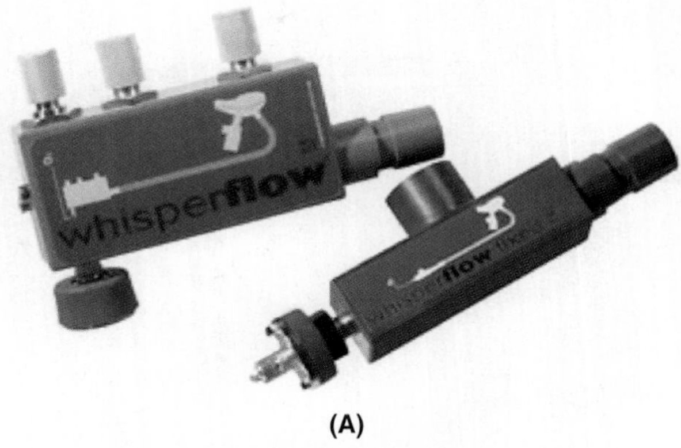

(A)

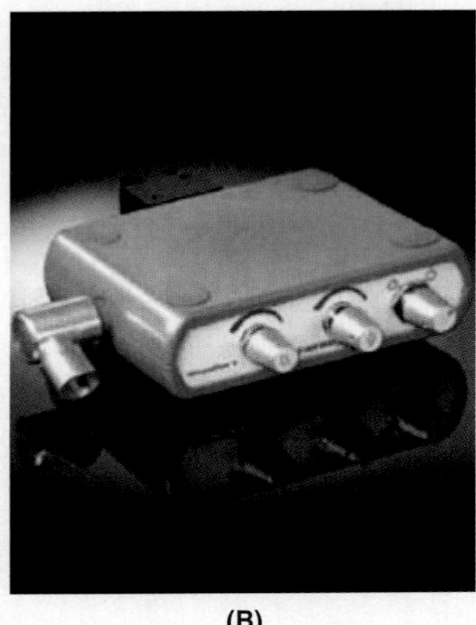

(B)

FIGURE 14-20 (**A**) WhisperFlow Fixed and Variable High Flow Generators. (**B**) WhisperFlow 2 Variable High Flow Generator.

Downs Flow Generator and Caradyne WhisperFlow

High-flow adaptations of the classic air-entrainment device that provides gas mixing are the Philips Respironics WhisperFlo and WhisperFlo 2 (**Figure 14-20**). These compact high performance Venturi-tubes are designed to provide high gas flows in situations in which downstream resistance occurs, such as freestanding CPAP systems.[36] This is in contrast to the air-entrainment nebulizer systems discussed earlier, which can provide high flows only in low-FIO_2 situations and are affected by downstream resistance. The high-flow generators can give gas flows (>100 L/min) to meet high inspiratory flow demand of tachypneic patients over a full FIO_2 range (0.3 to 1).

The mechanism by which the flow generator increases the FIO_2 is by redirecting the O_2 inlet flow in increasing amounts away from the jet. As greater proportions of the 100% O_2 are shifted away from the jet, less room air is entrained and the FIO_2 increases. The higher flow of O_2 (which directly enters the device's output gas flow) compensates for lesser amounts of entrained room air; thus, the FIO_2 increases and total device output flow is maintained. The needle valve at the top of the tube controls the total amount of source oxygen into the system and is adjusted to supply the appropriate total flow of mixed gas. Disadvantages of the Downs high-flow generator include high gas consumption and noise levels. A bacterial filter can be fitted over the air inlet port to reduce noise.

Air–Oxygen Blending Using Dual Flow Meters

Dual flow meters are the simplest and most economical method of delivering a specific FIO_2 and total flow. Two flow meters, one for air and one for O_2, can be used to mix and deliver precise oxygen concentrations (**Figure 14-21**). Instead of the standard 0 to 16 L/min Thorpe tube clinical flow meters, high-flow flow meters (0 to 75 L/min) would need to be used for many applications. The gas flow delivered to the patient through large-bore corrugated tubing is simply the sum of the flows from the two flow meters. Refer to **Equation 14-2** for a sample calculation using basic algebra and the previously mentioned volume × concentration relationship. Once the gases are mixed, they would be humidified before being delivered to the patient. The patient interface can be the standard aerosol mask, tent, tracheostomy mask, or Briggs adapter with tubing reservoir.[30]

Air–Oxygen Blenders (Proportioners)

Air–oxygen blenders, sometimes referred to as *mixers* or *proportioners* (**Figure 14-22**), provide a convenient, compact device for dialing in a specific FIO_2; however, they are expensive in comparison with dual flow meter manual techniques. The principal component of the

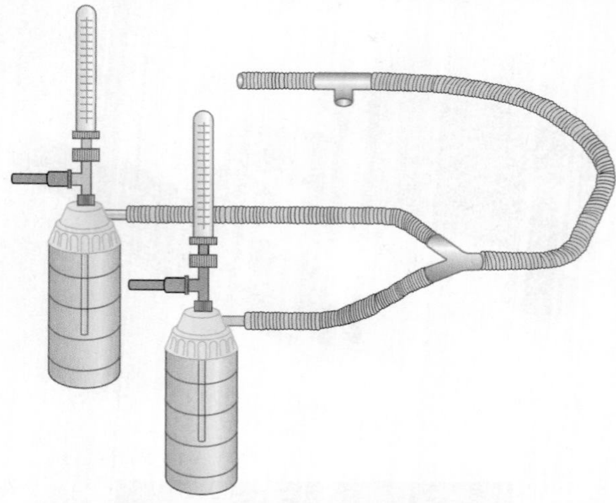

FIGURE 14-21 High-flow oxygen delivery system using two flow meters.

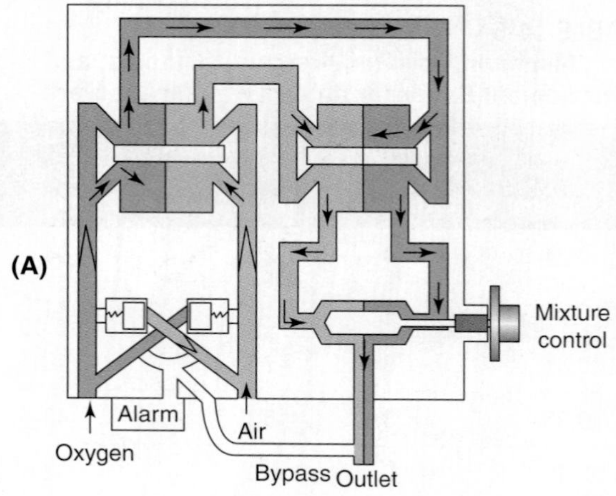

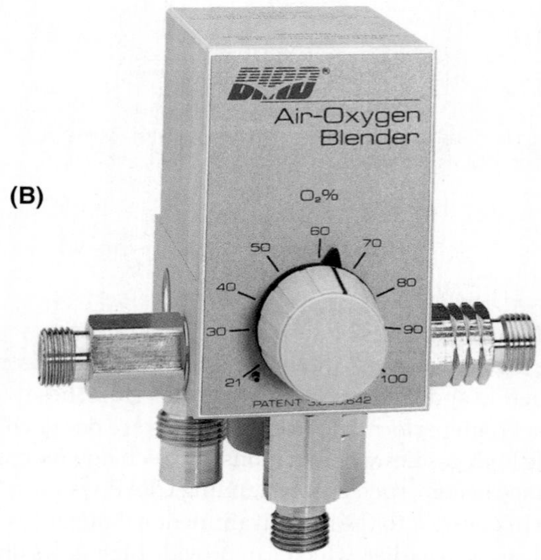

FIGURE 14-22 (A) Air–oxygen blender or proportioner. (B) Commercially available air–oxygen blender.

(A) modified from Ward JJ. Equipment for mixed gas and oxygen therapy. In: Barnes TA, ed. *Core Textbook of Respiratory Care Practice*. 2nd ed. Mosby; 1994; (B) reproduced with permission from CareFusion.

blender is a proportioning module, in which a 50-psig source of air and O_2 is proportioned to produce the required F_{IO_2}. The blender outlet usually produces 50 psig of the mixed gas, which can then be directly attached to devices by using a flow meter.

EQUATION 14-2

High-Flow Dual Flow Meter System

Problem

How should the O_2 and airflow meters be set to achieve 80 L/min and F_{IO_2} of 0.7?

Solution

$$\dot{V}_1 \times C_1 = \dot{V}_2 \times C_2 + \dot{V}_3 \times C_3$$

where $\dot{V}_1 = \dot{V}_{tot}$ = desired flow of 80 L/min; $\dot{V}_2 = O_2$ flow; $\dot{V}_3$ = airflow, and C represents concentrations (i.e., fractions of oxygen): $C_1 = 0.7$; $C_2 = 1.0$; $C_3 = 0.21$

Mixing equation adapted for mixing oxygen and air:

$$\dot{V}\text{tot desired} \times F_{IO_2} \text{ desired} = \dot{V}_{O_2} \times F_{IO_2} + \dot{V}\text{air} \times F_{IO_2}$$

Insert known data; note two unknowns:

$$80 \text{ L/min} \times 0.7 = \dot{V}_{O_2} \times 1 + \dot{V}\text{air} \times 0.21$$

Substitute for $\dot{V}_{O_2}$, because $\dot{V}\text{tot} = \dot{V}_{O_2} + \dot{V}\text{air}$, $\dot{V}_{O_2} = \dot{V}\text{tot} - \dot{V}\text{air} = 80 - \dot{V}\text{air}$

$$80 \text{ L/min} \times 0.7 = (80 - \dot{V}\text{air}) \times 1 + 0.21 \times \dot{V}\text{air}$$

$\dot{V}\text{air} = 24/0.79 = 30$ L/min and, therefore, $\dot{V}_{O_2} = 50$ L/min

Air–oxygen proportioners receive each gas separately from a pipeline or compressed gas cylinder. Ideally, the supply pressures of both gases are nearly equal, usually 50 psig. In clinical practice, this does not always occur, so blenders have internal pressure-regulating systems. Once the pressures for air and oxygen are sufficiently similar, a dual-orifice needle valve controls the amount of each gas flowing out of the orifices. For higher concentrations, the valve would simultaneously open for more O_2 flow as it decreases the airflow. Blender manufacturers provide built-in alarm systems and sometimes pressure gauges that allow the respiratory therapist to confirm the proper inlet pressures.

Aside from imbalances in the inlet gas pressure supply lines, another common problem is contamination of one gas supply by another because of retrograde flow. This problem has been reported when blenders are connected to gas inlets but are not running to patient systems.

The higher-pressure gas (usually oxygen) can flow into the medical air gas lines if inlet check valves are defective. When blenders are not in use, the path of least resistance for the higher-pressure oxygen is the piped air system. Contaminates from gas lines can prevent these pressure valves from sealing properly. Corrosion due to moisture and particulate matter can build up and restrict flow or prevent sealing of check valves. Routine inspection and cleaning twice a year are recommended. Replacement of inlet sintered metal filters and use of water trap filters should reduce this problem. In more serious cases, more complex filter systems may be required.

It is difficult for manufacturers to build blenders with the desired accuracy over the complete range of flows needed clinically. Low-flow blenders are most accurate at low-flow applications requiring less than about 20 L/min. High-flow blenders must be accurate in providing controlled F_{IO_2} levels at flows in the 80 to 100 L/min range. High-flow blenders tend to be more inaccurate at low flow rates, and low-flow blenders at high flows. Evaluations of commercially available medical air–oxygen blenders have found that all blenders were quite accurate when both inlet pressures were 50 psig.

Given the above technical challenges to the accuracy of air–oxygen blenders, it is important that all blenders be calibrated initially and verified periodically by O_2 analyzers. Although the devices are relatively reliable and the air–oxygen mixing equations are valid, inaccurately calibrated equipment and calculation errors may affect the delivered F_{IO_2}. To avoid potentially lethal medical mistakes, all fixed-performance devices and air–oxygen blender systems should always have the F_{IO_2} confirmed by direct oxygen analysis.

Oxygen Enclosures

Placing the patient into an oxygen-enriched environment was one of the earliest methods of O_2 administration. Adult **oxygen tents**, infant incubators, and pediatric croup tents were all introduced between the mid-1920s and the 1940s. The adult tent was widely used for both oxygen administration and high-humidity therapy through the 1960s. Today enclosures are used primarily in infant and pediatric applications and include hoods, incubators, and croup tents. Oxygen and aerosol tents, even for children, have been virtually abandoned.

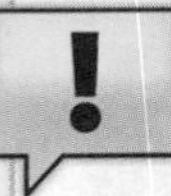

Respiratory Recap

Oxygen Enclosures

- O_2 enclosures include O_2 tents and hoods.
- HBO therapy is currently indicated for treatment of carbon monoxide poisoning, wounds (especially those infected by anaerobic bacteria), air embolism, and decompression sickness.

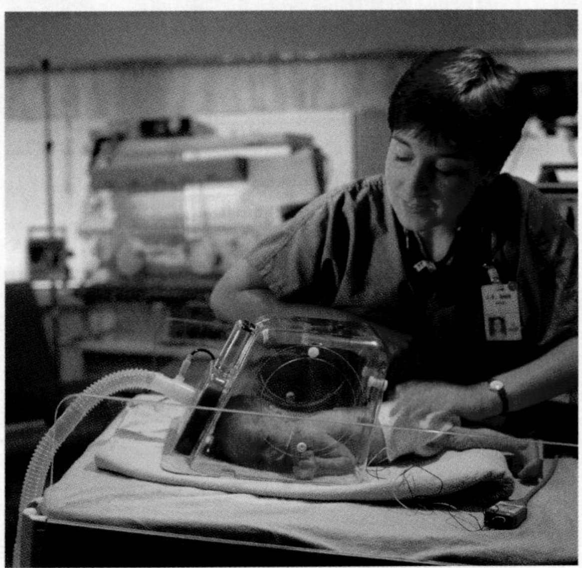

FIGURE 14-23 Oxygen hood.

Infant **oxygen hoods** are used, but infant nasal cannulas are being used increasingly as an alternative. The hood covers only the head, allowing access to the infant's lower body while still permitting use of a standard incubator or radiant warmer. The oxygen hood (**Figure 14-23**) is a round or rectangular, bottomless, clear rigid plastic device with a half-moon cutout that allows it to be placed over an infant's neck to enclose the entire head. O_2 is delivered to the hood through either a blender with a heated humidifier or a heated air-entrainment nebulizer. Providing a minimum flow of 6 to 8 L/min is necessary to prevent the accumulation of CO_2. Frequent or continuous monitoring of the O_2 concentration and internal hood temperature also is necessary.

Hyperbaric Oxygen Therapy

Hyperbaric oxygen (HBO) therapy involves administration of gas at an increased atmospheric pressure; its use in medicine has varied over the years. HBO patients are placed inside an airtight chamber that can be pressurized to several times the normal atmospheric pressure of 760 mm Hg. The goal of HBO is to dissolve more gas (particularly O_2) into the blood and body tissues of the patient. The increased O_2 dissolved in blood and body tissues facilitates metabolism in the absence of HbO_2 (when used for CO poisoning) and exposes anaerobic bacteria to a fatal level of O_2 (for treatment of wounds with *Clostridium* infections, such as gas gangrene).

Hyperbaric chambers can contain several patients and caretakers or can be designed to contain only one patient, with the care personnel remaining outside. Smaller HBO apparatuses designed to enclose individual affected limbs are also in use. There are many significant differences between conventional O_2 therapy and HBO therapy, and thus specialized training of respiratory therapy personnel involved with HBO is required. For example, gas volumes differ in relation to the chamber pressure, and O_2 toxicity occurs in both a pulmonary and cerebral form that occur much more rapidly under HBO conditions.

Because hyperbaric treatment is indicated for clinical situations arising from recreational or occupational diving accidents, many of the available HBO chambers are found in coastal areas or on rescue ships. Divers are trained to incrementally gas-off by ascending slowly or in stages, but when divers surface too rapidly, they may develop decompression sickness and air embolisms. In these cases, the affected divers are returned to their lowest depth pressure and decompressed more slowly in the chamber. Because of the frequent use of HBO equipment in diving accidents, gauges are calibrated in feet of seawater (fsw); 33 fsw = 1 atm = 10 msw. Treatment of recreational or occupational decompression sickness does not necessarily involve use of supplemental oxygen.

HBO treatment is indicated for carbon monoxide poisoning,[37] *Clostridium* myonecrosis (gas gangrene), air embolism (the bends), decompression sickness (N_2 narcosis, rapture of the deep), and accelerating healing of selected wounds, grafts, burns, or infections. Because of the biochemical complexity of CO poisoning, the advantages of HBO therapy in comparison to normobaric, ambient 100% oxygen therapy continue to be debated. HBO treatment for decompression sickness (the bends; nitrogen coming out of solution in the joints of the body) is not questioned.

Monitoring the Physiologic Effects of Oxygen

O_2 therapy is often initiated in response to patient complaints of shortness of breath. The actual symptoms of hypoxia, however, are cognitive impairment, cardiac rhythm and conduction dysfunction, and renal dysfunction. The signs of hypoxia may include high respiratory frequency, cyanosis, chest pain, low Pa_{O_2}, and low Sa_{O_2}. Effective oxygen treatment of these conditions requires careful monitoring.

Blood Gases and Oximetry

Assessment of patients' clinical signs and the results of arterial blood gas analysis are the gold standards for documenting physiologic indices of oxygenation, ventilation, and acid–base balance. Knowledge of the actual or *best estimate* of delivered FI_{O_2} is helpful to provide a baseline to evaluate the physiologic response to supplemental oxygen therapy. Measurement of Pa_{O_2}, Sp_{O_2}, Hb, and cardiovascular function (pulse, ECG, and blood pressure) are also useful to allow an informed differential diagnosis of the cause(s) of hypoxemia and/or hypoxia. Patient condition can rapidly change, however, and intermittent measurements may not reflect the status of dynamic patients. Continuous pulse oximetry monitoring is appropriate in unstable patients.

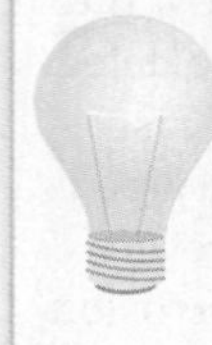

STOP AND THINK

The hospital where you work is opening a new critical care wing. You are asked to verify the function of the air and oxygen outlets. How would you approach this task?

Pulse oximetry has become the most common form of continuously monitoring oxygen saturation (Sp_{O_2}) and is the standard of care in the operating or recovery room, pulmonary function or sleep laboratory, intensive care unit, emergency room, and other clinical areas throughout the hospital. Its noninvasive approach, ease of use, and real-time feedback have led to its widespread acceptance in titrating oxygen levels to ventilated and spontaneously breathing patients. It may be used to spot check or continuously measure patients' condition. Pulse oximetry has some limitations, however. Most clinical oximeters only use two wavelength measurement, which cannot identify carboxyhemoglobinemia or other abnormal hemoglobins. More importantly, the pulse oximeter is a poor monitor of ventilation. If patients are breathing supplemental oxygen, this can further delay detection of elevated carbon dioxide levels and provide a false sense of security even when patients are in hypercapnic respiratory failure.[38]

Oxygen Analysis

Oxygen analyzers are used to measure the concentration of oxygen (O_2%) administered to patients (**Figure 14-24**). Analysis is routinely performed in infant oxygen hoods, incubators, mechanical ventilators, anesthetic circuits, and some fixed-performance oxygen administration devices (e.g., an aerosol-entrainment

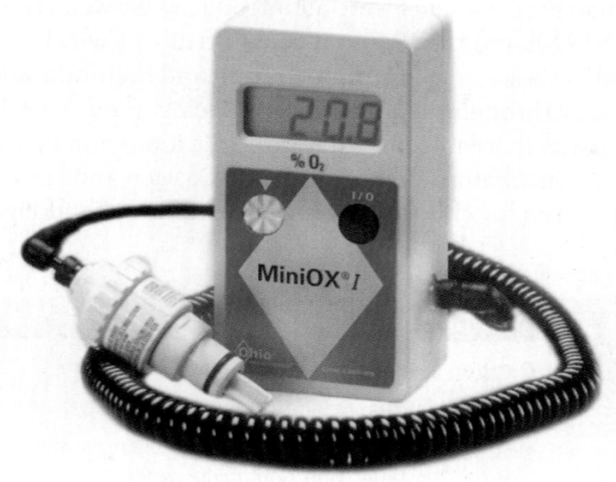

FIGURE 14-24 Oxygen analyzer.
Courtesy of Amvex Corporation.

T piece). Clinicians should check dual air–oxygen flow meters and blenders to confirm the desired oxygen concentrations. Monitoring can consist of spot samples, periodic checks, or continuous monitoring with high-low limit alarms.

Polarographic analyzers use a Clark electrode to measure oxygen. Galvanic cell analyzers, like polarographic analyzers, use an electrochemical principle. Although both analyzers actually measure P_{IO_2}, they display O_2%. Analyzers used at high altitudes therefore require recalibration. Calibration is usually accomplished by exposing the electrode to room air (21% oxygen) and then to 100% oxygen. The O_2 analyzer is then adjusted to read the two calibrating gas concentrations correctly. Inability to calibrate the analyzer usually means that the electrolyte in the electrode needs to be changed. O_2 analyzers should be checked relatively frequently for calibration and should be repaired if they are unable to read within ±2%.

Clinical Application of Oxygen Therapy

Respiratory therapists are frequently asked to integrate patient information and recommend a medical gas therapy. This process begins with patient assessment and is usually based on clinical circumstances or specific signs or symptoms that suggest hypoxemia or hypoxia. Sometimes laboratory data (e.g., blood gases) reveal an unnoticed problem. After determining that the patient has a problem that oxygen or other gas therapy may treat, the decision process is made complex by the many factors related to oxygen transport. For instance, there may be problems with ventilation, oxygen content of arterial blood, or perfusion. **Figure 14-25** shows factors to be considered in the decision-making process for O_2 therapy.

> **Respiratory Recap**
>
> **Evaluation of Oxygen Therapy**
>
> - Arterial blood gas measurements are the best way of evaluating hypoxemia.
> - Pulse oximetry provides a real-time, noninvasive estimate of oxygenation.
> - O_2 analyzers are used to measure the O_2 concentration of a gas mixture.

A complete history and laboratory profile are commonly absent when a patient has acute problems indicating medical gas therapy, and thus clinical signs

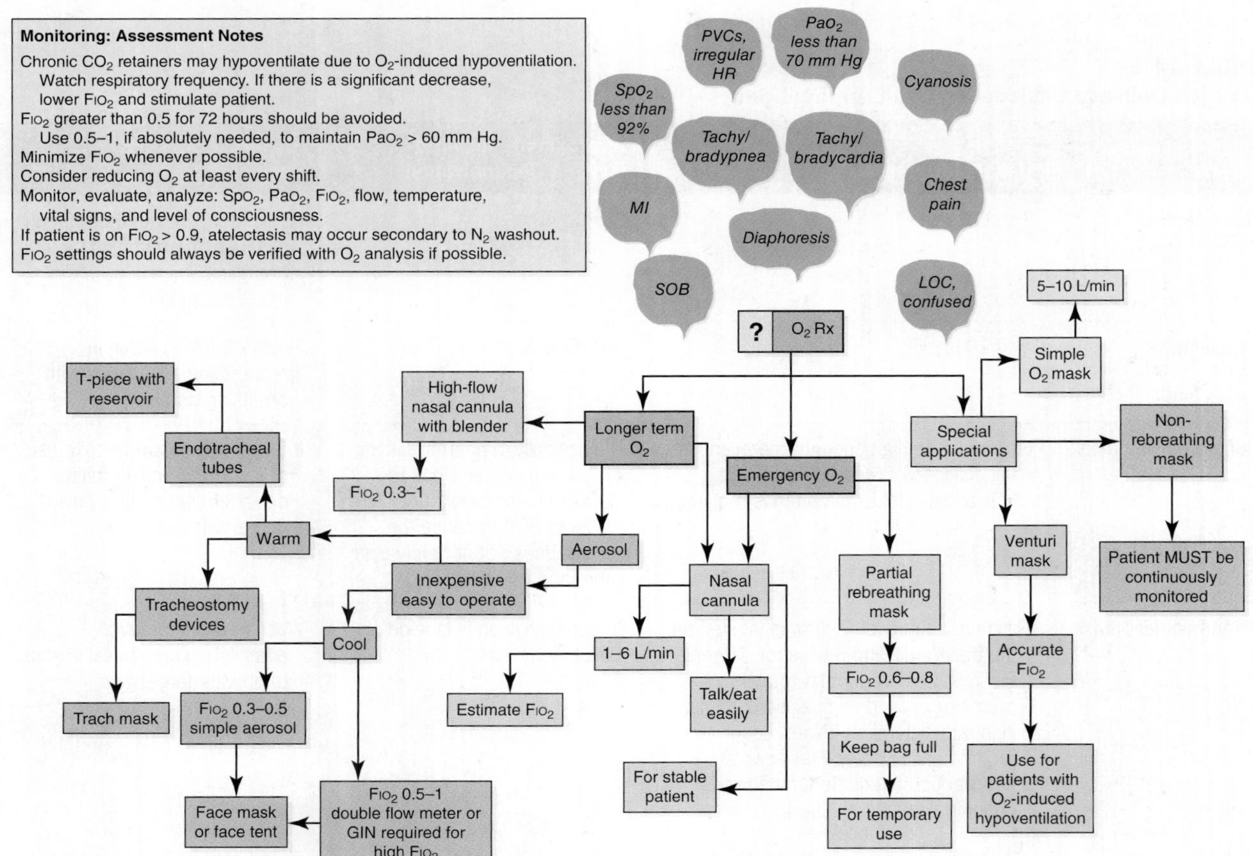

FIGURE 14-25 Oxygen administration guide.

and symptoms may be the clinician's only guides. As a general guideline, it is usually safer to provide liberal flows and concentrations than to restrict oxygen. There are always exceptions, but side effects of O_2 therapy are usually less significant than the profound brain damage secondary to hypoxia. In the past there has been inappropriate emphasis on withholding oxygen because of a relatively small number of COPD patients with chronic hypercarbia who may hypoventilate when O_2 is administered.

The initial assessment may also provide information about the cause of the dyspnea or hypoxemia. In the case of partial upper airway obstruction caused by severe acute asthma, heliox may allow time to further evaluate the pathology, prepare a definitive therapy, or await effects of pharmacologic therapy. Following initial assessment, clinicians should determine whether the patient requires hyperbaric O_2 therapy or traditional ambient medical gas therapy. Severe carbon monoxide poisoning can be treated with hyperbaric therapy if there is immediate access.

The next decision is the initial concentration of oxygen and appropriate O_2 therapy device (**Table 14-6**). Respiratory therapists often apply oxygen based on bedside assessment and clinical judgment. An O_2 mask is often more uncomfortable than a nasal cannula, but a mask may be more appropriate if the O_2 requirement is high. A room air blood gas analysis is quite valuable if it can be obtained without significant delay to assist with diagnosis and guide selection of the level of oxygen concentration needed. An O_2 therapy system should be selected based on the F_{IO_2} and inspiratory flow requirement. High-flow devices allow more consistent levels for patients who have rapid respiratory rates and those who require a high F_{IO_2}. Inspired O_2 is then titrated to achieve a Pa_{O_2} above 60 mm Hg or an Sp_{O_2} above 90%. Pulse oximetry can be useful for the initial O_2 titration. It should also be kept in mind that O_2 therapy alone may not correct hypoxemia in all patients. Patients with hypercapnia and hypoxemia frequently require ventilatory support. For patients with a large right-to-left shunt, O_2 therapy will not result in improvements in Pa_{O_2} or Sp_{O_2} regardless of the F_{IO_2} applied.

Respiratory therapists should be conservative when reducing F_{IO_2} and liberal when increasing it. A common guideline is to reduce the F_{IO_2} in decrements of 0.05, monitoring Pa_{O_2} or Sp_{O_2} as the F_{IO_2} is decreased and allowing at least 20 minutes to reflect the actual physiologic response to any F_{IO_2}. Patients with severe lung diseases may take even longer to equilibrate to changes in F_{IO_2}. For increases in F_{IO_2}, it is always wise to overshoot or exceed the predicted Pa_{O_2} or Sp_{O_2} and then titrate down.

Therapist-driven protocols and clinical pathways (**Figure 14-26**) allow clinicians to apply oxygen therapy within a predetermined decision-making algorithm.

TABLE 14-6
Oxygen Delivery Devices for Adult Applications

Device	Usual Flow Range	Approximate Inspired Oxygen Concentration	Comments
Nasal cannula	1 to 6 L/min	24% to 40%	F_{IO_2} is reduced with tachypnea, nasal obstruction, and mouth breathing; F_{IO_2} varies with breathing pattern.
Simple mask	5 to 10 L/min	30% to 60%	Flows <5 L/min result in rebreathing; F_{IO_2} varies with breathing pattern.
Nonrebreathing mask	Flow must be high enough to prevent full collapse of reservoir bag during inhalation; >12 L/min often is required.	Theoretically, a nonrebreathing mask will deliver close to 100% O_2. In reality, it delivers 60% to 80% because the mask does not fit tightly over the face.	If Sp_{O_2} remains low despite use of a nonrebreathing mask, consider using a high-flow O_2 delivery device.
Air-entrainment mask	Minimum source jet O_2 flow is labeled on the mask's diluting device for differing F_{IO_2} mixtures. Verify that total flow meets or exceeds a specific patient's inspiratory demand. (Note: some recommended source jet flows do not produce adequate total flows for critically ill adults.)	O_2 concentration is labeled on dilution device(s).	When mask is removed, administer O_2 by nasal cannula to provide target Sp_{O_2}.
High-flow oxygen system	40 L/min, or 3 times the patient's minute ventilation.	24% to 100%, set by air and O_2 flow meters or blender.	Gas should be humidified with high-flow system.

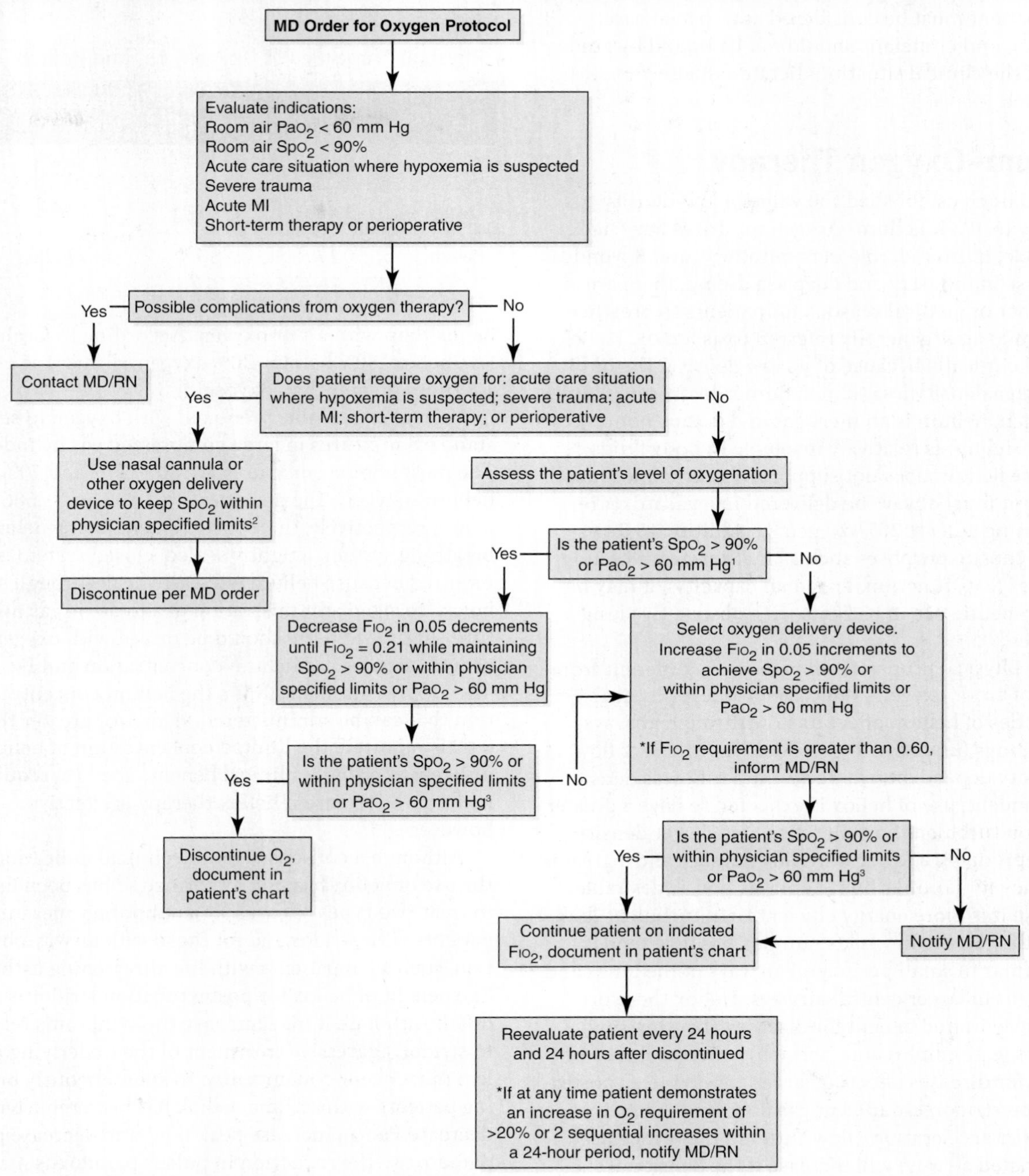
MD Order for Oxygen Protocol
Evaluate indications:
Room air PaO_2 < 60 mm Hg
Room air SpO_2 < 90%
Acute care situation where hypoxemia is suspected
Severe trauma
Acute MI
Short-term therapy or perioperative
Possible complications from oxygen therapy?
Yes
No
Contact MD/RN
Does patient require oxygen for: acute care situation where hypoxemia is suspected; severe trauma; acute MI; short-term therapy; or perioperative
Yes
No
Use nasal cannula or other oxygen delivery device to keep SpO_2 within physician specified limits[2]
Discontinue per MD order
Assess the patient's level of oxygenation
Is the patient's SpO_2 > 90% or PaO_2 > 60 mm Hg[1]
Yes
No
Decrease FIO_2 in 0.05 decrements until FIO_2 = 0.21 while maintaining SpO_2 > 90% or within physician specified limits or PaO_2 > 60 mm Hg
Select oxygen delivery device. Increase FIO_2 in 0.05 increments to achieve SpO_2 > 90% or within physician specified limits or PaO_2 > 60 mm Hg
*If FIO_2 requirement is greater than 0.60, inform MD/RN
Is the patient's SpO_2 > 90% or within physician specified limits or PaO_2 > 60 mm Hg[3]
Yes
No
Discontinue O_2, document in patient's chart
Is the patient's SpO_2 > 90% or within physician specified limits or PaO_2 > 60 mm Hg[3]
Yes
No
Continue patient on indicated FIO_2, document in patient's chart
Notify MD/RN
Reevaluate patient every 24 hours and 24 hours after discontinued
*If at any time patient demonstrates an increase in O_2 requirement of >20% or 2 sequential increases within a 24-hour period, notify MD/RN

[1] If ABG available, check correlation of SpO_2 with ABG saturation
[2] Oxygen device should be appropriate for patient's pathophysiology
[3] Acceptable FIO_2 may vary with the clinical situation or physician

FIGURE 14-26 Protocol for oxygen administration.

Each patient must be considered as a special case, however, and clinicians should not be bound by guidelines if the clinical situation dictates an alternative approach.

Helium–Oxygen Therapy

Since Barach established the value of low-density gas therapy in 1934, helium–oxygen mixtures have had a notable, if limited, role in respiratory care. Beyond their use in industry and deep sea diving, there are a number of medical reasons for patients to breathe these mixtures, generally referred to as **heliox**. Heliox is used clinically because of its low density. The only gas with a density less than helium is hydrogen. Unlike hydrogen, helium is an inert gas and is thus nonreactive. Helium is relatively insoluble in body fluids. Because helium does not support life, for clinical applications it must always be delivered in a gas mixture containing at least 20% oxygen. In addition to its use for diagnostic purposes such as measurement of lung volumes (e.g., functional residual capacity), it may be of therapeutic use in patients with obstructive lung diseases.[39–45]

The physical properties of helium are different from those of air or oxygen (**Table 14-7**). These physical properties of helium affect its flow through airways of the lungs (**Equation 14-3**). Because turbulent flow is density dependent, whereas laminar flow is density independent, use of heliox is expected to have a greater effect on turbulent flow. Because of its lower density heliox produces a lower Reynolds number and a greater tendency for laminar flow. Laminar flow is desirable because it is more energy efficient than turbulent flow. According to the Reynolds number, gas flow tends to be laminar in small peripheral airways of the lungs and turbulent in larger central airways. Heliox therefore may have limited benefit for diseases affecting small airways (e.g., emphysema, asthma), whereas it may be useful for diseases affecting larger airways (e.g., postextubation stridor, croup). For gas flow through an orifice (i.e., axial acceleration), flow through the orifice (e.g., constricted airway) will increase if the density of the gas decreases (e.g., heliox). Because of the Bernoulli principle, less pressure is required to produce flow with heliox than with air or oxygen. According to Graham's law, heliox (80% helium/20% oxygen) diffuses at a rate 1.8 times greater than oxygen.

TABLE 14-7
Physical Properties of Oxygen, Air, and Helium

Gas	Density (g/L)	Viscosity (μpoise)	Thermoconductivity (μcal × cm × 5 × °K)
Air	1.293	170.8	58.0
Oxygen	1.429	192.6	58.5
Helium	0.179	188.7	352.0

Helium is available premixed with oxygen in several standard mixtures in large compressed gas cylinders. The most popular mixtures are 80%/20% and 70%/30% helium–oxygen. The densities are 1.805 and 1.586 less dense, respectively, than pure oxygen. In any heliox breathing system, a tightly sealed, closed system is required because helium will easily leak through small holes. To avoid administration of a hypoxic gas mixture, 20% O_2/80% He should be mixed with oxygen to provide the desired helium concentration and F_{IO_2}. The F_{IO_2} requirement limits the helium concentration that can be administered. If an F_{IO_2} greater than 0.40 is required, the limited concentration of helium is unlikely to produce clinical benefit. The F_{IO_2} requirement may decrease if heliox therapy is effective, however.

Although a consensus on the clinical indications for the use of heliox has not yet formed, it has been used to treat two types of cases: as a temporary measure for patients with stridor and for those with airway obstruction, such as in patients with life-threatening asthma. The benefit of heliox for postextubation stridor is anecdotal. Although it may improve the symptoms related to stridor, aggressive treatment of the underlying problem must occur concurrently. In spontaneously breathing patients with asthma, heliox has been reported to decrease Pa_{CO_2}, increase peak flow, and decrease pulsus paradoxus. The reduction in pulsus paradoxus may be particularly important because it reflects a reduction in inspiratory muscle work. Heliox has also been used with intubated and mechanically ventilated asthmatic patients, in whom it reportedly produces a reduction in Pa_{CO_2} with a lower peak airway pressure and an improvement in oxygenation. The role of heliox in the treatment of COPD is unclear. COPD is a disease of the small airways, a region of the lungs in which flow is density independent.

Nonintubated patients may receive therapy via a well-fitting simple mask or a mask with a reservoir bag (**Figure 14-27**). A Y piece attached to the mask allows concurrent delivery of aerosolized medications. Sufficient flow is required to keep the reservoir bag inflated. This is often 12 to 15 L/min and requires

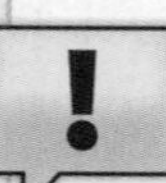

Respiratory Recap

Heliox

- Therapeutic benefits are related to the low density of heliox.
- Use of heliox is beneficial in some patients with partial upper airway obstruction or asthma.
- Heliox adversely affects the function of equipment such as flow meters, nebulizers, and ventilators.

EQUATION 14-3

Physical Principles That Explain the Benefits of Heliox Therapy

For turbulent flow, the Hagen-Poiseuille equation predicts that flow is affected by the radius of the conducting tube, the pressure gradient, the density of the gas (ρ), and the length of the conducting tube (l) as follows:

$$\dot{V} = (4\pi r^5 \Delta P)/(\rho l)$$

where $\dot{V}$ is flow and ΔP is the pressure gradient.

Whether flow is laminar or turbulent is determined by the Reynolds number (Re), as follows:

$$\text{Re} = \text{Inertial forces/Viscous forces} = (vr\rho)/\eta$$

where v is the velocity of gas movement, r is the radius, and η is viscosity. A low Reynolds number causes flow to be laminar.

For gas flow through an orifice (e.g., axial acceleration), flow has only a weak dependence on the Reynolds number and is affected by density as follows:

$$\dot{V}^2 = (\Delta P)/\rho$$

In other words, flow through an orifice (e.g., constricted airway) will increase if the density of the gas decreases (e.g., heliox).

The Bernoulli principle states that the pressure required to produce flow is affected by the mass of the gas as follows:

$$(P_1 - P_2) = ½ \times m \times (v_2^2 - v_1^2)$$

where $(P_1 - P_2)$ = pressure required to produce flow, $(v_2^2 - v_1^2)$ = difference in velocity between P_1 and P_2, and m = mass of the gas. In other words, less pressure is required to produce flow with heliox than with air or oxygen.

Graham's law states that the rate of diffusion is inversely related to the square root of gas density. Thus, heliox (80% He/20% O_2) will diffuse at a rate 1.8 times faster than oxygen, which explains why the flow of heliox through an oxygen flow meter is 1.8 times faster than the indicated flow.

According to wave speed theory, flow through an airway cannot be greater than the flow at which gas velocity equals wave speed. Wave speed is the speed at which a small disturbance travels in a compliant tube filled with a fluid. The wave speed (c) in an airway depends on the cross-sectional area of the airway (A), the density of the fluid, and the slope of the pressure–area curve of the airway (dP/dA), as follows:

$$c^2 = A/\rho \times dP/dA$$

Note that maximal flow ($\dot{V}_{max}$) is the product of the fluid velocity at wave speed and the airway area (cA). If $\dot{V}_{max}$ = cA, then the following occurs:

$$\dot{V}_{max} = (A/\rho \times dP/dA)^{1/2}$$

According to wave speed theory, $\dot{V}_{max}$ increases as gas density decreases. Wave speed theory is useful only when gas flow is density dependent, however. In small airways, and particularly at low lung volumes, gas flow is density independent, and viscous flow limitation becomes more important than wave speed.

three to six H-size cylinders per day. Using an oxygen-calibrated flow meter for heliox therapy causes the flow of heliox (80% helium/20% oxygen) to be 1.8 times greater than the indicated flow. Accurate flows are not required in administering helium–oxygen mixtures. The objective when using a reservoir bag and mask is to keep the reservoir bag nearly full at all times.

Heliox administration during mechanical ventilation can be problematic. Ventilators are designed to deliver a mixture of air and oxygen. The density, viscosity, and thermal conductivity of helium can affect the delivered tidal volume and the measurement of exhaled tidal volume. With some ventilators, no reliable tidal volume is delivered with heliox. Use of other ventilators may result in a much higher delivered tidal volume than desired. A number of ventilators are currently approved for heliox delivery.

Several studies reported improved aerosol penetration and deposition in the lungs with the nebulizer powered with heliox rather than air, but studies reported no benefit with the use of heliox-driven nebulizer therapy. Heliox can affect nebulizer function, resulting

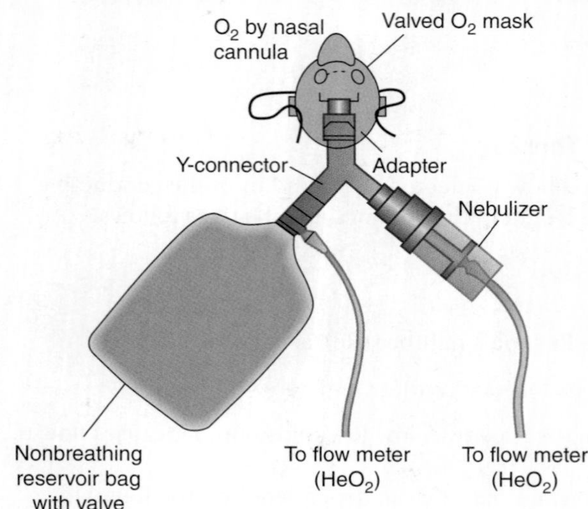

FIGURE 14-27 Equipment for heliox administration to spontaneously breathing patients.

in a smaller particle size, reduced output, and longer nebulization time. When heliox (rather than air or oxygen) is used to power the nebulizer, the flow should be increased by 50% to 100% to ensure adequate output from the nebulizer. Heliox has been shown also to improve aerosol delivery during mechanical ventilation.

In patients with COPD, heliox might reduce Pa_{CO_2}, dyspnea, and work of breathing to a greater extent than oxygen alone. Outcome studies have not shown an improvement in patient outcomes when using a combination of noninvasive ventilation and heliox, however.

Carbon Dioxide Therapy

Therapeutic applications are quite limited or controversial. Carbon dioxide therapy has several dangerous side effects, and its efficacy remains unproved in many of the following applications. Historically, it was thought that increasing inspired CO_2 levels could treat hysterical hyperventilation (anxiety attacks) by lessening syncopal attacks due to hypocarbia. Five percent carbon dioxide in oxygen (**carbogen**) or rebreathing into a paper bag or tubing reservoir was used. Breathing into a paper bag might still relieve anxiety attacks, but current treatment standards recommend treating most cases with anxiolytic medications.

Carbogen historically was also used to stimulate spontaneous breathing in postoperative patients to hasten the removal of volatile anesthetics and to prevent atelectasis, but this practice has been abandoned. Treatment of hiccoughs (singultus) with carbogen or by rebreathing exhaled CO_2 is occasionally successful, but the mechanisms by which such treatment works are unknown. Carbogen has also been used to terminate seizures (petit mal) by the mechanism of decreasing brain excitability. CO_2 was also used in the past to improve regional blood flow by dilating vessels in the brain for the treatment of strokes. More recently, carbogen has been used to encourage ophthalmic artery blood flow.

Because expired air normally contains approximately 5% CO_2 (normal $F\bar{E}_{CO_2}$ is approximately 0.05), rebreathing that gas can provide CO_2 gas therapy. The paper bag is the simplest device. The Adler rebreather and Dale-Schwartz tube are commercial adaptations. Premixed high-pressure gas cylinders can provide administration of specific mixtures of carbon dioxide. Regulators that attach to the cylinder valves must be specific for the concentration used. Most common are mixtures of 5% CO_2 and 95% O_2 and of 7% CO_2 and 93% O_2, although no more than 5% CO_2 is normally used. CO_2 concentrations greater than 10% are not recommended because of the risk of rapidly developing side effects.

A nonrebreathing mask is used for administration devices for CO_2/O_2 gas therapy. Administration times are normally limited to fairly short periods of 5 to 15 minutes. Patients on carbogen therapy must be carefully monitored for pulse, respiratory rate, blood pressure, and mental state. Pulse rate, minute ventilation, and blood pressure usually increase somewhat when carbogen treatments are administered, but significant changes in any of these should prompt the discontinuance of the therapy. Carbogen therapy may also depress the patient's mental state and can result in convulsions, coma, and ultimately death.

Nitric Oxide Therapy

In 1987, it was found that **nitric oxide (NO)** is normally biosynthesized in vascular endothelial cells and is an important mediator of physiologic function, including vasodilation, neurotransmission, long-term memory, and immunologic defense. The NO molecule is highly diffusible and lipid soluble. Its half-life ranges from 3 to 50 seconds as it converts to nitrates, nitrites, and higher oxides of nitrogen. Nitric oxide is a ubiquitous, highly reactive, gaseous, diatomic radical that is important physiologically at low concentrations (**Box 14-1**). Atmospheric concentrations of NO usually range from 10 to 100 ppb.

L-Arginine is the substrate for NO synthesis in biologic systems. NO is produced in the presence of nitric

BOX 14-1

Typical Expression of Concentration of Nitric Oxide and Nitrogen Dioxide

Concentrations are usually expressed in parts per million (ppm) or parts per billion (ppb).

% = 1:100
ppm = 1:1,000,000
10,000 ppm = 1%
1000 ppb = 1 ppm

oxide synthase (NOS). NO is lipophilic and readily diffuses across cell membranes to adjacent cells, thus serving as a local messenger molecule. It typically diffuses from its cell of origin to a neighboring cell, where it binds with guanylate cyclase. Activation of guanylate cyclase results in the production of cyclic guanosine 3′,5′-monophosphate (cGMP) from guanosine triphosphate (GTP), which produces a biologic effect within the cell (e.g., smooth muscle relaxation).

The term *selective pulmonary vasodilation* is used to indicate two physiologic phenomena (**Figure 14-28**). First, selective pulmonary vasodilators reduce pulmonary vascular resistance without affecting systemic vascular resistance. Second, a selective pulmonary vasodilator affects vascular resistance only near ventilated alveoli. Inspired vasodilators are delivered to those lung units that are ventilated. NO is not a selective pulmonary vasodilator but becomes one when inhaled. Inhaled NO selectively improves blood flow to ventilated alveoli and produces a reduction in intrapulmonary shunt and improved arterial oxygenation.[46] The selective pulmonary vasodilation demonstrated by inhaled NO is due to the high affinity of hemoglobin for NO, which is about 10^6 times as great as the affinity of hemoglobin for O_2. In contrast to inhaled NO, intravenous vasodilators (e.g., sodium nitroprusside, nitroglycerin, prostacyclin) are not selective. Although intravenous vasodilators lower pulmonary artery pressure, they also lower systemic blood pressure. These agents increase blood flow to both ventilated and unventilated lung units, resulting in an increased intrapulmonary shunt and a lower Pa_{O_2}.

Multicenter, randomized, double-blind, placebo-controlled studies of inhaled NO for persistent

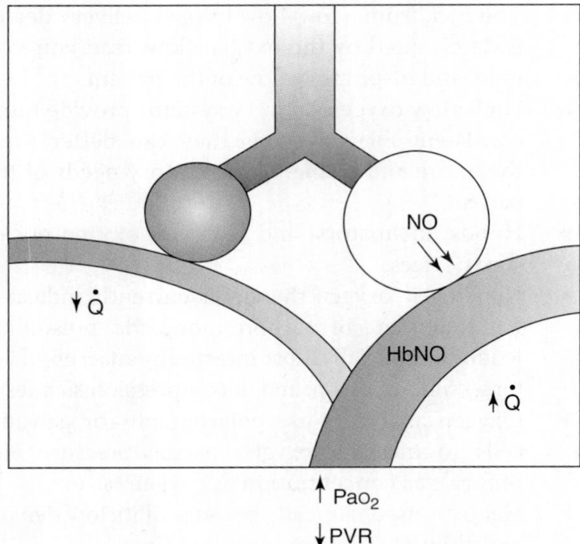

FIGURE 14-28 Inhaled nitric oxide is a selective pulmonary vasodilator because vasodilation occurs primarily in parts of the lungs that are ventilated and because systemic vasodilation does not occur.

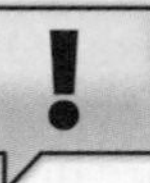

Respiratory Recap

Inhaled Nitric Oxide

- Inhaled nitric oxide is a selective pulmonary vasodilator.
- Inhaled nitric oxide is an FDA-approved treatment of hypoxic respiratory failure of the newborn.
- Toxicity is low at usual clinical doses.
- Inhaled NO is administered via a specially designed delivery system.

pulmonary hypertension of the newborn (PPHN) have reported improvements in Pa_{O_2} and a reduction in the requirement for extracorporeal life support with the use of inhaled NO.[47–49] These studies established a role for inhaled NO in term infants with PPHN and led to approval by the FDA in 1999 for use of inhaled NO:

> INO_{max}, in conjunction with ventilatory support and other appropriate agents, is indicated for the treatment of term and near-term (>34 weeks) neonates with hypoxic respiratory failure associated with clinical or echocardiographic evidence of pulmonary hypertension, where it improves oxygenation and reduces the need for extracorporeal membrane oxygenation.

This is the only FDA-approved indication for inhaled NO, and all other uses are off-label. Nitric oxide should not be used for hypoxemic newborns with congenital cardiac defects who are dependent upon right-to-left shunt. The usual starting dose of inhaled NO is 20 ppm. This dose is then weaned to the lowest effective dose (e.g., 5 ppm) and continued until the condition of the baby is improved. Inhaled NO produces an initial improvement in Pa_{O_2} for patients with ARDS, but this effect is lost after several days. Randomized multicenter trials in ARDS failed to report improvements in important patient outcomes such as mortality with the use of inhaled NO.[50–52]

The toxicity of inhaled NO appears to be low when administered by clinicians familiar with its use. Nitrogen dioxide (NO_2) is produced spontaneously from NO and O_2. The conversion rate of NO to NO_2 is determined by the O_2 concentration, NO concentration, and the residence time of NO with O_2. The Occupational Safety and Health Administration (OSHA) has set safety limits for NO_2 at 5 ppm, but airway reactivity and parenchymal lung injury have been reported with inhalation of 2 ppm NO_2 or less. Methemoglobin production after NO exposure is uncommon at the NO doses used for therapeutic inhalation (20 ppm or less). Inhibition of platelet adhesion,

AGE-SPECIFIC ANGLE

The only FDA-approved indication for inhaled nitric oxide is hypoxic respiratory failure of the newborn.

aggregation, and agglutination has been reported with inhaled NO. At high doses (40 to 80 ppm), inhaled NO reportedly decreases pulmonary vascular resistance and increases pulmonary capillary wedge pressure in some patients with severe left ventricular dysfunction.

Withdrawal of inhaled NO is problematic for some patients. In some cases, the degree of hypoxemia and pulmonary hypertension is greater after discontinuation of NO than at baseline, leading to hemodynamic instability. Reinstitution of NO inhalation promptly corrects the hemodynamic instability, and NO withdrawal is postponed until the patient is less severely ill. The reasons for rebound are not known but may relate to feedback inhibition of NOS activity. The following guidelines may prevent the deleterious effects of rebound during withdrawal of inhaled NO:

1. Use the lowest effective NO dose (5 ppm or less).
2. Do not withdraw inhaled NO until the patient's clinical status has improved sufficiently.
3. Set the NO dose at 1 ppm for a short time (30 min to 1 hour) before discontinuing NO.
4. Increase the FIO_2 before withdrawal of inhaled NO and prepare to support the patient's hemodynamics if necessary.

The INOmax DS and INOblender (**Figure 14-29**) allow for operator-determined concentrations of inhaled NO without excessive inhaled NO_2. These devices can be used with neonatal ventilators, adult ventilators, and anesthesia machines and with spontaneously breathing patients. The system is configured for 0 to 80 ppm with an 800-ppm NO source cylinder. These cylinders are either D size or size 88 (1963 L at 2000 psig), are constructed of aluminum alloy, and have threaded connections specific for NO (CGA 626). NO is stored as nitrogen gas. The injection module of the INOvent is inserted into the inspiratory circuit at the outlet of the ventilator. The injection module consists of a hot-film flow sensor and a gas injection tube. Flow in the ventilator circuit is precisely measured, and NO is injected proportional to that flow to provide the desired NO dose. The delivery system includes gas monitoring of O_2, NO, and NO_2 downstream from the point of injection.

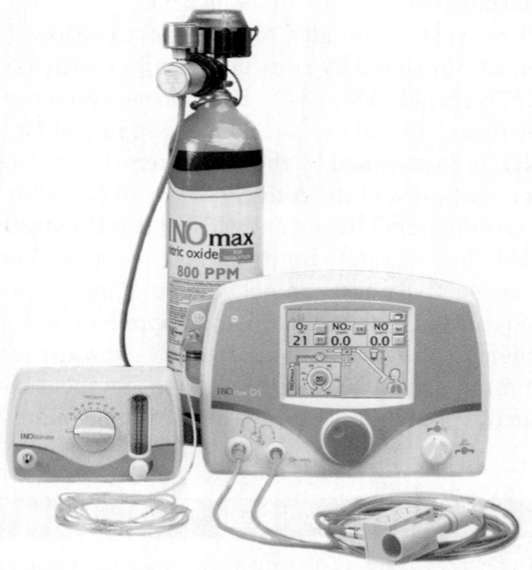

FIGURE 14-29 INOmax DS.
Courtesy of IKARIA.

Key Points

- Supplemental oxygen is indicated to treat hypoxemia as determined by scenario, clinical exam, pulse oximetry, or arterial blood analysis.
- O_2 therapy is used for perioperative conditions, COPD, ARDS, CPR, MI, pulmonary edema, CO poisoning, and traumatic brain injury.
- O_2 is not explosive but increases the combustibility of other flammable materials.
- Supplemental oxygen is a relatively benign drug. However, complications of O_2 therapy include oxygen toxicity, nitrogen washout atelectasis, oxygen-induced hypoventilation, retinopathy of prematurity, and failure of ductus closure in infants with congenital heart disease.
- O_2 may be of limited usefulness for anemia, low cardiac output, or right-to-left shunt >10%.
- Flow control devices include flow restrictors, Bourdon gauges, and Thorpe tubes.
- Back-pressure-compensated Thorpe tubes are accurate regardless of downstream resistance when powered by 50-psig sources.
- Nasal cannulas, simple masks, partial rebreathing masks, and nonrebreathing masks are low-flow oxygen delivery devices, and delivered FIO_2 can vary with patient breathing patterns.
- The FIO_2 from a low-flow oxygen delivery device is determined by the oxygen flow, reservoir volume, and inspiratory flow of the patient.
- High-flow oxygen delivery systems provide more consistent FIO_2 levels as they can better meet the entire and changing inspiratory needs of the patient.
- Hoods, incubators, and tents are oxygen enclosure devices.
- Hyperbaric oxygen therapy is currently indicated for treatment of carbon monoxide poisoning, wounds (especially those infected by anaerobic bacteria), air embolism, and decompression sickness.
- Oxygen analyzers use polarography or galvanic cells to measure oxygen partial pressure and report it as concentration as oxygen %.
- Heliox is used clinically because of its low density and ability to prevent turbulent flow.
- Therapeutic applications of CO_2 therapy are limited or controversial.
- Inhaled nitric oxide is a selective pulmonary vasodilator.

References

1. Criner GJ. Ambulatory home oxygen: what is the evidence for benefit, and who does it help? *Respir Care.* 2013;58:48–64.
2. Owens RL. Supplemental oxygen needs during sleep. Who benefits? *Respir Care.* 2013;58:32–47.
3. Nonoyama ML, Brooks D, Lacasse Y, et al. Oxygen therapy during exercise training in chronic obstructive pulmonary disease. *Cochrane Database of Systematic Reviews.* 2007;(2):CD005372.
4. Mehta V, Vasu TS, Phillips B, Chung F. Obstructive sleep apnea and oxygen therapy: a systematic review of the literature and meta-analysis. *J Clin Sleep Med.* 2013;9:271–279.
5. Hedenstierna G, Rothen HU. Atelectasis formation during anesthesia: causes and measures to prevent it. *J Clin Monit.* 2000;16: 329–335.
6. Togioka B, Galvagno S, Sumida S, et al. The role of perioperative high inspired oxygen therapy in reducing surgical site infection: a meta-analysis. *Anesth Analg.* 2012;114:334–342.
7. Guérin C, Reignier J, Richard JC, Pascal Beuret P, et al. Prone positioning in severe acute respiratory distress syndrome. *N Engl J Med.* 2013;368:2159-2168. http://www.nejm.org/doi/full/10.1056/NEJMoa1214103.
8. O'Driscoll BR, Howard LS, Davison AG, and British Thoracic Society. BTS guideline for emergency use in adult patients. *Thorax.* 2008;(Suppl VI):vi1–vi68.
9. Berg RA, Hemphill R, Abella BS, et al. Part 5: Adult basic life support: 2010 American Heart Association guidelines for cardiopulmonary resuscitation and emergency cardiovascular care. *Circulation.* 2010;122(Suppl 3):S685–S705.
10. SUPPORT Study Group of the Eunice Kennedy Shriver NICHD Neonatal Research Network. Target ranges of oxygen saturation in extremely preterm infants. *N Engl J Med.* 2010;362:1959–1969.
11. Dexter F, Reasoner DK. Theoretical assessment of normobaric oxygen therapy to treat pneumocephalus. *Anesthesiology.* 1996;84: 442–447.
12. Annane D, Troche G, Delisle F, et al. Effects of mechanical ventilation with normobaric oxygen therapy on the rate of air removal from cerebral arteries. *Crit Care Med.* 1994;22:851–857.
13. Martini RP, Deem S, Yanez ND, et al. Management guided by brain tissue oxygen monitoring and outcome following severe traumatic brain injury. *J Neurosurg.* 2009;111:644–649.
14. Nortje J, Gupta AK. The role of tissue oxygen monitoring in patients with acute brain injury. *Br J Anaesth.* 2006;97:95–106.
15. Kallet RH, Matthay MA. Hyperoxic acute lung injury. *Respir Care.* 2013;58:123–141.
16. Ingrassia TS, Ryu JH, Trastek VF, Rosenow EC. Oxygen-exacerbated bleomycin pulmonary toxicity. *Mayo Clin Proc.* 1991; 66:173–178.
17. Crossley DJ, McGuire GP, Barrow PM, Houston PL. Influence of inspired oxygen concentration on deadspace, respiratory drive, and $Paco_2$ in intubated patients with chronic obstructive pulmonary disease. *Crit Care Med.* 1997;25:1522–1526.
18. Aubier M, Murciano D, Milic-Emili J, et al. Effects of the administration of O_2 on ventilation and blood gases in patients with chronic obstructive pulmonary disease during acute respiratory failure. *Am Rev Respir Dis.* 1980;122:747–754.
19. Dunn WF, Nelson SB, Hubmayr RD. Oxygen-induced hypercarbia in obstructive pulmonary disease. *Am Rev Respir Dis.* 1991;144:526–530.
20. Hanson CW, Marshall BE, Frasch HF, Marshall C. Causes of hypercarbia with oxygen therapy in patients with chronic obstructive pulmonary disease. *Crit Care Med.* 1996;24:23–28.
21. Robinson TD, Freiberg DB, Regnis JA, Young IH. The role of hypoventilation and ventilation-perfusion redistribution in oxygen-induced hypercapnia during acute exacerbations of chronic obstructive pulmonary disease. *Am J Respir Crit Care Med.* 2000;161:1524–1529.
22. The BOOST II United Kingdom, Australia, and New Zealand Collaborative Groups. Oxygen saturation and outcomes in preterm infants. *N Engl J Med.* 2013;368:2094–2104.
23. Tálosi G, Katona M, Rácz K, et al. Prostaglandin E1 treatment in patent ductus arteriosus dependent congenital heart defects. *J Perinat Med.* 2004;32:368–374.
24. Bazuaye EA, Stone TN, Corris PA, Gibson GJ. Variability of inspired oxygen concentration with nasal cannulas. *Thorax.* 1992;47:609–611.
25. Dunlevy CL, Tyl SE. The effect of oral versus nasal breathing on oxygen concentrations received from nasal cannulas. *Respir Care.* 1992;37:357–360.
26. Ooi R, Joshi P, Soni N. An evaluation of oxygen delivery using nasal prongs. *Anaesthesia.* 1992;47:591–593.
27. Sim MAB, Dean P, Kinsella J, et al. Performance of oxygen delivery devices when the breathing pattern of respiratory failure is simulated. *Anaesthesia.* 2008;63:938–940.
28. Shigeoka JW, Bonekat HW. The current status of oxygen-conserving devices. *Respir Care.* 1985;30:833–836.
29. Gibson RL, Comer PB, Beckham RW, McGraw CP. Actual tracheal oxygen concentrations with commonly used oxygen equipment. *Anesthesiology.* 1976;44:71–73.
30. Markovitz GH, Colthurst J, Storer TW, et al. Effective inspired oxygen concentrations measured via transtracheal and oral gas analysis. *Respir Care.* 2010;55:453–459.
31. Estey W. Subjective effects of dry versus humidified low flow oxygen. *Respir Care.* 1980;25:1143–1144.
32. Campbell EJ, Baker MD, Crites-Silver P, et al. Subjective effects of humidification of oxygen for delivery by nasal cannula. A prospective study. *Chest.* 1988;93:289–293.
33. Ward JJ. High-flow oxygen administration by nasal cannula for adult and perinatal patients. *Respir Care.* 2013;58:98–120.
34. Jensen AG, Johnson A, Sandstedt S. Rebreathing during oxygen treatment with face mask. The effect of oxygen flow rates on ventilation. *Acta Anaesthesiol Scand.* 1991;35:289–292.
35. Wettstein RB, Shelledy DC, Peters JI. Delivered oxygen concentrations using low-flow and high-flow nasal cannulas. *Respir Care.* 2005;50:604–609.
36. Campbell DJ, Fairfield MC. The delivery of oxygen by a venturi T piece. *Anaesthesia.* 1996;51:558–560.
37. Weaver LK, Hopkins RO, Chan KJ, et al. Hyperbaric oxygen for acute carbon monoxide poisoning. *N Engl J Med.* 2002;347: 1057–1067.
38. Fu ES, Downs JB, Schweiger JW, et al. Supplemental oxygen impairs detection of hypoventilation by pulse oximetry. *Chest.* 2005;126:1552–1558.
39. Myers TR. Use of heliox in children. *Respir Care.* 2006;51: 619–631.
40. Fink JB. Opportunities and risks of using heliox in your clinical practice. *Respir Care.* 2006;51:651–660.
41. Hess DR, Fink JB, Venkataraman ST, et al. The history and physics of heliox. *Respir Care.* 2006;51:608–612.
42. McGarvey JM, Pollack CV. Heliox in airway management. *Emerg Med Clin North Am.* 2008;26:905–920.
43. Colebourn CL, Barber V, Young JD. Use of helium-oxygen mixture in adult patients presenting with exacerbations of asthma and chronic obstructive pulmonary disease: a systematic review. *Anaesthesia.* 2007;62:34–42.
44. Valli G, Paoletti P, Savi D, et al. Clinical use of heliox in asthma and COPD. *Monaldi Arch Chest Dis.* 2007;67:159–164.
45. Hess DR. Heliox and noninvasive positive-pressure ventilation: a role for heliox in exacerbations of chronic obstructive pulmonary disease? *Respir Care.* 2006;51:640–650.
46. Koh Y, Hurford WE. Inhaled nitric oxide in acute respiratory distress syndrome: from bench to bedside. *Int Anesthesiol Clin.* 2003;41:91–102.
47. Arul N, Konduri GG. Inhaled nitric oxide for preterm neonates. *Clin Perinatol.* 2009;36:43–61.
48. Soll RF. Inhaled nitric oxide in the neonate. *J Perinatol.* 2009;29:(Suppl 2):S63–S67.

49. Lorch SA, Cnaan A, Barnhart K. Cost-effectiveness of inhaled nitric oxide for the management of persistent pulmonary hypertension of the newborn. *Pediatrics*. 2004;114:417–426.
50. Griffiths MJ, Evans TW. Inhaled nitric oxide therapy in adults. *N Engl J Med*. 2005;353:2683–2695.
51. Adhikari NK, Burns KE, Friedrich JO, et al. Effect of nitric oxide on oxygenation and mortality in acute lung injury: systematic review and meta-analysis. *BMJ*. 2007;334:779.
52. Creagh-Brown BC, Griffiths MJ, Evans TW. Bench-to-bedside review: inhaled nitric oxide therapy in adults. *Crit Care*. 2009;13:221.

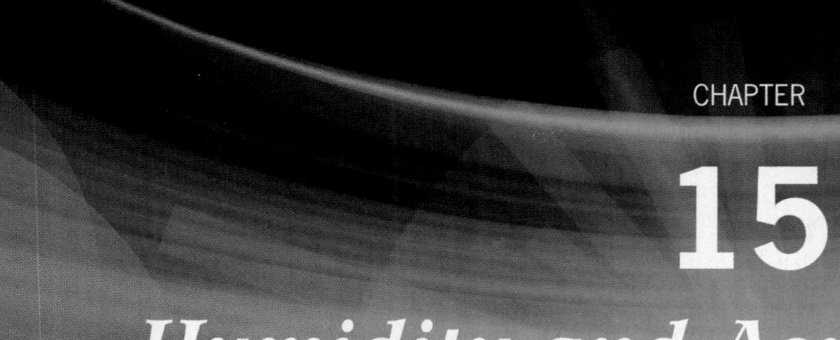

CHAPTER

15

Humidity and Aerosol Therapy

Dean R. Hess

OUTLINE

OBJECTIVES

1. Describe the normal gas warming and humidification functions of the upper airway.
2. List the goals of aerosol and humidity therapy.
3. Compare active and passive humidifiers.
4. Compare heated and unheated humidifiers.
5. Compare jet nebulizers, ultrasonic nebulizers, and mesh nebulizers.
6. Compare nebulizers, pressurized metered dose inhalers, and dry powder inhalers for aerosol drug administration.
7. Distinguish between spacers and valved holding chambers.
8. Discuss issues involved in the selection of a device for aerosol delivery.
9. Discuss issues pertinent to aerosol drug delivery during mechanical ventilation.

KEY TERMS

active humidifier
aerosol
artificial nose
bland aerosol therapy
bubble humidifier
dry powder inhaler (DPI)
geometric standard deviation (GSD)
gravitational sedimentation
humidity therapy
isothermic saturation boundary (ISB)
jet nebulizer
large-volume nebulizer
mass median aerodynamic diameter (MMAD)
mesh nebulizer
nebulizer
passive humidifier
passover humidifier
pressurized metered dose inhaler (pMDI)
Respimat soft mist inhaler
spacer
ultrasonic nebulizer
valved holding chamber

Introduction

Administration of humidity and aerosol therapy is a common task for the respiratory therapist. Humidification of inspired gas is particularly important in the care of mechanically ventilated patients, and many respiratory drugs are administered as aerosols. The selection of appropriate devices for humidity and aerosol production may have an important impact on the outcome of the patient's condition.

Humidity

The interface between the atmosphere and the lungs is mediated through the fluid lining of the airways. Water in inspired gas is essential to a healthy respiratory tract. Administration of dry, cold gas bypassing the upper airway can change the balance of the fluid lining the airways and may result in either short-term or irreversible structural damage of the airway.[1,2] Exposure of the airways to cold, dry air from the ambient environment increases mucus production and thickening of secretions, reduces the motility of the cilia, and increases airway irritability. Administration of dry gases via an endotracheal tube can damage the tracheal epithelium. **Humidity therapy** is the addition of water to the gas delivered to the airways.

The nose, which adds heat and humidity to the inspired gas, is an efficient humidifier. The respiratory mucosa lining the sinuses, trachea, and bronchi assists in heating and humidifying inspired gas. The respiratory mucosa is covered by secretions produced by mucous glands, goblet cells, and transudation of fluid through cell walls (**Figure 15-1**). Heat is transferred from capillary beds close to the surface of the mucosa. The nasal mucosa is particularly well suited for this function, having the highest concentration of mucous glands in the airway and a rich vascular bed close to the surface that provides heat and water. The turbinates and conchae provide a convoluted path for gas to travel, creating turbulent flow and a large surface area for contact with respiratory gases. This large surface area gives up heat and moisture to inspired gas and efficiently recovers heat and water on exhalation.

Normal Heat and Moisture Exchange

By the time inspired gas reaches the lung parenchyma, it is fully saturated with water vapor at body temperature (44 mg/L at 37° C). See **Figure 15-2**. The point at which this occurs is known as the **isothermic saturation boundary (ISB)**, which is approximately 5 cm below the carina at the level of the third-generation airways. Above the ISB, temperature and humidity fall during inspiration and rise during exhalation. Below the ISB, temperature and relative humidity do not fluctuate.

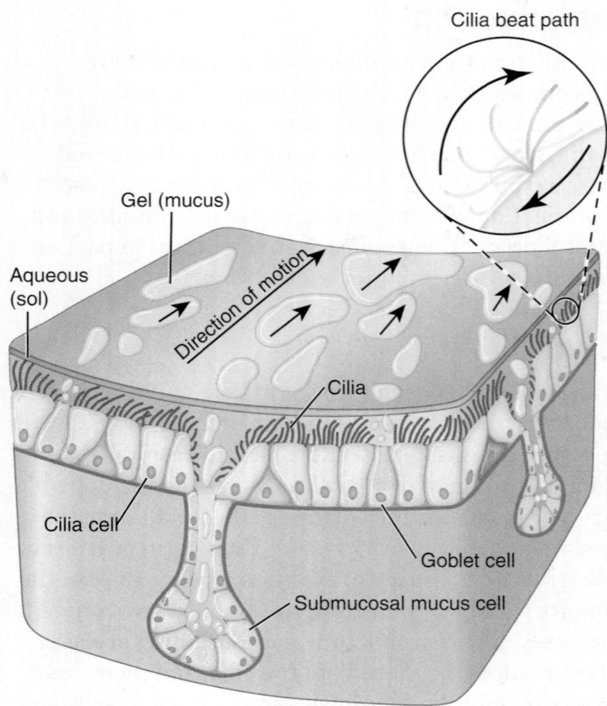

FIGURE 15-1 The cellular, aqueous, and mucous components of the airway mucosa.

Adapted from Williams R, Rankin N, Smith T, et al. Relationship between humidity and temperature of inspired gas and the function of the airway mucosa. *Crit Care Med.* 1996;24:1920–1929.

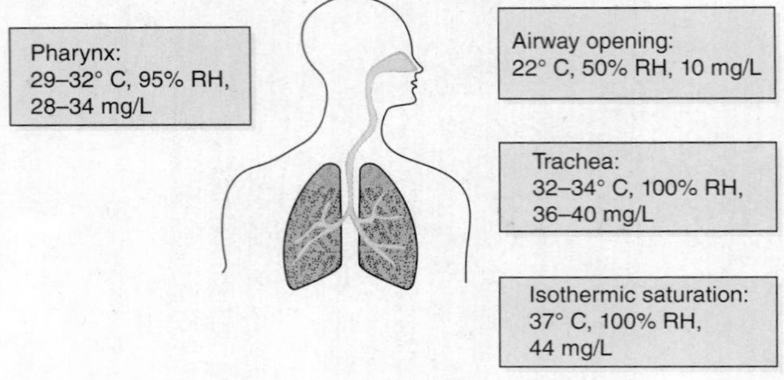

FIGURE 15-2 Normal temperature and humidity of gas at various points along the respiratory tract.

A drop in environmental temperature and humidity, mouth breathing, an increase in tidal volume, or endotracheal intubation (which bypasses the upper airway) moves the ISB deeper into the lungs, although it never reaches the level of the respiratory bronchioles or alveoli.

At the end of inspiration, the temperature of the nasal mucosa is 31° C (87.8° F) or lower because of heat loss caused by turbulent convection and loss of the latent heat of vaporization. As inspired gas warms, water vapor is transferred by evaporation from the mucosal lining through the latent heat of vaporization. Warming and humidification continue until the inspired gas is fully saturated at body temperature. Although the latent heat of vaporization remains as water vapor and does not contribute to warming of gases, the loss of latent heat of vaporization does cause the mucosa to cool. During exhalation, heat is transferred from exhaled gas to the cooler tracheal and nasal mucosa by convection. As these gases cool, their capacity to hold water vapor diminishes, and condensation occurs. Water accumulates on the tracheal surfaces, where the mucus reabsorbs it. Heat is transferred back to the mucosa, resulting in warming and rehydration. Latent heat and water are held until the next inspiration. With mouth breathing, the flow is more laminar, requiring heat transfer by radiation. Because air is a poor conductor of heat, the mouth is less efficient than the nose at heating inspired air.

The temperature and water vapor at the oropharynx during oral and nasal breathing of room air is about 22° C, with a relative humidity (RH) of 15% to 39%. At the pharynx, the temperature difference between

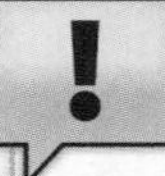

Respiratory Recap

Normal Heat and Moisture Exchange

- The upper airway is an effective humidifier.
- The isothermic saturation boundary (ISB) is the point at which inspired gas reaches body temperature and humidity.
- Breathing dry gas moves the ISB deeper into the respiratory tract.

inspired and expired gas is 4° C during nose breathing and 7° C during mouth breathing. The inspired gas temperature increases 5° C during mouth breathing and 9° C during nose breathing. The RH is 95% at the oropharynx during inspiration with nose breathing, and 75% during mouth breathing. On exhalation, the RH is nearly 95% at the pharynx and 90% at the airway opening. This suggests that the normal airway can condition inspired gas to add humidity with either nose or mouth breathing. More heat and moisture are lost with exhalation in mouth breathing than with exhalation in nose breathing. Even with mouth breathing, the ISB is not typically lower than the third generation of the bronchi.

Heat and moisture normally are lost from the mucosa above the ISB, from a surface area of approximately 300 cm^2 that is covered by 240 μL of airway lining fluid 8 μm deep. With normal tidal volume for an adult male, 22 μL of water and 61 J of heat are required to condition each breath from normal ambient conditions to 100% RH at body temperature. The water and heat losses per breath are 15 μL and 42 J, respectively. Over a 24-hour period, these losses total 250 mL of water and 726 kJ.

When dry, cold gases are inhaled, the ISB is shifted deeper into the respiratory tract, and ciliary function and mucus production are compromised. Bypassing the upper airway eliminates the normal efficient mechanisms used to retain heat and humidity in the lungs. Recruitment of airways that are less efficient for humidification changes their mucosal characteristics. The lower gas temperature farther down the airways reduces ciliary activity within 10 minutes. Once compromised, ciliary function can take several weeks to recover. Respiratory secretions become thicker, contributing to mucous plugging and inability to maintain normal bronchopulmonary hygiene. When absolute humidity drops below 24 mg/L in the inhaled gas, the beat frequency of the cilia is reduced.

Goals of Humidity Therapy

The primary goal of humidity therapy is to maintain normal physiologic conditions by providing adequate heat and humidity to inspired gas to approximate normal inspiratory conditions (**CPG 15-1**). Administration of heat and humidity is also advocated, with fewer supporting data, for the treatment of hypothermia, reactive airway response to cold air, and thickened secretions.

Medical gases are processed to remove all water vapor. When this gas is delivered to the nose and mouth, ideally it should be heated and humidified to normal ambient room air conditions (22° C at 50% RH or an absolute humidity of 10 mg/L). For gas delivered to the trachea through an endotracheal or tracheotomy tube, heat and humidity should be at least 32° to 35° C at 100% RH (absolute humidity of 36 to 40 mg/L).

For premature and newborn infants, a neutral thermal environment should be maintained, with adequate warmth and humidity to minimize insensible heat and water loss. Low-birth-weight infants provided adequate heat and humidity showed a reduced morbidity rate compared with infants breathing colder and dryer inspired gas. The body loses considerable heat through normal ventilation. For hypothermic patients, rewarming and reduction of further heat loss can be facilitated

CLINICAL PRACTICE GUIDELINE 15-1

Recommendations for Humidification During Invasive and Noninvasive Mechanical Ventilation

1. Humidification is recommended on every patient receiving invasive mechanical ventilation.
2. Active humidification is suggested for noninvasive mechanical ventilation, as it may improve adherence and comfort.
3. When providing active humidification to patients who are invasively ventilated, it is suggested that the device provide a humidity level between 33 mg H_2O/L and 44 mg H_2O/L and gas temperature between 34° C and 41° C at the circuit Y piece, with a relative humidity of 100%.
4. When providing passive humidification to patients undergoing invasive mechanical ventilation, it is suggested that the HME provide a minimum of 30 mg H_2O/L.
5. Passive humidification is not recommended for noninvasive mechanical ventilation.
6. When providing humidification to patients with low tidal volumes, such as when lung-protective ventilation strategies are used, HMEs are not recommended because they contribute additional dead space, which can increase the ventilation requirement and Pa_{CO_2}.
7. It is suggested that HMEs are not used as a prevention strategy for ventilator-associated pneumonia.

Reproduced from Restrepo RD, Walsh BK. Humidification during invasive and noninvasive mechanical ventilation: 2012. *Respir Care.* 2012:57:782–788.

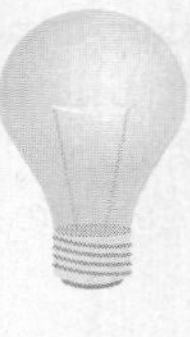

STOP AND THINK

A hypothermic patient arrives in your emergency department. You are asked to provide warm, humidified gas to speed rewarming. How effective do you think that will be?

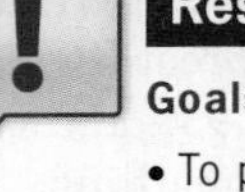

Respiratory Recap

Goals of Humidity Therapy

- To provide adequate heat and humidity
- To treat hypothermia
- To prevent airway response to cold air
- To aid removal of thick secretions

by heating the inspired gases. However, this technique is less useful than other warming treatments (e.g., wrapping the patient in blankets and warming intravenous solutions). Individuals with reactive airways develop increased airway resistance when they breathe cold air. This response can be diminished by warming of the inspired gases and provision of gas humidified with at least 20 mg/L of water at 23° C.

Heated humidity has been used in the treatment of patients with thick, tenacious secretions. No studies have reported a benefit from the use of external humidifiers to try to improve the character and mobilization of thick secretions. Most patients with an artificial airway require humidification of inspired gas to prevent the formation of thick, tenacious secretions. However, evidence is lacking to support the use of humidity therapy (i.e., cool mist or heated aerosol) for patients with an intact upper airway. Cooler than room temperature humidified gases and aerosols commonly are used in the treatment of upper airway inflammation caused by croup, epiglottitis, and swelling resulting from extubation. The cold gas promotes localized vasoconstriction, thereby reducing swelling and relieving the discomfort associated with upper airway inflammation.

Excessive humidity is defined as a level greater than 100% RH at body temperature. The water volume of a vapor stream is 20 to 50 μL of water per liter of air and is unlikely to cause overhumidification. To exceed that water volume, gas temperatures would have to be grossly in excess of body temperature. Humidification of inspired gas reduces insensible water loss from the airway but is unlikely to add significant water to the body. Inspired gas warmer than 45° C may cause thermal injury to the airway.

Devices Used for Humidification

A humidifier adds molecular water to gas.[3–5] An **active humidifier** adds water or heat or both to the inspired gas. A **nebulizer** produces an **aerosol**, or suspension of particles in gas. A **passive humidifier** uses exhaled heat and moisture to humidify inspired gas; heat and moisture exchangers are passive humidifiers. The American National Standards Institute (ANSI) recommends that heated humidifiers have a water output level of at least 30 mg/L (100% RH at 30° C). This is considered the minimum level of humidity to avoid mucosal damage and inspissation of secretions for patients who have a bypassed upper airway (i.e., an endotracheal or tracheostomy tube). The Emergency Care Research Institute (ECRI) recommends that active humidifiers have an output of 37 mg of water per liter of inspired gas (85% RH at body temperature or 100% RH at 34° C). Active heated water humidifiers are the devices of choice for intubation, tracheostomy, and long-term mechanical ventilation. The ANSI recommends a water output of 10 mg/L for unheated humidifiers; this provides approximately 50% RH at 22° C ambient conditions, which enhances the dissipation of static electricity to prevent fires. This humidity level is thought to be the lowest acceptable level to minimize mucosal damage to the upper airway in a variety of environments.

Active Humidifiers

A **passover humidifier** (**Figure 15-3**) directs gas over the surface of a body of water (Figure 15-3A and Figure 15-3B). The passover wick humidifier incorporates a wick of absorbent paper or cloth that draws

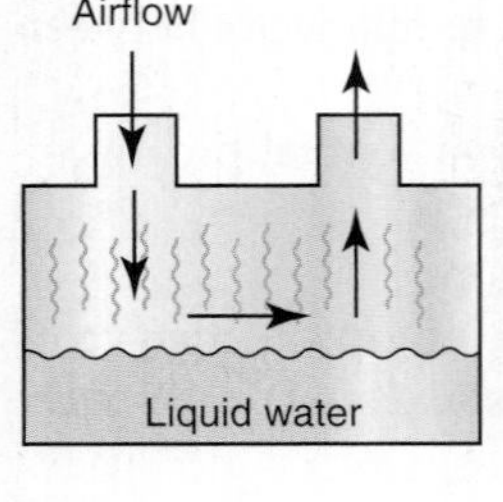

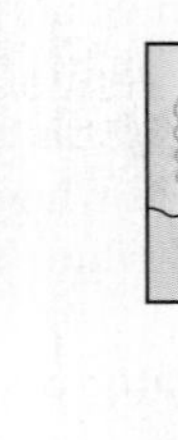

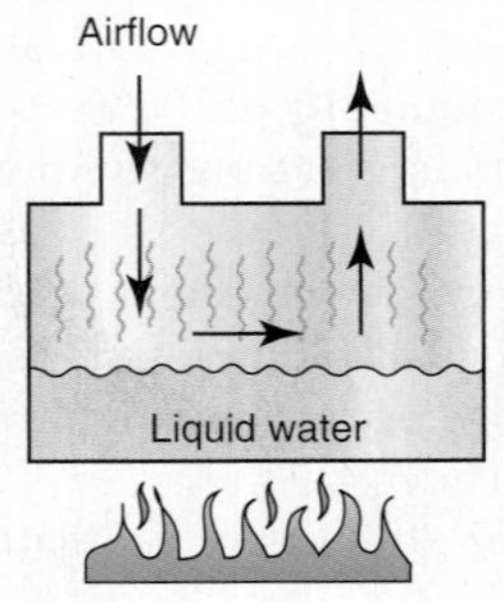

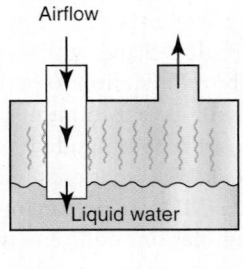

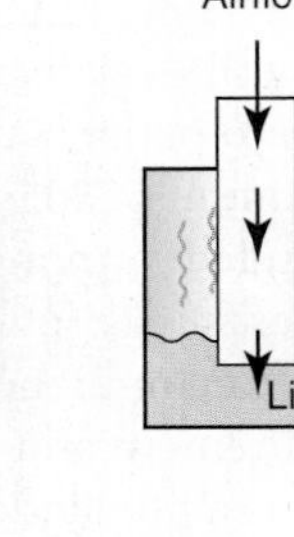

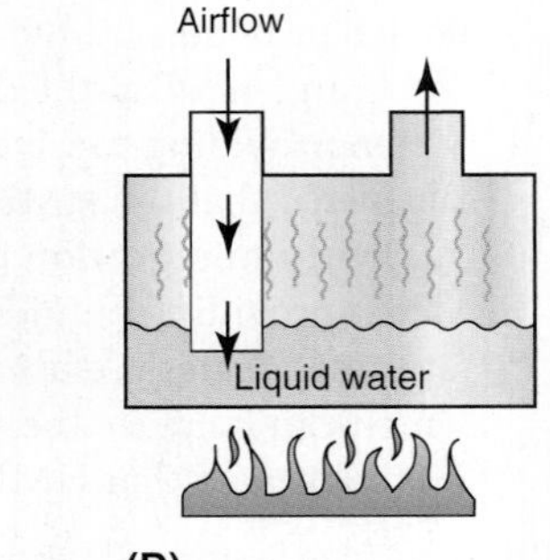

FIGURE 15-3 (**A**) Passover humidifier. (**B**) Heated passover humidifier. (**C**) Bubble humidifier. (**D**) Heated bubble humidifier.

(**A–D**) adapted from Peterson BD. Heated humidifiers. *Respir Care Clin North Am.* 1998;4:243–260.

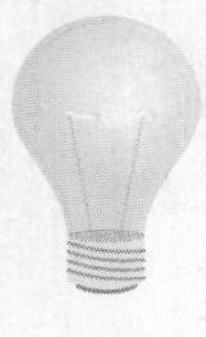

STOP AND THINK

A patient receiving low-flow oxygen therapy by cannula complains of nasal drying. Do you think a bubble humidifier will help? What other options might you suggest?

water from the reservoir and becomes saturated; the wick comes in contact with the gas stream. A passover/barrier humidifier uses a hydrophobic barrier that allows water molecules, but not droplets, to cross from the water reservoir into the gas stream.

In a **bubble humidifier**, dry gas is directed toward the bottom of a water-filled reservoir, where the stream of gas is broken up (diffused) into bubbles, which gain humidity as they rise through the water (Figure 15-3C). This commonly is accomplished with a tube that directs gas beneath the surface of the water; with a tube that has small holes along its length; or with a tube that is attached to a diffuser made of plastic foam, sintered metal, or mesh that breaks the stream of gas into small bubbles. Bubble humidifiers typically are not heated and are used with simple oxygen delivery devices. The higher the flow through a bubble humidifier, the lower the water vapor content and temperature of the gas leaving the device. Commercially available bubble humidifiers are capable of humidifying dry medical gas to an absolute humidity of 10 to 20 mg/L at flows of 2 to 10 L/min. Bubble humidifiers are most efficient at flows of 5 L/min or less. When flows greater than 10 L/min are required, other humidifying options should be considered. At flows under 10 L/min, bubble humidifiers are safe for extended single-patient use without risk of infection. Heating the reservoir improves the efficiency of these humidifiers; however, the small-bore tubing used to connect the humidifier to the administration appliance is easily obstructed by condensate as the humidified gas cools en route to the patient. Low-flow, unheated bubble humidifiers typically have a gravity or spring-loaded pressure-relief valve to protect against obstructed or kinked tubing and an alarm that sounds when a pressure of 2 psi or higher develops in the humidifier.

The addition of humidity to low-flow medical gas is not an evidence-based practice, and eliminating the use of humidifiers for low-flow oxygen reduces the cost of routine oxygen administration. Humidification of the inspired gas should be considered for patients who complain of discomfort associated with nasal dryness or irritation. Devices that are more efficient than simple bubble humidifiers better accomplish this. Topical application of water-based lubricants to the nostrils may be a reasonable response to complaints of dryness.

Heated bubble humidifiers (Figure 15-3D) can be used with intubated patients. These humidifiers can accommodate flows of 10 to 120 L/min and use tubing with a 22-mm inside diameter (ID). These devices use corrugated 22-mm ID tubing between the humidifier and the patient. At high flows bubble humidifiers produce aerosols that may transmit bacteria from the humidifier's reservoir to the patient. Heated passover humidifiers are used most commonly during mechanical ventilation (**Figure 15-4**).

A **jet nebulizer** (**Figure 15-5**) uses compressed gas that passes through a restricted orifice, creating a low-pressure area near the tip of a narrow tube. Fluid is drawn from a reservoir and sheared or shattered into droplets by the airstream. Jet nebulizers incorporate baffles to minimize aerosol exiting particle size and use the aerosol in the device to maximize surface contact with the gas. Because jet nebulizers pose a risk of infection from bacteria that might colonize the reservoir, they should always be filled with sterile fluids and residual fluids should be discarded before refilling.

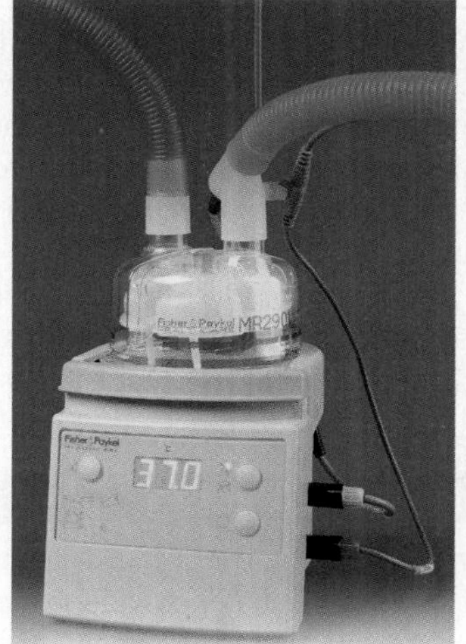

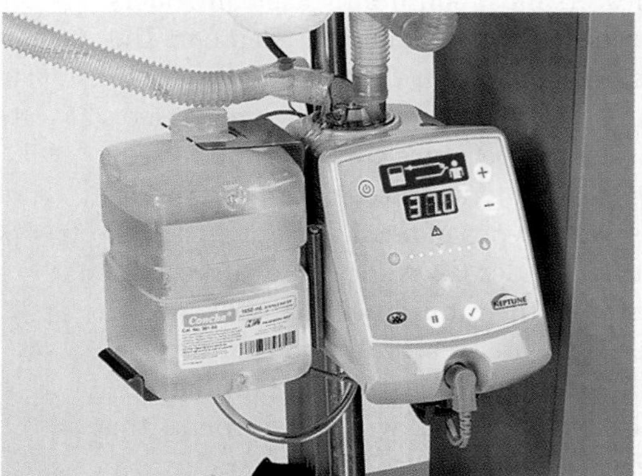

FIGURE 15-4 Commercially available heated humidifiers used during mechanical ventilation.

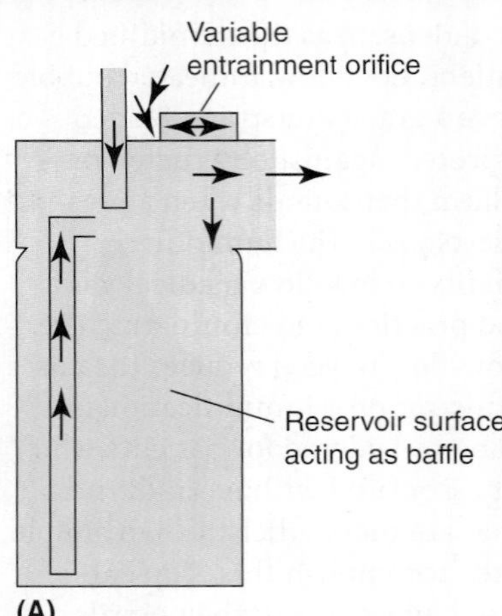

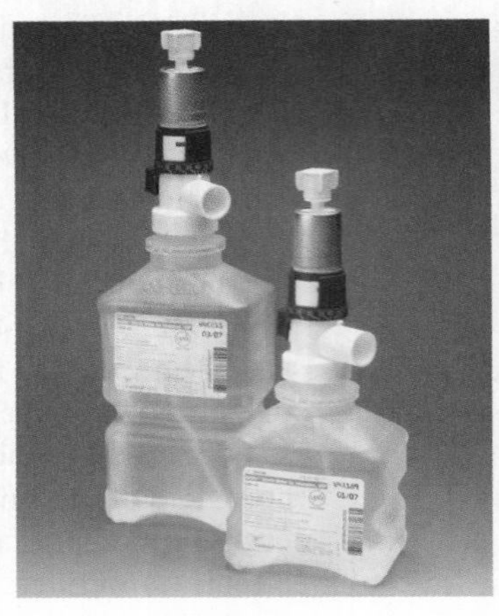

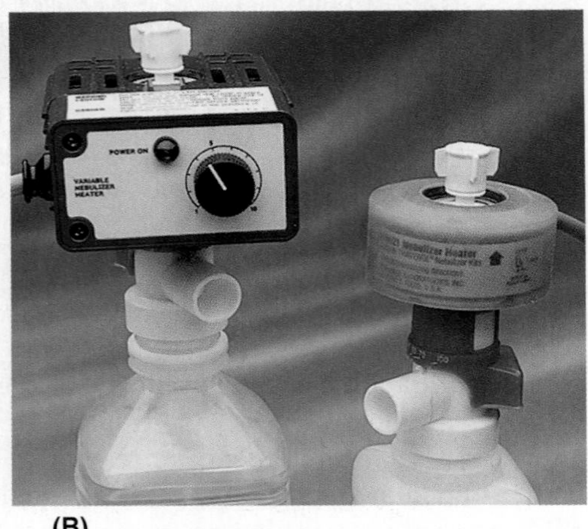

FIGURE 15-5 (**A**) Schematic drawing of large-volume jet nebulizer. (**B**) Commercially available large-volume nebulizers.
(**A**) modified from Cohen N, Fink J. Humidity and aerosols. In: Eubanks DH, Bone RC, eds. *Principles and Applications of Cardiorespiratory Care Equipment.* Mosby; 1994; (**B**) courtesy of Cardinal Health.

Systems used to replace the water in the humidifier should ensure continuity of therapy and minimize disruption of gas flow to the patient. Continuous-feed systems are desirable because the water is replenished without operator intervention or interruption of gas flow to the patient. These systems often rely on gravity, usually consisting of a mounted reservoir external to the humidifier mechanism and most commonly with flotation controls and level-compensated reservoirs. Continuous feed systems typically maintain a constant compressible volume, which is important when they are used in the neonatal or pediatric ventilator circuit.

Intermittent-fill systems have disadvantages compared with continuous-feed systems. Changing the water level in a fixed-volume container changes the compressible volume in both the humidifier and the ventilator, resulting in fluctuations in the delivered tidal volume. This problem is of greatest concern for mechanically ventilated newborns and pediatric patients. Open intermittent-fill systems are more susceptible to contamination of the reservoir. With humidifiers that do not have alarms for low water levels, the humidifier chamber must be checked regularly or it can become empty, reducing the humidity and temperature of gas delivered to the patient.

Humidifier heaters most commonly use controllers to regulate electrical power to the heater element. The most basic units do not monitor the temperature of the heater, providing power to the heating element based on the setting of the temperature control knob rather than the patient's airway temperature. Active humidifiers use one of several types of heating elements: a heating plate located under the reservoir, a curved element wrapped around the humidifier chamber, a yoke or collar between the water reservoir and the active mechanism of the nebulizer, a plate or rod immersed in the water reservoir, or a set of wires or elements that heat an absorbent wick or tubes containing water.

Servo-controlled humidifiers monitor the temperature of gas delivered to the patient, adjusting the power to the heating elements according to the temperature monitored by a thermistor probe placed downstream from the humidifier, near the patient's airway connection. When the temperature at the patient's airway is lower than desired, the controller supplies more power to the heater. As this distal temperature nears or exceeds the set temperature, power to the heating system is reduced. Thermistor probes are best placed in the inspiratory limb of the ventilator circuit, far enough from the patient that the temperature of the exhaled gas is not detected. The sensor probe in the inspiratory limb must be located outside the heated environment to allow the heated-wire controller to maintain the desired temperature and water content of inspired gases (**Figure 15-6**).

As heated and humidified gas cools, its ability to hold water vapor declines, and condensation (rain out) occurs. The amount of condensate is affected by the ambient temperature, gas flow, and the patient's airway temperature and by the length, diameter, and thermal mass of the tubing between the humidifier and the patient. In a traditional ventilator circuit, the humidifier is heated to 50° C or higher and saturated gas contains more than 80 mg of water per liter. As the gas cools to 35° C en route to the patient, it can hold only 40 mg of water per liter; therefore, any amount over that condenses in the tubing. The circuit must be drained frequently to prevent pooling condensate from obstructing the gas flow or inadvertently pouring into the patient's airway.

Often the ventilator circuit, and subsequently condensate, becomes contaminated with bacteria from the patient within the first hour that the patient is attached

AGE-SPECIFIC ANGLE

The temperature probe of a humidifier should not be placed inside an incubator or under a radiant heater because the surrounding air temperature affects humidifier function.

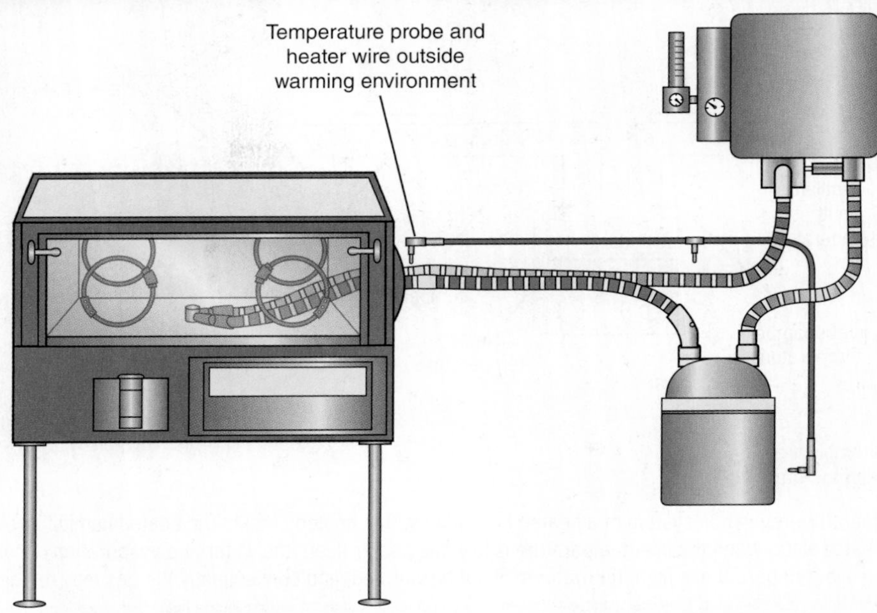

FIGURE 15-6 Position of temperature probe outside of incubator when using heated humidification system.
Adapted from Peterson BD. Heated humidifiers. *Respir Care Clin North Am.* 1998;4:243–260.

to the ventilator. The tubing should be positioned such that drainage is away from the patient's airway to avoid accidental lavage of the airway. Condensate presents a risk to the staff and should always be treated and disposed of as contaminated waste. Water traps placed in dependent positions in both the inspiratory and expiratory limbs drain condensate from the ventilator circuit, reducing the obstruction to gas flow. Water traps should minimize changes in circuit compliance and allow emptying without disrupting ventilation of the patient.

Techniques used to reduce the formation of condensate include an increase in the thermal mass of the circuit, use of a coaxial circuit with the inspiratory limb surrounded by the expiratory limb, and addition of heated wires to the circuit. Increasing the passive thermal mass of the circuit with thick tubing or wrapping the tubing with insulating material insulates the gas inside the tubing from ambient air. Surrounding the inspiratory limb of the circuit with the expiratory limb in a coaxial manner uses the patient's exhaled gas as a heated air bath surrounding the inspiratory limb.

Placing heated wires in the inspiratory and expiratory tubing of the ventilator circuit heats the gas in the circuit, reducing the temperature differential between humidifier and patient. The humidifier operates at a lower temperature with heated-wire circuits than it does with conventional circuits. The humidifier's RH control regulates the temperature differential between the humidifier and the circuit temperature. When the humidifier is cooler than the gas in the inspiratory limb, the absolute humidity remains the same although the relative humidity is decreased, and the circuit has no condensate (**Figure 15-7**). An increase in inlet chamber temperature induced by high ambient temperature reduces the performance of heated-wire humidifiers, leading to a risk of endotracheal tube occlusion (**Figure 15-8**).[6]

When inlet chamber temperature is high, the humidifier heater plate stops heating. The water contained in the chamber remains too cold for evaporation to occur, leading to low levels of humidity. Inlet chamber temperature is influenced by both ambient temperature and ventilator output temperature. High ambient temperature prevents the gas from cooling

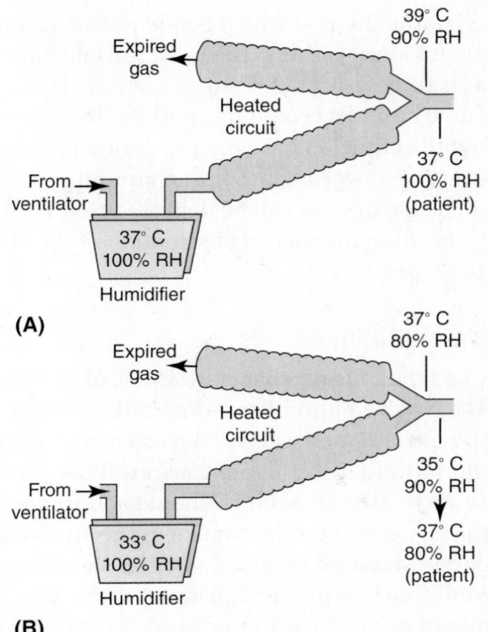

FIGURE 15-7 (**A**) Appropriate settings for a heated-wire circuit, such that gas delivered to the patient is 100% body humidity. (**B**) Settings too low for a heated-wire circuit, such that gas delivered to the patient is too dry.

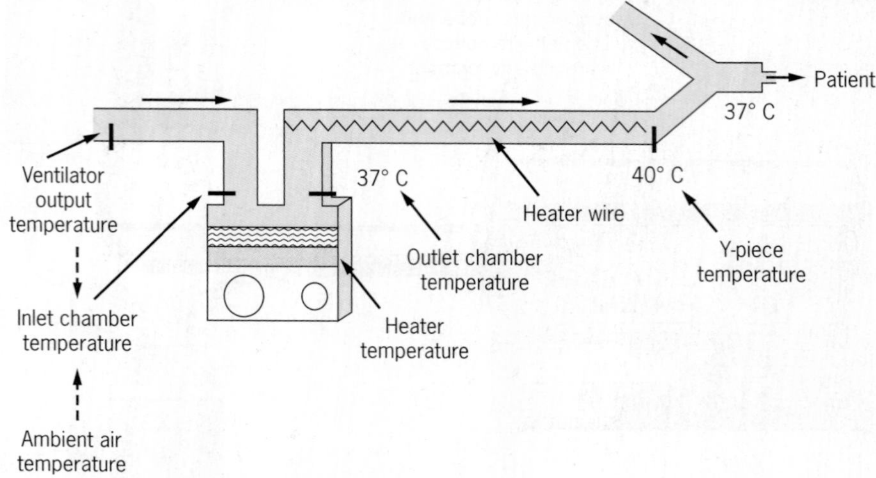

FIGURE 15-8 The temperature regulation system of a heated humidifier with a heated circuit. The heated humidifier outlet temperature is regulated through the heater plate. When the inlet temperature is low, the heater heats the water and evaporation occurs, ensuring sufficient humidification. When the inlet temperature is high, the water may not be warmed, and consequently the gas may remain dry.

in the circuit between the ventilator output and the humidification chamber. Ventilator output gas temperature is also influenced by minute ventilation. To avoid overhumidification, the temperature of gas delivered under conditions of induced hypoventilation should be set to the patient's core body temperature.[7]

When no condensate is visible in the inspiratory limb of the ventilator circuit, it is impossible to know whether the gas is being humidified without direct humidity measurements. To ensure humidification of the inspired gas, the temperature differential should be adjusted to the point at which condensation forms near the patient's airway; this is the most reliable indicator that gas is fully saturated. If no condensate is visible, the relative humidity could be anything from zero to 99%, and the clinician has no way of knowing what it is without using a hygrometer. If the humidity control is set incorrectly, dry gas can be delivered to the patient's airway, resulting in mucous obstruction of the airway (refer to Figure 15-7).

Passive Humidifiers

A heat and moisture exchanger (HME), or **artificial nose**, is a passive humidifier.[8] The HME captures exhaled heat and moisture and transfers part of that heat and humidity to the next inspired breath (**Figure 15-9**). The ideal HME should add minimal dead space, weight, and resistance to the airway, should incorporate standard connections, and should operate at 70% efficiency or higher. Efficiency is the ratio of the humidity of exhaled gas to the humidity returned to the patient by the HME.

HMEs include condensers, hygroscopic condensers, and hygrophobic condensers. Condenser humidifiers are constructed of metallic gauze, corrugated metal, or parallel metal tubes that provide high thermal conductivity. The condenser cools to room temperature during inspiration. During exhalation, saturated gas cools as it contacts the condenser, water condenses and collects on the elements of the condenser, and the temperature of the condenser core rises. On the next inspiration, air is warmed and humidified by the condenser through evaporation of water from the surface. Condenser humidifiers usually are only about 50% efficient.

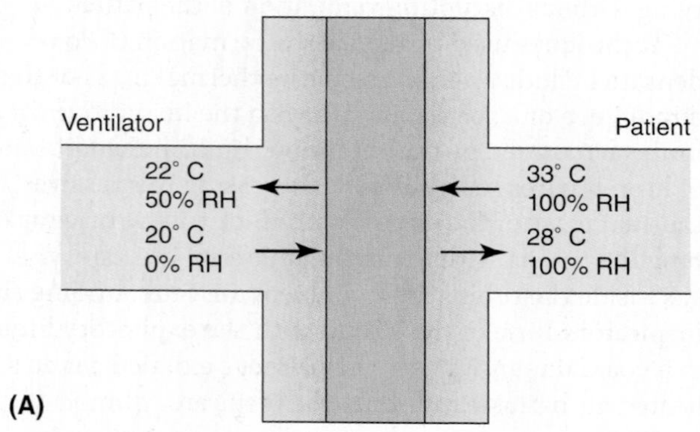

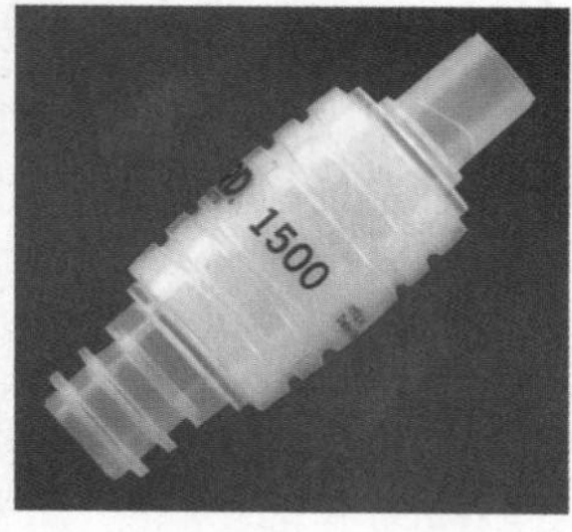

FIGURE 15-9 (**A**) Function of heat and moisture exchanger. (**B**) Commercially available heat and moisture exchanger.

Respiratory Recap

Assessment of Adequate Humidity Delivery

The delivered relative humidity is 100% if condensate is seen in the delivery tubing near the patient's airway.

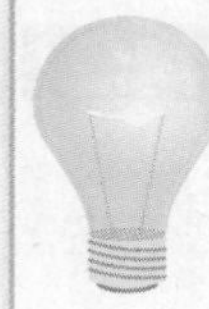

STOP AND THINK

A mechanically ventilated patient has a respiratory acidosis. How might an HME contribute to this problem?

Hygroscopic condenser humidifiers contain materials of low thermal conductivity (meaning that heat from conduction and the latent heat of condensation are not dissipated), such as paper, wool, or foam, which are impregnated with a hygroscopic chemical such as calcium chloride or lithium chloride. During exhalation, warm saturated gas precipitates water on the cool condenser element while water molecules bind to the salt without transition from vapor to liquid state. During inspiration, the lower water vapor pressure in the inspired gas liberates water molecules from the hygroscopic compound without a fall in temperature from vaporization. The efficiency of these devices can be as high as 70%.

Hydrophobic condenser humidifiers use a water-repellent element with a large surface area and low thermal conductivity. During exhalation, the condenser temperature rises to about 25° C. On inspiration, cool gas and evaporation cool the condenser to about 10° C. This large temperature shift results in more water condensation in the humidifier on exhalation, and this water is used to humidify the next inspiration. These devices are about 70% efficient. Hydrophobic humidifiers can also serve as efficient microbiologic filters.

The efficiency of HMEs declines as the tidal volume, inspiratory flow, or fraction inspired oxygen (FIO_2) increases. Resistance through the HME increases as the water load of the device increases. When the HME is dry, resistance across the device is minimal, but after several hours of use, resistance may increase as water is absorbed onto a hygroscopic HME. The increased work of breathing imposed by HMEs may not be well tolerated by patients. HMEs also increase mechanical dead space. This is particularly problematic with lung-protective mechanical ventilation, where the lower tidal volume coupled with the additional mechanical dead space can result in hypercapnia.[9–12]

The HME forms a barrier between the patient and the ventilator circuit. However, the value of the HME as a filter, in terms of patient outcomes and the safety of the healthcare provider, is unclear. A clinical algorithm can be used to guide the use of HMEs (**Figure 15-10**). Although manufacturers recommend that these devices be changed daily, current evidence suggests that they can be safely used for at least 48 hours.[13,14]

The choice of an HME should be based on efficiency, dead space, weight, and cost. In a study of 48 HMEs,[15] it was reported that the humidity efficiency of the devices ranged from 38% to 91%. Several HMEs performed so poorly that they should not be used. The resistance of these devices ranged from a maximum of 4 cm H_2O/L/s to a minimum of 0.4 cm H_2O/L/s, and the dead space ranged from 22 mL to 95 mL. It is important to appreciate the heterogeneity of the humidification performance of HMEs; in other words, some perform much better than others. HMEs are an inexpensive alternative to active humidifiers, but cost alone should not be the determining factor in the decision to use these devices.

Contraindications for HME use include the presence of thick, copious, or bloody secretions; a large leak, such as might occur with a large bronchopleural fistula, a leak around the endotracheal tube cuff, or a leak around the interface with noninvasive ventilation; a body temperature below 32° C; and a minute ventilation greater than 10 L/min. Of concern is the fact that the dead space of the HME can result in an increase in $PaCO_2$ or ventilatory requirement, or both, in the patient with a low tidal volume as part of a lung-protective ventilation strategy. Hazards associated with the use of HMEs include impaction of pulmonary

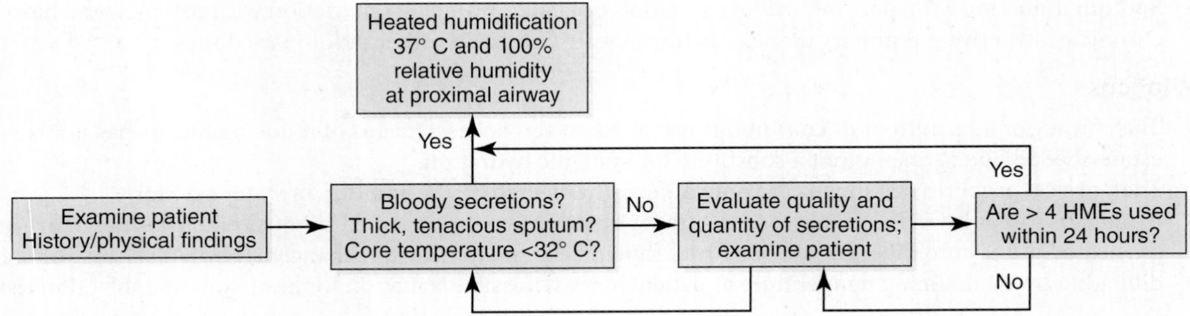

FIGURE 15-10 Clinical algorithm for use of heat and moisture exchanger.

Adapted from Branson RD, Campbell RS. Humidification in the intensive care unit. *Respir Care Clin North Am.* 1998;4:305–320.

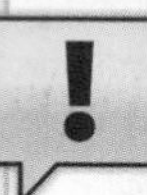

Respiratory Recap

Heat and Moisture Exchangers

- Efficiency declines as the tidal volume, inspiratory flow, and FIO_2 increase.
- HMEs increase dead space and resistive work of breathing.
- HMEs do not need to be changed more often than every 48 hours.

secretions, higher resistive work of breathing, mucous plugging, hypercapnia, and hypothermia. During aerosol administration, the HME must be removed or bypassed. Alternatively, the aerosol generator is placed between the HME and the patient.

With use of an HME, the circuit remains dry, and some HMEs are effective filters. This has led some to recommend that an HME can be used as part of a ventilator-associated pneumonia (VAP) prevention program. Recent studies, however, have not found that HME use is effective in prevention of VAP compared with active humidification.[16–19]

Bland Aerosol Therapy

Bland aerosol therapy provides humidification with solutions such as saline for therapeutic and diagnostic purposes (**CPG 15-2**). Large-volume pneumatic nebulizers and ultrasonic nebulizers are commonly used for these purposes. Large-volume pneumatic nebulizers, which have reservoir volumes greater than 100 mL,

CLINICAL PRACTICE GUIDELINE 15-2

Bland Aerosol Administration

Indications

- The presence of upper airway edema (cool bland aerosol)
- Laryngotracheobronchitis (LTB)
- Subglottic edema
- Postextubation edema
- Postoperative management of the upper airway
- The presence of a bypassed upper airway
- The need for sputum specimens or mobilization of secretions

Contraindications

- Bronchoconstriction
- History of airway hyperresponsiveness

Hazards and Complications

- Wheezing or bronchospasm
- Bronchoconstriction when artificial airway is employed
- Infection
- Overhydration
- Patient discomfort
- Caregiver exposure to droplet nuclei of *Mycobacterium tuberculosis* or other airborne contagious microorganisms produced as a consequence of coughing, particularly during sputum induction
- Edema of the airway wall
- Edema associated with decreased compliance and gas exchange and with increased airway resistance
- Sputum induction by hypertonic saline inhalation can cause bronchoconstriction with patients who have chronic obstructive pulmonary disease, asthma, cystic fibrosis, or other pulmonary diseases

Limitations

- The efficacy of intermittent or continuous use of bland aerosol as a means of reducing mucus has not been established. Bland aerosol is not a substitute for systemic hydration.
- The physical properties of mucus are only minimally affected by the addition of water aerosol.
- Bland aerosol for humidification when the upper airway has been bypassed is not as efficient or effective as are heated water humidifiers or adequately designed heat and moisture exchangers (HMEs) because of the difficulties in maintaining temperature at patient airway, possible irritation to the airway, and infection risk.

Modified from AARC clinical practice guideline: bland aerosol administration—2003 revision and update. *Respir Care.* 2003;48:529–533. Reprinted with permission.

are commonly used to aerosolize solutions such as normal saline (0.9% NaCl), half normal saline (0.45% NaCl), and distilled water for prolonged periods. They are primarily indicated to provide humidification of medical gases for patients with bypassed upper airways, as treatment of upper airway inflammation with cold mist for local vasoconstriction, to prevent occlusion of airway stents, and to induce sputum production for diagnostic purposes. There is little evidence to support the use of bland aerosols to hydrate lower respiratory tract secretions. For humidification of inspired gases, a large-volume nebulizer offers little advantage over alternative methods such as heated wick humidifiers.

Humidification to Tracheostomy

Heated humidity, bland aerosol, or HME can provide humidification of the inspired gas in patients with a tracheostomy who are breathing spontaneously. In patients who are not hospitalized, an HME might be more convenient. The configuration of HMEs for tracheostomized patients with spontaneous breathing differs from applications for mechanically ventilated patients. They typically have less dead space than the devices used with mechanical ventilation. Some HMEs have a port for delivering oxygen to hypoxemic patients, which may decrease the temperature and absolute humidity of inspired gas. The absolute humidity may not be affected by respiratory rate, but it can be strongly affected by tidal volume and oxygen supplementation. With 3 L/min of oxygen supplied through HMEs equipped with oxygen ports, absolute humidity may be inadequate.[20] As a general rule, heated humidity is superior to HME for spontaneously breathing patients with tracheostomy.

Device Selection for Humidity Therapy

Table 15-1 compares the relative attributes of common humidification systems. The authors of a Cochrane Review concluded that there is little evidence of an overall difference between HMEs and active heated humidifiers.[21] Selection of an appropriate humidification device should include consideration of the following questions:

- What source, temperature, and humidity of gas is the patient breathing?
- What is the point of entry of gas into the airway?
- What is the rate of inspiratory flow or minute volume?
- Does the patient have an intact or a bypassed upper airway?
- Does the patient have normal or diseased lungs?
- Is there evidence of increased, thick secretions or a humidity deficit?
- Are special needs imposed by dead space or the patient's size, age, ability to tolerate administration, or sensitivity to changes in the work of breathing?

TABLE 15-1
Comparison of Common Humidification Systems

Parameter	Bubble Humidifiers*	Passover Humidifiers†	Unheated Nebulizers	Heated Nebulizers	Heat and Moisture Exchangers
Output (mg/L)	15–20	30–50	15–30	20–40	13–32
Temperature (° C)	10–20	30–40	10–20	22–28	22–30
Flow limitation	Yes	No	Yes	Yes	Yes
Retains body temperature	No	Yes	No	Yes	Yes
Infection risk	Yes	No	Yes	Yes	No
Potential for overheating	No	Yes	No	Yes	No
Potential for overhydration	No	No	Yes	Yes	No
Potential for underhydration	Yes	No	Yes	No	Yes
Increases work of breathing	No	No	No	No	Yes
Possible electrical hazard	No	Yes	No	Yes	No

*Unheated.

†Heated.

Aerosol Drug Administration

Aerosol drug therapy has a number of advantages over other routes of administration: a smaller dose can be targeted to the site of action, the onset of action occurs more quickly, and the therapeutic effect is achieved with fewer systemic side effects.[22–24] When aerosolized drugs are delivered directly to the airways, systemic absorption is limited, systemic side effects are minimized, and a high therapeutic index is achieved compared with systemic administration. In contrast, a variety of medications, including peptides and other macromolecules, can be targeted to the lung parenchyma for systemic administration across the alveolar-capillary membrane into the pulmonary vascular bed. Aerosol devices can deliver a wide variety of medications, from bronchodilators to insulin, and many types of devices are used, including nebulizers, pressurized metered dose inhalers, and dry powder inhalers.[22–27] For medical use, aerosol generators produce particles with a mass median aerodynamic diameter of 1 to 5 μm.

Basic Concepts of Aerosol Therapy

An aerosol is composed of particles suspended in air. The time that particles can remain suspended depends on their low terminal settling velocity (v_t), or the velocity at which the aerosol particles fall in air because of gravity, a value related to the size and density of the particle. The geometric size of the particles is commonly expressed as the **mass median aerodynamic diameter (MMAD)**. The deposition of inhaled aerosols onto airway surfaces varies with the size of the particles. For example, the v_t of a 5-μm water droplet is 0.074 cm/s, almost 22 times greater than a 1-μm water droplet but one-fourth that of a 10-μm water droplet.

Half the mass of particles in an aerosol is less than the MMAD, and the other half is greater. Relatively few particles larger than the median particle diameter comprise the mass above the MMAD, with a much greater number of particles less than the median particle diameter required to reach comparable mass. **Geometric standard deviation (GSD)** is a measure of the magnitude of variation of particle size distribution. A monodisperse aerosol, in which all particles are basically the same size, has a GSD under 1.2, whereas a heterodisperse aerosol, with a wider range of particle sizes, has a GSD of more than 1.2. Most therapeutic aerosols are heterodisperse.

Respiratory Recap

Primary Factors Affecting Aerosol Delivery

- Deposition
- Inertia
- Gravity
- Diffusion

Inertia is the tendency of an object with mass, once it is in motion, to travel in a straight line. The greater the mass and velocity of a particle, the greater is the inertia that keeps it in motion. Inertial impaction is the primary mechanism of deposition of aerosol particles 5 μm or larger and an important mechanism for particles as small as 2 μm. As aerosol is inhaled and the stream of gas is diverted in the airway, particles tend to continue along their initial trajectory, impacting and depositing on the airway. The higher the inspiratory flow, the greater the velocity and inertia of the particles, which increases the tendency of smaller particles to impact and deposit in airways. Turbulent flow, complex passageways, bifurcation of the airways, and inspiratory flows greater than 30 L/min increase the impaction of particles larger than 2 μm in larger airways.

Gravitational sedimentation occurs when aerosol particles settle out of suspension because of gravity. The greater the mass of the particle, the faster it settles. Very small particles (those less than 0.5 μm in diameter) do not settle at all. Breath holding for 4 to 10 seconds after inhalation of an aerosol lengthens the residence time for particles in the lungs, increasing the time for deposition through gravitational sedimentation, especially in the last six generations of the airway. Breath holding increases deposition of aerosol by as much as 10%, with up to a fourfold increase in peripheral distribution. This marginal increase in deposition explains why breath holding has not been demonstrated to significantly improve the clinical response to aerosolized medications conducted to targeted airways.

Diffusion, or Brownian movement, is the primary mechanism of deposition of particles less than 3 μm in the airway. As gas reaches the distal regions of the lungs, its flow stops. Aerosol particles bouncing against air molecules and each other deposit on contact with the airway surfaces. Preferential deposition for particles 0.5 to 3 μm is divided between the central and peripheral airways. Coalescence, the attraction of particles to each other, occurs when particles come within a distance 25 times or less their diameter.

Aerosol droplets in the respirable range (1 to 5 μm) are more likely to deposit in the lower respiratory tract than are larger or smaller particles. For particles larger than 0.5 μm, the depth of penetration into the lungs is inversely proportional to the particle size. Particles between 0.1 and 1 μm are so small that a significant proportion of those that enter the lungs may be exhaled. Particles larger than 5 μm impact in the upper airway.

Respiratory Recap

Characterization of Aerosols

- Mass median aerodynamic diameter (MMAD)
- Geometric standard deviation (GSD)

Aerosol Deposition, Targeting, and Translocation

Once an aerosol deposits on the airway, it must translocate across the mucous barrier and retain bioactivity to be effective as a therapeutic agent. The optimum site of action depends on the agent administered. Bronchodilators and steroids must reach the epithelium to be effective. Aerosolized antibiotics and mucokinetic agents are most effective when dispersed in infected airway secretions at sites of maximum airway obstruction. Gene transfer therapy not only must access the epithelium through the mucous barrier but also must then gain access to the submucous glands or basal (progenitor) cells of the epithelium.

Particle charge, solubility, and size and the biophysical properties of secretions all affect the ability of an aerosol to penetrate the mucous barrier. Turbulent flow and airway obstruction affect the airway deposition pattern. Other factors that limit efficacy, especially of macromolecules, include binding to constituents of mucus, including mucin and deoxyribonucleic acid (DNA), and the breakdown of bioactive molecules by proteases and other enzymes. Molecular weight and particle diffusion through mucus are inversely related. The antibiotic diffusion barrier represented by mucin may be significant in vitro, particularly for aerosol antibiotics. Translocation of macromolecules can be further compromised by the hypersecretion that accompanies inflammation and chronic pulmonary disease. These secretions can act as a barrier to the penetration of an aerosol.

Factors that promote translocation of medicated aerosols to the airway include an effective surfactant layer and increased particle retention time. Mucus discontinuity in the airway may assist deposition and translocation. The translocation of particles through the mucous layer depends partly on the presence of bronchial surfactant. Pulmonary surfactant promotes the displacement of some particles from air to the aqueous phase. The extent of particle immersion depends on the surface tension of the surface-active film. For particles smaller than 100 μm, the surface tension force is several orders of magnitude greater than forces related to gravity.

Factors Affecting Drug Dose Distribution

Dosing of aerosolized medication is imprecise. It is unclear how much drug is delivered to targeted areas of the lung with progressive disease states and during acute exacerbations. These factors reduce aerosol deposition in the respiratory tract. There is no established correlation between tidal volume and aerosol effectiveness. Theoretically, larger breaths capture more aerosol, but this relationship has not been shown clinically. This may be the result of partitioning of the tidal volume, which is regulated both by the delivered volume and by the airway dimensions. High inspiratory flow increases aerosol impaction in larger airways, whereas low inspiratory flow may result in a reduced amount of medication being available for inhalation from a dry powder inhaler. Humidity also influences the delivery of aerosol medications. Droplets of solution evaporate or grow, depending on the water content and temperature of the gas, and powder can clump or aggregate in high humidity.

Drug formulations dictate, in part, which aerosol options are available for a specific medication. Most solutions can be nebulized if the medication is soluble, but the physical characteristics of the solution (or suspension) can affect particle size and nebulizer output. Furthermore, some macromolecules may not enter suspension well and can be shattered into nonbioactive forms by the force of air required to generate an aerosol.

Aerosol Generators

Jet Nebulizers

Pneumatic jet nebulizers use the Bernoulli principle to drive a high-pressure gas through a restricted orifice across the top of a capillary tube, with the bottom of the tube immersed in the solution (**Figure 15-11**). An aerosol is formed when the jet stream shears fluid from

(A)
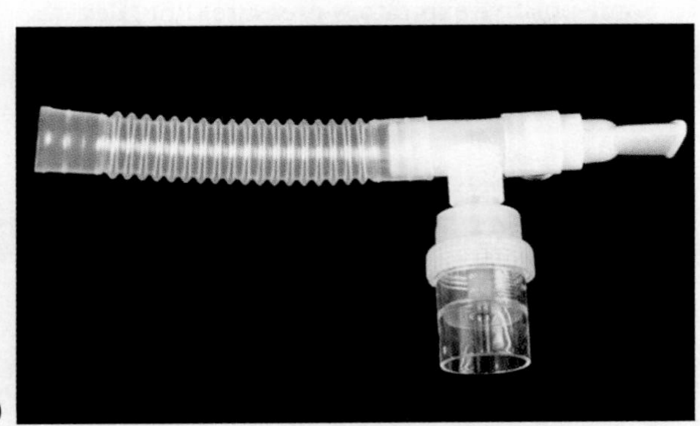

(B)
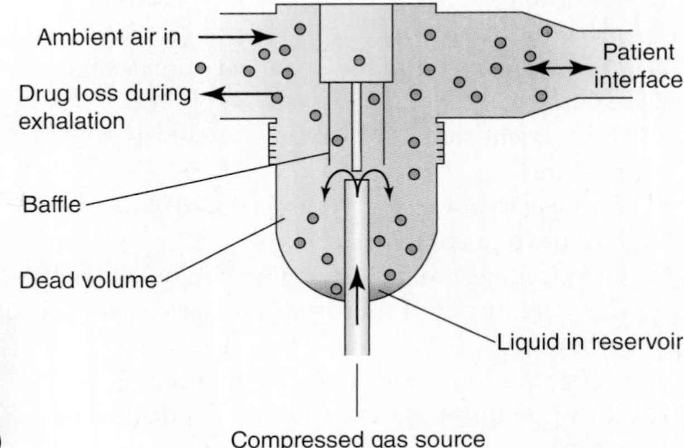

FIGURE 15-11 (**A**) Small-volume jet nebulizer for drug delivery. (**B**) Schematic drawing of small-volume jet nebulizer.

BOX 15-1

Factors That Affect Aerosol Delivery by Nebulizer

- Technical factors
- Manufacturer
- Gas flow
- Fill volume
- Solution characteristics
- Characteristics of driving gas
- Designs to enhance output
- Continuous versus intermittent delivery
- Patient factors
- Breathing pattern
- Nose versus mouth breathing
- Characteristics of gas
- Airway obstruction
- Positive pressure delivery
- Artificial airway and mechanical ventilation

the capillary tube and drives the particles against a solid or liquid surface that acts as a baffle. Impaction against a baffle removes larger particles from suspension and allows them to return to the reservoir, whereas smaller particles remain suspended in the gas and travel from the nebulizer. A number of factors affect the delivery of aerosols by nebulizer (**Box 15-1**). **Box 15-2** describes the technique for the use of a medication nebulizer.

BOX 15-2

Technique for Use of a Jet Nebulizer

1. Assemble tubing, nebulizer cup, and mouthpiece (or mask).
2. Place medicine into the nebulizer cup; use fill volume of 4 to 5 mL.
3. The patient should be seated in an upright position.
4. Connect to power source; use a flow of 6 to 8 L/min or a compressor.
5. Have patient breathe normally with occasional deep breaths until sputter or no more aerosol is produced.
6. Keep nebulizer vertical during treatment.
7. Rinse nebulizer with sterile water and allow to air dry.

An effective small-volume pneumatic nebulizer should deliver more than 50% of its total dose as aerosol in the respirable range (1 to 5 μm) in 10 minutes or less of nebulization time. Nebulizer performance varies with fill volume, flow, gas density, and nebulizer model.[27] The amount of drug nebulized increases as the fill volume increases. The residual volume of solution (dead volume) that remains in commercial small-volume nebulizers varies from 0.5 to 1.5 mL, depending on the specific device. Increasing the fill volume therefore allows a greater proportion of the medication to be nebulized. For example, with a 1-mL residual volume, a fill of 2 mL provides only 50% of the nebulizer charge available for nebulization. A fill of 4 mL makes 3 mL, or 75%, of the medication available for nebulization. Droplet size and nebulization time vary inversely with flow. Within the design limits of the nebulizer, the higher the flow to the nebulizer, the smaller the particle size generated and the shorter the time required to nebulize the full dose. Most nebulizers function best at a flow of 6 to 8 L/min, although some are designed for lower flows, such as those for continuous aerosol therapy.

Gas density affects both aerosol generation and delivery of aerosol to the lungs. This is most evident with low-density helium–oxygen mixtures (heliox).[28] A carrier gas of lower density produces less turbulent flow, reducing aerosol impaction losses during inspiration and improving delivery of aerosol to the lungs. When heliox is used to drive a jet nebulizer, however, aerosol output is reduced, requiring a twofold increase in flow to produce a comparable respirable aerosol output per minute.[29] The benefit of heliox for aerosol delivery in patients with acute asthma is unclear, with some reports of benefit[30,31] and others reporting no benefit.[32] Available evidence does not support routine use of heliox for aerosol delivery.

Humidity and temperature affect the particle size and concentration of drug remaining in the nebulizer. Evaporation of water and adiabatic expansion of gas reduce the temperature of the aerosol more than 5° C (41° F) below the ambient temperature. Aerosol particles entrained into a warm and water-saturated gas stream may increase in size. These larger particles tend to coalesce, increasing the MMAD.

Some positive expiratory pressure (PEP) devices allow concomitant administration of aerosols by nebulizer. Devices that obstruct the aerosol pathway

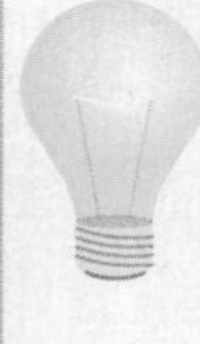

STOP AND THINK

You are asked to instruct a 4-year-old child with asthma, and the child's parents, on the proper use of a nebulizer and compressor for home therapy. How would you approach this assignment?

produce a significantly smaller particle size aerosol and a significant decrease of patient dose.[33] If a PEP device is used with a nebulizer, the nebulizer should be placed between the device and the patient airway.[34]

Clinicians and patients commonly tap a nebulizer periodically to shake droplets of medication from the walls of the nebulizer into the reservoir. Drug delivery from the nebulizer effectively stops with the onset of sputtering. Continuation past the point of initial jet nebulizer sputter is ineffective and should indicate an end of the treatment. Because the nebulizer selected affects aerosol delivery, a nebulizer should be chosen that reliably delivers specific medications. When a compressor is used to power the nebulizer, the performance of the compressor also is important.

Nebulizers commonly are operated continuously—that is, throughout the patient's respiratory cycle. This wastes the aerosol produced during the expiratory phase. A typical inspiration-to-expiration ratio of 1:3 results in 75% of the aerosol emitted from the nebulizer being lost to the atmosphere. This is a major factor in the poor efficiency associated with pneumatic nebulizers. If 50% of the nominal dose is emitted, 50% in the respirable range, and 25% of that is inhaled by the patient, then 12.5% of the nominal dose is inhaled by the patient and 20% of that is exhaled. This results in the 10% deposition observed with in vivo measurements.

A reservoir on the expiratory limb of the nebulizer conserves drugs by collecting some of the nebulizer output that otherwise would be wasted to the atmosphere. A reservoir can be created through placement of 15 cm of aerosol tubing on the expiratory side of the nebulizer. As an alternative, commercial devices such as simple bag reservoirs (**Figure 15-12**) provide a greater volume reservoir in which the smaller aerosol particles remain in suspension for inhalation and larger particles rain out.

Vented breath-enhanced nebulizer systems (**Figure 15-13**) allow the patient to inhale additional air through the nebulizer, increasing drug delivery on inspiration. The inlet vent closes on exhalation, and aerosol exits via a one-way valve in the mouthpiece.

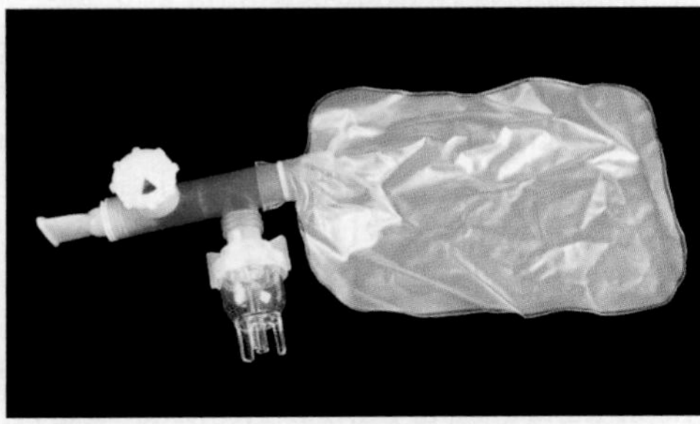

FIGURE 15-12 Nebulizer with reservoir bag to capture aerosol during the expiratory phase.

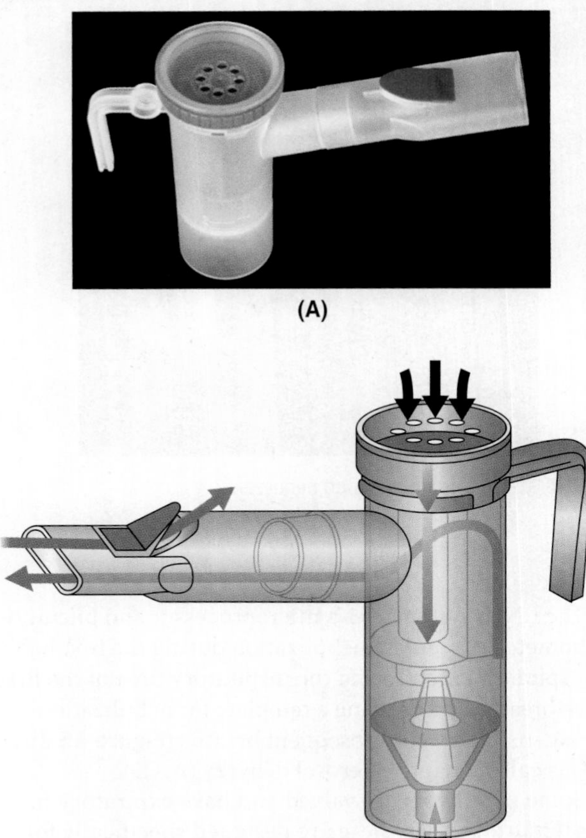

FIGURE 15-13 (**A**) Vented breath-enhanced nebulizer. (**B**) Schematic drawing of a vented breath-enhanced nebulizer.

This design reduces aerosol waste and increases the inhaled dose by as much as 50% without increasing the treatment time.

Breath-actuated nebulization synchronizes aerosol generation with inspiration, increasing the amount of drug available for inspiration by up to fourfold. The inhaled aerosol per breath is similar, but the amount of drug inhaled and the treatment time increase by a factor of four. Inspiratory phase nebulization can be accomplished with a thumb control port that allows the patient to manually direct gas to the nebulizer only on inspiration. This improves the efficiency of the nebulizer if the patient has good hand–breath coordination. More effective systems do not require hand–breath coordination and operate by synchronizing aerosol production to the patient's inspiratory phase. The Monaghan AeroEclipse (**Figure 15-14**) is a pneumatic breath-actuated nebulizer that responds to the patient's inspiratory flow, producing aerosol during inspiration and ending nebulization when the inspiratory flow drops below a threshold.[35–37]

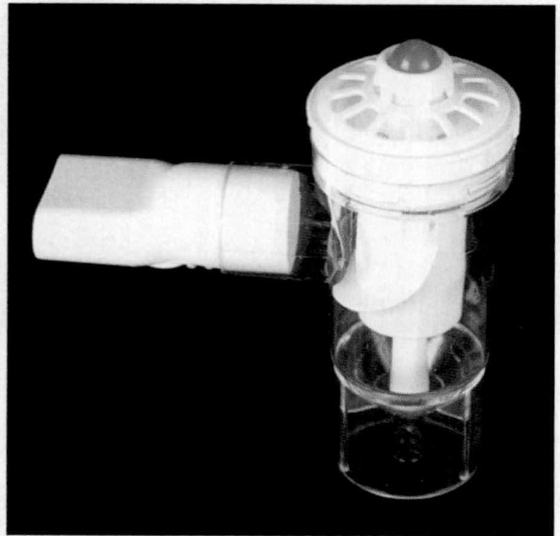

FIGURE 15-14 Breath-actuated nebulizer.

The I-Neb system uses a microprocessor and pneumotachometer to regulate nebulization during the first half of inspiration, monitoring the inspiratory time of the first three breaths and creating a template for nebulization during inspiration of subsequent breaths (**Figure 15-15**). This is called adaptive aerosol delivery (AAD).

Some nebulizers are valved and have expiratory filters (**Figure 15-16**); these are designed specifically for the delivery of pentamidine. The filter minimizes ambient contamination with the aerosol and the patient's exhaled gases. These nebulizers also produce very small particles to enhance parenchymal deposition.

Single patient use plastic nebulizers may show degradation of performance after many uses. Between treatments, nebulizers should be rinsed with sterile water and air-dried, or replaced. Contamination of

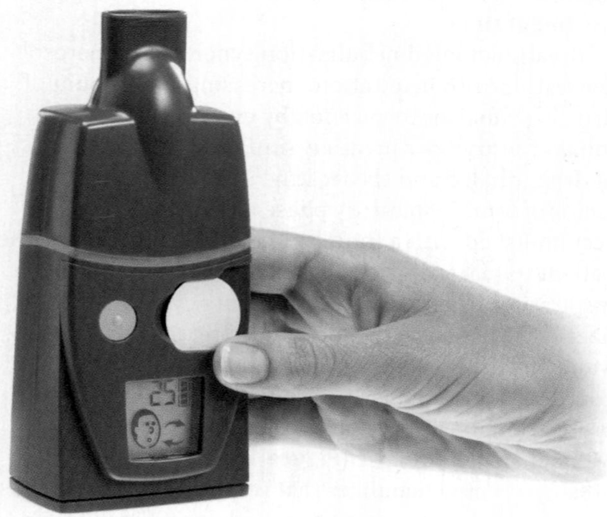

FIGURE 15-15 Adaptive aerosol delivery system.
Courtesy of Philips Respironics.

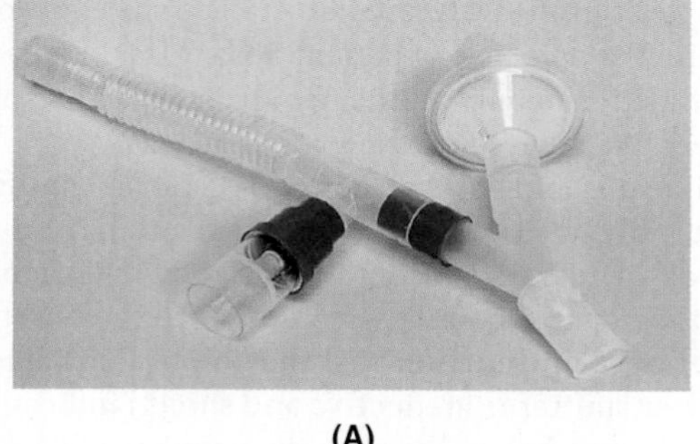

(A)

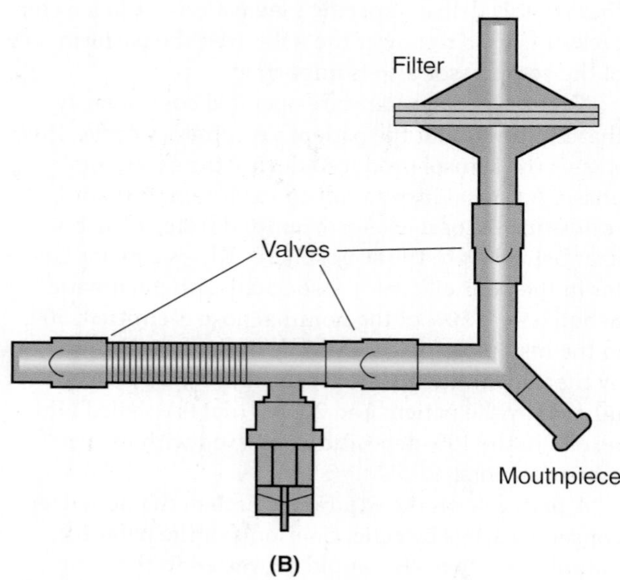

(B)

FIGURE 15-16 (**A**) Respirgard nebulizer for pentamidine administration (Marquest). (**B**) Schematic drawing of Respirgard nebulizer.

nebulizer solutions is related to storage of multiple-dose solutions at room temperature and reuse of syringes to measure the solution. Refrigerating solutions and disposing of syringes every 24 hours eliminates bacterial contamination.

For patients who cannot use a mouthpiece, the nebulizer can be fitted to an appropriate mask. No difference in clinical response has been found between mouthpiece and close-fitting mask treatment. Patient compliance and preference, therefore, should guide selection of the device. If a mask is used, care should be taken to avoid aerosol delivery in the eyes (**Figure 15-17**).[38–41] A mouthpiece enhances medication delivery to the airways in adults. Crying is a long exhalation preceded by a very short and rapid inhalation. This prevents lower airway deposition of an aerosol. Thus, aerosols should not be administered to a crying child. It is more efficient to deliver medication by close-fitting mask when the child is asleep. Blow-by, in which the clinician directs the aerosol from the nebulizer toward the patient's nose and mouth, is usually ineffective due to

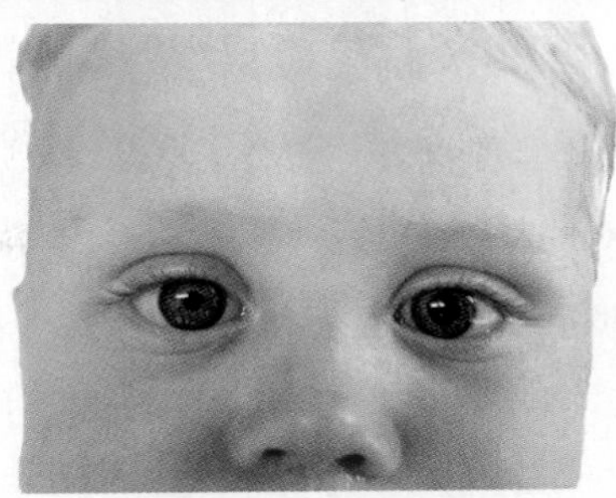

FIGURE 15-17 Unilateral left dilated pupil, which did not react to light, caused by the inadvertent aerosolization of ipratropium bromide into the eye.

Reproduced from Brodie T. and Adalat S. *Arch Dis Child.* 2006;91:961. With permission from BMJ Publishing Group Ltd.

the incremental aerosol drop-off with increasing distances from the face.[42,43] At a distance of 4 cm from the face, however, blow-by can be an effective means of drug delivery with the appropriate nebulizer system.[44]

The small particle aerosol generator (SPAG) is a jet-type aerosol generator used to administer ribavirin (**Figure 15-18**). It uses a secondary drying chamber that reduces the MMAD to 1.2 μm with a GSD of 1.4. The SPAG reduces the 50-psi of line-pressure medical gas to 26 psi, connected to two flow meters that control flow to the nebulizer and the drying chamber. The aerosol generated in the medication reservoir enters the long cylindrical drying chamber, where additional flow of dry gas reduces the size of the aerosol particles through evaporation. The flow to the nebulizer is adjusted to a maximum of 7 L/min, with a total flow from both flow meters of 15 L/min.

The administration of ribavirin has highlighted concerns about secondhand exposure of healthcare workers to aerosol, and thus open-air administration should be avoided. To protect clinical staff, ribavirin administration should be limited to a negative pressure, single-patient room with six air exchanges per hour. Procedures used to reduce the release of ribavirin into the environment include containment of the aerosol with a canopy over the delivery device (**Figure 15-19**),[45] use of a scavenging system, and filtering of the expiratory limb of the circuit of a mechanically ventilated patient. Practices that reduce caregiver exposure include the turning off of the nebulizer 5 minutes before opening the tent or 1 minute before disconnecting the ventilator and the use of personal protective equipment, including goggles, a respirator, gown, and gloves. Administrative policies should prevent pregnant or lactating women and staff members who have had reactions to the drug from coming into contact with ribavirin. Caution must be used when ribavirin is administered during mechanical ventilation because of the drug's tendency to occlude filters, valves, and endotracheal tubes. Tandem filters placed in series in the expiratory limb of the ventilator reduce expiratory valve occlusion but require frequent changing. Aerosol from the SPAG is entrained into the ventilator circuit distal to the output of the humidifier through a one-way valve. A high-pressure alarm in the circuit alerts the clinician to an excessive baseline pressure should expiratory occlusion occur.

If the symptoms of a patient with acute asthma are not relieved with standard bronchodilator dosing, continuous aerosol can be provided at a controlled rate of medication delivery.[46-48] Doses of albuterol between 7.5 and 15 mg/h have proved effective in treating acute exacerbations of asthma. One strategy is to use an intravenous infusion pump to deliver a premixed bronchodilator solution into a jet nebulizer (**Figure 15-20**).

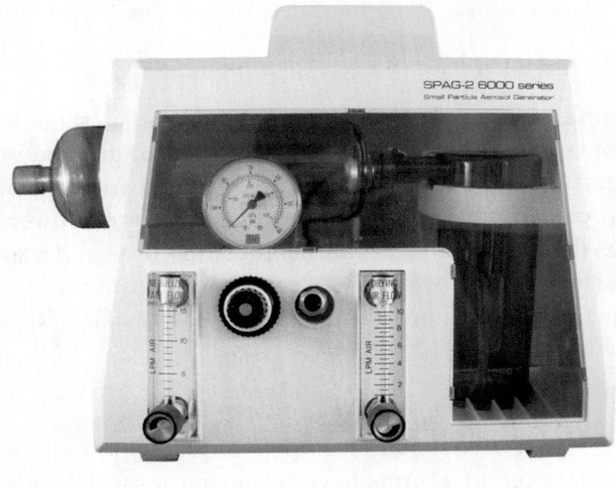

(A)

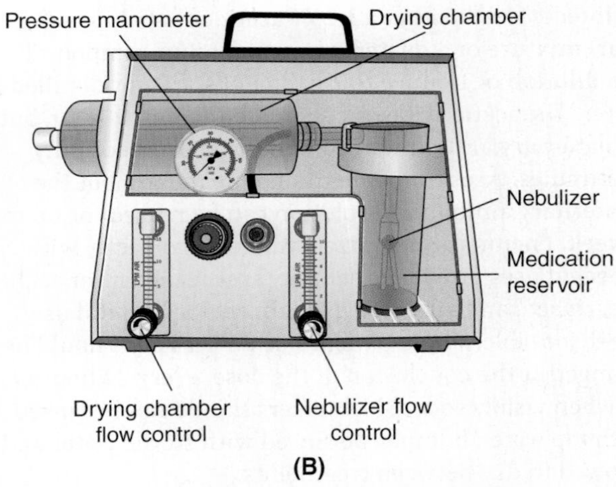

(B)

FIGURE 15-18 **(A)** Small particle aerosol generator (SPAG) for ribavirin administration. **(B)** Schematic drawing of SPAG.

(A) courtesy of Valeant Pharmaceuticals; **(B)** adapted from Scanlan CL, et al. *Egan's Fundamentals of Respiratory Care.* 7th ed. Mosby; 1999.

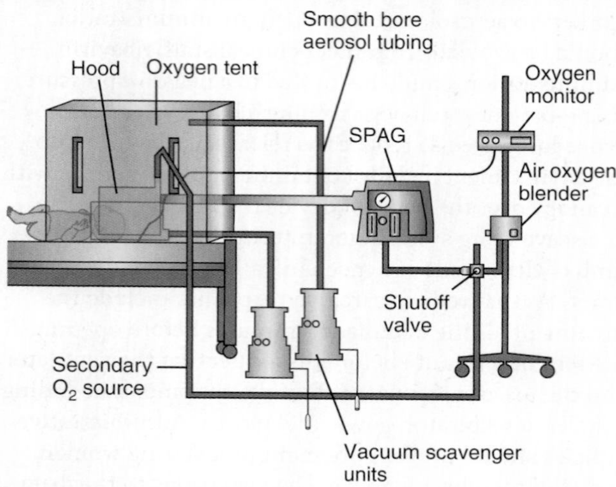

FIGURE 15-19 Scavenging system for ribavirin administration.

Modified from Kacmarek RM, Kratohvil J. Evaluation of a double-enclosure double-vacuum unit scavenging system for ribavirin administration. *Respir Care.* 1992;37:37–45. Reprinted with permission.

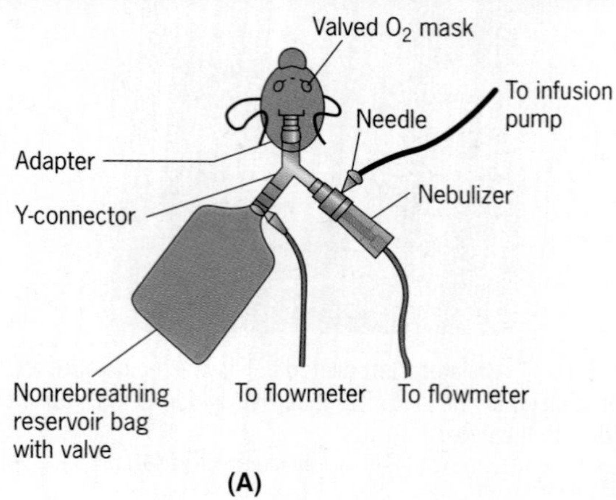

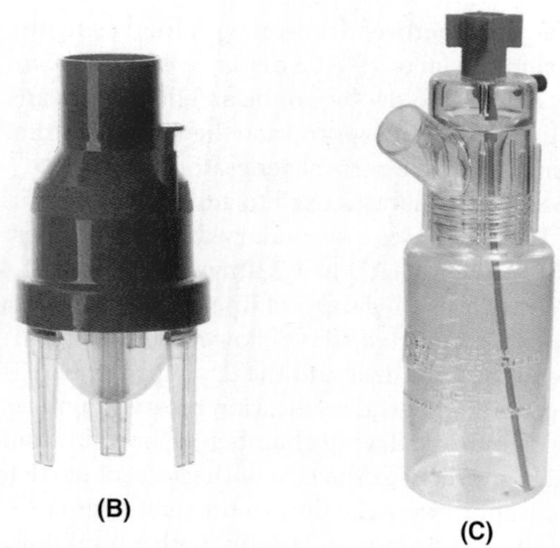

FIGURE 15-20 (**A**) Delivery systems for continuous aerosolized bronchodilator by continuous infusion of medications into a standard small-volume nebulizer. (**B**) Commercially available nebulizer for continuous aerosol administration. (**C**) Commercially available nebulizer for continuous aerosol administration.

(**A**) modified from Moler FW, et al. Continuous versus intermittent nebulized terbutaline: plasma levels and effects. *Am J Respir Crit Care Med.* 1995;151:602–606. The American Journal of Respiratory and Critical Care Medicine is an official journal of the American Thoracic Society. Reprinted with permission of the American Thoracic Society. Copyright © 2015 American Thoracic Society; (**B**) courtesy of Westmed, Inc.; (**C**) courtesy of B&B Medical Technologies.

Another strategy is to use a **large-volume nebulizer** that delivers a consistent output of medication at a specific flow. Albuterol solution and saline are mixed in the reservoir, and the nebulizer is operated at a flow recommended by the manufacturer to deliver the desired dose. The aerosol can be delivered with a mask, nasal cannula, or in-line with a ventilator circuit. The use of a nasal cannula interface[49–52] for continuous aerosol therapy is effective, particularly in an uncooperative child. For patients with moderately severe asthma, continuous or intermittent therapy has a similar effect with either low- or high-dose β-agonists.

Patients should be taught how to disinfect their nebulizers used in the home. After each treatment, the patient should shake the remaining solution from the nebulizer cup. The nebulizer cup should be rinsed with either sterile or distilled water and left to air dry on an absorbent towel. Once or twice a week, the nebulizer should be disassembled, washed in soapy tap water, and disinfected with either a 1.25% acetic acid (white vinegar) mixture or a quaternary ammonium compound at a dilution of 1 ounce to 1 gallon of sterile or distilled water. The acetic acid soak should be at least 1 hour, but a quaternary ammonium compound soak needs only 10 minutes. Acetic acid should not be reused, but the quaternary ammonium solution can be reused for up to 1 week. Pneumatic nebulizers function correctly with repeated uses provided that they are cleaned after each use, rinsed, and air-dried. Nebulizers for hospital use are disposable, single-patient-use devices and should be changed at the conclusion of the dose, every 24 hours, or when visibly soiled. Nebulizers should not be rinsed with tap water, but may be rinsed with sterile water and allowed to dry between treatments.

Compressed air or oxygen is needed for jet nebulizers. Compressors are the only available flow source at home and may also be used in the hospital. Although not commonly considered, the compressor gas flow and pressure can affect nebulizer performance in terms of droplet size distribution and drug output rate. Lower gas flows result in a longer nebulization time and larger particle size aerosols. There can be important differences in performance among compressors of different manufacturers.[53–57]

Mesh Nebulizers

Several manufacturers have developed aerosol devices that use a mesh or plate with multiple apertures to produce an aerosol (**Figure 15-21** and **Box 15-3**).[58–60] **Mesh nebulizers** use a vibrating mesh or a vibrating horn. For the vibrating mesh (e.g., Aerogen Aeroneb, Pari eFlow Technology), contraction and expansion of a vibrational element produces an upward and downward movement of a domed aperture plate. The aperture plate contains up to 4000 tapered holes. The holes have a tapered shape with a larger cross section on the liquid side and a smaller cross section on the side the droplets emerge. The medication is placed in a reservoir above the domed aperture plate. Sound pressure is built up in the vicinity of the membrane, creating a pumping action that extrudes solution through the holes in the plate to produce an aerosol. The aerosol particle size and flow are determined by the exit diameter of the aperture holes. The size of the holes in the plate can be modified for specific clinical applications. eFlow Technology combines a vibrating mesh with an aerosol mixing chamber; eFlow Technology devices are drug-specific and are linked to one drug. The Altera nebulizer system uses eFlow technology to deliver inhaled Cayston (aztreonam) in patients with cystic fibrosis.

In the vibrating horn system (e.g., Omron) a piezoelectric crystal vibrates at a high frequency when electrical current is applied, and the vibration is transmitted to a transducer horn that is in contact with the solution. Vibration of the transducer horn forces the liquid passes through the apertures in the plate and forms an aerosol.

The output of a mesh nebulizer is dependent on fluid characteristics.[61,62] These nebulizers may be unsuitable for viscous fluids, which suggests that matching the

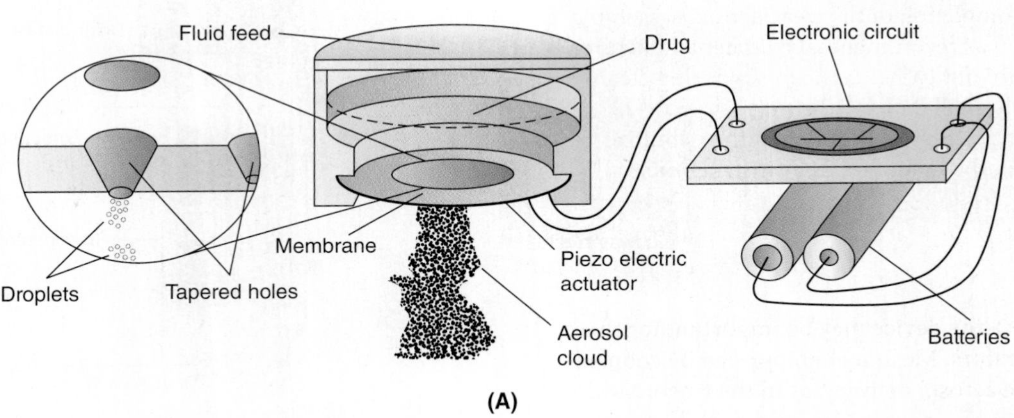

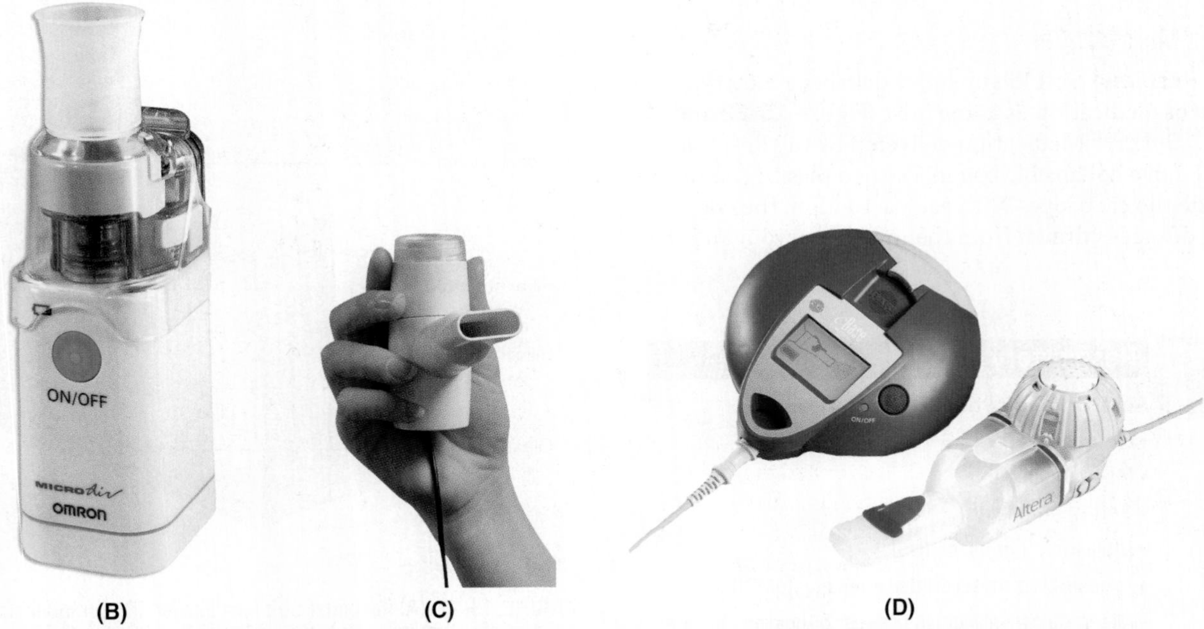

FIGURE 15-21 Mesh nebulizers. (**A**) Principle of operation. (**B–D**) Representative commercially available mesh nebulizers.

(**A**) adapted from Hess DR. Aerosol delivery devices in the treatment of asthma. *Respir Care*. 2008;53:699–725; (**B**) courtesy of Omron Healthcare. (**C**) courtesy of evo Medical Solutions; (**D**) courtesy of eFlow LLC [PARI Pharma GmbH].

BOX 15-3

Technique for Use of a Mesh Nebulizer

1. Correctly assemble the equipment.
2. Follow the manufacturer's instructions to perform a functionality test prior to the first use of a new device and after each disinfection to verify proper operation.
3. Pour the solution into the medication reservoir. Do not exceed the volume recommended by the manufacturer.
4. Turn on the power.
5. Hold the nebulizer in the position recommended by the manufacturer.
6. Breathe normally with occasional deep breaths.
7. If the treatment must be interrupted, turn off the unit to avoid waste.
8. At the completion of the treatment, disassemble and clean as recommended by the manufacturer.
9. Be careful not to touch the mesh during cleaning, as this will damage the unit.
10. Once or twice a week, disinfect the nebulizer following the manufacturer's instructions.

formulation to the device may be important for these aerosol generators. Mesh technology can be coupled with adaptive aerosol delivery, as in the I-neb. Mesh nebulizers can also be used for continuous aerosol administration.

Soft Mist Inhaler

The **Respimat Soft Mist Inhaler** delivers a metered dose of medication as a fine mist (**Figure 15-22** and **Box 15-4**).[63,64] Medication delivered by the Respimat is stored in a collapsible bag in a sealed plastic container inside the cartridge. With each actuation, the correct dosage is drawn from the inner reservoir, and the

Respiratory Recap

Aerosol Medication Delivery Devices

- Jet nebulizer
- Mesh nebulizer
- Soft mist inhaler
- Ultrasonic nebulizer (USN)
- Pressurized metered dose inhaler (pMDI)
- Metered dose inhaler with spacer or holding chamber
- Dry powder inhaler (DPI)

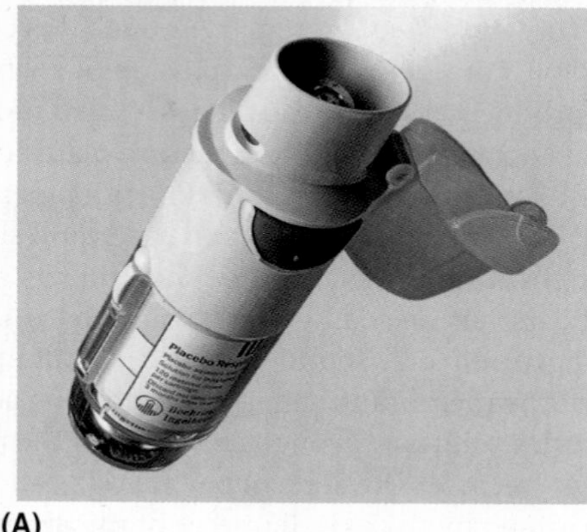

(A)

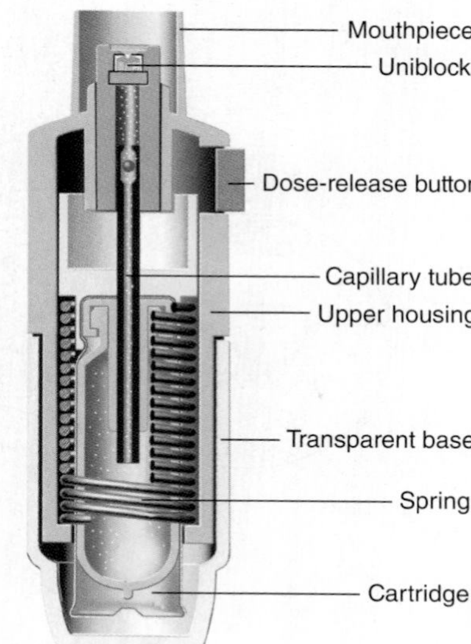

(B)

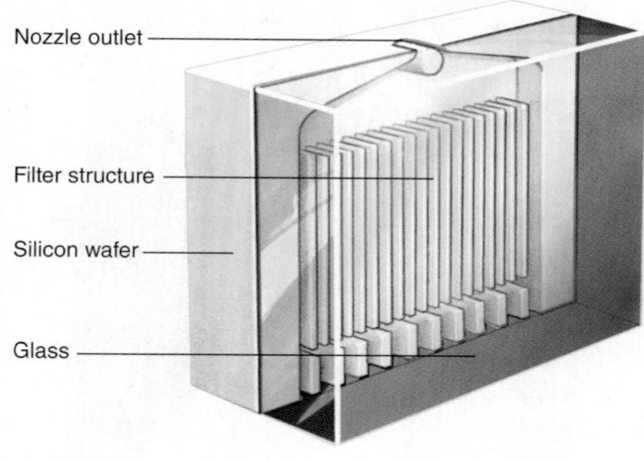

(C)

FIGURE 15-22 (**A**) Respimat Soft Mist Inhaler. (**B**) Components of the Respimat. (**C**) The uniblock, which is the core element of the Respimat.

BOX 15-4

Technique for Use of Respimat Inhaler

First Time Use

1. With the cap closed, press the safety catch while pulling off the clear base. Be careful not to touch the piercing element located inside the bottom of the clear base.
2. Write the discard by date on the label of the inhaler, which is the date 3 months from the date the cartridge is inserted into the inhaler.
3. Take the cartridge out of the box. Push the narrow end of the cartridge into the inhaler. The base of the cartridge will not sit flush with the inhaler. About 1/8 of an inch will remain visible when the cartridge is correctly inserted. The cartridge can be pushed against a firm surface to ensure that it is correctly inserted. Do not remove the cartridge once it has been inserted into the inhaler.
4. Put the clear base back into place. Do not remove the clear base again. The inhaler should not be taken apart after you have inserted the cartridge and put the clear base back.

Prime for First Time Use

The following steps are needed to prime the dosing system and will not affect the number of doses available. After preparation and initial priming, the inhaler will deliver 120 doses. Proper priming is important to make sure the correct amount of medicine is delivered.

1. Hold the inhaler upright, with the cap closed, to avoid accidental release of the dose. Turn the clear base in the direction of the white arrows on the label until it clicks (half turn).
2. Flip the cap until it snaps fully open.
3. Point the inhaler downward (away from your face). Press the dose release button. Close the cap.
4. Repeat these steps until a spray is visible. Once the spray is visible, repeat these steps three more times to make sure the inhaler is prepared for use.

Daily Dosing

1. Hold the inhaler upright with the cap closed to avoid accidental release of a dose. Turn the clear base in the direction of the white arrows on the label until it clicks (half turn).
2. Flip the cap until it snaps fully open.
3. Breathe out slowly and fully.
4. Close your lips around the end of the mouthpiece without covering the air vents.
5. Point the inhaler to the back of your throat.
6. While taking in a slow, deep breath through the mouth, press the dose release button and continue to breathe in slowly for as long as possible.
7. Hold your breath for 10 seconds or for as long as comfortable.
8. Close the cap until you use the inhaler again.
9. If the inhaler has not been used for more than 3 days, spray 1 puff toward the ground to prepare the inhaler for use.
10. If the inhaler has not been used for more than 21 days, repeat the priming process until a spray is visible. Then repeat three more times to prepare the inhaler for use.

When to Replace the Inhaler

The Respimat contains 120 doses. The dose indicator shows approximately how much medicine is left. When the pointer enters the red area of the scale, there is enough medicine for 7 days. Discard the inhaler 3 months after insertion of the cartridge into inhaler, even if all the medicine has not been used, or when the inhaler is locked (after 120 puffs), whichever comes first.

flexible bag contracts accordingly. A twist of the inhaler's base compresses a spring. A tube slides into a canal in the cartridge, and the dose is drawn through the tube into a micropump. When the dose-release button is pressed, the energy released from the spring forces the solution through the uniblock, and a slow-moving aerosol is released. A dose indicator shows how many doses are left.

The fine nozzle system of the uniblock is the core element of the Respimat. When the medication solution is forced through the nozzle system, two jets of liquid emerge and converge at an optimized angle, and the impact of these converging jets generates the aerosol. The aerosol produced by the Respimat moves much slower and has a more prolonged duration than an aerosol cloud from a **pressurized metered dose inhaler (pMDI)**.[65] Compared with a pMDI, lung deposition is doubled and oropharyngeal deposition reduced. Low deposition on the face, and especially in the eyes, occurs when the Respimat is fired accidentally outside the body or is fired at the same time as the patient exhales.[66] A high level of patient satisfaction has been reported with the Respimat.[67] A prototype adapter for use of the Respimat during mechanical ventilation has been described.[68]

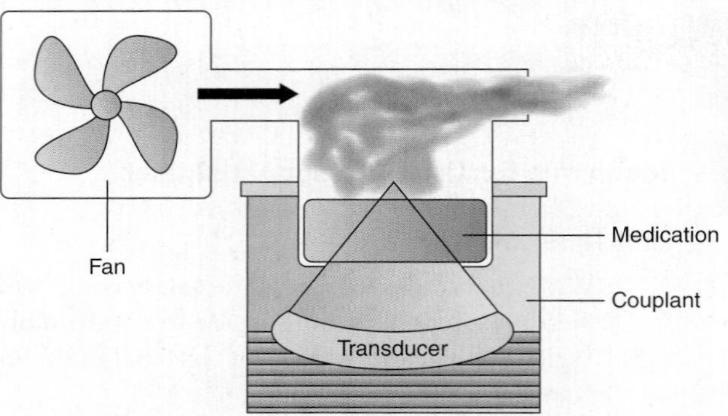

FIGURE 15-23 Schematic drawing of ultrasonic nebulizer.
Adapted from Cohen N, Fink J. Humidity and aerosols. In: Eubanks DH, Borne RC, eds. *Principles and Applications of Cardiorespiratory Care Equipment*. Mosby; 1994.

Ultrasonic Nebulizers

The **ultrasonic nebulizer** (USN) uses a piezoelectric crystal that vibrates at a high frequency to convert electricity to sound waves, creating standing waves in the liquid immediately above the transducer and disrupting the liquid's surface, forming a geyser of droplets (**Figure 15-23**). Because electronics are not readily sterilized, disposable medication cups with a flexible diaphragm are commonly used, with the sound waves communicated through a layer of water acting as a couplant. The USN is capable of greater aerosol output (0.4 to 5 mL/min) with greater aerosol density than conventional jet nebulizers. Particle size is determined by frequency, and output by the amplitude of the signal. Within limits, the particle size is inversely proportional to the frequency and is not user adjustable. USN can operate at different frequencies (1.24 to 2.25 MHz), producing a range of MMAD (2.5 to 6 μm).

The large-volume USN, which is used primarily for bland aerosol therapy or sputum induction, incorporate air blowers to carry the mist to the patient. An inverse relationship exists between the aerosol density emitted by the USN and the flow of gas through the nebulizer. Because of the energy required, the temperature of the solution in a USN increases by as much as 15° C (59° F) over 15 minutes. As the temperature rises, the drug concentration also rises, increasing the likelihood of undesirable side effects such as denaturing proteins.

Small-volume ultrasonic nebulizers are available for aerosol drug delivery (**Figure 15-24**). These systems may or may not use a water-filled couplant compartment, with the medication placed in a cup or directly onto the transducer connected to a battery-powered power source. The patient's inspiratory flow draws aerosol from the nebulizer into the lungs. As the USN operates, the aerosol remains in the medication cup or chamber until a flow of gas pushes or pulls the aerosol

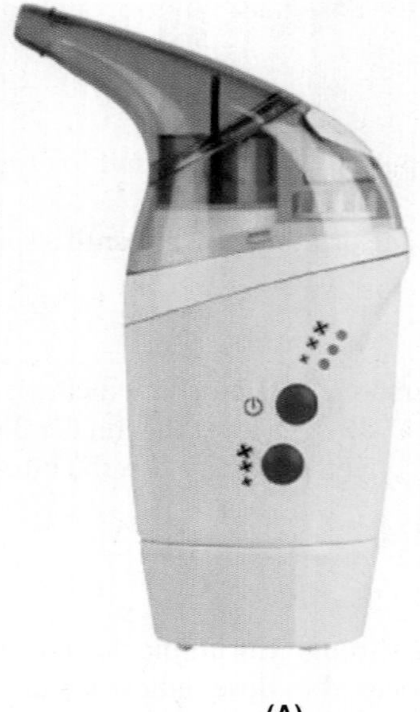

(A)

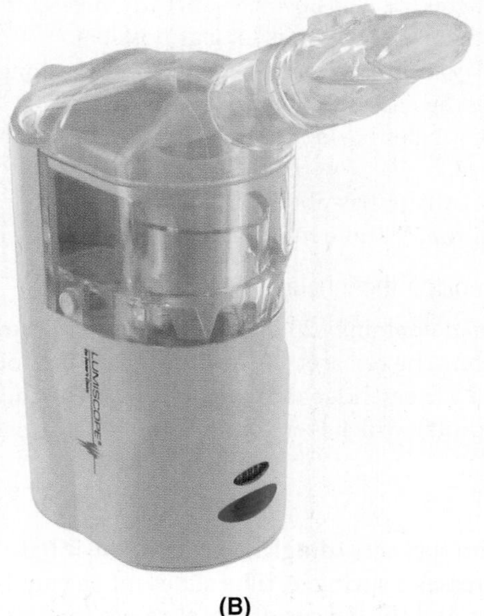

(B)

FIGURE 15-24 (**A**) Minibreeze ultrasonic nebulizer. (**B**) Lumiscope® ultrasonic nebulizer.
(**A**) courtesy of Briggs Healthcare; (**B**) courtesy of GF Health Products, Inc.

from the nebulizer. If a USN creates aerosol continuously, the patient draws aerosol from the nebulizer during inspiration and clears aerosol from the chamber during exhalation, with aerosol collecting in the chamber between end expiration and through inspiration. If exhalation is diverted away from the medication chamber, there is minimal waste to atmosphere and more available drug for inhalation.

Small-volume USNs may have less dead volume than small-volume nebulizers. The contained portable power source provides convenience and mobility. Advantages of ultrasonic nebulizers may be offset by their high cost relative to standard jet nebulizers. USNs have been promoted for administration of a wide variety of formulations ranging from bronchodilators to anti-inflammatory agents and antibiotics, but they are less effective than other delivery devices, especially with suspensions.

The Optineb (**Figure 15-25**) uses an ultrasonic nebulizer to deliver treprostinil inhalation solution for the treatment of pulmonary arterial hypertension. It incorporates filters to minimize ambient contamination with the drug. The device prompts the patient to use correct inhalation technique. The recommended prescribed dose of treprostinil is up to 9 breaths (54 micrograms) per treatment session and up to 4 treatment sessions per day.

Overhydration has been associated with prolonged bland aerosol treatment by USN in children and patients with renal insufficiency. The high-density aerosol from USN may precipitate bronchospasm. An acoustic power output above 50 watts/cm^2 has been associated with disruption of the structure of some molecules. USNs have drawn attention for the administration of aerosols during mechanical ventilation because they do not require the addition of a driving gas flow to the circuit. Disadvantages of the USN in the ventilator circuit include weight, position dependency, a tendency to heat medications, and the need for water couplants.

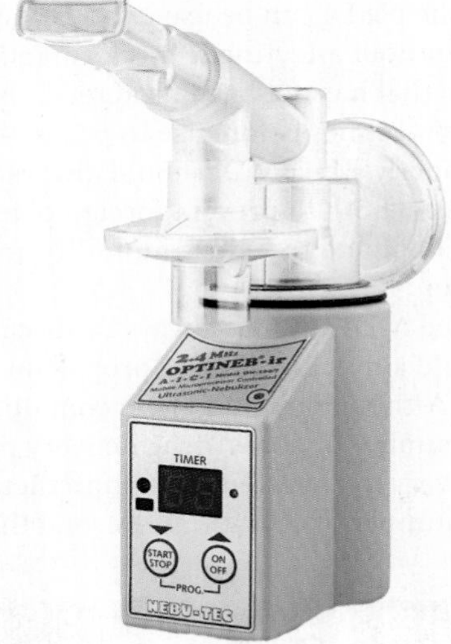

FIGURE 15-25 The Optineb uses an ultrasonic nebulizer to deliver treprostinil inhalation solution for the treatment of pulmonary arterial hypertension.

Courtesy of United Therapeutics Corporation, used with permission.

Pressurized Metered Dose Inhalers

The pressurized metered dose inhaler (**Figure 15-26**) is the most commonly prescribed method of aerosol delivery. Pressurized MDIs are used to administer

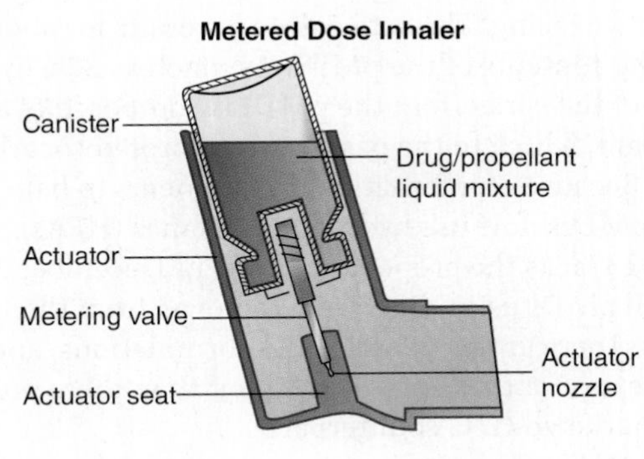

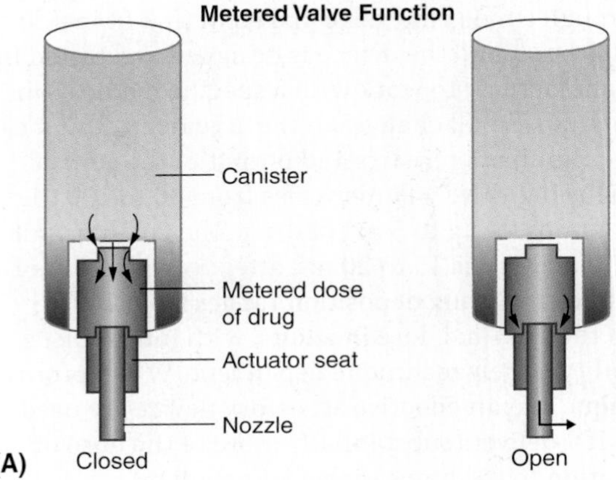

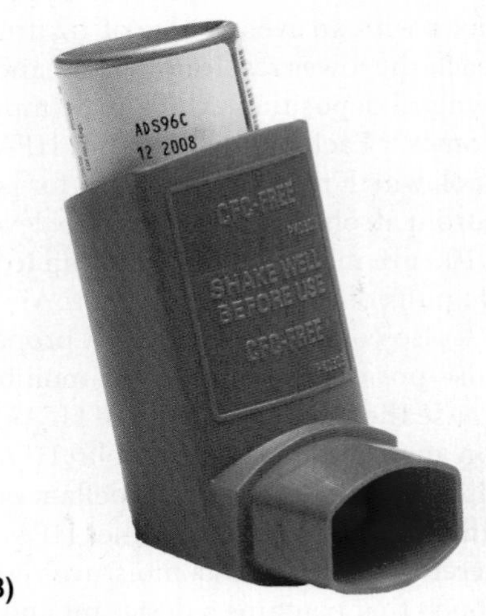

FIGURE 15-26 (**A**) Schematic drawing of metered dose inhaler. (**B**) Commercially available metered dose inhaler.

(**A**) adapted from Rau JL Jr. *Respiratory Care Pharmacology*, 5th ed. Mosby; 1998; (**B**) © M. Dykstra/ShutterStock, Inc.

bronchodilators, anticholinergics, anti-inflammatory agents, and steroids.[69,70] When properly used, pMDIs are at least as effective for drug delivery as other nebulizers.

A pMDI consists of a pressurized canister containing a drug in the form of a micronized powder or solution that is suspended with a mixture of propellants, surfactant, preservatives, flavoring agents, and dispersing agents. The concentrations of the dispersing agents are equal to or greater than that of the medication, and dispersing agents may be associated with coughing and wheezing. The active drug accounts for about 1% of the contents of the pMDI. As much as 80% by weight of the spray from the pMDI is composed of a propellant, which in the past was a chlorofluorocarbon (CFC). Because of international agreements to ban CFCs, pMDIs now use hydrofluoroalkanes (HFAs), such as HFA133a, as the propellant.[71,72] As of December 31, 2013, all pMDI using CFC were removed from the U.S. market. There are no generic HFA formulations, and thus the cost of these pMDI is higher than there previously marketed CFC counterparts.

In a pMDI, the mixture is released from the canister through a metering valve and stem that fit into an actuator boot, and the device is designed and tested by the manufacturer to work with a specific medication formulation. Small changes in the actuator's design can change the characteristics and output of the aerosol. The metering valve volume varies from 30 to 100 μL and contains 20 μg to 5 mg of drug. The volume emitted by the pMDI is 15 to 20 mL after volatilization of the propellant. Lung deposition ranges from 10% to 25% of the nominal dose in adults, with intersubject variability largely technique dependent. When proper technique and an effective accessory device are used, the pMDI delivers substantially more of the dose of medication to the lungs than a jet nebulizer.

HFA steroid inhalers were engineered to generate aerosol particles with an average size of 1.2 μm, to more effectively reach the lower respiratory tract and have less oropharyngeal deposition, which may improve clinical outcomes.[73] Each puff of Proventil HFA releases 4 μL of ethanol, which may be of concern for patients who abstain from alcohol. A breath alcohol level of up to 35 μg per 100 mL may be detected for up to 5 minutes after two puffs of Proventil HFA.[74] ProAir HFA and Xopenex HFA also contain ethanol. HFA propellant may cause false-positive readings in gas-monitoring systems, because the infrared spectra of HFAs overlap with common anesthetic gases.[75] Ventolin HFA contains no excipients other than the propellant but has a greater affinity for moisture than other HFA inhalers and is therefore packaged in a moisture-resistant protective pouch that contains a desiccant and has a limited shelf life once it is removed from the pouch. Clogging of HFA pMDI albuterol actuators has been reported.[76] They should be cleaned at least once a week by removing the metal canister, running warm water through the plastic actuator for 30 seconds, shaking the actuator to remove water, and then allowing it to air dry. The actuator should be cleaned more frequently if a reduction in the force of emitted spray is noted.

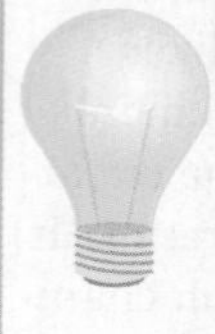

STOP AND THINK

You are caring for a patient in the emergency department who has severe acute asthma. Albuterol administration by pMDI has been prescribed, but the patient is demonstrating difficulty using the device effectively. What would you do to improve this patient's care?

The nominal dose of medication with the pMDI is much smaller than that with a nebulizer. The amount of albuterol exiting the actuator nozzle of a pMDI is 100 μg with each actuation, or 90 μg from the opening of the actuator boot; this is how pMDI aerosol actuations are characterized in the United States. Thus, a dose of two to four actuations (200 to 400 μg nominal dose) usually is used. In ambulatory patients, 10% deposition may deliver a dose of 20 to 40 μg for an effective bronchodilation response.

Effective use of the pMDI is technique dependent. Many patients who use pMDIs and health professionals who teach pMDI use do not perform the procedure properly.[77–80] **Box 15-5** lists the steps for administering a bronchodilator with a pMDI. Good patient instruction can take 10 to 30 minutes and should include demonstration, practice, and confirmation of the patient's performance. Demonstration placebo units are available for this purpose. Repeated instruction improves performance. Infants, young children, the elderly, and patients in acute distress may not be able to use a pMDI effectively. The pMDI can be used as often as every 30 seconds without affecting its performance. A new pMDI or one that has not been used recently should be actuated several times before use to prime the metering chamber properly. The pMDI should always be stored with the cap on, both to prevent foreign objects from entering the boot and to reduce humidity and microbial contamination.

Pressurized MDIs should always be discarded when empty to avoid administration of propellant without medication. Although many pMDIs contain more than the labeled number of doses, drug delivery per actuation may be very inconsistent and unpredictable after the labeled number of actuations. Beyond the labeled

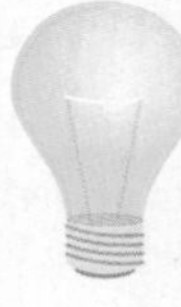

STOP AND THINK

You are asked to help a patient who is having difficulty using her pMDI. What would you do to help her improve her inhaled technique?

BOX 15-5

Technique for Use of a Pressurized Metered Dose Inhaler

1. Hold the pressurized metered dose inhaler (pMDI) in your hand to warm it.
2. Remove the mouthpiece cover.
3. Inspect the mouthpiece for foreign objects.
4. Hold the pMDI in a vertical position.
5. Shake the pMDI.
6. If the pMDI is new or has not been used recently, prime it by shaking and pressing the canister to deliver a dose into the room. Repeat several times.
7. Breathe out normally.
8. Open your mouth and keep your tongue from obstructing the mouthpiece.
9. Hold the pMDI in a vertical position, with the mouthpiece aimed at your mouth.
10. Place the mouthpiece between your lips or position it two finger widths from your mouth.
11. Breathe in slowly and press the pMDI canister down once at the beginning of inhalation.
12. Continue to inhale until your lungs are full.
13. Move the mouthpiece away from your mouth and hold your breath for 10 seconds (or as long as you comfortably can).
14. Wait at least 30 seconds between doses.
15. Repeat for the prescribed number of doses.
16. Recap the mouthpiece.
17. Rinse your mouth if using inhaled steroids.
18. Keep count of the number of uses so that you know when the canister is empty.
19. Clean the pMDI once a week and as needed.

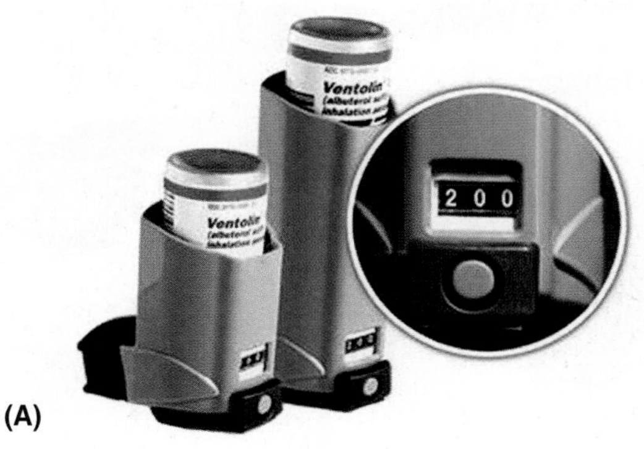

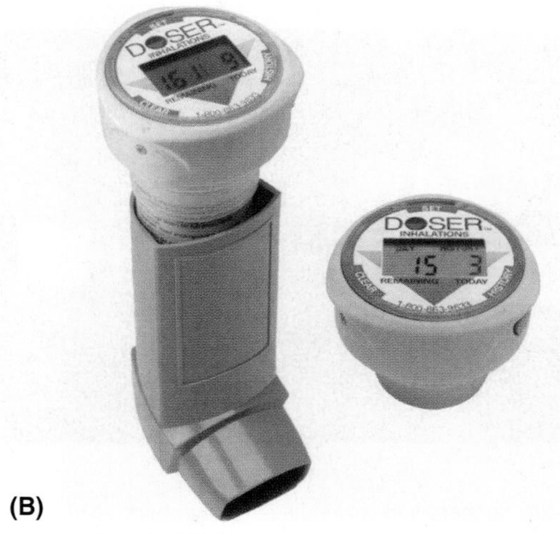

FIGURE 15-27 (**A**) Dose counter on a hydrofluoroalkane (HFA) pressurized metered dose inhaler (Ventolin HFA). (**B**) Doser.
(**A**) © GlaxoSmithKline. Used with permission; (**B**) courtesy of Doser-MediTrack Products.

number of actuations, propellant can release an aerosol plume that contains little or no drug, a phenomenon called tail-off. A practical problem for patients who use pMDIs is the difficulty of determining the number of doses remaining in the device. Ideally the patient knows the number of doses in a full pMDI and keeps track of how many actuations have been used. Many patients are unaware of the number of doses in a full pMDI, however, and most do not know how to determine when their pMDI is empty. Floating the canister in water has been suggested as a way to determine when it is depleted, but this method is unreliable and should not be used.[81,82] The Food and Drug Administration now recommends that manufacturers integrate a dose-counting device into new pMDIs, and several pMDIs have integrated dose counters (e.g., Ventolin HFA, Flovent HFA). Add-on devices can also be used that count down the number of puffs released from a pMDI (**Figure 15-27**).

AGE-SPECIFIC ANGLE

Infants, young children, the elderly, and patients in acute distress may not be able to use a pMDI effectively.

Spacers and Valved Holding Chambers

Spacers and valved holding chambers (**Figure 15-28**) are accessory devices that reduce oropharyngeal deposition of drugs, ameliorate the bad taste of some medications, eliminate the cold Freon effect, and, in the case of valved holding chambers, reduce the need for hand–breath coordination. These devices reduce the pharyngeal dose of aerosol from the pMDI 10-fold to 15-fold. This reduces the total body dose from swallowed medications, which is an important consideration with steroid administration. For the very young, the very old, or others unable to use the device with a mouthpiece, a face mask can be used (**Figure 15-29**).

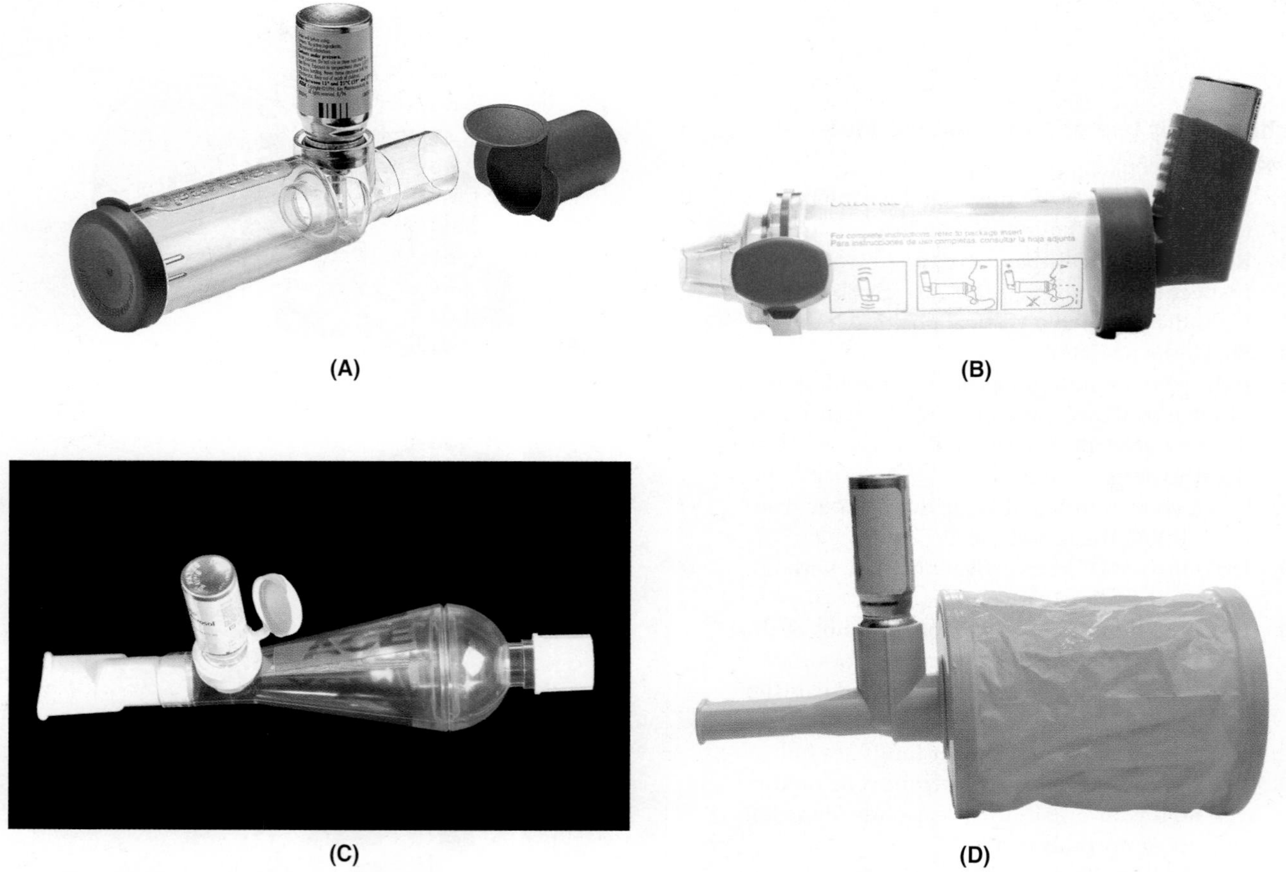

(A)

(B)

(C)

(D)

FIGURE 15-28 Spacers and valved holding chambers.
(**A**) courtesy of Philips Respironics; (**B**) © Rob Byron/ShutterStock, Inc.; (**D**) © Robeo/Dreamstime.com.

A **spacer** is a simple open-ended tube or bag that, with sufficiently large device volume, provides space for the pMDI plume to expand by allowing the propellant to evaporate. To perform this function, a spacer must have an internal volume of more than 100 mL and provide a distance of 10 to 13 cm between the pMDI nozzle and the first wall or baffle. Smaller, inefficient spacers can reduce the respiratory dose by 60% and offer no protection against poor coordination of actuation and breathing pattern. Spacers with internal volumes greater than 100 mL generally provide some protection against early firing of the pMDI, although exhalation immediately after the actuation clears most of the aerosol from the device, wasting the dose.

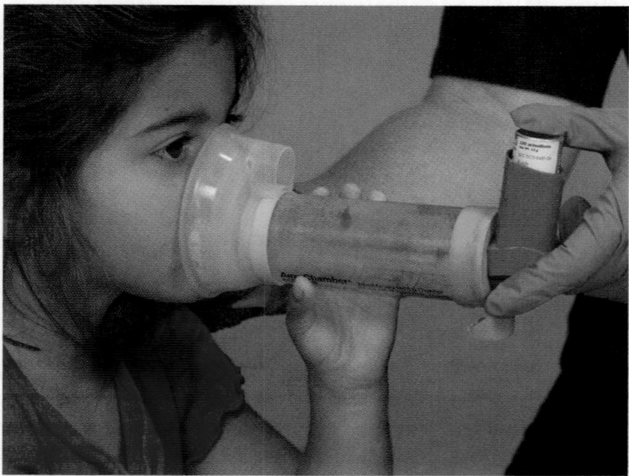

FIGURE 15-29 Valved holding chamber with face mask.
© Jones & Bartlett Learning. Courtesy of MIEMSS.

A **valved holding chamber** (usually 140 to 750 mL in volume) allows the plume from the pMDI to expand and incorporates a one-way valve that permits the aerosol to be drawn from the chamber during inhalation only, diverting the exhaled gas to the atmosphere and not disturbing remaining aerosol suspended in the chamber. Patients with small tidal volumes may empty the aerosol from the chamber with five to six breaths except when there is an exceptionally large dead space. A valved holding chamber (VHC) can also incorporate a mask for use with an infant, a child, or a patient unable to use a mouthpiece because of size, age, coordination, or mental status. With infants these masks must have minimal dead space and must be comfortable on the child's face, and the chamber must have a valve that opens or closes with the low inspiratory flow generated by the patient.

Box 15-6 describes the optimal technique for use of a valved holding chamber. The high oropharyngeal drug deposition with steroid pMDIs can increase the risk of oral yeast infections (thrush). Rinsing the mouth after steroid use can reduce this problem, but most pMDI steroid aerosol impaction occurs deeper in the pharynx, which is not easily rinsed. For this reason, steroid pMDIs should always be used in combination with a valved holding chamber.

Electrostatic charge acquired by the aerosol when generated, or present on the surface of the inhaler or add-on device, decreases aerosol delivery from VHCs.[83,84] Electrostatic charge may be particularly important with a delay in aerosol inhalation after actuation. VHCs made from conducting materials, such as stainless steel or aluminum, avoids this problem. Priming by firing 20 doses into a new spacer coats the inner surface with surfactant and minimizes static charge, but this is not practical because it uses more than 10% of the doses in a new pMDI canister. Washing a nonconducting VHC with detergent is a commonly used method to reduce surface electrostatic charge, and detergent washing is now incorporated in most manufacturer instructions. Detergent washing greatly improves drug delivery and is easy for the patient to perform. After washing, the VHC should not be towel dried, which could impart electrostatic charge; instead, the device should be allowed to drip dry in ambient air. The Food and Drug Administration requires manufacturers of add-on devices to recommend that patients rinse them in clean water after washing in detergent, to avoid patient contact with detergent-coated surfaces, which could result in contact dermatitis. VHCs manufactured from transparent, charge-dissipative polymers, as an alternative to opaque conducting materials such as stainless steel or aluminum, have become available in recent years.[84,85]

Accessory devices either use the manufacturer-designed boot that comes with the pMDI or incorporate a universal canister adapter to fire the pMDI canister. Different formulations of pMDI drugs operate at different pressures and have different-sized orifices in the boot designed by the manufacturer for use

BOX 15-6

Technique for Use of a Pressurized Metered Dose Inhaler with a Spacer or Valved Holding Chamber

1. Hold the pressurized metered dose inhaler (pMDI) in your hand to warm it.
2. Assemble the apparatus and check for foreign objects.
3. Remove the mouthpiece cover.
4. Shake the pMDI.
5. If the pMDI is new or has not been used recently, prime the device by shaking it and pressing the canister to deliver a dose into the room.
6. Repeat several times.
7. Hold the canister in a vertical position.
8. Breathe out normally.
9. Open your mouth and keep your tongue from obstructing the mouthpiece.
10. Place the mouthpiece into your mouth (or place the mask completely over your nose and mouth).
11. Breathe in slowly through your mouth and press the pMDI canister once at the beginning of inspiration.
12. If the device produces a "whistle," your inspiration is too rapid.
13. Allow 15 seconds between puffs.
14. Move the mouthpiece away from your mouth and hold your breath for 10 seconds (or as long as you comfortably can).
15. The technique is slightly different for a device with a collapsible bag:
16. Open the bag to its full size.
17. Remove the canister from the pMDI mouthpiece and insert it into the mouthpiece attached to the collapsible bag.
18. Press the pMDI canister immediately before inhalation and inhale until the bag is completely collapsed (if you have difficulty emptying the bag, you can breathe in and out of the bag several times to evacuate the medication).
19. Rinse your mouth if using inhaled steroids.
20. Clean the holding chamber every 2 weeks and as needed.
21. Keep count of the number of uses so that you know when the canister is empty.

> **AGE-SPECIFIC ANGLE**
>
> When using holding chambers with children, consideration should be given to mask fit and dead space volume.

exclusively with that pMDI. The output characteristics of a pMDI change if an adapter with a different-sized orifice is used. For this reason, spacers or holding chambers with universal canister adapters should be avoided, and only those with a universal boot adapter should be used.

Particularly in young children, use of a VHC requires a face mask. When using a face mask, an adequate seal is necessary, and five to six breaths are taken through the chamber to deliver the full dose. Drug delivery decreases when dead space increases, and drug delivery increases with smaller VHC volume and lower tidal volume. Rigid masks with large a large dead space volume might not be not suitable for use in children, especially if discomfort from the stiff mask makes its use less acceptable to the child.[86]

Dry Powder Inhalers

Dry powder inhalers (DPIs) create aerosols by drawing air through a dose of powdered medication. The powder contains micronized drug particles (less than 5 μm MMAD) with larger lactose or glucose particles (over 30 μm in diameter) or micronized drug particles bound into loose aggregates.[87,88] Micronized particles adhere strongly to each other and to most surfaces. Adding the larger particles of the carrier diminishes cohesive forces in the micronized drug powder so that separation into individual respirable particles (deaggregation) occurs more readily. The carrier particles, thus, aid the flow of the drug powder from the device. Carriers also act as fillers by adding bulk to the powder when the unit dose of a drug is very small. The drug particles usually are loosely bound to the carrier and are stripped from the carrier by the energy provided by the patient's inhalation (**Figure 15-30**). The release of respirable particles of the drug requires inspiration at relatively high flow (30 to 120 L/min). A high inspiratory flow results in pharyngeal impaction of the larger carrier particles that make up the bulk of the aerosol. The oropharyngeal impaction of carrier particles gives the patient the sensation of having inhaled a dose.

Commercially available DPIs are either multidose (the device contains a month's prescription) (**Figure 15-31**) or single dose (the patient loads a single-dose capsule prior to each use) (**Figure 15-32**). With single-dose devices, it is important to instruct the patient that the capsules are not to be ingested; they should be administered only via inhalation, with the appropriate delivery device. Moreover, the capsules should be used only in the intended device and should

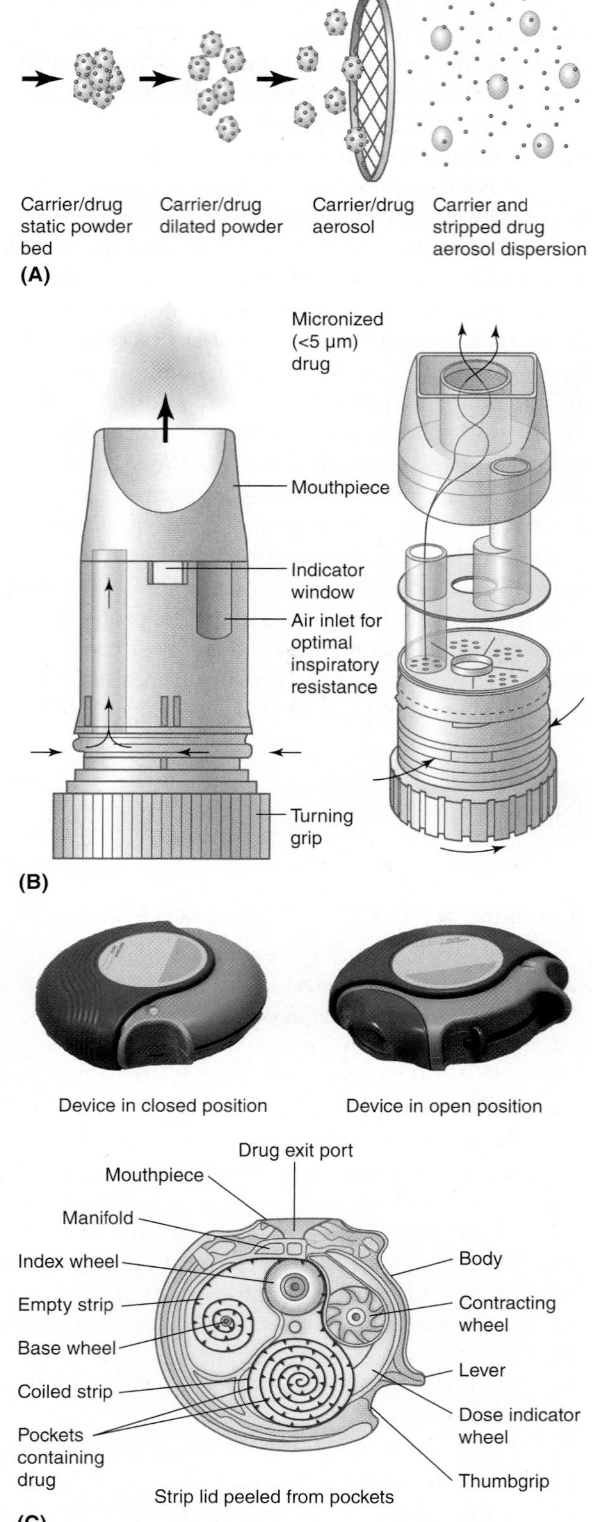

FIGURE 15-30 (**A**) Aerosolization of dry powder. (**B**) Component parts of Flexhaler. (**C**) Component parts of Diskus.

(**A**) modified from Dhand R, Fink JB. Dry powder inhalers. *Respir Care*. 1999;44:940–951. Reprinted with permission; (**B**) modified from Crompton GK. Delivery systems. In: Kay AB., ed. *Allergy and Allergic Diseases*. London: Blackwell Science; 1997:1440–1450.

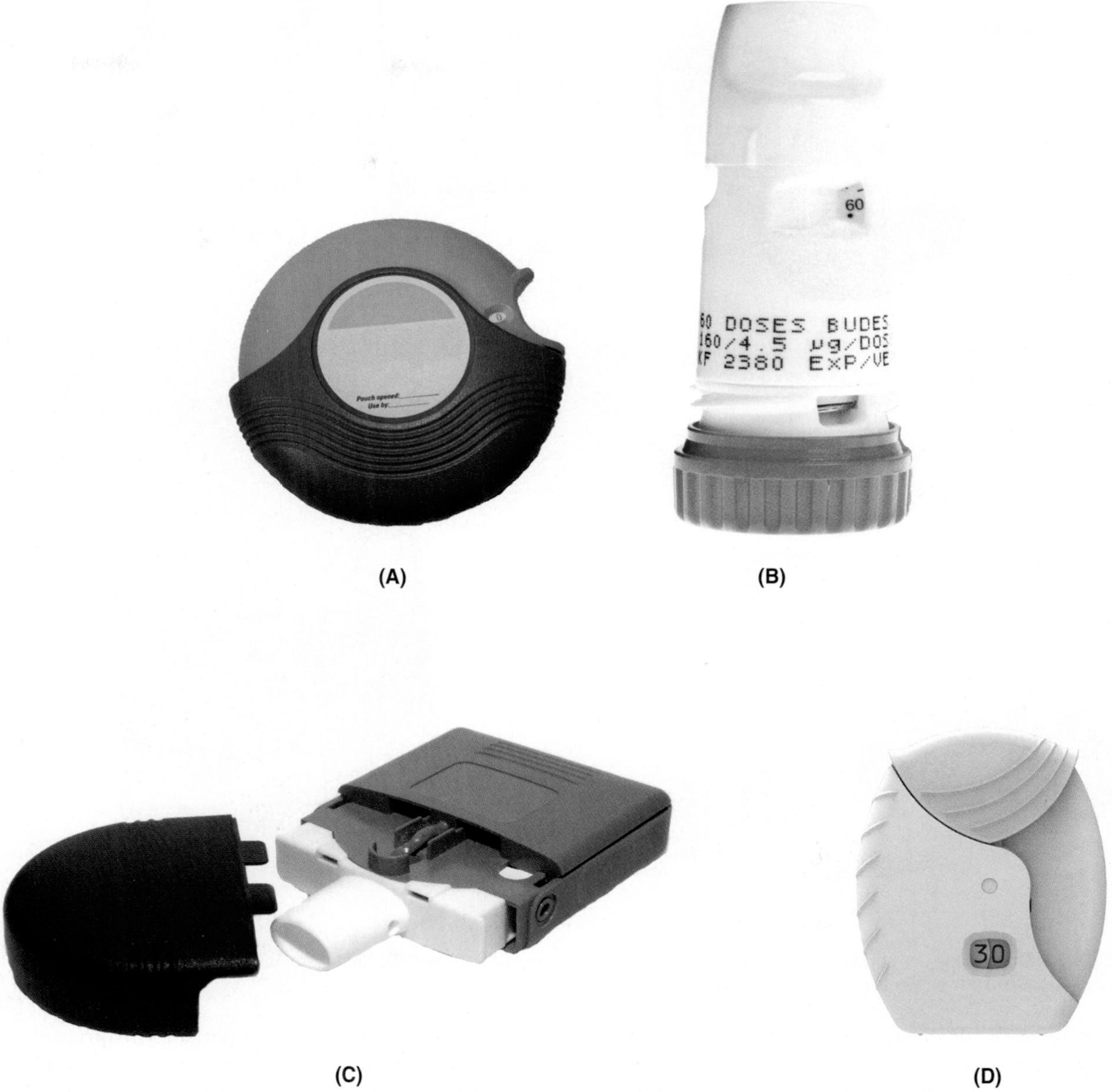

(A) (B)

(C) (D)

FIGURE 15-31 Multiple-dose dry powder inhalers. (**A**) Diskus. (**B**) Flexhaler. (**C**) Diskhaler. Single-dose dry powder inhalers. (**D**) Ellipta.

not be administered in another device. For example, formoterol capsules should not be administered in the HandiHaler, and the powder should never be dumped from the capsule into a nebulizer for administration. Currently available DPIs are all passive systems, meaning that the patient must provide the energy to disperse the powder from the device. A primary advantage of DPIs is coordination of actuation with inspiration, because they are breath actuated. A primary disadvantage of unit-dose DPIs is the time needed to load a dose for each use. Another disadvantage of DPIs is that each operates differently from the others in loading and priming.

The internal geometry of the DPI device influences the resistance offered to inspiration and the inspiratory flow required to deaggregate the medication. Devices with higher resistance require a higher inspiratory flow to produce a dose. Inhalation through high-resistance DPIs may improve drug delivery to the lower respiratory tract compared with pMDIs, provided the patient can reliably generate the required flow rate. High-resistance devices have not been shown to improve either deposition or bronchodilation compared with low-resistance DPIs. DPIs with several components require correct assembly of the apparatus

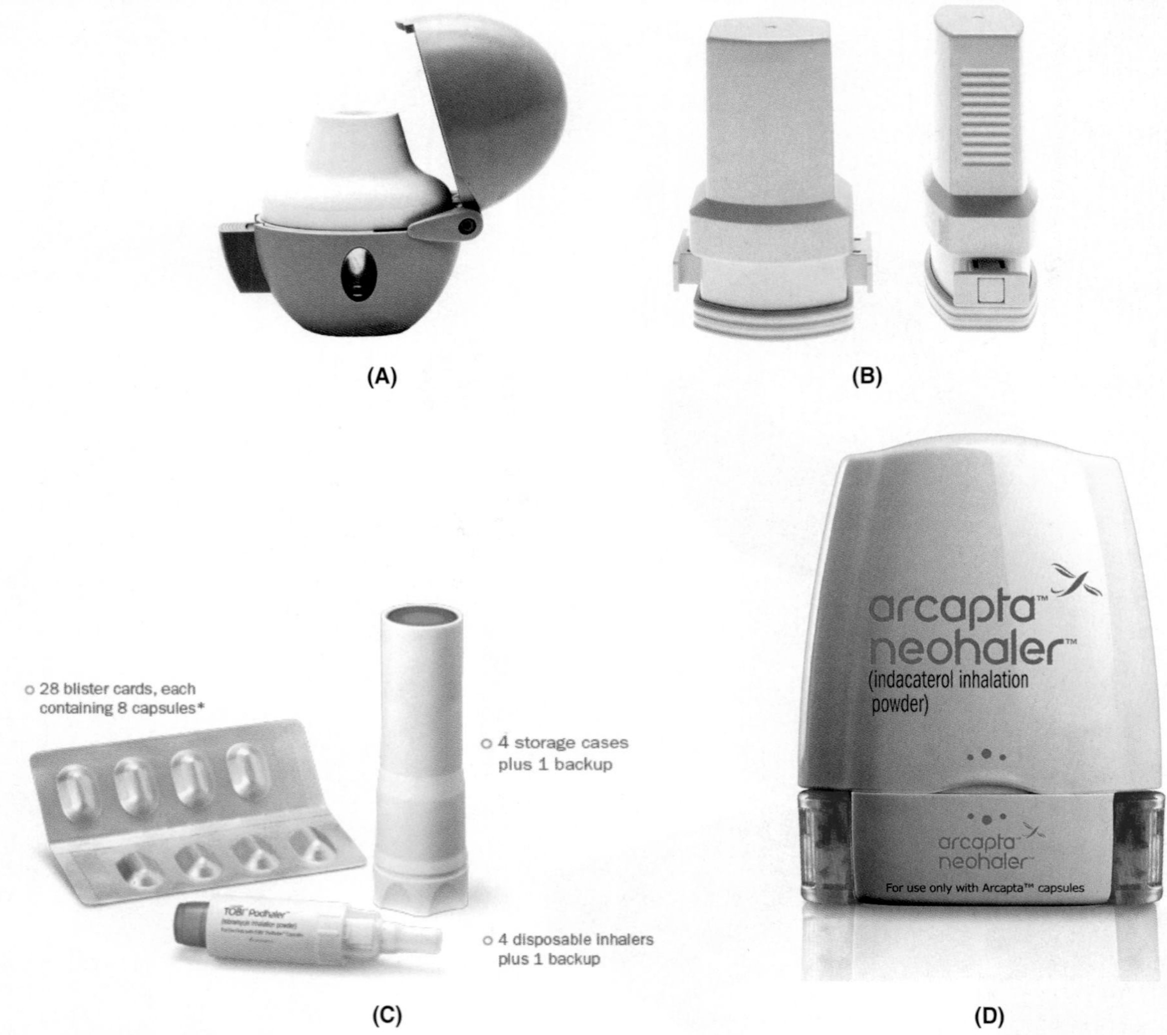

FIGURE 15-32 Single-dose dry powder inhalers. (**A**) Handihaler. (**B**) Aerolizer. (**C**) Podhaler. (**D**) Neohaler.

(**A**) © mayer kleinostheim/ShutterStock, Inc.; (**B**) © Silentiger/Dreamstime.com; (**C**) and (**D**) courtesy of Novartis Pharmaceuticals Corporation.

and priming of the device to ensure aerosolization of the dry powder. Some DPIs require periodic brushing to remove any residual powder that has accumulated in the device.

DPIs produce aerosols in which most of the drug particles are in the respirable range, with the distribution of particle sizes differing significantly among various DPIs. High ambient humidity causes the dry powder to clump, creating larger particles that are not as effectively aerosolized. Air with high moisture content is less efficient at deaggregating particles of dry powder than dry air, such that high ambient humidity increases the size of drug particles in the aerosol and may reduce drug delivery to the lungs. High ambient humidity also can result from exhalation into a DPI; from bringing a DPI into a warm indoor environment from the cold outdoors or a cold car, causing condensation to form inside the device; or from using a DPI in a warm, humid environment. Newer DPIs contain individual doses that are better protected from humidity. Humidity also can accumulate if the DPI is stored with the cap off.

Because the energy from the patient's inspiratory flow disperses the drug powder, the magnitude and duration of the patient's inspiratory effort influences aerosol generation from a DPI. Failure to perform inhalation at a sufficiently fast inspiratory flow reduces the dose of the drug emitted by the DPI and increases the distribution of particle sizes within the aerosol. Research on active DPI delivery devices is under way. These devices use either a small motor and impeller or compressed gas propulsion to disperse the powder. With active DPIs, aerosol production and airway deposition are less influenced by the patient's inspiratory flow than with DPIs that rely solely on patient effort for aerosol production.

Breath coordination is also important during use of a DPI. Exhalation into a DPI blows out the powder from the device and reduces drug delivery. Moreover, the humidity in the exhaled air reduces subsequent aerosol generation. For these reasons, patients must be instructed not to exhale into a DPI. Because DPIs are breath actuated, they reduce the problem of coordinating inspiration with actuation. Using a DPI (**Box 15-7**)

BOX 15-7

Technique for Use of Dry Powder Inhalers

Diskus

1. Open the device.
2. Slide the lever.
3. Breathe out normally; do not exhale into the device.
4. Place the mouthpiece into your mouth and close your lips tightly around the mouthpiece.
5. Keep device level while inhaling dose with a rapid and steady flow.
6. Remove the mouthpiece from your mouth and hold your breath for 10 seconds (or as long as you comfortably can).
7. When you exhale, be sure that you are not exhaling into the device.
8. Store the device in a cool, dry place.
9. Observe the counter for the number of doses remaining, and replace when appropriate.

Flexhaler

1. Twist and remove cap.
2. Hold inhaler upright (mouthpiece up).
3. In order to load the correct dose, the Flexhaler must be held in the upright position (mouthpiece up) whenever a dose of medication is being loaded. Do not hold the mouthpiece when you load the inhaler.
4. Twist the brown grip fully in one direction as far as it will go. Twist it fully back again in the other direction as far as it will go (it does not matter which way you turn it first). You will hear a click during one of the twisting movements.
5. Breathe out normally—do not exhale into the device. If you accidentally blow into your inhaler after loading a dose, simply follow the instructions for loading a new dose.
6. Place the mouthpiece into your mouth and close your lips tightly around the mouthpiece. Do not bite or chew on the mouthpiece.
7. Inhale dose with a rapid and forceful flow.
8. Remove the mouthpiece from your mouth and hold your breath for 10 seconds (or as long as you comfortably can).
9. When you exhale, be sure that you do not exhale into the device.
10. Replace the cover and twist to close. Store the device in a cool, dry place.
11. The dose indicator shows how many doses remain in the inhaler. Look at the middle of the window to find out how many doses are left in the inhaler. The dose indicator starts with either the number 60 or 120 when full, depending upon the strength of the product. The indicator is marked in intervals of 10 doses, alternating numbers and dashes. The dose indicator counts down each time a dose is loaded, not when a dose is inhaled. The grip will still twist and click even when the inhaler is empty, and you may still hear a sound if you shake it.

Aerolizer

1. Remove the mouthpiece cover.
2. Hold the base of the inhaler and twist the mouthpiece counterclockwise.
3. Remove capsule from foil blister immediately before use; do not store the capsule in the device.
4. Place the capsule in the chamber in the base of the inhaler.
5. Hold the base of the inhaler and turn it clockwise to close.
6. Simultaneously press both buttons; this pierces the capsule.
7. Keep your head in an upright position.
8. Breathe out normally; do not exhale into the device.
9. Hold the device horizontal, with the buttons on the left and right.
10. Place the mouthpiece into your mouth and close your lips tightly around the mouthpiece.
11. Breathe in rapidly and as deeply as possible.
12. Remove the mouthpiece from your mouth and hold your breath for 10 seconds (or as long as you comfortably can).
13. When you exhale, be sure that you are not exhaling into the device.

(continues)

BOX 15-7 *(continued)*

14. Open the chamber and examine the capsule; if there is powder remaining, repeat the inhalation process.
15. After use, remove and discard the capsule.
16. Close the mouthpiece and replace the cover.
17. Store the device in a cool, dry place.

HandiHaler

1. Immediately before using the HandiHaler, peel back the aluminum foil and remove a capsule; do not store capsules in the HandiHaler.
2. Open the dust cap by pulling it upward.
3. Open the mouthpiece.
4. Place the capsule in the center chamber; it does not matter which end is placed in the chamber.
5. Close the mouthpiece firmly until you hear a click; leave the dust cap open.
6. Hold the HandiHaler with the mouthpiece up.
7. Press the piercing button once and release; this makes holes in the capsule and allows the medication to be released when you breathe in.
8. Exhale normally; do not exhale into the device.
9. Place the mouthpiece into your mouth and close your lips tightly around the mouthpiece.
10. Keep your head in an upright position.
11. Breathe in slowly, at a rate sufficient to hear the capsule vibrate, until your lungs are full.
12. Remove the mouthpiece from your mouth and hold your breath for 10 seconds (or as long as you comfortably can).
13. When you exhale, be sure that you are not exhaling into the device.
14. To ensure you get the full dose, repeat the inhalation from the HandiHaler.
15. Open the mouthpiece, tip out the used capsule, and dispose of it.
16. Close the mouthpiece and dust cap for storage of the HandiHaler.

Diskhaler

1. Remove the mouthpiece cover.
2. Pull the tray out from the device.
3. Place the disk on the wheel (numbers up).
4. Rotate the disk by sliding the tray out and in.
5. Lift the back of the lid until fully upright so that the needle pierces both sides of the blister.
6. Breathe out normally; do not exhale into the device.
7. Place the mouthpiece into your mouth and close your lips tightly around the mouthpiece.
8. Keep the device level while inhaling the dose with a rapid and steady flow.
9. Remove the mouthpiece from your mouth and hold your breath for 10 seconds (or as long as you comfortably can).
10. When you exhale, be sure that you are not exhaling into the device.
11. Store the device in a cool, dry place.
12. Replace the disk when all of the blisters have been punctured.
13. Once every week, brush off any powder remaining within the device.

Ellipta

1. Open the cover of the inhaler. Slide the cover down to expose the mouthpiece. You should hear a click. The counter will count down by 1 number.
2. While holding the inhaler away from your mouth, breathe out fully. Do not breathe out into the mouthpiece.
3. Put the mouthpiece between your lips, and close your lips firmly around it. Take one long, steady, deep breath in through your mouth. Do not block the air vent with your fingers. Remove the inhaler from your mouth and hold your breath for about 3 to 4 seconds (or as long as comfortable for you).
4. Breathe out slowly and gently. You may not taste or feel the medicine, even when you are using the inhaler correctly. Do not take another dose from the inhaler even if you do not feel or taste the medicine.
5. Close the inhaler. You can clean the mouthpiece if needed, using a dry tissue, before you close the cover. Routine cleaning is not required. Slide the cover up and over the mouthpiece as far as it will go.

6. Rinse your mouth with water after you have used the inhaler and spit the water out. Do not swallow the water.
7. When you have less than 10 doses remaining in your inhaler, the left half of the counter shows red as a reminder to get a refill. After you have inhaled the last dose, the counter will show 0 and will be empty. Throw the empty inhaler away in your household trash out of reach of children and pets.

Neohaler

1. Pull off cap.
2. Hold the base of the inhaler firmly and tilt the mouthpiece to open the inhaler.
3. Prepare capsule. Separate one of the blisters from the blister card by tearing along the perforation. Take one blister and peel away the protective backing to expose the foil.
4. Capsules should always be stored in the blister and only removed immediately before use. With dry hands, remove one capsule from the blister by pushing the capsule through the foil. Do not swallow the capsule.
5. Place the capsule into the capsule chamber. Do not place a capsule directly into the mouthpiece.
6. Close the inhaler fully. You should hear a click as it fully closes.
7. Hold the inhaler upright. Press both buttons fully one time. You should hear a click as the capsule is being pierced. Do not press the piercing buttons more than one time.
8. Release the buttons fully.
9. Before placing the mouthpiece in your mouth, breathe out fully. Never blow into the mouthpiece.
10. Inhale the medicine. Before breathing in, place the mouthpiece in your mouth and close your lips around the mouthpiece. Hold the inhaler with the buttons to the left and right (not up and down). Breathe in rapidly and steadily, as deeply as you can. Do not press the piercing buttons. As you breathe in through the inhaler, the capsule spins around in the chamber and you should hear a whirring noise. If you do not hear a whirring noise, the capsule may be stuck in the capsule cavity. If this occurs, open the inhaler and carefully loosen the capsule by tapping the base of the device. Do not press the piercing buttons to loosen the capsule. Repeat steps 9 and 10 if needed.
11. Continue to hold your breath as long as comfortably possible while removing the inhaler from your mouth. Then breathe out. Open the inhaler to see if any powder is left in the capsule. If there is powder left in the capsule, close the inhaler and repeat steps 9 to 11. Most people are able to empty the capsule in one or two inhalations. Some people may cough soon after inhaling the medicine. But as long as the capsule is empty, you have received the full dose.
12. Remove capsule. After you have finished taking your daily dose, open the mouthpiece again, remove the empty capsule by tipping it out, and discard it. Close the inhaler and replace the cap. Do not store capsules in the device.

Podhaler

1. Hold the base of the Podhaler and unscrew the lid in a counter-clockwise direction. Set the lid aside.
2. Stand the Podhaler upright in the base of the case.
3. Hold the body of the Podhaler and unscrew the mouthpiece in a counter-clockwise direction. Set the mouthpiece aside on a clean, dry surface.
4. Take 1 blister card and tear the pre-cut lines along the length, and then tear at the pre-cut lines along the width.
5. Peel (by rolling back) the foil that covers 1 TOBI Podhaler capsule on the blister card. Always hold the foil close to where you are peeling.
6. Take out 1 TOBI Podhaler capsule from the blister card. Only remove one capsule at a time just before you are going to use it in the device.
7. Immediately, place the TOBI Podhaler capsule in the capsule chamber at the top of the Podhaler device. Do not put the capsule directly into the top of the mouthpiece.
8. Put the mouthpiece back on your Podhaler and screw the mouthpiece in a clockwise direction until it is tight. Do not overtighten.
9. Hold the Podhaler with the mouthpiece pointing down. Put your thumb on the blue button and press the blue button all the way down. Let go of the blue button. Do not press the blue button more than 1 time. The chances of the capsule breaking into pieces will be increased if the capsule is accidentally pierced more than once. You will need to inhale at least twice from each capsule in order to get the full dose.

(continues)

BOX 15-7 *(continued)*

10. Breathe out all the way. Do not blow or exhale into the mouthpiece.
11. Place your mouth over the mouthpiece and close your lips tightly around it.
12. Inhale deeply with a single breath.
13. Remove the Podhaler from your mouth, hold your breath for about 5 seconds, and then exhale normally away from the Podhaler.
14. Take a few normal breaths away from the Podhaler device. Do not blow or exhale into the mouthpiece.
15. For your second inhalation, repeat steps 10 through 13 using the same capsule.
16. Unscrew the mouthpiece and remove the TOBI Podhaler capsule from the capsule chamber.
17. Look at the used capsule. It should be pierced and empty. There will be a fine coating of powder remaining on the inside of the capsule. If it is pierced and empty, throw it away and go to step 18. If the capsule is pierced but still contains more than just a fine coating of powder, put the capsule back into the Podhaler device capsule-chamber with the pierced side of the capsule pointing down. Repeat steps 10 to 13. If the capsule does not look pierced, put the capsule back into the Podhaler capsule-chamber. Repeat steps 9 to 17. If the capsule still does not look pierced and still has some powder in it, use the reserve Podhaler provided in the TOBI Podhaler package and repeat steps 1 to 3, and then 7 to 17.
18. Repeat steps 6 to 17 for 3 more times until your whole dose (4 capsules) has been taken.
19. Throw away all the empty TOBI Podhaler capsules. Do not store the TOBI Podhaler capsules in the Podhaler device.
20. Put the mouthpiece back on to your Podhaler and twist the mouthpiece in a clockwise direction until it is tight. Do not overtighten.
21. Wipe the mouthpiece with a clean, dry cloth. Do not wash the Podhaler with water. Your Podhaler needs to stay dry at all times to work the right way.
22. Place your Podhaler back in the storage case base.
23. Place the lid back on the storage case base and screw the cover in a clockwise direction until it is tight. Store your Podhaler and blister-packaged capsules at room temperature between 68°F and 77°F (20°C and 25°C). Keep the TOBI Podhaler capsules and device in a dry place. Store the Podhaler tightly closed in its case when you are not using it.

Except for the mouthpiece, do *not* clean DPIs.

differs in important respects from the technique used to inhale drugs from a pMDI. Although DPIs are easier to use than pMDIs, as many patients use them improperly. DPIs are critically dependent on inspiratory airflow to generate the aerosol; therefore, they should be used with caution, if at all, in very young or ill children, the weak, the elderly, and those with altered mental status. Patients may need repeated instruction before they can master the use of a DPI, and periodic assessment is necessary to ensure that patients continue to use optimum technique.

Aerosol Delivery During Invasive Mechanical Ventilation

Aerosolized drugs are administered to mechanically ventilated patients using nebulizer or pMDI.[89–93] DPI cannot be used in intubated mechanically ventilated patients. A number of factors affect aerosol delivery during mechanical ventilation (**Figure 15-33**). **Box 15-8** and **Box 15-9** present the techniques used to deliver aerosolized bronchodilators during mechanical ventilation by jet nebulizer and pMDI, respectively.

Ventilator circuits are designed to heat and humidify the inspired gas. Humidity can increase particle size and reduce deposition during mechanical ventilation. Humidification of inhaled gas reduces aerosol deposition by approximately 40%, probably because of an increase in particle loss in the ventilator circuit. Some clinicians recommend bypassing the humidifier during aerosol administration. Nebulizers require as long as 30 minutes to complete aerosolization, however, and inhalation of dry gas for this length of time can damage the airway. In addition, disconnection of the ventilator circuit, which is required to bypass the humidifier,

Ventilator Related
- Mode of ventilation
- Tidal volume
- Respiratory rate
- Duty cycle
- Inspiratory waveform
- Breath-triggering mechanism

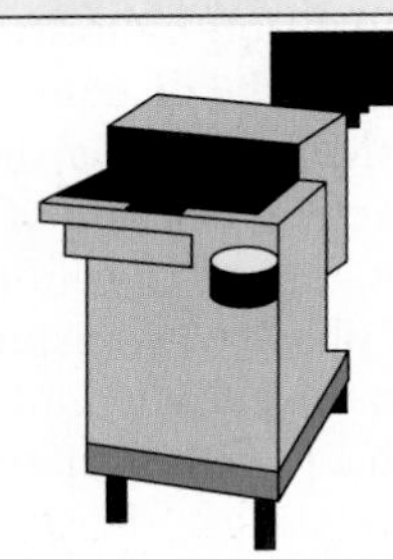

Circuit Related
- Endotracheal tube
- Inhaled gas humidity
- Inhaled gas density

Device Related—pMDI
- Type of spacer or adapter used
- Position of spacer in circuit
- Timing of pMDI actuation

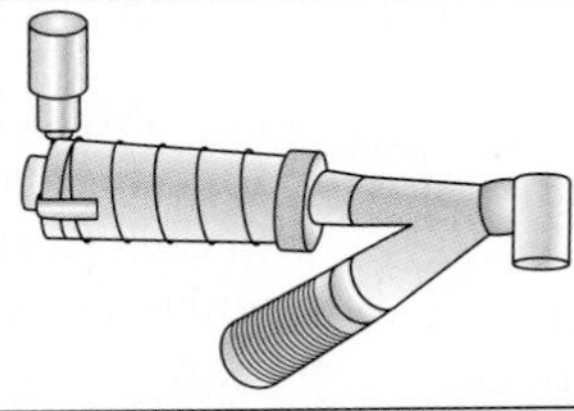

Device Related—nebulizer
- Type of nebulizer used
- Continuous/intermittent operation
- Duration of nebulization
- Position in the circuit

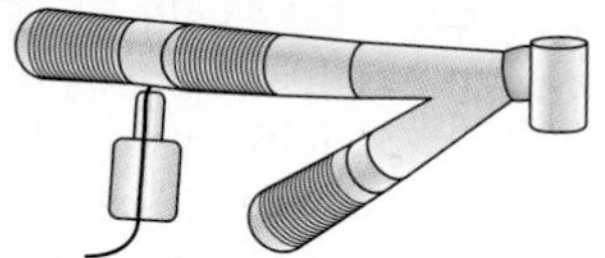

Drug Related
- Dose
- Aerosol particle size
- Duration of action

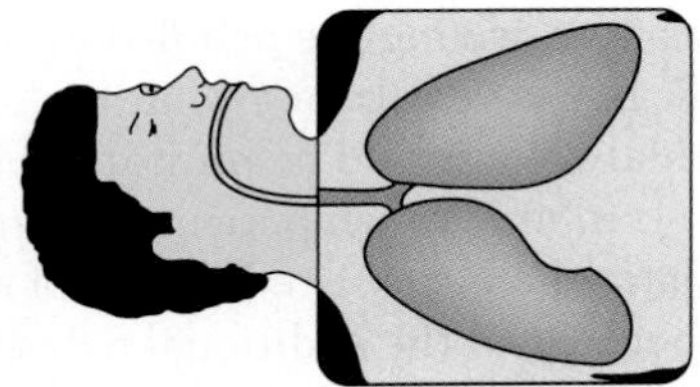

Patient Related
- Severity of airway obstruction
- Mechanism of airway obstruction
- Presence of dynamic hyperinflation
- Patient–ventilator synchrony

FIGURE 15-33 Summary of factors affecting delivery of aerosols during mechanical ventilation.
Adapted from Dhand R, et al. Bronchodilator delivery by metered-dose inhaler in ventilator supported patients. *Eur Respir J.* 1996;9:585–595.

BOX 15-8

Technique for Aerosol Delivery by Jet Nebulizer During Mechanical Ventilation

1. Fill the nebulizer with the drug solution to the optimum fill volume.
2. Place the nebulizer in the inspiratory line at least 30 cm from the patient's Y piece.
3. Ensure that the flow through the nebulizer is 6 to 8 L/min. Continuous gas flow from an external source or the nebulizer control of the ventilator can be used to power the nebulizer.
4. The nebulizer may be operated continuously or only during inhalation. Some ventilators provide inspiratory gas flow to the nebulizer.
5. Adjust tidal volume as necessary.
6. Turn off the bias flow on the ventilator if possible and remove (or bypass) the heat and moisture exchanger if present.
7. Check the nebulizer for adequate aerosol generation throughout its use.
8. Disconnect the nebulizer when all the medication has been nebulized or when no more aerosol is being produced. Store the nebulizer under aseptic conditions.
9. Reconnect the ventilator circuit and reinstate the original ventilator settings.

BOX 15-9

Technique for Use of a Pressurized Metered Dose Inhaler During Mechanical Ventilation

1. Place a spacer situated in the inspiratory limb of the ventilator circuit. It is preferable to use a spacer that remains in the ventilator circuit so that the circuit need not be disconnected for each bronchodilator treatment.
2. Shake the pressurized metered dose inhaler (pMDI) canister vigorously.
3. Actuate the pMDI to synchronize with the precise onset of inspiration by the ventilator. Actuate the pMDI once only.
4. Repeat actuations at 30-second intervals until the total dose has been delivered.

interrupts ventilation and may increase the risk of ventilator-associated pneumonia.[94]

Placement of a jet nebulizer 30 cm from the endotracheal tube is more efficient than placement between the inspiratory limb and the patient Y piece because the inspiratory ventilator tubing acts as a spacer for the aerosol to accumulate during the expiratory phase. Operating the nebulizer only during inspiration is more efficient for aerosol delivery than continuous aerosol generation.

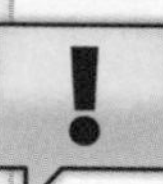

Respiratory Recap

Aerosol Delivery During Mechanical Ventilation

- Either a pMDI or nebulizer can be used.
- Careful attention to technique is important.

The gas flow driving the nebulizer produces additional flow in the ventilator circuit, requiring adjustment of tidal volume and inspiratory flow when the nebulizer is in use. When patients are unable to trigger the ventilator during assisted modes of mechanical ventilation (because of the additional nebulizer gas flow), hypoventilation can result. Longer inspiratory times allow a higher proportion of the aerosol generated by the nebulizer to be inhaled with each breath. Because nebulizers generate aerosol over several minutes, longer inspiratory times have a cumulative effect in improving aerosol delivery. Nebulizers placed in-line in the ventilator circuit can become contaminated with bacteria, which are then carried as microaerosols directly to the lower respiratory tract and can be the source of ventilator-associated pneumonia.

Because the pMDI cannot be used in the ventilator circuit with the actuator designed by the manufacturer, a third-party actuator is required (**Figure 15-34**). The size, shape, and design of these actuators affect the amount of respirable drug available to the patient and may vary with different pMDI formulations. A pMDI with a spacer in the inspiratory limb of the ventilator circuit produces a fourfold to sixfold greater delivery of aerosol than a pMDI connector that lacks a chamber.

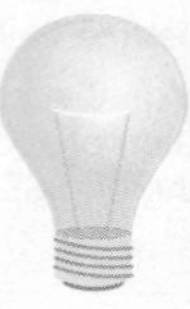

STOP AND THINK

You are asked if inhalers are better than nebulizers in mechanically ventilated patients. What would be your response?

When pMDIs are used with a collapsible cylindric spacer, the ventilator circuit need not be disconnected with each treatment. Leaving a pMDI noncollapsible chamber device in-line is not practical because of the increased compressible volume it adds to the circuit.

Actuation of the pMDI out of phase with inspiratory flow delivers very little aerosol to the patient. Unlike nebulizer use, dose delivery from a pMDI is relatively constant regardless of ventilator settings.[95] With use of pMDI during mechanical ventilation, delivery of a large tidal volume, use of an end-inspiratory pause, and use of a slow inspiratory flow have little effect on aerosol delivery and deposition.[96–98] If an HME is used, it must either be removed, or a specially designed HME that allows the HME to be bypassed during aerosol therapy can be used (**Figure 15-35**). No studies have demonstrated contamination problems with administration of aerosol from a pMDI during mechanical ventilation.

Depending on the FIO_2 and the propellant gas volume, an inline pMDI actuation theoretically may result in a hypoxic gas mixture to an infant receiving a tidal volume less than 100 mL. The large dead space volume

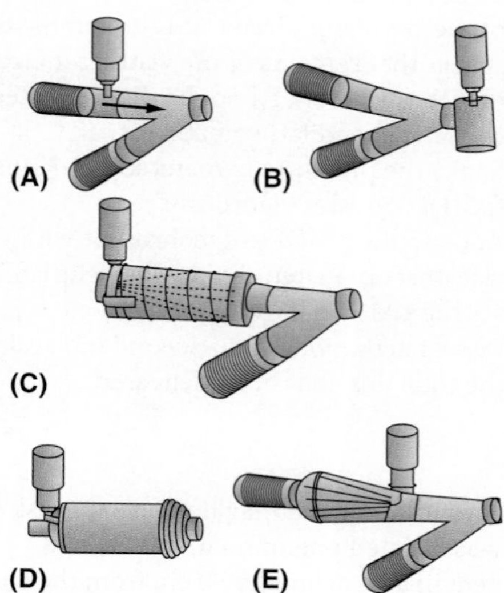

FIGURE 15-34 Devices to adapt a metered dose inhaler to a ventilator circuit. (**A**) Inline device. (**B**) Elbow device. (**C**) Collapsible chamber device. (**D**) Chamber device. (**E**) Chamber device in which aerosol is directed retrograde into the ventilator circuit.

Reproduced from Dhand R, et al. Bronchodilator delivery by metered-dose inhaler in ventilator supported patients. *Eur Respir J.* 1996;9:585–595. Reproduced with permission of the European Respiratory Society.

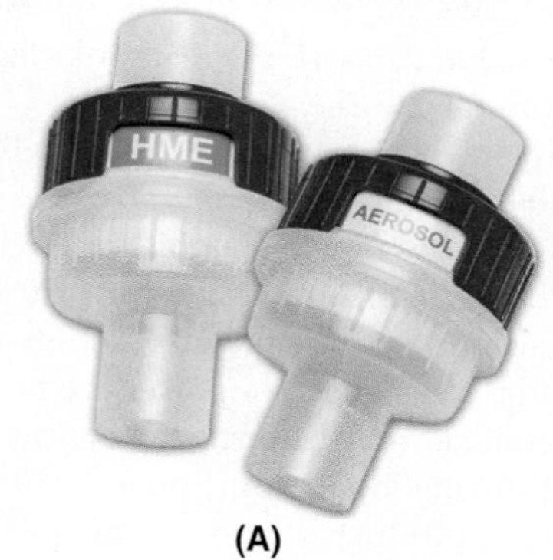

(A)

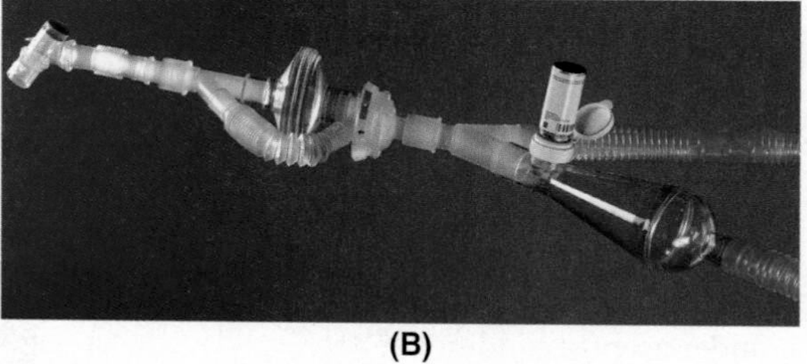

(B)

FIGURE 15-35 Devices that allow a heat and moisture exchanger to be bypassed during aerosol delivery.

(**A**) courtesy of Teleflex Incorporated. Unauthorized use prohibited; (**B**) courtesy of Smiths Medical.

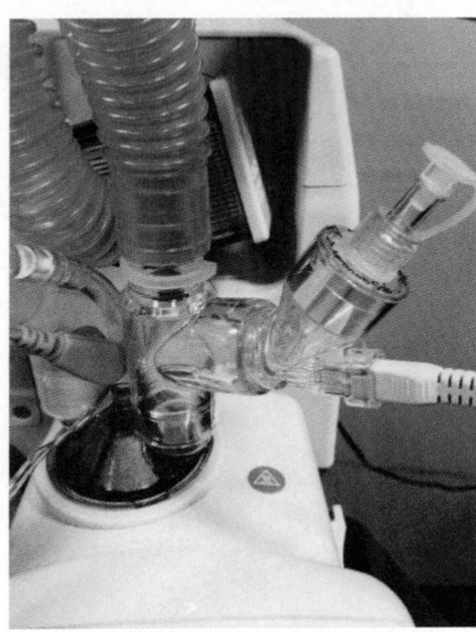

FIGURE 15-36 Mesh nebulizer at inlet of humidifier in ventilator circuit.

of a spacer or chamber at the end of the endotracheal tube must also be considered during administration of pMDI medications to an infant.

Stable mechanically ventilated patients with chronic obstructive pulmonary disease (COPD) achieve near-maximum bronchodilation after administration of four puffs of albuterol with a pMDI or 2.5 mg with a nebulizer. With proper technique, nebulizers and pMDIs produce similar therapeutic effects in mechanically ventilated patients. Aerosol delivery by pMDI is easy to administer, involves less personnel time, provides a reliable dose of the drug, is free of the risk of bacterial contamination, and adds no additional flow to the circuit.

The vibrating mesh nebulizer overcomes some of the issues associated with the jet nebulizer because it adds no gas flow into the circuit and the device can remain in the circuit between treatments. It is placed between the ventilator and the humidifier (**Figure 15-36**). Aerosol delivery is more efficient with the mesh nebulizer compared to the jet nebulizer. Because of the cost of HFA pMDI formulations, the vibrating mesh nebulizer is being used increasingly during mechanical ventilation.[99–101]

Aerosol Delivery During Noninvasive Ventilation

Aerosol therapy during noninvasive ventilation (NIV) can be delivered effectively by pressurized metered dose inhaler with a spacer or nebulizer.[102,103] Alternatively, the patient can be removed from NIV and the inhaled medication administered in the usual manner,[104] but this has the disadvantage of interrupting NIV.

A number of factors affect aerosol delivery during NIV, and these include the type of ventilator, mode of ventilation, circuit conditions, type of interface, type of aerosol generator, drug-related factors, breathing parameters, and patient-related factors (**Figure 15-37**). When a critical care ventilator is used for NIV, factors affecting aerosol delivery are much the same as the factors affecting aerosol delivery with invasive ventilation. Despite the impediments to efficient aerosol delivery with a bilevel ventilator, due to the continuous gas flow and leaks, therapeutic effects are achieved after inhaled bronchodilator administration to patients with asthma and COPD. Careful attention to the technique of drug administration is required to optimize therapeutic effects of inhaled drugs during NIV. The nebulizer should be placed near the mask rather than at the outlet of the ventilator during NIV (**Figure 15-38**). A metered dose inhaler should be used with a spacer. A mesh nebulizer can be incorporated directly into the mask for NIV (**Figure 15-39**).[105] Care must be taken to ensure an adequate mask fit so that aerosol is not directed into the eyes of the patient.

Ventilator related
Critical care ventilator
NIV ventilator
Home care ventilator

Circuit related
Type of circuit
Position of leak port
Inhaled gas humidity
Inhaled gas density

Device related - pMDI
Type of spacer/adapter used
Timing of pMDI actuation
Position of pMDI/spacer

Drug related
Dose
Aerosol particle size
Duration of action

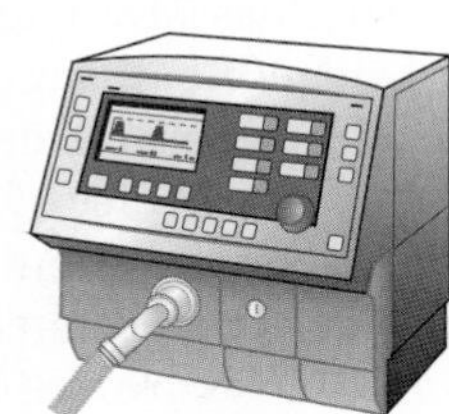

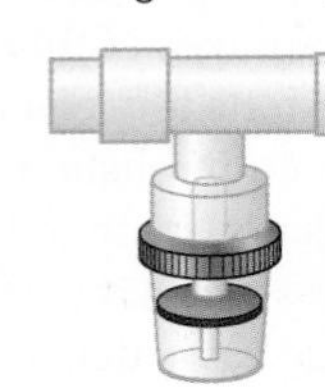

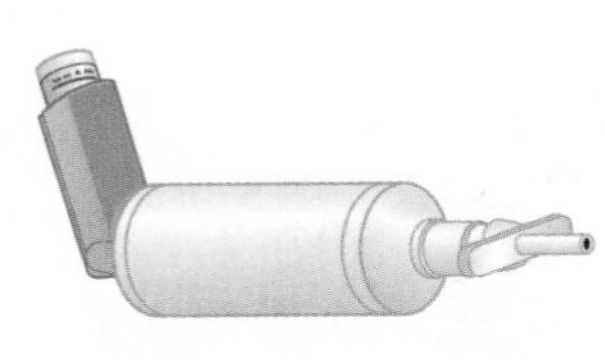

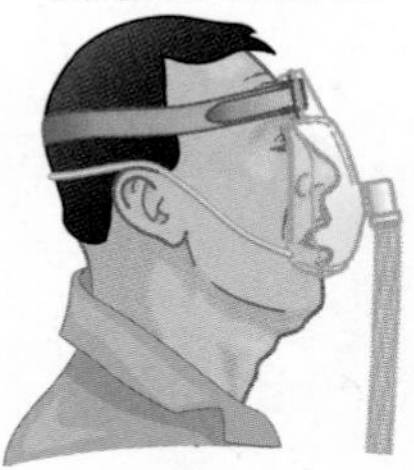

Breathing parameters
Mode of ventilation
Tidal volume
Respiratory rate
Inspiratory air flow
Pressure settings

Type of interface
Face mask
Nasal cannula

Device related - nebulizer
Type of nebulizer used
Continuous/intermittent operation
Duration of nebulization
Position of the circuit

Patient related
Severity of airway obstruction
Mechanism of airway obstruction
Presence of intrinsic PEEP
Patient-ventilator synchrony

FIGURE 15-37 Factors influencing aerosol delivery during noninvasive ventilation.

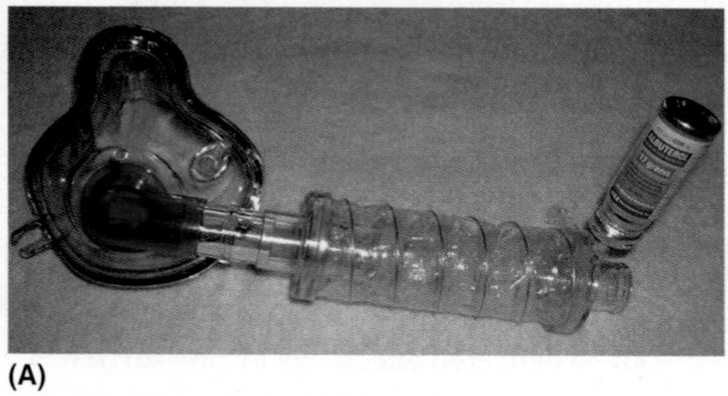

(A)

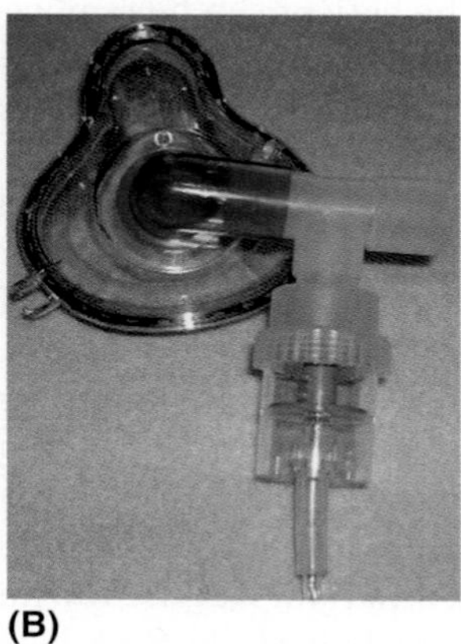

(B)

FIGURE 15-38 Insertion site for nebulizer and inhaler for use with a bilevel ventilator during NIV.

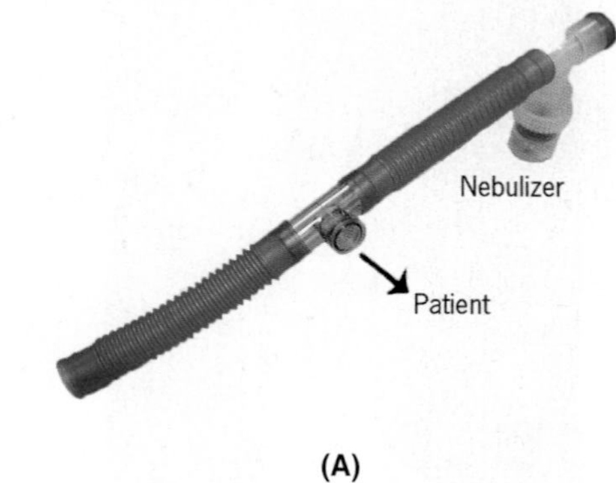

(A)

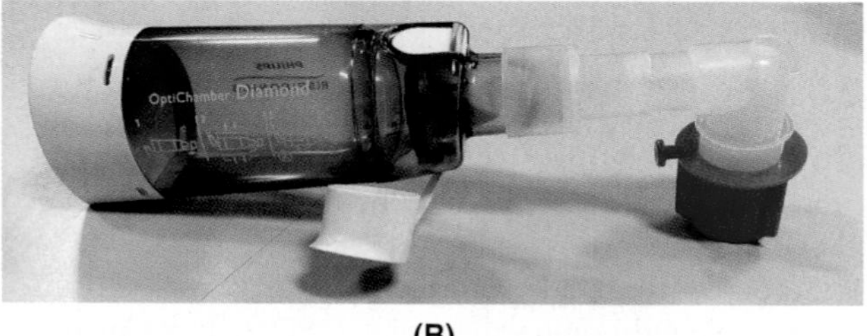

(B)

FIGURE 15-40 Equipment for aerosol delivery to tracheostomy. (A) Nebulizer. (B) Spacer for pMDI delivery by tracheostomy.

Aerosol Delivery by Tracheostomy

Inhaled albuterol is occasionally used in spontaneously breathing patients with a tracheostomy tube.[106–111] A measurable amount of albuterol aerosol can be delivered through the tracheostomy tube during spontaneous breathing, whether a nebulizer or a pMDI with spacer is used. Delivery of albuterol aerosol into a high gas flow is inefficient for the nebulizer, and use of a T piece for albuterol delivery is more effective than use of a tracheostomy mask. The efficiency is greater for a pMDI with valved holding chamber than for a nebulizer, and the pMDI is most efficient when a valved T piece is used and the valve is placed proximal rather than distal to the spacer. Figure 15-40 shows the proper equipment for aerosol delivery by nebulizer and pMDI for spontaneously breathing patients with a tracheostomy. Aerosol delivery through a tracheostomy tube may be greater with assisted ventilation compared to spontaneous breathing. The use of a manual resuscitation bag for aerosol delivery in spontaneously breathing patients with tracheostomy is not a standard practice, however.

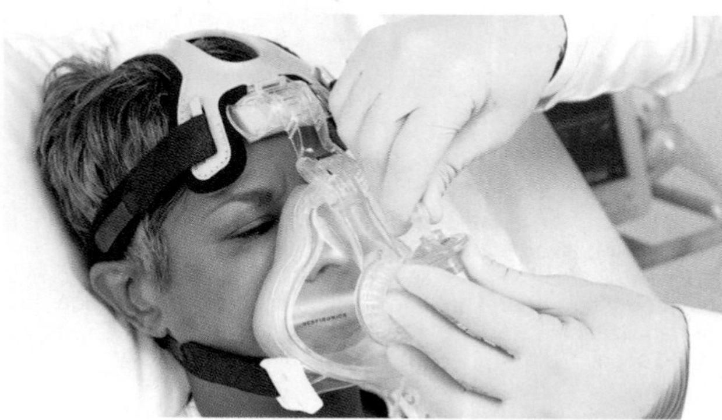

FIGURE 15-39 NIV mask incorporating mesh nebulizer.

Selection of an Aerosol Delivery Device

Each type of aerosol delivery device has advantages and disadvantages (Table 15-2).[112] Evidence-based recommendations for selection of an aerosol delivery device have been published (CPG 15-3).[113] The choice of device often is determined by patient preference or clinician bias. In some cases the choice of device is dictated by the drug to be delivered (e.g., antibiotics are available only for nebulizer delivery).[114] In some cases, the FDA has cleared drugs for use with a specific nebulizer (Table 15-3). Whenever possible, patients should use only one type of aerosol delivery device. The technique for the use of each device is different, and repeated instruction is necessary to ensure that the patient uses the device appropriately. Using different devices can be confusing for patients and may reduce their compliance

TABLE 15-2
Advantages and Disadvantages of Various Aerosol Delivery Devices

Device	Advantages	Disadvantages
Jet nebulizer	Patient coordination is not required Effective with tidal breathing High doses can be given Dose modification is possible Can be used with supplemental O_2 Can deliver combination therapies if drugs are compatible Some are breath actuated	Expense Device is not portable Pressurized gas source is required Lengthy treatment time Contamination is possible Device preparation required Not all medications are in solution form Performance variability
Mesh nebulizer	Patient coordination is not required Effective with tidal breathing High doses can be given Dose modification is possible Some are breath actuated Small dead volume Quiet Faster delivery than jet nebulizer Less drug is lost during exhalation Battery operated Portable and compact Dose reproducibility is high	Expense Contamination is possible Device preparation is required Not all medications are in solution form
Respimat Soft Mist Inhaler	Low velocity of emitted aerosol No propellant Dose counter	Expense May be difficult for some patients to use device Limited medications available
Ultrasonic nebulizer	Patient coordination is not required High doses are possible Small dead volume Quiet Faster delivery than jet nebulizer Less drug is lost during exhalation Some are breath actuated	Expense Need for electrical power Contamination is possible Prone to malfunction Possible drug degradation Does not nebulize suspensions well Device preparation is required Potential for airway irritation exists Not all medications are in solution form
Pressurized metered dose inhaler (pMDI)	Portable and compact No drug preparation is required Dose reproducibility is high Device is difficult to contaminate Treatment time is short Some have a dose counter	Patient coordination is essential Patient actuation is required Large pharyngeal deposition occurs High doses are difficult to deliver Not all medications available
Metered dose inhaler with holding chamber	Less patient coordination is required Less pharyngeal deposition occurs	More complex for some patients More expensive than a pMDI alone Less portable than a pMDI
Dry powder inhaler	Less patient coordination is required Propellant is not required Breath activated Small and portable Short treatment time	Requires moderate to high inspiratory flow Some units are single dose High pharyngeal deposition is possible Not all medications available High doses are difficult to deliver

CFC, chlorofluorocarbon.

Adapted from AARC consensus statement: aerosols and delivery devices. *Respir Care.* 2000;45:589–595; and Dolovich MB, Ahrens RC, Hess DR, et al. Device selection and outcomes of aerosol therapy: evidence-based guidelines. *Chest.* 2005;127:335–371.

CLINICAL PRACTICE GUIDELINE 15-3

Recommendations Related to Selection of Aerosol Delivery Device

- It is recommended that selection of the appropriate aerosol generator and interface be made based on the patient's age, physical and cognitive ability, cost, and the availability of the prescribed drug for use with a specific device.
- Nebulizers and pressurized metered dose inhalers (pMDIs) with valved holding chambers are suggested for use with children < 4 years of age and adults who cannot coordinate the use of pMDI or dry-powder inhaler (DPI).
- It is suggested that administration of aerosols with DPIs be restricted to patients > 4 years of age who can demonstrate sufficient flow for the specific inhaler.
- For patients who cannot correctly use a mouthpiece, aerosol masks are suggested as the interface of choice.
- It is suggested that blow-by not be used for aerosol administration.
- It is suggested that aerosol therapy be administered with a relaxed and nondistressed breathing pattern.
- Unit dose medications are suggested to reduce the risk of infection.
- It is suggested that nebulizer/drug combinations should be used as approved by the FDA.
- It is recommended that healthcare providers know the correct use of aerosol generators; they should teach and periodically re-teach patients about how to use aerosol devices correctly.
- It is suggested that intermittent positive-pressure breathing should not be used for aerosol therapy.
- It is recommended that either nebulizer or pMDI can be used for aerosol delivery during noninvasive ventilation.

Modified from Ari A, Restrepo RD. Aerosol delivery device selection for spontaneously breathing patients: 2012. *Respir Care.* 2012;57:613–626.

TABLE 15-3
Approved Devices for Specific Drug Formulations

Formulation	FDA-Approved Device
Tobramycin (TOBI)	Pari LC
Dornase alfa (Pulmozyme)	Hudson T Up-draft II, Marquest Acorn II, Pari LC, Durable Sidestream, Pari Baby
Pentamadine (NebuPent)	Marquest Respirgard II
Ribavirin (Virazole)	Small Particle Aerosol Generator (SPAG)
Iloprost (Ventavis)	I-neb Adaptive Aerosol Delivery (AAD) System
Aztreonam (Cayston)	Altera nebulizer system
Treprostinil (Tyvaso)	Optineb

with therapy. When patients must use different devices, it is important to teach the proper inspiratory flow with each. A commercially available device can be used to facilitate this teaching (**Figure 15-41**).

Each of the aerosol delivery devices can work equally well provided that patients can use them correctly. When selecting an aerosol delivery device, the following questions should be considered:[114]

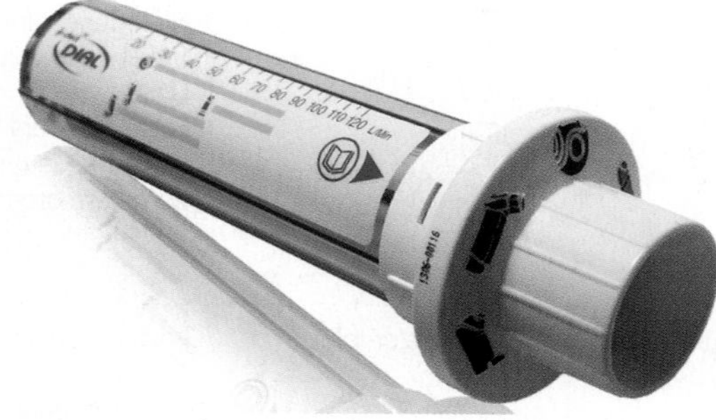

FIGURE 15-41 In-Check DIAL inhaler technique training and assessment device. It enables clinicians to train patients to the proper inspiratory technique considering force and flow rate to achieve optimal deposition of the medication being inhaled into the lungs.
Courtesy of Alliance Tech Medical, Inc.

- In what devices is the desired drug available?
- What device is the patient likely to be able to use properly, given the patient's age and the clinical setting?
- For which device and drug combination is reimbursement available?
- Which devices are the least costly?
- Can all types of inhaled asthma/COPD drugs that are prescribed for the patient be delivered with the same type of device? Using the same type of device for all inhaled drugs may facilitate patient teaching and decrease the chance of confusion among devices that require different inhalation techniques.

- Which devices are the most convenient for the patient, family (outpatient use), or medical staff (acute care setting) to use, given the time required for drug administration and device cleaning and the portability of the device?
- How durable is the device?
- Does the patient or clinician have any specific device preferences?

Proper patient education is critical. Respiratory therapists, physicians, and nurses caring for patients with respiratory diseases should be familiar with issues related to performance and with the correct use of aerosol delivery devices. If the selected delivery device should fail to provide satisfactory treatment, another option should be considered.

To improve adherence, aerosol therapy should be administered with some easily remembered activity of daily living. For twice-daily administration, medications can be kept with the toothbrush and inhaled just before teeth brushing. Commercially available devices can also be used to remind patients when to use their inhalers (**Figure 15-42**). This also reduces aerosol corticosteroid deposition in the oropharynx. It is always best to avoid regular use of medication at school, because the inconvenience can significantly reduce compliance and may be an embarrassment to some children. Rescue medication must be available at school or daycare or the caretaker's home. It helps to prepare written guidelines for use of the medication, and the guidelines must be distributed to all places where the child stays, such as home, school, or the residences of both parents in cases of divorce or separation.

Lack of response to inhaled asthma medication can be related to a number of factors, including incorrect inhalation technique, inhalation from an empty canister, failure to take preventive medications as prescribed, a change in the patient's environment, or perhaps misdiagnosis. For example, children who have aspirated a foreign body or who have gastroesophageal reflux disease or psychogenic wheeze have a poor response to asthma therapy, and infants with tracheomalacia or bronchopulmonary dysplasia may even worsen after inhaling a bronchodilator aerosol because of increased dynamic airway collapse.

Aerosol Delivery for Systemic Disease

Aerosols are usually inhaled for treatment of pulmonary disease; however, there is also interest in using the lungs to deliver inhaled drugs to the systemic circulation. One example is inhaled insulin. Afrezza is rapid-acting inhaled insulin indicated to improve glycemic control in adult patients with diabetes mellitus; it is taken at the beginning of a meal. It is not recommended for patients who smoke or those with lung disease. Afrezza is available in two strengths; 4 units (blue cartridge) and 8 units (green cartridge). The manufacturer provides a conversion table to allow the clinician and the patient to determine the number of Afrezza cartridges equivalent to injected mealtime insulin. As many as three cartridges might be required. The Afrezza inhaler is shown in **Figure 15-43**. The steps for use are shown in **Box 15-10**.

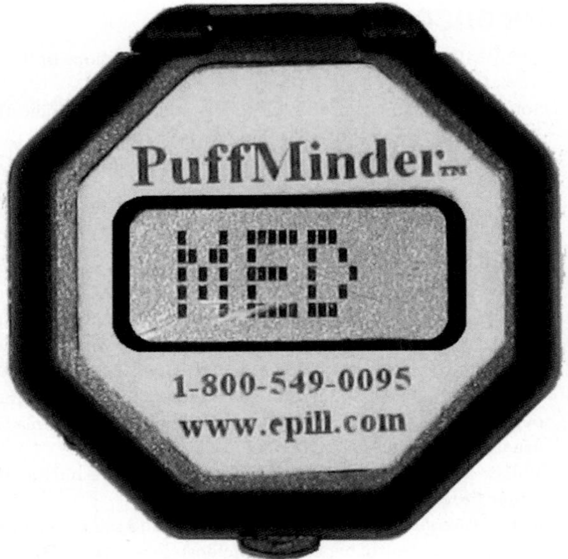

FIGURE 15-42 The Puffminder device that can be used to remind patients when to use their inhaler.
Courtesy of e-pill Medication Reminders.

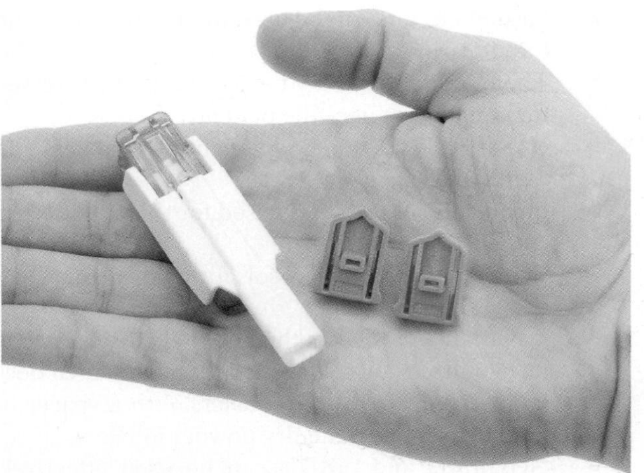

FIGURE 15-43 The Afrezza inhaler.
Courtesy of Mannkind Corporation.

BOX 15-10

Technique for Use of Afrezza Inhaler

Step 1. Select the correct number of Afrezza cartridges for the dose. Remove a cartridge from the strip by pressing on the clear side to push the cartridge out. Remove the correct number of cartridges for the dose. Pushing on the cup will not damage the cartridge. Afrezza cartridges in an opened strip must be used within 3 days.

Step 2. Loading a cartridge. Hold the inhaler level in one hand with the white mouthpiece on the top and purple base on the bottom. Open the inhaler by lifting the white mouthpiece to a vertical position. Before placing the cartridge into the inhaler, be sure it has been at room temperature for 10 minutes (cartridges are stored in a refrigerator). Hold the cartridge with the cup facing down. The pointed end of the cartridge should line up with the pointed end in the inhaler. Place the cartridge into the inhaler. Be sure that the cartridge lies flat in the inhaler. Lower the mouthpiece to close the inhaler, which will open the drug cartridge. Once the cartridge is loaded, it should be held level to avoid loss of the powder. There is a snap when the inhaler is closed.

Step 3. Inhaling Afrezza. Remove the mouthpiece cover. Hold the inhaler away from the mouth and exhale. Place the mouthpiece into the mouth and tilt the inhaler down toward your chin. Close lips around the mouthpiece to form a seal. Tilt the inhaler downward while keeping head level. Inhale deeply through the inhaler. Breath hold as long as comfortable and remove inhaler from the mouth. After the breath hold, resume normal breathing.

Step 4. Remove used cartridge. Place the purple mouthpiece cover back onto the inhaler. Open the inhaler by lifting up the white mouthpiece. Remove the cartridge from the purple base. Discard the used cartridge.

Repeat steps 2 through 4 for each Afrezza cartridge needed for the prescribed dose. Use one inhaler at a time. Discard the inhaler after 15 days.

Key Points

- The upper airway is an efficient humidifier.
- The primary goal of humidity therapy is to maintain normal physiologic conditions by providing heat and humidity in the inspired gas.
- Humidifiers can provide active or passive humidification.
- Active humidifiers may be heated or unheated.
- Heated circuits can be used to maintain heat and humidity in gas delivery.
- The humidity delivery device should be assessed for condensate near the patient.
- Use of HMEs is limited by their effectiveness and their dead space.
- Bland aerosol therapy is used for therapeutic and diagnostic purposes.
- The particle size of aerosols for medical purposes should be 1 to 5 μm.
- Devices used to deliver therapeutic aerosols include jet nebulizers, ultrasonic nebulizers, metered dose inhalers, metered dose inhalers with a spacer or holding chamber, and dry powder inhalers.
- Nebulizers and pMDIs can be used effectively in patients receiving mechanical ventilation and in spontaneously breathing patients with a tracheostomy.
- Either a nebulizer, pMDI, pMDI with a spacer or valved holding chamber, or DPI can be used effectively if the patient uses good technique.

References

1. Shelly MP. The humidification and filtration functions of the airways. *Respir Care Clin North Am.* 2006;12:139–148.
2. Sottiaux TM. Consequences of under- and over-humidification. *Respir Care Clin North Am.* 2006;12:233–252.
3. Rathgeber J. Devices used to humidify respired gases. *Respir Care Clin North Am.* 2006;12:165–182.
4. Peterson BD. Heated humidifiers. *Respir Care Clin North Am.* 1998;4:243–260.
5. Züchner K. Humidification: measurement and requirements. *Respir Care Clin North Am.* 2006;12:149–163.
6. Lellouche F, Taillé S, Maggiore SM, et al. Influence of ambient and ventilator output temperatures on performance of heated-wire humidifiers. *Am J Respir Crit Care Med.* 2004;170:1073–1079.
7. Lellouche F, Qader S, Taille S, et al. Under-humidification and over-humidification during moderate induced hypothermia with usual devices. *Intensive Care Med.* 2006;32:1014–1021.
8. Wilkes AR. Heat and moisture exchangers: structure and function. *Respir Care Clin North Am.* 1998;4:261–279.
9. Prin S, Chergui K, Augarde R, et al. Ability and safety of a heated humidifier to control hypercapnic acidosis in severe ARDS. *Intensive Care Med.* 2002;28:1756–1760.
10. Hinkson CR, Benson MS, Stephens LM, Deem S. The effects of apparatus dead space on Pa_{CO_2} in patients receiving lung-protective ventilation. *Respir Care.* 2006;51:1140–1144.

11. Lellouche F, Pignataro C, Maggiore SM, et al. Short-term effects of humidification devices on respiratory pattern and arterial blood gases during noninvasive ventilation. *Respir Care*. 2012;57: 1879–1886.
12. Campbell RS, Davis K Jr, Johannigman JA, Branson RD. The effects of passive humidifier dead space on respiratory variables in paralyzed and spontaneously breathing patients. *Respir Care*. 2000;45: 306–312.
13. Hess D. Prolonged use of heat and moisture exchangers: why do we keep changing things? *Crit Care Med*. 2000;28:1667–1668.
14. Hess DR, Kallstrom TJ, Mottram CD, et al. Care of the ventilator circuit and its relation to ventilator-associated pneumonia. *Respir Care*. 2003;48:869–879.
15. Lellouche F, Taillé S, Lefrançois F, et al. Humidification performance of 48 passive airway humidifiers: comparison with manufacturer data. *Chest*. 2009;135:276–286.
16. Lacherade JC, Auburtin M, Cerf C, et al. Impact of humidification systems on ventilator-associated pneumonia: a randomized multicenter trial. *Am J Respir Crit Care Med*. 2005;172: 1276–1282.
17. Ricard JD, Boyer A, Dreyfuss D. The effect of humidification on the incidence of ventilator-associated pneumonia. *Respir Care Clin North Am*. 2006;12:263–273.
18. Siempos II, Vardakas KZ, Kopterides P, Falagas ME. Impact of passive humidification on clinical outcomes of mechanically ventilated patients: a meta-analysis of randomized controlled trials. *Crit Care Med*. 2007;35:2843–2851.
19. Kola A, Eckmanns T, Gastmeier P. Efficacy of heat and moisture exchangers in preventing ventilator-associated pneumonia: meta-analysis of randomized controlled trials. *Intensive Care Med*. 2005;3:5–11.
20. Chikata Y, Oto J, Onodera M, Nishimura M. Humidification performance of humidifying devices for tracheostomized patients with spontaneous breathing: a bench study. *Respir Care*. 2013;58: 1442–1448.
21. Kelly M, Gillies D, Todd DA, Lockwood C. Heated humidification versus heat and moisture exchangers for ventilated adults and children. *Cochrane Database Syst Rev*. 2010:CD004711.
22. Gardenhire DS, Ari A, Hess DR, Myers TR. *A Guide to Aerosol Delivery Devices or Respiratory Therapists*. 3rd ed. Irving, TX: American Association for Respiratory Care; 2013.
23. Dolovich MB, Dhand R. Aerosol drug delivery: developments in device design and clinical use. *Lancet*. 2011;377:1032–1045.
24. Rau JL. The inhalation of drugs: advantages and problems. *Respir Care*. 2005;50:367–382.
25. Hess DR. Aerosol delivery devices in the treatment of asthma. *Respir Care*. 2008;53:699–725.
26. Rau JL. Design principles of liquid nebulization devices currently in use. *Respir Care*. 2002;47:1257–1278.
27. Hess DR. Nebulizers: principles and performance. *Respir Care*. 2000;45:609–622.
28. Kim IK, Saville AL, Sikes KL, Corcoran TE. Heliox-driven albuterol nebulization for asthma exacerbations: an overview. *Respir Care*. 2006;51:613–618.
29. Hess DR, Acosta FL, Ritz RH, et al. The effect of heliox on nebulizer function using a beta-agonist bronchodilator. *Chest*. 1999;115: 184–189.
30. Alcoforado L, Brandão S, Rattes C, et al. Evaluation of lung function and deposition of aerosolized bronchodilators carried by heliox associated with positive expiratory pressure in stable asthmatics: a randomized clinical trial. *Respir Med*. 2013;107:1178–1185.
31. Brandão DC, Britto MC, Pessoa MF, et al. Heliox and forward-leaning posture improve the efficacy of nebulized bronchodilator in acute asthma: a randomized trial. *Respir Care*. 2011;5: 947–952.
32. Bigham MT, Jacobs BR, Monaco MA, et al. Helium/oxygen-driven albuterol nebulization in the management of children with status asthmaticus: a randomized, placebo-controlled trial. *Pediatr Crit Care Med*. 2010;11:356–361.
33. Berlinski A. In-vitro evaluation of positive expiratory pressure devices attached to nebulizers. *Respir Care*. 2014;59:216–222.
34. Mesquita FO, Galindo-Filho VC, Neto JL, et al. Scintigraphic assessment of radio-aerosol pulmonary deposition through acapella device with different nebulizer configurations. *Respir Care*. 2014;59:328–323.
35. Arunthari V, Bruinsma RS, Lee AS, Johnson MM. A prospective, comparative trial of standard and breath-actuated nebulizer: efficacy, safety, and satisfaction. *Respir Care*. 2012;57:1242–1247.
36. Haynes JM. Randomized controlled trial of a breath-activated nebulizer in patients with exacerbation of COPD. *Respir Care*. 2012;57:1385–1390.
37. Sabato K, Ward P, Hawk W, et al. Randomized controlled trial of a breath-actuated nebulizer in pediatric asthma patients in the emergency department. *Respir Care*. 2011;56:761–770.
38. Harris KW, Smaldone GC. Facial and ocular deposition of nebulized budesonide: effects of face mask design. *Chest*. 2008;133:482–488.
39. Smaldone GC, Sangwan S, Shah A. Facemask design, facial deposition, and delivered dose of nebulized aerosols. *J Aerosol Med*. 2007;20(Suppl 1):S66–S75.
40. Bisquerra RA, Botz GH, Nates JL. Ipratropium-bromide-induced acute anisocoria in the intensive care setting due to ill-fitting face masks. *Respir Care*. 2005;50:1662–1664.
41. Brodie T, Adalat S. Unilateral fixed dilated pupil in a well child. *Arch Dis Child*. 2006;91:961.
42. Lin HL, Restrepo RD, Gardenhire DS, Rau JL. Effect of face mask design on inhaled mass of nebulized albuterol, using a pediatric breathing model. *Respir Care*. 2007;52:1021–1026.
43. Rubin BK. Bye-bye, blow-by. *Respir Care*. 2007;52:981.
44. Mansour MM, Smaldone GC. Blow-by as potential therapy for uncooperative children: an in-vitro study. *Respir Care*. 2012; 57:2004–2011.
45. Kacmarek RM, Kratohvil J. Evaluation of a double-enclosure double-vacuum unit scavenging system for ribavirin administration. *Respir Care*. 1992;37:37–45.
46. Krebs SE, Flood RG, Peter JR, Gerard JM. Evaluation of a high-dose continuous albuterol protocol for treatment of pediatric asthma in the emergency department. *Pediatr Emerg Care*. 2013;29: 191–196.
47. Peters SG. Continuous bronchodilator therapy. *Chest*. 2007;131:286–289.
48. Camargo CA Jr, Spooner CH, Rowe BH. Continuous versus intermittent beta-agonists in the treatment of acute asthma. *Cochrane Database Syst Rev*. 2003;CD001115.
49. Perry SA, Kesser KC, Geller DE, et al. Influences of cannula size and flow rate on aerosol drug delivery through the Vapotherm humidified high-flow nasal cannula system. *Pediatr Crit Care Med*. 2013;14:e250–256.
50. Longest PW, Walenga RL, Son YJ, Hindle M. High-efficiency generation and delivery of aerosols through nasal cannula during noninvasive ventilation. *J Aerosol Med Pulm Drug Deliv*. 2013;26:266–279.
51. Ari A, Harwood R, Sheard M, et al. In vitro comparison of heliox and oxygen in aerosol delivery using pediatric high flow nasal cannula. *Pediatr Pulmonol*. 2011;46:795–801.
52. Bhashyam AR, Wolf MT, Marcinkowski AL, et al. Aerosol delivery through nasal cannulas: an in vitro study. *J Aerosol Med Pulm Drug Deliv*. 2008;21:181–188.
53. Standaert TA, Bohn SE, Aitken ML, Ramsey B. The equivalence of compressor pressure-flow relationships with respect to jet nebulizer aerosolization characteristics. *J Aerosol Med*. 2001;14: 31–42.
54. Standaert TA, Vandevanter D, Ramsey BW, et al. The choice of compressor effects the aerosol parameters and the delivery of tobramycin from a single model nebulizer. *J Aerosol Med*. 2000;13: 147–153.
55. Reisner C, Katial RK, Bartelson BB, et al. Characterization of aerosol output from various nebulizer/compressor combinations. *Ann Allergy Asthma Immunol*. 2001;86:566–574.

56. de Boer AH, Hagedoorn P, Frijlink HW. The choice of a compressor for the aerosolisation of tobramycin (TOBI) with the PARI LC PLUS reusable nebuliser. *Int J Pharm.* 2003;268:59–69.
57. Awad S, Williams DK, Berlinski A. Longitudinal evaluation of compressor/nebulizer performance. *Respir Care.* 2014;59:1053–1061.
58. Dhand R. Nebulizers that use a vibrating mesh or plate with multiple apertures to generate aerosol. *Respir Care.* 2002;47:1406–1416.
59. Lass JS, Sant A, Knoch M. New advances in aerosolised drug delivery: vibrating membrane nebuliser technology. *Expert Opin Drug Deliv.* 2006;3:693–702.
60. Knoch M, Keller M. The customised electronic nebuliser: a new category of liquid aerosol drug delivery systems. *Expert Opin Drug Deliv.* 2005;2:377–390.
61. Ghazanfari T, Elhissi AM, Ding Z, Taylor KM. The influence of fluid physicochemical properties on vibrating-mesh nebulization. *Int J Pharmacol.* 2007;339:103–111.
62. Zhang G, David A, Wiedmann TS. Performance of the vibrating membrane aerosol generation device: Aeroneb Micropump Nebulizer. *J Aerosol Med.* 2007;20:408–416.
63. Dalby R, Spallek M, Voshaar T. A review of the development of Respimat Soft Mist Inhaler. *Int J Pharmacol.* 2004;283:1–9.
64. Dalby RN, Eicher J, Zierenberg B. Development of Respimat® Soft Mist™ Inhaler and its clinical utility in respiratory disorders. *Med Devices (Auckl).* 2011;4:145–155.
65. Hochrainer D, Holz H, Kreher C, et al. Comparison of the aerosol velocity and spray duration of Respimat Soft Mist inhaler and pressurized metered dose inhalers. *J Aerosol Med.* 2005;18: 273–282.
66. Newman SP, Steed KP, Reader SJ, et al. An in vitro study to assess facial and ocular deposition from Respimat Soft Mist inhaler. *J Aerosol Med.* 2007;20:7–12.
67. Ferguson GT, Ghafouri M, Dai L, Dunn LJ. COPD patient satisfaction with ipratropium bromide/albuterol delivered via Respimat: a randomized, controlled study. *Int J Chron Obstruct Pulmon Dis.* 2013;8:139–150.
68. Dellweg D, Wachtel H, Höhn E, et al. In vitro validation of a Respimat® adapter for delivery of inhaled bronchodilators during mechanical ventilation. *J Aerosol Med Pulm Drug Deliv.* 2011;24:285–292.
69. Hess DR. Metered-dose inhalers and dry powder inhalers in aerosol therapy. *Respir Care.* 2005;50:1376–1383.
70. Fink JB. Metered dose inhalers, dry powder inhalers, and transitions. *Respir Care.* 2000;45:623–625.
71. Leach CL. The CFC to HFA transition and its impact on pulmonary drug development. *Respir Care.* 2005;50:1201–1208.
72. Hendeles L, Colice GL, Meyer RJ. Withdrawal of albuterol inhalers containing chlorofluorocarbon propellants. *N Engl J Med.* 2007;356:1344–1351.
73. Cheng YS, Fu CS, Yazzie D, Zhou Y. Respiratory deposition patterns of salbutamol pMDI with CFC and HFA-134a formulations in a human airway replica. *J Aerosol Med.* 2001;14:255–266.
74. Barry PW, O'Callaghan C. New formulation metered dose inhaler increases breath alcohol levels. *Respir Med.* 1999;93:167–168.
75. Levin PD, Levin D, Avidan A. Medical aerosol propellant interference with infrared anaesthetic gas monitors. *Br J Anaesth.* 2004;92:865–869.
76. Bamber MG. Difficulties with CFC-free salbutamol inhaler. *Lancet.* 1996;348:1737.
77. Sanchis J, Corrigan C, Levy ML, Viejo JL; ADMIT Group. Inhaler devices—from theory to practice. *Respir Med.* 2013;107:495–502.
78. Price D, Bosnic-Anticevich S, Briggs A, et al. Inhaler competence in asthma: common errors, barriers to use and recommended solutions. *Respir Med.* 2013;107:37–46.
79. Batterink J, Dahri K, Aulakh A, Rempel C. Evaluation of the use of inhaled medications by hospital inpatients with chronic obstructive pulmonary disease. *Can J Hosp Pharm.* 2012;65:111–118.
80. Vargas O, Martinez J, Ibanez M, et al. The use of metered-dose inhalers in hospital environments. *J Aerosol Med Pulm Drug Deliv.* 2013;26:287–296.
81. Cain WT, Oppenheimer JJ. The misconception of using floating patterns as an accurate means of measuring the contents of metered dose inhaler devices. *Ann Allergy Asthma Immunol.* 2001;87:417–419.
82. Rubin BK, Durotoye L. How do patients determine that their metered-dose inhaler is empty? *Chest.* 2004;126:1134–1137.
83. Mitchell JP, Coppolo DP, Nagel MW. Electrostatics and inhaled medications: influence on delivery via pressurized metered-dose inhalers and add-on devices. *Respir Care.* 2007;52:283–300.
84. Rau JL, Coppolo DP, Nagel MW, et al. The importance of nonelectrostatic materials in holding chambers for delivery of hydrofluoroalkane albuterol. *Respir Care.* 2006;51:503–510.
85. Coppolo DP, Mitchell JP, Nagel MW. Levalbuterol aerosol delivery with a nonelectrostatic versus a nonconducting valved holding chamber. *Respir Care.* 2006;51:511–514.
86. Shah SA, Berlinski AB, Rubin BK. Force-dependent static dead space of face masks used with holding chambers. *Respir Care.* 2006;51:140–124.
87. Dhand R, Fink JB. Dry powder inhalers. *Respir Care.* 1999;44: 940–951.
88. Atkins PJ. Dry powder inhalers: an overview. *Respir Care.* 2005;50:1304–1312.
89. Dhand R. Aerosol delivery during mechanical ventilation: from basic techniques to new devices. *J Aerosol Med Pulm Drug Deliv.* 2008;21:45–60.
90. Dhand R, Guntur VP. How best to deliver aerosol medications to mechanically ventilated patients. *Clin Chest Med.* 2008;29:277–296.
91. Dhand R. Inhalation therapy in invasive and noninvasive mechanical ventilation. *Curr Opin Crit Care.* 2007;13:27–38.
92. Dhand R, Mercier E. Effective inhaled drug administration to mechanically ventilated patients. *Expert Opin Drug Deliv.* 2007;4: 47–61.
93. Ari A, Fink JB, Dhand R. Inhalation therapy in patients receiving mechanical ventilation: an update. *J Aerosol Med Pulm Drug Deliv.* 2012;25:319–332.
94. Hess DR, Kallstrom TJ, Mottram CD, et al. Care of the ventilator circuit and its relation to ventilator-associated pneumonia. *Respir Care.* 2003;48:869–879.
95. Hess DR, Dillman C, Kacmarek RM. In vitro evaluation of aerosol bronchodilator delivery during mechanical ventilation: pressure-control vs. volume control ventilation. *Intensive Care Med.* 2003;29:1145–1150.
96. Mouloudi E, Katsanoulas K, Anastasaki M, et al. Bronchodilator delivery by metered dose inhaler in mechanically ventilated COPD patients: influence of tidal volume. *Intensive Care Med.* 1999;25:1215–1221.
97. Mouloudi E, Katsanoulas K, Anastasaki M, et al. Bronchodilator delivery by metered dose inhaler in mechanically ventilated COPD patients: influence of end-inspiratory pause. *Eur Respir J.* 1998;12:165–169.
98. Mouloudi E, Prinianakis G, Kondili E, et al. Effect of inspiratory flow rate on b-agonist-induced bronchodilation in mechanically ventilated COPD patients. *Intensive Care Med.* 2001;27:42–46.
99. Berlinski A, Willis JR. Albuterol delivery by 4 different nebulizers placed in 4 different positions in a pediatric ventilator in vitro model. *Respir Care.* 2013;58:1124–1133.
100. Ari A, Atalay OT, Harwood R, et al. Influence of nebulizer type, position, and bias flow on aerosol drug delivery in simulated pediatric and adult lung models during mechanical ventilation. *Respir Care.* 2010;55:845–851.
101. Ari A, Areabi H, Fink JB. Evaluation of aerosol generator devices at 3 locations in humidified and non-humidified circuits during adult mechanical ventilation. *Respir Care.* 2010;55:837–844.
102. Dhand R. Aerosol therapy in patients receiving noninvasive positive pressure ventilation. *J Aerosol Med Pulm Drug Deliv.* 2012;25: 63–78.
103. Hess DR. The mask for noninvasive ventilation: principles of design and effects on aerosol delivery. *J Aerosol Med.* 2007;20(Suppl 1):S85–S98; discussion S98–S99.

104. Mukhopadhyay A, Dela Pena E, Wadden B, et al. Effects of inhalational bronchodilator treatment during noninvasive ventilation in severe chronic obstructive pulmonary disease exacerbations. *J Crit Care.* 2009;24:474, e471–e475.
105. White CC, Crotwell DN, Shen S, et al. Bronchodilator delivery during simulated pediatric noninvasive ventilation. *Respir Care.* 2013;58:1459–1466.
106. Piccuito CM, Hess DR. Albuterol delivery via tracheostomy tube. *Respir Care.* 2005;50:1071–1076.
107. Mir M, Dhand R. Nebulized drug delivery in patients breathing spontaneously through an artificial airway. *Respir Care.* 2012;57:1195–1196.
108. Ari A, Harwood RJ, Sheard MM, Fink JB. An in vitro evaluation of aerosol delivery through tracheostomy and endotracheal tubes using different interfaces. *Respir Care.* 2012;57:1066–1070.
109. Berlinski A. Nebulized albuterol delivery in a model of spontaneously breathing children with tracheostomy. *Respir Care.* 2013;58:2076–2086.
110. Berlinski A, Chavez A. Albuterol delivery via metered dose inhaler in a spontaneously breathing pediatric tracheostomy model. *Pediatr Pulmonol.* 2013;48:1026–1034.
111. Willis LD, Berlinski A. Survey of aerosol delivery techniques to spontaneously breathing tracheostomized children. *Respir Care.* 2012;57:1234–1241.
112. Myers TR. The science guiding selection of an aerosol delivery device. *Respir Care.* 2013;58:1963–1973.
113. Ari A, Restrepo RD. Aerosol delivery device selection for spontaneously breathing patients: 2012. *Respir Care.* 2012;57:613–626.
114. Dolovich MB, Ahrens RC, Hess DR, et al. Device selection and outcomes of aerosol therapy: evidence-based guidelines. *Chest.* 2005;127:335–371.

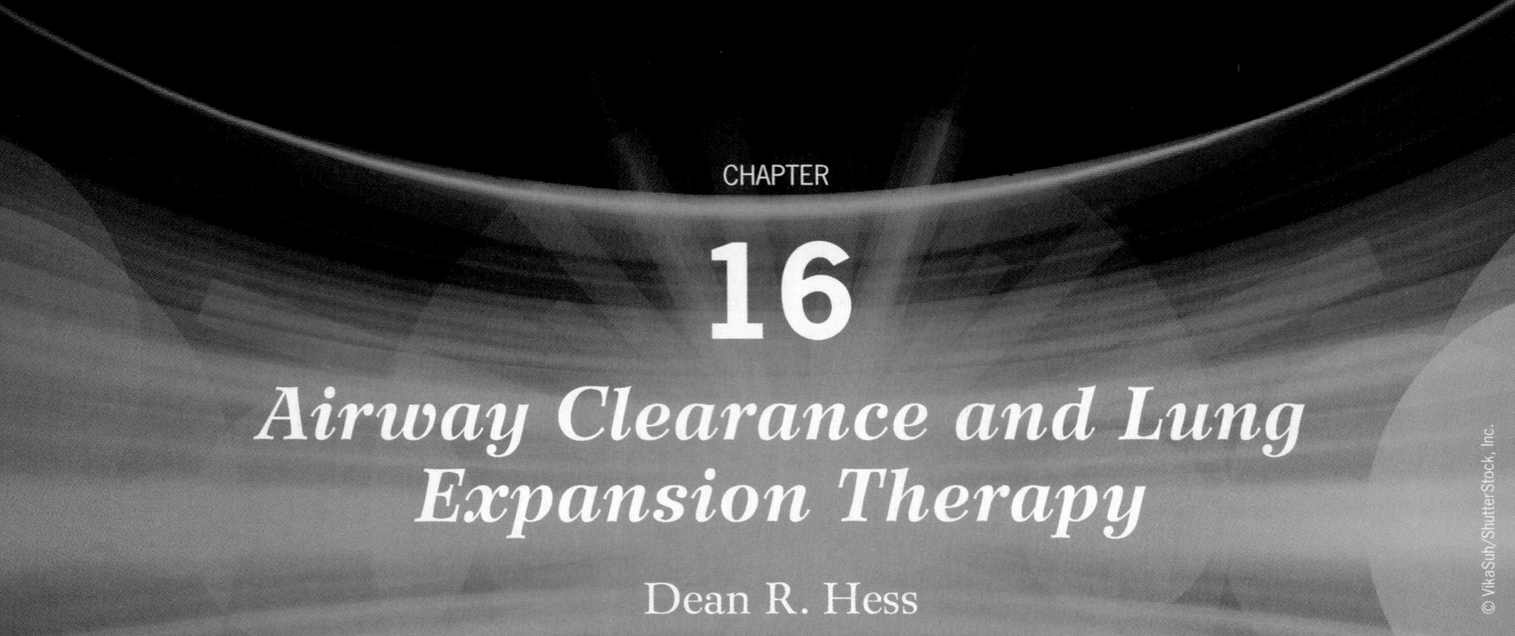

CHAPTER

16

Airway Clearance and Lung Expansion Therapy

Dean R. Hess

OUTLINE

Normal Mechanisms of Mucociliary Transport
Airway Clearance
Sputum Collection
Lung Expansion Therapy

OBJECTIVES

1. Describe the mechanism of normal mucus transport in the lungs.
2. Demonstrate the techniques of nasotracheal suctioning, mechanical insufflation–exsufflation, postural drainage, manually assisted coughing, active cycle of breathing, autogenic drainage, incentive spirometry, intermittent positive pressure breathing, positive expiratory pressure, oscillatory positive expiratory pressure, and high-frequency techniques.
3. List indications, contraindications, hazards, and precautions for nasotracheal suctioning, mechanical insufflation–exsufflation, postural drainage, manually assisted coughing, active cycle of breathing, autogenic drainage, incentive spirometry, intermittent positive pressure breathing, positive expiratory pressure, oscillatory positive expiratory pressure, and high-frequency techniques.
4. Compare the advantages and disadvantages of various secretion clearance techniques.
5. Compare the following methods of sputum collection: cough, induced sputum, tracheal aspiration, bronchoscopy, mini-bronchoalveolar lavage, transtracheal aspiration.
6. Compare techniques of lung inflation therapy.

KEY TERMS

active cycle of breathing
autogenic drainage
chest physiotherapy (CPT)
forced expiratory technique (FET)
high-frequency chest wall compression (HFCWC)
high-frequency chest wall oscillation (HFCWO)
huff coughing
incentive spirometry (IS)
intermittent positive pressure breathing (IPPB)
intrapulmonary percussive ventilation (IPV)
mechanical insufflation–exsufflation
minibronchoalveolar lavage (mini-BAL)
nasotracheal suctioning
percussion therapy
positive expiratory pressure (PEP)
postural drainage (PD)
sputum induction
vibration therapy

Introduction

Many acute and chronic respiratory diseases are associated with retained airway secretions due to increased mucus production, impaired mucociliary transport, or a weak cough. In normal lungs, mucociliary activity, breathing, and coughing are the primary mechanisms used to remove secretions. With disease, changes in volume and character of secretions, dyskinesia of the cilia, and instability of the airway reduce the ability to clear secretions from the airway. Difficulty with secretion clearance commonly occurs at the end of life.[1] A variety of breathing maneuvers and mechanical devices have been used to assist patients in mobilizing secretions from the lower respiratory tract. This chapter describes these maneuvers and devices.

Normal Mechanisms of Mucociliary Transport

Secretions from the submucosal glands and surface secretory cells cover the ciliated epithelium of the airway (**Figure 16-1**). The relatively thin and watery sol layer, through which the cilia normally beat, arises from serous cell secretions. The thicker, superficial gel layer is formed from the more viscous secretions contributed by mucous cells and surface goblet cells, possibly enriched by components from the sol layer as

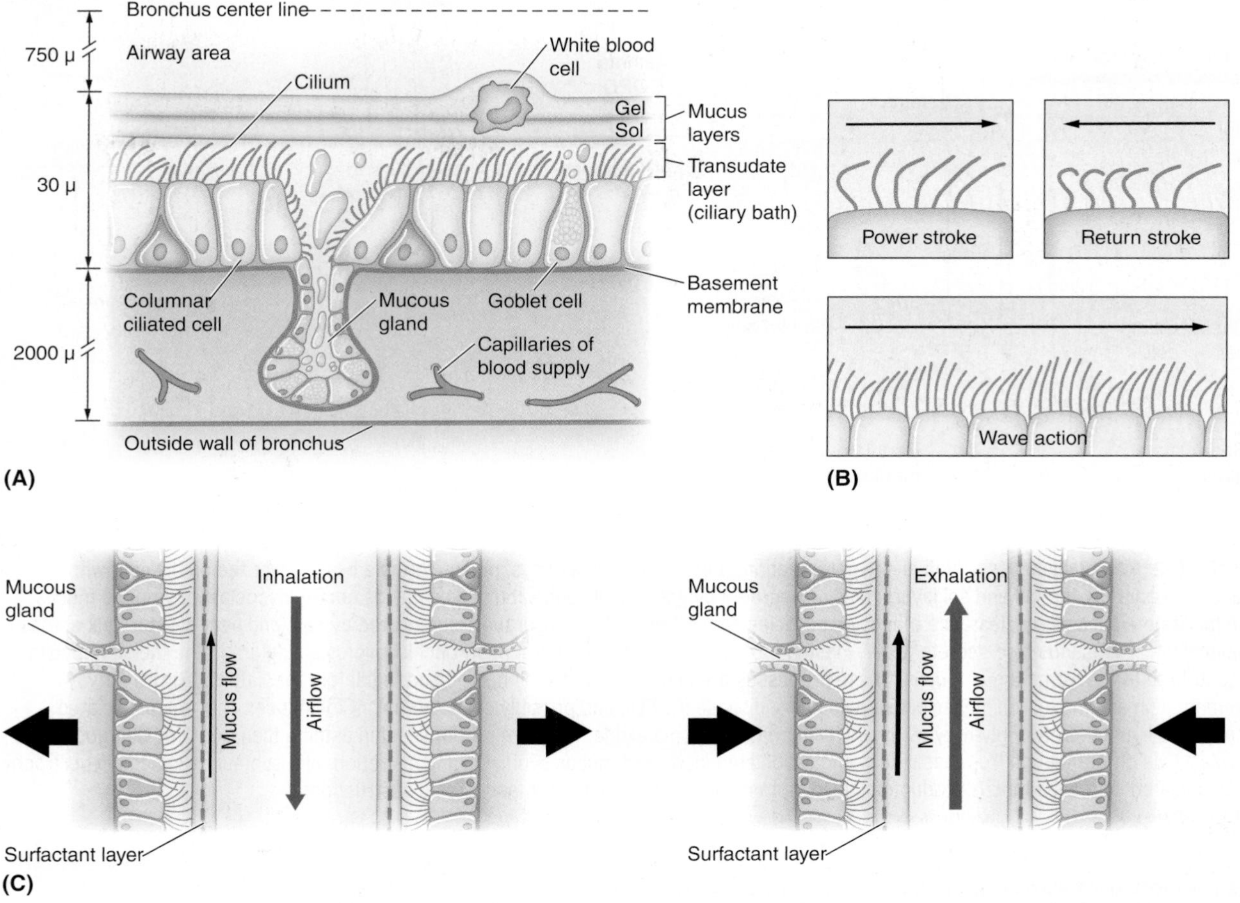

FIGURE 16-1 (**A**) Drawing of the surface of a typical ciliated epithelium. (**B**) Drawing of cilia at each phase of beat cycle. (**C**) Cephalad airflow bias. With normal mucociliary function, greater energy is applied to the mucous layer during expiration than during inspiration because of airway narrowing during expiration.

(**C**) reproduced from Fink JB. Forced expiratory technique, directed cough, and autogenic drainage. *Respir Care.* 2007;52:1210–1223. Reprinted with permission.

water evaporates. This gel layer traps and holds dust, pollens, contaminants, and microorganisms. In the central airways, the majority of the secretory capacity is attributed to submucosal glands rather than surface secretory cells.

The cilia beat in a coordinated wavelike motion through the sol layer, with the tips of the cilia extending to the gel layer, propelling it toward the pharynx during the forward power stroke. This action is followed by a return recovery stroke in which the cilia return to their starting position, closer to the cell surface and at a slower speed.[1–3] The normal respiratory tract produces about 100 mL of mucus per day, some of which is absorbed as the secretions converge on the trachea, the remainder being expelled from the respiratory tract and swallowed. This serves as a first-line defense and is protective of the lower respiratory tract. With airway mucus hypersecretion, the amount of mucus produced is abnormal, which is pathologic and no longer protective. In the case of mucus hypersecretion, there is submucosal gland hypertrophy, goblet cell hyperplasia, and increased mucin synthesis. There also is plasma exudation, decreased mucociliary transport, mucostasis, and mucous plugs (**Figure 16-2**).

Mucociliary transport is dependent on the rheologic properties of mucus.[3,4] The interaction of mucus and airflow can alter these properties. Mucous gel properties are primarily dependent on the concentration and molecular characteristics of the mucous glycoproteins (mucins). Deoxyribonucleic acid (DNA) and actin fibers resulting from infection and inflammation can contribute additional cross-linking to the mucous gel. The purulent sputum from adult patients with cystic fibrosis (CF) has higher elasticity and viscosity than nonpurulent sputum from normal subjects.[5]

Cough and other high-airflow maneuvers reduce the cross-linking of mucus when airflow linear velocities are high enough (3 L/s in the trachea) to cause wave formation in the mucous layer.[6] Reduced mucus viscosity during the cough maneuver may improve sputum clearance. Mucus acts as a low-viscosity fluid during the short time of the rapidly changing, turbulent airflow associated with effective cough but resumes its high-viscosity character after cessation of the cough and

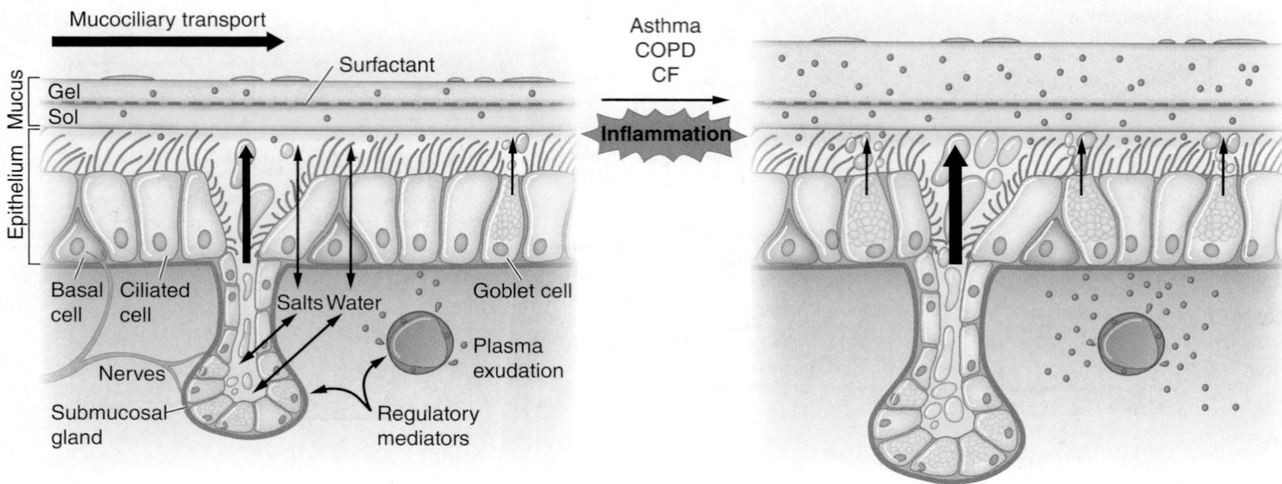

FIGURE 16-2 Airway mucus secretion and hypersecretion. (**Left**) In healthy airways, mucus forms a bilayer over the epithelium, with surfactant separating the gel and sol layers. Mucins secreted by goblet cells and submucosal glands confer viscoelasticity on the mucus, which facilitates mucociliary clearance of inhaled particles and irritants. Mucus hydration is regulated by salt (and hence water) flux across the epithelium. The glands also secrete water. Plasma proteins exuded from the tracheobronchial microvasculature bathe the submucosa and contribute to the formation of mucus. These processes are under the control of nerves and regulatory mediators. (**Right**) Airway inflammation (in asthma, chronic obstructive pulmonary disease [COPD], and possibly cystic fibrosis [CF]) induces changes associated with a mucus hypersecretory phenotype, including increased plasma exudation (more predominant in asthma than COPD or CF), goblet cell hyperplasia via differentiation from basal cells and associated increased mucus synthesis and secretion, and submucosal gland hypertrophy (with associated increased mucus production), leading to increased luminal mucus (and airway obstruction).

Adapted from Rogers DF. Physiology of airway mucus secretion and pathophysiology of hypersecretion. *Respir Care.* 2007;52:1134–1149.

does not flow backward under the influence of gravity. Airflows associated with tidal breathing have no effect on mucus viscoelasticity.

Cephalad airflow bias is responsible for the movement of mucus in airways during normal ventilation.[7,8] Airway diameters normally increase on inspiration and narrow on expiration. The narrowing of airways on exhalation increases the velocity and shearing forces in the airway, creating a cephalad airflow bias with tidal breathing. This bias is amplified during coughing, when increased transmural pressure causes the airways to fold and constrict, increasing airflow velocity even further. During mechanical ventilation, a peak expiratory flow greater than peak inspiratory flow favors mucus transport toward the airway opening (**Figure 16-3**).[8,9]

In healthy individuals the mucociliary escalator is the primary mechanism of mucus clearance from the lung. In acute airway diseases leading to ciliary dysfunction and/or mucus hypersecretion, cough is the primary mechanism for mucus clearance from the central airways, and cephalad airflow contributes increasingly to peripheral airway clearance. In chronic airway diseases involving mucus hypersecretion, these latter mechanisms become the major mechanisms responsible for keeping the airways patent. Gravity is not a primary mechanism for normal mucociliary transport because the viscosity of the normal mucous blanket is sufficient to resist flow of mucus into gravity-dependent terminal bronchioles.

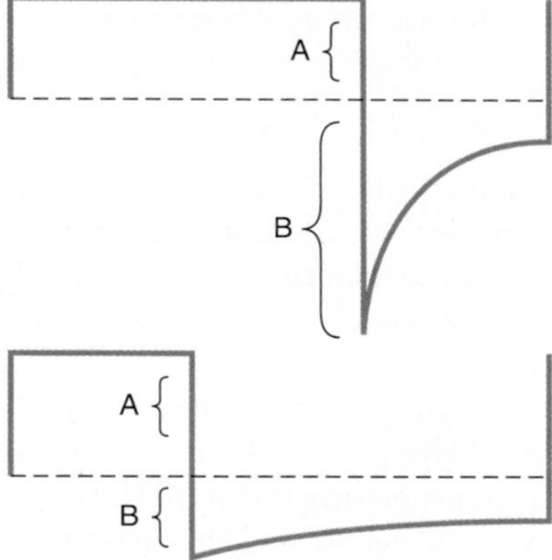

FIGURE 16-3 Method of determining expiratory–inspiratory flow difference and ratio. The upper panel displays an example of a flow pattern that gives a positive value for the expiratory–inspiratory flow difference (i.e., B – A > 0) and the expiratory–inspiratory flow ratio (B/A > 1), which would create an expiratory flow bias and therefore tend to expel mucus. In this example, intrinsic positive end-expiratory pressure might be generated by the ventilator settings. The lower panel shows a flow pattern in which B – A < 0 and B/A < 1, which favors mucus retention because of inspiratory flow bias and increased expiratory resistance. In this example, intrinsic positive end-expiratory pressure is generated by impedance, as in chronic obstructive pulmonary disease.

Reproduced from Volpe MS, Adams AB, Amato MB, Marini JJ. Ventilation patterns influence airway secretion movement. *Respir Care.* 2008;53:1287–1294. Reprinted with permission.

Cough is one of the most common respiratory symptoms for which patients seek medical attention.[10] During a normal cough, the expiratory airflow rises to a maximum along with narrowing of the intrathoracic airways. The narrowing of the airways is a product of high airflows and pressure differentials across the lung. Airflow velocity varies inversely with the cross-sectional area of the airways, creating high linear velocities, increased turbulence, high shearing forces within the airway, and high kinetic energy. These forces shear secretions and debris from the airway walls, propelling them toward the central and upper airway, where they are expectorated or swallowed. A rapid series of coughs improves airway clearance. A number of complications are associated with excessive cough (**Table 16-1**).[11] In chronic obstructive pulmonary disease (COPD), narrowing airways may close prematurely, trapping gas, reducing expiratory flow rates, and limiting the effectiveness of the cough. There is an important balance between compression and collapse of airways; with collapse of the airway, clearance is inhibited.

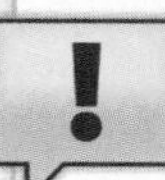

Respiratory Recap

Airway Clearance

- Coughing
- Forced expiratory technique
- Manually assisted coughing
- Active cycle of breathing
- Autogenic drainage
- Mechanical insufflation–exsufflation

Airway Clearance

Deep Breathing and Coughing

The normal mechanism for lung expansion and bronchial hygiene is spontaneous deep breathing (including yawn and sigh maneuvers) and an effective cough. Instructing and encouraging the patient to take sustained deep breaths is among the safest, most effective, and least expensive strategies to keep the lungs expanded and secretions moving.[12] The negative intrathoracic pressure generated during spontaneous deep breathing tends to better inflate the less compliant, gravity-dependent areas of the lung than mechanical methods relying on lung inflation by application of positive airway pressure. A deep breath is a key component of a normal effective cough.

An effective cough is the most important component of bronchial hygiene therapy (**Box 16-1**). The normal cough involves the taking of a deep breath, closure of the glottis, and compression of abdominal and thoracic muscles generating pressures in excess of 80 mm Hg, followed by an explosive release of gas as the glottis opens (**Figure 16-4**). In addition to mobilizing and expelling secretions, the high inspiratory volume generated during a cough may be an important factor in reexpanding lung tissue. Coughing is associated with a number of untoward effects (refer to Table 16-1). In the patient with unstable airways, high pleural pressures cause dynamic compression of airways, trapping gas and secretions and rendering the cough ineffective. A variety of breathing techniques enhance cephalad airflow bias.

Forced Expiratory Technique

For patients unable to generate an effective cough, sharp forced exhalations without glottis closure (**huff coughing**) may be the maneuver of choice. Huff coughing is a **forced expiratory technique (FET)** that is performed through sharp exhalation from high to mid lung volumes through an open glottis. The individual takes in a slow, deep breath, followed by a 1- to 3-second breath hold, and then performs short, quick forced exhalation with the glottis open. Toddlers can also be taught blowing games (e.g., pinwheel, bubbles) to encourage prolonged exhalation maneuvers.[13]

Manually Assisted Cough

The manually assisted cough involves thrusts with hands and arms positioned on the patient's abdomen, coordinated with expiration (**Figure 16-5**). Compression of the lateral aspect of the chest also can be effective. Often this technique is augmented with manual hyperinflation for patients with a low vital capacity. This technique requires a cooperative patient, good coordination between patient and clinician, and a clinician with sufficient physical strength to reliably perform the maneuver. Efficacy is limited for patients with significant scoliosis and osteoporosis of the rib cage. This technique is used most commonly in patients with neuromuscular disease or quadriplegia and is sometimes called *quad coughing*.

Active Cycle of Breathing

Active cycle of breathing technique is a combination of breathing control, thoracic expansion control, and forced expiration technique (**Box 16-2** and **Figure 16-6**). Breathing control is described as gentle breathing with the lower chest. With the upper chest and shoulders relaxed, the patient breathes at normal tidal volume and rate. The patient should feel a swelling around the waist on inspiration, which subsides while breathing out. Breathing control is the default maneuver between the more active techniques. Thoracic expansion exercises are large breaths with active inspiration (involving both diaphragm and rib cage musculature) and relaxed expiration. Increasing lung volume increases flow through small airways and collateral ventilation channels, increasing the volume of gas available to help mobilize secretions on expiration. This is limited to three or four deep breaths to avoid fatigue and hyperventilation. The FET consists of one or two forced expirations or huffs,

TABLE 16-1
Complications of Excessive Cough

Cardiovascular	Arterial hypotension Bradyarrhythmias and tachyarrhythmias Dislodgement/malfunctioning of intravascular catheters Loss of consciousness Rupture of subconjunctival, nasal, and anal veins, and massive intraocular suprachoroidal hemorrhage during pars plana vitrectomy
Constitutional symptoms	Excessive sweating, anorexia, exhaustion
Gastrointestinal	Gastroesophageal reflux events Gastric hemorrhage following percutaneous endoscopic gastrostomy Hepatic cyst rupture Herniations (e.g., inguinal, through abdominal wall, small bowel through laparoscopic trocar site) Malfunction of gastrostomy button Mallory-Weiss tear Splenic rupture
Genitourinary	Inversion of bladder through urethra Urinary incontinence
Musculoskeletal	From asymptomatic elevations of serum creatine phosphokinase to rupture of rectus abdominus muscles Diaphragmatic rupture Rib fractures Sternal wound dehiscence
Neurologic	Acute cervical radiculopathy Cerebral air embolism Cerebral spinal fluid rhinorrhea Cervical epidural hematoma associated with oral anticoagulation Cough syncope Dizziness Headache Malfunctioning ventriculoatrial shunts Seizures Stroke due to vertebral artery dissection
Ophthalmologic	Spontaneous compressive orbital emphysema of rhinogenic origin
Psychosocial	Fear of serious disease Lifestyle changes Self-consciousness
Quality of life	Decreased
Respiratory	Exacerbation of asthma Herniations of the lung (e.g., intercostal, supraclavicular) Hydrothorax in peritoneal dialysis Laryngeal trauma (e.g., laryngeal edema, hoarseness) Pulmonary interstitial emphysema, with potential risk of pneumatosis intestinalis, pneumomediastinum, pneumoperitoneum, pneumoretroperitoneum, pneumothorax, and subcutaneous emphysema Tracheobronchial trauma (e.g., bronchitis, bronchial rupture)
Skin	Petechiae and purpura Disruption of surgical wounds

Reproduced from Irwin RS. Complications of cough: ACCP evidence-based clinical practice guidelines. *Chest.* 2006;129(Suppl 1):54S–58S, with permission from the American College of Chest Physicians.

combined with a period of controlled breathing. A normal breath is taken in, and then the air is squeezed out by contraction of the chest wall and abdominal muscles. The mouth and glottis are kept open. The huff should not be a violent or explosive exhalation.

Autogenic Drainage

Autogenic drainage aims to achieve the highest possible airflow in the different generations of bronchi to move secretions without forced expirations (**Figure 16-7**).[14]

BOX 16-1

Procedure for Directed Cough

1. Explain to the patient that deep breathing and coughing will help to keep the lungs expanded and clear of secretions.
2. Assist the patient to a sitting position or to a semi-Fowler position if sitting position is not possible.
3. Directed cough procedure:
   a. Instruct patient to take a deep breath, then hold the breath, using abdominal muscles to force air against a closed glottis, and then cough with a single exhalation.
   b. Have the patient take several relaxed breaths before the next cough effort.
   c. Document teaching accomplished, procedures performed, and patient response in the patient record.
4. Huff cough procedure (forced expiratory technique):
   a. Instruct patient to take three to five slow, deep breaths, inhaling through the nose, exhaling through pursed lips, using diaphragmatic breathing. Have the patient take a deep breath and hold it for 1 to 3 seconds.
   b. Instruct patient to exhale from mid-to-low lung volume (to clear secretions from peripheral airways). Have the patient take a normal breath in and then squeeze it out by contracting the abdominal and chest wall muscles, with the mouth (and glottis) open during exhalation. Repeat several times.
   c. As secretions enter the larger airways, have the patient exhale from high-to-mid lung volume to clear secretions from more proximal airways. Repeat maneuver two to three times.
   d. Instruct patient to take several relaxed diaphragmatic breaths before the next cough effort.
   e. Document teaching accomplished, procedures performed, and patient response in the patient record.
5. Modified directed cough procedures:
   a. Patients who have had abdominal or thoracic surgery: Instruct patient to place hand or a pillow over the incision site and apply gentle pressure while coughing. Caregiver may assist with incision support during coughing. Support chest tubes as necessary.
   b. Quadriplegic patients: Clinician places palms on the patient's abdomen, below the diaphragm, and instructs the patient to take three deep breaths. On exhalation of the third breath, clinician pushes forcefully inward and upward as the patient coughs (similar to abdominal thrust maneuver performed on an unconscious patient with an obstructed airway). This technique depends on staged breathing at different lung volumes, starting with small tidal breaths from expiratory reserve volume (ERV), repeated until secretions are felt gathering in the central airways. At that point the cough is suppressed, and a larger tidal volume is taken for a series of 10 to 20 breaths, followed by a series of larger (approaching vital capacity) breaths, followed by several huff coughs. Although this technique is effective, it requires a great deal of patient cooperation.

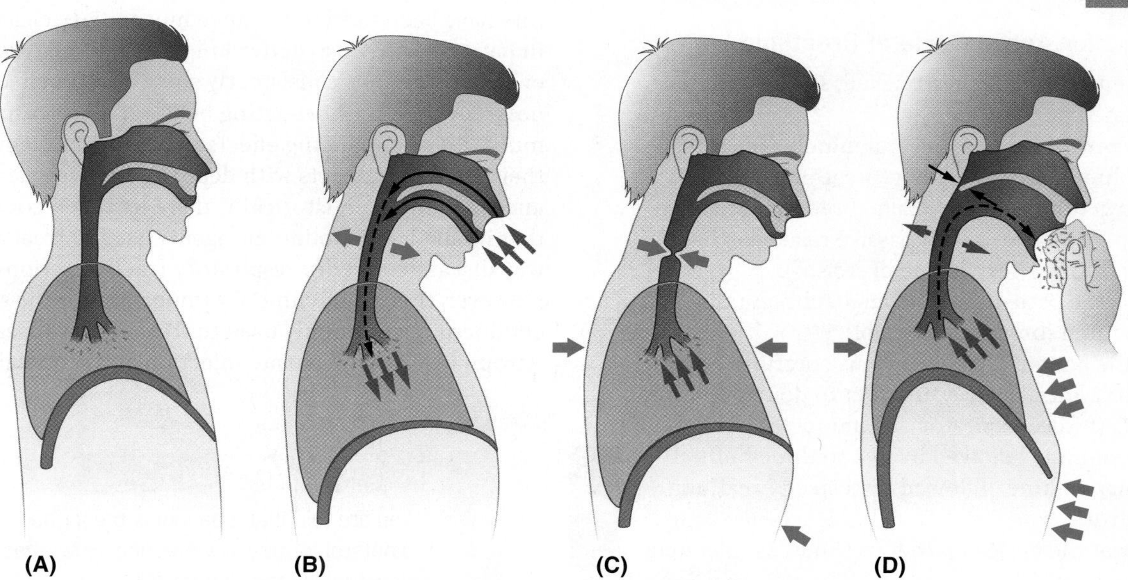

FIGURE 16-4 The cough reflex. (**A**) Irritation. (**B**) Inspiration. (**C**) Compression. (**D**) Expulsion.

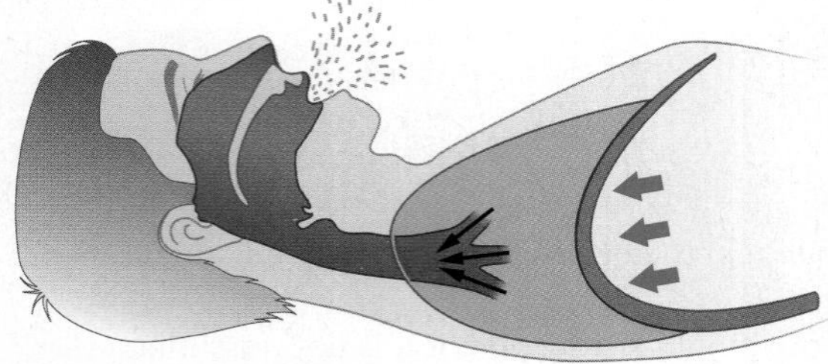

FIGURE 16-5 To produce manually assisted (quad) coughing, external abdominal pressure is applied under the diaphragm during exhalation following maximal inspiration, resulting in an increased expiratory flow and secretion clearance.

Mechanical Insufflation-Exsufflation

The mechanical insufflator-exsufflation (MIE), also called the Cough Assist, is a device (**Figure 16-8**) that inflates the lungs with positive pressure followed by a negative pressure to simulate a cough.[15] Treatment consists of five cycles of **mechanical insufflation–exsufflation** followed by 20 to 30 seconds of normal breathing, with repetitions until secretions are cleared. For each cycle the inspiratory pressure is 25 to 35 cm H_2O for 1 to 2 seconds, followed by an expiratory pressure of −30 to −40 cm H_2O for 1 to 2 seconds. The MIE can be used with an oronasal mask or with a mouthpiece, or it can be attached to an artificial airway. Combining manual abdominal thrusts with expiration can help to increase expiratory flow expulsion of secretions. This procedure is effective in patients with neuromuscular disease. In patients with bulbar disease, use of the MIE can be limited by upper airway closure during the active negative pressure expiratory phase.[16]

BOX 16-2

Procedure for Active Cycle of Breathing

1. Patient should be in a relaxed, sitting, or reclined position.
2. Have the patient do several minutes of relaxed diaphragmatic breathing (breathing control).
3. Instruct the patient to take three to four active deep inspirations with passive relaxed exhalation (thoracic expansion exercises).
4. Have the patient do relaxed diaphragmatic breathing (breathing control).
5. As the patient feels secretions entering the larger central airway, instruct to do two to three huffs (forced expiratory technique) starting at low volume, followed by two to three huffs at higher volume, followed by relaxed breathing control.
6. Repeat the cycle two to four times, as tolerated.

Aerosol Therapy

Aerosolized antibiotics and mucolytics are effective when dispersed in infected airway secretions at sites of maximal airway obstruction. Mucus is a nonhomogeneous, adhesive, viscoelastic gel consisting of high-molecular-weight, cross-linked glycoproteins mixed with serum, cellular proteins, lipids, and water. The antibiotic diffusion barrier represented by mucin may be significant in vitro, particularly for nebulized antibiotics. Translocation of macromolecules can be further compromised by the hypersecretion that accompanies inflammation and chronic pulmonary disease. Airway secretions can be a barrier to aerosol penetration.

Sputum is expectorated mucus mixed with inflammatory cells, cellular debris, polymers of DNA and F-actin, and bacteria. Recombinant human deoxyribonuclease (dornase alfa) was the first approved mucoactive agent for the treatment of CF. The efficacy of dornase alfa has not been demonstrated in treatment of other chronic airway diseases. Acetylcysteine (*N*-acetyl-L-cysteine sodium; Mucomyst) has been administered by aerosol or direct instillation based on its in vitro ability to break disulfide bonds of mucoprotein. Evidence does not support its in vivo efficacy, however. Mucomyst is an airway irritant that can induce bronchospasm, and it has a nauseating smell and taste. Hypertonic saline (7%) has been shown to improve outcomes in patients with CF,[17] but might not be useful for COPD.[18] Aerosolized isotonic saline from a small volume nebulizer is not an effective airway clearance therapy. Most guidelines for management of COPD do not advocate treatment with inhaled mucolytics.[19]

The involvement of the cholinergic and adrenergic neural pathways in the pathophysiology of mucus hypersecretion suggests the potential therapeutic role of bronchodilators as mucoactive agents. Although anticholinergics and adrenergic agonist bronchodilators have been used to enhance mucociliary clearance in patients with obstructive lung disease, the existing evidence does not consistently show clinical effectiveness.[20] Although short-acting beta-adrenergics have mucociliary-enhancing effects in healthy individuals, their effect in subjects with depressed airway clearance is minimal. Historically, there has been concern that inhaled anticholinergic agents used to treat airway disease could dry respiratory tract secretions. However, this is not clinically important for the anticholinergics commonly used to treat airway disease. Atropine or glycopyrrolate injection and scopolamine

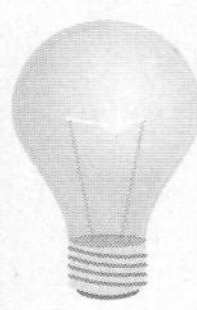

STOP AND THINK

You are told that a patient is prescribed albuterol for airway clearance. How effective do you think this therapy is?

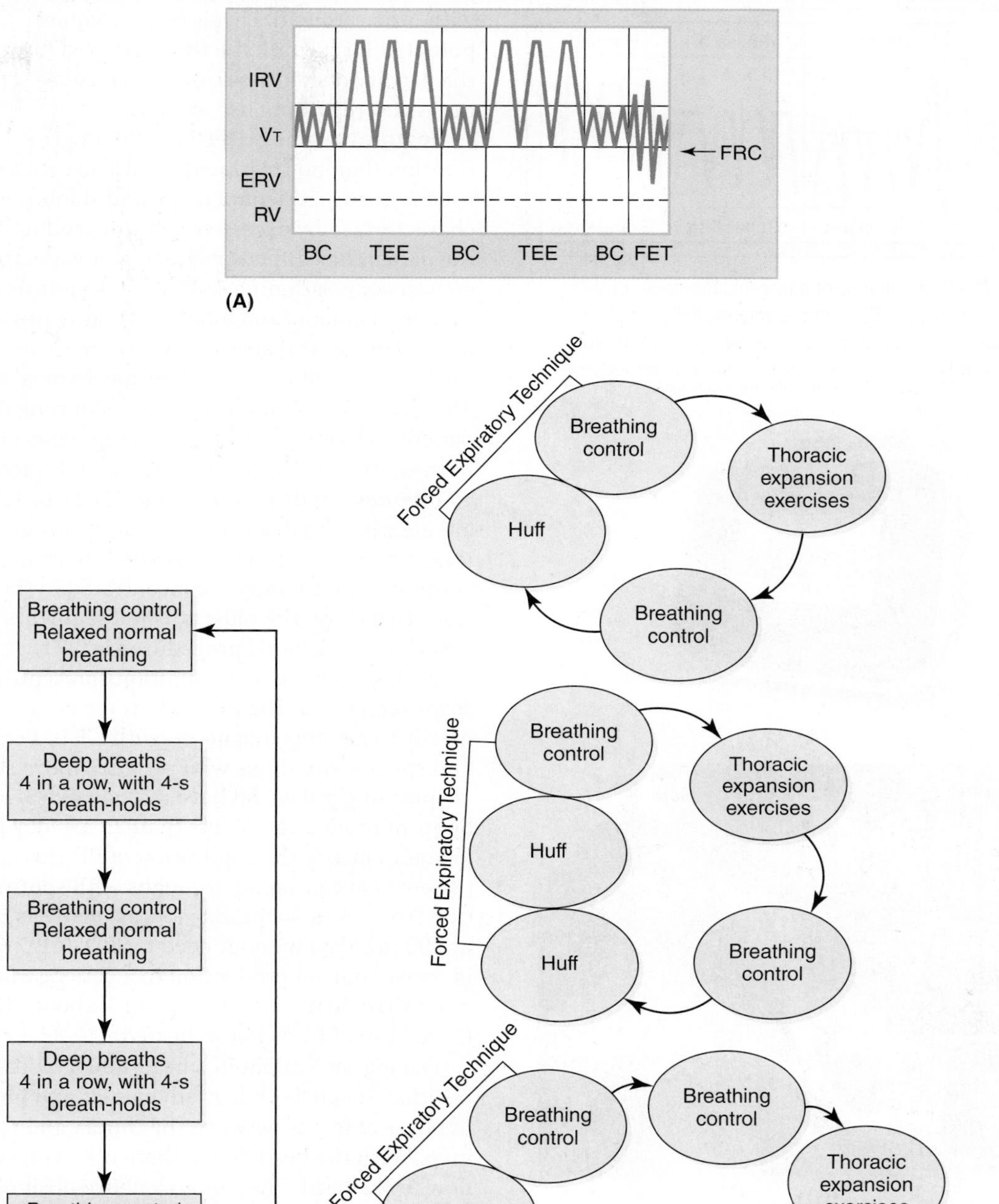

FIGURE 16-6 (**A**) Lung volumes during active cycle of breathing technique. (**B**) Active cycle of breathing technique. (**C**) Three active cycle of breathing routines.

Reproduced from Fink JB. Forced expiratory technique, directed cough, and autogenic drainage. *Respir Care.* 2007;52:1210–1223. Reprinted with permission.

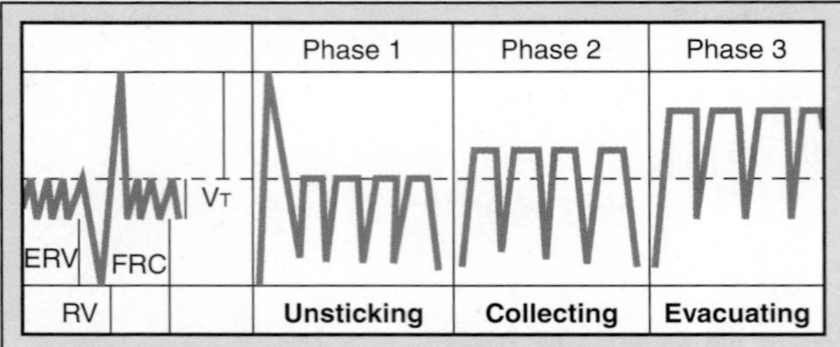

FIGURE 16-7 The three phases of autogenic drainage. ERV, expiratory reserve volume; RV, reserve volume; FRC, functional residual capacity; IRV, inspiratory reserve volume; VT, tidal volume.

Reproduced from Fink JB. Forced expiratory technique, directed cough, and autogenic drainage. *Respir Care.* 2007;52:1210–1223. Reprinted with permission.

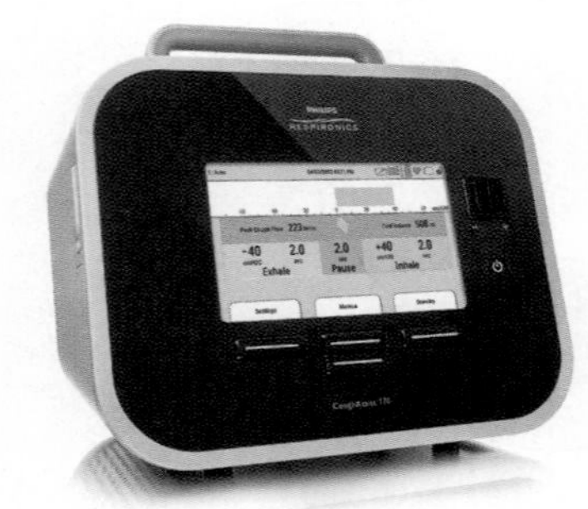

(A)

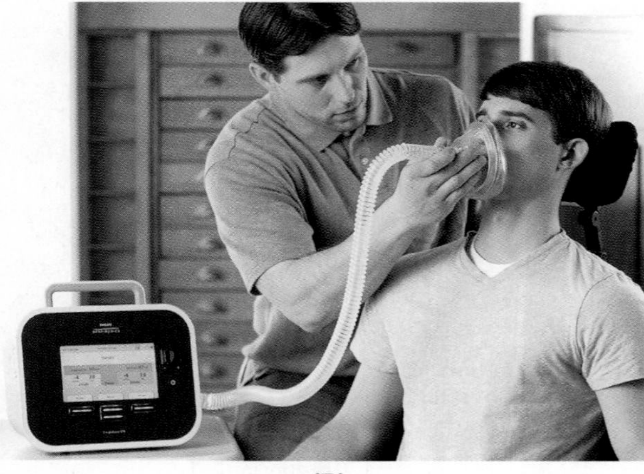

(B)

FIGURE 16-8 Cough Assist mechanical insufflation–exsufflation device.

patch are used to reduce cholinergic symptoms such as sialorrhea, bronchorrhea, and excessive pharyngeal secretions. Aerosolized anticholinergics, however, are minimally effective in drying respiratory tract secretions.

Conventional Chest Physiotherapy

Conventional **chest physiotherapy (CPT)** consists of a combination of forced exhalation (directed cough or huff), postural drainage, percussion, and/or shaking.[21] Conventional CPT has become the standard to which all other bronchial hygiene techniques are compared. Patient satisfaction with conventional CPT is less than with other bronchial hygiene techniques.[22] Given the potential for hazard, the time required for therapy, and the paucity of evidence to support its use,[23] prudence is necessary regarding use of CPT.

Postural drainage (PD) results in greater expectoration than no treatment in patients with CF. PD is used in the treatment of acute and stable conditions characterized by excessive sputum production that the patient has difficulty clearing or expectorating. It consists of positioning so that secretions drain from specific segments and lobes of the lung toward gravity-dependent central airways, where they can be more readily removed with cough or mechanical aspiration. This action is accomplished by positioning of the patient so that the affected lung segments are superior to the carina, with each position maintained for 5 to 10 minutes (**Figure 16-9**). Typically, 11 to 12 positions are identified to drain all areas of the lungs, requiring at least 1 hour for a complete session. Because of this time commitment, therapy is concentrated in those positions that drain the most affected segments. **Box 16-3** describes the general procedure for CPT.

PD has no benefit in conditions presenting with scant secretions. The indications for PD are limited primarily to patients diagnosed with CF or bronchiectasis, and specifically those who produce more than 30 mL of sputum per day and have difficulty clearing that. Sputum production of less than 25 mL/day is insufficient to justify the application of PD therapy. Some patients have productive coughs with sputum production from 15 to 30 mL/day (occasionally as high as 70 or 100 mL/day) without need for PD. If PD does not increase sputum production in a patient who produces more than 30 mL/day of sputum without PD, the continued use of PD is not indicated.

Placing the patient in a head-down or Trendelenburg position affects both hemodynamics and interaction of physical forces between the thorax and the abdomen. With the head down, there is increased blood flow to the head. The Trendelenburg position therefore should be avoided in patients with head injury, uncontrolled hypertension, or gross hemoptysis. Shifting of abdominal and thoracic contents with gravity in the Trendelenburg position may be deleterious in patients at risk for aspiration, with distended abdomens, or after recent esophageal surgery. Reverse Trendelenburg position may be hazardous for patients with hypotension or those receiving vasoactive medication.

During PD therapy, care should be taken to identify hypoxemia, bronchospasm, acute hypotension,

Respiratory Recap

Conventional Chest Physiotherapy

- Postural drainage
- May be combined with percussion and vibration

Upper and Middle Lobes

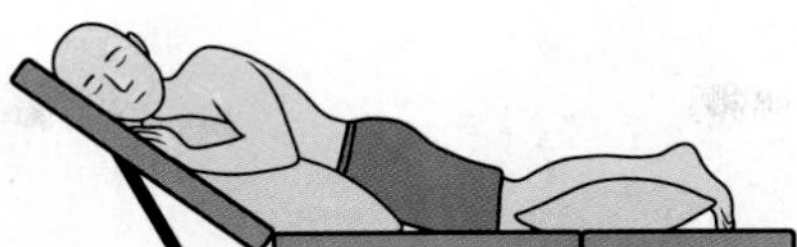
Apical posterior segment, left upper lobe

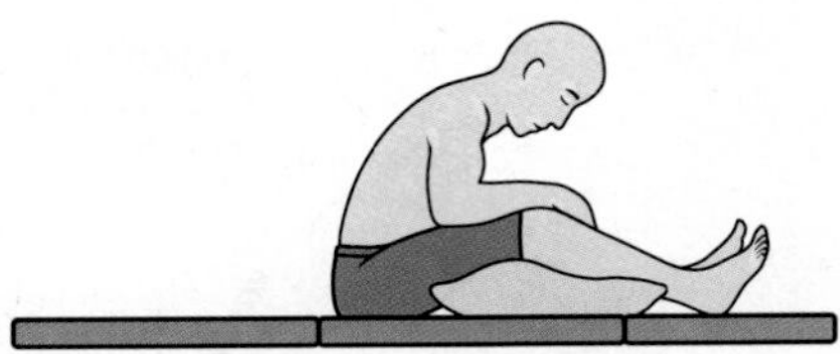
Apical segment, right upper lobe

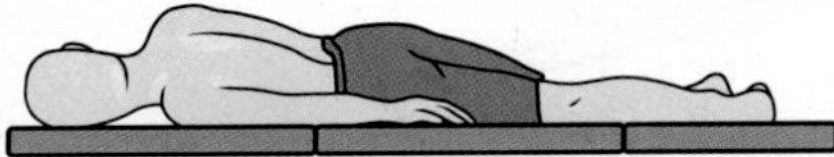
Posterior segment, right upper lobe

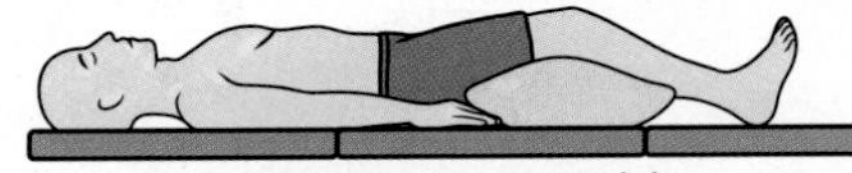
Anterior segments, upper lobes

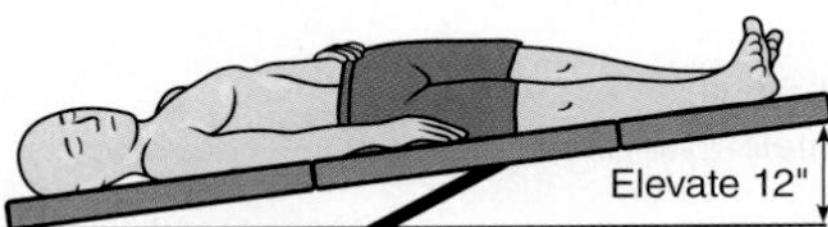

Left upper lobe, lingula

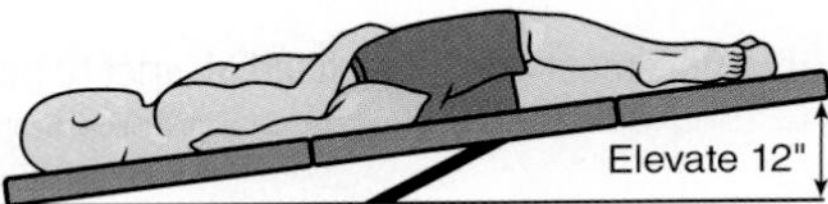

Right middle lobe

Lower Lobes

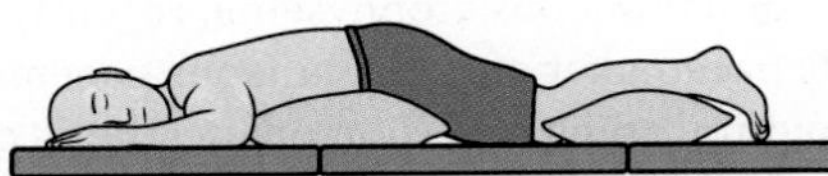
Superior segments, lower lobes

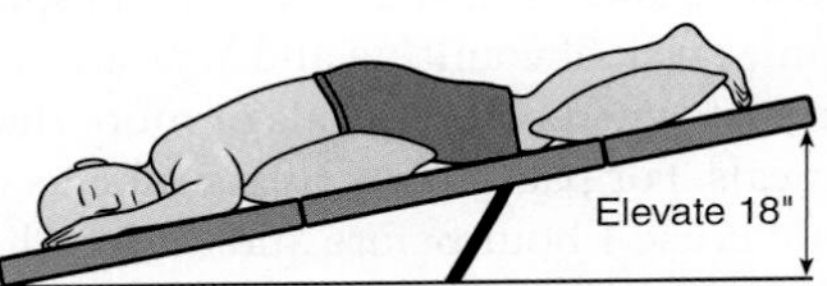

Posterior basal segments, lower lobes

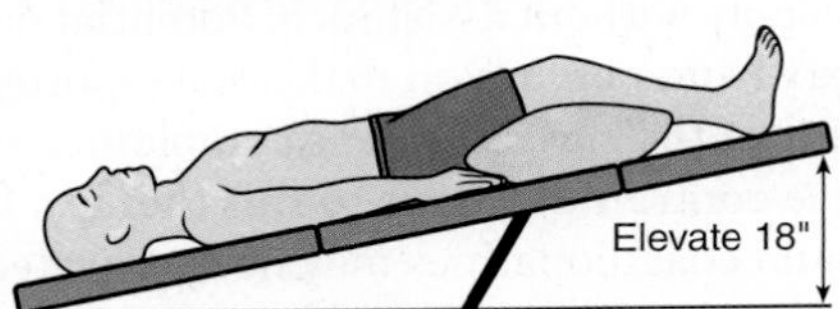

Right anterior basal and left anterior medial basal segments, lower lobes

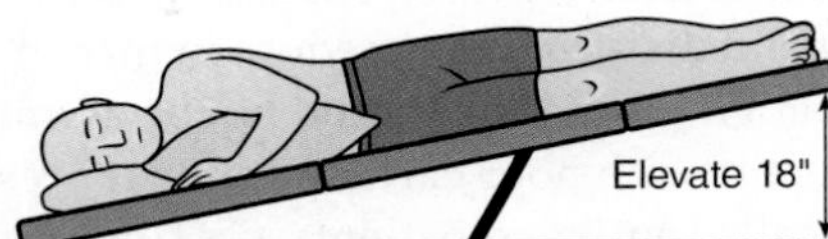

Lateral basal segment, left lower lobe

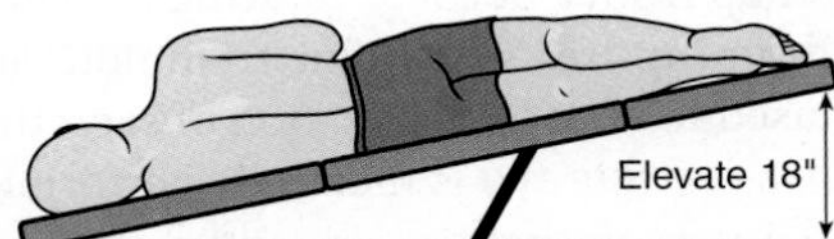

Lateral basal segment, right lower lobe

FIGURE 16-9 Positions for postural drainage.

BOX 16-3

Procedure for Chest Physiotherapy

1. Assess patient and need for chest physiotherapy.
2. Gather appropriate equipment: bed or table that can assume range of positions, pillows to support patient, light towel to cover chest percussion area, tissues or basin for secretions.
3. Explain therapy to patient and instruct patient in proper cough techniques.
4. Assist patient to each position and maintain for 5 to 10 minutes.
5. Assess patient response in each position; modify position if necessary.
6. Perform chest percussion and vibration over the affected area if necessary.
7. Encourage patient to take slow, deep breaths and cough between positions; note character of cough and secretions.
8. Document procedure and response to therapy in the medical record; communicate adverse effects to physician.

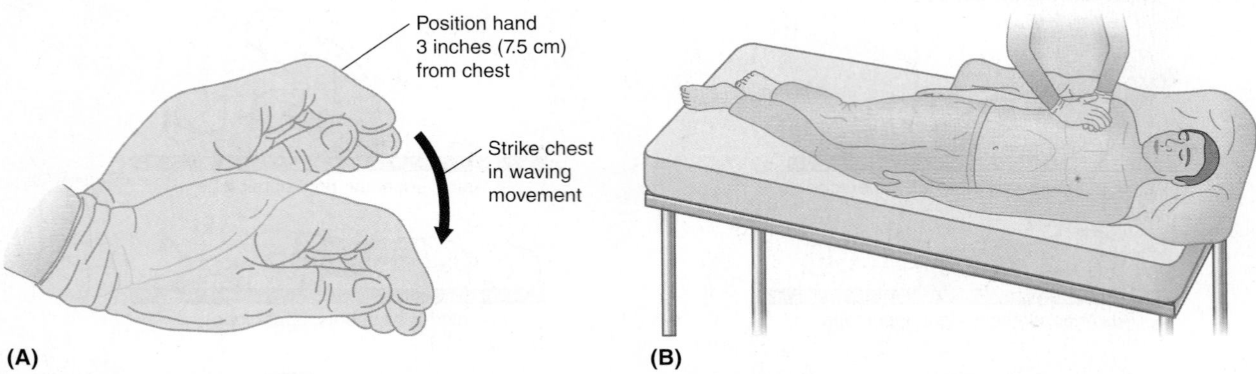

FIGURE 16-10 (**A**) Movement of cupped hand at wrist to percuss chest. (**B**) Chest vibration.
Reproduced from *Egan's Fundamentals of Respiratory Care*, Seventh Edition. Scanlan CL, Wilkins RL, Stoller JK. Copyright Elsevier (Mosby) 1999.

increased intracranial pressure, hemoptysis, pain or injury to the tissue, and vomiting with risk of aspiration. To minimize risk of vomiting and aspiration, therapy should be performed before meals or more than 1 hour after meals. For patients receiving tube feedings, feedings should cease 1 hour before and during therapy. For patients with a history of bronchospasm, bronchodilators are commonly administered before PD therapy.

Percussion therapy is a technique involving rapid clapping, cupping, or striking of the external thorax directly over the lung segment being drained, with either cupped hands or a mechanical device (**Figure 16-10**). Percussion has been advocated to assist secretion mobilization by shaking loose secretions, similar to the shaking of ketchup from a bottle. Vibrating the chest wall over the draining area with a fine tremulous action also has been used to assist mobilization of secretion during PD. **Vibration therapy** is manually performed by pressing in the direction that the ribs and soft tissue of the chest normally move during exhalation. Mechanical devices can be used to perform chest percussion and vibration. These devices may be more convenient for the caregiver, but data are lacking that these devices improve airway clearance.

Percussion and vibration appear to be relatively ineffective and do not add to the effectiveness of the combination of coughing, breathing exercises, and PD.[24] Little evidence exists that percussion alone, without positioning of the patient, is of any value. Although the clinical efficacy of percussion and vibration is questionable, the techniques are associated with a number of potential hazards and complications. A variety of conditions may be exacerbated by performance of percussion or vibration to the thorax, such as irregularities of the skin (e.g., burns, open wounds, skin infections, recent skin grafts), subcutaneous emphysema, recently placed transvenous pacemaker or subcutaneous pacemaker, or recent epidural spinal infusion of anesthetic of the spinal type. Percussion and vibration are difficult for patients to apply without assistance. Potential damage to the thorax from percussion makes osteoporosis and osteomyelitis of the ribs, as well as complaints of chest pain, relative contraindications to this therapy. Lung contusion and coagulopathies may be aggravated by percussion, resulting in increased bruising or bleeding of the chest wall or in the lungs.

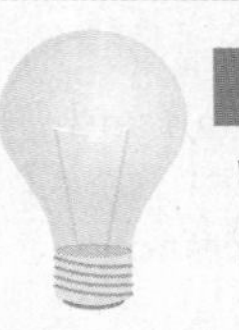

STOP AND THINK

When would you recommend chest physiotherapy for a patient?

Conventional CPT has been suggested as the most stimulating and disturbing procedure in mechanically ventilated patients and thus should not be administered to patients with poor cardiopulmonary reserve. In mechanically ventilated patients, CPT may be accompanied with manual hyperinflation. This practice is discouraged, however, because it may result in dangerously high airway pressures and tidal volumes in patients with acute lung injury.[25] In patients with CF, tolerance for CPT may be improved when combined with noninvasive pressure support.[26] Conventional CPT is overused in many hospitals, and efforts to reduce its unnecessary use have been successfully implemented without adversely affecting patient outcomes.[27]

Positive Expiratory Pressure

Positive expiratory pressure (PEP) therapy is performed with the patient seated comfortably and with elbows resting on a table (**Box 16-4**).[28] Equipment consists of a soft transparent mask or mouthpiece, T assembly with a one-way valve, a variety of fixed orifice resistors (or an adjustable expiratory resistor), and a manometer (**Figure 16-11**). The subject is instructed

BOX 16-4

Procedure for Positive Expiratory Pressure Therapy

1. The patient should sit comfortably upright while holding the mask firmly over the nose and mouth or the mouthpiece tightly between the lips (a nose clip may be necessary).
2. Adjust the expiratory resistor dial to the prescribed setting.
3. Have the patient breathe from the diaphragm, taking in a larger than normal tidal breath, but not to total lung capacity.
4. Have the patient gently exhale, maintaining a prescribed pressure of 5 to 20 cm H_2O.
5. Exhalation time should last approximately three times longer than inhalation.
6. Patient should perform 10 to 20 positive expiratory pressure breaths, and then perform two to three forced exhalation maneuvers or huffs.
7. Repeat steps 3 to 6 until secretions are cleared or until the predetermined treatment period has elapsed.

Reproduced from Myers TR. Positive expiratory pressure and oscillatory positive expiratory pressure therapies. *Respir Care.* 2007;52:1308–1327. Reprinted with permission.

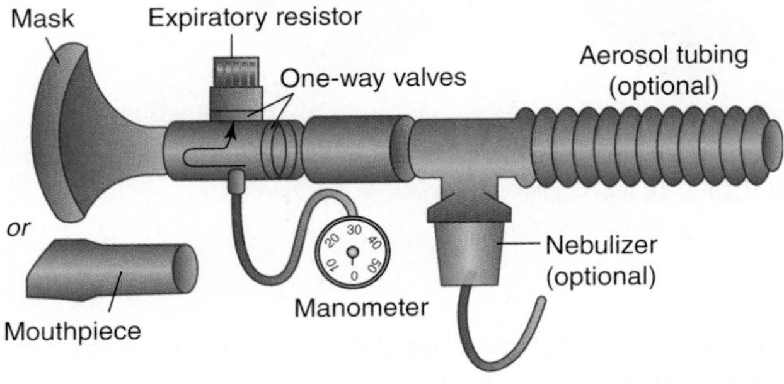

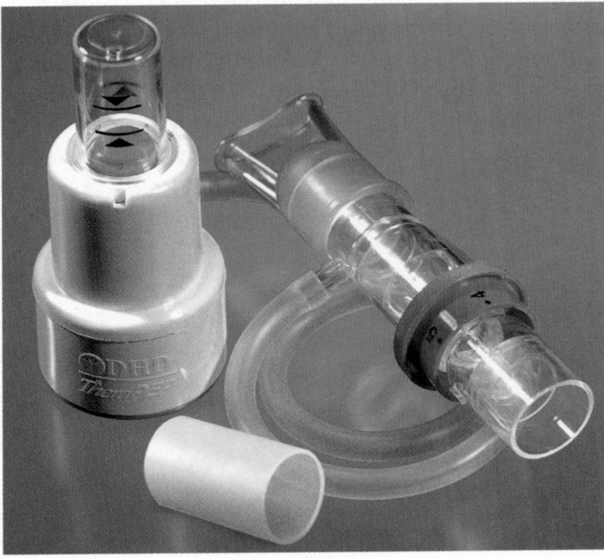

FIGURE 16-11 **(A)** Equipment for positive expiratory pressure (PEP) therapy. **(B)** Commercially available PEP device.

(A) adapted from Mahlmeister MJ, Fink JB, Hoffman GL, Fifer LF. Positive expiratory pressure mask therapy: theoretical and practical considerations and a review of the literature. *Respir Care.* 1991;36:1218–1229; **(B)** courtesy of Smiths Medical.

to relax while performing diaphragmatic breathing, inspiring a volume of air larger than normal tidal volume, but not to the level of total lung capacity, through the one-way valve. Exhalation to functional residual capacity (FRC) is active, but not forced, through the resistor chosen to achieve a peak airway pressure of 10 to 20 cm H_2O during exhalation. A series of 10 to 20 breaths is performed with the mask or mouthpiece in place. The mask (or mouthpiece) is then removed, and the patient performs several coughs to raise secretions. This sequence of 10 to 20 breaths, followed by huff coughing, is repeated four to six times per PEP therapy session. Each session requires 10 to 20 minutes and may be performed one to four times per day as needed. For lung expansion, patients should be encouraged to take 10 to 20 breaths every hour while awake.

Selection of an appropriate resistance is necessary for proper technique. The therapeutic goal is to achieve a PEP of 10 to 20 cm H_2O, with an inspiration-to-expiration (I:E) ratio of 1:3 to 1:4. When a fixed orifice is used, most adults achieve this pressure range with an orifice of 2.5 to 4.0 mm in diameter. A manometer is placed in-line to measure the expiratory pressure while the appropriate-sized orifice is selected. Once the proper resistor orifice has been determined, the manometer may be removed from the system. Selection of a resistor with too large an orifice produces a short exhalation, with failure to achieve the proper expiratory pressure. Too small an orifice prolongs the expiratory phase, elevates the pressure above 20 cm H_2O, and increases the work of breathing. Performing a PEP session for more than 20 minutes may lead to fatigue. During periods of exacerbation, individuals are encouraged to increase the frequency with which PEP is performed, rather than extending the length of individual sessions.

Although no absolute contraindications to the use of PEP therapy have been reported, common sense dictates that patients with acute sinusitis, ear infection, epistaxis, or recent facial, oral, or skull injury or surgery should be carefully evaluated before a decision is made to initiate PEP mask therapy. Patients experiencing active hemoptysis or those with unresolved pneumothorax should avoid using PEP therapy.

Oscillatory (or Vibratory) Positive Expiratory Pressure

Oscillatory, or vibratory, PEP combines the purported benefits of PEP with airway vibrations or oscillations.[28] Oscillations may decrease the viscoelastic properties of mucus, which makes it easier to mobilize mucus up the airways, and may create short bursts of increased expiratory airflow that assist in mobilizing secretions up the airways. The patient forcing exhalation through the device or with subsequent coughing and/or huffing techniques facilitates secretion removal.

The Flutter device is a pipe-shaped device with a steel ball in a bowl loosely covered by a perforated cap (**Figure 16-12**). The weight of the ball serves as a PEP device (approximately 10 cm H_2O), whereas the internal shape of the bowl allows the ball to flutter, generating oscillations of about 15 Hz (2 to 32 Hz), varying with the position of the device. Use of the Flutter device is gravity dependent, whereas other devices have become available that are gravity independent.

The Acapella (**Figure 16-13**) uses a counterweighted plug and magnet to create airflow oscillations during expiratory flow. The Quake (**Figure 16-14**) has a manually operated rotating handle that creates the oscillations; the oscillation frequency is controlled by how quickly the handle is rotated. Rotating the handle slowly creates a low-frequency oscillation and a higher pulsatile expiratory pressure. Rotating the handle quickly provides faster oscillations while decreasing the pulsatile expiratory pressure.

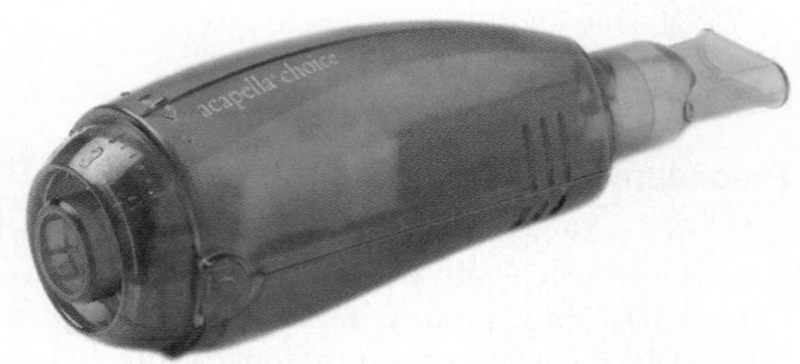

FIGURE 16-13 Acapella device.
Courtesy of Smiths Medical.

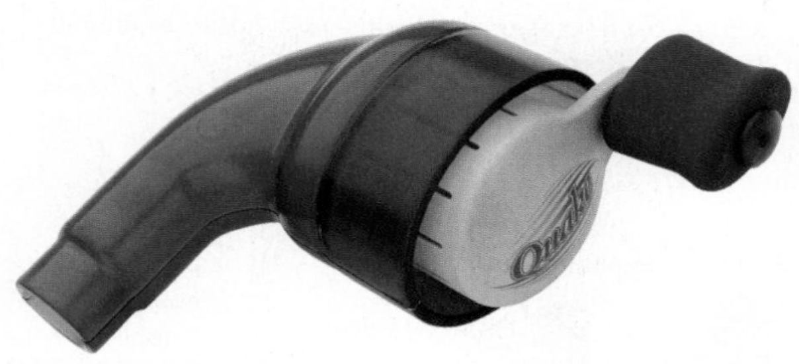

FIGURE 16-14 Quake device.
Courtesy of Thayer Medical Corporation.

With the RC-Cornet (**Figure 16-15**), therapy is fine-tuned by twisting the mouthpiece from the starting position for five changes to pressure and flow characteristics. It can be used as combined PEP, which is characterized as continuous positive pressure above baseline with applied pressure changes, or dynamic

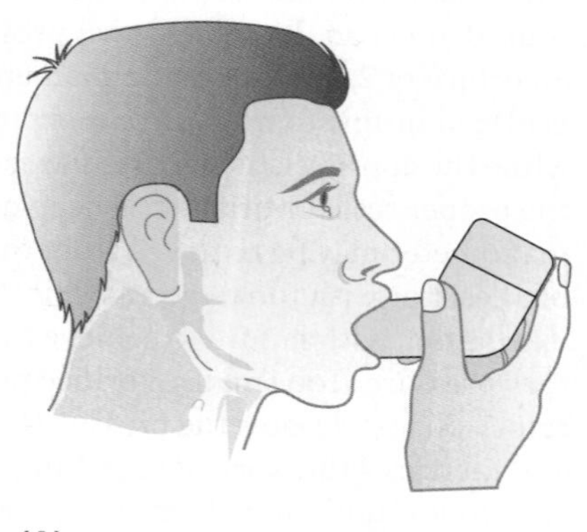

(A)

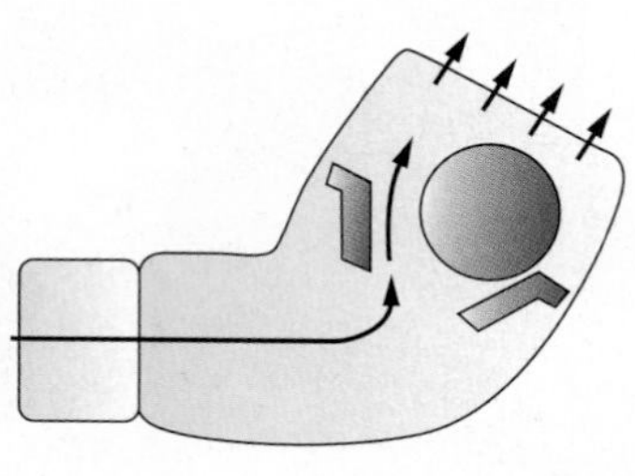

(B)

FIGURE 16-12 (**A**) Position of Flutter valve in patient's mouth. (**B**) During exhalation, the position of the steel ball is the result of an equilibrium between the pressure of the exhaled gas, the force of gravity on the ball, and the angle of the cone where the contact with the ball occurs. As the steel ball rolls and bounces up and down, it creates oscillations in the airway.

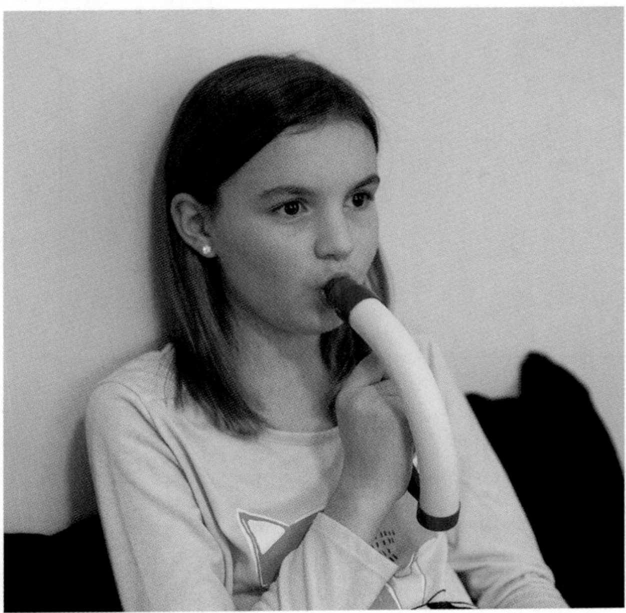

FIGURE 16-15 RC-Cornet device.
Courtesy of Curaplex.

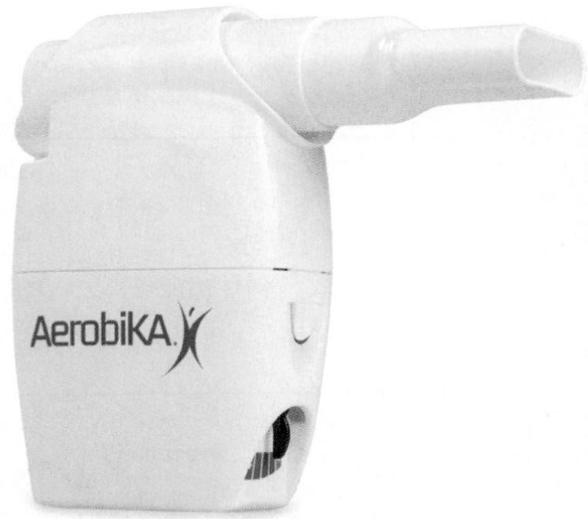

FIGURE 16-16 Aerobika Oscillating PEP device.
Courtesy of Monaghan Medical.

PEP, which is characterized by a pressure increase from zero to maximum with a drop back to zero. The Aerobika Oscillating PEP device (**Figure 16-16**) has five resistance settings. Selection of the proper resistance setting will produce the desired I:E flow ratio of 1:3 or 1:4 for 10 to 20 minutes without excess fatigue.

High-Frequency Chest Wall Compression

High-frequency chest wall compression (HFCWC) generates negative changes in transpulmonary pressure difference by compressing the chest externally (i.e., body surface pressure goes positive relative to the pressure at the airway opening, which remains at atmospheric pressure) to cause short, rapid expiratory flow pulses and relies on chest wall elastic recoil to return the lungs to functional residual capacity. HFCWC is accomplished by encasing the chest in an inflatable vest.[29] A high-output compressor rapidly inflates and deflates the vest. On inflation, pressure is exerted on the body surface (range 5 to 20 cm H_2O), which forces the chest wall to compress and generates a short burst of expiratory flow. Pressure pulses are superimposed on a small (about 12 cm H_2O) positive pressure baseline. On deflation, the chest wall recoils to its resting position, causing inspiratory flow.

The Vest Airway Clearance System (**Figure 16-17**) operates at 2 to 25 Hz and generates esophageal pressure and airflow oscillations as shown in **Figure 16-18**. HFCWC can generate volume changes of 17 to 57 mL and flows up to 1.6 L/s. This produces mini-coughs to mobilize secretions. HFCWC causes a decrease in end-expiratory lung volume, but the consequences of that decrease are debatable.[30] Other commercially available HFCWC devices include the InCourage system and the SmartVest (Figure 16-17). **Box 16-5** describes the procedure for use of HFCWC.

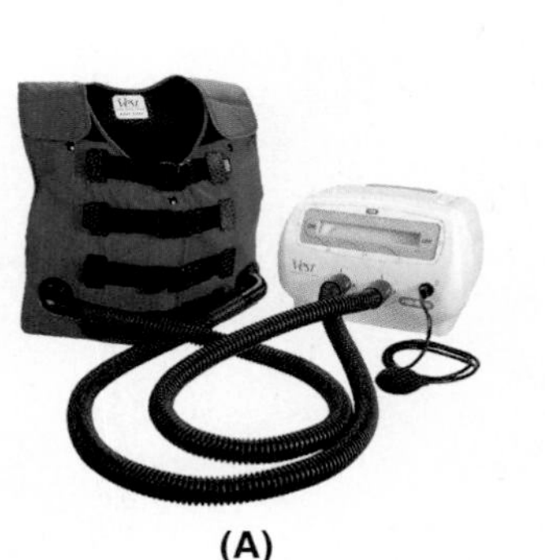

(A)

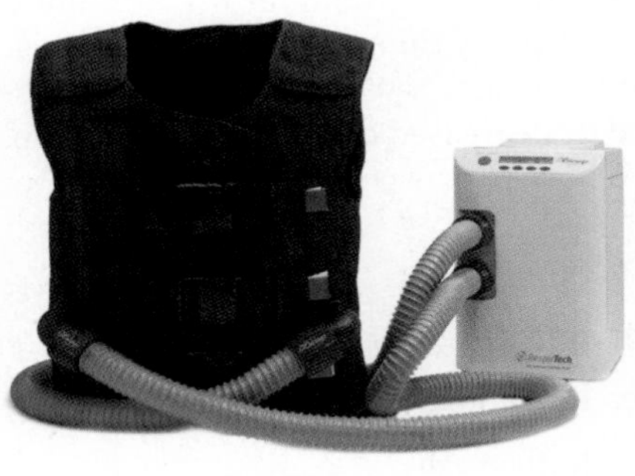

(B)

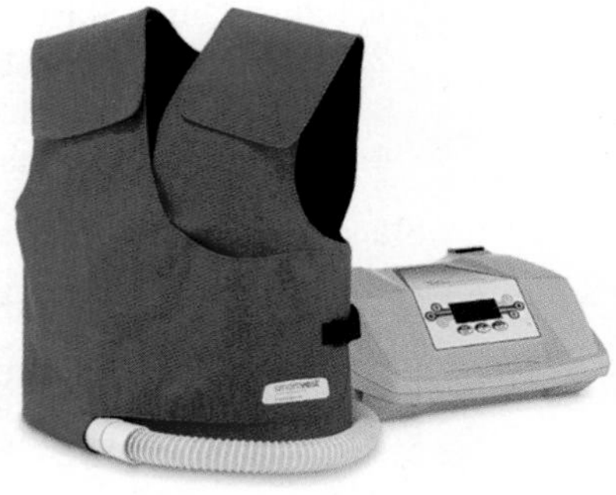

(C)

FIGURE 16-17 (**A**) Vest® Airway Clearance System. (**B**) InCourage device for high-frequency chest wall compression (HFCWC). (**C**) SmartVest device for HFCWC.
(**A**) © 2010 Hill-Rom Services PTE Ltd. Reprinted with permission. All rights reserved; (**B**) courtesy of RespirTech.; (**C**) courtesy of Electromed, Inc.

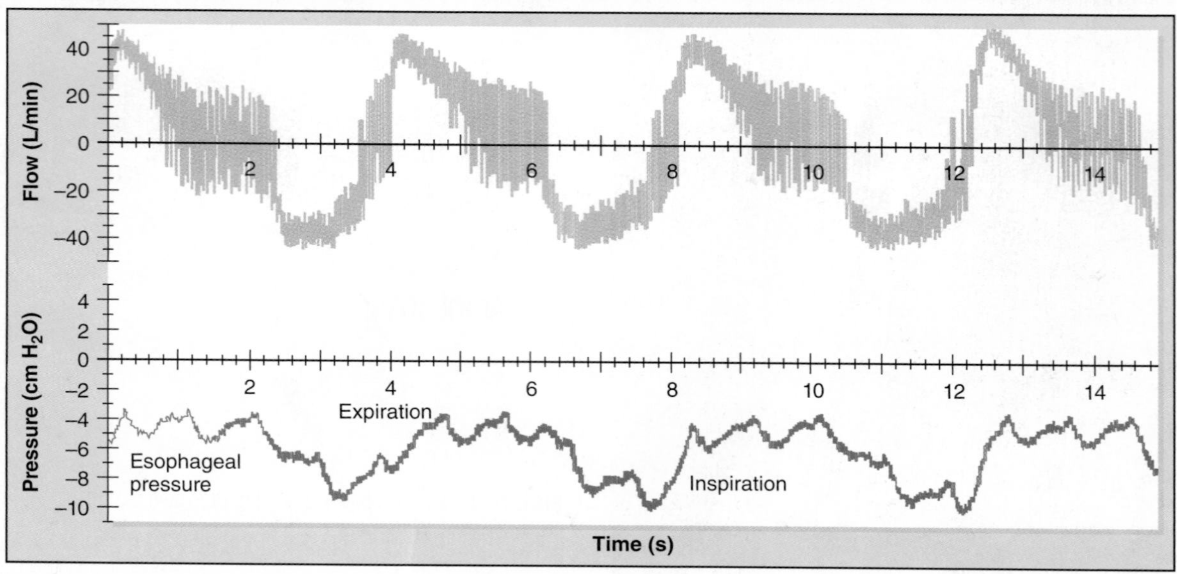

FIGURE 16-18 Flow, airway pressure, and esophageal pressure waveforms while breathing with the Vest Airway Clearance System.
Reproduced from Fink JB, Mahlmeister MJ. High-frequency oscillation of the airway and chest wall. *Respir Care*. 2002;47:797–807. Reprinted with permission.

BOX 16-5

Procedure for High-Frequency Chest Wall Compression

Ramping Session Using Hill-Rom Vest

Frequency	Pressure	Time
6, 8, 10 Hz	10	5 minutes at each frequency Pause machine and cough three times Resume session
16, 18, 20 Hz	6	5 minutes at each frequency Pause machine and cough three times Resume session

Therapy Session with InCourage

1. Push Quick Start button to initiate preprogrammed 30-minute automatic ramping session.
2. Pause button may be pushed at any time to allow for coughing.
3. Push Run button to resume therapy.
4. Pressure can be increased or decreased during therapy session.

Standard Protocol for SmartVest

Frequency	Duration
10 Hz	10 minutes, then huff cough
12 Hz	10 minutes, then huff cough
14 Hz	10 minutes, then huff cough

Reproduced from Lester MK, Flume PA. Airway-clearance therapy guidelines and implementation. *Respir Care*. 2009;54:733–753. Reprinted with permission.

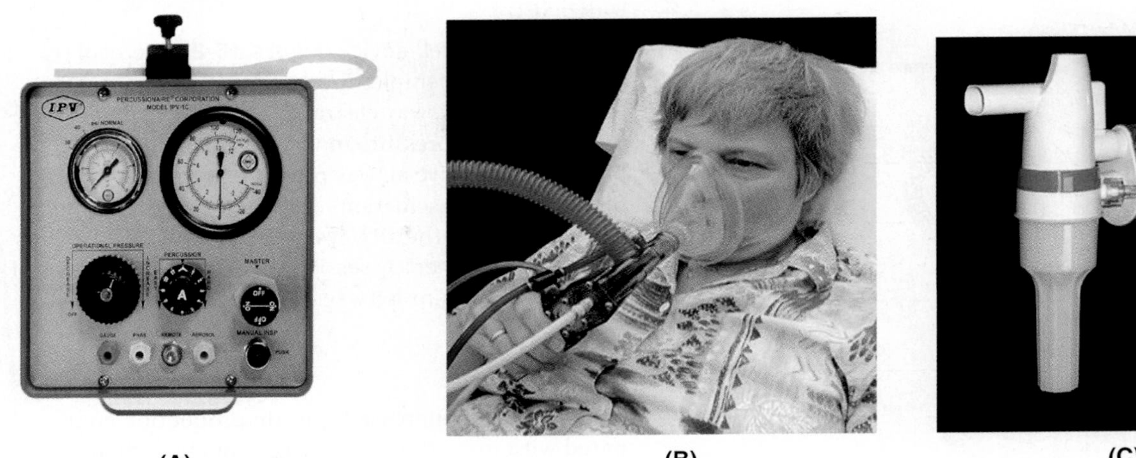

FIGURE 16-19 (**A**) Percussionaire Percussionator. (**B**) Patient using Percussionator. (**C**) VORTRAN® PercussiveNeb.
(**A** and **B**) courtesy of Dr. Pamela Bird, Percussionaire Corporation; (**C**) courtesy of VORTRAN® Medical Technology 1, Inc., Sacramento, CA.

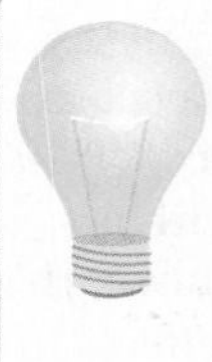

STOP AND THINK

You are asked to recommend an airway clearance therapy for a patient with neuromuscular disease. Which therapy do you think would be most beneficial?

Intrapulmonary Percussive Ventilation

Intrapulmonary percussive ventilation (IPV) creates positive changes in transrespiratory difference by injecting short, rapid inspiratory flow pulses into the airway opening and relies on chest wall elastic recoil for passive exhalation.[29] It delivers high-flow mini-bursts of air, along with an aerosolized medication to the lungs, at a rate of 300 to 400 per minute. The Percussionator (**Figure 16-19**) operates at 1.7 to 5 Hz. Treatments last about 15 to 20 minutes. It can be used with a mouthpiece or mask. Similar devices include the Breas IMP2, which operates at about 1 to 6 Hz and can also deliver aerosol medication, and the single-patient-use PercussiveNeb. The PercussiveNeb operates at frequencies of 11 to 30 Hz and can also deliver an aerosolized medication. It cannot be used with a ventilator. All three devices produce roughly comparable pressure waveforms (**Figure 16-20**). Each device delivers flow oscillations with normal spontaneous breathing.

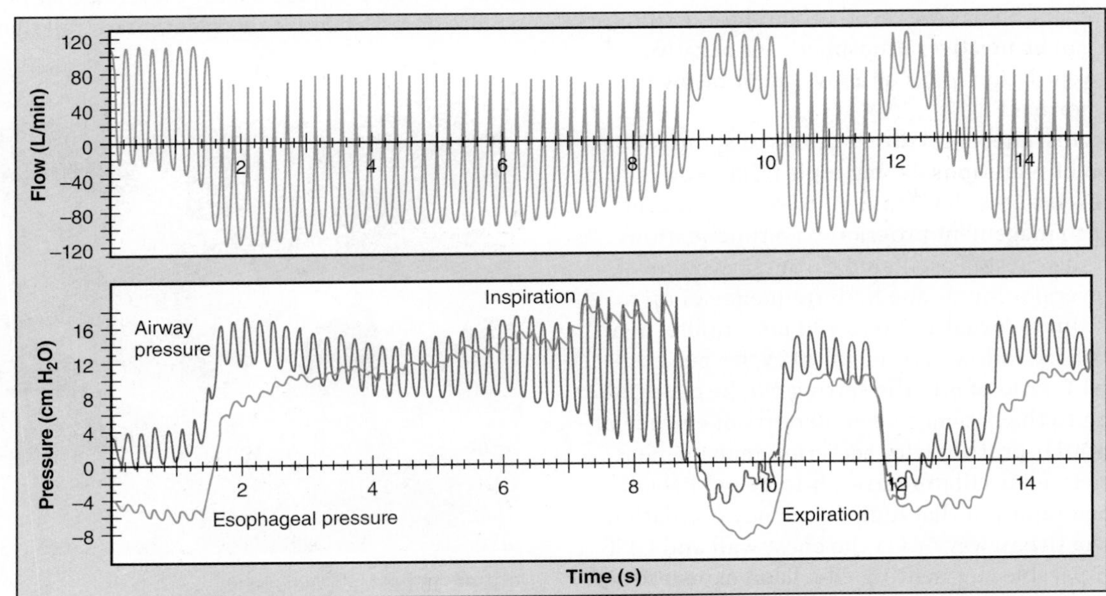

FIGURE 16-20 Flow, airway pressure, and esophageal pressure waveforms while breathing with an intrapulmonary percussive ventilator.
Reproduced from Fink JB, Mahlmeister MJ. High-frequency oscillation of the airway and chest wall. *Respir Care*. 2002;47:797–807. Reprinted with permission.

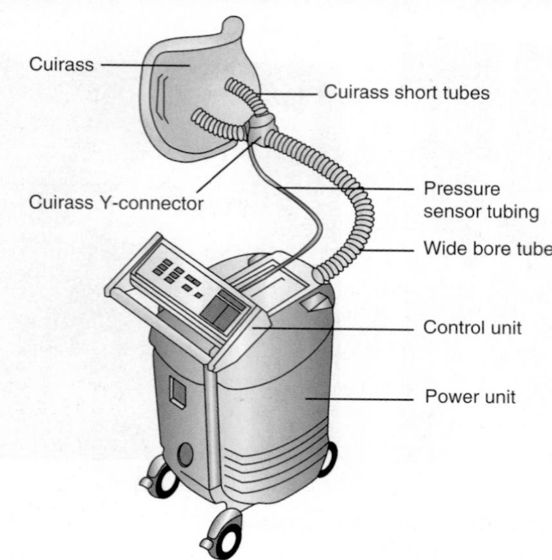

FIGURE 16-21 Schematic drawing of the Hayek oscillator.
Adapted from materials courtesy of Breasy Medical Equipment, Stamford, CT.

High-Frequency Chest Wall Oscillation

High-frequency chest wall oscillation (HFCWO) uses a chest cuirass to generate biphasic changes in transrespiratory pressure difference.[29] The Hayek oscillator is an electrically powered, microprocessor-controlled, noninvasive oscillator ventilator that uses an external flexible chest enclosure (cuirass) to apply negative and positive pressure to the chest wall to deliver noninvasive oscillation to the lungs (**Figure 16-21**). The negative pressure generated in the cuirass causes the chest wall to expand for inspiration, whereas positive pressure compresses the chest to produce a forced expiration. Both inspiratory and expiratory phases may be active and not reliant on passive recoil of the chest. Expiratory pressure can be positive, atmospheric, or negative, allowing ventilation to occur above, at, or below the patient's normal FRC.

Clinicians' anecdotal observations of spontaneous expulsion of secretions during high-frequency ventilation have led to the development of several discrete secretion management program recommendations in which the chest is oscillated through two sets of cycles: several minutes at a high frequency of up to 999 per minute (usually 600 to 720 per minute) at an I:E ratio of 1:1, followed by 60 or 90 cycles per minute at an I:E ratio of 5:1. The setting can be changed according to the patient's need. Reports of efficacy of this or similar protocols for secretion management with the Hayek oscillator have yet to be published. It has been reported that high-frequency oscillation applied via the airway or via the chest wall and CPT have comparable augmenting effects on expectorated sputum.[31]

MetaNeb

With the MetaNeb device (**Figure 16-22**), aerosol is delivered with therapies intended to improve lung expansion and airway clearance. In the continuous positive expiratory pressure mode, aerosol delivery is combined with positive airway pressure. In the continuous high frequency oscillation mode, aerosol is delivered while oscillating the airways with pulses of positive pressure. A typical therapy session consists of 10 minutes of alternating sessions between the two modes.

Exercise

Exercise causes increased sputum production compared with rest.[32,33] Exercise augments bronchial hygiene and should be encouraged as tolerated; however, it should not substitute for other bronchial hygiene regimens.

Selection of Airway Clearance Technique

Several Cochrane reviews have evaluated airway clearance techniques for patients with cystic fibrosis.[34–40] In a review that compared chest physiotherapy with no chest physiotherapy for cystic fibrosis, it was shown that airway clearance techniques have short-term effects in terms of increasing mucus transport; no evidence was found on which to draw conclusions concerning the long-term effects.[41] A review that compared conventional CPT with other airway clearance techniques for cystic fibrosis was unable to demonstrate any advantage of conventional CPT over other airway clearance techniques in terms of respiratory function, but there was a trend for participants to prefer self-administered airway clearance techniques.[39] Another review concluded that there was no clear evidence that PEP was a more or less effective intervention overall than other

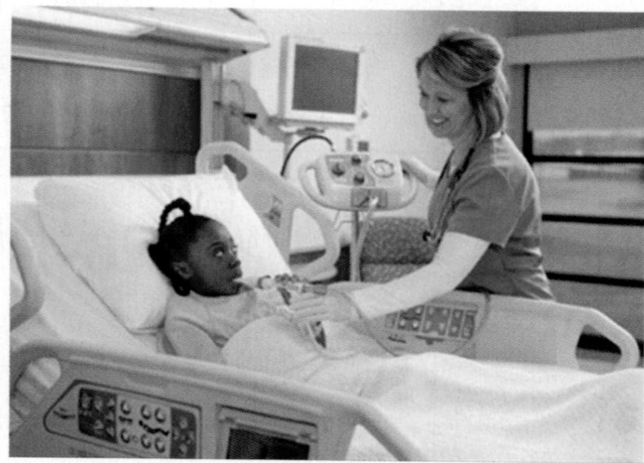

FIGURE 16-22 MetaNeb device.

forms of physiotherapy, but there was limited evidence that PEP was preferred by participants compared with other techniques. Similarly, there was no clear evidence that oscillation was a more or less effective intervention overall than other forms of physiotherapy.[40]

Guidelines of the Cystic Fibrosis Foundation recommend that airway clearance be performed on a regular basis in all patients with cystic fibrosis.[42] There is no airway clearance therapy, however, that has been demonstrated to be superior to others. For the individual, one form of airway clearance therapy may be superior to the others. The prescription of airway clearance therapy thus should be individualized based on factors such as age, patient preference, and adverse events, among others. Aerobic exercise is recommended for patients with cystic fibrosis as an adjunctive therapy for airway clearance and its additional benefits to overall health. One of the important considerations in selection of an airway clearance technique is the age of the patient (**Figure 16-23**), because some therapies are not appropriate for all age groups.

Guidelines of the British Thoracic Society (BTS) and the Association of Chartered Physiotherapists in Respiratory Care (ACPRC) have provided recommendations regarding airway clearance.[43] For patients in the intensive care unit, recommendations for airway clearance have been made by the European Respiratory Society and the European Society of Intensive Care Medicine Task Force on Physiotherapy for Critically Ill Patients.[44]

The American Association for Respiratory Care has published Clinical Practice Guidelines on the effectiveness of nonpharmacologic airway clearance therapies in hospitalized patients.[45] These guidelines were developed from a systematic review[46] with the purpose of determining whether the use of nonpharmacologic airway clearance therapy (ACT) improves oxygenation, reduces length of time on the ventilator, reduces stay in the ICU, resolves atelectasis/consolidation, and/or improves respiratory mechanics versus usual care. For hospitalized adult and pediatric patients without cystic fibrosis, (1) CPT is not recommended for the routine treatment of uncomplicated pneumonia; (2) ACT is not recommended for routine use in patients with COPD; (3) ACT may be considered in patients with COPD with symptomatic secretion retention, guided by patient preference, toleration, and effectiveness of therapy; (4) ACT is not recommended if the patient is able to mobilize secretions with cough, but instruction in effective cough technique may be useful. For adult and pediatric patients with neuromuscular disease, respiratory muscle weakness, or impaired cough, (1) cough assist techniques should be used in patients with neuromuscular disease, particularly when peak cough flow is < 270 L/min; CPT, positive expiratory pressure, intrapulmonary percussive ventilation, and high-frequency chest wall compression cannot be recommended, due to insufficient evidence. For postoperative adult and pediatric patients, (1) incentive spirometry is not recommended for routine, prophylactic use in postoperative patients; (2) early mobility and ambulation are recommended to reduce postoperative complications and promote airway clearance; (3) ACT is not recommended for routine postoperative care.

It has been suggested that the following hierarchy of questions might be asked when considering secretion clearance therapy for a patient.[45,47–49]

1. Is there a pathophysiologic rationale for use of the therapy? Is the patient experiencing difficulty clearing secretions? Are retained secretions affecting lung function in an important way, such as gas exchange or lung mechanics? Note that the production of large amounts of sputum does not necessarily mean that the patient is experiencing difficulty clearing sputum.
2. What is the potential for adverse effects from the therapy? Which therapy is likely to provide the greatest benefit with the least harm?

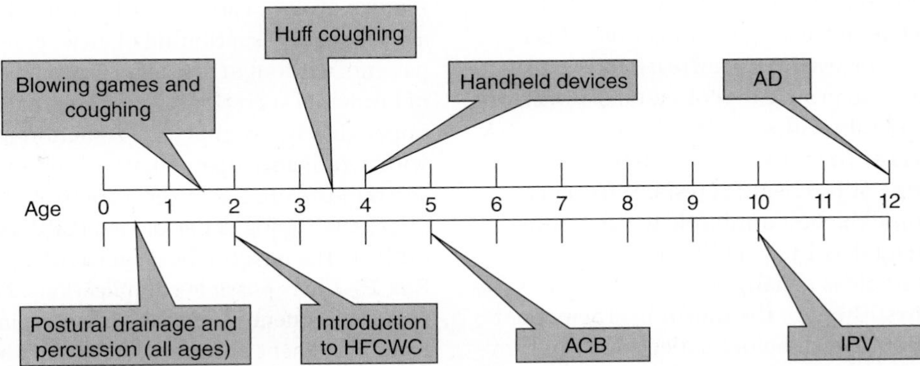

FIGURE 16-23 Various airway clearance techniques based on the patient's age and ability to perform the therapy. ACB, active cycle of breathing; AD, autogenic drainage; HFCWC, high frequency chest wall compression; IPV, intrapulmonary percussive ventilation.

Reproduced from Lester MK, Flume PA. Airway-clearance therapy guidelines and implementation. *Respir Care.* 2009;54:733–753. Reprinted with permission.

3. What is the cost of the equipment for this therapy? The cost of the device may not be covered by third-party insurers, resulting in considerable out-of-pocket expense for the patient or the hospital.
4. What are the preferences of the patient? Lacking evidence that any technique is superior to another, patient preference is an important consideration.

When a clinical decision is made to try a secretion clearance technique, a simple clinical trial can be conducted (*n*-of-1 trial).[50–52] Imagine that a decision is made to try PEP therapy for a patient with chronic obstructive pulmonary disease. The clinician and patient agree that a clinically useful outcome measure is fewer symptoms related to chest congestion and coughing up phlegm. A randomized controlled trial is designed. PEP is used for 2 weeks, a sham device is used for 2 weeks, and this process is repeated three times. The patient, who is naïve to the therapy, does not know which device is potentially therapeutic. The order of treatments is randomized (the patient flips a coin), and the sequence is repeated four times. Each day, the sputum produced during the therapy session is weighed. A diary also is kept, in which events such as chest infections and other symptoms are logged. At the end of 12 weeks, the results are analyzed (which may include statistical analysis), reviewed together by the clinician and patient, and a collaborative decision is made regarding the benefit of the therapy. In this manner, an objective decision is made regarding the benefits of this therapy for this individual patient.

Sputum Collection

A sputum sample can be used as a diagnostic test for pulmonary infection or cancer. A sputum culture is a test to detect and identify bacteria or fungi that are infecting the lungs. A sputum sample is placed into a sterile container and then sent to the microbiology laboratory for Gram stain, culture, and sensitivity. If there is no growth of bacteria or fungi, the culture is negative. If pathogenic organisms grow, the culture is positive and the type of bacteria or fungus is identified. Additional tests are done to determine which antibiotics are most effective in treating the infection. This is called *susceptibility* or *sensitivity testing*. Bacteria usually need 2 to 3 days to grow, fungi often take a week or longer to grow, and tuberculosis may take 6 weeks to grow. Any bacteria or fungi that grow will be identified under a microscope or by chemical tests. Sensitivity testing to determine the best antibiotic to use against the organism often takes 1 to 2 additional days.

The sputum sample is usually collected by coughing, most often first thing in the morning. The patient should not use mouthwash before collecting a sputum sample because it may contain antibacterial agents. Other factors that can affect the results of sputum culture include recent use of antibiotics, contamination of the sputum sample, an inadequate sputum sample, and waiting too long to deliver the sample to the laboratory.

Sputum cytology can be done when lung cancer is suspected or to detect certain noncancerous lung conditions. However, it is not used as a screening test for people at risk for developing lung cancer, such as smokers.

Induced Sputum

Aerosols of bland solutions, such as hypertonic saline, are used to stimulate cough and sputum production. Such therapy is used for diagnostic **sputum induction**. Hypertonic saline (e.g., 3% sodium chloride) is commonly used to induce sputum. Hypertonic saline on the mucosa moves water via osmosis from the airway into the secretions. This action causes a bronchorrhea, diluting the secretions and increasing their bulk to ease expectoration. The delivery of hypertonic saline by ultrasonic nebulizer is used to induce sputum for the diagnoses of *Pneumocystis carinii*, tuberculosis (acid-fast bacilli), *Legionella* species, and Mycobacteria atypical infections. The procedure involves the patient breathing hypertonic saline until about 5 mL of sputum is produced. It is important to instruct the patient to expectorate sputum from the lower respiratory tract; expectoration of saliva is not helpful. It is important for the respiratory therapist to observe appropriate infection control procedures during the procedure. Sputum induction is often repeated over 3 days. Induced sputum contains a higher proportion of viable cells than spontaneously produced sputum. Sputum induction is safe and well tolerated for patients with asthma and COPD.[53]

Tracheal Aspirate

When secretions in the airway cannot be effectively expelled with a cough, mechanical aspiration may be required. Tracheal aspiration for sputum collection uses a Lukens trap. This is a plastic collection unit designed for specimens collected from the lungs during suction (**Figure 16-24**). Patients with artificial airways almost always require suctioning of airway secretions. Some patients without artificial airways may need suctioning of bronchial secretions. To remove secretions from the upper airway, oropharyngeal suction may be performed with a Yankauer tip or suction catheter. To remove secretions from the lower respiratory tract, **nasotracheal suctioning** is performed (**CPG 16-1**). **Box 16-6** outlines the nasotracheal suctioning procedure; **Box 16-7** lists possible complications. Patients who require frequent nasotracheal suctioning may benefit from placement of a nasopharyngeal airway to reduce the trauma of repeated catheter insertion. Many patients respond to nasopharyngeal insertion of the catheter with a cough, which effectively removes secretions.

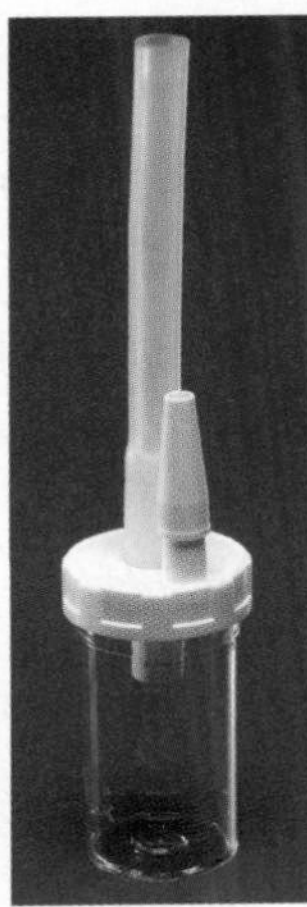

FIGURE 16-24 Lukens trap for sputum collection during tracheal suctioning.
Courtesy of Covidien. Used with permission.

Bronchoscopy

Diagnostic bronchoscopy is used with bronchoalveolar lavage (BAL) or protected specimen brush to obtain respiratory secretions for diagnostic purposes. This is commonly performed in the setting of suspected ventilator-associated pneumonia (VAP). Therapeutic bronchoscopy is used for removal of retained secretions, such as in hospitalized patients with new atelectasis or collapse of a lung segment, when less invasive procedures have failed.

Minibronchoalveolar Lavage

Minibronchoalveolar lavage (mini-BAL) is a nonbronchoscopic bedside method of performing a small-volume BAL for quantitative culture results to guide antibiotic therapy prescribed for patients suspected of VAP. These catheters are smaller in diameter than a bronchoscope, so the risk of complications is minimized. The procedure typically only requires the sampling catheter to be in the airway for 1 to 2 minutes. Moreover, lavage volumes are significantly smaller than those used in bronchoscopy, so there is less residual fluid in the lung, resulting in faster postprocedure patient recovery time.

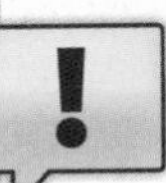

Respiratory Recap

Collection of Sputum for Diagnosis

- Cough
- Induced sputum
- Tracheal aspiration
- Bronchoscopy
- Mini-bronchoalveolar lavage
- Transtracheal aspiration

Some mini-BAL catheters are directional, meaning that they can be theoretically directed into one lung or the other. However, the procedure is blind, so the user has no means of confirming the actual catheter location. It also has been shown that a blindly inserted protected catheter yields similar results as a bronchoscopically directed catheter. Some mini-BAL catheters have a plugged tip to avoid upper airway contamination. In this design, there is a polyethylene-glycol tip that protects the inner sampling catheter from contamination (**Figure 16-25**). The mini-BAL procedure typically uses a small lavage volume of 20 to 60 mL in one to three aliquots. Mini-BAL performed by respiratory therapists has results comparable to bronchoscopy and is less costly (**Box 16-8**).[54–58]

Transtracheal Aspiration

Transtracheal aspiration, or transtracheal wash, is a technique in which a needle is inserted through the skin overlying the trachea and through the cricothyroid ligament. A catheter is introduced into the trachea and passed to the level of the tracheal bifurcation. Saline is then injected, withdrawn, and sent to the laboratory for histologic and microbiologic examination.

Lung Expansion Therapy

Incentive Spirometry

Incentive spirometry (IS) is a technique designed to mimic natural sighing or yawning maneuvers, also referred to as *sustained maximal inspiration* (**CPG 16-2**).[59] Because postoperative patients often adopt a pattern of rapid, shallow breathing, they should be encouraged to take 5 to 10 deep breaths every hour. IS provides patients with sensory feedback to quantify the depth of the breath. IS should provide patients with an objective comparison to the volumes (of flows) they were generating preoperatively, with the goal of attaining or returning to that preoperative volume in spite of the pain experienced. In addition, the IS device instruction should ideally include recording how long breaths are to be held, how many times the breaths were attempted, and how many times the patient succeeded in meeting his or her volume goals (**Box 16-9**).

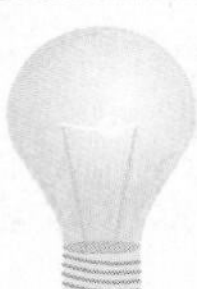

STOP AND THINK

You are asked for your suggestions to prevent postoperative pulmonary complications in the surgical ward. Would you recommend incentive spirometry? IPPB? Something else?

CLINICAL PRACTICE GUIDELINE 16-1

Nasotracheal Suctioning

Indications

- The need to maintain a patent airway and remove saliva, pulmonary secretions, blood, vomitus, or foreign material from the trachea in the presence of:
  - Inability to clear secretions when audible or visible evidence of secretions in the large/central airways persists in spite of patient's best cough effort (evidenced by one or more of the following: visible secretions in the airway; chest auscultation of coarse, gurgling breath sounds, rhonchi; or diminished breath sounds)
  - Feeling of secretions in the chest (increased tactile fremitus)
  - Suspected aspiration of gastric or upper airway secretions
  - Clinically apparent increased work of breathing
  - Deterioration of arterial blood gas values suggesting hypoxemia or hypercarbia
  - Chest radiographic evidence of retained secretions resulting in atelectasis or consolidation
- To stimulate cough or for unrelieved coughing
- To obtain a sputum sample for microbiologic or cytologic analysis

Contraindications

- Occluded nasal passages
- Nasal bleeding
- Epiglottitis or croup (absolute)
- Acute head, facial, or neck injury
- Coagulopathy or bleeding disorder
- Laryngospasm
- Irritable airway
- Upper respiratory tract infection
- Tracheal surgery
- Gastric surgery with high anastomosis
- Myocardial infarction
- Bronchospasm

Hazards and Complications

- Mechanical trauma
  - Laceration of nasal turbinates
  - Perforation of the pharynx
  - Nasal irritation/bleeding
  - Tracheitis
  - Mucosal hemorrhage
  - Uvular edema
- Hypoxia/hypoxemia
- Cardiac dysrhythmias/arrest
- Bradycardia
- Increase in blood pressure
- Hypotension
- Respiratory arrest
- Uncontrolled coughing
- Gagging/vomiting
- Laryngospasm
- Bronchoconstriction/bronchospasm
- Discomfort and pain
- Nosocomial infection
- Atelectasis
- Misdirection of catheter
- Increased intracranial pressure, intraventricular hemorrhage, exacerbation of cerebral edema
- Pneumothorax

Modified from AARC clinical practice guideline: nasotracheal suctioning—2004 revision and update. *Respir Care.* 2004;49:1080–1084. Reprinted with permission.

BOX 16-6

Procedure for Nasotracheal Suctioning

1. Assess patient and preoxygenate.
2. Assemble equipment and select appropriate suction pressure.
3. Determine which nasal passage is most patent.
4. Lubricate suction catheter.
5. Gently insert catheter through the nose to the level of the glottis; if obstruction is encountered, use other nostril.
6. During inspiration, pass the catheter into the trachea.
7. Assess for signs that the catheter is in the trachea: airflow through the catheter (listening over thumb port), patient coughing.
8. If catheter is not in the trachea, withdraw to the level of the pharynx, assess patient, and re-advance catheter.
9. Insert catheter until resistance is met, then withdraw by 1 to 2 cm, apply suction for 1 to 2 seconds, release suction, withdraw catheter several centimeters, and repeat until catheter is withdrawn from the airway; do not exceed 15 seconds.
10. Assess patient and need to repeat procedure.

BOX 16-7

Complications of Nasotracheal Suctioning

Trauma to upper airway and pain
Hypoxemia
Cardiac dysrhythmia, bradycardia, cardiac arrest
Hypertension or hypotension
Respiratory arrest
Uncontrolled coughing
Gagging/vomiting
Laryngospasm or bronchospasm
Nosocomial infection
Misdirection of catheter
Increased intracranial pressure

Objectives of IS are to increase transpulmonary pressure and inspiratory volumes to near-preoperative vital capacity, improve inspiratory muscle performance, and reestablish the normal pattern of periodic deep breathing. It should not be used as the sole treatment for major lung collapse or consolidation, but rather as a part of a more comprehensive program of lung reexpansion. Because IS requires patient cooperation, as well as the ability to understand and demonstrate proper use of the device, it is not a viable therapeutic option for the obtunded, confused, or uncooperative patient.

Most IS devices direct the patient's inspiratory flow through a tube to lift one or more light balls (or disks). The higher the patient's inspiratory flow, the higher the ball is raised or the greater the number

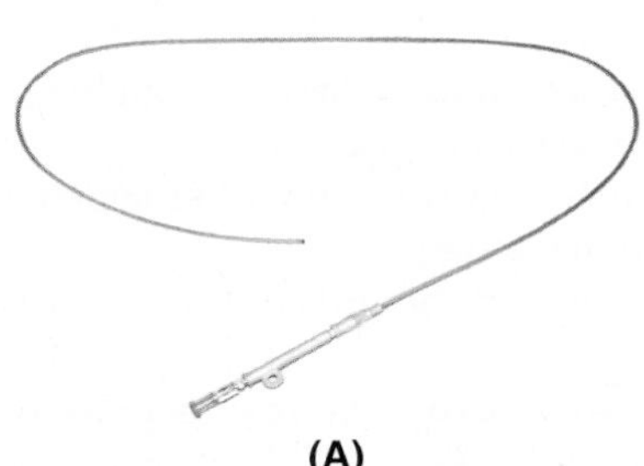

(A)

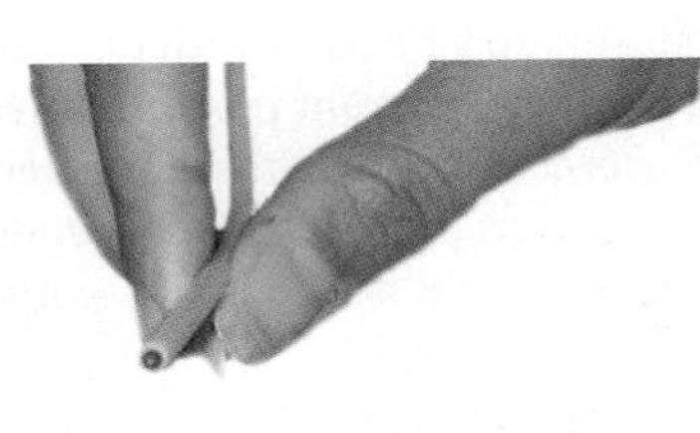

(B)

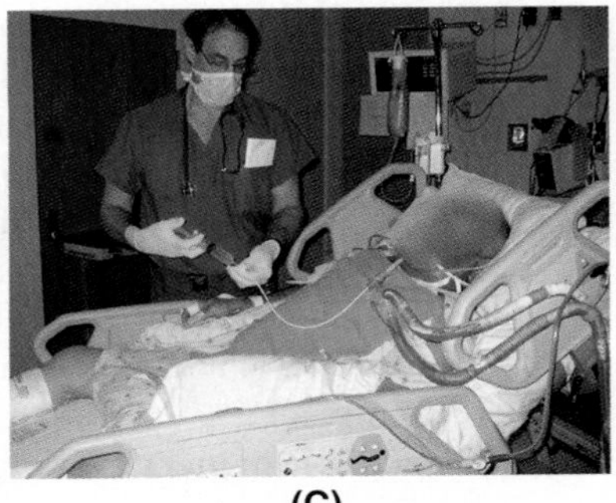

(C)

FIGURE 16-25 (**A**) Protected catheter for minibronchoalveolar lavage (mini-BAL). (**B**) Catheter tip. The red plug is removed to allow the inner protected catheter to exit. (**C**) Respiratory therapist performing mini-BAL procedure.

(**A**) courtesy of Prodimed; (**B** and **C**) courtesy of KOL Bio-Medical Instruments, Inc.

BOX 16-8

Procedure for Minibronchoalveolar Lavage

1. Place the patient on 100% oxygen.
2. Assess for sedation level; if patient is agitated, obtain order for sedation.
3. Place the bronchoscopy adapter on the end of the endotracheal tube.
4. Suction if there are a lot of tracheal secretions.
5. Place the bed in the flat position. This makes it easier and keeps the instilled saline from moving away from the catheter tip.
6. Open the catheter using aseptic technique, but do not remove from packaging.
7. Open the sterile field.
8. Open three syringes onto the sterile field.
9. Open the bottle of saline solution and pour it into a sterile bowl. Don the sterile gloves.
10. Pick up one of the syringes and fill it with 20 mL sterile saline and a 10 mL air bolus. Repeat with the other two syringes.
11. Insert the blunt end of the catheter (the end with the red plug) into the endotracheal tube via the bronchoscopy adapter. As you advance the catheter, remove the polyethylene sheath covering the white outer catheter, taking care not to dislodge the spacer for the inner cannula.
12. Slowly advance the catheter into the lungs until you feel a resistance. The CombiCath should usually be advanced past the 40-cm mark to pass the carina.
13. Pull the catheter back about 3 cm.
14. Remove the spacer at the proximal end of the catheter by sliding it off from the side channel.
15. Gently push the newly exposed inner cannula into the white portion of the catheter up to the hub of the Luer connector.
16. Connect the saline-filled syringe to the catheter.
17. Instill all 20 mL of the saline along with the 5 mL air bolus to ensure that all of the saline is pushed through the catheter.
18. Draw back on the syringe and retrieve the aspirate sample. *Note:* The size of the sample will be approximately 3 to 5 mL. A high-quality sample will have stable bubbles at the top of the meniscus, representing the presence of surfactant.
19. Assess the patient's vital signs.
20. Repeat with syringes 2 and 3. The procedure should be stopped if the patient is decompensating or the first or second instillation provided a good-quality sample.
21. Gently withdraw the entire catheter and syringe, taking care not to lose the sample.
22. Decant the samples into a sterile sputum trap. Send to laboratory for appropriate analysis.
23. Suction the patient if necessary. Return the bed to its original position. Return the ventilator to the original settings.
24. Document procedure.

CLINICAL PRACTICE GUIDELINE 16-2

Incentive Spirometry

The following recommendations are made regarding the use of incentive spirometry.

1. Incentive spirometry alone is not recommended for routine use in the preoperative and postoperative settings to prevent postoperative pulmonary complications.
2. It is recommended that incentive spirometry be used with deep breathing techniques, directed coughing, early mobilization, and optimal analgesia to prevent postoperative pulmonary complications.
3. It is suggested that deep breathing exercises provide the same benefit as incentive spirometry in the preoperative and postoperative setting to prevent postoperative pulmonary complications.
4. Routine use of incentive spirometry to prevent atelectasis in patients after upper-abdominal surgery is not recommended.
5. Routine use of incentive spirometry to prevent atelectasis after coronary artery bypass graft surgery is not recommended.
6. It is suggested that a volume-oriented device be selected as an incentive spirometry device.

Modified from AARC clinical practice guideline: incentive spirometry. *Respir Care*. 2011;56:1600–1604. Reprinted with permission.

BOX 16-9

Procedure for Incentive Spirometry

1. Explain to the patient the importance of deep breathing and coughing.
2. Establish the volume goal for incentive spirometry.
3. Assist the patient to a sitting or semi-Fowler position.
4. Instruct or assist the patient to splint incision when appropriate.
5. Instruct patient to do the following:
   a. Place the spirometer on a flat surface or hold in an upright position.
   b. Place lips firmly around the mouthpiece.
   c. After a normal exhalation, inhale slowly through the mouthpiece, raising the flow/volume indicator while taking as deep a breath as possible.
   d. Hold breath for 3 to 5 seconds.
   e. Remove mouthpiece and exhale normally.
   f. Relax and breathe normally for several breaths.
   g. Repeat the maneuver for 10 breaths each session.
6. Have patient repeat series of breaths once each hour while awake.
7. Visit patient periodically to reinforce instruction.
8. Document procedure and patient response in the medical record.

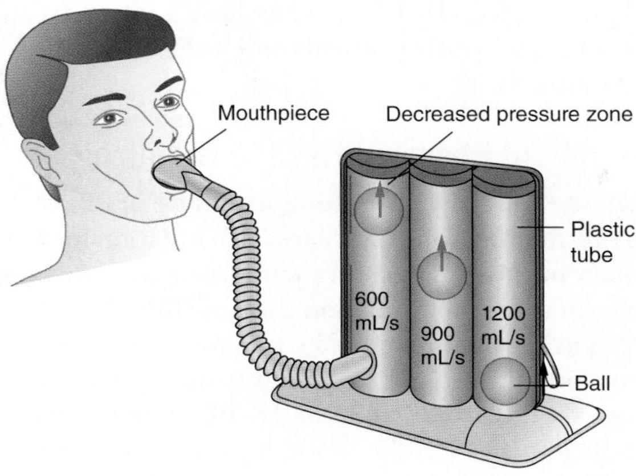

(A)

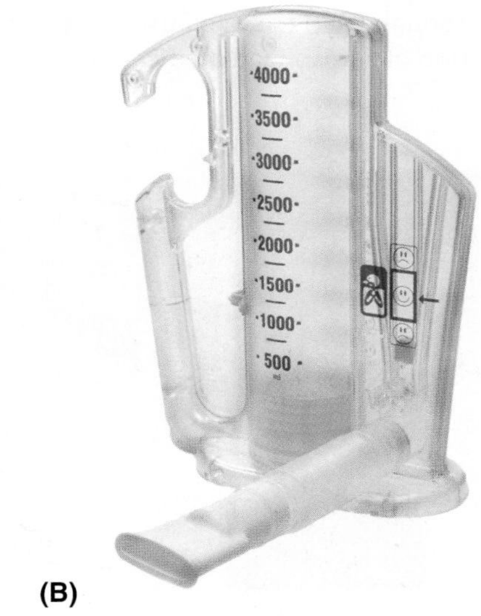

(B)

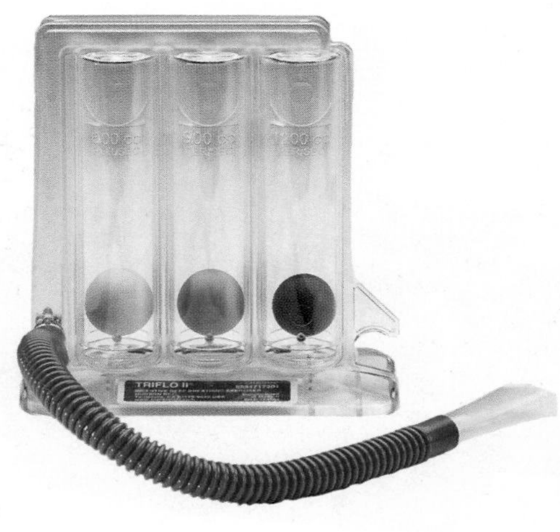

(C)

FIGURE 16-26 (**A**) Flow-oriented incentive spirometer. (**B** and **C**) Commercially available incentive spirometers.

(**A**) adapted from Eubanks DH, Bone RC. *Comprehensive Respiratory Care.* Mosby; 1985; (**B**) © Robert Byron/Dreamstime.com; (**C**) courtesy of Teleflex Incorporated. Unauthorized use prohibited.

of balls that are raised (**Figure 16-26**). The longer the flow is maintained, the larger the volume, so the patient is encouraged to take slow, deep breaths. Unfortunately, high flows can be generated (with low volumes) to raise the flow indicator to target levels without the patient meeting therapeutic volume or breath-holding objectives.

Evidence suggests that deep breathing alone, without mechanical aids, may be as beneficial as IS in preventing or reversing pulmonary complications, and controversy exists concerning overuse of IS. Mounting

Respiratory Recap

Inflation Therapy

- Incentive spirometry
- Intermittent positive pressure breathing

evidence suggests that IS may not have a role in treatment of postoperative patients and it should not be used routinely.[45,59]

Intermittent Positive Pressure Breathing

Intermittent positive pressure breathing (IPPB) is short-term or episodic mechanical ventilation for the primary purpose of assisting ventilation and providing short-duration hyperinflation therapy (**CPG 16-3**).[60] IPPB is usually administered with pneumatically driven, pressure-triggered, and pressure-cycled ventilators (**Figure 16-27** and **Box 16-10**). IPPB was first described in 1947. In the 1950s, it gained popularity as a method to treat and prevent postoperative atelectasis. In the 1960s, IPPB became a popular therapy for patients with pulmonary disease. In the 1970s, IPPB came under scrutiny both scientifically and by health-care payers. Although IPPB has been used as a method for administration of aerosolized medication, it has no advantage over nebulizers or metered dose inhalers. All of the mechanical effects of IPPB are short lived, lasting an hour or less after the treatment. Efficacy of IPPB for ventilation and aerosol delivery is technique dependent (e.g., coordination, breathing pattern, selection of appropriate inspiratory flow, peak pressure, inspiratory hold). Efficacy is dependent on the design of the device (e.g., flow, volume, pressure capability) and on the aerosol output and particle size.

Assessment of the need for IPPB should include evidence of atelectasis, reduced pulmonary function precluding an effective cough, neuromuscular disorders, or kyphoscoliosis with decreased lung volumes. IPPB may be applicable in situations of fatigue or muscle weakness with impending respiratory failure, in the presence of acute severe bronchospasm, and in COPD exacerbation that fails to respond to other therapy. IPPB should be volume oriented, with tidal volume during IPPB adjusted to deliver breaths that are at least

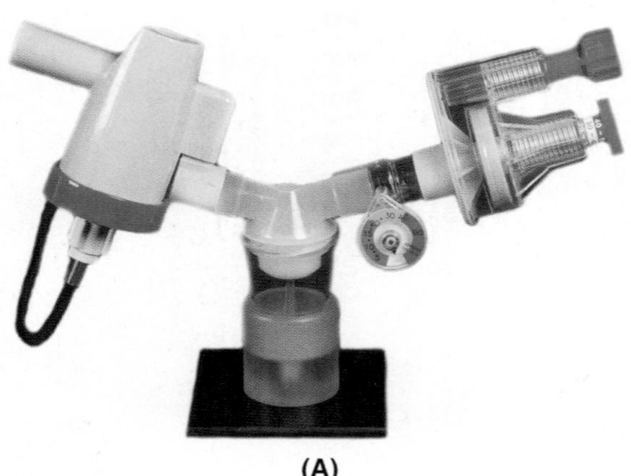

(A)

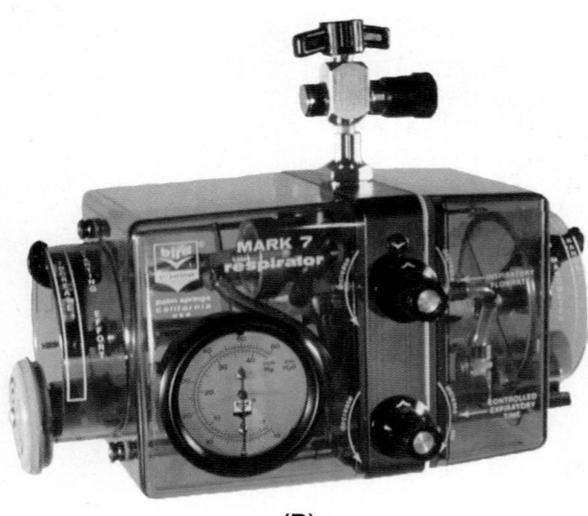

(B)

FIGURE 16-27 (**A**) VORTRAN® intermittent positive pressure breathing (IPPB) device. (**B**) Bird Mark 7 for IPPB therapy.

(A) courtesy of VORTRAN® Medical Technology 1, Inc., Sacramento, CA; (B) courtesy of Dr. Pamela Bird, Percussionaire Corporation.

BOX 16-10

Procedure for Intermittent Positive Pressure Breathing (IPPB) Therapy

1. Assess the need for IPPB and determine whether another therapy might be equally efficacious or superior.
2. Assemble necessary equipment.
3. Explain therapy to patient.
4. Determine appropriate interface: mouthpiece, lip seal, or mask.
5. Instruct patient to do the following:
   a. Sit comfortably.
   b. If using a mask, apply it tightly but comfortably over the nose and mouth; if mouthpiece is used, place lips firmly around it and breathe through mouth.
   c. Begin breathing to trigger the IPPB machine.
   d. Allow the machine to passively inflate the lungs to a volume that is larger than normal.
6. Make appropriate adjustments on the IPPB machine:
   a. Flow for I:E ratio of approximately 1:3
   b. Pressure to deliver an appropriate volume
7. Monitor inspiratory time and observe patient to prevent hyperventilation.
8. Encourage the patient to rest and cough as needed; do not exceed 20 minutes of treatment.
9. Rinse mouthpiece or mask, nebulizer, and manifold assembly with sterile water.
10. Document settings used, volume achieved, and patient response.

CLINICAL PRACTICE GUIDELINE 16-3

Intermittent Positive Pressure Breathing

Indications

- The need to improve lung expansion; the presence of clinically important pulmonary atelectasis when other forms of therapy have been unsuccessful (e.g., incentive spirometry, chest physiotherapy, deep breathing exercises, positive airway pressure) or the patient cannot cooperate; inability to clear secretions adequately because of pathologic process that severely limits the ability to ventilate or cough effectively; and failure to respond to other modes of treatment.
- The need for short-term ventilatory support for patients who are hypoventilating as an alternative to tracheal intubation and continuous ventilatory support.
- The need to deliver aerosol medication. Intermittent positive pressure breathing (IPPB) may be used to deliver aerosol medications to patients with fatigue as a result of ventilatory muscle weakness or chronic conditions in which intermittent ventilatory support is indicated.

Contraindications

- Pneumothorax
- Intracranial pressure >15 mm Hg
- Hemodynamic instability
- Recent surgery to face or mouth or skull
- Tracheoesophageal fistula
- Recent esophageal surgery
- Active hemoptysis
- Nausea
- Air swallowing
- Active untreated tuberculosis
- Radiographic evidence of bleb
- Singultations (hiccups)

Hazards and Complications

- Increased airway resistance
- Barotrauma
- Nosocomial infection
- Hypocarbia
- Hemoptysis
- Hyperoxia when oxygen is the gas source
- Gastric distention
- Impaction of secretions associated with inadequately humidified gas mixture
- Psychologic dependence
- Impedance of venous return
- Exacerbation of hypoxemia
- Hypoventilation
- Increased mismatch of ventilation and perfusion
- Air trapping

Modified from AARC clinical practice guideline: incentive spirometry. *Respir Care*. 2003;48:540–546. Reprinted with permission.

25% larger than the patient's tidal volume. The effects of IPPB can be assessed by improved secretion clearance, breath sounds, chest x-ray film, and dyspnea. IPPB has not been shown to have any benefit greater than other lung expansion techniques in spontaneously breathing patients. Its use for lung expansion should be considered only after other alternatives have been exhausted.

Key Points

- Mucociliary transport is responsible for normal clearance of secretions from the lower respiratory tract.
- Cough is responsible for secretion clearance in acute and chronic respiratory disease.
- Conventional chest physiotherapy consists of postural drainage, percussion, and vibration.
- Active cycle of breathing techniques consist of breathing control, thoracic expansion control, and forced expiratory technique.
- Autogenic drainage aims to achieve the highest possible airflow in different generations of bronchi to move secretions.
- Positive expiratory pressure, oscillating positive expiratory pressure, intrapulmonary percussive ventilation, and external chest wall compression are techniques that can be used for airway clearance.
- Techniques for sputum collection include cough, induced sputum, tracheal aspiration, bronchoscopy, mini-bronchoalveolar lavage, and transtracheal aspiration.
- Airway suctioning, nasotracheal suctioning, and bronchoscopy are used to mechanically clear secretions from the lower respiratory tract.
- Incentive spirometry is used to facilitate deep breathing in postoperative patients.
- Intermittent positive pressure breathing is used for short-term hyperinflation therapy.

References

1. Rogers DF. Physiology of airway mucus secretion and pathophysiology of hypersecretion. *Respir Care*. 2007;52:1134–1149.
2. Van der Schans CP. Bronchial mucus transport. *Respir Care*. 2007;52:1150–1158.
3. King M. Viscoelastic properties of airway mucus. *Fed Proc*. 1980;39:3080–3085.
4. King M. Rheological requirements for optimal clearance of secretions: ciliary transport versus cough. *Eur J Respir Dis*. 1980;110(Suppl):39–45.
5. King M. Is cystic fibrosis mucus abnormal? *Pediatr Res*. 1981;15:120–122.
6. King M, Kelly S, Cosio M. Alteration of airway reactivity by mucus. *Respir Physiol*. 1985;62:47–59.
7. Warwick WJ. Mechanisms of mucus transport. *Eur J Resp Dis*. 1983;127(Suppl 64):162–167.
8. Volpe MS, Adams AB, Amato MB, Marini JJ. Ventilation patterns influence airway secretion movement. *Respir Care*. 2008;53:1287–1294.
9. Li Bassi G, Saucedo L, Marti JD, et al. Effects of duty cycle and positive end-expiratory pressure on mucus clearance during mechanical ventilation. *Crit Care Med*. 2012;40:895–902.
10. Irwin RS, Madison JM. The diagnosis and treatment of cough. *N Engl J Med*. 2000;343:1715–1721.
11. Irwin RS. Complications of cough: ACCP evidence-based clinical practice guidelines. *Chest*. 2006;129(Suppl 1):54S–58S.
12. Fink JB. Forced expiratory technique, directed cough, and autogenic drainage. *Respir Care*. 2007;52:1210–1223.
13. Lester MK, Flume PA. Airway-clearance therapy guidelines and implementation. *Respir Care*. 2009;54:733–753.
14. Miller S, Hall DO, Clayton CB, et al. Chest physiotherapy in cystic fibrosis. A comparative study of autogenic drainage and the active cycle of breathing techniques with postural drainage. *Thorax*. 1995;50:165–169.
15. Homnick DN. Mechanical insufflation–exsufflation for airway mucus clearance. *Respir Care*. 2007;52:1296–1305; discussion 1306–1307.
16. Sancho J, Servera E, Díaz J, Marín J. Efficacy of mechanical-insufflation-exsufflation in medically stable patients with amyotrophic lateral sclerosis. *Chest*. 2004;125:1400–1405.
17. Elkins MR, Robinson M, Rose BR, et al. A controlled trial of long-term inhaled hypertonic saline in patients with cystic fibrosis. *N Engl J Med*. 2006;354:229–240.
18. Valderramas SR, Atallah AN. Effectiveness and safety of hypertonic saline inhalation combined with exercise training in patients with chronic obstructive pulmonary disease: a randomized trial. *Respir Care*. 2009;54:327–333.
19. Rogers DF. Mucoactive agents for airway mucus hypersecretory diseases. *Respir Care*. 2007;52:1193–1197.
20. Restrepo RD. Inhaled adrenergics and anticholinergics in obstructive lung disease: do they enhance mucociliary clearance? *Respir Care*. 2007;52:1159–1173.
21. van der Schans CP. Conventional chest physical therapy for obstructive lung disease. *Respir Care*. 2007;52:1198–1209.
22. Oermann CM, Swank PR, Sockrider MM. Validation of an instrument measuring patient satisfaction with chest physiotherapy techniques in cystic fibrosis. *Chest*. 2000;118:92–97.
23. Wallis C, Prasad A. Who needs chest physiotherapy? Moving from anecdote to evidence. *Arch Dis Child*. 1999;80:393–397.
24. van der Schans CP, Peris DA, Postma DS. Effect of manual percussion on tracheobronchial clearance in patients with chronic airflow obstruction and excessive tracheobronchial secretion. *Thorax*. 1986;41:448–452.
25. Clarke RCN, Kelly BE, Convery PN, et al. Ventilatory characteristics in mechanically ventilated patients during manual hyperventilation for chest physiotherapy. *Anaesthesia*. 1999;54:936–940.
26. Fauroux B, Boule M, Lofaso F, et al. Chest physiotherapy in cystic fibrosis: improved tolerance with nasal pressure support ventilation. *Pediatrics*. 1999;103:658–659.
27. Alexander E, Weingarten S, Mohsenifar Z. Clinical strategies to reduce utilization of chest physiotherapy without compromising patient care. *Chest*. 1996;110:430–432.
28. Myers TR. Positive expiratory pressure and oscillatory positive expiratory pressure therapies. *Respir Care*. 2007;52:1308–1327.
29. Chatburn RL. High-frequency assisted airway clearance. *Respir Care*. 2007;52:1224–1237.
30. Dosman CF, Jones RL. High-frequency chest compression: a summary of the literature. *Can Respir J*. 2005;12:37–41.
31. Scherer TA, Barandun J, Martinez E, et al. Effect of high-frequency oral airway and chest wall oscillation and conventional chest physical therapy on expectoration in patients with stable cystic fibrosis. *Chest*. 1998;113:1019–1027.
32. Zach MS, Purrer B, Oberwaldner B. Effect of swimming on forced expiration and sputum clearance in cystic fibrosis. *Lancet*. 1981;ii:1201–1203.
33. Bilton D, Dodd M, Webb AK. Evaluation of exercise as an adjunct to physiotherapy in the treatment of cystic fibrosis. *Thorax*. 1989;44:859.
34. van der Schans C, Prasad A, Main E. Chest physiotherapy compared to no chest physiotherapy for cystic fibrosis. *Cochrane Database Syst Rev*. 2000;2:CD001401.

35. Jones AP, Rowe H. Bronchopulmonary hygiene physical therapy for chronic obstructive pulmonary disease. *Cochrane Database Syst Rev*. 2000;2:CD000045.
36. van der Schans C, Prasad A, Main E. Conventional chest physiotherapy compared to any form of chest physiotherapy for cystic fibrosis. *Cochrane Database Syst Rev*. 2000;2.
37. Flenady VJ, Gray PH. Chest physiotherapy for preventing morbidity in babies being extubated from mechanical ventilation. *Cochrane Database Syst Rev*. 2000;2:CD000283.
38. Yang M, Yan Y, Yin X, et al. Chest physiotherapy for pneumonia in adults. *Cochrane Database Syst Rev.* 2013;2:CD006338.
39. Elkins MR, Jones A, van der Schans C. Positive expiratory pressure physiotherapy for airway clearance in people with cystic fibrosis. *Cochrane Database Syst Rev*. 2006;19:CD003147.
40. Morrison L, Agnew J. Oscillating devices for airway clearance in people with cystic fibrosis. *Cochrane Database Syst Rev.* 2009;1:CD006842.
41. Oberwaldner B. Physiotherapy for airway clearance in paediatrics. *Eur Respir J*. 2000;15:196–204.
42. Flume PA, Robinson KA, O'Sullivan BP, et al. Cystic fibrosis pulmonary guidelines: airway clearance therapies. *Respir Care*. 2009;54:522–537.
43. Bott J, Blumenthal S, Buxton M, et al. Guidelines for the physiotherapy management of the adult, medical, spontaneously breathing patient. *Thorax*. 2009;64(Suppl 1):1–51.
44. Gosselink R, Bott J, Johnson M, et al. Physiotherapy for adult patients with critical illness: recommendations of the European Respiratory Society and European Society of Intensive Care Medicine Task Force on Physiotherapy for Critically Ill Patients. *Intensive Care Med*. 2008;34:1188–1199.
45. Strickland SL, Rubin BK, Drescher GS, et al. AARC clinical practice guideline: effectiveness of nonpharmacologic airway clearance therapies in hospitalized patients. *Respir Care*. 2013;58:2187–2193.
46. Andrews J, Sathe NA, Krishnaswami S, McPheeters ML. Nonpharmacologic airway clearance techniques in hospitalized patients: a systematic review. *Respir Care*. 2013;58:2160–2186.
47. Hess DR. The evidence for secretion clearance techniques. *Respir Care*. 2001;46:1276–1293.
48. Hess DR. Secretion clearance techniques: absence of proof or proof of absence? *Respir Care*. 2002;47:757–758.
49. Hess DR. Airway clearance: physiology, pharmacology, techniques, and practice. *Respir Care*. 2007;52:1392–1396.
50. Hess DR. The evidence for secretion clearance techniques. *Respir Care*. 2001;46:1276–1293.
51. Hess DR. Secretion clearance techniques: absence of proof or proof of absence? *Respir Care*. 2002;47:757–758.
52. Hess DR. Airway clearance: physiology, pharmacology, techniques, and practice. *Respir Care*. 2007;52:1392–1396.
53. Bhowmik A, Seemungal TA, Sapsford RJ, et al. Comparison of spontaneous and induced sputum for investigation of airway inflammation in chronic obstructive pulmonary disease. *Thorax*. 1998;53:953–956.
54. Kollef MH, Bock KR, Richards RD, et al. The safety and diagnostic accuracy of minibronchoalveolar lavage in patients with suspected ventilator-associated pneumonia. *Ann Intern Med*. 1995;122:743–748.
55. Campbell GD Jr. Blinded invasive diagnostic procedures in ventilator-associated pneumonia. *Chest*. 2000;117(Suppl 2):207S–211S.
56. Fujitani S, Cohen-Melamed MH, Tuttle RP, et al. Comparison of semi-quantitative endotracheal aspirates to quantitative non-bronchoscopic bronchoalveolar lavage in diagnosing ventilator-associated pneumonia. *Respir Care*. 2009;54:1453–1461.
57. Tuttle RP, Cohen MH, Augustine AJ, et al. Utilizing simulation technology for competency skills assessment and a comparison of traditional methods of training to simulation-based training. *Respir Care*. 2007;52:263–270.
58. Boots RJ, Phillips GE, George N, Faoagali JL. Surveillance culture utility and safety using low-volume blind bronchoalveolar lavage in the diagnosis of ventilator-associated pneumonia. *Respirology*. 2008;13:87–96.
59. Restrepo RD, Wettstein R, Wittnebel L, Tracy M. Incentive spirometry: 2011. *Respir Care*. 2011;56:1600–1604.
60. Sorenson HM, Shelledy DC. AARC clinical practice guideline. intermittent positive pressure breathing—2003 revision and update. *Respir Care*. 2003;48:540–546.

CHAPTER

17

Airway Management

John D. Davies, Alexander S. Niven, Dean R. Hess

OUTLINE

OBJECTIVES

1. Demonstrate use of manual airway maneuvers.
2. Compare oropharyngeal and nasopharyngeal airways.
3. Demonstrate the techniques for inserting oropharyngeal and nasopharyngeal airways.
4. Describe the construction of an endotracheal tube.
5. Identify key roles and responsibilities for the airway management team.
6. Describe the technique for orotrachea and nasotracheal intubation.
7. Demonstrate the technique used to secure an endotracheal tube.
8. Demonstrate the technique used to measure cuff pressure.
9. Discuss the approach to evaluation and management of the difficult airway
10. Compare conventional and percutaneous tracheostomy.
11. Compare various designs of tracheostomy tubes.
12. Compare conventional and closed suction catheters.
13. Describe techniques used to prevent complications from suctioning.
14. Discuss the important points of extubation and decannulation.

KEY TERMS

airway cuff
bite block
cricothyrotomy
decannulation
endotracheal intubation
endotracheal tube
extraglottic airway
extubation
gum elastic bougie
laryngeal mask airway (LMA)
laryngoscope
nasopharyngeal airway
nasotracheal intubation
oropharyngeal airway
orotracheal intubation
speaking valve
suction catheter
team resource management
tracheostomy tube
tube exchanger
video laryngoscope

Introduction

Airway management is an important aspect of respiratory care. Manual airway maneuvers, intubation and airway maintenance can be high risk and unpredictable, underlining the importance of a thoughtful, interdisciplinary approach to maximize patient outcomes and safety. This chapter provides a systematic overview of the planning, preparation, teamwork, and technical skills required to effectively care for patients with airway issues.

Oropharyngeal Airways

The **oropharyngeal airway** is useful to promote airway patency in patients without a gag reflex. It is inserted into the mouth between the lips and teeth and extends from the lips to the pharynx, following the natural curvature of the tongue and palate, without entering the larynx or esophagus (**Figure 17-1**). Oropharyngeal airways are usually made of hard plastic and are relatively rigid.

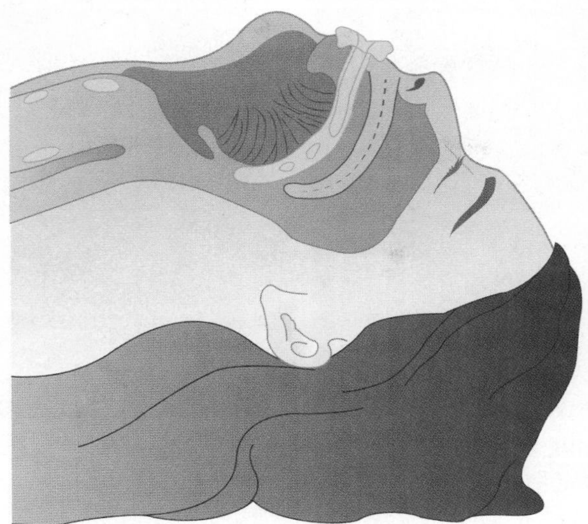

FIGURE 17-1 Oropharyngeal airway in place.

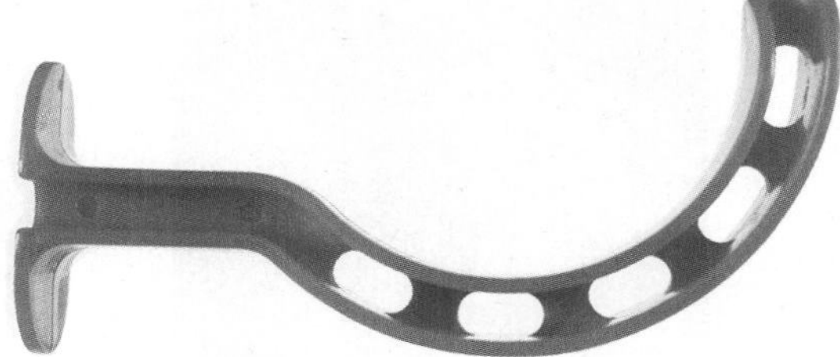

FIGURE 17-2 Berman airway.

They generally consist of a flange, a bite portion (body), and an air channel. The flange at the mouth opening prevents the airway from falling back and obstructing the airway. It also provides a means to stabilize the jaw against the lips or teeth. The bite portion, which fits between the upper and lower teeth or gums, is straight and firm enough to prevent the patient from obstructing airflow by biting down. The air channel, or curved portion, extends upward and backward along the curve of the tongue, pulling it and the epiglottis away from the posterior pharyngeal wall to improve airway patency.

Oropharyngeal airways are designed to open and stabilize the airway by preventing the tongue from falling into the hypopharynx and partly or completely obstructing the upper airway. Use of an oropharyngeal airway may be indicated during mask or mouth-to-tube ventilation. Oropharyngeal airways allow ready access to the mouth and pharynx for suctioning and may be inserted instead of a **bite block** to prevent a patient from biting an oral **endotracheal tube**. These airways also may help to optimize mask ventilation by improving airway patency. It is important to note that because of its placement location, an oropharyngeal airway may gag a semicomatose or an alert patient, which could induce vomiting and increase the risk of aspiration.

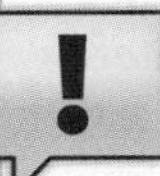

Respiratory Recap

Oropharyngeal Airways

- Prevent upper airway obstruction
- May be used as a bite block
- May make mask ventilation more effective
- Should not be used in semicomatose or alert patients

Types

The Berman airway (**Figure 17-2**) has a flange at the oral end, a rigid support beam through the center, and open sides. The open sides allow suctioning and serve as air channels. The center may have openings for suctioning should the airway become lodged sideways in the mouth. The advantages of the Berman airway are ease of cleaning and the dual side air channels, which are less likely to be obstructed by mucus or foreign bodies. Because the Berman airway is uniformly rigid throughout, it is less susceptible to airway occlusion by a patient's bite than the Guedel airway.

The Guedel airway (**Figure 17-3**) has a large flange at the oral end and a supportive bite section, and the curved portion that follows the curve of the tongue is made of a semirigid material. The Guedel airway differs from the Berman airway in that it is reinforced only in the bite region. This may pose a problem if a patient bites down on the Guedel airway before it is completely inserted, both preventing complete insertion and creating the possibility of the unreinforced portion occluding the airway. The Guedel airway also differs from the Berman airway in that it has an enclosed tubular channel to facilitate air exchange and suctioning.

Insertion

Before inserting an oropharyngeal airway, there should be an assessment for proper sizing. This is

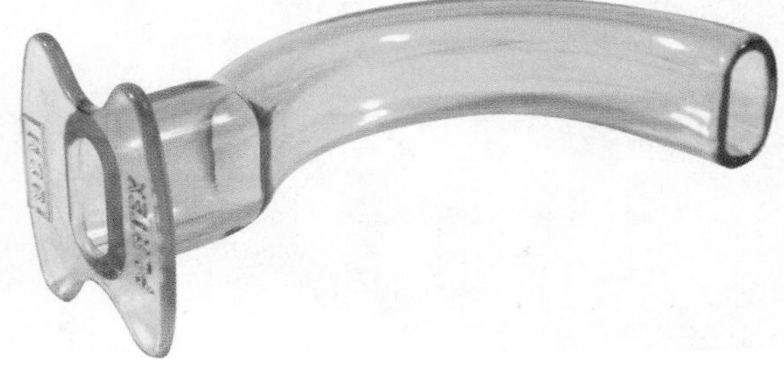

FIGURE 17-3 Guedel airway.

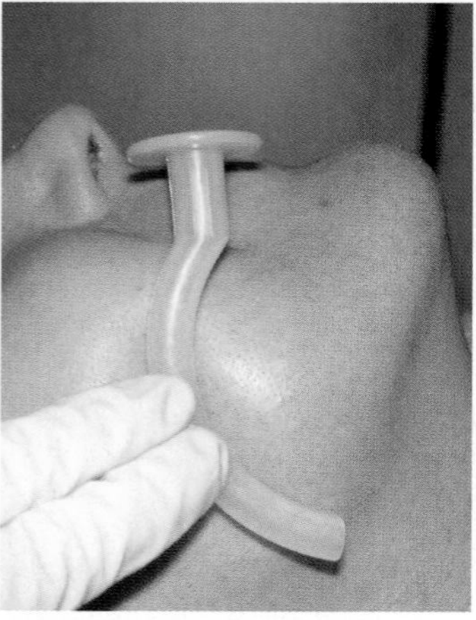

FIGURE 17-4 Sizing the oropharyngeal airway.

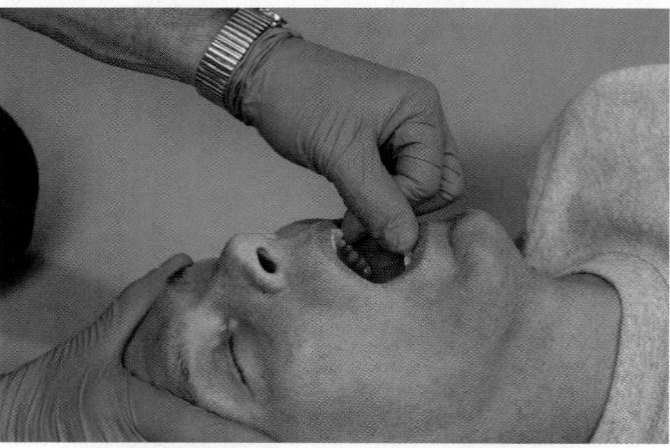

FIGURE 17-6 Cross-finger technique to open the mouth.

accomplished by placing the device on the patient's cheek with the flange parallel to his or her front teeth. The tip of the oropharyngeal airway should reach no further than the pinna of the ear (**Figure 17-4**). If the oropharyngeal airway selected is too large, its tip may press the epiglottis against the posterior pharyngeal wall or the larynx, obstructing both the device and the patient's airway. If the airway is inserted improperly or is too small, the tongue may be pushed against the posterior pharynx, causing obstruction. Oropharyngeal airways come in a variety of different sizes to accommodate adults, children, and infants (**Figure 17-5**).

To insert an oropharyngeal airway, stand at the patient's head, hyperextend the head and neck, and use the cross-finger technique to open the mouth (**Figure 17-6**). One method of insertion is to turn the airway 180 degrees from its resting position as it is passed over the tongue to avoid pushing the tongue back into the pharynx. When the tip of the airway reaches the uvula, the airway is rotated 180 degrees so that the tip is positioned behind the tongue and facing the larynx (**Figure 17-7 A**). A second method is, the airway can be inserted from the lateral aspect of the mouth followed by a 90 degree rotation to the position in which it will rest (**Figure 17-7 B**). Once it is in place, the airway should be assessed for proper size and position through determination of whether it facilitates unobstructed breathing.

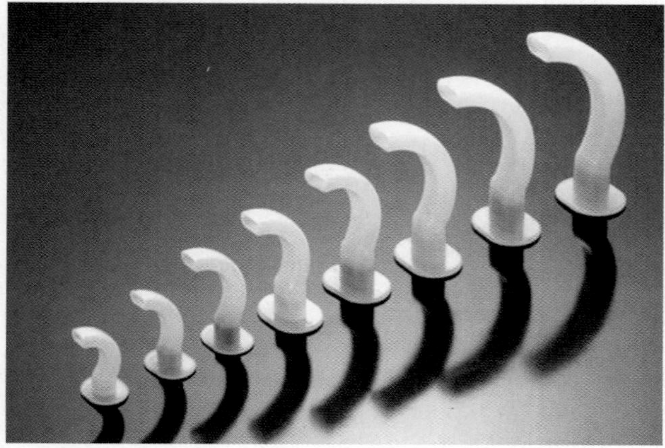

FIGURE 17-5 Different sizes of Guedel airway.

Complications

Regurgitation and aspiration are the major risks of oropharyngeal airway placement. Oropharyngeal airways can also cause coughing and laryngospasm in the awake patient. Coughing and laryngospasm can also occur when the device is too long and comes into contact with the epiglottis or vocal cords. Teeth can also be broken or torn forcibly from the mouth if the patient bites down on the oral airway. Oropharyngeal airways should be used judiciously if the patient has dental disease, decay, caps, crowns, and other dental appliances. In such cases, a **nasopharyngeal airway** or bite block may be indicated instead. When the oropharyngeal airway is in place the lip may also be damaged if it becomes pinched between the teeth and the airway. In the comatose patient continuous chewing motions may damage the tongue. Pressure necrosis of the tongue can occur if the airway is left in place for a prolonged period.

Nasopharyngeal Airways

The nasopharyngeal airway (**Figure 17-8**) is an alternative to the oropharyngeal airway. Nasopharyngeal airways are inserted into the nose and directed along the floor of the nose parallel to the hard palate. They are curved to follow the anatomy of the nasopharynx so that the tip rests behind the tongue, just above the epiglottis. These airways are made of plastic or rubber and resemble a shortened endotracheal tube. All types have some degree of flange at the nasal end to facilitate

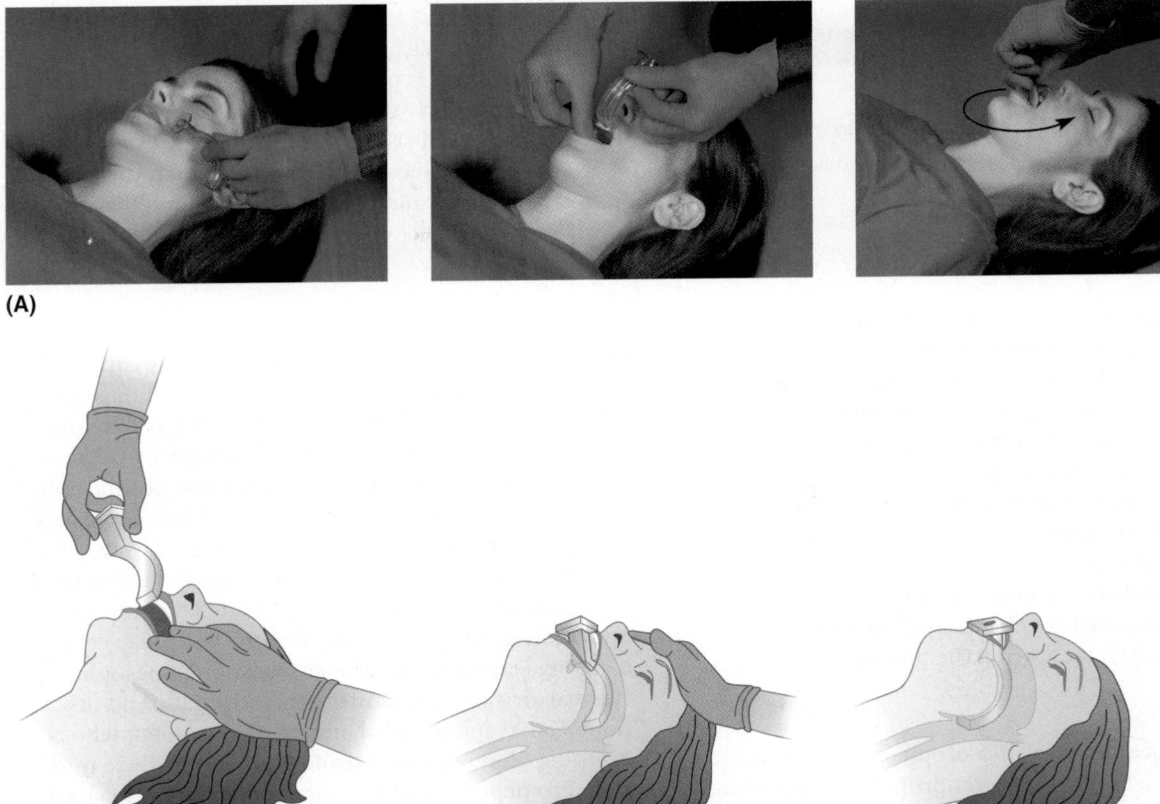

FIGURE 17-7 (**A**) Anti-anatomic insertion of an oral airway. (**B**) Insertion of an oral airway from the side of the mouth.
(**A**) © Jones & Bartlett Learning. Courtesy of MIEMSS; (**B**) adapted from Cairo JM, Pilbeam SP. *Mosby's Respiratory Care Equipment.* 7th ed. Mosby; 2004.

insertion and prevent accidental aspiration of the tube. The proper length of airway can be determined by measurement of the distance from the tip of the nose to the meatus of the ear or from the tip of the nose to the tragus of the ear plus 2 cm (**Figure 17-9**).

The nasopharyngeal airway can be an alternative to the oropharyngeal airway to help maintain airway patency. In some situations the mouth cannot be opened, an active gag reflex limits the use of an oral

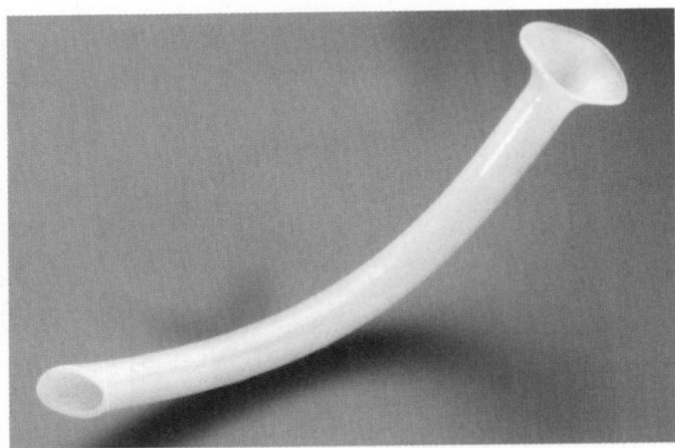

FIGURE 17-8 Nasopharyngeal airway.
Courtesy of Smiths Medical.

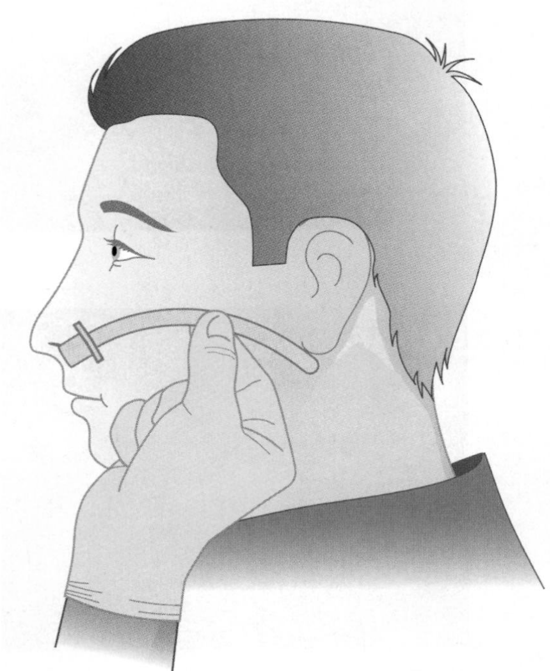

FIGURE 17-9 Sizing the nasopharyngeal airway.

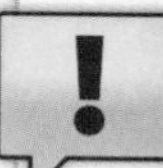

Respiratory Recap

Nasopharyngeal Airways

- May be used to bypass an upper airway obstruction
- Reduce trauma caused by repeated nasotracheal suctioning

airway (and actually can lead to vomiting and aspiration), or an oral airway does not relieve the obstruction. A nasopharyngeal airway is better tolerated and more comfortable than an oropharyngeal airway in a semi-awake patient, and it eliminates the risk of tongue and tooth trauma. Nasopharyngeal airways can provide easy access to the trachea for nasotracheal suctioning and protect the nasopharyngeal mucosa from the traumatic effects of repeated nasotracheal suctioning. A nasopharyngeal airway may also serve as a conduit for oxygenation during bronchoscopy if an upper airway obstruction is created during the procedure.[1]

Insertion

Nasopharyngeal airways, like oropharyngeal airways, come in a variety of sizes. After proper measurement, the nasopharyngeal airway first should be lubricated with a water-soluble gel. It is then introduced into the naris, and the end is pointed parallel to the hard palate. It is advanced gently to prevent trauma and bleeding (**Figure 17-10**). If resistance is met, the airway should be redirected. If excessive resistance is met, the attempt should be aborted and repeat attempts should either be made through the other nostril or using a smaller airway.

Complications

Incorrect sizing of a nasopharyngeal airway carries risks. Laryngospasm and coughing can be induced by insertion of a nasopharyngeal airway that is too long and comes into contact with the epiglottis or vocal cords. Epistaxis can occur from insertion of a nasopharyngeal airway, particularly if it is too large, and excessive force can also result in lacerations to the superior aspect of the soft palate. These airways should be used with caution in patients with low platelet counts or undergoing anticoagulation therapy because excessive bleeding can occur. Improper insertion of nasopharyngeal airways may damage the turbinate, and insertion of a nasopharyngeal airway into a patient who is draining blood or cerebrospinal fluid may cause infection. Prolonged use of this airway may result in sinus

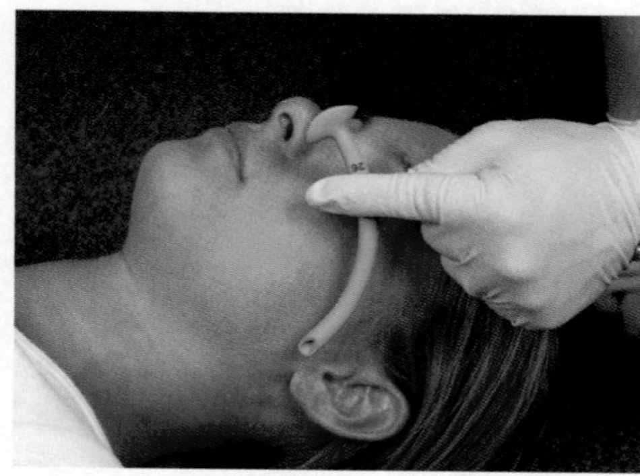

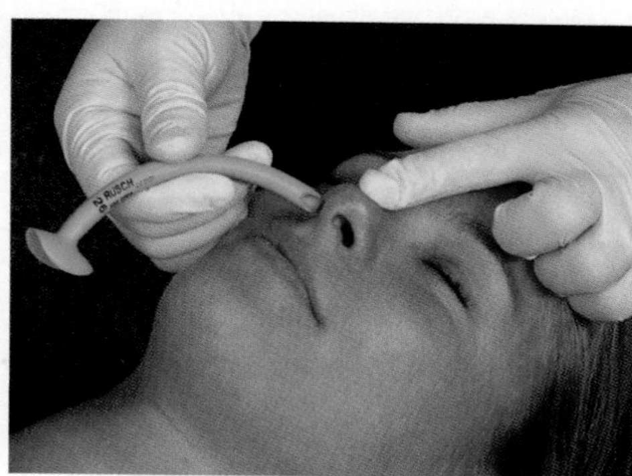

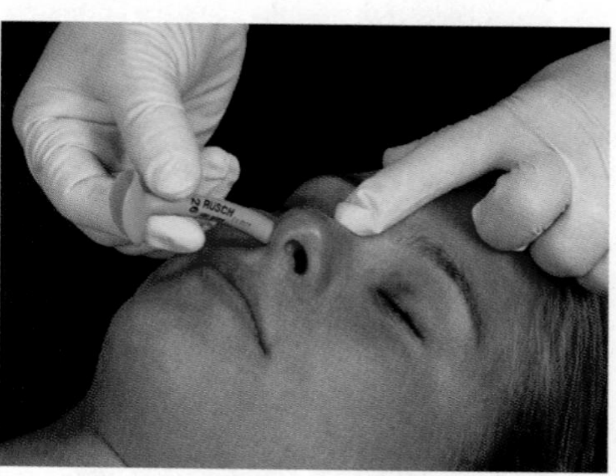

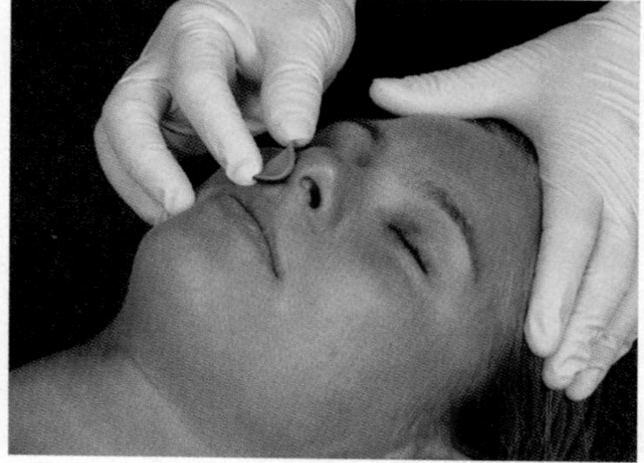

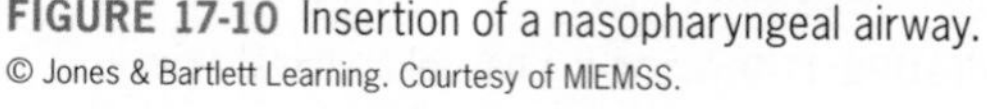

FIGURE 17-10 Insertion of a nasopharyngeal airway.

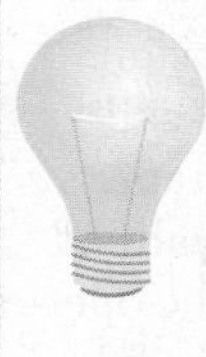

STOP AND THINK

A patient needs an artificial airway and intubation equipment is not readily available. The patient does not arouse but does cough. Which airway would you use?

infection. In patients with severe facial or head trauma, insertion of a nasopharyngeal airway may result, in rare cases, in cranial vault intubation, the risk being greatest in patients with basilar skull fractures.

History of Intubation

The use of tracheotomy to relieve upper airway obstruction dates to Asclepiad's first surgical tracheostomy in approximately 100 BC, which followed several hundred years of crude attempts with swords or other instruments. In the mid-1600s, Robert Hooke performed an experiment in which he kept animals alive by blowing air into their lungs with a bellows using a tracheotomy.[2] In the early 1700s, Trendelenburg fitted an inflatable cuff to a tracheostomy tube, creating the prototype for current airway devices. In the 1880s, MacEwen,[3] O'Dwyer,[4] and Fell[5] all described the use of **endotracheal intubation** for delivery of positive pressure ventilation. The fundamental design of current endotracheal tubes was established in 1941 by Murphy and was further refined in the early 1970s with the introduction of low-pressure, high-compliance cuffs to reduce the risk of tracheal injury.[6]

Selection and Training of Personnel

Understanding the concepts of airway management and becoming proficient in the techniques used to establish and maintain a patent airway are paramount in the practice of respiratory care. The airway should never be taken for granted. At times, a simple maneuver to reestablish a patent airway may prove to be life-saving. The major objectives of airway education are to (1) recognize the need for airway management, (2) properly identify airway anatomy and identify high risk patients, (3) develop skills in mask ventilation, laryngoscopy, and intubation, (4) develop strategies for the difficult airway, and (5) maintain ongoing proficiency in airway management.

The literature offers very little guidance on who should manage the airway, and as a result, regional practices vary considerably. In the surgical areas, anesthesiologists and certified registered nurse anesthetists usually manage the airway. In the nonhospital setting, most regions are comfortable with paramedics performing endotracheal intubation. Airway management of hospitalized patients outside of the operating room is generally considered high risk, with an approximately 10% incidence of difficult airways and higher complication rates even in the hands of experienced airway managers.[7,8] In support of current guidelines, there is a growing body of literature that demonstrates that an interdisciplinary team approach to airway management that emphasizes airway assessment, preoxygenation, and a preplanned airway management strategy can maximize intubation success and significantly reduce both patient complications and the need for surgical airways.[9–12]

Respiratory therapists are essential members of the airway management teams and frequently are the primary airway manager in the absence of more highly trained personnel. The National Board for Respiratory Care (NBRC) includes endotracheal intubation in its examination outline for registered respiratory therapists, and most respiratory therapy training programs instruct their students in the technique of endotracheal intubation.

Given the risk associated with unsuccessful airway management, many experts advocate training and proficiency in a relatively comprehensive set of skills for basic competence in airway management (**Table 17-1**).[13] Unfortunately, here again evidence to support specific training strategies is limited.

Opportunities to practice live intubations tend to be limited in the clinical setting, prompting many programs to provide learners with initial training followed by a controlled experience performing 10 to 15 intubations in the operating room closely supervised by an anesthesiologist.[14,15] After the operating room experience, a set number of supervised intubations is generally required before a trainee is considered competent in airway management. How many intubations are required to reach competence depends greatly on the experience level and psychomotor skills of the learner and the training they receive. In one small but well-designed study, 20 novice airway managers received formal airway instruction followed by practice performing 20 intubations using airway task trainers. Following this training they performed sequential endotracheal intubations in the operating room under the direct supervision of an experienced anesthesiologist, who evaluated their performance with the aid of a standardized checklist.

TABLE 17-1
Recommended Skills for Basic Airway Management

Face mask ventilation, airway positioning
Extraglottic airways (including intubating LMA)
Oral endotracheal intubation (direct laryngoscopy)
Simple maneuvers to improve glottis visualization
Use of stylet, gum elastic bougie
Rapid sequence induction
Fiberoptic intubation via conduit (oropharyngeal airway, LMA)
Percutaneous cricothyrotomy

Reproduced from Goldmann K, Ferson DZ. Education and training in airway management. *Best Pract Res Clin Anaesthesiol.* 2005;19:717–732.

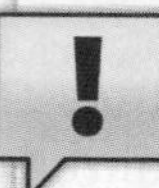

Respiratory Recap

Healthcare Workers Who Perform Endotracheal Intubation

- Anesthesia personnel (anesthesiologists and nurse anesthetists)
- Critical care and emergency physicians
- Paramedics
- Respiratory therapists

The authors demonstrated that the probability of a good intubation reached the 90% threshold after approximately 50 intubations.[16] The use of a videolaryngoscope to assist in initial airway instruction may accelerate progression to competence based on other small studies, possibly because this tool provides learners with better visualization and subsequent understanding of anatomic structures involved in the procedure.[17,18]

Incorporating simulation based training improves learner satisfaction and confidence with airway management skills but has not been clearly associated with more rapid psychomotor proficiency in these procedures even when human cadavers have been employed.[19] On the other hand, growing evidence supports the use of a simulated clinical environment to build teamwork skills and gain experience with a systematic approach to patient and equipment preparation using realistic clinical scenarios. A carefully designed iterative performance improvement program in airway management showed that a combined team approach, which included intensive simulation-based airway skills for physicians, **team resource management** training, use of a mandatory checklist during each intubation, and postevent debriefing, significantly improved the safety of airway management in that facility.[12]

Skill decay is a concern in many institutions where intubations may not be commonplace, and lack of regular procedures may lead to competency erosion. It therefore is very important to have a periodic skill maintenance program. Trained respiratory therapists should perform 10 intubations a year to be requalified or should undergo a repeat training course in the operating room. If the requirement for intubation outside the operating room is infrequent, training may need to be limited to supervisors or designated members of the airway or code team to achieve continued competence.

Anatomy of the Upper Airway and Airway Assessment

A thorough understanding of basic upper airway anatomy is essential to airway management, regardless of the technique used. The airway consists of five regions: the nose and nasopharynx, oral cavity and oropharynx, hypopharynx, larynx, and tracheobronchial tree (**Figure 17-11**).

The nose and nasopharynx region consist of the nasal cavity, turbinates, nasal septum, and adenoids. Warming, humidification, and filtering of inspired air are the primary functions of the nasopharyngeal structures, which are well suited to these tasks because of the region's large mucosal surface area and rich blood supply. If these nose functions are bypassed with the use of an endotracheal tube, these important functions must be substituted artificially. The vascular supply to the area is received from the ethmoid artery and the maxillary artery. Sensory innervation is supplied by the trigeminal nerve through the pterygopalatine branches of the maxillary division. Openings to the paranasal sinuses also are present in the nasal cavity, and drainage of these sinuses may be interrupted if they are occluded by an endotracheal tube or nasogastric tube and may result in sinusitis. Endotracheal intubation also interferes with the sense of olfaction.

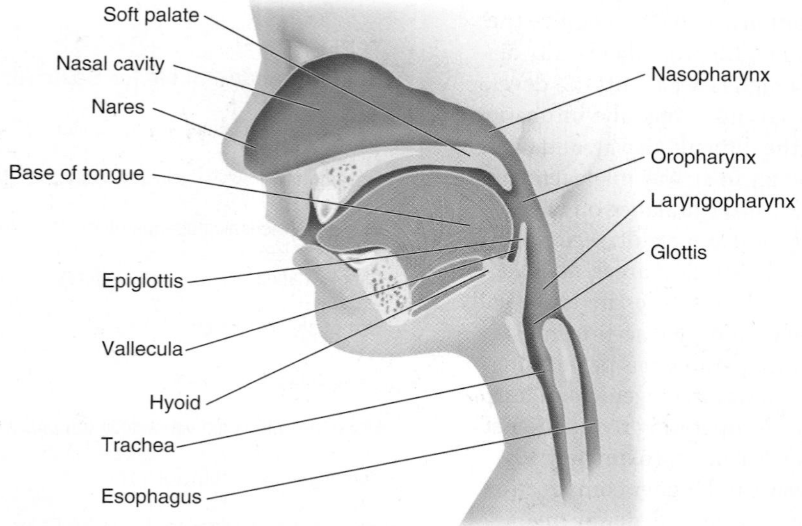

FIGURE 17-11 Anatomy of the upper airway.

The oral cavity and oropharynx consist of the teeth, tongue, buccal mucosa, faucial pillars, hard palate, soft palate, uvula, tonsils, and posterior pharyngeal wall. Functionally these structures are important for mastication, taste, phonation, humidification, and warming of inspired gas. As swallowing occurs, the soft palate closes the inferior aspect of the nasopharynx. The oropharynx has a rich mucosal blood supply, and innervation is complex, involving mandibular branches of the trigeminal, facial, and glossopharyngeal nerves. The mandible houses the tongue, and the temporomandibular joint (TMJ) and determines the ability to mobilize these structures. Reduced TMJ mobility may make direct laryngoscopy difficult or impossible. Prominent upper incisors may also impede glottis visualization using direct laryngoscopy. Dental appliances should be removed prior to intubation attempts to prevent damage and possible migration of the device into the trachea.

Below the oropharynx and above the larynx is the hypopharynx. This area contains the epiglottis and the opening to the esophagus. It is an extension of the oropharynx and the position where a laryngeal mask airway seats. The larynx is a complex structure composed of nine cartilages, seven muscles, and the vocal ligaments (**Figure 17-12**). The space between the vocal cords is the glottis; in adults this is the narrowest part of the upper airway, whereas in children the narrowest point is the cricoid ring. The vocal cords protect the lower airway from aspiration of foreign objects and allow phonation. The cartilaginous structures and complex muscle groups of the larynx are responsible for the intricate vocal abilities of human beings. Nerve or muscle damage can result in a damaged or paralyzed vocal cord, which can increase the risk of aspiration and present additional challenges to avoid damage during intubation.

The trachea is inferior to the larynx, starting just below the cricoid ring. C-shaped cartilaginous rings connected by fibromuscular tissue extend approximately 10 to 12 cm to where the trachea bifurcates into the left and right main stem bronchi at the carina. The carina usually is located at the level of the fourth thoracic vertebra. Posteriorly the tracheal cartilage rings are incomplete, and are bridged by a membranous wall formed by a longitudinal fibromuscular band. This allows for inward expansion of the trachea when food traverses down the esophagus.

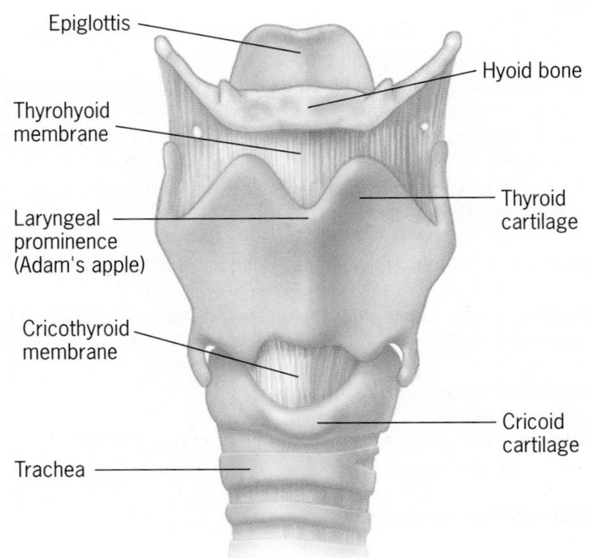

FIGURE 17-12 Anatomy of the larynx.

> **AGE-SPECIFIC ANGLE**
>
> In adults the glottis is the narrowest point of the upper airway, whereas in children the cricoid ring is the narrowest point.

Indications for Endotracheal Intubation

Conditions requiring airway management include respiratory failure due to inadequate oxygenation and/or ventilation, the need for airway protection due to obstruction, or inability to maintain a patent airway due to other patient factors (depressed level of consciousness and the subsequent risk of aspiration). Artificial airways, in addition to providing an intact airway conduit, can also facilitate airway secretion clearance and hyperventilation in the setting of increased intracranial pressure and herniation. **Box 17-1** lists specific conditions that require emergency endotracheal intubation.

Maintaining a patent airway is a vital and most basic intervention without which meaningful survival is impossible. Endotracheal intubation remains the gold standard to establish a definitive artificial airway, although it is important to recognize that both extraglottic devices and surgical airways can serve as effective temporizing bridges in an emergency situation when patient oxygenation and ventilation are compromised.

Noninvasive ventilation (NIV) and continuous positive airway pressure (CPAP) can be used to effectively manage patients with self-limited conditions such as exacerbations of chronic obstructive pulmonary disease or congestive heart failure without the use of an endotracheal tube.[20–24] Endotracheal intubation, however, remains the preferred initial management in these patients in the setting of significant alterations of consciousness, hemodynamic instability, severe

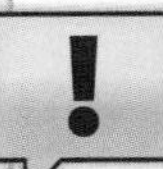

> **Respiratory Recap**
>
> **Indications for Endotracheal Intubation**
>
> - Bypass an upper airway obstruction
> - Apply positive pressure ventilation
> - Correct hypoxemia and/or respiratory acidosis
> - Reduce the risk of large volume aspiration
> - Aid clearance of secretions

BOX 17-1

Indications for Emergency Intubation

Persistent apnea
Traumatic upper airway obstruction
Accidental extubation of a patient unable to maintain adequate spontaneous ventilation
Obstructive angioedema
Massive uncontrolled upper airway bleeding
Coma with potential for increased intracranial pressure
Infection-related upper airway obstruction (e.g., epiglottitis, acute uvular edema, tonsillopharyngitis or retropharyngeal abscess, supportive parotitis)
Laryngeal and upper airway edema
Absence of airway protective reflexes
Cardiopulmonary arrest
Massive hemoptysis
Neonatal or pediatric disorders (e.g., perinatal asphyxia, severe tonsillar hypertrophy, severe laryngomalacia, bacterial tracheitis, neonatal epignathus, obstruction from abnormal laryngeal closure caused by arytenoid masses, mediastinal tumors, congenital diaphragmatic hernia, thick and/or particulate meconium in the amniotic fluid)

Reproduced from Hess DR. Indications for translaryngeal intubation. *Respir Care*. 1999;44:604–609. Reprinted with permission.

derangements of oxygenation or ventilation, or a failure to improve with noninvasive therapy.

When high oxygen concentrations are required to correct hypoxemia, placement of an endotracheal tube may be necessary. Most oxygen delivery devices fall well short of a 100% oxygen concentration because of air entrainment caused by poorly fitting devices or inadequate flow delivery. Tight-fitting masks work well for high oxygen delivery if the inspiratory flows are high enough, but patients find these devices uncomfortable and often remove them, dropping the F_{IO_2} to potentially dangerous levels. When high oxygen concentrations are needed, administration is usually required for several hours; therefore, the use of positive pressure through an endotracheal tube can be used to reduce the levels of inspired oxygen.

Aspiration is a major mechanism for pneumonia and respiratory failure, and can result in significant morbidity and mortality. Although not completely effective, placement of an endotracheal tube in the trachea minimizes the risk of large volume aspiration in the setting of a patient with a decreased level of consciousness (Glasgow Coma Scale <8).[25,26]

Initial Approach to Airway Management

A systematic approach to airway assessment, patient and equipment preparation, and procedure planning is essential to maximize success of an intubation procedure. **Table 17-2** displays a tool to ensure that these important steps are performed consistently with every intubation.

TABLE 17-2
The ACCP APPROACH to Airway Management

Assess the airway – it's all in your **HAND** **H**istory of difficult intubation **A**natomic considerations 3-3-2 rule Modified Mallampati Classification Other risk factors for airway distortion, obstruction **N**eck Mobility **D**ifficult airway should be considered if concerns with any of the factors above
Preoxygenate using 100% oxygen, bag valve mask with PEEP valve
Prepare Patient: Sniffing position, headboard off and patient head just below intubator's xyphoid process Medications: Free flowing IV, premedication, induction, paralytic, and vasopressor agents Right side: Suction, endotracheal tube with stylet and syringe attached Left side: Laryngoscope handle, blades, oral and nasal airways, end-tidal CO_2 detector
Review team member roles, primary and backup intubation plans
Oxygen cut offs: Identify signals to abort, reinitiate bag valve mask ventilation
Administer medication, if indicated
Confirm endotracheal tube placement using two indicators (including end-tidal CO_2)
Hold endotracheal tube until secured

Adapted with permission from the American College of Chest Physicians Airway Management Program Curriculum, 2013.

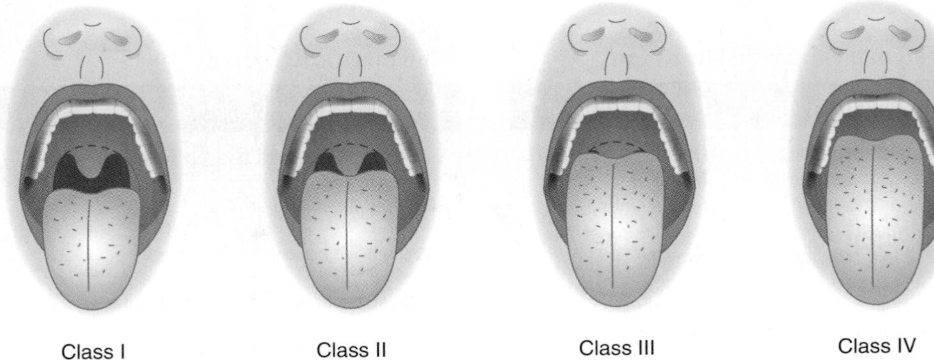

FIGURE 17-13 Mallampati classification.

Adapted from Mallampati SR, et al. *Can Anaesth Soc J.* 1985;32:429–434; and Samsoon GLT, Young JRB. *Anesthesiology.* 1987;42:487–490.

Airway Assessment

Figure 17-13 and **Table 17-3** represent difficulty-class scales based on visualization of airway structures during direct laryngoscopy. **Table 17-4** represents a difficulty-class scale based on structures visualized during an oropharyngeal examination. Prediction of the ability to perform direct laryngoscopy and intubation is also associated with structural and anatomic factors (**Table 17-5**). It must be noted that although many of these factors seem obvious, some are subtle and often are not appreciated in an emergency situation.

Although this variety of anatomic characteristics has been identified as being predictive of difficult intubation, the reality is that the sensitivity and specificity of each of these findings in isolation is relatively poor.[27] Combining several factors improves the predictive value of the airway assessment, such as the popular 3-3-2 rule. This assessment tool suggests that a difficult airway may be present if one or more of the following conditions are not met: (a) the patient's mouth should open adequately to permit three fingers to be placed between the upper and lower teeth; (b) three fingers should fit under the chin between the tip of the jaw and the beginning of the neck, and (c) there should be space for two fingers between the thyroid notch and the floor of the mandible.

The MACOCHA score, a seven-item prediction tool developed from the experience in 1,000 consecutive intubations and then prospectively validated in 400 additional procedures in outside institutions, is a recently published resource shown to effectively identify patients through higher scores who are at risk for a difficult airway (**Table 17-6**). The risk of difficult intubation and serious procedure-related complications increases proportionally with the MACOCHA score. It is important to emphasize that the value of all these tools is in their positive predictive value; given the

TABLE 17-3
Cormack-Lehane Difficulty Classification Based on Structures Visible on Direct Laryngoscopy

Class	Visible Structures
I	Supraglottic structures Laryngeal inlet Vocal cords
II	Epiglottis Laryngeal inlet Posterior aryepiglottic folds
III	Epiglottis only
IV	Epiglottis not visible

Reproduced from Watson CB. Prediction of difficult intubation: methods for successful intubation. *Respir Care.* 1999;44:777–796. Reprinted with permission.

TABLE 17-4
Modified Mallampati Difficulty Classification Based on Structures Visible During the Oropharyngeal Examination

Class	Visible Structures
I	Tongue Hard palate Soft palate Uvula Posterior pharynx
II	Tongue Hard palate Soft palate Part of the uvula and the posterior pharynx
III	Tongue Hard palate Soft palate Posterior pharynx not visible
IV	Anterior tongue Hard palate

Reproduced from Watson CB. Prediction of difficult intubation: methods for successful intubation. *Respir Care.* 1999;44:777–796. Reprinted with permission.

TABLE 17-5
Complicating Anatomic Factors in Intubation

Factor	Common Condition	Primary Problem
Disproportionate soft tissues	Lingual hypertrophy Down syndrome Lingual tonsillar hypertrophy Marked obesity Supraglottic inflammation Previous neck dissection Expanding neck hematoma	Oversized tongue Mass effect Redundant soft tissue Swelling Torsion Deviation Obstructive edema
Distorted anatomy	Peritonsillar abscess Pharyngeal mass and brachial cleft cyst Thyroid tumor or goiter Developmental craniofacial anomalies Spinal subluxation or osteophytes Maxillofacial trauma	Lateral compression and risk of rupture Deviated larynx or trachea Bony incongruity and disproportionate anatomy Extrinsic mass effect Displacement or bleeding or both
Inadequate jaw mobility	Temporomandibular joint dysfunction Short mandibular ramus Trauma Malignant hyperthermia Myotonic crisis Neuroleptic-malignant syndrome Drug intoxication Infections	Fixed or limited motion Inadequate hinge length Trismus or locked jaw or both Masseter tetanus and generalized rigidity Rigidity, trismus, tetanus
Inadequate neck mobility	Degenerative cervical arthritis Morbid obesity Facial or neck burn scarring Dwarfism Hydrocephalus Cranial dysplasia Cervical meningomyelocele Cervical trauma Fractures Thoracic kyphosis	Fused or irregular intervertebral joints Tissue limits movement Fusion and contractures Short, thick neck Limited neck extension Inadequate space External fixation Fractures Hematoma Limited cervical extension

Reproduced from Watson CB. Prediction of difficult intubation: methods for successful intubation. *Respir Care.* 1999;44:777–796. Reprinted with permission from *RESPIRATORY CARE* and The American Association for Respiratory Care.

incidence of 10% difficult airways in patients undergoing intubation in the hospital, providers should never omit the development of a backup airway management plan because of a reassuring score on a prediction tool.

TABLE 17-6
The MACOCHA Score

Factors	Points
Factors related to the patient	
Mallampati score III or IV	5
Diagnosis of obstructive sleep apnea	2
Reduced mobility of the cervical spine	1
Limited mouth opening <3 cm	1
Factors related to pathology	
Coma	1
Severe hypoxemia (Spo_2 <80%)	1
Factors related to the operator	
Nonanesthesiologist	1
TOTAL	12

Reproduced with kind permission from Springer Science + Business Media from De Jong A, Clavieras N, Conseil M et al. Implementation of a combo videolaryngoscope for intubation in critically ill patients: a before-after comparative study. *Intensive Care Med.* 2013;39:2144–2152.

Endotracheal Tubes

The construction of endotracheal tubes (ETTs) is dictated by the standards of the American Society for Testing and Materials (ASTM) (**Figure 17-14**).[28,29] The tubes usually are made of polyvinyl chloride (PVC). PVC is rigid, to facilitate insertion of the tube, but becomes softer at body temperature. The material used in endotracheal tubes is implant tested (i.e., it does not react with tissue), and it is smooth, to facilitate passage of a **suction catheter**. The distal end of the tube is beveled and rounded to minimize trauma on insertion. Endotracheal tubes usually have a Murphy eye near the distal tip, which allows the passage of gas if the end of the tube becomes occluded by secretions or the wall of the patient's airway. Near its distal end the tube has a cuff, which can be inflated by a pilot tube that extends past the proximal end of the tube and terminates with a pilot balloon and spring-loaded valve. A radiopaque line is molded into the tube to allow visualization of the tube on radiography.

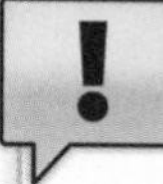

Respiratory Recap

Components of a Typical Endotracheal Tube

- Cuff
- Pilot balloon
- Radiopaque line
- Proximal 15-mm connector

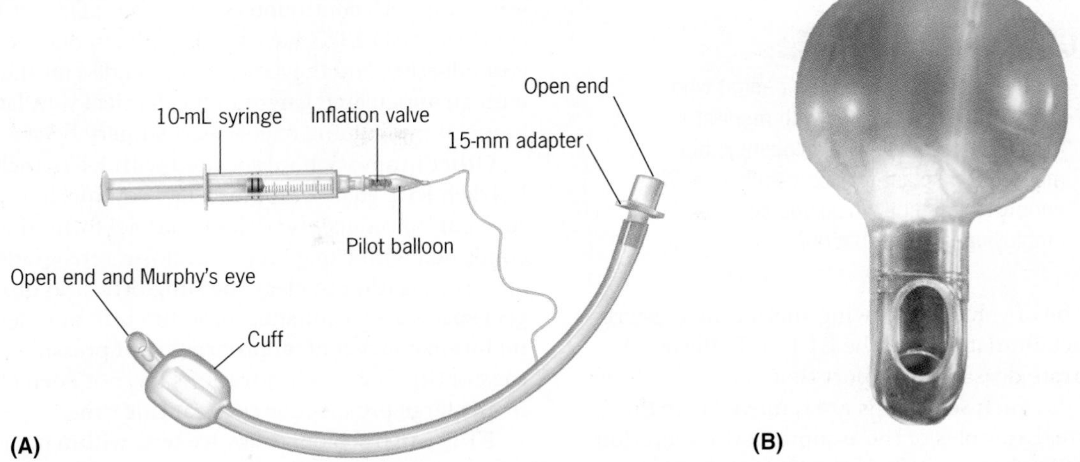

FIGURE 17-14 (**A**) Endotracheal tube. (**B**) Distal end of endotracheal tube showing cuff, beveled end, and Murphy eye.

The tube's inner diameter (ID) and outer diameter (OD) measurements (in millimeters) are marked on it, as are the distance from the distal tip (in centimeters), the manufacturer's name, whether the tube is for oral or nasal use (an oral tube has a 45-degree angle at the tip; a nasal or oronasal tube has a 60-degree angle), and an indication that the tube material has been implant tested (IT). The proximal end of the tube is fitted with a standard 15-mm OD connection for respiratory and anesthesia equipment. By convention, the size of the endotracheal tube is given by its ID measurement.

There are several variations in the design of the ETT. Tubes for selective endobronchial intubation (**Figure 17-15**), for example, are used during thoracic surgery (such as pneumonectomy) and for the rare cases of independent lung ventilation. The anode tube has a steel reinforcing wire that is wound spirally within the wall of the tube. This allows the tube to be made of a softer material, yet prevents kinking when the tube must be bent at an angle to clear the surgical field or for bronchospirometry. The Endotrol allows the practitioner to control the direction of the distal tip of the endotracheal tube during intubation by pulling a loop near the tube's proximal end. A flexible, spiral stainless steel tube called the Laser-Flex can be used for laser surgery.

Given the importance of preventing ventilator-associated pneumonia (VAP), several design modifications have emerged to address potential contributing factors associated with endotracheal tube devices. These innovations generally address either methods to reduce the drainage of subglottic secretions or to reduce the development of biofilm within endotracheal tube lumen that might subsequently drain or be introduced into the lung.[30]

Modified ETTs that facilitate either continuous or intermittent drainage of subglottic secretions can

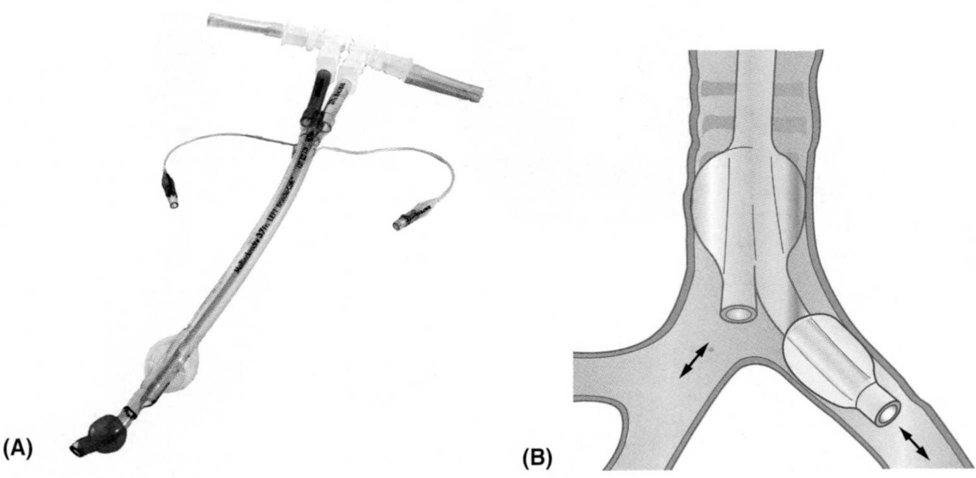

FIGURE 17-15 Double-lumen tube.

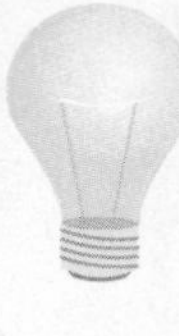

STOP AND THINK

You are asked to intubate a patient who is transferred to the ICU with respiratory failure 10 days following allogeneic bone marrow transplant for acute leukemia. What endotracheal tube would you consider employing in this situation?

potentially be of value by allowing suctioning of secretions that accumulate above the ETT cuff. These tubes have a separate dorsal lumen port that opens above the cuff, through which secretions are removed using negative pressure. Examples of these supraglottic secretion drainage (SSD) devices include the Hi Lo Evac tube (**Figure 17-16**) and the Seal Guard or Taper Guard.

The use of SSD devices remains controversial, despite two meta-analyses—the most recent including 13 prospective randomized trials and 2,442 patients—that show a significant reduction in VAP, shorter duration of mechanical ventilation, and possible shorter ICU length of stay.[31,32] The controversy surrounds the fact that these VAP reductions have not been shown to be associated with decreased mortality, and the high observed mechanical failure rate of SSD devices has caused some to question if these improvements are simply due to the fact that several of these tubes have PUC cuffs. The cause of this mechanical failure has been shown in some cases to be due to suctioned tracheal mucosa, raising additional concerns about the risk of tracheal injury especially with continuous suctioning.[33] Despite these concerns, SSD ETTs have been shown in one study to be cost effective, and they are recommended for individuals with an anticipated length of mechanical ventilation >72 hours or undergoing major heart surgery.[34–36]

Other innovations associated with ETTs include a Lotrach ETT that combines a low volume, low pressure cuff to reduce the risk of channel formation; SSD combined with capability to perform retrograde upper airway irrigation to clear the subglottic and oropharyngeal space; and a constant pressure inflation device to maintain consistent, appropriate cuff pressure. The efficacy of this array of innovations has not been examined in any large prospective trials at this time.[37]

ETTs can be colonized by bacteria within hours of insertion, and the same organisms isolated in cases of VAP can frequently be identified in the endoluminal biofilm of the patient's ETT. ETTs impregnated with antibiotics do not effectively penetrate this biofilm, but ETTs lined with a silver coating are thought to produce an enhanced antimicrobial activity in addition to blocking bacterial adhesion to the tube itself.[38–40] A large prospective randomized trial performed at 54 centers across the United States demonstrated both a significant reduction in VAP and a delayed onset in the cases that did develop (4.8% vs 7.5%), but no reductions in mechanical ventilation duration or ICU or hospital length of stay.[40] Despite a high individual cost, these silver impregnated ETTs might be cost effective and could be considered in ICUs with VAP concerns that persist after standard VAP prevention measures have been implemented.

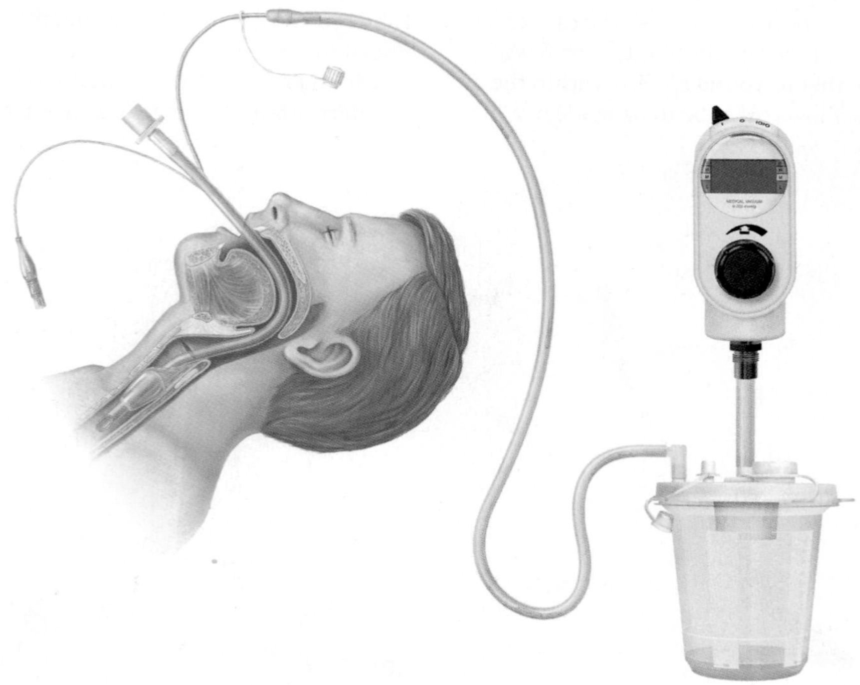

FIGURE 17-16 Hi Lo Evac endotracheal tube with subglottic suction.

Preoxygenation

Preoxygenation using effective mask ventilation technique and high flow oxygen replaces the normal mixture of nitrogen, oxygen, and carbon dioxide in the central and segmental airways with 100% oxygen. Adequate preoxygenation functionally converts the respiratory dead space into an oxygen reservoir, providing the intubator with more time to visualize the glottis and appropriately place the ETT before the development of clinically significant hypoxemia. Use of a positive end-expiratory pressure (PEEP) valve and noninvasive positive pressure ventilation (NIV) has also been shown to delay critical desaturation during intubation attempts, even after standard measures improve oxygen saturations above 90%.[41] Preoxygenation in a 25 degree upright position can also increase the duration of apneic normoxia in obese patients and is likely also helpful in patients with atelectasis and reduced lung compliance.[42]

Endotracheal Intubation: Preparation and Performance

Endotracheal intubation is the establishment of an artificial airway by placement of a tube through the mouth or nose, through the glottis, and into the trachea. This procedure can be performed electively under preplanned conditions or on an emergency basis if sudden respiratory failure occurs. The type of endotracheal tube and the placement technique are determined by the factors dictating its use. Instrumentation of the airway stimulates intense reflexive responses in all individuals except severely obtunded patients. For this reason, preplanning is imperative whenever possible, including a combination of topical application of local anesthetics, establishment of an intravenous line, intravenous induction and paralytic medications, electrocardiographic monitoring, oximetry, suction capability, and availability of various types of equipment to meet unforeseen circumstances. If mask ventilation can be performed with a bag-valve-mask system while some of this equipment is gathered, the chances of successful intubation increase.

Procedure of Endotracheal Intubation

Technique for Orotracheal Intubation

Once it has been determined that endotracheal intubation is required, proper preparation must follow. Each institution should have an emergency airway kit or cart designed by the healthcare workers most likely to use it. The equipment assembled in this kit should be checked on a regular basis to ensure its proper function in an emergency situation. A difficult airway may be encountered unexpectedly, or a marginal airway may deteriorate rapidly, leaving little time to obtain an item from elsewhere.

It is imperative that the process of intubation be approached calmly. Frantic and rushed attempts often result in failure and deterioration of the clinical scenario. Preoxygenation should be provided while the following preparatory steps are taken. Obtaining a brief history is important, and the few seconds this requires may prevent surprises during the process. This is especially important when there have been prior intubations. A previously difficult airway or visualization could be uncovered, and the clinician can take the appropriate steps to be prepared for the scenario.

Positioning is a key aspect of preparation. The patient should be positioned as optimally as possible within the limits of the environment. Some positioning tips include moving the bed away from the wall and raising its height, bringing the patient as close to the head of the bed as possible to limit the amount of reaching, adjusting the patient into an even supine position (or elevating the head of bed to 30 degrees if the patient is obese), and placing a folded blanket or towel under the head to achieve the sniffing position (**Figure 17-17**), which aligns the oral, pharyngeal, and laryngeal axes for optimum visualization of the larynx. In essence, this is flexion of the lower cervical spine and extension of the upper cervical spine and can also be further facilitated by placing a rolled towel or blanket under the shoulders as well. This position is contraindicated in a patient with a confirmed or suspected neck injury. In such cases an assistant should maintain the head and neck in a neutral position as intubation is attempted. Suction must be ready, preferably with a tonsil-tip suction apparatus, and a functioning intravenous line must be in place before any attempts at intubation are made.

Sedation or neuromuscular blocking agents may be necessary in a responsive patient to facilitate the intubation process, along with fluids and vasopressor agents to counteract any potential hypotension that may occur with the use of these medications. The use of paralytic agents has clearly been shown to provide superior glottis visualization, but elimination of spontaneous ventilation will also shorten the available intubation time, eliminate airway reflexes, and potentially further compromises airway patency.

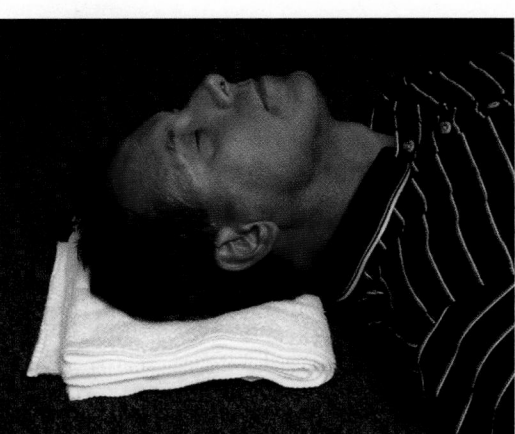

FIGURE 17-17 Sniffing position.

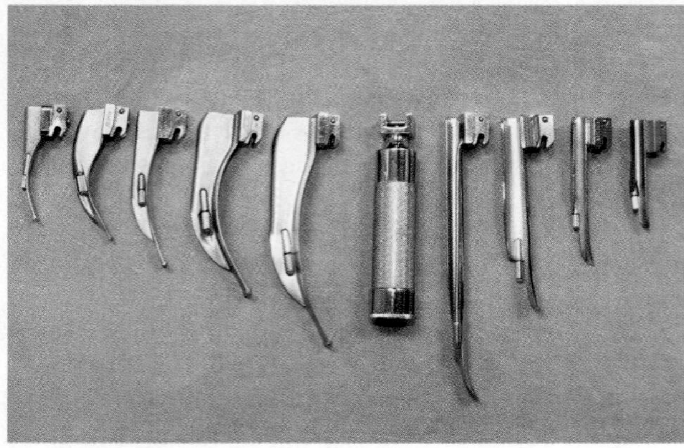

FIGURE 17-18 Laryngoscope handle (center), curved (MacIntosh) blades (left), and straight (Miller) blades (right).

When all preparations are complete, the procedure can be started. **Orotracheal intubation** is most commonly performed with a **laryngoscope**. The laryngoscope is composed of a handle and a blade. The handle may be made of metal or plastic, may be disposable or nondisposable, and may have a detachable or permanently affixed blade (**Figure 17-18**). Batteries in the body of the handle provide power to a lighting device in the blade or the handle. When the lighting mechanism is in the handle, a fiberoptic bundle in the blade transmits light to the distal end of the blade. The fiberoptic laryngoscope has several advantages over the traditional type. Because the light bulbs are in the handle in fiberoptic laryngoscopes, they do not contact the patient and cannot be dislodged into the airway. Also, fewer bulbs are needed because a laryngoscopy set with a handle and several blades requires only one light bulb, whereas the older system requires a bulb in each blade. The proper function of the handle and its bulb and batteries must be determined before use.

Laryngoscope blades vary in construction and are available in several shapes and sizes. The three standard blades are the curved (MacIntosh) blade, the straight (Wisconsin) blade, and the straight with a slightly curved tip (Miller) blade. Many specialty blades also are available, all designed for the occasional unusual circumstance that requires a minor variation of these standard blades. The operator's preference, training, and experience determine which blade is used. Most clinicians choose the blade they have used most often, but an experienced intubator is comfortable with all three types so that when one does not work, an alternative is available. Nearly all blades come in sizes 0 through 4, a range that accommodates neonates up through large adults.

The laryngoscope is introduced into the mouth from the right side, displacing the tongue to the left. This maneuver is used with either a curved or straight blade to prevent the tongue from reducing visualization of the glottis. As the posterior pharyngeal wall comes into view, the person performing the intubation looks for the epiglottis (**Figure 17-19**). When a curved blade is being used, the laryngoscope is gently readjusted once the epiglottis is visualized to place the tip of the blade into the vallecula (the junction of the base of the tongue and the epiglottis; **Figure 17-20**). This results in lifting of the epiglottis to reveal the glottis. If a straight blade is used, the laryngoscope is readjusted to directly lift the tip of the epiglottis (**Figure 17-21**). The proper motor action of readjustment of the laryngoscope is to direct a force on a vector caudal and anterior without a prying action, the latter of which increases the likelihood of dental damage during the procedure. The above maneuvers usually

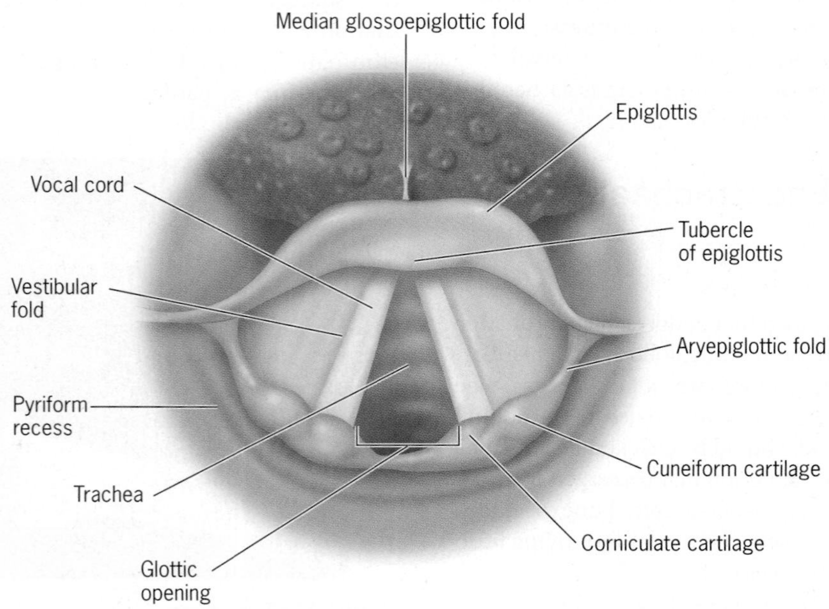

FIGURE 17-19 View of the glottis.

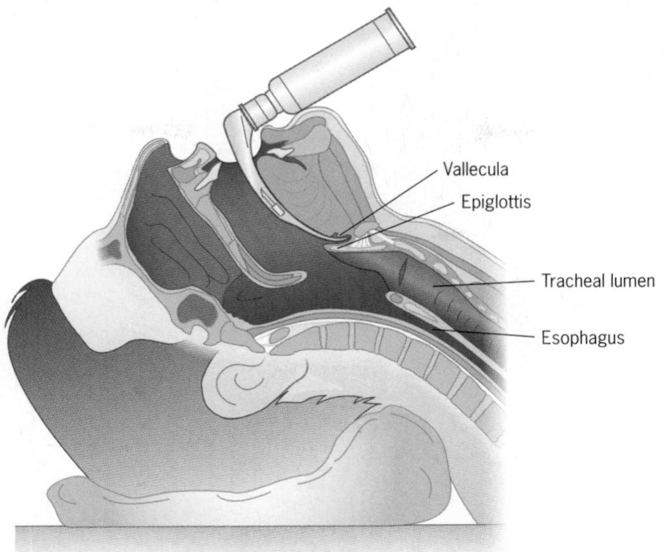

FIGURE 17-20 Use of curved blade.

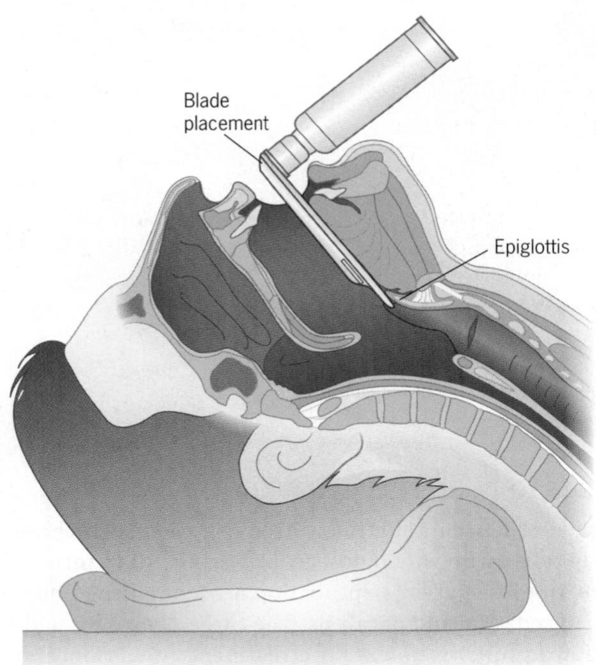

FIGURE 17-21 Use of straight blade.

bring the glottis into view, with the opening into the lower airway between the vocal cords. With spontaneous ventilation, the appropriately sized endotracheal tube is introduced gently between the vocal cords during inspiration. A stylet is generally used to help guide the ETT though the vocal cords and can be shaped to aid in the passage to the trachea. This may be of particular importance in the case of anterior airway presentation.

In adults, a 7- to 7.5-mm ID endotracheal tube is used for women and an 8- to 8.5-mm ID tube is used for men. The tube is advanced 2 to 4 cm below the level of the vocal

Respiratory Recap

Equipment Required for Endotracheal Intubation

- Correct size endotracheal tube
- Lubricant
- Suction
- Syringe
- Laryngoscope
- Stylet
- Carbon dioxide detector
- Bag-valve-mask device
- Oxygen
- Sedative and paralytic agents
- Fluids and vasopressor agents
- PEEP valve
- Oral and nasal airways
- Tape to secure tube

cords into the trachea, and bilateral breath sounds are then verified by auscultation. Correct placement is then checked by other means, such as measurement of expired carbon dioxide, negative auscultation of air movement over the epigastrium, and chest radiograph. As a general rule, the tube should be secured at the 21-cm mark (at the teeth) in women and at the 23-cm mark in men until chest x-ray confirmation is obtained. The tube is secured to the upper lip and maxilla, and another check is made for bilateral breath sounds. An appropriate oxygen delivery and ventilation system is then connected.

Technique for Nasotracheal Intubation

Nasotracheal intubation generally is used for specific indications and has some special considerations compared with orotracheal intubation. Nasotracheal intubation is useful when access to the mouth is unavailable, as in oral surgery or oral trauma, or when the mouth cannot be opened adequately, as in trauma, TMJ dysfunction, or mandibular fixation. Movement of the endotracheal tube in the trachea is one of the determining factors in airway trauma from intubation and, in this light, nasotracheal intubation may be less likely to cause tracheal injury.

Some experts feel that a nasotracheal tube is more easily tolerated once inserted. A nasotracheal tube is more stable because of the immobility of the nose and maxilla in contrast to mandibular movement, which can affect an orotracheal tube. Because the lips are not distorted, communication with the patient and oral care are easier. Uncooperative patients often bite on an orotracheal tube, causing occlusion of the tube and difficulty with mechanical ventilation. This is avoided with nasotracheal intubation.

There are some clinical issues associated with nasotracheal intubation. Development of sinusitis due to blockage of sinus drainage by the ETT often occurs in nasotracheally intubated patients. This, in turn, leads to an increased risk of VAP. Although the nasotracheal tube may be easier to secure, it is more difficult to suction secretions through this tube.

For nasotracheal intubation, as with orotracheal intubation, equipment for oxygen delivery, manual ventilation, and suction is required. A Magill forceps and a fiberoptic laryngoscope also are useful. When access to the mouth is difficult, spontaneous breathing should not be suppressed, but light sedation is beneficial. A topical anesthetic spray or jelly and a vasoconstricting spray are applied to the nares and nasopharynx to minimize sensation, trauma, and bleeding. The nasal passage can be gently dilated with lubricated, soft nasopharyngeal airways to facilitate introduction of the firmer and larger endotracheal tube. The endotracheal tube should be inserted with an initial upward motion until it just passes into the naris and then continued on a course parallel to the palate with firm, gentle pressure. As the tip of the tube reaches the posterior wall of the nasopharynx, resistance is met. Slightly increasing the gentle pressure usually causes the tip to deflect downward. If it does not, rotating the tube slightly usually works. It is important not to use excessive force, or a false passage may be created in the pharyngeal wall, causing trauma and bleeding. As an alternative, the other naris can be tried. As the tube is directed toward the glottis, the intubator should listen for air passing in and out of the tube. As long as air is heard, the tube should be superior to the larynx. The tube is inserted into the glottis during inspiration (when the vocal cords are the widest apart), and as it passes the cords, a cough usually is produced. If the tube does not blindly pass into the glottis, it can be directed fiberoptically or directly with a Magill forceps and laryngoscope if the mouth can be opened (**Figure 17-22**). When the tube has been inserted to the appropriate depth, verification of breath sounds, carbon dioxide measurement, and verification of placement by chest radiograph should be performed.

Nasotracheal intubation may be contraindicated in some cases. Alternate techniques should be considered for cases involving a suspected basilar skull fracture, nasal fracture, nasal polyps, epistaxis, coagulopathy, or planned thrombolysis. Nasotracheal intubation with a basilar skull fracture is very controversial, although there is an increase in the complication rate with this condition.[43] Epistaxis is the most common complication of nasotracheal intubation and usually can be easily managed in patients with normal coagulation processes. Because the tube causes mucosal trauma and edema, the opening to the maxillary sinuses may become occluded, with subsequent development of sinusitis.

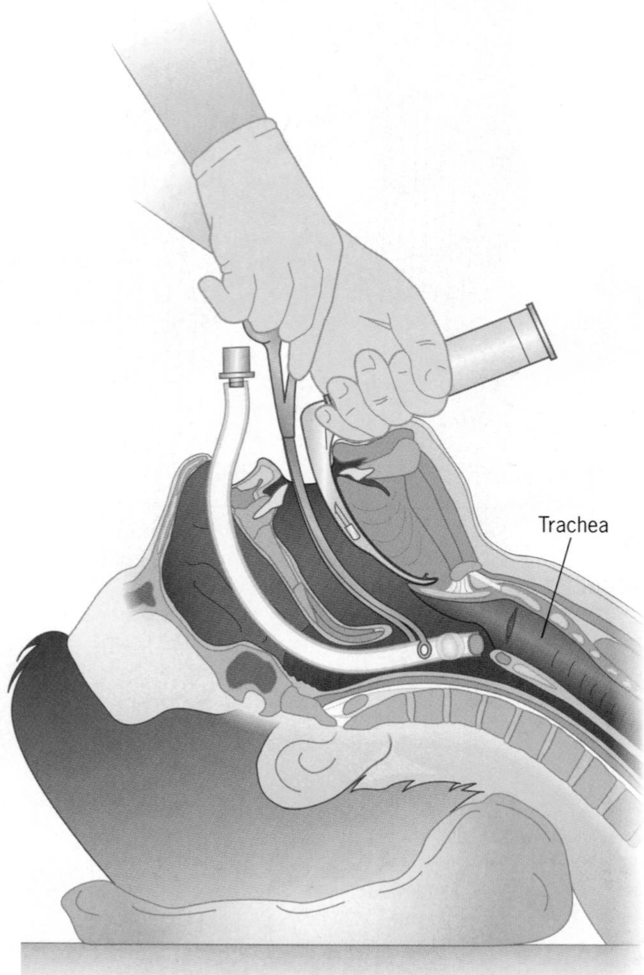

FIGURE 17-22 Use of Magill forceps.

Drugs to Facilitate Intubation

Rapid sequence intubation is used in patients who have a gag reflex who would otherwise be difficult to intubate. In these patients, intubation is accomplished by use of sedation and paralysis. The three phases of medication administration are pretreatment, induction, and paralysis. The patient is preoxygenated for 3 to 5 minutes. Pretreatment agents are used to lessen the physiologic response to laryngoscopy and include lidocaine, opioid analgesic (fentanyl, sufentanil, alfentanil), atropine, and defasciculating agents. As both opioids and lidocaine can be associated with increased intracranial pressure (ICP), esmolol can also be helpful to blunt the sympathetic tone commonly associated with intubation in neurosurgery and head trauma patients with ICP concerns (**Table 17-7**).

Induction agents are employed to provide sedation, upper airway relaxation, and an amnestic response in patients during intubation. Common induction agents used in the ICU include propofol, etomidate, ketamine,

TABLE 17-7
Common Pretreatment Agents Utilized in Endotracheal Intubation

Drug	Dose, Common Indications	Cautions
Fentanyl	2–3 μg/kg IV, 1–2 min CAD, aneurysm, increased ICP	Hypotension Masseter, chest wall rigidity
Esmolol	2–3 mg/kg IV Neurosurgery, head injury	Bradycardia Hypotension, bronchospasm
Lidocaine	1.5 mg/kg IV, 2–3 min Asthma, COPD, increased ICP	Hypotension

and midazolam (**Table 17-8**). Propofol appears to provide the best glottic visualization of these agents at full induction doses, but its use is frequently limited by significant, dose dependent hypotension. It is also contraindicated in patients with egg allergy due to its lipid-based medium. Etomidate has similar pharmacokinetic properties to propofol, with less associated hypotension and myocardial depression than the latter drug. Ketamine provides similar intubating conditions and outcomes to etomidate when combined with succinylcholine using a rapid sequence induction technique. Ketamine's effects are slightly slower in onset and longer in duration than the other two agents, and can increase both heart rate and blood pressure in standard doses. The dysphoric emergence phenomenon often associated with ketamine use is uncommon after a single induction dose, and empiric treatment with benzodiazepines is not generally necessary. Midazolam has been shown in previous prospective randomized trials to be an inferior agent to propofol both in airway relaxation and sedation and can be associated with significant hypotension at full induction doses. Because of these features it is a less preferred agent in the critical care setting.

In many instances propofol is used in conjunction with a paralytic to optimize intubating conditions. The most commonly used paralytic agent is succinylcholine, a depolarizing muscle relaxant with a rapid onset of action and very short duration. In situations where succinylcholine may be considered unsafe (**Table 17-9**), the nondepolarizing muscle relaxant rocuronium will provide a similar onset of action but a much longer duration of paralysis (**Table 17-10**).

TABLE 17-8
Common Induction Agents Utilized in Endotracheal Intubation

Agent	Onset (seconds)	Duration (minutes)	Dose
Propofol	9–50	3–10	0.5–2 mg/kg
Etomidate	30–60	3–5	0.15–0.3 mg/kg
Ketamine	60–120	5–15	2 mg/kg

TABLE 17-9
Contraindications to Succinylcholine

History of malignant hyperthermia
Hyperkalemia
Upper, lower motor neuron lesions
Myopathy
Crush injury
Severe burns (>24 hours)
Prolonged immobility

Complications of Endotracheal Intubation

A number of complications have been associated with endotracheal intubation (**Box 17-2**). These have been classified temporally as complications that occur during the intubation procedure, those that occur while the endotracheal tube is in place, those that occur during and immediately after **extubation**, and those that occur late after extubation. The risk of complications associated with endotracheal intubation is reduced by meticulous attention to care of the airway in intubated patients.

Securing the Endotracheal Tube

Securing the endotracheal tube is an extremely important aspect of airway management. Although not well established, the reported rates of unplanned extubation (accidental extubation or self-extubation) range from 2% to 13%.[44–49] Although reintubation is not necessary in every case of unplanned extubation, it is more likely than with planned extubation and may occur under more dire circumstances due to patient instability. Unplanned extubation may result in serious complications and even death. Factors associated with unplanned extubation include chronic respiratory failure, orotracheal intubation, lack of intravenous sedation, and securing of the endotracheal tube with only thin adhesive tape.

TABLE 17-10
Common Paralytic Agents Utilized in Endotracheal Intubation

Agent	Onset (seconds)	Duration (minutes)	Dose
Succinylcholine	30–60	5–15	1.0–1.5 mg/kg
Rocuronium	45–60	45–70	0.8–1.2 mg/kg

BOX 17-2

Complications of Intubation

During the Intubation Procedure

- Cardiac arrest
- Nasal and oral trauma
- Pharyngeal and hypopharyngeal trauma
- Laryngeal and tracheal trauma
- Main bronchus intubation
- Pulmonary aspiration
- Esophageal intubation

While the Endotracheal Tube Is in Place

- Nasal and oral ulceration (oral cellulitis)
- Sinus effusions and sinusitis
- Otitis
- Laryngeal injury
- Tracheal injury
- Pulmonary complication
- Self-extubation
- Mechanical problems with the tube or cuff
- Patient discomfort

During and Immediately After Extubation

- Sore throat
- Stridor
- Hoarseness
- Odynophagia
- True vocal cord immobility
- Pulmonary aspiration
- Cough

Late Complications After Extubation

- Laryngeal injury
- Stenosis
- Granuloma formation
- Tracheal injury
- Stenosis

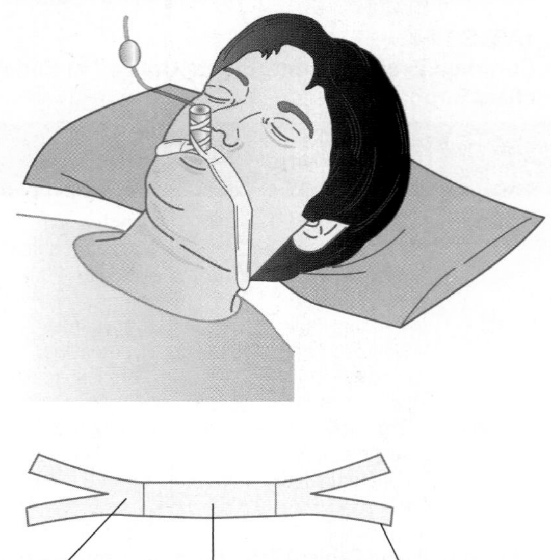

FIGURE 17-23 Securing the endotracheal tube (Lillehei technique).

Guidelines of the American Heart Association recommend the use of either tape or commercial devices to secure the endotracheal tube.[50] The traditional method used to secure an endotracheal tube has been to apply benzoin to the skin and secure the tube with adhesive tape (Lillehei technique) (**Figure 17-23**). Tape 2.5 cm wide is cut long enough to go around the circumference of the patient's head one and one-half to two times. A second piece of tape is cut long enough to fit over the mid-portion of the first piece, thus preventing the tape from sticking to the patient's neck. The tape is then placed around the patient's neck. The skin surface is dried, and tincture of benzoin is placed on both of the patient's cheeks where the tape will come into contact with the skin. The tape is pulled snug against the patient's neck and applied on the patient's cheeks to the edge of the endotracheal tube. The remaining tape is split longitudinally so that at least 5 cm of tape is available to be wrapped around the endotracheal tube at the lips. Later removal of the tape can be facilitated if the end of the tape is folded back on itself to form a tab. Some clinicians wrap both ends of the split tape around the tube, whereas others wrap one piece around the tube and pass the other piece over the lip and fasten it to the contralateral cheek. The tape is applied snugly but not so tight as to cause breakdown of the facial skin. The advantage of this method is that tape passes completely around the neck, which is preferable to techniques in which one or two pieces of tape are used to tape the tube to the patient's cheeks. A similar method can be used for nasally placed tubes. The endotracheal tube, gastric tube, and oral airway (if present) should be taped separately. In this way, one device can be repositioned or removed without affecting the other. The tube should not be taped to the mandible, because this increases the likelihood of tube movement if the jaw is moved.

Adhesive tape can pose some problems. Mouth care is difficult when too much tape is used. When an oral airway is added for stabilization and to prevent the patient from biting the tube, airway care becomes even more difficult. The patient's oral cavity and lips and the skin around the mouth must be carefully observed for signs of complications. The skin around the mouth of

Respiratory Recap

Means of Securing Endotracheal Tubes

- Adhesive tape
- Twill tape
- Commercially available devices

debilitated or immunosuppressed patients may become excoriated by tape on the face. In addition, the tape has been shown to promote bacterial growth. Although there are methods of securing tape for patients with beards and moustaches, tape securement of the endotracheal tube is probably not the best method. Commercially available devices specifically designed to anchor the endotracheal tube in place are optimal in these cases.

Twill tape is another common means to secure the endotracheal tube. With this method, a 1-m length of twill tape is folded in half and looped around the endotracheal tube. The ends are brought through this loop and tightened around the tube. One end of the twill tape is passed around the patient's head below one ear, and the other end is passed above the other ear. The two ends are tied in a bow on the cheek. This technique sometimes is repeated with a second piece of twill tape so that two ties are used to secure the endotracheal tube.

Tube movement is considered a cause of airway trauma. Movement of the tube against the tracheal mucosa causes a scraping motion along the soft tissues of the airway. The contact is greatest at the pressure points of the lips, posterior pharynx, and posterior of the glottis and at the site of the cuff. In adults, the tip of the endotracheal tube should be positioned 3 to 7 cm above the carina when the neck is in a neutral position. Flexion of the neck causes the distal tip to move toward the carina, and extension of the neck causes the tube to move toward the glottis (**Figure 17-24**). If the tube advances too far distally, it may enter a main stem bronchus (usually the right). If the tube moves proximally with the cuff inflated, laryngeal damage may occur.

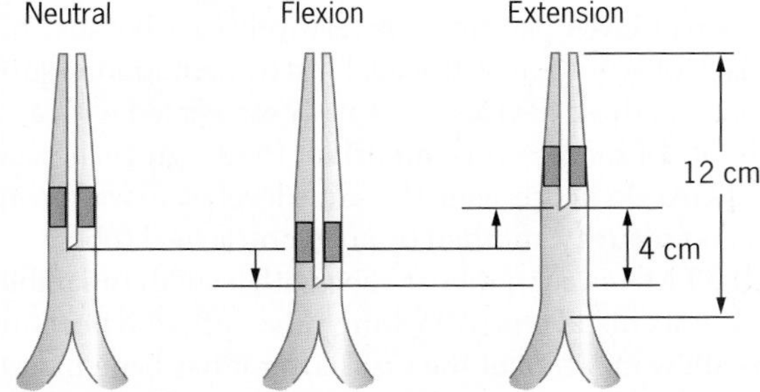

FIGURE 17-24 Movement of the distal endotracheal tube tip with flexion and extension of the head.

Reproduced from Conrardy PA, Goodman LR, Lainge F, et al. Alteration of endotracheal tube position: flexion and extension of the neck. *Crit Care Med.* 1976;4:8–12. Reprinted with permission from Wolters Kluwer Health.

Displacement into the esophagus or pharynx may result in gastric insufflation and inadequate lung ventilation.

There are a number of nontape devices available for securing endotracheal tubes. No one retention device has been universally accepted. Many nontape devices tend to be large, which could hinder mouth and facial care. The ideal nontape appliance should allow minimal tube migration, be comfortable for the patient, allow oral hygiene, preserve skin integrity and allow for safe and rapid tube repositioning. Finally an optimal nontape endotracheal tube holder should also be easy to apply and require minimal maintenance time. The one drawback to these holders is that they are cost prohibitive. They are more expensive than traditional taping methods and tend to be reserved for use with patients in which taping may not be sufficient for adequate anchoring (presence of beards, unusual facial anatomy, facial sores where the tape would be attached).

The endotracheal tube should be repositioned in the mouth periodically to allow provision of mouth care and to prevent pressure sores of the lips, gums, and mouth. Two people should be present when the endotracheal tube is unsecured for this care. One person is responsible for maintaining the tube's position, and the other person is responsible for providing mouth care and resecuring the tube. In some units it is common practice to trim the excess endotracheal tube length. This may reduce the risk of tube malposition or kinking. It is important to ensure that the tube is properly positioned before it is trimmed, however. A swivel connector should be used between the endotracheal tube and the breathing circuit, and the breathing circuit should be supported so that it does not promote tube movement.

A bite block can be placed between the teeth to prevent the patient from biting an orotracheal airway or from biting the tongue or lips, causing bleeding and trauma to the mouth. The material should be tough but not rigid and may have channels for air passage. A variety of materials and adaptations of other airways have been used as bite blocks. Oropharyngeal airways are sometimes used but may damage the teeth. Also, the complications of oropharyngeal airways when endotracheal tubes are in place for prolonged periods are problematic. Oral airways have been modified for this purpose by removal of the pharyngeal portion. An airway gag was developed for patients receiving electroconvulsive therapy. The device, a wedge-shaped piece of surgical rubber, consists of a body with air channels, a flange, and a tongue depressor and retractor that hold the tongue in place but do not extend into the pharynx deep enough to induce a gag reflex.

In patients with an endotracheal tube, bite blocks may be used to prevent occlusion due to either active biting or large teeth. Oropharyngeal tubes also can be used to serve this purpose. However, they tend to be somewhat large, may be difficult to position and anchor and have the potential to cause dental or mucosal damage. Another

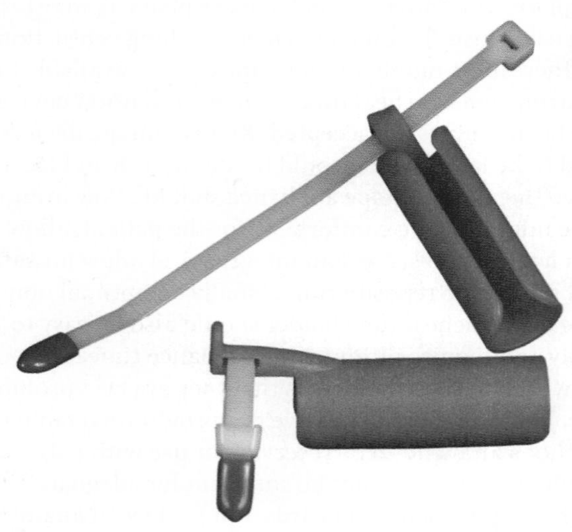

FIGURE 17-25 Universal bite block.
Courtesy of B&B Medical Technologies.

option is a device that surrounds a portion of the endotracheal tube to prevent occlusive biting but has minimal impact on surrounding tissue (**Figure 17-25**). Once placed around the appropriate portion of the endotracheal tube, it can be secured to minimize slippage. Devices such as these have the advantages of being smaller and of posing less risk of migrating away from the tube as well as of causing unwanted gag stimulation. The position of this type of bite block needs to be checked on a regular basis as it does have the potential to kink the pilot line of the endotracheal tube.[51]

The Difficult Airway: Assessment and Strategy

The American Society of Anesthesiologists (ASA) Task Force on Management of the Difficult Airway has described a difficult airway as a "clinical situation in which a conventionally trained anesthesiologist experiences difficulty with face mask ventilation of the upper airway, difficulty with tracheal intubation, or both."[9] In emergency situations an individual with much less experience than a conventionally trained anesthesiologist may have to perform endotracheal intubation and may encounter a difficult airway. The difficult airway has been blamed as the primary source of airway complications in the ICU. Hypoxemia from inadequate ventilation, difficult tracheal intubation, or inadvertent esophageal intubation remains the most common cause of injury lawsuits from anesthesia care. For all these reasons, training in the recognition and management of a difficult airway must occur concomitantly with training in basic intubation.

The incidence of difficult direct laryngoscopy and intubation has been reported to be approximately 10% in two large studies, with complication rates significantly higher than reported operating room outcomes.[7,8]

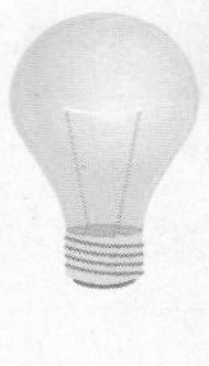

STOP AND THINK

You are intubating an obese patient. What positioning and additional techniques could you employ to maximize preoxygenation, and what approach and tools would you consider using in this situation?

The ASA task force has recommended preintubation assessment as a guide to plan intubation; use of awake techniques if direct laryngoscopy is likely to be difficult; selection of alternative airways and techniques in a methodical fashion when direct laryngoscopy is unexpectedly difficult; and use of an airway management algorithm (**Figure 17-26**) to improve the outcome.[9]

When difficult airway risk factors are present, an awake intubation might be attempted by an anesthesiologist. For the patient who is in respiratory distress and rapidly deteriorating, critical factors that drive the airway management plan include (a) the ability to preoxygenate the patient and stabilize the situation; (b) the ability to maintain adequate ventilation and oxygenation once the patient has received induction agents and/or paralytics; and (c) the ability to visualize the glottis and place the endotracheal tube.

Extraglottic Airways

Extraglottic airways (EGAs), sometimes called supraglottic airways, have evolved over a relatively short time and are currently in wide use both for routine airway management during general anesthesia and as an adjunct to manage difficult and emergency airways. The **laryngeal mask airway (LMA)** was invented in 1981, and subsequent modifications of more than 100 prototypes have resulted in the current device.[52,53]

Properly placed, EGAs like the LMA bypass upper airway soft tissue with a mask that forms a seal around the glottic aperture, with the tip engaging the proximal esophageal sphincter posterior to the cricoid cartilage. These devices provide superior ventilation to bag-valve-mask devices, with decreased risk of gastric insufflation and aspiration, and are relatively easy to place. Training for correct LMA placement is relatively easy because of the lack of laryngeal or tracheal instrumentation requirements and these devices are usually associated with a high rate of success. It is important to recognize, however, that EGAs do not provide the same level of airway protection and security afforded by an endotracheal tube.[52]

The LMA is a large-bore tube with a small inflatable mask at its distal end. A locking valve inflation port and tube allow inflation of the mask after it has been inserted and placed. The proximal end has the standard 15-mm adapter for connection to a ventilating or gas delivery device. The LMA is available in a range of sizes, from neonate to large adult. A No. 5 LMA is used for large adults, and sizes 3 and 4 are most often appropriate for

1. Assess the likelihood and clinical impact of basic management problems:
   A. Difficult Ventilation
   B. Difficult Intubation
   C. Difficulty with Patient Cooperation or Consent
   D. Difficult Tracheostomy

2. Actively pursue opportunities to deliver supplemental oxygen throughout the process of difficult airway management

3. Consider the relative merits and feasibility of basic management choices:

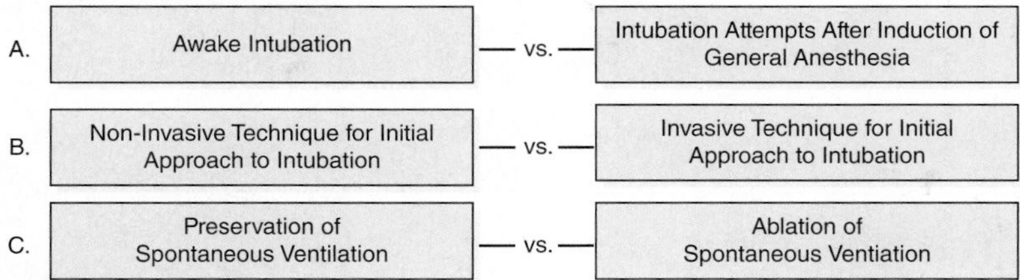

4. Develop primary and alternative strategies:

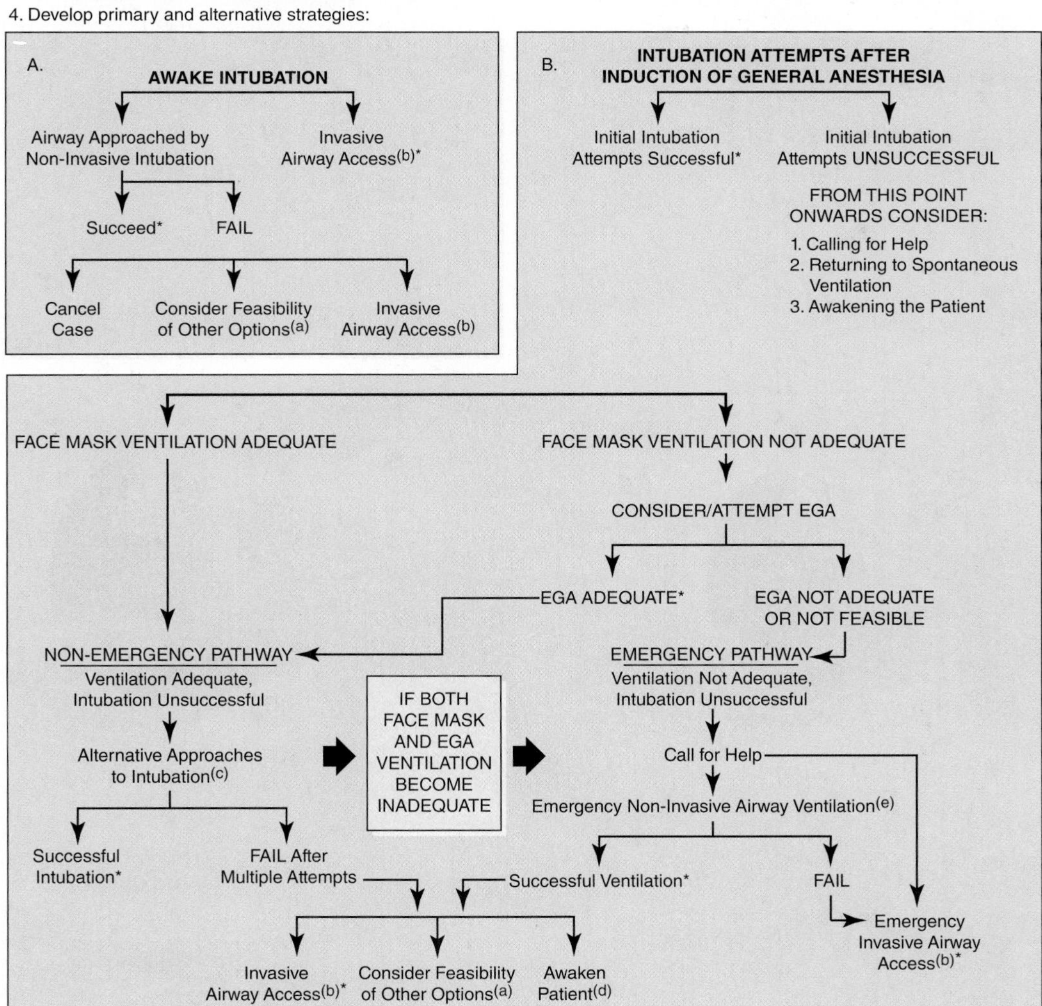

***Confirm ventilation, tracheal intubation, or EGA placement with exhaled CO_2**

a. Other options include (but are not limited to): surgery utilizing face mask or EGA anesthesia, local anesthesia infiltration, or regional nerve blockade. Pursuit of these options usually implies that mask ventilation will not be problematic. Therefore, these options may be of limited value if this step in the algorithm has been reached via the Emergency Pathway.

b. Invasive airway access includes surgical or percutaneous tracheostomy or cricothyrotomy.

c. Alternative non-invasive approaches to difficult intubation include (but are not limited to): use of different laryngoscope blades, EGA as an intubation conduit (with or without fiberoptic guidance), fiberoptic intubation, intubating stylet or tube changer, light wand, retrograde intubation, and blind oral or nasal intubation.

d. Consider repreparation of the patient for awake intubation or canceling surgery.

e. Options for emergency noninvasive airway ventilation include (but are not limited to): rigid bronchoscope, esophageal-tracheal combitube ventilation, or transtracheal jet ventilation.

FIGURE 17-26 Algorithm for a difficult airway.

Reproduced from American Society of Anesthesiologists. Practice Guidelines for management of the difficult airway. *Anesthesiology.* 2003;98:1269–1277. Reproduced with permission.

small to average-sized adults. The technique for insertion of an LMA is shown in **Figure 17-27**.

The LMA has made a significant contribution to the management of the difficult airway and is featured prominently in the ASA Difficult Airway Algorithm. An LMA has been shown to be effective as a primary rescue tool in an airway emergency when effective ventilation and oxygenation cannot be established and as a backup plan when definitive endotracheal intubation cannot be performed using direct laryngoscopy.[52,53]

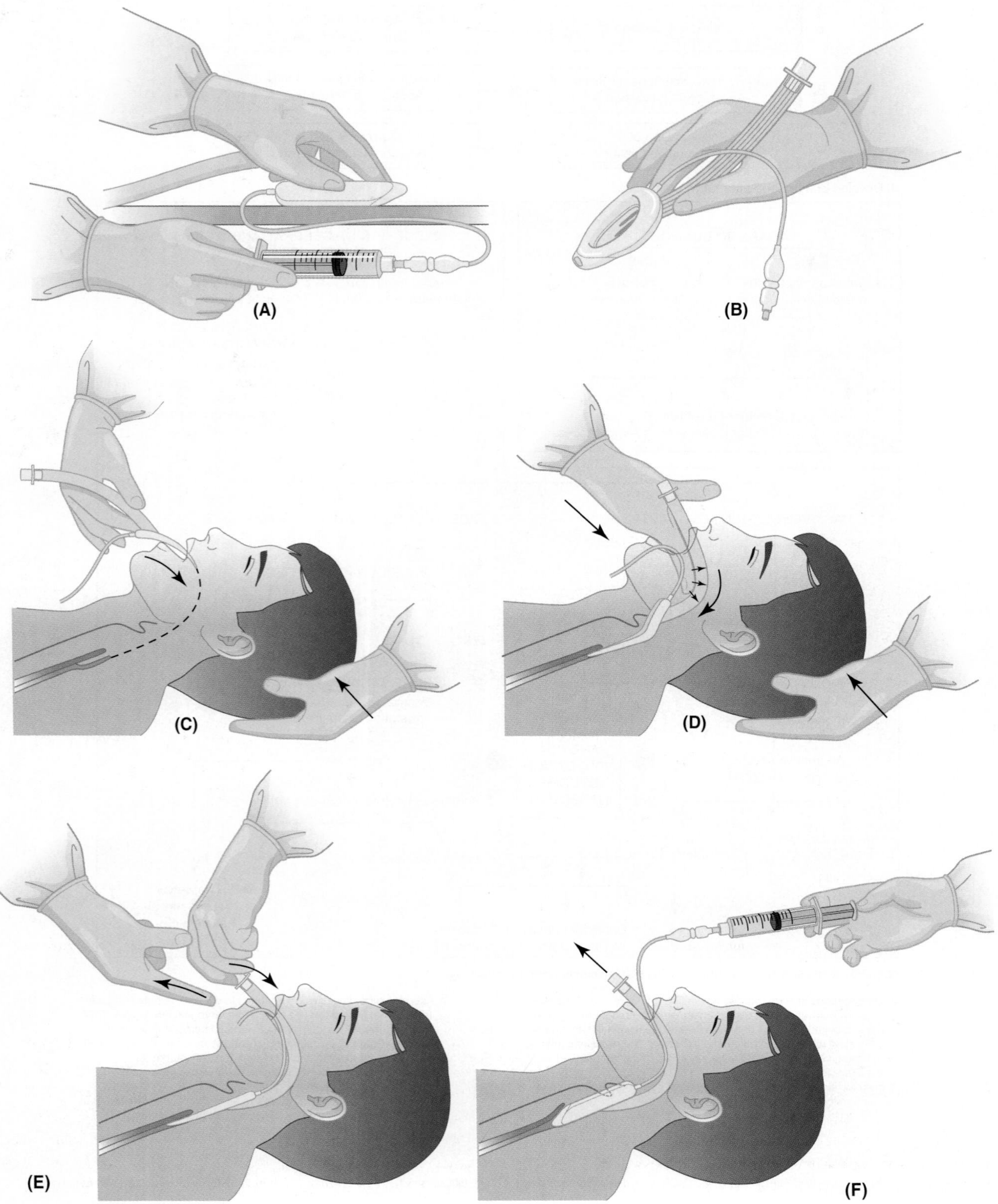

FIGURE 17-27 Insertion technique for laryngeal mask airway.
Courtesy of LMA North America, Inc.

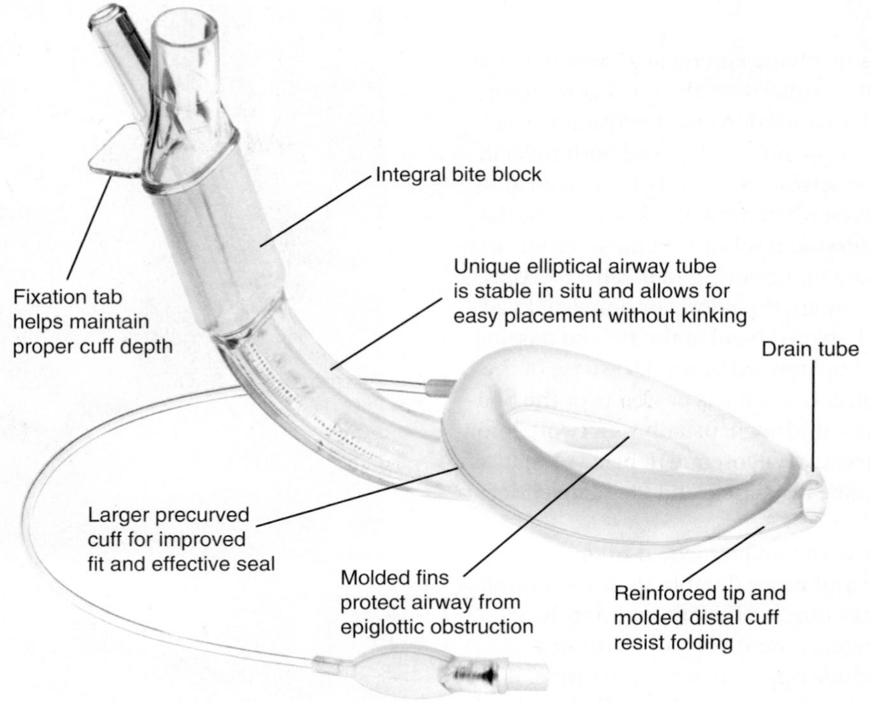

FIGURE 17-28 LMA Supreme.
Courtesy of LMA North America, Inc.

Other EGAs have been developed to improve on the basic LMA for specific indications and to offer a disposable device. Specific modifications were made to (1) provide portals for evacuation of gastric contents while the device is in place (**Figure 17-28**),[54–56] (2) provide for temperature monitoring, (3) enhance the anatomic shape of the device, and (4) offer opportunities for endotracheal intubation. Conditions limiting the use of supraglottic devices include morbid obesity, known gastric contents, oropharyngeal swelling, airway trauma, tumors, and distorted facial anatomy.

The widespread use of EGAs and their inclusion in the difficult airway algorithm has prompted the development of special intubating EGAs that can be found on many difficult-airway carts. The LMA Fastrach (iLMA) has a curved metal shaft and handle to facilitate midline oropharyngeal placement with the patient's head in a neutral position and provides a rigid, preformed, larger lumen to facilitate endotracheal tube passage. Sizes 4 and 5 typically provide optimal intubating conditions in adult women and men, accommodating size 7.5 and 7.5–8.0 endotracheal tubes, respectively.[56] A disposable form of the device is also commercially available. After the iLMA is placed and adequate ventilation is confirmed, a wire reinforced silicone endotracheal tube manufactured with the LMA Fastrach can be placed either blindly or with fiberoptic guidance, and a pusher provided with the device is used to stabilize the tube during iLMA removal after successful endotracheal intubation.

If ventilation is inadequate following initial placement or resistance is encountered during endotracheal tube passage, the iLMA can be repositioned using either the up-down or Chandy maneuvers. The up-down maneuver usually corrects down folding of the esophagus and involves pulling out the iLMA approximately 6 cm with the cuff inflated and then reinserting it into the hypopharynx. The two-step Chandy maneuver includes gentle manipulation of the iLMA handle in the horizontal and sagittal planes. This helps to adjust positioning during hand ventilation and identify the position in which airway resistance is at a minimum. The iLMA handle can then be lifted anteriorly to displace the device away from the posterior pharyngeal wall. Both components of the Chandy maneuver attempt to align the iLMA mask orifice to optimize tracheal intubation.

A number of other similar intubating EGA devices are commercially available, including the Cookgas airQ and intubating laryngeal airway (ILA) and the Ambu Aura-i. The I-gel is a disposable cuffless intubating EGA with a mask made of a thermoplastic elastomer that expands and adapts to the patient's airway following insertion that is growing in popularity because of its ease of use.[52] Intubation through this device and other extraglottic airways designed to allow intubation has proven successful both following failed direct laryngoscopy and as a more rapid primary approach in patients with a predicted difficult airway.

Gum Elastic Bougie

In recent large trials involving emergent airway management, the **gum elastic bougie** was the most commonly employed airway adjunct used to effectively manage a difficult intubation.[7] This tool can be used both to facilitate intubation in the setting of a poorly visualized glottis and to act as a guide when difficulties advancing the endotracheal tube into the trachea are encountered. The gum elastic bougie is a blunt-ended, malleable rod that is commonly passed through the poorly or nonvisualized larynx by putting a J-shaped bend at the tip and passing it blindly in the midline upward beyond the base of the epiglottis. The endotracheal tube is passed over the bougie and the bougie is withdrawn, usually as a two-person procedure with a direct laryngoscope in place to reduce upper airway soft tissue resistance and facilitate endotracheal tube passage.

A similar device is the endotracheal **tube exchanger**. Longer and more flexible than the bougie, this device facilitates quick, efficient endotracheal tube exchange or replacement with or without a laryngoscope to reduce upper airway resistance. It is constructed of flexible material and usually has depth marks to aid precise placement. Some tube exchangers have an internal lumen that allows for spontaneous breathing during the tube exchange.

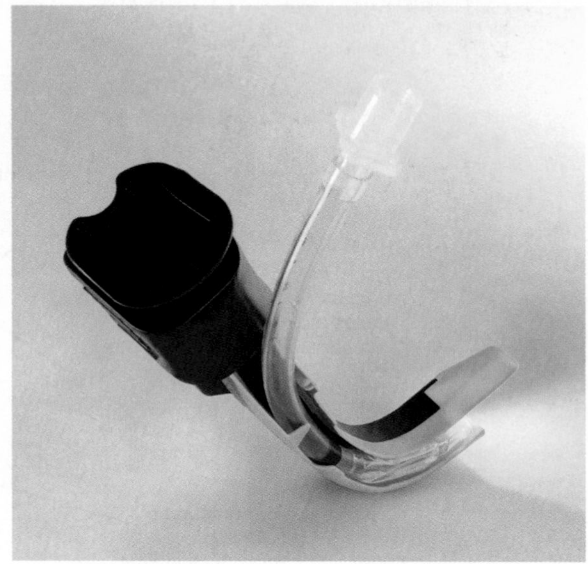

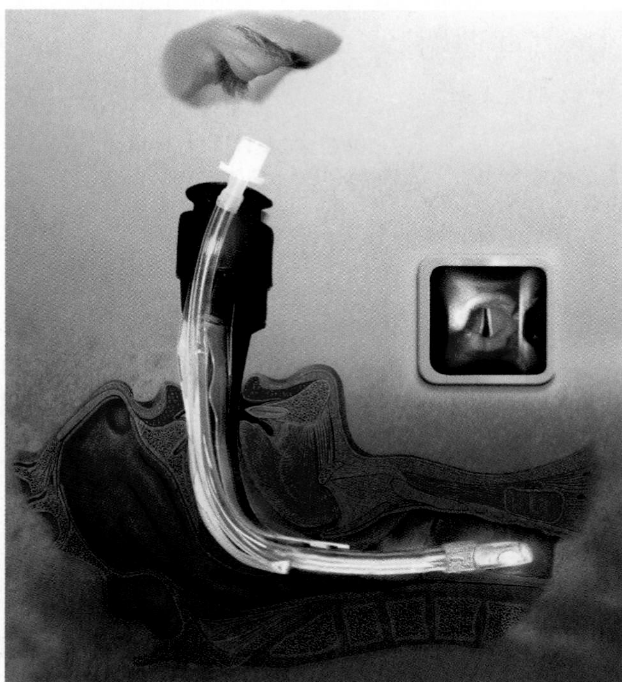

FIGURE 17-29 Airtraq laryngoscope with a tracheal tube in place in the side channel.

Courtesy of Airtraq LLC, www.airtraq.com. Used with permission.

Video Laryngoscopy Devices

Recent years have seen the development of a wide array of commercially available indirect optical devices and **video laryngoscopes**, the characteristics and technical use of which have been recently and extensively reviewed.[57–59] These devices have gained significant popularity despite limited data supporting their utility over standard direct laryngoscopy. They generally provide a digitally produced real-time view of the larynx without having to directly view through the patient's open mouth. The image is displayed on a screen attached to the scope or on a separate monitor and is particularly useful in difficult airway situations such as limited mouth opening, neck positioning, or following failed intubation attempts.

Several manufacturers have developed video laryngoscopes, and some are in common use today. The Airtraq by King Systems is a single-use device that is battery powered and portable. It has an L-shaped design and two channels, one for the optics and one a delivery channel for introduction of the endotracheal tube (**Figure 17-29**). The Airtraq is introduced above the epiglottis similar to a MacIntosh laryngoscope blade, and the endotracheal tube is advanced into the glottis under visualization and then moved out of the channel as the Airtraq is removed. Comparative studies with the MacIntosh laryngoscope have shown superior viewing with the Airtraq.[60–62]

Two multiple-use devices with single-use blade covers are the GlideScope (**Figure 17-30**) and McGrath video laryngoscopes (**Figure 17-31**). The McGrath is more portable because its small LCD screen is mounted directly on the handle, but the small size of the screen limits the view clarity at times. The view obtained with the McGrath is slightly better than the view obtained with the Airtraq, and the LCD screen is also adjustable to some degree. The GlideScope has a larger monitor attached by a video cable, which improves the

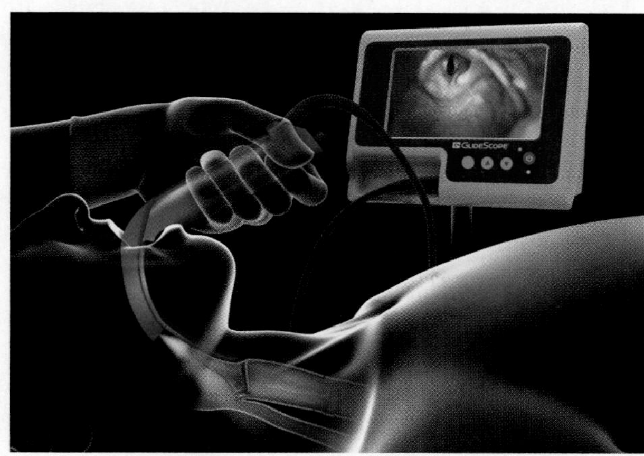

FIGURE 17-30 GlideScope video laryngoscope.
Courtesy of Verathon, Inc.

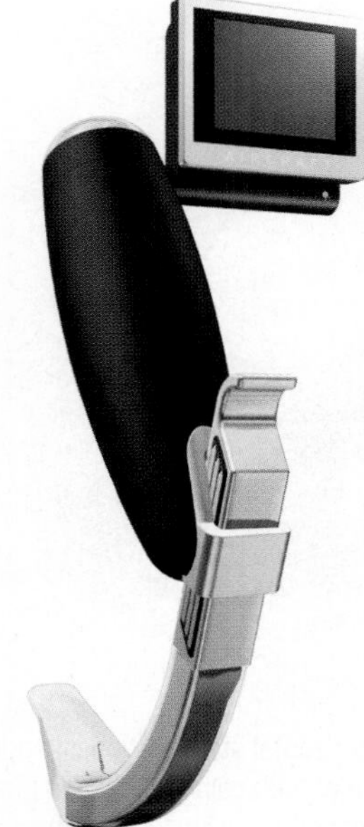

FIGURE 17-31 McGrath video laryngoscope.
Courtesy of LMA North America, Inc.

quality and size of the image but limits its portability. A more portable version is the GlideScope Ranger (**Figure 17-32**), which has a handheld monitor that can be placed on the patient's chest during intubation for easier viewing. Several other manufacturers have developed variations of the three mentioned devices, and most are functional and improve visualization over the classic direct laryngoscopy, particularly in difficult visualization situations.

A growing body of evidence suggests that video laryngoscopes provide better glottic visualization than direct laryngoscopy, reducing the incidence of difficult intubation in both low risk and difficult airways especially in the hands of less experienced airway managers.[63–66] Severe complications and patient outcomes, however, have not been consistently demonstrated.

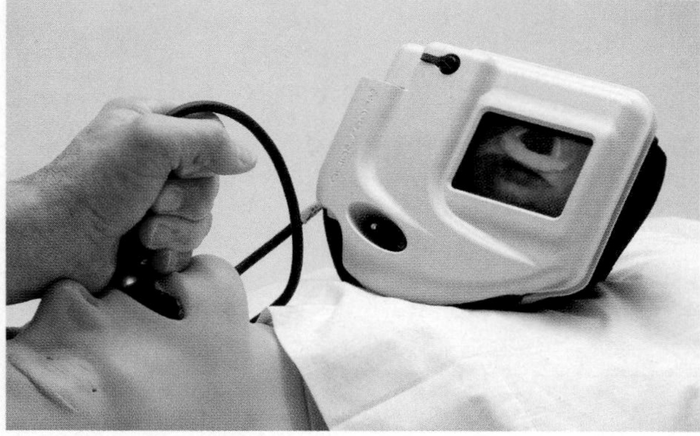

FIGURE 17-32 GlideScope Ranger.
Courtesy of Verathon, Inc.

This is perhaps because the indirect glottis view afforded by modern devices can translate into slower intubation times compared to direct laryngoscopy, especially in patients without difficult airway features.[67,68] In patients with difficult airway risk factors or failed airway attempts using direct laryngoscopy, however, several studies have now demonstrated high rates of intubation success with several video laryngoscopes.[69–71] The Airtraq optical laryngoscope has performed less favorably in difficult airways in the prehospital setting, but the generalizability of these results to the inpatient setting remains unclear.[72]

Cricothyrotomy

Creating an airway through the cricothyroid membrane is called a **cricothyrotomy**. Surgical cricothyroidotomy is an uncommon procedure generally reserved for the emergency airway situation when an extraglottic airway cannot be effectively employed due to upper airway abnormalities, blood, or secretions that obviate proper placement and function. It is also an important rescue strategy in the setting of the failed airway, especially when ventilation and oxygenation are inadequate. Cricothyroidotomy can be performed most rapidly with minimal surgical skills using a rapid four-step technique (RFST): (1) palpation of the cricothyroid membrane, (2) making of a vertical or horizontal incision (3–4 cm), (3) insertion of a dilator, and (4) intubation with a tracheostomy tube (**Figure 17-33**). A modified RFST, performed by inserting a bougie into the trachea through the incision to serve as a guide for a standard endotracheal tube, has also been shown to be successful in the hands of the novice nonsurgeon.[73] A cricothyroidotomy kit that utilizes a Seldinger approach is commercially available, too, but has been associated with longer time to placement.[74] Access can also be gained by passing a 12- to 16-gauge over-the-needle catheter (needle cricothyrotomy) through the cricothyroid membrane. Once access to the trachea is gained, the needle is removed and the catheter can then be attached to an oxygen/ventilation source.

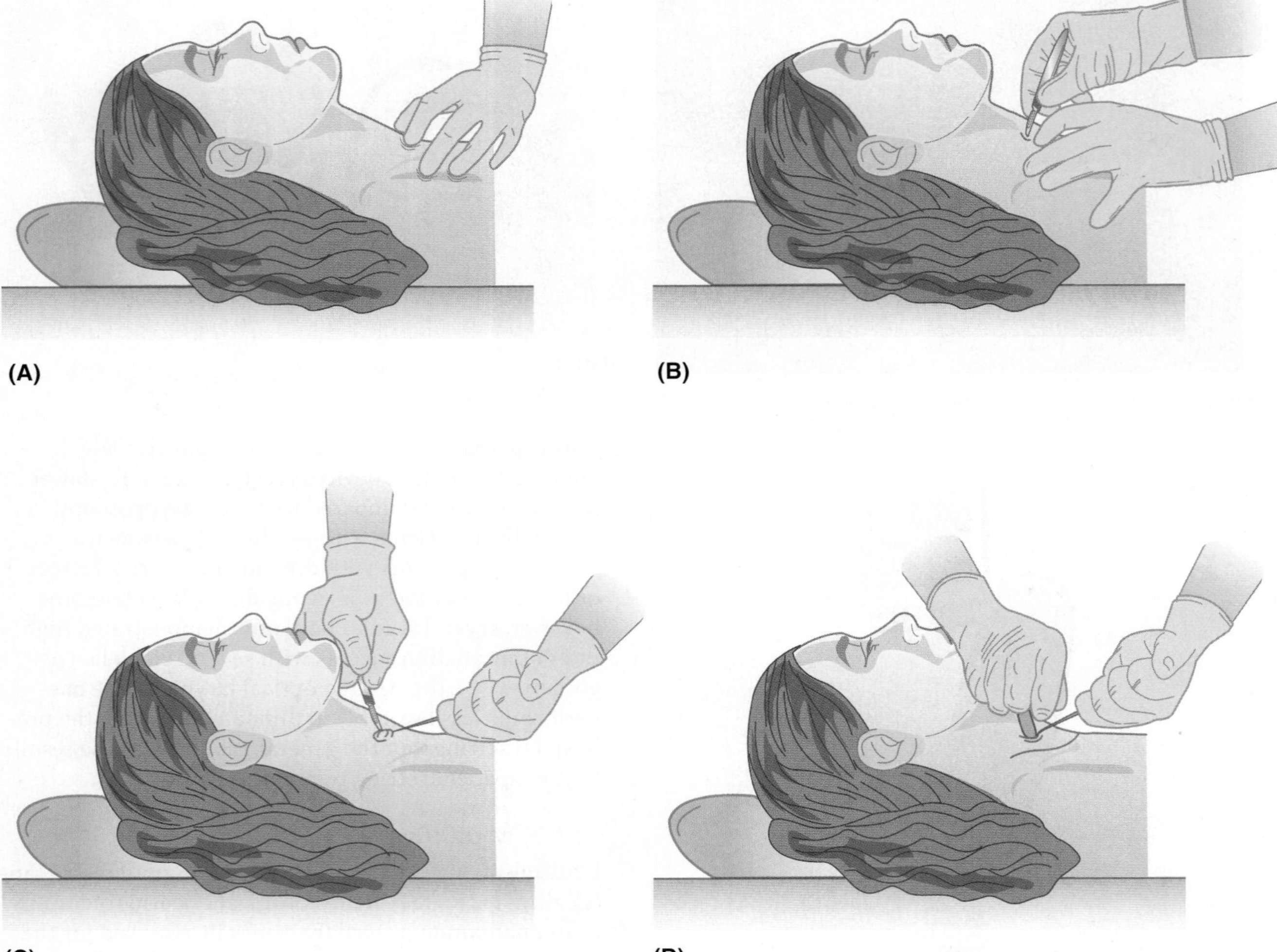

FIGURE 17-33 Approach to cricothyrotomy. (**A**) The operator palpates the cricoid membrane. (**B**) A horizontal stab incision is made into the inferior aspect of the cricothyroid membrane. (**C**) The tracheal hook is placed flush against the caudal surface of the scalpel blade and pushed into the trachea. The scalpel is removed, and traction is maintained. (**D**) A cuffed tracheostomy or endotracheal tube is inserted into the incision.

Adapted from Brofeldt T, Panacek EA, Richards JR. *Acad Emerg Med.* 1996;3:1060–1063.

Of the four available techniques described, surgical cricothyroidotomy with a cuffed tube or a commercially available kit that allows placement of a wide bore cannula over a needle or wire is probably more appropriate than a needle cricothyroidotomy with low pressure or jet ventilation in the ICU. Major complications of the procedure include esophageal perforation, subcutaneous emphysema, and bleeding.

Another airway technique that is used on rare occasions is retrograde intubation. In a retrograde intubation, the cricothyroid membrane again is accessed with a through-the-needle catheter or a guidewire. The catheter or guidewire is then passed from the larynx back up to the oral cavity. An endotracheal tube is passed over the guidewire to the larynx and trachea.[75] This technique is rarely used because of its invasiveness and complexity.

Extubation

Extubation is defined as the removal of an endotracheal tube (**CPG 17-1**). Because endotracheal tubes are considered a temporary measure, clinicians must determine the appropriate time to remove them from patients. Some patients require a permanent artificial airway, but these should receive a tracheostomy. The patient is considered ready to be extubated when the initial reason for intubation has been corrected. Several criteria must also be met, however. These criteria include the ability to protect the lower airway from aspiration, the ability to clear secretions (cough strength), the nature of secretions (quantity and character), and the ability to prevent obstruction of the upper airway. Quantity of secretions is assessed by suction frequency, and strength of cough can be assessed by peak cough flow using a peak flow meter attached to

CLINICAL PRACTICE GUIDELINE 17-1

Removal of the Endotracheal Tube

Indications

- When the airway control afforded by the endotracheal tube is deemed to be no longer necessary for the continued care of the patient, the tube should be removed. Subjective or objective determination of improvement of the underlying condition impairing pulmonary function and/or gas exchange capacity is made prior to extubation. To maximize the likelihood for successful extubation, the patient should be capable of maintaining a patent airway and generating adequate spontaneous ventilation. In general, this requires the patient to possess adequate central inspiratory drive, respiratory muscle strength, cough strength to clear secretions, laryngeal function, nutritional status, and clearance of sedative and neuromuscular blocking effects.
- Occasionally, acute airway obstruction of the artificial airway due to mucus or mechanical deformation mandates immediate removal of the artificial airway. Reintubation or other appropriate techniques for reestablishing the airway (i.e., surgical airway management) must be used to maintain effective gas exchange.
- Patients in whom an explicit declaration of the futility of further medical care is documented may have the endotracheal tube removed despite failure to meet the above indications.

Contraindications

- There are no absolute contraindications to extubation; however, to maintain acceptable gas exchange after extubation, some patients may require one or more of the following: noninvasive ventilation, continuous positive airway pressure, high FIO_2, or reintubation. Airway protective reflexes may be depressed immediately following and for some time after extubation. Therefore, measures to prevent aspiration should be considered.

Assessment of Extubation Readiness

- The endotracheal tube should be removed as soon as the patient no longer requires an artificial airway. Patients should demonstrate some evidence for the reversal of the underlying cause of respiratory failure and should be capable of maintaining adequate spontaneous ventilation and gas exchange. The determination of extubation readiness may be individualized using the following guidelines.
- Patients with an artificial airway to facilitate treatment of respiratory failure should be considered for extubation when they have met established extubation readiness criteria.
- Resolution of the need for airway protection may be assessed by, but is not limited to, appropriate level of consciousness, adequate airway protective reflexes, and easily managed secretions.
- Issues that should be considered in all patients prior to extubation are no immediate need for reintubation anticipated; known risk factors for extubation failure; presence of upper airway obstruction or laryngeal edema as detected by diminished gas leak around the endotracheal tube with positive pressure breaths; evidence of stable, adequate hemodynamic function; evidence of stable nonrespiratory functions; electrolyte values within normal range; and evidence of malnutrition decreasing respiratory muscle function and ventilatory drive. Anesthesia literature indicates the patient must have no intake of food or liquid by mouth for a period of time prior to airway manipulation. The continuation of transpyloric feedings during an extubation procedure remains controversial.
- Prophylactic medication prior to extubation to avoid or reduce the severity of postextubation complications (e.g., steroids).

Hazards and Complications

- Hypoxemia after extubation may result from, but is not limited to, failure to deliver adequate inspired oxygen fraction through the natural upper airway, acute upper airway obstruction secondary to laryngospasm, postobstruction pulmonary edema, bronchospasm, atelectasis, pulmonary aspiration, and hypoventilation.
- Hypercapnia after extubation may be caused by, but is not limited to, upper airway obstruction resulting from edema of the trachea, vocal cords, or larynx; respiratory muscle weakness; excessive work of breathing; and bronchospasm.
- Death may occur when medical futility is the reason for removing the endotracheal tube.

Adapted from AARC clinical practice guideline: removal of the endotracheal tube—2007 revision and update. *Respir Care.* 2007;52:81–93. Reprinted with permission.

the endotracheal tube. It has been shown that patients with a cough peak flow of 60 L/min or less were nearly five times as likely to fail extubation.[76] Patients with secretions of more than 2.5 mL/h were three times as likely to fail. Patients who were unable to complete four simple tasks (i.e., open eyes, follow with eyes, grasp hand, stick out tongue) were more than four times as likely to fail as those who completed the four commands. The failure rate was 100% for patients with all three risk factors (cough, secretions, inability to complete four simple tasks) compared with 3% for those with no risk factors.

In some cases the upper airway is at risk for swelling and inflammation during the period of intubation. Before extubation can be performed in these patients, the absence of these conditions is often assessed as the amount of leakage around the endotracheal tube during positive pressure ventilation with the cuff deflated. Qualitatively, the leak test is performed by deflating the cuff, and then assessing for the presence of leak through the upper airway. Quantitatively, the leak can be assessed as the volume of the leak or the percentage of the tidal volume that leaks. The value of the leak test is controversial because false positives and false negatives are common.[77,78] Also, the cuff leak test increases the risk of aspiration because secretions located on the superior surface of the cuff may have a clear path to the lower respiratory tract with the cuff down. When upper airway edema is suspected, prophylactic administration of corticosteroids decreases the risk of postextubation stridor and reintubation.[79,80]

Two methods have been described for extubation, each intended to reduce the risk of aspiration of subglottic secretions. They are the trailing suction catheter method and the subglottic purge maneuver. The trailing suction catheter method uses a suction catheter passed through the endotracheal tube. The cuff is then deflated, and suction is applied as the tube is removed. For the subglottic purge maneuver, a positive pressure hyperinflation is provided followed by cuff deflation. The concept is that secretions in the subglottic space are propelled upward into the oral pharynx where they can be cleared.

Extubation failure, or the need to reintubate, occurs in 5% to 15% of cases for a variety of reasons.[81,82] Most commonly, the patient cannot sustain adequate spontaneous ventilation. Reintubation is not benign and has been associated with increased morbidity and mortality. Conversely, unwarranted delay in extubation resulting in prolonged intubation is also associated with increased morbidity and mortality. Some patient populations may be at a higher risk of extubation failure; therefore, equipment and preparations for a timely reintubation should be present. Because some risk of extubation failure exists in all patients, it is important that a clinician who can perform reintubation be present at the time of extubation.

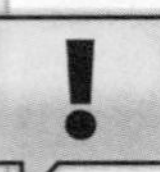

Respiratory Recap

Extubation

- Extubation is the removal of an endotracheal tube.
- Adequacy of airway clearance and ability to protect the airway must be assessed before extubation.
- Prophylactic corticosteroids decrease the risk of postextubation stridor and reintubation.

Tracheostomy

Advantages and Disadvantages of Tracheostomy

Tracheostomy is the surgical introduction of a tube into the trachea. It is among the most commonly conducted procedures in critically ill patients. A tracheostomy is usually done for three main reasons: to bypass an upper airway obstruction, to aid in removal of secretions from the airway, and to provide long-term mechanical ventilation.

Compared with endotracheal intubation, a tracheostomy has the advantages of lowering airway resistance, causing less tube movement in the trachea, affording greater patient comfort, and allowing the patient to swallow secretions and nourishment. The patient can communicate by moving the lips and can even talk with the aid of special **tracheostomy tubes** and devices. If accidental decannulation occurs, the tube can be reinserted into the mature stoma more easily than reintubation with an endotracheal tube can be accomplished after accidental extubation. Because the tracheostomy tube is shorter than an endotracheal tube, more of the airway below the cuff may be suctioned with greater efficiency. Tracheostomy also avoids the oral, nasal, pharyngeal, and laryngeal complications of translaryngeal intubation.

A tracheostomy also has disadvantages. It is a surgical procedure and has greater morbidity and mortality risks than endotracheal intubation. Additional risks include incisional hemorrhage, subcutaneous emphysema, pneumothorax, and pneumomediastinum. Tracheal stenosis is common, and a permanent scar is unavoidable. As with endotracheal intubation, the tracheostomy tube bypasses normal defense mechanisms

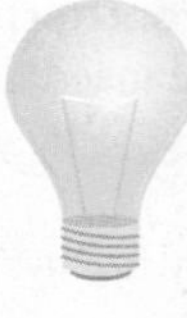

STOP AND THINK

You are helping to care for a patient with severe ARDS. It is day six of mechanical ventilation and the question arises about tracheostomy. What would be some of the advantages and disadvantages of performing a tracheostomy at this time?

and impedes an effective cough because the glottis is bypassed. Many of the complications experienced during conventional tracheostomy may be avoided if the surgery is performed by a skilled surgeon as an elective procedure under optimum conditions when the patient's airway has already been stabilized, rather than at the bedside as an emergency effort.

Timing of Tracheostomy

The timing of tracheostomy in patients receiving prolonged mechanical ventilation is controversial. On one hand, earlier tracheostomy avoids complications of prolonged endotracheal intubation, improves patients' ability to communicate, and makes nursing care easier. The procedure is not without risk, however. Several studies compared early versus late tracheostomy in mechanically ventilated patients.[83,84] Tracheostomy performed within the first week of mechanical ventilation was not associated with an improvement in ventilator-associated pneumonia, mortality, or other important secondary outcomes. There is no question that early tracheostomy should be performed in patients who go on to require prolonged mechanical ventilation, but the decision for early tracheostomy depends on the clinician's ability to predict which patients will require extended ventilatory support, a difficult prediction to make.

Open Tracheostomy

An open tracheostomy can be done in the intensive care unit at the bedside, under local anesthesia, or under general anesthesia in the operating room. The patient's head is hyperextended over a shoulder roll (unless there is a contraindication). A vertical or horizontal surgical incision is made, usually between the second and third tracheal ring, and the tube is inserted into the trachea. If accidental decannulation occurs within the first several days following open tracheostomy, the stomal tract is immature and the patient should be reintubated orally.

Percutaneous Dilational Tracheostomy

A common technique is the percutaneous dilational tracheostomy (PDT). PDT is a comparatively new procedure that is less traumatic than the conventional surgical method.[85] The patient is positioned with the neck extended, and the skin in the area of puncture and incision is infiltrated with a local anesthetic with epinephrine. A small incision is made midway between the cricoid cartilage and the sternal notch, and a 14-gauge cannula is inserted into the trachea between the first and second tracheal rings. A guide wire is introduced into the trachea under direct bronchoscopic observation, and the stoma is dilated with increasing sizes of specially designed plastic dilators by use of the Seldinger catheter-over-wire technique (**Figure 17-34**). Once the dilation is

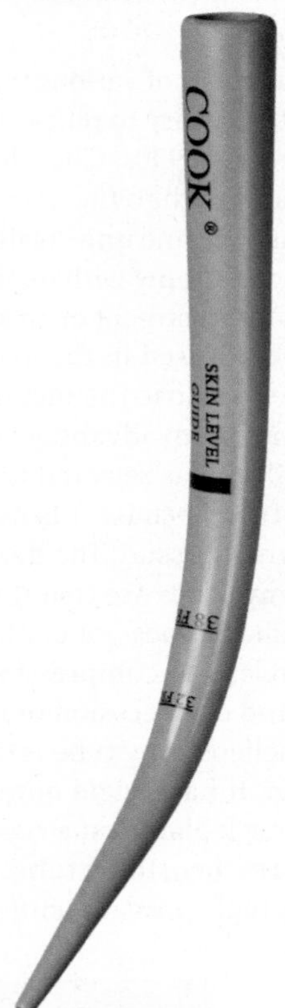

FIGURE 17-34 Dilator to form stoma for placement of percutaneous tracheostomy tube.
Courtesy of Cook Medical.

complete, an appropriately sized tracheostomy tube is inserted over a small dilator and placed in position in the trachea.

The advantages of PDT are that it can be performed at the bedside in the intensive care unit, eliminating the risks involved in moving a high-risk patient to the operating room, and that it greatly reduces the potential for hemorrhage. The dilation creates an opening that fits tightly around the tracheostomy tube for several days, rather than the large, secured opening created during a conventional tracheostomy. Once the airway is secure, the tract can be explored, the guidewire and dilators replaced, and the tracheostomy tube reinserted.

Long-term problems with PDT, such as tracheal stenosis, have not yet been seen. In fact, the quality of the stoma is often better following PDT than with open tracheostomy. Compared with surgical tracheostomy procedures, PDT has a lower incidence of pneumothorax, bleeding complications, and stenosis. With bronchoscopic guidance, PDT can be considered for patients with a difficult anatomy due to morbid obesity or abnormalities of the neck.

If accidental decannulation occurs within the first several days following PDT, the patient should be reintubated orally. The tracheostomy tube can usually be safely changed or downsized 5 days after PDT.

Metal Tracheostomy Tubes

Metal tracheostomy tubes of various types were used throughout the 19th century to relieve upper airway obstruction. In the early 1930s, Chevalier Jackson developed a systematic approach to the management of airway obstruction that became universally accepted. This approach made tracheostomy with double-lumen silver tubes the standard for treatment of airway obstruction.

Silver has long been used in the manufacture of tracheostomy tubes because the metal walls can be kept very thin, which is an advantage when the inner cannula is used. Silver was selected for construction of the tracheostomy tube because it is nonreactive when in contact with human tissue. The disadvantages of silver for tracheostomy tubes are that it is expensive and rigid. The curved shape does not conform well to the trachea, which can lead to compression damage along the tracheal wall and even erosion of major vessel walls.

The Jackson tracheostomy tube is constructed completely of silver. It has a rigid outer cannula with an attached fixed neck plate and a rigid inner cannula. These metal tracheostomy tubes are cuffless, but a rubber, reusable, high-pressure cuff can be added to prevent leaks during mechanical ventilation. The size of the metal tubes is identified by the Jackson system, which uses the outer tube diameter. Disadvantages of metal tracheostomy tubes are their narrow IDs, the rigid structure of the neck plate, and the lack of a 15-mm adapter for connection to most ventilatory devices. Problems associated with the reusable high-pressure cuffs are nonuniform expansion along the tracheal wall, lack of cuff strength, and the danger of the cuff slipping over the end of the tracheostomy tube, causing airway occlusion. Metal tracheostomy tubes are available in pediatric and adult sizes. However, because of improvements in material design, clinical use of metal tracheostomy tubes is almost nonexistent.

Current Construction of Tracheostomy Tubes

Tracheostomy tubes may be made of metal, rubber, silicone, Teflon, polyethylene, and PVC materials.[86,87] Like endotracheal tubes, tracheostomy tubes must satisfy ASTM requirements. Because the tubes are in direct contact with body tissue, the ideal material is nontoxic and determined by implant testing. Modern tracheostomy tubes (**Figure 17-35**) are available in sizes 2.5 to

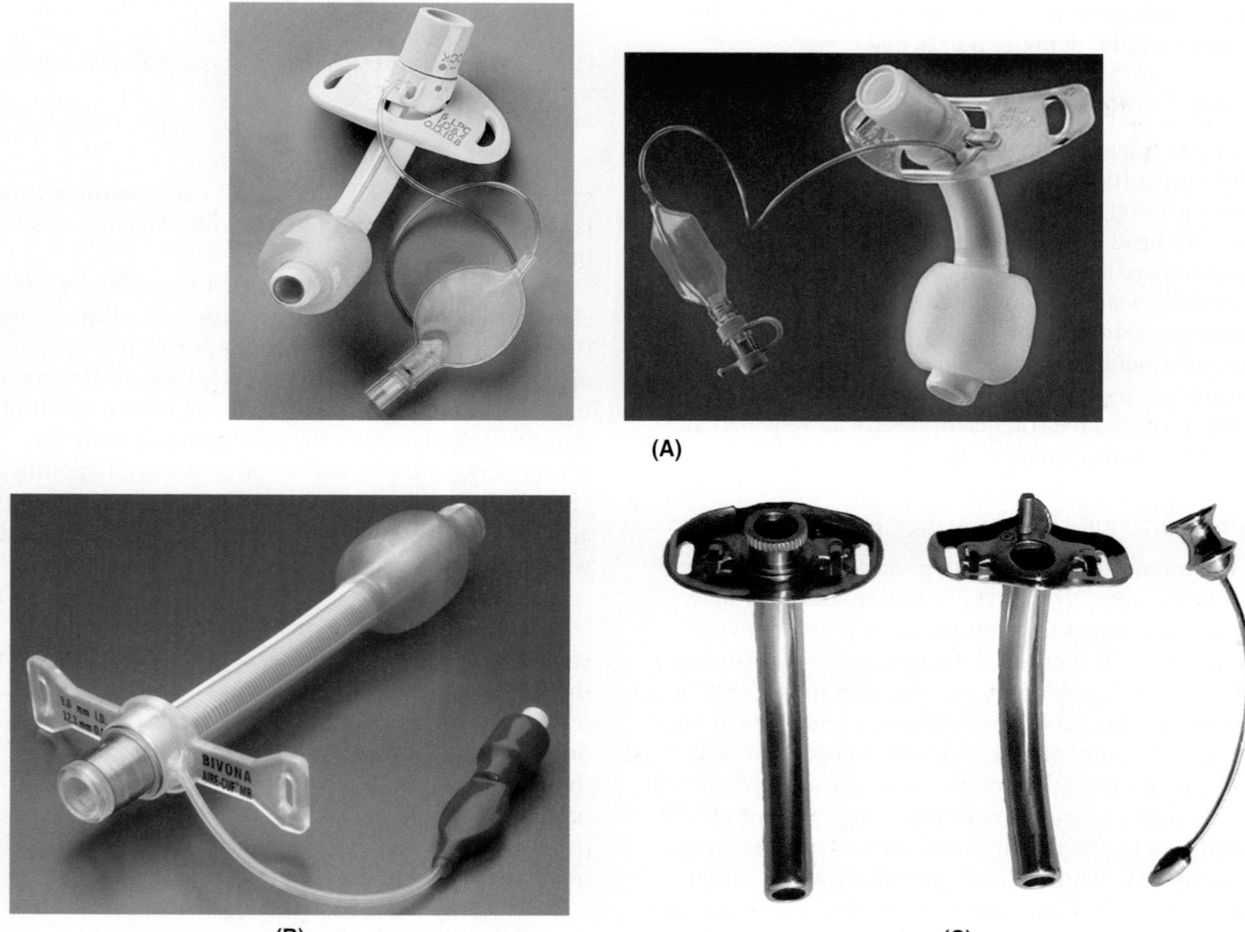

FIGURE 17-35 (**A**) Standard cuffed tracheostomy tubes. (**B**) Flexible tracheostomy tube. (**C**) Metal tracheostomy tubes.
(**A**) courtesy of Smiths Medical; (**B**) courtesy of Smiths Medical; (**C**) courtesy of the Department of Otolaryngology-Head and Neck Surgery, Johns Hopkins Medicine.

11.5 mm according to their ID. The manufacturer should mark both the ID and the OD as a guide for the user. Besides materials, standard requirements cover surface characteristics, dimensions, tolerances, cuff characteristics, and labeling of tubes and packages.

When selecting a tracheostomy tube, the ID, OD, and length must be considered. If the ID is too small, it will increase the resistance through the tube, making airway clearance more difficult. A smaller ID may also result in a smaller OD, which increases the cuff pressure required to create a seal in the trachea. If the OD is too large, the leak with the cuff deflated will be decreased and this will affect the ability to use the upper airway with cuff deflation for speech. A tube with a larger OD will also be more difficult to pass through the stoma. A 10 mm OD tube is usually appropriate for adult women and an 11 mm OD tube is usually appropriate for adult men as an initial tracheostomy tube size. A difference in tracheostomy tube length between tubes of the same ID, but from different manufacturers, is not commonly appreciated and this can have important clinical implications.

The shape of the tracheostomy tube should conform as closely as possible to the anatomy of the airway. Two main types of tracheostomy tubes are available—those that are curved, and those that are angled to fit the trachea at one end and the area between the skin and the trachea at the other end. Curved tracheostomy tubes usually have an inner cannula that can be removed for cleaning while the outer cannula remains in place. The outer cannula may have a window, or fenestration, to allow for speech when the inner cannula is removed. Because the trachea is mostly straight, the curved tracheostomy tube often does not conform to the shape of the trachea, which may allow compression of the membranous part of the trachea, and the tip may traumatize the anterior portion. These tubes may also damage the area of the stoma.

Extended-length tracheostomy tubes (**Figure 17-36**) are angled and provide extra length in the proximal or distal portions of the tube for a more customized fit. Extra length in the proximal portion accommodates patients with thick necks who have increased skin-to-tracheal-wall distances. Extra length in the distal portion of the tube is used to compensate for conditions such as tracheal stenosis or malacia.

Uncuffed Tracheostomy Tubes

Standard uncuffed tracheostomy tubes have the same basic design as those described previously. On the flange attachment of some uncuffed adult tracheostomy tubes, UNCUFFED designates that the tube is uncuffed, and FEN indicates that the tube is fenestrated. If the tracheostomy tube chosen uses a removable inner cannula, the package of the inner cannula should list the size and make of the tube into which it is intended to fit.

Uncuffed tracheostomy tubes are used primarily in pediatric patients, in whom the cricoid ring is narrower than the glottis. Because the tissues anterior to the trachea in infants are thinner and the laryngeal and tracheal cartilages are softer, use of cuffed tracheostomy tubes in infants and children up to 6 years of age makes them susceptible to tracheal deformation. In children, especially infants, the shape of the neck plate of the tracheostomy tube is important. The usual straight neck plate does not fit well because of anatomic differences between infants and adults. The newer, flexible, soft, swivel-neck flange on most current tracheostomy tubes

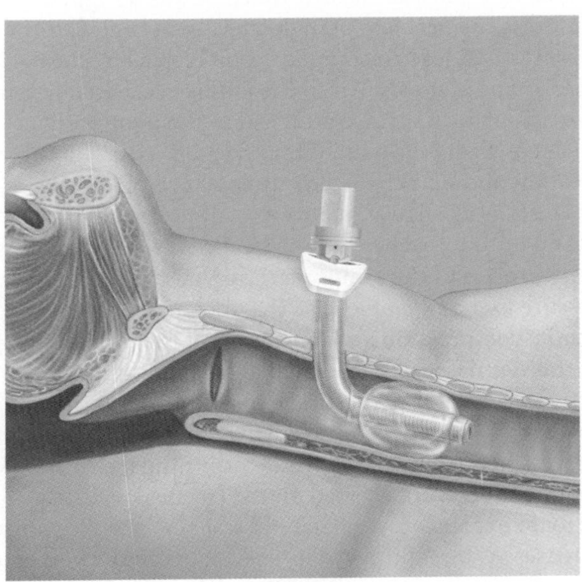

(A)

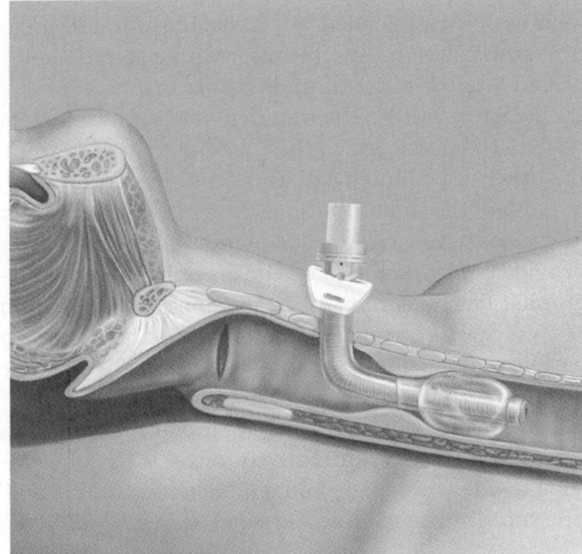

(B)

FIGURE 17-36 Examples of extra length angled tracheostomy tubes. (**A**) Increased proximal length. (**B**) Increased distal length.

AGE-SPECIFIC ANGLE

Uncuffed tracheostomy tubes are used primarily for pediatric patients.

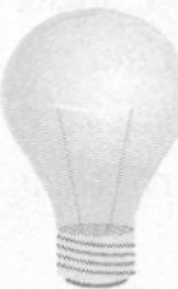

STOP AND THINK

A patient has recurrent obstruction of his tracheostomy tube. What might you do to address this problem?

solves this problem. Uncuffed tracheostomy tubes are intended to allow a small leak during ventilation. Unfortunately, some clinicians tend to use a tube that fits rather snugly to reduce this leak. The large stomal opening required to accommodate the tube increases the chances of stomal stenosis. Silastic tubes with a single lumen that do not require an inner cannula are available for pediatric patients.

In adults, uncuffed tracheostomy tubes are used primarily after laryngectomy and in patients with neuromuscular disease who need frequent suctioning but not mechanical ventilation. Uncuffed tubes have also been used as a method of weaning from the tracheostomy tube. Progressively smaller diameters of uncuffed tubes are used to allow suctioning and maintenance of the stoma while allowing the patient to adapt to the normal airway. The absence of a cuff on a tracheostomy tube does not help prevent aspiration, and this type of tube should not be used in unconscious patients or in those in whom airway defenses have been lost.

Cuffed Tracheostomy Tubes

Like the uncuffed standard tracheostomy tubes, the typical cuffed tracheostomy tube is composed of outer and inner cannulas. The outer cannula forms the primary structure of the tube and also has the cuff assembly attached to its distal end. A standard 15-mm adapter is present on the proximal end of the tube. Also at the proximal end are the inflation tube and pilot balloon with spring-loaded valve assembly for cuff inflation and deflation. An obturator with a rounded tip is placed into the outer cannula before insertion of the tracheostomy tube. The rounded obturator tip extends beyond the distal end of the tube far enough to round the otherwise blunted end; this minimizes trauma to the mucosa of the tracheal wall during insertion of the tube. The tubes have a radiopaque marker on the distal tip to provide confirmation of the tube's position on radiographs. Tracheostomy tubes are constructed primarily of PVC or other synthetic materials and are tissue compatible as determined by acceptable implant test methods. Modern tracheostomy tubes are disposable and offer the practitioner a variety of models ranging from a standard system similar to the silver tracheostomy tube to one with single and double fenestrations and pressure-limiting automatic relief valves.

Dual-Cannula Tracheostomy Tube

A controversy in the selection of the proper tracheostomy tube involves the choice of a single-lumen tube or a tube with an inner cannula. With a dual-cannula tracheostomy tube, the inner cannula can be removed for cleaning. In some cases, the ventilator connection is to the inner cannula. It is important to appreciate that an inner cannula (dual-cannula design) results in a decrease in the inner diameter of the tube or an increase in the outer diameter of the tube. An inner cannula is necessary to block the opening in a fenestrated tracheostomy tube.

Subglottic Suction Port

Tracheostomy tubes are available that provide a suction port above the cuff. One such design is the Blom tracheostomy tube (**Figure 17-37**). The subglottic suctioning cannula is located on the exterior surface of the cannula as a separate lumen, which can be connected to intermittent or continuous suction. The subglottic suctioning cannula is intended for the evacuation of secretions situated above the tracheostomy tube cuff. Subglottic suction with tracheostomy tubes may reduce the risk of ventilator-associated pneumonia, but the evidence is not mature.[88]

Foam Cuff Tracheostomy Tubes

The Bivona foam cuff consists of a large-diameter, high-residual-volume cuff composed of polyurethane foam covered by a silicone sheath. This cuff was designed to address the problem of high lateral tracheal wall pressures that lead to complications such as tracheal necrosis and stenosis. Air in the cuff is evacuated before insertion using a syringe attached to the pilot port, which contracts the foam (**Figure 17-38**). This allows insertion of the tracheostomy tube. Once the tube is in place, the syringe is removed to allow the cuff to re-expand until it reaches the tracheal wall. The pilot tube remains open to the atmosphere so that the intracuff pressure is at ambient levels. The open pilot port also permits compression and expansion of the cuff during the ventilatory cycle, which allows intermittent perfusion of the tracheal tissue in contact with the tube without loss of volume during ventilation. The degree of foam expansion is a determining factor in the amount of pressure exerted on the tracheal wall. As the foam expands further, lateral tracheal wall pressure increases. When the device is used properly, however, this pressure rarely exceeds 20 mm Hg.

When a foam cuff tracheostomy tube is selected, the proper size is important to maintain a seal and still benefit from the pressure-limiting advantages of the

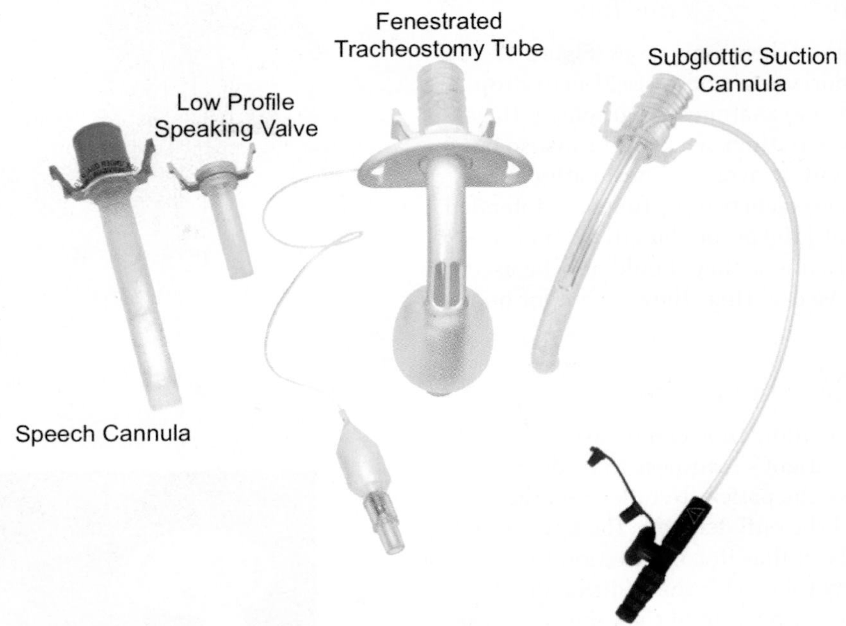

FIGURE 17-37 Blom® tracheostomy tube system.
Courtesy of Pulmodyne.

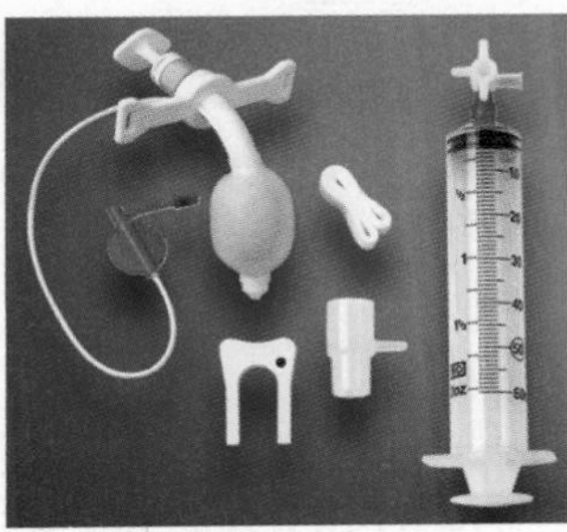

FIGURE 17-38 Foam cuff trach tube kit.
Courtesy of Smiths Medical.

foam-filled cuff. If the tube is too small, the foam will inflate to its unrestricted size and the cuff may leak, causing loss of ventilation and loss of protection against aspiration. If the tube is too large, the foam is unable to expand properly to provide the desired cushion, with resultant increased pressure against the tracheal wall. If air is injected into the cuff to increase the lateral wall pressure and provide a seal, the purpose and pressure-limiting benefits of the foam cuff are defeated and the cuff may leak, which can result in a loss of ventilator volume during inspiration. The manufacturer recommends periodic cuff deflation to assess the integrity of the cuff and prevent the silicone sheath from adhering to the tracheal mucosa.

Tight-to-Shaft Cuff Tracheostomy Tubes

The tight-to-shaft tracheostomy tube is used for patients requiring short-term cuff inflation, such as avoidance of aspiration during feeding or nocturnal-only ventilation. When the silicone cuff is totally deflated, it adds no distinguishable dimension to the outer diameter of the tube's shaft. This cuff is unique because it is inflated with water rather than air.

Sleep Apnea Tracheostomy Tubes

These tubes are uncuffed tubes designed for use in patients with obstructive sleep apnea who do not tolerate continuous positive airway pressure (CPAP) therapy. They have a flexible all-silicone construction that improves patient comfort and minimizes skin irritation, encrustation, and mucus occlusion. These tubes have a low-profile design and are easily capped and concealed during waking hours. They also are used when airway access for pulmonary hygiene and suctioning is required. These tubes cannot be used in patients who require invasive ventilator assistance.

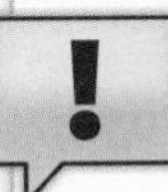

Respiratory Recap

Types of Tracheostomy Tubes

- Uncuffed
- Cuffed
- Dual cannula
- Subglottic suction
- Foam cuff
- Tight to shaft cuff
- Sleep apnea tubes
- Adjustable flange tubes
- Fenestrated tubes
- Talking trach tubes

Adjustable Flange Tracheostomy Tubes

Adjustable neck flange tracheostomy tubes (**Figure 17-39**) can be adjusted for horizontal and vertical shaft drop to accommodate unusual anatomy or pathology. They are used for patients with thick necks and can also be used to position the cuff to avoid tracheal pathology. Adjustable neck flange tracheostomy tubes are intended for temporary use until the proper length fixed neck flange tube can be obtained. They should only be used in a clinically supervised setting. They are not for home care use.

Fenestrated Tracheostomy Tubes

A fenestrated tracheostomy tube can be useful in the assessment of a patient's readiness to be decannulated, and it allows the patient to talk when the tube is occluded and the cuff deflated. The fenestrated tracheostomy tube is similar in construction to a regular tracheostomy tube, with the addition of an opening in the posterior portion of the tube above the cuff (**Figure 17-40**). Fenestrated tubes are composed of a tracheostomy tube with a fenestration, a removable inner cannula, and a plastic plug. When the inner cannula is removed, the cuff deflated, and normal air passage occluded with the plug, the patient can inhale and exhale through the fenestration and around the tube. This allows for assessment of the patient's ability to breathe through the normal oral/nasal route (preparing the patient for decannulation) and permits air to pass by the vocal cords, creating phonation.

Healthcare workers must be properly trained in the use of fenestrated tracheostomy tubes. If the patient has been receiving humidified, oxygen-enriched air via the tube, an alternate source must be provided, such as a nasal cannula. Also, before the proximal end is blocked, the cuff must be completely deflated by evacuating all of the air. The tracheal cap is then put in place to allow the patient to breathe through the fenestrations and around the tube. If the cuff is left inflated during the capping procedure, airway resistance will be excessive, and the patient will experience respiratory distress. The patient must be observed carefully for aspiration of secretions or oral fluids while the cuff is deflated. This type of tube should be considered only for patients with normal upper airway reflexes.

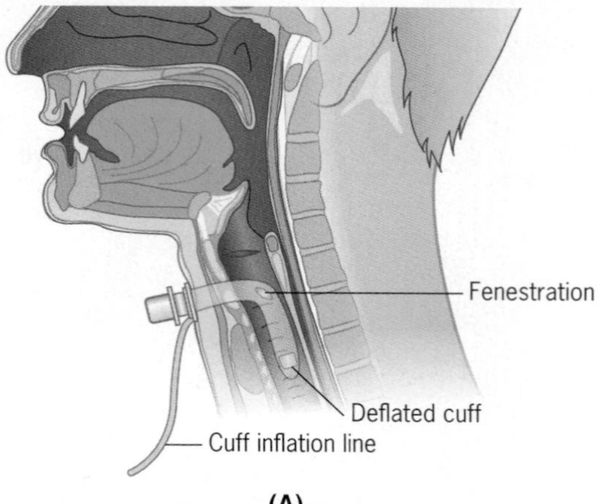

(A)

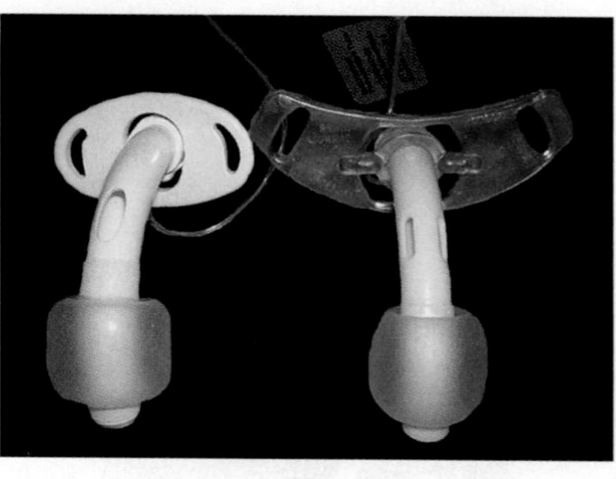

(B)

FIGURE 17-40 Fenestrated tracheostomy tubes.

Talking Tracheostomy Tubes

Specialized tracheostomy tubes allow communication for ventilator-dependent patients. The talking tracheostomy tube (**Figure 17-41**) operates using an external gas flow (4–6 L/min) that is routed through the larynx via a separate flow line with a thumb port. When the thumb port is occluded, gas passes though the larynx and can be used for phonation. The cuff stays inflated, separating speech from ventilation. A couple of drawbacks to this system are that a specialized tube has to be placed (perhaps replacing the existing tube) and that someone must be available to occlude the thumb port (e.g., the caregiver or, in some instances, the patients themselves).

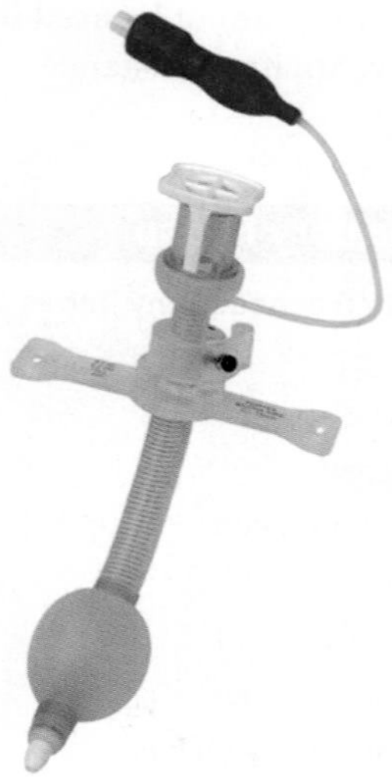

FIGURE 17-39 Adjustable flange tracheostomy tube.
Courtesy of Smiths Medical.

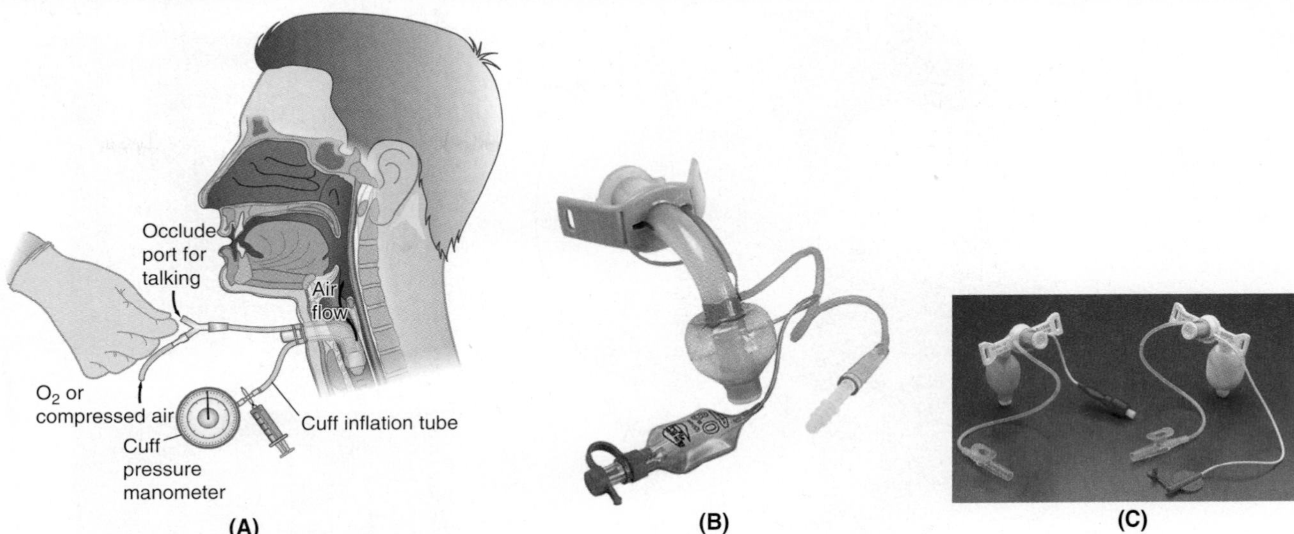

FIGURE 17-41 Talking tracheostomy tubes.
(B) and (C) courtesy of Smiths Medical.

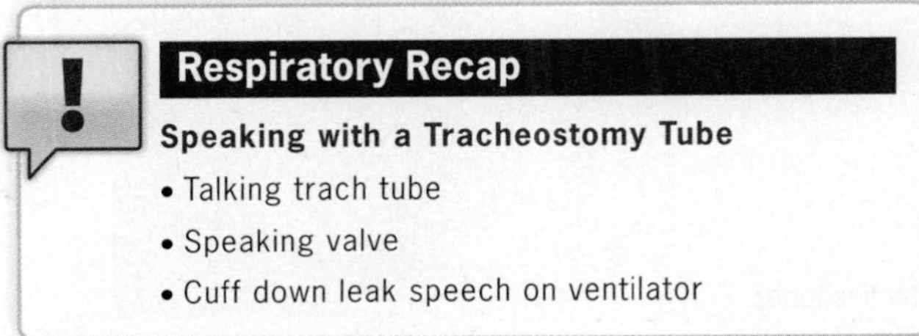

Respiratory Recap

Speaking with a Tracheostomy Tube

- Talking trach tube
- Speaking valve
- Cuff down leak speech on ventilator

The Blom fenestrated tracheostomy tube has a speech cannula, which is made of silicone and has two valves.[89] Inspiratory pressure opens the flap valve and closes the bubble valve, which seals the fenestration so that all of the inspiratory air goes to the lungs. As inspiration ends, the flap valve closes. Expiratory pressure collapses the bubble valve, which unblocks the fenestration and directs all the exhaled air to the upper airway to allow phonation (**Figure 17-42**). The exhaled volume reservoir is a separate component that assists in preventing false low-expiratory volume alarms that would occur because the exhaled breath is directed through the upper airway instead of back to the ventilator. The exhaled volume reservoir is a small silicone bellows system that expands and traps gas during inspiration, and then returns the gas to the ventilator to be measured as exhaled volume during exhalation.

Speaking Valves

The tracheostomy **speaking valve** (**Figure 17-43**) is designed to eliminate the need for finger occlusion to communicate by speaking.[90] The valve attaches to the 15-mm universal adapter of all tracheostomy tubes and can be used in adult and pediatric patients. The valve opens on inspiration, with air passing through to the lungs, and closes on expiration, with the air directed

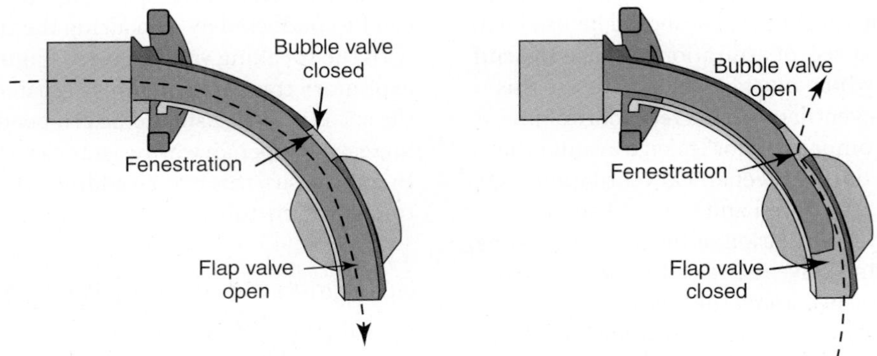

FIGURE 17-42 The Blom speech cannula. Inspiratory pressure opens the flap valve and closes (expands) the bubble valve, which seals the fenestration so that all the tidal volume goes to the lungs. As inspiration ends, the flap valve closes. Expiratory pressure collapses the bubble valve, which unblocks the fenestration and directs all the exhaled air to the upper airway to allow phonation.
Reproduced from Kunduk M, Appel K, Tunc M, et al. Preliminary report of laryngeal phonation during mechanical ventilation via a new cuffed tracheostomy tube. *Respir Care.* 2010;55:1661–1670.

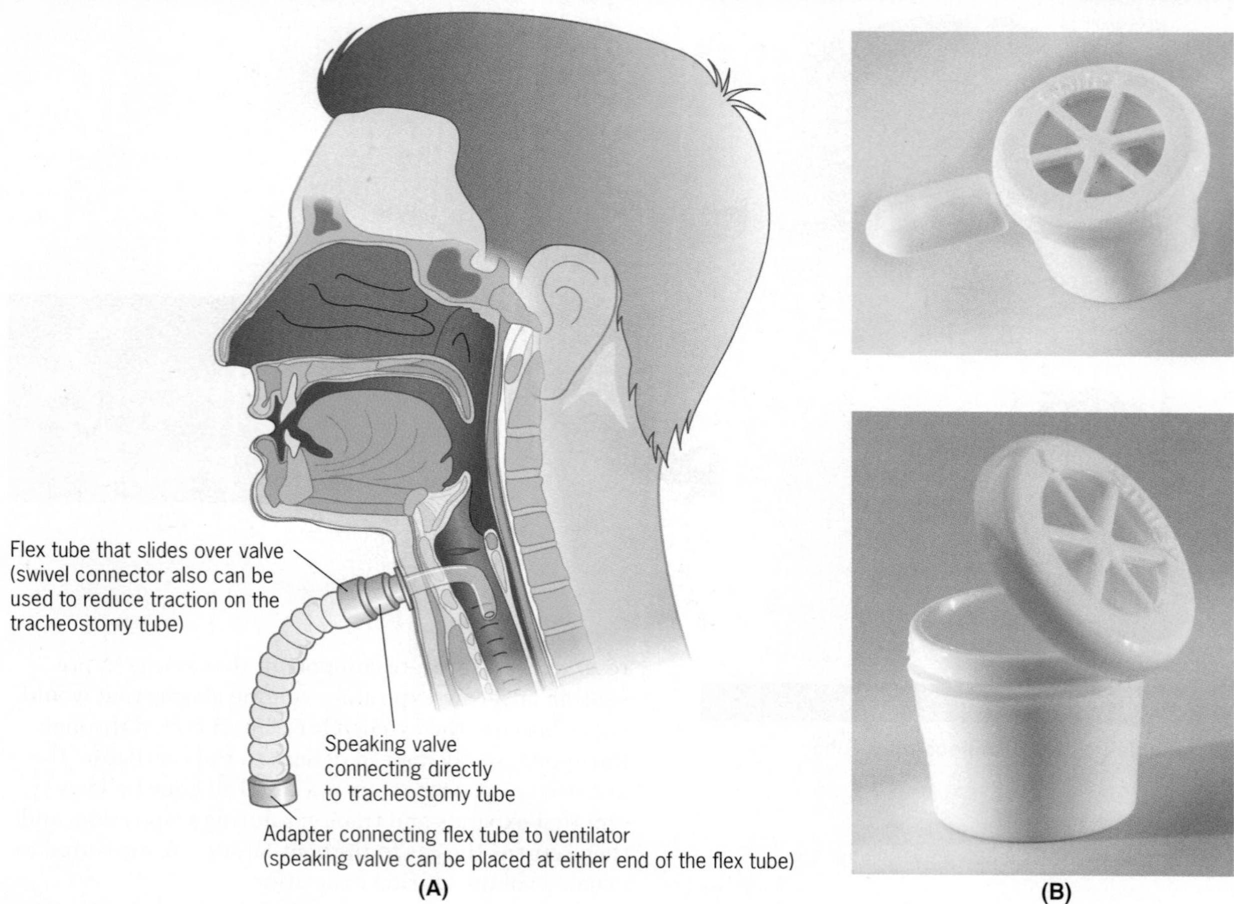

FIGURE 17-43 (**A**) Speaking valve in-line during mechanical ventilation. (**B**) Speaking valves.

into the trachea and up past the vocal cords to permit speech. This device can be used in either spontaneously breathing or ventilator-dependent patients. Some patients may immediately adjust to breathing with the valve in place. Others may need to gradually increase the time the valve is worn.

Breathing out with the valve in place is harder work than breathing through the tracheostomy tube, and some patients may need to build up strength and ability to use the valve. The speaking valve should be used with caution in patients at risk of aspiration because the cuff of the tracheostomy tube must be deflated to use this device. Increases in ventilator-delivered tidal volume may be needed to compensate for leakage around the tracheostomy tube during mechanical ventilation. After the speaking valve is removed and the tracheostomy cuff is reinflated, overventilation of the patient must be avoided. The speaking valve may also be used to wean patients from the tracheostomy tube as a means to reorient them to use of the upper airway for breathing.

Contraindications to the use of a speaking valve include an unconscious or comatose patient, situations in which the cuff cannot be deflated, use with a foam cuffed tube, copious secretions, and severe upper airway obstruction. Humidity and oxygen can both be delivered with the valve in place. The valve must be removed during the administration of aerosolized medications, because these may cause the valve to stick or not work well. It is important to consider the input of the speech-language pathologist to assess the patient's ability to produce voice in different situations that may include using a speaking valve. Also important is assessment of upper airway resistance when the cuff is deflated and the speaking valve is in place. This can be conducted by measuring the tracheal pressure with the speaking valve in place (**Figure 17-44**).[91] If the expiratory tracheal pressure is greater than 10 cm H_2O, the speaking valve should be removed and causes of increased upper airway resistance should be explored. In most cases, this can be addressed by downsizing the tracheostomy tube.

Speaking in Ventilator-Dependent Patients with a Tracheostomy Tube

In mechanically ventilated patients, speech can be provided by the use of a talking tracheostomy tube, using a cuff-down technique with a speaking valve, and using a cuff-down technique without a speaking valve.[92] Simple manipulations of the ventilator allow the patient to speak

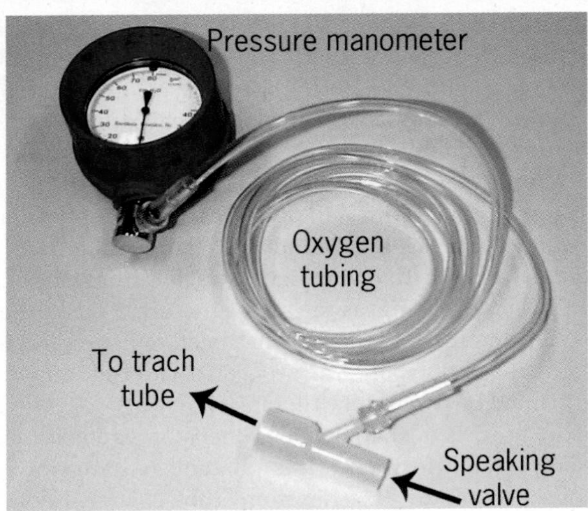

FIGURE 17-44 Equipment used to measure tracheal pressure with a speaking valve in place.

during both the inspiratory phase and expiratory phase. Moreover, the lack of a speaking valve may increase safety should the upper airway become obstructed. If the cuff is deflated, gas can escape through the upper airway during the inspiratory phase. If the leak is excessive, the cuff can be partially inflated. This leak results in the ability to speak during the inspiratory phase.

Increasing the inspiratory time setting on the ventilator increases the leak. If the positive end-expiratory pressure (PEEP) setting on the ventilator is zero, most of the exhaled gas exits through the ventilator circuit rather than the upper airway. In this situation, there is little ability to speak during the expiratory phase. If PEEP is set on the ventilator, then expiratory flow is more likely to occur through the upper airway, which increases speaking rate. Longer inspiratory time and higher PEEP are additive in their ability to improve speaking rate. Tracheal pressure (important for speech) is similar with the use of PEEP and the use of a speaking valve. By prolonging the inspiratory time and using PEEP, mechanically ventilated patients with a tracheostomy may be able to use 60% to 80% of the breathing cycle for speaking. Such patients may be able to speak throughout the entire ventilatory cycle without any pauses for breathing. This is unlike normal subjects without tracheostomy tubes, who speak only during the expiratory phase.

The ventilator is normally flow cycled during pressure support. In the presence of a leak through the upper airway, the ventilator may fail to cycle appropriately and thus result in a prolonged inspiratory phase. Although this would usually be considered undesirable, it might facilitate speech

Eating with a Tracheostomy

Having a tracheostomy usually does not affect the patient's eating or swallowing patterns. Sometimes there are changes in swallowing dynamics that require adjusting to, but it is rare not to be able to overcome such issues in a short period of time. If swallowing problems do occur, they are usually due to limited elevation of the larynx or to poor closure of the epiglottis and vocal cords, which allows food or liquids into the trachea. A speech pathologist can be consulted for an evaluation, which may include a videofluoroscopic swallowing study or other procedures to make sure the patient is swallowing safely. If the patient eats by mouth, it is recommended that the tracheostomy tube be suctioned prior to eating. This often prevents the need for suctioning during or after meals, which may stimulate excessive coughing and could result in vomiting. Always observe the patient while eating to be sure food does not get into the trachea.

Trach and Stoma Buttons

Tracheostomy (Trach) buttons and stoma buttons (**Figure 17-45**) are used to maintain the tracheostomy stoma. They are temporary appliances generally made of Teflon or silicone. Some consist of a hollow outer cannula and an inner solid cannula. The device fits from the skin to just inside the anterior wall of the trachea. They should be used when the tracheostomy stoma must be maintained, either for later replacement

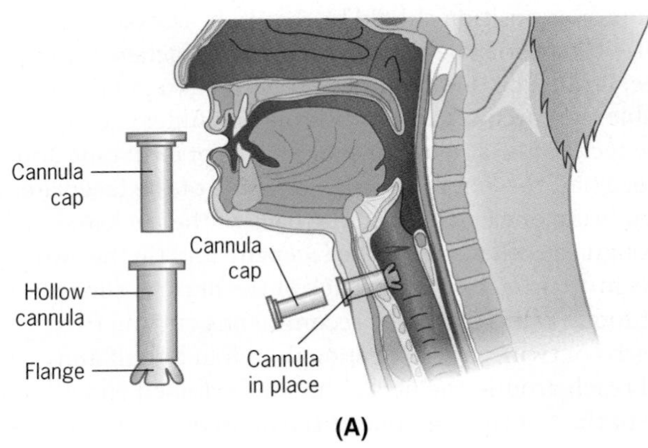

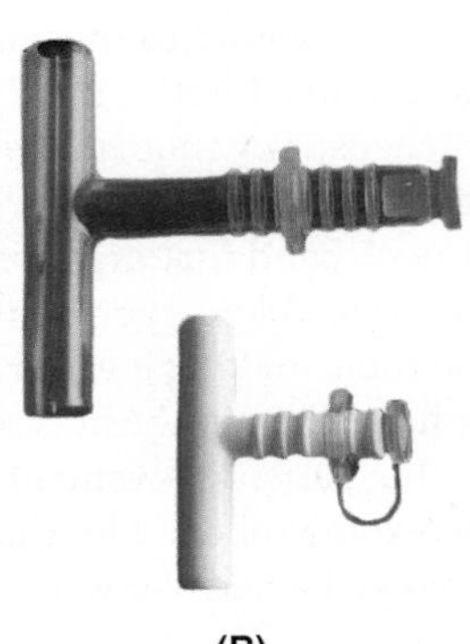

FIGURE 17-45 (**A**) Tracheostomy button. (**B**) Montgomery Standard Safe-T-Tube.

(**B**) courtesy of Boston Medical Products, Inc.

of a tracheostomy tube or for suctioning. A button does not have a cuff and, therefore, it is of limited value in cases involving a risk of aspiration or during positive pressure ventilation.

The Montgomery Safe-T-Tube is a silicone T-shaped tube with internal and external limbs. Its primary indication is to maintain a patent airway in instances of tracheal stenosis, after laryngeal injuries such as crushing or laryngeal fractures, and after tracheal reconstruction and reanastamosis. It ranges in size from 6 to 16. The most common adult sizes are 11 to 13. The external limb can be gently tilted to allow the suction catheter to pass beyond the 45-degree angle of the tube. Ring washers assist in preventing posterior displacement. Several versions are available for specific patient needs. It is important to provide constant humidification to avoid obstruction of the tube by secretions. Capping the tube allows normal humidification and phonation.

Securing Tracheostomy Tubes

A major complication of tracheostomy is accidental decannulation. It is important to secure the tube appropriately while maintaining patient comfort by minimizing friction and pressure on the neck. It is also important to ensure that the tracheostomy tube is properly aligned in the trachea. A 10% rate of tracheostomy tube malposition has been reported, suggesting that proper position should be regularly assessed.[93]

Twill tape may be used to secure the tracheostomy tube. It must be tied securely, yet with enough give to enable the caregiver to slip two fingers under the tape. One technique is to use one long piece of twill tape and thread half the length through one side of the faceplate. Then bring one end around the back of the neck and through the other side of the faceplate and tie the two ends in a triple knot at the back of the neck. A second technique using twill tape recommends cutting two lengths of twill, each long enough to fold in half and still reach around the neck. Thread the folded end of one of the ties through one of the holes on the tracheostomy tube until it forms a loop, pulling it tightly. Repeat on the other side of the tracheostomy tube. Bring the loose ends of both ties around to the back of the neck and tie them together in a knot.

Specialized tracheostomy tube holders, such as the Dale tracheostomy holder, are available. This holder has a wider diameter neck band that distributes pressure and prevents skin irritation. Velcro-type hook fasteners are used to secure the tube, making it easier and faster to apply. The holder has elastic in the back, promoting tube security and allowing patient movement. Regardless of the type of tracheostomy tube holder that is used, the device must be changed whenever wet or soiled.

Changing the Tracheostomy Tube

The tracheostomy tube may be changed to another one for a number of reasons: to reduce the size of the tube, to change the length of the tube if it is malpositioned, because it is obstructed with secretions, because it is broken (e.g., cuff leak), to change the type of tube, or as a routine change with a chronic tracheostomy.[94] The first tracheostomy tube change carries some risk and should be performed by a skilled operator in a safe environment; this will often be supervised by the clinical service that initially placed the tube. The risk associated with changing the tracheostomy tube diminishes over time as the stoma matures. When the stoma is mature and the tube has been replaced previously without incident, the procedure can be safely performed by respiratory therapists.

The process of changing a tracheostomy tube is usually straightforward.[94] It is advisable to have two people present for a tracheostomy tube change. Prior to removing the old tube, all components of the new tracheostomy tube should be checked for integrity, the obturator should be placed into the tube, and the cuff should be inflated to check for leaks and then deflated prior to insertion. Water-soluble lubricant is placed on the tube. The patient is placed either supine or semirecumbent, with the neck extended. Retaining sutures, if present, are removed, the tube is gently withdrawn, the new tracheostomy tube inserted, and the obturator removed. Removal of a tube through a tight stoma with a bulky cuff can be facilitated using lidocaine jelly or water-soluble lubricant inserted around the stoma/tube interface. Once the new tube is in place, its position in the trachea is confirmed by airflow through the tube if the patient is breathing spontaneously or the presence of bilateral breath sounds during positive pressure ventilation. Of concern is that the tube may be placed into a false track outside of the trachea. The presence of carbon dioxide in the exhaled gas confirms that the tube is in the trachea. Bronchoscopy and chest radiography can also be used to confirm tube placement.

The new tracheostomy tube can usually be inserted using the obturator packaged with the tube. If difficulty is anticipated during a tracheostomy tube change, a tube exchanger or suction catheter can be used to facilitate this procedure. The tube exchanger is passed through the tube into the trachea. The tube is then withdrawn while keeping the tube changer in place and the new tube is then passed over the tube changer into the trachea. In these cases, it is also important that an individual skilled in endotracheal intubation is available in the event that the tracheostomy tube cannot be replaced. If difficulty changing the tube is anticipated, it is advisable that a clinician skilled in endotracheal intubation is present, or that the tube is changed in the operating room. Generally, the tracheostomy tube should be changed in a clinical unit (ICU, ward, clinic). It is not recommended to change the tracheostomy tube in the patient's home, where monitoring is suboptimal and the ability to adequately respond to loss of the airway is inadequate.

Bleeding can occur during the tracheostomy tube change, particularly if the patient is anticoagulated or if there is granulation tissue at the stoma. Of greatest concern is inability to insert the new tube. It is advisable to have a backup tube of smaller size available in case this should occur. An algorithm to manage failure to replace a tracheostomy tube during a routine change is shown in **Figure 17-46**.

It is commonly recommended that the initial tracheostomy tube change should occur between day 7 and 14 postinsertion. If the tube is changed before day 7, that might lead to earlier use of a speaking valve and earlier oral intake.[95] The need for routine tracheostomy tube changes is unclear. Fewer complications due to granulation tissue may occur with more frequent tracheostomy tube changes.[96] Manufacturers include recommendations for routine changes of tracheostomy tubes in their package inserts. Shiley recommends changing their polyvinyl chloride (PVC) tracheostomy tubes every 29 days. The Portex Blue Line package insert recommends 30 days as the maximum recommended period of use. The Portex Bivona tube package insert recommends it be used for up to 29 days. Many manufacturers recommend that a tube with an inner cannula should not be used for more than 30 days. Several studies have reported material breakdown of tracheostomy tubes over time.[96–98]

Decannulation

Decannulation is the removal of the tracheostomy tube once the patient no longer needs it. The patient should be alert and responsive to commands, no longer dependent on a ventilator for assisted breathing, and no longer requiring frequent suctioning for removal of tracheal secretions. Weaning from the tracheostomy tube typically is done through placement of a smaller tracheostomy tube, perhaps one that is fenestrated or cuffless; patients should not have breathing difficulty in the presence of this tube. The smaller tracheostomy tube can then have either a speaking valve or cap placed on it for several hours to assess the patient's ability to talk and clear his or her own secretions with no evidence of breathing difficulty. An algorithm for decannulation assessment is shown in **Figure 17-47**.

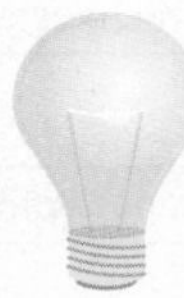

STOP AND THINK

A patient received a tracheostomy 30 days ago. You are asked to develop a care plan to result in decannulation of the patient. How would you approach this assignment?

It has been reported that physicians and respiratory therapists based their decision to recommend decannulation on patients' level of consciousness, cough effectiveness, secretions, and oxygenation.[99] Most clinicians defined decannulation failure as the need to reinsert an artificial airway within 48 to 96 hours of planned tracheostomy removal. Once this process is tolerated, the patient is placed supine in bed, the tube is removed, and the opening in the neck is covered with sterile gauze and tape is placed over the gauze. Decannulation should be done in the hospital where there is emergency support should it be needed.

Accidental Decannulation

Accidental decannulation occurring in a patient with a mature stoma and with normal neck anatomy should

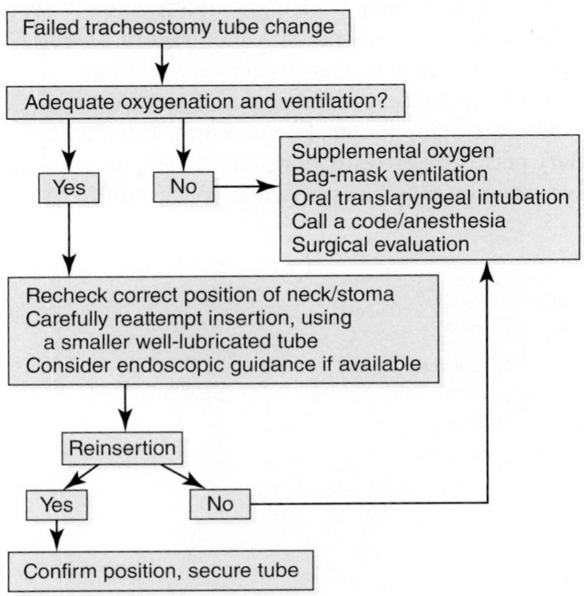

FIGURE 17-46 Algorithm to manage failure to replace a tracheostomy tube during a routine change.

Reproduced from White AC, Kher S, O'Connor HH. When to change a tracheostomy tube. *Respir Care*. 2010;55:1069–1075.

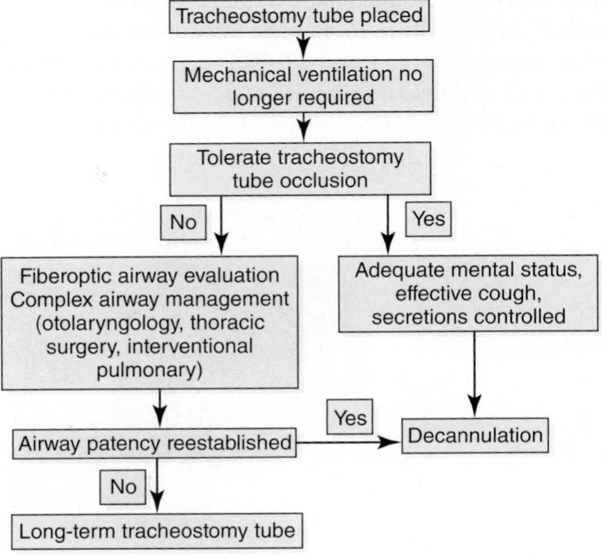

FIGURE 17-47 Algorithm for decannulation assessment.

Reproduced from O'Connor HH, White AC. Tracheostomy decannulation. *Respir Care*. 2010;55:1076–1081.

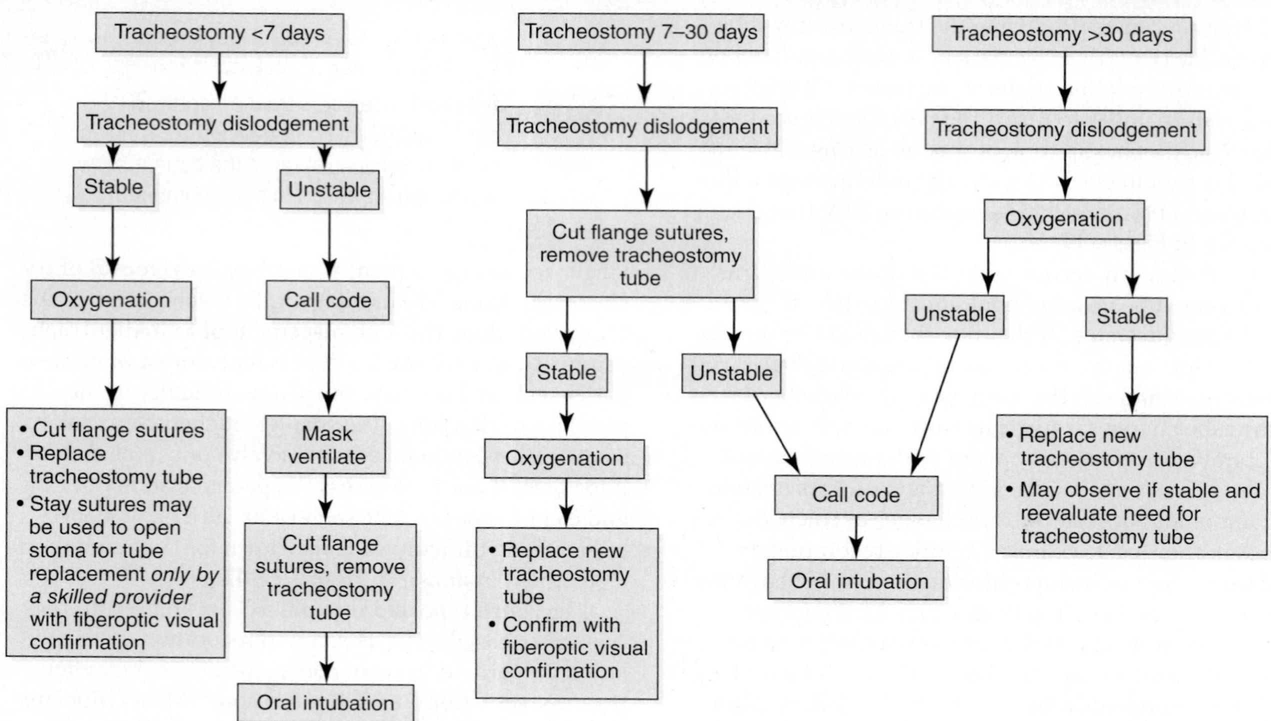

FIGURE 17-48 Algorithm to manage unplanned decannulation.
Reproduced from O'Connor HH, White AC. Tracheostomy decannulation. *Respir Care.* 2010;55:1076–1081.

be a benign event because the tracheostomy tube can usually be easily reinserted. Accidental decannulation may result in morbidity and mortality, however, when it occurs in patients with a recently placed tracheostomy tube and in those with substantial airway pathology, increased neck circumference, marginal oxygenation, or in whom the tracheostomy tube is essential for mechanical ventilation. In these situations, airway patency must be quickly reestablished in order to avoid prolonged hypoxemia, organ failure, or death.[100] An algorithm to manage unplanned decannulation is shown in **Figure 17-48**.[101] Factors associated with accidental decannulation include mental status changes, increased secretions, and change of shift.[102] Interventions to reduce the rate of accidental decannulation include increased availability of telemetry and oximetry and signage to identify patients at high risk of accidental decannulation.

Airway Cuff Concerns

An **airway cuff** is classified as a high-volume, low-pressure cuff or a low-volume, high-pressure cuff (**Figure 17-49**). Because high tracheal wall pressures exerted by an inflated cuff can injure the tracheal mucosa, most cuffs used today are high-volume, low-pressure. The tracheal capillary perfusion pressure normally is 25 to 35 mm Hg. Because the pressure transmitted from the cuff to the

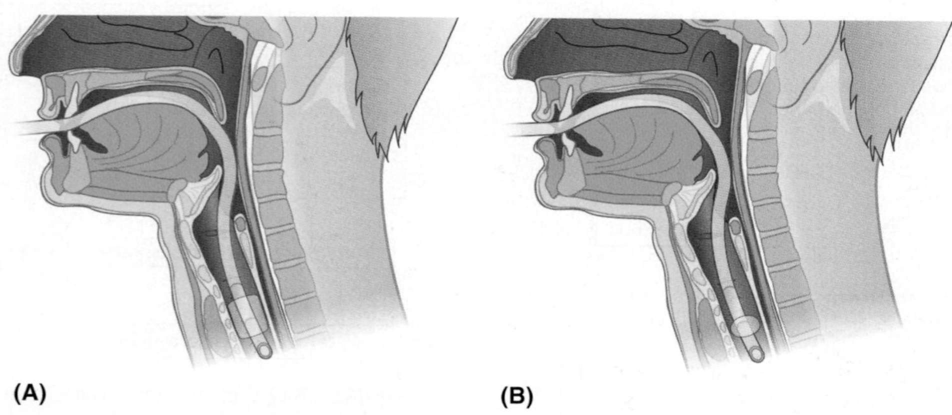

FIGURE 17-49 (**A**) High-volume, low-pressure cuff. (**B**) High-pressure, low-volume cuff.

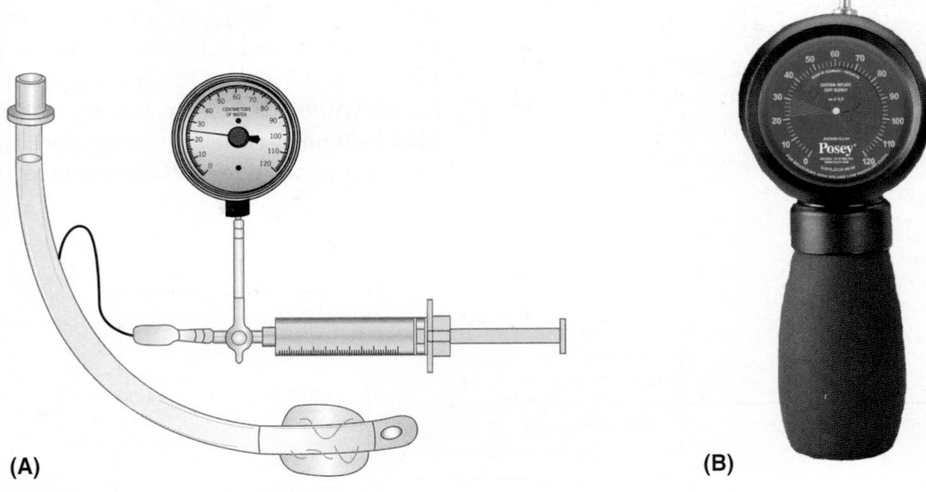

FIGURE 17-50 Equipment to measure cuff pressure.
(**B**) courtesy of Posey Company.

tracheal wall usually is less than the pressure in the cuff, it is generally agreed that 30 cm H_2O is the maximum acceptable intracuff pressure. If the cuff pressure is too low (<20 cm H_2O), microaspiration is more likely. It therefore is reasonable to maintain cuff pressures at 20 to 30 cm H_2O to minimize the risks of tracheal wall injury and aspiration.

The cuff can be inflated with a minimum occlusion pressure or minimum leak technique. With the minimum occlusion pressure method, the cuff is inflated to a volume that just eliminates an end-inspiratory leak during positive pressure ventilation. With the minimum leak technique, the cuff is inflated to a volume that allows a small leak to occur at end-inspiration. With either method, leakage around the cuff is assessed by auscultation over the suprasternal notch or the lateral neck. With either of these approaches, the cuff pressure should be maintained between 20 and 30 cm H_2O.

Monitoring of the cuff pressure is standard respiratory care practice. The intracuff pressure should be monitored and recorded at least once per shift and more often if the tube position is changed, if the volume of air in the cuff is changed, or if a leak occurs. Cuff pressure is measured with a syringe, stopcock, and manometer (**Figure 17-50**). With this method, the cuff pressure can be measured simultaneously with adjustment of the cuff volume. Methods in which the manometer is attached directly to the pilot balloon are discouraged, because they cause air to escape from the cuff to pressurize the manometer.

A common cause of high cuff pressure is a tube that is too small, which results in overfilling of the cuff to achieve a seal in the trachea. If the volume of air in the cuff required to achieve a seal exceeds the cuff's nominal volume, the tube is too small. The nominal cuff volume is the volume below which the cuff pressure is less than 20 cm H_2O ex vivo. Another common cause of high cuff pressure is incorrect positioning of the endotracheal tube, particularly a cephalad position in which the cuff is inflated in the larynx and pharynx. Other causes of high cuff pressure are overfilling of the cuff, tracheal dilation, and use of a low-volume, high-pressure cuff.

Occasionally the pilot tube may become severed. To correct this problem, a short, blunt needle can be passed into the pilot tube and a stopcock attached to the needle hub to add and maintain air in the cuff until the tube can be replaced (**Figure 17-51**). Cuff leaks also can occur, and a continuous flow of gas into the cuff can be used to temporarily maintain cuff inflation until the tube can be changed. Interestingly, a large number of endotracheal tubes removed for presumed cuff rupture were flawless, and it has been speculated that incorrect tube positioning may be the explanation for this finding.

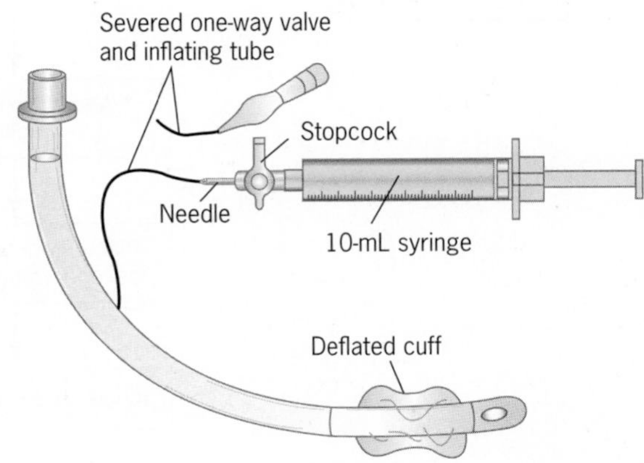

FIGURE 17-51 Technique to inflate cuff with severed inflating tube.
Adapted from Sills J. *Respir Care.* 1986;31:199–201.

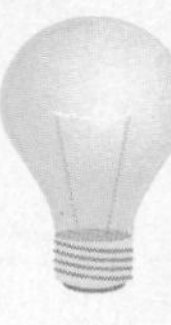

STOP AND THINK

You are repeatedly being called by the nurse to address a cuff leak. You notice that exhaled tidal volumes have dropped on the ventilator. How would you address this issue?

A simple method can be used to assess cuff rupture. If a leak occurs during a cuff inflation maneuver, there may be a ruptured cuff or an ineffective pilot balloon valve. This is assessed by clamping the pilot tube. If a leak occurs without the clamp, but not with the clamp, the pilot balloon or valve is incompetent. **Figure 17-52** presents an algorithm for cuff management. Occasionally an

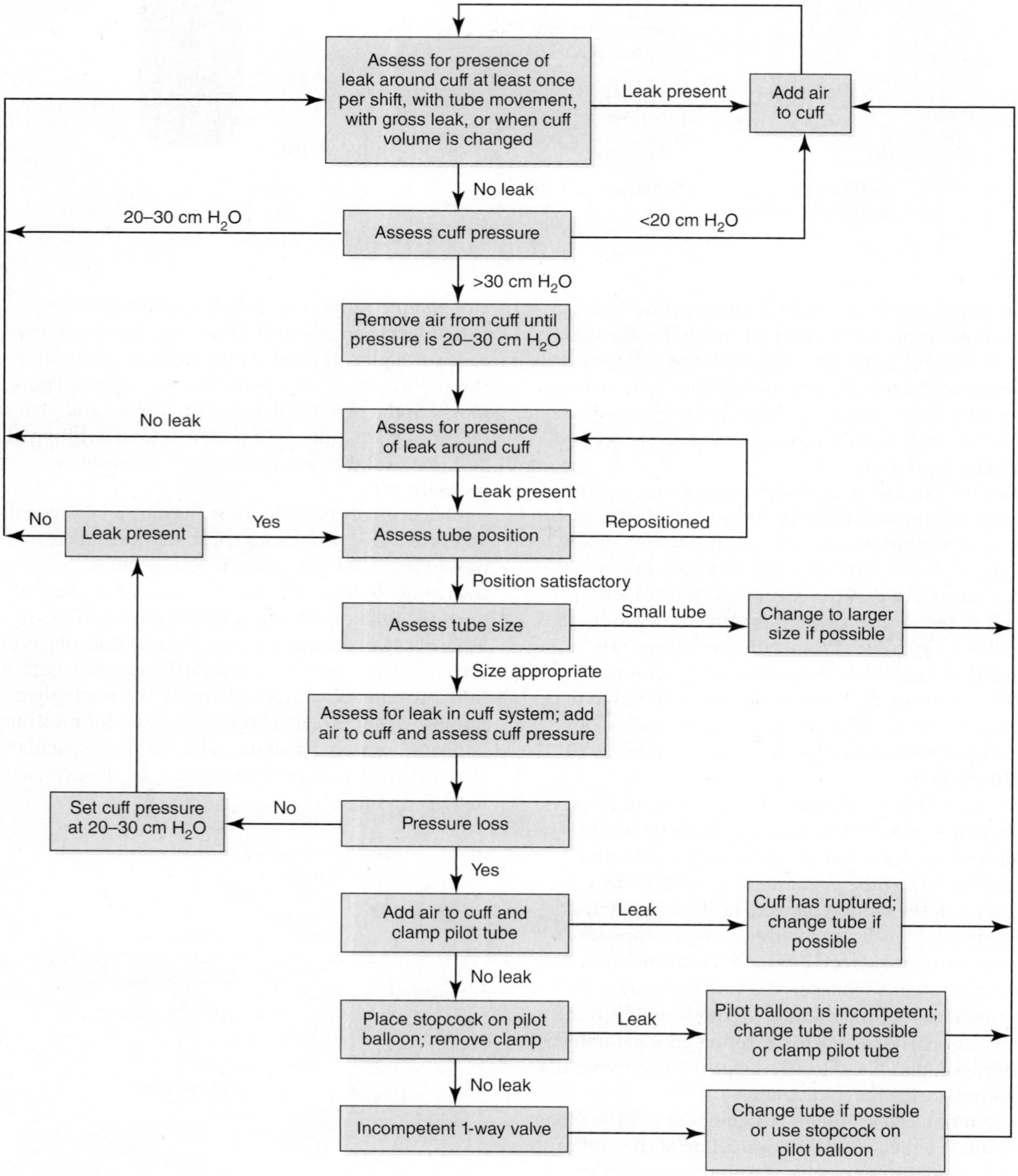

Assess for presence of leak around cuff at least once per shift, with tube movement, with gross leak, or when cuff volume is changed
Leak present
Add air to cuff
No leak
20–30 cm H_2O
Assess cuff pressure
<20 cm H_2O
>30 cm H_2O
Remove air from cuff until pressure is 20–30 cm H_2O
No leak
Assess for presence of leak around cuff
Leak present
No
Leak present
Yes
Assess tube position
Repositioned
Position satisfactory
Assess tube size
Small tube
Change to larger size if possible
Size appropriate
Assess for leak in cuff system; add air to cuff and assess cuff pressure
Set cuff pressure at 20–30 cm H_2O
No
Pressure loss
Yes
Add air to cuff and clamp pilot tube
Leak
Cuff has ruptured; change tube if possible
No leak
Place stopcock on pilot balloon; remove clamp
Leak
Pilot balloon is incompetent; change tube if possible or clamp pilot tube
No leak
Incompetent 1-way valve
Change tube if possible or use stopcock on pilot balloon

FIGURE 17-52 Algorithm to address issues with an artificial airway cuff leak.

Reproduced from Hess DR. Managing the artificial airway. *Respir Care.* 1999;44(7):759–772. Reprinted with permission.

endotracheal tube must be changed, such as when the cuff has ruptured. A tube changer can be used to facilitate this procedure. The tube changer is passed through the endotracheal tube into the trachea, and the endotracheal tube is withdrawn while the tube changer is kept in place. The new endotracheal tube then is passed over the tube changer into the trachea.

Secretions that collect on top of ETT cuffs can leak into the lungs and are considered a risk factor for VAP. Cuff pressures of up to 60 cm H_2O may be needed to minimize the risk of these secretions from leaking around the ETT cuff, but sustained pressures at this level have been associated with the risk of tracheal mucosal injury. High volume–low pressure (HVLP) cuffs that can provide good tracheal seals at 30 cm H_2O were developed to alleviate this problem, but secretion leakage has been shown to still occur through channels that form due to folding of these cuffs within the trachea. A novel HVLP ETT has been developed with an ultrathin polyurethane cuff (PUC), which demonstrates less leakage than a standard polyvinyl (PVC) comparison, and can provide a good seal with pressures of 8 to 12 cm H_2O with associated VAP reduction. Other PUC cuff manufacturers have experimented with the effect of tapered cuff shapes. PUC cuffs are considerably more expensive than standard PVC ETTs, but no cost-effectiveness data are currently available. Commercially available systems can also be used to measure cuff pressure. Continuous cuff monitoring to ensure a consistent ETT cuff pressure of 25 cm H_2O has been shown to reduce the risk of microaspiration.[103] There is increased interest in devices that can monitor cuff pressures continuously, but their cost-effectiveness is yet to be evaluated.

Airway Clearance

Open Suction

Suctioning is a procedure that uses negative pressure to remove secretions from the trachea, pharynx, nose, or mouth either through the natural orifice (nose or mouth) or artificial airways such as endotracheal tubes, tracheostomy tubes, or nasal or oral airways. Suctioning should be considered whenever physical examination reveals secretions in the airway or whenever secretions are suspected and may be hindering oxygenation and ventilation or increasing the work of breathing. Suspected secretions can be identified through direct auscultation or from visual clues on the expiratory flow graphic display on the ventilator (sawtooth pattern).

Because tracheal suctioning is uncomfortable for the patient and carries some risk, it should be performed only when indicated and not at fixed intervals. The presence of the catheter in the trachea can induce coughing and may stimulate bronchospasm in patients with reactive airways. In the absence of an artificial airway, nasotracheal suctioning can be performed if secretions need to be removed. In this scenario a suction catheter can be passed through a naris and into the trachea. This can be even more uncomfortable due to the added irritation of the nasal passage. If repeated nasotracheal suctioning is required in the absence of an endotracheal tube, a nasopharyngeal airway can be inserted and left in place to reduce trauma in future procedures. This procedure is used on patients who have a decreased or absent cough reflex. **CPG 17-2** lists indications and contraindications for endotracheal suctioning. If suctioning is required in the absence of an endotracheal tube and nasotracheal suctioning is not an option (trauma, occlusion), suctioning assist devices may be an option. These devices generally provide rigid support so the patient cannot bite the suction catheter and they may be contoured to help guide the catheter into the trachea.

The upper airway should be suctioned periodically to remove oral secretions. **Figure 17-53** depicts the Yankauer mouth/pharyngeal suctioning device. This is generally used when secretions are visible in the oral cavity or prior to extubation. For suctioning through artificial airways, a suction catheter is used. A suction catheter must be long enough to enter the main stem bronchi and various sizes are available to accomplish this procedure (**Figure 17-54**). A thumb port at the proximal end controls suction to the catheter. The catheter must be rigid enough to allow passage through an artificial airway but flexible enough to prevent damage

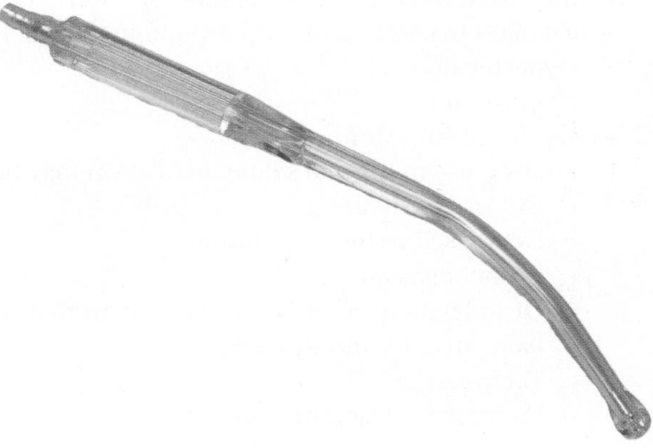

FIGURE 17-53 Yankauer mouth/pharyngeal suction.
Courtesy of Covidien. Used with permission.

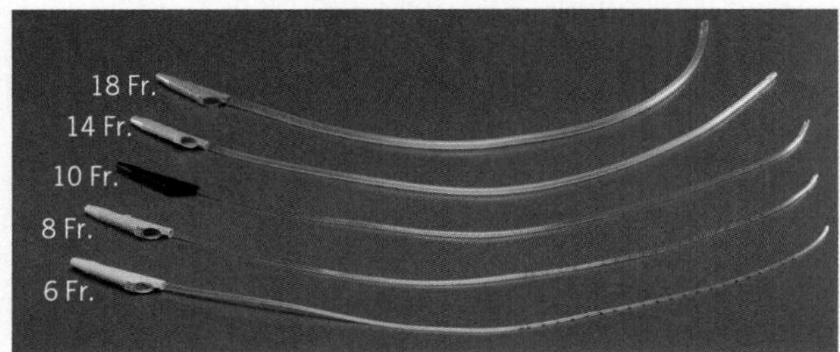

FIGURE 17-54 Suction catheter.
Courtesy of Covidien. Used with permission.

CLINICAL PRACTICE GUIDELINE 17-2

Endotracheal Suctioning of Mechanically Ventilated Patients with Artificial Airways

Indications

- The need to maintain the patency and integrity of the artificial airway
- The need to remove accumulated pulmonary secretions as evidenced by one of the following: (1) sawtooth pattern on the flow–volume loop on the monitor screen of the ventilator and/or the presence of coarse crackles over the trachea are strong indicators of retained pulmonary secretions; (2) increased peak inspiratory pressure during volume-controlled mechanical ventilation or decreased tidal volume during pressure-controlled ventilation; (3) deterioration of oxygen saturation and/or arterial blood gas values; (4) visible secretions in the airway; or (5) patient's inability to generate an effective spontaneous cough, acute respiratory distress, or suspected aspiration of gastric or upper airway secretions
- The need to obtain a sputum specimen to rule out or identify pneumonia or other pulmonary infection or for sputum cytology

Contraindications

- Endotracheal suctioning is a necessary procedure for patients with artificial airways. Most contraindications are relative to the patient's risk of developing adverse reactions or worsening clinical condition as a result of the procedure. When indicated, there is no absolute contraindication to endotracheal suctioning because the decision to withhold suctioning in order to avoid a possible adverse reaction may, in fact, be lethal.

Hazards and Complications

- Decrease in dynamic lung compliance and functional residual capacity
- Atelectasis
- Hypoxia/hypoxemia
- Tissue trauma to the tracheal and/or bronchial mucosa
- Bronchoconstriction/bronchospasm
- Increased microbial colonization of lower airway
- Changes in cerebral blood flow and increased intracranial pressure
- Hypertension
- Hypotension
- Cardiac dysrhythmias
- Routine use of normal saline instillation may be associated with the following adverse events:
  - Excessive coughing
  - Decreased oxygen saturation
  - Bronchospasm
  - Dislodgement of the bacterial biofilm that colonizes the endotracheal tube into the lower airway
  - Pain, anxiety, and dyspnea
  - Tachycardia
  - Increased intracranial pressure

Recommendations

The following recommendations are made following the Grading of Recommendations Assessment, Development, and Evaluation (GRADE) criteria.

- It is recommended that endotracheal suctioning should be performed only when secretions are present and not routinely (1C).
- It is suggested that preoxygenation be considered if the patient has a clinically important reduction in oxygen saturation with suctioning (2B).
- Performing suctioning without disconnecting the patient from the ventilator is suggested (2B).
- Use of shallow suction is suggested instead of deep suction, based on evidence from infant and pediatric studies (2B).
- It is suggested that routine use of normal saline instillation prior to endotracheal suction should *not* be performed (2C).

(continues)

Clinical Practice Guideline 17-2 *(continued)*

- The use of closed suction is suggested for adults with high F_{IO_2} or PEEP or who are at risk for lung derecruitment (2B) and neonates (2C).
- Endotracheal suctioning without disconnection (closed system) is suggested in neonates (2B).
- Avoidance of disconnection and use of lung-recruitment maneuvers are suggested if suctioning-induced lung derecruitment occurs in patients with acute lung injuries (2B).
- It is suggested that a suction catheter is used that occludes less than 50% of the lumen of the ETT in children and adults, and less than 70% in infants (2C).
- It is suggested that the duration of the suctioning event be limited to less than 15 seconds (2C).

Reproduced from AARC clinical practice guideline: endotracheal suctioning of mechanically ventilated patients with artificial airways. *Respir Care.* 2010;55(6):758–764. Reprinted with permission.

to the airway mucosa. Also to prevent damage to the airway mucosa, the catheter should have smooth, molded ends, one or more side holes near the catheter tip, and minimum frictional resistance when passed through the airway. The catheter should be transparent so that the aspirated secretions can be assessed.

The suction pressure should be no greater than that required to remove secretions adequately. It should not exceed 100 mm Hg in infants, 125 mm Hg in children, and 150 mm Hg in adults. Suction catheters are available in a variety of sizes. The catheter size is determined by its OD in French (Fr) units, which refers to the circumference of the tube. Because circumference equals 3.14 (π) $\times$ diameter, the French size is estimated by multiplication of the diameter by 3. The OD of the suction catheter should not exceed one-half to two-thirds the ID of the artificial airway. A 14 Fr catheter usually is acceptable for adults.

Although viewed as a beneficial therapeutic procedure, suctioning is not without risks to the patient. Potential complications associated with suctioning include hypoxemia, atelectasis, hyperinflation (if a manual resuscitator is used), airway trauma, contamination of the lower respiratory tract, arrhythmias, and increased intracranial pressure.

A number of factors contribute to suction-related hypoxemia, including interruption of mechanical ventilation during the suctioning procedure (i.e., loss of ventilation, inspired oxygen, and PEEP), aspiration of gas from the respiratory tract during the application of suction, entrainment of room air into the lungs, the duration of suctioning, and suction-related atelectasis. To prevent suction-related hypoxemia, the patient should be hyperoxygenated prior to the procedure. This most commonly is accomplished by an increase in the F_{IO_2} to 1.

Atelectasis can occur during suctioning as the result of evacuation of gases from the lower respiratory tract. This is more likely to occur when excessive suction pressures are used and when the size of the suction catheter is large in relation to the size of the endotracheal or tracheostomy tube. Derecruitment of lung units will then lead to some hypoxemia. The duration of suctioning also affects the degree of hypoxemia. A suctioning attempt should be as brief as possible to achieve the desired effect, which is removal of secretions, but should last no longer than 15 seconds.

Hyperinflation or hyperventilation (or both) to prevent suction-related hypoxemia should be used cautiously because of the hazards of overdistension lung injury. In some critical care units a manual ventilator (resuscitator) is used for hyperinflation and hyperoxygenation during suctioning procedures. The use of a manual resuscitator (especially without a pressure gauge) poses a significant threat of lung hyperinflation, which increases the potential risks of barotrauma.

Airway edema, hyperemia, mucosal ulceration, hemorrhage, and diminished mucociliary transport can occur with suctioning. These effects are related to operator technique and the amount of suction pressure used. Intermittent, rather than continuous, suctioning may be less traumatic to airway mucosa, but little evidence is available regarding this issue. The catheter tip should be smooth, molded, and atraumatic, and side holes near the tip of the catheter can minimize trauma to the airway mucosa. In infants, the suction catheter should not be inserted more than 1 cm beyond the tip of the endotracheal tube. A similar practice should be used for patients who have had a recent tracheal reconstructive surgery or pneumonectomy.

Contamination of the lower respiratory tract can occur during tracheal suctioning. This complication can be avoided with the use of sterile technique during the procedure. Care must be taken during suctioning to avoid contamination of the suction catheter, the ventilator circuit or the valve of the manual ventilator, and the clinician performing the procedure. Bedside manual ventilators can also be a source of contamination of the lower respiratory tract, which may increase

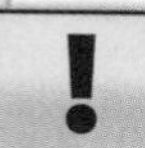

Respiratory Recap

Complications of Suctioning

- Hypoxemia
- Atelectasis
- Hyperinflation
- Airway trauma
- Contamination of the lower respiratory tract
- Arrhythmias
- Increased intracranial pressure
- Preferential suctioning of the right bronchus

AGE-SPECIFIC ANGLE

Pneumothorax that occurred secondary to bronchial perforation by a suction catheter has been reported in infants.

the chance of pulmonary infection. Arrhythmias may occur during tracheal suctioning as a result of hypoxemia or vagal stimulation. This complication often can be avoided by hyperoxygenation of the patient during suctioning.

Because the left main stem bronchus has a smaller diameter than the right bronchus and leaves the trachea at a more acute angle, the suction catheter is more likely to enter the right main stem bronchus. Secretions therefore are more likely to be suctioned from the right lung than the left. Several techniques can be used for selective endobronchial suctioning, particularly of the left bronchus, including use of curved-tip catheters, turning the patient's head to the side (e.g., turning of the head to the right to facilitate suctioning of the left bronchus), and lateral positioning (turning of the patient onto the left side to facilitate passage of the catheter into the left main stem bronchus). Use of a curved-tip catheter (**Figure 17-55**) has proved to be the best means to accomplish endobronchial suctioning. When a curved-tip catheter with a guide mark is used for this purpose, successful endobronchial placement may occur in as many as 90% of cases. Factors that affect the success of the selective introduction of a catheter into a main stem bronchus include the anatomy of the carinal bifurcation, the patient's head and body positions, the route of tracheal tube placement (endotracheal or tracheostomy), the shape and direction of the endotracheal tube's bevel, the configuration and rigidity of the suction catheter, and the location of the tip of the endotracheal tube. Curved-tip catheters may be more effective with tracheostomy tubes than with endotracheal tubes.

An increase in intracranial pressure (ICP) can occur during tracheal suctioning, which may be clinically important in patients with a closed head injury. If a patient's ICP is being monitored, it should be watched closely during suctioning. Preoxygenation, hyperventilation, and pharmacologic support may be necessary for suctioning patients with an elevated ICP.

Closed Suction

With the closed suction system (**Figure 17-56**), the catheter becomes part of the ventilator circuit.[104–107] Closed suction and conventional suction catheters are equally effective at secretion clearance. The closed system may cause significantly fewer physiologic disturbances, such as dysrhythmias and desaturation, however, and environmental contamination is lower with the closed system. Perhaps the main advantage of a closed system is the minimization of circuit breaks, thus maintaining end-expiratory lung volume. A potential problem with closed suction catheters involves the catheter remaining in the airway after suctioning or migrating into the airway between suctioning procedures. This may be of particular concern during pressure ventilation, because the patient's tidal volume may be considerably compromised. Care must also be taken to avoid accidental patient lavage (which may wash some pathogens to the lower respiratory tract) when the catheter is rinsed with saline. Prolonged use of closed suction catheters does not affect the rate of ventilator-associated pneumonia, and they do not need to be changed at regular intervals.[107–109]

Saline Instillation

Although saline may be instilled into the airway as part of the suctioning procedure to facilitate the removal of

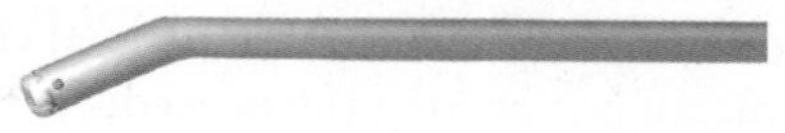

FIGURE 17-55 Curved-tip suction catheter.
Image reproduced with kind permission of Pennine Healthcare.

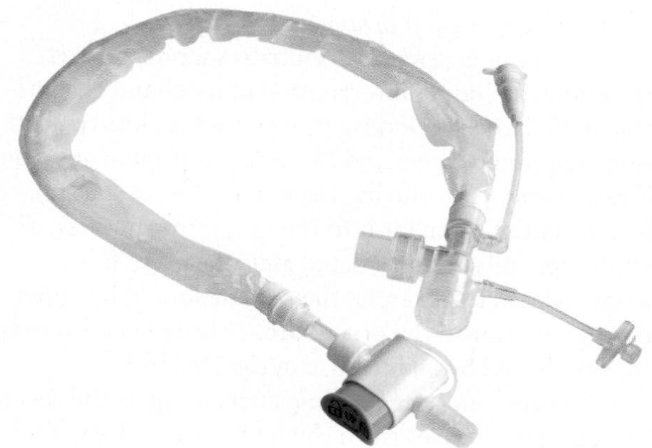

FIGURE 17-56 Closed suction catheter.
Courtesy of medisize, www.medisize.com.

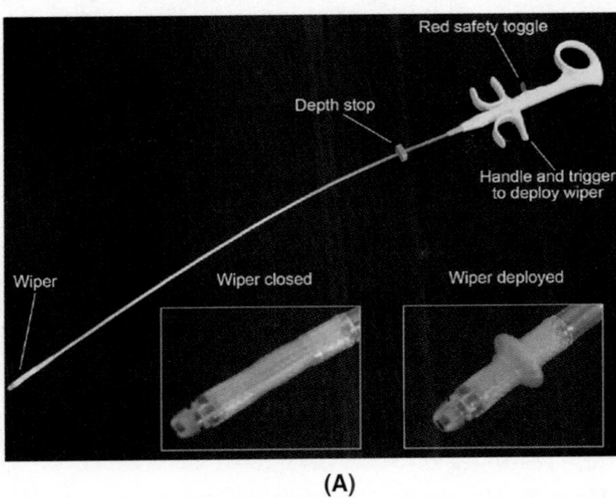

(A)

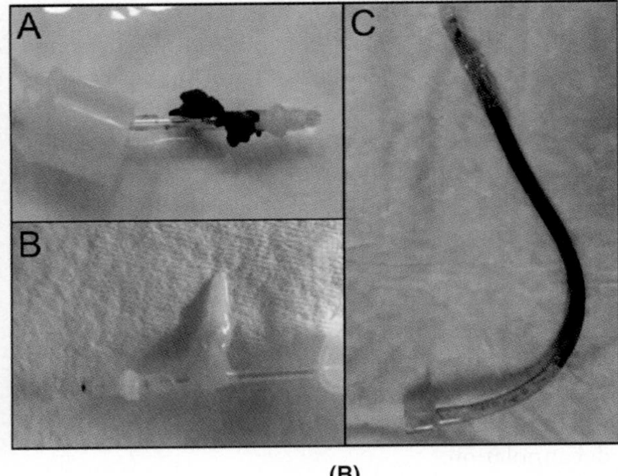

(B)

FIGURE 17-57 (**A**) The endOclear endotracheal tube-cleaning device. (**B**) Case A: Tip of the endOclear device with dried secretions after endotracheal tube (ETT) cleaning. Case B: Tip of the endOclear device with a large mucus plug after ETT cleaning. Case C: An occluded ETT from an ICU burn patient. Standard suctioning and emergency bronchoscopy did not maintain normal gas exchange and ventilation. The patient had to be reintubated to resume oxygenation and ventilation.

Reproduced from Mietto C, Foley K, Salerno L, et al. Removal of endotracheal tube obstruction with a secretion clearance device. *Respir Care.* 2014;59:e122–e126.

secretions, this practice is controversial.[110,111] Typically, more saline is instilled than is retrieved by the suctioning, which may result in an increase in the volume of secretions and worsening of airway obstruction. Saline instillation during suctioning may have an adverse effect on arterial oxygen saturation and may dislodge large numbers of bacteria from the lumen of the endotracheal tube, which may increase the likelihood of organisms being washed from the endotracheal tube into the lower respiratory tract. In a very few patients, saline instillation may be useful to loosen and remove thick secretions. This practice should be used judiciously, however, and should *not* be a routine procedure each time a patient is suctioned.

There has been recent concern about the potential buildup of secretions on the intraluminal wall of the endotracheal tube. Secretion buildup can lead to varying occlusion levels leading to an increased work of breathing and possibly increased weaning times. Additionally secretion buildup on the walls of the endotracheal tube often serves as a source of continuous aspiration of microorganisms into the lungs. Several devices have been recently introduced that consist of a catheter designed to enter the endotracheal tube with a balloon or net on its distal end (**Figure 17-57**).[112] Once the catheter is advanced into the endotracheal tube, the balloon is inflated (or the net is opened) and the catheter is pulled back out of the endotracheal tube carrying with it the secretions from the intraluminal wall. One recent, small study showed that the Mucus Shaver appears to be safe and does remove secretions from the interior walls of the endotracheal tubes.[113] More investigation needs to be done with these devices in terms of ventilator-associated pneumonia reduction, effects on the duration of mechanical ventilation, and weaning times.

Key Points

- Oropharyngeal airways extend from the lips to the pharynx, following the natural curvature of the tongue, without entering the larynx or esophagus.
- Nasopharyngeal airways follow the anatomy of the nasopharynx so that the tip rests behind the tongue just above the epiglottis.
- The airway consists of five regions: the nose and nasopharynx, oral cavity and oropharynx, hypopharynx, larynx, and tracheobronchial tree.
- Anesthesia personnel have the highest level of intubation skills, but in the hospital setting, the clinician with the highest level of experience and training outside the operating room may be the respiratory therapist.
- Indications for endotracheal intubation include bypassing of an upper airway obstruction, protection of the airway from aspiration, application of positive pressure ventilation, facilitation of secretion clearance, and delivery of high oxygen concentrations.
- Endotracheal intubation is the establishment of an artificial airway by use of a tube passed through the mouth or nose, then through the glottis, and into the trachea.
- Endotracheal intubation should be approached calmly; frantic and rushed attempts at intubation often result in failure and worsening of the situation.
- Nasotracheal intubation generally is used for specific indications.
- The shape and design of the laryngeal mask airway allows it to form a seal around the glottic opening that excludes the esophageal opening from the airway.
- The risk of complications associated with endotracheal intubation is reduced by meticulous attention to care of the airway in intubated patients.

- The traditional method used to secure an endotracheal tube is to apply benzoin to the skin and secure the tube with adhesive tape, but commercial holding systems also are available.
- A bite block is placed between the teeth to prevent the patient from biting an orotracheal airway.
- The primary reason to perform a tracheostomy is to maintain a secure airway in patients who require long-term intubation.
- Percutaneous dilational tracheostomy is a comparatively new procedure that is less traumatic than the conventional tracheostomy.
- The fenestrated tracheostomy tube can be useful for assessment of a patient's readiness for decannulation.
- The primary goal of a talking tracheostomy tube is to allow cognitively intact, ventilator-dependent patients to communicate by speaking.
- Speaking valves are designed to eliminate the need for finger occlusion for oral communication.
- Tracheal buttons are used to maintain tracheostomy stomas.
- Cuff pressure should be kept at 20 to 30 cm H_2O to minimize the risks of tracheal wall injury and aspiration.
- Intubated patients should be suctioned whenever a physical examination reveals secretions in the airway.
- Numerous complications are possible with airway suctioning.
- With the closed suction system, the catheter becomes part of the ventilator circuit.
- Saline instillation during suctioning should be used judiciously and should not be performed each time a patient is suctioned.
- The most frequent cause of extubation failure is inability of the patient to sustain adequate spontaneous ventilation.

References

1. Chhajed PN, Aboyoun C, Malouf MA, et al. Management of acute hypoxemia during flexible bronchoscopy with insertion of a nasopharyngeal tube. *Chest.* 2002;121:1350–1354.
2. Hooke R. [title unknown.] *Phil Trans Roy Soc.* 1667;2:539.
3. MacEwen W. Clinical observations on the introduction of tracheal tubes by the mouth instead of performing tracheostomy or laryngotomy. *Br Med J.* 1880;2:122–124, 163–165.
4. O'Dwyer J. Intubation of the larynx. *N Y Med J.* 1885;4:145.
5. Fell GE. Forced respiration in opium poisoning: its possibilities and the apparatus best adapted to produce it. *Buffalo Med Surg J.* 1887;28:145.
6. Murphy FJ. Two improved intratracheal catheters. *Anesth Analg.* 1941;27:102–105.
7. Martin LD, Mhyre JM, Shanks AM, et al. 3,423 Emergency tracheal intubations at a university hospital. Airway Outcomes and Complications. *Anesthesiology.* 2011;114:42–48.
8. Simpson GD, Ross MJ, McKeown DW, Ray DC. Tracheal intubation in the critically ill: a multi-centre national study of practice and complications. *Br J Anaesth.* 2012;108:792–799.
9. American Society of Anesthesiologists. Practice guidelines for management of the difficult airway: an updated report by the American Society of Anesthesiologists Task Force on Management of the Difficult Airway. *Anesthesiology* 2003;98:1269–1277.
10. Jaber S, Jung B, Corne P, et al. An intervention to decrease complications related to endotracheal intubation in the intensive care unit: a prospective, multiple-center study. *Intensive Care Med.* 2010;36:248–255.
11. Berkow LC, Greenberg RS, Kan KH, et al. Need for emergency surgical airway reduced by a comprehensive difficult airway program. *Anesth Analg.* 2009;109:1860–1869.
12. Mayo PH, Hegde A, Eisen LA, et al. A program to improve the quality of emergency endotracheal intubation. *J Intens Care Med.* 2011;26:50–56.
13. Goldmann K, Ferson DZ. Education and training in airway management. *Best Pract Res Clin Anaesthesiol.* 2005;19(4):717–732.
14. Bishop MJ. Who should perform intubation? *Respir Care.* 1999;44:750–758.
15. Bishop MJ, Michalowski P, Hussey JD, et al. Recertification of respiratory therapists' intubation skills one year after initial training: analysis of skill retention and retraining. *Respir Care.* 2001;46:234–237.
16. Mulcaster JT, Mills J, Hung OR, et al. Laryngoscopic intubation: learning and performance. *Anesthesiology.* 2003;98:23–27.
17. Howard-Quijano KJ, Huang YM, Matevosian R. Video-assisted instruction improves the success rate for tracheal intubation by novices. *Br J Anaesth.* 2008;101:568–572.
18. Nouruzi-Sedeh P, Schumann M, Groeben H. Laryngoscopy via Macintosh blade versus GlideScope: success rate and time for endotracheal intubation in untrained medical personnel. *Anesthesiology.* 2009;110:32–37.
19. Kennedy CC, Cannon EK, Warner DO. Advanced airway management simulation training in medical education: a systematic review and meta-analysis. *Crit Care Med.* 2014 Jan;42:169–178.
20. Vital FM, Saconato H, Ladeira MT, et al. Non-invasive positive pressure ventilation (CPAP or bilevel NPPV) for cardiogenic pulmonary edema. *Cochrane Database Syst Rev.* 2008;3:CD005351.
21. Ram FSF, Picot J, Lightowler J, Wedzicha JA. Non-invasive positive pressure ventilation for treatment of respiratory failure due to exacerbations of chronic obstructive pulmonary disease. *Cochrane Database Syst Rev.* 2004;3:CD004104.
22. Nava S, Hill N. Noninvasive ventilation in acute respiratory failure. *Lancet.* 2009;374:250–259.
23. Hess DR. The evidence for noninvasive positive-pressure ventilation in the care of patients in acute respiratory failure: a systematic review of the literature. *Respir Care.* 2004;49:810–829.
24. Keenan SP, Mehta S. Noninvasive ventilation for patients presenting with acute respiratory failure: the randomized controlled trials. *Resp Care.* 2009;54:116–124.
25. Kollef MH. What is ventilator-associated pneumonia and why is it important? *Respir Care.* 2005;50:714–772.
26. Coffin SE, Klompas M, Classen D, et al. Strategies to prevent ventilator-associated pneumonia in acute care hospitals. *Infect Control Hosp Epidemiol.* 2008;19:S31–S40.
27. Pearce A. Evaluation of the airway and preparation for difficulty. *Best Pract Res Clin Anaesthesiol.* 2005;19:559–579.
28. Dunn PF, Goulet RL. Endotracheal tubes and airway appliances. *Int Anesth Clin.* 2000;38:65–94.
29. Jaeger JM, Durbin CG. Special-purpose endotracheal tubes. *Respir Care.* 1999;44:661–683.
30. Fernandex JF, Levine SM, Restrepo MI. Technology advances in endotracheal tubes for the prevention of ventilator-associated pneumonia. *Chest.* 2012;142:231–238.
31. Dezfulian C, Shojania K, Collard HR, et al. Subglottic secretion drainage for preventing ventilator associated pneumonia: a meta-analysis. *Am J Med.* 2005;118:11–18.
32. Muscedere J, Rewa O, McKechnie K, et al. Subglottic secretion drainage for the prevention of ventilator-associated pneumonia: a systematic review and meta-analysis. *Crit Care Med.* 2011;39:1985–1991.

33. Dragoumanis CK, Vretzakis GI, Papaioannou VE, et al. Investigating the failure to aspirate subglottic secretions with the Evac endotracheal tube. *Anesth Analg.* 2007;105:1083–1085.
34. Shorr AF, O'Malley PG. Continuous subglottic suctioning for the prevention of ventilator-associated pneumonia: potential economic implications. *Chest.* 2001;119:228–223;.
35. Dezfulian C, Shojania K, Collard HR, et al. Subglottic secretion drainage for preventing ventilator associated pneumonia: a meta-analysis. *Am J Med.* 2005;118:11–18.
36. Bouza E, Pérez MJ, Muñoz P , et al. Continuous aspiration of subglottic secretions in the prevention of ventilator-associated pneumonia in the postoperative period of major heart surgery. *Chest.* 2008;134:938–946.
37. Fletcher AJW, Ruffell AJ, Young PJ. The Lo Trach system: its role in the prevention of ventilator-associated pneumonia. *Nurs Crit Care.* 2008;13:260–268.
38. Olson ME, Harmon BG, Kollef MH. Silver-coated endotracheal tubes associated with reduced bacterial burden in the lungs of mechanically ventilated dogs. *Chest.* 2002;121:863–870.
39. Kollef MH, Afessa B, Anzueto A, et al. Silver-coated endotracheal tubes and incidence of ventilator-associated pneumonia: the NASCENT randomized trial. *JAMA.* 2008;300:805–813.
40. Shorr AF, Zilberberg MD, Kollef M. Cost-effectiveness analysis of a silver-coated endotracheal tube to reduce the incidence of ventilator-associated pneumonia. *Infect Control Hosp Epidemiol.* 2009;30:759–763.
41. Ballard C, Fosse JP, Sebbane M, et al. Noninvasive ventilation improves preoxygenation before intubation of hypoxic patients. *Am J Respir Crit Care Med.* 2006;174:171–177.
42. Dixon BJ, Dixon JB, Carden JR, et al. Preoxygenation is more effective in the 25° head-up position than in the supine position in severely obese patients. a randomized controlled study. *Anesthesiology.* 2005;102:1110–1115.
43. Rosen CL, Wolfe RE, Chew SE, et al. Blind nasotracheal intubation in the presence of facial trauma. *J Emerg Med.* 1997;15:141–145.
44. Tominga GT, Rudzwick H, Scannell G, et al. Decreasing unplanned extubations in the surgical intensive care unit. *Am J Surg.* 1995;170: 586–590.
45. Boulain T. Unplanned extubations in the adult intensive care unit: a prospective multicenter study. *Am J Respir Crit Care Med.* 1998;157:1131–1137.
46. Christie JM, Dethlefsen M, Cane RD. Unplanned endotracheal extubation in the intensive care unit. *J Clin Anesth.* 1996;8:289–293.
47. Atkins PM, Mion LC, Mendelson W, et al. Characteristics and outcomes of patients who self-extubate from ventilatory support: a case-control study. *Chest.* 1997;112:1317–1323.
48. Betbese A, Perez M, Rialp G, et al. A prospective study of unplanned endotracheal extubation in intensive care unit patients. *Crit Care Med.* 1998;26:1180–1186.
49. Kapadia FN, Bajan KB, Raje KY. Airway accidents in intubated intensive care unit patients: an epidemiological study. *Crit Care Med.* 2000;28:659–664.
50. 2005 American Heart Association guidelines for cardiopulmonary resuscitation and emergency cardiovascular care. *Circulation.* 2005;112:IV-19–IV-34.
51. Adams JR, Hoffman J, Lavelle J, Mireles-Cabodevila E. Pilot balloon malfunction caused by endotracheal tube bite blocker. *Respir Care.* 2014;59:e22–e24.
52. Asai T, Morris S. The laryngeal mask airway: its features, effects, and roles. *Can J Anaesth.* 1994;41:930–960.
53. Hernandez MR, Klock PA, Ovassapian A. Evolution of the extraglottic airway: a review of its history, applications, and practical tips for success. *Anesth Analg.* 2012;114:349–368.
54. Verghese C, Ramaswamy B. LMA-Supreme—a new single-use LMA with gastric access: a report on its clinical efficiency. *Br J Anaesth.* 2008;101:405–410.
55. Theiler LG, Kleine-Brueggeney M, Kaiser D, et al. Crossover comparison of the Laryngeal Mask Supreme and the i-gel in simulated difficult airway scenario in anesthesized patients. *Anesthesiology.* 2009;111:55–62.
56. LMA North America, Inc. LMA Fastrach instruction manual. February 2006. Available at: http://www.lmana.com/pwpcontrol.php?pwpID=6342. Accessed on February 18, 2014.
57. Niforopoulou P, Pantazopoulos I, Demesthia T, et al. Video-laryngoscopes in the adult airway management: a topical review of the literature. *Acta Anaesthesiol Scand.* 2010;54:1050–1061.
58. Ahmed-beringer A. Videolaryngoscopy. *Curr Anaesthesia Crit Care.* 2010;21:199–205.
59. Behringer EC, Kristensen MS. Evidence for benefit vs novelty in new intubation equipment. *Anaesthesia.* 2011;66(Suppl. 2): 57–64.
60. Maharaj CH, O'Croinin D, Curley G, Harte BH, Laffey JG. A comparison of tracheal intubation using the Airtraq or the MacIntosh laryngoscope in routine airway management: a randomized, controlled clinical trial. *Anaesthesia.* 2006;61:1093–1099.
61. Maharaj CH, Buckley E, Harte BH, Laffey JG. Endotracheal intubation in patients with cervical spine immobilization: a comparison of Macintosh and Airtraq laryngoscopes. *Anesthesiology.* 2007;107:53–59.
62. Maharaj CH, Costello JF, McDonnell JG, Harte BH, Laffey JG. The Airtraq as a rescue device following failed direct laryngoscopy: a case series. *Anaesthesia.* 2007;62:598–601.
63. De Jong A, Clavieras N, Conseil M et al. Implementation of a combo videolaryngoscope for intubation in critically ill patients: a before-after comparative study. *Intensive Care Med.* 2013;39: 2144–2152.
64. Yeatts DJ, Dutton RP, Hu PF et al. Effect of video laryngoscopy on trauma patient survival: a randomized controlled trial. *J Trauma Acute Care Surg.* 2013;75:212–219.
65. Griesdale DE, Chau A, Isac G et al. Video-laryngoscopy versus direct laryngoscopy in critically ill patients: a pilot randomized trial. *Can J Anaesth.* 2012;59:1032–1039.
66. Larsson A, Dhonneur G. Videolaryngoscopy: towards a new standard method for tracheal intubation in the ICU? *Intensive Care Med.* 2013;39:2220–2222.
67. Mihai R, Blair E, Kay H, et al. A quantitative review and meta-analysis of performance of non-standard laryngoscopes and rigid fibreoptic intubation aids. *Anaesthesia.* 2008;63:745–760.
68. Meininger D, Strouhal U, Weber CF, et al. Direct laryngoscopy or C-MAC video laryngoscopy? Routine tracheal intubation in patients undergoing ENT surgery. *Anaesthesist.* 2010;59: 806–811.
69. Noppens RR, Mobus S, Heid F, et al. Evaluation of the McGrath Series 5 Videolaryngoscope after failed direct laryngoscopy. *Anaesthesia.* 2010;65:716–720.
70. Noppens RR, Geimer S, Eisle N et al. Endotracheal intubation using the C-MAC® video laryngoscope or the Macintosh laryngoscope: a prospective, comparative study in the ICU. *Crit Care.* 2012;16:R103.
71. Mosier JM, Stolz U, Chiu S, et al. Difficult airway management in the emergency department: Glidescope videolaryngoscopy compared to direct laryngoscopy. *J Emerg Med.* 2012;42: 629–634.
72. Trimmel H, Kreutziger J, Fertsak G, et al. Use of the Airtraq laryngoscope for emergency intubation in the prehospital setting: a randomized control trial. *Crit Care Med.* 2011;39:489–493.
73. Hill C, Reardon R, Joing S, et al. Cricothyroidotomy technique using gum elastic bougie is faster than standard technique: a study of emergency medicine residents and medical students in an animal lab. *Acad Emerg Med.* 2010;17:666–669.
74. Schaumann N, Lorenz V, Schellongowski P, et al. Evaluation of Seldinger technique emergency cricothyroidotomy versus standard surgical cricothyroidotomy in 200 cadavers. *Anesthesiology.* 2005 Jan;102:7–11.
75. Blanda M, Gallo UE. Emergency airway management. *Emerg Med Clin North Am.* 2003;21:1–26.

76. Salam A, Tilluckdharry L, Amoateng-Adjepong Y, Manthous CA. Neurologic status, cough, secretions, and extubation outcomes. *Intensive Care Med*. 2004;30:1334–1339.
77. Kriner EJ, Shafazand S, Colice GL. The endotracheal tube cuff leak test as a predictor for post-extubation stridor. *Respir Care*. 2005;50:1632–1638.
78. Shin SH, Heath K, Reed S, et al. The cuff leak test is not predictive of successful extubation. *Am Surg*. 2008;74:1182–1185.
79. Jaber S, Jung B, Chanques G, Bonnet F, Marret E. Effects of steroids on reintubation and post-extubation stridor in adults: meta-analysis of randomized controlled trials. *Crit Care*. 2009; 13(2):R49.
80. Fan T, Wang G, Mao B, et al. Prophylactic administration of parenteral steroids for preventing airway complications after extubation in adults: meta-analysis of randomized controlled trials. *BMJ*. 2008;337:a1841.
81. Esteban A, Alia I, Gordo F, et al. Extubation outcome after spontaneous breathing trials with T-tube or pressure support ventilation. *Am J Respir Crit Care Med*. 1997;156:459–465.
82. Epstein SK, Ciubotaru RL. Independent effects of etiology of failure and time to reintubation on outcome for patients failing extubation. *Am J Respir Crit Care Med*. 1998;158:489–493.
83. Terragni PP, Antonelli M, Fumagalli R, et al. Early vs late tracheotomy for prevention of pneumonia in mechanically ventilated adult ICU patients: a randomized controlled trial. *JAMA*. 2010;303:1483–1489.
84. Young D, Harrison DA, Cuthbertson BH, Rowan K, TracMan Collaborators. Effect of early vs late tracheostomy placement on survival in patients receiving mechanical ventilation: the TracMan randomized trial. *JAMA*. 2013;309:2121–2129.
85. Hsia DW, Ghori UK, Musani AI. Percutaneous dilational tracheostomy. *Clin Chest Med*. 2013;34:515–526.
86. Hess DR. Tracheostomy tubes and related appliances. *Respir Care*. 2005;50:497–510.
87. Hess DR, Altobelli NP. Tracheostomy tubes. *Respir Care*. 2014;59:956–973.
88. Souza CR, Santana VT. Impact of supra-cuff suction on ventilator-associated pneumonia prevention. *Rev Bras Ter Intensiva*. 2012;24:401–406.
89. Kunduk M, Appel K, Tunc M, et al. Preliminary report of laryngeal phonation during mechanical ventilation via a new cuffed tracheostomy tube. *Respir Care*. 2010;55:1661–1670.
90. Hess DR. Facilitating speech in the patient with a tracheostomy. *Respir Care*. 2005;50:519–525.
91. Johnson DC, Campbell SL, Rabkin JD. Tracheostomy tube manometry: evaluation of speaking valves, capping and need for downsizing. *Clin Respir J*. 2008;3:8–14.
92. Hoit JD, Banzett RB, Lohmeier HL, Hixon TJ, Brown R. Clinical ventilator adjustments that improve speech. *Chest*. 2003;124:1512–1521.
93. Schmidt U, Hess D, Kwo J, et al. Tracheostomy tube malposition in patients admitted to a respiratory acute care unit following prolonged ventilation. *Chest*. 2008;134:288–294.
94. White AC, Kher S, O'Connor HH. When to change a tracheostomy tube. *Respir Care*. 2010;55:1069–1075.
95. Fisher DF, Kondili D, Williams J, et al. Tracheostomy tube change before day 7 is associated with earlier use of speaking valve and earlier oral intake. *Respir Care*. 2013;58:257–263.
96. Yaremchuk K. Regular tracheostomy tube changes to prevent formation of granulation tissue. *Laryngoscope*. 2003;113:1–10.
97. Bjorling G, Axelsson S, Johansson UB, et al. Clinical use and material wear of polymeric tracheostomy tubes. *Laryngoscope*. 2007;117:1552–1559.
98. Backman S, Bjorling G, Johansson UB, et al. Material wear of polymeric tracheostomy tubes: a six-month study. *Laryngoscope*. 2009;119:657–664.
99. Stelfox HT, Crimi C, Berra L, et al. Determinants of tracheostomy decannulation: an international study. *Crit Care*. 2008;12:R26.
100. White AC, Purcell E, Urquhart MB, et al. Accidental decannulation following placement of a tracheostomy tube. *Respir Care*. 2012;57:2019–2025.
101. O'Connor HH, White AC. Tracheostomy decannulation. *Respir Care*. 2010;55:1076–1081.
102. White AC, Purcell E, Urquhart MB, et al. Accidental decannulation following placement of a tracheostomy tube. *Respir Care*. 2012;57:2019–2025.
103. Nseir S, Zerimech F, Fournier C, et al. Continuous control of tracheal cuff pressure and microaspiration of gastric contents in critically ill patients. *Am J Respir Crit Care Med*. 2011;184:1041–1047.
104. Rabitsch W, Kostler WJ, Fiebiger W, et al. Closed suctioning system reduces cross-contamination between system and gastric juices. *Anesth Analg*. 2004;99:886–892.
105. Maggiore SM, Lellouche F, Pigeot J, et al. Prevention of endotracheal suctioning-induced alveolar derecruitment in acute lung injury. *Am J Respir Crit Care Med*. 2003;167:1215–1224.
106. Cereda M, Villa F, Colombo E, et al. Closed system endotracheal suctioning maintains lung volume-controlled mechanical ventilation. *Intensive Care Med*. 2001;27:648–654.
107. Vonberg RP, Eckmanns T, Welte T, Gastmeier P. Impact of the suctioning system (open vs. closed) on the incidence of ventilation-associated pneumonia: meta-analysis of randomized controlled trials. *Intensive Care Med*. 2006;32:1329–1335.
108. AARC clinical practice guideline: endotracheal suctioning of mechanically ventilated patients with artificial airways. *Respir Care*. 2010;55:758–764.
109. Stoller JK, Orens DK, Fatica C, et al. Weekly versus daily changes of in-line suction catheters: impact on rates of ventilator-associated pneumonia and associated costs. *Respir Care*. 2003;48:494–499.
110. Ji YR, Kim HS, Park JH. Instillation of normal saline before suctioning in patients with pneumonia. *Yonsei Med J*. 2002;43:607–612.
111. Caruso P, Denari S, Ruiz SA, Demarzo SE, Deheinzelin D. Saline instillation before tracheal suctioning decreases the incidence of ventilator-associated pneumonia. *Crit Care Med*. 2009;37:32–38.
112. Mietto C, Foley K, Salerno L, et al. Removal of endotracheal tube obstruction with a secretion clearance device. *Respir Care*. 2014;59:e122–e126.
113. Berra L, Coppadoro A, Bittner EA, et al. A clinical assessment of the Mucus Shaver: a device to keep the endotracheal tube free from secretions. *Crit Care Med*. 2012;40:119–124.

CHAPTER

18

Cardiopulmonary Resuscitation

Rhonda Bevis, Christine J. Moore, William F. Galvin

OUTLINE

Cardiopulmonary Resuscitation
Basic Life Support
Advanced Cardiovascular Life Support
Ethical Concerns

OBJECTIVES

1. Define cardiopulmonary resuscitation (CPR).
2. Provide a brief historical account of the evolution and development of CPR.
3. List and explain the chain of survival.
4. Identify and briefly explain risk factors for sudden death.
5. Explain techniques of basic life support for adults, children, and infants.
6. Describe CABD sequence of applying basic life support.
7. Compare one-rescuer and two-rescuer cardiopulmonary resuscitation.
8. Describe emergency management of foreign body airway obstruction for adults, children, and infants.
9. Explain techniques of advanced cardiovascular life support.
10. Identify and explain actions of advanced cardiovascular life support medications.
11. Explain patient care and support after resuscitation.
12. Explain ethical issues and concerns of cardiopulmonary resuscitation.

KEY TERMS

advanced cardiovascular life support (ACLS)
automated external defibrillator (AED)
basic life support (BLS)
CABD sequence
cardiac arrest
cardiopulmonary resuscitation (CPR)
chest compressions
defibrillation
face shield
foreign body obstruction (FBO)
impedance threshold valve (ITV)
manual resuscitator
rapid response team
respiratory arrest

Introduction

Resuscitation of patients in cardiopulmonary arrest requires assessment of the problem, proper training, and an organized response system. Code teams and rapid response teams are the primary vehicle or mechanism by which effective and successful resuscitation efforts occur and respiratory therapists are always vital members of this team. This chapter emphasizes the critical role played by the RT as well as essential elements in the CPR process. Specifically, it addresses a definition and explanation of cardiopulmonary resuscitation; a brief historical account of contemporary events and milestones in the evolution of CPR; the principles and application of **basic life support (BLS)** for adults, children, and infants; the use of **automated external defibrillation (AED)**; the principles and application of **advanced cardiovascular life support (ACLS)**; post–cardiac arrest care and management; and the ethical issues and concerns of cardiopulmonary resuscitation. In addition, the chapter highlights new developments in resuscitation science with the release of the 2005 and 2010 American Heart Association (AHA) Guidelines for Cardiopulmonary Resuscitation (CPR) and Emergency Cardiovascular Care (ECC).

Cardiopulmonary Resuscitation

Definitions

Cardiopulmonary resuscitation (CPR) can be defined as a series of life-saving actions that can improve the chance of survival following cardiac arrest.[1] **Cardiac arrest** is defined as cessation of cardiac mechanical activity and is confirmed by the absence of signs of circulation.[2] Cardiopulmonary resuscitation is also viewed as a procedure to support and maintain breathing and circulation for a neonate, infant, child, or adult who has stopped breathing (**respiratory arrest**) and/or whose heart has stopped. The authors of the 2005 AHA CPR and ECC guidelines recognized the potential confusion regarding age delineation and arrived at a consensus decision for the ease of teaching and practicing BLS and ACLS for healthcare providers. Because there is no one anatomic or physiologic characteristic that distinguishes an infant from a child, they defined an infant to include neonates (those in the first 28 days of life) and patients less than approximately 1 year of age and a child as a patient from 1 year of age to the onset of puberty (about 12 to 14 years of age or more precisely breast development in females and the presence of axillary hair in males). Adults are considered patients at and beyond puberty.[3]

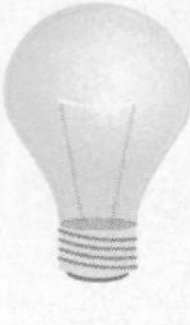

STOP AND THINK

You've heard the grim statistics for CPR survival. In your opinion, what would need to occur for a significant improvement in survival for out-of-hospital CPR? What about for in-hospital CPR?

Incidence and Epidemiology

There are approximately 360,000 out-of-hospital cardiac arrests in the United States every year accounting for about 15% of all deaths.[4] Approximately 60% of out-of-hospital cardiac arrests are treated by emergency medical services (EMS) personnel.[5] While survival data are highly variable, one study demonstrated that survival from out-of-hospital arrest ranged from 1.0% to 16.3%.[6] Another study indicated that survival to hospital discharge in 2010 (after EMS-treated nontraumatic cardiac arrest with any first recorded rhythm) for adults was 9.8% and for children was 7.8%.[7]

Extrapolation of the incidence of in-hospital cardiac arrest in the United States suggests that each year 209,000 people are treated for in-hospital cardiac arrest. According to these same investigators, 23.9% of adults and 40.2% of children (excluding neonates) survived to discharge.[8] A subsequent Consensus Statement from the American Heart Association published in 2013 reflected a median hospital survival rate from adult cardiac arrest at 18% (interquartile range of 12% to 22%) and pediatric cardiac arrest at 36% (interquartile range of 33% to 49%).[9]

Numerous factors impact in-hospital survival. Among them are the locations within the institution as well as time of day. There is a 9% survival rate at night for patients in unmonitored settings compared to nearly 37% survival in the operating room or postanesthesia care units during the day. Additionally, survival rates for the in-hospital setting between 7 AM and 11 PM is >20% and only 15% between 11 PM and 7 AM.[10] In-hospital resuscitation outcomes are also associated with the initial cardiac rhythm, time to initiate CPR, time to defibrillate, duration of CPR, and whether or not the arrest was witnessed. With properly trained caregivers, the survival rates for a witnessed ventricular fibrillation (VF) increases to 49% to 74%.[11] Proper training includes rapid recognition of the cardiopulmonary arrest, rapid response, CPR, and early defibrillation (within 5 minutes).[11]

History, Evolution, and Milestones

While the roots of CPR date back centuries, considerable evidence suggests the genesis of *contemporary* cardiopulmonary resuscitation began in 1960 when the Maryland Medical Society formally introduced chest compression and rescue breathing as key elements to successful resuscitation.[12] In 1966, the first CPR guidelines were published recommending the training of medical personnel in external chest compressions.[13] This training was extended to the broader community through a milestone event: the introduction of the Resusci Anne mannequin.[14] The mannequin was created by Asmund Laerdal, a plastic-toy company owner, who was so moved by the death of a young unnamed girl who drowned in the Seine River that he went on to collaborate with anesthesiologists in the development and manufacture of a low cost but highly effective human model. This revolutionized the way resuscitation training was delivered. It was closely followed by another milestone event in the 1970s—the world's first mass citizen training program. This training program was championed by Drs. Cobb, Kopass, Eisenberg, and colleagues and occurred in Seattle, Washington, where over 100,000 people were trained within a 2 year period to perform layperson CPR.[15] In1979, advanced cardiovascular life support (ACLS) was introduced and in 1983 the AHA convened a national conference on pediatric resuscitation and later developed guidelines for pediatric advanced life support (PALS) and neonatal advanced life support (NALS). The 1990s saw the Early Public Access Defibrillation (PAD) programs providing training and resources to the lay public in the use of the automated external defibrillator (AED), which further facilitated the successful resuscitation of sudden cardiac arrest victims in the community.[16]

In 2005, the AHA developed the Family & Friends® CPR Anytime Kit designed to allow anyone to learn the core skills of CPR in just 20 minutes.[17] Additionally, the AHA released the 2005[18] Guidelines, which revealed a new compression-to-ventilation ratio as well as changes to AED usage. Most recently, the AHA celebrated the 50-year anniversary of contemporary cardiopulmonary

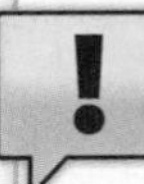

Respiratory Recap

Milestones in Contemporary CPR

1960s - Publication of first CPR Guidelines
Manufacture of Resusci Anne mannequin
1970s - Mass citizen training in Seattle, WA
Introduction of ACLS
1980s - Introduction of PALS and NALS
1990s - Early Public Access Defibrillation (PAD) programs
2000s - AHA Family and Friends' CPR Anytime Kit
2010s - Change in sequence from "A-B-C" to "C-A-B"

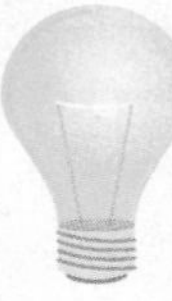

STOP AND THINK

What does the future hold for CPR? What new innovations or developments will we see with the next release of AHA CPR Guidelines? How about in the next 50 years?

resuscitation with the release of the 2010[11,19] AHA Guidelines for Cardiopulmonary Resuscitation (CPR) and Emergency Cardiovascular Care (ECC). The newest development of these 2010 Guidelines was the change in sequence from "A-B-C" to "C-A-B," making them the most comprehensive and state-of-the-art advances and innovations in the art and science of cardiopulmonary resuscitation.

Current Guideline Developments

Recommendations and guidelines for resuscitation procedures are provided by the AHA and are based on recommendations from the ECC Committee. Over the years, ECC Committees evaluated the sequence, priorities, and steps of BLS and ACLS to determine which factors were most likely to have the greatest positive effect on the successful resuscitation of individuals who suffered a cardiopulmonary arrest. The 2005 Guidelines were based on research indicating that during the first few minutes of a cardiac arrest with ventricular fibrillation, management of the airway, oxygenation, and ventilation are probably not as important as chest compressions. This is because the total amount of oxygen delivered to the vital organs is limited more by the amount of arterial blood flow to the organs than by the oxygen content of the arterial blood itself. During resuscitation, chest compressions are responsible for restoring blood flow to vital organs, and any interruption results in a lower perfusion pressure for the coronary and cerebral arteries and a higher rate of deaths for patients following a cardiac arrest.[19–21]

In 2010,[19] the American Heart Association eliminated "Look, Listen, and Feel" from the algorithm, and it implemented a change in sequence from "A-B-C" to "C-A-B" for adults and children. It stressed the need for high-quality compressions and a minimization of interruptions to chest compressions to facilitate better perfusion to the patient's vital organs. Additionally, the AHA has made several changes in the ratio of ventilations to compressions for CPR.

Healthcare providers commonly provide excessive ventilation and chest compressions that are inadequate and frequently interrupted during the resuscitation. Laypersons commonly provide ventilations ineffectively, are reluctant to do mouth-to-mask ventilations, and lack assessment skills sufficient to evaluate an arrest victim's ventilatory efforts. Compression-only CPR therefore is currently taught to laypersons[22] and the current 2010 Guidelines continue to emphasize chest compressions rather than ventilation during CPR.

The 2010 Guidelines reinforced the value of an integrated team of trained healthcare providers. Thus emphasis was placed on recognizing team building and re-delegation of roles as each member arrives to the site of the arrest.[11]

Chain of Survival

The chain of survival illustrates an integrated set of coordinated actions that improves the rate of survival after cardiac arrest (**Figure 18-1**). It includes individual

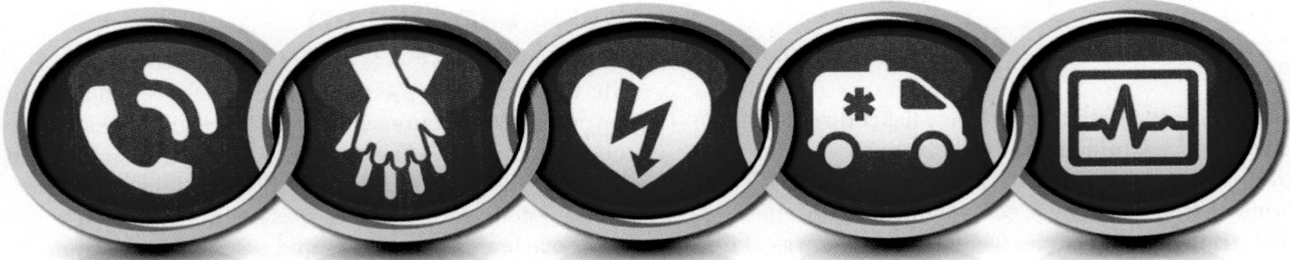

FIGURE 18-1 Chain of survival.

Reproduced from 2010 American Heart Association Guidelines for Cardiopulmonary Resuscitation and Emergency Cardiovascular Care. Part 4: CPR Overview. *Circulation.* 2010;122:S768–S786.

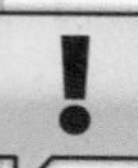

Respiratory Recap

Chain of Survival

- Immediate recognition and activation of emergency response system
- Early CPR
- Rapid defibrillation
- Effective ACLS
- Integrated post–cardiac arrest care

links that are interdependent, with the success of each link being dependent on the effectiveness of those links that precede it.[23] The five links are: (1) immediate recognition of cardiac arrest and activation of the emergency response system, (2) early CPR with emphasis on chest compression, (3) rapid defibrillation, (4) effective advanced life support, and (5) integrated post–cardiac arrest care.

CPR should be initiated immediately if the victim is unresponsive and not breathing, or not breathing normally. This should be coupled with activation of the emergency management system. Chest compressions should be high-quality, meaning at a rate of at least 100/min; at a compression depth of at least 2 inches for adults, at least one-third the anterior-posterior diameter of the chest for infants and children (or about 1½ inches for infants or 2 inches for children); allow for complete chest recoil after each compression; minimize interruptions; and avoid excessive ventilation. Rapid defibrillation remains the cornerstone for ventricular defibrillation and pulseless ventricular tachycardia and data suggest that with each passing moment of untreated ventricular fibrillation, the likelihood of survival is reduced by 7% to 10%.[14]

Advanced life support entails advanced airway management, rhythm recognition, and pharmacologic intervention. Postcardiac care emphasizes optimizing cardiopulmonary function and vital organ perfusion. All of these links in the chain of survival will be addressed in more detail in subsequent sections of this chapter, but note that the highest hospital discharge rate is when CPR is initiated within 4 minutes of arrest and advanced life support is initiated within 8 minutes.

Risk Factors

Sudden death related to coronary heart disease (CHD) is the most prominent medical emergency in the United States. **Box 18-1** lists risk factors for CHD. A prudent heart lifestyle is considered a highly effective strategy and includes weight control, physical fitness, smart eating habits, and avoidance of stress and cigarette smoking. The most important risk factor for CHD is cigarette smoking. The CHD death rate is 70% greater for smokers than nonsmokers, and the risk from smoking increases when combined with other factors (most notably elevated cholesterol and hypertension).

BOX 18-1

Risk Factors for Coronary Heart Disease

Factors That Cannot Be Changed

Heredity
Gender
Increasing Age

Factors That Can Be Changed

Cigarette Smoking
Hypertension
Lack of Exercise
Obesity
Excessive Stress
Diabetes
Blood Cholesterol Level

Clinical Practice Guidelines

Each hospital defines their respiratory therapists' involvement on rapid response teams and code teams. Therapists utilize their skills and expertise in patient assessment, airway management, oxygen therapy, mechanical ventilation, electrocardiograph (ECG) recognition, chest compressions, defibrillation, hemodynamic monitoring, and administration of ACLS drugs. This chapter summarizes the BLS and ACLS responsibilities of respiratory therapists who work in these capacities. The clinical practice guidelines (CPG) of the American Association for Respiratory Care (AARC) describe the role of respiratory therapists in providing patient support (**CPG 18-1**). Healthcare workers and respiratory therapists should modify their sequence of actions based on their location, whether or not immediate help is available, and their hospital or department protocol.

Basic Life Support

BLS includes all aspects of care required to treat life-threatening events (sudden cardiac arrest, acute myocardial infarction, stroke, and foreign body airway obstruction), CPR, and **defibrillation** with an automated external defibrillator.[11] Respiratory therapists, nurses, and physicians work together as members of rapid response teams providing rapid assessment and quick intervention or as code teams providing BLS and ACLS in healthcare settings. A **rapid response team**, also called a *medical emergency team*, is a team of clinicians who bring critical care expertise to the patient's side

CLINICAL PRACTICE GUIDELINE 18-1

Resuscitation and Defibrillation in the Healthcare Setting

Specialty resuscitation teams trained to meet the needs of different hospital populations are desirable in emergency situations (e.g., trauma, stroke). The development of emergency response teams, proper education and training, and a way to quickly and simultaneously notify members of the team greatly improve patient care in emergency situations. All hospital workers are required to know how to activate the hospital's emergency response system when appropriate emergency situations arise.

Level I

- *Training:* All Level I personnel should be trained, evaluated by performance checks, and retrained as necessary in basic life support (BLS) and the use of automated external defibrillators (AEDs) at frequent intervals that do not exceed 2 years.
- *Responsibilities:* First responders must be able to recognize that the patient is unresponsive, apneic, and/or pulseless. They should be able to activate the emergency response system, attach automated defibrillator electrodes, and operate AEDs. Level I personnel also assist the primary (Level II) members of the resuscitation team by (l) assessing patients for respiratory and/or cardiac arrest, (2) activating the resuscitation team, (3) administering BLS, (4) providing mouth-to-mask ventilation, (5) attaching electrocardiogram (ECG) and automatic defibrillator electrodes, (6) assisting with tracheal intubation, (7) defibrillating with automatic electronic defibrillators, (8) attaching pulse oximeter and capnograph, (9) preparing a written record of resuscitation effort, and (10) collecting arterial blood for analysis.

Level II

- *Training:* Level II personnel should be trained, evaluated by skills performance, and retrained as necessary in emergency cardiac care (ECC) and advanced cardiac life support (ACLS) as appropriate at intervals that should not exceed 2 years.
- *Responsibilities:* Level II health professionals should be capable of serving as primary members of the resuscitation team and as team leader when they are the best-qualified respondents. They are skilled in the use of all adjunctive equipment and special techniques for ECC/ACLS. They have the skills of Level I personnel and the following capabilities: (1) advanced ECG monitoring and dysrhythmia recognition, (2) tracheal intubation, (3) capability to deliver shocks with defibrillators, (4) use of mechanical ventilators, (5) preparation and administration of cardiac drugs, (6) stabilization of patients in the postarrest period, (7) provision of access for rapid administration of intravenous fluids, (8) management of ventilation via transtracheal catheter and cricothyrotomy, (9) emergency treatment of tension pneumothorax or hemothorax with large-bore needle, (10) interpretation of hemodynamic data, and (11) evaluation of oxygenation, ventilation, and acid–base balance from blood gas reports.

Adapted from AARC clinical practice guideline: resuscitation and defibrillation in the health care setting—2004 revision and update. *Respir Care.* 2004;49:1085–1099. Reprinted with permission.

wherever and whenever it is needed. In many situations, rapid response teams can prevent the patient's deterioration to the point where BLS or ACLS is not needed to resuscitate the patient.

Indications for CPR are cardiac arrest, respiratory arrest, or both. Cardiac arrest is usually secondary to ventricular fibrillation (VF) but may be the result of other arrhythmias (i.e., supraventricular tachycardia, ventricular tachycardia). Recognition of VF is particularly important because prompt defibrillation and return to a spontaneous perfusing rhythm greatly improves the success of CPR. Respiratory problems causing respiratory arrest include an obstructed airway (partial or complete), interference with the respiratory drive mechanism (spinal cord or head injury), and pulmonary disorders (COPD, pulmonary edema or pulmonary embolus), or gas transport (anemia, shock).

The Initial Steps

The initial step of cardiopulmonary resuscitation is a quick assessment of whether or not the patient truly needs to be resuscitated (**Algorithm 18-1**). The healthcare

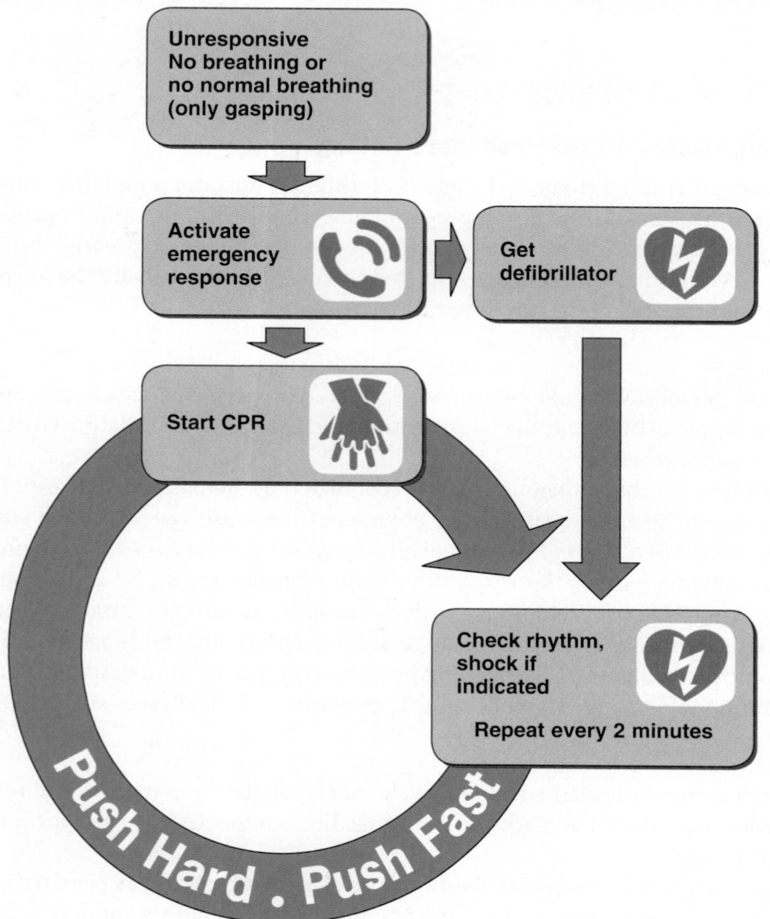

ALGORITHM 18-1 Simplified Basic Life Support Algorithm.

Reproduced from 2010 American Heart Association Guidelines for Cardiopulmonary Resuscitation and Emergency Cardiovascular Care. Part 5: Adult Basic Life Support. *Circulation.* 2010;122:S685–S705. © 2010 American Heart Association, Inc.

provider checks for responsiveness by tapping the patient and asking in a loud voice, "Are you all right?" If there is no response, he/she activates the emergency response system according to the guidelines of the institution. This is followed by quickly and safely placing the patient in a supine position on a hard surface and positioning yourself where you can do CPR by either standing or kneeling at the level of the patient's upper chest.

A respiratory arrest is considered to be present when the patient's respirations are completely absent or when there is evidence that they are clearly inadequate to maintain adequate ventilation or oxygenation, or both. The agonal gasps that may occur in the first few minutes after a cardiac arrest should not be interpreted as adequate breathing. A cardiac arrest is considered to be present when the pulse is absent or when it is insufficient to support perfusion of vital organs. Either of these situations requires quick and effective action by the rescuers.

CABD Sequence

Traditionally, opening the airway was the first step in providing CPR. In 2010, however, this changed from ABCD (airway, breathing, circulation, and defibrillation) to CABD (circulation, airway, breathing, and defibrillation).[11] The AHA Guidelines indicate that chest compressions are the foundation for CPR, and the AHA recommends that chest compressions are done before opening the airway and providing ventilation by following the **CABD sequence**. The rationale for initiation of CPR with chest compressions ensures that the victim receives this critical intervention early. Additionally, the 2010 Guidelines recognize the varying levels of rescuer proficiency by stressing the need for the untrained rescuer to provide hands-only (compressions-only) CPR, whereas healthcare providers incorporate rescue breathing, use of an AED, defibrillation if necessary, and coordinated teamwork[23] (**Box 18-2**). **Algorithm 18-2** represents the adult BLS healthcare

BOX 18-2

CABD: Circulation, Airway, Breathing, and Defibrillation

Primary CABD Sequence (Basic Life Support Sequence)

1. Check the patient for responsiveness and presence/absence of normal breathing or gasping.
2. Activate emergency response system and call for defibrillator.
3. Check pulse for no more than 10 seconds. If no pulse detected, start chest compressions.
4. **Compressions:** start 30 chest compressions at a depth of at least 2 inches and a rate of 100/min.
5. **Airway:** open airway.
6. **Breathing:** give two slow breaths.
7. Immediately resume chest compressions.
8. **Defibrillator:** attach automated external defibrillator (AED) when available and use if indicated.
9. Immediately resume chest compressions.

Secondary CABD Sequence (Advanced Cardiac Life Support Algorithm)

1. **Compressions:** Continue chest compressions immediately after defibrillation.
2. Initiate oxygen, IV, monitor, and fluids.
   - Monitor vital signs: temperature, blood pressure, heart rate, respirations.
3. **Airway:** Provide advanced airway as soon as possible.
   - If possible do not interrupt compressions if ventilation and oxygenation can be accomplished adequately with a bag/mask.
   - Confirm endotracheal tube placement; use two methods to confirm.
   - Do primary physical examination criteria *plus* secondary confirmation device (qualitative and quantitative measures of end-tidal CO_2).
   - Secure tracheal tube.
     - Prevent dislodgement; purpose-made tracheal tube holders are recommended over tie-and-tape approaches.
     - If the patient with suspected cervical injury requires transport or movement, a cervical collar and backboard are recommended.
4. **Breathing: After every 30 compressions, deliver two breaths sufficient to cause the chest to raise**
   - Confirm initial oxygenation and ventilation.
     - End-tidal CO_2 monitor.
     - Oxygen saturation monitor.
5. **Differential diagnosis**:
   - Search for a possible cause and treat appropriately.

Adapted from Adult basic life support. *Circulation.* 2010;102:1–22; and 2010 American Heart Association Guidelines for Cardiopulmonary Resuscitation and Emergency Cardiovascular Care. Part 5: Adult Basic Life Support. *Circulation.* 2010;122:S685–S705.

provider algorithm where the boxes bordered with dashed lines are steps performed by healthcare providers and not by lay rescuers.

Circulation

The presence of a heartbeat for an adult or child is determined by palpation of the carotid artery on the side of the neck nearest to the rescuer (**Figure 18-2**). The rescuer should take no more than 10 seconds to do this. If a pulse is not present, or if there is uncertainty, immediately administer 30 chest compressions.[24] According to the 2010 AHA Guidelines, chest compressions delivered to patients subsequently found not to be in cardiac arrest rarely lead to significant injury.[25] If the patient is on a soft surface, a firm surface should be placed under the patient. Compressions should not be withheld while waiting for a firm surface, however. When possible, safely and quickly move a sitting patient to a flat hard surface before beginning compressions.

Chest compressions are the rhythmic application of pressure on the lower half of the sternum to facilitate blood flow by compressing the heart. When performed properly they produce a low arterial blood flow, which delivers critically needed oxygen to the brain and

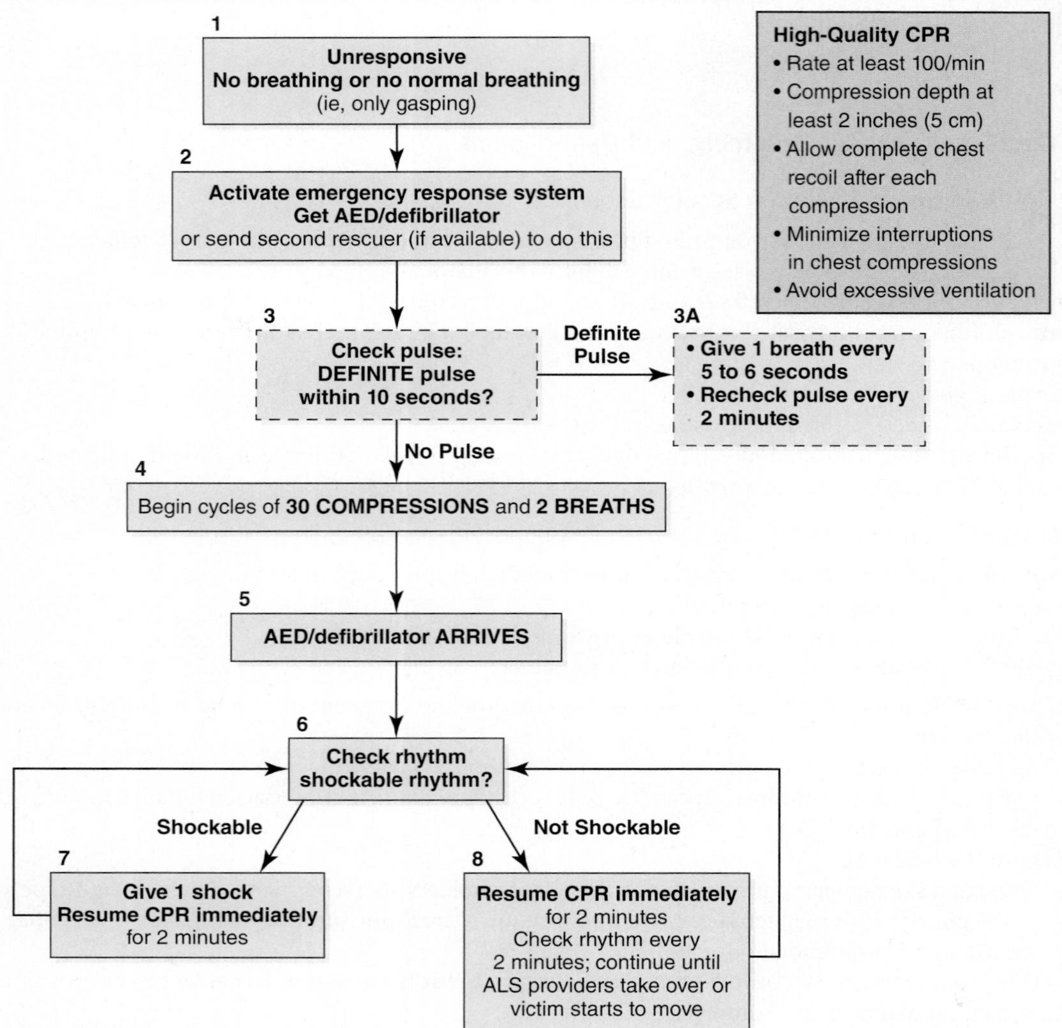
1
Unresponsive
No breathing or no normal breathing
(ie, only gasping)
2
Activate emergency response system
Get AED/defibrillator
or send second rescuer (if available) to do this
High-Quality CPR
• Rate at least 100/min
• Compression depth at least 2 inches (5 cm)
• Allow complete chest recoil after each compression
• Minimize interruptions in chest compressions
• Avoid excessive ventilation
3
Check pulse:
DEFINITE pulse
within 10 seconds?
Definite Pulse
3A
• Give 1 breath every 5 to 6 seconds
• Recheck pulse every 2 minutes
No Pulse
4
Begin cycles of 30 COMPRESSIONS and 2 BREATHS
5
AED/defibrillator ARRIVES
6
Check rhythm
shockable rhythm?
Shockable
Not Shockable
7
Give 1 shock
Resume CPR immediately
for 2 minutes
8
Resume CPR immediately
for 2 minutes
Check rhythm every
2 minutes; continue until
ALS providers take over or
victim starts to move
Note: The boxes bordered with dashed lines are performed
by healthcare providers and not by lay rescuers

ALGORITHM 18-2 BLS Healthcare Provider.

Reproduced from 2010 American Heart Association Guidelines for Cardiopulmonary Resuscitation and Emergency Cardiovascular Care. Part 5: Adult Basic Life Support. *Circulation.* 2010;122:S685–S705. © 2010 American Heart Association, Inc.

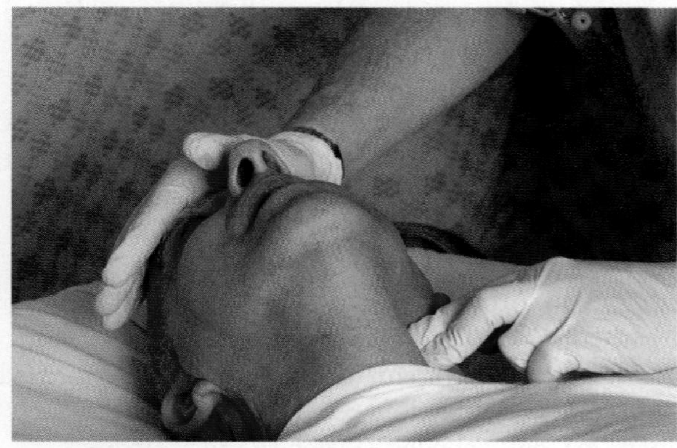

FIGURE 18-2 Carotid pulse check.

© Jones & Bartlett Learning. Courtesy of MIEMSS.

myocardium. Recently, several studies have reported that healthcare providers did not provide a sufficient number or an adequate depth of compressions. These same studies reported that ventilation was frequently excessive after the patient's airway was secured. The combination of inadequate compressions, interruptions in compressions for ventilation, and excessive ventilation rates resulted in lower than expected blood flow to vital organs.[26–28] Due to the importance of chest compressions, lay rescuers are encouraged to perform compressions-only CPR.

The 2005 and 2010 Consensus Conferences promulgated the following guidelines regarding chest compressions.[18,19] External chest compressions are

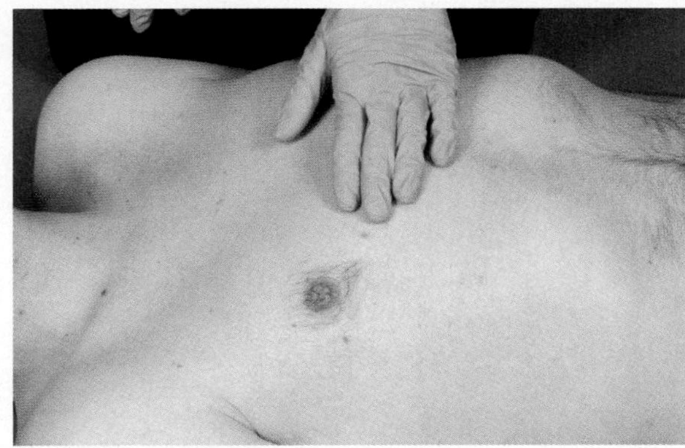

FIGURE 18-3 Identifying proper hand position for chest compressions. Chest compressions are performed on the lower half of the sternum, above the notch where the ribs meet the lower sternum or between the nipples.

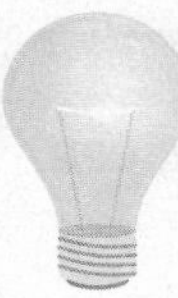

STOP AND THINK

Comment on performance of CPR in the ocean, in a telephone booth, on a trampoline.

performed on the lower half of the adult sternum, above the notch where the ribs meet the lower sternum or between the nipples (**Figure 18-3**). The heel of the first hand is placed on the lower half of the sternum, with the second hand on top of the hand on the sternum. The fingers are extended or interlaced to keep them up and off the chest. The rescuer's arms are kept straight, with the elbows locked and the shoulders of the rescuer directly over the patient's sternum. Pressure is exerted downward to depress the sternum at least 2 inches (5 cm) at a rate of at least 100 per minute (**Figure 18-4**). The rescuer's hands should not be removed from the chest between compressions (during relaxation of the heart and recoil of the chest).

Compression of the xiphoid process can cause laceration of the liver, which causes severe internal bleeding. Rib fractures and costochondral separation can occur if the rescuer's hand placement deviates from midline or if pressure is placed on the rib cage with the fingers during compressions. The broken ends of a rib can in turn cause lacerations of the lungs. Elderly patients, patients on chronic steroids, or patients with calcium deficiencies are the most susceptible to these injuries. If cracking of the ribs is felt or heard, the rescuer doing compressions should check his or her hand position, make corrections if necessary, and continue to compress as quickly as possible.

Another complication of closed chest compression is the formation of fat emboli, which may occur without

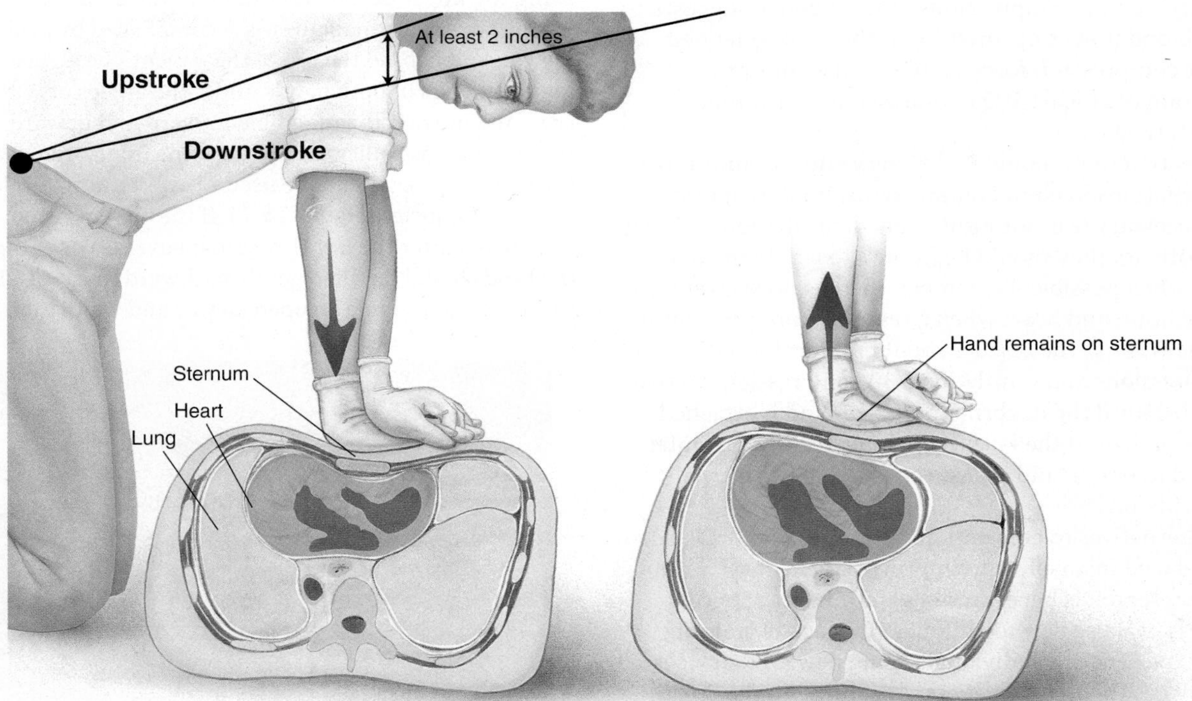

FIGURE 18-4 Body position for chest compressions. The hands remain on the sternum but allow complete chest recoil between compressions.

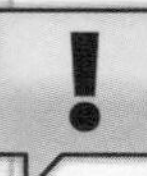

Respiratory Recap

Primary Circulation Management During CPR

- Press hard and fast
- Compress over the lower half of the sternum
- Remove weight from chest after each compression allowing for recoil and the heart to refill
- Do not interrupt chest compression
- Use a compression-to-ventilation ratio of 30:2
- Defibrillate as soon as possible if indicated

evidence of overt fractures. Compressing bones such as the rib cage and sternum may lead to microfractures within the medulla of the ribs and sternum and an increase in marrow pressure. Fat may enter the venous circulation from the marrow. Cerebral fat emboli can cause mental deterioration after successful resuscitation of a patient who has suffered an arrest.[28]

When doing chest compressions at a rate of at least 100 per minute, it is important to press hard and fast and then to quickly take the weight off your arms after each compression. This relieves the pressure on the chest wall, allowing it to recoil and the heart to refill with blood before the next compression.[29–31] Chest compression and chest recoil/relaxation times should be almost equal.[30] The effectiveness of chest compressions should be evaluated by a second person who palpates the carotid or femoral arteries for a pulse during compressions. The evidence suggests that blood flow is optimal when the recommended chest compression force is used and a compression rate of at least 100 compressions per minute is maintained.

Resuscitators should make every effort to minimize interruptions in chest compressions. If interruptions are necessary (e.g., for intubation, defibrillation, moving the patient), they should be limited to less than 10 seconds when possible. Remember, there is no blood flow to the brain and heart when a rescuer is not performing compressions. The rescuer should perform five cycles of compressions and ventilations (30 compressions to two breaths) until the defibrillator arrives and is attached to the patient. If the rescuer is alone, CPR can be interrupted to obtain and attach the automated external defibrillator.

Alternatives to conventional compressions have been introduced in an effort to improve patient survival, but more research is necessary to determine the successfulness of these new techniques. The lack of training and experience by individuals using new CPR devices influences their effectiveness. According to the 2010 Guidelines, no adjunct or devices other than a defibrillator have consistently proven to improve long-term survival from out-of-hospital cardiac arrest.[23]

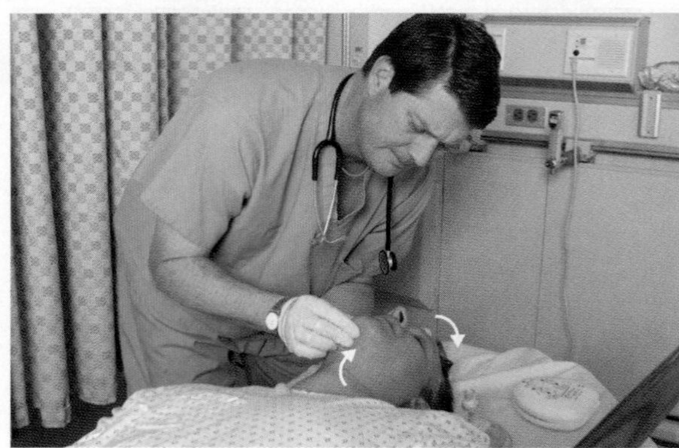

FIGURE 18-5 Opening the airway using the head tilt–chin lift method.

Airway

Opening the airway can be done using one of two methods—the head tilt–chin lift maneuver or the jaw-thrust maneuver—depending on whether there is a possibility of a cervical spine injury. It is estimated that approximately 2% of all victims of blunt trauma have a spinal cord injury; this risk increases threefold if the patient has a craniofacial injury.[32]

The head tilt–chin lift method is performed by standing to the side of the patient and placing the palm of one hand on the patient's forehead and the fingers of the other hand under the bony part of the lower jaw near the chin. The head is then tilted backward using the palm of one hand while the chin is lifted forward using the finger of the other hand (**Figure 18-5**).

The jaw-thrust maneuver is accomplished by positioning yourself behind the top of the patient's head, placing the fingers of both hands under the angles of both jaws, and moving the mandible forward and upward. If there is a possibility of cervical spine injury, the jaw-thrust maneuver should be used to avoid the possibility of further injuries (**Figure 18-6**). If the airway remains obstructed after the jaw-thrust maneuver is performed, the head should be tilted gently backward until the airway opens to provide an open airway and ventilation.

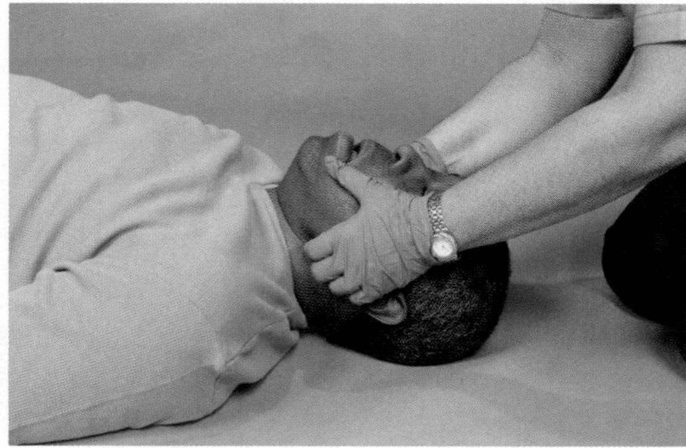

FIGURE 18-6 Jaw-thrust maneuver.

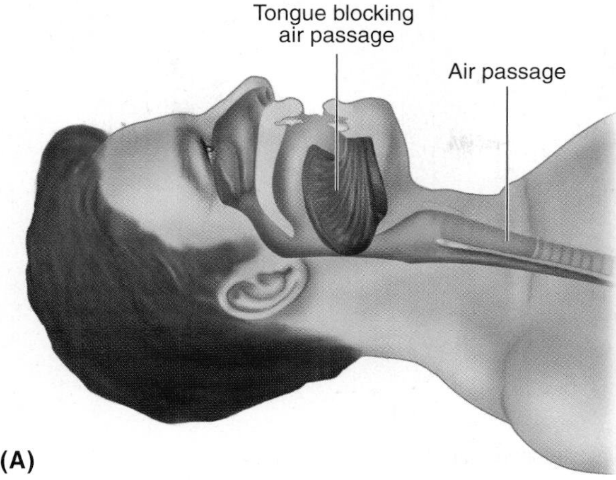

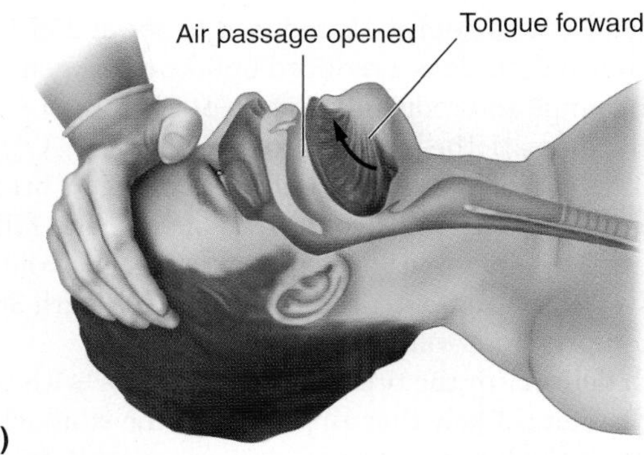

FIGURE 18-7 (**A**) Obstruction of upper airway by the tongue in an unconscious patient. (**B**) Opening the airway by tilting the head backward.

Posterior displacement of the tongue is the most common cause of airway obstruction in the unconscious person (**Figure 18-7**). Loss of control of the submandibular muscles allows the tongue to drop and obstruct the oropharynx. Because the tongue is attached to the lower jaw, movement of the jaw forward using either maneuver moves the tongue up and away from the posterior pharynx, which facilitates opening of the airway. Because positioning of the head can block the airway and prevent adequate breathing, in some patients opening the airway may allow the patient to resume sufficient breathing without the rescuer having to take further actions. Once the mouth is open, the upper airway can be inspected for foreign objects, vomit, or blood. If foreign objects are seen, they should be removed using a finger sweep or by suctioning, being careful not to push the object further into the airway.

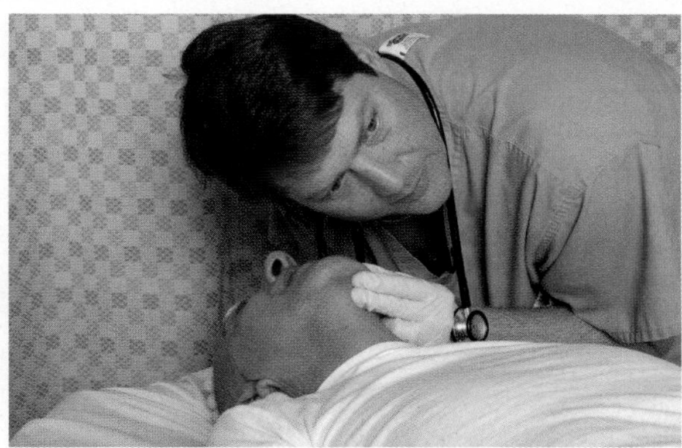

FIGURE 18-8 Opening the airway and checking for apnea.

Breathing

Traditionally, the "look, listen, and feel" technique had been taught to assess whether the patient is breathing. It entailed placing your ear over the patient's mouth and nose, listening for air movement, and looking for chest wall movement. While it is illustrated in **Figure 18-8**, a major change was made to the 2010 CPR Guidelines in which the "look, listen, and feel" technique was removed from the algorithm. Instead quick observations are used, and if the patient is breathing, he or she is placed in the recovery position and the rescuer continues to monitor (**Figure 18-9**).

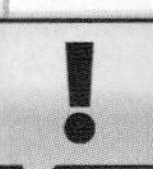

Respiratory Recap

Primary Airway Management During CPR

- Posterior displacement of tongue obstructs airway.
- Use head tilt–chin lift maneuver to open airway.
- Use jaw-thrust maneuver with spinal injury.
- Clean foreign objects from airway.

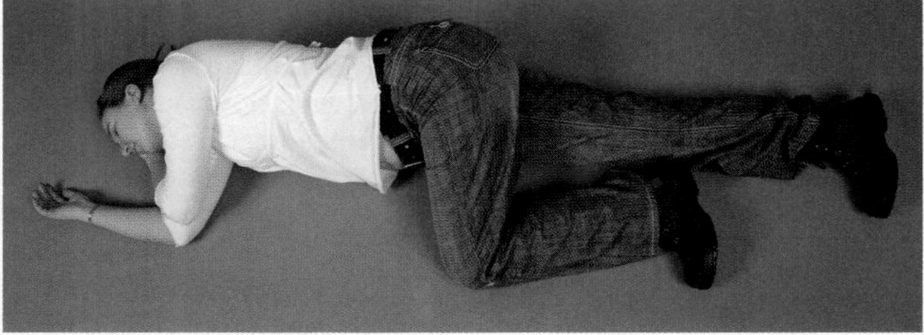

FIGURE 18-9 Recovery position.

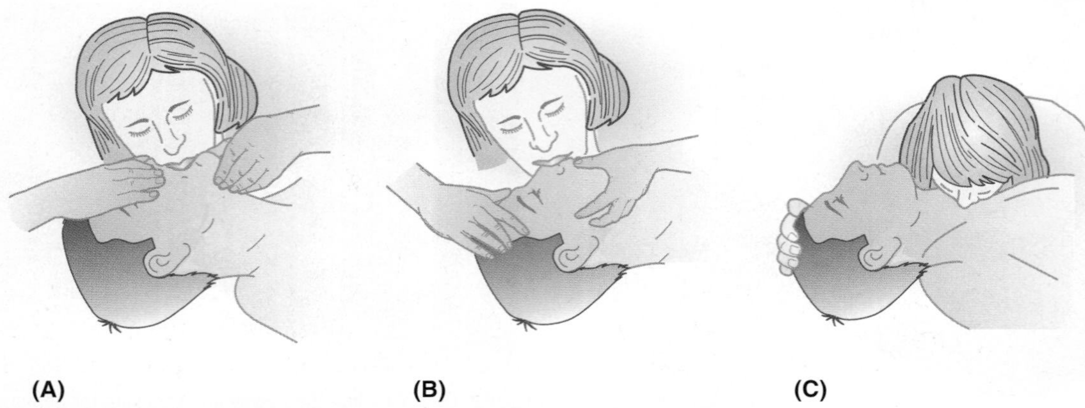

FIGURE 18-10 (A) Mouth-to-mouth ventilation. (B) Mouth-to-nose ventilation. (C) Mouth-to-stoma ventilation.

After 30 chest compressions and opening the airway, emergency ventilation should be provided for the patient with agonal breathing or apnea. Provide two breaths lasting no more than 1 second each, using the mouth-to-mouth, mouth-to-mask, mouth-to-stoma, or bag-to-mask method, to deliver enough air to cause a rise of the patient's chest (**Figure 18-10** and **Figure 18-11**). If the first breath does not achieve chest rise, reposition the airway and attempt to deliver a second breath. Usually tidal volumes of 6 to 7 mL/kg are sufficient for normal oxygenation and ventilation during CPR.[33]

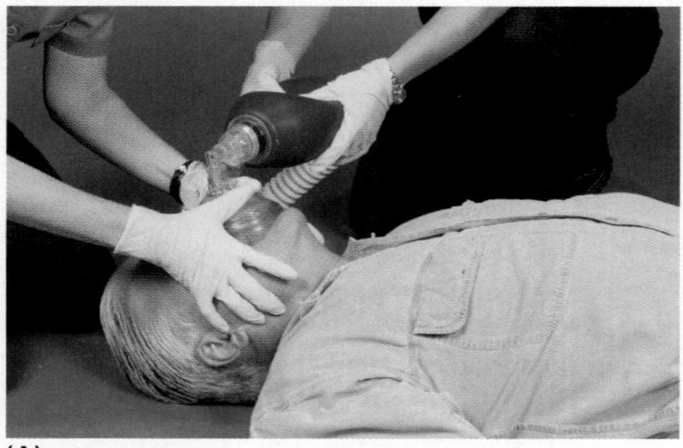

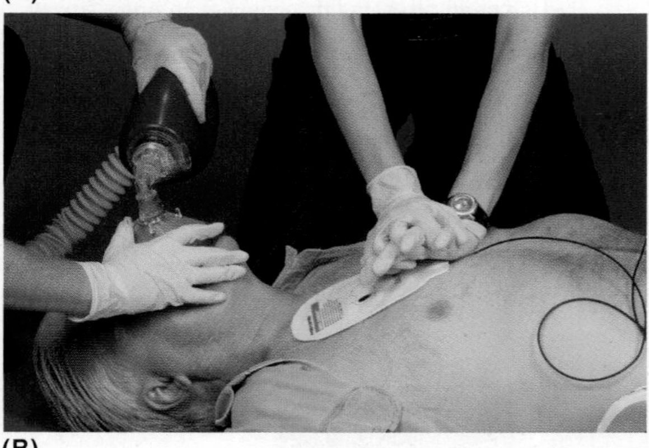

FIGURE 18-11 (A) Two-person bag-mask ventilation. (B) One-person bag-mask ventilation.

Because cardiac output is reduced to about 25% to 33% of normal, there is a reduced uptake of oxygen from the lungs and reduced delivery of carbon dioxide to the lungs.[34] The emphasis of the 2005 AHA Guidelines is that the volume delivered during a breath should be just enough to produce visible rise and fall of the chest. The guidelines not only recommend avoiding excessive ventilation but also beginning CPR with 30 chest compressions followed by 2 ventilations.

With delivery of the breaths too quickly or with too much force, it is likely that air will enter the stomach rather than the lungs and cause gastric inflation to occur.[21] Gastric inflation is the result of a breath that is too large, resulting in an airway pressure that exceeds the esophageal opening pressure and allowing air to enter the stomach. This can result in serious complications such as vomiting, aspiration, and the later development of pneumonia.

Mouth-to-mouth breathing is done by the rescuer holding the patient's mouth open with one hand, pinching the nose with the other hand, taking in a breath, placing his or her mouth over the patient's mouth to make a seal, and blowing air directly into the patient's mouth to cause a chest rise.[34]

When necessary, the rescuer can modify the delivery of breaths by doing mouth-to-nose or mouth-to-stoma breaths. Mouth-to-nose ventilation is necessary when it becomes impossible to ventilate through the patient's mouth in situations in which the mouth cannot be sealed or opened or the mouth is injured. To perform mouth-to-nose ventilation, the mouth is closed with the hand that normally maintains the jaw thrust; then the rescuer makes a seal with his or her mouth over the patient's nose and blows air into the nose while watching for a chest rise. In patients with a tracheal stoma, mouth-to-stoma ventilation is provided using a seal made over the stoma to inflate the lungs. With mouth-to-mouth, mouth-to-nose, or mouth-to-stoma ventilation, after the delivery of a breath, the rescuer quickly removes his or her mouth from the patient's airway to allow the patient to exhale and the rescuer to

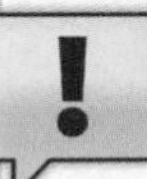

Respiratory Recap

Primary Breathing Management During CPR

- Mouth to mouth, mouth to nose, mouth to stoma
- Face shield
- Mouth to mask
- Bag-valve-mask ventilation
- Tidal volume 6 to 7 mL/kg
- Slow inflation

inhale another breath. The most common cause of difficulty providing ventilation for an apneic patient is an improperly opened or an occluded airway.

The risk of infection from CPR is very low, but the Occupational Safety and Health Administration (OSHA) requires that all healthcare workers use standard precautions in the workplace anytime there is exposure to blood or bodily fluids (e.g., saliva). These standard precautions include using barrier devices such as a face shield, face mask, or a bag-mask device (**Figure 18-12**). **Face shields** are clear plastic sheets that reduce direct contact between the patient and the rescuer. They do not prevent contamination of the rescuer if used incorrectly and may increase the resistance to flow. The rescuer should use face mask or bag-mask ventilation as soon as possible.

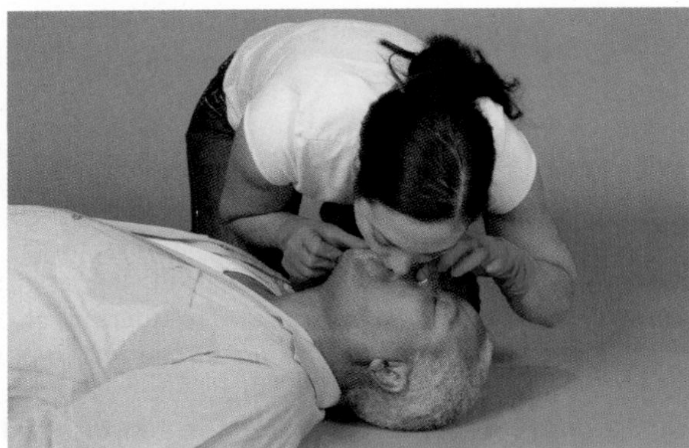

(A)

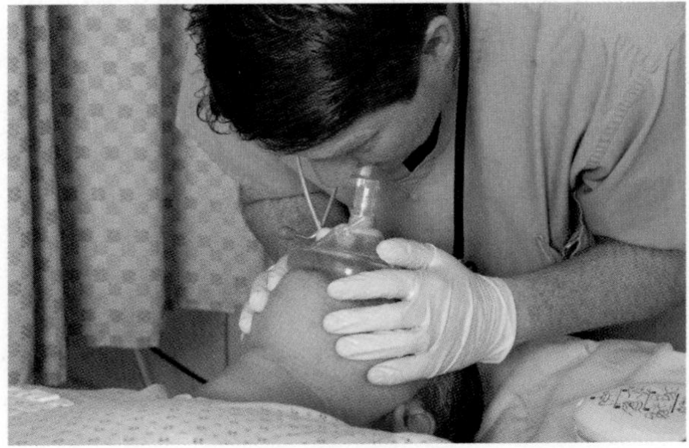

(B)

FIGURE 18-12 Barrier devices. **(A)** Face shield with duckbill valve. **(B)** Mouth-to-mask ventilation device.

Mouth-to-mask devices are very effective for delivering adequate ventilation. These masks have a one-way valve that diverts the patient's exhaled air away from the rescuer's face. Some of these masks have an oxygen inlet that allows the use of supplemental oxygen. To use the mask, the rescuer is positioned at the patient's head and to the side, the airway is opened, and the mask is placed over the patient's nose and mouth using the bridge of the patient's nose as a guide. The mask is held in place using the thumbs and first fingers of each hand on top of the mask pressing firmly around the outside of the mask against the patient's face to create a seal, while the remaining fingers lift the jaw up and into the mask as the head is tilted back. The exhaled gas of the individual doing rescue breathing contains approximately 14% to 17% oxygen and 4% carbon dioxide. Mouth-to-mask or mouth-to-mouth breathing is a quick and effective way to provide sufficient oxygen to the patient for a short time until a manual resuscitator and mask can be provided.

Manual resuscitators (bag-mask devices) consist of a self-inflating bag, a nonjamming air intake valve, a nonrebreathing valve, an oxygen inlet nipple, and an oxygen reservoir (**Figure 18-13**). A variety of manufacturers produce disposable manual resuscitator bags capable of ventilating patients during CPR. They are designed so that one end of the nonrebreathing valve connects to the self-inflating bag and the other end is connected to the face mask. The masks should be made of a transparent material to allow the rescuer to detect whether the patient regurgitates into the mask. When the bag is compressed, the nonrebreathing valve directs gas from the bag through the mask and to the patient. When the bag is released, the exhaled gas is directed through the exhalation port, and at the same time the bag reinflates. During a cardiac arrest, it is important to administer the highest oxygen concentration possible. When oxygen is available, the flow device should provide a minimum oxygen flow rate of 10 to 12 L/min.

One rescuer providing manual ventilation by bag-valve-mask device may not provide adequate tidal volumes. This is improved when ventilation is performed by two persons simultaneously: one who opens the airway and holds the mask in place with two hands and one who squeezes the bag with two hands (see Figure 18-11). Both rescuers should watch for a rise and fall of the patient's chest.[30] Manual ventilation may be less effective when performed by a single operator with little training or experience than it would be in the hands of a skilled clinician (e.g., respiratory therapist, nurse anesthetist, anesthesiologist). It is difficult to deliver an adequate tidal volume that produces a sufficient rise of the chest with one hand compressing the bag and the other hand holding the airway open and creating a seal with the mask.

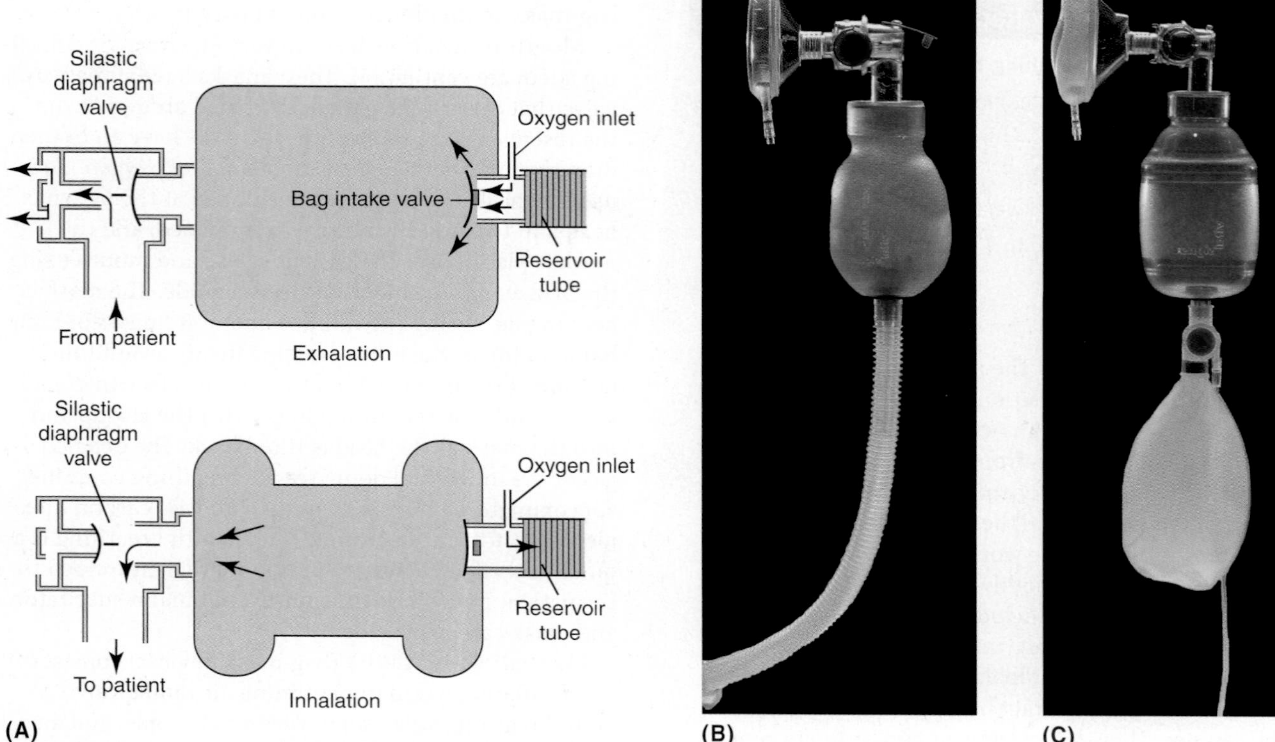

FIGURE 18-13 (**A**) Manual resuscitator with gas intake located at the bottom of the bag. (**B**) Manual resuscitator with tube reservoir. (**C**) Manual resuscitator with bag reservoir.

(**A**) this article was published in *Respiratory Therapy Equipment*. 4th ed. McPherson SP. Copyright Elsevier (Mosby) 1990; (**B**) and (**C**) © Vital Signs, Inc. Used with permission of GE Healthcare. All Rights Reserved.

The use of a bag-valve device to provide oxygen for a spontaneously breathing patient is discouraged because of the increased effort required to breathe through the nonrebreathing valve of a self-inflating manual resuscitator. In an adult patient with a depressed level of consciousness (i.e., with no cough or gag reflex), it is important to secure the airway as quickly as possible to prevent gastric contents from being regurgitated into the hypopharynx and then aspirated back into the trachea.

According to the 2010 AHA Guidelines, the Sellick maneuver (application of pressure to the cricoid cartilage) is no longer recommended and should not be routinely performed. In special circumstances, however, the Sellick maneuver may be useful as it aids in moving the glottis downward and improving visualization of the vocal cords during tracheal intubation (**Figure 18-14**).

Opening the patient's airway and delivering the two initial breaths should take between 5 and 10 seconds. According to the 2005 AHA Guidelines and supported in the 2010 AHA Guidelines, when adequate ventilation and chest rise can be accomplished using mouth-to-mask or bag-mask ventilation, early placement of an endotracheal tube is not as important as providing compressions for circulation when necessary.

Automated External Defibrillation

There is a strong relationship between the speed with which defibrillation current is administered and the survival of patients requiring defibrillation. The length of time from which a patient collapses to the time he or she is electrically defibrillated is one of the most important determinants of survival from cardiac arrest for the following reasons. When a patient has a witnessed sudden cardiac arrest, the most common initial rhythm is ventricular fibrillation (VF).[35] When the heart is in VF, it physically quivers and does not pump blood to

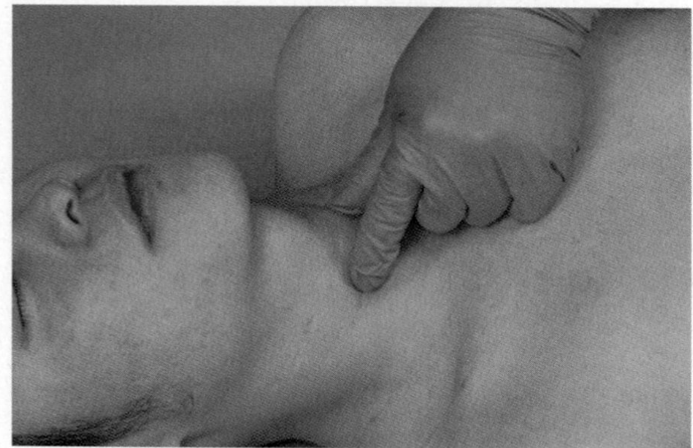

FIGURE 18-14 Sellick maneuver.

© Jones & Bartlett Learning. Courtesy of MIEMSS.

the other vital organs of the body. The most effective treatment for VF is to deliver an electrical shock to the heart (electrical defibrillation) to momentarily stop the heart and allow it to regain a more normal pacing. The electrical current is passed through the heart in an attempt to eliminate the chaotic asynchronous activity of the heart that causes the ventricular fibrillation. If the defibrillation is successful, the cardiac cells will depolarize and then repolarize in a uniform manner with the resumption of a more coordinated cardiac contraction. If VF is not treated quickly or the defibrillation is not successful, the heart's electrical rhythm quickly deteriorates to asystole.[35] Providing good CPR until electrical defibrillation can be done improves the patient's chances for survival from ventricular fibrillation and cardiac arrest.

The automated external defibrillator (AED) is a computerized device that is attached to a breathless, pulseless patient's chest with adhesive pads, and if the computer recognizes a heart rhythm that can be treated with defibrillation, it delivers an electrical shock to the patient's heart (**Figure 18-15**). The defibrillator then incorporates the rhythm recognition and analysis function with either fully automated or semiautomated shock delivery. When using the AED, it is useful to remember the mnemonic P-A-I-D:

- **P**ower on: The first step is to turn on the power. This will usually activate voice prompts for all subsequent steps. With some of the newer AEDs the power will automatically come on when the case or lid is opened.
- **A**ttach leads: The first voice prompt is to attach the leads. Choose the correct-size electrode pads (child or adult) for the patient and peel the protective backing from the pads. Quickly wipe the patient's chest if it is wet with water or sweat, attach one electrode pad to the patient's upper-right chest in the area to the right of the sternum and just below the collarbone, and attach the second electrode pad on the left of the nipple and just below the left armpit.
- **I**nterpret/analyze: The second voice prompt indicates the beginning of the analysis of the patient's cardiac rhythm. This instructs you to make sure no one is touching or moving the patient, allowing the AED's internal computer to analyze the patient's cardiac rhythm without the interference of chest compressions or ventilation by rescuers. The analysis process will usually take 5 to 15 seconds; afterward, the AED's third voice prompt will instruct you whether analysis of the patient's cardiac rhythm indicates that a shock is indicated.
- **D**efibrillate: If the AED advises that a shock is indicated, the next prompt will be for you to make sure the patient is "clear" to avoid injury to yourself and other rescuers. You should loudly state "clear" and visually check to ensure that others are not touching or manually bagging the patient before you press the Shock button. Immediately after the shock produces a sudden contraction of the patient's skeletal muscles, the rescuers should restart chest compressions.[18,35] After a period of 2 minutes (five sets of 30 compressions and two breaths), the AED should be used to reanalyze the patient to determine whether subsequent shocks are indicated.

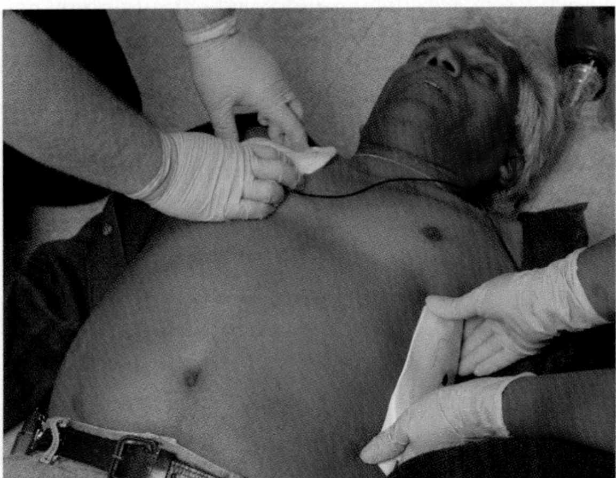

FIGURE 18-15 Pad placement for automated external defibrillation.

In the lone-rescuer situation, where only one person is present to do resuscitation, research has shown that doing CPR before obtaining the AED did not improve outcomes.[35,36] If two or more individuals are present, CPR should be performed by one individual while the other obtains and attached the AED.

Relief for a Choking Adult

Aspiration of a foreign body can cause mild, severe, or total airway obstruction, which results in a patient's inability to breathe and eventually in death if not quickly alleviated. This is an uncommon but preventable cause of death. The key to helping a choking adult patient is early recognition of airway obstruction and taking quick steps to correct the patient's situation. The signs and symptoms of choking include inability to breathe, poor or ineffective air exchange, a high-pitched sound while the patient is inhaling or the patient being unable to make any sounds or speak, possible cyanosis, and the universal sign of choking, in which patients use their own hands to clutch their neck (**Figure 18-16**).

If patients are choking, their own coughing is the most effective way for their airway to be cleared. So, if they are coughing, allow them to continue. If their coughing is weak or ineffective, however, the rescuer can assist the patient using the Heimlich maneuver (abdominal thrust) on adults and children. To successfully relieve an airway obstruction may require

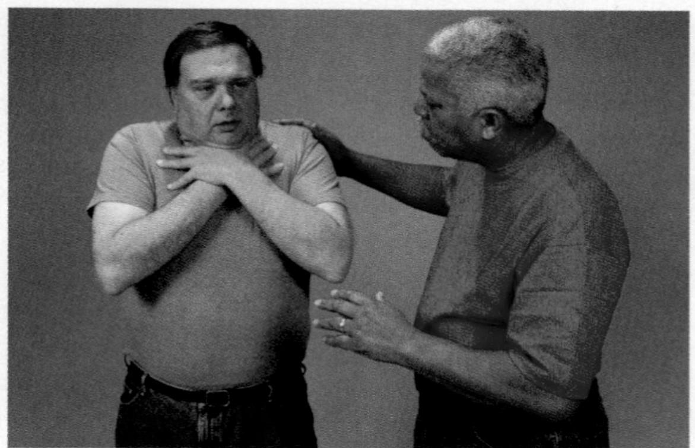

FIGURE 18-16 Universal choking sign.

the rescuer to repeat the Heimlich maneuver several times. Performing the abdominal thrust improperly or with too much force can result in damage to internal organs. It has been reported that approximately 50% of all choking episodes caused by airway obstruction were not relieved by a single abdominal thrust, and that the likelihood of success was increased when a combination of back blows, abdominal thrusts, and chest thrusts were used. It is important to assess for possible damage to the patient after any of these methods have been used to relieve the airway obstruction.

To perform the Heimlich maneuver, the rescuer should stand behind the adult patient and wrap his or her arms around the patient's waist, making a fist with one hand and placing the thumb side of the fist against the patient's middle abdomen slightly above the navel but well below the breastbone, then grasp the fist with the other hand and, using a quick upward thrust, press their fists into the patient's abdomen and quickly release the pressure (**Figure 18-17**). This is repeated until the object is expelled from the airway or the patient becomes unresponsive. The possibility that a cardiac arrest or unresponsiveness will be caused by an unsuspected foreign body airway obstruction is very low. If the patient's airway cannot be cleared and the patient becomes unconscious and unresponsive, however, the rescuer should support the patient to the ground and perform an abdominal thrust maneuver (**Figure 18-18**).

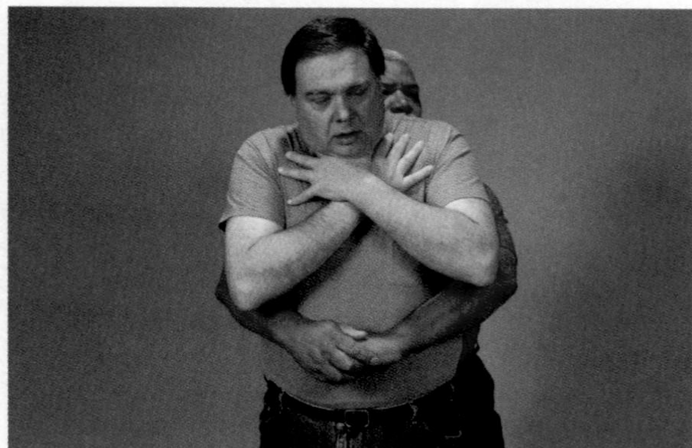

FIGURE 18-17 Heimlich maneuver.

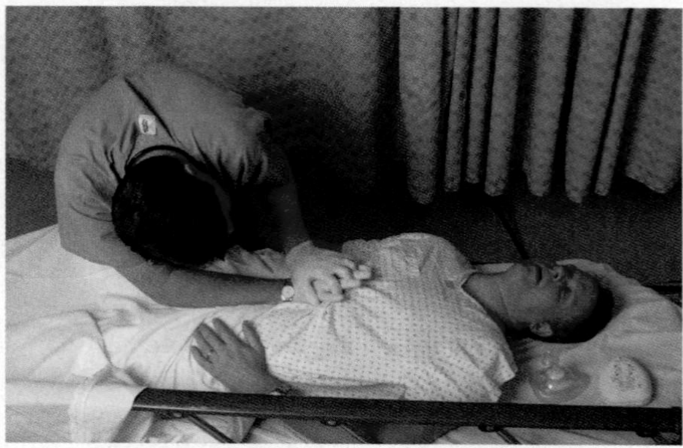

FIGURE 18-18 Abdominal thrust for foreign body airway obstruction.

If the patient becomes unresponsive or is found unresponsive, the rescuer should activate his or her emergency response system, open the airway, and if the obstruction is seen in the oropharynx, remove it and begin basic life support. Each time the rescuer provides a breath for the patient, the rescuer should open the patient's mouth, look to see whether the obstruction is now visible, and if possible remove it. Remember, if the airway is blocked, the breaths will not enter the lungs or cause a rise and fall of the chest. In the past, guidelines have recommended using a blind finger sweep for relieving airway obstructions. Case study reports have reported harm to the patient or rescuer with blind sweeps, so they are no longer done.

Difficult Bag-Mask Ventilation

The ability to safely manage a patient's airway is central to the role of the respiratory therapist. This includes airway opening maneuvers, placement of oropharyngeal and nasopharyngeal airways, the placement of advanced airways such as endotracheal tubes, laryngeal airway mask, Combitubes, and optimum bag-mask ventilation. The skill of bag-mask ventilation is the most fundamental and essential of airway management because it is used to preoxygenate/ventilate the patient prior to the placement of an advanced airway and it

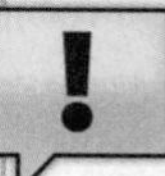

Respiratory Recap

Choking Adult

- Coughing is the most effective way to clear the airway.
- Heimlich maneuvers are used on adults and children.
- Do not perform blind sweeps of the airway.

is the necessary rescue skill used when attempts at advanced airway placement are unsuccessful.

Airway management is usually learned through some form of formal training, and then it is improved, refined, and retained with regular practice. Techniques such as keeping dentures in the patient's mouth and placing an oropharyngeal airway in patients with small chins to achieve a tight seal on patients with abnormal anatomy are simply learned through practice in the clinical setting. Several problems identified as predictors of difficult mask ventilation (DMV) are inability to create an adequate mask seal causing an excessive gas leak and excessive resistance to gas entering the airway.

DMV occurs when the individual using positive pressure mask ventilation cannot maintain the oxygen saturation >90% using 100% oxygen and positive pressure ventilation or prevent or reverse the signs of inadequate ventilation.[37] Other signs of inability to effectively ventilate with a mask include cyanosis, absence of exhaled CO_2, absence of adequate breath sounds, absence of chest movement, auscultatory signs of severe airway obstruction, gastric air entry, or dilation and hemodynamic changes associated with hypoxemia or hypercarbia (i.e., hypertension, tachycardia, arrhythmias).[37] These are life-threatening situations requiring rapid assessment and action by the respiratory therapist, and the ability to predict DMV is important for patient safety.

Research has identified several different patient physical factors that are significantly associated with DMV.[38,39] They include age older than 55 years, BMI more than 30, history of snoring, male gender, Mallampati Class III or IV, lack of teeth, and presence of a beard.[38,39] Difficult mask ventilation is also associated with upper and lower airway obstruction. In the upper airway the most common causes include a large tongue or a small pharyngeal space, tonsillar hyperplasia, excessive tissue in the oropharyngeal space or oropharyngeal collapse, trauma, morbid obesity, and neck or oral tumors. In the lower airway, tracheal, bronchial, and mediastinal tumors, severe bronchial spasms, noncompliant lungs, and bronchopleural fistula have also been associated with DMV. A mnemonic often used to predict potentially difficult bag mask ventilation is "MOANS," where "M" represents mask seal, male gender, or Mallampati Class III or IV, "O" represents obesity or obstruction, "A" represents age greater then 55, "N" indicates the patient has no teeth, and "S" represents a stiff lung or a patient that snores (**Box 18-3**).[39]

Common equipment problems associated with DMV include masks that do not seal properly because of improper size or a partially deflated mask cushion. The patient's inappropriate head and neck position or the need to place a properly sized oropharyngeal airway may also result in DMV. Patients with multiple

BOX 18-3

Difficult Bag-Mask Ventilation Mnemonic: MOANS

M – mask seal/male gender/Mallampati Class III or IV
O – obesity/obstruction
A – age >55 years
N – no teeth
S – stiff lung/snoring

indicators of DMV may require additional assistance and changing to two-person ventilation, possibly moving more quickly to placement of an advanced airway using fiberoptic intubation.

Cardiopulmonary Resuscitation for a Child

The major causes of pediatric cardiopulmonary arrest are often respiratory failure, sudden infant death syndrome (SIDS), sepsis, neurologic diseases, and trauma.[40] Attempts to prevent injury can reduce childhood death and disability, especially when prevention strategies are geared toward the six most common types of severe childhood injuries: motor vehicle passenger injuries, pedestrian injuries, bicycle injuries, submersion injuries, fire- and burn-related injuries, and firearm injuries. Even after 20 years of educational efforts to prevent such injuries, studies found that when compared with white children, American Indian/Alaska Native and African American children consistently have a higher rate of injury deaths. Hispanic children have comparable rates of injury-related deaths, and Asian/Pacific Islanders have a significantly lower rate of death than white children.[41]

When resuscitating a child, just as with an adult, the rescuer begins with a quick assessment for responsiveness. If the patient is found to be unresponsive, the rescuer should activate the emergency system, call for

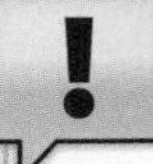

Respiratory Recap

Child CPR

- Begin CPR with pulse below 60 beats/min
- Compression-to-breath ratio of 30 compressions to two breaths for one rescuer and 15 compressions to two breaths for two rescuers
- Chest compressions at midsternum between the nipples
- Fast and hard compressions

AGE-SPECIFIC ANGLE

- Most cardiac arrests in children are *not* caused by ventricular arrhythmias.

AGE-SPECIFIC ANGLE

- The treatment for a child older than 1 year who is choking is similar to that for an adult.

an AED, and then check for breathing. If apneic, the next step is to perform 30 chest compressions, followed by two ventilations. The sequence should be CABD as the "look, listen, and feel for breathing" sequence was removed in the 2010 Guidelines.

The rescuer should then check for the pulse for less than 10 seconds (same as an adult), at the carotid or femoral arteries. In the 2010 Guidelines, however, there is deemphasis of the pulse check. Chest compressions are performed at midsternum between the nipples at a depth of one-third of the anterior-posterior diameter of the chest; about 2 inches (5 cm) in most children. The compression-to-breath ratio for a child is 30 compressions to two breaths if there is only one rescuer and 15 compression to two breaths if there are two rescuers.[23] When doing the compressions, the rescuer should push fast and hard, making sure that any interruptions, including those for the two breaths, are kept shorter than 10 seconds.

Most cardiac arrests in children are *not* caused by ventricular arrhythmias. The time necessary for using an AED (attaching the leads to the patients and analyzing the rhythm) delays or interrupts the vitally important rescue breathing and chest compressions.[42] If the child's arrest occurs outside of the hospital or is unwitnessed, the AED should be placed on the child after rescuers have completed five cycles of 15 compressions and two breaths, which should take about 2 minutes. If the child's arrest occurs inside a hospital or is witnessed, however, the AED should be placed on the child as soon as available and used appropriately for the child.

If the AED is designed for both adults and children, change to the appropriate adult or child shock dose. When the child is younger than 8 years, the rescuer should use electrode pads designated for children and select the appropriate child shock dose. If the child is older than 8 years, however, this shock may not be sufficient for the desired effect.[42] For children older than 8 years, the rescuer should use the adult shock dose and the adult electrode pads.[42] If a shock is indicated, immediately after the shock is delivered the rescuers should begin chest compressions for 2 minutes and then recheck for a pulse. The algorithm for pediatric BLS is depicted in **Algorithm 18-3**.

Relief for a Choking Child

The most common causes of a child choking are balloons, small objects, and food such as hot dogs, round candies, nuts, and grapes.[43] The treatment for a child older than 1 year who is choking is similar to that for an adult. While evaluating the child, the rescuers should try to determine whether the obstruction is mild or severe.

The signs of mild **foreign body obstruction (FBO)** include a sudden onset of respiratory distress associated with coughing, stridor, or unilateral wheezing. When possible, the rescuer should allow the child to clear his or her own airway by coughing. The patient with severe obstruction may not be able to cough or make sounds, however. In this situation it is imperative that rescuers be able to recognize the difference and be prepared to intervene if necessary. Subdiaphragmatic abdominal thrusts (Heimlich maneuvers) are recommended for relief of airway obstruction in children. The sequence of intervention used to treat a child with an obstructed airway is similar to that for an adult.[44] When abdominal thrusts are delivered to a child who is unconscious or who becomes unconscious, the heel of one hand is used rather than a two-handed fist.

The exception to use of the Heimlich maneuver is a situation in which the rescuer is alone and the child becomes unresponsive. If this should occur, the rescuer should open the airway and remove the object if it is seen. If the object cannot be removed from the airway, or if the child does not start breathing after the object has been removed, the rescuer should begin basic life support. He or she should then do five cycles of compressions and breaths and activate the emergency response system if the rescuer has not already done so.

Cardiopulmonary Resuscitation for an Infant

According to the AHA, the term *infant* refers to neonatal patients from the time they leave the delivery room until they are 12 months old. The term *newly born* applies specifically to an infant at the time of birth undergoing intrauterine to extrauterine transition. Approximately 10% of newly borns require some assistance to begin breathing at birth and a rapid assessment entailing 3 questions is generally performed.[45] The three questions assess whether the *newly born* infant: (1) is of gestational term, (2) is crying or breathing, and (3) has good muscle tone. If the answer is "Yes," then no resuscitation is needed. If the answer to any of these queries is "no," the infant should receive one or more of the following four categories of actions: initial steps in stabilization, ventilation, chest compression, and/or administration of epinephrine or volume expanders. **Algorithm 18-4** provides the unique steps in the resuscitation of the newly born. General measures for the resuscitation of infants not considered newly born follow.

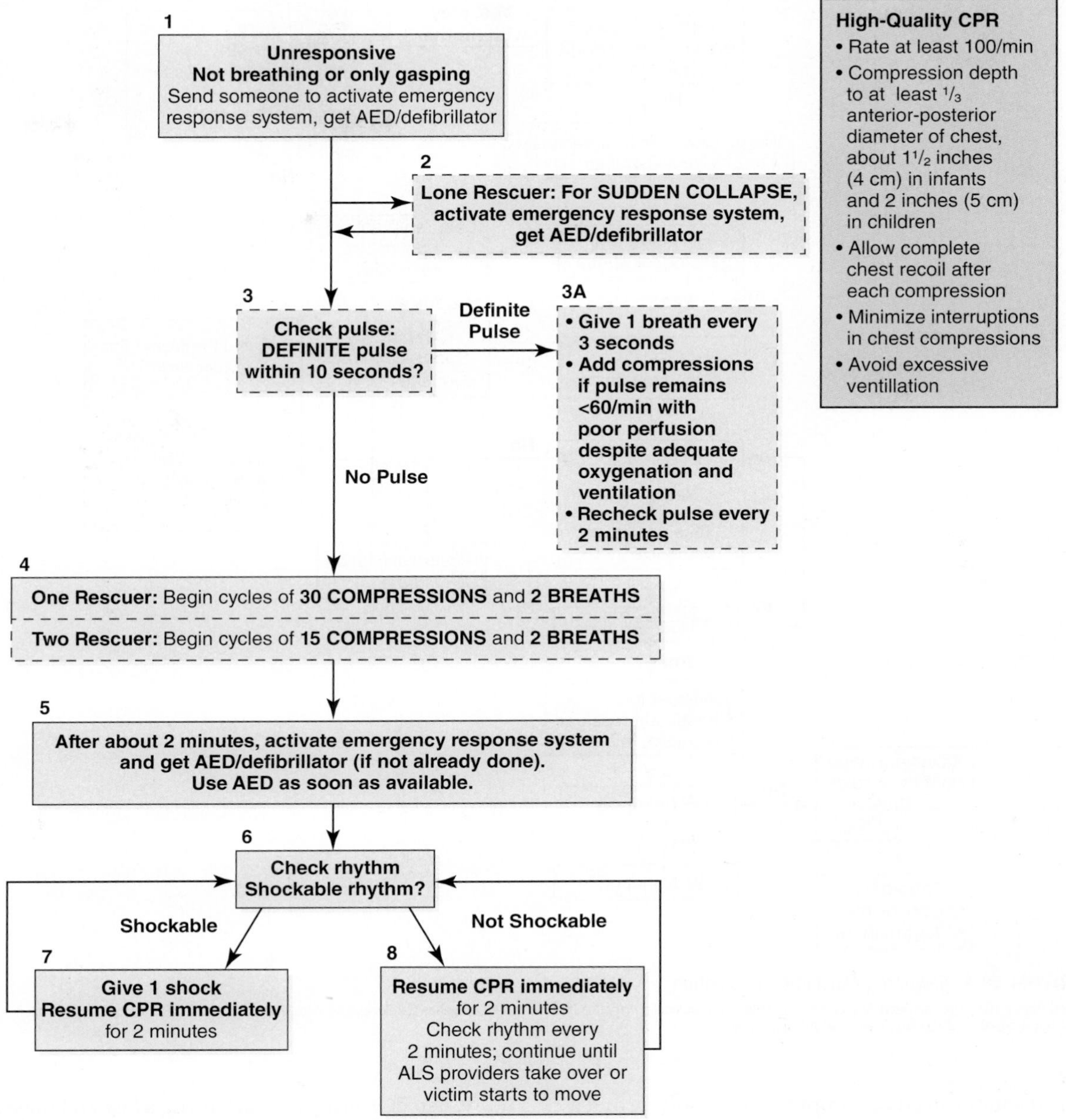

1
Unresponsive
Not breathing or only gasping
Send someone to activate emergency response system, get AED/defibrillator
2
Lone Rescuer: For SUDDEN COLLAPSE, activate emergency response system, get AED/defibrillator
3
Check pulse: DEFINITE pulse within 10 seconds?
Definite Pulse
3A
• Give 1 breath every 3 seconds
• Add compressions if pulse remains <60/min with poor perfusion despite adequate oxygenation and ventilation
• Recheck pulse every 2 minutes
No Pulse
4
One Rescuer: Begin cycles of 30 COMPRESSIONS and 2 BREATHS
Two Rescuer: Begin cycles of 15 COMPRESSIONS and 2 BREATHS
5
After about 2 minutes, activate emergency response system and get AED/defibrillator (if not already done). Use AED as soon as available.
6
Check rhythm
Shockable rhythm?
Shockable
Not Shockable
7
Give 1 shock
Resume CPR immediately for 2 minutes
8
Resume CPR immediately for 2 minutes
Check rhythm every 2 minutes; continue until ALS providers take over or victim starts to move
High-Quality CPR
• Rate at least 100/min
• Compression depth to at least 1/3 anterior-posterior diameter of chest, about 1 1/2 inches (4 cm) in infants and 2 inches (5 cm) in children
• Allow complete chest recoil after each compression
• Minimize interruptions in chest compressions
• Avoid excessive ventillation
Note: The boxes bordered with dashed lines are performed by healthcare providers and not by lay rescuers

ALGORITHM 18-3 Pediatric BLS Algorithm.

Infants and children who develop cardiac arrest usually do so secondary to pulmonary disease or pulmonary arrest. As with the adult or child, first determine whether the infant needs resuscitation, and then activate the emergency response system and place the patient on a firm, flat surface. The next step is to perform 30 chest compressions. The sequence should be compressions–airway–breathing. ("Look, listen, and feel for breathing" was removed in the 2010 Guidelines.) Then open the infant's airway using the head tilt–chin lift method, being careful not to press the fingers too deeply into the soft tissue underneath the infant's chin. The most common structure causing airway obstruction for an infant is the tongue, which becomes flaccid and falls backward into the throat. Improper opening of the infant's airway by a rescuer is the most common cause of inadequate ventilation during resuscitation. If the rescuer tilts the infant's head back more than what would resemble a neutral or sniffing position, the infant's airway may become blocked. The rescuer may need to reposition the head several times using the head tilt–chin lift maneuver to deliver two effective breaths.

A bag-mask device or a T-piece resuscitator (Neopuff) can be used to give rescue breaths to an infant.

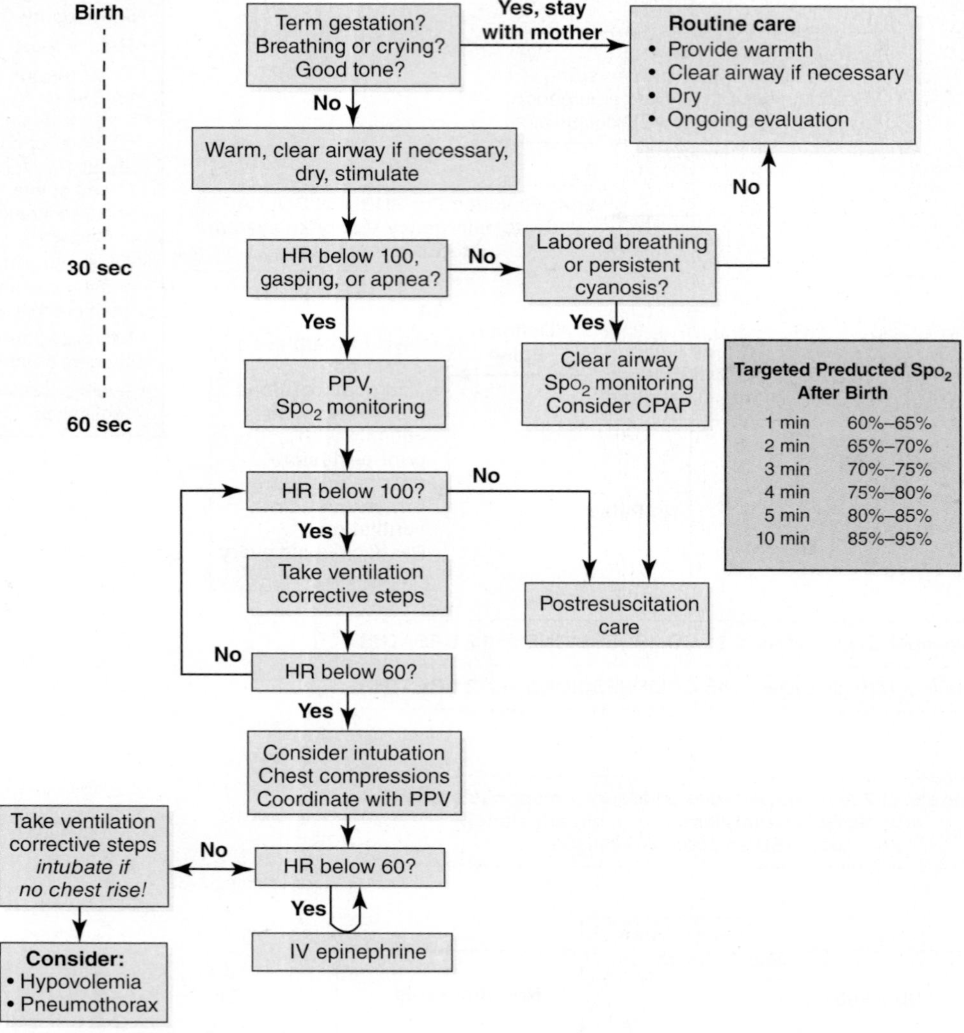

ALGORITHM 18-4 Newborn Resuscitation Algorithm.

Reproduced from 2010 American Heart Association Guidelines for Cardiopulmonary Resuscitation and Emergency Cardiovascular Care. Part 15: Neonatal Resuscitation. *Circulation.* 2010;122:S909–S919. © 2010 American Heart Association, Inc.

This resuscitator needs a compressed gas source and a tight face mask seal (**Figure 18-19**). Only trained clinical professionals should use the T-piece resuscitator because it is a flow-controlled, pressure-limited manual ventilator.[46] The T-piece resuscitator has six parts: gas inlet, gas outlet, inspiratory pressure control, patient T-piece with positive end-expiratory pressure (PEEP) cap, circuit pressure gauge, and maximum pressure-relief control.[47] Advantages of the T-piece resuscitator include its ability to deliver a consistent pressure and a reliable concentration of 100% oxygen, with no fatigue for rescuers from bagging. Some disadvantages include the need for a readily available compressed gas source, the need for a tight face seal, the time necessary for the rescuers to set pressure prior to use, and the time necessary for changing pressures while the resuscitator is in use. Whenever the T-piece resuscitator is being used, rescuers should make sure a backup self-inflating bag is available.

When delivering a breath using a bag and mask, it is important that the rescuer take the time to choose the appropriate-sized bag and mask. The face mask should be able to cover the patient's mouth and nose completely

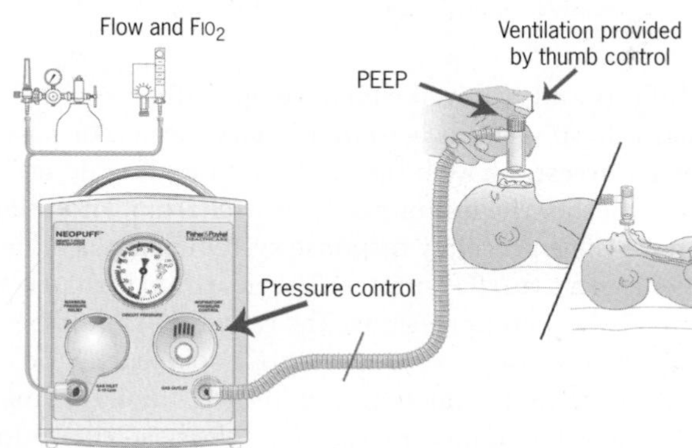

FIGURE 18-19 Neopuff for neonatal resuscitation.

Courtesy of Fisher & Paykel Healthcare.

without covering the eyes or without extending beyond the infant's chin. The patient's airways should be opened using the head tilt–chin lift maneuver, the mask pressed against the face, making sure to protect the eyes, and the jaw lifted to create a seal. The mask should not be pressed down onto the infant's face to create the seal.

The rescuer should check for the brachial pulse by placing his or her index and middle fingers on the inside of the infant's upper arm (**Figure 18-20**). The size of the neck in an infant younger than 1 year makes palpation of the carotid artery very difficult. In the 2010 Guidelines, however, there is deemphasis of the pulse check. The infant is considered to be in a cardiac arrest if the infant's heart rate is absent or less than 60 beats/min and the infant shows signs of poor perfusion (i.e., cyanosis, pallor) despite oxygenation and ventilation.[23]

The rescuer should perform compressions by placing the tips of two fingers between the nipple line and compressing approximately one-third of the anterior-posterior diameter of the chest.[48] An alternative to the two-finger compression technique is the two-thumb compression technique, in which the rescuer encircles the infant's chest with both hands and compresses the chest using his or her thumbs (**Figure 18-21**). The compression-to-breath ratio for an infant is 30 compressions to two breaths if there is only one rescuer and 15 compressions to two breaths if there are two rescuers. It is important for rescuers to keep the tips of the fingers on the infant's chest after compressions and to make sure they release the pressure on the sternum to allow for chest recoil. There is no recommendation for use of an AED for an infant younger than 1 year.[42]

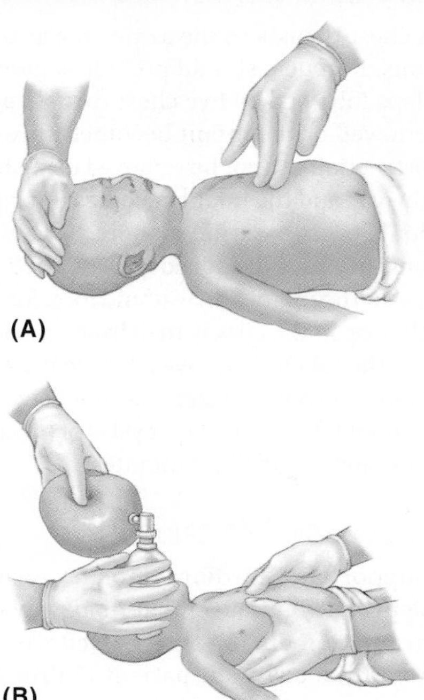

FIGURE 18-21 (**A**) Two-finger chest compressions. (**B**) Two-thumb chest compressions.

Relief for a Choking Infant

Liquids are the most common cause of an infant choking.[44] The abdominal thrusts used on an adult and child are not used on a choking infant; instead, rescuers use a series of back slaps and chest thrusts (**Figure 18-22**). If the infant is responsive, the rescuer should kneel or sit with the infant in his or her lap and then place the infant in a prone position with the head slightly lower than the chest resting on the rescuer's forearm and hand, while being careful not to compress the soft tissues of the infant's throat. The rescuer should provide five forceful back blows using the heel of his or her hand to the middle of the infant's back in the area located between the infant's shoulder blades. If this does not dislodge the obstruction, the rescuer should place his or her free hand under the infant's back and neck, using the palm to support the head, and turn the infant onto his or her back, keeping the head slightly lower than the trunk, and then provide five quick

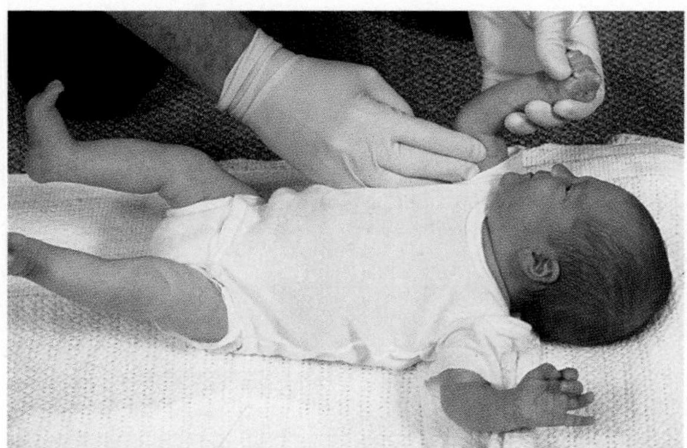

FIGURE 18-20 Brachial pulse check.

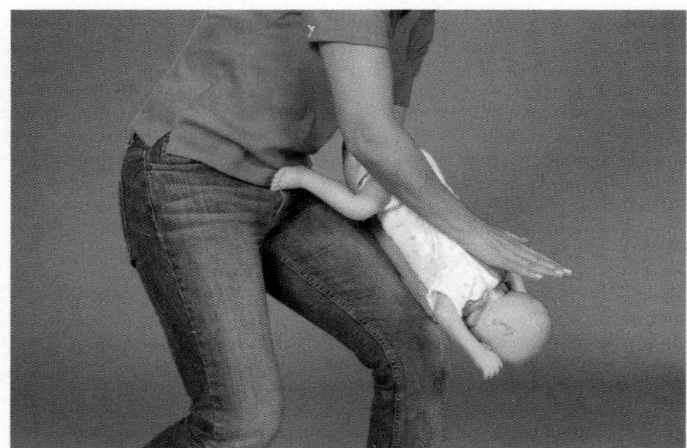

FIGURE 18-22 Back blows in infant foreign body obstruction.

downward chest thrusts to the same area as used for compressions. Rescuers should provide sequences of five back slaps followed by five chest thrusts until the object is removed or the infant becomes unresponsive.

If the obstruction cannot be removed using back blows and chest thrusts and the infant becomes unresponsive, rescuers should begin basic life support. Because the chest compressions may have dislodged the obstruction, rescuers should open the infant's airway and look for the object each time they open the airway to deliver a breath. If they see an object, they should remove it before breath delivery. If the emergency response system has not been activated, the rescuer should do so after five cycles of breaths to compressions (approximately 2 minutes).

Summary of Basic Life Support

Basic life support and cardiopulmonary resuscitation include the primary management of airway, breathing, and circulation during the resuscitative effort for an adult, child, or infant patient (**Table 18-1**). Respiratory therapists' knowledge of guidelines and good assessment skills make them an ideal part of most hospital resuscitation teams. After a patient succumbs to a cardiopulmonary arrest, the most important determinant of the patient's survival is the presence of a trained rescuer who is ready, willing, and able to do basic life support. The 2010 American Heart Association recommendations are simple guidelines that will not apply to all patients in all situations. Members of resuscitation teams must use their knowledge, experience, and skills to adapt these guidelines to each patient's unique situation. Basic life support is usually followed by advanced cardiovascular life support. Together they provide a comprehensive outline that can be followed by teams during highly stressful events such as a patient's cardiopulmonary arrest and resuscitation.

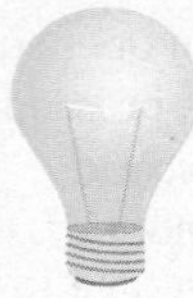

STOP AND THINK

What are the major differences between CPR performed by a layperson versus a healthcare provider?

TABLE 18-1
Comparison of Basic Life Support Techniques for Adults, Children, and Infants

Maneuver	Adolescent and Older	1 Year to Adolescent	Infant Younger Than 1 Year
Pulse check (≤10 seconds)	Carotid	Carotid	Brachial or femoral
Compression landmarks	Lower half of sternum, between nipples	Lower half of sternum, between nipples	Just below nipple line (lower half of sternum)
Compression method (push hard and fast; allow complete recoil)	Heel of one hand, other hand on top, fingers interlaced	Heel of one hand or as for adults	Two or three fingers, or two thumbs with hands encircling the infant's chest
Compression depth	At least 2 inches	Approximately one-third the depth of the chest	
Compression rate	At least 100/minute		
Compression-to-ventilation ratio	30:2 (one or two rescuers)	30:2 (single rescuer); 15:2 (two rescuers)	
Airway	Head tilt–chin lift (with suspected spinal trauma, use jaw thrust)		
Breathing			
Initial	2 breaths at 1 s/breath		
With advanced airway	8 to 10 breaths/min (approximately)		
Foreign body airway obstruction	Abdominal thrusts	Abdominal thrusts	Back slaps and chest thrusts
Defibrillation			
AED	Use adult pads; do not use child pads	Use AED after five cycles of CPR (out of hospital)	Not recommended

CPR, cardiopulmonary resuscitation; AED, automated external defibrillator. *Note*: The correct sequence is compressions–airway–breathing.

Advanced Cardiovascular Life Support

Advanced cardiovascular life support (ACLS) encompasses multiple links in the chain of survival, which includes intervention to prevent cardiac arrest, treating cardiac arrest, and improving outcomes for patients who achieve a return of spontaneous circulation (ROSC) after a cardiac arrest.[23] The 2010 Guidelines continue to emphasize the importance of successful transition from BLS to ACLS by stressing the necessity of providing good chest compressions. In ACLS advanced airway placement, vascular access, and drug delivery should not result in a delay of chest compressions or defibrillation.

Most respiratory therapists are required to be certified in ACLS as part of their work. Although BLS is still the foundation for all ACLS algorithms, nothing in ACLS is as important as maintaining good BLS throughout the resuscitation. Typically, ACLS skills include recognition of the cardiac rhythm and determining which algorithm should be followed, insertion and management of advanced airways, insertion of intravenous or intraosseous lines, knowledge of cardiac pharmacology, and the ability to make a differential diagnosis to determine and reverse the cause of cardiopulmonary arrest.

Four different cardiac rhythms can produce a pulseless cardiac arrest: ventricular fibrillation, pulseless rapid ventricular tachycardia (VT), pulseless electrical activity (PEA), and asystole (**Algorithm 18-5**, **Algorithm 18-6**, and **Algorithm 18-7**). **Table 18-2** lists drugs commonly administered during CPR.

Airway Management

Although the most recent AHA recommendations for cardiopulmonary resuscitation place a greater emphasis on chest compressions, successful management of the airway, oxygenation, and ventilation is still an important part of the resuscitation process. It is important for all respiratory therapists to be trained and skilled in airway management. Because the placement of advanced airways requires an interruption in chest compressions, the skills necessary to manage the airway using less invasive methods have gained importance given the 2005 and 2010 AHA Guidelines. The rescuer's use of effective bag-mask ventilation during the first few minutes of resuscitation will facilitate uninterrupted chest compressions and defibrillation until an advanced airway is placed.

The rescuer should open the airway using a chin lift or jaw thrust, insert a nasopharyngeal or oropharyngeal airway if necessary, and deliver two breaths using a volume of ventilation that is sufficient to produce a chest rise (approximately 6 to 7 mL/kg, or 500 to 600 mL).[49] Each breath is delivered during a very brief pause in compressions and takes less than 1 second. If not used appropriately, bag-valve ventilation can result in air trapping.

Patients with obstructive lung disease are very susceptible to this problem because of their increased airway resistance. The air trapping can further reduce their cardiac output. If the patient develops hypotension during bag-valve ventilation, ventilation should be stopped for 20 to 30 seconds. If blood pressure is restored during this period of apnea, it suggests the presence of air trapping, and ventilation should be resumed less aggressively. To prevent air trapping, rescuers should deliver a slow respiratory rate (6 to 8 breaths/min), which allows more time for the patient to exhale. Once an advanced airway has been placed, the rescuer should deliver 10 to 12 breaths/min, and there is no longer the need to pause compressions to deliver the breaths.

Several different types of advanced airway adjuncts can be used during resuscitation. In field studies, it has been reported that 6% to 14% of endotracheal tubes were misplaced when postmortem exams were done.[50,51] In part because of these studies, the AHA stresses training prehospital providers to use several different advanced airways and suggests that it is important to remember that there is no evidence that placing an advanced airway in a prehospital situation improves survival.[49] It is equally important for the individual managing the airway to use multiple techniques to verify that the placement is correct. The 2010 AHA Guidelines recommend quantitative waveform capnography (P_{ETCO_2}) as a means to confirm and monitor endotracheal tube placement, CPR quality, and the return of spontaneous circulation (ROSC).[19]

Indications for emergency endotracheal intubation include the inability of the rescuers to adequately ventilate with a bag-mask device, the inability of a patient to protect his or her own airway (i.e., an unconscious patient), and the presence of a rescuer who is adequately trained to do the procedure. Advantages of inserting an endotracheal tube include securing the airway from aspiration, keeping the airway patent, permitting the suctioning of the lower airway, and providing an alternative route for administration of some resuscitative drugs.

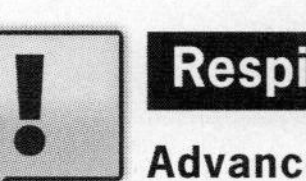

Respiratory Recap

Advanced Life Support

- Optimize compressions
- Use of airways and ventilation equipment
- ECG monitoring
- Insertion of intravenous lines
- Drug therapy

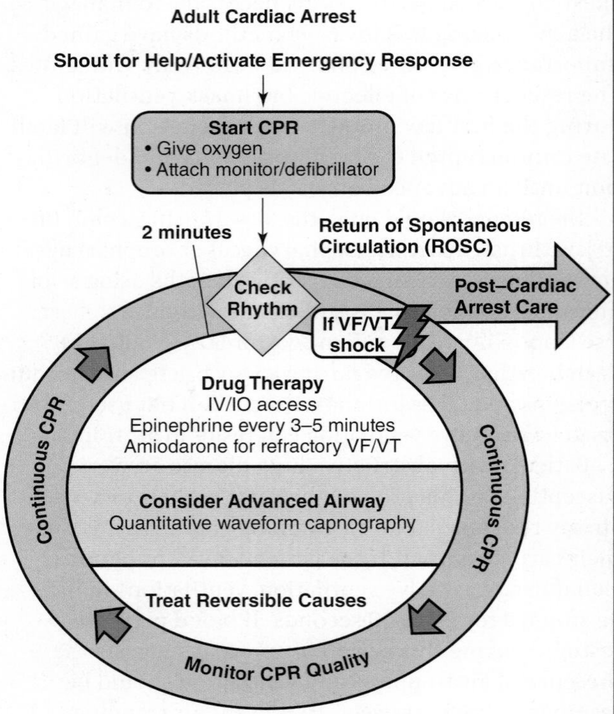

Adult Cardiac Arrest

Shout for Help/Activate Emergency Response

Start CPR
- Give oxygen
- Attach monitor/defibrillator

2 minutes

Return of Spontaneous Circulation (ROSC)

Check Rhythm

If VF/VT shock

Post–Cardiac Arrest Care

Drug Therapy
IV/IO access
Epinephrine every 3–5 minutes
Amiodarone for refractory VF/VT

Consider Advanced Airway
Quantitative waveform capnography

Treat Reversible Causes

Continuous CPR

Continuous CPR

Monitor CPR Quality

CPR Quality
- Push hard (≥2 inches [5 cm]) and fast (≥100/min) and allow complete chest recoil
- Minimize interruptions in compressions
- Avoid excessive ventilation
- Rotate compressor every 2 minutes
- If no advanced airway, 30:2 compression-ventilation ratio
- Quantitative waveform capnography
  – If P_{ETCO_2} <10 mm Hg, attempt to improve CPR quality
- Intra-arterial pressure
  – If relaxation phase (diastolic) pressure <20 mm Hg, attempt to improve CPR quality

Return of Spontaneous Circulation (ROSC)
- Pulse and blood pressure
- Abrupt sustained increase in P_{ETCO_2} (typically ≥40 mm Hg)
- Spontaneous arterial pressure waves with intra-arterial monitoring

Shock Energy
- **Biphasic:** Manufacturer recommendation (eg, initial dose of 120–200 J); if unknown, use maximum available. Second and subsequent doses should be equivalent, and higher doses may be considered.
- **Monophasic:** 360 J

Drug Therapy
- **Epinephrine IV/IO Dose:** 1 mg every 3–5 minutes
- **Vasopressin IV/IO Dose:** 40 units can replace first or second dose of epinephrine
- **Amiodarone IV/IO Dose:** First dose: 300 mg bolus. Second dose: 150 mg

Advanced Airway
- Supragiottic advanced airway or endotracheal intubation
- Waveform capnography to confirm and monitor ET tube placement
- 8–10 breaths per minute with continuous chest compressions

Reversible Causes
- **H**ypovolemia
- **H**ypoxia
- **H**ydrogen ion (acidosis)
- **H**ypo-/hyperkalemia
- **H**ypothermia
- **T**ension pneumothorax
- **T**amponade, cardiac
- **T**oxins
- **T**hrombosis, pulmonary
- **T**hrombosis, coronary

ALGORITHM 18-5 Advanced Cardiovascular Life Support Cardiac Arrest Circular Algorithm.

Reproduced from 2010 American Heart Association Guidelines for Cardiopulmonary Resuscitation and Emergency Cardiovascular Care. Part 8: Adult Advanced Cardiovascular Life Support. *Circulation.* 2010;122:S729–S767. © 2010 American Heart Association, Inc.

Complications include trauma to the oropharynx, interruption of compressions and ventilations, and failure of the rescuer to recognize the misplacement of a tube. The interruption in compressions for intubation should be only during the time the rescuer needs to visualize the vocal cords. If the first attempt to intubate is unsuccessful, the rescuer doing the intubation should stop the procedure, provide ventilation and oxygenation, and allow time for others to do compressions before attempting intubation again.

Esophageal-tracheal Combitubes are relatively easy to place compared with an endotracheal tube. They are more effective than a face mask at isolating the airway and reducing the risk of aspiration, and they enable rescuers to provide ventilation and oxygenation. Another advantage of using a Combitube is the ease of training healthcare providers to insert the tube.[19] Complications associated with the Combitube include esophageal trauma, lacerations, bruising,[52] and fatalities that may occur when the position of the tube is not confirmed by the rescuers.

A laryngeal mask airway provides a more secure and reliable means of ventilation than the bag-mask device.[53] The advantages of using a laryngeal mask are its relative ease of insertion, simpler training for rescuers (rescuers do not have to visualize the vocal cords), better protection against aspiration than with a face mask, and the ability to insert the airway when a patient has the possibility of an unstabilized neck injury.

Impedance Threshold Valve

The **impedance threshold valve (ITV)** increases the negative intrathoracic pressure in the chest by creating a vacuum pressure that essentially "pulls" venous blood

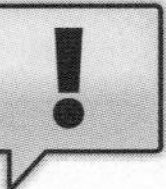

Respiratory Recap

Equipment for Emergency Airway Management
- Endotracheal tube
- Oropharyngeal airway
- Nasopharyngeal airway
- Esophageal-tracheal Combitube
- Laryngeal mask airway

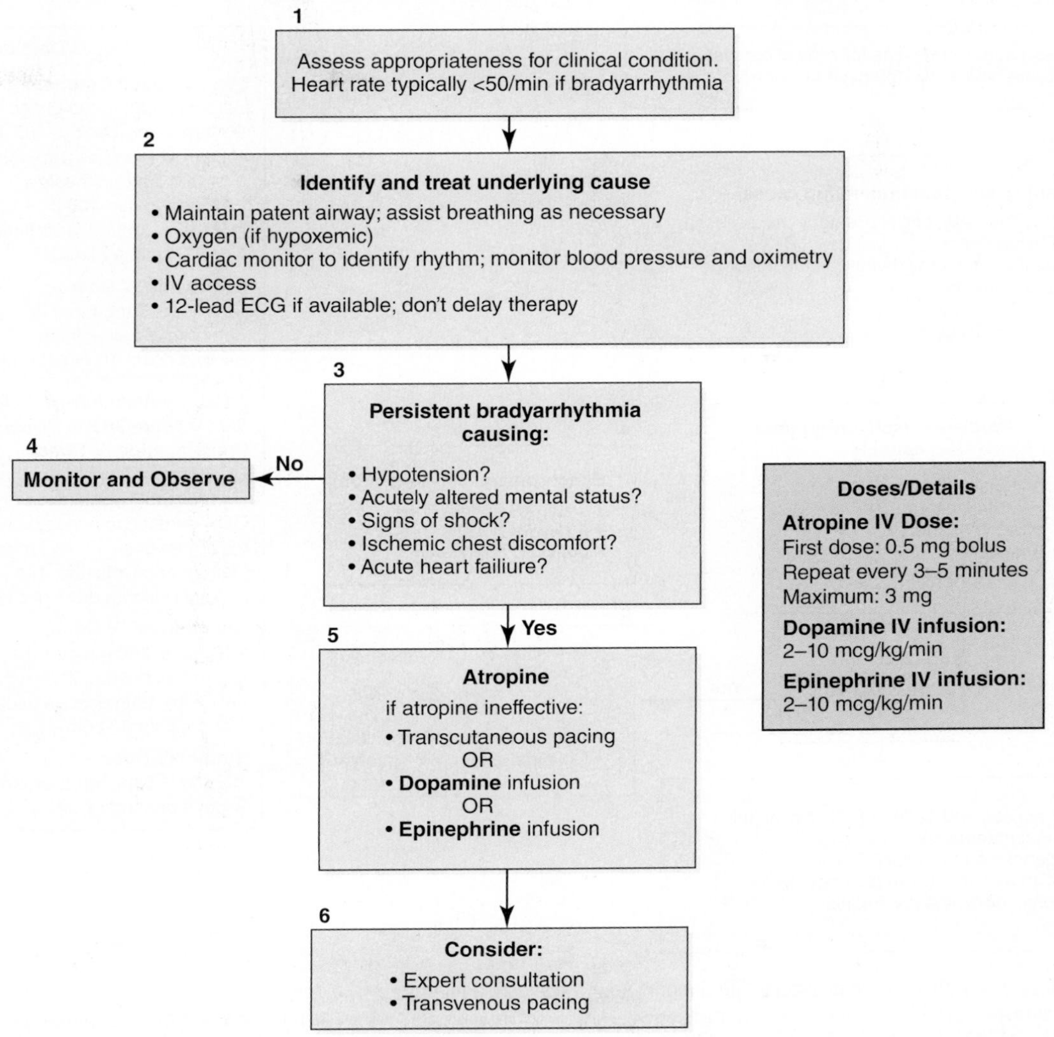

1
Assess appropriateness for clinical condition.
Heart rate typically <50/min if bradyarrhythmia
2
Identify and treat underlying cause
• Maintain patent airway; assist breathing as necessary
• Oxygen (if hypoxemic)
• Cardiac monitor to identify rhythm; monitor blood pressure and oximetry
• IV access
• 12-lead ECG if available; don't delay therapy
3
Persistent bradyarrhythmia causing:
• Hypotension?
• Acutely altered mental status?
• Signs of shock?
• Ischemic chest discomfort?
• Acute heart failiure?
No
4
Monitor and Observe
Yes
5
Atropine
if atropine ineffective:
• Transcutaneous pacing
OR
• Dopamine infusion
OR
• Epinephrine infusion
6
Consider:
• Expert consultation
• Transvenous pacing
Doses/Details
Atropine IV Dose:
First dose: 0.5 mg bolus
Repeat every 3–5 minutes
Maximum: 3 mg
Dopamine IV infusion:
2–10 mcg/kg/min
Epinephrine IV infusion:
2–10 mcg/kg/min

ALGORITHM 18-6 Advanced Cardiovascular Life Support Adult Bradycardia Algorithm.

Reproduced from 2010 American Heart Association Guidelines for Cardiopulmonary Resuscitation and Emergency Cardiovascular Care. Part 8: Adult Advanced Cardiovascular Life Support. *Circulation*. 2010;122:S729–S767. © 2010 American Heart Association, Inc.

back into the chest during expansion of the chest after compression, thereby enhancing venous return and cardiac output (**Figure 18-23**).[54] During resuscitation, cardiac output is dependent on both the amount of venous return to the heart and the physical compression of the heart. Venous return is partially dependent on the degree of negative intrathoracic pressures. This device is contraindicated in patients with pulmonary edema or congestive heart failure because it can exacerbate these conditions.

The ITV attaches to a resuscitator bag and limits air entry into the chest during chest recoil after each compression. This reduces the intrathoracic pressures and thereby increases venous return to the heart during the chest decompression phase of compressions. In several studies it has been successfully used with a laryngeal mask airway, cuffed endotracheal tube, and even a face mask if the rescuers can maintain a tight seal with the mask.[55–59]

During a cardiac arrest, use of the impedance threshold valve decreased intrathoracic pressures by 6 to 8 mm Hg.[58] When the valve is used during active compression–decompression resuscitation, it has resulted in a greater than 50% increase in coronary perfusion pressures, improved 24-h patient survival, and improved neurologic function following cardiac arrest.[60]

Because the ITV reduces negative intrathoracic pressures during recoil of the chest following compressions, there are concerns about the possibility of an increase in the work of breathing, especially for patients who are using the valve with a mask to treat orthostatic hypotension.[61] In healthy individuals, the imposed work of breathing was increased, but not excessively.[43,61]

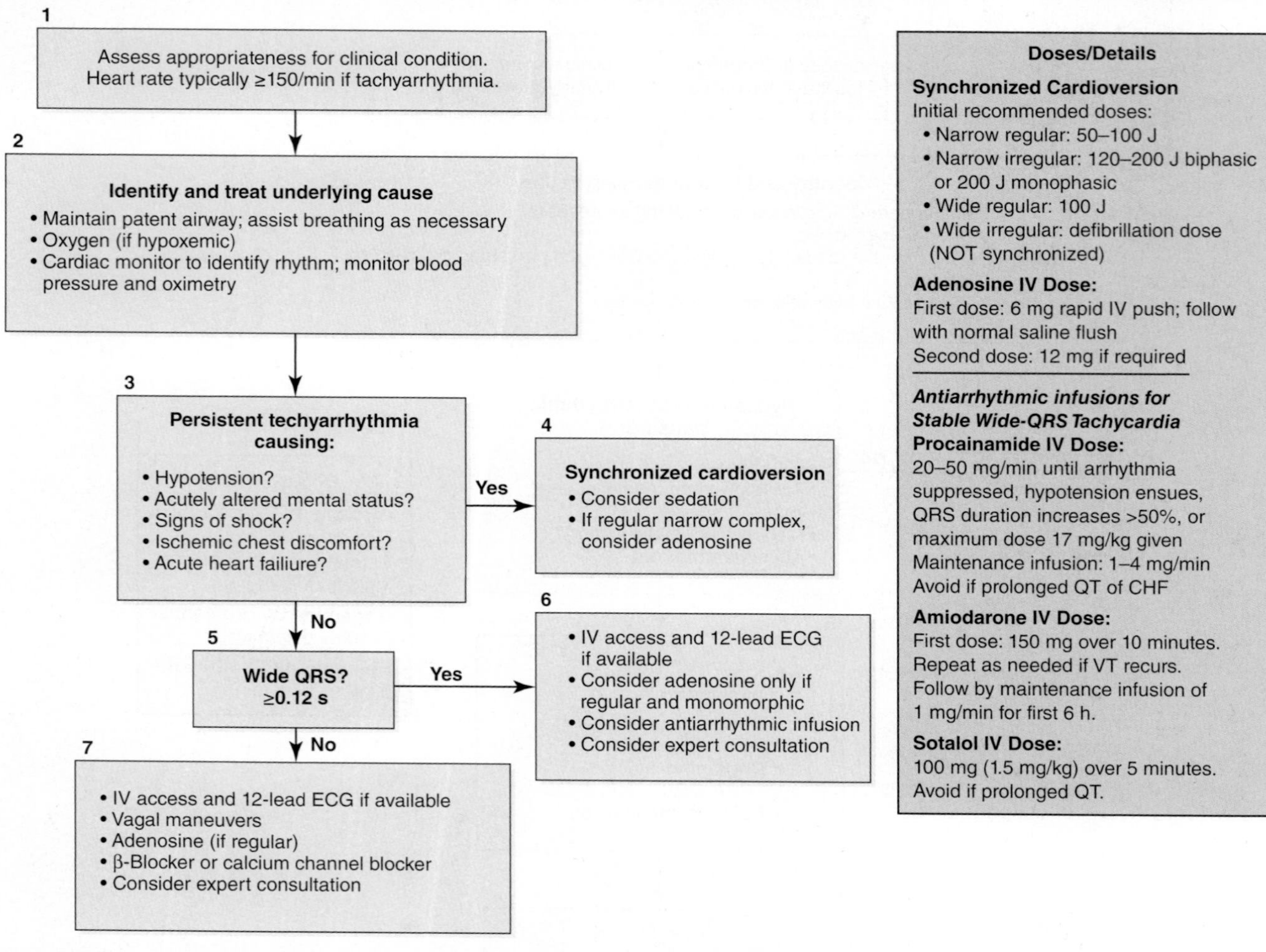

ALGORITHM 18-7 Advanced Cardiovascular Life Support Adult Tachycardia Algorithm.

Reproduced from 2010 American Heart Association Guidelines for Cardiopulmonary Resuscitation and Emergency Cardiovascular Care. Part 8: Adult Advanced Cardiovascular Life Support. *Circulation.* 2010;122:S729–S767. © 2010 American Heart Association, Inc.

Post–Cardiac Arrest Care

The postresuscitation period is a period of time during which multiorgan dysfunction can occur. According to the 2005 AHA Guidelines, most postresuscitation deaths occur during the first 24 hours after a cardiac arrest.[62] These patients require respiratory support, management of cardiac arrhythmias, monitoring and management of hemodynamic instability using mechanical or pharmacologic agents or both, and monitoring and management of metabolic abnormalities.[23] According to the 2010 AHA Guidelines,[63] survival for victims of cardiac arrest who are admitted to the hospital can be improved by implementing a comprehensive, structured, integrated, and multidisciplinary system of post–cardiac arrest care. The key issues to be addressed in this post–cardiac care are (1) optimize cardiopulmonary function and vital organ perfusion after return of spontaneous circulation; (2) transport/transfer to an appropriate hospital or critical care unit with a comprehensive post–cardiac arrest treatment system of care; (3) identify and treat ACS and other reversible causes; (4) control temperature to optimize neurologic recovery; and (5) anticipate, treat, and prevent multiple organ dysfunction, which includes avoiding excessive ventilation and hyperoxia. Clinicians should try to identify the precipitating cause of the arrest, prevent the recurrence of the arrest, and optimize cardiopulmonary functions and systemic perfusion (especially to the brain) to improve long-term survival with neurologic function intact.

Studies have indicated that a mild degree of therapeutic hypothermia may play an important role in the postresuscitative period. In these studies, patients were cooled to a range of 33° C to 34° C for 12 to 24 hours after resuscitation from ventricular fibrillation or pulseless electrical activity or asystole rhythms.[64–67] It is suggested that only a subset of cardiopulmonary arrest patients may benefit from induced hypothermia at this time. In the future, others may benefit as well.[68] In some older studies, external cooling techniques

Table 18-2
ALS Drugs

Drug	Indication	Dosage
Epinephrine	Shock, refractory VF and pulseless VT, asystole, PEA	*Cardiac arrest* 1 mg IV push (10 mL of 1:10,000 solution) Repeat 1 mg every 3–5 min Endotracheal dose = 2 to 2.5 times intravenous dose *Symptomatic bradycardia* 2–10 mcg/min
Vasopressin	VF/pulseless VT, asystole, PEA	*Any pulseless patient* 40 units IV single dose—1 time only To replace first or second dose of epinephrine
Atropine	Symptomatic bradycardia	*Bradycardia* 0.5 mg every 3–5 min Repeat to total dose of 0.04 mg/kg Endotracheal dose = 2 to 2.5 times IV dose
Amiodarone	VF/pulseless VT	300 mg IV push in cardiac arrest (VF/VT) 150 mg IV push for tachycardia with pulse (give over 10 minutes); can repeat *one* dose of 150 mg in 5 min
Lidocaine	VT (with pulse—stable), VF/pulseless VT	*VF or pulseless VT* 1–1.5 mg/kg; repeat at 0.5–0.75 mg/kg in 3–5 min, for total dose of 3 mg/kg *VT with pulse* 0.5–0.75 mg/kg; repeat in 3–5 min, for total dose of 3 mg/kg
Procainamide	Stable monomorphic VT, SVT, tachycardia of unknown origin	20 mg/min IV infusion; in urgent situations, up to 50 mg/min (max 17 mg/kg)
Magnesium	Cardiac arrest only if torsades is present or low magnesium is suspected	1–2 g per 10 mL D5W over 1–2 s
Adenosine	Stable SVT, undefined stable narrow complex tachycardia	6 mg IV over 1–3 s followed by 20 mL saline flush, then elevate arm; repeat 12 mg IV rapid push
Sodium bicarbonate	Preexisting hyperkalemia, drug overdose, known ketoacidosis, prolonged cardiac arrest with adequate ventilation	1 mmol/kg IV bolus

ALS, advanced life support; VF, ventricular fibrillation; VT, ventricular tachycardia; PEA, pulseless electrical activity; SVT, supraventricular tachycardia; D5W, 5% dextrose in water.

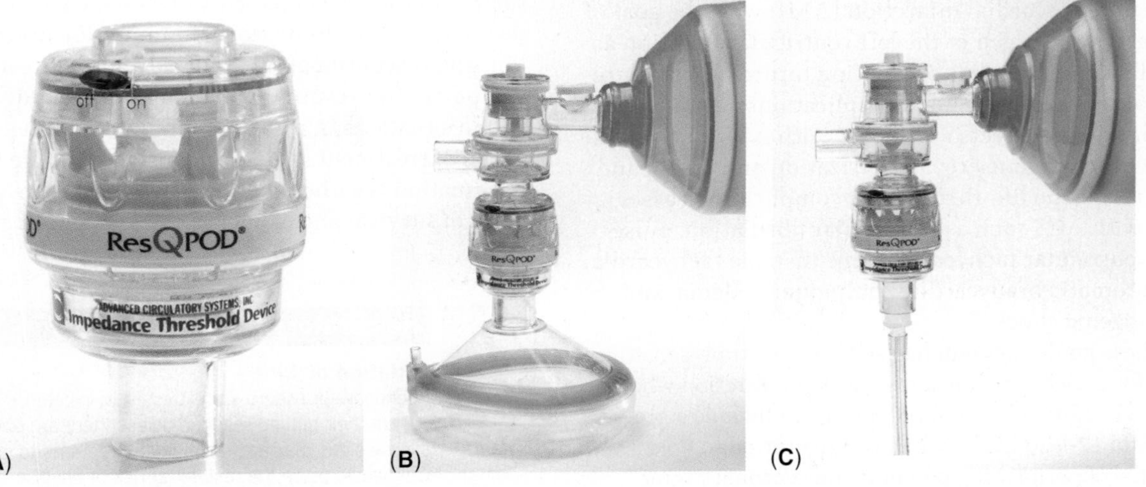

FIGURE 18-23 **(A)** Impedance threshold valve device (ITV). **(B)** ITV attached to mask. **(C)** ITV between bag-valve resuscitator and endotracheal tube.

Courtesy of Advanced Circulatory System, Inc.

(e.g., cooling blankets, ice bags) have taken several hours to reach the desired level of hypothermia; the newer studies suggest that internal cooling techniques (e.g., cold saline, endovascular cooling catheters) may also be used and result in less time to reach the desired temperatures and better patient outcomes.[69] Commercially available devices use pads placed on the patient that contain channels of circulating water that cool the body.

Therapeutic hypothermia has potential complications. The patient's temperature should be continuously monitored, and clinicians should watch for these complications very closely during this period. If the patient's temperature drops below the desired range, coagulopathy and arrhythmias may develop. An increased number of patients develop pneumonia and/or sepsis and hyperglycemia with hypothermia after therapeutic hypothermia.[70] During this process the temperature on the humidifier of the ventilator should be set at the target core temperature of the patient.[71]

Normal blood gas values should be maintained during the postresuscitation period. Studies have determined that during this time, hyperventilation of the patient, increased airway pressures, and intrinsic positive end-expiratory pressures may cause increased cerebral vasoconstriction, increased intracranial pressures, increased cerebral ischemia, and ultimately ischemic brain injury.[72]

Stabilization of Acute Coronary Care Patients

In 2010, the AHA Guidelines defined the scope of practice for patients with suspected or definite signs of acute coronary syndrome (ACS), within the first hour after the onset of symptoms.[23] The primary therapeutic goals are: (1) to limit and reduce the amount of myocardial necrosis that occurs in patients suffering an acute myocardial infarction (AMI) with the goal of preserving as much of the left ventricular function as possible and therefore preventing future heart failure and other cardiovascular complications; (2) to prevent major adverse effects associated with ASC, such as the need for emergency revascularization and death; and (3) to treat the life-threatening complications associated with ACS such as ventricular fibrillation, pulseless ventricular tachycardia, any unstable tachycardia, symptomatic bradycardias, pulmonary edema, and cardiogenic shock.

These guidelines emphasized specific, time-sensitive care for patients having a myocardial infarction who have ST segment elevation (STEMI) to include a prehospital 12-lead ECG, which is transmitted to hospitals capable of performing percutaneous coronary interventions and care. During the past decade, the AHA Guidelines have recommended the importance of rapid reperfusion with fibrinolysis. The 2010 Guidelines focused on the need to decrease the time from initial event to treatment by the use of ECG and triage prior to patient's arrival in the hospitals.[73–75] **Algorithm 18-8** addresses adult immediate post–cardiac arrest care.

Summary of Advanced Cardiovascular Life Support

The successful resuscitation of patients suffering from cardiopulmonary arrest requires teams of rescuers with advanced skills and knowledge. The institutions determine the role of respiratory therapists on these teams where they work. The 2005 and 2010 AHA Guidelines provide algorithms to determine appropriate actions for a variety of different situations. No guidelines can detail the actions necessary to be taken for each and every individual patient, however. Good assessment skills, airway management skills, a sufficient knowledge base, and the ability to learn new skills help prepare therapists to function in a range of situations from preventive early response teams to postarrest support teams when managing cardiopulmonary arrest patients.

Ethical Concerns

Healthcare providers are expected to initiate CPR as part of their duty to respond unless there are obvious clinical signs of irreversible death, attempts to perform CPR would place the rescuer at risk of physical injury, or the patient or his or her surrogate has indicated with an advance directive (do-not-resuscitate order) that resuscitation is not desired.[76] Respiratory therapists have a responsibility to know the resuscitation status of patients under their care. Unlike other medical interventions, CPR is initiated without a physician's order, based on implied consent for emergency treatment. A physician's order is necessary to withhold CPR. A physician may also determine that continued care is futile, such as in the case of patients in whom CPR would not restore effective circulation. Noninitiation of resuscitation and discontinuation of life-sustaining treatment during or after resuscitation are ethically equivalent, and in situations in which the prognosis is uncertain, a trial of treatment should be considered while further information is gathered to help determine the likelihood of survival and expected clinical course.

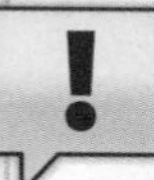

Respiratory Recap

Initiation of CPR

Healthcare providers are expected to initiate CPR as part of their duty to respond unless there are obvious clinical signs of irreversible death, attempts to perform CPR would place the rescuer at risk of physical injury, or the patient or the patient's surrogate has indicated with an advance directive that CPR is not desired.

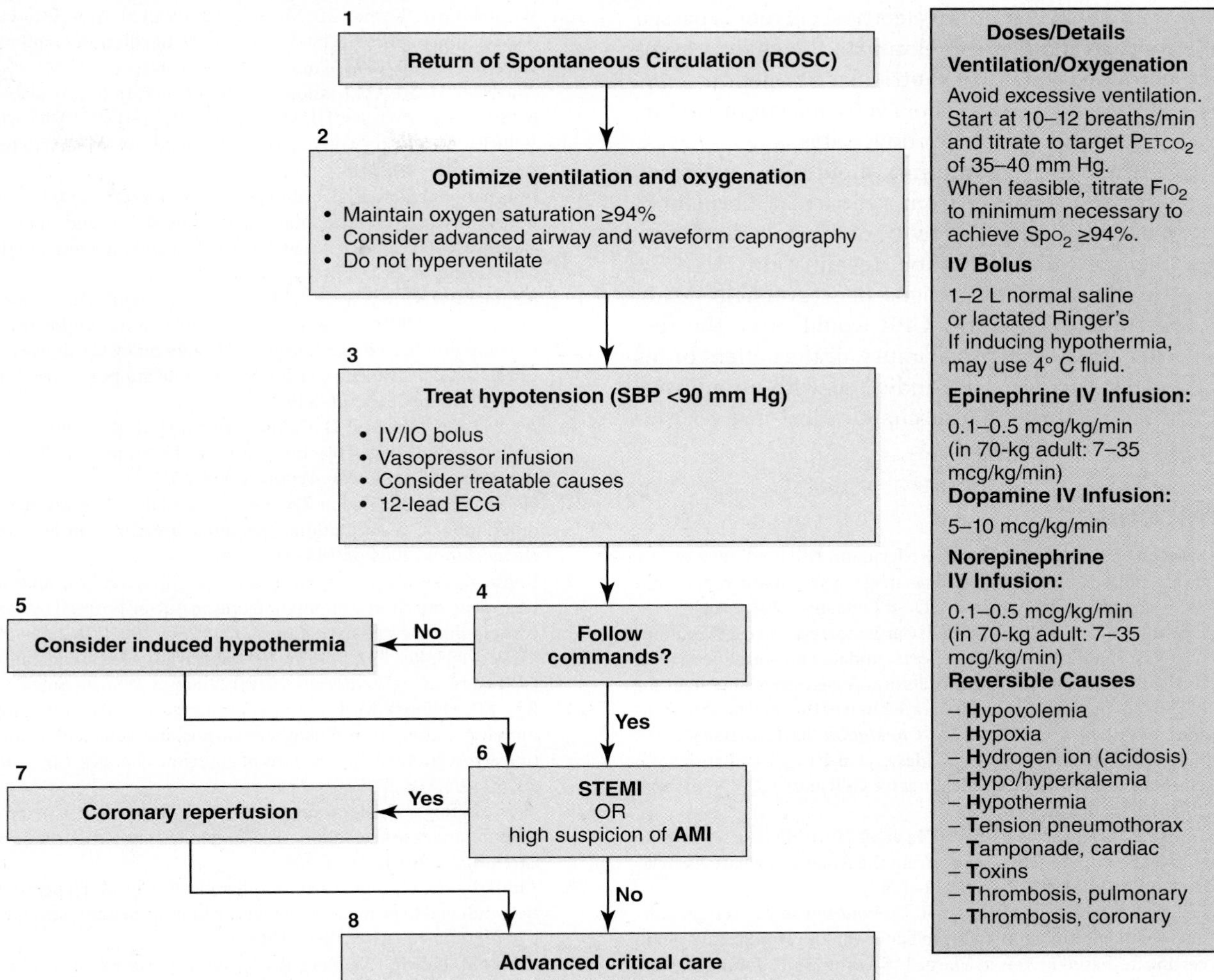

ALGORITHM 18-8 Post–Cardiac Arrest Care Algorithm.

Reproduced from 2010 American Heart Association Guidelines for Cardiopulmonary Resuscitation and Emergency Cardiovascular Care. Part 9: Post-Cardiac Arrest Care. *Circulation.* 2010;122:S768–S786. © 2010 American Heart Association, Inc.

All patients in cardiac arrest should receive CPR unless the patient has a valid do-not-resuscitate order, the patient has signs of irreversible death (e.g., rigor mortis, decapitation, decomposition, dependent lividity), or no physiologic benefit can be expected because vital functions have deteriorated despite maximal therapy (e.g., progressive septic, cardiogenic shock).

The decision to terminate resuscitative efforts rests with the treating physician in the hospital and is based on consideration of many factors, including time to CPR, time to defibrillation, comorbid disease, pre-arrest state, and initial arrest rhythm.

Key Points

- CPR is a series of life-saving actions that can improve the chance of survival following cardiac arrest.
- Factors related to resuscitation outcomes after CPR include the initial rhythm, time elapsed before initiation of CPR, time elapsed before defibrillation of ventricular fibrillation or pulseless ventricular tachycardia, duration of CPR, and whether arrest was witnessed.
- The CABD sequence has replaced the ABCD sequence and consists of circulation, airway, breathing, and defibrillation.
- With two-rescuer CPR, one person performs chest compressions and the other person performs ventilation and assesses cardiopulmonary function.
- Masks, face shields, or bag-mask devices should be used for emergency ventilation.
- In airway management, there is no substitute for tracheal intubation.
- Manual ventilation with a bag-mask-valve device may not provide adequate tidal volumes if performed incorrectly.
- The abdominal thrust maneuver is recommended to relieve airway obstruction.
- During cardiac arrest, it is important to administer the highest oxygen concentration possible.
- When intravenous access is delayed, some drugs can be administered through the tracheal tube.

- With defibrillation, an electrical current is passed through the heart to eliminate the chaotic asynchronous activity of ventricular fibrillation.
- The impedance threshold valve may improve cardiac output during low flow states.
- Therapeutic hypothermia should be considered after resuscitation from ventricular fibrillation, pulseless electrical activity, or asystole rhythms.
- General guidelines for termination of CPR are obvious clinical signs of irreversible death, attempts to perform CPR would place the rescuer at risk of physical injury, or the patient or his or her surrogate has indicated with an advance directive (do-not-resuscitate order) that resuscitation is not desired.

References

1. Sassoon C, Rogers MA, Dahl J, Kellermann AL. Predictors of survival from out-of-hospital cardiac arrest: a systematic review and meta-analysis. *Circ Cardiovasc Qual Outcomes*. 2010;3:63–81.
2. Jacobs I, Nadkarni V, Bahr J, et al. Cardiac arrest and cardiopulmonary resuscitation outcome reports: update and simplification of the Utstein templates for resuscitation registries; a statement for healthcare professionals from a task force of the international liaison Committee on Resuscitation. *Circulation*. 2004;110:3385–3397.
3. Berg M, Schexnayder M, Chameides L, et al. Part 13: Pediatric Basic Life Support: 2010 AHA Guidelines for CPR and ECC. *Circulation*. 2010;122(Suppl 3);S862–S875.
4. Go AS, Mozaffarian D, Roger VL, et al. Heart disease and stroke statistics–2013 update: a report from the American Heart Association. *Circulation*. 2013;127:1342–1350.
5. Chugh SS, Jui J, Gunson K, et al. Current burden of sudden cardiac death: multiple source surveillance versus retrospective death certificate-based review in a large U.S. community. *J Am Coll Cardiol*. 2004;44:1268–1275.
6. Nichol G, Thomas E, Callaway CW, et al. Regional variation in out-of-hospital cardiac arrest incidence and outcome. *JAMA*. 2008; 300:1423–1431.
7. Go AS, Mozaffarain D, Roger VL, et al. American Heart Association Statistics Committee and Strokes Statistics Committee. Heart disease and stroke statistics–2013 update: a report from the American Heart Association. *Circulation*. 2013;127:e6–e245.
8. Merchant RM, Yang L, Becker LB, et al. Incidence of treated cardiac arrest in hospitalized patients in the United States. *Crit Care Med*. 2011;39:2401–2406.
9. Meaney PA, Bobrow BJ, Mancini JC, et al. Cardiopulmonary resuscitation quality: improving cardiac resuscitation outcomes both inside and outside the hospital: a consensus statement from the American Heart Association. *Circulation*. 2013;128:417–435.
10. Peberdy MA, Ornato JP, Larkin GL, et al. Survival from in-hospital cardiac arrest during nights and weekends. *JAMA*. 2008;299: 785–792.
11. Field JM, Hazinski MF, Sayre MR, et al. 2010 American Heart Association guidelines for cardiopulmonary resuscitation and emergency cardiovascular care. *Circulation*. 2010;122(Suppl 3):S640–S656.
12. Eisenberg M. *Resuscitate! How Your Community Can Improve Survival from Sudden Cardiac Arrest*. Seattle: University of Washington Press; 2009.
13. Safar P. History of cardiopulmonary resuscitation. In Kaye W, Bircher N, eds. *Cardiopulmnary Resuscitation*. New York: Churchill Livingston; 1989:1–53.
14. Cooper JA, Cooper JD, Cooper J. CPR: history, current practice and future direction. *Circulation*. 2006;114:2839–2849.
15. Cobb LA, Alvanez H, Kopass MK. A Rapid Response System for out-of-hospital cardiac emergencies. *Med Clin North Am*. 1976; 60:283–290.
16. Weisfeldt ML, Kerper RE, McGoldrick RP, et al. American Heart Association report on Public Access Defibrillation Conference December 8–10, 1994. *Circulation*. 1995; 92:2740–2747.
17. American Heart Association. *History of CPR*. (n.d.). Available at: http://www.heart.org/HEARTORG/CPRAndECC/WhatisCPR/CPRFactsandStats/History-of-CPR_UCM_307549_Article.jsp. Accessed July 19, 2014.
18. International Liaison Committee on Resuscitation. 2005 international consensus on cardiopulmonary resuscitation and emergency cardiovascular care science with treatment and recommendations. *Circulation*. 2005;112:III-I–III-136.
19. Neumar RW, Otto CW, Link MS, et al. Part 8: Adult Cardiovascular Life Support: 2010 American Heart Association Guidelines for Cardiopulmonary Resuscitation and Emergency Cardiovascular-Care. Part B: Advanced Cardiovascular Life Support. *Circulation*. 2010;122(Suppl 3):S729–S767.
20. Azar D, Chamberlain D, Colquhoun M, et al. Randomized controlled trials of staged teaching for basic life support: skill acquisition at bronze stage. *Resuscitation*. 2004;5:7–15.
21. Heidenreich JW, Higdon TA, Kern KB, et al. Single-rescuer cardiopulmonary resuscitation: "two quick breaths"—an oxymoron. *Resuscitation*. 2004;62:283–289.
22. Bohm K, Rosenqvist M, Herlitz J, et al. Survival is similar after treatment and chest compression only in out-of-hospital bystander cardiopulmonary resuscitation. *Circulation*. 2007;116:2908–2912.
23. Travers AH, Rea TD, Bobrow B, et al. Part 4: AHA Guidelines for CPR and ECC. *Circulation*. 2010;122(Suppl 3):S676–S684.
24. Rea TD, Helbock M, Perry S, et al. Increasing use of cardiopulmonary resuscitation during out-of-hospital ventricular fibrillation arrest survival implications of guideline changes. *Circulation*. 2006;114:2760–2765.
25. White L, Rogers J, Bloomingdale M, et al. Dispatcher-assisted cardiopulmonary resuscitation: risks for patients not in cardiac arrest. *Circulation*. 2010;121:91–97.
26. Aufderheide TP, Sigurdsson G, Pirrallo RG, et al. Hyperventilation-induced hypotension during cardiopulmonary resuscitation. *Circulation*. 2004;109:1960–1965.
27. Kern KB, Hilwig RW, Berg RA, et al. Importance of continuous chest compressions during cardiopulmonary resuscitation: improved outcomes during a simulated single lay-rescuer scenario. *Circulation*. 2003;108:2575–2594.
28. Handley AJ. Teaching hand placement for chest compressions—a simpler technique. *Resuscitation*. 2002;53:29–36.
29. Aufderheide TP, Pirrallo RG, Yannopoulos D, et al. Incomplete chest wall decompression: a clinical evaluation of CPR performance by EMS personnel and assessment of alternative manual chest-compression-decompression techniques. *Resuscitation*. 2005;64:353–362.
30. Aufderheide TP, Pirrallo RG, Yannopoulos D, et al. Incomplete chest wall decompression: A Clinical Evaluation of CPR performance by trained laypersons and an assessment of alternative manual chest compression-decompression techniques. *Resuscitation*. 2006;71:341-351.
31. Yannopoulos D, McKnite S, Aufderheide TP, et al. Effects of incomplete chest wall decompression during cardiopulmonary resuscitation on coronary and cerebral perfusion pressures in a porcine model of cardiac arrest. *Resuscitation*. 2005;64:363–372.
32. Hackl W, Hausberger K, Sailer R, et al. Prevalence of cervical spine injuries in patient with facial trauma. *Oral Surg Oral Med Oral Pathol Oral Radiol Endod*. 2001;92:370–376.
33. Dorges V, Ocker H, Hagelberg S, et al. Smaller tidal volumes with room air are not sufficient to ensure adequate oxygenation during bag-mask ventilation. *Resuscitation*. 2000;44:37–41.
34. American Heart Association in collaboration with International Liaison Committee on Resuscitation. Guidelines 2000 for cardiopulmonary resuscitation and emergency cardiovascular care: international consensus on science, part 3: adult basic life support. *Circulation*. 2000;102(Suppl I):I-22–I-59.
35. Baker PW, Conway J, Cotton C, et al. Defibrillation or cardiopulmonary resuscitation first for patients with out-of-hospital cardiac

arrest found by paramedics to be in ventricular fibrillation? A randomized control trial. *Resuscitation.* 2008;79:424–431.

36. Rea TD, Shah S, Kudenchuk PF, et al. Automated external defibrillators: to what extent does the algorithm delay CPR? *Ann Emerg Med.* 2005;46:132–141.
37. Kheterpal S, Han R, Tremper KK, et al. Incidence and predictors of difficult and impossible mask ventilation. *Anesthesiology.* 2006:105:885–891.
38. El-Orbany M, Woechlck H. Difficult mask ventilation. *Anesth Analg.* 2009;109:1870–1880.
39. Walls RM, Murphy MF. *Emergency Airway Manual*, 4th ed. Philadelphia, Penn.: Lippincott Williams & Wilkins; 2012:5–6.
40. Centers for Disease Control and Prevention. Web-Based Injury Statistics Query and Reporting System (WISQARS). National Center for Injury Prevention and Control, Centers for Disease Control and Prevention (producer). Available at: http://www.cdc.gov/injury/wisqars/index.html. Accessed July 19, 2014.
41. Centers for Disease Control and Prevention. *Injury Fact Book.* Atlanta, Ga.: U.S. Department of Health and Human Services; 2006.
42. Samson R, Berg R, Bingham R, et al. Use of automated external defibrillators for children: an update. An advisory statement from the Pediatric Advanced Life Support Task Force, International Liaison Committee on Resuscitation. *Resuscitation.* 2003;57:237–243.
43. Morley RE, Ludemann JP, Moxham JP, et al. Foreign body aspiration in infants and toddlers: recent trends in British Columbia. *J Otolaryngol.* 2004;33:37–41.
44. Vilke GM, Smith AM, Rau LU, et al. Airway obstruction in children aged less than 5 years: the prehospital experience. *Prehosp Emerg Care.* 2004;8:196–199.
45. Kattwinkel J, Perlman JM, Aziz K. Part 15: Neonatal Resuscitation 2010 AHA Guidelines for CPR and ECC. *Circulation.* 2010;122(Suppl 3):S909–S919.
46. Zaichkin Z, *Neonatal Resuscitation Manual.* 6th ed. Elk Grove Village, Ill.: American Academy of Pediatrics; 2011.
47. Finer NN, Rich W, Craft A, Henderson C. Comparison of methods of bag and mask ventilation for neonatal resuscitation. *Resuscitation.* 2001;49:299–305.
48. Clemets F, McGowan J. Finger position for chest compression in cardiac arrest in infants. *Resuscitation.* 2000;44:43–46.
49. Dorges V, Ocker H, Hagelberg S, et al. Smaller tidal volumes with room-air are not sufficient to ensure adequate oxygenation during bag-valve mask ventilation. *Resuscitation.* 2000;44:37–41.
50. Jones JH, Murphy MP, Dickerson RL, et al. Emergency physician–verified out-of-hospital intubations: miss rates by paramedics. *Acad Emerg Med.* 2004;11:707–709.
51. Katz SH, Falk JL. Misplaced endotracheal tubes by paramedics in an urban emergency medical services system. *Ann Emerg Med.* 2001;37:32–37.
52. Vezina D, Lessard MR, Bussieres J, Topping CA. Complications associated with the use of esophageal tracheal Combitube. *Can J Anaesth.* 1998;45:76–80.
53. Stone BJ, Chantler PJ, Baskett PJ. The incidence of regurgitation during cardiopulmonary resuscitation: a comparison between the bag valve mask and the laryngeal mask airway. *Resuscitation.* 1998;38:3–6.
54. Ahamed HI, Convertino VA, Ratliff DA, et al. Imposed power of breathing associated with use of an impedance threshold device. *Respir Care.* 2007;52:177–183.
55. Plaisance P, Lurue JG, Payen D. Inspiratory impedance during active compression-decompression cardiopulmonary resuscitation: a randomized evaluation in patients in cardiac arrest. *Circulation.* 2000;101:989–994.
56. Plaisance P, Soleil C, Lurie KG, et al. Use of an inspiratory impedance threshold device on a face mask and endotracheal tube to reduce intrathoracic pressures during the decompression phase of active compression-decompression cardiopulmonary resuscitation. *Crit Care Med.* 2005;33:990–994.
57. Wolcke BB, Mauer DK, Schoefmann MF, et al. Comparison of standard cardiopulmonary resuscitation versus the combination of active compression–decompression cardiopulmonary resuscitation and an inspiratory impedance threshold device for out-of-hospital cardiac arrest. *Circulation.* 2003;108:2201–2205.
58. Aufderheide TP, Pirrallo RG, Provo TA, Lurie KG. Clinical evaluation of an inspiratory impedance threshold device during standard cardiopulmonary resuscitation in patients with out-of-hospital cardiac arrest. *Crit Care Med.* 2005;33:734–740.
59. Pirrallo RG, Aufderheide TP, Provo TA, Lurie KG. Effect of an inspiratory impedance threshold device on hemodynamics during conventional manual cardiopulmonary resuscitation. *Resuscitation.* 2005;66:13–20.
60. Lurie KG, Zeilinski T, McKnite S, et al. Use of an inspiratory impedance valve improves neurologically intact survival in a porcine model of ventricular fibrillation. *Circulation.* 2002;105:124–129.
61. Concertion VA, Ratliff DA, Crissey J, et al. Effects of inspiratory impedance on hemodynamic responses to a squat-stand test in human volunteers: implications for treatment of orthostatic hypotension. *Eur J Appl Physiol.* 2005;94:392–399.
62. Laurent I, Monchi M, Chiche JD, et al. Reversible myocardial dysfunction in survivors of out-of-hospital cardiac arrest. *J Am Coll Cardiol.* 2002;40:2110–2116.
63. Pederby MA, Callway CW, Neumar RW. Part 9; Post-Cardiac Arrest Care. 2010 American Heart Association Guidelines for Cardiopulmonary Resuscitation and Emergency Cardiovascular Care. *Circulation.* 2010;122(Suppl 3):S768–S786.
64. Part 7. 5: Postresuscitation Support. 2005 American Heart Association Guidelines for Cardiopulmonary Resuscitation and Emergency Cardiovascular Care. *Circulation.* 2005;112:IV-84–IV-88.
65. Hypothermia After Cardiac Arrest Study Group. Mild therapeutic hypothermia to improve the neurological outcomes after the cardiac arrest. *N Engl J Med.* 2002;346:549–556.
66. Bernard SA, Gray TW, Buist MD, et al. Treatment of comatose survivors of out-of-hospital cardiac arrest. *N Engl J Med.* 2002;346:549–556.
67. Hachimi-Idressi S, Corne L, Ebinger G, et al. Mild hypothermia induced by helmet device: a clinical feasibility study. *Resuscitation.* 2001;51:275–281.
68. Langhelle A, Tyvold SS, Lexow K, et al. In-hospital factors associated with improved outcomes after out-of-hospital cardiac arrest: a comparison between four regions in Norway. *Resuscitation.* 2003;56:247–263.
69. Bernard S, Buist M, Monteiro O, Smith K. Induced hypothermia using large volume, ice-cold intravenous fluid in comatose survivors of out-of hospital cardiac arrest: a preliminary report. *Resuscitation.* 2003;56:9–13.
70. Bernard S, Buist M, Monteiro O, Smith K. Induced hypothermia using large volume, ice-cold intravenous fluid in comatose survivors of out-of hospital cardiac arrest: a preliminary report. *Resuscitation.* 2003;56:9–13.
71. Lellouche F, Qader S, Taille S, et al. Under-humidification and over-humidification during moderate induced hypothermia with usual devices. *Intensive Care Med.* 2006;32:1014–1021.
72. Afolabi BA, Novaro GM, Pinski SL, et al. Use of the prehospital ECG improves door-to-balloon times in ST segment elevation myocardial infarction irrespective of time or day of week. *Emerg Med J.* 2007;24:588–591.
73. Afolabi BA, Novaro GM, Pinski SL, et al. Use of the prehospital ECG improves door-to-balloon times in ST segment elevation myocardial infarction irrespective of time or day of week. *Emerg Med J.* 2007;24:588–591.
74. Terkelsen CJ, Lassen JF, Norgaard BL, et al. Reduction of treatment delay in patients with ST-elevation myocardial infarction: impact of pre-hospital diagnosis and direct referral to primary percutaneous coronary intervention. *Eur Heart J.* 2005;26:770–777.
75. Dhruva VN, Abdelhadi SI, Anis A, et al. ST-segment analysis using wireless technology in acute myocardial infarction (STAT-MI) trials. *J Am Coll Cardiol.* 2007:50:509–513.
76. Morrison LJ et al. Part 3: Ethics: 2010 American Heart Association Guidelines for Cardiopulmonary Resuscitation and Emergency Cardiovascular Care. *Circulation.* 2010;122(Suppl 3):S665–S675.

CHAPTER

19

Mechanical Ventilators: Classification and Principles of Operation

Robert L. Chatburn, Teresa A. Volsko

OUTLINE

Basic Concepts
Understanding Ventilator Technology
Taxonomy of Mechanical Ventilation
Comparing Modes of Mechanical Ventilation

OBJECTIVES

1. Define a mechanical ventilator.
2. Differentiate between resuscitators and mechanical ventilators.
3. Describe the key design features of mechanical ventilators.
4. Describe how 10 maxims are used to develop a standardized ventilator taxonomy.
5. Describe the operating characteristics of mechanical ventilators used in the critical care, home care, and transport environments.
6. List four basic ways to present monitored data.
7. State the three main goals of mechanical ventilator support.

KEY TERMS

assisted breath
breath
continuous mandatory ventilation (CMV)
continuous spontaneous ventilation (CSV)
control system
cycle
elastic load
equation of motion
intermittent mandatory ventilation (IMV)
mandatory breath
mode
resistive load
spontaneous breath
synchronization window
trigger
trigger window
ventilator
ventilatory pattern

Introduction

Mechanical **ventilators** are more than simple machines designed to support the work of the respiratory system and improve or stabilize gas exchange.[1] These machines have evolved significantly over the past three decades and are now complex computers with sophisticated software and artificial intelligence. Their complex design and advanced monitoring capabilities make it possible to deliver mechanical breaths from conventional to high-frequency rates, monitor lung mechanics, and administer specialty gas therapy, such as heliox, nitric oxide, and subambient oxygen concentrations. Many types of ventilators are used along the continuum of care, from transport to critical care and home or long-term care settings.

There are a wide variety of **modes** of ventilation offered by these sophisticated machines. Some modes have similar names but function differently. Others have very different names and function similarly. It therefore is essential for the respiratory therapist to understand ventilator design and mode classification in order to safely and effectively match a ventilator's capability to the patient's physiologic need. This chapter presents mechanical ventilator terminology and mode classification along with the basic principles for ventilator design.

Basic Concepts

A ventilator is an automatic machine designed to provide all or part of the work required to ventilate or move gas into and out of the lungs. Ventilators are often confused with manual or mechanical resuscitators. Devices such as resuscitation bags or T-piece resuscitators (mechanical resuscitators used for infants) are used to assist breathing. These devices are not automatic, however, and require a clinician to supply the energy to either push gas into the lungs through the mouth and nose or control the direction of gas flow to the patient. Automating the ventilator requires three basic components:

1. A source of input energy to drive the device
2. A means of converting input energy into output energy in the form of pressure and flow waveforms to control the timing and size of **breaths**
3. A means of monitoring the output performance of the device and the condition of the patient

Today, ventilators are incredibly complex mechanical devices controlled by multiple microprocessors running sophisticated software. All tasks but the most rudimentary maintenance of ventilators is now the responsibility of specially trained biomedical engineers. Because the design of ventilators has changed, the approach to describing ventilator design has changed as well. Rather than focusing on descriptions of individual components (valves, pistons, circuits, etc.), attention now shifts to a more generalized model of a ventilator as a black box, a device for which the clinician supplies an input and expects a certain output.[2] The reason for this change is that the internal operations of the ventilator have become so complex that they are now largely unknowable and unimportant to most clinicians. Here only a brief overview of the key design features of mechanical ventilators is presented with an emphasis on input power requirements, transfer functions (pneumatic and electronic **control systems**), and outputs (pressure, volume, and flow waveforms). Interactions between the operator and the ventilator (the operator interface) and various types of ventilator output displays are also discussed.

This brief introduction to ventilator design will enable the respiratory therapist to concentrate on the interaction between the ventilator and the patient. Ultimately, the application of mechanical ventilation involves selecting a mode of ventilation. The term "mode of ventilation" means a preset pattern of interaction between the ventilator and the patient. The word *mode* and many other words associated with mechanical ventilation, however, are used without definition and often in illogical ways both in the research literature and in ventilator operator manuals. To understand the technology and terminology associated with modes, 10 basic concepts are explained, starting with how a breath is defined and ending with a classification system for modes of ventilation.

> **Respiratory Recap**
>
> **A Ventilator**
>
> - Has input power
> - Can convert input energy into output energy
> - Is able to monitor the output performance of the device and the condition of the patient

Power Inputs

The input power for ventilators comes from electricity or compressed gas. Electricity comes either from wall outlets (e.g., 100 to 240 volts A/C, at 50/60 Hz) or from batteries (e.g., 10 to 30 volts DC) and is used to run compressors or blowers of various types. Batteries are a common power source for patient transport or emergency backup when electrical power failures occur in the hospital or the home. The length of time the internal or external battery source will provide power to the ventilator varies. In an evaluation of portable ventilators used for mechanical ventilatory support in the home, Blakeman et al. found a significant difference in the battery duration among the ventilators tested. The type of drive mechanism and type of battery (lithium ion, nickel metal hydride, lead/acid batteries) made a difference in battery duration, which ranged from 1.8 to 9.4 hours.[3] Lithium ion and nickel metal hydride batteries were smaller, lighter, had a higher power for a given size, and shorter charging time than lead/acid batteries. Battery duration may also be affected by ventilator settings (pressure vs. volume control) and the patient's pulmonary characteristics. The literature supports that an increased patient load (high airways resistance, and/or low lung compliance) coupled with the use of PEEP, delivery of high concentrations of oxygen, and use of pressure control modes of ventilation may significantly shorten the expected battery life.[4]

Alternatively, the power to expand the lungs is supplied by compressed gas from tanks, electric compressors (i.e., air compressor), or wall outlets in the hospital (e.g., 30 to 80 pounds per square inch, psi). Some transport and emergency ventilators use compressed gas to power both lung inflation and the control circuitry. When this type of ventilator is used, knowledge of gas consumption is critical because the compressed gas source will be limited by what is supplied in the cylinders. Depending on the type of transport, the size of the cylinder (i.e., E, M, etc.) and the number of cylinders are limited. More stringent restrictions exist for the number of a particular size of cylinders used for air medical transport than ground transport. The total weight of the patient, clinical crew, and equipment must be taken into consideration before a medical air transport occurs, which may put additional restrictions on compressed gas resources. Because the supply of gas is limited, the respiratory therapist must be able to calculate the compressed gas needs to make sure the gas supply in the cylinders does not deplete and cause a mechanical ventilator failure during the patient transport.

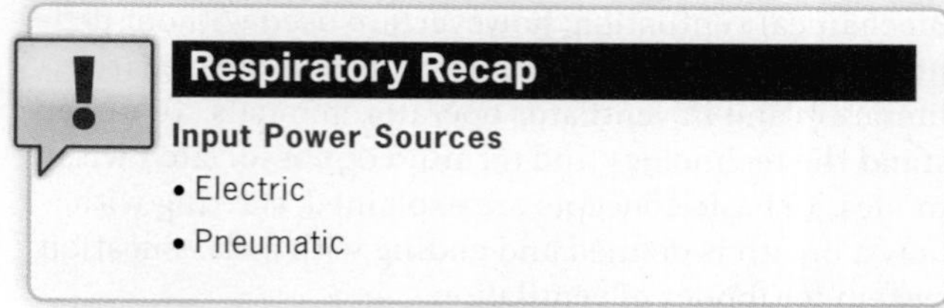

Respiratory Recap

Input Power Sources

- Electric
- Pneumatic

Ventilators used in the critical care setting are powered by separate sources of compressed air and compressed oxygen. This permits the delivery of a range of oxygen concentrations to support the needs of sick patients. Ventilators operated by pressurized gas typically have internal reducing regulators so the normal operating pressure (e.g., 20 psi) is lower than the source gas pressure (50 psi). This feature permits uninterrupted operation from piped gas sources that are subject to periodic fluctuations. Because compressed air and oxygen are in abundant supply in the hospital setting, ventilators used in the intensive care unit (ICU) are designed to use the energy stored in pressurized gas to drive flow but depend on electrical energy to power their computerized control mechanisms. As with portable ventilators, some ICU ventilators have internal batteries that will function for a limited amount of time during interruptions in electrical power. It is also important to note that compressed gas has all moisture removed; the gas delivered to the patient must be warmed and humidified in order to avoid drying out the lung tissue.

Conversion Subsystems

Input power must be converted to get the desired outputs of pressure, volume, and flow. Electrically powered ventilators use a compressor or blower to generate the required pressure and flow. A compressor is a machine for moving a relatively low flow of gas at ambient pressure to a storage container at a higher level of pressure (e.g., 20 psi). Compressors are generally found on intensive care ventilators. A blower is a machine for generating relatively larger flows of gas as the direct ventilator output (rather than filling a storage container) with a relatively moderate increase of pressure (e.g., 2 psi). Blowers are incorporated into portable ventilators used in the home and/or long-term care setting or for transport. Blowers are smaller and typically consume less electrical power than compressors, making them more suitable for portable ventilation devices.

Flow Control Valves

Ventilators use different kinds of flow control valves to manipulate the flow of gas from the ventilator to the patient. The simplest valve is a fixed orifice flow resistor that permits setting a constant flow to the external tubing that conducts the gas to the patient, called the *patient circuit*. Manually adjusted variable orifice flow meters allow the clinician to set constant flows in a range of values. This provides a simple means, for example, of adjusting inspired volume during assisted ventilation. Fixed and adjustable flow valves are used in some transport ventilators and resuscitation devices. Inexpensive microprocessors became available in the 1980s and led to development of digital control of flow valves (**Figure 19-1**), which are now used in most of the current generation of intensive care ventilators. Digital control allows

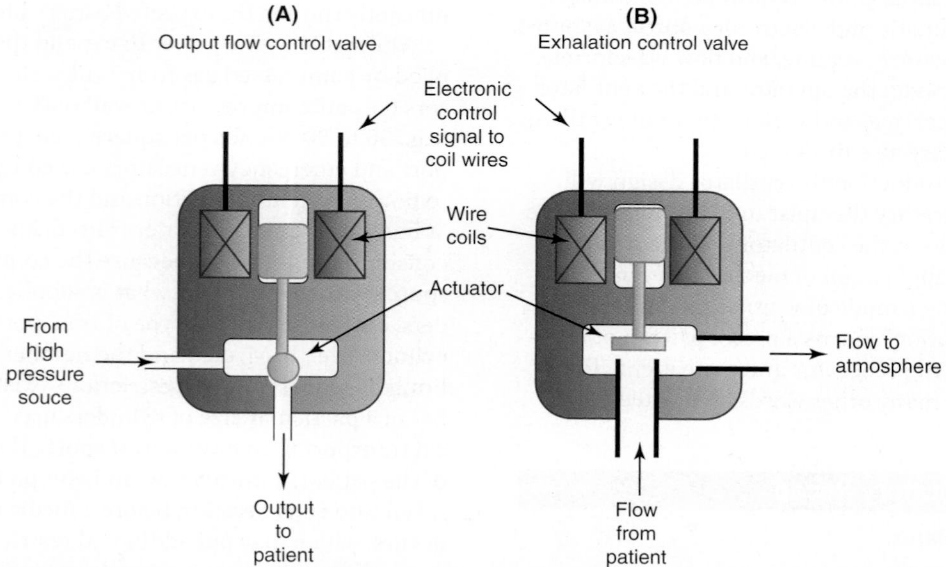

FIGURE 19-1 (**A**) Simplified schematic of a general flow control valve. Such a valve is controlled by an electronic signal (usually a digital signal from a microcontroller). The signal energizes electrical coils comprising an electro magnet that moves the actuator. The movement of the actuator changes the diameter of the flow path from a high-pressure source (e.g., air or oxygen) and thereby changes the flow waveform. (**B**) Simplified schematic of a general exhalation valve. The valve is controlled by an electronic signal as with the flow control valve. The movement of the actuator changes the diameter of the flow path from the patient's lungs and thereby allows exhalation and also the control of PEEP.

flexibility in shaping the ventilator's output pressure, volume, and flow.[5]

Delivering flow to the patient requires the coordination of the output flow control valve and an expiratory valve or exhalation manifold. When inspiration is triggered, the output control valve opens (allowing flow from the source), the expiratory valve closes (so the gas does not escape to the atmosphere), and the gas is delivered through the only path left into the patient. When inspiration is cycled off, the output valve closes and flow from the ventilator ceases. At the same time, the exhalation valve opens and the patient exhales out through the expiratory valve (Figure 19-1). The exhalation valve also controls the level of positive end-expiratory pressure (PEEP). The most sophisticated ventilators employ a complex interaction between the output flow control valve and the exhalation valve such that many different pressure, volume, and flow waveforms may be generated to promote patient safety and comfort.

Control Systems

A ventilator's control system generates the signals that operate the output valve and the exhalation manifold. Control systems may be based on mechanical, pneumatic, fluidic, or electronic components. Mechanical components include levers, pulleys, cams, etc.[6] Pneumatic control circuits use gas pressure to operate diaphragms, jet entrainment devices, pistons, etc. Fluidic circuits are like electronic logic circuits, but they operate with gas instead of electricity.[7] Both pneumatic and fluidic control systems are unaffected by electromagnetic interference. Ventilators that use this type of control system are safe to use in close proximity to magnetic resonance imaging equipment.[8] Most ventilators, however, use electronic control circuits with microprocessors and complex software algorithms to manage monitoring (e.g., from pressure and flow sensors) and control functions.

The differences among ventilators are due to the control system software as much as to the hardware. Software determines mode capabilities, which influence how the ventilator interacts with the patient. The description of ventilator control systems is essentially a discussion about mode capabilities and classifications. But in order to understand modes, discussing some fundamental concepts beyond the constructs of input and output is important.

Pressure, Volume, and Flow Outputs

The outputs of a mechanical ventilator are the pressure, volume, and flow waveforms it generates in supporting the patient's work of breathing along with measured or calculated data it generates and displays to the operator. The best way to begin to learn this subject is to use idealized waveforms or waveforms that would exist in an ideal world with perfect machines and no interferences from leaks or patient breathing efforts. Such waveforms can be generated for educational purposes by using graphs of mathematical models. An understanding of idealized waveforms can help you interpret waveforms displayed on ventilators in the clinical setting.

Idealized Pressure, Volume, and Flow Waveforms

Many ventilators allow the display of pressure, volume, and flow waveforms. Some limit the number of waveforms that can be displayed at a time. If only two waveforms are available for display at a time, the pressure and flow waveforms usually provide the most useful information. By convention, the horizontal axis is time for pressure, volume, and flow waveforms. The vertical axis displays either pressure, volume, or flow in appropriate units (e.g., cm H_2O, mL, and L/min). When interpreting waveforms, it is important to pay attention to the relative magnitudes of each of the variables and evaluate how the value of one affects or is affected by the values of the others.

Typical waveforms available on modern ventilators are illustrated in **Figure 19-2**. The waveforms displayed in this figure are idealized, meaning that they were generated by mathematical equations and are meant to characterize the operation of the ventilator's control system. They do not show the minor deviations, or noise, often seen during actual ventilator use. This noise can be caused by extraneous factors such as vibration and flow turbulence. Of course, scaling of the horizontal and vertical axes can affect the appearance of actual waveforms considerably. Interferences from leaks, vibrations, flow turbulence, or patient-breathing efforts can also affect the shape of the waveform and make waveform interpretation more difficult.

Patient Circuits

The patient circuit is the tubing that connects the ventilator to the patient. There is an endless diversity of circuits but only three basic configurations (**Figure 19-3**). Some portable ventilators use only one tube, called a single limb circuit (Figure 19-3 top). Near the end that connects to the patient, there is a pneumatically controlled exhalation valve in line with the flow to the patient. The exhalation valve is switched on and off by a pressure signal from the ventilator, conveyed through small-bore tubing. When the pressure signal goes high, the valve closes and flow is directed from the ventilator to the patient. When the pressure signal goes low, the valve opens and the patient exhales to the atmosphere. Often there is a residual pressure in the valve that sets the PEEP level.

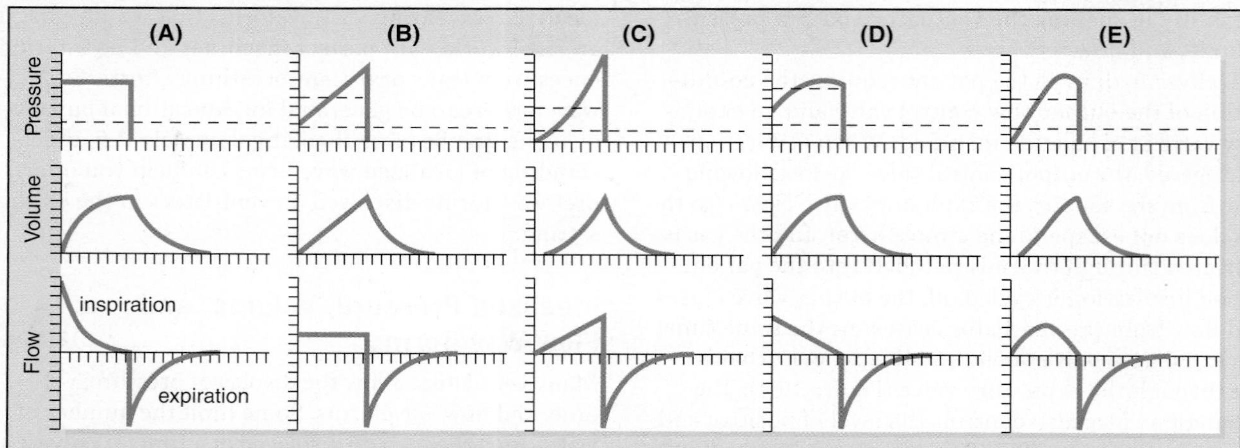

FIGURE 19-2 Idealized ventilator output waveforms. (**A**) Pressure-controlled inspiration with a rectangular pressure waveform. (**B**) Volume-controlled inspiration with a rectangular flow waveform. (**C**) Volume-controlled inspiration with an ascending-ramp flow waveform. (**D**) Volume-controlled inspiration with a descending-ramp flow waveform. (**E**) Volume-controlled inspiration with a sinusoidal flow waveform. The short dashed lines represent mean inspiratory pressure, and the long dashed lines represent mean pressure for the complete respiratory cycle (i.e., mean airway pressure). Note that mean inspiratory pressure is the same as the pressure limit in A. These waveforms were created as follows: (1) defining the control waveform using a mathematical equation (e.g., an ascending-ramp flow waveform is specified as Flow = Constant × Time), (2) specifying the tidal volume for flow- and volume-control waveforms, (3) specifying the resistance and compliance, (4) substituting the preceding information into the equation of motion for the respiratory system, and (5) using a computer to solve the equation for the unknown variables and plotting the results against time.

Reproduced from Chatburn RL. *Fundamentals of Mechanical Ventilation*. Cleveland Heights,Ohio: Mandu Press Ltd., 2003:143.

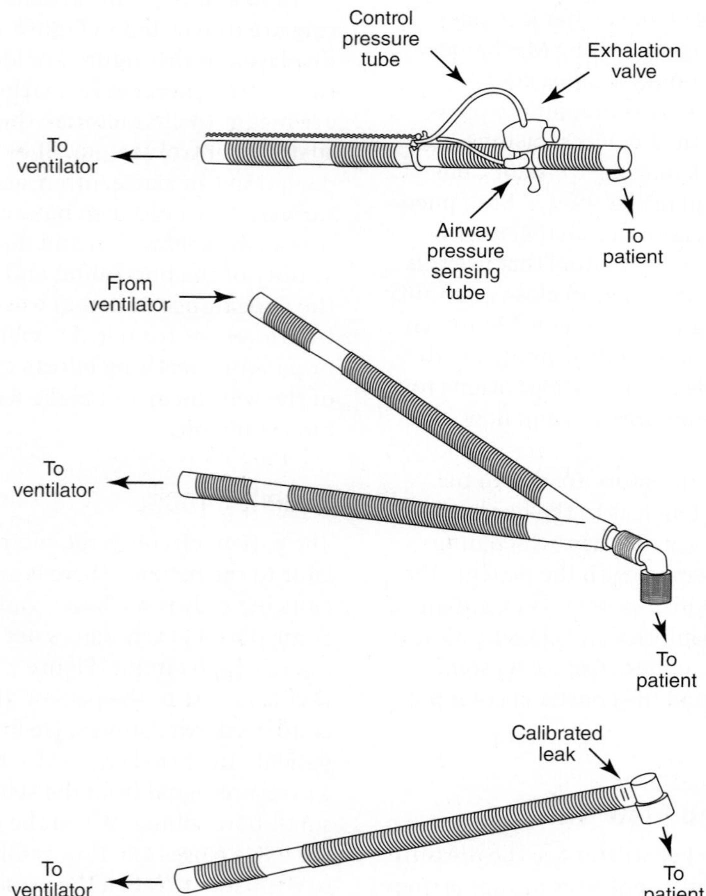

FIGURE 19-3 Three basic types of patient circuit. **Top:** Single-limb circuit with exhalation valve often used on home care or transport ventilators. **Middle:** Double-limb circuit usually used on intensive care ventilators. **Bottom:** Single-limb circuit without exhalation valve used on noninvasive ventilators.

Most intensive care ventilators have the exhalation valve built into the ventilator and are connected to the patient with a double-limb circuit (Figure 19-3 middle). Ventilators designed for noninvasive ventilation, using a mask instead of an artificial airway, often have single-limb circuits that are used without an exhalation valve (Figure 19-3 bottom). The circuit may have a small fitting that has a carefully sized opening or port. The port provides a known leak and the relationship between circuit pressure and leak flow is programmed into the ventilator's microcontroller. By measuring the pressure in the circuit, calculating the leak flow, and deducting that from the total flow delivered by the blower, the ventilator thus can estimate the flow and hence volume delivered to the patient. Sometimes the leak port is in the mask instead of the patient circuit.

Some intensive care ventilators measure flow at the airway opening using a small, usually disposable sensor. There are two basic types of flow sensors used with ventilators. One is called a pneumotachometer (**Figure 19-4**). It has a flow resistive element such as a screen or plastic flap in the flow path. The pressure on both sides of the resistor is conducted to pressure sensors in the ventilator through small diameter tubing. The difference between the two pressures is proportional to flow. The second type of flow sensor is called a hot wire anemometer. Very thin wires are placed in the flow path and heated. The flow carries away the heat. The amount of energy required to maintain the heat in the wires therefore is proportional to flow.

Some ventilator manufacturers require the use of a proprietary circuit, or one that is manufactured specifically for use with a particular ventilator. This is most commonly seen with portable ventilators. The ventilator's operator manual will provide useful information regarding not only the circuit type but the need for a proprietary circuit. Although the circuit configuration may make it extremely difficult to use the wrong type, it is important to note that ventilator malfunction may occur if the wrong type of circuit configuration is used.

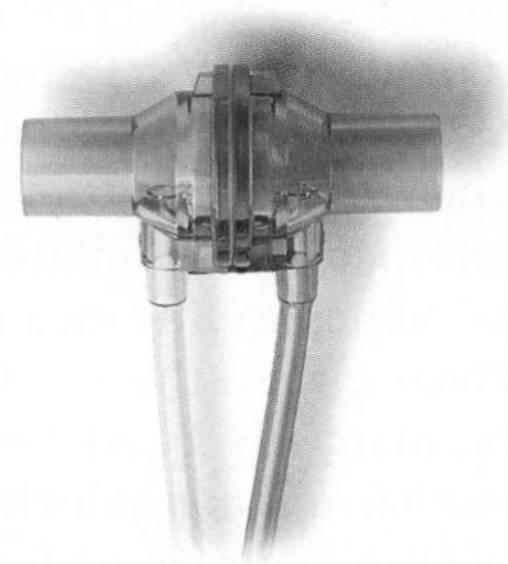

FIGURE 19-4 Example of a disposable flow sensor (pneumotachometer) that uses the pressure difference across a flow resistive element to generate a signal proportional to flow.
Courtesy of Hamilton Medical.

Ventilator Alarm Systems

Ventilator alarms have increased in number and complexity. There is no generally agreed upon classification system for alarms, but MacIntyre and Branson[9] have proposed that alarms be categorized by the events that they are designed to detect (**Table 19-1**). Level 1 events include life-threatening situations.

TABLE 19-1
A Hierarchical Classification of Ventilator Alarms Based on the Significance of the Event Triggering and Audible and Visual Signals

Alarm Level	Description	Examples of Alarm Triggers	Alarm Characteristics
Level 1	Life-threatening situations	Loss of input power Ventilator malfunction that would provide excessive or no flow of gas to the patient	Mandatory Redundant Noncanceling
Level 2	Significant and may contribute to life-threatening situations	Blender failure High and low airway pressure I:E ratio	Self-canceling
Level 3	Changes in patient condition that influence ventilator function or ventilatory support requirements	High respiratory rate	Self-canceling
Level 4	Changes in patient condition as detected by noninvasive monitors	High or low heart rate, respiratory rate, or blood pressure detected by a cardiorespiratory monitor High or low Sp_{O_2} High or low P_{ETCO_2}	Self-canceling

The alarms in this category are critical and necessitate immediate attention by the respiratory therapist. Alarms at this level should be mandatory, noncanceling, and redundant, using multiple sensors and circuits to prevent inadvertent failure of the audible and visual alarm. Noncanceling means the alarm continues to activate even if the event has corrected and must be reset manually. Level 2 events can lead to significant patient harm if not quickly corrected. They may also warn of suspicious ventilator settings such as an I:E ratio greater than 1:1, or autotriggering though a high respiratory rate alarm. High-pressure alarms may alert clinicians to occlusions in the ventilator circuit or tracheal tube. Low-pressure alarms may signify a disruption in the circuit integrity from a disconnection or leak (crack in the circuit or humidifier chamber). Alarms for level 2 events may be self-canceling, meaning that the alarm is automatically inactivated if the event ceases to occur. Level 3 events are those that may influence the level of support provided such as changes in patient lung mechanics, changes in patient respiratory drive, and autoPEEP. Alarm performance at this level is similar to that of level 2 alarms. Level 4 events reflect the patient condition alone rather than ventilator function. Stand-alone monitors such as oximeters and cardiac monitors usually detect these events. Alarm performance at this level is also similar to that of level 2 alarms. As ventilators have become more sophisticated, they have incorporated some stand-alone monitor functionality, such as esophageal pressure monitoring, pulse oximetry, and volumetric or end-tidal carbon dioxide monitoring.

Ventilator Displays

Display Types

Ventilator output displays have also advanced tremendously in the last 30 years, evolving from simple lights and dials to digital readouts, to full graphic user interfaces with touch screens. There are four basic ways to present the monitored data: as alphanumeric values (numbers or text), waveforms, trend lines, and in the form of abstract graphic symbols.

Alphanumeric Values

Measured or calculated data are most commonly represented as numeric values such as F_{IO_2}, peak, plateau, mean, and baseline airway pressures, inhaled/exhaled tidal volume, minute ventilation, and frequency. Depending on the ventilator, a wide range of calculated parameters may also be displayed, including resistance, compliance, time constant, percent leak, I:E ratio, and peak inspiratory/expiratory flow, to name just a few. Text messages are now common on ventilator displays. They are used for explaining alarm conditions and also for giving brief instructions to the operator about settings. An example of an alphanumeric ventilator display is shown in **Figure 19-5**.

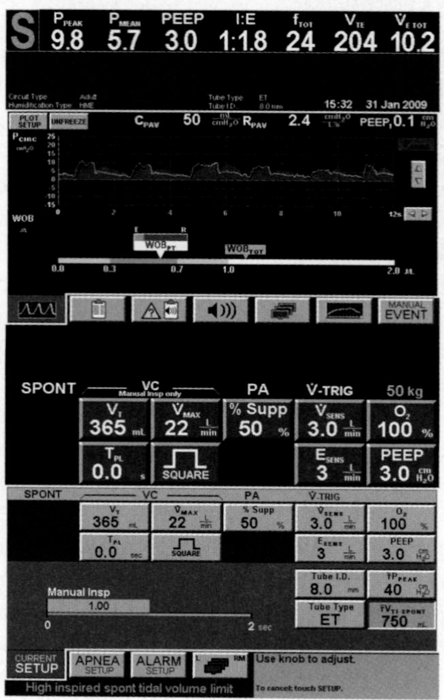

FIGURE 19-5 Example of an alphanumeric ventilator screen display.

Trends

The basic display of all ventilators shows the current state of the device. Clinicians are often interested in how parameters related to mechanical support change over time, however. Many ventilators provide trend graphs of just about any parameter that can be measured or calculated. These graphs show how the monitored parameters change over long periods of time (**Figure 19-6**). Significant events or gradual changes in patient condition can be easily identified. In addition, ventilators often provide an alarm log. This is usually a text-based list documenting such things as the date, time, alarm type, urgency level, and events associated with alarms, including when activated and when canceled. Such a log could be invaluable in the event of a ventilator failure and may be used as evidence in a legal investigation if a patient harm occurred.

Waveforms and Loops

Most ventilators display graphical depictions of pressure, volume, and flow waveforms. These waveforms are quite useful for adjusting ventilator settings or evaluating respiratory system mechanics.[10,11] They are essential for assessing sources of patient–ventilator asynchrony, such as missed triggers, flow asynchrony,

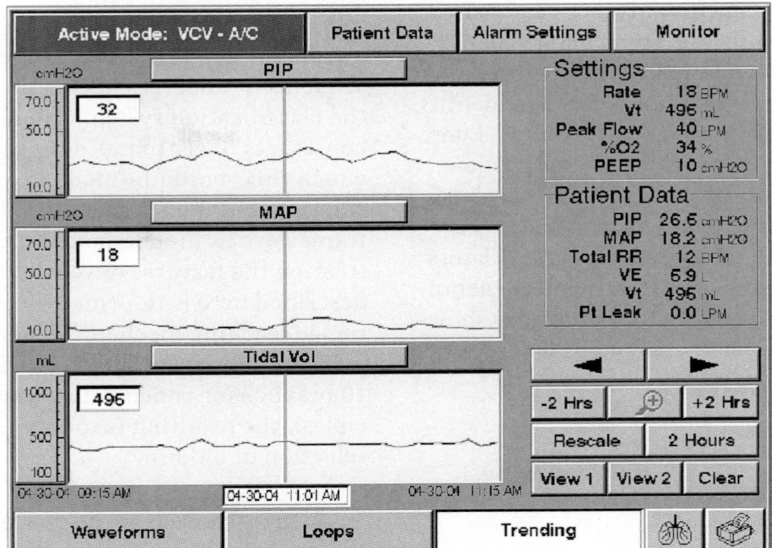

FIGURE 19-6 Example of a ventilator trend display.

Reproduced with permission from Philips Healthcare.

and delayed/premature cycling, and making appropriate corrections.[12] Sometimes it is more useful to plot one variable against another as an x-y or loop display. Pressure–volume loop displays (i.e., Paw–V displayed on the top left-hand corner of **Figure 19-7**) are useful for identifying optimum PEEP levels (to avoid atelectrauma) and optimum tidal volume (to avoid volutrauma).[13] Ideally, loop displays for such usage should be made with patients who are paralyzed or heavily sedated (to avoid errors due to patient effort effects) and with very slow inflations (i.e., quasistatic curve). Caution must be exercised because ventilators display

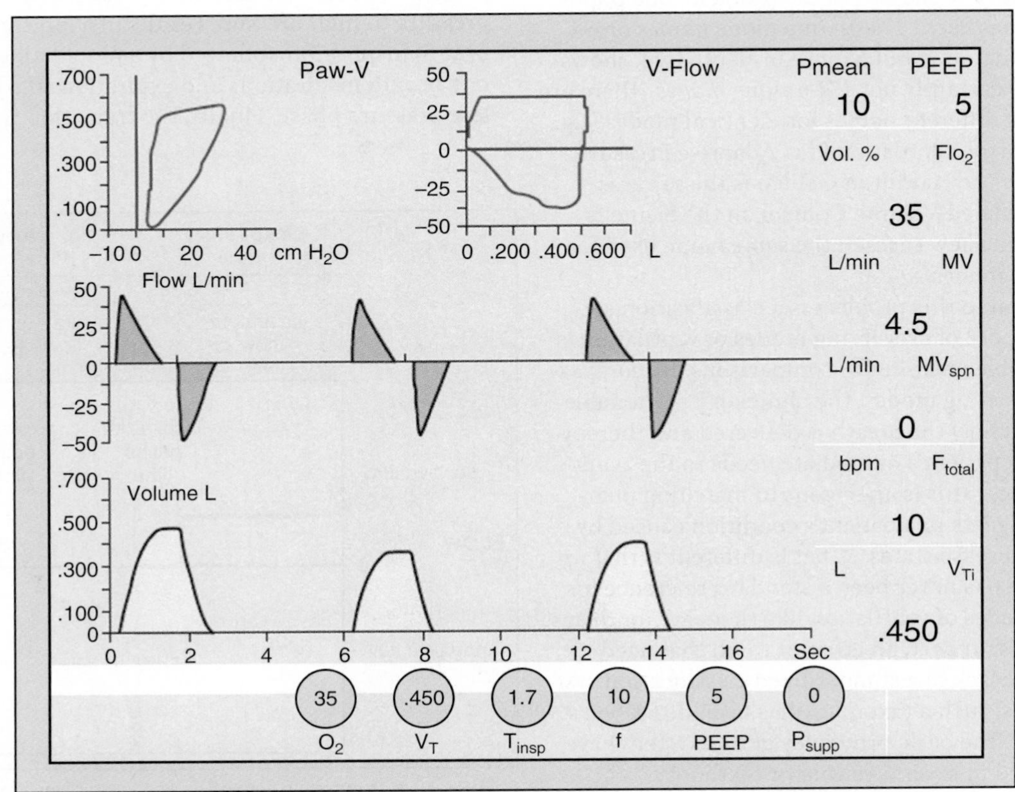

FIGURE 19-7 Example of a ventilator display with alphanumeric, waveform, and loop displays.

Reproduced with permission from Mandu Press Ltd., Cleveland, OH.

loops under any ventilating circumstances and hence the display may be meaningless. For example, loop displays for pressure control modes (with relatively square pressure waveforms) cannot be used to identify either optimum PEEP or optimum tidal volume. Loop displays for volume control modes (with square flow waveforms) can show overdistention and so may be used to adjust tidal volume. Flow–volume loops are useful for identifying the response to bronchodilators (i.e., V-Flow displayed on the top right-hand corner of Figure 19-7). An example of a composite display showing numeric values, waveforms, and loops is shown in Figure 19-7.

Understanding Ventilator Technology

Ventilator manufacturers provide resource materials for clinicians, such as operator manuals. But manuals are often wrought with detail and cumbersome to read. In contrast, manufacturer's specification sheets do not provide sufficient detail and often skim over important elements of ventilator function. There is an even bigger problem, however, as there is no standardization in either vocabulary or format among manuals created by different manufacturers. This makes comparison of modes among different ventilators very difficult.

To get an idea of the size of the problem, one popular textbook has listed 174 unique mode *names* on 34 different ventilators.[14] But a more in-depth look shows that there are certainly not 174 unique *modes*. There are many cases of different names for identical modes (e.g., Pressure-Control Ventilation Plus Adaptive Pressure Ventilation on the Hamilton Galileo is the same as Pressure Regulated Volume Control on the Siemens Servo 300) and a few cases of the same name used for very different modes.

The solution to this problem is a classification system. The purpose of classifying modes of ventilation is to make possible meaningful comparisons. By comparing and contrasting modes, the clinician is better able to understand how the breath is delivered and thereby match a given patient's immediate needs to the available technology. This is analogous to matching pharmacological agents to a patient's condition caused by one or more disease states. What is different is that up till now, there has never been a standard reference for classifying modes of ventilation like there are for drugs. This chapter is, in part, an attempt to fill that need.

Despite the lack of a standardized classification system for modes, such a taxonomy has been described previously.[15,16] The basic principles of this system have been described in several ventilator textbooks.[17–20] What has been lacking, up till now, is a systematic approach for teaching ventilator technology. This section provides the basic structure for such a system.

Ten Fundamental Maxims

Taxonomy can be viewed as the last step in a sequence of theoretical constructs that comprise the classification system. There are 10 fundamental constructs of ventilator design and function upon which this ventilator mode taxonomy is based. These concepts build on one another to yield a practical framework for understanding, comparing, and contrasting the features of ventilators. The approach described here is informed by over 30 years of experience teaching mechanical ventilation and the data from an international survey.[21] After describing these 10 maxims (or concise statements of scientific principles), the resulting taxonomy is applied to guide the selection of modes.

1. A breath is one cycle of positive flow (inspiration) and negative flow (expiration) defined in terms of the flow–time curve.

The most basic function of a ventilator is to deliver a breath. The most basic definition of a breath is one **cycle** of inspiratory flow followed by a matching expiratory flow (**Figure 19-8**). These flows are paired by size, meaning approximately equal inspiratory and expiratory volumes. For some modes of ventilation, inspiration is not necessarily followed immediately by the matching expiration. For example, during airway pressure release ventilation, the transition from low pressure to high pressure results in a large **mandatory breath** inspiration, followed by a few small **spontaneous breath** inspirations and expirations during the low-pressure phase. Finally, the transition from high

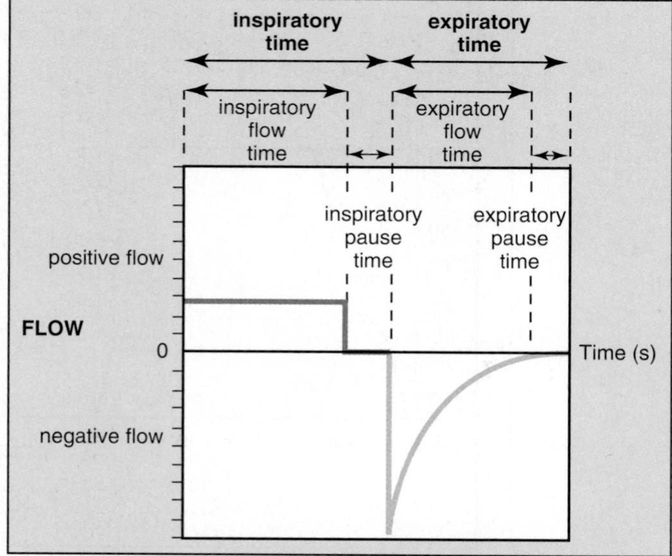

FIGURE 19-8 A breath is defined as one cycle of inspiratory flow followed by a matching expiratory flow, yielding approximately the same volumes.
Courtesy of Mandu Press Ltd.

pressure to low pressure results in the matching mandatory exhalation. It is also possible to have many small mandatory breaths superimposed on larger spontaneous breaths, as seen during high-frequency oscillatory ventilation.

The two most basic definitions in reference to a breath are inspiratory time and expiratory time. Inspiratory time is the period from the start of inspiratory flow to the start of expiratory flow. Inspiratory time equals inspiratory flow time plus inspiratory hold time. Inspiratory hold time (pause time) is the period from the cessation of inspiratory flow (into the airway opening) to the start of expiratory flow during mechanical ventilation. On some ventilators, inspiratory hold time is set directly. On others, hold time is the difference between the preset inspiratory time and the inspiratory flow time due to the preset tidal volume at the preset inspiratory flow (i.e., Inspiratory flow time = Tidal volume/Inspiratory flow). Inspiratory hold time is often used to increase mean airway pressure and improve oxygenation or to create a static airway pressure (called plateau pressure). During an inspiratory pause, flow of gas to and from the patient ceases, and the pressure displayed during the inspiratory pause or plateau pressure is used to calculate respiratory system resistance and compliance. Expiratory time is the period from the start of expiratory flow to the start of inspiratory flow. Figure 19-8 is the basis for several mathematical equations relevant to ventilator settings (**Table 19-2**).

TABLE 19-2
Equations for Breath Timing

Parameter	Symbol	
Volume (L)	V	
Flow (L/min)	$\dot{V}$	
Time (s)	t	
Frequency (breaths/min)	f	
Parameter	**Symbol**	**Equation**
Inspiratory time (s)	T_I	$(60/f)-T_E$ or $(60 \times I)/[f \times (I+E)]$
Expiratory time (s)	T_E	$(60/f)-T_I$ or $(60 \times E)/[f \times (I+E)]$
Total cycle time or period (s)	T_{TOT}	$T_I + T_E$ or $60/f$
Inspiratory to expiratory time ratio	I:E	T_I: T_E or $D/(100\% - D)$
Duty cycle (%)	D	$(T_I/T_{tot}) \times 100\%$ or $100\% \times I/(I + E)$
Mean inspiratory flow	$\bar{\dot{V}}_I$	V_T/T_I
Tidal volume	V_T	$\bar{\dot{V}} \times T_I$

Courtesy of Mandu Press Ltd.

2. A breath is assisted if the ventilator provides some or all of the work of breathing.

The main purpose of a ventilator is to assist with the patient's work of breathing. Work is a function of the pressure necessary to deliver the tidal volume to the respiratory system. Pressure is generated either by patient's inspiratory muscles (Pmus) or the ventilator (Pvent). Either way, there is an increase in the pressure difference across the respiratory system that is termed inspiratory pressure.[22] During inspiration, volume increases. An **assisted breath** can be recognized on a ventilator graphic display by examining the pressure waveform during inspiration. During an assisted breath, there is a positive change in flow (as defined in maxim #1), and airway pressure rises above baseline (end-expiratory pressure). If airway pressure falls below baseline pressure during inspiration, the patient is doing some work on the ventilator and the breath is termed loaded rather than assisted. Some loading is unavoidable because ventilators cannot control airway pressure perfectly; some pressure drop is necessary for triggering a breath, and there are electrical/mechanical delays between sensing a patient effort and the start of inspiratory flow.[12]

3. A ventilator assists breathing using either pressure control or volume control based on the equation of motion for the respiratory system.

A ventilator provides assistance either by maintaining a desired waveform for inspiratory pressure (called *pressure control*) or inspiratory flow (called *volume control*). The theoretical foundation for this assertion is a mathematical model of patient–ventilator interaction known as the **equation of motion** for the respiratory system (**Figure 19-9**):[23]

$$\text{Pvent}(t) = EV(t) + R\dot{V}(t) \quad (1)$$

where Pvent(t) is inspiratory pressure generated by the ventilator as a function of time (see #2 above), E is the

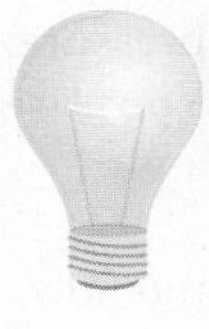

STOP AND THINK

Use the equation of motion to describe how the tidal volume can increase or decrease with pressure-controlled ventilation. Now use the equation of motion to describe how the airway pressure can increase or decrease during volume-controlled ventilation.

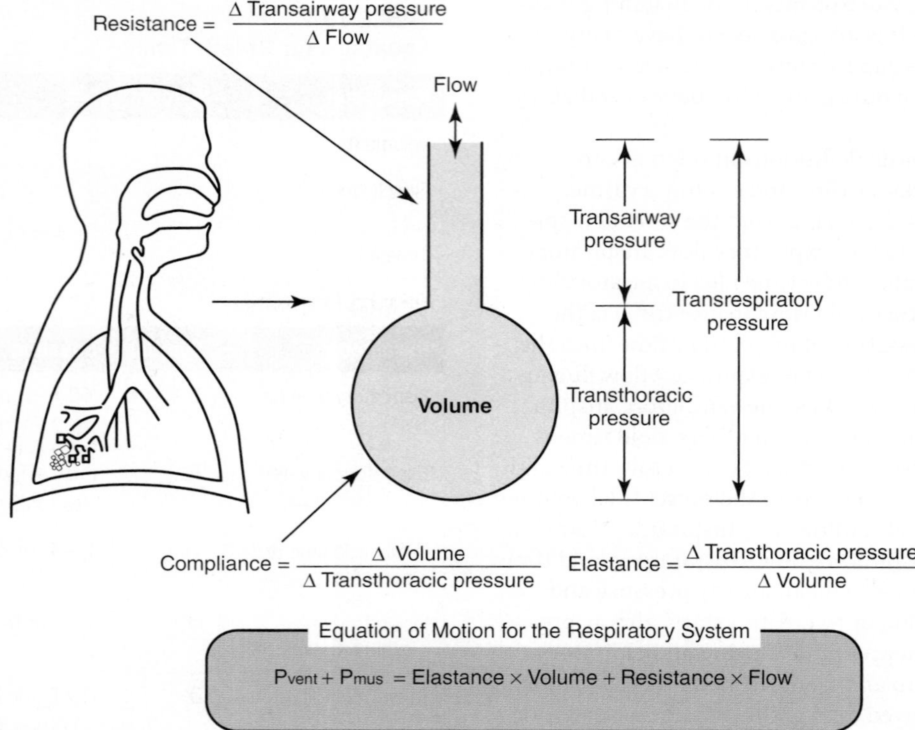

FIGURE 19-9 The study of the respiratory system mechanics is based on graphical and mathematical models. The respiratory system can be modeled as a single flow-conducting tube connected to a single elastic compartment. This physical model can be described as a mathematical model called the equation of motion for the respiratory system, where pressure, volume, and flow are variables (i.e., functions of time) while resistance and compliance are constants.

elastance of the respiratory system (lungs and chest wall), V(t) is volume as a function of time, R is respiratory-system resistance, $\dot{V}(t)$ is flow as a function of time. *Note that all these variables are measured relative to their end-expiratory values.* Under normal circumstances these values are Pvent = set PEEP, V = end-expiratory lung volume (functional residual capacity if PEEP = 0), and $\dot{V} = 0$.

In the Equation of Motion, the term EV(t) has the units of pressure and is called the ***elastic load.*** The term $R\dot{V}(t)$ also has the units of pressure and is called the ***resistive load.*** Hence, the term "breath unloading" means that the ventilator supplies some portion of the work to deliver volume and flow against these loads.

A plot of Pvent(t) versus time gives the airway pressure waveform seen on ventilator displays. If the shape of this waveform is predetermined by the ventilator settings and not affected by resistance and compliance, the ventilator is providing pressure control (PC). One very confusing issue with PC is that sometimes the operator sets the magnitude of the pressure waveform relative to atmospheric pressure (called peak inspiratory pressure) and other times the magnitude is set relative to positive end-expiratory pressure (PEEP), in this case simply termed "inspiratory pressure."[24]

A plot of the V(t) and $\dot{V}(t)$ yields the volume and flow waveforms. If the shape of these waveforms is predetermined by the ventilator settings and not affected by resistance and compliance, the ventilator is providing volume control (VC). Note that direct control of the flow waveform (e.g., with a flow control valve) implies indirect control of volume because volume is the integral of flow with respect to time. It is also true that direct control of the volume waveform (e.g., with a piston) implies indirect control of flow because flow is the derivative of volume with respect to time. For historical reasons, the term "volume control" is used rather than "flow control."

In summary:

- *Volume control* means that *both* volume and flow are preset prior to inspiration. Setting tidal volume is a necessary but not sufficient criterion for declaring volume control because some modes of pressure control allow the operator to set a *target* tidal volume but allow the ventilator to determine the flow (see adaptive targeting schemes below). Similarly, setting flow is also a necessary but not sufficient criterion; some pressure control modes allow the operator to set the maximum inspiratory flow but the tidal volume depends on the inspiratory pressure target and respiratory system mechanics. In a passive patient, after setting the form of the flow function (i.e., the flow and volume waveforms), the airway pressure waveform depends on *E* (respiratory-system elastance) and *R* (respiratory-system resistance).
- *Pressure control* means that inspiratory pressure as a function of time is predetermined. In practice, this currently means presetting a particular

waveform, for example, P(t) = constant, or inspiratory pressure is set to be proportional to patient inspiratory effort, measured by various means. For example, P(t) = NAVA level × EAdi(t), where NAVA stands for neurally adjusted ventilatory assist and EAdi stands for electrical activity of the diaphragm; see the Servo targeting scheme below. In a passive patient, after setting the form of the pressure function (i.e., the waveform), volume and flow depend on E (respiratory-system elastance) and R (respiratory-system resistance).
- *Time control* (TC) is a general category of ventilator modes for which inspiratory flow, inspiratory volume, and inspiratory pressure are all dependent on respiratory system mechanics. As no parameters of the pressure, volume, or flow waveforms are preset, the only control of the breath is the timing, i.e., inspiratory and expiratory times. Examples of this are high-frequency oscillatory ventilation (CareFusion 3100 ventilator) and Volumetric Diffusive Respiration (Percussionaire).

The algorithm for determining the control variable for a given mode of ventilation is shown in **Figure 19-10**. Common pressure, volume, and flow waveforms produced by ventilators are shown in Figure 19-2. **Figure 19-11**

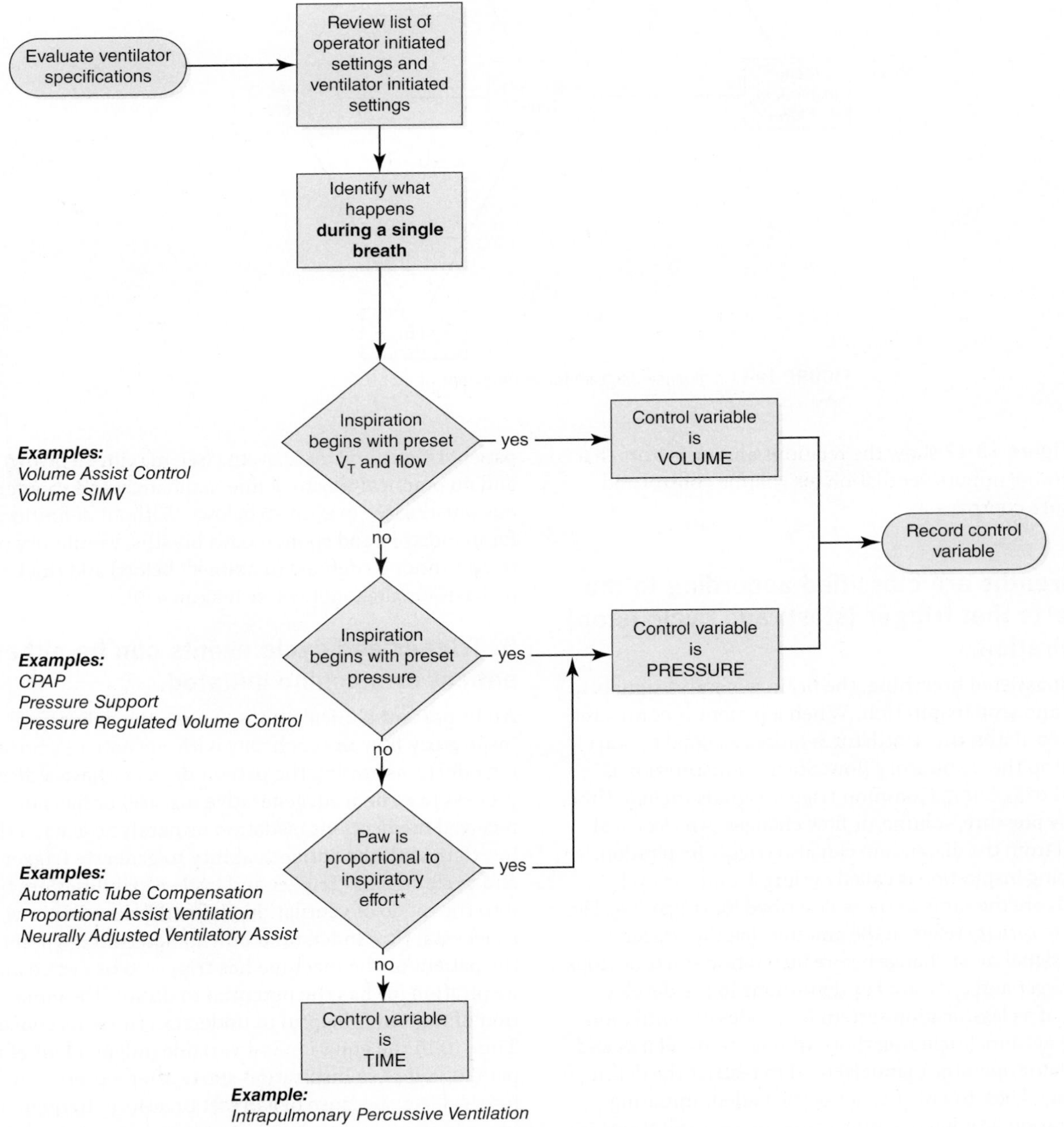

FIGURE 19-10 Algorithm for determining the control variable of a mode.
Courtesy of Mandu Press Ltd.

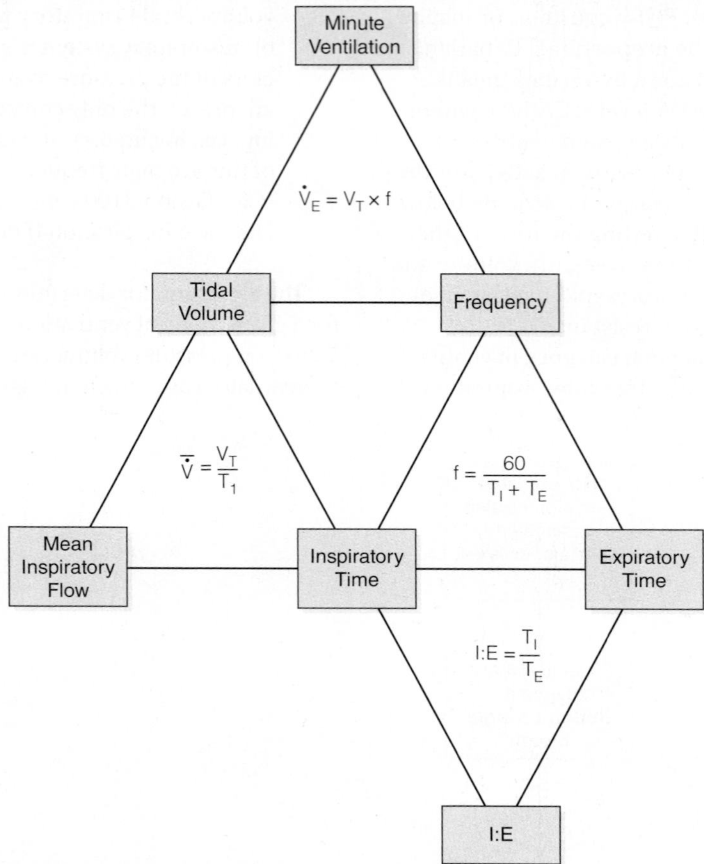

FIGURE 19-11 Influence diagram for volume control.
Courtesy of Mandu Press Ltd.

and **Figure 19-12** show the relations among factors that determine minute ventilation for volume control and pressure control.

4. Breaths are classified according to the criteria that trigger (start) and cycle (stop) inspiration.

For unassisted breathing, the brain generates signals to start and stop inspiration. When a patient is connected to a ventilator, the ventilator requires a signal to start and stop the inspiratory flow. Starting inspiration is called **triggering**. Common trigger signals include time, airway pressure, volume, or flow changes. An electrical signal from the diaphragm can also trigger inspiration. Stopping inspiration is called cycling. Common cycle signals are the same as those described for triggering. The term *sensitivity* refers to the amount that the trigger or cycle signal must change before inspiration starts or stops.

Trigger and *cycle* are key definitions in the development of a classification system for modes of ventilation. Some authors (including those who write standards and ventilator operator manuals) tend to restrict the definition of trigger to only the act of the patient initiating inspiration, leaving machine initiation of inspiration undefined. As a result, there is no convenient method of distinguishing machine trigger and cycle events from patient trigger and cycle events (see maxim #5 below) and no practical way to define mandatory and spontaneous breaths (see maxim #6 below). Without definitions for mandatory and spontaneous breaths, ventilatory patterns cannot be defined (maxim #7 below) and there is no basis for a taxonomy (see maxim #10).

5. Trigger and cycle events can be either patient or machine initiated.

An important clinical aim is to keep the delivery of inspiratory flow in synchrony with the patient's breathing efforts, assuming the patient does not have a disease process (e.g., neurodegenerative disease) or has not received medications (sedation or paralytic agents) that interfere with the patient's ability to generate trigger and cycle signals. Trigger and cycle capabilities are built into the mode of ventilation, defined below. For now, it is necessary to understand how to determine whether the patient or the machine has triggered or cycled an inspiration (or has the potential to do so). The equation of motion is helpful in understanding this concept. Time (t) in the equation is a variable independent of the patient. Suppose inspiration starts after a preset time interval (e.g., because of a preset breathing frequency) or ends after a preset inspiratory time or a preset tidal volume (the integral of flow with respect to time). In this instance, inspiration has started or stopped

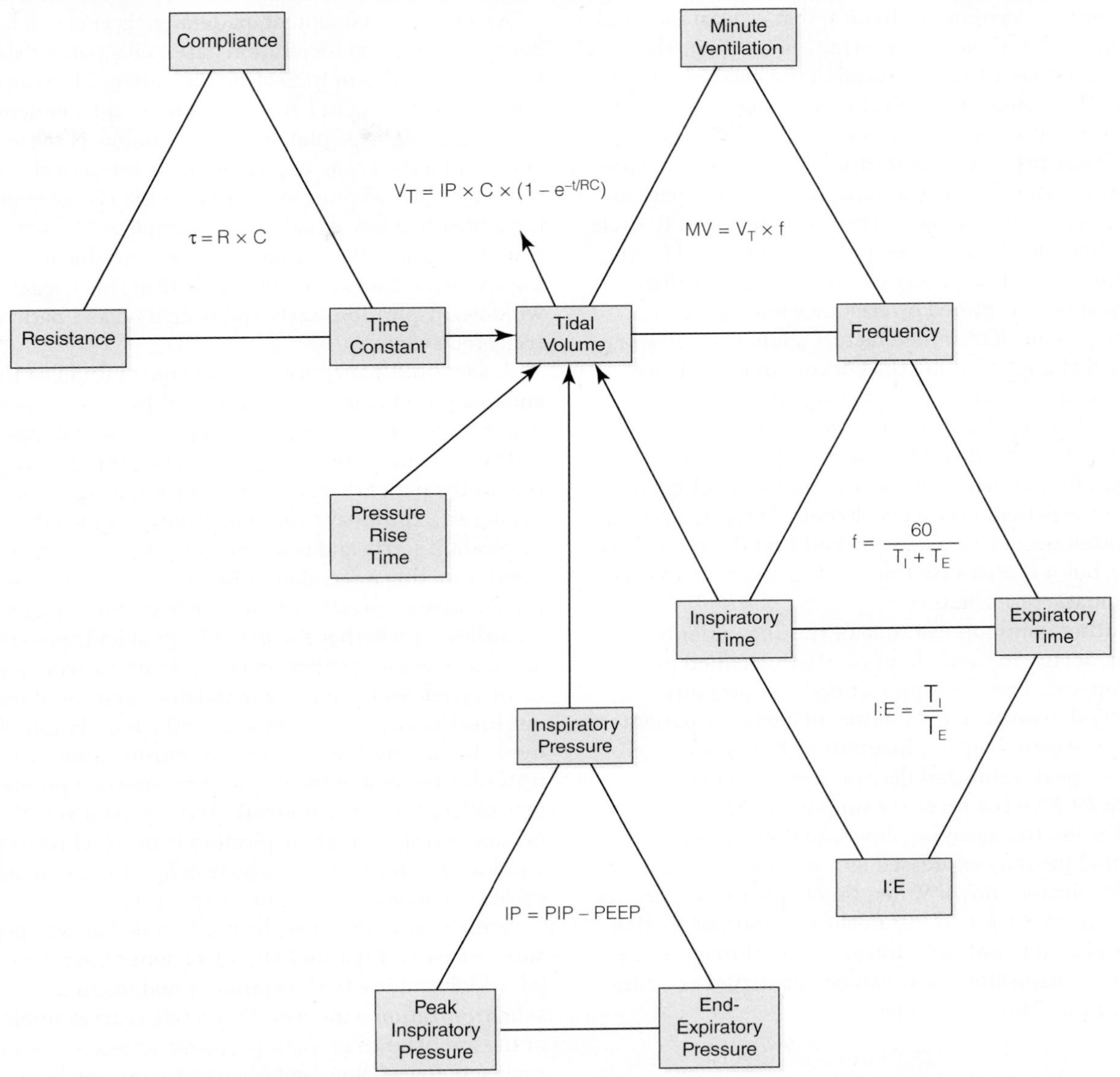

FIGURE 19-12 Influence diagram for pressure control.
Courtesy of Mandu Press Ltd.

regardless of any inspiratory or expiratory efforts made by the patient (i.e., changes in Pmus). During this breath, therefore, inspiration is machine triggered and machine cycled. The trigger and cycle signal for inspiration is time, due to a preset frequency. Another signal the ventilator can use to trigger inspiration is minute ventilation threshold. Minute ventilation is calculated by dividing the tidal volume by the time for one breath cycle (equivalent to multiplying tidal volume by frequency). Some ventilators allow the clinician to set a minimum threshold for minute ventilation. In this case, if minute ventilation drops below a preset threshold, then inspiration is triggered.

Cycling can be due to a variety of signals as well. Cycling due to a preset tidal volume is called *volume cycling*. Cycling due to a preset inspiratory time (or inspiratory pause time) is time cycling. Cycling due to a preset decay in inspiratory flow is termed *flow cycling*.

Patient triggering or cycling implies that inspiration starts or stops independently of any preset trigger or cycle signals generated by the ventilator. In the equation of motion, Pmus, elastance, and resistance are all patient determined. If inspiration starts or stops because of one or more of these factors, then inspiration is patient triggered or cycled. For example, if the patient makes an inspiratory effort (positive change in Pmus), then the ventilator may detect this by a change in airway pressure, volume, or flow. On some ventilators inspiratory effort is detected by electrical signals derived from the movement of the diaphragm (e.g., NAVA) or expansion of the chest wall (e.g., electrical impedance tomography). When the ventilator detects an inspiratory effort signal, inspiration is triggered on. Similarly, if the patient makes an expiratory effort (negative change in Pmus), then inspiration may be cycled off. The patient thus can actively pressure, volume, or flow trigger and cycle inspiration.

Respiratory system mechanics, that is, elastance and resistance, play a role in triggering and cycling. These factors are easiest to understand in the passive patient (Pmus = 0). Consider first cycling of inspiration. If the ventilator delivers a constant inspiratory flow, then peak airway pressure is determined by not only the preset flow but the elastance and resistance of the patient's respiratory system. Suppose the ventilator is set to cycle inspiration off when a preset pressure threshold is met; for a given preset inspiratory flow, the time for this threshold is determined by elastance and resistance. If these patient-determined factors change, inspiratory time will change. Cycling thus occurs independently of any preset machine generated signal and inspiration is patient cycled. Pressure cycling therefore is a form of patient cycling. Of course, if the patient makes an expiratory effort, Pmus may also cause cycling, in which case patient cycling is obvious. Pressure cycling most often occurs as an alarm condition (high pressure alarm), but it is also a routine cycling mechanism used in automatic resuscitators.[25]

Another common example of routine patient cycling occurs for a mode of ventilation called pressure support. Pressure support delivers pressure-controlled breaths. For example, in a passive patient during pressure control, inspiratory flow starts out at its peak value and decays exponentially (Figure 19-2A). For pressure support, inspiration is cycled when the decaying flow signal meets a preset threshold (usually expressed as a percentage of the peak inspiratory flow). When this happens determines the inspiratory time. If P(t) in the equation of motion is set to be constant (i.e., preset constant inspiratory pressure), inspiratory flow can be calculated as a function of time. The solution is:

$$\dot{V}(t) = \frac{\Delta P}{R}(e^{-t/RC}) \qquad (2)$$

A plot of Equation 2 will yield the flow waveform shown in Figure 19-2A. The term RC in Equation 2 is called the time constant. The time constant is the time at which an exponential function attains 63% of its steady-state value in response to a step input (ΔP). In other words, in this case, it is the time necessary for inspiratory flow to drop 63% of its peak value. The time constant, for a passive patient, thus determines how long it takes to reach the cycle threshold and it determines the inspiratory time independent of any cycle signal generated by the ventilator. It is possible for even a passive patient to cycle inspiration. Interestingly, a passive patient can trigger inspiration by the same mechanism. Except in this case the cycle threshold is based on the decay of expiratory pressure (an exponential flow through a constant expiratory resistance gives an exponential pressure waveform). This is the mechanism used in some automatic resuscitators.[25]

As a further refinement, patient triggering can be defined as starting inspiration based on a patient signal (i.e., a measurement indicating the patient's breathing motion) occurring in a ***trigger window***, independent of a machine trigger signal. A trigger window is the period comprising the entire expiratory time minus a short refractory period required to reduce the risk of triggering a breath before exhalation is complete. If a signal from the patient (i.e., some measured variable indicating an inspiratory effort) occurs within this trigger window, inspiration starts and is defined as a patient-triggered event.

A ***synchronization window*** is a short period, at the end of a preset expiratory time or at the end of a preset inspiratory time, during which a patient signal may be used to synchronize the beginning or ending of inspiration to the patient's actions. If the patient signal occurs during an expiratory time synchronization window, inspiration starts and is defined as a machine-triggered event initiating a mandatory breath. This is because the mandatory breath would have been time triggered regardless of whether the patient signal had appeared and because the distinction is necessary to avoid logical inconsistencies in defining mandatory and spontaneous breaths (see below), which are the foundation of the mode taxonomy. Sometimes a synchronization window is used at the end of the inspiratory time of a pressure controlled, time cycled breath. If the patient signal occurs during such an inspiratory time synchronization window, expiration starts and is defined as a machine-cycled event, ending a mandatory breath.

Some ventilators offer the mode called airway pressure release ventilation (APRV), or something similar, which can use both expiratory and inspiratory synchronization windows. This mode is an example of the importance of distinguishing between trigger/cycle windows (allowing for patient-triggered breaths) and synchronization windows (allowing for patient-synchronized, machine-triggered breaths). APRV is intended to provide a set number of releases or drops from a high-pressure level to a low-pressure level. Spontaneous breaths are possible at the high- and low-pressure levels (although there may not be enough time to accomplish this if the duration of the low pressure is too short). Using the standardized vocabulary, these releases (paired with their respective rises) are actually mandatory breaths because, as originally described, they were time triggered and time cycled. On some newer ventilators, synchronization windows have been added to both the expiratory time (to synchronize the transition to the high pressure with a patient inspiratory effort) and the inspiratory time (to synchronize cycling with the expiratory phase of a spontaneous breath taken during the high pressure level). If both triggering and cycling occurred with patient signals in the synchronization window, and if these events were called patient-triggered and patient-cycled, the result would be the ambiguous possibility of having *spontaneous breaths* (i.e., synchronized) *occurring during spontaneous breaths* (unsynchronized breaths during the high pressure level).

Another example occurs with a ventilator like the CareFusion Avea that allows the operator to set a flow cycle criterion for PC-IMV. Every inspiration thus is patient cycled. If any synchronized (SIMV) breaths were considered to be patient triggered, it would imply that these mandatory breaths were really spontaneous breaths. This would be misleading, because the preset mandatory breath frequency would then be larger than what was counted as mandatory breaths when observing the patient. On modes that are classified as forms of IMV (such as APRV), the operator must distinguish between the mandatory minute ventilation and the spontaneous minute ventilation (to gauge the level of mechanical support); this cannot be done if the definitions of mandatory and spontaneous breaths are in any way ambiguous.

In summary:

- *Patient triggering* means starting inspiration based on a patient signal independent of a machine trigger signal.
- *Machine triggering* means starting inspiratory flow based on a signal (usually time) from the ventilator, independent of a patient trigger signal.
- *Patient cycling* means ending inspiratory time based on signals representing the patient determined components of the equation of motion, (i.e., elastance, or resistance and including effects due to inspiratory effort). Flow cycling is a form of patient cycling because the rate of flow decay to the cycle threshold, and hence the inspiratory time, is determined by patient mechanics.
- *Machine cycling* means ending inspiratory time independent of signals representing the patient determined components of the equation of motion.

6. Breaths are classified as spontaneous or mandatory based on both the trigger and cycle events.

Whether the ventilator or the patient triggers and cycles has clinical relevance because these events determine the extent to which the patient retains control over the timing of the breath. A *spontaneous breath* is a breath for which the patient retains substantial control over timing. This means that the patient, independent of any machine settings for inspiratory time and expiratory time, determines the start and end of inspiration. That is, the patient both triggers and cycles the breath. A spontaneous breath may occur during a mandatory breath (e.g., airway pressure release ventilation).

Some authors use the term *spontaneous breath* to refer only to unassisted breaths. But that is an unnecessary limitation that prevents the word from being used as a key term in the mode taxonomy. The definition given here applies for assisted and unassisted breathing. For unassisted breathing, the brain provides the trigger and cycle signals. For assisted breathing, the signals may come from the brain or the ventilator.

A mandatory breath is a breath for which the patient has lost control over timing (i.e., frequency or inspiratory time). This means a breath for which the start or end of inspiration (or both) is determined by the ventilator, independent of the patient. In other words, the machine triggers and/or cycles the breath. A mandatory breath can occur during a spontaneous breath (e.g., High Frequency Jet Ventilation). A mandatory breath is, by definition, assisted.

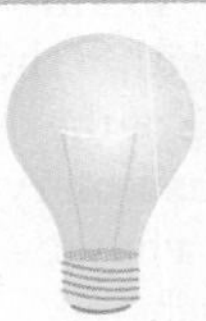

STOP AND THINK

You are examining the breath delivery for a new ventilator mode. How would you determine if the breath type is spontaneous or mandatory?

7. There are three basic breath sequences: continuous mandatory ventilation, intermittent mandatory ventilation, and continuous spontaneous ventilation.

A breath sequence is a particular pattern of spontaneous and/or mandatory breaths. The three possible breath sequences are: **continuous mandatory ventilation (CMV)**, **intermittent mandatory ventilation (IMV)**, and **continuous spontaneous ventilation (CSV)**. Continuous mandatory ventilation, commonly known as Assist/Control, is a breath sequence for which spontaneous breaths are not possible between mandatory breaths because every patient trigger signal in the trigger window produces a machine-cycled inspiration (i.e., a mandatory breath). Machine-triggered mandatory breaths may also be delivered at a preset frequency. In contrast to IMV, the mandatory breath frequency for CMV may be higher than the set frequency but never below it (i.e., the set frequency is a minimum value). In some pressure controlled modes on ventilators with an active exhalation valve, spontaneous breaths may occur during mandatory breaths, but the defining characteristic of CMV is that spontaneous breaths are not permitted between mandatory breaths. Note that trigger windows are used in CMV only and synchronization windows are use in IMV only.

There are three variations of IMV:

1. Mandatory breaths are always delivered at the set frequency (e.g., Covidien's SIMV Volume Control) and spontaneous breaths are permitted between mandatory breaths. If a synchronization window is used, the actual ventilatory period for a mandatory

breath may be shorter than the set period. Some ventilators will add the difference to the next mandatory period to maintain the set mandatory breath frequency (e.g., Dräger Evita XL).

2. Mandatory breaths are delivered only when the spontaneous breath frequency falls below the set frequency (e.g., Philips Respironics BiPAP S/T mode).
3. Mandatory breaths are delivered only when the measured minute ventilation (i.e., product of breath frequency and tidal volume) drops below a preset threshold (examples include Dräger's Mandatory Minute Volume Ventilation mode and Hamilton's Adaptive Support Ventilation mode). In contrast to CMV, with IMV the mandatory breath frequency therefore can never be higher than the set rate, but it may be lower (i.e., the set frequency is a maximum value).

Note that use of the definitions for mandatory and spontaneous breaths for determining the breath sequence (i.e., CMV, IMV, CSV) assumes normal ventilator operation. For example, coughing during VC-CMV may result in patient cycling for a patient-triggered breath due to the pressure alarm limit. While inspiration for that breath is both patient triggered and patient cycled, this is not normal operation and the sequence does not turn into IMV.

The algorithm for determining the breath sequence of a given mode is shown in **Figure 19-13.**

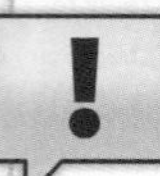

Respiratory Recap

Ten Fundamental Axioms of Mechanical Ventilators

1. A breath is one cycle of positive flow (inspiration) and negative flow (expiration).
2. A breath is assisted if the ventilator provides some or all of the work of breathing.
3. A ventilator assists breathing based on the equation of motion for the respiratory system.
4. Breaths are classified according to the criteria that trigger and cycle inspiration.
5. Trigger and cycle events can be either patient or machine initiated.
6. Breaths are classified as spontaneous or mandatory based on trigger and cycle events.
7. There are only three breath sequences: CMV, IMV, and CSV.
8. There are five basic ventilatory patterns: VC-CMV, VC-IMV, PC-CMV, PC-IMV, PC-CSV.
9. Within each ventilatory pattern there are types distinguished by their targeting schemes (set-point, dual, biovariable, servo, adaptive, optimal, and intelligent).
10. A mode of ventilation is classified according to control variable, breath sequence, and targeting scheme.

8. There are five basic ventilatory patterns: VC-CMV, VC-IMV, PC-CMV, PC-IMV, and PC-CSV.

There are two control variables and three breath sequences. Combining the two concepts results in a simple mode classification scheme called a ***ventilatory pattern***. These ventilatory patterns are VC-CMV, VC-IMV, PC-CMV, PC-IMV, PC-CSV. Note that VC-CSV is not a valid pattern because presetting the tidal volume implies machine cycling that makes spontaneous breaths (both triggered and cycled by the patient) impossible. For completeness, we should also include the possibility of a time-control ventilatory pattern such as TC-IMV. Although this is uncommon and nonconventional, it is possible as demonstrated by the modes like High Frequency Oscillatory Ventilation and Intrapulmonary Percussive Ventilation. Because any mode of ventilation can be associated with one and only one ventilatory pattern, the ventilatory pattern serves as a simple mode classification system.

This simple way of referring to modes frees the clinician from having to use names coined by various ventilator manufacturers and offers practical advantages in clinical situations. For example, when a patient is anesthetized during surgery, there may be no need to accommodate inspiratory efforts and thus VC-CMV may be the most convenient mode. Postoperatively, when the patient is receiving ventilatory support and care in the postanesthesia care unit (PACU) or the ICU, a ventilator mode change to pressure control will allow unrestricted inspiratory flow when the effects of anesthesia wear off and the patient begins to make some breathing effort.

Continuous mandatory ventilation may be required (i.e., PC-CMV) to ensure adequate ventilation in case of apnea, while allowing the patient some freedom over breath timing by permitting patient triggered breaths. When the patient is evaluated for extubation, a spontaneous breathing trial may be attempted using PC-CSV (e.g., Pressure Support). Referring to modes in terms of breathing patterns instead of specific names on particular ventilators simplifies both verbal communication and documentation in the patient's health care record.

9. Within each ventilatory pattern there are several types distinguished by their targeting schemes (set-point, dual, bio-variable servo, adaptive, optimal, and intelligent).

The five ventilatory patterns serve as simple but useful tags for classifying hundreds of mode names. To distinguish among the fairly large number of modes within the same category, however, a deeper understanding of the feedback control schemes used by engineers is necessary to construct the mode. **Figure 19-14** illustrates a basic schematic of a closed loop or feedback control scheme. The operator sets a desired input, for example, inspiratory pressure. The software reads the instruction and

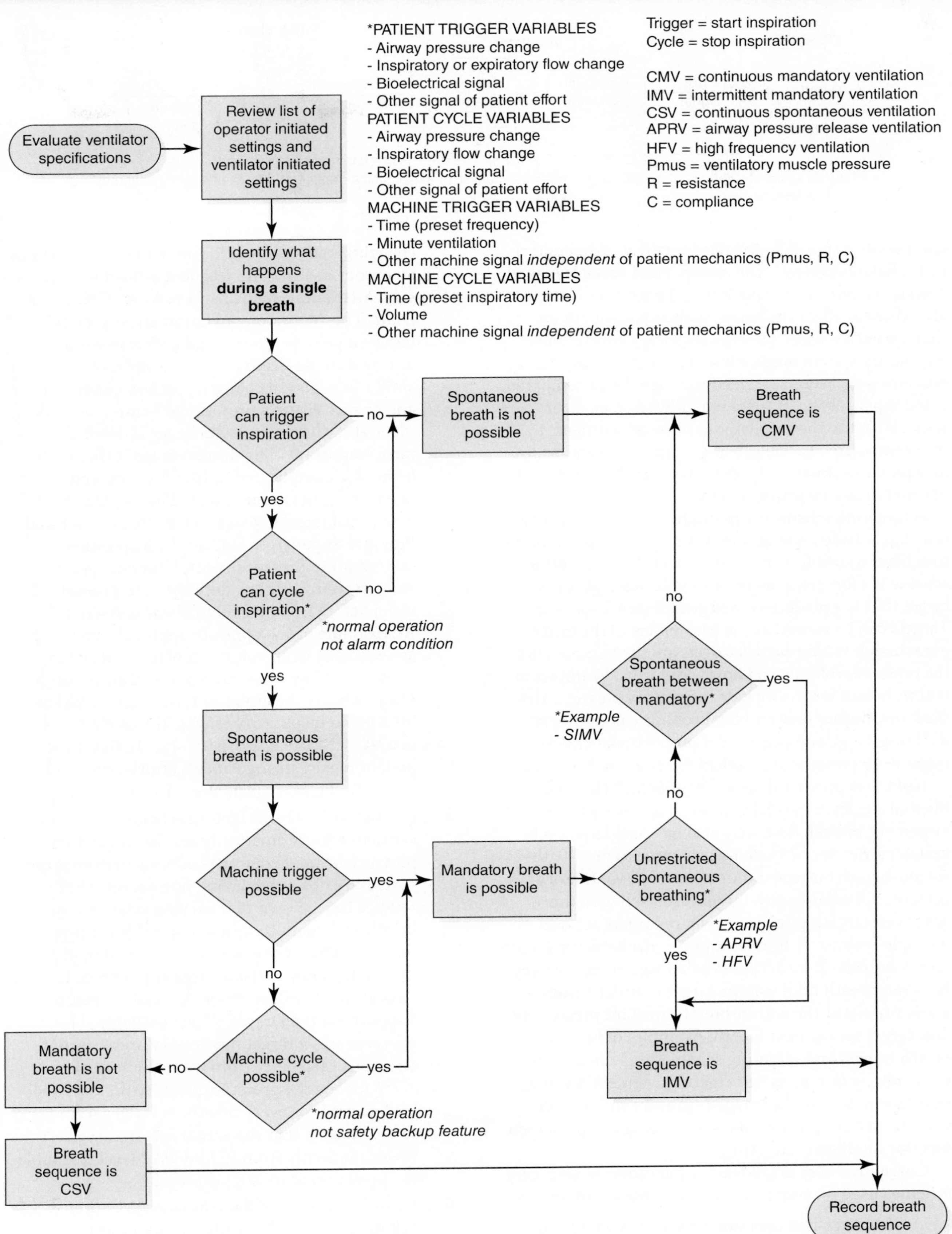

FIGURE 19-13 Algorithm for determining the breath sequence of a mode.

Courtesy of Mandu Press Ltd.

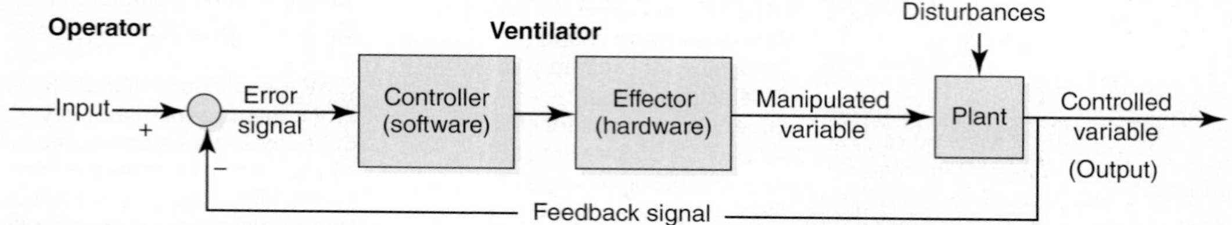

FIGURE 19-14 Schematic of closed loop or feedback control of a mechanical ventilator (e.g., the targeting scheme).
Courtesy of Mandu Press Ltd.

sends control signals to the hardware (e.g., flow control and exhalation valves). The manipulated variable (usually flow) is delivered to the plant (i.e., the patient). Various disturbances affect the result, such as patient circuit characteristics, leaks, patient ventilatory efforts, and respiratory system mechanics. The resulting inspiratory pressure is measured as a feedback signal and compared to the input setting. If there is a difference, an error signal is sent to the ventilator to make adjustments to the manipulated variable, bringing the resultant inspiratory pressure closer to the desired value. This system is referred to as a targeting scheme.

A targeting scheme is essentially a model of the relationship between operator inputs and ventilator outputs to achieve a specific ventilatory pattern. The targeting scheme is a key component of a mode description. A target thus is a predetermined goal of ventilator output. Targets can be viewed as the parameters of the targeting scheme. *Within-breath targets* are the parameters of the pressure, volume, and flow waveforms. Examples of within-breath targets include inspiratory pressure, rise time, inspiratory flow and tidal volume (set-point and dual targeting), and constant of proportionality between inspiratory pressure and patient effort (servo targeting).

Note that preset values *within a breath* that end inspiration, such as tidal volume, inspiratory time, or percent of peak flow, may also be considered cycle variables. *Between-breath targets* serve to modify the within-breath targets and/or the overall ventilatory pattern. Between-breath targets are used with more advanced targeting schemes, where targets act over multiple breaths. A simple example of a between-breath target is to compare actual exhaled volume to a preset between-breath tidal volume target in order to automatically adjust the within-breath constant pressure or flow target for the next breath. Examples of between-breath targets and targeting schemes include average tidal volume (for adaptive targeting), percent minute ventilation (for optimal targeting) and combined P_{CO_2}, volume, and frequency values describing a zone of comfort (for intelligent targeting).

Currently, there are at least seven different targeting schemes used on commercially available ventilators:[26]

1. *Set-point:* The operator sets all parameters of the pressure waveform (pressure control modes) or volume and flow waveforms (volume control modes). The advantage is simplicity. The disadvantage is that changing patient condition may make the settings inappropriate, making frequent adjustment necessary. An example mode name is Assist/Control.
2. *Dual:* The ventilator can automatically switch between volume control and pressure control during a single inspiration. The advantage is the ability to adjust to changing patient condition and ensure either a preset tidal volume or peak inspiratory pressure—whichever is deemed most important. The disadvantage is that some forms are complicated, difficult to set, and need constant readjustment. The original mode using dual targeting was called Volume Assured Pressure Support. In this mode, inspiration started off in pressure control but changed to volume control if flow decayed to the preset value before the tidal volume was delivered.[27] An example of the opposite approach, such as switching from volume control to pressure control, is Flow Adaptive Volume Control on the Maquet Servo-i ventilator. If the patient makes little or no inspiratory efforts, the mode looks like VC-CMV (e.g., Assist/Control). But if the patient makes strong enough efforts, the mode looks like PC-CSV (e.g., Pressure Support).[28]
3. *Bio-variable:* This targeting scheme allows the ventilator to automatically set the inspiratory pressure or tidal volume randomly to mimic the variability observed during normal breathing. Studies have shown that varying tidal volume breath-by-breath to mimic normal breathing improves short term outcomes.[29,30] Currently this biologically variable targeting scheme is only available in one mode, Variable Pressure Support, on the Dräger V500 ventilator. The operator sets a target inspiratory pressure and a percent variability from 0% to 100%. A setting of 0% means the preset inspiratory pressure will be delivered for every breath. A 100% variability setting means that the actual inspiratory pressure varies randomly from PEEP/CPAP level to double the preset pressure support level.
4. *Servo:* The output of the ventilator (pressure/volume/flow) automatically follows a varying input. In current modes, the varying input is some measure of the patient's inspiratory effort. The advantage is that assistance is proportional to the

patient's inspiratory effort; the more assistance the patient demands, the more the ventilator delivers. No other targeting scheme does this. The disadvantage is that it requires estimates of artificial airway and/or respiratory system mechanical properties or special equipment to monitor the respiratory effort signal. Example mode names include, Automatic Tube Compensation (ATC), Proportional Assist Ventilation (PAV), and Neurally Adjusted Ventilatory Assist (NAVA).

5. *Adaptive:* The ventilator automatically sets target(s) between breaths in response to varying patient conditions. The advantage is that it can adjust to changing patient lung mechanics (including inspiratory effort). The disadvantage is that the automatic adjustment may be inappropriate if the algorithm assumptions are violated or they do not match the patient's actual physiology.[31] The first mode to use this was called Pressure Regulated Volume Control.
6. *Optimal:* The ventilator automatically adjusts the targets of the ventilatory pattern to either minimize or maximize some overall performance characteristic. The advantage is that it can adjust to changing patient condition. The disadvantage is that the automatic adjustment may be inappropriate if the algorithm assumptions are violated or they do not match the patient's actual physiology. The only mode currently using this is Adaptive Support Ventilation (ASV).
7. *Intelligent:* A targeting scheme that uses artificial intelligence programs such as fuzzy logic, rule based expert systems, and artificial neural networks. The advantage is that it can adjust to changing patient condition. The disadvantage is that the automatic adjustment may be inappropriate if the algorithm assumptions are violated or they do not match the patient's actual physiology. The only modes currently using this scheme are SmartCare/PS and IntelliVent (not available in the United States). Information for identifying the targeting schemes associated with various control variables is given in **Table 19-3**.

As targeting schemes have evolved, they have become more automated and thus more complicated. More is not always better, however. Automation schemes rely on various assumptions, for example, that compliance and resistance are linear or that a patient's carbon dioxide production is a particular number of milliliters per minute. If the underlying assumptions of a targeting scheme are violated, unexpected and possibly unwanted results may result. An example is set-point targeting that assumes constant respiratory system mechanics. If respiratory system mechanics change rapidly, either peak airway pressure (during volume control) or tidal volume (during pressure control) may become unstable and drift out of acceptable ranges.

Dual targeting assumes that mechanics may change but may be useless without careful setting of the criteria for switching between volume and pressure control breaths. Servo control requires accurate data for respiratory system mechanical properties, such as resistance and elastance; if the data are unavailable, the mode cannot be used. Some forms of adaptive targeting assume that changes in respiratory system mechanics are only related to compliance. The ventilator cannot distinguish between patient inspiratory effort and an increase in compliance, however, thus fooling the targeting scheme into decreasing support when the patient needs it most.[31]

Optimal targeting is based on mathematical models (e.g., the relations among power of breathing, lung mechanics, frequency, and tidal volume). When the models do not match the actual physiology of the patient, they may instruct the ventilator to do inappropriate things (e.g., hyper/hypoventilate the patient or increase risk of ventilator induced lung damage).

Intelligent targeting systems may rely on rules in the form of "if the patient does this, the ventilator should do this" derived from the consensus of clinical experts. Yet these rules, at present, cover a very small set of actual clinical scenarios. Therefore, asumptions upon which the artificial intelligence system are based may easily be violated by the actual conditions of the patient. For example, the targeting scheme might assume that the patient can be aggressively weaned when in fact the patient is not ready. These drawbacks of ventilator technology should alert the clinician to fully understand both the capabilities and limitations of the modes used.

10. A mode of ventilation is classified according to its control variable, breath sequence, and targeting scheme(s).

A *mode of ventilation* can be defined in the most general sense as a predefined pattern of interaction between the ventilator and the patient. Historically, modes have been referred to only by the names coined by their creators and it may be important for ventilator manufacturers to have a unique name for the mode features on their respective ventilators. As a consequence, there are now so many different names that understanding and comparing all modes has become nearly impossible. The solution is to use a classification system, or taxonomy, to simplify modes.

The use of a taxonomy may make it easier (1) to compare research reports, facilitating the development of evidence-based clinical practice; (2) for clinicians to select the most appropriate modes, making optimal ventilator management more likely; and (3) for manufacturers to communicate with clients, thus improving the effectiveness of both sales and training. The classification of modes is based on the concepts of the control variable, the breath sequence, and the targeting scheme, as described in the previous nine maxims.

TABLE 19-3
Targeting schemes

Name	Abbreviation	Description	Advantage	Disadvantage	Example Mode Name	Ventilator	Manufacturer
Set-point	s	The operator sets all parameters of the pressure waveform (pressure control nodes) or volume and flow waveforms (volume control modes)	Simplicity	Changing patient condition may make settings inappropriate	Volume Control Continuous Mandatory Ventilation	Evita Infinity 500	Dräger
Dual	d	The ventilator can automatically switch between volume control and pressure control during a single inspiration	Can adjust to changing patient condition and ensure either a preset tidal volume or peak inspiratory pressure, whichever is deemed most important	May be complicated to set for some modes	Volume Control	Servo-i	Maquet
Servo	r	The output of the ventilator (pressure/volume/flow) automatically follows a varying input	Support by the ventilator is proportional to inspiratory effort	Requires estimates of artificial airway and/or respiratory system mechanical properties	Proportional Assist Ventilation Plus	PB 840	Covidien
Adaptive	a	The ventilator automatically sets target(s) between breaths in response to varying patient conditions	Can maintain stable tidal volume delivery with pressure control for changing lung mechanics or patient inspiratory effort	Automatic adjustment may be inappropriate if algorithm assumptions are violated or they do not match physiology	Pressure Regulated Volume Control	Servo-i	Maquet
Bio-variable	b	The ventilator automatically adjusts the inspiratory pressure or tidal volume randomly	Simulates the variability observed during normal breathing and may improve oxygenation or mechanics	Manually set range of variability may be inappropriate to achieve goals	Variable Pressure Support	Evita Infinity 500	Dräger
Optimal	o	The ventilator automatically adjusts the targets of the ventilatory pattern to either minimize or maximize some overall performance characteristic (e.g., work rate of breathing)	Can adjust to changing lung mechanics or patient inspiratory effort	Automatic adjustment may be inappropriate if algorithm assumptions are violated or they do not match physiology	Adaptive Support Ventilation	G5	Hamilton Medical
Intelligent	i	Targeting scheme that uses artificial intelligence programs such as fuzzy logic, rule based expert systems, and artificial neural networks	Can adjust to changing lung mechanics or patient inspiratory effort	Automatic adjustment may be inappropriate if algorithm assumptions are violated or they do not match physiology	SmatCare/PS	Evita Infinity 500	Dräger

Taxonomy of Mechanical Ventilation

A taxonomy (classification system) is typically a hierarchy (outline) of concepts starting with the most general and progressing to more specific with each successive level of the outline. The ventilator mode taxonomy has four hierarchical levels similar to the Order, Family, Genus, and Species used in biology:[15,32,33]

1. Control variable (pressure or volume)
    A. Breath sequence (CMV, IMV, or CSV)
        i. Primary breath targeting scheme (for CMV or CSV)
            a. Secondary breath targeting scheme (for IMV)

The primary breath is either the only breath there is (mandatory for CMV and spontaneous for CSV) or it is the mandatory breath in IMV. An example of how this taxonomy can be used to compare the modes of two common intensive care ventilators is shown in **Table 19-4**. The table is sorted by control variable, breaths sequence, and targeting scheme. This illustrates how modes that are essentially the same or very similar are given very different names. You can see that modes are most practically compared using their *tags* (taxonomic attribute groupings) rather than by their given *names* or ad-hoc pseudo classifications (e.g., VC-CMV is often referred to as assist/control in the adult literature, but it means PC-CMV in the pediatric literature).

Note that a four level hierarchy does not distinguish among all possible modes. Adding a fifth level that could be called variety can accommodate minor differences in modes. As an example, there are three varieties of PC-CSV using servo targeting. One makes inspiratory pressure proportional to the square of inspiratory flow (Automatic Tube Compensation); one makes it proportional to the electrical signal from the diaphragm (Neurally Adjusted Ventilatory Support), and one makes it proportional to the patient's spontaneous volume and flow (Proportional Assist Ventilation). The first can only support the resistive load of breathing, while the other two can support both the elastic and resistive loads.

Respiratory Recap

Three Goals of Mechanical Ventilation

- Safety
- Comfort
- Liberation

Comparing Modes of Mechanical Ventilation

Classifying modes of ventilation provides a means for comparing and contrasting the technological capabilities of the devices used for life support. The use of taxonomy is an important step in this process. It allows clinicians to distinguish the tools in the toolbox in order to appropriately match the technology to the patients' needs. It therefore is important to know not only what tool to use but how to use it. Understanding the technological capabilities of a given mode of ventilation can assist clinicians in determining which mode can be used to provide the best patient care.

The three main goals of mechanical ventilatory support are safety (adequate gas exchange and hemodynamics while avoiding atelectrauma and volutrauma), comfort (optimum synchrony between patient and ventilator), and liberation (shortest duration of ventilation with fewest adverse events).[34] These general goals can be further refined into specific objectives and clinical aims that may be applied to individual patients. Goals, objectives, and aims are the product of clinical assessment. Having assessed the patient's needs, the next step is to match those needs to the technological capabilities of the available modes of ventilation. The framework for matching patient need with treatment options is shown in **Table 19-5**.

Table 19-6 is a list of the names and tags of the unique modes provided by current intensive care ventilators (i.e., only one name was selected from a group of mode names identified by the taxonomy). These modes have been grouped according to the three goals of ventilation. The basic idea is that the available mode that has the most technological capabilities meeting the goals for a particular patient is the most appropriate mode to use. A full description of this system is beyond the scope of this chapter but is available in the literature.[34]

The above system of matching patient needs to available technology should be applied cautiously. In order to compare modes it is important to consider the best-case scenario, in which the modes are functioning under conditions that do not violate their underlying design assumptions (see the discussion about targeting schemes above). *The clinician must appropriately identify the patient's condition, assess ventilatory needs, and rule out any mode features that may be inappropriate.* The conceptual tools provided in this chapter may assist clinicians in selecting the mode that meets the patient's ventilatory need.

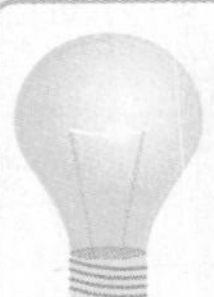

STOP AND THINK

Why do you think that it is important for all clinicians to use similar terminology when describing a ventilator mode?

TABLE 19-4
Comparison of the Modes of Two Intensive Care Ventilators

Manufacturer	Model	Manufacturer's Mode Name	Primary Control Variable	Breath Sequence	Primary Breath Target Scheme	Secondary Breath Target Scheme	Tag
Hamilton	G5	Adaptive Pressure Ventilation Controlled Mandatory Ventilation	pressure	CMV	adaptive	N/A	PC-CMVa
Maquet	Servo-i	Pressure Regulated Volume Control	pressure	CMV	adaptive	N/A	PC-CMVa
Hamilton	G5	Pressure Controlled Mandatory Ventilation	pressure	CMV	set-point	N/A	PC-CMVs
Maquet	Servo-i	Pressure Control	pressure	CMV	set-point	N/A	PC-CMVs
Maquet	Servo-i	Volume Support	pressure	CSV	adaptive	N/A	PC-CMVa
Maquet	Servo-i	Neurally Adjusted Ventilatory Assist	pressure	CSV	servo	N/A	PC-CMVr
Hamilton	G5	Pressure Support (SPONT)	pressure	CSV	set-point	N/A	PC-CSVs
Hamilton	G5	Noninvasive Ventilation	pressure	CSV	set-point	N/A	PC-CMVs
Maquet	Servo-i	Pressure Support/CPAP	pressure	CSV	set-point	N/A	PC-CMVs
Hamilton	G5	Adaptive Pressure Ventilation Synchronized Intemittent Mandatory Ventilation	pressure	IMV	adaptive	set-point	PC-IMa,s
Maquet	Servo-i	Synchronized Intermittent Mandatory Vertilation (Pressure Regular)	pressure	IMV	adaptive	set-point	PC-IMa,s
Maquet	Servo-i	Automode (Pressure Regulated Volume Control to Volume Support)	pressure	IMV	adaptive	adaptive	PC-IMa,a
Hamilton	G5	Adaptive Support Ventilation	pressure	IMV	optimal	optimal	PC-IMo,o
Hamilton	G5	Pressure Synchronized Intermittent Mandatory Ventilation	pressure	IMV	set-point	set-point	PC-IMs,s
Hamilton	G5	Duo Positive Airway Pressure	pressure	IMV	set-point	set-point	PC-IMs,s
Hamilton	G5	Airway Pressure Release Ventilation	pressure	IMV	set-point	set-point	PC-IMs,s
Maquet	Servo-i	Synchronized Intermittent Mandatory Ventilation (Pressure Control)	pressure	IMV	set-point	set-point	PC-IMs,s
Maquet	Servo-i	Bi-Vent	pressure	IMV	set-point	set-point	PC-IMs,s
Maquet	Servo-i	Automode (Pressure Control to Pressure Support)	pressure	IMV	set-point	set-point	PC-IMs,s
Hamilton	G5	Synchronized Controlled Mandatory Ventilation	volume	CMV	set-point	N/A	VC-CMVs
Maquet	Servo-i	Volume Control	volume	IMV	dual	set-point	VC-IMd,s
Maquet	Servo-i	Synchronized Intermittent Mandatory Ventilation (Volume Control)	volume	IMV	dual	set-point	VC-IMd,s
Maquet	Servo-i	Automode (Volume Control to Volume Support)	volume	IMV	dual	adaptive	VC-IMd,a
Hamilton	G5	Synchronized Intermittent Mandatory Ventilation	volume	IMV	set-point	set-point	VC-IMs,s

TABLE 19-5
Goals of Mechanical Ventilation

Objectives Serving Goals
Aims of Clinical Management
Capabilities of Ventilators
Features of Specific Modes

1. SAFETY

Optimize ventilation/perfusion of the lungs

Maximize alveolar ventilation

Automatic adjustment of minute ventilation target

Ventilator set minute ventilation or CO_2 target

Example mode: INTELLiVENT (G5, Hamilton Medical)

Explanation: Clinician inputs patient condition. Ventilator monitors mechanics and end-tidal CO_2 and automatically adjusts minute ventilation to keep end-tidal CO_2 within target range.

Example mode: VPAP Adapt (S9 VPAP Adapt, ResMed)

Explanation: VPAP Adapt algorithm adapts to the patient's ventilation needs on a breath-by-breath basis by automatically calculating a target ventilation (90% of the patient's recent average ventilation) and adjusting the pressure support to achieve it.

Automatic adjustment of support in response to changing respiratory mechanics

Ventilator set inspiratory pressure to achieve target minute ventilation

Example mode: Automode with Pressure Regulated Volume Control and Volume Support (Servo-i, Maquet)

Explanation: Target minute ventilation is based on the set tidal volume and rate. It uses intermittent mandatory ventilation to synchronize mandatory breaths (PRVC) and spontaneous breaths (volume support). It uses an adaptive pressure targeting scheme where the ventilator monitors tidal volume and automatically adjusts inspiratory pressure between breaths to achieve average exhaled tidal volume equal to set target. If the spontaneous respiratory rate does not achieve the minimum minute ventilation, mandatory breaths are triggered.

Ventilator set inspiratory pressure to achieve target tidal volume

Example mode: Pressure Regulated Volume Control (Servo-i, Maquet)

Explanation: PRVC is a pressure control mode, but the clinician sets a target tidal volume. Ventilator monitors tidal volume and automatically adjusts inspiratory pressure between breaths to achieve average exhaled tidal volume equal to set target.

Automatic adjustment of minute ventilation parameters (f, V_T)

Ventilator set mandatory breath frequency

Example modes: Volume Control Mandatory Minute Volume Ventilation (Evita Infinity V500, Dräger), AutoMode (Servo-i, Maquet)

Explanation: Clinician inputs minute ventilation target. If total minute ventilation created by mandatory and spontaneous breaths falls below target, the ventilator triggers mandatory breaths.

Manual adjustment of minute ventilation parameters

Clinician set tidal volume and frequency

Example mode: Volume Control (Servo-i, Maquet)

Explanation: Clinician sets tidal volume and frequency to meet predicted minute ventilation requirement.

Maximize oxygenation

Automatic adjustment of oxygen delivery

Ventilator set F_{IO_2}

Example mode: INTELLiVENT (G5, Hamilton Medical)

Explanation: Operator inputs patient condition. Ventilator monitors Sp_{O_2} and automatically adjusts F_{IO_2} to keep oxygenation within target range.

Automatic adjustment of end-expiratory lung volume

Ventilator set PEEP

Example mode: INTELLiVENT (G5, Hamilton Medical)

Explanation: Clinician inputs patient condition. Ventilator automatically adjusts PEEP to keep Sp_{O_2} within target range.

Optimize pressure/volume curve

Minimize risk of volutrauma

Automatic adjustment of lung protective limits

Ventilator set safety limits on ventilation parameters

Example mode: Adaptive Support Ventilation (G5, Hamilton Medical)

Explanation: Clinician inputs patient weight and % of predicted minute ventilation to support. Ventilator monitors mechanics and automatically sets minimum and maximum values for tidal volume, mandatory breath frequency, inspiratory pressure, and inspiratory/expiratory times.

Automatic adjustment of minute ventilation parameters (f, V_T)

Ventilator set tidal volume and frequency

Example mode: Adaptive Support Ventilation (G5, Hamilton Medical)

Explanation: Clinician inputs patient weight and % of predicted minute ventilation to support. Ventilator monitors mechanics and then automatically adjusts tidal volume and frequency to minimize work rate. The effect is to decrease tidal volume as compliance decreases, consistent with a lung-protective ventilation strategy.

(*continues*)

TABLE 19-5
Goals of Mechanical Ventilation (*continued*)

Minimize tidal volume
Ventilatory frequencies above 150/min
Example mode: High Frequency Jet Ventilation (LifePulse, Bunnell)
Explanation: High frequency modes allow lowest possible tidal volume.

Minimize risk of atelectrauma
Automatic adjustment of end-expiratory lung volume
Ventilator set PEEP
Example mode: INTELLiVENT (G5, Hamilton Medical)
Explanation: Clinician inputs patient condition. Ventilator automatically adjusts PEEP to keep Spo_2 within target range.

Biologically variable tidal volume
Ventilator adjusts inspiratory pressure randomly
Example mode: Variable Pressure Support (Evita Infinity V500, Dräger)
Explanation: Clinician inputs the desired target Pressure Support level and the desired percentage of pressure variation. Ventilator automatically adjusts Pressure Support level for individual breaths randomly within a range equal to the set Pressure Support plus or minus the set percentage.

Optimize alarm settings
Minimize time spent in unsafe conditions
Automatic selection of optimum alarm variables
Nothing available yet

Minimize false alarms
Automatic adjustment of optimum alarm thresholds
Nothing available yet

2. COMFORT
Optimize patient–ventilator synchrony
Maximize trigger/cycle synchrony
All breaths are spontaneous with sufficient patient trigger effort
All breaths are patient triggered and patient cycled
Example mode: Pressure Support (Covidien PB 840)
Explanation: Pressure support delivers breaths that are pressure or flow triggered and flow cycled.

Trigger/cycle based on signal representing chest wall/diaphragm movement
Trigger/cycle based on diaphragm electromyogram
Example mode: Neurally Adjusted Ventilatory Support (Servo-i, Maquet)
Explanation: Ventilator monitors electrical activity of the diaphragm (Edi). Clinician sets Edi trigger threshold and ventilator sets default Edi cycle threshold.

Coordination of mandatory and spontaneous breaths
Spontaneous breaths suppress mandatory breaths
Example mode: Spont/T (V200, Philips)
Explanation: Clinician sets a breath frequency. Ventilator delivers time or patient triggered, pressure limited, flow cycled, breaths. Breaths are machine triggered only if the spontaneous respiratory rate is below the set threshold.
Spontaneous breaths permitted between mandatory breaths
Example mode: Volume Control Synchronized Intermittent Mandatory Ventilation (PB 840, Covidien)
Explanation: Spontaneous breaths with or without pressure support permitted between volume control mandatory breaths.
Pressure control mandatory breaths with unrestricted inspiration and expiration
Example mode: BiLevel (PB 840, Covidien)
Explanation: BiLevel is a form of pressure control synchronized intermittent mandatory ventilation. However, as opposed to conventional PC-SIMV on this ventilator, spontaneous breaths are allowed during mandatory breaths in BiLevel only.

Minimize autoPEEP
Automatic limitation of autoPEEP
Ventilator set minimum expiratory time
Example mode: Adaptive Support Ventilation (G5, Hamilton Medical)
Explanation: Clinician inputs patient weight and % of predicted minute ventilation to support. Ventilator monitors respiratory mechanics and automatically adjusts mandatory breath frequency, keeping expiratory time at least three time constants long to minimize autoPEEP.

Maximize flow synchrony
Unrestricted inspiratory flow
Pressure control mandatory breaths with unrestricted inspiration
Example mode: Pressure Control (Servo-i, Maquet)
Explanation: Inspiration is pressure controlled. Ventilator delivers flow to maintain the inspiratory pressure setting as the patient inhales.

TABLE 19-5
Goals of Mechanical Ventilation (*continued*)

Ventilator automatically switches from volume control to pressure control
Example mode: Volume Control (Servo-i, Maquet)
Explanation: During volume control modes, ventilator automatically switches from constant flow delivery to constant pressure delivery to meet the patient's inspiratory flow demand (i.e., dual targeting scheme). If inspiration was patient triggered, this action may turn a mandatory breath into a flow cycled spontaneous breath, and hence the breath sequence is intermittent mandatory ventilation, IMV.

Automatic adjustment of flow based on frequency
Ventilator maintains constant I:E ratio in volume control
Example mode: Adaptive Flow and I Time (iVent, Versamed)
Explanation: In volume control modes, ventilator automatically adjusts inspiratory flow and inspiratory time to deliver the preset tidal volume and maintain I:E ratio at 1:2.

Coordinate ventilator work output with patient demand
Automatic adjustment of support to maintain specified breathing pattern
Ventilator set pressure support to keep patient in a predefined ventilatory pattern
Example mode: SmartCare/PS/PS (Evita XL, Dräger)
Explanation: SmartCare/PS/PS is a form of pressure control continuous spontaneous ventilation (e.g., Pressure Support). Ventilator automatically adjusts the level of pressure support to keep the patient within a "zone of comfort" based on end-tidal CO_2, tidal volume, and frequency.
Ventilator set pressure support to maintain frequency target
Example mode: Mandatory Rate Ventilation (Taema-Horus, Air Liquide)
Explanation: This mode is a form of pressure control continuous spontaneous ventilation (e.g., Pressure Support). Unlike conventional Pressure Support, the clinician sets a target frequency and the ventilator adjusts the pressure support in proportion to difference between the target and actual frequencies. The assumption of the targeting scheme is that when the pressure support is correctly adjusted, the patient will have a comfortable ventilatory frequency (e.g., 15–25 breaths/min).

Automatic adjustment of support to meet patient demand
Ventilator set inspiratory pressure in proportion to inspiratory effort
Example mode: Proportional Assist Ventilation Plus (PB 840, Covidien)
Explanation: Clinician sets the percent support of total work of inspiration and ventilator delivers inspiratory pressure in proportion to both inspiratory volume and flow according to the equation of motion for the respiratory system.
Example mode: Automatic Tube Compensation (Evita XL, Dräger)
Explanation: Clinician sets percent support of resistive work of breathing based on size of artificial airway. Ventilator delivers pressure in proportion to the square of spontaneous inspiratory flow.

3. LIBERATION
Optimize weaning experience
Minimize duration of ventilation
Ventilator led weaning of support
Ventilator initiated reduction of pressure support and evaluation of patient response
Example mode: SmartCare/PS (Evita XL, Dräger)
Explanation: SmartCare/PS is a form of pressure control continuous spontaneous ventilation (e.g., Pressure Support). Ventilator automatically adjusts the level of pressure support to keep the patient within a predefined ventilatory pattern based on end-tidal CO_2, tidal volume, and frequency.

Ventilator recommends liberation
Ventilator initiated spontaneous breathing trial
Example mode: SmartCare/PS (Evita XL, Dräger)
Explanation: SmartCare/PS is a form of pressure control continuous spontaneous ventilation (e.g., Pressure Support) with a rule-based expert system. Ventilator automatically conducts spontaneous breathing trial and, if passed, recommends liberation.

Automatic reduction of support in response to increased patient effort
Ventilator reduces inspiratory pressure as inspiratory effort increases to maintain preset tidal volume target
Example mode: Continuous Mandatory Ventilation with AutoFlow (Evita XL, Dräger)
Explanation: Pressure control mode but clinician sets target tidal volume. Ventilator monitors tidal volume and automatically adjusts inspiratory pressure between breaths to achieve average exhaled tidal volume equal to set target. Increased patent effort results in reduced inspiratory pressure.

Minimize adverse events
Monitor probability of failure
Nothing available yet
Identify adverse event
Nothing available yet

TABLE 19-6
Technological Capabilities of Unique Modes of Ventilation

Mode Name	Mode Tag	Automatic adjustment of minute ventilation target	Automatic adjustment of support in response to changing respiratory mechanics	Automatic adjustment of minute ventilation parameters (f, V_T)	Manual adjustment of minimum minute ventilation parameters (f, V_T)	Automatic adjustment of oxygen delivery	Automatic adjustment of end-expiratory lung volume	Automatic adjustment of ventilation parameters within lung-protective limits	Minimize tidal volume	**Safety Capabilities**	All breaths are spontaneous with patient effort	Trigger/cycle based on signal representing chest wall/diaphragm movement	Coordination of mandatory and spontaneous breaths	Automatic limitation of autoPEEP	Unrestricted inspiratory flow	Automatic adjustement of flow based on frequency	Automatic adjustemnt of support to maintain specific breathing pattern	Automatic adjustment of support proportional to patient demand	**Comfort Capabilities**	Ventilator initiated weaning of support	Ventilator recommends liberation	Automatic reduction of support in response to increased patient effort	**Liberation Capabilities**	Total
INTELLIVENT-ASV	PC-IMVoi,oi	✓	✓	✓		✓	✓	✓		6	✓		✓	✓	✓				4	✓	✓	✓	3	13
Adaptive Support Ventilation	PC-IMVoi,oi		✓	✓				✓		3	✓		✓	✓	✓				4			✓	1	8
SmartCare/PS	PC-CSVi		✓							1	✓				✓		✓		3	✓	✓	✓	3	7
Automode (Pressure Regulated Volume Control to Volume Support)	PC-IMVa,a		✓	✓	✓					3	✓		✓		✓				3			✓	1	7
Automode (Volume Control to Volume Support)	VC-IMVd,a		✓	✓	✓					3	✓		✓		✓				3			✓	1	7
Mandatory Minute Volume with Pressure Limited Ventilation[3]	VC-IMVd,a			✓	✓					2	✓		✓		✓				3			✓	1	6
Adaptive Pressure Ventilation Synchronized Intermittent Mandatory Ventilation	PC-IMVa,s		✓		✓					2			✓		✓				2			✓	1	5
Mandatory Minute Volume Ventilation	VC-IMVa,s			✓	✓					2	✓		✓						2			✓	1	5

TABLE 19-6
Technological Capabilities of Unique Modes of Ventilation (*continued*)

Mode Name	Mode Tag	Automatic adjustment of minute ventilation target	Automatic adjustment of support in response to changing respiratory mechanics	Automatic adjustment of minute ventilation parameters (f, V_T)	Manual adjustment of minimum minute ventilation parameters (f, V_T)	Automatic adjustment of oxygen delivery	Automatic adjustment of end-expiratory lung volume	Automatic adjustment of ventilation parameters within lung-protective limits	Minimize tidal volume	**Safety Capabilities**	All breaths are spontaneous with patient effort	Trigger/cycle based on signal representing chest wall/diaphragm movement	Coordination of mandatory and spontaneous breaths	Automatic limitation of autoPEEP	Unrestricted inspiratory flow	Automatic adjustement of flow based on frequency	Automatic adjustemnt of support to maintain specific breathing pattern	Automatic adjustment of support proportional to patient demand	**Comfort Capabilities**	Ventilator initiated weaning of support	Ventilator recommends liberation	Automatic reduction of support in response to increased patient effort	**Liberation Capabilities**	Total
Neurally Adjusted Ventilatory Support	PC-CSVr									0	✓	✓			✓			✓	4				0	4
Volume Support	PC-CSVa		✓							1	✓				✓				2			✓	1	4
Mandatory Rate Ventilation	PC-CSVa			✓						1	✓				✓		✓		3				0	4
Pressure Regulated Volume Control	PC-CMVa		✓		✓					2					✓				1			✓	1	4
Synchronized Intermittent Mandatory Ventilation (Volume Control)[1]	VC-IMVd,s				✓					1			✓		✓				2				0	3
Proportional Assist Ventilation	PC-CSVr									0	✓				✓			✓	3				0	3
High Frequency Oscillatory Ventilation	TC-IMVs,s								✓	1			✓		✓				2				0	3
Volume Control Synchronized Intermittent Mandatory Ventilation (Adaptive Flow & Time)[2]	VC-IMVa,s				✓					1			✓			✓			2				0	3
Volume Control Synchronized Intermittent Mandatory Ventilation	VC-IMVs,s				✓					1			✓						1				0	2

(*continues*)

TABLE 19-6
Technological Capabilities of Unique Modes of Ventilation (*continued*)

Mode Name	Mode Tag	Automatic adjustment of minute ventilation target	Automatic adjustment of support in response to changing respiratory mechanics	Automatic adjustment of minute ventilation parameters (f, V_T)	Manual adjustment of minimum minute ventilation parameters (f, V_T)	Automatic adjustment of oxygen delivery	Automatic adjustment of end-expiratory lung volume	Automatic adjustment of ventilation parameters within lung-protective limits	Minimize tidal volume	Safety Capabilities	All breaths are spontaneous with patient effort	Trigger/cycle based on signal representing chest wall/diaphragm movement	Coordination of mandatory and spontaneous breaths	Automatic limitation of autoPEEP	Unrestricted inspiratory flow	Automatic adjustement of flow based on frequency	Automatic adjustemnt of support to maintain specific breathing pattern	Automatic adjustment of support proportional to patient demand	Comfort Capabilities	Ventilator initiated weaning of support	Ventilator recommends liberation	Automatic reduction of support in response to increased patient effort	Liberation Capabilities	Total
Pressure Support	PC-CSVs									0	✓				✓				2				0	2
Airway Pressure Release Ventilation	PC-IMVs,s									0			✓		✓				2				0	2
Pressure Control Synchronized Intermittent Mandatory Ventilation	PC-IMVs,s									0			✓		✓				2				0	2
Continuous Mandatory Ventilation with Pressure Limited[3]	VC-CMVd				✓					1					✓				1				0	2
Pressure Control Assist Control	PC-CMVa									0					✓				1				0	1
Volume Control Assist/Control	VC-CMVs				✓					1									0				0	1

[1]*Maquet Servo-i ventilator*

[2]*GE Healticare/Versamed iVent 201 ventilator*

[3]*Unrestricted inspiratory flow (but no expiratory) flow after Pmax threshold is met*

PC = pressure control, VC = volume control, TC = time control, CMV = continuous mandatory ventilation, IMV = intermittent mandatory ventilation, CSV = continuous spontaneous ventilation

Targeting scheme abbreviations: s = set-point, d = dual, r = servo, a = adaptive, o = optimal, i = intelligent

Modified with permission from Mireles-Cabodevila E, Chatburn RL. A rational basis for comparing modes of mechanical ventilation. *Respir Care* 2013;58:348–366.

Key Points

- The equation of motion is the basic model for describing patient–ventilator interaction. It relates the variables pressure, volume, and flow to the model parameters of elastance (or compliance) and resistance.
- During pressure control, pressure is the independent variable and the shapes of the volume and flow waveforms depend on the shape of the pressure waveform and respiratory system mechanics (elastance, resistance, and inspiratory effort represented by muscle pressure, Pmus).
- During pressure control, changes in respiratory system mechanics affect peak inspiratory flow and tidal volume.
- During volume control, volume is the independent variable and the shape of the pressure waveform depends on the shape of the volume waveform and respiratory system mechanics (elastance, resistance, and inspiratory effort represented by muscle pressure, Pmus).
- During volume control, changes in respiratory system mechanics affect mean and peak inspiratory pressure.
- Patient circuit configuration may affect ventilator function, so it is important to use the manufacturer's recommenced circuit configuration. The ventilator's operator manual will provide information regarding the type of configuration to use as well as any requirements for a proprietary circuit.
- There are several different levels of ventilator alarms, whose levels are numbered in order of the critical nature of the event. Life-threatening events are typically when Levels 1 and 2 alarms are violated.
- A ventilator may display monitored data as numbers or texts, waveforms, trend lines, or in the form of abstract graphic symbols.
- A breath can be defined in terms of the flow–time curve.
- A breath is assisted if pressure rises above baseline during inspiration or falls below baseline during expiration.
- A ventilator can control only one variable at a time: pressure or volume.
- Breaths are classified according to the criteria that trigger (start) and cycle (stop) inspiration.
- Inspiration can be triggered by the patient or the ventilator.
- Breaths are classified as spontaneous or mandatory based on both the trigger and cycle events.
- Ventilators deliver only three basic breath sequences: continuous mandatory ventilation (CMV), intermittent mandatory ventilation (IMV), and continuous spontaneous ventilation (CSV).
- Two control variables and three breath sequences combine to form the five basic ventilatory patterns: VC-CMV, VC-IMV, PC-CMV, PC-IMV, and PC-CSV.
- A targeting scheme is a model of the relationship between operator inputs and ventilator outputs to achieve a specific ventilatory pattern and is a key component of a mode description.
- The seven different targeting schemes used on commercially available ventilators include set-point, dual, biovariable, servo, adaptive, optimal, and intelligent.
- The control variable, breath sequence, and targeting scheme are used to classify the mode of ventilation.

References

1. Mushin WW, Rendell-Baker L, Thompson PW, et al. *Automatic Ventilation of the Lungs*. Philadelphia: FA Davis; 1980.
2. Chatburn RL, Mireles-Cabodevila E. Basic principles of ventilator design and operation. In: Tobin MJ, ed. *Principles and Practice of Mechanical Ventilation*. 3rd ed. New York: McGraw-Hill; 2012: 65–97.
3. Blakemen TC, Rodriquez D, Hanseman D, Branson RD. Bench evaluation of 7 home-care ventilators. *Respir Care*. 2011;56:1791–1798.
4. Campbell RS, Johannigman JA, Branson RD, et al. Battery duration of portable ventilators: effects of control variable, positive end-expiratory pressure, and inspired oxygen concentration. *Respir Care*. 2002;47:1173–1183.
5. Sanborn WG. Microprocessor-based mechanical ventilation. *Respir Care*. 1993;38:72–109.
6. Morch ET. History of mechanical ventilation. In: Kirby RR, Smith RA, Desautels DA, eds. *Mechanical Ventilation*. New York: Churchill Livingstone; 1985:1–58.
7. Russell IF, Ross DG, Manson HJ. Fluidic cycling devices for inspiratory and expiratory timing in automatic ventilators. *J Biomed Eng*. 1983;5:227–234.
8. Chatburn RL. Classification of mechanical ventilators. In: Branson RD, Hess DR, Chatburn RL, eds. *Respiratory Care Equipment*. Philadelphia: Lipponcott Williams & Wilkins; 1999:359–393.
9. MacIntyre NR, Branson RD. *Mechanical Ventilation*. 2nd ed. St. Louis: Saunders Elsevier; 2009:153–156.
10. de Wit M. Monitoring of patient-ventilator interaction at the bedside. *Respir Care*. 2011;56:61–72.
11. Henderson WR, Sheel AW. Pulmonary mechanics during mechanical ventilation. *Respir Physiol Neurobiol*. 2012;180:162–172.
12. Sassoon CSH. Triggering of the ventilator in patient-ventilator interactions. *Respir Care*. 2011;56:39–48.
13. Grooms DA, Sibole SH, Tomlinson JR, et al. Customization of an open-lung ventilation strategy to treat a case of life-threatening acute respiratory distress syndrome. *Respir Care*. 2011;56:514–519.
14. Cairo JM, Pilbeam SP. *Mosby's Respiratory Care Equipment*. 8th ed. St. Louis: Mosby; 2010.
15. Chatburn RL, Khatib, ME, Mireles-Cabodevila E. A Taxonomy for Mechanical Ventilation: 10 Fundamental Maxims. *Respir Care*. 2014;59:1747–1763.
16. Chatburn RL. Understanding mechanical ventilators. *Expert Rev Respir Med*. 2010;4:809–819.
17. Cairo JM. *Pilbeam's Mechanical Ventilation. Physiological and Clinical Applications*. 5th ed. St. Louis: Mosby; 2012.
18. Fedor K. Mechanical ventilators. In: Walsh BK, Czervinske MP, DiBlasi RM, eds. *Perinatal and Pediatric Respiratory Care*. 3rd ed. St. Louis: Saunders; 2010:267–304.
19. Hess DR, Kacmarek RM. *Essentials of Mechanical Ventilation*. 3rd ed. New York: McGraw-Hill; 2014.
20. Chatburn RL. Classification of mechanical ventilators and modes of ventilation. In: Tobin MJ, ed. *Principles and Practice of Mechanical Ventilation*. 3rd ed. New York: McGraw-Hill; 2012.

21. Chatburn RL, Volsko TA, Hazy J, et al. Determining the basis for a taxonomy of mechanical ventilation. *Respir Care.* 2012;57:514–524.
22. Chatburn RL, Daoud EG. Ventilation. In: Kacmarek RM, Stoller JK, Heuer AH, eds. *Egan's Fundamentals of Respiratory Care.* 10th ed. St. Louis: Mosby Elsevier; 2012:225–249.
23. Rodarte JR, Rehder K. Dynamics of respiration. In: Fishman AP, Macklem PT, Mead J, Geiger SR. *Handbook of Physiology. The Respiratory System. Volume III, Mechanics of Breathing, Part 1.* Bethesda, Md.: American Physiological Society; 1986:131–144.
24. Chatburn RL, Volsko TA. Documentation issues for mechanical ventilation in pressure-control modes. *Respir Care.* 2011;55: 1705–1716.
25. Babic MD, Chatburn RL, Stoller JK. Laboratory evaluation of the Vortran Automatic Resuscitator Model RTM. *Respir Care.* 2007;52:1718–1727.
26. Chatburn RL, Mireles-Cabodevila E. Closed-loop control of mechanical ventilation: description and classification of targeting schemes. *Respir Care.* 2011;56:85–102.
27. Amato MB, Barbas CS, Bonassa J, et al. Volume-assured pressure support ventilation (VAPSV). A new approach for reducing muscle workload during acute respiratory failure. *Chest.* 1992;102: 1225–1234.
28. Volsko TA, Hoffman J, Conger A, Chatburn RL. The effect of targeting scheme on tidal volume delivery during volume control mechanical ventilation. *Respir Care.* 2012;57:1297–1304.
29. Mutch WA, Harms S, Ruth GM, et al. Biologically variable or naturally noisy mechanical ventilation recruits atelectatic lung. *Am J Respir Crit Care Med.* 2000;162:319–323.
30. Spieth PM, Güldner A, Beda A, et al. Comparative effects of proportional assist and variable pressure support ventilation on lung function and damage in experimental lung injury. *Crit Care Med.* 2012;40:2654–2661.
31. Mireles-Cabodevila E, Chatburn RL. Work of breathing in adaptive pressure control continuous mandatory ventilation. *Respir Care.* 2009;54:1467–1472.
32. Chatburn RL, Volsko TA. Mechanical ventilators. In: Kacmarek RM, Stoller JK, Heuer AH, eds. *Egan's Fundamentals of Respiratory Care.* 10th ed. St. Louis: Mosby Elsevier; 2012:1006–1040.
33. Chatburn RL, Volsko TA. Mechanical ventilators: classification and principles of operation. In: Hess DR, MacIntyre NR, Mishoe SC, Galvin WF, Adams AB, Saposnick AB, eds. *Respiratory Care: Principles and Practice.* Philadelphia: Saunders; 2012.
34. Mireles-Cabodevila E, Chatburn RL. A rational basis for comparing modes of mechanical ventilation. *Respir Care.* 2013;58:348–366.

CHAPTER

20 Mechanical Ventilation

Dean R. Hess, Neil R. MacIntyre

OUTLINE

OBJECTIVES

1. List the indications for and complications of mechanical ventilation.
2. Discuss issues related to ventilator-associated lung injury.
3. Select appropriate ventilator settings.
4. List parameters that should be monitored during mechanical ventilation.
5. Discuss issues related to liberation from mechanical ventilation.

KEY TERMS

adaptive pressure control
adaptive support ventilation (ASV)
airway pressure release ventilation (APRV)
auto-PEEP
compressible volume
continuous mandatory ventilation (CMV)
continuous positive airway pressure (CPAP)
flow triggering
high-frequency oscillatory ventilation (HFOV)
intermittent mandatory ventilation (IMV)
lung-protective ventilator strategy
mean airway pressure ($\bar{P}aw$)
neurally adjusted ventilatory assist (NAVA)
oxygen toxicity
patient–ventilator asynchrony
peak inspiratory pressure (PIP)
permissive hypercapnia
plateau pressure (Pplat)
positive end-expiratory pressure (PEEP)
pressure control (PC)
pressure support (PS)
pressure triggering
proportional assist ventilation (PAV)
spontaneous breathing trial (SBT)
synchronized intermittent mandatory ventilation (SIMV)
tube compensation (TC)
ventilator-induced lung injury (VILI)
volume control (VC)
weaning parameters

Introduction

Mechanical ventilation is an important life support technology that is an integral component of critical care. Mechanical ventilation can be applied as negative pressure to the outside of the thorax (e.g., the iron lung) or, most often, as positive pressure to the airway. The desired effect of positive pressure ventilation is to maintain adequate levels of Pa_{O_2} and Pa_{CO_2} while also unloading the inspiratory muscles. Mechanical ventilation is a life-sustaining technology, but recognition is growing that when used incorrectly, it can contribute to morbidity and mortality. Positive pressure ventilation is provided in intensive care units (ICUs), subacute facilities, long-term care facilities, and the home. Positive pressure ventilation can be invasive (i.e., with an endotracheal tube or tracheostomy tube) or noninvasive (e.g., with a face mask). This chapter addresses invasive positive pressure ventilation as it is applied in adults with acute respiratory failure. Modern ventilators used in the intensive care unit are microprocessor controlled and available from several manufacturers (**Figure 20-1** and **Figure 20-2**).

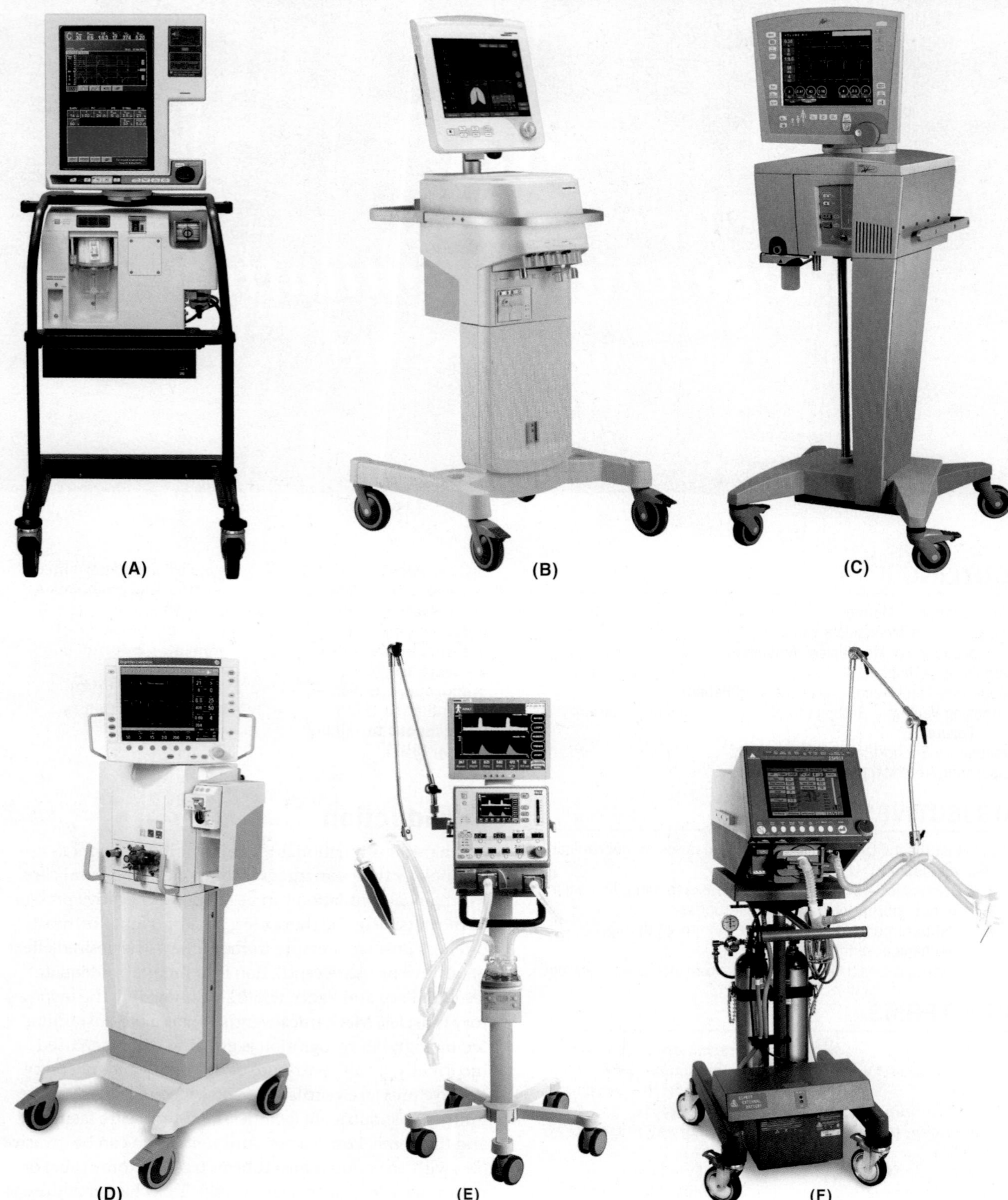

FIGURE 20-1 Examples of mechanical ventilators commonly used in critical care in the United States.

(**A**) © 2014 Covidien. All rights reserved. Used with the permission of Covidien; (**B**) courtesy of Hamilton Medical, Inc.; (**C**) reproduced with permission from CareFusion; (**D**) image courtesy of GE HealthCare, used with permission; (**E**) image courtesy of Newport Medical Instruments, Inc.; (**F**) courtesy of Philips Respironics.

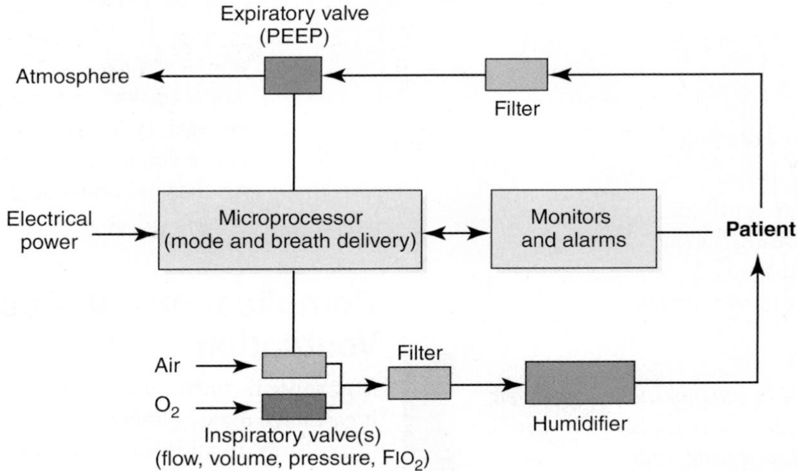

FIGURE 20-2 Modern ventilators are electronically and pneumatically controlled. The inspiratory valves control flow, pressure, and FIO_2 to the patient. The expiratory valve is closed during the inspiratory phase and the inspiratory valve is closed during the expiratory phase. The expiratory valve controls positive end-expiratory pressure (PEEP). The inspiratory and expiratory valves are controlled by the microprocessor. Sensors measure pressure and flow, which are displayed as numeric and graphic data and determine when an alarm condition is generated.

The Equation of Motion

Positive pressure, when applied at the airway opening, interacts with respiratory system (lung and chest wall) compliance, airways resistance, respiratory system inertance, and tissue resistance to produce gas flow into the lung. The interactions of airway pressure (Paw), respiratory muscle pressure (Pmus), flow, and volume with respiratory system mechanics can be expressed as the equation of motion:

$$\text{Paw} + \text{Pmus} = (\text{Flow} \times \text{Resistance}) + (\text{Volume/Compliance}) + \text{Applied PEEP} + \text{auto-PEEP}$$

For spontaneous breathing, Paw = 0 and all of the pressure required for ventilation is provided by the respiratory muscles. For full ventilatory support, Pmus = 0 and all of the pressure required for ventilation is provided by the ventilator. For partial ventilatory support, both the ventilator and the respiratory muscles contribute to ventilation.

For full ventilatory support, the ventilator controls either the pressure or the flow (volume) applied to the airway. The equation of motion predicts that Paw will vary for a given resistance and compliance if flow and volume are controlled, as in **volume control (VC)**. The equation of motion also predicts that flow and volume will vary for a given resistance and compliance if Paw is controlled, as in **pressure control (PC)**.

An important point to remember in considering the equation of motion is that, in the setting of high minute ventilation, long inspiratory-to-expiratory time ratios, and prolonged expiratory time constants (e.g., as seen in obstructive lung disease), the lungs may not return to the baseline circuit pressure during exhalation. This creates **auto-PEEP**, which must be counteracted by Pmus and Paw in the equation of motion to affect flow and volume delivery. The effects of other factors, such as inertance and tissue resistance, are small and their effects are usually ignored.

Indications for Mechanical Ventilation

Mechanical ventilation is indicated in many situations (**Box 20-1**). Goals of mechanical ventilation are shown in **Box 20-2**. Although these conditions are useful in the determination of whether mechanical ventilation is needed, clinical judgment is as important as strict adherence to absolute guidelines. One indication for mechanical ventilation is imminent acute respiratory failure; in such cases, initiating mechanical ventilation may prevent overt respiratory failure and respiratory arrest. On the other hand, depression of respiratory drive from drug overdose or from anesthesia involved with major surgery is an indication that does not

BOX 20-1

Indications for Mechanical Ventilation

Apnea
Acute ventilatory failure (e.g., rising $PaCO_2$ with acidosis, respiratory muscle dysfunction, excessive ventilatory load, altered central ventilatory drive)
Impending ventilatory failure
Severe oxygenation deficit

BOX 20-2

Goals of Mechanical Ventilation

Provide adequate oxygenation
Provide adequate alveolar ventilation
Avoid alveolar overdistention
Maintain alveolar recruitment
Promote patient–ventilator synchrony
Avoid auto-PEEP
Use the lowest possible F_{IO_2}
When choosing appropriate goals of mechanical ventilation for an individual patient, consider the risk of ventilator-induced lung injury.

involve primary respiratory system failure. In short, mechanical ventilation is required when the patient's capabilities to ventilate the lung and/or effect gas transport across the alveolocapillary interface are compromised to the point that the patient's life is threatened.

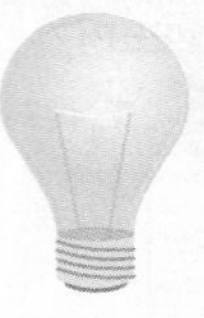

STOP AND THINK

You are asked to see a patient in acute respiratory failure. What findings might cause you to recommend intubation and mechanical ventilation?

Complications of Mechanical Ventilation

Mechanical ventilation is not a benign therapy, and it can have major effects on the body's homeostasis (**Box 20-3**). In addition to the serious complications reviewed here associated with positive pressure applied to the lungs, intubated mechanically ventilated patients also are at risk for complications associated with the use of artificial airways, the most serious being accidental disconnection and the development of pneumonia from compromised natural airway defenses. Mechanically ventilated patients are also at risk for gastrointestinal bleeding and often are given antacids, proton pump inhibitors, or histamine (H_2) blockers to prevent this complication. The nutritional needs of mechanically ventilated patients play an important role in preventing or promoting complications.

BOX 20-3

Complications of Mechanical Ventilation

Airway Complications

Laryngeal edema
Tracheal mucosal trauma
Contamination of the lower respiratory tract
Loss of humidifying function of the upper airway

Mechanical Complications

Accidental disconnection
Leaks in the ventilator circuit
Loss of electrical power
Loss of gas pressure

Pulmonary Complications

Ventilator-induced lung injury
Barotrauma
Oxygen toxicity
Atelectasis
Nosocomial pneumonia
Inflammation
Auto-PEEP
Asynchrony
Dyspnea

Cardiovascular Complications

Reduced venous return
Reduced cardiac output
Hypotension

Gastrointestinal and Nutritional Complications

Gastrointestinal bleeding
Malnutrition

Renal Complications

Reduced urine output
Increase in antidiuretic hormone (ADH) and decrease in atrial natriuretic peptide (ANP)

Neuromuscular Complications

Sleep deprivation
Increased intracranial pressure
Critical illness weakness

Acid–Base Complications

Respiratory acidosis
Respiratory alkalosis

Undernourished patients are at risk for respiratory muscle weakness and pneumonia. An excessive caloric intake, on the other hand, may increase carbon dioxide production, which can markedly increase the patient's ventilatory requirements. Sleep deprivation also occurs in mechanically ventilated patients.[1]

Ventilator-Induced Lung Injury

The application of positive pressure to the airways can create lung injury under a variety of circumstances. Pulmonary barotrauma (e.g., subcutaneous emphysema, pneumothorax, pneumomediastinum) is one of the most serious complications of excessive pressure and volume delivery to the lung and is a consequence of alveolar overdistention to the point of rupture (**Figure 20-3**). However, even when the lung is not distended to the point of rupture, excessive transpulmonary stretching pressures (lung stress) beyond the normal maximum (i.e., 20 to 25 cm H_2O) can produce a parenchymal lung injury not associated with extra-alveolar air (**ventilator-induced lung injury [VILI]**).[2] Importantly, it is the physical stretching and distention of alveolar structures that causes the injury. This concept has been demonstrated in numerous animal models in which limiting alveolar expansion (e.g., with chest strapping) prevents lung injury even in the face of very high airway pressures.

Clinical trials have confirmed these animal observations and indicate that ventilator strategies exposing injured human lungs to transpulmonary pressures in excess of 25 cm H_2O are associated with lung injury.[3] In patients with normal chest wall mechanics, this translates to a plateau pressure (Pplat) >30 cm H_2O. Of note is that this injury is likely more than simply the result of excessive end-inspiratory alveolar stretch. Excessive tidal stretch (i.e., lung strain associated with repetitive tidal volumes greater than 6 mL/kg), even in the setting of maximal transpulmonary pressures less than 30 cm H_2O, may contribute to VILI.[4–7] This provides the rationale for using **lung-protective ventilator strategies** that limit tidal volume and end-inspiratory distending pressures. Importantly, this approach may require acceptance of less than normal values for pH and Pa_{O_2} in exchange for lower (and safer) distending pressures.

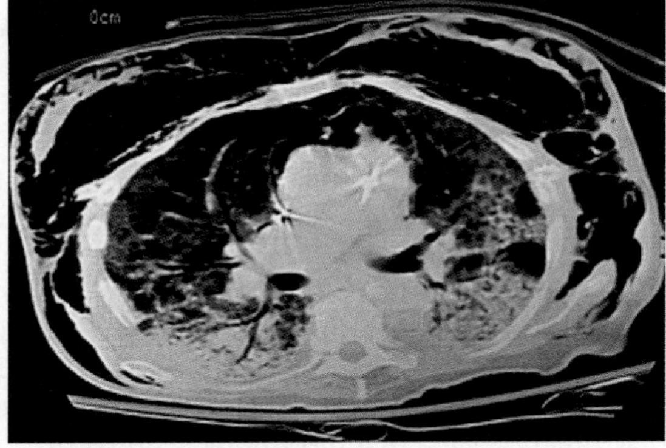

FIGURE 20-3 Computed tomography scan of the thorax of a mechanically ventilated patient with severe barotrauma. Note the presence of pneumothorax, pneumomediastinum, and subcutaneous emphysema.

Respiratory Recap

Types of Ventilator-Induced Lung Injury

- Volutrauma
- Atelectrauma
- Biotrauma
- Oxygen toxicity

VILI also can result from the cyclical opening of an alveolus during inhalation and closure during exhalation (cyclical atelectasis producing atelectrauma).[8,9] Indeed, pressures at the junction between an open and a closed alveolus may exceed 100 cm H_2O during this process (sometimes called a raiser or stress multiplier).[10] This injury is reduced with the use of smaller tidal volumes and may be ameliorated by optimal lung recruitment and an expiratory pressure (PEEP) that prevents alveolar derecruitment. **Positive end-expiratory pressure (PEEP)**, however, can be a two-edged sword. If an increase in PEEP results in an increase in alveolar recruitment and lung compliance, then the stress in the lungs is reduced. But if an increase in PEEP increases end-inspiratory transpulmonary pressure, then the stress on the lungs is increased.[6] Other ventilatory pattern factors may also be involved in the development of VILI. These include frequency of stretch[11] and the acceleration or velocity of stretch.[12] Vascular pressure elevations may also contribute to VILI.[13]

VILI is manifest pathologically as diffuse alveolar damage, and it increases inflammatory cytokines in the lungs (biotrauma).[14–16] VILI is also spillage of inflammatory cytokines from the lungs into the blood stream and bacterial translocation,[17] which are implicated in the systemic inflammatory response with multiorgan dysfunction that increases mortality. The way in which the lungs are ventilated may therefore play a role in systemic inflammation (**Figure 20-4**).

Oxygen Toxicity

Oxygen concentrations approaching 100% are known to cause oxidant injuries in airways and lung parenchyma.[18] Many of the data supporting the concept of **oxygen toxicity**, however, have come from animals that often have quite different tolerances to oxygen than humans. It is unclear what the safe oxygen concentration or duration of exposure is in sick humans, such as those with acute respiratory distress syndrome (ARDS). Many authorities have argued that a fraction of inspired oxygen (F_{IO_2}) less than 0.4 is safe for prolonged periods of time and that a F_{IO_2} greater than 0.80 should

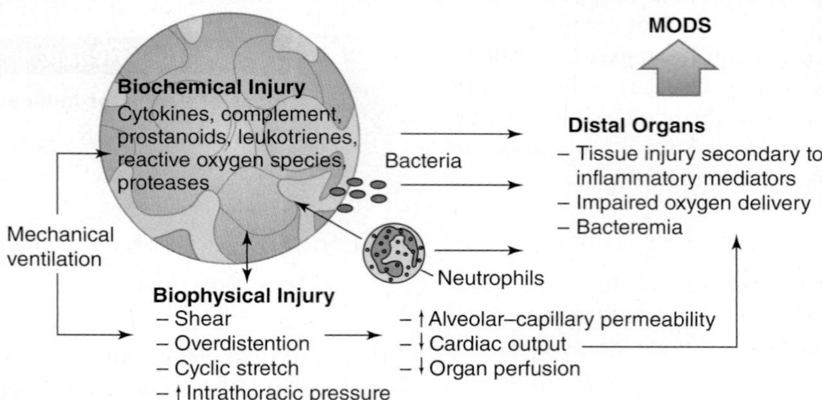

FIGURE 20-4 Mechanical ventilation can result in biochemical and biophysical injury to the lungs, which may result in multisystem organ failure. MODS, multiple organ dysfunction syndrome.

Adapted from Slutsky AS, Trembly L. Multiple system organ failure: is mechanical ventilation a contributing factor? *Am J Respir Crit Care Med.* 1998;157:1721–1725.

be avoided. The relative toxicities of VILI and oxygen are not clear. In one large study (ARDSnet), however, survival was greater in patients with ARDS who were ventilated with a lower tidal volume, presumably avoiding significant VILI, despite the fact that the required FIO_2 was higher in the group receiving the lower tidal volumes.[3]

Ventilator-Associated Pneumonia

An endotracheal tube compromises the natural laryngeal mechanism that protects the lower respiratory tract from aspiration. This permits oropharyngeal debris to leak into the airways, even in the presence of a cuff seal. The endotracheal tube also impairs the cough reflex and serves as a potential portal for pathogens to enter the lungs. The underlying disease process makes the lungs prone to infection. In addition, heavy antibiotic use in the ICU and the presence of very sick patients in close proximity are risk factors for antibiotic-resistant infection.

Preventing ventilator-associated pneumonia (VAP) is important because VAP is associated with morbidity and mortality.[19] VAP prevention has become an important priority in the mechanically ventilated patient. Hand washing, elevating the head of the bed, oral care, and carefully choosing antibiotic regimens can have important preventive effects. Circuit changes only when visibly contaminated is a helpful strategy.[20] Endotracheal tubes that provide continuous drainage of subglottic secretions, endotracheal tubes with specialized cuff designs, and endotracheal tubes made with antimicrobial materials are other ways of reducing lung contamination with oropharyngeal material. However, these tubes are more expensive and their cost-effectiveness is controversial.[21,22]

Auto-PEEP

As described above, auto-PEEP (also known as intrinsic PEEP or air trapping) is the result of the lungs not returning to the baseline proximal airway pressure at end-exhalation.[23] The determinants of auto-PEEP are high minute volume, long inspiratory-to-expiratory time relationships, and long expiratory time constants (i.e., obstructed airways and high-compliance alveolar units). Because it results in dynamic hyperinflation, auto-PEEP raises all intrathoracic pressures, which can affect gas delivery, hemodynamics, end-inspiratory distention (and thus VILI), and patient breath triggering. Although sometimes desired in long inspiratory time ventilatory strategies, auto-PEEP is generally to be avoided because it is difficult to recognize and to predict its effects.

Hemodynamic Effects of Positive Pressure Ventilation

Because positive pressure ventilation increases intrathoracic pressure, it can reduce venous return and increase right ventricular afterload, which may result in decreased cardiac output and a drop in arterial blood pressure. Fluid administration and drug therapy (such as with vasopressors and inotropes) may be necessary to maintain cardiac output, blood pressure, and urine output under these circumstances. Mechanical ventilation also can cause an increase in plasma antidiuretic hormone (ADH) and a decrease in atrial natriuretic peptide (ANP), which may reduce urine output and promote fluid retention.

The effect of reduced cardiac filling on cardiac output may be partially counteracted by better left ventricular function due to elevated intrathoracic pressures, which reduce left ventricular afterload. In patients with fluid overload and left heart failure, the reduced cardiac filling and reduced left ventricular afterload effects of elevated intrathoracic pressure may actually improve cardiac function such that intrathoracic pressure removal may produce left ventricular failure.

Intrathoracic pressure can also influence distribution of perfusion, as described by the West model

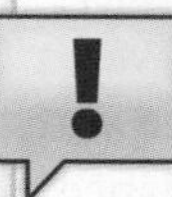

Respiratory Recap

Indications for and Complications of Mechanical Ventilation

- Mechanical ventilation supports gas exchange in patients with acute respiratory failure.
- A number of complications are possible with mechanical ventilation, and efforts must be made to minimize these complications.

of pulmonary perfusion. In the supine human lung, blood flow is greatest in zone 3. As intra-alveolar pressure rises, there is an increase in zone 2 and zone 1 (dead space) regions, creating high ventilation-perfusion ($\dot{V}/\dot{Q}$) units. Dyspnea, anxiety, and discomfort associated with inadequate ventilatory support can lead to stress-related catecholamine release, with increases in myocardial oxygen demands and risk of dysrhythmias. In addition, coronary blood flow can be compromised by inadequate gas exchange from the lung injury coupled with low mixed venous Po_2 due to high oxygen consumption demands by the inspiratory muscles.

Ventilator Settings

Terminology

The terminology used to describe ventilator modes has grown complicated over the years. Manufacturers have coined different names for the same modes and individual clinicians have developed their own pet jargon. This is particularly problematic when ventilators from different manufacturers are used in the same hospital and when clinicians (respiratory therapists and physicians) use different words to mean the same thing.

The positive pressure ventilators of the late 1960s and early 1970s only provided volume-controlled breaths (e.g., Emerson Post-Op) and could not be triggered by the patient. These breaths were termed *controlled* and the mode was called *controlled mechanical ventilation.* Importantly, patients could not interact with these breaths and often needed deep sedation, sometimes with paralysis, to suppress breathing efforts. As appreciation grew that spontaneous breathing efforts should not be fully suppressed, the ability for patients to breathe spontaneously, without any ventilator assistance, between mandatory breaths was developed and **intermittent mandatory ventilation (IMV)** was introduced.

Terminology became confusing when patient triggering of mandatory breaths was introduced to improve synchrony. This mode of ventilation became known as assist-control (A/C) ventilation. If the patient did not trigger the breath, this was called controlled ventilation. If the patient triggered the breath, this was called assisted ventilation, implying that the ventilator was assisting the patient's breathing with pressure-controlled or volume-controlled breaths. Confusion developed because the term *control* was now being used to describe triggering as well as to describe the primary variable the ventilator targeted during breath delivery. This led to some clinicians arguing that it is incorrect to refer to breaths that are not patient triggered as *controlled breaths*, because breath delivery such as VC or PC is *controlled* exactly the same by the ventilator whether triggered by the patient or not. Making this even more confusing, some clinicians began referring to the patient-triggered breaths as the *patient assisting*, which was unfortunate because the ventilator assists the patient, not vice versa.

Breath types are called *mandatory* when the ventilator delivers the same breath type with every cycle, regardless of whether triggered by the patient or ventilator. When every breath is a mandatory breath (VC or PC), the mode is *continuous mandatory ventilation* (CMV). This is commonly called *assist-control* by clinicians and manufacturers when patient triggering is possible, and the terms CMV and A/C are used interchangeably to mean the same thing. Note that the contemporary CMV (*continuous mandatory ventilation*) is different from the original *controlled mechanical ventilation.*

When the ventilator requires every breath to be triggered and cycled by the patient, these are called *spontaneous* breaths, meaning that a spontaneous respiratory drive of the patient is required to determine breath timing. This is what occurs with continuous positive airway pressure (CPAP) and with pressure support (PS); the patient triggers every breath, but the ventilator either maintains a baseline pressure (PEEP; CPAP) or assists the patient's breathing by applying pressure to the airway during the inspiratory phase to unload inspiratory muscles (PS)—just as mandatory breaths do. Depending on the settings, PS potentially can unload respiratory muscles either more or less than patient triggered mandatory breaths. The distinction is not the amount of respiratory muscle unloading by the breath type, but whether or not the patient must trigger and cycle the breath.

For everyday clinical speak, the breath type may be combined with the mode. For example, when the breath type is VC and the mode is A/C (CMV), some would call this VC-CMV, whereas others might call it VACV. Similarly, what some would call PC-CMV, others might call PACV (PC with A/C). And others have probably adapted their own pet jargon to describe these terms. Thus it is important to understand exactly how breath delivery occurs from the specific ventilator used so as not to introduce confusion—and potentially clinical error—from misinterpretation of the language used by different clinicians and different manufacturers.

Volume-Control Versus Pressure Control

The ventilator controls either flow or pressure with each breath delivery. Although many breath types exist on modern ventilators, they all derive from ventilator control of either flow or pressure during the inspiratory phase.

With VC, the ventilator controls the inspiratory flow (**Figure 20-5**). Tidal volume is determined by the settings of flow and the inspiratory time. In practice, however, the flow and tidal volume are set on the ventilator. Because flow and volume delivery are fixed with VC, airway pressure varies with changes in resistance and compliance. Flow and tidal volume are the independent variables, and pressure is the dependent variable. With VC, the tidal volume is delivered regardless of patient effort, resistance, or compliance, provided

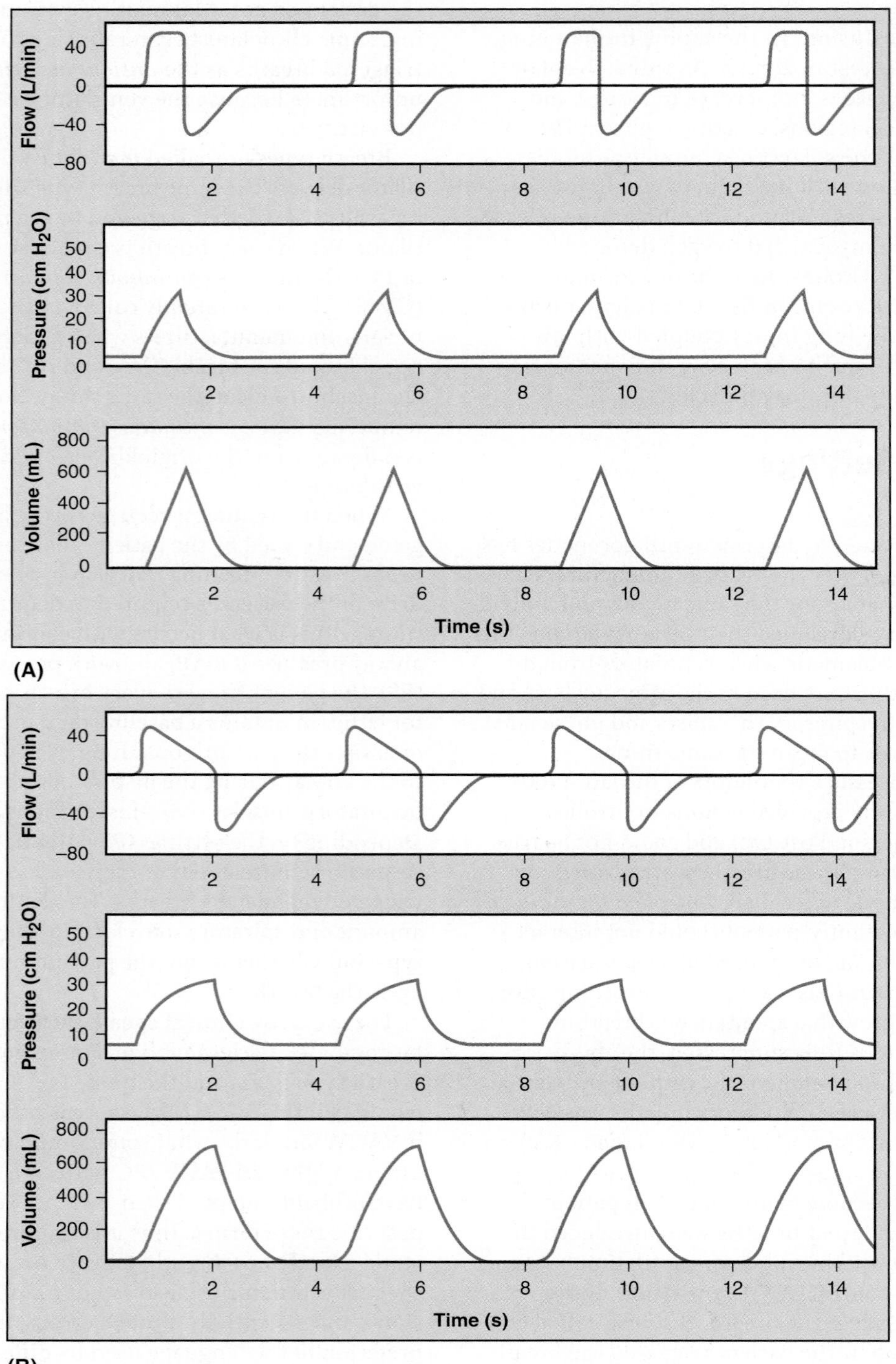

FIGURE 20-5 (**A**) Constant-flow (square wave) volume control. (**B**) Descending ramp flow with volume control.

BOX 20-4

Factors That Affect Peak Inspiratory Pressure (PIP) with Volume Control

Peak inspiratory flow setting: A higher flow setting increases the PIP.
Inspiratory flow pattern: PIP is lower with descending ramp flow.
Positive end-expiratory pressure (PEEP): An increase in PEEP increases the PIP.
Auto-PEEP: Auto-PEEP increases the PIP.
Tidal volume (VT): An increase in VT results in a higher PIP.
Resistance: Greater airways resistance results in a higher PIP.
Compliance: Decreased compliance results in a higher PIP.

that the high-pressure alarm limit is not reached, and the peak airway pressure varies (**Box 20-4**). VC should be used whenever a constant tidal volume is important in the maintenance of a desired Pa_{CO_2}. Because inspiratory flow is fixed, VC can be associated with **patient–ventilator asynchrony**, particularly if the inspiratory flow is set too low. With VC, the set flow can be constant or a descending ramp. A descending ramp flow pattern produces a longer inspiratory time unless the peak flow is increased.

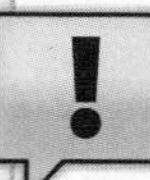

Respiratory Recap

Volume Control Versus Pressure Control

- *Volume control*: Ventilation remains constant with changes in respiratory mechanics or effort, but airway and plateau pressures can fluctuate.
- *Pressure control*: Ventilation fluctuates with changes in respiratory mechanics or effort, but pressure is limited to the peak pressure set on the ventilator.

With PC (**Figure 20-6**), airway pressure is set and remains constant despite changes in effort, resistance, and compliance. The pressure set is the independent variable, and the flow and tidal volume are the dependent variables. **Box 20-5** lists factors that affect the tidal volume with PC. PC generally prevents localized alveolar overdistention with changes in resistance and compliance, because the peak alveolar pressure cannot be greater than the pressure set on the ventilator. It must be remembered that patient effort during PC can result in additional tidal volume and end-inspiratory transpulmonary pressure.

Because the flow can vary with PC, this mode might improve patient–ventilator synchrony during patient-triggered breaths in some patients,[24] but this benefit is limited when attempts are made to constrain the tidal volume during lung-protective ventilation.[25] The choice of VC or PC is often determined by clinician or institutional bias, and both modes have advantages and

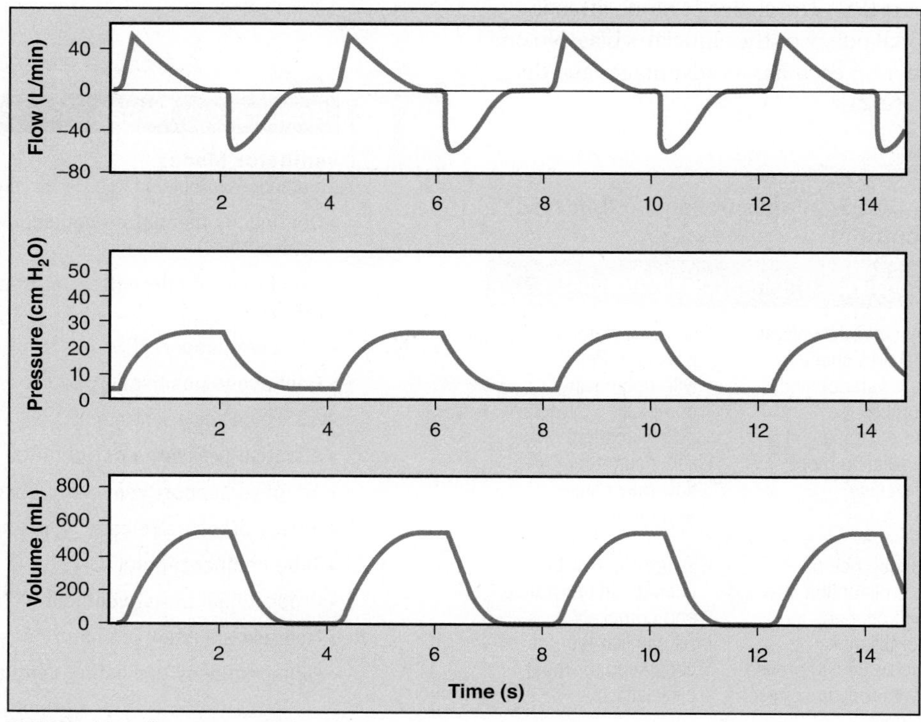

FIGURE 20-6 Pressure control.

BOX 20-5
Factors That Affect Tidal Volume (V_T) with Pressure Control

Driving pressure: A higher driving pressure (difference between peak inspiratory pressure and PEEP) increases the V_T.
Auto-PEEP: An increase in auto-PEEP reduces the V_T.
Inspiratory time: An increase in inspiratory time increases the V_T if inspiratory flow is present; after flow decreases to zero, further increases in the time do not affect the V_T.
Compliance: Decreased compliance decreases the V_T.
Resistance: Increased resistance decreases the V_T; after flow decreases to zero, resistance no longer affects the delivered V_T.
Patient effort: Greater inspiratory effort by the patient increases the V_T.

disadvantages (**Table 20-1**).[26] Whichever breath type is chosen, the principles of lung-protection ventilation should be observed (volume and pressure limitation with appropriate levels of PEEP).

Ventilator Mode

Options for breath delivery are referred to as *modes of ventilation*.[27] Traditional modes include continuous mandatory ventilation (CMV), also called assist-control (A/C), synchronized intermittent mandatory ventilation (SIMV), and pressure support (PS). The choice of mode often is based on institutional policy or the clinician's bias. No one mode is clearly superior; each has its advantages and disadvantages (**Table 20-2**).

TABLE 20-1
Advantages and Disadvantages of Volume Control and Pressure Control

Type	Advantages	Disadvantages
Volume control	Constant tidal volume (V_T) with changes in resistance and compliance Type of ventilation familiar to most clinicians	Increased plateau pressure (Pplat) with decreasing compliance (alveolar overdistention) Fixed inspiratory flow may cause asynchrony
Pressure control	Reduced risk of overdistention with changes in compliance Variable flow improves synchrony in some patients	Changes in V_T with changes in resistance and compliance Less familiar type of ventilation for most clinicians

Continuous mandatory ventilation (CMV) (or A/C) delivers VC or PC (could be adaptive pressure control with a volume target) and a set minimum respiratory rate (**Figure 20-7**). The patient can trigger additional breaths above the minimum rate, but the set volume or pressure, and inspiratory time, remain constant. When mechanical ventilation is initiated, it often is best to use CMV (A/C) to produce nearly complete respiratory muscle rest (i.e., full ventilatory support). Regardless of the mode used, the goal is to strike a balance between excessive respiratory muscle rest, which promotes atrophy, and excessive respiratory muscle activity, which promotes fatigue. Or, put simply, to avoid the extremes of too much rest or too much exercise.

Continuous positive airway pressure (CPAP) is a spontaneous breathing mode with a constant positive pressure throughout the breathing cycle (**Figure 20-8**). CPAP is commonly used as a means of maintaining alveolar recruitment in mild to moderate forms of pulmonary edema and parenchymal lung injury. CPAP often is used to evaluate a patient's ability to breathe spontaneously before extubation.

Pressure support (PS) is a breathing mode in which the patient's spontaneous effort is augmented by a clinician-determined level of pressure (**Figure 20-9**).[28] Although the clinician sets the level of pressure support, the patient sets the respiratory rate and inspiratory flow. Inspiratory time is determined by a flow cycle mechanism. The pressure support level, the amount of patient effort, the flow cycle criteria, and the resistance and compliance of the respiratory system determine V_T.

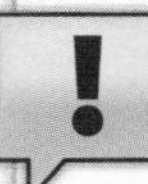

Respiratory Recap

Ventilator Modes
Commonly available on virtually all ventilators:

- Continuous mandatory ventilation (CMV); assist-control (A/C)
- Synchronized intermittent mandatory ventilation (SIMV)
- Pressure support (PS)
- Continuous positive airway pressure (CPAP)

Available on some ventilators:

- Adaptive pressure control (APC)
- Adaptive support ventilation (ASV)
- Airway pressure release ventilation (APRV)
- Tube compensation (TC)
- Proportional assist ventilation (PAV)
- Neurally adjusted ventilatory assist (NAVA)
- High-frequency oscillatory ventilation (HFOV)

TABLE 20-2
Advantages and Disadvantages of Common Modes of Mechanical Ventilation

Mode of Ventilation	Advantages	Disadvantages
Continuous mandatory ventilation (CMV)	Guaranteed volume (or pressure) with each breath Low patient workload if sensitivity and inspiratory flow set correctly	High mean airway pressure Respiratory alkalosis and auto-PEEP if patient triggers at rapid rate Respiratory muscle atrophy possible
Synchronized intermittent mandatory ventilation (SIMV)	Lower mean airway pressure Prevents respiratory muscle atrophy	Asynchrony if rate set too low High work of breathing with older ventilators
Pressure support (PS)	Variable flow may improve synchrony in some patients Overcomes tube resistance Prevents respiratory muscle atrophy	Requires spontaneous respiratory effort Fatigue and tachypnea with PS too low Activation of expiratory muscles with PS too high
Adaptive pressure control	Ventilator maintains tidal volume with changes in respiratory system mechanics Variable flow may improve synchrony in some patients	Does not precisely control tidal volume Support is taken away if the patient's tidal volume consistently exceeds target
Adaptive support ventilation (ASV)	Ventilator adapts settings to patient's physiology	May not precisely control tidal volume
Airway pressure release ventilation (APRV)	Allows spontaneous breathing at any time during the ventilator cycle May improve ventilation to dependent lung zones May improve oxygenation in patients with ARDS	May be uncomfortable for some patients May result in large tidal volumes, depending on $P_{high} - P_{low}$ difference May be large transpulmonary pressure swings during spontaneous breathing
Tube compensation (TC)	Overcomes resistance through artificial airway	Effect is usually small and may not affect patient outcomes
Proportional assist ventilation (PAV)	Pressure applied to the airway is determined by respiratory drive and respiratory mechanics	Not useful with weak drive or weak respiratory muscles Clinician has little control over tidal volume or respiratory rate
Neurally adjusted ventilatory assist (NAVA)	Pressure applied to the airway is determined by diaphragm activity	Requires insertion of special gastric tube to measure diaphragm EMG Not useful with weak respiratory drive or motor neuron disease

PEEP, positive end-expiratory pressure; P_{high}, high airway pressure setting; P_{low}, pressure release level; ARDS, acute respiratory distress syndrome; EMG, electromyelogram.

Pressure support is a frequently used mode of mechanical ventilation. Because it is patient triggered, however, PS is not an appropriate mode for patients who do not have an adequate respiratory drive. PS normally is flow cycled, with secondary cycling mechanisms of pressure and time. Although PS often is considered a simple mode of ventilation, it can be quite complex (**Figure 20-10**). First, the ventilator must recognize the patient's inspiratory effort, which depends on the ventilator's trigger sensitivity and the amount of auto-PEEP. Second, the ventilator must deliver an appropriate flow at the onset of inspiration. A flow that is too high can produce a pressure overshoot, and a flow that is too low can result in patient flow starvation and asynchrony. Third, the ventilator must appropriately cycle to the expiratory phase without the need for active exhalation.

The flow at which the ventilator cycles to the expiratory phase during PS can be a fixed absolute flow, a flow based on the peak inspiratory flow, or a flow based on peak inspiratory flow and elapsed inspiratory time. With airflow obstruction, the inspiratory flow decreases slowly during PS, and the flow necessary to cycle may not be reached. This can result in excessive inspiratory time and auto-PEEP or active exhalation to pressure cycle the breath. The problem increases with higher levels of PS and with higher levels of airflow obstruction. On newer ventilators, the flow cycle criteria can be adjusted to a level appropriate for the patient (**Figure 20-11**).

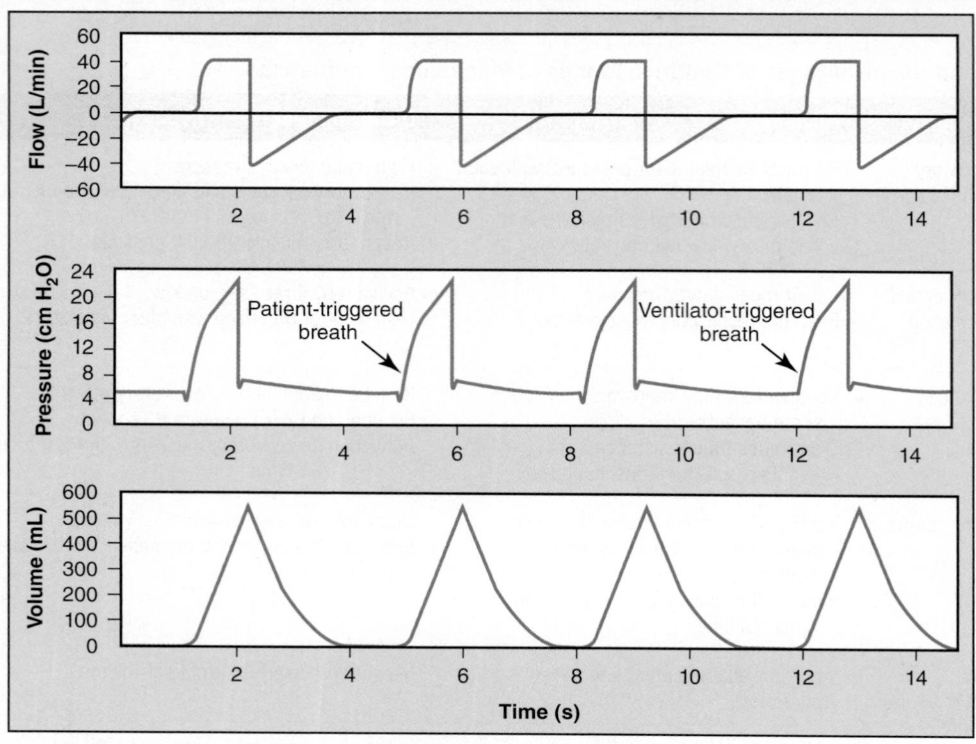

FIGURE 20-7 Continuous mandatory ventilation illustrating ventilator-triggered and patient-triggered breaths.

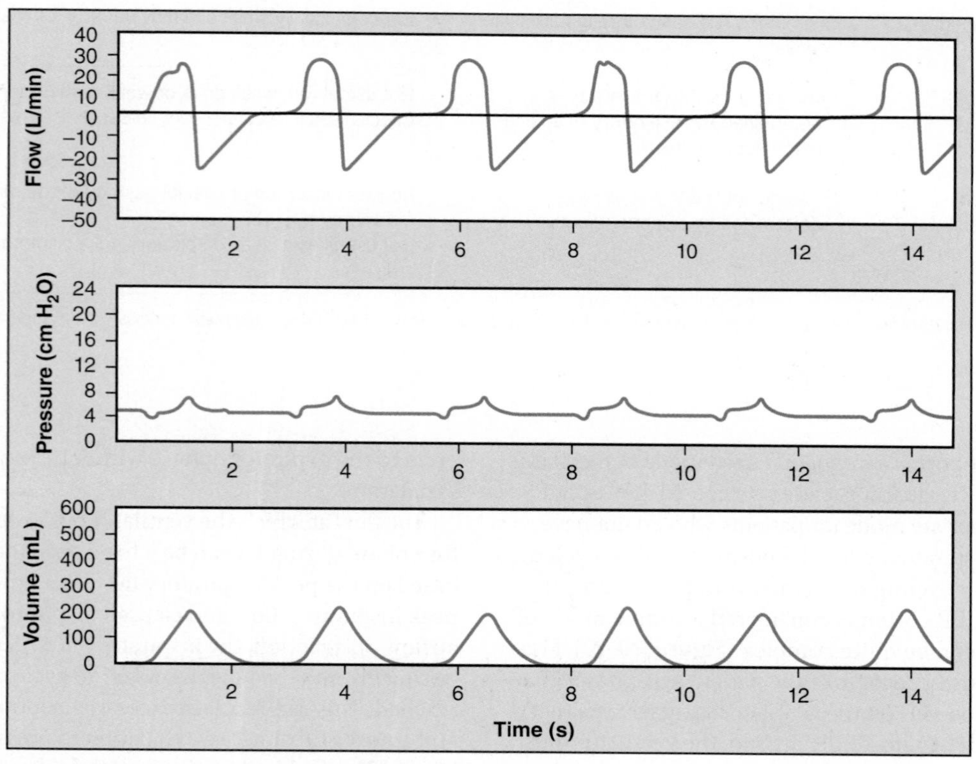

FIGURE 20-8 Continuous positive airway pressure.

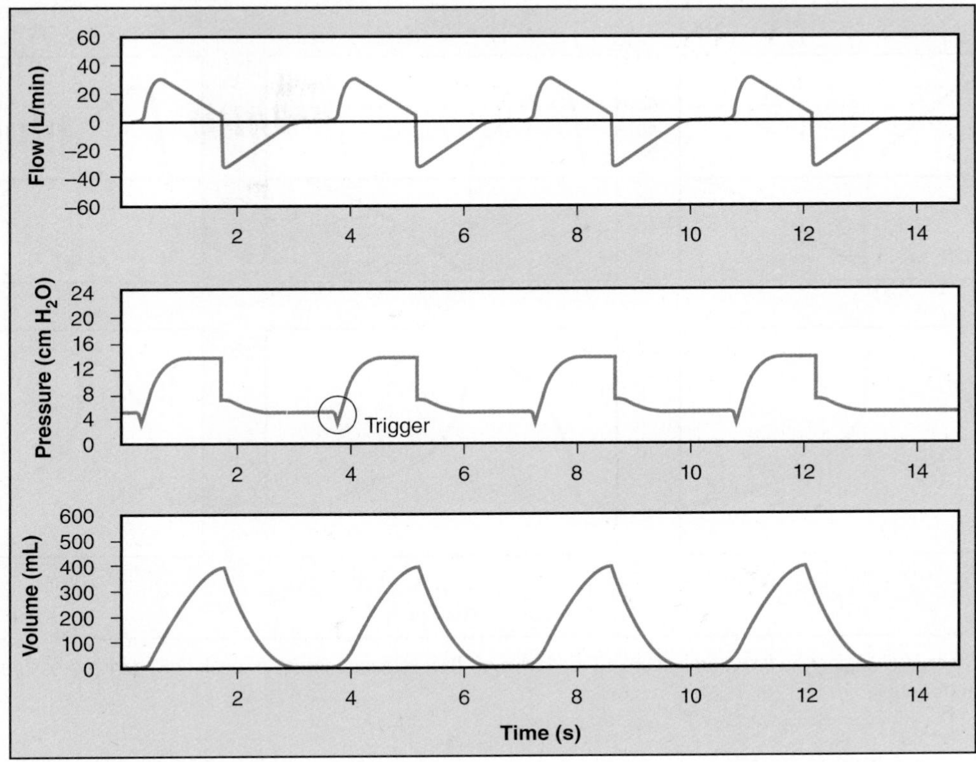

FIGURE 20-9 Pressure support.

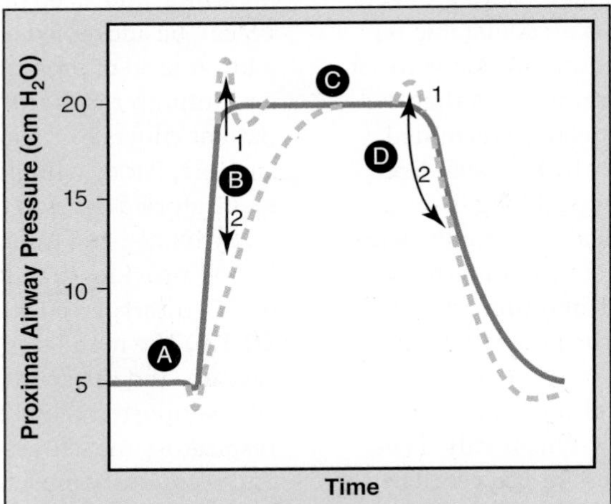

FIGURE 20-10 Design characteristics of a pressure-supported breath. In this example, baseline pressure (i.e., PEEP) is set at 5 cm H_2O and pressure support is set at 15 cm H_2O (PIP 20 cm H_2O). The inspiratory pressure is triggered at point A by a patient effort resulting in an airway pressure decrease. Demand valve sensitivity and responsiveness are characterized by the depth and duration of this negative pressure. The rise to pressure (line B) is provided by a fixed high initial flow delivery into the airway. Note that if flows exceed patient demand, initial pressure exceeds set level (B1), whereas if flows are less than patient demand, a very slow (concave) rise to pressure can occur (B2). The plateau of pressure support (line C) is maintained by servo control of flow. A smooth plateau reflects appropriate responsiveness to patient demand; fluctuations would reflect less responsiveness of the servo mechanisms. Termination of pressure support occurs at point D and should coincide with the end of the spontaneous inspiratory effort. If termination is delayed, the patient actively exhales (bump in pressure above plateau) (D1); if termination is premature, the patient will have continued inspiratory efforts (D2).

Modified from McIntyre N, Nishimura M, Usada Y, et al. The Nagoya conference on system design and patient-ventilator interactions during pressure support ventilation. *Chest.* 1990;97:1463–1466, with permission from the American College of Chest Physicians.

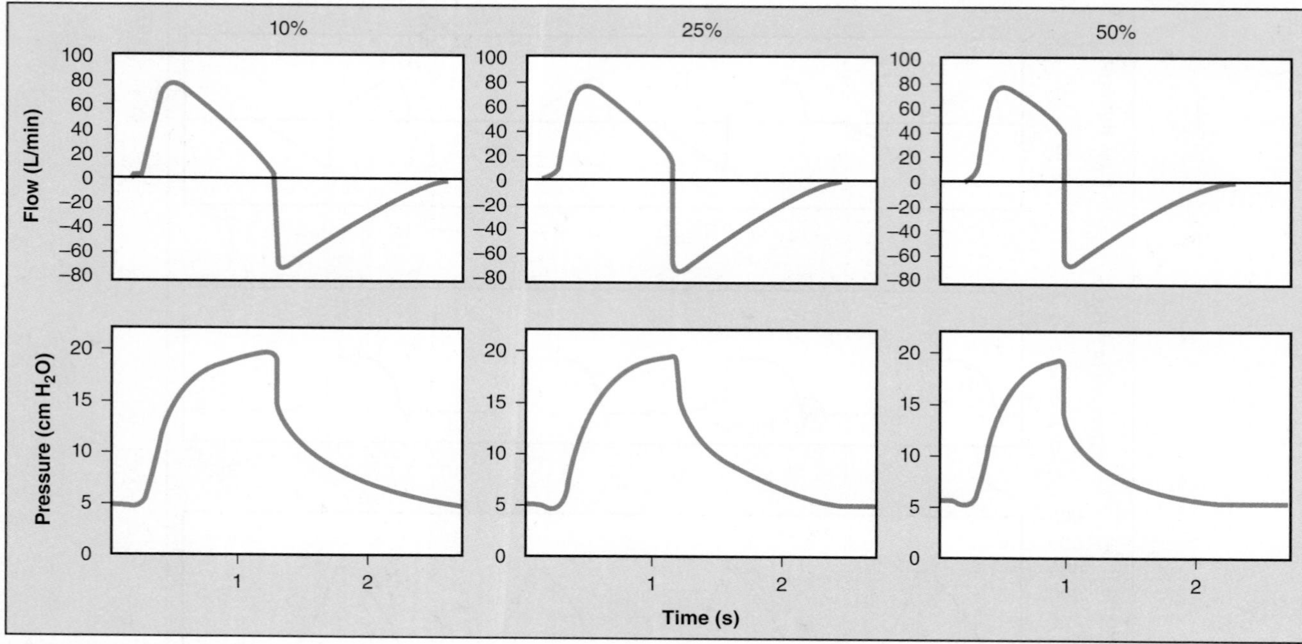

FIGURE 20-11 Effect of changing the flow termination criteria (cycle off flow as a percentage of peak flow) during pressure support. Note the effect on inspiratory time.

Another concern with PS is leaks, such as with a bronchopleural fistula, uncuffed airway, or mask leak with noninvasive ventilation. If the leak exceeds the termination flow at which the ventilator cycles, either active exhalation occurs to terminate inspiration, or a prolonged inspiratory time is applied. With a leak, either PC or a ventilator that allows an adjustable termination flow should be used. Another option is to set a maximum inspiratory time during PS such that the breath can be time cycled at a clinician-determined setting. This secondary cycle typically has been fixed at a time to prevent untoward effects of long inspiratory times. Note that this is identical to using PC with the set rate set very low, in which case all breaths are patient triggered, pressure limited, and time cycled. Some new ventilators allow both the flow cycle and time cycle to be set.

The flow at the onset of the inspiratory phase may also be important during PC or PS. This is called *rise time* and refers to the time required for the ventilator to reach the set pressure at the onset of inspiration. Flows that are too high or too low at the onset of inspiration can cause asynchrony. For example, with a high inspiratory flow at the onset of inspiration, and an excessive inspiratory flow, the inspiratory phase may be prematurely terminated during PS if the ventilator cycles to the expiratory phase at a flow that is a fraction of the peak inspiratory flow.[29] Most ventilators allow adjustment of the pressure rise time during PS and PC (**Figure 20-12**). Rise time should be adjusted to patient comfort, and ventilator graphics may be useful as a guide to this setting—the target being a smooth square wave of inspiratory pressure.

Sleep fragmentation may be more likely during PS than during CMV because there is no backup rate.[30] Central apnea during PS results in an alarm, which awakens the patient. The pattern of awakening and breathing with sleeping and apnea results in periodic breathing and sleep disruption. This complication of PS can be addressed by switching to CMV or by using a lower level of pressure support. With CMV, there is a minimum respiratory rate set, while still allowing patient efforts to trigger. With a lower level of pressure support, $Paco_2$ will likely be greater, and the associated respiratory drive will decrease the risk of apnea.

Synchronized intermittent mandatory ventilation (SIMV) provides mandatory breaths that are either VC or PC, interspersed with spontaneous breaths (**Figure 20-13**). The mandatory breaths are delivered at the set rate, and the spontaneous breaths may be pressure supported (**Figure 20-14**). The intent is to provide respiratory muscle rest during mandatory breaths and respiratory muscle exercise with the intervening breaths. However, it has been shown that considerable inspiratory effort occurs with both the mandatory breaths and the intervening spontaneous breaths.[31] As the level of SIMV support is reduced, the work of breathing increases for both mandatory and spontaneous breaths (**Figure 20-15**). This effect can be ameliorated with the addition of pressure support, which results in unloading of spontaneous breaths. The addition of pressure support might result in a reduction in respiratory drive and thereby also unloading the patient-triggered mandatory breaths.

Newer ventilators have a volume feedback mechanism for pressure control or pressure support.[32,33] This is

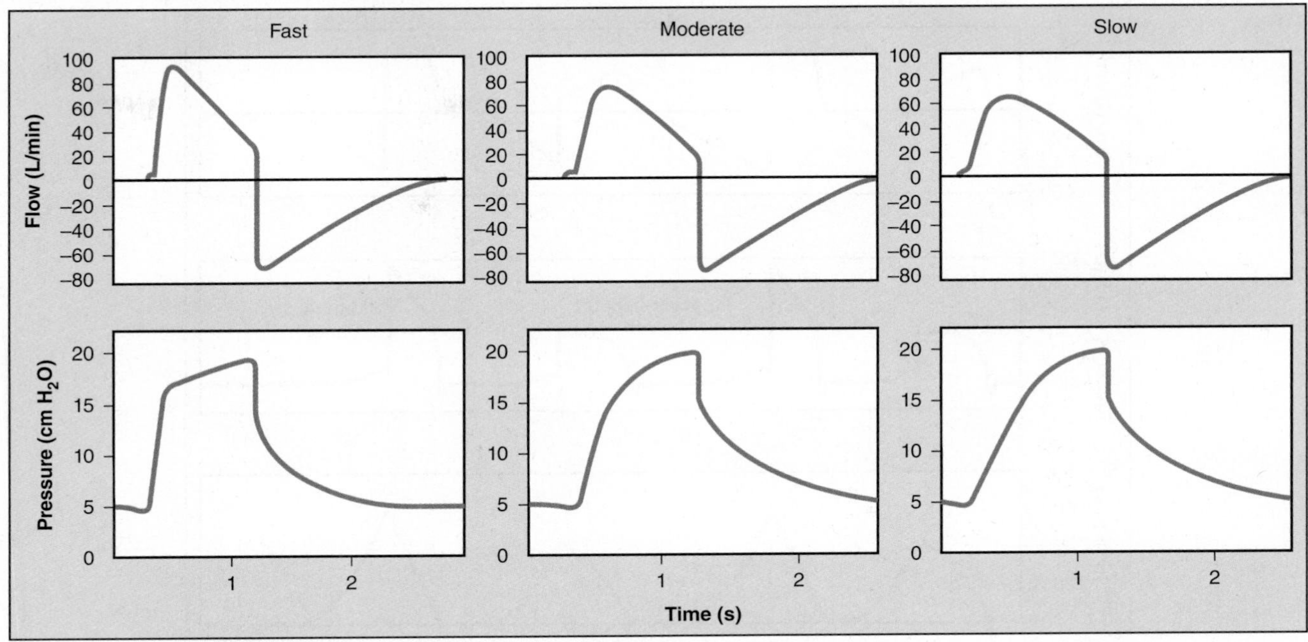

FIGURE 20-12 Effect of changing rise time during pressure support. Note the effect on peak flow.

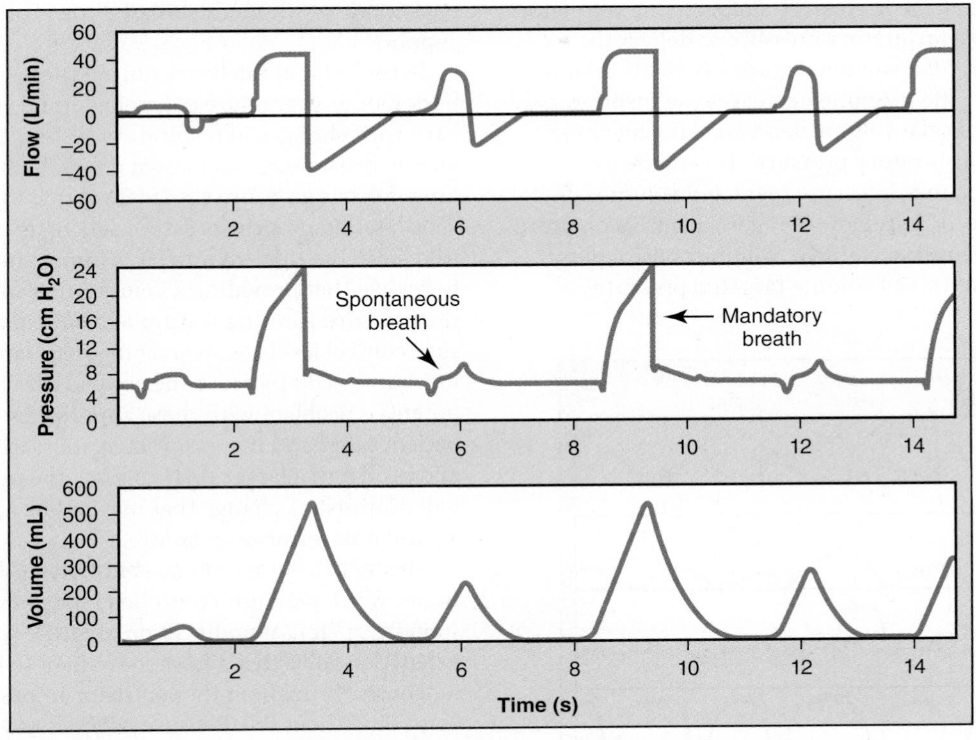

FIGURE 20-13 Synchronized intermittent mandatory ventilation illustrating spontaneous and mandatory breaths.

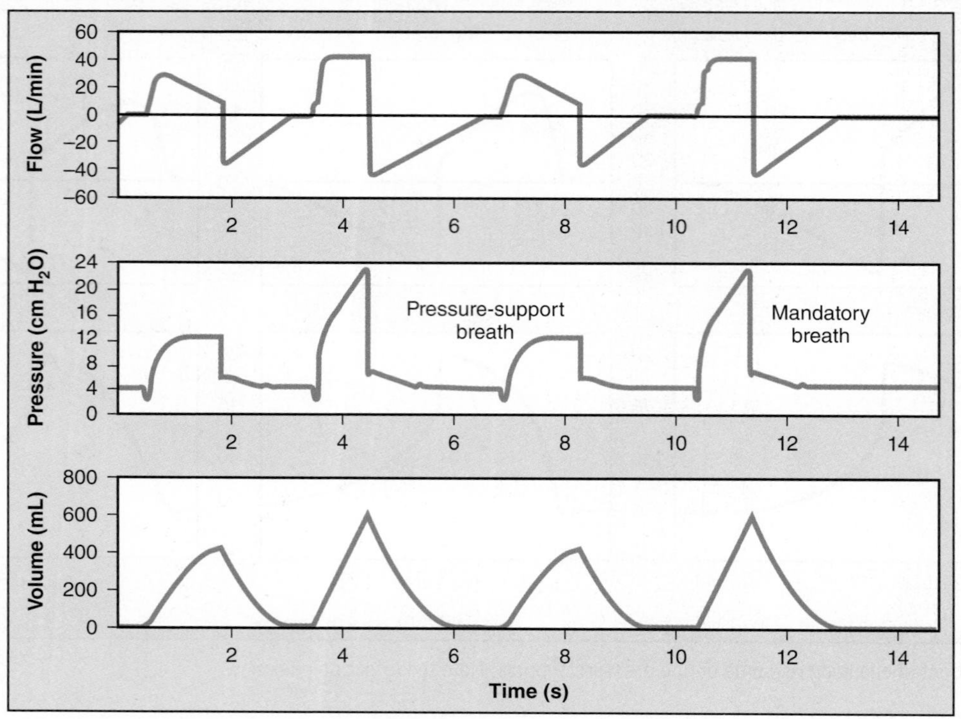

FIGURE 20-14 Synchronized intermittent mandatory ventilation with pressure support of spontaneous breaths.

called **adaptive pressure control**. The desired tidal volume is set on the ventilator, but the breath type is actually pressure control or pressure support. The ventilator then adjusts the inspiratory pressure to deliver the set minimal target tidal volume (**Figure 20-16**). If tidal volume increases, the machine decreases the inspiratory pressure, and if tidal volume decreases, the machine increases the inspiratory pressure. This mode goes by the following names: pressure regulated volume control (Maquet Servo-i), AutoFlow (Dräger), adaptive pressure ventilation (Hamilton Galileo), volume control plus (Puritan Bennett), and volume targeted pressure control or pressure controlled volume guaranteed (General Electric). Volume support is a volume feedback mode in which the breath type is only pressure support.

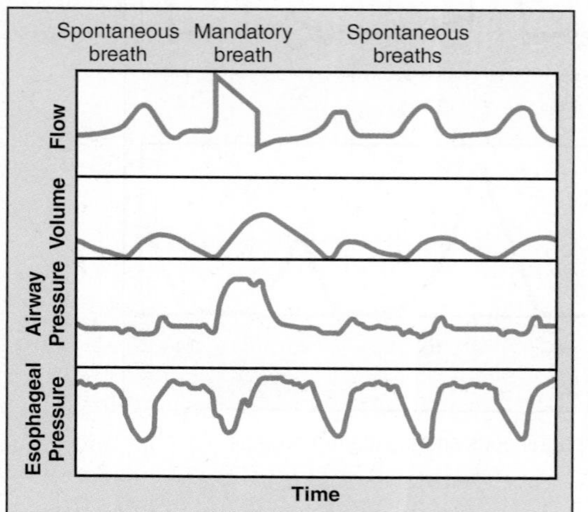

FIGURE 20-15 Synchronized intermittent mandatory ventilation. Note that the esophageal (i.e., pleural) pressure change for the mandatory breath is nearly as great as that for the spontaneous breaths.

Because breath delivery during these volume feedback modes is pressure controlled, tidal volume will vary with changes in respiratory system compliance, airway resistance, and patient effort. If changes in lung mechanics cause the tidal volume to change, the ventilator adjusts the pressure setting in an attempt to restore the tidal volume. It is important, however, to realize that providing a volume guarantee negates the pressure-limiting feature of a clinician-set pressure control level (i.e., worsening respiratory system mechanics will increase the applied pressure). Another potential problem with these approaches is that if the patient's demand inappropriately increases (e.g., pain) and produces a larger tidal volume, the pressure level will diminish, a change that may not be appropriate for a patient in respiratory failure.[34,35]

Airway pressure release ventilation (APRV) is a time-cycled, pressure-controlled mode of ventilatory support.[36,37] It is a modification of SIMV with an active exhalation valve that allows the patient to breathe spontaneously throughout the ventilator-imposed pressures (with or without PS). Because APRV is often used with a long inspiratory-to-expiratory timing pattern, most of the spontaneous breaths will occur during the long lung inflation period (**Figure 20-17**). APRV is available under a variety of proprietary trade names: APRV (Dräger), BiLevel (Puritan Bennett), BiVent (Siemens), BiPhasic (Avea), PC+ (Dräger), and DuoPAP (Hamilton).

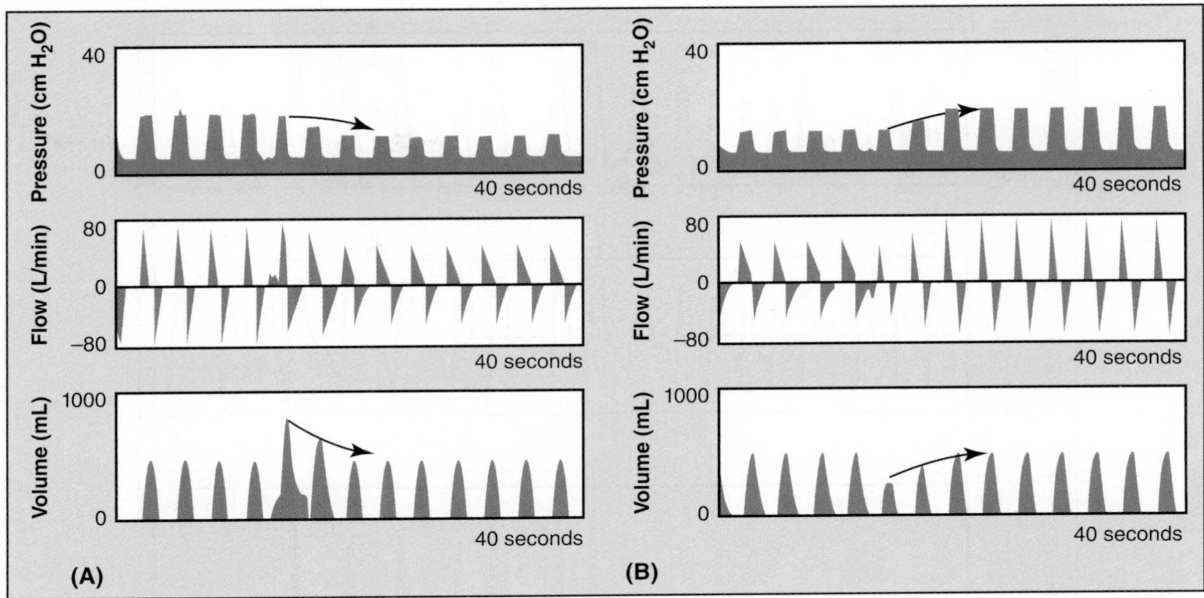

FIGURE 20-16 (**A**) Effect of adaptive pressure control with a compliance increase or respiratory effort increase. (**B**) Effect of adaptive pressure control with a compliance decrease or respiratory effort decrease.

Reproduced from Branson RD, Johannigman JA. The role of ventilator graphics when setting dual-control modes. *Respir Care* 2005;50[2]:187–201. Reprinted with permission.

APRV uses different terminology to describe breath delivery phases. Lung inflation depends on the high airway pressure setting (P_{high}). The duration of this inflation is termed T_{high}. P_{high}, T_{high}, and F_{IO_2} thus heavily influence oxygenation. The magnitude and duration of lung deflation are determined by the pressure release level (P_{low}) and the release time (T_{low}). The ventilator-determined tidal volume is therefore dependent on lung compliance, airways resistance, and the duration and timing of this pressure release maneuver. The timing and magnitude of this tidal volume coupled with the patient's spontaneous breathing determine alveolar ventilation (Pa_{CO_2}). As noted earlier, T_{high} is usually much greater than T_{low}; thus, in the absence of spontaneous breathing, APRV is functionally the same as pressure-controlled inverse ratio ventilation. To sustain optimal recruitment with APRV, the greater part of the total time cycle (80% to 95%) usually occurs at P_{high}, whereas in order to minimize derecruitment, the time spent at P_{low} is brief (0.2 to 0.8 s in adults). Because T_{low} is very short, exhalation is often incomplete and intrinsic PEEP results.

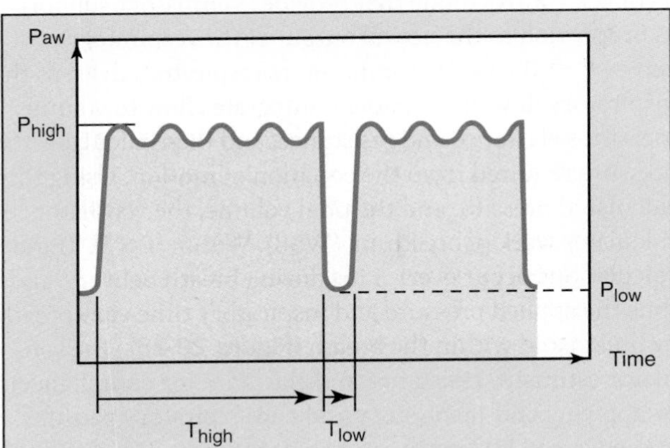

FIGURE 20-17 Airway pressure release ventilation.

Spontaneous breathing during APRV results from diaphragm contraction, which should result in recruitment of dependent alveoli, thus reducing shunt and improving oxygenation. The spontaneous efforts also may enhance both recruitment and cardiac filling as compared with other controlled forms of support. The long inflation phase also recruits more slowly filling alveoli and raises mean airway pressure without increasing applied PEEP. Improved gas exchange, often with lower maximal set airway pressures than CMV, has been demonstrated with APRV. The end-inspiratory alveolar distention (transpulmonary pressure) in APRV is not necessarily less than that provided during other forms of support, and it could be substantially higher, because spontaneous tidal volumes can occur while the lung is fully inflated with the APRV set pressure. Evidence is lacking for improved outcomes when APRV is used.[38–42]

Adaptive support ventilation (ASV) automatically selects tidal volume and frequency for mandatory breaths and the tidal volume for spontaneous breaths on the basis of the respiratory system mechanics and target minute ventilation. ASV delivers pressure-controlled breaths using an adaptive scheme, in which the mechanical work of breathing is minimized. The ventilator selects a tidal volume and frequency that the patient's brain stem would theoretically select. The ventilator calculates the required minute ventilation based on the patient's ideal body weight and estimated dead space

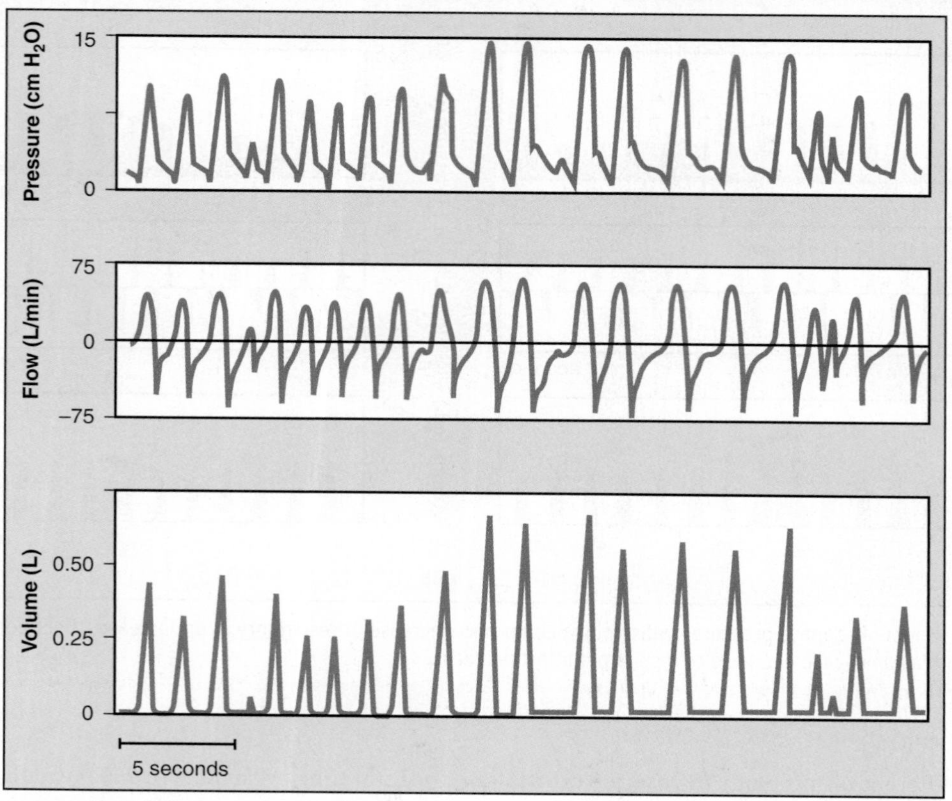

FIGURE 20-18 Proportional assist ventilation.

Reproduced from Marantz S, Patrick W, Webster K, et al. Response of ventilator-dependent patients to different levels of proportional assist. *J Appl Physiol.* 1996;80:397–403. Reprinted with permission.

volume (2.2 mL/kg). The clinician sets a target percentage of the target minute ventilation of 0.1 L/min/kg that the ventilator will support. A target minute ventilation is set to more than 100% if the patient has increased ventilatory requirements (e.g., sepsis or increased dead space) or less than 100% during ventilator liberation. The ventilator measures the expiratory time constant and uses this along with the estimated dead space to determine an optimal breathing frequency in terms of the work of breathing. The target tidal volume is calculated as the minute ventilation divided by the frequency, and the pressure limit is adjusted to achieve an average delivered tidal volume equal to the target. The ventilator also adjusts the inspiration-to-expiration (I:E) ratio to avoid air trapping. Importantly, in the presence of patient triggering, ASV resembles volume support.

ASV has been shown to supply reasonable ventilatory support in a variety of patients with respiratory failure,[43–48] but tidal volumes might exceed 10 mL/kg ideal body weight in near normal or mildly injured lungs. Importantly, outcome data are lacking. It may have a role in units where staffing is suboptimal.

Intellivent expands on the concept of ASV by adding closed loop control of oxygenation to closed loop control of ventilation. Control of ventilation is primarily based on ASV, but with the option of additional control based on end-tidal P_{CO_2}. End-tidal P_{CO_2} algorithms for normal lungs, ARDS, head injury, and COPD are available. Oxygenation is based on the ARDSnet PEEP/F_{IO_2} tables utilizing the Sp_{O_2} to adjust PEEP and F_{IO_2}.[49]

Tube compensation (TC) is designed to overcome the flow-resistive work of breathing imposed by an endotracheal tube or tracheostomy tube.[50–53] It measures the resistance of the artificial airway and applies a pressure proportional to that resistance. The clinician can set the fraction of tube resistance for which compensation is desired (e.g., 50% compensation rather than full compensation). Although it has been shown that TC can effectively compensate for resistance through the artificial airway, it has not been shown to improve outcome.[53]

Proportional assist ventilation (PAV) is a positive-feedback control mode that provides ventilatory support in proportion to the neural output of the respiratory center.[54–56] The ventilator monitors respiratory drive as the inspiratory flow of the patient, integrates flow to volume, measures elastance and resistance, and then calculates the pressure required from the equation of motion. Using this calculated pressure and the tidal volume, the ventilator calculates work of breathing (WoB): $WoB = \int P \times V$. These calculations occur every 5 ms during breath delivery, and thus the applied pressure and inspiratory time vary breath by breath and within the breath (**Figure 20-18**). The ventilator estimates resistance and elastance (or compliance) by applying end-inspiratory and end-expiratory pause maneuvers of 300 ms every 4 to 10 seconds. The clinician adjusts the percentage of support (from 5% to 95%), which allows the work to be partitioned between the ventilator and the patient. Typically, the percentage of support is set so that the work of breathing is in the range of 0.5 to 1.0 joules per liter. If the percentage of support is high, patient work of breathing may be inappropriately low and excessive volume and pressure may be applied (runaway phenomenon). If the percentage of support is too low, patient work of breathing may be excessive. Importantly, unlike conventional interactive modes like PS, there is no minimal support level. Thus alarms and backup modes are important with the use of PAV.

PAV applies a pressure that will vary from breath to breath depending upon changes in the patient's compliance, resistance, and flow demand. This differs from PS or PC, in which the level of applied pressure is constant regardless of demand, and from VC, in which the level of pressure decreases when demand increases (**Figure 20-19**). The cycle criterion for PAV is flow and is adjustable by the clinician, similar to pressure support. PAV requires the presence of an intact ventilatory drive and a functional neuromuscular system. PAV is available on one ventilator in the United States for invasive ventilation (PAV+, Puritan Bennett 840) and another for noninvasive ventilation (Philips Respironics V60). PAV may be more comfortable compared with other modes, and it may be associated with better patient–ventilator synchrony and sleep.[56] Whether PAV improves clinical outcomes remains to be determined.

Neurally adjusted ventilatory assist (NAVA) is triggered, limited, and cycled by the electrical activity of the diaphragm (diaphragmatic EMG).[56,57] The neural drive is transformed into ventilatory output (neuroventilatory coupling). The diaphragmatic EMG is measured by a multiple-array esophageal electrode, which is amplified to determine the support level (NAVA gain). The cycle-off is commonly set at 80% of peak inspiratory activity. The level of assistance is adjusted in response to changes in neural drive, respiratory system mechanics, inspiratory muscle function, and behavioral influences.

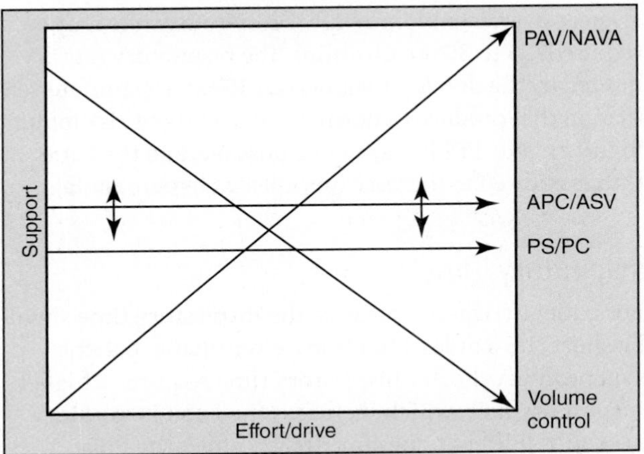

FIGURE 20-19 Effect of patient effort on the amount of support provided with various ventilator modes.

Because the trigger is based on diaphragmatic activity rather than pressure or flow, triggering is not adversely affected in patients with flow limitation and auto-PEEP. NAVA is only available on the Servo-i ventilator. Small clinical studies have demonstrated improved trigger and cycle synchrony with NAVA, but data demonstrating improved outcomes are lacking. Another concern with NAVA is the expense associated with the esophageal catheter and the invasive nature of its placement. Like PAV, there is no minimal support level and thus alarms and backup modes are important.

High-frequency oscillatory ventilation (HFOV) uses very high breathing frequencies (up to 900 breaths/min in the adult) coupled with very small tidal volumes to provide gas exchange in the lungs. HFOV vibrates a bias flow of gas delivered at the proximal end of the endotracheal tube and effects gas transport through complex nonconvective gas transport mechanisms. At the alveolar level, the substantial mean pressure functions as high-level CPAP. The potential advantages to HFOV are twofold. First, the very small alveolar pressure swings minimize overdistention and derecruitment. Second, the high mean airway pressure maintains alveolar patency and prevents derecruitment. Experience with HFOV in neonatal respiratory failure is generally positive. Its routine use in patients with ARDS is not supported by available evidence[58–61] but might be considered for refractory hypoxemic respiratory failure in centers experienced with its use. Whether its use is associated with better patient outcomes for severe refractory hypoxemic respirator failure is yet to be determined.

Breath Triggering

Positive pressure breaths can be either time triggered (breaths delivered according to a clinician-set rate or timer) or patient triggered (breaths triggered by either a change in circuit pressure or flow resulting from patient effort). The patient effort required to trigger the ventilator is an imposed load for the patient. **Pressure triggering** occurs because of a pressure drop in the system (**Figure 20-20**). The pressure level at which the ventilator is triggered is set so that the trigger effort is minimal but auto-triggering is unlikely (typically this is 1 to 2 cm H_2O below the PEEP or CPAP setting).

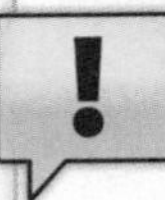

Respiratory Recap

Conventional Ventilator Triggering

- Ventilator self-triggers when a set time is reached.
- Patient triggers the ventilator through changes in pressure or flow.

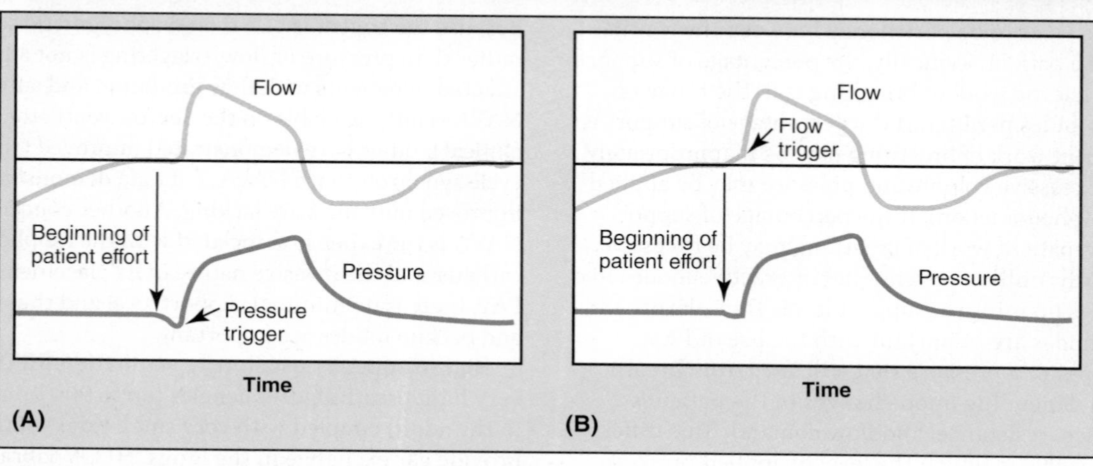

FIGURE 20-20 (A) Pressure-triggered breath. (B) Flow-triggered breath.

Flow triggering is an alternative to pressure triggering. With flow triggering the ventilator responds to a change in flow rather than a drop in pressure at the airway. With some ventilators, a pneumotachometer is placed between the ventilator circuit and the patient to measure inspiratory flow. In other ventilators, a background or base flow and flow sensitivity are set. When the flow in the expiratory circuit decreases by the amount of the flow sensitivity, the ventilator is triggered. For example, if the base flow is set at 10 L/min and the flow sensitivity is set at 3 L/min, the ventilator triggers when the flow in the expiratory circuit drops to 7 L/min (the assumption is that the patient has inhaled at 3 L/min). Neither pressure triggering nor flow triggering may be effective if significant auto-PEEP is present. Regardless of whether pressure triggering or flow triggering is used, the current generation of ventilators is more responsive to patient effort, and differences between pressure and flow triggering are minor.

Tidal Volume

Tidal volume is selected to provide an adequate Pa_{CO_2} but avoid alveolar overdistention, decreased cardiac output, and auto-PEEP.[62] Tidal volume is directly set in VC, but is determined by the driving pressure and inspiratory time in PC and PS. Large tidal volumes increase mortality in patients with ARDS and increase the risk of developing ARDS in patients with previously normal lungs.[63–67] A tidal volume should be chosen that maintains **plateau pressure (Pplat)** below 30 cm H_2O (assuming a near-normal chest wall compliance), or perhaps higher if chest wall compliance is severely reduced (e.g., morbid obesity, anasarca, ascites, abdominal compartment syndrome). Tidal volume should be selected based on ideal body weight (IBW), sometimes called predicted body weight, which is determined by height and sex:

Male patients: IBW = 50 + 2.3 × [Height (inches) – 60]

Female patients: IBW = 45.5 + 2.3 × [Height (inches) – 60]

A reasonable starting point for most patients with respiratory failure is 6 mL/kg IBW.

> **STOP AND THINK**
>
> You select a lower tidal volume for a patient intubated following drug overdose. A colleague challenges you, suggesting that large tidal volumes are acceptable if the patient has normal lungs. How would you defend your selection of a tidal volume of 6 mL/kg?

Respiratory Rate

Respiratory rate is chosen to provide acceptable minute ventilation:

$$\dot{V}_E = V_T \times f_b$$

where f_b is the respiratory rate, $\dot{V}_E$ is the minute ventilation, and V_T is the tidal volume. A rate of 15 to 25 breaths/min is often used when mechanical ventilation is initiated. If a smaller tidal volume is selected to prevent alveolar overdistention, a higher respiratory rate may be required (25 to 35 breaths/min). The respiratory rate is limited by the development of auto-PEEP. The minute ventilation that produces a normal Pa_{CO_2} without risk for lung injury or auto-PEEP may not be possible, and the Pa_{CO_2} thus is allowed to increase (**permissive hypercapnia**).

Inspiratory Time

For patient-triggered breaths, the inspiratory time should be short (1.5 s or less) to improve ventilator–patient synchrony. A shorter inspiratory time requires a higher inspiratory flow, which increases the **peak inspiratory pressure (PIP)** but does not greatly affect the Pplat. Increasing the inspiratory time increases the **mean airway pressure ($\bar{P}aw$)**, which may improve oxygenation

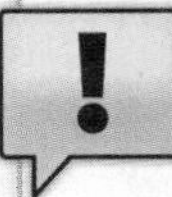

Respiratory Recap

Settings for Tidal Volume, Respiratory Rate, and Inspiratory Time

- *Tidal volume*: Set to avoid overdistention
- *Respiratory rate*: Set for desired partial pressure of arterial carbon dioxide ($Paco_2$)
- *Inspiratory time*: Set to avoid auto-PEEP and hemodynamic compromise

in some patients with ARDS. When long inspiratory times are used (over 1.5 s) and spontaneous breaths are not permitted, paralysis or sedation (or both) often is required. Long inspiratory times also can cause auto-PEEP and may result in hemodynamic instability. Although inverse ratio ventilation has been advocated to improve oxygenation, unless it is coupled with the ability to spontaneously breathe (see the discussion of APRV earlier in this chapter), this extreme (and potentially hazardous) form of ventilation is seldom necessary to achieve adequate oxygenation.

The I:E ratio is the relationship between inspiratory time and expiratory time. For example, an inspiratory time of 2 s with an expiratory time of 4 seconds produces an I:E ratio of 1:2 and a respiratory rate of 10 breaths/min. With VC, the peak inspiratory flow, flow pattern, and tidal volume are the principal determinants of inspiratory time and the I:E ratio. With PC, the inspiratory time, I:E ratio, or percentage inspiratory time are set directly. In both VC and PC, the principal determinant of expiratory time is the respiratory rate.

Inspiratory Flow Pattern

For VC, the inspiratory flow pattern can be constant or descending ramp. For the same inspiratory time, the PIP is greater with constant flow than with descending ramp flow; $\overline{P}aw$ is greater with ramp flow than with constant flow. Gas distribution may be better with a descending ramp flow pattern, but the effect on gas exchange in small. Some clinicians believe that patient–ventilator synchrony is better in some patients with a descending ramp flow pattern, but evidence to support this belief is lacking. An end-inspiratory pause can be set to improve distribution of ventilation, but this prolongs inspiration and may have a deleterious effect on hemodynamics and auto-PEEP. Experimental evidence suggests greater potential of lung injury with a descending ramp flow pattern, but this has not been studied in humans. Clinicians prefer the lower peak pressure with a descending ramp flow pattern, but the alveolar pressure is the same whether a constant flow or a descending ramp of flow is set.

The inspiratory flow decreases exponentially with PC and PS. The peak flow and rate of flow decrease depend on the driving pressure, airways resistance, lung compliance, and patient effort. With high resistance, flow decreases slowly. With low respiratory system compliance, flow decreases more rapidly, and a period of zero flow may be present at end-inhalation (**Figure 20-21**).

Positive End-Expiratory Pressure

Because critical care patients are often immobile and supine, with compromised cough ability, it is common to use low-level PEEP (3 to 5 cm H_2O) with all mechanically ventilated patients to prevent atelectasis. In patients with ARDS, more substantial levels of PEEP may be required to maintain alveolar recruitment. An appropriate level of PEEP to maintain alveolar recruitment is also part of a lung-protective ventilation strategy. PEEP should be used cautiously in patients with unilateral disease, because it may overdistend the more compliant lung, causing shunting of blood to the less compliant lung.

PEEP might also be useful to improve triggering by patients experiencing auto-PEEP.[68] Auto-PEEP functions as a threshold pressure that must be overcome before the pressure (or flow) decreases at the airway to trigger

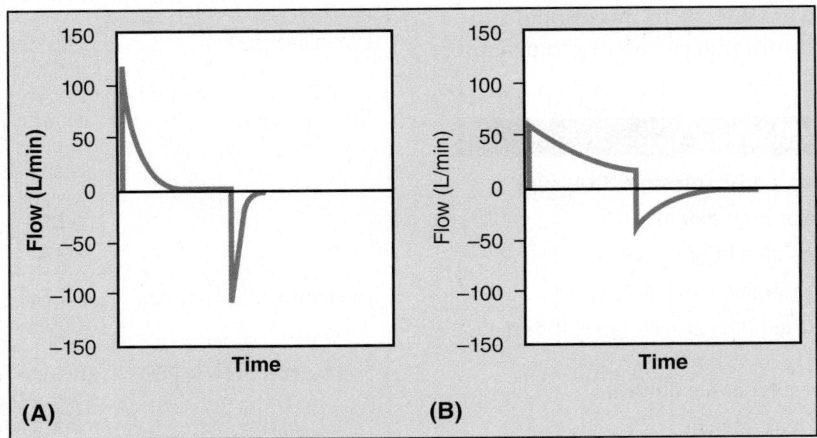

FIGURE 20-21 Flow waveforms during pressure control: low resistance and low compliance (**A**), and high resistance and high compliance (**B**).

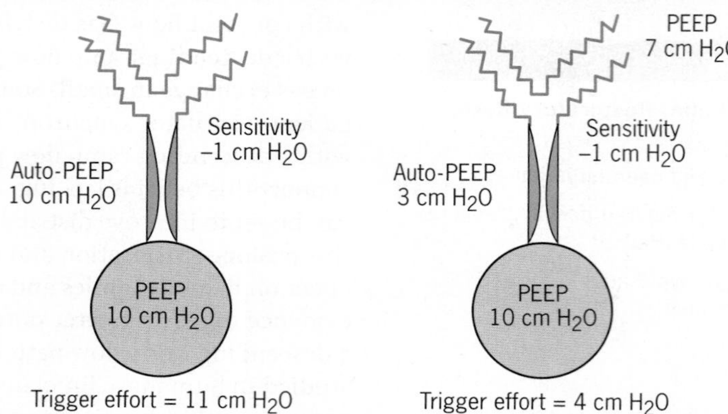

FIGURE 20-22 Trigger effort is increased when auto-PEEP is present. To trigger the ventilator, the patient's effort must first overcome the level of auto-PEEP that is present. Increasing the set PEEP level may raise the trigger level closer to the total PEEP, thus improving the ability of the patient to trigger the ventilator. This method should not be used, however, if raising the set PEEP level results in an increase in the total PEEP.

the ventilator. Increasing the set PEEP to a level near the auto-PEEP may improve the patient's ability to trigger the ventilator (**Figure 20-22**). Whenever PEEP is used to overcome the effect of auto-PEEP on triggering, PIP and Pplat must be monitored to ensure that increasing the set PEEP does not contribute to further hyperinflation.

Other uses of PEEP include preload and afterload reduction in the setting of left heart failure, reducing microaspiration around the cuff of the artificial airway, pneumatic splinting in the setting of airway malacia, and facilitation of leak speech with cuff deflation in patients with a tracheostomy.

Mean Airway Pressure

Across all modes, oxygenation and cardiac effects of mechanical ventilation often correlate best with the mean airway pressure ($\bar{P}aw$). $\bar{P}aw$ is a key component of the oxygenation index ($OI = 100 \times [\bar{P}aw \times FIO_2]/PaO_2$) that often is used as a more accurate reflection of gas transport impairment. Factors that affect the $\bar{P}aw$ during mechanical ventilation are the PIP, PEEP, I:E ratio, respiratory rate, and inspiratory flow pattern. Most patients can be managed with mean $\bar{P}aw$ values of 10 to 20 cm H_2O.

Recruitment Maneuvers

A recruitment maneuver (RM) is an intentional transient increase in transpulmonary pressure to promote reopening of unstable collapsed alveoli and thereby improve gas exchange.[69] Although use of the maneuver is physiologically reasonable, there is no high level evidence demonstrating an outcome benefit from this improvement in gas exchange. RMs are probably best reserved for the setting of refractory hypoxemia in patients with ARDS.[70] Although generally safe, hypotension and hypoxemia might occur during application of the recruitment maneuver.[71] A variety of techniques have been described as recruitment maneuvers (**Table 20-3**). It is uncertain whether any one approach is superior to the others. After performing an RM, it is important to set PEEP to a level that retains recruitment. If the lungs are already maximally recruited as the result of PEEP, the benefits of an RM are likely minimal.

> **Respiratory Recap**
>
> **Uses of Positive End-Expiratory Pressure**
>
> - Maintain alveolar recruitment
> - Counterbalance auto-PEEP
> - Reduce cardiac preload and afterload
> - Reduce microaspiration around the cuff of the artificial airway
> - Pneumatic splinting of the airway
> - Facilitation of leak speech

TABLE 20-3
Different Lung Recruitment Maneuvers

Recruitment Maneuver	Method
Sustained high-pressure inflation	Sustained inflation delivered by increasing PEEP to 30–50 cm H_2O for 20–40 s
Intermittent sigh	Sighs with a tidal volume reaching Pplat of 45 cm H_2O
Extended sigh	Stepwise increase in PEEP by 5 cm H_2O with a simultaneous stepwise decrease in tidal volume over 2 min leading to a CPAP level of 30 cm H_2O for 30 s
Intermittent PEEP increase	Intermittent increase in PEEP from baseline to higher level
Pressure control with PEEP	Pressure control of 10–15 cm H_2O with PEEP of 25–30 cm H_2O to reach a peak inspiratory pressure of 40–45 cm H_2O for 1–2 min

Respiratory Recap

Setting the F_{IO_2}

- Initiate mechanical ventilation with 100% oxygen.
- Titrate the F_{IO_2} to maintain acceptable arterial oxygen saturation by pulse oximetry.

Inspired Oxygen Concentration

An F_{IO_2} of 1.0 is commonly used when mechanical ventilation is initiated. Pulse oximetry (Sp_{O_2}) is useful to guide titration of the F_{IO_2} (and PEEP) provided periodic blood gas measurements are obtained to confirm the pulse oximetry results. A target Sp_{O_2} of 88% or higher usually provides a partial pressure of arterial oxygen (Pa_{O_2}) of 60 mm Hg or higher. A target Sp_{O_2} of 88% to 95% (Pa_{O_2} 55 to 80 mm Hg) is usually appropriate, and excessive F_{IO_2} should be avoided.[72] Although it is common practice to wait 20 to 30 minutes after the F_{IO_2} is changed before arterial blood gas measurements are obtained, 10 minutes may be adequate unless the patient has obstructive lung disease, which requires a longer equilibration time.

Sigh

Some ventilators are capable of providing periodic sigh volumes. The rationale for use of sighs is that the periodic hyperinflation reduces the risk of atelectasis. Indeed, a sigh is actually a very brief RM. For many years the use of sighs during mechanical ventilation was not considered important. Improved alveolar recruitment in patients with ARDS has reported with the use of sighs.[73]

Alarms

It is particularly important that all alarms be correctly set on the ventilator. The most important alarm is the patient-disconnect alarm, which can be a low-pressure alarm or a low exhaled volume alarm (or both). Exhaled CO_2 can also be used as a disconnect alarm. A sensitive alarm should detect not only disconnection but also leaks in the system. The ability to detect a leak depends on the site where the volume is measured (**Figure 20-23**). Other alarms set on the ventilator include those for high pressure, I:E ratio, F_{IO_2}, and loss of PEEP. To detect changes in resistance and compliance, the peak airway pressure alarm is important with VC, and the low exhaled volume alarm with PC or PS.

Circuit

Because of the gas compression in the ventilator circuit and the compliance of the ventilator circuit tubing, as much as 3 to 5 mL/cm H_2O can be compressed in the ventilator circuit. In other words, at an airway pressure of 25 cm H_2O above PEEP, about 100 mL of the gas delivered from the ventilator is not delivered

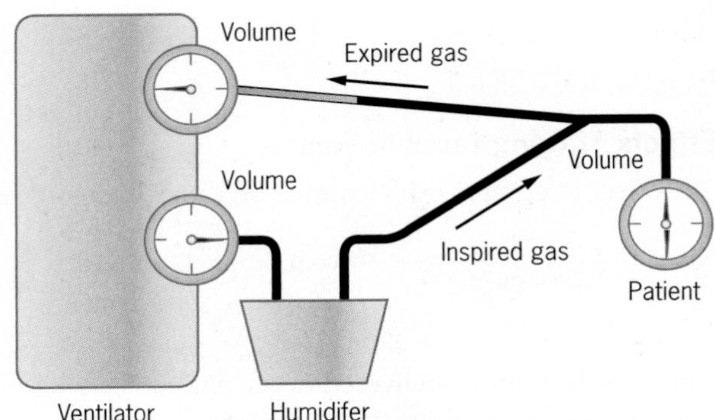

FIGURE 20-23 The ability to detect a leak depends on the site where volume is measured. If the volume on the inspiratory limb is greater than the volume on the expiratory limb, then there is a leak in the system (circuit or patient). If the inspired volume at the patient is greater than the expired volume at the patient, there is a leak in the patient (e.g., around the cuff of the endotracheal tube or a bronchopleural fistula).

to the patient. Most modern ventilators adjust for the effects of **compressible volume** such that the volume chosen by the clinician is the actual delivered V_T after correction for the effect of compressible volume. The effects of compressible volume on the delivered V_T, auto-PEEP, plateau pressure, and mixed exhaled partial pressure of carbon dioxide ($P\bar{E}_{CO_2}$) are shown in **Equation 20-1**.

Mechanical dead space is that part of the ventilator circuit through which the patient rebreathes and thus becomes an extension of the patient's anatomic dead space. Alveolar ventilation is zero if the sum of the volume loss in the circuit and the mechanical dead space is greater than the V_T set on the ventilator. The effect of mechanical dead space is particularly important with lung-protective ventilation, where the small tidal volume coupled with excessive dead space might lead to unnecessary hypercapnia.[74]

Humidification

Because the function of the upper airway is bypassed when endotracheal and tracheostomy tubes are used, the inspired gas must be filtered, warmed, and humidified before delivery to the patient. All ventilator circuits include a filter in the inspiratory limb and an active or passive humidifier. An active humidifier typically

Respiratory Recap

Methods of Humidification with Mechanical Ventilation

- *Active humidification*: Heated humidifier
- *Passive humidification*: Artificial nose
- The presence of condensate in the inspiratory circuit near the patient indicates adequate humidification.

EQUATION 20-1

Effects of Compressible Volume

The effect of compressible volume on the delivered tidal volume (VT) can be expressed as follows:

$$V_T pt = \frac{1}{1 + (Cpc / Crs)} \times V_T vent$$

where:

$V_T pt$ = Tidal volume delivered to the patient
Cpc = Compliance of the ventilator circuit
Crs = Compliance of the respiratory system
$V_T vent$ = Tidal volume from the ventilator circuit

The effect of compressible volume on auto-PEEP (positive end-expiratory pressure) can be expressed as follows:

$$\text{auto-PEEP} = \frac{Crs + Cpc}{Crs} \times \text{Measured auto-PEEP}$$

where auto-PEEP is the patient's actual auto-PEEP (positive end-expiratory pressure).

The effect of compressible volume on the Pplat (plateau pressure) can be expressed as follows:

$$Pplat = \frac{Crs + Cpc}{Crs} \times \text{Measured Pplat}$$

where Pplat is the patient's actual plateau pressure.

The effect of compressible volume on $P\bar{E}CO_2$ can be expressed as follows:

$$P\bar{E}CO_2 = P\bar{E}CO_2 vent \times \frac{V_T vent}{V_T pt}$$

where:

$P\bar{E}CO_2$ = Patient's actual $P\bar{E}CO_2$
$P\bar{E}CO_2 vent$ = $P\bar{E}CO_2$ from the ventilator circuit
$V_T vent$ = Tidal volume from the ventilator circuit
$V_T pt$ = Tidal volume delivered to the patient

humidifies the inspired gas by passing it over or bubbling it through a heated water bath. When an active humidifier is used, the ventilator circuit may be heated to prevent excessive condensation in the circuit. A passive humidifier uses an artificial nose (heat and moisture exchanger) to collect heat and humidity from the patient's exhaled gas and returns that to the patient on the next inhalation. Regardless of the humidification technique used, condensation should be seen in the inspiratory ventilator circuit or the proximal endotracheal tube or both, which indicates that the inspired gas is fully saturated with water vapor.

Monitoring the Mechanically Ventilated Patient

Physical Assessment

Asymmetric chest motion may indicate main stem (endobronchial) intubation, pneumothorax, or atelectasis. Paradoxical chest motion may be seen with flail chest or respiratory muscle dysfunction. Retractions may occur if the inspiratory flow or sensitivity is inappropriately set or if the airway is obstructed. If the patient is not breathing in synchrony with the ventilator (i.e., bucking the ventilator), the settings on the ventilator may not be appropriate or the patient may need sedation or analgesia or both. A patient respiratory rate greater than the ventilator rate indicates that auto-PEEP is compromising triggering. In conjunction with inspection, the chest can be palpated to assess the symmetry of chest movement. Palpation of the tracheal position can help detect pneumothorax. Crepitation indicates subcutaneous emphysema. Percussion can be useful in the detection of unilateral hyperresonance or tympany with a pneumothorax. Unilateral decreased breath sounds may indicate bronchial intubation, pneumothorax, atelectasis, or pleural effusion. An end-inspiratory squeak over the trachea usually indicates insufficient air in the artificial airway cuff.

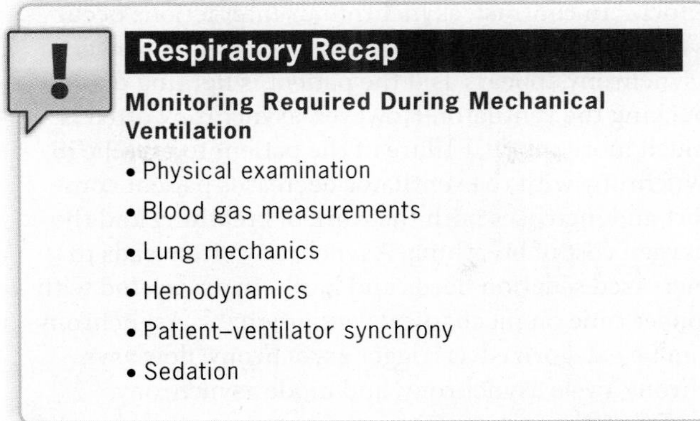

Respiratory Recap
Monitoring Required During Mechanical Ventilation
• Physical examination
• Blood gas measurements
• Lung mechanics
• Hemodynamics
• Patient–ventilator synchrony
• Sedation

Blood Gas Measurements

The earliest indicators of hypoxemia often are changes in the patient's clinical status (e.g., restlessness and confusion, changes in level of consciousness, tachycardia or bradycardia, changes in blood pressure, tachypnea, bucking the ventilator, cyanosis). The most commonly used assessment of oxygenation is the Pa_{O_2}. A low Pa_{O_2} indicates hypoxemia and dysfunction in the lungs' ability to oxygenate arterial blood. In mechanically ventilated patients, a number of factors can affect the Pa_{O_2}, such as F_{IO_2}, PEEP, or the patient's lung function (**Figure 20-24**). The mixed venous oxygenation ($P\bar{v}_{O_2}$ or $S\bar{v}_{O_2}$) is a better indicator of tissue oxygenation. A $P\bar{v}_{O_2}$ less than 35 mm Hg (or $S\bar{v}_{O_2}$ less than 70%) indicates tissue hypoxia.

Pa_{CO_2} is determined by carbon dioxide production ($\dot{V}_{CO_2}$) and the alveolar ventilation ($\dot{V}_A$). If $\dot{V}_{CO_2}$ is constant, the Pa_{CO_2} varies inversely with the $\dot{V}_A$. Minute ventilation ($\dot{V}_E$) affects Pa_{CO_2} indirectly because of the relationship between the $\dot{V}_E$ and the $\dot{V}_A$. An increase in the $\dot{V}_E$ decreases the Pa_{CO_2}, and a decrease in the $\dot{V}_E$ increases the Pa_{CO_2}. This is illustrated by the following relationship:

$$Pa_{CO_2} = (\dot{V}_{CO_2} \times 0.863) / (\dot{V}_E \times [1 - V_D/V_T])$$

Note that 0.863 is replaced with barometric pressure (e.g., 760 mm Hg) in this equation if the units and conditions of all measurements are the same. **Figure 20-25** shows the factors that determine the Pa_{CO_2} during mechanical ventilation.

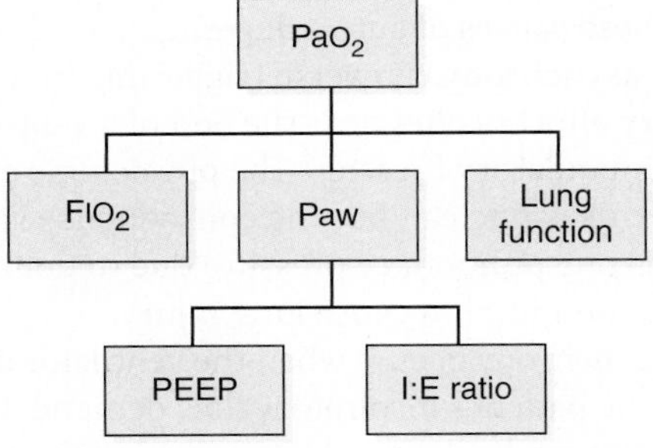

FIGURE 20-24 Factors affecting Pa_{O_2} during mechanical ventilation.

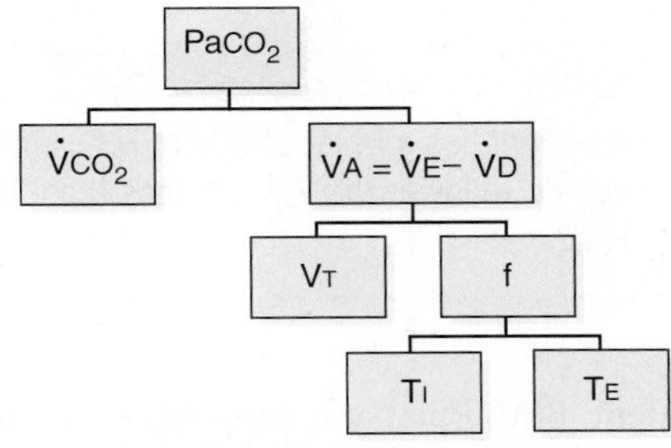

FIGURE 20-25 Factors affecting Pa_{CO_2} during mechanical ventilation.

The use of noninvasive monitors may reduce the need for arterial blood gas determinations, because they allow continuous assessment between blood gas measurements. Pulse oximetry can be used to titrate an appropriate F_{IO_2} and PEEP. Continuous pulse oximetry has become the standard of care in mechanically ventilated patients. End-tidal P_{CO_2} is used to monitor carbon dioxide levels noninvasively. In patients with normal lungs, end-tidal P_{CO_2} closely approximates the Pa_{CO_2}. In patients with an elevated V_D/V_T, however, there can be a large and inconsistent gradient between the Pa_{CO_2} and the end-tidal P_{CO_2}. For this reason, monitoring end-tidal P_{CO_2} is of limited value for the assessment of the Pa_{CO_2} during mechanical ventilation.

Plateau Pressure and Auto-PEEP

Pplat is measured by application of an end-inspiratory pause of 0.5 to 1.5 seconds, and auto-PEEP is determined by application of an end-expiratory pause of 0.5 to 1.5 seconds (**Figure 20-26**). During PC the inspiratory flow often decreases to a no-flow period at end-inspiration. In this case, the peak pressure and Pplat

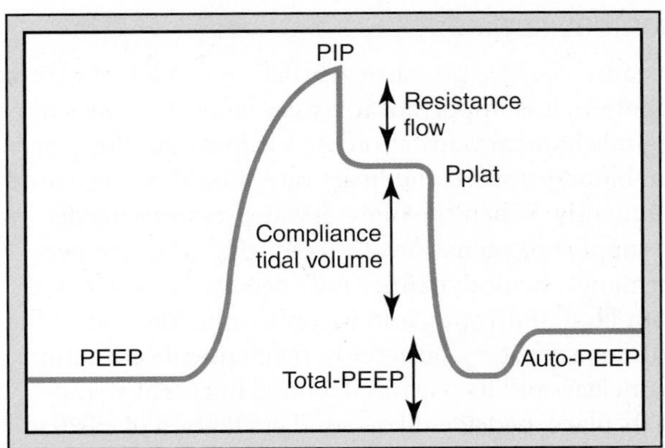

FIGURE 20-26 Airway pressure waveform during volume control. An end-inspiratory and an end-expiratory breath hold is applied to measure plateau pressure and auto-PEEP. Note that the difference between peak inspiratory pressure and plateau pressure is determined by the flow setting on the ventilator and airways resistance. Note that the difference between plateau pressure and total PEEP is determined by the tidal volume setting on the ventilator and the total level of PEEP (including auto-PEEP).

STOP AND THINK

A patient has a Pplat of 40 cm H_2O. What can you do to lower the Pplat to less than 30 cm H_2O?

are equivalent. Both Pplat and auto-PEEP can be accurately measured only when the patient is not actively breathing.

To avoid overdistention lung injury, the goal is to maintain Pplat below 30 cm H_2O (and lower if possible). Circuit measurements of respiratory system pressures all assume normal chest wall compliance in order for them to be a reasonable estimate of transpulmonary pressures (i.e., a normal chest wall compliance will have little effect on the measured airway pressures). In the setting of abnormal, very low chest wall compliance (e.g., obesity, ascites, abdominal compartment syndrome), these airway pressure measurements may be profoundly affected by chest wall stiffness and these effects need to be subtracted from the airway pressure to determine true transpulmonary pressure. This can be done with an esophageal pressure measurement or estimated by an experienced clinician.

The presence of auto-PEEP has manifestations that can be monitored. The patient's breathing pattern can be observed; if exhalation is still occurring when the next breath is delivered, auto-PEEP is present. Inspiratory efforts that do not trigger the ventilator suggest the presence of auto-PEEP. From the flow graphics on the ventilator, it can be observed that expiratory flow does not return to zero before the subsequent breath is delivered when auto-PEEP is present.

Hemodynamics

Because positive pressure ventilation can affect cardiac function, it is important to assess hemodynamics during mechanical ventilation. At a minimum, the arterial blood pressure and heart rate should be measured frequently. When the high airway pressures needed to support oxygenation adversely affect cardiac performance, hemodynamics may need to be supported with fluid, inotropes, and vasopressors. The role of the pulmonary artery catheter in mechanical ventilation is unclear, and its use has declined in recent years. In its place, bedside ultrasound evaluation of cardiac function has grown rapidly in popularity.

Patient–Ventilator Interaction

During any patient-triggered breath, the patient's effort must interact with the ventilator's gas delivery algorithm. These interactions are considered synchronous when ventilator breath delivery is in phase with patient effort.[75] In contrast, asynchronous interactions occur when these processes are out of phase. At its worse, asynchrony appears as if the patient is fighting or bucking the ventilator. However, asynchrony often is much more subtle. Failure of the patient to breathe in synchrony with the ventilator decreases patient comfort and increases both the work of breathing and the oxygen cost of breathing. Asynchrony often leads to increased sedation needs and has been associated with longer time on mechanical ventilation.[76,77] Asynchrony can be categorized as trigger asynchrony, flow asynchrony, cycle asynchrony, and mode asynchrony.

Trigger asynchrony occurs when the patient has difficulty triggering the ventilator, or the ventilator auto-triggers. The ventilator trigger sensitivity should be as sensitive as possible without causing auto-triggering. Inability of the patient to trigger can be caused by an insensitive trigger setting on the ventilator, which can be corrected by reduction of the pressure or flow required for the patient to trigger the ventilator. Inability to trigger also can be due to respiratory muscle weakness. Perhaps the most common cause of failure to trigger is auto-PEEP in patients with obstructive airway disease. Auto-PEEP can be reduced by lowering minute ventilation, shortening the I:E ratio, or reducing airway obstruction through administration of bronchodilators and clearing of secretions. Using PEEP to counterbalance auto-PEEP and thus reduce the triggering load can be effective for patients with COPD, but this technique is not effective if the auto-PEEP is primarily the result of a high minute ventilation and insufficient expiratory time. Whenever PEEP is used to counterbalance auto-PEEP, care must be taken to avoid hyperinflation with the PEEP. When the attempt is to counterbalance auto-PEEP with PEEP, the clinician should monitor the peak inspiratory pressure as PEEP is increased. If the PIP rises above the desired threshold or increases by a value greater than the increase in PEEP, overdistention should be suspected.

Another form of trigger asynchrony is auto-triggering. Auto-triggering causes the ventilator to trigger in response to an artifact. One artifact that can produce auto-triggering is cardiac oscillations.[78] This is addressed by adjusting the trigger sensitivity. Other causes of auto-triggering include excessive water condensation in the ventilator circuit and leaks in the circuit. Draining the circuit and correcting the leak address these causes of auto-triggering. Another form of trigger asynchrony is reverse triggering, in which an inspiratory effort occurs near the end of a ventilator-triggered mandatory breath.[79] The physiologic explanation of this is unclear, but the consequence is an increased transpulmonary pressure due to double triggering and potential to cause lung injury.

Flow asynchrony occurs when the ventilator does not meet the patient's inspiratory flow demand. Lack of synchrony can be detected by evaluating the airway

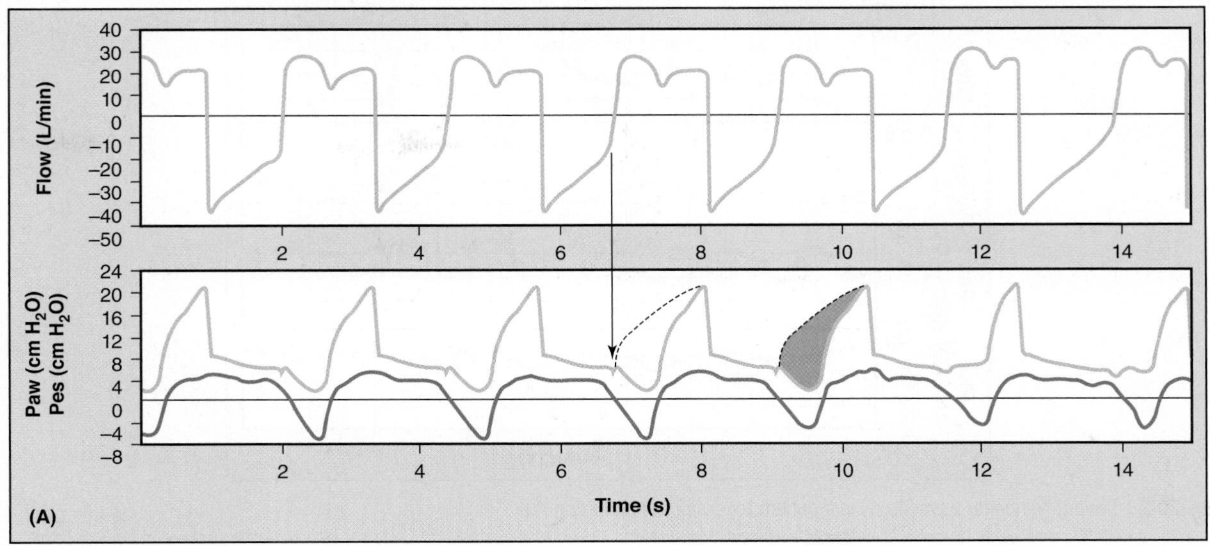

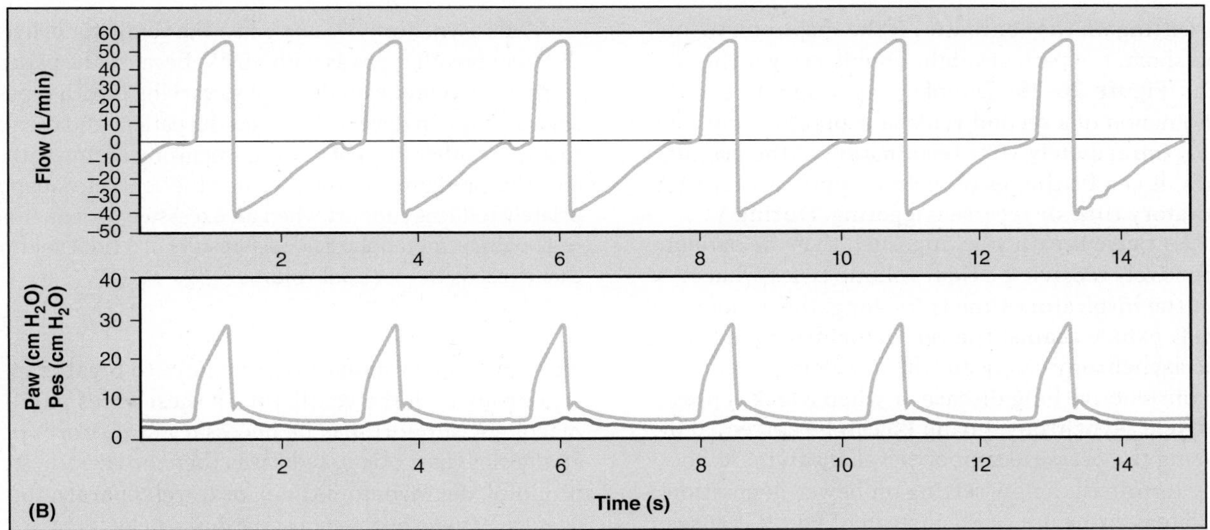

FIGURE 20-27 (**A**) The inspiratory effort of the patient is not met by fixed flow from the ventilator during volume control. The dashed line represents the airway pressure curve that would result from passive inflation, and the shaded area represents the work done by the patient against the insufficient flow from the ventilator. (**B**) When the flow setting of the ventilator is increased, the patient is more synchronous with the ventilator.

pressure waveform. With asynchrony, the pressure waveform with each breath differs from every other, and there is breath-to-breath variability in the peak airway pressure (**Figure 20-27**). A good way to detect asynchrony is to compare patient-triggered breaths with a breath delivered via the manual breath control. Comparing the shape of the patient-triggered and the machine-triggered breaths on the pressure–time waveform can demonstrate the effects of patient effort (i.e., a vigorous patient effort literally sucks the airway pressure graphic downward). Clinical signs of flow asynchrony include tachypnea, retractions, and chest-abdominal paradox. Flow asynchrony can be corrected by an increase in the flow setting or change in the inspiratory flow pattern during VC, by changing from VC to PC or PS,[24] or by an increase in the pressure setting or the rise time setting during PC or PS. Although flow asynchrony is more commonly reported with VC, asynchrony can also occur with PC (**Figure 20-28**).[25] For patients who have a high respiratory drive because of anxiety or pain, flow asynchrony may be improved by appropriate use of sedation or analgesia.[80]

Cycle asynchrony occurs when the neural inspiratory time of the patient does not match the inspiratory

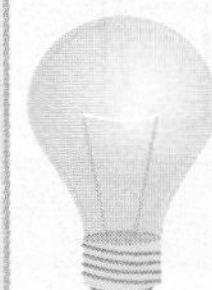

STOP AND THINK

You observe that a patient is not breathing in synchrony with the ventilator. What can you do to remedy this situation?

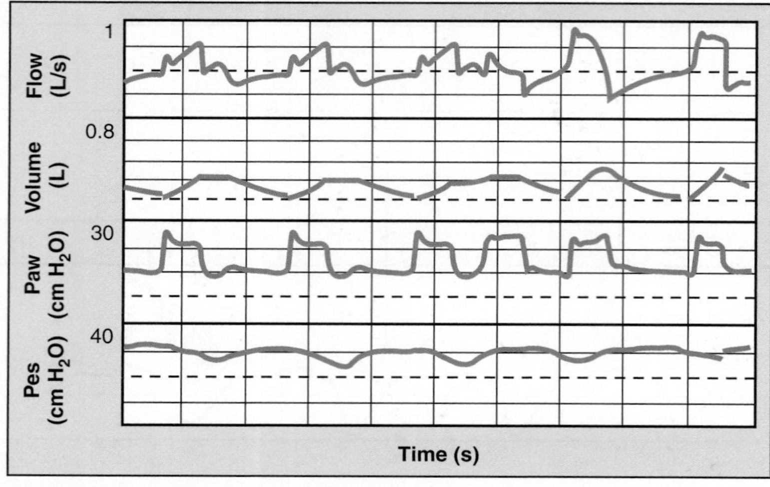

FIGURE 20-28 Patient–ventilator asynchrony in a patient receiving pressure control.

Reproduced from Kallet RH, Campbell AR, Dicker RA, et al. Work of breathing during lung-protective ventilation in patients with acute lung injury and acute respiratory distress syndrome: a comparison between volume and pressure-regulated breathing modes. *Respir Care.* 2005;50[12]:1623–1631. Reprinted with permission.

time setting on the ventilator. If the inspiratory time is too short, the patient might double-trigger the ventilator (**Figure 20-29**). Double triggering refers to the phenomenon of a second ventilator breath occurring almost immediately after termination of the original breath. It can be the result of an inappropriately short inspiratory time or reverse triggering. During VC, this can cause breath stacking, such that the patient is effectively receiving a tidal volume twice what is set. If the inspiratory time is too long, the patient will actively exhale against the ventilator-delivered breath. Cycle asynchrony can occur during PS in patients with obstructive lung disease or when a leak is present. Cycle asynchrony during PS can be corrected by lowering the pressure support level, by an increase in the termination flow setting on newer-generation ventilators, or by use of PC instead of PS (PC causes inspiration to be time cycled rather than flow cycled). Cycle asynchrony is recognized as activation of the expiratory (abdominal) muscles during the inspiratory phase; this can be detected clinically by palpation of the patient's abdomen. Cycle asynchrony can also be detected by observation of the ventilator graphics (**Figure 20-30**).

Mode asynchrony occurs when the ventilator delivers different breath types as with SIMV. Because the patient's respiratory center cannot adapt to varying breath types, asynchrony can develop between the patient and the ventilator. Another form of mode asynchrony occurs with adaptive pressure control, in which the ventilator inappropriately reduces support when an excessive patient effort (e.g., pain or metabolic acidosis) results in a tidal volume that exceeds the set tidal volume.[35,81]

Sedation

Anxiety is a common cause of failure to breathe in synchrony with the ventilator. In these cases pharmacologic support may be necessary in the form of analgesics (narcotics), sedatives (benzodiazepines, propofol, dexmedetomidine), or (rarely) paralyzing agents. When short-term sedation is necessary to bring a patient into synchrony with the ventilator, propofol may be useful. Dexmedetomidine results in attenuation of the stress response with no significant respiratory depression and has been reported to result in earlier liberation for mechanical ventilation when compared to midazolam.[82] When ventilation requires long inspiratory times and high airway pressures,

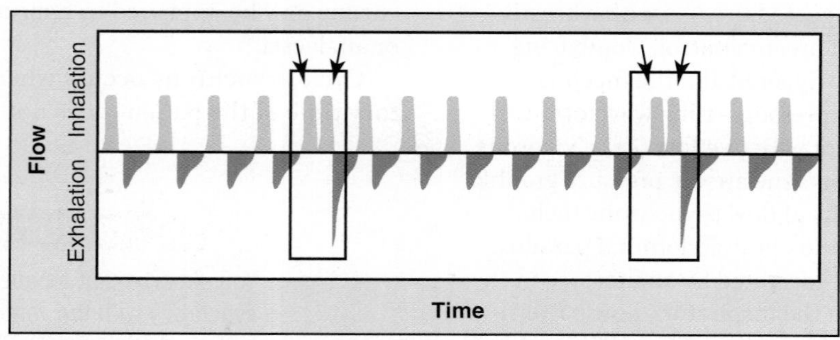

FIGURE 20-29 Double triggering. Note that the patient receives two breaths in rapid succession.

Adapted from Pohlman MC, et al. Excessive tidal volume from breath stacking during lung-protective ventilation for acute lung injury. *Crit Care Med.* 2008;36:3019–3023.

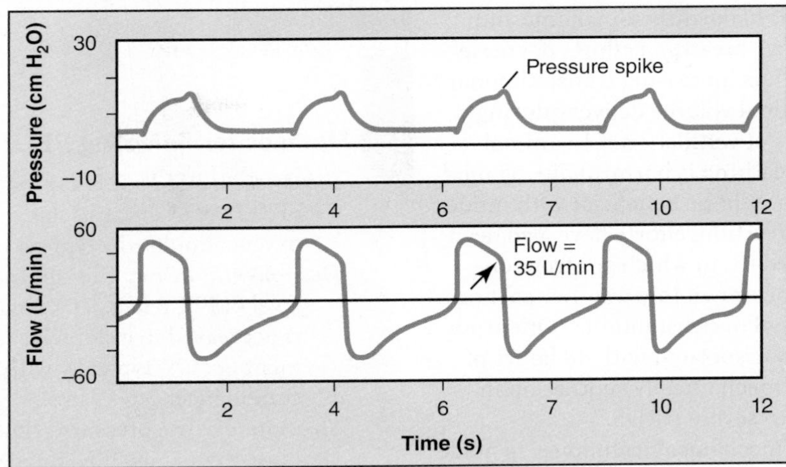

FIGURE 20-30 Airway pressure and flow waveforms illustrating active exhalation during pressure support. Note that the flow does not decelerate to the flow termination criterion of the ventilator (5 L/min for this specific ventilator). Also note the presence of a pressure spike at the end of each inspiration, indicating that the ventilator is pressure cycling rather than flow cycling.

Modified from Branson RD. Modes of ventilator operation. In: MacIntyre NR, Branson RD, eds. *Mechanical Ventilation*. Philadelphia: WB Saunders; 2000. Copyright Elsevier 2000.

pharmacologic control of the patient's breathing is almost always necessary.

All forms of respiratory suppression are associated with adverse side effects. It is most important that disconnect alarms be properly set when the patient's ability to breathe spontaneously is pharmacologically suppressed. Significant problems with pharmacologic suppression of respiration have been reported, such as long-term respiratory muscle weakness after use of paralyzing agents during mechanical ventilation.[83,84] It has been shown that assessment of the patient's response to a daily trial of sedation cessation significantly reduces the days of mechanical ventilation.[85] This suggests that many mechanically ventilated patients are excessively sedated and that this excessive sedation prolongs the course of mechanical ventilation.[86]

Choosing Ventilator Settings for Different Forms of Respiratory Failure

Acute Respiratory Distress Syndrome (ARDS)

With ARDS, lung volume is decreased and lung compliance is low. It is important to realize, however, that there are often marked regional differences in the degree of alveolar involvement. Whereas some alveoli may be collapsed or consolidated, others may be hyperinflated and others may be normal. The tidal volume will go to the regions with the more normal mechanics. A normal tidal volume may thus be distributed preferentially to the healthier regions of the lungs, resulting in potential for regional overdistention injury. Parenchymal injury can also affect the airways, which can contribute to reduced regional ventilation to injured lung units. Gas exchange abnormalities with ARDS are a consequence of alveolar flooding and/or collapse, resulting in $\dot{V}/\dot{Q}$ mismatch and shunt. The low-$\dot{V}/\dot{Q}$ regions result in hypoxemia, and the high-$\dot{V}/\dot{Q}$ regions result in increased dead space and hypercarbia.

Frequency–tidal volume settings for ARDS focus on limiting end-inspiratory alveolar stretch, which has been shown to improve patient outcomes.[3,87] This has been most convincingly demonstrated by the ARDS Network Trial, which reported a 10% absolute reduction in mortality with a ventilator strategy using a V_T of 6 mL/kg ideal body weight compared with 12 mL/kg.[3] Thus, initial V_T should be 6 mL/kg and should be based on ideal body weight. Moreover, strong consideration should be given to further reducing the V_T if Pplat, adjusted for the effect of excessive chest wall stiffness, exceeds 30 cm H_2O. Evidence is accumulating that suggests that Pplat should be as low as possible, and at levels of 25–30 cm H_2O might cause regional overdistention.[4,5] V_T can be increased to 8 mL/kg if there is marked asynchrony or severe acidosis, provided that the Pplat does not exceed 30 cm H_2O.

Respiratory rate is adjusted to control pH. The potential for air trapping in parenchymal lung injury is low if the breathing frequency is less than 35 breaths/min. An increased inspiratory time, and even inverse ratio ventilation (e.g., APRV), can be used to increase Pa_{O_2} with refractory hypoxemia. The mechanisms for improved oxygenation with inverse ratio ventilation include longer gas mixing time, recruitment of slowly filling alveoli, and development of auto-PEEP.

Whether or not spontaneous breathing efforts should be permitted in patients with severe ARDS is an area of controversy. Allowing spontaneous breathing efforts might avoid issues such as prolonged weakness during recovery. On the other hand, it can contribute to asynchrony and might make difficult volume and pressure limitation. Active breathing efforts decrease intrathoracic pressure, thus increasing transpulmonary pressure and adding to tidal volume delivery during pressure-targeted modes of ventilation.[88] In animal models, spontaneous breathing is harmful during models of severe ARDS, but might be beneficial with milder ARDS.[89] Spontaneous breathing efforts have also been shown to produce pendelluft, in which gas from one region of the lungs can be drawn into another part of the lungs, causing regional overdistention.[90] One study reported lower mortality associated with 48 hours of paralysis at the onset of mechanically ventilation in patients with moderate to severe ARDS.[91]

Although imaging or mechanical techniques to guide proper PEEP settings have physiologic appeal, they are technically challenging and not practical for routine use. Most clinicians thus rely on various gas exchange criteria to guide PEEP and F_{IO_2} titrations. This involves the use of tables designed to provide adequate oxygenation (Pa_{O_2} 55 to 80 mm Hg or Sp_{O_2} of 88% to 95%) while minimizing F_{IO_2} and limiting Pplat. Two examples are from the National Institutes of Health's ARDS Network, one emphasizing PEEP over F_{IO_2} (high or aggressive PEEP) and one emphasizing F_{IO_2} over PEEP (low or conservative PEEP).[3,92]

Randomized controlled trials have compared various gas exchange strategies for setting PEEP in conjunction with low V_T strategies and have reported that both aggressive (i.e., 13 to 15 cm H_2O PEEP) and conservative (i.e., 7 to 9 cm H_2O) approaches have comparable outcomes.[92–94] In terms of hospital survival, however, a meta-analysis of these studies suggests that higher levels of PEEP may be beneficial for patients with moderate and severe ARDS (Pa_{O_2}/F_{IO_2} ≤200 mm Hg), whereas higher levels of PEEP are not beneficial (and may produce harm) in patients with mild ARDS (Pa_{O_2}/F_{IO_2} 200 mm Hg).[95] The appropriate setting of PEEP demands a careful consideration of the benefits of alveolar recruitment balances against the risks of overdistention. The results of one study suggests that the use of a table such as that used by the ARDSnet might best accomplish this goal.[96]

Some mechanical approaches to setting PEEP are used in ICUs where the staff has considerable experience managing ARDS (**Box 20-6**).[97] These include titration to the highest compliance, titration to a pressure greater than the lower inflection point of the pressure–volume curve, the best stress index, and incorporation of esophageal pressure measurements in settings of abnormal chest wall compliance. PEEP should be avoided that results in a Pplat above 30 cm H_2O (unless there is abnormal chest wall mechanics). Higher levels of PEEP should be reserved for cases where lung recruitment can be demonstrated. In the setting of refractory hypoxemia, recruitment maneuvers may be used, followed by a level of PEEP to maintain alveolar recruitment. When setting PEEP in patients with ARDS, the hemodynamic effects of the increased intrathoracic pressure should also be monitored.

BOX 20-6

Methods for Selecting PEEP

Incremental PEEP: This approach uses combinations of PEEP and F_{IO_2} to achieve the desired level of oxygenation or the highest compliance.

Decremental PEEP: This approach begins with a high level of PEEP (e.g., 20 cm H_2O), after which PEEP is decreased in a stepwise fashion until derecruitment occurs, typically with decreases in Pa_{O_2} and compliance.

Stress index: The pressure–time curve is observed during constant-flow inhalation for signs of tidal recruitment and overdistention.

Esophageal pressure: This method estimates the intrapleural pressure by using an esophageal balloon to measure the esophageal pressure and subsequently determine the optimal level of PEEP required to counterbalance pleural pressure.

Pressure–volume curve: PEEP is set slightly greater than the lower inflection point.

Obstructive Lung Disease

Respiratory failure from airflow obstruction is due to increases in airway resistance. This increases the pressure required for flow, which may overload inspiratory muscles, producing a ventilatory pump failure with spontaneous minute ventilation inadequate for gas exchange. In addition, the narrowed airways create regions of lung that cannot properly empty, and auto-PEEP occurs. These regions of overinflation create dead space and put inspiratory muscles at a substantial mechanical disadvantage, which further worsens muscle function. Overinflated regions may also compress more healthy regions of the lung, impairing $\dot{V}/\dot{Q}$ matching. Regions of air trapping and intrinsic PEEP also function as a threshold load to trigger mechanical breaths.

Noninvasive ventilation (NIV) is standard first-line therapy in patients with COPD and has been shown to improve outcomes by reducing the need for endotracheal intubation and improving survival in this patient population.[98] NIV has also been used in other forms of obstructive lung disease (e.g., asthma, cystic fibrosis), but there is less evidence for better outcomes in these patient populations. Invasive ventilatory support is usually reserved for those who fail NIV or in those in whom NIV is contraindicated.

Tidal volume should be sufficiently low (e.g., 6 mL/kg) to ensure that Pplat values are below 30 cm H_2O. The set rate is used to control pH. The elevated airways resistance and the low elastic recoil pressure with emphysema increase the potential for air trapping, however, and this limits the range of breath rates available. Permissive hypercapnia may be an appropriate trade-off to limit overdistention. The inspiratory time in obstructive lung disease is set as low as possible to minimize the development of air trapping. Judicious application of PEEP (up to 75% to 85% of auto-PEEP) can counterbalance auto-PEEP to facilitate triggering.[99] Use of a low-density gas (e.g., helium–oxygen mixtures [heliox]) is another technique that can be used to decrease auto-PEEP, but this is technically challenging and its impact on outcome is unknown.

Neuromuscular Disease

The risk of VILI is generally less in a patient with neuromuscular failure, because lung mechanics are often near normal and regional overdistention is thus less likely to occur. Accumulating evidence supports that a target tidal volume of 6 mL/kg is appropriate even in patients with normal lungs. One study reported increased risk of developing ARDS when higher tidal volumes are used in patients with spontaneous intracerebral hemorrhage.[100] A low level of PEEP is often beneficial for preventing atelectasis. If patients with neuromuscular disease develop ARDS, they should be managed using ventilator strategies incorporating lower tidal volumes and higher levels of PEEP. Lung-protective ventilation is also recommended for brain dead patients who are potential donors for lung transplantation.[101]

Intraoperative and Postoperative Mechanical Ventilation

Progressive atelectasis occurs during anesthesia, and the use of high VT was recommended many years ago to combat this problem.[102] Although large VT might recruit collapsed alveoli, this strategy without the application of PEEP might promote cyclical alveolar collapse and reopening. Following elective coronary artery bypass surgery, a lung-protective strategy with a VT of 6 mL/kg attenuated postoperative pulmonary dysfunction,[103] and VT >10 mL/kg IBW was a significant risk factor for multiorgan failure and prolonged stay in the ICU.[104] As compared with a practice of nonprotective mechanical ventilation, the use of a lung-protective ventilation strategy in intermediate-risk and high-risk patients undergoing major abdominal surgery was shown to improve clinical outcomes.[105] A smaller VT to avoid overdistention and PEEP to maintain alveolar recruitment are lung protective, even in patients with normal lung function such as in the intraoperative and postoperative periods.

Ventilatory Support Involves Trade-Offs

To provide adequate support yet minimize VILI, mechanical ventilation goals must involve trade-offs. Thus the need for potentially injurious ventilating pressures, volumes, and supplemental O_2 must be weighed against the benefits of better gas exchange. Accordingly, pH goals as low as 7.15 and Pa_{O_2} goals as low as 55 mm Hg are often considered acceptable if necessary to protect the lungs from VILI. Ventilator settings are thus selected to provide an adequate, but not necessarily normal, level of gas exchange while meeting the goals of enough PEEP to maintain alveolar recruitment and avoidance of a PEEP–tidal volume combination that unnecessarily overdistends alveoli at end-inspiration. This has led to ventilatory strategies such as permissive hypercapnia, permissive hypoxemia, and permissive atelectasis.

Liberation from Mechanical Ventilation

An important aspect of the management of patients receiving mechanical ventilation is recognizing when the patient is ready to be liberated from the ventilator and extubating the patient at that point. Evidence-based clinical practice guidelines have been published related to liberation from mechanical ventilation. **Box 20-7** lists the recommendations from these guidelines.[106]

Respiratory Muscles

For successful liberation from the ventilator, the load placed on the respiratory muscles must be balanced by the muscles' ability to meet that load (**Figure 20-31**). Respiratory muscle fatigue occurs if the load placed on the muscles is excessive, if the muscles are weak, or if the duty cycle (the inspiratory time relative to total cycle time) is too long. Common causes of a high load are high airways resistance, low lung compliance, and high minute ventilation. In addition, malposition of the diaphragm from dynamic hyperinflation compromises inspiratory muscle function. Diminished respiratory muscle function may also be the result of systemic disease, disuse, malnutrition, hypoxia, or electrolyte imbalance. The clinical signs of respiratory muscle fatigue are tachypnea, abnormal respiratory movements (respiratory alternans and abdominal paradox), and an increase in Pa_{CO_2}.[107]

Because the maximum inspiratory pressure (PI_{max}, sometimes termed negative inspiratory force or NIF) is a good indicator of overall respiratory muscle strength, a low PI_{max} may predict respiratory muscle fatigue. The PI_{max} is measured by attachment of an aneroid manometer to the endotracheal or tracheostomy tube. The patient then forcibly inhales after maximum exhalation. When the PI_{max} is measured, it is recommended that a unidirectional valve be used and that the airway be completely obstructed for 20

BOX 20-7

Evidence-Based Guidelines for Discontinuing Ventilatory Support

***Recommendation 1*:** In patients requiring mechanical ventilation for more than 24 hours, a search for all the causes that may be contributing to ventilator dependence should be undertaken. This is particularly true in the patient who has failed attempts at withdrawing the mechanical ventilator. Reversing all possible ventilatory and nonventilatory issues should be an integral part of the ventilator discontinuation process.

***Recommendation 2*:** Patients receiving mechanical ventilation for respiratory failure should undergo a formal assessment of discontinuation potential if the following criteria are satisfied: (1) evidence for some reversal of the underlying cause for respiratory failure, (2) adequate oxygenation and pH, (3) hemodynamic stability, and (4) the capability to initiate an inspiratory effort.

***Recommendation 3*:** Formal discontinuation assessments for patients receiving mechanical ventilation for respiratory failure should be performed during spontaneous breathing rather than while the patient is still receiving substantial ventilatory support. An initial brief period of spontaneous breathing can be used to assess the capability of continuing onto a formal spontaneous breathing trial (SBT). The criteria with which to assess patient tolerance during SBTs are the respiratory pattern, the adequacy of gas exchange, hemodynamic stability, and subjective comfort. The tolerance of SBTs lasting 30 to 120 minutes should prompt consideration for permanent ventilator discontinuation.

***Recommendation 4*:** The removal of the artificial airway from a patient who has successfully been discontinued from ventilatory support should be based on assessments of airway patency and the ability of the patient to protect the airway.

***Recommendation 5*:** Patients receiving mechanical ventilation for respiratory failure who fail an SBT should have the cause for the failed SBT determined. Once reversible causes for failure are corrected, subsequent SBTs should be performed every 24 hours.

***Recommendation 6*:** Patients receiving mechanical ventilation for respiratory failure who fail an SBT should receive a stable, nonfatiguing, comfortable form of ventilatory support.

***Recommendation 7*:** Anesthesia/sedation strategies and ventilator management aimed at early extubation should be used in postsurgical patients.

***Recommendation 8*:** Weaning/discontinuation protocols that are designed for nonphysician healthcare professionals should be developed and implemented by intensive care units. Protocols aimed at optimizing sedation also should be developed and implemented.

***Recommendation 9*:** Tracheostomy should be considered after an initial period of stabilization on the ventilator when it becomes apparent that the patient will require prolonged ventilator assistance. Tracheostomy then should be performed when the patient appears likely to gain one or more of the benefits ascribed to the procedure. Patients who may derive particular benefit from early tracheostomy are those requiring high levels of sedation to tolerate a translaryngeal tube; those with marginal respiratory mechanics (often manifested as tachypnea) in whom a tracheostomy tube having lower resistance might reduce the risk of muscle overload; those who may derive psychological benefit from the ability to eat orally, communicate by articulated speech, and experience enhanced mobility; and those in whom enhanced mobility may assist physical therapy efforts.

***Recommendation 10*:** Unless there is evidence for clearly irreversible disease (e.g., high spinal cord injury or advanced amyotrophic lateral sclerosis), a patient requiring prolonged mechanical ventilatory support for respiratory failure should not be considered permanently ventilator dependent until 3 months of ventilator liberation attempts have failed.

***Recommendation 11*:** Critical care practitioners should familiarize themselves with facilities in their communities, or units in hospitals they staff, that specialize in managing patients who require prolonged dependence on mechanical ventilation. Such familiarization should include reviewing published peer-reviewed data from those units, if available. When medically stable for transfer, patients who have failed ventilator discontinuation attempts in the intensive care unit should be transferred to those facilities that have demonstrated success and safety in accomplishing ventilator discontinuation.

***Recommendation 12*:** Ventilator liberation strategies in the prolonged mechanical ventilation patient should be slow paced and should include gradually lengthening self-breathing trials.

Modified from MacIntyre NR, Cook DJ, Ely EW Jr, et al. Evidence-based guidelines for weaning and discontinuing ventilatory support: a collective task force facilitated by the American College of Chest Physicians; the American Association for Respiratory Care; and the American College of Critical Care Medicine. *Chest.* 2001;120:375S–396S, with permission from the American College of Chest Physicians.

Minute Ventilation
Pain and anxiety
Sepsis
Increased dead space
Excessive feeding

Increased Resistive Load
Bronchospasm
Secretions
Small endotracheal tube

Increased Elastic Load
Low lung compliance
Low chest wall compliance
Auto-PEEP

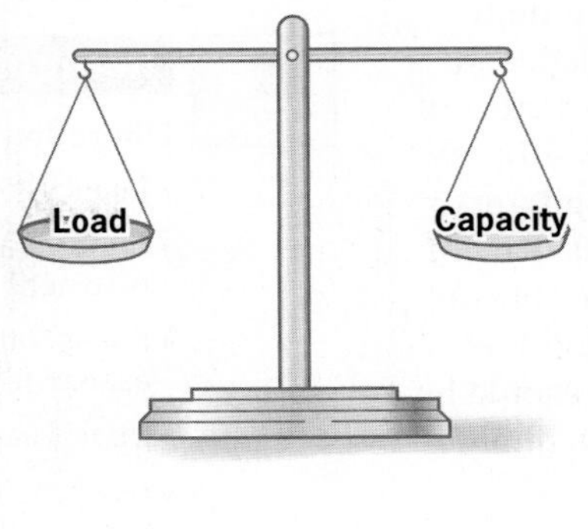

Depressed Respiratory Drive
Sedative drugs
Brain stem lesion

Neuromuscular Disease
Cervical spine injury
Phrenic nerve injury
Critical illness polyneuropathy
Prolonged neuromuscular blockade
Hyperinflation (COPD)
Malnutrition
Electrolyte disturbance
Primary neuromuscular disease

Thoracic Wall Abnormality
Flail chest
Pain

FIGURE 20-31 Respiratory muscle performance is determined by the balance between the load that is placed on the respiratory muscles and the ability of the muscles to meet that load.

to 25 seconds (**Figure 20-32**). A PI_{max} more negative than –20 cm H_2O suggests adequate inspiratory muscle strength. If the patient has high airways resistance or low compliance, however, even a PI_{max} of –20 cm H_2O might not be adequate for unassisted breathing.

The respiratory muscles should be rested if fatigue occurs, and a rest period of 24 hours may be required.[108] Appropriate respiratory muscle rest usually is provided by ventilatory support high enough to provide patient comfort and still allow some inspiratory efforts. Importantly, total rest (i.e., no inspiratory muscle activity with controlled mechanical ventilation) can also be harmful, because muscle atrophy has been shown to develop in as little as 24 hours under these conditions. If respiratory muscle fatigue is the result of an excessive load, the load should be reduced before attempts are made to liberate the patient from the ventilator. This is done with provision of therapies that can increase lung compliance or reduce airways resistance.

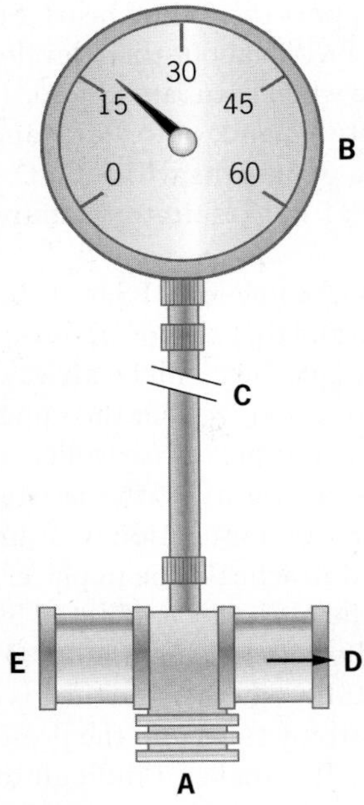

FIGURE 20-32 The one-way valve system used to measure maximum inspiratory pressure. The patient is connected at A, the manometer (B) is connected at C, and the patient exhales through D. In this way, maximum inspiratory pressure is measured at functional residual capacity.

Reproduced from Kacmarek RM, Cycyk-Chapman MC, Young PJ, Romagnoli DM. Determination of maximal inspiratory pressure: a clinical study and literature review. *Respir Care.* 1989;34:868–878.

Assessing Readiness for Liberation

A number of factors should be improved before an attempt is made to liberate the patient from the ventilator (**Box 20-8**). **Weaning parameters**[109,110] often are used to assess liberation potential and are divided into two categories: parameters affected by lung mechanics, and gas exchange parameters. The spontaneous VT

BOX 20-8

Criteria Assessed to Determine Readiness for Ventilator Discontinuation (Liberation)

1. Evidence for some reversal of the underlying cause for respiratory failure
2. Adequate oxygenation (e.g., PaO_2/FIO_2 >150 to 200; PEEP = 8 cm H_2O; $FIO_2 \leq 0.4$ to 0.5) and pH (e.g., >7.25)
3. Hemodynamic stability, defined as absence of active myocardial ischemia and absence of clinically significant hypotension (i.e., requiring no vasopressor therapy or therapy with only low-dose vasopressors)
4. The capability to initiate an inspiratory effort

(5 mL/kg), respiratory rate (30 breaths/min), minute ventilation (12 L/min), vital capacity (15 mL/kg), and the PI_{max} (–20 cm H_2O) have been used as predictors of success. The rapid shallow breathing index (RSBI)[111] is calculated by division of the spontaneous respiratory rate by the V_T (in liters). An RSBI less than 105 has been used as predictive of successful ventilator liberation, and an RSBI greater than 105 has been used to predict failure. An increase in V_D/V_T (which should be less than 0.6) and an increase in V_{CO_2} and V_{O_2} imply an increased ventilatory requirement.

Despite the many weaning parameters that have been reported, no single criterion is better at predicting extubation readiness than a **spontaneous breathing trial (SBT)** with an integrated assessment focusing on the respiratory pattern, gas exchange, hemodynamics, and comfort. Overreliance on weaning parameters may result in prolonged stay on the ventilator.[112] It also is important to reduce or temporarily discontinue sedation in preparation of ventilator liberation; this has been reported to decrease both days of ventilation and mortality.[85,113]

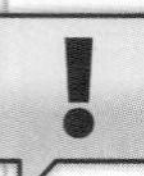

Respiratory Recap

Liberation from Mechanical Ventilation

- Regularly assess for liberation readiness.
- Perform a spontaneous breathing trial to assess readiness for extubation.
- If a spontaneous breathing trial is not tolerated, assess for causes of failure.
- Do not use SIMV as a weaning mode.
- Use protocols to improve successful liberation.

Approaches to Liberation

Two prospective, randomized, controlled trials compared IMV weaning (i.e., gradual reduction in mandatory breath rate), PS weaning (i.e., gradual reduction in the level of PS), and daily (or twice daily) SBT.[114,115] In these studies, after meeting screening criteria, an SBT was performed. Both studies reported that the majority of patients were successfully extubated after the first SBT. In those who failed the initial SBT, no difference in outcome (duration of ventilation) was seen between the T-piece and PS methods. Both the SBT and PS methods were superior to IMV in both studies. Although newer-generation ventilators feature modes intended to facilitate weaning (e.g., SmartCare, adaptive support ventilation, volume support), evidence is lacking that they hasten ventilator liberation compared with use of a daily SBT.

The traditional approach to an SBT uses a T-piece, in which the patient is removed from the ventilator, and humidified supplemental oxygen is provided. Humidified gas typically is provided as a heated or cool aerosol of water from a large-volume nebulizer. For patients with reactive airways, this aerosol may induce bronchospasm. In such cases a humidification system that does not generate an aerosol should be used, such as a heated passover humidifier. Passive humidifiers (e.g., artificial noses, heat and moisture exchangers) should be avoided because of their dead space and resistive workload.

The SBT can be conducted without removal of the patient from the ventilator, and this approach has several advantages. No additional equipment is required, and if the patient fails the SBT, ventilatory support can be quickly reestablished. All the monitoring functions and alarms on the ventilator are available during the SBT, which may allow prompt recognition that the patient is failing the SBT. Most of the literature related to ventilator liberation studies used a traditional SBT, although several studies allowed performance of the SBT with the patient attached to the ventilator.[116–118]

The SBT can be performed with no positive pressure applied to the airway, with a low level of CPAP (5 cm H_2O), with a low level of PS (5 to 8 cm H_2O), or with the use of inspiratory pressure automatically titrated to overcome endotracheal tube resistance (i.e., tube compensation). Proponents of the CPAP approach argue that this maintains functional residual capacity at a level similar to that after extubation. It is argued that, in a patient with obstructive lung disease, this low level of CPAP maintains airway patency if the patient cannot control exhalation because of the presence of the artificial airway. In patients with marginal left ventricular function, however, a low level of positive intrathoracic pressure may support the failing heart. Such patients may tolerate a CPAP trial but then develop congestive heart failure when extubated. Also, a low level of CPAP may counterbalance auto-PEEP and facilitate breath triggering in patients with COPD, resulting in a successful SBT but respiratory failure soon after extubation.

Proponents of the low-level PS (or tube compensation) approach argue that this overcomes the resistance to breathing through the artificial airway. However, this argument fails to recognize that the upper airway of an intubated patient typically is swollen and inflamed, such that, at least in one study, the resistance through the upper airway after extubation was similar to that seen with the endotracheal tube in place.[119] Resistance through the artificial airway is affected by many factors, including the patient's inspiratory flow, the inner diameter of the tube, whether the tube is an endotracheal or tracheostomy tube, and the presence of secretions in the tube. This makes it difficult to choose an appropriate level of pressure support to overcome tube resistance. One study reported similar outcomes when the SBT was performed with a T-piece and with 7 cm H_2O PS.[120] Similar outcomes of an SBT have also been reported with or without the use of tube compensation during an SBT.[121,122] Whether an on-ventilator or off-ventilator approach is used, it is generally best to

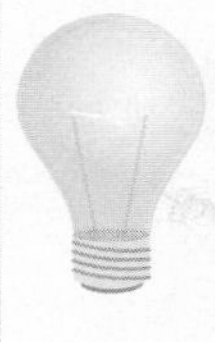

STOP AND THINK

You are caring for a patient who has been intubated for the past 3 days. How would you know if the patient is ready for liberation from mechanical ventilation?

perform the SBT with no additional support.[123,124] Even low levels of support can produce false-positive results.

Similar outcomes are likely with a 2-hour SBT or a 30-minute SBT.[125] In the acute care setting, tolerance of an SBT of 30 minutes to 2 hours duration should prompt consideration for extubation. For chronically ventilator-dependent patients with a tracheostomy, the length of each SBT is increased, with alternating periods of ventilatory support and SBT. In this case, the goal may be daytime liberation with nocturnal ventilation.

Recognition of a Failed Spontaneous Breathing Trial

A failed SBT is discomforting for the patient and may induce significant cardiopulmonary distress. Commonly listed criteria for discontinuation of an SBT include tachypnea (respiratory rate over 35 breaths/min for 5 min or longer); hypoxemia (Spo_2 below 90%); tachycardia (heart rate over 140 beats/min or a sustained increase above 20%); bradycardia (sustained decrease in the heart rate of over 20%); hypertension (systolic blood pressure over 180 mm Hg); hypotension (systolic blood pressure under 90 mm Hg); and agitation, diaphoresis, or anxiety. In some patients the last three factors are not caused by SBT failure and can be appropriately treated with verbal reassurance or pharmacologic support. When SBT failure is recognized, ventilatory support should be promptly reestablished.

Causes of a Failed Spontaneous Breathing Trial

When a patient fails an SBT, the reason should be identified and corrected before another SBT is performed. There are a variety of physiologic and technical reasons why patients fail an SBT. An excessive respiratory muscle load may be the cause. High airways resistance and low compliance contribute to the increased effort necessary to breathe. Auto-PEEP may delay liberation in patients with COPD, because it increases the pleural pressure needed to initiate inhalation. Electrolyte imbalance may cause respiratory muscle weakness. Inadequate levels of potassium, magnesium, phosphate, and calcium impair ventilatory muscle function. Appropriate nutritional support often improves the ventilator discontinuation process, but care should be taken to avoid overfeeding, because excessive caloric ingestion elevates carbon dioxide production. Failure of any major organ system can result in failure to liberate the patient from the ventilator. Fever and infection are of particular concern because they increase both oxygen consumption and carbon dioxide production, resulting in an increased ventilatory requirement. Cardiac dysfunction can delay liberation until appropriate management of cardiovascular status has occurred.

Once the patient has been judged to no longer need mechanical ventilatory support, attention then turns to the need for the artificial airway. This requires a different set of assessments that focus on the patient's ability to protect the natural airway. Key parameters include cough strength and the need for suctioning (i.e., suctioning requirements exceeding every 2 h should preclude extubation). Although the ability to follow commands is desirable before extubation, it is not essential in patients otherwise able to protect the airway.

In appropriately selected patients (e.g., those recovering from a COPD exacerbation), extubation to NIV may reduce the duration of mechanical ventilation.[126] Extubation to NIV can also be considered to prevent extubation failure in patients at risk, such as those with COPD, cardiac disease, or others at risk for extubation failure. NIV is generally not recommended to rescue a failed extubation, however, except in patients with hypercapnic respiratory failure. There is no role for routine use of postextubation NIV.

Ventilator Discontinuation (Weaning) Protocols

Ventilator discontinuation (weaning) protocols have become increasingly popular in recent years, and respiratory therapists and nurses typically implement these protocols. Studies have reported improved outcomes when protocols are used.[127,128] **Figure 20-33** presents the elements of an effective protocol. From these elements incorporating best evidence, a specific protocol can be developed that meets the local culture of the ICU. Note that the use of an SBT is central to the protocol.

Sedation

Critically ill mechanically ventilated patients often receive sedatives in the form of benzodiazepines and analgesics in the form of opioids to ensure comfort, minimize distress, and make invasive procedures tolerable. Oversedation may be responsible for prolonged mechanical ventilation and increased ICU length of stay.

One approach to manage sedation is to conduct daily interruptions of sedative infusions, called a spontaneous awakening trial (SAT). These have been shown to shorten the duration of mechanical ventilation. Evidence supports a protocol in which an SAT is coupled to an SBT.[85] Unless contraindicated (active seizures, alcohol withdrawal, escalating sedative doses due to agitation, receiving neuromuscular blockers, evidence of active myocardial ischemia in the previous 24 hours, or evidence of increased intracranial pressure), an SAT should be conducted on a daily basis.

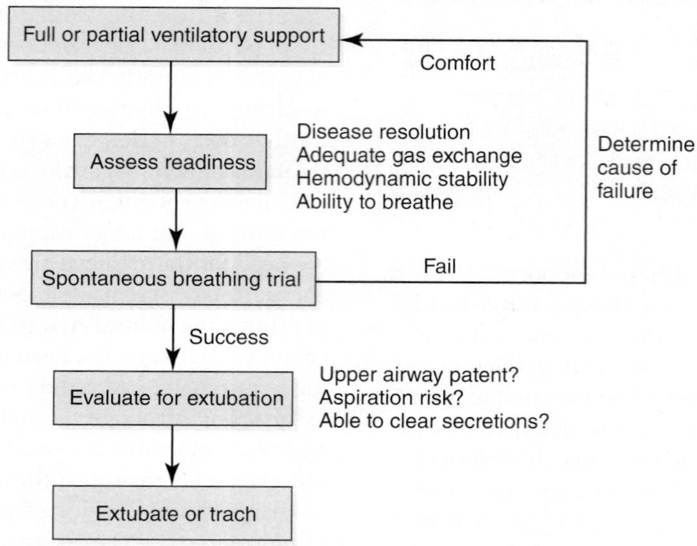

FIGURE 20-33 An evidence-based approach to ventilator discontinuation and extubation.

If the patient does not tolerate the SAT (anxiety, agitation, pain, a tachypnea, desaturation, acute cardiac dysrhythmia, respiratory distress), sedatives are restarted at half of the previous dose. If the patient tolerates the SAT, an SBT is conducted.

ABCDE Bundle

ICU-acquired weakness affects up to half of critically ill patients and prolongs mechanical ventilation. Early mobilization, including ambulation, of mechanically ventilated patients is safe and feasible and may result in better functional outcomes. Combining protocols for early mobility and sedation management may have synergistic benefits, as do combined protocols for sedation and SBTs. This has informed the ABCDE bundle:[129,130]

A. Awakening: spontaneous awakening trials
B. Breathing: spontaneous breathing trials
C. Choice of appropriate sedation and analgesia
D. Delirium monitoring
E. Early mobility

Key Points

- Efforts should be made to avoid complications during mechanical ventilation.
- Forms of ventilator-induced lung injury include alveolar overdistention and repetitive opening and closing.
- Volume control maintains minute ventilation but allows airway pressure and plateau pressure to fluctuate.
- Pressure control allows minute ventilation to fluctuate, but airway pressure is limited to the peak pressure set on the ventilator.
- Modes on modern ventilators include continuous mandatory ventilation (A/C), synchronized intermittent mandatory ventilation, pressure support, continuous positive airway pressure, adaptive pressure control, adaptive support ventilation, airway pressure release ventilation, tube compensation, proportional assist ventilation, neurally adjusted ventilatory assist, and high-frequency oscillatory ventilation.
- The tidal volume should be set to avoid overdistention lung injury: 6 mL/kg IBW is a suggested initial setting.
- The respiratory rate and I:E ratio are set to control the $Paco_2$ and to avoid hemodynamic compromise and auto-PEEP.
- The Fio_2 initially should be set at 1 and then weaned per pulse oximetry to maintain an Spo_2 >88%.
- PEEP should be set to avoid alveolar derecruitment for patients with ARDS and to counterbalance auto-PEEP in patients with COPD.
- The following should be monitored in the mechanically ventilated patient: physical signs and symptoms, blood gas measurements, lung mechanics, hemodynamics, patient–ventilator synchrony, and sedation.
- The most important aspect of liberation from mechanical ventilation is assessment for readiness.
- A spontaneous breathing trial identifies most patients who are ready for liberation from mechanical ventilation.
- The poorest outcomes from the ventilator discontinuation process have been reported with SIMV.
- For patients who do not tolerate a spontaneous breathing trial, ventilatory support should be reestablished, sedation targets reassessed, and the cause of the failure identified.
- Early mobility of mechanically ventilated patients can lead to improved functional outcomes.

References

1. Parthasarathy S, Tobin MJ. Sleep in the intensive care unit. *Intensive Care Med.* 2004;30:197–206.
2. Slutsky AS, Ranieri VM. Ventilator-induced lung injury. *N Engl J Med.* 2013;369:2126–2136.
3. NIH ARDS Network. Ventilation with lower tidal volumes as compared with traditional tidal volumes for acute lung injury and the acute respiratory distress syndrome. *N Engl J Med.* 2000;342:1301–1308.
4. Terragni PP, Filippini C, Slutsky AS, et al. Accuracy of plateau pressure and stress index to identify injurious ventilation in patients with acute respiratory distress syndrome. *Anesthesiology.* 2013;119:880–889.
5. Terragni PP, Rosboch G, Tealdi A, et al. Tidal hyperinflation during low tidal volume ventilation in acute respiratory distress syndrome. *Am J Respir Crit Care Med.* 2007;175:160–166.
6. Chiumello D, Carlesso E, Cadringher P, et al. Lung stress and strain during mechanical ventilation for acute respiratory distress syndrome. *Am J Respir Crit Care Med.* 2008;178:346–355.
7. Hager DN, Krishnan JA, Hayden DL, Brower RG, ARDS Clinical Trials Network. Tidal volume reduction in patients with acute lung injury when plateau pressures are not high. *Am J Respir Crit Care Med.* 2005;172:1241–1245.
8. Webb HJH, Tierney DF. Experimental pulmonary edema due to intermittent positive pressure ventilation with high inflation pressures: protection by positive end-expiratory pressure. *Am Rev Respir Dis.* 1974;110:556–565.
9. Crotti S, Mascheroni D, Caironi P, et al. Recruitment and derecruitment during acute respiratory failure. *Am J Respir Crit Care Med.* 2001;164:131–140.
10. Mead J, Takishima T, Leith D. Stress distribution in lungs: a model of pulmonary elasticity. *J Appl Physiol.* 1970;28:596–608.
11. Vaporidi K, Voloudakis G, Priniannakis G, et al. Effects of respiratory rate on ventilator-induced lung injury at a constant $Paco_2$ in a mouse model of normal lung. *Crit Care Med.* 2008;36: 1277–1283.
12. Rich BR, Reickert CA, Sawada S, et al. Effect of rate and inspiratory flow on ventilator induced lung injury. *J Trauma.* 2000;49: 903–911.
13. Marini JJ, Hotchkiss JR, Broccard AF. Bench-to-bedside review: microvascular and airspace linkage in ventilator-induced lung injury. *Crit Care (London).* 2003;7:435–444.
14. Trembly L, Valenza F, Ribiero SP, Li J, Slutsky AS. Injurious ventilatory strategies increase cytokines and c-fos m-RNA expression in an isolated rat lung model. *J Clin Invest.* 1997;99:944–952.
15. Ranieri VM, Suter PM, Tortorella C, et al. Effect of mechanical ventilation on inflammatory mediators in patients with acute respiratory distress syndrome: a randomized controlled trial. *JAMA.* 1999;282:54–61.
16. Slutsky AS, Trembly L. Multiple system organ failure: is mechanical ventilation a contributing factor? *Am J Respir Crit Care Med.* 1998;157:1721–1725.
17. Nahum A, Hoyt J, Schmitz L, et al. Effect of mechanical ventilation strategy on dissemination of intertracheally instilled *E. coli* in dogs. *Crit Care Med.* 1997;25:1733–1743.
18. Kallet RH, Matthay MA. Hyperoxic acute lung injury. *Respir Care.* 2013;58:123–141.
19. Kollef MH. Prevention of hospital-associated pneumonia and ventilator-associated pneumonia. *Crit Care Med.* 2004;32:1396–1405.
20. Han J, Liu Y. Effect of ventilator circuit changes on ventilator-associated pneumonia: a systematic review and meta-analysis. *Respir Care.* 2010;55:467–474.
21. Gentile MA, Siobal MS. Are specialized endotracheal tubes and heat-and-moisture exchangers cost-effective in preventing ventilator associated pneumonia? *Respir Care.* 2010;55:184–196.
22. Deem S, Treggiari MM. New endotracheal tubes designed to prevent ventilator-associated pneumonia: do they make a difference? *Respir Care.* 2010;55:1046–1055.
23. Marini JJ. Dynamic hyperinflation and auto-positive end-expiratory pressure: lessons learned over 30 years. *Am J Respir Crit Care Med.* 2011;184:756–762.
24. Yang L-Y, Huang Y-CT, MacIntyre NR. Patient-ventilator synchrony during pressure-targeted versus flow-targeted small tidal volume assisted ventilation. *J Crit Care.* 2007;22:252–257.
25. Kallet RH, Campbell AR, Dicker RA, et al. Work of breathing during lung-protective ventilation in patients with acute lung injury and acute respiratory distress syndrome: a comparison between volume and pressure-regulated breathing modes. *Respir Care.* 2005;50:1623–1631.
26. MacIntyre NR, Sessler CN. Are there benefits or harm from pressure targeting during lung-protective ventilation? *Respir Care.* 2010;55:175–180.
27. Chatburn RL. Classification of ventilator modes: update and proposal for implementation. *Respir Care.* 2007;52:301–323.
28. Hess DR. Ventilator waveforms and the physiology of pressure support ventilation. *Respir Care.* 2005;50:166–186.
29. Jubran A. Inspiratory flow: more may not be better. *Crit Care Med.* 1999;27:670–671.
30. Parthasarathy S, Tobin MJ. Effect of ventilator mode on sleep quality in critically ill patients. *Am J Respir Crit Care Med.* 2002;166:1423–1429.
31. Hess DR. Ventilator modes: where have we come from and where are we going? *Chest.* 2010;137:1256–1258.
32. Branson RD, Chatburn RL. Controversies in the critical care setting. Should adaptive pressure control modes be utilized for virtually all patients receiving mechanical ventilation? *Respir Care.* 2007;52:478–488.
33. Mireles-Cabodevila E, Diaz-Guzman E, Heresi GA, Chatburn RL. Alternative modes of mechanical ventilation: a review for the hospitalist. *Cleve Clin J Med.* 2009;76:417–430.
34. Jaber S, Delay J-M, Matecki S, et al. Volume-guaranteed pressure-support ventilation facing acute changes in ventilatory demand. *Intensive Care Med.* 2005;31:1181–1188.
35. Mireles-Cabodevila E, Chatburn RL. Work of breathing in adaptive pressure control continuous mandatory ventilation. *Respir Care.* 2009;54:1467–1472.
36. Daoud EG, Farag HL, Chatburn RL. Airway pressure release ventilation: what do we know? *Respir Care.* 2012;57:282–292.
37. Habashi NM. Other approaches to open-lung ventilation: airway pressure release ventilation. *Crit Care Med.* 2005;33(Suppl 3): S228–S240.
38. Varpula T, Valta P, Niemi R, et al. Airway pressure release ventilation as a primary ventilatory mode in acute respiratory distress syndrome. *Acta Anaesth Scand.* 2004;48:722–731.
39. Varpula T, Valta P, Markkola A, et al. The effects of ventilatory mode on lung aeration assessed with computer tomography: a randomized controlled study. *J Intensive Care Med.* 2009;24:122–130.
40. Maung AA, Schuster KM, Kaplan LJ, et al. Compared to conventional ventilation, airway pressure release ventilation may increase ventilator days in trauma patients. *J Trauma Acute Care Surg.* 2012;73:507–510.
41. Maxwell RA, Green JM, Waldrop J, et al. A randomized prospective trial of airway pressure release ventilation and low tidal volume ventilation in adult trauma patients with acute respiratory failure. *J Trauma.* 2010;69:501–510; discussion 511.
42. González M, Arroliga AC, Frutos-Vivar F, et al. Airway pressure release ventilation versus assist-control ventilation: a comparative propensity score and international cohort study. *Intensive Care Med.* 2010;36:817–827.
43. Gruber PC, Gomersall CD, Leung PE, et al. Randomized controlled trial comparing adaptive-support ventilation with pressure-regulated volume-controlled ventilation with automode in weaning patients after cardiac surgery. *Anesthesiology.* 2008;109:81–87.
44. Jaber S, Sebbane M, Verzilli D, et al. Adaptive support and pressure support ventilation behavior in response to increased ventilatory demand. *Anesthesiology.* 2009;110:620–627.

45. Sulemanji D, Marchese A, Garbarini P, et al. Adaptive support ventilation: an appropriate mechanical ventilation strategy for acute respiratory distress syndrome? *Anesthesiology*. 2009;111: 863–870.
46. Chen C-W, Wu C-P, Dai Y-L, et al. Effects of implementing adaptive support ventilation in a medical intensive care unit. *Respir Care*. 2011;56:976–983.
47. Kirakli C, Ozdemir I, Ucar ZZ, et al. Adaptive support ventilation for faster weaning in COPD: a randomised controlled trial. *Eur Respir J*. 2011;38:774–780.
48. Burns KEA, Lellouche F, Lessard MR. Automating the weaning process with advanced closed-loop systems. *Intensive Care Med*. 2008;34:1757–1765.
49. Branson RD. Modes to facilitate ventilator weaning. *Respir Care* 2012;57:1635–1648.
50. Guttmann J, Haberthür C, Mols G, Lichtwarck-Aschoff M. Automatic tube compensation (ATC). *Minerva Anesthesiol*. 2002;68:369–377.
51. Cohen JD, Shapiro M, Grozovski E, et al. Extubation outcome following a spontaneous breathing trial with automatic tube compensation versus continuous positive airway pressure. *Crit Care Med*. 2006;34:682–686.
52. Elsasser S, Guttmann J, Stocker R, et al. Accuracy of automatic tube compensation in new-generation mechanical ventilators. *Crit Care Med*. 2003;31:2619–2626.
53. Haberthür C, Mols G, Elsasser S, et al. Extubation after breathing trials with automatic tube compensation, T-tube, or pressure support ventilation. *Acta Anaesthesiol Scand*. 2002;46:973–979.
54. Gay PC, Hess DR, Hill NS. Noninvasive proportional assist ventilation for acute respiratory insufficiency. Comparison with pressure support ventilation. *Am J Respir Crit Care Med*. 2001;164: 1606–1611.
55. Bosma K, Ferreyra G, Ambrogio C, et al. Patient-ventilator interaction and sleep in mechanically ventilated patients: pressure support versus proportional assist ventilation. *Crit Care Med*. 2007;35:1048–1054.
56. Kacmarek RM. Proportional assist ventilation and neurally adjusted ventilatory assist. *Respir Care*. 2011;56:140–148; discussion 149–152.
57. Verbrugghe W, Jorens PG. Neurally adjusted ventilatory assist: a ventilation tool or a ventilation toy? *Respir Care*. 2011;56:327–335.
58. Ferguson ND, Cook DJ, Guyatt GH, et al. High-frequency oscillation in early acute respiratory distress syndrome. *N Engl J Med*. 2013;368:795–805.
59. Young D, Lamb SE, Shah S, et al. High-frequency oscillation for acute respiratory distress syndrome. *N Engl J Med*. 2013;368:806–813.
60. Goffi A, Ferguson ND. High-frequency oscillatory ventilation for early acute respiratory distress syndrome in adults. *Curr Opin Crit Care*. 2014;20:77–85.
61. Gupta P, Green JW, Tang X, et al. Comparison of high-frequency oscillatory ventilation and conventional mechanical ventilation in pediatric respiratory failure. *JAMA Pediatr*. 2014;168:243–249.
62. MacIntyre NR. Is there a best way to set tidal volume for mechanical ventilatory support? *Clin Chest Med*. 2008;29:225–231.
63. Gajic O, Dara SI, Mendez JL, et al. Ventilator-associated lung injury in patients without acute lung injury at the onset of mechanical ventilation. *Crit Care Med*. 2004;32:1817–1824.
64. Ahmed AH, Litell JM, Malinchoc M, et al. The role of potentially preventable hospital exposures in the development of acute respiratory distress syndrome: a population-based study. *Crit Care Med*. 2014;42:31–39.
65. Biehl M, Kashiouris MG, Gajic O. Ventilator-induced lung injury: minimizing its impact in patients with or at risk for ARDS. *Respir Care*. 2013;58:927–937.
66. Serpa Neto A, Cardoso SO, Manetta JA, et al. Association between use of lung-protective ventilation with lower tidal volumes and clinical outcomes among patients without acute respiratory distress syndrome: a meta-analysis. *JAMA*. 2012;308:1651–1659.
67. Serpa Neto A, Nagtzaam L, Schultz MJ. Ventilation with lower tidal volumes for critically ill patients without the acute respiratory distress syndrome: a systematic translational review and meta-analysis. *Curr Opin Crit Care*. 2014;20:25–32.
68. MacIntyre NR, McConnell R, Cheng KC. Applied PEEP reduces the inspiratory load of intrinsic PEEP during pressure support. *Chest*. 1997;1111:188–193.
69. Hess DR, Bigatello LM. Lung recruitment: the role of recruitment maneuvers. *Respir Care*. 2002;47:308–318.
70. Fan E, Wilcox ME, Brower RG, et al. Recruitment maneuvers for acute lung injury: a systematic review. *Am J Respir Crit Care Med*. 2008;178:1156–1163.
71. Fan E, Checkley W, Stewart TE, et al. Complications from recruitment maneuvers in patients with acute lung injury: secondary analysis from the lung open ventilation study. *Respir Care*. 2012;57:1842–1849.
72. Rachmale S, Li G, Wilson G, et al. Practice of excessive FIO_2 and effect on pulmonary outcomes in mechanically ventilated patients with acute lung injury. *Respir Care*. 2012;57:1887–1893.
73. Badet M, Bayle F, Richard JC, Guérin C. Comparison of optimal positive end-expiratory pressure and recruitment maneuvers during lung-protective mechanical ventilation in patients with acute lung injury/acute respiratory distress syndrome. *Respir Care*. 2009;54:847–854.
74. Hinkson CR, Benson MS, Stephens LM, Deem S. The effects of apparatus dead space on $PaCO_2$ in patients receiving lung-protective ventilation. *Respir Care*. 2006;51:1140–1144.
75. Gilstrap D, MacIntyre N. Patient-ventilator interactions. Implications for clinical management. *Am J Respir Crit Care Med*. 2013;188:1058–1068.
76. de Wit M, Miller KB, Green DA, et al. Ineffective triggering predicts increased duration of mechanical ventilation. *Crit Care Med*. 2009;37:2740–2745.
77. Thille AW, Rodriguez P, Cabello B, et al. Patient-ventilator asynchrony during assisted mechanical ventilation. *Intensive Care Med*. 2006;32:1515–1522.
78. Imanaka H, Nishimura M, Takeuchi M, et al. Autotriggering caused by cardiogenic oscillation during flow-triggered mechanical ventilation. *Crit Care Med*. 2000;28:402–407.
79. Akoumianaki E, Lyazidi A, Rey N, et al. Mechanical ventilation-induced reverse-triggered breaths: a frequently unrecognized form of neuromechanical coupling. *Chest*. 2013;143:927–938.
80. Hess DR, Thompson BT. Patient-ventilator dyssynchrony during lung protective ventilation: what's a clinician to do? *Crit Care Med*. 2006;34:231–233.
81. Branson RD, Johannigman JA. The role of ventilator graphics when setting dual-control modes. *Respir Care*. 2005;50:187–201.
82. Riker RR, Shehabi Y, Bokesch PM, et al. Dexmedetomidine vs midazolam for sedation of critically ill patients: a randomized trial. *JAMA*. 2009;301:489–499.
83. Levine S, Nguyen T, Taylor N, et al. Rapid disuse atrophy of diaphragm fibers in mechanically ventilated humans. *N Engl J Med*. 2008;358:1327–1335.
84. Hermans G, De Jonghe B, Bruyninckx F, Van den Berghe G. Clinical review: critical illness polyneuropathy and myopathy. *Crit Care*. 2008;12:238.
85. Girard TD, Kress JP, Fuchs BD, et al. Efficacy and safety of a paired sedation and ventilator weaning protocol for mechanically ventilated patients in intensive care (Awakening and Breathing Controlled trial): a randomised controlled trial. *Lancet*. 2008;371:126–134.
86. Strøm T, Martinussen T, Toft P. A protocol of no sedation for critically ill patients receiving mechanical ventilation: a randomised trial. *Lancet*. 2010;375:475–480.
87. Amato MB, Barbas CSV, Medievos DM, et al. Effect of a protective ventilation strategy on mortality in ARDS. *N Engl J Med*. 1998;338:347–354.
88. Richard JCM, Lyazidi A, Akoumianaki E, et al. Potentially harmful effects of inspiratory synchronization during pressure preset ventilation. *Intensive Care Med*. 2013;39:2003–2010.

89. Yoshida T, Uchiyama A, Matsuura N, et al. The comparison of spontaneous breathing and muscle paralysis in two different severities of experimental lung injury. *Crit Care Med*. 2013;41:536–545.
90. Yoshida T, Torsani V, Gomes S, et al. Spontaneous effort causes occult pendelluft during mechanical ventilation. *Am J Respir Crit Care Med*. 2013;188:1420–1427.
91. Papazian L, Forel J-M, Gacouin A, et al. Neuromuscular blockers in early acute respiratory distress syndrome. *N Engl J Med*. 2010;363:1107–1116.
92. Brower RG, Lanken PN, MacIntyre N, et al. Higher versus lower positive end-expiratory pressures in patients with the acute respiratory distress syndrome. *N Engl J Med*. 2004;351:327–336.
93. Meade MO, Cook DJ, Guyatt GH, et al. Ventilation strategy using low tidal volumes, recruitment maneuvers, and high positive end-expiratory pressure for acute lung injury and acute respiratory distress syndrome: a randomized controlled trial. *JAMA*. 2008;299:637–645.
94. Mercat A, Richard JC, Vielle B, et al. Positive end-expiratory pressure setting in adults with acute lung injury and acute respiratory distress syndrome: a randomized controlled trial. *JAMA*. 2008;299:646–655.
95. Briel M, Meade M, Mercat A, et al. Higher vs lower positive end-expiratory pressure in patients with acute lung injury and acute respiratory distress syndrome: systematic review and meta-analysis. *JAMA*. 2010;303:865–873.
96. Elmer J, Hou P, Wilcox SR, et al. Acute respiratory distress syndrome after spontaneous intracerebral hemorrhage. *Crit Care Med*. 2013;41:1992–2001.
97. Hess DR. Approaches to conventional mechanical ventilation of the patient with acute respiratory distress syndrome. *Respir Care*. 2011;56:1555–1572.
98. Nava S, Hill N. Non-invasive ventilation in acute respiratory failure. *Lancet*. 2009;374:250–259.
99. Medoff BD. Invasive and noninvasive ventilation in patients with asthma. *Respir Care*. 2008;53:740–750.
100. Elmer J, Hou P, Wilcox SR, et al. Acute respiratory distress syndrome after spontaneous intracerebral hemorrhage. *Crit Care Med*. 2013;41:1992–2001.
101. Mascia L, Pasero D, Slutsky AS, et al. Effect of a lung protective strategy for organ donors on eligibility and availability of lungs for transplantation: a randomized controlled trial. *JAMA*. 2010;304:2620–2627.
102. Hess DR, Kondili D, Burns E, et al. A 5-year observational study of lung-protective ventilation in the operating room: a single-center experience. *J Crit Care*. 2013;28:533.e9–15.
103. Chaney MA, Nikolov MP, Blakeman BP, Bakhos M. Protective ventilation attenuates postoperative pulmonary dysfunction in patients undergoing cardiopulmonary bypass. *J Cardiothorac Vasc Anesth*. 2000;14:514–518.
104. Lellouche F, Dionne S, Simard S, et al. High tidal volumes in mechanically ventilated patients increase organ dysfunction after cardiac surgery. *Anesthesiology*. 2012;116:1072–1082.
105. Futier E, Constantin J-M, Paugam-Burtz C, et al. A Trial of intraoperative low-tidal-volume ventilation in abdominal surgery. *N Engl J Med*. 2013;369:428–437.
106. MacIntyre NR, Cook DJ, Ely EW Jr, et al. Evidence-based guidelines for weaning and discontinuing ventilatory support: a collective task force facilitated by the American College of Chest Physicians; the American Association for Respiratory Care; and the American College of Critical Care Medicine. *Chest*. 2001;120(Suppl 6): 375S–395S.
107. Cohen CA, Zagelbaum G, Gross D, et al. Clinical manifestations of inspiratory muscle fatigue. *Am J Med*. 1982;73:308–316.
108. Laghi F, D'Alfonso N, Tobin MJ. Pattern of recovery from diaphragmatic fatigue over 24 hours. *J Appl Physiol*. 1995;79: 539–546.
109. Epstein SK. Weaning parameters. *Respir Care Clin North Am*. 2000;6:253–301.
110. Meade M, Guyatt G, Cook D, et al. Predicting success in weaning from mechanical ventilation. *Chest*. 2001;120(Suppl 6):400S–424S.
111. Yang KL, Tobin MJ. A prospective study of indices predicting the outcome of trials of weaning from mechanical ventilation. *N Engl J Med*. 1991;324:1445–1450.
112. Tanios MA, Nevins ML, Hendra KP, et al. A randomized, controlled trial of the role of weaning predictors in clinical decision making. *Crit Care Med*. 2006;34:2530–2535.
113. Kress JP, Pohlman AS, O'Connor MF, et al. Daily interruption of sedative infusions in critically ill patients undergoing mechanical ventilation. *N Engl J Med*. 2000;342:1471–1477.
114. Esteban A, Frutos F, Tobin MJ, et al. A comparison of four methods of weaning patients from mechanical ventilation. *N Engl J Med*. 1995;6:345–350.
115. Brochard L, Rauss A, Benito S, et al. Comparison of three methods of gradual withdrawal from ventilatory support during weaning from mechanical ventilation. *Am J Respir Crit Care Med*. 1994;150:896–903.
116. Ely EW, Baker AM, Dunagan DP, et al. Effect of the duration of mechanical ventilation on identifying patients capable of breathing spontaneously. *N Engl J Med*. 1996;335:1864–1869.
117. Ely EW, Bennett PA, Bowton DL, et al. Large-scale implementation of a respiratory therapist-driven protocol for ventilator weaning. *Am J Respir Crit Care Med*. 1999;159:439–446.
118. Robertson TE, Mann HJ, Hyzy R, et al. Multicenter implementation of a consensus-developed, evidence-based, spontaneous breathing trial protocol. *Crit Care Med*. 2008;36:2753–2762.
119. Straus C, Louis B, Isabey D, et al. Contribution of the endotracheal tube and the upper airway to breathing workload. *Am J Respir Crit Care Med*. 1998;157:23–30.
120. Esteban A, Alia I, Gordo F, et al. Extubation outcome after spontaneous breathing trials with T-tube or pressure-support ventilation. *Am J Respir Crit Care Med*. 1997;156:459–465.
121. Figueroa-Casas JB, Montoya R, Arzabala A, Connery SM. Comparison between automatic tube compensation and continuous positive airway pressure during spontaneous breathing trials. *Respir Care*. 2010;55:549–554.
122. Oto J, Imanaka H, Nakataki E, et al. Potential inadequacy of automatic tube compensation to decrease inspiratory work load after at least 48 hours of endotracheal tube use in the clinical setting. *Respir Care*. 2012;57:697–703.
123. Tobin MJ. Extubation and the myth of "minimal ventilator settings." *Am J Respir Crit Care Med*. 2012;185:349–350.
124. Bien M-Y, Shui Lin Y, Shih C-H, et al. Comparisons of predictive performance of breathing pattern variability measured during T-piece, automatic tube compensation, and pressure support ventilation for weaning intensive care unit patients from mechanical ventilation. *Crit Care Med*. 2011;39:2253–2262.
125. Esteban E, Alia I, Tobin MJ, et al. Effect of spontaneous breathing trial duration on outcome of attempts to discontinue mechanical ventilation. *Am J Respir Crit Care Med*. 1999;159: 512–518.
126. Hess DR. The role of noninvasive ventilation in the ventilator discontinuation process. *Respir Care*. 2012;57:1619–1625.
127. Girard TD, Ely EW. Protocol-driven ventilator weaning: reviewing the evidence. *Clin Chest Med*. 2008;29:241–252.
128. Haas CF, Loik PS. Ventilator discontinuation protocols. *Respir Care*. 2012;57:1649–1662.
129. Pandharipande P, Banerjee A, McGrane S, Ely EW. Liberation and animation for ventilated ICU patients: the ABCDE bundle for the back-end of critical care. *Crit Care*. 2010;14:157.
130. Morandi A, Brummel NE, Ely EW. Sedation, delirium and mechanical ventilation: the "ABCDE" approach. *Curr Opin Crit Care*. 2011;17:43–49.

CHAPTER

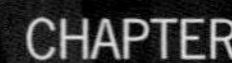

21 Noninvasive Ventilation and Continuous Positive Airway Pressure

Dean R. Hess

OUTLINE

Interfaces
Noninvasive Positive Pressure Ventilation
Continuous Positive Airway Pressure
Negative Pressure Ventilation, Rocking Beds, and Pneumobelts

OBJECTIVES

1. Compare noninvasive positive pressure ventilation, negative pressure ventilation, and continuous positive airway pressure.
2. Describe interfaces and ventilators for noninvasive ventilation (NIV) and continuous positive airway pressure (CPAP).
3. List selection criteria for noninvasive positive pressure ventilation (inclusion and exclusion).
4. Discuss acute care applications of CPAP.
5. Discuss the use of CPAP to treat obstructive sleep apnea.
6. Discuss the role of humidification in the application of NIV and CPAP.
7. Discuss issues of compliance with CPAP for treatment of obstructive sleep apnea.
8. Describe the operation and use of auto-positive airway pressure devices.
9. Describe the principles of negative pressure ventilation, rocking beds, and pneumobelts.

KEY TERMS

auto-positive airway pressure (APAP)
continuous positive airway pressure (CPAP)
cuirass
expiratory positive airway pressure (EPAP)
helmet
inspiratory positive airway pressure (IPAP)
iron lung
nasal mask
nasal pillow
negative pressure ventilation
noninvasive ventilation (NIV)
oronasal mask
pneumobelt
rocking bed
total face mask

Introduction

Noninvasive ventilation (NIV) provides ventilatory support without an endotracheal tube or tracheostomy tube. Both positive pressure and negative pressure approaches can be used to provide NIV. With **continuous positive airway pressure (CPAP)**, a pressure greater than atmospheric pressure is applied to the airway throughout the respiratory cycle. This chapter covers the clinical and technical aspects of the application of CPAP and NIV.

Interfaces

The interface distinguishes invasive from noninvasive ventilation. Similar interfaces are used for CPAP and NIV.[1,2] **Figure 21-1** compares NIV and CPAP. The interface has a major impact on patient comfort and compliance during NIV. A poorly fitting interface decreases clinical effectiveness and patient compliance. A number of interfaces are available, each of which has advantages and disadvantages (**Table 21-1**). The most commonly used interfaces are **oronasal** and **nasal masks**. Other interfaces include **nasal pillows**, mouthpieces, **total face masks**, hybrid masks, and helmets (**Figure 21-2**). A variety of sizes and designs are commercially available. Desirable features of a mask include low dead space, transparency, light weight, being easy to secure, having an adequate seal with low facial pressure, being disposable or easy to clean, being nonirritating to the skin, and low cost.

The mask cushion produces the seal between the mask and the patient (**Figure 21-3**). Although it should minimize air leakage, small leaks are common and may

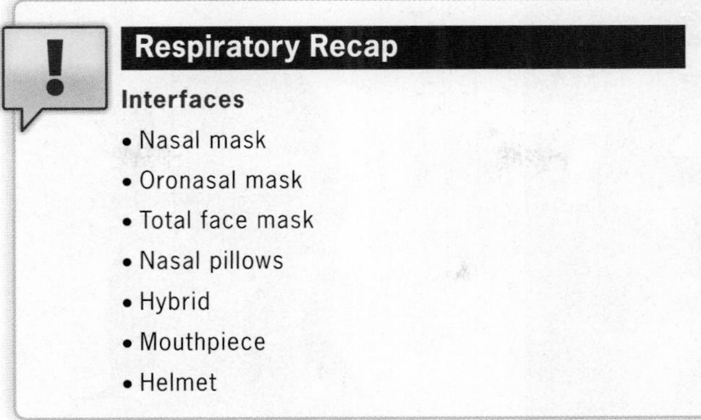

Respiratory Recap

Interfaces

- Nasal mask
- Oronasal mask
- Total face mask
- Nasal pillows
- Hybrid
- Mouthpiece
- Helmet

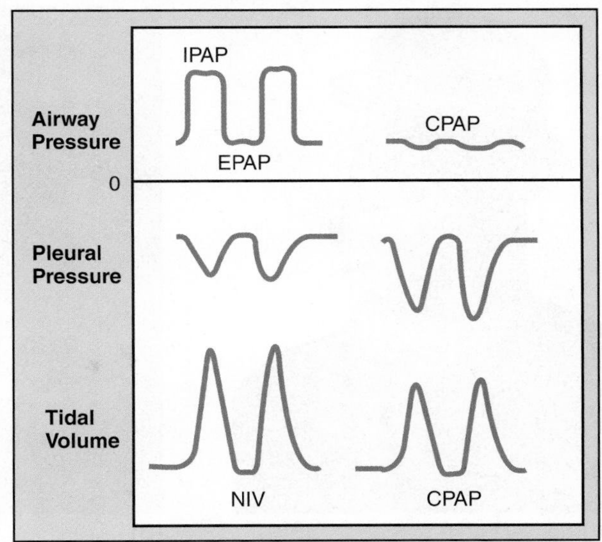

FIGURE 21-1 A comparison of the physiologic effects of NIV and CPAP. Both increase airway pressure, but NIV, unlike CPAP, also provides respiratory muscle unloading.

not necessarily compromise the effectiveness of CPAP or NIV. Nasal or oronasal masks designed specifically for NIV often use an open cushion with an inner lip, in which pressure inside the mask pushes the cushion against the face. The mask cushion should be soft and

TABLE 21-1
Advantages and Disadvantages of Various Types of Interfaces for Noninvasive Ventilation

Interface	Advantages	Disadvantages
Nasal mask	Less risk for aspiration Easier secretion clearance Less claustrophobia Easier speech May be able to eat Easy to fit and secure Less dead space	Mouth leak Higher resistance through nasal passages Less effective with nasal obstruction Nasal irritation and rhinorrhea Upper airway dryness with mouth leak
Nasal pillows	Lower profile allows wearing eye glasses Less facial skin breakdown Simple headgear Easy to fit	Mouth leak Higher resistance through nasal passages Less effective with nasal obstruction Nasal irritation and rhinorrhea Upper airway dryness with mouth leak
Oronasal mask	Better oral leak control More effective in mouth breathers	Increased dead space Increased aspiration risk Increased difficulty speaking and eating Asphyxiation with ventilator malfunction
Mouthpiece	Less interference with speech Very little dead space May not require headgear	Less effective if patient cannot maintain mouth seal Usually requires nasal or oronasal interface at night Nasal leak Potential for orthodontic injury
Hybrid	Eliminates mouth leak Lower profile allows wearing eye glasses Less facial skin breakdown	Increased aspiration risk Increased difficulty speaking and eating Asphyxiation with ventilator malfunction
Total face mask	May be more comfortable for some patients Easier to fit Less facial skin breakdown	Potentially greater dead space Potential for drying of the eyes Cannot deliver aerosolized medications
Helmet	May be more comfortable for some patients Easier to fit (one size fits all) Less facial skin breakdown	Rebreathing Poorer patient–ventilator synchrony Less respiratory muscle unloading Asphyxiation with ventilator malfunction Cannot deliver aerosolized medications

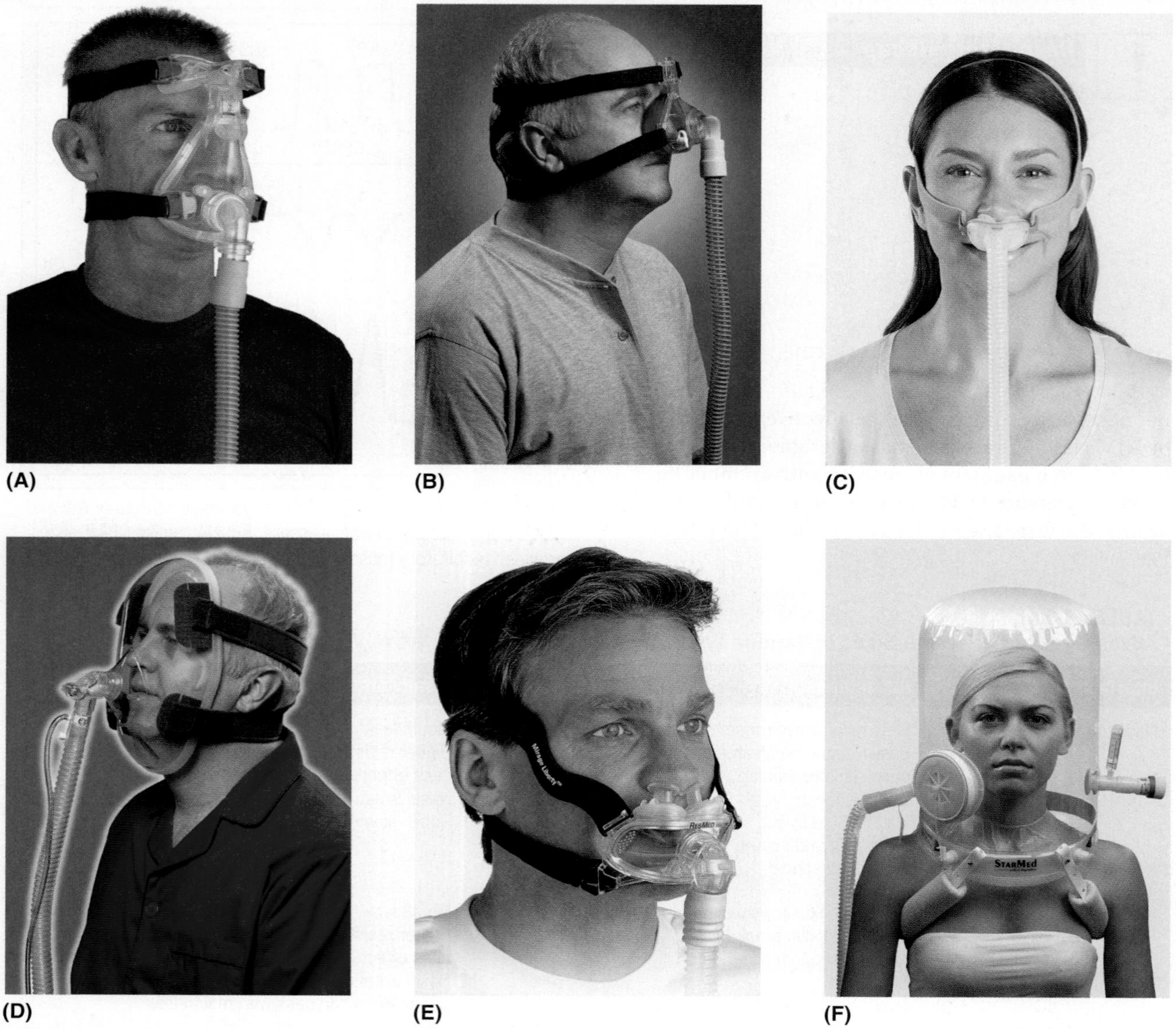

(A) (B) (C)

(D) (E) (F)

FIGURE 21-2 Interfaces for NIV and CPAP. (**A**) Oronasal mask. (**B**) Nasal mask. (**C**) Nasal pillows. (**D**) Total face mask. (**E**) Hybrid. (**F**) Helmet.
(**A**) and (**E**) © ResMed 2010. Used with permission; (**B**) and (**D**) courtesy of Philips Respironics; (**C**) © ResMed 2014. Used with permission; (**F**) courtesy of StarMed SpA.

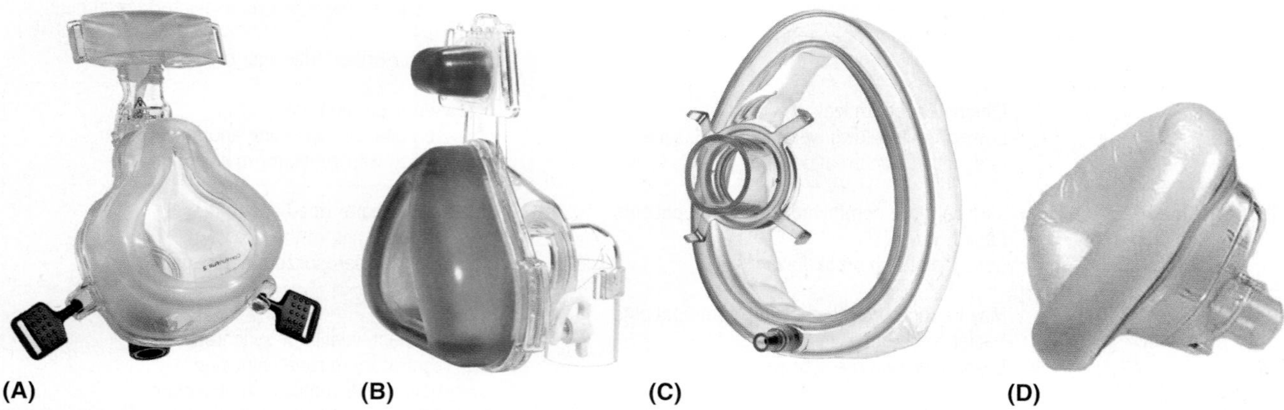

FIGURE 21-3 Styles of cushions on masks for NIV and CPAP. (**A**) Inner flap. (**B**) Gel. (**C**) Air-filled. (**D**) Foam-filled.
(**A**), (**B**), and (**C**) courtesy of Philips Respironics; (**D**) courtesy of Med Systems.

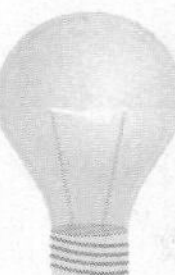

STOP AND THINK

Which do you think is better, a nasal interface or an oronasal interface? Explain why.

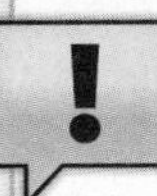

Respiratory Recap

Choosing an Interface

- Use the proper interface for the patient.
- Avoid an interface that is too large.
- Avoid strapping the mask too tightly.

malleable to the facial anatomy. Anesthesia and resuscitation masks are not desirable for NIV. Some masks have an inflatable cushion, and some masks are gel filled. A correctly sized mask minimizes leak, improves comfort, and improves effectiveness. Masks for use with a bilevel ventilator or CPAP machine may incorporate a leak port and an antiasphyxia port that opens if flow is lost from the ventilator (**Figure 21-4**). Masks used with a conventional ventilator have a standard elbow without a leak port. Commercial oronasal masks also have quick-release features so that the mask can be removed quickly if necessary. The hybrid interface is a combination of nasal pillows and a mask that fits over the mouth. The total face mask fits over the entire face of the patient.

The **helmet**, a transparent, latex-free polyvinyl chloride cylinder linked by a metallic ring to a soft collar that seals the helmet around the neck, has been proposed as an effective alternative to conventional face masks for NIV in patients with acute respiratory failure. One concern with the use of the helmet is the risk of rebreathing. The helmet has may be less effective in unloading inspiratory muscles compared with a standard face mask and has been associated with patient–ventilator asynchrony.

The nasal mask should fit just above the junction of the nasal bone and cartilage, directly at the sides of the nares, and just below the nose above the upper lip. The oronasal mask should fit just above the junction of the nasal bone and cartilage to just below the lower lip. Sizing gauges are available to properly fit masks. These are mask specific and cannot be interchanged between manufacturers or different mask styles of the same manufacturer.

A common mistake is to choose a mask that is too large. This results in leaks, decreased effectiveness, and patient discomfort. Leaks through the mouth are common when using a nasal mask. Unsuccessful NIV has been associated with mouth leak. When mouth leak interferes with the effectiveness of ventilation with a nasal mask, a chinstrap can be tried. Upper airway dryness may occur with use of a nasal mask and mouth leak. This can be addressed by using an oronasal mask or heated humidification; a heat and moisture exchanger should not be used with NIV. For many patients with acute respiratory failure, the oronasal mask or total face mask is better tolerated than a nasal interface.

Appropriate headgear is needed to maintain correct position of the mask. Most masks designed specifically for NIV and CPAP use cloth straps and Velcro to secure the mask. The cloth straps fit through attachments at the sides and top of the mask. Use of Velcro to secure the mask allows nearly infinite adjustments of the headgear. A common mistake is to fit the headgear too tightly. It should be possible to pass one or two fingers between the headgear and the face. Fitting the headgear too tightly may not improve the fit and always decreases patient comfort and compliance. The design of most masks for NIV is such that the top of the mask is secured on the forehead rather than at the bridge of the nose. Forehead spacers and an adjustable bridge on the mask are used to decrease pressure on the bridge of the nose.

Pressure sores on the bridge of the nose are a common complaint during NIV. Fortunately, ulceration and skin breakdown are avoided in most patients. Measures to reduce pressure injury should be taken as soon as signs of soreness occur at the bridge of the nose. Correct mask fit and size should be reassessed. The tension of the headgear should be reduced. A different

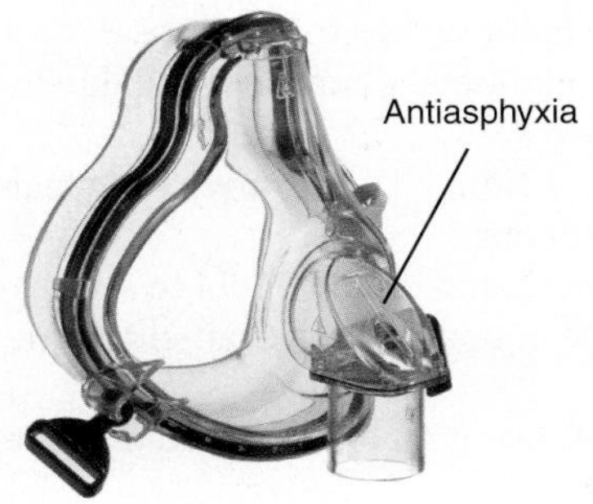

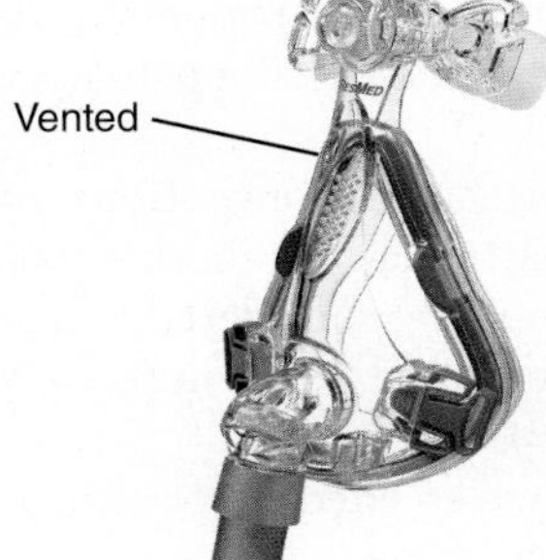

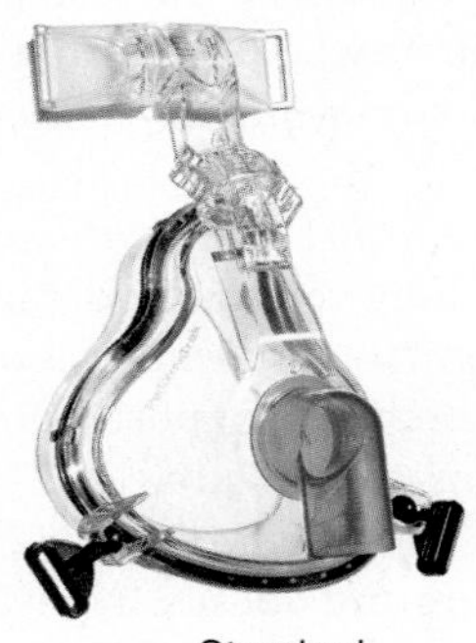

FIGURE 21-4 Masks with antiasphyxia valve, leak ports, and standard elbow.
(**A**) and (**C**) courtesy of Philips Respironics; (**B**) © ResMed 2014. Used with permission.

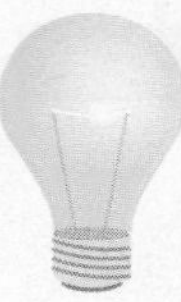

STOP AND THINK

A patient receiving noninvasive ventilation is developing facial skin breakdown. What would you do to remedy this problem?

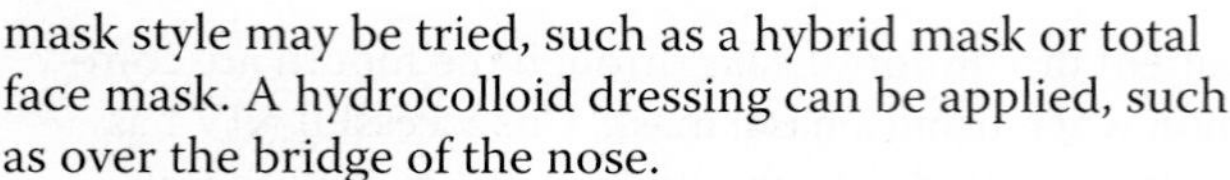

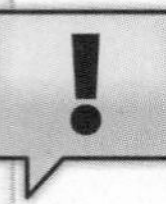

Respiratory Recap

Benefits of NIV for Acute Respiratory Failure

- Decreased intubation rate
- Improved survival
- Decreased pneumonia rates

mask style may be tried, such as a hybrid mask or total face mask. A hydrocolloid dressing can be applied, such as over the bridge of the nose.

Noninvasive Positive Pressure Ventilation

Acute Care Applications

NIV is commonly used in the treatment of patients with acute respiratory failure (**Box 21-1**).[3–6] In appropriately selected patients, NIV decreases the need for endotracheal intubation, decreases the risk of nosocomial pneumonia, and improves survival. The strongest evidence supportive of the use of NIV has been seen in patients with COPD exacerbation and acute cardiogenic pulmonary edema. NIV is also useful in patients with respiratory failure following solid organ transplantation and in those who are immunocompromised. It is being used increasingly to prevent extubation failure.[7]

BOX 21-1

Strength of Evidence Supporting Use of Noninvasive Ventilation for Acute Respiratory Failure

COPD exacerbations: NIV is first-line therapy and standard of care.

Acute cardiogenic pulmonary edema: NIV or CPAP is first-line therapy and standard of care.

Prevention of extubation failure: Accumulating evidence supports extubating patients directly to NIV who are at risk for extubation failure.

Transplantation, immunocompromised: Evidence supports the use of NIV in patients who develop respiratory failure following transplantation and in those who are immunocompromised.

Respiratory failure following lung resection: Evidence supports the use of NIV in patients who develop respiratory failure following lung resection surgery.

Acute hypoxemic respiratory failure: Evidence does not support the use of NIV for patients with acute hypoxemic respiratory failure, such as those with acute lung injury or acute respiratory distress syndrome.

Asthma: The role of NIV in acute asthma is unclear because there have been few high-level studies for this application.

Patients with Do Not Intubate or Do Not Resuscitate orders: In this patient population, NIV may be indicated in patients with COPD or cardiogenic pulmonary edema; it is not useful for malignancy except for patients in whom it is used for palliation.

Failed extubation: The results of high-level studies do not support the use of NIV to prevent reintubation in patients who fail a planned extubation, except in patients with hypercapnic respiratory failure.

Community-acquired pneumonia: The benefit of NIV in patients with pneumonia is controversial due to high failure rates.

Preoxygenation before intubation: Compared with conventional preoxygenation, NIV improves oxygenation and lung volume before intubation, particularly in morbidly obese patients.

Postoperative respiratory failure: NIV should be considered as a prophylactic and curative tool to improve gas exchange in postoperative patients, and it might improve outcome in postoperative patients with respiratory failure.

Obesity hypoventilation syndrome: NIV was an effective treatment for patients with hypercapnic respiratory failure and obesity hypoventilation syndrome.

Bronchoscopy: NIV might decrease the risk of complications in patients with severe refractory hypoxemia, postoperative respiratory distress, or severe COPD.

COPD, chronic obstructive lung disease; NIV, noninvasive ventilation; CPAP, continuous positive airway pressure.

BOX 21-2

Selection of Appropriate Patients for Noninvasive Ventilation

Step 1: Patient needs mechanical ventilation, such as

Respiratory distress with dyspnea, use of accessory muscles, abdominal paradox
Respiratory acidosis; pH <7.35 with $Paco_2$ >45 mm Hg
Tachypnea; respiratory rate >25 breaths/min
Diagnosis shown to respond well to noninvasive ventilation (e.g., chronic obstructive pulmonary disease, cardiogenic pulmonary edema)

Step 2: No exclusions for noninvasive ventilation, such as

Airway protection: respiratory arrest, unstable hemodynamics, high aspiration risk, copious secretions
Unable to fit mask: facial surgery, craniofacial trauma or burns, anatomic lesion of upper airway
Uncooperative patient; anxiety
Patient wishes

Box 21-2 lists inclusion and exclusion criteria for NIV. The initial response to NIV may predict success or failure. A more rapid decrease in $Paco_2$ occurs in patients for whom NIV is successful. Unsuccessful nasal NIV has been associated with greater severity of illness, greater mouth leak, and increased difficulty acclimating to NIV. Greater mouth leak has been associated with patients who are edentulous, have excess secretions, and use pursed-lip breathing. Success of NIV also has been reported to be greater for patients with higher baseline pH levels, perhaps because low pH was considered a marker of more severe illness. A good level of consciousness also has been associated with successful responses to NIV for patients with COPD and acute hypercapnic respiratory failure. If a patient does not improve on NIV within 1 to 2 hours of initiation, alternative therapy such as intubation should be considered. Consideration should also be given to transfer of the patient using NIV to a monitored unit such as an intensive care unit (ICU).[8] **Figure 21-5** presents an algorithm for use of NIV.

Aerophagia commonly occurs with NIV, but this is usually benign because the airway pressures are less than the esophageal opening pressure. A gastric tube, therefore, is not routinely necessary for mask ventilation. A gastric tube might interfere with the effectiveness of mask ventilation in several ways. It may be more difficult to achieve a mask seal if a gastric tube is present. Compression of the gastric tube against the face by the mask may increase the likelihood of facial skin breakdown. A nasogastric tube will increase resistance to nasal gas flow, which may decrease the effectiveness of mask ventilation—particularly nasal ventilation.

Chronic Applications

NIV is used for chronic respiratory failure resulting from restrictive lung disease, COPD, and nocturnal hypoventilation.[9] In many patients receiving chronic NIV, however, the therapy is administered only at night. Common goals of this therapy are to improve symptoms (e.g., fatigue, morning headache), to decrease $Paco_2$, and to decrease the degree of nocturnal arterial oxygen desaturation. **Box 21-3** lists recommended clinical indications for the use of NIV in chronic applications.[9,10] Chronic NIV use is most common with neuromuscular respiratory failure, where it is used as an alternative to tracheostomy and can be used for full-time ventilatory support. Some patients with neuromuscular disease can use a mouthpiece or nasal pillows during the daytime and a mask at night. The use of NIV for chronic stable COPD is controversial and is not common.

Ventilators for Noninvasive Positive Pressure Ventilation

Critical care ventilators are designed primarily for invasive ventilation but can be used for NIV. An issue with the use of critical care ventilators for NIV is that many are leak intolerant. However, newer generations of critical care ventilators feature NIV modes, and some compensate well for leaks.[11–14] Intermediate ventilators are typically used for patient transport or home care ventilation (**Figure 21-6**). Older generations of these ventilators only provided volume control continuous mandatory ventilation and were used for nasal, oronasal, or mouthpiece ventilation. Early studies of nocturnal NIV in patients with neuromuscular disease

Respiratory Recap

Goals of Chronic Use of NIV

- Improve symptoms
- Decrease $Paco_2$
- Decrease degree of nocturnal oxygen desaturation

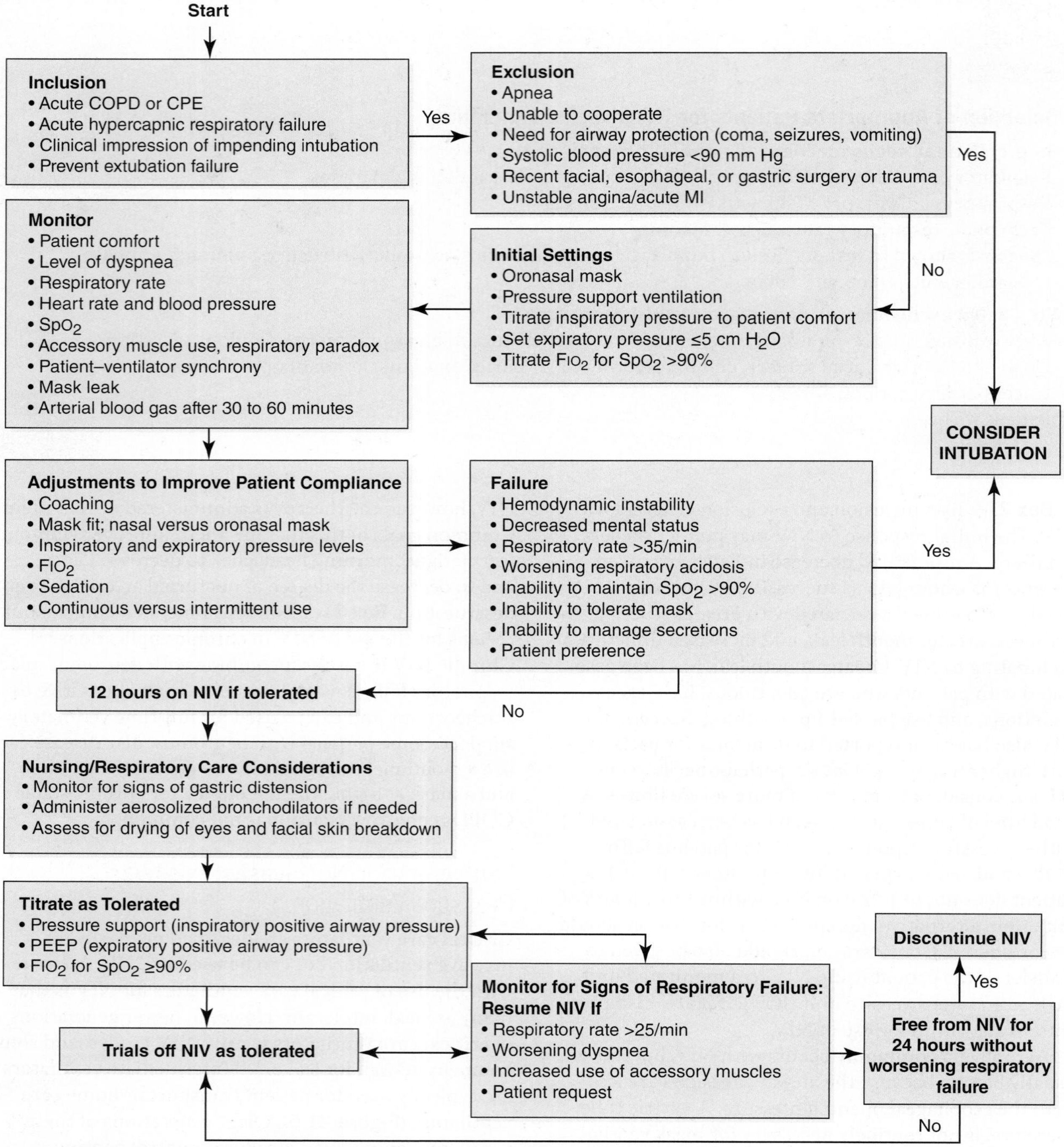

Start

Inclusion
- Acute COPD or CPE
- Acute hypercapnic respiratory failure
- Clinical impression of impending intubation
- Prevent extubation failure

Yes →

Exclusion
- Apnea
- Unable to cooperate
- Need for airway protection (coma, seizures, vomiting)
- Systolic blood pressure <90 mm Hg
- Recent facial, esophageal, or gastric surgery or trauma
- Unstable angina/acute MI

Yes → CONSIDER INTUBATION

No →

Initial Settings
- Oronasal mask
- Pressure support ventilation
- Titrate inspiratory pressure to patient comfort
- Set expiratory pressure ≤5 cm H_2O
- Titrate FIO_2 for SpO_2 >90%

Monitor
- Patient comfort
- Level of dyspnea
- Respiratory rate
- Heart rate and blood pressure
- SpO_2
- Accessory muscle use, respiratory paradox
- Patient–ventilator synchrony
- Mask leak
- Arterial blood gas after 30 to 60 minutes

Adjustments to Improve Patient Compliance
- Coaching
- Mask fit; nasal versus oronasal mask
- Inspiratory and expiratory pressure levels
- FIO_2
- Sedation
- Continuous versus intermittent use

Failure
- Hemodynamic instability
- Decreased mental status
- Respiratory rate >35/min
- Worsening respiratory acidosis
- Inability to maintain SpO_2 >90%
- Inability to tolerate mask
- Inability to manage secretions
- Patient preference

Yes → **CONSIDER INTUBATION**

No →

12 hours on NIV if tolerated

Nursing/Respiratory Care Considerations
- Monitor for signs of gastric distension
- Administer aerosolized bronchodilators if needed
- Assess for drying of eyes and facial skin breakdown

Titrate as Tolerated
- Pressure support (inspiratory positive airway pressure)
- PEEP (expiratory positive airway pressure)
- FIO_2 for SpO_2 ≥90%

Trials off NIV as tolerated

Monitor for Signs of Respiratory Failure: Resume NIV If
- Respiratory rate >25/min
- Worsening dyspnea
- Increased use of accessory muscles
- Patient request

Free from NIV for 24 hours without worsening respiratory failure

Yes → **Discontinue NIV**

No → Trials off NIV as tolerated

FIGURE 21-5 Clinical algorithm for application of NIV in the acute care setting.

typically used these ventilators. Newer generations of intermediate ventilators provide volume control, pressure control, and pressure support. Some are designed for either invasive or noninvasive ventilation. They vary in their ability to compensate for leaks, but most compensate well; some compensate for leaks in either pressure-targeted or volume-targeted modes. Most have internal batteries.

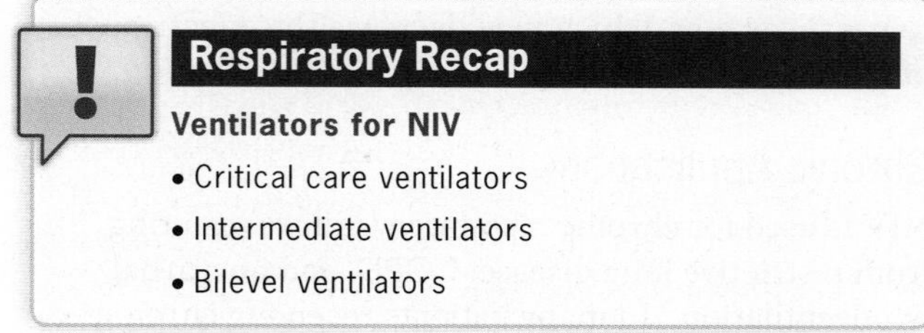
!
Respiratory Recap
Ventilators for NIV
• Critical care ventilators
• Intermediate ventilators
• Bilevel ventilators

BOX 21-3

Clinical Indications for Noninvasive Positive Pressure Ventilation in Chronic Respiratory Failure

Restrictive Thoracic Disorders

Examples: Sequelae of polio, spinal cord injury, neuropathies, myopathies and dystrophies, amyotrophic lateral sclerosis (ALS), chest wall deformities, kyphoscoliosis

Symptoms: Fatigue, dyspnea, morning headache

Physiologic criteria: Paco_2 ≥45 mm Hg, nocturnal oximetry demonstrating oxygen saturation ≤88% for 5 consecutive minutes, maximal inspiratory pressure > –60 cm H_2O or forced vital capacity <50% of predicted

Chronic Obstructive Pulmonary Disease

Examples: Chronic bronchitis, emphysema, bronchiectasis, cystic fibrosis

Symptoms: Fatigue, dyspnea, morning headache

Physiologic criteria: Paco_2 ≥55 mm Hg, Paco_2 of 50 to 54 mm Hg and nocturnal oximetry demonstrating oxygen saturation ≤88% for 5 consecutive minutes while receiving oxygen therapy ≥2 L/min, Paco_2 of 50 to 54 mm Hg, and hospitalization related to recurrent episodes of hypercapnic respiratory failure

Information from Clinical indications for noninvasive positive pressure ventilation in chronic respiratory failure due to restrictive lung disease, COPD, and nocturnal hypoventilation—a consensus conference report. *Chest.* 1999;16:521–534.

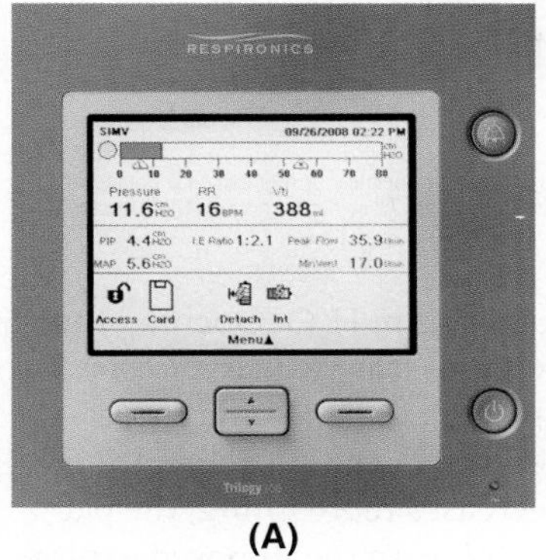

(A)

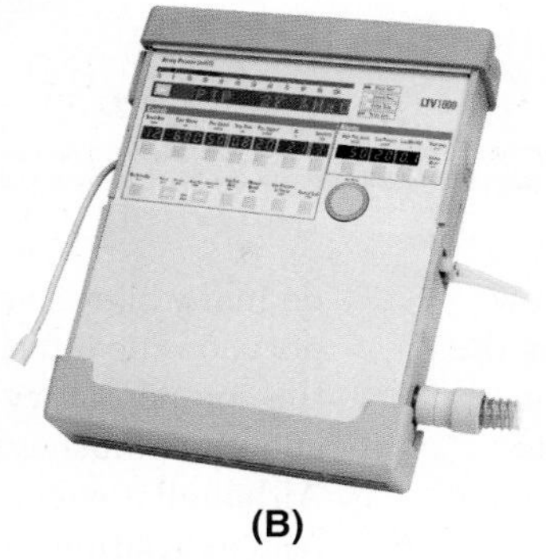
(B)

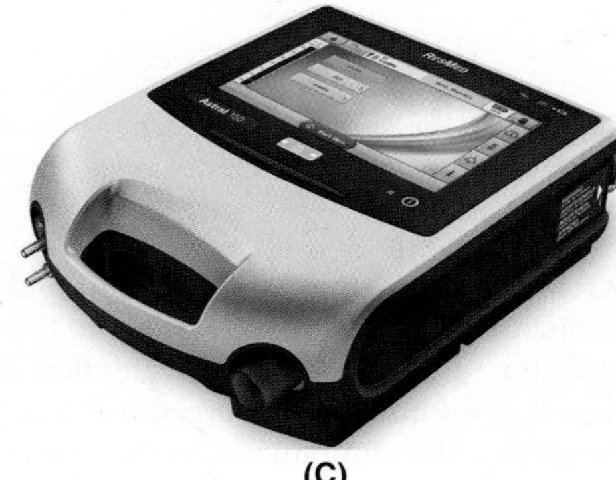
(C)

FIGURE 21-6 Intermediate ventilators that can be used for NIV.

(**A**) courtesy of Philips Respironics; (**B**) reproduced with permission from CareFusion; (**C**) © ResMed 2014. Used with permission.

Bilevel ventilators are blower devices that deliver inspiratory and expiratory pressures (**Figure 21-7**). They are designed to function in the presence of a leak. Bilevel ventilators use a single limb circuit. A leak port is present, which serves as a passive exhalation port for the patient (**Figure 21-8**). In some configurations, the leak port is incorporated into the circuit near the patient. In other configurations, the leak port is incorporated into the interface. Bilevel ventilators typically provide pressure support or pressure control. Pressure applied to the airway is a function of flow and leak. For a given leak, more flow is generated if the pressure setting is increased. For a given pressure setting, more flow is also required if the leak increases.

Intermediate ventilators use a single limb circuit with an active exhalation valve near the patient (Figure 21-8), although some use a passive leak port similar to bilevel devices. Newer generations of intermediate ventilators provide volume control, pressure control, and pressure support. Critical care ventilators have a dual limb circuit with inspiratory and expiratory valves and separate hoses for the inspiratory gas and the expiratory gas (Figure 21-8).

A concern with the use of single limb circuits that have a passive exhalation port is the potential for rebreathing. If the expiratory flow of the patient exceeds the flow capacity of the leak port, then it is possible to exhale into the single limb circuit and rebreathe on the subsequent inhalation. Several steps can be taken to minimize this risk. Rebreathing is decreased if the leak port is in the mask rather than the hose,[15,16] if oxygen is titrated into the mask rather than into the hose,[17] with a higher level of expiratory pressure, and with a plateau exhalation valve. Major determinants

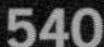

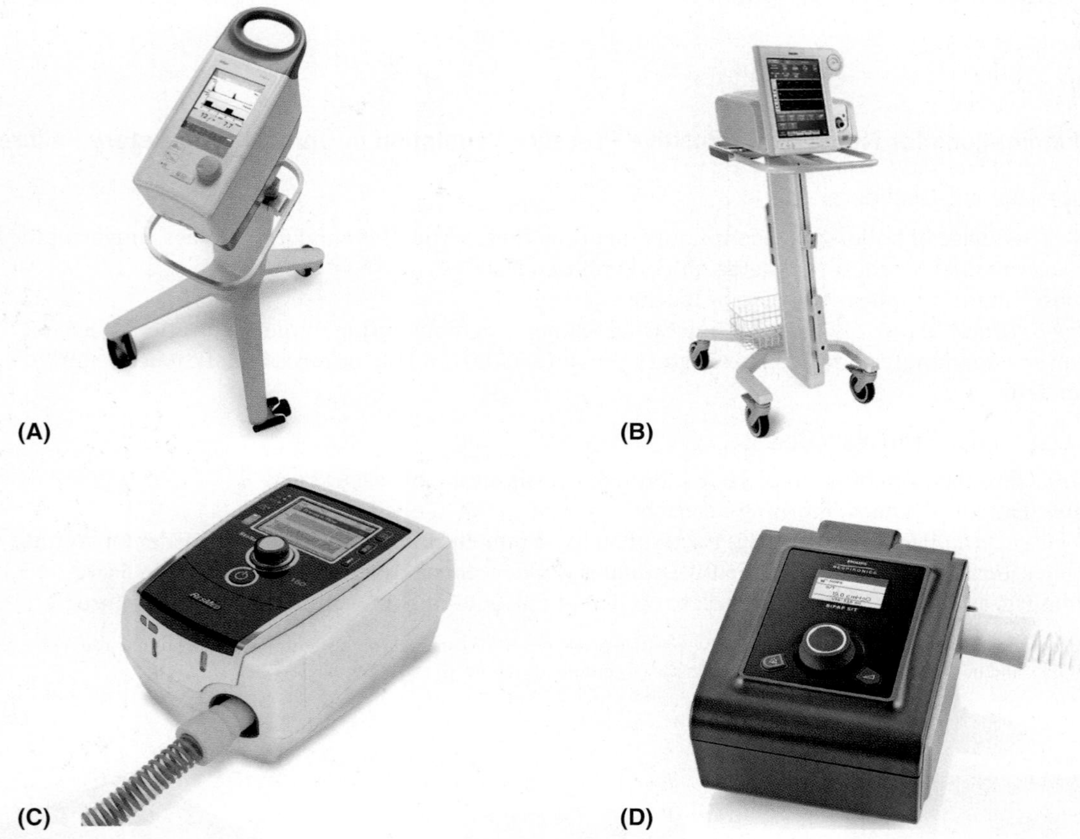

FIGURE 21-7 Bilevel ventilators that can be used for NIV.

of rebreathing are the expiratory time and the flow through the circuit during exhalation. Increasing the expiratory pressure requires greater flow and thus decreases the amount of rebreathing. It is for this reason that the minimum expiratory pressure setting on many bilevel ventilators is 4 cm H_2O. Opening the ports on the interface increases leak, which increases the compensatory flow through the hose and more effectively flushes the hose and decreases rebreathing. Although it effectively decreases rebreathing, the plateau exhalation valve may increase the imposed expiratory resistance.

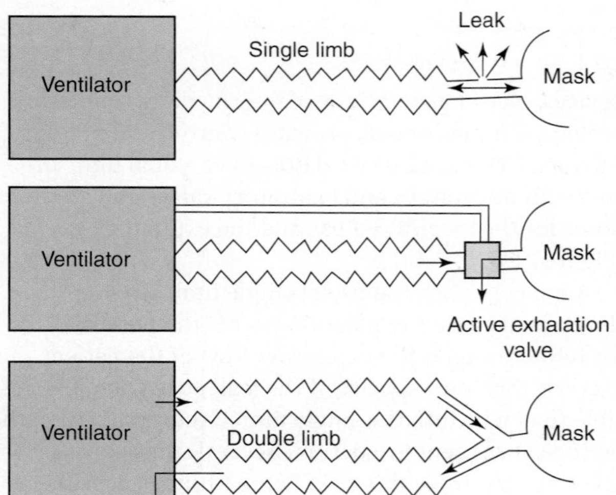

FIGURE 21-8 Circuit configurations for noninvasive ventilation.

Reproduced from Hess DR. Noninvasive ventilation for acute respiratory failure. *Respir Care.* 2013;58:950–972.

Some ventilators are able to detect unintentional leak (e.g., leak due to a poorly fitting interface) and adjust flow to accommodate the leak. Some bilevel ventilators allow the user to enter the interface that will be used to allow more precise identification of the unintentional leak. This approach, however, requires the use of an interface provided by the manufacturer of the ventilator. Other bilevel ventilators allow the user to test the leak port as part of the pre-use procedure.

If the leak is great, the patient may breathe from the leak rather than producing a flow or pressure change that will trigger the start of the breath. On the other hand, the leak could produce a pressure or flow drop that produces auto-triggering. Leaks also can affect the ventilator's ability to cycle to exhalation. Unintentional leaks should be minimized, and use of a ventilator with good leak compensation is ideal. All ventilators have a maximum inspiratory time during pressure support (typically 3 s), and the maximum inspiratory time is adjustable on some ventilators. Some ventilators allow the flow cycle criteria to be adjusted, which may be useful if a leak is present.

For acute care applications, it is desirable to use a ventilator with a blender allowing precise F_{IO_2} administration from 0.21 to 1.0. Bilevel ventilators used outside the acute care setting generally do not have a blender, but rather provide supplemental oxygen by titration into the circuit or interface.[17,18] This results in a delivered oxygen concentration that is variable, and only modest concentrations can be achieved (e.g., <60%). With oxygen titration, the F_{IO_2} is not easily predictable and is affected by the site of the oxygen titration, type of exhalation port, ventilator settings, oxygen flow, breathing pattern, and leak.

Pressure support is used most commonly for NIV.[19] With a critical care ventilator, the level of pressure support is applied as a pressure above the baseline positive end-expiratory pressure (PEEP). The approach, however, is different with bilevel ventilators, in which an **inspiratory positive airway pressure (IPAP)** and **expiratory positive airway pressure (EPAP)** are set. In this configuration, the difference between the IPAP and EPAP is the level of pressure support (**Figure 21-9**). With pressure support, the pressure applied to the airway is fixed for each breath, but there is no backup rate or fixed inspiratory time. Rise time (pressurization rate) is the time required to reach the inspiratory pressure at the onset of the inspiratory phase with pressure support or pressure control.[20] This can be adjusted on many ventilators used for NIV. With a fast rise time, the inspiratory pressure is reached quickly, whereas with a slow rise time it takes longer to reach the inspiratory pressure. A faster rise time may better unload the respiratory muscles of patients with COPD, but this may be accompanied by substantial air leaks and poor tolerance.[21] In patients with neuromuscular disease, a slower rise time is often better tolerated. Rise time should be set to maximize patient comfort.

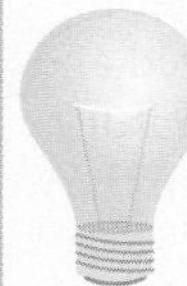

STOP AND THINK

Do you prefer a bilevel ventilator, intermediate ventilator, or critical care ventilator for noninvasive ventilation. Why?

Pressure control is similar to pressure support in that the ventilator applies a fixed level of support with each breath. Trigger and rise time are similar in pressure support and pressure control.[22] The primary differences between pressure control and pressure support are that (1) there is a backup rate with pressure control, and (2) the inspiratory time is fixed with pressure control. The backup rate is theoretically beneficial in the setting of apnea or periodic breathing, which may occur with pressure support. The fixed inspiratory time of pressure control is beneficial when the inspiratory phase is prolonged during pressure support due to leak or lung mechanics (e.g., COPD).[23–25]

Bilevel ventilators typically provide pressure support with a mode called *spontaneous*. In the spontaneous mode, IPAP and EPAP are set, but there is no backup rate. For safety, a backup rate should be provided. This is the case with the spontaneous/timed (S/T) mode on bilevel ventilators. The patient receives pressure support if the rate is greater than the set rate. If the patient becomes apneic, however, the ventilator will deliver flow-cycled or time-cycled breaths at the rate set on the ventilator. For critical care ventilators set for pressure support, the backup ventilation rate and alarms occur if the patient becomes apneic. A backup rate is also important to prevent periodic breathing. Central apnea is more prevalent with pressure support in normal subjects using a nasal mask,[26] in intubated patients,[27] and in patients being evaluated in an outpatient sleep laboratory.[28] For these reasons, a backup rate is recommended during NIV, particularly with nocturnal

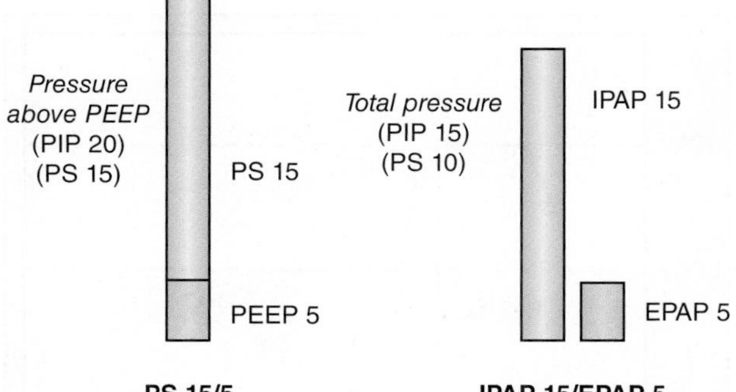

FIGURE 21-9 Comparison of pressure support, such as with a critical care ventilator, and inspiratory positive airway pressure (IPAP) with a bilevel ventilator. Note that the IPAP is the peak inspiratory pressure (PIP) and includes the expiratory positive airway pressure (EPAP), whereas pressure support is provided on top of the positive end-expiratory pressure (PEEP).

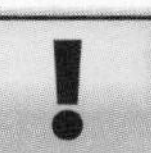

Respiratory Recap

Bilevel Ventilators for NIV

- Use blower devices
- Allow adjustment of IPAP and EPAP to produce pressure support
- Typically have modes such as spontaneous, spontaneous/timed, and timed
- Some have new modes such as AVAPS and adaptive servo-ventilation
- Use a single limb circuit with potential for rebreathing
- Some have a blender; others provide F_{IO_2} by titration

applications. Some bilevel ventilators have a timed mode. With this mode, the ventilation is triggered and cycled by the ventilator at the set rate and inspiratory time. This mode allows little interaction between the patient and the ventilator.

With volume control, the ventilator delivers a fixed tidal volume and inspiratory flow with each breath. Volume control has been used during NIV primarily in the home setting.[29,30] Volume control for home NIV is provided with an intermediate ventilator. Volume control has also been used to provide mouthpiece ventilation.[31,32] A low-pressure alarm is prevented during mouthpiece ventilation by producing enough circuit back pressure with sufficient peak inspiratory flow against the restrictive mouthpiece according to the set tidal volume. The ventilator rate is also set at a low level to prevent an apnea alarm. Some intermediate ventilators provide modes to specifically facilitate mouthpiece ventilation. Breath stacking maneuvers can be provided with volume control, but not with pressure control or pressure support. **Table 21-2** lists the advantages and disadvantages of pressure-targeted versus volume-targeted ventilation during NIV.

Average volume assured pressure support (AVAPS) is a feature available on the latest generation of Philips Respironics bilevel ventilators.[33] It helps patients maintain a tidal volume equal to or greater than the target tidal volume by automatically controlling the pressure support. The IPAP level is varied between the minimum and maximum IPAP settings. AVAPS averages tidal volume over time and changes the IPAP gradually over several minutes. If patient effort decreases, AVAPS automatically increases IPAP to maintain the target tidal volume. On the other hand, if patient effort increases, AVAPS will reduce IPAP. AVAPS functions much like adaptive pressure control modes such as volume support. With AVAPS-AE mode, the device monitors the patient's upper airway resistance and automatically adjusts the EPAP to maintain airway patency; the device will adjust the back-up breath rate based on the patient's spontaneous respiratory rate. A similar mode on the ResMed device is iVAPS.

A feature on the ResMed bilevel ventilator is adaptive servo-ventilation (adapt SV). With adapt SV, the algorithm uses three factors to achieve synchronization between pressure support and the patient's breathing: the patient's average respiratory rate; the direction, magnitude, and rate of change of the patient's airflow; and a backup respiratory rate of 15 breaths/min. When central apnea or hypopnea occurs, support initially continues to reflect the patient's breathing pattern. If apnea or hypopnea persists, the ventilator uses the backup respiratory rate. When breathing resumes and ventilation exceeds the target, pressure support is reduced to the minimum of 3 cm H_2O. A similar mode, AutoSV, is available from Philips Respironics. These servo modes are intended for use in the treatment of complex sleep apnea.

Ramp is used to reduce the pressure and then gradually increase it to the pressure setting. A ramp is used primarily in patients receiving CPAP or bilevel ventilation for sleep apnea, the objective being to allow the patient to fall asleep more comfortably. The role of a ramp during NIV is unclear. Particularly for acute care applications, this feature may be undesirable because it delays application of therapeutic pressure setting.

A feature on the Philips Respironics bilevel ventilators, Bi-Flex, inserts a small amount of pressure relief during the latter stages of inspiration and the beginning part of exhalation (**Figure 21-10**). High-level evidence supporting the use of Bi-Flex with NIV is lacking. A similar feature on ResMed bilevel ventilators is expiratory pressure relief.

Use of alarms during NIV is a balance between patient safety and annoyance. The extent of alarms necessary depends on the underlying condition of the patient and the ability of the patient to breathe without support. For example, consider the patient with neuromuscular disease receiving near full support by NIV. This patient is unable to reattach the interface or circuit should it become disconnected. In this case,

TABLE 21-2
Comparison of Volume Ventilators and Bilevel Pressure Ventilators for Noninvasive Ventilation

Volume Ventilators	Pressure Ventilators
More complicated to use	Simple to use
Wide range of alarms	Limited alarms
Constant tidal volume	Variable tidal volume
Breath stacking possible	Breath stacking not possible
No leak compensation with older models	Leak compensation
Can be used without PEEP	PEEP (EPAP) always present
Rebreathing minimized	Rebreathing possible

PEEP, positive end-expiratory pressure; EPAP, expiratory positive airway pressure.

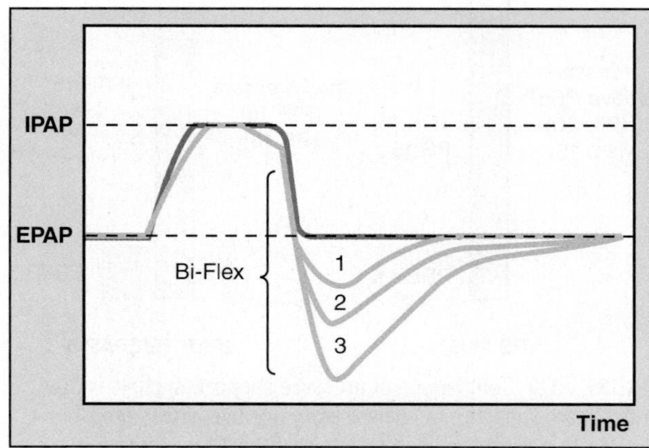

FIGURE 21-10 Bi-Flex mode inserts a small pressure relief during the latter stages of inspiration and at the beginning of exhalation.
Courtesy of Philips Respironics.

disconnect alarms and alarms indicating large leaks or changes in ventilation are desirable. Similar alarms are desirable in a patient with acute respiratory failure receiving NIV. On the other extreme, in the case of a patient using daytime mouthpiece ventilation, alarms may be an annoyance. When there is a question of the extent of alarms necessary, one should err on the side of patient safety. Ventilators for NIV have increasing capability to monitor the patient's breathing. Display of tidal volume, respiratory rate, and leak is useful for titrating settings. Many ventilators also display waveforms of pressure, flow, and volume. These waveforms can be useful in titrating settings to improve patient–ventilator synchrony.

Ventilators for NIV can be battery powered for safety and increased portability. Some have an internal battery, whereas others can be powered with an external battery or uninterruptible power supply. Many bilevel ventilators can be powered with a direct current (DC) converter. This allows the ventilator to be powered by the auxiliary power source in a vehicle. Bilevel ventilators can also be powered by a lead-acid battery such as a deep cycle or marine battery. Here an inverter is used to convert battery power into mains power. The duration of the battery is determined by the size of the battery, ventilator settings, amount of leak, and whether or not a humidifier is used. When using a battery, it is generally best not to use a humidifier if possible, as this will extend the life of the battery. It is also best to avoid use of the humidifier when the bilevel ventilator is made portable to avoid accidentally spilling water into the ventilator.

Humidity is added by placement of a humidifier between the ventilator and the patient interface. A cool, ambient-temperature, passover humidifier chamber adds a small amount of water vapor to the air flowing to the patient. Because of the velocity and volume of airflow, the limited surface area of the water chamber, and the evaporative cooling effect, however, the water content of the air being delivered to the patient increases only slightly. For some patients this may be enough to minimize nasal mucous membrane drying. For others a heated humidifier may be necessary. Heating the water in the reservoir counters the effects of evaporative cooling and raises the temperature of the air passing through the humidifier, allowing it to carry more water content.

Clinical Application

The application of NIV requires caregiver patience and skills with both the technical aspects of mechanical ventilation and patient coaching to adapt to the mask and ventilator. In many cases the appropriate settings for NIV are determined largely by trial and error, with appropriate feedback from the patient. The primary goal in the initiation of NIV is patient comfort and not an improvement in arterial blood gas values per se. An improvement in blood gas values usually follows if patient comfort and respiratory muscle unloading are achieved. Important steps in the clinical application of NIV are as follows:

1. Select patients for NIV who are most likely to benefit (e.g., those experiencing a COPD exacerbation or acute cardiogenic pulmonary edema).
2. Choose a ventilator capable of meeting patient needs.
3. Choose the correct interface; avoid a mask that is too large.
4. Explain the therapy to the patient.
5. Silence alarms and choose low settings.
6. Initiate NIV while holding mask in place.
7. Secure mask, avoiding a tight fit.
8. Titrate inspiratory pressure to patient comfort.
9. Titrate F_{IO_2} to Sp_{O_2} greater than 90%.
10. To minimize gastric insufflation, avoid inspiratory pressure above 20 cm H_2O.
11. Titrate expiratory pressure per trigger effort and Sp_{O_2}.
12. Continue to coach and reassure patient; make adjustments to improve patient compliance.

Complications of NIV are usually minor and include leaks, facial skin breakdown, mask discomfort, eye irritation, sinus congestion, oropharyngeal drying, patient–ventilator asynchrony, gastric insufflation, and hemodynamic compromise.[34] Approaches to improve asynchrony during NIV are listed in **Box 21-4**.[35] **Box 21-5** lists parameters that should be monitored during NIV. For acute care applications, NIV should be provided in a setting where the patient can be adequately monitored. If the patient does not improve within 1 to 2 hours after initiation of NIV, endotracheal intubation should be considered. The best weaning approach for NIV is unclear. The patient may request removal of the mask. If the patient's condition deteriorates after removal of the mask, then the therapy should be resumed.

Continuous Positive Airway Pressure

CPAP has applications in both the acute care and chronic care of patients. In acute care, noninvasive (mask) CPAP is used to administer intermittent lung expansion therapy, to treat acute hypoxemic respiratory failure, and to treat acute cardiogenic pulmonary edema. In chronic care, CPAP is used to treat obstructive sleep apnea (OSA).

Acute Care Applications

Mask CPAP is an effortless, painless type of respiratory care to prevent postoperative atelectasis.[36] It has been used in patients with acute hypoxemic respiratory failure to improve Pa_{O_2}.[37] Although mask CPAP can produce an initial improvement in Pa_{O_2}, it may not improve important outcomes such as intubation rate

BOX 21-4

Monitoring the Effect of Noninvasive Positive Pressure Ventilation

Assessment of Response

Physiologic: Arterial blood gases, pulse oximetry
Objective: Respiratory rate, hemodynamics
Subjective: Dyspnea, comfort, neurologic status

Mask

Fit
Comfort
Leak
Skin breakdown

Respiratory Muscle Unloading

Accessory muscle use
Thoracoabdominal paradox

Abdomen

Gastric distention
Expiratory muscle activation

Reproduced from Hess DR. Patient-ventilator interaction during noninvasive ventilation. *Respir Care.* 2011;56:153–165; discussion 165–167.

BOX 21-5

Strategies to Improve Synchrony with Noninvasive Ventilation

Trigger Synchrony

Adjust trigger sensitivity for the best balance between trigger effort and auto-triggering
Increase PEEP (expiratory positive airway pressure) to counterbalance auto-PEEP
Minimize unintentional leak with appropriate fitting of the interface
Treat underlying disease process (e.g., bronchodilators to decrease airways resistance and air trapping)

Flow Synchrony

Use pressure-targeted or volume-targeted ventilation per patient comfort
Adjust inspiratory pressure with pressure-targeted ventilation; adjust flow and tidal volume with volume-control
Adjust rise time (pressurization rate) per patient comfort
Minimize unintentional leak with appropriate fitting of the interface
Reduce respiratory drive (e.g., increase ventilation to treat acidosis)

Cycle Synchrony

Minimize unintentional leak with appropriate fitting of the interface
Use time-cycled (pressure control) rather than flow-cycled (pressure support) ventilation
Adjust flow cycle setting
Reduce pressure support setting
Treat underlying disease process (e.g., bronchodilators to decrease airways resistance)

Mode Synchrony

Use backup rate if apnea or periodic breathing occurs

Reproduced from Hess DR. Patient-ventilator interaction during noninvasive ventilation. *Respir Care.* 2011;56:153–165; discussion 165–167.

or hospital mortality. The strongest evidence for the use of mask CPAP is for patients with acute cardiogenic pulmonary edema. In these patients the increase in intrathoracic pressure decreases preload, decreases afterload, improves lung compliance, decreases intrapulmonary shunt, and increases Pa_{O_2}. A typical CPAP level of 5 to 10 cm H_2O is used. Mask CPAP, similar to NIV, decreases the intubation rate and improves survival rate in patients with acute cardiogenic pulmonary edema.[38]

A bilevel ventilator set to the CPAP mode is commonly used to provide mask CPAP for acute care applications. Otherwise, a CPAP circuit can be used. The CPAP circuit (**Figure 21-11**) consists of a high-flow gas source and an expiratory valve that maintains pressure in the circuit at the desired level (5 to 20 cm H_2O). CPAP requires a relatively high gas flow to maintain the desired positive airway pressure.

CPAP valves are classified as threshold resistors or fixed orifices. Threshold resistors maintain a constant pressure in the circuit, regardless of flow. A pressure exceeding the threshold opens the valve and allows expiration, whereas pressures below threshold allow the valve to close, sealing the circuit and stopping the flow of gas. Commonly used threshold resistor devices use spring tension to produce CPAP (**Figure 21-12**). With the fixed-orifice device, a restricted opening of a fixed size is placed at the end of the expiratory limb of a breathing circuit. The resistance through the fixed orifice produces backpressure, which is CPAP pressure produced in the circuit. For a given flow, a higher pressure is generated with a smaller orifice. Expiratory pressure is flow dependent, so pressure decreases as flow decreases. The fixed-orifice resistor has been abandoned in adult respiratory care but remains in use in neonatal care.

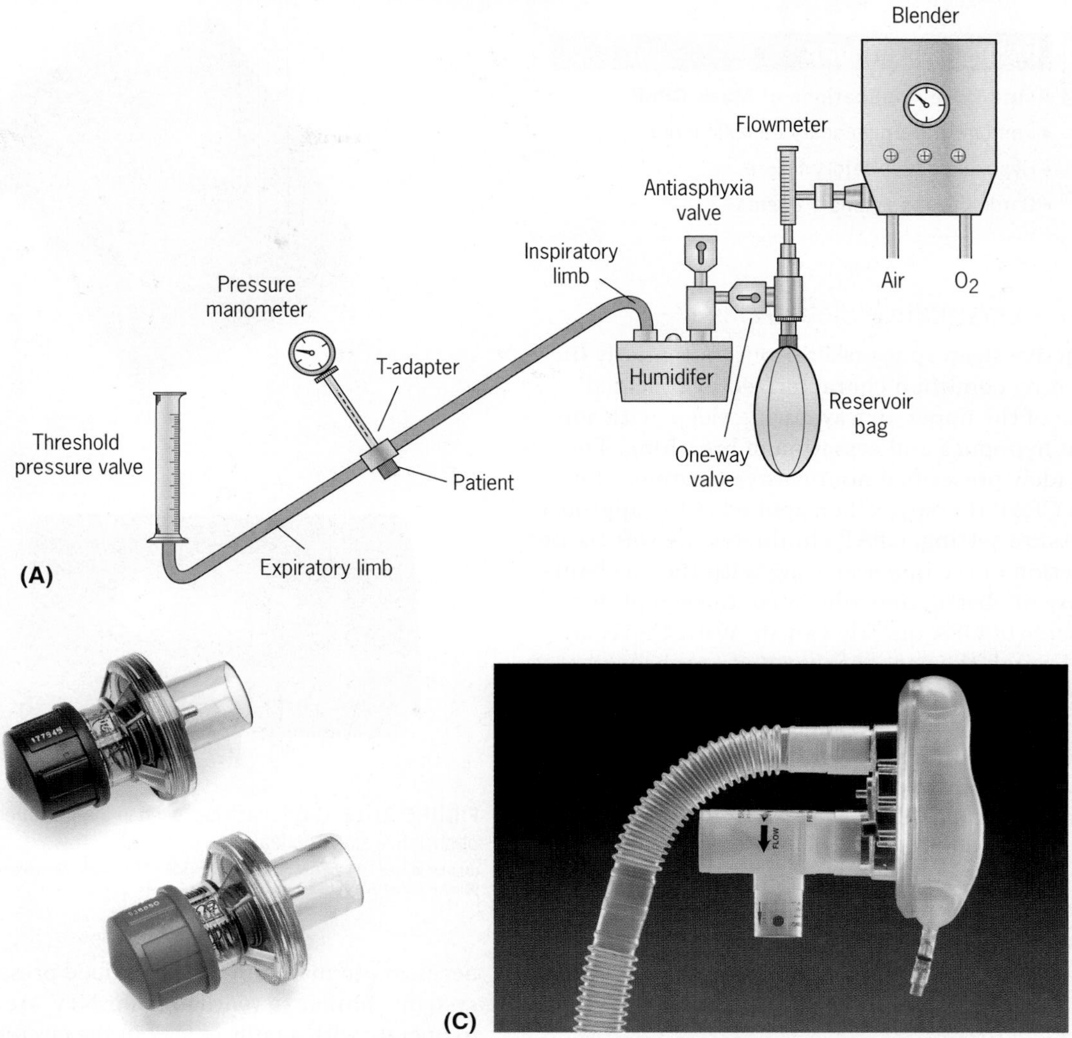

FIGURE 21-11 (**A**) CPAP circuit for acute respiratory failure. (**B**) Commercially available CPAP/PEEP valves. (**C**) Commercially available system for CPAP.

(**A**) adapted from Branson RD. Spontaneous breathing systems: IMV and CPAP. In: Branson RD, Hess DR, Chatburn RL, eds. *Respiratory Care Equipment*. 2nd ed. JB Lippincott; 1999; (**B**) courtesy of Ambu, Inc.; (**C**) © Vital Signs, Inc. Used with permission of GE Healthcare. All Rights Reserved.

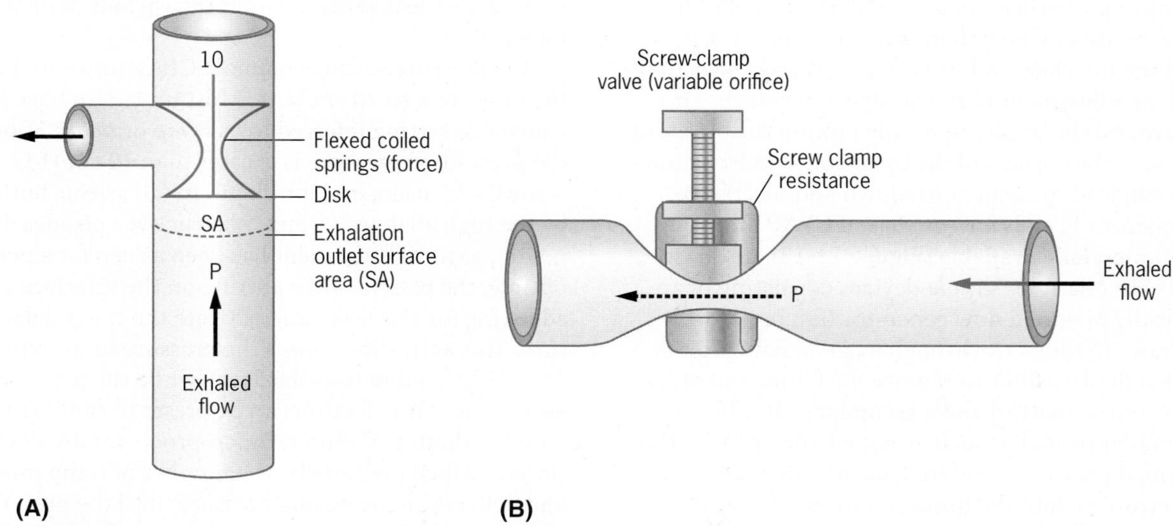

FIGURE 21-12 (**A**) Threshold resistor CPAP valve. (**B**) Fixed-orifice CPAP valve.

Adapted from Banner MJ, Lampotang S. Expiratory pressure valves. In: Branson RD, Hess DR, Chatburn RL, eds. *Respiratory Care Equipment*. 2nd ed. JB Lippincott; 1999.

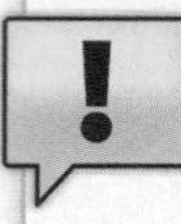

Respiratory Recap

Acute Care Applications of Mask CPAP

- Postoperative pulmonary complications
- Hypoxemic respiratory failure
- Cardiogenic pulmonary edema

CPAP for Obstructive Sleep Apnea

Obstructive sleep apnea is a serious, potentially life-threatening condition characterized by repeated collapse of the upper airway during sleep, with subsequent hypopnea and cessation of breathing. The most widely prescribed noninvasive treatment for OSA is CPAP therapy. When applied at the appropriate pressure setting, CPAP eliminates the soft tissue obstruction of the upper airway. With the mechanical cause of obstruction alleviated, the symptoms and effects of OSA quickly vanish. With CPAP, air flows through the nasopharynx and oropharynx at a preset pressure to maintain a constant positive pressure within the upper airway. This action has the effect of splinting the soft tissue, preventing its collapse into the airway during sleep and the subsequent obstruction. CPAP pressure is prescribed after a sleep study during which the pressure is slowly increased (titrated) until the pressure necessary to significantly eliminate the apneas and hypopneas has been achieved.

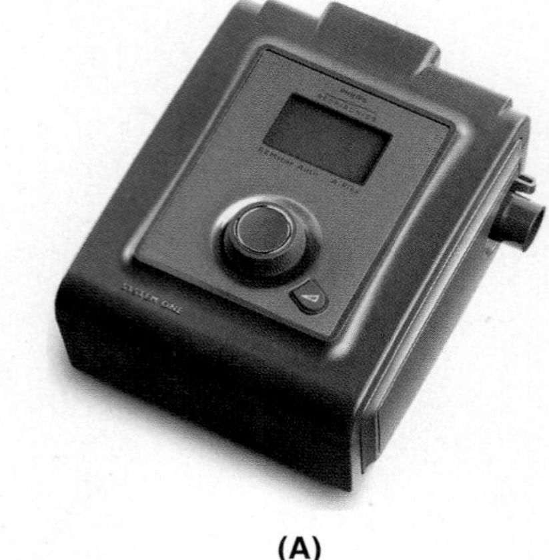

(A)

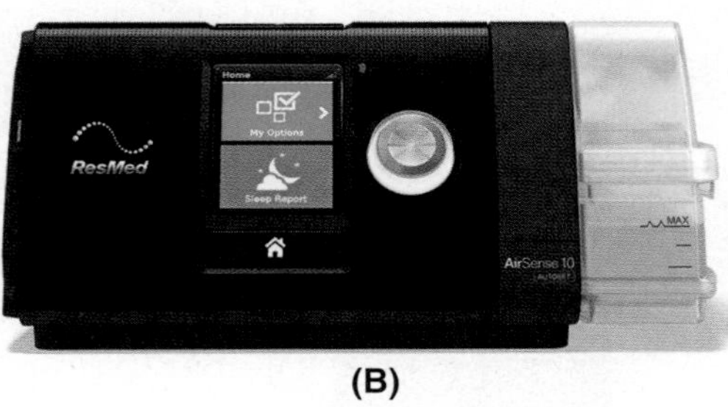

(B)

FIGURE 21-13 CPAP machines used in the treatment of obstructive sleep apnea.

(A) reproduced with the permission of Koninklijke Philips N.V. All rights reserved; (B) © ResMed 2014. Used with permission.

CPAP Equipment for OSA

The patient interface used for nocturnal CPAP therapy is the same as that used for NIV. Selecting the most appropriate interface and the correct size for each individual patient is one of the most important factors determining whether a patient will be successful in long-term use of CPAP therapy. Inappropriate selection of the interface and its size, or incorrect selection, fitting, or adjustment of the headgear, results in air leaks around the mask (especially around the bridge of the nose at the corners of the eyes) and skin irritation, which can lead to tissue breakdown and ulceration.

Numerous brands and models of CPAP machines are commercially available (**Figure 21-13**). The basic models are relatively simple devices consisting of an electrically operated flow generator (fan or turbine) that draws in room air through a particulate filter (a gross particulate filter to remove dust, lint, and other large airborne matter) and a secondary filter (to capture smaller particles, such as pollen and spores). The prescribed pressure is entered, usually through digital electronics, into the unit's microprocessor, which causes the flow generator to deliver the flow of air necessary to maintain the prescribed pressure. CPAP systems, similar to ventilators for NIV, are designed to operate with a built-in leak in the circuit. This leak port usually is found in the mask or between the tubing and mask. Because the system is designed to automatically compensate for this leak and to maintain the designated pressure, it also accommodates other small to moderate leaks that occur at the various patient interfaces.

The pressure settings on most CPAP units are in the range of 3 to 20 cm H_2O. Most units also have an adjustable setting referred to as *ramp* or *delay*. When the prescribed pressure is greater than 10 cm H_2O, some CPAP users find it difficult to fall asleep, bothered by the high airflow. Because obstructive episodes do not occur until the patient has been asleep for a period of time, the patient, after putting on the interface and adjusting for any leaks, can activate the ramp/delay feature. This activation causes the pressure to drop to 4 to 6 cm H_2O, a more tolerable level, while the patient falls asleep. The ramp feature can be preset to range from 5 to 45 minutes. The unit's microprocessor divides the set prescribed pressure by the number of ramp minutes and delivers an increasing pressure until the prescribed level is reached.

Improving Patient Compliance with CPAP for OSA

Table 21-3 lists common problems, and usual solutions, associated with the use of CPAP for OSA.[39] Respiratory therapists commonly encounter patients with OSA who use CPAP and should be able to assist such patients with these problems. Patients should be reminded of the benefits of CPAP in the setting of OSA. Some patients have difficulty adjusting to their interface and/or therapeutic pressure after their CPAP titration in the sleep lab. These patients may benefit from desensitization. CPAP can be applied with a lower than therapeutic CPAP to help the patient adjust

TABLE 21-3
Common Problems During the Use of CPAP for Obstructive Sleep Apnea

Problem	Cause	Solution
Nasal irritation, congestion, or rhinorrhea	Dry air Chronic rhinitis Nasal allergies	Heated humidification Nasal decongestants Nasal steroids Antihistamines
Dry throat and/or mouth	Dry air Mouth leak	Heated humidification Chin strap Oronasal or full-face interface
Painful pressure in ears	High airway pressure Nasal congestion	Verify CPAP level Decrease CPAP level Trial on auto or bilevel mode Nasal decongestants Nasal steroids
Gastric bloating and/or chest discomfort	Air swallowing High airway pressure	Decrease CPAP level Trial on auto or bilevel mode
Claustrophobia	Anxiety Interface	Desensitization Anxiolytics Optimize interface fit
Nasal pressure sores	Poor interface fit	Readjust headgear Change interface size or style Apply skin protection Reassess patient education on interface fit
Eye irritation	Interface air leak	Readjust headgear Change interface size or style Reassess patient education on interface fit
Skin creases	Improperly adjusted headgear	Readjust headgear Change interface size or style Reassess patient education on interface fit
Skin irritation	Sensitivity to interface Improperly adjusted headgear Heat rash	Trial using nasal pillows Readjust headgear Lower temperature on humidifier Trial using nasal pillows or skin protector
Air leaks	Excessive interface/headgear wear Poor interface fit Improperly adjusted headgear Excessive air pressure Facial hair interference	Replace interface and/or headgear Change interface Readjust headgear Verify pressure setting Consider pressure change Consider auto or bilevel mode Trial with nasal pillows Shave

CPAP, continuous positive airway pressure.

Reproduced from Allen KY, Bollig S, Selecky PA, Smalling T. *The Clinician's Guide to PAP Adherence*. Irving, Tx.: American Association for Respiratory Care; 2009. Reprinted with permission from the American Association for Respiratory Care.

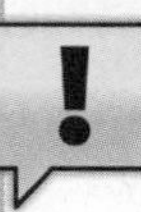

Respiratory Recap

Factors Affecting CPAP Compliance

- Poor patient education and understanding
- Improper interface size, selection, and fit
- Drying of nose and mouth
- High inward flow during exhalation

to the pressure. When the patient has adapted to the lower pressure, the pressure is gradually increased to the prescribed level. The patient can be encouraged to continue acclimation exercises by performing practice-breathing sessions with the interface and pressure for short periods during a distraction such as watching television, listening to music, or reading a book. Patients should use CPAP when they take a nap and should be encouraged to use it during the first 4 to 5 hours of sleep, with the ultimate goal of using CPAP throughout the night.

Upper airway discomforts of dryness of the nasal passages and/or the mouth, epistaxis, nasal congestion, and rhinitis are frequent complaints of CPAP users. The flow of air through the nasal passages during CPAP therapy, especially when high pressures are required, leads to drying and inflammation of the mucous membranes. The inflamed nasal mucosa restricts airflow, increasing nasal airway resistance, which is especially problematic in patients who sleep with their mouths open. The use of a chinstrap (**Figure 21-14**) to help keep the mouth closed may be helpful to lessen this problem in some patients. Heated humidification during CPAP therapy improves comfort and compliance.

A number of manufacturers have incorporated into their units the capability to record, and hold in memory, data such as the date, time on and off, time at pressure, leak, and use of a ramp. Some units identify and report apnea hypopnea index (AHI) and periodic breathing. The stored data can be downloaded to a computer. The raw data are uploaded to a computer program that displays the data in various graphic and tabular formats. This information is valuable to the equipment provider, referring physician, sleep laboratory, and insurer because it provides details of ongoing patient compliance and helps identify problems requiring intervention.

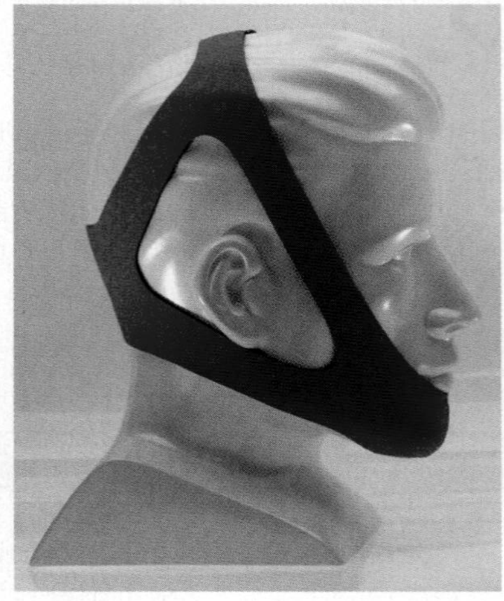

(A)

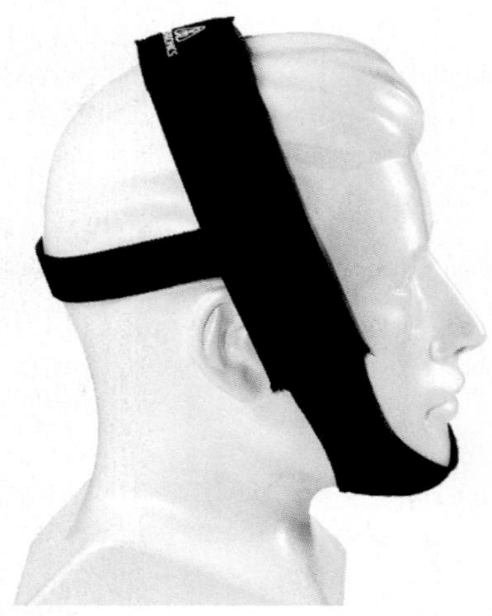

(B)

FIGURE 21-14 Chin straps used to prevent mouth leak.
(**A**) courtesy of SP Medical; (**B**) courtesy of Philips Respironics.

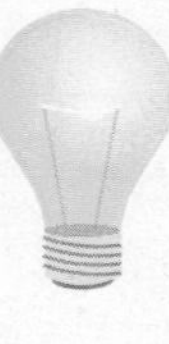

STOP AND THINK

A patient is admitted to the hospital for routine surgery. You are asked to see the patient because he is intolerant of CPAP, which has been prescribed for severe OSA. What strategies might you recommend to improve the patient's tolerance for this therapy?

Some patients find exhaling against the CPAP difficult, creating a feeling of discomfort and anxiety. Bilevel positive airway pressure systems are an alternative for individuals unable to tolerate CPAP therapy. With a bilevel device, the IPAP and EPAP are adjusted independently. The IPAP level is set at a point that eliminates the sleep-disordered breathing (apneas, hypopneas, snoring). The EPAP is set at a lower pressure to allow the patient to exhale against less resistance yet maintain airway splinting and patency. The use of bilevel therapy causes the mean airway pressure to be lower, which may increase comfort and tolerance.

The pressure required to prevent airway collapse varies in most patients from night to night and from

BOX 21-6

Recommendations for the Use of Auto-Positive Airway Pressure (APAP) from the Standards of Practice Committee of the American Academy of Sleep Medicine

Positive airway pressure (PAP) devices are not recommended to diagnose obstructive sleep apnea (OSA).

Patients with congestive heart failure; patients with significant lung disease, such as chronic obstructive pulmonary disease (COPD); patients expected to have nocturnal oxygen desaturation due to conditions other than OSA (e.g., obesity hypoventilation syndrome); patients who do not snore (either naturally or as a result of palate surgery); and patients who have central sleep apnea syndromes are not candidates for APAP titration or treatment.

APAP devices are not currently recommended for split-night titration.

Certain APAP devices may be used during attended titration with polysomnography to identify a single pressure for use with standard continuous positive airway pressure (CPAP) for treatment of moderate to severe OSA.

Certain APAP devices may be initiated and used in the self-adjusting mode for unattended treatment of patients with moderate to severe OSA without significant comorbidities (congestive heart failure [CHF], COPD, central sleep apnea syndromes, or hypoventilation syndromes).

Certain APAP devices may be used in an unattended way to determine a fixed CPAP treatment pressure for patients with moderate to severe OSA without significant comorbidities (CHF, COPD, central sleep apnea syndromes, or hypoventilation syndromes).

Patients being treated with fixed CPAP on the basis of APAP titration or being treated with APAP must have close clinical follow-up to determine treatment effectiveness and safety.

A reevaluation and, if necessary, a standard attended CPAP titration should be performed if symptoms do not resolve or the APAP treatment otherwise appears to lack efficacy.

Reproduced from Morgenthaler TI, Aurora RN, Brown T, et al. Practice parameters for the use of autotitrating continuous positive airway pressure devices for titrating pressures and treating adult patients with obstructive sleep apnea syndrome: an update for 2007. An American Academy of Sleep Medicine report. *Sleep*. 2008;31:141–147. Reprinted with permission of American Academy of Sleep Medicine; permission conveyed through Copyright Clearance Center, Inc.

hour to hour throughout any night because of changes in body position, level and stage of sleep, ingestion of alcohol or caffeine, and airway congestion. Several devices actively monitor one or more airway variables during sleep and respond to upper airway changes by automatically adjusting the pressure within a range of 4 to 20 cm H_2O.[40] These auto-titrating devices are called **auto-positive airway pressure (APAP)**. One or more of the following parameters are monitored: pharyngeal wall vibration (snoring), inspiratory flow limitation, hypopnea, and apnea. The APAP algorithms used by different manufacturers are proprietary and may vary greatly in their response to respiratory events. The system responds automatically when it senses an impending respiratory event by slowly increasing the pressure in a stepwise pattern until airway patency is reestablished. After a few minutes the pressure slowly decreases to the lowest pressure possible to maintain airway stability. APAP devices are potentially useful for patients who require different pressures in different sleep positions or sleep stages or for patients who have weight loss or return of daytime sleepiness and require assessment of their CPAP settings. These devices report useful information such as AHI and periodic breathing. Use of APAP devices is controversial, however, particularly if used in lieu of a formal sleep study, and guidelines for the appropriate use of these devices have been published (**Box 21-6**).[41]

Expiratory pressure relief (C-Flex), similar to the Bi-Flex mode, has been shown to be associated with similar outcomes to standard CPAP, but this feature improved adherence for those patients with low compliance.[42] This type of embellishment allows for a slight decrease in pressure at the beginning of exhalation. Although the feature is primarily designed to address the patient's comfort level and perception that exhalation against a positive pressure is difficult, the actual amount of pressure decrease varies from one manufacturer to another.

Negative Pressure Ventilation, Rocking Beds, and Pneumobelts

Negative pressure ventilation (body ventilators) provide intermittent subatmospheric pressure around the thorax and abdomen.[43,44] Typically the patient is partially enclosed in a chamber, with the ventilator providing negative pressure to the area between the chamber and the chest wall. This subatmospheric pressure

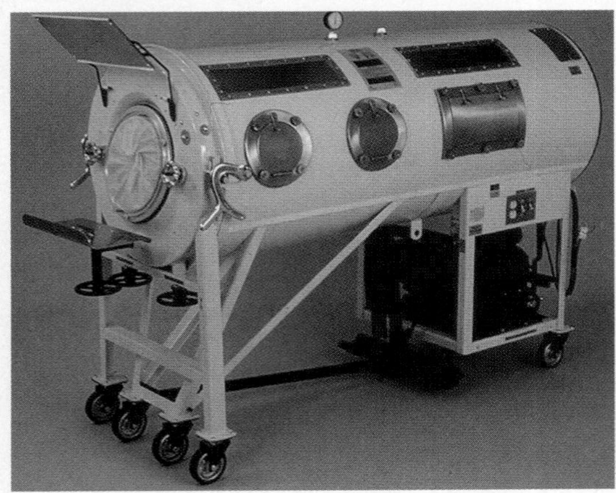

FIGURE 21-15 Iron lung.
Courtesy of Philips Respironics.

is transmitted to the pleural space, which promotes gas flow into the lungs. The prototype negative pressure ventilator was the **iron lung** (or tank ventilator), which was popular during the 1952 polio epidemic and remains in limited use today (**Figure 21-15**). The **cuirass** (also called the chest shell or turtle shell) consists of a lightweight rigid dome that fits over the anterior chest wall (**Figure 21-16**) and connects to a negative pressure generator. Other versions of negative pressure ventilators include wrap devices (ponchos, body suits, and pneumosuits) that fit over the patient, surround a semicylindrical grid, and attach to a negative pressure generator.

Given the increased popularity of NIV, negative pressure devices are no longer in common use. They do provide a treatment option for patients who cannot use NIV, however. Negative pressure devices are more complex and bulky than NIV devices. In addition, negative pressure devices can produce upper airway obstruction and thus are contraindicated in patients with obstructive sleep apnea. **Table 21-4** outlines selection criteria for body ventilators; **Table 21-5** lists typical settings.

An unconventional ventilation device is the **rocking bed** (**Figure 21-17**). The action of the rocking bed has been compared to a piston in a cylinder. As the patient's head moves down, the piston-like viscera and diaphragm slide cephalad within the cylinder-like chest

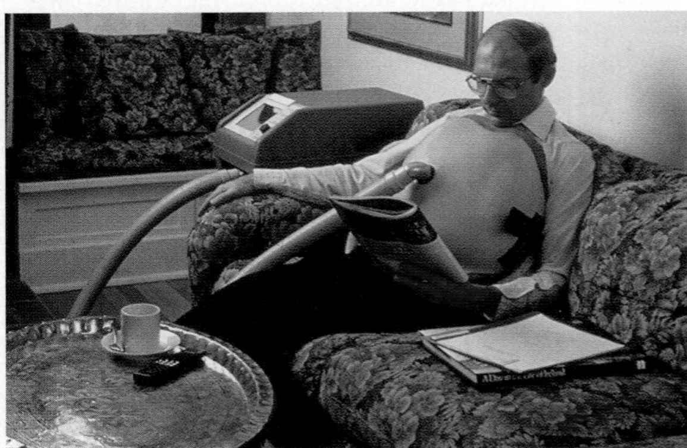

(A)

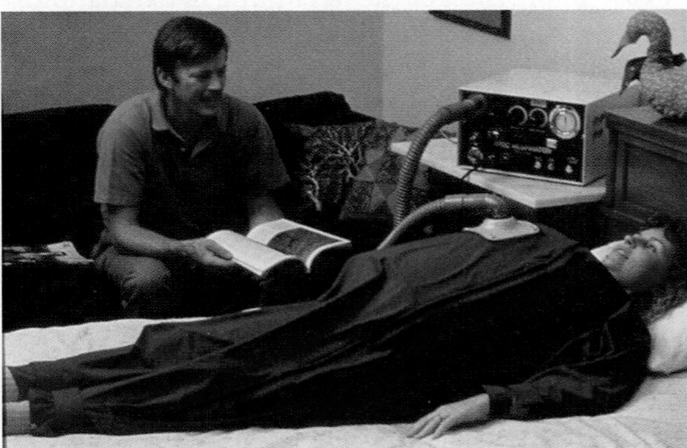

(B)

FIGURE 21-16 (**A**) Chest shells (cuirasses) to provide negative pressure ventilation. (**B**) Pneumosuit.
(**A**) and (**B**) courtesy of Philips Respironics.

TABLE 21-4
Selection Criteria for Body Ventilators

Considerations	Possible Solutions
Patient Preference	
Portability	Wrap, cuirass, pneumobelt
Convenience	Rocking bed, cuirass
Freedom of hands and face	Rocking bed, pneumobelt
Efficiency and reliability	Iron lung
Diagnosis	
Bilateral diaphragm paralysis	Rocking bed, pneumobelt
High spinal cord lesion	Pneumobelt
Obstructive sleep apnea	Noninvasive positive pressure ventilation
Body Habitus	
Marked kyphoscoliosis or obesity	Noninvasive positive pressure ventilation, iron lung

TABLE 21-5
Typical Settings for Body Ventilators

Ventilator	Rate (breaths/min)	Pressure (cm H_2O)
Iron lung	12 to 24	–10 to –35
Porta lung	12 to 24	–10 to –35
Wrap	14 to 28	–15 to –45
Shell	14 to 28	–15 to –45
Pneumobelt	12 to 24	+15 to +50
Rocking bed	12 to 24	40-degree tilt

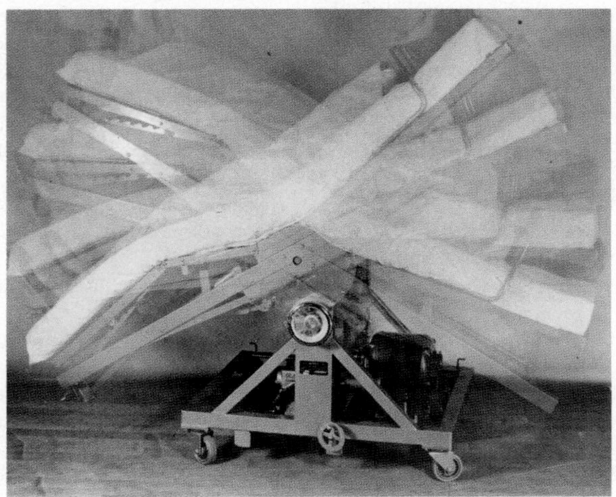

FIGURE 21-17 Rocking bed.
Courtesy of Division of Medicine and Science, National Museum of American History/Smithsonian Institution.

wall, assisting exhalation. In the foot-down position the abdominal contents and diaphragm slide caudad, assisting inhalation. Another unconventional ventilation device is the **pneumobelt** (**Figure 21-18**). It consists of an inflatable rubber bladder held over the abdomen by an adjustable corset and assists diaphragmatic motion by causing piston-like motions of the abdominal viscera.

Key Points

- Noninvasive ventilation (NIV) for acute respiratory failure has been demonstrated to decrease intubation rate, decrease pneumonia rate, and increase survival rates.
- Some patients—particularly those with neuromuscular disease—may benefit from chronic nocturnal NIV.

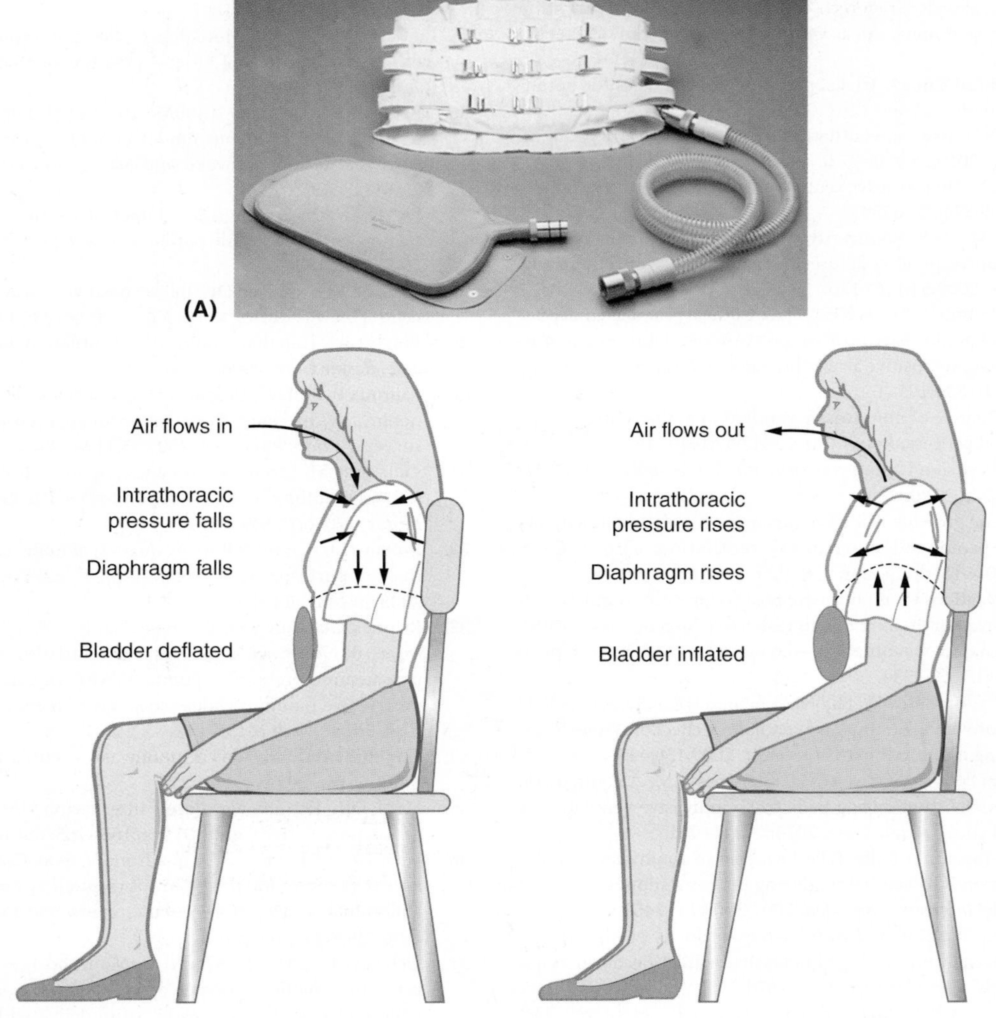

FIGURE 21-18 (**A**) Pneumobelt. (**B**) Mode of action of pneumobelt.
(**A**) courtesy of Philips Respironics; (**B**) adapted from Gilmartin ME. Body ventilators. Equipment and techniques. *Respir Care Clin North Am.* 1996;2:195–222.

- Nasal and oronasal interfaces are available for NIV.
- Any ventilator can be used to provide NIV, but bilevel ventilators are most commonly used.
- Clinician and patient preference determine the choice of interface, ventilator, and ventilator mode for NIV.
- Mask continuous positive airway pressure (CPAP) can be used in acute care applications to prevent postoperative pulmonary complications and to treat cardiogenic pulmonary edema.
- Mask CPAP is used to treat obstructive sleep apnea.
- CPAP compliance can be improved by use of an appropriate interface, by humidification of the gas flow, by use of the ramp function, by use of expiratory pressure relief, and by use of bilevel therapy.
- Auto-CPAP units vary pressure by monitoring changes in upper airway obstruction.
- Negative pressure devices are no longer in common use.

References

1. Nava S, Navalesi P, Gregoretti C. Interfaces and humidification for noninvasive mechanical ventilation. *Respir Care*. 2009;54:71–84.
2. Nava S. Behind a mask: tricks, pitfalls, and prejudices for noninvasive ventilation. *Respir Care*. 2013;58:1367–1376.
3. Hess DR. Noninvasive ventilation for acute respiratory failure. *Respir Care*. 2013;58:950–972.
4. Nava S, Hill N. Non-invasive ventilation in acute respiratory failure. *Lancet*. 2009;374:250–259.
5. Keenan SP, Mehta S. Noninvasive ventilation for patients presenting with acute respiratory failure: the randomized controlled trials. *Respir Care*. 2009;54:116–126.
6. Keenan SP, Sinuff T, Burns KEA, et al. Clinical practice guidelines for the use of noninvasive positive-pressure ventilation and noninvasive continuous positive airway pressure in the acute care setting. *CMAJ*. 2011;183:E195–E214.
7. Hess DR. The role of noninvasive ventilation in the ventilator discontinuation process. *Respir Care*. 2012;57:1619–1625.
8. Hill NS. Where should noninvasive ventilation be delivered? *Respir Care*. 2009;54:62–70.
9. Hess DR. The growing role of noninvasive ventilation in patients requiring prolonged mechanical ventilation. *Respir Care*. 2012;57:900–918, discussion 918–920.
10. Clinical indications for noninvasive positive pressure ventilation in chronic respiratory failure due to restrictive lung disease, COPD, and nocturnal hypoventilation—a consensus conference report. *Chest*. 1999;16:521–534.
11. Ferreira JC, Chipman DW, Hill NS, Kacmarek RM. Bilevel vs ICU ventilators providing noninvasive ventilation: effect of system leaks: a COPD lung model comparison. *Chest*. 2009;136:448–456.
12. Oto J, Chenelle CT, Marchese AD, Kacmarek RM. A comparison of leak compensation during pediatric noninvasive ventilation: a lung model study. *Respir Care*. 2014;59:241–251.
13. Vignaux L, Tassaux D, Jolliet P. Performance of noninvasive ventilation modes on ICU ventilators during pressure support: a bench model study. *Intensive Care Med*. 2007;33:1444–1451.
14. Carteaux G, Lyazidi A, Cordoba-Izquierdo A, et al. Patient-ventilator asynchrony during noninvasive ventilation: a bench and clinical study. *Chest*. 2012;142:367–376.
15. Schettino GP, Chatmongkolchart S, Hess DR, Kacmarek RM. Position of exhalation port and mask design affect CO_2 rebreathing during noninvasive positive pressure ventilation. *Crit Care Med*. 2003;31:2178–2182.
16. Saatci E, Miller DM, Stell IM, Lee KC, Moxham J. Dynamic dead space in face masks used with noninvasive ventilators: a lung model study. *Eur Respir J*. 2004;23:129–135.
17. Thys F, Liistro G, Dozin O, Marion E, Rodenstein DO. Determinants of F_{IO_2} with oxygen supplementation during noninvasive two-level positive pressure ventilation. *Eur Respir J*. 2002;19:653–657.
18. Schwartz AR, Kacmarek RM, Hess DR. Factors affecting oxygen delivery with bi-level positive airway pressure. *Respir Care*. 2004;49:270–275.
19. Hess DR. Noninvasive ventilation in neuromuscular disease: equipment and application. *Respir Care*. 2006;51:896–912.
20. Hess DR. Ventilator waveforms and the physiology of pressure support ventilation. *Respir Care*. 2005;50:166–186.
21. Prinianakis G, Delmastro M, Carlucci A, Ceriana P, Nava S. Effect of varying the pressurisation rate during noninvasive pressure support ventilation. *Eur Respir J*. 2004;23:314–320.
22. Williams P, Kratohvil J, Ritz R, et al. Pressure support and pressure assist/control: are there differences? An evaluation of the newest intensive care unit ventilators. *Respir Care*. 2000;45:1169–1181.
23. Hotchkiss JR Jr, Adams AB, Stone MK, et al. Oscillations and noise: inherent instability of pressure support ventilation? *Am J Respir Crit Care Med*. 2002;165:47–53.
24. Hotchkiss JR, Adams AB, Dries DJ, et al. Dynamic behavior during noninvasive ventilation: chaotic support? *Am J Respir Crit Care Med*. 2001;163:374–378.
25. Adams AB, Bliss PL, Hotchkiss J. Effects of respiratory impedance on the performance of bi-level pressure ventilators. *Respir Care*. 2000;45:390–400.
26. Parreira VF, Delguste P, Jounieaux V, et al. Effectiveness of controlled and spontaneous modes in nasal two-level positive pressure ventilation in awake and asleep normal subjects. *Chest*. 1997;112:1267–1277.
27. Parthasarathy S, Tobin MJ. Effect of ventilator mode on sleep quality in critically ill patients. *Am J Respir Crit Care Med*. 2002;166:1423–1429.
28. Johnson KG, Johnson DC. Bilevel positive airway pressure worsens central apneas during sleep. *Chest*. 2005;128:2141–2150.
29. Benditt JO. Full-time noninvasive ventilation: possible and desirable. *Respir Care*. 2006;51:1005–1012.
30. Fauroux B, Boffa C, Desguerre I, Estournet B, Trang H. Long-term noninvasive mechanical ventilation for children at home: a national survey. *Pediatr Pulmonol*. 2003;35:119–125.
31. Toussaint M, Steens M, Wasteels G, Soudon P. Diurnal ventilation via mouthpiece: survival in end-stage Duchenne patients. *Eur Respir J*. 2006;28:549–555.
32. Boitano LJ, Benditt JO. An evaluation of home volume ventilators that support open-circuit mouthpiece ventilation. *Respir Care*. 2005;50:1457–1461.
33. Briones Claudett KH, Briones Claudett M, Chung Sang Wong M, et al. Noninvasive mechanical ventilation with average volume assured pressure support (AVAPS) in patients with chronic obstructive pulmonary disease and hypercapnic encephalopathy. *BMC Pulm Med*. 2013;13:12.
34. Gay PC. Complications of noninvasive ventilation in acute care. *Respir Care*. 2009;54:246–258.
35. Hess DR. Patient-ventilator interaction during noninvasive ventilation. *Respir Care*. 2011;56:153–165; discussion 165–167.
36. Ferreyra GP, Baussano I, Squadrone V, et al. Continuous positive airway pressure for treatment of respiratory complications after abdominal surgery: a systematic review and meta-analysis. *Ann Surg*. 2008;247:617–626.
37. Delclaux C, L'Her E, Alberti C, Mancebo J, et al. Treatment of acute hypoxemic nonhypercapnic respiratory insufficiency with continuous positive airway pressure delivered by a face mask: a randomized controlled trial. *JAMA*. 2000;284:2352–2360.
38. Peter JV, Moran JL, Phillips-Hughes J, et al. Effect of non-invasive positive pressure ventilation (NIPPV) on mortality in patients with

acute cardiogenic pulmonary oedema: a meta-analysis. *Lancet*. 2006;367:1155–1163.

39. Allen KY, Bollig S, Selecky PA, Smalling T. *The Clinician's Guide to PAP Adherence*. American Association for Respiratory Care; 2009. Available at: http://www.aarc.org/education/pap_adherence.
40. Brown LK. Autotitrating CPAP. *Chest*. 2006;130;312–314.
41. Morgenthaler TI, Aurora RN, Brown T, et al. Practice parameters for the use of autotitrating continuous positive airway pressure devices for titrating pressures and treating adult patients with obstructive sleep apnea syndrome: an update for 2007. An American Academy of Sleep Medicine report. *Sleep*. 2008;31:141–147.
42. Pepin JL, Muir JF, Gentina T, et al. Pressure reduction during exhalation in sleep apnea patients treated by continuous positive airway pressure. *Chest*. 2009;136:490–497.
43. Hill NS. Use of negative pressure ventilation, rocking beds, and pneumobelts. *Respir Care*. 1994;39:532–549.
44. Hill NS. Clinical applications of body ventilators. *Chest*. 1986;90:897–905.

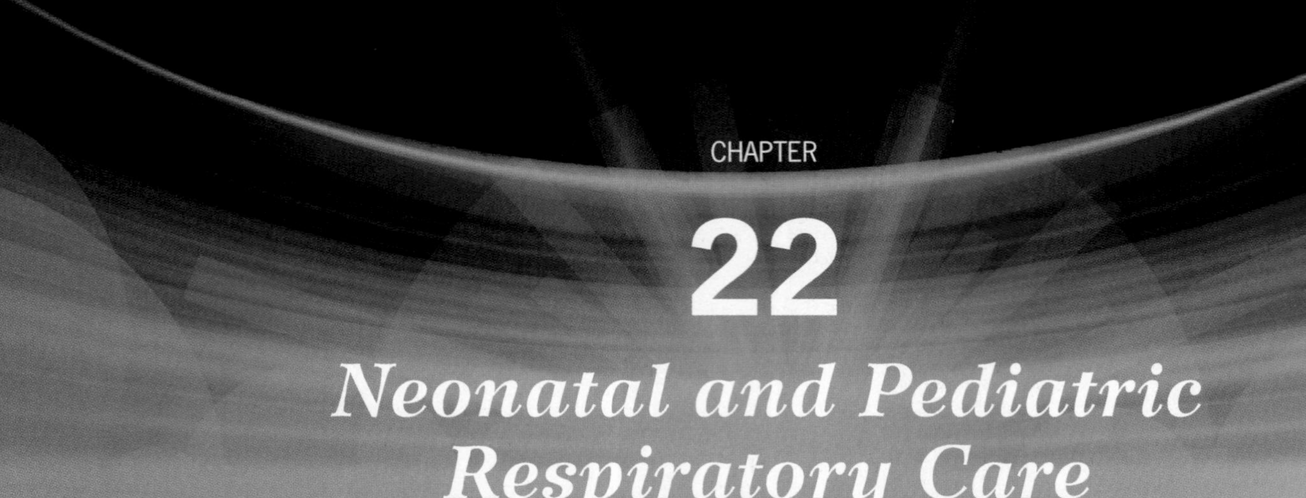

CHAPTER

22

Neonatal and Pediatric Respiratory Care

Melissa K. Brown

OUTLINE

OBJECTIVES

1. Identify and describe some of the risk factors for developing respiratory distress syndrome.
2. List the five components of the Apgar score.
3. Identify and describe the signs of respiratory distress in the neonate.
4. Describe the hazards associated with oxygen use in premature infants.
5. Describe oxygen administration techniques for infants and children.
6. Compare the use of flow-inflating and self-inflating manual ventilation devices.
7. Describe the proper position for oral endotracheal tubes in neonates and children.
8. Describe the use of nasal continuous positive airway pressure in neonates.
9. Discuss issues related to artificial airway care of neonates and children.
10. List indications for mechanical ventilation of neonates and children.
11. List the usual settings for conventional mechanical ventilation of neonates and children.
12. List the hazards and complications of conventional neonatal and pediatric mechanical ventilation.
13. Discuss approaches to weaning neonates and children from mechanical ventilation.
14. Compare the four general types of high-frequency ventilation of neonates and children.
15. Discuss issues related to surfactant administration in neonates and children.

KEY TERMS

Apgar score
bronchopulmonary dysplasia (BPD)
flow-inflating bag
hertz (Hz)
high-frequency flow interrupter ventilation (HFFIV)
high-frequency jet ventilation (HFJV)
high-frequency oscillatory ventilation (HFOV)
high-frequency positive pressure ventilation (HFPPV)
high-frequency ventilation (HFV)
lecithin-to-sphingomyelin (LS) ratio
mean airway pressure
nasal continuous positive airway pressure (NCPAP)
neutral thermal environment
noninvasive ventilation (NIV)
pressure amplitude
primary apnea
retinopathy of prematurity (ROP)
secondary apnea
self-inflating bag
surfactant
transillumination

Introduction

Neonates and children may require respiratory therapy for a variety of reasons. Regardless of the pathologic condition, the goal is to achieve adequate gas exchange while minimizing risks and complications. Many factors influence the respiratory management of neonates and children, and no single approach is ideal for all patients. Maintaining adequate support of ventilation and oxygenation by continual reassessment is essential to prevent complications.

Neonatal Assessment

Awareness and understanding of maternal risk factors are crucial for the identification of newborns at risk for life-threatening complications in the perinatal period (**Box 22-1**). Clinicians must be prepared to resuscitate infants with serious problems at birth or soon after. One of the most common problems other than congenital birth defects is preterm birth (prior to 38 weeks' gestation). Infants born prematurely are at risk of developing respiratory distress syndrome (RDS).

Laboratory tests have been developed to assist with the assessment of lung maturity. By assessing the amniotic fluid for the **lecithin-to-sphingomyelin (LS) ratio**, lung maturity can be determined. Lecithin (dipalmitoyl phosphatidylcholine) is the most plentiful phospholipid found in surfactant. Generally, babies with an LS ratio of more than 2:1 are considered to have mature lungs. Usually, the LS ratio will approach 2:1 at approximately 34 to 35 weeks' gestation. Babies with ratios of less than 2:1 are considered at higher risk for developing RDS. Infants of diabetic mothers may develop RDS even with LS ratios greater than 2:1. Phosphatidylglycerol (PG) is the second most plentiful phospholipid in surfactant. PG increases closer to term. When PG is present in the amniotic fluid, the infant is less likely to develop RDS.

The maternal history and laboratory test results may prepare the clinician for what to expect in the delivery room, but once the baby is born a thorough assessment must be done. The American Academy of Pediatrics Neonatal Resuscitation Program (NRP) outlines a specific sequence of events.[1] If the newborn is term gestation, breathing or crying, and displaying good muscle tone, then the infant should remain with the mother and be kept warm with ongoing observation. If the newborn does not display one of the above assessments, then the steps of stabilization should be initiated. The infant is dried and warmed, and the airway is opened and cleared of secretions.

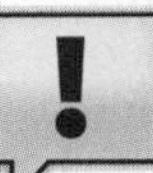

Respiratory Recap

Neonatal Assessment

- Infants with LS ratios of less than 2:1 are considered at higher risk for RDS.
- The Apgar score evaluates heart rate, respiratory effort, muscle tone, reflex irritability, and color.
- Apnea is a cessation of breathing for longer than 20 seconds.
- Signs of respiratory distress include expiratory grunting, retracting, nasal flaring, and tachypnea.
- Capillary blood gas values are minimally invasive measures of pH and Pco_2.

BOX 22-1

Maternal Risk Factors for Perinatal Complications

Preterm birth
Postterm birth
Multiple birth
Maternal tobacco, alcohol, or drug abuse
Hypertension
Polyhydramnios (too much amniotic fluid volume)
Oligohydramnios (too little amniotic fluid volume)
Diabetes mellitus
Infectious diseases
Premature rupture of the membranes
Placenta and umbilical cord abnormalities
Breech or cesarean delivery

The baby should respond to stimulation with adequate depth and rate of respirations. Infants with absent or ineffective ventilations should immediately receive positive pressure ventilation and oxygen saturation monitoring (Spo_2). After evaluation of respirations, the heart rate is assessed by either feeling the infant's pulse by holding the base of the umbilical cord or by listening with a stethoscope to the apical pulse. If the newborn has adequate respirations and a heart rate of at least 100 beats/min, the newborn's color should be assessed. Many newborns have acrocyanosis (blue extremities) in the first few minutes of life as a result of poor circulation. If central cyanosis persists or labored breathing is present with adequate ventilation and a heart rate greater than 100 beats/min, then Spo_2 monitoring and continuous positive airway pressure (CPAP) is indicated.

Apgar Score

The **Apgar score**, introduced in 1952 by Virginia Apgar, evaluates five factors: heart rate, respiratory effort, muscle tone, reflex irritability, and color (**Table 22-1**). The score is assigned at 1, 5, and 10 minutes of life. Therapeutic interventions should not be delayed in order to assign the 1-minute score. The 1-minute score is intended to provide an immediate evaluation of the infant and guide appropriate intervention. When the score is less than 7 at 5 minutes, an additional score is usually assigned at 10 minutes. If the Apgar score remains 0 after 10 minutes of resuscitation, it is unlikely the infant will survive.[2]

The Apgar score is not as useful for babies born prematurely. Three of the assessment criteria—muscle tone, respiratory effort, and reflex irritability—are related to the neonate's developmental maturity. Muscle tone may be absent and respiratory effort may be poor in neonates of less than 28 weeks' gestation.

TABLE 22-1
Apgar Scoring

Parameter	Points		
	0	1	2
Heart rate	None	<100 beats/min	>100 beats/min
Respiratory effort	None	Weak, irregular	Strong cry
Color	Pale blue	Body pink, extremities blue	Completely pink
Reflex (irritability to suction)	No response	Grimace	Cry, cough, or sneeze
Muscle tone	Limp	Some flexion	Well flexed

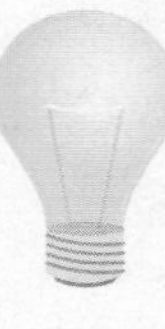

STOP AND THINK

At one minute after birth a neonate is limp, apneic, and has a heart rate of 85 beats/min. He is completely cyanotic and shows no response to suctioning. What Apgar score would you assign and what would be your next response?

Gestational Age

Gestational age should be assessed by the time the infant is 12 hours old. Gestational age is assessed using several factors: the mother's last menstrual cycle, prenatal ultrasound findings, and postnatal physical and neurologic findings, which are included in the Ballard score (**Figure 22-1**). After gestational age assessment, the newborn's weight, length, and head circumference are plotted on a grid. An infant whose weight is below the 10th percentile is considered small for gestational age (SGA); an infant above the 90th percentile is considered large for gestational age (LGA). Infants born weighing less than 2500 grams are considered low birth weight (LBW), those less than 1500 grams are very low birth weight (VLBW), and those less than 1000 grams are extremely low birth weight (ELBW). Neonates who fall into one of these categories are more likely to be at risk for morbidity and mortality.

Physical Assessment

The normal infant heart rate is 120 to 160 beats/min. A stressed infant from overstimulation or pain may temporarily have a heart rate greater than 200 beats/min. During deep sleep, the infant heart rate may drop to 80 to 90 beats/min. Right-to-left shunting from a patent ductus arteriosis (PDA) can result in bounding peripheral pulses. **Table 22-2** lists normal ranges for neonatal vital signs.

All newborns have an irregular respiratory breathing pattern, but the respiratory rate of a term newborn usually averages 40 to 60 breaths/min. It is common for premature infants to have periodic breathing, which consists of intermittent respiratory pauses that last longer than 5 seconds. When breathing stops for longer than 20 seconds, or for shorter periods in combination with bradycardia, cyanosis, or pallor, it is called *apnea*. Stressed newborns will often have a period of rapid breathing followed by a period of gasping or no breathing called **primary apnea**. While in primary apnea, tactile stimulation of the infant will cause breathing to resume. If the infant continues in this pattern without interruption, however, an irregular breathing pattern will follow the primary apnea and the patient will enter into **secondary apnea**. For the patient in secondary apnea, positive pressure ventilation is required to restore spontaneous ventilation. As children mature, their normal respiratory rates decline until they become teenagers, at which point their respiratory rates mimic those of adults (**Table 22-3**).[3]

The Silverman scoring system assesses the magnitude of the respiratory distress of the infant (**Figure 22-2**). Signs of respiratory distress include expiratory grunting, retracting, nasal flaring, and tachypnea. Expiratory grunting is caused by the closing of the glottis during expiration in an attempt to maintain lung volume and expand alveoli. It is a common sign of RDS. Retractions are a visible sinking in of the chest wall on inspiration. Retractions are usually a sign of decreased chest compliance but can also be a sign of airway obstruction. They are usually observed between the ribs (intercostal), in the area above the clavicle (superclavicular), below the xiphoid process (substernal), and below the ribcage (subcostal). Retractions are more commonly observed in neonates than in adults due to the soft, pliable chest wall and thoracic cage of the neonate. Seesaw respirations, also indicative of severe respiratory distress, occur when the chest moves in and the abdomen pushes out on inspiration. Infants may have nasal flaring to decrease the resistance to air entry. Tachypnea is usually one of the first signs of respiratory distress. Infants and children have difficulty increasing their tidal volume and instead will increase

Neuromuscular Maturity

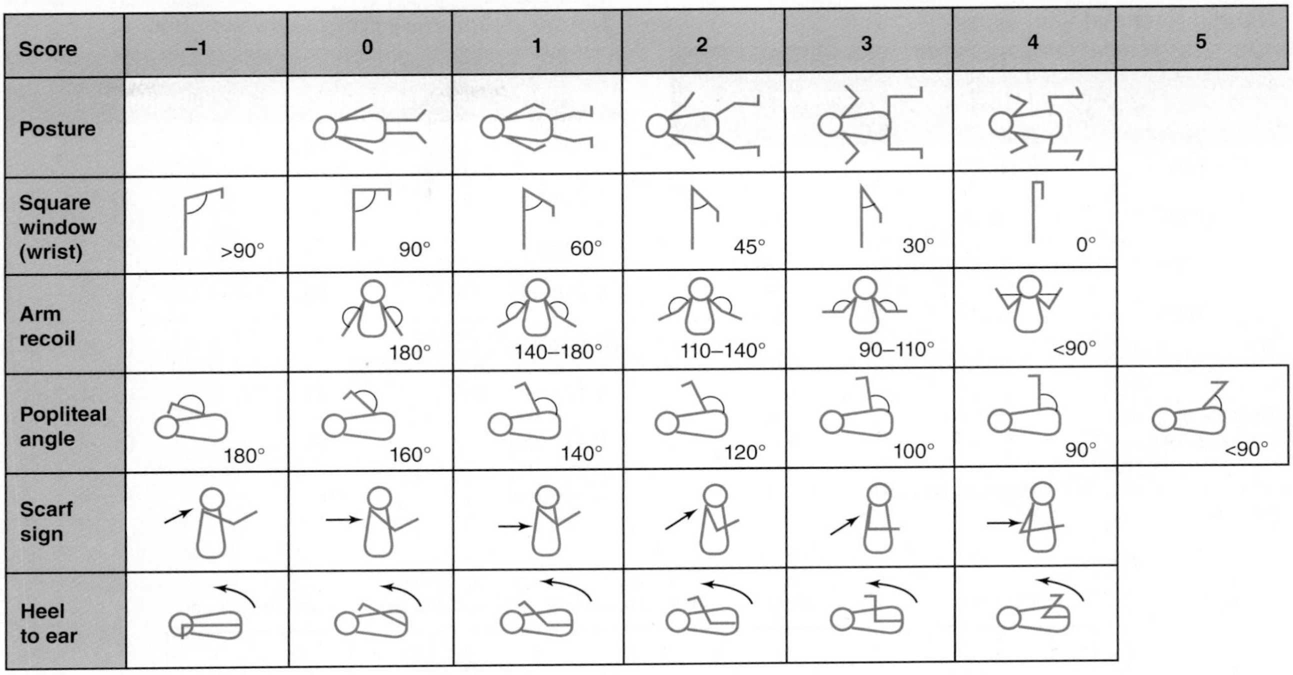

Score	–1	0	1	2	3	4	5
Posture							
Square window (wrist)	>90°	90°	60°	45°	30°	0°	
Arm recoil		180°	140–180°	110–140°	90–110°	<90°	
Popliteal angle	180°	160°	140°	120°	100°	90°	<90°
Scarf sign							
Heel to ear							

Physical Maturity

Skin	Sticky, friable, transparent	Gelatinous, red, translucent	Smooth, pink; visible veins	Superficial peeling and/or rash; few veins	Cracking, pale areas; rare veins	Parchment, deep cracking; no vessels	Leathery, cracked, wrinkled
Lanugo	None	Sparse	Abundant	Thinning	Bald areas	Mostly bald	
Plantar surface	Heel-toe 40–50 mm: –1 <40 mm: –2	>50 mm, no crease	Faint red marks	Anterior transverse crease only	Creases anterior 2/3	Creases over entire sole	
Breast	Imperceptible	Barely perceptible	Flat areola, no bud	Stippled areola, 1–2 mm bud	Raised areola, 3–4 mm bud	Full areola, 5–10 mm bud	
Eye/Ear	Lids fused loosely: –1 tightly: –2	Lids open; pinna flat; stays folded	Slightly curved pinna, soft slow recoil	Well curved pinna, soft but ready recoil	Formed and firm, instant recoil	Thick cartilage, ear stiff	
Genitals (male)	Scrotum flat, smooth	Scrotum empty, faint rugae	Testes in upper canal, rare rugae	Testes descending, few rugae	Testes down, good rugae	Testes pendulous, deep rugae	
Genitals (female)	Clitoris prominent, labia flat	Clitoris prominent, small labia minora	Clitoris prominent, enlarging minora	Majora and minora equally prominent	Majora large, minora small	Majora cover clitoris and minora	

Maturity Rating

Score	Weeks
–10	20
–5	22
0	24
5	26
10	28
15	30
20	32
25	34
30	36
35	38
40	40
45	42
50	44

FIGURE 22-1 New Ballard score for estimating gestational age to include extremely premature infants.

Reproduced from Ballard JL. New Ballard score, expanded to include extremely premature infants. *J Pediatr.* 1991;119:417–423, with permission from Elsevier.

TABLE 22-2
Normal Neonatal Vital Signs

Birth Weight (g)	Systolic/Diastolic Blood Pressure (mm Hg)	Mean Blood Pressure (mm Hg)
>600	42/20	25
>1000	48/25	35
>2000	50/30	40
>3000	50/35	45
>4000	65/40	50
Neonate older than 12 hours	75/50	60

Normal respiratory rate: 30–60 breaths/min; normal heart rate: 120–160 beats/min.

TABLE 22-3
Normal Respiratory Rates in Awake Children

Age	Mean (breaths/min)	Range (breaths/min)
6–12 months	64	58–75
1–2 years	35	30–40
2–4 years	31	23–42
4–6 years	26	19–36
6–8 years	23	15–30
8–10 years	21	15–31
10–12 years	21	15–28
12–14 years	22	18–26

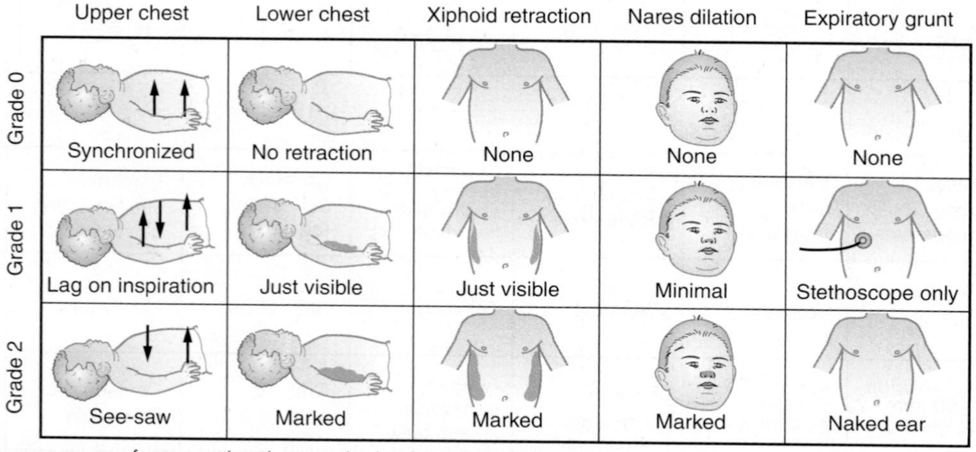

FIGURE 22-2 Silverman score for assessing the magnitude of respiratory distress.

their respiratory rate in order to increase their minute ventilation.

Auscultation of infants and small children can be difficult. Their chests are small, and sounds sometimes transmit from one lung region to another. Infants and children often cry and hold their breath during examination, making assessment difficult. Symmetric assessment from left to right is crucial and will help identify asymmetric disease such as a pneumothorax or a poorly positioned endotracheal tube. Rhonchi are coarse breath sounds that come from air moving through fluid in the large airways. Usually, suctioning will eliminate the secretions and the rhonchi. Crackles, also known as rales, are indicative of fluid in the small airways and alveoli and are commonly heard on inspiration in infants with RDS, pneumonia, or pulmonary edema and in normal infants soon after birth. Wheezes are high-pitched musical sounds that can be heard on inspiration or expiration and are caused by a narrowing of the conducting airways. Wheezes are most commonly heard in children with asthma. Wheezing over an isolated area can indicate foreign body aspiration. Stridor is a high-pitched squeaking sound heard on inspiration. Stridor indicates a large upper airway obstruction as can occur in patients with croup, tracheomalacia, and postextubation laryngeal edema. Stridor can be easily distinguished from other sounds by placing the stethoscope over the neck region and isolating the sound. Neonates with RDS, atelectasis, and pulmonary interstitial edema (PIE) may also have diminished breath sounds. In the neonate, **transillumination** of the chest wall can be used to identify a suspected pneumothorax. A fiberoptic light source is placed on the chest wall in a darkened room. A large pneumothorax will glow, or seem very pink and illuminated, in comparison with the other areas of the chest.

Noninvasive and Hemodynamic Monitoring

In addition to physical assessment, chest radiography and blood gas measurements are vital in the respiratory assessment of the patient. Noninvasive monitoring of oxygenation and ventilation is widely used in the care of infants and children. Spo_2 and transcutaneous monitoring ($Ptco_2$ and $Ptcco_2$) are used to closely track the oxygenation and ventilation status of patients and are correlated with blood gas values when appropriate. Poor tissue perfusion interferes with the accuracy of noninvasive monitoring. Patient movement can make the reliable measurement of pulse oximetry challenging in neonates and pediatrics.

Blood gas samples can be obtained from umbilical artery catheters (UACs) or umbilical venous catheters (UVCs) in neonates and from peripheral arterial lines in older children. Capillary blood gases are a less invasive way to measure the pH and Pco_2 of an infant, but are not always reliable in determining oxygenation. Poor sampling technique can greatly influence the results of capillary blood gases. Umbilical cord blood gases are often drawn after the birth of the child to document whether the infant was in severe distress in utero. The cord blood gas values are not used to treat the infant after birth. Blood gas results should be interpreted in the context of the gestational age, the disease state of the patient, and the risk for complications with additional respiratory support. For the newborn, time may be necessary to transition to extrauterine life. **Table 22-4** provides normal blood gas values.

UACs and arterial lines are used for blood pressure monitoring. The UVC or central venous catheter is primarily used for the administration of fluids and drugs to the central circulation and for central venous pressure (CVP) monitoring. CVP monitoring allows measurement of the right atrial pressure and assessment of the patient's fluid volume. Normal CVP is 2 to 7 mm Hg. Pulmonary artery catheters are used to assess left ventricular function, fluid status, and pulmonary artery pressure (PAP). Normal mean PAP is 10 to 20 mm Hg.

Oxygen Therapy

Indications

The goal of oxygen therapy is to prevent or correct hypoxemia and to provide oxygen to the tissues with the lowest possible concentration of oxygen. Preterm babies, term babies, and children have different oxygen requirements depending on their gestational age or disease state. Children and term infants with a Pao_2 below 80 mm Hg and an oxygen saturation of less than 95% are generally considered to have hypoxemia. In preterm infants, Pao_2 and oxygen saturation goals are lower than those for term babies and are based on corrected gestational age.

Hazards

The hazards of oxygen therapy for the preterm infant include **retinopathy of prematurity (ROP)**. ROP is a potentially blinding disease caused by the abnormal development of the retina in premature infants. Generally, babies born weighing less than 1500 grams or at less than 32 weeks' gestational ages are monitored for ROP. Oxygen therapy directed toward Pao_2 goals of 50 to 80 mm Hg is usually considered safe.[4] Other factors that contribute to the severity of ROP include gestational age, low birth weight, blood transfusion, respiratory distress, PDA, and the overall health of the infant. Excessive use of oxygen also can lead to the development of **bronchopulmonary dysplasia (BPD)**, which is generally defined as the need for supplemental oxygen at 36 weeks' postmenstrual age or 28 days of life.[5]

The delivery of 100% oxygen can lead to absorption atelectasis as alveolar nitrogen is replaced by oxygen. There also can be cardiovascular effects from the delivery of high concentrations of oxygen, such as pulmonary vasodilation and the constriction of the ductus arteriosus. In patients with hypoplastic left heart disease, the increase in pulmonary blood flow that occurs with oxygen therapy can flood the lungs with blood and decrease systemic circulation. The closing of the PDA can further decrease the flow of blood to the systemic circulation and create a life-threatening situation.

TABLE 22-4
Normal Cord, Neonatal, and Pediatric Blood Gas Values

Parameter	Umbilical Artery	Umbilical Vein	Newborn	Infant to Toddler	Child to Adult
pH	7.24	7.32	7.3–7.4	7.3–7.4	7.35–7.45
Pco_2 (mm Hg)	49	38	30–40	30–40	35–45
Po_2 (mm Hg)	16	27	60–90	80–100	80–100
HCO_3^- (mmol/L)	19	20	20–22	20–22	22–24

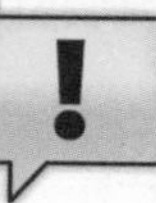

Respiratory Recap

Oxygen Therapy

- Oxygen therapy directed toward Pa_{O_2} goals of 50 to 80 mm Hg is usually considered safe.
- Excessive oxygen use could lead to retinopathy of prematurity and bronchopulmonary dysplasia in the premature infant.
- F_{IO_2} should be adjusted to meet oximetry goals for the patient based on gestational age.

Delivery Devices

Supplemental oxygen can be delivered using many different devices. The best device to use is the one that most closely suits the needs of the individual patient. The clinician should contemplate several factors before choosing an oxygen delivery device, including what fraction of inspired oxygen (F_{IO_2}) is required, whether a precise F_{IO_2} is required, what gas temperature and humidity is needed, how the equipment will affect the nursing care and handling of the infant or child, and what will make the patient the most comfortable. Oxygen therapy should be administered according to the Sp_{O_2} goal. If the patient consistently requires more than 50% oxygen, additional respiratory support may be indicated.

In the neonatal intensive care unit (NICU), low-flow meters with flows that span 25 mL/min to 3 L/min are commonly used. In most cases, these flow meters should be connected to a 100% oxygen source and flows titrated to meet oximetry goals. On neonatal patients requiring high flows, such as 2 L/min, an air–oxygen blender should be used and the F_{IO_2} adjusted to meet the Sp_{O_2} goal for the patient. The most frequently used oxygen delivery devices include the conventional nasal cannula, high-flow nasal cannula, entrainment mask, oxygen hood, and incubator; each of which has advantages and disadvantages (**Table 22-5**).

Mechanical Ventilation

Regardless of the pathologic condition, the goal is to achieve adequate gas exchange while minimizing the risks and complications associated with mechanical ventilation. Many factors influence the respiratory management of neonates and children, and no single approach is ideal for all. Maintaining adequate support of ventilation and oxygenation by reassessment of the patient and adjustment of the ventilator is essential to prevent complications. Mechanical ventilation in the intensive care environment is an art form. It is practiced differently throughout the world, and the method chosen depends on the strategies adopted by the institution.

Manual Ventilation

Positive pressure ventilation (PPV) usually begins as manual bag-mask ventilation (BMV), often in the delivery room. Immediately after birth, the infant is placed under a warmer and dried, positioned, and provided with tactile stimulation. BMV is indicated if the infant is apneic or gasping or has a heart rate below 100 beats/min. Appropriate use of positive pressure can make a significant difference in the infant's course. During the initial resuscitation, administration of oxygen should be titrated to specific preductal Sp_{O_2} goals based on the

TABLE 22-5
Supplemental Oxygen Delivery Devices

Device	Patient Age	Oxygen Delivered	Advantages	Disadvantages
Nasal cannula	Premature infant to pediatric	Flows of 25 mL/min to ≤2 L/min	Comfortable, good access to patient, easy to apply	F_{IO_2} not precise
High-flow nasal cannula	Premature infant to pediatric	≥2 L/min	Comfortable, good access to patient, easy to apply	F_{IO_2} not precise, possible inadvertent PEEP, low relative humidity unless heated and humidified
Air entrainment mask	Children	Up to 100%	High F_{IO_2}, precise F_{IO_2}	Confining, uncomfortable, low relative humidity
Oxygen hoods (tot huts, care cubes)	Premature infants to 6 months	21% to 100%	Precise F_{IO_2}, heated and humidified	Poor access to patient, excessive noise, must maintain flow to wash out CO_2, gas layering
Incubators	Neonates	21% to 40%	Neutral thermal environment	Poor access to patient, difficult to maintain precise F_{IO_2}

TABLE 22-6
Targeted Preductal Spo_2 After Birth

1 min	60%–65%
2 min	65%–70%
3 min	70%–75%
4 min	75%–80%
5 min	80%–85%
10 min	85%–95%

Reproduced from 2010 American Heart Association Guidelines for Cardiopulmonary Resuscitation and Emergency Cardiovascular Care. Part 15: Neonatal Resuscitation. 2010;122:S909–S919. © 2010 American Heart Association, Inc. and American Academy of Pediatrics. Reproduced with permission.

newborn's minutes of life (see **Table 22-6**). Pure (100%) oxygen administration was recommended in the past, but current evidence suggests that exposure to excess oxygen is harmful.[1] Once pulse oximetry is initiated, both the high and low Spo_2 alarms should be set to reduce the risks of hyperoxia and hypoxia.

Manual resuscitators are classified as self-inflating or flow-inflating (**Figure 22-3**).[6] A **self-inflating bag** inflates automatically and does not need an external gas source to provide positive pressure. These bags usually have a reservoir to deliver 100% oxygen with a flow of 5 to 10 L/min. Most self-inflating bags incorporate a pressure-limiting device and a pop-off valve that releases pressure at a preset level. The pop-off valve reduces the risk of excessive pressure being applied, but it can be manually overridden when delivery of high pressures

Respiratory Recap

Neonatal Manual Resuscitators

- Self-inflating bags inflate automatically.
- Flow-inflating bags require a continuous gas flow.

is indicated. Self-inflating bags generally do not allow maintenance of positive end-expiratory pressure (PEEP) unless an external PEEP valve is added.

A **flow-inflating bag** requires a continuous flow from an external gas source. The flow and the pressure release valve determine pressure. Wide ranges of peak inspiratory pressure (PIP) and PEEP are attainable with flow-inflating bags. Continuous flow at the patient connection makes the device suitable for the delivery of continuous positive airway pressure (CPAP) and a convenient method to deliver oxygen short term to spontaneously breathing infants. Flow-inflating bags are well suited to the needs of neonates. Clinicians responsible for resuscitating neonates should be familiar with self-inflating and flow-inflating bags and with the specific characteristics of the bags used in their institution.

BMV is ineffective if the mask is not the correct size. A variety of masks are available that fit infants of all sizes. The mask should fit over the infant's nose and mouth, with the edge of the infant's chin resting on the rim of the mask. As the mask is applied to the face, a seal is created by encircling the mask with the thumb and index finger and applying a gentle pressure (**Figure 22-4**). The infant's face should be pulled into the mask to open the airway. The ring finger can be used to hold the chin in the mask. Positioning of the infant is critical to achieve effective BMV; slight extension of the neck, often accomplished by placement of a blanket roll under the shoulders, aligns the airway to allow effective ventilation.

Knowledge of the infant's gestational age and prenatal history may be helpful during initiation of BMV. Premature infants are likely to need higher ventilating pressures (more than 35 cm H_2O) during the initial breaths to overcome the surface tension in surfactant-deficient lungs. Depending on lung

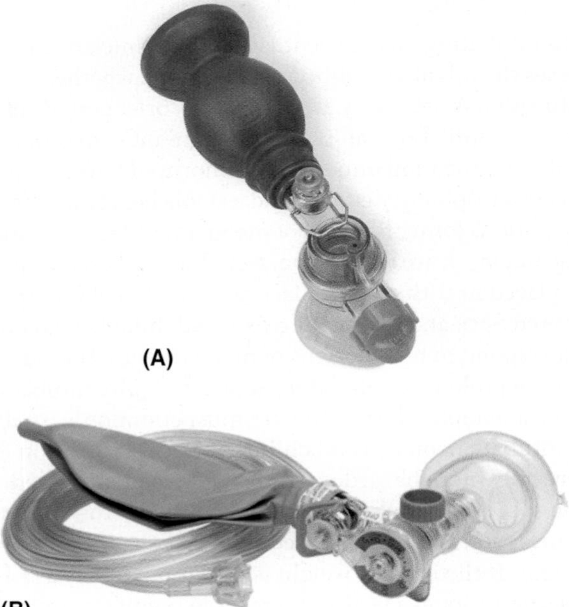

FIGURE 22-3 (**A**) Self-inflating neonatal resuscitation bag. (**B**) Flow-inflating neonatal resuscitation bag.
Courtesy of Mercury Medical.

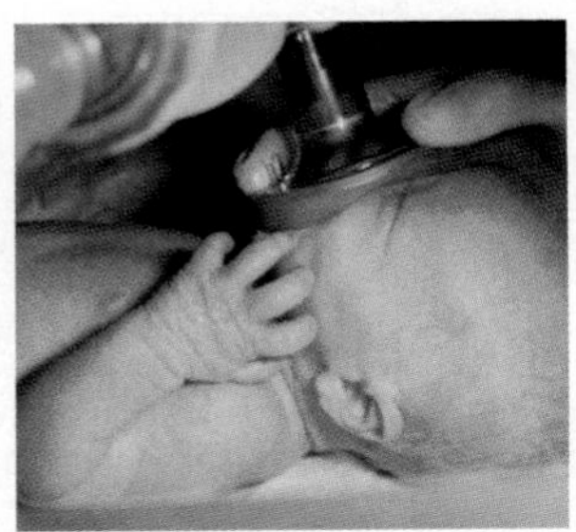

FIGURE 22-4 Positioning of the mask for bag-mask ventilation.
Courtesy of David J. Burchfield, MD.

maturity, successive breaths may require less pressure as lung volume is established. The pressure used to ventilate should be that needed to cause the infant's chest to rise. Maintaining PEEP throughout the respiratory cycle aids in the maintenance of lung volume. Observing chest movement while the bag is being squeezed is essential for correct application of pressure. Common reasons for poor chest movement are an inadequate mask seal, airway obstruction caused by improper head position, secretions in the airway, fingers on the patient's neck, or inadequate ventilating pressure. Inadequate pressure leads to low lung volume, inability to oxygenate, and hemodynamic compromise. Excessive pressure can result in pneumothorax and further respiratory and hemodynamic compromise. An in-line pressure manometer should be used to monitor the applied peak airway pressure and PEEP levels. A disposable carbon dioxide detector can be placed between the resuscitation bag and mask to verify the presence of exhaled carbon dioxide. **Table 22-7** lists factors to consider with BMV.

An apneic or distressed infant typically requires a respiratory rate of 40 to 60 breaths/min with an inspiratory time of 0.4 to 0.5 second. Administration of oxygen during the initial resuscitative effort should be titrated to Spo_2. Improvement in the skin color, heart rate, and hemodynamics should be apparent after a brief period. If the patient shows no sign of improvement, the adequacy of the delivery system should be reviewed. Oxygen disconnection or inadequacy of the gas source, mask seal, or head position should be considered.

Infants with evidence of meconium on the skin or in the airway, and who are not vigorous at birth, should have the mouth and trachea suctioned before positive pressure ventilation. A vigorous infant is one that has a heart rate above 100 beats/min, strong respiratory efforts, and good muscle tone. A 12 F or 14 F suction catheter should be used to clear the mouth and posterior pharynx of meconium so that the cords may be visualized. Intubation with the largest possible endotracheal tube is recommended to facilitate the removal of meconium from the airway. Clearing of meconium in the airway is attempted with a meconium aspirator. The aspirator is attached to the endotracheal tube, suction is applied at 100 mm Hg, and the endotracheal tube is withdrawn. Reintubation is performed with a new tube, and the process is repeated until no particulate meconium is present or the baby's heart rate indicates that resuscitation is required. After the meconium has been cleared, positive pressure ventilation can be provided by BMV or through an endotracheal tube. Insertion of a gastric tube to clear meconium from the stomach may reduce the risk of further meconium aspiration.

Mask positive pressure ventilation is contraindicated in infants who have or are suspected of having a congenital diaphragmatic hernia. BMV can promote the entry of air into the gastrointestinal tract and further impair gas exchange. These infants should be intubated and ventilated through an endotracheal tube.

TABLE 22-7
Bag-Mask Ventilation of the Neonate

Problem	Solutions
No seal between mask and face	Reposition mask; consider different mask size.
No chest movement	Check head position; do not overextend neck or push head forward with mask pressure.
	Check for secretions in airway.
	Check for fingers on the neck.
Pressure too low (flow-inflating bag)	Check flow; adjust flow meter; check manometer connections.
Pressure too low (self-inflating bag)	Ensure pop-off valve is active; consider need to override the valve.

Airway Management

Oral and nasal airways can be used to assist with maintaining an open airway. Oral airways are generally used only in unconscious patients who do not have a gag reflex. The clinician must select an oral airway large enough to keep the tongue from obstructing the pharynx but not so large that the tube itself is an airway obstruction. Nasal airways are generally better tolerated and can be used in awake patients, but they can become occluded with secretions or cause nasal trauma with insertion or removal.

Endotracheal Intubation

After initiating manual ventilation, the clinician reassesses the infant's condition to determine whether intubation is necessary. In some cases, brief periods of manual ventilation can stabilize the infant's condition, making intubation unnecessary. Improved Spo_2, spontaneous respiratory efforts, and a stable heart rate are indications for withdrawal of manual ventilation. As the bag and mask are withdrawn, free-flowing oxygen can be placed near the infant's face as needed to obtain the desired Spo_2 and the infant reassessed. Infants who do not respond to brief periods of manual ventilation or who require prolonged ventilatory support require intubation.

Oral endotracheal tubes are most commonly used to intubate neonates and children. Nasal intubation is generally more hazardous and is not frequently used. The appropriate tube size (**Table 22-8**) and the distance of insertion can be estimated based on the infant's weight. If the infant's weight is not immediately available, gestational age also is a reliable predictor for tube size (**Table 22-9**).

Unlike adults and large children, the narrowest point of an infant's airway is at the cricoid cartilage;

TABLE 22-8
Suggested Neonatal Endotracheal Tube Size Based on Body Weight

Weight (g)	Tube Size*
Less than 1000	2.5
1000 to 2000	3.0
2000 to 3000	3.5
More than 3000	3.5 to 4

*Tube size is given as the inside diameter in millimeters.

TABLE 22-9
Suggested Endotracheal Tube Size Based on Gestational Age

Gestational Age (Weeks)	Tube Size*
Less than 30	2.5
30 to 35	3.0
More than 35	3.5

*Tube size is given as the inside diameter in millimeters.

this characteristic allows the use of uncuffed airways. Although a complete seal is not always obtained, the cricoid cartilage provides a functional cuff. Despite some leakage, adequate ventilation can be achieved with an appropriate-sized uncuffed endotracheal tube. Also, use of an uncuffed tube prevents cuff-related tracheal injury in these patients. For these reasons, cuffed tubes are rarely used in neonates.

The correct endotracheal tube (ETT) size for children 1 to 10 years old can be estimated by using the child's age:

Endotracheal tube size (mm internal diameter) = (Age in years / 4) + 4

The clinician should have an ETT one-half size larger and smaller than the estimated size available if needed. ETT size can also be estimated by using a child's length. Length-based tapes are available and are generally considered useful for children up to 35 kg.

Cuffed ETTs can be as safe as uncuffed tubes for infants and children in the hospital setting.[7] There are circumstances in which a cuffed ETT is useful, such as when lung compliance is low and high airway pressures are needed. When cuffed ETT tubes are used, cuff inflation pressures should be kept below 20 cm H_2O.[8]

The approximate distance to insert the ETT, measured from the lips, can be estimated by the addition of 6 cm to the infant's weight in kilograms. In children, adding 10 to the child's age estimates this. These formulas can be used to estimate initial tube placement, but bilateral auscultation of the chest is essential. A disposable CO_2 detector can be placed between the resuscitation device and the endotracheal tube, and is a quick and easy way to confirm that the ETT is in the trachea. Because false positives and negatives are possible with the device, when bilateral breath sounds are noted, the tube should be secured and its position confirmed by chest radiograph. The tube then can be cut to minimize additional dead space and reduce the risk of inadvertent extubation. In addition, a gastric tube should be inserted and suction applied to decompress the stomach of air inadvertently delivered during mask ventilation.

Respiratory Recap

Endotracheal Intubation

- Oral tubes are most commonly used in neonates and children.
- Neonatal tubes are uncuffed.
- Pediatric tubes are sometimes cuffed.

Suctioning

Suctioning should be performed secondary to clinical assessment and not as a routine procedure. Suctioning can cause hypoxia, atelectasis, infection, tissue damage, and changes in the heart rate, blood pressure, and intracranial pressure. The need for suctioning is generally related to the underlying pathologic condition. Infants intubated because of respiratory distress syndrome, persistent pulmonary hypertension, or apnea require less suctioning than infants with meconium aspiration, sepsis, or pulmonary hemorrhage. Indications for suctioning include evidence of secretions in the endotracheal tube, diminished breath sounds, decreased tidal volume (during pressure ventilation), or increased peak inspiratory pressure (during volume ventilation). An obstructed airway or endotracheal tube should always be considered when acute desaturation occurs, particularly in infants with meconium aspiration, pulmonary hemorrhage, or pneumonia. Increases in carbon dioxide may also be a sign that the airway is obstructed and suctioning should be attempted. Providing adequate humidity can reduce the risk of tube obstruction, but plugging of artificial airways in infants with thick or abundant secretions is always a concern given the small internal diameter of the tube.

Oral or nasopharyngeal suctioning of infants is most often accomplished with a bulb syringe or other noninvasive technique to minimize airway trauma and edema. For the intubated patient, an inline suction catheter (**Figure 22-5**) offers several advantages over single-use catheters, and their use has become a routine practice in intensive care units (ICUs). With the inline catheter, the child can be suctioned without ventilator disconnection. Maintaining a closed system can reduce the risk of lung volume loss during suctioning. An

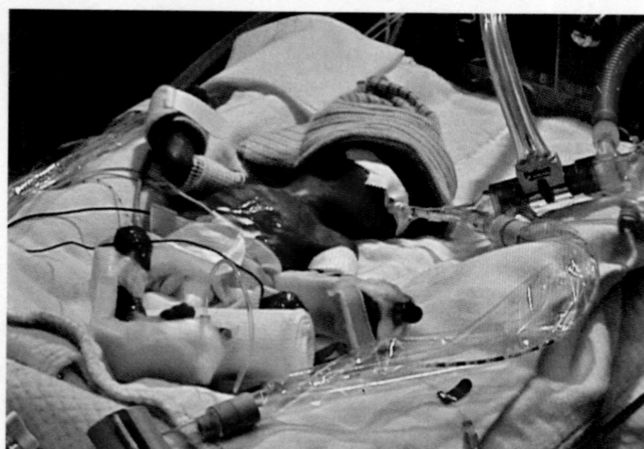

FIGURE 22-5 Neonatal inline suction catheter.
Courtesy of Melissa Brown BS RRT-NPS.

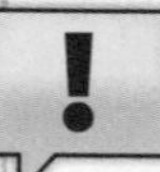

Respiratory Recap

Suctioning

- The recommended suction level is as low as will effectively remove secretions.
- Select a catheter with a French size two times the size of the inner diameter (in millimeters) of the endotracheal tube.

inline catheter that connects directly to the ETT with minimum dead space is ideal.

Selection of the suction catheter size is based on the size of the ETT. A common rule of thumb is to select a catheter with a French size two times the size of the inner diameter (in millimeters) of the ETT. The distance the catheter is inserted should be determined before the procedure to avoid airway trauma.[9] With the ETT in proper position, the distance is measured from the lips to the tip of the inline catheter fully withdrawn. The catheter is then inserted 0.5 cm farther than this distance. The recommended suction level is no greater that 75 to 100 mm Hg for infants (some recommend 60 to 80 mm Hg) and 100 to 125 mm Hg for children (some recommend 80 to 100 mm Hg). The suction pressure should be limited to the lowest level that effectively removes secretions and should be applied intermittently during withdrawal of the catheter. In neonates, an increase in FIO_2 of 0.1 for 30 to 60 seconds prior to and during the suction procedure is generally needed to maintain arterial oxygen saturation. For larger pediatric patients, the use of 100% oxygen to preoxygenate is considered safe.[10]

The duration of each suctioning event should be limited to 15 seconds. The patient must be assessed throughout the procedure. Decreases in the heart rate or significant arterial oxygen desaturation during suctioning is an indication to remove the catheter and support the child as needed. If further suctioning is

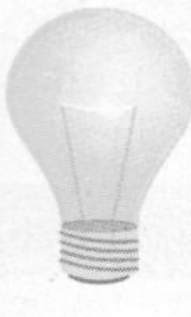

STOP AND THINK

You are caring for a 28-week gestational age, 1-kg premature infant who requires intubation. What size endotracheal tube would you select? At what centimeter marking should you initially secure the tube? What size suction catheter would be appropriate for the tube selected?

indicated, additional oxygen may be required before the procedure continues. After the procedure is completed, reassessment of the heart rate, oxygen saturation, color, chest expansion, and breath sounds is indicated. Ventilator adjustments and changes in the oxygen concentration may be needed to keep the oxygen saturation within the desired range.

Nasal Continuous Positive Airway Pressure

Infants who show adequate spontaneous efforts but whose clinical presentation indicates the potential for low lung volumes and associated hypoxemia may benefit from **nasal continuous positive airway pressure (NCPAP)**. The infant who is grunting will likely benefit from a trial of NCPAP. NCPAP can be applied via a variety of different nasal prongs and masks and with different pressure-generating devices (**Figure 22-6**). It can serve as an oxygen delivery source and aid in lung recruitment. NCPAP also is used to minimize airway collapse in patients with tracheomalacia.[11,12]

The CPAP level is started at 4 to 6 cm H_2O, and the child is reevaluated with pulse oximetry, transcutaneous monitoring, and arterial, venous, or capillary blood gas measurements. Breath sounds confirm airflow into the lungs. Appropriately sized nasal prongs are needed to achieve the desired benefit. Prongs that are too large can cause skin breakdown at the nares, and prongs that

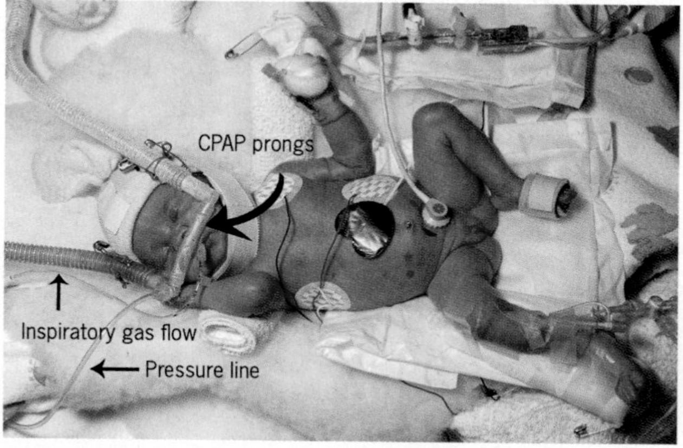

FIGURE 22-6 Setup for neonatal nasal continuous positive airway pressure (NCPAP) therapy.

are too small allow the infant to breathe around the device, making continuous airway pressure difficult to maintain. Nasal masks are also available and can be used with some CPAP devices. Nasal masks can be a good alternative to nasal prongs when skin breakdown is an issue and for larger children. The CPAP flows must be adequate to meet the patient's inspiratory demand, but not so large as to create significant work of breathing. Insertion of an orogastric tube is strongly advised to minimize air accumulation in the gastrointestinal tract. The circuit used to deliver NCPAP must be heated and humidified, because it becomes the major portion of the child's inspired air. Inadequately humidified gas can increase the risk of airway obstruction, and inadequately heated gas may result in difficulty in maintaining the infant's neutral thermal environment.

Nasal cannulas, variable-flow nasal CPAP generators, bubble CPAP setups, and nasal prongs and masks in conjunction with a conventional mechanical ventilator are used to provide NCPAP in neonatal and pediatric ICUs in the United States. These devices have advantages, disadvantages, and attendant difficulties. Problems of delivering nasal CPAP, regardless of device used, include difficulty in obtaining a seal and maintaining pressure, tubes becoming blocked and preventing pressure from being delivered to the lungs, and nasal trauma and breakdown. Some of the devices also have issues regarding inaccurate or absent pressure monitoring and increased work of breathing due to the design of the device.

Nasal cannulas are primarily used to deliver supplemental oxygen. In many hospitals, high-flow nasal cannulas (HFNCs) are being used as substitute NCPAP devices. Although there is not complete agreement as to what constitutes high flow, cannulas with flows of 1 to 8 L/min are frequently described as HFNCs in the neonatal environment.[13] An air–oxygen blender is used in combination with the cannula to titrate the F_{IO_2} delivered to the patient. The advantages of using nasal cannulas as nasal CPAP devices are that they are low in cost, easy to set up, readily available, and usually well tolerated by neonates. Unlike conventional nasal CPAP devices, however, the nasal cannula does not have a mechanism to monitor or regulate the generation of positive airway pressure. Due to variability in cannula sizes, patient sizes, and disease processes, it is difficult to predict what, if any, airway pressure is being delivered. There are also doubts about whether infants who use HFNCs have a comparable outcome to those infants who use other delivery devices.[14]

Variable-flow nasal CPAP devices, sometimes called flow drivers (FDs), generate CPAP at the airway unlike continuous-flow CPAP devices such as bubble CPAP. One example of this type of device (**Figure 22-7**) uses the Bernoulli effect and dual injector jets directed toward each nasal passage to maintain a constant pressure. If the infant needs more flow, the Venturi action

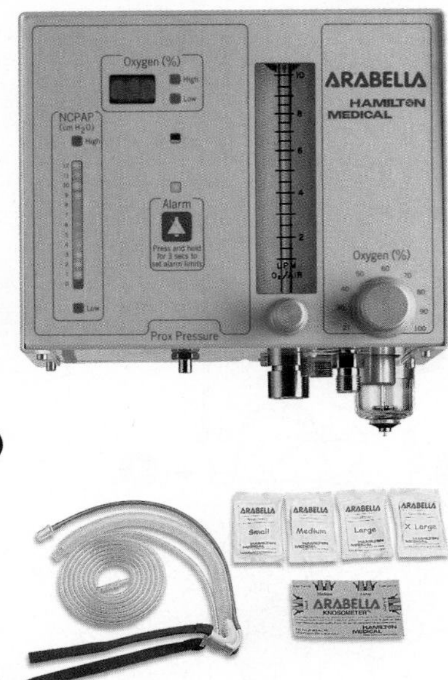

FIGURE 22-7 (**A**) The Arabella continuous positive airway pressure system. (**B**) The Arabella Universal Generator and nasal prongs.
Courtesy of Hamilton Medical, Inc.

of the jets will entrain additional flow. The infant can exhale without added work because the expiratory flow is shunted out the expiratory outlet that is open to ambient air. Continuous positive pressure is maintained throughout the respiratory cycle by residual gas pressure. The nasal prongs used can be of a much larger diameter than traditional prongs. They are made of a thin, soft material that flares out during inspiration, increasing the internal diameter and decreasing the leaking around them. No mechanical valves are used, and the intranasal airway pressure can be continuously monitored. The variable-flow capability of the FD assists with spontaneous breathing and creates more stable pressure delivery, which leads to improved functional residual capacity (FRC). NCPAP has demonstrated that it creates less work of breathing, and the infant using NCPAP has less thoracoabdominal asynchrony.[15]

Homemade bubble CPAP systems are popular in the United States (**Figure 22-8**). These systems comprise a heater/humidifier, a fresh gas source at a flow of up to 10 L/min, a separate inspiratory and expiratory length

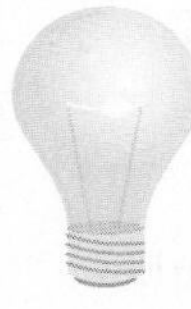

STOP AND THINK

You are caring for an infant on bubble NCPAP. The infant has acutely developed central cyanosis and oxygen desaturation. Upon inspection of the circuit you visualize adequate bubbling of the water column. What are the potential patient sources of the infant's oxygenation problem?

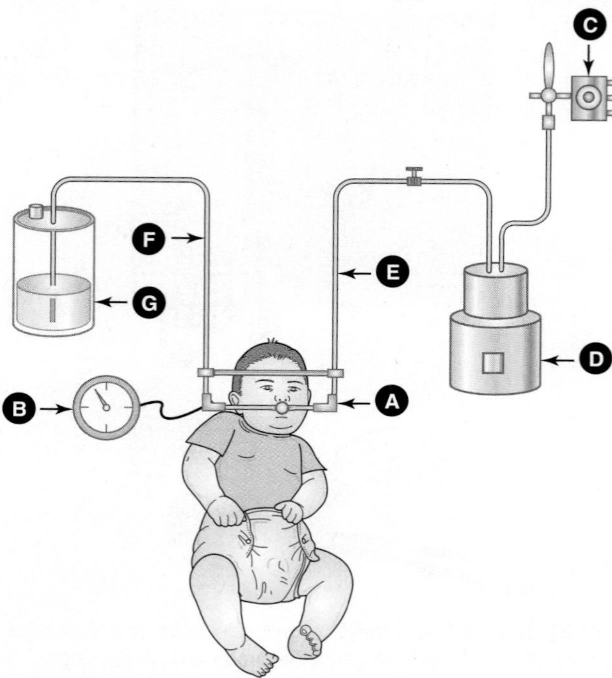

FIGURE 22-8 Schematic of bubble NCPAP delivery system. (**A**) Prongs. (**B**) Manometer. (**C**) Oxygen blender with flowmeter. (**D**) Heated humidifier. (**E**) Inspiratory tubing. (**F**) Expiratory tubing. (**G**) Underwater bubble chamber.

Adapted from Liptsen E, et al. Work of breathing during nasal continuous positive airway pressure in preterm infants: a comparison of bubble vs variable-flow devices. *J Perinatology*. 2005;25:453–458.

of tubing, a nasal prong interface, a pressure manometer, and a water seal column of sterile H_2O plus 0.25% acetic acid. Most of this equipment is found in any respiratory therapy department. The CPAP level is set by submerging the end of the expiratory tubing under the surface of the liquid to a depth in centimeters that is marked on the side of the column.[16] The pressure delivered is measured in centimeters of water (cm H_2O). The amount of pressure delivered is also influenced by the amount of flow through the system, so a pressure manometer should be placed as close to the nasal interface as possible.[17,18] The absence of bubbling in the water column suggests a leak. The clinician needs to assess the circuit and nasal interface for leaks, or possibly utilize a chinstrap to close the patient's mouth to maintain airway pressure. Some suggest that the oscillations that come from bubble CPAP may improve gas exchange, whereas others dispute this.[17]

Noninvasive Positive Pressure Ventilation

Mechanical ventilation can also be provided without an artificial airway, called **noninvasive ventilation (NIV)**. One of the main advantages of NIV is the ability to provide mechanical support for patients without exposing them to the risks involved with intubation. In addition, support can be provided for a short period of time, intermittently as needed, or for longer periods of time if necessary. The patient interface can be a nasal mask, an oronasal mask, or nasal prongs for infants. The patient interface can be connected to either a noninvasive mechanical ventilator or a standard mechanical ventilator. Although CPAP can be delivered, more frequently this type of ventilation is used in a bilevel mode that combines positive pressure breaths with PEEP. The goals of NIV include mechanical stenting of the airway with tracheomalacia and treatment of acute respiratory failure. NIV is frequently used for obstructive sleep apnea, RDS, and postextubation respiratory failure.[17,19,20] It is also used in acute asthma and with respiratory failure associated with cystic fibrosis. The patient must be monitored for facial skin breakdown due to excessive pressure from the mask or prongs.

Conventional Infant and Pediatric Ventilation

Indications

Mechanical ventilation is required for a variety of clinical presentations in neonates and children.[21] Full-term infants who require mechanical ventilation can have complex presenting symptoms that often include intrapulmonary and intracardiac shunting. Infants with congenital heart disease have particularly complex circulatory alterations. Some of these patients depend on the fetal blood flow that normally occurs only in utero. Maintaining patency of a ductus arteriosus or septal defect may save a life. During mechanical ventilation, abrupt changes in hemodynamics, normoxia, and hyperoxia can be fatal to these infants. Blood flow through these shunts is sometimes the primary means to maintain blood flow to the systemic circulation. Until corrective procedures can be performed, oxygen concentrations at or below room air can alter intracardiac shunts and ensure the patient's survival. An understanding of various cardiac anomalies is essential for appropriate ventilator management.

Providing adequate oxygenation and ventilation in conditions such as pneumonia, meconium aspiration, and congenital diaphragmatic hernia often is difficult. Nonhomogeneous lung disease increases the risk of barotrauma because the most compliant alveoli become overdistended. These underlying conditions often cause difficulty in the maintenance of adequate oxygenation and ventilation and lead to pulmonary vasoconstriction and significant pulmonary hypertension. As a result, shunting occurs through a patent ductus arteriosus or patent foramen ovale, making oxygenation more difficult.

Persistent pulmonary hypertension of the neonate (PPHN) can appear as a primary condition and be extremely difficult to manage. In infants with PPHN, the pulmonary vasculature has increased tone and abnormal responsiveness to vasodilators or the pulmonary arteries are muscularized, with a decreased

Respiratory Recap

Preductal and Postductal Spo_2 Monitoring

- Used to detect right-to-left shunting
- Preductal site: Generally the right arm
- Postductal site: Left arm or either lower extremity

cross-sectional area. In either condition blood flow is restricted, pulmonary artery pressure increases, and intracardiac shunting occurs. Because limited blood flow reaches the pulmonary vasculature to participate in gas exchange, ventilator adjustments in this population have little effect. Deoxygenated blood is shunted through a patent foramen ovale or a patent ductus arteriosus, making it difficult to achieve adequate arterial oxygen saturation. The pulmonary vasculature responds to hypoxia with further vasoconstriction, creating the possibility of greater amounts of blood being shunted and worsening oxygenation. Definitive diagnosis of PPHN generally is done by cardiac ultrasound. Clinically, right-to-left shunting is detected when oxygen saturation by Spo_2 is monitored at a site receiving preductal blood (generally the right arm) and compared with a simultaneously monitored postductal site (left arm or right or left lower extremity). A difference in the oxygen saturation values from these two sites (preductal value higher than the postductal value) indicates right-to-left shunting, often a result of pulmonary hypertension.

Infant Ventilators

Infant ventilators fall into two major categories: conventional ventilators and high-frequency ventilators. A conventional ventilator offers a variety of modes, alarms, and other options. Selection of the appropriate mode and other ventilator options is based on the infant's underlying condition and the desired effect of ventilatory support during both spontaneous and ventilator-initiated breaths.

Historically, a neonatal ventilator has been continuous flow, time cycled, and pressure limited. This is very similar to pressure control, with the rapid rise of gas flow and pressurization of the circuit leading to very early tidal volume delivery and then decelerating flow.[22] The first ventilators of this type did not allow for patient triggering. Current infant-only ventilators offer volume-limited and pressure-limited options, as well as patient-triggered and non-patient-triggered modes. Most modern mechanical ventilators have the ability to ventilate all patient types: premature infants, pediatric patients, and adults. These are called cradle-to-grave ventilators. Most ICU ventilators can be set up for neonates or children such that the trigger sensitivity and delivered pressures and volumes are suitable to respond to these patient populations. ICU ventilators evaluated in a 2009 study were capable of responding to neonatal inspiratory efforts and providing initial gas as effectively as traditional infant ventilators.[23]

When initiating ventilation, the clinician must select a pressure and/or tidal volume, respiratory rate, ventilator mode, inspiratory time or inspiration-to-expiration (I:E) ratio, PEEP, flow, and fraction of inspired oxygen (Fio_2). **Table 22-10** shows initial ventilator settings.

Pressure Limit and Tidal Volume

In neonatal time-cycled, pressure-limited ventilation, the clinician selects a pressure limit and inspiratory time that result in the delivery of a desired tidal volume. The tidal volume varies depending on the PIP, inspiratory time, and lung compliance. For example, if the lungs are less compliant, as in RDS, a higher PIP is needed to obtain a desired tidal volume. On the other hand, a lower PIP is needed if the lungs are more compliant. It should also be noted that, unlike most adult ventilators, the pressure set on a neonatal ventilator is the PIP—not the pressure above PEEP. The tidal volume thus is determined by the difference between the set pressure and PEEP. For this reason, an increase in PEEP may reduce the tidal volume unless the pressure limit is increased by an equivalent amount.

In the volume-targeted mode, the delivered tidal volume is preset and the PIP varies. The clinician presets the maximum pressure delivered. Volume ventilation has been found to reduce ventilator days and decrease the risk of pneumothorax and grades 3 and 4 intraventricular hemorrhage (IVH), and has shown a trend toward a reduced incidence of BPD.[24] Monitoring of the delivered tidal volume at the airway opening is essential to assess the effect of leaks (**Figure 22-9**). The uncuffed endotracheal tube can be a concern in volume ventilation in neonates because leaks of greater than 60% can limit the effectiveness of volume ventilation. The placement of an appropriate-sized endotracheal tube is key for success with volume-targeted ventilation for neonates.

TABLE 22-10
Initial Ventilator Settings for Conventional Ventilation

Setting	Instructions for Use
Peak inspiratory pressure (PIP)	As needed to provide a tidal volume of 4 to 6 mL/kg
PEEP	4 to 6 cm H_2O
Respiratory rate	20 to 40 breaths/min
Inspiratory time	0.3 to 0.5 s
Fio_2	As needed to maintain Spo_2 based on gestational age
Flow	6 to 12 L/min

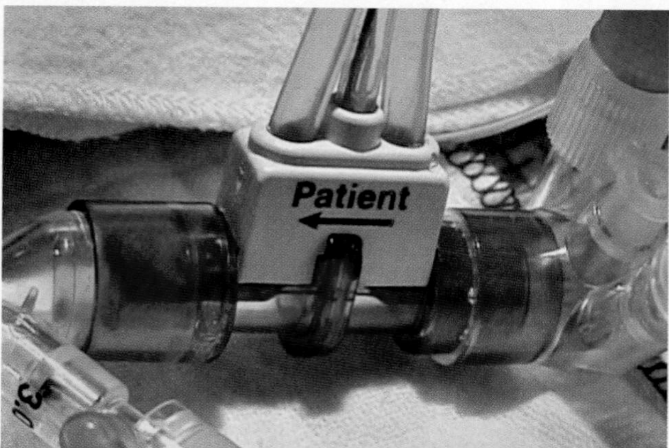

FIGURE 22-9 Flow sensor at airway to measure delivered tidal volume.

Courtesy of Melissa Brown BS RRT-NPS.

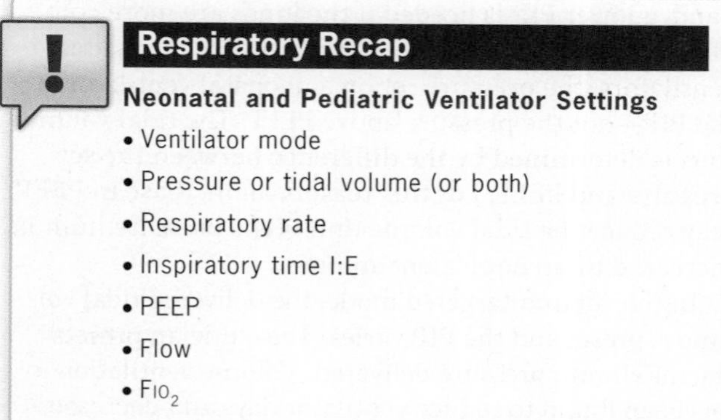

Respiratory Recap

Neonatal and Pediatric Ventilator Settings

- Ventilator mode
- Pressure or tidal volume (or both)
- Respiratory rate
- Inspiratory time I:E
- PEEP
- Flow
- F_{IO_2}

Pressure-limited ventilation with a target tidal volume is a common approach to neonatal and pediatric ventilation. Whether volume-limited, pressure-limited, or dual ventilation control is selected, a tidal volume of 4 to 6 mL/kg is generally targeted for neonates. For children, 6 to 8 mL/kg is acceptable.[25] As changes in tidal volume occur, clinical assessment determines the best intervention (**Table 22-11**). Adaptive pressure control (APC) can be used. With APC, the clinician sets a target tidal volume. The ventilator uses either pressure control or pressure support, but the pressure is increased or decreased as necessary to achieve the target tidal volume.

A practical issue with the ventilation of neonates is the effect of circuit compliance and compressible volume. These can substantially reduce the tidal volume available, particularly with volume ventilation. For this reason, a noncompliant, low-volume circuit typically is used. Because of the high resistance through this smaller-bore tubing, it is important to monitor airway pressure and flow directly at the Y piece of the ventilator circuit.[24]

Respiratory Rate

After a tidal volume is established, the respiratory rate becomes the primary adjustment for the achievement of desired minute ventilation. Spontaneously breathing neonates normally take 40 to 60 breaths/min to maintain a normal partial pressure of arterial carbon dioxide (Pa_{CO_2}). During mechanical ventilation, delivery of a larger than normal tidal volume (>4 to 6 mL/kg) at a lower respiratory rate can be more effective at eliminating carbon dioxide because a greater percentage of each tidal volume participates in gas exchange. Higher rates at lower tidal volumes result in a higher percentage of dead space ventilation and may result in less effective ventilation.

The ventilator rate should target a desired Pa_{CO_2}. The required rate depends on the target Pa_{CO_2}, the degree of lung disease (i.e., the amount of dead space), carbon dioxide production, the ventilator mode, and the amount of spontaneous breathing.

TABLE 22-11
Changes in Tidal Volume During Pressure Ventilation

Tidal Volume Change	Possible Causes	Solutions
Increase	Increased compliance, decreased resistance, decreased PEEP, increased inspiratory time, decreased leak	Reduce peak inspiratory pressure.
Decrease	Decreased compliance, increased resistance, decreased peak inspiratory pressure, increased PEEP, decreased inspiratory time, increased leak	Suction airway. Reposition infant. Administer surfactant. Increase inspiratory pressure. Perform transillumination to check for pneumothorax. Auscultate to detect pneumothorax or main stem intubation. Obtain chest radiograph. Check tube position.

Mode

In continuous mandatory ventilation (CMV or assist/control) mode, a minimum respiratory rate is set. Each spontaneous respiratory effort triggers a ventilator-assisted breath, and the preset pressure or volume is delivered. The inspiratory time is preset, and the patient determines the total respiratory rate above the set rate.

In synchronized intermittent mandatory ventilation (SIMV) mode, a minimum respiratory rate is set. Between the mandatory breaths the patient can breathe spontaneously. Spontaneous efforts are unassisted, and the rate, inspiratory time, and tidal volume are determined by the patient. The patient's inspiratory efforts trigger the mandatory breaths. The mandatory breaths may be pressure or volume limited. If the patient becomes apneic, the SIMV rate is delivered. Intermittent mandatory ventilation (IMV) mode is similar to SIMV except that the mandatory breaths are not synchronized to patient effort. This mode is almost never used anymore because of the large number of complications that can result from the patient's lack of synchrony with the ventilator.

With pressure support (PS), all breaths are triggered by the patient. A pressure limit is set to achieve a target tidal volume. The total rate, inspiratory time, expiratory time, and tidal volume are determined by the patient. Because inspiration normally is flow cycled with PS, leaks around the endotracheal tube can prolong inspiratory time unless the ventilator has a mechanism to terminate flow in leak situations. Most ventilators offer mechanisms to adjust the flow cycle, preventing prolonged inspiratory times with a leak. Pressure support may improve patient–ventilator synchrony in some patients by allowing flows and inspiratory times more consistent with the infant's needs. Improved patient–ventilator synchrony can lead to greater patient comfort, reduce the need for sedation, and potentially reduce the time the infant stays on mechanical ventilation.[20,21] Frequent apnea and periodic breathing are contraindications to this mode.

Inspiratory Trigger and Expiratory Cycle

Patient effort may trigger a breath in two primary ways. Depending on the ventilator, the patient-initiated breaths may be flow triggered, pressure triggered, or volume triggered. The signal for neonatal flow triggering typically occurs from a pneumotachometer positioned close to the infant's airway. A change in flow through the pneumotachometer triggers the ventilator. The amount of flow change required to trigger the ventilator is called the flow-trigger sensitivity, which is set by the clinician at a level that allows the least trigger effort without auto-triggering. Pressure triggering occurs with a change in the baseline pressure. The amount of pressure change required to trigger the ventilator is the pressure-trigger sensitivity, set in centimeters of water. At a sensitivity of 1 cm H_2O, a patient effort that reduces the baseline system pressure by 1 cm H_2O below PEEP will trigger a breath. The specifics of the trigger mechanism vary from ventilator to ventilator. Some ventilators will flow trigger in one mode and pressure trigger in other modes. Volume triggering uses the integral of the flow signal for triggering. Because this is an averaging of the flow signal over time, signal noise is reduced. This gives volume triggering a theoretic advantage over flow triggering.

An adjustable expiratory flow cycle is incorporated into some patient-triggered, pressure-limited modes. The expiratory flow cycle is based on a percentage of the peak flow. This cycle produces a variable inspiratory time, much like pressure support, which may reduce ventilator asynchrony. Familiarity with the inspiratory trigger and expiratory cycle mechanisms of the ventilator is essential to determine the appropriate settings for an individual patient.

Inspiratory Time

The inspiratory time is set in conjunction with the respiratory rate. The inspiratory time and the respiratory rate determine the I:E ratio. For example, if the respiratory rate is 30 breaths/min, each breathing cycle takes 2 seconds. If the inspiratory time is 0.5 second, the I:E ratio is 1:3. Ventilator graphics should be used to determine the best inspiratory time for each patient's current clinical condition.[26]

An inspiratory time that is too short can compromise both oxygenation and ventilation. The **mean airway pressure** is affected by the inspiratory time. A lower mean airway pressure may result in a loss of lung volume or inability to establish lung volume, causing a decrease in the Pa_{O_2}. Decreased ventilation, resulting in less carbon dioxide elimination and a higher Pa_{CO_2}, occurs if a shortened inspiratory time reduces the delivered tidal volume.

An inspiratory time that is too long may shorten the expiratory time and result in auto-PEEP, which may cause alveolar overdistention, increasing the risk of pneumothorax. Alveolar overdistention may also interfere with pulmonary blood flow, increase dead space ventilation, and reduce carbon dioxide elimination. Inspiratory times that are too long can also cause a patient to perform a forced exhalation maneuver, potentially causing excessive pressure, poor tidal volume delivery, and ventilator asynchrony (**Figure 22-10**). A typical inspiratory time with conventional positive pressure ventilation for the neonate is 0.3 to 0.5 of a second. Pediatric patients will have longer inspiratory times, frequently as long as 1 second. Monitoring the expiratory flow with graphics (**Figure 22-11**) or expiratory flow monitors and adjustment of the respiratory rate and inspiratory time can help prevent complications related to the I:E ratio such as air trapping and auto-PEEP.

Positive End-Expiratory Pressure

PEEP is routinely set in all ventilator modes to prevent alveolar collapse during expiration. PEEP usually is started at 4 to 6 cm H_2O. In the neonate, lung volumes are assessed by chest radiograph, with the ideal lung volume expansion being to eight or nine ribs bilaterally. PEEP and PIP are adjusted if the lungs appear underinflated or overinflated. Higher PEEP levels may be indicated for patients with a persistently low lung volume. Low levels of PEEP are indicated with evidence of pulmonary interstitial emphysema or persistent air leakage after barotraumas. The delivered tidal volumes should be assessed when PEEP levels are adjusted. In pressure-limited ventilation, the change in the PEEP setting may result in a change in the delivered tidal volume. The pressure limit may need to be adjusted to maintain the volume target.

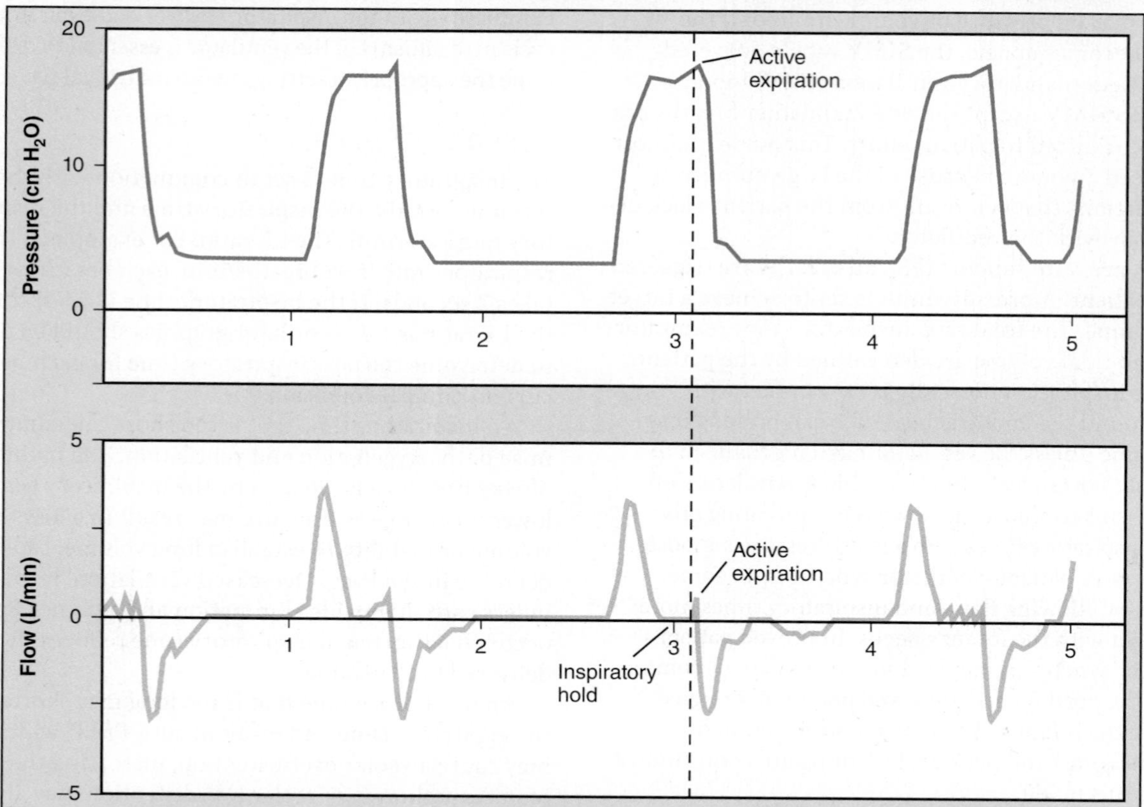

FIGURE 22-10 Excessive inspiratory time scalars. The pressure and flow scalars show an excessive inspiratory time, which can cause active exhalation. The inspiratory time is too long, and this causes a spiked appearance at the completion of each breath. This patient is forcibly exhaling.

Reproduced from Waugh JB, Deshpande VM, Brown MK, Harwood R. *Rapid Interpretation of Ventilator Waveforms*, 2nd, © 2006. Reprinted by permission of Pearson Education, Inc., Upper Saddle River, NJ.

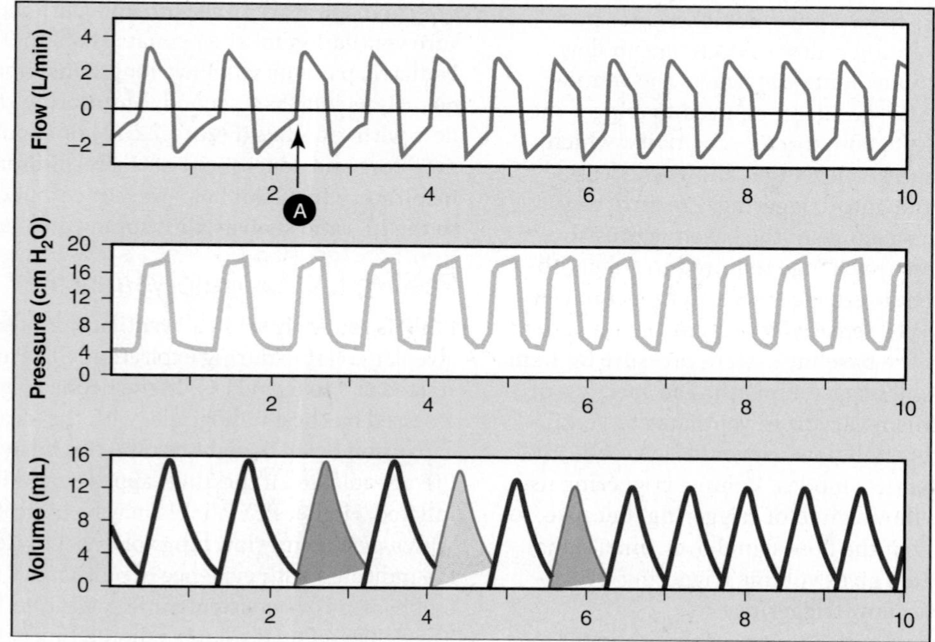

FIGURE 22-11 A ventilator rate set too high can cause breath stacking to occur, resulting in air trapping or auto-PEEP. Point A shows how the flow does not reach baseline before the next breath is delivered. Notice on the volume scalar how tidal volumes are decreasing due to air trapping.

Reproduced from Waugh JB, Deshpande VM, Brown MK, Harwood R. *Rapid Interpretation of Ventilator Waveforms*, 2nd, © 2006. Reprinted by permission of Pearson Education, Inc., Upper Saddle River, NJ.

Humidification

Adequate humidification of the inspired gas is critical to the maintenance of airway patency. A decrease in humidity can lead to dried secretions and atelectasis and may result in partial or complete airway obstruction. This risk is particularly high in neonates because of their small airways. An appropriately humidified circuit shows moisture throughout both the inspiratory and the expiratory limbs. Circuits should be inspected routinely for evidence of humidity. Adequate humidification is also important to maintain the **neutral thermal environment** of the newborn, particularly the premature newborn. Breathing a cool, dry gas may stress the metabolic demands on the newborn, resulting in increased oxygen consumption.

One issue with the neonatal ventilator circuit involves the position of the temperature sensor.[27] Critically ill neonates usually are in an incubator or under a radiant heater. If the temperature sensor in the circuit is placed in the incubator or under the radiant heater, it may be affected by a temperature other than the temperature of the gas in the ventilator circuit. This could result in malfunction of the humidification system. For this reason, the temperature sensor is placed at a point in the circuit outside the incubator or radiant heater, or it is otherwise shielded from the effects of the ambient temperature in these devices.

Hazards and Complications

Complications from mechanical ventilation in the neonatal and pediatric population can be substantial. Ventilator-associated pneumonia can occur. Tracheal damage from endotracheal tubes can create long-term problems. A neuropathologic consequence of reduced cerebral blood flow known as periventricular leukomalacia (PVL) has been associated with ventilator-induced hypocarbia in preterm infants.

Some neonates who survive the newborn course are left with varying degrees of chronic lung disease, a condition called bronchopulmonary dysplasia. The contribution of mechanical ventilators and oxygen therapy to this condition is not entirely known, but indiscriminate use of high pressure and exposure to high oxygen concentrations over time are thought to be factors. Neonates with BPD have a chronic oxygen requirement, chronic carbon dioxide retention, and pulmonary hypertension. These neonates also have an increased susceptibility to pulmonary infections.[5,20]

Weaning

Consideration of weaning from ventilatory support should begin as soon as the patient's condition has stabilized from the disorder that required support. The patient's hemodynamic, pulmonary, neurologic, and nutritional status must be assessed. Also, weaning must not be confused with readiness for extubation. Rather, weaning should be an ongoing process of support adjustment to a level that maintains adequate gas exchange without requiring significantly increased work of breathing. No single approach to weaning can be applied to all patients. The goal is to provide appropriate support by continuous assessment of the patient's total needs and recognize when weaning is indicated.

In infants and children, weaning is generally done in the SIMV or a PS mode or a combination of both. In SIMV mode, the set respiratory rate is lowered to assess the patient's ability to breathe spontaneously and maintain adequate minute ventilation. Pressure-support levels can also be reduced gradually, as the patient is able to support an adequate tidal volume on his or her own. The presence of an endotracheal tube reduces the airway size and leaves the patient at risk for increased work of breathing. For this reason, infants generally are not expected to demonstrate the ability to breathe without any assistance before extubation. The pressure or volume limit is adjusted to keep the tidal volume in the range of 4 to 6 mL/kg. Premature infants <500 grams may need tidal volumes closer to 6 mL/kg to overcome the dead space of the ventilator flow sensor at the airway and maintain adequate gas exchange.[24] The PEEP level usually is maintained at a minimum of 4 to 6 cm H_2O to prevent loss of lung volume.

The patient's breathing effort and the ventilatory pattern are continually assessed during weaning. Periods of apnea are common in premature infants. In infants whose condition otherwise is stable, respiratory stimulants such as caffeine may be beneficial in the reduction of apnea during weaning. Pulse oximetry, transcutaneous monitoring, apnea, respiratory rate, and minute ventilation monitoring can help alert the clinician to changes in the patient's respiratory status. Infants with persistent tachypnea, retractions, and an increased oxygen requirement during the weaning process use calories needed for normal growth and development. Adequate gas exchange may be achieved, but the caloric expense to the patient can be far greater than the benefit. Continual assessment of the patient's tolerance for weaning from a multisystem perspective is essential throughout the weaning process.

Extubation is considered when no contraindications exist from the neurologic or other nonrespiratory systems, when the patient shows the ability to maintain a stable respiratory and heart rate, and when oxygen saturation is acceptable, with an F_{IO_2} of 0.3 or lower. The ability to feed and the infant's growth pattern also play a role in the decision to extubate. Because of the effects of the endotracheal tube on lung volume and work of breathing, extubation of the neonate often occurs with ventilator settings of 10 to 20 breaths/min, a PIP of 10 to 18 cm H_2O, and a PEEP of 4 to 5 cm H_2O. Ventilator settings prior to extubation of the pediatric patient are similar to the neonate, with the exceptions that a higher PIP is acceptable and expected and that lower rates may be tolerated. Readiness for extubation should be assessed daily in all ventilated patients.

High-Frequency Ventilation

High-frequency ventilation (HFV) is an accepted mode of mechanical ventilation in neonatal and pediatric critical care. HFV is defined as positive pressure ventilation at a respiratory rate more than 150 breaths/min and tidal volumes approximating anatomic dead space.[28] The advantage of this technique over conventional mechanical ventilation is its ability to deliver an adequate minute ventilation with a lower airway pressure, often when conventional mechanical ventilation has failed. Treatment with a high mean airway pressure often is better tolerated with HFV than with conventional mechanical ventilation. With conventional mechanical ventilation, the alveolar volume is the difference between tidal volume and the dead space volume. Tidal volumes near the dead space volume produce little alveolar ventilation. The fact that gas exchange occurs with HFV, at times more efficiently than with CMV, is intriguing. HFV is used daily throughout the country, but the exact mechanism by which it accomplishes adequate gas exchange is not completely understood.

Classification

The four general types of HFV are high-frequency positive pressure ventilation, high-frequency jet ventilation, high-frequency flow interrupter ventilation, and high-frequency oscillatory ventilation.

High-frequency positive pressure ventilation (HFPPV) is conventional positive pressure ventilation at a high respiratory rate (more than 150 breaths/min) and small tidal volumes.[29] The inspiratory time is short to facilitate the increased respiratory rate. Exhalation is passive. The use of airway graphics to closely monitor changes in mean airway pressure is essential with HFPPV. Although HFPPV laid the foundation for modern high-frequency ventilation, its use has declined with the availability of high-frequency ventilators.

High-frequency jet ventilation (HFJV) delivers short pulses of gas directly into the trachea through a narrow-bore cannula or jet injector. Jet ventilators can maintain oxygenation and ventilation over a wide range of patient sizes. These systems have negligible compressible gas volume and operate effectively at rates of 150 to 600 breaths/min. Exhalation is passive. The tidal volume often is equal to or slightly less than the dead space volume. The high-flow jet pulse produces a jet mixing effect that creates an area of negative pressure and entrains additional gas into the airway. The high gas velocities and gas mixing effects make pressure monitoring difficult. Jet ventilators are used with a conventional ventilator that provides PEEP, entrained gas, and intermittent sighs.

High-frequency flow interrupter ventilation (HFFIV) delivers inspiratory flow to the patient in short bursts by means of a rotating ball valve or microprocessor-controlled solenoid valve. These ventilators produce breath rates of 2 to 22 Hz (1 **hertz [Hz]** equals 60 breaths/min). HFFIV is similar to high-frequency oscillatory ventilation in that inspiration and exhalation are both active. Active exhalation is defined as a drop in airway pressure during exhalation to accelerate exhaled gas flow.[30] Background mandatory breaths may or may not be used to maintain lung volume.

High-frequency oscillatory ventilation (HFOV) essentially uses airway vibrators, usually with piston pumps or vibrating diaphragms that operate at frequencies ranging from 400 to 2400 breaths/min.[31] During HFOV, inspiration and expiration are both active. Oscillators produce little if any bulk gas delivery. A continuous flow of fresh gas (bias flow) provides inspired gas and clears carbon dioxide from the system. Pressure oscillations in the airway produce tiny tidal volumes around a constant mean airway pressure. The tidal volume is determined by the amplitude of airway pressure oscillations, determined by the stroke of the device producing the oscillations.

Gas Transport Theories

Several theories have been proposed to explain gas transport at high respiratory frequencies. The mechanisms of gas exchange during HFV are not completely understood, and several effects interact during HFV.[32]

In *spike formation* (**Figure 22-12**), a high-energy wave impulse of gas penetrates the center of the airway, enhancing bulk flow of gas in the upper airway and providing a more expansive area of gas mixing in the more distal lung. In the more compliant airway of the premature infant, spike formation is less effective. It is possible that turbulence increases with a more compliant airway, limiting spike effectiveness.

Helical diffusion (**Figure 22-13**), a variant of the spike theory, also may play a role in HFV. Fresh gas enters the lung through a spike generated in the center of the airway while gas exits the lung circumferentially along the periphery of the airway (coaxial flow).[33] This theory assumes that carbon dioxide removal occurs in a spiral fashion, producing a whirlpool effect, whereby fresh gas moves through the center of the airway while gas simultaneously exits the lungs.

Taylor dispersion (**Figure 22-14**) is the augmented diffusion of gas in situations of parabolic gas flow

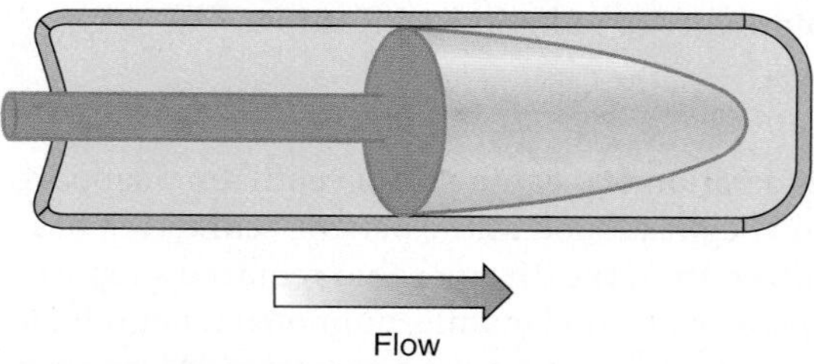

FIGURE 22-12 Spike formation in the airway during high-frequency ventilation.

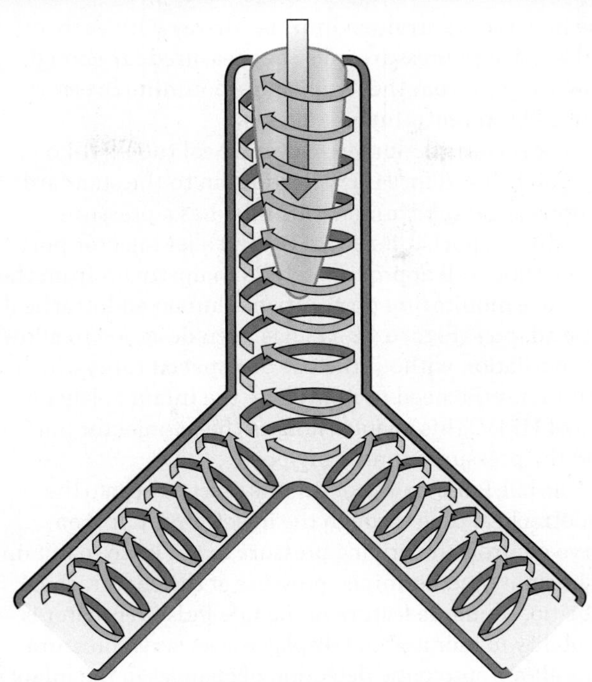

FIGURE 22-13 Helical diffusion during high-frequency ventilation.
Adapted from Karp TB, et al. High frequency ventilation: a neonatal nursing perspective. *Neonatal Netw.*. 1986;4:43.

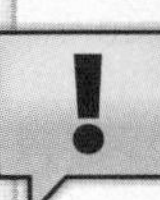

Respiratory Recap

Categories of High-Frequency Ventilation

- High-frequency positive pressure ventilation (HFPPV)
- High-frequency jet ventilation (HFJV)
- High-frequency flow interrupter ventilation (HFFIV)
- High-frequency oscillatory ventilation (HFOV)

resulting in high energy spikes.[34] This augmented diffusion can occur wherever two gas streams meet, such as in coaxial flow in larger airways and convective streaming more distal in the lung. The increased surface area between two gas streams during HFV facilitates this diffusion process. These high-energy jet spikes probably result in the delivery of more total fresh gas to distal respiratory units before significant contamination of the inflow gas occurs. This preserves the diffusion gradient needed to remove carbon dioxide from the blood.

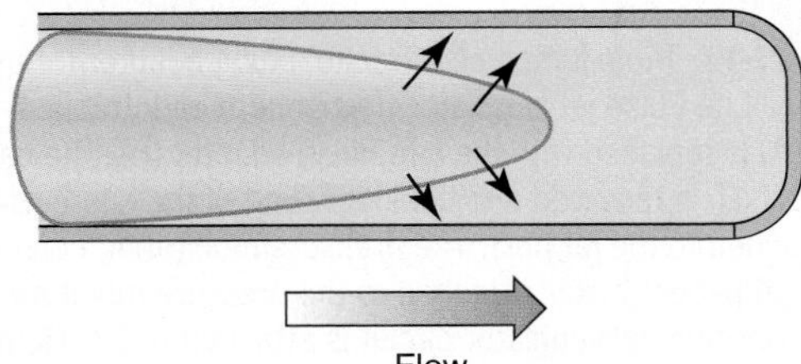

FIGURE 22-14 Taylor dispersion during high-frequency ventilation.

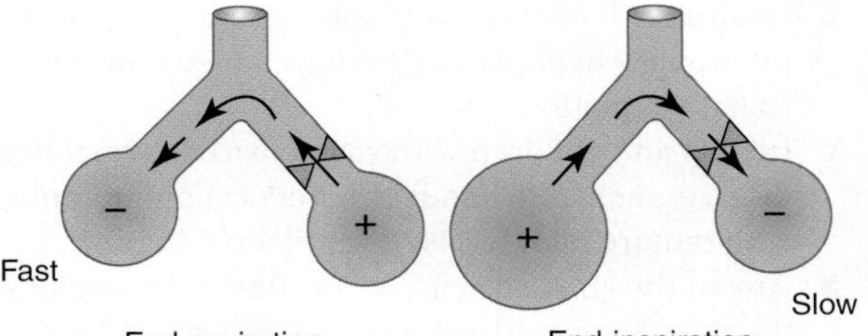

FIGURE 22-15 Pendelluft during high-frequency ventilation.

Pendelluft ventilation (**Figure 22-15**) is the result of gas mixing between lung regions that have different time constants; this is also called out-of-phase ventilation. When parallel lung units have different time constants, resistance tends to dominate the rate of filling and emptying at rapid respiratory rates.[32] At the end of a rapid inspiration, gas flows from the fast unit, which is beginning to empty, to the slow unit, which is still filling. This motion of gas between two neighboring units during phasic ventilation is called pendelluft.[32]

Molecular diffusion is a transport mechanism derived from random thermal oscillation of a molecule. So long as the molecules have a constant temperature, molecular diffusion always occurs. Molecular diffusion is responsible for gas exchange at the level of the alveolocapillary membrane.[32] Molecular diffusion is altered during HFV. The rapid kinetic motion of oxygen and carbon dioxide molecules during HFV and the process of gas exchange at the alveolar level are speculative at this time.

Patient Selection

Specific strategies for the use of HFV depend on the institution. The question of when to use HFV in neonatal and pediatric patients, therefore, is not easily answered. Should HFV be implemented early in the treatment of respiratory failure, or should conventional ventilation be used first and HFV applied only if this approach fails? Some centers are very aggressive and institute HFV without trying conventional ventilation, seeking to protect the patient from pulmonary barotrauma at the onset of ventilation. Others try conventional ventilation before HFV.

Use of HFV is considered in the following situations:

- Preterm infants with severe hyaline membrane disease requiring a PIP of more than 30 cm H_2O and children with acute respiratory distress syndrome (ARDS) requiring a PIP of more than 40 cm H_2O
- Infants with severe meconium aspiration syndrome and persistent pulmonary hypertension that does not respond to maximum ventilatory support with a PIP of more than 35 cm H_2O
- Infants and children with air leak syndrome, including progressive pulmonary interstitial emphysema, recurring pneumothorax, and pneumopericardium

- Infants with congenital diaphragmatic hernia or pulmonary hypoplasia who have failed conventional ventilation
- Infants and children with severe parenchymal lung disease, such as group B streptococci pneumonia, who require high levels of ventilatory support
- Any of the above disease states that may preclude the use of conventional ventilation and that indicate the need to institute HFV as an initial point of care
- A patient in need of inhaled nitric oxide (iNO), who might benefit from the improved gas distribution properties of HFV

High-Frequency Ventilators

The Bunnell Life Pulse jet ventilator (**Figure 22-16**) is a microprocessor-controlled system capable of delivering and monitoring 240 to 660 breaths/min. It is used in conjunction with a conventional ventilator that provides a source of continuous gas flow, PEEP, and low-rate IMV. The Life Pulse ventilator is approved for clinical use in neonates and infants. It appears to be most effective in disorders in which hypercarbia is the major problem. With HFJV, carbon dioxide removal is achieved at lower airway pressures than with other types of high-frequency ventilators. When managed properly, HFJV can acutely improve oxygenation and the oxygen index in infants with PPHN and other associated pulmonary conditions.

The patient box is an integral component of the Life Pulse ventilator. This box contains the pressure transducer and inhalation pinch valve necessary for operation. The patient box is placed close to the patient's head to provide accurate monitoring and delivery of gas to the patient. The pinch valve regulates gas flow. The Life Pulse controls the PIP, respiratory rate, jet valve on-time (inspiratory time), and on/off ratio (I:E ratio). The jet ventilator delivers short pulses of pressurized gas directly into the airway through a narrow-bore cannula or jet injector. The system has negligible compressible volume, and exhalation is always passive. The tidal volume is difficult to measure but is equal to or slightly greater than the dead space volume. Gas surrounding the injector is entrained into the airway with each jet pulse. Airway pressure must be measured far enough downstream from the jet injector to minimize errors caused by air entrainment effects.

A special triple-lumen endotracheal tube (Hi-Lo Jet) can be used for HFJV. In addition to the standard endotracheal tube lumen, this tube has a pressure monitoring port at its distal tip and a jet injector port in the tube wall approximately 7 cm upstream from the pressure monitoring port. A triple-lumen endotracheal tube adapter (**Figure 22-17**) has been designed to allow jet ventilation without the use of a special tube, which eliminates the need to reintubate the infant solely for use of HFJV. This adapter houses the jet injector port and the pressure monitoring port.

The Life Pulse ventilator delivers its jet pulse into the endotracheal tube through the injector port. It then servo controls the driving pressure to the jet to maintain a constant predetermined pressure at the endotracheal tube tip. A unique feature of the Life Pulse ventilator is its ability to monitor and display the jet servo pressure. This allows automatic detection of changes in the infant's lung compliance and airway resistance. Servo pressure is proportional to the lung volume being ventilated. For example, as lung compliance or airway resistance (or both) improves, servo pressure increases. This is typically used as an indicator to begin weaning the patient from high-frequency ventilation. Conversely, a decrease in

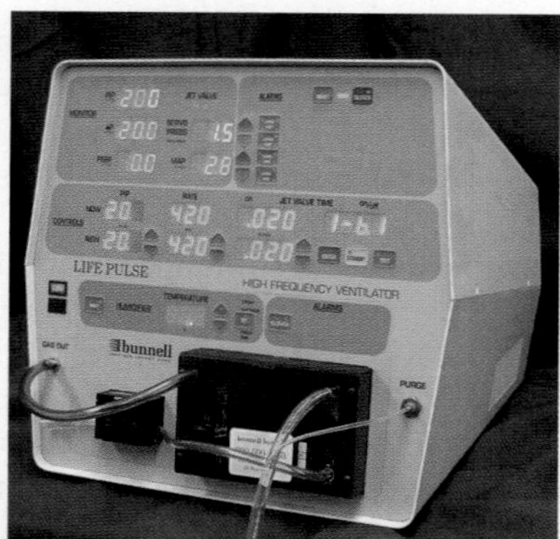

FIGURE 22-16 Bunnell Life Pulse ventilator.
Courtesy of Bunnell Incorporated.

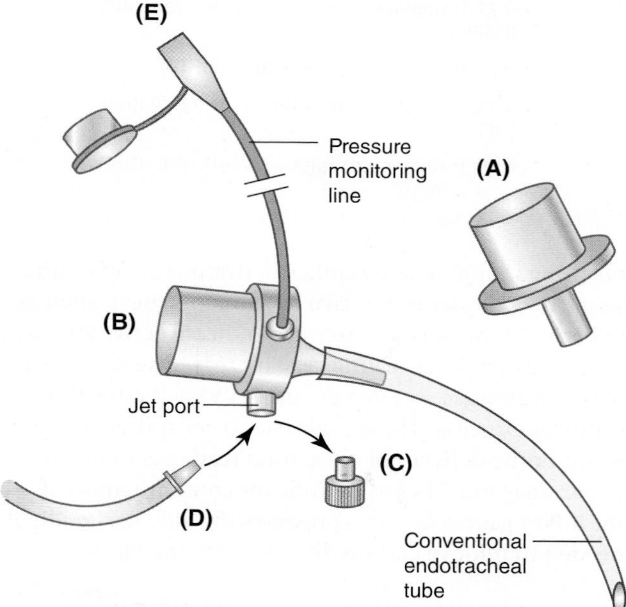

FIGURE 22-17 Triple lumen endotracheal tube adapter for use with the Bunnell Life Pulse jet ventilator. The 15 mm endotracheal tube adapter (**A**) is replaced with the Life Pulse adapter (**B**). The cap on the jet port (**C**) is removed and the luer fitting of the Life Pulse circuit (**D**) is attached to the jet port. The pressure monitoring connector from the jet patient box is attached to the pressure monitoring line (**E**). The conventional ventilator circuit is attached to the 15 mm port of the Life Pulse adapter.
Modified from Aloan CA, Hill TV. *Respiratory Care of the Newborn and Child.* 2nd ed. Lippincott Williams & Wilkins; 1997.

servo pressure indicates that lung compliance or airway resistance has worsened, the endotracheal tube has become obstructed, a tension pneumothorax has developed, or the patient requires suctioning. Respiratory therapists and other clinicians find servo pressure helpful for assessing the patient's pulmonary status.

The SensorMedics 3100A (CareFusion, San Diego, CA) is an electronically controlled oscillatory ventilator (**Figure 22-18**). Its 365-mL oscillatory driver is a diaphragmatically sealed piston with adjustable displacement, frequency, and I:E ratio. It produces 3- to 15-Hz pressure waves superimposed on an adjustable level of mean airway pressure. The SensorMedics 3100A is distinguished from other types of high-frequency ventilators by its active expiratory phase. It is used for ventilatory support and for treatment of respiratory failure and barotrauma in neonates and small pediatric patients.

The primary therapeutic effects are obtained with just two controls: the oscillatory **pressure amplitude** (ΔP) and the mean airway pressure. In some cases, changing the frequency (hertz) or the percent inspiratory time or both may provide additional benefits to those patients who do not respond to initial standard settings.

End-expiratory lung volume is determined by the mean airway pressure and remains relatively constant during the respiratory cycle. The SensorMedics 3100A does not require use of a special endotracheal tube. It has fewer control settings than other high-frequency ventilators, and once the patient's condition has been stabilized, the ventilator settings are changed infrequently.

The mean airway pressure on the SensorMedics 3100A can be adjusted from 3 to 45 cm H_2O. The mean airway pressure limit can be operated in two modes. In the safety limit mode, the mean airway pressure limit is set to a level higher than the range of normal mean airway pressures to protect the patient from accidental overpressure. In the controlled mode, the mean airway pressure limit is set to a level below that which would otherwise exist through the adjustment of the mean pressure control. In this mode, the mean airway pressure remains constant regardless of changes in bias flow, the percent inspiratory time, or frequency settings. With HFOV the mean airway pressure is the most important determinant of oxygenation. It dictates whether the patient can be weaned from the potentially harmful effects of an elevated F_{IO_2}. The mean airway pressure is maximized initially, with close attention paid to hyperinflation and monitoring of the chest radiograph to maintain lung volume at the level of ribs T8 to T9.

Bias flow is necessary to maintain oxygenation, the mean airway pressure, and an oscillatory waveform. The system must be charged with flow to operate effectively. Standardized bias flow settings are 10 to 20 L/min. A common rule of thumb is that the smaller the child, the lower the bias flows. Manipulations of the Pa_{CO_2} level are made primarily with the amplitude or power control (ΔP). Increasing the amplitude increases displacement of the bellows, which increases tidal volume delivery. This is measured as increased pressure amplitude at the airway opening and results in a lower Pa_{CO_2}. Frequent arterial blood gas measurements or monitoring of the transcutaneous P_{CO_2} is necessary to titrate the Pa_{CO_2}.

The respiratory rate on the SensorMedics 3100A is measured in hertz. The concept of active inspiration and active expiration allows the delivery of very rapid respiratory rates without air trapping. The rate can be set from 3 to 15 Hz. The higher the respiratory rate, the smaller the tidal volume, partly because of the short cycle time at the higher rate. Conversely, the lower the rate, the larger the tidal volume, because of the longer cycle and the ability to move more volume through the circuit. The respiratory therapist must recognize that the delivered tidal volumes are very small and are equal to or less than the dead space volume. As a rule of thumb, larger babies (more than 2 kg) fall into the lower rate category (8 to 10 Hz), whereas smaller infants (less than 2 kg) fall into the smaller tidal volume requirement category and hence require a higher rate (12 to 15 Hz). The selection of rate among hospitals may vary, however, and often the rate will be adjusted based on the resonance frequency of the particular patient (e.g., how well the chest shakes on the particular hertz setting).

The inspiratory time on the SensorMedics 3100A is nearly always set at 33%, which has been determined to

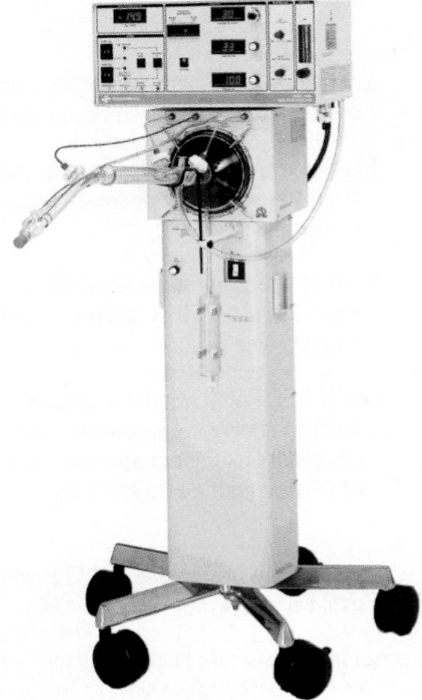

FIGURE 22-18 SensorMedics 3100A.
Reproduced with permission from CareFusion.

Respiratory Recap

High-Frequency Ventilators

- Bunnell Life Pulse jet ventilator
- SensorMedics 3100A

be the standard inspiratory time setting for this ventilator. Only in extreme cases (e.g., with a large patient with a severely elevated physiologic dead space) is the percent inspiratory time increased to improve carbon dioxide elimination. As with slowing of the respiratory rate, an increase in the percent inspiratory time allows a longer inspiratory phase, thus increasing the delivered tidal volume. The inspiratory time can be adjusted from 33% to 50% in 1% increments.

Management Strategies

Management strategies are divided into two categories: high lung volume and low lung volume. Most patients fall into the high lung volume management category. This means that the ventilator parameters are maximized at the clinician's discretion. The only disease that would preclude this approach is air leak syndrome. Establishing lung volume and restoring it to an acceptable level is a critical component of HFV. Because the delivered tidal volumes are small, the mean lung volume does not change dramatically during inspiration. PEEP is the primary contributor to mean airway pressure and end-expiratory lung volume during HFV.

The Bunnell Life Pulse HFV is used with a conventional ventilator. **Table 22-12** shows general management strategies for high-frequency jet ventilation. The conventional ventilator is responsible for controlling the PEEP level. Hence, the mean airway pressure is controlled by the conventional ventilator, and the PIP, respiratory rate, inspiratory time, and I:E ratio are controlled by the HFJV. Once the infant's condition has

TABLE 22-12
Patient Management Guidelines for Life Pulse High-Frequency Ventilation

1. HFV ΔP (PIP – PEEP) is the primary determinant of $Paco_2$. High-frequency ventilation (HFV) rate is secondary.
2. Resting lung volume (FRC supported by set PEEP) and mean airway pressure are crucial determinants of Pao_2.
3. Avoid hyperventilation and hypoxemia by using optimal PEEP.
4. Minimize IMV at all times using very low rates (typically 0–3 breaths/min) unless IMV is being used to dilate airways or *temporarily* recruit collapsed alveoli. In general, keep IMV PIP 10–30% < HFV PIP.
5. To overcome atelectasis, IMV rates up to 5 breaths/min can be used for 10–30 min. Thereafter, IMV rate should be decreased to 0–3 breaths/min. In general, keep IMV inspiratory time at 0.4–0.6 s.
6. If lowering IMV rate worsens oxygenation, PEEP is probably too low. Higher PEEP and lower IMV rates reduce the risk of lung injury.
7. Decrease Fio_2 before PEEP until Fio_2 is less than 0.4.

Setting	Usual	When to Raise	When to Lower
HFV PIP	Whatever produces desired $Paco_2$	To lower $Paco_2$	To increase $Paco_2$ (increase PEEP simultaneously to keep aw and Pao_2 constant)
HFV rate	420 breaths/min (neonates) or 300 breaths/min (children)	To decrease $Paco_2$ in *smaller* patients or to increase aw and Pao_2	To eliminate inadvertent PEEP or hyperinflation by lengthening exhalation time or to increase $Paco_2$
HFV inspiratory time	0.02 s	To enable jet to reach PIP at low HFJV rates in *larger* patients (>15 kg)	Keep at the minimum of 0.02 s in most cases
IMV rate	0–3 breaths/min	To reverse atelectasis or dilate restricted airways (3–5 breaths/min)	To minimize volutrauma (especially when air leaks are present) or decrease hemodynamic compromise
IMV PIP	PIP necessary to get adequate chest rise	To reverse atelectasis or dilate airways; PIP may be greater or less than HFJV PIP	To minimize volutrauma (especially when air leaks are present) or decrease hemodynamic compromise
IMV inspiratory time	0.4 s	To reverse atelectasis or dilate airways	To minimize volutrauma (especially when air leaks are present) or decrease hemodynamic compromise
PEEP	7–12 cm H_2O (neonates) or 10–15 cm H_2O (children)	To improve oxygenation and decrease hyperventilation; to find optimal PEEP increase PEEP until Spo_2 stays constant when switching from IMV to CPAP	Lower PEEP only when it appears that cardiac output is being compromised or when oxygenation is adequate and when decreasing PEEP does not decrease Pao_2
Fio_2	<0.60	Increase as needed after optimizing PEEP	Lower Fio_2 in preference to PEEP when weaning until Fio_2 <0.4

Special air leak considerations: (1) Minimize IMV by using HFV + adequate CPAP, and (2) if oxygenation is compromised, increase PEEP even if the lungs appear to be overdistended on chest radiograph. PIP, peak inspiratory pressure; PEEP, positive end-expiratory pressure; CPAP, continuous positive airway pressure; Fio_2, fraction inspired oxygen; HFV, high-frequency ventilation; HFJV, high-frequency jet ventilation; IMV, intermittent mandatory ventilation; $\bar{P}aw$, mean airway pressure.
Modified with permission from materials courtesy of Bunnell, Inc., Salt Lake City, UT.

stabilized, efforts are made to reduce the mean airway pressure. The PIP may be reduced gradually and the respiratory rate dropped to 250 to 300 breaths/min. The PEEP may also be decreased if the Pao_2 is acceptable and the patient tolerates the change.

Management of the infant on HFOV is more straightforward than with HFJV. **Table 22-13** shows general management strategies for HFOV. HFOV decouples (separates) ventilation and oxygenation. The mean airway pressure and Fio_2 control oxygenation, whereas amplitude, the percent inspiratory time, and respiratory rate determine ventilation. This simplistic approach to HFOV benefits both clinician and patient. Initially, the mean airway pressure and Fio_2 are maximized. Ventilation may be more difficult to control because the patient's size and disease determine what settings are chosen. The smaller the patient, the higher the rate setting; the percent inspiratory time is set at 33%. Amplitude (ΔP) is a more discretional setting, and the respiratory therapist must be judicious in determining it. Amplitude is what ventilates or moves the chest with HFOV. Although the setting of ΔP is arbitrary, what happens to the patient is not. The higher the amplitude setting, the more vigorously the chest wall moves or wiggles; this is called the chest wiggle factor. The clinician must determine what degree of chest wiggle is acceptable for the patient. The patient's compliance determines how aggressive the clinician is with ΔP.

One of the differences between HFOV and HFJV is that higher rather than lower mean airway pressures are required to maintain oxygenation with HFOV. Higher mean airway pressure settings are used early in the ventilatory course and weaned as tolerated when the Pao_2 level is acceptable. In HFOV the mean airway pressure is increased in increments of 1 to 2 cm H_2O, provided there is no air leak, until the Spo_2 rises above 95%, which indicates adequate lung recruitment. A chest radiograph must be obtained to ensure that inflation is adequate, to the level of the eighth to the ninth rib. Hyperinflation can adversely affect hemodynamics, and the mean airway pressure should be reduced if hyperinflation occurs.[28] Hyperinflation also poses an increased risk of air leakage. As the patient on HFOV improves, the Fio_2 should be weaned to 0.6 before the mean airway pressure is reduced, unless hyperinflation is noted by chest radiograph. When the mean airway pressure has been reduced 10 to 12 cm H_2O, the clinician should consider transferring the patient back to CMV or continue weaning to extubation on HFOV.

TABLE 22-13
General Guidelines for Use of High-Frequency Oscillatory Ventilation

Clinical Indicators	Therapeutic Intervention	Treatment Rationale
Fio_2 below 0.70 High $Paco_2$ with: Pao_2 satisfactory Pao_2 low Pao_2 high	Increase ΔP Increase aw, ΔP, Fio_2 Increase ΔP; decrease Fio_2	Increase ΔP to achieve optimum $Paco_2$ Adjust aw and Fio_2 to improve O_2 delivery Decrease Fio_2 to minimize O_2 exposure
Fio_2 below 0.70 Normal $Paco_2$ with: Pao_2 satisfactory Pao_2 low Pao_2 high	Take no action Increase aw, Fio_2 Decrease Fio_2	Take no action Adjust aw and Fio_2 to improve O_2 delivery Decrease Fio_2 to minimize O_2 exposure
Fio_2 below 0.70 Low $Paco_2$ with: Pao_2 satisfactory Pao_2 low Pao_2 high	Decrease ΔP Increase aw, Fio_2; decrease ΔP Decrease Fio_2, ΔP	Decrease ΔP to achieve optimum $Paco_2$ Adjust aw and Fio_2 to improve O_2 delivery Decrease Fio_2 to minimize O_2 exposure
Fio_2 above 0.70 High $Paco_2$ with: Pao_2 satisfactory Pao_2 low Pao_2 high	Increase ΔP Increase Fio_2, ΔP Increase ΔP; decrease aw	Increase ΔP to achieve optimum $Paco_2$ Increase Fio_2 to improve Pao_2 Decrease aw to reduce Pao_2
Fio_2 above 0.70 Normal $Paco_2$ with: Pao_2 satisfactory Pao_2 low Pao_2 high	Take no action Increase Fio_2 Decrease aw, Fio_2	Take no action Increase Fio_2 to improve Pao_2 Decrease aw and Fio_2 to reduce Pao_2
Fio_2 above 0.70 Low $Paco_2$ with: Pao_2 satisfactory Pao_2 low Pao_2 high	Decrease ΔP Increase Fio_2; decrease ΔP Decrease aw, ΔP	Decrease ΔP to achieve optimum $Paco_2$ Increase Fio_2 to improve Pao_2 Decrease aw and Fio_2 to minimize O_2 exposure

Fio_2, fraction inspired oxygen; $Paco_2$, partial pressure of arterial carbon dioxide; Pao_2, partial pressure of arterial oxygen; ΔP, pressure amplitude; aw, mean airway pressure.
Reproduced with permission from CareFusion.

Complications

Complications associated with HFV include tracheal injury, atelectasis, pulmonary overdistention, acute respiratory alkalosis, hypotension, decreased cardiac output, and a displaced or disconnected endotracheal tube.[35] In early uses of HFV, tracheal

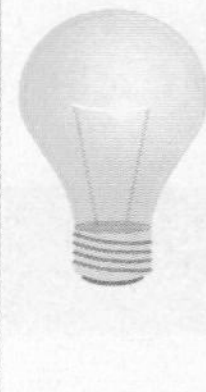

STOP AND THINK

You are caring for a pediatric patient on HFOV. You realize that the patient is hypocarbic and is not within the ordered parameters. The patient's oxygenation status is satisfactory. What ventilator change would you recommend?

injury was reported in some cases, but improved humidification has eliminated this complication. Atelectasis may occur as a result of mucous plugging or low airway pressures leading to alveolar collapse, which can be prevented through maintenance of an adequate mean airway pressure. Pulmonary overdistention and cardiac compromise can result from failure to wean excessive mean airway pressures. Overdistention can cause acute lung injury, pneumothorax, and increased physiologic shunt. Patients must be monitored closely for signs of decreased systemic perfusion when HFV is initiated. A high mean airway pressure may not be tolerated. If myocardial dysfunction occurs, inotropic therapy may be indicated. Minimizing the adverse effects of an increased intrathoracic environment is an essential component of the care of the child on HFV.

An issue related to HFV is the noise of the ventilator, which contributes to the noise level in the neonatal and pediatric intensive care unit.[36] Newer models have been designed to operate more quietly, so this should be less of an issue as hospitals acquire new equipment.

Adjuncts to Neonatal and Pediatric Mechanical Ventilation

Preterm infants (those less than 34 weeks of gestational age) have varying degrees of lung maturity, and the respiratory needs of these infants may be significantly different from those of a full-term infant with mature lungs. Infants born at less than 35 weeks' gestation often have a surfactant deficiency. Surfactant production begins about week 23 of gestation, and the fetal lungs reach maturity at week 35. Between weeks 23 and 35, lung maturity may be enhanced in utero by administration of corticosteroids. Corticosteroids often are given to mothers at risk for premature delivery. Infants who receive corticosteroids in utero are likely to have greater lung maturity than infants of similar gestational age who were not treated with steroids in utero. Many infants are born prematurely with either partial treatment or no treatment with steroids and have a surfactant deficiency, however.

Surfactant Administration

Surfactant is a combination of lipoproteins found in mature alveoli that reduces surface tension at the alveolar air–fluid interface.[37] Alveoli with low surface tension require less pressure to stabilize lung volume and avoid alveolar collapse. Infants with a surfactant deficiency often show signs of respiratory distress syndrome. The clinical findings associated with RDS are tachypnea, intercostal and sternal retractions, nasal flaring, expiratory grunting, decreased compliance, and an oxygen requirement. The typical chest radiograph of an infant with RDS has a ground glass appearance and low lung volumes. Administration of exogenous surfactant has been shown to prevent and treat RDS (**Table 22-14**). Surfactant can be given as a rescue therapy after clinical signs of RDS have developed, or prophylactic surfactant can be given in the delivery room to try to prevent the development of RDS or minimize its effects (**CPG 22-1**).[38] The available evidence suggests that NCPAP initiated in the delivery room, followed by mechanical ventilation only when necessary, is a reasonable alternative to prophylactic surfactant treatment for preterm infants.[39]

Surfactant is given endotracheally (**Box 22-2**). In infants, with clinical signs of RDS and impending respiratory failure, intubation and early administration of surfactant are recommended. Before the surfactant is administered, the infant's lung compliance is reduced significantly. It may be necessary to use high pressures to ventilate a surfactant-deficient infant. Reassessment of the infant's ventilatory needs after administration of surfactant is vital. Adjustments to the ventilator are indicated as compliance increases and oxygenation improves. Maintenance of a delivered tidal volume of 4 to 6 mL/kg is achieved by a reduction in the PIP or volume setting. The F_{IO_2} must be adjusted to keep the arterial oxygen saturation in the desired range. Attention to these details is essential to reduce the risk of ventilator-induced complications.

Inhaled Nitric Oxide

Administration of inhaled nitric oxide (iNO) has been shown to improve oxygenation in neonates

TABLE 22-14
Commercial Surfactant Preparations

Surfactant	Description	Route of Administration	Dose (mL/kg)
Survanta	Bovine lung extract	Endotracheal	4.0
Curosurf	Isolated from minced pig lungs	Endotracheal	2.5
Infrasurf	Calf lung surfactant	Endotracheal	3.0
Surfaxin	Synthetic	Endotracheal	5.8

CLINICAL PRACTICE GUIDELINE 22-1

Surfactant Replacement Therapy

The following recommendations are made regarding surfactant replacement therapy.

1. Administration of surfactant replacement therapy is strongly recommended in a clinical setting where properly trained personnel and equipment for intubation and resuscitation are readily available.
2. Prophylactic surfactant administration is recommended for neonatal respiratory distress syndrome in which surfactant deficiency is suspected.
3. Rescue or therapeutic administration of surfactant after the initiation of mechanical ventilation in infants with clinically confirmed respiratory distress syndrome is strongly recommended.
4. A multiple surfactant dose strategy is recommended over a single dose strategy.
5. Natural exogenous surfactant preparations are recommended over laboratory derived synthetic suspensions at this time.
6. It is suggested that aerosolized delivery of surfactant not be utilized at this time.

Modified from Walsh BK, Daigle B, DiBlasi RM, Restrepo RD. AARC Clinical Practice Guideline. Surfactant replacement therapy: 2013. *Respir Care.* 2013;58:367–375. Reprinted with permission.

with hypoxemia and pulmonary hypertension.[40] The primary mechanism is thought to be lowering of pulmonary vascular resistance by vasodilation of the pulmonary vasculature, resulting in decreased right-to-left shunting of blood. Inhaled NO is selective to the pulmonary vasculature and has not been associated with a lowering of systemic blood pressure. Inhaled NO can be administered with either a conventional or high-frequency ventilator. Although the optimum dose of iNO is not entirely clear, 20 ppm or less usually is sufficient. Because administration of iNO can cause methemoglobinemia, this value should be monitored during therapy.

NO and oxygen can combine to produce nitrogen dioxide (NO_2). The NO and NO_2 levels should be monitored during therapy, but a high NO_2 level usually can be prevented with proper delivery equipment. The NO concentration is reduced once oxygenation is stable. Continuous monitoring with pulse oximetry as the NO concentration is reduced is essential. Before NO is discontinued, the F_{IO_2} can be increased by 10% to 20% to prevent a rebound effect. During the administration of NO, the manual resuscitation bag at the bedside should be adapted to provide NO in the event manual ventilation is required to avoid abrupt withdrawal of NO and rebound. NO should not flow into the reservoir of the resuscitation bag until needed to avoid production of NO_2.

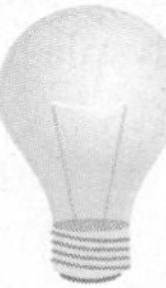

STOP AND THINK

You are caring for a 24-week, 0.5 kg premature neonate. The physician would like you to administer a dose of Curosurf surfactant after intubation. How much medication should you prepare to administer and how would you proceed with the administration procedure?

Key Points

- Awareness and understanding of maternal risk factors are crucial for the identification of newborns at risk for life-threatening complications.
- A specific sequence of events for neonatal resuscitation is outlined in the American Academy of Pediatrics Neonatal Resuscitation Program (NRP).

BOX 22-2

Administration of Surfactant

Determine the surfactant preparation to be used and the dose.
Allow the drug to reach room temperature.
Confirm the position of the endotracheal tube.
Instill the drug directly into the endotracheal tube.
Continuously monitor the heart rate and oxygen saturation as measured by pulse oximetry (Sp_{O_2}) during administration; also monitor for endotracheal tube obstruction.
Monitor tidal volume and Sp_{O_2} immediately after dose is given.
Adjust ventilator support as compliance changes.

- Excessive use of oxygen could lead to retinopathy of prematurity and bronchopulmonary dysplasia in the premature infant.
- Positive pressure ventilation usually begins with bag-mask ventilation.
- Nasal CPAP and NIV are used to aid lung recruitment and to minimize airway collapse.
- Uncuffed oral endotracheal tubes are most commonly used in neonates.
- Infant ventilators are either conventional or high-frequency ventilators.
- Traditional conventional neonatal ventilators are continuous flow, time cycled, and pressure limited.
- High-frequency ventilators are classified as high-frequency positive pressure ventilation, high-frequency jet ventilation, high-frequency flow interrupter ventilation, and high-frequency oscillatory ventilation.
- High lung volume and low lung volume management styles are used for high-frequency ventilation.
- Adjuncts to neonatal mechanical ventilation include surfactant administration and inhaled nitric oxide.

References

1. Kattwinkel J, Perlman JM, Aziz K, et al. Part 15: neonatal resuscitation: 2010 American Heart Association Guidelines for Cardiopulmonary Resuscitation and Emergency Cardiovascular Care. *Circulation*. 2010;122(Suppl 3):S909–S919.
2. Thebaud B, Mercier JC, Dinh-Xuan AT. Congenital diaphragmatic hernia: a cause of persistent pulmonary hypertension of the newborn which lacks an effective therapy. *Biol Neonate*. 1998;74: 323–336.
3. Iliff A, Le VA. Pulse rate, respiratory rate, and body temperature of children between two months and eighteen years of age. *Child Dev*. 1952;23:237.
4. American Academy of Pediatrics, American College of Obstetricians and Gynaecologists. *Guidelines for Perinatal Care*. 4th ed. Elk Grove Village, Ill.: American Academy of Pediatrics; 1997.
5. Deakins KM. Bronchopulmonary dysplasia. *Respir Care*. 2009;54:1252–1262.
6. Mondolfi AA, Grenier BM, Thompson JE, et al. Comparison of self-inflating bags with anesthesia bags for bag-mask ventilation in the pediatric emergency department. *Pediatr Emerg Care*. 1997;13:312–316.
7. Pediatric advanced life support. 2010 American Heart Association Guidelines for Cardiopulmonary Resuscitation and Emergency Cardiovascular Care. *Circulation*. 2010;122(Suppl 3): S876–S908.
8. Parwani VHI-H, Hsu B, Hoffman RJ. Experienced emergency physicians cannot safely or accurately inflate endotracheal tube cuffs or estimate endotracheal tube cuff pressure using standard technique. *Acad Emerg Med*. 2004;11:490–491.
9. Hess DR. Managing the artificial airway. *Respir Care*. 1999;44: 759–772.
10. American Association of Respiratory Care. Endotracheal suctioning of mechanically ventilated patients with artificial airways 2010. *Respir Care*. 2010;55:758–764.
11. Davis S, Jones M, Kisling J, et al. Effect of continuous positive airway pressure on forced expiratory flows in infants with tracheomalacia. *Am J Respir Crit Care Med*. 1998;158:148–152.
12. Panitch HB, Allen JL, Alpert BE, et al. Effects of CPAP on lung mechanics in infants with acquired tracheobronchomalacia. *Am J Respir Crit Care Med*. 1994;150:1341–1346.
13. Walsh BK, Brooks TM, Grenier BM. Oxygen therapy in the neonatal care environment. *Respir Care*. 2009;54:1193–1202.
14. Finer NN, Mannino FL. High-flow nasal cannula: a kinder, gentler CPAP? *J Pediatr*. 2009;154:160–162.
15. Gupta S, Sinha S, Tin W, Donn S. A randomized controlled trial of post-extubation bubble continuous positive airway pressure versus infant flow driver continuous positive airway pressure in preterm infants with respiratory distress syndrome. *J Pediatr*. 2009;154:645–650.
16. Diblasi RM. Nasal continuous airway pressure (CPAP) for the respiratory care of the newborn infant. *Respir Care*. 2009;54: 1209–1235.
17. Courtney SE, Barrington KJ. Continuous positive airway pressure and noninvasive ventilation. *Clin Perinatol*. 2007;34:73–92.
18. Kahn DJ, Habib RH, Courtney SE. Effects of flow amplitudes on intraprong pressures during bubble versus ventilator generated nasal continuous positive airway pressure in premature infants. *Pediatrics*. 2008;122:1009–1013.
19. Loh LE, Chan YH, Chan I. Noninvasive ventilation in children: a review. *J Pediatr (Rio J)*. 2007;83(Suppl 2):S91–S99.
20. Ramanathan R. Optimal ventilatory strategies and surfactant to protect the preterm lungs. *Neonatology*. 2008;93:302–308.
21. AARC clinical practice guidelines: neonatal time-triggered, pressure-limited, time-cycled mechanical ventilation. *Respir Care*. 1994;39:808–816.
22. Donn SM, Boon W. Mechanical ventilation of the neonate: should we target volume or pressure? *Respir Care*. 2009;54:1236–1243.
23. Marchese AD, Chipman D, de la Oliva P, Kacmarek RM. Adult ICU ventilators to provide neonatal ventilation: a lung simulator study. *Intensive Care Med*. 2009;35:631–638.
24. Brown MK, Diblasi RM, Mechanical ventilation of the premature neonate. *Respir Care*. 2011;56:1298–1311.
25. Cheifetz IM. Invasive and noninvasive pediatric mechanical ventilation. *Respir Care*. 2003;48:442.
26. Waugh JB, Deshpande VM, Brown MK, Harwood RJ. *Rapid Interpretation of Ventilator Waveforms*. 2nd ed. Upper Saddle River, N.J.: Pearson, Prentice Hall; 2007.
27. Chatburn RL. Physiologic and methodologic issues regarding humidity therapy. *J Pediatr*. 1989;114:416–420.
28. Courtney SE, Asselin JM. High-frequency jet and oscillatory ventilation for neonates: which strategy and when? *Respir Care Clin North Am*. 2006;12:453–467.
29. Sjostrand UH. Review of the physiological rationale for and development of high-frequency positive pressure ventilation. *Acta Anaesthesiol Scand*. 1977;64:7–27.
30. Hess D, Mason S, Branson R. High-frequency ventilation design and equipment issues. *Respir Care Clin North Am*. 2001;7:577–598.
31. Smith R. Ventilation at high respiratory frequencies. *Anaesthesia*. 1982;37:1011–1018.
32. Chunk HK. Mechanisms of gas transport during ventilation by high-frequency oscillation. *J Appl Physiol*. 1984;56:553–563.
33. Fredberg JJ, Glass GM, Boynton BR, et al. Features influencing mechanical performance of neonatal high-frequency ventilators. *J Appl Physiol*. 1987;62:2485–2490.
34. Taylor GI. Dispersion of matter in turbulent flow through a pipe. *Proc R Soc Lond B Biol Sci*. 1954;223:446–448.
35. Boros SJ, Mammel MC, Lewullen PK, et al. Necrotizing tracheobronchitis: a complication of high-frequency ventilation. *J Pediatr*. 1986;109:95–100.
36. Hoehn T, Busch A, Krause ME. Comparison of noise levels caused by four different high-frequency ventilators. *Intensive Care Med*. 2000;26:84–87.
37. Been JV, Zimmermann LJI. What's new in surfactant? *Eur J Pediatr*. 2007;166:889–899.
38. Walsh BK, Daigle B, Diblasi RM, Restrepo RD. AARC clinical practice guidelines: surfactant replacement therapy: 2013. *Respir Care*. 2013;58:367–375.
39. Finer NN, Carlo WA, Walsh MC, et al. Early CPAP versus surfactant in extremely preterm infants. *N Engl J Med*. 2010;362:1970–1979.
40. Diblasi RM, Myers TR, Hess DR. Evidence-based clinical practice guideline: inhaled nitric oxide for neonates with acute hypoxic respiratory failure. *Respir Care*. 2010;55:717–745.

CHAPTER

23

Extracorporeal Life Support for Respiratory Failure

Kyle J. Rehder, David A. Turner

OUTLINE

OBJECTIVES

1. Describe basic principles of extracorporeal membrane oxygenation (ECMO).
2. Review common applications of ECMO and contraindications to its use.
3. Appraise data supporting the use of ECMO for acute respiratory failure.
4. Discuss factors associated with the increase in ECMO utilization for adult respiratory failure.
5. Review common complications of ECMO support and their impact on patient outcomes.
6. Discuss ECMO management techniques.
7. Review adjunctive therapies coupled with ECMO for respiratory failure.
8. Assess technological achievements and advancements of ECMO support and safety.
9. Describe novel applications of ECMO, including inter-hospital transport of ECMO patients.
10. Discuss ECMO trends and advances expected in the next decade.

KEY TERMS

ECMO circuit
Extracorporeal Life Support Organization (ELSO)
extracorporeal membrane oxygenation (ECMO)
oxygenator
pumpless extracorporeal lung assist (PECLA)
respiratory dialysis
sweep gas
venoarterial (VA) ECMO
venovenous (VV) ECMO

Introduction

Despite continued advancements in conventional therapies, acute hypoxemic respiratory failure continues to carry a high disease burden. Severe acute respiratory distress syndrome (ARDS) mortality is approximately 40% in adults.[1–3] In both adults and pediatrics, ARDS survivors often face a prolonged recovery, long-term morbidity, and disability.[4]

The strategy that has made the greatest impact on survival in ARDS is lung-protective ventilation.[5] Lung-protective ventilation helps to mitigate ventilator-induced lung injury (VILI), which occurs early after the initiation of mechanical ventilation even in healthy lungs.[6] In diseased lungs, this injury is further exacerbated and additive to the initial insult. Minimizing VILI through limitation of tidal volume and ventilation pressure is an important priority in the management of critically ill patients, giving them the best chance for recovery.[5,7]

Gas exchange in some patients may be too compromised to allow appropriate limitation of conventional ventilator support, however. When a patient progresses to refractory respiratory failure and gas exchange targets cannot be met using conventional support, therapeutic options are limited. Many of the strategies that have been attempted for refractory ARDS have not demonstrated improved survival in clinical trials including high-frequency oscillatory ventilation, airway pressure release ventilation, exogenous surfactant, steroids, nitric oxide, and others.[1–3,8–11]

Extracorporeal methods of gas exchange represent a mechanism to mitigate VILI and allow clinicians to meet clinical goals, and there is increasing interest in this approach. **Extracorporeal membrane oxygenation**

(ECMO) is the most common type of extracorporeal support, and this technique has been successfully used for over 40 years in neonates, children, and adults. While ECMO may be used for either cardiac or respiratory indications, this chapter will focus primarily on ECMO for respiratory failure. This chapter reviews basic ECMO principles, available data, trends in its utilization, recent advances in strategies and technology, and future directions.

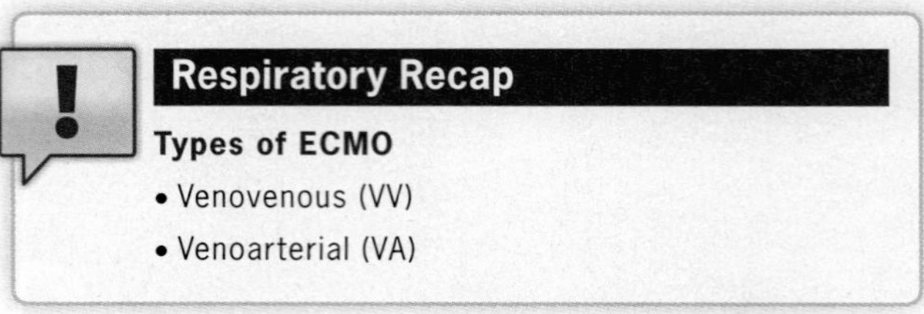

Respiratory Recap

Types of ECMO

- Venovenous (VV)
- Venoarterial (VA)

ECMO Basics

ECMO is accomplished by inserting a large-bore cannula into a central vein, passively draining blood from the patient, pumping that blood through an artificial gas exchanger (**oxygenator**), and returning the oxygenated/ventilated blood to the patient. An oxygen/air mixture (**sweep gas**) is passed through the oxygenator to provide gas exchange. The blood is oxygenated through exposure of red blood cells to the large surface area of the artificial membrane. Carbon dioxide removal occurs through passive diffusion from the blood into the sweep gas and is so efficient that a low concentration of carbon dioxide often needs to be added to the sweep gas to avoid severe hypocapnia.

Blood may be returned either to the venous (**venovenous**, or **VV ECMO**) or arterial (**venoarterial**, or **VA ECMO**) system (**Figure 23-1**). Under optimal conditions, a large portion of the patient's cardiac output flows through the **ECMO circuit**. In adults, flows exceed 4 L/min for VV ECMO and higher for VA ECMO. In general, the higher the blood flow, the more effective the oxygenation.

VV ECMO acts as a third lung to augment gas exchange, while VA ECMO provides this lung support along with directly supporting cardiac output. VV ECMO is typically the preferred method of support in respiratory failure, both for simplicity as well as its more favorable safety profile. VA ECMO may be required for direct cardiac support or for anatomic reasons in smaller children and neonates.

Primary sites of cannulation include the right internal jugular vein and/or femoral vessels in pediatric and adult patients, but subclavian and axillary vessels have also been used. Improvements in cannula technology have led to an increase in double-lumen cannula use, with almost one-half of adults and children receiving

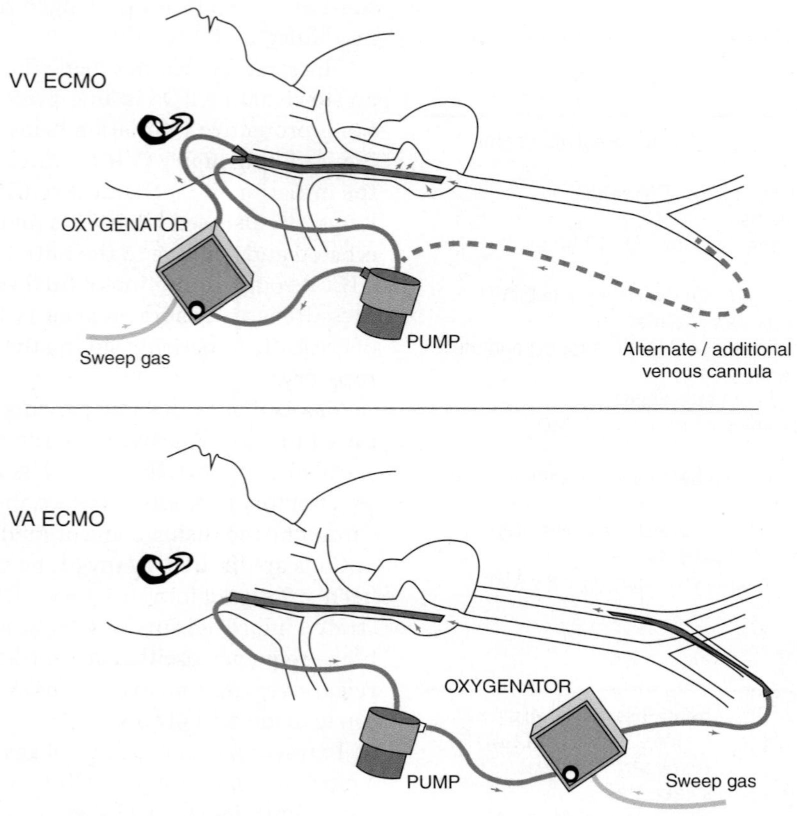

FIGURE 23-1 Schematic of VV and VA ECMO.

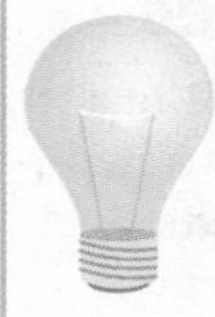

STOP AND THINK

Which is the right patient for ECMO support? When should you consider ECMO? What patient factors increase mortality risk?

VV ECMO being managed with a double lumen cannula in 2012.[12] Use of a double-lumen cannula allows for single site cannulation, reduces vessel trauma and infection risk, and potentially allows for increased wakefulness and mobility of ECMO patients.[13,14] The femoral vein may be accessed as an alternative, or if necessary, an additional efferent cannulation site. Most patients with respiratory failure supported with ECMO do not need an additional venous drainage cannula, making single (usually internal jugular) site cannulation a common approach. When VA ECMO support is indicated in adolescents and adults, the most common arterial access is the femoral artery. The carotid artery is typically used for neonates and younger children requiring VA ECMO, either for cardiac support or inability to technically place a double lumen venous cannula in an inadequately sized internal jugular vein (in neonates). In emergent cases, open chest cannulation may be performed with direct access to the right atrium and aorta.

Indications and Contraindications

In patients with severe hypoxemic respiratory failure, the challenge is to select the optimal therapy that maximizes benefit and minimizes risk. Conceptually, like invasive mechanical ventilation, ECMO is a method to support patients while they recover from their underlying illness or insult. As such, ECMO should be reserved for patients with a reversible process, or in cases of end-stage lung disease, patients who can be successfully bridged to lung transplant. In balancing the risks and benefits of ECMO, the toxicity of conventional therapies, the risks of ECMO, and other known comorbidities must be carefully considered.

Traditionally, ECMO has been reserved for respiratory failure refractory to conventional therapy. There is wide variety in the level of conventional support attempted prior to initiating ECMO, however. Much of this variation in ECMO timing may be attributed to differing levels of experience and comfort with ECMO, as well as variable conventional practices and implementation of other rescue therapies. The **Extracorporeal Life Support Organization (ELSO)** has published guidelines recommending initiation of ECMO, once predicted mortality reaches 50% to 80%.[15] In adults, a 50% mortality rate corresponds to a PaO_2/FIO_2 of <150 on FIO_2 >0.9 and/or a Murray score of 2 to 3, while an 80% mortality corresponds to a PaO_2/FIO_2 of <80 on FIO_2 >0.9 and/or a Murray score of 3 to 4.[15,16] Other data in adults demonstrate clear mortality benefit to lung-protective ventilation, keeping tidal volumes ≤6 mL/kg ideal body weight and plateau pressure ≤30 cm H_2O.[5] As such, if clinical goals cannot be met within these lung-protective settings, ECMO should be considered.

Oxygenation index ($[\overline{P}aw \times FIO_2 \times 100]/PaO_2$) is another useful calculation that may guide providers regarding the timing of ECMO initiation in hypoxemic respiratory failure. In contrast to PaO_2/FIO_2, the oxygen index (OI) accounts for the support provided by the ventilator to achieve a particular PaO_2. ELSO recommends initiation of ECMO in neonates between an OI of 20 to 40,[15] and one study found a cutoff of OI ≥33 as an indicator for when the risk of lung injury outweighs the risk of ECMO in neonates.[17] Similar OI values are commonly used as indications for ECMO initiation in children and adults.[18–20]

As the primary purpose of respiratory ECMO is to allow adequate gas exchange while minimizing VILI, it is also important to consider when irreversible lung injury has occurred prior to initiating ECMO. Current guidelines suggest that mechanical ventilation at high settings (FIO_2 >0.9, Pplat >30 cm H_2O) for 7 days or more is a contraindication to ECMO.[15] While more than 7 days of mechanical ventilation has historically been used as an exclusion criteria for ECMO candidacy in many centers, emerging data would suggest that the window of time to initiate ECMO may be increasing, likely due to improved lung-protective ventilation strategies. Recent studies demonstrate the mortality does not significantly increase until at least 10 to 14 days of pre-ECMO mechanical ventilation.[21–23] Because survival may decrease with each additional day of mechanical ventilation prior to ECMO, however,[24,25] identification of patients who will require ECMO early in their disease course is an important goal. Furthermore, the levels of ventilatory support may be more important than actual duration of ventilation as providers attempt to determine reversibility of lung injury.

Direct and indirect lung injuries are not the only indications for respiratory ECMO. ECMO should also be considered for patients with other reversible causes of inadequate gas exchange refractory to conventional

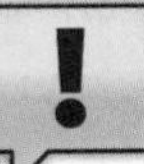

Respiratory Recap

Indications for ECMO for Respiratory Failure

- Severe reversible respiratory failure associated with:
  - Persistent pulmonary hypertension of the newborn
  - ARDS
  - Congenital airway anomalies
  - Status asthmaticus
  - Pulmonary embolism
  - Airway compression due to mediastinal masses
  - Air leak syndromes

management, including status asthmaticus, pulmonary embolism, airway compression due to mediastinal masses, air leak syndromes, persistent pulmonary hypertension of the newborn, and congenital airway anomalies. Many of these disease processes have the best outcomes on ECMO,[12,23,25] as they may not be associated with the multiorgan dysfunction that may be present with hypoxemic respiratory failure and ARDS.

Absolute contraindications to ECMO are rare and relate to the ability to successfully initiate and manage the extracorporeal device. These contraindications may include irreversible coagulopathy and inability to cannulate due to anatomic reasons. As with any medical therapy, futility should also be considered an absolute contraindication to initiation or continuation of ECMO, but determination of futility in the acutely deteriorating patient can be challenging. Known risk factors for poor outcomes in ECMO patients should be considered when estimating disease reversibility and survivability. ELSO suggests preexisting conditions that affect the quality of life as a relative contraindication to ECMO, but many patients with significant nonpulmonary comorbidity can be successfully supported with ECMO.[12] Central nervous system status is an important consideration and severe neurologic injury is commonly considered a contraindication to ECMO.[26] The delineation of severe injury allows a wide range of interpretation, however, and this exclusion is controversial.

A final factor in the decision to initiate ECMO is resource allocation. ECMO is a resource intensive therapy, both in terms of financial cost and manpower. Most centers will be limited regarding the number of ECMO circuits they can run simultaneously. It is therefore imperative that providers consider the likelihood for meaningful survival when assessing patients for ECMO candidacy, and the potential for other patients who, in turn, may require but not be able to receive ECMO.

ECMO Utilization and Outcomes

The first successful utilization of ECMO in 1971 in a young man with trauma-related ARDS demonstrated the promise of this technology. However, the first randomized trial of ECMO in adults in 1979 demonstrated dismal outcomes (10% survival) for both the ECMO and conventional arms.[27] A repeat study 15 years later showed improved survival but still failed to demonstrate a difference between ECMO and conventional management.[28] In the face of these negative studies, ECMO use remained minimal in adults during these early years. Meanwhile, ECMO for neonates with respiratory failure demonstrated very promising outcomes, and the use in this population rapidly increased throughout the 1980s (**Figure 23-2**).

Any complex technology has a steep learning curve to achieve optimal outcomes, and ECMO centers were able to gain key experience during these early years with neonates. Self-limited diseases such as persistent pulmonary hypertension of the newborn and meconium aspiration responded well to ECMO, with survival rates as high as 80% to 90%.[12,29] Randomized trials in neonates supported the mortality advantage and cost effectiveness of ECMO support, and its use slowly spread into the management armamentarium for pediatric respiratory failure. As other conventional therapies such as inhaled nitric oxide and high-frequency ventilation emerged and were able to rescue many neonates and children without ECMO, the population of patients requiring ECMO grew and continues to grow more complex and at higher risk for mortality.[12,23,25,30,31]

Over the last two decades, as providers came to understand the importance of lung-protective ventilation, ECMO conceptually made sense as a therapy for hypoxemic respiratory failure and ARDS. The use of an

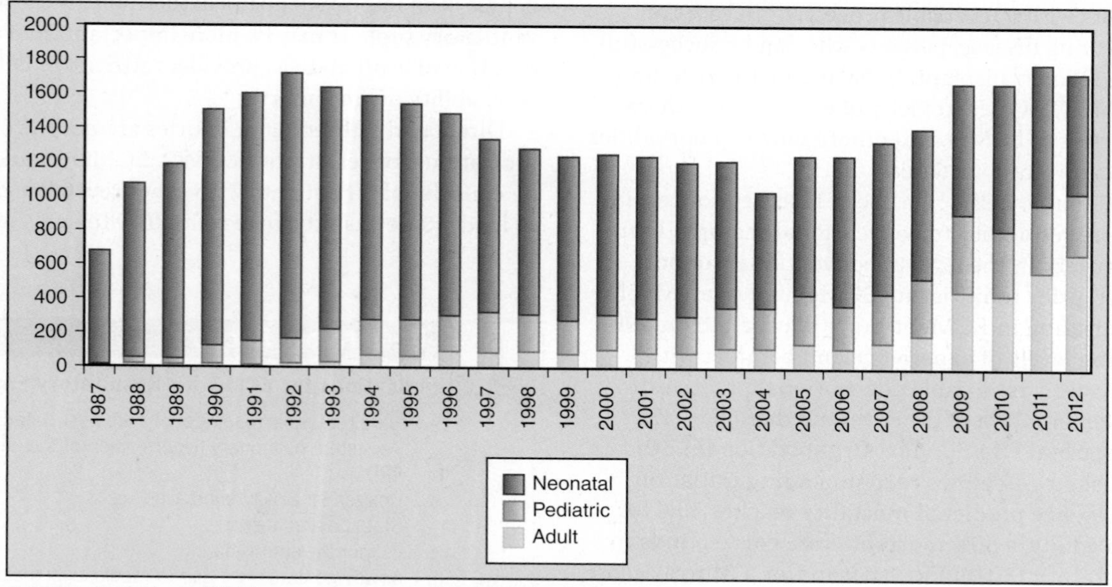

FIGURE 23-2 Yearly ECMO cases reported to the ELSO database, by age group.
Information from *ECLS Registry Report*. Ann Arbor, Mich.: Extracorporeal Life Support Organization; January 2013.

oxygenator as a third lung allows providers to reduce ventilator settings and rest the native lungs, minimizing further VILI. Despite this theoretical advantage of ECMO, there remained a lack of data supporting its widespread use in adults with refractory respiratory failure until very recently, with two simultaneous events changing the outlook for adult respiratory ECMO in the late 2000s. The first was the outbreak of the novel H1N1 influenza virus in 2008 to 2009, which affected an inordinate number of young, healthy adults. Institutions from multiple countries reported survival rates in young adults infected with H1N1 supported with ECMO exceeding 70% in a cohort of patients with a much higher predicted mortality.[20,32,33] The second event was the publication of the Conventional Ventilatory Support versus ECMO for Severe Adult Respiratory Failure (CESAR) trial from the United Kingdom.[34] In this investigation, adult patients with severe respiratory failure were randomized to either transfer to a single ECMO center or to remain at the referral center to receive conventional therapy. This investigation demonstrated an improved disability-free survival at 6 months (63% vs. 47%) for the group randomized to ECMO referral. As is common in ECMO referral centers,[33,35] 18% of the patients randomized to ECMO referral were not supported with ECMO because they were stabilized on conventional therapy.[34] While outcomes were improved, five patients in the ECMO group died before arrival at the ECMO center (3 prior to transport and 2 during transport), demonstrating the challenges in transferring unstable patients between hospitals. Both this randomized trial and the reports of success treating H1N1-related severe ARDS led to a resurgence of interest in adult ECMO. Since that time, there has been a rapid rise in ECMO utilization in adults, with adult ECMO now exceeding neonatal ECMO cases for the first time since it began being used in the 1970s (Figure 23-2).[12]

Cumulative survival for all respiratory ECMO patients is 61%, and survival rates decrease with age.[12,23,25] **Table 23-1** summarizes reported outcomes for the most common respiratory ECMO indications. Several studies have demonstrated a consistent mortality for ECMO patients over time, despite an increasingly complex patient population.[23,25,36] While adult data are limited, when controlling for comorbidities and risk factors, survival for children on ECMO without comorbidities has significantly increased from 57% in 1993 to 72% in 2007.[23] This improved survival is largely due to refinement in techniques and technological advancements.[12,23,25,30,31]

Known pre-ECMO risk factors for poor outcomes include lower pH, higher Pco_2, increased days of mechanical ventilation, and increased age.[23,25] Comorbidities that negatively affect survival include renal failure, liver failure, chronic lung disease, cardiac dysfunction or arrest, and immunodeficiency (primary or acquired).[23] Of particular note, patients with a history of hematopoietic stem cell transplantation who are on ECMO have a less than 5% survival rate.[23]

TABLE 23-1
Reported ECMO Outcomes

Primary Disease	Survival (%)		
	Neonates	Children	Adults
Viral pneumonia	—	64–70	66
Bacterial pneumonia	57	58	61
Aspiration pneumonitis/ pneumonia	—	67	63
Acute respiratory distress syndrome	—	52–60	50–55
Status asthmaticus	—	83	79
Sepsis	75	40–79	45
Primary pulmonary hypertension	77	—	—
Meconium aspiration	94	—	—
Congenital diaphragmatic hernia	51	—	—

— = Data not available.

Patients on VV ECMO consistently have improved survival when compared to patients on VA ECMO, across all indications.[23,25] Some of this survival difference is likely secondary to self-selection for less severely ill patients and/or patients with reasonable cardiac function being supported with VV ECMO. The survival difference is significant, however, with a 5% to 15% mortality advantage of VV ECMO across age groups,[12] and this survival advantage may persist when controlling for severity of illness.[37] It is also important to note that while VV ECMO does not provide any direct cardiac support, data demonstrate similar ability to wean vasopressors for patients on VV ECMO compared to VA ECMO, suggesting that improved oxygen delivery with VV ECMO may improve hemodynamics.[38] Also, VV ECMO patients have lower neurologic complication rates that are likely attributable to the protection of the arterial system and lower risk of arterial thromboembolism with VV ECMO.

Another important population of patients receiving VV ECMO is the group with end-stage lung disease being bridged to lung transplant. These patients have historically had poor outcomes, with high mortality and prolonged hospital stays following lung transplant.[39] These poor outcomes likely result from significant deconditioning that exists in these patients secondary to deep sedation and immobility while on ECMO. Emerging data demonstrate improved outcomes in these patients using a novel awake and ambulatory ECMO strategy.[13,40] In keeping patients awake, the negative effects of sedation and immobility may be

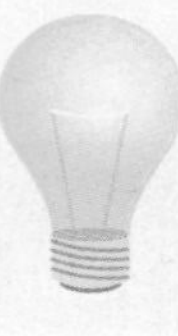

STOP AND THINK

What are the major complications of ECMO? Are these complications directly attributable to the technology, or are they common in patients with respiratory failure?

avoided. These awake patients may also participate in early rehabilitation, which likely contributes to quicker recovery from critical illness.[14,41] While most of these data have been exclusively collected in the population bridging to lung transplant, the lessons learned also have implications for the general respiratory ECMO population.

Complications

ECMO represents a complex system and is certainly not without risk. While some complications, such as bleeding from anticoagulation, are directly related to ECMO, other organ dysfunction makes it difficult to differentiate effects of the patient's overall severity of illness from complications related to ECMO. The most common complications encountered in ECMO patients are summarized in **Table 23-2**.

Bleeding

Bleeding is the most frequent complication in ECMO patients, most commonly at cannulation or other surgical site(s), and is typically manageable with local measures. Bleeding at other sites, including intracranial, gastrointestinal, and pulmonary, is associated with increased morbidity and mortality.[12,25] Significant bleeding may be addressed through administering fresh frozen plasma to replace coagulation factors and maintaining the platelet count above 100,000 per microliter.

Neurologic Injury

Complications involving the central nervous system carry the greatest risk of morbidity and mortality for ECMO patients. Intracranial hemorrhage is the most significant of these complications and often necessitates terminal discontinuation of ECMO. Seizures are often underappreciated neurologic complications of ECMO, particularly in the younger ages. As these seizures may often be subclinical, providers should consider electroencephalogram monitoring for heavily sedated or paralyzed ECMO patients.

Infection

ECMO patients are at risk for infection given their critical illness, ventilator status, and indwelling cannula. Culture proven infections in respiratory ECMO are relatively common (occurring in up to 20% of adult ECMO

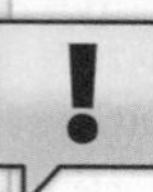

Respiratory Recap

Complications of ECMO

- Bleeding
- Neurologic injury
- Infection
- Multiorgan dysfunction
- Ischemia

cases) and are associated with increased mortality.[12,42,43] Risk factors for infection include increasing age, VA ECMO use, and increased days on ECMO.[42] As intensive care units continue to focus on reducing hospital acquired conditions such as catheter-associated blood stream infection and ventilator-associated pneumonia, however, the incidence of infections appears to be decreasing over time. No data exist to support the use of prophylactic antibiotics for ECMO patients.

Multiorgan Dysfunction

Similar to infection risk, development of multiorgan dysfunction (MOD) in ECMO patients is difficult to delineate from the baseline risk of MOD in patients with severe refractory hypoxic respiratory failure. As with conventional therapies, hepatic and renal dysfunction for patients receiving ECMO are individually associated with increased mortality. Fortunately, the great majority of survivors with renal dysfunction on ECMO will have normal renal function by 6 months.[26]

Ischemia

While limb ischemia is often not a significant issue in VV ECMO patients, when arteries supplying blood flow to limbs are used for VA ECMO, the arterial cannula has the potential to occlude the vessel and create limb ischemia. A distal perfusion cannula or surgical jump graft may be required to perfuse the distal extremity. Similarly, in femoral artery cannulation, the coronaries and head vessels may be primarily perfused by the heart's native ejection rather than by ECMO flow, and therefore may also be at risk for ischemia. If adequate pulmonary venous saturations cannot be achieved through native lung oxygenation, an additional arterial cannula (typically via the axillary artery) may be required to provide oxygenated blood flow to these critical structures.

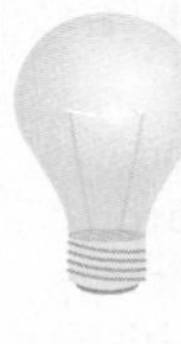

STOP AND THINK

How is an ECMO patient managed differently than a typical patient with respiratory failure? What therapies are beneficial in conjunction with ECMO? How do you know when it is time to discontinue ECMO support?

TABLE 23-2
Complications Associated with ECMO

Complication During ECMO	Neonates		Children		Adult	
	Incidence (%)	Survival (%)	Incidence (%)	Survival (%)	Incidence (%)	Survival (%)
Intracranial hemorrhage	7	44	6	23	4	19
Pulmonary hemorrhage	4	43	8	30	8	36
Cannulation site hemorrhage	7	64	17	52	16	51
Hemorrhage (other)	2–11	39–64	4–17	25–52	4–16	25–43
Circuit clots	3–17	44–67	4–11	45–55	3–12	43–56
Mechanical/ component failure*	0.3–12	53–70	0.4–15	44–53	0.3–15	30–47
Cardiac tamponade	0–0.6	36–55	0.3–2	22–41	0.2–3	47–75
Renal failure (creatinine >3.0 mg/dL)	1	37	4	29	12	41
Infection (culture proven)	6	53	18	46	20	45
Seizures (EEG or clinically determined)	1–9	50–61	2–6	34–38	0.3–1	45

Information from *ECLS Registry Report.* Ann Arbor, Mich.: Extracorporeal Life Support Organization; January 2013.

*Rate of complication varies depending on specific circuit component

Strategic Considerations

While ELSO has published guidelines regarding ECMO management,[15,26] these guidelines primarily focus on broad recommendations and leave ample room for individualization. As such, there is wide variation in utilization of specific ECMO techniques across centers, often with limited data to support many specific strategies. While in-depth management discussion lies outside the scope of this chapter, highlighted here are some of the more common and often controversial topics in ECMO patient management.

Monitoring

Patient monitoring typically includes frequent blood sampling to ensure adequate gas exchange and monitoring of hemoglobin, platelets, and anticoagulation status. Oxygenation measured by arterial blood gas analysis may need to be interpreted with caution in VA ECMO, however, as arterial cannula placement sometimes causes flow streaming and unequal distribution of oxygenated blood to all extremities. In cases of disparate oxygen saturations, systemic oxygen delivery should be assessed using other invasive or noninvasive measures such as mixed venous oxygen saturation or near-infrared spectroscopy. Pump monitoring for clots may include visual inspection of the circuit tubing, cannula, and oxygenator as well as pressure monitoring for increased resistance to flow. The pump must also be checked for integrity of the circuit, including potential sites of air embolus. Other monitoring components may include sonographic flow probes, continuous blood gas analyzers,[44] bubble detectors to identify air embolus, and emergency clamps to stop flow if air is detected.

Anticoagulation

The immune system of the patient will react to the foreign surfaces on the ECMO circuit and trigger the inflammatory response and coagulation cascade.[45–47] As such, the pump must be maintained with systemic anticoagulation and must be monitored closely for clot formation. While ELSO recommends maintaining activated clotting time (ACT) at 1.5 times the normal range, ECMO centers use a number of different techniques to monitor anticoagulation. In addition to following ACTs and activated partial thromboplastin times (aPTTs), other tests that are becoming more commonly used include anti-Factor Xa levels and thromboelastography (TEG).[48,49]

When faced with significant bleeding, providers may also consider lowering anticoagulation goals, balancing the risk of bleeding with that of thrombosis. Data regarding hemorrhagic complications in relation to anticoagulation strategy are limited. Recombinant Factor VII has been used for severe hemorrhage, but also carries significant thrombosis risk, and should be reserved for life-threatening bleeding refractory to other measures.[50,51] Heparin-coated ECMO circuits may also allow providers to use minimal or no heparin for a limited period of time for refractory bleeding or invasive procedures.

Ancillary Therapies

Data are limited regarding use of specific ancillary therapies while patients are on ECMO. The primary role of ECMO is to provide gas exchange while giving the lungs time to recover; other therapies should be directed at the underlying disease process. Unfortunately, there is a paucity of data demonstrating the clinical effectiveness of most ancillary therapies in acute lung injury and ARDS, irrespective of whether ECMO is implemented. Optimizing lung rest therefore should remain the primary focus during ECMO support. While no data support improved outcomes with their use, ancillary therapies such as bronchoscopy and surfactant appear to be safe on ECMO, if clinically indicated.

Timing of ECMO Decannulation

Knowing when to liberate a patient from the ECMO circuit can be an even more difficult decision than the choice to initiate ECMO. The decision to remove a patient from ECMO is a risk–benefit analysis including multiple factors. Crucial considerations include: Has the underlying or initial disease process resolved? Is the patient suffering undue morbidity or complication from ECMO, or is he/she stable without complications?

Mean duration of ECMO support for select disease processes is listed in **Table 23-3**. These values provide only an estimate of the time a specific patient may require ECMO support, however. Outcomes for repeat courses of ECMO are predictably poor,[23] so it is generally preferable to remove a patient from ECMO on less than maximal support. Similarly, the avoidance of VILI that is the primary advantage of ECMO may be negated if the patient is transitioned from ECMO to toxic ventilator settings. Finally, if it becomes clear that the patient has no meaningful chance of survival, then the only ethical choice is to discontinue ECMO rather than continue to provide futile care.

TABLE 23-3
Mean Duration of Support for Common ECMO Indications

	Mean ECMO Run (Days)		
Primary Disease	**Neonates**	**Children**	**Adults**
Viral pneumonia	—	13	12
Bacterial pneumonia	10	11.5	10
Aspiration pneumonitis/ pneumonia	—	11.5	8
Acute respiratory distress syndrome	—	12.5	11.5
Sepsis	6	—	—
Primary pulmonary hypertension	6	—	—
Meconium aspiration	5.5	—	—
Congenital diaphragmatic hernia	10.5	—	—

— = Data not available.

Information from *ECLS Registry Report*. Ann Arbor, Mich.: Extracorporeal Life Support Organization; January 2013.

Technological Advancements

The state of the art in ECMO technology has benefited from several recent advancements in key circuit components. These advancements in oxygenators, circuit pumps, and cannulas have led to a decrease in mechanical complications and failures in the modern era.[52]

Roller-head pumps, previously the standard for most ECMO centers, are being increasingly replaced with centrifugal pumps.[12,52] Roller-head pumps are large mechanical pumps that create a higher risk for circuit rupture than centrifugal pumps due to direct mechanical shear on the circuit tubing. Newer centrifugal (or axial) pumps use a magnetic impeller to drive flow, resulting in smaller pumps, lower priming volumes, and quicker setup times (**Figure 23-3**). Some data also suggest that these axial pumps may cause less red blood cell shear and hemolysis.[53,54]

Newer cannulas and circuit tubing are often coated with a heparin or heparin-like substance that helps mediate the inflammatory response from serum exposure to artificial surfaces as well as reduce the risk of clotting and factor deposition on these surfaces. Each of these actions may allow for less systemic anticoagulation and might assist with reduced blood product administration.

Other cannula advancements include the development of percutaneously placed ECMO cannula and new double lumen cannula with directional outflow. Older

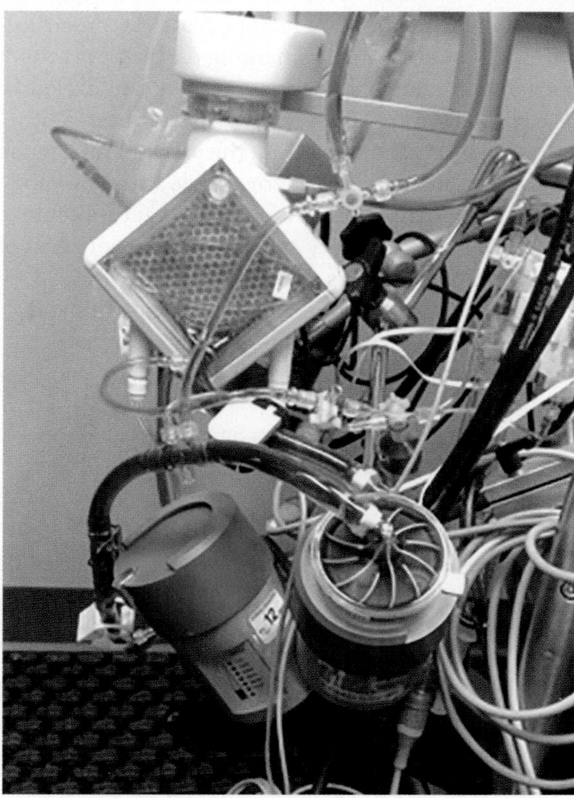

FIGURE 23-3 Saline primed centrifugal pump and oxygenator.

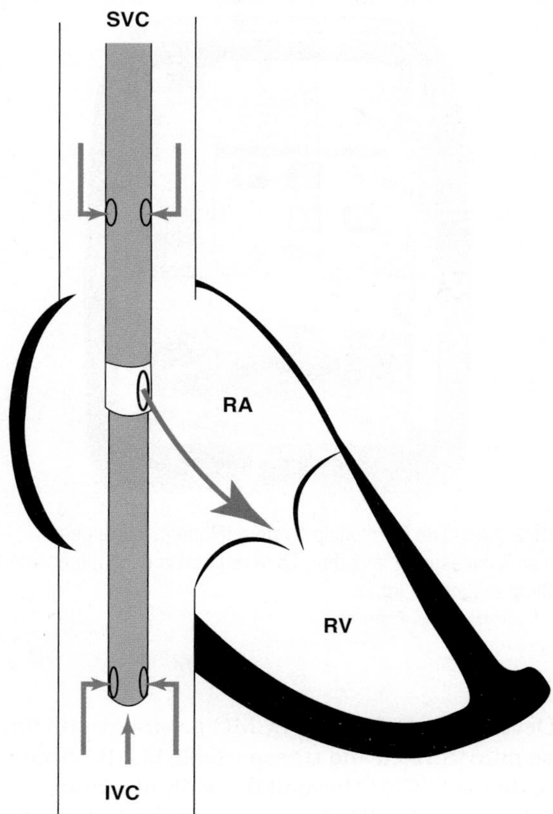

FIGURE 23-4 Example of a double lumen venovenous ECMO cannula. The oxygenated blood returning from the ECMO circuit is directed toward the tricuspid valve, allowing for higher flow rates with minimal recirculation (reuptake of oxygenated blood into venous ports).

versions of dual lumen cannulas commonly demonstrated recirculation, in which the oxygenated blood retuning from the ECMO pump would drain into the venous ports before it could pass into the pulmonary circulation. This incidence of recirculation commonly limited dual lumen cannula use to infants and young children. Newer cannulas direct the flow returning to the patient toward the tricuspid valve, dramatically reducing the risk of recirculation and allowing for single-site, dual lumen cannula use in adolescents and adults (**Figure 23-4**). To ensure return flow is correctly directed at the tricuspid valve, these cannulas are often placed with assistance of echocardiography or fluoroscopy.

First generation silicone oxygenators required large fill volumes, were slow to prime, caused a significant inflammatory response, and had limited life spans. The newest generation of polymethylpentene hollow-fiber oxygenators have improved flow characteristics, rapid priming times, superior gas exchange, reduced inflammatory response, and lengthened life spans.[55,56] All of these technical advances contribute to safer, lower-maintenance, and more efficient ECMO circuits. Certainly, the technology will rapidly progress over the next few years, continuing to expand the utility and adaptability of ECMO for a wide range of clinical scenarios.

ECMO Transport

The technological advances in recent years have also led to the development of smaller and miniaturized ECMO circuits (**Figure 23-5**) that have been successfully used to transport patients between hospitals.[55–57] Due to the resources needed to run an ECMO program, support with ECMO remains largely limited to large hospitals and regional referral centers. Emerging data suggest that regionalization of ECMO care to high-volume centers may also provide a mortality advantage.[58] Patients with refractory respiratory failure may present to any hospital, however, and these patients may face a high risk of mortality during transport to the closest ECMO center. The two patients in the CESAR trial who died during transport highlight this danger.[34]

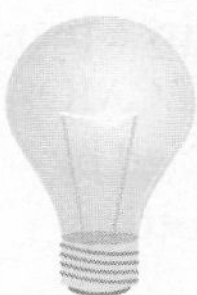

STOP AND THINK

How might extracorporeal support for respiratory failure change in the next few years?

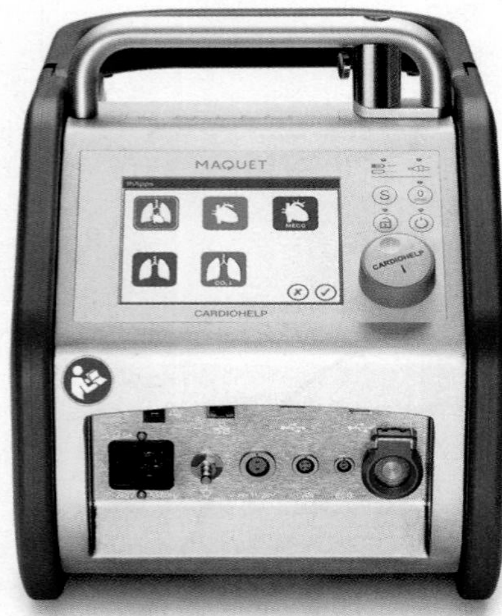

FIGURE 23-5 The Cardiohelp System (Maquet, Hirrlingen, Germany), measuring less than 18 in (50 cm) in each dimension and weighing around 10 kg.
Courtesy of Maquet Medical Systems.

Development of mobile ECMO programs utilizing these miniaturized and transportable ECMO circuits has extended ECMO beyond the walls of tertiary care centers. Critically ill patients can now be placed on ECMO at the referring center, stabilized, and then transferred for continued management. In some transport models, the receiving center will send a team of ECMO specialists to perform the cannulation. This model of ECMO stabilization prior to transport is supported by data demonstrating few complications during these transports.[59–61] It is likely that the number of centers offering mobile ECMO will continue to increase over the next several years.

Expectations for the Coming Years

Despite its importance in the management of respiratory failure, much of ECMO management is unfortunately driven by experience and anecdotal evidence. The vast majority of published literature consists of retrospective reviews and small single center trials.[62] As such, significant variability in practice exists in ECMO management. Increased standardization of ECMO, both within and across centers, is needed to better assess, study, and define those key strategic variables that can drive improved patient outcomes.[63]

A key example of practice variability driven by a paucity of data is anticoagulation management for ECMO patients. Traditionally, anticoagulation was guided by activated clotting time, a test of whole blood clotting accounting for coagulation factors, platelets, procoagulants, and anticoagulants. Emerging data support the consideration of other tests that may better correlate to the patient's anticoagulation status, however. With these conflicting data regarding the optimal testing for anticoagulation, currently there is wide variability to anticoagulation management on ECMO across centers.[64] Considering the frequency and potential seriousness of bleeding and thrombosis as a complication of ECMO, research into optimal anticoagulation strategies and subsequent standardization of this process across centers will be crucial to reducing bleeding and thrombosis complications.

Technological advancements have continued to make ECMO safer, easier to use, and more flexible in its application. Undoubtedly, advancements in oxygenators, pumps, cannulas, circuitry, and monitoring equipment will continue to drive ECMO use and improve outcomes. Other forms of extracorporeal respiratory support also are beginning to see increasing use in respiratory failure. The **pumpless extracorporeal lung assist (PECLA)** device uses an oxygenator attached to the patient's arterial and venous systems. Instead of pumping blood through the oxygenator from the venous system to the arterial, this device uses the patient's own arterial pressure as the driving force for blood flow through the pump and then returning the blood to the venous system. When compared to VV ECMO, PECLA devices have decreased gas exchange and are associated with increased cardiac work,[65] making their use limited to hemodynamically stable patients with respiratory failure. Experience with this device in patients with ARDS has demonstrated inferior outcomes to ECMO, with reported survival of 33% to 45%.[66,67] The simplicity of the device has generated interest for select populations, however, including its use as an adjunct to avoid mechanical invasive ventilation altogether.[68]

Another strategy of low-flow extracorporeal carbon dioxide removal, commonly referred to as **respiratory dialysis**, mimics VV ECMO in its use of a double lumen catheter to remove the patient's blood, pass the blood through a gas exchanger, and return it to the patient. Limited data with respiratory dialysis demonstrate adequate carbon dioxide removal to avoid invasive mechanical ventilation in chronic obstructive pulmonary disease (COPD) patients failing noninvasive mechanical ventilation.[69] Both respiratory dialysis and the PECLA device support lower flow rates than traditional ECMO[65] and are therefore more useful for carbon dioxide removal than oxygenation. Each of these novel devices require further study to determine safety and efficacy for respiratory failure.

Recent years have brought increasing recognition of the deleterious effects of sedation and immobility of ICU patients. In the same manner that ECMO may be used to avoid VILI, there is a growing body of literature demonstrating the use of awake and ambulatory ECMO to avoid the long-term morbidities associated with intubation, sedation, and ICU deconditioning.[13,14,40,41,70] While much of this work has been done in the context of patients being bridged to lung transplant, it is almost certain that the future will bring increased utilization of this strategy to avoid non-ventilator-associated morbidities in other ECMO patients.

One controversy that remains to be answered is the optimal time to initiate ECMO. While ECMO is almost exclusively used as support for refractory respiratory failure, some have questioned if ECMO should be considered earlier in the course of ARDS.[71] Given the advantages of lung protection provided with ECMO and the mortality of increased ventilation days prior to ECMO, it is reasonable to theorize that earlier application of ECMO may benefit patients with severe hypoxemic respiratory failure. This concept is supported by the improved functional outcomes seen in ECMO patients during the randomized CESAR trial. The debate is further compounded by the emerging data around awake ECMO, which in some cases is used to avoid intubation and invasive mechanical ventilation altogether. It remains unclear at what point the risks of invasive mechanical ventilation outweigh the risks of ECMO, however, and how best to identify the subset of patients with respiratory failure who would most greatly benefit from early application of ECMO.

Key Points

- ECMO acts as a third lung to augment gas exchange in patients with respiratory failure.
- VV ECMO is the preferred modality for patients with respiratory failure.
- ECMO use for adult respiratory failure is steadily increasing, likely secondary to support from a randomized controlled trial and favorable outcomes during a worldwide viral pandemic.
- Predictors of ECMO mortality include increasing age, multiorgan dysfunction, and culture proven infections.
- Indications for ECMO associated with improved survival include viral pneumonia and status asthmaticus.
- Bleeding is the most common complication related to ECMO, and further research is ongoing to determine optimal anticoagulation strategies.
- Technological advancements have made ECMO safer, easier, and more versatile.
- There remains a paucity of data to clarify optimal ECMO management strategies.
- Mobile ECMO is becoming more common as a way to stabilize and transport critically ill respiratory failure patients between hospitals.
- Awake and ambulatory ECMO shows promise as a method to avoid critical-illness-related weakness and long-term morbidity and represents a method to rehabilitate end-stage respiratory failure patients for lung transplant.
- There is growing interest in using ECMO and other extracorporeal forms of gas exchange earlier in the course of ARDS, potentially even to avoid invasive mechanical ventilation.

References

1. Ferguson ND, Cook DJ, Guyatt GH, et al. High-frequency oscillation in early acute respiratory distress syndrome. *N Engl J Med.* 2013;368:795–805.
2. Young D, Lamb SE, Shah S, et al. High-frequency oscillation for acute respiratory distress syndrome. *N Engl J Med.* 2013;368: 806–813.
3. Santa Cruz R, Rojas JI, Nervi R, et al. High versus low positive end-expiratory pressure (PEEP) levels for mechanically ventilated adult patients with acute lung injury and acute respiratory distress syndrome. *Cochrane Database Syst Rev.* 2013;6:CD009098.
4. Griffiths RD, Hall JB. Intensive care unit-acquired weakness. *Crit Care Med.* 2010;38:779–787.
5. Ventilation with lower tidal volumes as compared with traditional tidal volumes for acute lung injury and the acute respiratory distress syndrome. The Acute Respiratory Distress Syndrome Network. *N Engl J Med.* 2000;342:1301–1308.
6. Gajic O, Dara SI, Mendez JL, et al. Ventilator-associated lung injury in patients without acute lung injury at the onset of mechanical ventilation. *Crit Care Med.* 2004;32:1817–1824.
7. Plataki M, Hubmayr RD. The physical basis of ventilator-induced lung injury. *Expert Rev Respir Med.* 2010;4:373–385.
8. Alhazzani W, Alshahrani M, Jaeschke R, et al. Neuromuscular blocking agents in acute respiratory distress syndrome: a systematic review and meta-analysis of randomized controlled trials. *Critical Care.* 2013;17:R43.
9. Roch A, Hraiech S, Dizier S, Papazian L. Pharmacological interventions in acute respiratory distress syndrome. *Ann Intensive Care.* 2013;3:20.
10. Willson DF, Thomas NJ, Tamburro R, et al. Pediatric calfactant in acute respiratory distress syndrome trial. *Pediatr Crit Care Med.* 2013;14:657–665.
11. Daoud EG, Farag HL, Chatburn RL. Airway pressure release ventilation: what do we know? *Respir Care.* 2012;57:282–292.
12. *ECLS Registry Report.* Ann Arbor, Mich.: Extracorporeal Life Support Organization. Available at http://www.elso.org/index.php?option=com_content&view=article&id=68&Itemid=435. Accessed July 27, 2014.
13. Fuehner T, Kuehn C, Hadem J, et al. Extracorporeal membrane oxygenation in awake patients as bridge to lung transplantation. *Am J Respir Crit Care Med.* 2012;185:763–768.
14. Turner DA, Cheifetz IM, Rehder KJ, et al. Active rehabilitation and physical therapy during extracorporeal membrane oxygenation while awaiting lung transplantation: a practical approach. *Crit Care Med.* 2011;39:2593–2598.
15. ELSO Patient Specific Guidelines. Available at http://www.elsonet.org/. Accessed November 11, 2013.

16. Murray JF, Matthay MA, Luce JM, Flick MR. An expanded definition of the adult respiratory distress syndrome. *Am Rev Respir Dis.* 1988;138:720–723.
17. Bayrakci B, Josephson C, Fackler J. Oxygenation index for extracorporeal membrane oxygenation: is there predictive significance? *J Artif Organs.* 2007;10:6–9.
18. Smalley N, MacLaren G, Best D, Paul E, Butt W. Outcomes in children with refractory pneumonia supported with extracorporeal membrane oxygenation. *Intensive Care Med.* 2012;38:1001–1007.
19. Trachsel D, McCrindle BW, Nakagawa S, Bohn D. Oxygenation index predicts outcome in children with acute hypoxemic respiratory failure. *Am J Respir Crit Care Med.* 2005;172:206–211.
20. Turner DA, Rehder KJ, Peterson-Carmichael SL, et al. Extracorporeal membrane oxygenation for severe refractory respiratory failure secondary to 2009 H1N1 influenza A. *Respir Care.* 2011;56:941–946.
21. Mehta NM, Turner D, Walsh B, et al. Factors associated with survival in pediatric extracorporeal membrane oxygenation—a single-center experience. *J Pediatr Surg.* 2010;45:1995–2003.
22. Nehra D, Goldstein AM, Doody DP, et al. Extracorporeal membrane oxygenation for nonneonatal acute respiratory failure: the Massachusetts General Hospital experience from 1990 to 2008. *Arch Surg.* 2009;144:427–432; discussion, 432.
23. Zabrocki LA, Brogan TV, Statler KD, et al. Extracorporeal membrane oxygenation for pediatric respiratory failure: survival and predictors of mortality. *Crit Care Med.* 2011;39:364–370.
24. Nance ML, Nadkarni VM, Hedrick HL, et al. Effect of preextracorporeal membrane oxygenation ventilation days and age on extracorporeal membrane oxygenation survival in critically ill children. *J Pediatr Surg.* 2009;44:1606–1610.
25. Brogan TV, Thiagarajan RR, Rycus PT, et al. Extracorporeal membrane oxygenation in adults with severe respiratory failure: a multi-center database. *Intensive Care Med.* 2009;35:2105–2114.
26. ELSO General Guidelines. Available at http://www.elsonet.org. Accessed July 27, 2014.
27. Zapol WM, Snider MT, Hill JD, et al. Extracorporeal membrane oxygenation in severe acute respiratory failure. A randomized prospective study. *JAMA.* 1979;242:2193–2196.
28. Morris AH, Wallace CJ, Menlove RL, et al. Randomized clinical trial of pressure-controlled inverse ratio ventilation and extracorporeal CO_2 removal for adult respiratory distress syndrome. *Am J Respir Crit Care Med.* 1994;149:295–305.
29. Bahrami KR, Van Meurs KP. ECMO for neonatal respiratory failure. *Semin Perinatol.* 2005;29:15–23.
30. Rehder KJ, Turner DA, Bonadonna D, et al. State of the art: strategies for extracorporeal membrane oxygenation in respiratory failure. *Expert Rev Respir Med.* 2012;6:513–521.
31. Rehder KJ, Turner DA, Bonadonna D, et al. Technological advances in extracorporeal membrane oxygenation for respiratory failure. *Expert Rev Respir Med.* 2012;6:377–384.
32. Davies A, Jones D, Bailey M, et al. Extracorporeal membrane oxygenation for 2009 influenza A(H1N1) acute respiratory distress syndrome. *JAMA.* 2009;302:1888–1895.
33. Noah MA, Peek GJ, Finney SJ, et al. Referral to an extracorporeal membrane oxygenation center and mortality among patients with severe 2009 influenza A(H1N1). *JAMA.* 2011;306:1659–1668.
34. Peek GJ, Mugford M, Tiruvoipati R, et al. Efficacy and economic assessment of conventional ventilatory support versus extracorporeal membrane oxygenation for severe adult respiratory failure (CESAR): a multicentre randomised controlled trial. *Lancet.* 2009;374:1351–1363.
35. Patroniti N, Zangrillo A, Pappalardo F, et al. The Italian ECMO network experience during the 2009 influenza A (H1N1) pandemic: preparation for severe respiratory emergency outbreaks. *Intensive Care Med.* 2011;37:1447–1457.
36. Fliman PJ, deRegnier RA, Kinsella JP, et al. Neonatal extracorporeal life support: impact of new therapies on survival. *J Pediatr.* 2006;148:595–599.
37. Skinner SC, Iocono JA, Ballard HO, et al. Improved survival in venovenous vs venoarterial extracorporeal membrane oxygenation for pediatric noncardiac sepsis patients: a study of the Extracorporeal Life Support Organization registry. *J Pediatr Surg.* 2012;47:63–67.
38. Roberts N, Westrope C, Pooboni SK, et al. Venovenous extracorporeal membrane oxygenation for respiratory failure in inotrope dependent neonates. *ASAIO J.* 2003;49:568–571.
39. Organ Procurement and Transplantation Network Data Reports. Available at: http://optn.transplant.hrsa.gov/data. Accessed July 26, 2014.
40. Rehder KJ, Turner DA, Hartwig MG, et al. Active rehabilitation during extracorporeal membrane oxygenation as a bridge to lung transplantation. *Respir Care.* 2013;58:1291–1298.
41. Olsson KM, Simon A, Strueber M, et al. Extracorporeal membrane oxygenation in nonintubated patients as bridge to lung transplantation. *Am J Transplant.* 2010;10:2173–2178.
42. Bizzarro MJ, Conrad SA, Kaufman DA, Rycus P. Infections acquired during extracorporeal membrane oxygenation in neonates, children, and adults. *Pediatr Crit Care Med.* 2011;12:277–281.
43. Aubron C, Cheng AC, Pilcher D, et al. Infections acquired by adults who receive extracorporeal membrane oxygenation: risk factors and outcome. *Infect Control Hospital Epidemiol.* 2013;34:24–30.
44. Schreur A, Niles S, Ploessl J. Use of the CDI blood parameter monitoring system 500 for continuous blood gas measurement during extracorporeal membrane oxygenation simulation. *J Extra Corpor Technol.* 2005;37:377–380.
45. Oliver WC. Anticoagulation and coagulation management for ECMO. *Semin Cardiothorac Vasc Anesth.* 2009;13:154–175.
46. Peek GJ, Firmin RK. The inflammatory and coagulative response to prolonged extracorporeal membrane oxygenation. *ASAIO J.* 1999;45:250–263.
47. Vallhonrat H, Swinford RD, Ingelfinger JR, et al. Rapid activation of the alternative pathway of complement by extracorporeal membrane oxygenation. *ASAIO J.* 1999;45:113–114.
48. Khaja WA, Bilen O, Lukner RB, et al. Evaluation of heparin assay for coagulation management in newborns undergoing ECMO. *Am J Clin Pathol.* 2010;134:950–954.
49. Nankervis CA, Preston TJ, Dysart KC, et al. Assessing heparin dosing in neonates on venoarterial extracorporeal membrane oxygenation. *ASAIO J.* 2007;53:111–114.
50. Dunne B, Xiao P, Andrews D. Successful use of factor VIIa to control life-threatening post-operative haemorrhage in a patient on extra-corporeal membrane oxygenation. *Heart Lung Circ.* 2012;21:229–230.
51. Syburra T, Lachat M, Genoni M, Wilhelm MJ. Fatal outcome of recombinant factor VIIa in heart transplantation with extracorporeal membrane oxygenation. *Ann Thorac Surg.* 2010;89:1643–1645.
52. Sivarajan VB, Best D, Brizard CP, et al. Improved outcomes of paediatric extracorporeal support associated with technology change. *Interact Cardiovasc Thorac Surg.* 2010;11:400–405.
53. Curtis JJ, Walls JT, Wagner-Mann CC, et al. Centrifugal pumps: description of devices and surgical techniques. *Ann Thorac Surg.* 1999;68:666–671.
54. Lawson DS, Ing R, Cheifetz IM, et al. Hemolytic characteristics of three commercially available centrifugal blood pumps. *Pediatr Crit Care Med.* 2005;6:573–577.
55. Horton S, Thuys C, Bennett M, et al. Experience with the Jostra Rotaflow and QuadroxD oxygenator for ECMO. *Perfusion.* 2004;19:17–23.
56. Peek GJ, Killer HM, Reeves R, et al. Early experience with a polymethyl pentene oxygenator for adult extracorporeal life support. *ASAIO J.* 2002;48:480–482.
57. Roch A, Hraiech S, Masson E, et al. Outcome of acute respiratory distress syndrome patients treated with extracorporeal membrane oxygenation and brought to a referral center. *Intensive Care Med.* 2014;40:74–83.
58. Freeman CL, Bennett TD, Casper TC, et al. Pediatric and neonatal extracorporeal membrane oxygenation: does center volume impact mortality? *Crit Care Med.* 2014;42:512–519.
59. Forrest P, Ratchford J, Burns B, et al. Retrieval of critically ill adults using extracorporeal membrane oxygenation: an Australian experience. *Intensive Care Med.* 2011;37:824–830.

60. Coppola CP, Tyree M, Larry K, DiGeronimo R. A 22-year experience in global transport extracorporeal membrane oxygenation. *J Pediatr Surg.* 2008;43:46–52; discussion, 52.
61. Foley DS, Pranikoff T, Younger JG, et al. A review of 100 patients transported on extracorporeal life support. *ASAIO J.* 2002;48:612–619.
62. Rehder KJ, Turner DA, Cheifetz IM. Extracorporeal membrane oxygenation for neonatal and pediatric respiratory failure: an evidence-based review of the past decade (2002–2012). *Pediatr Crit Care Med.* 2013;14:851–861.
63. Dalton HJ, Dodge-Khatami A, MacLaren G. Pediatric mechanical circulatory support: future directions. *Pediatr Crit Care Med.* 2013;14(suppl 1):S94–S95.
64. Bembea MM, Annich G, Rycus P, et al. Variability in anticoagulation management of patients on extracorporeal membrane oxygenation: an international survey. *Pediatr Crit Care Med.* 2013;14:e77–84.
65. Kopp R, Bensberg R, Wardeh M, et al. Pumpless arterio-venous extracorporeal lung assist compared with veno-venous extracorporeal membrane oxygenation during experimental lung injury. *Br J Anaesth.* 2012;108:745–753.
66. Florchinger B, Philipp A, Klose A, et al. Pumpless extracorporeal lung assist: a 10-year institutional experience. *Ann Thorac Surg.* 2008;86:410–417; discussion, 417.
67. Nierhaus A, Frings D, Braune S, et al. Interventional lung assist enables lung protective mechanical ventilation in acute respiratory distress syndrome. *Minerva Anestesiol.* 2011;77:797–801.
68. Kluge S, Braune SA, Engel M, et al. Avoiding invasive mechanical ventilation by extracorporeal carbon dioxide removal in patients failing noninvasive ventilation. *Intensive Care Med.* 2012;38:1632–1639.
69. Mani RK, Schmidt W, Lund LW, Herth FJ. Respiratory dialysis for avoidance of intubation in acute exacerbation of COPD. *ASAIO J.* 2013;59:675–678.
70. Malagon I, Greenhalgh D. Extracorporeal membrane oxygenation as an alternative to ventilation. *Curr Opin Anaesthesiol.* 2013;26:47–52.
71. Checkley W. Extracorporeal membrane oxygenation as a first-line treatment strategy for ARDS: is the evidence sufficiently strong? *JAMA.* 2011;306:1703–1704.

CHAPTER

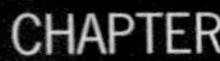

24 Pulmonary Rehabilitation

Neil R. MacIntyre, Rebecca H. Crouch

OUTLINE

OBJECTIVES

1. Define pulmonary rehabilitation.
2. List the team members that comprise a pulmonary rehabilitation program.
3. Compare intensive programs, maintenance programs, and perioperative programs.
4. Identify candidates for a pulmonary rehabilitation program.
5. Describe the components of patient assessment in a comprehensive pulmonary rehabilitation program.
6. Describe the role of education in a pulmonary rehabilitation program.
7. Discuss the benefits of upper and lower extremity exercise training in a pulmonary rehabilitation program.
8. Explain the guidelines used to prescribe an exercise training program.
9. Discuss the roles of the following in a pulmonary rehabilitation program: respiratory therapies, psychological therapies, physical therapy, individualized instruction, nutrition counseling, and pharmacologic therapy.

KEY TERMS

breathing retraining
chronic lung disease
exercise assessment
exercise capacity
exercise training
exertional dyspnea
healthcare utilization
intensive program
maintenance program
perioperative program
pulmonary rehabilitation
Rating of Perceived Exertion (Modified Borg Scale)

Introduction

Comprehensive **pulmonary rehabilitation** is a concept that has evolved steadily over the last 50 years.[1–4] Prior to that time, the standard therapy for patients with **chronic lung disease** was rest and avoidance of physical activity. In the early 1960s, however, studies challenged this standard therapy by demonstrating that exercise training in patients with chronic obstructive pulmonary disease (COPD) not only resulted in training effects similar to those observed in normal subjects but also promoted a state of well-being.[5–9] Numerous investigations followed that supported these initial findings. Almost universally, the early investigations supported three conclusions:

1. Exercise training in patients with COPD increases **exercise capacity**.
2. Exercise training improves the patient's psychological state.
3. Exercise training *does not* improve pulmonary function.

As a consequence of these developments, the American College of Chest Physicians (ACCP) in 1974 and the American Thoracic Society (ATS) in 1981 both formally recognized the effectiveness of pulmonary rehabilitation and offered the following definition:

Pulmonary rehabilitation can be defined as an art of medical practice wherein an individually tailored multidisciplinary program is formulated, which, through accurate diagnosis, therapy, emotional support, and education, stabilizes or reverses both the physio- and psychopathology of pulmonary diseases and attempts to return the patient to the highest possible functional capacity allowed by his pulmonary handicap and overall life situation.[1]

Since the 1970s, there has been a steady growth in the number of pulmonary rehabilitation programs. These programs have become increasingly multidisciplinary and comprehensive, incorporating psychological, nutritional, and vocational support; oxygen therapy; bronchial hygiene; education; and exercise.[4,10,11] Along with this growth has come the development of professional societies (e.g., the American Association of Cardiovascular and Pulmonary Rehabilitation [AACVPR]), professional standards, accreditation and certification programs, and ongoing efforts to obtain proper third-party reimbursement.[1–4,11]

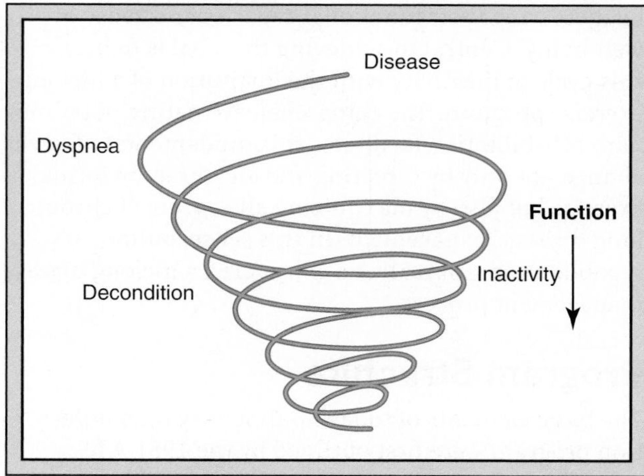

FIGURE 24-1 The downward spiral of functional loss induced by lung disease and accelerated by resulting inactivity.

Mechanisms of Functional Deterioration in Patients with Chronic Lung Disease

Much of the research on functional deterioration in chronic lung disease has been done in patients with chronic obstructive pulmonary disease (COPD).[12] In these patients, unlike cardiac patients, there is a long, slow, downhill course often punctuated by acute exacerbations. The underlying chronic inflammation of COPD progressively damages lung tissue and airways and, over a period of years, ultimately results in a depletion of ventilatory reserves.[12] Complicating this physiologically are abnormalities in gas exchange and elevations in pulmonary vascular pressures that lead to right ventricular dysfunction. Finally, data have demonstrated that an ongoing systemic inflammatory process from COPD can impair skeletal muscle function.[13,14] All these factors contribute to the sensation of dyspnea and the resultant limitation on physical activity.

As dyspnea and exercise capacity worsen, the need for medical care increases and the patient's ability for self-care decreases; a confusing combination of functional limitations, complex medical regimens, and dependence on others is thrust on the patient. The net effect is a profound sense of loss of control, with consequent depression and anxiety.

These factors are further worsened by the vicious cycle of inactivity (**Figure 24-1**). The cycle begins when the patient starts to associate **exertional dyspnea** with the disease and no longer recognizes dyspnea as a normal response to exertion. In this setting, exertional dyspnea promotes increased levels of anxiety, depression, and fear of exertion, all of which generally lead to an exertion phobia and a reduction in physical activity. The lack of exercise, in turn, leads to both central and peripheral deconditioning and, ultimately, to decreased endurance and weakness, and often to muscular atrophy.[13,14] As a result of deconditioning, the patient experiences greater dyspnea, an even greater intolerance to exertion, and further loss of functional capacity. As the cycle continues, the patient's exercise capacity spirals progressively downward while the levels of fear, anxiety, and depression increase unabated. As the patient becomes progressively more physically and psychologically incapacitated, the consumption of medical resources increases dramatically. The progressive loss of exercise capacity resulting from the vicious cycle of inactivity is superimposed on the underlying functional reduction caused by the lung disease.

Other chronic lung diseases (e.g., interstitial lung disease, pulmonary hypertension), while operating through different pathophysiologic mechanisms and at different disease trajectories, produce similar deteriorations in functional impairment over time. Because of this, non-COPD patients are being increasingly referred for pulmonary rehabilitation.[15–23]

The goal of pulmonary rehabilitation is to improve the quality of life of patients with chronic lung disease

Respiratory Recap

Pulmonary Rehabilitation

- Pulmonary rehabilitation is a multidisciplinary, multifaceted approach to chronic lung disease management.
- Pulmonary rehabilitation has been endorsed by all of the major respiratory societies.

Respiratory Recap

Goal of Pulmonary Rehabilitation

- Functional loss in chronic lung disease is multifactorial and involves respiratory dysfunction as well as cardiovascular, skeletal muscle, and metabolic factors.
- The goal of pulmonary rehabilitation is to improve functional capacity by addressing all of these factors.

by increasing their functional capacity and sense of well-being. Central to achieving this goal is to break this cycle of inactivity with the institution of a lifelong exercise program. The comprehensive nature of pulmonary rehabilitation facilitates this fundamental lifestyle change not only by directing and encouraging formal exercise but also by maximizing all aspects of chronic lung disease management. In this sense, pulmonary rehabilitation can really be considered a lifelong disease management process.

Program Structure

The basic elements of today's pulmonary rehabilitation program were first outlined by the 1981 ATS statement on pulmonary rehabilitation[1] and later formalized in the AACVPR guidelines and program certification process.[4,11] Even within these established guidelines, however, the potential exists for diversity in the structure of pulmonary rehabilitation programs. This potential diversity results from consideration of several factors at the time the pulmonary rehabilitation program is under development, including the patient population, the available physical facilities, and the available pool of health professionals.

The pulmonary rehabilitation team is usually a multidisciplinary team that consists of a pulmonary physician and a number of other health professionals that can include respiratory therapists, physical therapists, psychologists, nutritionists, occupational therapists, social workers, and pulmonary nurses, among others. Although this implies the necessity for a large, diverse team, the recommended services for pulmonary rehabilitation may be provided by far fewer personnel if the individuals are appropriately trained in the evaluation and management of pulmonary disease patients. The ultimate provider of the essential services depends on the health professionals available to the program and the size of the facility and will likely vary from program to program.

Pulmonary rehabilitation programs often provide at least two types of programs: a short-term intensive program that provides an intense focus on pulmonary rehabilitation; and a long-term maintenance program that is less time consuming.

> **Respiratory Recap**
>
> **Pulmonary Rehabilitation Programs**
>
> - Pulmonary rehabilitation programs are based on exercise training, education, and psychosocial support.
> - Pulmonary rehabilitation is a lifelong process, with formal programs usually being either several weeklong intensive programs or lifelong maintenance programs.
> - In recent years, pulmonary rehabilitation programs focusing on perioperative patients have emerged.

Intensive Programs

Intensive programs generally provide two to five sessions per week for periods of 4 to 12 weeks. The emphasis of the intensive program is on exercise training, education, medication optimization, bronchial hygiene, and psychosocial support. In addition to respiratory therapists and physical therapists, healthcare specialists who contribute regularly to the program through the educational component could include a clinical pharmacist, a nutritionist, a pulmonary nurse clinician, an occupational therapist, and a psychosocial counselor. Individual consultations with specialists in nutrition, psychology, and smoking cessation are common. The intense focus of this program produces recognized benefits sooner than less intensive programs—a factor that enhances patient motivation.

Maintenance Programs

Maintenance programs serve primarily as medically supervised facility- or home-based programs for pulmonary disease patients who reside locally. Enrollment is usually limited to patients who have successfully completed the intensive program. Programs are generally open daily, and participants select their own schedules. Although program emphasis is on exercise conditioning, all intensive program services are available to these participants as needed. Long-term social interaction with peers and the formation of support groups are major advantages of the maintenance program.

Perioperative Programs

In recent years, another type of program has emerged in some centers that focuses on the perioperative management of patients receiving lung cancer surgery, lung volume reduction surgery, or lung transplantation.[15,16,18,19,22–25] In **perioperative programs**, the preoperative period functions much like the intensive program described above and is designed to optimize a patient's functional status and education prior to surgery. In the postoperative period, these programs are designed to restore and improve function as the patient recovers from the surgery.

The Process of Pulmonary Rehabilitation

Patient Selection

Any patient with stable chronic respiratory disease who is symptomatic and experiences dyspnea on exertion should be considered a candidate for pulmonary rehabilitation. In addition, candidates must be free of acute illness (including unstable medical conditions such

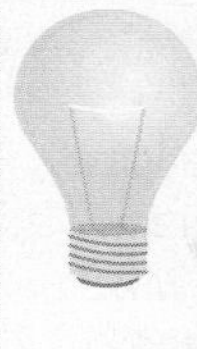

STOP AND THINK

You are caring for a patient with COPD who is considering enrolling in a pulmonary rehabilitation program. He asks you what is involved in the program. How would you respond?

as ischemic coronary disease) and motivated to lead a more active life.

The clinical description of patients who potentially may benefit from pulmonary rehabilitation has broadened over the years. In the original position statement published by the ATS in 1981, the section on patient selection mentioned only patients with COPD.[1] Recent evidence, however, has demonstrated that multidisciplinary pulmonary rehabilitation programs are also of value in the management of patients with restrictive and other pulmonary diseases.[15,17,20,25] These findings should encourage acceptance of patients with non-COPD pulmonary diseases as well as those with COPD into pulmonary rehabilitation programs.

The observation that patients with limited ventilatory capacity may be unable to exercise with sufficient intensity to receive a training effect has raised concern over whether they could derive benefits from a comprehensive pulmonary rehabilitation program. Although evidence of a true training effect in this group of patients remains controversial, at a minimum they can benefit from a program designed to improve coordination, muscle strength, functional activities, and a state of well-being. Even exercise capacity may be improved in patients with limited ventilatory capacity, because the standard training effect is only one of several ways in which exercise capacity is known to increase.[6,14,26]

Concern that exercise might precipitate respiratory failure by overloading weakened respiratory muscles leads to speculation that exercise training might be contraindicated in hypercapnic COPD patients. It has been shown, however, that hypercapnic COPD patients with severe ventilatory impairment and respiratory muscle weakness tolerate exercise and benefit significantly from intensive pulmonary rehabilitation.[5–8] Similarly, exercise hypoxemia has been considered by some to be a contraindication to an exercise program. Appropriate supplemental oxygen and proper monitoring (e.g., oximetry), however, allow such patients to participate fully in all aspects of the exercise program.[27] Finally, concerns about cardiac dysrhythmias and right ventricular dysfunction in patients with pulmonary hypertension have often limited participation of these patients in pulmonary rehabilitation. Recent data, however, suggest that appropriate exercise strategies (see below) and proper monitoring can allow pulmonary hypertension patients to benefit from pulmonary rehabilitation.[17]

Despite the broadening of criteria for participation in pulmonary rehabilitation, it appears only the minority of eligible patients are entering programs.[28,29] Moreover, many who enter programs fail to finish.[29] One approach to increasing pulmonary rehabilitation usage has been to use the teachable moment of an acute exacerbation to introduce the concept of pulmonary rehabilitation and the associated disease management features of the program.[30]

Patient Assessment

A comprehensive patient evaluation is essential to attaining the goals of pulmonary rehabilitation and is the foundation on which the individually tailored program is constructed. Any condition or attitude that potentially limits the patient's ability to perform desired activities or grasp essential information must be identified by the healthcare team, assessed, and ultimately addressed. All members of the rehabilitation team are vital participants in the process of gathering and evaluating information from patient questionnaires, interviews, and a variety of clinical evaluations.

The first step in this assessment is to make an accurate diagnosis of the patient's pulmonary problem and any complicating medical problems. The diagnosis should be substantiated by history, physical examination, pulmonary function testing (especially spirometry), and, as needed, chest roentgenograph and other laboratory tests. Other diseases or medical problems that may have a potential impact on the rehabilitation process also must be identified. These include rhinitis/sinusitis, hypertension, gastrointestinal conditions, and arrhythmias or coronary artery disease. Other potentially complicating diseases include diabetes, obesity, osteoporosis, and stroke. Once proper diagnoses are made, an appropriate medication regimen can be established.

Exercise assessment is a critical component of participants prior to entering a rehabilitation program. These assessments perform two functions: they quantitate the level of disability and provide information for setting initial exercise loads (see below) and program expectations, and they provide insight into the various cardiorespiratory factors that are involved in the functional disabilities. This permits focused therapies to be done. For instance, detecting exercise hemoglobin oxygen desaturation would lead to oxygen therapy, detecting exercise bronchospasm would lead to better bronchodilator therapy, and detecting exercise cardiac dysrhythmias would prompt a more thorough cardiovascular exam.

In the Duke University program, symptom-limited maximal exercise assessment for many years was often performed on incoming pulmonary rehabilitation patients.[26] Over the years, these tests have detected hemoglobin oxygen desaturation with exercise in 34% of patients. In the non-oxygen-requiring patients, ventilation limitations (exercise ventilation/maximal ventilatory volume >0.7 or rising Pa_{CO_2}) were present in 27%, and cardiovascular limitations (maximum heart rate >80% of predicted maximum) were present in 37%. These data illustrate the wide variety of physiologic derangements of these patients and the importance of designing exercise therapy regimens appropriate to the patient's limitations.

More recently, walk tests, especially 6-minute walk tests (6MWT), have become the method of choice to assess exercise capacity both before and after pulmonary rehabilitation.[31] The 6MWT is simple to perform at the rehabilitation site and walk distance is closely linked to functional performance. In addition, heart rate, pulse oximetry, blood pressure, perceived exertion, and ventilation response can all be assessed during the test.

Because psychological disturbances are common in patients with chronic lung disease, psychosocial assessment is important prior to participation in a pulmonary rehabilitation program.[32–34] The most common emotional consequences of COPD are depression and anxiety, which can further reinforce social isolation and inactivity. Cognitive function has also been shown to be impaired in these patients, perhaps as a consequence of chronic hypoxemia. Medications and psychotherapy can be provided as necessary.

Other assessments necessary prior to beginning pulmonary rehabilitation include physical therapy evaluations, nutritional evaluations, occupational therapy evaluations (especially activities of daily living), and an educational assessment for the patient's knowledge and understanding of the disease process and its management. A particularly important assessment is tobacco usage. Although it is reasonable to allow current smokers to participate in a rehabilitation program, formal efforts should be made to persuade the patient to discontinue smoking through participation in smoking cessation-counseling sessions with program staff. These may be done on either an individual or group basis.

Education

A primary purpose of the educational component of pulmonary rehabilitation is to provide the framework for self-care. Through an educational process of instruction, supervision, and practice, patients can acquire an awareness of their disease and its management that allows them to take responsibility for their own care. A spouse, family member, or close friend who participates in the educational activities can provide familial understanding of the disease process and can reinforce the recommended self-care techniques in the home setting.

The educational process usually consists of a combination of lectures, discussions, demonstrations, and practice sessions.[35] During all program activities, the patient's knowledge and ability to perform self-management techniques are continually reinforced. Topics typically covered in formal lectures and discussion sessions include the anatomy and physiology of the lung, the pathophysiology of chronic lung disease, pulmonary medications, nutrition, physiologic responses to exercise, sexual concerns, travel concerns, coping with chronic lung disease, early recognition and management of infections and exacerbations, and psychosocial issues.

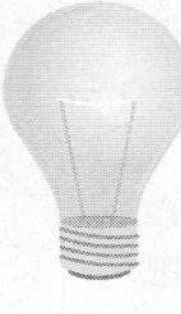

STOP AND THINK

You are asked to provide patient education as part of a pulmonary rehabilitation program. What information would you cover and what strategies would you use to maximize the effectiveness of your teaching?

Medication management is a critical component of the educational process. The array of inhaled medication options can be bewildering to patients. This bewilderment is further amplified by the complexity of aerosol delivery systems associated with proprietary medications. Considerable education time may be required to ensure that patients have a good working knowledge of their medication regimens.

Another key educational component is the management of COPD exacerbations.[36–38] The cost of treating exacerbations is the single most expensive aspect of caring for the COPD patient. Importantly, patients can be taught to recognize signs and symptoms of an exacerbation developing. An action plan under these circumstances can include transient increased dosing of bronchodilators, prompt initiation of antibiotics, and pulse steroid therapy. Aborting an exacerbation early can lead to reduced need for hospitalizations and a faster return to baseline function.

Respiratory therapy and physical therapy techniques are more appropriately presented in either individual or group demonstrations and in practice sessions. These topics include cleaning and care of equipment; proper use of metered dose inhalers and spacers; stress management; and supplemental oxygen therapy. Airway clearance techniques may include instruction in controlled coughing, postural drainage, percussion, vibration, and the use of vibratory positive end pressure devices and vest therapy to facilitate secretion mobilization. Educational material in the form of pamphlets, booklets, and books are available from a multitude of sources, including various websites and the American Lung Association. This additional information should be used to support and reinforce the information the patient receives in the lectures, discussions, and demonstrations.

Breathing retraining traditionally has been a key aspect of the educational component of a pulmonary rehabilitation program.[4,35] Pursed-lip breathing, diaphragmatic breathing, and paced breathing are commonly used concomitantly to reduce shortness of breath and improve gas exchange. By using pursed-lip breathing, patients may be able to maintain adequate oxygenation without supplemental oxygen.

The success of the program's educational process may be assessed by providing testing on didactic information before and after instruction and by requiring each patient to satisfactorily demonstrate the recommended management techniques.

Exercise

In general, the **exercise training** experience provided by the pulmonary rehabilitation program should expose the patient to a balance of three types of exercise: stretching and flexibility exercises, strengthening exercises, and endurance exercises. Stretching and flexibility exercises are usually part of a floor exercise routine that improves range of motion and helps provide a general warm-up. Strength training may be obtained as part of the floor exercise routine by performing exercises with dumbbells, cuff weights, or a stretch band. Pulmonary patients also do well with free weights and weight machines for strength training. Strengthening exercises for the pulmonary population should be prescribed at lower weights and higher repetitions initially. General endurance training involves exercises that produce a cardiopulmonary stress that results in elevated heart rate (HR) and ventilation. Such exercises include walking, rowing, swimming, water aerobics, cycling (arm or leg), and stair climbing. Endurance training is of lower intensity and higher frequency. Interval training, with higher work intensities alternating with rest breaks, results in lower perceived exertion scores and improved exercise continuity while demonstrating comparable exercise training to continuous endurance training.[39]

The benefits of exercise training are, for the most part, specific to the muscles and tasks involved in training.[4–7,40] For instance, a walking program will produce significant improvement in walking performance but not in swimming or biking performance. It is important, therefore, to consider the particular mode of exercise in conjunction with the needs and goals of the patient. If a patient has a stated goal that requires improvement in stair climbing, this should be one of the modes of exercise in the prescription. Walking is generally considered an essential exercise because of its prevalence in daily activities; probably for that reason, most exercise training prescriptions use predominantly lower extremity exercises.

Many patients with chronic airway obstruction experience marked shortness of breath when they use their arms for even simple tasks. Arm exercise may contribute to the dyspnea by contributing to ventilatory muscle fatigue, by placing a load on an already stressed system, and by placing a nonventilatory demand on shoulder girdle muscles that have been recruited to act as accessory muscles of respiration. Improvement in upper extremity function as a result of specific upper extremity exercises has been demonstrated in patients with COPD.[4,40]

Improvement in upper extremity function has been observed to carry over to self-care, leisure, and other arm activities. Combining arm and leg exercises in a training program for patients with chronic airway obstruction has been shown not only to increase exercise performance in both upper and lower extremities but also to significantly improve patients' state of well-being, which was greater in the combined training than in either arm or leg training alone.[4,40]

Upper extremity exercise training may be accomplished through activities that use the arms at or above shoulder height (e.g., passing an object overhead) or gravity-resistive exercises (e.g., lifting objects to chest level or overhead and walking a short distance). Upper extremity strength training may be achieved by performing exercises with free weights, pulley systems, or weight machines. Arm endurance training may be accomplished with an arm ergometer, rowing machine, combined arm/leg bicycle, or cross-country ski machine.

Well-established guidelines exist for prescribing the intensity of endurance exercise for normal subjects as well as for cardiac patients. These guidelines are based on target exercise heart rates expressed as a percentage of the predicted maximum HR. Application of these guidelines, however, may not always be appropriate to pulmonary patients because gas exchange and/or ventilatory impairments may prevent the patient from reaching the predicted maximum HR.[6,7,41]

The initial load prescription should be of sufficiently low intensity that it can be accomplished by the patient without discomfort. Nothing destroys a patient's motivation faster than failure to complete the initial exercise or experiencing significant discomfort during or after the first exercise session. Should a symptom-limited stationary bicycle Graded Exercise Test (GXT) be performed prior to program entry, the initial exercise prescription workloads are normally based on the maximum workloads achieved during the test. The Duke University Pulmonary Rehabilitation Program uses 50% to 80% of the maximum watts achieved for the stationary bicycle workload prescription and 30% to 40% for the arm ergometer prescription.

Other approaches to determine the exercise prescription are often based on perceived physical exertion and breathing effort (dyspnea). Perceived physical exertion and breathing effort are commonly quantified using the Modified Borg Scale, a visual analogue scale easy for patients to understand (**Figure 24-2**).[42] Because this scale is used to rate both perceived physical exertion and breathing effort, it is important to instruct the patient on the difference. We have found that separating perceived physical exertion

0	Nothing at all
0.5	Very, very light
1	Very light
2	Fairly light
3	Moderate
4	Somewhat hard
5	Hard
6	
7	Very hard
8	
9	
10	Very, very hard (maximal)

FIGURE 24-2 The Modified Borg Scale for Rating of Perceived Exertion or breathing effort (dyspnea).

and breathing effort allows a more complete assessment of patient difficulties when performing exercise and allows therapies to be more focused. In general, if perceived physical exertion and breathing effort fall between 4 and 6 on the Modified Borg Scale, the patient's effort and exercise prescription are considered adequate.

The exercise prescription in pulmonary patients must also take into account the cardiac response (i.e., heart rate) and oxygenation status. Work from Cassaburi and colleagues suggests that training intensity should be pushed to a training effect (i.e., up to 70% to 80% predicted maximal heart rate) if at all possible.[7] Even patients with ventilatory or gas exchange limitations who cannot reach these target heart rates also appear to benefit from higher rather than lower levels of exercise, however. Finally, all exercise training should be performed under conditions of adequate arterial oxygenation (Pao_2 >55 mm Hg, Spo_2 >88%).[3,4] This ensures both patient safety as well as allows the otherwise hypoxemic patient to exercise for a longer duration at a higher intensity, enhancing the beneficial effects of the exercise. If the initial patient assessment has determined that the resting oxygenation is low or that significant desaturation occurs with exertion, supplemental oxygen must be provided to the patient to maintain adequate oxygen saturation. This may require complex mask and oxygen reservoir systems in patients with severe exercise hypoxemia. When adequate oxygenation cannot be maintained, either the intensity of the exercise must be reduced or the patient must be instructed to stop exercising until oxygenation is again adequate. An interesting additional application for supplemental oxygen may be in patients who have some degree of rest or exercise hemoglobin desaturation but who do not fall to critical levels that impair cardiac function or oxygen delivery (i.e., they remain above Pao_2 values of 60 mm Hg or Spo_2 values above 90%). In this group, oxygen therapy will have little impact on cardiac function or oxygen delivery but may reduce carotid body (i.e., oxygen receptor) output, thereby reducing dyspnea and allowing exercise training at a higher level.[27] This concept needs further study.

The recommended minimum duration and frequency of endurance exercise is no less than 20 minutes three times per week.[3,4] Increasing the duration and frequency beyond this minimum must take into consideration the motivation and goals of the patient, and balance the time spent in training against the benefits derived from a more intense, and less frequent, training regimen.

When transitioning from lower initial loads to higher target loads, the Modified **Rating of Perceived Exertion (Modified Borg Scale)** is used as a measure of perceived stress, and the exercise heart rate and oxygen saturation as a measure of cardiopulmonary stress.[20] Using these parameters, if the patient is capable of performing a given load for the duration of the exercise session (e.g., 20 minutes), the Modified Borg Scale values are <4, the heart rate is <80% predicted maximum, and the oxygen saturation is at an acceptable level, the load is increased for 3 to 5 minutes to the next highest workload, and then reduced to the previous workload for the remainder of the prescribed time. This pattern of advancement is repeated at graduated intervals until the patient is able to achieve the higher workload for the prescribed time period (e.g., 20–30 minutes). To encourage improvement in ambulation endurance, patients may be given a distance goal within a predetermined amount of time or a simple time goal (e.g., one-half mile in 20 minutes or ambulate without rest stops for 30 minutes). After approximately six exercise sessions, most patients will have attained an exercise level representing a high percentage of the target workload.

Whenever the patient experiences significant symptoms of fatigue or dyspnea, instead of stopping exercise, the load is reduced, or the patient is allowed to take a rest break and encouraged to complete the exercise following a recuperation period. The duration of the rest period is considered part of the exercise period. The short-term goal then becomes reducing the number and length of rest breaks during the exercise period.

Other Interventions

Other focused interventions often depend on the individual patient. Patients with clinically important depression or anxiety may need focused psychological therapies; patients with orthopedic impairments may benefit from physical therapy; patients with specific educational needs (e.g., medication understanding, equipment operation, airway clearance procedures)

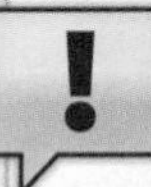

Respiratory Recap

The Process of Pulmonary Rehabilitation

- Patients appropriate for pulmonary rehabilitation are those with stable chronic lung disease and resulting functional impairment.
- Patient assessment should include a general physical exam, a medication review, an exercise assessment, a psychosocial assessment, and a search for comorbidities that would impair exercise training.
- Program content should include comprehensive educational services (e.g., lectures, demonstrations, practice sessions), intensive exercise training (with careful monitoring), psychosocial support sessions, and the availability of consultative services such as psychosocial counseling and nutrition.

may need individualized instruction; patients with nutritional issues may need nutrition counseling.

Physician review of the medication regimen is particularly important. Chronic medical therapy for COPD and other chronic lung diseases is constantly evolving, and the array of medications (e.g., short- and long-acting beta agonists, short- and long-acting anticholinergics, inhaled and oral steroids, oxygen) can be very confusing to chronically ill patients. As noted previously, patients should also be instructed on an action plan in the event of an exacerbation.

Outcomes from a Pulmonary Rehabilitation Program

In 1997, the ACCP/AACVPR published a landmark comprehensive evidence-based review on the effectiveness of pulmonary rehabilitation.[43] Ten years later, over 1000 new publications were reviewed, and recommendations were updated.[4] In 2010, the Canadian Thoracic Society Clinical Practice Guideline for Optimizing Pulmonary Rehabilitation for Chronic Obstructive Pulmonary Disease added to the body of knowledge and recommendations for pulmonary rehabilitation.[44] Moreover, the widely referenced Global Obstructive Lung Disease (GOLD) Initiative has been publishing updated evidence-based recommendations, with the most recent in 2014.[40] In the GOLD report, conclusions and recommendations were graded on the strength of the evidence: Grade A conclusions were based on scientific evidence provided by well-designed, well-conducted, controlled trials with statistically significant and consistent findings. Grade B conclusions were based on scientific evidence provided by randomized controlled trials with less consistent results. Grade C conclusions were based on observational trials and nonrandomized trials. Grade D conclusions were based on expert opinions or consensus groups because

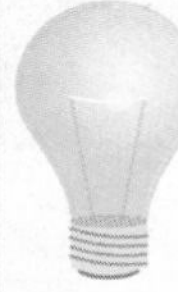

STOP AND THINK

You recommend pulmonary rehabilitation for a patient with COPD. The patient's physician asked what is the evidence to support this. How would you respond?

available scientific evidence did not present consistent results or evidence was lacking.

Evidence supporting the benefits of exercise training in chronic lung disease is compelling and received Grade A (lower extremity) and Grade B (upper extremity) support in the most recent GOLD review.[40] Lower extremity exercise programs consistently improved walk distance and maximal workload in all studies reviewed. Proposed mechanisms of improvement include improved aerobic capacity (in those who can reach cardiovascular training levels), increased motivation, desensitization to the sensation of dyspnea, improved ventilatory muscle function, and improved techniques of performance. Data from upper extremity exercise programs were less extensive but did support the concept that upper extremity exercise might improve the thoracic cage muscles of ventilation and improve activities of daily living.[40] Finally, exercise aimed only at inspiratory muscle training is less compelling and resulted in only a Grade B from GOLD.[40]

Evidence supporting the effectiveness of pulmonary rehabilitation in reducing dyspnea also received a Grade A rating in the GOLD report.[40] This was a consistent finding using any number of dyspnea grading scales (e.g., visual analogue scales, baseline dyspnea index, transitional dyspnea index, other respiratory questionnaires). The mechanisms of reduced dyspnea are no doubt multifactorial but would include better exercise tolerance (and reduced ventilation for a given load), better breathing patterns, better medications, and a better comprehension by the patient of his or her disease and how it can be effectively managed.[45]

Many studies have demonstrated that improved psychosocial function occurs as a result of pulmonary rehabilitation.[32–35] Much of this benefit may come from improved exercise tolerance, reduced dyspnea, informal patient support groups and interactions, and a better understanding of the disease process and management by the patient. Indeed, the recent GOLD report gave a Grade A rating for the evidence supporting reduced anxiety and depression in COPD from pulmonary rehabilitation. Little evidence, however, supports a routine formal psychosocial component in a pulmonary rehabilitation program. This should not be interpreted as evidence stating that psychosocial support through less formal processes is unimportant or that selected patients would not benefit from focused therapies or medications, however.

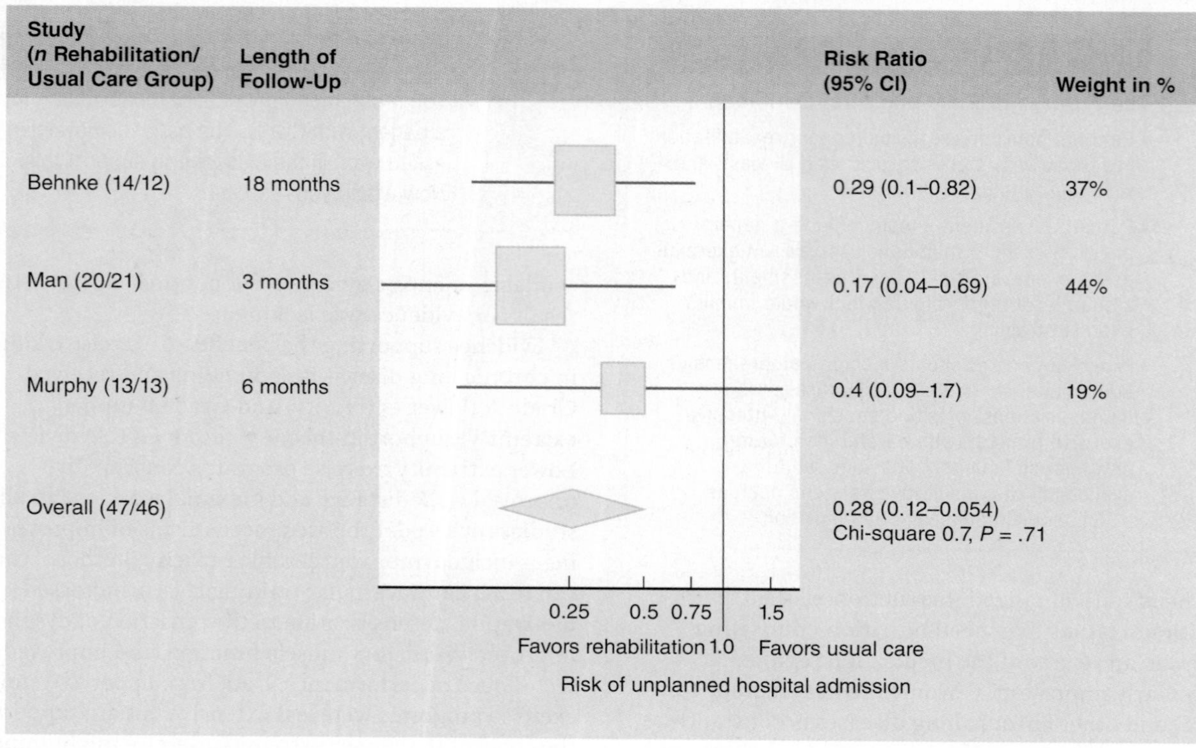

Study
(n Rehabilitation/
Usual Care Group)
Length of
Follow-Up
Risk Ratio
(95% CI)
Weight in %
Behnke (14/12)
18 months
0.29 (0.1–0.82)
37%
Man (20/21)
3 months
0.17 (0.04–0.69)
44%
Murphy (13/13)
6 months
0.4 (0.09–1.7)
19%
Overall (47/46)
0.28 (0.12–0.054)
Chi-square 0.7, P = .71
0.25
0.5 0.75
1.5
Favors rehabilitation 1.0
Favors usual care
Risk of unplanned hospital admission

FIGURE 24-3 A meta-analysis depicting significant reductions in exacerbations of COPD from pulmonary rehabilitation.
Reproduced from Puhan MA, Scharplatz M, Troosters T, et al. *Respir Res.* 2005;6:54. © 2005 licensee BioMed Central Ltd. Courtesy of Milo A. Puhan, Johns Hopkins Bloomberg School of Public Health.

Quality of life (QOL) indicators have consistently shown benefit from pulmonary rehabilitation. Recent evidence has raised this to a Grade A rating in the GOLD report.[40] Like improvements in dyspnea and psychosocial function, the mechanisms for improved QOL following pulmonary rehabilitation are probably multifactorial.

An important benefit of pulmonary rehabilitation is a reduction in **healthcare utilization** and costs. Several recent trials supporting this concept have resulted in a Grade A rating by the GOLD report (**Figure 24-3**).[36–38,40]

Finally, evidence supporting a survival benefit for pulmonary rehabilitation is largely inferential.[46] This potential effect thus only received a Grade B rating in the GOLD report.[40] This should not be surprising, because the goals of pulmonary rehabilitation are not to reverse the disease process but rather to improve the patient's functional capabilities within the constraints of the reduced lung function.

> **Respiratory Recap**
>
> **Outcomes of Pulmonary Rehabilitation**
>
> - A growing body of evidence supports that pulmonary rehabilitation improves exercise tolerance, dyspnea, and quality of life and reduces healthcare costs.
> - Evidence-based reviews have all given this growing evidence base the highest ratings.

Recording and reporting outcomes is increasingly important in today's healthcare environment. To this end the American Association of Cardiovascular and Pulmonary Rehabilitation has published a useful approach to measuring and recording important outcomes from pulmonary rehabilitation.[47]

The outcome benefits noted earlier are largely evaluated at the conclusion of short-term programs (i.e., up to 12 weeks). Important questions remain involving the durability of these benefits over time and the role (if any) of maintenance programs in preserving beneficial effects.[48–50] Long-term studies are few and show variable patterns with some maintaining improved function and others deteriorating.[51,52] Continued adherence to regular exercise can forestall this deterioration, but adherence can be difficult in a chronic disease that is punctuated by exacerbations and the development or worsening of comorbidities.[29,51–54] Interestingly, despite functional loss, QOL benefits from pulmonary rehabilitation appear more durable.[50] Refresher programs, regular maintenance programs, and even simple routine follow-up encouragement phone calls may help,[48–55] although none of these approaches has been well studied.

Reimbursement Issues

Obtaining proper reimbursement for pulmonary rehabilitation is an ongoing challenge. Until recently in the United States, pulmonary rehabilitation was not a specifically identified Medicare benefit and thus funding programs had to be done as incident to physician services. This led to considerable ambiguity and variability in reimbursement rules around the United States. In 2003, the National Emphysema Treatment Trial evaluating lung volume reduction surgery (partially funded by Medicare) required perioperative pulmonary rehabilitation.[24,25] This opened the doors to three new Medicare G billing codes that were used for a number of years to fund many programs. In 2010, pulmonary rehabilitation was finally added as an official Medicare benefit, which provides opportunities for more appropriate levels of reimbursement both from Medicare and other third parties, who often follow Medicare practices. Under these new rules the billing code is G0424 for a session of pulmonary rehabilitation. This code represents a bundled service (including physician supervision) and can be used a maximum of twice daily. One session must be >30 minutes of exercise in duration, two sessions on the same day must be >90 minutes of exercise in duration. Importantly, this new billing code applies only to patients with moderate to severe COPD at the present time. Pulmonary rehabilitation services for patients with other lung diseases and mild COPD must still be billed using other strategies including physical therapy billing codes (CPT series) or respiratory therapy billing codes (G0237, G0238, G0239).

Future Directions

While pulmonary rehabilitation has clearly been shown to improve outcomes in many patients with chronic lung disease, much still remains to be done for it to reach its full potential as a comprehensive disease management strategy. To this end, important efforts going forward are aimed at enhancing access and developing adjuncts to promote exercise in the most limited of patients.

As noted above, only a small fraction of chronic lung disease patients actually enroll in pulmonary rehabilitation programs. To reduce barriers, programs are now focusing on patient-centered operations including convenient program locations, operating hours, and reimbursement support. In addition, programs are being integrated into in-hospital early mobility programs, discharge planning processes, established disease management programs, and home-based operations.[56,57] Even with the best of operations, however, a persistent challenge is convincing patients of the benefit of committing to the concept of lifelong pulmonary rehabilitation. Aggressive marketing, enlisting family support, developing financial rewards, and taking advantage of teachable moments like acute exacerbation episodes can all help in this regard.

There are also interesting developments designed to assist exercise in the most severely debilitated patients. High-flow nasal oxygen devices provide a means to greatly enrich inspired O_2 through a comfortable nasal cannula in patients with severe hypoxemia.[58] These devices also likely reduce dead space and can provide a small amount of continuous positive airway pressure to assist in oxygenation. Unfortunately, the need for a heated humidifier limits the portability of these devices, but future designs will likely address this. Noninvasive ventilation has been used as a technique to unload (rest) ventilatory muscles at night in order to assist patients who have ventilatory limits to exercise.[59] Unfortunately, these devices are cumbersome and often uncomfortable and thus are difficult to use during an exercise session. Addressing these limitations has been the development of a novel wearable ventilator that can attach to the patient's belt. This device delivers positive pressure breaths through a comfortable nasal interface using a clever entrainment system linked to a small portable source of O_2.[60] Finally, in the most severe patients, usually on a wait list for lung transplant, the use of venovenous extracorporeal oxygenation systems can allow ambulation and other exercises.[61]

Both scientific rationale and abundant clinical evidence support physiologic and psychological mechanisms that explain the functional benefits derived from pulmonary rehabilitation. Incorporating these principles into structured programs has repeatedly been shown to improve exercise tolerance and quality of life and reduce the healthcare costs associated with chronic lung disease. Indeed, pulmonary rehabilitation is actually a form of comprehensive disease management. All of the important professional societies have endorsed these concepts. However, regulatory and political barriers persist for proper reimbursement. Continued political advocacy is required to ensure access to these important services for all patients limited by chronic lung disease.

Key Points

- Pulmonary rehabilitation programs are comprehensive and multidisciplinary.
- The goal of pulmonary rehabilitation is to improve quality of life and increase functional capacity and sense of well-being.
- Individuals with stable chronic respiratory disease who are symptomatic, experience dyspnea on exertion, are free from acute illness, and are motivated to lead a more active life are candidates for a pulmonary rehabilitation program.
- Patient education and self-care are critical components of a pulmonary rehabilitation program.
- Exercise training generally entails the enhancement of upper and lower extremity function.
- In the establishment of an exercise training prescription, the initial load should be of sufficiently low intensity that the patient can accomplish it without undue discomfort.
- Both rationale and evidence exist for consideration of physiologic and psychological mechanisms for the functional benefits derived from pulmonary rehabilitation.

References

1. American Thoracic Society. ATS official statement: pulmonary rehabilitation. *Am Rev Respir Dis.* 1981;124:663–666.
2. Ries AL. Position paper of the American Association of Cardiovascular and Pulmonary Rehabilitation: scientific basis of pulmonary rehabilitation. *J Cardiopulm Rehabil.* 1990;10:418–441.
3. Nici I, Donner C, Wouters E, et al. American Thoracic Society/European Respiratory Society statement on pulmonary rehabilitation. *Am J Respir Crit Care Med.* 2006;173:1390–1413.
4. Ries AL, Bauldoff GS, Carlin BW, et al. Pulmonary rehabilitation: joint ACCP/AACVPR evidence-based clinical practice guidelines. *Chest.* 2007;131(Suppl 5):4S–42S.
5. Belman MJ. Exercise in patients with COPD. *Thorax.* 1993;48: 936–946.
6. Ries AL, Archibald CJ. Endurance exercise training at maximal targets in patients with chronic obstructive pulmonary disease. *J Cardiopulm Rehabil.* 1987;7:594–601.
7. Cassaburi R, Petessio A, Ioli F, et al. Reductions in exercise lactic acidosis and ventilation as a result of training in patients with obstructive lung disease. *Am Rev Respir Dis.* 1991;143:9–18.
8. Lacasse Y, Wong E, Guyatt GH, et al. Meta-analysis of respiratory rehabilitation in COPD. *Lancet.* 1996;348:1115–1119.
9. O'Donnell DE, McGuire M, Samis L, et al. The impact of exercise reconditioning on breathlessness in severe chronic airflow limitation. *Am J Respir Crit Care Med.* 1995;152(6 pt 1):205–213.
10. Nici L, Raskin J, Rochester C, et al. Pulmonary rehabilitation: what we know and what we need to know. *J Cardiopulm Rehabil.* 2009;29:141–151.
11. Reis AL. ACCP/AACVPR evidence-based guidelines for pulmonary rehabilitation. *J Cardiopulm Rehabil.* 2007;27:233–236.
12. Mannino DM. The natural history of chronic obstructive pulmonary disease. *Pneumonol Alergol Pol.* 2011;79:139–143.
13. MacIntyre NR. Muscle dysfunction associated with COPD. *Respir Care.* 2006;51:840–848.
14. American Thoracic Society and European Respiratory Society Task Force. Skeletal muscle dysfunction in chronic obstructive pulmonary disease. A statement of the American Thoracic Society and European Respiratory Society. *Am J Respir Crit Care Med.* 1999;159:S1–S40.
15. Foster S, Thomas HM III. Pulmonary rehabilitation in lung disease other than chronic obstructive pulmonary disease. *Am Rev Respir Dis.* 1990;141:601–604.
16. Bradley A, Marshall A, Stonehewer L, et al. Pulmonary rehabilitation programme for patients undergoing curative lung cancer surgery. *Eur J Cardiothoracic Surg.* 2013;44:2266–2271.
17. Zafrir B. Exercise training and rehabilitation in pulmonary arterial hypertension: rationale and current data evaluation. *J Cardiopulm Rehabil Prev.* 2013;33:263–273.
18. Florian J, Rubin A, Mattiello R, et al. Impact of pulmonary rehabilitation on quality of life and functional capacity in patients on waiting lists for lung transplantation. *J Bras Pneumol.* 2013;39:349–356.
19. Sterzi S, Cesario A, Cusumano G, et al. Post-operative rehabilitation for surgically resected non-small cell lung cancer patients: serial pulmonary functional analysis. *J Rehabil Med.* 2013;45:911–915.
20. Johnson-Warrington V, Williams J, Bankart J, et al. Pulmonary rehabilitation and interstitial lung disease: aiding the referral decision. *J Cardiopulm Rehabil Prev.* 2013;33:189–195.
21. Crouch R, MacIntyre NR. Pulmonary rehabilitation of the patient with nonobstructive lung disease. *Respir Care Clin N Am.* 1998;4:59–70.
22. Li M, Mathur S, Chowdhury NA, et al. Pulmonary rehabilitation in lung transplant candidates. *J Heart Lung Transplant.* 2013;32: 626–632.
23. Stefanelli F, Meoli I, Cobuccio R, et al. High-intensity training and cardiopulmonary exercise testing in patients with chronic obstructive pulmonary disease and non-small-cell lung cancer undergoing lobectomy. *Eur J Cardiothoracic Surg.* 2013;44:e260–e265.
24. National Emphysema Treatment Trial Steering Committee. Rationale and design of the National Emphysema Treatment Trial. *Chest.* 1999;116:1750–1761.
25. Ries AL, Make BJ, Lee SM, et al; National Emphysema Treatment Trial Research Group. The effects of pulmonary rehabilitation in the National Emphysema Treatment Trial. *Chest.* 2005;128:3799–3809.
26. Plankeel JF, McMullen B, MacIntyre NR. Exercise outcomes after pulmonary rehabilitation depend on the initial mechanism of exercise limitation among non-oxygen-dependent COPD patients. *Chest.* 2005;127:110–116.
27. Emtner M, Porszasz J, Burris M, et al. Benefits of supplemental oxygen in exercise training in nonhypoxemic chronic obstructive pulmonary disease patients. *Am J Respir Crit Care Med.* 2003;169:1034–1042.
28. Johnston K, Young M, Grimmer K, et al. Frequency of referral to and attendance at a pulmonary rehabilitation program amongst patients admitted to a tertiary hospital with chronic obstructive pulmonary disease. *Respirology.* 2013;18:1089–1094.
29. Hayton C, Clark A, Olive S, et al. Barriers to pulmonary rehabilitation: characteristics that predict patient attendance and adherence. *Respir Med.* 2013;107:401–407.
30. Jones SE, Green SA, Clark AL, et al. Pulmonary rehabilitation following hospitalization for acute exacerbation of COPD: referrals, uptake and adherence. *Thorax.* 2013;69:181–182.
31. Chandra D, Wise RA, Kulkarni HS, et al. Optimizing the 6-min walk test as a measure of exercise capacity in COPD. *Chest.* 2012;142:1545–1552.
32. Emery CF, Leatherman NE, Burker EJ, et al. Psychological outcomes of a pulmonary rehabilitation program. *Chest.* 1991;100:613–617.
33. Ries AL, Kaplan RM, Linberg TM, et al. Effects of pulmonary rehabilitation on physiological and psychological outcomes in patients with COPD. *Ann Intern Med.* 1995;122:823–832.
34. Tselebis A, Bratis D, Pachi A, et al. A pulmonary rehabilitation program reduces levels of anxiety and depression in COPD patients. *Multidiscip Respir Med.* 2013;8:41.
35. Stoilkova A, Janssen DJ, Wouters EF. Educational programmes in COPD management interventions: a systematic review. *Respir Med.* 2013;107:1637–1650.
36. Bourbeau J, Julien M, Maltais F, et al. Reduction of hospital utilization in patients with chronic obstructive pulmonary disease: a disease-specific self-management intervention. *Arch Intern Med.* 2003;163:585–591.
37. Puhan MA, Scharplatz M, Troosters T, et al. Respiratory rehabilitation after acute exacerbation of COPD may reduce risk for readmission and mortality—a systematic review. *Respir Res.* 2005;6:54.
38. Burtin C, Decramer M, Gosselink R, et al. Rehabilitation and acute exacerbations. *Eur Resp J.* 2011;38:702–712.
39. Mador MJ, Krawza M, Alhajhusian A, et al. Interval training versus continuous training in patients with chronic obstructive pulmonary disease. *J Cardiopulm Rehabil Prev.* 2009;29:126–132.
40. World Health Organization. Global Initiative for Chronic Obstructive Lung Disease. *Global Strategy for the Diagnosis, Management, and Prevention of Chronic Obstructive Pulmonary Disease.* 2014. Available at: http://www.goldcopd.com. Accessed July 27, 2014.
41. Garvey C, Fullwood MD, Rigler J. Pulmonary rehabilitation exercise prescription in chronic obstructive lung disease: US survey and review of guidelines and clinical practices. *J Cardiopulm Rehabil Prev.* 2013;33:314–322.
42. Borg GA. Psychophysical bases for perceived exertion. *Med Sci Sports Exerc.* 1982;14:377–381.
43. ACCP/AACVPR Pulmonary Rehabilitation Guidelines Panel. Pulmonary rehabilitation: evidence based guidelines. *Chest.* 1997;112:1363–1396.
44. Marciniuk D, Brooks D, Butcher S, et al. Optimizing pulmonary rehabilitation in chronic obstructive pulmonary disease—practical issues: A Canadian Thoracic Society Clinical Practice Guideline. *Can Respir J.* 2010;17:159–168.

45. Wadell K, Webb KA, Preston ME, et al. Impact of pulmonary rehabilitation on the major dimensions of dyspnea in COPD. *COPD.* 2013;10:425–435.
46. Troosters T, Gosselink R, Paepe KD. Pulmonary rehabilitation improves survival in COPD patients with a recent severe acute exacerbation. *Am J Respir Crit Care Med.* 2002;165:A16.
47. Peno-Green L, Verrill G, Vitcenda M, et al. Patient and program outcome assessment in pulmonary rehabilitation. *J Cardiopulm Rehabil.* 2009;29:402–410.
48. Behnke M, Taube C, Kirsten D, et al. Home-based exercise is capable of preserving hospital-based improvements in severe chronic obstructive pulmonary disease. *Respir Med.* 2000;94:1184–1191.
49. Foglio K, Bianchi L, Ambrosino N. Is it really useful to repeat outpatient pulmonary rehabilitation programs in patients with chronic airway obstruction? A 2-year controlled study. *Chest.* 2001;119:1696–1704.
50. Ries AL, Kaplan RM, Myers R, et al. Maintenance after pulmonary rehabilitation in chronic lung disease: a randomized trial. *Am J Respir Crit Care Med.* 2003;167:880–888.
51. Soicher J, Mayo NE, Gauvin L, et al. Trajectories of endurance activity following pulmonary rehabilitation in COPD patients. *Eur Resp J.* 2012;39:272–278.
52. Ochmann U, Jorres R, Nowak D. Long-term efficiency of pulmonary rehabilitation. *J Cardiopulm Rehabil.* 2012;32:117–126.
53. Thorpe O, Johnston K, Kumar S. Barriers and enablers to physical activity participation in patients with COPD: a systematic review. *J Cardiopulm Rehabil Prev.* 2012;32:359–369.
54. Heerema-Poelman A, Stuive I, Wempe JB. Adherence to a maintenance exercise program 1 year after pulmonary rehabilitation: what are the predictors of drop-out? *J Cardiopulm Rehabil Prev.* 2013;33:419–426.
55. Griffiths TL, Phillips CJ, Davies S, et al. Cost effectiveness of an outpatient multidisciplinary pulmonary rehabilitation program. *Thorax.* 2001;56:779–784.
56. Man WD, Polkey MI, Donaldson N, et al. Community pulmonary rehabilitation after hospitalisation for acute exacerbations of chronic obstructive pulmonary disease: randomised controlled study. *BMJ.* 2004;329:1209–1215.
57. Murphy N, Bell C, Costello RW. Extending a home from hospital care programme for COPD exacerbations to include pulmonary rehabilitation. *Respir Med.* 2005;99:1297–1302.
58. Ward JJ. High-flow oxygen administration by nasal cannula for adult and perinatal patients. *Respir Care.* 2013;58:98–122.
59. McEvoy RD, Pierce RJ, Hillman D, et al; Australian trial of non-invasive Ventilation in Chronic Airflow Limitation (AVCAL) Study Group. Nocturnal non-invasive nasal ventilation in stable hypercapnic COPD: a randomised controlled trial. *Thorax.* 2009;64:561–566.
60. Porszasz J, Cao R, Morishige R, et al. Physiologic effects of an ambulatory ventilation system in chronic obstructive pulmonary disease. *Am J Respir Crit Care Med.* 2013;188:334–342.
61. Rehder KJ, Turner DA, Hartwig MG, et al. Active rehabilitation during extracorporeal membrane oxygenation as a bridge to lung transplantation. *Respir Care.* 2013;58:1291–1298.

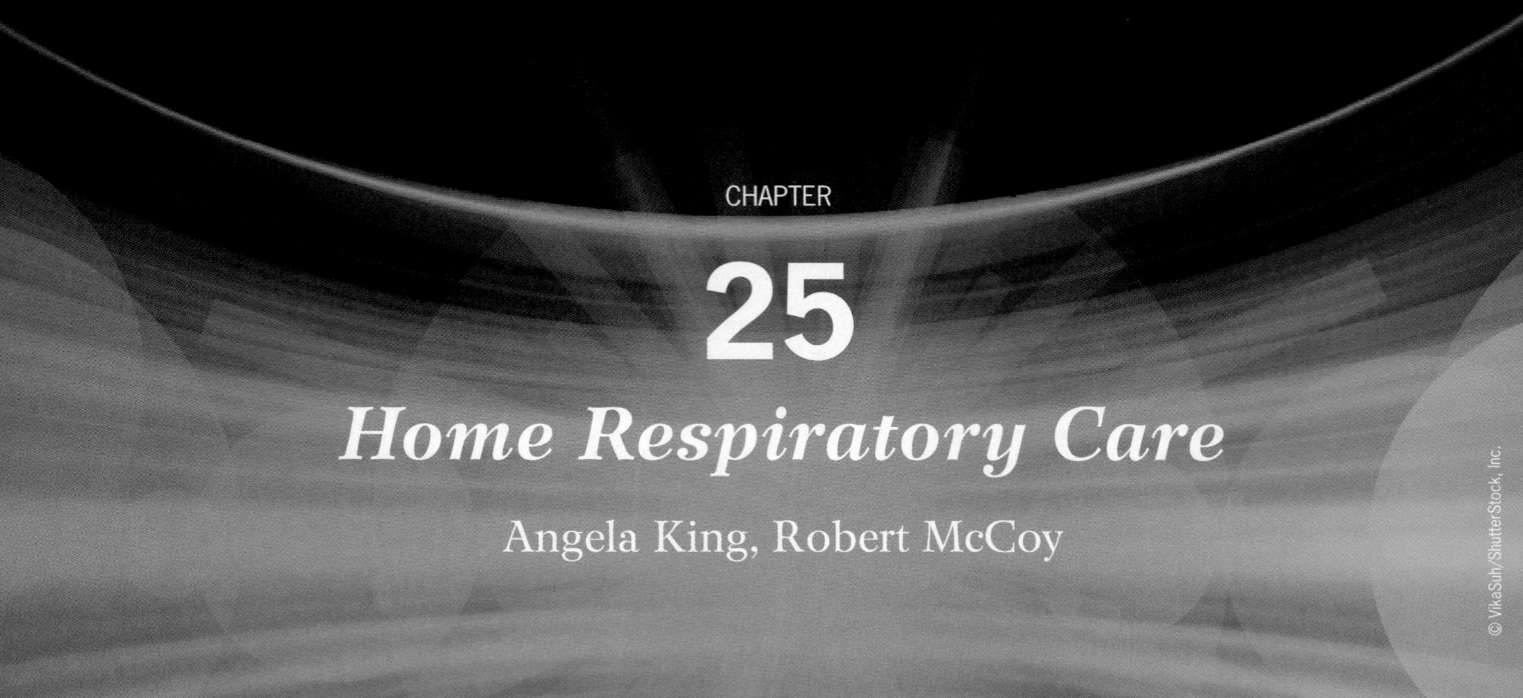

CHAPTER
25
Home Respiratory Care
Angela King, Robert McCoy
© VikaSuh/ShutterStock, Inc.

OUTLINE

OBJECTIVES

1. Discuss factors leading to the increase in home respiratory care.
2. Describe the role of the home medical equipment company.
3. Discuss the reimbursement system for home care in the United States.
4. Discuss issues related to home oxygen administration.
5. Compare home oxygen administration systems.
6. Compare mechanical ventilation in the hospital to that provided in the home.
7. List key safety considerations for the ventilator-assisted individual at home.

KEY TERMS

backup ventilator
bag technique
clinical respiratory services
compressed gas system
continuous-flow oxygen (CFO)
demand delivery device
durable medical equipment (DME) company
emergency plan
equipment management service
go-bag
ground circuit detector
home medical equipment (HME) company
home respiratory care
intermittent-flow device
intermittent-flow oxygen
liquid oxygen (LOX) storage system
long-term oxygen therapy (LTOT)
Medicaid
Medicare
nasal high flow (NHF)
noninvasive open ventilation (NIOV)
oxygen concentrator
oxygen-conserving device (OCD)
portable oxygen concentrator (POC)
pulse flow
remote alarm
transtracheal oxygen

Introduction

The American Association of Respiratory Care defines **home respiratory care** as "[t]hose prescribed respiratory care services provided in a patient's personal residence." Prescribed respiratory care services may include patient assessment and monitoring, such as listening to breath sounds; observing the patient's respiratory rate, chest excursion, and skin tone; and evaluating the patient's sputum. Respiratory care services may involve diagnostic and therapeutic modalities, such as observing the patient's pulse oximetry and transcutaneous carbon dioxide (CO_2) values and performing airway clearance therapy. Importantly, home respiratory care services may include providing education regarding respiratory equipment, disease management, and health-promoting behaviors for the patient and the family caregiver(s). This chapter covers issues related to home respiratory care, with specific emphasis on home oxygen (O_2) therapy and home mechanical ventilation.

Home Care Services

The patient's home may be a single-family residence, a multifamily dwelling, an assisted living facility or group home, a retirement community, or a skilled nursing facility.[1] The four types of home care services are home medical equipment services, episodic home health care, hospice home health care, and chronic home care services.[2]

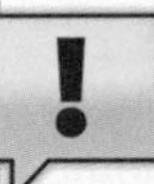

Respiratory Recap

Individuals Providing Services for DME Companies

- Technician
- Respiratory therapist
- Qualified nurse

Depending on the equipment ordered, **home medical equipment (HME) companies**, also called **durable medical equipment (DME) companies**, can provide service by a technician, respiratory therapist (RT), or a qualified nurse. A hospital bed would most likely be set up by a technician, whereas a suction machine and a mechanical ventilator would be set up by an RT. Episodic home health care is often ordered for the time period immediately following the patient's hospital stay and is usually provided for a finite period of time. Hospice care is provided for the terminally ill and provides palliative end-of-life care. Chronic home care services, sometimes referred to as *private duty*, are typically provided on an hourly basis and may involve nurses, health aides, chore providers, and companions.

Improved medical equipment has resulted in an increase in home respiratory care. The Medicare prospective payment system encourages earlier hospital discharge.[3] Modern therapies for the treatment of newborns have resulted in more infants and pediatric patients requiring home O_2 and home mechanical ventilation.[4] Another factor driving the increase in home care is the proportion of the population older than 65 years, which is projected to increase to 19.6% of the total population in 2030.[5] In the United States, approximately 80% of all persons over age 65 have at least one chronic condition, and 50% have at least two. Since the early 1990s, accumulating data have supported the cost-effectiveness of home care for respiratory patients (**Table 25-1**).[6,7] Medicare and other healthcare providers began encouraging the transition of technology-dependent patients from the acute care setting to less costly environments of care.[8] In addition to technological advances, changing demographics, and economic pressures, another key factor increasing home respiratory care is that most patients prefer to be cared for at home if possible.

TABLE 25-1
Hospital Cost Versus Home Care Cost, Per Patient, Per Month

Condition	Hospital Cost	Home Care Cost	Savings
Adult, ventilator dependent*	$21,570	$7,050	$14,520
Pediatric, oxygen dependent†	$12,090	$5,250	$6,840

*Information from Bach JR. The ventilator-assisted individual: cost analysis of institutional vs. rehabilitation and in-home management. *Chest.* 1992;101:26–30.
†Information from Field AI. Home care cost-effectiveness for respiratory technology-dependent children. *Am J Dis Child.* 1991;145:729–733.
Adapted from National Association for Home Care and Hospice. *Basic Statistics About Home Care: Updated 2008.* Washington, DC: The National Association for Home Care and Hospice; 2008.

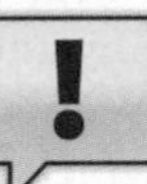

Respiratory Recap

Goals of Home Care

- Achieve the optimum level of patient function
- Educate patients and their caregivers
- Administer diagnostic and therapeutic services
- Conduct disease management and promote health

Goals of Home Care

The goals of home respiratory care are to achieve the optimum level of patient function through goal setting, educate patients and their caregivers, administer diagnostic and therapeutic modalities and services, conduct disease management, and promote health.[1] The general goals of home care for individuals with a respiratory disorder are to increase survival, decrease morbidity, improve function and quality of life, support independence and self-management, encourage positive health behaviors, and, for children with lung disease, promote optimal growth and development; for patients with a terminal illness, the goals are to provide physical and psychological comfort and to make it possible for the patient to die at home.[2]

The Medicare Program

As part of the Social Security Amendments of 1965, **Medicare** was established to provide a health insurance program for aged persons to complement the retirement, survivors, and disability insurance benefits under Title II of the Social Security Act. The Medicare program began on July 1, 1966. In 1973, persons who were entitled to Social Security or Railroad Retirement disability benefits for at least 24 months, persons with end-stage renal disease, and certain other persons became eligible for Medicare benefits. Persons with amyotrophic lateral sclerosis (ALS) were allowed to waive the 24-month waiting period after passage of Public Law 106-554, the Medicare, Medicaid, and SCHIP Benefits Improvement and Protection Act of 2000.

Hospital insurance is known as Medicare Part A. Part A covers inpatient care, skilled nursing facility care, and hospice care. Supplementary medical insurance is known as Part B. Most people have to pay a premium for Part B coverage. Part B includes medical services typically delivered in the outpatient setting and includes tests, lab services, and various health screenings. Part B also includes home health services, which are defined as medically necessary, reasonable, and part-time care and services such as skilled nursing care, home health aide services, physical and occupational therapies, speech and language pathology therapy, and medical social services. Part B also includes certain prescribed medical supplies and durable medical equipment, such as wheelchairs, hospital beds, home O_2 devices and mechanical ventilators, and related equipment. The Medicare Advantage program, also known as Part C, was established by Public Law 105-33, the Balanced Budget Act of 1997, which expanded options for beneficiaries to participate in private-sector healthcare plans. All Part C plans are run by private companies. Part C plans often offer extra benefits to beneficiaries, but they do not offer Hospice benefits. The newest part of Medicare is prescription drug coverage, also known as Part D. The Medicare Prescription Drug Improvement and Modernization Act of 2003 authorized this legislation. It provides seniors and people with disabilities a prescription drug benefit.

To qualify for Medicare skilled nursing services, the patient must (1) be under the care of a physician; (2) receive services under a plan of care established and periodically reviewed by a physician; (3) be in need of skilled nursing care, physical therapy, occupational therapy, and/or speech and language pathology therapy on an intermittent basis; and (4) be homebound, meaning that the patient is confined to the home or that leaving the home is a major effort that is seldom undertaken. For example, the patient may leave the home to get therapeutic or psychosocial care or to attend a funeral, graduation, or other infrequent event. Skilled nursing services must be provided by a registered nurse or by a licensed practical nurse under the supervision of a registered nurse. Unfortunately, respiratory therapists are not included in the Medicare home health services benefit.

Medicare Part B covers medically necessary durable medical equipment such as O_2 concentrators, nebulizer compressors, and mechanical ventilators, but there is no separate reimbursement for the respiratory therapist's professional expertise. Twenty years ago, a patient with chronic obstructive pulmonary disease (COPD) who was prescribed home O_2 would have received a home safety evaluation and equipment instruction, as well as periodic respiratory assessments, from a home care respiratory therapist. Unfortunately, as Medicare reimbursement for home O_2 has steadily declined over the years, the number of DME providers using technicians, as opposed to respiratory therapists, to set up and monitor the home respiratory equipment has increased dramatically. The majority of home O_2 patients today do not receive in-home clinical monitoring from a therapist. In addition, because many patients on home O_2 therapy leave the home frequently to attend religious services or social outings or to go shopping, they do not qualify for Medicare skilled nursing services either.

> **Respiratory Recap**
>
> **Medicare Benefits**
>
> - Part A: hospital insurance
> - Part B: supplementary medical insurance
> - Part C: alternative to Medicare run by private companies
> - Part D: prescription drug coverage

Medicaid Coverage for Home Medical Equipment

Many patients who need respiratory-related durable medical equipment but who are not eligible for Medicare may receive DME through the **Medicaid** program. For example, a child on a mechanical ventilator whose parents do not have private medical insurance will most likely receive coverage from the Medicaid program. In many cases, the DME provider must obtain prior authorization from the Medicaid program to determine whether a specific piece of equipment is covered. The coverage determination criteria for a given piece of respiratory equipment within the Medicaid program can vary by state. For example, one northeastern state does not cover a noninvasive ventilator used with a mouthpiece for a patient with Duchenne muscular dystrophy (DMD) but covers that same ventilator if the patient undergoes a tracheostomy. The best strategy to help the home patient obtain coverage for a given item is to proactively work with the Medicaid case worker, offering relevant published research papers and a detailed letter of medical necessity from the patient's physician. In many cases, appealing a negative coverage decision and presenting additional supporting documentation will result in a favorable outcome. In the case of the patient with DMD mentioned earlier, the Medicaid program did agree to cover the ventilator upon appeal after receiving information about the increased life expectancy of DMD patients when ventilated with noninvasive ventilation and presented with data showing that noninvasive ventilation was a more cost-effective alternative than a tracheostomy.

Requirements for Home Medical Equipment Companies

Depending on state respiratory care laws and regulations, and depending on the types of services offered, an HME company may require some or all of the following: retail license, HME license, a bedding supplier license, and an O_2 manufacturer/distributor license and possibly other licenses/permits as required by the state. Medicare also requires that all HME companies obtain a surety bond of at least $50,000. A surety bond is issued by an entity on behalf of a second party. It guarantees that the second party will fulfill an obligation to a third party. In the event that the obligation is not met, the third party will recover its losses via the bond. Medicare also requires all HME companies to have liability insurance.

Beginning in September 2009, Medicare began requiring all HME companies to be accredited by an approved agency. **Box 25-1** lists the Medicare supplier standards.

BOX 25-1

Medicare Home Medical Equipment Supplier Standards

1. A supplier must be in compliance with all applicable federal and state licensure and regulatory requirements.
2. A supplier must provide complete and accurate information on the DMEPOS supplier application. Any changes to this information must be reported to the National Supplier Clearinghouse within 30 days.
3. An authorized individual (one whose signature is binding) must sign the application for billing privileges.
4. A supplier must fill orders from its own inventory or must contract with other companies for the purchase of items necessary to fill the order. A supplier may not contract with any entity that is currently excluded from the Medicare program, any state health care programs, or from any other federal procurement or nonprocurement programs.
5. A supplier must advise beneficiaries that they may rent or purchase inexpensive or routinely purchased durable medical equipment, and of the purchase option for capped rental equipment.
6. A supplier must notify beneficiaries of warranty coverage and honor all warranties under applicable state law and repair or replace free of charge Medicare-covered items that are under warranty.
7. A supplier must maintain a physical facility on an appropriate site.
8. A supplier must permit Centers for Medicare and Medicaid Services (CMS) or its agents to conduct on-site inspections to ascertain the supplier's compliance with these standards. The supplier location must be accessible to beneficiaries during reasonable business hours and must maintain a visible sign and posted hours of operation.
9. A supplier must maintain a primary business telephone listed under the name of the business in a local directory or a toll free number available through directory assistance. The exclusive use of a beeper, answering machine, or cell phone is prohibited.
10. A supplier must have comprehensive liability insurance in the amount of at least $300,000 that covers both the supplier's place of business and all customers and employees of the supplier. If the supplier manufactures its own items, this insurance must also cover product liability and completed operations. Failure to maintain required insurance at all times will result in revocation of the supplier's billing privileges retroactive to the date the insurance lapsed.
11. A supplier must agree not to initiate telephone contact with beneficiaries, with a few exceptions allowed. This standard prohibits suppliers from calling beneficiaries in order to solicit new business.
12. A supplier is responsible for delivery and must instruct beneficiaries on use of Medicare-covered items and maintain proof of delivery.
13. A supplier must answer questions and respond to complaints of beneficiaries and maintain documentation of such contacts.
14. A supplier must maintain and replace at no charge or repair directly, or through a service contract with another company, Medicare-covered items it has rented to beneficiaries.
15. A supplier must accept returns of substandard (less than full quality for the particular item) or unsuitable items (inappropriate for the beneficiary at the time it was fitted and rented or sold) from beneficiaries.
16. A supplier must disclose these supplier standards to each beneficiary to whom it supplies a Medicare-covered item.
17. A supplier must disclose to the government any person having ownership, financial, or control interest in the supplier.
18. A supplier must not convey or reassign a supplier number; that is, the supplier may not sell or allow another entity to use its Medicare Supplier Billing Number.
19. A supplier must have a complaint resolution protocol established to address beneficiary complaints that relate to these standards. A record of these complaints must be maintained at the physical facility.

(*continues*)

Box 25-1 *(continued)*

20. Complaint records must include the name, address, telephone number and health insurance claim number of the beneficiary, a summary of the complaint, and any actions taken to resolve it.
21. A supplier must agree to furnish CMS any information required by the Medicare statute and implementing regulations.
22. All suppliers must be accredited by a CMS-approved accreditation organization in order to receive and retain a supplier billing number. The accreditation must indicate the specific products and services for which the supplier is accredited in order for the supplier to receive payment of those specific products and services (except for certain exempt pharmaceuticals).
23. All suppliers must notify their accreditation organization when a new DMEPOS location is opened.
24. All supplier locations, whether owned or subcontracted, must meet the DMEPOS quality standards and be separately accredited in order to bill Medicare.
25. All suppliers must disclose upon enrollment all products and services, including the addition of new product lines for which they are seeking accreditation.
26. Must meet the surety bond requirements specified in 42 C.F.R. 424.57(c).
27. A supplier must obtain oxygen from a state-licensed oxygen provider.
28. A supplier must maintain ordering and referring documentation consistent with provisions found in 42 C.F.R. 424.516(f).
29. A supplier is prohibited from sharing a practice location with other Medicare providers and suppliers.
30. A supplier must remain open to the public for a minimum of 30 hours per week except physicians (as defined in section 1848 (j) (3) of the Act) or physical and occupational therapists or a DMEPOS supplier working with custom made orthotics and prosthetics.

Note: This list is an abbreviated version of the application certification standards that every Medicare DMEPOS supplier must meet in order to obtain and retain their billing privileges. These standards, in their entirety, are listed in 42 Code of Federal Regulations (CFR), part 424, section 57. The new supplier standards were effective on September 27, 2010.

Reproduced from Centers for Medicare and Medicaid Services. *Medicare Enrollment Application: Durable Medical Equipment, Prosthetics, and Orthotics Supplies (DMEPOS) Suppliers, Form CMS-855S.* Available at: http://www.cms.hhs.gov/cmsforms/downloads/cms855s.pdf.

Accreditation of Home Medical Equipment Companies

Home care providers must be accredited by one of several accreditation agencies approved by the Medicare program, similar to accreditation for hospitals. There are generally two types of accreditation: Equipment Management Services and Clinical Respiratory Services. Accreditation in Clinical Respiratory Services includes everything required for accreditation in equipment management, plus additional requirements governing actual hands-on patient care and clinical personnel qualifications and requirements.

Not all home medical equipment companies are accredited for Clinical Respiratory Services, and that specific accreditation is not required by Medicare to participate in the program. If a company provides hands-on patient care such as performing patient assessment, administering treatment, providing disease management education, and/or monitoring respiratory status, however, it must be accredited for Clinical Respiratory Services.[9] Several accreditation agencies are approved by Medicare, including, but not limited to, the Joint Commission (formerly known as the Joint Commission on Accreditation of Healthcare Organizations), Community Health Accreditation Program (CHAP), and Accreditation Commission for Health Care (ACHC). The accreditation survey is normally repeated every 3 years, but the interval may vary based on the accrediting agency.

Equipment Management Services Versus Clinical Respiratory Services

Equipment management services are not hands-on patient care services. In other words, the patient is not touched by the RT for the purpose of providing care. The RT checks the home medical equipment, such as the percent oxygen from the O_2 concentrator or the ventilator settings and alarms, makes prescribed setting changes, delivers additional supplies, and performs similar equipment-related duties. The therapist does not perform diagnostic or therapeutic procedures. Equipment management services require a physician's order for the home medical equipment and settings. If the RT provides professional services in the home beyond equipment management, the RT is performing **clinical respiratory services**, which include performing clinical assessments and diagnostic procedures,

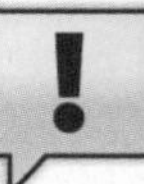

Respiratory Recap

Accreditation of Home Medical Equipment Companies

- Equipment Management Services
- Clinical Respiratory Services

Respiratory Recap

Types of Respiratory Care Services

- Equipment management services
- Clinical respiratory services

administering treatments or medications, providing patient education, and monitoring the patient's respiratory status. If patient education involves more than education on the use of the equipment, the RT is considered to be providing clinical respiratory services.

Orders for Clinical Respiratory Services

Orders for clinical respiratory services are considered a part of the care plan and should be included in the HME company's care plan as well as the home health agency's nursing care plan, if applicable. The home care RT should coordinate the care plan with that of the home health agency's personnel (nursing; physical, occupational, or speech therapy) to encourage a collaborative approach. The plan of care describes the planned treatments, education, and services and must be approved and signed by the patient's physician.

The Respiratory Therapist as Home Care Provider

By virtue of education, training, and competency testing, the respiratory therapist is the most competent healthcare professional to provide home respiratory care. Home respiratory care, particularly for ventilator-assisted individuals, can be highly complex; therefore, the risk of a negative outcome is great if the services are not performed by a highly skilled professional.[1]

Requirements for the Respiratory Therapist Providing Home Respiratory Care

Table 25-2 lists some of the key characteristics required of the home care respiratory therapist. The ability to assess many different aspects of the patient is probably the most important skill for a home care therapist.[10]

TABLE 25-2
Key Characteristics Required of the Home Care Respiratory Therapist

Objective Requirements	
Licensed or certified (as applicable per state)	All reputable DME providers hire only licensed/certified therapists. Note: If the therapist will visit patients in multiple states, a current license is required for each state.
Driver's license	Most DME providers will obtain an annual copy of the therapist's driving record, and employment is often contingent upon maintaining a clean driving record.
Automobile insurance	Most DME providers will require proof that the therapist has adequate automobile insurance coverage.
Subjective Requirements	
Highly skilled at patient assessment	The therapist often is the only clinician visiting the patient's home, or the patient may be seen by other clinicians only sporadically. The respiratory therapist must be skilled at respiratory assessment for patients ranging from preterm infants to geriatric patients.
Highly skilled at home safety assessment	The therapist often will be the only clinician assessing the patient's home for safety and the proper use of the medical equipment.
Excellent critical thinking ability	On occasion, the therapist will need to call the patient's physician or protective services on an emergent basis. The therapist requires excellent judgment and decision-making skills in order to appropriately handle such situations.
Good teacher	The bulk of the home care therapist's job is to teach patients and families. Most DME providers offer equipment and service to a wide variety of patient populations, from preterm infants to geriatric patients; thus, the therapist must be skilled at teaching diverse patient populations.
Respects people from other cultures and socioeconomic backgrounds	The home care therapist will most likely be visiting patients from a variety of backgrounds, with diverse belief systems and ways of doing things. The therapist must keep in mind that he or she is a guest in the patient's home and treat all patients and families with respect.
Good communication skills	The therapist will need good communication skills, both verbal and written, to work with a wide variety of patients, families, coworkers, other home care providers (e.g., nursing, PT, OT, SLP, MSW, HHA), and physicians.
Intrinsically motivated	The home care therapist will most often be working without direct supervision.
Good organizational skills	The home care therapist must be organized regarding prioritizing and planning home visits, ensuring that all required equipment and supplies are ordered and stocked in his or her vehicle, and that all required paperwork is completed in a timely fashion.

DME, durable medical equipment; PT, physical therapist; OT, occupational therapist; SLP, speech-language pathologist; MSW, master of social work; HHA, home health aide.

The RT must be able to assess respiratory and overall physical status. The home RT is often the first to note a deterioration in the patient's physiologic condition. He or she also needs to evaluate the patient's and family caregiver's ability to learn and retain new information and maintain the prescribed medical equipment. The home care RT teaches pediatric, adult, and geriatric patients and their families and must be able to work with patients from diverse cultures and economic backgrounds. The RT must be able to assess the family and social support available as well as the safety and appropriateness of the patient's home environment. The RT must also be aware of the requirements of insurance coverage for commonly prescribed home medical equipment. Organization skills are important because coverage of a large geographic area means that making a trip back to the office to retrieve a forgotten item is often impossible.

The daily routine of a home care RT is much different from that of a hospital-based therapist. Although home care RTs see a variety of patients and families each day, they do not enjoy the same camaraderie with their coworkers as experienced by RTs working in a hospital. The home care RT often is on call 24 hours a day, 7 days a week. On the positive side, the home care therapist often develops long-term relationships with patients and their families.

The Initial Home Visit

The tasks completed during the initial home visit vary depending on the equipment and services ordered (clinical respiratory services versus equipment management services) and on the policies and procedures of the HME company. For a patient on a ventilator at home, the initial home visit must not be the first time the therapist makes face-to-face contact with the patient. The home environment evaluation should always be done prior to discharge so that any safety issues or inadequacies are identified and corrected prior to the patient's return home. Equipment can be set up in the home days prior to discharge, but billing for the equipment cannot be started prior to the patient's discharge to the home.

During the initial home visit, the RT has several important tasks to complete:

- Establish a rapport with the patient and family.
- Evaluate the home environment.
- Complete the equipment setup and instruction.
- Perform any ordered patient assessments and diagnostic or therapeutic procedures.
- Determine if there are unmet needs and make a plan for addressing those needs.
- Communicate, as appropriate, with other professional caregivers (e.g., home health nurse, physical therapist, physician).
- Complete the required admission paperwork.

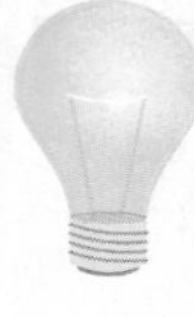

STOP AND THINK

You are caring for a patient with ALS who is about to receive a tracheostomy, followed by discharge home. What considerations will be important when preparing the patient and her family for discharge home?

The RT should have a company photo identification card visible to allay any security concerns. The RT should address the patient and family using the appropriate titles (e.g., Mrs., Ms., Mr.) unless invited to do otherwise. RTs must keep in mind that, although performing a professional role in the patient's home, they also are guests in the home. The RT should use an alcohol-based handrub in view of the patient and family caregivers.

The patient rights and responsibilities document explains to the patient some important points about the planned services. For example, the patient has the right to refuse service, the right to make a complaint without fear of retaliation, and the right to know how much the services being provided are going to cost. In addition, this document explains some of the patient's responsibilities while receiving services. For example, the responsibility for open and honest communication, for using the equipment in the manner prescribed, for maintaining the equipment properly, and for paying any deductible or copayment as required by regulation or law or the terms of an insurance contract.

The patient should also receive a copy of the company's complaint procedure form. This form outlines the procedure the patient needs to follow in order to file a complaint and lists contact numbers the patient can call to issue a complaint, including Medicare, Medicaid, and the accreditation agency by which the company is accredited. The document also includes an overview of the actions the company will take to resolve the issue.

If the patient has not already completed an advance directive, he or she should be given written information about advance directives and an explanation. Obtaining a copy of the patient's advance directive for the medical record is crucial so that the RT, or any other caregiver in the home, knows how to respond to a cardiopulmonary arrest.

The patient must receive information on the HME company's methods for ensuring Health Insurance Portability and Accountability Act (HIPAA) compliance. This document will inform the patient about how medical information is stored and who will have access to it.

If the patient qualifies for Medicare, the advance beneficiary notice (ABN) and the assignment of benefits (AOB) forms must be completed. The ABN form is to help patients make an informed choice about whether or not they want to receive items or services, knowing that there might be an additional personal cost if the items and services are not covered by their insurance plan. The AOB gives the patient's authorization to the HME company to assign Medicare, Medicaid, or insurance benefits to the company for all covered medical equipment and supplies; for direct billing to Medicare, Medicaid, or other insurers; and for release of personal health information (PHI) to Medicare, Medicaid, or other valid insurance companies and to other healthcare providers.

The home environment must be evaluated specific to the type of home medical equipment being provided. For example, if the patient will be receiving home O_2, the RT or technician will need to ensure there are no sources of open flame in the home when O_2 is being used and that a working smoke detector is installed. If the patient will be receiving postural drainage therapy, the RT must evaluate the home to determine whether there is a suitable bed to perform the therapy.

The RT may provide the patient and family with additional information, such as a list of community resources. This resource list may include agencies and services such as the American Lung Association (ALA), Better Breather's Clubs, Meals on Wheels, the Area Agency on Aging, hospice services, free or reduced-cost medical clinics in the area, domestic violence hotline information, poison control hotline information, and the closest ALS or muscular dystrophy clinic.

If home medical equipment has been prescribed, the therapist will set up the equipment and instruct the patient and family caregivers in the proper use and care of the equipment. The instructional checklist should include common troubleshooting tips and maintenance requirements for the equipment delivered. The instructional checklist may also include instructions for the patient to follow to order additional O_2 or supplies, as well as what to do in the event of home medical equipment failure or patient emergency.

All insurance companies, Medicare, and Medicaid require proof of delivery of the equipment and supplies. Generally, the delivery ticket lists the patient's name and demographic information and specifies the quantity, manufacturer, and serial number (if applicable) of the home medical equipment provided. For some high-tech equipment, such as mechanical ventilators, it is crucial that the serial number be properly recorded and tracked in the event there is a recall of the equipment.

After assessing the home environment and teaching the patient and caregivers about the equipment, the RT will have an idea of the patient's needs and goals. If the patient is receiving only equipment management services, information can be documented on a progress note or any other document that can be incorporated into the patient's medical record. Alternatively, if the patient is on a home ventilator and is receiving clinical respiratory services, a goal might be for the patient to be able to speak. The therapist would document this goal on the patient's plan of care, which must be signed by the physician. For example, the therapist may request an order to determine the patient's ability to tolerate cuff deflation, and, if successful, attempt the use of a speaking valve.

Bag Technique

It is important for home care RTs to determine whether **bag technique** should be incorporated into their routine.[11] Most home care RTs carry a bag containing their handrub, stethoscope, blood pressure cuff, pulse oximeter, CO_2 monitor, peak flow meter, and other necessary implements. Because the RT will be traveling from home to home, it is prudent that the therapist minimize the likelihood of disease transmission. Stethoscopes and other items can be contaminated with various pathogens.[12] It is also important for patients receiving both nursing and RT visits to receive the same standard of care from each discipline.

Bag technique means keeping the bag and its contents as clean as possible. The bag should not rest on an unclean area, such as the floor or on the patient's unmade bed. Depending on the space available in the home environment, it may be easiest for the therapist to use a barrier, such as a blue pad or sheet of newspaper, to serve as a clean resting place for the bag. Using a blue pad also helps protect the patient's furniture from damage, which communicates that the RT is respectful of the patient's home. Hand hygiene should be performed before reaching into the bag. Everything needed for the visit should be removed at one time, prior to beginning patient care. When the visit is finished, anything that may have been soiled should be wiped clean before being replaced in the bag.

Home Environment Evaluation

The home care RT is responsible for evaluating the home environment to ensure that it is appropriate for the planned equipment and services. Some components of the home environment evaluation apply to all patients, such as ensuring that there are adequate means of egress and no fall hazards.

Environmental Issues for Patients on Home Oxygen Therapy

Patients who receive O_2 at home are exposed to the risk of improper storage and handling of O_2 cylinders, unsafe usage of O_2 in the kitchen or workshop, improper transfer of liquid O_2, inadequate ventilation, and smoking or other unsafe flames. It is important for the RT to evaluate whether there are smoking materials and other fire safety risks, such as candles or open flames, in the home and whether the home has functional smoke detectors.[13] Patients receiving O_2 may also be exposed to risk from not securing portable O_2 properly while driving or riding in an automobile. It is crucial that the cylinders be secured in the event the car brakes suddenly or is involved in an accident.

Environmental Issues for Patients on Home Mechanical Ventilation

If the patient will receive a home ventilator, the environment evaluation should include verifying the adequacy of the home electrical system. Home medical equipment that is double insulated generally does not require grounding. Most home medical equipment companies do not have a biomedical engineer on staff to verify the electrical safety of each piece of medical equipment, however; and thus it is prudent for the therapist to ensure that the electrical outlets used for home medical equipment are properly grounded.[13] Most hardware stores stock a **ground circuit detector** that can be purchased inexpensively. These devices typically use red and amber bulbs to indicate the outlet status, although the therapist must read the instructions for the particular brand of ground circuit detector being used. In the case of the ground circuit detector shown in **Figure 25-1**, the outlet is properly grounded if the two amber bulbs illuminate. If the red bulb or a single amber bulb illuminates, there is a problem with the outlet that must be remedied before that outlet can be safely used.

Another important aspect of electrical safety in the home is ensuring that the electrical circuit is not overloaded. Most ventilator patients have several pieces of electrical equipment (e.g., ventilator, heated humidifier, nebulizer, O_2 concentrator, suction machine) within the same room in addition to the standard household items. It is easy to overload the electrical circuit. Sometimes the homeowner will have a diagram detailing which outlets are on the same circuit, but usually testing must be done. To determine which outlets are on the same circuit, turn off the circuit breaker for that room and then insert the ground circuit detector into each outlet. If the ground circuit detector does not illuminate (no bulbs light), that outlet is controlled by the circuit breaker that was turned off. If the bulbs on the outlet circuit detector illuminate, that outlet is on a different circuit. The therapist should be careful not to plug too many devices into the same circuit. If concerned, the therapist can total the amperes of each item he or she intends to plug into a particular circuit and compare that total to the rated amperage of the circuit breaker. This information can usually be found in the operator's manual for each piece of equipment. Note that some ventilators draw more current on startup and then drop back after the ventilator is operating.[14]

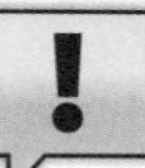

Respiratory Recap

Environmental Issues

- Safe storage of oxygen
- Electrical safety
- Backup electrical/battery power
- Emergency plan
- Alarms and communication
- Local EMS and firefighters

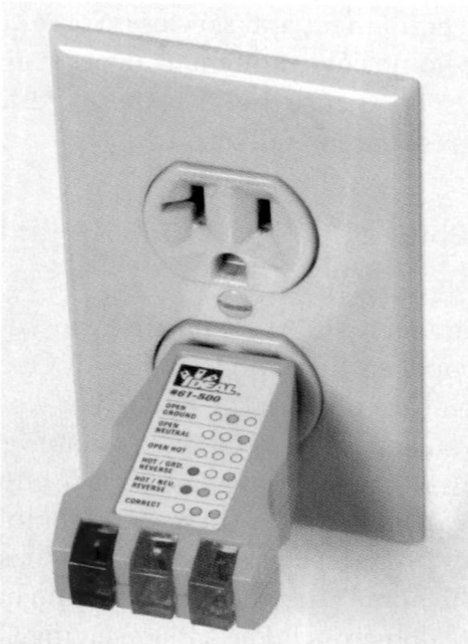

FIGURE 25-1 Two LEDs indicating a properly grounded outlet.
Courtesy of Ideal Industries, Inc.

The therapist should avoid the use of extension cords for the home medical equipment if at all possible. In practical application, however, there will be times when an extension cord is needed. If an extension cord must be used, ensure that the cord is of high quality, in good condition, and includes three prongs rated appropriately to carry the anticipated amperage. Of course, the extension cord must be plugged into an outlet that the therapist has already tested with the ground circuit detector. Some new extension cords include a ground fault interrupter (GFI), which can add an additional measure of safety when properly used. Of course, when there is any concern about the home's electrical system, it is imperative that a licensed electrician provides the final word on the home's electrical safety.

Some patients who are on home O_2 and/or a home mechanical ventilator will be concerned about the anticipated increase in their electric bill. If the patient expresses a significant concern about the bill, the RT can help the patient estimate the additional electric consumption and the increased cost.[15] See **Figure 25-2** for a sample calculation.

Some electric companies allow patients who are dependent on a mechanical ventilator to be placed on a priority restoration service in the event of a power failure. If the patient's electric company offers this service, the therapist should forward a letter to the electric company including the patient's name, address, and reason for the priority designation along with a request signed by the patient and physician. Even if priority

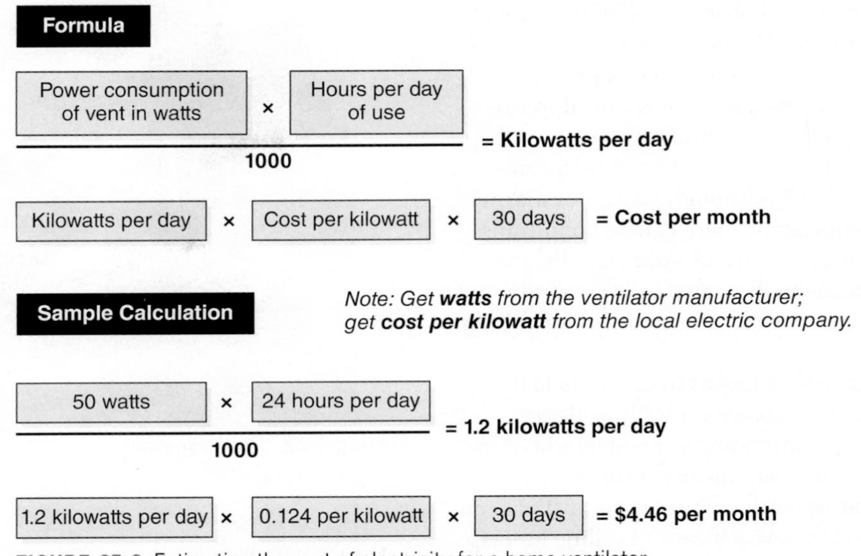

Formula
Power consumption of vent in watts
×
Hours per day of use
1000
= Kilowatts per day
Kilowatts per day
×
Cost per kilowatt
×
30 days
= Cost per month
Sample Calculation
Note: Get watts from the ventilator manufacturer; get cost per kilowatt from the local electric company.
50 watts
×
24 hours per day
1000
= 1.2 kilowatts per day
1.2 kilowatts per day
×
0.124 per kilowatt
×
30 days
= $4.46 per month

FIGURE 25-2 Estimating the cost of electricity for a home ventilator.
Information from Turner J. *Handbook of Adult and Pediatric Respiratory Home Care.* Mosby; 1994.

designation is granted, however, the patient must be cautioned that it is not always possible for the electric company to restore service promptly, and alternate plans must be put into place for whenever electrical power is interrupted.

The RT must work with the patient and family to determine the optimal **emergency plan** for handling a power failure. Some families choose to obtain a generator. Generators vary in complexity of operation. Some generators automatically turn on when necessary, and even perform self-tests at scheduled intervals. However, some generators are difficult to start and may require physical strength and agility to pull-start. It is imperative that this type of generator be started periodically, per the manufacturer's guidelines. It is wise for the family to identify and train several people who are usually available and able and willing to start the generator should the need arise.

All patients who depend on a ventilator should have a battery system in case of emergency and for mobility purposes.[16] Each patient's need for battery duration must be evaluated individually. For example, a patient who has no spontaneous breathing capability and who lives in an area with frequent power outages will require much longer battery duration than a patient capable of spontaneous ventilation who uses a ventilator only at night. A patient attending school daily will require longer battery duration than a patient who is homebound. All home ventilator manufacturers offer various battery types and sizes. Richardson Products (Frankfort, IL) makes a product called the PowerTech Vent Power Center that allows the patient to operate the ventilator from a power wheelchair battery (**Figure 25-3**). Many patients also have a DC power cord; in an absolute emergency, the patient could use the ventilator in the car. In some communities, the local fire department may allow the patient to wait out a power outage at the fire station if it has power. Firefighter personnel may also help operate the patient's generator if previous arrangements have been made. Determining the optimal plan for handling power outages requires an understanding of the patient's needs, the family's capabilities, and the community services available.

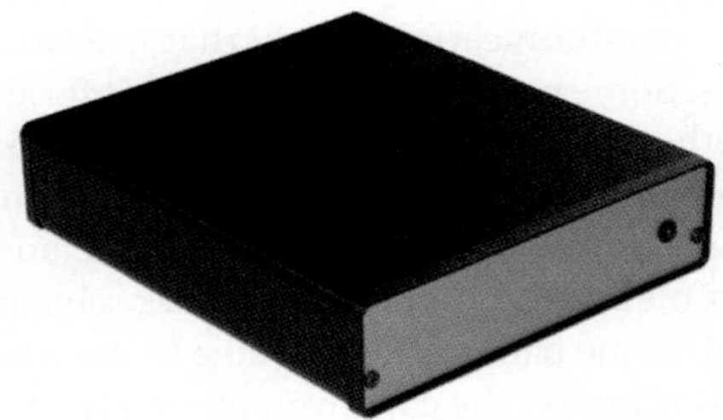

FIGURE 25-3 The PowerTech Vent Power Center.
Courtesy of Richardson Products, Inc.

An important aspect of the home environmental assessment is to ensure that the ventilator alarms can be heard by the caregiver in all areas of the home.[17] It is not uncommon for the alarms to be inaudible in the basement, or even in the main living areas if a dishwasher, window air conditioner unit, or other appliance is running. Most ventilator manufacturers offer **remote alarms** that can be placed strategically to ensure that the ventilator alarm is heard throughout the home. Because these alarms work in conjunction with the ventilator, the patient and caregiver can be confident that the alarm has been tested thoroughly. Some families also use commercially available baby monitors in order to hear the patient and ventilator alarms in another room. Some of the latest monitors allow visual observation as well as auditory monitoring of the patient and ventilator. These have served some patients and caregivers well.[18]

A caregiver's direct visual observation of the patient offers the most security for the home mechanical ventilator patient; however, it is not always practical or even preferable. Caregivers sometimes need to use the restroom, and patients often prefer their privacy. It therefore is crucial that the patient be able to summon assistance if needed.[17] Although ventilator alarms usually activate appropriately, there can be conditions in which the alarm does not sound. Additionally, the patient may have a problem or need that is not ventilator related; hence the patient needs a mechanism for calling the caregiver.

Finally, the patient needs a means to call for help if something happens to the caregiver. Ideally, patients should have a means of summoning a caregiver who is in the home with them as well as a means of summoning 911 services. It may be especially important for patients on mouthpiece ventilation to have a means of calling for help because these patients often do not have a low-pressure or disconnect alarm set on their ventilator because the mouthpiece is not in the mouth all of the time.

It is important for the RT to recognize that there is no single communication system that will work for all patients. Some patients are able to shout for help, whereas others cannot speak, or more often, cannot speak loudly enough to be heard in another room. Part of the RT's assessment of the patient should include evaluating what method or methods may work reliably for the patient. Some patients may be able to use a wireless doorbell to summon the caregiver, placing the button with the patient and the chimer with the caregiver. It is important to test the range of the device. Other patients use a cellular phone that is programmed to dial their own home landline telephone so that the home phone will ring, alerting the caregiver,[18] although this method is dependent on the cellular phone battery being properly charged, having sufficient plan minutes, and having a good signal. Unfortunately, both of these methods require a degree of finger strength and dexterity.

The E-Z Call and the PA-1 portable alarm (Med Labs, Goleta, CA) are available for the patient who has very limited movement or strength (**Figure 25-4**). The E-Z Call can be connected to a hospital call system or can be used in conjunction with the PA-1 portable alarm. The E-Z Call features a square pad that can be placed on the patient's tray-table. The pad is very sensitive, so that a very light tap on the pad will trigger the PA-1 alarm. If the patient can move only his or her head, the alarm pad can be clipped to the pillow. The PA-1 alarm will sound by pressing the head onto the pad. Another model, called the Bite-or-Puff, uses a straw-like device that the patient bites or puffs into in order to trigger an alarm.

Some DME companies require the family of home-ventilated patients to have a landline telephone system instead of, or in addition to, a cellular phone. The rationale is that cell phones may not be as reliable (for reasons previously mentioned) and that caregivers may take the cell phone with them if they leave the patient in the care of the nurse, potentially leaving the home nurse without a means to summon emergency services should the need arise. Another important reason for the requirement of a landline is that emergency service providers may be able to more quickly pinpoint the address and location of the individual calling for help when the call comes from a landline.

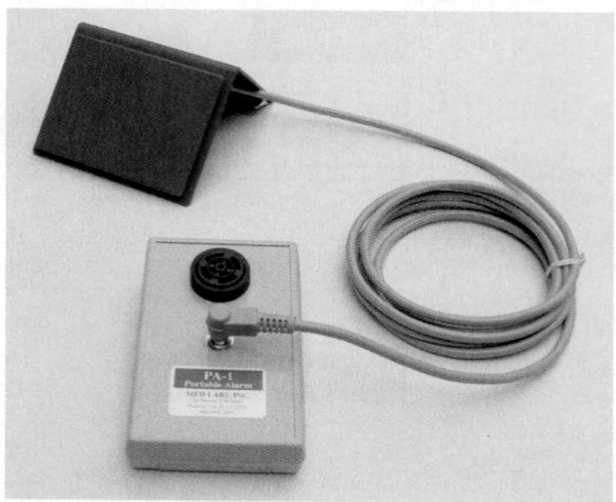

FIGURE 25-4 E-Z Call and PA-1.
Courtesy of Med Labs, Inc.

X10 (Renton, WA) makes a relatively inexpensive product called the Personal Assistance Voice Dialer that may be helpful for some patients (**Figure 25-5**). It consists of a base unit connected to the home telephone. It can be activated by pressing a button that can be mounted on the patient's wheelchair tray or worn like a wristwatch or pendant. When activated, the device flashes its lights, sounds a siren alarm, and dials up to four preprogrammed telephone numbers. When the dialed party answers, the Personal Assistance Voice Dialer plays the prerecorded outgoing voice message and then allows the dialed party to listen into the patient's home.

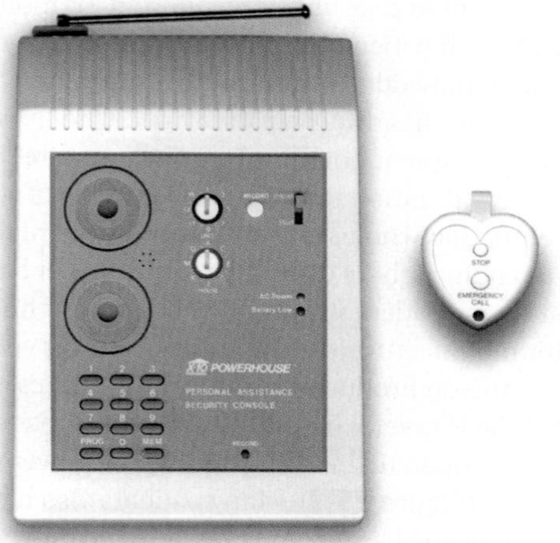

FIGURE 25-5 X10 Personal Assistance Voice Dialer.
Courtesy of x10.com.

Working with Local Emergency Medical Services and Firefighters

It is a good idea for some home care patients, particularly O_2 and ventilator patients, to meet with their local emergency medical services (EMS) personnel or firefighters before there is any type of emergency. In most communities, EMS personnel or firefighters will visit the patient's home, free of charge, to help perform the home environment evaluation. This visit also allows them to learn where the patient's home is, to note if the house numbers are sufficiently visible, and to learn about any special conditions or needs. If the patient has a Do Not Resuscitate order, it should be discussed with the EMS squad during the visit. In some communities, the EMS squad may ask that a copy of the order be taped over the patient's bed, placed on the refrigerator, or worn on an alert bracelet so that it is easily visible should they be called to the home in an emergency situation.

The Physician Order

The initial order for home respiratory equipment often comes to the DME company on a prescription from a physician's pad or on a discharge note from the hospital. If the patient is in the Medicare program, an additional document called a certificate of medical necessity (CMN) may be required. If the patient is to receive clinical respiratory services, a concise description of the planned services must be documented and signed for by the physician. Some therapists refer to these physician-signed orders as a *care plan*, which is the same terminology used by home health nurses. Other therapists refer to the signed orders as a *plan of treatment*, and still others refer to the orders as *the prescription*. Unfortunately, there is no standardized terminology across all home care disciplines.

In recent years, guided self-management has become more commonplace.[19] Guided self-management means that patients or caregivers have appropriate knowledge or are adequately trained so that they know when they can make adjustments to the treatment plan, what adjustments they can make, and when they need to seek medical attention.[20] For the patient who is mechanically ventilated at home, it is now relatively common for a range of ventilator settings to be prescribed by the physician, allowing the patient or caregiver to make adjustments within the prescribed range in order to meet the patient's changing needs.

Long-Term Oxygen Therapy

The Evidence Supporting Home Oxygen Therapy

Oxygen therapy in the home or alternate-site healthcare facility is indicated for the treatment of hypoxemia and has been shown to significantly improve survival in hypoxemic patients with COPD.[21] The Nocturnal Oxygen Therapy Trial (NOTT) and Medical Research Council (MRC) multicenter studies created the foundation for studies showing that continuous use of O_2 improves survival.[22,23] A later review of the NOTT study (**Figure 25-6**) reported that home **long-term oxygen therapy (LTOT)** reduced healthcare costs by reducing hospitalizations.[24]

Key Issues in Oxygen Therapy

The goal for efficient O_2 delivery is proper arterial O_2 saturation at all activity levels.[25,26] The degree of pulmonary disease is the major determinant of a patient's inspired O_2 requirement. It is important to note that saving O_2 is considered accomplished only *after* the patient is adequately oxygenated and is a secondary

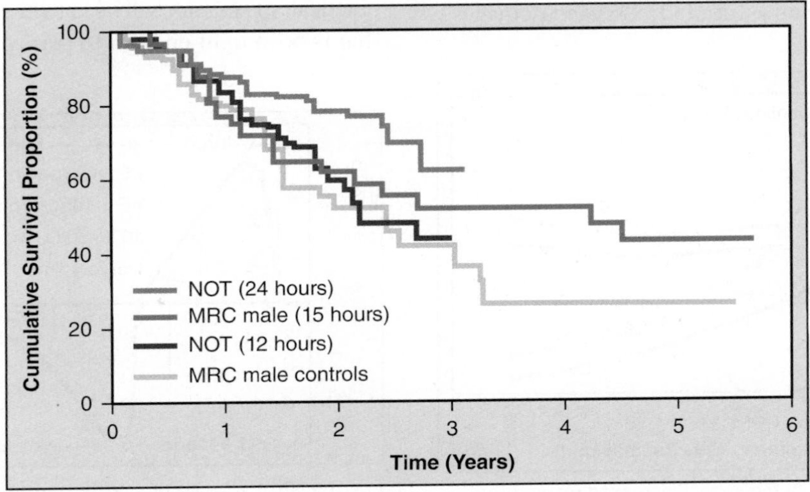

FIGURE 25-6 Nocturnal Oxygen Therapy Trial study results.

Reproduced from Petty TL, McCoy RW, Doherty DE. *Long Term Oxygen Therapy (LTOT) History, Scientific Foundations, and Emerging Technologies: Sixth Oxygen Consensus Conference Recommendations*. National Lung Health Education Program; August 2005.

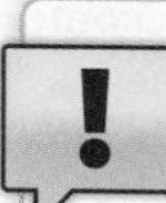

Respiratory Recap

Long-Term Oxygen Therapy

- The goal is to maintain adequate arterial O_2 saturation.
- Studies show that O_2 therapy is life prolonging in patients with COPD.
- Respiratory rate affects the amount of O_2 the patient receives.

objective for device performance. Even if an O_2 delivery device is providing consistent O_2 delivery, results can vary for an individual patient from moment to moment, and between groups of patients using similar devices.

Increased respiratory rate will shorten inspiratory time and may reduce the amount of O_2 a patient will receive (**Figure 25-7**). In the past, the general rule of thumb was to double the patient's flow rate (e.g., from 2 L/min to 4 L/min) during exercise. Any change in respiratory rate or pattern may affect the patient's oxygenation. The lack of attention to this variable in the past has created the misperception that some O_2 delivery devices, especially conserving devices, are not effective. Oxygen-dependent patients should be tested on their O_2 system at different activity levels reflecting real-life conditions: sleep, rest, and exercise, as well as at altitude. A titration test is the standard method of measuring patients' O_2 needs with exercise. There is no standard for O_2 titration. Most clinicians use a simple method that only requires an oximeter and exercise. If a patient will be doing more strenuous activity, every attempt should be made to simulate that activity to see whether the device properly oxygenates the user. Overnight oximetry is strongly recommended for intermittent-flow O_2 delivery devices to determine whether the device is triggering with each breath and maintaining patient Sp_{O_2}.[21]

Altitude has an impact on the pressure of O_2 and not necessarily on the amount of O_2. Oxygen delivery devices deliver approximately the same volume of O_2 at higher altitudes (or in an airplane), but the pressure at different altitudes may have an impact on blood oxygenation. It is important to understand that if an O_2 system is able to meet a patient's O_2 needs at a lower altitude, it is possible that that same system may not be able to meet the patient's needs at a higher altitude. It is generally unfeasible to test patients on their O_2 systems at pressures that they would be experiencing at varying altitudes. A common practice is to double the setting when the patient is at altitude. However, if the O_2 system the patient is using is already running at or near its top setting at a lower altitude, another system should be considered for use at higher altitudes.

By selecting one breathing pattern and one breath rate, a delivered dose volume of O_2 can be made equivalent to the volume taken in during continuous flow of O_2.[27] As a result, manufacturers select a volume of O_2 for a given oxygen-conserving device setting that they feel would be equivalent to **continuous-flow oxygen (CFO)** and make that the flow setting on their device. This only works if the patient never changes his or her breathing pattern, however. Most oxygen-conserving devices have a number on the selector dial and, though they claim to deliver O_2 equivalently to CFO at that same setting, are not equivalent to CFO, let alone another conserving device at that setting (**Figure 25-8**). There is a wide variety in F_{IO_2}, and no device can be considered to have delivered therapy equivalent to CFO.

Patients on home O_2 therapy need to stay active to maintain a healthy lifestyle and prevent complications associated with a sedentary lifestyle.[24] Activity is important to health, yet patients requiring supplemental O_2 are challenged by the need to carry or transport the O_2 necessary to maintain proper oxygenation. In the hospital, patients are requested to stay in their beds, and when transportation is necessary, an assistant carries the O_2 and moves patients to their destinations within the hospital. In the home, this is not possible or practical, so patients will need to be provided an O_2 system that is both light enough to transport and capable of

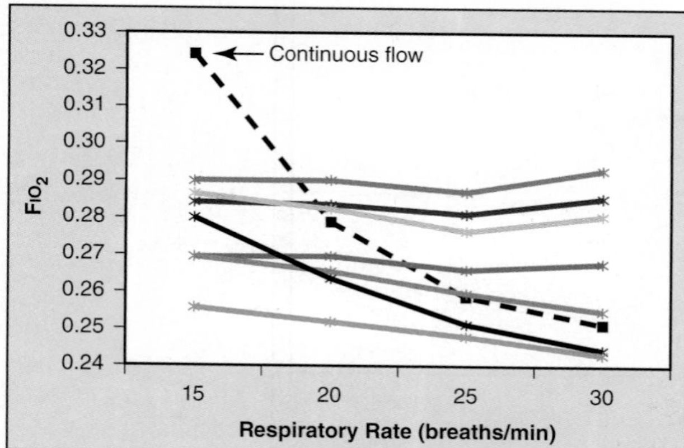

FIGURE 25-7 An example of the impact increased respiratory rate has on F_{IO_2} between continuous flow and a variety of oxygen-conserving devices.

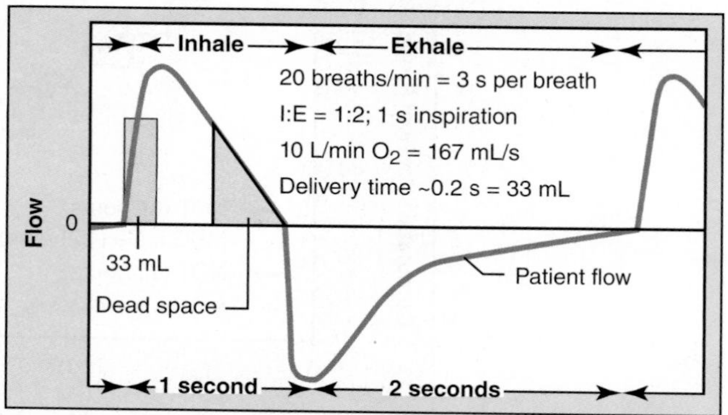

FIGURE 25-8 Increasing peak flow on an oxygen-conserving unit can provide more gas delivery to useful sections of the lung, preventing delivery of oxygen to dead space.

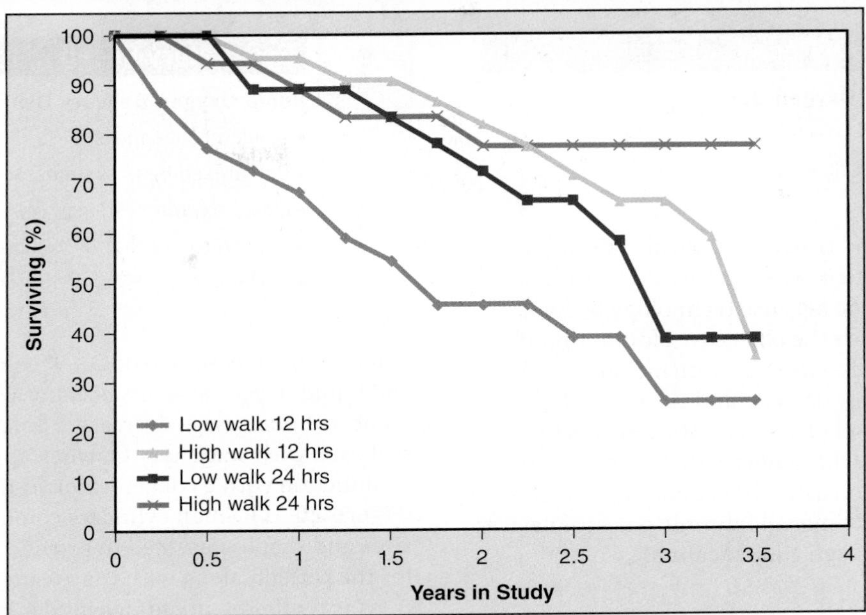

FIGURE 25-9 A retrospective analysis of the Nocturnal Oxygen Therapy Trial data shows the value of exercise to the survival of patients on long-term oxygen therapy. Eighty patients matched for age, treatment group, and FEV_1. They were spilt into activity groups by walking level measured by pedometer at baseline study. No oxygen during 1-week trial. Medial level was 0.68 miles per day.

Reproduced from Petty TL, McCoy RW, Doherty DE. *Long Term Oxygen Therapy (LTOT) History, Scientific Foundations, and Emerging Technologies: Sixth Oxygen Consensus Conference Recommendations*. National Lung Health Education Program; August 2005.

providing the required O_2 to meet their needs with activity. In the NOTT study, patients who were high walkers with 12 hours of O_2 had a higher survival than low walkers on 24 hours of O_2 (**Figure 25-9**). This finding indicated that activity had a greater impact on survival than continuous-flow O_2 delivery.

Methods of Oxygen Delivery

Continuous-flow O_2 delivery is the standard for O_2 delivery in the hospital and in institutional settings with unlimited O_2 supply, typically from an industrial liquid O_2 source. This is the simplest form of O_2 delivery because the only requirements are a device to meter the flow of O_2 and a patient interface. With an unlimited supply of O_2, simply increasing flow when patient O_2 demands an increase is a viable solution. With a limited supply of O_2, however, alternatives are required. In the home, stationary O_2 from a concentrator (**Figure 25-10**) can be thought of as unlimited because the O_2 source is dependent only on electricity, which is usually available. If a packaged gas is used, such as liquid oxygen or compressed gas, refill and distribution issues as well as cost become a consideration.

Intermittent-flow oxygen was a technical challenge until the mid-1980s, when the first intermittent-flow O_2 delivery system was introduced.[28] Sensing a patient's

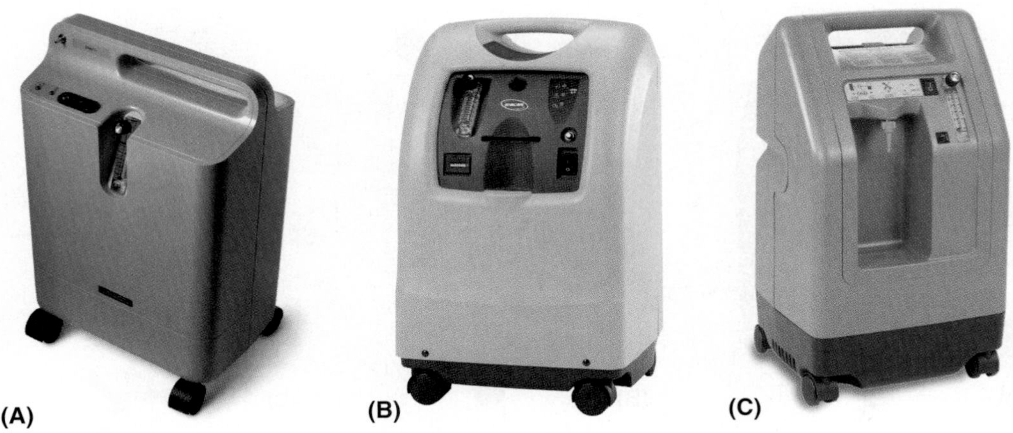

FIGURE 25-10 Example of three stationary oxygen concentrators.

(**A**) courtesy of Philips Respironics; (**B**) courtesy of Invacare Corporation; (**C**) courtesy of DeVilbiss Healthcare.

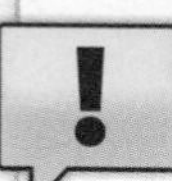

Respiratory Recap

Methods of Oxygen Delivery

- Continuous flow
- Intermittent flow

inspiratory effort and triggering a dose of O_2 at the beginning of the patient's inspiratory cycle was an engineering challenge because technology had not evolved to accomplish the objective. Fluidic amplifiers and sensitive pressure switches were included in the first intermittent-flow devices, and the technology has evolved to a high level of sophistication at this time. The challenge to provide a device that is as sensitive as possible to trigger consistently, yet not too sensitive to auto-trigger. At this time, all intermittent-flow devices sense breathing through a nasal cannula.

Home Oxygen Delivery Devices

Oxygen concentrators have been the standard for stationary O_2 delivery in the home for decades. The convenience of producing O_2 in the home eliminated the need to refill package gas systems such as high-pressure cylinders and liquid O_2. Using pressure swing adsorption (PSA) methodology, O_2 is separated from nitrogen, and the net result is an F_{IO_2} of 0.93 ± 0.03. Over the years these systems have become more reliable and smaller, and consume less electricity than previous models. Today's typical home stationary O_2 concentrator weighs about 35 pounds (16 kg) and can provide up to 5 L/min continuous-flow O_2. These smaller systems produce less noise and heat, which had been an issue in years past. Stationary concentrators have become the anchor for most home O_2 programs, yet for an ambulatory patient, a portable O_2 system must be provided.

Compressed gas systems were the standard for home O_2 therapy until other options became available. Large cylinders were used in both the hospital and the home as the only source of O_2. When concentrators and liquid oxygen systems became available for the home, cylinder usage decreased. Small cylinders are still used with stationary O_2 when appropriate and in conjunction with a concentrator transfilling system (**Figure 25-11**). Small cylinders come in a variety of sizes and shapes designed to provide the lightest system for the patient, along with the greatest operating range. A typical fill pressure for a cylinder is 2000 psig, yet 3000 psig is available for newer cylinders designed for that operating pressure. Cylinders that are transfilled from a home concentrator will be at a purity equal to the source concentrator, which typically produces 93% ± 3% O_2. Cylinders filled at an industrial gas supplier are at 99% purity.

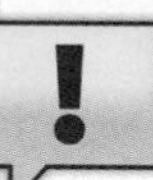

Respiratory Recap

Home Oxygen Delivery Devices

- Oxygen concentrators
- Compressed gas systems
- Liquid oxygen systems
- Concentrators that fill compressed gas systems
- Portable oxygen concentrators

Liquid oxygen (LOX) storage systems have the greatest storage capacity for O_2 (**Figure 25-12**). Most hospitals use large cryostats to supply the large volume of O_2 gas required by the hospital. Home LOX systems became available in the mid-1960s when Union Carbide introduced the first home LOX system. The benefit of the home LOX system is the ability to transfill a smaller, lightweight, portable O_2 system. Liquid O_2 has an 860:1 expansion ratio, so 1 liter of LOX will expand to 860 liters of gaseous O_2 with more efficiency and greater weight-to-operating-time ratio than packaged gas. LOX became the choice for patients who were highly ambulatory and required more functionality from their portable O_2 system. Limitations of a LOX system

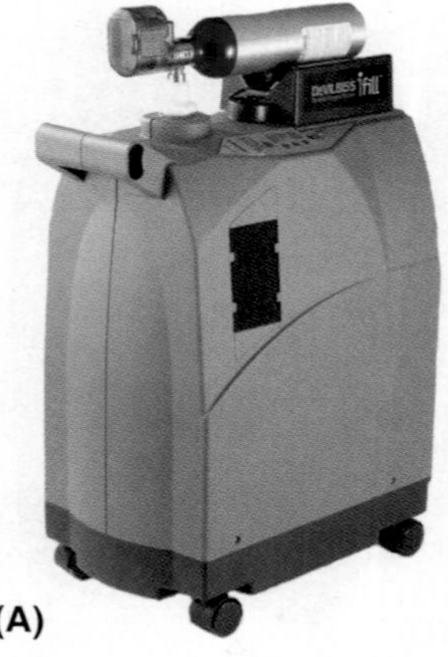
(A)

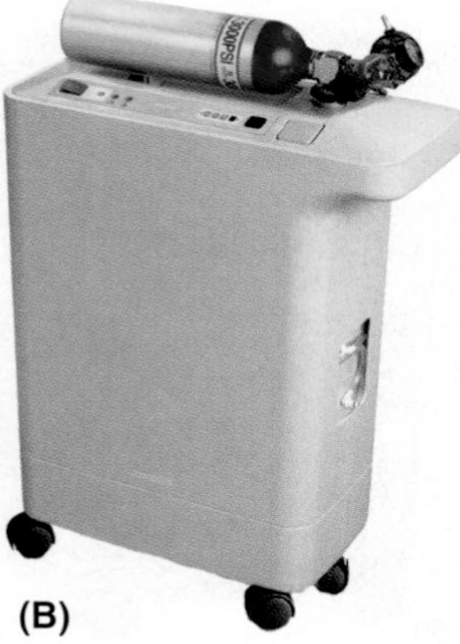
(B)

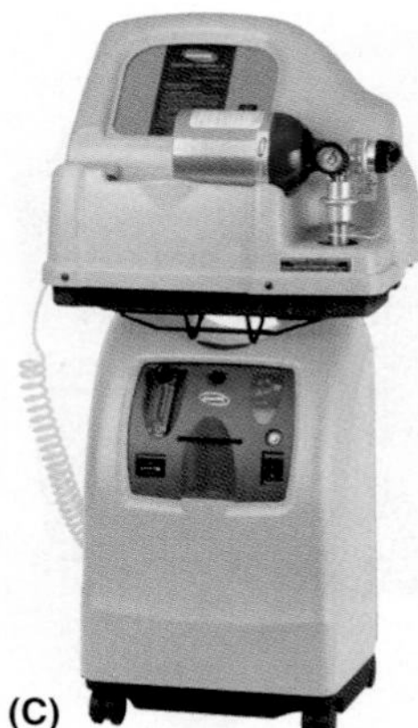
(C)

FIGURE 25-11 Transfilling concentrators.

(**A**) courtesy of DeVilbiss Healthcare; (**B**) courtesy of Philips Respironics; (**C**) courtesy of Invacare Corporation.

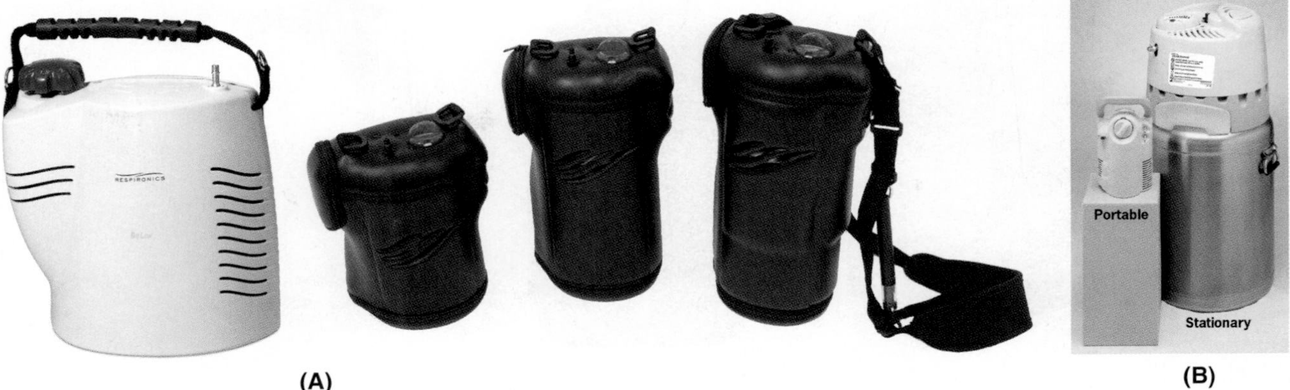

FIGURE 25-12 (**A**) Portable liquid oxygen units. (**B**) A liquid oxygen base unit with a portable.
(left) Courtesy of Philips Respironics; (middle and right) Courtesy of Chart, Inc.

are that it has a finite amount of gas and requires refilling from a larger base unit. Both the base units and portable units come in a variety of sizes, allowing for refilling options for both patients and O_2 distributors.

Concentrators that fill compressed gas cylinders in the home entered the market a few years ago. Models differ among manufacturers, but the principles remain the same. A concentrator generates O_2 and then transfers the O_2 as compressed gas to the portable cylinder. O_2 monitoring equipment ensures gas purity. This allows patients to refill cylinders themselves, and it saves the home care provider from visiting patients' homes to exchange cylinders. Concentrators that fill LOX portables have just become available for commercial use. The concentrator generates O_2 for the portable, but rather than pressurizing the gas, it is liquefied and transfills to the portable. This allows patients the advantage of both a lightweight and long-term-use portable.

O_2 purity in the portable that is transfilled, with both compressed gas and LOX, is about 94% due to the concentrator being the source gas. The variable with these systems is often the conserving device used with the portable because the source gas for all the systems is similar. Options available for a transfilling system are interchangeable regulators with postvalve cylinders, pressure ranges that affect operating times with 2000- and 3000-psig fill pressures, and an option for a combined or separate gas pumping unit for cylinders.

Portable oxygen concentrators (POCs) manufacture O_2; they do not store O_2 (**Figure 25-13**). This requires the POC to produce enough O_2 per minute to allow for an acceptable dose of O_2 to the patient with each breath. POC O_2 production is similar to the larger stationary systems, used in the home since the mid-1970s, which use PSA technology to generate O_2. POC manufacturers have been able to reduce the size of the sieve bed, improve compressor performance, utilize O_2-conserving technology, and integrate sophisticated battery systems to make these systems as small as possible. Each manufacturer has determined how much O_2 the device will produce, which determines maximum O_2 delivery, weight, and operating time.[29] These differences will have an impact on patient therapy, and the clinician needs to know the capabilities of a POC to determine the appropriate device to use for the patient. Patient needs vary as much as the POCs, so there is no one right POC for all patients. Knowing the capabilities of the POC, the needs of the patient, and the activities the patient will be doing while using the POC are important points of information for the clinician to consider when working with the patient to determine therapy options.

Recommendation 8 from the 1987 LTOT Consensus Conference states, "Clinical evaluation should include regular assessments of patients' compliance with prescribed therapy, potential complications, potential hazards and the need for continued education. Patients receiving LTOT share responsibility with the prescribing physicians for remaining in communication with their physician in order to assure continued appropriate care for their condition."[30] This recommendation emphasizes that patients be titrated on the O_2 system they will be using at all activity levels at which they will be using the device. Portable O_2 concentrators have the potential to be used at rest, exercise, sleep, and altitude. Each one of these situations needs to be evaluated with the patient and the specific POC.

Portable O_2 concentrators provide the benefit of making O_2 rather than storing it, which allows patients to use electricity to charge batteries so as to use the concentrator when they travel from home. These advantages are tempered by other constraints on the system's operation. Portable O_2 concentrators use the same technology as stationary O_2 concentrators, only in smaller sizes. That means that the maximum O_2 produced and the dosing of the O_2 differ by concentrator. These two variables restrict the system because the concentrator cannot make more O_2 than it was originally intended

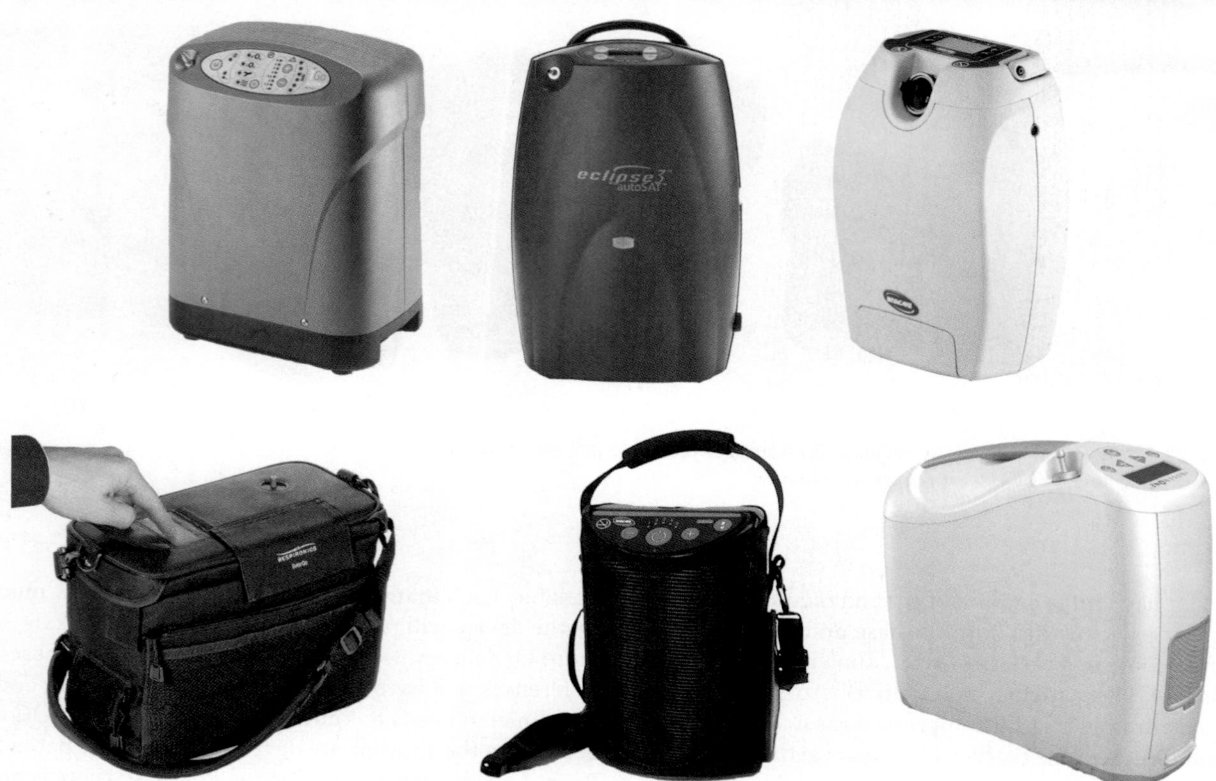

FIGURE 25-13 Portable oxygen concentrators. The units on top are greater than 10 lbs, and the units on the bottom are less than 10 lbs.
(top row, left to right) Courtesy of DeVilbiss Healthcare; SeQual Technologies, Inc.; and Invacare Corporation. (bottom row, left to right) courtesy of Philips Respironics; Invacare Corporation; and courtesy of Inogen.

to produce. If the patient increases the demand with a higher dose setting or respiratory rate, either delivered dose, O_2 purity, or both will decrease.[31] These limitations must be considered when prescribing and monitoring patients on this system, as well as any portable O_2 system, due to the limited maximum amount of O_2 that can be provided (**Figure 25-14**). Systems weighing less than 10 pounds (4.5 kg) only use oxygen-conserving technology and therefore are suitable for use in a car, airplane, or wheelchair (patient seated); they may have variable effectiveness with exercise. Systems weighing more than 10 pounds (4.5 kg) are capable of

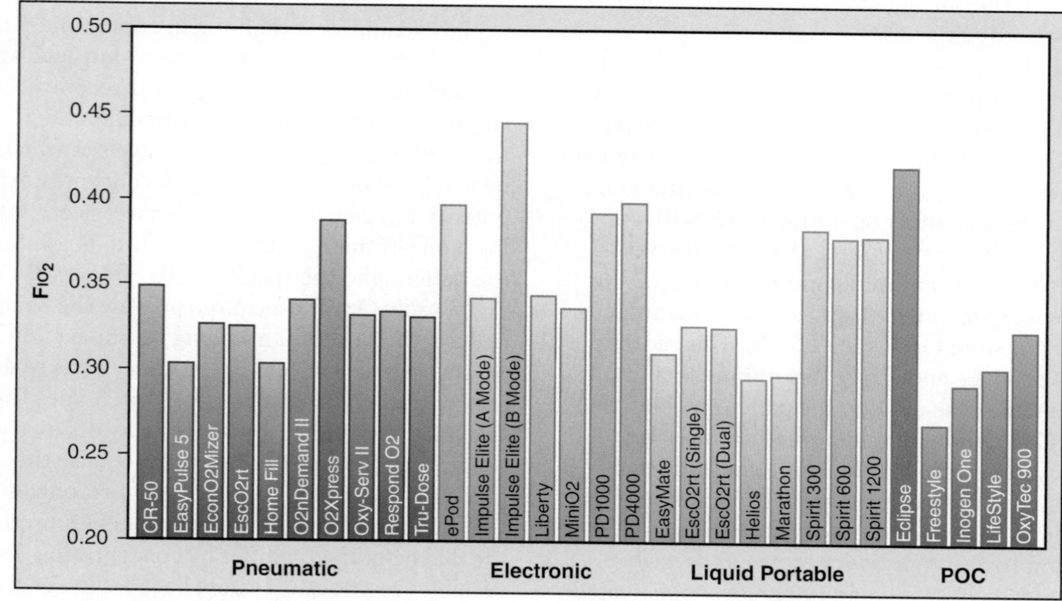

FIGURE 25-14 Maximum F_{IO_2} delivery among a variety of home portable oxygen systems.

continuous-flow and O_2-conserving and can be used for most purposes, including exercise and sleep.

Oxygen-Conserving Devices

In the past, patients were prescribed a default setting of 2 L/min continuous flow for O_2 delivery. If the patient's O_2 levels were appropriate, rarely did the clinician test to determine whether a lower setting would accomplish the same objective. Doing so would have conserved some O_2.[32] With the introduction of **oxygen-conserving devices (OCDs)**, regular CFO therapy from O_2 cylinders is being used much less than in the past for home care applications.

Reservoir cannulas, often referred to as moustache or pendant cannulas depending on the design and use characteristics, have approximately 20 mL of reservoir space that stores O_2 during exhalation (**Figure 25-15**). On inhalation, the patient receives that stored O_2, essentially adding a bolus volume to the ongoing continuous-flow delivery. These devices are simple, effective, and, when used properly, can allow a patient to receive the same therapy at a lower CFO flow rate, thus conserving O_2. Although they are effective, their appearance has been a limiting factor.

Intermittent-flow devices operate by turning O_2 delivery on during some portion of inhalation and off for the balance of the breathing cycle. In this way, O_2 that would otherwise be wasted as the patient exhales is conserved. This often allows a supply of O_2 to last two to four times as long as it would if it were delivered continuously.

One benefit of the use of intermittent-flow conserving devices is that a smaller O_2 supply may be carried. With intermittent-flow devices, the way in which O_2 is delivered to the patient differs greatly from one device to another, and no device delivers O_2 in the same way as continuous-flow devices. Intermittent-flow devices can be separated into two broad categories, pulse and demand, and within these categories there are many variants.

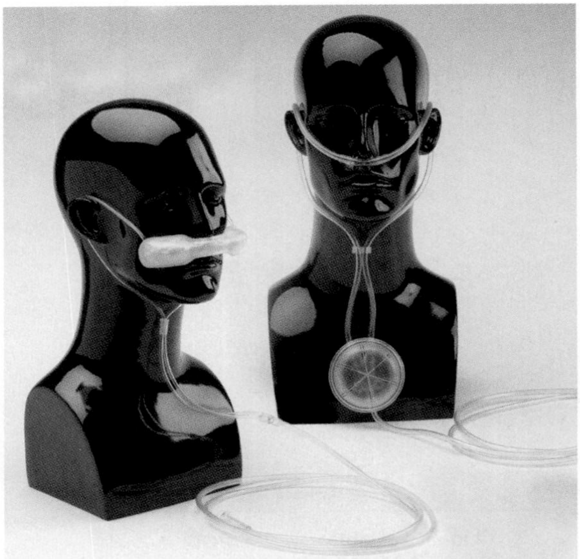

FIGURE 25-15 Reservoir cannulas.
Courtesy of Inovo/Chad Therapeutics.

Pulse flow is defined as the device responding to the patient's inspiratory effort and terminating flow at a predetermined time that is controlled electronically.[33] Pulse delivery devices deliver O_2 in the form of a relatively high flow rate bolus beginning early in inhalation. Some pulse delivery devices vary the dose of O_2 by changing the duration of the bolus. Others increase the peak flow rate at which the dose is delivered as the user increases the setting number. Some devices do a combination of both. Most pulse delivery devices deliver volumes at a given setting regardless of the breathing rate. As respiratory rate increases, the volume of O_2 inhaled from a CFO device over time does not change. With a typical pulse delivery device, however, the bolus volume is always the same, and so the O_2 volume inhaled per minute increases as the breath rate increases (assuming the entire bolus volume is inhaled; at high rates and/or high settings this may not be the case). As a patient moves from rest to activity and his or her breath rate increases, a pulse device operating in this manner may maintain oxygenation better than a continuous-flow or a demand device. This has not been proven clinically and it is impossible to say that pulse-type delivery is equivalent to continuous-flow delivery across a wide variety of breathing patterns. Device manufacturers, however, label their products with the same setting numbers used for continuous flow (1, 2, 3, etc.), and so there is often confusion about why a conserving device set at 2 is not oxygenating a patient like a continuous-flow device at 2 L/min. Pulse systems typically need a power source, so batteries are a factor to consider.

Demand delivery devices have evolved from the initial idea of creating an oxygen-conserving device that uses the patient's breathing to turn on the device during inhalation and off during exhalation. Demand flow senses the patient's inspiratory effort, yet flow is terminated on exhalation. The amount of O_2 delivered will vary with inspiratory time. These units are not as efficient as pulse-flow devices in utilization of O_2, yet have the advantage of not requiring batteries. Most demand systems use a dual-lumen cannula, with one

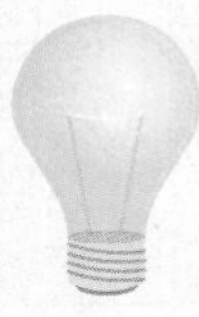

STOP AND THINK

You are asked to see a patient with interstitial lung disease who is using nasal cannula O_2 at a flow of 5 L/min. During ambulation, his Spo_2 drops from 92% to 80%. How would you decide on a more appropriate O_2 delivery system for mobility?

channel of the cannula sensing inspiration and the other channel delivering O_2. A set rate of O_2 is delivered over the entire inhalation cycle only. These devices are sometimes called hybrids because they act like both a pulse and demand device, delivering a fixed pulse volume at the onset of inhalation and then continuing to deliver O_2 until the device senses the beginning of exhalation.

Transtracheal oxygen (**Figure 25-16**) uses a catheter that is placed during a surgical procedure to bypass the upper airway.[34] The catheter is placed through a small hole made in the front of the neck and into the trachea. O_2 conservation is achieved because the patient is usually able to be given the equivalent of CFO therapy with nasal breathing at a lower continuous-flow setting. A single-lumen intermittent-flow conserving device can be used with transtracheal delivery, but the O_2 savings are about the same as using nasal breathing with that same intermittent-flow device. A benefit of transtracheal O_2 therapy is an increase in patient compliance with therapy because it is hidden from others to see the catheter.

With the manufacturers focusing on O_2 savings rather than patient oxygenation, OCDs have had an acceptance problem.[35] Because the devices differ in dose delivery (**Figure 25-17**), patients should be tested on the unit they will be using in the home and at the activity levels at which they will use the device. Clinicians need to be informed about the performance capabilities of each piece of equipment that a patient uses. A respiratory-rate-regulated OCD monitors the patient's respiratory rate and has an algorithm that switches the dose setting to a higher dose with a higher respiratory rate. As the patient breathes faster, the dose will increase; as the patient breathes slower, the dose will return to a lower setting. This technique allows the patient to increase the dose of O_2 with demand without manually changing the dose setting. An oximeter-regulated OCD monitors the patient's Spo_2. An algorithm in the device changes the O_2 dose based on Spo_2. There is an

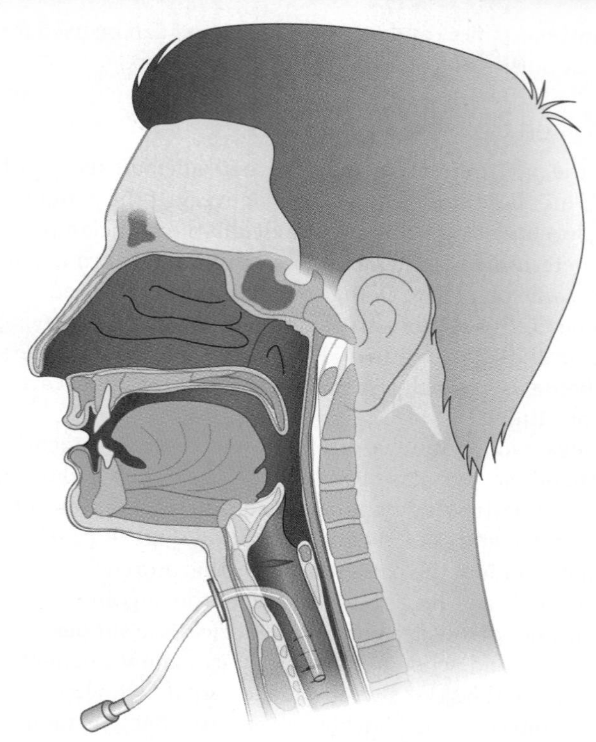

FIGURE 25-16 Transtracheal placement of oxygen delivery catheter.

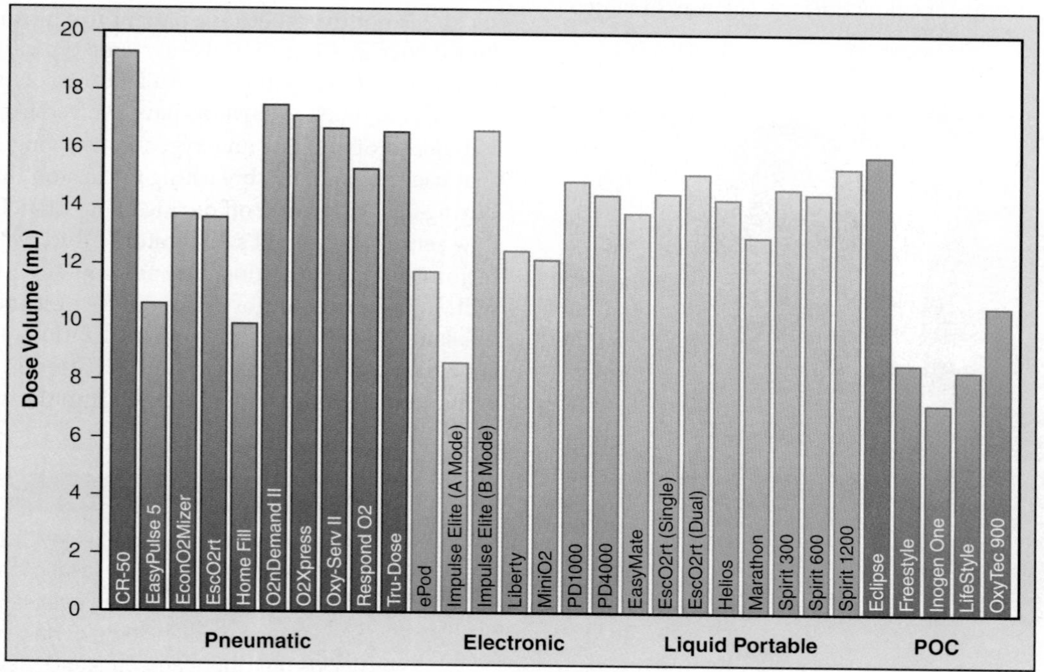

FIGURE 25-17 The average dose volume per setting for a variety of oxygen-conserving devices, indicating the high variability of dose volume among products.

Respiratory Recap

Oxygen-Conserving Devices

- Reservoir cannulas
- Intermittent-flow devices
- Pulse-flow devices
- Demand delivery devices
- Transtracheal oxygen

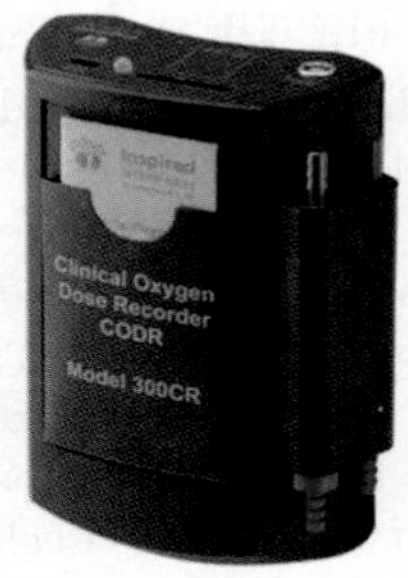

FIGURE 25-18 Clinical Oxygen Dose Recorder system.
Courtesy of Inspired Technologies, Inc.

approved product with this feature, but it is not currently commercially available. A motion-regulated OCD senses movement and changes the O_2 dose to a higher setting. When movement stops, the OCD then switches back to the lower dose setting. An approved product featuring this ability to change dose setting as a result of movement is currently on the market.

High-Flow Oxygen Delivery in the Home

Typically, home O_2 therapy is provided in a range of 1 to 6 L/min, yet flows of up to 10 L/min are possible from some O_2 concentrators. Home LOX systems can provide up to 15 L/min with units designed for that flow. Industrial LOX units can be used for flows higher than 15 L/min. Home portable O_2 systems can operate at higher flows, yet for a very short time. Patients requiring high-flow portable O_2 typically use a LOX system for the efficient operation. Special delivery tubing and cannulas need to be used for higher-flow systems to compensate for the resistance to the higher flows.

Diagnostics Systems for Long-Term Oxygen Therapy

Personal oximeters are used to assess a patient's Spo_2. Small simple-to-operate units can be used by patients to assess O_2 status. Patients' ability to understand the oximeter values and the variability of both the oximeter and the O_2 delivery system have caused some concern, yet many patients are purchasing personal oximeters. Education is key to the safe and effective use of a personal oximeter, and clinicians should take every opportunity to reinforce the issues related to their use.

Home care providers check continuous-flow units with devices that monitor O_2 concentration and flow. A simple liter meter can verify flow in the home and determine whether the O_2 delivery device is providing the flow correctly or whether extended O_2 supply tubing has created a drop in flow. There is a device that monitors both flows and O_2 concentrations. Basic O_2 monitors are also used for doing routine checks on home O_2 equipment. Pulse-dose O_2 delivery from an oxygen-conserving device requires a test unit that can measure volume rather than flow. These O_2 systems deliver a specific amount (mL) of O_2 that can be measured to determine whether the device is operating within specifications. Each oxygen-conserving device provides a different volume of O_2 at a specific setting, so the manufacturer's specific value is needed to determine whether the device is working within the specifications.

A system has been developed that can monitor both the O_2 delivery device and the patient (**Figure 25-18**). This unit can determine the delivery capabilities of the O_2 system and how the patient is responding. Given the great variability of performance in portable O_2 systems, this unit can help clinicians determine which home O_2 system should be used based on patient requirements.

Oxygen Delivery Accessory Items

Carts have helped patients be more mobile with their O_2 systems. Originally O_2 carts were the same as those used in the hospital, with weight and aesthetics being an issue. Now lightweight functional carts are available for the home O_2 patient's use. Backpacks became a request of patients who wanted to have more free use of their hands. A user-friendly backpack allows for more mobility for an active LTOT patient performing the activities of daily living than is typically possible with a shoulder strap. Shoulder straps have also evolved to more comfortable, aesthetically pleasing options. Some shoulder straps are made of elastic material that can act as a shock absorber for the pressure transferred to the shoulder.

Liter meters are devices that are used to spot-check the continuous flow from a low-flow O_2 device. These devices are used by home care providers to check the accuracy of the flow setting, yet patients can do the same spot check with proper training and availability of the tool. Pulse meters are devices that check the pulse volume of a pulse-style intermittent-flow device. These products are used by home care providers yet are more expensive than a liter meter, so may not be an option for patient purchase and use.

Batteries are an option for POCs because the operation time of a POC away from an AC or DC source is determined by the use time of the battery. If necessary, additional batteries can extend use time and are an important factor for air travel. Pulse-style conserving devices have a set battery life, so extra batteries should be available for the system as a backup.

Patient Delivery Interface Devices

The nasal cannula has been the standard for low-flow O_2 delivery. Cannula options have included multiple lengths for specific applications, different materials (e.g., plastic, silicone) different-diameter nasal prong lumens, and accessories for comfort. Lumen size and tubing length have an impact on O_2 delivery, and if the cannula is changed to a different capability, the flow and patient oximetry should be checked. Single-lumen cannulas are typical and account for the majority of cannula options. Dual-lumen cannulas are used with demand flow-conserving devices and can be used for other gas monitoring, such as CO_2 monitoring.

Headset low-flow O_2 delivery was originally designed to provide an alternative to the cannula putting pressure on the ears and cheeks. Headsets are used with prolonged phone use, so they appear to be a good option for patients using home O_2. Oxygen glasses have the same potential as the headset (**Figure 25-19**). The oxygen glasses also add an aesthetic value because often patients using these devices are not known to be wearing oxygen.

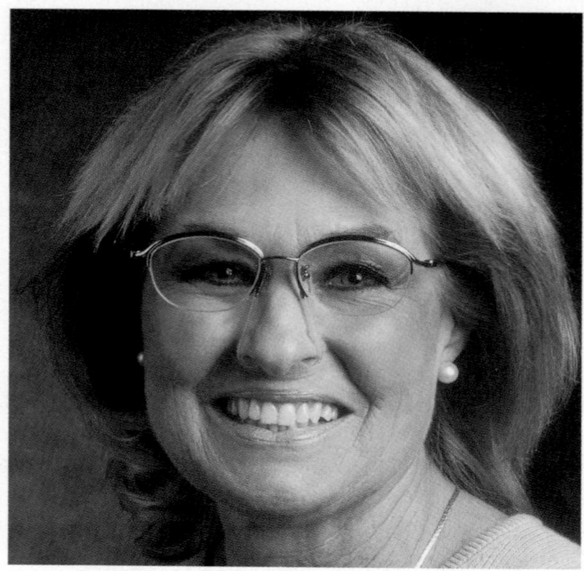

FIGURE 25-19 Oxy-View glasses.
Courtesy of Oxy-View, Inc.

Nasal masks are an alternative to the cannula. The nasal mask cups O_2 around the nose to eliminate the prongs entering the nose. If the nasal cannula prongs are causing irritation, the nasal mask can be used as an option. The nasal mask must be used with continuous-flow O_2 because the conserving-type systems would not be able to sense an inspiration and function properly.

Newer Home Therapies

The Breathe Technologies **NIOV (noninvasive open ventilation)** system is a 1-pound, battery operated, portable ventilator and a nasal pillows interface (**Figure 25-20**). Incorporating the Venturi principle at its nasal pillows interface, and a 50-psi oxygen gas source, the NIOV system augments the adult patient's tidal volume with supplemental oxygen and ambient air. The NIOV system has been shown to relieve dyspnea, increase oxygenation, reduce respiratory muscle activation, and increase patient activity and exercise endurance.[36] The FDA created a new ventilator code for the NIOV system, ONZ, for a volume assist ventilator intended for adult patients with respiratory insufficiency.

Nasal high flow (NHF) is a relatively new therapy that delivers high flows of blended, heated, and humidified oxygen through a specially designed nasal cannula. A home version of the therapy is available as the Fisher & Paykel My Airvo System. The device is a combination flow generator, air/oxygen blender, and heated humidifier used with the Fisher & Paykel Optiflow nasal cannula (**Figure 25-21**). A temperature sensor is built into the breathing circuit, keeping the device uncomplicated for home use. The flow generator can deliver up to 63% oxygen at flows of 15 to 45 L/min. Although an oxygen

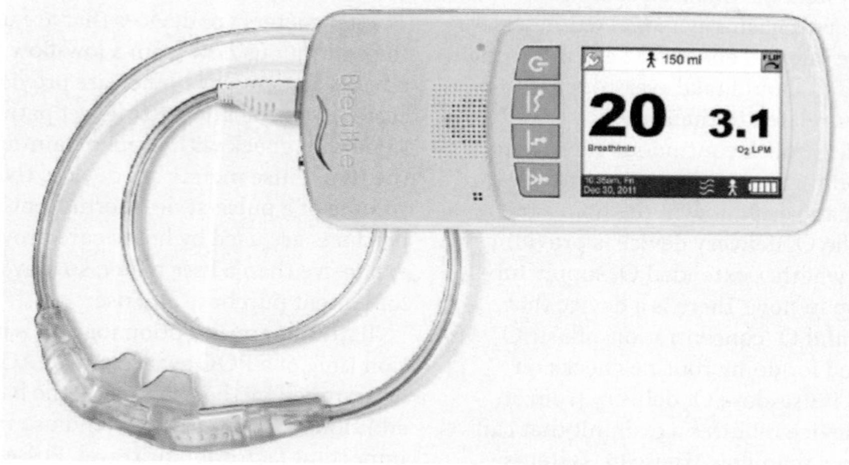

FIGURE 25-20 Breathe Technologies NIOV (noninvasive open ventilation) system.
Courtesy of Breathe Technologies.

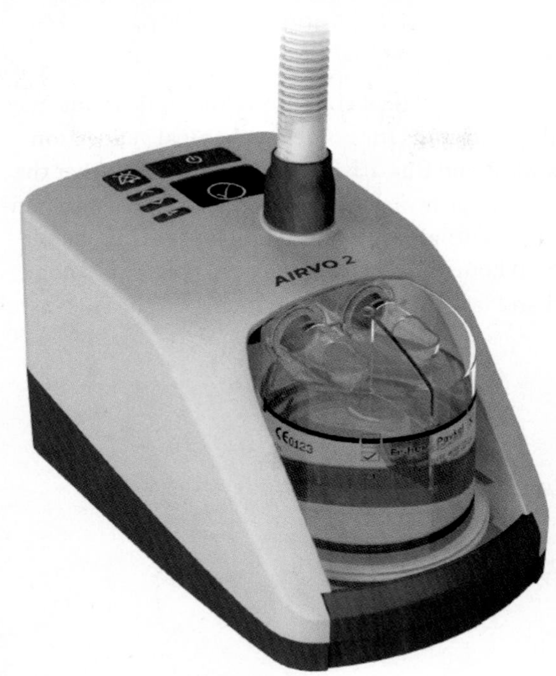

FIGURE 25-21 Fisher & Paykel My Airvo System.
Courtesy of Fisher & Paykel Healthcare, Inc.

source is required, the device eliminates the need for a compressor. The benefits of the system include the delivery of higher oxygen concentrations than can typically be achieved with a traditional nasal cannula, flushing of anatomic dead space, positive airway pressure during the respiratory cycle, and optimized mucociliary clearance.

Home Mechanical Ventilation

There is no general agreement on the definition of a home mechanical ventilator. Some clinicians refer to a bilevel flow generator that includes a backup rate, known in Medicare parlance as a *respiratory assist device* (RAD), as a mechanical ventilator. Other clinicians reserve the term *mechanical ventilator* for devices that include an exhalation valve (as opposed to a passive exhalation port) and the ability to set a breath rate and alarms. The Medicare program has categorized devices with exhalation valves, adjustable breath rates, and alarms as mechanical ventilators and places them in the group of devices requiring frequent and substantial service. Medicare will rent a mechanical ventilator for qualified patients as long as medical necessity exists. Medicare places respiratory assist devices in the capped rental category, however. For capped rental equipment, the DME provider receives a monthly rental fee for 13 months, after which the ownership of the equipment is transferred to the Medicare beneficiary. It is imperative for the home care RT to periodically reevaluate patients receiving any type of home ventilation, including those who are using respiratory assist devices. Some patients with deteriorating conditions such as ALS or Duchenne muscular dystrophy who are using a respiratory assist device may ultimately need to transition to a mechanical ventilator with appropriate alarms, patient monitoring, and emergency power supply. The plan for managing the patient's respiratory needs throughout the disease process should be discussed in advance with the patient and the physician as well as the patient's family when appropriate.

The Food and Drug Administration (FDA) classifies mechanical ventilators as described in **Table 25-3**. Note that all of the home ventilators classified by the FDA as life-support ventilators have been placed in the Medicare category that requires frequent and substantial service. The FDA has created an additional code, NOU, for home mechanical ventilators. The code's purpose is to clarify that home mechanical ventilators must be tracked by the home medical equipment company so that, in the event of a recall, the device can be located. The FDA broadly defines the intended use of each device; individuals who need noninvasive home mechanical ventilation for respiratory insufficiency are often placed on a MNS or NOU device, depending on the acuity of the patient's condition and the expected course of the disease and the physician's preference. Conversely, patients who have a tracheostomy and require home ventilation are almost always placed on a NOU device.

An accurate count of the number of individuals receiving home mechanical ventilation in the United States is unknown. In 1998 there were an estimated 10,000 to 20,000 patients on home mechanical ventilation.[17] Unlike many European countries, the United States does not have a central registry or database tracking individuals receiving either invasive or noninvasive home mechanical ventilation. Medicare claims data from 2010 indicate approximately 3172 patients on

TABLE 25-3
FDA Classification of Mechanical Ventilators

FDA Code	FDA Definitions	Common Use Description
CBK	Continuous facility use	Life support ventilator* for patients with respiratory failure
NOU	Continuous home use	Life support ventilator* for patients with respiratory failure
MNS	Continuous, non–life supporting; nonactive exhalation valve	Non–life support, for patients with respiratory insufficiency or obstructive sleep apnea

*The term *life support ventilator* generally refers to a device that can be used invasively or noninvasively and will support apneic patients; it includes alarms, exhaled volume monitoring, and an internal battery.

home mechanical ventilation using an invasive interface and 899 patients on home mechanical ventilation with a noninvasive interface. There are approximately 36,117 patients using a RAD without a backup rate, and 7793 patients using a RAD with a backup rate. Taking these numbers together, it appears that roughly 47,981 Medicare patients are receiving some form of home ventilation. Of the total Medicare population using some form of RAD or ventilator, only approximately 6.6% are using invasive ventilation.[37]

Diagnoses and Indications for Home Mechanical Ventilation

A number of medical conditions and indications may result in the need for home mechanical ventilation (**Box 25-2** and **Box 25-3**). Note in particular that the indication for invasive ventilation (as opposed to noninvasive ventilation) for individuals requiring more than 20 hours of ventilatory support per day is not a hard and fast rule. Some individuals can be successfully

BOX 25-2

Medical Conditions That May Be Appropriate for Home Mechanical Ventilation

Central Nervous System Disorders

- Arnold-Chiari malformation
- Central nervous system trauma
- Cerebrovascular disorders
- Congenital and acquired central control of breathing disorders
- Myelomeningocele
- Spinal cord traumatic injuries

Neuromuscular Disorders

- Amyotrophic lateral sclerosis
- Guillain-Barré syndrome
- Myotonic dystrophy
- Muscular dystrophies
- Myasthenia gravis
- Phrenic nerve paralysis
- Polio and postpolio sequelae
- Spinal muscle atrophy

Skeletal Disorders

- Kyphoscoliosis
- Thoracic wall deformities
- Thoracoplasty

Cardiovascular Disorders

- Acquired and congenital heart disease

Respiratory Disorders

- Upper airway
  - Pierre-Robin syndrome
  - Tracheomalacia
  - Vocal cord paralysis
- Lower airway
  - Bronchopulmonary dysplasia
  - Chronic obstructive pulmonary disease
  - Cystic fibrosis
  - Complications of infectious pneumonias
  - Pulmonary fibrotic diseases

Adapted from Make BJ, Hill NS, Goldberg AI, et al. Mechanical ventilation beyond the intensive care unit: report of a consensus of the American College of Chest Physicians. *Chest*. 1998;113(5 suppl):289S–344S.

BOX 25-3

Indications for Home Mechanical Ventilation

Indications for Noninvasive Ventilation

Patient has chronic stable or slowly progressive respiratory failure:

- Significant CO_2 retention ($Paco_2$ ≥50 mm Hg) with appropriately compensated pH *or*
- Mild daytime nocturnal CO_2 retention ($Paco_2$ 45 to 50 mm Hg) with symptoms attributable to hypoventilation (e.g., morning headaches, restless sleep, nightmares, enuresis, daytime hypersomnolence)
- Significant nocturnal hypoventilation or oxygen desaturation

The following conditions have been met:

- Patient has had optimal medical therapy for underlying respiratory disorders
- Patient is able to protect airway and adequately clear secretions
- Patient's reversible contributing factors have been treated (e.g., obstructive sleep apnea, congestive heart failure, severe electrolyte disturbance)

The diagnosis is appropriate.

Indications for Invasive Ventilation

Patient meets indications for noninvasive ventilation and has the following:

- Uncontrollable airway secretions despite use of noninvasive expiratory aids *or*
- Impaired swallowing leading to chronic aspiration and repeated pneumonias

Patient has persistent symptomatic respiratory insufficiency and fails to tolerate or improve with noninvasive ventilation.

Patient needs round-the-clock (>20 hours per day) ventilatory support because of severely weakened or paralyzed respiratory muscles (e.g., high spinal cord injury or end-stage neuromuscular disease) and patient or provider prefers invasive ventilation.

Adapted from Make BJ, Hill NS, Goldberg AI, et al. Mechanical ventilation beyond the intensive care unit: report of a consensus of the American College of Chest Physicians. *Chest*. 1998;113(5 suppl):289S–344S.

ventilated with noninvasive methods for 24 hours per day for many years.[38] Some patients prefer invasive ventilation if the need for support is continuous or almost continuous, however. Also note that the indications listed are similar to, but not exactly the same as, the Centers for Medicare and Medicaid Services (CMS) requirements for coverage of respiratory assist devices. The American Association of Respiratory Care and the American College of Chest Physicians both have drafted goals for the management of mechanical ventilation in the home (**Table 25-4**).

TABLE 25-4
Goals for Home Mechanical Ventilation

American College of Chest Physicians	American Association for Respiratory Care
Provide an environment that enhances the individual's potential Improve physical and physiologic function Reduce morbidity Extend life Provide cost-effective care	Sustain and extend life Enhance the quality of life Reduce morbidity Improve or sustain physical and psychological function of all VAIs and enhance growth and development in pediatric VAIs Provide cost-effective care

VAI, ventilator-assisted individual.
Adapted from Make BJ, Hill NS, Goldberg AI, et al. Mechanical ventilation beyond the intensive care unit: report of a consensus of the American College of Chest Physicians. *Chest*. 1998;113(5 suppl):289S–344S.

Discharge Planning for the Patient Going Home with a Mechanical Ventilator

If a hospitalized patient is prescribed home mechanical ventilation, a comprehensive team approach to discharge planning is required (**CPG 25-1**). Most home care RTs suggest a minimum of 2 weeks of preparation to ensure that the home environment is appropriate and that all required education has been performed.

Most home care companies require that a minimum of two family or lay caregivers be identified and trained prior to discharge of the home mechanically ventilated patient. Appropriately trained lay caregivers must be

CLINICAL PRACTICE GUIDELINE 25-1

Oxygen Therapy in the Home or Alternate-Site Healthcare Facility

Indications

- Long-term oxygen therapy (LTOT) in the home or alternate-site healthcare facility is normally indicated for the treatment of hypoxemia. LTOT has been shown to significantly improve survival in hypoxemic patients with chronic obstructive pulmonary disease (COPD). LTOT has been shown to reduce hospitalizations and lengths of stay.
- Laboratory indications: Documented hypoxemia in adults, children, and infants older than 28 days as evidenced by (1) Pa_{O_2} less than or equal to 55 mm Hg or Sa_{O_2} less than or equal to 88% in subjects breathing room air or (2) Pa_{O_2} of 56 to 59 mm Hg or Sa_{O_2} or Sp_{O_2} less than or equal to 89% in association with specific clinical conditions (e.g., cor pulmonale, congestive heart failure, erythrocythemia with hematocrit above 56).
- Some patients may not demonstrate a need for oxygen therapy at rest (normoxic) but will be hypoxemic during ambulation, sleep, or exercise. Oxygen therapy is indicated during these specific activities when the Sa_{O_2} is demonstrated to fall to 88% or below.
- Oxygen therapy may be prescribed by the attending physician for indications outside of those noted above or in cases where strong evidence may be lacking (e.g., cluster headaches) on the order and discretion of the attending physician.
- Patients who are approaching the end of life frequently exhibit dyspnea with or without hypoxemia. Dyspnea in the absence of hypoxemia can be treated with techniques and drugs other than oxygen. Oxygen may be tried in these patients at 1 to 3 liters per minute to obtain subjective relief of dyspnea.
- All oxygen must be prescribed and dispensed in accordance with federal, state, and local laws and regulations.

Contraindications

No absolute contraindications to oxygen therapy exist when indications are present.

Precautions and Possible Complications

- There is a potential in some spontaneously breathing hypoxemic patients with hypercapnia and chronic obstructive pulmonary disease for oxygen administration to lead to an increase in Pa_{CO_2}.
- Undesirable results or events may result from noncompliance with physicians' orders or inadequate instruction in home oxygen therapy.
- Complications may result from use of nasal cannulas or transtracheal catheters.
- Fire hazard is increased in the presence of increased oxygen concentrations.
- Bacterial contamination associated with certain nebulizers and humidification systems is a possible hazard.
- Possible physical hazards can be posed by unsecured cylinders, ungrounded equipment, or mishandling of liquid oxygen. Power or equipment malfunction and/or failure can lead to an interruption in oxygen supply.

Modified from AARC clinical practice guideline: oxygen therapy in the home or alternative site health care facility. *Respir Care.* 2007;52:1063–1068. Reprinted with permission.

able to explain and demonstrate the proper use, troubleshooting, and routine maintenance of the ventilator and all related equipment (**Table 25-5**). The caregiver must know how and when to order supplies and must be able to maintain good infection control processes. Importantly, the caregiver must verbalize and demonstrate the proper response to emergencies such as power failures, equipment failures, or serious patient events such as accidental decannulation.[39]

Ideally, the home care RT works with the appropriate hospital staff to complete an instructional checklist to ensure that the patient and family are properly trained (**Table 25-6**). Education of the patient and of family caregivers should promote positive interactions in a low-key manner.[40] Depending on the patient's condition and on family caregiver availability, it helps if each educational session is limited to 30- to 60-minute time periods over several days. These sessions may be taught by the RT and reinforced by the hospital nursing staff, or vice versa. It is also crucial that patients (when able), as well as family caregivers, perform return demonstrations without prompting.

TABLE 25-5
Common Home Medical Equipment and Supplies for a Patient Ventilated at Home

Home Medical Equipment		
Bedside ventilator and wheelchair ventilator Wheelchair Heated humidifier Portable suction machine (stationary suction machine optional) External battery and charger or universal power supply (UPS) Oximeter	Stationary oxygen concentrator Portable oxygen system Nebulizer compressor and/or 50-psi compressor Hospital bed Portable battery and charger End-tidal or transcutaneous CO_2 monitor Resuscitation bag	Enteral pump & pole stand Special mattress surface (to promote skin integrity and to avoid pneumonia) Cough assist device Intermittent percussive ventilator (IPV) Lymphedema pump Remote ventilator alarm and/or patient monitoring system
Supplies		
Oxygen tubing Oximeter probe Tracheostomy tubes and inner cannulas (patient size and one size smaller) Flex tubing (tracheostomy tube to ventilator circuit) Tracheostomy care kits Heat and moisture exchangers Bacterial filters for ventilator and cough assist Water traps (if not using heated tubing) MDI and/or nebulizer ports	Suction tubing and canister End-tidal or transcutaneous monitor supplies Syringes (for cuff maintenance) Ventilator circuits Tracheostomy ties Humidifier chambers Tubing for cough assist Enteral pump sets	Nebulizer cups Gloves Suction catheters Speaking valve Elbows (tracheostomy tube to flex tubing) Distilled or sterile water for humidifier (per prescription) IPV circuits Lymphedema stockings

TABLE 25-6
Predischarge Joint Instructional Plan for Home Mechanical Ventilation

Instructions for form completion: 1. List the topic that will be covered. 2. Jointly determine whether the hospital RN, hospital RT, or home care RT is responsible for instruction of each topic. 3–6. Record the instructor's name, the date(s) of the verbal instruction, and the date(s) of the demonstration. Record your initials and date in column 5 if the patient/family demonstrated with verbal assistance and in column 6 if patient/family demonstrated skill completely independently.

1. Topic	2. Person Responsible for Instruction	3. Verbal Instruction Provided *(Also note "WM" if written materials provided)*	4. Demonstration Provided	5. Patient/ Family Performed Satisfactory Demonstration with Verbal Assistance	6. Patient/ Family Performed Satisfactory Demonstration Without Assistance
Use of resuscitation bag • When to use • Connect to O_2 • Adjusting O_2 flow • How hard to squeeze bag • Rate of squeeze					
Suctioning • Check suction pressure • Supplies used at home (glove[s], kit) • When to suction • Preoxygenation • Remove from ventilator • Insert catheter • Remove catheter • Number of passes • Back on ventilator					

Home care RTs usually recommend a minimum 24-hour live-in demonstration, during which the family caregivers perform all of the patient's care without help from the RT or hospital staff, as the final indication that the patient and family are ready for discharge.

Evolution of Positive Pressure Home Mechanical Ventilators

The first generation of positive pressure home care ventilators were piston driven and offered only volume control (**Table 25-7**). These ventilators weighed over

TABLE 25-7
Evolution of Positive Pressure Home Mechanical Ventilators

	Generation 1		Generation 2				Generation 3			
Name	LP-3 to LP-20	PLV Series	T-Bird Series	LTV Series	HT 50	Achieva	Astral 150	PB 540	Trilogy 100	Vivo 50
Current manufacturer	Covidien (Boulder, CO)	Phillips Respironics (Murrysville, PA)	CareFusion (San Diego, CA)	CareFusion (San Diego, CA)	Newport Medical (Costa Mesa, CA)	Covidien (Boulder, CO)	ResMed (San Diego, CA)	Covidien (Boulder, CO)	Philips Respironics (Murrysville, PA)	Breas (Charlottesville, VA)
Weight (lb)	34	28.9	34	14.5	15	32	7.1	9.9	11.5	5.2 (kg)
Dimensions (in.)	9.75 × 14.5 × 13.25	9 × 12.25 × 12.25	13.0 × 11.0 × 13.5	3.25 × 10.5 × 13.5	10.63 × 7.87 × 10.24	10.75 × 13.30 × 15.60	11.22 × 8.47 × 3.66	6.0 × 9.2 × 12.4	4.5 × 6.88 × 9.5	348 × 120 × 264 (mm)
Flow generator	Piston	Piston	Turbine	Turbine	Dual pistons	Piston	Turbine	Turbine	Turbine	Turbine
FDA approval date	1977	10/20/83	5/3/96	10/30/98	8/4/00	10/18/00	6/4/14	10/31/08	3/13/09	6/18/13
FDA code	CBK	CBK	CBK	CBK	CBK	CBK	CBK/NOU	CBK	CBK	NOU/CBK
Minimum patient weight (kg)	Not specified	Not specified	10	5	10	5	5	5	5	10
Modes	A/C vol; A/C vol. with press. limit; SIMV vol.; SIMV vol. with press. limit; press. cycle	Control vol.; A/C vol.; SIMV vol.	Control (vol. or press.); A/C (vol. or press.); SIMV (vol. or press.); CPAP; pressure support	A/C (vol. or press.); SIMV (vol. or press.), pressure support, CPAP	A/C (vol. or press.); SIMV (vol. or press.); spontaneous	A/C (vol. or press.); SIMV (vol. or press.); spontaneous, CPAP, PS+CPAP	(A)CV, P(A)CV, P-SIMV, V-SIMV, PS, CPAP, (S)T, P(A)C	CPAP; PS; A/C (vol. or press.); SIMV (vol. or press.)	Pres. modes: CPAP; S; S/T; PC; PC-SIMV Vol. modes: A/C; SIMV + PS; CV	PSV; PSV (TgV); PCV; PCV (TgV); PCV(A); PCV(A + TgV); VCV; VCV(A); CPAP
Single-limb passive	No	No	No	No	No	No	Yes	Yes	Yes	Yes
Single-limb valve	Yes	Yes	No	No	Yes	Yes	Yes	Yes	Yes	Yes
Dual-limb valve	No	No	Yes	Yes	No	No	Yes	Yes	No	No
Tidal volume (mL)	100–2200	200–3000	50–2000	50–2000	100–2200	50–2200	50–2500	50–2000	50–2000	100–2500
Breath rate (breaths/min)	1–38	2–40	2–80	0–80	1–99	1–80	0-80	1–60	1–60	4–40
Pressure control (cm H_2O)	No	No	1–100	1–99	5–60	No	50	0–60	4–50	4–50
Pressure support (cm H_2O)	No	No	1–60	1–60	0–60	0–50	0–50	5–55	0–30	4–40
Inspiratory time	0.5– 5.5 s	10–120 L/min	0.3–10 s	0.3–9.9 s	1.1–3.0 s	0.2–5.0 s	0.3–5.0 s	0.3–6.0 s	0.3–5.0 s	0.3–5.0 s
Trigger	Pressure	Pressure	Flow	Flow	Pressure	Flow and pressure	Flow/pressure	Flow	Flow	Flow

A/C, assist/control; SIMV, synchronized intermittent mandatory ventilation; CPAP, continuous positive airway pressure; PS, pressure support; S, spontaneous; S/T, spontaneous-timed; T, timed; PC, pressure control; CV, control ventilation; PRVC, pressure-regulated volume control; VC, volume control; PC, pressure control.

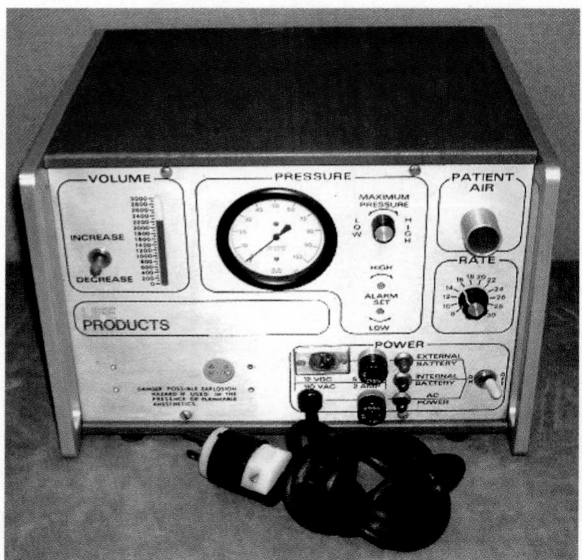

FIGURE 25-22 Life Products LP3.

30 pounds (14 kg) and had very limited internal battery duration. First-generation devices had few options for external batteries other than large, sealed lead-acid batteries. Bulky external positive end-expiratory pressure (PEEP) valves also contributed to the lack of easy portability. First-generation home care ventilators included the Life Products LP-3 (**Figure 25-22**) and Lifecare Services PLV-100 portable ventilators. Surprisingly, some patients still use first-generation devices.

With a few exceptions, the second generation of home ventilators switched from piston driven to turbine driven. Another major difference between first- and second-generation ventilators was the addition of modes such as pressure control, pressure support, and synchronized intermittent mandatory ventilation (SIMV). The second-generation ventilators also offered significant improvements in battery options, as well as enhanced portability. Most of the second-generation ventilators allow supplemental O_2 to be connected to a port directly on the ventilator rather than titrated into the patient circuit. Additionally, most of the second-generation devices changed from using an external PEEP control to a PEEP control integrated into the ventilator. There are many patients still using second-generation devices.

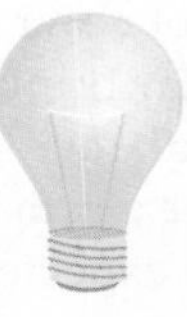

STOP AND THINK

You are asked to help a patient select a ventilator. He has a tracheostomy and requires ventilation secondary to cervical spine injury. What are important considerations in the selection of a ventilator that best meets his needs?

Almost all of the third-generation ventilators are turbine driven and include significant advances in portability and features. Some allow the use of both passive circuits (such as found on a traditional bilevel device) and active circuits (which include an exhalation valve rather than an exhalation port). Most third-generation ventilators allow optional direct exhaled volume monitoring (rather than a software algorithm that estimates the exhaled volume). Additionally, the portability of the third-generation ventilators has increased significantly, and the first hot-swappable battery was introduced. Third-generation home ventilators are also the first to offer hybrid modes that deliver pressure breaths while guaranteeing delivery of a target tidal volume. The latest home ventilators also feature graphics (**Figure 25-23**) and have integrated software to allow various reports to be downloaded and printed, including waveforms, ventilator settings, alarm history, patient compliance data, oximetry, and summary reports (**Figure 25-24**). These additional data are quite helpful for the RT when troubleshooting ventilator problems such as excessive leaks, hypoventilation, and/or desaturations.[41]

Backup Ventilator and Emergency Supplies

There is wide variation across the United States with regard to when a **backup ventilator** is provided to the patient. The Medicare system generally does not pay for a backup ventilator but may pay for a secondary ventilator when medically indicated.[42] Generally, in order for Medicare to consider coverage for a secondary ventilator, there must be documentation from the physician stating that the patient cannot maintain spontaneous ventilation for 4 or more hours, that a ventilator is required on the patient's wheelchair or mobility device as part of the patient's rehabilitation plan, or that the expected response time from emergency services is greater than 2 hours. Unfortunately, lack of reimbursement often means that patients who have a clearly demonstrated clinical requirement for a second ventilator do not receive one.

All home mechanically ventilated patients should have a **go-bag** prepared to accompany them on any trips outside the home. The detail-oriented RT should

Respiratory Recap

Home Mechanical Ventilators

- All first-generation ventilators were piston driven and offered only volume-controlled breaths.
- Most second-generation ventilators switched from piston driven to turbine driven and offered a variety of modes.
- Most third-generation ventilators are turbine driven and include significant advances in portability, modes, and features.

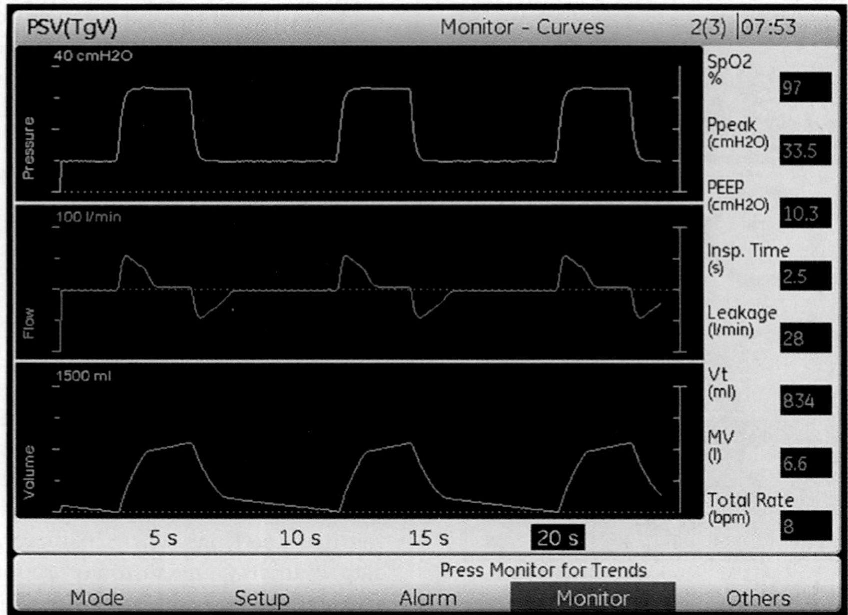

FIGURE 25-23 Breas Vivo 50 home care ventilator screen.

Courtesy of Breas Medical.

include a check of the go-bag during each visit to the patient's home. The most important item in the go-bag is a manual resuscitation bag. It must be stressed to the patient and family that the resuscitation bag *always* goes with the patient. Other important items for the go-bag may include the following:

For Patients Receiving Invasive or Noninvasive Ventilation

- Resuscitation bag
- Copy of prescription including vent settings
- Copy of important phone numbers, including referring physician
- Second power supply for ventilator (external battery or DC power cord)
- Handrub
- Flashlight
- Ventilator circuit (including metered dose inhaler and/or nebulizer port if applicable)
- Extra patient interface (mask) and headgear (if noninvasive)
- Cylinder wrench (if on O_2)
- O_2 tubing (if on O_2)
- Battery-operated nebulizer and medications (if applicable)
- Inhaler(s)

For Patients Receiving Invasive Ventilation

- Spare tracheostomy tube (one size smaller)
- Tracheostomy ties and split gauze
- Syringes for cuff inflation/deflation
- Spare heat and moisture exchangers
- Battery-operated suction machine with canister, tubing, and catheters
- Normal saline vials (if prescribed)
- Spare flex tube

Setting Ventilator Alarms

Unfortunately, patients sometimes die at home from accidental ventilator disconnections, even patients who have been home for a long period of time and presumably have experienced caregivers.[43] Continuous visual monitoring of the home mechanically ventilated patient is best, but there are times when the family caregiver must rely on the audible alarms.[44] One of the most important and problematic tasks faced by the RT is determining appropriate alarm settings. Some RTs may simply duplicate the alarm settings that were in use at the hospital prior to the patient's discharge. This method of alarm setting may not be adequate at home, however. While in the hospital, the patient's Spo_2, respiratory rate, and heart rate were undoubtedly monitored via a central monitoring system that added another layer of protection above and beyond the ventilator alarms. Many payers, however, do not cover a home continuous-use pulse oximeter. RTs may think that because the doctor signed off on the ventilator settings, the therapist is not responsible for the alarm settings. Realistically, the physician cannot be expected to know the intricacies of every home ventilator. Clearly, the RT is the expert on the ventilator and must make appropriate recommendations to the physician if the proper orders are not received.

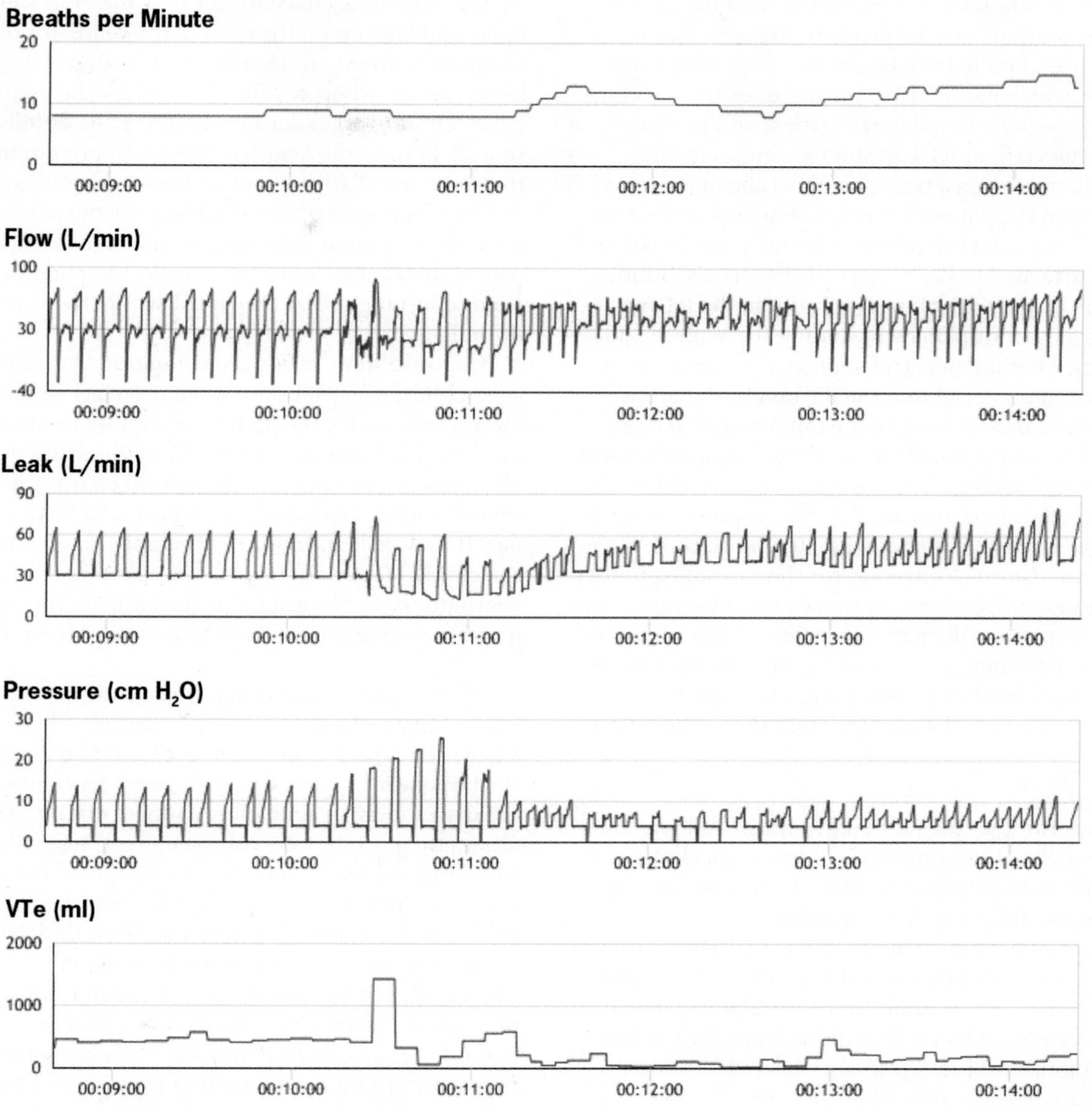

FIGURE 25-24 Sample report downloaded and printed from the Trilogy ventilator.
Courtesy of Philips Respironics.

Particularly for pediatric patients, there has been a move toward the use of pressure control. While in the hospital, if the patient partially decannulates, the low Spo_2 alarm and perhaps the high respiratory rate alarm will alert the staff, even if the ventilator did not sound a low-pressure alarm. Many of the second- and third-generation home ventilators have high flow capabilities and are able to reach the pressure control setting even in the face of significant leaks. At home, a patient who decannulates in pressure ventilation, particularly if the diameter of the tracheostomy tube is small, may not trigger a low-pressure ventilator alarm because the ventilator will most likely be able to achieve the prescribed pressure control setting. In this situation, a properly set low exhaled volume alarm,[44] low exhaled minute volume alarm, high inspired volume alarm, or high inspired minute volume alarm would most likely sound.

Another problematic situation can occur for patients who are prone to mucous plugging and who are on pressure control at home. If the patient develops a mucous plug that occludes a significant portion of the lung, or even a plug that completely blocks the tracheostomy tube, a high-pressure alarm will not sound. The same situation can develop if the heat and moisture exchanger becomes occluded or if the patient rolls over on the ventilator circuit.[45] In these situations, a properly set low exhaled volume alarm, low exhaled minute volume alarm, low inspired volume alarm, or low inspired minute volume alarm would most likely sound.

The RT should test the ventilator alarms per the manufacturer's instructions during every home visit, but some additional tests beyond the manufacturer's recommendations may be prudent. Many pediatric patients use uncuffed tracheostomy tubes with varying leaks, which complicates the use of exhaled volume alarms. Especially for pediatric patients on pressure control, the vigilant RT can simulate an accidental decannulation using a tracheostomy tube one size smaller than the patient's usual tube to ensure that an alarm will sound if the tube accidentally comes out and remains attached to the Y-piece of the circuit. If indicated for the patient's clinical condition, the RT may simulate a mucous plug by occluding the Y-piece and observing whether an alarm sounds. If an alarm does not sound, it is crucial that the RT obtain the proper order to take one or more of the following actions as appropriate: adjust the alarm settings, change the ventilator settings, change the ventilator to one that has the necessary alarm, or provide a cardio-respiratory monitor and/or a pulse oximeter with audible alarms. When there is no insurance coverage for the cardiorespiratory monitor or a pulse oximeter, the RT must become a vigorous advocate for the patient's safety. Often a letter to the insurance company describing the potential safety issues, signed by the physician and the respiratory therapist, may help the family obtain the needed device.

Safety Tips

It is important that the RT make frequent and regular visits to the ventilator patient's home to check the ventilator and related equipment. These visits are especially important for pediatric patients because they provide an opportunity to observe the patient's growth and development and how that may affect the respiratory care plan. For example, most ventilator-dependent infants are placed in a crib while sleeping for the first several months of life. Typically, a heated humidifier rests on a table near the crib.

One possible safety hazard can occur when parents allow the infant to play and crawl while on the floor. The vigilant therapist needs to make sure the parents understand that the baby should never be placed below the heated humidifier. Similarly, as the infant becomes stronger, care must be taken to prevent the infant from pulling the ventilator down off a table or bureau, perhaps sustaining an injury in the process or damaging the ventilator.

Respiratory Recap

Setting Ventilator Alarms

- A balance between safety and nuisance should be maintained.
- The RT should test ventilator alarms, with special caution for pediatric pressure ventilation.

The lighted O_2 concentrator flow meter as well as the lights and buttons on the front of the ventilator often fascinate toddlers, and inadvertent setting changes can be the result. Another safety hazard for the pediatric patient is accidental decannulation as the toddler tries to walk beyond the length of the ventilator circuit. Note that some ventilator manufacturers offer longer circuits to allow increased physical activity for the patient. Also, most parents know they have to secure the pediatric patient in a car seat while in a vehicle, but parents also need to be taught that they must secure the ventilator as well.

There are some safety considerations for school-aged children as well. A resuscitation bag should always travel with the patient, including on the school bus. Some schools may allow the patient to keep an extra power cord and/or battery and charger at the school, rather than carry them back and forth each day. It may be helpful for the therapist to offer to visit the child's classroom to give a simple talk on what the ventilator is and how it helps the patient. The school nurse may appreciate a brief overview of the ventilator as well.

Older children who hang their ventilator on the back of their wheelchair must be cautioned not to hang a heavy backpack over their ventilator and not to allow the backpack to block the ventilator's air intake. Older children may also appreciate a longer circuit, which allows them to shower while keeping the ventilator a safe distance away. Note that special ventilator covers can be purchased to protect the ventilator from moisture (Freedom Vent Systems, West End, NC). Care must be taken to prevent water from entering into or around the tracheostomy tube. A tracheostomy mask or sheet of plastic wrap placed over the area may be helpful. Active children may have trouble with their ventilator circuit disconnecting from the tracheostomy tube. A number of commercial products are available to secure the circuit. **Figure 25-25** shows one patient's ingenuity. Each day she chooses a grosgrain ribbon, color coordinated with her outfit, to secure her circuit.

Caregiver Burden

There is a high incidence of depression among family caregivers.[46] The home care RT should be mindful that the family caregiver may be at risk for depression and may consider discussing with the physician the use of a depression screening tool for caregivers, such as the Center for Epidemiological Studies Depression Screening Index (CES-D). When appropriate, the RT may consider querying the caregiver about his or her quality and amount of sleep, as well as reviewing the ventilator alarm logs, to determine whether excessive ventilator alarms are interrupting the caregiver's sleep. The RT should also be knowledgeable about local nursing services, respite programs, daycare facilities that accept ventilator patients, camps for

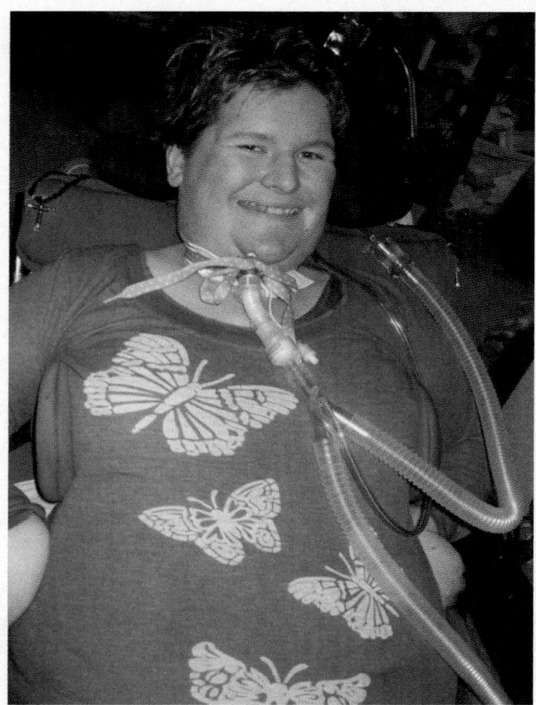

FIGURE 25-25 Example of patient and caregiver ingenuity: MJ uses a color-coordinated ribbon to secure her trach tube.

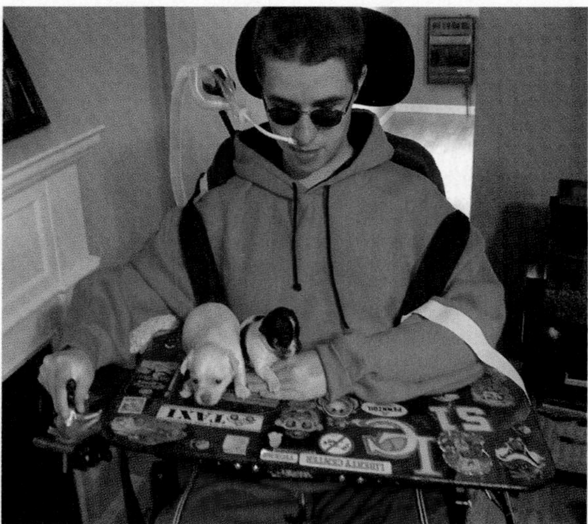

FIGURE 25-26 This young adult uses mouthpiece ventilation all day and mask ventilation at night. He works part time and enjoys raising puppies.

ventilator-dependent children, or other agencies that may provide some respite for the family caregiver.

Ventilator User's Quality of Life

Many healthcare workers underestimate the ventilator user's quality of life.[38] In a report of 621 ventilator users with neuromuscular conditions, it was found that about one-third of patients were employed; a few others reported they were active on a daily basis as volunteers or students. Healthcare professionals underestimated the satisfaction of severely disabled, ventilator-assisted people. The RT who has internalized that ventilator-dependent patients can have meaningful, productive lives can have a significant positive impact on the patient and family's quality of life (**Figure 25-26**).

Key Points

- Depending on the equipment ordered, durable medical equipment (DME) companies can provide service by a technician, respiratory therapist, or qualified nurse.
- The goals of home respiratory care are to achieve the optimum level of patient function through goal setting, educate patients and their caregivers, administer diagnostic and therapeutic modalities and services, conduct disease management, and promote health.
- Unfortunately, respiratory therapists are not included in the Medicare home health services benefit.
- A DME or home medical equipment (HME) company may be required to have a retail license, HME license, a bedding supplier license, an O_2 manufacturer/distributor license, and/or possibly other licenses/permits as required by the state.
- There are generally two types of accreditation for a DME or HME: Equipment Management Services and Clinical Respiratory Services.
- The respiratory therapist is the most competent healthcare professional to provide home respiratory care.
- The home environment must be evaluated specific to the type of home medical equipment.
- Bag technique means that the respiratory therapist's bag and its contents must be kept as clean as possible.
- Patients who receive O_2 at home are exposed to the risk of improper storage and handling of O_2 cylinders, unsafe usage of O_2, improper transfer of O_2, inadequate ventilation, and smoking or other unsafe flames.
- The environmental evaluation should verify the adequacy of the home electrical system for patients with a home ventilator.
- An important aspect of the home environmental assessment is to ensure that the caregiver in all areas of the home can hear alarms.
- It is a good idea for some home care patients, particularly O_2 and ventilator patients, to meet with their local EMS personnel and/or firefighters before there is any type of emergency.
- For patients with COPD, long-term O_2 therapy prolongs life and decreases overall cost of care.
- The goal for efficient O_2 delivery is proper arterial O_2 saturation at all activity levels.

- Methods of O_2 delivery in the home include continuous-flow oxygen and intermittent-flow oxygen.
- Home O_2 delivery devices include oxygen concentrators, compressed gas systems, liquid O_2 systems, concentrators that fill compressed gas systems, and portable O_2 concentrators.
- Oxygen-conserving devices include reservoir cannulas, intermittent-flow devices, pulse-flow devices, demand delivery devices, and transtracheal O_2.
- Medicare categorizes devices with exhalation valves, adjustable breath rates, and alarms as mechanical ventilators.
- The indication for invasive ventilation (rather than noninvasive ventilation) for individuals requiring more than 20 hours per day of support is not a hard and fast rule.
- A comprehensive team approach to discharge planning is required.
- The first generation of positive pressure home care ventilators was piston driven and offered only volume-controlled breaths.
- Most of the second generation of home ventilators switched from piston driven to turbine driven and offered additional modes.
- Most of the third-generation ventilators are turbine driven and include significant advances in modes, portability, and features.
- One of the most important and problematic tasks faced by the respiratory therapist is determining appropriate ventilator alarm settings.
- There is a high incidence of depression among family caregivers of patients ventilated at home.
- Many healthcare workers underestimate the ventilator user's quality of life.

References

1. American Association for Respiratory Care. Position statement: home respiratory care services. Available at: http://www.aarc.org/resources/position_statements/hrcs.html. Published December 14, 2000. Updated July 2010. Accessed July 21, 2014.
2. American Thoracic Society Documents. Statement on home care for patients with respiratory disorders. *Am J Respir Crit Care Med.* 2005;171:1443–1464.
3. Gay EG. Increasing home health services referrals, boon or bane? *Home Health Care Serv Q.* 1994;14:49–67.
4. Halliday H. History of surfactant from 1980. *Biol Neonate.* 2005;87:317–322.
5. U.S. Census Bureau. *2012 National Population Projections.* Available at: http://www.census.gov/population/projections/. Accessed August 1, 2014.
6. Bach JR, Intintola P, Alba AS, Holland IE. The ventilator-assisted individual. Cost analysis of institutionalization vs. rehabilitation and in-home management. *Chest.* 1992;101:26–30.
7. Field AI, Rosenblatt A, Pollack MM, Kaufman J. Home care cost-effectiveness for respiratory technology-dependent children. *Am J Dis Child.* 1991;145:729–733.
8. Lewarsksi JS, Gay PC. Current issues in home mechanical ventilation. *Chest.* 2007;132:671–676.
9. The Joint Commission. *2010 Standards for Home Medical Equipment, Rehabilitation Technology Services, and Clinical Respiratory Services.* Oakbrook Terrace, Ill.: Joint Commission; 2009.
10. Dunne PJ, McInturff SL. *Respiratory Home Care: The Essentials.* Philadelphia: FA Davis; 1998.
11. Posey SC, Aaltonen PM, DePalma RA, Femea P. Use of the public health nursing bag reexamined. *Public Health Nursing.* 2007;4:111–113.
12. Merlin MA, Wong ML, Pryor PW, et al. Prevalence of methicillin-resistant *Staphylococcus aureus* on the stethoscopes of emergency medical services providers. *Prehosp Emerg Care.* 2009;13:71–74.
13. Wolf A. When health care moves home. *NFPA J.* 1998;92(1). Available at: http://findarticles.com/p/articles/mi_qa3737/is_199801/ai_n8773480/?tag=content;col.
14. Pulmonetic Systems. *LTV 1000 Operator's Manual.* Minneapolis, Minn.: Pulmonetic Systems; 2005.
15. Turner J, McDonald GJ, Larter NL. *Handbook of Adult and Pediatric Respiratory Home Care.* St. Louis: Mosby; 1994.
16. American Association for Respiratory Care. Clinical practice guideline: long-term invasive mechanical ventilation in the home. *Respir Care.* 2007;52:1056–1062.
17. Make BJ, Hill NS, Goldberg AI, et al. Mechanical ventilation beyond the intensive care unit: report of a consensus of the American College of Chest Physicians. *Chest.* 1998;113(Suppl 5):289S–344S.
18. Stuban S. Safety issues generate practical solutions. *Ventilator-Assisted Living.* 2007;21:1–3.
19. Dunbar H, Wensley D. Guided self-management. In: Silverman M, O'Callaghan C, eds. *Practical Paediatric Respiratory Medicine.* London: Arnold; 2001:265–274.
20. Partridge MR. Self-management plans: uses and limitations. *Br J Hosp Med.* 1996;55:120–122.
21. AARC clinical practice guideline: oxygen therapy in the home or alternate site health care facility—2007 revision and update. *Respir Care.* 2007;52:1066–1068.
22. Nocturnal Oxygen Therapy Trial Group. Continuous or nocturnal oxygen therapy in hypoxemic chronic obstructive lung disease: a clinical trial. *Ann Intern Med.* 1980;93:391–398.
23. Report of the Medical Research Council Working Party: long-term domiciliary oxygen therapy in chronic hypoxic cor pulmonale complicating chronic bronchitis and emphysema. *Lancet.* 1981;1:681–686.
24. Petty TL, Bliss PL. Ambulatory oxygen therapy, exercise and survival with advanced COPD (the Nocturnal Oxygen Therapy Trial revisited). *Respir Care.* 2000;45:204–213.
25. Doherty DE, Petty TL, Bailey W, et al. Recommendations of the 6th Long-Term Oxygen Therapy Consensus Conference. *Respir Care.* 2006;51:519–525.
26. McCoy R. Options for home oxygen therapy equipment: storage and metering of oxygen in the home. *Respir Care.* 2013;58:65–85.
27. Bliss PL, McCoy RW, Adams AB. A bench study comparison of demand oxygen delivery systems and continuous flow oxygen. *Respir Care.* 1999;44:925–931.
28. Dunne PJ. The clinical impact of new long term oxygen therapy technology. *Respir Care.* 2009;54:1100–1111.
29. McCoy B, Gay P, Petty T, et al. Portable oxygen concentrating device comparison during exercise. Abstract 556; ATS International Conference, 2007.
30. Further recommendations for prescribing and supplying long-term oxygen therapy. Summary of the Second Conference on Long-Term Oxygen Therapy held in Denver, Colorado, December 11–12, 1987. *Am Rev Respir Dis.* 1988;138:745–747.
31. Diesem R, Voss G, McCoy R. A bench study to compare the performance characteristics of portable oxygen concentrators [Abstract]. *Respir Care.* 2007;51:1327.
32. McCoy R. Oxygen-conserving techniques and devices. *Respir Care.* 2000;45:95–103.

33. Valley Inspired Products. *Your 2007 Guide to Understanding Oxygen Conserving Devices*. Apple Valley, Minn.: Valley Inspired Products; 2007.
34. Christopher KL, Spofford BS, Goodman JR. A program for transtracheal oxygen delivery, assessment of safety and efficacy. *Ann Intern Med.* 1987;6:802–808.
35. Block AJ. Intermittent flow oxygen devices—technically feasible, but rarely used [Editorial]. *Chest.* 1984;86:657–658.
36. Porszasz J, Cao R, Morishige, et al. Physiologic effects of an ambulatory ventilation system in chronic obstructive pulmonary disease. *Am J Respir Crit Care Med.* 2013;188:334–342.
37. King A. Long term home mechanical ventilation in the United States. *Respir Care.* 2012;57:921–932.
38. Bach JR, Tzeng AC. *Guide to the Evaluation and Management of Neuromuscular Disease.* Philadelphia: Hanley & Belfus; 1999:134–137.
39. Tearl DK, Hertzog JH. Home discharge of technology-dependent children: evaluation of a respiratory therapist driven family education program. *Respir Care.* 2007;52:171–176.
40. Stegmaier J. The role of patient education in compliance. *Focus: J Respir Care Sleep Med.* 2005;22(Winter):85.
41. Pasquina P, Adler D, Farr P, et al. What does built-in software of home ventilators tell us? An observational study of 150 patients on home ventilation. *Respiration.* 2012;83:293–299.
42. Hanna S. Working down denials: EO463 pressure support ventilator. *HomeCare,* October 16, 2009.
43. Gilgoff RL, Gilgoff IS. Long-term follow-up of home mechanical ventilation in young children with spinal cord injury and neuromuscular conditions. *J Pediatr.* 2003;142:476–480.
44. ECRI. Leaving ventilator-dependent patients unattended. *Health Devices.* 1986;15:102-103.
45. Kun SS, Nakamura CT, Ripka JF, et al. Home ventilator low-pressure alarms fail to detect accidental decannulation with pediatric tracheostomy tubes. *Chest.* 2001;119:562–564.
46. Gelinas D, O'Connor P, Miller RG. Quality of life for ventilator-dependent ALS patients and their caregivers. *J Neurol Sci.* 1998;160(Suppl 1):S134–S136.

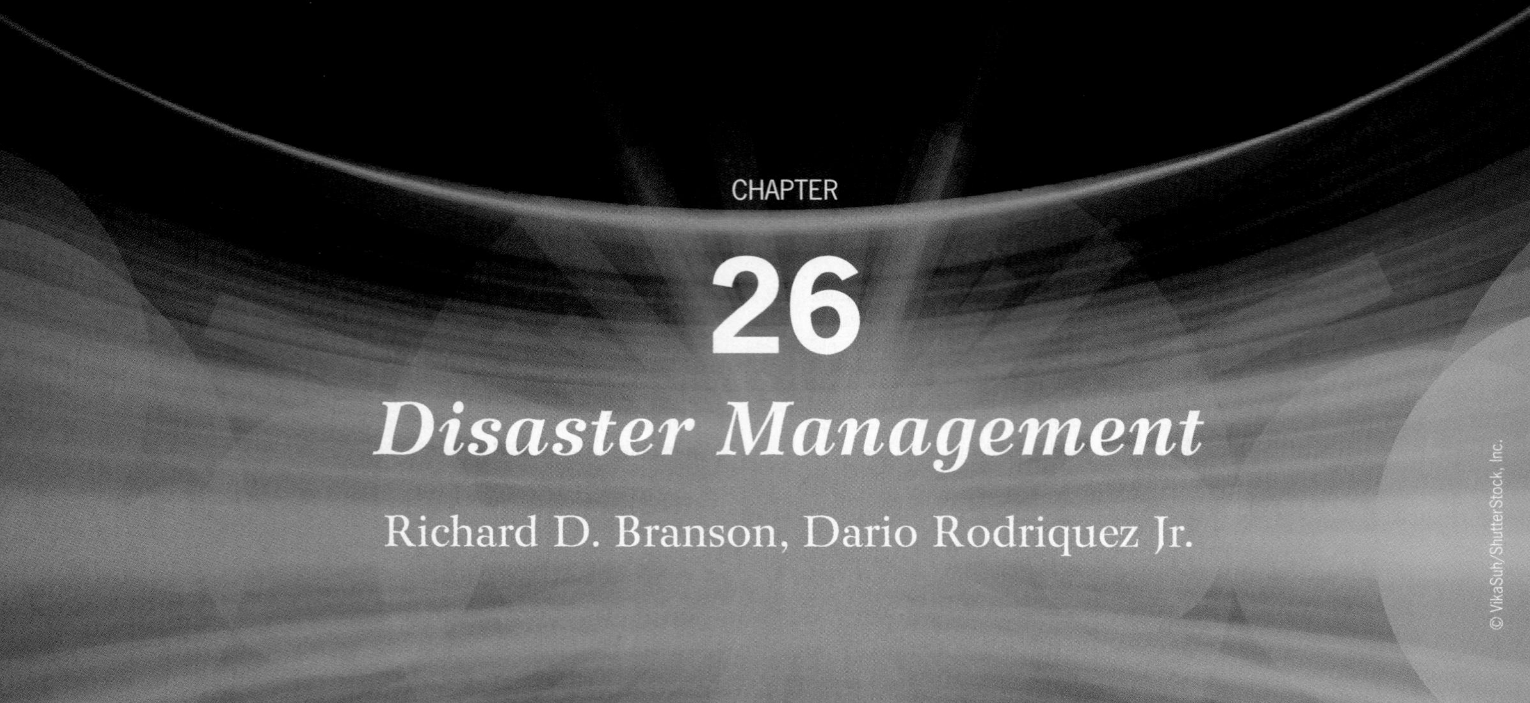

CHAPTER

26 Disaster Management

Richard D. Branson, Dario Rodriquez Jr.

OUTLINE

History
The Threat
Planning for Mass Casualty Respiratory Failure
Personal Protective Equipment
Ventilator Performance Characteristics
Ventilators for Mass Casualty Respiratory Failure
Triage

OBJECTIVES

1. Define mass casualty respiratory failure.
2. List the most likely disaster scenarios to result in mass casualty respiratory failure.
3. Describe the characteristics of devices required to provide ventilation in mass casualty respiratory failure.
4. Describe issues related to respiratory consumables and oxygen in mass casualty respiratory failure.
5. Discuss the role of the respiratory therapist in a disaster.
6. Justify a system for triage of patients based on severity of illness in a mass casualty respiratory failure event.

KEY TERMS

automatic resuscitator
chemical agent
critical care ventilator
disaster management plan
electrically powered portable ventilator
EMS portable ventilator
epidemic
mass casualty respiratory failure (MCRF)
noninvasive ventilation (NIV)
personal protective equipment (PPE)
pneumatically powered portable ventilator

Introduction

Recent history is rife with natural disasters, the threat of terrorism, and outbreaks of severe febrile respiratory illness, including H1N1 influenza and severe acute respiratory syndrome (SARS). Outbreaks of Middle East Respiratory Syndrome (MERS), emerging flu strains (H7N9, and Ebola hemorrhagic fever) continue to challenge disaster preparation. These real and perceived threats have focused healthcare planners, hospitals, and communities on how to care for large numbers of critically ill patients. Planning requires not only space for the care of patients but also adequate equipment and staff.[1] This chapter focuses specifically on the concerns related to and requirements for **mass casualty respiratory failure (MCRF)**, which is defined as an event resulting in patients requiring mechanical ventilation in excess of the space to care for them and devices to provide ventilatory support.[2–4]

History

Mass casualty respiratory failure (MCRF) has an interesting, yet mostly unimpressive past. The most illuminating instance occurred in the 1950s during the European poliomyelitis epidemic. The care of patients at a hospital in Copenhagen at the height of the epidemic is instructive.[5] During the summer of 1952, the hospital owned five negative pressure ventilators. In the same time frame over 100 patients required mechanical ventilation. This surge of patients relative to available ventilators had not been seen before or since. The hospital staff devised a clever solution to the problem. Instead of negative pressure ventilation with an iron lung, they performed tracheostomy and enlisted medical students to perform manual ventilation in 4-hour shifts. Using a non–self-inflating bag and rebreathing system incorporating a carbon dioxide absorber, they were able to use very low flows of oxygen to sustain ventilation and oxygenation. Interestingly, manual ventilation was also used following Hurricane Katrina, when electricity failed at Charity Hospital in New Orleans.[6]

Terrorist attacks using nerve agents have been attempted, but in each case the number of patients requiring mechanical ventilation was fewer than 10 individuals. The SARS epidemic was an example of a natural febrile respiratory illness that resulted in significant morbidity and mortality. SARS highlighted the impact of international travel on the spread of disease and the importance of caregiver protection. In Toronto, a number of patients with SARS were nurses and respiratory therapists who had cared for patients prior to recognition of the risk. In 2009, while the world awaited an anticipated H5N1 (avian flu) outbreak, a novel H1N1 virus originated in Mexico. The resulting pandemic taxed intensive care units (ICUs) around the world with severe respiratory failure in pediatric, obese, and obstetric patients. The H1N1 epidemic is a lesson in the unpredictability of viruses. H1N1 did not overwhelm hospitals, but did result in ICUs full of critically ill patients. In 2013, H1N1 again resulted in a number of patients with severe hypoxemic respiratory failure requiring heroic measures to treat many. There were no reports of ventilator or bed shortages, but the severity of acute respiratory distress syndrome (ARDS) associated with H1N1 infection spurred a renewed interest in rescue therapies for refractory hypoxemia.[7]

Fortunately for the U.S. population, neither natural nor human-made events have resulted in a surge of critically ill patients requiring mechanical ventilation and exceeding the capacity for space, stuff, or staff. Alternatively, each small event provides lessons from which the medical community can learn. What seems clear is that whatever mass casualty event occurs, it is likely to be unexpected and unpredictable.

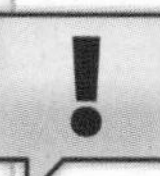

Respiratory Recap

Disasters Causing Mass Casualty Respiratory Failure

- Traumatic injury
- Chemical weapons
- Epidemics and febrile respiratory illness

The Threat

In the United States, the *National Planning Guidelines* of the Department of Homeland Security coordinates and prioritizes emergency preparedness efforts at all response levels. Contained within the guidelines are 15 national planning scenarios. At least two-thirds of these may result in MCRF.[8]

The medical impact of a mass casualty event will depend on the disaster's characteristics (e.g., lethality of exposure, numbers of persons exposed) and interaction with the exposed population's and medical response systems' capabilities and vulnerabilities. Only in disasters likely to result in exposed victims developing ARDS will mechanical ventilation potentially be a limiting factor for survival. Disaster characteristics that may influence the demand for ventilators include the number of victims, the time from exposure to development of ARDS, and the duration of ARDS. It is possible that victims requiring mechanical ventilation may far outnumber normal mechanical ventilator capacity. If this were to occur, many patients with potentially reversible disease would likely die. Each scenario considers the expected number of victims requiring mechanical ventilation, the time from injury until need for mechanical ventilation, the pathophysiology necessitating mechanical ventilation, and the geographic area affected.

Accommodating potentially large numbers of pediatric patients should be an added consideration to disaster planning given that few facilities are well prepared for pediatric emergencies nor do they possess the requisite population-specific equipment to support their needs.[9]

Traumatic Injury

Traumatic injury may result on a local level from fire, explosion, or terrorist attack. These events typically result in fewer than 100 casualties. The Israeli experience with homicide bombers suggests that most incidents result in 20 to 30 casualties, with half of these patients being hospitalized and half of those admitted to ICUs, the majority for life-saving mechanical ventilation. Traumatic injury also may result from a natural disaster such as an earthquake or tsunami. These events occur over a wider area, damaging infrastructure and impeding response. Mechanical ventilation may be required following near drowning, crush injuries, and chest trauma.[8]

- *Expected number of victims*: In a local explosion or fire, typically fewer than 100 victims require hospitalization and fewer require mechanical ventilation.
- *Time from injury to need for mechanical ventilation*: The severity of trauma may require immediate mechanical ventilation for survival (e.g., head injury, blast lung injury), whereas others only require ventilation after operative repair.
- *Pathophysiology*: Traumatic injuries resulting in a need for mechanical ventilation include closed head injury, hemothorax, pneumothorax, pulmonary contusion, flail chest, traumatic amputation, blood loss, and blast injury.
- *Area affected:* In an explosion or fire, the affected area is usually finite. The result is a defined local area in which casualties are limited and local infrastructure can handle the surge in patients easily. A larger natural event may affect greater numbers of patients and result in damage to hospitals and transportation systems. In these instances, critically ill victims at the scene are likely to expire.

Chemical Weapons

Injuries following exposure to chemical weapons vary with the agent. **Chemical agents** are classified as lung-damaging agents, blood agents, blister agents, and nerve agents. These agents include chlorine, phosgene, and ammonia, all of which are commonly used in industrial processes and readily available. Nerve agents causing paralysis have been used recently. Mustard gas is perhaps the best-known blister agent, and cyanide is the most likely blood agent.

- *Expected number of victims*: Under the appropriate environmental conditions, population density, and dispersion, chemical agents may result in thousands of victims. Despite this prediction, however, to date the number of victims has been in the hundreds and the number of victims requiring mechanical ventilation has been less than a dozen.
- *Time from injury to need for mechanical ventilation*: The time until respiratory failure requires mechanical ventilation varies with the agent and exposure. Pulmonary agents can cause sudden death as a result of laryngeal obstruction or severe respiratory failure days after exposure. Nerve agents causing paralysis may require ventilation to be performed at the scene. Historically, those patients who survive exposure to nerve agents require only short-term mechanical ventilation (<8 hours).[10]
- *Pathophysiology*: Chemical weapons enter the body through the respiratory system and skin. Blistering and choking agents result in bronchospasm and, over time, ARDS. Cyanide poisons mitochondria and prevents cellular respiration, resulting in death from cellular hypoxia. Nerve agents result in flaccid paralysis and apnea but also produce significant bronchorrhea and bronchospasm. Thus, although patients exposed to nerve agents may have normal lung compliance, airway resistance may be elevated.
- *Area affected*: The optimum effectiveness of these agents as a weapon requires exposure of a large number of victims in a closed space. These exposures therefore are limited to a small geographic area.

Epidemics and Febrile Respiratory Illness

Epidemics and febrile illness may result from both natural and human-made causes. SARS and pandemic flu are good examples of diseases that traveled around the world in short order. Anthrax and botulism exposure are most likely to be the result of bioterrorism, although botulism poisoning can occur from improperly preserved foods. Anthrax, caused by the bacillus *Anthracis*, has been used in the United States as a weapon, infecting 22 people and killing five. Anthrax, however, is not contagious; that is, it cannot be passed from one person to another.

- *Expected number of victims*: Epidemics have the possibility of involving people from all over the world, affecting tens of thousands of people. Weaponized botulism and anthrax have the ability to infect similar numbers of people.
- *Time from injury to need for mechanical ventilation*: Epidemics are likely to result in the greatest number of casualties, and typically the time from exposure until respiratory failure develops is prolonged (days to weeks). In these cases, patients will likely arrive at the hospital with early signs of respiratory distress.
- *Pathophysiology:* Pandemic flu and SARS result in ARDS in the worst cases. Botulism results in neuromuscular ventilatory failure from paralysis and may require prolonged mechanical ventilation. Anthrax results in hemorrhagic mediastinitis, hemoptysis, sepsis, profound hypoxemia, and acute respiratory failure.
- *Area affected*: Natural epidemics and bioterrorism agents in this class have the ability to infect entire regions, depending on the length of the incubation period and the continued presence of the contagion. These events may be limited to a municipality or may include an entire city. In the case of pandemic flu, entire portions of a country may be affected.

Planning for Mass Casualty Respiratory Failure

Respiratory therapists play an important role during disasters, and even more so during MCRF scenarios. This role includes managing staff, providing personal protective equipment, assuming additional duties, ensuring an adequate supply of disposables (e.g., ventilator circuits, suction catheters, heat and moisture exchangers), arranging for appropriate oxygen reserves, and devising a plan for additional mechanical ventilators—all this in addition to normal duties.

Staffing

Any MCRF scenario results in an exponential need for mechanical ventilation and will dramatically increase the need for ICU nurses, respiratory therapists, and physicians. This is a particular challenge considering

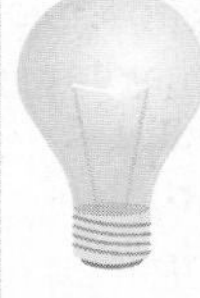

STOP AND THINK

What are some ways that you can think of to improve availability of respiratory therapists during a mass casualty respiratory failure event?

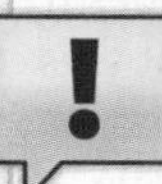

Respiratory Recap

Planning for Mass Casualty Respiratory Failure

- Staffing
- Personal protective equipment
- Oxygen
- Disposables
- Ventilators

that many ICUs have lost beds due to staffing shortages. In an MCRF scenario the respiratory therapist will be overwhelmed by responsibility. Staffing will be based on patient acuity and caregiver availability, and may be supplemented with in-place memorandums of understanding with cooperating facilities.

A plan for respiratory extenders has been developed but has yet to be put to use. The major issue is identifying the appropriately trained people. Occupational and physical therapists, veterinarians, and prehospital providers have all been discussed. Additionally, the duties these individuals would be assigned is unclear.[11] On the other hand, in the event of a mass casualty incident not involving large numbers of patients with respiratory failure, the respiratory therapist should be prepared to aid physicians, nurses, and other professionals in duties not normally in the scope of respiratory care. In the event staff is requested to perform duties outside their general scope of practice, assurances should be provided that they will be afforded legal protection.[12]

Reassignment of those in administrative duties, outpatient services, and/or ward units should be considered to augment critical care staff. Those with expertise in vent management should be used as a force multiplier and could oversee less experienced staff, creating synergy to manage greater numbers of patients.[13] Also, assigning those vaccinated or deemed immune to areas with infected patients may be beneficial.[13]

The respiratory therapy department should be involved in the community and hospital **disaster management plan**. Surge-capacity-specific protocols should be established to optimize resource utilization.[14] A plan for notifying department members via text, email, or phone is vital. An essential personnel list should be established to avoid confusion when recalling staff. Disaster planning cannot be done in isolation.

Personal Protective Equipment

Several of the febrile respiratory illnesses associated with MCRF are highly contagious. **Personal protective equipment (PPE)** is a critical component of mass casualty care in this setting. Availability of PPE is important because it allows caregivers to feel safe during patient interactions. In the absence of sufficient PPE, concerns about personal and family health may lead to employees avoiding the workplace. Adequate supplies are not enough; proper use of PPE must be taught and evaluated. The risk of secondary transmission is likely greater in the ICU as a result of the number of interventions causing aerosolization of infectious material. Procedures such as endotracheal intubation, open circuit suctioning, and bronchoscopy are associated with increased probability of secondary transmission. The risk associated with procedures such as noninvasive ventilation, administration of medications by nebulizer, and manual ventilation is unclear. Some have advocated higher levels of respiratory protection for those engaging in high-risk interventions such as use of powered air-purifying respirators for bronchoscopy. Also, use of negative-pressure rooms should be prioritized for those with the most severe illness.[15]

The SARS experience showed that correct use of recommended PPE among healthcare workers is highly efficacious in limiting disease spread. Ensuring correct use of PPE, however, especially during a prolonged response, remains a challenge. Reports from the SARS outbreak reveal that compliance with PPE regimens was below 70% in Hong Kong and U.S. healthcare workers caring for infected patients.[16]

The use of filters in the ventilator circuit on the inspired or expired side, or both, or inside a heat and moisture exchanger (HME) appears to be suggested by common sense, but data are lacking. Ventilators that use room air for gas delivery to the patient should have a filter on the inspiratory inlet. Filters are used in the expiratory limb of the ventilator circuit to protect the delicate, expensive flow and pressure monitoring components rather than for infection control. It is unknown whether there is any risk of secondary infection in caregivers from expired gas from intubated patients. Clearly, the risk is greatest in the unintubated patient capable of coughing or sneezing droplets into the environment. The use of an HME with a filter (HMEF) has not been shown to reduce the rate of ventilator-associated pneumonia or to alter contamination of the environment. The presence of a filter in the HME, however, increases the risk of airway obstruction. If used, filters in the expiratory limb of the circuit should be inspected frequently for signs of obstruction to avoid complications secondary to air trapping (barotrauma, hypotension). An important rule of personal protection is proximity. An N-95 mask worn by a caregiver is much more effective than depending on a filter in the ventilator circuit to prevent infection.

Oxygen

Oxygen is readily available in liquid form at most hospitals. Under normal circumstances the liquid system of a hospital can provide gas for approximately 3 weeks. In part because of the threat of disaster, most hospitals request that the liquid oxygen vessel never be allowed

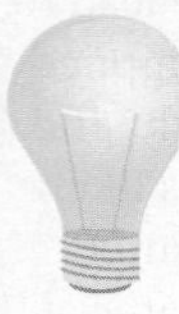

STOP AND THINK

In your hospital, what are ways that oxygen can be conserved during a mass casualty respiratory failure event?

to fall below half-full. Systems are typically filled at night to prevent interference with workflow and reduce the risk of accidents. A typical liquid system has 6000 to 9000 gallons of liquid oxygen, which evaporates to nearly 30,000,000 gaseous liters of oxygen. It has been estimated that a 500-bed hospital uses 1.5 million liters of oxygen per day.[17] Of particular note, most systems incorporate their reserves in direct connection to the main supply line. Such a setup places the entire supply in jeopardy if the primary source is damaged.[18]

Cylinders, portable liquid systems, and concentrators can also supply oxygen. Note that most concentrators are only capable of producing 93% oxygen from room air. Most hospitals do not have space to house sufficient numbers of cylinders to prove useful in a disaster. Concentrators can provide low-flow oxygen and may be considered for critically ill ventilated patients in a resource-constrained environment with adequate training. Liquid systems are the standard, and portable, truck-mounted systems are available for emergencies, assuming the roads are passable. Additional consideration may be given to chemically generated oxygen; although it offers limited stores per unit, it, however, is a potential resource.

During a disaster, oxygen conservation can be helpful. This includes use of reservoir or pendant cannulas, turning off flow to manual resuscitators, switching from heated aerosols to HMEs, and accepting lower levels of oxygen saturation in patients. Although the Strategic National Stockpile maintains equipment and medications, it does not provide for any oxygen reserves, and neither FEMA nor the CDC specifies plans for sourcing oxygen needs.[18] Planning factors should include a contingency for loss of facility oxygen as well as consideration of use of alternate facility oxygen capabilities in particular for those patients who are less acute and require minimal support, such as power for their home concentrators. Additionally, a variety of multipatient oxygen distribution systems have been designed to address oxygen needs during an MCRF.

Disposables

A frequently overlooked aspect of MCRF is availability of disposable equipment. Ventilators require circuits, HMEs or humidifiers, and suction catheters. Oxygen requires delivery tubing, cannulas, masks, and other appliances. In keeping with cost containment, these devices are commonly kept at a level sufficient for several weeks of supply. In MCRF, most experts suspect that the disposables will be among the first supplies to run out. Reuse of circuits has been suggested, but this should only be considered as a last resort. Ventilators from the SNS include an adult and pediatric ventilator circuit within the delivered case. At tidal volumes suggested by a lung-protective approach, the smaller diameter (13 mm ID) pediatric circuit can be used in adult patients.

Ventilators

Ventilators may be needed following a disaster in three distinct scenarios: (1) in the field to move patients from the scene of an accident to definitive care, (2) between facilities (decompressing a localized event), and (3) for in-hospital care of critically ill and injured patients. The movement of patients from the scene may be accomplished with oxygen, manual ventilation, or use of a portable ventilator under the purview of the emergency medical services (EMS) director. In scenarios such as pandemic flu, patients are likely to seek relief of flu symptoms long before they require mechanical ventilation. In these cases, the need for large numbers of EMS ventilators will be unnecessary. Special consideration must be given to the mechanism of transport to accommodate resource planning for ground transport or allowances for ventilator capabilities in a hypobaric environment.

The second and third scenarios involve the care of critically ill patients with respiratory failure and ARDS requiring mechanical ventilation. Ventilators used for interfacility transport and ICU care are under the purview of the critical care team, including an intensivist and respiratory therapist. Evidence-based management of the patient with ARDS is founded in the success of the Acute Respiratory Distress Syndrome Network (ARDSnet) trial.[19] The principles of ARDS management are straightforward:

- Tidal volume 4–8 mL/kg of ideal body weight
- Ability to give a constant tidal volume
- Plateau pressure (Pplat) less than or equal to 30 cm H_2O
- Stable inspired oxygen concentration (F_{IO_2}) from 0.21 to 1.0
- Continuous mandatory ventilation (CMV)
- Positive end-expiratory pressure (PEEP) to maintain alveolar recruitment

On the first day of the ARDSnet trial, the patients in the low-tidal-volume arm of the trial received PEEP of 6 to 13 cm H_2O, an F_{IO_2} of 0.35 to 0.75, and a minute ventilation of 10 to 16 L/min. On day 7, PEEP was an average of 8 cm H_2O, F_{IO_2} was 0.50, and minute ventilation averaged about 14 L/min. These data provide standard requirements for the functional performance of ventilators to be stockpiled for use in MCRF. Ventilators for MCRF should be capable of PEEP from 6 to 13 cm H_2O, F_{IO_2} from 0.35 to 0.75, and a minute ventilation of 10 to 18 L/min. Assuming ideal body weight of 62 to 90 kg (males with a height of 65 inches to 77 inches, or 5 feet 5 inches to 6 feet 5 inches), tidal volumes of 375 to 540 mL (6 mL/kg) are required. It is important to note that the desired tidal volume is based on ideal patient weight, not lung compliance or actual weight.

There are many opinions about what kind of ventilator should be stockpiled for MCRF, ranging from a minimalist approach of just replacing the manual resuscitator to the ICU approach that every possible option must be available. At a minimum, ventilators stockpiled for MCRF *must* be capable of delivering a respiratory frequency of 6 to 35 breaths/min, a tidal volume of 350 to 600 mL (the adjustment of respiratory rate and tidal volume must be separate), F_{IO_2} of 0.35 to 0.75, and PEEP of 5 to 15 cm H_2O. Ventilators unable to produce these settings are not suitable for in-hospital MCRF. **Figure 26-1** shows examples of suitable ventilators.

Ventilator Performance Characteristics

Operational characteristics of ventilators for MCRF have been suggested by the American Association for Respiratory Care (AARC).[20] Some explanation and clarification of these characteristics are in order.[21,22] **Table 26-1** lists the desirable characteristics of ventilators for MCRF. The optimal ranges for operation remain to be determined but represent the minimum required characteristics as well as characteristics that might provide added benefit. Physical characteristics of ventilators for MCRF, which are more difficult to quantify, are clearly just as important. A ventilator for MCRF should be rugged and portable, withstand shock and vibration, and continue to operate if dropped. There is a military specification for these characteristics, but it is unclear whether ventilators for MCRF must meet this standard. Clearly, meeting the military standard would be desirable. Portability is important. A weight of less than 5 kg is often the goal. A portable device is one that a respiratory therapist or nurse can pick up with one hand (with or without a carrying case) and move without difficulty.

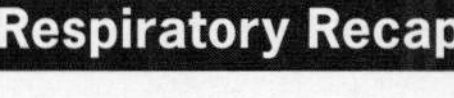

Respiratory Recap

Performance Characteristics of a Ventilator for Mass Casualty Respiratory Failure

- Rugged
- Portable
- Low gas consumption
- Adequate battery life
- Minimal imposed work of breathing

Ideally, a ventilator for MCRF should have low gas consumption. That is, oxygen should not be wasted. Pneumatic or fluidic control, continuous flow for triggering, pressure relief from blenders, and internal leaks affect gas consumption of ventilators. Although this has not been well studied, ideally 90% of the gas entering the ventilator should go to the patient as part of the minute ventilation. Equally important is battery life. Battery life is affected by age of the battery, temperature, and the battery's charging history regardless of the ventilator. Ventilator characteristics that decrease battery life include the mode of ventilation, F_{IO_2}, and PEEP. Patient characteristics can also affect battery life: the greater the load (lower compliance, higher airway resistance), the shorter the duration of operation.

The ventilator should be easy to trigger and have an acceptable imposed work of breathing. Most current-generation portable ventilators meet this requirement. Cost should be less than $10,000. In large purchases, such as those made by the government for mass casualty care, significant price reductions can be realized. The ventilator should be intuitive and easy to use. In addition, the manufacturer should provide training in person and via multimedia (DVD or Web based). Maintenance, including battery charging and replacement, is also an important issue. Ventilator maintenance should be able to be accomplished by trained technicians on site, and requirements for battery charging should be explicitly detailed.

Vendor support and longevity are critical. The manufacturer should have a technical support line that operates all day, every day of the year. There is some advantage to purchasing ventilators made in the United States because in a pandemic situation both shipping times and the loyalty of foreign manufacturers may create a problem.

Ventilators for Mass Casualty Respiratory Failure

For the purposes of describing ventilators for MCRF, their operation and application lead to categorization based on functional characteristics. These categories include automatic resuscitators, EMS ventilators,

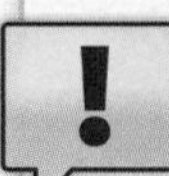

Respiratory Recap

Ventilators for Mass Casualty Respiratory Failure

- Automatic resuscitators
- EMS ventilators
- Pneumatically powered portable ventilators
- Electrically powered pneumatic ventilators
- Critical care ventilators
- Noninvasive ventilators

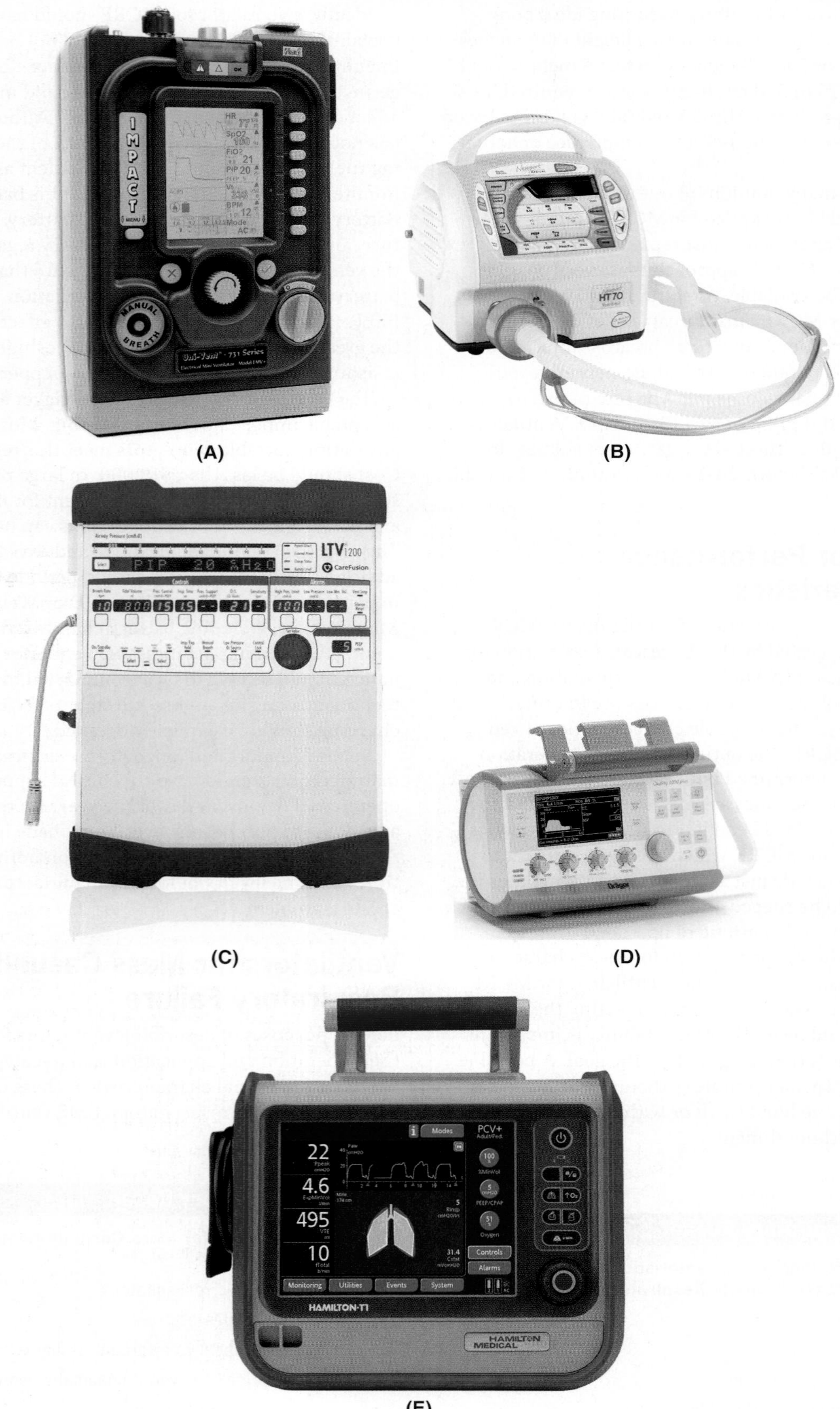

FIGURE 26-1 Examples of ventilators that might be used in the setting of mass casualty respiratory failure.

(A) courtesy of ZOLL®, formerly Impact Instrumentation; (B) © 2014 Covidien. All rights reserved. Used with the permission of Covidien; (C) reproduced with permission from CareFusion. (D) © Drägerwerk AG & Co. KGaA, Lubeck. All rights reserved. No portion hereof may be reproduced, saved or stored in a data processing system, electronically or mechanically copied or otherwise recorded by any other means without our express prior written permission; (E) courtesy of Hamilton Medical, Inc.

TABLE 26-1
Suggested Performance Characteristics of Ventilators for Mass Casualty Respiratory Failure

Characteristic	Rationale	Mandatory and Desirable Characteristics	
		Mandatory	**Desirable**
FDA approved for adults and pediatrics	Natural disasters, pandemics, and chemical/bioterrorism attacks will also affect children	Ventilate 10-kg patient	Ventilate 5-kg patient
Ability to operate without 50-psig compressed gas	The redundancy for electrical power in hospitals far exceeds oxygen stores and redundancy In the absence of high-pressure oxygen, low-flow oxygen from a flow meter can be used to increase F_{IO_2}	Operate without 50-psig input F_{IO_2} from 0.21 to 1.0	Operate with or without 50-psig input alone
Battery life of 4 hours or greater	Allow for transport from facility to facility Provide continuous support during intermittent power failure	4 hours of operation at nominal settings	Greater than 4 hours operation at nominal settings
Constant volume delivery	Meet guidelines for tidal volume delivery as dictated by ARDSnet protocol Reduce potential for ventilator-induced lung injury Provide age-appropriate settings	Volume control (350 to 600 mL)	Pressure control and volume control
Mode	Meet ARDSnet guidelines Ensure minimum ventilation in a situation of multiple patients and a shortage of caregivers	CMV	CMV, IMV, and pressure support
Positive end-expiratory pressure (PEEP)	Meet ARDSnet guidelines Prevent ventilator-induced lung injury Reverse hypoxemia	Adjustable from 5 to 15 cm H_2O	Adjustable from 5 to 20 cm H_2O
Separate controls for respiratory rate and tidal volume	Meet ARDSnet guidelines Ensure minute ventilation in apneic patients	Respiratory rate from 6 to 35 breaths/min	Respiratory rate from 6 to 75 breaths/min (for pediatric patients)
Monitor airway pressures and tidal volume	Meet ARDSnet guidelines Provide assessment of patient's lung compliance Patient safety (prevent overdistension)	Monitor peak inspiratory pressure and delivered tidal volume	Monitor plateau pressure and patient tidal volumes
Alarms	Patient safety Improve ability to monitor large numbers of patients with reduced staff	Alarms for: Circuit disconnect High airway pressure Low airway pressure (leak) Loss of electric power Loss of high-pressure source gas	Alarms for: High tidal volume in pressure modes Low minute ventilation Remote alarms

ARDSnet, Acute Respiratory Distress Syndrome Network; CMV, continuous mandatory ventilation; IMV, intermittent mandatory ventilation.

pneumatically powered portable ventilators, electrically powered portable ventilators, full-feature critical care ventilators, and noninvasive ventilators.

Automatic Resuscitators

An **automatic resuscitator** is designed to replace the need for manual ventilation. These devices are predominantly pneumatically powered and pressure cycled. Automatic resuscitators have few to no alarms, cannot provide a constant tidal volume, cannot set rate and tidal volume separately, and commonly provide 100% source gas or a lower concentration with the use of a Venturi. Most manuals of automatic resuscitators start with the warning, "Do not leave the patient unattended," which is problematic in a scenario in which there are too many patients and not enough caregivers. These devices are inexpensive but fail to meet the demands of patients with ARDS and are not suitable for stockpiling to treat MCRF.

EMS Portable Ventilators

An **EMS portable ventilator** is used in patient transport, typically in emergency care via ambulance. These devices are more reliable and rugged and have greater functionality than automatic resuscitators. The functionality and cost in this group of ventilators are variable. Some devices set tidal volume and respiratory rate via a single control. Others have separate controls for both settings. PEEP is usually set on an external valve. F_{IO_2} is commonly provided by 100% O_2 source gas or a single lower concentration with use of an air entrainment system. Most of these devices are pneumatically powered, with or without electronic control. Monitoring and alarms are limited. These devices require a 50-psig input; this, along with the limited alarms and monitoring, limits their usefulness in the stockpile.

Pneumatically Powered Portable Ventilators

Sophisticated **pneumatically powered portable ventilators** have the ability to provide continuous mandatory ventilation (CMV) and intermittent mandatory ventilation (IMV), set PEEP, possess a low imposed work of breathing, and allow separate control of tidal volume and respiratory rate. These devices meet most of the performance characteristics for MCRF. The limitations of these devices are related to the pneumatic power source. In the absence of a 50-psig gas source, these devices cannot operate. F_{IO_2} is typically limited to 100% source gas, which wastes oxygen. Few alarms are also a weakness.

Electrically Powered Portable Ventilators

Electrically powered portable ventilators often are used for home care and for in-hospital transport. Electrically powered, sophisticated portable ventilators meet the performance characteristics required of a ventilator for MCRF. There is some significant difference in the weight of these devices (ranging from 5 to 15 kg). Battery life and gas consumption vary depending on the driving system of the ventilator. A number of commercially available ventilators in this category have been stockpiled by the Centers for Disease Control and Prevention and by state disaster management teams for MCRF.

Critical Care Ventilators

Critical care ventilators are capable of managing all types of respiratory failure. These devices have not been recommended for MCRF because of their large size, cost (over $30,000), and complexity. The plethora of modes and options provided by a critical care ventilator is an advantage in routine use by critical care respiratory therapists and intensivists but becomes a liability in a mass casualty situation.

Noninvasive Ventilators

Noninvasive ventilation (NIV) is a standard of care for respiratory failure in patients with chronic obstructive pulmonary disease (COPD) under normal circumstances. The use of NIV in MCRF, however, has significant limitations.

- NIV is not the treatment of choice for ARDS, commonly seen in MCRF.
- The significant time commitment (1–2 hours) spent by the respiratory therapist at the bedside at initiation is impractical in MCRF.
- NIV failure may require emergency intubation, which is a more difficult scenario when there are too many patients and too few caregivers.
- In infectious disease, the ability of the patient to cough and the high flows associated with NIV may spread infectious agents into the ambient air.

Noninvasive ventilators tend to be inexpensive and smaller than many invasive devices but have limitations that preclude recommendation for stockpiling, such as lack of battery backup, limited monitoring, limited alarms, and inability to provide volume control (most devices provide pressure-targeted ventilation). Despite the limitations of noninvasive ventilators, many hospitals have these devices available. In an MCRF situation, noninvasive ventilators can be repurposed for use as invasive ventilators. **Table 26-2** lists possible sources of additional ventilators during an MCRF scenario.

Triage

A commonsense approach to ventilator allocation should be made at the site of care. A number of the ventilators in the SNS provide consistent ventilation but do not have the monitoring or work of breathing characteristics of the modern ICU ventilators. The respiratory therapist should triage the current hospital ventilators to the sickest patients, using the SNS ventilators for patients who are not as sick and who need minimal support.

No discussion of MCRF is complete without mentioning triage of mechanical ventilation. This is an ethical dilemma that the modern world has not yet had to face. In MCRF, all patients will receive care based on the likelihood of survival. These systems are being developed by national societies to allow the most good to be done for the most patients with the best possible outcome. All patients will receive care in a mass casualty situation, even if it is only comfort care. Additional planning factors should consider air transport for capabilities outside those immediately available.[23] Survival outcomes have illustrated improvements when patients have been triaged to treatment facilities with greater assets. This also aids in freeing up resources.

TABLE 26-2
Sources of Additional Ventilators for a Mass Casualty Respiratory Failure Scenario

Source	Method	Problems
Affected hospital	Cancel elective surgeries Repurpose anesthesia workstations as mechanical ventilators and ICU monitors (during nontrauma disasters)	Numbers of anesthesia machines are limited. If the duration of mechanical ventilation is prolonged, anesthesia machines will be needed when surgeries and other procedures are reinitiated.
Unaffected hospitals	Redistribution of available equipment from unaffected hospitals to those in need	There are few extra available ventilators at most hospitals even during usual conditions. Delayed situational awareness may reduce the willingness of unaffected hospitals to share equipment.
Mechanical ventilator rental services	Provision of additional ventilators by a rental company	The same company may have contracts with a number of affected hospitals, so the total number of additional ventilators may be limited. Logistical delays may be encountered when sending ventilators from distant geographic areas.
Strategic national stockpile	Deployment of mechanical ventilators to states or cities in need	Delay in distribution may occur because most states still have limited capacity to distribute equipment from the strategic national stockpile. It is unclear how distribution will be prioritized when multiple hospitals are requesting ventilators at the same time.

Key Points

- At least two-thirds of potential disasters result in mass casualty respiratory failure (MCRF).
- Traumatic injury may result on a local level from fire, explosion, or terrorist attack.
- Chemical agents are classified as lung-damaging agents, blood agents, blister agents, and nerve agents.
- Epidemics and febrile illness may result from both natural and human-made causes.
- Personal protective equipment is a critical component of mass casualty care in the disaster setting.
- During a disaster, oxygen conservation can be helpful.
- Ventilators may be needed following a disaster in three distinct scenarios: (1) in the field to move patients from the scene of an accident to definitive care, (2) between facilities (decompressing a localized event), and (3) for in-hospital care of critically ill and injured patients.
- Operational characteristics of ventilators for MCRF have been suggested by the American Association for Respiratory Care.
- Ventilators for MCRF include automatic resuscitators, EMS ventilators, pneumatically powered portable ventilators, electrically powered portable ventilators, critical care ventilators, and noninvasive ventilators.
- Respiratory therapists play an important role during disasters, and even more so during MCRF.

References

1. Hotchkin DL, Rubinson L. Modified critical care and treatment space consideration for mass casualty critical illness and injury. *Respir Care*. 2008;53:67–74.
2. Rubinson L, Nuzzo JB, Talmor DS, et al. Augmentation of hospital critical care capacity after bioterrorist attacks or epidemics: recommendations of the Working Group on Emergency Mass Critical Care. *Crit Care Med*. 2005;33:2393–2403.
3. Rubinson L, O'Toole T. Critical care during epidemics. *Crit Care*. 2005;9:311–313.
4. Rubinson L, Branson RD, Pesik N, Talmor D. Positive-pressure ventilation equipment for mass casualty respiratory failure. *Biosecur Bioterror*. 2006;4:183–194.
5. Lassen HCA. *Management of Life-Threatening Poliomyelitis. Copenhagen, 1952–1956, with a Survey of Autopsy-Findings in 115 Cases*. Edinburgh: Livingstone; 1956.
6. deBoisblanc BP. Black Hawk, please come down: reflections on a hospital's struggle to survive in the wake of Hurricane Katrina. *Am J Respir Crit Care Med*. 2005;172:1239–1240.
7. Tang JW, Shetty N, Lam TT. Features of the new pandemic influenza A/H1N1/2009 virus: virology, epidemiology, clinical and public health aspects. *Curr Opin Pulm Med*. 2010;16:235–241.
8. Federal Emergency Management Agency (FEMA). *National Preparedness*. Available at: http://www.fema.gov/national-preparedness. Accessed July 31, 2014.
9. Branson RD. Disaster planning for pediatrics. *Respir Care*. 2011;56;1457–1465.
10. Muskat P. Mass casualty chemical exposure and implications for respiratory failure. *Respir Care*. 2008;53:58–63.
11. Hanley ME, Bogdan GM. Mechanical ventilation in mass casualty scenarios. Augmenting staff: project XTREME. *Respir Care*. 2008;53:176–188.
12. Sprung CL, Zimmerman JL, Christian MD, et al. Recommendations for intensive care unit and hospital preparations for an influenza epidemic or mass disaster: summary report of the European Society of Intensive Care Medicine's Task Force for intensive care unit triage during an influenza epidemic or mass disaster. *Intensive Care Med*. 2010:36:428–443.
13. Manuell ME, Co MDT, Ellison RT III. Pandemic influenza: implications for preparation and delivery of critical care services. *J Intensive Care Med*. 2011:26:347–367.
14. Hick JL, Christian MD, Sprung CL. Chapter 2. Surge capacity and infrastructure considerations for mass critical care. *Intensive Care Med*. 2010:36(Suppl 1):S11–S20.
15. Westfall GP, Paraskeva M. H1N1 influenza: critical care aspects. *Seminars in Respiratory and Crit Care Med*. 2011: 32:400–408.

16. Daugherty E, Branson RD, Desai A, Rubinson L. Infection control in mass respiratory failure: preparing to respond to H1N1. *Crit Care Med.* 2010;38(Suppl 4):e103–109.
17. Ritz RH, Privitera JE. Oxygen supplies during a mass casualty situation. *Respir Care.* 2008;53:215–224.
18. Blakeman TC, Branson RD. Oxygen Supplies in Disaster Management. *Respir Care.* 2013:58:173–183.
19. NIH ARDS Network. Ventilation with lower tidal volumes as compared with traditional tidal volumes for acute lung injury and the acute respiratory distress syndrome. *N Engl J Med.* 2000;342:1301–1308.
20. American Association for Respiratory Care. *Guidelines for Acquisition of Ventilators to Meet Demands for Pandemic Flu and Mass Casualty Incidents.* 2010. Available at: http://www.alliedhpi.com/images/mcv200_aarc_guidelines.pdf.
21. Branson RD, Johannigman JA, Daugherty EL, Rubinson L. Surge capacity mechanical ventilation. *Respir Care.* 2008;53:78–90.
22. Daugherty EL, Branson RD, Rubinson L. Mass casualty respiratory failure. *Curr Opin Crit Care.* 2007;13:51–56.
23. Blakeman TC, Branson RD. Inter- and intra-hospital transport of the critically ill. *Respir Care.* 2013:58:1008–1023.

CHAPTER

27

Respiratory Care of the Elderly

William F. Galvin, Helen M. Sorenson

OUTLINE

The Demography of Aging
Terms Associated with Aging
Aging Pulmonary Anatomy and Physiology
Geriatric Patient Assessment
Atypical Disease Presentation
Geriatric Pharmacotherapy
Communicating with Older Adults
Pulmonary Disease After Age 65 Years
Role of RT in Caring for Elderly

OBJECTIVES

1. Discuss the importance of gerontology and geriatric principles in respiratory care practice.
2. Explain how demographics of aging will affect healthcare professionals.
3. Define terms associated with aging.
4. Describe age-associated changes in pulmonary anatomy and physiology.
5. Compare the physical assessment and geriatric assessment in elderly individuals.
6. Explain reasons why older patients may not present with typical complaints when ill.
7. List common atypical symptoms of the elderly.
8. Elaborate on issues surrounding medication management in older adults.
9. Discuss adverse consequences of miscommunication with elderly patients.
10. Compare asthma and chronic obstructive pulmonary disease in older adult patients.
11. Describe beneficial effects of the aging population adhering to healthy lifestyle choices.
12. Explain the role of the respiratory therapist in caring for the elderly.

KEY TERMS

baby boomer
frailty
geriatrics
gerontology
hypothermia
immunosenescense
life expectancy
life span
longevity
orthostatic hypotension
sarcopenia

Introduction

Respiratory care of the elderly is pervasive and omnipresent in the day-to-day practice of the respiratory therapist. Most respiratory therapists care for patients who are 70, 80, 90, and even some who are older than 100 years. The American Association for Respiratory Care (AARC) has initiated measures to address the needs of the elderly population. In 1997, they developed a position statement on age-appropriate care, which specifically addressed the elderly and encouraged the development of a **gerontology** module and clinical training at long-term care and rehabilitation facilities to provide students with the opportunity to learn how to appropriately plan for and provide respiratory care services for geriatric patients.[1] The AARC has created and supported a roundtable in gerontology, which informs, educates, and lobbies on behalf of respiratory therapists who are involved in the care and well-being of this population.

Over the past 25 years the AARC sponsored numerous educational consensus conferences to forecast its future and the needs of the populations it services.

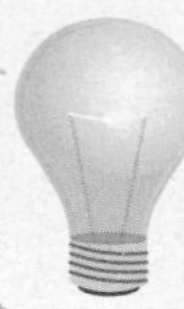

STOP AND THINK

What actions can be taken to highlight the critical role of gerontology to the RT?

Virtually all of these consensus conferences alluded to the significant impact that the aging population will have in shaping its future scope of practice. The first educational consensus conference identified aging of the population as a major trend affecting the profession.[2] The second stated that programs should better prepare students in geriatrics and gerontology,[3] and the third, and most recent, affirmed the findings of the first two, adding that health care will undergo marked changes as the country adjusts to the increasing population of **baby boomers** turning 65 years old.[4]

The primary factor preventing a greater role for **geriatrics** in respiratory care education is an already crowded curriculum. Future forecast for an expanding curriculum should address this shortcoming. Virtually all AARC professional meetings offer educational programs related to this theme.

In addition to the educational issues are the needs of the clinical arena and the daily experiences of practicing respiratory therapists. Respiratory problems, both chronic and acute, multiple comorbidities, and adverse drug events are more common in the elderly. Respiratory disease is the second most common cause of severe disability in older adults, second only to musculoskeletal disorders.[5] Pneumonia is a leading cause of morbidity and mortality in older adults.

Fragile bones, thin skin, altered thermoregulatory mechanisms, weaker immune systems, and age-related changes in organ systems are hallmarks of the elderly. Thirty years ago, it is likely that less than 50% of pulmonary patients were over the age of 65 years. Today there is a much larger pool of older patients who suffer from both acute and chronic disease. As noted by Petty, "Almost no one reaches the age of 65 without some disease or associated illness."[6] Gerontology and geriatrics have a prominent role in the life of the respiratory therapist. Gaining an understanding and appreciation of the uniqueness of the elderly and the aging process will be essential in the provision of safe, effective, and quality respiratory care.

This chapter covers the demography of aging and terms associated with aging, identifying the normal aging process and highlighting the normal and abnormal pulmonary anatomy and physiology of the elderly. Additionally, it covers the components of a physical assessment and a comprehensive geriatric assessment. Finally, the chapter addresses atypical disease presentation, geriatric pharmacology, effective communication strategies with older adults, and common pulmonary diseases occurring after age 65 years.

Respiratory Recap

- Pneumonia is a leading cause of morbidity and mortality in older patients.

The Demography of Aging

The current growth in the number and proportion of older adults in the United States is unprecedented. By 2015, it is anticipated that Americans aged 65 or older will number nearly 89 million—more than double the number in 2010[7]—and they are getting older by a number of measures. For example, the median age of the American population (the age at which half the population is younger and half older) increased from 22.9 in 1900 to 35.3 in 2000 and is predicted to reach 39.0 by 2030.[8] The increase was also accompanied by an increase in life expectancy at birth, from 47 years in 1900 to 78 years in 2005. The increase in older adults rose sharply in 2011 when the baby boomers (defined as those born between 1946 and 1964) officially entered the old-age category. This launched an unprecedented phenomenon whereby each day for the next 15 to 20 years, roughly 10,000 adults will celebrate their 65th birthday and become eligible for Medicare. In 2030, when the last of the baby boomers turns 65, the demographic landscape of our nation will have changed significantly and approximately one in every five Americans will be an older adult.[7]

This boom in the aging population, often referred to as the graying of America, is not just an American phenomenon. Among both developed and undeveloped nations, in America and worldwide, the older population is growing. The U.S. Census Bureau has compiled actual and projected growth charts for the aging population (**Table 27-1**).[9] Global projected populations of adults over age 65 years have also been compiled by the U.S. Census Bureau (**Table 27-2**).[10]

The aging population has been categorized into three component groups: the young old represented by the 65- to 74-year-olds; the aged who are 75 to 84; and the oldest old represented by those 85 and older.[11] Adults over the age of 85 years are the fastest-growing segment of the population in the United States. **Figure 27-1** provides a chart of the actual and projected population change of adults 65–74 years, 75–84 years, and over 85 years in the United States from 1900 to 2050 and highlights the magnitude of this oldest of the old cohort of the aging population.[12]

Respiratory Recap

- Baby boomers will increase in number by approximately 10,000 per day starting in 2011 and continue until approximately 2030.

TABLE 27-1
Aging Population in United States, 1900–2050 (Projected)

	1900	1950	2000	2020	2050 (Projected)
Total population (in millions)	76.0	150.5	276.2	325.9	392.0
Percentage of population age 65 years and older	4.1%	8.1%	12.6%	16.5%	20.4%
Percentage of population age 85 years and older	0.2%	0.4%	1.6%	2.0%	4.8%

U.S. Bureau of the Census. *Current Population Reports, Special Studies, P23-190, 65+ in the United States*. Washington, DC: U.S. Government Printing Office. Available at: https://www.census.gov/prod/1/pop/p23-190/p23-190.pdf. Accessed August 5, 2014.

TABLE 27-2
Global Percentage of Adults Over the Age of 65 Years, 2010–2030 (Projected)

	World	Europe	North America	Latin America	Asia	Sub-Saharan Africa
2010	7.6	16.2	13.2	6.9	6.7	3.2
2030 (projected)	11.7	22.4	20.2	12.1	11.6	3.8

Information from Lam D, Leibbrandt M. Global demographic trends and their implications for employment: background research paper. Submitted to the High Level Panel on the Post-2015 Development Agenda, May 2013.

Respiratory Recap

- Adults over the age of 85 are the fastest-growing segment of the U.S. population.

Whether we are talking about the young old, the aged, or the oldest old, all three groups will be characterized by chronic health conditions. The type, number, and severity of chronic health conditions can vary from one person to another and can affect multiple physiologic systems and often require multiple interventions. On average, 80% of adults ages 65 and over have at least one chronic condition and 50% have at least two.[13] Almost every medical specialty will be affected by this phenomenon. The leading causes of morbidity and mortality in adults over the age of 65 are cardiac, cerebrovascular, and pulmonary diseases as well as musculoskeletal disorders and malignancies. There is a significant shift in the nature of disease as six of the seven leading causes of death in the United States

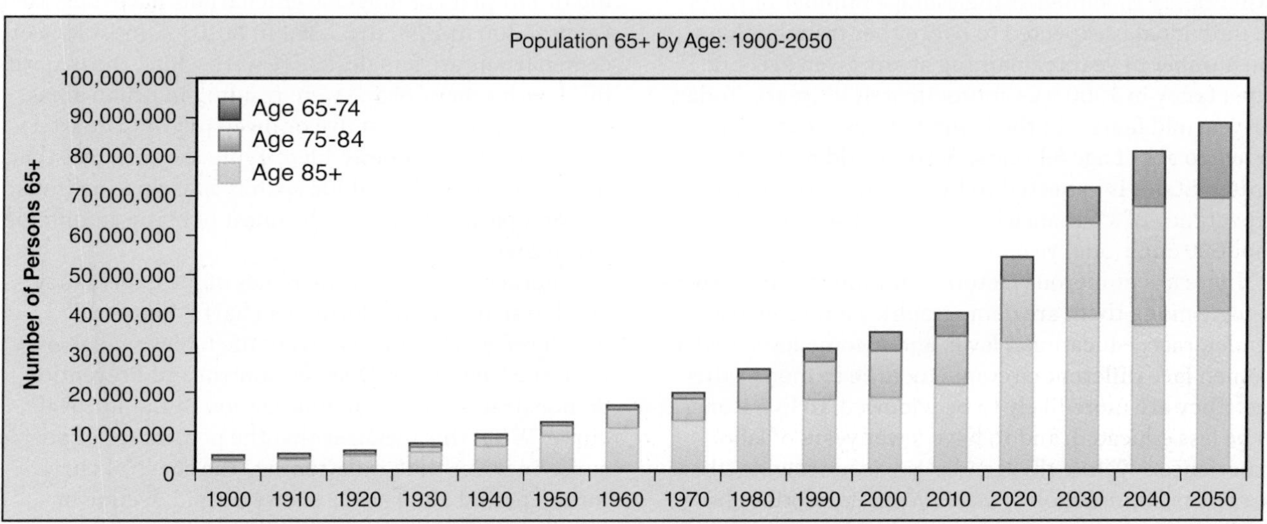

FIGURE 27-1 Actual and projected population of adults ages 65–74 years, 75–84 years, and over 85 years in the United States, 1900–2050.
Data from Department of Health and Human Services, Administration on Aging. Available at: http://www.aoa.gov/Aging_Statistics/future_growth/future_growth.aspx#age.

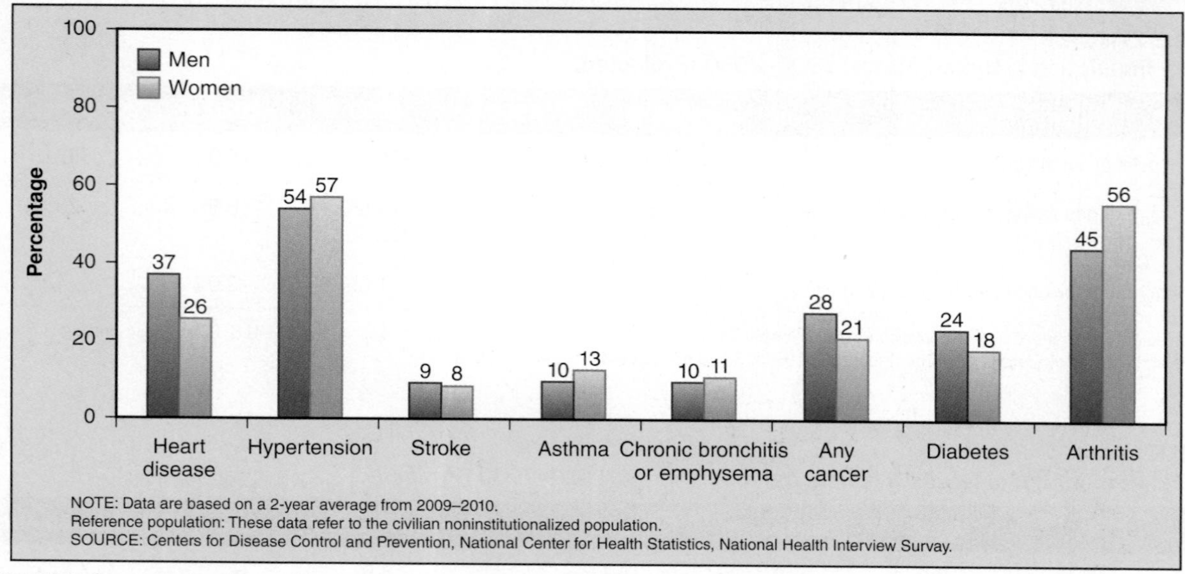

FIGURE 27-2 Common chronic conditions among men and women aged 65 years and older (expressed in percentages), 2009–2010.
Courtesy of Federal Interagency Forum on Aging-Related Statistics. *Older Americans 2012: Key Indicators of Well-Being*. Federal Interagency Forum on Aging-Related Statistics. Washington, DC: U.S. Government Printing Office. June 2012. Retrieved from http://www.agingstats.gov/Main_Site/Data/2012_Documents/docs/EntireChartbook.pdf.

fall into these categories of chronic and debilitating conditions. The most common chronic conditions among elderly men and women are shown in **Figure 27-2**.[14] Given the role of RTs across the continuum of care and particularly in the chronic and home care markets, understanding the delivery of healthcare to older adults will be essential.

Terms Associated with Aging

The terms *life expectancy* and *life span* often are interchanged both in conversation and in printed materials, but they are decidedly different concepts. **Life expectancy** is defined as the average number of years an individual is expected to live, either from birth or the number of years remaining at any given age. Life expectancy in 1900 was approximately 47 years. Today, a 1-year-old female in the United States is expected to live to about age 83 years. A 1-year-old male in the United States is expected to live to age 76 years. The life expectancy of a female who reaches 63 years of age is about 20 additional years.

There are numerous factors that influence life expectancy; among them are demographic factors such as gender, race, educational level, and income level. Older women face different circumstances than men as they age. They are more likely to be widowed, to live alone, to be less educated, and to have fewer years of labor experience.[15] While this gender gap is narrowing, there is a term, *feminization of later life*, that describes how women predominate at older ages and how the proportions increase with advancing age. In addition to demographics, environmental factors (such as exposure to pollutants), clean water, and sanitation play roles. However, lifestyle choices, such as diet, exercise, use of tobacco and alcohol, have clearly been found to be major influences

Life span, on the other hand, is species specific and defined as the typical length of time a species is expected to live. The life span of a housefly is 21 days, and that of a mouse is 3 to 4 years. The life span of humans is currently considered to be 122 years, based on the age to which Jean Calment survived in France. The 2010 U.S. Census Bureau reported only 1.73 per 10,000 to be centenarians,[16] and approximately 1 person out of 5 million will become a super-centenarian by living to 110 years or longer. Centenarians have increased from 37,306 in 1990 to 53,364 in 2010.[9] Almost 83% of centenarians are female, 82.5% were white, the majority lived with others, 85.7% were residing in urban areas, and, as expected, most live or dwell in group quarters such as nursing homes.[17] Identifying the variables that influence **longevity** and life span is a fascinating investigative topic and has been the quest of many gerontology researchers.

Another way to view the issues of life expectancy and life span is in the form of a chart.[18] **Figure 27-3**, which reflects the most current life tables available from the Centers for Disease Control and Prevention, demonstrates the rectangularization of the survival curve. What this means is that the percentage of people surviving over time is flattening. The survival curve for the period 1900–1902 shows a rapid decline in survival in the first few years of life and a relatively steady decline thereafter. In contrast, the survival curve for 2006 is nearly flat until about age 50 years,

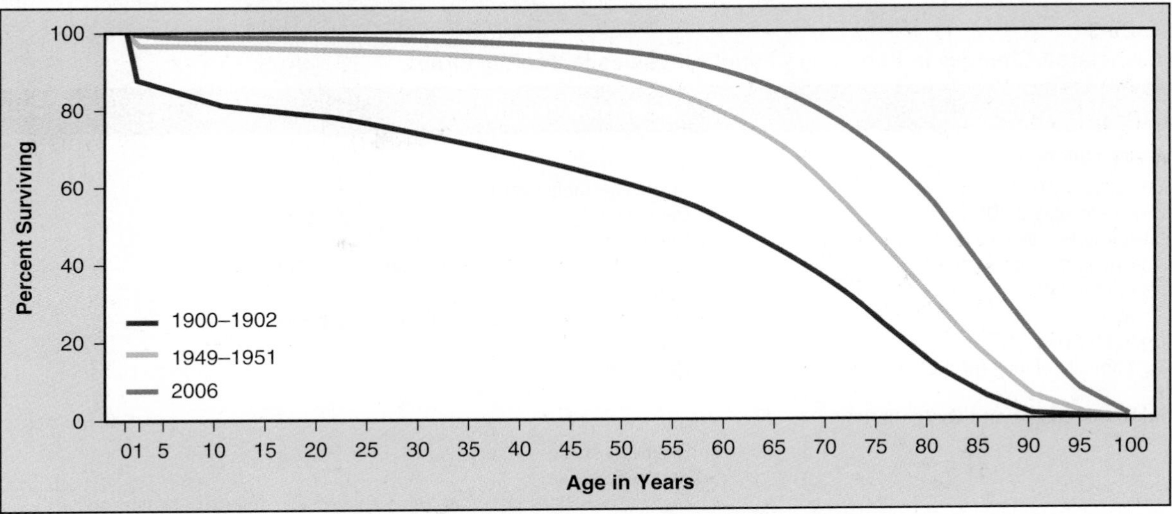

FIGURE 27-3 Percentage of persons surviving by age, 1900–1902, 1949–1951, and 2006.

Reproduced from Arias E. United States life tables, 2006. *National Vital Statistics Reports*. 2010;58:no 21. Hyattsville, MD: National Center for Health Statistics. http://www.cdc.gov/nchs/data/nvsr/nvsr58/nvsr58_21.pdf.

after which the decline in survival becomes more rapid. Improvements in survival between the periods 1900–1902 and 1949–1951 occurred at all ages, although the largest improvements were among the younger population. Between 1949–1951 and 2006, improvements occurred primarily for the older population. The survival curve has become increasingly flat in response to progressively lower mortality, particularly at the younger ages, and increasingly vertical at the older ages. This shows that life expectancy is increasing. Note, however, that at age 100 years there is little difference in survivability between 1900 and 2006, demonstrating that life span has not changed appreciably in the last century.[18]

Aging Pulmonary Anatomy and Physiology

Like other organ systems, the lungs, surrounding muscles, pulmonary vessels, and bony structure are all affected by age. Although the changes are not major, some subtle changes in structure and function occur that affect ventilation, perfusion, and diffusion in the elderly.

The lungs and the chest wall both have elastic properties. The thorax has the tendency to pull outward, and the lungs are inclined to recoil inward. Normally these opposing forces balance each other. With age the chest wall becomes stiffer, due in part to costal cartilage calcification, osteoporosis, changes in rib–vertebral articulations, and narrowing of the intervertebral disk, often resulting in settling of the vertebrae with age, and loss in height. While the chest wall becomes stiffer, the lungs become more compliant as a result of reduced elastic recoil pressure. The net effect is an overall decrease in compliance, which increases the work of breathing for older adults. Such changes make work of breathing almost twice for a 70-year old compared to a 20-year-old. The alterations in the lungs and chest wall also effect the anterior–posterior (AP) chest configuration. A normal ratio of AP to transverse diameter is 1:2; with advanced age, the AP to transverse diameter approaches 1:1.

Respiratory muscle strength declines with age. **Sarcopenia**, the age-related loss of muscle mass, starts to develop somewhere between ages 40 and 60 years for both sexes. Longitudinal studies have established the rate of decline to be between 1% and 3% per year after age 50 years.[19] All of the respiratory muscles, including inspiratory and expiratory accessory muscles, go through age-associated decremental change and many pulmonary flows, volumes, and capacities are altered with age (**Table 27-3**).

An additional change in the pulmonary system notable in the elderly is a reduction in the alveolar gas exchange surface area. Alveoli dilate and the pores of Kohn become larger, likely due to changes in elasticity in the parenchyma. Less surface area reduces the diffusion of pulmonary gases. The central and peripheral chemoreceptors are less responsive to changes in Pa_{O_2} and Pa_{CO_2}. The adaptation to low oxygen or high carbon dioxide in terms of ventilatory response in a 75-year-old is almost half of that noted in a 25-year-old adult.[20]

Respiratory Recap

- Sarcopenia, the age-related loss of muscle mass, develops between the ages of 40 and 60 years.

TABLE 27-3
Age-Associated Changes in Pulmonary Function Values in Healthy Elders

Value	Age-Related Change
Pulmonary Function	
Total lung capacity (TLC)	Relatively stable over time
Forced vital capacity (FVC)	Decreases 20–30 mL/year after age 20 years
Forced expiratory volume in 1 second (FEV_1)	Decreases
Functional residual capacity (FRC)	Increases (as a result of increased residual volume)
Residual volume (RV)	Increases
RV/TLC ratio	Increases from 20% to roughly 40% in old age
Peak expiratory flow (PEF)	Decreases
Diffusing capacity of lung for carbon monoxide (D_{LCO})	Decreases
Arterial Blood Gases and Oxygenation	
pH	Relatively stable
$Paco_2$	Relatively stable
Pao_2	Decreases slightly (<70 mm Hg is abnormal in otherwise healthy adults regardless of age) Supine Pao_2 5 mm Hg less than seated Pao_2
Spo_2	Relatively stable (<94% is abnormal in otherwise healthy adults; <90% in patients with COPD is treated)
$P(A - a)o_2$	Increases slightly

There are many reasons why understanding normal age-related physiologic changes in the pulmonary system are important. Well over half the patients seen by RTs are older than 65 years. Our patients not only have age-associated decremental change but also almost always have a disease process that we are treating. RTs must be able to distinguish age-related decline from pathology. Most notable is the tendency to falsely presume that older adults with a 1:1 AP to transverse chest diameter and enlarged alveoli have senile emphysema.

The implications for RTs may be more critical when caring for older adults in the intensive care unit. A weaker diaphragm, reduced vital capacity, and compromised cough mechanism must be taken into consideration post-extubation. Older patients may need closer monitoring and hyperinflation therapy to prevent atelectasis. Unfortunately, because of age-associated physiology, older adults are more likely to become ventilator dependent and to suffer the consequences associated with long-term mechanical ventilation. Liberating older patients from the ventilator in less than 48 hours is optimal, which may be facilitated by extubation to noninvasive ventilation.

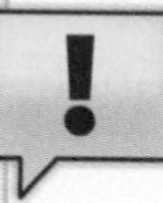

Respiratory Recap

Primary Age-Related Pulmonary Changes

- Loss of elasticity
- Loss of muscle strength
- Loss of alveolar gas exchange surface area
- Decreased responsiveness of the chemoreceptors

Geriatric Patient Assessment

Physical Assessment

Physical assessments include all systems, vital signs, skin, chest and back, sensory and motor function, mental acuity, and nutritional status. Consider this scenario: You walk into an elderly patient's room early morning to deliver therapy. You listen to lung sounds, gather vital signs, ask the patient a few questions, and ask if he or she can sit up in bed for you. While listening to lung sounds on the posterior thorax, you note that the scapulae are uneven and there is significant kyphosis. You also notice that the patient's skin is very dry and lacking the normal tension or fullness known as turgor. These are signs of a restrictive disease process and possible dehydration. How will this affect the patient's breathing? The lung sounds are decreased and you hear crackles in the bases. You also note that the patient is using accessory muscles to breathe. While auscultating the right upper lobe, you hear wheezes. Which of these findings are normal in an older adult? Because of an increased AP chest diameter, the lung sounds may be decreased. Crackles in the bases are not uncommon in older adults. This may indicate atelectasis, which often clears after you ask the patient to take a few good deep breaths. Crackles can also be due to congestive heart failure. The use of accessory muscles to breathe and the wheezes, however, are likely associated with pathology.

Did the patient complain of dizziness or lightheadedness when he or she sat up in bed? Changing position from being supine to being seated or standing can occasionally cause a drop in blood pressure. A decrease in systolic pressure of 20 mm Hg upon change in position is diagnostic for **orthostatic hypotension**. Although this may not affect a patient's pulmonary system, it will increase his or her risk of falling.

While checking the identification band on the patient's wrist, look to see whether clubbing is present. Clubbing, an enlargement of the terminal aspect of the fingers, is not age related and is usually not associated with COPD. If clubbing is present in your patient with COPD, suspect an additional comorbidity such as bronchiectasis, bronchogenic cancer, or asbestosis. Renal and cardiac disease have also been associated with clubbing.[21]

In less than 2 minutes, you have made a cursory assessment of the patient for breath sounds, dehydration, restrictive disease, orthostatic hypotension, and clubbing (comorbidities). Continuing on with the assessment, asking an open-ended question such as "How did you sleep last night?" or "What did you order for breakfast?" is instructive. The patient's response will give you information about the level of cognition and insight into nutritional or other habits.

Heart rate does not change appreciably with age. In sedentary older adults, it may be a little lower. RTs may notice stronger or bounding pulses in older patients, likely an effect of atherosclerotic changes in blood vessels. There is an age-associated decrease in the number of pacemaker cells in the sinoatrial node, which may lead to symptomatic bradyarrhythmias.[22] To get an accurate heart rate in elderly patients, it may be necessary to count their pulse for a full minute.

Note whether the patient feels warm or cold while palpating the pulse. Body temperature is often a little lower in older adults due in part to decreased metabolism. The thermoregulatory mechanism is also blunted with age, making older patients more susceptible to changes in environmental temperatures. How would a cold room (<65° F) affect your COPD patient? **Hypothermia**, defined as a core temperature of 95° F (35° C) or less, can develop in rooms where the temperature is maintained at 60° to 65° F. A pulmonary consequence of accidental hypothermia may be bradypnea, which can lead to hypoxemia or hypercapnia or both. Hypothermia that develops as a consequence of a surgical procedure can also affect immunity. Even mild hypothermia (core temperature decrease by 1° C) can cause significant alteration to the normal immune response.[23]

Do not assume that an afebrile patient is infection free. Fever may be blunted 20% to 30% of the time in a patient with an infection, which unfortunately contributes to diagnostic delays.[24] If elderly patients do have a fever, it is likely to be associated with a more serious viral or bacterial infection than fever in a younger adult.

Respiratory rate is stable across the adult life span. It is advisable to measure respiratory rate prior to starting therapy. When patients are actively involved in nebulizer or hyperinflation therapy, their respiratory rate will be altered. A normal respiratory rate in adults over 65 years remains in the range of 16 to 24 breaths per minute despite physiologic changes in the lungs. Dyspnea, however, is rarely normal. If patients have a resting respiratory rate greater than 25, there is likely some pathology associated with the increased work of breathing.

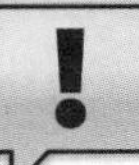

Respiratory Recap

Physical Assessment Findings in the Elderly

- Increased AP chest diameter
- Decreased lung sounds
- Atelectasis in the bases
- Increased pulse pressure
- Respiratory rate a little faster
- Heart rate normal or a little slower
- Bounding pulses
- Lower body temperature

Comprehensive Geriatric Assessment

History, Definition, and Components

The history of comprehensive geriatric assessment (CGA) dates back to the mid-1940s when neglected and bedridden elderly patients were cared for in a large, chronic disease hospital and systematically evaluated using assessments to determine who might benefit from medical and rehabilitation efforts.[25] Since that time, CGAs have evolved and become much more sophisticated. A CGA is a multidimensional, interdisciplinary diagnostic process to determine the medical, psychological, and functional capabilities of a frail elderly person in order to develop a coordinated and integrated plan for treatment.[26] Care of an older adult extends beyond the traditional medical management of illness. It requires evaluation of multiple issues including physical, cognitive, affective, social, financial, environmental, and spiritual components that influence an older adult's health.

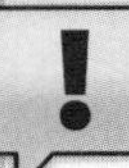

Respiratory Recap

Components of a Comprehensive Geriatric Assessment

- Physical
- Cognitive
- Affective
- Social
- Financial
- Environmental
- Spiritual

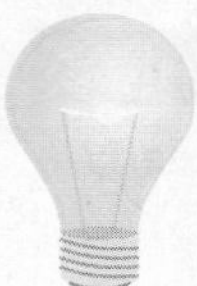

STOP AND THINK

How would you perform a comprehensive geriatric assessment?

Role of the RT in Geriatric Assessments

A comprehensive geriatric assessment does not generally fall under the duties of the RT. It is generally conducted by a geriatrician or family practitioner with a goal of uncovering treatable health problems or issues in community-dwelling older adults. The process involves screening patients, often those older than 75 to 80 years, for functional ability, geriatric syndromes, specific medical conditions, medication management, and support systems. It typically involves elderly individuals who are frail and disabled or have multiple interacting comorbid conditions.

Frailty

Frail elderly has been defined as "older adults who are lacking in general strength and are unusually susceptible to disease or other infirmity."[27] **Frailty** has attracted increased attention in the medical literature recently, likely corresponding with the increased numbers of frail individuals being admitted to healthcare institutions. In addition to assessing activities of daily living (ADLs) and instrumental activities of daily living (IADLs), the CGA involves screening for a myriad of potential disabilities. While there is no gold standard to assess frailty, the Mini-Mental Status Exam (MMSE), clock-drawing test, Geriatric Depression Scale (GDS), Mini-Nutritional Assessment (MNA), Snellen eye test, whispered voice test, Functional Assessment Staging (FAST), and the Hearing Handicap Inventory for the Elderly (HHIE) are just a few of the available instruments. In addition, the Caregiver Burden Interview may be valuable in heading off potential elder abuse before it becomes a reality (see **Appendix 28-1**).

Chronological age is sometimes used as a marker of frailty (e.g., only screening adults over the age of 75 or 80 years); however, there is a wide range of function in the older adult population. In a systematic review of the literature by Sternberg et al.,[28] three identifying components were noted to be most commonly associated with frailty (physical function, gait speed, and cognition) and three common outcomes (death, disability, and institutionalization).

As the aging population continues to grow, RTs who see the need for additional assessments in elderly pulmonary patients may need to take the lead in recommending a comprehensive assessment for the patient. Home care RTs may be in the best position to recommend screening services for their elderly patients.

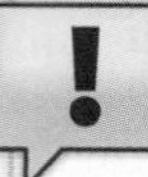

Respiratory Recap

Comprehensive Geriatric Assessment

- ADLs and IADLs
- Vision and hearing (Snelling eye test, HHIE, and whisper voice test)
- Mental status (MMSE and clock-drawing test)
- Geriatric Depression Scale (GDS)
- Nutrition (MNA) and nutritional health assessment
- Functional Assessment Staging (FAST)
- Caregiver Burden Interview (possible need for assistance)

Atypical Disease Presentation

Atypical or nonspecific clinical presentation of disease in the elderly is much like the diversity common in the whole population of older adults. There are no hard and fast specifics, but there are generalities about which healthcare professionals should be knowledgeable. In older adults, the first signs of an acute illness or an exacerbation of a chronic disease may be functional decline, cognitive impairment, or both. Because symptoms are not always typical, older adults may not recognize subtle changes as being associated with a disease process. Atypical symptoms may be ignored, may be denied, often out of fear, or may simply be regarded as one of the joys of aging. Well elders are more likely to present with fewer atypical symptoms. Nonspecific symptoms, which are more difficult to diagnose, are more common in frail elders, in particular women over the age of 80 years.

Unfortunately, the lines between aging and ailing are often blurred and there is compelling evidence that older people are not treated purely on the basis of their physiological condition and their wishes but on age per se.[5] The medical profession is often unduly pessimistic about the outcomes in older adults and is either overtreating when palliative care would have been preferred by the patient or undertreating because of the physician's expectation of a poor outcome.

Aches and pains may be caused by chronic osteoarthritis, overexertion, exercise, the weather, lack of activity, medications, or pathology. A change in gait or new onset of tripping or running into furniture may be related to infection, medications, or dehydration. A new onset of confusion in a formerly cognitive, sapient individual may be related to infection or hypoxemia. Weak nonproductive cough may be a side effect of drugs (e.g., angiotensin-converting enzyme inhibitors) or a pulmonary disorder. RTs are accustomed to looking for usual symptoms, such as pain, fever, cough, dyspnea, and nausea/vomiting, in patients as signs of illness. In the elderly, it may be better to ask about dizziness, syncope, abdominal pain, and fatigue.

TABLE 27-4
Normal Age-Related Changes in Various Organ Systems

Cardiac	Cardiac muscle thickens, leading to enlarged left ventricle. Arterial walls stiffen with age; aorta becomes dilated and elongated. Aortic knob calcification (crescent-shaped ring on top of aorta) is noted in about 30% of older adults but has no pathologic significance. Systolic blood pressure increases more than diastolic, leading to increased pulse pressure and isolated systolic hypertension.
Pulmonary	Diaphragm loses strength, up to 25% by age 75–80 years. At age 20 years, alveolar surface area is about 70 m^2; at age 70 years, it is reduced to about 60 m^2.
Brain/central nervous system	Cell loss in some areas of the brain is stable; profound loss in other areas. The weight of the brain gradually decreases with age (approximately 10% from age 30 years to age 90 years).
Kidneys	Renal mass slowly diminishes (from about 250–270 g in young adults to about 180–200 g in adults older than 80 years).

Two major reasons why symptoms in the elderly are not typical are age-associated changes in the immune system and normal age-related change in various organ systems (**Table 27-4**). The reasons why older adults do not present with classic symptoms are poorly understood but are likely multifactorial. Age-associated changes in physiology, a reduced response to hypoxemia and hypercapnia, and alterations in the cardiac conduction system are all likely contributors. Also suggested is a decreased peripheral sensitivity that can reduce the sensation of pain.[29] The immune system undergoes age-related functional decline. The thymus gland decreases in size and function. The T-lymphocyte response to antigens decreases. **Immunosenescense**, defined as aging of the immune system, progresses as we grow older, reducing both cell-mediated and humoral immunity. These factors combined may be the reason why elderly persons are susceptible to respiratory infections from all causes.[6]

The presentation of symptoms may also be disproportionate to the severity of illness, causing further diagnostic confusion. A temperature of 99.6° F (38° C) in an older adult may be recorded and noted as a little elevated, but not associated with disease. Consider, however, that this same patient has a usual body temperature of 96.8° F (36° C) and that the temperature is elevated 3° F (2° C). Would this justify an intervention? The importance of monitoring body temperature on a regular basis in the elderly cannot be overstated. Early intervention is needed to keep our older patients from suffering repeated exacerbations of chronic or acute disease.

Some of the more common cardiorespiratory diseases and disorders that present atypically in older adults are pneumonia,[30] myocardial infarction,[31–33] congestive heart failure (CHF),[29,34] tuberculosis,[35] and depression.[29] The atypical symptoms and important age-related considerations for each are presented here.

Pneumonia

- Presentation may be latent and come with or without a chill
- Cough and expectoration are slight.
- Physical findings are ill defined and changeable.
- Constitutional symptoms occur out of proportion to the extent of the local lesion.
- Classic symptoms of fever, cough, sputum production, dyspnea, and pleuritic chest pain may be absent or diminished.
- The elderly may present with more slowly progressive, nonspecific features of ill health.
- Key clinical features might include unexplained confusion, falls, decreased appetite, or headache.
- Clinical features may be as general as widespread aches or fatigue.

Myocardial Infarction

- Patients may present with syncope, confusion, palpitations, stroke, vertigo, nausea.
- Dyspnea is the most common symptom.
- In women, the most common prodromal (>1 month prior) symptoms are fatigue, sleep disturbance, and dyspnea. Acute chest pain was absent in 43% of older women.
- Chest pain in adults younger than 65 years occurs 89% of the time.
- Chest pain in adults older than 65 years occurs 66% of the time.
- Chest pain in adults older than 85 years occurs 33% of the time.
- Silent presentation is not uncommon.

Congestive Heart Failure

- New-onset pulmonary edema (a classic sign of CHF) may be confounded by comorbid conditions.
- Orthopnea (difficulty breathing in a flat position) may be hidden if the patient has a habit of sleeping on two to three pillows.
- Dyspnea on exertion may be absent in older adults who have little exertion on a daily basis.
- Patients may present with complaints of tiredness, decreased appetite, weight gain of 2 to 3 pounds (0.9 to 1.4 kg), fatigue and generalized weakness, and/or a nonproductive cough and complaints of poor sleep.

Tuberculosis

- Adults older than 65 years are much less likely to present with typical symptoms of hemoptysis, fever, or night sweats.
- Older adults may present with hepatosplenomegaly (enlarged liver and spleen), weight loss, abnormal liver function tests, and/or anemia.
- A high index of suspicion is recommended if a patient presents with cough or pneumonia unresponsive to conventional therapy.
- Tuberculosis infection is four times higher for nursing home residents than for community-dwelling older adults.
- Mortality rates from tuberculosis are highest in the elderly.

Depression

- Depression is the most commonly occurring mental health problem for the older adult population and while not truly a cardiorespiratory disease, it is listed because of its close association to COPD.
- The ageist attitude that older adults usually complain of feeling sad, tired, or depressed may make depression hard to recognize.
- Screening for depression in high-risk groups is recommended, including alcoholics; drug addicts; and adults with dementia, stroke, cancer, hip fracture, myocardial infarction, COPD, or Parkinson disease.
- The Geriatric Depression Scale is a useful instrument.

Geriatric Pharmacotherapy

While medication management is a major public health issue, it is particularly problematic for older adults. As a result of their increased incidence of both acute and chronic illness, older adults are the highest users of medication compared with all other age groups. Although the elderly make up on average 12% to 13% of the total population of the United States, they consume about 33% of all prescription drugs and about 25% of all over-the-counter drugs. A report by the U.S. Department of Health and Human Services estimates that 76% of adults ages 60 and older are taking two or more medications and 37% use five or more prescription drugs.[36] Among the issues related to geriatric pharmacotherapy are medication safety, adverse drug events, inappropriate medication use, underprescribing and overprescribing, and the rising cost of drugs.

Medication Safety

Medication safety—cited almost 15 years ago by the IOM[37]—continues to be a serious medical problem for all medical professionals with appropriate prescribing for older adults presenting unique challenges. Some of the biological reasons why older adults are more likely than younger adults to have adverse drug reactions are smaller body size and different body composition (reduced lean muscle mass), reduced ability of the kidneys and liver to metabolize and clear drugs out of the body, decrease in gastric motility, and decline in gastric pH.

To fully understand the effect age-associated physiology has on drugs, it is instructive to consider the half-life of drugs. The liver is the primary site of drug metabolism. With age, the liver volume, mass, and blood flow decline. Hepatic metabolism of drugs decreases up to 25% over the life span.[20] The duration of drug action is determined by the metabolic rate and is measured in terms of half-life. Consider the following:

- The half-life of diazepam (Valium) in a younger adult is about 24 hours; the half-life of diazepam in an older adult is about 82 hours.
- The half-life of flurazepam (Dalmane) in a younger adult is about 74 hours; the half-life of flurazepam in an older adult is about 106 hours.

If the dosing is not adjusted, significant amounts of drug can accumulate in the body.

Despite that drug safety is a concern, newer medications have saved countless lives, and few would argue against their benefit. In older adult patients, however, caution must be exercised. The advice to start low and go slow regarding dosing of medications for the elderly is a prudent course of action.

Adverse Drug Reactions

The World Health Organization (WHO) defines an adverse drug reaction (ADR) as a noxious response to a medication that is unintended at doses usually administered for diagnosis, prophylaxis, or treatment.[38] ADRs are common in the elderly, but what is most

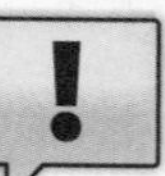

Respiratory Recap

Diseases That May Present Atypically in Older Adults

- Pneumonia
- Myocardial infarction
- Congestive heart failure
- Tuberculosis
- Depression

AGE-SPECIFIC ANGLE

Whereas the half-life of Valium in a 20-year-old is approximately 24 hours, in an 80-year-old the half-life is approximately 82 hours.

concerning is that many are preventable and in most cases safe alternatives are generally available. A drug that will effectively treat a 40-year-old patient may not be indicated for an 80-year-old patient. Drugs that are successful in treating a specific disease process may not be appropriate for an older patient who is already on multiple drugs for other comorbidities. The more medication an individual takes, the greater the potential for an adverse effect.

Unfortunately, few drug studies are done on healthy elders, so prescribing appropriately for sick elders can sometimes be a challenge. One excellent resource is the *American Geriatrics Society Updated Beers Criteria for Potentially Inappropriate Medication Use in Older Adults*. The criteria were updated most recently in 2012.[39] The final criteria include 53 individual medications or medication classes that are divided into three categories: potentially inappropriate medications and classes to avoid in older adults, potentially inappropriate medications and classes to avoid in older adults with certain diseases and syndromes that the drugs listed can exacerbate, and finally medications to be used with caution in older adults. The guidelines list the drug, the rationale, the quality of evidence, and the strength of recommendation. This most recent update uses an evidence-based approach of the Institute of Medicine standards and the development of a partnership to regularly update the criteria. Thoughtful application of the criteria will allow for closer monitoring of drug use, application of real-time e-prescribing and interventions to decrease adverse drug events in older adults, and better patient outcomes.[39] Anyone who works with older adults is advised to access the tables in the guidelines as a reference.

Medication Undertreatment and Overtreatment

Medication undertreatment in the elderly is another troubling reality in many long-term care facilities. A multicenter survey of a stratified random sample of 193 residential care and assisted living facilities in four states (2104 residents older than 65 years) revealed the following: of 328 subjects with CHF, 204 (62%) were not receiving an angiotensin-converting enzyme inhibitor; of 172 subjects with a prior history of myocardial infarction, 60.5% were not receiving aspirin and 76% were not receiving beta blockers; and of 435 subjects with a prior history of stroke, only 37.5% were receiving an anticoagulant or antiplatelet agent.[40] Although drugs must be administered judiciously to older adults, failure to prescribe appropriate drugs that decrease morbidity as established in clinical trials is also inappropriate.

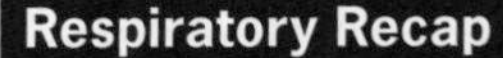

Respiratory Recap

Adverse Drug Reactions (ADRs) Are Common in the Elderly

- ADRs are preventable.
- Safe drug alternatives are generally available.

The self-medication habits of older adults, although harder to track, have some commonalities. Many older adults continue to take medications and consume alcohol at the same time. Healthcare literacy issues may be a factor, but willful noncompliance with recommended dosing instructions is also a reality. Many older adults regularly depend on over-the-counter (OTC) cold medicine, pain relievers, and vitamins. The number of OTC medications has grown exponentially to over 300,000 marketed products[41]and they are not always perceived to be real medicine. Older adults thus continue to self-dose while on prescription medications. As one example, the OTC medication diphenhydramine (e.g., Benadryl), which is used for short-term insomnia and allergies is included in both combination cough and cold and combination pain products, is among the most common but unsafe medications taken by the general older adult population.[42] Diphenhydramine has been shown to produce cognitive impairment in healthy adults, leading to excessive cognitive deficits and increased falls risk. Further, OTC medications such as diphenhydramine can lead to poorer control of chronic conditions such as arthritis, sleep, and depression. Potentially more safe and effective prescription medications are available under healthcare provider guidance.[43]

Drug Expenditures

Prescription drug costs have risen exponentially in the past few years. In a study conducted in 2011 by Chiu and associates, Medicaid spending on antiasthmatic medication from 1991 to 2009 rose by 595%, from $180.7 million to $1.3 billion. The authors cite a fourfold increase in the average price per prescription for antiasthmatic medications. While the following does not represent a fourfold increase, an example is for a medication regime common to the elderly asthmatic (an inhaled corticosteroid/long-acting beta agonist) costing $119.60 in 2001 that increased to $208.77 in 2009.[44] Older adults on fixed incomes or with incomes that have dwindled due to the changes in the economy are finding it harder to afford medications. Medicare Part D offers some help, as do other prescription drug plans, but not all older adults have coverage. Compounding the problem is the fact that prescription drugs may cost more in poor areas. Although chain pharmacies are often less expensive, they are not always located in poor areas. Prescription drugs can cost up to 15% more from independent pharmacies in poor zip codes.[45] Although there are independent pharmacies in poor zip codes that do not inflate costs, issues of finances, transportation, and health literacy limit consumers from shopping around. When older adults cannot access medication, and thus cannot control their disease process, they will end up in emergency departments, adding to the burden of escalating healthcare costs.

Communicating with Older Adults

Most RTs have encountered frustrating situations in which communication with the patient seems nonexistent. Language barriers, hearing deficits, poststroke aphasia, Alzheimer disease, and even patients on mechanical ventilators pose a challenge. Knowing that patient cooperation will increase the effectiveness of therapy makes communication more important in any of these situations. Taking the time to establish some measure of mutual understanding, however, is not always possible. In today's healthcare environment, time constraints create barriers to effective communication. When busy, the amount of time spent with each patient decreases, and communication gets lost in the hustle. What is important to remember, though, is that effective communication benefits more than just the patient. RTs who sense that their encounter with a patient was successful will feel that they have accomplished something and will be more rewarded by the whole process.

Communication Defined

Communication implies two things: a message delivered and a message understood. Although some people appear to be better at relaying information than others, most can be taught this skill; thus, we often refer to it as the art of communication. Communication is a dynamic, two-way process of imparting data or information between two or more individuals. Communication can be verbal or nonverbal, in written or sign language. Transfer of information likewise can be formal or informal. What is essential is that the information delivered has been received and comprehended. Talking to patients in a language foreign to them is delivering the message, but if they do not understand, there has been no communication.

Effective Communication

Successful transfer of information with an elderly patient is challenging at times. Actually, effective communication often starts with attitude. An RT who is tired and frustrated at the end of his or her shift may not communicate well with an older patient. Nonverbal communication may interfere. An observation attributed to Ralph Waldo Emerson states, "Who you are speaks so loudly, I can't hear what you're saying." When dealing with older adults, RTs must be careful not to send mixed messages. Sitting in a chair reading a paper while a patient is taking a treatment devalues both the patient and the therapy you are delivering.

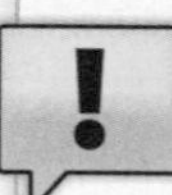

Respiratory Recap

Communication Is Dependent on Two Variables

- Message delivered
- Message understood

Another useful tactic in effective communication is the expression of empathy instead of sympathy to patient concerns. Although saying "I'm sorry" appears to be kind, it may be better to try to understand what the patient is going through. A statement such as "I can see that this is really distressing for you" does not imply that you can fix anything, just that you acknowledge the patient's feelings. Often this is enough to calm the patient down a little.

The Angry Patient

Patrick Everett, an 82-year-old patient with COPD, is angry much of the time. Staff members have come to accept the fact that he can be grumpy and difficult to handle. Today when you enter his room to deliver his medication, he snarls, "I don't need that, and I don't need you bothering me today either." How will you respond? Your choices are as follows:

1. "Yes you do need this medicine, and if I don't give it to you, who will?"
2. "What's the matter, Mr. Everett?"
3. "I'm just following the doctor's orders and he wants you to take this medicine."
4. Turn and walk angrily out of the room without responding.

Depending on the time of day and the existing patient load, RTs may be inclined to say or do any of the above. What is important to remember, however, is that most likely the patient's mood is not about us. Patients often lash out at caregivers when they are struggling with something that has nothing to do with other people. In this situation, perhaps the best response is to just say, "What's the matter, Mr. Everett?" He may or may not share his problem with you, but at the very least you have not caused an escalation of the situation.

Contrary to what we are accustomed to hearing, "Don't just do something, stand there" may be an effective way of communicating. Giving patients time to collect their thoughts and tell you what is bothering them, or giving them time to rethink the angry words they have spoken, may open doors to more effective communication.

The Verbally Abusive Patient

You are delivering therapy to Miss Rory, a patient with COPD and Alzheimer disease (AD) who is continually cursing at you. How will you respond? Your choices are as follows:

1. Curse back at her and let her know how it feels.
2. Respond by saying, "You need to change your nasty behavior—let's work on it together."

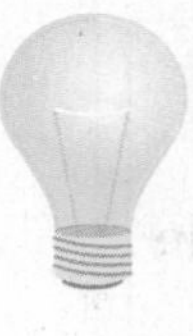

STOP AND THINK

How would you handle a patient situation in which you were confronted with anger, belligerence, or some other emotional outburst?

3. Say, "I'm sorry you feel like this, but I don't care to be spoken to in that manner."
4. Step back, look out the window, and say, "It sure is nice today."

One unfortunate characteristic of patients with AD is that dementia robs them of the ability to control their behavior. When AD begins to develop, the frontal part of the brain is damaged, and subsequently destroyed, causing lack of impulse control. Thus, AD patients may swear and use words that make us uneasy.

When caring for patients with dementia, sometimes there are no effective solutions, but therapy still needs to be delivered. If faced with a situation like this, remain calm and do not attempt to argue or correct such patients. Back off a little, perhaps try to distract them, and continue to proceed with the task at hand.

Decreased communication skills have been well documented in AD. Patients who cannot accurately report symptoms are at increased risk for developing more serious complications from a disease process. Asking questions may not always generate accurate information, especially if they are yes-or-no questions. Patients with AD may answer yes or no without understanding the question. RTs need to be aware that a change in behavior such as restlessness, decreased activity, decreased appetite, or anything out of the ordinary for the patient may be a clue of physical impairment or illness. The Alzheimer's Association[46] offers these communication tips for caregivers to more effectively engage and converse with the patient suffering from dementia:

- *Identify yourself.* Approach the person from the front and say who you are. Keep good eye contact; if the person is seated or reclined, go down to that level.
- *Call the person by name.* It helps orient the person and gets his or her attention.
- *Use short, simple words and sentences.* Lengthy requests or stories can be overwhelming. Ask one question at a time.
- *Speak slowly and distinctively.* Be aware of speed and clarity. Use a gentle and relaxed tone—a lower pitch is more calming.
- *Patiently wait for a response.* The person may need extra time to process what you said.
- *Repeat information or questions as needed.* If the person doesn't respond, wait a moment. Then ask again.
- *Turn questions into answers.* Provide the solution rather than the question. For example, say, "The bathroom is right here," instead of asking, "Do you need to use the bathroom?"
- *Avoid confusing and vague statements.* If you tell the person to "Hop in!" he or she may interpret your instructions literally. Instead, describe the action directly: "Please come here. Your shower is ready." Instead of using "it" or "that," name the object or place. For example, rather than "Here it is," say "Here is your hat."
- *Turn negatives into positives.* Instead of saying, "Don't go there," say, "Let's go here."
- *Give visual cues.* To help demonstrate the task, point or touch the item you want the individual to use or begin the task for the person.
- *Avoid quizzing.* Reminiscing may be healthy but avoid asking, "Do you remember when ... ?"
- *Write things down.* Try using written notes as reminders if the person is able to understand them.
- *Treat the person with dignity and respect.* Avoid talking down to the person or talking as if he or she isn't there.
- *Convey an easygoing manner.* Be aware of your feelings and attitude that you may be communicating through your tone of voice. Use positive, friendly facial expressions and nonverbal communication.

Pulmonary Disease After Age 65 Years

Obstructive Disease

Obstructive pulmonary diseases (COPD and asthma) are commonly diagnosed in older adult patients. The prevalence of COPD rises with age for both men and women throughout most of the life span and is highest among men aged 75 to 84 (11.2%) and women aged 65 to 74 (10.4%) and 75 to 84 (9.7%)[47] (**Figure 27-4**). This has huge implications for RTs. By nature of its chronicity, COPD develops over a long period of time; thus, many patients afflicted with this disease are older. Additionally, many former smokers who have the disease may never be diagnosed until age-associated decline is coupled with tobacco-related damage, making the disease process more obvious. Because both

Respiratory Recap

Obstructive Pulmonary Diseases

- The prevalence of COPD rises with age for both men and women.
- COPD is highest among men aged 75–84 and women aged 65–74 and 75–84.

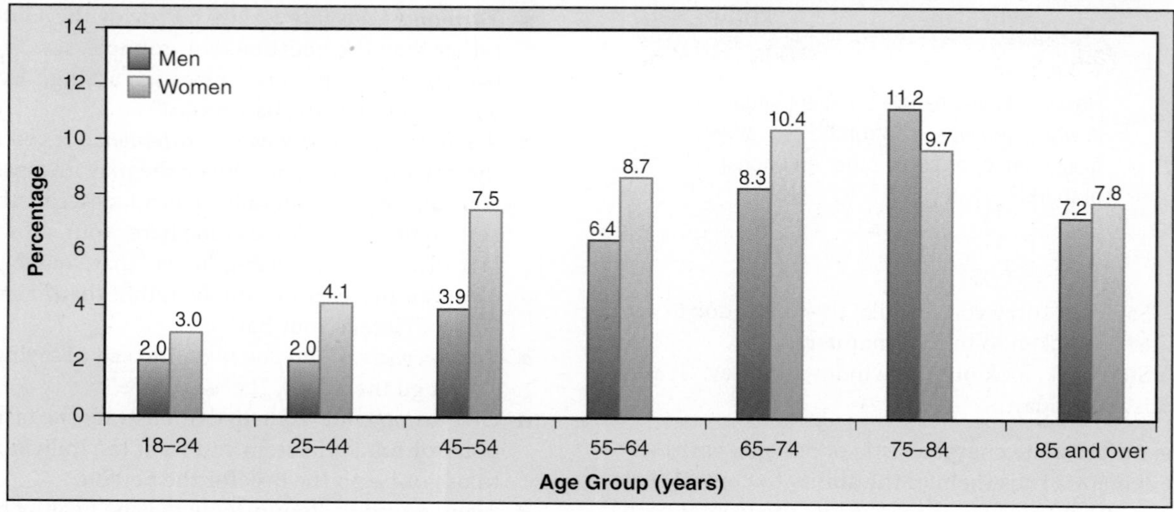

FIGURE 27-4 Prevalence of COPD by age and sex, U.S. annual average 2007–2009.

Reproduced from Akinbami LJ, Liu X. *Chronic obstructive pulmonary disease among adults aged 18 and over in the United States, 1998–2009.* NCHS data brief, no. 63. Hyattsville, MD: National Center for Health Statistics. 2011. Available at: http://www.cdc.gov/nchs/data/databriefs/db63.htm.

diseases present with similar symptoms, and some symptoms present simultaneously, it is sometimes difficult to determine whether the patient has asthma, COPD, or both. Because the diseases are treated differently, it is important to try to determine the primary problem. **Table 27-5** may be helpful in identifying features that favor asthma or COPD.[48]

Geriatric patients admitted to the hospital with COPD or an acute respiratory infection, or both, should be given special attention. The presence of an acute respiratory infection places the COPD patient at increased risk for a more complicated hospital stay. Infection control measures, although always important, are imperative in hospitalized elders. Chronic mucus production is a strong predictor of the incidence of respiratory infection and is also a strong predictor of death from COPD.[49]

Based on both disease- and age-associated physiologic changes in the lungs, hospitalized elders with COPD must be considered extremely susceptible to adverse events and should be monitored closely. Many of our regular patients with COPD—those known well to pulmonary services—may not desire special attention and may resist monitoring. To treat them the same as younger adults, however, would be a mistake. Their lives may depend on our diligence. Once the acute phase of their disease is controlled and the patient has stabilized, the focus needs to be on disease management. Smoking cessation, nutrition, exercise (pulmonary rehabilitation), a review of their medications and delivery devices, recognition of the signs and symptoms of an exacerbation, and social support networks are important aspects of patient education. RTs should review these with every patient with COPD prior to discharge, regardless of how many admissions and discharges the patient has had.

TABLE 27-5
Differentiation of Asthma from COPD in Older Adults

Favors Asthma	Favors COPD
• Onset before age 20 years	• Onset after age 40 years
• Variation in symptoms over minutes, hours, or days • Symptoms worse during the night or early morning • Symptoms triggered by exercise, emotions, including laughter, dust, or exposure to allergens	• Persistence of symptoms despite treatment • Good and bad days but always daily symptoms and exertional dyspnea • Chronic cough and sputum precede onset of dyspnea, unrelated to triggers
• Record or variable airflow limitation (spirometry, peak flow)	• Record of persistent airflow limitation (postbronchodilator FEV_1/FVC <0.7)
• Lung function normal between symptoms • Previous doctor diagnosis of asthma • Family history of asthma and other allergic condition	• Lung function abnormal between symptoms • Previous doctor diagnosis of COPD, chronic bronchitis, or emphysema • Heavy exposure to a risk factor: tobacco smoke, biomass fuels
• No worsening of symptoms over time. Symptoms vary either seasonally or from year to year • May improve spontaneously or have an immediate response to BD or to ICS over weeks	• Symptoms slowly worsening over time (progressive course over years) • Rapid-acting bronchodilator treatment provides only limited relief
• Normal chest radiograph	• Severe hyperinflation on chest radiograph

BD, bronchodilators; ICS, inhaled corticosteroids.

Information from Petty TL, Seebass JS, eds. Pulmonary Disorders of the Elderly. Philadelphia: American College of Physicians; 2007 and Sin BA, Akkoca Ö, Öner F, et al. Differences between asthma and COPD in the elderly. *J Invest Allerg Clin Immunol.* 2006;16:44-50.

Elderly patients with asthma, likewise, are at risk for developing complications. Unfortunately, asthma is often underdiagnosed or misdiagnosed as COPD, CHF, or GERD, and thus not managed appropriately. Elderly patients with asthma may also have a more severe form of the disease or may be affected more seriously. Despite better medications, asthma action plans, and a better understanding of the pathophysiology of the disease, mortality is still increasing. Patients over the age of 65 have the highest asthma mortality rate of any age group, accounting for over 50% of all asthma deaths.[50] Asthma in the elderly is not a benign disease, and care must be taken to ensure appropriate disease management.

Pharmacotherapy for the adult with asthma depends on the severity of the disease. Inhaled corticosteroids remain the medication of choice for persistent asthma. For moderate and severe persistent asthma, the addition of a long-acting beta agonist (LABA) to inhaled corticosteroids is recommended. The long-acting anticholinergic tiotropium is useful for many patients with COPD. Unfortunately, guidelines are not always followed.

Restrictive Disease

Many disease processes are capable of contributing to less compliant lungs in older adults. Restrictive disease is characterized by smaller lungs, reduced total lung compliance, and reduced volumes. The precipitating factors may be an alteration in the lung parenchyma or pathology in the pleura, chest wall, or neuromuscular function. If the cause is parenchymal lung disease, as in asbestosis, diffusion of gases will also be impaired. Because airflows and airway resistance are relatively normal, pulmonary function testing will show a restrictive pattern: FEV_1/FVC normal or above normal, with all lung volumes reduced. Causes of pulmonary restrictive disease in the elderly can be divided into three categories: intrinsic lung disease, extrinsic disorders, and idiopathic fibrotic disease.

Intrinsic lung diseases comprise the largest number of etiologic factors. The estimated incidence and prevalence increase from 7 and 14 per 100,000 per year for the general population to approximately 70 and 270 per 100,000 per year for the elderly.[51] Included in the intrinsic category are collagen vascular diseases; diseases caused by certain drugs, organic dust exposure, or inorganic dust exposure; and unclassified diseases. The collagen vascular diseases most often associated with the development of a restrictive pulmonary component are scleroderma, polymyositis, dermatomyositis, systemic lupus erythematosus, ankylosing spondylitis, and perhaps the most common, rheumatoid arthritis. The pharmaceutical agents implicated in the development of intrinsic lung disease are drugs such as amiodarone, bleomyocin, and methotrexate, which damage lung tissue. Organic dust exposure over time may cause restrictive lung disease and is usually occupation related.

Byssinosis (cotton worker's disease) and farmer's lung disease are two examples of pulmonary diseases caused by organic dusts. Inorganic dusts such as silicon, asbestos, and hard metal dust are causative agents in the development of fibrosis, and their inhalation may also be occupation related. The final category of intrinsic lung disease includes unclassified diseases such as sarcoidosis, alveolar proteinosis, and bronchiolitis obliterans with organizing pneumonia (BOOP).

The extrinsic category of restrictive pulmonary diseases includes both primary and secondary kyphoscoliosis, postpolio syndrome, pleural effusions, and morbid obesity (defined as more than 130% of desired weight),[20] all of which cause a restrictive component.

Idiopathic fibrotic disorders are a challenge. The rate of disease progression is highly variable, and disease does not always respond to therapy. The prognosis for older adults who do not respond to therapy is poor. Lung transplantation is an optional therapy but is not always available to the elderly (those younger than 65 years usually qualify). The scope of this chapter does not allow for a full explanation of treating the myriad of intrinsic and extrinsic disorders; however, corticosteroids are often prescribed. Because treatment differs, however, it is important on diagnosis to determine, based on pulmonary function values, whether the disorder is intrinsic or extrinsic.

Healthy Aging Strategies

Most of the advertisements targeted at the elderly are selling youth with the right diet, the appropriate exercises, the newest antiaging serums, or cosmetic surgery. Many older adults, however, are not all that concerned about looking or acting younger. Issues such as paying bills, dealing with chronic diseases, finding transportation, and caring for younger family members often take precedence. Having time to do things that are enjoyable and being able to spend time with family and friends are important to older adults; thus, maintaining adequate health to allow for these activities is the goal of many.

Biological aging is a process of change and takes its toll on tissues and organs. Functional decline is a factor of advanced age, even in the absence of disease, but can be slowed. Healthy lifestyle choices or the avoidance of health-damaging behaviors may ultimately result in preserved functionality for an extended period of time.

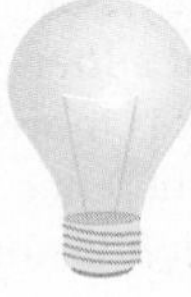

STOP AND THINK

Do you think that scientist Olshansky at 130 years or Austad at 150 years will likely be correct regarding the optimum life span of humans?

Although the human life span is currently 120 years, two renowned scientists are betting that in the year 2150, someone will be alive at either 130 years (Olshansky's bet) or 150 years (Austad's bet). The heirs of the scientist who wins the bet will collect the prize, estimated to be about $500 million in 2150. The scientists are basing their claims on the progress in aging research, including cloning technology, and stem cell research. They both agree that better understanding of the fundamental processes of aging, newer pharmaceuticals, and gene therapy may be able to combat aging within the next few decades.[52]

Health-Damaging Behaviors

There seems no better way to conclude a chapter on caring for the elderly than to address the issue of health behaviors that support a long and fruitful life. Gerontologists and specialists on aging have long sought the magic ingredients to longevity and extending life. The literature supports the notion that genetics represents approximately 20% of the determinants of health with use and access to the healthcare system and environment representing 20% and 10%, respectively. That leaves approximately 50% for lifestyle behaviors. There are a number of health-damaging behaviors that elders should avoid to improve the quality of their lives and avoid or postpone some of the chronic diseases or conditions noted earlier in the chapter. Some of the more popular are tobacco use, excessive use of alcohol, limited physical activity, poor diet and nutrition, and obesity. An interesting study investigated the extent to which adherence to recommendations regarding health behaviors among older adults were likely to result in aging successfully.[53] The results revealed that as the number of adherent behaviors increased so did the likelihood of aging successfully and that adherence to some health behavior clusters was more closely associated with successful aging than adherence to others. The focus was on exercise, alcohol consumption, cigarette smoking, adherence to a Mediterranean diet, and body mass index (BMI). Adherence to each of the five health behaviors varied from 28.6% adherence to exercise recommendations, 83.9% adherence to smoking recommendations, 29.2% adherence to a prescribed BMI, 31.1% adherence to a Mediterranean diet, and 39.4% adherence to a moderate alcohol recommendation. Additionally, 4.9% of participants adhered to none of the health behaviors, 28.4% adhered to only one, 31.4% adhered to two, 22.1% adhered to three, 10.3% adhered to four, and 2.8% of the sample adhered to all five health behaviors. There were other elements to the study, but the conclusion supported the central theme that adherence to more health behavior recommendations is more highly associated with successful aging than adherence to fewer health behaviors. They also suggest that it is not critical for all people to adhere to all of these behaviors, as there are multiple pathways to successful aging.[53]

Tobacco Use

Tobacco use remains the single largest preventable cause of death and disease in the United States. Cigarette smoking kills more than 480,000 Americans each year, with more than 41,000 of these deaths from exposure to secondhand smoke. In 2012, an estimated 18.1% (42.1 million) U.S. adults were current cigarette smokers. Of these, 78.4% (33.0 million) smoked every day, and 21.6% (9.1 million) smoked some days. Although the incidence of smoking is lower in older adults, the 65 years and older group represents 8.9% of the adult smoking population.[54]

Older adults who have smoked for a long time will often refuse to even consider quitting, arguing that "the damage has been done, so why quit now?" Smoking has become so much of a habit that many have no desire to quit or, having tried, find they are sad and depressed and thus resume smoking. This is more often the case when they try to quit cold turkey. Nicotine works as an antidepressant, and in its absence, addicted smokers suffer.

Smoking has many negative effects that can exacerbate already existing comorbidities in older adults. The two main components of tobacco smoke are tar and nicotine. The nicotine causes an increase in blood pressure and an increase in the incidence of arrhythmias. The myriad of chemicals in tar, many of which are known to cause cancer, are associated with an increase in damage to the arteries and malignancy. Information regarding smoking cessation programs designed to help older adults can be found at http://www.lung.org/stop-smoking/about-smoking/facts-figures/smoking-and-older-adults.html.

Alcohol Abuse

Alcohol abuse is another health-damaging behavior that is not uncommon in the elderly population. Loneliness, depression, and loss of a spouse are all contributing factors. If asked, many older adults will deny that they have a problem and may become defensive. Approaching alcohol use from a healthcare standpoint and not addressing drinking as a moral issue may be more productive. Adverse complications of excessive alcohol consumption that may affect the pulmonary system are pulmonary edema, esophageal varices, altered electrolyte levels, and decreased hemoglobin. Additionally, the immune system is weakened and malnutrition is more likely in alcoholics. Lack of medication compliance (under- or overdosing) is a dangerous

Respiratory Recap

- Healthy lifestyle choices or the avoidance of health-damaging behaviors may ultimately result in preserved functionality for an extended period of time.

consequence of alcohol consumption, and when drugs are taken with alcohol, the effects or side effects of the drugs may be altered, leading to disastrous results.

Physical Activity

Physical activity, although recommended for every age group, is of particular importance in older adults. Regular exercise can help prevent or delay the onset of chronic conditions and can improve endurance, strength, and flexibility, all of which decrease the incidence of falls. Lack of activity today is partly a result of social change in the past 50 years. Computers, television, remote controls, cars, and desk jobs have all had a part in engineering routine daily physical activity out of the lives of many. By age 75 years, few older adults engage in regular physical activity. Many health-related organizations have recommended walking programs for seniors as a means of increasing physical activity. It should be noted that previously sedentary older adults should consult with a physician prior to starting an exercise program. Once the go-ahead is given, recruiting friends to participate in activities may provide the support and encouragement needed to keep active. Many communities have senior centers or a local YMCA that may have specially designed programs for well elders.

Diet/Nutrition

The importance of nutrition in older adults cannot be overemphasized, in particular, older adults with COPD. It has been estimated that as many as 25% to 30% of patients with COPD are malnourished.[55] Malnutrition is not just a factor of being underweight; it also can be applied to individuals who are grossly overweight. In both cases, nutrition is poor. Being underweight with

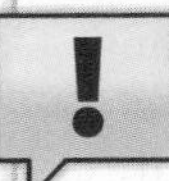

Respiratory Recap

- Older adults with COPD are advised to eat small, frequent meals with nutrient-dense foods that are easy to prepare.

COPD can make symptoms worse and further reduce the effectiveness of the immune system. Older adults with COPD are advised to eat small, frequent meals with nutrient-dense foods that are easy to prepare in the microwave. Nutritional supplements are also recommended, not to replace meals but rather as a supplement after or between meals to add calories.

Obesity

Obesity in older adults has risen dramatically in the past 20 years and is associated with functional decline, ill health, dependency, and a reduced quality of life. **Obesity** is defined as a body mass index (BMI) of greater than 30. Data from the 2007–2010 National Health and Nutrition Examination Survey indicated that about 35% of individuals over the age of 65 are obese, representing over 8 million adults between the ages of 65 and 74 and 5 million ages 75 and over[56] (**Figure 27-5**).

Respiratory Recap

- Obesity, which is defined as a body mass index (BMI) of greater than 30, is estimated to occur in about 35% of individuals over the age of 65, representing over 8 million adults between the ages of 65 and 74 and 5 million ages 75 and over.

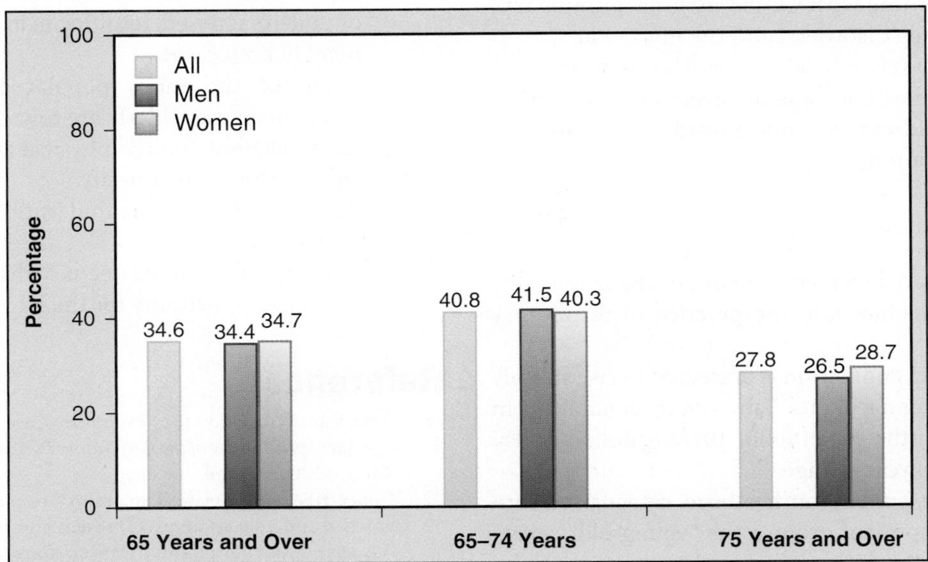

FIGURE 27-5 Prevalence of obesity among adults aged 65 and over, by age and sex, U.S. 2007–2010.

Reproduced from Fakhouri TH, Ogden CL, Carroll MD, et al. *Prevalence of obesity among older adults in the United States, 2007–2010*. NCHS data brief, no 106. Hyattsville, MD: National Center for Health Statistics. 2012.

Obesity in the elderly must be monitored to prevent major nutrient loss and worsening of existing comorbidities. Given the already marginal health status of many older adults, health-damaging behaviors will add to the incidence of exacerbations and frequency of hospitalizations and will be an increased drain on the already strained healthcare budget.

Preventive Services

Unfortunately, there is an underutilization of preventive services in the elderly population. Whether because of cost, transportation, or healthcare literacy, older adults do not always have access to the preventive screenings and educational interventions that would be useful. To find out which disease-specific screenings are currently recommended for older adults, search specific diseases at the CDC's website.

Role of the RT in Caring for the Elderly

Considering that 10,000 65-year-olds are entering the Medicare system on a daily basis and will continue to do so till at least 2029, a tremendous increase in the number of elderly will create a significant financial impact on the U.S. economy. Chronic and debilitating diseases (especially cardiorespiratory in nature) will plague the healthcare system. Couple this with the long-term projection for a significant decline in adult primary physicians and a regrettable disinterest on the part of medical school graduates to enter the specialty area of gerontology, a dearth of healthcare professionals to care and manage the growing elderly population will manifest and befall the U.S. healthcare system. Such factors will create opportunity for a physician extender, an RT trained to address the complexity of care for the older adult presenting with COPD, asthma, pulmonary hypertension, sleep disorders, and the myriad of cardiorespiratory-related conditions. The respiratory care profession must continue to develop its knowledge and skill set to address the unique needs of this growing elderly population.

Key Points

- Geriatrics is a vital component of the respiratory care curriculum and the practice of respiratory care.
- The elderly population is projected to rise sharply with the aging of the baby boom generation in 2011, with the potential of 10,000 adults per day turning 65 years of age.
- The aging population has been categorized into three component groups: the "young old" represented by the 65- to 74-year-olds; the "aged" who are 75 to 84; and the oldest old represented by those 85 and older.
- There has been a significant shift in the patterns of disease, and the leading causes of death among the elderly are now chronic in nature.
- Physical assessments in older adults may require more time, but they are extremely important as they uncover subtle but unique differences.
- A comprehensive geriatric assessment (CGA) is a multidimensional, interdisciplinary diagnostic process to determine the medical, psychological, and functional capabilities of a frail elderly person in order to develop a coordinated and integrated plan for treatment.
- Hand-grip strength may be a marker of frailty in the oldest-old.
- Two major reasons why symptoms in the elderly are not typical are (1) age-associated changes in the immune system and (2) normal age-related change in various organs.
- Depression is the most commonly occurring mental health problem in older adults.
- Although the elderly make up (on average) about 13% of the total U.S. population, they consume 33% of prescription drugs and 25% of all over-the-counter drugs.
- Medication safety is a serious medical problem and presents unique challenges in the elderly population.
- Adverse drug reactions in the elderly are highly preventable, and in most cases safe alternative medications are generally available.
- Drug expenditures have risen exponentially in the past few years, for example, a fourfold increase for some antiasthmatic medications.
- Communication can be particularly challenging with older adults, and expressing empathy can be a useful tactic.
- Elderly patients with asthma are often misdiagnosed or underdiagnosed, resulting in inappropriate treatment in both cases.
- Some of the more popular health-damaging behaviors in the elderly are tobacco use, excessive use of alcohol, limited physical activity, poor diet and nutrition, and obesity.
- Preventive services are underutilized in the elderly population.
- Caring for the unique needs of the elderly provides a unique opportunity for the RT.

References

1. American Association for Respiratory Care. *Position Statement, Age Appropriate Care of the Respiratory Patient.* Irving, TX: AARC. Revised 2005, Retired.
2. Douce HF, et al. A critical analysis of respiratory care scope of practice and education: past, present and future. In: American Association for Respiratory Care. *Delineating the Educational Direction for the Future Respiratory Care Practitioners: Proceedings of a National Consensus Conference on Respiratory Care Education.* Dallas, TX: AARC; 1992.

3. American Association for Respiratory Care. *An Action Agenda: Proceedings of the Second National Consensus Conference on Respiratory Care Education*. Dallas, TX: Author; 1993.
4. Kacmarek RM, Durbin CG, Barnes TA, et al. Creating a vision for respiratory care in 2015 and beyond. *Respir Care.* 2009;54(3): 375–389.
5. Dyer C. The interaction of ageing and lung disease. *Chron Respir Dis*. 2012;9:63–67.
6. Petty TL, Seebass JS, eds. *Pulmonary Disorders of the Elderly*. Philadelphia: American College of Physicians; 2007.
7. Centers for Disease Control and Prevention. *The State of Aging and Health in America 2013*. Atlanta, GA: Centers for Disease Control and Prevention, U.S. Department of Health and Human Services; 2013.
8. National Center for Health Statistics. Table 26. In *Health Status and Determinants, United States, 2008*. Available at: http://www.cdc.gov/nchs/data/hus/hus08.pdf#listtables. Accessed August 5, 2014.
9. U.S. Bureau of the Census. *Current Population Reports, Special Studies, P23-190, 65+ in the United States*. Washington, DC: U.S. Government Printing Office. Available at: https://www.census.gov/prod/1/pop/p23-190/p23-190.pdf. Accessed August 5, 2014.
10. Lam D, Leibbrandt M. *Global Demographic Trends and their Implications for Employment: Background Research Paper*. Submitted to the High Level Panel on the Post-2015 Development Agenda, May 2013. Available at: http://www.post2015hlp.org/wp-content/uploads/2013/05/Lam-Leibbrandt_Global-Demographic-Trends-and-their-Implications-for-Employment.pdf. Accessed August 5, 2014.
11. Schneider MJ. *Introduction to Public Health*. 3rd ed. Sudbury, MA: Jones and Bartlett; 2011.
12. Department of Health and Human Services, Administration on Aging. *Projected Future Growth of the Older Population.* Available at: http://www.aoa.gov/Aging_Statistics/future_growth/future_growth.aspx#age. Accessed August 5, 2014.
13. Centers for Disease Control and Prevention. Healthy aging: helping people to live long and productive lives and enjoy a good quality of life. 2011. Available at: http://www.cdc.gov/chronicdisease/resources/publications/aag/aging.htm. Accessed August 5, 2014.
14. Federal Interagency Forum on Aging-Related Statistics. *Older Americans 2012: Key Indicators of Well-Being.* Washington, DC: U.S. Government Printing Office; June 2012. Available at: http://www.agingstats.gov/Main_Site/Data/2012_Documents/docs/EntireChartbook.pdf. Accessed August 5, 2014.
15. U.S. Department of Commerce. *Women in America: Indicators of Economic and Social Well-Being*. March 2011. Available at: http://www.esa.doc.gov/sites/default/files/reports/documents/womeninamerica.pdf. Accessed August 5, 2014.
16. U.S. Census Bureau. *2010 Census Special Report, Centenarians: 2010*. C2010 SR-03. Washington, DC: US Government Printing Office; 2012.
17. Brandon E. What people who live to be 100 have in common. *U.S. News & World Report*. January 7, 2013. Available at: http://money.usnews.com/money/retirement/articles/2013/01/07/what-people-who-live-to-100-have-in-common?page=2. Accessed August 5, 2014.
18. Arias E. Percentage of persons surviving by age, 1900–1902, 1949–1951, and 2006. *Natl Vital Stat Rep*. 2010;58(21):5. Available at: http://www.cdc.gov/nchs/data/nvsr/nvsr58/nvsr58_21.pdf. Accessed August 5, 2014.
19. Doherty TJ. Aging and sarcopenia. *J Appl Physiol*. 2003; 95:1717–1727.
20. Beers MH, Jones TV, eds. *The Merck Manual of Geriatrics* [Online]. 3rd ed. Available at: http://www.merck.com/mkgr/mmg/home.jsp. Accessed August 5, 2014.
21. Finesilver C. Pulmonary assessment: what you need to know. *Prog Cardiovasc Nursing*. 2003;18:83–92.
22. Sebastian JL, Pfeifer KJ. Cardiac disorders. In: Duthie EH, Katz PR, Malone ML, eds. *Practice of Geriatrics*. 4th ed. Philadelphia: Saunders-Elsevier; 2007.
23. Harris SN. Anesthetic considerations for geriatric surgery. In: Rosenthal RA, Zenilman ME, Katlic MR, eds. *Principles and Practices of Geriatric Surgery*. New York: Springer-Verlag; 2000.
24. Normal DC. Fever in the elderly. *Clin Infect Dis*. 2000;31:148–151.
25. Warren MW. Care of the chronic aged sick. *Lancet*. 1946; i:841-843.
26. Ellis G, Whitehead MA, O'Neill D, et al. Comprehensive geriatric assessment for older adults admitted to hospital. *Cochrane Database Syst Rev.* 2011, Issue 7.
27. Bergman H, Ferrucci L, Guralnik J, et al. Frailty: an emerging research and clinical paradigm—issues and controversies. *J Gerontol Med Sci.* 2007;62A:731–737.
28. Sternberg SA, Wershof Schwartz A, Karunananthan S, et al. The identification of frailty: a systematic review. *Am Geriatric Soc.* 2011;59:2129–2138.
29. Amella EJ. Presentation of illness in older adults: if you think you know what you're looking for, think again. *Am J Nursing*. 2004;104: 40–51.
30. Malin A. Pneumonia in old age. *Chron Respir Dis.* 2011;8:207–210.
31. McSweeney JC, Cody M, O'Sullivan P, et al. Women's early warning symptoms of acute myocardial infarction. *Circulation.* 2003;108:2619–2623.
32. Woon VC, Lim KH. Acute myocardial infarction in the elderly—the differences compared with the young. *Singapore Med*. 2003;44: 414–418.
33. Alfredo R, Manuel B, Vicente B, et al. Management and risk factors for mortality in very elderly patients with acute myocardial infarction. *Geriatr Gerontol Int*. 2013;13:146–151.
34. Emmett KR. Nonspecific and atypical presentation of disease in the older patient. *Geriatrics*. 1998;53:50–52, 58–60.
35. Chmura K, Chan ED. Tuberculosis in the elderly: keep a high index of suspicion. *J Respir Dis*. 2006;27:307–315.
36. Gu Q, Dillon CF, Burt VL. *Prescription drug use continues to increase: U.S. prescription drug data for 2007–2008*. NCHS data brief, no 42. Hyattsville, MD: National Center for Health Statistics. 2010.
37. Kohn LT, Corrigan J, Donaldson MS. *To Err Is Human: Building a Safer Health System*. Washington, DC: National Academy Press; 2000.
38. Nebeker JR, Barach P, Samore MH. Clarifying adverse drug events: a clinician's guide to terminology, documentation, and reporting. *Ann Intern Med*. 2004;140:795–801.
39. Campanelli CM. American geriatrics society updated Beers criteria for potentially inappropriate medication use in older adults: the American Geriatrics Society 2012 Beers Criteria Update Panel. *J Am Geriatr Soc*. 2012:60:616–631.
40. Sloane PD, Gruber-Baldini AL, Zimmerman S, et al. Medication undertreatment in assisted living settings. *Arch Intern Med.* 2004;164:2031–2037.
41. U.S. Food and Drug Administration. *Drug Applications for Over-the-Counter (OTC) Drugs*. 2012. Available at: http://www.fda.gov/drugs/developmentapprovalprocess/howdrugsaredevelopedandapproved/approvalapplications/over-the-counterdrugs/default.htm. Accessed May 30, 2014.
42. Thorpe JM, Kennelty KA. Potentially inappropriate medication use in community-dwelling dementia patients and their informal caregivers. *Gerontologist.* 2009;49:500.
43. Chui MA, Stone JA, Thorpe JM, Martin BA. Work system barriers to providing safe over-the-counter (OTC) medication recommendations for older adults. In: *Proceedings of the Human Factors and Ergonomics Society Annual Meeting*. 2013:57:1098.
44. Chiu S, Guo JJ, Lin AC, et al. Utilization, spending, and price trends for short- and long-acting beta-agonists and inhaled corticosteroids in the Medicaid Program, 1991–2010. *Am Health Drug Health.* 2011;4:140–149.
45. Gellad WF. Variation in drug prices at pharmacies: are prices higher in poorer areas? *Health Services Res*. 2008;44(2 Pt. 1):606–617.

Available at: http://www.ncbi.nlm.nih.gov/pmc/articles/PMC2677057/. Accessed August 5, 2014.

46. Alzheimer's Association. *Communication Tips for Caregivers*. Available at: http://www.alz.org/care/dementia-communication-tips.asp. Accessed August 5, 2014.

47. Akinbami LJ, Liu X. *Chronic Obstructive Pulmonary Disease Among Adults Aged 18 and Over in the United States, 1998–2009*. NCHS data brief, no 63. Hyattsville, MD: National Center for Health Statistics; 2011. Available at: http://www.cdc.gov/nchs/data/databriefs/db63.htm. Accessed August 5, 2014.

48. Global Initiative for Asthma. *Diagnosis of Diseases of Chronic Airflow Limitation: Asthma COPD and Asthma-COPD Overlap Syndrome (ACOS)*. 2014. Available at: http://www.goldcopd.org/uploads/users/files/AsthmaCOPDOverlap.pdf. Accessed August 5, 2014.

49. Sadowska AN. N-Acetylcysteine mucolysis in the management of chronic obstructive pulmonary disease. *Ther Adv Respir Dis*. 2012;6:127–135.

50. Baptist AP, Deol BB, Reddy RC, et al. Age-specific factors influencing asthma management by older adults. *Qual Health Res*. 2010;20:117–124.

51. Myer KC. Management of interstitial lung disease in elderly patients. *Curr Opin Pulm Med*. 2012;18:483–492.

52. Gresh LH, Weinberg RE. *The Science of Supervillains*. Hoboken, NJ: Wiley; 2005:120–121.

53. Pruchno R, Wilson-Genderson M. Adherence to clusters of health behaviors and successful aging. *J Aging Health*. 2012;24:1279–1297.

54. Centers for Disease Control and Prevention. Current cigarette smoking among adults—United States, 2005–2012. *Morbid Mortal Wkly Rep*. 2014;63:29–34.

55. Rennard SI. Patient information: chronic obstructive pulmonary disease (COPD) treatments. Last updated June 2, 2014. *UpToDate*. Available at: http://www.uptodate.com/contents/chronic-obstructive-pulmonary-disease-copd-treatments-beyond-the-basics. Accessed August 5, 2014.

56. Fakhuri THI, Ogden CL, Carroll MD, et al. Prevalence of obesity among adults aged 65 and over. Centers for Disease Control. *NCHS Data Brief*. 2012:No. 106. Available at: http://www.cdc.gov/nchs/data/databriefs/db106.pdf. Accessed August 5, 2014.

APPENDIX 27-1 RESOURCES FOR SCREENING TESTS IN THE ELDERLY

Test	Website
Hearing Handicap Inventory for the Elderly (HHIE)	http://www.audiologyonline.com
Mini-Nutritional Assessment (MNA)	http://www.mna-elderly.com/mna_forms.html
Functional Assessment Staging (FAST)	http://www.ec-online.net/Knowledge/articles/alzstages.html

The following instruments can be accessed on the University of Iowa's Geriatric Education website (http://www.medicine.uiowa.edu/igec/tools/default.asp):

- Snellen eye test (visual acuity)
- Whispered voice test (hearing loss)
- Nutritional health assessment
- Clock-drawing test
- Geriatric Depression Scale (GDS)
- Mini-Mental Status Exam (MMSE)
- Activities of daily living (ADL)
- Instrumental activities of daily living (IADL)
- Caregiver Burden Interview

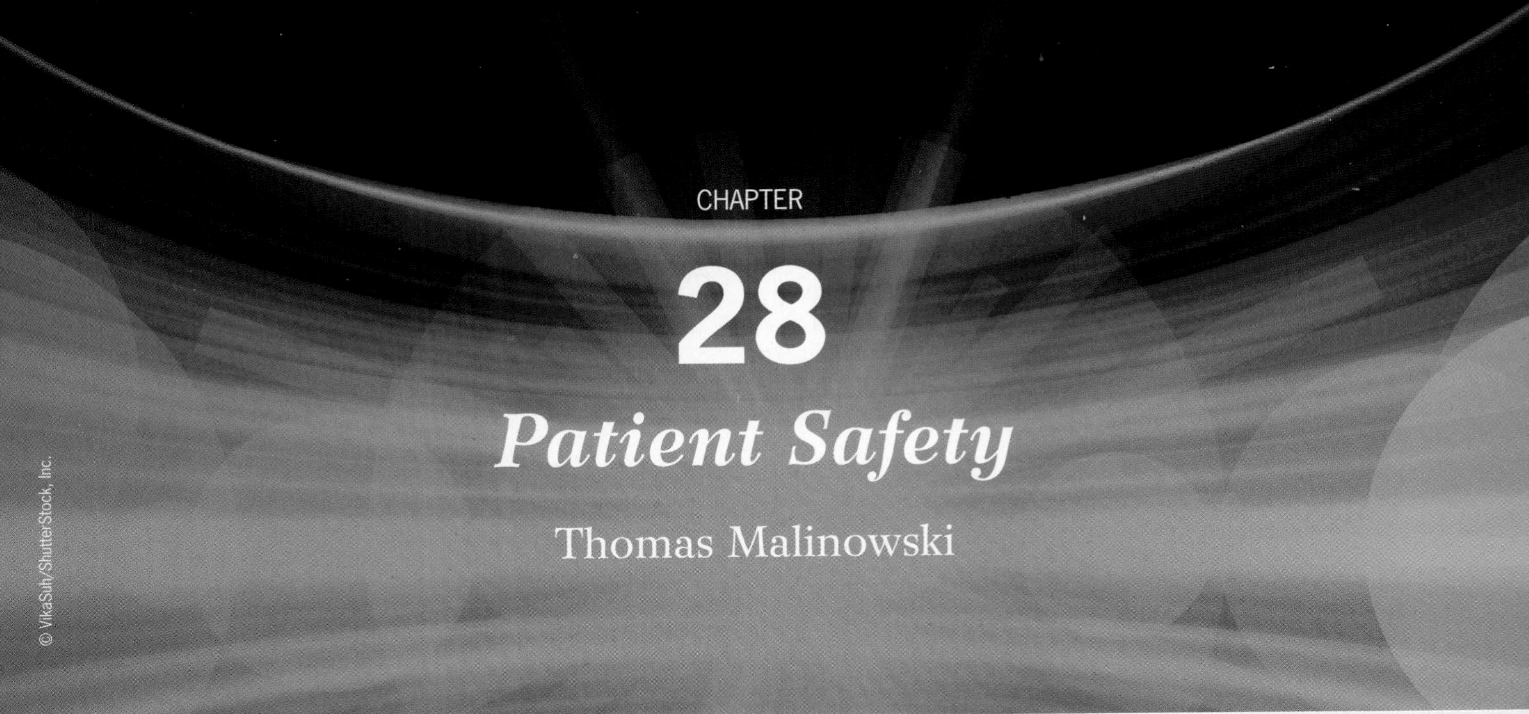

CHAPTER

28

Patient Safety

Thomas Malinowski

OUTLINE

OBJECTIVES

1. Explain the concept and characteristics of high-reliability organizations.
2. Explain the term culture of safety as it applies to the issues of high risk/high reliability, safe harbor, teamwork, and commitment.
3. Define the concept of robust process improvement and identify the tools that are incorporated within the concept.
4. Define root cause analysis and explain its relationship to active and latent errors.
5. Describe the purpose and process of filing an incident report.
6. Identify and provide examples of the Joint Commission's 2014 National Patient Safety Goals as they apply to respiratory care.
7. Explain the role, purpose, and composition of rapid response teams.
8. Describe the role of the respiratory therapist in safe medication practice.
9. Explain how shift report, patient handoffs, and alarm fatigue pose potential safety consequences to the patient.
10. Explain Universal Protocol and its application to respiratory care.
11. Identify the specific conditions that comprise healthcare-associated infections and magnitude of ventilator-associated events.
12. Describe the impact of respiratory protocols on patient safety.
13. Describe the rationale for documenting respiratory care activities.
14. List the elements of a patient medical record.
15. Identify medical record documentation standards.
16. List respiratory care information commonly recorded in the medical record.
17. Describe a properly transcribed verbal order.
18. Describe the rationale for the electronic medical or health record.
19. Explain the legal implications of the medical record.
20. Explain the concept of patient confidentiality.

KEY TERMS

active error
alarm fatigue
confidentiality
culture of safety
electronic health record (EHR)
electronic medical record (EMR)
electronic signature
handoff
healthcare-associated infection (HAIs)
Health Insurance Portability and Accountability Act (HIPAA)
high-reliability organization (HROs)
incident report
I-PASS
latent error
medical record
medication reconciliation
National Patient Safety Goals
rapid response team
robust process improvement (RPI)
root cause analysis (RCA)
safe harbor
situation, background, assessment, recommendation (SBAR)
sentinel event
Universal Protocol
ventilator-associated events (VAE)
ventilator-associated pneumonia (VAP)

Introduction

Patient safety issues have gained increased attention and importance in recent years. Regrettably, numerous documented examples of unsafe practices and patient harm have resulted in reports and directives from the National Institutes of Health, the Joint Commission, and other organizations.

This chapter provides a detailed account of patient safety as these concepts apply to the practice of respiratory care. It specifically addresses the rationale and standards of patient safety issues, including high-reliability organizations, the creation of a culture of safety, robust process improvement, and **incident reporting**. Additionally, safety initiatives related to the practice of respiratory care are addressed, including the role of monitoring, rapid response teams, safe medication practices, handoffs, discharge education and planning, and healthcare-associated infections. It concludes by addressing the importance of the **medical record** and the respiratory therapist's responsibility for charting and documentation.

Patient Safety

Medical errors have been implicated in the premature deaths of 98,000 patients per year, accounting for between $17 billion and $29 billion in costs annually.[1] Millions of people suffer from medication errors, associated infections, and other adverse effects of care. Errors often transpire during the transition of responsibility from one healthcare provider to another.[2] Respiratory therapists play an essential role in preventing or reducing errors and improving overall healthcare quality. Learning and practicing safe respiratory care is therefore extremely important for all respiratory therapists. A clinician's decision to practice safe care is a choice and is influenced by the present circumstance or situation as well as knowledge, skills, and previous experiences.

High-Reliability Organizations

The concept of a **culture of safety** originated outside healthcare, in what are described as **high-reliability organizations (HROs)**—organizations that consistently minimize adverse events despite carrying out intrinsically complex and hazardous work (e.g., commercial airlines, nuclear power generating plants, aircraft carriers). HROs adjust quickly to changing situations and are adept at building safeguards against failure of high-risk processes and solutions for possible failures. Hospitals and departments are attempting to adapt and apply the principles and characteristics of HROs,[3] but the change has been difficult because the situations and circumstances encountered in health care are more variable than in other industries. Five characteristics consistent within HROs are their preoccupation with failure, reluctance to simplify interpretations, sensitivity to operations, commitment to resilience, deference to expertise.[4] **Table 28-1** lists the characteristics of HROs and briefly describes each of them.

TABLE 28-1
Characteristics of Highly Reliable Organizations (HROs)

Characteristic	Description
Preoccupation with failure	HROs do not focus on broadcasting successes; in fact, they continually look for failures or problems and implement ways to resolve them. They realize there are always areas to improve, and they relentlessly seek out these difficulties.
Reluctance to simplify interpretations	HROs recognize the complexity of the issues being dealt with, and do not oversimplify. They seek out differences in perspectives and avoid the pitfalls of groupthink.
Sensitivity to operations	HROs focus on unexpected events and latent failures, a term that describes loopholes in safeguards or a system's defenses. Latent failures are often only identified after a safety event has occurred. Latent failures are often attributable to training, process, or management deficiencies.
Commitment to resilience	HROs know that any operation is not perfect, but respond to errors without overreacting or becoming paralyzed or disabled.
Deference to expertise	Diversity brings different perspectives, which helps identify complexity and consequently aids problem solving. Problem identification and solution move to those individuals most familiar and expert and are not dependent on hierarchy or rank.

Adapted from Weick KE, Sutcliffe KM. *Managing the Unexpected: Assuring High Performance in an Age of Complexity.* San Francisco: Jossey-Bass. 2001:10–17.

Culture of Safety

In 2009 the Joint Commission began to require healthcare leaders to create and maintain a culture of safety.[5] Many hospitals now assess the safety culture by conducting staff and physician surveys. Unfortunately, many facilities have not yet moved to the next phase of taking actions that propagate a culture of safety. A purposeful and appropriate goal for any provider or department is to continually strive to achieve a highly reliable level of safety practice and to help others achieve the same goal. Organizations that embrace this safety philosophy create a culture of safety. Safe cultures are relentless in their pursuit of fewer errors and critical events. They also are realistic about the complexity of the work environment and the inevitability of the occurrence of errors.

Respiratory Recap

Medical Errors

- Medical errors have been implicated in the premature deaths of 98,000 patients per year, accounting for between $17 billion and $29 billion in costs annually.

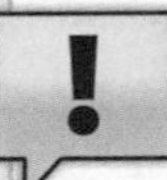

Respiratory Recap

Culture of Safety

- Health care is complex and variable, and safety-related issues are a frequent occurrence.
- Healthcare workers should feel comfortable addressing and escalating safety issues.
- All members of the healthcare team need to work together, at all times, to safely provide care.
- Organizations (departments, institutions, professional associations) need to relentlessly advocate and work to address patient safety.

They recognize that many problems are process oriented and work to resolve those issues.

The following characteristics are commonly seen in highly engaged safety cultures and serve as a foundation for establishing a safety-focused culture within a respiratory department:

- Recognition of the high-risk nature of an organization's activities and the determination to achieve consistently safe operations (high risk/high reliability)
- An environment in which individuals are able to report errors or near misses without fear of reprimand or punishment (**safe harbor**)
- Collaboration within and between disciplines to seek solutions to patient safety problems (teamwork)
- Organizational commitment to addressing safety issues (commitment)

High Risk/High Reliability

Respiratory care by its very nature requires operation in high-risk environments (e.g., transport, rapid response teams, resuscitation, emergency care, trauma) as well as areas of lower urgency. Our actions and behaviors in these environments often determine the success of the outcome. Practitioners need to be continually diligent, for errors and mistakes can occur with the most basic and simplistic tasks (e.g., connecting a cannula to an air flow meter in lieu of an oxygen flow meter for a newly admitted patient in a dark room at 3:00 a.m.) as well as the more critical tasks, such as initiating inhaled nitric oxide for the first time in 5 months. Safe cultures initiate process improvements that reduce the probability of error. In the night-shift nasal cannula example, two practitioners (a respiratory therapist and registered nurse) might be used to verify the proper connection of oxygen, or a lights on for safety policy might be used for all night admissions. For those low frequency–high risk procedures (e.g., application of nitric oxide or inhaled prostacyclin), mock drills conducted every 4 to 6 weeks would help maintain skill sets and confidence.

Safe Harbor

A culture of blame can impair the advancement of a culture of safety. Hospitals often underreport or fail to respond to the safety events that occur because healthcare providers feel uncomfortable or intimidated for escalating the observed safety issues. Some circumstances are a result of individual accountability, but more often safety events occur as a result of breakdown in processes. Practitioners should be rewarded for good catches, that is, identification of situations or events that could have been a problem. Staff should be encouraged to describe problems that they have observed and should be solicited for solutions. In addition, these problems should be highlighted to all staff, through methods such as bulletin boards and start-of-shift huddles.

This is not to say that practitioners are not responsible for their actions. When organizations focus on identifying and understanding the causes of unsafe behavior and simultaneously hold individuals accountable for reckless behavior, they develop a just culture. In a just culture, the response to an error or near miss is predicated on the type of behavior associated with the error, not the severity of the event. For example, reckless behavior such as refusing to perform a duplicate patient ID check prior to performing an arterial blood gas assessment or assisting with a bronchoscopy would merit punitive action, even if no patients were harmed.

When healthcare workers are exposed to intimidating behavior there is a reduction in the frequency of reporting of safety issues. The Institute of Safe Medical Practices conducted surveys in 2004 and 2013 of over 6200 healthcare workers and has identified the extent that disrespectful and intimidating behavior exists in health care.[6,7] The most commonly encountered intimidating behaviors are not verbal outbursts or rants, but are more subtle, such as the use of condescending language, impatience during discussion, or failure to respond to phone calls or pages. Physicians are not the sole providers of intimidating behaviors; these traits are reported across disciplines and teams as well. Staff will often develop solutions to avoid confrontations with intimidating providers, including asking other healthcare workers to clarify medication orders or help order interpretation to avoid contacting the culprit. All of these alternative work-arounds suppress safe practice and perpetuate unsafe conditions.

Teamwork

Safe healthcare requires highly trained individuals with differing perspectives to act together for the common interest of the patient. Communication barriers across hierarchies, failure to acknowledge human fallibility, and lack of situational awareness combine to cause poor teamwork and can lead to clinical adverse events.

Highly integrated teams minimize rank and position and deliberately encourage all members to contribute, regardless of title. In HROs this consistent structured team behavior is focused on safety and standardized operations and includes checklists and other tools to provide consistent behavior. This structured team behavior is known as crew resource management (CRM).[3]

Teamwork training is intended to minimize the potential for error by training each team member to respond appropriately in acute situations. Teamwork training focuses on respect, responsibility, and communication. It is intended to enhance cohesion among team members and to create an atmosphere in which all personnel feel comfortable speaking up when they suspect a problem. Highly integrated teams have been shown to improve the staff's perception of safety and to significantly improve safety processes.[8]

Team members are trained to crosscheck each other's actions, offer assistance when needed, and address errors in a nonjudgmental fashion. Debriefing and providing feedback, particularly after critical incidents, are important parts of teamwork training.

Respiratory care departments can apply the principles of teamwork training in multiple areas of clinical training and practice. Applications include all aspects of departmental orientation, start-of-shift safety huddles, transport teams, rapid response teams, and **handoffs** or transfer of care to other providers. Many departments are using more structured handoff methods such as SBAR (situation, background, assessment, recommendation) or I-PASS (illness, patient summary, action list, situation awareness and contingency, synthesis by receiver) to standardize the report process.

Commitment

Fundamentally, in order to improve the safety culture, the underlying problem areas must be identified and solutions constructed to target each specific problem. Although many organizations assess safety culture at the institutional level (commonly by employee or physician surveys), significant variations in safety culture may exist within an organization. For example, the perception of a culture of safety may be high in one unit within a hospital and low in another unit, or high among senior leadership and low among frontline workers. These variations likely contribute to the mixed record of interventions intended to improve safety climate and reduce errors.

There is an increasing interest to apply lessons learned by HROs to the medical community. Many of these lessons are intended to prevent communication breakdowns, a frequent source of errors and mistakes. **Table 28-2** lists examples of commonly applied tools and techniques used within the aviation industry, a HRO, and how those would apply to a respiratory care application.

TABLE 28-2
HRO Tools and Techniques Used Within Airline Industry and Corollaries to Respiratory Care Profession

Aviation Application	Respiratory Care Application
Briefings	Shift Huddles. Start-of-shift, contact by RC supervisor with MSET team leader as to anticipated high risk patients. Avoidance of one-way dialogue.
Checklist	Pre-procedural list of key must-haves prior to transport, bronchoscopy, high-risk delivery, etc.
Cross-Checks	Two person check-off for more complex or low frequency/high risk procedures (e.g., continuous bronchodilator infusion pump, aerosolized prostacyclin, NIV in the operating room)
Sterile Cockpit	Zero interruptions during critical procedures (two patient identifiers, drawing up medications)
Read back	Repeating back of verbal order or directive with acknowledgment
Challenge rules	Time out by anyone regardless of position within the procedural area if they are unsure or unclear of directive or request
Environmental Human Factors	Design and placement of monitors and displays to reduce fatigue, ambiguity, false alarms
Industry Learning	System-wide process to share information on mistakes and opportunities with limited liability

Adapted from Ornato JP, Peberdy MA. Applying lessons from commercial aviation safety and operations to resuscitation. *Resuscitation.* 2014;85:173–176.

Robust Process Improvement

Robust process improvement (RPI) is a method proposed by the Joint Commission to help address the low reliability and safety issues facing health care.[9] RPI represents the next generation in process improvement beyond the standard PDCA (plan, do, check, act) model that has been used during the previous decades. RPI incorporates three sets of process improvement tools; Lean, Six Sigma, and Change Management, in attempts to improve safety processes.[10] Combined, the processes provide a more systematic attention to finding the true cause of process failures. These approaches identify specific causes, measure prevalence, and direct methods and efforts to eliminate the true causes of many failures. Often in the past the tendencies have been to try and simplify the issues, and this has led to failures of process improvement solutions. RPI has directly resulted in improvements in projects including hand hygiene, handoff communication, and wrong site surgery at sites where applied.[11]

Root Cause Analysis

Root cause analysis (RCA) is a structured method used to identify underlying problem issues or analyze serious adverse events. The process was initially developed to help analyze industrial accidents but now is widely used in healthcare to analyze errors. RCA is used to get to the source of a problem. RCA can identify both **active errors** (errors occurring when practitioners apply processes) and **latent errors** (the hidden problems that increase the probability of error). The reason to use RCA is to prevent future harm by eliminating the active and latent errors that frequently are the cause of adverse events. The Joint Commission has mandated use of RCA to analyze **sentinel events.**[12]

RCAs generally follow a protocol that begins with data collection and reconstruction of the event in question through record review and participant interviews. A multidisciplinary team is often assembled to analyze the sequence of events leading to the error, with the goals of identifying how the event occurred (through identification of active errors) and why the event occurred (through systematic identification and analysis of latent errors). **Table 28-3** describes examples of latent errors in respiratory care.

TABLE 28-3
Examples of Latent Error Factors in Respiratory Care

Type of Factor	Example
Organizational/ Management	A respiratory student detects a medication error, but the preceptor therapist discourages the student from reporting it.
Work environment	Lacking appropriate gas storage space, medical gases are kept in the same storage location as nonmedical gas. A gas cylinder of acetylene was found mixed in the heliox gas cylinders transferred to an ICU location.
Team environment	A physician insists on continuing with a bronchoscopy even though the consent form has not been completed. The patient has already received sedation and the physician does not want to reschedule the procedure.
Staffing	A department has three sick calls for the shift, and no additional staff members are available to call in. A therapist makes a decision to triage care without having assessed a patient, and the patient has a history of severe COPD.
Task related	A respiratory therapist fails to follow proper procedure and complete the transport checklist prior to departing with a ventilator patient to MRI. The patient self-extubates during transfer in the imaging room, and no resuscitator mask is available to bag the patient prior to intubation.
Patient characteristics	An elderly patient with COPD fails to follow proper directions and is taking his long-acting beta-adrenergic inhaler six times a day.

Incident Reports

Incident reports, sometimes called safety reports, become an important way for associates to escalate safe care and describe the specific details of an undesirable event. When an untoward event occurs, an incident report may be filed to initiate tracking of the event. For example, an incident report should be completed when a patient receives an incorrect medication or when a patient accidentally falls when getting out of bed. The individual who observes or discovers the incident should begin the documentation process. An occurrence report may include specifics such as patient name and identification number; date, time, and description of the incident; the immediate action taken; and the signature of the reporting employee and additional individuals involved in the incident.

A supervisor should always be notified when an untoward incident is observed, and the written reporting procedure should address how and to whom incident reports should be routed. The process includes an evaluation of the incident and follow-up action. Some state laws protect incident reports from discovery in litigation and address the state's protection of the report if it is qualified or limited in any way. Access to patient-identifiable incident report information is limited to designated individuals.

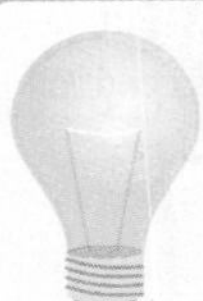

STOP AND THINK

What is a scenario in which an incident report would be required?

Safety Initiatives and Respiratory Care Applications

Over the last decade, the Joint Commission has described a series of safety initiatives that, if fully implemented, would profoundly improve the quality of patient care. These initiatives are periodically updated to include new areas of focus. The **National Patient**

TABLE 28-4
2014 National Patient Safety Goals as Applied to Respiratory Services

National Patient Safety Goal	Practical Respiratory Therapy Examples
Identify Patients Correctly	• Use 2 patient identifiers before initiating care (ask patient name, check patient ID band)
Improve Staff Communication	• Use I-PASS or SBAR with collaborative communication, read back of orders
Use Medications Safely	• Pharmacy review of all orders • Aerosol compatibility charts for staff to access
Use Alarms Safely	• Establish pulse oximetry thresholds to minimize clinically irrelevant alarms.
Prevent Infections	• Hand hygiene surveillance • Monitor ventilator settings to identify ventilator-associated events
Identify Patient Safety Risks	• Revisit high-risk/low-frequency procedures multiple times during year to maintain skills • Develop skin breakdown monitoring process for high-risk patients (e.g., NIV mask, nasal cannulas behind ears, nasal CPAP in infants)

Information from The Joint Commission. 2014 National Patient Safety Goals Hospital Program. Available at: http://www.jointcommission.org/standards_information/npsgs.aspx. Accessed August 1, 2014.

Safety Goals are monitored by the Joint Commission when performing surveys of care.[13] **Table 28-4** lists the Joint Commission's National Patient Safety Goals for 2014 and provides examples of respiratory therapy applications. The following subsections provide more information on specific applications for some previously identified goals, including rapid response teams; medication safety; communication and handoffs; discharge education and planning; and healthcare-associated infections.

Rapid Response Teams

Rapid response teams (sometimes known as emergency response or medical safety emergency teams) are designed to intervene during the critical pre-arrest period when patients often demonstrate clinical warning signs of pending demise. When summoned to the bedside, the rapid response team immediately assesses and treats the patient with the goal of preventing intensive care unit transfer, cardiac arrest, or death. At some hospitals, patients or family members are encouraged to activate the team response when certain clinical signs or symptoms are present. Rapid response teams were identified in 2008 and 2009 as a Joint Commission National Patient Safety Goal. Team composition varies from institution to institution but often includes a respiratory therapist, a critical care nurse, and occasionally a house physician. The respiratory therapist is extraordinarily valuable to the rapid response team. **Table 28-5** describes model criteria for the composition and activation of a rapid response team.

Patient safety is enhanced when the respiratory therapist anticipates which patients may be at higher risk for complications and takes steps to prevent decompensation from occurring. The postoperative patient population is particularly at risk for life-threatening respiratory complications, often as a result of IV analgesic use during postoperative care. The incidence of respiratory complications from postoperative anesthetic complications in academic institutions has been reported at two events per 1000 anesthetic administrations.[14] Considering the number of surgical events, the respiratory therapist will most likely encounter a postoperative complication from analgesics. The first 12 to 24 hours provide the highest risk for activation of the rapid response team for these types of events.[14,15]

TABLE 28-5
Typical Rapid Response Staffing Model and Activation Criteria

Model	Personnel	Duties
Rapid Response Team	Critical care nurse, respiratory therapist, and physician (critical care specialist) backup	• Respond to emergencies • Follow up on patients discharged from the ICU • Proactively evaluate high-risk ward patients • Educate and act as liaison toward staff
Any staff member may call the team if one of the following criteria is met: • Heart rate over 140 beats/min or less than 40 beats/min • Respiratory rate over 28 breaths/min or less than 8 breaths/min • Systolic blood pressure greater than 180 mm Hg or less than 90 mm Hg • Oxygen saturation less than 89% despite oxygen supplementation • Acute change in mental status • Urine output less than 50 mL over 4 hours • Staff member has significant concern about the patient's condition • Chest pain unrelieved by nitroglycerin • Airway patency • Seizure • Symptoms of stroke		

Preoperative opioid use, heart disease, hemodynamic instability, and obstructive sleep apnea risk are all associated with a higher risk of postoperative complications requiring rapid response team activation. In addition, patients recently transferred out of the intensive care unit are more likely to experience respiratory or hemodynamic compromise within 24 hours of discharge requiring activation of the rapid response team.

In spite of the absence of clear outcomes benefit (mortality, length of stay), most hospitals have continued to apply the rapid response team and incorporate it into their daily clinical response models.

Safe Medication Practices

When patients are admitted for exacerbation of their conditions, they may receive new medications or use aerosol delivery methods different from their preexisting home medications. As a result, the new medication regimen prescribed at the time of discharge may inadvertently omit needed medications that patients have been receiving for some time.

Such unintended inconsistencies in medication regimens may occur at any point of transition in care (e.g., transfer from an intensive care unit to a general ward), not just at hospital admission or discharge. More than 50% of patients discharged have an unintended medication discrepancy.[16] **Medication reconciliation** is reviewing the patient's complete medication regimen at the time of admission, transfer, and discharge and comparing it with the regimen being considered for the new setting of care.

Safe medication use is a 2014 National Patient Safety Goal by the Joint Commission across the continuum of care. Respiratory therapists most commonly deal with reconciliation issues on a patient's admission to the facility or during discharge education. It is important that the medications and delivery systems explained to the patient be the same that the patient will receive on discharge.

Reports and Handoffs

Patients are inevitably cared for by different providers during their hospitalization. Respiratory therapists and nurses may change shifts every 8 to 12 hours, and physicians (particularly hospitalists) typically change service coverage as well. These shift changes create opportunities for error when clinical information is not accurately transferred between providers.

A handoff, or transition in a patient's care from one provider to another, involves the transfer of information, primary responsibility, and authority between providers. In hospitals, handoffs take place in multiple activities and locations, such as on admission, during shift and unit changes, before and after procedures, and at discharge. A hospital with 400 bed occupancy will probably experience between 1 million and 1.4 million handoffs a year.

Communication problems cause almost 70% of sentinel events in accredited healthcare organizations,

Respiratory Recap

Handoffs

- Transitions in care from one provider to another
- Involve the transfer of information, primary responsibility, and authority between providers

and between 50% and 80% of communication breakdowns take place during handoffs.[17] Care handoff has been identified by the World Health Organization and the Joint Commission as a risk factor associated with increased errors, and consequently has been a National Patient Safety Goal since 2007.[17–19] Respiratory care is not immune to this area of potential errors. The seemingly straightforward act of communicating important information beyond a treatment-due time is not uniformly practiced in most facilities.

Current report mechanisms may vary from department to department or from area to area (e.g., the intensive care unit vs. general care floors). Guidelines for safe reporting recommend standardizing the report process. If handoffs are ineffective, this leads to a progressive reduction in the quality. Omissions and inaccuracies will lead to errors and risks. A variety of mnemonics, templates, and checklists have been developed to help standardize the process.[20]

Need for Conversation at Handoffs

One key safety item related to the handoff is the need to move away from the one-way transmission of information, telegraphing reports.[21] Handoffs should be co-constructed and inclusive of dialogue between both parties. Remedies such as read-back may be helpful with specific orders (e.g., initial ventilator settings, medication orders) but of limited help when looking to provide guidance on escalation of care. The effectiveness of communication in changing and directing action is dependent on the knowledge states, prior experience, and the training of participants, and this required dialogue between both parties.[22,23]

I-PASS is a mnemonic developed as a resident handoff bundle and based on best practices in the literature. I-PASS is presently being studied for effectiveness in reducing medical errors in 10 pediatric institutions.[22] **Table 28-6** identifies the elements of the I-PASS mnemonic, and **Table 28-7** provides an example of a verbal handoff using I-PASS.

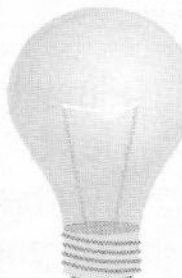

STOP AND THINK

You are caring for a mechanically ventilated patient with ARDS. During handoff, what specifically should be shared with regard to the patient and the mechanical ventilator?

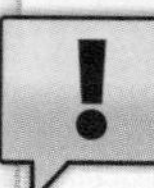

Respiratory Recap

Guidelines Effective in Improving Communication

- Ensuring that communication is interactive
- Limiting interruptions
- Providing a process for verification
- Providing an opportunity to review historical data

TABLE 28-6
Elements of the I-PASS Mnemonic

I	Illness Severity	Stable, watcher, unstable
P	Patient Summary	• Summary statement • Events leading up to admission • Hospital course • Ongoing assessment • Plan
A	Action List	• To do list • Time line and ownership
S	Situation Awareness and Contingency Planning	• Know what is going on • Plan for what might happen
S	Synthesis by Receiver	• Receiver summarizes what was heard • Asks questions • Restates key action/to do items

Reproduced with permission from Starmer AJ, Spector ND, Srivastava AD, et al. I-Pass: a mnemonic to standardize verbal hand-offs. *Pediatrics.* 2012;129:201, © by the AAP.

SBAR is an acronym **(situation, background, assessment, recommendation)** used to describe key points about a patient and the present environmental context in which the patient is being treated. It has become widely accepted not only as a sign-out tool but as a structured method for all communications between providers. **Table 28-8** provides an example of an SBAR report process for respiratory care.

TABLE 28-8
Example of an SBAR Report Process for Respiratory Care

SBAR (Situation, Background, Assessment, Recommendations)
Situation: A patient has been on the ventilator for 3 days and is slated to go to CT today for a scan between 10 AM and 12 noon.
Background: The patient meets the Berlin definition of ARDS criteria, and we have been using lung-protective strategies to guide a low-tidal volume ventilator strategy and PEEP. He has been extremely agitated for 2 days, requiring frequent boluses for sedation. Blood pressure has been labile and requiring pressors to maintain >60 mm Hg mean. The patient is very PEEP-dependent and desaturates rapidly when disconnected from the vent, turned, or moved.
Assessment: This patient is very unstable and a transport today, while necessary, will be difficult and require careful attention by experienced staff.
Recommendation: Contact the team leader and let them know about the transport so they may help you prior to your arrival. Make sure the most experienced RT travels with the patient. Use the transport check-off list. Use the capnograph, pulse oximeter, and a transport ventilator with PEEP capability.

TABLE 28-7
Sample I-PASS Verbal Handoff

I	Illness Severity	This is one of your sickest patients.
P	Patient Summary	17-yr-old male with previous history of asthma admissions. He presented to the ED this AM with chest tightening and worsening dyspnea nonresponsive to home albuterol treatments. He was started on solumedrol, albuterol, and magnesium in the ED. He has 6 known admissions in the past 2 years, 2 of which required NIV and one requiring intubation and mechanical ventilation. He presently is on continuous bronchodilator therapy and heliox. His asthma severity score is 7 and his pulse ox is 94% on 30% O_2.
A	Action List	Please check on him within the hour and reassess his asthma severity score. He will need backup heliox cylinders replaced before midnight, and a new continuous bronchodilator mixture sent up from Pharmacy at 04:00. Please verify with the bedside nurse the continuous infusion mixture concentration and rate of infusion into the nebulizer.
S	Situation Awareness and Contingency Planning	If the asthma score does not change or worsens, call the pediatric hospitalist. You may need to be ready to apply NIV.
S	Synthesis by Receiver	OK, so this 17-yr-old severe asthmatic with an asthma score of 7 is on continuous bronchodilators, heliox, IV steroids, and magnesium. He has a history of requiring NIV and ventilator support. I need to reassess him in one hour and obtain heliox cylinders. Pharmacy should be sending up the new bag of bronchodilator for the continuous neb at 04:00, and I'll reach out to the bedside nurse to double-check the infusion. I think I got it. Did I miss anything?

Reproduced with permission from Starmer AJ, Spector ND, Srivastava AD, et al. I-Pass: a mnemonic to standardize verbal hand-offs. *Pediatrics.* 2012;129:201, © by the AAP.

Other guidelines have been equally effective in helping improve communication;[23,24] examples include ensuring that communication is interactive (e.g., reading back an order), limiting interruptions (pagers, phones), providing a processes for verification (e.g., making rounds on ventilators during report time to verify), and providing an opportunity to review historical data (chart review).

Clinical Alarms and Equipment

Alarms help alert caregivers to important medical conditions, including adverse or dangerous changes in clinical condition. Unfortunately, the prevalence and numerous clinical alarms create an oversaturation to both visible and auditory alarm conditions. Multiple studies have demonstrated that most alarms are not clinically significant, and this occurrence reduces the attentiveness of staff and the patient safety intended to be preserved. This phenomenon is known as **alarm fatigue.**[25] The challenge falls between the need to have a high level of sensitivity for an alarm to activate (often sought by manufacturers) and high specificity so that it alarms only at a critical moment (desired by bedside clinicians). In 2014 the Joint Commission required hospital leaders to start establishing alarm system safety as a hospital priority. Hospitals will be required to review practices and risks and identify best practices in 2014–2015 that help to reduce erroneous alarms and insure response by the appropriate individuals. By 2016 they are required to develop processes that identify the who, how, what, and why of alarm settings; parameter changes; alarm conditions; and verification of alarm function. Studies have demonstrated that a typical medical/surgical ICU nurse may have over 100 alarms within a standard shift, that less than 7% of ICU alarms are clinically important requiring intervention, that 25% of alarms are attributable to erroneous detection, and over 60% are not relevant to safe care.[25,26]

Alarms are not the only source of equipment-related issues. The ECRI identified the top 10 health technology hazards for 2014 and five in that list have potential respiratory care applications. **Table 28-9** lists the applications to respiratory care.[27]

TABLE 28-9
Top Health Technology Hazards Applicable to Respiratory Care

Hazard	Implications for Respiratory Care
Alarm Hazards	• Pulse oximetry, capnometry, ventilator alarms, low specificity, high false alarm rate, clinical relevance
Infusion Pump Medication Errors	• Continuous infusion of aerosolized agents (e.g., bronchodilators, prostacyclin) during transport
Inadequate Reprocessing of Endoscopes	• Bronchoscope cleaning and processing
Pediatric Risks for Adult Technologies	• Default apnea settings are not adjusted for pediatric application after a ventilator had previously been applied to adult
Neglecting Change Management for Networked Services	• A new computerized order-set for COPD used in the emergency department does not include a communication order to respiratory care

© ECRI Institute 2013, reprinted with permission from ECRI Institute. Top 10 Health Technology Hazards for 2014. Available at https://www.ecri.org/Documents/Secure/Health_Devices_Top_10_Hazards_2013.pdf. Accessed Accessed August 1, 2014.

Universal Protocol

The **Universal Protocol** was created to address the continuing occurrence of wrong site, wrong procedure, and wrong person surgery. It is used to verify the correct procedure, for the correct patient, at the correct site. When possible, it should involve the patient in the verification process. It should also use a standardized list to verify the availability of items for the procedure. The Universal Protocol is required for procedures such as diagnostic bronchoscopy or a tracheostomy tube change. However, it is not required for minor procedures such as arterial puncture.

An invasive procedure should not be started until all questions or concerns are resolved. A time-out should be conducted immediately before starting the procedure. A designated member of the team starts the time-out, which involves all immediate members of the procedure team, including the respiratory therapist as appropriate. All relevant members of the procedure team, including the respiratory therapist, actively communicate during the time-out. During the time-out, the team members agree, at a minimum, on the correct patient identity, correct site, and the procedure to be done. Completion of the time-out must be documented.

Discharge Education and Planning

Safe care transitions (e.g., from hospital to home) require a systematic approach. One of the most problematic areas is discharge education and management for chronic respiratory conditions (e.g., chronic obstructive pulmonary disease, asthma) in the event of symptom escalation. Proper discharge education ensures a higher probability of compliance, which reduces readmissions and untoward safety events. CMS has identified in 2014 that COPD readmissions will be a targeted readmissions group and intends to reduce or eliminate reimbursement to facilities that have higher than acceptable readmission rates. Nationwide, COPD readmission rates average 25%. The respiratory therapist can assist the healthcare team by reviewing three key areas prior to discharge:

- *Medication administration:* Review the patient's medications to ensure that maintenance and rescue medications are appropriate.
- *Structured discharge communication:* Inform the patient of medication changes, pending tests and studies, and follow-up appointments. Communicate with outpatient physician offices whenever possible.
- *Patient education:* Patients and their families must understand their diagnosis, medications, equipment and techniques, and steps to take in case of exacerbation of symptoms after discharge.

The RT should access the available tools from the AARC for aerosol delivery and the COPD Foundation to help with discharge training, education, teaching, and feedback.

Healthcare-Associated Infections

Healthcare-associated infections (HAIs) are the most common complication of hospital care. According to the Centers for Disease Control and Prevention (CDC), nearly 1.7 million HAIs occur yearly, leading to approximately 99,000 deaths every year.[28,29] Recent efforts have demonstrated that relatively simple measures can prevent the majority of common HAIs. Five specific infections together account for the majority of all HAIs: surgical site infections (SSIs), catheter-associated urinary tract infections (CAUTIs), central venous catheter-related bloodstream infections (CRBSIs), **ventilator-associated pneumonia (VAP)**, and *Clostridium difficile*–associated disease (CDI).[28,29] Reducing the risk of HAI is one of the Joint Commission's National Patient Safety Goals.[29] The goal specifically requires adherence to hand hygiene practices and also considers death or serious disability due to HAI to be a sentinel event. Appropriate hand hygiene, influenza vaccination for healthcare workers, and prevention of VAE, CRBSI, and SSI are among the National Quality Forum's Safe Practices for Better Healthcare.[30] HAIs have resulted in considerable regulatory attention. The Centers for Medicare and Medicaid Services will not reimburse hospitals for the costs of care associated with certain HAIs, including SSIs, CRBSIs, and CAUTIs.[31] Although all of these are important to the respiratory therapist, VAE is an especially prominent concern.

Ventilator-Associated Events

One important challenge in using public reporting and payment policies to catalyze efforts to decrease HAIs is that the definitions are complex and may be subject to interpretation. Prior to 2013 VAP was the only condition monitored by the NHSN. Currently, however, there is no valid, reliable definition for VAP, and even the most widely used VAP criteria and definitions are neither sensitive nor specific. Bronchoalveolar lavage has not demonstrated superiority to standard nonquantitative culture techniques.[32] In 2011 the Centers for Disease Control assembled a working group that included representation from the AARC to develop an alternative surveillance tool for **ventilator-associated events (VAE)** and pneumonia. The VAE surveillance definition algorithm developed by this group was initiated in January 2013. The algorithm is based on objective and streamlined criteria that will identify many conditions and complications occurring in mechanically ventilated adult patients.[33] The respiratory therapist should know how to apply the VAE surveillance definition algorithm.

There are three definition tiers within the VAE algorithm: (1) ventilator-associated condition (VAC) (**Figure 28-1**); (2) infection-related ventilator-associated complication (IVAC) (**Figure 28-2**); and (3) possible

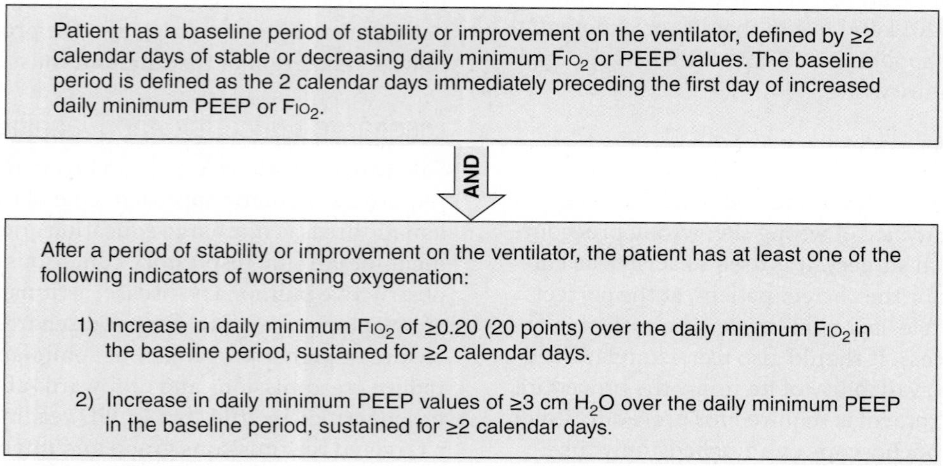

Patient has a baseline period of stability or improvement on the ventilator, defined by ≥2 calendar days of stable or decreasing daily minimum F_{IO_2} or PEEP values. The baseline period is defined as the 2 calendar days immediately preceding the first day of increased daily minimum PEEP or F_{IO_2}.

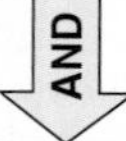

After a period of stability or improvement on the ventilator, the patient has at least one of the following indicators of worsening oxygenation:

1) Increase in daily minimum F_{IO_2} of ≥0.20 (20 points) over the daily minimum F_{IO_2} in the baseline period, sustained for ≥2 calendar days.

2) Increase in daily minimum PEEP values of ≥3 cm H_2O over the daily minimum PEEP in the baseline period, sustained for ≥2 calendar days.

FIGURE 28-1 Ventilator-associated condition.

Reproduced from *CDC Guidelines Device Associated Events: Ventilator Associated Events [VAE]*. January 2013. http://www.cdc.gov/nhsn/PDFs/pscManual/10-VAE_FINAL.PDF.

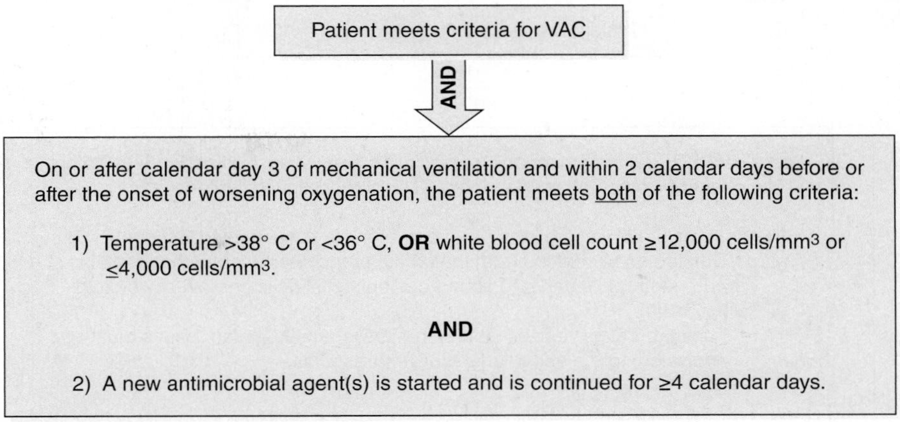

Patient meets criteria for VAC

On or after calendar day 3 of mechanical ventilation and within 2 calendar days before or after the onset of worsening oxygenation, the patient meets both of the following criteria:

1) Temperature >38° C or <36° C, **OR** white blood cell count ≥12,000 cells/mm^3 or ≤4,000 cells/mm^3.

AND

2) A new antimicrobial agent(s) is started and is continued for ≥4 calendar days.

FIGURE 28-2 Infection-related ventilator-associated condition.
Reproduced from *CDC Guidelines Device Associated Events: Ventilator Associated Events [VAE]*. January 2013. http://www.cdc.gov/nhsn/PDFs/pscManual/10-VAE_FINAL.PDF.

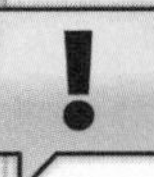

Respiratory Recap

Safe Practices for Better Health Care

- Appropriate hand hygiene
- Influenza vaccination for healthcare workers
- Prevention of central venous catheter-related bloodstream infections, ventilator-associated pneumonia, catheter-associated urinary tract infections, and surgical site infections
- RT involvement in VAE screening

and probable VAP (**Figure 28-3**). Algorithms to detect ventilator-associated complications can make use of electronic medical records and identify events that are clinically important and impact ICU and hospital length of stay and mortality.

Respiratory Protocols and Patient Safety

Respiratory protocols have gained wide acceptance for their positive impact on quality of care. Protocol application has consequently been associated with an improvement in the delivery of safe care. **Table 28-10** provides examples of how respiratory protocols have impacted patient safety. Ventilator protocols have resulted in reductions in duration of mechanical ventilation, weaning duration, and ICU stay, known contributors to patient mortality.[34,35]

Management of Medical Information

The medical record is a crucial element in preventing and minimizing potential adverse consequences. It also serves as a primary source of information for describing what transpired when an event occurred, and the subsequent actions taken. This is particularly important when performing root cause and risk analysis. Medical records that are poorly maintained, incomplete, inaccurate, or illegible or altered create questions of fact regarding the treatment given to a patient and increase the liability risk for a hospital or healthcare provider.

Rationale

Documentation within the medical record serves many purposes, but its primary function is to describe information pertinent to the patient (e.g., assessment, history, diagnostics, response to care) and provide for continuity in information about the patient's medical treatment. The patient's medical record is a permanent document, intended for use both inside and outside the hospital. Other key uses of the medical record include the following: a method for evaluating the quality of care provided; a basis for financial reimbursement to hospitals, healthcare providers, and patients; a tool for evaluating resource allocation (e.g., staffing, supplies, equipment); and a legal document for use in other legal proceedings.

Some respiratory therapists may consider documentation to be a burden or an afterthought, but documentation is an essential element of the provision of care. Documentation provides a reference on the status of the patient's condition prior to intervention, a record

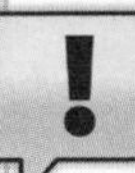

Respiratory Recap

Key Uses for Medical Record

- Describe information pertinent to the patient
- Provide for continuity in information about patient treatment
- Act as a method for evaluating quality of care
- Serve as a basis for reimbursement
- Function as a tool for evaluating resource allocation
- Serve as a legal document

Patient meets criteria for VAC and IVAC

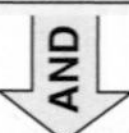

On or after calendar day 3 of mechanical ventilation and within 2 calendar days before or after the onset of worsening oxygenation, ONE of the following criteria is met:

1) Purulent respiratory secretions (from one or more specimen collections)
   - Defined as secretions from the lungs, bronchi, or trachea that contain ≥25 neutrophils and ≤10 squamous epithelial cells per low power field [lpf, ×100].
   - If the laboratory reports semi-quantitative results, those results must be equivalent to the above quantitative thresholds.

OR

2) Positive culture (qualitative, semi-quantitative, or quantitative) of sputum,* endotracheal aspirate,* bronchoalveolar lavage,* lung tissue, or protected specimen brushing*

Excludes the following:
- Normal respiratory/oral flora, mixed respiratory/oral flora or equivalent
- *Candida* species or yeast not otherwise specified
- Coagulase-negative *Staphylococcus* species
- *Enterococcus* species

Patient meets criteria for VAC and IVAC

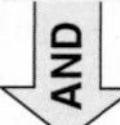

On or after calendar day 3 of mechanical ventilation and within 2 calendar days before or after the onset of worsening oxygenation, ONE of the following criteria is met:

1) Purulent respiratory secretions (from one or more specimen collections—and defined as for possible VAP)

AND one of the following:
- Positive culture of endotracheal aspirate,* ≥10^5 CFU/mL or equivalent semi-quantitative result
- Positive culture of bronchoalveolar lavage,* ≥10^4 CFU/mL or equivalent semi-quantitative result
- Positive culture of lung tissue, ≥10^4 CFU/g or equivalent semi-quantitative result
- Positive culture of protected specimen brush,* ≥10^3 CFU/mL or equivalent semi-quantitative result

**Same organism exclusions as noted for possible VAP.*

OR

2) One of the following (without requirement for purulent respiratory secretions):
- Positive pleural fluid culture (where specimen was obtaind during thoracentesis or initial placement of chest tube and NOT from an indwelling chest tube)
- Positive lung histopathology
- Positive diagnostic test for *Legionella* spp.
- Positive diagnostic test on respiratory secretions for influenza virus, respiratory syncytial virus, adenovirus, parainfluenza virus, rhinovirus, human metapneumovirus, coronavirus

FIGURE 28-3 Possible ventilator-associated pneumonia.

Reproduced from *CDC Guidelines Device Associated Events: Ventilator Associated Events [VAE]*. January 2013. Available at: http://www.cdc.gov/nhsn/PDFs/pscManual/10-VAE_FINAL.PDF.

TABLE 28-10
Examples of How Respiratory Protocols Impact Patient Safety

Protocol Type	Impact on Safety
Liberation from mechanical ventilation*	• Reduction in duration of mechanical ventilation • Reduction in duration of weaning • Reduction in ICU length of stay
Lung-protective ventilation strategies in patients without ARDS**	• Reduction in lung injury • Reduction in mortality • Reduction in lung infections • Reduction in occurrence of atelectasis

*Information from Blackwood B, Alderdice F, Burns K, et al. Use of weaning protocols for reducing duration of mechanical ventilation in critically ill adult patients: Cochrane systematic review and meta-analysis. Available at: http://www.ncbi.nlm.nih.gov/pmc/articles/PMC3020589/pdf/bmj.c7237.pdf. Accessed August 1, 2014.

**Information from Serpa Neto A, Cardoso SO, Manetta JA, et al. Association between use of lung-protective ventilation with lower tidal volumes and clinical outcomes among patients without acute respiratory distress syndrome. A meta-analysis. *JAMA*. 2012;308:1651–1659.

of key steps associated with the provision of care, an account of the effectiveness of care, an opportunity to record recommendations or modifications to the care, and a record of the educational materials provided to the patient, along with his or her ongoing needs and the discharge plan.

Elements of a Patient Medical Record

The medical record includes documentation of commonly used clinical data, including the patient assessment, problem identification, care plans, treatments, and outcomes. Technologic options include the use of multiple forms of digital media, including images and recordings. Healthcare providers should only document factual and objective information from their own treatment or observation of the patient. When documenting information derived from other sources (e.g., other healthcare providers, other medical records, or entries in the same medical record), be sure to reference the source of that information. **Table 28-11** includes examples of elements of the medical record and the types of media that may be considered part of such a record.[36]

Medical Record Documentation Standards

Consistent, current, and complete documentation in the medical record is an essential component of quality patient care. Regulatory and standards organizations have developed guidelines for the essential elements a medical record should contain.[36] **Box 28-1** reflects a set of commonly accepted standards for medical record documentation. Organizations use these standards to

TABLE 28-11
Elements of a Patient Medical Record

Elements	Examples
Progress notes	Notes of daily assessment and progress by physician or other members of the healthcare team
Physician orders	All medical orders written by physician or recorded as verbal orders by authorized individuals
Discharge summary	Summary of patient condition on discharge, postdischarge instructions, and care plan
Flow sheets/graphic sheets	Input and output records, daily graph of vital signs, mechanical ventilation records, and therapy records
Laboratory reports	Clinical laboratory reports and pulmonary function laboratory reports
Medication administration	Medication log
Photographs	Digital images, photographs from specific procedures, such as ultrasound or bronchoscopy
Videotapes/audio recordings	Digital recordings, tapes from procedures, such as sleep studies or bronchoscopy
Radiology reports	Radiographs, scans, and images
Monitoring strips	Electrocardiogram strips
Admissions sheet	Demographics, pertinent patient information, admitting diagnosis, and physician information
History and physical	Body system review by physician and all pertinent history information
Consultation sheet	Review, impressions, and recommendations of patient by specialists consulted
Consent forms	Forms signed by patient or representative for special procedures, such as surgery or bronchoscopy
Surgical records	Recording of all events occurring immediately before, during, and after surgery

Adapted from Care First Blue Choice. *Medical Records Documentation Standards*. Available at: http://www.carefirst.com/providers/attachments/BOK5129.pdf. Accessed March 7, 2014.

BOX 28-1

Medical Record Documentation Standards

Elements of the record are organized.
Records are stored and maintained in a way to protect safety and confidentiality of information.
Patient name and ID appear on each page.
The record is legible to others.
All entries are dated.
All entries contain the author's identification (written or **electronic signature**).
Personal biographical data are included.
Contributory past medical history, family, and birth history are noted as appropriate.
Medication allergies and adverse reactions are prominently noted.
Personal habits—including smoking, alcohol, and substances history and sexual behavior—are noted.
Significant illnesses/medical conditions are indicated on the problem list.
Chief complaint or reason for visit is noted.
The history and physical examination identify appropriate information pertinent to patient's complaints and a working diagnosis consistent with the findings.
Treatment plans are consistent with diagnoses.
Medical record shows clear justification for diagnostic tests and therapies.
Unresolved problems from previous office visits are addressed in subsequent visits.
Follow-up care is noted when indicated.
Current medications are documented; long-term medications are reviewed at least annually.
Healthcare education is provided, noted, and updated as appropriate.
Immunization record (for children) is up to date or there is an appropriate history.
Evidence that preventive screening and services have been offered is noted.
Consultation requests are justified by medical records evidence.
Laboratory and diagnostic results reflect practitioner review.
Patients are notified of abnormal diagnostic results and recommended to follow up.
Evidence of continuity of care between primary care and specialist providers is noted.

Adapted from Care First Blue Choice. *Medical Records Documentation Standards*. Available at: http://www.carefirst.com/providers/attachments/BOK5129.pdf. Accessed August 1, 2014.

audit the quality and thoroughness of medical record documentation.

Essentials for Respiratory Care Documentation

Respiratory charting should represent the key elements of patient interventions and data. It should be organized and integrated into the other areas of the medical record.

It is primarily designed to reflect the presentation and status of the patient, yet it also needs to meet the needs of other end users of information. It should be structured in an organized manner that lends itself to ease of entry and of interpretation and analysis. Information should be organized for rapid access and presentation to be used to its fullest. Consequently, the respiratory care section of the medical record should be systematically designed to record the information clinically appropriate for the patient's presentation.

Respiratory therapists must possess the necessary skills to document, manage, and access patient information if they are to be effective clinicians. They also must remain informed about the various medical, ethical, legal, and financial roles that documentation and medical information play. Careless or insufficient documentation may result in misinterpretation and patient harm, penalties, lawsuits, and financial consequences. Departments should describe in policy and procedure manuals the key charting requirements for the various activities performed. **Table 28-12** describes respiratory care information commonly recorded in the medical record.

Orders

Physician-directed orders drive the course of care for all patients. Each healthcare system has specific policies and procedures governing who may write orders, who may accept verbal orders, and the procedure used to

TABLE 28-12
Respiratory Care Information Commonly Recorded in the Medical Record

Category	Examples of Data Recorded
Patient demographics	Patient identification, institution, medical record number, accession (hospital visit) number
Date/time	Date and time of assessment, therapeutic intervention, and documentation
Interview and respiratory history	Pulmonary history, contributory health, smoking history
Vital signs	Pulse, respiratory rate, blood pressure, temperature
Physical examination	Breath sounds, head and neck, thorax
Laboratory and blood gases	Blood gas values, hematology, chemistry, microbiology
Pulmonary function testing	FVC, SVC, IC, FEV_1, peak expiratory flow
Radiographic diagnostic information	Chest radiograph, CT, MRI
Essential monitoring data	Pulse oximetry; capnometry; ventilator settings; flow, volume, and pressure information; minute ventilation; cuff pressure; tube position
Medication administration	Aerosolized, airway instilled, intravenous
Risk assessment, severity, and triage scores	Mild to severe, ARDS risk, sepsis score
Therapeutic interventions	Aerosol, bronchial hygiene, lung inflation, ventilatory care
Other systems information	Nutritional, hemodynamic, neurologic
Therapeutic effectiveness/ readiness to progress	Response to applied adjuncts, readiness for liberation, extubate
Adverse reactions/actions taken	Unforeseen consequences, actions taken when identified
Patient education/discharge planning	Discharge asthma education instruction, tobacco cessation

FVC, forced vital capacity; SVC, slow vital capacity; IC, inspiratory capacity; FEV_1, forced expiratory volume in 1 second; CT, computed tomography; MRI, magnetic resonance imaging; ARDS, acute respiratory distress syndrome.

document the order in the medical record. All medical orders, whether written or verbally accepted, must be recorded accurately to ensure patient safety and accurate care.

The Joint Commission specifies standards for all medical orders. Verbal orders may be accepted by authorized individuals and transcribed by qualified personnel identified by title, state licensure and scope of practice, or category in the medical staff rules and regulations.[37] Respiratory therapists meet this requirement, but nonlicensed respiratory therapy students are not qualified to accept verbal orders; consequently, students require licensed respiratory therapists to take and transcribe orders during their clinical experiences. Qualified individuals must strictly follow the institution's procedure for recording of verbal orders. Respiratory therapists providing any clinical care of patients should understand and review the institution's procedures for acceptance and recording of verbal orders. **Figure 28-4** provides an example of a transcribed verbal order.

Electronic Medical or Health Records

Electronic medical record (EMR) and **electronic health record (EHR)** are two terms used synonymously to describe computerized systems that track and record patient information electronically. The premise of the EMR is that electronic capture of information speeds entry, improves the storage and retrieval of patient information, and subsequently improves the provision of care. The transition from paper to electronic records provides an extraordinary opportunity to reduce risk, improve quality and efficiency, and affect outcome. Properly designed and applied EMR systems can be robust tools to help with all manner of clinical applications and can be a great advantage to the respiratory therapist for respiratory charting, work assignments, triaging, and the application of clinical guidelines, protocols, or pathways.

Legal Implications of the Record

The medical record is a legal document that, when properly completed, represents an accounting of the assessment and care provided to a patient. When used haphazardly or inconsistently, it becomes a source of ambiguity, question, and error. In a courtroom setting, it may be likened to a witness whose memory is never lost. It serves to correlate, for all involved, important

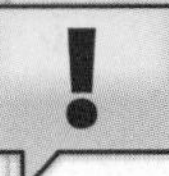

Respiratory Recap

Legalities of the Medical Record

- Medical records that are poorly maintained, incomplete, inaccurate, illegible, or altered increase liability risk for the hospital and healthcare provider.

Patient name and identification number
Date
Perform lung volumes and airways resistance study today 4 hours after 2 puffs of
albuterol inhaler have been administered via Metered Dose Inhaler with spacer.
v.o. Rory Agnes, MD
Patrick Everett, RRT, RPFT
3-7-14 01:10 PM

FIGURE 28-4 Example of a transcribed verbal order.

patient information regarding the treatment rendered and the patient's treatment plan and is the means by which a level of communication is achieved among all healthcare providers involved in the patient's care.

Patient Confidentiality Issues

Confidentiality is the right of an individual to have personal, identifiable medical information kept private. Medical information should be available only to the physician of record and other healthcare and insurance personnel as necessary. Patient confidentiality is protected by federal statute, namely, by the passage of the **Health Insurance Portability and Accountability Act (HIPAA)**.[38] HIPAA is intended to ensure the privacy and protection of personal records and data in an environment of electronic medical records and third-party insurance payers. HIPAA provides a uniform set of guidelines that apply to all providers and organizations.

All healthcare systems must have policies and procedures to protect patient confidentiality. Employees must be familiar with their system's information security plan, which outlines steps governing access to medical information. Practitioners should refrain from discussing patients in the hallways, cafeterias, and elevators. Practitioners should not review the confidential information of any patient unless it is directly essential to the provision of care. Engaging in discussions outside the care setting is unprofessional behavior and breaches patient confidentiality.

The release of patient information should always ensure confidentiality as the first premise. Patients must authorize the release of their health information in most situations. If the patient is unable to authorize release of information, other guidelines apply. The medical records department should be able to answer queries about whether a signed release is necessary.

Releasing only the specific medical information that is requested and authorized, and no more, is a good practice. Hospital departments generally involved with the release of medical information include medical records, risk management, quality management, and utilization management. These departments may coexist or be organized under a health information management division. Corporate offices or headquarters may serve as the institutional authority for an entire healthcare network within a state, regional, national, or international network.

The respiratory therapist is expected to practice the art of respiratory care with knowledge, skill, and a continuously professional attitude. It is equally important that the therapist understand that information, and the manner in which he or she imparts that information, affects the safety and sequential care the patient receives. All documentation and communication must be provided in a manner consistent with institutional

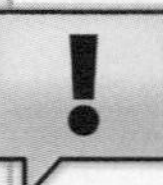

Respiratory Recap

Confidentiality

- The Health Insurance Portability and Accountability Act (HIPAA) is a federal mandate that ensures patient confidentiality. Respiratory therapy students and clinicians should carefully follow policies and procedures to protect patient confidentiality.

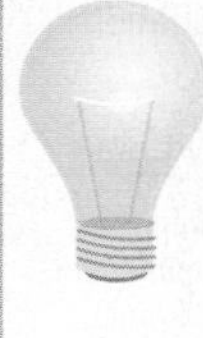

STOP AND THINK

Your cousin is on life support. Family members know you are an RT at the institution where he is being treated and that you have access to information related to his condition. How do you legally handle their inquiries to the specifics of his condition?

and regulatory standards for accuracy, clarity, and confidentiality. Technological advances will continue to drive many of the changes in the development, maintenance, and transfer of medical information over the coming years. The challenge of each respiratory therapist is to understand the basic principles and to apply them in the future to improve safe and effective patient care.

Key Points

- Safe care at all times should be a hallmark of every respiratory therapist.
- Respiratory therapists influence the culture of safety in their organization.
- Respiratory therapists should continually strive to achieve a highly reliable level of safe practice.
- Incident reports help escalate safe care and should be filed whenever an untoward event occurs.
- Rapid response teams have become commonplace in health care and are designed to encourage early intervention for adverse signs, symptoms, or conditions.
- Medication reconciliation is designed to pick up inconsistencies or discrepancies in a patient's medication regimen.
- Reports, handoffs, and rounds are the source of many medical errors in care. Collaborative communication and dialogue by both parties elevates the level of safety during report.
- A time-out should be conducted immediately before starting an invasive procedure.
- Proper discharge education ensures a higher probability of compliance and reduces readmission and untoward safety events.
- Healthcare-associated infections continue to be the source of numerous medical problems and complications, and regulatory interventions are exerting significant influence on healthcare institutions to reduce their incidence.
- Medical documentation serves many purposes: as a method to evaluate quality of care, a basis for financial reimbursement, a means to evaluate resources, and as a legal document.
- Regulatory and standards organizations have guidelines identifying essential elements of medical documentation.
- Respiratory charting should not be taken lightly because if it is careless or insufficient, it could result in patient harm, penalties, lawsuits, and financial consequences.
- Requirements for medical record entries vary based on setting and institution, but therapists must be knowledgeable about the policies and procedures for their respective clinical settings.
- The electronic medical record is gaining popularity: it speeds entry, improves storage and retrieval, and improves the provision of care.
- Confidentiality is the fundamental right for patients to have personal, identifiable medical information kept private and is protected by a federal statue known as HIPAA.

References

1. Kohn LT, Corrigan JM, Donaldson MS, eds. *To Err Is Human: Building a Safer Health System*. Washington, DC: National Academies Press; 2000.
2. Bodenheimer T. Coordinating care—a perilous journey through the health care system. *N Engl J Med*. 2008:358;1064–1071.
3. Ornato JP, Peberdy MA. Applying lessons from commercial aviation safety and operations to resuscitation. *Resuscitation*. 2014;85:173–176.
4. Weick KE, Sutcliffe KM. *Managing the Unexpected: Assuring High Performance in an Age of Complexity*. San Francisco: Jossey-Bass; 2001:10–17.
5. Schyve P. Leadership in Healthcare Organizations: A Guide to Joint Commission Leadership Standards. The Governance Institute. Available at: http://www.jointcommission.org/assets/1/18/wp_leadership_standards.pdf. Accessed August 1, 2014.
6. Institute for Safe Medication Practices. *Intimidation: Practitioners Speak Up on This Unresolved Problem. Part 1*. ISMP Medication Safety Alert. March 11, 2004. Available at: http://www.ismp.org/newsletters/acutecare/articles/20040311_2.asp. Accessed August 1, 2014.
7. Institute for Safe Medication Practices. *Unresolved Disrespectful Behavior in Healthcare. Practitioners Speak Up (Again). Part 1*. ISMP Medication Safety Alert. October 3, 2013. Available at: http://www.ismp.org/Newsletters/acutecare/showarticle.asp?id=60. Accessed August 1, 2014.
8. Weaver S. Promoting a culture of safety as a patient safety strategy—a systematic review. *Ann Intern Med*. 2013;158:369–374
9. Chassin MR, Loeb JM. High-reliability health care: getting there from here. *Milbank Q*. 2013:91:459–490.
10. The Joint Commission Center for Transforming Health Care. *Robust Process Improvement*. 2013. Available at: http://www.centerfortransforminghealthcare.org/about/rpi.aspx. Accessed August 1, 2014.
11. DelliFraine JL, Langabeer JR, Nembhard IM. Assessing the evidence of Six Sigma and Lean in the health care industry. *Qual Manag Health Care*. 2010;19:211–225.
12. The Joint Commission. Framework for Conducting Root Cause Analysis and Action Plan. March 22, 2013. Available at: http://www.jointcommission.org/Framework_for_Conducting_a_Root_Cause_Analysis_and_Action_Plan/. Accessed August 1, 2014.
13. The Joint Commission. *2014 National Patient Safety Goals Hospital Program*. Available at: http://www.jointcommission.org/standards_information/npsgs.aspx. Accessed August 1, 2014.
14. Weingarten TN, Venus SJ, Whalen FX, et al. Postoperative emergency response team activation at a large tertiary medical center. *Mayo Clin Proc*. 2012;87:41–49.
15. Ramachandran SK, Haider N, Saran KA, et al. Life-threatening critical respiratory events: a retrospective study of postoperative patients found unresponsive during analgesic therapy. *J Clin Anesth*. 2011;23:207–213.
16. Wong JD, Bajcar JM, Wong GG, et al. Medication reconciliation at hospital discharge: evaluating discrepancies. *Ann Pharmacother*. 2008;42:1373–1379.
17. Greenberg CC, Regenbogen SE, Studdert DM, et al. Patterns of communication breakdowns resulting in injury to surgical patients. *J Am Coll Surg*. 2007;204:533–540.
18. Joint Commission Center for Transforming Health Care. *Improving Transitions of Care – Hand-off Communications*. 2013. Available at: http://www.centerfortransforminghealthcare.org/assets/4/6/CTH_Hand-off_commun_set_final_2010.pdf. Accessed August 1, 2014.

19. World Health Organization for Patient Safety Initiatives. *Communication During Patient Hand-Overs*. 2007. Available at: http://www.who.int/patientsafety/solutions/patientsafety/PS-Solution3.pdf. Accessed August 1, 2014.
20. Riesenberg LA, Leitzsch L, Little BW. Systematic review of handoff mnemonics literature. *Am J Med Qual.* 2009;24:196–204.
21. Cohen MD, Hilligoss B, Kajdacsy-Balla Amaral AC. A Handoff is not a telegram: an understanding of the patient is co-constructed. *Crit Care.* 2012;16:303–308.
22. Starmer AJ, Spector ND, Srivastava R, et al. I-PASS a mnemonic to standardize verbal handoffs. *Pediatrics.* 2012;129:201–204.
23. Farhan M, Brown R, Wolosynowych M, Vincent C. The ABC of handover: a qualitative study to develop a new tool for handover in the emergency department. *Emerg Med J.* 2012;29:941–946.
24. Abraham J, Kannampallil T, Patel B, Almoosa K, Patel VL. Comparative evaluation of the content and structure of communication using two handoff tools: implications for patient safety [Abstract]. *J Crit Care.* 2014:29:311.
25. Voepel-Lewis T, Parker ML, Burke CN, et al. Pulse oximetry desaturation alarms on a general postoperative adult unit: a prospective observational study of nurse response time. *Int J Nurs Stud.* 2013;50:1351–1358.
26. Inokuchi R, Sato H, Nanjo Y, et al. The proportion of clinically relevant alarms decreases as patient clinical severity decreases in intensive care units: a pilot study. *BMJ Open.* 2013;3:e003354.
27. ECRI Institute. *Top 10 Health Technology Hazards for 2014*. Adapted from *Health Devices*, 2013:42(11). Available at: https://www.ecri.org/Forms/Documents/2014_Top_10_Hazards_Executive_Brief.pdf. Accessed August 1, 2014.
28. Klevens RM, Edwards JR, Richards CL Jr., et al. Estimating health care associated infections and deaths in U.S. hospitals, 2002. *Public Health Rep.* 2007;122:160–166.
29. Centers for Disease Control and Prevention. *The Direct Medical Costs of Healthcare-Associated Infections in U.S. Hospitals and the Benefits of Prevention*. Available at: http://www.cdc.gov/hai/pdfs/hai/scott_costpaper.pdf. Accessed August 1, 2014.
30. National Quality Forum. *Safe Practices for Better Healthcare: 2010 Update*. Available at: http://www.qualityforum.org/Publications/2010/04/Safe_Practices_for_Better_Healthcare_%E2%80%93_2010_Update.aspx. Accessed August 1, 2014.
31. Medicare.gov. The Official U.S. Government Site for Medicare. Healthcare-Associated Infections. Available at: http://www.medicare.gov/hospitalcompare/Data/Healthcare-Associated-Infections.html. Accessed December 17, 2014.
32. Canadian Critical Care Trials Group. A randomized trial of diagnostic techniques for ventilator associated pneumonia. *N Engl J Med.* 2006;355:2619–2630.
33. Centers for Disease Control and Prevention. Ventilator associated event. 2014. Available at: http://www.cdc.gov/nhsn/PDFs/pscManual/10-VAE_FINAL.pdf. Accessed August 1, 2014.
34. Blackwood B, Alderdice F, Burns, K, et al. Use of weaning protocols for reducing duration of mechanical ventilation in critically ill adult patients: Cochrane systematic review and meta-analysis. *BMJ.* 2011; 342c 7237. Available at: http://www.ncbi.nlm.nih.gov/pmc/articles/PMC3020589/pdf/bmj.c7237.pdf. Accessed August 1, 2014.
35. Serpa Neto A, Cardoso SO, Manetta JA, et al. Association between use of lung-protective ventilation with lower tidal volumes and clinical outcomes among patients without acute respiratory distress syndrome: a meta-analysis. *JAMA.* 2012;308:1651–1659.
36. Care First Blue Choice. *Medical Records Documentation Standards*. Available at: http://www.carefirst.com/providers/attachments/BOK5129.pdf. Accessed August 1, 2014.
37. The Joint Commission. *2012 Comprehensive Accreditation Manual for Hospitals: The Official Handbook*. Oak Brook, IL: Joint Commission Resources; 2011.
38. U.S. Department of Health and Human Services. *Understanding HIPPA Privacy for Covered Entities*. Available at: http://www.hhs.gov/ocr/privacy/hipaa/understanding/coveredentities/index.html. Accessed August 1, 2014.

Section III
Respiratory Diseases

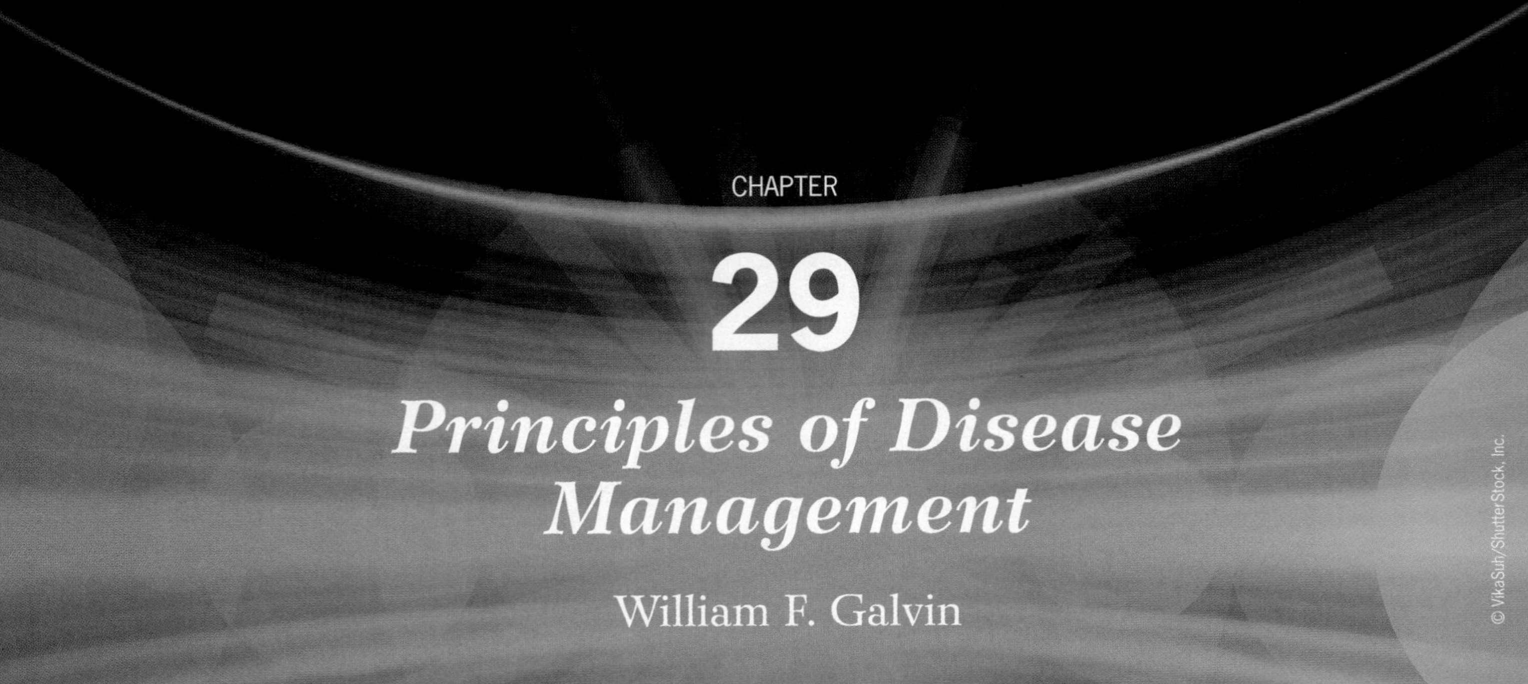

CHAPTER
29
Principles of Disease Management
William F. Galvin
© VikaSuh/ShutterStock, Inc.

OUTLINE

OBJECTIVES

1. Identify trends and future directions of healthcare delivery.
2. Define disease management and terms associated with care management.
3. Identify the forces driving disease management.
4. Explain the history and evolution of the disease management movement.
5. Explain the difference between case management and disease management.
6. Identify core components of disease management.
7. Explain goals of disease management.
8. List and explain the basic principles of disease management.
9. Identify diseases best suited for disease management programs.
10. Explain the development and implementation of disease management programs.
11. Define and explain respiratory protocols.
12. Explain the future of disease management.
13. Explain the role of respiratory therapists with regard to disease management.

KEY TERMS

care management
case management
chronic care model (CCM)
component management
demand management
disease management
evidence-based medicine
integrated care
pathway
protocol

Introduction

Meeting the healthcare needs of the sickest and most medically vulnerable segment of the population—those with multiple chronic conditions—is not only a challenge but a healthcare imperative. It is well documented that among the 15 chronic conditions of Medicare fee-for-service (FFS) beneficiaries, over two-thirds have two or more chronic conditions and 14% have six or more.[1] While the average spending for Medicare FFS beneficiaries was $9738, that number increases to $32,658 for individuals with six or more chronic conditions.[1] In addition, 1% of the nation's population account for over 20% of medical costs, 10% account for over 60%, and 20% account for an astounding 81.7% of medical costs.[2] Cost concentration thus rests in the hands of a relatively small percentage of individuals and places a tremendous financial burden on our healthcare system. A strategy to combat this problem is desperately needed. One such strategy is disease management.

This chapter addresses trends shaping healthcare delivery; defines the terms associated with disease management; describes forces driving disease management; explains the history and evolution of the disease management movement; addresses the goals, principles, and specific cardiopulmonary diseases targeted for disease management programs; explains the development and implementation of a disease management program; addresses respiratory protocols; and discusses the future of disease management. The chapter concludes with an explanation of the role of the respiratory therapist as a disease manager.

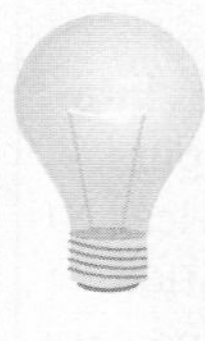

STOP AND THINK

Elaborate on the trends in how health care is perceived, and how it will be delivered in the future, with specific examples or explanations as to how they pertain to respiratory care practice.

Trends and Directions in Healthcare Delivery

The healthcare system is constantly evolving. This evolution is the result of a fundamental shift in emphasis and a change in mindset in how health is perceived. This new mindset is the impetus behind the disease management movement and is the theme of this chapter. It represents a new direction in the delivery of health care. **Table 29-1** illustrates a transformation and the trends and direction in how health care is perceived and how it will be delivered in the future.[3]

Terms and Concepts Associated with Disease Management

Care Management

Care management is a general term for the coordination of patient interventions. It is an umbrella term under which many loosely related terms are gathered. The more popular terms associated with care management are *component management, demand management, case management,* and *disease management.* Respiratory therapists must have an understanding of these terms because efforts are continuously under way to institute measures aimed at the coordination of the care and management of respiratory diseases.

Component Management

Component management is an approach to healthcare cost containment that involves trying to control individual components (e.g., a drug, hospitalization, or laboratory test). It is the opposite of disease management and is the predominant method that has been used to control healthcare costs since the 1980s. Its focus is cost control through limitation of the use of resources or services such as therapeutic procedures, diagnostic tests, medications, or hospital lengths of stay. Unfortunately, component management often results in lower quality of care and poorer clinical outcomes, and is an ineffective way to truly control costs.

The problem with component management is that each aspect of care—emergency room visits, physician services, medications—is managed separately and services are not integrated. In the case of the patient with asthma, all health plans cover emergency room visits, inpatient hospital stays, and physician services. Medications may or may not be covered. Few plans, however, provide coverage for patient education and counseling. Consequently, the limited coverage for medications and patient education leads to significantly higher costs in the form of more emergency room visits, inpatient hospitalizations, and physician office visits. When respiratory therapy departments were revenue generators, component care approaches allowed them to flourish. Component management is flawed, however; it is episodic and uncoordinated, emphasizes treatment instead of prevention, and provides little incentive to treat the entire disease.

TABLE 29-1
Trends and Directions in Healthcare Delivery

Illness → Wellness
Acute care → Primary care
Inpatient → Outpatient
Individual health → Community well-being
Fragmented care → Managed care
Independent institutions → Integrated systems
Service duplication → Continuum of services

Demand Management

Demand management entails any organized effort or program designed to guide healthcare consumers into the most appropriate level of healthcare service by involving them in their own care. It reduces the need for and use of costly, often unnecessary, medical services and arbitrary managed care interventions. The tools of demand management consist of patient **protocols**, clinical **pathways**, case management, and disease management. These tools were developed to enable clinicians to achieve better outcomes by making it easier to give patients what they need when they need it. The intention is to weed out inappropriate and unnecessary care.

Case Management

Case management is defined as a collaborative process that assesses, plans, implements, coordinates, monitors, and evaluates the options and services required to meet an individual's health needs, using communication and available resources to promote quality, cost, and effective outcomes, and that occurs across a continuum of care, addressing ongoing needs rather than being restricted to a single practice setting.[4] It is generally employed for the high-risk, high-cost patient who suffers repeated admissions, encounters significant variances, is unpredictable, and may be socioeconomically disadvantaged. Case management was built on the notion that 20% of patients were responsible for 80% of costs. The rationale was that focusing on the care of the 20% would reduce this 80% cost. Traditional case management is one-on-one care and is expensive. Case managers focus on an individual patient and assist in acquiring equipment and services, work with schools and other community-based organizations, provide technical support, conduct patient education, and identify and remove barriers to achieve effective implementation of the care plan.

Disease Management

Disease management is more innovative and exciting a concept. Numerous synonyms are associated with the concept. Some of the more popular are *disease state management, system-based disease management, total health management, medical management, population-based management, best practices, care mapping,* and *outcomes management.* The different terminology attempts to capture or highlight one or more of the numerous principles that drive the disease management movement.

Definitions for disease management are numerous and diverse, as shown by the following examples:

- A clinical management process of care that spans the continuum of care from primary prevention to ongoing long-term health maintenance for individuals with chronic health conditions or diagnoses[5]
- An approach to identify a specific subpopulation of patients at high risk for undesirable outcomes and intervene to modify that risk[6]
- The cure to high-cost conditions[5]
- Self-care with professional support, in which the patient has significant responsibility for his or her own health[3]
- An ongoing, comprehensive case management program for specific chronic diseases that is based on clearly defined, well-established best practices of care[7]

For purposes of this chapter, the definition provided by the Population Health Alliance (PHA; formerly Disease Management Association of America) will be used: disease management is a system of coordinated healthcare interventions and communications for populations with conditions in which patient self-care efforts are significant.[8]

Often the difference between case management and disease management is not apparent. **Table 29-2** compares conventional case management and disease management.

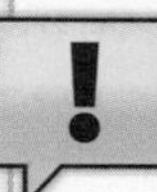

Respiratory Recap

Synonyms for Disease Management

- Disease state management
- System-based disease management
- Total health management
- Medical management
- Population-based management
- Best practices
- Care mapping
- Outcomes management

Integrated Care

The World Health Organization (WHO) defines **integrated care** as a "concept bringing together inputs, delivery, management and organization of services related to diagnosis, treatment, care, rehabilitation and health promotion."[9] Alternatively, integrated care can be considered as "an organizational process of coordination that seeks to achieve seamless and continuous care, tailored to the patient's needs, and based on a holistic view of the patient."[10] Integrated care and the chronic care model of disease management are so similar in concept that they may be considered

TABLE 29-2
Difference Between Case Management and Disease Management

Traditional/Catastrophic Case Management	Disease Management
Emphasis is on single patient	Emphasis is on population with a chronic illness
Early identification of people with acute catastrophic conditions (known high cost or known diagnoses that lead to high cost in the near term)	Early identification of all people with targeted chronic diseases (20–40) whether mild, moderate, or severe
Acuity level of catastrophic cases is high; acuity level of traditional cases is high to moderate	Acuity level is moderate
Applies to 0.5% to 1% of commercial membership	Applies to 15% to 25% of commercial membership
Value relies heavily on price negotiations and benefit flexing	Value is result of member and provider behavior change that results in improved health status
Requires plan design manipulation (e.g., adding more home care visits)	Requires plan design changes that reward enrollment in DM and shrink drug copays
Primary objective is to arrange for care using the least restrictive, clinically appropriate alternatives	Primary objective is to avoid hospitalization *and* modify risk factors, lifestyle, and medication adherence to improve health status
Episode is 60 to 90 days	Intervention is 365 days for most conditions
Site of interaction is primarily hospital, hospice, subacute facility, or home health care	Sites of interaction include work, school, and home
Driven by need for arrangement of support services, community resources, transportation	Driven by nonadherence to medical regimens
Outcome metrics are single-admission length of stay and cost per case	Outcome metrics are annual cost per diseased member and disease-specific functional status and gaps in care

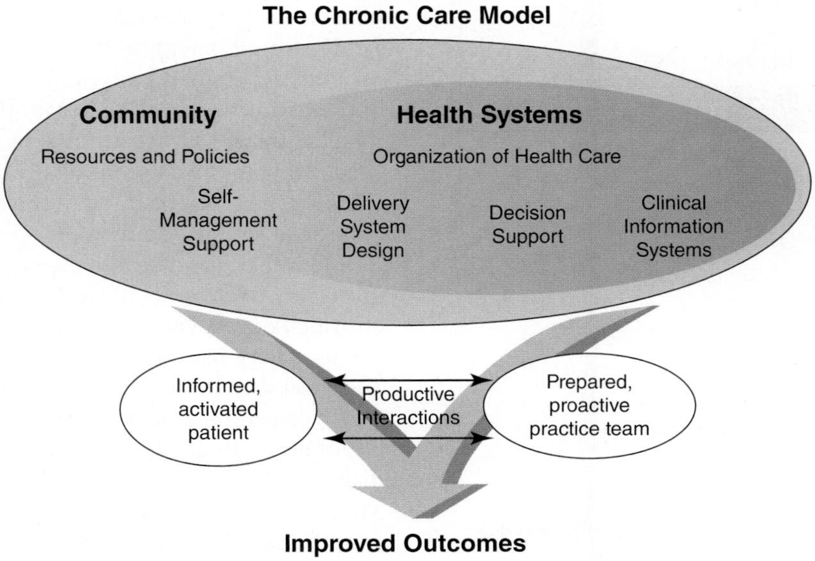

The Chronic Care Model

Community
Resources and Policies
Self-Management Support
Health Systems
Organization of Health Care
Delivery System Design
Decision Support
Clinical Information Systems
Informed, activated patient
Productive Interactions
Prepared, proactive practice team
Improved Outcomes

FIGURE 29-1 The chronic care model.

Reproduced from Chronic Disease Management: What Will It Take To Improve Care for Chronic Illness? Effective Clinical Practice, August/September 1998;1:2–4; permission conveyed through Copyright Clearance Center, Inc.

interchangeable. The term is included among the list due to its adoption by such professional organizations as the American Thoracic Society.[11]

Chronic Care Model

Wagner at the MacColl Institute designed the **chronic care model (CCM) for healthcare innovation** at the Group Health Cooperative of Puget Sound, Seattle. The chronic care model identifies the essential elements of a healthcare system that encourage high-quality chronic disease care. The elements comprising the model are the community, the health system, self-management support, delivery system design, decision support, and clinical information systems. While a more detailed explanation is forthcoming, the model entails evidence-based change concepts and fosters productive interactions between informed patients who take an active part in their care and providers with resources and expertise. The ultimate goal is improved patient outcomes[12] (**Figure 29-1**).

Forces Driving Disease Management

Cost and Changing Patterns of Disease

The primary forces driving disease management are cost (**Figure 29-2**) and the changing pattern of disease (**Table 29-3**), specifically, the increase in chronic,

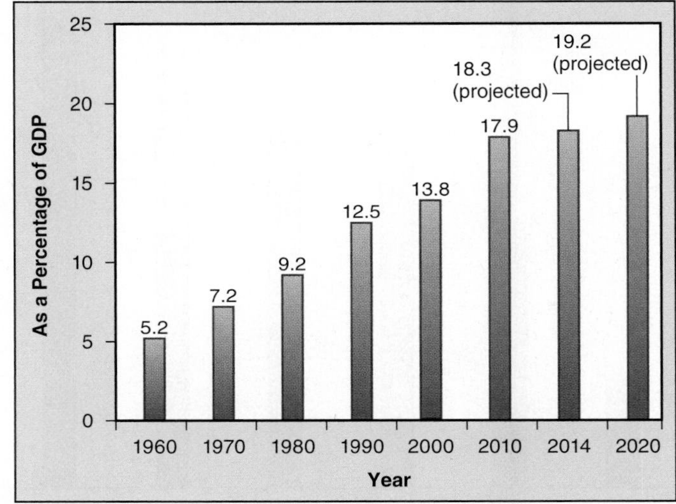

FIGURE 29-2 Healthcare expenditures as a percentage of gross domestic product (GDP).

Information from Centers for Medicare and Medicaid Services. Available at: http://www.cms.gov/Research-Statistics-Data-and-Systems/Statistics-Trends-and-Reports/NationalHealthExpendData/NationalHealthAccountsProjected.html.

TABLE 29-3
Changing Patterns of Disease: 1900–2010

1900	2010
Pneumonia	Heart disease
Tuberculosis	Cancer
Diarrhea and enteritis	Chronic lower respiratory disease
Heart disease	Stroke
Stroke	Accidents
Liver disease	Alzheimer disease
Injuries	Diabetes
Cancer	Nephritis, necrotic syndrome, and nephrosis
Senility	Influenza and pneumonia
Diphtheria	Suicide

Statistics for 1900 from Centers for Disease Control and Prevention. Control of infectious diseases, 1900–1999. *Morbid Mortal Wkly Dis.* 1999;45: 621–629. Statistics for 2010 from National Center for Health Statistics. *Health, United States, 2012.* Hyattsville, MD: Department of Health and Human Services; 2013:88.

debilitating disease. Healthcare cost as a component of the gross domestic product (GDP) shifted from 5.2% in 1960 to 17.9% in 2010.[13] This escalating increase in the healthcare component of the GDP is at the heart of efforts to reform and restructure the healthcare system. As illustrated in **Figure 29-3**, costs are concentrated on a relatively small percentage of individuals, with 1% of the nation's population accounting for over 20% of medical costs, 10% accounting for over 60%, and 20% accounting for an astounding 81.7% of medical costs.[2] Clearly, this is on the mind of the healthcare industry and the federal government.

The infectious diseases prevalent in 1900 have given way to chronic, lifestyle diseases. This issue of chronicity is especially important because chronic diseases have become the leading causes of death and disability in the United States. Almost 50% of Americans have at least one chronic illness[14] and 8.7 out of every 10 deaths are attributable to chronic disease.[15] According to the Centers for Medicare and Medicaid Services, the prevalence of multiple chronic conditions is high, with over two-thirds of beneficiaries having two or more chronic conditions and 14% having six or more (**Figure 29-4**). The most common chronic conditions among Medicare beneficiaries are high blood pressure, high cholesterol, ischemic heart disease, arthritis, and diabetes. Beneficiaries younger than 65 years of age (who are primarily disabled) are 1.8 times as likely to have asthma compared to aged beneficiaries.[1] A more complete list of common chronic conditions along with their respective percentages is illustrated in **Figure 29-5**.[1]

It is estimated that 75% of total health expenditures in the United States are attributable to the treatment of chronic conditions.[16] In 2011, total healthcare costs associated with the treatment of chronic diseases were

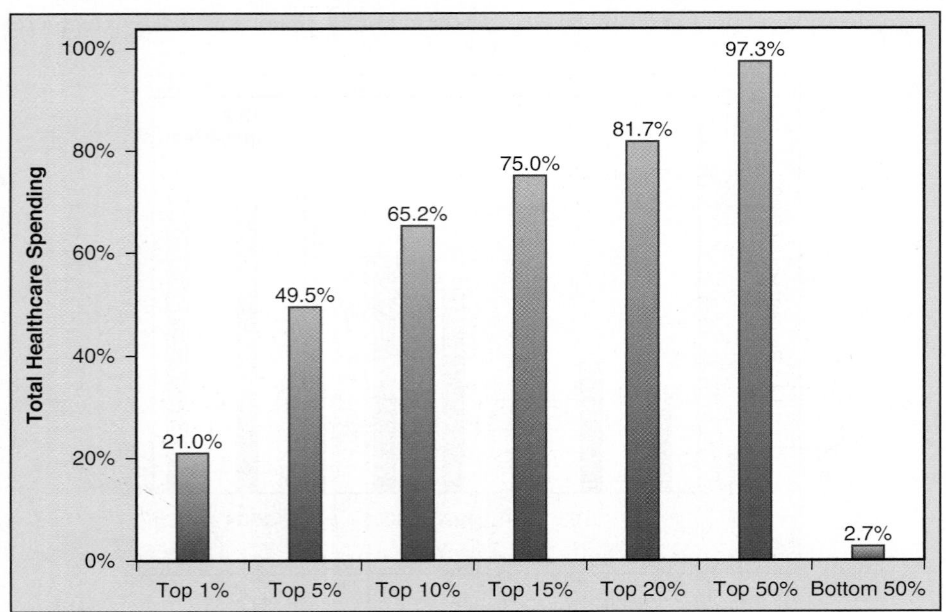

FIGURE 29-3 Concentration of healthcare spending in the U.S. population, 2010.

Reproduced from Kaiser Family Foundation using data from U.S. Department of Health and Human Services, Agency for Healthcare Research and Quality, Medical Expenditure Panel Survey (MEPS), Household Component, 2010.

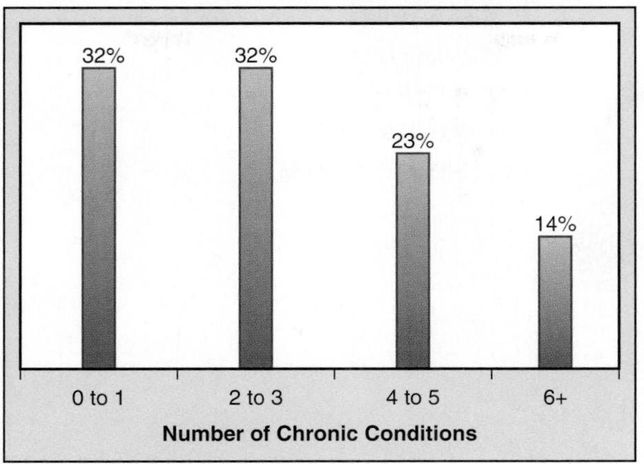

FIGURE 29-4 Percentage of Medicare beneficiaries by number of chronic conditions, 2010.

Reproduced from Centers for Medicare and Medicaid Services. *Chronic Conditions Among Medicare Beneficiaries*, Chartbook, 2012 Edition. Baltimore, MD. 2012. Available at: http://www.cms.gov/Research-Statistics-Data-and-Systems/Statistics-Trends-and-Reports/Chronic-Conditions/Downloads/2012Chartbook.pdf.

approximately $1.7 trillion.[16] Of particular concern is the projection that by 2020 the aging baby boomers will raise the percentage of Americans having multiple chronic conditions to 25%, with associated care costs projected at $1.07 trillion.[4]

Determinants of Health

It is interesting to note that of the four determinants[3] of one's health, lifestyle, which is reflected in an individual's health behaviors, clearly reflects the largest percentage. It accounts for about 50% of an individual's health status (**Figure 29-6**) and is associated with every leading cause of death in the United States. Its impact is even more pronounced when one views the leading causes of death from the perspective of the behavioral causes of death (**Table 29-4**). Of particular note is that tobacco use is at the top of the list, representing 18.1% of total deaths, and that poor diet and physical inactivity is at second position at 16.6%, with a strong likelihood of overtaking tobacco as the leading behavioral cause.[17]

The Epidemiology Triangle

Another view of disease occurrence is a tripartite model known as the epidemiology triangle (**Figure 29-7**).[3] It is truly epidemiologic in nature and consists of the host (genetic makeup, level of immunity, fitness, and personal habits and behaviors), an agent (chemical agents, radiation, tobacco smoke, dietary indiscretions, and nutritional deficiencies), and the environment (sanitation, air pollution, anthro-cultural beliefs, social equity, social norms, and economic status). The three entities obviously interact and disease prevention efforts should focus on a broad approach to mitigate or eliminate risk factors. The U.S. Department of Health and Human Services has published a list of behavioral risks and the percentage of the U.S. population with these

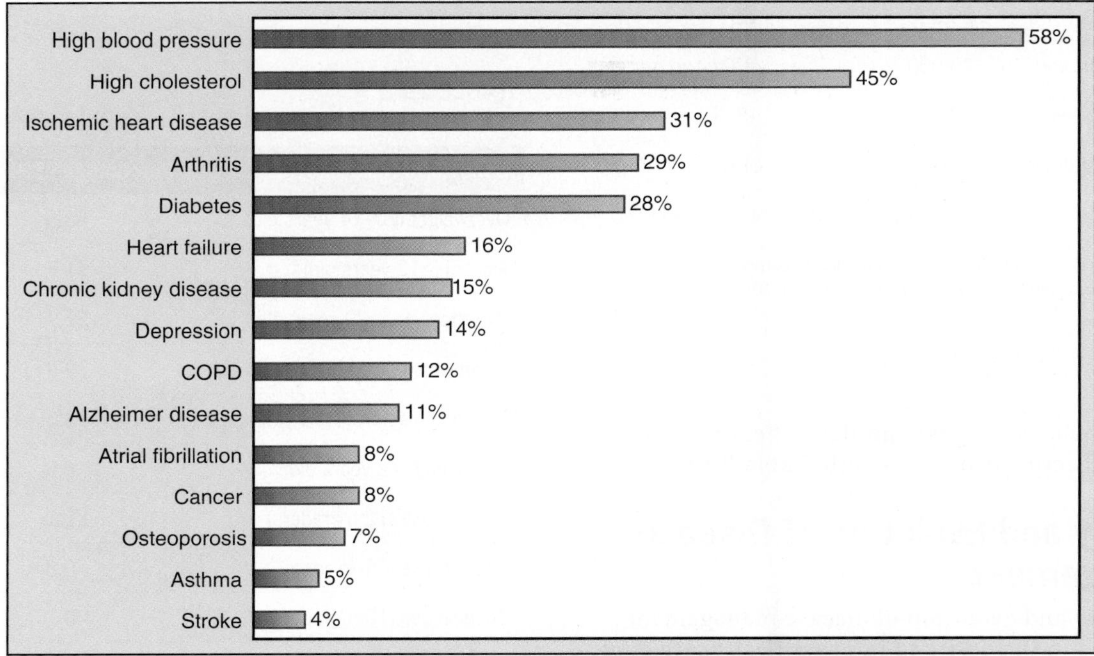

FIGURE 29-5 Common chronic conditions among Medicare beneficiaries, 2010.

Reproduced from Centers for Medicare and Medicaid Services. *Chronic Conditions Among Medicare Beneficiaries*, Chartbook, 2012 Edition. Baltimore, MD. 2012. Available at: http://www.cms.gov/Research-Statistics-Data-and-Systems/Statistics-Trends-and-Reports/Chronic-Conditions/Downloads/2012Chartbook.pdf.

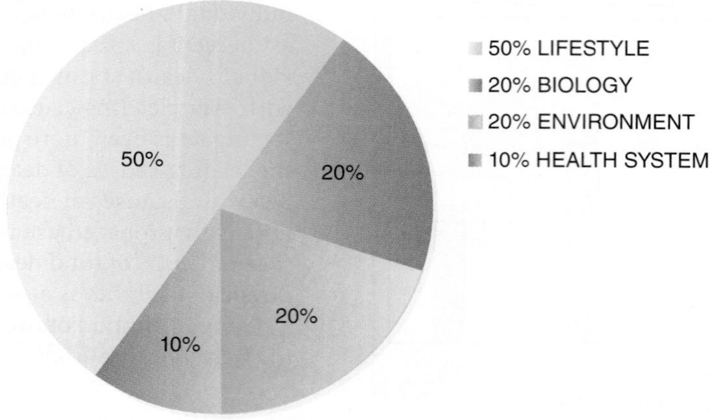

FIGURE 29-6 Determinants of health.
Adapted from Health and Healthcare 2010—Insitute for the Future, CDC, p. 23.

TABLE 29-4
Behavioral Causes of Death in the United States in 2000

Cause	Number of Total Deaths	Percentage of Total Deaths
Tobacco use	435,000	18.1
Diet/activity patterns	400,000	16.6
Alcohol	85,000	5.0
Microbial agents	75,000	3.1
Toxic agents	55,000	2.2
Firearms	29,000	1.2
Sexual behavior	20,000	<1.0
Motor vehicles	43,000	1.8
Illicit use of drugs	17,000	<1.0
Total	1,159,000	Approximately 50

Adapted from Mokdad AH, Marks JS, Stroup DF, Gerberding JL. Actual causes of death in the United States, 2000. *JAMA*. 2004;291(10):1238–1245.

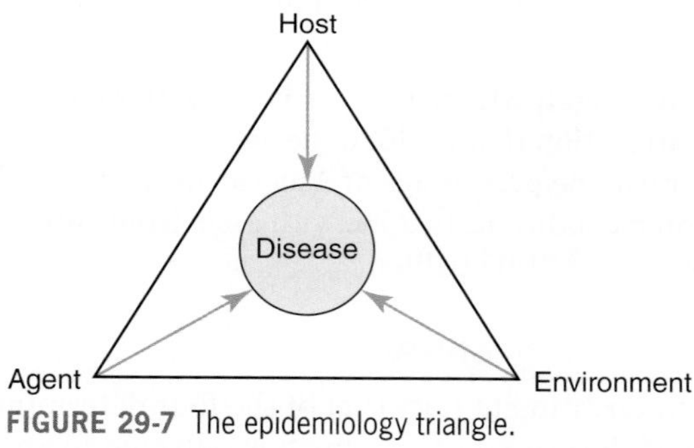

FIGURE 29-7 The epidemiology triangle.

TABLE 29-5
Percentage of U.S. Population with Behavioral Risks

Behavioral Risk (age)	Percentage of Population
Overweight (20–74 years old)	68.5
Alcohol (≥12 years old)	51.8
Hypertension (≥20 years old)	31.9
Cigarette smoking (≥18 years old)	19.0
Serum cholesterol (≥20 years old)	13.6
Marijuana (≥12 years old)	6.9
Cocaine use (12th graders)	1.1
Cocaine use (8th graders)	0.8
Cocaine use (10th graders)	0.7

Information from National Center for Health Statistics. *Health, United States, 2009*. Hyattsville, MD: Department of Health and Human Services; 2010:276, 281, 283, 292, 293, 301.

selected behavioral risks, similar to health determinants and actual causes of death (**Table 29-5**).[18]

History and Evolution of Disease Management

The origin and evolution of disease management are rooted in the desire to improve healthcare quality and contain healthcare costs. Disease management first became popular in 1993 when the Boston

Consulting Group introduced the term in its study of the pharmaceutical industry.[19] Since that time, every healthcare-related group or entity has been involved in some way with the evolution, development, and implementation of disease management (**Table 29-6**). Two groups in particular are considered responsible for spearheading the popularity of disease management: the pharmaceutical industry and managed care organizations. Their goals are to optimize profits, contain healthcare costs, and provide quality patient care.

Pharmaceutical Industry

Large pharmaceutical corporations purchased pharmaceutical benefits companies with the initial intention of capturing market distribution channels for managed care organizations and leveraging resources and contacts to develop state-of-the-art programs to manage the various diseases of these large populations.[20] Although pharmaceutical companies do not provide direct treatment, they do have extensive databases and can use them to influence the industry. Local pharmacies have a distinct advantage: they are strategically placed in the community and have access to the databases of both physicians and patients. This allows them to provide advice, guidance, and support; identify adverse drug interactions; adjust dosages and schedules; employ utilization review; and document compliance through knowledge of the refill and usage patterns of their customers.[21] Disease management provides them with an opportunity to demonstrate how appropriately selected and administered drug and device interventions may result in improved outcomes, patient satisfaction, and financial rewards.

TABLE 29-6
Selected List of Participants in the Disease Management Movement

Parent Group	Specific Organizations
Managed care organizations	Aetna U.S. Healthcare, Group Health Care of Puget Sound
Pharmaceutical firms	Merck, Smith Kline Beecham, Glaxo Wellcome
Integrated delivery systems	Lovelace Health System, Henry Ford Health System, Mayo Clinic
Specialty centers	National Jewish Center for Immunology and Respiratory Diseases, Memorial Sloan Kettering
Academic health centers/ systems	University of Pennsylvania Health System, Johns Hopkins Health System
Multihospital chains	Columbia HCA, Tenet, Intermountain Health Care
Employers and coalitions	Xerox, GTE, Digital, Business Health Care Action Group
Pharmaceutical benefit companies	Medco, PCS, DPS, Caremark, Value Rx
Independent disease management companies	Greenstone Health Care, Stuart Disease Management, AirLogix

Reproduced from Couch JB. *The Physician's Guide to Disease Management.* Gaithersburg, MD: Aspen; 1997:2.

Managed Care Organizations

The impetus for use of disease management programs by managed care organizations came from two sources: the employment benefits consultant community and the employer coalition community. The people who write the request for proposals (employee benefits managers) drive the market. The employer coalition community is bringing enormous numbers of employees to managed care, which serves to shape thought and acceptable standards.[5] Managed care organizations have strong motivation and strong financial incentives to cut resource consumption at all provider sites, and they tend to move aggressively to this end. They are at the forefront of adopting this approach because the shift from discounted fees to a prepaid per-member formula for enrollees drives demand to increase efficiencies, ensuring that providers are uniformly using the most effective procedures, drugs, and supplies.[22]

Disease management has become a way for pharmaceutical firms to sell more products, for managed care organizations to contain costs, and for healthcare professionals (e.g., respiratory therapists) to improve patient outcomes.[21] For disease management to be effective, a partnership must exist between the patient, health plan, and provider.

Population Health Alliance

The Population Health Alliance (PHA),[8] formerly known as the Disease Management Association of America (DMAA) and rebranded as the Care Continuum Alliance (CCA), is an organization representing population health, disease management, and wellness and prevention. It provides its members a fostering, evolving platform on which to share, collaborate, apply and advocate for evidence-guided knowledge, technological advances, and best practices that grow and strengthen population health efforts. It represents a way for its members—employers, providers, insurers, government agencies, advocates, and technologists—to improve the quality of care and reduce avoidable healthcare costs.[8]

BOX 29-1

Core Components of a Disease Management Program

Population identification processes
Evidence-based practice guidelines
Collaborative practice models to include physician and support-service providers
Patient self-management education (may include primary prevention, behavior modification programs, and compliance/surveillance)
Process and outcomes measurement, evaluation, and management
Routine reporting/feedback loop (may include communication with patient, physician, health plan and ancillary providers, and practice profiling)

Reproduced with permission of Care Continuum Alliance. Copyright by Care Continuum Alliance, 2010. http://www.populationhealthalliance.org/research/phm-glossary/d.html.

Core Components of Disease Management

According to Kongstvedt[4] there are six core components of a full-service disease management program (**Box 29-1**). Programs consisting of fewer than these six components are considered disease management support services.

Key Components of Chronic Care Model

Chronic care integrates services and therapies across settings and providers and tailors therapy to the individual needs of the patient. The model consists of six key components schematically addressed in Figure 29-1[12] and listed in **Box 29-2**. Additional detail will be addressed under the heading of Development and Implementation of a Disease Management Program.

BOX 29-2

Key Components of Chronic Care Model

- Community (Resources and Policies)
- Health Systems (Organization of Health Care)
- Self-Management Support
- Delivery System Design
- Decision Support
- Clinical Information Systems

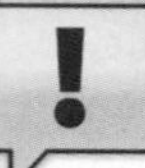

Respiratory Recap

Goals of Disease Management

- Achieve control of episodic cost of care
- Reduce morbidity
- Improve functional status
- Improve patient and physician satisfaction
- Acquire more meaningful outcomes data
- Develop an improved ability to bear financial risk for services

Goals of Disease Management

The goal of disease management is to prevent or delay comorbidities and complications arising from uncontrolled chronic conditions.[3] It is intended to take what was learned in epidemiology and research and incorporate that knowledge into everyday practice, while measuring the results and attempting to make improvements. The plan is never really finished but rather is under continuous quality improvement.[22]

The challenge is to apply a gradation of resources to members of the population in question so that each does not get too little (low quality) or too much (poor cost containment), but just the right amount of resources (high value).[23] In short, disease management attempts to achieve better control of the episodic cost of care, reduce mortality, improve functional status, improve patient and physician satisfaction, acquire meaningful outcomes data (e.g., medication compliance), and develop an improved ability to bear financial risk for services.[4]

Basic Principles of Disease Management

Years ago five underlying principles that characterize disease management were identified. They provide a deeper appreciation of the disease management movement and continue to hold value in today's world. **Box 29-3** lists the five principles and a brief description of each follows.[6]

Natural Course, Causes, and Cost Drivers of Disease

One of the more important principles of disease management is understanding the natural course of the disease, the causes of the disease, and the factors that typically drive costs.[24] The course and causes of most cardiopulmonary disease are fairly predictable and straightforward. Factors that drive the cost of disease may not be obvious. Cost drivers of disease are compliance, prevention, rapid resolution, acute flare-ups, and the 80/20 rule.

BOX 29-3

Principles Characterizing Disease Management

Understanding of the disease's natural course, causes, and cost drivers

Diagnosis and treatment based on the disease process rather than on reimbursement patterns

Patient education and compliance programs for chronic disease management

Management of treatment that cuts across care settings and provides full continuity of care

Directing resources toward the best and most cost-effective treatments and comparing outcomes among plans and treatments

Adapted from Zitter M. Disease management: a new approach to health care. *Med Interface*. 1994;7:70–76.

Tuberculosis is an example of a respiratory disease in which *noncompliance* with long-term pharmacologic management results in ineffective treatment, lack of resolution of the disease process, and risk of exposure and transmission to the public. Patients with tuberculosis typically require a regimen of multiple medications for a prolonged period of time (6 to 12 months). Patients often feel better shortly after initial treatment, however, and stop taking their medications. The result is a lack of eradication of the disease and potentially serious health consequences for the individual and the public. In short, compliance with the care plan results in a significant impact on cost containment.

With regard to *prevention*, many patients with acquired immune deficiency syndrome (AIDS) could have been spared disease by practicing safe sex. In other words, the high cost of treatment could have been prevented if the individuals had engaged in a healthy lifestyle practice. A high percentage of managed care organizations' disease management efforts are focused on treatment rather than prevention. In the future this is likely to shift; efforts will be directed at prevention rather than treatment.[5]

Rapidly resolving the disease or condition curtails healthcare costs. For example, a patient who develops a serious case of pneumonia should receive immediate treatment with antibiotics. Ideally, the invading organism is identified, the appropriate antibiotic ordered, and the patient adheres to the therapeutic care plan. Delays in a patient's seeking medical attention or inaccurate assessment and diagnosis will result in a more serious affliction and a condition that is protracted or sustained. A prolonged illness can result in an increase in the number and intensity of additional services, an increased length of stay, and ultimately increased healthcare costs. Efforts should always be directed at rapidly resolving the disease or condition.

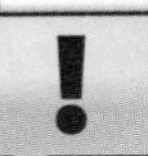

Respiratory Recap

Cost Drivers of Disease

- Compliance
- Prevention
- Rapid resolution
- Acute flare-ups
- The 80/20 rule

Asthma often is characterized by acute exacerbation of the disease. These *acute flare-ups* are preventable by identification of triggers, education on the action and use of medications, and instruction in the proper use of medication delivery devices. Hospitalization and frequent emergency room visits are extremely costly. Efforts directed at curtailing these acute flare-ups result in significant reduction of healthcare costs.

The 80/20 rule indicates that a high percentage of healthcare costs are represented by a relatively small number of conditions. This fact was identified in the introduction of the chapter[2] and using the 80/20 rule—targeting the at-risk population for prevention and treatment—can be an effective and efficient means to control cost drivers.[24]

Diagnosis and Treatment Based on Disease Rather Than Reimbursement Patterns

Fragmentation is a major problem within the healthcare system. The critically important functions of the provision of care and reimbursement for services rendered are fragmented and disharmonious. The provider network made up of physicians and other care providers is interested primarily in quality of care issues, whereas the payer network is concerned almost exclusively with the costs of services and the method and amount of reimbursement. The two seem to be going in different directions. Under a disease management program, the system is integrated and the primary focus is on diagnosing and treating the disease process, with emphasis on preventive measures.

Patient Education and Compliance Programs for Chronic Disease Management

With regard to disease management, strong patient education skills and abilities take on new meaning. A strategy such as motivational interviewing,[25] which is designed to better engage the patient at the bedside, is quite successful. The cost of nonadherence in the United States has been estimated at more than $100 billion each year,[26] and the problem of noncompliance is monumental. Thus, there is a critical need for patient education through scheduled inpatient

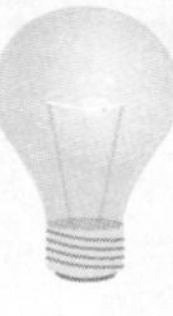

STOP AND THINK

Perform a literature search and investigate the basic components of motivational interviewing. Provide specific examples of how each component applies to respiratory care.

sessions at the bedside, counseling, telephone and mail prompts, home visits, or a combination of these strategies. Disease management programs emphasize and employ many of these measures on a more concerted basis.

Empowering the patient and stressing the importance of self-management of the disease process are emphasized. The patient needs to be more knowledgeable and better informed. In addition, patients must be held accountable for their actions. This often is difficult; however, patient involvement is key because one of the major measures of quality is patient satisfaction.

Management of Treatment Across the Full Continuum of Care

Disease management programs have the ability to coordinate all aspects of care across all elements of the healthcare delivery system and to individualize that care to the specific needs of the patient. Coordinating care across the continuum implies that healthcare settings are no longer confined to the hospital or the physician's office. Delivery settings have proliferated in response to the changing configuration of economic incentives, and disease management programs treat disease in a broader array of settings that include extended care (skilled nursing homes), acute care (hospitals), ambulatory care (physician offices and outpatient clinics), home care (hospice, durable medical equipment, home health visits), outreach (screening, information and referrals, telephone contact), wellness and health promotion (educational and exercise programs, support groups), and housing (assisted living, retirement communities).

Acute care is the most expensive form of care, whereas home care and self-care are significantly cheaper. This is especially true in the critical care areas, in which significant human and technologic resources are expended. In addition, most patients prefer the home care setting because it offers the added advantages of comfort, familiarity, and proximity to the family.

Funding for the Most Powerful Interventions

Disease management entails funding of the most powerful and successful interventions. It calls for physicians to discard their old, autonomous way of making decisions and substitute new group-tested approaches for the treatment of common conditions. It swaps medicine's tradition of independence for "group think."[22] The notion of group think has given rise to the term **evidence-based medicine**, an approach to practice and teaching that integrates pathophysiologic rationale, caregiver experience, and patient preferences with valid and current clinical research evidence.[27] It entails precise definition of the patient problem, proficient searching, and critical appraisal of relevant information from the literature, and subsequent incorporation of that information into medical practice. This prevents common conditions from spiraling out of control and creates a clinical road map for each targeted condition.[22]

Diseases Targeted for Disease Management Programs

A number of diseases and conditions are ideally suited for a disease management program. The Population Health Alliance[8] and the Agency for Healthcare Research and Quality[28] identify the top diseases/conditions as follows: ischemic heart disease, diabetes, chronic obstructive pulmonary disease (COPD), asthma, and heart failure. Many of the cardiorespiratory diseases are considered ideal illnesses for implementation of a disease management intervention.

Development and Implementation of a Disease Management Program

Numerous approaches exist for the development of a disease management program.[18] This chapter addresses four: the work of Ellrodt and colleagues,[27] the work of Lamb and Zazworsky,[29] the work of Kongstvedt,[4] and the chronic care model.[12]

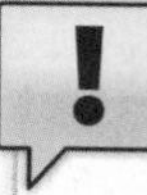

Respiratory Recap

Conditions Targeted for Disease Management: The Big Five

- Ischemic heart disease
- Diabetes
- COPD
- Asthma
- Heart failure

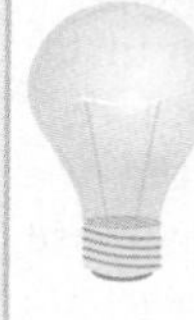

STOP AND THINK

Why do you think the diseases/conditions noted here are ideal for the implementation of disease management?

The Ellrodt and Colleagues Model

The approach suggested by Ellrodt and colleagues is of particular value because it is evidence based and well suited for respiratory care. The Ellrodt model includes the following steps in the development and implementation of a disease management program: a multidisciplinary team of healthcare workers to define the problem; a process to search, select, appraise, and summarize the relevant literature to develop practice guidelines, pathways, and algorithms; implementation of the guidelines, pathways, and algorithms; and development of a method to measure and report process and outcome measures that inform the quality improvement exercise (**Box 29-4**).[27]

The first step taken to create a disease management program in this model is to define the clinical and economic scope of the condition. What is the economic cost to society? How large a population is affected? Which patients should be included in the program? What critical interventions are likely to improve clinical and economic outcomes? What is the problem and what are the realistic goals or desired outcomes of the disease management process? Additionally, team composition is crucial, and involvement of all relevant caregivers should be ensured. Typically, the team includes a physician, a nurse, a respiratory therapist, a financial and actuarial professional, and individuals with marketing and communications expertise.

After the scope is defined and the team assembled, data must be garnered on current practice patterns, patient outcomes, and resource utilization. Ascertaining prevailing practices and accurately measuring the impact of the program is important. At this point in the process, the team needs to develop questions regarding clinical and economic measures related to the condition. In the case of asthma, what medications are appropriate? What modes of medication delivery are most effective? Which medications are most cost-effective? Critical and insightful questions must be asked.

The next step is literature reviews that are systematic, comprehensive, and rigorous. The results of the search require critical appraisal and finally a summary of the findings. The summary should include a description of the design, population, intervention, and outcomes of each study. The conclusions and recommendations are graded to indicate the quality of the evidence. After the summary, the team considers the anticipated benefits, harm, and costs in light of local practice and administrative constraints. In the absence of high-quality research, patient values are considered.

The team then attempts to gain consensus on the results of the effort and to format the findings into practice guidelines. The guidelines should reflect the best scientific evidence (from controlled clinical trials, the medical literature, and outcome-validated databases) concerning which clinical processes have achieved the best results for the best expenditure of resources. The guidelines and protocols should be user friendly and widely disseminated. The practice guidelines are converted to pathways that become timed and sequenced events. Algorithms entail conditional responses and are generally "if–then" statements.

The impact of the effort should be measured and a system of reporting the results determined. Key questions must be addressed. What will be measured? Who will do the measuring? Who will report the findings? How will it be reported? The intention is to compare the actual outcomes measured after the intervention with the original goals.

Another step in the development of a disease management program entails facilitation of the implementation of the guidelines, pathways, and algorithms into clinical practice. The intention is to communicate the intervention (guidelines, pathways, and algorithms) in a manner most likely to change clinical decision making. This step is often underrated. The most important variables are message content, the media for delivery, and feedback. Even the most rigorously validated evidence-based guidelines must be recast into an appropriate format to influence the clinical decision-making behavior of clinicians and patients.

Clinicians prefer to receive short manuals, executive summaries of guideline recommendations, or a synopsis of the supporting evidence and quantification of the expected benefits. Involving respected peers and

BOX 29-4

Steps in the Development and Implementation of a Disease Management Program (Ellrodt Model)

Formulate a clear definition of the disease, its scope, and its impact over time using a multidisciplinary team.

Develop comprehensive baseline information to understand current healthcare delivery and resource utilization.

Generate specific clinical and economic questions and search the literature.

Critically appraise and synthesize the evidence.

Evaluate the benefits, harms, and costs.

Develop evidence-based practice guidelines, clinical pathways, and algorithms.

Create a system for process and outcome measurement and reporting.

Implement the evidence-based guidelines, pathways, and algorithms.

Complete the quality improvement cycle.

opinion leaders is an important consideration used to gain acceptance and compliance; this has proven to be an effective way to change practice patterns.

Steps are essential to ensure compliance with the evidence-based practice guidelines. Compliance can be undermined for a number of reasons. Clinicians may be unaware of the guidelines, they may lack confidence in the recommendations because of controversy or divergence in the literature, or inefficiencies or barriers in the system may preclude their use. Updated literature searches and feedback on outcome measures should be periodically provided.

FAST Approach (Lamb and Zazworsky Model)

A second approach to disease management, known as the FAST approach, was proposed by Lamb and Zazworsky,[29] who identified four components of disease management. The FAST approach is action oriented and based on the assumption that to effectively care for at-risk populations, there must be a system in place for rapid identification, triage, monitoring, and communication.[30] The four components are find, assess, stratify, and treat/train/track.

The first component is to identify high risk, high-volume populations using multiple sources, including service use data, pharmacy data, and easy-access referral forms in physician offices. The second component is to conduct a brief assessment to determine the risk for hospitalization, severe complications of chronic illness, and skilled facility placement. The third component is stratification, in which the disease manager matches patients to clinical interventions according to risk level. The fourth component is to treat, train, and track. The disease manager should determine the appropriate treatment regimens as well as train patients to care for themselves and track the progression or regression of their condition. The FAST approach has been heralded as a systematic, organized, and simple process to follow in the implementation of a disease management program.[30]

Kongstvedt Model

Kongstvedt identified six core components.[4] The first was the population identification process where demographic characteristics, healthcare use, and expenditures are reviewed to identify individuals who could benefit from a disease management program. This was followed by evidence-based practice guidelines, which are based on clinical evidence to ensure consistency in treatment across the targeted population. Collaborative practice models entail the use of multidisciplinary teams, such as physicians, nurses, respiratory therapists, pharmacists, and others as needed to manage the disease or condition. Processes and outcomes, including the use of healthcare services, expenditures, and patient satisfaction surveys, need to be employed to measure the impact of the disease management program. Finally feedback to all parties (physician, patient, and all healthcare providers) must be ensured in order to inform, monitor, and manage effectiveness of care.

The work of Kongstvedt[4] went on to indicate that there are basically two primary delivery options in disease management: in-house programs and outsourced programs. Outsourced programs represent a larger market segment. The essential elements common to most programs are condition prioritization, participant identification, recruitment and engagement, interaction and management, documentation, information technology support, and reporting.

Condition prioritization entails claims analysis and understanding which major diagnostic categories are the largest drivers of claims. Feasibility analysis is performed and entails treatment decisions that are evidence based (the foundation for treatment decisions) and assurance that behavior modification can be accomplished at an acceptable overhead cost. Participants who are symptomatic are preferred because they are considered more motivated to change behaviors.

Participant identification occurs by applying algorithms that identify candidates projected to become high cost. Disease managers screen the resulting candidates, and a plan for intensity of outreach resources is developed. During the past few years, an additional layer of data mining has evolved whereby claim pattern recognition software is applied to scan for gaps in care. Attempts are made to identify whether a patient with a key diagnosis is absent a recommended prescription, not refilling prescriptions, or not visiting a physician in a timely manner. Claims analysis and reporting seek information that is actionable.

Recruitment and engagement occur either through an opt-in model, in which the candidate initiates enrollment, or an opt-out method, in which enrollment is automatic based on an algorithm, but the candidate can decline to participate.

Interaction and management are considered the most important activities of the disease manager. These elements entail a call center professional who interviews patients and motivates them to adhere to their medical regimen. The interaction and management phase can involve calls or mailings to participants or

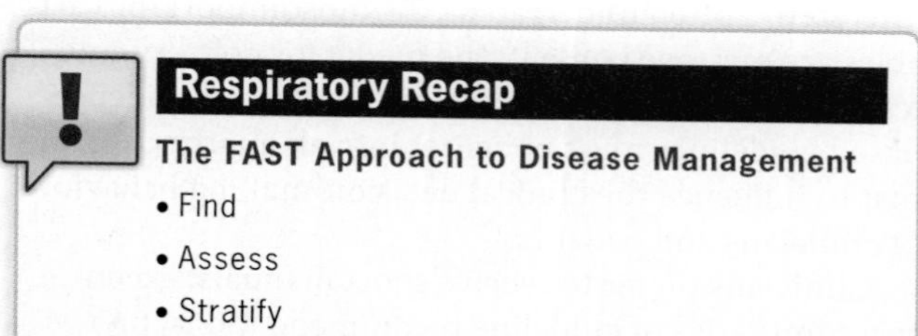

Respiratory Recap

The FAST Approach to Disease Management

- Find
- Assess
- Stratify
- Treat/train/track

BOX 29-5

Essential Elements Common to Most Disease Management Programs

Condition prioritization
Participant identification
Recruitment and engagement
Interaction and management
Documentation
Information technology support
Reporting

physicians, or both. Additionally, it could entail home monitoring and medication adherence technology.

The documentation phase entails documenting each participant's risk stratification and establishing a level of severity to determine call frequency. Information technology support is critical and entails creation of automated care plans, the disease manager's ability to view claim history, and the participants' electronic medical records.

The final phase is reporting, in which disease managers produce fulfillment reports, which include activity and participation (e.g., call frequencies, mailings).

Box 29-5 lists the essential elements common to most disease management programs.

Chronic Care Model or Integrated Care

Three issues were identified by Wagner,[12] who is credited with developing the chronic care model (CCM). They are: (1) primary care offices are set up to respond to acute illnesses rather than anticipate and respond proactively to patients' needs (which is what individuals with chronic illness need), (2) patients with chronic illness are not adequately informed about their conditions and are not supported in the self-care of their conditions beyond the physician's office, and (3) physicians are too busy to educate and support patients with chronic illness to the degree needed for them to stay healthy.[31] The American Thoracic Society developed a workshop report entitled *The Integrated Care of the COPD Patient*,[11] which parallels concepts of the chronic care model and attempts to capture some of these issues. The two models are considered interchangeable. (The reader is referred to Figure 29-1, as a brief description of the six key components addressed below.[12])

Self-management is cited as the first key element of the integrated care model. It consists of three components: education, behavioral support, and motivational support. The points of emphasis are soliciting the patient's active participation and promoting behavioral change. The workgroup suggest that this is accomplished by formulating treatment goals, encouraging patients to experiment with adaptive behaviors, encouraging problem solving and decision making, and promoting self-efficacy (the belief that they can actualize the goals).

The second component is *clinical information systems*. There are a number of challenges related to clinical information systems, and among them are identifying the population for proactive care, facilitating the plan, sharing information with the patient and the care team, providing timely reminders to the patient and provider, and measuring performance. The electronic medical record, call centers, and telemedicine have been particularly useful in facilitating the flow of information and overcoming the challenges.

The third component is *delivery system design*. It entails defining roles and distributing tasks among the care team, use of planned interactions to support evidence-based care, providing case management for more complex cases, ensuring follow-up by the care team, and giving care tailored to the patient's needs and abilities.

The fourth component is decision support, which consists of embedding and sharing evidence-based clinical practice guidelines; use of proven education strategies and techniques; and integrating specialist expertise and primary care. The workgroup indicated that evidence-based clinical practice guidelines were a critical component but had limitations in that most COPD patients had comorbidities and that guidelines did not always address multiple patient needs.

The final two components are health organizations and community resources. Health organizations can be national, state, or local organizations, such as the American Association for Respiratory Care (AARC), American Thoracic Society (ATS), and state lung association or a community "Better Breathers Club." Most patients are not aware of the vast number of such groups and yet they can be extremely valuable as a source of information as well as a support group.[11,12]

Respiratory Protocols

The value and importance of evidence-based medicine (EBM) in the planning, development, and implementation of a disease management program is well documented. Virtually every model addresses the criticality of EBM or practice guidelines that are scientifically proven and the accepted standard of care. Their role in medicine is well established and will be the topic of a single dedicated chapter at the end of this text. A variation or related component of this theme, however, is the

Respiratory Recap

Respiratory Protocols

- Respiratory protocols are defined as guidelines, usually written in algorithmic form, for providing respiratory care services.

current desire and emphasis placed on respiratory care departments to implement protocols as a medical standard in routine daily practice.

Respiratory protocols are defined as guidelines, usually written in algorithmic form, for providing respiratory care services.[32] Interest and need for respiratory care protocols grew from the misallocation of respiratory care services and the need to lower healthcare cost while maintaining high quality care. Their origin dates back to 1981 when Nielsen-Tietsort et al.[33] proposed "a new therapy delivery system: the Respiratory Care Protocol." In a landmark study in 1986, Zibrak et al.[34] reported that implementing protocols resulted in marked reductions in all categories of respiratory therapy. Since that time countless studies have been performed with compelling results reflecting value in implementing protocols for numerous respiratory therapy modalities. Misallocation and inappropriate care have been one of the major drivers of protocol development, with misallocation occurring in the overordering as well as the underordering of services. The AARC sees value in protocols and developed a Position Statement on Respiratory Therapy Protocols indicating their use to initiate or modify a patient care plan following a predetermined and structured set of physician orders.[35] Included should be instructions or interventions in which the respiratory therapist is allowed to initiate, discontinue, refine, transition, or restart therapy as the patient's condition dictates. They reiterated the need for the protocols to be based on scientific evidence and included guidelines and options at decision points along with clearly stated outcome objectives. The AARC strongly endorses and recommends that protocols be used by the respiratory therapist as the standard of care for providing respiratory therapy services under qualified medical direction.

The Future of Disease Management

Disease management will continue to play a central role in healthcare delivery of the future. Under the Affordable Care Act, however, disease management will likely take on added importance in the areas of health promotion and disease prevention, where more and more wellness programs will evolve. This will trigger interest in the premorbid population, where monitoring of high blood pressure, elevated levels of blood cholesterol, abnormal glucose levels, and decreases in flow rates, etc. will serve as early indicators of disease and trigger preventive measures. Experts speculate that this will create opportunities for healthcare professionals, namely, pharmacists and nonphysician practitioners who are in closest proximity to the patient. The former would be due to the frequency of interaction with the patient and the latter because of the decrease in cost (compared to physicians) but only for certain routine services.[4] Pay for performance to incentivize the physician community will continue as will consumer engagement through health savings accounts. The government's role through Medicare and Medicaid will continue to be substantial, and information technology in the form of metrics will be employed to assess quantitative and qualitative measures. Evidence-based medicine will continue to drive medical decision making, and patient accountability will be encouraged and demanded.

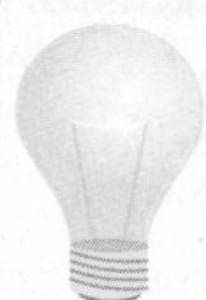

STOP AND THINK

How would you go about creating a protocol for inhaled bronchodilator therapy?

Respiratory Therapists as Disease Managers

The healthcare system will experience a significant increase in the aging population and with it a continuous increase in chronic debilitating disease. Many of these diseases will be cardiopulmonary in nature. Concurrently, the medical school literature projects a serious decline in the number of adult primary care physicians, some 20,000 to 40,000 by 2020. Healthcare needs will rise, supply of PCPs will decline, and opportunities for physician extenders will emerge. Respiratory therapists are bedside specialists in the care and treatment of the patient with cardiopulmonary disease. Their experience and expertise make them the ideal professionals to engage in cardiopulmonary disease management and care coordination. An opportunity exists for them to position themselves for such a role, and they would be wise to embrace the merits of the disease management movement.

Key Points

- A disproportionately small number of individuals consume a large amount of the healthcare budget: the chronically ill.
- The evolving healthcare system is undergoing significant change emphasizing wellness, primary care, outpatient and community settings, managed care, integrated health systems, and a continuum of services.
- Care management is an umbrella term for component management, demand management, case management, and disease management.
- Component management is episodic, uncoordinated, and focuses on treatment versus prevention.
- Tools of demand management are patient-driven protocols, clinical pathways, case management, and disease management.
- Case management focuses on an individual patient and is expensive.
- Disease management focuses on subpopulations of patients and emphasizes coordinated

comprehensive care along the continuum of disease and across healthcare delivery systems.

- Two major forces driving disease management are escalating healthcare costs and the changing patterns of cardiopulmonary diseases.
- Lifestyle is the dominant determinant of healthcare status.
- The origin and evolution of the disease management movement are rooted in the pharmaceutical industry and managed care organizations.
- Core components of disease management are: population identification, evidence-based practice guidelines, collaborative models, self-management and education, and process and outcomes measurements.
- Key components of the chronic care model are: self-management support, clinical information systems, delivery system design, decision support, healthcare organizations, and community services.
- The challenge of disease management is to apply a gradation of resources to members of the population so that each does not get too little (low quality) or too much (high cost), but just the right (high quality) amount of care.
- The basic principles of disease management include an understanding of the course, cause, and cost drivers of a disease; diagnoses and treatment based on the disease process; emphasis on patient education and compliance for chronic disease management; management across care settings with full continuity of care; and direction of resources to proven methodologies.
- The cost drivers of a disease are compliance, prevention, rapid resolution, acute flare-ups, and the fact that 80% of the costs are produced by 20% of diseases.
- Disease management programs entail assembly of a multidisciplinary team to define the problem, an extensive search of the literature, development of guidelines and protocols, implementation of the guidelines and protocols, and assessment of the process and outcomes measures.
- Considerable opportunities exist for respiratory therapists to serve as physician extenders and employ disease management strategies in their daily practice.

References

1. Centers for Disease Control and Prevention (CDC). *Chronic Conditions among Medicare Beneficiaries, Chartbook, 2012 Edition.* Baltimore, MD: CDC; 2012. Available at: http://www.cms.gov/Research-Statistics-Data-and-Systems/Statistics-Trends-and-Reports/Chronic-Conditions/Downloads/2012Chartbook.pdf. Accessed September 14, 2014.
2. Kaiser Family Foundation using data from U.S. Department of Health and Human Services, Agency for Healthcare Research and Quality, Medical Expenditure Panel Survey (MEPS, Household Component). 2010. *Concentration of Health Care Spending in the U.S. Population, 2010.* March 13, 2013. Available at: http://kff.org/health-costs/slide/concentration-of-health-care-spending-in-the-u-s-population-2010/. Accessed September 14, 2014.
3. Shi L, Singh DA. *Delivering Health Care in America: A Systems Approach.* 6th ed. Burlington, MA: Jones & Bartlett Learning; 2015.
4. Kongstvedt P. *Essentials of Managed Health Care.* 6th ed. Burlington, MA: Jones & Bartlett Learning; 2013.
5. Johnson SK. The state of disease state management. *Case Rev.* 1996;Fall:53–55.
6. Durbin CG. The role of the respiratory care practitioner in the continuum of disease management. *Respir Care.* 1997;42: 159–165.
7. Bunch D. Demand management tools help providers lower costs of care. *AARC Times.* 1996;20:24–27.
8. Population Health Alliance. PHA definition of disease management. Available at: http://www.populationhealthalliance.org.
9. World Health Organization. *The World Health Report 1998: Life in the 21st Century: A Vision of All.* Geneva: World Health Organization; 1998.
10. Mur-Veeman I, Hardy B, Steenbergen M, Wistow G. Development of the integrated care in England and the Netherlands: management across public boundaries. *Health Policy.* 2003;65: 227–241.
11. Nici L, ZuWallack R. An Official ATS Workshop report: the integrated care of the COPD patient. *Proc Am Thorac Soc.* 2012; 9:9–18.
12. Improving Chronic Illness Care. *The Chronic Care Model.* 2006. Available at: http://www.improvingchroniccare.org/index.php?p=Model_Elements&s=18. Accessed September 14, 2014.
13. Centers for Medicare and Medicaid Services, Office of the Actuary, National Health Statistics Group, at http://www.cms.hhs.gov/NationalHealthExpendData/ (see Historical; NHE summary including share of GDP, CY 1960–2010; file nhegdp10.zip). Accessed September 16, 2014.
14. Robert Wood Johnson Foundation. *Chronic Care: Making the Case for Ongoing Care.* 2010. Available at: http://www.rwjf.org/content/dam/farm/reports/reports/2010/rwjf54583. Accessed September 14, 2014.
15. World Health Organization (WHO). *Noncommunicable diseases country profiles.* 2014. Available at: http//www.who.int/nmh/countries/usa_en.pdf?ua=1. Accessed September 14, 2014.
16. Partnership to Fight Chronic Disease. *Almanac of Chronic Disease.* 2009. Available at: http://www.fightchronicdisease.org/resources/almanac-chronic-disease-0. Accessed September 15, 2014.
17. Modak AH, Marks JS, Stroup DF, Gerberding JL. Actual causes of death in the US, 2000. *JAMA.* 2004;291:1238–1245.
18. National Center for Health Statistics. *Health, United States, 2009.* Hyattsville, MD: U.S. Department of Health and Human Services; 2012:276, 281, 283, 292, 293, 301.
19. Boston Consulting Group. *The Changing Environment for Pharmaceuticals.* Boston: Boston Consulting Group; 1993.
20. Couch JB. *The Physician's Guide to Disease Management.* Gaithersburg, MD: Aspen; 1997.
21. Phillips L. Disease management: the next step in managed care depends on information sharing. *J AHIMA.* 1996;67:44–46.
22. Lumsdon K. Disease management: the heat and heartaches of retooling patient care create hard labor. *Hosp Health Networks.* April 5, 1995:34–42.
23. O'Brien K. Asthma management: a new paradigm. *Case Rev.* March/April 1998:16, 18, 59, 60.
24. Zitter M. Disease management: a new approach to health care. *Med Interface.* August 1994:70–76.
25. Miller WR, Rollnick S, Butler C. *Motivational Interviewing in Health Care: Helping Patients Change Behavior.* New York: Guilford Press; 2008.
26. Muma RD, Lyons BA. *Patient Education: A Practical Approach.* 2nd ed. Sudbury, MA: Jones & Bartlett Learning; 2012.
27. Ellrodt G, Cook D, Lee J, et al. Evidence-based disease management. *JAMA.* 1997;278:1687.

28. U.S. Department of Health and Human Services. Agency for Healthcare Research and Quality (AHRQ). *Chronic Disease Management Can Reduce Readmissions.* Available at: http://www.innovations.ahrq.gov/content.aspx?id=3867. Accessed September 15, 2014.
29. Lamb GS, Zazworsky D. Improving outcomes fast: the FAST approach to disease management. *Adv Providers Post-Acute Care.* 2000;3:28–29.
30. Cesta TG. *Survival Strategies for Nurses in Managed Care.* St. Louis: Mosby; 2002:392.
31. Lubkin IM, Larsen PD. *Chronic Illness: Impact and Intervention.* 8th ed. Burlington, MA: Jones & Bartlett Learning; 2013.
32. Modrykamien AM, Stoller JK. The scientific basis for protocol-directed respiratory care. *Respir Care.* 2013;58:1662–1668.
33. Nielsen-Tietsort J, Poole R, Creagh CE, Repsher LE. Respiratory care protocols: an approach to in-hospital respiratory therapy. *Respir Care.* 1981;26:430–436.
34. Zibrak JD, Rossetti P, Wood E. Effect of reductions in respiratory therapy on patient outcomes. *N Engl J Med.* 1986;315:292–295.
35. AARC Position Statement. Respiratory Therapy Protocols. Revised July 2007; reviewed May 2013. Available at: http://www.aarc.org/resources/position_statements/documents/respiratory_therapy_protocols2013.pdf. Accessed September 15, 2014.

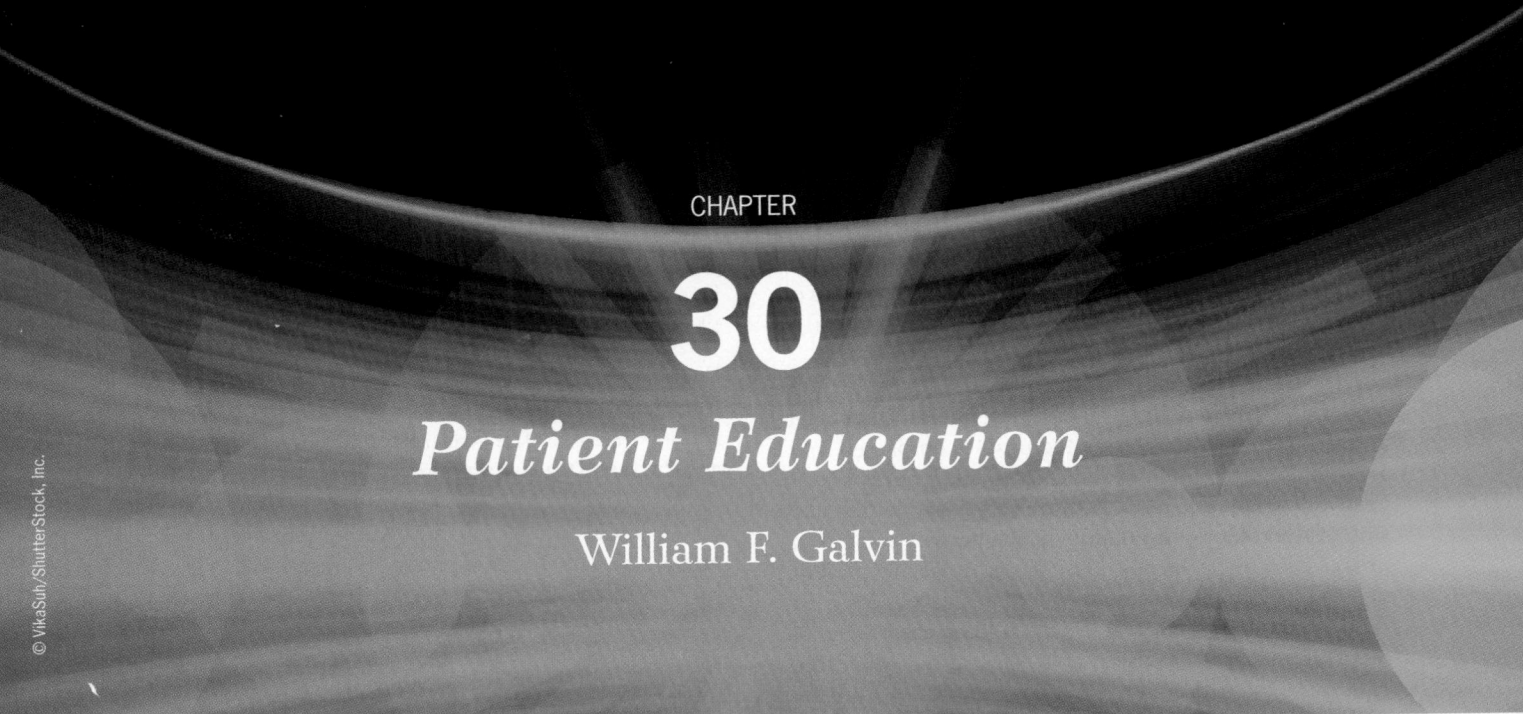

CHAPTER

30

Patient Education

William F. Galvin

OUTLINE

OBJECTIVES

1. State the rationale for patient education in the practice of respiratory care.
2. Define patient education and related terms.
3. Explain the critical role of effective therapeutic communication, to include the basic principles, the factors affecting communication, and the process of communication.
4. Identify and explain the skills of the sender and receiver and questioning techniques employed in communication encounters.
5. List the goals of patient education from the perspective of the patient and the provider.
6. Identify and explain the major components of the patient education process.
7. Assess the learning needs of the patient.
8. Identify the factors that can adversely affect learner readiness.
9. Discuss the planning phase of the patient education process, including the development of goals and objectives, use of learning domains, content development, and evaluation.
10. Identify and explain appropriate use of various teaching strategies in patient education.
11. Identify and discuss the basic principles of adult learning.
12. Discuss the evaluation phase of the patient education process.
13. Explain how patient education can be incorporated into asthma education, pulmonary rehabilitation, and smoking cessation.

KEY TERMS

affective domain
behavioral contracting
behavior modification
channel
clarification
client education
clinical practice guideline
closed-ended question
cognitive domain
compound question
confrontation
consumer education
decoding
dialogue
documentation
emotional filter
encoding
evaluation
facilitation
feedback
health belief model
health promotion
illness/wellness continuum
implementation
kinesics
leading question
locus of control
medium
message
motivation
motivational interviewing (MI)
nonverbal communication
nonverbal cue
open-ended question
paralinguistics
patient education
planning
PRECEDE-PROCEED model
prevention
programmed instruction
proxemics
psychomotor domain
self-instructional
teaching moment
verbal expression
wellness

Introduction

Today's healthcare system is undergoing unprecedented change. At the heart of this change is spiraling healthcare cost and demand for high quality care. While the chapter on healthcare economics addresses in considerable detail the more prominent forces driving our U.S. healthcare system, a more subtle issue central to our healthcare dilemma is the critical need for patients to assume a greater degree of responsibility and accountability for their care. Clearly, self-care has a vital role in any effective healthcare system. In order for this to occur, individuals must be taught about their health.

They must be actively engaged and receive proper and effective education and training about their specific healthcare disease or condition. This chapter addresses the important role that **patient education** holds in the changing and evolving healthcare system. It addresses self-management and empowerment. It provides a rationale for patient education and offers definitions of patient education terminology. It stresses the critical importance of effective therapeutic communication and the basic principles and factors affecting communication. It identifies the skills of the sender and receiver and the various questioning techniques employed in any patient encounter. It also explains the purpose and goals of patient education as well as a detailed discussion of the major components of the patient education process. Emphasis is placed on assessment of a patient's needs, planning for instruction, identification and removal of barriers to teaching and learning, implementing teaching/learning strategies, and acquisition of an understanding of the basic principles of adult learning. The chapter concludes with a brief description of how patient education can be incorporated into asthma education, pulmonary rehabilitation, and smoking cessation.

The Rationale for Patient Education

Self-Management and Self-Empowerment

The traditional view of health care was rather paternalistic, in that the healthcare provider was considered the expert and the only one capable of determining the care and management of the patient. This provider, usually a physician, was considered to know what was best for patients, was solely responsible for making decisions, and rarely shared information with or involved patients in their own care or treatment. Simply stated, the patient was outside the healthcare system and was not involved in the process. The experts controlled patients, by the system.

Although much of the practice of medicine clearly is the responsibility of the healthcare expert, more contemporary thinking supports the idea that there are many stakeholders in the provision of health care. Perhaps the most crucial stakeholders are the patients themselves. Patients must be educated and equipped to assume greater control over their health and well-being. They must come to understand that the healthcare system of the future requires personal responsibility, ownership, and a greater degree of self-empowerment. In short, health care requires self-control rather than other-control.

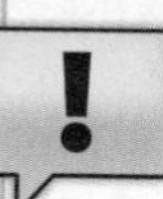

Respiratory Recap

Need for Patient Education

- The healthcare system of the future requires personal responsibility, accountability, ownership, and a greater degree of self-empowerment.
- In short, health care requires a greater degree of self-management.

Forces Affecting the Patient Education Movement

Enabling patients to assume greater responsibility for their healthcare is a theme that has taken on increasing importance over the years. Patient education programs are the fastest-growing component of the healthcare system. All hospitals in the United States have patient education programs and all healthcare institutions engage in some form of patient education activity. The increasing emphasis has been driven by economic, social, demographic, regulatory and legal, philosophic, and practical considerations (**Box 30-1**).

The current system clearly is driven by economic incentives to curtail costs and reduce a healthcare budget that is spiraling out of control. In 2013, healthcare expenditures in the United States represented 18% of the gross domestic product, over $2.9 trillion, and $9216 per person.[1] More and more, costs and risk are being shifted to the consumer and away from employers, insurers, and providers.

BOX 30-1

Rationale for Patient Education in Respiratory Care

Economic incentive: Reimbursement requirements are shifting to an emphasis on greater patient involvement and patient accountability.

Social incentive: The consumer education movement and a well-informed public have demanded such education.

Demographic incentive: Given the graying of America, the number of people requiring health care has risen, and the use of informal caregivers (families and friends) has increased. Decline of primary care physician population represents a strain on the healthcare system and a concomitant need for a physician extender to assume this role.

Regulatory and legal incentives: Patient education is a requirement of the Joint Commission.

Philosophic incentive: The wellness model of health care has become more popular than the traditional healthcare model, and self-management of one's own health has become an important issue.

Practical incentives: Patients prefer to care for themselves, and it is more sensible and easy for them to participate in their own care.

Demographic factors reflect an increasing number of people, namely, those of the baby boom generation, approaching their retirement years, often developing chronic, debilitating diseases that create significant healthcare needs. This places considerable economic tension on a healthcare delivery system that is already strained. The care and treatment of this elderly population will come from a variety of sources, among them informal caregivers, assisted living providers, and unskilled healthcare extenders. These new providers will require a more sophisticated understanding of the conditions and diseases affecting the elderly population. Additionally, data from a number of medical sources reflect grave concerns with the imminent shortage of primary care physicians and the physician community's ability to provide care to the significant number of previously uninsured and underinsured population.[2–4]

From legislative and social perspectives, more emphasis is being placed on consumer education. The public is becoming better informed through Internet sites and is demanding more information about the consequences of unhealthy lifestyle behaviors. Regulatory agencies, such as the Joint Commission, have established policies and requirements for patient education and withhold accreditation for serious neglect of such programs.

From a philosophical and practical view, **health promotion** and disease prevention appear to be logical, cost-effective ways to curtail healthcare costs. Adoption of a health promotion and disease prevention philosophy helps instill in patients some degree of responsibility for and ownership of their health and **wellness**. Assuming individual responsibility for and having a greater degree of involvement in one's own healthcare is simply good medicine. Likewise, increasing the number of well-informed patients and caregivers goes a long way toward improving the efficiency and effectiveness of healthcare in the United States. With these points in mind, it seems only logical that effective patient education should be considered an integral component of the healthcare system.

Role of the Respiratory Therapist

Bedside clinician, astute diagnostician, resourceful technical expert, and troubleshooter are the well-established roles of the respiratory therapist. The more contemporary view includes the roles of patient advocate, care coordinator, counselor, patient navigator, and patient educator.

The role of patient educator has been often de-emphasized, frequently misunderstood, seldom appreciated, and not uncommonly absent from the array of duties and responsibilities of today's respiratory therapist. Patient education is assuming new prominence and will be of paramount importance in future healthcare practice. Healthcare providers with sophisticated teaching skills and a savvy ability to assess patients' educational needs will be held in high esteem. Equally important will be the ability to develop educational goals, communicate accurately and effectively, and ensure that patients have an understanding of their disease and comply with treatment.

Respiratory Recap

Traditional and Contemporary Roles of Respiratory Therapists

Traditional
- Bedside clinician
- Diagnostician
- Technical expert
- Troubleshooter

Contemporary
- Patient advocate
- Care coordinator
- Counselor
- Patient navigator
- Patient educator

Respiratory therapists are considered the nonphysician experts in cardiorespiratory care. Their continual presence at the patient's bedside enables them to assume greater responsibility for effective patient education. Respiratory therapists must recognize that patient education is not a game of show-and-tell. It requires three important attributes: (1) savvy, sophisticated skills and knowledge of the teaching and learning process; (2) an understanding of motivational theory and what makes people tick; and (3) an appreciation of the principles of adult learning. Respiratory therapists must develop a greater appreciation for the significant role they play in the patient education movement.

Terms Associated with Patient Education

Client Education, Consumer Education, and Patient Education

Patient education is more than providing information about a disease or condition. It also is more than simple identification of common signs and symptoms and explanations of therapeutic interventions. Patient education is a process with succinct, discrete steps that must be followed to engage the patient effectively in the important function of self-management. Before describing this process, clarification of terminology is needed.

Two terms that are frequently associated with patient education are *client education* and *consumer education.* **Client education** is defined as the use of the educational process for individuals who are partners in the health education effort.[5] Inherent in this definition is the notion that the teacher and learner work together to identify the issues to be taught and the manner in which the teaching is to be carried out. The term implies that the learner has some degree of autonomy and is self-directed.

The term **consumer education** is closely related to client education but differs in that it involves a person or a group of people who are independent decision makers; they identify the health learning need and initiate the learning process. The teacher facilitates the learning process.[5]

Patient education has been defined in a number of ways with authors emphasizing or highlighting different components of their definitions. For example, one author defines it as the use of the educational process to aid individuals, their families, and other significant persons when they become dependent on the healthcare system for diagnosis, treatment, or rehabilitation.[5]

The three terms can be distinguished on the basis of the amount of teaching assistance *(level of dependence)* that learners require to make behavioral changes. In the case of consumer education, there is a relatively high level of *independence* and the learner is capable of exercising considerable self-responsibility, whereas patients are more *dependent* and require more teaching assistance; clients fall somewhere in between.

In both consumer and client education, the healthcare provider or professional serves as a facilitator, assists in decision making, acts as a resource person, and gives encouragement and support to ideas the individual already has. In patient education, the learner is highly dependent on the healthcare provider or professional and frequently has little if any knowledge of the content to be learned. In such situations the healthcare provider or professional may well need to direct the teaching process almost entirely.

Illness/Wellness Continuum

Another expression associated with patient education is the **illness/wellness continuum** proposed by Travis and Ryan.[6] In this model, health is viewed both from a medical perspective and a wellness perspective (**Figure 30-1**). The left side of the continuum represents the traditional medical model of health (illness or treatment paradigm); it starts at the neutral point, the center of the continuum. The neutral point represents the absence of any physical disease and at this point the individual is considered healthy. On moving to the left, the individual is exposed to certain risks, which can become signs and symptoms. If left untreated, they lead to disability and eventually to premature death.

The entire continuum reflects a wellness model of health. It signifies that health is more than the absence of disease; rather, it is a state of high-level wellness over which the individual has considerable control. The person can choose to follow a lifestyle that incorporates health promotion and disease prevention principles and measures. The individual who adopts the wellness model would become knowledgeable about healthy lifestyle practices, would be sufficiently motivated to incorporate such practices into his or her daily routine, would use **behavior modification** techniques as needed, and ultimately would enjoy a higher level of wellness and well-being.

An example from respiratory disease may help clarify the significance of this continuum. The traditional view of health holds that the absence of disease exists at the neutral point. A man who begins smoking has

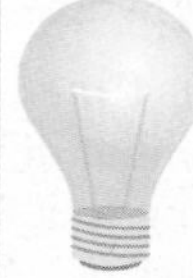

STOP AND THINK

Behavior modification is viewed as a strategy to aid in patient education. What is it? Provide examples of how it can be implemented.

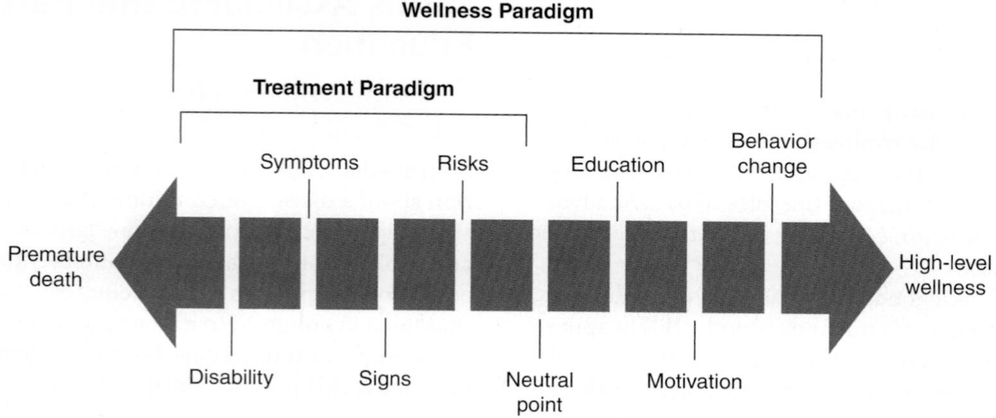

FIGURE 30-1 Illness/wellness continuum.

Adapted with permission from *Illness–Wellness Continuum in Wellness Workbook*. 3rd ed. Travis JW, Ryan RS. (Celestial Arts, 2004). © 1981, 1988, 2004 by John W. Travis. http://www.wellnessworkbook.com.

moved to the left and incurred a *risk* factor for chronic obstructive pulmonary disease (COPD). Continued use of cigarettes could lead to increased production of mucus and shortness of breath (i.e., the *signs and symptoms* of the disease—another move to the left). Continued and unabated use of cigarettes could lead to the man's inability to walk up a single flight of stairs, at which point he becomes a pulmonary cripple, having a *disability,* which is yet another move left. Progression of this process ultimately leads to *premature death.* Rather than living to age 79, the normal life expectancy of men in the United States,[7] this man might die at age 65.

In contrast to this scenario, let's say the individual as a boy or young man is taught *(educated)* that smoking is harmful to his health. If he accepts this and is *motivated* to ban smoking from his lifestyle, or if he did smoke and modified his smoking behavior (*changed behavior*), he will attain a state of well-being and ultimately *high-level wellness.* The critical step in the wellness model is education.

It is vital that patients be educated about their condition and about the ill effects of unhealthy lifestyle behaviors. Effective patient education can go a long way toward effectively engaging the patient in self-management, fostering a healthy lifestyle, and addressing health concerns.

Clinical Practice Guidelines

The American Association for Respiratory Care (AARC) defines patient education through its **clinical practice guideline (CPG 30-1)**.[8] According to the guideline, patient and caregiver training is a process initiated by the healthcare provider to help patients or caregivers acquire knowledge and skills that will help them understand the patient's medical condition and participate in its management. This training process should occur with every encounter.[8]

CLINICAL PRACTICE GUIDELINE 30-1

Providing Patient and Caregiver Training

Indications

- The presence of a patient population with the need to:
  - Increase knowledge and understanding of health status, disease pathophysiology, and therapy
  - Improve skills necessary for safe and effective health care (i.e., inability to perform needed therapy)
  - Foster a positive attitude, stronger motivation, and increase adherence to therapeutic modalities
  - Know the answers to "Ask Me 3": What is my main problem? What do I need to do? Why is it important for me to do this?

Contraindications

- There are no contraindications to patient and caregiver training when a need exists.

Hazards and Complications

- Omission of essential steps in care, inconsistency in information presented, or failure to validate the learning process can lead to untoward results
- Lack of cultural competence, materials in plain language, and information appropriate to the language needs of the patient and/or caregiver (including languages other than English and American sign language), which result in less than desirable outcomes
- Lack of trust by the patient, family, or care provider of the medical team, institution, or individual instructor

Limitations

- Patient limitations:
  - Lack of motivation or interest in acquiring knowledge or skills
  - Impairment (e.g., in hearing or vision; poor dexterity; decreased energy, strength, or stamina; learning defects; age-specific; pain; medication adverse effects)
  - Inability to comprehend or lack of awareness due to factors such as anxiety, depression, hypoxemia, or substance abuse, which may include denial
  - Negative response to past educational experiences or encounters
  - Lack of health literacy, despite level of education completed, which may include functional illiteracy in dealing with the healthcare process

(continues)

Clinical Practice Guideline 30-1 *(continued)*

  - A mind-set that leads to misapplication, misinterpretation, or rejection of instruction as irrelevant
  - Language that is different than that of the healthcare provider
  - Conflict of religious beliefs and/or cultural practices with material presented or manner in which it is presented
- Healthcare provider limitations:
  - Lack of positive attitude or adaptability
  - Limited understanding of knowledge or skill to be taught
  - Inadequate assessment of patient's need or readiness to learn as well as inability to individualize the instructional approach to the patient, including age-specific needs
  - Multiple patient needs and training goals to be met in the allotted time
  - Inappropriate or inadequate communication skills (e.g., unnecessary use of medical terminology, lack of listening skills)
  - Lack of documentation or discussion with other team members or inconsistency in information presented
  - Inadequate knowledge of cultural or religious practice that may affect educational process, communication, or adherence to the plan of care
  - Inadequate teaching skills of the healthcare provider/respiratory therapist conducting the training
- System limitations:
  - Hospital stay too brief
  - Absence of interdisciplinary cooperation and communication
  - Inconsistency in information provided
  - Failure to coordinate the assistance of family or community-based interpreters
  - Education and training started too late in the discharge planning process
- Psychosocial limitations:
  - Absence of support system
  - Reimbursement issues
- Environmental limitations:
  - Inadequate lighting, poor temperature control, uncomfortable seating, or inadequate space for demonstrations
  - Interruptions, distractions, and noise that interrupt the learning environment
  - Failure to use trained interpreters
- Failure to provide translated vital materials for language groups meeting the numerical threshold
- Poorly chosen resources, including inappropriate reading level and vocabulary

Recommendation

- It is suggested that respiratory therapists take an active role in educating patient, family, and caregivers in the management of their cardiopulmonary disease state.

Modified from AARC clinical practice guideline: providing patient and caregiver training. *Respir Care.* 2010;55:765–769. Reprinted with permission.

Critical Role of Communication in Patient Education

Communication is a complex and dynamic process at the heart of all human interaction. It can take the form of a **dialogue**, involving purposeful, reciprocal, and close or intimate expression between participants. Dialogue is particularly significant and valuable in patient education, in which meaningful communication must occur between therapist and patient. This is in contrast to a monologue, in which one party speaks and dominates the conversation. A monologue can obviously be highly ineffective and limit interaction.

Multidimensional Communication

Communication has a content dimension and a relationship dimension, meaning that any encounter entails the words, language, and information (content dimension), as well as the perceived relationship of one communicant to another (relationship dimension), which involves attitudes, feelings, and emotions.[9] For example, a therapist says to a patient, "Please take this treatment." Those words represent the content dimension and are fairly straightforward, whereas the relationship dimension refers to how the two get along or how they perceive their association. Is the relationship

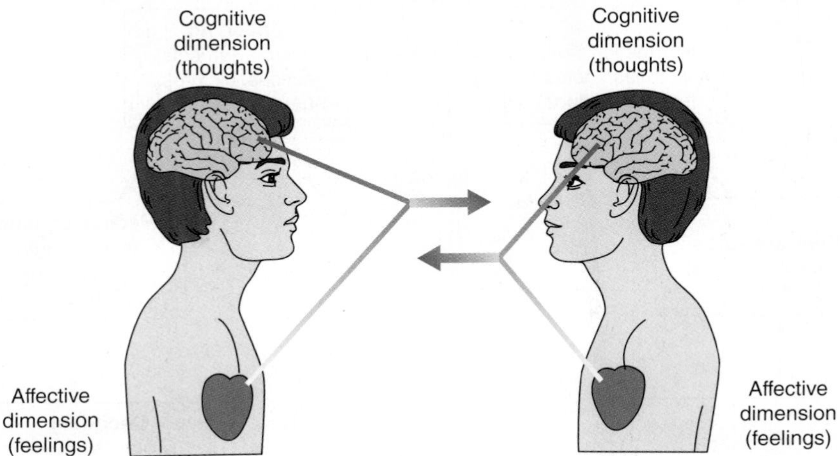

FIGURE 30-2 Cognitive and affective dimensions of communication.
Adapted from Balzer-Riley JW. *Communication in Nursing.* 7th ed. St. Louis: Elsevier; 2013.

one of support, care, concern, compassion, and mutual respect? Or is it strained, distant, hierarchical, directive, contemptuous, or disrespectful?

In addition, communication has a cognitive dimension (thoughts) and an affective dimension (emotions).[9,10] **Figure 30-2** is a graphic view of this phenomenon in which the cognitive dimension (thoughts) is represented by the head and the affective dimension (feelings or emotions) by the heart. Both the relationship dimension and the affective dimension are critical for successful communication. An amicable relationship built on honesty and trust goes a long way toward a patient adhering to suggested treatment regimens.

Transactional Communication

To say the communication is transactional simply means that each party is both a sender and a receiver. A reciprocal relationship, a give and take, exists in which each alternates between these two roles. When senders speak, they also receive **messages** from the listener; likewise, the listener does more than simply receive a message but also sends a message. This constant sending and receiving takes the form of **feedback** and can be done verbally or nonverbally. **Figure 30-3** illustrates a transactional relationship.

The Process of Communication

Communication is a process; meaning it involves separate and distinct components that are essential for successful communication.[9–12] This process can consist of as many as seven components, which are graphically represented in **Figure 30-4** and expressed in the following statement: "The *sender* transmits the *message,* which is *encoded* and sent through the *channel* for *decoding* by the *receiver* who then sends *feedback.*"[12]

The sender, or source, is the person initiating the interaction. In the case of patient education, the sender is the respiratory care educator communicating valuable advice or guidance to a patient or family member. The message consists of the information, facts, data, ideas, thoughts, feelings, or attitude conveyed. It is the content to be communicated. The message is **encoded** in the form of words, symbols, actions, pictures, numbers, or gestures and transmitted through a **channel**, or **medium**, which can be verbal or nonverbal and involves the senses. Messages can be transmitted through sound (speaking and listening), sight (seeing), touch (feeling), smell, and taste. **Decoding** is similar to encoding and entails interpretation of the words, symbols, actions, pictures, numbers, or gestures back into the thought, feeling, or attitude.

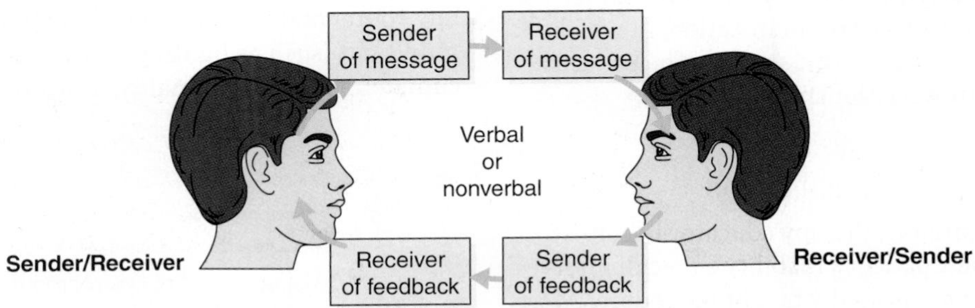

FIGURE 30-3 Transactional dimension of communication.
Adapted from Schuster P. *Communication: The Key to the Therapeutic Relationship.* Philadelphia: F.A. Davis; 2000:5.

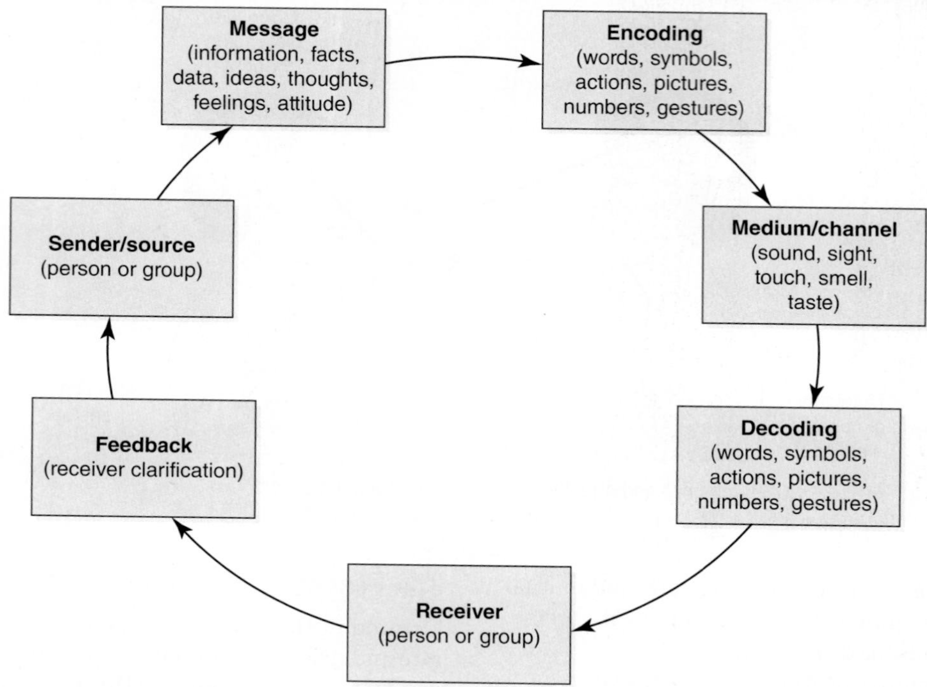

FIGURE 30-4 The communication process.

The receiver is the recipient of the sender's message. The receiver is the patient or family member receiving information, education, or training regarding treatment. Feedback is the final component in the process and occurs when the receiver and sender verify their perception of the message. The receiver encodes a return message either verbally or nonverbally through gestures.

With regard to the medium or channel, the therapist must be aware of the extensive and increasing use of electronic media. Voice mail, email, texting, and other electronic vehicles that offer real and significant advantages in speed and cost are replacing memos, letters, directives, bulletin boards, and other written formats. When using such media, the wise therapist follows the KISS acronym (keep it short and simple). The most important point, however, is to pick and choose the medium most appropriate for the circumstances and situation at hand. *Short* and *simple* do not apply to every type of interaction. Therapists must recognize the importance of face-to-face communication, in which verbal and **nonverbal communication** can help clarify meaning and nurture relationships.

Factors Affecting Communication

Why does the respiratory therapy educator become frustrated with their patient's inability to recall information or perform a repeatedly taught procedure? Why was a message sent not received? The answer is complex and tied to a multitude of factors.[9,10,13] The major categories of factors affecting communication are listed in **Box 30-2** and illustrated in **Figure 30-5**.

BOX 30-2

Major Categories of Factors Affecting Communication

Environmental
Emotional and sensory
Verbal expressions
Nonverbal cues
Internal or intrapersonal
Physical appearance and status

Environmental Factors

Environmental factors can include physical surroundings (such as lighting, noise, temperature, and climate), a sense of formality, a lack of warmth, little

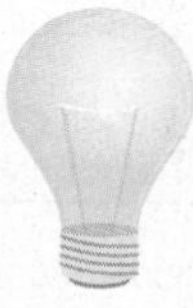

STOP AND THINK

Using the list of environmental factors noted in the text, provide one practical and everyday example for any five of the factors.

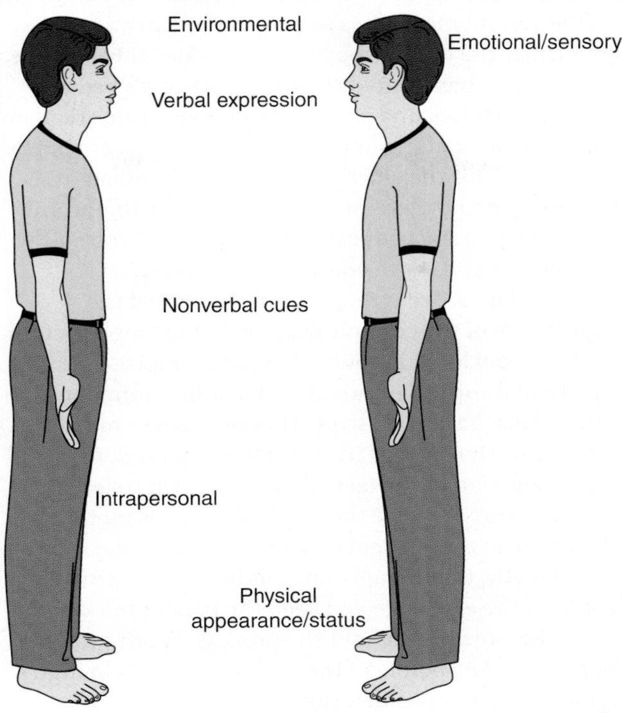

FIGURE 30-5 Factors influencing interpersonal communication.
Adapted from Balzer-Riley JW. *Communication in Nursing*. 4th ed. Mosby; 2000.

privacy, unfamiliarity with the surroundings, feelings of urgency and stress, loss of personal freedom, excessive constraints, uncomfortable distance or spacing between people, overcrowding, and uncomfortable or obstructed seating arrangements.

That environmental issues are significant in setting the stage for effective interaction should be apparent. Respiratory therapists and managers must be astute in identifying such factors and adept in correcting or optimizing them to enhance the relationships among subordinates, peers, and patients.

Emotional and Sensory Factors

A second major category affecting communication is emotional and sensory factors, which can consist of fear, stress, anxiety, and pain, as well as limited or compromised mental acuity, sight, hearing, or speech. The healthcare environment involves considerable stress and anxiety, and patients can exhibit these emotions because of loss of control, frustration, low self-esteem, or feelings of inadequacy. Patients often demonstrate fear for their own well-being or that of their family members. A patient suspecting lung cancer may be so distraught about the thought of imminent death and the inability to care for loved ones that the ability to communicate can be significantly impaired. Elderly patients are particularly susceptible to sensory limitations. The respiratory therapy educator must be vigilant in recognizing these factors and express understanding and empathy to the patient.

Verbal Expressions

A third major category affecting effective communication is **verbal expression**, which involves language, jargon, choice of words or questions, voice tone and quality, and feedback. Language is the basis of communication, and words are the tools or symbols for the exchange. For instance, highly technical medical jargon is rarely appropriate for patient–therapist interaction. Although the use of medical jargon has the potential to increase patient confidence and credibility, the loss of information and missed opportunity to build a rapport far outweigh such potential. Medical terms such as *stat*, *prn*, and *NPO*, are rarely understood by the layperson and should be avoided in any patient–therapist interaction.

Nonverbal Cues

Nonverbal cues are defined as a form of communication without words and include messages created through body motion (**kinesics**), the use and interpretation of space (**proxemics**), the use of sounds (**paralinguistics**), and touch. Nonverbal communication is powerful but learned. Individuals are not born knowing these cues but develop them through modeling or imitating the actions or gestures of parents and peers. Recognizing and interpreting such messages can be tricky, but nonverbal communication is considered an extremely reliable index of the real meaning of what is being said or communicated, because a person generally is unable to exert as much conscious control over this aspect of behavior.

Intrapersonal Factors

Intrapersonal factors are factors *within* the individual that affect communication. They make up the person's constitution and thus indirectly influence medical choices and decisions, but are not necessarily heard or seen. Intrapersonal factors are present in both the sender and the receiver and can entail developmental stage, language mastery, previous experiences, attitudes, values, cultural heritage, religious beliefs, convictions, preoccupations, feelings, interest, and relative state of health.

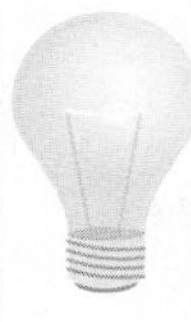

STOP AND THINK

Perform a literature search and identify three or four distance zones. Provide a brief explanation of each and explain the concept of invading space. What actions should the respiratory therapy educator employ when they invade space?

Physical Appearance and Status

Physical appearance and status involve age, gender, race, body size and shape, body movements, posture, dress, hair, body adornments, body smell, role, position, organizational status and influence, and professionalism.

Communication should always be age-appropriate. In general, the elderly require slower, more deliberate communication, with written materials enlarged and presented in bold print. Sensitivity should be exercised whenever communicating and interacting across genders. Large physical size can convey dominance. Posture and body movement can convey rigidity and being unapproachable or openness and receptiveness. Dress is an especially important point because people generally judge others based on attire. Fair or not, patients and other healthcare professionals do respond more favorably to a positive professional appearance. Therapists are advised to remain well groomed with minimal body adornments. In short, physical appearance and status can have a significant bearing on communication.

Skills of the Sender

To be an effective sender, the therapist should be aware of six simple measures that can enhance this aspect of the communication. The acronym SENDER can help recall the six measures: (1) set the stage, (2) enunciate clearly, (3) notify the receiver of the importance, (4) demand feedback, (5) eliminate the unnecessary, and (6) receiver-orient the message.

Setting the stage simply means that before commencing, the sender should decide what information is desired and decide on a time and an appropriate setting for the interaction. For example, for a patient education session, the intention is to assess learning needs, provide instruction, and evaluate understanding and performance. The choice of time and setting should entail a time free of interruptions and distractions in a quiet, comfortable room furnished with appropriate resources (e.g., blackboard, audiovisual aids, written materials). Such an environment may be the patient's room or a designated conference area.

> **Respiratory Recap**
>
> **Skills of the Sender**
>
> - Set the stage.
> - Enunciate clearly.
> - Notify the receiver of the importance of the message.
> - Demand feedback.
> - Eliminate the unnecessary.
> - Receiver-orient the message.

The second measure is to enunciate clearly. Frequently the therapist educator is under considerable pressure and has limited time at the patient's bedside. Avoiding fast talk and garbled, inaudible, or inarticulate speech is particularly important. This issue is especially problematic for the elderly, who may need added time to absorb and process information. Equally important is that the therapist educator does not speak too softly; he or she should try to energize the delivery.

A third measure is to notify the patient of the importance of the communication. For example, before a patient education session, the wise therapist educator would inform the patient of his or her imminent hospital discharge and stress that the patient must self-administer the pMDI thereafter. This statement is a strong motivating factor for the patient to learn the procedure, and the therapist educator is more likely to gain that patient's attention and cooperation. Additionally, the therapist may indicate the estimated length of the exchange and keep the patient informed about the time throughout the process. Finally, a summary of the key points of the exchange may help highlight important considerations.

Soliciting feedback also facilitates communication. The therapist educator may open the dialogue with a general statement inviting the patient to stop the instruction at any point with a question or concern. Periodic queries about whether the patient understands can help. Requiring a return demonstration from patients is an extremely effective way to obtain assurance of mastery and secure feedback.

The fifth measure is to eliminate the unnecessary. Research has found that most people use 30% more words than necessary. The therapist should be as clear and concise as possible, and when in doubt, should say something and wait for feedback. Further information can always be provided as needed. The acronym KISS is appropriate—keep it short and simple.

Finally, the therapist educator should orient the message for the patient. The therapist educator's focus should not be *me* but *we*. This focus helps instill an attitude of collaboration rather than one of superiority and authority. Whenever possible, information should be *shared* rather than *told*.

Skills of the Receiver

At one time or another every person has walked away from a conversation only to say, "I have no idea what was just said." The volume and tone of the sender were more than adequate, so the message was heard. The problem was not hearing, but listening. Hearing is a physical act that acknowledges sound, whereas listening is an intellectual and emotional act that includes understanding and requires active involvement. The five skills of active listening are: (1) listen to the content, (2) listen to the intent, (3) assess the sender's nonverbal communication, (4) monitor nonverbal communication and

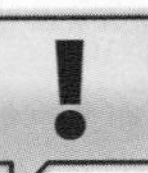

Respiratory Recap

Skills of the Receiver

- Listen to the content.
- Listen to the intent.
- Assess the sender's nonverbal communication.
- Monitor personal nonverbal communication and emotional filters.
- Listen without judgment and with empathy.

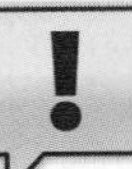

Respiratory Recap

Questioning Strategies and Techniques

- Closed-ended questions
- Open-ended questions
- Clarification
- Leading questions
- Compound questions
- Facilitation
- Confrontation
- Silence
- Support and reassurance

emotional filters, and (5) listen without judgment and with empathy.

Listening to the content means giving full attention to the speaker. A listener should eliminate internal and external distractions and, if needed, be prepared to take notes and physically move closer to the sender.

Listening to the intent means attempting to hear the whole message, not just what is implied. The intent includes the content, the nonverbal cues, the sender's background and biases, and any other factors that affect the issue at hand. Listening to the intent means listening to *why* the patient says something rather than just *what* is being said.

Assessing the sender's nonverbal communication involves body language and tone of voice and represents more than 90% of the message. Nonverbal elements also represent the *how* rather than the *what* and are considered a true reflection of the sender's innermost thoughts.

Skillful listeners monitor their own nonverbal cues and control their **emotional filters**, meaning simply that just as the sender sends nonverbal messages, so does the receiver. The receiver's messages may be supportive and encouraging, such as, "Yeah, I follow you; go on" or just the opposite, such as, "Yeah, right (*sarcasm*); no way that could be true." With emotional filters, both the sender and the receiver have a particular mind-set developed over years, consisting of personal biases, experiences, and expectations. The listener should check emotional filters and not allow them to interfere with listening to the whole message.

Empathetic listening simply means the return of feedback that reflects care about the receiver and the importance of that individual's message. Being nonjudgmental means being open-minded and not entering a situation with one's mind already decided. In essence, the listener reflects on the whole message and at the same time says, "I am here for you."

Questioning Techniques

Questioning techniques are a powerful way to obtain information, clarify uncertainties, facilitate learning, and resolve conflicts. Some of the more important questioning strategies and techniques used by the respiratory therapy educator are closed-ended questions, open-ended questions, clarification, leading questions, compound questions, facilitation, confrontation, silence, and support or reassurance.[9,10]

Closed-ended questions help obtain specific information, yield a limited number of possible answers, and generally can be answered with a simple *yes* or *no*. Although they are valuable in certain focused questioning sessions, in general they have limited value during the initial patient interview or assessment.

Open-ended questions are considered the most valuable form of questioning during the initial patient assessment. They yield the broadest amount of information and allow for more freedom of response. They generally involve short probes followed by periods of silence in which the interviewee is permitted more in-depth and personal responses. Such questions almost always begin with the words *what*, *why*, or *how*. Examples include "What brings you to the hospital?" or "How do you use your inhaler?" or "Tell me about your shortness of breath."

Clarification attempts to correct ambiguity and clear up the meaning of confusing responses. Patients may be asked to elaborate on an ambiguous or uncertain issue. Examples of clarifying questions include "What do you mean by the statement that you have a cold?" or "What exactly do you mean by shortness of breath?"

Leading questions are those phrased so that a predetermined or expected response is inevitable. Such questions reflect the bias of the interviewer and should not be asked because they can produce useless, unreliable, or inaccurate responses. Examples include "You've never smoked, have you?" or "You're feeling better today, aren't you?"

Compound questions ask more than one question at a time and do not allow adequate time for each answer. They are confusing and generally result in a response to the last part of the question only. Examples include "Tell me about yourself. How old are you? Are you married? What do you do for a living?" The interviewee is likely to hear "What do you do for a living?" In short, the interviewee is likely to answer the very last part of the question, which garners the interviewer little information about the other issues.

Facilitation is actually a technique whereby words, postures, or actions encourage more detail. Facilitation is a skill that must be performed with sincerity and genuineness, with examples including "Please go on ..." or "uh huh." Nonverbal actions that display sincerity, genuine interest, and attentiveness can include sitting forward or touching the patient.

Confrontation can be very tricky because the therapist educator would not want to close off communication and yet needs to be honest and bring a patient's behavior or emotional state to that individual's conscious awareness. Examples include "You said your breathing was fine, yet I noticed your respiratory rate was quite high and your breathing is labored."

Silence allows time for reflection and is an effective way for the patient to organize thoughts and feelings. Although silence takes many forms, the therapist educator must learn to deal with the difficulty of prolonged periods of utter stillness as the patient may simply need time to process and think through the information.

Finally, support and reassurance are valuable techniques in questioning. When the therapist educator expresses sensitivity and sincere understanding regarding the patient's reactions that is demonstrating support. The most important aspect of this technique is to be genuine and sincere. Even with sincerity and genuineness, the therapist is still likely to receive a curt rebuttal stating, "You have no idea what I am going through." As difficult as this response may be, a continued display of warmth, hope, dignity, empathy, and reassurance is recommended. Feelings of sympathy are feelings of sorrow *for* someone, whereas empathy describes feelings of sorrow *with* a person, meaning that the empathizer too has had similar experiences.

Teaching and Learning Aspects of Patient Education

Although patient education can be defined in numerous ways, it always entails teaching. Teaching, whether done formally or informally, is a process that facilitates learning. Learning is defined as a change in behavior (knowledge, attitudes, and/or skills) that can be observed or measured and that occurs at any time or in any place as a result of exposure to environmental stimuli.[14] This change in behavior ultimately results in patients living longer and more productively.

Unfortunately, too often healthcare providers think that teaching a patient or family member means telling them about the diagnosis or condition and what can be done about it. Certainly, explaining the facts about a diagnosis or condition is important, but it is not likely by itself to produce a change in the patient's behavior. Furthermore, this type of teaching generally is done hurriedly and at the convenience of the provider, not that of the patient or family members. Often little regard is shown for privacy or comprehension of the subject matter. The provider receives no assurance that learning has occurred.

Patient education should be viewed as an orderly, sequential process, whether done in the formal setting of a classroom or in an informal manner at the bedside. Healthcare educators must rid themselves of the notion that simply informing patients of their disease and the appropriate therapeutic interventions is effective patient education. Effective patient education can occur only when learning has occurred, resulting in a change in the patient's behavior. For learning to occur, teaching must entail a logical set of steps.

Goals in Patient Education

While the goals of patient education may seem obvious, they should be considered from two distinct perspectives—those of the patient or informal caregiver and those of the healthcare professional. The caregiver usually is a person who plays a crucial role in the patient's life; this often is a family member or significant other, although the caregiver may not be legally related to the patient. Important to note is that in most cases caregivers are not healthcare professionals; they usually are laypeople who are genuinely interested in the patient's health and well-being but who may not have a sophisticated understanding of the patient's disease or condition. The healthcare professional, on the other hand, does have an extensive knowledge of the particular health condition and has established some degree of competence in providing health care. The goals of these participants are different.

The goals of the patient and caregiver are to (1) obtain accurate information about the condition, (2) develop the ability to make appropriate health decisions, (3) learn skills and attitudes that foster self-care and appropriate use of health services, and (4) alleviate anxiety and increase satisfaction with health matters and healthcare.[14]

The goals of the healthcare provider or professional are to (1) provide more effective and efficient health care, (2) improve patient compliance, (3) increase the patient's satisfaction with health care, (4) obtain informed consent when necessary, and (5) meet professional practice requirements.[14]

These two sets of goals work together toward the ultimate goal of the patient education process, that is, to equip the patient and caregiver with the knowledge, skills, and attitudes to better understand the patient's condition and to more fully participate in health care. Teaching therefore is intended to foster change in the patient's adaptation to illness; it is a planned activity that is individualized to the learner's abilities, needs, resources, and support systems.[15]

Process of Patient Education

Most resource materials on patient education describe it as a process. And while there are numerous models, two of the more popular will be addressed—the ASSURE model and the APIE model.

Overview of the ASSURE Model

The ASSURE model was originally developed by Heinrich and colleagues and is a variation of the assess, plan, implement, and evaluate (APIE) model that will shortly follow. It includes analysis of the learner; statement of objectives; select, modify, design media and materials; utilize media and materials; require learner performance; and evaluate and revise the learning methods, media, materials, and teacher performance. It is an abbreviated and more simplified model and thus more attractive for the therapist facing a limited timeline and yet looking to maximize effort and benefits of teaching. **Table 30-1** lists the elements of the ASSURE model and some of the key points addressed in each element.[16]

TABLE 30-1
ASSURE Model of Instruction

	Element	Key Points
A	Analyze	• Define audience • Determine needs of learner • Determine characteristics of learner • Determine learning style
S	State objectives	• Outline goals and objectives • Partner with learner to establish goals and objectives • Determine level of mastery
S	Select media and materials	• Determine most appropriate tools • Determine best methodology to employ in facilitating learning
U	Utilize media and materials	• Preview and prepare materials, environment, and patient for teaching • Employ tools
R	Require learner performance	• Determine how performance will be assessed • Have patient demonstrate knowledge gained from teaching
E	Evaluate and Revise	• Evaluate patient's demonstration of learning • Evaluate and (as needed) revise methods, media, and materials employed • Evaluate teacher's performance

Information from Smaldino S, Lowther D, Russell J. *Instructional Technology and Media for Learning*. 10th ed. Upper Saddle River, NJ: Prentice Hall; 2012.

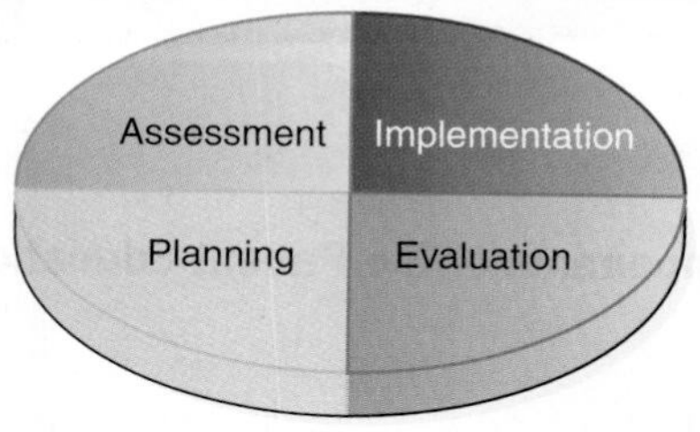

FIGURE 30-6 Major components of the patient education process.

Overview of the APIE Model

The APIE model is an acronym or mnemonic used to better recall the four major elements: assessment, planning, implementation, and evaluation (**Figure 30-6**). It is perhaps the most common and clearly most popular process employed in health practice. Considerable attention will be spent on illustrating each of the four major components.

Assessment is the process of collecting information to help plan and implement teaching activities. The healthcare provider must assess both the need for patient education and the readiness of the patient, or learner, to benefit from it. Assessment requires extensive collection of data, including information about (1) the learner's readiness and ability to learn, (2) the learner's current knowledge of the subject, (3) what the learner wants to know about the subject, (4) any incorrect information or misconceptions the learner may have, and (5) the educational needs of both the learner and the family.[15]

Planning is the next step in the process and involves construction of an individualized patient education program. Planning involves identification of goals, development of objectives, addressing learning domains, and creation, development, and refining of the information to be covered.

Implementation is the third major component. It is the actual process of teaching and requires the use of a variety of teaching methods and tools.

Evaluation, the last of the four major components, enables the teacher to determine whether learning has occurred. It basically is a feedback loop set up by the method of evaluation developed during the planning stage.

Box 30-3 presents a more detailed outline of the four components and specific steps involved in each. The way in which the process is used varies from practitioner to practitioner, and seldom does an orderly, sequential flow come about. In their zeal to jump in and get started, respiratory therapy educators often skip from one component to another. More often than not the assessment component is overlooked, and the educator consequently becomes frustrated and discouraged when obstacles to learning are uncovered later in the process. Gross errors in the practice of patient education occur with some regularity. Errors are frequently

thorough assessment is a valuable tool; omitting this first and crucial step can be catastrophic. A thorough assessment prevents backpedaling during the implementation phase, contributes to the development of an effective action plan, and aids the effort to have patients assume responsibility for their care.

Readiness to Learn

Assessing the patient's readiness to learn can be a bit tricky. Some patients may mask their denial of the need for education and training or their unwillingness to accept it. Other patients may be willing but physically or mentally incapable of learning. The educator's time limitations may compound these problems. Factors that can adversely affect learner readiness are lack of awareness of the diagnosis, previous knowledge and experience of the disease, intellectual ability, motivational level, physical condition, psychological state, and lack of a perceived need to learn. Other experts have identified similar problems of the learner, including lack of readiness, physical obstacles, emotional obstacles, language barriers, and lack of **motivation**.[15]

Patients must always be assessed to determine what they know about their condition. Healthcare educators should not assume that patients understand the nature of their disease. For example, patients with COPD often simply say that they have something wrong with their lungs. They may or may not fully understand the source and extent of their condition. A wise healthcare educator always starts with an open-ended question that allows patients to state what they know about the illness. Such a question might be, "What have you been told about your illness?"

The educator also should question patients closely about any previous knowledge or experience with the illness or condition. The educator might ask, "Did any family members have a similar problem? What do you remember about their experiences? Were they able to work? Were they hospitalized frequently? Were they severely debilitated?" These factors are likely to have influenced the way the patient views the condition and the way in which he or she deals with it.

The respiratory therapy educator also should take into account the patient's intellectual level, which affects the ability to comprehend the illness and determines the teaching approach. A plumber with COPD who needs frequent suctioning might be more responsive if the situation is compared to the clogging of a pipe, with the resultant drainage problem and obstruction of water flow. Asking a family member to breathe through a straw for a minute or so can be quite effective in having that person live the experience of severe bronchoconstriction. Most people do not understand the complicated jargon used to describe medical conditions; therefore, the teaching approach must match the patient's intellectual level.

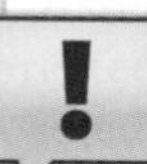

Respiratory Recap

Common Problems of the Learner

- Lack of readiness
- Physical obstacles
- Emotional obstacles
- Language barriers
- Lack of motivation

Health Literacy

Walking into a physician's office or through the doors of the emergency department does not ensure access to health care. For health care to be truly effective, the patient must understand what is being said and must be engaged in his or her care. Until recently, this lack of understanding and disengagement on the part of the patient had gone largely unrecognized. Numerous articles, surveys, reports, and publications have brought attention to this disturbing and alarming problem, however, resulting in a call to action and interest in the topic of health literacy.

Health literacy is the ability to obtain, process, and understand basic health information and services needed to make appropriate healthcare decisions and follow instructions for treatment.[17] The genesis of the health literacy issue dates back to 1993, with the federal government's release of the landmark report *Adult Literacy in America*. This report surveyed approximately 26,000 adults in the United States, asking them to perform tasks such as identifying a particular intersection on a street map, finding an expiration date on a license, or simply demonstrating the ability to sign one's name. Participants were categorized into literacy levels, and the results demonstrated that 49.5% (almost 50%) were either functionally illiterate or marginally illiterate; approximately 90 million Americans were estimated to have limited literacy skills.[18]

A sequel to this survey was performed in 2002 and entitled the National Assessment of Adult Literacy.[19] This survey consisted of approximately 19,000 individuals and was based on a comprehensive set of tasks to measure an individual's ability to read and understand text (prose literacy), interpret numbers (numeracy literacy), and interpret documents (document literacy).

Respiratory Recap

Definition of Health Literacy

- The ability to obtain, process, and understand basic health information and services needed to make appropriate healthcare decisions and follow instructions for treatment.

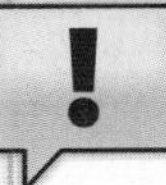

Respiratory Recap

Adult Literacy in America

- This landmark 1993 federal government report demonstrated that 49.5% (almost 50%) of adults in the United States were functionally or marginally illiterate.

The findings were similarly categorized and the results equally alarming, with some 36% of the group categorized at the basic or below basic level and considered by the surveyors to be problematic.

In 2003 the American Medical Association (AMA) and the AMA Foundation released a report entitled *Health Literacy: A Manual for Clinicians.*[20] The results of this report were equally alarming and quite revealing. Of particular note was the identification of risk factors for limited literacy as well as behaviors and responses that may indicate limited literacy, or what the authors call red flags. **Box 30-5** lists the key risk factors for limited literacy, and **Box 30-6** lists the behaviors and responses that indicate limited literacy.

The sequel to this first AMA/AMA Foundation publication was a 2007 publication entitled *Health Literacy and Patient Safety: Help Patients Understand.*[21] This document further substantiated the fact that we need to be more cognizant of the health literacy problem and more vigilant in our interaction with our patients, especially with regard to providing patient education.

The severity and magnitude of the health literacy problem caught the attention of the accreditation and regulatory agencies. In 2007, the Joint Commission published its own white paper, entitled *"What Did the Doctor Say? Improving Health Literacy to Protect Patient Safety."* The paper was considered a call to action for those who influence, develop, or carry out policies that lead the way to resolution of these issues.[22] Additionally, the Commission assembled a roundtable of experts, charging them with framing the issues that underlie the health literacy problem. The findings of these experts culminated in the development of the three recommendations highlighted in **Box 30-7**. The Commission indicated that effective communication is a cornerstone of patient safety and that Commission standards underscore the fundamental right and need for patients to receive information—both orally and written—about their care in a way in which they can understand.[22]

BOX 30-6

Behaviors and Responses That Indicate Limited Literacy

Patient registration forms that are incomplete or inaccurately completed
Frequently missed appointments
Noncompliance with medication regime
Lack of follow-through with test results or referrals to consultants
Aloofness or seeming disinterest
Patient indicates s/he is taking medications but lab tests and/or physiologic parameters do not reflect expected outcomes
Statements such as, "I forgot my glasses. I'll read this when I get home," "I forgot my glasses. Can you read this to me?" or "Let me bring this home so I can discuss it with my children"

Reproduced from Weiss B. *Help Patients Understand: A Manual for Clinicians.* 2nd ed. © 2007 American Medical Association Foundation and American Medical Association.

BOX 30-5

Key Risk Factors for Limited Literacy

Elderly
Low income
Unemployment
Did not finish high school
Minority ethnic group
Recent immigrant to United States who does not speak English
Born in United States but English is second language

Reproduced from Weiss B. *Help Patients Understand: A Manual for Clinicians.* 2nd ed. © 2007 American Medical Association Foundation and American Medical Association.

BOX 30-7

Three Recommendations of the Joint Commission That Underlie the Focus on the Health Literacy Problem

- Make effective communications an organizational priority to protect the safety of patients.
- Address patients' communication needs across the continuum of care.
- Pursue policy changes that promote improved practitioner–patient communications.

Adapted from The Joint Commission. *"What Did the Doctor Say?" Improving Health Literacy to Protect Patient Safety.* Oakbrook Terrace, IL: The Joint Commission; 2007.

Respiratory Recap

Ask Me 3

- What is my main problem?
- What do I need to know?
- Why is it important for me to do this?

A final report of considerable note was the publication *Ask Me 3,* developed by the Partnership for Clear Health Communication.[23] The purpose of the document was to aid physicians and other clinicians in gaining access to information, resources, and practical tools designed to enhance communication between patients and providers. The key point was to encourage patients to understand the answers to three key questions: What is my main problem? What do I need to do? and Why is it important for me to do this?

The literature suggests numerous solutions—some related to the patient, some to the provider, and some to the health literature or information provided. Although all three should be considered, there are six strategies that appear to be most effective in improving interpersonal communication with patients: slow down, use plain or nonmedical language, show or draw pictures, limit the amount of information provided and repeat it, use the teach-back or show-me technique, and create a shame-free environment.[20]

The first suggestion may seem simple; however, it is extremely profound. Slowing down is particularly important because many patients may be overwhelmed concerning their condition and require additional time to not only hear but to comprehend what is being said. Providers often find themselves repeating the same information over and over from patient to patient. This constant repetition can create a situation in which the provider goes on automatic pilot and repeats directives or information much like a recording. Patients' needs may not be met, and true understanding left unsatisfied. The provider simply needs to slow down and be more deliberate in his or her delivery.

The second strategy is to use plain, nonmedical language. This is another one of those simple and yet often overlooked issues. As respiratory therapists, we have our own unique vocabulary—our own language. Terms and language commonly understood between healthcare providers, such as PRN, STAT, QID, and so on, are not typically known or understood by the layperson. Virtually every discipline, whether it be accounting, computer science, or engineering, has its own jargon or discipline-specific terminology. It is imperative that we refrain from using such language when conversing with our patients.

A third strategy entails the use of drawings, pictures, charts, tables, brochures, and even video clips (such as on YouTube) to teach or illustrate a concept, principle, technique, or procedure. The old adage that "a picture is worth a thousand words" is particularly relevant when imparting knowledge, a skill, or a belief. Whereas some individuals may like to read the book, others may like to listen to the audiotape, and still others view the movie. This third strategy speaks to the learning style of the patient, and using multiple-sense learning is clearly more effective than any single-sense strategy.

The fourth strategy is to limit the amount of information provided at any one sitting and to repeat this information, especially the critical elements. It should be obvious that individuals can only absorb so much information at a time. The amount will vary from person to person but nonetheless will be limited to a certain amount. It is best to focus on what patients need to *do* rather than what they need to *know.* Clearly there are concepts that the patient should know; however, it is far more critical that they leave the session being able to perform the necessary tasks or procedures. Practitioners may be well intentioned in their effort to teach virtually every portion of the topic at hand. An extensive knowledge and understanding of the anatomy, physiology, and pathology of the respiratory system is not appropriate for the initial encounter, however. It is far more effective to provide such information in bits and pieces and to spread such a discussion and elaboration over a period of sessions. Additionally, spaced repetition—that is, constant repetition and reinforcement—is extremely effective in imparting a more thorough and comprehensive understanding of the information.

A fifth strategy is the teach-back or show-me technique. This is also known as *return demonstration* and simply means that once the information, technique, or concept is taught, the patient is required to give it back to the therapist educator to confirm the degree of understanding or mastery of the subject at hand. Therapist educators will frequently ask, "Do you understand?" which is often followed by an abrupt or quick transition to the next issue at hand. We seldom take the time to stop, listen, and truly engage in a dialogue that allows for confirmation or assurance of understanding. This technique is frequently employed in our respiratory care programs in the form of competency assessment. Respiratory care programs are mandated to prepare competent respiratory therapists. Program and clinical faculty will often begin by teaching theory, follow this with a show and tell or laboratory demonstration, which is followed by observation, practice, and reinforcement, finally culminating in a summative clinical evaluation or competency assessment. The teach-back or show-me technique entails requiring the patient to demonstrate mastery and can be expressed by statements such as, "I explained and demonstrated the correct way to use your pressurized metered dose inhaler (pMDI). There will obviously be occasions for you to use your pMDI without the aid of the instruction booklet or the presence of your therapist. So, I would like you to show me how to use your pMDI correctly and independently."

An anecdotal story associated with this technique concerns the renowned medical missionary Dr. Albert Schweitzer, who was often described as demanding that his patients repeat back to him the directions, instructions, or advice given by him in the care and management of their condition. Dr. Schweitzer recognized the value of this technique because he often experienced the poor and marginalized patients' unfamiliarity with modern medicine and the critical need for them to self-manage their condition. Simply stated, return demonstration ensures better understanding and greater likelihood of treatment compliance for the low-literate or less educated patient.

The sixth and final strategy is perhaps the most important: it is to create a shame-free environment. Personal experience, as well as documented evidence in the literature, suggests that patients may be ashamed and embarrassed by their lack of understanding of written materials, professional advice, guidance, or direction. Their hidden secret is known by few and may in fact never be shared with anyone, perhaps not even their spouse or family. They may feel stupid and will mask this inadequacy by feigning understanding, providing excuses, or modeling expected behaviors or conformity. The respiratory therapy educator must demonstrate patience, sensitivity, care, and compassion. It is best to use statements such as, "I teach the use of the pMDI to many people and often find that it can be difficult to master. I understand this and want you to know how hard it can be to learn. I want you to feel comfortable in asking me questions about this. I will help you master this procedure."

Simply stated, patients need to know that it is all right not to know something and acceptable to ask questions regardless of how simple or ridiculous the questions may seem. You as the respiratory therapy educator may be the first and only person who truly allowed them to express their feeling of inadequacy. Wouldn't it be morally wrong, callous, and extremely insensitive to say, "Boy, are you stupid" or "I can't believe you don't know how to take a simple breathing treatment"? An insightful quotation hangs in my office that says, "People don't care how much you know, until they know how much you care." It is important that we establish a rapport with our patients. If we are to address the issue of health literacy, we must build a relationship by demonstrating sensitivity, compassion, empathy, and cultivation of trust.

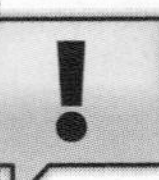

Respiratory Recap

Six Strategies to Improve Interpersonal Communication with Patients

- Slow down
- Use plain, nonmedical language
- Show or draw pictures
- Limit the amount of information provided and repeat it
- Use the teach-back or show-me technique
- Create a shame-free environment

Locus of Control

Educators also should determine whether patients are interested in changing any undesirable behaviors associated with their condition. Are they motivated to learn the best ways to deal with the condition? If so, what provides that motivation? For patients who want to quit smoking, is it because they want to prolong life, save money, live to see their grandchildren, or increase their physical activities (or all of those)? Is their motivation internal or external? Do they feel they have control over their actions, or do they believe they are helpless creatures of society or fate? These questions get at the issue of **locus of control** and reflect whether patients are willing to assume responsibility for their actions.

Many people are of the mind-set that their condition is the result of fate or happenstance. They believe that they are literally at the mercy of others, of the environment, or of the system. These people have an *external locus of control*. They may make little effort to watch their salt intake, for example, because they believe that there is nothing they can do about the condition or believe that they can indulge in an unhealthy practice and simply take a magic pill later to counteract any ill effects. They may not have an interest in preventing the problem or practicing healthy lifestyle behaviors. These individuals simply do not take ownership of their conditions, and they feel that they can do little to influence them. Individuals with an *internal locus of control* believe they can direct their destiny; they therefore are more likely to assume responsibility for their actions and comply with recommended treatments and interventions. This concept obviously is centered on the notion of self-care, and a number of health models deal with the issue.

Health Models

One of the more frequently cited theories of intrinsic motivation is the **health belief model**. This model proposes that **prevention** of disease and the taking of action depends on a person's perception of four issues: the person's level of susceptibility to the condition, the severity of the consequences of developing the condition, the possible benefits of the health action in preventing or reducing susceptibility, and the barriers or costs related to starting or continuing the proposed behavior.

An equally popular health model that deals more with planning and focuses on extrinsic motivation

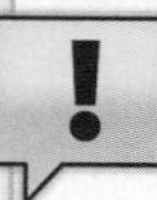

Respiratory Recap

Assessment of Readiness to Learn

- An aroused interest or motivation
- Relevant preparatory training
- Physiologic maturity

is the **PRECEDE-PROCEED model.**[24] The acronym *PRECEDE* stands for predisposing, reinforcing, and enabling constructs in educational/environmental diagnosis and evaluation. *PROCEED* stands for policy, regulatory, and organizational constructs in educational and environmental development. This model, which is widely used in health promotion, focuses on factors external to the individual that shape healthcare behavior.

A person's physical or psychological state also can have a major bearing on readiness to learn. Many patients are simply too sick to engage in any meaningful patient education or training. The respiratory therapy educator may have every good intention to inform, train, and educate, but patients may be too ill to absorb what is being said. They may be in pain, groggy from sedation, or just too weak or too tired. The educator must be adept at recognizing such situations and postpone intervention to a more appropriate time.

A mix of emotions also is likely to be a factor. Such feelings could include anxiety, fear, anger, or depression, or all of these. Given such a state of mind in a patient, attempts to teach may be met with rejection or hostility. The respiratory therapy educator must be astute at recognizing a need to learn. If the patient is unreceptive to the need to learn, any attempt to educate will fail. Simply stated, the patient must *want* to learn.

In short, readiness to learn depends on three major factors: an aroused interest or motivation, relevant preparatory training, and physiologic maturity.[25] Respiratory therapy educators not only must be experts on the subject matter but also must be able to read the patient effectively and follow the subtle cues provided to ensure that the patient learns.

Planning

After assessing the need for patient education and determining the individual's readiness to learn, the respiratory therapy educator can move on to planning, the second phase of the patient education process. Planning involves establishment of goals or learning outcomes and crafting of more specific learning objectives. It also requires an understanding and appropriate use of learning domains, the development of content and subject matter, and preliminary design and development of evaluation strategies. Although evaluation is the final major step in the patient education process, its framework should be developed earlier. The planning phase is an appropriate starting point for this step, and soliciting feedback from the patient and family members during the planning phase ensures harmony among all parties.

Goals

Goals are general statements of the expected outcomes of the teaching and learning process. The expected learning outcomes are tied to the real educational need identified during the assessment phase. The goal statement must center on the learner. Each learning goal should be tailor-made for the individual patient. The patient and family members should participate in the process of goal establishment. This collaboration promotes cooperation and buying in from all parties and is more likely to produce the desired change in behavior that drives the patient education activity. Goals give direction to the teaching and learning process. **Box 30-8** presents an example of a goal.

Objectives

Objectives are stated more specifically than goals and provide more detail; they are smaller steps along the path to goal achievement.

SMART Objectives

A well-written objective can be characterized as SMART: specific, measurable, attainable, relevant, and having timelines. General statements, such as "I will lose weight," are far too vague and should be avoided. Much better is the specification of an actual value, such as "I will lose 10 pounds in 6 months." Measurability is important because it allows the educator to determine whether the objective has been reached, and attainability ensures that the objective is reasonable and possible. Losing 30 pounds in 1 week is hardly likely, let alone healthy or desirable.

BOX 30-8

Example of a Goal

The goal of the National Asthma Education and Prevention Program Expert Panel Report 3 is to help people with asthma control their asthma so that they can be active all day and sleep well at night.

Reproduced from National Heart, Lung, and Blood Institute. *National Asthma Education and Prevention Program: Guidelines for the Diagnosis and Management of Asthma.* Bethesda, MD: National Health Institutes; October 2007. NIH Publication 08-5846.

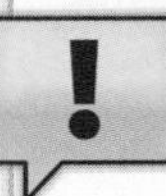

Respiratory Recap

SMART Objectives

- Specific
- Measurable
- Attainable
- Relevant
- Timelines

Relevancy simply means that the objective must relate to the goal. For example, losing weight and quitting smoking are two separate behaviors, even though a person may gain weight after quitting smoking. These are distinct behaviors and should be approached separately.

Timelines are an important part of an objective because they establish closure or an endpoint to the process.

ABCDs of Objectives

In addition to the SMART characteristics noted above, a well-written objective has elements that can be expressed as the ABCDs of objective development (**Table 30-2**).[14] *A* stands for audience and should reflect the "who" in the objective. The audience is the patient, the family member, or the informal caregiver. *B* is the behavior and signifies the "what," or the action to be achieved. An action word (e.g., *list, explain, apply, perform, express*) is the hallmark of this part of the objective. *C* stands for condition, which means any specific condition that must be present or met to complete the objective correctly. This part of the objective might be stated with phrases such as *after gathering the appropriate equipment, after viewing the tape*, or *from the handouts provided*. Conditions also could involve timelines in a phrase such as *at the end of the teaching session* or *by the end of the semester*. *D* stands for degree of performance or accuracy. It states how well the action or task is to be done, with phrases such as *with 100% accuracy, as specified in the policy and procedure manual*, or *identify at least three indications*. **Table 30-3** presents an example of an objective segmented according to the four elements listed.

TABLE 30-2
ABCDs of Objective Development

Acronym Letter	Word	Definition	Meaning
A	Audience	The "who"	Patient, family member, or informal caregiver
B	Behavior	The "what"	Action to be achieved
C	Condition	The "givens"	Any condition that must be present or met for the objective to be completed correctly (possibly also entailing timelines)
D	Degree	How well or by when	Degree to which the action or task must be done

Modified from Boyd M, Graham B, Gleit C, et al. *Teaching in Nursing Practice: A Professional Model*. 3rd ed. Stamford, CT: Appleton & Lange. © 1998. Adapted by permission of Pearson Education, Inc., Upper Saddle River, New Jersey

TABLE 30-3
Use of the ABCDs of Objective Development

Who (A)	What (B)	Under What Condition (C)	How Well or By When (D)
Patrick Everett	Will administer medication in his metered dose inhaler	After correctly assembling the device	By following all steps identified in the patient education packet; taking the medication twice daily

Modified from Boyd M, Graham B, Gleit C, et al. *Teaching in Nursing Practice: A Professional Model*. 3rd ed. Stamford, CT: Appleton & Lange. © 1998. Adapted by permission of Pearson Education, Inc., Upper Saddle River, New Jersey.

Learning Domains

The respiratory therapy educator must be familiar with the three learning domains: cognitive, psychomotor, and affective. The **cognitive domain** involves *knowing*, the **psychomotor domain** involves *doing*, and the **affective domain** involves *feeling*. When planning an individualized patient education program, the educator must consider using learning objectives from each of these three domains to obtain the desired learning outcome.

For example, an asthma education program clearly entails the use of all three domains. In teaching the patient about the signs, symptoms, pathophysiology, mechanism of action of medications, and adverse effects of the asthmatic condition, the respiratory therapy educator might best establish objectives that fall into the cognitive domain, because this is largely information that the patient must *know*.

When teaching the use of a metered dose inhaler, the educator is using the psychomotor domain and therefore should develop objectives that engage the patient in the actual performance of the maneuver; the patient must *do*.

Finally, when a family member is asked to show compassion, patience, or understanding for what the patient

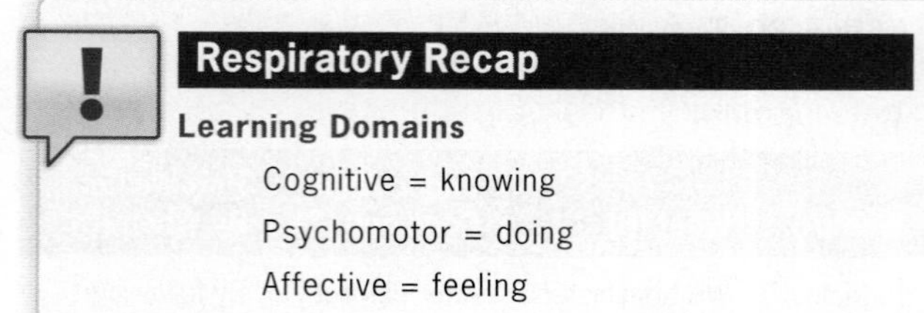

Respiratory Recap

Learning Domains

Cognitive = knowing
Psychomotor = doing
Affective = feeling

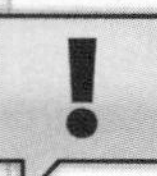

Respiratory Recap

Teaching Strategies for Patient Education

- Lecture
- Modified lecture (guided discussion)
- Demonstration
- Printed materials
- Case studies or simulations
- Role playing
- Problem solving
- Self-instructional materials and programmed instruction
- Drills
- Behavioral contracting

is experiencing, that person is exhibiting an affective quality, expressing *feelings*. Many patient educators are somewhat uncomfortable in dealing with the affective domain because it focuses on values, attitudes, and emotions. Although such issues are difficult to discuss, the key to writing affective objectives is to focus on measurable behaviors. For example, the educator can observe a person placing a hand on the patient's shoulder in an attempt to console and comfort; such a display represents affective behavior and is clearly measurable.

Content and Subject Matter

Obviously, content and subject matter vary according to the topic. A vast amount of material is available on almost every cardiorespiratory condition. The respiratory therapy educator should focus on the goals and objectives already determined and develop the specific content from these points. Programs such as Open Airways,[26] which was developed by the American Lung Association, and those described in the *Guidelines for the Diagnosis and Management of Asthma*,[27] written by a panel of experts under the guidance of the National Institutes of Health, are excellent models that can be used to plan and identify the detailed content of a patient education program.

Implementation

The third phase of the patient education process is implementation. In this phase, the respiratory therapy educator sets the teaching plan into action. The educator should not jump in too quickly; simply providing an explanation of the disease and its treatment does not constitute effective patient education or ensure understanding and compliance. Various teaching and learning strategies should be considered, and sending the message does not ensure reception, let alone understanding or adherence to the treatment plan.

Implementation of a teaching plan requires a dynamic, interactive encounter between the respiratory therapy educator and the patient, family member, or caregiver. Numerous techniques can be used. Some of the more popular ones are the lecture, the modified lecture or guided discussion, the demonstration, use of printed materials, case studies or simulations, role playing, problem solving, self-instructional materials or programmed instruction, drills, and behavioral contracting. Combining techniques can have a synergistic effect that can enhance the learning process.

Teaching Techniques

Lecture

Perhaps the single most popular teaching method is the lecture, which is also referred to as simply "talking to" or "talking at" the patient. The advantages of such an approach are that a considerable amount of material can be presented at one time, the presentation time can be controlled to the minute, many instructors can be used, topics can be specialized, additional questions and discussion can be elicited, and a certain degree of spontaneity and instantaneous modification of the subject matter can occur. Disadvantages include the potential for passivity on the part of the audience or recipient; the need for preparation on the part of the presenter; the need to avoid a lengthy, preachy approach that can result in boredom and resentment; and the risk that the patient simply will not use the information provided. The respiratory therapy educator must be astute in identifying problems and modifying this approach to better engage the patient in the learning process.

Demonstration

Another popular approach is the demonstration. Demonstrations allow the patient both to see and to hear the necessary information. More important, demonstrations allow the patient to engage in more active learning. Information can be provided simultaneously, and discussion and questioning can be enhanced.

Demonstrations can be more time consuming and resource dependent than lectures. They should follow a planned sequence, and dividing the tasks into smaller components generally results in a more successful encounter.

Of considerable importance is the return demonstration, which requires the learner to repeat for the instructor predetermined steps essential to the proper performance of the procedure in question. Demonstration should be followed by practice and skill refinement. Frequent repetition of the procedure, coupled with remediation and feedback, leads to a higher degree of competency.

Printed Materials

The use of printed materials—in the form of books, pamphlets, brochures, or handouts—is an especially effective teaching strategy. The use of such materials is especially valuable when the respiratory therapy educator has a limited amount of time. Printed materials can address a wide variety of topics at a variety of reading levels. They also can serve as reinforcement for other teaching strategies. The limitations of printed materials lie in the reading level and ability of the patient and in their expense, the lack of social contact and interaction between the educator and patient, and the need to evaluate the huge amount of material available.

Case Studies, Role Playing, and Problem Solving

Although used less often, case studies, role playing, and problem solving all have a place in patient education. They generally are effective in urging patients to think critically about problems and situations that could arise because of their condition. These techniques are inexpensive, usually take little time to implement, and require direct interaction with others. **Self-instructional** materials and **programmed instruction** allow patients to learn at their own pace, are helpful in clarifying complex issues, and require little time on the part of the instructor. Many of these materials provide direct feedback and reinforcement of critical information. Their limitations are that they require a motivated, disciplined patient; can be boring; may require resources; and are extremely impersonal.

Drills

Drills are valuable in that they are a quick way to learn sequences of a required skill or procedure, allow for repetition and reinforcement of tasks, and generally break down the specific elements of a task into separate elements. The disadvantages are that they require a high degree of patient cooperation and may require the continual presence of additional resources and equipment.

Behavioral Contracting

Behavioral contracting is a highly accountable technique. It can create a higher level of responsibility and call on the patient's integrity and autonomy. It has an added advantage of identifying expectations up front and creating a strong alliance between patient and instructor. However, some patients might refuse to use this technique or may be reluctant to assume responsibility for behavior change.

Aligning Teaching Strategies and Learning Domains

The respiratory therapy educator should make an effort to identify the teaching strategies that might be more effective for a particular learning domain. For example, if the educator is attempting to teach a cognitive objective, he or she could employ the lecture, group discussion, or printed materials, or a combination of these or other techniques. **Table 30-4** matches the teaching strategy or methodology with the learning domain of the objective. Additionally, it lists general characteristics of the learner's role and the teacher's role as well as the advantages and limitations of these strategies or methodologies.

Common Problems of the Provider

Like patients, educators face obstacles in the teaching and learning process (**Box 30-9**).[15] One of the more important problems, inadequate assessment, can arise for a number of reasons. It may be as simple as a burning desire on the part of educators to jump in and get started without acquainting themselves with patient or family conditions. Clinicians often assume that they know what is best for the patient and what needs to be taught. They fail to individualize the teaching program and to center it on the specific needs of the patient. They may overlook social or environmental issues, such as a broken family or cramped living conditions in the home. They may use poor communication skills or poor observational techniques and miss important information. The value of a thorough, complete assessment cannot be overstated. Vigilance in this first step is essential and goes a long way toward prevention of later problems.

Another problem cited by respiratory therapy educators is the financial limitations imposed by the institution, a form of inadequate support. A number of healthcare administrators and decision makers consider patient education a nonessential or at least less essential healthcare service. The Joint Commission and the consumer movement do not concur, however. Managed care organizations are demanding better patient outcomes. Patient education has been cited as a means to increase patient compliance and to reduce costs, the length of the hospital stay, and the need for

BOX 30-9

Common Problems of the Provider

- Inadequate assessment
- Cost limitations
- Inadequate support
- Time limitations
- Environmental limitations
- Sociocultural differences between teacher and learner
- Inadequate evaluation

TABLE 30-4
General Characteristics of Teaching Strategies or Instructional Methodologies

Method	Domain	Learner Role	Teacher Role	Advantages	Limitations
Lecture	Cognitive	Passive	Presents information	Cost effective Targets large groups	Not individualized
Group discussion	Cognitive Affective	Active—if learner participates	Guides and focuses discussion	Stimulates sharing ideas and emotions	Shy or dominant member High levels of diversity
One-to-one instruction	Cognitive Psychomotor Affective	Active	Presents information and facilities individualized learning	Tailored to individual's needs and goals	Labor intensive Isolates learner
Demonstration	Cognitive	Passive	Models skill or behavior	Preview of exact skill/behavior	Small groups needed to facilitate visualization
Return demonstration	Psychomotor	Active	Individualizes feedback to refine performance	Immediate individual guidance	Labor intensive to view individual performance
Gaming	Cognitive Affective	Active—if learner participates	Oversees pacing Referees Debriefs	Captures learner enthusiasm	Environment too competitive for some learners
Simulation	Cognitive Psychomotor	Active	Designs environment Facilitates process Debriefs	Practice reality in safe setting	Labor intensive Equipment costs
Role playing	Affective	Active	Designs format Debriefs	Develops understanding of others	Exaggeration or underdevelopment of role
Role modeling	Cognitive Affective	Passive	Models skills or behavior	Helps with socialization to role	Requires rapport
Self-instruction	Cognitive Psychomotor	Active	Designs package Gives individual feedback	Self-paced Cost effective Consistent	Procrastination Requires literacy
Computer-assisted instruction	Cognitive	Active	Purchases or designs program Provides individual feedback	Immediate and continuous feedback Private Individualized	Costly to design or purchase Must have hardware
Distance learning	Cognitive	Passive	Presents information Answers questions	Targets learners who are at varying distances from expert	Lack of personal contact Accessibility

more expensive acute care. The Joint Commission has developed standards that require patient education in all healthcare institutions; most institutions designate a department to ensure that the requirements are met. These mandates and the emergence of a savvier healthcare consumer likely will change the perception of patient education in the future and promote more widespread acceptance.

Environmental limitations, sociocultural differences, and inadequate evaluation are related to the educator's ability to function successfully as a teacher. Environmental limitations involve issues such as privacy, room temperature, lighting, noise, and distractions. Privacy can be dealt with if the educator shows sensitivity and awareness. Patients are not likely to share their innermost thoughts without some degree of privacy, confidence, and confidentiality. Sociocultural differences also must be recognized and require a caring, nonjudgmental demeanor on the part of the educator. Inadequate evaluation is always a concern because patient educators must be astute enough in their observations to note nonverbal and verbal cues that indicate the patient does not understand or accept the material.

Perhaps the most frequently cited problem of patient educators is the serious time limitation imposed by the high treatment load expected of healthcare providers. This is a recurrent theme as healthcare administrators are constantly reminding their workforce of the need to do more with less. Direct patient care will always win out over education, but greater appreciation is needed of the value of effective patient teaching. A strong argument can be made that effective patient education is cost effective because a well-informed, motivated patient places fewer demands on the healthcare system, especially emergency room visits. Ultimately, patient education can curtail the use of healthcare services and reduce healthcare costs.

Levels of Patient Education

When the respiratory therapy educator is faced with the problem of time limitations, the teaching plan can be modified according to the three levels of education (**Table 30-5**).[28]

Level 1 education is used in cases in which the educator is informed that the patient is leaving in 2 hours and must be educated about the condition. In such cases the teaching method is limited to literature in the form of a well-written fact sheet. This fact sheet must be written in language understandable to the patient, and the educator must read it in advance so as to circle or highlight key points and address questions before the patient is discharged.

Level 2 education is used when the educator has a few days to accomplish the teaching plan. It involves literature and reinforcement of the written material by some other means, such as a videotape. Educators should preview such material so that they or other members of the healthcare team can highlight key points and follow up with a discussion of the material.

TABLE 30-5
Levels of Patient Education

Level	Time Constraints	Teaching Method
1	Only a few hours available before patient is discharged	Provide literature, fact sheets, and teaching guides and discuss with patient to the extent possible.
2	A few days available for teaching	Provide literature and reinforce with an instructional videotape.
3	A considerable amount of time available for teaching	Use four-step process (assess, plan, implement, and evaluate). Use counseling skills (active listening, coaching, clarifying, summarizing).

Modified with permission from Winthrop E. *Patient Teaching Tips*. St. Louis: Mosby; 1995.

Level 3 education is used when the educator has considerable time for the program. This optimal situation allows for the incorporation of all four major components of the patient education process. Level 3 education includes a counseling role and is more likely to result in a successful intervention.

Principles of Adult Learning

The basic principles of adult learning are important elements of any patient teaching program. Numerous courses, books, and articles have been written on this topic, but a useful and meaningful delineation has been provided by Kroehnert,[29] who uses the mnemonic RAMP-2-FAME to represent nine critical principles of adult learning.

R stands for recency, which means that the principles or concepts taught last are most likely to be remembered best. This stems from human beings' tendency to remember material that was addressed most recently; this also is affected by the order in which material is presented (see information on primacy that follows). The implication for respiratory therapy educators is that they should plant important information in the patient's mind just before leaving the room. Keeping sessions short and summarizing often helps the patient remember essential information.

The second letter in the mnemonic, *A*, stands for appropriateness and signifies that learners engage in the learning process only if the material presented has meaning and relevance for their needs. Explaining the biochemistry of leukotriene inhibitors in the discussion of medication for the treatment of airway obstruction would be inappropriate and futile. Equally inappropriate would be a discussion of detailed respiratory anatomy, such as the pores of Kohn. A more appropriate discussion would be to explain the inflammatory reaction as being similar to sunburn or to describe bronchoconstriction as similar to breathing through a narrow straw. Such everyday examples have more meaning and more relevance. They are more likely to be received favorably.

The *M* stands for motivation. Patients must be moved to take action; they must want to learn. Imparting a sense of urgency or a strong need to learn the subject matter can create this motivation. For example, a parent whose child had recently experienced a serious asthmatic attack while playing soccer would be greatly motivated to learn the correct use of the child's metered dose inhaler. Patient educators must find the motivating factors and employ them in getting the point across and engaging the patient or family member in patient education.

The fourth letter, *P*, stands for primacy, meaning that the information the patient learns first is usually learned best. As with recency, patients are more attentive at both the beginning and end of a presentation, thus there is an emphasis on increased learning at these stages.

Primacy gets at the issue of first impressions and the need to deliver the most important information first. More often than not, the respiratory therapy educator has a receptive audience at the first meeting with the patient because the patient is curious about what the educator has to say. This is a golden opportunity for educators to make their case.

The numeral *2* in the mnemonic signifies the need for two-way communication. The conversation should be *with*, not *at*, the patient. Interaction should be encouraged.

The *F* stands for feedback, which should be given both to the patient and to the educator. People simply need to know how they are doing. Feedback provides the opportunity for both parties to validate their roles and their understanding of the interaction.

The second *A* stands for active learning, which entails participation in the learning process. This point is extremely important because patient passivity progresses to boredom, loss of concentration, and, ultimately, to very little learning.

The second *M* stands for multiple-sense learning, one of the most important points. Whenever another sense is brought into the learning process, the amount of material that will be remembered has been estimated to double. People learn in different ways, and educators should use as many different techniques as possible. Although explaining a procedure to patients may be effective, showing them a picture and letting them touch or handle the equipment adds considerable value to the learning experience; it clearly results in a heightened sense of understanding and ultimately to subject mastery.

The last letter, *E*, is exercise and refers to the value of the educator's repeating the new information over and over to better ensure retention. The repetition of the times tables in elementary school is a classic example of the power of repetition. The more often patients repeat the material, the more likely they are to remember it.

Respiratory Recap

Principles of Adult Learning: RAMP-2-FAME

- Recency
- Appropriateness
- Motivation
- Primacy
- 2-way communication
- Feedback
- Active learning
- Multiple-sense learning
- Exercise

Teaching Principles for Children Through the Elderly

In addition to the adult learning principles, respiratory therapy educators must also recognize the unique learning needs of all age groups (infants and toddlers through older adults). Whereas the teaching/learning process for infants and children will generally require more parental involvement, relatively shorter sessions, and techniques that are more concrete and interactive, the elderly have more sensory deficits and will generally require more involvement in the planning and decision-making process. **Table 30-6** notes age-related considerations across the population.

The Teaching Moment

The respiratory therapy educator must take advantage of the **teaching moment**, that is, any opportunity to impart meaningful information to a captive audience. Such an opportunity likely will occur only after a certain degree of trust, comfort, and mutual respect has been established between patient and educator. It behooves the respiratory therapy educator to establish this relationship as soon as possible and to be prepared to take advantage of teaching moments.

Evaluation

Evaluation, the last major component of the patient education process, involves measurement and **documentation** of the results of the interventions. It is the culmination of all the effort that has been expended throughout the patient–educator interaction. The evaluation component can be divided into two subcategories: process evaluation and evaluation of learning.

Process Evaluation

Process evaluation is a continuous reassessment of the effectiveness of all components of the teaching/learning interaction. Respiratory therapy educators must constantly ask themselves, "Did I gather all the information needed during the assessment phase? Did I achieve my goals and objectives? Was my decision to use a demonstration technique the right one? Did I use appropriate language?" and "Did I progress too quickly?"

Evaluation of Learning

Evaluation of learning requires the respiratory therapy educator to take a step back and look at each component of the teaching/learning interaction individually,

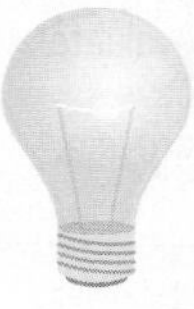

STOP AND THINK

Identify and discuss with your colleagues an example of when you experienced a teachable moment.

TABLE 30-6
Age-Related Considerations in Patient Teaching

Patient's Age	Teaching Considerations
Infant or toddler	Involvement of parents (key players) is important. Parents should be present to alleviate separation anxiety. Educator must establish a relationship with patient and caregiver (trust). Story reading, pictures, and puppets are useful tools. Terminology should be kept simple (concrete, nonthreatening). Familiar surroundings are comforting. Session should be kept short (2 to 5 minutes). Teaching session should be held close to the occurrence of the event. Activity should be incorporated into learning.
Preschool	Child may participate in planning. If possible, a choice between two options should be allowed. A group size of five to eight is best. Physical and visual stimuli are better than verbal stimuli. Neutral, concrete, and action-oriented words should be used whenever possible. A safe, secure environment for learning should be created. Sessions should be kept short (15 minutes or less) and slow paced; the focus should be present oriented. Tangible rewards work well and should be given immediately.
School age	Participation in activities is important. Repetition and summarizing are useful methods. This age group is responsive to modeling and to peer-group and mass-media influence. Decision making is based on simple scientific knowledge of cause and effect. Groups of friends of the same age are important. Safety and security are less important than with preschoolers. Sessions can be longer (15 to 30 minutes). Careful listening is important. This age group can be assisted to move from the concrete (how) to the abstract (why). These children often have misconceptions that may need clarification. Time is needed to clarify, validate, and expand the child's knowledge. Privacy is important. Praise is very effective.
Adolescent	Cognitive abilities allow for greater participation in learning and planning. Patient can begin to process future health implications. Written information is more meaningful and useful. Privacy is also important. Learning can be enhanced by use of group methods. Issues may need to be clarified. Reinforcement through recognition is a valuable motivator.
Adult	Independence in self-care and decision making should be promoted. Actions may be influenced by experience, economics, sociocultural factors, and values. Learning needs should be determined. Readiness to learn should be recognized. Relevancy should be maintained. Connecting to patient's knowledge and experience is important. Analogies can be used for complex ideas. Patient should be involved in planning and decision making.
Older adult	Distinct, large configurations should be used in visual aids. Good lighting and high-contrast colors are helpful. Educator should speak clearly, adjusting the rate and loudness as necessary. Short learning sessions involving a small amount of material work best. Adequate response time should be allowed. Repetition aids learning. Goals should be mutually established and reachable. New learning should be integrated with previously established information. Patient should be encouraged to participate in planning and decision making. Family involvement should be encouraged.

Modified from Boyd M, Graham B, Gleit C, et al. *Teaching in Nursing Practice: A Professional Model.* 3rd ed. Stamford, CT: Appleton & Lange. © 1998. Adapted by permission of Pearson Education, Inc., Upper Saddle River, New Jersey.

1.__ Remove the cap and hold the inhaler upright.
2.__ Shake the inhaler.
3.__ Tilt your head back slightly and breathe out slowly.
4.__ Position the inhaler.
5.__ Press down on the inhaler to release medication as you start to breathe in slowly.
6.__ Breathe in slowly (3 to 5 seconds).
7.__ Hold your breath for 10 seconds to allow the medicine to reach deep into your lungs.
8.__ Repeat puff as directed. Waiting 1 minute between puffs may permit a second puff to penetrate your lungs better.
9.__ Spacers/holding chambers are useful for all patients. They are particularly recommended for young children and older adults and for use with inhaled corticosteroids.

FIGURE 30-8 Example of a teaching checklist for use of a pressurized metered dose inhaler.

Reproduced from U.S. Department of Health and Human Services, National Institutes of Health, National Heart, Lung, and Blood Institute. *Practical Guide for the Diagnosis and Management of Asthma*. Bethesda, MD: National Institutes of Health; 1997. NIH Publication 97-4051.

with a view to corrective intervention and remediation. It often requires educators to ask themselves, "What did the patient learn?" or "How can I enhance teaching or learning?"

Evaluation of the patient's learning involves measurement of the learner's achievement, a task easily performed through rephrasing of the learning objectives as a series of oral questions or as questions on a written test, teaching checklist, or observational checklist that the patient completes. This evaluation must be as objective as possible, and judgments must be determined against an accepted standard. **Figure 30-8** is an example of a teaching checklist used to evaluate a patient's use of an inhaler.[27]

Documentation

Documentation of the patient education process is crucial and serves a number of purposes, including cataloguing the respiratory therapist's involvement in teaching; demonstrating a systematic, planned approach to teaching; serving as a means of communication among healthcare professionals; satisfying legal and regulatory requirements; reflecting patients' levels of understanding or misunderstanding of the subject matter; and providing patients the opportunity to express their responses to the intervention.[5]

Documentation can take many forms. Most institutions use electronic documentation, whereas others use such techniques as anecdotal chart entries, checklists, and standardized forms. An informal survey of a variety of institutions showed that almost all believed that documentation of patient education should be included as part of the patient's permanent record and that such documentation should be interdisciplinary. The following five key components were identified:

1. Date and time of the intervention
2. Initials of the healthcare provider
3. Subject matter or content addressed
4. Method of instruction
5. Response of the learner or the results of the learning

Figure 30-9 shows a sample interdisciplinary patient education/family education record.

For ease of charting, some institutions use a coded checklist. For example, under method of instruction, the educator would check off *E* for explanation, *D* for demonstration, *P* for printed materials, or *V* for video. Under response of the learner, *1* might stand for communicates understanding, *2* for return demonstration provided, *3* for requires reinforcement, *4* for referral indicated, or *5* for refused interaction. Almost all methods of documentation include a section for educator comments, and some have a more elaborate section for factors noted at the initial assessment, such as barriers

Interdisciplinary Patient Education/Family Education Record

Patient's name: ____________________

Date: ____________________ Time of intervention: ____________________

Subject matter/content addressed: ____________________

Method of instruction: ____________________

Response of learner/results of learning: ____________________

Initials/signature of healthcare provider: ____________________

FIGURE 30-9 Sample of an interdisciplinary patient education/family education record.

to learning and the patient's motivational level and learning preferences.

Above all, respiratory therapy educators must be mindful of the need to constantly update and refine their teaching skills. Observation of colleagues, formal training through academic and professional courses and programs, and practice can help the patient educator attain this goal and become a more effective teacher.

Examples of Patient Education Programs

It should be obvious that multiple opportunities for patient education abound within the profession of respiratory care. Three areas of practice are particularly applicable, namely, asthma education, pulmonary rehabilitation, and tobacco cessation. Although some redundancy occurs in the respective sections for these topics, a brief but pointed treatise is provided here as to how patient education can be incorporated within these topical areas.

Asthma Education

Asthma education represents one of the best examples of how respiratory therapists can incorporate their knowledge, skills, and abilities in fulfilling their role as patient educators. The landmark and most authoritative reference for the management of asthma is the NIH report entitled *National Asthma Education and Prevention Program, Expert Panel Report 3: Guidelines for the Diagnosis and Management of Asthma*. Embedded within this document is a detailed account of the four components of care for an asthma disease management program, namely, assessment and monitoring, education, control of environmental factors and comorbid conditions, and medications. **Table 30-7** provides an overview of the four components of care as well as the key clinical activities and action steps identified in the guidelines.[30] The four components addressed in this document are quite similar in design to the four components addressed in previous literature and expressed through the acronym ACME: assess, control, medicate, and educate. Incorporating the principles and concepts of patient education within the area of asthma management entails the theme of "Education for a Partnership in Care."[30]

An asthma education program using these guidelines stresses self-management, development of a written action plan, and the integration of education into all points of care. To be successful, the therapist must follow the educational process. We provide some commentary here on how respiratory therapy educators can incorporate these concepts into their teaching.

When the respiratory therapy educator begins the education process, it is critical that he or she avoid the temptation to begin the teaching/learning process by *telling* the patient about his or her asthma. Rather, the four components of the teaching process—assessment, planning, implementation, and evaluation (APIE)—should be followed. Assessment entails determining what patients know about their condition and, more important, assessing what they need to know. Where are the gaps in their knowledge and understanding of their asthma? What is needed in order for them to care for themselves?

Armed with this knowledge, the therapist educator develops a plan, often referred to as an asthma action plan, that is tailored to the unique needs of the patient.[27] **Figure 30-10** provides an example of an asthma action plan for schools and families. The action plan should address the goals of asthma care as well as specific objectives to achieve these goals. The respiratory therapy educator must be mindful that there are concepts that should be known and understood (cognitive objectives) as well as procedures and therapies that patients must be able to perform (psychomotor objectives) and beliefs or feelings that patients must possess (affective objectives) in order for them to effectively care for their asthma. In short, there are objectives that the patient should *know*, *do*, and *believe* or *feel*.

Development of the action plan is followed by implementation of the plan and the actual teaching and learning strategy. This could include a one-on-one presentation, a demonstration, and/or a group session. During the teaching session, the therapist educator must be mindful of learning styles and barriers to learning. Once the actual teaching has occurred, the therapist educator evaluates the effectiveness of the learning, perhaps through a quick question and answer session or through a return demonstration. It is critical that the therapist educator follow the process and equally important that he or she address the key teaching points. **Box 30-10** includes key teaching messages from the National Asthma Education and Prevention Program's guidelines that should be taught and reinforced at every opportunity.[27]

Respiratory Recap

Theme of Patient Education

- The theme of patient education as it relates to asthma education is "Education for a Partnership in Care."

Pulmonary Rehabilitation

Pulmonary rehabilitation is another area within the profession of respiratory care where patient education skills have a significant role. Perhaps the most obvious and prominent condition associated with pulmonary rehabilitation is COPD.

One of the more authoritative publications related to pulmonary rehabilitation is the clinical practice guidelines jointly developed by the American College

TABLE 30-7
Components of Care for an Asthma Disease Management Program

Clinical Issue	Key Clinical Activities	Action Steps
Assessment and monitoring	Assess asthma severity to initiate therapy. Assess asthma control to monitor and adjust therapy. Schedule follow-up care.	Use severity classification chart, assessing both domains of impairment and risk, to determine initial treatment. Use asthma control chart, assessing both domains of impairment and risk, to determine whether therapy should be maintained or adjusted (step up if necessary; step down if possible). Asthma is highly variable over time, and periodic monitoring is essential. In general, consider scheduling patients at 2- to 6-week intervals while gaining control; at 1- to 6-month intervals, depending on step of care required or duration of control, to monitor if sufficient control is maintained; at 3-month intervals if a step down in therapy is anticipated. Assess asthma control, medication technique, written asthma action plan, and patient adherence and concerns at every visit.
Control environmental factors and comorbid conditions	Recommend measures to control exposure to allergens and pollutants or irritants that make asthma worse. Treat comorbid conditions.	Determine exposures, history of symptoms in presence of exposures, and sensitivities (in patients who have persistent asthma, use skin or in vitro testing to assess sensitivity to perennial indoor allergens). Advise patients on ways to reduce exposure to those allergens and pollutants or irritants to which the patient is sensitive. Multifaceted approaches are beneficial; single steps alone are generally ineffective. Advise all patients and pregnant women to avoid exposure to tobacco smoke. Consider allergen immunotherapy, by specifically trained personnel, for patients who have persistent asthma and when there is clear evidence of a relationship between symptoms and exposure to an allergen to which the patient is sensitive. Consider especially allergic bronchopulmonary aspergillosis, gastroesophageal reflux, obesity, obstructive sleep apnea, rhinitis and sinusitis, and stress or depression. Recognition and treatment of these conditions may improve asthma control. Inhaled corticosteroids are the most effective long-term control therapy. When choosing among treatment options, consider domain of relevance to the patient (impairment, risk, or both), patient's history of response to the medication, and patient's willingness and ability to use the medication.
Medications	Select medication and delivery devices to meet patient's needs and circumstances.	Use stepwise approach to identify appropriate treatment options. Inhaled corticosteroids (ICSs) are the most effective long-term control therapy. When choosing among treatment options, consider domain of relevance to the patient (impairment, risk, or both), patient's history of response to the medication, and patient's willingness and ability to use the medication.
Education	Provide self-management education. Develop a written asthma action plan in partnership with patient. Integrate education into all points of care where health professionals interact with patients.	Teach and reinforce: Self-monitoring to assess level of asthma control and signs of worsening asthma (either symptom or peak flow monitoring shows similar benefits for most patients). Peak flow monitoring may be particularly helpful for patients who have difficulty perceiving symptoms, a history of severe exacerbation, or moderate or severe asthma. Using written asthma action plan (review differences between long-term control and quick-relief medication). Taking medication correctly (inhaler technique and use of devices). Avoiding environmental factors that worsen asthma. Tailor education to literacy level of patient. Appreciate the potential role of a patient's cultural beliefs and practices in asthma management. Agree on treatment goals and address patient concerns. Provide instructions for (1) daily management (long-term control medication, if appropriate, and environmental control measures) and (2) managing worsening asthma (how to adjust medication, and knowing when to seek medical care). Involve all members of the healthcare team in providing/reinforcing education, including physicians, nurses, pharmacists, respiratory therapists, and asthma educators. Encourage education at all points of care: clinics (offering separate self-management programs as well as incorporating education into every patient visit), emergency departments and hospitals, pharmacies, schools and other community settings, and patients' homes. Use a variety of educational strategies and methods.

Reproduced from National Heart, Lung, and Blood Institute. *National Asthma Education and Prevention Program, Expert Panel Report 3: Guidelines for the Diagnosis and Management of Asthma*. Bethesda, MD: National Institutes of Health; August 2007. NIH Publication 07-4051.

School Information | **Asthma Action Plan for Schools and Families** | Health Care Provider Information

Last Name: ______ First Name: ______
Date of Birth (mm/dd/yyyy): ______ Medical Record #: ______
School Name: ______ School Contact Phone #: ______
Parent/Guardian Name: ______ Parent/Guardian Phone #: ______
Emergency Contact: ______ **Emergency Phone #:** ______
Health Care Provider Name: ______ Health Care Provider Phone #: ______

To be completed by health care provider: **Asthma Severity:** ☐ Intermittent ☐ Mild Persistent ☐ Moderate Persistent ☐ Severe Persistent
Attention Parent/Guardian/School Personnel: ANY student with asthma (of any severity) can have a severe asthma attack.
Asthma symptoms are triggered by: ☐ Exercise ☐ Dust ☐ Animal dander ☐ Strong Odors or Fumes ☐ Mold ☐ ______

Green Zone **Personal Best Peak Flow (PF)** ______ Date: ______
Peak flow is between______ (80% of personal best) and ______ (100% of personal best)

1. Take CONTROLLER medication(s) (at home) EVERY DAY:
Take ______ (Name of Medicine) inhaler______ (How much) puffs ______ (How often) times/day.
Take ______ (Name of Medicine) inhaler ______ (How much) puffs ______ (How often) times/day.
If asthma is triggered by exercise (at school or home), take ☐ Albuterol or ______ (Name of Medicine) inhaler______ (How much) puffs at least ______ minutes before exercise. Restrictions or activity limitations: ______

Yellow Zone-Caution! DO NOT LEAVE STUDENT ALONE!
Peak flow is between______ (50% of personal best) and ______ (80% of personal best).

1. Begin QUICK RELIEF medication (at school or home) right NOW:
Take ☐ Albuterol or ______ (Name of Medicine) inhaler ______ (How much) puffs **OR** ______ (Name of Medicine) solution ______ (How much) ml by nebulizer.
- If symptoms are better or if the peak flow is improved within ☐ 15 minutes/______minutes, THEN repeat QUICK RELIEF MEDICATION (as listed above in 1) every ______ (Number) hours for ______ (Number) days.
- If symptoms are **NOT** better or if the peak flow is **NOT** improved, go to Red Zone.
  ☐ **Attention School: Call Parent/Guardian when quick relief medication has been administered by student and/or staff.**

2. Attention Parent/Guardian (Home Instructions):
☐ Call your child's Health Care Provider
☐ Continue to take CONTROLLER medication (at home) everyday as written above in *Green Zone* instructions.
☐ Increase CONTROLLER medication:
Take ______ (Name of Medicine) inhaler______ (How much) puffs ______ (How often) times/day for ______ (Number) days.

Red Zone-Medical Alert! Get Help! DO NOT LEAVE STUDENT ALONE! Peak flow is below______ (50% of personal best).

1. Take QUICK RELIEF medication (at school or home) right NOW:
Take ☐ Albuterol or ______ (Name of Medicine) inhaler ______ (How much) puffs **OR** ______ (Name of Medicine) solution ______ (How much) ml by nebulizer and **REPEAT EVERY 20 MINUTES UNTIL PARAMEDICS ARRIVE!**
- **Call 9-1-1 immediately and call Parent/Guardian**

2. Attention Parent/Guardian (Home Instructions):
☐ Call your child's Health Care Provider. ☐ Continue CONTROLLER medication (at home):
Take ______ (Name of Medicine) inhaler______ (How much) puffs ______ (How often) times/day for ______ (Number) days.
☐ And ADD______ (Name of Medicine) ______ (How much) mg orally once daily for______ (Number) days.

Authorization and Disclaimer from Parent/Guardian: I request that the school assist my child with the above asthma medications and the Asthma Action Plan in accordance with state laws and regulations. Yes ☐ No ☐
My child may carry and self-administer asthma medications and I agree to release the school district and school personnel from all claims of liability if my child suffers any adverse reactions from self-administration of asthma medications: Yes ☐ No ☐

______ Parent/Guardian Signature ______ Date

Health Care Provider: My signature provides authorization for the above written orders. I understand that all procedures will be implemented in accordance with state laws and regulations. Student may carry and self-administer asthma medications: Yes ☐ No ☐ (This authorization is for a maximum of one year from signature date.) ______ Healthcare Provider Signature ______ Date

1-24-07 California Asthma Public Health Initiative, California Department of Health Services

FIGURE 30-10 Asthma action plan for schools and families.

Reproduced from California Asthma Public Health Initiative. *Asthma Action Plan for Schools and Families*. Available at: http://www.scsdk8.org/wp-content/uploads/Asthma-Action-Plan.pdf. Courtesy of the California Asthma Public Health Initiative.

of Chest Physicians and the American Association of Cardiovascular and Pulmonary Rehabilitation entitled "Pulmonary Rehabilitation: Joint ACCP/AACVPR Evidence-Based Clinical Practice Guidelines." Among the many recommendations in this document is the statement that education should be an integral component of pulmonary rehabilitation and should include information on collaborative self-management and on the prevention and treatment of exacerbations.[31] Additionally, the *Guidelines for Pulmonary Rehabilitation Programs*, prepared by the American Association for Cardiovascular and Pulmonary Rehabilitation, supports the use and value of pulmonary rehabilitation.[32] These guidelines indicate that three key steps are essential in the education process: assessing the patient's educational needs, determining how the patient learns best, and selecting the approach or style that most benefits the patient.

The respiratory therapy educator must first determine the gaps in the patient's knowledge and understanding of his or her condition and contemplate a teaching plan. Assessing gaps in the patient's knowledge or understanding is best accomplished through a series of straightforward but nonthreatening questions. In developing the teaching plan, the therapist educator

BOX 30-10

Key Educational Messages for Asthma Education

Basic Facts About Asthma

The contrast between airways of a person who has and a person who does not have asthma; the role of inflammation

What happens to the airways in an asthma attack

Roles of Medications: Understanding the Difference Between the Following

Long-term control medications: prevent symptoms, often by reducing inflammation. Must be taken daily. Do not expect them to give quick relief.

Quick-relief medications: short-acting beta-2 agonists relax muscles around the airway and provide prompt relief of symptoms. Do not expect them to provide long-term asthma control. Using quick-relief medication on a daily basis indicates the need for starting or increasing long-term control medications.

Patient Skills

Taking medications correctly

- Inhaler technique (demonstrate to patient and have the patient return the demonstration)
- Use of devices, such as prescribed valved holding chamber (VHC), spacer, nebulizer

Identifying and avoiding environmental exposures that worsen the patient's asthma (e.g., allergens, irritants, tobacco smoke)

Self-monitoring

- Assess level of asthma control
- Monitor symptoms and, if prescribed, peak flow
- Recognize early signs and symptoms of worsening asthma

Using written asthma action plan to know when and how to

- Take daily actions to control asthma
- Adjust medication in response to signs of worsening asthma
- Seek medical care as appropriate

Reproduced from National Heart, Lung, and Blood Institute. *National Asthma Education and Prevention Program, Expert Panel Report 3: Guidelines for the Diagnosis and Management of Asthma*. Bethesda, MD: National Institutes of Health; August 2007. NIH Publication 07-4051.

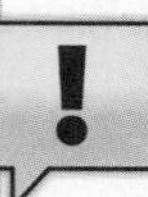

Respiratory Recap

Three Key Steps in Teaching Pulmonary Rehabilitation

1. Assessing the patient's educational needs
2. Determining how the patient learns best
3. Selecting the approach or style that most benefits the patient

must be mindful of the patient's demographic characteristics, such as age, cultural background, language, educational level, and previous life experiences. Active rather than passive participation should be stressed, and the use of repetition and reinforcement of key messages emphasized. Variation in presentation methods, meaning multiple-sense approaches in the form of visual, auditory, and tactile teaching techniques, is more effective. There is considerable value in providing patients written material to take home and share with their family and support persons. Ensuring coverage of key educational content is critical to the success of the patient education program. **Box 30-11** lists key educational topics for pulmonary rehabilitation.[32] Clinical competency guidelines for professionals engaged in the assessment and intervention stages of education and training have also been identified.[33]

BOX 30-11

Key Educational Topics for a Pulmonary Rehabilitation Program

Normal pulmonary anatomy and physiology
Chronic lung disease
Description and interpretation of medical tests
Breathing retraining
Bronchial hygiene
Medications
Benefits of exercise
Activities of daily living
Eating right
Irritant avoidance/Prevention and control of respiratory infections
Leisure activities
Coping with chronic lung disease and end-of-life planning

Adapted with permission from American Association for Cardiovascular and Pulmonary Rehabilitation. *Guidelines for Pulmonary Rehabilitation Programs.* 4th ed. Champaign, IL: Human Kinetics; 2011:24–25.

Tobacco Cessation

Clearly, one of the more exciting opportunities for respiratory therapists to have an impact and to practice as a patient educator involves tobacco cessation. The definitive document for tobacco cessation is the government's clinical practice guideline entitled *Treating Tobacco Use and Dependence: 2008 Update.*[34] Driving this need and opportunity for respiratory therapists' involvement was a 2004 directive from the Joint Commission that mandated that all patients diagnosed with acute myocardial infarction, heart failure, or pneumonia must receive some form of smoking cessation counseling. This counseling must be medically documented and can be in the form of advice, a brochure or handout, an aid (e.g., nicotine patch, gum), or the viewing of a video.[35] Just how seriously clinicians took this mandatory requirement was highly questionable, and the earnestness of interventions has been subjected to considerable criticism.

In 2011, the Joint Commission developed a new set of performance measures to encourage better assessment and treatment of tobacco dependence for all hospitalized patients. The new measures were implemented in 2012 and require acute care hospitals to identify all inpatients who use tobacco, to offer them counseling and medication, and to follow-up post discharge to maximize the benefits of in-hospital cessation interventions. The new tobacco use measures include: (1) tobacco use screening, (2) tobacco use treatment provided or offered during hospital stay, (3) tobacco use treatment provided or offered at discharge, and (4) tobacco use assessment after discharge. A detailed description of the tobacco measure set specifications appears in **Table 30-8**.

Although the effectiveness of intervention by the healthcare provider is debatable, it is apparent that opportunity abounds for someone to take this mandate

TABLE 30-8
Tobacco Measure Set Specifications

Set Measure ID#	Measure Short Name
TOB-1	Tobacco Use Screening
TOB-2	Tobacco Use Treatment Provided or Offered
TOB-2a	Tobacco Use Treatment
TOB-3	Tobacco Use Treatment Provided or Offered at Discharge
TOB-3a	Tobacco Use Treatment at Discharge
TOB-4	Tobacco Use: Assessing Status After Discharge

© Joint Commission Resources. Tobacco Measure Set Table, 2012. Reprinted with permission.

seriously and boldly move the antitobacco agenda forward. Respiratory therapists are well positioned and well qualified to take on this role and make a huge impact in the tobacco cessation movement.

The clinical practice guidelines provide guidance and direction for tobacco cessation by addressing such issues as the rationale for smoking cessation, patient readiness, and various strategies for effective intervention. The guidelines also indicate that tobacco use presents a rare confluence of circumstances; that is, it is a highly significant health threat, there is a disinclination among clinicians to intervene consistently, and there exist highly effective interventions.[34] **Box 30-12** outlines key clinical points for treating tobacco use and dependency provided in a 2011 update to the clinical practice guidelines.

Of profound importance is the fact that smoking tobacco is the leading cause of preventable morbidity and mortality in the United States. Tobacco use is no longer considered merely a habit but rather an addiction. This latter point is particularly critical because it reflects the need for both a behavioral and a pharmacologic intervention. The patient must be motivated to change, and thus stages of readiness have been identified, with intervention strategies associated with each stage. **Table 30-9** lists the stages of readiness as well as their characteristics and appropriate intervention techniques. Behavioral approaches entail individual, group, and telephone counseling; the literature indicates that effectiveness increases with treatment intensity.[34]

Clinicians specializing in tobacco cessation counseling can adopt a behavioral technique known as **motivational interviewing (MI)**. The overall spirit of motivational interviewing has been described as collaborative, evocative, and honoring of patient autonomy.[35] It is collaborative in that instead of an uneven power relationship in which the clinician assumes a superior position and directs the care, the patient assumes a more active role and participates with the clinician in the decision-making process. The MI process is evocative in that it seeks to motivate the patient to align his or her goals, dreams, desires, and aspirations with health behaviors that are in the patient's best interest. Finally, the MI process strives to honor the autonomy of the patient. Patients inherently strive for self-determination and freedom of choice. The MI process

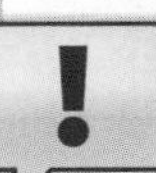

Respiratory Recap

Unique Considerations Related to Tobacco Cessation

- Smoking poses a highly significant health threat.
- There is a disinclination among clinicians to intervene consistently.
- Highly effective interventions exist.

BOX 30-12

Key Clinical Points for Treating Tobacco Use and Dependency

- Smoking will prematurely kill half of smokers who do not quit.
- At all visits, patients should be asked about smoking, and smokers should be encouraged to quit.
- For patients who are willing to try to quit, clinicians should discuss treatments for smoking cessation:
  - Deliver key counseling messages that will enhance the likelihood of successful cessation (set a quit date, review lessons from past quitting experiences, anticipate challenges to the upcoming attempt to quit, reduce or eliminate alcohol use, address other smokers in household).
  - Recommend consistent use of medications approved by the FDA for smoking cessation. Combination nicotine-replacement therapy (e.g., a nicotine patch plus bupropion) and varenicline result in the highest sustained cessation rates, and their use should be encouraged in patients without contraindications.
- For patients who are not yet willing to try to quit, clinicians should encourage the use of motivational interventions:
  - Use one of two types of counseling to boost the patient's motivation to quit: motivational interviewing techniques or five Rs counseling (a discussion of personally relevant reasons to quit, the risks associated with continued smoking, rewards for quitting, and roadblocks to successful quitting, with repetition of the counseling at subsequent clinic visits).
  - Encourage the use of a smoking-reduction intervention. For example, patients should use nicotine-replacement therapy while reducing the number of cigarettes they smoke per day and the locations where they smoke.
- For all patients who smoke, clinicians should refer them to adjuvant treatment resources: 1-800-QUIT-NOW, a national tobacco-cessation quit line, Online smoking-cessation resources, including www.smokefree.gov and www.women.smokefree.gov.

Information from Fiore M, Baker T. Treating smokers in the health care setting. *N Engl J Med.* 2011; 365:1222–1231. Available at: http://www.nejm.org/doi/full/10.1056/NEJMcp1101512.

TABLE 30-9
Stages of Readiness: Characteristics and Intervention Techniques

Stage	Characteristics	Intervention Techniques
Precontemplative	Uninterested, unaware, or unwilling to make a change May be in denial	Best to avoid arguing. Maintain a positive relationship. Demonstrate empathy. Ask thought-provoking questions such as, "What would have to happen for you to know there is a problem with your smoking?" Well-phrased questions will leave patients pondering and will move them along the process to change.
Contemplative	Considering a change Ambivalent about change	Continue to demonstrate empathy, praise, and encouragement. Consider having the patient weigh the benefits and costs of behavior change. Ask questions such as, "Why do you want to change?", "What are reasons for not changing?", and "What are the barriers that keep you from change?"
Preparation	Preparing to make a specific change	Continue to assist with problem-solving barriers. Strategies should shift from motivational to behavioral skills. Encourage small changes, such as switching to a different brand of cigarette.
Action	Practicing new behaviors Taking definitive action	Ask about successes and difficulties. Continue to provide praise and admiration.
Maintenance	Involves incorporating the new behavior over the long haul	Continue to ask about successes and difficulties. Continue to provide praise and admiration.
Relapse	Resumption of old behaviors May feel demoralized	Recognize that this is common. Explain that, despite relapses, they have learned something new about themselves, such as that it is best to avoid smoke-filled environments. Evaluate triggers. Focus on the successful part of the plan. Be supportive, and re-engage their efforts.

Information from Zimmerman G, Olsen C, Bosworth M. A "Stage of Change" approach to help patients change behavior. *Am Fam Physician.* 2000;61:1409–1416.

avoids being paternal and judgmental and is respectful of the patient's freedom to make choices and to self-manage his or her health.

Motivational interviewing entails four guiding principles: (1) resisting the righting reflex, (2) understanding and exploring the patient's own motivations, (3) listening with empathy, and (4) empowering the patient, encouraging hope and optimism.[35] Resisting the righting reflex simply means to avoid telling people what they should do. Although telling the patient what to do is admirable and seemingly the right thing to do, it will typically result in resistance from the patient and can be destructive to the relationship. The patient will likely defend his or her behavior and attempt to minimize or justify his or her actions. It is imperative that one avoid arguing. Little progress can occur when feelings of hostility are present, and thus it is more effective to express empathy and attempt to understand what motivates the patient's behavior. One should first *listen* to what patients have to say and elicit from them what they desire. In other words, actively listen with the intention of eliciting discrepancy (a gap) between desired behavior versus actual behavior. This can take the form of reflective and respectful listening in which one reserves judgment and avoids criticism. More often than not, the proper and appropriate actions are known and desired by the patient.

Finally, it is critical that the patient be empowered to actively come to the right choice and to essentially *own* his or her decision. The therapist should invite new perspectives and not impose his or her desires. The patient thus must be the source of finding answers and solutions. Patients must believe in the possibility of change and that they are *in control* and *have control* over their actions. The therapist's role is to affirm this view as well as provide assistance in appropriate interventions.

Table 30-10 provides some interviewing strategies and supporting strategies that pertain to each of the four guiding principles. These techniques are often

Respiratory Recap

Motivational Interviewing

- Collaborative
- Evocative
- Honoring of patient autonomy

TABLE 30-10
Selective Examples of Interviewing Strategies from the Four Guiding Principles of Motivational Interviewing

Guiding Principle	Interviewing Strategies	Statements Supporting Strategies
Resist the righting reflex	Back off and use reflection when the patient expresses resistance Express empathy Ask permission to provide information	"Sounds like you are feeling pressured about your smoking." "You are worried about how you would manage withdrawal symptoms." "Would you like to hear about some strategies that can help you address that concern when you quit?"
Understand your patient's motivations	Highlight the discrepancy between the patient's present behavior and expressed priorities, values, and goals Reinforce and support change talk and commitment language Build and deepen commitment to change	"It sounds like you are very devoted to your family. How do you think your smoking is affecting your children?" "So, you realize how smoking is affecting your breathing and making it hard to keep up with your kids." "It's great that you are going to quit when you get through this busy time at work." "There are effective treatments that will ease the pain of quitting, including counseling and many medication options." "We would like to help you avoid a stroke like the one your father had."
Listen with empathy	Use open-ended questions to explore: The importance of addressing smoking or other tobacco use Concerns and benefits of quitting Use reflective listening to seek shared understanding: Reflect words or meaning Summarize Normalize feelings and concerns Support the patient's autonomy and right to choose or reject change	"How important do you think it is for you to quit smoking?" "What might happen if you quit?" "So do you think smoking helps you to maintain your weight?" "What I have heard so far is that smoking is something you enjoy. On the other hand, your boyfriend hates your smoking, and you are worried you might develop a serious disease." "Many people worry about managing without cigarettes." "I hear you saying you are not ready to quit smoking right now. I'm here to help you when you are ready."
Empower the patient	Help the patient to identify and build on past successes Offer options for achievable small steps toward change: Call the quit line (1-800-QUIT-NOW) for advice and information Read about quitting benefits and strategies Change smoking patterns (e.g., no smoking in the home) Ask the patient to share his or her ideas about quitting strategies	"So you were fairly successful the last time you tried to quit."

Modified from Fiore MC, Jaen CR, Baker, TB, et al. *Treating Tobacco Use and Dependence: 2008 Update. Clinical Practice Guideline.* Rockville, MD: U.S. Department of Health and Human Services; May 2008:58.

represented in brief by the acronym RULE: resist, understand, listen, and empower.[35]

The practice guidelines provide considerable guidance regarding the steps to follow for the patient who is willing to change as well as the patient who is unwilling to change. **Table 30-11** provides a detailed account of the action and strategies for implementation of the five steps to follow for the patient willing to change. These five steps are also known as the five As and consist of the following: ask, advise, assess, assist, and arrange.

Figure 30-11 depicts the model for the treatment of tobacco use and dependence and demonstrates how these five steps can be employed in a tobacco cessation program.[36]

In the event the patient is not motivated or is unwilling to change, the guidelines recommend the use of the five Rs: relevance, risk, rewards, roadblocks, and repetition. **Table 30-12** provides a detailed account of the five Rs.

The practice guidelines also are helpful with regard to pharmacologic support. The guidelines recommend seven approved, first-line medications for the treatment of tobacco cessation. The seven consist of the five nicotine replacement therapies (NRTs)—nicotine gum, nicotine inhaler, nicotine lozenge, nicotine nasal spray, and the nicotine patch—as well as two non-nicotine-based products, bupropion SR and varenicline. The actions of each group are different. NRTs are intended to satisfy the craving for nicotine by replacing the nicotine provided by cigarettes with nicotine in the various forms just identified. The nicotine levels are gradually reduced in the body; in essence, the patient is weaned from nicotine by methodically and systematically decreasing the dose delivered.

Bupropion was the first nonnicotine drug. It is marketed as Wellbutrin as an antidepressant and as Zyban as a smoking cessation aid. It is considered to function

TABLE 30-11
The Five Steps of a Tobacco Cessation Program for Patients Willing to Quit (the 5 As)

Strategy	Action	Strategies for Implementation
1. Ask	Implement an officewide system that ensures that, for every patient at every clinic visit, tobacco use is queried and documented.	Expand the vital signs to include tobacco use, or use an alternative universal identification system.
2. Advise	In a clear, strong, and personalized manner, urge every tobacco user to quit.	Advice should be: *Clear:* "It is important that you quit smoking (or using chewing tobacco) now, and I can help you." "Cutting down while you are ill is not enough." "Occasional or light smoking is still dangerous." *Strong:* "As your clinician, I need you to know that quitting smoking is the most important thing you can do to protect your health now and in the future. The clinic staff and I will help you." *Personalized:* Tie tobacco use to current symptoms and health concerns, and/or its social and economic costs, and/or the impact of tobacco use on children and others in the household. "Continuing to smoke makes your asthma worse, and quitting may dramatically improve your health." "Quitting smoking may reduce the number of ear infections your child has."
3. Assess	Assess every tobacco user's willingness to make a quit attempt at this time.	Assess patient's willingness to quit: "Are you willing to give quitting a try?" If the patient is willing to make a quit attempt at this time, provide assistance. If the patient will participate in an intensive treatment, deliver such a treatment or link/refer to an intensive intervention. If the patient is a member of a special population (e.g., adolescent, pregnant smoker, racial/ethnic minority), consider providing additional information. If the patient clearly states that he or she is unwilling to make a quit attempt at this time, provide an intervention shown to increase future quit attempts.
4. Assist	Help the patient with a quit plan. Recommend the use of approved medication, except when contraindicated or with specific populations for which there is insufficient evidence of effectiveness (e.g., pregnant women, smokeless tobacco users, light smokers, adolescents). Provide practical counseling (problem-solving/skills training). Provide intratreatment social support. Provide supplementary materials, including information on quit lines. For the smoker unwilling to quit at this time	A patient's preparations for quitting: Set a quit date. Ideally, the quit date should be within 2 weeks. Tell family, friends, and coworkers about quitting, and request understanding and support. Anticipate challenges to the upcoming quit attempt, particularly during the critical first few weeks. These include nicotine withdrawal symptoms. Remove tobacco products from your environment. Prior to quitting, avoid smoking in places where you spend a lot of time (e.g., work, home, car). Make your home smoke-free. Recommend the use of medications found to be effective in this guideline. Explain how these medications increase quitting success and reduce withdrawal symptoms. The first-line medications include bupropion SR, nicotine gum, nicotine inhaler, nicotine lozenge, nicotine nasal spray, nicotine patch, and varenicline; second-line medications include clonidine and nortriptyline. There is insufficient evidence to recommend medications for certain populations (e.g., pregnant women, smokeless tobacco users, light smokers, adolescents). *Abstinence.* Striving for total abstinence is essential. Not even a single puff after the quit date. *Past quit experience.* Identify what helped and what hurt in previous quit attempts. Build on past success. *Anticipate triggers or challenges in the upcoming attempt.* Discuss challenges/triggers and how the patient will successfully overcome them (e.g., avoid triggers, alter routines). *Alcohol.* Because alcohol is associated with relapse, the patient should consider limiting/abstaining from alcohol while quitting. (Note that reducing alcohol intake could precipitate withdrawal in alcohol-dependent persons.) *Other smokers in the household.* Quitting is more difficult when there is another smoker in the household. Patients should encourage housemates to quit with them or to not smoke in their presence. Provide a supportive clinical environment while encouraging the patient in his or her quit attempt. "My office staff and I are available to assist you." "I'm recommending treatment that can provide ongoing support." *Sources:* Federal agencies, nonprofit agencies, national quit line network (1-800-QUIT-NOW), or local/state/tribal health departments or quit lines. *Type:* Culturally, racially, educationally, and age-appropriate for the patient. *Location:* Readily available at every clinician's workstation.

(*continues*)

TABLE 30-11
The Five Steps of a Tobacco Cessation Program for Patients Willing to Quit (the 5 As) (*continued*)

Strategy	Action	Strategies for Implementation
5. Arrange	Arrange for follow-up contacts, either in person or via telephone. For smokers unwilling to quit at this time	*Timing:* Follow-up contact should begin soon after the quit date, preferably during the first week. A second follow-up contact is recommended within the first month. Schedule further follow-up contacts as indicated. *Actions during follow-up contact:* For all patients, identify problems already encountered and anticipate challenges in the immediate future. Assess medication use and problems. Remind patients of quit line support (1-800-QUIT-NOW). Address tobacco use at next clinical visit (treat tobacco use as a chronic disease). For patients who are abstinent, congratulate them on their success. If tobacco use has occurred, review circumstances and elicit recommitment to total abstinence. Consider use of or link to more intensive treatment.

Modified from Fiore MC, Jaen CR, Baker TB, et al. *Treating Tobacco Use and Dependence: 2008 Update. Clinical Practice Guideline*. Rockville, MD: U.S. Department of Health and Human Services; May 2008:58.

by blocking the neuronal reuptake of dopamine and norepinephrine and by blockade of nicotinic acetylcholinergic receptors. Varenicline, marketed as Chantix, is also an antidepressant that was found to reduce the cravings for nicotine. Varenicline is said to work in two ways: it targets nicotine receptors in the brain, attaches to them, and blocks nicotine from reaching them. The blocking of nicotine results in reduction of craving, and thus smokers find little if any satisfaction in smoking and discontinue the smoking habit.

Finally, relapse is a serious issue related to success, and variables associated with abstinence have been identified. **Table 30-13** provides examples of variables associated with both high as well as low abstinence.

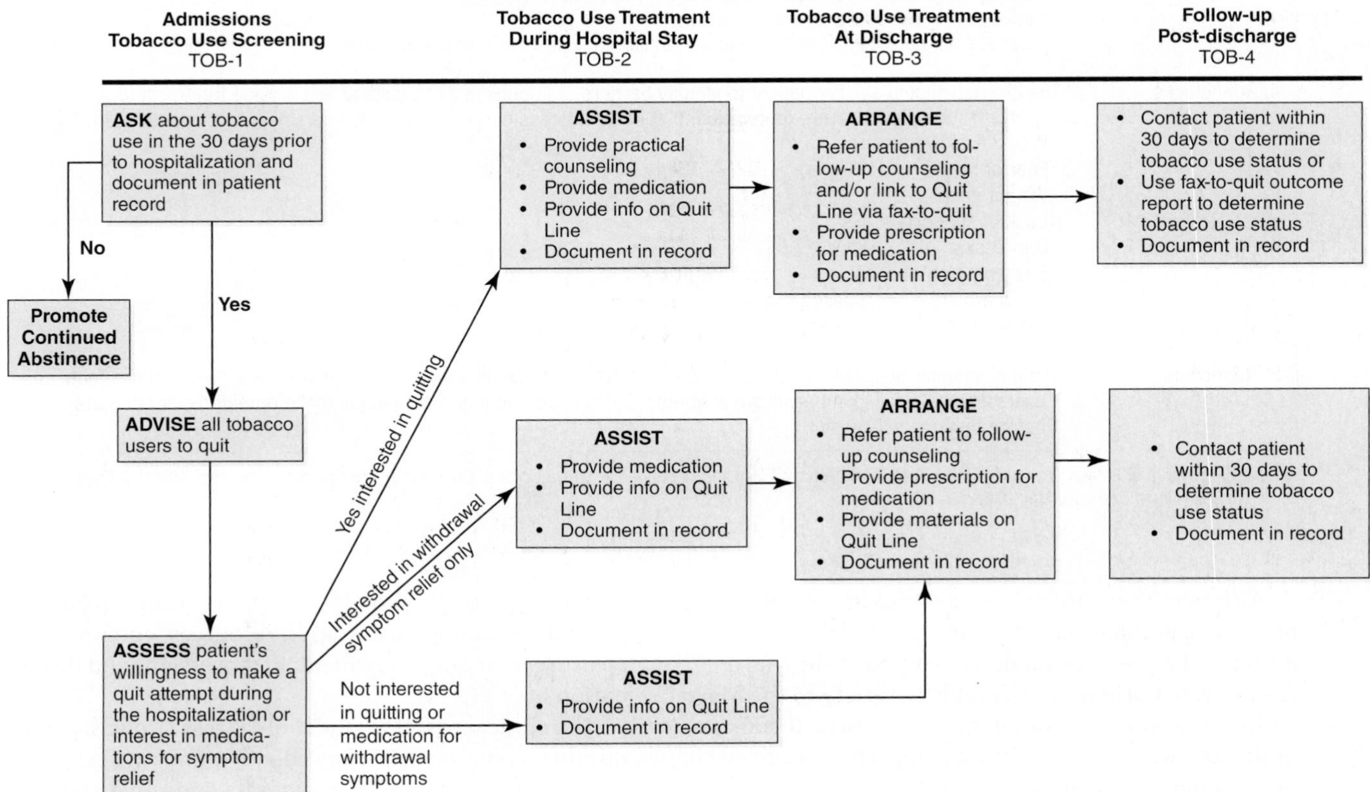

FIGURE 30-11 Tobacco Dependence Treatment Inpatient Flowsheet.

Reproduced from University of Wisconsin Center for Tobacco Research and Intervention. *Treating Tobacco Use and Dependence in Hospitalized Patients*. Available at: http://www.ctri.wisc.edu/HC.Providers/healthcare_hospitalmanual.html.

TABLE 30-12
The Five Steps of a Tobacco Cessation Program for Patients Unwilling to Quit (the 5 Rs)

Step	Explanation
1. Relevance	Encourage the patient to indicate why quitting is personally relevant, being as specific as possible. Motivational information has the greatest impact if it is relevant to a patient's disease status or risk, family or social situation (e.g., having children in the home), health concerns, age, gender, and other important patient characteristics (e.g., prior quitting experience, personal barriers to cessation).
2. Risk	The clinician should ask the patient to identify potential negative consequences of tobacco use. The clinician may suggest and highlight those that seem most relevant to the patient. The clinician should emphasize that smoking low-tar/low-nicotine cigarettes or use of other forms of tobacco (e.g., smokeless tobacco, cigars, pipes) will not eliminate these risks. Examples of risks are as follows. *Acute risks:* Shortness of breath, exacerbation of asthma, increased risk of respiratory infections, harm to pregnancy, impotence, infertility. *Long-term risks:* Heart attacks and strokes, lung and other cancers (e.g., larynx, oral cavity, pharynx, esophagus, pancreas, stomach, kidney, bladder, cervix, acute myelocytic leukemia), chronic obstructive pulmonary diseases (e.g., chronic bronchitis, emphysema), osteoporosis, long-term disability, and need for extended care. *Environmental risks:* Increased risk of lung cancer and heart disease in spouses; increased risk for low birth weight, sudden infant death syndrome (SIDS), asthma, middle ear disease, and respiratory infections in children of smokers.
3. Rewards	The clinician should ask the patient to identify potential benefits of stopping tobacco use. The clinician may suggest and highlight those that seem most relevant to the patient. Examples of rewards follow. Improved health Food will taste better Improved sense of smell Saving money Feeling better about oneself Home, car, clothing, and breath will smell better Setting a good example for children and decreasing the likelihood that they will smoke Having healthier babies and children Feeling better physically Performing better in physical activities Improved appearance, including reduced wrinkling/aging of skin and whiter teeth
4. Roadblocks	The clinician should ask the patient to identify barriers or impediments to quitting and provide treatment (e.g., problem-solving counseling, medication) that could address barriers. Typical barriers might include the following. Withdrawal symptoms Fear of failure Weight gain Lack of support Depression Enjoyment of tobacco Being around other tobacco users Limited knowledge of effective treatment options
5. Repetition	The motivational intervention should be repeated every time an unmotivated patient visits the clinic setting. Tobacco users who have failed in previous quit attempts should be told that most people make repeated quit attempts before they are successful.

Modified from Fiore MC, Jaen CR, Baker TB, et al. *Treating Tobacco Use and Dependence: 2008 Update. Clinical Practice Guideline*. Rockville, MD: U.S. Department of Health and Human Services; May 2008:59–60.

Although there are numerous smoking cessation programs, perhaps one of the most popular and authoritative is the program model developed at the Mayo Clinic. What brings considerable notoriety to the Mayo Clinic program is its comprehensive nature. It consists of the following components: a comprehensive tobacco use assessment, personalized treatment plans and educational materials appropriate for the patient's stage of readiness to change, different interventions at various stages of behavior change, individual counseling sessions, information on local support groups, relapse prevention strategies, cessation resources, outcome measurement and assessment, and oversight and distribution of NRT.[37]

The clinical practice guidelines stress two basic and minimal components of any effective smoking cessation program, namely, behavioral counseling and pharmacologic intervention. The guidelines also make a compelling case that a successful tobacco dependence treatment strategy must be tied to the healthcare

TABLE 30-13
Variables Associated with Higher and Lower Tobacco Abstinence

Variable	Examples
Higher Abstinence Rates High motivation Ready to change Moderate to high self-efficacy Supportive social network	Tobacco user reports a strong motivation to quit. Tobacco user is ready to quit within a 1-month period. Tobacco user is confident in his or her ability to quit. A smoke-free workplace and home; friends who do not smoke in the quitter's presence.
Lower Abstinence Rates High nicotine dependence Psychiatric comorbidity and substance use High stress level Exposure to other smokers	Tobacco user smokes heavily (≥20 cigarettes per day), and/or has first cigarette of the day within 30 minutes after waking in the morning. Tobacco user currently has elevated depressive symptoms, active alcohol abuse, or schizophrenia. Stressful life circumstances and/or recent or anticipated major life changes (e.g., divorce, job change). Other smokers in the household.

Modified from Fiore MC, Jaen CR, Baker TB, et al. *Treating Tobacco Use and Dependence: 2008 Update. Clinical Practice Guideline*. Rockville, MD: U.S. Department of Health and Human Services; May 2008:81.

system in which it is embedded, however.[34] It must include clinicians, administrators, insurers, and purchasers. One can clearly see that the role of the respiratory therapist as the frontline patient educator, patient advocate, and clinician is central to the smoking cessation movement.

Respiratory Recap

Critical Components of the Mayo Clinic Smoking Cessation Program

- A comprehensive tobacco use assessment
- Personalized treatment plans and educational materials appropriate for the patient's stage of readiness to change
- Different interventions at various stages of behavior change
- Individual counseling sessions
- Information on local support groups
- Relapse prevention strategies
- Cessation resources
- Outcome measurement and assessment
- Oversight and distribution of nicotine replacement therapy

Key Points

- Patient education plays an increasingly important role in healthcare delivery.
- Regulatory, social, demographic, economic, philosophic, and practical incentives drive patient education.
- The healthcare system must better prepare patients and informal caregivers to engage in preventive, maintenance, and restorative healthcare measures.
- Respiratory therapists must be aware of the highly dependent nature of patients.
- Effective communication is both multidimensional and transactional, meaning there is both content and emotion expressed in communication.
- Communication is a process involving sending and receiving the message through various channels where encoding and decoding take place, raising possibilities for significant miscommunication to occur.
- Multiple factors affect communication with patients, namely: environmental, emotional and sensory perceptions; verbal expressions; nonverbal cues; intrapersonal perceptions; and physical appearance and status.
- The goals and indications of patient education focus on the creation of behavior change.
- Patient education is a detailed, sequential process.
- Assessment is the first step; it involves determination of the patient's learning needs and readiness to learn.
- The planning phase involves development of goals, well-written objectives, and addressing the three learning domains.
- The implementation phase involves actual teaching, which requires a variety of strategies and techniques.
- Common barriers to learning include lack of readiness, physical and emotional obstacles, language barriers, and lack of motivation.
- The nine principles of adult learning produce the mnemonic RAMP-2-FAME: recency, appropriateness, motivation, primacy, two-way communication, feedback, active learning, multiple-sense learning, and exercise.
- Evaluation, the last phase in patient education, should be a continual process encompassing evaluation of the entire teaching process and of the effectiveness of the patient's learning.
- Respiratory therapy educators should always be alert to take advantage of the teaching moment.
- Examples of programs in which patient education skills can be incorporated within the practice of a respiratory therapist are asthma education, pulmonary rehabilitation, and smoking cessation programs.
- Patient education for a partnership is one of the four key components of asthma care.

- One of the major goals of any pulmonary rehabilitation program is teaching the patient how to care for himself or herself and to improve his or her quality of life.
- The Joint Commission mandates that all patients with certain conditions receive medically documented smoking cessation counseling.
- Effective smoking cessation entails behavioral counseling as well as pharmacologic intervention.
- Respiratory therapists possess the skill set to effectively serve as patient educators and should continue to endorse and welcome this critical role.

References

1. CMS.gov. Centers for Medicare and Medicaid Services. *National Health and Expenditure Data. Projected.* Available at: http://www.cms.gov/Research-Statistics-Data-and-Systems/Statistics-Trends-and-Reports/NationalHealthExpendData/NationalHealthAccountsProjected.html. Accessed August 3, 2014.
2. Lubell J. 2014 predicted to mark faster decline in primary care access. *Amednews.com.* May 6, 2013. Available at: http://www.amednews.com/article/20130506/government/130509969/6/. Accessed August 3, 2014.
3. Chen C, Petterson S, Phillips RL, et al. Toward graduate medical education (GME) accountability: measuring the outcomes of GME institutions. *Acad Med.* 2013;88:1267–1280.
4. Colwill JM, Cultice JM, Kruse RI. Will generalist physician supply meet demands of an increasing and aging population? *Health Aff.* 2008;27(3):w232–w241.
5. Boyd M, Graham B, Gleit C, et al. *Health Teaching in Nursing Practice: A Professional Model.* 3rd ed. Stamford, CT: Appleton & Lange; 1998.
6. Travis J, Ryan RS. *Wellness Workbook.* 2nd ed. Berkeley, CA: Ten Speed Press; 1988.
7. Hoyert DL, Xu JQ. *Deaths: Preliminary data for 2011.* National Vital Statistics Report; vol.61, no 6. Hyattsville, MD: National Center for Health Statistics; 2012.
8. American Association for Respiratory Care. Clinical practice guideline: providing patient and caregiver training. *Respir Care.* 2010;55:765–769.
9. Van Servellen G. *Communication Skills for the Health Care Professional: Concepts, Practice and Evidence.* Sudbury, MA: Jones & Bartlett; 2009.
10. Balzer-Riley JW. *Communication in Nursing.* 7th ed. St. Louis: Elsevier; 2013.
11. Schuster PM. *Communication: The Key to the Therapeutic Relationship.* Philadelphia: FA Davis; 2000.
12. Fink JB, Fink AK. *The Respiratory Therapist as Manager.* Chicago: Yearbook; 1986.
13. Arnold E, Boggs K. *Interpersonal Relationships: Professional Communication Skills for Nurses.* 6th ed. St. Louis: WB Saunders; 2011.
14. Bastable S, Gramet P, Jacobs K, et al. *Health Professional as Educator: Principles of Teaching and Learning.* Sudbury, MA: Jones & Bartlett; 2011.
15. Lubkin IM. *Chronic Illness: Impact and Intervention.* 8th ed. Burlington, MA: Jones & Bartlett Learning; 2013.
16. Smaldino S, Lowther D, Russell J. *Instructional Technology and Media for Learning.* 10th ed. Upper Saddle River, NJ: Prentice Hall; 2012.
17. Committee on Health Literacy, Institute of Medicine; Nelsen-Bohlman LN, Panzer AM, Kindig DA, eds. *Health Literacy: A Prescription to End Confusion.* Washington, DC: National Academies Press; 2004.
18. Kirsch I, Jungeblut A, Jenkins A. *Adult Literacy in America: A First Look at the Results of the National Adult Literacy Survey (NALS).* Washington, DC: National Center for Education Statistics, U.S. Department of Education; September 1993.
19. Kutner M, Greenberg E, Jin Y, Paulsen C. *The Health Literacy of America's Adults: Results from the 2003 National Assessment of Adult Literacy.* Washington, DC: National Center for Education Statistics, U.S. Department of Education; 2006.
20. American Medical Association Foundation. *Health Literacy: A Manual for Clinicians.* Chicago: American Medical Association Foundation and American Medical Association; 2003.
21. Weiss B. *Health Literacy and Patient Safety: Help Patients Understand.* Chicago: American Medical Association Foundation and American Medical Association; 2007.
22. The Joint Commission. *"What Did the Doctor Say?" Improving Health Literacy to Protect Patient Safety.* Oakbrook Terrace, IL: The Joint Commission; 2007.
23. Partnership for Clear Health Communication. National Patient Safety Foundation. *Ask Me 3: Program Implementation Guide for Health Care and Information Providers.* 2008. Available at: http://www.montgomerymedicine.org/members/learningdocs/AskMe3%20Pgm%20Guide%202008.pdf.
24. McKenzie J, Smeltzer J. *Planning, Implementing and Evaluating Health Promotion Programs: A Primer.* 2nd ed. Boston: Allyn & Bacon; 1997.
25. Miller M, Stoeckel P. *Client Education: Theory and Practice.* Sudbury, MA: Jones & Bartlett, 2011.
26. National Heart, Lung, and Blood Institute. *Open Airways: Asthma Self-Management Program.* Bethesda, MD: National Institutes of Health; 1984. NIH Publication 84-2365.
27. National Heart, Lung, and Blood Institute. *National Asthma Education and Prevention Program, Expert Panel Report 3: Guidelines for the Diagnosis and Management of Asthma.* Bethesda, MD: National Institutes of Health; August 2007. NIH Publication 07-4051. Available at: http://www.nhlbi.nih.gov/guidelines/asthma/asthgdln.htm. Accessed August 3, 2014.
28. Winthrop E. *Patient Teaching Tips.* St. Louis: Mosby; 1995.
29. Kroehnert G. *Basic Training for Trainers: A Handbook for Trainers.* 2nd ed. New York: McGraw-Hill; 1995.
30. National Heart, Lung, and Blood Institute. *National Asthma Education and Prevention Program, Expert Panel Report 3: Guidelines for the Diagnosis and Management of Asthma—Summary Report.* Bethesda, MD: National Institutes of Health; October 2007. NIH Publication 08-5846.
31. Ries AL, Bauldoff GS, Carlin BW, et al. Pulmonary rehabilitation: Joint ACCP/AACVPR evidence-based clinical practice guidelines. *Chest.* 2007;131(Suppl 5):4S–42S.
32. American Association for Cardiovascular and Pulmonary Rehabilitation. *Guidelines for Pulmonary Rehabilitation Programs.* 3rd ed. Champaign, IL: Human Kinetics; 2004:21.
33. Nici L, Limberg T, Hilling L, et al. Clinical competency guidelines for pulmonary rehabilitation professionals. *J Cardiopulm Rehabil Prev.* 2007;27:355–358.
34. Fiore MC, Jaén CR, Baker TB, et al. *Treating Tobacco Use and Dependence: 2008 Update. Quick Reference Guide for Clinicians.* Rockville, MD: U.S. Department of Health and Human Services; April 2009.
35. Rollnick S, Miller WR, Butler CC. *Motivational Interviewing in Health Care: Helping Patients Change Behavior.* New York: Guilford Press; 2008.
36. Fiore M, Baker T. Treating smokers in the health care setting. *N Engl J Med.* 2011;365:1222–1231.
37. Mayo Clinic Health Solutions. *Mayo Clinic Tobacco Quitline: Program Components.* Available at: https://www.healthtradition.com/wp-content/uploads/2012/02/TobaccoQuitline.pdf.

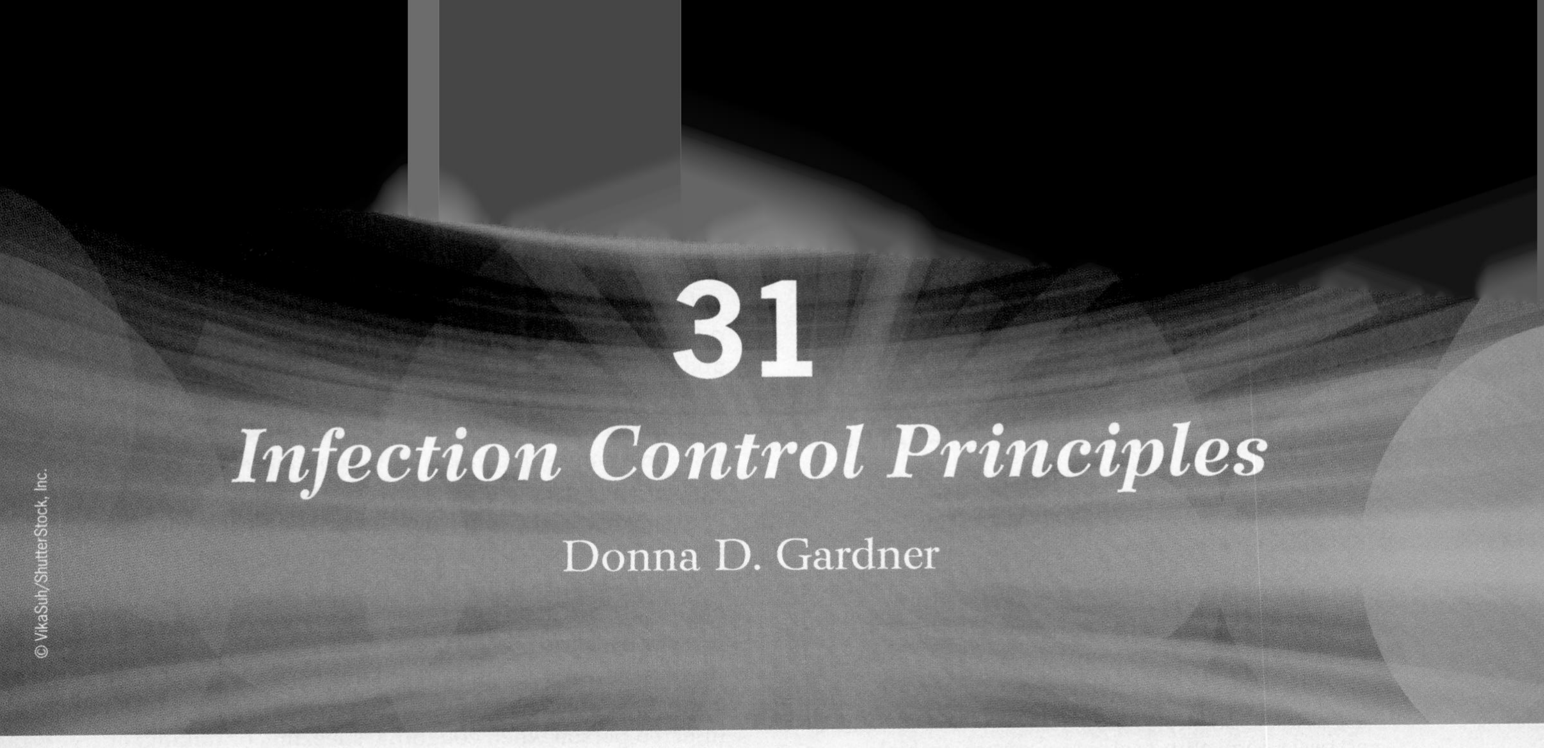

31 Infection Control Principles

Donna D. Gardner

OUTLINE

OBJECTIVES

1. Define healthcare-associated infection.
2. Compare the different methods of transmitting infections.
3. Describe the strategies for infection control.
4. Discuss the methods for processing equipment.
5. Explain the importance of a regular surveillance and monitoring program.
6. Explain the importance of hand hygiene.
7. Determine the appropriate isolation procedure for preventing transmission of infections.

KEY TERMS

airborne precautions
antisepsis
bactericidal
cleaning
contact precautions
cough etiquette
disinfection
droplet precautions
equipment surveillance
hand hygiene
healthcare-associated infections (HAIs)
infection control
nosocomial
pasteurization
personal protective equipment (PPE)
standard precautions
sterilization
vehicle transmission

Introduction

There are at least two million **healthcare-associated infections (HAIs)** each year, with about 100,000 deaths associated with these infections; a third of these infections are preventable.[1] HAIs cost $6.65 billion per year in the United States. HAIs are acquired during the delivery of care in any healthcare setting (e.g., hospital, long-term care facility, ambulatory setting, home care).[1] These infections are commonly known as **nosocomial** infections, but the Centers for Disease Control and Prevention (CDC) replaced the term *nosocomial infection* with *healthcare-associated infections* because patients move among and between different healthcare sites frequently. When an infection is present during two calendar days prior to the day of admission, the infection is considered present on admission (POA) and not a HAI. A number of factors contribute to HAIs. The development of progressive and complex medical procedures, invasive technology, and antimicrobial-resistant bacteria put patients at greater risk for contracting these infections.

Preventing these infections has become a priority in the United States as a result of initiatives led by the Joint Commission, professional organizations, government, legislators, regulators, payers, consumer advocacy groups, and guidelines from the CDC.[2,3] Reports suggest that HAIs can be prevented by implementing evidence-based best practices.[3] Bundling multiple concurrent interventions has synergistic effects in specific settings.[3] The Institute for Healthcare Improvement created the 5 Million Lives campaign to promote practices aimed at preventing HAIs.[4] More than 160 years ago, Semmelweis was able to decrease mortality related to puerperal fever by initiating a systematic hand washing protocol.[5] Hand hygiene remains the most important infection control measure.[5]

This chapter describes issues related to infection control, including methods of infection transmission, principles of infection control, and methods of sterilizing equipment.

Transmission of Infection

For the transmission of infectious agents, three conditions are necessary: (1) a source of infection, (2) a susceptible host with a portal of entry receptive to the agent, and (3) a mode of transmission for the agent. Infections are transmitted during patient care primarily via human contact or inanimate sources. Human sources include patients, healthcare personnel, family members, and visitors. Individuals may have active infections, they may be asymptomatic, or they may be carriers.[1] Individuals also may be colonized and become the source of their own infection. Respiratory care equipment, stethoscopes, bedside tables, and other inanimate objects can also be sources of infection.

A susceptible host is a person who is exposed to an infection and becomes an asymptomatic carrier or develops the disease. Others exposed to the same infection may be immune and will not develop the disease. Factors that can make a person more susceptible to infection include underlying diseases, recent surgery, anesthesia, indwelling catheters, antimicrobial or corticosteroid treatments, immunosuppressive agents, and age. Transplant recipients, patients undergoing chemotherapy or radiation, and patients with acquired immunodeficiency syndrome (AIDS) are immunocompromised hosts; these patients are extremely susceptible to any type of infection.[1] Patients who have their upper airways bypassed with an endotracheal tube or tracheostomy tube are also susceptible hosts. These tubes bypass the normal protective mechanisms of the upper airway, allowing microorganisms to easily gain access to the lower airway. Cross contamination may occur when suctioning artificial airways.[6]

Table 31-1 lists the most common routes for transmitting disease. Routes of transmission can be categorized as contact (direct, indirect, droplet) and noncontact (airborne vehicle, vector).

TABLE 31-1
Transmission Routes

Mode of Transmission	Examples
Contact	
Direct contact	Influenza, HIV, Ebola
Indirect contact	*Staphylococcus, Pseudomonas aeruginosa*, hepatitis B and C, HIV
Droplet	Rhinovirus, SARS, rubella
Noncontact	
Airborne	Legionellosis, tuberculosis, varicella
Vehicle	Waterborne: cholera Foodborne: salmonellosis and hepatitis
Vector-borne	Ticks: rickettsia, Lyme disease Mosquitoes: malaria

HIV, human immunodeficiency virus; SARS, severe acute respiratory syndrome.

Information from The Association of Faculties of Medicine of Canada. AFMC Primer on Population Health. Available at http://phprimer.afmc.ca/Part3-PracticeImprovingHealth/Chapter11InfectiousDiseaseControl/Modesandcontroloftransmission.

Direct contact transmission occurs when there is body surface–to–body surface contact between people in which a transfer of microorganisms occurs between a susceptible host and an infected or colonized individual. Transmission by direct transfer can occur during open suctioning of a patient if one is not wearing gloves and touches the secretions. Sexually transmitted infections can be transmitted via secretion transfer as well.[1]

Indirect contact transmission occurs when a susceptible host comes in contact with a contaminated object such as a needle or stethoscope. The hands of healthcare providers who touch a contaminated object or a patient and then touch a different patient are the most common cause of indirect contact transmission in the healthcare setting.

Droplet transmission occurs when droplets larger than 5 μm containing microorganisms are propelled a short distance (about 3 feet) through the air from an infected person when coughing, sneezing, or talking, or during procedures such as suctioning or bronchoscopy, and are deposited on another person's conjunctivae, nasal mucosa, or mouth. These droplets do not remain suspended in the air and therefore cannot be cleared with ventilation systems. The wearing of appropriate masks by healthcare providers is an important barrier to preventing droplet transmission.

Airborne transmission occurs by the spread of evaporated droplet nuclei smaller than 5 μm or dust particles containing microorganisms that remain suspended in the air for a long period of time. Microorganisms carried in this manner can be dispersed widely by air currents and may be inhaled by individuals within the same room. Preventing this type of transmission requires special handling and ventilation systems in which there are 12 air exchanges per hour for new construction and 6 air exchanges per hour for existing facilities. Air exhaust is directed to the outside or recirculated through high-efficiency particulate-arresting (HEPA) filtration before return. Two of the most common microorganisms transmitted in this way are the tuberculosis bacillus and the varicella virus. Personal respiratory protection via use of a National Institute for Occupational Safety and Health (NIOSH)–approved

Respiratory Recap

Routes of Infection Transmission

- Direct contact
- Indirect contact
- Droplet
- Airborne
- Vehicle
- Vector

N95 (or higher) respirator mask is required to prevent airborne transmission.

Types of airborne transmission of disease include obligate, preferential, and opportunistic.[7] An *obligate airborne transmission* is an infection, such as tuberculosis, acquired under natural conditions via aerosols deposited in the distal lung.[7] *Preferential airborne transmission* occurs through multiple routes but is predominantly via aerosols deposited in the distal airways.[7] Measles and smallpox can be acquired by either preferential or obligate airborne transmission. *Opportunistic airborne transmission* includes those organisms that naturally cause disease through other routes such as the gastrointestinal tract and can also initiate infection through the distal lung.[7] The severe acute respiratory syndrome (SARS) epidemic provided an opportunity for critical reevaluation of aerosol transmission routes of communicable respiratory diseases. SARS appears to have been transmitted predominately by having close interactions with the infected persons. Although respiratory secretions are the most likely source of infection, fecal transmission may have occurred by touching objects contaminated with stool in some settings.

Vehicle transmission occurs when contaminated food, water, medications, devices, or equipment transmits microorganisms. Vector-borne transmission occurs when vectors such as mosquitoes, flies, and other vermin transmit microorganisms.[6] Common examples of vector-borne disease include Lyme disease and Rocky Mountain spotted fever.

Strategies for Infection Control

Infection control procedures decrease the spread of infection. Infection control programs in the healthcare setting must have a commitment to patient and healthcare provider safety. Employers and employees must participate in practices to protect patients and healthcare providers by using protective equipment, participating in immunization programs, and offering safety training.

Healthcare providers must be immunized against certain communicable diseases. The Occupational Safety and Health Administration (OSHA) requires employees provide proof of hepatitis A and B vaccination and immunity against varicella, rubella, and measles. If the employee is not immune to these microorganisms, the employer must provide the immunizations. Employees are required to receive annual influenza vaccinations unless there are documented medical or religious exemptions.[6] In addition, employees should not report to work if they have a potentially infectious condition that could be transferred to patients (e.g., influenza and other acute viral respiratory infections, conjunctivitis, diarrheal diseases, chicken pox, mononucleosis, hepatitis A and B, group A streptococcal infection, herpetic whitlow, measles).

> **STOP AND THINK**
>
> What are some important practices that respiratory therapists can use to prevent the spread of infection within the hospital?

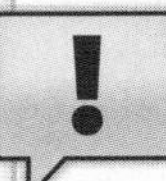

> **Respiratory Recap**
>
> **Levels of Equipment Processing**
>
> - *Critical (sterile)*: no viable (living) organisms
> - *Semicritical (disinfected)*: few organisms remaining, with spores and nonlipid viruses possibly remaining viable
> - *Noncritical (clean)*: grossly appreciable organic matter (dirt) removed

A rational approach to disinfection and sterilization of patient care equipment is the use of three levels of concern: critical, semicritical, and noncritical.[8,9] Critical equipment, such as a chest tube, comes directly into contact with sterile tissue such as the pleural space. This equipment *must* be sterile. Semicritical equipment touches mucosal surfaces, where transmission of an infective agent is relatively possible, requiring high-level disinfection of the equipment during processing. Most respiratory care equipment is semicritical. The components of a ventilator circuit have been categorized as semicritical in the Spaulding classification system because they come into direct or indirect contact with mucous membranes but do not ordinarily penetrate body surfaces. An exception is equipment passed through an endotracheal tube in which a protected passage to the lower airways is established that bypasses the relatively unclean upper airway. In this setting, use of sterile supplies such as suction catheters may decrease the infectious load introduced to the lower airways. Noncritical equipment touches only intact skin and must be cleaned only, although disinfection is usually performed.

Regulatory Agencies

The Environmental Protection Agency (EPA), Food and Drug Administration (FDA), and CDC are the agencies involved in creating the regulations that govern the sale, distribution, and use of disinfectants and sterile agents. The Joint Commission is a nongovernmental agency that devises standards of quality used to accredit hospitals. These standards are varied and include the responsibility of an employer to an employee in regard to employee education, safety, and ethics. The Joint Commision has mandated that all healthcare facilities have an infection control committee. OSHA enforces activities to reduce the occupational risk of bloodborne infections and to share standards on other exposures. One set of standards requires employers to provide hepatitis B vaccinations, personal protective equipment, and postexposure medical evaluation with follow-up. OSHA ensures healthcare facility compliance through periodic inspections.[1,6]

Cleaning, Disinfection, and Sterilization

Cleaning

To prevent cross contamination, respiratory care equipment surfaces are first cleaned and then disinfected or sterilized. Cleaning is part of the daily routine for respiratory therapists in the patient care setting. Equipment processing uses one or a combination of four modalities: cleaning, disinfection, antisepsis, and sterilization. **Cleaning** equipment removes gross contamination such as dirt, secretions, or other visible materials from a surface, reducing the number of microorganisms and removing much of their potential growth medium. Equipment should be cleaned according to the manufacturer's guidelines. Cleaning is generally a prerequisite for the other three modalities. Most respiratory care supplies, however, are disposable.

Respiratory care departments should have a designated area in which to clean equipment. This area should separate dirty equipment from clean equipment. In order for equipment to be cleaned, it must be disassembled and examined. It should be placed in a sink or basin filled with hot water, soap, detergent, or enzymatic cleaner. Water alone will not dissolve any secretions or other organic materials. Soap is not **bactericidal**, but many detergents are weak bactericidal agents against gram-positive bacteria. Adding a detergent can dissolve substances that are not soluble in water and therefore help to remove contamination. Equipment can be washed with a brush or placed into an ultrasonic washer to remove debris.

Equipment must be rinsed and dried after cleaning. Rinsing the equipment will remove any residue formed from the soap or detergent. Residue can irritate human tissues and may interfere with the sterilization and disinfection processes. Drying is also important to prevent bacterial growth on the equipment. Once the equipment is clean and dry, it should be packaged appropriately for the sterilization or disinfection process or taken to the clean area of the department and reassembled. Prior to reassembling the equipment, hand hygiene is important to prevent recontamination of the equipment.

Respiratory Recap

Equipment Processing

- Cleaning
- Disinfection
- Sterilization
- Monitoring and surveillance

Disinfection

Disinfection does not remove all microorganisms but reasonably reduces the number of potential infectious organisms by killing most of those present. Spores, mycobacteria, and viruses are the most resistant to being destroyed. The term **antisepsis** is sometimes used synonymously with *disinfection* but usually describes the use of chemical agents (antiseptics) to inhibit microbial growth. Microbes may not be killed with an antiseptic; however, the microbes' ability to replicate and produce toxins is impaired. Disinfection occurs through physical or chemical methods and is affected by several factors, such as prior cleaning of the object, type of contamination, temperature, and the pH of the disinfection solution. **Table 31-2** summarizes disinfecting agents.

Pasteurization is a common technique used to disinfect equipment. A pasteurizer is similar to a kitchen dishwasher. The equipment is immersed in water heated to just below its boiling point for a period of time. Respiratory care equipment is typically immersed in water of about 70° C for 30 minutes. Once the equipment is pasteurized, it is placed in a dryer.[1]

Chemical disinfectants are used on the contaminated surface of the equipment. The equipment is immersed in the disinfectant for a period of time. Contact time may range from 20 minutes to 3 hours. Once the time requirement for disinfection is met, the equipment is removed, rinsed in sterile water, and dried. Once the equipment is dried, it must be handled with sterile gloves and towels to prevent recontamination during reassembly and packaging. Examples of disinfectants include alcohol, chlorine, glutaraldehyde, iodophors, phenolics, quaternary ammonium compounds, acetic acid, hydrogen peroxide, and peracetic acid (a mixture of acetic acid and hydrogen peroxide).

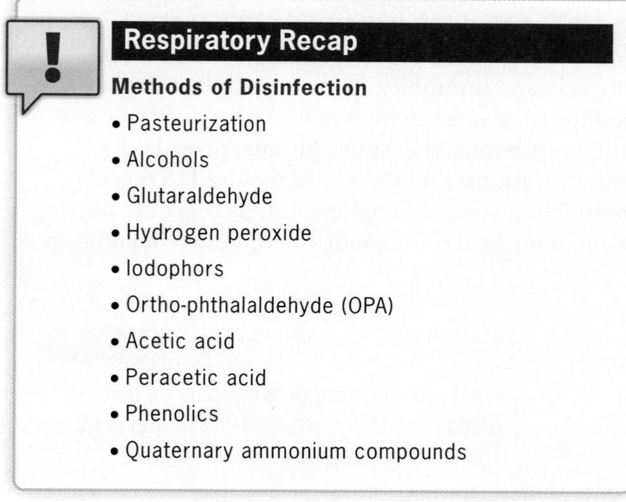

Respiratory Recap
Methods of Disinfection
• Pasteurization
• Alcohols
• Glutaraldehyde
• Hydrogen peroxide
• Iodophors
• Ortho-phthalaldehyde (OPA)
• Acetic acid
• Peracetic acid
• Phenolics
• Quaternary ammonium compounds

TABLE 31-2
Disinfecting Agents

Agent	Example of Use	Advantages	Disadvantages
Alcohols	Thermometers, scissors, stethoscopes	Easily accessible.	Damages the shellac mountings of instruments. Swells and hardens rubber and plastic tubing. Discolors rubber and plastic tiles.
Chlorine and chlorine compounds	Spot disinfection, CPR training manikins	Easily accessible.	Pungent odor. Do not mix with acidic solutions.
Glutaraldehyde	Spirometry tubing, anesthesia resuscitation bags	Can be reused for 14 to 20 days after activation. Relatively inexpensive. Excellent materials compatibility.	Respiratory tract irritation. Pungent and irritating odor. Relatively slow mycobactericidal activity. Allergic contact dermatitis. Monitoring recommended. Must use butyl gloves and well-ventilated area.
Hydrogen peroxide	Ventilator surfaces	No activation required. May enhance removal of organic matter. No disposal issues. Does not coagulate blood or fix tissue to surface.	Material compatibility concerns. Serious eye damage with contact.
Iodophors	Hydrotherapy tanks, thermometers	Does not stain. No activation required.	Should not be used to disinfect surfaces.
OPA	Endoscopes	Better than glutaraldehyde because it does not irritate the eyes or nasal passages. Fast acting. No activation required. Odor is not significant. Excellent materials compatibility.	Stains skin, mucous membranes, clothing, and environmental surfaces gray if used improperly. Repeated exposure may result in hypersensitivity in some patients. More expensive than glutaraldehyde. Eye irritation with contact. Slow sporicidal activity.
Peracetic acid	Endoscopes	Rapid sterilization cycle time (30–45 minutes). Low-temperature (50–55° C) liquid immersion sterilization. Environmentally friendly by-products. Fully automated. Single-use system eliminates need for concentration testing. Standardized cycle. May enhance removal of organic materials. No adverse health effects under normal operating conditions. Compatible with many materials and instruments.	Potential materials incompatibility. Used for immersible instruments only. Biological indicator may not be suitable for routine monitoring. Only one scope or a small number of instruments can be processed in a given time; thus, it is more expensive. Serious eye and skin damage is possible. Point-of-use system.
Phenols	Environmental surfaces such as bed rails, tables, and surfaces	Long history of being safe and of use in hospitals.	Do not use in nurseries; hyperbilirubinemia has been found.
Quaternary ammonium compounds	Floors, furniture, and walls; blood pressure cuffs	Long history of being safe and of use in hospitals.	May cause asthma exacerbation.

CPR, cardiopulmonary resuscitation; OPA, ortho-phthalaldehyde.

Modified from Rutala WA, Weber DJ, and the Health Infection Control Practices Advisory Committee. *Guideline for Disinfection and Sterilization in Healthcare Facilities 2008*. November 2008. Available at: http://www.cdc.gov/ncidod/dhqp/pdf/guidelines/Disinfection_Nov_2008.pdf.

Ethyl or isopropyl alcohol applied to the skin is used in healthcare settings to disinfect the skin prior to injections or drawing of blood samples. Alcohols can penetrate the cell wall and denature proteins or disrupt the hydrogen bonds. These agents are bactericidal, tuberculocidal, fungicidal, and virucidal. They do not kill spores and therefore are not recommended for sterilizing medical equipment. Alcohols may damage equipment made of rubber and plastic. They may be used to disinfect oral thermometers, pagers, scissors, and stethoscopes. Small alcohol pads are frequently used to disinfect the tops of medication vials.[8]

Chlorine and chlorine compounds are referred to as *hypochlorite* disinfectants. They are contained in the household bleach used in homes. Hypochlorite solutions are antimicrobial, do not leave any toxic residue on equipment, are inexpensive, and are fast acting. The CDC recommends using hypochlorite solutions in a 1:10 dilution of 5.25% concentration in water for routine environmental disinfection of blood spills and in rooms where patients are infected with *Clostridium difficile* after the surfaces are cleaned.[8] It is important to avoid mixing any hypochlorite solution with an acid because of the risk of creating toxic chlorine gas.[8]

Glutaraldehyde (Cidex, Sonacide, Sporicidin, Hospex, Omnicide, Matricide, Wavicide) is a high-level disinfectant. It is a colorless, oily liquid with a sharp pungent odor. It turns green when activated to a pH of 7.5 to 8.5. Glutaraldehyde can disinfect within 20 minutes and sterilize in 6 to 10 hours. Glutaraldehyde is safe to use with metal, rubber, or plastic equipment. It is also used to sterilize bronchoscopes and spirometry tubing. Because glutaraldehyde is toxic, the equipment must be rinsed with sterile water and usually dried. Although its use is limited to immersible equipment, glutaraldehyde is convenient because the solution may be kept in a small container and reused for 14 to 30 days. The solution should be monitored regularly for contamination.

Glutaraldehydes are toxic, and, therefore, healthcare providers need to use caution when working with this type of solution. Glutaraldehydes should be used in a designated area where there is adequate ventilation and where people and the cleaning process can be monitored. Glutaraldehyde should be stored in a tightly closed, properly labeled container in a cool, secure area. Activated glutaraldehyde is safe to use for 14 to 21 days. Glutaraldehyde can be disposed of with an abundant amount of cold water into a drain connected to a sanitary sewer. It should not be discarded into a septic system.

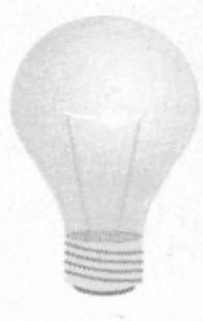

STOP AND THINK

What options are available to clean and disinfect respiratory care equipment used in the home? How would you decide on the best approach for an individual piece of equipment?

Side effects associated with glutaraldehyde exposure include epistaxis, rhinitis, and asthma exacerbations. Dermatitis, skin irritations, and mucous membrane irritation have also been reported with acute and chronic exposures to glutaraldehyde. To prevent these side effects from occurring, exhaust hoods should be used in the room where the agent is kept. Tight-fitting lids should be secured to the immersion baths, and personal protective equipment such as nitrile or butyl rubber gloves or polyethylene and spun-bonded polypropylene-coated gloves should be worn to protect the hands. An isolation gown or lab coat should be worn. Appropriate respirators should be worn to prevent exposure to glutaraldehyde vapors.

Hydrogen peroxide was added to the CDC guidelines for disinfection and sterilization in healthcare facilities as a safe disinfectant agent in a 2008 update.[8] Hydrogen peroxide is germicidal and active against bacteria, fungi, yeasts, and viruses and is available in 7.35%, 3.0%, and 1.0% solutions. Hydrogen peroxide produces destructive hydroxyl free radicals that attack the cell membrane. It is a safe disinfectant used on heat-sensitive medical devices such as bronchoscopes. Peroxides, however, are oxidizing chemicals and may cause cosmetic and functional damage to the scope.

Iodophor (povidone iodine) solutions or tinctures have been used as antiseptics on skin or tissue. Iodophors are germicidal because they penetrate the cell wall and disrupt protein/nucleic acid structure and synthesis.[8] Iodophors do not stain like the general iodines. This type of agent is reported to be bactericidal, mycobactericidal, and virucidal with long contact times.

Ortho-phthalaldehyde (OPA) has received clearance from the FDA as a high-level disinfectant. It is a clear, pale blue liquid with a pH of 7.5. OPA has advantages over glutaraldehyde in that it is more stable and does not irritate the eyes or nasal passages. OPA does not require exposure monitoring, has a slight odor, and requires no activation. It has excellent material compatibility. Because OPA stains proteins gray, unprotected skin will be stained by exposure. It is important to be trained to use this agent and to wear the proper personal protective equipment, including gown, gloves, and goggles. Exposure time is 12 minutes, and it is important to rinse the equipment with water.[8]

Acetic acid is white household vinegar, which is used exclusively in home care settings. Acetic acid with a pH of 2.0 or greater is bactericidal, lowers a microbe's intracellular pH, and inactivates energy-producing enzymes. The optimal concentration for acetic acid is 1.25%, which is equal to one part 5% white household vinegar and three parts water. Exposure time is 1 hour. It is an effective bactericidal agent against *Pseudomonas aeruginosa*, but its sporicidal and virucidal activity has not been established.

Peracetic acid is acetic acid with an additional oxygen atom. It acts rapidly against all microorganisms. It will inactivate gram-positive and gram-negative bacteria, fungi, and yeasts in less than 5 minutes. An advantage of this agent is that it lacks harmful decomposition products, which enhances the removal of organic material and leaves no residue. Little is known about the mechanism of action of this agent, but it is believed to denature proteins and disrupt cell wall permeability. A 35% peracetic acid solution is diluted to 0.2% with filtered water at 50° C. This method may be more expensive because an automated system requiring training must be installed.

Phenolics have been used in the healthcare settings for years. They are germicidal, antimicrobial, bactericidal, fungicidal, virucidal, and tuberculocidal at recommended dilutions. Phenolics in high concentrations penetrate and disrupt the cell wall, and in low concentrations they inactivate the essential enzyme system and leak metabolites from the cell wall. Phenolics are absorbed by porous material, and residual disinfectant can irritate the skin. These agents are used to disinfect environmental surfaces such as bedside tables or bed rails. Phenolics are not recommended in neonatal units because of a reported link to hyperbilirubinemia when phenolics were used to clean bassinets and incubators.[8]

Quaternary ammonium compounds (quats) are cationic detergents that dissolve the cell membranes of microorganisms. Quats are used as disinfectants and cleaning agents. Later-generation quats are considered fungicidal, bactericidal, and virucidal; however, they are not sporicidal.[8] Quats inactivate the enzymes and denature the cell proteins of the cell membrane. They are used to disinfect medical equipment that comes into contact with skin, such as blood pressure cuffs, and to clean floors, furniture, and walls in healthcare settings. In the home care setting, they can be used as an alternative to acetic acid at a dilution of 1 ounce to 1 gallon of sterile or distilled water for at least 10 minutes.

Sterilization

Sterilization is the complete destruction of all microorganisms, including spores. Sterilization prevents the transmission of diseases.[8] Sterilization processes are effective when healthcare providers adhere to the recommendations and instructions on the product labels. There are two types of sterilization: physical and chemical. Physical processes include steam and radiation. Chemical processes include ethylene oxide (ETO), hydrogen peroxide gas plasma, and peracetic acid. **Table 31-3** summarizes sterilization techniques.

TABLE 31-3
Sterilization Techniques and Uses

Agent	Example of Use	Advantages	Disadvantages
Steam (autoclave)	Critical and semicritical items that are heat and moisture resistant; respiratory therapy and anesthesia equipment; hemostats; surgery utensils; laboratory specimens	Nontoxic to patient, staff, and environment. Cycle is easy to control and monitor. Rapidly microbicidal. Least affected by organic/inorganic soils among sterilization processes.	Deleterious for heat-sensitive instruments. Damages microsurgical instruments. Potential for burns.
Hydrogen peroxide gas plasma	Materials that cannot tolerate high temperatures or humidity such as plastics and electrical devices	Safe for the environment. Cycle time is 28–75 minutes. Used for heat- and moisture-sensitive items (temperature <50° C). Simple to operate and install and monitor. Only requires electrical outlet.	Linens, paper, and liquids cannot be processed. Sterilization chamber size varies. Some medical devices with long or narrow lumens will not be processed in this system. Hydrogen peroxide can be toxic.
Ethylene oxide (ETO)	Critical items and some semicritical items that are moisture or heat sensitive and cannot be sterilized by steam sterilization	Penetrates packaging materials, device lumens. Single-dose cartridge and negative-pressure chamber minimize the potential for gas leak and ETO exposure. Simple to operate. Compatible with most medical materials.	Requires aeration time to remove ETO residue. Sterilization chamber size varies. ETO is toxic, carcinogenic, and flammable. ETO emission must be regulated. ETO cartridges must be stored in flammable liquid storage cabinet. Lengthy cycle aeration time.
Peracetic acid	Endoscopes	Rapid cycle time (30–45 minutes). Low-temperature immersion sterilization (50–55° C). Environmentally friendly by-products. Flows through the scopes.	Point-of-use system. No sterile storage. Biological indicator may not be suitable for routine monitoring. Used for immersible instruments only. Some materials incompatibility. Small number of instruments processed in the cycle. Potential for serious eye and skin damage with contact.

Modified from Rutala WA, Weber DJ, and the Health Infection Control Practices Advisory Committee. *Guideline for Disinfection and Sterilization in Healthcare Facilities 2008.* Available at: http://www.cdc.gov/ncidod/dhqp/pdf/guidelines/Disinfection_Nov_2008.pdf.

Critical items are those medical devices that come in contact with sterile body tissues or fluids. These critical items must be sterilized to prevent any possibility of transmitting diseases. Steam sterilization is recommended for equipment that is heat resistant. Those pieces of equipment that are sensitive to heat and moisture require a low-temperature process such as ETO, hydrogen peroxide gas plasma, or peracetic acid.[8]

Steam autoclave kills microorganisms by heat-denaturing microbial proteins. Effective sterilization requires adequate heat and time, but increases in pressure or the addition of moisture enhances and hastens killing. Moist heat in the form of saturated steam under pressure is the most commonly used method for sterilization of equipment. Autoclaves are similar to pressure cookers and range in size from a desktop unit to a walk-in closet. The autoclave is used to expose equipment to direct steam at the required temperature and pressure for a specific time. Autoclaving, therefore, has the advantage of being fast (typically 5 to 15 minutes plus cooling time), but it damages some types of equipment.[8]

Autoclaving is nontoxic, inexpensive, rapidly microbicidal, sporicidal, and penetrates fabrics. The four parameters that influence this process are steam, pressure, time, and temperature. The most common temperatures used are 121° C (250° F) and 132° C (270° F).[8] The temperatures must be maintained for a minimum time to kill organisms. All equipment must be cleaned before being placed in the steam sterilization process. The clean equipment is wrapped in linen, muslin, or paper wraps. Equipment exposed to steam heat for 30 minutes at 15 psi and 121° C or for 4 minutes at 15 psi and 132° C should be sterile.[8] The time and temperature used will be determined by the type of items being sterilized. Air is evacuated and is replaced with steam, which reaches a higher temperature than air. The high-temperature steam can surround and infiltrate the equipment, including all of the crevices.

The equipment must have time to air dry because water can become trapped in the wrappers or equipment itself. Mechanical, chemical, and biological indicators should monitor the autoclave process. Wrapped packages should have a piece of indicator tape placed on the seal of the wrapper before being placed in the autoclave. The indicator tape will change color when the equipment has been sterilized.

Respiratory Recap

Methods of Sterilization

- Steam (autoclaving)
- Ethylene oxide
- Hydrogen peroxide gas plasma
- Peracetic acid sterilization

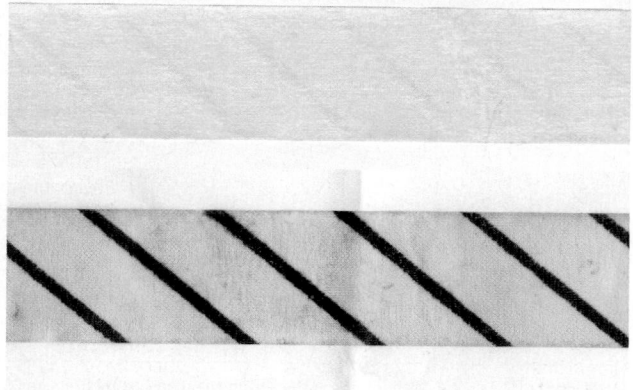

Flash sterilization is a modification of the steam sterilization process in which the flashed item is placed in an open tray at 132° C for 3 minutes at 27 psi.[8] It is not recommended as a routine sterilization method because there is no method for monitoring its performance. This type of process may be useful in surgical suites where this sterilizer is in close proximity to the site of use. It is considered acceptable for processing cleaned patient care items that cannot be packaged, sterilized, and stored before use. This process should not be used for convenience or as an alternative to the previous method discussed.

Low-temperature sterilization at temperatures below 60° C is used on equipment that is sensitive to heat and moisture. ETO, hydrogen peroxide gas plasma, and liquid peracetic acid chemicals all are examples of low-temperature sterilization techniques.

Ethylene oxide is a colorless, flammable, explosive, and toxic gas that has been used since the 1950s. Ethylene oxide is a dry gas that sterilizes without need for heat or moisture. It is used to process equipment that is unable to tolerate autoclaving or immersion. The equipment must be dry when placed in the ETO chamber to prevent ethylene glycol from forming. The equipment must be packaged in a moisture-permeable wrapping made of muslin, paper, or plastic made of polyethylene. Indicator tape similar to the tape used for the autoclave is used and will change color to indicate that proper conditions were met for sterilization (**Figure 31-1** and **Figure 31-2**). The chambers are controlled at temperatures between 50° C and 56° C and humidity between 30% and 70% to ensure optimum conditions for sterilization.[8] Approximately 3 to 4 hours of gas exposure are required, and processed equipment usually requires ventilation for 8 to 24 hours afterward.[8] Chronic exposure to ETO is associated with nausea, headache, dizziness, and airway inflammation. Residue from the ETO on equipment can lead to tissue inflammation and hemolysis. Contact of ethylene oxide with water produces ethylene glycol (antifreeze), which may persist on the equipment as a toxic, sticky residue. ETO also has carcinogenic, mutagenic, and teratogenic effects.

FIGURE 31-1 Indicator strips.

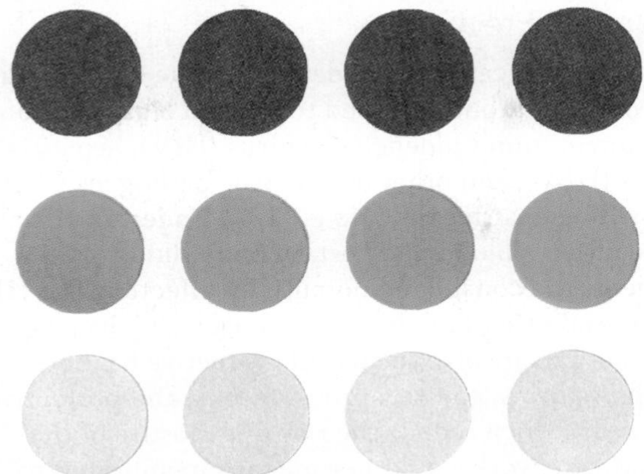

FIGURE 31-2 Indicator strips for sterilization via ethylene oxide, steam, and radiation methods.
Courtesy of QOSINA.

Hydrogen peroxide gas plasma is a new sterilization technology. Gas plasmas are generated in an enclosed chamber under deep vacuum using radio frequency or microwave energy to excite the gas molecules and produce charged free radicals.[8] The free radical production within a plasma field is capable of interacting with cell components and disrupting the metabolism of microorganisms.[8] The sterilization chamber is evacuated, and hydrogen peroxide solution is injected from a cassette and vaporized into the chamber.[8] It vaporizes in the chamber over the surfaces of the equipment, and an electrical field created by a radio frequency is applied to the chamber to create a gas plasma over 50 to 75 minutes.[8] The excess gas is then removed from the chamber, followed by depressurization. This is the preferred choice for sterilizing equipment that cannot tolerate high temperatures and humidity.

Peracetic acid sterilization is usually used on surgical and medical endoscopes. This method uses 35% peracetic acid and an anticorrosive agent in a single-dose container.[8] The container is punctured at the time of use and activated when the lid is closed. The peracetic acid is diluted with filtered water at 50° C and then circulated within the chamber and pumped through the equipment for 12 minutes. Once used, it is discarded into the sewer, and the instruments are rinsed with filtered water.

Ionizing radiation uses cobalt 60 gamma rays or electron accelerators. Radiation can sterilize tissues for transplantation, pharmaceuticals, and medical devices, but it is not an FDA-approved process for use by healthcare facilities.

Dry heat sterilizers should be used for equipment that might be damaged by moist heat or products that are impenetrable to moist heat, such as plastics or rubber. Dry heat is effective and usually used for laboratory glassware, surgical instruments, petroleum products, sharp instruments, and powders. Dry heat is nontoxic and does not harm the environment, yet the process is time consuming, requiring exposure for 60 minutes at 170° C.

Incineration is the simplest means of destroying microorganisms. Incineration is used when there is no other way of sterilizing equipment.

Equipment Surveillance and Monitoring

Maintaining a regular program of **equipment surveillance** and monitoring is important to ensure that sterile and disinfected equipment is being properly processed to meet the necessary levels of cleanliness. A surveillance program usually includes three components: monitoring equipment-processing procedures, sampling in-use equipment, and microbiologically identifying suspect pathogens.

Equipment in use can be sampled with a sterile cotton swab or aerosol impaction. The swabs can be used to sample easily accessible surfaces of respiratory care equipment. The microbiology laboratory then identifies the infectious organisms.

Although indicator tapes are regularly placed in autoclaves and gas sterilizers to indicate that proper heat and gas concentrations and duration have been achieved for each run, this action does not ensure that sterilization has actually taken place. Also, biologic tests are regularly run in each sterilizer. The tubes containing bacteria in growth media are subsequently cultured to ensure complete killing. Still, this step does not guarantee that the equipment itself is being sterilized. Inadequate cleaning before autoclaving, for example, may allow organisms to survive, requiring that the equipment itself be cultured periodically to verify sterility or to detect low bacterial counts for clean equipment. One of the following three methods is typically used:

- *Aspiration*: A quantity of sterile saline is drawn through the lumen of the equipment to be tested, after which the saline is cultured.
- *Plating*: To culture exterior surfaces, the equipment may be rolled directly onto a culture medium, usually a Petri dish filled with agar (the plate). The culture obtained may be qualitative (measuring only the presence and type of organism) or quantitative (measuring the level of infection by counting the number of colonies that grow on the agar surface).
- *Swabbing*: Irregular surfaces that are not easily rolled onto an agar plate may be rubbed with a sterile swab coated with culture medium. The swab may then be used to inoculate a plate.

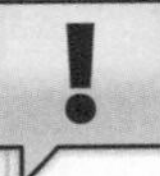

Respiratory Recap

Equipment Surveillance Methods

- Aspiration
- Plating
- Swabbing

Precautions

The healthcare setting is a place where respiratory therapists and other healthcare professionals can be exposed to patients' blood and body fluids. Protecting patients and ourselves against infection requires strict adherence to the standard and transmission-based precautions set out by the *Guideline for Isolation Precautions: Preventing Transmission of Infectious Agents in Healthcare Settings 2007* published by the CDC.[1] The CDC identifies two tiers of precautions to prevent transmission of infectious agents: standard precautions and transmission-based precautions. **Standard precautions** are applied to the care of all patients in all healthcare settings. Patients who are known or suspected of being infected or colonized with infectious agents require additional control measures in the form of transmission-based precautions.

Standard Precautions

Universal precautions, as defined by the CDC, are a set of precautions designed to prevent transmission of human immunodeficiency virus (HIV), hepatitis B virus (HBV), and other bloodborne pathogens when providing health care (**Table 31-4**). Under universal precautions, blood and certain body fluids of all patients are considered potentially infectious for HIV, HBV, and other bloodborne pathogens. Universal precautions involve the use of protective barriers such as gloves, gowns, aprons, masks, and protective eyewear, which reduce the risk of exposure of the healthcare worker's skin or mucous membranes to potentially infective materials. In addition, it is recommended that all healthcare workers take precautions to prevent injuries caused by needles, scalpels, and other sharp instruments or devices. In 1996, the

TABLE 31-4
Recommendations for Application of Standard Precautions for All Patients in All Healthcare Settings

Component	Recommendation
Hand hygiene	After touching blood, body fluids, secretions, excretions, contaminated items; immediately after removing gloves; between patient contacts.
Personal protective equipment (PPE)	
Gloves	For touching blood, body fluids, secretions, excretions, contaminated items; for touching mucous membranes and nonintact skin.
Gowns	During procedures and patient care activities when contact of clothing/exposed skin with blood, body fluids, secretions, and excretions is anticipated.
Masks, eye protection, face shields	During procedures and patient care activities likely to generate splashes or sprays of blood, body fluids, or secretions, especially suctioning and endotracheal intubation.
Patient placement	Prioritize for single-patient room if patient is at increased risk of transmission, is likely to contaminate the environment, does not maintain appropriate hygiene, or is at increased risk of acquiring infection or developing adverse outcome following infection.
Patient resuscitation	Use mouthpiece, resuscitation bag, or other ventilation devices to prevent contact with mouth and oral secretions.
Soiled patient care equipment	Handle in a manner that prevents transfer of microorganisms to others and to the environment; wear gloves if visibly contaminated; perform hand hygiene.
Textiles and laundry	Handle in a manner that prevents transfer of microorganisms to others and to the environment.
Environmental control	Develop procedures for routine care, cleaning, and disinfection of environmental surfaces, especially frequently touched surfaces in patient care areas.
Needles and other sharps	Do not recap, bend, break, or hand-manipulate used needles; if recapping is required, use a one-handed scoop technique only; use safety features when available; place used sharps in puncture-resistant container.
Respiratory hygiene/cough etiquette (source containment of infectious respiratory secretions in symptomatic patients, beginning at initial point of contact)	Instruct symptomatic persons to cover mouth/nose when sneezing/coughing; use tissues and dispose in no-touch receptacle; observe hand hygiene after soiling of hands with respiratory secretions; wear surgical mask if tolerated or maintain spatial separation >3 feet if possible.

Modified from Siegel JD, Rhinehart E, Jackson M, Chiarello L, and the Healthcare Infection Control Practices Advisory Committee. *Guideline for Isolation Precautions: Preventing Transmission of Infectious Agents in Healthcare Settings 2007*. Atlanta, GA: Centers for Disease Control and Prevention; 2007.

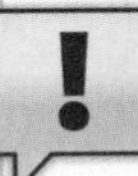

Respiratory Recap

Standard Precautions

- Hand hygiene
- Use of gloves, masks, and eye protection (goggles or face shield), depending on reasonably anticipated exposure to blood and body fluids
- Limit touching your face or adjusting PPE with contaminated gloves

CDC established standard precautions, which synthesized the major features of body substance isolation (a form of isolation precautions used before 1996) and universal precautions to prevent transmission of microorganisms.

Standard precautions include hand hygiene and the use of gloves, gowns, masks, and eye protection (goggles or face shield), depending on reasonably anticipated exposure to blood and body fluids. This also includes concerns about equipment in the patient environment that may be contaminated with infectious body fluids, which must be handled appropriately to prevent the transmission of diseases. The appropriate precautions to use (standard or transmission based) will be determined by the nature of the healthcare provider, the patient interaction, and the extent of the anticipated blood, body fluid, or pathogen exposure. For some interactions, only gloves are required. For other interactions, gloves, gowns, and eye protection will be required. Standard precautions are recommended in all healthcare settings, including hospitals, long-term acute care settings, rehabilitation hospitals, home care settings, doctor's offices, and clinics. Combining body substance isolation policies and universal precautions will reduce the risk of transmission of infections between patients and healthcare providers.

Hand Hygiene

Hand hygiene is the most important part of standard precautions. It is the single most important measure to reduce the transmission of microorganisms from one person to another or from one site to another on the same patient.[10,11] **Hand hygiene** refers to either hand washing with soap and water for 15 to 20 seconds or the use of alcohol-based gels, foams, or rubs that do not require water. In the absence of visible soiling of hands, approved alcohol-based products for hand disinfection are preferred over antimicrobial or plain soap and water because of their superior microbicidal activity, reduced drying of the skin, and convenience. Current guidelines for hand hygiene promote the use of alcohol-based antiseptic preparations. Competent hand rubbing requires that a sufficient volume of an alcohol-based rub be applied to cover all surfaces of the hands and fingers and that at least 15 seconds of rubbing be used before the hands are dry. Application of the hand rub is facilitated by placing the bottle in dispensers (**Figure 31-3**).

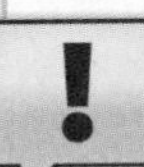

Respiratory Recap

Hand Hygiene

- Hand hygiene is the most important factor in the prevention of spread of infection.
- Alcohol-based hand rubs are an effective form of hand hygiene.
- Wash hands if soiled by blood, body fluids, or excrement.
- Hand hygiene effectiveness is reduced with long nails, extenders, and jewelry.

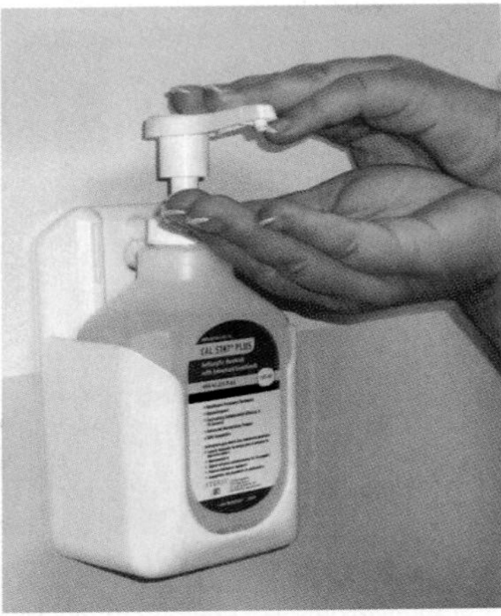

FIGURE 31-3 Hand hygiene dispenser, as found throughout healthcare facilities.

Hands should be washed with soap and warm water if they are soiled with blood, body fluids, or excrement. Hand hygiene effectiveness can be reduced by the type and length of fingernails, extenders, and jewelry. The use of artificial nails, extenders, and jewelry is discouraged for healthcare personnel who have contact with high-risk patients.

Personal Protective Equipment

Personal protective equipment (PPE) for healthcare providers refers to the various barriers and respirators used to protect the mucous membranes, skin, airways, and clothing from contact with infectious agents. The selection of PPE is based on the nature of the patient interaction and possible mode of transmission.

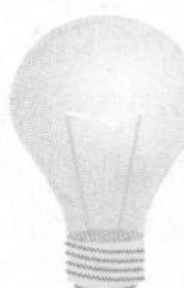

STOP AND THINK

Explain how you properly use various personal protective equipment and the situations in which you use that equipment.

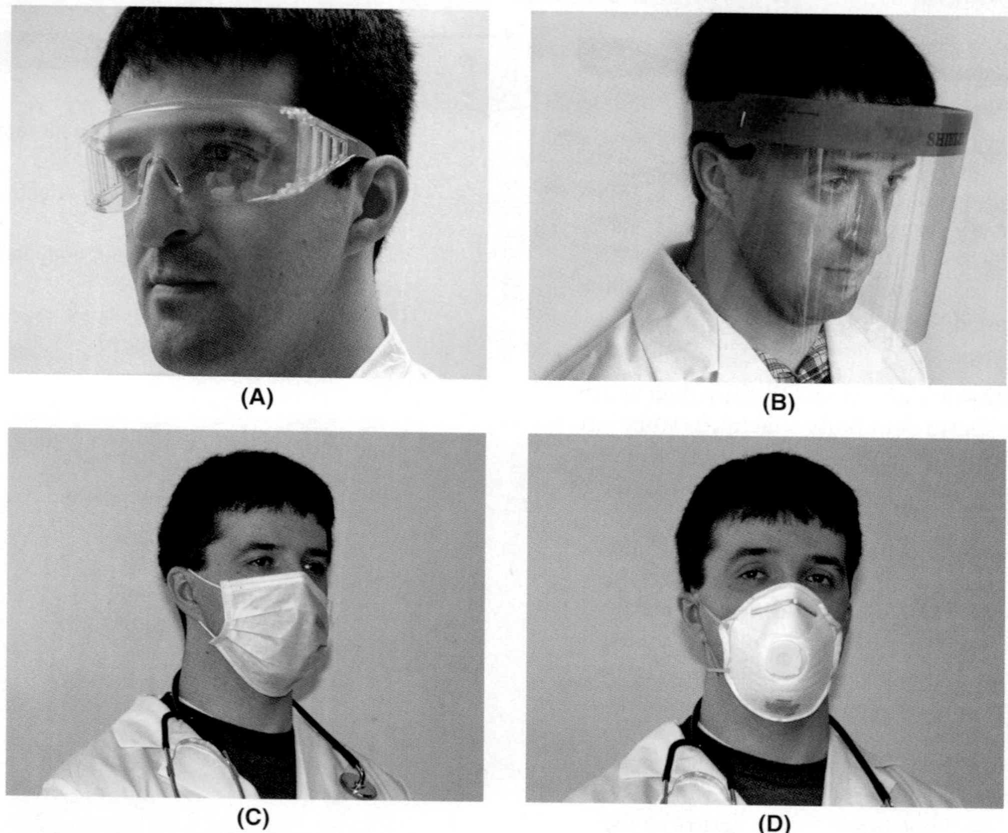

FIGURE 31-4 Personal protective equipment. (**A**) Goggles. (**B**) Face shield. (**C**) Surgical mask. (**D**) N95 respirator mask.

Specific PPE includes gloves, eye protection, face protection, gowns, and respiratory masks (**Figure 31-4** and **Figure 31-5**). Hand hygiene is performed after removing PPE. **Box 31-1** describes the order in which PPE is donned and removed.

Gloves are used to protect the patient and healthcare provider from pathogens that may be transmitted by direct contact with blood or body fluids, those who are colonized or infected with pathogens on the hands, and when handling patient equipment and environmental surfaces contaminated with pathogens.

Nonsterile gloves are made of a variety of materials, such as latex, vinyl, and nitrile for routine patient care. Healthcare facilities are moving toward a latex-free environment. Nonsterile gloves should be worn during any patient care. Sterile gloves should be worn when performing invasive procedures such as open suctioning or tracheostomy care. When gloves are worn in combination with other PPE, they should be put on last. When using an isolation gown, gloves should fit snugly around the wrist to cover the cuff of the gown and provide a more reliable barrier for the wrists and hands.

Gloves may need to be changed between patient procedures and after touching portable computers or mobile equipment because they are a means for contaminating you, other patients, and surfaces. Always

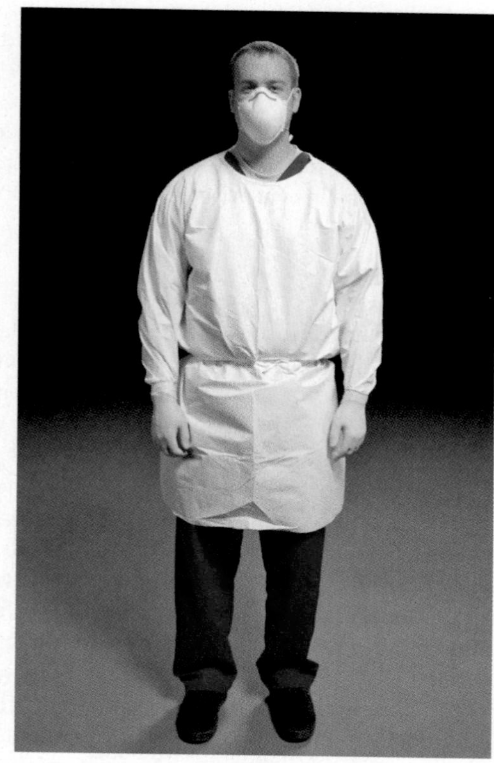

FIGURE 31-5 Mask, gown, and gloves for personal protection.
Courtesy of James Gathany/CDC.

BOX 31-1

Sequence for Donning and Removing Personal Protective Equipment

Sequence for Donning Personal Protective Equipment (PPE)

The type of PPE used will vary based on the level of precautions required.

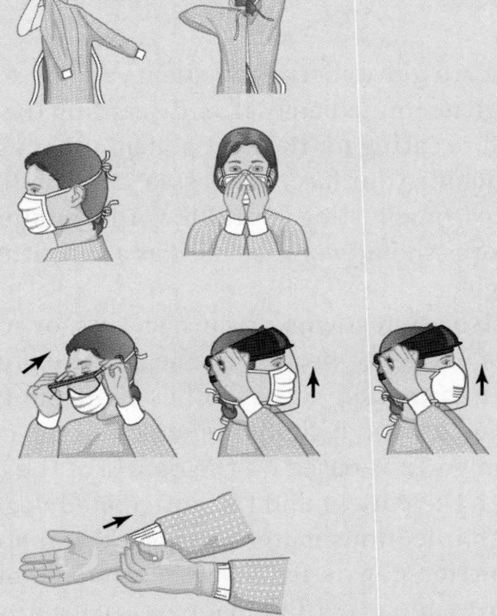

1. Gown
   Fully cover torso from neck to knees, arms to end of wrists, and wrap around the back.
   Fasten in back of neck and waist.
2. Mask or respirator
   Secure ties or elastic bands at middle of head and neck.
   Fit flexible band to nose bridge.
   Fit snug to face and below chin.
   Fit-check respirator.
3. Goggles or face shield
   Place over face and eyes and adjust to fit.
4. Gloves
   Extend to cover wrist of isolation gown.

Sequence for Removing Personal Protective Equipment (PPE)

Except for respirator, remove PPE at doorway or in anteroom. Remove respirator after leaving patient room and closing door.

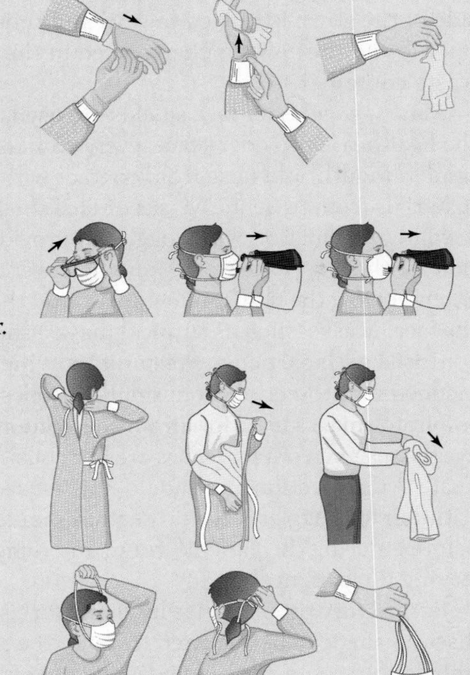

1. Gloves
   Outside of gloves is contaminated.
   Grasp outside of glove with opposite gloved hand and peel off.
   Hold removed glove in gloved hand.
   Slide fingers of ungloved hand under remaining glove at wrist.
   Peel glove off over first glove.
   Discard gloves in a waste container.
2. Goggles or face shield
   Outside of goggles or face shield is contaminated.
   To remove, handle by headband or ear pieces.
   Place in designated receptacle for reprocessing or in a waste container.
3. Gown
   Gown front and sleeves are contaminated!
   Unfasten ties.
   Pull away from neck and shoulders, touching inside of gown only.
   Turn gown inside out.
   Fold or roll into a bundle and discard.
4. Mask or respirator
   Front of mask/respirator is contaminated; do not touch.
   Grasp bottom and then top ties or elastics and remove. Discard in waste container.

Perform hand hygiene immediately after removing all PPE.

Modified from the CDC Sequence for Donning and Removing Personal Protective Equipment poster found in English and Spanish. December 2013. Available at: http://www.cdc.gov/HAI/pdfs/ppe/ppeposter1322.pdf.

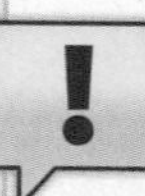

Respiratory Recap

Personal Protective Equipment (PPE)

- Gloves
- Eye protection
- Face protection
- Gowns
- Masks

discard gloves between patients and perform hand hygiene immediately after discarding the gloves and before caring for the next patient. Be cautious to avoid touching your face, eyeglasses, and environmental surfaces, or adjusting your PPE with contaminated gloves. Gloves should *never* be used as a substitute for hand hygiene.

Isolation gowns, aprons, jackets, or pants are used as a barrier to protect the healthcare provider from contamination of the clothes and from the patient's blood and body fluids. Selection of the type of isolation gown is based on the nature of the interaction with the patient and the anticipated degree of contact with infectious material or blood and body fluids. Isolation gowns are always worn in combination with gloves and other PPE. Gowns are usually the first PPE to be donned. Isolation gowns should be removed before leaving the patient care area to prevent contamination of the environment outside the patient's room. When removing the gown, the outer contaminated side of the gown is turned inward and rolled into a bundle and the gown is then placed in the correct waste container.

Masks, goggles, or face shields are used to protect the healthcare provider's face, eyes, skin, mucous membranes, mouth, and nose from contact with infectious materials from patients. Masks or face shields can be used in combination with goggles to provide protection for the face. Face shields should cover the forehead, extend below the chin, and wrap around the side of the face. Masks (such as surgical masks) should not be confused with particulate respirators, which are recommended for protection from small particles (e.g., N95 respirator masks used for airborne isolation). Personal eyeglasses and contact lenses are *not* considered adequate eye protection and should not be used as a substitution for goggles. Face protection should be donned before entering the patient's room and removed before leaving the patient's room.[12]

Respiratory protection is intended for use to prevent diseases that can be acquired through the airborne (inhalation) route. This includes the use of NIOSH-approved N95 or higher-level respirator masks that fit properly. OSHA broadly regulates respiratory protection for healthcare providers, which includes medical clearance to wear a respirator, fit testing for the respirator, and education on the use and periodic reevaluation of the respirator.[12]

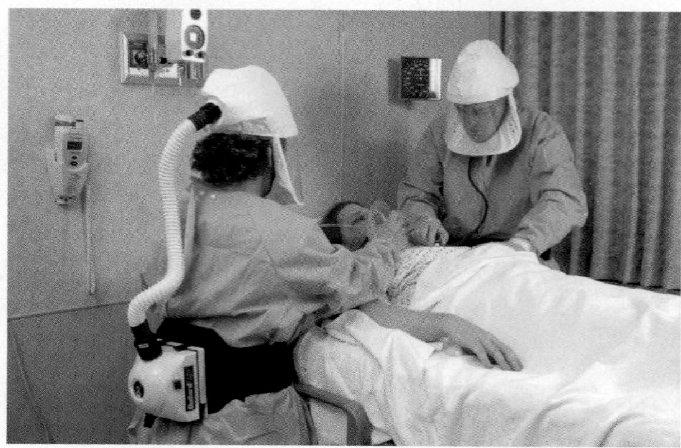

FIGURE 31-6 Powered air-purifying respirator (PAPR).
Courtesy of Bullard Company.

A powered air-purifying respirator (PAPR) is a device with a half- or full-face piece, breathing tube, battery-operated blower, and HEPA filters (**Figure 31-6**). A PAPR uses a blower to pass contaminated air through the HEPA filter, which removes the contaminant and supplies purified air to a face piece. However, it is not a true positive pressure device because it can be over breathed when inhaling. A face shield may be used in conjunction with a half-mask PAPR respirator for protection against body fluids. The most common use for a PAPR is in the case where an N95 respirator mask does not fit. It can also be used if the healthcare provider has facial hair or facial deformity that interferes with the mask-to-face seal. It might also be used when a N95 respirator mask is unavailable. Some prefer to use a PAPR for high-risk aerosol-generating procedures.

Accidental injuries associated with needle sticks and other sharp objects have been associated with transmission of hepatitis C, HIV, and other pathogens. Prevention of needle sticks and other sharps injuries is a major concern for healthcare providers. Healthcare providers must use caution when handling any and all sharp instruments, including needles and syringes. Needle protection devices should be used on arterial blood gas syringes, and a needle-free syringe should be used whenever possible (**Figure 31-7**). Needles should be properly disposed of in an appropriate sharps container (**Figure 31-8**). If a needle stick injury occurs, the area should be immediately washed with soap and water, and the incident should be reported to a supervisor, medical attention should be sought, and appropriate follow-up is necessary.

Patient Placement

When there is a concern about transmission of an infectious agent, patients should be placed in a single-patient room. Single-patient rooms are indicated for

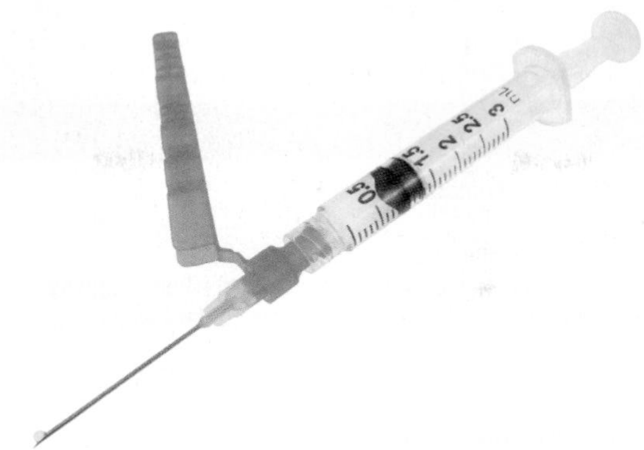

FIGURE 31-7 Syringe with needle guard.
© pancaketom/Dreamstime.com.

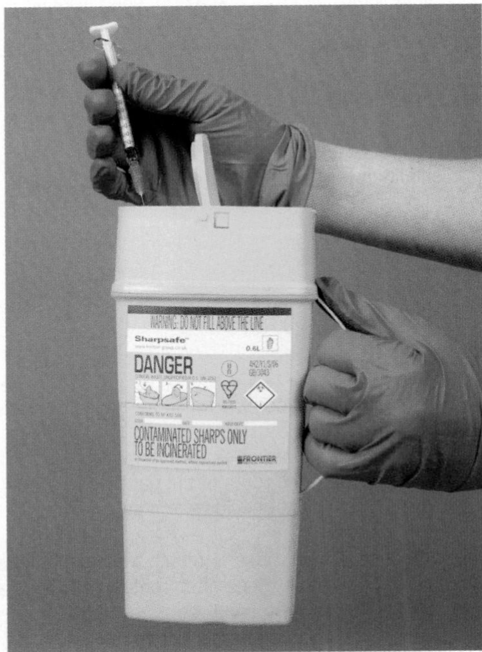

FIGURE 31-8 Sharps container.

patients requiring airborne isolation and those in need of a protective environment and are preferred for those requiring contact or droplet precautions. Patients may be placed in the same room if they have the same transmittable disease, however. Limiting the transport of patients with contagious diseases limits the risk of transmission. When they must be transported, it is imperative the patient wear barrier protection (gown, gloves, or mask) consistent with the route for transmission. An N95 respirator mask is not required for the patient. It is also imperative to notify the healthcare personnel in the area receiving the patient to ensure that precautions are taken to prevent transmission.

Patient equipment that has been contaminated should be placed into an impervious bag before removal from the patient's room. A single bag may be used if the contaminated equipment can be placed in the bag without contaminating the outer surface of the bag. Otherwise, the equipment must be double-bagged. The bags should be clearly labeled and are often colored red. These bags prevent exposure of healthcare providers and the environment to the contaminated equipment. The contaminated equipment should be processed according to OSHA procedures.

The need for respiratory hygiene and **cough etiquette** at the first point of contact became evident after reevaluating the SARS outbreaks, where failure to implement simple source control measures with patients, visitors, and healthcare personnel with respiratory symptoms may have contributed to SARS corona virus (SARS-CoV) transmission. This new strategy is targeted at patients, family members, and friends with undiagnosed transmissible respiratory infections and applies to any person with signs of illness that include cough, congestion, rhinorrhea, or increased production of respiratory secretions. Respiratory hygiene and cough etiquette includes educating staff, patients, and visitors; posting instructions for patients and family members in the appropriate language(s); source control measures such as covering the mouth and nose with a tissue when coughing and prompt disposal of used tissues; providing surgical masks for persons with a cough; hand hygiene after contact with respiratory secretions; and spatial separation, ideally more than 3 feet, between people with respiratory infection and those in the waiting areas. The main source of control is covering sneezes and coughs and applying a mask to a coughing person. These simple acts have been proven to prevent infected persons from dispersing secretions in the air. Measures such as these are important for infectious diseases such as the H1N1 influenza virus and other highly contagious respiratory infections.

Healthcare providers should observe droplet precautions and hand hygiene when caring for patients with signs and symptoms of respiratory infections. Those healthcare providers who have a respiratory infection are advised to avoid direct patient contact with high-risk patients. If this is not possible, the healthcare provider should wear a mask as well.

Transmission-Based Precautions

For some diseases, standard precautions are not enough to keep them from being spread to others or to other sites on the same patient. Therefore, standard precautions *and* one or more of the transmission-based precautions must be used. Remember that standard precautions are *always* used in the healthcare setting in interactions with all patients. Categories of transmission-based precautions include contact precautions, droplet precautions, and airborne precautions (**Table 31-5**).

TABLE 31-5
Isolation Precautions

Type	Selected Patients	Major Specifications
Standard	All patients	Hand hygiene before and after every patient contact. Gloves, gowns, eye protection as required. Safe disposal or cleaning of instruments and linen. Cough etiquette: Patients and visitors should cover their nose or mouth when coughing, promptly dispose of used tissues, and practice hand hygiene after contact with respiratory secretions.
Contact	MRSA, VRE, *C. difficile* Scabies Impetigo Noncontained abscesses or decubitus ulcers (especially for *Staphylococcus aureus* and group A streptococci)	In addition to standard precautions: Private room preferred; multipatient room allowed if necessary. Gloves required upon entering room. Change gloves after contact with contaminated secretions. Gown required if clothing may come into contact with the patient or environment surfaces, or if the patient has diarrhea. Patient wears gown during transport. Contact precautions plus: Wash hands after removing gown and before hand hygiene. Strict contact precautions: Must wear gown.
Droplet	Known or suspected: Influenza Meningococcal disease Epiglottitis (*Haemophilus influenzae*) Diphtheria Pneumonic plague Rubella Mumps Adenovirus Parvovirus	In addition to standard precautions: Private room preferred; multipatient room allowed if necessary. Wear a surgical mask when within 3 feet of the patient. Patient wears surgical mask during transport. Cough etiquette: Patients and visitors should cover their nose or mouth when coughing, promptly dispose of used tissues, and practice hand hygiene after contact with respiratory secretions.
Airborne	Known or suspected: Tuberculosis Smallpox Measles SARS	In addition to standard precautions: Place the patient in an AIIR (airborne infection isolation room), a monitored negative-pressure room with at least 6 to 12 air exchanges per hour. Room exhaust must be appropriately discharged outdoors or passed through a HEPA filter. An N95 respirator mask must be worn when entering the room of the patient. Transport of the patient should be minimized; the patient should wear a surgical mask if transported within the hospital. Cough etiquette: Patients and visitors should cover their nose or mouth when coughing, promptly dispose of used tissues, and practice hand hygiene after contact with respiratory secretions.

MRSA, methicillin-resistant *Staphylococcus aureus*; VRE, vancomycin-resistant *Enterococcus*; HEPA, high-efficiency particulate-arresting; SARS, severe acute respiratory syndrome.

Information from Siegel JD, Rhinehart E, Jackson M, Chiarello L, and the Healthcare Infection Control Practices Advisory Committee. *Guideline for Isolation Precautions: Preventing Transmission of Infectious Agents in Healthcare Settings 2007*. Atlanta, GA: Centers for Disease Control and Prevention; 2007.

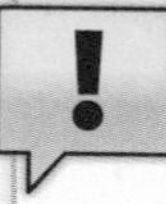

Respiratory Recap

Transmission-Based Precautions

- Contact
- Droplet
- Airborne

Contact precautions are used to prevent the transmission of infectious agents that are spread by direct or indirect contact with the patient or the patient's environment. This includes placing the patient in a single-patient room; if a multipatient room placement is unavoidable, there must be more than 3 feet of separation between beds to reduce the opportunity for sharing of items between the infected/colonized patient and other patients. Healthcare providers should wear a gown and gloves for *all* interactions that may involve contact with the patient or with potentially contaminated areas in the patient's environment. The PPE should be put on prior to entering the patient's room and discarded before exiting the patient's room. Examples of patients requiring contact precautions include those with methicillin-resistant *Staphylococcus aureus* (MRSA), vancomycin-resistant enterococci (VRE), herpes simplex, and herpes zoster.

A more strict form of contact precautions is contact precautions plus. This requires hand washing between the steps of removing the gown and hand hygiene with an alcohol-based rub. Contact precautions plus are used if the patient has *Clostridium difficile* diarrhea. Another form of contact precautions is strict contact precautions, used with vancomycin-insensitive *S aureus* (VISA) and vancomycin-resistant *S aureus* (VRSA). With strict contact precautions, a gown is required when entering the room (not just for patient contact).

Droplet precautions are used to prevent the transmission of pathogens spread by close respiratory or mucous membrane contact with respiratory secretions. Coughing and sneezing can generate droplets in the air. These pathogens are not typically transmissible over a distance greater than 3 feet. A single-patient room is preferred. Healthcare providers should wear a mask for all close contact with the patient. An N95 respirator mask is not required; a surgical mask is sufficient. The mask should be put on before entering the room. In the event the patient must be transported outside the room, the patient should wear a surgical mask and follow respiratory hygiene and cough etiquette. Examples of patients requiring droplet precautions include those with influenza, pertussis, adenovirus (in which case contact precautions should also be used), meningococcal disease, and *Haemophilus influenza* epiglottitis.

Airborne precautions are used to prevent the transmission of infectious agents over a long distance when suspended in the air. These patients must be placed in a private room that has monitored negative air pressure. The door must remain closed. Healthcare providers must wear a NIOSH-approved N95 respirator mask that has been fit-tested to ensure that the mask seals appropriately. The patient must wear a surgical mask during transport. Examples of patients requiring airborne precautions are those with tuberculosis, measles, smallpox, and viral hemorrhagic fevers, such as Ebola. Another form of airborne precautions is airborne/contact precautions, in which a gown is required if the healthcare provider has contact with the patient or the patient's environment. Airborne/contact precautions are used for chickenpox and herpes zoster if disseminated or in an immunocompromised patient.

A protective environment is designed to minimize fungal spore counts in the air and reduce the risk of invasive environmental fungal infections for allogeneic hematologic stem cell transplant (HSCT) patients. The air quality for HSCT patients is improved through a combination of environmental controls that include HEPA filtration of incoming air, directed room airflow, positive room air pressure relative to the corridor, well-sealed rooms to prevent the flow of air from the outside, ventilation to provide more than 12 air changes per hour, strategies to reduce dust, and the elimination of dried or fresh flowers and potted plants from the rooms of HSCT patients.[1]

Respiratory Recap

Precautions

- Precautions protect both the patient and the caregiver.
- Apply standard precautions for every patient encounter, assuming everyone is at risk.
- When body fluids (including significant aerosol) may be encountered, use appropriate barriers, including gloves, mask, eye protection, gowns, and booties.
- Use hand hygiene before and after contact with each patient.
- Remove personal protective equipment correctly.

Healthcare-Associated Infections Related to Respiratory Care Equipment

A primary issue in respiratory care is to prevent the introduction of infectious agents into the lungs. Although the majority of nosocomial pneumonia cases arise from microaspiration, respiratory care equipment itself can be a source of infection. It is imperative, therefore, that single-patient, disposable equipment be used when available. Otherwise, respiratory therapists must handle reusable equipment in a manner to prevent the spread of infection.

Ventilator-Related Issues

The CDC recommends that ventilator circuits *not* be changed routinely, but only when there is visual or known contamination of the circuit. Several studies have shown that less-frequent tubing changes may reduce infection rates, although the optimum frequency for ventilator tubing changes is still considered uncertain.[12,13]

Common practice is to fill the humidification chamber of the ventilator with sterile water to prevent the introduction of heat-resistant organisms, such as *Legionella* species, which may contaminate the device despite its high temperatures that inactivate most common respiratory pathogens. The efficacy of this practice has not been validated but appears prudent given the demonstrated danger of *Legionella* presence in hospital tap water.

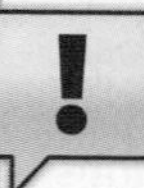

Respiratory Recap

Healthcare-Associated Sources of Respiratory Infection

- Ventilator circuit changes
- Condensate in ventilator tubing
- Humidifiers
- Nebulizers
- Suction catheters
- Pulmonary function testing equipment

Water condenses and accumulates in the ventilator circuit, which is a potential growth medium for microorganisms. Regardless of the humidification technique used, care should be taken to drain condensate and, when manipulating the tubing, to prevent the condensate from unintentionally pouring into the patient's airway via the endotracheal or tracheostomy tube.[12,13]

Suction catheters can introduce microorganisms into a patient's lower respiratory tract. The single-use open catheter system requires the therapist to maintain a sterile field while suctioning the airway. The inline closed suction system has an advantage because the circuit does not have to be broken when suctioning the patient. Although inline suction catheters become colonized with organisms originating from the patient's lower respiratory tract, the clinical importance of this is unclear.[12,13] Introduction of normal saline for suction lavage should be limited as this can also lead to infection by creating a host environment.[14]

Nebulizers

Rinse with sterile water (or saline) and air-dry, or replace, small-volume nebulizers between treatments on the same patient. Because they produce aerosols that can carry microorganisms into the lower respiratory tract, nebulizers should be changed at a frequency determined by the hospital infection control surveillance practices. Transmission of infection from contaminated nebulizers is particularly problematic in patients with cystic fibrosis.

Nebulizers placed in-line in the ventilator circuit can become contaminated by colonized condensate and increase the patient's risk of pneumonia. It is reasonable to use a metered dose inhaler rather than a nebulizer as an infection control measure, given that it is virtually impossible to contaminate the interior of a metered dose inhaler. Another acceptable practice is the use of a mesh nebulizer that is not removed from the ventilator circuit.

Spirometers and Pulmonary Function Testing Equipment

Pulmonary function testing (PFT) equipment is not believed to carry a high risk of infection, although cross contamination between patients is possible. The use of filters between the patient and PFT equipment has been advocated to trap aerosolized microbes.[12,13]

Key Points

- ▶ Healthcare-associated infections (HAIs) result in preventable suffering and lost lives.
- ▶ The common routes of disease transmission are by contact, vehicle, airborne, and vector routes; the most common routes are contact (direct and indirect), airborne, and vehicle-borne.
- ▶ Infection control methods include cleaning, disinfecting, and sterilizing the equipment.
- ▶ Isolation precautions assist with preventing the spread of HAIs.
- ▶ Primary precautions include hand hygiene, standard precautions, and personal protective equipment.
- ▶ The most important way to prevent transmission of infection is hand hygiene before and after patient contact.
- ▶ Transmission-based precautions include contact precautions, droplet precautions, and airborne precautions.
- ▶ Hospitals are implementing vaccination programs and monitoring as part of infection control programs.

References

1. Siegel JD, Rhinehart E, Jackson M, Chiarello L, and the Healthcare Infection Control Practices Advisory Committee. *Guideline for Isolation Precautions: Preventing Transmission of Infectious Agents in Healthcare Settings 2007.* Atlanta, GA: Centers for Disease Control and Prevention; 2007.
2. Yokoe DS, Mermel LA, Anderson DJ, et al. A compendium of strategies to prevent healthcare-associated infections in acute care hospitals. *Infect Control Hosp Epidemiol.* 2008;29(Suppl 1):S12–S21.
3. Yokoe D, Classen D. Improving patient safety through infection control: a new healthcare imperative. *Infect Control Hosp Epidemiol.* 2008;29(Suppl 1):S3–S11.
4. Institute for Healthcare Improvement. *Protecting 5 Million Lives From Harm.* Available at: http://www.ihi.org/IHI/Programs/campaign/campaign.htm?Tabld=2#PreventSrugicaglsiteinfection. Accessed March 30, 2009.
5. Eggimann P, Pittet D. Infection control in the ICU. *Chest.* 2001;120;2059–2093.
6. Sehulster LM, Chinn RYW, Arduino MJ, et al. *Guidelines for Environmental Infection Control in Healthcare Facilities. Recommendations from CDC and the Healthcare Infection Control Practices Advisory Committee (HICPAC).* Chicago: American Society for Healthcare Engineering/American Hospital Association; 2004.
7. Public Health Guidance for community level preparedness and response to Severe Acute Respiratory Syndrome (SARS). Version 2.

January 8, 2004. Available at: http://www.cdc.gov/sars/guidance/index.html. Accessed September 6, 2014.

8. Rutala WA, Weber DJ, and the Health Infection Control Practices Advisory Committee. *Guideline for Disinfection and Sterilization in Healthcare Facilities 2008*. November 2008. Available at: http://www.cdc.gov/hicpac/pdf/guidelines/disinfection_nov_2008.pdf. Accessed August 6, 2014.
9. Rutala WA, Weber DJ. Disinfection and sterilization in health care facilities: what clinicians need to know. *Clin Infect Dis*. 2004;39:702–709.
10. Rupp M, Fitzgerald T, Puumala S, et al. Controlled cross-over trial of alcohol-based hand gel in critical care units. *Infect Control Hosp Epidemiol*. 2008;29:8–15.
11. Calfee DP, Salgado CD, Classen D, et al. Strategies to prevent transmission of MRSA in acute care hospitals. *Infect Control Hosp Epidemiol*. 2008;29(Suppl 1):S62–S80.
12. Centers for Disease Control and Prevention. Guidelines for preventing healthcare-associated pneumonia, 2003. *MMWR Morbid Mortal Wkly Rep*. 2004;55(RR03):1–36.
13. Hess DR, Kallstrom TJ, Mottram CD, et al. Care of the ventilator circuit and its relation to ventilator-associated pneumonia. *Respir Care*. 2003;48:869–879.
14. Restrepo RD, Brown JM 2nd, Hughes JM. AARC Clinical Practice Guidelines. Endotracheal suctioning of mechanically ventilated patients with artificial airways 2010. *Respir Care*. 2010;55: 758–764.

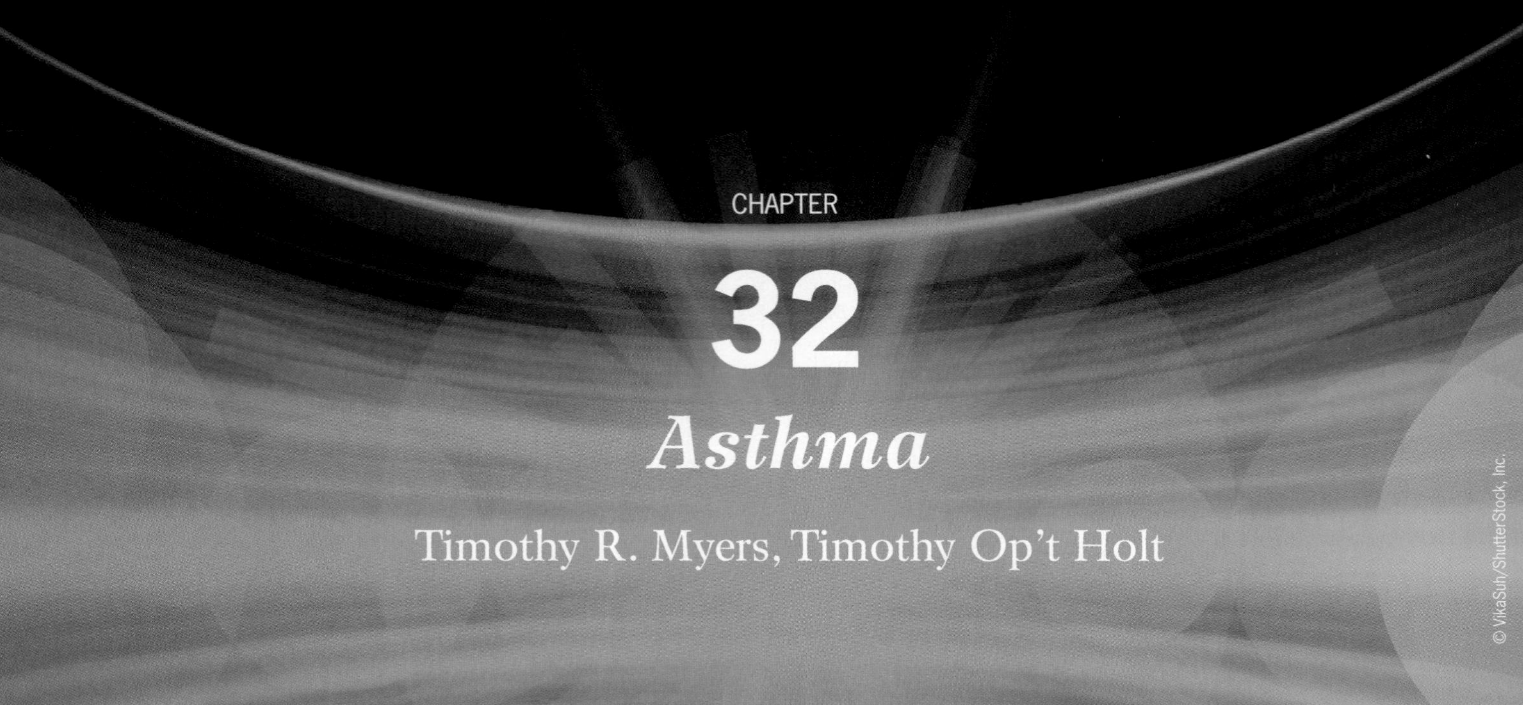

OUTLINE

Epidemiology
Pathophysiology
Pathogenesis
Risk Factors
Asthma Phenotypes
Disease Severity Classification
Assessing Control of Asthma
Objective Measurements
Pharmacologic Therapy
Aerosol Therapy
Adjunctive Treatments
Education
Case Studies

OBJECTIVES

1. Define asthma.
2. Discuss the epidemiology of asthma.
3. Discuss the pathophysiology of asthma.
4. List the risk factors for asthma.
5. Describe the clinical features of allergic asthma, nocturnal asthma, exercise-induced asthma, asthma associated with food and drugs, emotion-induced asthma, and occupational asthma.
6. Describe the disease severity classification from the National Asthma Education and Prevention Program.
7. Discuss how asthma control is assessed and classified.
8. Discuss the role of peak flow monitoring in the management of asthma.
9. Compare the role of controller medication and quick-relief medication in the management of asthma.
10. Compare the use of nebulizers, pressurized metered dose inhalers, and dry powder inhalers in the delivery of aerosols to the patient with asthma.
11. Discuss the role of alternative treatment modalities in the management of asthma.
12. List the goals of mechanical ventilation of the patient with asthma.
13. Discuss the role of education in the disease management of asthma.

KEY TERMS

airway hyperresponsiveness
airway inflammation
allergen
asthma
asthma education program
asthma trigger
bronchial challenge testing
controller medication
exercise-induced asthma (EIA)
exhaled nitric oxide (eNO)
heliox
intermittent asthma
mild persistent asthma
moderate persistent asthma
National Asthma Education and Prevention Program (NAEPP)
nocturnal asthma
peak flow meter
quick-relief medication
severe persistent asthma

Introduction

Asthma is one of the most common chronic diseases of the pulmonary system. The third expert panel report (EPR) from the **National Asthma Education and Prevention Program (NAEPP)** of the National Institutes of Health issued this working definition of **asthma**, which remains unchanged from previous EPR guidelines:

> Asthma is a chronic inflammatory disorder of the airways in which many cells and cellular elements play a role: in particular, mast cells, eosinophils, T lymphocytes, macrophages, neutrophils and epithelial cells. In susceptible individuals, this inflammation causes recurrent episodes of wheezing, breathlessness, chest tightness, and coughing, particularly at night or in the early morning. These episodes are usually associated with widespread but variable airflow obstruction that is often reversible either spontaneously or with treatment. The inflammation also causes an associated increase in the existing bronchial hyperresponsiveness to a variety of stimuli; reversibility of airflow limitation may be incomplete in some patients with asthma.[1]

In addition to the NAEPP, the Global Initiative for Asthma (GINA) works with healthcare professionals and public health officials around the world to reduce asthma prevalence, morbidity, and mortality.[2] This chapter presents issues related to the respiratory care of patients with asthma.

Epidemiology

Asthma is a common chronic disease that is increasing in prevalence and severity. The asthma literature frequently mentions epidemiology, prevalence, and incidence. Webster's ninth *New Collegiate Dictionary* defines *epidemiology* as a branch of medical science that deals with the incidence, distribution, and control of disease in a population. *Prevalence* refers to the number of individuals with a diagnosis at any given time (e.g., in 2014), whereas *incidence* refers specifically to the number of newly diagnosed cases that occur within a specific period of time (e.g., the past century).

The prevalence and incidence of asthma are difficult to estimate because of the inherent problems with surveys and the varying definitions for asthma. Asthma is prevalent in approximately 10% to 12% of the population in different countries. This represents an estimated 300 million cases globally, 22 million of which are in the United States (**Figure 32-1**).[3]

Despite recent advances in both pharmacologic and nonpharmacologic management strategies, the prevalence of asthma is increasing, particularly in developing and developed nations. Presently, prevalence in the United States is monitored in terms of prevalence of attacks per year. This increased in the period from 2003 to 2010 from 11 million to 13.9 million per year. Likewise, outpatient and physician office visits and emergency department visits increased, but fortunately deaths decreased (**Table 32-1**).[3]

Although asthma is more prevalent in males, it tends to be more severe in females. African Americans, especially those residing in urban areas, are three times more likely to be diagnosed with asthma in the United States. In the United States, asthma is the third leading cause of preventable hospitalization and resulted

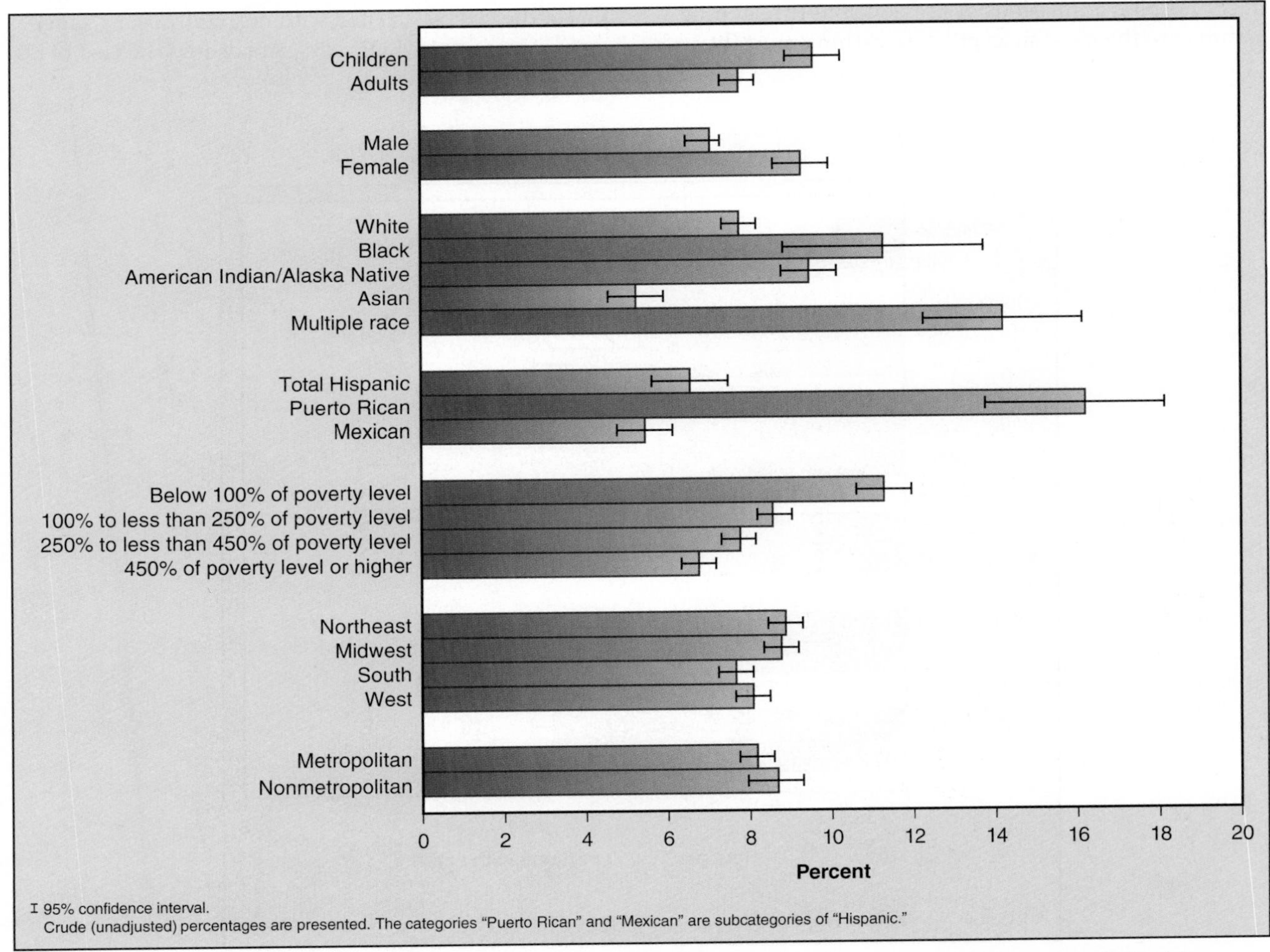

FIGURE 32-1 Current asthma prevalence, by age group, sex, race and ethnicity, poverty status, geographic region, and urbanicity: United States, average annual 2008–2010.

Reproduced from National Surveillance of Asthma: United States, 2001–2010. http://www.cdc.gov/nchs/data/series/sr_03/sr03_035.pdf.

TABLE 32-1
Changes in Asthma Prevalence, Number of Outpatient Visits, Emergency Department Visits, and Death, 2001–2009/10

	2001	2009–2010
Prevalence	20.3 M	25.7 M
Outpatient visits	1.3 M	1.2 M*
Emergency department visits	1.6 M	2.1M*
Deaths	4269	3388*

*2009

Information from *National Surveillance of Asthma: United States, 2001–2010.* http://www.cdc.gov/nchs/data/series/sr_03/sr03_035.pdf.

in 3388, down from 4269 in 2001, deaths in 2003.[2] There was no trend in hospitalization in the 2001–2009 period. People with asthma who are Puerto Rican have death rates that are four times higher than those of Caucasians (**Figure 32-2**).[3] Patients who have had frequent hospital admissions or previous life-threatening asthma are the most susceptible to asthma mortality.

AGE-SPECIFIC ANGLE

Death rates are greatest for people with asthma aged 18 years and older.

Misdiagnosis and inadequate treatment by disease severity are significant factors contributing to the increased incidence and prevalence of asthma. This makes accurate diagnosis of asthma, ruling out of asthma mimics, assessment of asthma severity, and assessment of asthma control all the more important.

The severity of acute episodes may vary from mild to life threatening within a given patient over the course of the disease or within a given year. In 2010, people with asthma lost 46.7 million school, work, and activity days because of their disease.[3] In 2009, there were 479,300 hospitalizations for asthma.

Along with the increasing prevalence of asthma is the economic burden that comes with this chronic condition. In the early 1990s, the cost to treat asthma was estimated to be approximately $6 billion per year, with 43% of the cost associated with hospitalizations, emergency department (ED) visits, and death. The cost of ED

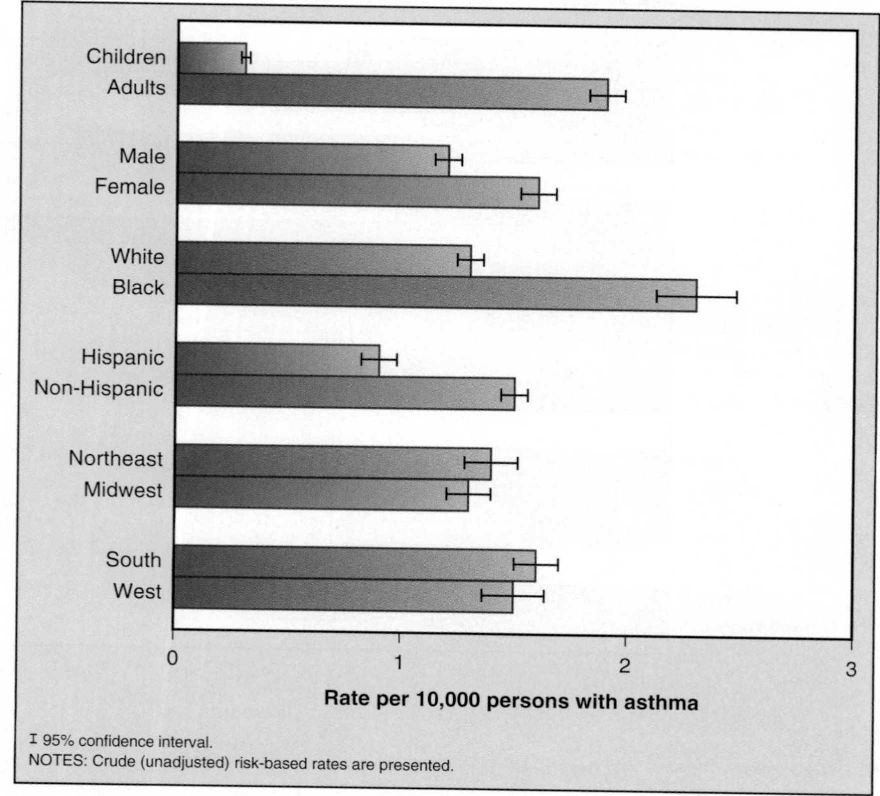

FIGURE 32-2 Asthma death rates (risk-based), by age group, sex, race and ethnicity, and geographic region: United States, average annual 2007–2009.

Reproduced from National Surveillance of Asthma: United States, 2001–2010. http://www.cdc.gov/nchs/data/series/sr_03/sr03_035.pdf.

> **AGE-SPECIFIC ANGLE**
>
> Asthma is increasing at the fastest rate in children younger than 5 years. Before puberty, asthma affects more boys than girls. This trend switches after puberty.

therapy for asthma in the same year was $270 million, which represented 8% of the total direct cost of caring for asthma.[4] By contrast, in 2007, the direct cost (hospitalization, physician visits, and drugs) to treat the 13 million asthmatics in the United States was $50.13 billion. With the additional billions in lost work and school days and productivity loss due to death, the total cost was $56.03 billion. This represents a healthcare expenditure of $3259 per person with asthma more than those without asthma.[5] The fastest-growing age segment with asthma is children, a fact that has been reported to have had a staggering impact on the cost to treat asthma. There are no studies within the last 15 years looking specifically at the economic burden of asthma in children in the United States. A study from 1997 suggested that hospitalization costs for children with asthma younger than 5 years of age reach approximately 74% of their healthcare costs.[6] Asthma therefore is an expensive disease, as it impacts both quality of life and financial variables.

The high cost associated with acute care treatment of asthma has led to the implementation of disease management programs which have had an impact on ED visits, admissions, cost of care, and length of stay.[7–9] The components of asthma disease management programs and asthma management programs for patients in different age groups and in different settings is addressed elsewhere.[10] It has been difficult to determine the effectiveness of disease management programs. It may be impossible to determine the impact of asthma disease management programs on outcomes because of differences in intervention components, study designs, and outcomes assessed. Few studies provided sufficient detail about physician-pharmacist-nurse interactions during and between office visits, nor did they provide detailed costs and other statistics necessary to determine cost effectiveness or effect size of the interventions.[11] Because of the high volume of asthma visits and admissions in most urban areas, disease management programs or clinical practice guidelines can reduce cost by eliminating practice variation in the emergency department or hospital in the treatment of asthma. Eliminating acute treatment that adds cost without degrading the overall quality of care can be an effective tool in the management of asthma.[12,13]

Although asthma is not a curable disease, it can be managed effectively. Asthma mortality, and to a lesser degree morbidity, is largely preventable. Appropriate medications based on disease severity and patient or caregiver adherence to a written asthma action plan can result in highly effective disease management. Patient education and awareness and control of environmental triggers also play a significant role in the overall management of the disease. Even with overall effective management from an educational, medical, and adherence standpoint, some patients develop severe persistent asthma with frequent exacerbations that may result in ED visits or hospitalizations.

Pathophysiology

The exact underlying cause of asthma is still unknown. Asthma is a multifactorial disease that has been associated with allergenic, hereditary, psychosocial, socioeconomic, environmental, and infectious causes. Asthma is not the only cause of wheezing. **Box 32-1** lists other potential causes or diagnoses associated with wheezing.

Even if the underlying cause of asthma is known in an individual, the trigger stimuli of an exacerbation may change over time. The pathophysiology of the disease is largely related to inflammation, hyperresponsiveness, and obstruction. **Figure 32-3** demonstrates the interrelationship of these three factors in the underlying mechanism of the disease.

Airway Inflammation

Regardless of the trigger mechanism or the underlying cause of asthma, **airway inflammation** plays an important role. Acute and chronic inflammation affects

> **BOX 32-1**
>
> **Differential Diagnosis of Wheezing**
>
> Small and Large Airway Obstruction
>
> Asthma
> Chronic obstructive pulmonary disease
> Airway tumors
> Bronchiolitis (in children)
> Cardiogenic pulmonary edema
> Cystic fibrosis
> Pneumonia; aspiration
> Bronchopulmonary dysplasia
>
> Large Airway Obstruction
>
> Airway and esophageal foreign bodies
> Pulmonary emboli
> Tumors
> Vascular rings
> Focal pneumonia
> Laryngeal webs or malacia
> Tracheal stenosis
> Lymphadenopathies
> Vocal cord dysfunction

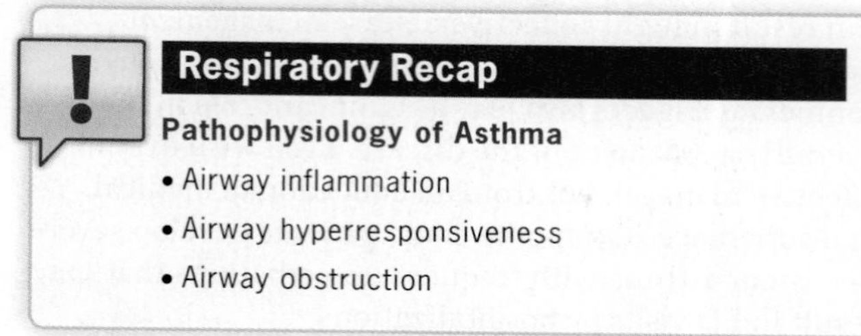

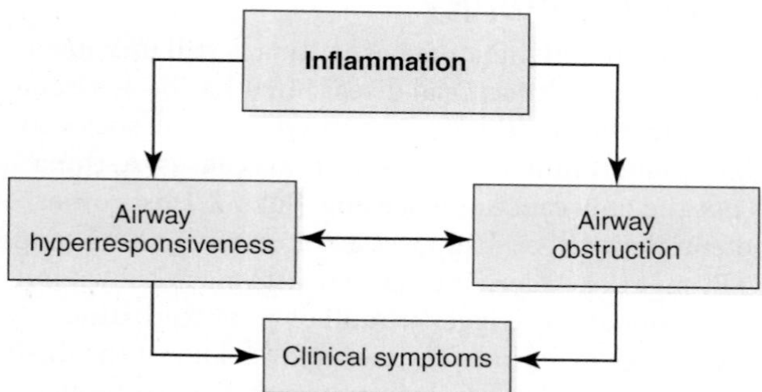

FIGURE 32-3 The interplay and interaction between airway inflammation and the clinical symptoms and pathophysiology of asthma.

Modified from National Asthma Education Program, National Heart, Lung, and Blood Institute. *Expert Panel Report 3: Guidelines for the Diagnosis and Management of Asthma. Full Report 2007*. Bethesda, MD: National Institutes of Health; 2007. NIH Publication 08-4051.

airway caliber, airflow, and underlying bronchial hyperresponsiveness, which enhance susceptibility to bronchospasm. Chronic inflammation may be associated with a permanent alteration in airway structure, known as *remodeling*. These structural changes can include thickening of the sub-basement membrane, subepithelial fibrosis, airway smooth muscle hypertrophy and hyperplasia, blood vessel proliferation and dilation, and mucous gland hyperplasia and hypersecretion. Once remodeling occurs, the patient's asthma is not responsive to current treatment. Control of inflammation therefore is a central feature of asthma therapy.

Inflammatory cells that appear to be the most significant are lymphocytes, dendritic cells, mast cells, eosinophils, macrophages, epithelial cells, and T helper 2 cells. Among the mediators of inflammation are chemokines, nitric oxide, IgE, interleukins, cytokines, histamine, granulocyte macrophage colony-stimulating factor (GM-CSF), and tumor necrosis factor-α (TNF-α). The release of inflammatory mediators results in recurrent exacerbations that manifest as wheezing, progressive shortness of breath, chest tightness, and coughing that may be more persistent nocturnally or in the early mornings. In most patients, these exacerbations are usually self-limiting or resolve rapidly to appropriate asthma treatment.

Airway Hyperresponsiveness

A marker associated with asthma is the increased sensitivity, or **airway hyperresponsiveness**, to both specific and nonspecific factors. These factors have little or no effect on people with normal airways.

Airway hyperresponsiveness is a mechanism in which the airways constrict too easily and frequently, an exaggerated bronchoconstrictor response to a wide variety of stimuli. Factors associated with hyperresponsive airways include environmental factors (both indoor and outdoor), exercise, allergens, and viral infections. The degree or level of airway hyperresponsiveness usually correlates with the clinical severity of the disease.[1] Control of inflammation can reduce airway hyperresponsiveness and improve asthma control.[1]

Bronchial challenge testing with methacholine or mannitol serves as a measure of responsiveness to general stimuli. Asthma is characterized by the reversibility of airflow obstruction. These challenge tests are usually administered in a pulmonary function laboratory. The methacholine or mannitol challenge test begins with spirometry. The patient then inhales five breaths of increasing concentrations of methacholine, or increasing doses of dry powder mannitol, each time followed by performance of spirometry. The methacholine or mannitol concentration at which a 20% decrease in FEV_1 (forced expiratory volume in 1 second) occurs (PC_{20}) is the endpoint. PC_{20} is reached sooner and with a lower dose of methacholine or mannitol in patients with asthma than in subjects without asthma. The test is followed (usually within 15 minutes) by administration of a short-acting β_2-agonist that should result in a 12% to 15% increase in FEV_1.

Airway Obstruction

The final component in the definition of asthma is airway obstruction, or the limitation of airflow through the airways. Airflow limitation is most commonly caused by the IgE-mediated release of inflammatory mediators into the airways, which come into contact with airway smooth muscles. More specifically, the mediators usually associated with an IgE response include histamine, tryptase, prostaglandin, and leukotrienes. When the airways are hyperresponsive, however, several stimuli can exacerbate bronchoconstriction (**Box 32-2**). The result of inflammation is an increase in airway wall thickness and increased secretions,

BOX 32-2

Changes That Lead to Airway Obstruction

Acute bronchoconstriction
Chronic mucous plug formation
Airway edema
Airway remodeling

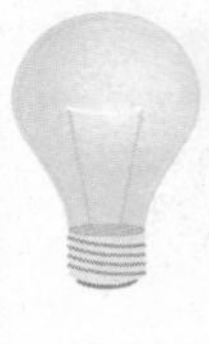

STOP AND THINK

You are caring for a patient with asthma who tells you that he was looking up information on the Internet about his disease and asks you to explain what the asthma triad means. How would you respond?

obstructing the airway. The airway hyperresponsiveness manifests itself as bronchospasm. This combination of inflammation, airway hyperresponsiveness, and secretions is often referred to as the asthma triad and is the object of therapy for asthma.

In most patients, the airflow limitation or bronchoconstriction will spontaneously resolve with the administration of a short-acting β_2-agonist. Inflammation in patients with persistent asthma is treated with corticosteroids, usually inhaled corticosteroids, and they may also receive long-acting β_2 adrenergic bronchodilators. Patients who have persistent disease or who have had asthma for a number of years may develop an incomplete response as a result of airway remodeling. These patients may have a history of smoking, so they are difficult to separate from the COPD population. Patients who continue to have symptoms after initiation of conventional therapy are considered to be in status asthmaticus. While this term is popular, it is not used in the EPR-3.

Pathogenesis

The factor that initiates the inflammatory process in the first place is unknown. It is known that the origins of asthma occur early in life, with the interplay of genetic and environmental factors as the immune system develops. This field of study, which emerged after the release of the second EPR, focuses on what has become known as the hygiene hypothesis.[1] Two types of T helper (Th) lymphocytes exist: Th1 and Th2. Th1 lymphocytes produce interleukin-2 and interferon-γ, which are important in response to infection. Th2 lymphocytes generate cytokines that mediate inflammation. At birth, Th2 is favored, and exposure to environmental stimuli such as infections will activate Th1 responses and balance Th1 and Th2. The imbalance in or favoring of Th2 favors the development of asthma. The favoring of Th2 is associated with the Western lifestyle: widespread use of antibiotics, an urban environment, diet, and sensitization to house-dust mites and cockroaches. The favoring of Th1 occurs when the child is exposed to other children or siblings, viral infection, and a rural environment. Our Western obsession with cleaning everything and eliminating microorganisms from the environment thus may not be doing our children any favors (the hygiene hypothesis). A review can be found elsewhere.[14] The hygiene hypothesis was first described in 1989 and had a significant following; however, recent evidence has made clinicians more skeptical.

Other factors affecting pathogenesis are genetics (asthma has an inheritable component), gender (asthma predominates in boys until puberty), environmental factors (which are important in the development, persistence, and severity of asthma), allergens (sensitivity and exposure to allergens are important to the development of asthma in children), respiratory infections (see the earlier discussion of the hygiene hypothesis), and other environmental exposures (especially tobacco). This interaction of host and environmental exposures early in life is related to development of asthma.

Risk Factors

The strongest identifiable predisposing factor for the development of asthma is atopy. Atopy is the familial or genetic predisposition to develop an IgE-mediated response to common allergens in the environment. Asthma in childhood is normally linked to atopic factors. Among the many phenotypes of asthma, this is called *atopic, pediatric*, or *allergic asthma.* A study of 6- to 32-year-olds in Tucson, Arizona, found a strong, direct correlation between serum IgE levels and the development or presence of asthma, and a weaker correlation between positive skin test reactions and the development or presence of asthma.

Atopic asthma is diagnosed by skin-prick testing, in which a multitude of known allergens are introduced to the patient's immune system through small pricks in the arms. A study of children in eight metropolitan areas indicated that the highest risk factors for atopic asthma in inner-city children were cockroach antigen, animal dander, and dust mites.[15]

Factors that may contribute to or enhance the development of asthma include environmental pollution, low birth weight, tobacco smoke, diet, and viral infections. Asthma has also been associated with sinusitis and gastroesophageal reflux.

Asthma Phenotypes

The term *phenotype* refers to the cause of asthma or to what an asthma flare is related. Common asthma phenotypes are allergic, irritant-related, emotion, food

Respiratory Recap

Risk Factors for Asthma

- Allergens
- Pollution
- Food and drug additives
- Viral agents

and drug additive–related, virus-related, nocturnal, exercise-induced, and occupational. Each is described here. Recently, therapy for asthma has become more related to phenotype rather than specifically to a level of severity, as in the use of immunomodulator drug and leukotriene modifier drugs. How to avoid an asthma flare is also related to phenotype. For example, nocturnal asthma may be related to presence of dust mites, so dust mite avoidance is important in the care of a person with nocturnal asthma.

Allergens

The majority of asthmatics suffer attacks exacerbated by inhalation of an **allergen**. Many allergens, both indoor (e.g., mold, animal dander, cockroach antigen, dust mites) and outdoor (e.g., grass and tree pollens), may trigger an exacerbation. Other allergens are found in certain foods such as dairy products, shellfish, nuts, mushrooms, and preservatives.

An allergic asthma exacerbation usually has two phases. The first phase is the acute phase. The presence of an **asthma trigger** on a hypersensitive airway causes rupture and degranulation of mast cells. Airway mast cells release mediators (leukotrienes, eosinophil chemotactic factor of anaphylaxis [ECF-A], prostaglandins, and histamine) into the tracheobronchial tree. These mediators all interact with the airway smooth muscle, resulting in bronchoconstriction, edema, vasodilation, and eosinophil release, and also may cause increased secretion production.

The second phase of an asthma attack is the inflammatory phase, occurring several hours after the first phase has resolved. Inflammatory mediators are released into the airway. Evidence suggests that airway inflammation is caused not by one particular type of inflammatory mediator but by an intricate cycle of complex interactions that develop between multiple mediators, inflammatory cells, and other cells and tissues commonly found in the airways. The inflammatory response usually results in the migration of these various inflammatory cells and mediators into the airways, where they cause direct injuries, such as alterations in epithelial integrity, abnormalities in autonomic neural control of airway tone, mucus hypersecretion, change in mucociliary function, and an increase in airway smooth muscle responsiveness.[1] The presence of the second phase of an asthma exacerbation is why a patient should be monitored for 4 to 8 hours after the initial phase has resolved, and why oral corticosteroids are considered for rapid relief in the emergency department for treatment of exacerbation. Oral corticosteroids help to control the severity of the second phase.

Allergens from indoor sources consist mainly of cockroach antigen, domestic dust mites, animal dander, and mold (*Alternaria*) or fungi. Indoor allergens appear to be a main trigger in industrialized, developed countries. In developed countries, insulated housing that has been heated, humidified, cooled, and carpeted is prone to increased levels of indoor allergenic sources.

Dust mites appear to be the major cause of asthma worldwide, especially when infants are exposed to high concentrations in the first 3 to 6 months of life. The predominant domestic mite is *Dermatophagoides* species. The allergens are located in the inhaled microscopic fecal pellets. Dust mites are found in common household products but are especially prominent in bedding, carpet, stuffed animals, and soft furnishings. Dust mites grow best in humid air at temperatures of 22° to 26° C (71.6° to 78.8° F). The best method for eradicating mites is to wash potential breeding material in hot water (>54.4° C; >130° F). One study indicated cockroach antigen as the leading allergenic cause of inner-city asthma.[16] Cockroach antigen is found in the microscopic excrement and powdered dried bodies of cockroaches and is inhaled by the sensitized patient.

Cats are highly allergenic. The principal source of allergen is found in cat excrement. Cat saliva has also been identified as a source of cat antigen. Dog sensitivity is not as well documented but has been found to contribute to allergenic sources.

Fungi and molds also have been identified as allergenic risks in specific individuals with moderate to severe asthma. Fungi are most commonly found to grow extremely well in areas used for heating, cooling, or humidification. Home humidifiers provide a special risk for indoor fungal growth and air contamination.

Outdoor allergen sources are primarily pollens. The sources of these pollens include grasses, trees, flowers, weeds, and fungi. Each season particular outdoor allergen sources appear as major contributing factors for initiating asthma exacerbations. In the early spring, trees are the prominent trigger in pollen-associated asthma attacks. As the temperatures warm in the late spring and early summer, grasses and flowers reign as the initiators. In early fall, weeds play an important role in eliciting asthma exacerbations. The fall season also initiates the mold-induced exacerbations, predominately from *Alternaria* and *Cladosporium* species.

AGE-SPECIFIC ANGLE

Dust mites are a major cause of asthma when infants are exposed to high concentrations in their first 3 to 6 months of life.

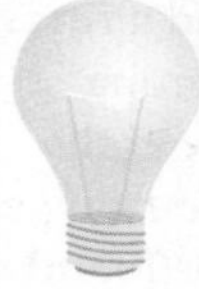

STOP AND THINK

You are caring for a patient who has recently been diagnosed with asthma. What allergens would you investigate as an asthma trigger?

Pollution and Environmental Irritants

The role of indoor and outdoor air pollution in the development or initiation of an asthma attack remains unproved and controversial. Air pollution often has been accused of being a viable source for the increase in prevalence of asthma, but research has failed to produce a direct link between air pollution and asthma. Outdoor types of pollution are mainly associated with industrialized nations that have a large amount of industrial or photochemical smog.

Indoor air pollutants have had a higher association with the development of respiratory symptoms. Maternal smoking during pregnancy results in harmful in utero exposure of the fetus and increases the risk of the child's developing recurrent wheezing in the first 5 years of life. It is well established that exposure to environmental tobacco smoke increases the severity of asthma, increases the risk of asthma-related ED visits and hospitalizations, and decreases the quality of life in both children and adults.[1] Other potential sources of indoor air pollution include nitric oxide, carbon dioxide, carbon monoxides, nitrogen oxides, sulfur dioxides, formaldehydes, cleaning chemicals, solvents and paint, perfumes or aerosol sprays, and biologic sources such as endotoxins.

Temperature changes often have been associated with eliciting asthma exacerbations. Although this appears to be largely unfounded, the roles of humidity in the summer months and cold air during winter months are still a mystery.

Emotion

In some patients, strong emotion, either happy or sad, will trigger bronchospasm. The mechanism of this is not well known but may relate to vagal excitation. In a clinical study, patients with asthma received a dose of placebo or ipratropium and then were shown both pleasant and disturbing images. Airway resistance increased for both placebo and ipratropium subjects; however, the resistance was not increased as much in the ipratropium group, due to muscarinic blockade by ipratropium.[17] This has not translated into a recommendation to give ipratropium in patients who have emotion-induced asthma. Present therapy is to promote relaxation techniques such as breathing exercises, yoga, and meditation, in addition to rescue medication.

Food and Drug Additives

Many patients with asthma who have allergies to specific foods increase their potential to develop exacerbations from intake of these foods. Foods that contain salicylates, some food-coloring agents, food preservatives (e.g., sulfites), and monosodium glutamate are substances known to be associated with asthma exacerbations.

Drugs may be associated with an increased likelihood of exacerbation. The primary risk is with nonsteroidal anti-inflammatory agents and aspirin. Patients who have sensitivity to aspirin have an increased risk of developing asthma later in life.

Viruses

Viral illness seasons (October through December and February through April) coincide with the most prevalent hospitalization periods for asthma in both children and adults. It has been reported that 37% of adult patients with acute asthma admitted over a 12-month period had evidence of recent respiratory tract infection.[18] The inflammatory responses to viral infections (especially in the lower respiratory tract) may start the cascade of symptomatic wheezing from inflammatory debris or excessive mucus production in the airways.

Induced sputum[19] has been used as a marker of the effects of natural colds and influenza on the airways of the lungs. Natural colds (by day 4) cause neutrophilic lower airway inflammation that is greater in people with asthma than in healthy subjects. The greater inflammatory response in people with asthma may be due to the changes associated with trivial eosinophilia or to the different viruses involved. As was stated earlier, exposure to viral infections early in life influences the development of the immune system, promoting a protective function.

The most prominent of these viral infections is respiratory syncytial virus (RSV). The population at highest risk for severe cases of RSV and other lower respiratory tract infections, namely, the indigent inner-city population, also is at high risk for asthma. Infants with RSV early in life who developed high titers of RSV IgE were three times more likely to have recurrent wheezing after 48 months.

The exact role that early childhood respiratory tract infections play in the development of asthma is unclear. Respiratory tract infections are a significant risk factor for the initiation of an asthma exacerbation that may or may not result in an individual seeking acute care. Infections should be identified to the patient with asthma as a trigger. Furthermore, written asthma treatment plans should include a component for increasing or stepping up therapy at the onset of symptoms. There is an advantage of hospitalization prevention when families of children with asthma had a written treatment plan that could initiate more aggressive outpatient management with the onset of coldlike symptoms.[20] All asthmatics should receive the annual flu vaccine, unless contraindicated.

AGE-SPECIFIC ANGLE

A relationship exists between respiratory viral infections in early childhood and the development of asthma.

Nocturnal Asthma

Nocturnal symptoms are quite common in people of all ages with asthma and even in patients who have intermittent or mild persistent asthma. Although **nocturnal asthma** is prevalent in up to 75% of all patients with asthma,[21] many do not correlate these nighttime symptoms with asthma. The presence of nocturnal asthma is a marker for uncontrolled or more severe asthma.[22–24]

A variety of mechanisms are interactive when nocturnal asthma is present.[25] The mechanisms seem to revolve around circadian alterations of body temperature, vagal tone, mediators, inflammation, epinephrine, and β_2-receptor function.[26,27] Other variables considered to be potential causes include gastroesophageal reflux, inhalation of cooler or drier air by mouth while sleeping, aspiration, sinusitis, increased mucus production, sleep apnea, and the normal decrease in lung function while sleeping.

Treatment is consistent with the stepwise approach discussed under asthma pharmacology. Comorbid conditions (e.g., obstructive sleep apnea, gastroesophageal reflux) must also be treated. Nighttime awakenings are a sign of persistence of asthma and loss of control, and are not to be tolerated.

Exercise-Induced Asthma

Exercise-induced asthma (EIA) is characterized by transient airway obstruction, typically occurring 5 to 15 minutes after strenuous exertion. EIA is prevalent in 90% of individuals with asthma. The prevalence of EIA among athletes is estimated to range between 3% and 11%.

There are cases of undiagnosed asthma that suddenly appears in competitive high school athletes.[28] Diagnosis of EIA may be made based on a history of symptoms (cough, wheeze, and chest tightness with exercise challenge testing). More traditionally or for definitive diagnosis, a fall of 10% or more in the FEV_1 or in peak expiratory flow (PEF) rate after exercise is diagnostic. Vocal cord dysfunction is commonly confused with EIA.[1]

The exact etiology of EIA is unclear. Theories range from temperature-related causes to inflammatory mediator release (**Box 32-3**). EIA symptoms typically appear during or after exercise, peak at 8 to 15 minutes after exercise, and eventually spontaneously resolve in about 20 to 30 minutes. Frequently, a refractory period (of up to 3 hours) occurs after initial recovery, during which repeat exercise causes less bronchospasm.

Appropriate treatment with anti-inflammatory medication reduces airway hyperresponsiveness and is associated with a reduction in the frequency and severity of EIA.[1] Other therapy for EIA includes the use of a short-acting β_2-agonist (SABA) 15 to 20 minutes before exercise; although a long-acting β_2-agonist (LABA) is also appropriate, frequent use may mask poorly controlled persistent asthma. Leukotriene receptor antagonists (LTRAs) can help in 50% of cases of EIA. Cromolyn may be effective but is not as good as SABAs and is only available as a solution for nebulization. A warm-up period before exercise and cool-down afterward may help attenuate EIA, as will a mask or scarf over the mouth and nose in cold weather. Coaches should be made aware of EIA in any student so a SABA can be used prior to exercise classes. Although prevention is the main objective in managing EIA, education regarding its nature and management is important.

BOX 32-3

Etiologic Theories for Exercise-Induced Asthma

Respiratory heat or water loss (or both) from the bronchial mucosa
Mucosal drying and increased osmolarity stimulating mast cell degranulation
Rapid airway rewarming after exercise, causing vascular congestion, increased permeability, and edema leading to obstruction
Hyperventilation, causing discharge of bronchospastic chemical mediators

Occupational Asthma

Occupational asthma is characterized by variable airway hyperresponsiveness in the workplace. The patient typically reports increased symptoms while at work or within several hours of the completion of a shift, with improvement on weekends or during vacations. In addition, the presence of sensitizing agents and the presence of similar symptoms in coworkers are suggestive of occupational asthma. Monitoring peak flow for 2 weeks in the workplace and 1 week away can make the diagnosis. Both new-onset asthma and exacerbations of preexistent asthma may occur as a result of occupational exposures. Occupational asthma is the most common occupational lung disease in developed countries.

Isocyanates are the most common etiologic agents. Inciting agents are divided into two broad categories: low-molecular-weight chemicals (e.g., trimellitic anhydride, formaldehyde), which require combination of

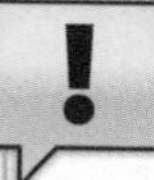

Respiratory Recap

Asthma Disease Severity Classification

- Intermittent
- Mild persistent
- Moderate persistent
- Severe persistent

the chemical, which is an incomplete antigen (i.e., a hapten), with a protein conjugate to produce a sensitizing neoantigen; and high-molecular-weight organic materials (e.g., grain dust, avian proteins), which may serve as complete antigens. Cigarette smoking is also an important risk factor for occupational asthma. The asthma educator may work with the onsite healthcare providers to discuss avoidance, ventilation, respiratory protection, and provision of a tobacco smoke-free environment. The list of all known causes of occupational asthma is long and beyond the scope of this chapter.[29]

Disease Severity Classification

Asthma is classified in terms of severity and control. *Severity* is defined as the intrinsic intensity of the disease process, wherein the patient's frequency and intensity of symptoms is evaluated. *Control* refers to the degree to which the manifestations of asthma are minimized and the goals of therapy are met. Both severity and control include the domains of current impairment (symptoms) and future risk (based on history of exacerbation and use of oral corticosteroids). Preferably, the patient's asthma should be classified before beginning controller therapy. Once classification has occurred, therapy is started based on a stepwise approach, to include recommended SABAs, LABAs, and inhaled corticosteroids. Once a patient has been on the recommended regimen and efforts have been made to control environmental factors, the patient is reevaluated for asthma control.

Patients are divided into three age categories by the EPR-3: children aged 0 to 4 years, children aged 5 to 11 years, and children aged 12 and older to adults. For the child 0 to 4 years of age, upon presentation, the child is evaluated for frequency of symptoms, nighttime awakenings, use of SABAs, and interference with normal activity (the elements of impairment) and risk (i.e., the number of exacerbations requiring oral corticosteroids in the past year and the frequency of exacerbations; **Figure 32-4**).[1] For the child aged 5 to 11 years, the same factors are used to assess impairment, plus spirometry is added, with particular attention to FEV_1 and the ratio of FEV_1 to percent forced vital capacity (FEV_1/FVC%); (**Figure 32-5**).[1] The same criteria are used for risk. In all patients older than 12 years, the same criteria are used to assess impairment, with age-specific ranges for FEV_1/FVC% (**Figure 32-6**). The same criteria are used for risk as with children.[1]

The NAEPP expert panel has developed a four-tiered system to classify disease severity.[1] The four categories are intermittent, mild persistent, moderate persistent, and severe persistent asthma. Classification of severity is usually done in patients who are steroid-naïve. Once steroid therapy has been implemented, control is assessed periodically. A patient may have a higher severity in one area versus another. When classifying the patient's asthma, the level of severity corresponds to the worst level of the patient's impairment or risk. For example, the patient may have symptoms on more than 2 days per week, but not daily, but has an FEV_1 less than 60% of predicted. This patient would be classified as having severe persistent asthma and treated accordingly.

Therapy is a stepwise approach, according to level of severity. Once the level of severity is established, the clinician selects a therapeutic step (steps 1 through 6, with step 6 being reserved for the most severe cases). **Figures 32-7** through **32-9** show the stepwise approach to pharmacologic therapy, by age group.

Intermittent

Intermittent asthma is the least severe of the four classes of disease severity. People with asthma in this category experience symptoms two or more times per week. These patients generally are expected to experience nocturnal symptoms of coughing, wheezing, or breathlessness no more than two times per month. They require SABAs no more than twice per week and do not require any controller medication. There is no interference with normal activity. These patients have normal pulmonary function tests between exacerbations, although their exacerbations are generally brief (from a few hours to a few days). They have required zero to one course of oral corticosteroids in the past year.

Although these patients may have the chronic component of their disease classified as intermittent, the periodic exacerbations that occur may vary in their intensity. Sometimes, although rarely, these exacerbations result in this class of patients needing to seek ED treatment or hospitalization.

Mild Persistent

People with **mild persistent asthma** experience symptoms of coughing or wheezing more than twice per week but less than once per day. These patients generally experience nocturnal symptoms of coughing, wheezing, or breathlessness more than two times per month. These patients may use their SABA more than twice per week, but not daily. These patients have symptoms that cause a minor limitation to normal activities of daily living. Pulmonary function is normal. Exacerbations may be more frequent.

Routine management of these patients generally consists of step 2 therapy: as-needed short-acting β_2-agonist with the addition of a controller medication. In all patients, the recommended controller medication is a low-dose inhaled corticosteroid (ICS), whereas in children aged 0 to 4 the options of cromolyn sodium or montelukast are indicated as

Classifying severity in children who are not currently taking long-term control medication.

Components of Severity		Classification of Asthma Severity (Children 0–4 years of age)			
		Intermittent	Persistent		
			Mild	Moderate	Severe
Impairment	Symptoms	≤2 days/week	>2 days/week but not daily	Daily	Throughout the day
	Nighttime awakenings	0	1–2/month	3–4/month	>1/week
	Short-acting beta$_2$-agonist use for symptom control (not prevention of EIB)	≤2 days/week	>2 days/week but not daily	Daily	Several times per day
	Interference with normal activity	None	Minor limitation	Some limitation	Extremely limited
Risk	Exacerbations requiring oral systemic corticosteroids	0–1/year	≥2 exacerbations in 6 months requiring oral steroids, or ≥4 wheezing episodes/1year lasting >1day AND risk factors for persistent asthma		
		← Consider severity and interval since last exacerbation. Frequency and severity may fluctuate over time. →			
		Exacerbations of any severity may occur in patients in any severity category			

- Level of severity is determined by both impairment and risk. Assess impairment domain by caregiver's recall of previous 2–4 weeks. Assign severity to the most severe category in which any feature occurs.
- At present, there are inadequate data to correspond frequencies of exacerbations with different levels of asthma severity. For treatment purposes, patients who had ≥2 exacerbations requiring oral corticosteroids in the past 6 months, or ≥4 wheezing episodes in the past year, and who have risk factors for persistent asthma may be considered the same as patients who have persistent asthma, even in the absence of impairment levels consistent with persistent asthma.

Classifying severity in patients after asthma becomes well controlled, by lowest level of treatment required to maintain control.*

Lowest level of treatment required to maintain control	Classification of Asthma Severity			
	Intermittent	Persistent		
		Mild	Moderate	Severe
	Step 1	Step 2	Step 3 or 4	Step 5 or 6

EIB, exercise-induced bronchospasm

*For population-based evaluations, clinical research, or characterization of a patient's overall asthma severity after control is achieved. For clinical management, the focus is on monitoring the level of control, not the level of severity, once treatment is established.

FIGURE 32-4 Classifying asthma severity in children 0–4 years of age.

Reproduced from National Asthma Education Program, National Heart, Lung, and Blood Institute. *Expert Panel Report 3: Guidelines for the Diagnosis and Management of Asthma. Full Report 2007.* Bethesda, MD: National Institutes of Health; 2007. NIH Publication 08-4051.

Classifying severity in children who are not currently taking long-term control medication.

Components of Severity		Classification of Asthma Severity (Children 5–11 years of age)			
			Persistent		
		Intermittent	Mild	Moderate	Severe
Impairment	Symptoms	≤2 days/week	>2 days/week but not daily	Daily	Throughout the day
	Nighttime awakenings	≤2/month	3–4/month	>1/week but not nightly	Often 7/week
	Short-acting beta$_2$-agonist use for symptom control (not prevention of EIB)	≤2 days/week	>2 days/week but not daily	Daily	Several times per day
	Interference with normal activity	None	Minor limitation	Some limitation	Extremely limited
	Lung function	Normal FEV_1 between exacerbations FEV_1 >80% predicted FEV_1/FVC >85%	FEV_1 >80% predicted FEV_1/FVC >80%	FEV_1 = 60–80% predicted FEV_1/FVC = 75–80%	FEV_1 <60% predicted FEV_1/FVC <75%
Risk	Exacerbations requiring oral systemic corticosteroids	0–1/year	≥2 in 1 year →		
		← Consider severity and interval since last exacerbation. Frequency and severity may fluctuate over time for patients in any severity category. →			
		Relative annual risk of exacerbations may be related to FEV_1			

- Level of severity is determined by both impairment and risk. Assess impairment domain by patient's/caregiver's recall of the previous 2–4 weeks and spirometry. Assign severity to the most severe category in which any feature occurs.
- At present, there are inadequate data to correspond frequencies of exacerbations with different levels of asthma severity. In general, more frequent and intense exacerbations (e.g., requiring urgent, unscheduled care, hospitalization, or ICU admission) indicate greater underlying disease severity. For treatment purposes, patients who had ≥2 exacerbations requiring oral systemic corticosteroids in the past year may be considered the same as patients who have persistent asthma, even in the absence of impairment levels consistent with persistent asthma.

Classifying severity in patients after asthma becomes well controlled, by lowest level of treatment required to maintain control.*

Lowest level of treatment required to maintain control	Classification of Asthma Severity			
		Persistent		
	Intermittent	Mild	Moderate	Severe
	Step 1	Step 2	Step 3 or 4	Step 5 or 6

EIB, exercise-induced bronchospasm; FEV_1, forced expiratory volume in 1 second; FVC, forced vital capacity; ICU, intensive care unit

*For population-based evaluations, clinical research, or characterization of a patient's overall asthma severity after control is achieved. For clinical management, the focus is on monitoring the level of control, not the level of severity, once treatment is established.

FIGURE 32-5 Classifying asthma severity in children 5–11 years of age.

Reproduced from National Asthma Education Program, National Heart, Lung, and Blood Institute. *Expert Panel Report 3: Guidelines for the Diagnosis and Management of Asthma. Full Report 2007.* Bethesda, MD: National Institutes of Health; 2007. NIH Publication 08-4051.

Classifying severity for patients who are not currently taking long-term control medications.

Components of Severity		Classification of Asthma Severity (Youths ≥12 years of age and adults)			
			Persistent		
		Intermittent	**Mild**	**Moderate**	**Severe**
Impairment Normal FEV_1/FVC: 8–19 yr 85% 20–39 yr 80% 40–59 yr 75% 60–80 yr 70%	Symptoms	≤2 days/week	>2 days/week but not daily	Daily	Throughout the day
	Nighttime awakenings	≤2/month	3–4/month	>1/week but not nightly	Often 7/week
	Short-acting $beta_2$-agonist use for symptom control (not prevention of EIB)	≤2 days/week	>2 days/week but not >1/day	Daily	Several times per day
	Interference with normal activity	None	Minor limitation	Some limitation	Extremely limited
	Lung function	Normal FEV_1 between exacerbations FEV_1 >80% predicted FEV_1/FVC normal	FEV_1 ≥80% predicted FEV_1/FVC normal	FEV_1 >60% but <80% predicted FEV_1/FVC = reduced 5%	FEV_1 <60% predicted FEV_1/FVC reduced >5%
Risk	Exacerbations requiring oral systemic corticosteroids	0–1/year	≥2/year →		
		← Consider severity and interval since last exacerbation. Frequency and severity may fluctuate over time for patients in any severity category. →			
		Relative annual risk of exacerbations may be related to FEV_1			

- Level of severity is determined by assessment of both impairment and risk. Assess impairment domain by patient's/caregiver's recall of previous 2–4 weeks and spirometry. Assign severity to the most severe category in which any feature occurs.
- At present, there are inadequate data to correspond frequencies of exacerbations with different levels of asthma severity. In general, more frequent and intense exacerbations (e.g., requiring urgent, unscheduled care, hospitalization, or ICU admission) indicate greater underlying disease severity. For treatment purposes, patients who had ≥2 exacerbations requiring oral systemic corticosteroids in the past year may be considered the same as patients who have persistent asthma, even in the absence of impairment levels consistent with persistent asthma.

Classifying severity in patients after asthma becomes well controlled, by lowest level of treatment required to maintain control.*

Lowest level of treatment required to maintain control	Classification of Asthma Severity			
		Persistent		
	Intermittent	**Mild**	**Moderate**	**Severe**
	Step 1	Step 2	Step 3 or 4	Step 5 or 6

EIB, exercise-induced bronchospasm; FEV_1, forced expiratory volume in 1 second; FVC, forced vital capacity; ICU, intensive care unit

*For population-based evaluations, clinical research, or characterization of a patient's overall asthma severity after control is achieved. For clinical management, the focus is on monitoring the level of control, not the level of severity, once treatment is established.

FIGURE 32-6 Classifying asthma severity in youths ≥12 years of age and adults.

Reproduced from National Asthma Education Program, National Heart, Lung, and Blood Institute. *Expert Panel Report 3: Guidelines for the Diagnosis and Management of Asthma. Full Report 2007.* Bethesda, MD: National Institutes of Health; 2007. NIH Publication 08-4051.

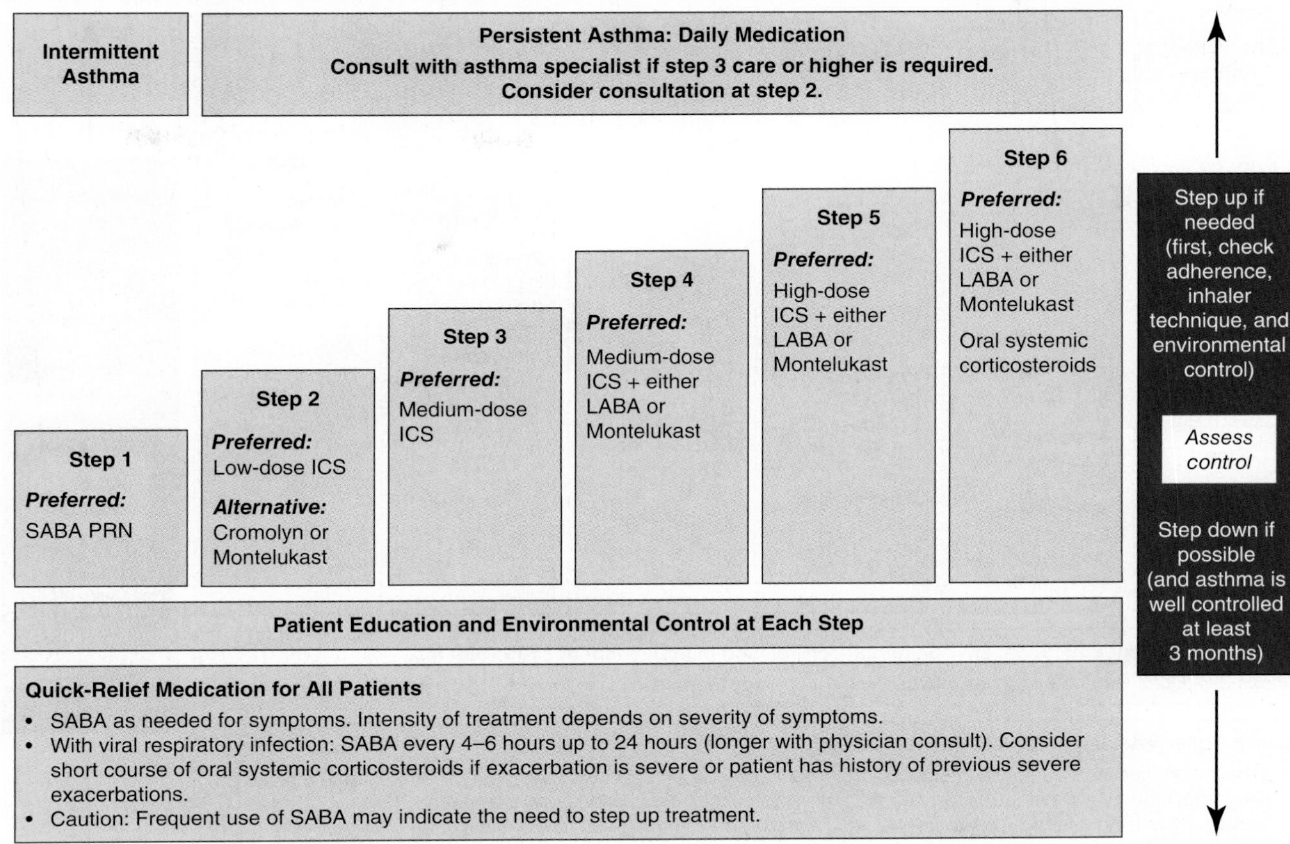
Intermittent Asthma
Persistent Asthma: Daily Medication
Consult with asthma specialist if step 3 care or higher is required.
Consider consultation at step 2.
Step 1
Preferred:
SABA PRN
Step 2
Preferred:
Low-dose ICS
Alternative:
Cromolyn or Montelukast
Step 3
Preferred:
Medium-dose ICS
Step 4
Preferred:
Medium-dose ICS + either LABA or Montelukast
Step 5
Preferred:
High-dose ICS + either LABA or Montelukast
Step 6
Preferred:
High-dose ICS + either LABA or Montelukast
Oral systemic corticosteroids
Step up if needed (first, check adherence, inhaler technique, and environmental control)
Assess control
Step down if possible (and asthma is well controlled at least 3 months)
Patient Education and Environmental Control at Each Step
Quick-Relief Medication for All Patients
• SABA as needed for symptoms. Intensity of treatment depends on severity of symptoms.
• With viral respiratory infection: SABA every 4–6 hours up to 24 hours (longer with physician consult). Consider short course of oral systemic corticosteroids if exacerbation is severe or patient has history of previous severe exacerbations.
• Caution: Frequent use of SABA may indicate the need to step up treatment.

FIGURE 32-7 Stepwise approach for managing asthma in children 0–4 years of age. National Asthma Education Program, National Heart, Lung, and Blood Institute.

Reproduced from National Asthma Education Program, National Heart, Lung, and Blood Institute. *Expert Panel Report 3: Guidelines for the Diagnosis and Management of Asthma. Full Report 2007*. Bethesda, MD: National Institutes of Health; 2007. NIH Publication 08-4051.

alternatives for inhaled corticosteroids. In children aged 5 to 11, alternatives include cromolyn, montelukast, or theophylline.

The alternatives are only used if there is a contraindication to ICS, because the ICS is actually controlling inflammation. The same therapy is used for those aged 12 years and older.

Although these patients may have the chronic component of their disease classified as mild persistent, the periodic exacerbations that occur also vary in their intensity. These exacerbations periodically result in this class of patients needing to seek ED treatment or occasionally result in hospitalization.

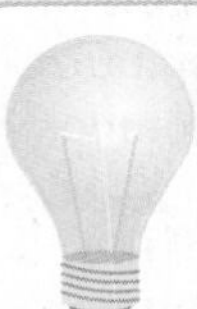

STOP AND THINK

What information would you need to classify the severity of a patient's asthma?

Moderate Persistent

People with **moderate persistent asthma** experience symptoms of coughing or wheezing on a daily basis. Moderate persistent asthma patients generally experience nocturnal symptoms of coughing, wheezing, or breathlessness more than once per week. SABA use is daily. These patients have symptoms that cause some interference with normal activities of daily living. Spirometry results show an FEV_1 above 60% but less than 80% of predicted, and FEV_1/FVC% is reduced by 5%.

Management of patients aged 0 to 4 years consists of step 3 or 4 therapy: SABA for exacerbations and medium-dose inhaled corticosteroid (step 3) in addition to LABA or montelukast (step 4) daily. In older children, step 3 therapy consists of low-dose ICS and either LABA, LRTA, or theophylline, or medium-dose ICS. Step 4 therapy is medium-dose ICS with a LABA or medium-dose ICS and either LRTA or theophylline. For those aged 12 and older, step 3 therapy is low-dose ICS and the addition of a LABA, or low-dose ICS with

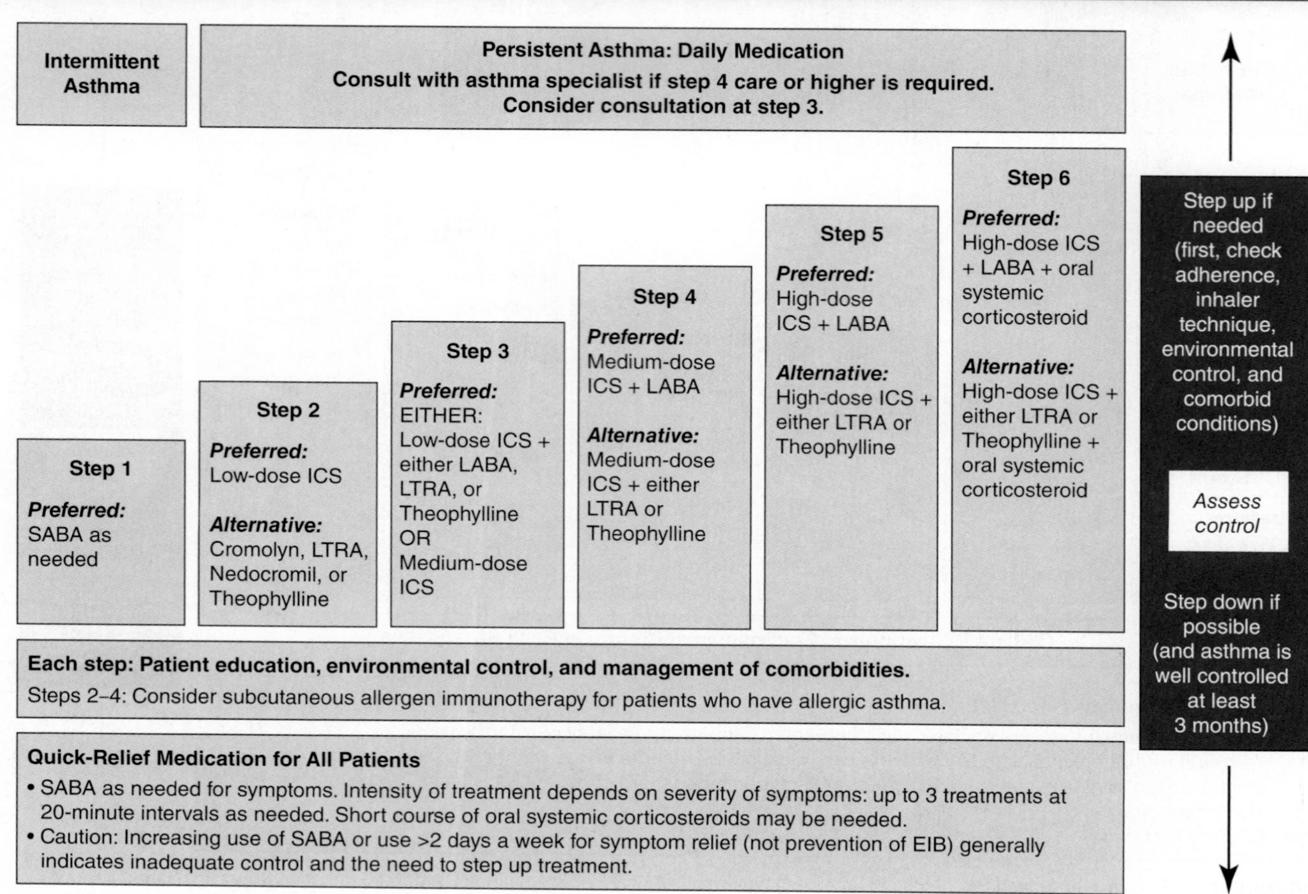

Intermittent Asthma
Persistent Asthma: Daily Medication
Consult with asthma specialist if step 4 care or higher is required.
Consider consultation at step 3.
Step 1
Preferred:
SABA as needed
Step 2
Preferred:
Low-dose ICS
Alternative:
Cromolyn, LTRA, Nedocromil, or Theophylline
Step 3
Preferred:
EITHER:
Low-dose ICS + either LABA, LTRA, or Theophylline
OR
Medium-dose ICS
Step 4
Preferred:
Medium-dose ICS + LABA
Alternative:
Medium-dose ICS + either LTRA or Theophylline
Step 5
Preferred:
High-dose ICS + LABA
Alternative:
High-dose ICS + either LTRA or Theophylline
Step 6
Preferred:
High-dose ICS + LABA + oral systemic corticosteroid
Alternative:
High-dose ICS + either LTRA or Theophylline + oral systemic corticosteroid
Step up if needed (first, check adherence, inhaler technique, environmental control, and comorbid conditions)
Assess control
Step down if possible (and asthma is well controlled at least 3 months)
Each step: Patient education, environmental control, and management of comorbidities.
Steps 2–4: Consider subcutaneous allergen immunotherapy for patients who have allergic asthma.
Quick-Relief Medication for All Patients
• SABA as needed for symptoms. Intensity of treatment depends on severity of symptoms: up to 3 treatments at 20-minute intervals as needed. Short course of oral systemic corticosteroids may be needed.
• Caution: Increasing use of SABA or use >2 days a week for symptom relief (not prevention of EIB) generally indicates inadequate control and the need to step up treatment.

FIGURE 32-8 Stepwise approach for managing asthma in children 5–11 years of age.

Reproduced from National Asthma Education Program, National Heart, Lung, and Blood Institute. *Expert Panel Report 3: Guidelines for the Diagnosis and Management of Asthma. Full Report 2007*. Bethesda, MD: National Institutes of Health; 2007. NIH Publication 08-4051.

an LRTA or theophylline. Step 4 therapy is medium-dose ICS with a LABA or medium-dose ICS with either LRTA or theophylline. These patients may routinely need to seek ED treatment or require hospitalization secondary to the chronic inflammatory component of their asthma.

Severe Persistent

This category is the highest level of the four classes of disease severity. Patients with **severe persistent asthma** experience symptoms of coughing or wheezing almost continually. Severe persistent asthma patients experience nocturnal symptoms of coughing, wheezing, or breathlessness almost every night. These patients may use their SABA several times daily, a dangerous practice that correlates with an increased incidence of death. These patients have symptoms that cause extremely limited activities of daily living. Spirometry results show an FEV_1 less than 60% of predicted and an $FEV_1/FVC\%$ reduced more than 5%.

Management of these patients consists of step 5 or 6 therapy: short-acting β_2-agonist for exacerbations for all age groups. Controller drugs for the 0- to 4-year age group are high-dose ICS in addition to either LABA or montelukast (step 5), or high-dose ICS with LABA or montelukast or oral corticosteroids (step 6). Step 5 therapy for the 5- to 11-year age group consists of high-dose ICS with a LABA, or high-dose ICS and LRTA or theophylline. Step 6 is high-dose ICS and LABA with consideration of oral corticosteroid, or high-dose ICS and LRTA or theophylline plus an oral corticosteroid. For those 12 and older, step 5 therapy is high-dose ICS in combination with a LABA and consideration of subcutaneous omalizumab (an immunomodulator drug) for those with allergies. In step 6, an oral corticosteroid is added to step 5 therapy and omalizumab is considered. These patients may frequently seek ED treatment and require hospitalization secondary to the chronic inflammatory component of their asthma.

Although patients may be classified in any of the four categories, periodic review of chronic symptoms

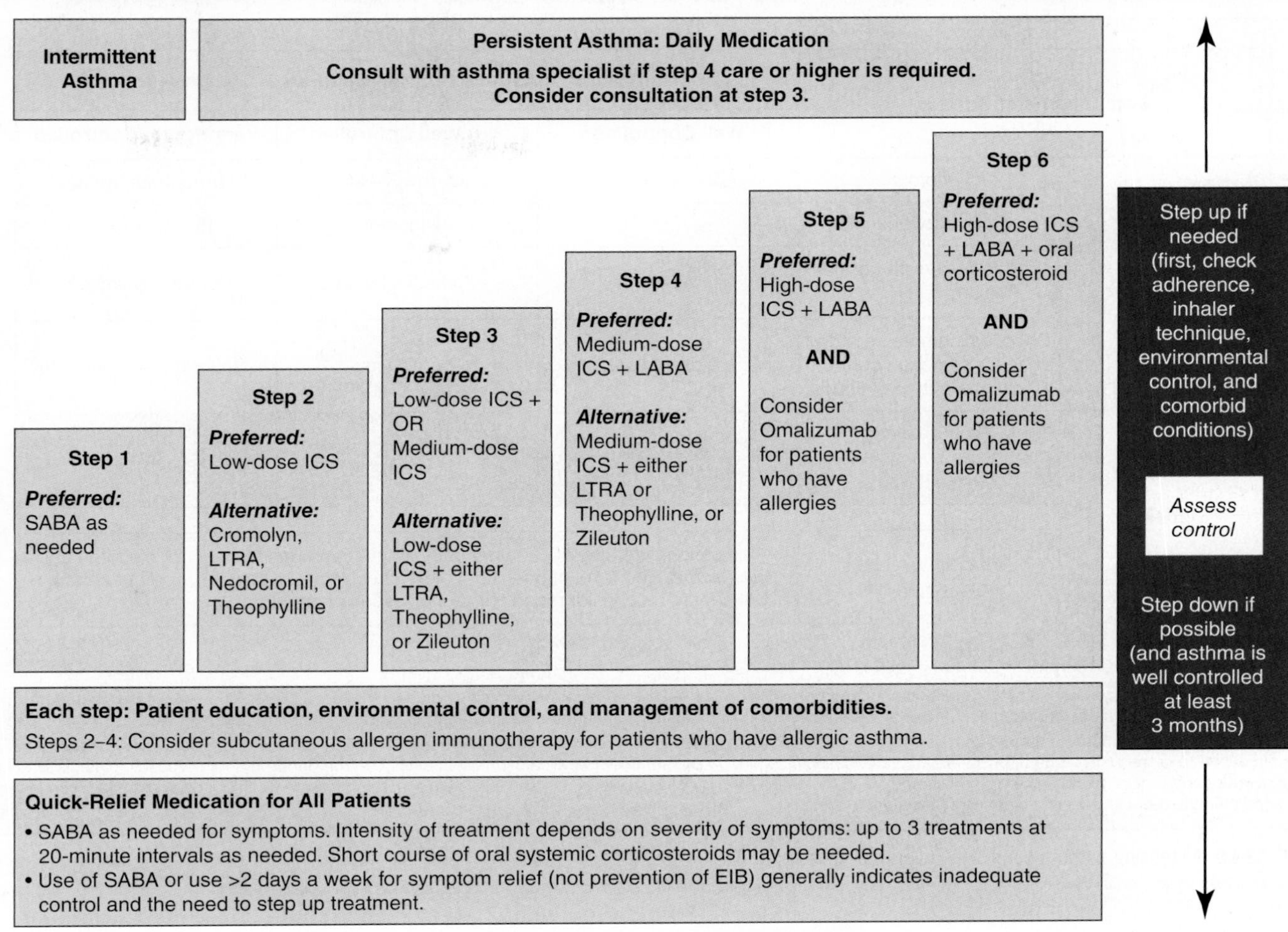
Intermittent Asthma
Persistent Asthma: Daily Medication
Consult with asthma specialist if step 4 care or higher is required.
Consider consultation at step 3.
Step 1
Preferred:
SABA as needed
Step 2
Preferred:
Low-dose ICS
Alternative:
Cromolyn, LTRA, Nedocromil, or Theophylline
Step 3
Preferred:
Low-dose ICS + OR Medium-dose ICS
Alternative:
Low-dose ICS + either LTRA, Theophylline, or Zileuton
Step 4
Preferred:
Medium-dose ICS + LABA
Alternative:
Medium-dose ICS + either LTRA or Theophylline, or Zileuton
Step 5
Preferred:
High-dose ICS + LABA
AND
Consider Omalizumab for patients who have allergies
Step 6
Preferred:
High-dose ICS + LABA + oral corticosteroid
AND
Consider Omalizumab for patients who have allergies
Step up if needed (first, check adherence, inhaler technique, environmental control, and comorbid conditions)
Assess control
Step down if possible (and asthma is well controlled at least 3 months)
Each step: Patient education, environmental control, and management of comorbidities.
Steps 2–4: Consider subcutaneous allergen immunotherapy for patients who have allergic asthma.
Quick-Relief Medication for All Patients
• SABA as needed for symptoms. Intensity of treatment depends on severity of symptoms: up to 3 treatments at 20-minute intervals as needed. Short course of oral systemic corticosteroids may be needed.
• Use of SABA or use >2 days a week for symptom relief (not prevention of EIB) generally indicates inadequate control and the need to step up treatment.

FIGURE 32-9 Stepwise approach for managing asthma in youths >12 years of age and adults.

Reproduced from National Asthma Education Program, National Heart, Lung, and Blood Institute. *Expert Panel Report 3: Guidelines for the Diagnosis and Management of Asthma. Full Report 2007.* Bethesda, MD: National Institutes of Health; 2007. NIH Publication 08-4051.

and adherence is necessary. Quite often asthma is controlled with appropriate medications, and compliance and treatment can be decreased to a lower severity class with a decrease in symptoms. From the opposite perspective, with increasing symptomatic data, it may be necessary to intensify the treatment regimen to address the increase in symptoms.

Assessing Control of Asthma

After initiating therapy according to the stepwise scheme, patients should be evaluated for control of asthma. Just as when initiating therapy, the practitioner evaluates the patient in the domains of impairment and risk, using the same criteria: frequency of symptoms, nighttime awakenings, interference with normal activity, SABA use, lung function (age 5 and older), validated questionnaires about quality of life (adults), number of exacerbations requiring oral corticosteroids, and treatment-related adverse effects (**Figures 32-10** through **32-12**).

Asthma is classified as well controlled, not well controlled, or very poorly controlled, according to the worst symptom or finding. If a patient's asthma is well controlled for at least 3 months, consideration is given to stepping therapy down one step. If the asthma is not well controlled, patient adherence is checked and consideration is given to stepping up one step, with reevaluation in 6 weeks. If asthma is very poorly controlled, a short course of oral corticosteroids is considered, as is stepping up one to two steps, in addition to checking adherence and evaluating side effects. In either case, alternative treatment options are considered in the presence of adverse effects. Each time control is assessed, the patient's adherence to the asthma action plan is checked: are they using the prescribed medications? Are they using the inhalers properly? Are they avoiding asthma triggers? If so, and they are not well controlled, a step-up is indicated. If not, further education about environmental control and inhaler use is indicated.

Components of Control		Classification of Asthma Control (Children 0–4 years of age)		
		Well Controlled	**Not Well Controlled**	**Very Poorly Controlled**
Impairment	Symptoms	≤2 days/week	>2 days/week	Throughout the day
	Nighttime awakenings	≤1/month	>1/month	>1/week
	Interference with normal activity	None	Some limitation	Extremely limited
	Short-acting beta$_2$-agonist use for symptom control (not prevention of EIB)	≤2 days/week	>2 days/week	Several times per day
Risk	Exacerbations requiring oral systemic corticosteroids	0–1/year	2–3/year	>3/year
	Treatment-related adverse effects	Medication side effects can vary in intensity from none to very troublesome and worrisome. The level of intensity does not correlate to specific levels of control but should be considered in the overall assessment of risk.		

EIB, exercise-induced bronchospasm; ICU, intensive care unit

- The level of control is based on the most severe impairment or risk category. Assess impairment domain by caregiver's recall of previous 2–4 weeks. Symptom assessment for longer periods should reflect a global assessment, such as inquiring whether the patient's asthma is better or worse since the last visit.
- At present, there are inadequate data to correspond frequencies of exacerbations with different levels of asthma control. In general, more frequent and intense exacerbations (e.g., requiring urgent, unscheduled care, hospitalization, or ICU admission) indicate poorer disease control. For treatment purposes, patients who had ≥2 exacerbations requiring oral systemic corticosteroids in the past year may be considered the same as patients who have not-well-controlled asthma, even in the absence of impairment levels consistent with persistent asthma.

FIGURE 32-10 Assessing asthma control in children 0–4 years of age.

Reproduced from National Asthma Education Program, National Heart, Lung, and Blood Institute. *Expert Panel Report 3: Guidelines for the Diagnosis and Management of Asthma. Full Report 2007*. Bethesda, MD: National Institutes of Health; 2007. NIH Publication 08-4051.

Status Asthmaticus

Severe attacks of asthma poorly responsive to adrenergic agents and associated with signs or symptoms of potential respiratory failure are referred to as *status asthmaticus*. The mechanisms of airflow obstruction and the principles of treatment for status asthmaticus are similar to those in which the asthma responds promptly to treatment. Although this term has been used for years when referring to a refractory asthma exacerbation, it is not used anywhere in the EPR-3, other than in a few references. Perhaps it is time to refer to this condition as a severe exacerbation or an exacerbation requiring admission to an intensive care unit.

Objective Measurements

One of the primary goals of asthma management and control is to maintain normal (or near normal) lung function. Objective assessment of the degree of variable airflow obstruction, hyperresponsiveness, and airflow reversibility is a fundamental component in the diagnosis of asthma. The precise measurement of airflow changes is important to evaluate the effectiveness of therapeutic maintenance or interventions.

The most familiar ways to diagnose and monitor airflow are pulmonary function testing (spirometry) and peak flow meters. In 1994 the American Thoracic Society (ATS) differentiated between diagnostic and monitoring devices.[30] Diagnostic evaluation by pulmonary function testing includes bronchial challenge, spirometry, lung volumes, and airway resistance.

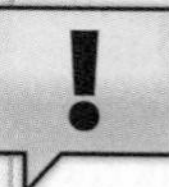

Respiratory Recap

Objective Measurements in Asthma

- Spirometry
- Lung volumes and airways resistance
- Peak flow
- Exhaled nitric oxide

Components of Control		Classification of Asthma Control (Children 5–11 years of age)		
		Well Controlled	Not Well Controlled	Very Poorly Controlled
Impairment	Symptoms	≤2 days/week but not more than once on each day	>2 days/week or multiple times on ≤2 days/week	Throughout the day
	Nighttime awakenings	≤1/month	≥2/month	≥2/week
	Interference with normal activity	None	Some limitation	Extremely limited
	Short-acting $beta_2$-agonist use for symptom control (not prevention of EIB)	≤2 days/week	>2 days/week	Several times per day
	Lung function • FEV_1 or peak flow • FEV_1/FVC	>80% predicted/personal best >80%	60–80% predicted/personal best 75–80%	<60% predicted/personal best <75%
Risk	Exacerbations requiring oral systemic corticosteroids	0–1/year	≥2/year (see note)	
		Consider severity and interval since last exacerbation		
	Reduction in lung growth	Evaluation requires long-term follow-up.		
	Treatment-related adverse effects	Medication side effects can vary in intensity from none to very troublesome and worrisome. The level of intensity does not correlate to specific levels of control but should be considered in the overall assessment of risk.		

EIB, exercise-induced bronchospasm; FEV_1, forced expiratory volume in 1 second; FVC, forced vital capacity; ICU, intensive care unit

- The level of control is based on the most severe impairment or risk category. Assess impairment domain by patient's/caregiver's recall of previous 2–4 weeks and by spirometry or peak flow measures. Symptom assessment for longer periods should reflect a global assessment, such as inquiring whether the patient's asthma is better or worse since the last visit.
- At present, there are inadequate data to correspond frequencies of exacerbations with different levels of asthma control. In general, more frequent and intense exacerbations (e.g., requiring urgent, unscheduled care, hospitalization, or ICU admission) indicate poorer disease control. For treatment purposes, patients who had ≥2 exacerbations requiring oral systemic corticosteroids in the past year may be considered the same as patients who have not-well-controlled asthma, even in the absence of impairment levels consistent with not-well-controlled asthma.

FIGURE 32-11 Assessing asthma control in children 5–11.

Reproduced from National Asthma Education Program, National Heart, Lung, and Blood Institute. *Expert Panel Report 3: Guidelines for the Diagnosis and Management of Asthma. Full Report 2007.* Bethesda, MD: National Institutes of Health; 2007. NIH Publication 08-4051.

A relatively new diagnostic tool for the inflammatory component of asthma is measurement of exhaled nitric oxide levels.

Spirometry

Studies have demonstrated that children as young as 3 years of age can perform spirometry approximately 20% of the time. The NAEPP recommends diagnostic spirometry at initial diagnosis and at least yearly after initial diagnosis, at the age of 5 or later. Abnormality of spirometry in asthma is classified by the EPR-3 according to decrements in $FEV_1/FVC\%$ by age according to the following scheme:

Age	Normal $FEV_1/FVC\%$
8–19 years	85%
20–39 years	80%
40–59 years	75%
60–80 years	70%

Components of Control		Classification of Asthma Control (Youths ≥12 years of age and adults)		
		Well Controlled	**Not Well Controlled**	**Very Poorly Controlled**
Impairment	Symptoms	≤2 days/week	>2 days/week	Throughout the day
	Nighttime awakenings	≤2/month	1–3/week	≥4/week
	Interference with normal activity	None	Some limitation	Extremely limited
	Short-acting beta$_2$-agonist use for symptom control (not prevention of EIB)	≤2 days/week	>2 days/week	Several times per day
	FEV_1 or peak flow	>80% predicted/personal best	60–80% predicted/personal best	<60% predicted/personal best
	Validated Questionnaires ATAQ ACQ ACT	 0 ≤0.75* ≥20	 1–2 ≥1.5 6–19	 3–4 N/A ≤15
Risk	Exacerbations	0–1/year	≥2/year (see note)	
		Consider severity and interval since last exacerbation		
	Progressive loss of lung function	Evaluation requires long-term follow-up care		
	Treatment-related adverse effects	Medication side effects can vary in intensity from none to very troublesome and worrisome. The level of intensity does not correlate to specific levels of control but should be considered in the overall assessment of risk.		

*ACQ values of 0.76–1.4 are indeterminate regarding well-controlled asthma.

EIB, exercise-induced bronchospasm; FEV_1, forced expiratory volume in 1 second.

- The level of control is based on the most severe impairment or risk category. Assess impairment domain by patient's recall of previous 2–4 weeks and by spirometry/or peak flow measures. Symptom assessment for longer periods should reflect a global assessment, such as inquiring whether the patient's asthma is better or worse since the last visit.
- At present, there are inadequate data to correspond frequencies of exacerbations with different levels of asthma control. In general, more frequent and intense exacerbations (e.g., requiring urgent, unscheduled care, hospitalization, or ICU admission) indicate poorer disease control. For treatment purposes, patients who had ≥2 exacerbations requiring oral systemic corticosteroids in the past year may be considered the same as patients who have not-well-controlled asthma, even in the absence of impairment levels consistent with not-well-controlled asthma.

FIGURE 32-12 Assessing asthma control in youths >12 years of age and adults.

Reproduced from National Asthma Education Program, National Heart, Lung, and Blood Institute. *Expert Panel Report 3: Guidelines for the Diagnosis and Management of Asthma. Full Report 2007.* Bethesda, MD: National Institutes of Health; 2007. NIH Publication 08-4051.

An FEV_1/FVC% less than the value denoted as normal for the age group indicates obstruction and is a part of the assessment of severity and control. The airflow obstructive component of asthma is caused primarily by a decrease in expiratory flows and/or a high airways resistance. The spirometry data of a patient with asthma with airflow obstruction may show a normal or slightly decreased FVC, a decreased or normal FEV_1, a decreased or normal PEF, and a decreased FEV_1/FVC%. The ATS has recommended a diagnosis of asthma when airflow reversibility achieves an increase in FEV_1 of 200 mL and 12%.[30] Patients with a history of smoking and limited or no reversibility are more likely to have COPD. Pre- and postbronchodilator testing is the hallmark intervention to decipher airflow reversibility. Normal spirometry with a suspected history of asthma symptoms may be an indication for bronchial challenge testing. During periods of acute exacerbations, people with asthma may have significant amounts of hyperinflation and air trapping that will suggest a restrictive disease and require the measurement of lung volumes for accurate diagnosis.

Lung Volumes and Airways Resistance

Body plethysmography is the diagnostic tool that is used to achieve measurements of airways resistance (Raw), airway conductance (Gaw), and static lung volumes. Static lung volumes are the primary test that differentiates restrictive diseases from obstructive diseases. Static lung volumes are useful also to detect the presence of hyperinflation. Raw may be normal in asymptomatic asthma, although Gaw may be decreased. Normally during acute exacerbations, Raw is increased. Bronchodilator effectiveness is accurately evaluated with measurements of Raw during acute exacerbations.

Peak Flow Meters

Peak flow meters (**Figure 32-13**) have been classified by the ATS as monitoring devices for the management of asthma.[30] The EPR-3 recommends that written asthma action plans be based on either symptoms or peak flow measurements.[1] Peak flow monitoring should be considered for patients who have moderate or severe persistent asthma, those classified as poor perceivers, or those with worsening asthma, an unexplained response to environmental or occupational exposures, and others at the discretion of the clinician and the patient. The patient's personal best peak flow should be known. The personal best is the highest peak flow of three

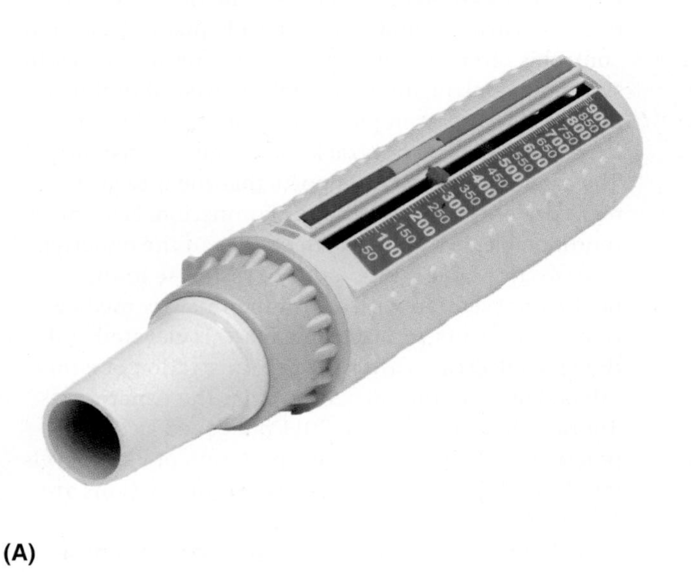

(A)

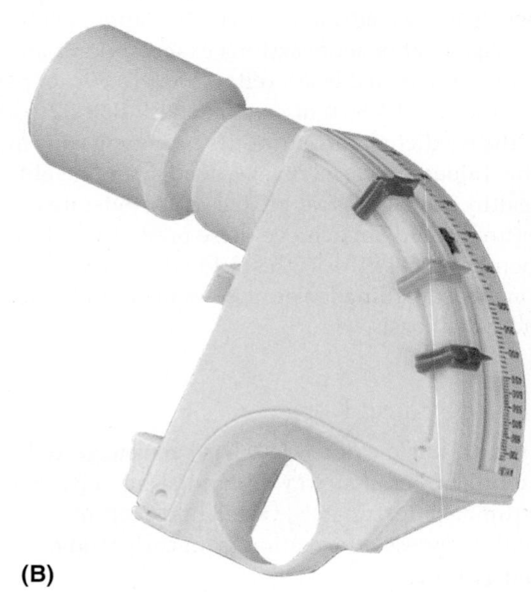

(B)

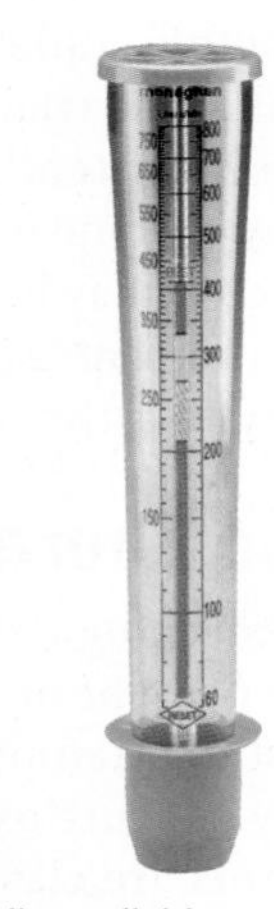

(C)

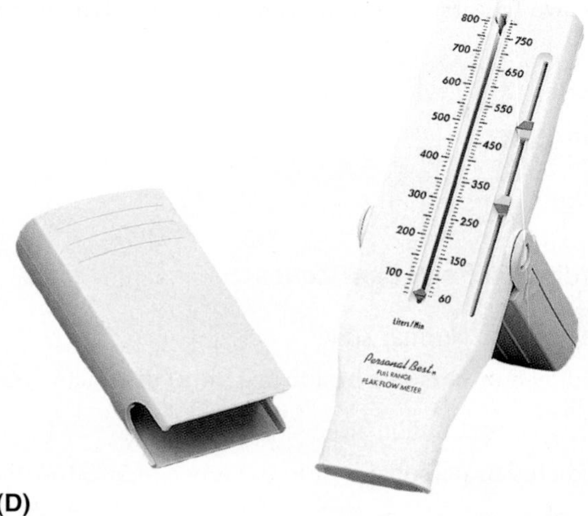

(D)

FIGURE 32-13 Commercially available peak flow meters.

(**A**) Reproduced with permission from CareFusion. (**B**) courtesy of nSpire Health, Inc. (**C**) courtesy of Invacare Corporation. (**D**) courtesy of Philips Respironics.

successive measurements, taken during an asymptomatic period.

The accuracy and reliability of different peak flow meters have been questioned. Variation occurs even within a manufactured brand of peak flow meter. For this reason, a patient should use a specific device for consistent readings. When analyzing peak flow data, one must realize the limitations of the measurements. Peak flow readings are extremely effort dependent and are an indicator of large airway obstruction. Often the mistake is made to attribute all low measurements to poor effort or lack of cooperation when there is airway obstruction present. Sometimes the clinician cannot differentiate between poor data or airway obstruction.

Consensus opinion from the NAEPP committee established a traditional three-zone approach to the management of acute asthma exacerbations: green (>80% of personal best), yellow (50% to 79% of personal best), and red (<50% of personal best; **Box 32-4**). Most of the predicted normal values or nomograms for peak flow values are based on age, gender, and height in healthy subjects. Most people with moderate to severe asthma could not achieve these predicted values on their best days. This is the rationale to develop a personal best reading for peak flows on an individual-by-individual basis.

Exhaled Nitric Oxide

Exhaled nitric oxide (eNO) has been suggested to be a useful marker of airway inflammation in patients with asthma. Unfortunately, varied protocols make it difficult to assess information from early studies on eNO and asthma.

An important issue is standardization of measurement techniques for eNO analysis. Measurement of the fraction of exhaled NO (FENO) can be complicated by two factors: contamination by nasal nitric oxide and variable expiratory flow rates. The FENO concentration can be up to 1000 times higher in the nasal cavity and paranasal sinuses than concentrations found in the lower airways. Turbulent gas mixing during exhalation allows nitric oxide contamination from the nasal cavity. The FENO is also highly flow dependent, allowing for measurement difficulty with variable flow rates. With high expiratory flow rates, nitric oxide levels will be lower than with a constant and slow expiratory maneuver. Techniques have been developed for measuring FENO that potentially overcome these factors.[31]

Exhaled nitric oxide is an important measurement of the inflammatory component of asthma in both children and adults. People with asthma who suffer from nocturnal asthma have higher FENO levels during the day and night than those who do not suffer from nocturnal symptoms.[32] The adequacy of asthma control is often, but imperfectly, measured by assessing symptom control, improvement in physical findings, and improvements in pulmonary function, because these outcomes do not track each other consistently.[33] The available evidence supports that the measurement of FENO is a marker of inflammation, is highly reproducible, is responsive to change in the underlying disease state, and is predictive of response to therapeutic intervention with anti-inflammatory medications. In patients with asthma, FENO is elevated and the FENO decreases after the administration of either inhaled or systemic corticosteroids. The American Thoracic Society (ATS) in 2011 published a clinical practice guideline on the interpretation of FENO levels for clinical applications. Their recommendations are in **Table 32-2**.[34]

Two devices are presently cleared for FENO measurement by the Food and Drug Administration (FDA). Reimbursement is presently very limited. The reluctance regarding third-party reimbursement was based on a review of several articles that concluded that methodology was heterogeneous and that there were different FENO cutoffs, differences in definition of outcomes, and conflicting trial conclusions. Perhaps as FENO is used more consistently with the ATS guidelines, its use may become more standardized and reimbursement for its use may become more common. Presently, FENO measurement is an adjunct in the diagnosis and management of asthma.

BOX 32-4

Traditional Peak Flow Zones

Green Zone: Normal Zone

Predicted or personal best in the range of 80% to 100%

Yellow Zone: Caution Zone

Predicted or personal best in the range of 50% to 79%

Red Zone: Danger Zone

Predicted or personal best less than 50%

Pharmacologic Therapy

The purpose of pharmacologic therapy in the treatment of asthma is to prevent or control asthma symptoms, or at least to attempt to reduce the frequency or severity of acute exacerbations. Medications for asthma are classified as either long-term controllers or quick relievers in the National Heart, Lung, and Blood Institute's (NHLBI) asthma guidelines released by the expert panel.[1] The

TABLE 32-2
ATS Recommendations on the Use of FENO in Patients with Asthma

- Recommend the use of FENO in the diagnosis of eosinophilic airway inflammation (strong recommendation, moderate quality of evidence).
- Recommend the use of FENO in determining the likelihood of steroid responsiveness in individuals with chronic respiratory symptoms possibly due to airway inflammation (strong recommendation, low quality of evidence).
- Suggest that FENO may be used to support the diagnosis of asthma in situations in which objective evidence is needed (weak recommendation, moderate quality of evidence).
- Suggest the use of cut points rather than reference values when interpreting FENO levels (weak recommendation, low quality of evidence).
- Recommend accounting for age as a factor affecting FENO in children younger than 12 years of age (strong recommendation, high quality of evidence).
- Recommend that low FENO less than 25 ppb (<20 ppb in children) be used to indicate that eosinophilic inflammation and responsiveness to corticosteroids are less likely (strong recommendation, moderate quality of evidence).
- Recommend that FENO greater than 50 ppb (>35 ppb in children) be used to indicate that eosinophilic inflammation and, in symptomatic patients, responsiveness to corticosteroids are likely (strong recommendation, moderate quality of evidence).
- Recommend that FENO values between 25 ppb and 50 ppb (20–35 ppb in children) should be interpreted cautiously and with reference to the clinical context (strong recommendation, low quality of evidence).
- Recommend accounting for persistent and/or high allergen exposure as a factor associated with higher levels of FENO (strong recommendation, moderate quality of evidence).
- Recommend the use of FENO in monitoring airway inflammation in patients with asthma (strong recommendation, low quality of evidence).
- Suggest using the following values to determine a significant increase in FENO: greater than 20% for values over 50 ppb or more than 10 ppb for values lower than 50 ppb from one visit to the next (weak recommendation, low quality of evidence).
- Suggest using a reduction of at least 20% in FENO for values over 50 ppb or more than 10 ppb for values lower than 50 ppb as the cut point to indicate a significant response to anti-inflammatory therapy (weak recommendation, low quality of evidence).

Reproduced from Dweik R, et al. An Official ATS Clinical Practice Guideline: Interpretation of Exhaled Nitric Oxide Levels (FENO) for Clinical Applications. *Am J Respir Crit Care Med.* 2011;184:602-615. Official Journal of the American Thoracic Society. Reprinted with permission of the American Thoracic Society. © 2015 American Thoracic Society.

long-term **controller medications** are taken prophylactically in order to decrease the degree or severity of inflammatory mediator release in the airways. These medications include inhaled corticosteroids, long-acting bronchodilators, combination products (long-acting β_2-agonist and inhaled corticosteroids), leukotriene modifiers, and immunomodulators.

Quick-relief medications are used to combat acute exacerbations of bronchoconstriction or provide quick, complete resolution of airflow obstruction and its accompanying symptoms of cough, wheezing, and chest tightness. This class of medications includes short-acting β_2-agonists and anticholinergics. Patients in all severity classes of asthma should at a minimum receive a prescription for quick-relief medications for use with signs and symptoms of asthma or during acute exacerbations.

Because the NHLBI asthma guidelines stress the importance of management and treatment of the inflammatory components of asthma, the following medication sections start with a description of the controller medications.

Controller Medications

Inhaled Corticosteroids

Corticosteroids are considered the most potent and consistent anti-inflammatory agents currently available by inhaled therapy in the long-term management of the inflammatory component of asthma. Anti-inflammatory medications, as supported by the evidence-based guidelines, are the recommended first-line medications for the treatment and management of asthma. All asthma severity classes that have been identified as having a persistent component are most effectively controlled with daily anti-inflammatory therapy.

Corticosteroids have been shown to suppress the release of certain inflammatory mediators. The use of corticosteroids in the management of asthma has been correlated with an overall reduction in asthma symptoms, an increase in lung function (as well as a decrease in the overall decline of FEV_1 with chronic disease), a decrease in airway hyperresponsiveness, a decrease in the frequency of acute exacerbations, and hypothetically a potential decrease in the amount or severity of airway remodeling in both adults and children.[35]

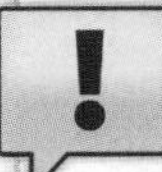

Respiratory Recap

Asthma Controller Medications

- Inhaled corticosteroids
- Long acting β_2-agonists
- Methylxanthines
- Leukotriene modifiers
- Immunomodulators
- Oral corticosteroids

The exact mechanism of action involved with corticosteroids and inflammation is not well understood. Several mechanisms appear to be actively and intimately involved. Corticosteroid therapy has provided evidence of an interference with the production of cytokines or suppression of cytokine release, a depression in the production of leukotrienes, and active recruitment of eosinophils. Clinical effects may take 2 to 3 weeks or more to bring forth baseline stability, but some of the more recent ICS agents have demonstrated improvement within 24 to 48 hours.

Dosage and frequency of corticosteroids can vary, depending on the specific type of product or delivery device (**Table 32-3**). Dosing to effect is patient and time dependent. The ability to eventually wean patients off corticosteroids also depends on patient physiology. An attempt to decrease the dose of ICS should be made only after asthma has been well controlled for 3 to 6 months. Patients who have moderate to severe persistent asthma often have persistent symptoms and a decline in lung function with attempts to wean or decrease the dose or use of corticosteroids.

The dose and frequency of ICS vary with the corticosteroid to be administered. Adherence to daily medication administration is enhanced as the frequency of doses per day decreases. Most controller preparations are formulated to be given once or twice daily. In cases of uncontrolled asthma or increasing disease severity, the dosage and frequency can be increased. It is important, however, to also review the patient's environmental control as well as medication adherence and technique before increasing the ICS dose.

The most common complications associated with the use of corticosteroids are persistent reflex cough, occasional dysphonia, sore throat, and oropharyngeal candidiasis. The majority of these short-term complications can be eliminated or greatly reduced with the use of an accessory device (valved holding chamber or spacer) and rinsing the mouth after inhalation. Systemic toxic effects are a rare occurrence with inhaled corticosteroids. The effect of corticosteroids on the linear growth of preadolescents who are taking this class of medications long term is controversial.[36,37] The EPR-3 states the following:[1]

- ICS are the preferred therapy for initiating long-term control therapy in children of all ages.

TABLE 32-3
Long-Term Controller Medications

Medication	Dose Strength	Adult Medium Daily Dose
Corticosteroids		
Metered dose inhalers (pMDI or DPI)		
Beclomethasone dipropionate (QVAR)	40 or 80 μg/puff	>240–480 μg
Budesonide (Pulmicort)	90, 180, or 200 μg/puff	>600–1200 μg
Fluticasone propionate (Flovent)	44, 110, or 220 μg/puff	>264–440 μg
Mometasone (Asmanex)	200 μg/puff	400 μg
Ciclesonide (Alvesco)	80 or 160 μg/puff	Starting dose in steroid-naive patients is 160 μg bid
Tablets		
Prednisone	1, 2.5, 5, 10, 20, 25, and 50 mg	40–60 mg/day for 3–10 days for control in exacerbation
Prednisolone	5 mg	40–60 mg/day for 3–10 days for control in exacerbation
Methylprednisolone	2, 4, 8, 16, 24, and 32 mg	7.5–60 mg/day or qod as needed for control
Long-Acting β_2-Agonists		
Dry powder inhalers		
Salmeterol (Serevent)	50 μg/puff	bid
Formoterol (Foradil)	12 μg/puff	bid
Methylxanthines (Oral)		
Theophylline (Slo-Bid, Theo-24, Theo-Dur, Uniphyl)	Various, depending on formulation	
Leukotriene Modifiers (Oral)		
Montelukast (Singulair)	10-mg tablets	qd
Combination Products		
Advair DPI or MDI (fluticasone/salmeterol)	100/50, 250/50, 500/50 (DPI) 45/21, 115/21, 230/21 HFA MDI	250/50 bid
Symbicort (budesonide/formoterol)	80/4.5, 160/4.5	160/4.5 bid
Immunomodulatars		
Omalizumab	Based on IgE level and weight	

bid, twice a day; qid, four times a day; qod, every other day; qd, daily; HFA, hydrofluoroalkane.

- ICS, especially at low doses, and even for extended periods of time, are generally safe.
- The potential for the adverse effect of low- to medium-dose ICS on linear growth is usually limited to a small reduction in growth velocity (approximately 1 centimeter in the first year of treatment) that is generally not progressive over time.
- The potential risks of ICS are well balanced by their benefits.
- High doses of ICS administered for prolonged periods of time (>1 year), particularly in combination with frequent courses of oral corticosteroid therapy, may be associated with adverse growth effects.

Long-Acting β_2-Agonists

This class of long-term controller medication is predominantly used to provide a longer duration of airway smooth muscle relaxation. This class of medication is not intended for relief of acute bronchospasm or for monotherapy (delivery without an ICS). LABAs have bronchodilation duration of approximately 12 hours but require a longer onset of action than SABAs for peak bronchodilatory protection. Two medications are in this class of controller: salmeterol and formoterol (refer to Table 32-3).

LABAs relax smooth muscle by stimulating the β_2 receptors, thereby increasing cyclic adenosine monophosphate (cAMP). LABAs have a 12-hour duration of effect; the molecule remains bound within the muscle cell wall because it is lipophilic. These medications work well as an adjunct therapy to anti-inflammatory medications in the long-term control of symptoms.[38] LABAs appear to work exceptionally well at controlling symptoms that occur at night[39] and at minimizing the risk of exercise-induced exacerbations.

The complications of long-acting β_2-agonists are still somewhat controversial. There are reports of sudden severe asthma attacks that could have been worsened or initiated with the use of salmeterol.[40] Two studies that looked closely at this issue in a large cohort of patients found a slight increase in deaths in patients who were taking salmeterol than in those who were not taking salmeterol.[41,42] On the basis of these data, clinicians need to pay close attention to properly educating patients who are using LABAs. LABAs should be used only as a supplement to inhaled corticosteroids and never as a quick-relief medication.

The EPR-3 recommendations for the use of LABAs are as follows:[1]

- LABAs are used as an adjunct to ICS therapy for providing long-term control of symptoms.
- LABAs are not recommended as monotherapy for long-term control of persistent asthma.
- The use of LABAs is not recommended to treat acute symptoms or exacerbation of asthma.
- LABAs may be used before exercise to prevent exercise-induced bronchoconstriction, but frequent and chronic use of LABAs for exercise-induced bronchoconstriction may indicate poorly controlled asthma, which should be managed with daily anti-inflammatory therapy.

Methylxanthines

Theophylline is an alternative, but not preferred, therapy in mild-to-moderate persistent asthma. Slow-release theophylline is used primarily as adjuvant therapy for nocturnal asthma (refer to Table 32-3). The exact mechanism of action of methylxanthines in asthma is not well established.[43,44] Theophylline acts as a nonselective phosphodiesterase inhibitor. This results in an increase in cyclic guanosine monophosphate levels and cAMP levels that inhibit inflammation cells and produce bronchodilation. Recent studies indicate that low serum concentrations of theophylline may act as a mild anti-inflammatory medication.[45] This is possible most likely because of the decreased mediator release from mast cells and reactive oxygen species and the inhibition of neutrophil activity.

Theophylline is relatively safe. Its use requires frequent monitoring of serum drug levels so that therapeutic, but not toxic, levels are achieved. Serum drug levels are affected by a patient's comorbidities and the presence of smoking and are therefore often difficult or impractical to manage with asthma on theophylline. Potential toxic side effects include tachycardia, nausea and vomiting, central nervous system stimulation, arrhythmias, headache, seizures, hyperglycemia, and hypokalemia. The therapeutic serum range is 5 to 15 mg/L to limit potential toxic effects. Pay close attention to other medications that patients using theophylline are receiving (e.g., antibiotics, β_2-blockers, quinolones).

Leukotriene Modifiers

Leukotriene modifiers also fall into the class of controller medications. This class of medications acts on the inflammatory cells known as leukotrienes. Leukotrienes are mediators that are released from mast cells, eosinophils, and basophils; they are responsible for airway bronchoconstriction, inflammatory cell recruitment, increased vascular permeability, and secretion production.

Montelukast is a leukotriene receptor antagonist (LTRA) that blocks the receptor sites on inflammatory cells for leukotrienes. Leukotriene receptor antagonists appear to work best in patients who have mild to moderate persistent asthma. Leukotriene receptor antagonists are an alternative, but not preferred, therapy to low- to medium-dose inhaled corticosteroids. Studies demonstrate a greater improvement in lung function and symptom scores with the use of ICS versus LTRA.[46] Regardless, LRTAs improve lung function, diminish asthma symptoms, and decrease the need for short-acting β_2-agonists, particularly in patients with allergies.[47]

Immunomodulators

There is currently one immunomodulator drug used for asthma: omalizumab, which has a trade name of Xolair. Omalizumab is a recombinant DNA-derived monoclonal antibody that inhibits the binding of IgE to the IgE receptor on the surface of mast cells and basophils. When the IgE receptors are bound by omalizumab, there is a reduction in surface-bound IgE, and therefore a decrease in the activation of mast cells and a decrease in the release of inflammatory mediators. Omalizumab is an alternate, but not preferred, drug in the treatment of moderate-to-severe persistent asthma in patients who have a positive skin test to aeroallergens and whose symptoms are inadequately controlled with ICS. It has been approved only for patients 12 years old and older.

Omalizumab is administered subcutaneously, and the dose is based on IgE level and patient weight. Omalizumab must be administered only in a closely observed clinic, because a rare adverse effect is anaphylaxis. The patient is directed to remain in the clinic for a period of observation following injection. Omalizumab has been shown to decrease the incidence of asthma exacerbations and emergency department visits, increase efficacy in patients with severe persistent allergic asthma who are already on high-dose ICS and LABA, and improve quality of life scores. Other than its adverse effects, the other drawback to omalizumab is its cost, which is approximately $1000 per month.[1]

Quick-Relief Medications

Short-Acting β_2-Agonists

This class of quick-relief medication is used predominantly to relieve airway bronchoconstriction and symptoms of cough, chest tightness, and wheezing. Short-acting β_2-agonists are the first-line medications used to treat an acute asthma exacerbation and for preventing exercise-induced bronchoconstriction. Before the 1990s, this was the first line of medications prescribed to result in overall control of asthma symptoms. Given the focus on the role of airway inflammation in the chronic management of asthma, SABAs have become quick-relief medications. The most common SABA medication is albuterol (**Table 32-4**).

The mechanism of action is to relax smooth airway muscle and cause quick resolution to airway obstruction. Bronchodilation occurs primarily through β_2-adrenergic receptor stimulation in bronchial smooth muscle. These receptors are also present in airway epithelium, airway smooth muscle, mucus glands, and mast cells. The onset of action for a short-acting β_2-agonist is approximately 5 to 15 minutes under most circumstances of mild-to-moderate acute exacerbations.

TABLE 32-4
Quick-Relief Medications

Medication	Dose	Frequency
Short-Acting β_2-Agonists		
Pressurized metered dose inhalers		
Racemic albuterol (Ventolin HFA, Proventil HFA, Pro-Air HFA)	90 μg/puff	prn; q4h–q6h
Levalbuterol (Xopenex HFA)	45 μg/puff	prn, q6h
Nebulization		prn, q4h–q6h
Racemic albuterol (Ventolin, Proventil, generic)	2.5 mg (0.5% solution	
Levalbuterol (Xopenex)	0.31 mg and 0.63 mg	prn; q4h–q6h
Metaproterenol (Alupent)	5% solution	
Oral tablets		
Albuterol (Repetabs, Volmax)	2 and 4 mg	
Metaproterenol	10 and 20 mg	prn; q4h–q6h
Syrup		
Albuterol	2 mg/5 mL	
Metaproterenol	10 mg/5 mL	prn; q4h–q6h
Subcutaneous injection		
Terbutaline	1 mg/mL injection	prn; q4h–q6h
Anticholinergics		
Pressurized metered dose inhalers		
Ipratropium bromide (Atrovent)	18 μg/puff	bid–qid
Nebulization		
Ipratropium bromide (Atrovent)	500-μg solution	bid–qid

HFA, hydrofluoroalkane; prn, as needed; bid, twice a day; qid, four times a day; q4h, every 4 hours; q6h, every 6 hours.

Complications from SABAs are usually mild and self-limiting upon stopping the medication. Potential side effects include tachycardia, nausea, vomiting, tremors, headache, palpitation, paradoxical bronchospasm, and hypokalemia. Some potential complications from high use or prolonged use over time include subsensitivity (reduction in bronchodilation effect), increased airways hyperreactivity, and life-threatening episodes with overuse. The frequency of SABA use or prescription refills can be used as a marker of disease worsening or to indicate an increased risk of death or near death.

Patients should be cautioned to use SABAs only as needed. If the patient uses a SABA more often than

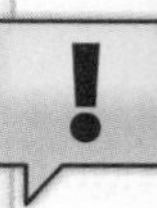

Respiratory Recap

Asthma Quick-Relief Medications

- Short-acting β_2-agonists
- Anticholinergics
- Systemic corticosteroids

twice per week, this indicates decreased asthma control. A red flag for the practitioner is if the patient uses more than one canister of SABA per month, because this indicates that the patient has used his or her SABA approximately three times per day. The need for this much SABA is an indication that the underlying inflammation has worsened. The patient should seek medical attention in this event.

Anticholinergics

This class of quick-relief medication is used predominantly as an adjunct to short-acting β_2-agonists in acute severe exacerbations of airway bronchoconstriction in the emergency department. The mechanism of action of anticholinergics is airway smooth muscle tone relaxation through cholinergic innervation. Ipratropium is the primary asthma medication in the anticholinergic class. Ipratropium is a derivative of atropine without the common side effects of atropine (refer to Table 32-4).

The overall effectiveness of ipratropium bromide in the management of asthma remains controversial.[48,49] Its effectiveness for long-term asthma management has not been demonstrated. Adult patients who have asthma and a component of chronic obstructive pulmonary disease apparently experience some beneficial outcomes.

Studies in children have demonstrated that the use of ipratropium in combination with β_2-agonists in patients with acute exacerbations or severe airway obstruction may be beneficial. Routine administration of this combination therapy does not appear to be beneficial.[50,51]

Systemic Corticosteroids

Systemic corticosteroids are usually combined with a short-acting β_2-agonist for a quick resolution of airway obstruction in an emergency department or hospital setting.[52] These drugs may be given either orally or intravenously. Normal dosage in this setting is 2 mg/kg (given every 6 hours, up to a maximum dose of 120 mg). The mechanism of action for systemic corticosteroids is the same as inhaled corticosteroids. The administration of a systemic corticosteroid in the ED is used to help prevent or ease the onset of the delayed (phase 2) asthmatic response. This phase 2 response is secondary to the event that led the patient to present to the ED. In the absence of a systemic corticosteroid, the patient may present to the ED again following discharge with more severe bronchospasm and inflammation than during the initial admission.

For outpatient use, systemic corticosteroids are prescribed for short-term burst therapy (once a day for 3 to 10 days). Normal dosing is prescribed at the lowest possible dose (0.5 to 2 mg/kg/day). Maximum dose is normally restricted to 60 mg daily for outpatient use. If chronic use of systemic corticosteroids is needed, a study has documented improved efficacy when the medication is given at 3 PM instead of in the morning.

Aerosol Therapy

The main routes of delivery for asthma medications are systemic or inhaled. The main routes of systemic delivery are oral (ingested) or parenteral (subcutaneous, intramuscular, or intravenous).[1] Oral medications are mainly in either pill or liquid form. Parenteral medications are usually limited to patients who either are in the emergency department or are admitted to the hospital.

The inhaled route is more convenient and common because of fewer side effects and quicker onset of action. The disadvantages of the inhaled route are associated with the delivery device and the factors that affect drug penetration and deposition in the lungs. The main factors involved in penetration and deposition are physical (sedimentation, inertial impaction, and diffusion) and clinical (particle size, ventilatory pattern, and lung function).[53]

Nebulizers, pressurized metered dose inhalers (pMDIs), and dry powder inhalers (DPIs) are used for inhaled medications. Opinions have varied on the best and most efficient method, but available evidence suggests that all three devices are equally effective in treating an acute exacerbation.[54]

Nebulizers

The small-volume jet nebulizer (SVN) is the most common device used to deliver medications to small children and patients requiring hospitalization. Although theoretically aerosol delivery and deposition in an asthmatic airway may be improved with a less

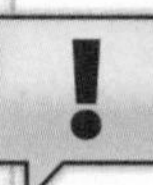

Respiratory Recap

Aerosol Delivery Devices for Patients with Asthma

- Small volume nebulizers (SVN)
- Jet nebulizer
- Pressurized metered dose inhaler
- Pressurized metered dose inhaler with accessory device
- Dry powder inhaler

dense gas (**heliox**),[55–58] there are potential problems with the use of nebulizers powered by it.[53] Heliox is best reserved for severe exacerbations that are refractory to conventional therapy. A number of factors affect SVN performance.[59–61] Deposition of appropriate particle size in the lower respiratory tract depends on ventilatory pattern. To ensure optimal deposition, a slow breath through the mouth to total lung capacity with an end-inspiratory breath hold is ideal. With proper breathing technique, aerosol delivery with an SVN is equally effective with a mask or mouthpiece, but a mouthpiece is preferred when possible as the nose acts as a filter for up to 40% of the delivery aerosol with a mask.[62]

Continuous Aerosols

In a severe asthma attack, aggressive intermittent aerosol therapy may fail to relieve symptoms. Studies have demonstrated that continuous bronchodilator therapy is as effective or more effective than intermittent therapy. Continuous aerosol bronchodilator therapy has become an accepted alternative to intermittent therapy in emergency departments for patients who fail to respond to less aggressive therapy. Current evidence supports the use of continuous bronchodilator administration in patients with severe acute asthma who present to the ED to increase their pulmonary functions and reduce hospitalization,[63] and it is safe and well tolerated.

Pressurized Metered Dose Inhalers

The pMDI is the most common device used to deliver medications in an ambulatory setting and is commonly used in hospitalized and ED treatment. The canister is activated by compressing it into a mouthpiece, which causes a metered dose of the drug to be delivered for inhalation.

A number of factors can affect pMDI performance and drug delivery. A potential factor that can interfere with appropriate metered dose delivery is using medications from one manufacturer with an actuator or accessory device from another manufacturer. Most of the factors that affect optimal delivery involve patient delivery technique; this is especially the case in the very young or elderly. Factors critical in the effectiveness of pMDI performance include timing of actuation, lung volume, pMDI position to the mouth (without spacer), inspiratory flow rate, and the ability to perform a breath hold.[53]

> **STOP AND THINK**
>
> In a hospitalized patient with asthma, do you think a jet nebulizer or pressurized metered dose inhaler should be used? Why?

Each type of pMDI has specific instructions on priming, so it is important to read the package insert to learn how many times a pMDI needs to be primed, and how and when to clean the pMDI actuator, so that this information may be taught to the patient.

The Respimat is a propellant-free soft-mist inhaler that utilizes mechanical energy in the form of a tensioned spring to generate the soft aerosol plume. Energy created by turning the device's base to the right one-half turn draws a predetermined metered volume of solution from the medication cartridge through a capillary tube into a micro-pump. When the dose release button is depressed, energy from the spring forces solution to the mouthpiece, creating a soft aerosol plume that lasts approximately 1.5 seconds.[64]

Spacers and Valved Holding Chambers

If patients find it difficult to properly use a pMDI or if an ICS pMDI is being used, patients should use a spacer or valved holding chamber to enhance optimal drug delivery. A spacer is a cylindrical or cone-shaped chamber that receives the pMDI actuator on one end and has a mouthpiece on the other. A valved holding chamber is a spacer with a one-way valve at the mouthpiece end that prevents the patient from exhaling into the chamber. Several of these devices also incorporate a flow signal that has an audible sound if the patient is inhaling too fast. With optimal MDI delivery technique, evidence exists (even with children) of no difference in deposition with or without a spacing device.[65]

With an accessory spacing device, a pMDI is actuated into the chamber, and the patient breathes the medication from a mouthpiece or mask attached to the chamber. For optimal medication availability, the valved holding chamber is preferred. This decreases the potential of medication being lost through the device on exhalation. Different spacing devices affect drug delivery,[53,66] and more studies are needed to evaluate new medications and spacing devices.

Another potential factor that may affect the amount of drug delivered with a spacing device is a static charge that occurs from washing the chamber. Antistatic chambers have also been developed. Generally, the device should be disassembled and washed in soapy water, rinsed, and allowed to air-dry before use. Manufacturers' instructions should be followed regarding appropriate device cleaning.

Dry Powder Inhalers

Two types of DPI exist: single-dose devices (e.g., Spiriva Handihaler, Foradil Aerolizer) and multidose devices (e.g., Advair discus, Pulmicort Flexhaler, Asmanex Twisthaler).[53] DPIs are breath activated with a high inspiratory flow generated at the mouthpiece.

Because of the requirement of a high inspiratory flow for actuation, DPIs are not indicated for use in children younger than 12 years. Several instructions are common to DPIs. The DPI must be kept level during inhalation, it must be kept in a dry location to prevent clumping of the powder, and the patient must not exhale into the DPI. Multidose DPIs have dose counters to alert the patient as to the remaining doses in the device.

Adjunctive Treatments

Oxygen, inhaled β_2-adrenergic agonists, and corticosteroids remain the cornerstones of therapy for asthma. This section discusses four alternative therapies to aerosolized medications in the treatment of a severe asthma exacerbation: helium–oxygen gas mixtures (heliox), magnesium sulfate, noninvasive ventilation, and invasive mechanical ventilation. Because of the risk of immediate respiratory decompensation, these therapies are normally administered in the confines of an intensive care unit or emergency department.

Heliox

Helium is a gas that is less dense than air, which may be beneficial in the treatment of asthma.[67] Heliox is not a stand-alone therapy to treat a severe asthma exacerbation but rather is supportive therapy before intubation to allow time for bronchodilators and corticosteroids to take effect.[68] A difficulty in the provision of heliox in nonintubated patients is that the available gas mixtures in concentrations may not provide adequate supplemental oxygen to achieve acceptable oxyhemoglobin saturations (80% helium to 20% oxygen or 70% helium to 30% oxygen).

The therapeutic benefits of heliox are controversial. Reports of the therapeutic benefits of heliox are isolated primarily to the management of pediatric asthma[56,57,68] or the management of adult patients who present to the ED with a respiratory acidosis and/or a short duration of symptoms.[69] Some studies have shown that the use of heliox has no effect on FEV_1.[70,71] Given the safety profile of heliox and the short time to achieve a positive response, a brief trial of heliox may serve as a therapeutic bridge until corticosteroid therapy has taken effect. One study documented a rapid resolution (less than 60 minutes) to respiratory acidosis by using heliox, especially in patients who had brief duration of symptoms (less than 24 hours) and a severely acidotic pH (7.20 or less) at presentation.[72] Randomized trials in patients with asthma have reported benefit with the use of heliox.[57,73] The EPR-3 cites a meta-analysis of six studies that did not find a statistically significant improvement in pulmonary function or other measured outcomes in patients receiving heliox compared with oxygen or air.[1] The EPR-3 recommends consideration of heliox-driven albuterol nebulization for patients who have life-threatening exacerbations and for those patients whose exacerbations remain in the severe category after 1 hour of intensive conventional therapy.[1]

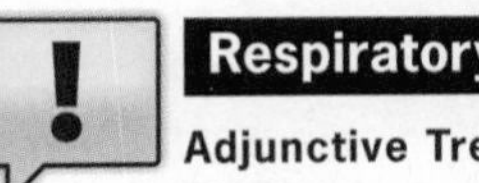

Respiratory Recap

Adjunctive Treatments for Asthma

- Heliox
- Magnesium sulfate
- Noninvasive ventilation
- Invasive ventilation

Magnesium Sulfate

Administration of magnesium sulfate is an alternative treatment for a severe asthma exacerbation.[74,75] The EPR-3 recommends intravenous magnesium sulfate in patients who have life-threatening exacerbations and in those whose exacerbations remain in the severe category after 1 hour of conventional therapy.[1] The mechanisms of action include calcium-channel blockade in the airway smooth muscle and inhibition of acetylcholine and histamine release. Magnesium may promote bronchodilation that would improve β_2-agonist delivery. A study comparing nebulized magnesium to salbutamol demonstrated a similar response,[75] but nebulized magnesium does not consistently have this bronchodilator effect. Other studies have documented no improvement in FEV_1 in patients who were treated with magnesium intravenously.[76–77]

The dose for intravenous magnesium is 2 g in adults and from 25 to 75 mg/kg up to 2 g in children administered over a half hour. The onset of action for magnesium can occur within minutes of administration. Potential side effects are usually minor (facial warmth and flushing). Magnesium can be toxic with high serum levels. Signs of magnesium toxicity include hypotension, dysrhythmias, areflexia, and muscle weakness. The use of magnesium sulfate in the treatment of severe exacerbations is not recommended as a first-line therapy. The treatment has no apparent value in exacerbations of lesser severity.[1]

Noninvasive Ventilation

The use of noninvasive positive pressure ventilation (NIV) has taken a role in the management of patients who are at high risk for intubation and mechanical ventilation. NIV offers a viable means of overcoming increased work of breathing without an endotracheal tube. Recent studies have demonstrated the use of noninvasive ventilation as a viable alternative to mechanical ventilation.[78,79] The key factor in the use of NIV is early initiation of the therapy in conjunction with bronchodilators and corticosteroids. Appropriate inspiratory flow is important to ensure patient comfort and

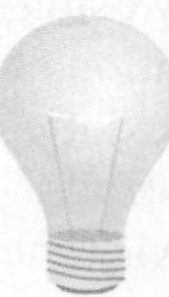

STOP AND THINK

When would you recommend the use of noninvasive ventilation for a patient with severe acute asthma?

to decrease the work of breathing. Avoiding delivery of excessive minute ventilation is important, because it could lead to hyperinflation and air trapping. The use of aerosolized medications with NIV is feasible.[80] NIV in patients with asthma is supportive and meant to be used in conjunction with established therapies. NIV may be useful in carefully selected patients with a severe exacerbation, even though there have been few trials of NIV in asthma.[81]

Invasive Ventilation

Invasive ventilation of patients with asthma is a treatment of last resort for patients experiencing respiratory failure because of severe airflow obstruction, increased mucus production, and/or severe airway inflammation.[81,82] Asthma resulting in intubation and mechanical ventilation is not a common event, occurring in less than 5% of patients treated. **Box 32-5** lists the general indications for mechanical ventilation in the patient with asthma. The obstructive nature of a severe exacerbation of asthma produces a ventilation-perfusion mismatch and increased work of breathing, but this rarely produces severe hypoxemia. The more difficult issue in the patient with acute asthma is optimizing the pH and $Paco_2$ because of bronchoconstriction, air trapping, and increased dead space.[83]

On intubation of a patient with acute asthma, full ventilatory support is usually provided (i.e., no spontaneous breathing by the patient). This allows optimization of the patient–ventilator interface under the best possible conditions. The principal goal of mechanical ventilation of the patient with asthma is to provide acceptable gas exchange while avoiding air trapping (auto-PEEP [positive end-expiratory pressure]). With auto-PEEP, alveolar overdistention may occur with concomitant hypotension and barotrauma.

BOX 32-5

Indications for Mechanical Ventilation of the Patient with Asthma

$Paco_2$ >40 mm Hg (especially if increasing)
Refractory hypoxemia (Pao_2 <60 mm Hg or Fio_2 ≥0.5)
Mental status deterioration
Decrease or loss of breath sounds
Apnea

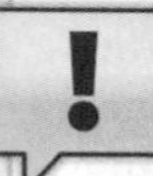

Respiratory Recap

Mechanical Ventilation of the Patient with Asthma

- Avoid strategies that cause air trapping and auto-PEEP.
- Consider PEEP to counterbalance auto-PEEP.
- Avoid plateau pressure above 30 cm H_2O.
- Permissive hypercapnia may be necessary.
- Inhaled bronchodilators can be administered using nebulizers or pMDIs.

The choice of ventilator mode is often based on clinical preference or institutional bias. Either volume or pressure control modes can be used, and advantages and disadvantages exist for both. With volume control, auto-PEEP results in increased plateau pressures and alveolar overdistention. With pressure control, auto-PEEP results in decreased tidal volumes and respiratory acidosis. In patients with asthma with severe airflow obstruction, it may be difficult to deliver an adequate tidal volume with pressure control. Regardless of the mode chosen, auto-PEEP and plateau pressures must be monitored closely.

The ultimate goal of tidal volume selection in severe asthma exacerbation is to avoid overdistention of the alveoli. Generally, tidal volumes are set in the 5 to 8 mL/kg range and adjusted to minimize overdistention (i.e., to avoid a plateau pressure of more than 30 cm H_2O). This often results in a ventilator strategy of permissive hypercapnia. With permissive hypercapnia, $Paco_2$ is allowed to rise and an acidic pH is tolerated. The limits of safe $Paco_2$ and pH are debated, but general consensus suggests that $Paco_2$ levels of 80 to 100 mm Hg and pH levels of 7.15 to 7.20 are acceptable.[84,85]

The use of positive end-expiratory pressure when ventilating the patient with asthma is controversial. PEEP as a means to prevent atelectasis or collapse is not necessary. PEEP has been used to combat auto-PEEP. The intent is to counterbalance auto-PEEP by applying PEEP so that the patient will be better able to trigger the ventilator. Care must be taken to avoid increased overdistention with the application of PEEP. PEEP has no role in counterbalancing auto-PEEP in the patient who is not attempting to trigger the ventilator.[86,87]

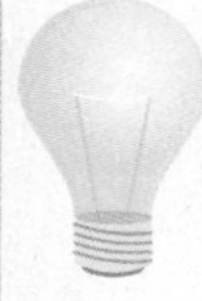

STOP AND THINK

What can be done to minimize air trapping in the mechanically ventilated patient with asthma?

One study observed that there are three different responses to PEEP in the setting of auto-PEEP. In the biphasic response, expiratory flow and lung volume remained constant during progressive PEEP steps until a threshold was reached, beyond which overinflation ensued. In the classic overinflation response, any increment of PEEP caused a decrease in expiratory flow and overinflation. In the paradoxical response, a drop in functional residual capacity during PEEP application was commonly accompanied by decreased plateau pressures and total PEEP, with increased expiratory flow.[88] Generally, no more than 10 cm H_2O PEEP is used to counterbalance auto-PEEP. Some auto-PEEP that occurs during mechanical ventilation of the patient with asthma may not be measurable in the usual manner because of complete airway closure during the expiratory phase.[88]

The inspiratory-to-expiratory (I:E) ratio in a patient with airflow obstruction is important to avoid air trapping. The I:E ratio is determined by the inspiratory time (flow and tidal volume for volume control) and respiratory rate. The goal when setting the I:E ratio in patients with asthma is to allow adequate expiratory time to minimize auto-PEEP. Use of prolonged expiratory times requires a low respiratory rate and a shortened inspiratory time in the range of 0.8 to 1.2 seconds (high flow). Typically, a respiratory rate of 15 per minute or less is used.

When aggressive therapy fails to stabilize a patient's asthma and intubation occurs, the need to provide aerosol therapy remains important in the resolution of the acute exacerbation. Aerosol therapy of the intubated patient has been an area of debate.[89] Some support either nebulizers or pMDIs as the most effective and efficient method from a clinical and financial standpoint. Aerosol delivery to intubated patients with either nebulizers or MDIs is less effective than when delivered to a spontaneously breathing patient. Many factors in intubated patients affect optimal aerosol delivery and deposition. Higher-than-standard doses may be necessary to elicit a desired response because of potential barriers involved with mechanically ventilated patients. Aerosol administration by both nebulizers and MDIs is an effective means of delivering medication to ventilated patients. Studies using both devices have demonstrated lung deposition efficiency of 5% to 15%.[90] Sufficient attention to detail, including the use of an efficient nebulizer and/or adapter and proper placement and operating method, is required to provide optimal delivery.

The use of heliox with mechanical ventilation may be beneficial when a patient with asthma is difficult to manage with traditional ventilator manipulations. Caution is warranted because the addition of heliox may result in ventilator malfunction. Many, but not all, of the current-generation ventilators are compatible with heliox. Inhalational anesthetics (e.g., enflurane, sevoflurane, or isoflurane) have a bronchodilatory effect and are used rarely in the most severe cases.

Mechanical ventilation of the patient with asthma may be a lifesaving measure, but it can also be associated with significant morbidity and mortality. The major complications of mechanical ventilation of the patient with asthma include overdistention, pneumothorax, hypotension, air trapping, patient–ventilator asynchrony, and neuromuscular blocking agent–related myopathies.[91–93]

Education

Asthma education begins at diagnosis and should be reinforced with each visit. The ability to modify morbidity and resource consumption through education has been well documented in asthma. Over the past 20 years, many programs and formats have been designed and implemented to demonstrate that asthma education is a main component of the overall successful management of the disease. The items in **Box 32-6** should be included in **asthma education programs.**[1]

Many studies of educational interventions are available in the literature, covering many different care settings. These include ambulatory clinics, allergy or pulmonary specialty clinics, emergency departments, hospitals, patient homes, and asthma camps. The impact of educational interventions has been evaluated regarding readmission rates, hospitalizations, compliance, ED visits, clinic follow-up rates, test scores, and behavior changes.

The rapid expansion of managed health care in the 1990s led to the study of the financial aspects of providing asthma education. Some of the earlier managed care education interventions assessed patients with asthma determined to be at high risk. Although these programs still exist, asthma educators are looking at ways to target a variety of patients with asthma because

BOX 32-6

Educational Recommendations of the NAEPP

- Teach basic facts about asthma
- Teach the necessary medication skills (techniques, delivery devices, and dosing regimens)
- Teach self-monitoring skills: symptom-based, peak flow monitoring
- Teach relevant environmental control/avoidance strategies
- Provide a written asthma exacerbation treatment plan

Modified from National Asthma Education Program, National Heart, Lung, and Blood Institute. *Expert Panel Report 3: Guidelines for the Diagnosis and Management of Asthma.* Bethesda, MD: National Institutes of Health; 2007. NIH Publication 07-4051.

AGE-SPECIFIC ANGLE

Children as young as 2 years can begin learning about asthma and its management.

of a regression-toward-the-mean concept. The theory of regression toward the mean implies that patients with chronic conditions do not have steady-state healthcare resource consumption year after year. One year's high-resource consumers do not necessarily translate into the next year's high-resource consumers. Therefore, these earliest managed care programs and interventions resulted in a shifting of the costs from group to group or from year to year (**Table 32-5**).

The asthma education program needs to take a proactive approach. An asthma education program should provide education to the patient with asthma and include all potential caregivers (spouses, parents, older children, day-care providers, teachers, coaches, group leaders, and counselors). The National Cooperative Inner City Asthma Study (NCICAS) reported that often a child has several care providers in the home.[94] This pediatric study demonstrated the importance of involving as many caregivers as possible in the asthma education to ensure consistent management. This study also identified that pediatric asthma has additional educational barriers. Often education providers overlook the child to concentrate their educational efforts on the caregivers. Children as young as 2 years can begin learning about their asthma and its management. As children age, the scope and the depth of the information will need to continue to grow. As children grow into adolescents, they should receive all asthma information themselves.[95]

Asthma education information should be repeated several times for maximum effect, and educational objectives should be reinforced with written materials targeted for age appropriateness. Asthma self-management education should be modified to the needs of each individual patient. Cultural beliefs and harmful practices should be approached and discussed with sensitivity and understanding. The education provider should be attentive and document the concerns of the patient and the family regarding medications and asthma management. Addressing concerns and explaining the rationale for treatment may be the overriding factor in patient compliance with chronic asthma management. The asthma educator also must be prepared to intervene and problem-solve in the areas of medications, level of treatment, trigger avoidance, compliance, and self-management skills.

One of the indicators of a chronic condition is the ability to modify or reduce morbidity and mortality risks through patient education. Asthma is a chronic disease condition that has demonstrated this ability. An unlimited number of approaches or interventions are readily available to provide effective and efficient asthma education to healthcare providers. Perhaps one method is not truly better than another. The important features are to provide the resources and information at diagnosis and consistently thereafter to each patient with asthma individually.

TABLE 32-5
Theoretic Look at Regression Toward the Mean

	Percentage of Resource Cost Consumption			
	Original Percentage of Patients	Year 1	Year 2	Year 3
High-resource consumers	10	80	10	4
Low-resource consumers	90	20	90	96

Case Studies

Case 1. Ambulatory Asthma Management

A 43-year-old woman with asthma presents to an inner-city emergency department with coughing, wheezing, and shortness of breath. She reports a respiratory viral infection within the last week that resolved with over-the-counter medicines in 3 or 4 days. Her initial physical examination reveals the following: respiratory rate of 36 breaths/min, labored; heart rate of 120 beats/min; blood pressure of 120/80 mm Hg; pulse oximetry of 93% in room air; inspiratory and expiratory wheezing upon auscultation; equal air exchange bilaterally; moderate intercostal retractions; and peak expiratory flow (PEF) of 290 L/min (60% of predicted). The initial treatment consists of six puffs of albuterol, administered via an MDI with a holding chamber. Each puff is given with the appropriate technique. Posttreatment PEF is 300 L/min (62% of predicted).

The woman reports that she stopped taking her beclomethasone about 2 months before this visit. The following additional information is acquired:

- *Reported medications*: Beclomethasone two puffs twice a day, and albuterol two puffs as needed and before exercise
- *Treatment before arrival*: None
- *Peak flow meter diary*: None
- *Unscheduled ED/MD visits in the past month*: 0
- *Unscheduled ED/MD visits in the past year*: 3
- *Hospital admissions in the past year*: 1
- *Prior intensive care unit (ICU) admissions*: 0
- *Cough or wheeze frequency*: Two times per week
- *Activity limitations*: Occasionally
- *Nocturnal cough or wheeze*: Two to three times per week
- *Work absenteeism*: 6 days per year

Approximately 20 minutes after the initial treatment, a second treatment is administered with six puffs of albuterol via pMDI and holding chamber as before. The patient is also given 60 mg of prednisolone. Posttreatment assessment reveals a respiratory rate of 24 breaths/min; heart rate of 100 beats/min; oxygen saturation of 95% breathing room air; inspiratory and expiratory wheezing upon auscultation; equal air exchange bilaterally; mild intercostal retractions; and PEF of 315 L/min (65% predicted).

Approximately 20 minutes after the second treatment, a third treatment of albuterol (six puffs) is administered, along with two puffs of Atrovent. Posttreatment assessment reveals a respiratory rate of 16 breaths/min; heart rate of 80 beats/min; oxygen saturation of 95% breathing room air; faint end-expiratory wheezes with auscultation and bilateral equal air exchange; no intercostal retractions; and PEF of 365 L/min (75% predicted).

The next β_2-agonist treatment is withheld, and she is reassessed in 60 minutes. The prior assessment response is sustained upon physical examination, and the woman is readied for discharge. Based on the self-reported asthma history, the woman's chronic asthma is determined to be moderate persistent asthma. She is instructed to continue her albuterol treatments with two puffs every 4 to 6 hours for the next several days. She also is told to resume her beclomethasone therapy of two puffs twice a day for chronic inflammatory control. She is given a peak flow meter and instructed in its proper use. She is also instructed in the use of an asthma action plan with a peak flow diary that illustrates meter readings in three color-coded zones to assist her in self-management. She is also instructed to call her primary care physician and to schedule a follow-up visit in the next week to 10 days.

Case 2. Life-Threatening Asthma Management

A 10-year-old boy with asthma presents to an inner-city ED with dyspnea at rest, talking in phrases, agitated, and dusky in color. The boy's mother reports having administered three nebulizer treatments before arrival in the emergency department. The child's initial physical examination reveals the following: respiratory rate of 48 breaths/min, labored; heart rate of 170 beats/min; blood pressure of 160/100 mm Hg; oxygen saturation of 89% breathing room air; breath sounds muffled to inaudible; severe intercostal and substernal retractions; and inability to perform a PEF.

The patient is then started on undiluted albuterol that was nebulized with 100% oxygen. An IV is placed and he is given 60 mg methylprednisolone. During the aerosol treatment, an asthma history is taken from the boy's mother. She reports that her child had been outside playing basketball with his friends for most of the afternoon. Before this episode, he was in good health. The following information is acquired:

- *Reported medications*: Albuterol two puffs as needed before exercise
- *Treatment before arrival*: Three nebulized treatments with albuterol
- *Peak flow meter diary*: None
- *Unscheduled ED/MD visits in the past month*: 0
- *Unscheduled ED/MD visits in the past year*: 1
- *Hospital admissions in the past year*: 1
- *Prior ICU admissions*: 1 (3 years ago)
- *Cough or wheeze frequency*: With respiratory infections
- *Activity or play limitations*: Always
- *Nocturnal cough or wheeze*: One to two times per week
- *School absenteeism*: Three to four days per year

While receiving continuous albuterol treatments, the child is assessed every 20 minutes. Electrocardiography and pulse oximetry are monitored continuously. After the initial 20 minutes, 0.5 mg of ipratropium is added to the aerosol. Thirty-five minutes after treatment was started, the boy's status is a respiratory rate of 20 breaths/min, labored; heart rate of 80 beats/min; blood pressure of 200/100 mm Hg; oxygen saturation of 88% on continuous nebulizer; inaudible breath sounds; severe intercostal and substernal retractions; inability to perform PEF; and lethargy and drowsiness. Arterial blood gas results are pH 7.29, $Paco_2$ 52 mm Hg, Pao_2 60 mm Hg, HCO_3^- 26 mmol/L, and oxygen saturation of 87%.

The decision is made to intubate the child. After atropine, ketamine, and succinylcholine are administered, he is intubated with a 6.0 mm cuffed endotracheal tube. Upon arrival in the pediatric intensive care unit, the child is placed on the following settings: volume control continuous mandatory ventilation (VC-CMV), tidal volume 350 mL (7 mL/kg), PEEP 3 cm H_2O, mandatory breath rate 10 breaths/min, I:E ratio of 1:5, and Fio_2 0.50. After 1 hour on the ventilator, the arterial blood gas results are pH 7.32, $Paco_2$ 46 mm Hg, Pao_2 120 mm Hg, HCO_3^- 22 mmol/L, and oxygen saturation 99%. The Fio_2 is weaned to 0.4. The patient is ventilated with permissive hypercapnia to prevent auto-PEEP and overdistention. Continuous ventilator waveform analysis is used to detect auto-PEEP, and the flow is increased to allow for a longer expiratory time. The patient is kept moderately sedated, and paralysis is not necessary at this time. The child is given albuterol and Atrovent through the ventilator circuit with a mesh nebulizer. The patient remains on IV methylprednisolone.

After 6 hours of this therapy, the albuterol treatments are changed to a frequency of every hour. After 12 hours of mechanical ventilation and pharmacologic therapy, blood gas results are pH 7.42, $Paco_2$ 33 mm Hg, Pao_2

95 mm Hg on FIO_2 of 0.25, HCO_3^- 24 mmol/L, and oxygen saturation 99%. He is awake and triggering at a rate of 6 to 10 breaths/min above the mandatory rate. A spontaneous breathing trial is successful, he is extubated to a 2 L/min nasal cannula, 5.0 mg nebulized albuterol every hour, and IV methylprednisolone and ipratropium 0.5 mg every 6 hours.

Key Points

- Asthma is a common chronic disease that is increasing in prevalence and severity.
- The pathophysiology of asthma is largely related to inflammation, hyperresponsiveness, and airway obstruction.
- The most identifiable predisposing factor for the development of asthma is atopy.
- Nocturnal symptoms of asthma are common.
- Exercise-induced asthma is characterized by transient airway obstruction after strenuous exercise.
- Occupational asthma is characterized by variable airway hyperresponsiveness in the workplace.
- The NAEPP has developed a four-tiered system to classify asthma disease severity.
- The most common ways to diagnose and monitor airflow obstruction in asthma are spirometry and peak flow meters.
- Asthma medications are classified as either long-term controllers or quick-relief medications.
- Inhaled medications are delivered by nebulizer, pressurized metered dose inhaler, or dry powder inhalers.
- Oxygen, inhaled β_2-agonists, and corticosteroids are the cornerstones of therapy for asthma.
- Mechanical ventilation is the treatment of last resort for patients with asthma and respiratory failure.
- Asthma education begins with diagnosis and should be reinforced with each visit.

References

1. National Asthma Education Program, National Heart, Lung, and Blood Institute. *Expert Panel Report 3: Guidelines for the Diagnosis and Management of Asthma*. Bethesda, MD: National Institutes of Health; 2007. NIH Publication 07-4051.
2. The Global Initiative for Asthma (GINA). http://www.ginasthma.org. Accessed September 2, 2014.
3. Moorman JE, Akinbami LJ, Bailey CM, et al. National Surveillance of Asthma: United States, 2001–2010. National Center for Health Statistics. *Vital Health Stat*. 2012;3(35). Available at: http://www.cdc.gov/nchs/data/series/sr_03/sr03_035.pdf. Accessed August 7, 2014.
4. Schaubel D, Johansen H, Mao Y, et al. Risk of preschool asthma: incidence, hospitalization, recurrence, and readmission probability. *J Asthma*. 1996;33:97–103.
5. Barnett SBL, Nurmagambebetov TA. Costs of asthma in the United States. *J Allergy and Clin Immunol*. 2011;127:145–152.
6. Smith D, Malone D, Lawson K, et al. A national estimate of the economic costs of asthma. *Am J Respir Crit Care Med*. 1997;156:787–793.
7. McFadden ER, Elsanadi N, Dixon L, et al. Protocol therapy for acute asthma: therapeutic benefits and cost savings. *Am J Med*. 1995;99:651–660.
8. Myers TR, Chatburn RL, Kercsmar CM. A pediatric asthma unit staff by respiratory therapists demonstrates positive clinical and financial outcomes. *Respir Care*. 1998;43:22–29.
9. McDowell KM, Chatburn RL, Myers TR, et al. A cost-saving algorithm for children hospitalized for status asthmaticus. *Arch Pediatr Adolesc Med*. 1998;152:977–984.
10. Jones M. Asthma self-management patient education. *Respir Care*. 2008;53:778–784.
11. Maciejewski ML, Chen SY, Au DH. Adult asthma disease management: an analysis of studies, approaches, outcomes and methods. *Respir Care*. 2009;54:878–886.
12. Mayo PH, Weinberg BJ, Kramer B, et al. Results of a program to improve the process of inpatient care of adult asthmatics. *Chest*. 1996;110:48–52.
13. Kwann-Ghett TS, Lozano P, Mullin K, et al. One-year experience with an inpatient asthma clinical pathway. *Arch Pediatr Adolesc Med*. 1997;151:684–689.
14. Brooks C, Pearce N, Douwes J. The hygiene hypothesis in allergy and asthma: an update. *Curr Opin Allergy Clin Immunol*. 2013;13:70–77.
15. Eggleston PA, Rosenstreich D, Lynn H, et al. Relationship of indoor allergen exposure to skin test sensitivity in inner-city children with asthma. *J Allergy Clin Immunol*. 1998;102:563–570.
16. Rosenstreich DL, Eggleston P, Kattan M, et al. The role of cockroach allergy and exposure to cockroach allergen in causing morbidity among inner-city children with asthma. *N Engl J Med*. 1997;336:1356–1363.
17. Ritz T, Kullowatz A, Goldman MD, et al. Airway response to emotional stimuli in asthma: the role of the cholinergic pathway. *J Appl Physiol*. 2010;108:1542–1549.
18. Teichtahl H, Buckmaster N, Pertnikovs E. The incidence of respiratory tract infection in adults requiring hospitalization for asthma. *Chest*. 1997;112:591–596.
19. Pizzichini MM, Pizzichini E, Efthimiadis A, et al. Asthma and natural colds. Inflammatory indices in induced sputum: a feasibility study. *Am J Respir Crit Care Med*. 1998;158:1178–1184.
20. Lieu TA, Quesenberry CP Jr, Capra AM, et al. Outpatient management practices associated with reduced risk of pediatric asthma hospitalization and emergency department visits. *Pediatrics*. 1997;100:334–341.
21. Martin RJ. Nocturnal asthma and the use of theophylline. *Clin Exp Allergy*. 1998;28:64–70.
22. Meijer GG, Postma DS, Wempe JB, et al. Frequency of nocturnal symptoms in asthmatic children attending a hospital out-patient clinic. *Eur Respir J*. 1995;8:2076–2080.
23. Di Stefano A, Lusuardi M, Braghiroli A, et al. Nocturnal asthma: mechanisms and therapy. *Lung*. 1997;175:53–61.
24. Fix A, Sexton M, Langenberg P, et al. The association of nocturnal asthma with asthma severity. *J Asthma*. 1997;34:329–336.
25. Martin RJ. *Nocturnal Asthma*. Mount Kisco, NY: Futura; 1993.
26. Silkoff PE, Martin RJ. Pathophysiology of nocturnal asthma. *Ann Allergy Asthma Immunol*. 1998;81:378–383.
27. Syabbalo N. Chronobiology and chronopathophysiology of nocturnal asthma. *Int J Clin Pract*. 1997;51:455–462.
28. Kukafka DS, Lang OM, Porter S, et al. Exercise-induced bronchospasm in high school athletes via a free running test: incidence and epidemiology. *Chest*. 1998;114:1613–1622.
29. Occupational Asthma Causing Agents. Adapted from: Chan-Yeung M. Malo JL. Aetiological agents in occupational asthma. *Eur Respiry J*. 1994;7:346–371. Available at: http://www.oem.msu.edu/userfiles/file/Resources/AsthmaCausingAgents.pdf. Accessed August 7, 2014.
30. American Thoracic Society. Standardization of spirometry: 1994 update. *Am J Respir Care Med*. 1995;152:1107–1136.
31. Silkoff PE, McClean PA, Slutsky AS, et al. Marked flow-dependence of exhaled nitric oxide using a new technique to exclude nasal nitric oxide. *Am J Respir Crit Care Med*. 1997;155:260–267.
32. ten Hacken NH, van der Vaart H, van der Malk TW, et al. Exhaled nitric oxide is higher both at day and night in subjects with nocturnal asthma. *Am J Respir Crit Care Med*. 1998;158:902–907.

33. Lim KG, Mottram C. The use of fraction of exhaled nitric oxide in pulmonary practice. *Chest.* 2008;133:1232–1242.
34. Dweik RA, Boggs PB, Erzurum SC, et al. An official ATS clinical practice guideline: interpretation of exhaled nitric oxide levels (FENO) for clinical applications. *Am J Respir Crit Care Med.* 2011;184:602–615.
35. Chauhan BF, Chartrand C, Ducharme FM. Intermittent versus daily inhaled corticosteroids for persistent asthma in children and adults. *Cochrane Database Syst Rev.* 2013 Feb 28;2:CD009611.
36. Russell G. Inhaled corticosteroid therapy in children: an assessment of the potential for side-effects. *Thorax.* 1994;49:1185–1188.
37. Bartholow AK, Deshaies DM, Skoner JM, Skoner DP. A critical review of the effects of inhaled corticosteroids on growth. *Allergy Asthma Proc.* 2013;34:391–407.
38. Chauhan BF, Ducharme FM. Addition to inhaled corticosteroids of long-acting beta2-agonists versus anti-leukotrienes for chronic asthma. *Cochrane Database Syst Rev.* 2014;1:CD003137.
39. Yates DH, Sussman HS, Shaw MJ, et al. Regular formoterol treatment in mild asthma. Effect of bronchial responsiveness during and after treatment. *Am J Respir Crit Care Med.* 1995;152:1170–1174.
40. Clark CE, Ferguson AD, Siddorn JA. Respiratory arrests in young asthmatics on salmeterol. *Respir Med.* 1993;87:227–228.
41. Castle W, Fuller R, Hall J, et al. Serevent nationwide surveillance study: comparison of salmeterol with salbutamol in asthmatic patients who require bronchodilator treatment. *BMJ.* 1993;306: 1034–1037.
42. Mann RD, Kubota K, Pearce G, et al. Salmeterol: a study by prescription-event monitoring in a UK cohort of 15,407 patients. *J Clin Epidemiol.* 1996;49:247–250.
43. Weinberger M, Hendeles L. Theophylline in asthma. *N Engl J Med.* 1996;334:1380–1388.
44. Hendeles L, Harman E, Huang D, et al. Theophylline attenuation of airway responses to allergen: comparison with cromolyn metered-dose inhaler. *J Allergy Clin Immunol.* 1995;95:505–514.
45. Kidney J, Dominguez M, Taylor PM, et al. Immunodilation by theophylline in asthma. *Am J Respir Crit Care Med.* 1995;151: 1907–1914.
46. Malmstrom K, Rodriguez-Gomez G, Guerra J, et al. Oral montelukast, inhaled beclomethasone, and placebo for chronic asthma. A randomized, controlled trial. Montelukast/Beclomethasone Study Group. *Arch Intern Med.* 1999;130:487–495.
47. Matsuse H, Kohno S. Leukotriene receptor antagonists pranlukast and montelukast for treating asthma. *Expert Opin Pharmacother.* 2014;15:353–363.
48. FitzGerald JM, Grunfeld A, Pare PD, et al. The clinical efficacy of combination nebulized anticholinergic and adrenergic bronchodilators vs nebulized adrenergic bronchodilator alone in acute asthma. Canadian Combivent Study Group. *Chest.* 1997;111:311–315.
49. Lanes SF, Garrett JE, Wentworth CE, et al. The effect of adding ipratropium bromide to salbutamol in the treatment of acute asthma: a pooled analysis of three trials. *Chest.* 1998;114:365–372.
50. Craven D, Kercsmar CM, Myers TR, et al. Ipratropium bromide plus nebulized albuterol for the treatment of hospitalized children with acute asthma. *J Pediatr.* 2001;138:51–58.
51. Qureshi F, Pestian J, Davis P, et al. Effect of nebulized ipratropium on the hospitalization rates of children with asthma. *N Engl J Med.* 1998;339:1030–1035.
52. Connett GJ, Warde C, Wooler E, et al. Prednisolone and salbutamol in the hospital treatment of acute asthma. *Arch Dis Child.* 1993;70:170–173.
53. Hess DR. Aerosol delivery devices in the treatment of asthma. *Respir Care.* 2008;53:699–725.
54. Raimondi AC, Schottlender J, Lombardi D, et al. Treatment of acute asthma with inhaled albuterol delivered via jet nebulizer, metered dose inhaler with spacer, or dry powder. *Chest.* 1997;112:24–28.
55. Kim IK, Saville AL, Sikes KL, Corcoran TE. Heliox-driven albuterol nebulization for asthma exacerbations: an overview. *Respir Care.* 2006;51:613–618.
56. Myers TR. Use of heliox in children. *Respir Care.* 2006;51:619–631.
57. Dolovich MB, Ahrens RC, Hess DR, et al. Device selection and outcomes of aerosol therapy: evidence-based guidelines. *Chest.* 2005;127:335–371.
58. Hess DR, Acosta FL, Ritz RH, et al. The effect of heliox on nebulizer function using a beta-agonist bronchodilator. *Chest.* 1999;115:184–189.
59. Hess DR, Fink JB, Venkataraman ST, et al. The history and physics of heliox. *Respir Care.* 2006;51:608–612.
60. Hoffman L, Smithline H. Comparison of Circulaire to conventional small volume nebulizer for the treatment of bronchospasm in the emergency department. *Respir Care.* 1997;42:1170–1174.
61. Hess D, Fisher D, Williams P, et al. Medication nebulizer performance. Effects of diluent volume, nebulizer flow, and nebulizer brand. *Chest.* 1996;110:498–505.
62. Rubin BK. Air and soul: the science and application of aerosol therapy. *Respir Care.* 2010;55:911–921.
63. Camargo CA Jr, Spooner CH, Rowe BH. Continuous versus intermittent beta-agonists in the treatment of acute asthma. *Cochrane Database Syst Rev.* 2003;4:CD001115.
64. Wise RA, Anzueto A, Calverley P, et al. The Tiotropium Safety and Performance in Respimat Trial (TIOSPIR), a large scale, randomized, controlled, parallel-group trial-design and rationale. *Respir Res.* 2013;14:40.
65. Newman SP. Principles of metered-dose inhaler design. *Respir Care.* 2005;50:1177–1190.
66. Barry PW, O'Callaghan C. Inhalational drug delivery from seven different spacer devices. *Thorax.* 1996;51:835–840.
67. Tobias JD. Heliox in children with airway obstruction. *Pediatr Emerg Care.* 1997;13:29–32.
68. Kudukis TM, Manthous CA, Schmidt GA, et al. Inhaled helium-oxygen revisited: effect of inhaled helium-oxygen during the treatment of status asthmaticus in children. *J Pediatr.* 1997;130:217–224.
69. Kass JE, Castriotta RJ. Heliox therapy in acute severe asthma. *Chest.* 1995;107:757–760.
70. Carter ER, Webb CR, Moffitt DR. Evaluation of heliox in children hospitalized with acute severe asthma. A randomized crossover trial. *Chest.* 1996;109:1256–1261.
71. Verbeek PR, Chopra A. Heliox does not improve FEV_1 in acute asthma patients. *J Emerg Med.* 1998;16:545–548.
72. Kass JE, Castratta RJ. Heliox therapy in acute severe asthma. *Chest.* 1995;107:757.
73. Kass JE, Terregino CA. The effect of heliox in acute severe asthma: a randomized controlled trial. *Chest.* 1999;116:296–300.
74. Ciarallo L, Sauer AH, Shannon MW. Intravenous magnesium therapy for moderate to severe pediatric asthma: results of a randomized placebo-controlled trial. *J Pediatr.* 1996;129:809–814.
75. Bloch H, Silverman R, Mancherje N, et al. Intravenous magnesium sulfate as an adjunct in the treatment of acute asthma. *Chest.* 1995;107:1576–1581.
76. Mangat HS, D'Souza GA, Jacob MS. Nebulized magnesium sulphate versus nebulized salbutamol in acute bronchial asthma: a clinical trial. *Eur Respir J.* 1998;12:341–344.
77. Hill J, Britton J. Dose-response relationship and time-course of the effect of inhaled magnesium sulphate on airflow in normal and asthmatic subjects. *Br J Clin Pharmacol.* 1995;40:539–544.
78. Gupta D, Nath A, Agarwal R, Behera D. A prospective randomized controlled trial on the efficacy of noninvasive ventilation in severe acute asthma. *Respir Care.* 2010;55:536–543.
79. Carson KV, Usmani ZA, Smith BJ. Noninvasive ventilation in acute severe asthma: current evidence and future perspectives. *Curr Opin Pulm Med.* 2014;20:118–123.
80. Pollack C, Fleisch K, Dowsey K. Treatment of acute bronchospasm with beta-adrenergic agonist aerosols delivered by a nasal bilevel positive airway pressure circuit. *Ann Emerg Med.* 1995;26:552–557.
81. Medoff BD. Invasive and noninvasive ventilation in patients with asthma. *Respir Care.* 2008;53:740–748.
82. Marquette CH, Saulnier F, Leroy O, et al. Long-term prognosis of new fatal asthma. A 6-year follow-up of 145 asthmatic patients who underwent mechanical ventilation. *Am Rev Respir Dis.* 1992;146: 76–81.

83. Leatherman J. Life-threatening asthma. *Clin Chest Med.* 1994;15: 453–479.
84. Feihl F, Perret C. Permissive hypercapnia: how permissive should we be? *Am J Respir Crit Care Med.* 1994;150:1722–1737.
85. Darioli R, Perret C. Mechanical controlled hypoventilation in status asthmaticus. *Am Rev Respir Dis.* 1984;129:385–387.
86. Ranieri VM, Grasso S, Fiore T, et al. Auto-positive end-expiratory pressure and dynamic hyperinflation. *Clin Chest Med.* 1996;17: 379–394.
87. Tuxen DV, Williams TJ, Scheinkestel CD, et al. Use of a measurement of pulmonary hyperinflation to control the level of mechanical ventilation in patient with acute severe asthma. *Am Rev Resp Dis.* 1992;146:1136–1142.
88. Caramez MP, Borges JB, Tucci MR, et al. Paradoxical responses to positive end-expiratory pressure in patients with airway obstruction during controlled ventilation. *Crit Care Med.* 2005;33:1519–1528.
89. Leatherman JW, Ravenscraft SA. Low measured auto-positive end-expiratory pressure during mechanical ventilation of patients with severe asthma: hidden auto-positive end-expiratory pressure. *Crit Care Med.* 1996;24:541–546.
90. Dhand R. Bronchodilator therapy in mechanically ventilated patients: patient selection and clinical outcomes. *Respir Care.* 2007;52:152–153.
91. Douglass JA, Tuxen DV, Horne M, et al. Myopathy in severe asthma. *Am Rev Respir Dis.* 1992;146:517–519.
92. Levy BD, Kitch B, Fanta CH. Medical and ventilatory management of status asthmaticus. *Intensive Care Med.* 1998;24:105–117.
93. Jain S, Hanania NA, Guntupalli KK. Ventilation of patients with asthma and obstructive lung disease. *Crit Care Clin.* 1998;14:685–705.
94. Wade S, Weil C, Holden G, et al. Psychosocial characteristics of inner-city children with asthma: a description of the NCICAS psychosocial protocol. National Cooperative Inner-City Asthma Study. *Pediatr Pulmonol.* 1997;24:263–276.
95. Wade SL, Islam S, Holden G, et al. Division of responsibility for asthma management tasks between caregivers and children in the inner city. *Dev Behav Pediatr.* 1999;20:93–98.

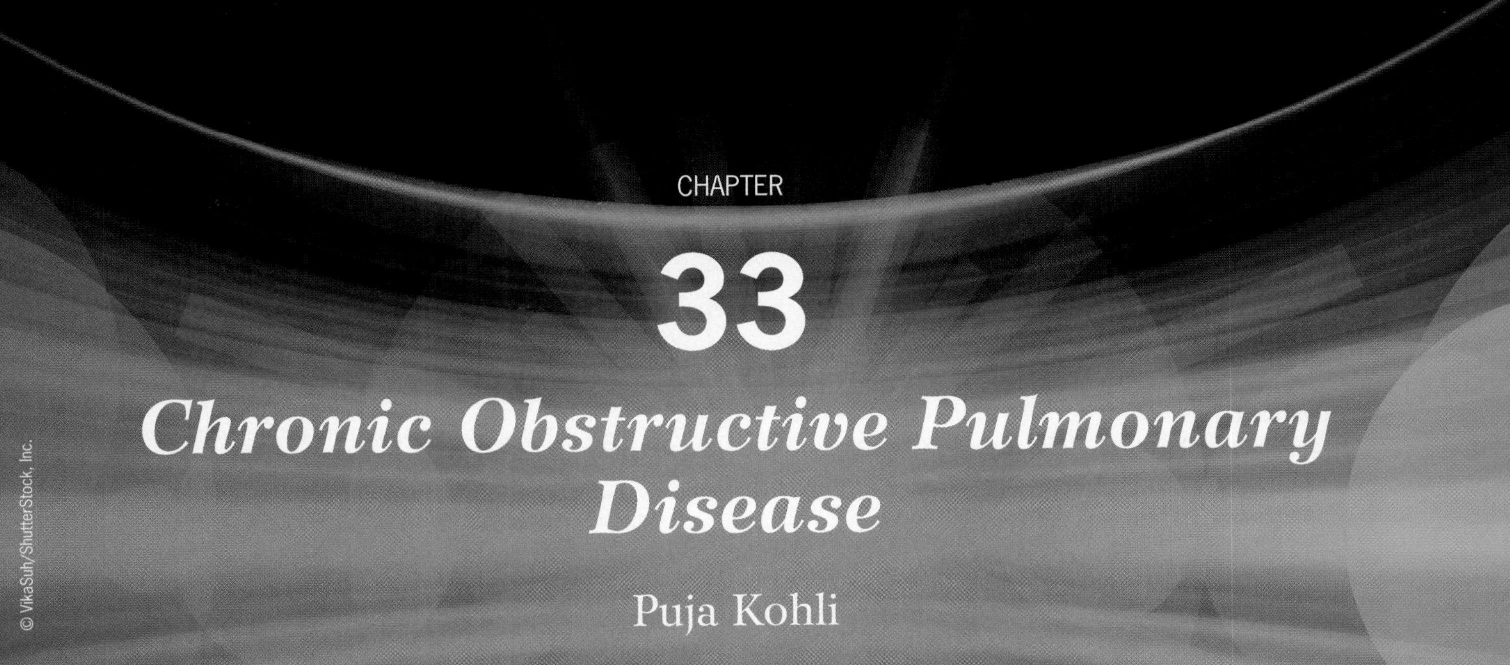

CHAPTER

33

Chronic Obstructive Pulmonary Disease

Puja Kohli

OUTLINE

OBJECTIVES

1. Define chronic obstructive pulmonary disease (COPD).
2. Describe the epidemiology, pathogenesis, and pathophysiology of COPD.
3. Compare therapeutic strategies for stable patients and patients experiencing an exacerbation in the ambulatory or inpatient setting.
4. Discuss the surgical approaches to improve lung function in COPD.
5. Identify important aspects of palliative and end-of-life care for patients with COPD.

KEY TERMS

air trapping
alpha$_1$-antitrypsin (AAT) deficiency
antibiotic
anticholinergic agent
bullae
bullectomy
chronic bronchitis
chronic obstructive pulmonary disease (COPD)
corticosteroid
dynamic airway compression
dynamic hyperinflation
dyspnea
elastic recoil
emphysema
exacerbation
hyperinflation
intrinsic positive end-expiratory pressure (auto-PEEP)
long-acting β_2-agonist
long-acting muscarinic antagonist (LAMA)
long-term oxygen therapy (LTOT)
lung transplantation
lung volume reduction surgery (LVRS)
methylxanthine
mucokinetic agent
noninvasive positive pressure ventilation (NIV)
pulmonary rehabilitation
short-acting β_2-agonist
sleep apnea hypopnea syndrome (SAHS)
smoking cessation

Introduction

Chronic obstructive pulmonary disease (COPD) has emerged as a major health condition worldwide, with 80 million people affected. In the United States, more than 12 million people carry a diagnosis of COPD and an equal number have the disease but have not yet been diagnosed.[1] This chapter provides a general discussion of the diagnosis and care of patients with COPD, with an emphasis on practical elements of management. It centers on the premise that respiratory therapists have the needed expertise to intercede at all stages of COPD to improve patients' functional status, quality of life, and the outcome of their disease.

Burden of Chronic Obstructive Pulmonary Disease

In both the United States and in the world, COPD is the third most common cause of death and will continue to increase in prevalence worldwide over the coming years.[2] The estimated prevalence of COPD varies from 7% to 19% in epidemiologic studies. In 2010, the direct and indirect costs of COPD in the United States amounted to $50 billion.[1] Unfortunately, COPD remains underdiagnosed in the United States.

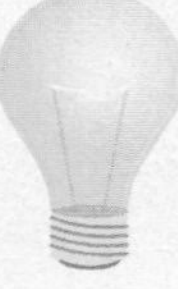

STOP AND THINK

You are explaining COPD to a member of your family. What would you say is the major risk factor for developing this disease?

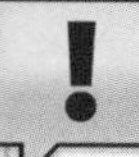

Respiratory Recap

Definition of COPD

- *COPD* refers to a group of preventable and treatable disorders characterized by progressive airflow limitation that is not fully reversible by bronchodilator or anti-inflammatory therapy.
- The term *chronic bronchitis* is less preferred because it incorrectly limits its focus to inflammatory changes observed in pathologic examinations of central airways (bronchi).
- Some degree of emphysema occurs in nearly all patients with COPD.
- Expiratory airflow limitation is defined by an FEV_1/FVC less than 0.70.

Many patients with long-term respiratory symptoms due to COPD first receive a diagnosis when they have far-advanced disease.

Regardless of the stage of the disease, COPD has important effects on health status. Early symptomatic disease decreases exercise capacity, causes work absenteeism, and interferes with vigorous lifestyle pursuits. More advanced COPD increases the risk of pneumonia, heart disease, metabolic syndrome, and lung cancer.[3] The association of COPD with dysfunction of body systems and organs other than the lung has reclassified COPD from a disorder of the lungs to a chronic condition characterized by systemic inflammation and degenerative effects on multiple organs that adversely affect the entire patient. Patients with severe COPD suffer from major limitations in activities of daily living and may experience progressive cachexia. Because of the chronic nature of COPD and its typically relentless progression, few conditions present such long-term and disabling burdens for personal health and well-being.

Definitions and Staging of Disease

The term *chronic obstructive pulmonary disease (COPD)* refers to a group of preventable and treatable disorders characterized by progressive airflow limitation that is not fully reversible by bronchodilator or anti-inflammatory therapy.[4] Airflow limitation is associated with an abnormal inflammatory response of the lungs to noxious particles or gases, especially cigarette smoking.[4] COPD also produces systemic inflammation and important nonpulmonary consequences, such as cachexia, skeletal muscle dysfunction, cardiovascular disease, osteoporosis, depression, fatigue, and cancer. The airflow limitation is caused by a combination of destruction of lung parenchyma (emphysema) and small airways disease (obstructive bronchiolitis), with the relative proportions of each varying in individual patients.[4] Other specific causes of chronic airflow limitation, such as cystic fibrosis, asthma, bronchiolitis obliterans, and bronchiectasis, are not categorized as types of COPD.

The broad term *airway disease* is used to define the pathologic and physiologic abnormalities observed in airways of patients with COPD because these changes occur both in central (bronchi) and small airways (bronchioles). The historical categorical term **chronic bronchitis** is less preferred because it incorrectly limits its focus to inflammatory changes observed in pathologic examinations of central airways (bronchi). *Chronic bronchitis* presents additional confusion because it defines a clinical condition wherein patients have a productive cough for at least 3 months of the year for 2 or more successive years. Some patients with chronic bronchitis diagnosed clinically might not have spirometric evidence of airflow obstruction and therefore do not fulfill the definition of COPD. The newer terminology of *airway disease* recognizes that mucus hypersecretion occurs in the proximal airways, but that the site of increased airway resistance in COPD is in the peripheral, small airways, where inflammation results in fibrosis and airway distortion.[5] The specific causative factors of airflow limitation in peripheral airways, however, have not been clearly defined, as indicated by the poor correlation between pathologic changes observed in the bronchioles and the degree of measured airflow limitation.

Some degree of **emphysema** occurs in nearly all patients with COPD, although the extent of emphysema observed varies widely between patients. *Emphysema* is a pathologic and not a clinical term. Emphysema is detected by histopathologic examination of lung tissue or by imaging studies, such as high-resolution computed tomography (HRCT), that can detect emphysema-related pathologic changes.[6] It has been defined by an expert panel as "a condition characterized by abnormal enlargement of the airspaces distal to the terminal bronchiole, accompanied by destruction of their walls, and without obvious fibrosis"[7] (**Figure 33-1**). This irreversible airspace enlargement occurs in the alveolar, alveolar duct, and respiratory bronchiolar regions of the lung where gas exchange occurs. Structural abnormalities in these regions cause uneven distribution of ventilation and hypoxemia, hypercapnia, and decreased lung diffusion as measured by the diffusing capacity for carbon monoxide (DLCO).

Airspace enlargements larger than 1 cm in diameter are termed **bullae** (**Figure 33-2**). Bullae can progressively enlarge and compress adjacent lung tissue,

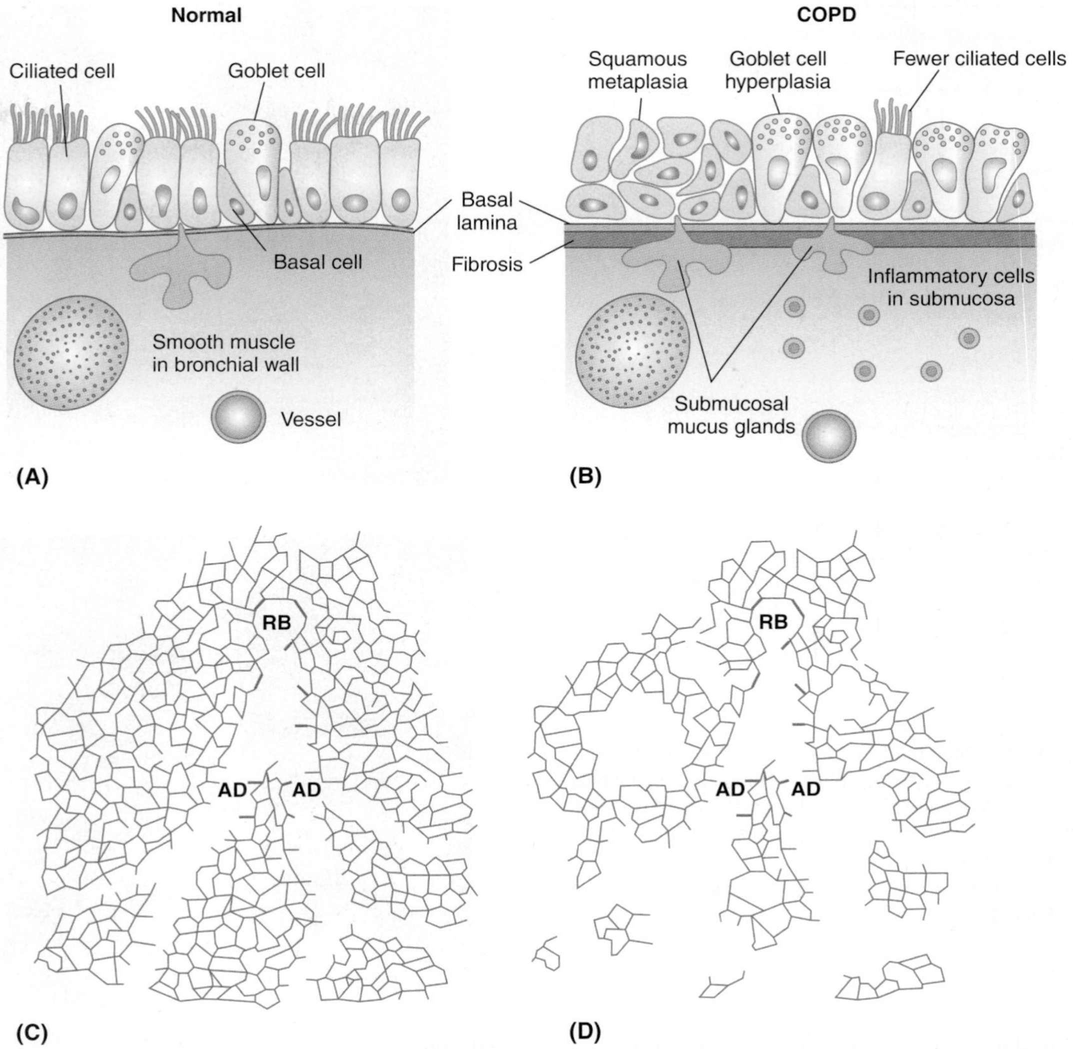

FIGURE 33-1 Schematic models showing the airways and lung parenchyma of normal individuals (**A** and **C**) and patients with COPD (**B** and **D**). Airways in COPD patients are characterized by hyperplasia of surface mucous cells, enlargement of tracheobronchial submucosal glands, excess mucus, loss of cilia and ciliary dyskinesia, and the presence of inflammatory cells. Compared with patients with normal lungs (C), patients with COPD have permanently enlarged airspaces distal to terminal bronchioles caused by alveolar wall destruction (D).

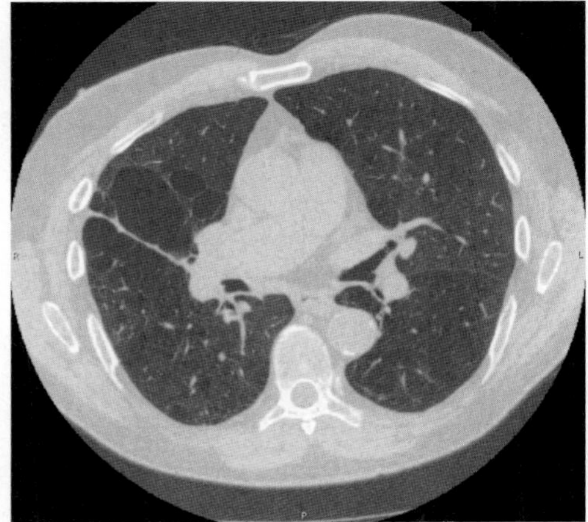

FIGURE 33-2 Computed tomography scan of a patient with severe emphysema. Note the multiple bullae throughout the lung parenchyma, which appears hyperlucent, indicating generalized loss of lung tissue and hyperinflation.

further impairing respiratory function. Emphysema contributes to airflow limitation by decreasing lung elastic recoil. During exhalation, positive intrathoracic pressure compresses airways that are no longer tethered open by surrounding normal lung tissue. This process is termed **dynamic airway compression**, which results in **air trapping** and **hyperinflation** (**Figure 33-3**). Hyperinflation with increased lung volumes may be apparent on chest radiographs (**Figure 33-4**) and chest computed tomography (CT) scans.

Limitation of maximal expiratory flow rate represents the cardinal abnormality associated with COPD and serves both to diagnose the presence of the disease and stage its severity. Simple spirometric measures of postbronchodilator forced expiratory volume in the first second of expiration (FEV_1) and the ratio of FEV_1 to forced vital capacity (FEV_1/FVC) provide the best measures of expiratory airflow limitation, with airflow

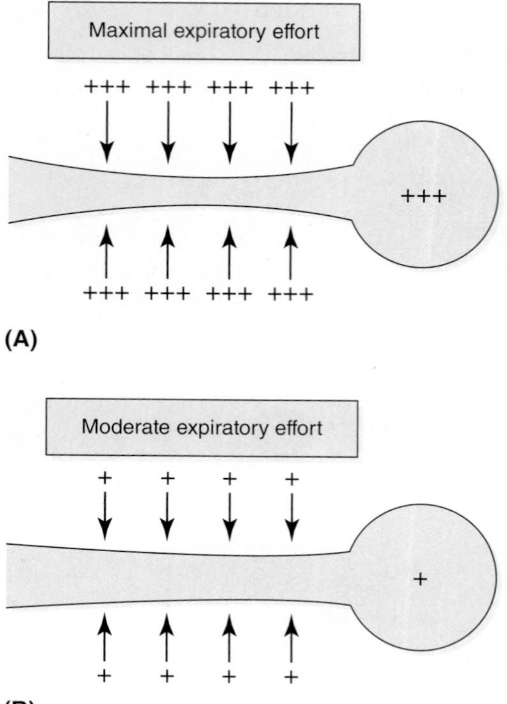

FIGURE 33-3 Schematic model demonstrating the morphologic changes associated with dynamic airway compression in patients with COPD. The loss of parenchymal tethering external to airways causes airway collapse during forced expiration. Maximal expiratory effort (**A**) creates more compressing pressure around airways and produces more dynamic compression as compared with moderate expiratory effort (**B**).

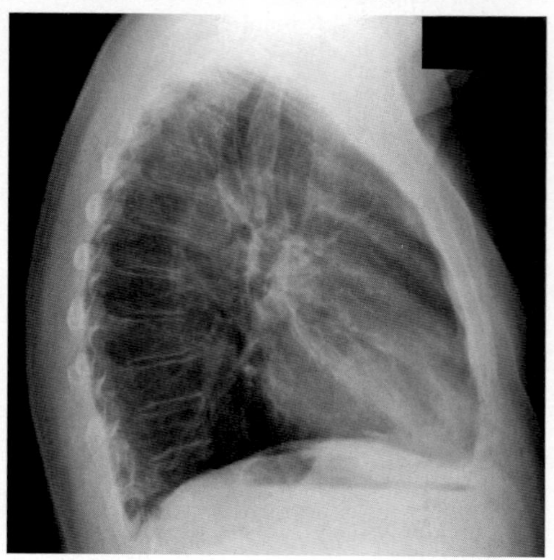

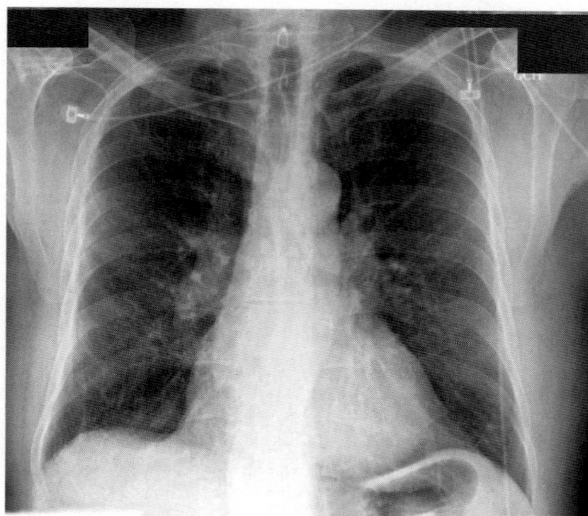

FIGURE 33-4 Chest radiograph of a patient with emphysema showing hyperinflation as evidenced by the flattening of the diaphragm, best observed on the lateral view, and hyperlucent lung fields.

obstruction defined by an FEV_1/FVC less than 0.70,[4] which is an abnormal finding in nearly all age groups. This FEV_1/FVC threshold, however, may overdiagnose COPD in elderly subjects because of the normally observed decrease in lung volumes and airflows with aging. The clinical practice guidelines of the Global Alliance for Chronic Obstructive Pulmonary Disease (GOLD) use spirometric values to classify the severity of COPD into four stages (**Table 33-1**).[4]

Spirometric values of FEV_1 and FVC alone, however, do not correlate well with severity of dyspnea and functional performance, survival, or response to therapy. Because hyperinflation has important effects on lung function, lung volume measurements, such as the ratio of the inspiratory capacity to the total lung capacity, are better predictors of survival than FEV_1. It has recently been recognized that the systemic nonpulmonary manifestations of COPD have important effects on prognosis. Multidimensional measures of dyspnea, body mass, and functional levels, which capture effects of these systemic manifestations, predict survival and response to therapy more accurately than FEV_1. The BODE index (body mass index, airflow obstruction, dyspnea, and exercise capacity) provides clinicians with

TABLE 33-1
Spirometric Classification of COPD Severity Based on Postbronchodilator FEV_1

Stage I: Mild	$FEV_1/FVC < 0.70$ $FEV_1 \geq 80\%$ predicted
Stage II: Moderate	$FEV_1/FVC < 0.70$ $50\% \leq FEV_1 < 80\%$ predicted
Stage III: Severe	$FEV_1/FVC < 0.70$ $30\% \leq FEV_1 < 50\%$ predicted
Stage IV: Very severe	$FEV_1/FVC < 0.70$ $FEV_1 < 30\%$ predicted *or* $FEV_1 < 50\%$ predicted plus chronic respiratory failure

FEV_1, forced expiratory volume in 1 second; FVC, forced vital capacity. Respiratory failure is defined as a Pao_2 less than 60 mm Hg with or without a $Paco_2$ greater than 50 mm Hg while breathing air at sea level.

TABLE 33-2
BODE Index

Variable	Points on BODE Index			
	0	1	2	3
FEV_1 (% predicted)	>65	50–64	36–49	≤35
Distance walked in 6 minutes (m)	>350	250–349	150–249	≤149
mMRC dyspnea scale*	0–1	2	3	4
Body mass index	>21	<21		

The total possible values range from 0 to 10. FEV_1, forced expiratory volume in 1 second.

*Scores on the Modified Medical Research Council (mMRC) dyspnea scale can range from 0 to 4, with a score of 4 indicating that the patient is too breathless to leave the house or becomes breathless when dressing or undressing.

a multidimensional measure of disease severity, prognosis, and response to therapy (**Table 33-2**).[8] Some clinicians now combine the BODE index with spirometry to stage COPD (**Table 33-3**). Similarly, in 2011, new GOLD criteria for the combined assessment of COPD were formulated in an effort to improve the management of COPD (**Table 33-4**).[4]

When assessing risk, choose the highest risk according to GOLD group or exacerbation history. One or more hospitalizations for COPD exacerbations should be considered high risk. Symptom burden is measured by the mMRC, Modified Medical Research Council questionnaire or the COPD Assessment Test (CAT).

Etiology of Chronic Obstructive Pulmonary Disease

Epidemiologic and experimental evidence demonstrates that smoking is the major cause of COPD. Nonsmokers, however, may also develop COPD when exposed to other risk factors,[9] which include passive exposure to cigarette smoke and nontobacco inhalational factors such as occupational dusts and chemicals and both indoor and outdoor air pollution.

Because not all smokers develop clinically apparent COPD, genetic factors must modify risk from tobacco inhalation. The best characterized genetic risk factor for COPD is **alpha$_1$-antitrypsin (AAT) deficiency**.

TABLE 33-3
Classification of COPD Severity Based on BODE Index and Spirometry

At risk	FEV_1/FVC <0.70 FEV_1 ≥80% predicted
Mild	FEV_1/FVC <0.70 FEV_1 <80% predicted BODE index 0–2
Moderate	FEV_1/FVC <0.70 FEV_1 <80% predicted BODE index 3–4
Severe	FEV_1/FVC <0.70 FEV_1 <80% predicted BODE Index 5–6
Very severe	FEV_1/FVC <0.70 FEV_1 <80% predicted BODE index 7–10

FEV_1, forced expiratory volume in 1 second; FVC, forced vital capacity; BODE, body mass index, airflow obstruction, dyspnea, and exercise capacity.

Modified with permission from Celli BR. Update on the management of COPD. *Chest.* 2008;133:1451–1462, with permission from the American College of Chest Physicians.

TABLE 33-4
Combined Assessment of COPD Using GOLD Criteria

Group A: Low Risk, Low Symptom Burden	FEV_1/FVC <0.70 Low symptom burden (mMRC of 0–1 OR CAT score <10) *AND* FEV_1 of 50% or greater (old GOLD 1–2) *AND* low exacerbation rate (0–1/year)
Group B: Low Risk, Higher Symptom Burden	FEV_1/FVC <0.70 Higher symptom burden (mMRC of ≥2 *OR* CAT of ≥10) *AND* FEV_1 of 50% or greater (old GOLD 1–2) *AND* low exacerbation rate (0–1/year)
Group C: High Risk, Low Symptom Burden	FEV_1/FVC <0.70 Low symptom burden (mMRC of 0–1 *OR* CAT score <10) *AND* FEV_1 <50% (old GOLD 3–4) *AND/OR* high exacerbation rate (≥2/year)
Group D: High Risk, Higher Symptom Burden	FEV_1/FVC <0.70 Higher symptom burden (mMRC of 2 or more *OR* CAT of ≥10) *AND* FEV_1 <50% (old GOLD 3–4) *AND/OR* high exacerbation rate (≥2/year)

This condition is a hereditary defect that occurs almost entirely in Caucasians and results from abnormal function or insufficient production of AAT.[10] Patients with AAT deficiency demonstrate an abnormal antiprotease response to proinflammatory effects of tobacco smoke. The resultant activation of proteases and toxic oxygen metabolites results in accelerated lung destruction and emphysema in early life. Individuals with AAT may remain healthy throughout their lives, but even nonsmokers with AAT deficiency may develop COPD symptoms, usually late in life. The most common abnormal gene for AAT is the Z allele. Normal genes are labeled M. The most common genotype associated with AAT is ZZ (also referred to as PiZ). There are about 100,000 people with the ZZ phenotype in the United States.

Males and females have an equivalent prevalence of COPD, although some studies suggest a greater risk of COPD among women smokers.[11] Prevalence of COPD is greater in smokers with lower socioeconomic status,[12] but this observation may result from associated differences in living conditions, exposure to environmental toxins, or smoking behaviors. Various occupational dusts, including coal and grain dusts; air pollution; indoor air pollution caused by cooking fuels or cigarette smoke; and childhood respiratory infections are additional risk factors for the development of COPD.

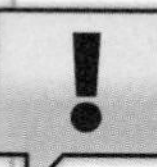

Respiratory Recap

Pathophysiology of COPD

- Most of the increase in airways resistance occurs in peripheral airways.
- Loss of pulmonary elasticity is due to destruction of alveolar structures.
- Decreased diameter of airways lowers the maximum expiratory airflow at all lung volumes.
- Flow limitation results in dynamic hyperinflation.
- Lung volume is more closely associated with dyspnea and functional limitation than spirometry.

Pathophysiology of Chronic Obstructive Pulmonary Disease

Recognition of the pathogenetic importance of impaired antiprotease defenses in AAT deficiency led to the protease–antiprotease theory for the etiology of smoking-related COPD. In this model, smoking and other noxious inhalants overwhelm the lungs' antioxidant and antiprotease defense mechanisms, allowing proteolytic digestion of lung tissue. Recently, different COPD-like phenotypes have been generated in animal models by targeting the immune system or causing disturbances of apoptotic control in pulmonary endothelium.[13] These observations have expanded the pathophysiologic understanding of COPD beyond protease–antiprotease mechanisms to include multiple immunogenetic disturbances that can combine in varying ways to produce unique COPD phenotypes in different patients. The convergence of these different mechanisms may explain why the COPD population has diverse clinical expressions.

The cardinal structural abnormalities that produce respiratory symptoms and functional limitations in COPD occur in the central and peripheral airways and the lung parenchyma. The central airways are the site of most of the increased mucus production in patients who raise excess sputum and carry the clinical diagnosis of chronic bronchitis. Mucous glands below the epithelial basement membrane in central airways secrete mucus that serves in health as a mechanical host defense mechanism against environmental particulate inhalants. Some, but not all, patients with COPD have moderate enlargement of mucous glands,[14] which correlates directly with cough and sputum production. Mucus-secreting goblet cells are nested among epithelial cells along all segments of the conducting airways. Descriptive studies suggest that goblet cells may expand in number in the central airways of patients with COPD and contribute to excess mucus production. Ciliary dyskinesia, loss of cilia, and epithelial metaplasia has also been observed in central airways (refer to Figure 33-1). Inflammation is present in the form of neutrophils, macrophages, and lymphocytes within the epithelium and submucosa of central airways and neutrophils and eosinophils within airway secretions.[15] Eosinophils are found in the airway submucosa during exacerbations of COPD. Nodules rich in both T and B cells develop in regions of abnormal lung tissue, lending support to an immunogenic etiology to COPD.[16] Altered T- and B-cell responses are also observed in the peripheral blood, indicating the systemic nature of the disease and the presence of immunodysregulation in nonpulmonary organs.[17]

In normal lungs, most of the resistance to airflow occurs in peripheral small airways. In COPD, most of the increase in airways resistance similarly occurs in peripheral airways, where multiple pathologic changes occur. Early in the course of COPD, brown-pigmented macrophages aggregate in respiratory bronchioles. As COPD progresses, a low-grade inflammatory response develops in membranous bronchioles, characterized by a modest influx of neutrophils, macrophages, and lymphocytes. In some patients, smooth muscle enlargement, minimal fibrosis, squamous cell metaplasia of airway epithelial cells, and goblet cell metaplasia develop. These changes combined with abnormalities of smooth muscle and connective tissue result in a narrowed caliber of the airway lumen both from a thickening of airway walls and a decrease in cross-sectional total airway diameter.

Although these pathologic abnormalities in peripheral airways contribute to the expiratory airflow limitation observed in COPD, they do not entirely explain the increased airways resistance. Other contributory factors, such as the loss of airway tethering caused by decreased elastic recoil of the lung parenchyma, airway secretions, changes in the properties of airway lining fluid, and smooth muscle contraction, interact in complex and poorly understood ways.[18] Among these factors, loss of elastic recoil plays an important role.

The term **elastic recoil** refers to the lung's natural tendency to deflate after inspiration. It is expressed by plotting lung volume as a function of transpulmonary pressure. **Figure 33-5** shows the comparative pressure–volume curves of a normal adult and a patient with emphysema. With loss of pulmonary elasticity from destruction of alveolar and interstitial structures, the patient with emphysema has increased lung compliance, as shown by a shift of the pressure–volume curve up and to the left. Increased lung compliance results is an attenuation of the tethering effect that normal lung parenchyma has on airways to resist airway narrowing during expiration. Consequently, the airways of patients with COPD decrease in caliber and resist expiratory airflow to a greater degree than normal (refer to Figure 33-3). Consequently, dynamic airway compression occurs during expiration as patients contract expiratory muscles and increase intrathoracic pressure, which is transmitted to the external walls of conducting airways. The relationship of flow to pressure during inspiration and expiration at a given lung volume is shown in **Figure 33-6**.

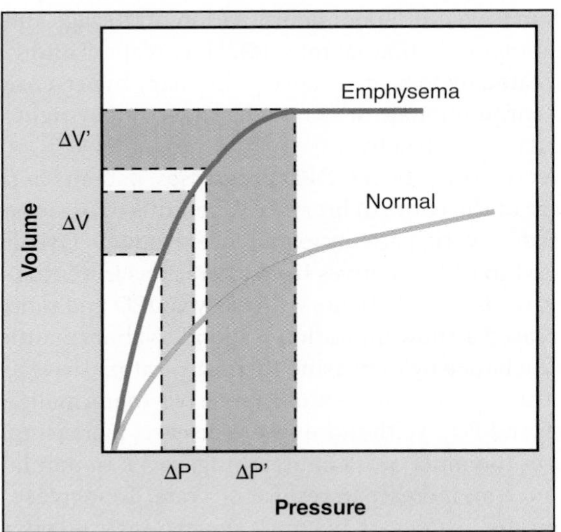

FIGURE 33-5 Volume–pressure relationships of individuals with normal lungs and patients with emphysema. Patients with emphysema experience a small increase in pressure (ΔP) with an increase in volume (ΔV) while breathing at low lung volumes. In contrast, patients with emphysema have large increases in pressure (ΔP′) for a similar change in volume (ΔV′) when breathing at high lung volumes, at which point their lungs become hyperinflated and stiff. Patients with emphysema have heterogeneous distribution of emphysema, so that normal regions of lung follow the normal volume–pressure curve and emphysematous regions follow the emphysema curve.

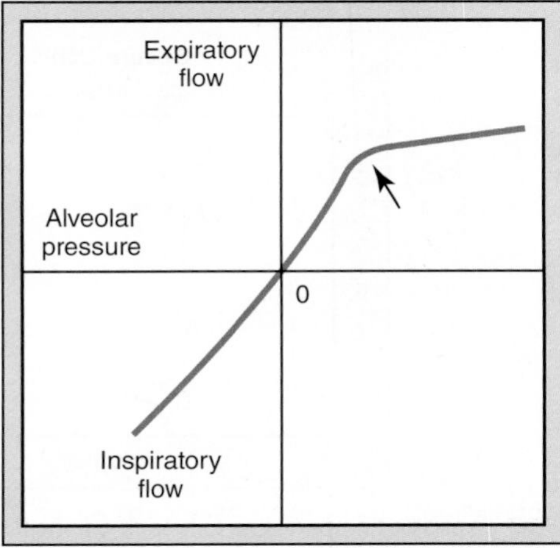

FIGURE 33-6 Relationship of flow to pressure during inspiration and expiration at a given lung volume. This relationship is linear during inspiration, but dynamic airway compression (arrow) causes expiratory flow to reach an early maximal value that does not increase with further increases in alveolar pressure.

Expiratory flow–volume curves present a visual image of these relationships (**Figure 33-7**). Individuals with normal lung function increase their expiratory airflow during forced expiratory maneuvers until dynamic airway compression occurs, at which point airflow does not increase with increased effort. During tidal breathing, expiratory airflow is much lower than during a maximal, forced expiration, indicating that patients in good health have considerable ventilatory reserve available for increasing minute ventilation ($\dot{V}_E$).

In patients with COPD, decreased diameter of conducting airways lowers the maximal expiratory airflow and airflow at all lung volumes compared with normal individuals. Because of the loss of lung elasticity and the collapsibility of airways in patients with emphysema, dynamic airway compression occurs at lower intrathoracic pressures. In patients with severe COPD, maximal airflow may be reached during minimal exercise and eventually at resting tidal breathing (refer to Figure 33-7). When maximal airflow is reached during tidal breathing, patients faced with increased ventilatory demands from exercise cannot increase airflow to recruit a larger tidal volume (V_T). To respond to exercise demands, therefore, they must increase $\dot{V}_E$ by generating higher respiratory rates. An increased respiratory rate decreases expiratory time, which promotes air trapping and increased intrathoracic pressures and further aggravates dynamic airway compression.[19]

As air trapping progresses, intra-alveolar pressure at end-expiration may remain positive rather

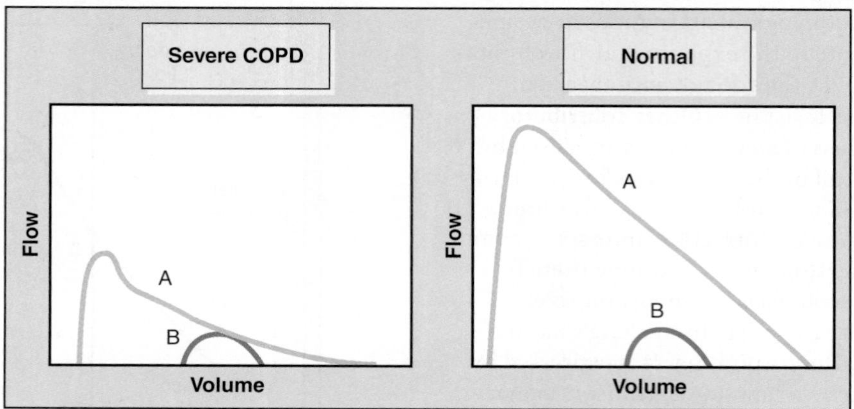

FIGURE 33-7 Expiratory flow–volume curves of a patient with severe COPD compared with an individual with normal lungs. The patient with COPD reaches maximal expiratory airflow during tidal breathing.

than equilibrating with ambient pressure as occurs in healthy patients. This condition is termed **intrinsic positive end-expiratory pressure (auto-PEEP)**. Auto-PEEP places an inspiratory threshold load that increases the work of breathing because patients must contract inspiratory muscles to negate auto-PEEP before they can create the necessary negative alveolar pressure that initiates inspiration. These changes result in patients breathing with a decreased V_T and increased respiratory rates at higher lung volumes. Higher lung volumes at end-expiration increase the inspiratory work of breathing because patients must overcome the increased elasticity of the chest wall and lungs that begin inspiration in an already expanded anatomic configuration.

Assess hyperinflation by measuring lung volumes, which demonstrate increased total lung capacity (TLC), functional residual capacity (FRC), and residual volume (RV) in patients with COPD. As FEV_1 and FVC decrease with progressive COPD, a corresponding increase in lung volumes occurs that maintains a close correlation.[20]

The severity of emphysema and airflow limitation in small airways varies between different regions of the lung. This heterogeneity causes regional variations in the distribution of ventilation, which results in mismatching of ventilation and perfusion. Although emphysematous regions of the lung are underventilated, perfusion is more severely decreased, so that ventilation-perfusion ratios ($\dot{V}/\dot{Q}$) increase. Consequently, emphysematous regions of the lung have increased dead space that causes hypoxemia and hypercapnia. In other regions of the lung, increased resistance or partial obstruction of airways that ventilate relatively normal alveolocapillary units generates decreased $\dot{V}/\dot{Q}$ ratios that cause venous admixture and hypoxemia. The combination of lung regions with high and low $\dot{V}/\dot{Q}$ alters gas exchange and places demands on the ventilatory capacity of patients, thereby increasing respiratory work.[21] Worsening $\dot{V}/\dot{Q}$ abnormalities eventually result in hypoxemia and, if ventilation is markedly impaired, hypercapnia, both of which are associated with a poor prognosis in patients with COPD. Shunts are notably absent in stable COPD, indicating the efficiency of collateral ventilation and hypoxic pulmonary vasoconstriction and the absence of complete airway obstruction.

Patients with COPD also experience abnormalities in the coordination of respiratory muscle function. During exercise and voluntary hyperventilation, patients demonstrate early fatigue of the exercising muscle groups combined with asynchrony of respiratory muscles with poor coordination of rib cage and diaphragm-abdominal muscles. Hypercapnia and untreated hypoxia can cause pulmonary hypertension and cor pulmonale, which is characterized by right ventricular hypertrophy.

As the severity of COPD progresses, patients become aware of the effort to breathe. When this effort is perceived as work, patients experience **dyspnea**. Dyspnea related to COPD derives from alterations in ventilatory mechanics. Patients with early COPD and mildly increased airflow limitation respond to abnormalities in gas exchange by increasing their respiratory drive and V_E through recruitment of a larger V_T to normalize P_{CO_2} and P_{O_2}. With more severe disease, increasing V_T causes too much work of breathing, so $\dot{V}_E$ is maintained through an increase in respiratory rate. To increase respiratory rate, patients must shorten their inspiratory time (T_I), resulting in a decreased fractional duration of inspiration (T_I/T_{TOT}) and an increased mean inspiratory flow rate (V_T/T_I).

An increased respiratory rate eventually decreases expiratory time to such a degree that airspace emptying cannot occur and further hyperinflation develops. Worsening hyperinflation shifts the pressure–volume curve of emphysematous lung units further upward and to the left, adding a restrictive pulmonary defect to the underlying airflow limitation. This produces the rapid and shallow respiratory pattern commonly observed in patients with severe COPD.

Rapid and shallow breathing places greater demands on respiratory muscles both in terms of the amount of pressure they need to generate for breathing (P_{breath}) and the proportion of the respiratory cycle during which muscle contraction is required to occur (TI/TTOT). Progressive dyspnea correlates both with increasing P_{breath} and TI/TTOT.[22] As P_{breath} approaches the maximal pressure that respiratory muscles can generate (PI_{max}), patients function near their limits of ventilatory reserve and fatigue threshold. Further demands on respiratory muscles, such as an exacerbation of COPD with increased airway resistance, can overburden compensatory mechanisms and cause acute respiratory failure.

Increasing evidence indicates that lung volumes are more closely associated with dyspnea and functional limitations of patients with advanced disease than spirometric measurements, such as FEV_1. As patients exercise, $\dot{V}E$ increases and expiratory airflow limitations produce **dynamic hyperinflation**, as expressed as the ratio of inspiratory capacity to total lung capacity. This ratio has been shown to predict survival better than FEV_1. Additionally, improvements in exercise capacity and dyspnea produced by inhaled bronchodilators, pulmonary rehabilitation, and lung volume reduction surgery are less closely associated with improvements in FEV_1 and more tightly linked to delaying dynamic hyperinflation.[23]

Diagnosis and Clinical Course

Patients who develop COPD from smoking have a prolonged initial subclinical course. Cough and eventually dyspnea with exertion represent early symptoms that patients often ascribe to expected consequences of smoking rather than an underlying lung disease. Many patients are first diagnosed when they experience an exacerbation of COPD and present with increased cough, dyspnea, and sputum production that may require hospitalization. Other patients may present with a complication of COPD and smoking, such as pneumonia. Patients may also present with an associated disorder that has an increased incidence in patients with COPD, such as cancer or heart disease.

Because early diagnosis helps patients consider smoking cessation and emerging data suggest that therapy may alter the course of the disease,[24] patients over 40 years old with respiratory symptoms (**Box 33-1**) who smoke should undergo spirometry. Once diagnosed by spirometry, patients with COPD follow a variable clinical course. Patients who continue to smoke have an accelerated decline in FEV_1 as compared with nonsmoking, age-matched individuals. Patients with moderate to severe COPD commonly experience exacerbations, each of which risks respiratory failure and a potentially irreversible decrement in lung function. Patients who have COPD with onset in the fifth decade of life or in the absence of a smoking history should be evaluated for AAT deficiency.

BOX 33-1

Symptoms That Suggest a Diagnosis of COPD

Dyspnea that progressively worsens over time, increases with exercise, persists on a daily basis, and feels to the patient like an "increased effort to breathe," "heaviness," or "gasping."

Chronic cough that may be persistent, intermittent, and/or nonproductive.

Chronic sputum production of any pattern or nature of sputum.

History of risk factors of tobacco smoke, occupational dusts or chemicals, and/or smoke from home cooking or heating fuels.

Reproduced with permission of the American Thoracic Society. Copyright © American Thoracic Society. Modified from Rabe KF, Hurd S, Anzueto A, et al. Global strategy for the diagnosis, management, and prevention of chronic obstructive pulmonary disease: GOLD executive summary. *Am J Respir Crit Care Med.* 2007;176:532–555.

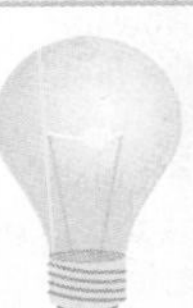

STOP AND THINK

You are assisting in the care of a patient with COPD. What are the treatment goals for this patient?

Outpatient Care of Stable Chronic Obstructive Pulmonary Disease

An integrated outpatient approach to the management of COPD provides opportunities to reduce symptoms and improve quality of life, slow the decline in lung function, prevent complications, avoid or minimize adverse effects of therapy, and prolong survival. Approaches recommended by clinical practice guidelines incorporate drug therapy, surgical interventions, rehabilitation, education, prophylactic measures, and supplemental oxygen. Chronic disease management models recommend collaborative care wherein clinicians partner with patients to ensure self-reliance and high personal esteem. Preventive care is a cornerstone of therapy that includes immunization with pneumococcal vaccine and yearly influenza vaccinations. Unfortunately, considerable gaps exist in primary care management of patients with COPD,

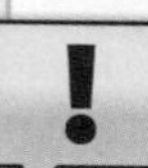

Respiratory Recap

Outpatient Care of the Patient with COPD

- Smoking cessation is indicated for all smokers.
- Encourage exercise and vaccinations for all patients with airflow limitation.
- Drug therapy is prescribed for all symptomatic patients; additional drugs are added as airflow limitation and functional impairment worsen.
- Long-term oxygen therapy improves survival.
- NIV improves outcomes for exacerbations; the benefit of chronic intermittent use in stable patients is uncertain.
- Sleep-disordered breathing should be considered.
- Pulmonary rehabilitation is beneficial.
- Evaluate patients with advanced disease and functional limitations for surgical options.

BOX 33-2

Health Benefits of Quitting Smoking

Longer Life

Decreased risk for lung cancer and other types of cancer, heart attack, and stroke
Reduction in risk for cardiac events
Improved circulation
Chronic cough improves
Lung function improves within 3 months
Dyspnea improves within 1 to 9 months
Improved sense of smell and taste
Improved functional abilities such as walking and climbing stairs

with many patients being both underdiagnosed and undermanaged.

Goals of treatment center on preventing deterioration of lung function, enhancing quality of life by diminishing symptoms, managing complications, and prolonging meaningful life. Survival benefits have been demonstrated for smoking cessation,[25] long-term oxygen therapy for hypoxic patients,[26] lung volume reduction surgery for patients with upper lobe emphysema and poor exercise capacity,[27] and **noninvasive positive pressure ventilation (NIV)** during episodes of exacerbations with acute respiratory failure.[28] Drug therapy improves symptoms of cough and dyspnea and lowers the risk of exacerbations. Other therapies, such as lung transplantation and pulmonary rehabilitation, improve functional levels, symptoms, and quality of life for patients with advanced COPD.[29]

Smoking Cessation

Smoking cessation is the only healthcare intervention clearly shown to slow the accelerated annual decline of FEV_1 experienced by patients with COPD. Although most smokers want to quit smoking, they face multiple barriers, which include the lack of training in smoking cessation self-reported by physicians. Respiratory therapists and other caregivers can assist patients in stopping smoking by addressing the issue, providing brief advice, and guiding patients toward smoking cessation resources. Brief interventions during hospitalization, however, have negligible effects.[30] Referral to counseling programs represents an effective tobacco use treatment strategy.[31] While delivering respiratory care to hospitalized patients, respiratory therapists and others should discuss the health benefits that smoking cessation can provide at any patient age (**Box 33-2**). Five-step interventions for promoting smoking cessation are shown in **Table 33-5** and **Box 33-3**.[32] The American College of Physicians has published a review of smoking cessation interventions that provides caregivers with information to guide patients toward available resources.

Combining pharmacotherapy with behavioral therapy and other interventions increases success rates for patients motivated to stop smoking (**Box 33-4**).

TABLE 33-5
Five As for Patients Willing to Quit Smoking

Ask about tobacco use	Identify and document tobacco use status for every patient at every visit.
Advise to quit	In a clear, strong, and personalized manner, urge every tobacco user to quit.
Assess willingness to make a quit attempt	Is the tobacco user willing to make a quit attempt at this time?
Assist in quit attempt	For the patient willing to make a quit attempt, offer medication and provide or refer for counseling or additional treatment to help the patient quit. For patients unwilling to quit at the time, provide interventions designed to increase future quit attempts.
Arrange follow-up	For the patient willing to make a quit attempt, arrange for follow-up contacts, beginning within the first week after the quit date. For patients unwilling to make a quit attempt at the time, address tobacco dependence and willingness to quit at next clinic visit.

BOX 33-3

Five Rs to Motivate Patients Unwilling to Quit Smoking

Encourage patient to think of the **relevance** of quitting smoking to their lives.
Assist patients in identifying the **risks** of smoking.
Assist the patient in identifying **rewards** of smoking cessation.
Discuss with patient **roadblocks** or barriers to attempting cessation.
Repeat the motivational intervention at all visits.

Nicotine replacement therapy reduces symptoms related to nicotine withdrawal and produces smoking cessation rates of 17% at 6 months as compared with 10% among control groups.[32] Only limited data support combination nicotine replacement therapy as being superior to a single route of nicotine replacement.[33] Other than cost, no differences exist in efficacy between the different forms of nicotine replacement therapy. Bupropion reduces cravings for cigarettes through unknown mechanisms. Insufficient comparative data with nicotine replacement therapy exist, but one study reported a doubling of quit rates at 1 year as compared with the nicotine patch.[34] Varenicline reduces cravings for cigarettes by binding to a nicotine receptor associated with the relaxing effects felt by smoking. Clinical trials of varenicline as compared with placebo or bupropion demonstrated higher abstinence rates for varenicline.[35] Limited evidence of efficacy exists for clonidine, nortriptyline, naltrexone, alprazolam, silver acetate, mecamylamine, and lobeline, and these agents are not FDA approved for smoking cessation. Clonidine and nortriptyline are recommended as second-line therapy for patients who fail first-line therapy or have contraindications to first-line drugs.

BOX 33-4

Pharmacologic Interventions to Assist Smoking Cessation

Nicotine Replacement Therapy

Gum: Increases cessation rates about 1.5 to 2 times control at 6 months
24-hour patch: Increases cessation rates about 1.5 to 2 times control at 6 months
Nasal sprays: Increase cessation rates about 1.5 to 2 times control at 6 months
Inhaler: Increases cessation rates about 1.5 to 2 times control at 6 months
Lozenges: Increase cessation rates about 1.5 to 2 times control at 6 months

Bupropion

Oral sustained-release formulation: Increases cessation rates about 2 times control at 1 year

Varenicline

Oral tablet: Increases cessation rates over 3.5 times control and almost 2 times bupropion at 12 weeks

Drug Therapy

Symptomatic patients with COPD benefit from pharmacologic therapy. Oral and inhaled medications are directed toward relieving symptoms, improving functional capacity and quality of life, decreasing hyperinflation, and preventing or reversing exacerbations and worsening of lung function. The modern approach to pharmacotherapy in COPD initiates drug therapy in a stepwise manner based on the severity of the disease and the efficacy of different drugs on various outcomes (**Box 33-5**). Mild disease (GOLD group A) with intermittent symptoms responds to occasional use of short-acting bronchodilators, either a short-acting β_2-agonist (SABA), a short-acting muscarinic agent (an anticholinergic, such as ipratropium), or both. Maintenance

BOX 33-5

Drug Therapy for COPD

First step: Short-acting β_2-agonists, short-acting muscarinic antagonist (anticholinergic), or both in combination as needed for symptoms.
Second step: Add long-acting β_2-agonists or long-acting muscarinic antagonist.
Third step: Use a combination of long-acting β_2-agonists and long-acting anticholinergics.
Fourth step: Add inhaled corticosteroids to the combination of long-acting β_2-agonists and long-acting muscarinic antagonist.
Fifth step: Consider adding theophylline to combination inhaled therapies.
Antibiotics: Use during exacerbations. Patients with coexisting bronchiectasis benefit from chronic or seasonal use of antibiotics to prevent exacerbations.
Systemic corticosteroids: Use only during exacerbations, for 7 to 10 days.

bronchodilator therapy with long-acting agents can be used for patients with moderate disease (GOLD group B), poorly controlled symptoms, or for those who rely on rescue therapy with more than one aerosol canister a month. Available long-acting agents include a once-daily **long-acting muscarinic antagonist (LAMA)** or twice-daily long-acting β_2-agonist (LABA). Evidence suggests that combining drugs from different classes (β_2-agonists, muscarinic antagonists, inhaled corticosteroids) has additive beneficial effects.[4,36]

These recommendations are based on observations that 80% of stable patients with COPD experience improved measured airflow with bronchodilator therapy,[1] and a larger proportion have improved symptoms and exercise capacity even in the absence of measured improvements in airflow due to mechanisms such as decreased air trapping.[22] The inhaled route with a metered dose inhaler (MDI), dry powder inhaler (DPI), or nebulizer is the preferred mode. Effectiveness of therapy is highly dependent on the ability of patients to use MDI or DPI aerosol devices correctly. Because long-acting inhaled bronchodilators are preferred over short-acting agents for maintenance therapy, patients who cannot coordinate use of portable devices may benefit from once-a-day or twice-a-day therapy with a home nebulizer.

Inhaled β_2-agonist drugs promote airway smooth muscle relaxation by stimulating airway β_2-receptors and increasing intracellular cyclic adenosine monophosphate. They also promote mucociliary clearance, inhibit cholinergic neurotransmission, and limit inflammatory mediator release from mast cells and basophils, although the clinical importance of these effects is uncertain.[37] Inhaled β_2-agonists are preferred over oral tablet forms because of a lower incidence of systemic adverse effects. Although these drugs bind preferentially to β_2-receptors, they have minimal binding to β_1-receptors in the heart and can produce hypertension, tachycardia, and other cardiac symptoms in some patients. Rarely, paradoxical bronchospasm has been reported with both oral and inhalational formulations of β_2-agonists.

Short-acting β_2-agonists have a peak bronchodilatory effect within 5 to 15 minutes and abate within 4 to 6 hours. Albuterol is the most commonly used SABA in the United States and comes in an MDI, as a solution for nebulization, and in pill and syrup formulations. The MDI is dosed with two puffs four times a day for management of intermittent symptoms in patients with mild COPD.[4] Levalbuterol is the R-enantiomer of albuterol, which has not been shown to have advantages as compared with albuterol, which comprises both the R- and S-enantiomers in a racemic form. SABAs have been shown to provide temporary improvements in FEV_1, lung volumes, dyspnea, and exercise endurance in COPD.[38] Other SABAs include pirbuterol and terbutaline. Frequent and regular use is discouraged because SABAs can down regulate β_2-receptors, causing tachyphylaxis.

Long-acting β_2-agonists are recommended as twice-a-day maintenance therapy for patients with persistent symptoms and moderate to very severe COPD.[4,39] The available drugs are salmeterol, formoterol, and arformoterol. Salmeterol and formoterol have been shown to temporarily improve FEV_1, decrease lung volumes, improve dyspnea, decrease adverse events, and improve quality of life.[38] One study demonstrated that salmeterol with or without an inhaled corticosteroid slows the annual decline of FEV_1 in patients with COPD.[24] Salmeterol binds to lipophilic β_2-agonist sites and has a time to onset of effect of 30 to 60 minutes and a duration of effect up to 12 hours. Formoterol binds both to amphiphilic and lipophilic receptor sites and has a rapid onset of action of 5 to 15 minutes and duration of 12 hours. Salmeterol and formoterol are available as a DPI formulation. Formoterol and arformoterol are available as a solution for nebulization. Initial experience with arformoterol indicates that patients can experience sustained benefit over 12 weeks of taking the drug.[40] Considerable clinical experience with both short-acting and long-acting β_2-agonists demonstrates their safety for patients with COPD.[41]

Anticholinergic agents decrease airflow limitation by blocking muscarinic (M) receptors on airway smooth muscle and submucosal gland cells. Stimulation of these receptors results in bronchoconstriction and increased mucus secretion. As with other inhaled drugs, symptomatic improvement results from a decrease in exercise-related dynamic hyperinflation. Ipratropium is a short-acting and relatively nonselective drug that blocks both M2 and M3 receptors. Blockage of M2 receptors increases acetylcholine release, whereas blockage of M3 causes bronchodilation, which is the dominant effect from ipratropium. Ipratropium has no effect on decreasing mucus secretion. At conventional doses, ipratropium provides greater bronchodilatory potency compared to β_2-agonists, although bioactivity is similar at maximal doses.[42] Ipratropium has been shown to improve FEV_1, reduce lung volumes and dyspnea, decrease adverse events, and improve exercise tolerance.[38] Long-term use does not promote tolerance. Usual doses with an MDI are two to four puffs every 6 or 8 hours, although some patients may tolerate higher doses. Ipratropium is available in an MDI, as a single agent or combined with albuterol, and as a solution for nebulization. Atropine-like adverse effects are typically mild, but patients should be observed for urinary retention, closed angle glaucoma, and constipation. Case-control studies suggest that ipratropium is associated with an increased risk of cardiovascular mortality among patients treated for COPD.[43]

Tiotropium is an inhaled long-acting anticholinergic agent available as a DPI that requires only once-a-day dosing. It blocks M_1, M_2, and M_3 receptors nonselectively, like ipratropium, but disassociates more rapidly from M_2 receptors than M_1 or M_3 receptors. The onset of peak bronchodilation ranges between 1 and 3 hours, so tiotropium is not used for acute relief of bronchospasm. It improves FEV_1, lung volumes, dyspnea, adverse events from COPD, and exercise endurance.[44] In contrast to ipratropium, tiotropium has been shown to improve quality of life and prevent exacerbations.[44] Tiotropium has also been shown to improve the effectiveness of pulmonary rehabilitation.[45] Exacerbation rates have recently been shown to be similar between tiotropium as compared with salmeterol combined with inhaled corticosteroids. Compared with LABAs, tiotropium produces better bronchodilation and greater improvements in dyspnea.[46]

Aclidinium inhalation powder recently became available for the long-term maintenance treatment of bronchospasm associated COPD. It is administered twice daily by DPI inhalation. Aclidinium is a long-acting agent that also exhibits selectivity for the M_3 muscarinic acetylcholine receptor, similar to tiotropium.[47,48] Clinical experience with this agent is limited.

Theophylline is a phosphodiesterase inhibitor that raises intracellular concentrations of cyclic adenosine monophosphate within smooth muscle cells. It has moderate bronchodilatory effects in addition to acting as a diuretic, stimulant of central respiratory drive, enhancer of diaphragmatic contractility, and reliever of diaphragmatic fatigue. It may alter genes that promote airway inflammation in COPD and provide an anti-inflammatory effect, although the clinical importance of this effect is uncertain.[49] It is available in sustained-release formulations for once- or twice-daily dosing. A meta-analysis of 18 primary studies reported that theophylline improves FEV_1 and FVC both during the trough and peak phases of its serum concentrations.

Theophylline has a narrow therapeutic window, however, and can cause serious adverse effects that include cardiac arrhythmias and seizures, which may be the initial manifestations of toxicity. Theophylline is now recommended as third-line therapy for patients with inadequate responses to inhaled bronchodilators and for patients who cannot use inhaler therapy optimally. Target drug serum concentrations are 8 to 13 mg/dL, which is achieved in most patients with a 300 mg dose once daily at bedtime.[4] Theophylline has multiple interactions with other drugs.

Roflumilast is an oral phosphodiesterase 4 inhibitor that decreases inflammation and may promote smooth muscle relaxation. The FDA-approved indication for roflumilast is for the reduction of exacerbations in patients with chronic bronchitis, severe or very severe airflow limitation, and a history of exacerbations. A meta-analysis of 23 randomized trials of roflumilast or cilomilast versus placebo showed that treatment with PDE4 inhibitors resulted in improvements in the FEV_1 and reduced exacerbation rates but had little effect on quality of life.[50] Whether roflumilast provides additional benefits when combined with other inhaled medications to reduce COPD exacerbation frequency is currently unknown.

Short-term administration of systemic **corticosteroids** for 5 to 14 days has a role in managing patients with exacerbations of COPD, but for patients with stable COPD, no measurable benefit is achieved by long-term use of oral corticosteroids. Moreover, corticosteroid therapy causes multiple adverse effects that include osteoporosis, diabetes, fluid retention, hypertension, cataracts, immunosuppression with risk of infection, integument changes, and redistribution of fat. A trial of oral corticosteroids does not predict which patients with COPD will benefit from inhaled corticosteroids.

Inhaled corticosteroids have anti-inflammatory effects on the airways and provide opportunities to improve symptoms and the clinical course of patients with COPD while avoiding many of the side effects associated with oral corticosteroids. Most multicenter trials have not shown benefit from inhaled corticosteroids in slowing the annual rate of decline of FEV_1 in COPD,[51,52] although reanalysis of data from one trial found a slower rate of decline for patients with moderate to severe COPD treated with inhaled fluticasone.[24] Several studies demonstrate that inhaled corticosteroids lower the rate of progressive loss of quality of life and the frequency of exacerbations among patients with advanced COPD. Because of these benefits, clinical guidelines recommend inhaled corticosteroids for patients with severe (GOLD group C or D) COPD and repeated exacerbations (e.g., three within the previous 3 years).[4]

Inhaled corticosteroids may cause oral thrush but have negligible risks for cataracts, muscle weakness, or osteoporosis. The effect on blood glucose among patients with diabetes is poorly defined. Two studies have noted a higher risk of pneumonia among patients treated with inhaled corticosteroids, but no increase in pneumonia-related deaths.

Combination therapy with inhaled and oral bronchodilators from different drug classes provides additive benefit. Adding theophylline to inhaled albuterol and ipratropium[53] or to salmeterol[54] improves FEV_1 as compared with each individual drug. The combination of salmeterol and ipratropium also has additive effects on spirometric values.[55] Combining once-a-day tiotropium and twice-a-day formoterol improved morning and evening FEV_1 and resting hyperinflation.[56] Additive benefit was also achieved when formoterol was dosed only once a day with tiotropium. Similar additive benefits have been observed with tiotropium combined with salmeterol and fluticasone. Tiotropium combined with a SABA has additive effects, but not when combined with ipratropium.[57] A large multicenter trial (the TORCH trial) demonstrated that salmeterol added to fluticasone improves FEV_1, exacerbation rate, and quality of life as compared with either drug alone, which is consistent with previous studies that examined the effects of adding inhaled corticosteroids to β_2-agonists.[58] A reanalysis of the TORCH trial data determined that the combination of salmeterol and fluticasone slowed the annual decline of FEV_1, although salmeterol had similar benefit in this study when given alone.[24]

Antibiotics are reserved for patients with COPD exacerbations characterized by fever, leukocytosis, purulent sputum, or chest radiographic changes consistent with bronchitis. Chronic use of antibiotics for stable patients has not been consistently shown to preserve lung function or prevent exacerbations. One study, however, demonstrated benefit in decreasing rates of exacerbations among patients treated with intermittent or continuous antibiotics during at-risk periods if they had a history of frequent exacerbations in the past.[59] For those patients who continue to have frequent exacerbations despite optimal therapy for COPD including bronchodilators and anti-inflammatory agents, antibiotic prophylaxis with azithromycin should be considered.[60]

Mucokinetic agents are intended to reduce mucus viscosity and assist with the mobilization of airway secretions. Iodinated glycerol has been demonstrated in a placebo-controlled trial to improve cough symptoms and sense of well-being, although objective markers of airflow limitation did not improve.[61] Because of these marginal benefits, mucokinetic agents are used empirically in occasional patients who have marked difficulty with expectoration of secretions despite maximal therapy. Oral *N*-acetylcysteine has the potential to break sulfhydryl bonds and provide antioxidant effects. The largest study to date, however, did not demonstrate efficacy.[62] Aerosolized surfactant has been shown to improve pulmonary function and ciliary sputum transport in patients with stable chronic bronchitis.[63] Inhaled ribonuclease benefits patients with cystic fibrosis but provides no benefit in COPD.[4]

Long-Term Oxygen Therapy

Long-term oxygen therapy (LTOT) for hypoxemic patients with COPD prolongs survival.[26] The mechanisms of benefit are unclear, although patients treated with LTOT for an average of 19 hours per day have a slower progression of pulmonary hypertension compared with those treated with 12 hours per day or less, suggesting a positive effect on pulmonary vasculature as the basis for improved survival.[26] LTOT also decreases dyspnea awareness, oxygen cost of breathing, pulmonary hypertension, disordered sleep, nocturnal dysrhythmias, exercise endurance, strength, and mental alertness.[64]

BOX 33-6

Indications for Long-Term Oxygen Therapy for Stable COPD

Continuous Oxygen Therapy

Pao_2 ≤55 mm Hg or oxygen saturation ≤88% at rest while breathing room air

Pao_2 between 56 and 59 mm Hg or oxygen saturation of 89% at any time during breathing of room air with one or more of the following:

- Polycythemia (Hct >56%)
- Pulmonary hypertension as evidenced by right heart dysfunction

Noncontinuous Oxygen Therapy

Pao_2 ≤55 mm Hg or oxygen saturation ≤88% during exertion or sleep while breathing room air

Patients are selected for oxygen therapy on the basis of specific indications derived from clinical and laboratory findings (**Box 33-6**).[1,4] Demonstration of hypoxemia should occur after a 4-week stable period when patients are receiving full medical therapy and are not smoking. Subsequent monitoring of oxygenation is performed on an individual basis. Up to 40% of patients initiated on LTOT experience improved oxygenation after 1 month of therapy and no longer fulfill the indications for supplemental oxygen.[65]

Vaccinations

Vaccinations are a central preventive measure in the management of patients with COPD. All caregivers interacting with patients should counsel them regarding their annual vaccination with trivalent influenza

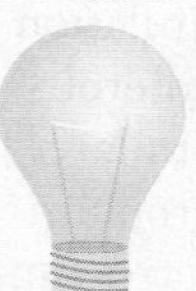

STOP AND THINK

You are asked to see a patient in the clinic who is having difficulty correctly using her COPD drugs. How would you assess for proper medication administration?

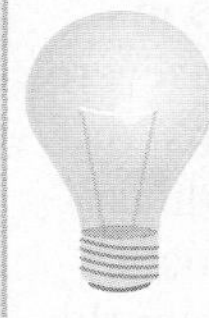

STOP AND THINK

Oxygen should be delivered to what target Spo_2 during COPD exacerbation. Why?

vaccine. Pneumococcal vaccination is recommended for patients with COPD regardless of age.

Ventilatory Support

The benefit of intermittent NIV in the outpatient management of patients with severe stable COPD is not clearly defined. The purpose of ventilator support is to unload respiratory muscles and treat or prevent muscle fatigue. Such therapy has been shown to benefit patients with chronic respiratory failure caused by restrictive lung diseases, such as kyphoscoliosis.[66] A systematic review of 15 studies of NIV observed that the 6 available randomized controlled trials (RCTs) demonstrated no improvement in gas exchange, but the 9 non-RCTs did report some other clinical improvements.[67] These improvements included health-related quality of life and dyspnea. The authors of the review concluded that a subset of patients on maximal medical treatment for severe stable COPD might receive benefit from bilevel noninvasive positive pressure ventilation when used as adjunctive therapy. Additional studies are needed, however, before recommending intermittent ventilation as standard therapy. Guidelines exist from Medicare for reimbursement for NIV for patients with COPD (**Box 33-7**).

Management of Sleep-Related Abnormalities

Patients with COPD are at risk for sleep-related disorders characterized by poor sleep quality and worsening hypoxia and hypercapnia at night.[67] Although the prevalence of sleep-related disorders among patients with varying severity of COPD is unknown, studies indicate that 45% of normoxic COPD patients develop significant oxyhemoglobin desaturation during sleep,[69] and 47% of hypercapnic COPD patients experience a 10 mm Hg increment in $Paco_2$ at night.[70] Multiple factors contribute to sleep-related breathing disorders in COPD, but alveolar hypoventilation is the predominant mechanism. Sleep-related increases in upper airway resistance, worsening of $\dot{V}/\dot{Q}$, and changes in oxygen consumption, carbon dioxide production, and cardiac output most likely play contributory roles. Alterations in sleep-related breathing patterns create greater changes in respiratory function for patients with COPD as compared with normal subjects because COPD patients have higher physiologic dead space at baseline. Patients with COPD also have abnormal respiratory system mechanics—with hyperinflation and diaphragmatic flattening—that amplify the effects of altered breathing patterns during sleep.

The coexistence of COPD with **sleep apnea hypopnea syndrome (SAHS)** occurs in approximately 10% of patients with a history of SAHS. Patients with the combined disorders develop more severe hypoxia during sleep as compared with other patients with SAHS.

It remains unresolved whether combined disease results from the coincidental occurrence of these two relatively common conditions in the same individual or whether COPD predisposes patients to SAHS. Affected patients may present with greater degrees of polycythemia and lower extremity edema than expected by the severity of their airway obstruction. A sleep study is indicated if patients have these findings or evidence of general symptoms of SAHS, such as daytime sleepiness, heavy snoring, or observed obstructed breathing during sleep.

Respiratory stimulants or other pharmacologic agents have not been shown to improve sleep architecture or reduce nocturnal oxygen desaturation in patients with COPD. Nasal continuous positive airway pressure (CPAP) remains the mainstay of therapy for patients with SAHS with or without COPD, although few data exist demonstrating the outcome of this therapy for patients with COPD.

BOX 33-7

Guidelines for Medicare Reimbursement for Noninvasive Positive Pressure Ventilation in Patients with COPD

1. Symptomatic despite optimal medical therapy.
2. Abnormal gas exchange:
   a. $Paco_2 \geq 52$ mmHg *and*
   b. Nocturnal hypoventilation with $Spo_2 < 89\%$ for ≥5 consecutive minutes while breathing usual Fio_2
3. Obstructive sleep apnea excluded at least on clinical grounds. If obstructive sleep apnea exists, CPAP is indicated initially.
4. Repeated hospital admissions for hypercapnic respiratory failure can be considered.

Pulmonary Rehabilitation

Enrollment of patients with moderate to severe COPD in outpatient **pulmonary rehabilitation** programs provides opportunities to restore patients to the highest possible level of independence and functioning in the community.[71] Components of an effective, multidisciplinary rehabilitation program include exercise training and conditioning, physical therapy, education for patients and family (e.g., nutrition, oxygen use, inhaler techniques), instruction in airway clearance techniques, energy conservation, vocational counseling, and psychological support (**Box 33-8**). The effectiveness of pulmonary rehabilitation has long been debated because of the limited outcomes data available to demonstrate measurable improvements in postrehabilitation endpoints. A systematic review of evidence concluded

BOX 33-8

Components of Pulmonary Rehabilitation for the Patient with COPD

Detailed history and physical examination
Measurement of spirometry before and after a bronchodilator drug
Assessment of exercise capacity
Measurement of health status and impact of breathlessness
Assessment of inspiratory and expiratory muscle strength and lower limb strength in patients with muscle wasting
Assessment of patient's advance planning needs

Reproduced with permission of the American Thoracic Society. Modified from Rabe KF, Hurd S, Anzueto A, et al. Global strategy for the diagnosis, management, and prevention of chronic obstructive pulmonary disease: GOLD executive summary. *Am J Respir Crit Care Med.* 2007;176:532–555.

TABLE 33-6
Giant Bullectomy Indications, Contraindications, and Ideal Candidate

Indications	Contraindications	Ideal Candidate
Severe functional limitation despite maximal medical therapy Nonsmoker or ex-smoker Little bronchodilator responsiveness Bulla occupies more than one-third of hemithorax Crowding of adjacent lung on CT angiogram Elevated trapped gas (elevated RV) on PFTs Normal or near-normal DLCO Normal Pa_{O_2} and Pa_{CO_2}	Substantial emphysema elsewhere in the lung	All of the preceding indications *and* • Bulla >50% of hemithorax • All of the preceding indications *without* • Chronic bronchitis or recurrent infections • Pulmonary hypertension • Comorbid illness • Older age • FEV_1 <35% of predicted

CT, computed tomography; RV, residual volume; PFT, pulmonary function test; DLCO, diffusing capacity of the lung for carbon monoxide; FEV_1, forced expiratory volume in 1 second.

Reproduced from Benditt JO. Surgical options for patients with COPD: sorting out the choices. *Respir Care.* 2006;51:173–182. Reprinted with permission.

that pulmonary rehabilitation is beneficial for patients with COPD.[71] Such evidence has resulted in approval by Medicare for payment of pulmonary rehabilitation services.

Surgery

Multiple surgical procedures have been evaluated over the last 50 years to improve lung function in COPD.[72] Presently, only giant bullectomy, lung volume reduction surgery, and lung transplantation have survived scientific scrutiny and demonstrated clinical utility for selected patients with COPD.

Giant Bullectomy

Giant bullae represent an unusual complication of emphysema that can cause pulmonary decompensation as bullae expand and compress adjacent functioning lung tissue. Patients are selected for **bullectomy** by estimating the degree of lung compression and the functional status of the compressed lung to determine the amount of improvement that can be anticipated by bullectomy. Patients with giant bullae who have limited amounts of potentially functioning compressed lung tissue, called vanishing lung syndrome, gain no benefit from bullectomy. CT scans can assess the size of bullae, the amount of compressed lung, and the severity of diffuse emphysema.[73] Pulmonary function tests (PFTs) determine the severity of underlying emphysema. Appropriate candidates for surgery have a restrictive rather than an obstructive PFT pattern because of lung compression by the bullae (**Table 33-6**). A severe obstructive pattern suggests the presence of advanced diffuse emphysema that will not improve with bullectomy. The gas volume of giant bullae can be calculated by subtracting the total lung volume (TLC) determined by helium dilution (which does not measure the volume of bullae) from the TLC measured by plethysmography (which includes the volume of bullae).

Lung Volume Reduction Surgery

The term **lung volume reduction surgery (LVRS)** refers to surgical procedures that resect the regions of lung tissue most severely affected by emphysema. After removal of 20% to 30% of an emphysematous lung, the remaining lung expands beyond its previous boundaries and gains increased recoil elasticity. The lung, chest wall, and diaphragm demonstrate improved mechanics, with higher expiratory airflow and less air trapping. The procedure can be performed through a midline sternotomy or by video-assisted thoracotomy, both of which allow stapled resection of tissue.[72]

The National Emphysema Treatment Trial (NETT) demonstrated improved short-term outcomes in carefully selected patients with COPD (**Table 33-7**). Patients with a heterogeneous upper lobe distribution of emphysema and low exercise capacity experienced improved long-term survival following LVRS as

TABLE 33-7
Lung Volume Reduction Surgery Indications, Contraindications, and Ideal Candidate

Indications	Contraindications	Ideal Candidate
Severe functional limitation despite maximal medical therapy Nonsmoker for at least 3 months Completed pulmonary rehabilitation (6–12 weeks) Postbronchodilator FEV_1 <45% of predicted RV >150% of predicted TLC >100% of predicted Pa_{O_2} >45 mm Hg Pa_{CO_2} <60 mm Hg Postpulmonary rehabilitation 6-min walk distance >140 m	Comorbid illness Substantial untreated cardiac disease Cancer other than basal cell or squamous cell skin cancer within the last 5 years Diseases in other organs increasing surgical risk BMI >31.1 kg/m² (males) or 32.3 kg/m² (females) FEV_1 <20% of predicted and either DLCO <20% of predicted or homogeneous emphysema on CT scan Pulmonary artery hypertension Systolic >45 mm Hg Mean >35 mm Hg Prednisone >20 mg/d	All of the preceding indications *and* • Upper lobe emphysema and cycle-ergometry exercise capacity <25 watts (women) or <40 watts (men) while breathing F_{IO_2} of 0.30 All of the preceding indications *without* • Older age • Comorbid illness • Pulmonary hypertension • Frequent respiratory tract infections or chronic bronchitis

FEV_1, forced expiratory volume in 1 second; RV, residual volume; TLC, total lung capacity; BMI, body mass index; DLCO, diffusing capacity of the lung for carbon monoxide; CT, computed tomography.

Reproduced from Benditt JO. Surgical options for patients with COPD: sorting out the choices. *Respir Care.* 2006;51:173–182. Reprinted with permission.

compared with continued medical therapy.[27] Patients without these preoperative characteristics did not benefit from LVRS and had either worse or similar survival as compared with medical management. In secondary subgroup analyses, patients with upper lobe distribution of emphysema and poor exercise capacity had improved quality of life and exercise capacity.

The long-term results of LVRS are not completely defined. Most studies report improved lung function and gas exchange for some patients up to 24 to 36 months after surgery.[74] Complications of LVRS include prolonged air leak, pneumonia, respiratory failure, postoperative ileus and colonic or cecal perforation, and cardiac ischemia.[75]

Extensive research is now examining nonsurgical alternatives to LVRS that achieve similar goals of reducing lung volume by deflating lung regions that are most affected by emphysema. Bronchoscopic insertion of one-way valves and biological substances into the airways occlude ventilation to emphysematous regions and allow other lung segments to expand.

Lung Transplantation

COPD is the most common indication for **lung transplantation**. In the absence of contraindications, patients are selected for transplantation if they have advanced COPD with an estimated survival of less than 2 years (**Table 33-8**).[72] It is difficult to estimate the survival of individual patients, but markers of high near-term mortality include an FEV_1 below 25% to 30% of predicted, a rapid decline in lung function, and severe hypoxemia, hypercapnia, and secondary pulmonary hypertension despite maximal medical therapy.[72] Recent Canadian guidelines on lung transplantation include the BODE index for patient selection (**Box 33-9**).[76]

TABLE 33-8
Lung Transplant Indications, Contraindications, and Ideal Candidate

Indications	Contraindications	Ideal Candidate
Advanced COPD • Symptomatic despite maximal medical therapy High risk of death within 2 to 3 years COPD-specific (one or more) FEV_1 <25% to 30% of predicted • Pulmonary artery hypertension • Right ventricular failure • Pa_{CO_2} >55 mm Hg Severe functional limitation, but preserved ability to walk Suggested age limitations • Age <55 for heart–lung transplantation candidates • Age <60 for bilateral lung transplantation candidates • Age <65 for single-lung transplantation candidates	Active malignancy within 2 years (except basal or squamous cell skin cancer) Substance addiction within 6 months Substantial dysfunction of extrathoracic organs HIV infection Hepatitis B antigen positive Hepatitis C with biopsy-proven evidence of liver disease	All of the preceding indications *and* • Highly motivated individual • Excellent social support All of the preceding indications *without* • Symptomatic osteoporosis • Oral steroids >20 mg/day • Invasive mechanical ventilation • Colonization with fungi, resistant organisms, or atypical mycobacteria

LVRS, lung volume reduction surgery; COPD, chronic obstructive pulmonary disease; FEV_1, forced expiratory volume in 1 second; HIV, human immunodeficiency virus.

Reproduced from Benditt JO. Surgical options for patients with COPD: sorting out the choices. *Respir Care.* 2006;51:173–182. Reprinted with permission.

BOX 33-9

Canadian Guidelines for Transplantation

Patients with a BODE index of 7 to 10 or at least one of the following:

- History of hospitalization for exacerbation associated with acute hypercapnia $Pa_{CO_2} > 50$ mm Hg
- Pulmonary hypertension or cor pulmonale, or both, despite oxygen therapy
- FEV_1 of less than 20% and either DLCO of less than 20% or homogeneous distribution of emphysema

FEV_1, forced expiratory volume in 1 second; DLCO, diffusing capacity of the lung for carbon monoxide.

Reproduced from Orens JB, Estenne M, Arcasoy S, et al. International guidelines for the selection of lung transplant candidates: 2006 update—a consensus report from the Pulmonary Scientific Council of the International Society for Heart and Lung Transplantation. *J Heart Lung Transplant.* 2006;25:745–755. Copyright © (2006). Reprinted with permission from Elsevier.

TABLE 33-9
Criteria for Selection of LVRS Versus Lung Transplant in Patients with COPD

Lung Transplant	LVRS	LVRS or Lung Transplant, or LVRS Followed by Lung Transplant
Purulent obstructive disease • Bronchiectasis • More than ¼ cup of phlegm per day Associated pulmonary artery hypertension and/or right heart failure Absence of hyperinflation: TLC <100% of predicted or RV <150% of predicted FEV_1 <20% of predicted with either homogeneous emphysema or DLCO <20% of predicted (NETT high-risk subgroup) Non-upper-lobe emphysema with low exercise capacity Pa_{CO_2} >55 mm Hg Pa_{O_2} <50 mm Hg 6-min walk distance <300 feet	Age >65, with upper lobe emphysema and low exercise capacity Age >65 with upper lobe disease and high exercise capacity Age >65, with non-upper-lobe disease and low exercise capacity Age <65 with FEV 30% to 40% of predicted but disabling symptoms present despite maximal medical therapy	Age <65 and meets criteria for both transplant and LVRS

LVRS, lung volume reduction surgery; COPD, chronic obstructive pulmonary disease; TLC, total lung capacity; RV, residual volume; FEV_1, forced expiratory volume in 1 second; DLCO, diffusing capacity of the lung for carbon monoxide; NETT, National Emphysema Treatment Trial.

Reproduced from Benditt JO. Surgical options for patients with COPD: sorting out the choices. *Respir Care*. 2006;51:173–182. Reprinted with permission.

Both single- and double-lung transplantations are performed for COPD, but single-lung procedures are most common because of the limited availability of donor lungs. Similar postoperative exercise functional capacities result from either procedure, but data suggest improved survival with double-lung transplantation. Double-lung transplantation also produces greater improvement in spirometric measures. Coexistence of bronchiectasis with associated purulent airway secretions requires double-lung transplantation to prevent infection of the allograft.[77] Single-lung transplantation is usually performed through a lateral thoracotomy incision. Bilateral lung transplantation is done most often through a median sternotomy or transverse thoracosternotomy clamshell incision. Bilateral lung transplantation may require cardiopulmonary bypass in 20% of patients. The selection of patients for lung volume reduction surgery versus lung transplantation is guided by the criteria in **Table 33-9**.

One-year survival for patients undergoing lung transplantation for COPD is 90%, with 5-year survival being 40% to 50%. Although lung transplantation in COPD has not been subjected to randomized trials to determine its effect on survival, analyses of retrospective data controlled for independent risk factors of death indicate improved survival compared with patients with severe COPD who have not received transplants. In contrast, other retrospective analyses reported similar survival between patients who received lung transplants and those who remained on the transplant list.[78] The primary rationale for lung transplantation centers on improvement of functional status and quality of life rather than survival benefits.[72] Nearly all studies demonstrate that patients experience improved pulmonary function,[79] exercise capacity,[80] and quality of life[81] after transplantation.

Complications of lung transplantation include infection, early allograft dysfunction that may progress to acute lung injury, hemorrhage, dehiscence of the bronchial anastomoses, and acute and chronic lung rejection. The development of acute postoperative allograft edema that requires mechanical ventilation in patients who have undergone single-lung transplantation complicates ventilator management. The overexpansion of the highly compliant native lung compared with the low-compliant allograft may necessitate independent lung ventilation with a double-lumen endotracheal tube.

Overview of Management of Stable Chronic Obstructive Pulmonary Disease

Clinical practice guidelines have proposed a stepwise initiation of increasingly more intensive therapy directed by the severity of airflow limitation as measured by FEV_1 (**Figure 33-8**). The introduction of the BODE index has provided a more comprehensive measure of patients' functional limitations from COPD and associated conditions than FEV_1 alone.[8] Clinicians are beginning to include such measures of functional limitations in their decisions for escalating therapeutic interventions. Based on clinical trials that demonstrate added benefit from combined inhaled medications, the stepwise management shown in **Figure 33-9** for patients with progressive disease and functional limitations has been proposed as a clinical approach.[38]

Managing Exacerbations

Patients with COPD are at risk for exacerbations of their airways disease that may require hospitalization. The GOLD guideline defines an **exacerbation** as "a change in a patient's baseline dyspnea, cough, and/or sputum that is beyond day-to-day variations, is acute in onset, and may warrant a change in regular medications."[4] Exacerbations are characterized by lung inflammation, which plays a central etiologic role and may cause irreversible decrements in lung function and functional status after each exacerbation. Bacterial or viral respiratory infections precipitate most exacerbations, although environmental pollutants and other undefined precipitants play a role.[82] Exacerbations may remain mild and respond to outpatient modifications of therapy or become severe and require ventilatory support. The mortality of hospitalized patients with

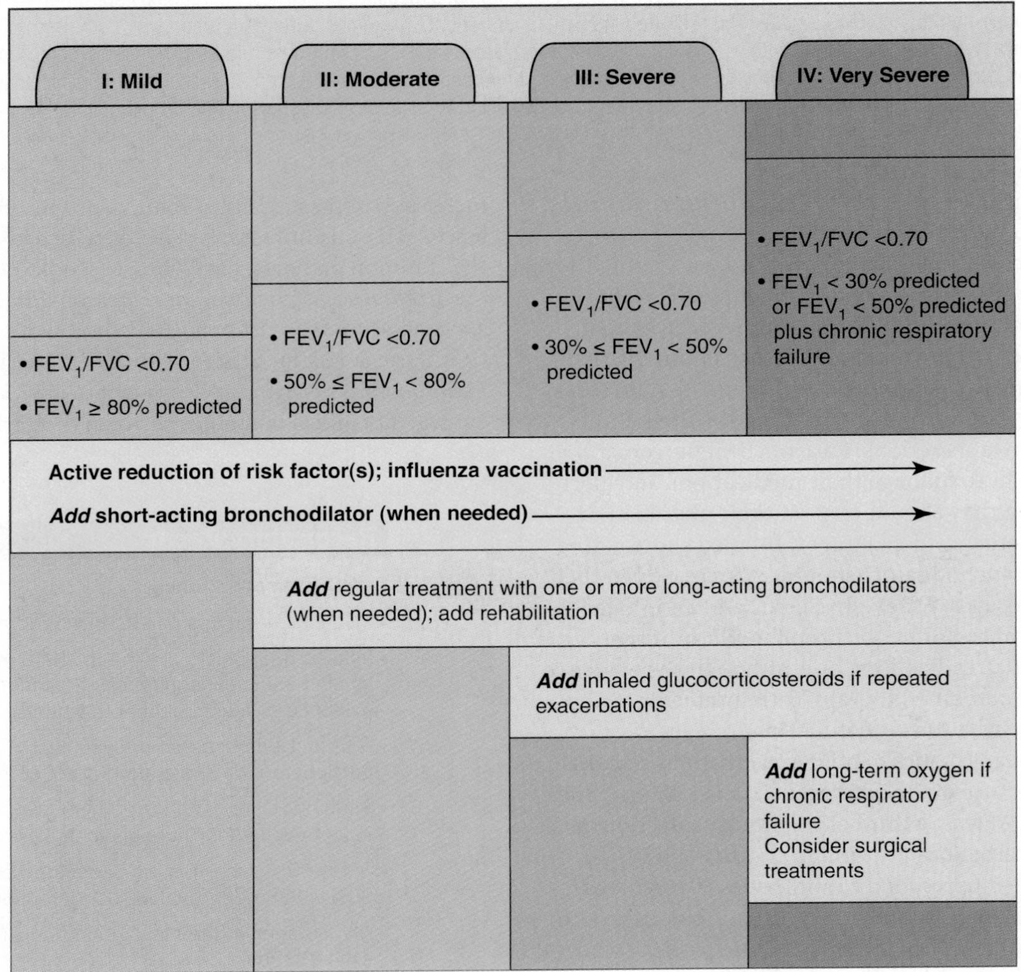

Postbronchodilator FEV1 is recommended for the diagnosis and assessment of severity of COPD.
I: Mild
II: Moderate
III: Severe
IV: Very Severe
• FEV1/FVC <0.70
• FEV1 ≥ 80% predicted
• FEV1/FVC <0.70
• 50% ≤ FEV1 < 80% predicted
• FEV1/FVC <0.70
• 30% ≤ FEV1 < 50% predicted
• FEV1/FVC <0.70
• FEV1 < 30% predicted or FEV1 < 50% predicted plus chronic respiratory failure
Active reduction of risk factor(s); influenza vaccination
Add short-acting bronchodilator (when needed)
Add regular treatment with one or more long-acting bronchodilators (when needed); add rehabilitation
Add inhaled glucocorticosteroids if repeated exacerbations
Add long-term oxygen if chronic respiratory failure
Consider surgical treatments

FIGURE 33-8 Therapy for COPD based on the GOLD stages of disease.

Reproduced with permission of the American Thoracic Society. Copyright © American Thoracic Society. From Rabe KF, Hurd S, Anzueto A, Barnes PJ, et al. Global strategy for the diagnosis, management, and prevention of chronic obstructive pulmonary disease: GOLD executive summary. *Am J Respir Crit Care Med.* 2007;176:532–555.

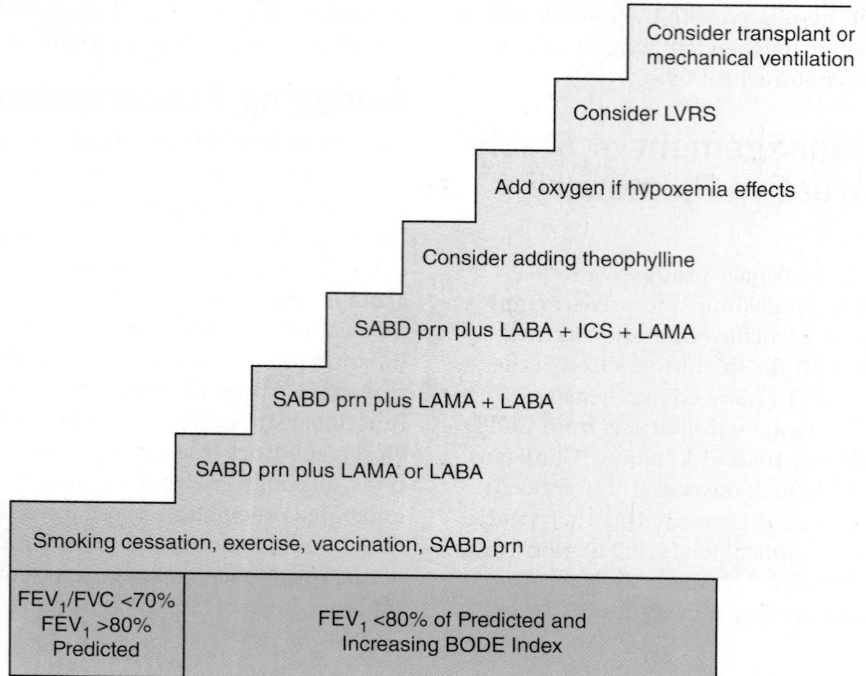

FIGURE 33-9 Stepwise progression of management of patients that combines measures of airflow limitation by spirometry and measures of functional impairment by the BODE index. The first step indicates that patients have mild airflow limitation with some symptoms, such as a cough, but have not become impaired with worsening dyspnea, exercise capacity, or symptoms related to systemic compromise. As the disease progresses from left to right, increasing airflow limitation and functional impairment occur. At each step, the clinician is looking for a response to the new intervention either in improved spirometric or BODE index values. SABD; short-acting bronchodilator.

Modified with permission from Celli BR. Update on the management of COPD. *Chest.* 2008;133:1451–1462, with permission from the American College of Chest Physicians.

exacerbations is 10%,[83] with 25% of patients requiring admission to the intensive care unit (ICU).

Mild exacerbations can be managed with home therapy in the absence of severe COPD, clinically important acute or chronic comorbidities, or other factors that present risk of hypercapnic respiratory failure. Patients should be encouraged to maintain adequate fluid intake to avoid dehydration and should monitor their ability to cough and raise secretions. Patients benefit from a written action plan to manage their medications and alert them to when they should contact their physician or go to the emergency department. Inhaled short-acting β_2-agonist bronchodilators should be increased to their maximum dosages. Many physicians add an inhaled short-acting anticholinergic bronchodilator if the patient is not already taking one, although the evidence of efficacy of combined therapy with ipratropium and a SABA in exacerbations is conflicting.

The role of antibiotics in mild exacerbations remains uncertain because of the heterogeneity of existing clinical trial designs. At least a third of respiratory infections that underlie exacerbations are viral in etiology and would not be expected to respond to antibiotics. Nevertheless, a recent meta-analysis concluded that antibiotics reduce mortality and treatment failures in those patients who require hospitalization.[84] The ATS COPD guidelines recommend the initiation of antibiotics for exacerbations if any two of the following three features are present: increased dyspnea, sputum volume, or sputum purulence.[8] An oral antibiotic is selected with activity against the common pathogens in COPD exacerbations, which are *Streptococcus pneumoniae, Haemophilus influenzae,* and *Moraxella catarrhalis.* Patients with severe COPD are at risk for gram-negative bacteria, including *Pseudomonas aeruginosa.* A systematic review observed equivalent clinical outcomes between drug trials that

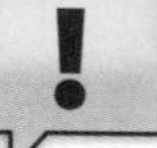

Respiratory Recap

COPD Exacerbations

- Mild exacerbations can be managed at home.
- Inhaled β_2-agonists are the first-line therapy. Inhaled anticholinergics may be added, but evidence of added benefit is limited.
- A 5- to 14-day course of systemic corticosteroids is standard practice.
- Antibiotics are used for patients with increased sputum volume or purulence and/or dyspnea.
- Titrate O_2 to maintain an adequate Spo_2 above 90% without aggravating CO_2 retention.
- NIV is useful in the management of COPD exacerbation.
- Life-threatening respiratory failure requires intubation and mechanical ventilation.

compared quinolones, macrolides, and amoxicillin-clavulonate.[85] Recently, the length of time after antibiotic therapy during which the patient avoids a subsequent exacerbation (termed *disease-free interval* [DFI]) has been used as an endpoint for studies of antibiotic efficacy. Studies using this endpoint suggest that quinolones are associated with longer DFIs.[85]

Numerous studies have examined the value of systemic corticosteroids in outpatients with mild exacerbations.[86] Thompson and colleagues treated outpatients with 9 days of prednisone versus placebo and observed more rapid and greater degrees of improvement in oxygenation and FEV_1 and fewer treatment failures with prednisone.[86] New guidelines recommend a dose of 30 to 40 mg of prednisone per day for 5 to 14 days for outpatients with an exacerbation, although there are insufficient data to provide firm conclusions concerning the optimal duration of corticosteroid therapy.[4]

Severe exacerbations occur in patients with moderate, severe, and very severe COPD and commonly alter gas exchange, which may result in acute respiratory failure. Baseline abnormalities in $\dot{V}/\dot{Q}$ worsen, intrapulmonary shunts develop, and hyperinflation increases with the onset or worsening of auto-PEEP.[87] These pathophysiologic factors require careful evaluation of patients for a need for hospitalization (**Box 33-10**) or admission to the ICU (**Box 33-11**).

Despite modern advances in respiratory care, the inpatient mortality of patients hospitalized for an exacerbation of COPD remains substantial, ranging from 6% to 30%.[84] Markers of increased mortality include advanced age, need for mechanical ventilation, ventricular dysrhythmia, atrial fibrillation, acute or chronic cardiac disease, associated nonpulmonary organ failure, high APACHE (Acute Physiology and Chronic Health Evaluation) III score, poor nutritional status, poor baseline health status, and an alveolar–arterial oxygen gradient on room air greater than 40 mm Hg or a low Pao_2/Fio_2.[84] Alternative diagnoses (**Box 33-12**), such as

BOX 33-11

Indications for Intensive Care Unit Admission of Patients with Exacerbations of COPD

Severe dyspnea that responds inadequately to initial emergency therapy
Changes in mental status (confusion, lethargy, coma)
Persistent or worsening hypoxemia (Pao_2 <40 mm Hg) and/or severe or worsening respiratory acidosis (pH <7.25) despite supplemental oxygen and noninvasive ventilation
Need for invasive mechanical ventilation
Hemodynamic instability—need for vasopressors

 From Rabe KF, Hurd S, Anzueto A, et al. Global strategy for the diagnosis, management, and prevention of chronic obstructive pulmonary disease: GOLD executive summary. *Am J Respir Crit Care Med.* 2007;176:532–555.

BOX 33-10

Indications for Hospital Assessment or Admission for Exacerbations of COPD

Marked increase in intensity of symptoms, such as sudden development of resting dyspnea
Severe underlying COPD
Onset of new physical signs such as cyanosis, peripheral edema
Failure of exacerbation to respond to initial medical management
Significant comorbidities
Frequent exacerbations
Newly occurring arrhythmias
Diagnostic uncertainty
Older age
Insufficient home support

 From Rabe KF, Hurd S, Anzueto A, et al. Global strategy for the diagnosis, management, and prevention of chronic obstructive pulmonary disease: GOLD executive summary. *Am J Respir Crit Care Med.* 2007;176:532–555.

BOX 33-12

Conditions That May Simulate an Exacerbation of COPD

Pneumonia
Pulmonary emboli
Myocardial infarction or ischemia
Congestive heart failure
Dysrhythmia
Pneumothorax
Aspiration
Neuromuscular weakness
Rib or vertebral body fractures
Metabolic acidosis or other electrolyte disturbance
Pleural effusion
Sedating drugs or beta-blocking drugs
Inappropriate use of oxygen with hyperoxia and retained CO_2
Other organ dysfunction, such as renal failure or gastrointestinal hemorrhage

heart failure, pulmonary emboli, and myocardial infarction, should be carefully considered and excluded if suggestive findings exist. Of note, 25% of patients with COPD hospitalized for severe exacerbations of uncertain etiologies have pulmonary emboli.

Severe exacerbations require a prompt acceleration of outpatient therapy. Supplemental oxygen should be administered routinely and titrated to a flow rate to maintain Pao_2 above 60 mm Hg and Spo_2 above 90% (**Figure 33-10**). Sampling of arterial blood gases is indicated within 30 to 60 minutes to ensure adequate oxygenation and the absence of progressive hypercapnia. Either an air entrainment mask or a nasal cannula is an acceptable oxygen delivery device, depending on patient tolerance.

Because of their rapid onset of action, SABAs represent preferred first-line therapy,[4] although systematic reviews report similar clinical benefit from inhaled ipratropium.[88] SABAs, but not anticholinergic agents, may transiently worsen hypoxia through pulmonary vascular effects.[89] Little evidence supports the combination of SABAs and ipratropium,[88] although this combination is commonly recommended in view of the absence of an increased risk of short-term adverse drug effects.[4]

A meta-analysis of randomized trials does not support the use of methylxanthine bronchodilators, such as aminophylline or theophylline, for the treatment of exacerbations of COPD.[90] Administration of **methylxanthines** was noted to increase adverse events of nausea and vomiting without demonstrated improvement of respiratory endpoints. The GOLD guideline, however, recommends methylxanthines as second-line therapy for patients who have inadequate response to SABAs.[4]

Systematic reviews report that systemic corticosteroids improve respiratory physiologic measures during the first 72 hours of care and reduce risk for 30-day treatment failure, although the incidence of hyperglycemia during steroid treatment is increased. It is

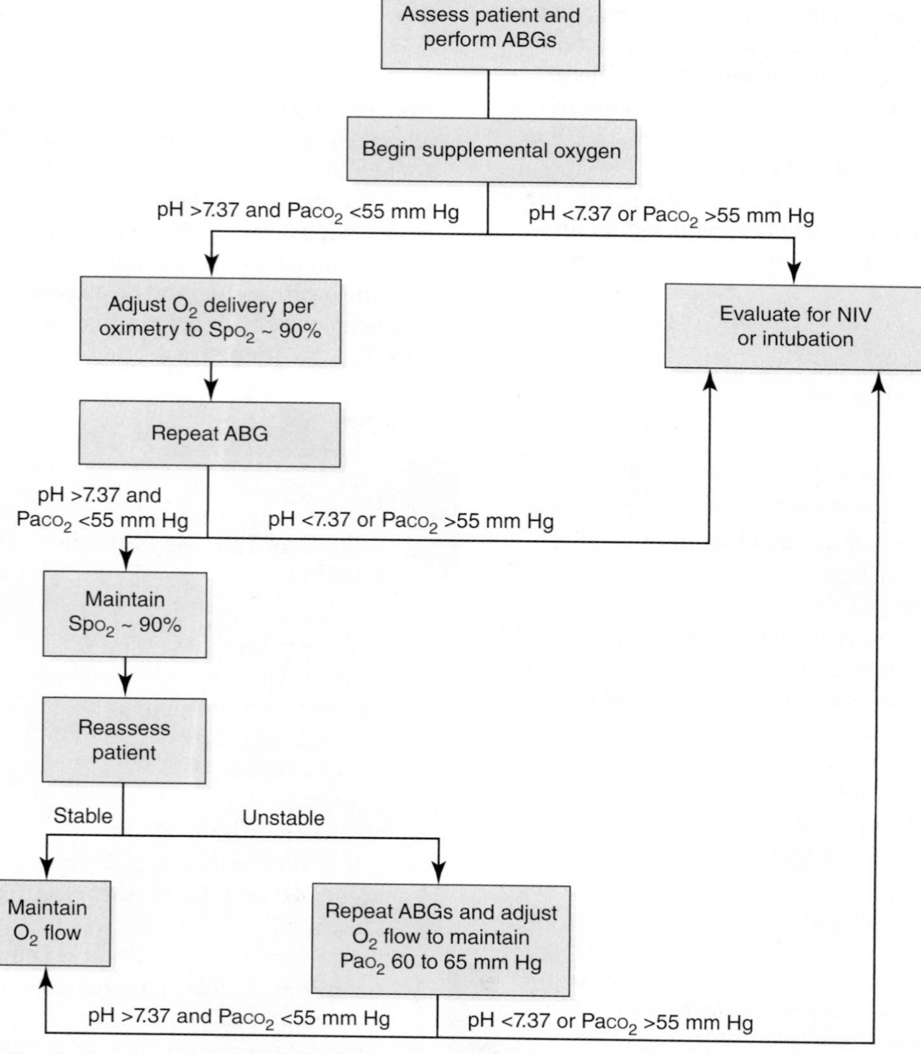

FIGURE 33-10 Algorithm for the management of supplemental oxygen in patients hospitalized for an exacerbation. ABGs, arterial blood gas values; Spo_2, arterial oxygen saturation by pulse oximetry; $Paco_2$, partial pressure of arterial carbon dioxide.

currently recommended that all hospitalized patients with exacerbations be treated with corticosteroids.[4] The recommended dose is 30 to 40 mg of oral prednisone or an equivalent dose of methylprednisolone intravenously for 5 to 14 days.[4,91,92] A response to corticosteroids during an acute hospitalization should not be interpreted as an indication for chronic corticosteroid therapy.

Recommendations for antibiotic therapy for patients hospitalized for severe exacerbations are similar to those for mild exacerbations (discussed earlier). Recent guidelines, however, have suggested stratifying patients according to their risk for treatment failure. Patients with worse lung function, increased frequency of exacerbations or office visits, ischemic heart disease, and other comorbidities may benefit from treatment with extended-spectrum antibiotics.

Hospitalized patients with exacerbations may present with acute respiratory failure or develop respiratory failure after a period of initial medical management. The cause of respiratory failure varies between patients, but a common scenario occurs when patients with moderate to severe airway obstruction increase their $\dot{V}_E$ and work of breathing in response to increased airways resistance due to worsening airway inflammation, edema, bronchospasm, and secretions. The increasing respiratory rate shortens expiratory time and causes dynamic hyperinflation and auto-PEEP. Other factors, such as pulmonary hypertension, poor nutrition with muscle weakness, disadvantageous chest wall mechanics from hyperinflated lungs, and baseline hypercapnia, may lower ventilatory reserve. As work of breathing continues to increase, the patient tires and acute respiratory failure ensues.

Patients with acute respiratory failure have fatigued respiratory muscles and benefit from ventilatory assistance. Goals of assisted ventilation include unloading of respiratory muscles to allow recovery from muscle fatigue, reduction of air trapping, and maintenance of $Paco_2$ at or near the patient's baseline value. Many patients develop acute respiratory failure in the setting of chronic compensated respiratory acidosis. It is important to adjust ventilatory support to the patient's baseline $Paco_2$, which can be estimated by the patient's serum bicarbonate level at admission or during a previous period of stability. Overventilation to a normal $Paco_2$ of 40 mm Hg if the patient is chronically hypercapnic results in renal loss of bicarbonate and uncompensated respiratory acidosis when the patient returns to the baseline level of hypercapnia during discontinuation of ventilatory support.

Ventilatory support can be delivered by invasive or noninvasive mechanical ventilation. NIV avoids potential complications of invasive ventilation, such as airway injury from intubation, requirements for sedation, and ventilator-associated pneumonia. Randomized clinical trials[28,93] and meta-analyses[84,94,95] have compared outcomes of NIV with standard care. The meta-analyses established benefit for patients with more severe disease in decreasing mortality and need for intubation.[84,94] A regression analysis of primary studies recommends NIV for patients with a pH less than 7.37 or a $Paco_2$ greater than 55 mm Hg.[95]

NIV may be delivered with either an oronasal or nasal mask, but a comfortable mask fit is important for patient acceptance. Most clinical trials have used NIV, but successful outcomes have been reported with CPAP.[96] Patients managed with NIV require close monitoring because up to 50% of patients may fail and require intubation.

Patients who fail NIV or have immediately life-threatening respiratory failure (severe hypoxemia, hypercapnia, hemodynamic instability, altered mental status, or increased work of breathing with impending apnea) require intubation and mechanical ventilation. Initial ventilator settings should limit the inspiratory effort necessary to trigger the ventilator to reduce work of breathing and allow recovery from respiratory muscle fatigue. The mode of ventilation, V_T, respiratory rate, and inspiratory flow rate should be adjusted to ensure that fatigued respiratory muscles are adequately unloaded and dynamic hyperinflation improved or eliminated.

Invasive ventilation presents the greatest risk in COPD for severe dynamic hyperinflation because the ventilator can deliver a V_T and $\dot{V}_E$ beyond the patient's expiratory capabilities if an insufficient expiratory time is provided (**Box 33-13**). The resulting air trapping and

BOX 33-13

Guidelines for Initial Ventilator Settings for Patients with COPD

- Set respiratory rate low, 8–12 breaths/min.
- Set initial tidal volume at 6–8 mL/kg.
- Start Fio_2 initially at 100%, obtain arterial blood gas values, and wean oxygen to provide an oxygen saturation of 90% to 92% with Fio_2 goals of 40%.
- Adjust PEEP between 0 and 5 cm H_2O to manage ventilator triggering and auto-PEEP.
- Set peak flow high to provide adequate expiratory time.
- Avoid overventilation and target baseline $Paco_2$.
- Monitor auto-PEEP, peak pressure, and plateau pressure to avoid dynamic hyperinflation and barotrauma.
- Consider early extubation to noninvasive positive pressure ventilation.

Fio_2, fraction inspired oxygen; $Paco_2$, partial pressure of arterial carbon dioxide; PEEP, positive end-expiratory pressure.

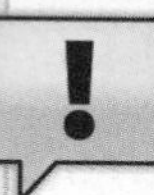

Respiratory Recap

Goals of Invasive Mechanical Ventilation in the Patient with COPD

- Unload ventilatory muscles and allow the patient to rest and recover from fatigue
- Provide an adequate expiratory time to avoid auto-PEEP and dynamic hyperinflation
- Prevent overventilation and respiratory alkalosis
- Prevent patient–ventilator asynchrony or excessive effort to trigger the ventilator

auto-PEEP cause lung overdistension, patient discomfort, and patient–ventilator asynchrony in addition to barotrauma-related complications (e.g., pneumothorax, hemodynamic instability). Hemodynamic instability occurs because auto-PEEP decreases venous return and cardiac output.[97]

Overdistention of lung regions can compress functional adjacent lung units and aggravate $\dot{V}/\dot{Q}$ mismatch, which may worsen hypoxia and paradoxically increase $Paco_2$ with further increases in $\dot{V}E$. Additionally, auto-PEEP increases inspiratory effort by increasing the amount of negative intrathoracic pressure necessary to trigger the ventilator.

The ventilator should be set to avoid dynamic hyperinflation. Respiratory rate, VT, inspiratory flow waveform, and inspiratory-to-expiratory (I:E) ratio should be set to allow a sufficient expiratory time. Some patients with extreme air trapping may require heavy sedation and paralysis to allow tolerance of a low respiratory rate that provides a longer expiratory time and permits less air trapping. Application of PEEP may improve dynamic hyperinflation by countering airway closure during exhalation. Applied PEEP theoretically stents open airways and increases expiratory flow. Multiple studies demonstrate that applied PEEP in this setting may have no effect, may decrease inspiratory flow, or may increase inspiratory flow with beneficial effects not occurring until applied PEEP approaches 80% of the auto-PEEP.[98] Determining the appropriate PEEP setting for an individual patient to avoid adverse effects remains a challenge with existing methods that employ an airway occlusion technique or an esophageal balloon. Some authorities discount the value of applied PEEP in stenting open airways, although evidence supports that it can reduce triggering effort. Some patients with air trapping may experience decreased auto-PEEP and work of breathing with application of helium–oxygen mixtures.[99]

After starting mechanical ventilation, caregivers should monitor patients for the presence of air trapping. Rising plateau pressures (Pplat), which should be low in patients with emphysema because of high lung compliance, suggest the pressure of auto-PEEP. The flow–time curves can also suggest the presence of auto-PEEP by demonstrating that expiratory flow continues to the initiation of inspiration. Quantifying actual values of auto-PEEP for spontaneously breathing patients remains challenging because minimal inspiratory or expiratory patient efforts have large effects on measured auto-PEEP values.[97]

Respiratory parameters measured at the bedside are poor predictors of extubation readiness.[100] Among patients with COPD who are difficult to liberate from mechanical ventilation, no differences exist between pressure support weaning versus spontaneous breathing trials.[101] Patients who fail a spontaneous breathing trial after 48 hours of ventilation have been shown to benefit from extubation to NIV.[102] In patients who pass a spontaneous breathing trial, extubation directly to NIV may prevent extubation failure.[103] Breathing a helium–oxygen mixture may decrease work of breathing after extubation but has not been shown to prevent extubation failure.[104] Elevation of *N*-terminal pro-brain natriuretic peptide blood levels in difficult-to-wean patients may identify patients with clinically occult heart failure as the cause of extubation failure.[105] Patients treated with corticosteroids for a COPD exacerbation are at risk for critical illness-related neuromuscular disease. One study reported that 9 of 26 patients ventilated for more than 48 hours and treated with more than 240 mg of methylprednisolone a day developed acute quadriplegic myopathy.[106] This respiratory muscle weakness may make ventilator liberation more difficult.

Prolonged weaning failure warrants consideration of a tracheostomy. Conversion of a translaryngeal endotracheal tube to a tracheostomy increases patient comfort, provides easier access for suctioning, enhances patient mobility, and may allow a more aggressive weaning approach.[107] Patients also may have an improved sense of well being because of the ability to speak with a tracheostomy in place. No data indicate that a tracheostomy must be performed after any specific duration of translaryngeal intubation. Patients with COPD are considered for tracheostomy after an initial 7 days of mechanical ventilation if successful ventilator discontinuation is not imminent. Earlier tracheostomy can be performed if the severity of the illness makes extubation unlikely within a reasonable time. Considering that most of the benefits of tracheostomy are comfort related, it is less compelling to perform an early tracheostomy in patients with depressed mental status who are otherwise tolerating translaryngeal intubation well. The decision regarding tracheostomy should be based on the individual needs of a specific patient rather than general guidelines that direct routine tracheotomy only after 21 days of intubation.[108]

Palliative and End-of-Life Care

Patients with COPD may experience progressively worsening symptoms and quality of life as their disease becomes more severe. Palliative care provides opportunities to prevent and relieve suffering by managing symptoms and providing support to both patients and their families. As defined by the World Health Organization, palliative care is "an approach that improves the quality of life of patients and their families facing the problems associated with life-threatening illness, through the prevention and relief of suffering by means of early identification and impeccable assessment and treatment of pain and other problems, including physical, psychosocial, and spiritual issues."[109] The ATS endorses the concept that palliative care should be available to patients at all stages of their illness and should be individualized based on the needs and preferences of the patient and the patient's family.[110] Caregivers of patients with COPD should have an understanding of palliative care and a willingness to consult with palliative care specialists to assist with special patient needs.

Most patients hospitalized for COPD exacerbations survive to hospital discharge. A subgroup of patients, however, present with acute respiratory failure as the terminal event. Intubation and life support are burdensome for this group of patients and may prolong their dying process. Unfortunately, clinical and laboratory findings available at the time of admission are poor discriminators between those patients who will survive their hospitalization and those who will not recover. In such circumstances, clinicians having a clear understanding of their patients' end-of-life wishes aid decisions about the withdrawal of life support. Patients can formulate their own decisions about the acceptability of life support by blending their life goals and values with their physicians' estimates of anticipated outcome from life support interventions. This process centers on a patient's ability to provide informed decision making and requires an ongoing dialogue among patients, families, and caregivers.

Nonphysician educators can supplement physician discussions on end-of-life issues to promote patients' abilities to provide informed decisions. Nurses, for instance, often have heightened sensitivities to their patients' needs and greater opportunities than physicians for discussing emotionally charged issues, such as advance planning. Although not yet studied, end-of-life discussions initiated by respiratory therapists may effectively introduce patients with COPD to topics of life support and advance planning during hospitalizations, home visits, and enrollment in pulmonary rehabilitation. Patients have demonstrated that they are willing to learn about advance planning from a wide range of nonphysician sources.[111] The Society of Critical Care Medicine encourages all members of the healthcare team, physicians and nonphysicians alike, to initiate discussions with their patients about end-of-life issues.

Patients with severe COPD who choose to forgo life supportive care in the terminal phases of their disease must be continuously reassured by all caregivers that they will not be medically or emotionally abandoned. Intensive comfort care and close monitoring to detect a need for aggressive pain, anxiety, and dyspnea relief are fundamentally important. In such settings, the principle of double effect ethically, morally, and legally allows the administration of sufficient sedatives and analgesics to relieve pain and suffering even if drug therapy accelerates the patient's death, as long as the intent is to relieve suffering.[110] Alternatives to acute care hospitalization do exist for patients with terminal COPD. COPD is recognized as a condition warranting hospice services by the National Hospice Organization, which has published guidelines to identify patients who qualify for hospice care (**Box 33-14**).

Case Studies

Case 1. Initial Presentation of Chronic Obstructive Pulmonary Disease

During a routine physical examination, a 62-year-old woman complains of increasing shortness of breath with exertion. She has a 40-year smoking history and presently smokes one pack of filtered cigarettes per day. She reports occasional nonproductive cough but denies ever having symptoms compatible with an exacerbation of COPD. Physical examination reveals bilateral breath sounds with no adventitious sounds. Respiratory rate and pattern are normal at rest. No cyanosis or edema is present, and the remainder of the history and physical examination are unremarkable. She is referred to the pulmonary clinic for consultation, pulmonary function testing, and arterial blood gas analysis.

Results of pulmonary function testing are an FVC of 2.10 L (80% predicted), FEV_1 of 1.20 L (65% of predicted), and FEV_1/FVC of 58%. After administration of inhaled β_2-agonist, the FEV_1 increases to 1.35 L (73% of predicted). Lung volumes (residual volume, functional residual capacity, and total lung capacity) reveal mild hyperinflation. Single-breath DLCO is 70% of predicted. Arterial blood gases on the breathing of room air are pH 7.42, $Paco_2$ 39 mm Hg, and Pao_2 72 mm Hg. A chest radiograph is unremarkable other than giving the suggestion of mild hyperinflation.

The patient is counseled in the office about the importance of stopping smoking and referred to a smoking cessation program. She receives influenza and pneumococcal vaccinations. Albuterol by MDI is prescribed every 4 to 6 hours as needed to relieve symptoms. She is told to use the MDI before exertion if she anticipates dyspnea. She is instructed in the proper use of inhalers with a valved holding chamber.

BOX 33-14

Parameters to Identify Patients Who Qualify for Hospice Services

Patients will be considered to be in the terminal stage of pulmonary disease (life expectancy of 6 months or less) if they meet the following criteria. The criteria refer to patients with various forms of advanced pulmonary disease who eventually follow a final common pathway for end-stage pulmonary disease. (Criteria 1 and 2 should be present. Criteria 3, 4, and 5 will lend supporting documentation.)

1. Severe chronic lung disease as documented by both a and b:
   a. Disabling dyspnea at rest, poor response or unresponsive to bronchodilators, resulting in decreased functional capacity (e.g., bed-to-chair existence), fatigue, and cough. (Documentation of FEV_1, after bronchodilator, less than 30% of predicted is objective evidence for disabling dyspnea, but is not necessary to obtain.)
   b. Progression of end-stage pulmonary disease, as evidenced by increasing visits to the emergency department or hospitalizations for pulmonary infections and/or respiratory failure or increasing physician home visits before initial certification. (Documentation of serial decrease of FEV_1 >40 mL/yr is objective evidence for disease progression, but is not necessary to obtain.)
2. Hypoxemia at rest on ambient air, as evidenced by Po_2 less than or equal to 55 mm Hg; or oxygen saturation less than or equal to 88% on supplemental oxygen determined either by arterial blood gases or oxygen saturation monitors; *OR* hypercapnia, as evidenced by Pco_2 ≥50 mm Hg. These values may be obtained from recent (within 3 months) hospital records.
3. Right heart failure secondary to pulmonary disease (cor pulmonale) (e.g., not secondary to left heart disease or valvulopathy).
4. Unintentional progressive weight loss of greater than 10% of body weight over the preceding 6 months.
5. Resting tachycardia >100/minute.

 From Lanken PN, Terry PB, Delisser HM, et al. An official American Thoracic Society clinical policy statement: palliative care for patients with respiratory diseases and critical illnesses. *Am J Respir Crit Care Med*. 2008;177:912–927.

Pulmonary rehabilitation is arranged. She is scheduled for a follow-up at 2 months to evaluate her symptoms and exercise capability after smoking cessation and rehabilitation. If she remains exercise limited, long-acting inhaled bronchodilator therapy will be presented as an opportunity to improve her symptoms and quality of life. The potential benefits of preventing exacerbations and diminishing her decline in lung function by long-acting bronchodilator therapy will also be discussed.

Case 2. Exacerbation of Chronic Obstructive Pulmonary Disease

A 72-year-old man with a history of severe COPD is admitted to the emergency department with progressively increasing dyspnea over the past 48 hours. He uses continuous home oxygen at 2 L/min. He also uses inhaled albuterol, fluticasone (a corticosteroid), and tiotropium by MDI. His sputum became purulent 3 days ago, and his primary care physician prescribed antibiotic therapy (azithromycin). The patient has a respiratory rate of 30 breaths/min with use of accessory muscles and pursed lip exhalation. Breath sounds are distant, but no adventitious sounds are present. The chest is hyperinflated. Mild neck vein distention and ankle edema are present. The electrocardiogram is normal, with the exception of a mild tachycardia (110 beats/min). The patient appears dyspneic, but he cooperates with the physical examination. Arterial blood gas values are obtained with the patient breathing oxygen at 2 L/min: pH 7.28, $Paco_2$ 78 mm Hg, and Pao_2 52 mm Hg.

A nebulizer treatment has been administered with albuterol and ipratropium. Prednisone is given at a dose of 40 mg, and an antibiotic (moxifloxacin) is started. NIV is initiated. An oronasal mask is necessary because of the patient's dyspnea and inability to maintain a closed mouth. After 30 minutes of ventilation, accessory muscle use decreases, respiratory rate improves, and dyspnea is reported by the patient to be better. Inspired oxygen is titrated to maintain a Spo_2 of 88% to 90%. Preparations are made to admit him to the ICU.

Two hours later, the patient is in the ICU. He continues on NIV, but appears more comfortable. Arterial blood gas values at this time are pH 7.36, $Paco_2$ 65 mm Hg, and Pao_2 66 mm Hg. Four hours later, the patient asks to have the mask removed. He initially appears comfortable, but after 1 hour he has increasing dyspnea and accessory muscle use. NIV is resumed at the previous settings, but with the use of a nasal mask instead of the oronasal mask. This pattern of failed attempts to discontinue NIV continues for the next 36 hours, at which time the patient remains comfortable after removal of the mask.

Six hours after discontinuation of NIV, his arterial blood gas values breathing 2 L/min of oxygen by nasal cannula are pH 7.37, $Paco_2$ 60 mm Hg, and Pao_2 62 mm Hg. The patient is transferred from the ICU to a general ward.

The following day, he continues to do well, and plans are made for discharge home. Options related to future exacerbations are discussed with the patient and his wife. He decides that NIV may be used for future exacerbations, but he elects not to be intubated or receive other resuscitative measures if he fails NIV. He completes a living will and advance directive for healthcare and ensures that his healthcare providers have future access to this information.

Key Points

- Chronic obstructive pulmonary disease is the fourth most common cause of death in the United States, and its prevalence is increasing worldwide.
- Airflow limitation defines the presence of COPD. Both central and peripheral airways are affected by inflammatory and immunologic changes, but most of the observed increased airway resistance occurs in the peripheral airways.
- Smoking is the cause of COPD in 85% to 90% of patients. The prognosis of this progressive disorder is improved at any age with smoking cessation.
- Although existing clinical practice guidelines stage the severity of COPD by FEV_1, patients' quality of life and prognosis relate more closely to multidimensional measures that assess both respiratory and systemic features of COPD.
- The BODE index (body mass index, airflow obstruction, dyspnea, and exercise capacity) provides clinicians with a comprehensive measure of the severity of disease and response to therapy.
- COPD is a treatable disease. Management is directed toward reducing symptoms and improving quality of life, reducing decline in lung function, preventing complications, preventing or minimizing adverse effects of therapy, and prolonging survival.
- NIV improves outcomes of patients with COPD exacerbation.
- Palliative care and end-of-life planning are important components in the management of patients with all stages of COPD.

References

1. National Heart, Lung and Blood Institute. *COPD: for Healthcare Professionals*. (ND). Available at: http://www.nhlbi.nih.gov/health/public/lung/copd/health-care-professionals/index.htm. Accessed August 9, 2014.
2. World Health Organization. *Chronic Respiratory Diseases. Burden of COPD*. Available at: http://www.who.int/respiratory/copd/burden/en/index.html. Accessed August 9, 2014.
3. Fabbri LM, Luppi F, Beghe B, Rabe KF. Complex chronic comorbidities of COPD. *Eur Respir J*. 2008;31:204–212.
4. Global Strategy for the Diagnosis, Management and Prevention of COPD, Global Initiative for Chronic Obstructive Lung Disease (GOLD) 2014. Available at: http://www.goldcopd.org/. Accessed August 9, 2014.
5. Speizer FE. The rise in chronic obstructive pulmonary disease mortality: overview and summary. *Am Rev Respir Dis*. 1989;140(Suppl 1): S106–S107.
6. Muller NL, Coxson H. Chronic obstructive pulmonary disease. Part 4: imaging the lungs in patients with chronic obstructive pulmonary disease. *Thorax*. 2002;57:982–985.
7. The definition of emphysema. Report of a National Heart, Lung, and Blood Institute, Division of Lung Diseases workshop. *Am Rev Respir Dis*. 1985;132:182–185.
8. Celli BR, Cote CG, Marin JM, et al. The body-mass index, airflow obstruction, dyspnea, and exercise capacity index in chronic obstructive pulmonary disease. *N Engl J Med*. 2004;350: 1005–1012.
9. Celli BR, Halbert RJ, Nordyke RJ, Schau B. Airway obstruction in never smokers: results from the Third National Health and Nutrition Examination Survey. *Am J Med*. 2005;118: 1364–1372.
10. Stoller JK, Fromer L, Brantly M, et al. Primary care diagnosis of alpha-1 antitrypsin deficiency: issues and opportunities. *Cleve Clin J Med*. 2007;74:869–874.
11. Silverman EK, Weiss ST, Drazen JM, et al. Gender-related differences in severe, early-onset chronic obstructive pulmonary disease. *Am J Respir Crit Care Med*. 2000;162:2152–2158.
12. Prescott E, Lange P, Vestbo J. Socioeconomic status, lung function and admission to hospital for COPD: results from the Copenhagen City Heart Study. *Eur Respir J*. 1999;13:1109–1114.
13. Churg A, Wright JL. Animal models of cigarette smoke-induced chronic obstructive lung disease. *Contrib Microbiol*. 2007;14:113–125.
14. Jeffery PK. Comparative morphology of the airways in asthma and chronic obstructive pulmonary disease. *Am J Respir Crit Care Med*. 1994;150(5 Pt 2):S6–S13.
15. Jeffery PK. Remodeling and inflammation of bronchi in asthma and chronic obstructive pulmonary disease. *Proc Am Thorac Soc*. 2004;1:176–183.
16. Curtis JL, Freeman CM, Hogg JC. The immunopathogenesis of chronic obstructive pulmonary disease: insights from recent research. *Proc Am Thorac Soc*. 2007;4:512–521.
17. Lee SH, Goswami S, Grudo A, et al. Antielastin autoimmunity in tobacco smoking-induced emphysema. *Nat Med*. 2007;13: 567–569.
18. Di Stefano A, Capelli A, Lusuardi M, et al. Severity of airflow limitation is associated with severity of airway inflammation in smokers. *Am J Respir Crit Care Med*. 1998;158:1277–1285.

19. O'Donnell DE. Ventilatory limitations in chronic obstructive pulmonary disease. *Med Sci Sports Exerc.* 2001;33(Suppl 1): S647–S655.
20. Dykstra BJ, Scanlon PD, Kester MM, Beck KC, Enright PL. Lung volumes in 4,774 patients with obstructive lung disease. *Chest.* 1999;115:68–74.
21. Parot S, Miara B, Milic-Emili J, et al. Hypoxemia, hypercapnia, and breathing patterns in patients with chronic obstructive pulmonary disease. *Am Rev Respir Dis.* 1982;126:882–886.
22. Killian K. Dyspnea. *J Appl Physiol.* 2006;101:1013–1014.
23. O'Donnell DE, Sciurba F, Celli B, et al. Effect of fluticasone propionate/salmeterol on lung hyperinflation and exercise endurance in COPD. *Chest.* 2006;130:647–656.
24. Celli BR, Thomas NE, Anderson JA, et al. Effect of pharmacotherapy on rate of decline of lung function in chronic obstructive pulmonary disease: results from the TORCH study. *Am J Respir Crit Care Med.* 2008;178:332–338.
25. Anthonisen NR, Skeans MA, Wise RA, et al. The effects of a smoking cessation intervention on 14.5-year mortality: a randomized clinical trial. *Ann Intern Med.* 2005;142:233–239.
26. Nocturnal Oxygen Therapy Trial Group. Continuous or nocturnal oxygen therapy in hypoxemic chronic obstructive lung disease: a clinical trial. *Ann Intern Med.* 1980;93:391–398.
27. Fishman A, Martinez F, Naunheim K, et al. A randomized trial comparing lung-volume-reduction surgery with medical therapy for severe emphysema. *N Engl J Med.* 2003;348: 2059–2073.
28. Bott J, Carroll MP, Conway JH, et al. Randomised controlled trial of nasal ventilation in acute ventilatory failure due to chronic obstructive airways disease. *Lancet.* 1993;341:1555–1557.
29. Nici L, Donner C, Wouters E, et al. American Thoracic Society/European Respiratory Society statement on pulmonary rehabilitation. *Am J Respir Crit Care Med.* 2006;173:1390–1413.
30. Rigotti NA, Munafo MR, Murphy MF, Stead LF. Interventions for smoking cessation in hospitalised patients. *Cochrane Database Syst Rev.* 2003;CD001837.
31. Fiore MC, Jaén CR, Baker TB, et al. *Treating Tobacco Use and Dependence: 2008 Update.* Clinical Practice Guideline. Rockville, MD: U.S. Department of Health and Human Services, Public Health Service; May 2008.
32. Silagy C, Lancaster T, Stead L, et al. Nicotine replacement therapy for smoking cessation. *Cochrane Database Syst Rev.* 2004; CD000146.
33. Blondal T, Gudmundsson LJ, Olafsdottir I, et al. Nicotine nasal spray with nicotine patch for smoking cessation: randomised trial with six year follow up. *BMJ.* 1999;318:285–288.
34. Jorenby DE, Leischow SJ, Nides MA, et al. A controlled trial of sustained-release bupropion, a nicotine patch, or both for smoking cessation. *N Engl J Med.* 1999;340:685–691.
35. Gonzales D, Rennard SI, Nides M, et al. Varenicline, an a4b2 nicotinic acetylcholine receptor partial agonist, vs sustained-release bupropion and placebo for smoking cessation: a randomized controlled trial. *JAMA.* 2006;296:47–55.
36. COMBIVENT Inhalation Aerosol Study Group. In chronic obstructive pulmonary disease, a combination of ipratropium bromide and albuterol is more effective than either agent alone. An 85-day multicenter trial. *Chest.* 1994;105:1411–1419.
37. Nelson HS. β-Adrenergic bronchodilators. *N Engl J Med.* 1995;333: 499–506.
38. Celli BR. Update on the management of COPD. *Chest.* 2008;133: 1451–1462.
39. Rennard SI, Anderson W, ZuWallack R, et al. Use of a long-acting inhaled β_2-adrenergic agonist, salmeterol xinafoate, in patients with chronic obstructive pulmonary disease. *Am J Respir Crit Care Med.* 2001;163:1087–1092.
40. Hanrahan JP, Hanania NA, Calhoun WJ, et al. Effect of nebulized arformoterol on airway function in COPD: results from two randomized trials. *COPD.* 2008;5:25–34.
41. Rodrigo GJ, Nannini LJ, Rodriguez-Roisin R. Safety of long-acting beta-agonists in stable COPD: a systematic review. *Chest.* 2008;133:1079–1087.
42. Easton PA, Jadue C, Dhingra S, et al. A comparison of the bronchodilating effects of a beta-2 adrenergic agent (albuterol) and an anticholinergic agent (ipratropium bromide), given by aerosol alone or in sequence. *N Engl J Med.* 1986;315:735–739.
43. Lee TA, Pickard AS, Au DH, et al. Risk for death associated with medications for recently diagnosed chronic obstructive pulmonary disease. *Ann Intern Med.* 2008;149:380–390.
44. Tashkin DP, Celli B, Senn S, et al. A 4-year trial of tiotropium in chronic obstructive pulmonary disease. *N Engl J Med.* 2008;359: 1543–1554.
45. Casaburi R, Kukafka D, Cooper CB, et al. Improvement in exercise tolerance with the combination of tiotropium and pulmonary rehabilitation in patients with COPD. *Chest.* 2005;127: 809–817.
46. Rodrigo GJ, Nannini LJ. Tiotropium for the treatment of stable chronic obstructive pulmonary disease: a systematic review with meta-analysis. *Pulm Pharmacol Ther.* 2007;20:495–502.
47. Fuhr R, Magnussen H, Sarem K, et al. Efficacy of aclidinium bromide 400 mcg twice daily compared with placebo and tiotropium in patients with moderate to severe COPD. *Chest.* 2012;141:745–752.
48. Karabis A, Lindner L, Mocarski M, et al. Comparative efficacy of aclidinium versus glycopyrronium and tiotropium, as maintenance treatment of moderate to severe COPD patients: a systematic review and network meta-analysis. *Int J Chron Obstruct Pulmon Dis.* 2013;8: 405–423.
49. Barnes PJ, Ito K, Adcock IM. Corticosteroid resistance in chronic obstructive pulmonary disease: inactivation of histone deacetylase. *Lancet.* 2004;363:731–733.
50. Chong J. Phosphodiesterase 4 inhibitors for chronic obstructive pulmonary disease. *Cochrane Database Syst Rev*, 2011.
51. Burge PS, Calverley PM, Jones PW, et al. Randomised, double blind, placebo controlled study of fluticasone propionate in patients with moderate to severe chronic obstructive pulmonary disease: the ISOLDE trial. *BMJ.* 2000;320:1297–1303.
52. The Lung Health Study Research Group. Effect of inhaled triamcinolone on the decline in pulmonary function in chronic obstructive pulmonary disease. *N Engl J Med.* 2000;343:1902–1909.
53. Karpel JP, Kotch A, Zinny M, et al. A comparison of inhaled ipratropium, oral theophylline plus inhaled beta-agonist, and the combination of all three in patients with COPD. *Chest.* 1994;105: 1089–1094.
54. ZuWallack RL, Mahler DA, Reilly D, et al. Salmeterol plus theophylline combination therapy in the treatment of COPD. *Chest.* 2001;119: 1661–1670.
55. van Noord JA, de Munck DR, Bantje TA, et al. Long-term treatment of chronic obstructive pulmonary disease with salmeterol and the additive effect of ipratropium. *Eur Respir J.* 2000;15:878–885.
56. van Noord JA, Aumann JL, Janssens E, et al. Effects of tiotropium with and without formoterol on airflow obstruction and resting hyperinflation in patients with COPD. *Chest.* 2006;129: 509–517.
57. Kerstjens HA, Bantje TA, Luursema PB, et al. Effects of short-acting bronchodilators added to maintenance tiotropium therapy. *Chest.* 2007;132:1493–1499.
58. Calverley PM, Boonsawat W, Cseke Z, et al. Maintenance therapy with budesonide and formoterol in chronic obstructive pulmonary disease. *Eur Respir J.* 2003;22:912–919.
59. Adams SG, Melo J, Luther M, Anzueto A. Antibiotics are associated with lower relapse rates in outpatients with acute exacerbations of COPD. *Chest.* 2000;117:1345–1352.
60. Albert RK. Azithromycin for prevention of exacerbations of COPD. *N Engl J Med.* 2011:365:689. Correction: 2012;366:1356.
61. Petty TL. The National Mucolytic Study. Results of a randomized, double-blind, placebo-controlled study of iodinated glycerol in chronic obstructive bronchitis. *Chest.* 1990;97:75–83.

62. Decramer M, Rutten-van Molken M, Dekhuijzen PN, et al. Effects of *N*-acetylcysteine on outcomes in chronic obstructive pulmonary disease (Bronchitis Randomized on NAC Cost-Utility Study, BRONCUS): a randomised placebo-controlled trial. *Lancet.* 2005;365:1552–1560.
63. Anzueto A, Jubran A, Ohar JA, et al. Effects of aerosolized surfactant in patients with stable chronic bronchitis: a prospective randomized controlled trial. *JAMA.* 1997;278:1426–1431.
64. Criner GJ, Celli BR. Ventilatory muscle recruitment in exercise with O_2 in obstructed patients with mild hypoxemia. *J Appl Physiol.* 1987;63:195–200.
65. Tarpy SP, Celli BR. Long-term oxygen therapy. *N Engl J Med.* 1995;333:710–714.
66. Simonds AK, Elliott MW. Outcome of domiciliary nasal intermittent positive pressure ventilation in restrictive and obstructive disorders. *Thorax.* 1995;50:604–609.
67. Kolodziej MA, Jensen L, Rowe B, Sin D. Systematic review of noninvasive positive pressure ventilation in severe stable COPD. *Eur Respir J.* 2007;30:293–306.
68. Krachman S, Minai OA, Scharf SM. Sleep abnormalities and treatment in emphysema. *Proc Am Thorac Soc.* 2008;5:536–542.
69. O'Donohue WJ Jr, Bowman TJ. Hypoxemia during sleep in patients with chronic obstructive pulmonary disease: significance, detection, and effects of therapy. *Respir Care.* 2000;45:188–191; discussion 192–193.
70. O'Donoghue FJ, Catcheside PG, Ellis EE, et al. Sleep hypoventilation in hypercapnic chronic obstructive pulmonary disease: prevalence and associated factors. *Eur Respir J.* 2003;21:977–984.
71. Ries AL, Bauldoff GS, Carlin BW, et al. Pulmonary rehabilitation: joint ACCP/AACVPR evidence-based clinical practice guidelines. *Chest.* 2007;131(suppl 5):4S–42S.
72. Benditt JO. Surgical options for patients with COPD: sorting out the choices. *Respir Care.* 2006;51:173–182.
73. Morgan MD, Denison DM, Strickland B. Value of computed tomography for selecting patients with bullous lung disease for surgery. *Thorax.* 1986;41:855–862.
74. Snyder ML, Goss CH, Neradilek B, et al. Changes in arterial oxygenation and self-reported oxygen use after lung volume reduction surgery. *Am J Respir Crit Care Med.* 2008;178:339–345.
75. Edelman JD, Kotloff RM. Surgical approaches to advanced emphysema. *Respir Care Clin North Am.* 1998;4:513–539.
76. Orens JB, Estenne M, Arcasoy S, et al. International guidelines for the selection of lung transplant candidates: 2006 update—a consensus report from the Pulmonary Scientific Council of the International Society for Heart and Lung Transplantation. *J Heart Lung Transplant.* 2006;25:745–755.
77. Schulman LL. Lung transplantation for chronic obstructive pulmonary disease. *Clin Chest Med.* 2000;21:849–865.
78. Hosenpud JD, Bennett LE, Keck BM, et al. Effect of diagnosis on survival benefit of lung transplantation for end-stage lung disease. *Lancet.* 1998;351:24–27.
79. Bavaria JE, Kotloff R, Palevsky H, et al. Bilateral versus single lung transplantation for chronic obstructive pulmonary disease. *J Thorac Cardiovasc Surg.* 1997;113:520–527; discussion 528.
80. Pellegrino R, Rodarte JR, Frost AE, Reid MB. Breathing by double-lung recipients during exercise: response to expiratory threshold loading. *Am J Respir Crit Care Med.* 1998;157:106–110.
81. Gross CR, Savik K, Bolman RMR, Hertz MI. Long-term health status and quality of life outcomes of lung transplant recipients. *Chest.* 1995;108:1587–1593.
82. Sethi S, Sethi R, Eschberger K, et al. Airway bacterial concentrations and exacerbations of chronic obstructive pulmonary disease. *Am J Respir Crit Care Med.* 2007;176:356–361.
83. Connors AF Jr, Dawson NV, Thomas C, et al. Outcomes following acute exacerbation of severe chronic obstructive lung disease. The SUPPORT (Study to Understand Prognoses and Preferences for Outcomes and Risks of Treatments) investigators. *Am J Respir Crit Care Med.* 1996;154:959–967.
84. Quon BS, Gan WQ, Sin DD. Contemporary management of acute exacerbations of COPD: a systematic review and metaanalysis. *Chest.* 2008;133:756–766.
85. Siempos II, Dimopoulos G, Korbila IP, et al. Macrolides, quinolones and amoxicillin/clavulanate for chronic bronchitis: a meta-analysis. *Eur Respir J.* 2007;29:1127–1137.
86. Thompson WH, Nielson CP, Carvalho P, et al. Controlled trial of oral prednisone in outpatients with acute COPD exacerbation. *Am J Respir Crit Care Med.* 1996;154:407–412.
87. Stevenson NJ, Walker PP, Costello RW, Calverley PM. Lung mechanics and dyspnea during exacerbations of chronic obstructive pulmonary disease. *Am J Respir Crit Care Med.* 2005;172:1510–1516.
88. McCrory DC, Brown CD. Inhaled short-acting β2-agonists versus ipratropium for acute exacerbations of chronic obstructive pulmonary disease. *Cochrane Database Syst Rev.* 2001;2.
89. Cazzola M, Spina D, Matera MG. The use of bronchodilators in stable chronic obstructive pulmonary disease. *Pulm Pharmacol Ther.* 1997;10:128–144.
90. Barr RG, Rowe BH, Camargo CAJ. Methylxanthines for exacerbations of chronic obstructive pulmonary disease: meta-analysis of randomised trials. *BMJ.* 2003;327:643.
91. Leuppi JD. Short-term vs conventional glucocorticoid therapy in acute exacerbations of chronic obstructive pulmonary disease: the REDUCE randomized clinical trial. *JAMA.* 2013: 309:2223–2231.
92. Walters JA. Different durations of corticosteroid therapy for exacerbations of chronic obstructive pulmonary disease. *Cochrane Database Syst Rev.* 2011.
93. Martin TJ, Hovis JD, Costantino JP, et al. A randomized, prospective evaluation of noninvasive ventilation for acute respiratory failure. *Am J Respir Crit Care Med.* 2000;161:807–813.
94. Keenan SP, Sinuff T, Cook DJ, Hill NS. Which patients with acute exacerbation of chronic obstructive pulmonary disease benefit from noninvasive positive-pressure ventilation? A systematic review of the literature. *Ann Intern Med.* 2003;138:861–870.
95. Peter JV, Moran JL. Noninvasive ventilation in exacerbations of chronic obstructive pulmonary disease: implications of different meta-analytic strategies. *Ann Intern Med.* 2004;141(5): W78–W79.
96. Goldberg P, Reissmann H, Maltais F, et al. Efficacy of noninvasive CPAP in COPD with acute respiratory failure. *Eur Respir J.* 1995;8:1894–1900.
97. Tuxen DV, Lane S. The effects of ventilatory pattern on hyperinflation, airway pressures, and circulation in mechanical ventilation of patients with severe air-flow obstruction. *Am Rev Respir Dis.* 1987; 136:872–879.
98. Dambrosio M, Cinnella G, Brienza N, et al. Effects of positive end-expiratory pressure on right ventricular function in COPD patients during acute ventilatory failure. *Intensive Care Med.* 1996;22:923–932.
99. Tassiopoulos AK, Kwon SS, Labropoulos N, et al. Predictors of early discharge following open abdominal aortic aneurysm repair. *Ann Vasc Surg.* 2004;18:218–222.
100. Alvisi R, Volta CA, Righini ER, et al. Predictors of weaning outcome in chronic obstructive pulmonary disease patients. *Eur Respir J.* 2000;15:656–662.
101. Reissmann HK, Ranieri VM, Goldberg P, Gottfried SB. Continuous positive airway pressure facilitates spontaneous breathing in weaning chronic obstructive pulmonary disease patients by improving breathing pattern and gas exchange. *Intensive Care Med.* 2000;26:1764–1772.
102. Nava S, Ambrosino N, Clini E, et al. Noninvasive mechanical ventilation in the weaning of patients with respiratory failure due to chronic obstructive pulmonary disease. A randomized controlled trial. *Ann Intern Med.* 1998;128:721–728.
103. Ferrer M, Sellarés J, Valencia M, et al. Non-invasive ventilation after extubation in hypercapnic patients with chronic respiratory disorders: randomised controlled trial. *Lancet.* 2009;374: 1082–1088.

104. Diehl JL, Mercat A, Guerot E, et al. Helium/oxygen mixture reduces the work of breathing at the end of the weaning process in patients with severe chronic obstructive pulmonary disease. *Crit Care Med.* 2003;31:1415–1420.
105. Grasso S, Leone A, De Michele M, et al. Use of *N*-terminal pro-brain natriuretic peptide to detect acute cardiac dysfunction during weaning failure in difficult-to-wean patients with chronic obstructive pulmonary disease. *Crit Care Med.* 2007;35: 96–105.
106. Amaya-Villar R, Garnacho-Montero J, Garcia-Garmendia JL, et al. Steroid-induced myopathy in patients intubated due to exacerbation of chronic obstructive pulmonary disease. *Intensive Care Med.* 2005;31:157–161.
107. Heffner JE. The role of tracheotomy in weaning. *Chest.* 2001;120: 477S–481S.
108. King C, Moores LK. Controversies in mechanical ventilation: when should a tracheotomy be placed? *Clin Chest Med.* 2008;29:253–263.
109. World Health Organization. Cancer. Palliative care is an essential part of cancer control. Available at: http://www.who.int/cancer /palliative/en. Accessed August 9, 2014.
110. Lanken PN, Terry PB, Delisser HM, et al. An official American Thoracic Society clinical policy statement: palliative care for patients with respiratory diseases and critical illnesses. *Am J Respir Crit Care Med.* 2008;177:912–927.
111. Heffner JE, Fahy B, Barbieri C. Advance directive education during pulmonary rehabilitation. *Chest.* 1996;109:2.

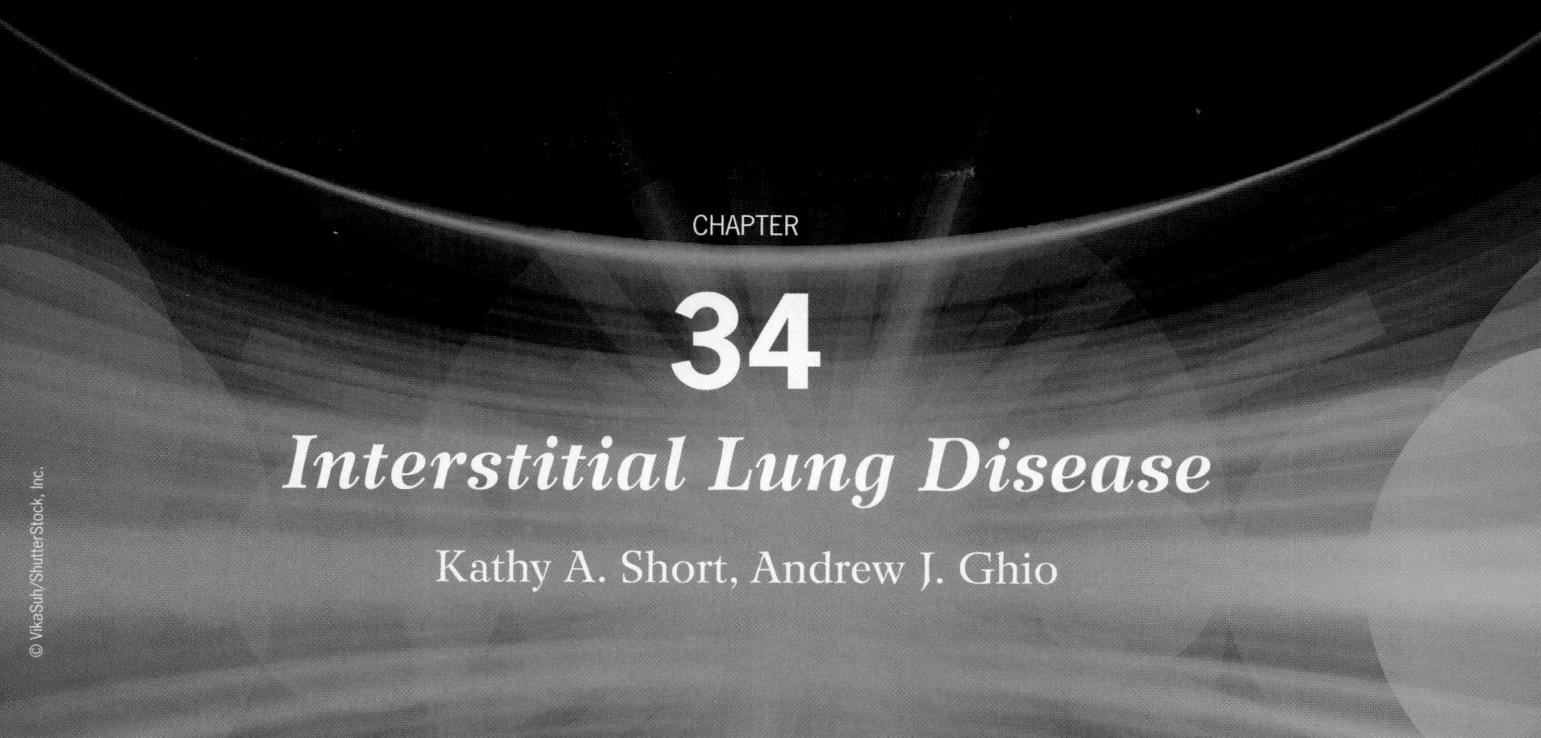

CHAPTER

34 Interstitial Lung Disease

Kathy A. Short, Andrew J. Ghio

OUTLINE

Pathophysiology
Classification
Clinical Presentation and Diagnostic Evaluation
Pathology
Prognosis
Management
Specific Interstitial Lung Diseases

OBJECTIVES

1. Describe the precipitating causes, clinical manifestations, and radiographic, laboratory, and pathophysiologic findings of interstitial lung disease.
2. Describe the diseases associated with pulmonary fibrosis.
3. Describe the management and therapy of interstitial lung disease.
4. Discuss the prognosis of interstitial lung disease.

KEY TERMS

bronchiolitis obliterans with organizing pneumonia (BOOP)
collagen vascular disease
eosinophilic granuloma
idiopathic pulmonary fibrosis (IPF)
interstitial lung disease (ILD)
pulmonary alveolar proteinosis (PAP)
respiratory bronchiolitis
sarcoidosis

Introduction

Interstitial lung disease (ILD) encompasses over 100 distinct diseases in which the interstitium is altered by some combination of inflammation and fibrosis. The interstitium of the lung includes the alveolar walls (and lumens), pulmonary microvasculature, interstitial macrophages, fibroblasts, myofibroblasts, and matrix components of the lungs (**Figure 34-1**). The inflammatory and fibrotic disorders of ILD can affect any of these components. The resulting infiltration of the acinar region by cellular and extracellular elements may either distort the alveolar and bronchiolar architecture or cause little associated damage (**Figure 34-2**).

ILD is an extremely diverse group of both acute and chronic disorders. Common clinical, radiographic, and pathophysiologic features form the basis for collective reference to this complex group of disorders as interstitial lung disease (**Box 34-1**). Most often the patient complains of dyspnea, a chest radiograph shows abnormal markings, and lung function tests demonstrate a loss of function including decreased volumes and reduced diffusing capacity. To make the diagnosis of ILD, the clinical presentation, radiographic findings, pulmonary function test results, laboratory values, and lung biopsy findings all must be correlated. In most cases, a definitive diagnosis cannot be made without a biopsy.

Pathophysiology

A common sequence of events that results in ILD begins when either a recognized or an unidentified agent induces alveolitis and vasculitis (**Box 34-2**). Persistence of this inflammatory lesion results in alveolar, capillary, and parenchymal cell injury. Abnormal repair leads to proliferation of mesenchymal cells, with the production of excess collagen and other extracellular matrix connective tissue elements. In the later stages of ILD, the normal architecture of the lung is replaced by cystic spaces separated by thick bands of fibrous tissue, a condition called *honeycomb lung*.

Although the end stage of the lung injury is histologically similar in many types of ILD, the alveolitis stage often is distinctive because of the number and

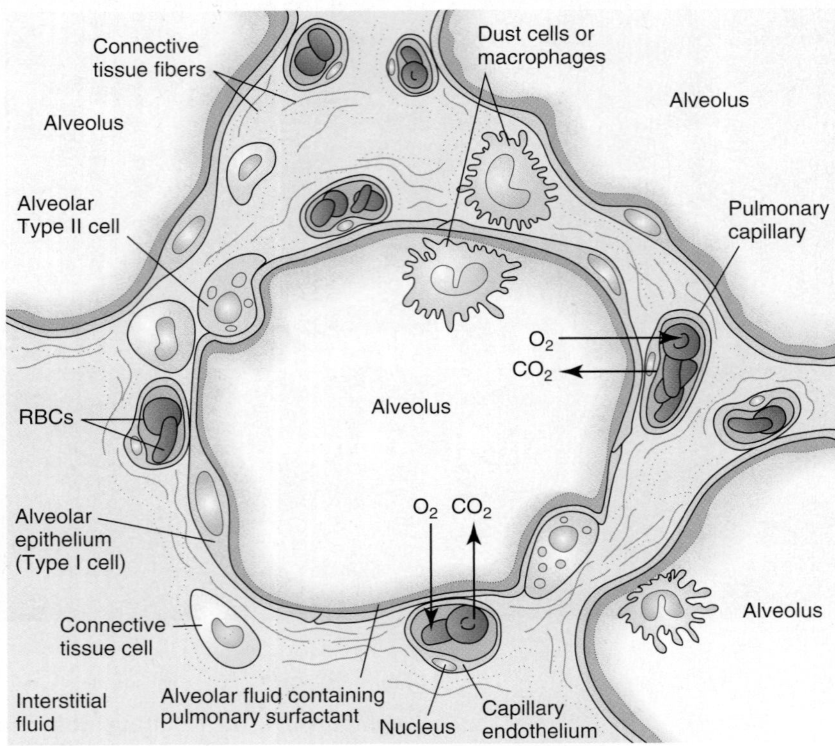

FIGURE 34-1 Schematic of lung illustrating components of the interstitium.

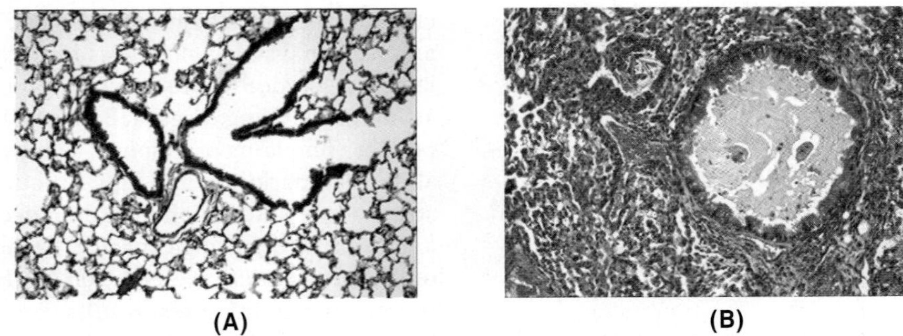

FIGURE 34-2 Micrographs showing (**A**) normal lung and (**B**) interstitial lung disease. In contrast to normal lung, there are alterations in the interstitium with an accumulation of inflammatory cells and subsequent widening. The stain is hematoxylin and eosin at a magnification of approximately 100.

BOX 34-1

Key Diagnostic Features of Interstitial Lung Disease

Dyspnea at rest or with exertion (or in both cases)

Bilateral diffuse interstitial infiltrates on chest radiograph

Physiologic abnormalities of a restrictive lung defect: decreased lung volumes, decreased diffusing capacity for carbon monoxide (DLCO), and abnormal difference between the alveolar and arterial oxygen pressure gradients ($P[A - a]O_2$) at rest and/or with exertion

Histopathologic features of inflammation or fibrosis (or both) of the pulmonary parenchyma

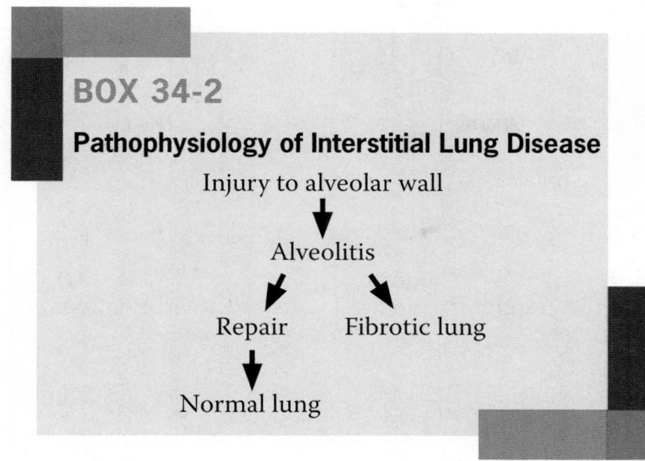

influence of various inflammatory and immune effector cells present, such as neutrophils, eosinophils, and lymphocytes. Oxidants (generated both exogenously and endogenously) and neutrophil proteases (e.g., elastase, collagenase, and cathepsins) are assumed to mediate some portion of tissue injury in many of these disorders. The alveolar macrophage was previously considered to coordinate this injury because of its release of reactive oxygen species, chemoattractants for neutrophils, and growth factors for mesenchymal cells, including fibronectin, platelet-derived growth factor, and insulin-like factor 1, which are involved in the progression to fibrosis. It has been demonstrated, however, that cells other than the alveolar macrophage, and resident in the lower respiratory tract, have a similar capacity to elaborate these same mediators and coordinate an inflammatory and fibrotic response to numerous agents.

BOX 34-2
Pathophysiology of Interstitial Lung Disease
Injury to alveolar wall
Alveolitis
Repair
Fibrotic lung
Normal lung

Classification

As a result of a lack of knowledge regarding causes of these diseases, a satisfactory classification system for ILD is not yet available. For practical purposes, it is useful to categorize the disorders by whether the cause is known or unknown (**Box 34-3**). An alternative criterion is the presence or absence of granulomas as a pathologic feature of the inflammatory process. Hypersensitivity pneumonitis, sarcoidosis, eosinophilic granuloma, Wegener granulomatosis, Churg-Strauss syndrome, and silicosis all are associated with the formation of granulomas. Idiopathic pulmonary fibrosis (IPF), connective tissue disorders, asbestosis, and disease caused by drugs, radiation, and toxic gas exposure are not associated with granulomas.

Clinical Presentation and Diagnostic Evaluation

Symptoms and Signs

Although some forms of ILD can present in an acute fashion, the most common presentation of ILD is a slowly progressive onset of dyspnea and a nonproductive cough. The dyspnea may occur on exertion at first but progresses to dyspnea at rest. The history is the most important tool in the identification of the cause of ILD. A thorough history limits the differential diagnosis and may preclude the need for biopsy. But even with a detailed history, the causative agent is identified in fewer than 20% to 30% of patients with ILD.[1]

To determine the causative agent of the ILD, the clinician must ask detailed questions and note specific symptoms. A list of all medications the patient has been taking should be compiled to detect drug-related causes of ILD. It should be remembered that patients can be vague about medications they are currently taking or may have been provided in the past. A detailed job history can help define occupational exposures and possible dusts, fumes, and antigens associated with ILD. Hobbies and environmental exposures (e.g., pigeon breeding, home saunas, heating and air conditioning units) should also be noted. Knowledge of the agents that can cause ILD can serve as a guide to the areas that should be emphasized in the occupational and environmental history. The patient should be repeatedly asked about the illicit use of recreational drugs because these may contribute to their ILD. Risk factors for infection with the human immunodeficiency virus (HIV) must be explored.

A review of systems must include attention to symptoms of fevers, chills, night sweats (e.g., hypersensitivity pneumonitis, vasculitis), arthralgia and myalgia (ILD with connective tissue disorders), sinusitis, hemoptysis (alveolar hemorrhage syndromes), and chest pain (ILD resulting from toxic gas exposure). A past medical history should inquire into episodes of pneumothorax. The family medical history should be reviewed closely to rule out a number of inherited disorders known to cause ILD, such as IPF, tuberous sclerosis, and neurofibromatosis. A history of cigarette smoking is important in the pathogenesis of some interstitial lung diseases,

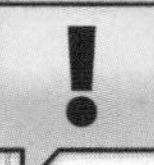

Respiratory Recap

Clinical History of Interstitial Lung Disease

- Dyspnea on exertion or at rest
- Cough
- Fevers, chills, and night sweats
- Medications taken
- Detailed work history
- Hobbies
- Environmental exposures
- Risk factors for infection with the human immunodeficiency virus (HIV)
- Past medical history of pneumothoraces
- Family medical history of interstitial lung disease
- Cigarette smoking

BOX 34-3

Classification of Interstitial Lung Disease

Known Cause

Infection

- Bacteria (*Legionella pneumophila*, *Bordetella pertussis*)
- Viruses (cytomegalovirus, human immunodeficiency virus, respiratory syncytial virus, adenovirus, influenza, parainfluenza, measles)
- *Mycoplasma* species
- *Mycobacterium* species
- Fungi (*Aspergillus* species)
- Parasites
- *Pneumocystis carinii* pneumonia

Occupational exposure

- Inorganic dusts (silicosis, asbestosis, talcosis, berylliosis, coal worker's pneumoconiosis, siderosis, baritosis)
- Microbial antigens (farmer's lung, humidifier lung, bird fancier's lung)
- Fumes (lung injury from exposure to chlorine gas, sulfuric acid, hydrochloric acid, nitrogen dioxide, or ammonia)

Neoplasm

- Bronchoalveolar carcinoma
- Leukemia
- Hodgkin disease
- Non-Hodgkin lymphoma

Congenital and metabolic causes

- Lipoidoses (Gaucher disease, Niemann-Pick disease)
- Storage disorders (Hermansky-Pudlak syndrome)
- Cystic fibrosis
- Radiation

Drug reactions
Recurrent aspiration
Lipoid pneumonia
Amyloidosis
Microlithiasis
Heart disease (congestive heart failure)
Liver disease (chronic active hepatitis, primary biliary cirrhosis)
Renal disease (renal failure)
Bowel disease (ulcerative colitis, Crohn disease)
Graft-versus-host disease
Pulmonary veno-occlusive disease
Acute respiratory distress syndrome (ARDS)
Acute eosinophilic pneumonia (parasitic infections, such as with *Strongyloides*, *Ascaris*, and *Ancylostoma* subspecies)

Unknown Cause

Idiopathic pulmonary fibrosis
Sarcoidosis
Vasculitides

- Wegener granulomatosis, Churg-Strauss angiitis, lymphomatoid granulomatosis, alveolar hemorrhage syndromes accompanied by capillaritis, microscopic polyangiitis, Behçet syndrome, Takayasu disease, Henoch-Schönlein purpura

Collagen vascular diseases
- Rheumatoid arthritis, systemic sclerosis, systemic lupus erythematosus (SLE), polymyositis, dermatomyositis, Sjögren syndrome, mixed connective tissue disease, ankylosing spondylitis

Diffuse alveolar hemorrhage syndromes
- Antiglomerular basement membrane antibody disease (Goodpasture syndrome), bleeding in patients with systemic necrotizing vasculitis (Wegener granulomatosis and microscopic polyangiitis) and collagen vascular diseases, hemorrhage in immunocompromised hosts and after administration of exogenous agents (trimellitic anhydride, cocaine, and penicillamine), idiopathic pulmonary hemosiderosis

Eosinophilic granuloma
Chronic eosinophilic pneumonia
Bronchiolitis obliterans with organizing pneumonia
Respiratory bronchiolitis
Pulmonary alveolar proteinosis
Lymphangioleiomyomatosis, tuberous sclerosis, and ataxia telangiectasia
Lymphoid interstitial pneumonitis
Acute interstitial pneumonitis

including eosinophilic granuloma, respiratory bronchiolitis, and alveolar hemorrhage syndromes.

The physical examination is frequently less helpful than the history in the determination of a specific diagnosis in ILD (**Table 34-1**). Bilateral, end-inspiratory, basilar crackles are a feature in several ILD diseases, including IPF, ILD with collagen vascular diseases, and asbestosis. Wheezes are rare except in Churg-Strauss syndrome. Other findings on the physical examination can assist in the differential diagnosis. Patients who have had severe disease for a protracted period may show evidence of pulmonary hypertension on the physical examination.

TABLE 34-1
Physical Examination Findings with Interstitial Lung Disease

Finding	Associated Disease
Digital clubbing	Idiopathic pulmonary fibrosis
Cutaneous lesions	Sarcoidosis, tuberous sclerosis, necrotizing vasculitis, dermatomyositis, collagen vascular diseases
Ocular signs	Sarcoidosis, ILD in systemic vasculitis, ILD with Sjögren syndrome or other connective tissue disorders
Polyarthritis	Sarcoidosis, ILD in systemic vasculitis, ILD with Sjögren syndrome or other connective tissue disorders
Peripheral lymphadenopathy	Sarcoidosis, lymphoid interstitial pneumonitis, ILD with connective tissue disorders
Hepatosplenomegaly	Sarcoidosis, amyloidosis, eosinophilic granuloma, chronic cor pulmonale
Neurologic manifestations	Tuberous sclerosis, systemic vasculitis, sarcoidosis, eosinophilic granuloma

ILD, interstitial lung disease.

Pulmonary Function Changes

The initial evaluation of pulmonary function in the patient with ILD should include spirometry, measurement of lung volumes and diffusing capacity (DLCO), inspiratory effort, maximum voluntary ventilation, arterial blood gas measurements, and exercise oxygen saturation. These studies characteristically reveal restriction with a decreased forced vital capacity (FVC), a decreased forced expiratory volume in the first second (FEV_1), and a normal or increased FEV_1 to FVC ratio. Total lung capacity (TLC) and the DLCO are decreased. The DLCO can sometimes be the most sensitive of the pulmonary function measures and may be abnormal even when lung volumes are preserved.[2]

A mild resting hypoxemia with significant arterial oxygen desaturation after exercise often is seen. The resting hypoxemia is the result of both ventilation-perfusion mismatch and shunt; the worsening of the condition with exercise may reflect diffusion restrictions in addition to mismatch and shunt. In patients with normal lung volumes or spirometry results, desaturation with ambulation may be a clue to the presence of pulmonary fibrosis.[2] A 6-minute walk test with pulse oximetry is well tolerated, provides a measure of oxygen requirements, and can be a quantifiable index of disease progression.[3]

Pulmonary function test results reflecting airway obstruction sometimes are seen in sarcoidosis, hypersensitivity pneumonitis, eosinophilic granuloma, Wegener granulomatosis, and lymphangioleiomyomatosis.

Radiographic Findings

The classic findings of ILD on a posteroanterior chest radiograph are those of a diffuse reticular, nodular, or reticulonodular pattern and reduced lung volume (**Figure 34-3**). Upper lobe predominance is seen in sarcoidosis, eosinophilic granuloma, silicosis, coal worker's pneumoconiosis, eosinophilic pneumonia, and ILD with ankylosing spondylitis. Lower lobe predominance is found in IPF, ILD with collagen vascular diseases, and asbestosis. The presentation usually is bilateral and symmetric but may be asymmetric and even unilateral, and alveolar infiltrates may be seen rather than small opacities. If the disorder has been long-standing, pulmonary hypertension may have developed and sometimes can be documented by the chest radiograph. An array of abnormalities can be seen on the chest radiographs of patients with ILD, which sometimes can be helpful in the determination of the differential diagnosis (**Table 34-2**).

High-resolution computed tomography (HRCT) is an important advance in the diagnosis and staging of ILD. Thin sections (1 to 2 mm) are used to portray two distinct patterns of disease: a ground glass increase in attenuation and a reticular pattern. The ground glass appearance is associated with a cellular histologic appearance of that area of lung, whereas the reticular pattern is found in patients whose subsequent lung biopsy confirms fibrosis. HRCT is significantly more sensitive and specific than a chest radiograph in the diagnosis of ILD and in the assessment of both the extent and severity of the disease.[4] It can identify disease before any abnormality is apparent on a chest radiograph. The distribution patterns and variability of involvement in ILD are more evident with HRCT and can be virtually pathognomonic for several forms of ILD, such as eosinophilic granuloma, IPF, lymphangioleiomyomatosis, lymphangitis carcinomatosa, sarcoidosis, and hypersensitivity pneumonitis.[5] The pattern of involvement observed on the CT scan of the chest also correlates very strongly with the histology of usual interstitial pneumonitis (UIP). In addition, HRCT has prognostic value in that a demonstration of honeycomb cysts indicates end-stage, irreversible fibrosis and loss of alveolar walls. Finally, HRCT can also guide parenchymal biopsy sites or direct the surgeon to lymph nodes for biopsy by mediastinoscopy.

Nuclear scintigraphy with gallium citrate Ga 67 has been proposed as a diagnostic and staging tool in the assessment of patients with ILD, particularly sarcoidosis and IPF. Gallium uptake is nonspecific, however, and this procedure has no clinical utility either in monitoring or predicting the clinical course of patients with ILD. Similarly, technetium-99 (^{99m}Tc) radionuclide scans and positron emission tomography (PET) scans currently have no clinical role in either the diagnosis or staging of ILD.

TABLE 34-2
Radiographic Findings with Interstitial Lung Disease

Finding	Associated Disease
Normal radiograph (10% of ILD cases)	Early IPF, sarcoidosis, and hypersensitivity pneumonitis
Spontaneous pneumothorax	Eosinophilic granuloma and lymphangioleiomyomatosis
Hilar or mediastinal lymphadenopathy	Sarcoidosis, berylliosis, and silicosis
Eggshell calcification	Silicosis
Pleural disease	Asbestos-related ILD, tuberculosis, ILD with collagen vascular disease, malignancies, and lymphangioleiomyomatosis
Honeycombing	IPF, eosinophilic granuloma, collagen vascular diseases, pneumoconioses, sarcoidosis

ILD, interstitial lung disease; IPF, idiopathic pulmonary fibrosis.

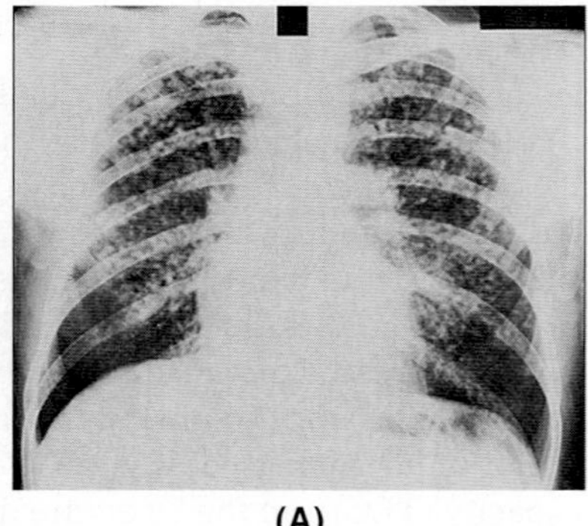

(A)

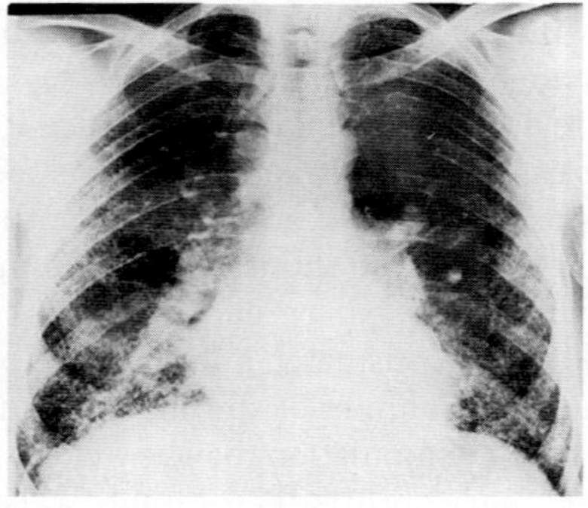

(B)

FIGURE 34-3 Chest radiographs demonstrating predominantly rounded opacities in the upper lung fields consistent with either silicosis or coal worker's pneumoconiosis (**A**). These are in contrast to the linear markings of asbestosis most commonly observed in the lower lung fields (**B**).

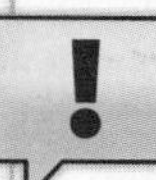

Respiratory Recap

High-Resolution Computed Tomography

- High-resolution computed tomography (HRCT) can aid in the diagnosis of idiopathic pulmonary fibrosis, eosinophilic granuloma, lymphangioleiomyomatosis, sarcoidosis, and hypersensitivity pneumonitis.

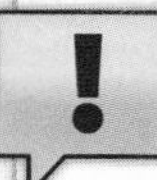

Respiratory Recap

Bronchoalveolar Lavage

- Bronchoalveolar lavage can assist in the diagnosis of lung infections, alveolar hemorrhage, pulmonary alveolar proteinosis, eosinophilic granuloma, and pneumoconiosis.

Laboratory Findings

Routine blood and serologic test results most often are unremarkable for patients with ILD. Many patients have a mild anemia and elevated erythrocyte sedimentation rate, reflecting inflammation. Serologic tests (including angiotensin-converting enzyme, antinuclear antibody, and antineutrophil cytoplasmic antibody determinations), hypersensitivity pneumonitis screening (serum precipitins), and complement fixation for fungi can be helpful in some patients.

Although nonspecific, laboratory results can support diagnoses and narrow the differential diagnosis in ILD. Evidence of renal insufficiency or hematuria raises the possibility of renal–pulmonary syndromes (e.g., Wegener granulomatosis, Goodpasture syndrome, systemic lupus erythematosus, and systematic necrotizing vasculitis), whereas abnormal results on liver function tests and high serum calcium levels are clues to the diagnosis of either sarcoidosis or metastatic malignancy.

Bronchoscopy

With ILD it is unusual to reach a specific diagnosis on the basis of the history, physical examination, pulmonary function test results, chest radiograph, and laboratory studies. After the HRCT scan, bronchoscopy with lavage and transbronchial lung biopsy usually follow. The exception to this order of investigation is the patient for whom bronchoscopy is thought to be more diagnostic; in such cases this procedure might be done before HRCT (**Figure 34-4**).

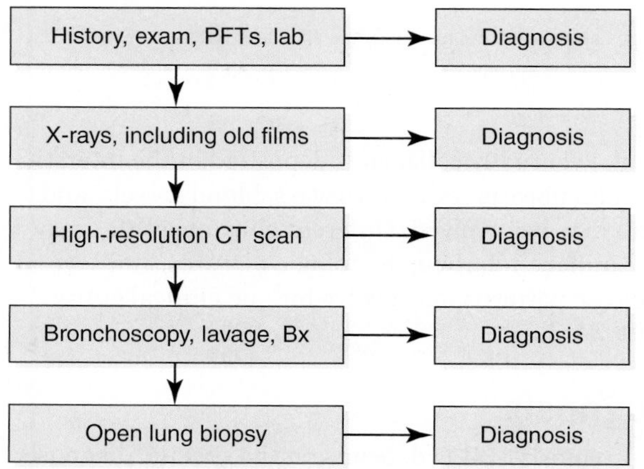

FIGURE 34-4 Approach to the evaluation of a patient with interstitial lung disease.

In the United States more than 60% of all patients with ILD undergo bronchoscopy.[1] In the evaluation of ILD, bronchoalveolar lavage samples cells and noncellular material from the lower respiratory tract.[6] Currently the clinical application of lavage in ILD is limited. Although the technique can be diagnostic (e.g., pulmonary alveolar proteinosis and pneumoconiosis), especially when particular cytologic or immunohistologic stains are applied (e.g., eosinophilic granuloma and alveolar hemorrhage syndromes), precise information is not obtained for most ILD disorders. Lavage can be extremely useful in the exclusion of specific etiologies and in the provision of supportive data to determine the differential diagnosis, however. The processing of lavage fluid should include cytologic studies and smears or cultures for acid-fast bacilli, fungi, *Pneumocystis carinii*, and viruses. This allows the clinician to exclude certain malignancies and specific infectious agents.

The cellular profiles obtained through analysis of the lavage fluid may indicate the underlying nature of the ILD. A lymphocytosis can be seen in sarcoidosis, berylliosis, and hypersensitivity pneumonitis. The CD4 (T helper) cells increase in sarcoidosis, with a ratio of CD4 to CD8 (T suppressor) cells of more than 3:5, whereas CD8 cells predominate with hypersensitivity pneumonitis. A lavage sample yielding more than 30% eosinophils supports a diagnosis of chronic or acute eosinophilic pneumonia. Neutrophils abound in several forms of ILD, including IPF and asbestosis.

Transbronchial biopsy (TBB) is particularly helpful if a primary lung neoplasm, infectious pneumonitis, or sarcoidosis is high in the differential diagnosis. TBB can sometimes diagnose Wegener granulomatosis, rheumatoid lung disease, lymphangioleiomyomatosis, eosinophilic granuloma, eosinophilic pneumonitis, pulmonary alveolar proteinosis, silicosis, hypersensitivity pneumonitis, lymphangitic spread of carcinoma, and Goodpasture syndrome. Several specimens (up to 6) should be obtained from both the upper and lower lobes of either the right or the left lung. If lavage and

Respiratory Recap

Transbronchial Biopsy

- Transbronchial biopsy can aid in the diagnosis of sarcoidosis, lung infection, cancer, and hypersensitivity pneumonitis.

TBB are not diagnostic, surgical lung biopsies should be considered in situations where clinical decisions will be based on pathologic findings.

Surgical Lung Biopsy

When lavage and transbronchial biopsy are nondiagnostic, surgical lung biopsies should be done unless specific contraindications exist. Lung biopsy is conventionally regarded as the gold standard used to determine a specific diagnosis for patients with ILD. In the United States, fewer than 50% of patients with ILD have a lung biopsy of some type for diagnostic purposes, although the decision to obtain a surgical lung biopsy must be individualized. There are several indications for surgical lung biopsy (**Box 34-4**). Examination of tissue can allow confirmation of a specific diagnosis, affect the development of a plan of treatment, predict response to therapy, and provide prognostic information.[7] It can also present insight into the pathogenesis of the ILD.

Lung biopsy through video-assisted thoracoscopic surgery (VATS) is tolerated extremely well and morbidity and mortality rates are low.[8] Biopsy specimens should be obtained from several sites, including apparently normal lung tissue adjacent to and remote from obviously involved tissue. HRCT can help determine the needed biopsy sites. Alveolar tissue is preferred. Tissue processing requirements include samples untreated for bacteriologic and virologic studies, fixed in 10% formalin, fixed in Methacarnoys solution for immunofluorescence, fixed in glutaraldehyde for electron microscopy, and cryopreserved for immunologic and molecular studies.

Pathology

The pathologic findings in ILD are remarkably similar.[9] Alveolitis (granulomatous or nongranulomatous) is initially observed, which may continue for a prolonged period. Eventually collagen is deposited in the interstitium, and fibrosis results. Airways, blood vessels, and pleura may be involved. Different clinical entities may have similar underlying histologic pictures, and several histologic patterns may evolve for one clinical entity (**Table 34-3**).

BOX 34-4

Indications for Surgical Lung Biopsy

Patient younger than 65 years
History of fevers, weight loss, and sweats
History of hemoptysis
Family history of interstitial lung disease
Symptoms and signs of peripheral vasculitis
History of pneumothorax
Normal chest radiograph despite clinical signs
Atypical radiographic features of idiopathic pulmonary fibrosis
Unexplained extrapulmonary manifestations
Unexplained pulmonary hypertension
Unexplained cardiomegaly
Rapidly progressive disease

TABLE 34-3
Histologic Patterns with Interstitial Lung Disease

Pattern	Associated Disease
Usual interstitial pneumonitis (UIP)	IPF, ILD with collagen vascular disease, asbestosis, sarcoidosis, hypersensitivity pneumonitis, radiation, drug reactions
Nonspecific interstitial pneumonitis (NSIP)	IPF, ILD with collagen vascular disease, drug reactions, hypersensitivity pneumonitis
Acute interstitial pneumonitis (AIP)	Acute respiratory distress syndrome, cytotoxic drugs, ILD with collagen vascular disease, Hamman-Rich syndrome
Cryptogenic organizing pneumonitis (COP)	IPF, ILD with collagen vascular disease, drug reactions, radiation, alveolar hemorrhage, eosinophilic pneumonia, hypersensitivity pneumonitis
Desquamative interstitial pneumonitis (DIP)	IPF, respiratory bronchiolitis, eosinophilic granuloma, drug reactions, lipoid pneumonia
Lymphocytic interstitial pneumonitis (LIP)	Infection, collagen vascular disease, immunodeficiency, drug reactions
Eosinophilic pneumonia	IPF, drug reactions, allergic granulomatosis of Churg-Strauss, tropical eosinophilia, hypereosinophilic syndrome
Diffuse alveolar hemorrhage	Vasculitis, ILD with collagen vascular disease, Goodpasture syndrome, idiopathic pulmonary hemosiderosis
Alveolar proteinosis	Pulmonary alveolar proteinosis, silicosis
Granulomas	Sarcoidosis, hypersensitivity pneumonitis, berylliosis, infections

IPF, idiopathic pulmonary fibrosis; ILD, interstitial lung disease.

Prognosis

The prognosis of ILD depends on the specific diagnosis, and most of the current information results from studies of IPF. Findings in the history, the chest radiograph,

Respiratory Recap

Factors Indicating an Improved Prognosis in Idiopathic Pulmonary Fibrosis

- Female patient
- Younger age
- Less dyspnea
- Greater cellular response in lavage

the pathology of the disease, and the response to therapy can provide prognostic information. In IPF, factors that predicted a better chance of survival in an untreated group were female gender and a younger age at presentation or at the onset of symptoms; the median survival among these patients was 4.5 years. In a treated group, factors associated with a better chance of survival were a younger age at the time of either presentation or onset of symptoms, less dyspnea, less impairment of diffusing capacity of carbon monoxide, less radiographic abnormality, a more cellular histologic appearance on biopsy, and an early response to corticosteroids. The response to steroids was closely linked with a more cellular appearance on biopsy.

HRCT has been used to predict response to treatment and outcome and is deemed more accurate than a chest radiograph.[10] A ground glass appearance was associated with 100% survival rate at 50 months after diagnosis of IPF, compared with a 50% survival rate for patients with disease that appeared with a more reticular pattern. Bronchoscopy with lavage also can provide prognostic information. An increased number of lymphocytes can be associated with a good response to corticosteroids and a better overall prognosis, compared with an elevated number of eosinophils and neutrophils, which predicts a poorer response to corticosteroids in IPF.

Management

Left untreated, the majority of the disorders included in the ILD diagnosis are progressive and result in death that occurs secondary to respiratory insufficiency and cor pulmonale. The most important tenet of therapy is to remove the agent of injury to the lung if possible, which may mean an exhaustive search for a causative agent.

If no agent is found, therapy can be directed toward suppression of inflammatory and cellular immune responses.[11] Agreement has never been reached on guidelines for standards of care and time of treatment for patients with ILD. The natural history of many with ILD is a steady progression and functional deterioration to the point where treatment is warranted. An important and challenging issue is when to start treatment. Many of the drugs used to treat ILD have the potential for serious side effects, which often is a disincentive to their use until no choice remains. By this time the patient has developed unequivocal breathlessness, and a considerable proportion of functional lung capacity has already been lost. It therefore is not surprising that meaningful improvements in lung function are uncommon and that often the best that can be achieved is stabilization of the disease to prevent further deterioration.

In ILD, few diseases are amenable to specific treatments. Corticosteroids can be curative in some ILDs (e.g., hypersensitivity pneumonitis, eosinophilic granuloma, and sarcoidosis). Lavage in pulmonary alveolar proteinosis is an exception and can restore the patient to health. Effective therapy is frequently not available, however, because the origin or mechanism of disease is not recognized. The alveolitis may be suppressed with corticosteroids and they are the initial therapy in the majority of patients treated for alveolitis. Corticosteroids can be associated with many adverse side effects. A few adequately controlled trials have assessed corticosteroid use in ILD and, among IPF patients, half experienced subjective improvement with steroids, yet only 15% to 20% improved by objective measures. The specific steroid regimen varies, but most commonly, therapy is initiated with prednisone 1 mg/kg, which is given for 3 to 6 months and then tapered over 4 to 6 months to 0.25 mg/kg. The efficacy of alternate-day regimens is not known.

Immunosuppressive or cytotoxic agents may be considered for patients for whom corticosteroids appear to have failed or for those who experience adverse side effects or have contraindications to corticosteroids, such as age, morbid obesity, insulin-dependent diabetes mellitus, or severe osteoporosis. Cyclophosphamide and methotrexate have been used in a number of disorders included in ILD. Methotrexate has been employed infrequently because pulmonary toxicity can occur in a significant number of patients. Azathioprine also has been used as a corticosteroid-sparing agent in diverse autoimmune disease and as therapy for sarcoidosis, IPF, and ILD with collagen vascular disease. This medication is given orally and is associated with fewer adverse side effects than methotrexate, and cyclophosphamide.

Meticulous supportive care can improve the quality of life of patients with ILD. Such therapy includes vaccines, antibiotics for episodes of purulent sputum, supplemental oxygen when the $Pa{O_2}$ drops below 55 mm Hg, bronchodilators for wheezing, psychosocial therapy, and pulmonary rehabilitation. Supplemental oxygen therapy can be used to relieve symptoms of dyspnea at rest and during exercise. A 6-minute walk test can help to determine adequate oxygen flows and concentrations to prescribe. Oxygen therapy may help patients with ILD maintain activities of daily living and help to increase exercise endurance, especially in patients with end-stage disease. Higher oxygen flow rates and oxygen-conserving devices may be needed as the ILD progresses and hypoxia-related complications occur.

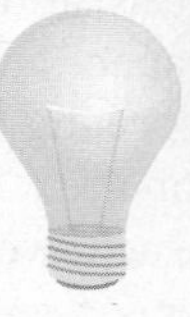

STOP AND THINK

You are asked to perform a 6-minute walk test for a patient with ILD. What are other ways that you, as a respiratory therapist, can help with the care of this patient?

Bronchodilators may be used to effect an increase in exercise capacity for patients with moderate to severe ILD and to reduce the increased work of breathing and feelings of breathlessness associated with ILD. Coupled with oxygen therapy, bronchodilators may promote physiologic improvements and subsequently improve quality of life among patients with severe symptoms from ILD.

Chronic lung conditions such as ILD can benefit from pulmonary rehabilitation programs. A comprehensive and individualized exercise training and education program can provide long-term health benefits and help to prevent and treat acute exacerbations. Rehabilitation programs can provide psychosocial support for patients, smoking cessation programs, and good nutrition guidance.

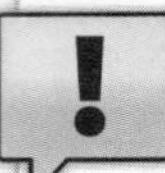

Respiratory Recap

Characteristics of Idiopathic Pulmonary Fibrosis

- Disease predominantly affects men in the fifth to seventh decades of life.
- History of exertional dyspnea is typical.
- Chest radiograph correlates poorly with clinical findings.
- High-resolution computed tomography shows the disease's highly distinctive distribution and pattern of lesions.
- Transbronchial biopsy usually is not diagnostic.
- Most patients require a surgical lung biopsy.
- Disease currently is diagnosed by histologic exclusion of other specific entities.
- Mortality rate is approximately 50% at 5 years.
- Initial trial of prednisone (40 to 60 mg given orally once a day for 3 months) is a reasonable treatment choice; continuation of therapy depends on an objective response.

Specific Interstitial Lung Diseases

Idiopathic Pulmonary Fibrosis

Idiopathic pulmonary fibrosis (IPF) predominantly affects males in the fifth to seventh decades of life.[12] No genetic basis has yet been determined. The pathogenesis is not known but is likely to reflect either an aberrant host response to injury at the alveolar epithelium and endothelium or a protracted response to the same. A history of a gradual onset of dyspnea with exercise is typical. More than 30% of patients experience constitutional symptoms such as weight loss, malaise, and easy fatigability. With progression of the disease, dyspnea at rest, clubbing of the fingers and toes, crackles in lung bases, and evidence of cor pulmonale become more prominent. The chest radiograph correlates poorly with clinical findings. In 10% of patients the radiograph is normal, but a reticulonodular pattern at the lung bases is characteristic in IPF. The distribution and pattern of the lesions are highly distinctive on HRCT scans, which show patchy subpleural and basilar lesions.

Pulmonary function tests show reduced lung volumes and a decrease in diffusing capacity. Laboratory values are nonspecific. Transbronchial biopsy is usually nondiagnostic. Most but not all patients with IPF ultimately require a surgical lung biopsy. Biopsies reveal a mixture of fibrosis and inflammatory cell infiltration in the pulmonary interstitium. IPF has no pathognomonic clinical, biochemical, or pathologic finding and therefore is currently diagnosed by histologic exclusion of other specific entities. As the lesions progress, the lung architecture is distorted, and respiratory failure ensues within 5 years. The mortality rate approximates 50% at 5 years. The prognosis is worse in men and for patients with honeycombing, severely depressed pulmonary function, and an absence of lymphocytes on lavage.

The decision as to which patients should be treated with steroids and/or cytotoxic agents is difficult. Most would agree with the treatment of patients who have significant gas exchange abnormalities and ILD symptoms. Corticosteroids have been associated with a favorable response in 10% to 30% of these patients. An initial trial of 40 to 60 mg by mouth daily for 3 months is reasonable. Continuation of therapy should depend on an objective response to these agents. Criteria and endpoints used to document a response are controversial. A 10% or greater increase in the FVC and FEV_1 or a 20% or greater increase in the DLCO is considered a favorable response. Responders should be tapered to 10 to 20 mg by mouth daily within 6 months. The optimum duration of therapy has not been determined. In nonresponders, the corticosteroid should be tapered and stopped. Immunosuppressive or cytotoxic agents (cyclophosphamide and azathioprine) should be considered for patients in whom corticosteroids appear to be ineffective or who are at risk of adverse effects from corticosteroids. Data show a low rate of response to alternative therapies in patients whose condition is resistant to steroids, however. Lung transplantation is an option for younger patients whose condition fails to respond to medical therapy.

Sarcoidosis

Sarcoidosis is a disorder in which multiple organ systems usually demonstrate noncaseating granulomas.[13] It is a common disorder and is the most prevalent ILD of

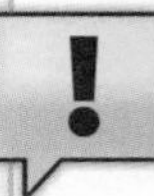

Respiratory Recap

Characteristics of Sarcoidosis

- Disease causes noncaseating granulomas in several organ systems.
- Sarcoidosis is the most common ILD of unknown origin.
- Most cases are seen in patients 20 to 45 years old.
- Disease is common in African Americans.
- Lung is the organ most frequently involved.
- Chest radiograph shows bilateral hilar lymph node enlargement (stage I), ILD with lymph node enlargement (stage II), and ILD alone (stage III).
- Adenopathy and ILD frequently regress spontaneously.
- Extrapulmonary involvement is common.
- Transbronchial biopsy demonstrates noncaseating granulomas.
- Thoracoscopic or open lung biopsy is rarely needed for diagnosis.
- Steroids are given with functional impairment of one or more organs.

unknown cause. The prevalence of sarcoidosis in North America is 10 to 20 cases per 100,000 people, and the rate in Scandinavia is approximately 80 per 100,000. The disorder is rare in Africa, South America, and Central America. Most cases occur between 20 and 45 years of age, and the disease is rare in children and the elderly. Sarcoidosis is more common among African Americans relative to Caucasians.

In sarcoidosis the lung is the organ most frequently involved. This high frequency of respiratory tract involvement may represent a response to an inhaled antigen. A significant proportion of individuals with sarcoidosis are asymptomatic (40% to 60%), but the chest radiograph is abnormal in more than 90%. The chest radiograph in sarcoidosis shows one of the following patterns: lymph node enlargement, which most frequently is bilateral and hilar (stage I disease); ILD with lymph node enlargement (stage II); or ILD alone (stage III). Most patients with stage II or stage III disease demonstrate restrictive results on pulmonary function tests. Some individuals with sarcoidosis may show a pattern of airway obstruction. Laboratories can demonstrate an increased serum concentration of angiotensin-converting enzyme (ACE) and hypercalcemia. The level of ACE may correspond to disease activity, and this measurement has been used as an index of granuloma burden.

Over time both the adenopathy and the ILD may regress spontaneously in about 60% of all patients (this occurs in 80% of patients in stage I, 40% in stage II, and 10% in stage III sarcoidosis). At the other extreme, however, the interstitial disease may progress to extensive scarring and end-stage lung disease, at which point the patient may have severe respiratory compromise. The course of the disease usually is dictated in the first 24 months, with almost all spontaneous remissions occurring during this time.

Extrapulmonary involvement is common in patients with sarcoidosis. Eye and skin involvement are particularly common manifestations of sarcoidosis, but the disease may also have cardiac, neuromuscular, hematologic, hepatic, endocrine, and peripheral lymph node effects. Mortality from sarcoidosis most often is the result of cardiac involvement.

The diagnosis can be made in several ways. The history, a physical examination, and chest radiography may provide the diagnosis in young African American women with bilateral hilar adenopathy. Transbronchial biopsy demonstrates noncaseating granulomas (which have a central core of histiocytes, epithelioid cells, and multinucleated giant cells) in as many as 90% of patients, because this process involves peribronchial and bronchiolar tissue. If bronchoscopy is not diagnostic, mediastinoscopy may be done to sample hilar and mediastinal lymph nodes. Biopsies of other involved tissues (skin, conjunctiva, salivary glands, or liver) can also provide a diagnosis. Thoracoscopic or open lung biopsy is rarely needed for diagnosis.

Treatment of sarcoidosis consists of steroid administration when evidence of progressive functional impairment of one or more vital organs is seen. Treatment of patients with mild symptoms or nonprogressive disease is inappropriate. Severe pulmonary dysfunction, hypercalcemia, and myocardial, nervous system, and eye involvement and disfiguring skin lesions necessitate corticosteroid treatment. The appropriate dose, duration, and tapering of the corticosteroid have not been defined. Response to the treatment is evident within 12 weeks, but the corticosteroid should be continued for at least 12 months at a minimally effective dose, because relapses of sarcoidosis occur often as the corticosteroid is tapered. Immunosuppressive agents (methotrexate and azathioprine) have been used for steroid-resistant cases, for steroid sparing, and for individuals who have contraindications to or who have had adverse effects from steroids. Transplantation has been used in end-stage lung disease with sarcoidosis.

Interstitial Lung Disease with Collagen Vascular Disease

Patients with a **collagen vascular disease** can develop ILD. Interstitial lung disease is one of the most serious pulmonary complications associated with collagen vascular disease and results in significant morbidity and mortality. Specific collagen vascular diseases associated with ILD include progressive systemic sclerosis,[14] systemic lupus erythematosus (SLE),[15] polymyositis and dermatomyositis, Sjögren syndrome, and mixed connective tissue disease.[16] Although progression of ILD with collagen vascular diseases is usually slower, the

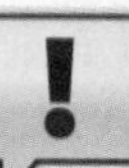

Respiratory Recap

Interstitial Lung Disease with Collagen Vascular Disease

- Progression of ILD with collagen vascular diseases is slow, but the clinical presentation is comparable to that of idiopathic pulmonary fibrosis, as is the histopathology.
- Diagnosis is assumed in patients with a known underlying collagen vascular disease and classic clinical features of ILD.
- Treatment involves administration of corticosteroids or immunosuppressive agents or both.

clinical presentation is comparable to that of IPF. The histopathologic features of ILD in this setting also correspond to those of IPF, with the additional features of lymphoid hyperplasia, cellular interstitial pneumonitis, lymphoid interstitial pneumonitis, diffuse alveolar damage, and bronchiolitis obliterans with organizing pneumonia. The diagnosis is assumed in patients with a known, underlying collagen vascular disease and classic clinical features of ILD (crackles, dyspnea, interstitial infiltrates, and restrictive results on pulmonary function tests). Before aggressive immunosuppressive therapy is begun, bronchoscopy with lavage and transbronchial biopsy should be performed to exclude alternative etiologies such as malignancy and infection. For patients with a deteriorating course, treatment involves administration of corticosteroids or immunosuppressive agents or both.

ILD shows a high association with progressive systemic sclerosis, and most patients with this disorder have ILD at some time during the course of their illness. There is an even greater prevalence of pulmonary hypertension (80% to 95%).

Eosinophilic Granuloma

Eosinophilic granuloma, also called *Langerhans cell granulomatosis*, was first described in 1953 as a bone disease having characteristics similar to those of Letterer-Siwe disease and Hand-Schüller-Christian disease.[17] Since then, it has been shown to be predominantly a pulmonary disorder. Eosinophilic granuloma is a rare disease that occurs almost exclusively in smokers or former smokers 10 to 40 years old. Although the cause remains unknown, eosinophilic granuloma probably is an inflammatory response by Langerhans cells to a component of tobacco smoke. Common presenting symptoms are a nonproductive cough, chest pain, and dyspnea on exertion. Weight loss, fever, and hemoptysis occasionally occur. Extrapulmonary features, including involvement of the posterior pituitary gland with the development of diabetes insipidus and lytic bony lesions, have frequently been described (20% of patients).

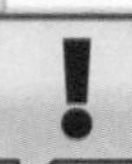

Respiratory Recap

Characteristics of Eosinophilic Granuloma

- Disease also is called Langerhans cell granulomatosis.
- Eosinophilic granuloma was first described as a bone disease but is now recognized as a predominantly pulmonary disorder.
- Disease occurs almost exclusively in smokers or former smokers 10 to 40 years old.
- Cause is unknown.
- Common presenting symptoms are a nonproductive cough, chest pain, and dyspnea on exertion.
- Extrapulmonary features include diabetes insipidus and lytic bony lesions.
- High-resolution computed tomography scans are highly distinctive.
- Light microscopy shows the cleft nuclei of the Langerhans cells and stellate pattern of fibrosis in 80% of patients.
- Spontaneous remissions are the rule.
- Patient must stop smoking if the disease is to resolve.

The physical examination often is unremarkable, but occasional wheezing may be heard. Pulmonary function tests show a decrease in lung volumes and diffusing capacity with normal or reduced expiratory flow rates. Radiographic findings of nodular densities in the upper and mid-lung fields with sparing of the lung bases are characteristic, but reticular, reticulonodular, and cystic lesions can be observed. Pleural effusions are uncommon. Pneumothorax occurs in approximately 10% of patients. The HRCT scans are highly distinctive, revealing numerous peribronchiolar nodular and cystic lesions.

As the disease progresses, the nodules are replaced by cysts that become confluent. Biopsy shows a mixture of inflammatory, cystic, nodular, and fibrotic lesions centered at or adjacent to bronchioles. Light microscopy shows the cleft nuclei of the Langerhans cells and the stellate pattern of fibrosis in 80% of patients. Aggregates of Langerhans cells can be demonstrated by immunostaining for S-100 protein or OKT6 antigen. Electron microscopy reveals Birbeck granules (X bodies) within these large, mononuclear phagocytes. As the inflammation progresses, alveolar architecture is destroyed and replaced by cysts and fibrosis.

In some cases TBB can provide the diagnosis. Spontaneous remissions are the rule, and no therapy beyond symptomatic and supportive care has been shown to be effective. Cigarette smoking must be stopped. There is progressive loss of pulmonary function in up to one-quarter of these individuals, who can die of respiratory failure. Corticosteroids often are used in severe and progressive disease, but no data are available on their efficacy.

Respiratory Bronchiolitis Interstitial Lung Disease

Respiratory bronchiolitis interstitial lung disease is a rare disorder that occurs exclusively in cigarette smokers.[18,19] Most of these individuals are asymptomatic, but they may have a mild cough, dyspnea, and sputum production. Crackles can be detected in some of these patients in the physical examination. The chest radiograph may demonstrate reticulonodular infiltrates at the bases, but it also may be normal. Pathologic studies reveal intracytoplasmic, golden-brown, granular pigment in alveolar macrophages in the respiratory and terminal bronchioles. The disease resolves in almost all patients after the person stops smoking.

Pulmonary Alveolar Proteinosis

Pathologically, **pulmonary alveolar proteinosis (PAP)** is characterized by filling of alveolar spaces with a lipoproteinaceous exudate and interstitial fibrosis.[20] The intra-alveolar phospholipid stains bright pink with periodic-acid Schiff (PAS) reagent. Although some patients are asymptomatic, most have dyspnea and cough, and alveolar infiltrates are seen on the chest radiograph. Laboratory values can verify hypoxemia. The disease spontaneously remits in one-third of patients. While the mortality rate was high in the past, death is now rare following introduction of whole-lung lavage of 20 to 40 L of saline as the treatment of choice. The cause remains unknown, but some patients have a history of exposure to silica and hydrocarbons.

Drug-Induced Interstitial Lung Disease

A number of different drugs can result in ILD.[21] The clinical and radiographic features differ depending on the implicated agent. Clinical presentations are specified as syndromes of acute pneumonitis, chronic interstitial pneumonitis, acute alveolar hemorrhage, or noncardiac pulmonary edema. A dose-related toxicity (e.g., as with antineoplastic agents) may be seen but often is not (such as with bleomycin), and the presentation may be that of an idiosyncratic reaction. Agents may be synergistic with each other, with radiation, or with oxygen exposure in the resultant lung toxicity.

A number of mechanisms are involved in drug-induced ILD, including cytotoxicity, hypersensitivity pneumonitis, and noncardiogenic pulmonary edema. Cytotoxic drug injury may occur with bleomycin, alkylating agents, and nitrosoureas. Previous chemotherapy or radiation therapy can amplify the risk of ILD with use of these drugs. The histopathologic features include type II pneumocyte proliferation with cellular atypia (large nuclei, prominent nucleoli, and bizarre chromatin patterns), inflammatory cell incursion, and fibrosis. Cytotoxic lung injury has a significant mortality rate (10% to 50% of patients, depending on the drug). Corticosteroids are most effective if given early, when a cellular rather than a fibrotic histology is present; the response is extremely variable and often negative with established disease. Methotrexate, nitrofurantoin, gold, and sulfasalazine are associated with hypersensitivity pneumonitis. Both acute and subacute forms manifest with fever, chest pain, and interstitial or alveolar infiltrates on the radiograph. The prognosis is good when the medication is stopped. Corticosteroids may hasten resolution. Salicylates, thiazides, narcotics, and cytarabine all can induce a noncardiac pulmonary edema.

Acute Interstitial Lung Disease

A number of interstitial lung diseases manifest in a more acute fashion. They include acute interstitial pneumonitis (Hamman-Rich syndrome), acute **bronchiolitis obliterans with organizing pneumonia (BOOP)**, acute eosinophilic pneumonia, and lymphoid interstitial pneumonitis.[22] The presentation of these diseases mimics an atypical pneumonia, with the patient reporting an unproductive cough, dyspnea, fever, and malaise. These patients may develop acute respiratory failure that requires mechanical ventilation.

Acute interstitial pneumonitis is a rapidly progressive form of interstitial pneumonitis thought either to exemplify an accelerated phase of IPF or to be a distinct entity of unknown origin. It has been described as an acute respiratory distress syndrome without an underlying precipitating injury. Acute interstitial pneumonitis is characterized by an epithelial cell injury that results in denudation of the epithelial lining of the alveolus and edema of the alveolar walls (i.e., diffuse alveolar damage). Intra-alveolar fibrin, edema accumulation, mild acute and chronic interstitial inflammation, and formation of intra-alveolar hyaline membranes also are frequently described. Collagen deposition by fibroblasts and honeycomb lung can follow. Hypoxemic respiratory failure is common, and the mortality rate is high. Patients are treated with corticosteroids, but the drugs' effectiveness is not known.

Acute BOOP appears to be a response of the lung to a variety of injuries that affect the smaller airways and alveoli as a unit. These injuries include infections, exposure to toxic gases, radiation therapy, drug toxicity, eosinophilic pneumonia, Wegener granulomatosis, and hypersensitivity pneumonitis. Acute BOOP manifests as an upper respiratory infection with a persistent cough and then dyspnea. Focal alveolar infiltrates are seen on the chest radiograph. Histologically, proliferating fibroblasts are noted in alveolar spaces, and polyps (inflammatory cells and fibrosis) project into the lumina of distal bronchioles. Extrapulmonary involvement does not occur. Treatment is administration of corticosteroids, with most individuals demonstrating good response. The idiopathic form of BOOP is classified as cryptogenic organizing pneumonia (COP) and the secondary form as secondary organizing pneumonia (SOP).[23]

Acute eosinophilic pneumonia is distinguished by fleeting pulmonary infiltrates and peripheral eosinophilia. Simple pulmonary eosinophilia (Löffler syndrome) is most commonly the result of infection with parasites such as *Strongyloides*, *Ascaris*, and *Ancylostoma* species but also can be caused by a drug reaction. The most common symptom is a dry cough. The infiltrates resolve within 2 weeks, and the peripheral eosinophilia is transitory. Treatment is directed at an identifiable underlying cause. Tropical eosinophilia can manifest as an acute eosinophilic pneumonia and is believed to be part of a hypersensitivity reaction to the filarial worm. Cough, fever, myalgia, and dyspnea are common. The histologic appearance is that of a cellular interstitial pneumonia with both infiltration of the interstitium and alveolar spaces by mononuclear cells and eosinophils and areas of BOOP. This can lead to respiratory failure requiring mechanical ventilation.

Various drugs have also been reported to produce acute eosinophilic pneumonia. In these cases the bronchoalveolar lavage shows a predominance of eosinophils. Treatment with corticosteroids cures the disease, and recurrences are unusual.

Allergic bronchopulmonary aspergillosis manifests as an acute eosinophilic pneumonia and is seen in asthmatics. Patients have a productive cough, eosinophilia, and a patchy infiltrate. Treatment is administration of corticosteroids.

Lymphoid interstitial pneumonitis is distinguished by dense lymphocytic infiltrates in the alveolar interstitium and lymphatics. The patient complains of cough and dyspnea. On the radiograph, bilateral reticular and reticulonodular infiltrates, dense alveolar infiltrates, or focal nodules are observed. The disease is considered a lymphoproliferative disorder. Lymphoid interstitial pneumonitis is associated most commonly with HIV infection (especially in children) but also with dysproteinemias, hypogammaglobulinemia, common variable immunodeficiency syndrome, monoclonal gammopathy, SLE, Sjögren syndrome, chronic active hepatitis, primary biliary cirrhosis, and bone marrow transplantation. Treatment is administration of corticosteroids, but no data are available on their effectiveness. The mortality rate for lymphoid interstitial pneumonitis is high.

Key Points

- Interstitial lung disease is a heterogeneous group of disorders classified together because of similarities in their clinical and pathologic presentation.
- The most common identifiable causes of interstitial lung disease are related to occupational or environmental exposure.
- A large number of ILD patients have interstitial lung disease of unknown origin, including idiopathic pulmonary fibrosis and sarcoidosis.
- Treatment of interstitial lung disease most often is supportive.

References

1. du Bois RM. Diffuse lung disease. An approach to management. *Br Med J.* 1994;309:175–179.
2. Martinez FJ, Flaherty K. Pulmonary function testing in idiopathic interstitial pneumonias. *Proc Am Thorac Soc.* 2006;3:315–321.
3. Eaton T, Young P, Milne D, Wells AU. Six-minute walk, maximal exercise tests: reproducibility in fibrotic interstitial pneumonia. *Am J Respir Crit Care Med.* 2005;171:1150–1157.
4. Sung A, Swigris J, Saleh A, Raoof S. High-resolution chest tomography in idiopathic pulmonary fibrosis and nonspecific interstitial pneumonia: utility and challenges. *Curr Opin Pulm Med.* 2007;13:451–457.
5. Mueller-Mang C, Grosse C, Schmid K, et al. What every radiologist should know about idiopathic interstitial pneumonias. *Radiographics.* 2007;27:595–615.
6. Nagai S, Handa T, Ito Y, et al. Bronchoalveolar lavage in idiopathic interstitial lung diseases. *Semin Respir Crit Care Med.* 2007;28:496–503.
7. Katzenstein AL, Mukhopadhyay S, Myers JL. Diagnosis of usual interstitial pneumonia and distinction from other fibrosing interstitial lung diseases. *Hum Pathol.* 2008;39:1275–1294.
8. Riley DJ, Costanzo EJ. Surgical biopsy: its appropriateness in diagnosing interstitial lung disease. *Curr Opin Pulm Med.* 2006;12:331–336.
9. Lai CK, Wallace WD, Fishbein MC. Histopathology of pulmonary fibrotic disorders. *Semin Respir Crit Care Med.* 2006;27:613–622.
10. Ryu JH, Daniels CE, Hartman TE, Yi ES. Diagnosis of interstitial lung diseases. *Mayo Clin Proc.* 2007;82:976–986.
11. Nathan SD. Therapeutic intervention: assessing the role of the international consensus guidelines. *Chest.* 2005;128(Suppl 1):533S–539S.
12. Walter N, Collard HR, King TE Jr. Current perspectives on the treatment of idiopathic pulmonary fibrosis. *Proc Am Thorac Soc.* 2006;3:330–338.
13. Judson MA. Sarcoidosis: clinical presentation, diagnosis, and approach to treatment. *Am J Med Sci.* 2008;335:26–33.
14. Fischer A, Swigris JJ, Groshong SD, et al. Clinically significant interstitial lung disease in limited scleroderma: histopathology, clinical features, and survival. *Chest.* 2008;134:601–605.
15. Cheema GS, Quismorio FP Jr. Interstitial lung disease in systemic lupus erythematosus. *Curr Opin Pulm Med.* 2000;6:424–429.
16. Vij R, Strek ME. Diagnosis and treatment of connective tissue disease-associated interstitial lung disease. *Chest.* 2013;143:814–824.
17. Abbott GF, Rosado-de-Christenson ML, Franks TJ, et al. From the archives of the AFIP: pulmonary Langerhans cell histiocytosis. *Radiographics.* 2004;24:821–841.
18. Vassallo R. Diffuse lung diseases in cigarette smokers. *Semin Respir Crit Care Med.* 2012;33:533–542.
19. Caminati A, Harari S. Smoking-related interstitial pneumonias and pulmonary Langerhans cell histiocytosis. *Proc Am Thorac Soc.* 2006;3:299–306.
20. Presneill JJ, Nakata K, Inoue Y, Seymour JF. Pulmonary alveolar proteinosis. *Clin Chest Med.* 2004;25:593–613.
21. Camus P, Fanton A, Bonniaud P, et al. Interstitial lung disease induced by drugs and radiation. *Respiration.* 2004;71:301–326.
22. Vourlekis JS. Acute interstitial pneumonia. *Clin Chest Med.* 2004;25:739–747.
23. Heffner JE. No matter how you push and squeeze, organizing pneumonia remains more than one disease. *Respir Care.* 2009;54:1020–1023.

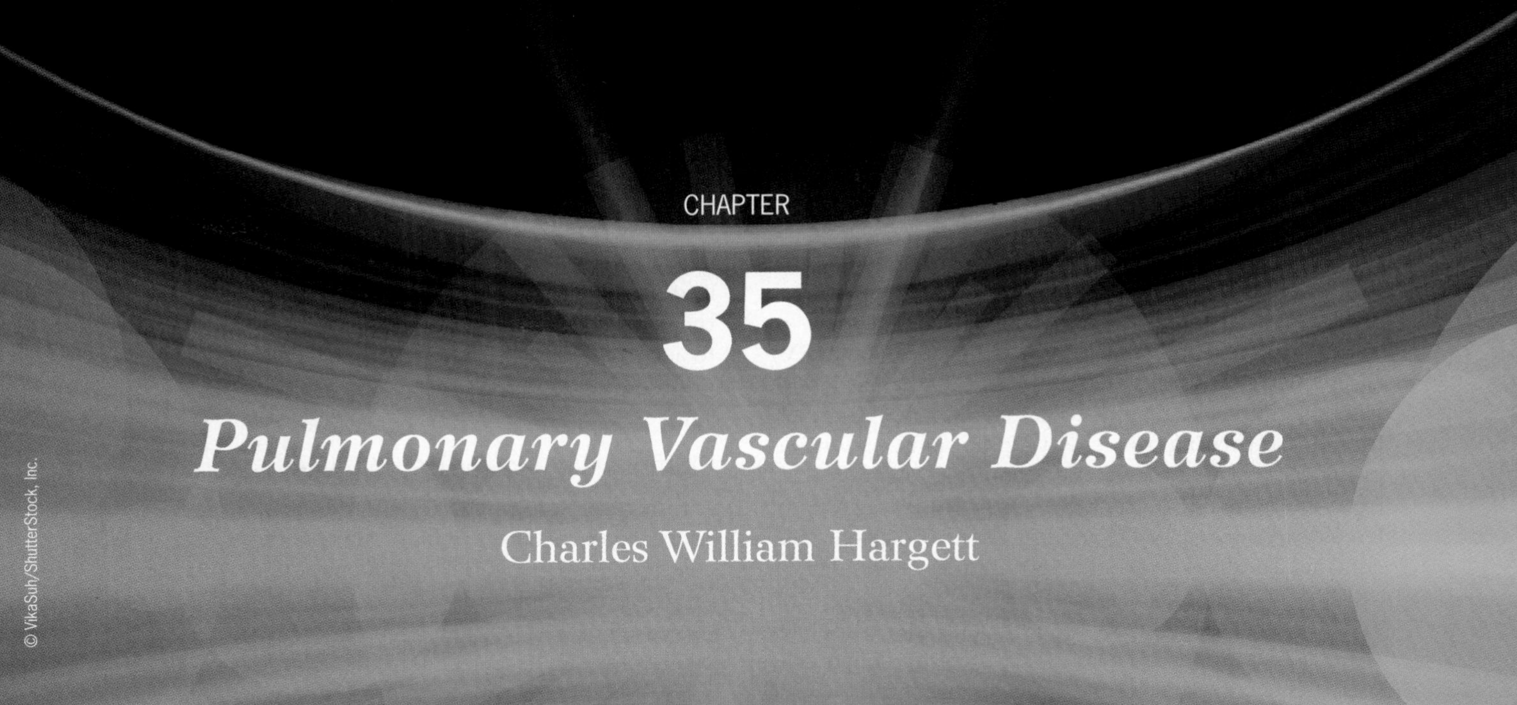

CHAPTER

35

Pulmonary Vascular Disease

Charles William Hargett

OUTLINE

OBJECTIVES

1. Describe the physiology of the pulmonary circulation and right ventricle in normal and disease states.
2. Describe the WHO Classification and various types of clinical pulmonary hypertension.
3. Describe the signs and symptoms of pulmonary vascular diseases, including those present in pulmonary embolism (PE), cor pulmonale, and idiopathic pulmonary arterial hypertension (IPAH).
4. Define the role of ventilation-perfusion scanning, computed tomographic angiography, and pulmonary angiography in the diagnosis of PE.
5. Discuss the role of anticoagulation, vena cava filters, and thrombolytic therapy in the management of acute PE.
6. Describe the pathogenesis and treatment of cor pulmonale.
7. Discuss the role of advanced therapies in the management of IPAH.

KEY TERMS

anticoagulation
computed tomographic angiography (CTA)
cor pulmonale
deep vein thrombosis (DVT)
hypoxic pulmonary vasoconstriction
idiopathic pulmonary arterial hypertension (IPAH)
inferior vena cava (IVC) filter
prostacyclin
pulmonary angiography
pulmonary arterial hypertension (PAH)
pulmonary artery pressure
pulmonary embolism (PE)
pulmonary hypertension (PH)
pulmonary vascular resistance (PVR)
thrombolytic therapy

Introduction

Pulmonary vascular disease is one of the major classifications of respiratory disorders and describes any condition that affects the blood vessels between the heart and lungs. Disorders of the pulmonary circulation include a large and heterogeneous group of conditions and are important because they can be severe and difficult to treat. Some pulmonary vascular diseases, such as pulmonary embolism, occur quite commonly, whereas others, such as idiopathic pulmonary arterial hypertension, are quite rare. Conditions which affect the movement of blood from the right side of the heart, to the lungs, and back to the left side of the heart may lead to pulmonary hypertension, or high blood pressure in the lungs, and subsequent right-sided heart failure. In fact, these disorders can perhaps most effectively be described in the framework of pulmonary hypertension, which represents a final common pathway of almost all forms of pulmonary vascular disease. In this chapter, the pathophysiology of pulmonary vascular disease is reviewed in the context of normal cardiopulmonary physiology and function. Features common to many forms of pulmonary vascular disease are described, in addition to issues related to the diagnosis and management of several specific disorders of the pulmonary circulation.

Pathophysiology

Normal Pulmonary Vascular Physiology

The principal function of the pulmonary circulation is gas exchange. Venous blood low in oxygen and rich in carbon dioxide passes through the pulmonary capillaries, where oxygen is absorbed and carbon dioxide is eliminated, thus allowing the left ventricle to return oxygenated blood to the rest of the body. Under normal circumstances, the pulmonary circulation is a low-pressure, high-flow system, providing little resistance to the right ventricular outflow. Mean **pulmonary artery pressure** and **pulmonary vascular resistance (PVR)** at rest are approximately one-sixth that of the systemic circulation.[1] Although the right ventricle (RV) is sensitive to the pulmonary vascular load, in a classic view the RV serves primarily as a capacitance chamber for blood returning from the systemic veins. As long as pulmonary vascular resistance is normal, blood flows from the right side of the heart through the lungs to the left side of the heart as a result of left heart action. The contraction of the left ventricle and interventricular septum pulls the free wall of the RV against the septum and augments the flow of blood through the pulmonary circulation.[2] The phasic changes in intrathoracic pressure that accompany respiration also direct the forward flow of blood from the RV through the pulmonary circulation.

Normally, the pulmonary vascular bed is able to accommodate large increases in blood flow without much change in pressure, thus effectively preventing RV overload. For example, cardiac output can increase substantially during exercise in normal individuals, with increases of up to fivefold in pulmonary blood flow.[2,3] The thin-walled RV is highly compliant and able to accommodate large volumes and filling pressures. Recruitment of vessels in the poorly perfused upper lung and distention of the compliant vessels in the dependent areas allow the pulmonary circulation to accommodate these increases in cardiac output and pulmonary blood flow.[4,5]

Pulmonary Vascular Pathophysiology

Although the pulmonary circulation is remarkable in adjusting to increases in blood flow, many pathologic conditions can give rise to **pulmonary hypertension (PH)**, or an increase in blood pressure in the lung vasculature (**Box 35-1**). PH is present when the mean pulmonary artery pressure exceeds 25 mm Hg and may occur as a result of intrinsic abnormalities of the pulmonary vessels, secondary to underlying cardiac or pulmonary disorders, or as a complication from obstructive embolization. PH was originally classified as secondary in the presence of a known cause and primary when no underlying etiology or risk factor could be identified.[6]

BOX 35-1

Selected Causes of Pulmonary Hypertension

Pulmonary Arterial Hypertension (PH Associated with Pulmonary Arterial Disease)

- Idiopathic and familial pulmonary arterial hypertension
- Connective tissue disease (e.g., scleroderma)
- Portal hypertension
- Human immunodeficiency virus (HIV)
- Congenital heart disease (e.g., Eisenmenger syndrome)
- Drugs (e.g., anorexic agents, methamphetamine)
- Persistent pulmonary hypertension of the newborn
- Pulmonary hypertension associated with left heart disease
- Left-sided systolic or diastolic dysfunction
- Left-sided valvular heart disease

Pulmonary Hypertension Associated with Lung Diseases and/or Hypoxemia

- Chronic obstructive pulmonary disease (COPD)
- Diffuse parenchymal lung diseases (e.g., idiopathic pulmonary fibrosis)
- Hypoventilation and sleep-disordered breathing

Pulmonary Hypertension Associated with Chronic Thrombotic and/or Embolic Disease

- Pulmonary embolism
- Other materials (e.g., parasites, tumor, foreign material)

Other Disorders

- Sarcoidosis
- Compression of pulmonary vessels (e.g., mediastinal lymphadenopathy)

Major advances in our understanding have led to the current classification, in which pulmonary hypertensive diseases are grouped into five categories according to cause and therapeutic strategy, with each category subdivided to reflect diverse underlying etiologies and sites of injury.[7] Although the underlying pulmonary vascular disease may differ for the various types of clinical PH, this phenotypic categorization is useful for understanding and managing these conditions.

Destruction or obliteration of the pulmonary vascular bed is likely to play a role in patients with chronic lung diseases, such as chronic obstructive pulmonary disease (COPD).[8] In contrast, **pulmonary arterial hypertension (PAH)** is characterized by vasoconstriction and vascular remodeling in the precapillary segments of the pulmonary vasculature due to an imbalance between endothelial mediators such as prostacyclin, thromboxane, and endothelin;[9,10] the histopathology may include plexogenic arteriopathy, thrombotic lesions, and medial hypertrophy with intimal fibrosis. Unexplained PAH is designated idiopathic pulmonary arterial hypertension (formerly primary pulmonary hypertension) and is the most well-studied form of PAH. In addition, in many individuals with pulmonary vascular diseases, chronic alveolar hypoxia and associated hypoxic pulmonary vasoconstriction contribute to the development of PH.

Once PH develops, independent of the inciting event, pulmonary vascular remodeling occurs, leading to medial hypertrophy and intimal fibrosis, which further reduces pulmonary vascular cross-sectional area and exacerbates PH. **Figure 35-1** illustrates vascular changes observed in a patient with PH. As right ventricular afterload increases with worsening PH, right ventricular hypertrophy, dilation, or failure can occur. When right heart failure is caused by a primary disorder of the respiratory system, it is classically named **cor pulmonale**, or pulmonary heart failure. COPD and idiopathic pulmonary fibrosis (IPF) are two diseases commonly associated with the development of cor pulmonale.

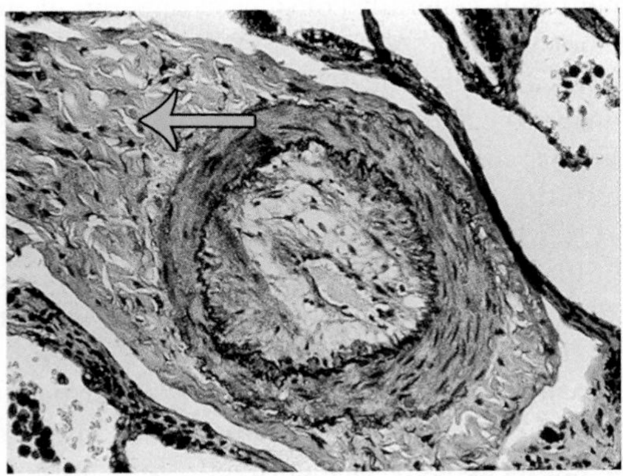

FIGURE 35-1 Arrow shows pulmonary arteriolar smooth muscle cell hypertrophy, with prominent thickening of the medial layer.

Pathophysiology of Acute Pulmonary Embolism

Venous thromboemboli that cause **pulmonary embolism (PE)** usually arise from **deep vein thrombosis (DVT)** in the lower extremities. When emboli acutely obstruct a significant portion of the pulmonary arterial bed, profound hemodynamic alterations occur. Hypoxemia occurs as a result of regions with low ventilation-perfusion ($\dot{V}/\dot{Q}$) ratios and shunting secondary to perfusion of atelectatic areas. The impact of the embolic event depends on the extent of reduction of the cross-sectional area of the pulmonary vasculature and on the presence or absence of underlying cardiovascular disease.[11] With massive emboli, cardiac output is diminished but may be sustained to a certain point. Increased pulmonary vascular resistance impedes right ventricular outflow and reduces left ventricular preload. More than 50% obstruction of the pulmonary arterial bed is usually present before substantial elevation of mean pulmonary artery pressure develops. When the extent of obstruction of the pulmonary circulation approaches 75%, a normal individual cannot generate the right ventricular systolic pressures in excess of 50 mm Hg, which is required to preserve pulmonary perfusion, and cardiac failure and death will occur.[12]

Epidemiology

Disorders of the pulmonary circulation include a diverse group of clinical conditions that result in substantial morbidity and mortality. Pulmonary embolism, for example, is recognized as the third most common cause of cardiovascular disease in the United States after ischemic heart disease and stroke.[13] Autopsy studies suggest that more than 600,000 patients in the United States develop DVT or PE or both each year, with over half of these cases not recognized before death. PE probably causes or contributes to the death of at least 100,000 of these patients each year.[12]

In addition, cor pulmonale appears to contribute substantially to mortality in patients with significant pulmonary parenchymal disease. The exact incidence and prevalence of cor pulmonale in COPD is not known, but recent estimates suggest that 10% to 40% of patients with COPD have evidence of right ventricular hypertrophy.[8] Cor pulmonale increases in prevalence with increased severity of lung disease and may occur in over 70% of COPD patients with a forced expiratory volume in the first second of expiration (FEV_1) of less than 0.6 L.[14] The development of cor pulmonale in these patients portends a significantly worse prognosis than in patients with normal right ventricular pressures. In patients with COPD, which causes an estimated 120,000 deaths each year in the United States, overt right heart failure is associated with a 5-year survival of only 30%.[8,15] Similarly, in patients with fibrotic lung disease, such as IPF, PH is also an important predictor of survival.[16,17]

Idiopathic pulmonary arterial hypertension (IPAH) is an uncommon disorder of the pulmonary vessels associated with severe elevation in pulmonary vascular resistance. The incidence of IPAH is unknown but is estimated at 2 to 6 cases per million people in the population.[10,18] IPAH is most common among younger patients (ages 20 to 40 years) and occurs at least three times as frequently in women. IPAH is a devastating disease and has traditionally been associated with poor prognosis, with a 5-year survival of only 34%.[19] Poor survival has been associated with worse functional class (III or IV) and reduced right ventricular hemodynamic function (specifically, elevated mean right atrial pressure, elevated mean pulmonary arterial pressure, and decreased cardiac index). Pulmonary vascular disease clinically and pathologically indistinguishable from IPAH can occur in association with a number of systemic illnesses, such as scleroderma and human immunodeficiency virus (HIV) infection, or in association with certain drugs, including appetite suppressants.[20–22] The appetite suppressants fenfluramine and dexfenfluramine have been found to significantly increase the risk of pulmonary hypertension (odds ratio of greater than 20 with more than 3 months of use).[22] Despite approval by the Food and Drug Administration of nine PAH drugs in four different classes over the past 20 years, PAH remains a severe condition, often leading to significant debility and death, and generally requires advanced medical and surgical treatments.

Diagnosis

Acute Pulmonary Embolism

The history, physical exam, arterial blood gas analysis, electrocardiogram (ECG), and chest radiograph often are useful in suggesting the presence or absence of pulmonary embolism. The clinical evaluation alone, however, is not a reliable guide to the diagnosis of PE, as is underscored by the high incidence of unsuspected PE in autopsy series.[23] PE should be considered whenever unexplained dyspnea occurs, but it also should be considered when a patient with another potential explanation for dyspnea, such as underlying cardiopulmonary disease, develops new or worsening symptoms. **Box 35-2** lists common risk factors for PE. The presence of one or more risk factors should increase the clinical suspicion. Unexplained dyspnea in association with pleuritic chest pain or hemoptysis is suggestive of PE, and PE must also be considered in the setting of unexplained syncope or sudden hypotension.

The physical examination may be unrevealing in patients with acute PE. Because patients with lower extremity DVT often do not exhibit pain, warmth, erythema, or swelling, the physical exam may not provide clues to the presence of an underlying DVT. An increased pulmonic component of the second heart sound has been reported in massive PE, but the nonspecific findings of tachypnea and tachycardia are the most common physical examination abnormalities described in PE.

BOX 35-2

Important Risk Factors for Pulmonary Embolism

- Recent surgery
- Acute medical illness
- Malignancy
- Pregnancy or postpartum
- Immobilization or paralysis
- Prior history of deep vein thrombosis or pulmonary embolism
- Hypercoagulable states such as:
  - Factor V Leiden mutation
  - Prothrombin gene mutation
  - Protein C or S deficiency
  - Antithrombin deficiency
  - Dysfibrinogenemia
  - Antiphospholipid syndrome
  - Heparin-induced thrombocytopenia

Hypoxemia is common in acute PE but is not universally present. Young patients without underlying lung disease may have a normal Pa_{O_2}. In a retrospective analysis of hospitalized patients with proven PE, the Pa_{O_2} was more than 80 mm Hg in 29% of patients younger than 40 years, compared with 3% in the older group.[24] The alveolar–arterial difference was abnormal in all patients, however. Thus, the diagnosis of acute PE cannot be excluded based on a normal Pa_{O_2}.

Laboratory tests that may be useful include testing for D-dimer, a breakdown product of cross-linked fibrin present in acute DVT and PE. Unfortunately, D-dimer may be present in patients with infections, cancer, and other disorders, rendering it nonspecific for acute venous thromboembolism. If the clinical suspicion of acute DVT or PE is low, however, a *negative* quantitative D-dimer test is generally considered sensitive enough to rule out VTE.

Electrocardiographic findings in acute PE are generally nonspecific and include T wave changes, ST segment abnormalities, and left or right axis deviation. Manifestations of acute right heart failure, including the S1 Q3 T3 pattern, right bundle branch block, P wave pulmonale, or right axis deviation, were present in only 32% of patients with massive PE in the Urokinase Pulmonary Embolism Trial (UPET).[25]

The majority of patients with PE have nonspecific abnormalities on chest radiographs, with common findings including atelectasis, pleural effusion, pulmonary infiltrates, and elevation of a hemidiaphragm.[26] Classic radiographic findings of pulmonary infarction such as

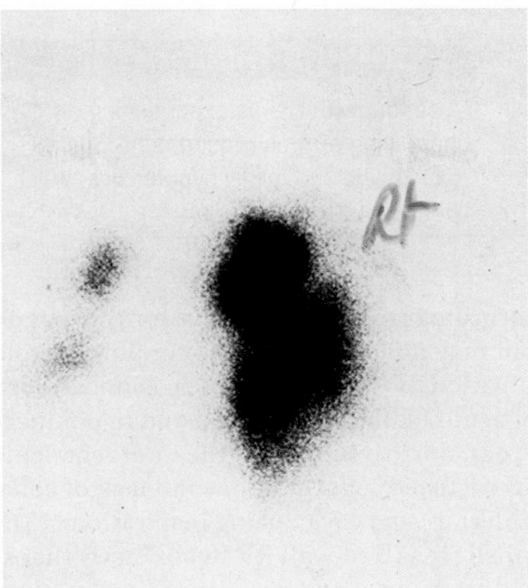

FIGURE 35-2 This perfusion scan (posterior view) reveals extensive pulmonary embolism with essentially absent flow to the left lung and perfusion defects in the right lung. The ventilation scan was normal.

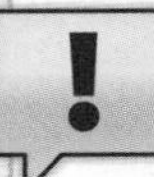

Respiratory Recap

Diagnosis of Pulmonary Embolism

- The physical exam may be unremarkable.
- Hypoxemia is common but not universally present.
- Electrocardiographic findings often are nonspecific.
- The chest radiograph is often unremarkable; a normal chest radiograph with dyspnea and hypoxemia (and without significant bronchospasm) is suggestive of PE.
- In patients with a low pretest probability for PE, a negative quantitative D-dimer assay result can be used to exclude PE.
- High-probability $\dot{V}/\dot{Q}$ scans are virtually diagnostic when acute PE is *clinically* likely.
- Chest computed tomographic angiography is the most common test employed to detect PE and is sensitive and specific.
- Pulmonary angiography is the most accurate diagnostic test for PE but is invasive.
- Echocardiography is insensitive for the diagnosis of PE but may play a role in evaluation and risk stratification.

wedge-shaped pleural density (Hampton's hump) or decreased vascularity (Westermark sign) are suggestive but infrequent. A normal chest radiograph in the setting of severe dyspnea and hypoxemia without evidence of bronchospasm or cardiac shunt is strongly suggestive of PE. In general, however, the chest radiograph cannot be used to conclusively prove or exclude PE.

Ventilation-perfusion scanning may be performed when PE is suspected. When abnormal, $\dot{V}/\dot{Q}$ scans are conventionally read as showing low, intermediate, or high probability for PE. Normal and high-probability scans are considered diagnostic. **Figure 35-2** illustrates a high-probability $\dot{V}/\dot{Q}$ scan in a patient with PE. In the Prospective Investigation of Pulmonary Embolism Diagnosis (PIOPED) study, the utility of $\dot{V}/\dot{Q}$ scanning combined with clinical assessment of patients with suspected PE was prospectively evaluated in more than 700 patients.[27] Patients with PE had scans that were high, intermediate, or low probability, but so did most patients without PE. Although the specificity of high-probability scans was 97%, the sensitivity was only 41%. Of interest, 33% of patients with intermediate-probability scans and 12% of patients with low-probability scans were diagnosed definitively with PE by pulmonary arteriography. When the clinical suspicion of PE was considered high, PE was found to be present in 96% of patients with high-probability scans, 66% of patients with intermediate-probability scans, and 40% of patients with low-probability scans. Additional diagnostic tests thus must be pursued when the $\dot{V}/\dot{Q}$ scan is of low or intermediate probability if the clinical scenario is suggestive of PE.

Over the past decade, $\dot{V}/\dot{Q}$ scanning has decreased in favor of contrast-enhanced **computed tomographic angiography (CTA)** of the chest, which may reveal emboli in the main, lobar, or segmental pulmonary arteries. The reported sensitivity and specificity of single-slice helical CTA has ranged from 53% to 100% and from 81% to 100%, respectively, but visualization of segmental and subsegmental pulmonary arteries is substantially better with newer multidetector scanners, as evidenced by the PIOPED II, where the specificity of chest CTA was 95% and the sensitivity 83%.[28,29] **Figure 35-3** illustrates chest CTA identification of a proximal pulmonary artery clot in a patient with PE. **Box 35-3** summarizes advantages and disadvantages of chest CTA in the diagnosis of PE.

In patients requiring additional testing, **pulmonary angiography** can be performed and remains

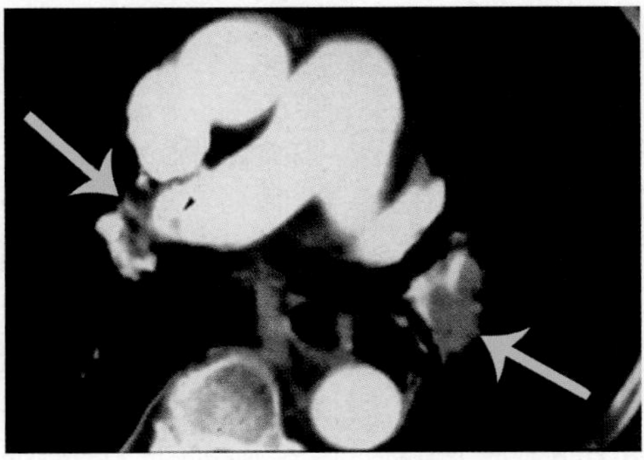

FIGURE 35-3 Computed tomographic angiogram in a patient with bilateral, proximal, acute pulmonary emboli (arrows).

BOX 35-3

Utility of Computed Tomographic Angiography of the Chest in the Diagnosis of Pulmonary Embolism

Advantages

- Excellent visualization of pulmonary arteries
- Noninvasive
- Relative rapidity of procedure
- Diagnosis of other (nonvascular) abnormalities

Disadvantages

- Experienced radiologist required to interpret results
- Adverse reactions to contrast (e.g., anaphylaxis, nephrotoxicity)
- Radiation exposure

the gold-standard diagnostic technique. **Figure 35-4** illustrates a pulmonary angiogram diagnostic of PE. Serious complications of pulmonary angiography occur infrequently (less than 0.5% incidence in most series), but respiratory failure, renal failure, significant bleeding, and death have been reported.[30] Angiography requires the presence of experienced physicians to perform the test and interpret the results; however, this test is rarely needed because CTA is very accurate and offers the potential for additional diagnoses. In selected stable patients with suspected acute PE and nondiagnostic lung scans, serial noninvasive lower extremity testing to rule out DVT may be a reasonable alternative approach because a positive lower extremity study requires treatment without further testing.[31]

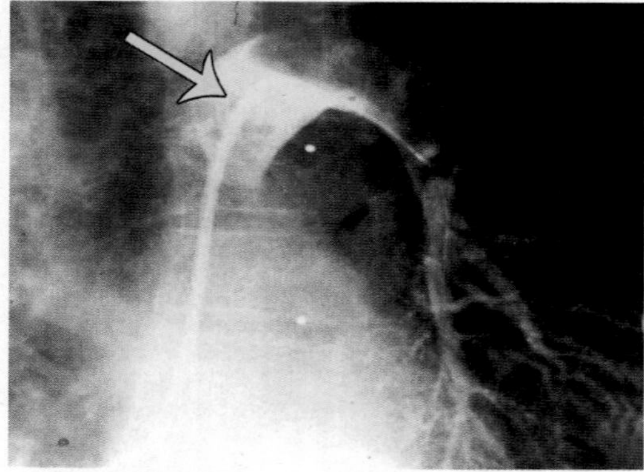

FIGURE 35-4 Pulmonary angiogram demonstrating acute pulmonary embolism. There is a large filling defect in the right pulmonary artery (arrow) and marked hypoperfusion to the right upper and middle lobes.

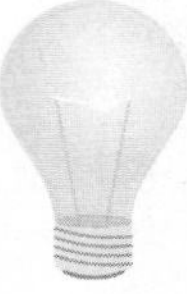

STOP AND THINK

A patient with DVT is experiencing an increasing oxygen requirement. She is tachypneic and mildly hypotensive. What would you suggest?

Echocardiography is insensitive for the diagnosis of PE but may nonetheless play an important role in the evaluation of PE. Transthoracic echocardiographic signs of acute PE include dilation and hypokinesis of the RV, paradoxical motion of the interventricular septum, tricuspid regurgitation, and lack of collapse of the inferior vena cava during inspiration.[32] The McConnell sign (free-wall RV hypokinesis that spares the apex) may be a more specific finding; rarely, direct visualization of a thrombus may guarantee the diagnosis.[33] The speed and portability of echocardiography make it particularly useful in patients who are suspected of having PE and are too unstable for further evaluation with CTA or $\dot{V}/\dot{Q}$ scan. Additionally, echocardiography has proven helpful for risk stratification in patients with proven PE, and serial exams may demonstrate interval change in cardiac function.[34,35] Echocardiography may also be useful in identifying other causes of shock, such as aortic dissection and cardiac tamponade.

Chronic Pulmonary Hypertension and Right Heart Failure

The manifestations of PH are generally nonspecific, so careful attention to the clinical history and physical examination can provide important clues to the presence of disease. In all patients, a careful history of current and prior medication use and concomitant medical conditions is essential.

Dyspnea is a common feature, and chest pain may also occur, but these symptoms may often be attributed to other more common conditions such as asthma, deconditioning, weight gain, panic attacks, coronary artery disease, or gastroesophageal reflux disease. This may significantly delay the diagnosis; in fact, patients in the IPAH registry had symptoms from 2 to 5 years prior to a formal diagnosis.[36] Raynaud phenomenon may occur in patients with IPAH but is much more common with PAH associated with connective tissue disease. Exertional presyncope and syncope may be due to the inability to increase cardiac output in response to the increased demand and suggests advanced PH with right heart failure.

Orthopnea is relatively common in patients with severe COPD, although it is not necessarily accompanied by worsening cardiac function. Orthopnea in these patients is related to hyperinflation of the lungs and the subsequent effects on ventricular function or

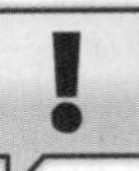

Respiratory Recap

Diagnosis of Pulmonary Hypertension

- Dyspnea is common but not specific.
- Chest pain may occur but generally with more advanced PH.
- Exertional presyncope or syncope or both may occur with advanced PH.
- A loud second heart sound (pulmonic valve closure) is common.
- Hypoxemia is often present in patients with advanced PH.
- Electrocardiographic findings consistent with right heart strain are commonly observed.
- Enlarged pulmonary arteries may be seen on the chest radiograph.
- Echocardiography may help determine the underlying cause of PH.
- Echocardiography is also useful in determining and following RV size and function.
- The gold standard for diagnosis of pulmonary hypertension is right heart catheterization.

reduction in venous return, or both. In patients with cor pulmonale and other forms of PH, increased venous and hepatic congestion can occur in advanced disease and lead to the development of early satiety, increasing lower extremity edema, and fluid overload.

The presence of a loud pulmonic valve closure sound is a common finding in patients with PH, independent of the cause. It may be accompanied by a parasternal or epigastric lift resulting from a hypertrophied RV. Tricuspid valvular regurgitation also develops because of dilation of the RV, which causes a prominent jugular V wave. Progressive signs of chronic right ventricular dilation and failure include pulmonic valve insufficiency, a right ventricular third heart sound, jugular venous distention, hepatojugular reflux, hepatomegaly, lower extremity edema, ascites, and eventually anasarca.

Patients with cor pulmonale and PH resulting from COPD also invariably have findings associated with their obstructive lung disease, including decreased breath sounds and hyperinflation. Individuals with cor pulmonale secondary to interstitial lung disease often have dry crackles at the lung bases. Auscultation of the lungs in IPAH is generally unremarkable. Clubbing also is a common finding in patients with pulmonary fibrosis, but not in PH alone.

Hypoxemia is frequently observed in patients with significant PH and cor pulmonale. Patients with IPAH may have normal arterial oxygen content until late in the disease. Pulmonary function tests may sometimes help identify the etiology of pulmonary vascular disease. The presence of significant PH and cor pulmonale with mild abnormalities in pulmonary function tests should suggest a diagnosis of primary pulmonary vascular disease.

In contrast to acute PE, in which nonspecific ECG changes are commonly observed, right heart strain, including P pulmonale, right axis deviation, and right ventricular hypertrophy, is typically present in patients with advanced pulmonary hypertension or cor pulmonale. For example, evidence of right heart strain ultimately occurs in approximately 80% of patients with IPAH.[36]

Patients with longstanding PH or cor pulmonale have markedly abnormal radiographs that suggest the presence of their disease. Enlarged pulmonary arteries with or without an enlarged RV are often evident. **Figure 35-5** illustrates severe bilateral pulmonary artery and RV enlargement in a patient with IPAH.

Echocardiography is quite useful in the diagnosis of PH.[37] The echocardiogram also helps establish secondary causes for PH, such as left ventricular dysfunction, mitral valve abnormalities, or congenital heart disease. Although echocardiography is not foolproof in the detection of mild to moderate PH, it is sensitive in the detection of severe elevations in pulmonary artery pressure. The majority of such patients have tricuspid regurgitation, thereby allowing a reasonably accurate estimate of pulmonary artery systolic pressure. Because echocardiography is noninvasive, it is generally used early to determine the presence and severity of PH in the presence or absence of cor pulmonale. It is also useful for serial monitoring of patients with established PH after therapeutic interventions. For evaluation of a patient with PH, $\dot{V}/\dot{Q}$ scanning is important in excluding chronic thromboembolic disease as a secondary cause of PH.[37]

The gold standard for the diagnosis of PH remains right heart catheterization, which should always be done prior to instituting therapy. This technique utilizes a thermodilution balloon catheter to measure right ventricular, pulmonary artery, and pulmonary

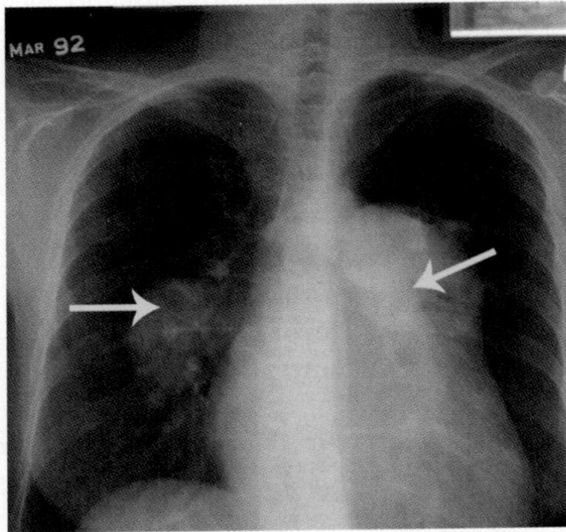

FIGURE 35-5 Chest radiograph in a patient with primary pulmonary hypertension. Enlarged right and left pulmonary arteries are evident (arrows).

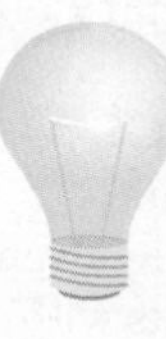

STOP AND THINK

Your patient with severe COPD has noted increasing lower extremity edema for the past month and now has been admitted to the hospital with an exacerbation. What do you suggest for further evaluation and management?

capillary wedge pressures.[38] Patients with IPAH have normal wedge pressures. The presence of an abnormal capillary wedge pressure suggests a left-sided cause of PH. In addition, right heart catheterization allows for comparisons between the oxygen saturation in the central veins, right atrium, right ventricle, and pulmonary artery. This determines whether left-to-right or right-to-left shunting is present. Right heart catheterization supplements the echocardiographic data in the diagnosis and evaluation of congenital heart disease. In many centers, exposure to a pulmonary vasodilator is done during cardiac catheterization to assess vascular reactivity.

In summary, in patients in whom PH is suspected based on the clinical history or physical exam, a reasonable diagnostic approach may begin with a chest radiograph and echocardiogram. A $\dot{V}/\dot{Q}$ scan should be performed to exclude PE in patients with evidence of PH. If PH is a high probability, then CTA, pulmonary arteriography, or both should be performed.

Management of Selected Pulmonary Vascular Diseases

Acute Pulmonary Embolism

Anticoagulation has been proven to reduce mortality in acute PE, and it should be immediately instituted unless contraindications are present. Although anticoagulants do not directly dissolve preexisting clots, they prevent thrombus extension and indirectly decrease clot burden by allowing the natural fibrinolytic system to proceed unopposed.[39] When there exists a high clinical suspicion for PE, anticoagulation is appropriate while diagnostic testing is under way unless the risk of therapy is deemed excessive. Standard therapy is parenteral anticoagulants (full-dose unfractionated heparin, low-molecular-weight heparin, or fondaparinux) followed by oral vitamin K antagonists (warfarin) or new direct oral anticoagulants (NOACs).

Unfractionated heparin (UFH) is usually delivered by continuous IV infusion, and therapy is monitored by measurement of the activated partial thromboplastin time (aPTT). Traditional, or physician-directed, dosing of heparin often leads to subtherapeutic aPTT; validated dosing nomograms are generally favored because they reduce the time to achieve therapeutic anticoagulation and may decrease the risk of recurrent thromboembolic events.[40–42] A heparin regimen consisting of a bolus of 80 units/kg followed by 18 units/kg/h has been recommended, and, following the institution of intravenous UFH, the aPTT should be followed at 6-hour intervals until it is consistently in the therapeutic range of 1.5 to 2.0 times control values.[43] Further adjusting of the heparin dose should be weight based.

Low-molecular-weight heparin (LMWH) is at least as safe and effective as UFH for the treatment of acute venous thromboembolism (VTE) and is now favored for most hemodynamically stable patients[44,45] with acute DVT or PE, except when the much shorter acting heparin is deemed more appropriate. LMWH preparations offer several advantages over UFH, including greater bioavailability, longer half-life, lack of need for an intravenous infusion, more predictable anticoagulant response to weight-based dosing, and a decreased risk of heparin-induced thrombocytopenia (HIT). These preparations can be administered once or twice per day subcutaneously and do not require monitoring of the aPTT. Monitoring of antifactor Xa levels is reasonable in certain settings such as morbid obesity, very small patients (<40 kg), pregnancy, renal dysfunction, or patients with unanticipated bleeding or recurrent VTE despite appropriate weight-based dosing.

Long-term treatment with warfarin (a vitamin K antagonist) is effective for preventing recurrent VTE, and therapy may be initiated after a heparin preparation is begun. Initial therapy with warfarin alone may cause a transient hypercoagulable state due to the abrupt decline in vitamin K–dependent coagulation inhibitors and may paradoxically increase the risk of recurrent PE or DVT. Warfarin therapy thus should be overlapped with therapeutic heparin for a minimum of 5 days and until two consecutive international normalized ratio (INR) values of 2.0 to 3.0 have been documented at least 24 hours apart.[46] The duration of anticoagulation depends on the presence or persistence of risk factors, but in all cases, documented PE should be treated with anticoagulation for at least 3 months. In some cases, however, with underlying hypercoagulable states (refer to Box 35-2), lifetime anticoagulation may be indicated. Oral warfarin therapy must take into account many drug and food interactions, as well as genetic variations in drug metabolism, and careful monitoring is warranted.

Other, newer agents may be useful in the treatment of VTE. Fondaparinux is a heparin-derived synthetic polysaccharide that catalyzes factor Xa activation. Direct thrombin inhibitors such as lepirudin and argatroban have an important niche in the treatment of HIT, but their anticoagulant effect is not readily reversible. New direct oral anticoagulants such as rivaroxaban and dabigatran demonstrate comparable efficacy to warfarin and may have a lower risk of bleeding complications.[47]

Complications of heparin include bleeding and heparin-induced thrombocytopenia. The rates of major bleeding in trials using heparin by continuous infusion are less than 5%.[48] Heparin-induced thrombocytopenia (defined as a platelet count that drops by greater than 50% or to less than 100,000 mm^3) typically develops 5 to 10 days after the initiation of heparin therapy, occurring in 3% to 5% of patients. The syndrome is caused by heparin-dependent IgG antiplatelet antibodies and can result in either paradoxical thrombosis or bleeding.[49] If a patient is placed on heparin for venous thromboembolism and the platelet count progressively decreases to 100,000/mm^3 or less, heparin therapy should be discontinued. It is important to realize that HIT can occur with a platelet count of higher than 100,000/mm^3. Several anticoagulants have been approved for use in the setting of HIT.

Inferior vena cava (IVC) filter placement can be undertaken to prevent lower extremity thrombi from embolizing to the lungs.[50] These devices have been widely used for over two decades. The primary indications for filter placement include contraindications to anticoagulation, significant bleeding complications during anticoagulation, and recurrent embolism while on adequate therapy. Filters are sometimes placed in the setting of massive PE when it is believed that any further emboli might be lethal. A randomized study suggested that filter placement in patients with new DVT reduces the risk of acute PE at day 12 but increases the risk of recurrent DVT at 2 years.[51] A number of filter designs exist, and temporary, removable filters are widely used currently. Filters can be inserted via the jugular or femoral vein. These devices are effective, and complications are unusual but may include perforation of the IVC, filter migration, and IVC obstruction due to filter thrombosis. In general, anticoagulation is continued when a filter is placed unless it is contraindicated.

The National Institutes of Health consensus guidelines for PE thrombolysis issued in 1980 suggested that **thrombolytic therapy** was appropriate for patients with obstruction of blood flow to a lobe or multiple pulmonary segments and for patients with hemodynamic compromise, regardless of the size of the PE.[52] Current guidelines also favor the use of thrombolytic therapy in patients with hemodynamic instability (hypotension) or severely compromised oxygenation. Risk stratification is important in acute PE, and more stable patients with a significant embolic load are considered on an individual basis, with thrombolytic therapy being considered in the absence of absolute or relative contraindications. Such settings might include severe hypoxemia, significant RV dysfunction by echocardiography, elevated troponin values, or a combination of these.

Acceleration of clot lysis in PE with thrombolytic therapy was documented in several trials.[25,53] One trial demonstrated that thrombolysis was accelerated in patients receiving urokinase compared with those on heparin when pulmonary arteriograms and lung perfusion scans were examined 24 hours after treatment. At present, tissue plasminogen activator (100 mg intravenous infusion delivered over 2 hours) may be the most commonly employed protocol when thrombolysis is used in PE.[54] Heparin should be withheld until the thrombolytic infusion is completed.

Some patients deemed candidates for thrombolytic therapy based on the severity of their PE might have contraindications such as bleeding or high risk of bleeding (e.g., recent surgery). In such cases, surgical removal of clot (pulmonary embolectomy) can be considered.

Chronic Cor Pulmonale

Cor pulmonale describes RV dysfunction caused by diseases affecting the lung or its vasculature. The treatment of patients with cor pulmonale focuses on treatment of the underlying lung disease, with efforts toward improving oxygenation, decreasing pulmonary vascular resistance, and improving RV function. In the case of COPD, β-receptor agonists (e.g., albuterol, salmeterol) and anticholinergics (e.g., ipratropium, tiotropium) are inhaled bronchodilators used in patients with airflow obstruction. Theophylline is also a bronchodilator but may offer additional beneficial effects such as improved cardiac contractility, mild pulmonary vasodilation, and enhanced diaphragm endurance. Finally, inhaled or systemic corticosteroids, or both, appear to benefit a subset of patients with COPD.

Because **hypoxic pulmonary vasoconstriction** is thought to contribute to the pathogenesis of PH in patients with cor pulmonale, supplemental oxygen therapy is often employed. Supplemental oxygen reduces hypoxic pulmonary vasoconstriction, thereby reducing pulmonary artery pressures and decreasing the workload of the right ventricle. Two large trials have demonstrated a survival benefit of supplemental oxygen therapy in COPD patients with hypoxemia and cor pulmonale.[55,56] Based on the results of these and other studies, long-term oxygen therapy is recommended in patients with a Pao_2 of 55 mm Hg or less or in patients with a Pao_2 of 60 mm Hg or less and evidence of cor pulmonale or secondary polycythemia.

There are only limited data regarding the use of inotropic agents or pulmonary vasodilators in cor pulmonale. Digoxin does not improve RV function in patients with COPD and cor pulmonale without concomitant left ventricular failure.[57] Diuretic therapy may improve right heart function by decreasing the RV filling volume in cases of significant volume overload. Traditional pulmonary vasodilators (e.g., hydralazine, calcium channel blockers) have not shown sustained benefits

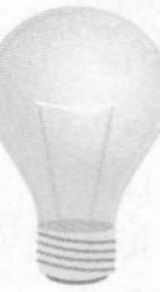

STOP AND THINK

A patient with severe idiopathic pulmonary fibrosis is admitted for worsening dyspnea and hypoxemia. The plan is to administer intravenous prostacyclin for treatment of pulmonary hypertension. Would you anticipate any challenges with this therapy or have any additional suggestions?

and may be associated with deleterious effects resulting from systemic vasodilation.

More advanced therapy (e.g., sildenafil, epoprostenol) may be considered in selected patients with persistent PH and a poor functional status despite maximal primary therapy. There is little direct evidence, however, supporting advanced therapy in cor pulmonale. The treatment of PH with systemic pulmonary artery vasodilator therapy may actually worsen gas exchange in patients with significant parenchymal lung disease due to the release of regional hypoxic pulmonary vasoconstriction, the loss of which leads to worsening ventilation-perfusion mismatch. The use of inhaled selective pulmonary vasodilators (e.g., inhaled nitric oxide, inhaled prostacyclin) may attenuate this likelihood by producing pulmonary vasodilation in those relative lung areas receiving ventilation, and thus diverting blood flow away from nonventilated areas and decreasing intrapulmonary shunting. These PH-specific treatment approaches remain controversial and should be considered on a case-by-case basis at specialized centers. Lung transplantation should be considered for eligible patients refractory to treatment.

Pulmonary Arterial Hypertension

Initial therapeutic trials in PAH focused on the use of calcium channel blockers to treat PH, and an improvement in pulmonary hemodynamics occurs in a minority of treated patients.[58] A sustained improvement is less common, and these agents also may have significant adverse effects such as hypotension. As in patients with cor pulmonale, traditional therapies such as supplemental oxygen and diuretics are useful. These forms of therapies for PAH are generally insufficient and advanced therapies are needed.

Prostacyclin (epoprostenol, PGI_2) is a pulmonary vasodilator that has proven to be the most effective therapy available in the treatment of patients with IPAH. Because prostacyclin has a short half-life and is rapidly inactivated by the low gastric pH, it is given as a continuous intravenous infusion via a permanent indwelling catheter with a portable infusion pump. A large, prospective, randomized, multicenter trial compared prostacyclin plus conventional therapy with conventional therapy alone in patients with class III and class IV IPAH.[59] The patients treated with prostacyclin had significant improvements in exercise capacity, hemodynamics, and survival. Long-term benefits are likely due to the vasodilation, antiplatelet, and antiproliferation properties of prostacyclin. Prostacyclin analogues, such as treprostinil and iloprost, are also beneficial in the management of PAH;[60,61] treprostinil has proved effective when delivered via the subcutaneous, intravenous, and inhaled routes, and iloprost is effective via the intravenous or inhaled route.

Extraordinary advances in the understanding of PH have led to the development of other treatment regimens for PAH. Endothelin is a potent vasoconstrictor and smooth muscle mitogen, and oral endothelin receptor antagonists (bosentan, ambrisentan) have been shown to improve hemodynamics and functional status in patients with PAH.[62,63] Oral phosphodiesterase-5 inhibitors (sildenafil, tadalafil) prolong the vasodilatory effects of endogenous nitric oxide and are also effective therapies.[64,65] There is also emerging evidence that combination therapy is useful in the treatment of PAH. Finally, lung transplantation is appropriate in carefully selected patients with PAH who fail medical therapy.

Because microscopic thrombi and frank VTE are associated with PAH, systemic anticoagulation has been suggested to improve survival in patients with IPAH.[66] When warfarin is used, an INR of 1.5 to 2.5 is considered therapeutic. The risk–benefit ratio must be considered on an individual basis when considering anticoagulant therapy.

Other Classes of Pulmonary Hypertension

Other classes of PH should be managed with primary therapy directed at the underlying cause of the PH as described previously. For example, the treatment of PH resulting from cardiac disease is aimed at the treatment of the underlying cardiac defect (i.e., mitral stenosis, left ventricular systolic or diastolic failure, sleep apnea). In general, treatment of any underlying disease that may be contributing to the development of PH and the use of supplemental oxygen to alleviate hypoxic pulmonary vasoconstriction remain important goals of therapy. Following treatment, the severity of PH may be reassessed and more advanced therapy considered on a case-by-case basis by physicians who are experienced in the evaluation and management of PH at a specialized center.

Recent consensus statements by the World Health Organization convening at Nice, France, in 2013, have offered detailed evidence-based recommendations for the treatment of PH. These include having a low threshold to refer patients to PH centers with expertise in treating this disease.[66]

Case Studies

Case 1. Acute Right Ventricular Failure

A 50-year-old man with a history of arthritis 5 days after left hip replacement suddenly developed shortness of breath and hypotension. The patient previously had been healthy and well. His postoperative course was uncomplicated, and warfarin had been started for thromboembolism prophylaxis. The patient had just gotten out of bed to go to the bathroom when he suddenly felt short of breath and dizzy. On examination he looked pale and in moderate respiratory distress. Blood pressure was 85 systolic, heart rate 120 beats/min, respiratory rate 30 breaths/min, and oxygen saturation 90% on 15 L/min oxygen via nonrebreathing mask. Physical exam was notable for clear lungs, an elevated jugular venous pressure with a prominent V wave, tachycardia with a prominent S_2 sound, a systolic murmur at the left sternal border, and an S_3 sound that was augmented with inspiration. The left leg was edematous. An arterial blood gas revealed a pH of 7.45, a $Pa\text{CO}_2$ of 28 mm Hg, and a $Pa\text{O}_2$ of 59 mm Hg on supplemental O_2 at 15 L/min. An ECG revealed tachycardia with a new right bundle branch pattern, and a chest radiograph disclosed bilateral lower lobe atelectasis.

The patient has had an acute event resulting in hypoxemia, hypotension, and signs of right heart failure. Given his recent hip surgery, the most likely etiology is acute PE. Hypotension is likely from acute right-sided heart failure. This results from an acute rise in the pulmonary vascular resistance leading to a decrement in RV stroke volume and an increase in the RV end diastolic volume. This increase has multiple detrimental effects, including increased oxygen demands resulting in ischemia and decreased left ventricular compliance via ventricular interdependence. The result is decreased cardiac performance and shock.

The approach to this patient will involve prompt, accurate diagnosis and treatment. Diagnostically, the patient could have a $\dot{V}/\dot{Q}$ scan or a chest CTA. Given the instability of the patient, a CTA, the faster test, is preferred. The options for treatment include anticoagulation with UFH or LMWH, anticoagulation plus inferior vena cava filter placement, or fibrinolytic therapy. In the meantime the patient will require transfer to an intensive care unit for hemodynamic and respiratory support. His oxygen requirement is high, and he is hypotensive. Fluids should be administered, and vasopressor therapy should follow if the blood pressure remains low. This patient would meet the indications for thrombolytic therapy, but recent surgery (less than 1 week ago) increases the risk for bleeding complications. A careful assessment of the risks and benefits of fibrinolytic therapy is necessary in this case. Pulmonary embolectomy could be considered if thrombolytics were deemed contraindicated.

Case 2. Idiopathic Pulmonary Arterial Hypertension

A 30-year-old woman developed progressive dyspnea over a 6-month period. The patient had been previously healthy and active until approximately 6 months before presentation, when she noted dyspnea when walking to her third-floor apartment. This was associated with occasional sharp chest pains but no wheezing or fever. The dyspnea had progressed over the next few months such that the patient was getting short of breath after climbing only a few stairs or walking on a hill. An evaluation had disclosed a normal chest radiograph, normal spirometry, a decreased diffusion capacity at 55% of predicted, and an ECG consistent with strain on the right ventricle. An echocardiogram disclosed a dilated, hypokinetic RV with an estimated RV systolic pressure of 76 mm Hg. The left ventricle had normal size and function. No shunts were evident when contrast bubbles were injected.

On presentation, the patient reports dyspnea with short walks on a flat surface. She had had a syncopal episode about 1 week before presentation. Further review of the history disclosed no history of prior lung disease, connective tissue disease (or unexplained arthritis or skin abnormalities), diet pill use, exotic travel, or previous thromboembolic disease. She had no history of smoking and a noncontributory family history. Her oxygen saturation was 89% on room air. She had clear lungs on auscultation. Her cardiac exam was notable for elevated neck veins and a prominent RV heave. On auscultation she had a loud P_2 with a right-sided S_3. A prominent systolic murmur was detectable at the left lower sternal border that increased in intensity with inspiration (tricuspid regurgitation). The patient also had 2+ edema of her lower extremities. A full laboratory evaluation was notable for normal rheumatologic serologies, a negative HIV test, normal coagulation profile, and normal liver function. The chest radiograph was clear with prominent central pulmonary arteries. A $\dot{V}/\dot{Q}$ scan disclosed only small peripheral defects and was considered low probability for PE.

The patient was diagnosed with IPAH and referred to a PH specialist for additional diagnostic workup and consideration for prostacyclin therapy.

Key Points

- The low-pressure pulmonary circulation normally offers little resistance to the flow of blood out of the right ventricle.
- Pulmonary vascular disease leads to pulmonary hypertension and increased pulmonary vascular resistance. When sustained over time, elevations in pulmonary vascular resistance lead to right ventricular hypertrophy, dilation, and failure.
- The diagnosis of pulmonary vascular disease based on clinical examination is often difficult because many signs and symptoms are nonspecific. Therefore, when pulmonary embolism (PE) or pulmonary hypertension (PH) is suspected, additional diagnostic testing is indicated.

- ▶ Chest computed tomographic angiography (CTA) often is the first diagnostic study employed in patients with suspected PE.
- ▶ Anticoagulation with unfractionated heparin or low-molecular-weight heparin is the primary therapy in acute PE, except in cases with hemodynamic instability or severe hypoxemia, where thrombolytic therapy may be indicated.
- ▶ Treatment of cor pulmonale is directed at the reduction of hypoxic pulmonary vasoconstriction and the treatment of any underlying pulmonary disease that may be contributing to the PH.
- ▶ Prostacyclin decreases pulmonary vascular resistance and improves survival in patients with idiopathic pulmonary arterial hypertension.
- ▶ Other new therapies, including endothelin receptor antagonists and phosphodiesterase inhibitors, can be considered for treatment of pulmonary arterial hypertension.

References

1. Schulman DS, Matthay RA. The right ventricle in pulmonary disease. *Cardiol Clin.* 1992;10:111–135.
2. Weber KT, Janicki JS, Shroff SG, et al. The right ventricle: physiologic and pathophysiologic considerations. *Crit Care Med.* 1983;11:323–328.
3. Damato AN, Galante JG, Smith WM. Hemodynamic response to treadmill exercise in normal subjects. *J Appl Physiol.* 1966;21:959–966.
4. Epstein SE, Beiser GD, Stampfer M, et al. Characterization of the circulatory response to maximal upright exercise in normal subjects and patients with heart disease. *Circulation.* 1967;3:1049–1062.
5. Fishman AP. State of the art: chronic cor pulmonale. *Am Rev Respir Dis.* 1976;114:775–794.
6. Hatano S, Strasser T, eds. *Primary Pulmonary Hypertension. Report on a WHO Meeting.* Geneva: World Health Organization; 1975:7–45.
7. Simonneau G, Gatzoulis MA, Adatia I, et al. Updated clinical classification of pulmonary hypertension. *J Am Coll Cardiol.* 2013;62(Suppl 25):D34–D41. Erratum, *J Am Coll Cardiol.* 2014;63:746.
8. Klinger JR, Hill NS. Right ventricular dysfunction in chronic obstructive pulmonary disease. Evaluation and management. *Chest.* 1991;99:715–723.
9. Christman BW, McPherson CD, Newman JH, et al. An imbalance between the excretion of thromboxane and prostacyclin metabolites in pulmonary hypertension. *N Engl J Med.* 1992;327:70–75.
10. Rubin LJ. Primary pulmonary hypertension. *N Engl J Med.* 1997;336:111–117.
11. McIntyre KM, Sasahara AA. The ratio of pulmonary arterial pressure to pulmonary vascular obstruction: index of preembolic cardiopulmonary status. *Chest.* 1977;71:692–697.
12. Dalen JE, Alpert JS. Natural history of pulmonary embolism. *Prog Cardiovasc Dis.* 1975;17:259–270.
13. Giuntini C, Di Ricco G, Marini C, et al. Pulmonary embolism: epidemiology. *Chest.* 1995;107(Suppl 1):3S–9S.
14. Renzetti AD Jr, McClement JH, Litt BD. The Veterans Administration cooperative study of pulmonary function. 3. Mortality in relation to respiratory function in chronic obstructive pulmonary disease. *Am J Med.* 1966;41:115–129.
15. McFadden E, Brunwald E. Cor pulmonale. In: Braunwald E, ed. *Heart Disease: A Textbook of Cardiovascular Medicine.* 3rd ed. Philadelphia: Saunders; 1988:1597–1616.
16. Bishop JM, Cross KW. Physiological variables and mortality in patients with various categories of chronic respiratory disease. *Bull Eur Physiopathol Respir.* 1984;20:495–500.
17. Behr J, Ryu JH. Pulmonary hypertension in interstitial lung disease. *Eur Respir J.* 2008;31:1357–1367.
18. Humbert M, Sitbon O, Chaouat A, et al. Pulmonary arterial hypertension in France: results from a national registry. *Am J Respir Crit Care Med.* 2006;173:1023–1030.
19. D'Alonzo GE, Barst RJ, Ayres SM, et al. Survival in patients with primary pulmonary hypertension. Results from a national prospective registry. *Ann Intern Med.* 1991;115:343–349.
20. Petitpretz P, Brenot F, Azarian R, et al. Pulmonary hypertension in patients with human immunodeficiency virus infection. Comparison with primary pulmonary hypertension. *Circulation.* 1994;89:2722–2727.
21. Brenot F, Herve P, Petitpretz P, et al. Primary pulmonary hypertension and fenfluramine use. *Br Heart J.* 1993;70:537–541.
22. Abenhaim L, Moride Y, Brenot F, et al. Appetite-suppressant drugs and the risk of primary pulmonary hypertension. International Primary Pulmonary Hypertension Study Group. *N Engl J Med.* 1996;335:609–616.
23. Goldhaber SZ, Hennekens CH, Evans DA, et al. Factors associated with correct antemortem diagnosis of major pulmonary embolism. *Am J Med.* 1982;73:822–826.
24. Green RM, Meyer TJ, Dunn M, Glassroth J. Pulmonary embolism in younger adults. *Chest.* 1992;101:1507–1511.
25. The Urokinase Pulmonary Embolism Trial. A national cooperative study. *Circulation.* 1973;47(Suppl 2):II1–II108.
26. Stein PD, Terrin ML, Hales CA, et al. Clinical, laboratory, roentgenographic, and electrocardiographic findings in patients with acute pulmonary embolism and no pre-existing cardiac or pulmonary disease. *Chest.* 1991;100:598–603.
27. Value of the ventilation/perfusion scan in acute pulmonary embolism. Results of the prospective investigation of pulmonary embolism diagnosis (PIOPED). The PIOPED Investigators. *JAMA.* 1990;263:2753–2759.
28. Rathbun SW, Raskob GE, Whitsett TL. Sensitivity and specificity of helical computed tomography in the diagnosis of pulmonary embolism: a systematic review. *Ann Intern Med.* 2000;132:227–232.
29. Stein PD, Fowler SE, Goodman LR, et al. Multidetector computed tomography for acute pulmonary embolism. *N Engl J Med.* 2006;35:2317–2327.
30. Stein PD, Athanasoulis C, Alavi A, et al. Complications and validity of pulmonary angiography in acute pulmonary embolism. *Circulation.* 1992;85:462–468.
31. Stein PD, Hull RD, Pineo G. Strategy that includes serial noninvasive leg tests for diagnosis of thromboembolic disease in patients with suspected acute pulmonary embolism based on data from PIOPED. Prospective Investigation of Pulmonary Embolism Diagnosis. *Arch Intern Med.* 1995;155:2101–2104.
32. Goldhaber SZ. Echocardiography in the management of pulmonary embolism. *Ann Intern Med.* 2002;136:691–700.
33. McConnell MV, Solomon SD, Rayan ME, et al. Regional right ventricular dysfunction detected by echocardiography in acute pulmonary embolism. *Am J Cardiol.* 1996;78:469–473.
34. Grifoni S, Olivotto I, Cecchini P, et al. Short-term clinical outcome of patients with acute pulmonary embolism, normal blood pressure, and echocardiographic right ventricular dysfunction. *Circulation.* 2000;101:2817–2822.
35. Kucher N, Rossi E, De Rosa M, Goldhaber SZ. Prognostic role of echocardiography among patients with acute pulmonary embolism and a systolic arterial pressure of 90 mm Hg or higher. *Arch Intern Med.* 2005;165:1777–1781.
36. Rich S, Dantzker DR, Ayres SM, et al. Primary pulmonary hypertension. A national prospective study. *Ann Intern Med.* 1987;107:216–223.
37. D'Alonzo GE, Bower JS, Dantzker DR. Differentiation of patients with primary and thromboembolic pulmonary hypertension. *Chest.* 1984;85:457–461.
38. Swan HJ, Ganz W, Forrester J, et al. Catheterization of the heart in man with use of a flow-directed balloon-tipped catheter. *N Engl J Med.* 1970;283:447–451.
39. Hirsh J, Dalen JE, Deykin D, Poller L. Heparin: mechanism of action, pharmacokinetics, dosing considerations, monitoring, efficacy, and safety. *Chest.* 1992;102(Suppl 4):337S–351S.

40. Raschke RA, Reilly BM, Guidry JR, et al. The weight-based heparin dosing nomogram compared with a "standard care" nomogram. A randomized controlled trial. *Ann Intern Med.* 1993;119:874–881.
41. Hull RD, Raskob GE, Brant RF, et al. Relation between the time to achieve the lower limit of the APTT therapeutic range and recurrent venous thromboembolism during heparin treatment for deep vein thrombosis. *Arch Intern Med.* 1997;157:2562–2568.
42. Hull RD, Raskob GE, Brant RF, et al. The importance of initial heparin treatment on long-term clinical outcomes of antithrombotic therapy. The emerging theme of delayed recurrence. *Arch Intern Med.* 1997;157:2317–2321.
43. Hull RD, Raskob GE, Rosenbloom D, et al. Optimal therapeutic level of heparin therapy in patients with venous thrombosis. *Arch Intern Med.* 1992;152:1589–1595.
44. van Dongen CJ, van den Belt AG, Prins MH, Lensing AW. Fixed dose subcutaneous low molecular weight heparins versus adjusted dose unfractionated heparin for venous thromboembolism. *Cochrane Database Syst Rev.* 2004;4:CD001100.
45. Quinlan DJ, McQuillan A, Eikelboom JW. Low-molecular-weight heparin compared with intravenous unfractionated heparin for treatment of pulmonary embolism: a meta-analysis of randomized, controlled trials. *Ann Intern Med.* 2004;140:175–183.
46. Kearon C, Kahn SR, Agnelli G, et al. Antithrombotic therapy for venous thromboembolic disease: American College of Chest Physicians Evidence-Based Clinical Practice Guidelines. 8th ed. *Chest.* 2008;133(Suppl 6):454S–545S.
47. van der Hulle T, Kooiman J, den Exter PL, et al. Effectiveness and safety of novel oral anticoagulants as compared with vitamin K antagonists in the treatment of acute symptomatic venous thromboembolism: a systematic review and meta-analysis. *J Thromb Haemost.* 2014;12:320–328.
48. Clagett GP, Anderson FA Jr, Heit J, et al. Prevention of venous thromboembolism. *Chest.* 1995;108(Suppl 4):312S–334S.
49. Kelton JG, Sheridan D, Santos A, et al. Heparin-induced thrombocytopenia: laboratory studies. *Blood.* 1988;72:925–930.
50. Greenfield LJ. Vena caval interruption and pulmonary embolectomy. *Clin Chest Med.* 1984;5:495–505.
51. Decousus H, Leizorovicz A, Parent F, et al. A clinical trial of vena caval filters in the prevention of pulmonary embolism in patients with proximal deep-vein thrombosis. Prevention du Risque d'Embolie Pulmonaire par Interruption Cave Study Group. *N Engl J Med.* 1998;338:409–415.
52. Thrombolytic therapy in thrombosis: a National Institutes of Health consensus development conference. *Ann Intern Med.* 1980;93:141–144.
53. Miller GA, Gibson RV, Honey M, Sutton GC. Treatment of pulmonary embolism with streptokinase. A preliminary report. *Br Med J.* 1969;1:812–815.
54. Goldhaber SZ, Kessler CM, Heit J, et al. Randomised controlled trial of recombinant tissue plasminogen activator versus urokinase in the treatment of acute pulmonary embolism. *Lancet.* 1988;2:293–298.
55. Nocturnal Oxygen Therapy Trial Group. Continuous or nocturnal oxygen therapy in hypoxemic chronic obstructive lung disease: a clinical trial. *Ann Intern Med.* 1980;93:391–398.
56. Long term domiciliary oxygen therapy in chronic hypoxic cor pulmonale complicating chronic bronchitis and emphysema. Report of the Medical Research Council Working Party. *Lancet.* 1981;1:681–686.
57. Mathur PN, Powles P, Pugsley SO, et al. Effect of digoxin on right ventricular function in severe chronic airflow obstruction. A controlled clinical trial. *Ann Intern Med.* 1981;95:283–288.
58. Rich S, Brundage BH. High-dose calcium channel-blocking therapy for primary pulmonary hypertension: evidence for long-term reduction in pulmonary arterial pressure and regression of right ventricular hypertrophy. *Circulation.* 1987;76:135–141.
59. Barst RJ, Rubin LJ, Long WA, et al. A comparison of continuous intravenous epoprostenol (prostacyclin) with conventional therapy for primary pulmonary hypertension. The Primary Pulmonary Hypertension Study Group. *N Engl J Med.* 1996;334:296–302.
60. Tapson VF, Gomberg-Maitland M, McLaughlin VV, et al. Safety and efficacy of IV treprostinil for pulmonary arterial hypertension: a prospective, multicenter, open-label, 12-week trial. *Chest.* 2006;129:683–688.
61. Olschewski H, Simonneau G, Galie N, et al. Inhaled iloprost for severe pulmonary hypertension. *N Engl J Med.* 2002;347:322–329.
62. Rubin LJ, Badesch DB, Barst RJ, et al. Bosentan therapy for pulmonary arterial hypertension. *N Engl J Med.* 2002;346:896–903.
63. Galie N, Olschewski H, Oudiz RJ, et al. Ambrisentan for the treatment of pulmonary arterial hypertension: results of the Ambrisentan in Pulmonary Arterial Hypertension, Randomized, Double-Blind, Placebo-Controlled, Multicenter, Efficacy (ARIES) Study 1 and 2. *Circulation.* 2008;117:3010–3019.
64. Galie N, Ghofrani HA, Torbicki A, et al. Sildenafil citrate therapy for pulmonary arterial hypertension. *N Engl J Med.* 2005;353:2148–2157.
65. Galie N, Brundage BH, Ghofrani HA, et al. Tadalafil therapy for pulmonary arterial hypertension. *Circulation.* 2009;119:2894–2903.
66. Galiè N, Corris PA, Frost A, et al. Updated treatment algorithm of pulmonary arterial hypertension. *J Am Coll Cardiol.* 2013;62(Suppl 25):D60–D72.

CHAPTER

36

Pneumonia

Nicholas Wysham, Morgan Mullaney, Bryan D. Kraft

OUTLINE

OBJECTIVES

1. Define pneumonia.
2. Compare and contrast community-acquired pneumonia and nosocomial pneumonia.
3. Discuss the etiology, initial management, treatment, and prognosis of community-acquired pneumonia.
4. Describe the clinical, radiographic, and microbiologic methods to diagnose pneumonia.
5. Discuss the diagnosis and treatment of aspiration and anaerobic pneumonia.
6. Discuss the differences between healthcare-associated, hospital-acquired, and ventilator-associated pneumonia.
7. Discuss the prevention and treatment of ventilator-associated pneumonia.
8. Describe the clinical and radiographic findings, diagnostic procedures, causes, and therapeutic considerations for pneumonia in the immunocompromised host.
9. Describe the management of pneumonia in patients with HIV infection.
10. Discuss the risk factors for viral, mycobacterial, and fungal pneumonia.
11. Discuss the clinical presentations and diagnosis of viral, mycobacterial, and fungal pneumonia.
12. Discuss the management of pneumonia in children.

KEY TERMS

antigen detection
aspiration pneumonia
atypical organisms
atypical pneumonia
bacteremia
biomarkers
bronchoalveolar lavage (BAL)
community-acquired pneumonia (CAP)
empyema
fungal pneumonia
hospital-acquired pneumonia (HAP)
human immunodeficiency virus (HIV)
nontuberculous mycobacterial infection (NTM)
nosocomial pneumonia
sputum gram stain and culture
tuberculosis (TB)
typical pneumonia
ventilator-associated pneumonia (VAP)
viral pneumonia

Introduction

Pneumonia is the third leading cause of death worldwide, resulting in over 3 million deaths per year.[1–3] In the United States, pneumonia hospitalizations are projected to increase significantly over the coming decades as the population ages.[4] The vast majority of these pneumonia cases will be due to *Streptococcus pneumoniae,* the most common cause of pneumonia in the world. Moreover, pneumonia due to multidrug-resistant bacteria and opportunistic pathogens is also increasing as patients with complex medical conditions and/or compromised immune systems are more frequently treated outside of the hospital. As a result, respiratory therapists and other healthcare providers will see regularly many forms of pneumonia and must have a strong command of pneumonia types, pathogenesis, diagnosis, prognosis, treatment, and prevention.

Definition and Classification of Pneumonia

Pneumonia is the inflammation and consolidation of lung tissue, most frequently due to an infection. Pathogens may gain access to the lower respiratory tract via aspiration of gastric, oropharyngeal, or nasopharyngeal secretions, inhalation of infectious droplets or aerosols, hematogenous dissemination, or direct spread from the pleural space. The human lung has a number of innate defenses against invading microorganisms, including cough, lining epithelial cells, mucus production, mucociliary transport, and alveolar macrophages. While these defenses are adept at protecting the lung from infection, they can become weakened or overwhelmed, allowing the entry of pathogens into the lower respiratory tract leading to pneumonia. Symptoms of pneumonia vary but generally include fever or chills; cough productive of purulent, green, or rust-colored sputum; shortness of breath; pleuritic chest pain; fatigue; and myalgia. Signs of pneumonia may include tachypnea, tachycardia, increased work of breathing, hypoxemia, change in white blood cell (WBC) count, and infiltrate on chest radiograph (**Box 36-1**).

Pneumonia can be classified a number of ways, including by place of acquisition (community-acquired vs. hospital-acquired), type of pathogen (viral vs. bacterial), clinical features (typical vs. atypical), type of insult (infectious vs. noninfectious), and immune-status (immunocompetent vs. immunocompromised). Accurate classification of pneumonia is critical. Depending on pneumonia type, the pathogens, treatment, and prognosis vary greatly. **Community-acquired pneumonia (CAP)** refers to pneumonia in patients *without* recent exposure to a healthcare facility, such as a hospital or skilled nursing home (**Table 36-1**). **Nosocomial pneumonia** refers to pneumonia developing in hospitalized or healthcare-exposed patients and is more likely to be caused by multidrug-resistant (MDR) microorganisms, such as methicillin-resistant *Staphylococcus aureus* (MRSA), *Pseudomonas aeruginosa*, and *Acinetobacter* species. As a result, these pathogens demand special consideration when choosing initial antibiotic therapy.

TABLE 36-1
Classification of Pneumonia

Type	Definition
Community-acquired	Occurs in patients who lack risk factors for nosocomial pneumonia.
Healthcare-associated	Occurs in nonhospitalized patients with current or recent healthcare exposure, including: • Hospitalization for >2 days within the last 90 days; • Use of hemodialysis, wound care, or intravenous therapy within 30 days; • Residents of skilled-nursing or long-term care facilities.
Hospital-acquired	Occurs after 48 hours of hospitalization and is not incubating at time of admission.
Ventilator-associated	Occurs in mechanically ventilated patients after 2–4 days.

Information from Kollef MH, Shorr A, Tabak YP, et al. Epidemiology and outcomes of healthcare-associated pneumonia: results from a large US database of culture-positive pneumonia. *Chest.* 2005;128:3854–3862.

Community-Acquired Pneumonia

CAP is a significant cause of morbidity and mortality in the United States and abroad. In adults aged 65 years or older, the average incidence is 14 cases per 100,000 person-years, but can be up to fourfold higher in patients with certain risk factors.[5] Known risk factors for CAP include age (infants, young children, and adults ≥65 years), male sex, tobacco smoking, chronic cardiovascular, pulmonary, liver or kidney disease, diabetes mellitus, immunosuppression (e.g., HIV/AIDS, chronic corticosteroid use), functional or anatomic asplenia (e.g., sickle cell disease), immune dysregulation (e.g., celiac disease, rheumatoid arthritis), cancer, neurologic disorders (e.g., dementia, stroke/transient ischemic attacks, multiple sclerosis, Parkinson disease, and cerebrospinal fluid shunts), cochlear implants, osteoporosis, and hospitalization within the last 2 years for pneumonia.[5,6] Time of year is also a risk factor,

BOX 36-1

Clinical Signs and Symptoms of Pneumonia

Constitutional: Fever, chills, night sweats, fatigue, and/or myalgias
Respiratory: Productive cough, shortness of breath, and/or pleuritic chest pain
Laboratory: Leukocytosis, increased % bands (immature neutrophils), or leukopenia
Radiology: Infiltrate(s) on chest radiograph and/or CT scan

AGE-SPECIFIC ANGLE

The incidence of CAP is highest in infants, young children, and adults ≥65 years old.

as nearly all cases of viral CAP occur between October and May.[7]

Etiology

CAP is most commonly caused by bacterial pathogens (>50%), but up to 40% of cases may be due to respiratory viruses, and up to 11% of cases may be mixed bacterial and viral infections.[7] The presenting signs and symptoms of CAP can provide clues as to the etiology. **Typical pneumonias** are characterized by the abrupt onset of shaking chills (rigors), high fever, pleuritic chest pain, and cough productive of rusty or purulent sputum. Physical exam findings generally include signs of consolidation such as bronchial breath sounds and inspiratory crackles. The WBC count is usually elevated. The chest radiograph demonstrates lobar or segmental consolidation with air bronchograms. *S pneumoniae* is the most common cause of typical pneumonia and CAP in general, accounting for up to 50% of total cases. Other common pathogens include *P aeruginosa, Haemophilus influenzae, S aureus,* Enterobacteriaceae (e.g., *Klebsiella pneumoniae*), and *Moraxella catarrhalis.*[5]

Atypical pneumonia is more common in young adults and is characterized by a flu-like illness with dry cough, rhinorrhea, myalgias, malaise, and moderate fever. Rigors are generally absent. Unlike lobar pneumonias, the WBC count is usually normal. The chest radiograph shows diffuse interstitial or peribronchial opacities. Common causes of atypical pneumonia include *Mycoplasma pneumoniae, Chlamydophila psittaci, Chlamydophila pneumoniae, Coxiella burnetii, Legionella pneumophila,* and respiratory viruses. These organisms are not detectable on sputum gram stain and do not grow on standard bacteriologic media, making the diagnosis more difficult. The etiology of CAP is modified by patient-specific variables and risk factors, such as the patient's age, comorbidities, geographic location, and time of year (**Table 36-2**).

TABLE 36-2
Etiology of Pneumonia by Risk Factor

Risk Factor	Pathogen
COPD	*S pneumoniae, H influenzae, M catarrhalis, P aeruginosa*
Alcohol abuse	*S pneumoniae, K pneumoniae,* aspiration pneumonia, anaerobic lung abscess
Cystic fibrosis	*P aeruginosa, S aureus, H influenzae*
Neurologic impairment	Aspiration pneumonia
HIV/AIDS	*S pneumoniae, Pneumocystis* pneumonia, TB
Travel	*Coccidioides immitis* (Southwest U.S.); *Histoplasma capsulatum* (Ohio River Valley); *Blastomyces dermatitidis* (Southeast and Midwest U.S.); *Mycobacteria tuberculosis* (developing countries)
Time of year	*Legionella* (Summer/Fall); Respiratory viruses, esp. influenza (Winter)
Animal exposure	*C psittaci* (birds); *C burnetii* (farm animals); *Cryptococcus neoformans* (birds, esp. pigeons); *Histoplasma capsulatum* (birds, bats); *Francisella tularensis* (rabbits)
IV drug abuse	*S pneumoniae, S aureus*
Post-influenza	*S pneumoniae, S aureus, H influenzae*
Frequent antibiotics	Enterobacteriaceae, *P aeruginosa*

Information from Mandell LA, Wunderink RG, Anzueto A, et al. Infectious Diseases Society of America/American Thoracic Society consensus guidelines on the management of community-acquired pneumonia in adults. *Clin Infect Dis.* 2007;44(Suppl 2):S27–S72.

Gram-Positive Bacteria

Streptococcus pneumoniae

Risk factors for *S pneumoniae* infection include anatomic or functional asplenia, **human immunodeficiency virus (HIV)** infection, alcoholism, liver cirrhosis, hypogammaglobulinemia, and COPD. Complications can include lung abscess, empyema, septic shock, pericarditis, endocarditis, and meningitis. First-line treatment is a third-generation cephalosporin, although vancomycin may be required for resistant strains.

AGE-SPECIFIC ANGLE

Atypical pneumonia is more common in younger patients.

Staphylococcus aureus

The incidence of community-acquired *S aureus* pneumonia has been steadily increasing, and methicillin-resistant *S aureus* (MRSA) pneumonia is a small (2%) but significant cause of morbidity and mortality.[8] The risk factors for *S aureus* pneumonia include intravenous drug use, recent antibiotic use, recent or concurrent viral respiratory infection (especially influenza), liver cirrhosis, recent healthcare exposure, history of MRSA infection, close contact in the last month with someone with a skin infection, and immunosuppressed state.[8,9]

Common clinical features of *S aureus* pneumonia include hemoptysis, necrotizing pneumonia, hypotension, comatose state, multilobar infiltrates, and empyema.[8,10,11] Nearly all patients with *S aureus* pneumonia require hospitalization, and as many as 65% develop acute respiratory failure requiring mechanical ventilation. Mortality may be as high as 40%.[10] The first-line antibiotics for methicillin-sensitive *S aureus* (MSSA) pneumonia are nafcillin or first-generation cephalosporin, whereas the treatment of MRSA pneumonia is generally vancomycin or linezolid.

Gram-Negative Bacteria

Haemophilus influenzae

H influenzae naturally inhabits the human pharynx. *H influenzae* serotype b is the most significant cause of infection, and can cause pneumonia, meningitis, epiglottitis, arthritis, and bacteremia. Risk factors for *H influenzae* pneumonia include COPD, defects in B-cell function, functional and anatomic asplenia, and HIV infection. The typical chest radiograph finding is bronchopneumonia. *H influenzae* is treated with ampicillin or amoxicillin. If beta-lactamase-producing *H influenzae* is suspected, treatment with amoxicillin-clavulanate, fluoroquinolones, or second- and third-generation cephalosporins is preferred.

Moraxella catarrhalis

Moraxella catarrhalis is also a natural inhabitant of the human pharynx. The most common risk factor is structural lung disease, such as COPD or bronchiectasis. The chest radiograph usually reveals a bronchopneumonia. Most *M catarrhalis* strains produce beta-lactamases necessitating treatment with amoxicillin-clavulanate, ampicillin-sulbactam, fluoroquinolones, macrolides, trimethoprim-sulfamethoxazole, or second- and third-generation cephalosporins.

Atypical Organisms

Legionella Species

Most *Legionella* infections are caused by *L pneumophila.* This **atypical organism** colonizes domestic water and cooling systems, which have been implicated as sources of outbreaks of Legionnaires' disease. Symptoms can include cough, fever, dyspnea, confusion, abdominal pain, and diarrhea. Complications of infection include pericarditis, myocarditis, encephalomyelitis, Guillain-Barré syndrome, rhabdomyolysis, acute renal failure, paralytic ileus, and pancreatitis. *Legionella* pneumonia can be severe and frequently precipitates acute hypoxic respiratory failure. The first-line treatment is either fluoroquinolones or macrolides.

Mycoplasma pneumoniae

M pneumoniae is acquired by inhalation of respiratory droplets and occurs more frequently in close-quartered populations, such as boot camps, boarding schools, and college dormitories. Symptoms can include fever, malaise, headache, and cough. Complications can include myringitis and hemolytic anemia due to cold hemagglutinins. Treatment is generally with fluoroquinolones, tetracyclines, or macrolides.

Chlamydophila psittaci

C psittaci causes psittacosis and can be acquired by close contact with birds. Symptoms can include fever, cough, dyspnea, headache, and myalgia. Extrapulmonary manifestations are common and involve the skin, blood, kidney, liver, central nervous system, and heart. The treatment of choice is doxycycline.

Chlamydophila pneumoniae

Outbreaks of *C pneumoniae* infection have occurred in schools, military institutions, and within families. The clinical manifestations include fever, cough, and pharyngitis. Extrapulmonary manifestations of *C pneumoniae* can include arthritis, meningoencephalitis, myocarditis, endocarditis, coronary artery disease, and Guillain-Barré syndrome. Treatment includes fluoroquinolones, doxycycline, or macrolides.

Coxiella burnetii

The main reservoirs for *C burnetii,* which causes Q-fever, are cattle, goats, and sheep. The clinical manifestations can include fever, chills, cough, fatigue, myalgia, and diarrhea. The nonpulmonary manifestations can include endocarditis, hepatitis, meningoencephalitis, and osteomyelitis. Tetracyclines or fluoroquinolones are used for treatment.

Diagnostic Workup

Pneumonia is a clinical diagnosis based on a constellation of characteristic signs and symptoms, radiographic findings, and microbiologic results. Simply put, no single test can diagnose pneumonia. Determining the causative pathogen is helpful and allows for narrowing and

Respiratory Recap

Community-Acquired Pneumonia (CAP)

- The most common cause of CAP is *Streptococcus pneumoniae*.
- Pneumonia can be classified in many different ways.
- Patient risk factors, comorbidities, exposures, and seasonal and geographic variations influence the type of pathogen(s) that cause pneumonia.
- Antibiotics are chosen based on the most likely pathogen(s) for which each patient is at risk.

simplification of the antibiotic regimen. Unfortunately, the etiology of CAP may not be found in up 60% of cases despite aggressive evaluation.[7] The general principles of CAP diagnosis apply broadly to all other types of pneumonia (e.g., nosocomial, viral, TB) and will be discussed here. Diagnostic considerations unique to specific types of pneumonia will be discussed later.

Radiology

Chest imaging should be performed routinely in patients suspected of having pneumonia, not only because a lung infiltrate is a necessary component of the diagnosis but also because imaging can help exclude other causes for the patient's symptoms (e.g., pneumothorax). The infiltrate is frequently visible on the chest radiograph (**Figure 36-1**) but occasionally will only be seen with computed tomography (CT) of the chest (**Figure 36-2**). Different causes of pneumonia will usually have different radiographic appearances: *S pneumoniae* frequently causes lobar consolidation with air bronchograms, *H influenzae* frequently causes bronchopneumonia, and *M pneumoniae* frequently causes diffuse, interstitial opacities.

Microbiology

The cornerstone of the microbiologic diagnosis of pneumonia is **sputum gram stain and culture**. Samples that grow $\geq 10^6$ colony-forming units (CFU) per milliliter of a respiratory pathogen are considered positive.

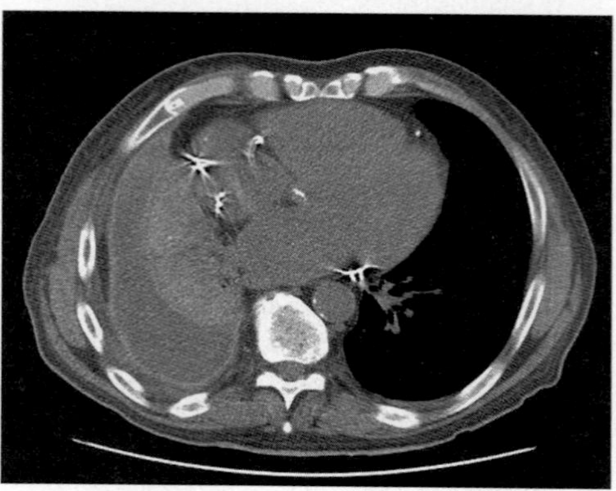

FIGURE 36-2 Computed tomography of the chest of a patient with right-sided pneumococcal empyema.

Culture results must be interpreted cautiously though, as inadequate collection methods or recent antibiotic administration may cause false-negative results, and oropharyngeal flora contamination or microbial colonization of the lower respiratory tract may cause false-positive results.

Blood may also be collected and cultured for pathogens. **Bacteremia** develops in up to 14% of hospitalized patients with CAP and may be as high as 30% in patients with pneumococcal pneumonia.[12] Ideally, blood should be collected from two separate sites prior to antibiotic administration. Because bacteremia is an intermittent rather than continuous phenomenon, blood cultures lack sensitivity but when positive are highly specific.

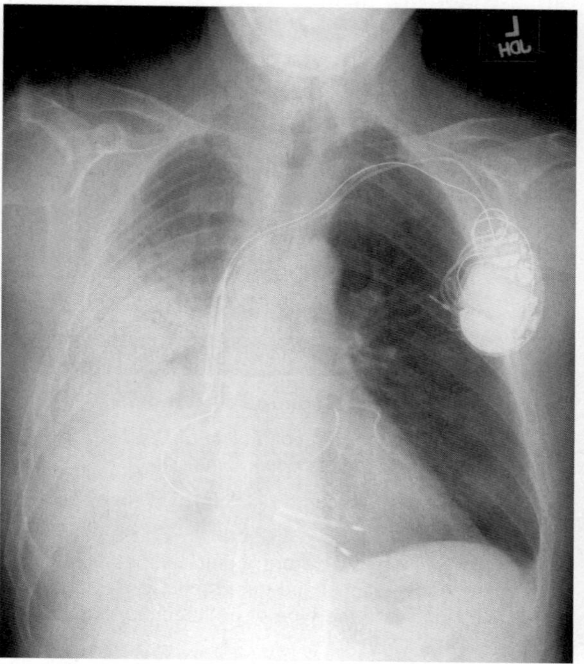

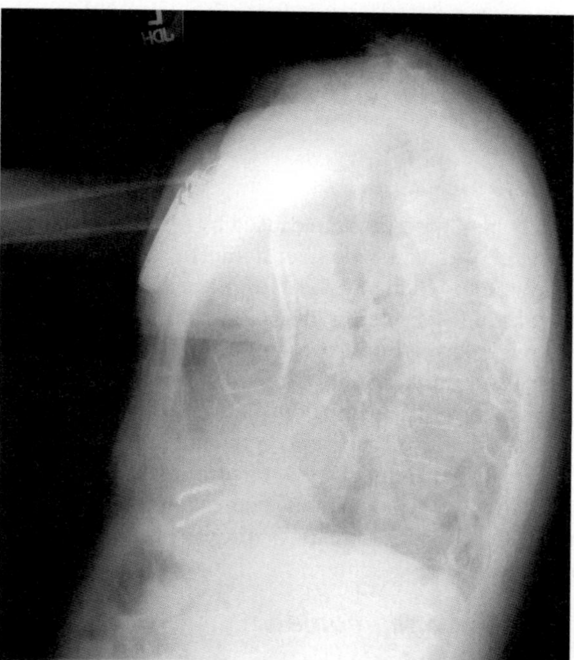

FIGURE 36-1 Posteroanterior and lateral chest radiographs of a patient with pneumococcal pneumonia and empyema showing right lower lobe and right middle lobe consolidation and right pleural effusion.

Serologic testing provides retrospective confirmation (or exclusion) of infection by certain pathogens. Paired serum samples from the acute (generally within 1 week of symptom onset) and convalescent (generally after 2 to 3 weeks of symptom onset) periods are tested for the presence and concentration (titers) of pathogen-specific antibodies. A rise in convalescent titers by approximately two- to threefold, depending on the pathogen, confirms a recent infection. This diagnostic method is usually of limited clinical value because results are not available until after completion of antibiotic therapy.

Another indirect method, **antigen detection**, is a rapidly evolving diagnostic modality that employs polymerase chain reaction (PCR) and other molecular tests to detect pathogen-specific molecular markers (antigens) such as proteins, polysaccharides, and nucleic acids. Unlike microbial cultures, PCR does not require the presence of live pathogens and is therefore unaffected by antibiotic administration. Antigen detection is useful for identifying atypical pathogens (e.g., *L pneumophila*, *M pneumoniae*, *C pneumoniae*, respiratory viruses) as well as common pathogens such as *S pneumoniae*. The pneumococcal antigen test is performed on urine and has a sensitivity of 50% to 80% and a specificity of ≥90%. False-positive results may occur in children colonized with or recently vaccinated against pneumococcus. After an episode of pneumococcal CAP, the antigen may be detectable for up to 3 months. The *Legionella* urinary antigen assay has a sensitivity of 70% to 90% and a specificity of nearly 99%. A negative test result does not exclude *Legionella* pneumonia, however, because only *L pneumophila* serogroup 1 is tested. While this is the most common serotype, up to 20% of *Legionella* pneumonia cases are caused by other serogroups and will therefore falsely test negative. The *Legionella* urinary antigen may be detectable for weeks after the acute illness.[12]

Diagnostic Procedures

Pleural effusions commonly develop in patients with pneumonia and require fluid sampling (thoracentesis) to exclude **empyema**. At minimum, the pleural fluid analysis should include pH, total protein, lactate dehydrogenase, glucose, and gram stain and bacterial culture, although additional tests may be necessary depending on the clinical suspicion.

Bronchoscopy and **bronchoalveolar lavage (BAL)** are appropriate to aid the diagnosis of pneumonia in several clinical scenarios: in patients with severe pneumonia requiring intubation, when there is concern for unusual microorganisms, in patients who are immunocompromised, and in patients unable to produce sputum. In order to determine the best site for BAL, clinicians should incorporate available chest imaging to identify the most abnormal lung, lobe, segment, or subsegment. The threshold for a positive BAL fluid culture is $\geq 10^4$ CFU/mL, although oropharyngeal contamination in nonintubated patients or the use of lidocaine for topical anesthesia (bacteriostatic) may temper the results. Transbronchial biopsy can also improve diagnosis, especially in immunocompromised hosts, although it is rarely performed in patients receiving positive pressure ventilation due to the higher risk of pneumothorax.

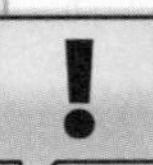

Respiratory Recap

Diagnostic Methods

- Sputum gram stain and culture
- Blood culture
- Serology and PCR
- Thoracentesis
- Bronchoscopy

Choice of diagnostic method is patient-specific and depends on risks, benefits, availability, expertise, severity of illness, and cost effectiveness.

Choosing Diagnostic Methods

Choosing the right diagnostic tests for a given patient requires consideration of patient-specific (risk vs. benefit, severity of illness) and hospital-specific (availability, expertise, cost-effectiveness) factors. In a patient with mild pneumonia who does not require hospitalization, sputum gram stain and culture may be the only necessary test. In contrast, critically ill patients with severe pneumonia may require more extensive and invasive testing.

Risk Stratification

The overall mortality from CAP is 12% to 14%[5,13,14] but can be as high as 40% to 50% in patients admitted to the intensive care unit (ICU).[5,14,15] A number of factors are known to confer a higher risk of dying from CAP, such as hyperglycemia,[16] admission from a skilled nursing facility, nonambulatory status, and malignancy.[14] As such, patients with CAP should be assessed for these and other risk factors to guide prognosis and location of treatment (i.e., outpatient vs. inpatient treatment).[12] Several scoring systems have been developed to help healthcare providers make these decisions, including CURB-65 and the Pneumonia Severity Index score. In a landmark 1997 study, Fine et al. derived the Pneumonia Severity Index (PSI or PORT score), a prediction rule designed to risk-stratify patients with CAP.[17] The PSI assigns points based on the patient's age and the presence of 19 additional risk factors which are independently associated with mortality (**Box 36-2**). The risk class is dependent on the number of points earned, with higher risk classes predicting a higher risk of mortality (**Table 36-3**). Based on the associated mortality risks, patients in risk classes I and II are usually treated as outpatients, those in risk class III

BOX 36-2

The Pneumonia Severity Index (PSI) Criteria

Presence of Coexisting Illnesses

Age	+1 point per year
Female sex	−10 points
Nursing home residence	+10 points
Presence of coexisting illnesses	
Neoplastic disease	+30 points
Congestive heart failure	+10 points
Cerebrovascular disease	+10 points
Renal disease	+10 points
Liver disease	+20 points

Physical Examination Findings

Altered mental status	+20 points
Pulse ≥125 per minute	+10 points
Respiratory rate ≥30 per minute	+10 points
Systolic blood pressure <90 mm Hg	+20 points
Temperature <35° C or ≥40° C	+15 points

Laboratory or Radiographic Findings

Blood urea nitrogen ≥30 mg/dL	+20 points
Glucose ≥250 mg/dL	+10 points
Hematocrit <30%	+10 points
Sodium <130 mmol/L	+20 points
Pao_2 <60 mm Hg	+10 points
Arterial pH <7.35	+30 points
Presence of pleural effusion	+10 points

Information from Chastre J, Fagon JY. Ventilator-associated pneumonia. *Am J Respir Crit Care Med*. 2002;165:867–903.

BOX 36-3

The CURB-65 Criteria

- Confusion
- Blood urea nitrogen (BUN) ≥20 mg/dL
- Respiratory rate ≥30 breaths/min
- Systolic blood pressure <90 mm Hg or diastolic ≤60 mm Hg
- Age ≥65 years

Information from Lim WS, van der Eerden MM, Laing R, et al. Defining community acquired pneumonia severity on presentation to hospital: an international derivation and validation study. *Thorax*. 2003;58:377–382.

TABLE 36-3
Risk of Mortality in Patients with CAP According to the Pneumonia Severity Index Score

Risk Class (# of points)	Mortality (%)	ICU Admission (%)	Hospital Length of Stay (median, days)
I*	0.1	4.3	5.0
II (≤70)	0.6	4.3	6.0
III (71–90)	0.9	5.9	7.0
IV (91–130)	9.3	11.4	9.0
V (≥130)	27.0	17.3	11.0

*Patients without any risk factors were included in risk class I.
Information from Fine MJ, Auble TE, Yealy DM, et al. A prediction rule to identify low-risk patients with community-acquired pneumonia. *N Engl J Med*. 1997;336:243–250.

usually require observation or hospitalization, and those in risk class ≥IV require hospitalization and frequently require ICU-level care.[12,17]

In a 2003 study, Lim et al. reported the CURB-65 score, which is based on five risk factors (1 point each) associated with increased mortality in patients with CAP (**Box 36-3**).[18] In patients with a score of 0, the 30-day mortality was 0.7%. Scores of 1, 2, 3, 4, and 5 were associated with mortality rates of 3.2%, 3%, 17%, 41.5%, and 57%, respectively. As a result, patients with a CURB-65 score of 0 to 1 are most likely able to be treated as outpatients, while a score of 2 likely requires hospitalization, and a score of ≥3 requires hospitalization and possibly ICU-level care.[18]

While these scoring systems have greatly improved the ability of healthcare providers to assess risk in patients with CAP, they have several limitations. The PSI can be burdensome to calculate, and the necessary variables may not always be available. Conversely, the CURB-65 score consists of only five variables that are readily available but may *incorrectly* classify high risk patients as being low risk.[19] No scoring system is perfect and healthcare providers must incorporate all available clinical data when determining an individual patient's prognosis. More recently, studies have investigated the use of biological markers or **biomarkers** in predicting the risk of severe CAP and mortality. Biomarkers are substances (e.g., hormones, proteins, and cytokines) produced by the body that are indicative of certain conditions (e.g., cancer, infections). A number of biomarkers have been studied for this purpose, including C-reactive protein, procalcitonin, and pro- and anti-inflammatory cytokines (e.g., IL-6, IL-10, CXCL8, TNF-α). Most of these biomarkers are not yet clinically available but show promise when used in combination with the PSI and CURB-65 to improve pneumonia risk stratification.[20]

BOX 36-4

IDSA/ATS Criteria for Severe Community-Acquired Pneumonia

Major

Invasive mechanical ventilation
Septic shock

Minor

Respiratory rate ≥30 breaths/min
$Pa{O_2}/F{IO_2}$ ≤250 mm Hg
Multilobar infiltrates
Confusion/disorientation
Uremia with blood urea nitrogen ≥20 mg/dL
Leukopenia <4000 cells/mm^3
Thrombocytopenia with platelet count <100,000 cells/mm^3
Hypothermia with core temperature <36° C
Hypotension requiring aggressive fluid resuscitation

Information from Mandell LA, Wunderink RG, Anzueto A, et al. Infectious Diseases Society of America/American Thoracic Society consensus guidelines on the management of community-acquired pneumonia in adults. *Clin Infect Dis.* 2007;44(Suppl 2): S27–S72.

The IDSA and ATS have also jointly published guidelines on risk stratifying patients for admission to the ICU. ICU admission is recommended for patients meeting one major criterion or three minor criteria for severe CAP (**Box 36-4**).[12] Additionally, $Pa{CO_2}$ <35 mm Hg or >45 mm Hg within 24 hours of hospital admission predicts a higher risk of transfer to the ICU and a higher 30-day mortality.[21]

Antibiotic Therapy

The mainstay of CAP treatment is appropriate antimicrobial therapy. As discussed earlier, the initial (empiric) antimicrobial drugs are directed toward the pathogens for which the patient is most likely at risk. Not only does this require knowing a patient's risk factors for certain pathogens but it also requires knowledge of local antibiotic susceptibility patterns for specific bacteria.[12] Appropriate antibiotics should be given within 6 hours if possible, as further delays are associated with an increased hospital length of stay and a higher mortality.[22]

The 2007 IDSA/ATS consensus guidelines recommend specific antibiotic regimens for empiric treatment of CAP according to treatment location (e.g., outpatient, inpatient, ICU).[12] For previously healthy patients without risk factors for drug-resistant *S pneumonia* (DRSP), macrolides (e.g., azithromycin, clarithromycin) are first-line therapy for outpatient treatment of CAP, although doxycycline may be adequate. Risk factors for DRSP include age ≤2 years or ≥65 years, antibiotic therapy within the last 3 months, chronic medical comorbidities such as heart disease, lung disease, liver disease, or kidney disease, diabetes mellitus, malignancy, immunosuppressed state, alcoholism, and asplenia, and exposure to a child in day care. For patients with DRSP risk factors, first-line therapy includes (1) a respiratory fluoroquinolone (e.g., moxifloxacin, levofloxacin), or (2) a beta-lactam (high-dose amoxicillin or amoxicillin-clavulanate) WITH a macrolide (doxycycline could be substituted for a macrolide if indicated). In regions where macrolide-resistant *S pneumonia* is highly prevalent, patients should be given one of the above alternatives.[12]

For patients hospitalized on the medical ward, first-line therapy for CAP includes (1) a respiratory fluoroquinolone, or (2) a beta-lactam (ceftriaxone, cefotaxime, or ampicillin preferred, ertapenem reasonable in selected patients) WITH a macrolide (or doxycycline). For patients admitted to the ICU, a beta-lactam (cefotaxime, ceftriaxone, or ampicillin-sulbactam) PLUS either azithromycin or a respiratory fluoroquinolone is recommended. Penicillin-allergic patients should be treated with a respiratory fluoroquinolone and aztreonam.[12]

Some patients with severe CAP who require ICU admission have risk factors for multidrug-resistant organisms (e.g., MRSA, *Pseudomonas*), such as structural lung disease (e.g., COPD, bronchiectasis) or frequent antibiotic use. If *Pseudomonas* is a concern, patients should be given: (1) a beta-lactam active against *Pseudomonas* (piperacillin/tazobactam, cefepime, imipenem, or meropenem) PLUS an antipseudomonal fluoroquinolone (ciprofloxacin or levofloxacin), or (2) a beta-lactam as above PLUS an aminoglycoside PLUS either azithromycin, moxifloxacin, or levofloxacin. In patients with a penicillin allergy, aztreonam should be substituted for the beta-lactam.[12] If MRSA is a concern, patients should be given vancomycin or linezolid as part of the antibiotic regimen,[12] although a retrospective study of patients with CAP due to MSSA and MRSA found that treatment with a toxin-inhibiting drug such as linezolid or clindamycin was associated with improved survival.[10]

Once the etiology of CAP has been identified in hospitalized patients, the antibiotic regimen should be changed to a single antibiotic, preferably the most narrow spectrum to which the pathogen is sensitive. Patients should be switched from intravenous to oral

STOP AND THINK

A 65-year-old male is admitted to the hospital for pneumonia. This is his second admission in 2 months. He has a history of diabetes mellitus and bronchiectasis. For which pathogens is the patient most at risk? Which antibiotic(s) should this patient receive?

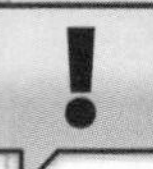

Respiratory Recap

Management of Pneumonia

- Differentiate between community-acquired and nosocomial pneumonia.
- Identify the organisms for which the patient is most at risk.
- Promptly administer appropriate, empiric antibiotics.
- Provide supportive care.
- Administer pneumococcal and influenza vaccinations to at-risk patients.

therapy when they are clinically stable or improving (e.g., afebrile, normotensive, no longer tachycardic or tachypneic, not requiring supplemental oxygen, exhibiting normal mentation, and tolerating oral intake). The same criteria may be used to identify patients who are candidates for discharge from the hospital.[12] Antibiotic treatment should continue for a minimum of 5 days and may go as long as 14 days depending on the pathogen and the patient's immune function.

Complications of Community-Acquired Pneumonia

The median time for hospitalized patients with CAP to achieve clinical stability is 3 days. Patients failing to respond to the initial antibiotic regimen, which occurs in up to 15% of cases, have a higher mortality compared with responders.[12,23] Clinical deterioration usually occurs within the first 72 hours of hospital admission,[23] and manifests as acute respiratory failure and/or shock. Such patients require transfer to the ICU, further diagnostic testing, and escalation of antibiotic coverage. There are numerous risk factors associated with initial treatment failure, including congestive heart failure, higher CURB-65 score,[23] higher PSI score, liver disease, necrotizing pneumonia, multilobar infiltrates, leukopenia, *Legionella* or gram-negative pneumonia, and inappropriate initial antibiotic coverage.[12] Patients failing CAP treatment also deserve consideration for alternative diagnoses such as pulmonary embolism, congestive heart failure, and ARDS.

Another cause of CAP treatment failure is pneumonia-associated pleural disease. Pneumonia commonly causes the accumulation of benign, sympathetic pleural fluid (parapneumonic effusion), which is transudative and self-resolving. In more severe cases, however, the pleural fluid becomes exudative and is characterized by a low pH (<7.2), low glucose (<40 mg/dL), elevated LDH (>1000 units/L),[24] and/or pleural space loculations. These complicated parapneumonic effusions occur in up to 7% of patients with CAP. In addition to antibiotics, treatment can require fluid drainage via tube thoracostomy. When the pleural space becomes grossly infected, it is known as an *empyema*. Empyema occurs in up to 1.5% of cases and is diagnosed by either visualization of frank pus on pleural fluid aspiration, or the identification of pathogens on pleural fluid gram stain and/or culture.[24] When a complicated effusion or empyema is present, morbidity and hospital length of stay are significantly increased, and the risk of transfer to the ICU is elevated threefold.[24] For these reasons, pneumonia-associated pleural fluid should always be sampled via thoracentesis to rule out significant pleural disease. Empyema almost always requires drainage via tube thoracostomy, a prolonged course of antibiotics (up to 6 weeks or more), and, in refractory cases, surgical debridement.

Prevention

Numerous studies have shown that immunization against *S pneumoniae* reduces the likelihood of hospitalization and improves survival.[25–28] There are two pneumococcal vaccines currently approved for use in adults: the pneumococcal conjugate vaccine (PCV13) and the pneumococcal polysaccharide vaccine (PPSV23). PCV13 is recommended for ages ≥19 years with any of the following conditions: immunosuppressed states (e.g., HIV infection, corticosteroids, radiation therapy, chronic renal failure or nephrotic syndrome, solid organ transplant, malignancy, congenital immunodeficiency), functional or anatomic asplenia, cerebrospinal fluid (CSF) leaks, or cochlear implants. PPSV23 targets 12 of the 13 pneumococcal serotypes in PCV13, plus 11 other serotypes, and is recommended for (1) all adults ≥65 years, and (2) adults ages 19 to 64 who qualify for the PCV13, or who have chronic heart disease (e.g., heart failure), lung disease (e.g., COPD, asthma), liver disease (e.g., cirrhosis), diabetes mellitus, alcohol abuse, or tobacco abuse.[29] Influenza vaccination has also been found to reduce the severity of pneumonia during peak influenza season.[30]

Aspiration and Anaerobic Pneumonia

Aspiration pneumonia is caused by inhalation of bacteria-rich oropharyngeal or gastric secretions. Predisposing risk factors for aspiration pneumonia include decreased level of consciousness, anesthesia, neurologic disorders, immobility, poor dental hygiene, gastroesophageal reflux, esophageal disorders, and oropharyngeal dysphasia. In community-dwelling, healthy patients, oropharyngeal flora is normally composed of viridans streptococci, *H influenzae*, and anaerobic bacteria.[31] The anaerobes most commonly implicated in aspiration pneumonia include *Bacteroides melaninogenicus*, *Fusobacterium nucleatum*, and *Peptostreptococcus* species. These and other anaerobes seldom cause infections by themselves but rather act synergistically with other pathogens to cause polymicrobial infections. Samples from patients with anaerobic infections are frequently foul smelling due to the microbial production of volatile short-chain fatty acids.[32] In contrast to community-dwelling patients, the oropharyngeal flora of hospitalized patients shifts from anaerobes to gram-negative rods. These infections are approached similarly to nosocomial pneumonia.

Aspiration pneumonia is a clinical diagnosis. It is supported by patient-specific risk factors, microbiology, and chest imaging. The chest radiograph most commonly shows involvement in the lungs' dependent areas. In the supine position, these are the posterior segments of the upper lobes and the superior segments of the lower lobes. In the sitting position, this is more commonly the lower lobes.[32]

Once aspiration pneumonia is suspected, providers should promptly initiate treatment. As shown in several studies, clindamycin is an effective drug for anaerobic lung infections. Other antibiotics such as beta-lactams with beta-lactamase inhibitors (e.g., amoxicillin-clavulanate, ampicillin-sulbactam), carbapenems, and moxifloxacin have also been shown to be effective. Metronidazole has poor activity against *Streptococcus* species and is therefore only adequate in combination with a beta-lactam.[32] If the anaerobic lung infection remains untreated, it will eventually (after 7 to 14 days) cause necrosis, lung abscess, bronchopleural fistula, and empyema.

Actinomycosis

Actinomyces species are anaerobic, gram-positive rods and are normal inhabitants of the human oropharynx, gastrointestinal tract, and female genital tract. Most commonly, these anaerobes gain access to the lungs via aspiration, although infection can also follow penetrating trauma. Patients with structural lung disease or alcohol abuse are at increased risk. Pulmonary actinomycosis is an indolent disease. Initial symptoms can be similar to TB or lung cancer and include cough, fever, hemoptysis, chest pain, weight loss, and malaise. The chest radiograph may reveal mass-like consolidation with cavitation or chest wall involvement. In fact, one of the hallmarks of pulmonary actinomycosis is the direct invasion of surrounding structures such as adjacent lung tissue, pleura, bone, and soft tissue. Ultimately, this can lead to formation of a bronchocutaneous fistula. Diagnosis of pulmonary actinomycosis can be difficult to establish and requires the integration of available clinical, radiographic, microbiologic, and histopathologic data. Classic histopathologic findings include granulomatous inflammation and sulfur granules.[33] First-line treatment for pulmonary actinomycosis is high-dose intravenous penicillin for 2 to 6 weeks followed by oral penicillin for 6 to 12 months. Patients who do not respond to antibiotic therapy alone may require surgical debridement.[33,34]

Nosocomial Pneumonia

Pneumonia occurring in hospitalized patients is called *nosocomial pneumonia*. Nosocomial pneumonia differs significantly from CAP in regards to risk factors (e.g., mechanical ventilation) and microbiology (i.e., more commonly caused by multidrug-resistant [MDR] organisms). MDR pathogens (or potentially MDR pathogens) are notable because they (can) rapidly acquire resistance to antibiotics, which complicates diagnosis, treatment, and prognosis. Nosocomial pneumonia is comprised of three major subtypes: *hospital-acquired pneumonia* (HAP), *ventilator-associated pneumonia* (VAP), and the recently recognized *healthcare-associated pneumonia* (HCAP), discussed in more detail below.

Healthcare-Associated Pneumonia

The term "healthcare-associated pneumonia" was first introduced by the 2005 ATS/IDSA guidelines on nosocomial pneumonia.[35] It refers broadly to pneumonia in nonhospitalized patients with current or recent healthcare exposure, including hospitalization for more than 2 days in the last 90 days, use of hemodialysis, wound care, or intravenous therapy (e.g., chemotherapy, antibiotic infusions) within the last 30 days, and residing at a skilled nursing or long-term care facility.[35]

Most studies find that HCAP is more severe than CAP. Patients with HCAP are more likely to have bilateral infiltrates and a higher pneumonia severity class by PSI or CURB-65.[36] Moreover, the short-term (<30 days) and long-term (180–365 days) mortality rates for HCAP patients are at least twofold higher.[36–39] However, this difference may reflect the higher burden of comorbidities in patients with HCAP.[39]

Hospital-Acquired Pneumonia

As defined by the 2005 ATS/IDSA guidelines, **hospital-acquired pneumonia (HAP)** is pneumonia that (1) occurs in patients hospitalized for more than 48 hours, and (2) is not incubating at the time of admission.[35] HAP is the second most common nosocomial infection,[35] occurring in 3.5% of hospitalized patients.[40] HAP increases mean hospital stay by 7 to 9 days and healthcare costs by more than $40,000 per patient.[35]

A number of risk factors for HAP have been identified, including malnutrition (albumin <2 mg/dL), chronic kidney disease, anemia (hemoglobin <10 g/dL), altered consciousness, Charlson comorbidity index ≥3, previous hospitalization, and thoracic surgery.[41] Additionally, the use of proton-pump inhibitors (PPIs) has been associated with a 30% increased odds of HAP.[40]

Complications of HAP are frequent and may occur in more than 50% of patients. In one study, HAP-associated complications included respiratory failure (52.9%), septic shock (10.1%), acute kidney injury (7.6%), pleural effusion or empyema (9.2%), transfer to the ICU (9.2%), and initiation of mechanical ventilation (5.8%). The mean length of stay was approximately 26 days, and only a third of patients were discharged home. The other two-thirds were either discharged to a skilled nursing facility (33%) or did not survive the hospitalization (33%).[41]

Ventilator-Associated Pneumonia

Ventilator-associated pneumonia (VAP) is pneumonia occurring in patients receiving mechanical ventilation after 48 hours of endotracheal intubation. VAP occurs in approximately 15% to 26% of intubated patients,[42,43] with an incidence of 7 to 28 episodes per 1000 ventilator-days.[44,45] One episode of VAP nearly doubles the cost of hospitalization for a given patient due to longer length of stay. Median duration of intubation is increased 5 days, ICU stay is increased 10.5 days, and hospital stay is increased 12.5 days.[46] Mortality estimates for VAP range from 35% in middle-aged patients to 51% in the elderly.[47,48]

Pathogenesis of VAP

The pathogenesis of VAP relies on four major factors: the patient, healthcare devices, the hospital environment, and bacterial colonization. Bacterial colonization by aerobic gram-negative and gram-positive microbes (including MRSA) occurs universally in mechanically ventilated patients. The most colonized sites are the oropharynx, sinuses, and stomach. These are also common sites for indwelling healthcare devices (e.g., nasogastric or orogastric tubes), which allow for biofilm formation. Biofilms also form on the endotracheal tube, allowing pathogens direct entry into the lower respiratory tract via leakage around the tube (despite the inflated cuff) or through the tube. The endotracheal tube also circumvents the patient's host defenses by impairing the cough reflex, damaging the tracheal epithelial barrier, and impeding mucociliary clearance.[31] Other healthcare devices which can deposit bacteria into the lower airways are fiberoptic bronchoscopes and endotracheal suction catheters.[49] Patient factors known to increase the risk of VAP include cigarette smoking, postsurgery, reintubation, supine position, malnutrition, enteral feeding, use of sedatives/paralytics, use of proton-pump inhibitors, transport out of the ICU, and bacterial sinusitis.[31,49] Finally, VAP can arise from a contaminated hospital environment. For example, *Legionella* has been isolated from hospital water supplies and is a reported cause of epidemic VAP.[31]

Diagnosis of VAP

The diagnosis of VAP is traditionally based on a combination of clinical signs and symptoms of respiratory infection, chest imaging (new or worsening lung infiltrates), and microbiology data (positive qualitative or quantitative respiratory specimen cultures). Signs and symptoms of VAP can include fever, leukocytosis, altered mental status, purulent tracheobronchial secretions, and/or hypoxia. In a study of 827 patients with HAP or VAP, 77% had worsening hypoxia, 72% had purulent/changing respiratory secretions, and 69% had a new fever.[50] Other studies, however, have found that these criteria lack sensitivity and specificity for VAP when compared with autopsy findings.[51,52]

A widely used tool to diagnosis VAP is the clinical pulmonary infection score (CPIS). CPIS was developed in a cohort of 28 patients and uses temperature, white blood cell count, tracheobronchial secretions, Pa_{O_2}, chest radiographic findings, and respiratory culture data to predict the likelihood of VAP (**Box 36-5**).[53] While the CPIS was initially promising, subsequent studies revealed it to be imprecise and neither sensitive nor specific.[54] Still, CPIS may be useful in identifying patients who have responded to VAP treatment, thereby helping clinicians de-escalate antibiotic therapy.[55]

This failure of CPIS and other tools to improve VAP diagnosis is in part due to the lack of an objective, universally accepted VAP definition. Many questions need to be answered before a successful definition can be attained. Is pneumonia within the first 24 hours of mechanical ventilation the same as pneumonia after 5 days? How can pneumonia be distinguished from ARDS on chest radiograph? What constitutes infection versus colonization? In an attempt to answer these and other questions, representatives from numerous pulmonary, critical care, infectious disease, respiratory care, and epidemiological professional societies, as well as governmental organizations such as the National Institutes of Health (NIH), Centers for Disease Control and Prevention (CDC), and Department of Health and Human Services (HHS), convened to formulate a unified and objective VAP definition used for VAP surveillance.[56] The proposed definition is an algorithm designed to detect a broad range of ventilator-associated complications, including but not limited to VAP. There is a new minimum period for which a patient on a ventilator must be stable or improving (≥2 days), followed by a minimum

BOX 36-5

The Clinical Pulmonary Infection Score (CPIS)

1. Temperature in °C
   36.5–38.4 = 0
   38.5–38.9 = 1
   ≥39 or ≤36 = 2
2. White blood cell count per liter
   $4 \times 10^9 - 11 \times 10^9 = 0$
   $<4 \times 10^9$ or $>11 \times 10^9 = 1$
   + band form $\geq 0.5 \times 10^9 = 1$
3. Tracheal secretions
   Absence of tracheal secretions = 0
   Presence of nonpurulent tracheal secretions = 1
   Presence of purulent tracheal secretions = 2
4. Oxygenation, $Pa{O_2}/F{I}{O_2}$, mm Hg
   >240 or ARDS = 0
   ≤240 and no evidence of ARDS = 2
5. Chest radiograph
   No infiltrate = 0
   Diffuse or patchy infiltrate = 1
   Localized infiltrate = 2
6. Progression of pulmonary infiltrate
   No radiographic progression = 0
   Radiographic progression (after exclusion of CHF and ARDS) = 2

ARDS, acute respiratory distress syndrome; CHF, congestive heart failure.
Information from Pugin J, Auckenthaler R, Mili N, et al. Diagnosis of ventilator-associated pneumonia by bacteriologic analysis of bronchoscopic and nonbronchoscopic "blind" bronchoalveolar lavage fluid. *Am Rev Respir Dis.* 1991;143:1121–1129.

period for which a patient must display worsening hypoxemia (≥2 days) (ventilator-associated complication). In parallel, patients must demonstrate signs of an infection (e.g., fever or abnormal WBC count) and initiate antibiotics (infection-related ventilator-associated complication). If patients meeting these broader categories of ventilator-associated events also have purulent secretions or a positive respiratory culture, they will be considered to have possible VAP, and if they have both, they have probable VAP. Patients with neither of these signs can still qualify for probable VAP if they have a positive pleural fluid culture, positive lung histopathology, positive *Legionella* test, or positive respiratory viral test. By definition, therefore, a patient will not meet criteria for VAP (possible or probable) until at least ventilator day 4 (**Figure 36-3**).

Notably absent from the new definition is the requirement of a chest radiograph. This is largely because of the high variability in radiographic image quality, interpretation, and accuracy. Chest radiographs are not sensitive for pneumonia, missing up to 25% of lung infiltrates.[48] In a study comparing chest radiograph and autopsy findings (the gold standard for VAP diagnosis), radiographic infiltrates did not correlate well with lung histopathology.[57] In fact, there are many conditions that cause infiltrates in ventilated patients that could be mistaken for pneumonia, such as atelectasis, chemical pneumonitis (aspiration), pulmonary edema (heart failure), pulmonary embolism, alveolar hemorrhage, and ARDS.[58] While it is yet to be determined how this new surveillance definition will affect diagnosis of VAP at the bedside, it is a step forward in developing a unified definition.

Microbiology

The microbiology of nosocomial pneumonia differs from that of CAP. Nosocomial pneumonia is more commonly caused by MDR or potentially MDR pathogens. This is especially true for late-onset nosocomial pneumonia, which is defined as occurring more than 4 to 5 days after hospitalization or intubation. Conversely, early-onset nosocomial pneumonia occurs within 4 days of hospitalization or intubation and is more frequently caused by antibiotic-sensitive bacteria and usually carries a better prognosis (**Table 36-4**).[35,48,59]

The most common (potentially) MDR pathogens causing nosocomial pneumonia include: (1) the gram-positive coccus *S aureus*, (2) the enteric gram-negative rods (e.g., *E coli*, *Proteus*, *Serratia*, *Enterobacter*, *Citrobacter*, and *Klebsiella* species), and (3) the nonenteric gram-negative rods (e.g., *Pseudomonas*, *Stenotrophomonas*, and *Acinetobacter* species). Of these, Koulenti et al. found that *S aureus* (26%), *Pseudomonas* (23%), and *Acinetobacter* (19%) predominated.[50] One recently identified risk factor for MDR VAP is tracheobronchial colonization with *Candida* species, a relatively common phenomenon in intubated patients.[60]

The association of HCAP and MDR (or potentially MDR) pathogens is more controversial. Several studies have found that HCAP is more commonly caused by MRSA, *Pseudomonas*, and other (potentially) MDR gram-negative rods compared with CAP,[61,62] whereas CAP is more commonly caused by *S pneumoniae*, *Legionella*, and *Haemophilus*.[62] However, other studies have found no difference in the microbiology of HCAP and CAP.[38,39,63] In an effort to more accurately predict which patients with HCAP have MDR organisms, investigators have started to identify patient-specific risk factors to enable risk stratification of individual patients. One study found that nursing home residents were more likely to have MDR HCAP only if they were

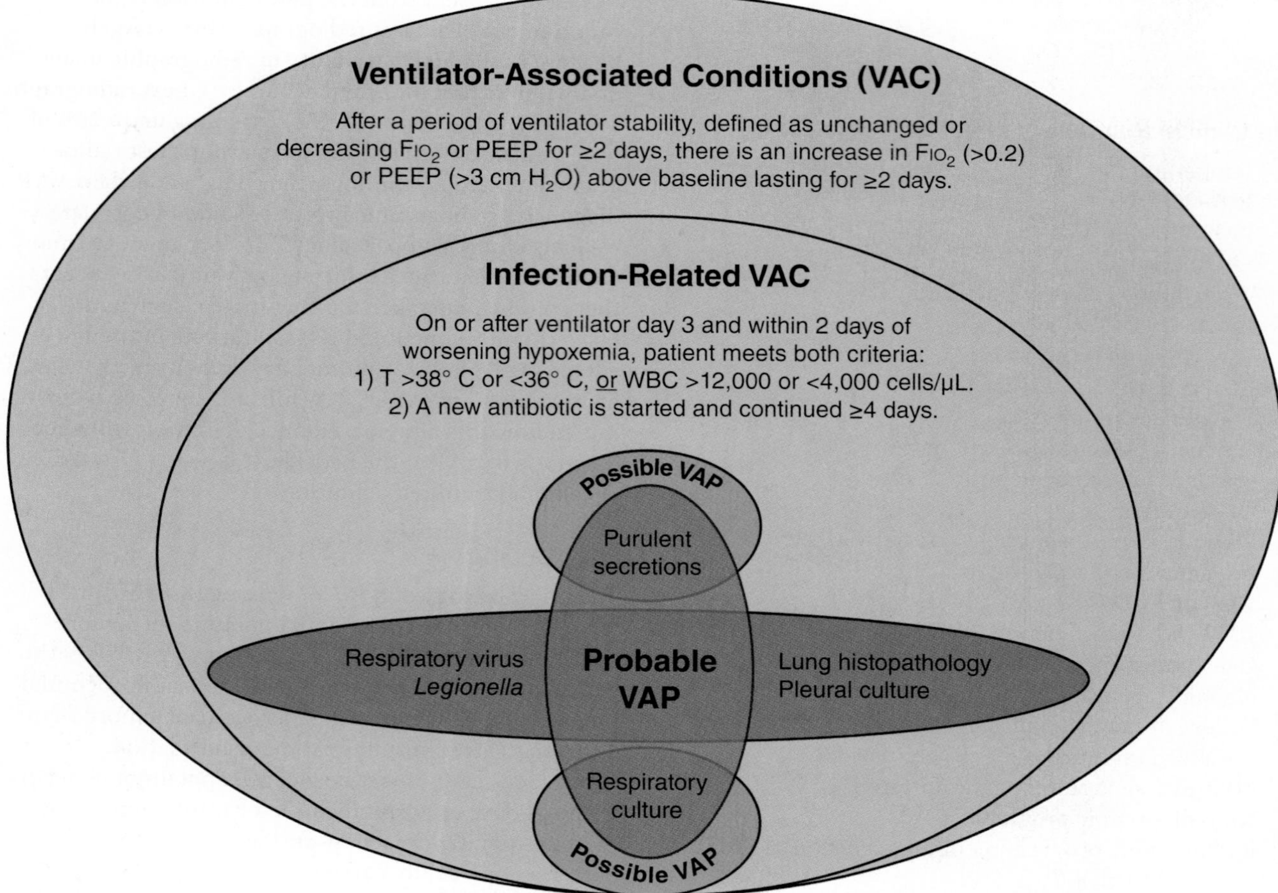

FIGURE 36-3 Venn diagram for surveillance of ventilator-associated events. PEEP, positive end-expiratory pressure; F_{IO_2}, fraction of inspired oxygen; T, temperature; VAP, ventilator-associated pneumonia.

Information from Magill SS, Klompas M, Balk R, et al. Executive summary: developing a new, national approach to surveillance for ventilator-associated events. *Ann Am Thorac Soc.* 2013;10:S220–S223.

immunosuppressed, used gastric-acid-suppressing medications, were nonambulatory, or used tube feeding.[64] Additional HCAP studies are necessary so that the risk of MDR HCAP can be more accurately assessed for an individual patient.

TABLE 36-4
Most Likely Etiologies of Ventilator-Associated Pneumonia

Early Onset and No Risk for MDR Pathogens	Late Onset or At Risk for MDR Pathogens
Streptococcus pneumoniae *Haemophilus influenzae* Methicillin-sensitive *S aureus* *E coli* *Klebsiella pneumoniae* *Enterobacter spp.* *Proteus spp.* *Serratia spp.*	Methicillin-resistant *S aureus* Multidrug-resistant enteric and nonenteric gram-negative rods (e.g., *Acinetobacter, Pseudomonas, Stenotrophomonas*) ESBL or KPC-producing organisms Early-onset pathogens

MDR, multidrug resistant; ESBL, extended-spectrum beta-lactamase; KPC, *K pneumoniae* carbapenemase.

Of particular concern are the emerging *Klebsiella pneumoniae* carbapenemase (KPC)-producing organisms (named for its initial discovery in *Klebsiella*) that are resistant to all beta-lactams, cephalosporins, monobactams, and carbapenems. While *Klebsiella* pneumonia is the most prevalent bacteria to carry KPC, it has been identified in a number of other enteric and nonenteric bacteria. Carbapenems are among the broadest-spectrum antibiotics manufactured to date, so infection with KPC-producing bacteria significantly complicates treatment and is associated with an increased mortality.[65]

Determining whether pathogens isolated from the lower respiratory tract are in fact the source of the infection (as opposed to merely being colonizers) can be difficult. Either quantitative or semiquantitative microbiological techniques can be used to help answer this question. The semiquantitative method provides an estimated colony count (e.g., moderate, or 3+), whereas the quantitative method provides an exact colony count (e.g., 2×10^5 CFU/mL). Standardized quantitative cutoffs exist for the microbiologic diagnosis of VAP for BAL

BOX 36-6

Thresholds for the Diagnosis of Ventilator-Associated Pneumonia

Endotracheal aspirates	$\geq 10^5$–10^6 CFU/mL
Bronchoalveolar lavage	$\geq 10^4$ CFU/mL
Protected specimen brush	$\geq 10^3$ CFU/mL

CFU, colony-forming unit.

($>10^4$ CFU/mL) and PSB ($>10^3$ CFU/mL). A cut-off of ≥3+ by semiquantitative count, which generally corresponds to 10^5 CFU/mL by quantitative count, has been proposed for endotracheal aspirate. This cut-off is more sensitive but less specific than a higher cut-off of ≥4+ or 10^6 CFU/mL. Any of these methods are likely valid for interpreting respiratory specimen bacterial growth (**Box 36-6**).[48]

Treatment

According to the 2005 IDSA/ATS recommendations, patients with suspected or confirmed nosocomial pneumonia, especially those at risk for MDR pathogens, should receive early, empiric, combination antibiotic therapy. Combination therapy will increase the likelihood that (potential) MDR pathogens are treated with a drug to which they are susceptible. Specifically, patients should be given one antibiotic from each of the following three antibiotic categories: (A) an antipseudomonal cephalosporin (e.g., cefepime, ceftazidime), carbapenem (e.g., imipenem, meropenem), or penicillin/beta-lactamase inhibitor (e.g., piperacillin/tazobactam), (B) an antipseudomonal fluoroquinolone (e.g., ciprofloxacin, levofloxacin) or aminoglycoside (e.g., gentamicin, tobramycin), and (C) an anti-MRSA antibiotic (e.g., vancomycin, linezolid) (**Box 36-7**). Patients with early-onset VAP who do not have identifiable risk factors for MDR pathogens can be given a more limited-spectrum antibiotic regimen. In all cases, the choice of antibiotics for a given patient should be guided by the patient's previous antibiotic exposure, allergies/sensitivities, historical culture data, and local patterns of pathogen prevalence and antibiotic susceptibility.[35] Knowledge of the local resistance patterns and pathogen prevalence is especially critical, as studies have found a significantly higher mortality in patients who receive inappropriate, initial antibiotics.[66]

In patients with suspected or confirmed MRSA nosocomial pneumonia, there are emerging data on the choice of antibiotics. In one study, patients with MRSA HCAP treated with linezolid experienced similar clinical cure rates and mortality compared to vancomycin. However, treatment with linezolid was associated with a lower incidence of renal failure (8% vs. 18%).[67] In a prospective, nonblinded study of patients with MRSA VAP, trends were found for improved clinical cure rate, duration of ventilation, hospital and ICU length of stay, and survival in patients treated with linezolid compared to vancomycin.[68] While these data are encouraging for the use of linezolid, the issue is far from settled and deserves further study. Several new antibiotics with activity against MRSA are now FDA-approved for HCAP (the glycopeptide, televancin) and CAP (ceftaroline, a fifth-generation cephalosporin). Additional

BOX 36-7

Empiric Antibiotic Treatments for Ventilator-Associated Pneumonia

Early Onset and No Risk for MDR

Ceftriaxone *or*
Levofloxacin or moxifloxacin or ciprofloxacin *or*
Ampicillin/sulbactam *or*
Ertapenem

Late Onset or High Risk for MDR

Antipseudomonal cephalosporin (cefepime or ceftazidime) *or* antipseudomonal carbapenem (imipenem or meropenem) *or* beta-lactam/beta-lactamase inhibitor (piperacillin-tazobactam)

and

Antipseudomonal fluoroquinolone (ciprofloxacin, levofloxacin) or aminoglycoside (amikacin, gentamicin, or tobramycin)

and

AntiMRSA antibiotics (e.g., linezolid, vancomycin)

MDR, multidrug resistance; MRSA, methicillin-resistant *S aureus*.

antibiotics with activity against MRSA are in the pipeline. How and when these newer antibiotics should be used is not clear and in need of further study.

Patients with nosocomial pneumonia due to a KPC-producing organism generally require combination antibiotic therapy with tigecycline, aminoglycosides, and/or polymixins. Until recently, polymixins (e.g., colistin, polymixin B) were used rarely due to higher rates of nephrotoxicity and neurotoxicity. With the increasing prevalence of KPC, however, polymixin use is also on the rise.[65]

An emerging concept for treating patients with MDR VAP, particularly those with KPC-producing organisms, is the use of nebulized antibiotics. Experimental pneumonia models indicate that nebulized antibiotics are deposited in high concentrations in the lung. Given the increasing need for systemic, toxic antibiotics (e.g., colistin), nebulized antibiotics may effectively treat pneumonia but avoid systemic toxicity. To date, two randomized-controlled trials have evaluated the use of nebulized antibiotics in patients with MDR VAP. Lu et al. treated patients with confirmed *Pseudomonas* VAP with either nebulized or intravenous ceftazidime and amikacin combination therapy and found no differences in treatment failure or super-infection. However, the nebulized drugs caused obstruction of the ventilator's expiratory filter in three patients, one of which suffered a cardiopulmonary arrest as a direct result.[69] In a study by Rattanaumpawan et al., patients with MDR VAP (mostly due to *Acinetobacter* and *Pseudomonas*, including KPC-producing strains) who were already receiving systemic antibiotic therapy were randomized to inhaled colistin or placebo/saline. In this study, adjunctive inhaled colistin treatment did not improve clinical cure rates or mortality compared with placebo, although it did result in more bronchospasm (7.8% vs. 2%).[70] These data, therefore, do not support the use of nebulized antibiotics for the treatment of nosocomial pneumonia.

Once the susceptibilities of the isolated pathogens are known, the antibiotic regimen should be de-escalated to the most narrow-spectrum drug(s) possible. This is to reduce the development of resistance to the broad-spectrum antibiotics. Moreover, in patients who have not had any changes to their antibiotic regimen for >72 hours, a negative respiratory specimen culture supports the discontinuation of antibiotics altogether in an otherwise stable patient.[35]

Duration of Antibiotic Treatment

In addition to narrowing the antibiotic regimen, there is also evidence to shorten the duration of antibiotic exposure. For the treatment of VAP, two prospective, randomized clinical trials have found that there is no difference between a short (8 days) and long (15 days) antibiotic course in regards to clinical cure rate or mortality.[35,59,71] The one caveat may be in regards to patients with *Pseudomonas* and other nonenteric pathogens, or MRSA, which may require a longer duration of therapy than 8 days.[35,59,71]

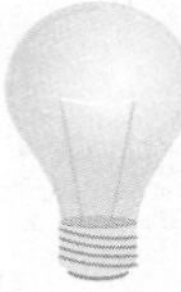

STOP AND THINK

You are caring for a 71-year-old male undergoing mechanical ventilation for an exacerbation of COPD. On ventilator day 6 he is requiring more oxygen and has a new fever. What is the differential diagnosis? What test should be ordered to help determine the diagnosis?

Reasons for Deterioration or Nonresolution

Even with the initiation of appropriate antibiotics for suspected VAP, patients may not improve clinically until day 3. Because of this, the antibiotic regimen should generally not be changed before this time unless there is significant clinical deterioration or there are new respiratory culture data on which to act. Patients with nosocomial pneumonia who do not improve, or worsen, by day 3 of antibiotics are considered to have failed therapy. In one study, up to 31.8% of patients with VAP failed to improve by day 3. Independent predictors of clinical failure were lack of improvement in $Pa{O_2}/F{IO_2}$ and persistent fever by day 3.[72]

There are a number of possible explanations for clinical failure. First, assuming the diagnosis and the antibiotic choice(s) are correct, the antibiotic dose or dosing frequency could be incorrect, there could be a drug–drug interaction causing rapid metabolism or poor absorption of the antibiotic, or there could be poor penetration of the antibiotic into the site of infection. Second, the diagnosis may be correct, but the pathogen may be resistant to the antibiotic(s). Third, the diagnosis may be incorrect, where instead of VAP, the patent has atelectasis, ARDS, pulmonary hemorrhage, congestive heart failure, pulmonary embolus with infarction, lung contusion, or chemical pneumonitis, all of which can mimic pneumonia. Fourth, there could be host factors, such as immunosuppression, that may delay clinical improvement. Fifth, there could be other pulmonary sites of infection, such as empyema or lung abscess, or nonpulmonary sites such as sinusitis, central venous catheter-related infections, pseudomembranous colitis, or urinary tract infections present that delay clinical improvement.[35]

Prevention of VAP

Ventilator-Care Bundles

A number of practices have been identified that improve outcomes in mechanically ventilated patients. These ventilator bundles focus on reducing exposure to mechanical ventilation (e.g., use of noninvasive positive

BOX 36-8

Ventilator Bundle

Elevation of the head of the bed to 45 degrees
Daily awakening trial and assessment of readiness for extubation
Peptic ulcer disease prophylaxis
Deep venous thrombosis prophylaxis
Daily oral care with chlorhexidine

pressure ventilation), reducing the duration of mechanical ventilation (e.g., accelerated weaning protocols, daily sedation vacations, daily spontaneous breathing trials), reducing aspiration of contaminated secretions (e.g., oral care with chlorhexidine, endotracheal cuff pressure 20–30 cm H_2O, continuous aspiration of subglottic secretions, elevation of the head of the bed to 45 degrees—especially during enteral feeding), and reducing nonventilator complications (e.g., DVT prophylaxis with unfractionated or low-molecular-weight heparin and GI prophylaxis with H_2 blockers or sucralfate). ICUs should also incorporate into their individualized VAP prevention policies staff education, infection control, and microbiologic surveillance (**Box 36-8**).[55]

Early Versus Late Tracheostomy

One suggested strategy to reduce the frequency of VAP in orotracheally intubated patients is to perform early tracheostomies (within 2 to 4 days), rather than after the usual practice of 10 to 16 days. Rumbak et al. found that patients randomized to early tracheostomy had significantly decreased mortality, VAP, duration of mechanical ventilation and time in the ICU, and damage to mouth and larynx compared with late tracheostomy.[73] Subsequent randomized controlled trials found no reduction in mortality or VAP.[74,75] Terragni et al. found early tracheostomy increased successful ventilator liberation and ICU discharge.[75] These studies employed slightly different inclusion criteria, making generalizability difficult, although a meta-analysis found similar findings to Terragni.[76] It seems likely that early tracheostomy benefits some patients and not others, but how to determine which patients are which is currently unclear.

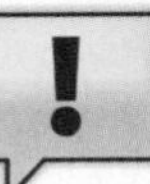

Respiratory Recap

Nosocomial Pneumonia

- Nosocomial pneumonia is very common and increases morbidity, mortality, and healthcare costs.
- Nosocomial pneumonia is more likely to be caused by multidrug-resistant organisms.
- The number one risk factor for nosocomial pneumonia is an endotracheal tube.
- Guidelines for the management of nosocomial pneumonia emphasize appropriate, empiric antibiotic therapy, de-escalation of initial antibiotic therapy, and shortening the duration of antibiotic therapy to the minimum effective period.
- VAP prevention should focus on avoiding mechanical ventilation, reducing duration of ventilation, and minimizing aspiration of contaminated secretions.

AGE-SPECIFIC ANGLE

Influenza rates are highest in young children. Hospital admission and mortality rates are highest among the elderly.

Viral Pneumonia

Respiratory viruses cause the vast majority of upper respiratory tract infections (URIs). Growing evidence suggests these viruses also account for a significant number of pneumonia cases as well. In fact, among patients admitted to the ICU with pneumonia, up to one-third may be due to viruses.[77] The viruses most commonly associated with pneumonia are influenza, parainfluenza, human metapneumovirus, adenovirus, rhinovirus, and respiratory syncytial virus (RSV). Other viruses that can cause pneumonia in immunocompromised hosts are cytomegalovirus (CMV), varicella zoster virus (VZV), and herpes simplex virus (HSV). Rare but often fatal causes of **viral pneumonia** include hantavirus, measles, and the emerging Middle-Eastern respiratory syndrome coronavirus (MERS-CoA).

Influenza Virus

Seasonal influenza infection causes nearly 1 million hospitalizations annually[78] and traditionally peaks in the winter months. Those particularly susceptible are young children, the elderly, and patients with chronic medical conditions. Influenza infection is frequently complicated by secondary bacterial pneumonia, usually due to *S aureus* or *S pneumoniae*, and portends a worse prognosis.[79]

In contrast to the seasonal influenza virus, which mutates slightly from year to year, several novel influenza strains have recently circulated causing pandemics. These viruses most likely arose after human influenza strains combined with avian or porcine strains, hence the names bird flu for the H5N1 pandemic of 2003 to 2006, and swine flu for the H1N1 pandemics of 2009 and 2013. Unlike seasonal influenza,

STOP AND THINK

You are caring for an elderly woman hospitalized for influenza pneumonia. Which precautions should be taken to protect yourself and others?

these outbreaks were unpredictable and targeted both chronically ill patients as well as previously healthy, young adults,[80] with mortality rates as high as 60%.[81] The elderly were relatively protected from the H1N1 pandemic perhaps because of antigenic similarities to prior influenza strains.[82] Obesity and pregnancy (or postpartum status) are unique risk factors for severe H1N1 infection, as these patients have higher rates of H1N1-associated complications and mortality.[83]

The diagnosis of influenza is based on clinical symptoms (e.g., high fevers, chills, pharyngitis, malaise, myalgias) and viral testing. Rapid influenza detection assays are nearly 100% specific but only 40% to 50% sensitive in adults and only slightly higher in children.[84] Viral culture and PCR have near perfect performance characteristics but are more expensive, not universally available, and can take several days to complete.[85] Influenza is normally spread via aerosolized respiratory droplets, so once influenza is suspected or confirmed, patients should be isolated to avoid infecting others. Healthcare practitioners can reduce their risk of exposure by wearing a surgical mask. Standard treatment of influenza infection includes antiviral therapy (i.e., the neuraminidase-inhibitors oseltamivir and zanamivir) and supportive care.[86] To be most effective, antiviral medications should be given within 48 hours of symptom onset.

Approximately 60% of influenza infections are prevented annually by the influenza vaccine.[87] As a result, the vaccine is now recommended for everyone over 6 months of age. In the past, the influenza vaccine was contraindicated in patients with chicken egg allergies, although this has since been revised for patients with nonanaphylactic reactions. Reactions are also less likely with the attenuated vaccine compared with the live vaccine.[88]

Viral Pneumonias in Children

RSV is the most common cause of lower respiratory tract infections in children under age 1 year and an infrequent cause of pneumonia in adults.[81] RSV peaks in the winter months like influenza but, unlike influenza, causes significantly more wheezing and acute bronchiolitis. Treatment includes aerosolized ribavirin and epinephrine, as well as supportive care. Other common respiratory viruses include parainfluenza, adenovirus, and rhinovirus. These viruses are common causes of conjunctivitis and URIs[81] and rising causes of pneumonia in children.[89] The vast majority of these viral pneumonias are self-limited, but some do progress to severe acute respiratory failure. There are no specific treatments available other than supportive care.

AGE-SPECIFIC ANGLE

RSV infection is frequent in children, particularly in the winter months.

Human metapneumovirus (hMPV) is an emerging pathogen in children. Similar to rates of influenza and parainfluenza, hMPV causes one childhood hospitalization per thousand in the United States. Fifty percent of those hospitalized with hMPV infections are diagnosed with pneumonia. Compared with RSV, hMPV generally infects older children up to age 3.[90]

Viral Pneumonias in the Immunosuppressed

Patients with impaired immune function are at risk for pneumonia caused by varicella virus (VZV), herpes simplex virus (HSV), and cytomegalovirus (CMV). These viruses are from the Herpesviridae family and are commonly acquired during childhood or adolescence. CMV can also be contracted from blood products or tissues from a CMV-positive donor. After the self-limited infection resolves, these viruses remain dormant in the body forever and can reactivate if the immune system is weakened. While impaired immune function is the most significant risk factor, recent studies have suggested that CMV reactivation may also occur in nonimmunocompromised, critically ill patients. This is associated with increased duration of mechanical ventilation, ICU length of stay, and mortality.[91]

Signs and symptoms of pneumonia due to a Herpesviridae virus may be nonspecific and include fever, dry cough, tachypnea, and hypoxemia. Chest imaging commonly shows diffuse nodular or interstitial infiltrates. Diagnosis generally requires microbiologic and histopathologic confirmation of infection.

Treatment includes antiviral medications and supportive care. CMV pneumonitis is treated with ganciclovir or foscarnet. Varicella and herpes simplex pneumonias are treated with acyclovir, vidarabine, or foscarnet. The best treatment of course is prevention. Varicella vaccination is now recommended during childhood. While there is no vaccine for CMV, prophylactic ganciclovir or valganciclovir can be administered to immunocompromised patients at risk of reactivation.

Other Viral Pneumonias

The measles virus is now an exceedingly rare cause of viral pneumonia due to the highly effective MMR vaccine. Unfortunately, fabricated research from the 1990s claiming an association between MMR and autism has caused many parents to defer vaccinating their children.[92] This falsity has been perpetuated by certain celebrities and popular media, resulting in outbreaks of this highly contagious virus in areas with lower vaccination rates. Signs and symptoms of measles pneumonia generally include the classic measles rash followed by prolonged fever, cough, and progressive respiratory failure requiring mechanical ventilation. Intravenous ribavirin has been used to treat measles; however, most cases resolve with supportive care alone.

Hantavirus is transmitted by aerosolized droppings of the deer mouse, which is native to the southwestern United States.[93] Infection causes an influenza-like illness with fever and myalgia, followed by dyspnea, hypoxemia, pulmonary edema, hemorrhage, and shock. There is no specific therapy for this virus and it is often fatal.

Two novel coronavirus strains have recently emerged that cause severe pneumonia. Severe acute respiratory syndrome coronavirus (SARS-CoV) and MERS-CoV.[94] These viruses are hypothesized to have migrated from animals to humans, although the precise animal reservoir remains controversial. Unlike other zoonotic infections, however, these viruses can also be transmitted *between* humans.[94,95] The SARS-CoV epidemic was responsible for nearly 800 deaths between 2002 and 2004.[81] MERS-CoV has been less widespread to date, but pandemic potential still exists. Both infections cause an influenza-like illness progressing to profound respiratory failure. There is no known antiviral therapy and reported mortality is 50%.[94]

Mycobacterial Pneumonia

Tuberculosis

Tuberculosis (TB) is caused by *Mycobacterium tuberculosis* complex (MTB) and is a major cause of morbidity and mortality worldwide. In fact, one-third of the world's population has been infected with MTB.[96] In 2012, there were 1.3 million TB-related deaths. One-third of these occurred in India and South Africa, largely due to their burden of HIV infection. With the institution of an aggressive public health campaign, the global burden of disease is declining by approximately 2% per year. Still, adequate MTB control has not yet been realized, and MTB continues to represent a major public health threat.[97]

Initial infection

Tuberculosis is transmitted by cough-induced dispersal of infected droplets. These droplets are then inhaled by exposed persons into the small airways where infection is established. The initial TB infection, also known as primary TB, is usually asymptomatic, although some may experience fever, malaise, or other respiratory symptoms. In most cases, primary TB is contained by the host immune responses via granuloma formation, scarring, and calcification. This calcified area of lung on chest radiograph is called a Ghon focus, and when present with a calcified ipsilateral, hilar lymph node, it is called a Ranke complex. Patients able to contain their initial TB infections are said to have latent TB.

When MTB avoids initial containment it causes active primary TB. Patients with active primary TB may present with middle or lower lobe pneumonia and pleural effusion or hematogenous dissemination due to miliary TB. Miliary TB is characterized by innumerable, small pulmonary nodules and can be seen in patients with severe immune compromise, such as in end-stage HIV.

Latent TB

Patients with TB infection who are without signs or symptoms of active disease (including by chest radiography) are said to have latent TB. Latent TB is diagnosed by an immunologic test such as a tuberculin skin test (TST) or IFN-γ release assays (IGRA). A TST will be positive in up to 30% of patients exposed to MTB. Latent TB represents a state of equilibrium between the host defenses and MTB. The infection is merely contained, but not eradicated. If the host becomes weakened, MTB can progress to active disease.[98] Because of this risk, patients with latent TB are generally treated for 6 to 12 months with isoniazid (INH) and/or a rifamycin (e.g., rifampin, rifabutin, rifapentine). This prophylactic treatment can reduce the subsequent risk of developing reactivation TB by up to 90%.[99]

Post-Primary TB

Patients who do develop reactivation of latent TB are said to have post-primary TB. This is characterized by upper lobe cavity formation with a productive cough or hemoptysis and B symptoms such as malaise, anorexia, fever, night sweats, and weight loss (**Figure 36-4**). Rarely, post-primary TB can develop in patients with repeated primary MTB infection. Post-primary TB only occurs when the host immune defenses are weakened, such as with HIV/AIDS (CD4 count >300 cells/mm ^{3}), organ transplantation,[100] severe malnutrition,[101] use of immunosuppressive drugs,[102] or malignancy.[103] Post-primary TB develops in 5% to 10% of TB-exposed patients and usually occurs within 2 years of initial infection. Diagnosis of post-primary TB requires microbiologic confirmation, usually accomplished by isolation of MTB from cultured sputum. Occasionally, confirmation of the diagnosis requires bronchoscopy.

Treatment of TB

Treatment of TB consists of ≥6 months of INH and rifampin (RIF), and 2 months of ethambutol (EMB) and pyrazinamide (PZA). Longer treatment courses are given to patients with certain high-risk features,

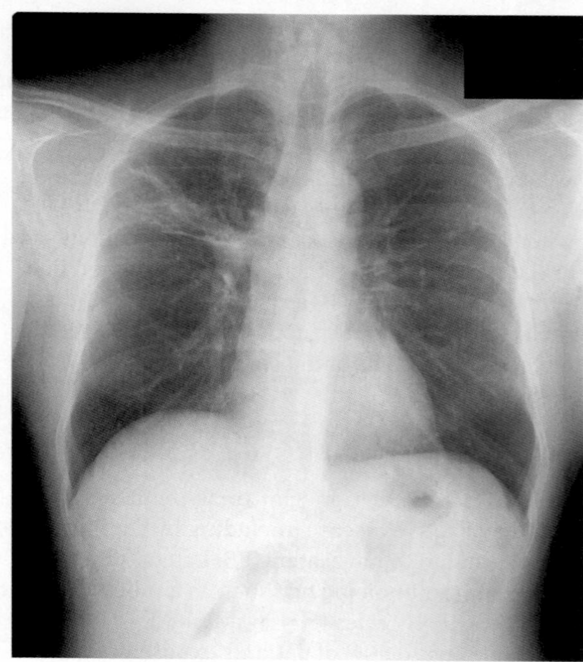

FIGURE 36-4 Posteroanterior chest radiograph of a patient with active tuberculosis pneumonia showing right upper lobe consolidation and volume loss.

including persistently positive sputum cultures after 2 months, presence of a lung cavity, or lack of PZA during initial phase.[99]

The increasing prevalence of TB resistance to INH and RIF (MDR TB) poses a public health threat. MDR TB occurs in 3.5% of incident TB cases, and 20% of patients with previously treated TB. Nine percent of patients with MDR TB are believed to have extensively drug-resistant TB (XDR TB), defined as MDR TB that is also resistant to a fluoroquinolone and an injectable anti-TB drug. Mortality rates for patients with MDR TB are as high as 15%. In 2012, the FDA approved the first anti-TB drug with a novel mechanism of action since 1971, bedaquiline. Bedaquiline is approved (as part of combination therapy) for patients with MDR TB. While this is an encouraging step forward in the treatment of MDR TB, additional studies are necessary to fully define the role of this new drug.[104]

Infection Control

Exposure to TB can occur in a variety of settings, including household contacts of infected individuals, endemic areas, correctional facilities, homeless shelters, and healthcare facilities. Healthcare exposures can occur during routine patient examination or during invasive procedures such as bronchoscopy.[105] Patients suspected of having TB should be isolated in a negative pressure room. Additionally, TB transmission can be reduced 56% by placing surgical masks on patients suspected of having the infection.[106]

Nontuberculous Mycobacteria

In contrast to *M tuberculosis*, **nontuberculous mycobacteria (NTM)** are noninfectious mycobacterial microorganisms found in soil and water. This diverse group of mycobacteria comprises more than 100 species. The most common NTM in humans is *Mycobacterium avium* complex (MAC), which is composed of two organisms, *M avium* and *M intracellulare.*

The two major risk factors for NTM infection are impaired immunity and structural lung disease. Examples of structural lung diseases include cystic fibrosis, chronic obstructive pulmonary disease (COPD), previous TB, pneumoconiosis—especially silicosis, alveolar proteinosis, and bronchiectasis.[107] Bronchiectasis in particular appears to have a bidirectional relationship with NTM. It is both a risk factor for, and consequence of, NTM infection. Another recognized NTM pulmonary syndrome is fibrocavitary disease. Fibrocavitary disease is usually due to MAC and is more common in middle-aged or elderly males with a history of alcohol abuse and/or COPD.

The diagnosis of NTM is clinical. Patients must have suggestive symptoms, chest imaging, microbiology, and/or histopathology to confirm the diagnosis (**Box 36-9**). Treatment of NTM generally requires long-term (>12 months) combination antimicrobial therapy. The most common treatment regimen for MAC consists of a macrolide, rifampin, and ethambutol. Other NTM may require a combination of fluoroquinolones, aminoglycosides, imipenem, sulfonamides, cefoxitin, clarithromycin, and/or linezolid. If the treatment regimen fails or is stopped prematurely due to medication intolerance, surgical resection can be considered.[108]

Fungal Pneumonia

Aspergillosis

Aspergillus species are ubiquitous, spore-forming molds. Inhalation of *Aspergillus* spores by susceptible hosts (i.e., immunocompromised patients) can cause a necrotizing, hemorrhagic respiratory infection called invasive pulmonary aspergillosis (IPA). The most common cause of IPA is *Aspergillus fumigatus.*

The predominant risk factor for IPA is impaired host immunity. This is most commonly due to neutropenia. Neutropenia can occur in a number of conditions including post-chemotherapy, post-solid organ transplant or hematopoietic stem cell transplant (HSCT), and hematologic malignancy. Among patients with HSCT or hematologic malignancies, the reported IPA prevalence ranges from 0.8% to 8%.[109,110]

Signs and symptoms of pulmonary IPA include fever, pleuritic chest pain, dyspnea, cough, and hemoptysis. The diagnosis of IPA is largely clinical. Healthcare providers must incorporate the patient's signs and symptoms with radiologic, microbiologic, and histopathologic data. Patients should have compatible signs

BOX 36-9

American Thoracic Society Diagnostic Criteria for Pulmonary Disease Caused by Nontuberculous Mycobacteria

Clinical (both required)

1. Pulmonary symptoms, nodular or cavitary opacities on chest radiograph, or a high-resolution computed tomography scan that shows multifocal bronchiectasis with multiple small nodules

and

2. Appropriate exclusion of other diagnoses

Microbiologic

1. Positive culture results from at least two separate expectorated sputum samples. If the results from (1) are nondiagnostic, consider repeat sputum AFB smears and cultures

or

2. Positive culture result from at least one bronchial wash or lavage

or

3. Transbronchial or other lung biopsy with mycobacterial histopathologic features (granulomatous inflammation or AFB) and positive culture for NTM or biopsy showing mycobacterial histopathologic features (granulomatous inflammation or AFB) and one or more sputum or bronchial washings that are culture positive for NTM
4. Expert consultation should be obtained when NTM are recovered that are either infrequently encountered or that usually represent environmental contamination
5. Patients who are suspected of having NTM lung disease but do not meet the diagnostic criteria should be followed until the diagnosis is firmly established or excluded
6. Making the diagnosis of NTM lung disease does not, per se, necessitate the institution of therapy, which is a decision based on potential risks and benefits of therapy for individual patients

AFB, acid-fast bacilli; NTM, nontuberculous mycobacteria.

 From Griffith DE, Aksamit T, Brown-Elliott BA, et al. An official ATS/IDSA statement: diagnosis, treatment, and prevention of nontuberculous mycobacterial diseases. Griffith, DE. *Am J Respir Crit Care Med.* Feb 2007;175:367–416.

and symptoms, chest imaging, and a positive diagnostic test for IPA, such as detection of indirect laboratory markers (e.g., galactomannan), isolation of *Aspergillus* from culture, and/or identification of *Aspergillus* on a biopsy specimen.[111]

Patients suspected of having IPA should be treated promptly. First-line therapy is voriconazole for 6 to 12 weeks. In patients who fail voriconazole, salvage antifungal therapy may include amphotericin B, posaconazole, itraconazole, caspofungin, or micafungin. If IPA invades the chest wall, great vessels, or other critical structures, surgical resection may be necessary. Treatment may also be rendered more effective by reducing concurrent immunosuppressive drugs.[111]

Zygomycosis

Mucor is an order of fungi that includes *Mucor, Rhizopus, Rhizomucor,* and *Cunninghamella* species. These molds are found in soil and decaying organic matter. *Mucor* can cause a severe, necrotizing, angioinvasive pneumonia called zygomycosis (or mucormycosis) when inhaled by immunocompromised hosts. Patients at risk for *Mucor* are the same as those at risk for *Aspergillus* infection. Moreover, these patients commonly take voriconazole for prophylaxis against fungal infections. While this can be effective against *Aspergillus* infections, *Mucor* species are inherently resistant to this drug. As a result of this positive selective pressure, the incidence of *Mucor* infections is rising. Zygomycosis requires a three-pronged treatment plan: (1) maximally reduce immunosuppressive drugs, (2) surgically debride the necrotic tissue, and (3) use antifungal drugs such as amphotericin B or posaconazole.[112] Even despite optimal therapy, the mortality of zygomycosis is very high. In one study of HSCT patients with zygomycosis, only 50% were alive at 1 month and 30% were alive at 3 months.[113]

Histoplasmosis

Histoplasma capsulatum is a dimorphic fungus endemic to the Ohio and Mississippi River valleys. Exposure occurs by the inhalation of *H capsulatum* spores found in soil and bird or bat droppings. Certain activities are associated with *H capsulatum* exposure such as construction, chopping contaminated wood, and spelunking.

Most individuals exposed to *H capsulatum* are asymptomatic. However, immunocompromised hosts or individuals exposed to a large inoculum may develop acute pulmonary histoplasmosis. Acute pulmonary histoplasmosis can range from a mild, influenza-like illness occurring several weeks to months after exposure, to severe acute respiratory failure and/or extrapulmonary dissemination. Rare complications include broncholithiasis and fibrosing mediastinitis.

The diagnosis of acute pulmonary histoplasmosis requires isolation of *H capsulatum* from blood or body fluid and is supported by detection of *H capsulatum* antigen in urine, blood, or BAL fluid. Treatment depends on the duration of symptoms, host immune function, and severity of disease. Itraconazole is indicated for mild-to-moderate disease lasting more than 1 month. Amphotericin B is indicated for severe respiratory failure or dissemination. Methylprednisolone may also be used as an adjunctive therapy.[112]

Blastomycosis

Blastomyces dermatitidis is a dimorphic fungus endemic to the southern and midwestern United States. *B dermatitidis* growth in soil is favored by decaying organic debris and high humidity. Blastomycosis is acquired via inhalation of spores and can be transmitted sexually.

Acute pulmonary blastomycosis is characterized by fever, chills, myalgias, and productive cough. Chronic blastomycosis presents with similar symptoms as well as weight loss and hemoptysis and can involve the skin, bones, joints, and central nervous system. The diagnosis is made by identification on fungal stains and/or cultures from sputum, bronchial lavage, pleural fluid, skin lesions, cerebrospinal fluid, or urine. Blastomycosis is treated with itraconazole or amphotericin B for 6 to 12 months.[112]

Cryptococcosis

Cryptococcus neoformans is a yeast found worldwide in soil contaminated with bird (especially pigeon) droppings. *C neoformans* is the most common cause of human disease, although *C gattii* is an emerging pathogen in the U.S. Pacific Northwest and Canada. *Cryptococcus* spores can become aerosolized and inhaled, leading to infection. While most infections are asymptomatic, disease can occur in immunocompromised or normal hosts. Normal hosts usually develop a self-limited pneumonia without extrapulmonary manifestations. Symptoms of pulmonary cryptococcosis include dry cough, dyspnea, and chest pain. Immunocompromised hosts more frequently experience disseminated disease, most commonly to the meninges, but virtually any other organ can be involved. The diagnosis of pulmonary cryptococcosis requires microbiologic confirmation. *Cryptococcus* can be cultured from sputum, BAL fluid, or tissue or directly observed on histopathology stains. The cryptococcal antigen test is a noninvasive test that can be used in patients with disseminated disease. Treatment includes amphotericin B with or without flucytosine for patients with severe cryptococcal pneumonia, extrapulmonary disease, or immunosuppression. Patients without these risk factors can be treated with fluconazole.[112]

Coccidioidomycosis

Coccidioides immitis lives in soil and is endemic in areas with arid climates such as the southwestern United States, Mexico, and areas of South and Central America. Infection occurs following inhalation of *Coccidioides* spores. For unclear reasons, the incidence of pulmonary coccidioidomycosis increased nearly eightfold from 1998 to 2011. This might be due to higher temperatures, drought, or disruption of soil due to construction.[114]

Signs and symptoms of pulmonary coccidioidomycosis include fever, malaise, anorexia, myalgia, cough, hemoptysis, rash, and chest pain, although infection is asymptomatic in the majority of cases. The chest radiograph may demonstrate patchy alveolar infiltrates, nodules, cavitation, or a miliary pattern consistent with dissemination. Hematogenous dissemination is more common in African Americans and Filipinos.
A minority of patients may develop chronic, progressive, pulmonary coccidioidomycosis characterized by apical fibronodular infiltrates. The diagnosis of pulmonary coccidioidomycosis requires isolation of the organism from cultures of sputum, BAL fluid, or lung tissue. In a patient with a compatible clinical presentation, the diagnosis is supported by a positive complement fixation test and positive serologies.

Pulmonary coccidioidomycosis is usually a self-limited infection that does not require antifungal therapy. However, therapy may be indicated in patients with the following risk factors: structural lung disease, chronic kidney disease, congestive heart failure, diabetes mellitus, pregnancy, African American or Filipino American heritage, HIV infection, and use of TNF-α inhibitors. Treatment includes fluconazole or itraconazole for mild-to-moderate disease or amphotericin B for severe respiratory failure.

Candidiasis

Candida species are yeasts and part of normal human flora. These organisms colonize the skin, the gastrointestinal and female genital tracts, and the oropharynx. As a result, invasive candidiasis, predominantly due to candidemia, is a common nosocomial infection in the United States.[112] Candida pneumonia (pulmonary candidiasis) is significantly less common but can occur via one of two mechanisms: (1) aspiration of oropharyngeal secretions causing a primary pneumonia, or (2) hematogenous dissemination to the lungs, causing a secondary pneumonia. Of these two mechanisms, hematogenous dissemination is the most common and, when present, affects other organs as well.

Aspiration is the other mechanism by which *Candida* gains access to the lung. *Candida* is frequently isolated from lower respiratory tract specimens of intubated patients. However, aspiration of *Candida* rarely causes primary pneumonia. In one autopsy study of 135 patients who died with pneumonia in the ICU (30% of whom were immunocompromised), not a single case of pulmonary candidiasis was found. This is despite isolating *Candida* from premortem respiratory specimens in 57% of the patients.[115] In another autopsy study of 351 immunocompromised patients with proven pulmonary candidiasis, 9% were due to primary pneumonia, whereas 91% were due to secondary pneumonia. In this study, the overall prevalence of primary pulmonary candidiasis among 7725 autopsies performed over 20 years was 0.4%.[116] Because of the high frequency in which patients become colonized with *Candida* relative to the low frequency of primary pulmonary candidiasis, the diagnosis requires histopathologic confirmation.

When present, primary pulmonary candidiasis causes a hemorrhagic, necrotizing pneumonia. Treatment is based on local epidemiologic data, the patient's clinical status, likelihood of drug toxicity, and prior exposure to antifungal drugs. Antifungal therapy can include amphotericin B, an echinocandin (e.g., micafungin), fluconazole, or voriconazole.[112]

Pneumonia in Immunocompromised Patients

Immunocompromised patients are at risk for both infectious and noninfectious causes of lung disease. Impaired immune function predisposes to infection from typical pathogens (e.g., pneumococcus) and opportunistic pathogens (e.g., CMV). Moreover, these patients commonly have other comorbidities and frequently use high-risk medications, increasing their risk for noninfectious pulmonary complications such as diffuse alveolar hemorrhage, pneumonitis due to drug toxicity, pulmonary edema, and progression of their underlying disease. As a result, immunocompromised patients with suspected pneumonia require a thorough (and at times, invasive) workup to differentiate between infectious and noninfectious diseases and to identify the causative pathogen when infection is present.

Clinical Considerations

In immunocompromised patients with pneumonia, the presenting history can provide clues regarding the causative pathogen. Two relevant components of the history are the *timing of illness* and the *acuity of symptom onset*. The timing of the illness refers to when the symptoms started in relation to other events such as recent chemotherapy administration, diagnostic procedures, or organ transplantation. For example, within 30 days of HSCT, pneumonia is more frequently due to nosocomial bacteria, *Candida*, and HSV, whereas at 100 days post-HSCT, pneumonia is more frequently due to *Nocardia*, *Listeria*, encapsulated bacteria, *Pneumocystis*, endemic fungi, CMV, VZV, and Epstein-Barr virus. Pathogens that overlap these periods include *Aspergillus*, molds, and respiratory viruses.[117] Acuity of symptom onset refers to the rapidity in which the symptoms develop and peak. For example, pneumococcal pneumonia causes abrupt symptom onset and peaks within 1–2 days, whereas symptoms of *Pneumocystis* pneumonia (PCP) in an immunocompromised patient may develop and peak over 6 weeks. In contrast, symptoms due to post-primary TB develop and peak over months.

Once signs and symptoms of pneumonia do develop, they may differ between immunocompromised and immunocompetent patients. For example, dry cough may be the only presenting symptom in an immunocompromised patient with pulmonary aspergillosis, whereas immunocompetent patients may have a productive cough, fever, dyspnea, and chest pain. This is largely because signs and symptoms are produced by inflammation—a process that in immunosuppressed states is impaired. Immunocompromised patients are also more likely to present with disseminated disease. Furthermore, the pattern of organ system involvement may provide clues as to the causative pathogen. For example, a rash can be seen in patients with pulmonary blastomycosis, whereas meningitis may be seen in patients with pulmonary cryptococcosis.

A third relevant component of the patient's history is the type of immune defect that is present. Different defects in immune function cause varying degrees of immunosuppression and confer risks to different opportunistic pathogens. For example, asplenic patients are at increased risk for infections caused by encapsulated bacteria (e.g., *S pneumoniae*, *Klebsiella*, and *Neisseria meningitidis*), whereas neutropenic patients are at increased risk for invasive fungal infections.

Radiologic Considerations

The clinical differential diagnosis in immunocompromised patients with pneumonia is usually quite broad but can be narrowed with the appropriate use of thoracic imaging. Radiographic findings of one type of infection may be quite different than another type.

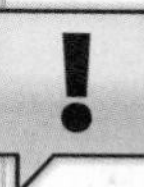

Respiratory Recap

Immunocompromised Patients with Pneumonia

- Different immune defects predispose to different types of pneumonia.
- Early, invasive diagnostic procedures are indicated for most immunocompromised patients with pneumonia.
- Approximately 25% of lung infiltrates are due to noninfectious diseases.

For example, in a study of HIV-negative immunocompromised patients by Vogel et al., PCP more frequently caused homogenous and sharply demarcated ground glass opacities (GGO) in the upper lung zones, whereas CMV pneumonia more frequently caused poorly demarcated GGO with centrilobular nodules and consolidation.[118]

Diagnostic Considerations

Essential to the management of pneumonia in an immunocompromised patient is diagnosing the cause of the infection. Once the causative pathogen is known, a more focused antimicrobial regimen can be instituted to reduce the patient's exposure to toxic antimicrobial drugs. Because many of the microbes can only be identified by culture and/or histopathology, immunocompromised patients must frequently undergo invasive procedures such as bronchoscopy. Numerous studies have evaluated the role of bronchoscopy in this clinical setting and have found mixed results. However, early bronchoscopy (within 48 to 72 hours of presentation) is generally recommended over empiric therapy. When bronchoscopy is performed, the combination of BAL, protected specimen brush (PSB) sampling, and transbronchial biopsy increases the diagnostic yield from 38% (BAL alone) to 86%.[119] This may be due to the inadequate diagnostic power of BAL for viral and **fungal pneumonia**, because these pneumonias often require further histopathologic confirmation of tissue invasion. This concept was underscored by Brownback et al., who found that reticular or nodular patterns on chest CT, which are more commonly due to viral and fungal infections, were associated with a lower diagnostic yield from BAL compared to consolidation, ground glass, or tree-and-bud patterns of infiltrate.[120]

Treatment Considerations

Antimicrobial therapy in immunocompromised patients with pneumonia must be started promptly, broadly, and concurrently with an early invasive diagnostic workup. Delayed or inadequate antibiotics have been associated in numerous studies with increased mortality.

Pneumonia and HIV/AIDS

In 2012, an estimated 35.3 million people worldwide were HIV-positive. Developing regions such as sub-Saharan Africa continue to be disproportionally affected, accounting for 70% of new infections. Incident HIV infections are also rising in Eastern Europe, Central Asia, the Middle East, and North Africa. Because these resource-poor areas carry much of the disease burden, only one-third of those eligible for antiviral therapy actually receive it.[121] In the United States, there are over 1 million HIV-infected persons, and nearly one in five are undiagnosed.[122] As a result, the prevalence of untreated HIV and end-stage AIDS will continue to rise, as will the associated infectious complications.

The most common infection among HIV-infected persons is pneumonia. The etiology of pneumonia is largely influenced by the degree of immune suppression as measured by the CD4 count. For example, CD4 counts of <200 cells/mm^3 (and even 200–499 cells/mm^3) confer a significantly increased risk of bacterial pneumonia and PCP.[123,124] Other factors influencing pneumonia etiology include geographic location, use of anti-*Pneumocystis* prophylaxis, history of prior infections, route of HIV exposure, virulence of the infecting microorganism, and use of highly active antiretroviral therapy (HAART).[123,125] Prior to the development of HAART, the most common cause of pneumonia among HIV-infected patients in the United States was the fungus *Pneumocystis jirovecii*. Since the introduction of HAART along with anti-*Pneumocystis* prophylaxis, however, rates of PCP in the United States have declined. The top three pulmonary infections among HIV-infected persons in the United States (in descending order) are now bacterial pneumonia, PCP, and TB.

Bacterial Pneumonia

HIV infection is associated with a more than 10-fold increased risk of bacterial pneumonia.[125] The most common cause of bacterial pneumonia in patients with HIV/AIDS is *S pneumoniae*, followed by *H influenzae*, *P aeruginosa*, and *S aureus*.[124,125] Risk factors for bacterial pneumonia in HIV-infected persons include cigarette smoking, intravenous drug use, detectable HIV viral load, prior episodes of bacterial pneumonia, and poor adherence to HAART.[125] Less common causes of bacterial pneumonia include *Rhodococcus* and *Nocardia*. These pathogens cause indolent pneumonia, which can mimic lung cancer, and are characterized by alveolar infiltrates or nodules with necrosis or cavitation, pleural effusions, and mediastinal/hilar lymphadenopathy.[126]

Pneumocystis Pneumonia (PCP)

While the incidence of PCP is declining, it remains the second leading cause of pneumonia in HIV-infected persons in developed countries.[125,127] PCP is caused by the yeast-like fungus *Pneumocystis jirovecii*. Infection is likely acquired via inhalation, although the exact mechanism and source of exposure is unknown.

When inhaled by a susceptible host, *Pneumocystis* causes a subacute pneumonia. Patients typically report gradually worsening dyspnea over 4 to 8 weeks, along with fever, chills, malaise, and a dry cough. In the early phase of illness, the chest radiograph can be normal. More commonly, the chest radiograph shows perihilar or diffuse, bilateral interstitial opacities (**Figure 36-5**). These can rapidly progress to diffuse, bilateral alveolar opacities and the acute respiratory distress syndrome (ARDS). Additional radiographic findings can include pneumothorax due to ruptured cysts. Notable laboratory findings generally include significant arterial hypoxemia with an elevated alveolar-arterial oxygen tension gradient as well as elevated serum lactate dehydrogenase.[127]

Diagnosis of PCP requires confirmation of the organism. Because *P jirovecii* cannot be cultured in vitro, the organism must be directly visualized in sputum, BAL fluid, or lung tissue. Identification of *P jirovecii* can be aided by using special stains such as methenamine silver. Respiratory specimens can also be sent for *Pneumocystis* DNA PCR. Because the diagnostic yield of induced sputum is variable, the gold standard for obtaining respiratory specimens to diagnose PCP is bronchoscopy.[127]

The mainstay of PCP treatment is trimethoprim-sulfamethoxazole. For patients with moderate to severe hypoxemia, prednisone has also been shown to reduce the risk of respiratory failure and death.[128] In patients who do not improve after 5 to 7 days, switching from standard treatment to salvage therapy (clindamycin and primaquine) may be appropriate.[127]

Primary PCP prophylaxis should be given to all HIV-infected persons with the following risk factors: previous history of PCP, history of any opportunistic infection, CD4 count less than 200 cells/mm^3, oral candidiasis, or unexplained constitutional symptoms. The most effective prophylactic regimen is one double-strength trimethoprim-sulfamethoxazole tablet taken orally three times weekly, although alternative drugs are available.[127]

MTB and HIV Infection

TB is the third leading cause of pneumonia among HIV-infected persons in the United States, but globally it is number one. Worldwide nearly half of the notified TB cases in 2012 were HIV-positive.[97] While the risk of developing active TB among immunocompetent hosts is 10% over a lifetime, among HIV-infected persons it is 10% *per year*.

The signs and symptoms of TB in HIV-infected persons can vary. Some patients may have little or no TB symptoms at all. In one cohort study, 8.5% of HIV-infected patients were found to have active, but asymptomatic TB.[129] Co-infected patients are also more likely to present with extrapulmonary TB, most commonly involving the lymphatic and pleural spaces. Other frequently involved sites include the thoracic spine, joints, psoas muscle, central nervous system, and pericardium.[130]

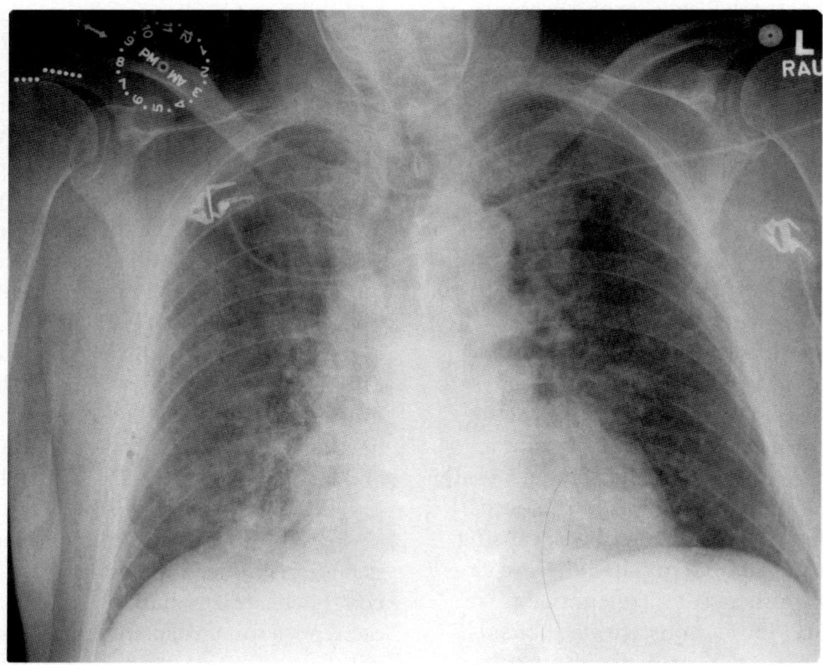

FIGURE 36-5 Portable anteroposterior chest radiograph of a patient with AIDS and *Pneumocystis* pneumonia showing bilateral diffuse infiltrates.

The radiographic appearance of TB among HIV-infected persons is dependent on the level of immune suppression. HIV-infected persons with a CD4 count >350 to 400 cells/mm³ generally present with post-primary TB and have upper-lobe cavitary lung disease. Patients with a CD4 count <200 cells/mm³, however, more commonly present with primary TB and have middle or lower lung zone infiltrates, a pleural effusion, and mediastinal/hilar lymphadenopathy.[125] The diagnosis of TB requires microbiologic confirmation, similar to HIV-negative persons. This can be difficult, however, as up to 75% of HIV-infected persons with active TB are AFB smear-negative, leading to delays in diagnosis.[129]

Treatment of TB in HIV-infected persons includes the same anti-TB four-drug regimen as in HIV-negative persons, although there are some special considerations. First, the World Health Organization (WHO) recommends that all HIV-TB co-infected patients receive HAART, which has been shown to improve survival.[97] Unfortunately, concurrent therapy has associated risks, such as a large daily pill burden, potential for overlapping drug toxicity or drug–drug interactions, and risk of immune reconstitution syndrome.[130] Therefore, this may not be possible in all patients. Second, the WHO recommends starting trimethoprim/sulfamethoxazole 1 month after initiation of anti-TB drugs, which also may reduce the risk of death.[97] Finally, patients with CD4 counts <100 cells/mm³ are at high risk of TB recurrence and require a longer duration of therapy.

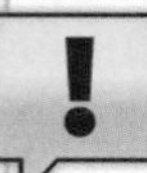

Respiratory Recap

Pneumonia in HIV-Infected Patients

- HIV-infected patients with pneumonia require aggressive workup similar to other immunosuppressed patients.
- *S pneumoniae* is a leading cause of pneumonia in HIV-infected persons.
- *Pneumocystis* pneumonia can cause severe ARDS.
- HIV infection is the most significant risk factor for TB.
- HIV-infected persons with TB may present with primary TB rather than post-primary.

AIDS-Defining Pneumonias

An HIV-infected person is said to have AIDS when one of the following is present: CD4 count <200 cells/mm³, CD4 cells <14% of total T-cells, or the presence of an AIDS-defining illness. Many of the AIDS-defining illnesses are pneumonias, such as recurrent bacterial pneumonias, PCP, and TB. As previously mentioned, TB and recurrent bacterial pneumonias can occur at virtually any CD4 count, whereas PCP generally occurs at CD4 counts <200 cells/mm³. Several other pneumonias qualify as AIDS-defining illnesses and generally occur at CD4 counts <50 cells/mm³, including pulmonary candidiasis, HSV pneumonia, and CMV pneumonia.[126]

Fungal pneumonias such as coccidioidomycosis, histoplasmosis, and cryptococcosis are considered AIDS-defining illnesses only when they are extrapulmonary. Cryptococcosis is one of the most common fungal infections in HIV-infected persons and generally disseminates when the CD4 count is <100 cells/mm³. Dissemination usually involves the meninges, causing meningitis. The diagnosis of disseminated disease can be made with a high cryptococcal serum antigen.[126]

Extrapulmonary NTM infections are also considered AIDS-defining illnesses. MAC is the most common cause, and dissemination generally occurs at CD4 counts <100 cells/mm³. Common sites of dissemination include liver, spleen, and bone marrow. Symptoms can include fever, weight loss, night sweats, malaise, and diarrhea.[126] NTM can be cultured from blood or bone marrow, confirming the diagnosis. MAC prophylaxis with a macrolide antibiotic is recommended for patients with CD4 counts <50 cells/mm³.

Pneumonia in Children

Pneumonia is a leading cause of death worldwide among children younger than 5 years old, accounting for 1.5 million deaths in 2008.[131] Most of these infections are due to *S pneumoniae*, a pathogen responsible for up to 11% of total deaths in this age group.[132] Prevention of pneumonia is the most effective strategy, and vaccines are available against *S pneumoniae*, *Haemophilus influenzae* type b, *Bordetella pertussis*, and influenza.[133,134]

Another pneumonia prevention strategy is identifying (and reducing) modifiable risk factors, such as lack of exclusive breastfeeding, malnutrition, indoor air pollution, passive smoking, low birth weight, and prematurity. These issues can be partially addressed through education and improved access to prenatal care. Nonmodifiable risk factors for childhood CAP include male sex, congenital lung disease, asthma,[135] congenital heart disease, neurologic impairment, and immunocompromised state.

The clinical presentation of pneumonia in children differs from that of adults due to their immature immune system and developing anatomy. Children have smaller airways, more compliant chest walls, and less efficient respiratory muscles. The diagnosis of pneumonia in children is based almost entirely on the history and physical exam. Pneumonia should be suspected in children with any of the following: dyspnea, cough, chest pain, high fever (≥38.5° C), hypoxemia, tachypnea for age, costal retractions, and abnormal chest auscultation.[136,137] Abdominal pain may be the predominant symptom in children under 5 years old

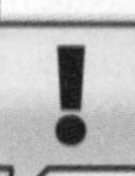

Respiratory Recap

Pneumonia in Children

- The differential diagnosis includes asthma, bronchiolitis, bronchitis, bronchiectasis, foreign body aspiration, pulmonary sequestration, and atelectasis.
- No pathogen is identified in approximately 50% of cases of pneumonia in children.
- Most children recover fully.

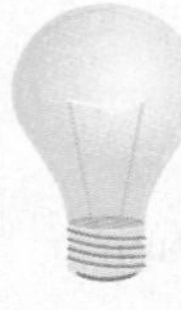

STOP AND THINK

You are caring for a 10-month-old infant with tachypnea in the emergency department. Which signs and symptoms would be consistent with pneumonia? Which signs and symptoms would suggest the need for hospitalization?

with lower lobe pneumonia.[134,138] Pulse oximetry should be measured in all children with a febrile, respiratory illness, as hypoxemia suggests the need for hospitalization.[134] The absence of fever, respiratory distress, tachypnea, and abnormal breath sounds make pneumonia less likely.[137] Moreover, children with wheezing, but without fever are also unlikely to have pneumonia.[138]

Viruses and bacteria are the most common causes of CAP in children (**Box 36-10**). RSV is a significant cause of pneumonia, particularly in children <3 years old, accounting for 14% to 35% of pneumonia cases.[139] *M pneumoniae* and *C pneumoniae* infections are more common in children >5 years old. Noninvasive diagnostic tests (e.g., PCR) often identify multiple pathogens in the same patient, including viral/bacterial co-infections. Mycobacterial and fungal pneumonias are rare in immunocompetent children, particularly in the developed world.[134]

BOX 36-10

Pathogens Causing Pneumonia in Children According to Age

Neonate

Group B streptococci
Escherichia coli
Staphylococcus aureus
Chlamydia trachomatis

1 Month to 2 Years

Respiratory syncytial virus
Parainfluenza
Influenza
Streptococcus pneumoniae
Haemophilus influenzae

2 to 12 Years

Streptococcus pneumoniae
Mycoplasma pneumoniae
Chlamydophila pneumoniae
Human metapneumovirus

Similar to in adults, pneumonia is a clinical diagnosis and incorporates laboratory testing, blood cultures, and chest imaging. However, much of this workup can be avoided in children who are well enough to be treated as outpatients.[134] Conversely, a workup in children requiring hospitalization is appropriate. A chest radiograph can confirm the diagnosis and rule out congenital abnormalities, and blood cultures are positive in 40% of neonates and 10% to 20% of older children. Testing for the pneumococcal or *H influenzae* type b antigens is not recommended in children due to high false-positive rates.[134] Nasopharyngeal aspirates from children younger than 18 months should be sent for viral antigen detection and viral culture. Even after extensive investigation, no pathogen is identified in 20% to 60% of cases.[139]

While severity of illness scores have not been as rigorously studied in children compared to adults,[134] the British Thoracic Society has outlined specific criteria for hospitalizing children with pneumonia. Of these criteria, hypoxia and respiratory distress are emphasized the most (**Box 36-11**).

Treatment of pneumonia includes antibiotics and supportive care. Several factors affect the choice of antibiotic, such as age, severity of illness, and likely pathogens. Oral antibiotics such as amoxicillin are adequate for most mild-to-moderate bacterial pneumonias, whereas parenteral antibiotics are indicated for severe bacterial pneumonia. Neonates should receive parenteral antibiotics that cover Group B *Streptococcus* and gram-negative bacteria. A macrolide is appropriate for school-aged children with severe pneumonia or when an atypical pathogen is suspected.[134,140]

Most children with pneumonia recover fully, although *Mycoplasma* and adenovirus pneumonias can cause permanent lung damage. As in adults, childhood pneumonia can be complicated by parapneumonic effusion and empyema. Routine follow-up chest radiography for uncomplicated CAP is also not recommended, unless there is evidence of recurrent pneumonias or structural lung disease.[136]

HCAP in Children

While CAP is the most common form of pediatric pneumonia, children with extensive healthcare

BOX 36-11

The British Thoracic Society Criteria for Hospital Admission of Children with Pneumonia

For Infants

- Temperature >38.5° C
- Respiratory rate >70 breaths/min
- Moderate-to-severe costal retractions
- Cyanosis
- Intermittent apnea or grunting
- Not feeding
- Tachycardia (adjusted for age and temperature)
- Capillary refill time >2 seconds
- Family not able to provide appropriate observation or supervision

For Older Children

- Temperature >38.5° C
- Respiratory rate >50 breaths/min
- Severe work of breathing
- Nasal flaring
- Cyanosis
- Grunting
- Dehydration
- Tachycardia (adjusted for age and temperature)
- Capillary refill time >2 seconds
- Family not able to provide appropriate observation or supervision

Information from British Thoracic Society guidelines for the management of community acquired pneumonia in childhood. *Thorax*. 2002;57(Suppl 1):1–24.

exposure can develop nosocomial pneumonia. The microbiology of pediatric nosocomial pneumonia is similar to that of adults. Risk factors for pediatric HAP/VAP include use of sedatives/analgesics, gastric tubes/enteral feeding, re-intubation, use of metoclopramide, new chest radiographic finding, and increasing number of ventilator days. HAP and VAP are associated with longer length of stay and high mortality.[141,142]

Case Studies

Case 1. Community-Acquired Pneumonia

A 44-year-old male presents to the local emergency department for a productive cough. He was in his usual state of health until 3 days ago when he developed a cough productive of yellow sputum. One day ago he developed subjective fevers and chills. He also noticed dyspnea with minimal exertion and right-sided chest pain with deep inspiration. He denies weight loss, night sweats, and exposure to tuberculosis. He has a history of alcohol abuse and has smoked a pack of cigarettes every day for the last 15 years.

The following vital signs are recorded by the nurse: temperature—102.1° F (38.9° C), respiratory rate—34 breaths/min, blood pressure—125/79 mm Hg, heart rate—125 beats/min, and oxygen saturation 93% breathing room air. On physical examination, he is in mild respiratory distress. Auscultation of the chest demonstrates rales over the right lower lung field with associated dullness to percussion and increased tactile fremitus. Laboratory studies show the WBC count is 16,000 cells/mm^3 and differential is 20% banwd neutrophils, 70% neutrophils, and 10% lymphocytes. Serum protein is 7 g/dL, and lactate dehydrogenase (LDH) is 210 units/L. Serum electrolytes, creatinine, liver function panel, hemoglobin, and platelet count are unremarkable. A chest radiograph demonstrates consolidation involving the right middle and right lower lobes with a right-sided pleural effusion.

Blood and sputum samples are collected and sent to the microbiology lab for gram stain and culture. The patient is given intravenous azithromycin and ceftriaxone and admitted to the General Medicine service. A diagnostic thoracentesis is performed and pleural fluid analysis demonstrates the following: pH 7.37, WBC count 1000 cells/mm^3 (95% neutrophils), total protein 5 g/dL, and LDH 198 units/L. Pleural fluid gram stain is negative, however, sputum gram stain reveals 3+ gram-positive, lancet-shaped diplococci.

On the second hospital day, the patient's cough and dyspnea are slightly improved. He is given a nicotine patch to help with cigarette cravings and is counseled about the importance of alcohol and tobacco cessation. On the third hospital day, the sputum and blood cultures collected in the emergency department grow *S pneumoniae* sensitive to amoxicillin. The antibiotic regimen is switched from intravenous ceftriaxone and azithromycin to intravenous ampicillin. On the fourth hospital day, the patient continues to improve, and the intravenous ampicillin is changed to oral amoxicillin. On the fifth hospital day, he is discharged home with oral amoxicillin to complete an 8-day antibiotic course. Prior to discharge, he receives an influenza vaccine and a pneumococcal (PPSV23) vaccine. The patient is given an appointment to follow up at an outpatient clinic in one week. The patient will need a follow-up chest radiograph in 4 to 8 weeks to ensure complete resolution of the radiographic abnormalities.

Case 2. Pneumonia in an Immunocompromised Host

A 26-year-old female is hospitalized for dyspnea. She reports significant weight loss (approximately 15 kg over a 3-month period) and cough for 5 weeks. The cough was initially dry, but became productive of brown sputum about 1 week ago. Over the last week, she also has noticed worsening dyspnea, subjective fever, and chills. She denies exposure to TB. She has no past medical history, but does remote report high-risk sexual encounters.

The following vital signs are recorded by the nurse: temperature—101.2° F (38.4° C), respiratory rate—39 breaths/min, blood pressure—90/55 mm Hg, heart rate—145 beats/min, and Spo_2 82% breathing room air and 94% on 6 L O_2 via nasal cannula. On physical examination, the patient is in moderate respiratory distress. There are diffuse rales on chest auscultation. The serum electrolyte values were normal. The hematocrit is 23%, the platelet count is 85,000 cells/mm^3, the WBC count is 5000 cells/mm^3, and the differential is 10% bands, 80% neutrophils, and 10% lymphocytes. Serum protein is 8 g/dL, albumin is 1.5 g/dL, and LDH is 900 units/L. A chest radiograph shows diffuse interstitial opacities with focal consolidation in the right upper lobe. Blood cultures are collected. Sputum is induced with 3% saline and sent for the following microbiological tests: gram stain, bacterial culture, KOH preparation and fungal culture, AFB stain and mycobacterial culture, and silver stain to evaluate for *Pneumocystis jirovecii*.

The patient is given intravenous azithromycin, ceftriaxone, and vancomycin for severe CAP. There is also concern for *Pneumocystis* pneumonia and intravenous trimethoprim-sulfamethoxazole and oral prednisone are initiated. On the second hospital day, the patient's condition worsens and she is transferred to the medical ICU for severe hypoxemic respiratory failure. Her Pao_2 is 65 mm Hg (breathing 100% O_2) and she undergoes endotracheal intubation and initiation of mechanical ventilation. Bronchoscopy is performed and BAL fluid is sent for the following tests: gram stain and culture, KOH preparation and fungal culture, AFB stain, MTB PCR, mycobacterial culture, cytology, WBC count and differential, and *Pneumocystis* PCR. On the third hospital day, the *Pneumocystis* PCR returns positive. The BAL fluid AFB smear and MTB PCR tests are also positive. TB treatment is initiated with INH, rifampin, pyrazinamide, and ethambutol. On hospital day four, the HIV ELISA and Western blot return positive. Her CD4 count is 10 cells/mm^3 and she is initiated on HAART. Over the next 3 weeks, the patient's condition gradually deteriorates. She has multiple complications including MRSA bacteremia, an upper gastrointestinal hemorrhage, and acute kidney injury requiring dialysis. On the 35th hospital day, she dies of multiple organ failure.

Key Points

- Pneumonia is the inflammation and consolidation of lung tissue caused by an infection.
- The most common cause of pneumonia worldwide is *Streptococcus pneumoniae*.
- Community-acquired pneumonia (CAP) occurs outside the hospital.
- Hospital-acquired pneumonia (HAP) and ventilator-associated pneumonia (VAP) are acquired in the hospital.
- Healthcare-associated pneumonia (HCAP) is acquired from healthcare or hospital exposure.
- Pneumonia diagnosis involves both noninvasive and invasive procedures.
- Organisms causing pneumonia include gram-positive, gram-negative, atypical, and anaerobic bacteria, viruses, mycobacteria, and fungi.
- Prognosis and treatment location for CAP can be determined from pneumonia severity scores.
- Pneumonia is the second most common nosocomial infection.
- Multidrug-resistant organisms are common causes of nosocomial pneumonia.
- VAP is associated with increased morbidity and mortality.
- Guidelines for the management of HCAP, HAP, and VAP emphasize early combination antibiotic therapy, de-escalation of initial antibiotic therapy, and shortening the duration of therapy to the minimum effective period.
- The endotracheal tube is the main risk factor for VAP. Prevention should focus on avoiding intubation, rapidly weaning, and minimizing aspiration of contaminated secretions.
- Pulmonary infections are common in immunocompromised patients, and bronchoalveolar lavage is often required for diagnosis.
- PCP and TB are common causes of mortality in patients with HIV.
- Children usually recover fully from pneumonia, and no pathogen is identified in about half of all cases.
- Delayed initiation of appropriate antibiotics for pneumonia increases mortality.

References

1. Walker CL, Rudan I, Liu L, et al. Global burden of childhood pneumonia and diarrhoea. *Lancet*. 2013;381:1405–1416.
2. World Health Organization. *The top 10 causes of death (factsheet no. 310)*. 2013. Available at: http://www.who.int/mediacentre/factsheets/fs310/en/. Accessed August 13, 2014.
3. Heron M. Deaths: leading causes for 2010. *Natl Vital Stat Rep*. 2013;62:1–97.
4. Wroe PC, Finkelstein JA, Ray GT, et al. Aging population and future burden of pneumococcal pneumonia in the United States. *J Infect Dis*. 2012;205:1589–1592.
5. Vila-Corcoles A, Ochoa-Gondar O, Rodriguez-Blanco T, et al. Epidemiology of community-acquired pneumonia in older adults: a population-based study. *Respir Med*. 2009;103:309–316.
6. Vinogradova Y, Hippisley-Cox J, Coupland C. Identification of new risk factors for pneumonia: population-based case-control study. *Br J Gen Pract*. 2009;59:e329–e338.
7. Johnstone J, Majumdar SR, Fox JD, Marrie TJ. Viral infection in adults hospitalized with community-acquired pneumonia: prevalence, pathogens, and presentation. *Chest*. 2008;134:1141–1148.

8. Moran GJ, Krishnadasan A, Gorwitz RJ, et al. Prevalence of methicillin-resistant staphylococcus aureus as an etiology of community-acquired pneumonia. *Clin Infect Dis.* 2012;54:1126–1133.
9. Fleming V, Buck B, Nix N, et al. Community-acquired pneumonia with risk for drug-resistant pathogens. *South Med J.* 2013;106:209–216.
10. Li HT, Zhang TT, Huang J, et al. Factors associated with the outcome of life-threatening necrotizing pneumonia due to community-acquired *Staphylococcus aureus* in adult and adolescent patients. *Respiration.* 2011;81:448–460.
11. Thomas R, Ferguson J, Coombs G, Gibson PG. Community-acquired methicillin-resistant *Staphylococcus aureus* pneumonia: a clinical audit. *Respirology.* 2011;16:926–931.
12. Mandell LA, Wunderink RG, Anzueto A, et al. Infectious Diseases Society of America/American Thoracic Society consensus guidelines on the management of community-acquired pneumonia in adults. *Clin Infect Dis.* 2007;44(Suppl 2):S27–S72.
13. Fine MJ, Smith MA, Carson CA, et al. Prognosis and outcomes of patients with community-acquired pneumonia. A meta-analysis. *JAMA.* 1996;275:134–141.
14. Ewig S, Birkner N, Strauss R, et al. New perspectives on community-acquired pneumonia in 388 406 patients. Results from a nationwide mandatory performance measurement programme in healthcare quality. *Thorax.* 2009;64:1062–1069.
15. Woodhead M, Welch CA, Harrison DA, et al. Community-acquired pneumonia on the intensive care unit: secondary analysis of 17,869 cases in the ICNARC Case Mix Programme Database. *Crit Care.* 2006;(Suppl 2):S1.
16. Lepper PM, Ott S, Nuesch E, et al. Serum glucose levels for predicting death in patients admitted to hospital for community acquired pneumonia: prospective cohort study. *BMJ.* 2012;344:e3397.
17. Fine MJ, Auble TE, Yealy DM, et al. A prediction rule to identify low-risk patients with community-acquired pneumonia. *N Engl J Med.* 1997;336:243–250.
18. Lim WS, van der Eerden MM, Laing R, Boersma WG, et al. Defining community acquired pneumonia severity on presentation to hospital: an international derivation and validation study. *Thorax.* 2003;58:377–382.
19. Myint PK, Sankaran P, Musonda P, et al. Performance of CURB-65 and CURB-age in community-acquired pneumonia. *Int J Clin Pract.* 2009;63:1345–1350.
20. Menendez R, Martinez R, Reyes S, et al. Biomarkers improve mortality prediction by prognostic scales in community-acquired pneumonia. *Thorax.* 2009;64:587–591.
21. Laserna E, Sibila O, Aguilar PR, et al. Hypocapnia and hypercapnia are predictors for ICU admission and mortality in hospitalized patients with community-acquired pneumonia. *Chest.* 2012;142:1193–1199.
22. Menendez R, Torres A, Reyes S, et al. Initial management of pneumonia and sepsis: factors associated with improved outcome. *Eur Respir J.* 2012;39:156–162.
23. Ott SR, Hauptmeier BM, Ernen C, et al. Treatment failure in pneumonia: impact of antibiotic treatment and cost analysis. *Eur Respir J.* 2012;39:611–618.
24. Chalmers JD, Singanayagam A, Murray MP, et al. Risk factors for complicated parapneumonic effusion and empyema on presentation to hospital with community-acquired pneumonia. *Thorax.* 2009;64:592–597.
25. Griffin MR, Zhu Y, Moore MR, et al. US hospitalizations for pneumonia after a decade of pneumococcal vaccination. *N Engl J Med.* 2013;369:155–163.
26. Kawakami K, Ohkusa Y, Kuroki R, et al. Effectiveness of pneumococcal polysaccharide vaccine against pneumonia and cost analysis for the elderly who receive seasonal influenza vaccine in Japan. *Vaccine.* 2010;28:7063–7069.
27. Johnstone J, Marrie TJ, Eurich DT, Majumdar SR. Effect of pneumococcal vaccination in hospitalized adults with community-acquired pneumonia. *Arch Intern Med.* 2007;167:1938–1943.
28. Maruyama T, Taguchi O, Niederman MS, et al. Efficacy of 23-valent pneumococcal vaccine in preventing pneumonia and improving survival in nursing home residents: double blind, randomised and placebo controlled trial. *BMJ.* 2010;340:c1004.
29. Centers for Disease Control and Prevention. Use of 13-valent pneumococcal conjugate vaccine and 23-valent pneumococcal polysaccharide vaccine for adults with immunocompromising conditions: recommendations of the Advisory Committee on Immunization Practices (ACIP). *Morbid Mortal Wkly Rep.* 2012;61:816–819.
30. Tessmer A, Welte T, Schmidt-Ott R, et al. Influenza vaccination is associated with reduced severity of community-acquired pneumonia. *Eur Respir J.* 2011;38:147–153.
31. Safdar N, Crnich CJ, Maki DG. The pathogenesis of ventilator-associated pneumonia: its relevance to developing effective strategies for prevention. *Respir Care.* 2005;50:725–739; discussion 739–741.
32. Bartlett JG. Anaerobic bacterial infection of the lung. *Anaerobe.* 2012;18:235–239.
33. Mabeza GF, Macfarlane J. Pulmonary actinomycosis. *Eur Respir J.* 2003;21:545–551.
34. Japanese Society of Chemotherapy Committee on guidelines for treatment of anaerobic infections; Japanese Association for Anaerobic Infection Research. Chapter 2-12-1. Anaerobic infections (individual fields): actinomycosis. *J Infect Chemother.* 2011;17(Suppl 1):119–120.
35. American Thoracic Society; Infectious Diseases Society of America. Guidelines for the management of adults with hospital-acquired, ventilator-associated, and healthcare-associated pneumonia. *Am J Respir Crit Care Med.* 2005;171:388–416.
36. Venditti M, Falcone M, Corrao S, et al. Outcomes of patients hospitalized with community-acquired, health care-associated, and hospital-acquired pneumonia. *Ann Intern Med.* 2009;150:19–26.
37. Hsu JL, Siroka AM, Smith MW, et al. One-year outcomes of community-acquired and healthcare-associated pneumonia in the Veterans Affairs healthcare system. *Int J Infect Dis.* 2011;15:e382–e387.
38. Polverino E, Torres A, Menendez R, et al. Microbial aetiology of healthcare associated pneumonia in Spain: a prospective, multicentre, case-control study. *Thorax.* 2013;68:1007–1014.
39. Ewig S, Klapdor B, Pletz MW, et al. Nursing-home-acquired pneumonia in Germany: an 8-year prospective multicentre study. *Thorax.* 2012;67:132–138.
40. Herzig SJ, Howell MD, Ngo LH, Marcantonio ER. Acid-suppressive medication use and the risk for hospital-acquired pneumonia. *JAMA.* 2009;301:2120–2128.
41. Sopena N, Heras E, Casas I, et al. Risk factors for hospital-acquired pneumonia outside the intensive care unit: a case-control study. *Am J Infect Control.* 2014;42:38–42.
42. Rello J, Afonso E, Lisboa T, et al. A care bundle approach for prevention of ventilator-associated pneumonia. *Clin Microbiol Infect.* 2013;19:363–369.
43. Nseir S, Zerimech F, Fournier C, et al. Continuous control of tracheal cuff pressure and microaspiration of gastric contents in critically ill patients. *Am J Respir Crit Care Med.* 2011;184:1041–1047.
44. Koff MD, Corwin HL, Beach ML, et al. Reduction in ventilator associated pneumonia in a mixed intensive care unit after initiation of a novel hand hygiene program. *J Crit Care.* 2011;26:489–495.
45. Valles J, Peredo R, Burgueno MJ, et al. Efficacy of single-dose antibiotic against early-onset pneumonia in comatose patients who are ventilated. *Chest.* 2013;143:1219–1225.
46. Restrepo MI, Anzueto A, Arroliga AC, et al. Economic burden of ventilator-associated pneumonia based on total resource utilization. *Infect Control Hosp Epidemiol.* 2010;31:509–515.
47. Blot S, Koulenti D, Dimopoulos G, et al. Prevalence, risk factors, and mortality for ventilator-associated pneumonia in middle-aged, old, and very old critically ill patients. *Crit Care Med.* 2014;42:601–609.
48. Craven DE, Hudcova J, Lei Y. Diagnosis of ventilator-associated respiratory infections (VARI): microbiologic clues for tracheobronchitis (VAT) and pneumonia (VAP). *Clin Chest Med.* 2011;32:547–557.
49. Chastre J, Fagon JY. Ventilator-associated pneumonia. *Am J Respir Crit Care Med.* 2002;165:867–903.
50. Koulenti D, Lisboa T, Brun-Buisson C, et al. Spectrum of practice in the diagnosis of nosocomial pneumonia in patients requiring mechanical ventilation in European intensive care units. *Crit Care Med.* 2009;37:2360–2368.

51. Fabregas N, Ewig S, Torres A, et al. Clinical diagnosis of ventilator associated pneumonia revisited: comparative validation using immediate post-mortem lung biopsies. *Thorax.* 1999;54:867–873.
52. Tejerina E, Esteban A, Fernandez-Segoviano P, et al. Accuracy of clinical definitions of ventilator-associated pneumonia: comparison with autopsy findings. *J Crit Care.* 2010;25:62–68.
53. Pugin J, Auckenthaler R, Mili N, et al. Diagnosis of ventilator-associated pneumonia by bacteriologic analysis of bronchoscopic and nonbronchoscopic "blind" bronchoalveolar lavage fluid. *Am Rev Respir Dis.* 1991;143:1121–1129.
54. Zilberberg MD, Shorr AF. Ventilator-associated pneumonia: the clinical pulmonary infection score as a surrogate for diagnostics and outcome. *Clin Infect Dis.* 2010;51(Suppl 1):S131–S135.
55. Nair GB, Niederman MS. Nosocomial pneumonia: lessons learned. *Crit Care Clin.* 2013;29:521–546.
56. Magill SS, Klompas M, Balk R, et al. Executive summary: developing a new, national approach to surveillance for ventilator-associated events. *Ann Am Thorac Soc.* 2013;10:S220–S223.
57. Wunderink RG, Woldenberg LS, Zeiss J, et al. The radiologic diagnosis of autopsy-proven ventilator-associated pneumonia. *Chest.* 1992;101:458–463.
58. Koenig SM, Truwit JD. Ventilator-associated pneumonia: diagnosis, treatment, and prevention. *Clin Microbiol Rev.* 2006;19:637–657.
59. Capellier G, Mockly H, Charpentier C, et al. Early-onset ventilator-associated pneumonia in adults randomized clinical trial: comparison of 8 versus 15 days of antibiotic treatment. *PloS One.* 2012;7:e41290.
60. Hamet M, Pavon A, Dalle F, et al. *Candida* spp. airway colonization could promote antibiotic-resistant bacteria selection in patients with suspected ventilator-associated pneumonia. *Intensive Care Med.* 2012;38:1272–1279.
61. Quartin AA, Scerpella EG, Puttagunta S, Kett DH. A comparison of microbiology and demographics among patients with healthcare-associated, hospital-acquired, and ventilator-associated pneumonia: a retrospective analysis of 1184 patients from a large, international study. *BMC Infect Dis.* 2013;13:561.
62. Micek ST, Kollef KE, Reichley RM, et al. Health care-associated pneumonia and community-acquired pneumonia: a single-center experience. *Antimicrob Agents Chemother.* 2007;51:3568–3573.
63. Woodhead M. Pneumonia classification and healthcare-associated pneumonia: a new avenue or just a cul-de-sac? *Thorax.* 2013;68: 985–986.
64. Shindo Y, Ito R, Kobayashi D, Ando M, et al. Risk factors for drug-resistant pathogens in community-acquired and healthcare-associated pneumonia. *Am J Respir Crit Care Med.* 2013;188:985–995.
65. Arnold RS, Thom KA, Sharma S, et al. Emergence of *Klebsiella pneumoniae* carbapenemase-producing bacteria. *South Med J.* 2011;104:40–45.
66. Kollef KE, Schramm GE, Wills AR, et al. Predictors of 30-day mortality and hospital costs in patients with ventilator-associated pneumonia attributed to potentially antibiotic-resistant gram-negative bacteria. *Chest.* 2008;134:281–287.
67. Wunderink RG, Niederman MS, Kollef MH, et al. Linezolid in methicillin-resistant *Staphylococcus aureus* nosocomial pneumonia: a randomized, controlled study. *Clin Infect Dis.* 2012;54:621–629.
68. Wunderink RG, Mendelson MH, Somero MS, et al. Early microbiological response to linezolid vs vancomycin in ventilator-associated pneumonia due to methicillin-resistant *Staphylococcus aureus*. *Chest.* 2008;134:1200–1207.
69. Lu Q, Yang J, Liu Z, et al. Nebulized ceftazidime and amikacin in ventilator-associated pneumonia caused by *Pseudomonas aeruginosa*. *Am J Respir Crit Care Med.* 2011;184:106–115.
70. Rattanaumpawan P, Lorsutthitham J, Ungprasert P, et al. Randomized controlled trial of nebulized colistimethate sodium as adjunctive therapy of ventilator-associated pneumonia caused by gram-negative bacteria. *J Antimicrob Chemother.* 2010;65:2645–2649.
71. Chastre J, Wolff M, Fagon JY, et al. Comparison of 8 vs 15 days of antibiotic therapy for ventilator-associated pneumonia in adults: a randomized trial. *JAMA.* 2003;290:2588–2598.
72. Shorr AF, Cook D, Jiang X, et al. Correlates of clinical failure in ventilator-associated pneumonia: insights from a large, randomized trial. *J Crit Care.* 2008;23:64–73.
73. Rumbak MJ, Newton M, Truncale T, et al. A prospective, randomized, study comparing early percutaneous dilational tracheotomy to prolonged translaryngeal intubation (delayed tracheotomy) in critically ill medical patients. *Crit Care Med.* 2004;32:1689–1694.
74. Trouillet JL, Luyt CE, Guiguet M, et al. Early percutaneous tracheotomy versus prolonged intubation of mechanically ventilated patients after cardiac surgery: a randomized trial. *Ann Intern Med.* 2011;154:373–383.
75. Terragni PP, Antonelli M, Fumagalli R, et al. Early vs late tracheotomy for prevention of pneumonia in mechanically ventilated adult ICU patients: a randomized controlled trial. *JAMA.* 2010;303:1483–1489.
76. Griffiths J, Barber VS, Morgan L, Young JD. Systematic review and meta-analysis of studies of the timing of tracheostomy in adult patients undergoing artificial ventilation. *BMJ.* 2005;330:1243.
77. Choi SH, Hong SB, Ko GB, et al. Viral infection in patients with severe pneumonia requiring intensive care unit admission. *Am J Respir Crit Care Med.* 2012;186:325–332.
78. Cox CM, D'Mello T, Perez A, et al. Increase in rates of hospitalization due to laboratory-confirmed influenza among children and adults during the 2009–10 influenza pandemic. *J Infect Dis.* 2012;206:1350–1358.
79. Rice TW, Rubinson L, Uyeki TM, et al. Critical illness from 2009 pandemic influenza A virus and bacterial coinfection in the United States. *Crit Care Med.* 2012;40:1487–1498.
80. Lee N, Chan PK, Lui GC, et al. Complications and outcomes of pandemic 2009 influenza A (H1N1) virus infection in hospitalized adults: how do they differ from those in seasonal influenza? *J Infect Dis.* 2011;203:1739–1747.
81. Ruuskanen O, Lahti E, Jennings LC, Murdoch DR. Viral pneumonia. *Lancet.* 2011;377:1264–1275.
82. Xie H, Li X, Gao J, et al. Revisiting the 1976 "swine flu" vaccine clinical trials: cross-reactive hemagglutinin and neuraminidase antibodies and their role in protection against the 2009 H1N1 pandemic virus in mice. *Clin Infect Dis.* 2011;53:1179–1187.
83. Siston AM, Rasmussen SA, Honein MA, et al. Pandemic 2009 influenza A (H1N1) virus illness among pregnant women in the United States. *JAMA.* 2010;303:1517–1525.
84. Chartrand C, Leeflang MM, Minion J, et al. Accuracy of rapid influenza diagnostic tests: a meta-analysis. *Ann Intern Med.* 2012;156:500–511.
85. Boggild AK, McGeer AJ. Laboratory diagnosis of 2009 H1N1 influenza A virus. *Crit Care Med.* 2010;38:e38–e42.
86. Erlikh IV, Abraham S, Kondamudi VK. Management of influenza. *Am Fam Physician.* 2010;82:1087–1095.
87. Osterholm MT, Kelley NS, Sommer A, Belongia EA. Efficacy and effectiveness of influenza vaccines: a systematic review and meta-analysis. *Lancet Infect Dis.* 2012;12:36–44.
88. Centers for Disease Control and Prevention. Prevention and control of influenza with vaccines: recommendations of the Advisory Committee on Immunization Practices (ACIP)—United States, 2012–13 influenza season. *Morbid Mortal Wkly Rep.* 2012;61:613–618.
89. Cao B, Huang GH, Pu ZH, et al. Emergence of community-acquired adenovirus type 55 as a cause of community-onset pneumonia. *Chest.* 2014;145:79–86.
90. Edwards KM, Zhu Y, Griffin MR, et al. Burden of human metapneumovirus infection in young children. *N Engl J Med.* 2013;368:633–643.
91. Limaye AP, Boeckh M. CMV in critically ill patients: pathogen or bystander? *Rev Med Virol.* 2010;20:372–379.
92. Deer B. How the case against the MMR vaccine was fixed. *BMJ.* 2011;342.
93. Duchin JS, Koster FT, Peters CJ, et al. Hantavirus pulmonary syndrome: a clinical description of 17 patients with a newly recognized disease. *N Engl J Med.* 1994;330:949–955.
94. Assiri A, McGeer A, Perl TM, et al. Hospital outbreak of Middle East respiratory syndrome coronavirus. *N Engl J Med.* 2013;369: 407–416.

95. Memish ZA, Zumla AI, Al-Hakeem RF, et al. Family cluster of Middle East respiratory syndrome coronavirus infections. *N Engl J Med.* 2013;368:2487–2494.
96. Getahun H, Gunneberg C, Granich R, Nunn P. HIV infection-associated tuberculosis: the epidemiology and the response. *Clin Infect Dis.* 2010;50(Suppl 3):S201–S207.
97. World Health Organization. *Global Tuberculosis Report 2013.* Geneva, Switzerland: World Health Organization; 2013. Available at: http://www.who.int/tb/publications/global_report/en/. Accessed August 13, 2014.
98. Lin PL, Flynn JL. Understanding latent tuberculosis: a moving target. *J Immunol.* 2010;185:15–22.
99. Blumberg HM, Burman WJ, Chaisson RE, et al. American Thoracic Society/Centers for Disease Control and Prevention/Infectious Diseases Society of America: treatment of tuberculosis. *Am J Respir Crit Care Med.* 2003;167:603–662.
100. Subramanian AK, Morris MI; AST Infectious Diseases Community of Practice. *Mycobacterium* tuberculosis infections in solid organ transplantation. *Am J Transplant.* 2013;13(Suppl 4):68–76.
101. Jaganath D, Mupere E. Childhood tuberculosis and malnutrition. *J Infect Dis.* 2012;206:1809–1815.
102. Xie X, Li F, Chen JW, Wang J. Risk of tuberculosis infection in anti-TNF-alpha biological therapy: from bench to bedside. *J Microbiol Immunol Infect.* 2014:268–274.
103. Kamboj M, Sepkowitz KA. The risk of tuberculosis in patients with cancer. *Clin Infect Dis.* 2006;42:1592–1595.
104. Mase S, Chorba T, Lobue P, et al. Provisional CDC guidelines for the use and safety monitoring of bedaquiline fumarate (Sirturo) for the treatment of multidrug-resistant tuberculosis. *Morbid Mortal Wkly Rep.* 2013;62(RR-9):1–12.
105. Jensen PA, Lambert LA, Iademarco MF, et al. Guidelines for preventing the transmission of *Mycobacterium* tuberculosis in health-care settings, 2005. *MMWR Recomm Rep.* 2005;54(RR-17): 1–141.
106. Dharmadhikari AS, Mphahlele M, Stoltz A, et al. Surgical face masks worn by patients with multidrug-resistant tuberculosis: impact on infectivity of air on a hospital ward. *Am J Respir Crit Care Med.* 2012;185:1104–1109.
107. Sexton P, Harrison AC. Susceptibility to nontuberculous mycobacterial lung disease. *Eur Respir J.* 2008;31:1322–1333.
108. Griffith DE, Aksamit T, Brown-Elliott BA, et al. An official ATS/IDSA statement: diagnosis, treatment, and prevention of nontuberculous mycobacterial diseases. *Am J Respir Crit Care Med.* 2007;175:367–416.
109. Auberger J, Lass-Florl C, Ulmer H, et al. Significant alterations in the epidemiology and treatment outcome of invasive fungal infections in patients with hematological malignancies. *Int J Hematol.* 2008;88:508–515.
110. Kurosawa M, Yonezumi M, Hashino S, et al. Epidemiology and treatment outcome of invasive fungal infections in patients with hematological malignancies. *Int J Hematol.* 2012;96:748–757.
111. Walsh TJ, Anaissie EJ, Denning DW, et al. Treatment of aspergillosis: clinical practice guidelines of the Infectious Diseases Society of America. *Clin Infect Dis.* 2008;46:327–360.
112. Limper AH, Knox KS, Sarosi GA, et al. An official American Thoracic Society statement: treatment of fungal infections in adult pulmonary and critical care patients. *Am J Respir Crit Care Med.* 2011;183:96–128.
113. Xhaard A, Lanternier F, Porcher R, et al. Mucormycosis after allogeneic haematopoietic stem cell transplantation: a French multicentre cohort study (2003–2008). *Clin Microbiol Infect.* 2012;18:E396–E400.
114. Centers for Disease Control and Prevention. Increase in reported coccidioidomycosis—United States, 1998–2011. *Morbid Mortal Wkly Rep.* 2013;62:217–221.
115. Meersseman W, Lagrou K, Spriet I, et al. Significance of the isolation of *Candida* species from airway samples in critically ill patients: a prospective, autopsy study. *Intensive Care Med.* 2009;35: 1526–1531.
116. Haron E, Vartivarian S, Anaissie E, et al. Primary *Candida* pneumonia. Experience at a large cancer center and review of the literature. *Medicine (Baltimore).* 1993;72:137–142.
117. Harris B, Lowy FD, Stover DE, Arcasoy SM. Diagnostic bronchoscopy in solid-organ and hematopoietic stem cell transplantation. *Ann Am Thorac Soc.* 2013;10:39–49.
118. Vogel MN, Brodoefel H, Hierl T, et al. Differences and similarities of cytomegalovirus and pneumocystis pneumonia in HIV-negative immunocompromised patients thin section CT morphology in the early phase of the disease. *Br J Radiol.* 2007;80:516–523.
119. Jain P, Sandur S, Meli Y, et al. Role of flexible bronchoscopy in immunocompromised patients with lung infiltrates. *Chest.* 2004;125:712–722.
120. Brownback KR, Simpson SQ. Association of bronchoalveolar lavage yield with chest computed tomography findings and symptoms in immunocompromised patients. *Ann Thorac Med.* 2013;8:153–159.
121. UNAIDS. *Global Report: UNAIDS Report on the Global AIDS Epidemic 2013.* Geneva, Switzerland: UNAIDS: Geneva, Switzerland; 2013. Available at: http://www.unaids.org/en/media/unaids/contentassets/documents/epidemiology/2013/gr2013/unaids_global_report_2013_en.pdf. Accessed August 13, 2014.
122. Centers for Disease Control and Prevention. Monitoring selected national HIV prevention and care objectives by using HIV surveillance data—United States and 6 U.S. dependent areas—2010. *HIV Surveillance Supplemental Report.* 2012;17 (No. 3, part A).
123. Wallace JM, Hansen NI, Lavange L, et al. Respiratory disease trends in the pulmonary complications of HIV infection study cohort. *Am J Respir Crit Care Med.* 1997;155:72–80.
124. Crothers K, Huang L, Goulet JL, et al. HIV infection and risk for incident pulmonary diseases in the combination antiretroviral therapy era. *Am J Respir Crit Care Med.* 2011;183:388–395.
125. Benito N, Moreno A, Miro JM, Torres A. Pulmonary infections in HIV-infected patients: an update in the 21st century. *Eur Respir J.* 2012;39:730–745.
126. Rosen MJ. Pulmonary complications of HIV infection. *Respirology.* 2008;13:181–190.
127. Miller RF, Huang L, Walzer PD. *Pneumocystis* pneumonia associated with human immunodeficiency virus. *Clin Chest Med.* 2013;34:229–241.
128. Bozzette SA, Sattler FR, Chiu J, et al. A controlled trial of early adjunctive treatment with corticosteroids for *Pneumocystis carinii* pneumonia in the acquired immunodeficiency syndrome. *N Engl J Med.* 1990;323:1451–1457.
129. Oni T, Burke R, Tsekela R, et al. High prevalence of subclinical tuberculosis in HIV-1-infected persons without advanced immunodeficiency: implications for TB screening. *Thorax.* 2011;66:669–673.
130. Sterling TR, Pham PA, Chaisson RE. HIV infection-related tuberculosis: clinical manifestations and treatment. *Clin Infect Dis.* 2010;50(Suppl 3):S223–S230.
131. Black RE, Cousens S, Johnson HL, et al. Global, regional, and national causes of child mortality in 2008: a systematic analysis. *Lancet.* 2010;375:1969–1987.
132. O'Brien KL, Wolfson LJ, Watt JP, et al. Burden of disease caused by *Streptococcus pneumoniae* in children younger than 5 years: global estimates. *Lancet.* 2009;374:893–902.
133. Pavia M, Bianco A, Nobile CG, et al. Efficacy of pneumococcal vaccination in children younger than 24 months: a meta-analysis. *Pediatrics.* 2009;123:e1103–e1110.
134. Bradley JS, Byington CL, Shah SS, et al. The management of community-acquired pneumonia in infants and children older than 3 months of age: clinical practice guidelines by the Pediatric Infectious Diseases Society and the Infectious Diseases Society of America. *Clin Infect Dis.* 2011;53:e25–e76.
135. Jung JA, Kita H, Yawn BP, et al. Increased risk of serious pneumococcal disease in patients with atopic conditions other than asthma. *J Allergy Clin Immunol.* 2010;125:217–221.
136. Harris M, Clark J, Coote N, et al. British Thoracic Society guidelines for the management of community acquired pneumonia in children: update 2011. *Thorax.* 2011;66(Suppl 2):ii1–23.

137. Neuman MI, Monuteaux MC, Scully KJ, Bachur RG. Prediction of pneumonia in a pediatric emergency department. *Pediatrics.* 2011;128:246–253.
138. Mathews B, Shah S, Cleveland RH, et al. Clinical predictors of pneumonia among children with wheezing. *Pediatrics.* 2009;124:e29–e36.
139. Harris M, Clark J, Coote N, et al. British Thoracic Society guidelines for the management of community acquired pneumonia in childhood. *Thorax.* 2002;57(Suppl 1):i1–24.
140. Ambroggio L, Taylor JA, Tabb LP, et al. Comparative effectiveness of empiric beta-lactam monotherapy and beta-lactam-macrolide combination therapy in children hospitalized with community-acquired pneumonia. *J Pediatr.* 2012;161:1097–1103.
141. Casado RJ, de Mello MJ, de Aragao RC, et al. Incidence and risk factors for health care-associated pneumonia in a pediatric intensive care unit. *Crit Care Med.* 2011;39:1968–1973.
142. Srinivasan R, Asselin J, Gildengorin G, et al. A prospective study of ventilator-associated pneumonia in children. *Pediatrics.* 2009;123:1108–1115.

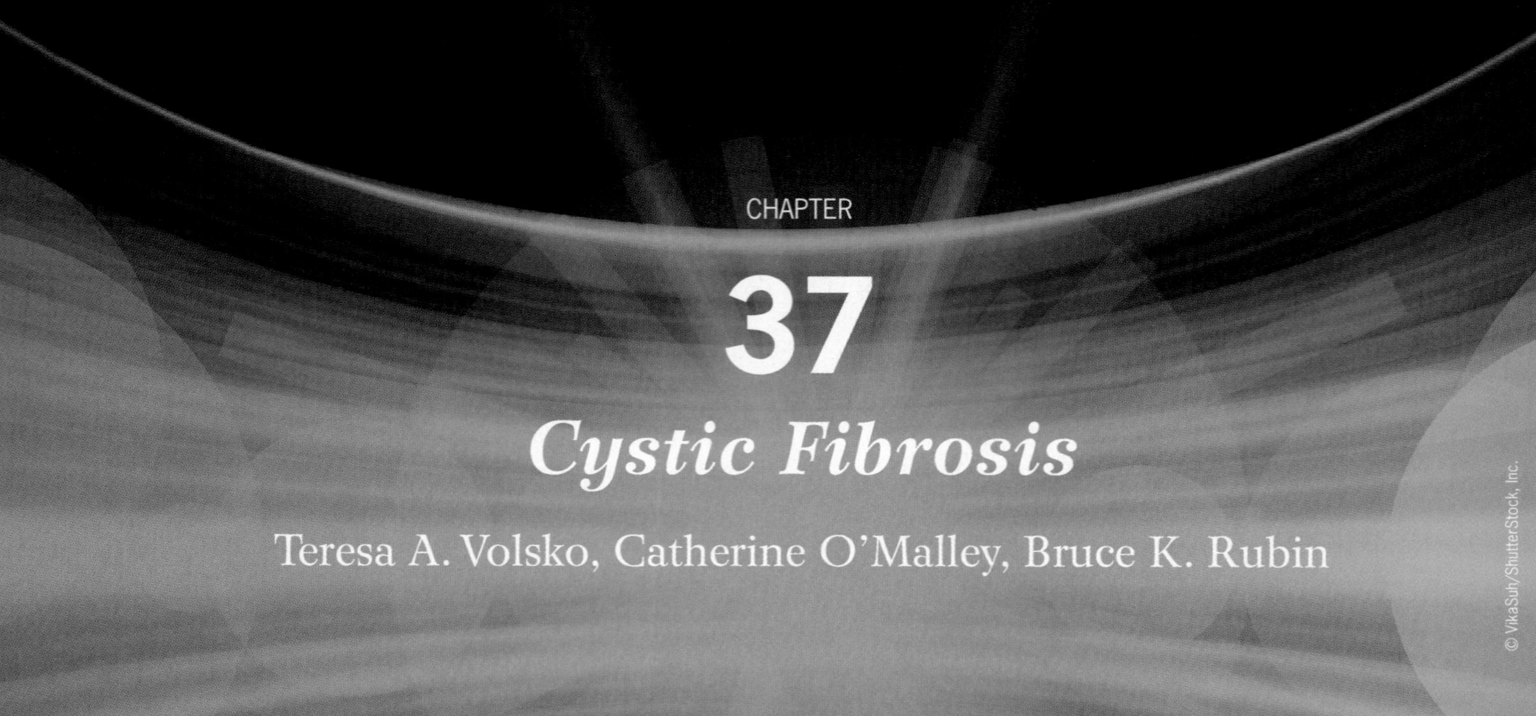

CHAPTER

37 Cystic Fibrosis

Teresa A. Volsko, Catherine O'Malley, Bruce K. Rubin

OUTLINE

History
Pathogenesis
Diagnosis
Extrapulmonary Manifestations
Respiratory Manifestations
Major Respiratory Complications
Standard Therapy of Lung Disease

OBJECTIVES

1. Describe the inheritance pattern of cystic fibrosis.
2. Describe the pathogenesis of cystic fibrosis.
3. List the diagnostic criteria for cystic fibrosis.
4. Describe the numerous extrapulmonary manifestations of cystic fibrosis.
5. Describe typical respiratory manifestations of cystic fibrosis.
6. Discuss the approach to common life-threatening respiratory complications of cystic fibrosis.
7. Describe the principles of preventive care for cystic fibrosis.
8. Outline an approach to the management of an acute exacerbation of cystic fibrosis lung disease.
9. Describe the role that lung transplantation plays in the management of cystic fibrosis.

KEY TERMS

bronchial artery embolization (BAE)
cepacia syndrome
cystic fibrosis (CF)
cystic fibrosis–related diabetes (CFRD)
cystic fibrosis transmembrane conductance regulator (CFTR)
distal intestinal obstruction syndrome (DIOS)
lung transplantation
meconium ileus
steatorrhea
sweat test

Introduction

Cystic fibrosis (CF) is an autosomal recessive genetic disorder, passed from parents to their children. Each parent must be a carrier of the gene defect if the children are to be affected. The disease does not affect parents who are carriers. Each child has a 25% chance of inheriting CF. Children who do not inherit the disease may be carriers of the altered gene or have a normal genetic pattern. This chapter addresses the care of a patient with CF.

History

Dorothy H. Andersen and Guido Fanconi first described CF as a distinct disease entity in the late 1930s independently. Fanconi described the connection among bronchiectasis, malabsorption, and pancreatic changes associated with CF.[1] Andersen described *cystic fibrosis of the pancreas* as a distinct disease entity in 1938.[2] Andersen conducted a pathology study, describing affected infants who presented with intestinal obstruction or malnutrition as a consequence of malabsorption.[3] In those days, the diagnosis was based on the patient's clinical presentation, and effective treatment was unavailable. Children with CF usually died in the first year of life. Postmortem studies revealed obstruction of pancreatic ducts and the gut with abnormally tenacious mucus, prompting the term *mucoviscidosis*.[3]

In the 1950s, di Sant'Agnese and colleagues investigated cases of severe dehydration in children with CF during a summer heat wave in New York City and recognized that excessive salt loss occurred through sweat.[4] This observation led to the development of the use of pilocarpine iontophoresis to stimulate the sweat glands and induce localized sweating in order to measure the concentration of salt in the sweat.[5] A salt concentration of 60 milliequivalents per liter (mEq/L) or higher is a positive test result for CF in children. The pilocarpine iontophoresis sweat test, described by Gibson and Cooke in 1959, remains a standard diagnostic test for CF. In 1989 the gene responsible for CF was discovered and cloned, and its protein product was named the **cystic fibrosis transmembrane conductance regulator (CFTR)**.[6]

Today CF is recognized as the most common life-shortening genetic disease in the white population. In North America one in 29 Caucasians carries a mutant CFTR allele, and one in 3300 live births is affected with CF. Other ethnic populations have lower mutation carrier rates, and thus lower incidences of CF disease. The Hispanic birth incidence is 1 in 9500; for Native Americans it is 1 in 11,200; African Americans, 1 in 15,300; and in the U.S. Asian population, 1 in 32,100 live births. Survival now commonly extends into adulthood, with a median life expectancy of 41 years (**Figure 37-1**).[7] Close to 28,000 patients with CF have been identified in the United States, and 49% are older than 18 years. This chapter describes the pathogenesis, diagnosis, and clinical manifestations of CF. Although CF is a multisystem disease, the management of acute and chronic respiratory complications is emphasized.

Pathogenesis

Genetics of Cystic Fibrosis

CF is a monogenetic classic Mendelian disorder that is inherited in an autosomal recessive pattern. Persons who carry a single mutated *CFTR* gene along with a normal CFTR allele are termed *carriers* and have few or no symptoms attributable to CF. Each offspring conceived from two CF carriers therefore has a one in four chance of being affected with CF, and a two in four chance of being a CF carrier.

The *CFTR* gene belongs to a family of membrane ATP-binding cassette (ABC) proteins that serve as molecular pumps. CFTR is a cAMP-regulated chloride channel in epithelial tissues. Since the discovery of the *CFTR* gene in 1989, more than 1800 individual mutations have been identified,[8] although the most common mutation (*F508del*) accounts for 66% of CF alleles reported worldwide, and thus about half of all persons with CF are homozygous for this mutation.[9] The exact prevalence of individual mutations also varies according to the ethnic group being studied, with the *F508del* mutation being less common among nonwhite populations.

Mutations in the *CFTR* gene have been categorized into five groups reflecting the mechanism for decreased or loss of CFTR function (**Table 37-1**). Class I mutations result in the loss of protein production and thus absence of full-length CFTR. Class II mutations result in abnormal protein processing between the cell nucleus and plasma membrane. This class of mutations includes the common *F508del* mutation, in which improper protein glycosylation and folding prevents normal transport to the apical cell membrane. Most of this abnormal protein is degraded in the endoplasmic reticulum. Class III mutations in the CFTR gene affect the regulation or activation of the CFTR chloride channel, although the channel itself successfully reaches the plasma membrane but does not open fully to chloride transport. These mutations tend to produce milder disease. Class IV mutations also reach the plasma membrane but affect the conductance of chloride through the channel pore. Class V *CFTR* mutations decrease the abundance of mature CFTR mRNA and protein levels and may include mutations in gene promoters or

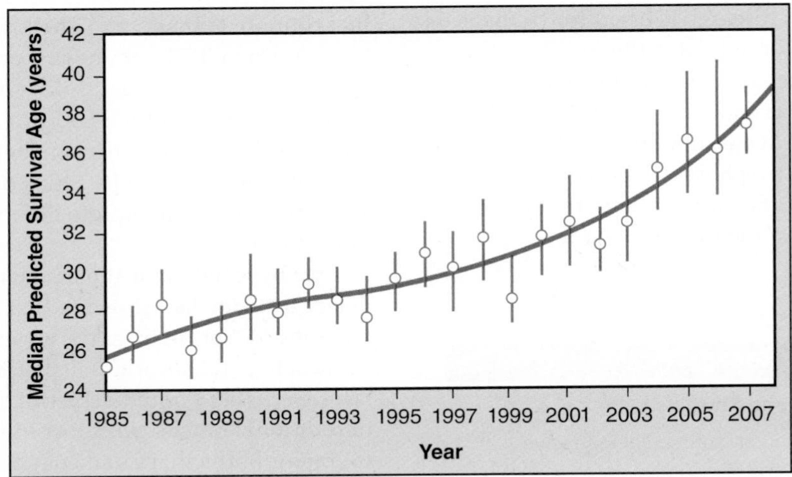

FIGURE 37-1 The median predicted survival age by life table analysis was 41 years for 2012. This represents the age to which half of the current cystic fibrosis (CF) registry population would be expected to survive, given the ages of the CF patients in the registry and the age distribution of the deaths in 2012. Ninety-five percent confidence bounds for the survival estimates are shown, indicating that for the 5-year band from 2008–2012 the median predicted survival was 37.8 years.

Reproduced from Patient Registry Annual Data Report for 2012. Bethesda, MD: Cystic Fibrosis Foundation; 2013.

TABLE 37-1
Consequences of *CFTR* Mutations by Class

Class	Problem	Examples	Features
I	No synthesis of mature protein	*G542X; 394delTT*	Mutations cause premature stop codons (e.g., frameshift, nonsense) or unstable mRNA.
II	Block in processing	*ΔF508; N1303K*	Mutations cause improper intracellular processing (folding, glycosylation), so protein may not reach plasma membrane.
III	Abnormal regulation	*G551D; G551S*	Protein reaches plasma membrane but is not activated properly; mutation may be mild or severe.
IV	Altered conductance	*R117H; R347P*	Ion conductance of the channel is altered. Partially functioning channel is often associated with pancreatic sufficiency.
V	Reduced synthesis	*3489+10kbC >7T*	Altered mRNA splicing sites result in reduced synthesis of normal protein; low levels of preserved synthesis often confer a milder phenotype.

regions that influence mRNA splicing. These mutations may permit the production of adequate CFTR levels to confer a less severe disease phenotype.[10]

Predicting an individual patient's clinical phenotype has been difficult based on the specific *CFTR* mutations present. Some genotype–phenotype correlation has been noted, principally among a group of mutations associated with pancreatic exocrine sufficiency, milder lung disease, and borderline or even normal sweat chloride values.[10,11] In addition, certain mutations have been found in men who present solely with infertility resulting from the congenital bilateral absence of the vas deferens (CBAVD), often without other symptoms of CF disease.[12] The manifestations of CF in an individual depend on other genetic factors (i.e., modifier genes) and environmental factors.

Current research in CF is investigating specific CFTR defects and determining ways to treat it. A successful outcome of this research is ivacaftor (Kalydeco), the first available CFTR modulator therapy drug that targets the underlying cause of CF. Kalydeco is an oral medication that was approved for use in 2012 for people with CF 6 years of age and older with the CFTR gene mutation *G551D*, which is a Class III mutation.[13] This medication is classified as a potentiator because it improves (*potentiates*) the function of the CFTR protein on the cell surface by allowing it to open to chloride transport.[13] Patients on this medication show marked improvement in lung function and weight gain, which are strong predictors of life expectancy in CF. Only 4% of people with CF have the *G551D* mutation.[14,15] Further research is studying other CFTR modulator therapies that may treat the other 96% of the CF population.

> **!** **Respiratory Recap**
>
> **Genetics of Cystic Fibrosis**
>
> - CF is inherited in an autosomal recessive pattern.
> - *CFTR* is the gene responsible for CF.
> - It is difficult to predict phenotype from *CFTR* mutation because of modifier genes and gene–environment interactions.

CFTR Functions and Host Defense

CFTR is a chloride channel expressed in the apical membrane of epithelial cells lining the lung, pancreas, gut, sweat duct, and reproductive tract (also kidney, liver, submucosal gland, etc). As its name implies, however, CFTR regulates several ion conductance pathways,[16] including the ENaC or epithelial sodium channels,[17] chloride channels other than CFTR,[18] potassium channels, and, importantly, bicarbonate transport.[19] The loss of a normally functioning CFTR can have a profound impact on epithelial ion transport. In the lung, the absence of CFTR causes increased sodium absorption from the airway lumen[20] and a diminished capacity to secrete chloride ions via CFTR. This combination alters the local milieu, and adequate defense against invading microbes is lost.

One hypothesis for the mechanism underlying this defect rests on data showing that increased isotonic volume absorption from the airway lumen (driven by sodium hyperabsorption) depletes the periciliary liquid layer. Periciliary liquid depletion results in disruption of rotational mucus transport in vitro and is predicted to impair both ciliary and cough clearance of airway secretions in vivo.[21] Reduced airway clearance and retention of mucus plaques will in turn cause airway obstruction and allow the establishment of bacterial infection. Mucociliary clearance is preserved in the nose of persons with CF, however. The middle ear and eustachian tube are also cleared by mucociliary clearance, but persons with CF do not usually develop chronic or persistent otitis media. Furthermore, persons with primary ciliary dyskinesia (PCD) have congenital absence of mucociliary transport but much milder lung disease than persons with CF. Despite absent ciliary function, cough clearance is not compromised in patients with PCD.[22]

A second hypothesis proposes that NaCl concentrations in airway surface liquid (ASL) are normally low (<50 mM NaCl) but are high in CF (>100 mM) because of the inability to absorb chloride through CFTR. Elevated NaCl concentrations in ASL may inhibit the antimicrobial effects of defensins, which are small, salt-sensitive peptides produced by airway epithelia.[23] Challenges to this hypothesis are the scarcity of defensins in ASL relative to other salt-insensitive antimicrobial molecules (e.g., lactoferrin, lysozyme)[24] and the absence of a physiologic mechanism for the generation of hypotonic fluids across the water-permeable airway epithelium.

Because CFTR expression in the lung is greatest within submucosal glands lining proximal conducting airways,[25] perhaps an alteration in glandular secretion resulting from absent CFTR is a cause of altered airway defense in CF. Indeed, CFTR is involved in generating airway surface liquid via submucosal glands in proximal airways.[26] A third hypothesis relating CFTR function and host defenses therefore emphasizes that deficient secretion of fluid containing sodium chloride or sodium bicarbonate from submucosal glands or serous cells lining small airways may lead to a volume-depleted ASL layer, an ASL layer with an altered composition, or both.

Other hypotheses relate to the pathogenesis of CF lung disease. It has been proposed that because there is less intact mucin (mucus) in the CF airway, this may leave the airway more vulnerable to chronic bacterial infection and to the development of bacterial biofilms by organisms in the airway.[27] In addition to hypotheses describing differences in airway mucins,[28] others relate to the CF immune response.[29] These do not tightly link CFTR function with the resulting disease process and in some cases rest on observations that may be secondary to infection. Most therapies focus on airway clearance and fighting chronic bacterial infection and on modulating the hyperimmune and inflammatory response in the airway.

Diagnosis

The diagnosis of CF is based on the combination of one or more typical phenotypic features and evidence of CFTR malfunction (**Box 37-1**).[30] Knowledge of the broad range of clinical features that may be present in CF and appropriate access to specialized diagnostic testing are essential for an accurate diagnosis. Among the clinical features assessed are the presence of obstructive lung disease leading to bronchiectasis and infection with typical pathogens, chronic sinus disease with or without nasal polyposis, exocrine pancreatic insufficiency or recurrent pancreatitis, intestinal obstruction either at birth (meconium ileus) or later in life (distal intestinal obstruction syndrome, formerly called meconium ileus equivalent), rectal prolapse, chronic liver disease, nutritional deficiencies including protein/caloric malnutrition and complications of fat-soluble vitamin deficiency, electrolyte abnormalities such as acute salt depletion or chronic metabolic alkalosis, absence of the vas deferens resulting in obstructive azoospermia in males, and digital clubbing. A family history of CF should also be sought in support of a clinical CF diagnosis.

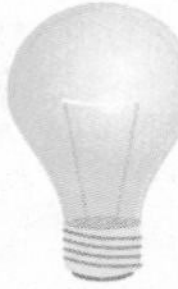

STOP AND THINK

A patient has a sweat chloride of 80 mmol/L. What would you include in the differential diagnosis?

Newborn screening (NBS) now includes screening for CF in every state in the United States. This test is called the IRT (immunoreactive trypsinogen), which analyzes a drop of blood taken from the baby's heel within the first few days of life.[31] Newborn screening for CF is not standardized in that not all states use IRT. Some directly test for common genetic abnormalities. Other states will use IRT screening and, if positive, go directly to genetic screening. If the IRT level is high, then the test is repeated. If it remains high, then sweat testing is needed to confirm a diagnosis of CF. Early diagnosis of CF through newborn screening has been adopted throughout the United States and Canada as well as Europe and Australia. Research demonstrates that early diagnosis and treatment preserves the rate of decline in lung function; enhances growth, nutritional status, and survival with less intensive therapy; and reduces cost of care.[32] The IRT method of newborn screening has lead to the identification of infants with milder forms of CFTR dysfunction. In these infants there is an elevated IRT on NBS, but the diagnostic criteria for CF is not met. The United States CF Foundation uses the term *cystic fibrosis transmembrane conductance regulator related metabolic syndrome (CRMS)* to describe the infants who have evidence of CFTR dysfunction but do not meet the diagnostic criteria for CF.[33] In a recent study by Ren and colleagues, CRMS patients were more likely to be pancreatic sufficient as assessed by fecal elastase measurement and had a normal weight for age percentile at birth. CRMS patients presented with milder clinical courses than CF infants and were less likely to receive oral antibiotics and be hospitalized for pulmonary symptoms.[34] The CF Foundation

BOX 37-1

Diagnostic Criteria for Cystic Fibrosis

Phenotypic Feature

Chronic sinopulmonary disease

- Persistent infection with typical cystic fibrosis pathogens (e.g., *Staphylococcus aureus, Pseudomonas aeruginosa, Burkholderia cepacia complex,* atypical *Mycobacteria*)
- Chronic cough, especially with sputum expectoration
- Persistent chest radiographic abnormality (e.g., bronchiectasis, hyperinflation, atelectasis)
- Airway obstruction pattern on pulmonary function testing
- Nasal polyps and chronic sinus (but not middle ear) involvement
- Digital clubbing

Gastrointestinal or nutritional abnormality

- *Intestinal*: meconium ileus, rectal prolapse, distal intestinal obstruction syndrome
- *Pancreatic*: pancreatic insufficiency, recurrent pancreatitis (in older children and adults)
- *Hepatic*: focal biliary cirrhosis
- *Nutritional*: malnutrition, hypoproteinemia, fat-soluble vitamin deficiency

Salt loss syndrome

- Acute salt depletion, especially with water loss, such as during exercise in heat
- Chronic metabolic alkalosis

Male urogenital abnormality

- Obstructive azoospermia resulting from congenital bilateral absence of the vas deferens (CBAVD)

CFTR Abnormality

Sweat chloride test

- Result >60 mmol/L on two occasions (minimum 75 mg of sweat collected during 30 minutes) without other causes for high sweat chloride (e.g., anorexia nervosa, atopic dermatitis)

CFTR mutational analysis

- Two identified mutant CFTR alleles

Nasal potential difference (PD) testing

- Higher basal PD
- Greater amiloride-sensitive PD
- Absent or minimal change in PD after isoproterenol in chloride-free perfusion solution

The combination of one or more phenotypic abnormalities (or CF in a sibling, or a positive newborn screening test) with evidence of a CFTR abnormality constitutes a CF diagnosis. CFTR, cystic fibrosis transmembrane conductance regulator.

addressed the need for monitoring and medical management guidelines for CRMS to assist clinicians with the most appropriate management based on the evidence in the literature, which include recommendations for well-baby and CF clinic visits as well as parental education on the symptoms of exacerbations and the importance of adhering to immunization guidelines.[33]

Evidence of CFTR dysfunction is typically provided by **sweat testing** with a chloride concentration of more than 60 mmol/L on two or more occasions in children over 6 months of age.[35] Values greater than 40 mmol/L are considered borderline and are more suggestive of CF in infants. Values between 60 and 80 mmol/L can also be seen in individuals with diseases other than CF. Laboratory errors are common with this technique, and even a small amount of water vapor loss from the collected sweat can concentrate ions and cause a false-positive test result. All positive and borderline tests thus should be repeated at a Cystic Fibrosis Foundation–accredited center.

A complementary approach to sweat testing is the use of CFTR mutational analysis to identify CF alleles. The identification of two disease-causing *CFTR*

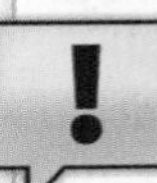

Respiratory Recap

Diagnosis of Cystic Fibrosis

- Abnormal newborn screening result
- CMRS vs. CF
- Clinical features consistent with the disease
- Family history
- Sweat testing
- Mutational analysis to identify CF alleles
- Nasal epithelial potential difference measurements in response to specific pharmacologic agents

mutations is highly specific for the diagnosis of CF, but this approach lacks sensitivity. *CFTR* mutational analysis usually screens for 32 to 70 common mutations and detects up to 95% of CF alleles. The use of mutation panels customized for a given ethnic group or clinical situation (e.g., African American, pancreatic sufficient) may increase the likelihood of the identification of CF alleles. No commercially available screening panel can rule out the diagnosis of CF, however, because no test for all of the known mutations capable of causing CF currently exists. Also, many mutations may have no functional consequences.

When sweat testing and *CFTR* mutational analysis are inconclusive, the measurement of nasal epithelial potential difference (PD) in response to various pharmacologic agents can be useful.[36] This test is only available at a few specialized research centers, however.

Extrapulmonary Manifestations

Upper Respiratory Tract

Nearly all patients with CF have radiographic opacification of the paranasal sinuses,[37] and a large fraction report symptoms attributable to either nasal obstruction or chronic sinusitis.[38] Symptomatic nasal polyps are particularly common toward the end of the first and during the second decade of life and occur in about 20% to 48% of all patients with CF.[39] This variation in prevalence may be attributed to differences in diagnostic method used. Manifestations include severe nasal airflow obstruction, rhinorrhea, and occasionally, widening of the bridge of the nose.

Severity of lung disease is reportedly less among children with CF presenting with recurrent nasal polyps and has been attributed to a proliferative airway repair mechanism.[40] Despite the universal presence of radiographic abnormalities, symptoms attributable to sinusitis occur in fewer than 10% of children[41] and approximately 24% of adults.[42] The kind of bacteria isolated in CF sinus disease varies with age and may be similar to those cultured from the lower respiratory tract. *Staphylococcus aureus* and *Haemophilus influenzae* are commonly found in younger children, whereas *Pseudomonas aeruginosa* appears more frequently at a later age. Unfortunately, recurrence of polyps and sinus symptoms is extremely common after surgical interventions. Patients thus must be carefully selected when a surgical intervention for nasal or sinus disease is considered.

Exocrine and Endocrine Pancreas

Exocrine pancreatic insufficiency is present from birth in most patients with CF.[43] Enzyme deficiency results in fat and protein maldigestion, producing **steatorrhea**. Uncorrected malabsorption results in failure to gain weight and ultimately a failure of linear growth. Exocrine pancreatic insufficiency and malnutrition are managed with oral pancreatic enzyme supplementation and dietary supplements. Impaired absorption of fat-soluble vitamins (A, D, E, and K) occasionally produces symptoms of vitamin deficiency, which can be prevented with adequate supplementation. Symptoms of pancreatitis are encountered in fewer than 1% of identified adolescent and adult CF patients and are limited to those who have retained some exocrine pancreatic function.[44] Recurrent non-ethanol-induced pancreatitis has been associated with mutations in *CFTR*, however, and may be the presenting symptom in adults with CF.[45]

Although the exocrine pancreas is frequently affected from birth, the gradual loss of insulin production from the endocrine pancreas occurs slowly over time in patients with CF. In the United States, the overall incidence of **cystic fibrosis–related diabetes (CFRD)** or glucose intolerance is reported to be 15% to 30% of adult patients with CF as defined by requiring chronic insulin therapy.[46] Because of the insidious onset of CFRD, screening is suggested for individuals aged 14 years and older. Measurements of 2-hour plasma glucose values obtained during an oral glucose tolerance test are a more reliable screening tool than random plasma glucose or glycosylated hemoglobin A1c measurement, performed alone or in combination.[47] Manifestations of CFRD may include failure to gain or maintain weight despite nutritional intervention, poor growth, or an unexplained chronic decline in pulmonary function.[48]

Insulin is the preferred hypoglycemic agent in CFRD, because limited islet cell reserve exists in most

AGE-SPECIFIC ANGLE

Exocrine pancreatic insufficiency is present from birth in most patients with CF. About 18% of newborns with CF have meconium ileus; these babies uniformly have pancreatic insufficiency.

cases. Other facets of CFRD management, however, differ substantially from that of either type 1 or 2 diabetes mellitus. Because all CF patients require a high-energy intake and generally malabsorb fat even with appropriate pancreatic enzyme supplementation, a high-calorie diet consisting of 40% fat is recommended. Caloric restriction never should be used to aid management of blood glucose in CF except in the rare pancreatic-sufficient and obese patent with CF with chronic type 2 diabetes. Insulin dosage is instead matched to the calorie and carbohydrate intake, and the presence of intercurrent infections is factored in as needed.[49] Patients also are at risk for the usual microvascular complications of diabetes;[46] therefore, similar glucose targets are used as with type 1 and type 2 diabetes mellitus. Equally important, however, is the maintenance of optimal nutrition and growth, the avoidance of severe hypoglycemia, and the need to fit this additional treatment burden within the patient's CF regimen.

Gastrointestinal Tract

Meconium ileus occurs in about 18% of newborns with CF, and true meconium ileus (as opposed to the meconium plugs commonly seen in very premature infants) is nearly diagnostic for CF.[50] A barium enema usually demonstrates a small colon, and a site of ileal obstruction may be identified. Intestinal obstruction can also be diagnosed by fetal ultrasound toward the end of pregnancy.

Later in life, intestinal obstruction may be caused by the **distal intestinal obstruction syndrome (DIOS)**, formerly referred to as "meconium ileus equivalent." This occurs in approximately 20% of patients and usually presents with constipation, right lower quadrant abdominal pain, anorexia, nausea, vomiting, and sometimes fever.[48] As with meconium ileus, obstruction usually occurs in the terminal ileum and is associated with copious, incompletely digested intestinal contents. DIOS has been associated with poor adherence to taking pancreatic enzyme therapy and with dietary indiscretions.

Other causes of abdominal pain include simple constipation, intussusception, intestinal adhesions from previous abdominal surgery (including for meconium ileus), or chronic appendicitis that has been partially suppressed by antibiotic therapy. Rectal prolapse occurs in up to 20% of children but is an infrequent event for adults with CF.[51] Excessive pancreatic enzyme dosages have been associated with the occurrence of fibrosing colonopathy, especially in those patients taking 6000 units or more of lipase per kilogram per meal.[52] Pancreatic enzyme dosages of 2500 units or less of lipase per kilogram per meal are recommended to avoid this complication. Gastroesophageal reflux disease is common and should be recognized and treated because this process may exacerbate lung disease, just as lung disease and chronic cough can worsen gastroesophageal reflux.[53]

> **Respiratory Recap**
>
> **Extrapulmonary Manifestations of Cystic Fibrosis**
>
> - Upper airway
> - Exocrine and endocrine pancreas
> - Gastrointestinal tract
> - Hepatobiliary system
> - Reproductive tract
> - Sweat glands

Hepatobiliary System

Focal biliary cirrhosis is characteristic of CF but produces symptoms in fewer than 5% of CF patients and is the cause of death in about 2%.[54] Unlike many complications of CF, hepatic disease has a peak incidence during adolescence and a decreased prevalence in patients older than 20 years.[55] Hepatic abnormalities can present as hepatosplenomegaly or as a persistent elevation of hepatic enzymes (particularly alkaline phosphatase). Rarely, patients may present with esophageal varices and hemorrhage resulting from portal hypertension. Fatty liver is also common and may improve with adequate nutrition. Dysfunctional gallbladders or gallstones are present in 10% to 30% of patients.[56]

Reproductive Tract

More than 98% of male patients with CF have azoospermia resulting from obstruction of the vas deferens.[57] In fact, absence of a palpable vas deferens is a useful clue to the diagnosis of CF during the evaluation of a male patient with otherwise unexplained lung disease or other manifestation of CF. Semen analysis may be required to identify the very rare man with CF who is fertile. The volume of ejaculate is usually one-third to one-half of normal, void of spermatozoa, and has a number of chemical abnormalities of seminal fluid that reflect the absence of secretions from the seminal vesicles.[58] Because spermatozoa do develop in the testis of patients with CF, despite being absent in the ejaculate, epididymal sperm microaspiration coupled with intracytoplasmic oocyte injection may allow successful conception.[57]

Although male infertility is nearly universal, female infertility is only about 20%.[57] Some women with CF are anovulatory because of chronic lung disease and malnutrition. In addition, mucus in the cervical os has abnormal electrolyte concentration and can present an obstacle to conception by impeding normal sperm migration.[57] Nevertheless, hundreds of pregnancies in women with CF have been reported. A longitudinal

AGE-SPECIFIC ANGLE

Young children with CF are most at risk for episodes of salt loss, especially in hot, arid climates and in the setting of concomitant salt/volume loss.

study of 325 pregnant women with CF reported 258 live births (79%) and 67 therapeutic abortions. Pregnancy in women with CF did not have a negative effect on pulmonary status or mortality over 2 years.[57] It is important for women with CF to consider their own health and expected life span in the context of family planning.

Sweat Glands

Sweat chloride is elevated in most CF patients because of reduced NaCl reabsorption in the sweat duct.[58] This abnormality forms the basis for the diagnostic sweat chloride test and may predispose patients to salt depletion. Young children are most at risk for episodes of salt loss, especially in hot, arid climates and in the setting of concomitant salt/volume loss resulting from vomiting, diarrhea, or exercise. These children usually present with lethargy, anorexia, and hypochloremic alkalosis. Presentation with hypochloremic alkalosis is rare in older children and adults.[58] Salt restriction is never indicated in CF, and increased salt intake should be encouraged when environmental or clinical circumstances place a patient at increased risk for salt depletion.

Respiratory Manifestations

Symptoms

Newborns with CF appear to have normal lung function, although studies in the CF pig suggest that there may be abnormal intrauterine airway development. Clinical symptoms or evidence of increased airways resistance and gas trapping often develop very early in life, although they may not be apparent until adulthood in a minority of patients. Respiratory symptoms typically include a cough that becomes persistent and productive of purulent sputum over time. Periods of clinical stability are inevitably interrupted by typical exacerbations, characterized by increased cough, sputum, fatigue, anorexia, weight loss, and decreased lung function. These exacerbations require more intensive therapy, with the goal of alleviating symptoms and restoring lost lung function through the use of antibiotics and airway clearance maneuvers. Over time exacerbations become more frequent, respond less well to interventions, and eventually result in respiratory failure.

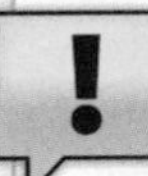

Respiratory Recap

Respiratory Manifestations of Cystic Fibrosis

- Clinical symptoms: cough, sputum, fatigue, anorexia, and weight loss are characteristic of an exacerbation of lung disease
- Chest radiograph: hyperinflation, progressing to bronchiectasis that is more prominent in the upper lobes
- Pulmonary function: airflow obstruction
- Respiratory microbiology: airways become persistently infected with gram-negative pathogens such as *P aeruginosa* and resistant *S aureus*

Chest Radiography

Chest radiographs in CF often are normal early in the course of disease. Hyperinflation may be the first radiographic finding in children, followed by increased interstitial markings. These increased interstitial markings progress to the typical findings of cystic bronchiectasis, which is usually most pronounced in the upper lobes. The right upper lobe is more frequently and severely affected than the left for unclear reasons. Despite high densities of bacteria in airways, findings of an alveolar filling process typical of bacterial pneumonia are not generally seen even during periods of acute illness. Segmental or subsegmental atelectasis and lobar collapse are common radiographic findings related to airway obstruction and retained secretions. Although the chest radiograph demonstrates the chronic progression of lung destruction and is useful for the detection of important complications such as lobar collapse and pneumothorax, there can be little correlation between the radiograph and acute clinical changes later in the course of disease.

High-resolution computed tomography (CT) scans of the chest may be useful to detect bronchiectasis and other early pathologic changes that are not visible on routine chest radiographs, especially during the evaluation of a patient with chronic cough and sputum production who is not otherwise known to have bronchiectasis.[59] Chest CT also may be useful in the CF patient with persistent atypical or nontuberculous

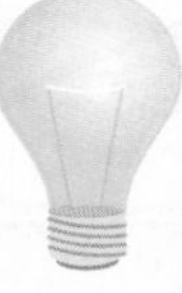

STOP AND THINK

A patient presents to the CF clinic for a routine evaluation. She has experienced increased dyspnea, cough, and sputum production with a decreased appetite over the past 5 days. What diagnostic testing would you recommend?

mycobacteria (NTM) infection, because the presence of multiple, small parenchymal nodules (so-called tree-in-bud nodules) predominating in the middle and lower lobes and patchy airspace disease are evidence of true NTM infection.[60]

Pulmonary Function

Pulmonary function testing is a reliable method used to evaluate the severity of CF lung disease and is an objective means to determine when a patient's clinical status has deteriorated and requires more intensive therapy. The first abnormality detected is obstruction of small airways, as indicated by reduced flow at low lung volumes (e.g., $FEF_{25-75\%}$) and gas trapping with an increase in the ratio of residual volume to total lung capacity (RV/TLC).[61] Later in the course of disease, pulmonary function tests demonstrate progressive reduction in FEV_1, followed by decreased functional vital capacity (FVC). The FEV_1 is the accepted indicator of disability and is somewhat predictive of length of survival.[62] An FEV_1 of about 30% of predicted often is used as an indication to initiate lung transplant evaluation, although other factors also should be considered.[63]

Well before spirometric abnormalities appear, bronchiectatic changes and airways obstruction may be evident on CT scans although chest X-rays may appear normal in young children. Newer tests of gas trapping, such as the lung clearance index (LCI), are more sensitive in the early stages of CF and are easier for younger patients to perform.[64] LCI is measured by performing an inert gas washout using a low concentration of an inert gas. In the future this technique may become a standard means for evaluating the severity of early CF lung disease.

As airway obstruction worsens, hypoxemia develops due to ventilation-perfusion mismatching. Even when oxygenation is adequate at rest, the clinician should be aware that hypoxemia may occur during sleep or with exercise in the setting of moderate-to-severe lung disease and should screen for it with exercise and sleep oximetry recordings.[65] Although significant hypoxemia tends to occur in patients with more advanced lung disease, pulmonary function test results can be a poor predictor of the need for oxygen therapy.[64] Supplemental oxygen may improve exercise performance in patients found to desaturate during exercise[66] and is generally effective in delaying the progression of pulmonary hypertension and cor pulmonale.[67]

Severe airway disease causes carbon dioxide retention due to an increased dead space to tidal volume ratio, which in turn may worsen hypoxemia. Carbon dioxide retention usually does not occur until severe airway obstruction is present. Along with resting hypoxemia, it is a predictor of end-stage lung disease and decreased survival.[68]

Respiratory Microbiology

The respiratory tract of newborns often becomes infected with typical CF pathogens early in life.[69] Once chronic infection is established, it is rarely eradicated and consists of characteristic age-related bacteria (**Figure 37-2**). *Staphylococcus aureus* and

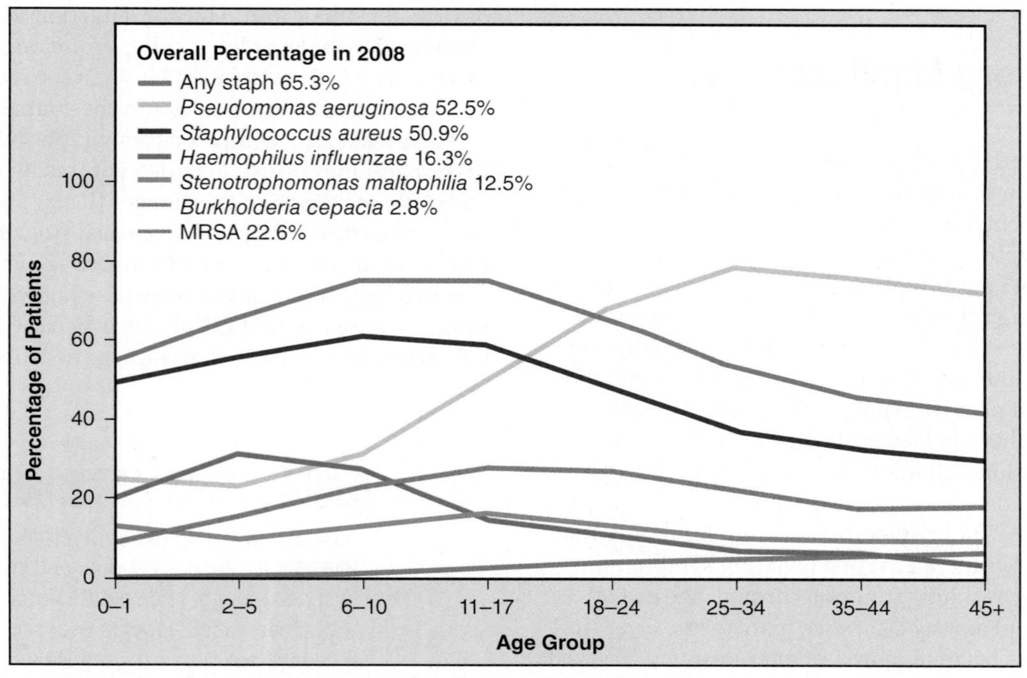

FIGURE 37-2 The prevalence of common bacterial organisms in different age groups.

Reproduced from Patient Registry Annual Data Report for 2012. Bethesda, MD: Cystic Fibrosis Foundation; 2013.

AGE-SPECIFIC ANGLE

The respiratory tract of a child with CF often becomes infected with bacteria early in life.

Haemophilus influenzae are often the first organisms detected, although *H influenzae* rarely persists beyond childhood.[70] *S aureus* may not persist after its initial isolation during childhood or may be isolated for the first time during the adult years. The prevalence of *S aureus* is nearly 60% in children less than 2 years of age peaks at approximately 80% in children aged 6 to 10 years, and then gradually decreases after the age of 17. *S aureus* resistant to available β-lactam antibiotics is referred to as multiply or methicillin-resistant *S aureus* (MRSA). MRSA strains are becoming increasingly more prevalent in persons with CF. In 2002, the mean MRSA infection rate at CF centers was reported to be 22.6%, an increase from 7% in 2001, and in 2012, the overall prevalence of MRSA was 26.5%.[7] Infection with MRSA is associated with more rapid decline in pulmonary function, more frequent exacerbations than infection with *Pseudomonas*,[71] and decreased survival.[72]

For unclear reasons, the airways of CF patients have a propensity to become persistently infected with otherwise uncommon gram-negative pathogens. These form bacterial biofilms in the airway, making eradication particularly difficult. Among these, *Pseudomonas aeruginosa* is the most common and clinically significant, with the prevalence ranging from approximately 25% during the first year of life to nearly 80% in adulthood[7] and overall prevalence is 49.6%. With the progression of lung disease, *P aeruginosa* is often the only organism recovered from sputum and may be present in several types of colonies, often with different antibiotic sensitivity patterns. The recovery of *P aeruginosa*, particularly the mucoid and biofilm form, from the lower respiratory tract of a child or young adult with chronic lung symptoms is highly suggestive of CF. Infection with *P aeruginosa* is a predictor of worse lung function and survival,[73] making avoidance of initial infection desirable. In Denmark, for example, CF clinics segregate infected patients from those who have never grown *P aeruginosa* in sputum cultures.[74] Along similar lines of reasoning, the feasibility and efficacy of the eradication of *Pseudomonas* on its initial isolation is being investigated. The Early *Pseudomonas* Infection Control (EPIC) large multicenter trials, for example, are currently under way to examine treatment strategies for early *Pseudomonas* infections in the airways of young children with CF.[75]

Burkholderia cepacia complex is highly transmissible among patients with CF and is difficult to treat because it is often resistant to antimicrobial drugs. *B cepacia* complex currently consists of 17 distinct species, with the overall prevalence of *B cepacia* complex in the United States being 2.6%.[7,76] The two most common species in patients with CF are *B cenocepacia* and *B multivorans*, accounting for approximately 45% and 40% of infections, respectively.[75] A subset of patients will manifest the **cepacia syndrome**,[77] a rapid clinical decline with fever and sepsis after initial infection, although the precise pathogen and host factors that trigger this dramatic and often fatal decompensation are unknown. It may be that the *B cenocepacia* strain is more virulent and transmissible than the other strains.[78] Because strong evidence exists that person-to-person spread of *B cepacia* complex occurs, particularly with highly transmissible strains expressing the cable pilus,[79] stringent infection control measures are now advocated wherever CF care is provided.[80] Several infection prevention and control measures, such as segregating infected patients, closing CF summer camps, a strong emphasis on hand hygiene, and contact isolation, have been successful at decreasing the transmission of this pathogen.[81]

Other gram-negative rods that may cause lung infection in CF include emerging pathogens, such as *Achromobacter xylosoxidans* and *Stenotrophomonas maltophilia*.[68] The prevalence of these bacterial species in patients in CF centers in the United States is 6.4% for *A xylosoxidans* and 13.4% for *S maltophilia*. The impact these infections have on the progression of disease in CF is unclear. There is little evidence of cross infection, and the source of infection may be the environment.[82] Because these organisms are often multidrug resistant, infection prevention and control measures are usually used.

Fungi and molds are frequently cultured from the respiratory secretions of CF patients. Invasive aspergillosis has only rarely been reported in CF, but allergic bronchopulmonary aspergillosis (ABPA) develops in 2% to 11% of CF patients.[83] The prevalence of ABPA is tracked by the CF Foundation's patient registry. Data gathered from 25,651 patients in the 2012 registry report found 4.7% had complications of ABPA.[7] Other fungi may colonize the airways and evoke similar allergic responses. The diagnosis of ABPA is based on the presence of clinical features such as new infiltrates, wheezing, increased cough, expectoration of brown plugs, or an unexplained deterioration in lung function. The combination of these clinical findings plus evidence for immunologic sensitivity to *Aspergillus* or other fungi, including elevated titers of *Aspergillus* precipitating antibodies and high total IgE levels above 500 IU, should prompt consideration of this diagnosis. Therapy includes systemic corticosteroids and antifungal medications.

Isolation of nontuberculous mycobacteria from appropriately processed CF sputum is relatively common and may occur in as many as 20% of adult CF patients.[84] Preliminary data from a multicenter study suggest an overall prevalence of about 13%, with *Mycobacterium avium* complex being most common; however, there is a significant prevalence of both

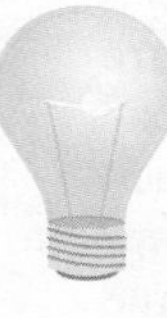

STOP AND THINK

Five hospitalized CF patients are ordered to receive HFCWC four times per day, but the facility only has three HFCWC units. What would you do to prevent the risk of cross contamination?

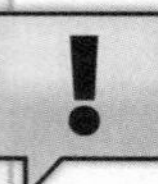

Respiratory Recap

Major Complications of Cystic Fibrosis

- Hemoptysis
- Pneumothorax
- Respiratory failure

M abscessus and *M fortuitum*. *M abscessus* is thought to be more virulent and to cause more severe and invasive disease.[85,86] The Cystic Fibrosis Foundation Registry reports an overall prevalence rate of 11.8% for nontuberculous mycobacteria.[7] Patients with high mycobacterial burdens and symptoms refractory to treatment of typical bacteria may benefit from antimycobacterial therapy.

Infection Control Recommendations

The sources of pathogens in CF include nature, contaminated objects, healthcare facilities, and respiratory care equipment, and there is strong epidemiologic evidence suggesting that people with CF can transmit pathogens to others with CF. Infection control practices have been successful in preventing transmission and include hand hygiene, respiratory hygiene, care of respiratory equipment, and keeping patients with CF apart from each other. In addition to standard precautions and transmission-based precautions, contact precautions are recommended for the care of all patients with CF because they can potentially harbor pathogens in their respiratory secretions.

Major Respiratory Complications

Hemoptysis, pneumothorax, and respiratory failure are major pulmonary complications that tend to occur in association with more severe lung disease. In the adult CF population, major hemoptysis and pneumothorax each occurs in about 1% of patients annually. Most patients who suffer massive hemoptysis or pneumothorax can be treated successfully. Respiratory failure, as the result of progressive airway obstruction and destruction, is the cause of death in 94% of CF patients. Although improved therapies have delayed the development of respiratory failure, at this time respiratory failure can only be treated by **lung transplantation**.

Hemoptysis

Hemoptysis in CF may range from minor blood streaking of the sputum, requiring little intervention, to massive bleeding (more than 240 mL in 24 hours). Minor hemoptysis is common and usually self-limited, although it may indicate an exacerbation of lung disease. Massive hemoptysis in CF almost invariably comes from the bronchial artery circulation, which is at systemic arterial pressure. The new occurrence of any amount of bleeding may signal the presence of an increased infectious or inflammatory burden and the need for intensified treatment. The approach to a minor amount of hemoptysis therefore is to determine whether the patient requires treatment with antibiotics and whether medications (e.g., NSAIDs, aspirin, penicillin) or vitamin K deficiency may be contributing to the new onset of bleeding.

Hemoptysis greater than 240 mL in 24 hours occurs in approximately 5% of patients[87] and may lead to airway obstruction and asphyxiation. Hypotension, anemia, and inflammation also may result from massive hemoptysis. Less voluminous hemoptysis that persists for several days (e.g., 100 mL/day for 3 days) also should be considered a major bleeding event, because it may herald massive bleeding. In addition to the correction of any hemostatic defects that are present, these patients should be hospitalized and treated with antibiotics based on recent sputum culture results. Cough suppression and bed rest may be used during the acute presentation to lessen the likelihood of further bleeding but should not be continued for prolonged periods in patients with advanced lung disease who are likely to suffer from inadequate airway clearance.

When bleeding is rapid, positioning the patient with the bleeding lung in a dependent position may help prevent soiling of the nonbleeding lung. Endotracheal intubation may be required if the patient is unable to maintain a patent airway. A large orotracheal tube, which can be advanced into the main bronchus serving the nonbleeding lung, is preferable to double-lumen tubes because the small lumens of these latter devices limit airway suctioning. Attempts to localize the site of bleeding with chest radiography, CT scanning, and bronchoscopy may help direct invasive therapies aimed at the control of bleeding but often are not diagnostic and may delay therapy.

With massive bleeding, **bronchial artery embolization (BAE)** is the therapy of choice and is usually directed at tortuous and hypertrophied bronchial arteries.[88] Nonbronchial systemic collateral vessels are also frequently involved, especially in cases of recurrent hemoptysis after BAE.[89] The use of nonionic contrast material and of embolizing particles large enough to prevent distal tissue ischemia and the avoidance of sclerosant agents have made BAE relatively safe and successful in experienced hands. Rebleeding after BAE is not uncommon and may require further attempts at BAE to achieve a successful outcome.[90] Studies have demonstrated a higher risk for rate of decline in lung function, need for lung transplantation, and death among adults with CF treated with BAE for hemoptysis.[91] Surgical resection is occasionally required for bleeding refractory to repeated attempts at BAE in patients with adequate pulmonary reserve.

Pneumothorax

Subpleural air cysts are probably responsible for the increased incidence of spontaneous pneumothorax in CF. The incidence of pneumothorax is approximately 1% per year overall, but it increases with age. Pneumothorax occurs in 16% to 20% of adult patients.[89] Most patients complain of a sudden increase in dyspnea or chest discomfort, although others are asymptomatic. The presence of a newly detected pneumothorax usually mandates hospitalization, whether or not chest tube insertion is planned at the outset. Asymptomatic pneumothoraces that occupy less than 20% of the hemithorax may be observed with clinical monitoring to assess progression.

Larger pneumothoraces leading to symptoms should be treated with small tube thoracostomy. Chest tubes may be removed once the pneumothorax has resolved and the air leak stopped. Additional tubes may be required when significant air collections persist after the initial tube placement. Chest tubes to evacuate air should generally be placed to water-seal rather than to suction because the negative pressure may inhibit the air leak from sealing. Chest tubes used to evacuate air are usually smaller than those needed to drain a parapneumonic effusion. Chest tubes should be removed as soon as practical as discomfort from the tube can impair effective coughing and airway clearance.

Further interventions may be necessary when an air leak results in recurrent or persistent pneumothorax. Talc pleurodesis has been used to cause an inflammatory reaction that leads to obliteration of the pleural space. Although in the past pleurodesis was a relative contraindication for eventual lung transplantation, this is no longer considered to be true. A surgical approach, with either a small transaxillary thoracotomy or a thoracoscopic procedure, is usually used. Stapling across ruptured pleural blebs and pleural abrasion can be performed with a relatively low rate of recurrence.[90,92]

Respiratory Failure

Hypoxemic and hypercapnic respiratory failure occurs in the late stages of CF and accounts for most deaths. Treatment of hypoxemia may improve both the quality and duration of life while delaying the development of cor pulmonale.[93] As infection and inflammation progress, airway obstruction and parenchymal destruction worsen, causing ventilation-perfusion mismatch and hypoxemia. Other mechanisms also may contribute to hypoxemia, including an increased partial pressure of carbon dioxide, intrapulmonary shunt, reduced mixed venous saturation resulting from increased oxygen consumption, malnutrition, and weakness.

The use of noninvasive mechanical ventilation (NIV) may be effective to improve ventilation and this can be used with supplemental oxygen therapy as needed. NIV can improve nocturnal ventilation, oxygenation, peak exercise capacity, exertional dyspnea, and sleep quality.[94,95] Treatment of hypoxemic respiratory failure is first aimed at correcting reversible processes. This includes optimization of the treatment of airway infection, clearance of retained secretions, improving nutrition, and treating other complications that may be present. Supplemental oxygen by nasal cannula should be prescribed with the goal of maintaining a Spo_2 of 90% or above. Even when daytime oxygen saturation is adequate, hypoxemia during sleep or exercise may occur and should be assessed, especially in the setting of severe lung disease ($FEV_1 \leq 30\%$ of predicted), low resting Spo_2 ($\leq 90\%$), or when signs of cor pulmonale are present. Because spirometry poorly predicts the occurrence of exercise- or sleep-induced hypoxemia, a low threshold for screening should exist.[64] This approach to the treatment of hypoxemic respiratory failure in CF can improve exercise capacity,[65] delay the development of cor pulmonale, and improve survival.[66]

Hypercapnic respiratory failure is the result of alveolar hypoventilation, primarily from airway obstruction and increased dead space ventilation. In addition, respiratory muscle weakness in association with muscle fatigue and malnutrition may be an important contributor. Acidosis that develops gradually from hypercapnia usually is compensated by renal mechanisms, such that an adequate acid–base balance is maintained. Acute elevations in the Pco_2 will lead to acidosis and an impaired sensorium. Although hypercarbia is often the result of slowly progressive lung disease, a search for treatable causes of respiratory failure should be performed. Ventilatory assistance can be provided by NIV or with endotracheal intubation. The decision to use assisted ventilation with intubation should be based on the baseline severity of lung disease, presence of a reversible precipitating process, and whether the patient has been accepted for lung transplantation.[96]

In the setting of an acute, reversible process such as pneumothorax, severe hemoptysis, or suboptimal treatment of the underlying CF lung disease, assisted ventilation may buy time needed to treat the acute, superimposed process. Once the decision to ventilate a patient has been made, airway clearance, suctioning, and antibiotics should be used. Therapy for muscle weakness with nutrition and exercise (including ambulation with assisted ventilation) should be started. Successful liberation from mechanical ventilation depends primarily on the extent of the underlying lung disease rather than the severity of the acute respiratory event. In the patient awaiting lung transplantation who has accrued enough seniority to make organ availability a possibility within days or weeks, a trial of mechanical ventilation and intensive therapy may be reasonable, with the understanding that prolonged support may not be possible. This period of support may provide a bridge to successful transplantation or may allow the patient and family to address end-of-life issues with greater control.

Patients with irreversible respiratory insufficiency are unlikely to benefit from invasive mechanical ventilation without the possibility of imminent lung transplantation. The debilitating nature of advanced lung disease makes the probability of liberation from mechanical support very low. NIV may relieve acute dyspnea and other symptoms of hypoventilation such as morning headaches, exertional dyspnea, and daytime lethargy.[97] NIV may also be useful as a bridge to transplantation for patients with decompensated respiratory failure.[97] In CF patients with severe airflow limitation and chronic respiratory failure, the use of nocturnal NIV was well tolerated and reduced complaints of daytime respiratory muscle fatigue, and dyspnea, with no concomitant improvement in lung function.[98] Studies examining the use of NIV in CF have yielded mixed results in terms of improved quality of life, daytime gas exchange, respiratory muscle function, and quality of sleep. As with conventional mechanical ventilation, NIV may help sustain patients with respiratory failure who are waiting for lung transplantation.[98] Because of these mixed results, NIV use should be individualized and closely monitored. Polysomnography should be used to document the degree of gas exchange deterioration during sleep and the frequency of respiratory disturbances and to titrate airway pressures.

Standard Therapy of Lung Disease

Treatment of CF lung disease can be broadly categorized as therapies used to prevent deterioration of lung function and those used to treat acute exacerbations. Although therapies are being introduced that are aimed at the correction of either the gene defect or the ion transport abnormalities that characterize CF epithelia, most of the available therapies either promote the physical removal of airway secretions or reduce airway infection and inflammation. Several types of therapy are often combined to provide optimal care for patients.

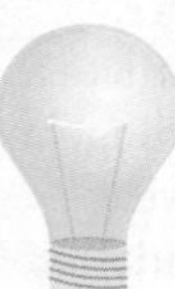

STOP AND THINK

A patient with an FEV_1 of 27% predicted is awaiting lung transplantation. The physician discussed NIV as a therapeutic option, but the patient is unclear about the rationale for therapy. How would you explain the risks and benefits to the patient?

TABLE 37-2
Airway Clearance and Medications

Agent	Rationale
Dornase alfa	Decreases secretion tenacity by degrading DNA polymers
Bronchodilator (β-adrenergic agonist)	May protect against bronchospasm induced by expectorants and/or antibiotics. No proven effect on airway clearance
Hypertonic saline or mannitol	May improve airway surface fluid hydration, increase mucin secretion, and increase effective coughing
Airway clearance maneuvers and devices	Methods should be individualized to the patient and used more frequently when the patient is acutely sick
Antibiotic (TOBI, Cayston)	Deposition may be enhanced during or after airway clearance

When multiple expensive and labor-intensive treatment modalities are prescribed, attention should be paid to appropriate use and adherence (**Table 37-2**).

Although not addressed in detail here, nutritional support to achieve and maintain ideal body weight and treatment of complications such as CF-related diabetes are integral parts of the multidisciplinary care of patients and may directly affect the severity of lung disease and survival. The development of specialized CF care centers where expertise from multiple disciplines is applied in an integrated fashion has greatly improved survival. **Box 37-2** lists typical respiratory therapist roles in the management of patients with CF.

BOX 37-2

Respiratory Therapist Roles in Cystic Fibrosis Management

- Evaluating the need for O_2 therapy
- Monitoring oxygenation status and titrating O_2 flow or FIO_2
- Administering aerosol therapies
- Providing assisted ventilation (via mask or endotracheal tube)
- Performing airway clearance maneuvers
- Performing spirometry and other pulmonary function testing
- Evaluating exercise tolerance
- Educating patients
  - Proper use of inhaled medications
  - Instruction on airway clearance techniques
  - Respiratory equipment care and maintenance

Maintenance Therapy

CF airway secretions are difficult to clear because of their lower viscosity and higher tenacity. This is probably caused by inflammation and the presence of DNA/F-actin copolymers in sputum. If left untreated, retained phlegm leads to progressive airway obstruction and serves as a nidus for ongoing infection and inflammation. In an attempt to treat the progression of infection, inflammation, and lung destruction, airway clearance techniques have been developed to promote the expectoration of airway secretions. These techniques continue to be a cornerstone of CF therapy (**Table 37-3**).

Several means of airway clearance are available to patients with CF, with little other than systematic, individual trials and expert opinion to guide clinicians to the best choice for a given patient. Chest physical therapy (CPT) by hand percussion over the chest wall, the traditional means used to clear secretions, is usually effective, although this form of therapy is considered time and labor intensive, and adherence is poor. CPT has been shown to improve mucus clearance and pulmonary function in otherwise stable patients.[99] This method requires a caregiver capable of performing the therapy correctly. There is strong evidence against the head down postural drainage positions because of the increase risk of gastroesophageal reflux.[100]

Alternative airway clearance therapies include breathing techniques such as autogenic drainage (AD) and the active cycle of breathing technique (ACBT), positive airway pressure adjuncts such as positive expiratory pressure (PEP)[101] and oscillatory PEP (OPEP),[102] and mechanical devices that deliver high-frequency chest wall compression (HFCWC).[103] These offer alternatives to traditional CPT and can be effectively self-administered, allowing for more independence. Also, the treatment times are typically less than that required for CPT. Because no single method has been shown to be consistently superior and great variability exists between patients, different methods should be tried until the patient identifies those that he or she is willing and able to use.[104]

To achieve good patient outcomes, it is essential for the respiratory therapist to understand the operation and limitations of the airway clearance devices available for use.[105] The patient's age, ability to cooperate and to properly perform the therapy, level of motivation, and degree of pulmonary impairment must be taken into consideration. The use of airway clearance protocols helps match therapeutic goals to clinical needs and guides selection and sequencing of therapy.

TABLE 37-3
Airway Clearance Techniques

Technique	Description	Performed Independently?
Chest physical therapy (CPT)	CPT includes manual or mechanical percussion and vibration applied over individual lung segments. Mechanical percussors provide limited patient autonomy and may decrease fatigue in the caregiver. The head down postural drainage positioning (tipping) should be avoided due to evidence of reflux and/or aspiration, particularly in infants. There is no proven benefit to adding postural draining to CPT chest percussion.	No
Active cycle of breathing technique (ACBT)	Technique alternates (1) gentle breathing with the lower chest, (2) deep breathing with emphasis on inspiration, and (3) forced exhalation technique (FET) using the abdominal muscles and an open mouth/glottis (huff). ACBT may be combined with posture positions.	Yes
Autogenic drainage (AD)	Technique alternates (1) breathing at low lung volumes to loosen peripheral secretions, (2) breathing at low to mid lung volumes to collect mucus from central airways, and (3) mucus evacuation by breathing at mid to high lung volumes. It is performed in the sitting position and requires significant teaching and practice.	Yes
Positive expiratory pressure (PEP)	Pressure (10–20 cm H_2O) is applied via an expiratory resistor attached to a mask or mouthpiece. Tidal breathing with slightly active exhalation is used. Forced expirations and cough follow PEP to evacuate mucus. Nebulized medications may be delivered in conjunction with PEP device.	Yes
Oscillatory PEP (OPEP)	A handheld device delivers airflow oscillations in addition to positive expiratory pressure. It is essential to achieve sufficient airflow and pressure through the device, and patients with very severe lung disease may not be able to perform this technique. Technique is tiring and adherence is poor. Some devices allow nebulized medications to be delivered in conjunction with OPEP therapy.	Yes
High-frequency chest wall compression (HFCWC)	An inflatable vest linked to a compressed air delivery system provides air pulses at high frequency. Therapy is given over 20 to 30 minutes, with the patient sitting in an upright position.	Yes

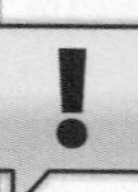

Respiratory Recap

Maintenance Therapy for Cystic Fibrosis

- Airway clearance techniques
- Aerosolized dornase alfa
- Other mucus-modifying agents
- Antibiotics
- Anti-inflammatory medications

Patient and family education should include how to perform the therapy as well as how to use and clean the equipment.[105,106] Effective strategies for integrating multiple lengthy therapy sessions into the patient's daily schedule should also be reviewed.[107] Patient acceptance of a technique is crucial if adherence is to be expected. In general, airway clearance therapies are some of the most time intensive used for CF with among the lowest rates of consistent adherence.

Exercise has been shown to enhance an airway clearance regimen and assist secretion removal. Beneficial effects on health and well-being have been well documented.[108] The need for supplemental oxygen during exercise should be assessed periodically in those patients with severe airway obstruction.

Another strategy used to aid secretion removal is to modify the transportability of phlegm. Because DNA is the major polymer in CF secretions, human recombinant DNase I (dornase alfa; Pulmozyme) was developed and approved for use in CF in 1994.[109] In a well-controlled 6-month study, once-daily use of dornase improved FEV_1 by 6% above baseline and decreased the frequency of respiratory exacerbations by 28%. The response to dornase is variable, with some patients showing clear benefit and others showing no change or actually worsening. Careful monitoring of the response therefore is warranted. Because most patients who benefit show a response within 1 to 3 months of starting the drug, a therapeutic trial should be considered for up to 3 months while the patient is monitored for improvement in lung function and clinical symptoms.

The efficacy of dornase over longer time periods is not reported. The timing of dornase alfa has been debated as well. In a recent Cochrane Review, 99 trial reports representing 48 studies providing data on 122 participants were reviewed to determine if the timing of dornase alfa administration (before or after airway clearance therapy) affected clinical outcomes of patients with CF.[110] The current evidence derived from a small number of participants in this meta-analysis did not indicate that inhalation of dornase alfa after airway clearance techniques is more or less effective than the traditional recommendation to inhale nebulized dornase alfa 30 minutes before airway clearance techniques.[111] The investigators reported, however, that for a small subset of children with well-preserved lung function, inhalation of dornase alfa before airway clearance may be more beneficial for small airway function than inhalation after airway clearance therapy.[110] The studies included in their analysis relied on measures with high degrees of variability and that variability was also present in patient follow-up.[110] The authors concluded that there was no strong evidence to indicate that one timing regimen was better and that the timing of dornase alfa inhalation was most likely largely based on pragmatic reasons or individual preference with respect to the time of airway clearance and time of day.[110]

The DNA polymer network copolymerizes with filamentous actin (F-actin) from effete airway and inflammatory cells and from neutrophil extracellular traps (NETs).[111] This increases the rigidity of these polymers. F-actin depolymerizing agents such as thymosin beta 4 have been shown to be both effective as mucolytics and synergistic with dornase alfa in vitro, but these have not been studied in patients with CF.[112]

Several mucolytics have been used in CF, although none has been shown to improve lung function or other clinical outcomes. Among these agents, *N*-acetylcysteine (Mucomyst) is perhaps the most commonly used. This agent breaks disulfide bonds in mucins, thus making them less viscous. Unfortunately, this agent may increase epithelial inflammation. Although irritation can induce coughing, aerosol *N*-acetylcysteine has not been shown to be beneficial for persons with CF. Other mucolytic agents also have been used but have not been shown to have benefit for CF. Recent studies indicate that oral administration of N-acetylcysteine may act more as an antioxidant than a mucolytic.[113,114]

Hypertonic saline has been used to promote hydration of periciliary fluid, induce coughing, and increasing mucus secretion. Studies examining the acute effect of hypertonic saline (3% to 12%) on mucociliary clearance[115] and studies of lung function suggest benefit.[116] Some CF patients with coexistent asthma may not tolerate hypertonic solutions because of bronchospasm.[116] Similarly, inhaled dry powder mannitol has been shown to improve the biophysical and transport properties of CF sputum.[117]

Because chronic airway infection causes progression of CF lung disease, oral and inhaled antibiotics are important parts of a standard CF care regimen. In general, oral antibiotics are used episodically, when new respiratory symptoms develop or a minor decline in lung function is detected. Scheduled cycles of oral antibiotics also may be used prophylactically in the patient having frequent exacerbations. Continuous use of an oral antibiotic designed to suppress infection with *S aureus* has been a common practice, especially in Europe. Long-term use of ciprofloxacin, the primary oral agent with good activity against *P aeruginosa*, should be avoided because of the rapid emergence of resistance after 3 to 4 weeks of use.

Because of the limited number of oral antibiotics available to treat *P aeruginosa*, inhaled aminoglycosides have been used. This route of administration has the benefit of achieving high drug levels in proximal airway secretions, with minimal systemic levels or toxicity. High drug concentrations in secretions may be particularly helpful in the treatment of organisms that are resistant to antibiotic concentrations that may be achieved via the intravenous route. Because of the natural concentration gradient of antibiotic in the airways distal secretions are exposed to progressively lower concentrations, inevitably leading to the development of antimicrobial resistance.

The best data for inhaled antibiotic efficacy exist for high-dose tobramycin. A preservative-free, concentrated preparation of tobramycin solution for inhalation (TOBI, Novartis) 300 mg twice a day taken during alternate months improves lung function and lessens the relative risk of hospitalization or treatment with intravenous antibiotics.[118] Tobramycin inhalation powder is also available for administration using the podhaler device. An alternative to inhaled tobramycin is aztreonam lysine (AZLI, Cayston), which has good in vitro activity against *P aeruginosa*.[119]

An alternative approach embraced by the Danish CF Centre stresses measures aimed at delaying the acquisition of *P aeruginosa* and aggressive antibiotic treatment once this organism is cultured from sputum. These measures include the segregation of patients by microbiologic status and attempts to eradicate pseudomonas when initially cultured in a patient.[70] Scheduled courses of intravenous antibiotics are also given every 3 months for patients who are chronically infected with *Pseudomonas*. This center claims that there is improved survival using this approach compared with historical controls.[120] Significant concerns include the earlier development of bacterial antibiotic resistance, the lack of proven efficacy by controlled trials, the enormous healthcare resources involved, and the personal impact this approach has on patients.

Bronchodilators, especially those delivered via the inhaled route, are commonly prescribed in CF. Approximately one-quarter of patients have bronchial hyperreactivity.[121] In these patients, bronchodilators may improve respiratory symptoms and airway secretion clearance. Whether these agents provide long-term benefit in CF is unknown. In general, inhaled β-adrenergic agents are used in patients with documented reversibility on spirometry or in those who receive symptomatic benefit. Inhaled anticholinergic agents, especially ipratropium bromide, may also have a role in CF.[122] Oral preparations, including theophylline, are not routinely used, have not been shown to be beneficial, and must be monitored carefully because of pharmacokinetic variability.

There is a clear rationale for using anti-inflammatory agents to decrease neutrophilic inflammation and the harmful effects of neutrophil products. Initial studies designed to test this approach used high doses of corticosteroids. Although patients receiving 1 to 2 mg/kg of prednisolone on alternate days had a slowed decline in lung function (ΔFEV_1 of –2% versus –6% in placebo group, at 48 months), there were unacceptable side effects.[123] Glucose metabolism abnormalities and delayed linear growth limit chronic therapy with oral corticosteroids. The risk–benefit ratio may favor their use in patients with ABPA. Inhaled steroids also have been studied in CF, but studies clearly suggest that with the exception of patients who have concomitant asthma, there are few if any benefits and some possible risks.[124]

An alternative means to decrease neutrophilic inflammation is high-dose ibuprofen. In a 4 year study, young patients (5 to 13 years) with mild lung disease (FEV_1 ≥60% of predicted) benefited from twice-daily ibuprofen at doses sufficient to achieve peak blood levels of 50 to 100 mg/L. In those who adhered to therapy, the annual rate of change in FEV_1 was –1.5%, versus –3.5% in the placebo group. Nutritional status and radiographic indices of disease activity also were improved in the treated group, and few side effects were encountered.[125]

Low-dose macrolide antibiotics (especially azithromycin) are effective as immunomodulatory medications and can decrease neutrophil-dominated airway inflammation and improve pulmonary function in patients with CF.[126] A large multicenter study demonstrated significant lung function improvement and fewer intravenous antibiotic courses in subjects with CF on azithromycin.[127] A meta-analysis of four studies with 296 participants concluded that there is a small but significant treatment effect for azithromycin in improving pulmonary function in persons with CF.[128]

Exacerbations

The course of CF lung disease is punctuated by periodic episodes of increased airway infection and inflammation with worsened lung function. These exacerbation episodes occur more frequently and become more

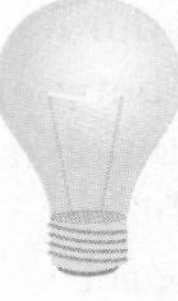

STOP AND THINK

A patient with FEV_1 of 95% predicted reports that he does not adhere to his airway clearance therapy, complaining that the therapy is time consuming and he sees no benefit. How would you explain the benefits of airway clearance to the patient?

difficult to treat as lung disease progresses and bacterial resistance develops. When exacerbations inevitably occur, an aggressive approach should be taken to reclaim lost lung function and to prevent early relapse with its associated risks.

Access to a CF center for early detection and treatment of an exacerbation is critically important. It has been reported that children with better lung function actually had *more* office sick visits, which implies that they were able to be treated promptly for pulmonary problems.[129] Typical features of an infectious exacerbation of CF lung disease include an increase in the frequency of cough and amount of sputum, diminished appetite, weight loss, fatigue, and a decrease in the FEV_1. Fever is not common, and high fever should prompt the search for other etiologies, including infection with *B cepacia* complex or atypical organisms (e.g., respiratory viruses, mycobacteria) or indwelling catheter infection. Leukocytosis is typically mild to moderate, and chest radiographs usually show little or no acute change.

During the initiation of therapy for a CF exacerbation, consideration of potential precipitating causes should include the presence of environmental allergens or irritants, inadequate airway clearance measures, allergic bronchopulmonary aspergillosis, and therapeutic nonadherence. The adequacy of airway clearance at home, the severity of the exacerbation, the baseline severity of lung disease, and the complexity of the treatment regimen being instituted should be weighed during consideration of whether home therapy with intravenous antibiotics may be an option. In either environment, airway clearance maneuvers should be intensified, preferably to include airway clearance therapy at least four times daily to clear the airways. Antibiotics should be selected based on recent, pretreatment culture and sensitivity testing whenever possible. Every isolated organism is targeted when feasible, although patients often improve even when only selected organisms are targeted.

There appears to be very little relationship between organisms cultured in sputum and therapeutic response to antimicrobials including those to whom they are resistant. *P aeruginosa*, *B cepacia* complex, and other gram-negative organisms (e.g., *S maltophilia*, *A xylosoxidans*) should be treated with two antibiotics from different complementary drug classes. When both a gram-negative organism and *S aureus* are cultured, antistaphylococcal therapy must be added. The duration of therapy is typically around 2 or 3 weeks but may be longer when the clinical response is slow. Pulmonary function testing near the end of a planned antibiotic course may be useful as an objective measure of the adequacy of therapy. Although some further improvement in lung function may occur even after completion of the antibiotic course, the return of lung function to pre-exacerbation levels is reassuring.

Lung Transplantation

Lung transplantation has become an accepted therapy for end-stage CF lung disease. The relative paucity of donor organs and subsequent long waiting times before organ availability mandate that patients be referred to transplant centers on a timely basis. With waiting times exceeding 2 years at some centers, close attention should be paid to clinical and testing results that predict a 2-year survival probability of 50%. These predictors include an FEV_1 of less than 30% of predicted, the rate of decline in lung function, and hypercapnia ($Paco_2$ ≥45 mm Hg). The presence of an accelerated clinical decline, characterized by more frequent exacerbations that respond incompletely to aggressive therapy, recurrent pneumothoraces, massive hemoptysis, or panresistant organisms, should prompt consideration for earlier referral.[62,130] Optimal transplant candidates should not have significant nonpulmonary organ dysfunction (e.g., kidney, liver, heart), should be motivated and adherent with therapy, and should have adequate psychosocial support.

The surgical approach now preferred is sequential, bilateral transplantation rather than heart–lung transplantation. Alternatively, when a patient is not likely to survive until a cadaveric transplant can be performed, living donor lobar transplantation can be performed at some centers when healthy donors of sufficient size and correct blood type are available.[131] In either case, survival after transplantation appears no different in CF than in transplantation for other indications. The 5-year survival rate is approximately 48% and is limited primarily by opportunistic infections and chronic graft rejection, manifesting as bronchiolitis obliterans.[132]

Key Points

- Cystic fibrosis is a prevalent inherited disorder that causes significant morbidity and premature mortality in those who suffer from it.
- Cystic fibrosis is the most common lethal genetic disease affecting the white population; it is autosomal recessive.
- Mutations in the *CFTR* gene result in several ion transport abnormalities, which in turn impair cough clearance and lung defense.
- Chronic infection and inflammation lead to progressive lung damage and respiratory failure in most patients.
- Improvements in care, including better antibiotics and nutritional support, have greatly extended survival.
- Cystic fibrosis is a multiorgan disease, with a broad spectrum of clinical manifestations.
- The combination of a typical CF clinical manifestation with evidence for abnormal CFTR is required for the diagnosis of cystic fibrosis.

- Preventive care is the cornerstone of effective CF management.
- Close monitoring of lung function, therapies aimed at airway clearance and minimization of infection, and nutritional support are necessary elements in CF care.
- Lung transplantation is an appropriate therapy for patients with severe CF lung disease. Evaluation for transplant in appropriate candidates should occur before the local waiting time for donor availability exceeds the anticipated survival time.

References

1. Lobitz S, Velleuer E. Guido Fanconi (1892–1979): a jack of all trades. *Nat Rev Cancer*. 2006;6:893–898.
2. Andersen DH. Cystic fibrosis of the pancreas and its relation to celiac disease: a clinical and pathologic study. *Am J Dis Child*. 1938;56:344–399.
3. Farber S. Some organic digestive disturbances in early life. *J Mich Med Sci*. 1945;44:587–594.
4. di Sant'Agnese PA, Darling RC, Perera GA, et al. Abnormal electrolyte composition of sweat in cystic fibrosis of the pancreas. *Pediatrics*. 1953;12:549–563.
5. Gibson LE, Cooke RE. A test for concentration of electrolytes in sweat in cystic fibrosis on the pancreas utilizing pilocarpine by iontophoresis. *Pediatrics*. 1959;23:545–549.
6. Riordan JR, Rommens JM, Kerem B-T, et al. Identification of the cystic fibrosis gene: cloning and characterization of complementary DNA. *Science*. 1989;245:1066–1073.
7. Cystic Fibrosis Foundation. *Patient Registry Annual Data Report for 2012*. Bethesda, MD: Cystic Fibrosis Foundation; 2013.
8. Cystic Fibrosis Mutation Database. *CFMDB Statistics*. Available at: http://www.genet.sickkids.on.ca/cftr/StatisticsPage.html. Accessed August 17, 2014.
9. Population variation of common cystic fibrosis mutations. The Cystic Fibrosis Genetic Analysis Consortium. *Hum Mutat*. 1994;4:167–177.
10. Zielenski J, Tsui LC. Cystic fibrosis: genotypic and phenotypic variations. *Annu Rev Genet*. 1995;29:777–807.
11. The Cystic Fibrosis Genotype-Phenotype Consortium. Correlation between genotype and phenotype in patients with cystic fibrosis. *N Engl J Med*. 1993;329:1308–1313.
12. Dork T, Dworniczak B, Aulehla-Scholz C, et al. Distinct spectrum of CFTR gene mutations in congenital absence of vas deferens. *Hum Genet*. 1997;100:365–377.
13. Rowe SM, Borowita DS, Burns JL, et al. Progress in cystic fibrosis and the CF therapeutics development network. *Thorax*. 2012;67:882–890.
14. Deeks ED. Ivacaftor: a review of its use in patients with cystic fibrosis. *Drugs*. 2013;73:1595–1604.
15. Kotha K, Clancy JP. Ivacaftor treatment of cystic fibrosis patients with the G551D mutation: a review of the evidence. *Ther Adv Respir Dis*. 2013;7:288–296.
16. Greger R, Mall M, Bleich M, et al. Regulation of epithelial ion channels by the cystic fibrosis transmembrane conductance regulator. *J Mol Med*. 1996;74:527–534.
17. Mall M, Bleich M, Kuehr J, et al. CFTR-mediated inhibition of epithelial Na^1 conductance in human colon is defective in cystic fibrosis. *Am J Physiol*. 1999;277:G709–G716.
18. Kunzelmann K, Mall M, Briel M, et al. The cystic fibrosis transmembrane conductance regulator attenuates the endogenous Ca^{21} activated Cl^- conductance of *Xenopus* oocytes. *Pflugers Arch*. 1997;435:178–181.
19. McNicholas CM, Guggino WB, Schwiebert EM, et al. Sensitivity of a renal K^1 channel (ROMK2) to the inhibitory sulfonylurea compound glibenclamide is enhanced by coexpression with the ATP-binding cassette transporter cystic fibrosis transmembrane regulator. *Proc Natl Acad Sci USA*. 1996;93:8083–8088.
20. Cotton CU, Stutts MJ, Knowles MR, et al. Abnormal apical cell membrane in cystic fibrosis respiratory epithelium. An in vitro electrophysiologic analysis. *J Clin Invest*. 1987;79:80–85.
21. Matsui H, Grubb BR, Tartan R, et al. Evidence for periciliary liquid layer depletion, not abnormal ion composition, in the pathogenesis of cystic fibrosis airways disease. *Cell*. 1998;95:1005–1015.
22. Lindström M, Camner P, Falk R, et al. Long-term clearance from small airways in patients with cystic fibrosis. *Eur Respir J*. 2005;25:317–323.
23. Smith JJ, Travis SM, Greenberg EP, et al. Cystic fibrosis airway epithelia fail to kill bacteria because of abnormal airway surface fluid. *Cell*. 1996;85:229–236.
24. Travis SM, Conway BA, Zabner J, et al. Activity of abundant antimicrobials of the human airway. *Am J Respir Cell Mol Biol*. 1999;20:872–879.
25. Engelhardt JF, Yankaskas JR, Ernst SA, et al. Submucosal glands are the predominant site of CFTR expression in the human bronchus. *Nat Genet*. 1992;2:240–248.
26. Ballard ST, Trout L, Bebok Z, et al. CFTR involvement in chloride, bicarbonate, and liquid secretion by airway submucosal glands. *Am J Physiol*. 1999;277:L694–L699.
27. Henke MO, Renner A, Huber RM, et al. MUC5AC and MUC5B mucins are decreased in cystic fibrosis airway secretions. *Am J Respir Cell Mol Biol*. 2004;31:86–91.
28. Davril M, Degroote S, Humbert P, et al. The sialylation of bronchial mucins secreted by patients suffering from cystic fibrosis or from chronic bronchitis is related to the severity of airway infection. *Glycobiology*. 1999;9:311–321.
29. Bonfield TL, Konstan MW, Berger M. Altered respiratory epithelial cell cytokine production in cystic fibrosis. *J Allergy Clin Immunol*. 1999;104:72–78.
30. Farrell PM, Rosenstein BJ, White TB, et al. Guidelines for the diagnosis of cystic fibrosis in newborns through older adults: Cystic Fibrosis Foundation consensus report. *J Pediatr*. 2008;153(Suppl):S4–S14.
31. Castellani C, Massie J. Emerging issues in cystic fibrosis newborn screening. *Curr Opin Pulm Med*. 2010;16:584–590.
32. Kleven DT, McCudden CR, Willis MS. Cystic fibrosis: newborn screening in America. *MLO Med Lab Obs*. 2008;40:16–18, 22, 24–27.
33. Borowitz D, Parad RB, Sharp JK, et al. Cystic Fibrosis Foundation practice guidelines for the management of infants with cystic fibrosis transmembrane conductance regulator-related metabolic syndrome during the first two years of life and beyond. *J Pediatr*. 2009;155(Suppl):S106–S116.
34. Ren CL, Desai H, Platt M, Dixon M. Clinical outcomes in infants with cystic fibrosis transmembrane conductance regulator (CFTR) related metabolic syndrome. *Pediatr Pulmonol*. 2011;46:1079–1084.
35. Farrell PM, Rosenstein BJ, White TB, et al. Guidelines for diagnosis of cystic fibrosis in newborns through older adults: Cystic Fibrosis Foundation consensus report. *J Pediatr*. 2008;153(Suppl):S4–S14.
36. Knowles MR, Paradiso AM, Boucher RC. In vivo nasal potential difference: techniques and protocols for assessing efficacy of gene transfer in cystic fibrosis. *Hum Gene Ther*. 1995;6:445–455.
37. Gharib R, Allen RP, Joos HA, et al. Paranasal sinuses in cystic fibrosis: incidence of roentgen abnormalities. *Am J Dis Child*. 1964;108:499–502.
38. Stern RC, Jones K. Nasal and sinus disease. In: Yankaskas JR, Knowles MR, eds. *Cystic Fibrosis in Adults*. Philadelphia: Lippincott-Raven; 1999:221–231.
39. Gysin C, Alothman GA, Papsin BC. Sinonasal disease in cystic fibrosis: clinical characteristics, diagnosis and management. *Pediatr Pulmonol*. 2000;30:481–489.

40. Robertson JM, Friedman EM, Rubin BK. Nasal and sinus disease in cystic fibrosis. *Paediatr Respir Rev*. 2008;9:213–219.
41. King VV. Upper respiratory disease, sinusitis and polyposis. *Clin Rev Allergy*. 1991;9:143–157.
42. Jaffe BF, Strome M, Khaw KT, et al. Nasal polypectomy and sinus surgery for cystic fibrosis—a 10-year review. *Otolaryngol Clin North Am*. 1977;10:81–90.
43. Durie PR, Forstner GG. The exocrine pancreas. In: Yankaskas JR, Knowles MR, eds. *Cystic Fibrosis in Adults*. Philadelphia: Lippincott-Raven; 1999:261–287.
44. Shwachman H, Lebenthal E, Khaw KT. Recurrent acute pancreatitis in patients with cystic fibrosis with normal pancreatic enzymes. *Pediatrics*. 1975;55:86–95.
45. Sharer N, Schwarz M, Malone G, et al. Mutations of the cystic fibrosis gene in patients with chronic pancreatitis. *N Engl J Med*. 1998;339:645–652.
46. Alves Cde A, Aquias RA, Alves AC, Santana MA. Diabetes mellitus in patients with cystic fibrosis. *J Bras Pneumol*. 2007;33:213–221.
47. Lanng S. Glucose intolerance in cystic fibrosis patients. *Paediatr Respir Rev*. 2001;2:253–259.
48. Marshall BC, Butler SM, Stoddard M, et al. Epidemiology of cystic fibrosis-related diabetes. *J Pediatr*. 2005;146:681–687.
49. Fischmann D, Nookala VK. Cystic fibrosis-related diabetes mellitus: etiology, evaluation and management. *Endoc Pract*. 2008;14:1169–1179.
50. di Sant'Agnese PA, Hubbard VS. The gastrointestinal tract. In: Taussig LM, ed. *Cystic Fibrosis*. New York: Thieme-Stratton; 1984:212–229.
51. Robertson MB, Choe KA, Joseph PM. Review of the abdominal manifestations of cystic fibrosis in the adult patient. *Radiographics*. 2006;26:679–690.
52. Stevens JC, Maguiness KM, Hollingsworth J, et al. Pancreatic enzyme supplementation in cystic fibrosis patients before and after fibrosing colonopathy. *J Pediatr Gastroenterol Nutr*. 1998;26:80–84.
53. Ledson MJ, Tran J, Walshaw MJ. Prevalence and mechanisms of gastro-esophageal reflux in adult cystic fibrosis patients. *J R Soc Med*. 1998;91:7–9.
54. Colombo C, Crosignani A, Battezzati PM. Liver involvement in cystic fibrosis. *J Hepatol*. 1999;31:946–954.
55. Scott-Jupp R, Lama M, Tanner MS. Prevalence of liver disease in cystic fibrosis. *Arch Dis Child*. 1991;66:698–701.
56. King L, Scurr E, Murugan N, et al. Hepatobiliary and pancreatic manifestations of CF: MR imaging appearances. *Radiographics*. 2000;20:767–777.
57. Lyon A, Bilton D. Fertility issues in cystic fibrosis. *Paediatr Respir Rev*. 2002;3:236–240.
58. Nussbaum E, Boat TF, Wood RE, et al. Cystic fibrosis with acute hypoelectrolytemia and metabolic alkalosis in infancy. *Am J Dis Child*. 1979;133:965–966.
59. Linnane B, Robinson P, Ranganathan S, Stick S, Murray C. Role of high-resolution computed tomography in the detection of early cystic fibrosis lung disease. *Paediatr Respir Rev*. 2008;9: 168–174.
60. Fujiuchi S, Matsumoto H, Yamazaki Y, et al. Analysis of chest CT in patients with *Mycobacterium avium* complex pulmonary disease. *Respiration*. 2003;70:76–81.
61. Wagener JS, Headley AA. Cystic fibrosis: current trends in respiratory care. *Respir Care*. 2003;48:234–245.
62. Konstan MW, Morgan WJ, Butler SM, et al. Scientific Advisory Group and the Investigators and Coordinators of the Epidemiologic Study of Cystic Fibrosis: risk factors for rate of decline in forced expiratory volume in one second in children and adolescents with cystic fibrosis. *J Pediatr*. 2007;151:134–139.
63. Boehler A. Update on cystic fibrosis: selected aspects related to lung transplantation. *Swiss Med Wkly*. 2003;133:111–117.
64. Davies JC, Cunningham S, Alton EW, Innes JA. Lung clearance index in CF: a sensitive marker of lung disease severity. *Thorax*. 2008;63:96–97.
65. Bradley S, Solin P, Wilson J, et al. Hypoxemia and hypercapnia during exercise and sleep in patients with cystic fibrosis. *Chest*. 1999;116:647–654.
66. Marcus CL, Bader D, Stabile MW, et al. Supplemental oxygen and exercise performance in patients with cystic fibrosis with severe pulmonary disease. *Chest*. 1992;101:52–57.
67. Tonelli AR. Pulmonary hypertension survival effects and treatment options in cystic fibrosis. *Curr Opin Pulm Med*. 201;19:1651–1661.
68. Kerem E, Reisman J, Corey M, et al. Prediction of mortality in patients with cystic fibrosis. *N Engl J Med*. 1992;326:1187–1191.
69. Grasemann H, Ratjen F. Early lung disease in cystic fibrosis. *Lancet Respir Med*. 2013;1:148–157.
70. Gilligan PH. Microbiology of cystic fibrosis lung disease. In: Yankaskas JR, Knowles MR, eds. *Cystic Fibrosis in Adults*. Philadelphia: Lippincott-Raven; 1999:93–114.
71. Dasenbrook EC, Merlo CA, Diener-West M, et al. Persistent methicillin-resistant *Staphylococcus aureus* and rate of FEV_1 decline in cystic fibrosis. *Am J Respir Crit Care Med*. 2008;178: 814–821.
72. Vanderhelst E, De Meirleir L, Verbanck S, et al. Prevalence and impact on FEV(1) decline of chronic methicillin-resistant *Staphylococcus aureus* (MRSA) colonization in patients with cystic fibrosis. A single-center, case control study of 165 patients. *J Cyst Fibros*. 2012;11:2–7.
73. Saiman L, Siegel J. Infection control in cystic fibrosis. *Clin Microbiol Rev*. 2004;17:57–71.
74. Frederiksen B, Koch C, Hoiby N. Changing epidemiology of *Pseudomonas aeruginosa* infection in Danish cystic fibrosis patients (1974–1995). *Pediatr Pulmonol*. 1999;28:159–166.
75. Li Z, Kosorok MR, Farrell PM, et al. Longitudinal development of mucoid *Pseudomonas aeruginosa* infection and lung disease progression in children with cystic fibrosis. *JAMA*. 2005;293:581–588.
76. LiPuma JJ. Update on the *Burkholderia* nomenclature and resistance. *Clin Microbiol Newsletter*. 2007;29:65–69.
77. Lewin LO, Byard PJ, Davis PB. Effect of *Pseudomonas cepacia* colonization on survival and pulmonary function of cystic fibrosis patients. *J Clin Epidemiol*. 1990;43:125–131.
78. Aris R, Routh J, LiPuma J, et al. *Burkholderia cepacia* complex in cystic fibrosis patients after lung transplantation: survival linked to genomovar type. *Am J Respir Crit Care Med*. 2001;164:2102–2106.
79. Holmes A, Nolan R, Taylor R, et al. An epidemic of *Burkholderia cepacia* transmitted between patients with and without cystic fibrosis. *J Infect Dis*. 1999;179:1197–1205.
80. Goldstein R, Sun L, Jiang RZ, et al. Structurally variant classes of pilus appendage fibers co-expressed from *Burkholderia (Pseudomonas) cepacia*. *J Bacteriol*. 1995;177:1039–1052.
81. Saiman L, Siegel J. Infection control in cystic fibrosis. *Clin Microbiol Rev*. 2004;17:57–71.
82. Davies JC, Rubin BK. Emerging and unusual gram-negative infections in cystic fibrosis. *Semin Respir Crit Care Med*. 2007;28:312–321.
83. Thia LP, Balfour Lynn IM. Diagnosing allergic bronchopulmonary aspergillosis in children with cystic fibrosis. *Paediatr Respir Rev*. 2009;10:37–42.
84. Kilby JM, Gilligan PH, Yankaskas JR, et al. Nontuberculous mycobacteria in adult patients with cystic fibrosis. *Chest*. 1992;102:70–75.
85. Oliver KN. Nontuberculosis mycobacteria. I: multicenter prevalence study in cystic fibrosis. *Am J Respir Crit Care Med*. 2003;167:828–834.
86. Esther CR Jr. *Mycobacterium abscessus* infection in young children with cystic fibrosis. *Pediatr Pulmonol*. 2005;40:39–44.
87. Flume PA, Yankaskas JR, Ebeling M, Hulsey T, Clark LL. Massive hemoptysis in cystic fibrosis. *Chest*. 2005;128:729–738.
88. Barben JU, Ditchfield M, Carlin JB, et al. Major haemoptysis in children with cystic fibrosis: a 20-year retrospective study. *J Cyst Fibros*. 2003;2:105–111.
89. Flume PA, Mogayzel PJ Jr, Robinson KA, Rosenblatt RL, Quittell L, Marshall BC, et al. Cystic fibrosis pulmonary guidelines: pulmonary

complications: hemoptysis and pneumothorax. *Am J Respir Crit Care Med.* 2010;182:298–306.
90. Barben JU, Ditchfield M, Carlin JB, et al. Major haemoptysis in children with cystic fibrosis: a 20 year retrospective study. *J Cyst Fibros.* 2003;2:105–111.
91. Vidal V, Therasse E, Berthiaume Y, et al. Bronchial artery embolization in adults with cystic fibrosis: impact on the clinical course and survival. *J Vasc Interv Radiol.* 2006;17:953–958.
92. Yankaskas JR, Egan TM, Mauro MA. Major complications. In: Yankaskas JR, Knowles MR, eds. *Cystic Fibrosis in Adults.* Philadelphia: Lippincott-Raven; 1999:175–193.
93. Spier S, Rivlin J, Hughes D, et al. The effect of oxygen on sleep, blood gases, and ventilation in cystic fibrosis. *Am Rev Respir Dis.* 1984;129:712–718.
94. Wedzicha JA, Muir JF. Noninvasive ventilation in chronic obstructive pulmonary disease, bronchiectasis and cystic fibrosis. *Eur Respir J.* 2002;20:777–784.
95. Young AC, Wilson JW, Kotsimbos TC, Naughton MT. Randomised placebo controlled trial of non-invasive ventilation for hypercapnia in cystic fibrosis. *Thorax.* 2008; 63:72–77.
96. Vedam H, Moriarty C, Torzillo PJ, et al. Improved outcomes of patients with cystic fibrosis admitted to the intensive care unit. *J Cyst Fibros.* 2004;3:8–14.
97. Young AC, Wilson JW, Kotsimbos TC, Naughton MT. Randomised placebo controlled trial of non-invasive ventilation for hypercapnia in cystic fibrosis. *Thorax.* 2008;63:72–77.
98. Flight WG, Shaw J, Johnson S, et al. Long-term non-invasive ventilation in cystic fibrosis—experience over two decades. *J Cyst Fibros.* 2012;11:187–192.
99. van der Schans CP. Conventional chest physical therapy for obstructive lung disease. *Respir Care.* 2007;52:1198–1209.
100. Button BM, Heine RG, Catto-Smith AG, et al. Chest physiotherapy in infants with cystic fibrosis: to tip or not? A five-year study. *Pediatr Pulmonol.* 2003;35:208–213.
101. Myers TR. Positive expiratory pressure and oscillatory positive expiratory pressure therapies. *Respir Care.* 2007;52:1308–1327.
102. Volsko TA, DiFiore J, Chatburn RL. Performance comparison of two oscillating positive expiratory pressure devices: Acapella vs Flutter. *Respir Care.* 2003;48:124–130.
103. Chatburn RL. High frequency assisted airway clearance. *Respir Care.* 2007;52:1224–1237.
104. Volsko TA. Airway clearance therapy: finding the evidence. *Respir Care.* 2013; 58:1669–1678.
105. Volsko TA. The value of conducting laboratory investigations on airway clearance devices. *Respir Care.* 2008;53:311–313.
106. Lester ML, Flume PA, Gray SL, et al. Nebulizer use and maintenance by cystic fibrosis patients: a survey study. *Respir Care.* 2004;49:1504–1508.
107. Homnick DN. Making airway clearance successful. *Paediatr Respir Rev.* 2007;8:40–45.
108. Havermans T, De Boeck K. Cystic fibrosis: a balancing act? *J Cyst Fibros.* 2007;6:161–162.
109. Fereday J, MacDougall C, Spizzo M, et al. "There's nothing I can't do—I just put my mind to anything and I can do it": a qualitative analysis of how children with chronic disease and their parents account for and manage physical activity. *BMC Pediatr.* 2009;9:1–16.
110. Fuchs HJ, Borowitz DS, Christiansen DH, et al. Effect of aerosolized recombinant human DNase on exacerbations of respiratory symptoms and on pulmonary function in patients with cystic fibrosis. The Pulmozyme Study Group. *N Engl J Med.* 1994;331:637–642.
111. Dentice R, Elkins M. Timing of dornase alfa inhalation for cystic fibrosis. *Cochrane Database Syst Rev.* 2013 Jun 5;6:CD007923.
112. Voynow JA, Rubin BK. Mucus, mucins, and sputum. *Chest.* 2009;135:505–512.
113. Kater A, Henke MO, Rubin BK. The role of DNA and actin polymers on the polymer structure and rheology of cystic fibrosis sputum and depolymerization by gelsolin or thymosin beta 4. *Ann N Y Acad Sci.* 2007;1112:140–153.
114. Nair GB, Ilowite JS. Pharmacologic agents for mucus clearance in bronchiectasis. *Clin Chest Med.* 2012;33:363–370.
115. Jones AM, Helm JM. Emerging treatments in cystic fibrosis. *Drugs.* 2009;69:1903–1910.
116. Wark P, McDonald VM. Nebulised hypertonic saline for cystic fibrosis. *Cochrane Database Syst Rev.* 2009;(2):CD001506.
117. Daviskas E, Anderson SD, Jaques A, Charlton B. Inhaled mannitol improves the hydration and surface properties of sputum in patients with cystic fibrosis. *Chest.* 2010;137:861–868.
118. Daviskas E, Rubin BK. Effect of inhaled dry powder mannitol on mucus and its clearance. *Expert Rev Respir Med.* 2013;7:65–75.
119. Ramsey BW, Pepe MS, Quan JM, et al. Intermittent administration of inhaled tobramycin in patients with cystic fibrosis. Cystic Fibrosis Inhaled Tobramycin Study Group. *N Engl J Med.* 1999;340:23–30.
120. Hutchinson D, Barclay M, Prescott WA, Brown J. Inhaled aztreonam lysine: an evidence-based review. *Expert Opin Pharmacother.* 2013;14:2115–2124.
121. Hordvik NL, Sammut PH, Judy CG, et al. Effects of standard and high doses of salmeterol on lung function of hospitalized patients with cystic fibrosis. *Pediatr Pulmonol.* 1999;27:43–53.
122. Konig P, Poehler J, Barbero GJ. A placebo-controlled, double-blind trial of the long-term effects of albuterol administration in patients with cystic fibrosis. *Pediatr Pulmonol.* 1998;25:32–36.
123. Eigen H, Rosenstein BJ, Fitzsimmons S, et al. A multicenter study of alternate-day prednisone therapy in patients with cystic fibrosis. Cystic Fibrosis Foundation Prednisone Trial Group. *J Pediatr.* 1995;126:515–523.
124. Lai HC, FitzSimmons SC, Allen DB, et al. Risk of persistent growth impairment after alternate-day prednisone treatment in children with cystic fibrosis. *N Engl J Med.* 2000;342:851–859.
125. Balfour-Lynn IM, Welch K. Inhaled corticosteroids for cystic fibrosis. *Cochrane Database Syst Rev.* 2009;(1):CD001915.
126. Kabra SK, Pawaiya R, Lodha R, et al. Long-term daily high and low doses of azithromycin in children with cystic fibrosis: a randomized controlled trial. *J Cyst Fibros.* 2010;9:17–23.
127. López-Boado YS, Rubin BK. Macrolides as immunomodulatory medications for the therapy of chronic lung diseases. *Curr Opin Pharmacol.* 2008;8:286–291.
128. Saiman LB, Marshall C, Mayer-Hamblett N, et al. for the Macrolide Study Group. Azithromycin in patients with cystic fibrosis chronically infected with *Pseudomonas aeruginosa*: a randomized controlled trial. *JAMA.* 2003;290:1749–1756.
129. Southern KW, Barker PM, Solis A. Macrolide antibiotics for cystic fibrosis. *Cochrane Database Syst Rev.* 2004;CD002203.
130. Padman R, McColley SA, Miller DP, et al. Infant care patterns at epidemiologic study of cystic fibrosis sites that achieve superior childhood lung function. *Pediatrics.* 2007;199:531–537.
131. Rosenblatt RL. Lung transplantation in cystic fibrosis. *Respir Care.* 2009:54:777–787.
132. Yankaskas JR, Mallory GB Jr. Lung transplantation in cystic fibrosis: consensus conference statement. *Chest.* 1998;113:217–226.

CHAPTER

38

Acute Respiratory Distress Syndrome

Craig R. Rackley, Christopher E. Cox, Michael A. Gentile

OUTLINE

Definition
Incidence
Etiology
Clinical Manifestations
Pathobiology
Management
Outcomes

OBJECTIVES

1. Define acute respiratory distress syndrome (ARDS).
2. List common risk factors for ARDS.
3. Recognize the clinical, radiographic, and pathophysiologic features of ARDS.
4. Describe the pathobiology of ARDS.
5. Discuss pharmacologic and nonpharmacologic therapies for ARDS.
6. Describe ventilation strategies for ARDS.
7. Describe how ARDS affects long-term physical functioning and quality of life.

KEY TERMS

acute respiratory distress syndrome (ARDS)
ARDS network (ARDSnet)
extracorporeal life support (ECLS)
lung injury score
lung-protective ventilation
mechanical ventilation
oxygenation index (OI)
Pao_2/Fio_2
plateau pressure
positive end-expiratory pressure (PEEP)
primary ARDS
prone position
secondary ARDS

Introduction

Acute respiratory distress syndrome (ARDS) is characterized by diffuse damage to the alveolar-capillary membrane leading to noncardiogenic pulmonary edema and hypoxemia. ARDS is a worldwide public health issue with significant morbidity and mortality that affects both medical and surgical patients of all ages. Respiratory therapists play an essential role in the early recognition of ARDS and contribute to the multidisciplinary team approach required to manage this life-threatening condition. Having an understanding of the epidemiology, diagnosis, and management of ARDS is essential in the care of these critically ill patients.

Definition

The first clinical description of ARDS was in 1967, when Ashbaugh et al.[1] identified 12 patients with trauma, aspiration, and pulmonary infection who presented with acute dyspnea, hypoxia, diffuse pulmonary infiltrates, and decreased pulmonary compliance. This was initially termed adult respiratory distress syndrome to distinguish it from neonatal acute respiratory failure that had similar physiologic derangements but was due to inadequate surfactant production in immature lungs.[2] Later, the name was changed to acute respiratory distress syndrome as it became apparent that diffuse lung injury from a variety of causes could affect both adult and pediatric populations.

In 1994, the American-European Consensus Conference (AECC) defined ARDS as "an acute clinical illness characterized by the development of bilateral pulmonary infiltrates on chest radiograph and severe hypoxemia with a **Pao_2/Fio_2** of less than 200 mm Hg in the absence of congestive heart failure."[3] The AECC also recognized a less severe form of ARDS, **acute lung injury (ALI)**, with similar clinical findings but with a Pao_2/Fio_2 less than 300. The AECC definitions have been widely used to identify patients with ALI and

Respiratory Recap

Acute respiratory distress syndrome (ARDS)

- Abrupt onset of respiratory distress
- Hypoxemia
- Bilateral pulmonary opacities

ARDS for enrollment in clinical trials. These broad and simplistic definitions do not take into account important physiologic factors affecting PaO_2/FIO_2 (i.e., positive airway pressure and FIO_2 levels), and they ignore both etiologic and host factors that likely affect the biochemical and cellular pattern of the illness.

Besides the PaO_2/FIO_2, two other widely used severity indices in ARDS are the **lung injury score** and **oxygenation index (OI)**. The lung injury score incorporates the **positive end-expiratory pressure (PEEP)**, PaO_2/FIO_2, extent of chest radiograph abnormality, and static lung compliance into a summary score that stratifies lung injury into either mild to moderate or severe.[4] The oxygenation index incorporates FIO_2 and mean airway pressure ($\bar{P}aw$) into its calculation:

$$OI = [(\bar{P}aw \times FIO_2)/PaO_2)] \times 100$$

The oxygenation index has been suggested as a severity score for initiation of methods such as high-frequency oscillatory ventilation (HFOV) and **extracorporeal life support (ECLS)**.[5,6]

More recently the ARDS Definition Task Force convened in Berlin in 2011 to refine the definition of ARDS. These investigators initially proposed three mutually exclusive categories of ARDS based on degree of hypoxemia in addition to four other variables reflecting clinical characteristics: radiographic severity, respiratory system compliance, positive end-expiratory pressure (PEEP), and corrected expired volume per minute. While the degree of hypoxemia was associated with increased mortality and increased duration of mechanical ventilation, the ancillary clinical variables were not predictive of outcomes. The final Berlin definition of ARDS therefore stratifies patients as mild (PaO_2/FIO_2 201 to 300 mm Hg), moderate (PaO_2/FIO_2 101 to 200 mm Hg), or severe (PaO_2/FIO_2 <100 mm Hg) ARDS (**Table 38-1**).[7]

In the future, it is likely that newer methods and measurements will be able to better characterize ARDS. These may include cytokine profiles, inflammatory cellular responses, genetic expression patterns, comorbidities, and accompanying organ injuries, which all have the potential to better stratify the various clinical phenotypes of ARDS.

TABLE 38-1
AECC and Berlin Definitions of ALI and ARDS

	AECC Definition	Berlin Definition
Timing	Acute onset	Onset within 1 week of a known clinical insult or new or worsening respiratory symptoms
Chest imaging	Bilateral infiltrates	Bilateral opacities not fully explained by effusions, lobar/lung collapse, or nodules
Origin of edema	PAWP ≤18 mm Hg or no clinical evidence of left atrial hypertension	Respiratory failure not fully explained by cardiac failure or fluid overload. Need objective assessment to exclude hydrostatic edema if no ARDS risk factor present
Category: PaO_2/FIO_2	ALI: ≤300 mm Hg regardless of PEEP or CPAP ARDS: ≤200 mm Hg regardless of PEEP or CPAP	Mild: 201–300 mm Hg with PEEP or CPAP 5 cm H_2O Moderate: 101–200 mm Hg with PEEP or CPAP 5 cm H_2O Severe: ≤100 mm Hg with PEEP or CPAP 5 cm H_2O

AECC, American-European Consensus Conference; ALI, acute lung injury; ARDS, acute respiratory distress syndrome; PAWP, pulmonary artery wedge pressure; PEEP, positive end-expiratory pressure; CPAP, continuous positive airway pressure.

Reproduced from Bernard GR, Artigas A, Brigham KL, et al. The American–European Consensus Conference on ARDS: definitions, mechanisms, relevant outcomes, and clinical trial coordination. *Am J Respir Crit Care Med.* 1994;149:818–824; Information from acute respiratory distress syndrome: the Berlin definition. ARDS Definition Task Force. *JAMA.* 2012;307(23):2526–2533.

Incidence

Efforts to determine the prevalence of ARDS have resulted in widely varying estimates. An initial report by the National Institutes of Health in 1972 estimated 75 cases of ARDS per 100,000 population (approximately 150,000 cases of ARDS per year) in the United States.[8] Other studies have often found lower estimates, ranging from 3 to 13.5 cases per 100,000 population.[9–11] The most recent study suggested a range of 79 to 86 per 100,000 person-years.[12] Approximately 10% to 15% of patients admitted to the intensive care unit (ICU) meet the diagnostic criteria for ARDS.[13]

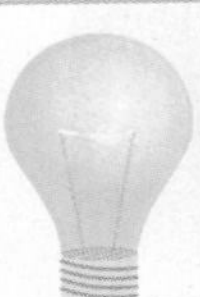

STOP AND THINK

You are caring for a patient with hypoxemic respiratory failure who was recently intubated. How would you know if the patient has ARDS?

Etiology

Multiple clinical conditions have been associated with the development of ARDS (**Box 38-1**).[14] Risk factors can be described as those that cause *direct* injury to the lungs (such as pneumonia, aspiration of gastric contents, inhalation of toxic gases, or pulmonary contusion)—so-called **primary ARDS**—and those that cause *indirect* injury to the lung (such as sepsis, multiple trauma, pancreatitis, or transfusion of blood products)—so-called **secondary ARDS**. In the case of indirect injury, ARDS is thought to be the result of systemic inflammation, which results in the release of proinflammatory mediators and neutrophil migration to the alveoli. Overall, patients with sepsis are those at the highest risk to develop ARDS, with a 40% incidence.[15] Secondary risk factors such as low serum pH, chronic lung disease, and chronic alcohol abuse have been associated with an increased risk for ARDS.[16] If patients with ARDS from a direct lung injury subsequently develop sepsis or shock, they can develop an indirect lung injury as well. The distinction between direct and indirect injury thus is often blurred.

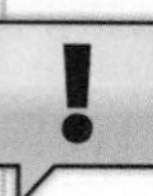

Respiratory Recap

Risk Factors for ARDS

- Direct injury to the lungs such as pneumonia or aspiration.
- Indirect injury to the lungs such as sepsis, multiple trauma, or acute pancreatitis.

BOX 38-1

Clinical Disorders Associated with ARDS

Direct Lung Injury (Primary Lung Injury)

Common causes

- Pneumonia
- Aspiration of gastric contents

Less common causes

- Pulmonary contusion
- Fat emboli
- Near-drowning
- Inhalation injury
- Reperfusion pulmonary edema after cardiopulmonary bypass

Indirect Lung Injury (Secondary Lung Injury)

Common causes

- Sepsis
- Trauma with shock and blood product transfusion

Less common causes

- Drug overdose
- Cardiopulmonary bypass
- Acute pancreatitis
- Transfusion of blood products

Reproduced from Ware LB, Matthay MA. The acute respiratory distress syndrome. *N Engl J Med*. 2000;342:18:1334–1348. © 2000 Massachusetts Medical Society. Reprinted with permission from Massachusetts Medical Society.

Clinical Manifestations

Patients with ARDS are symptomatic with progressive dyspnea and acutely abnormal oxygenation. Hypoxemia is primarily the result of shunt caused by atelectasis and alveolar flooding. In addition, disturbance of the normally protective mechanism of hypoxic pulmonary vasoconstriction contributes to shunt and hypoxemia. Patients in the first few days of ARDS experience a decrease in lung compliance, partly because of alveolar and interstitial edema, but also due to surfactant function impairment. Decreased compliance and hypoxemia together lead to rapid, shallow breathing with increased minute ventilation and an increased work of breathing. Many patients with ARDS require **mechanical ventilation**.

Chest radiographic findings show bilateral opacities reflecting inflammatory exudates and noncardiogenic pulmonary edema (**Figure 38-1**). The opacities may be confluent, patchy, or asymmetric and can be complicated by pleural effusions and heart failure. Because ARDS can represent a myriad of disease processes, the

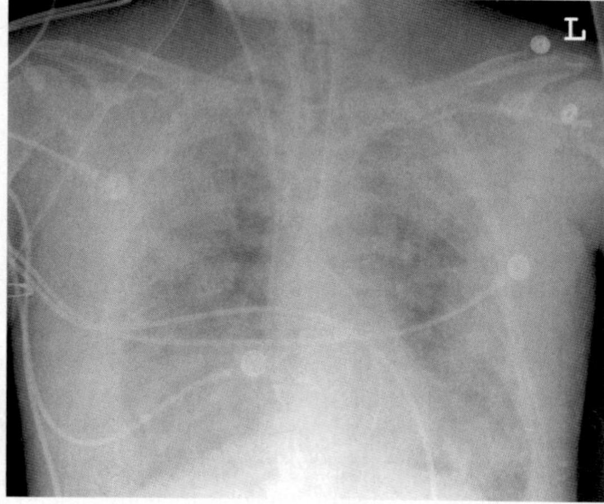

FIGURE 38-1 Anteroposterior supine radiograph of a patient with acute respiratory distress syndrome.

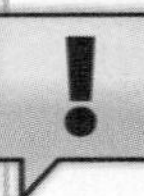

Respiratory Recap

Clinical Manifestations of ARDS

- Profound hypoxemia early in the disease course
- Decreased lung compliance
- Rapid shallow breathing pattern
- Increased dead space
- Bilateral opacities on chest x-ray
- Heterogeneity of disease on chest CT; dependent atelectasis

chest radiograph may also range from mild infiltrates to diffuse, dense consolidation, both extremes meeting the radiographic criteria for a diagnosis of ARDS. Chest radiographs in patients requiring higher levels of positive pressure ventilation may reveal evidence of barotrauma such as pneumothorax, pneumomediastinum, or pneumatoceles.[17]

Despite the appearance of diffuse infiltrates on the frontal chest radiograph, ARDS is not a homogeneous process. Although not necessary for the diagnosis of ARDS, computed tomography (CT) of the chest better demonstrates the heterogeneity of this disease (**Figure 38-2**).[18,19] More dependent portions of the lungs often demonstrate greater atelectasis than the more nondependent areas. This helps explain the different effects of positive airway pressure seen in these different regions of the lung.[19,20]

Some patients with ARDS longer than 3 to 7 days enter the fibroproliferative phase. Profound hypoxemia may subside, but poor compliance often continues, in part because of the development of fibrosis. Rather than intrapulmonary shunting, the problem at this phase is increasing dead space (high-$\dot{V}/\dot{Q}$ regions) resulting in increasing minute ventilation requirements. Dead space in excess of 70% may occur and has been associated with high mortality.[21] These patients may ultimately develop pulmonary hypertension and, in some cases, right heart dysfunction.[22]

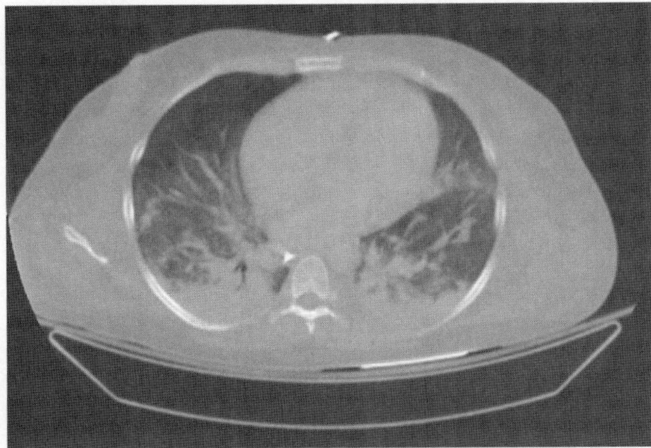

FIGURE 38-2 Computed tomography (CT) of the chest of a patient with acute respiratory distress syndrome.

Pathobiology

ARDS is characterized by acute alveolar inflammation, neutrophil activation, surfactant deficiencies, damage to the alveolar-capillary membrane (increased permeability, neutrophil and bacterial migration), and development of proteinaceous pulmonary edema and alveolar collapse.[23]

Destruction of the type I alveolar epithelial cells leads to detachment from their underlying basement membrane. This results in impairment of the normal anatomic barrier, which leads to increased permeability and resultant influx of protein-rich edema fluid into the interstitium and alveolar space (**Figure 38-3**). This denuded basement membrane becomes covered with a layer of fibrin, known as the hyaline membrane. These findings are described pathologically as diffuse alveolar damage. In patients with persistent lung injury (3 to 7 days after initial lung injury), the disease process progresses to a stage at which the basement membrane is replaced with a more fibrotic material enhanced by proliferation of alveolar type II cells. Additional destruction of the pulmonary vasculature is caused by fibrosis and microthrombi in the capillary bed.[24,25]

Although no clinically available marker exists that correlates with lung injury, bronchoalveolar lavage (BAL) results have provided a better understanding of the inflammation occurring in the alveolar space.[26–28] Analysis of BAL fluid in patients with early ARDS reveals a high percentage of neutrophils, usually present in only trace amounts in a normal lung lavage. As lung injury progresses, neutrophils tend to be replaced with alveolar macrophages and lymphocytes. A higher mortality in patients with persistence of alveolar neutrophils is found, however, due to their destructive nature and release of cellular debris.[29,30]

Management

Management of patients with ARDS involves a multidisciplinary approach. Early detection and treatment of the underlying and causative pathophysiology is paramount. This includes hemodynamic management, appropriate use of antibiotics, and surgical intervention when required. These actions are used in conjunction with supportive care involving lung-protective mechanical ventilation strategies and prevention of nosocomial infection. Of note is that many of our current management approaches have been a product of several large clinical trials conducted by the National Institutes of Health **ARDS Network (ARDSnet)**, a multicenter research consortium first assembled in 1994. ARDSnet trial results are detailed in many of the sections below.

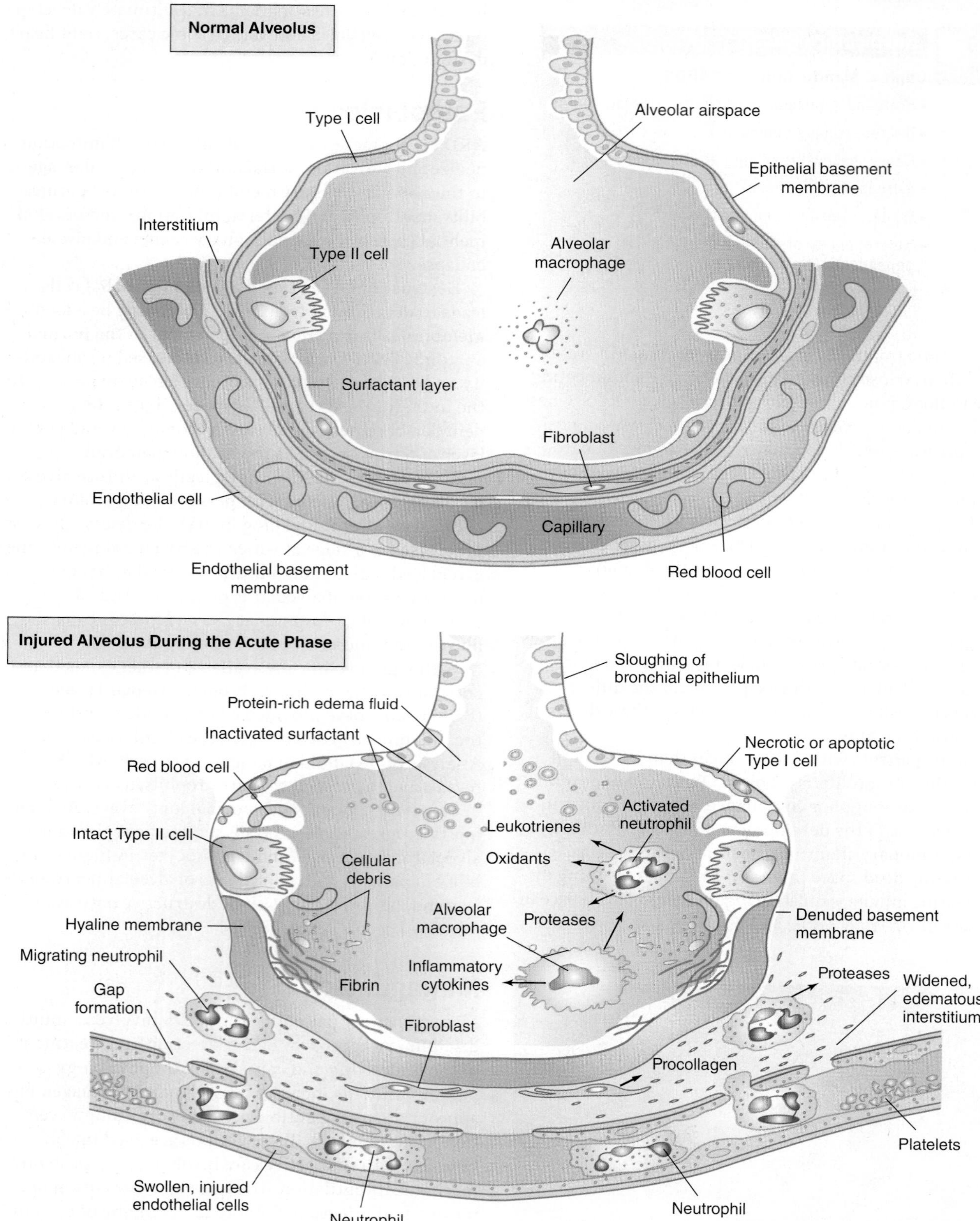

FIGURE 38-3 (**A**) Normal alveolus and (**B**) the injured alveolus in the acute phase of the acute respiratory distress syndrome. Neutrophils are shown adhering to the injured capillary endothelium and marginating through the interstitium into the airspace, which is filled with protein-rich edema fluid. In the airspace, an alveolar macrophage is secreting inflammatory cytokines, which act locally to stimulate chemotaxis and activate neutrophils. Macrophages also secrete other cytokines. Neutrophils can release oxidants, proteases, leukotrienes, and other proinflammatory molecules, such as platelet-activating factor. A number of anti-inflammatory mediators are also present in the alveolar milieu. The influx of protein-rich edema fluid into the alveolus has led to the inactivation of surfactant.

Adapted from Ware LB, Matthay MA. The acute respiratory distress syndrome. *N Engl J Med.* 2000;342:1334–1348.

Mechanical Ventilation

Patients with ARDS are first seen in either respiratory distress or respiratory failure (i.e., patients with symptomatic but not life-threatening physiology versus patients with life-threatening physiology). For respiratory distress, dyspnea and hypoxemia should be treated with supplemental oxygen and preparations made for escalation of care, including endotracheal intubation. Because the course of ARDS may include hemodynamic instability, sedation usage, and multisystem organ failure, many patients are not candidates for noninvasive ventilation (NIV). Endotracheal intubation should be performed before a patient progresses to full acute respiratory failure.

Mechanical ventilation is often required due to the severity of hypoxemia and can be life saving for patients with ARDS. The goal of mechanical ventilation for these patients is support of gas exchange without inducing further injury to the lungs. Because of the heterogeneity of the lungs of patients with ARDS, mechanical ventilation strategies include alveolar recruitment while avoiding overdistention of normal lung units.

Prolonged exposure to large tidal volumes (VT) and high transpulmonary pressures can overdistend alveoli and contribute to a cascade of lung and systemic inflammatory responses that can worsen the underlying lung injury (ventilator-induced lung injury, or VILI). VILI can manifest as air leak (barotrauma), diffuse alveolar damage by overinflation (volutrauma), or shear stress when collapsed lung units repeatedly open and close (atelectrauma). Growing appreciation for VILI has placed an emphasis on avoiding alveolar overdistention and cyclic alveolar collapse and re-expansion.

For much of the 20th century, VT was set at 10 to 15 mL/kg of body weight to normalize gas exchange. What has been termed **lung-protective ventilation** reduces the VT to near-normal ranges (4 to 8 mL/kg ideal body weight), thus decreasing the injurious alveolar stretch and subsequent release of inflammatory mediators. The use of a lung-protective ventilation strategy reduces mortality and should be employed in all patients with ARDS.[31–37]

The best evidence supporting lung-protective ventilation comes from the ARDSnet study of higher versus lower VT.[37] In this study, 861 patients were randomized to a VT of 6 mL/kg (lung protective) or 12 mL/kg (traditional), based on ideal body weight, rather than actual body weight. **Plateau pressure** was limited to 30 cm H_2O in the lung-protective group and 50 cm H_2O in the traditional group. A significant mortality difference was noted: 31% in the lung-protective group compared with 40% in the traditional group. In addition, levels of plasma interleukin-6, an important inflammatory cytokine, were noted to be lower in the lung-protective group. These data support the hypothesis that alveolar stretch can propagate systemic inflammation and can subsequently lead to multiple organ dysfunction and death.[37] For patients with ARDS, the ventilator should be set to achieve the lowest possible plateau pressure.

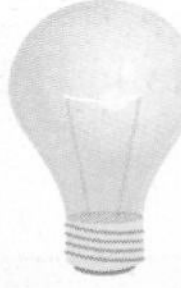

STOP AND THINK

You are caring for a mechanically ventilated patient with ARDS. How do you select an appropriate tidal volume and PEEP?

Raising F_{IO_2} improves Pa_{O_2} in low-$\dot{V}/\dot{Q}$ units but has little effect on Pa_{O_2} in the presence of shunt. Moreover, high F_{IO_2} can cause lung damage through free radical formation (oxygen toxicity). Efforts thus should be made to minimize F_{IO_2} exposure.[38,39] PEEP improves oxygenation by maintaining alveolar recruitment and thereby reducing shunt. Increased alveolar recruitment with PEEP also improves lung compliance and likely reduces VILI from shear forces that result when alveoli repetitively open and close.[20,31] PEEP has some potential negative effects as well, however. By increasing intrathoracic pressure, it can decrease venous return and cardiac output. Additionally, PEEP can result in overdistention of open alveoli and cause VILI and barotrauma.[40] Overdistention can increase resistance to blood flow in ventilated areas, resulting in increased dead space.

Investigators have proposed various mechanical (e.g., pressure–volume curve, stress index, best compliance, esophageal pressure) or radiographic (e.g., CT) approaches to optimize PEEP and F_{IO_2} settings. These approaches may be impractical for routine use. Balancing PEEP and F_{IO_2} to provide adequate oxygenation (e.g., Pa_{O_2} of 55 to 80 mm Hg) thus is often empiric. PEEP–F_{IO_2} tables were developed to assist clinicians in selecting the appropriate combinations of PEEP and F_{IO_2} (**Table 38-2**).

Attention to blood pressure, tidal volume, plateau pressure, and cardiac output (directly or by assessment of end-organ perfusion) is also important. Large multicenter randomized trials have evaluated higher versus moderate PEEP levels and have failed to show superiority of higher PEEP levels.[41–43] The results of a subsequent meta-analysis of these trials suggest that higher levels of PEEP are more effective in moderate to severe ARDS, whereas modest levels of PEEP are more effective in mild ARDS.[44] PEEP should be reduced slowly as an abrupt reduction in PEEP may be associated with alveolar derecruitment and rapid arterial oxygen desaturation.

High-frequency oscillatory ventilation (HFOV) delivers small VT, increased $\overline{P}aw$, and frequencies of 1 to 15 Hz (1 Hz = 60 breaths/min). Oxygenation is related to $\overline{P}aw$, facilitating the maintenance of end-expiratory lung volume, which may minimize VILI.[45] An observational study of adult patients with severe ARDS failing conventional ventilation reported a decrease in OI after starting HFOV.[46] Another study reported that early institution of HFOV was a significant factor for improved mortality.[47] Recently, two large multicenter randomized controlled trials were performed comparing the use of HFOV to standard lung-protective

TABLE 38-2
ARDSnet Mechanical Ventilation PEEP/FIO_2 Tables

Lower PEEP Strategy

FIO_2	0.3	0.4	0.4	0.5	0.5	0.6	0.7	0.7	0.7	0.8	0.9	0.9	0.9	1.0
PEEP	5	5	8	8	10	10	10	12	14	14	14	16	18	18–24

(A)

Higher PEEP Strategy

FIO_2	0.3	0.3	0.3	0.3	0.3	0.4	0.4	0.5	0.5	0.5–0.8	0.8	0.9	1.0	1.0
PEEP	5	8	10	12	14	14	16	16	18	20	22	22	22	24

(B)

ventilation in patients with ARDS. One study demonstrated no difference in mortality, whereas the other demonstrated increased mortality in the HFOV group.[48,49] Based on these results, routine use of HFOV is not recommended. It might be considered in the setting of severe refractory hypoxemia, but it should only be used at centers with extensive experience with this modality.

Another mode of ventilation that is increasingly being utilized is airway pressure release ventilation (APRV), which aims to increase the $\bar{P}aw$ through long inflation times in order to improve oxygenation.[50] APRV is a form of inverse ratio ventilation (IRV) but differs from older approaches to IRV in that spontaneous breathing is allowed during the inflation. In concept, this allows for better gas mixing and improved patient tolerance. No large clinical trials are available that demonstrate a significant clinical benefit to this mode of ventilation, however.

Extracorporeal Life Support

Despite maximal supportive care with mechanical ventilation, some patients with ARDS experience severe refractory hypoxemia. Extracorporeal life support (ECLS), also called extracorporeal membrane oxygenation (ECMO), uses venoarterial and venovenous approaches to remove CO_2 and add O_2 to blood. Venoarterial systems can provide complete cardiopulmonary bypass, whereas the simpler venovenous systems provide only partial support. Extracorporeal techniques provide adequate gas exchange with a lower inspired FIO_2 and reduced ventilation pressures. Complications include clot formation in the circuit, bleeding due to systemic anticoagulation, and technical failure leading to hemodynamic compromise. These complications are more common with venoarterial ECLS. Several studies have reported benefit with the use of ECLS in patients with ARDS and severe respiratory failure.[51,52] One study reported improvement in survival without severe disability at 6 months in patients transferred to a specialist center for consideration of ECLS treatment compared with continued conventional ventilation.[52] While the complexity and thoughtfulness of this study are notable, some aspects of its design have been criticized, therefore making the ideal role of ECLS in severe ARDS unclear.

Pharmacologic Agents

Neuromuscular blockade with cisatracurium during early, severe ARDS may reduce mortality. Patients with a PaO_2/FIO_2 of <150 were randomized to either receive 48 hours of cisatracurium or placebo. Mortality was reduced in the cisatracurium group, and notably, there was no long-term difference in muscle weakness between survivors in each group, which has previously been a major concern with the use of neuromuscular blocking agents in critically ill patients.[53] A follow-up meta-analysis confirmed these findings, but it was largely influenced by the aforementioned trial.[54] The improvement in mortality is likely related to better patient–ventilator synchrony and reduced early ventilator-induced lung injury. The use of neuromuscular blocking agents should be considered early in patients with ARDS in whom patient–ventilator synchrony is difficult to achieve despite adequate sedation.

Given the inflammatory response in ARDS, the use of corticosteroids, potent inhibitors of inflammation, has been proposed, but an appropriate balance of proinflammatory and anti-inflammatory mediators must be maintained.[55] Corticosteroids used early in the course of ARDS have not proven beneficial.[56–58] A randomized controlled trial sponsored by the ARDSnet addressed the potential benefits of corticosteroids in late-stage ARDS.[59]

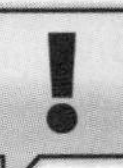

Respiratory Recap

Management of ARDS

- Most pharmacologic interventions have not proven to be useful
- Evidence does not support the routine use of steroids
- Prone position improves oxygenation and may improve outcome in patients with severe ARDS
- Effective ventilatory strategies include PEEP to maintain alveolar recruitment and low tidal volumes to avoid alveolar overdistention
- The timing and management of enteral feeding are controversial
- The role of extracorporeal life support in severe ARDS is unclear
- A conservative fluid management strategy may result in a shorter ventilator duration
- Early, short-term use of neuromuscular blockade may reduce mortality

Patients with ARDS of at least 7 days duration were randomized to either intravenous methylprednisolone or placebo. Although there appeared to be earlier extubations in the treated patients, at 60 days the hospital mortality rate and number of ventilator-free days were the same in each group. These results do not support the routine use of methylprednisolone for persistent ARDS.

Other anti-inflammatory agents such as ibuprofen, ketoconazole, and lisophylline have been shown to be ineffective in large randomized trials.[60,61] Some trials have investigated treatment with surfactant therapy.[62,63] Several different surfactant replacement products and delivery devices have been evaluated, but studies to date have not reported an improvement in survival.

Interventions with antioxidants (vitamin E or *N*-acetylcysteine) have been pursued with varying results.[64–66] In a randomized controlled study by the ARDSnet comparing standard enteral feeding to a formula supplemented with antioxidants along with omega-3 fatty acids and gamma-linoleic acid, the investigators reported that the group receiving the supplement had no improvement in outcomes and trended toward worse outcomes.[67]

Inhaled nitric oxide (iNO) can decrease pulmonary artery pressure, improve right ventricular function, and improve ventilation-perfusion matching, leading to improved oxygenation.[68–70] Despite these potential advantages, randomized controlled trials of iNO in patients with ARDS did not show an effect on mortality or any other meaningful outcomes.[71,72] Its routine use is discouraged, especially given the significant expense associated with iNO. Other inhaled vasodilators, such as prostacyclin, improve gas exchange in patients with ARDS, but the effect of these agents on patient outcomes is unknown.[73,74]

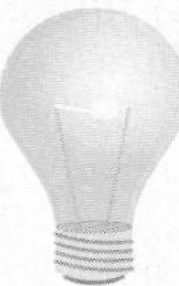

STOP AND THINK

What options are available to address refractory hypoxemic respiratory failure in a patient with ARDS?

Nutrition

Although few would argue that adequate nutrition is not important for recovery in critically ill patients, the timing and management of enteral feeding in ARDS have been controversial. On the one hand, aggressive attempts to rapidly reach nutrition goals would seem reasonable. Such a strategy may raise the risk of aspiration. An alternative approach is trickle feeding where the goal is to only supply enough enteral feeding to maintain gut epithelial function. An ARDSnet study compared lower-volume trophic feeding with full enteral feeding for the initial 6 days of mechanical ventilation for ARDS and found no differences in any clinically important outcome.[75]

Patient Position

Changes in body position may improve ventilation-perfusion matching and oxygenation, particularly in patients with very asymmetric disease. The use of the **prone position** is based on restoration of ventilation to dorsal areas of the lung that are collapsed in the supine position. Physiologic data suggest that gas exchange is improved in the prone position,[76] presumably because it improves shunt.[77–79] Prone positioning was not shown to significantly improve mortality in a combined group of patients with either moderate or severe ARDS.[80] In a group of patients with more severe ARDS (PaO_2/FIO_2 <150), however, prone positioning led to an absolute reduction in mortality of 16.8% compared to standard low tidal volume ventilation.[81]

While prone positioning is an important tool in the management of patients with severe ARDS, it should be performed in a facility that is familiar with the procedure and that has the resources to safely perform the maneuver. Complications include inadvertent removal of tubes and lines, pressure necrosis, and ocular injury.

Fluid Management

Because the pathophysiology of ARDS is characterized by lung edema formation, there has been long-standing interest in how best to manage fluids in these patients. While fluid restriction and diuresis may improve gas exchange and mechanical function, increased fluid volume would be expected to improve cardiac output and oxygen delivery. An ARDSnet study showed that a strategy of even fluid balance led to shorter ventilator duration compared with a traditional strategy that usually results in 1 liter or more positive fluid balance per day. Importantly, this conservative fluid strategy did not increase the incidence of shock or renal failure.[82]

Outcomes

ARDS mortality rates declined from a range of 60% to 70% in the early 1980s to 30% to 40% in the mid-1990s.[83,84] Examination of the mortality rate throughout the ARDSnet trials has demonstrated that the mortality rate associated with ARDS has decreased from 36% in 1996 to 22% in 2006.[85] While these trials may not be an exact representation of the general ARDS population, they do demonstrate the progress that has been made in the care of these patients.

Approximately one-third of the mortality occurs within the first 72 hours after onset. The cause of death in these patients is usually related to their underlying risk, such as sepsis or trauma. Only a minority (15%) of patients die from respiratory failure. The majority of ARDS mortality is in the setting of sepsis or multisystem organ failure.[86,87]

Assessments of pulmonary function, neuropsychiatric testing, and quality of life are important markers of outcome. Pulmonary function tests performed within 2 weeks of extubation have shown substantial restrictive impairments and impaired diffusing capacities.[86] This abnormal diffusing capacity is consistent with the known vascular destruction that occurs as part of the acute process of ARDS. In these patients, pulmonary function improved at 3 months, and further improvement was seen at 6 months. Little additional improvement was noted after that time, and no further gains were noted at 1 year. At the end of 1 year, most pulmonary function tests had returned to normal or had mild to moderate restriction, with an abnormal diffusing capacity being most common. Whereas many patients require oxygen at the time of hospital discharge, a persistent gas exchange abnormality at 1 year is uncommon, except for oxygen desaturation occasionally seen with exercise. Ultimate lung function is most consistently associated with the severity of the original lung injury and with duration of mechanical ventilation.

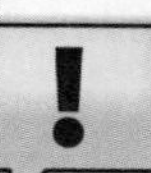

Respiratory Recap

ARDS Outcomes

- Mortality can be as high as 30% to 40%
- About one-third of patients who die do so within the first 72 hours
- Mortality is usually not due to inability to support lung function
- Most patients' lung function returns to near-normal within one year of discharge
- Many ARDS survivors have a lower than expected health-related quality of life and cognitive function

The impact of ARDS on quality of life was assessed by comparison of these patients with non-ARDS patients with similar levels of critical illness.[87] ARDS survivors were noted to have lower health-related quality of life scores. Decrements in perceived quality of life may persist for over a year. When tested at the 1-year interval, one-third of the patients had generalized cognitive decline, and 75% had at least one impairment in memory, attention, concentration, or mental processing speed.[88]

Although the outcome measures of pulmonary function, quality of life, and cognitive functioning are not as clearly defined or as readily attainable as mortality rates, they do represent a significant impact on the lives of the survivors.[89] Better understanding of these deficits will allow future research efforts to focus on these issues and will direct appropriate resources toward the care of these patients.

Key Points

- Current practice uses the Berlin definition of ARDS.
- Because of differences in definitions and study design, no clear national or worldwide incidence of ARDS can be estimated at this time.
- The most common risk factors for ARDS are sepsis, aspiration of gastric contents, transfusions, and severe trauma.
- ARDS is a heterogeneous disease and is characterized by alveolar inflammation and increased permeability of the alveolocapillary membrane.
- There are no proven effective drug therapies for ARDS.
- The most important therapeutic advance for treatment of ARDS has been the identification of lung-protective ventilatory strategies.
- Use a tidal volume of 6 mL/kg ideal body weight and a plateau pressure of less than 30 cm H_2O (lower if possible).
- Use PEEP to maintain alveolar recruitment.
- Mortality for ARDS patients has decreased significantly since the 1980s.
- ARDS survivors have mild to moderate pulmonary restriction and decreased diffusing capacity at 1 year.
- Decrements in quality of life and cognitive function are noted in ARDS survivors.

References

1. Ashbaugh DG, Bigelow DB, Petty TL, et al. Acute respiratory distress in adults. *Lancet*. 1967;12:319–323.
2. Petty TL, Ashbaugh DG. The adult respiratory distress syndrome; clinical features, factors influencing prognosis and principles of management. *Chest*. 1971;233–239.
3. Bernard GR, Artigas A, Brigham KL, et al. The American–European consensus conference on ARDS: definitions, mechanisms, relevant outcomes, and clinical trial coordination. *Am J Respir Crit Care Med*. 1994;149:818–824.

4. Murray JF, Matthay MA, Luce JM, et al. An expanded definition of the adult respiratory distress syndrome. *Am Rev Resp Dis.* 1988;138:720–723.
5. Mehta S, Granton J, MacDonald RJ, et al. High-frequency oscillatory ventilation in adults. *Chest.* 2004;126:518–527.
6. Monchi M, Bellenfant F, Cariou A, et al. Early predictive factors of survival in the acute respiratory distress syndrome. A multivariate analysis. *Am J Respir Crit Care Med.* 1998;158:1076–1081.
7. ARDS Definition Task Force. Acute respiratory distress syndrome: the Berlin definition. *JAMA.* 2012;307:2526–2533.
8. National Heart and Lung Institutes. *Task Force Report on Problems, Research Approaches, Needs.* Washington, DC: U.S. Government Printing Office; 1972:167–180.
9. Villar J, Slutsky AS. The incidence of the adult respiratory distress syndrome. *Am Rev Respir Dis.* 1989;140:814–816.
10. Lewandowski K, Metz J, Deutschmann C, et al. Incidence, severity, and mortality of acute respiratory failure in Berlin, Germany. *Am J Respir Crit Care Med.* 1995;151:1121–1125.
11. Thomsen GE, Morris AH. Incidence of the adult respiratory distress syndrome in the state of Utah. *Am J Respir Crit Care Med.* 1995;152:965–971.
12. Rubenfeld GD, Caldwell E, Peabody E, et al. Incidence and outcomes of acute lung injury. *N Engl J Med.* 2005;353:1685–1693.
13. Frutos-Vivar F, Nin N, Estaban A. Epidemiology of acute lung injury and acute respiratory distress syndrome. *Curr Opin Crit Care.* 2004;10:1–6.
14. Ware LB, Matthay MA. The acute respiratory distress syndrome. *N Engl J Med.* 2000;432:1334–1348.
15. Hudson LD, Milberg JA, Anardi D, et al. Clinical risks for development of the acute respiratory distress syndrome. *Am J Respir Crit Care Med.* 1995;151:293–301.
16. Doyle RL, Szaflarski N, Modin GW, et al. Identification of patients with acute lung injury. Predictors of mortality. *Am J Respir Crit Care Med.* 1995;152:1818–1824.
17. Steinberg KP. Diffuse pulmonary infiltrates and acute respiratory distress syndrome. In: Root RK, ed. *Clinical Infectious Diseases: A Practical Approach.* New York: Oxford University Press; 1999:557–564.
18. Gattinoni L, Caironi P, Valenza F, et al. The role of CT-scan studies for the diagnosis and therapy of acute respiratory distress syndrome. *Clin Chest Med.* 2006;27:559–570.
19. Gattinoni L, Caironi P, Cressoni M, et al. Lung recruitment in patients with the acute respiratory distress syndrome. *N Engl J Med.* 2006;354:1775–1786.
20. Gattinoni L, Pelosi P, Crotti S, et al. Effects of positive end-expiratory pressure on regional distribution of tidal volume and recruitment in adult respiratory distress syndrome. *Am J Respir Crit Care Med.* 1995;151:1807–1814.
21. Nuckton TJ, Alonso JA, Kallet RH, et al. Pulmonary dead-space fraction as a risk factor for death in the acute respiratory distress syndrome. *N Engl J Med.* 2002;346:1281–1286.
22. Brower RG, Ware LB, Berthiaume Y, et al. Treatment of ARDS. *Chest.* 2001;120:1347–1367.
23. Piantadosi CA, Schwartz DA. The acute respiratory distress syndrome. *Ann Intern Med.* 2004;141:460–471.
24. Artigas A, Bernard GR, Carlet J, et al. The American–European Consensus Conference on ARDS. Part 2. Ventilatory, pharmacologic, supportive therapy, study design strategies, and issues related to recovery and remodeling. *Am J Respir Crit Care Med.* 1998;157:1332–1347.
25. Idell S. Endothelium and disordered fibrin turnover in the injured lung: newly recognized pathways. *Crit Care Med.* 2002;30(Suppl 5):S274–S280.
26. Pugin J, Verghese G, Widmer M, et al. The alveolar space is the site of intense inflammatory and profibrotic reactions in the early phase of acute respiratory distress syndrome. *Crit Care Med.* 1999;27:237–238.
27. Goodman RB, Strieter RM, Martin DP, et al. Inflammatory cytokines in patients with persistence of the acute respiratory distress syndrome. *Am J Respir Crit Care Med.* 1996;154:601–611.
28. Martin TR. Lung cytokines and ARDS. *Chest.* 1999;116(Suppl 1):2S–8S.
29. Steinberg KP, Milberg JA, Martin TR, et al. Evolution of bronchoalveolar cell populations in the adult respiratory distress syndrome. *Am J Respir Crit Care Med.* 1994;150:113–122.
30. Meduri GU, Headley S, Kohler G, et al. Persistent elevation of inflammatory cytokines predicts a poor outcome in ARDS. Plasma IL-1 and IL-6 levels are consistent and efficient predictors of outcome over time. *Chest.* 1995;107:1062–1073.
31. Webb HH, Tierney DF. Experimental pulmonary edema due to intermittent positive pressure ventilation with high inflation pressures: protection by positive end-expiratory pressure. *Am Rev Respir Dis.* 1974;110:556–565.
32. Dreyfuss D, Saumon G. Role of tidal volume, FRC, and end-inspiratory volume in the development of pulmonary edema following mechanical ventilation. *Am Rev Respir Dis.* 1993;148:1194–1203.
33. Brochard L, Roudot-Thoraval F, Roupie E, et al. Tidal volume reduction for prevention of ventilator-induced lung injury in acute respiratory distress syndrome. The Multicenter Trial Group on Tidal Volume Reduction in ARDS. *Am J Respir Crit Care Med.* 1998;158:1831–1838.
34. Stewart TE, Meade MO, Cook DJ, et al. Evaluation of a ventilation strategy to prevent barotrauma in patients at high risk for acute respiratory distress syndrome. *N Engl J Med.* 1998;338:355–361.
35. Amato MB, Barbas CS, Medeiros DM, et al. Effect of a protective-ventilation strategy on mortality in the acute respiratory distress syndrome. *N Engl J Med.* 1998;338:347–354.
36. Ranieri VM, Suter PM, Tortorella C, et al. Effect of mechanical ventilation on inflammatory mediators in patients with acute respiratory distress syndrome: a randomized controlled trial. *JAMA.* 1999;282:54–61.
37. The Acute Respiratory Distress Syndrome Network. Ventilation with lower tidal volumes as compared with traditional tidal volumes for acute lung injury and the acute respiratory distress syndrome. *N Engl J Med.* 2000;342:1301–1318.
38. Singer MM, Wright F, Stanley LK, et al. Oxygen toxicity in man. A prospective study in patients after open-heart surgery. *N Engl J Med.* 1970;283:1473–1478.
39. Frank L, Roberts RJ. Endotoxin protection against oxygen-induced acute and chronic lung injury. *J Appl Physiol.* 1979;47:577–581.
40. Rouby JJ, Lu Q, Goldstein I. Selecting the right level of positive end expiratory pressure in patients with acute respiratory distress syndrome. *Am J Respir Crit Care Med.* 2002;165:1182–1186.
41. Brower RG, Lanken PN, MacIntyre N, et al. Higher versus lower positive end-expiratory pressures in patients with the acute respiratory distress syndrome. *N Engl J Med.* 2004;351:327–336.
42. Meade MO, Cook DJ, Guyatt GH, et al. Ventilation strategy using low tidal volumes, recruitment maneuvers, and high positive end-expiratory pressure for acute lung injury and acute respiratory distress syndrome: a randomized controlled trial. *JAMA.* 2008;299:637–645.
43. Mercat A, Richard JC, Vielle B, et al. Positive end-expiratory pressure setting in adults with acute lung injury and acute respiratory distress syndrome: a randomized controlled trial. *JAMA.* 2008;299:646–655.
44. Briel M, Meade M, Mercat A, Brower RG, et al. Higher vs lower positive end-expiratory pressure in patients with acute lung injury and acute respiratory distress syndrome: systematic review and meta-analysis. *JAMA.* 2010;303:865–873.
45. Pillow JJ. High-frequency oscillatory ventilation: mechanisms of gas exchange and lung mechanics. *Crit Care Med.* 2005;33(Suppl 3):S135–S141.
46. Fort P, Farmer C, Westerman J, et al. High frequency oscillatory ventilation for adult respiratory distress syndrome—a pilot study. *Crit Care Med.* 1997;25:937–947.
47. Mehta S, Lapinsky SE, Hallett DC, et al. Prospective trial of high-frequency oscillation in adults with acute respiratory distress syndrome. *Crit Care Med.* 2001;29:1360–1369.
48. Young D, Lamb SE, Shah S, et al. High-frequency oscillation for acute respiratory distress syndrome. *N Engl J Med.* 2013;368:806–813.

49. Ferguson ND, Cook DJ, Guyatt GH, et al. High-frequency oscillation in early acute respiratory distress syndrome. *N Engl J Med.* 2013;368:795–805.
50. Maung AA, Kaplan LJ. Airway pressure release ventilation in acute respiratory distress syndrome. *Crit Care Clin.* 2011;27;501–509.
51. The Australia and New Zealand Extracorporeal Membrane Oxygenation Influenza Investigators. Extracorporeal membrane oxygenation for 2009 influenza (H1N1) acute respiratory distress syndrome. *JAMA.* 2009;302:1535–1545.
52. Peek GJ, Mugford M, Tiruvoipati R, et al. Efficacy and economic assessment of conventional ventilatory support versus extracorporeal membrane oxygenation for severe adult respiratory failure (CESAR): a multicentre randomised controlled trial. *Lancet.* 2009;374:1351–1363.
53. Papazian L, Forel JM, Gacouin A, et al. Neuromuscular blockers in early acute respiratory distress syndrome. *N Engl J Med.* 2010;363:1107–1116.
54. Alhazzani W, Alshahrani M, Jaeschke R, et al. Neuromuscular blocking agents in acute respiratory distress syndrome: a systematic review and meta-analysis of randomized controlled trials. *Crit Care.* 2013;17:R43.
55. Martin TR. Cytokines and the acute respiratory distress syndrome (ARDS): a question of balance. *Nature Med.* 1997;3:272–273.
56. Lefering R, Neugebauer EA. Steroid controversy in sepsis and septic shock: a meta-analysis. *Crit Care Med.* 1995;23:1294–1303.
57. Cronin L, Cook DJ, Carlet J, et al. Corticosteroid treatment for sepsis: a critical appraisal and meta-analysis of the literature. *Crit Care Med.* 1995;23:1430–1439.
58. Meduri GU, Headley AS, Golden E, et al. Effect of prolonged methylprednisolone therapy in unresolving acute respiratory distress syndrome: a randomized controlled trial. *JAMA.* 1998;280:159–165.
59. Steinberg KP, Hudson LD, Goodman RB, et al. Efficacy and safety of corticosteroids for persistent acute respiratory distress syndrome. *N Engl J Med.* 2006;354:1671–1684.
60. The Acute Respiratory Distress Syndrome Network. Ketoconazole for early treatment of acute lung injury and acute respiratory distress syndrome: a randomized controlled trial. The ARDS Network. *JAMA.* 2000;283:1995–2002.
61. Bernard GR, Wheeler AP, Russell JA, et al. The effects of ibuprofen on the physiology and survival of patients with sepsis. The Ibuprofen in Sepsis Study Group. *N Engl J Med.* 1997;336:912–918.
62. Weg JG, Balk RA, Tharratt RS, et al. Safety and potential efficacy of an aerosolized surfactant in human sepsis-induced adult respiratory distress syndrome. *JAMA.* 1994;272:1433–1438.
63. Gregory TJ, Steinberg KP, Spragg R, et al. Bovine surfactant therapy for patients with acute respiratory distress syndrome. *Am J Respir Crit Care Med.* 1997;155:1309–1315.
64. Domenighetti G, Suter PM, Schaller MD, et al. Treatment with *N*-acetylcysteine during acute respiratory distress syndrome: a randomized, double-blind, placebo-controlled clinical study. *J Crit Care.* 1997;12:177–182.
65. Jepsen S, Herlevsen P, Knudsen P, et al. Antioxidant treatment with *N*-acetylcysteine during adult respiratory distress syndrome: a prospective, randomized, placebo controlled study. *Crit Care Med.* 1992;20:918–923.
66. Suter PM, Domenighetti G, Schaller MD, et al. *N*-acetylcysteine enhances recovery from acute lung injury in man. *Chest.* 1994;105:190–194.
67. Rice TW, Wheeler AP, Thompson BT, et al. Enteral omega-3 fatty acid, gamma-linolenic acid, and antioxidants supplementation in acute lung injury. *JAMA.* 2011;306:1574–1581.
68. Rossaint R, Falke KJ, Lopez F, et al. Inhaled nitric oxide for the adult respiratory distress syndrome. *N Engl J Med.* 1993;328:399–405.
69. Frostell CG, Blomqvist H, Hedenstierna G, et al. Inhaled nitric oxide selectively reverses human hypoxic pulmonary vasoconstriction without causing systemic vasodilation. *Anesthesiology.* 1993;78:427–435.
70. Gerlach H, Rossaint R, Pappert D, et al. Time-course and dose-response of nitric oxide inhalation for systemic oxygenation and pulmonary hypertension in patients with adult respiratory distress syndrome. *Eur J Clin Invest.* 1993;23:499–502.
71. Dellinger RP, Zimmerman JL, Taylor RW, et al. Effects of inhaled nitric oxide in patients with acute respiratory distress syndrome: results of a randomized phase II trial. Inhaled Nitric Oxide in ARDS Study Group. *Crit Care Med.* 1998;26:15–23.
72. Michael JR, Barton RG, Saffle JR, et al. Inhaled nitric oxide versus conventional therapy: effect on oxygenation in ARDS. *Am J Respir Crit Care Med.* 1998;157:1372–1380.
73. Siobal MS, Hess DR. Are inhaled vasodilators useful in acute lung injury and acute respiratory distress syndrome? *Respir Care.* 2010;55:144–161.
74. Sawheny E, Ellis AL, Kinasewitz GT. Iloprost improves gas exchange in patients with pulmonary hypertension and ARDS. *Chest.* 2013;144:55–62.
75. Rice TW, Wheeler AP, et al. Initial trophic vs full enteral feeding in patients with acute lung injury: the EDEN randomized trial. *JAMA.* 2012;307:795–803.
76. Albert RK, Hubmayr RD. The prone position eliminates compression of the lungs by the heart. *Am J Respir Crit Care Med.* 2000;161: 1660–1665.
77. Lamm WJE, Graham MM, Albert RK. Mechanism by which the prone position improves oxygenation in acute lung injury. *Am J Respir Crit Care Med.* 1994;150:184–193.
78. Nakos G, Tsangaris I, Kostanti E, et al. Effect of the prone position on patients with hydrostatic pulmonary edema compared with patients with acute respiratory distress syndrome and pulmonary fibrosis. *Am J Respir Crit Care Med.* 2000;161:360–368.
79. Jolliet P, Bulpa P, Chevrolet J. Effects of the prone position on gas exchange and hemodynamics in severe acute respiratory distress syndrome. *Crit Care Med.* 1998;26:1977–1985.
80. Taccone P, Pesenti A, Latini R, et al. Prone positioning in patients with moderate and severe acute respiratory distress syndrome: a randomized controlled trial. *JAMA.* 2009:302:1977–1984.
81. Guerin C, Reignier J, Richard JC, et al. Prone positioning in severe acute respiratory distress syndrome. *N Engl J Med.* 2013;368: 2159–2168.
82. Wheeler AP, Bernard GR, Thompson BT, et al. Pulmonary-artery versus central venous catheter to guide treatment of acute lung injury. *N Engl J Med.* 2006;354:2213–2224.
83. Montgomery AB, Stager MA, Carrico CJ, et al. Causes of mortality in patients with the adult respiratory distress syndrome. *Am Rev Respir Dis.* 1985;132:485–489.
84. Milberg JA, Davis DR, Steinberg KP, et al. Improved survival of patients with acute respiratory distress syndrome (ARDS): 1983–1993. *JAMA.* 1995;273:306–309.
85. Matthay MA, Ware LB, Zimmerman GA. The acute respiratory distress syndrome. *J Clin Invest.* 2012;122:2731–2740.
86. McHugh LG, Milberg JA, Whitcomb ME, et al. Recovery of function in survivors of the acute respiratory distress syndrome. *Am J Respir Crit Care Med.* 1994;150:90–94.
87. Herridge MS, Cheung AM, Tansey CM, et al. One-year outcomes in survivors of the acute respiratory distress syndrome. *N Engl J Med.* 2003;348:683–693.
88. Hopkins RO, Weaver LK, Pope D, et al. Neuropsychological sequelae and impaired health status in survivors of severe acute respiratory distress syndrome. *Am J Respir Crit Care Med.* 1999;160:50–56.
89. Cox CE, Docherty SL, Brandon DH, et al. Surviving critical illness: acute respiratory distress syndrome as experienced by patients and their caregivers. *Crit Care Med.* 2009;37:2702–2708.

CHAPTER

39

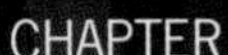

Postoperative Respiratory Care

Mark Simmons, Priscilla Simmons

OUTLINE

OBJECTIVES

1. List the steps in preoperative assessment and management.
2. Identify factors that increase the risk of postoperative pulmonary complications.
3. List the studies commonly performed during preoperative testing.
4. Identify the intraoperative factors that contribute to postoperative pulmonary complications.
5. Describe the common assessment and management practices employed to combat postoperative respiratory failure.
6. Discuss the etiology, risk factors, clinical manifestations, diagnostic findings, and management of postoperative atelectasis.
7. Discuss the etiology, risk factors, clinical manifestations, diagnostic findings, and management of postoperative thromboembolic disease and pulmonary embolism.
8. Discuss the etiology, risk factors, clinical manifestations, diagnostic findings, and management of postoperative pneumonia.

KEY TERMS

atelectasis
deep vein thrombosis (DVT)
heparin
myocardial ischemia
partial thromboplastin time (PTT)
patient-controlled analgesia (PCA)
pneumonia
pulmonary embolism (PE)
thrombolytic
tissue plasminogen activator (TPA)
total enteral nutrition (TEN)
total parenteral nutrition (TPN)

Introduction

Postoperative pulmonary complications (PPCs) can be defined as unexpected postoperative pulmonary abnormalities that produce identifiable disease or dysfunction that is clinically significant and requires therapeutic intervention. PPCs occur more frequently than postoperative cardiac complications and are a leading cause of postoperative morbidity and mortality.[1] PPCs also result in longer times spent in the ICU and increased hospital stays.[2] Most patients having thoracic or upper abdominal surgery will have a decrease in pulmonary function after surgery as a result of decreased lung volumes (atelectasis), diaphragmatic dysfunction, and ventilation-perfusion ($\dot{V}/\dot{Q}$) or gas exchange abnormalities. In addition, anesthesia may depress the postoperative respiratory drive. Inhibition of cough and impaired airway clearance of secretions can contribute to risk of infection. Many of these patients compensate for any decrease in pulmonary function with their pulmonary reserves, however. PPCs occur in approximately 7% of patients with normal preoperative lung function. Postoperative respiratory failure is rare without preexisting cardiopulmonary or neuromuscular disorders. In patients with increased risk factors, however, pulmonary complications have been reported to be as high as 70%. Postoperative reintubation is rare (about 0.5%).[3] This chapter addresses some of the preoperative and intraoperative factors that increase the

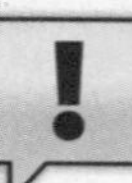

Respiratory Recap

Key Considerations in Preoperative Assessment and Management

- History and physical exam
- Detailed planning of surgery and postsurgical care and complications
- Patient education

risk of PPCs. Also included is management of the postoperative patient to prevent PPCs.

Preoperative Assessment and Management

The goal of preoperative evaluation is to identify patients who are at risk for intraoperative or postoperative complications. Multiple factors have been identified as risk factors for postoperative complications (**Box 39-1**).[4–7]

An important first step in preoperative management of nonemergent surgeries is obtaining a patient history. The history and physical may identify conditions that increase the risk of PPCs and identify indications for preoperative screening tests. Detailed preoperative planning of the surgery is necessary, including considerations for postoperative care. Nonelective and emergency procedures place the patient at higher risk because preoperative evaluation may not be completed and the surgery may need to be done regardless of the risk.

If a patient at risk is identified, the next step is to determine how complications can be prevented. In some cases this may mean postponement of surgery or a change in the anesthesia or surgical plan. Other interventions include modification of risk factors such as smoking. The use of pulmonary medications and deep breathing exercises also may be appropriate for the prevention of postoperative complications.

BOX 39-1

Patient Factors Increasing the Risk of Postoperative Pulmonary Complications

Age >60 years
Smoking history
Preexisting pulmonary disease
Obstructive sleep apnea (OSA)
Upper respiratory tract infection
Low Spo_2
Anemia
Heart failure
ASA ≥2
Functional dependence
Nutritional status

AGE-SPECIFIC ANGLE

The elderly are at increased risk for postoperative respiratory complications.

Age

When compared with patients younger than 50 years, aged patients have an increased chance of postoperative pulmonary complications. Postoperative complications occur in half of patients older than 70 years. Narcotics and sedatives can further compromise postoperative ventilatory function, leading to respiratory failure. Cardiopulmonary, hepatic, renal, and central nervous system reserves are reduced in the elderly, which increases their susceptibility to PPCs. Patients older than 75 years also have an increased inflammatory response. These factors result in increased postoperative mortality rates.[4,8–12]

Box 39-2 lists pulmonary changes seen in the elderly patient. Because of these changes, the use of supplemental oxygen is recommended after any operative procedure in the elderly. The increased work of breathing that accompanies increased age compromises the capacity to meet the additional workload demand following surgery and may contribute to postoperative respiratory failure.

The elderly also have a decreased cardiac stress response and an increased association with coronary artery disease, placing them at high risk for cardiac complications. Factors influencing cardiovascular function (e.g., hypotension, fluid volume, positive pressure ventilation) can have greater effects on the elderly than they do on the young. Each of these factors increases the probability of pulmonary complications after surgery in the elderly.

Smoking History

A patient with a 20-pack-year or greater smoking history has a higher incidence of postoperative complications when compared to a patient with a lower pack-year history. Smoking cessation is beneficial in decreasing pulmonary complications of general anesthesia and surgery. Smoking cessation for 8 weeks prior to surgery results in a significant decrease in pulmonary complications compared with those who continue to smoke. Persons who have stopped smoking for more than 6 months have complication rates similar to those who never smoked. Heavy smokers have a higher rate of pulmonary complications than light smokers and may benefit from

AGE-SPECIFIC ANGLE

Operative factors affecting cardiovascular function have a greater effect on the elderly.

BOX 39-2

Changes in the Pulmonary and Thoracic Systems of Elderly Individuals

Increased chest wall rigidity
Increased expenditure of energy to move chest wall
Decreased respiratory muscle strength (by 20% at age 70 years)
Decreased functional surface area for gas exchange (by 15% at age 70 years)
Increased $\dot{V}/\dot{Q}$ mismatch and decreased Pao_2
Diminished response to hypoxemia and hypercapnia
Decreased vital capacity
Increased closing volume

refraining from smoking for even 1 day before surgery. This allows carboxyhemoglobin levels to decrease and improves blood oxygen-carrying capacity.[8,9,12–18]

Preexisting Lung Disease

Patients with severe asthma and chronic obstructive pulmonary disease (COPD) are at increased risk for postoperative complications. Chronic lung disease has been identified as the most significant factor for increased risk of postoperative pulmonary complications, including respiratory failure. Patients with COPD have an increase in postoperative complications ranging from 26% to 78%, and patients with symptomatic asthma also have an increased risk of morbidity from anesthesia. Surgery on these patients should occur when they are symptom free or when their symptoms are well controlled. There is no increased postoperative risk for patients with well-controlled asthma.[4,9,12–14]

Increased residual volume, decreased forced expiratory volume in the first second (FEV_1), decreased diffusing capacity of the lung for carbon monoxide (DLCO), and excessive sputum production are predictive for postoperative pulmonary complications. Preoperative dyspnea also has been shown to correlate with increased postoperative complications. The use of antibiotics, bronchodilators, and steroids can reduce the risk of postoperative complications in high-risk patients. Antibiotics should be reserved for patients with infection, however.[19] Current evidence suggests increased PPCs in patients with recent upper airway infections (one month prior to surgery). It may be prudent to defer elective surgery in this patient population until the infection has resolved.[10,11,19]

Heart Disease

Coronary artery disease is common in the surgical population, with up to 50% of postoperative deaths resulting from cardiac events. Most of these events are ischemic. Catecholamine release during surgery can predispose the patient to arrhythmias and possible coronary artery plaque rupture. Recent data indicate that use of beta blockers during the perioperative period can decrease ischemia and the incidence of myocardial infarction. Heart failure has been shown to be a significant risk factor for postoperative pulmonary complications.[4] Stable heart function and careful management are required for patients undergoing surgery.

Obesity

Surgical mortality is not increased in obese patients, but morbidly obese patients are at increased risk for complications such as reduced lung volumes, atelectasis, $\dot{V}/\dot{Q}$ mismatch, and persistent hypoxemia. Comorbid conditions such as diabetes, asthma, and heart conditions commonly exist in the obese patient. Obesity has not consistently been shown to be a risk factor for postoperative complications, however.[4] The discrepancy among reports may be due to inadequate distinguishing of obesity itself from comorbid conditions. Although obesity alone is not currently identified to be a significant risk factor for postoperative pulmonary complications, delaying surgery in morbidly obese patients may be appropriate until some weight loss can be achieved.

Bariatrics is the branch of medicine that deals with the prevention, control, and treatment of obesity. Bariatric surgery should be an elective procedure. Although weight-related comorbidities (diabetes and hypertension) are more prevalent in bariatric patients, they do not appear to increase surgical risk if they are managed preoperatively.[20,21]

Obstructive sleep apnea (OSA) is also common in bariatric patients, and some evidence links OSA with perioperative complications. The STOP-BANG questionnaire was validated as a screening modality for OSA in the preoperative setting.[22–24]

- **S**noring? Do you snore loudly (louder than talking or loud enough to be heard through closed doors)?
- **T**ired? Do you often feel tired, fatigued, or sleepy during the daytime?

- **O**bserved? Has anyone observed you stop breathing during your sleep?
- **P**ressure? Do you have or are being treated for high blood pressure?
- **B**ody Mass Index more than 35?
- **A**ge older than 50 years?
- **N**eck size large? Do you have a neck that measures more than 16 inches (40 cm) around (measure at Adam's apple)?
- **G**ender = Male?

The OSA risk is high if 5 to 8 of these are answered yes, intermediate for 3 to 4, and low for 0 to 2. It is reasonable to recommend the continuation of postoperative continuous positive airway pressure (CPAP) in these patients who use CPAP for sleep. It is also reasonable to initiate CPAP in the perioperative period for those at high risk as determined by STOP-BANG.

Postoperative treatment for bariatric patients includes a head-up position to improve lung volumes and decrease atelectasis and shunting. Although mortality rates are low immediately following bariatric surgery, one of the leading causes of death is pulmonary embolus. Prophylactic use of lower extremity compression devices (compression stocking and pneumatic boots), anticoagulation therapy, and early ambulation should be considered. The placement of a vena caval filter (a device which prevents clots from reaching the lungs) is recommended in patients who have a history of a hypercoagulable condition.[12,19,25]

General Health Status

Functional dependence (exercise limitation) has been identified as a predictor of PPCs. Exercise studies are suggested for some patients prior to surgery.[26–28] Low Spo_2 and anemia have also been identified as increasing the risk of PPCs. Spo_2 less than 90% and hemoglobin levels less than 10 g/dL increase the likelihood of PPCs. Transfusion of blood products should be used with caution because lung transfusion injury can be significant, however.[8,10,11,19,29]

ASA Status Classification

The American Society of Anesthesiology (ASA) has developed a physical status classification scale that is used to help determine risk of PPCs. A classification of 3 or more suggests significant increased risk for PPCs.[8–11,19,30] **Box 39-3** shows the ASA scoring system.

Nutritional Status

Poor nutritional status in critically ill patients undergoing major surgery is associated with reduced systemic immunity and an exaggerated stress response. Weight loss (more than 10% from baseline), low ideal body weight (less than 85%), hypoalbuminemia, and protein-calorie malnutrition are all predictors of increased postoperative complications such as infection, organ system failure, delayed wound healing, and delayed functional recovery. Patients with at least one of these abnormalities have a significant increase in incidence of overall surgical complications, major complications, and increased length of stay when compared with patients who have normal markers.

Serum albumin levels less than 35 g/L (3.5 g/dL) place the patient at risk for postoperative complications. Patients with a serum albumin value less than 2.5 g/dL or those with more than 10% weight loss should have nutritional repletion for 7 to 10 days before surgery. If diet alone cannot correct the problem, nutritional support may be indicated. Preoperative **total parenteral nutrition (TPN)** (i.e., intravenous administration of

BOX 39-3

ASA Physical Status Classification

ASA Class	Class Definition	Rates of PPCs by Class, %
I	A normal healthy patient	1.2
II	A patient with mild systemic disease	5.4
III	A patient with severe systemic disease that is not incapacitating	11.4
IV	A patient with an incapacitating systemic disease that is a constant threat to life	10.9
V	A moribund patient who is not expected to survive 24 h with or without operation	NA

NA = not available.

Reproduced from Qaseem A, Snow V, Fitterman N, et al. Risk assessment for and strategies to reduce perioperative pulmonary complications for patients undergoing noncardiothoracic surgery: a guideline form the American college of physicians. *Ann Intern Med.* 2006;144:575–580.

nutrition) for malnourished patients is only indicated in selected patients. On the other hand, **total enteral nutrition (TEN)** (i.e., gastrointestinal administration of nutrition) is well tolerated as long as the patient has adequate gastric motility and emptying.[10,11,14,31,32]

Patient Education

Preoperative patient education is important. The patient should be informed about the type of surgery planned, the pain intensity expected postoperatively, and the type of respiratory therapy that may be required after surgery. Clearly, preoperative instruction about planned postoperative respiratory care procedures is important for effectiveness following surgery.[4] When patients are educated about postoperative expectations, they may require less analgesia in the postoperative period.

Preoperative Testing

Millions of surgical operations and procedures are performed in the United States each year, with estimated billions of dollars being spent on preoperative laboratory and diagnostic studies. These studies should be performed for specific clinical indications and not as a routine preoperative screen unless they will influence patient treatment and outcome. Although the following tests are appropriate in known cases of lung and heart disease, little evidence supports routine screening of healthy patients with electrocardiograms (ECGs), chest radiographs, pulmonary function tests (PFTs), echocardiograms, or blood chemistry panels.[9,26,27] As stated previously, a complete history and physical are very important parts of the preoperative assessment. It is during this time that significant risk factors should be identified. Following the history and physical, the need for appropriate screening tests can be determined.

Electrocardiogram

A preoperative ECG is important for the patient with a history of circulatory and cardiac problems. An ECG should not be performed as a routine preoperative screen or based on patient age alone. **Box 39-4** lists clinical indications for preoperative ECG. Exercise testing along with ECG monitoring is being done more frequently prior to surgery in some patient populations, especially in older patients. Evidence does not support its routine use in evaluation of patients prior to general surgery, however.[27,28,33]

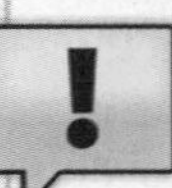

Respiratory Recap

Preoperative Laboratory and Diagnostic Studies

- Electrocardiogram
- Chest radiograph
- Arterial blood gas measurements
- Pulmonary function testing

BOX 39-4

Clinical Indications for Preoperative Electrocardiogram

Hypertension
Congestive heart failure
Diabetes
Chest pain
Dizziness
Syncope
Cerebral and peripheral vascular disease
Shortness of breath
Palpitations
Ankle edema
Abnormal valvular murmurs

Chest Radiograph

A chest radiograph is not recommended as part of a routine protocol in healthy patients.[9,32] Chest radiographs should be individualized and based on clinical indications. Chest radiographs are indicated in patients with acute, progressive, or chronic cardiopulmonary disease and in patients at high risk for developing postoperative pulmonary complications. Abnormal chest radiographs are more frequent in older patients. It is reasonable to perform chest radiography on patients older than 50 years who are undergoing high-risk surgical procedures. **Box 39-5** lists indications for preoperative chest radiographs.

BOX 39-5

Indications for Preoperative Chest Radiograph

Pneumonia
Pulmonary edema
Atelectasis
Aortic aneurysm
Mediastinal or pulmonary masses
Tracheal deviation
Cardiomegaly
Pulmonary hypertension
Chronic obstructive pulmonary disease
Pulmonary embolism
Dextrocardia

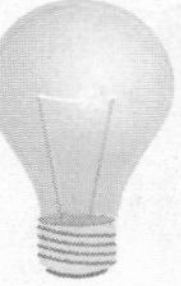

STOP AND THINK

You are paged by the preadmission testing area and asked to see a man who is 68 years old, weighs 280 pounds, and is a current smoker. When you see the patient, what information would you gather to assess the patient's operative risk? What advice would you provide for the patient and the care team?

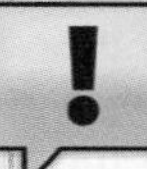

Respiratory Recap

Intraoperative Factors Contributing to Postoperative Pulmonary Complications

- Surgical incision site
- Duration of surgery
- Type of anesthesia
- Monitoring during anesthesia
- Intraoperative fluid management
- Ventilator settings—tidal volume and PEEP

Arterial Blood Gas Measurements

Arterial blood gas measurements are not recommended as a general preoperative screening test but are indicated in patients with new or changing lung disease and in patients at high risk for lung disease. Patients with an increased Pa_{CO_2} have an increased incidence of postoperative pulmonary complications. A chronically elevated Pa_{CO_2} greater than 45 mm Hg predicts a high risk for pulmonary complications or death. A Pa_{O_2} below 50 mm Hg may be a relative contraindication to surgery. Measurement of oxyhemoglobin saturation via pulse oximetry as a quick, easy, and noninvasive procedure has become the standard of care for screening arterial oxygenation. Sp_{O_2} <90% is associated with increased PPCs.[19]

Pulmonary Function Tests

All patients who are candidates for lung resection should have pulmonary function testing. Pulmonary function testing as a general preoperative screen for the presence of pulmonary disease in patients without a suggestive clinical history is not indicated and should not be done to predict postoperative pulmonary complications, however. For abdominal and cardiac surgery, the predictive value of spirometry and determination of lung volumes is unproven. Spirometry should be obtained before the initiation of general anesthesia if the patient's respiratory symptoms have changed. Spirometry is indicated in patients with severe pulmonary dysfunction to assess whether pulmonary rehabilitation is indicated to improve the pulmonary condition prior to surgery. Pulmonary function testing is also recommended in patients with neuromuscular disease, chest wall and spinal deformities, and morbid obesity. In patients with COPD, pulmonary function testing may help to assess the probability of early extubation.[9,11,32]

Intraoperative Risk Factors

Several intraoperative factors contribute to postoperative pulmonary complications. These include surgical incision site, duration of surgery, type of anesthesia used during surgery, monitoring, and fluid management.

Surgical incision site is the most important factor in predicting the overall risk of postoperative pulmonary complications. Thoracic incisions have been shown to have the greatest negative effect on pulmonary function and carry the highest rate of postoperative pulmonary complications (19% to 59%). The use of muscle-sparing thoracotomy and video-assisted thoracotomy (VAT) procedures help to preserve postoperative muscle strength and lung function. PPCs occur in up to 5% of lower abdominal surgeries. Upper abdominal and thoracic surgeries carry a 20% to 70% pulmonary complication rate, compared with a 4% pulmonary complication rate after urologic and orthopedic surgery. Aortic surgery, head and neck surgery, neurosurgery, and abdominal aortic aneurysm surgery are also listed as high-risk procedures.[10,11,30,34,35]

Reduced lung volume is a major factor contributing to postoperative pulmonary complications following surgery. Vital capacity can be reduced by 50% to 60% and remain decreased for up to a week. Supine positioning decreases the functional residual capacity (FRC) by 10% to 15%. General anesthesia can further decrease the FRC up to 30%. Postoperative complications double if surgery lasts longer than 3 hours.[8,10–13,19,30,32,35]

Although there are conflicting data, it appears that patients who receive general anesthesia are at higher risk for pulmonary complications than those who receive epidural or spinal anesthesia, with or without general anesthesia. Patients receiving epidural or spinal anesthesia have a 40% reduction in the risk of pneumonia and a 60% reduction in the risk of respiratory depression.[36] Long-acting neuromuscular blockers lead to a higher incidence of pulmonary complications than shorter-acting agents.[11]

Intraoperative monitoring may decrease risks for cardiopulmonary compromise during anesthesia, thus reducing postoperative complications. Intraoperative use of pulse oximetry and capnography has improved postoperative outcomes.

Proper fluid management is important for maintaining renal function, ensuring gastrointestinal integrity, and maintaining oxygen delivery. Blood loss and inadequate fluid replacement can lead to hypotension, poor organ perfusion, and insufficient oxygen delivery.

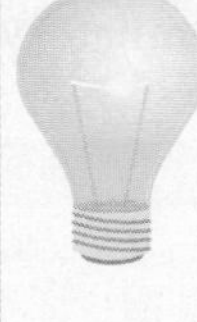

STOP AND THINK

An anesthesiologist asks if you think lung-protective ventilation has a role in the operating room. What would be your response? What tidal volume and PEEP should be used during surgery?

Intraoperative blood loss greater than 1200 mL has been associated with increased pulmonary complications. Excessive fluids, however, may lead to edema, congestive heart failure, and hypertension.[37] Massive volume resuscitation can result in abdominal compartment syndrome (high intra-abdominal pressure), in which the increased intra-abdominal pressure results in increased work of breathing and decreased renal blood flow.

Ventilator settings during surgery may affect postoperative outcomes. Lower tidal volumes (less than 10 mL/kg of ideal body weight and perhaps as low as 6 mL/kg) and the use of positive end-expiratory pressure (PEEP) of 5 to 10 cm H_2O is recommended.[38,39]

Postoperative Respiratory Failure: Assessment and Management

Postoperative pulmonary complications are common and contribute to postoperative morbidity and mortality. Common postoperative complications include atelectasis, infection, respiratory failure, exacerbation of underlying chronic lung disease, and bronchospasm. The goal is to prevent these complications. Postoperative respiratory management includes pain control, mobilization, deep breathing, airway clearance, ventilator liberation, nutritional support, and oxygen therapy.[18]

Hypoxemia

Mild hypoxemia is treated with low concentrations of oxygen, most commonly by nasal cannula. Severe hypoxemia requires more aggressive therapy with the use of CPAP or mechanical ventilation with positive end-expiratory pressure (PEEP). Atelectasis is a major contributor to postoperative hypoxemia, and lung volume expansion therapies such as mobilization, incentive spirometry, positive expiratory pressure (PEP), or CPAP may be required.[40] Intermittent positive pressure breathing (IPPB), although once a primary form of treatment, is rarely used. The benefit of incentive spirometry has also been called into question.[41]

Respiratory Recap

Components of Postoperative Management

- Pain control
- Mobilization
- Lung expansion therapy
- Airway clearance
- Ventilator liberation
- Nutritional support
- Oxygen therapy

Hypercapnia

If the central respiratory drive is blunted, increased $Paco_2$ may occur. The use of anesthetics and analgesics during and after surgery is the major cause of short-term acute respiratory failure following surgery. Once sedation has been terminated and the drug is metabolized or excreted, most postoperative patients ventilate appropriately if pain control measures are used. Treatment is aimed at the underlying etiology. Mechanical ventilation can be maintained until the respiratory failure is reversed. The use of respiratory stimulants is controversial and not recommended.

Motor neuron disorders, respiratory muscle weakness, chest wall abnormalities, and diaphragmatic or abdominal conditions also can result in hypercapnia. Postoperative respiratory failure resulting from ventilatory muscle dysfunction is uncommon except with preexisting preoperative factors. Diaphragmatic paralysis can occur after some surgeries and may contribute to respiratory failure, however. Muscle weakness may result from drugs used intraoperatively or during the postoperative period. Pain can also be a factor preventing the normal use of the respiratory muscles. Treatment is directed toward the underlying disorder, and mechanical ventilation both invasive and noninvasive can be used for supportive care.

Nutrition

The integrity of the gut affects immune defenses and organ function. If a patient is unable to eat, initiation of enteral nutrition (EN) may be desirable. Generally EN is well tolerated and improves postoperative morbidity and mortality better than parenteral nutrition. **Box 39-6** lists the positive aspects of enteral nutrition. When compared with subjects who received no feedings, nutritional intervention in the perioperative period has shown a benefit of reduced postoperative morbidity. A group of trauma patients receiving EN for 5 to 7 days had a lower rate of sepsis compared with a group receiving intravenous fluid administration. Patients with liver transplantation had a lower viral infection rate with administration of TEN. It should be noted, however, that the routine use of a nasogastric tube following surgery increases the risk of aspiration pneumonia and atelectasis. Nasogastric tubes should be used only when indicated.[8,10,11,42,43]

Pain Management

The use of analgesics is essential after surgery, particularly following thoracic and abdominal surgery. Effective

BOX 39-6

Advantages of Total Enteral Nutrition Compared with Total Parenteral Nutrition in the Postoperative Patient

Increased integrity of gastrointestinal system
Improved immune defenses
Improved organ function
Decreased nosocomial infections
Improved return of cognitive function
Decreased mortality
Less expensive
Decreased septic complications

pain control will encourage early ambulation and deep breathing. Ineffective pain management may lead to serious pulmonary complications. Analgesia can be delivered orally, parenterally (intravenous), or via epidural catheters. For epidural catheterization, the tip of a needle is positioned within the epidural space in the spinal column.[44] Once positioned, a thin catheter is threaded through the needle, and the needle is removed. The catheter is secured to the patient and is used to administer intermittent or continuous analgesia.

Patient-controlled analgesia (PCA) is a popular method of pain control. PCA allows the patient to titrate the amount of analgesic he or she receives by simply pressing a button. A limit set on the delivering device prevents the patient from overdosing. PCA can be used along with IV or epidural analgesic administration. The benefits of PCA include active involvement of the patient, lesser amounts of drug usage, more rapid analgesic action, and better pain control with minimal side effects.[45]

Narcotic sensitivity is widely variable and some patients can have respiratory depression even with low doses by PCA. Respiratory monitoring is necessary and is sometimes facilitated with the use of capnography. Due to concerns related to respiratory depression with opioids, alternatives such as IV acetaminophen may be used.

Patient Temperature

Postoperative hypothermia causes vasoconstriction and may decrease tissue perfusion, resulting in metabolic acidosis. Shivering will increase oxygen consumption and carbon dioxide production. This may increase the risk of **myocardial ischemia** and hypercapnic ventilatory failure.

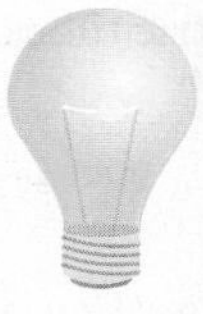

STOP AND THINK

A patient is to receive a PCA device following surgery. What are the main points you will want to emphasize to enhance the patient's understanding of the device?

Muscle Strength

Postoperative sedation may lead to respiratory depression as a result of muscle weakness. The diaphragm is the last muscle to become paralyzed and the first to recover from neuromuscular blockade. A 5-second head-lift or leg-lift evaluation may be a good indicator of a patient's ability to maintain an adequate airway. If a previously sedated patient who is alert and following commands can lift their extremities for 5 seconds, the diaphragm should be functional and they should be able to protect their airway. The 5-second lift test has correlated well with the maximal inspiratory pressure, which checks respiratory muscle strength.

Lung Expansion

Pulmonary complications are the most common form of postoperative morbidity experienced by patients who undergo general surgical abdominal and thoracic procedures. The high incidence of pulmonary complications in the postoperative period is likely due to pain and the inability to take deep breaths because of decreased diaphragmatic function, chest wall dysfunction, and alterations in chest wall mechanics. Some studies have shown that forced vital capacity and peak flow can be decreased by as much as 50%. Functional residual capacity may be decreased by as much as 10% to 15% in lower abdominal surgery, 30% in upper abdominal surgery, and 35% in thoracic surgery in the postoperative period and may not return to normal for 3 to 6 days. Transdiaphragmatic pressure has been shown to decrease by as much as 70% in abdominal surgery, and normal function may not return for 1 week. In some cases, adequate pain management does not reduce this impairment, which seems to occur from diaphragmatic dysfunction itself.

Another important element in the etiology of postoperative respiratory complications is the lung volume at which airway closure occurs. Factors that increase closing volumes include increased age, tobacco use, fluid overload, bronchospasm, and airway secretions. With a decreased FRC or increased closing volume, the lungs are predisposed to airway closure and atelectasis, leading to $\dot{V}/\dot{Q}$ mismatch, hypoxemia, retained secretions, and respiratory failure. Deep breathing exercises and pulmonary hygiene are important postoperative considerations for preventing pulmonary complications. Several techniques for lung expansion are available, including IPPB, incentive spirometry, PEP devices, flutter valves, deep breathing and coughing, CPAP, and others. Pulmonary complications, specifically atelectasis, pneumonia, respiratory failure, and pulmonary

embolism, represent the leading causes of postoperative morbidity and mortality.[46–54]

Atelectasis

Etiology and Risk Factors

Atelectasis is the collapse of previously expanded lung tissue. Collapse may be minimal and diffuse. It may be difficult to see on chest radiograph (microatelectasis) or it may involve whole segments, lobes, or a lung and be easily seen on chest x-rays. Atelectasis is one of the most common noninfectious pulmonary complications after surgery. Studies have reported that 20% to 25% of lung tissue in the basal lung areas collapses after induction with general anesthesia. Furthermore, the use of high concentrations of oxygen (more than 40%) contributes to collapse.[27] Atelectasis is reported to be present in 90% of anesthetized patients.[52] The incidence of clinically significant atelectasis after abdominal surgery is 15% to 20%, with the left lower lobe being the most common area for atelectasis.

Atelectasis may be caused by many factors, including small tidal volumes, inadequate lung-distending forces, airway obstruction with gas absorption, and reduction in surfactant levels. These conditions are likely in postoperative patients who are sedated, have significant pain, and often have poor clearance of airway secretions. Any condition that interferes with the generation of negative pleural pressure predisposes the lung to the development of atelectasis. Examples include weak inspiratory muscles because of sedation, advanced age, obesity, chest wall deformities, pulmonary fibrosis, abdominal and thoracic surgery, and pain.

Retained secretions may be the common factor in the development of postoperative atelectasis when the patient has an inadequate cough. Furthermore, anesthetics and a lack of humidity can diminish airway mucus transport during the intraoperative period. Surfactant levels may also be decreased in the lungs of postoperative patients as a result of the anesthetic, high concentrations of oxygen, and the absence of deep breathing. Intraoperative aspiration may also contribute to airway compromise.

Clinical Manifestations and Diagnostic Findings

Some of the signs and symptoms of atelectasis include fine late inspiratory crackles, bronchial-type breath sounds, diminished breath sounds, increased breathing frequency and dyspnea, increased heart rate, and hypoxemia due to $\dot{V}/\dot{Q}$ mismatch and shunt. The significance of each of these findings depends on the degree of atelectasis present. Atelectasis also can lead to respiratory failure and pneumonia. The presence of a fever in a patient with atelectasis is most often associated with infection resulting from retained secretions. Contrary to common teaching, atelectasis without infection does not result in fever.

Atelectasis is one of the most commonly encountered abnormalities on chest radiograph. At times it may be overlooked and at other times may be confused with other intrathoracic pathology such as **pneumonia**. Some of the radiographic signs of atelectasis include localized increase in density or opacity, presence of air bronchograms, displacement of lobar fissures, elevation of the diaphragm, mediastinal shift, hilar displacement, regional change in rib spacing, hyperinflation of surrounding lung, and generalized volume reduction. Differentiating atelectasis from a pneumothorax is important. With a pneumothorax and loss of lung volume, the visceral pleura will pull away from the parietal pleura creating an actual pleural space. This does not happen with atelectasis.

With atelectasis, pulmonary function tests reveal a decreased FRC, a decreased vital capacity, and decreased compliance. An arterial blood sample often shows an uncompensated respiratory alkalosis with hypoxemia. The hypoxemia is a result of $\dot{V}/\dot{Q}$ mismatch and areas of right-to-left shunt. The normal lung will divert blood away from areas of atelectasis by constricting blood vessels in these areas due to low Po_2 values. General anesthesia inhibits hypoxic pulmonary vasoconstriction, which further contributes to $\dot{V}/\dot{Q}$ mismatch and increased work of breathing.

AGE-SPECIFIC ANGLE

Elderly patients are at greater risk for atelectasis.

Management

Treatment for atelectasis depends on the severity and etiology of the problem. Preventive treatment is best. Preoperative patient education and training when the patient is alert, responsive to instruction, and without pain may play a significant role in preventing postoperative complications. Smoking cessation at least 8 weeks before surgery has also been shown to improve postoperative outcomes. Intraoperative lung recruitment

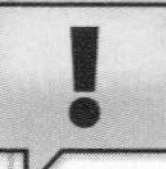

Respiratory Recap

Signs and Symptoms of Postoperative Atelectasis

- Inspiratory crackles
- Bronchial breath sounds
- Diminished breath sounds
- Tachypnea
- Dyspnea
- Tachycardia
- Hypoxemia

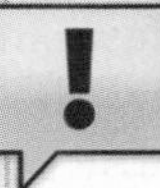

Respiratory Recap

Management of Postoperative Atelectasis

- Prevention
- Patient education
- Smoking cessation
- Spontaneous coughing
- Deep breathing exercises
- Mobilization
- Oxygen therapy
- CPAP therapy
- Mechanical ventilation
- The roles of incentive spirometry, IPPB, PEP, and airway clearance therapy are unclear and controversial

maneuvers and PEEP have been shown to reduce postoperative atelectasis.[21,38,39]

With minimal postoperative atelectasis, no special intervention is needed. Spontaneous coughing, deep breathing, and mobilization (walking) should be sufficient to reverse any pulmonary impairment. In moderate cases, incentive spirometry, IPPB, PEP therapy, and CPAP may be used to help prevent or reverse atelectasis.[38] IPPB and incentive spirometry were once commonly used to prevent and treat postoperative atelectasis. Guidelines no longer recommend routine postoperative incentive spirometry.[41,50] Airway clearance therapy and inhaled bronchodilators may improve bronchial hygiene in some patients, but these are usually not indicated in this patient population.[55,56] Deep breathing and coughing may be as effective as other modes of therapy for the treatment of atelectasis. No individual approach to lung inflation therapy is significantly superior to another. A bundle approach might be more effective than a single therapy.[57]

Low-risk surgical patients probably do not need respiratory therapy, but even with therapy, an estimated 25% of high-risk patients will have postoperative pulmonary complications. Short-term oxygen therapy is often indicated. In rare severe cases, mechanical ventilation with PEEP, lung recruitment maneuvers, and high oxygen levels may be indicated to re-inflate collapsed areas and support oxygenation until the patient has improved. Therapeutic fiberoptic bronchoscopy may be indicated to remove mucus plugs if they are the cause of airway obstruction and atelectasis.

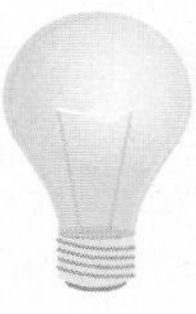

STOP AND THINK

A patient is at risk for developing post-op atelectasis. What therapeutic innervations may be used to prevent or treat post-op atelectasis? How would you choose the best approach for an individual patient?

Pulmonary Emboli and Pulmonary Thromboembolic Disease

Etiology and Risk Factors

The most common cause of **pulmonary embolism (PE)** is venous thromboembolism. Blood clots formed in the leg or pelvic veins travel to the lungs, where they obstruct pulmonary vessels. Blood clotting in the legs and pelvis, **deep vein thrombosis (DVT)**, occurs as a result of venostasis in surgical patients and from other causes of immobility. It may also occur due to damage to the endothelial wall of the blood vessels and in hypercoagulability states. Although not the most common PPC, PE is the third most common cause of death from cardiovascular disease after heart attack and stroke.[52] Risk factors associated with DVT include age greater than 65 years, obesity, congestive heart failure, presence of malignancies, use of estrogen-containing drugs, postoperative states, and patients genetically predisposed to abnormal clotting.

Clinical Manifestations and Diagnostic Findings

Signs and symptoms of acute PE include abrupt onset of cough, pleuritic chest pain, anxiety, and tachycardia. Tachypnea and dyspnea are the most common findings present, even in patients without hypoxemia. This is thought to be due to stimulation of J-receptors or juxtacapillary receptors, which respond to inflammation and increased pulmonary-capillary pressure. Lung auscultation may reveal wheezing or crackles. Hemoptysis may occasionally occur. The lower extremities may reveal some tenderness or swelling associated with DVT, but PE sometimes occurs as the first sign of DVT.

The severity of symptoms and degree of compromise depend on the magnitude of occlusion of the pulmonary vessels and the amount of preexisting cardiopulmonary disease. As a result of venous occlusion, hypoxemia usually occurs. This is due to $\dot{V}/\dot{Q}$ mismatch, bronchoconstriction, decreased surfactant production, atelectasis, and shunting. In healthy patients, right-sided heart dysfunction does not usually occur unless occlusion of 50% or more (massive occlusion) of the pulmonary vasculature occurs. In patients with cardiopulmonary disease, hemodynamic collapse can occur even with less than massive occlusion. Although pulmonary occlusion can be extensive, pulmonary infarction is uncommon because the lung receives oxygen from three sources: pulmonary circulation, bronchial circulation, and the alveolar gas.

PE can occur with few symptoms, or it may be mistaken for other diseases or coexist with them. PE is commonly mistaken for pneumonia. The diagnosis of PE includes clinical suspicion, physical exam, chest radiograph, ECG, and arterial blood gas measurements.

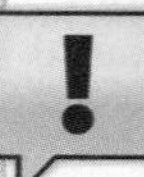

Respiratory Recap

Signs and Symptoms of Postoperative Pulmonary Embolism

- Abrupt onset of cough
- Pleuritic chest pain
- Anxiety
- Tachycardia
- Hypoxemia

Respiratory Recap

Management of Postoperative Pulmonary Embolism

- Prophylaxis/prevention of DVT
- Anticoagulation therapy
- Thrombolytic therapy
- Insertion of IVC filters
- Surgery

Chest radiographs may be normal, or an infiltrate may be present. X-rays are often not specific enough to be of great help. In some cases a wedge-shaped density called a Westermark sign may be present. A CT scan is often needed to document a PE. The ECG may have nonspecific alterations. Arterial blood gas values often show a respiratory alkalosis and hypoxemia.

A screening blood test to determine if a clot is present is the D-dimer. The D-dimer is highly sensitive in excluding acute DVT and PE with a value below 500 μg/L in patients with low clinical probability. A noninvasive test used to diagnose DVT is compression ultrasound. The invasive study for diagnosis is venography. Contrast venography is the gold standard in the diagnosis of DVT. The hazard associated with venography is mobilization of the clot, however. Because of this serious hazard, venography has been largely replaced by ultrasound.

To diagnose PE, the $\dot{V}/\dot{Q}$ scan can be used to evaluate perfusion defects combined with areas of normal ventilation. Another test, the pulmonary angiogram, although once considered the gold standard to determine the presence of PE, is invasive and carries with it a higher risk of complications than the $\dot{V}/\dot{Q}$ scan. Because of the increased risk of complications, pulmonary angiography is often used as a last resort. Because of its widespread availability, CT angiography with intravenous contrast is now being used to diagnose suspected PE.[52]

Management

Prophylaxis of PE involves prevention of DVT, including compression wraps (stockings) or pneumatic boots with intermittent inflation and early ambulation and leg exercises. Anticoagulation therapy is also indicated. Anticoagulation therapy (example: **heparin**) is considered therapeutic if the clotting time or **partial thromboplastin time (PTT)** is 2 to 2.5 times the control. If venous thrombosis is present, anticoagulants will prevent further clot formation but will not dissolve clots already present.

Warfarin is another anticoagulant used by patients who are at risk for thromboembolism. These at-risk conditions include atrial fibrillation, presence of prosthetic heart valves, and previous thromboembolism.[48] Although bleeding from the surgical site is a risk when using anticoagulants, withholding or reducing anticoagulants may increase the risk of thromboembolism, including stroke. Embolic strokes will not occur from DVTs, however. Blood clots in the venous circulation or from the right side of the heart will be filtered by the lungs. Only clots arising from the left heart chambers (e.g., atrial fibrillation) or left heart valves will embolize to the brain causing an embolic stoke.

Several factors influence the risk of bleeding in patients using anticoagulants. These include patient age, disease presence, type of surgery, other drug use such as aspirin or antiplatelet agents, and the degree of anticoagulation as determined by the international normalized ratio (INR). The INR is used to determine the degree of anticoagulation in patients who are on oral (warfarin) anticoagulation therapy. Once the INR is below 2.0, surgery can be performed with relative safety. The INR is normally kept between 2.0 and 3.0 for optimal therapeutic levels.

If clots are already present, **thrombolytic** therapy will help dissolve clots. Common thrombolytics include **tissue plasminogen activator (TPA)**, streptokinase, and urokinase. The use of thrombolytic therapy must be balanced against the risk of bleeding in postoperative patients. An inferior vena caval (IVC) filter (Greenfield or bird's nest filter) can be inserted to prevent clots originating in the lower extremities from reaching the lungs. These implanted filters intercept clots, thus preventing PE. Surgical removal of the embolus (embolectomy) may rarely be attempted. Supportive therapy includes supplemental oxygen and, in severe cases of acute respiratory failure, mechanical ventilation with PEEP and high oxygen levels may be used. ECMO (extracorporeal membrane oxygenation) can also be used.

Pneumonia

Etiology and Risk Factors

Hospital-acquired pneumonia (HAP), ventilator-associated pneumonia (VAP), and healthcare-associated pneumonia (HCAP) are important causes of morbidity and mortality in the healthcare setting. Nosocomial pneumonia (hospital acquired after more than 48 hours following admission) accounts for 15% of all hospital-acquired infections, with half occurring in surgical

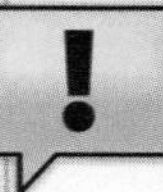

Respiratory Recap

Signs and Symptoms of Postoperative Pneumonia

- Fever
- Shaking chills
- Cough
- Hemoptysis
- Tachypnea
- Dullness to percussion
- Crackles
- Purulent sputum
- Pleuritic chest pain

patients. Postoperative pneumonia has been reported to occur in 18% of patients undergoing elective upper or lower abdominal and thoracic surgery. Pneumonia carries the highest mortality rate of hospital-acquired infections. It is the most common cause of death among surgical patients, with a reported mortality rate of 20% to 50% and up to 90% mortality in patients with acute respiratory distress syndrome.

Risk factors for development of pneumonia include immunosuppression, malnutrition, COPD, and age greater than 65 years. Additional risk factors for development of nosocomial pneumonia include major thoracic and upper abdominal surgery, greater than 1200 mL blood loss during surgery, altered protective effects of the glottic area, ineffective cough, inhibition of ciliary motion, and impaired consciousness leading to increased chance of aspiration. Postoperative patients are at high risk especially when they are intubated, have a nasogastric tube in place, have had general anesthesia, have swallowing difficulties, or have regurgitation of gastric contents.

Clinical Manifestations and Diagnostic Findings

Signs and symptoms of pneumonia include fever, shaking chills, cough, hemoptysis, tachypnea, dullness to percussion, crackles, purulent sputum production, and pleuritic chest pain. Some of the usual clinical manifestations are often unclear, however, and may be overshadowed by an underlying illness when pneumonia develops while a patient is in the hospital. When a bacterial pneumonia is present, laboratory data include increased white blood cell count (leukocytosis), increased granulocytes (neutrophilia), and an increased percentage of immature neutrophils (referred to as a shift to the left). Arterial blood gas measurements show hypoxemia with respiratory alkalosis. Chest radiographs vary according to the type of pneumonia present. Lobar pneumonia presents as a homogeneous infiltrate with air bronchograms. Nonhomogeneous, patchy, nonlobar densities occur with bronchopneumonia. A diffuse bilateral reticular pattern (bilateral network of patchy densities—ground glass appearance) often indicates a viral infection.

Management

Prevention is the best course of action. Proper hand hygiene is essential. Early mobilization and chest physiotherapy may decrease pulmonary infections. Deep breathing maneuvers and coughing are indicated for secretion removal.[53] Bronchodilator therapy and airway clearance therapies are usually not indicated for consolidative pneumonia. Administration of surgical antimicrobial prophylaxis, although controversial, may be associated with a decrease in the incidence of early-onset (less than 96 hours) postsurgical pneumonia.[54,58]

Once an infection has been suspected, rapid administration of appropriate antibiotics has a significant effect on outcomes. If isolation of the causative agent is possible, culture and sensitivity tests should direct proper antimicrobial use. If the agent cannot be isolated, initial general antimicrobial therapy (empiric therapy) includes the following drug options: extended-spectrum penicillins (piperacillin, tazobactam) or a cephalosporin (cefepime), plus a fluoroquinolone (levofloxacin) or an aminoglycoside (tobramycin), plus vancomycin or an oxazolidinone (linezolid). The beta-lactams, carbapenem and ertapenem, can also be considered. The actual drug regimen will vary depending on suspected microbial infection and other complicating patient factors and can be modified based on knowledge of local pathogens and their susceptibility to antibiotics. Oxygen is often needed for hypoxemia. In severe cases, mechanical ventilation with PEEP may be indicated.

Mechanical ventilation places a patient at risk for development of pneumonia, however. VAP occurs in 9% to 27% of mechanically ventilated patients, and mortality rates vary from 27% to 50%. A set of procedures used to prevent VAP is included in what is known as a *ventilator bundle*. The ventilator bundle for prevention of VAP includes elevating the head of the bed by at least 30 degrees, providing sedation vacations for assessment of extubation potential, peptic ulcer prophylaxis, oral care with chlorhexidine to decrease microbial flora, and DVT prophylaxis. Use of noninvasive ventilation (NIV) in select patient populations may also help reduce VAP. Other procedures that may help decrease VAP include use of protective covers for suction and resuscitation

Respiratory Recap

Management of Postoperative Pneumonia

- Antibiotics
- Oxygen
- Mechanical ventilation with PEEP

equipment, decontamination of the stomach, use of silver-coated endotracheal tubes,[59] and continuous subglottic suction with specially designed endotracheal tubes. Some of these techniques and devices need more study before their effectiveness in reducing VAP is known. The goal is to prevent VAP and thereby reduce medical costs along with reducing patient morbidity and mortality.

Mechanical Ventilation for Respiratory Failure

Postoperative mechanical ventilation is occasionally required, most commonly due to the residual respiratory depressant effects of anesthesia. This often involves several hours of ventilatory support in the postanesthesia care unit, after which the patient is extubated. After cardiac surgery, the patient is mechanically ventilated in the intensive care unit for several hours, after which fast-track ventilator discontinuation protocols are used to rapidly liberate the patient from the ventilator. After neurosurgery, mechanical ventilation may be needed because of respiratory depression and to assist with the control of intracranial pressure. After thoracic surgery, mechanical ventilation is often required because of the extent of surgical trauma to the thorax.

The principles of mechanical ventilation are similar for the postoperative patient as for other patients requiring this therapy. Appropriate ventilatory support is provided, with attention to the prevention of iatrogenic injuries (an injury occurring due to medical care) such as overdistention, auto-PEEP, and hemodynamic compromise. Some postoperative patients (e.g., after neurosurgery) may have relatively normal lungs and chest wall. Others may have relatively normal lung function but surgical chest wall trauma (e.g., after cardiac surgery). Thoracic surgery patients may be difficult to manage because they have surgical chest wall trauma, lung resection with risk of pneumothorax, and underlying lung disease such as COPD. A tidal volume of 6 to 8 mL/kg of ideal body weight, respiratory rate titrated to a normal Pa_{CO_2}, PEEP 5 to 8 cm H_2O, and F_{IO_2} for Sp_{O_2} >92% is usually sufficient.

Evidence supports the use of NIV in patients who develop respiratory failure in the postoperative period following abdominal surgery, thoracic surgery, cardiac surgery, thoracoabdominal surgery, bariatric surgery, and solid organ transplantation.[60,61] CPAP may be helpful in patients who develop postoperative hypoxemic respiratory failure, likely because it improves atelectasis.[38,47]

> **STOP AND THINK**
>
> You are called to see a patient in the postanesthesia care unit in respiratory failure. Would you recommend that the patient is intubated or would you try NIV? What settings would you choose on the ventilator, whether it is invasive or noninvasive ventilation?

Key Points

- An important first step in preoperative management is obtaining a patient history.
- Age, smoking history, preexisting lung disease, and poor nutritional status are risk factors for postoperative respiratory complications.
- Little evidence exists that routine screening of healthy patients with ECGs, chest radiographs, PFTs, echocardiograms, or blood chemistry panels significantly alters outcomes.
- Intraoperative factors that affect postoperative pulmonary complications include surgical incision site, duration of surgery, type of anesthesia, monitoring during anesthesia, and intraoperative fluid management.
- Postoperative respiratory management includes pain control, early mobilization, deep breathing, airway clearance therapy, early ventilator liberation, early feeding, and oxygen therapy, as indicated.
- Atelectasis, pneumonia, and respiratory failure are common postoperative problems.

References

1. Shander A, Fleisher L, Barie P, et al. Clinical and economic burden of postoperative pulmonary complications: patient safety summit on definition, risk-reducing interventions, and preventive strategies. *Crit Care Med.* 2011;39:2163–2172.
2. Feeney C, Reynolds J, Hussey J. Preoperative physical activity levels and postoperative pulmonary complications poet-esophagectomy. *Dis Esophagus.* 2011;24:489–494.
3. Brueckmann B, Villa-Uribe JL, Bateman BT, et al. Development and validation of a score for prediction of postoperative respiratory complications. *Anesthesiology.* 2013;118,1276–1285.
4. Smetana GW, Lawrence VA, Cornell JE. Preoperative pulmonary risk stratification for noncardiothoracic surgery: systematic review for the American College of Physicians. *Ann Intern Med.* 2006;144:581–595.
5. Bapoje SR, Whitcker JF, Schulz T, et al. Preoperative evaluation of the patient with pulmonary disease. *Chest.* 2007;13:1637–1645.
6. Sigworth S. Preoperative evaluation of hospitalized patients. *Mt Sinai J Med.* 2008;75:442–448.
7. Kanat F, Golcuk A, Teke T, Golcuk M. Risk factors for postoperative pulmonary complications in upper abdominal surgery. *ANZ J Surg.* 2007;77:135–141.
8. Thanavaro J, Foner B. Reducing risks for noncardiac surgery. *Nurse Pract.* 2013;38:38–47.
9. Agostini P, Cieslik H, Rathinam S. Postoperative pulmonary complications following thoracic surgery: are there any modifiable risk factors? *Thorax.* 2010;65:815–818.
10. Canet J, Gallart L, Gomar C, et al. Prediction of postoperative pulmonary complications in a population-based cohort. *Anesthesiology.* 2010;113:1338–1350.
11. Qaseem A, Snow V, Fitterman N, et al. Risk assessment for and strategies to reduce perioperative pulmonary complications for patients undergoing noncardiothoracic surgery: a guideline from the American College of Physicians. *Ann Intern Med.* 2006;144:575–580.
12. Guldner A, Pelosi P, Gama de Abreu M. Nonventilatory strategies to prevent postoperative pulmonary complications. *Curr Opin Anesthesiol.* 2013;26:141–151.

13. Grigorakos L, Sotiriou E, Koulendi D, et al. Preoperative pulmonary evaluation (PPE) as a prognostic factor in patients undergoing upper abdominal surgery. *Hepatogastroenterology*. 2008;55:1229–1232.
14. Smetana G, Lawrence V, Cornell J. Preoperative risk stratification for noncardiothoracic surgery: systematic review for the American college of physicians. *Ann Intern Med*. 2006;144:581–595.
15. Lindstrom D, Sadr AO, Wladis A, et al. Effects of a perioperative smoking cessation intervention on postoperative complications: a randomized trial. *Ann Surg*. 2008;5:739–745.
16. Theadom A, Cropley M. Effects of preoperative smoking cessation on the incidence and risk of intraoperative and postoperative complications in adult smokers: a systematic review. *Tob Control*. 2006;5:352–358.
17. Moller A, Tonnesen H. Risk reduction: perioperative smoking intervention. *Best Pract Res Clin Anaesthesiol*. 2006;2:237–248.
18. Lawrence V, Cornell J, Smetana G. Strategies to reduce postoperative pulmonary complications after noncardiothoracic surgery: systematic review for the American College of Physicians. *Ann Intern Med*. 2006;144:596–608.
19. Canet J, Gallart L. Predicting postoperative pulmonary complications in the general population. *Curr Opin Anesthesiol*. 2013;26:107–115.
20. Reiss KP, Baker MT, Lambert PJ, et al. Effect of preoperative weight loss on laparoscopic gastric bypass outcomes. *Surg Obes Related Dis*. 2008;4:704–708.
21. Talab H, Zabani I, Abdelrahman H, et al. Intraoperative ventilatory strategies for prevention of pulmonary atelectasis in obese patients undergoing laparoscopic bariatric surgery. *Anesth Analg*. 2009;109:1511–1516.
22. Singh M, Liao P, Kobah S, et al. Proportion of surgical patients with undiagnosed obstructive sleep apnoea. *Br J Anaesth*. 2013;110:629–636.
23. Chung F, Subramanyam R, Liao P, et al. High STOP-Bang score indicates a high probability of obstructive sleep apnoea. *Br J Anaesth*. 2012;108:768–775.
24. Liao P, Luo Q, Elsaid H, et al. Perioperative auto-titrated continuous positive airway pressure treatment in surgical patients with obstructive sleep apnea: a randomized controlled trial. *Anesthesiology*. 2013;119:837–847.
25. McGlinch BP, Que FG, Nelson JL, et al. Perioperative care of patients undergoing bariatric surgery. *Mayo Clin Proc*. 2006;81(Suppl 10):S25–S33.
26. Salati M, Brunelli A. Preoperative assessment of patients for lung cancer surgery. *Curr Opin Pulm Med*. 2012;18:289–294.
27. Young E, Karthikesalingam A, Huddart S, et al. A systematic review of the role of cardiopulmonary exercise testing in vascular surgery. *Eur J Vasc Endovasc Surg*. 2012;44:64–71.
28. Ridgway Z, Howell S. Cardiopulmonary exercise testing: a review of methods and applications in surgical patients. *Eur J Anaesthesiol*. 2010;27:858–865.
29. Nobili C, Marzano E, Oussoultzogloy E, et al. Multivariate analysis of risk factors for pulmonary complications after hepatic resection. *Ann Surg*. 2012;225:540–550.
30. Bapoje S, Whitaker J, Chu E, Albert R. Preoperative evaluation of the patient with pulmonary disease. *Chest*. 2007;132:1637–1645.
31. Lunardi A, Miranda C, Silva K, et al. Weakness of expiratory muscles and pulmonary complications in malnourished patients undergoing upper abdominal surgery. *Respirology*. 2012;17:108–113.
32. Duggan M, Kavanagh B. Perioperative modifications of respiratory function. *Best Pract Res Clin Anaesthesiol*. 2010;24:145–155.
33. Smith T, Stonell C, Purkayastha S, Paraskevas P. Cardiopulmonary exercise testing as a risk assessment method in non cardio-pulmonary surgery: a systematic review. *Anaesthesia*. 2009;64:883–893.
34. Sachdev G, Napolitano L. Postoperative pulmonary complications: pneumonia and acute respiratory failure. *Surg Clin N Am*. 2012;92:321–344.
35. Silva D, Gazzana M, Knorst M. Merit of preoperative clinical finding and functional pulmonary evaluation as predictors of postoperative pulmonary complications. *Rev Assoc Med Bras*. 2010;56:551–557.
36. Rodgers A, Walker N, Schug S, et al. Reduction of postoperative mortality and morbidity with epidural or spinal anesthesia: results from overview of randomized trials. *BMJ*. 2000;321:1493.
37. Rosenthal MH. Intraoperative fluid management—what and how much? *Chest*. 1999;115(Suppl 5):130S–137S.
38. Hess DR, Kondili D, Burns E, et al. A 5-year observational study of lung-protective ventilation in the operating room: a single-center experience. *J Crit Care* 2013;28:533.e9–e15.
39. Futier E, Constantin JM, Paugam-Burtz C, et al. A trial of intraoperative low-tidal-volume ventilation in abdominal surgery. *N Engl J Med*. 2013;369:428–437.
40. Squadrone V, Coha M, Cerutti E, et al. Continuous positive airway pressure for treatment of postoperative hypoxemia: a randomized trial. *JAMA*. 2005;293:589–595.
41. Restrepo RD, Wettstein R, Wittnebel L, Tracy M. Incentive spirometry: 2011. *Respir Care*. 2011;56:1600–1604.
42. Smith P, Baig M, Brito V. Postoperative pulmonary complications after laparotomy. *Respiration*. 2010;80:269–274.
43. Lawrence V, Cornell J, Smetana G. Strategies to reduce postoperative pulmonary complications after noncardiothoracic surgery: systematic review for the American College of Physicians. *Ann Intern Med*. 2006;144:596–608.
44. Sitsen E, van Poorten F, van Alphen W, et al. Postoperative epidural analgesia after total knee arthroplasty with sufentanil 1 microg/ml combined with ropivacaine 0.2%, ropivacaine 0.125%, or levobupivacaine 0.125%: a randomized, double-blinded comparison. *Reg Anesth Pain Med*. 2007;6:475–480.
45. Ballantyne J, Kupelnick B, McPeek B, Lau J. Does the evidence support the use of spinal and epidural anesthesia for surgery? *J Clin Anesth*. 2005;5:382–391.
46. Reinius H, Jonsson L, Gustafsson S, et al. Prevention of atelectasis in morbidly obese patients during general anesthesia and paralysis. *Anesthesiology*. 2009;111:979–987.
47. Ferreyra G, Baussano I, Squadrone V, et al. Continuous positive airway pressure for treatment of respiratory complications following abdominal surgery: a systematic review and meta-analysis. *Ann Surg*. 2008;247:617–626.
48. Douketis J, Berger P, Dunn A, et al. The perioperative management of antithrombotic therapy: American College of Physicians evidence-based clinical practice guidelines (8th edition). *Chest*. 2008;133(Suppl 6):299S–399S.
49. Herbst-Rodrigues M, Carvalho V, Abrahao L, et al. Alveolar recruitment maneuver in refractory hypoxemia and lobar atelectasis after cardiac surgery: a case report. *J Cardiothorac Surg*. 2012;7:58–61.
50. Guimaraes M, El Dib R, Smith A, Matos D. Incentive spirometry for prevention of postoperative pulmonary complications in upper abdominal surgery (review). *Cochrane Database Syst Rev*. 2009 July 8;(3):CD006058pub2. Update in *Cochrane Database Syst Rev*. 2014;2:CD006058.
51. Edmark L, Auner U, Endlund M, et al. Oxygen concentration and characteristics of progressive atelectasis formation during anaesthesia. *Acta Anaesthesiol Scand*. 2011;55:75–81.
52. Goldhaber S, Bounameaux H. Pulmonary embolism and deep vein thrombosis. *Lancet*. 2012;379:1835–1846.
53. Tusman G, Bohm S, Warner D, Sprung J. Atelectasis and perioperative pulmonary complications in high-risk patients. *Curr Opin Anesthesiol*. 2012;25:1–10.
54. Diez-Sebastian J, Herruzo R, Garcia-Caballero J. Prevention of early-onset pneumonia in surgical patients by chemoprophylaxis. *Am J Surg*. 2012;204:441–446.
55. Strickland SL, Rubin BK, Drescher GS, et al. AARC Clinical Practice Guideline: effectiveness of nonpharmacologic airway clearance techniques in hospitalized patients. *Respir Care*. 2013;58:2187–2193.

56. Andrews J, Sathe NA, Krishnaswami S, McPheeters ML. Nonpharmacologic airway clearance techniques in hospitalized patients: a systematic review. *Respir Care.* 2013;58:2150–2186.
57. Branson RD. The scientific basis for postoperative respiratory care. *Respir Care.* 2013;58:1974–1984.
58. Li Q, Yao G, Zhu X. High-dose Ambroxol reduces pulmonary complication in patients with acute cervical spinal cord injury after surgery. *Neurocrit Care.* 2012;16:267–272.
59. Rello J, Kollef M, Diaz E, et al. Reduced burden of bacterial airway colonization with a novel silver-coated endotracheal tube in a randomized multiple-center feasibility study. *Crit Care Med.* 2006;34:2766–2672.
60. Jaber S, Chanques G, Jung B. Postoperative noninvasive ventilation. *Anesthesiology.* 2010;112:453–461.
61. Pelosi P, Jaber S. Noninvasive respiratory support in the perioperative period. *Curr Opin Anaesthesiol.* 2010;23:233–238.

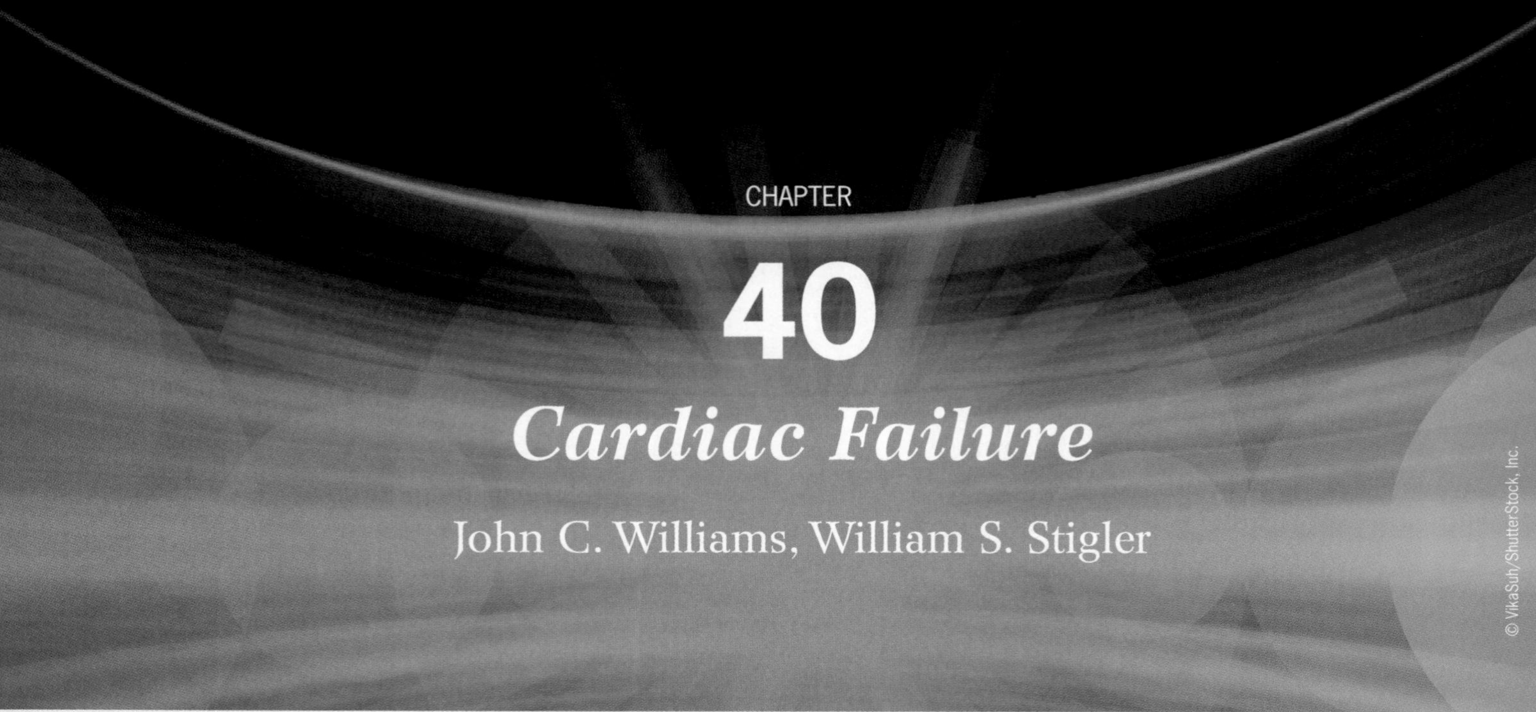

Cardiac Failure

John C. Williams, William S. Stigler

OUTLINE

OBJECTIVES

1. Discuss the epidemiology and etiology of cardiac failure.
2. Describe the physiology of normal cardiac function, the pathophysiology of abnormal cardiac function, and the pathophysiology of pulmonary edema.
3. Describe the determinants of ventricular function.
4. List the symptoms and signs of cardiac failure.
5. Discuss the basic ways in which the heart and lungs interact.
6. Discuss the common causes and treatment of cardiac failure.
7. Discuss the treatment of chronic and acute cardiac failure.
8. Discuss issues related to noninvasive and invasive ventilation of patients with cardiac failure.

KEY TERMS

afterload
cardiac failure
cardiac output ($\dot{Q}c$)
cardiomyocytes
cardiomyopathy
contractility
coronary angiography
coronary artery bypass surgery
diastole
diastolic dysfunction
echocardiography
hepatojugular reflux
intra-aortic balloon pump (IABP)
oncotic pressure
orthopnea
percutaneous coronary intervention (PCI)
preload
pulmonary edema
pulmonary vascular resistance (PVR)
Starling's law of cardiac function
stroke volume
systole
systolic dysfunction
venous return
ventricular interdependence

Introduction

Cardiac failure is the final common pathway of almost all forms of heart disease. The high prevalence of heart disease has made cardiac failure one of the most common problems encountered in hospitalized patients. Cardiac failure results in a broad range of symptoms and presentations and, in extreme cases, respiratory failure requiring mechanical ventilation. Mechanical ventilation of these patients can be challenging because of the complexity of the cardiopulmonary interactions and concomitant cardiac problems such as myocardial ischemia. Proper care of the ventilated patient with cardiac failure requires knowledge of the clinical manifestations and an understanding of the basic pathophysiology.

Definition

Cardiac failure is defined by the American College of Cardiology and American Heart Association as a complex clinical syndrome that can result from any structural or functional cardiac disorder that impairs the ventricle from filling with or ejecting blood. The cardinal manifestations of cardiac failure are dyspnea and fatigue, which may limit exercise tolerance, and fluid retention, which may lead to pulmonary congestion and peripheral edema.[1] Because cardiac failure is a complex syndrome, others define it in various ways, including an inability for cardiac function to meet the body's metabolic demands without increasing filling pressures.

Epidemiology

Cardiac failure is a common cause of morbidity and mortality in the United States and worldwide, accounting for 12 million to 15 million office visits and 6.5 million hospital days each year in the United States. In recent years, the number of hospitalizations due to cardiac failure has increased substantially, probably due to the aging of the U.S. population and improved survival after acute myocardial infarction. In 2012, the estimated direct and indirect costs for heart failure were about $31 billion.[2] Cardiac failure is linked closely with cardiovascular diseases such as coronary artery disease, hypertension, and diabetes mellitus.

Incidence

An estimated 5.7 million American adults (2.8% of the U.S. adult population) have been diagnosed with cardiac failure, and each year there are over a million hospitalizations for cardiac failure. Cardiac failure disproportionally affects the elderly; the incidence is 10 persons per 1000 population after age 65 years, and the rate continues to increase with age. Despite improved therapeutic interventions for many of the underlying diseases leading to cardiac failure, the incidence has not declined over the last two decades. People who are diagnosed with heart failure tend to live longer than they did in the past, probably due to improved recognition and evidence-based treatment guidelines.

Mortality

Establishing mortality due to cardiac failure is difficult because the syndrome is a manifestation of myriad underlying processes. Cardiac failure is an associated cause in 1 in 9 deaths, however; 52.3 per 1000 deaths are attributable entirely to cardiac failure. Data from the Framingham Heart Study cohort demonstrate that 80% of men and 70% of women who are diagnosed with heart failure at a relatively young age (less than 65 years) will still die of heart failure within 8 years of diagnosis. The mortality of cardiac failure approaches that observed in cancer, with 1-year and 5-year mortality rates of 22% and 42%, respectively.[3]

Etiology

Cardiac failure results from a large number of primary cardiac diseases as well as systemic diseases. The most common etiologies include coronary artery disease (CAD), hypertension, alcohol, and idiopathic dilated **cardiomyopathy**. **Box 40-1** lists many of the possible etiologies of cardiac failure.

Cardiac Physiology

The heart is a mechanical pump that circulates blood through the pulmonary and systemic circulations. The intact performance of the heart requires a complex series of events that coordinates excitation at the individual

BOX 40-1

Diagnoses Associated with Cardiac Failure

- Acute ischemia
- Dilated cardiomyopathy
  - Chronic ischemic disease
  - Idiopathic
  - Tachycardia induced
  - Myocarditis (e.g., viral, giant cell)
  - Chagas disease
  - Toxin or drug mediated (e.g., Adriamycin [doxorubicin], cobalt, ethanol, cocaine)
  - Sarcoidosis
  - Hemochromatosis
  - Thyroid disease
  - Heredity
- Restrictive cardiomyopathy
  - Hypertrophic cardiomyopathy
  - Infiltrative disorders (amyloid, malignancy)
  - Idiopathic
- Valvular or mechanical disease
  - Aortic stenosis
  - Aortic insufficiency (acute and chronic)
  - Mitral stenosis
  - Mitral regurgitation (acute and chronic)
  - Ventricular septal defect (acute and chronic)
  - Free wall rupture
- Arrhythmia
  - Tachycardia
  - Bradycardia
- Pericardial disease
  - Constrictive pericarditis
  - Constrictive/effusive pericarditis
  - Pericardial tamponade
- Right heart failure
  - Valvular (pulmonary stenosis/insufficiency, tricuspid regurgitation)
  - Eisenmenger syndrome (e.g., atrial septal defect)
  - Pulmonary hypertension (e.g., pulmonary embolism, primary)
- High-output failure
  - Arteriovenous shunting
  - Paget disease
  - Thyroid disease
  - Beriberi
  - Chronic anemia
- Miscellaneous
  - Vasculitis (e.g., Churg-Strauss, Wegener)
  - Carcinoid
  - Scleroderma
  - Eosinophilic cardiomyopathy (Löffler endocarditis)

myocyte to contraction of the heart muscle itself. To generate an adequate cardiac output, the heart must contract and pump blood out (systolic function) and also relax and refill the chambers with blood (diastolic function). Overall cardiac function is regulated by numerous neurohumoral and mechanical factors that can be manipulated with various pharmacologic agents.

Cellular Biology and Biochemistry of Cardiac Function

The heart is composed of cardiac muscle cells (**cardiomyocytes**) organized into linear series called *myofibers*. The myocytes contain the sarcomere, the basic contractile apparatus of the heart, as well as numerous mitochondria for energy production. In addition, the heart has specialized myocytes that initiate and propagate the action potential that causes contraction of the muscle cells.

The smallest unit of muscle that contracts is the sarcomere. Contraction of the myocyte is initiated by cell membrane depolarization. The conducting cells of the heart initiate the action potential that propagates to the muscle cells. When stimulated, myocytes release calcium; the calcium interacts with actin and myosin, the proteins forming the sarcomere, stimulating shortening and therefore contraction of the cells. Through an active process, calcium is again stored in the cell, allowing for relaxation. Both the contraction and the relaxation of the myocyte are energy-dependent functions.[4]

Cardiac Pump Function

The heart rhythmically contracts and continually empties and fills with blood, thus propelling blood through the circulation. The cardiac cycle consists of a period of contraction (**systole**), during which the heart pumps blood into the pulmonary and systemic circulation, followed by a relaxation period (**diastole**), during which venous blood returns to the heart. With each cardiac cycle, a volume of blood is ejected, termed the **stroke volume** of the heart. The product of the stroke volume and heart rate (in beats per minute) gives the **cardiac output** ($\dot{Q}c$), expressed as L/min.

After the blood is ejected, the heart quickly fills with blood from the venous circulation, termed **venous return**. In the steady state the venous return must equal the $\dot{Q}c$. The concept of matched venous return and $\dot{Q}c$ is important in the determination of overall function, because processes that affect the venous return must then affect $\dot{Q}c$, and vice versa.

Additionally, the left ventricle (LV) and the right ventricle (RV) interact with one another through a complex interplay termed **ventricular interdependence**. This concept introduces greater complexity because an understanding of LV function must take into account changes in RV dimensions and function. These aspects of the RV vary with alterations of venous return, pulmonary vascular resistance, and intrathoracic pressure changes.[5]

Determinants of Ventricular Function

Preload

Mechanical factors affect myocyte and myocardial contraction. **Starling's law of cardiac function** states that the longer the initial sarcomere length, the greater the force generated with contraction. The degree of precontraction stretch of the sarcomere is termed the **preload**. In general, $\dot{Q}c$ increases as preload increases, a function known as the Frank-Starling relationship. As preload continues to increase, however, the $\dot{Q}c$ eventually reaches a plateau and can decline if too great of a load is placed on the cardiac myocyte. The preload of the ventricle may be approximated by the ventricular end-diastolic volume (EDV) (**Figure 40-1**). Unfortunately,

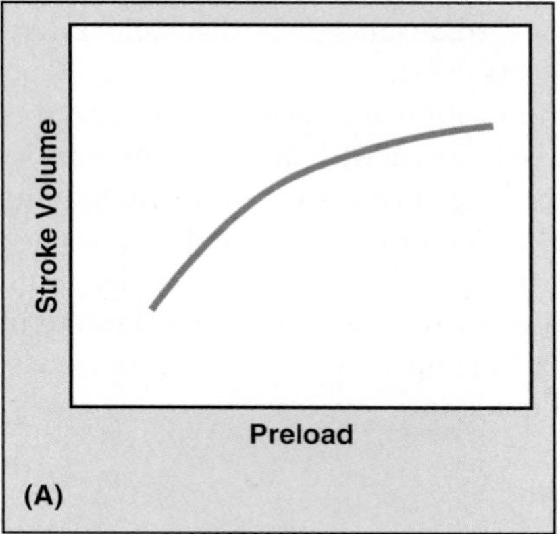

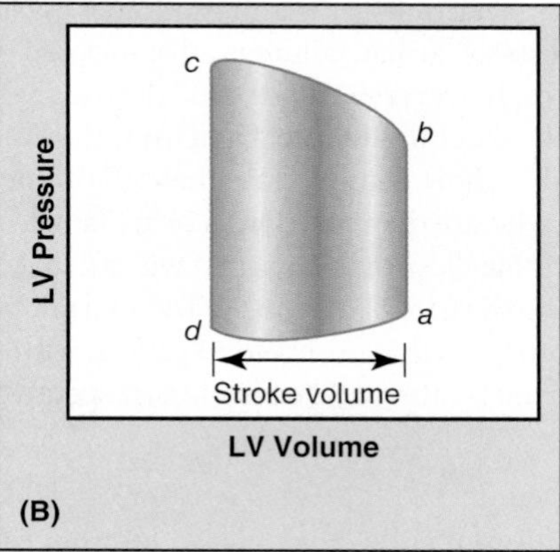

FIGURE 40-1 (**A**) Relationship between preload and stroke volume. (**B**) The pressure–volume loop. For a single cardiac cycle, left ventricular (LV) pressure is plotted against LV volume. Point a represents end-diastole and the start of isovolemic contraction. Ventricular pressure increases without a change in volume until ejection starts at point b, which represents the opening of the aortic valve. During ejection, ventricular volume decreases. Point c represents end-systole and the start of isovolumic relaxation. The aortic valve closes near end-systole. Ventricular pressure continues to fall until ventricular filling starts with the opening of the mitral valve at point d. Ventricular pressure increases very slightly during diastolic filling.

Modified from Wannenburg T, Little WC. Regulation of cardiac output. In: Brown DL, ed. *Cardiac Intensive Care*. WB Saunders; 2010.

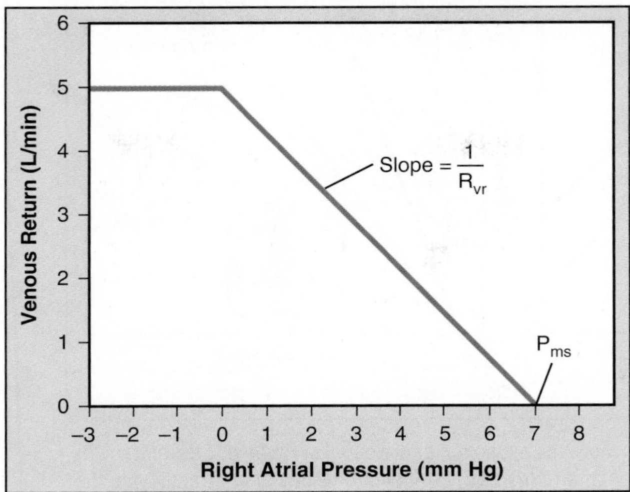

FIGURE 40-2 Normal venous return curve. Relationship between right atrial pressure and the venous return. R_{vr}, resistance to venous return; P_{ms}, mean systemic pressure.

Modified from Brienza N, et al. Peripheral control of venous return in critical illness: role of the splanchnic vascular compartment. In: Dantzker DR, Scharf SM, eds. *Cardiopulmonary Critical Care*. 3rd ed. Saunders; 1998.

this is a difficult variable to measure clinically, and the end-diastolic pressure (EDP) is often used as a surrogate. The ventricular diastolic filling pressure also represents a back pressure limiting venous return (**Figure 40-2**). The relationship between preload and $\dot{Q}c$ requires consideration of both intrinsic ventricular function and venous return (**Figure 40-3**).

Afterload

The load that opposes myocardial shortening is called the **afterload**. There is an inverse relationship between the force which must be generated by the cardiac muscle against a load and the degree and velocity of muscle shortening. As the afterload is increased at any fixed degree of contractility, there is less myocardial shortening and decreased cardiac output, a concept demonstrated graphically in **Figure 40-4**. Afterload is not easily quantified. For clinical purposes, the mean arterial blood pressure (MAP) is a reasonable estimate of afterload.

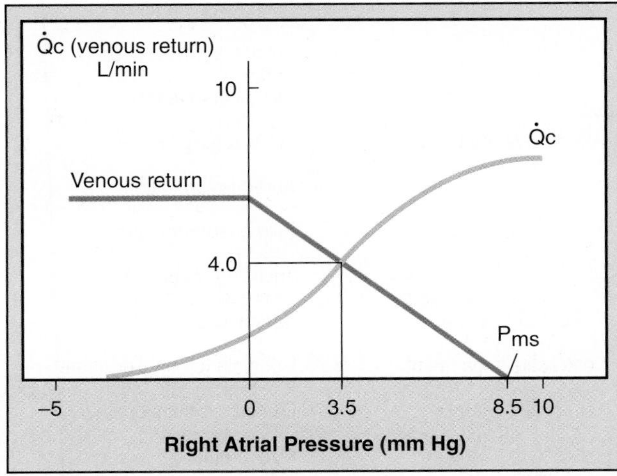

FIGURE 40-3 Venous return and cardiac output as a function of right atrial pressure. The intersection of the two curves represents the steady-state cardiac output of the heart under the given loading conditions.

Reproduced with kind permission from Springer Science+Business Media. *Can J Anesth.* The role of the vasculature in venous return and cardiac output: historical and graphical approach,1997;44:849–867. Jacobsohn E, Chorn R, O'Connor M.

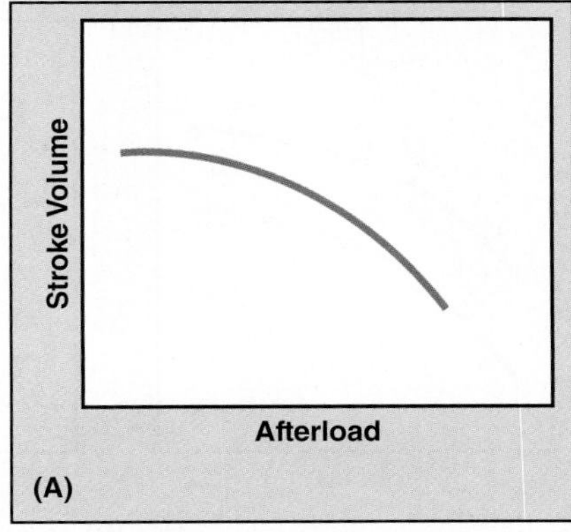

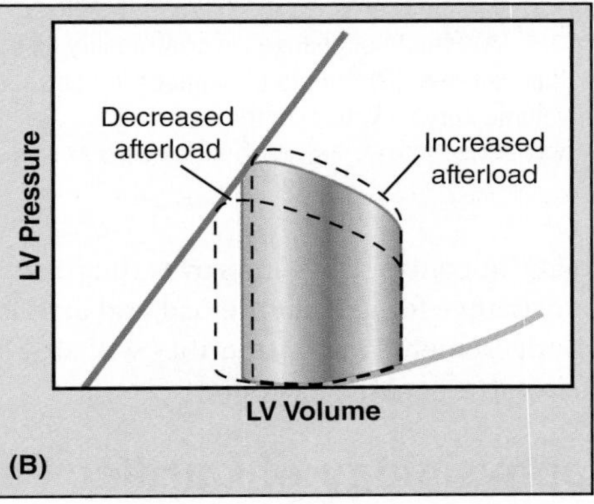

FIGURE 40-4 (**A**) Effects of afterload on stroke volume. (**B**) Effects of afterload on the pressure–volume curve of the left ventricle (LV).

Modified from Wannenburg T, Little WC. Regulation of cardiac output. In: Brown DL, ed. *Cardiac Intensive Care*. WB Saunders; 2010.

Contractility

Contractility defines the intrinsic strength of contraction independent of preload and afterload. The myocardium can alter contractility in many ways. In general, measures that increase the concentration or availability of cellular calcium ions increase the contractility. The effect of changes in contractility can be demonstrated graphically as a change in the relationship between stroke volume and preload or afterload (**Figure 40-5**).

Respiratory Recap

Determinants of Ventricular Function

- Preload
- Afterload
- Contractility

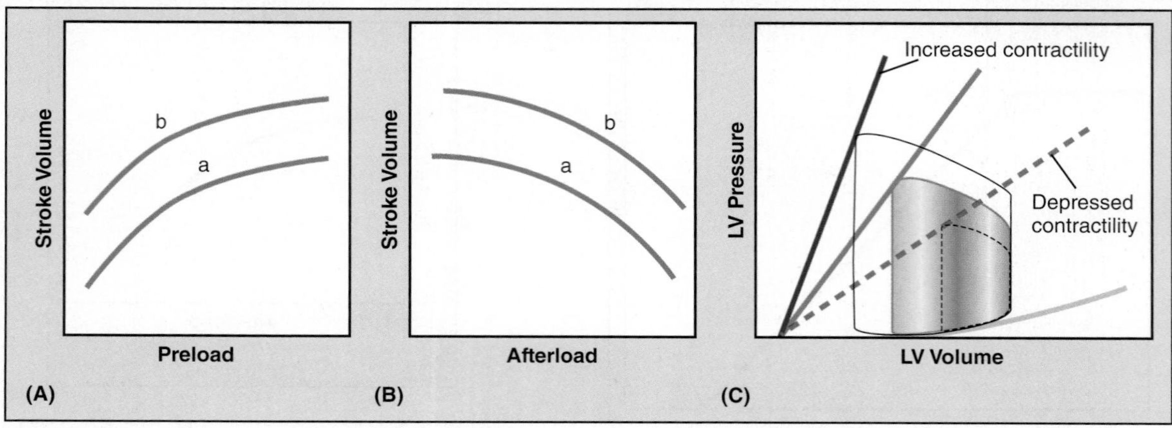

FIGURE 40-5 (**A**) Effects of changes in contractility on stroke volume as shown as a function of preload. For curve b, the contractility is greater than curve a. (**B**) Effects of changes in contractility as a function of afterload. (**C**) Effects of changes of contractility on the pressure–volume curve. LV, left ventricle.

Modified from Wannenburg T, Little WC. Regulation of cardiac output. In: Brown DL, ed. *Cardiac Intensive Care*. WB Saunders; 2010.

An increase in contractility improves the relative cardiac performance for a given preload and afterload. Similarly, decrements in contractility will alter this relationship in a negative fashion.

Pathophysiology of Cardiac Failure

Cardiac failure is defined as the inability of the heart to meet the metabolic needs of the body or the inability to meet those needs without an elevation in filling pressures. The complex interplay of various phenomena results in normal cardiac function. Valvular competence, synchronization of the cardiac cycle, and coordination of cardiac contraction with venous filling are all required. Abnormalities of any of these components can eventually lead to cardiac failure.

Mechanisms

Impairment of contractile function can be due to rhythm disorders like atrial fibrillation or due to disorders of muscular contraction. **Table 40-1** lists common cardiac disorders that can lead to heart failure. In these disorders, the primary problem is the inability of the heart to pump because of either direct impairment in the force of contraction or in the frequency of contractions (as in arrhythmias). This form of heart failure is often called **systolic dysfunction** and can be represented graphically as a shift in the Starling curve downward (**Figure 40-6**).

Many forms of heart disease impose an excessive load on the heart (Table 40-1). This load can be in the form of either an excess pressure requirement or an excess volume requirement. The load may occur as an acute overload that rapidly causes deterioration in cardiac function or as a chronic load that slowly leads to cardiac failure.

An example of an acute volume overload is papillary muscle rupture and acute mitral regurgitation. In this

TABLE 40-1
Pathophysiology of Cardiac Failure with Clinical Examples

Pathophysiology	Clinical Examples
Restricted filling	Restrictive cardiomyopathy
	Constrictive pericarditis
	Tamponade
	Hypertrophic cardiomyopathy
	Mitral stenosis
	Tricuspid stenosis
Pressure overload	Hypertension
	Aortic stenosis
	Pulmonary embolism
	Pulmonary hypertension
	Pulmonary stenosis
Volume overload	Mitral regurgitation
	Aortic regurgitation
	Pulmonary regurgitation
	Tricuspid regurgitation
	Septal defects
Contractile impairment	Ischemia (chronic or acute)
	Dilated cardiomyopathy
	Myocarditis
Arrhythmia	Tachycardia
	Bradycardia

Reproduced from Timmis AD, Nathan AW. *Essentials of Cardiology*. Oxford: Blackwell Scientific; 1993.

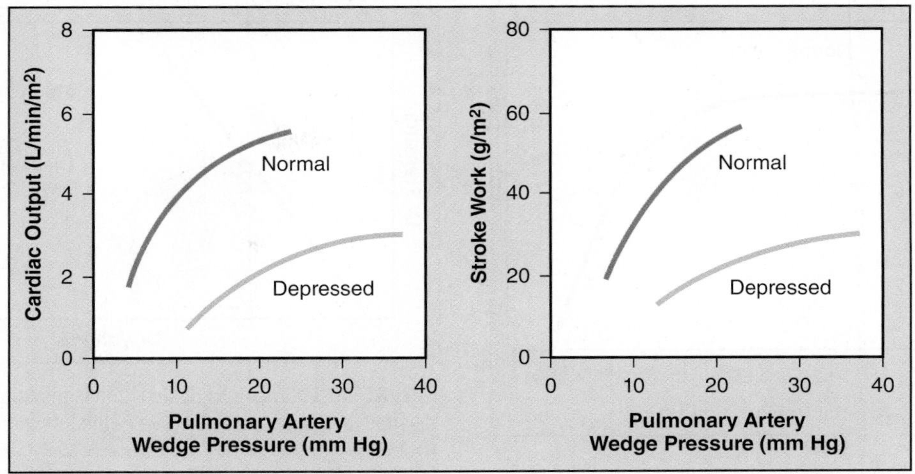

FIGURE 40-6 The effect of a decrease in contractility on the Starling relationship.

Reproduced from Little WC, Braunwald E. Assessment of cardiac function. In: Braunwald E, ed. *Heart Disease: A Textbook of Cardiovascular Medicine*. 5th ed. Copyright Elsevier (WB Saunders) 1997.

situation, the heart suddenly ejects a large amount of blood from the left ventricle through the mitral valve into the left atrium during systole, thus reducing the forward $\dot{Q}c$ to the systemic circulation and increasing left atrial pressure. Compensation via increased contractility may not adequately augment forward stroke volume because the low pressure of the left atrium relative to the systemic circulation preferentially directs blood flow through the injured valve. These patients thus will often present with hypotension and shock from low $\dot{Q}c$ and pulmonary edema from increased left atrial pressure.

Chronic volume overload results from disorders such as progressive aortic valve regurgitation, in which initially a small portion of the stroke volume is regurgitated into the ventricle. The result is a decrease in the true forward $\dot{Q}c$ at a given left ventricular end-diastolic volume (LVEDV). Under such conditions the slow progression of the degree of regurgitation allows the heart to compensate with slow dilation and an increase in mass, which helps to normalize wall stress and preserve the forward stroke volume (**Figure 40-7**), although this leads to a chronic increase in LVEDV and LV wall thickness.

In acute pressure overload, a high afterload reduces the forward output of the heart. Because of the acute nature of the overload, the compensatory mechanisms of the heart (increased LVEDV and increased contractility) may be inadequate to augment forward flow, leading to elevated filling pressures with pulmonary edema. Acute pressure overload is typified by hypertensive emergency, a process in which there is a sudden and severe increase in systemic blood pressure. **Figure 40-8** illustrates the relationship between $\dot{Q}c$ and arterial pressure.

Chronic pressure overload, as exemplified by chronic hypertension and aortic stenosis, results in a sustained increase in afterload and ventricular wall stress. Over time the cardiomyocytes will adapt to this stress by

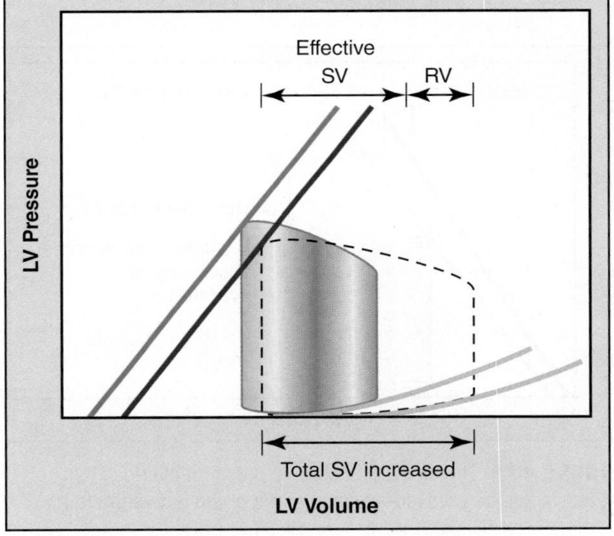

FIGURE 40-7 The effect of a chronic volume overload on the pressure–volume curve of the left ventricle (LV).

Modified from Wannenburg T, Little WC. Regulation of cardiac output. In: Brown DL, ed. *Cardiac Intensive Care*. WB Saunders; 2010.

hypertrophy, and clinically this adaptation can result in thickened ventricular walls. A pressure overload such as aortic stenosis can be demonstrated graphically as shown in **Figure 40-9**.

As the increased load continues, adaptive mechanisms will eventually fail to compensate and the signs of cardiac failure will become evident. The end result is systolic dysfunction. This process differs from the previously described mechanism because the original cause of the dysfunction is not a primary disorder of the contractile apparatus but, ultimately, is caused by exhausted compensation.

Alteration of ventricular filling may accompany a number of different cardiac disorders (refer to Table 40-1). The disorders range from myocardial valvular disease to

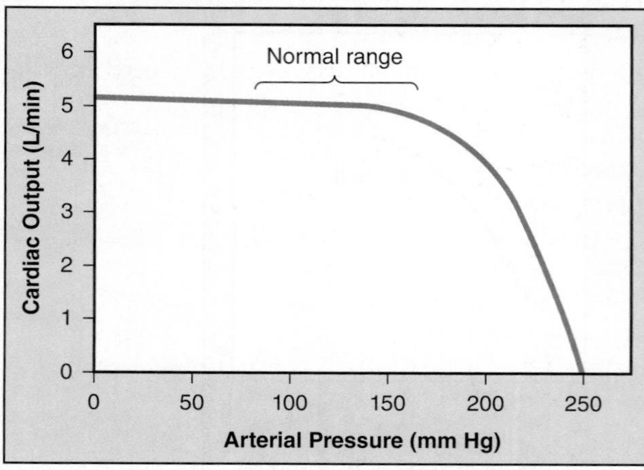

FIGURE 40-8 Constancy of cardiac output up to a pressure level of 160 mm Hg. Only when the arterial pressure rises above the normal operating pressure range does the pressure load cause the cardiac output to fall.

Reproduced from Guyton AC, Hall JE. *Textbook of Medical Physiology*. 10th ed. Copyright Elsevier (WB Saunders) 2000.

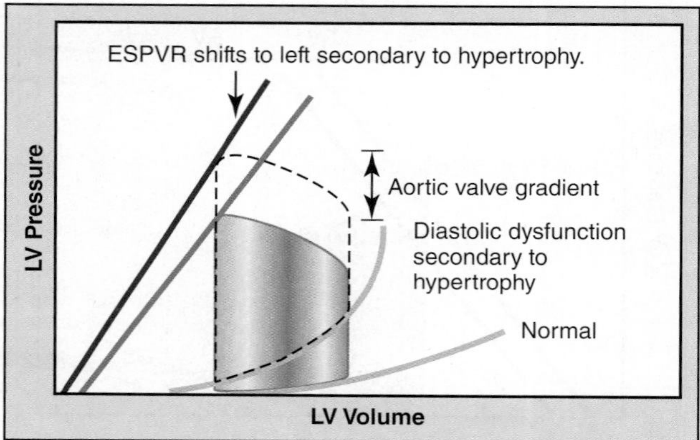

FIGURE 40-9 The effect of a chronic pressure overload (aortic stenosis) on the pressure–volume curve of the left ventricle (LV).

Modified from Wannenburg T, Little WC. Regulation of cardiac output. In: Brown DL, ed. *Cardiac Intensive Care*. WB Saunders; 2010.

pericardial disease. In these disorders, the abnormally high filling pressures are required to achieve the preload necessary to deliver an adequate stroke volume.[4]

The failure of the cardiac muscle to relax normally is often called **diastolic dysfunction** or heart failure with preserved ejection fraction (HFpEF) and represents a common and significant cause of cardiac failure. HFpEF results in elevated filling pressures and symptoms of pulmonary and systemic congestion despite normal systolic function. HFpEF is caused by processes that affect the active (energy-dependent) and passive (compliance) relaxation of the ventricle.[6,7] Many conditions cause diastolic dysfunction. As previously noted, early in diastole the ventricular relaxation is an energy-requiring process, so cardiac ischemia is a common cause of both diastolic and systolic dysfunction. Volume overload can cause relative diastolic dysfunction by increasing the LVEDV, thus increasing the LV filling

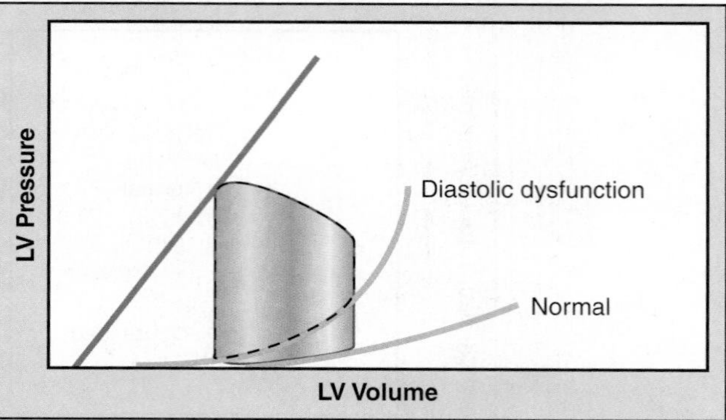

FIGURE 40-10 Diastolic dysfunction leads to an elevation of the diastolic pressure–volume curve of the left ventricle (LV).

Modified from Wannenburg T, Little WC. Regulation of cardiac output. In: Brown DL, ed. *Cardiac Intensive Care*. WB Saunders; 2010.

pressures because of a shift of the diastolic pressure–volume curve into a less compliant region (**Figure 40-10**). Diastolic dysfunction may also occur with an increase in afterload. With hypertrophy of the myocardium or in conditions of abnormal infiltration of the myocardium, the ventricles are less compliant, and the diastolic pressure volume curve will shift upward (Figure 40-10). Extrinsic compression of the heart does not affect the intrinsic relaxation of the myocardium but reduces the distensibility of the heart and thus displaces the pressure–volume curve upward.

Classification

The temporal course of cardiac failure is an important etiologic consideration. Myocardial infarction, myocarditis, and pulmonary emboli may cause acute cardiac failure. An acute, severe change in cardiac function can cause pulmonary edema and shock resulting from the inability of the heart to adapt rapidly to loss of

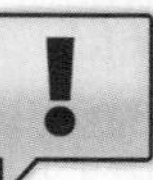

Respiratory Recap

Mechanisms of Cardiac Failure

- Primary impaired myocardial contractile function
- Excessive ventricular load (pressure or volume)
- Restricted ventricular filling

Note: These mechanisms of cardiac failure are not mutually exclusive, and many forms of heart disease show components of all three pathways.

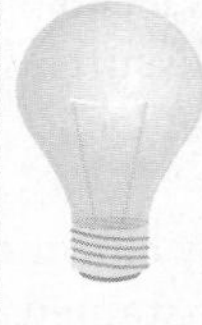

STOP AND THINK

Your patient with signs and symptoms of heart failure has normal systolic function on the echocardiogram. What are some other mechanisms by which this patient can have heart failure?

myocardium or a dramatic increase in load. Chronic cardiac failure is seen in conditions such as coronary artery disease, hypertensive heart disease, and chronic valvular disease. Long-standing compensation can often lead to chronic cardiac failure in later years. As opposed to the severe symptoms of acute changes in cardiac function, chronic cardiac failure may manifest only relatively mild symptoms until late in the disease process because of the compensatory mechanisms.

The clinical effects of isolated left ventricular failure are largely attributed to venous congestion of the lungs. Similarly, right ventricular failure leads to symptoms caused by congestion of the systemic veins. RV failure can occur in isolation (as with pulmonary embolism) or concurrent with LV failure (biventricular failure). RV failure most commonly results from LV failure. In cases of biventricular failure a patient may manifest symptoms of predominantly right or left ventricular failure, or both.

Most forms of cardiac failure are characterized by a reduction in the $\dot{Q}c$ either at rest or with exercise. In certain uncommon conditions, the tissue demand for oxygen cannot be met despite a high $\dot{Q}c$. This is called *high-output failure* and is seen in conditions of increased metabolic rate, reduced oxygen-carrying capacity of blood (e.g., anemia), and arteriovenous shunting, which reduces the effective $\dot{Q}c$ because a portion of the $\dot{Q}c$ bypasses systemic end-organ capillaries as shunted blood moves directly from arteries to the venous return.

Adaptive Mechanisms

The ventricle remodels in response to the load placed on it. This remodeling can be in several different forms: (1) concentric hypertrophy, (2) eccentric hypertrophy, or (3) changes in chamber geometry (usually more spherelike) (**Figure 40-11**). A prolonged pressure load on the myocardium leads to fundamental changes in cardiac muscle. In experimental models, increased systolic wall stress upregulates growth factors that increase the number of mitochondria and increase myofibril mass. The new myofibrils are usually laid down in parallel, leading to myocyte hypertrophy and, ultimately, to a concentrically thicker ventricle. Physiologically, a thicker ventricle serves to normalize increased wall stress. Wall stress can be calculated by the law of Laplace:

$$\text{Wall stress} = (\text{Pressure} \times \text{Radius})/(2 \times \text{Wall thickness})$$

The pressure the ventricle contracts against is thus directly proportional to wall stress. As the ventricle increases its thickness, wall stress decreases, which in turn improves cardiac performance to a point. This improved performance is at the price of increased oxygen demand and possible diastolic dysfunction. At a certain point the thickened myocardium will be prone to supply/demand mismatch, which can lead to myocardial necrosis and, over time, to overt systolic dysfunction.

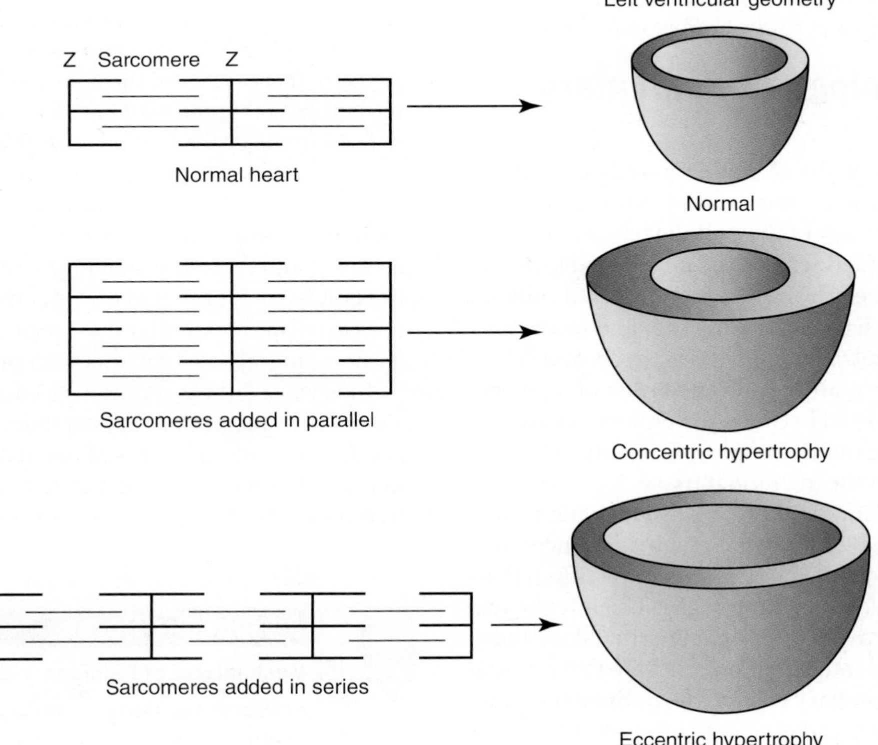

FIGURE 40-11 Remodeling of the ventricle.

Reproduced by permission from Macmillan Publishers Ltd from Gjesdal O, Bluemke DA and Lima JA. Cardiac remodeling at the population level—risk factors, screening, and outcomes. *Nature Rev Cardiol.* 2011;8:673–685.

STOP AND THINK

Your patient tells you that he was diagnosed with hypertension many years ago but never took antihypertensives or followed up with a physician. He now has shortness of breath and leg swelling. What is the most likely cause of his symptoms? What might his echocardiogram show?

The dilated ventricle has increased diastolic wall stress caused by increased diastolic volume (due to an increased radius). In an effort to accommodate the increased volume, myocytes increase the number of sarcomeres in series, thus increasing the radius and length of the ventricle. As the chamber radius increases, so does systolic wall stress, and the ventricle is therefore stimulated to increase in thickness. Volume overload thus induces ventricular dilation and hypertrophy to compensate for the increased diastolic wall stress. This adaptation initially allows compensation for increased diastolic load at normalized wall stress.

The ventricle changes in shape in response to the specific, chronic load placed on it in order to optimize function. Chronic pressure loads induce thickened ventricles with small cavities, whereas chronic volume loads cause dilation of the ventricle. These ventricular shape changes have effects on both systolic and diastolic performance as well as on oxygen use. These adaptive compensatory changes may become ineffective if the heart thickens or dilates excessively, and cardiac failure may ensue.[4]

Pathophysiology of Pulmonary Edema

Pulmonary edema is the accumulation of excess fluid in the interstitial and alveolar spaces in the lung. The large capillary network of the pulmonary circulation has extensive interaction with the air-filled alveoli. The interstitium between the capillary endothelial cells and the alveolar epithelial cells is quite thin and made up of a basement membrane, connective tissue, and cellular elements. Normally a continuous flux of fluid and proteins is transported between the pulmonary circulation and the lung interstitium, with a net flow from the capillaries into the interstitial tissue. Excess fluid is removed from the interstitium by the lymphatic system. Pulmonary edema develops when there is an increase in the flux of fluid going into the lung interstitium that overwhelms the lymphatic drainage. Normally the lymphatic drainage actively takes up interstitial fluid and removes it from the interstitial space at about 20 mL/hour. With chronic pulmonary edema, the pulmonary lymphatics hypertrophy and increased amounts of fluid can be removed (up to 200 mL/hour).

Pulmonary edema can result from any of a number of causes that create an increased influx of fluid to the interstitium. These mechanisms include increased pulmonary capillary pressure as in cardiac failure, decreased blood oncotic pressure, and increased capillary permeability. The forces that affect fluid dynamics in the lungs are summarized in Starling's equation:

$$J_v = K_f[P_c - P_i] - \sigma[\pi_c - \pi_i]$$

where:

- J_v is the net fluid movement between compartments; if J_v is positive, fluid will leave the capillary.
- $[P_c - P_i] - \sigma[\pi_c - \pi_i]$ is the net driving force
- P_c is the capillary hydrostatic pressure
- P_i is the interstitial hydrostatic pressure
- π_c is the capillary oncotic pressure
- π_i is the interstitial oncotic pressure
- K_f is the filtration coefficient—a proportionality constant
- σ is the reflection coefficient

Capillary hydrostatic pressure is directly influenced by left ventricular function and is increased in patients with heart failure. Capillary oncotic pressure is the osmotic pressure exerted by plasma proteins that acts to pull fluid from the interstitium into the circulatory system. Increased fluid flux into the interstitium eventually overwhelms the lymphatic drainage, and fluid initially collects in the most compliant regions of the interstitium around vessels and airways. With increased accumulation, fluid begins to collect in the alveolocapillary membrane and eventually floods the alveoli.

Gravity directs the majority of lung blood flow toward the most dependent regions of the lung. Pulmonary perfusion pressure and pulmonary venous pressure increase from the apex to the base in the upright lung (**Figure 40-12**). Edema thus is most likely to form in the dependent regions (West zone III). As interstitial pressure increases, the lumen of the pulmonary vessels may be compressed in the dependent regions, leading to a decrease in their perfusion (West zone IV) and redistribution of the blood flow into the nondependent regions. This is the cause of the increased apical vascular markings commonly seen on chest radiographs of patients with pulmonary edema.

In cardiac failure, pulmonary edema results from elevation in the pulmonary capillary pressure. This is a direct result of increased downstream pressure in the pulmonary veins, left atrium, and left ventricle that results from the various causes of heart failure.

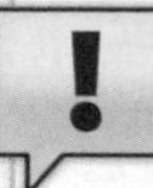

Respiratory Recap

Mechanisms of Pulmonary Edema

- Increased pulmonary capillary pressure as in cardiac failure
- Decreased blood oncotic pressure
- Increased capillary permeability

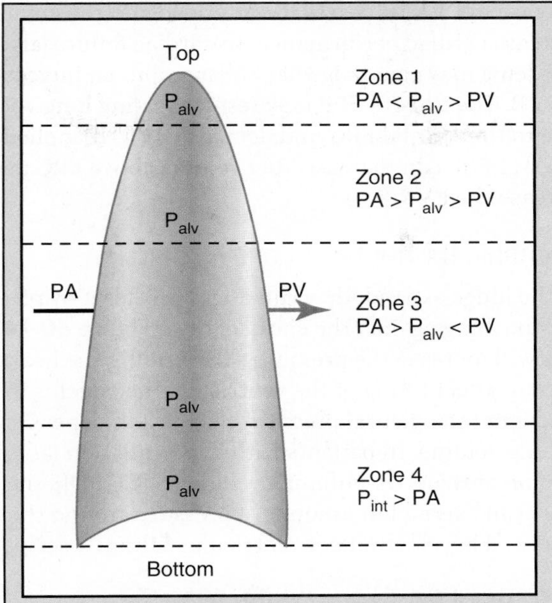

FIGURE 40-12 The four perfusion zones of the lung. The heights of the thick black lines represent pulmonary arterial (PA) and pulmonary venous (PV) pressures.

Modified from Gaine SP, et al. Pathophysiology of the pulmonary vascular bed. In: Dantzker DR, Scharf SM, eds. *Cardiopulmonary Critical Care*. 3rd ed. WB Saunders; 1998.

The development of pulmonary edema depends on the relationship between the capillary pressure, the **oncotic pressures**, and the lymphatic drainage.

As the pulmonary capillary pressure rises, there is an increase in the caliber of vessels and engorgement of the lungs with blood. This increases the elasticity of the lung and commonly is associated with a sense of dyspnea. As edema forms in the interstitium, there is a further increase in lung elasticity. Ventilation–perfusion inequalities appear, leading to increased work of breathing and problems with oxygen uptake. As edema worsens and fluid begins to flood alveoli, early dependent airway closure and associated lung collapse occur. This leads to further abnormalities in gas exchange and a dramatic increase in elasticity and work of breathing. In addition, engorged blood vessels may reduce the caliber of small airways and increase airways resistance. This can then cause a decreased vital capacity and air trapping. Often the airway edema predisposes patients to bronchospasm, and they may develop wheezing, sometimes called cardiac asthma. Gas exchange abnormalities may be quite severe, with hypoxemia followed by hypercapnia as the patient begins to fatigue. In acute severe pulmonary edema, the patient may rapidly progress to respiratory failure. Rapid diagnosis and application of therapy can be lifesaving and often can avoid the use of mechanical ventilation.

Heart–Lung Interactions

The heart and lungs are pressure-driven systems that share the primary responsibility for oxygen uptake and delivery to the body. They also share a common space (the thorax) and thus are linked anatomically. The heart and lung interactions based on these physiologic links often have profound consequences in critical illness. With each breath the lungs and thorax change in volume, thereby changing intrathoracic pressure. These fluctuations can affect cardiac function by inducing changes in the heart rate, preload, afterload, venous return, and contractility of the heart. The heart–lung interactions in cardiac failure can be especially challenging because the heart is less likely to tolerate fluctuations in these physiologic variables. A basic understanding of these interactions is important in the guidance of therapy such as mechanical ventilation.

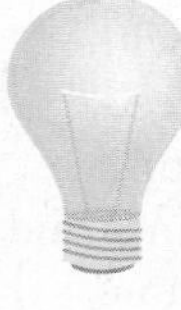

STOP AND THINK

Your patient has a tension pneumothorax and has developed severe hypotension and pronounced jugular venous distension. What is the reason for this, and how should he be treated?

Changes in Intrathoracic Pressure

The changes in pleural pressure with ventilation affect the pressures at the heart's surface. The cardiac surface pressure will affect cardiac filling pressures based on the compliance of the myocardium. In addition, cardiac filling volume is dependent on the transmural pressure, or the distending stress across the wall of the cardiac chamber. The pleural pressure swings during respiration therefore can affect preload and afterload of the heart. For example, a decrease in pleural pressure during inspiration will be transmitted to the surface of the heart. During inspiration, the right atrial pressure falls relative to the systemic extrathoracic venous circulation, and venous filling of the right atrium is enhanced. This leads to an increase in venous return and right atrial volume during inspiration. Similarly, assuming a constant arterial pressure, a decrease in the pleural pressure that also lowers cardiac surface pressure will increase afterload by increasing the LV transmural pressure. An increase in intrathoracic pressure can decrease afterload by a similar

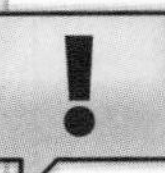

Respiratory Recap

Heart–Lung Interactions

- Intrathoracic pressure changes
- Lung volume changes
- Pulmonary vascular resistance
- Mechanical effects of lung expansion
- Abdominal pressure changes
- Ventricular interdependence

mechanism. Normally these are small changes, but if there are large swings in the pleural pressure (as with respiratory distress) or if cardiac function is reduced, the effects can be more significant. The cardiac surface pressure also depends on the pericardial compliance and pressure, which is sensitive to changes in the volume of the cardiac chambers. The change in cardiac surface pressure with a change in pleural pressure thus can be quite variable.

Changes in Lung Volume

Changes in lung volume can influence cardiovascular performance by a number of different mechanisms. These mechanisms include changes in autonomic tone, changes in **pulmonary vascular resistance (PVR)**, direct mechanical compression of the cardiac fossa, increases in intra-abdominal pressure, and ventricular interdependence. Such effects are manifest with every breath and can become quite significant during periods of sustained inflation as with mechanical ventilation and high positive end-expiratory pressure (PEEP).

Changes in Pulmonary Vascular Resistance

The major determinants of pulmonary blood flow are RV systolic performance and the PVR. The PVR is highly dependent on the volume of the lungs. As alveoli expand, the vessels surrounding them are compressed, thus increasing the resistance to flow. Vessels outside of the alveoli are pulled open during lung inflation by radial traction, which decreases vascular resistance. The net effect of the opposing changes is that PVR is lowest at the functional residual capacity (FRC) of the lungs. Decreases or increases in resting lung volume cause an increase in the PVR (**Figure 40-13**). An increase in PVR increases RV afterload and thus may decrease cardiac performance. In cardiac failure, alveolar edema may cause alveolar collapse and an increase in PVR. The use of PEEP may restore resting lung volume to the normal FRC and decrease PVR. If applied in excess, PEEP can increase lung volume above FRC and increase the PVR.[8,9]

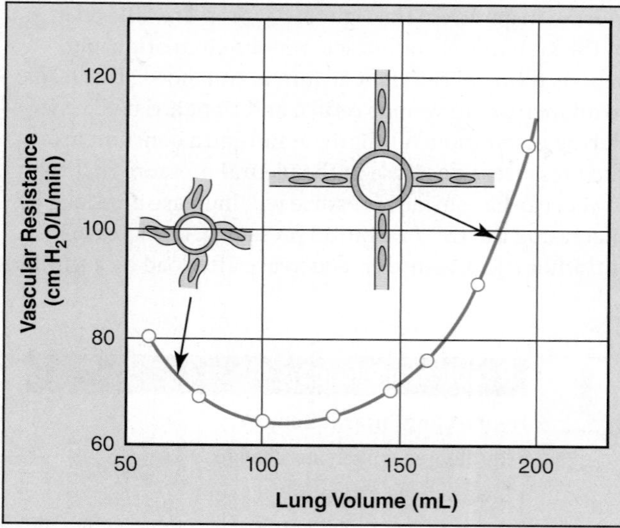

FIGURE 40-13 Effect of lung volume on the pulmonary vascular resistance. The effect of lung volume on the caliber of extra-alveolar vessels also is shown.

Reproduced from West JB. Respiratory Physiology: The Essentials. Lippincott (Wolters Kluwer Health). 2011.

Mechanical Effects of Lung Expansion

As the lungs expand, they can affect the heart by physically pushing against the cardiac fossa (**Figure 40-14**). This will increase the pressure surrounding the heart and can affect filling of the ventricles. The effect is independent of the pleural pressure change and dependent on lung volume. In patients with hyperinflation (as with chronic obstructive pulmonary disease [COPD]), the lungs can exert a fair amount of pressure around the heart and adversely affect ventricular filling.

Abdominal Pressure Changes

The descent of the diaphragm with respiration compresses the abdominal compartment and increases abdominal pressure. This increases the abdominal vascular pressures and increases the driving pressure for venous return. If the patient is receiving positive pressure ventilation, the increase in abdominal pressure may partially compensate for the increase in right atrial pressure induced by the positive pressure. The application of PEEP thus can have complicated effects on the venous return depending on the change in abdominal pressure and previous filling pressure of the ventricle (**Figure 40-15**).

Ventricular Interdependence

Although not a true heart–lung interaction, ventricular interdependence is often discussed in this setting.

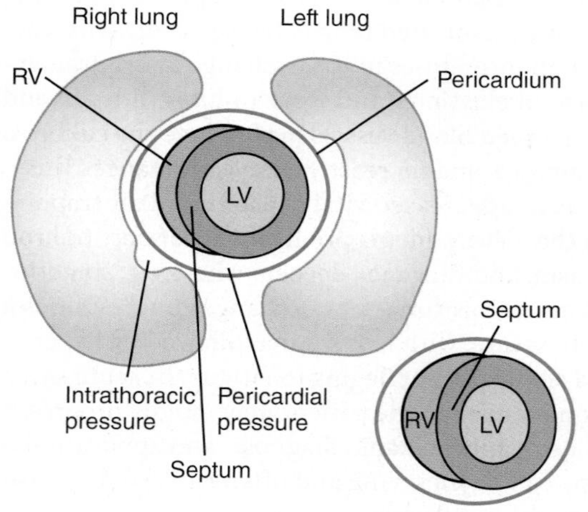

FIGURE 40-14 The anatomic relationship between the heart and lungs. RV, right ventricle; LV, left ventricle.

Reproduced from Scharf SM. Mechanical cardiopulmonary interactions in critical care. In: Dantzker DR. Scharf SM, eds. *Cardiopulmonary Critical Care*. 3rd ed. Copyright Elsevier (WB Saunders) 1998.

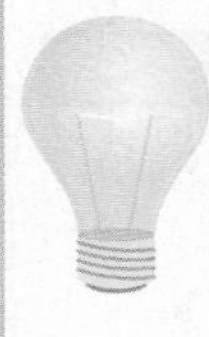

STOP AND THINK

Your patient just had a large pulmonary embolism and has an enlarged right ventricle on echocardiogram. Give two reasons why her cardiac output is decreased.

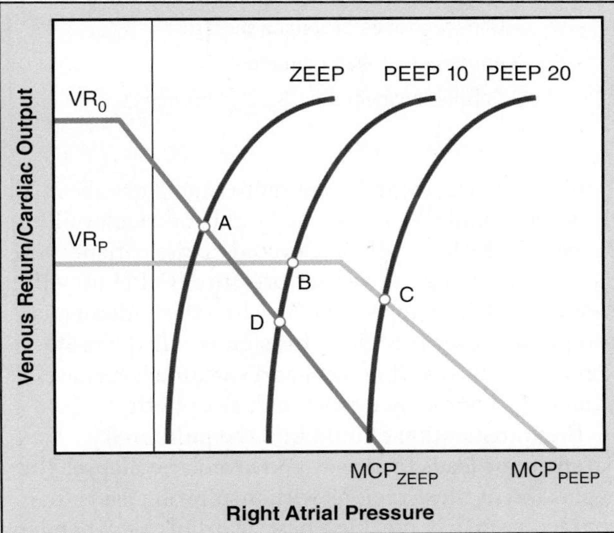

FIGURE 40-15 Effects of positive end-expiratory pressure (PEEP) on the determinants of venous return. VR_0, venous return curve with zero PEEP (ZEEP); VR_P, venous return with PEEP; MCP, mean circulatory pressure.

Reproduced from Scharf SM. Mechanical cardiopulmonary interactions in critical care. In: Dantzker DR, Scharf SM, eds. *Cardiopulmonary Critical Care*. 3rd ed. Copyright Elsevier (WB Saunders) 1998.

Changes in the volume and performance of one ventricle will affect the other ventricle through two general mechanisms. The filling of the LV depends on the output of the RV. A reduction in RV performance, therefore, will reduce LV output by reducing LV preload. This is often called the *series interaction*. In addition, the ventricles are both surrounded by the relatively nondistensible sac called the pericardium, and both ventricles share a common intraventricular septum. This anatomic coupling results in parallel interactions in which an increase in the volume of one ventricle reduces the compliance of the other. For instance, the rise in the RVEDV that often accompanies an acute increase in the PVR will act to decrease LV compliance via effects on the septum. The net effect is a reduction in the LV preload and a decreased $\dot{Q}c$.

Clinical Aspects of Cardiac Failure

The clinical manifestations of cardiac failure are related to inadequate organ perfusion and venous congestion from elevated ventricular filling pressures. The circulatory system has many compensatory mechanisms so that the signs and symptoms of cardiac failure may be manifest only during times of physiologic stress, such as with exercise or illness.

Symptoms

The increased pulmonary capillary pressure and resulting interstitial edema seen in cardiac failure commonly leads to difficulty in breathing or an increased awareness of breathing. Most of the dyspnea can be attributed to an increased work of breathing resulting from decreased pulmonary function and increased ventilatory drive. Pulmonary edema increases lung elastance and can increase airways resistance, thus increasing the pressure changes needed to move air in and out of the lungs. Ventilation and perfusion abnormalities lead to hypoxemia and hypercapnia, which increase the drive to breathe. With extreme decreases in $\dot{Q}c$, respiratory muscle fatigue can develop as a result of poor oxygen delivery to the respiratory muscles and further exacerbate the patient's dyspnea. Dyspnea thus may be caused by either pulmonary congestion leading to impaired gas exchange or a low-output state leading to tissue hypoxemia and muscle fatigue.

The breathlessness of cardiac failure can manifest in many different ways. Most commonly the patient with cardiac failure has dyspnea on exertion. This symptom can be a slowly progressive process, so it is important to ascertain the changes in the patient's exercise tolerance over time. As cardiac failure progresses, the patient may develop breathlessness when recumbent (**orthopnea**). This symptom likely results from decreased pooling of blood in the lower extremities in the supine position. This displaces blood into the central circulation, increases filling pressures, and increases interstitial edema. The patient may report a change in the number of pillows required to sleep or, in severe cases, the need to sleep in a chair. Breathlessness can occur suddenly during sleep, so-called paroxysmal nocturnal dyspnea (PND). Patients will relate terrifying episodes of air hunger during the night requiring them to sit upright. PND may result from sudden bronchospasm related to airway edema. Often the symptoms resolve once the patient is upright for a period of time. Finally, in its most severe forms, cardiac failure will lead to dyspnea at rest and, in acute situations, fulminant respiratory failure.

Patients commonly complain of a reduction in their exercise capacity. The limitation can be primarily caused by shortness of breath or muscle fatigue. An insufficient

Respiratory Recap

Symptoms of Cardiac Failure

- Dyspnea
- Reduced exercise capacity
- General fatigue, weakness, nocturia
- Peripheral edema

augmentation of the stroke volume and heart rate leads to inadequate oxygen delivery to the working muscle. The resulting oxygen debt leads to muscle fatigue. Patients may complain of leg pain or fatigue with exertion that resolves with rest.

A multitude of nonspecific symptoms are commonly seen in patients with cardiac failure. These include general fatigue, weakness, and frequent nocturnal urination. Occurrences of mental status changes or confusion are signs of a drastically reduced $\dot{Q}c$. Patients with right heart failure, either isolated or resulting from left heart failure, will commonly complain of peripheral edema. The legs are involved most commonly, but these patients can develop fluid accumulation in the abdomen in more severe cases.

Isolated right heart failure often results from abnormalities in the parenchyma or vasculature of the lung, which lead to increased pressures in the pulmonary artery and the syndrome known as cor pulmonale. Patients with isolated right heart failure due to diseases like pulmonary arterial hypertension, obstructive sleep apnea, or severe COPD often have similar symptoms to those with left heart failure or biventricular failure, but they rarely develop overt pulmonary edema because their left ventricular systolic function is usually normal.

Functional Classification

The New York Heart Association has developed a classification of patients with heart disease based on the severity of their symptoms.[10]

Class I: No limitation with ordinary activity

Class II: Slight limitation of physical activity; no symptoms at rest, but ordinary activity will result in fatigue, dyspnea, palpitation, or angina

Class III: Marked limitation of physical activity; less than ordinary activity results in symptoms, but comfortable at rest

Class IV: Inability to carry on any physical activity without discomfort; symptoms present at rest

Physical Examination

The physical signs of cardiac failure are often nonspecific, and many findings may be absent in patients, even with severe chronic heart failure. In the correct clinical setting, signs of elevated cardiac filling pressures can be diagnostic of cardiac failure. The following physical signs are suggestive of cardiac failure.

Fluid retention and elevated right filling pressures can lead to the extravasation of fluid into the extravascular space, which is usually seen in the legs or back. Commonly the edema is symmetrical and manifests over several days. An enlarged and/or pulsatile liver can result from elevated filling pressures and tricuspid regurgitation. Ascites can be seen in severe cases. In a recumbent patient with the head of bed at 45 degrees, the upper excursion of the pulsations in the internal jugular vein are normally not more than 3 cm above the sternal angle. With elevated right ventricular filling pressures, the level will be elevated. Some patients will have a normal jugular venous pressure (JVP) but will elevate the JVP inappropriately when the abdomen is compressed over the liver. This sign is called **hepatojugular reflux** and, if present and sustained, suggests altered RV compliance or RV failure or both.

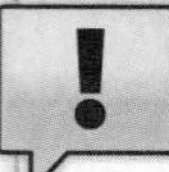

Respiratory Recap

Physical Examination in Cardiac Failure

- Peripheral edema
- Congestive hepatomegaly
- Elevated jugular venous pressure
- Pulmonary auscultation: dependent lung crackles and wheezes
- Cheyne-Stokes breathing pattern
- Abnormal cardiac palpation
- Cardiac auscultation: S_3, S_4, murmurs

The transudation of fluid into the pulmonary parenchyma leads to airway and alveolar collapse. The expansion of these regions with inspiration leads to characteristic wet crackles, best heard in the dependent regions. The presence of airway edema with bronchospasm will create high-pitched wheezes similar to those in patients with asthma. Crackles and wheezes together in a patient with sudden-onset shortness of breath are highly suggestive of pulmonary edema. Cheyne-Stokes respirations are occasionally seen in cardiac failure. This characteristic pattern of alternating hyperpnea and apnea results from a slow circulation time between the lungs and brain combined with exaggerated responses to high or low carbon dioxide levels. Patients are often unaware of the breathing pattern, and it may manifest only during sleep.

The contraction of the heart can normally be felt as a small impulse on the chest below the left nipple. With enlargement of the left ventricle, this point of maximal impulse will be displaced inferiorly and laterally on the chest. The impulse may become quite enlarged and diffuse with severe LV dilation. With hypertrophy of the left ventricle, the impulse may feel stronger and more sustained. The right ventricular impulse is not usually felt, but with RV strain or dilation, a lift may be felt just to the left of the sternum. This parasternal lift is suggestive of RV enlargement or failure. With pulmonary hypertension, a tap may be felt over the left base of the heart, a sign known as a pulmonary artery (PA) tap. Finally, severe murmurs can occasionally be palpated as thrills over the precordium.

The presence of a third heart sound (S_3) after the closure of the aortic and pulmonary valves is suggestive of cardiac failure. The sound likely represents the deceleration of blood in the right or left ventricle during

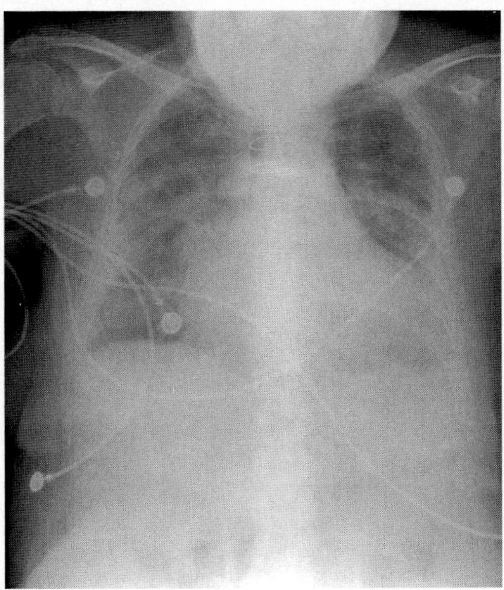

FIGURE 40-16 Anteroposterior chest radiograph of a patient with cardiac failure.

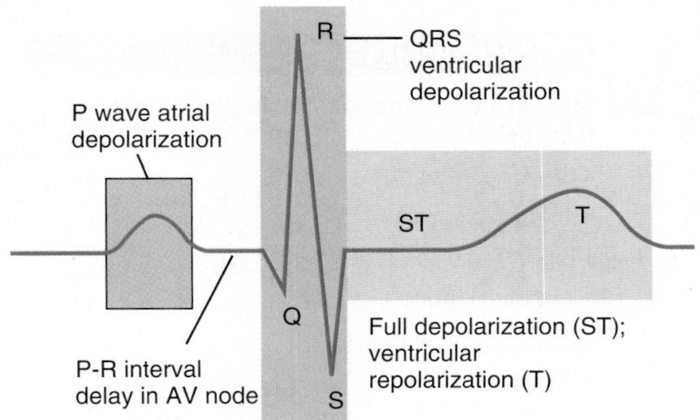

FIGURE 40-17 Normal electrocardiogram waveform. AV, arteriovenous.

early diastole. A fourth heart sound (S_4) occurring in late diastole is found in patients with thick, noncompliant ventricles and likely results from vibrations during atrial contraction. Other cardiac sounds, such as murmurs, which result from turbulent flow, can result from stenosis or regurgitation of any of the four valves. The presence of murmurs can provide clues to the etiology of cardiac failure.

Radiography

The chest radiograph (**Figure 40-16**) provides a relatively inexpensive and easy way to assess the lung fields and the size of the heart. Pulmonary edema is often evident on a chest radiograph as basilar infiltrates with pulmonary vascular redistribution. The infiltrates range from subtle interstitial markings to frank alveolar exudates. As blood flow is redistributed to the nondependent vessels, the upper lobe vasculature appears plump and indistinct. Bilateral pleural effusions and enlargement of the cardiac silhouette also are commonly seen. In chronic cardiac failure, the chest radiograph may be quite unremarkable apart from cardiomegaly. In addition, radiographic changes may lag behind clinical changes. Nevertheless, the chest radiograph remains a cornerstone for the diagnosis and follow-up of cardiac failure.

Measurement and Monitoring of Cardiac Function

Electrocardiography

The electrocardiogram (ECG) records the electrical impulses propagated in the heart (**Figure 40-17**). The impulses are recorded in two planes and at 12 different positions (leads). By examining the resulting complexes, one can determine the heart rate, the rhythm, and whether there are any abnormalities in conduction or repolarization. In addition, the patterns on the ECG may be diagnostic of certain cardiac disorders. Most notably, the syndrome of cardiac ischemia or infarction can be diagnosed by certain abnormalities on the electrocardiogram.

Echocardiography

Echocardiography is a noninvasive form of cardiac imaging used extensively to diagnose a variety of valvular and myocardial diseases. The images provide a wealth of information about cardiac pump function as well as valvular and pericardial disease. Many forms of cardiac disease can be definitively diagnosed with echocardiography. Injection of small air bubbles into a vein provides contrast within the cardiac chambers. Crossover of bubbles into the left-sided chambers allows identification of intracardiac and intrapulmonary shunts.

Exercise Stress Test

The exercise stress test is used to diagnose cardiac ischemia resulting from CAD as a cause of chest pain or cardiac dysfunction. The patient is exercised on a treadmill with electrocardiographic and blood pressure monitoring. ECG changes indicative of ischemia are a reasonably reliable method used to detect CAD.

Radionucleotide Imaging

The sensitivity and specificity of exercise ECG stress testing can be increased by imaging of myocardial perfusion with a radioisotope. The isotope is injected during peak exercise, and the heart is imaged with a gamma camera. The heart is then reimaged at rest and compared with the exercise images. Alternatively, images can be taken during infusion of a chemical agent, such as dobutamine or adenosine, which induces ischemia or changes in myocardial perfusion. Areas of myocardium that have altered perfusion caused by ischemia or infarction will not take up the isotope.

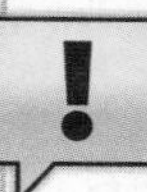

Respiratory Recap

Measurement and Monitoring of Cardiac Function

- Electrocardiogram
- Echocardiogram
- Exercise stress test
- Radionucleotide imaging
- Coronary angiography
- CT angiography
- Hemodynamic monitoring

At rest those areas that were ischemic during exercise (or chemical infusion) now perfuse and take up isotope.

Coronary Angiography

Direct imaging of the coronary arteries is possible by cardiac catheterization (**coronary angiography**). This technique is used to assess the extent and severity of CAD as a cause for chest pain or cardiac dysfunction. Special catheters are inserted into the aorta and into the origins of the right and left coronary arteries. Contrast dye is injected as radiographic images are obtained. The information obtained can identify atherosclerotic lesions as well as coronary anomalies, areas of spasm, and acute thrombi. Contrast dye also can be injected into the left ventricle and, with subsequent imaging, the cardiac pump function (ejection fraction) can be assessed. In addition, valvular disease can be diagnosed and quantified by imaging and direct pressure measurements.

Computed Tomographic Angiography

Computed tomographic (CT) angiography is an emerging imaging technique for assessment of risk of coronary artery disease. Use of CT imaging in cardiac disease includes both assessment of coronary calcium and CT angiography for evaluation of obstructing lesions in the coronary vessels. The exact use of CT angiography continues to evolve as the technology allows for higher-resolution visualization of the coronary anatomy. At the present time, patients with a low likelihood of having coronary artery disease are candidates for CT angiography, but high-risk individuals or those with known coronary artery disease should undergo traditional angiography.[11]

Hemodynamic Monitoring

Direct measurements of the intracardiac and pulmonary vascular pressures are possible through the use of the pulmonary artery catheter. This catheter is equipped with a balloon on the tip that allows it to float from a central vein (internal jugular, subclavian, or femoral) into the right atrium, right ventricle, pulmonary artery, and then into a pulmonary artery occlusion position (where it can measure the wedge pressure). A column of fluid within the catheter allows pressure fluctuations to be transmitted to a transducer and then displayed graphically for analysis. **Figure 40-18** shows a normal set of tracings.

The pulmonary artery occlusion technique creates a static column of blood in a section of the pulmonary vasculature. The measured pressure is a pulmonary venous pressure or wedge pressure, which closely approximates left atrial pressure. The mean left atrial pressure also estimates the pressure in the pulmonary capillary circulation. If elevated, fluid may move from the capillaries into the pulmonary interstitium, thereby creating pulmonary edema. These catheters also have the ability to perform measurements of the $\dot{Q}c$ using the thermodilution technique.

Determination of the filling pressures and $\dot{Q}c$ can provide a wealth of information in the setting of pulmonary edema or hypotension. In the case of pulmonary edema, an elevated pulmonary artery occlusion pressure suggests a cardiac cause for the edema, whereas a low occlusion pressure suggests a capillary leak syndrome (as with acute respiratory distress syndrome

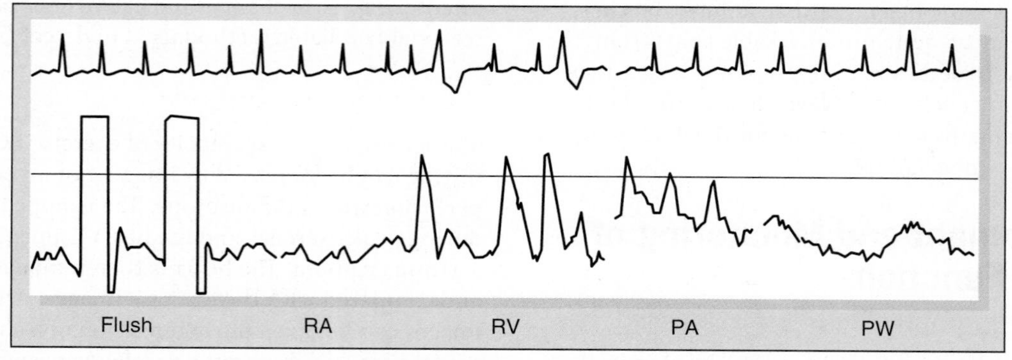

FIGURE 40-18 Normal tracing from a pulmonary artery catheter as it is advanced from the right atrium (RA), right ventricle (RV), pulmonary artery (PA), and into the occlusion or wedge (PW).

Reproduced from Leatherman JW, Marini JJ. 1998. Pulmonary artery catheterization: interpretation of pressure recordings. In: Tobin MJ, ed. *Principles and Practice of Intensive Care Monitoring*. McGraw-Hill, New York. (© The McGraw-Hill Companies, Inc.)

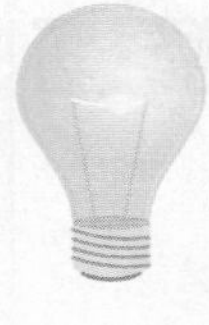

STOP AND THINK

Your patient with systolic heart failure had several extra servings of barbecue and iced tea yesterday at a Fourth of July picnic, and now she is short of breath. What is the cause of her increased dyspnea, and what medication could you give her to provide rapid relief of her symptoms?

[ARDS]). In the setting of hypotension, a low $\dot{Q}c$ with high filling pressures is suggestive of cardiogenic failure or cardiogenic shock.

Treatment Guidelines for Chronic Cardiac Failure

The initial approach to the patient with cardiac failure is to identify the underlying cause and, if possible, treat or remove it. Unfortunately, in the majority of cases of cardiac failure, the underlying cause cannot be easily reversed, so treatment of symptoms is a major goal of therapy. The management of cardiac failure is, however, no longer confined to symptom relief. Treatment to prevent or delay progression of disease and LV remodeling is now the primary focus of many interventions.

The goals of therapy are twofold. The first goal is symptom control and improvement in quality of life. Relieving circulatory congestion and increasing oxygen delivery are the major mechanisms employed to improve symptoms. The second goal is to prevent or delay the progression of the cardiac dysfunction and to prevent the complications that increase mortality. The following discussion is a brief overview of general treatment measures.

Nonpharmacotherapy

In general, lifestyle modification should consist of attempts to optimize diet and exercise, patient education regarding their disease, and avoidance of items that might exacerbate heart failure. In most patients, a modest sodium restriction can be helpful in preventing volume expansion that can lead to pulmonary edema and peripheral edema. Additionally, patients should be taught to weigh themselves frequently because even minor changes in weight can precede obvious clinical signs of volume overload and deterioration of cardiac failure. Although the benefits of exercise have not been proven in studies, experts generally recommend physical activity to prevent physical deconditioning. Patients are instructed to avoid toxins and medications that can either worsen their underlying cardiac disease or exacerbate the symptoms of cardiac failure. For example, alcohol should be avoided, especially when the etiology of the cardiac failure is a nonischemic alcohol-induced cardiomyopathy, because patients can have some recovery of function with cessation. Smoking cessation is also a priority given the association of smoking with cardiovascular disease. Obesity has been linked to many cardiac risk factors, including hypertension and diabetes, and patients should be encouraged to lose weight via lifestyle changes such as diet and exercise. Bariatric surgery can be considered in the morbidly obese with significant comorbidities. Aggressive treatment of other cardiovascular comorbidities like hypertension is also important.

Pharmacotherapy

The treatment of chronic cardiac failure has progressed greatly in the last several decades. Treatment is directed not only at symptom control but also at long-term reductions in morbidity and mortality. Many treatments have been shown to delay or prevent progression of cardiac dysfunction and improve mortality. Even asymptomatic patients with LV dysfunction thus require thorough evaluation and aggressive treatment.

Angiotensin-Converting Enzyme Inhibitors and Angiotensin Receptor Blockers

Angiotensin-converting enzyme (ACE) inhibitors have become the mainstay of treatment for chronic cardiac failure. They are one of the most studied classes of agents for heart failure and have multiple proposed benefits. Hemodynamic effects include vasodilation leading to a reduction in afterload and an increase in $\dot{Q}c$. ACE inhibitors are also believed to have beneficial effects on cardiac remodeling, thereby helping to prevent decompensation related to the adaptive mechanisms described previously. Overall, data support the claim that this class of medications improves symptoms and reduces hospital admissions and death. Unless a patient with reduced systolic function has a contraindication or experiences a severe adverse effect, he or she should be prescribed an ACE inhibitor.

Although ACE inhibitors are now a first-line therapy in cardiac failure, angiotensin receptor blockers (ARBs) are considered a reasonable alternative in patients unable to tolerate an ACE inhibitor. One common side effect of ACE inhibitors is a cough stimulated by increased bradykinin; this effect can be avoided with ARBs. Often the cough is severe enough to limit the use of an ACE inhibitor. Although the research evidence is not nearly as extensive as that regarding ACE inhibitors, ARBs have proven benefits similar to ACE inhibitors and should be used in patients who cannot tolerate ACE inhibitors due to allergy or cough.

β-Blockers

β-blockers have been used to treat heart failure caused by cardiac ischemia and diastolic dysfunction for many years. Although they slow relaxation, clinically they control symptoms of diastolic heart failure by slowing the heart rate and providing overall more time for filling during diastole. The use of β-blockers in systolic dysfunction seems counterintuitive because of their negative inotropic effects and decrease in contractility but is clearly effective. Initial studies in the 1970s suggested that β-blockade improved symptoms and cardiac function in patients with systolic heart failure. Smaller studies in the 1980s confirmed these results,[12,13] but β-blockade to treat cardiac failure caused by LV dysfunction did not become accepted therapy until more recently. One reason for this is the lack of a mechanistic consensus on how β-blockers are beneficial in cardiac failure. β-blockers alter the sympathetic axis and affect the β-receptor signaling cascade. Because excessive, sustained neurohumoral activation is common in cardiac failure and contributes to myocyte dysfunction and deleterious chamber remodeling, blockade of this pathway actually improves cardiac function in the long term by inhibiting adverse remodeling.[14]

Because of early reports of increased bronchospasm in patients with underlying reactive airways (both asthma and COPD), there is often concern about administering β-blockers to these patients. With the development of the more specific cardioselective β-blockers, which act preferentially on the β_1 receptor, however, there is little evidence to suggest an increased risk of exacerbating asthma or COPD with this class of β-blocker. A large meta-analysis concluded that cardioselective β-blockers do not produce significant adverse effects in patients with reactive airways, and in fact they may actually be beneficial.[15,16]

Diuretics

Diuretics are a class of drugs that prevent sodium reabsorption in the kidney and promote sodium loss in the urine. This effect increases salt and water excretion and in heart failure helps reduce circulatory congestion. The physiologic effect of reduced circulating volume is a reduction in filling pressures and thus less transudation of fluid from the systemic and pulmonary circulation. There are several classes of diuretics, but the one most commonly used for cardiac failure is the loop diuretic. Commonly used loop diuretics are furosemide and torsemide. Another frequently used class is the thiazide diuretic, although this class is more frequently used in heart failure as an adjunct to loop diuretics or in patients who also have difficult-to-control blood pressure. Diuretics are effective in both diastolic and systolic heart failure and can produce a rapid improvement in symptoms.

Aldosterone Antagonists

In select populations, the addition of an aldosterone antagonist such as spironolactone or eplerenone can be considered. Aldosterone antagonists work in the same pathway as ACE inhibitors, thereby having the similar hemodynamic effect of decreasing afterload. They also have a weak diuretic effect. This class of medications has proven beneficial in patients with heart failure symptoms and in those with LV dysfunction following myocardial infarction.[17] Patients must be monitored closely, however, for development of potentially life-threatening hyperkalemia, and use of aldosterone antagonists should be avoided in the setting of severe renal dysfunction.

Respiratory Recap

Pharmacotherapy for Cardiac Failure

- ACE inhibitors
- β-blockers
- Diuretics
- Aldosterone antagonists
- Hydralazine and nitrates
- Digoxin

Hydralazine and Nitrates

Hydralazine is an effective vasodilator that when combined with isosorbide dinitrate has been shown to modestly improve survival in selected patients with cardiac failure, particularly African Americans. Hydralazine is primarily an arterial vasodilator whose mechanism of action is unclear. Nitrates such as isosorbide dinitrate release nitric oxide. They are venodilators at low doses and arterial vasodilators at higher doses. The venodilation effect acts to decrease preload, thereby improving $\dot{Q}c$. The combination of hydralazine and nitrates should be considered in patients who cannot tolerate either ACE inhibitors or ARBs. A frequent indication is in the patient who develops hypotension and renal failure during treatment with an ACE inhibitor.

Digoxin

Derived from the leaves of the digitalis plant, digoxin is one of the oldest medications in use. This cardiac glycoside is a potent inhibitor of sodium and potassium exchange across the cardiac cell membranes. The excess sodium available within the cell increases calcium flux into the cell. The increased availability of cytosolic calcium increases the velocity and force of muscle shortening. Digoxin thus has a positive inotropic effect. Digoxin also increases the sensitivity of the baroreceptors, leading to a decrease in the sympathetic activation seen in cardiac failure.

The benefit of digoxin therapy is counterbalanced by the risk for toxicity. Increased serum levels of digoxin are associated with mental status changes, arrhythmias, and sinus arrest. Moreover, the drug has numerous interactions with other medications and has a reduced clearance in patients with renal failure. Studies of digoxin therapy in patients with systolic dysfunction have failed to show a mortality benefit, although digoxin did reduce symptoms and hospitalizations. In patients who have failed to respond appropriately to other treatment modalities, digoxin can be a useful adjunct therapy.[18]

Percutaneous Coronary Intervention

Percutaneous coronary intervention (PCI) consists primarily of either balloon angioplasty or placement of stents in occluded or stenotic coronary arteries. In conjunction with coronary angiography, in which contrast dye is used to evaluate the coronary circulation, PCI can be used to improve flow through affected arteries. The clearest indication for PCI is in the setting of acute coronary syndrome; however, there can be a role in cardiac failure if there is evidence of viable myocardium on radionucleotide imaging or in acute decompensated heart failure. Patients with a new diagnosis of cardiac failure generally should undergo coronary angiography to assess for evidence of ischemic disease and consideration of intervention to improve functional ability.[19–21]

Surgical Treatments

Coronary Revascularization

Coronary revascularization with **coronary artery bypass surgery** can improve myocardial function by reducing ischemia. In some cases so-called hibernating myocardium (myocardium rendered hypocontractile because of chronic hypoperfusion) can return to normal contractile function after restoration of normal blood flow. Other surgical procedures considered for patients with cardiac failure include valvular repairs or replacements and limited septal myomectomies for patients with hypertrophic obstructive cardiomyopathy.

Heart Transplantation

Advances in the techniques of heart transplantation and immunosuppression have improved survival. Patients who undergo transplantation experience a near-normal quality of life but remain at risk for rejection, increased rates of infection, and a unique coronary vasculopathy that leads to severe CAD. The major limitation in cardiac transplantation is organ availability.

Treatment Guidelines for Acute Cardiac Failure

Acute cardiac failure is notable for an acute deterioration of symptoms usually characterized by pulmonary congestion and often constitutes a medical emergency. Etiologies of acute cardiac failure are discussed in previous sections, but in general terms common precipitants in patients with preexisting cardiac dysfunction include nonadherence to therapy or diet recommendations, hypertensive crisis, and cardiac ischemia. As opposed to the extensive data supporting many of the therapies in chronic cardiac failure, therapy for acute cardiac failure is largely empiric while focusing on similar pathophysiologic variables, including alteration of preload, afterload, and contractility. Because acute cardiac failure can result in fulminant respiratory failure, patients often require support with positive pressure ventilation, either noninvasive ventilation or intubation.[18]

Pharmacologic Therapy

In the patient with acute severe pulmonary edema and volume overload, intravenous dosing of a loop diuretic may be necessary for rapid treatment of symptoms. Bolus dosing is usually effective; however, continuous drips may be more effective and have been associated with fewer side effects in some studies. If loop diuretics alone are not effective, then the addition of a thiazide diuretic may be useful. In patients who experience restlessness, anxiety, chest pain, and severe dyspnea, morphine can relieve some of these symptoms in addition to causing mild vasodilation and reduction of preload. For patients who are not hypotensive, vasodilators can be beneficial in acute cardiac failure because they decrease both afterload and preload. Frequently, IV nitrates are used. Nitroglycerin is primarily a venodilator and can affect preload, whereas nitroprusside can reduce both preload and afterload.

Tailored Therapy

In patients with severely decompensated heart failure, aggressive intravenous therapy with diuretics and vasodilators can be administered with concurrent hemodynamic monitoring. A pulmonary arterial catheter can provide important information regarding serial determination of filling pressures and allow optimal titration of vasodilators and volume status. Occasionally, intravenous inotropes such as dobutamine or milrinone are needed to augment the cardiac output and help optimize hemodynamics. Tailored therapy remains a useful intervention in patients with severe cardiac failure.

Intra-Aortic Balloon Pump

The **intra-aortic balloon pump (IABP)** uses the principle of counterpulsation to support the failing heart. The catheter-based balloon is inserted into the descending

Respiratory Recap

Treatments for Acute Cardiac Failure

- Pharmacologic therapy
- Tailored therapy
- Intra-aortic balloon pump (IABP)

aorta just below the aortic arch. The balloon is then inflated during diastole, causing increased coronary blood flow, and deflated during systole, causing decreased afterload. An IABP is especially effective in cardiogenic shock caused by myocardial ischemia because it decreases myocardial oxygen demand while increasing coronary perfusion. IABPs can be inserted safely in emergency situations and often can bridge a critically ill patient to corrective surgery.

Acute Myocardial Infarction

Acute myocardial infarction occurs when there is partial or complete occlusion of the coronary circulation. Infarction occurs most commonly when there is rupture of a plaque in one of the coronary arteries, resulting in thrombosis and obstruction of blood flow to the tissue it supplies. The end result of absent or reduced blood flow is tissue hypoxia and cell death unless blood flow is improved quickly. Acute coronary syndrome can manifest itself clinically in a variety of ways; however, the most common complaints are severe chest pain radiating to the left arm and jaw, dyspnea, nausea, and a sense of impending doom. Often the patient will appear uncomfortable and diaphoretic. The diagnosis can be confirmed by ECG and measurement of serum cardiac biomarkers such as troponin.

There are many subclassifications of acute coronary syndromes, but the most urgent is the ST-elevation myocardial infarction (STEMI), which warrants prompt intervention to prevent irreversible damage to the myocardium. Initial treatment involves the administration of aspirin and other anticoagulants such as heparin and clopidogrel to help prevent platelet adhesion and thrombosis; nitroglycerin to assist with coronary vasodilation; supplemental oxygen to alleviate tissue hypoxia; and often morphine if the patient has persistent chest pain. In centers where cardiac catheterization is available or can be obtained within 120 minutes, the patient should undergo PCI with angioplasty or placement of a stent to obtain revascularization of the affected artery. If PCI is unavailable, then medical thrombolysis can be attempted.[22]

Ventilatory Support of the Patient with Cardiac Failure

Pulmonary edema is associated with increased lung elastance, increased airway resistance, and lung collapse. Thus, pulmonary edema from any cause leads to increased work of breathing and hypoxemia. The large negative intrathoracic pressure swings may increase afterload for the strained left ventricle. Hypoxic pulmonary vasoconstriction will increase afterload of the right ventricle. In severe cases the patient may not be able to maintain adequate ventilation and oxygen delivery. This can then further exacerbate myocardial dysfunction because of cellular hypoxia and acidosis, especially when the heart failure is caused by cardiac ischemia. The increased work of the respiratory muscles also may steal oxygen from the working myocardium. Combined cardiac failure and respiratory distress thus begets more cardiac failure.

If the cycle of respiratory failure can be temporarily interrupted, therapy aimed at treating the cardiac abnormalities can be used and the process can be reversed. Positive pressure ventilation is an ideal mechanism used to stabilize the acutely decompensated patient. Positive pressure ventilation improves oxygenation by recruiting collapsed lung and decreases the work of breathing by unloading the respiratory muscles. In addition, positive intrathoracic pressure may improve forward $\dot{Q}c$. Chronic therapy with noninvasive positive pressure ventilators may have a role in selected patients with sleep-disordered breathing and heart failure.

Noninvasive Ventilation

In the past, many patients with respiratory failure caused by cardiac failure were intubated for mechanical ventilation. Experience with noninvasive ventilation (NIV) by face mask has provided encouraging results. In some cases the patient can be stabilized and endotracheal intubation can be prevented by the use of mask continuous positive airway pressure (CPAP) at 5 to 10 cm H_2O. Inspiratory pressure also can be applied to further unload the respiratory muscles. A systematic review of the use of NIV as compared with conventional medical therapy for acute cardiopulmonary edema found that NIV (consisting of CPAP or bilevel NIV) outperformed medical therapy in terms of mortality, intubation rates, and physiologic parameters.[23]

In patients with active cardiac ischemia, heavy sedation and controlled mechanical ventilation through an endotracheal tube significantly reduces the work of breathing, reduces the work of the myocardium, and allows the most effective oxygen delivery to the ischemic myocardium. Patients with hemodynamic instability, arrhythmias, and a depressed mental status or some patients undergoing invasive procedures (such as cardiac catheterization) should be managed with intubation and mechanical ventilation.

Invasive Mechanical Ventilation

Intubation of the patient with cardiac failure may prove challenging because of underlying hemodynamic abnormalities. The necessary sedation for this procedure can potentially cause hypotension and arrhythmias. Monitoring of the rhythm and blood pressure therefore is essential. Very few sedating medications do not have some cardiovascular depressive actions. One exception is etomidate, which is a hypnotic agent with minimal cardiovascular depressant actions. Etomidate is the recommended induction agent for intubation of patients with cardiovascular instability. After intubation the

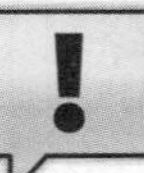

Respiratory Recap

Mechanical Ventilation for Cardiac Failure

- A mode should be chosen that is effective and comfortable for the patient.
- Avoid plateau pressure above 30 cm H_2O.
- Use an initial tidal volume of 6 mL/kg.
- Use an initial inspiratory time of 0.8 to 1.2 seconds.
- An initial FiO_2 of 1.0 should be chosen.
- An initial PEEP of 5 cm H_2O should be chosen.

patient may require intermittent doses or continuous infusion of opiates for analgesia.

No controlled trials on various modes of ventilation in cardiac failure have been conducted. The clinician should use the mode that provides the most effective and comfortable ventilation for the patient. Patients with mild or chronic cardiac failure and significant pulmonary edema may be managed with minimal ventilatory support and spontaneous ventilation with a mode such as pressure support. Most patients with severe cardiac failure will benefit from full ventilatory support. Pressure control or volume control can be used for cardiac failure as long as adequate ventilation and oxygenation are maintained without hyperinflation or significant lung collapse. Pressure support or pressure control may allow patients to set their own inspiratory flows and may permit less sedation by providing a comfortable form of ventilation. Tidal volume should be 6 to 8 mL/kg with an inspiratory time of 0.8 to 1.2 seconds. Setting the tidal volume at 6 to 8 mL/kg is based on the premise that larger tidal volumes can lead to ventilator-induced lung injury (VILI). Using a tidal volume of 6 to 8 mL/kg has been shown to be protective against VILI in clinical trials, although more studies are ongoing to confirm this finding.[24] Plateau pressure should be monitored and kept below 30 cm H_2O. An adequate rate should be provided if heavy sedation is used. FiO_2 should be set at 1.0 and then decreased to the lowest level that maintains SpO_2 above 90%. PEEP is initially set at 5 cm H_2O and titrated as needed for oxygenation if tolerated hemodynamically.

Cardiac Effects of Mechanical Ventilation

Positive pressure ventilation has many potential effects on the cardiovascular system. The filling of the ventricles is highly dependent on the pressures surrounding the heart. Cardiac surface pressure depends on the pericardial pressure, intrathoracic pressure, and lung volume around the heart. Changes in lung volume also will affect PVR and thus RV performance. In turn, RV performance can affect LV performance via series and parallel interactions. The overall effects of the application of positive pressure ventilation in the individual patient thus are highly unpredictable and can be beneficial (reduced work of breathing, reduced edema, increased $\dot{Q}c$) or potentially detrimental (hypotension, hyperinflation, ischemia). Therefore, a careful titration of respiratory support during monitoring of all available aspects of cardiovascular performance (i.e., blood pressure, heart rate, filling pressures, $\dot{Q}c$, arterial blood gases, electrocardiogram) may be the optimal method of ventilation in the patient with cardiac failure.

The most effective means to increase intrathoracic positive pressure is the application of PEEP. In addition to potentially reducing afterload and preload, PEEP prevents alveolar derecruitment. Collapsed lung units increase intrapulmonary shunt, increase PVR, and induce hyperinflation in open lung units by reducing the amount of lung available to accommodate the delivered tidal volume. In addition, cyclic opening and closure of alveoli over each ventilatory cycle can be injurious. Optimal ventilatory settings should prevent derecruitment by ventilating above the closing pressures of the lung units.

In patients with dilated cardiomyopathy, PEEP has been shown to improve $\dot{Q}c$ without increasing the oxygen requirements of the LV. It is widely believed that this effect is from a reduced afterload on the LV induced by the positive intrathoracic pressure. The afterload on the heart can be estimated by the transmural pressure across the LV, and since PEEP can increase cardiac surface pressure, it will reduce afterload, assuming the arterial pressure does not increase. This increase in $\dot{Q}c$ is not seen in patients with normal cardiac function or normal volume status, however, suggesting that the mechanism of benefit may not be as simple as a reduced afterload. It is hypothesized that the increase that occurs in patients with cardiac failure when placed on positive pressure ventilation may be caused by displacement of blood from the thorax leading to reduced ventricular volumes and improved contraction due to less pericardial constraint. In addition, PEEP may be beneficial by redistributing edema to the perivascular spaces and reducing PVR by limiting lung collapse. Based on the complex effects of PEEP, a careful increase in pressure is recommended, while simultaneously monitoring oxygenation, blood pressure, the electrocardiogram, and the $\dot{Q}c$ if possible.

Discontinuing Mechanical Ventilation

Acute respiratory failure from pulmonary edema is often rapidly reversible and does not usually require prolonged mechanical ventilation. Often the patient can be extubated without a prolonged weaning of support. Sudden loss of positive pressure in the thorax can lead to acute edema and rapid failure in fragile patients. If loss of positive pressure is a concern, patients can be placed on zero PEEP prior to extubation to assess their response, or they can be placed on bilevel NIV immediately after extubation. Ongoing cardiac ischemia is associated with failure to wean and should be corrected before ventilatory support is removed.

Chronic Noninvasive Ventilation in Sleep-Disordered Breathing

Many patients with chronic cardiac failure have sleep-disordered breathing, including Cheyne-Stokes respiration and sleep apnea. Perhaps as many as 40% to 50% of patients with cardiac failure also have obstructive sleep apnea (OSA) or Cheyne-Stokes respiration with central sleep apnea (CSR-CSA). In patients with cardiac failure, the presence of sleep-disordered breathing is associated with a poor prognosis and a higher mortality. **Box 40-2** lists the extensive cardiovascular effects of apneic episodes.

These effects work in concert to increase afterload and overload the myocardium. It has been suggested that these pathophysiologic effects may contribute to the progression of cardiac failure. There is increasing evidence that treatment of these disorders with nocturnal mask CPAP is associated with marked improvements in cardiac function and the symptoms of cardiac failure.

The assessment of all patients with cardiac failure should include questions about sleep disorders and symptoms of sleep deprivation, snoring, and apneas.

BOX 40-2

Effects of Obstructive Sleep Apnea on Cardiovascular Function

Negative Intrathoracic Pressure

Increased left ventricular systolic transmural pressure (i.e., afterload)
Reduced stroke volume and cardiac output

Hypoxemia and Hypercapnia

Increased respiratory drive and sympathetic nervous system activity
Pulmonary vasoconstriction and hypertension leading to increased right ventricular afterload
Systemic vasoconstriction and hypertension
Cardiac arrhythmias (bradycardia, heart block, ventricular and supraventricular tachycardias)

Arousal

Increased central sympathetic nervous system activity
Increased systemic blood pressure
Increased heart rate

Any suggestion of sleep-disordered breathing should prompt a thorough evaluation with a sleep study and treatment if indicated.[25]

Case Studies

Case 1. Ischemic Congestive Heart Failure

A 55-year-old man (80 kg) with a history of CAD and prior infarction presented with chest pain and shortness of breath. The patient presented with an anterior myocardial infarction (MI) 6 months ago and underwent emergent coronary angioplasty with stent placement to his left anterior descending (LAD) coronary artery. His LV function after MI was moderately impaired at an LVEF of 40%. He was managed with aspirin, β-blockers, and an ACE inhibitor. Over the last 2 weeks he has noted return of his chest pain with exertion, and on the day of presentation he had two 20-minute episodes of pain at rest. The last one was associated with some mild dyspnea. Shortly before presenting he developed severe crushing chest pain and became quite dyspneic.

An ambulance was called, and he was taken to the emergency department. On presentation he was in respiratory distress, sitting upright, and sweating, with marked use of accessory muscles. His respiratory rate was 36 breaths/min, heart rate 110 beats/min, and blood pressure 150/100 mm Hg, and oxygen saturation was 91% on 15 L/min oxygen via face mask. On exam the patient appeared to have distended neck veins. His chest had diffuse crackles and wheezes throughout. Cardiac exam was notable for tachycardia and a summation gallop. An ECG showed T-wave inversions and ST depression in leads V_2 to V_6, and a chest radiograph showed moderate pulmonary edema.

Critical Thinking Questions

- What is the cause of this patient's respiratory failure?
- What would be your first steps in management?
- What is the definitive treatment for the underlying problem?

The patient clearly has congestive heart failure (CHF) from myocardial ischemia. In this case, the lack of

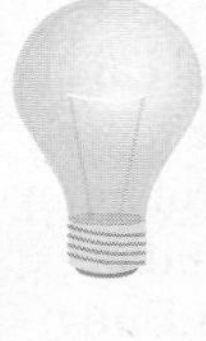

STOP AND THINK

Your patient was intubated due to respiratory failure from a large myocardial infarction (MI), and her echocardiogram after the MI shows that she has a reduced ejection fraction of 25%. She has passed her spontaneous breathing trial. What could you do to help prevent reintubation after she is extubated?

oxygen delivery to the working myocardium led to depletion in ATP and dysfunction of both contraction and relaxation of cardiac muscle. This insult resulted in elevated LV filling pressures and pulmonary edema. The patient has evidence of a marked increase in work of breathing that is likely contributing to the ischemia by increasing his oxygen delivery requirements. If the patient begins to retain carbon dioxide, the resulting acidosis may lead to further myocardial dysfunction and increase the risk of arrhythmias. Efforts to restore oxygen supply to the heart might be more successful if the patient were intubated and heavily sedated.

The therapeutic strategy is to intubate the patient and provide full mechanical ventilatory support. Pressure or volume ventilation so that the tidal volume is 6 mL/kg ideal body weight (420 mL) and inspiratory time is 1 second with a rate of 20 breaths/min is a good starting point. The F_{IO_2} should be 1.0 to start. PEEP of 5 cm H_2O should be applied, and if the blood pressure tolerates this, a slow increase to 10 cm H_2O could be attempted. In the meantime the patient should be treated with anticoagulation (aspirin, heparin, a II/IIIa inhibitor), intravenous nitroglycerin, and diuretics. Consultation with a cardiologist for possible cardiac catheterization also should be obtained.

Case 2. Acute Aortic Valve Insufficiency

A 28-year-old man complains of fevers, chills, and shortness of breath. The patient has a history of rheumatic fever as a child but has otherwise been in good health. Three days before presentation he injected intravenous heroin with a dirty needle. The day before presentation he noted chills and sweats. On the morning of presentation he had a rapid progression of dyspnea and nausea. He felt weak when standing and finally collapsed in his home. The patient was brought to the emergency department awake but in respiratory distress.

His blood pressure was 110/40 mm Hg, heart rate 120 beats/min, respiratory rate 30 breaths/min, temperature 102° F (40° C), and oxygen saturation 88% on 10 L/min oxygen by face mask. Physical exam was notable for signs of increased work of breathing and crackles on chest auscultation. His cardiac exam disclosed an elevated JVP, a hyperdynamic precordium on palpation, tachycardia, and a loud diastolic murmur at the left lower sternal border on auscultation. A summation gallop also was noted. The patient's extremities were cool and without edema. Laboratory evaluation disclosed an elevated white count; an ECG showed tachycardia with some nonspecific T-wave changes. The chest radiograph showed pulmonary edema. An urgent echocardiogram showed 4+ aortic regurgitation with LV dilation. LV systolic function appeared intact. A large vegetation was seen on one of the aortic cusps, and the other cusps appeared thickened.

Critical Thinking Questions

- What is the underlying cause of his respiratory failure?
- What interventions should be done acutely to treat his respiratory failure?
- What other interventions will be needed to address the underlying cause?

This patient has acute aortic valve endocarditis, likely from a staphylococcal infection. The infection was probably acquired from his IV drug use and involved his aortic valve, which may have been damaged previously from the episode of rheumatic fever. The infection has eroded his aortic valve and produced acute aortic insufficiency. In this case the LV acutely has a large regurgitant volume load. When the aortic valve eroded, there was an acute increase in diastolic volume caused by regurgitation of blood from the aorta. This led to LV dilation and increased diastolic wall stress and elevated filling pressures. The elevated filling pressures led to pulmonary edema and dyspnea. The $\dot{Q}c$ is decreased because of the regurgitation of blood into the LV, but the heart has partially compensated by increasing its rate and augmenting its stroke volume. Unfortunately, the $\dot{Q}c$ is not adequate to meet the body's demands, and the patient is developing tissue hypoperfusion and cardiogenic shock.

Management in this case begins with stabilization of the respiratory system. Oxygen delivery and respiratory muscle unloading are required. Positive pressure ventilation also may help cardiac function by reducing the afterload and the amount of blood regurgitated into the LV. A trial of noninvasive ventilation with PEEP may be attempted in this case. If the patient does not tolerate this intervention, he may require intubation, sedation, and ventilation with PEEP. PEEP can be started at 5 cm H_2O and increased as tolerated to support oxygenation and reduce afterload. In the meantime, antibiotic therapy and intravenous afterload reducers (such as sodium nitroprusside) can be administered. The patient should be considered for urgent surgical replacement of the aortic valve given the severity of heart failure.

Case 3. Diastolic Dysfunction from Hypertension

An 80-year-old woman with a long history of hypertension and COPD presented with a fractured hip after a fall. She underwent surgical fixation of the fracture that evening. Postoperatively she was observed to develop atrial fibrillation with a rapid ventricular response. Shortly afterward she complained of shortness of breath. The patient was sitting upright in bed, was diaphoretic, and was in moderate respiratory distress. Blood pressure was 180/100 mm Hg, heart rate was 140 to 160 beats/min and irregular, and temperature was

101° F (38.3° C). Spo_2 was 90% on 8 L/min oxygen via nasal cannula. Physical exam disclosed slight wheezing and crackles on chest auscultation. A chest radiograph was consistent with pulmonary edema. An ECG revealed atrial fibrillation without ischemic changes. An echocardiogram disclosed a thickened and hyperkinetic LV with normal chamber dimensions and ejection fraction.

Critical Thinking Questions

- Why did this patient develop pulmonary edema even though she has a normal ejection fraction?
- How should her atrial fibrillation be treated?
- Could a slow heart rate (bradycardia) cause the same problem?

This patient has pulmonary edema from diastolic dysfunction. The cause of her pulmonary edema is multifactorial. First, the heart is thickened from long-standing hypertension and likely has baseline abnormalities in relaxation. With atrial fibrillation, the contribution to ventricular filling from the atrial contraction was lost. Normally, atrial contraction serves to increase LVEDP without a large concurrent rise in mean left atrial pressure (LAP). Loss of atrial contraction causes a rise in the mean LAP and can contribute to pulmonary edema. The rapid ventricular rate that results from atrial fibrillation also may impede diastolic function by limiting the diastolic interval available for filling.

In this case, therapy should be directed at restoration of a normal sinus rhythm. The respiratory status is reasonably stable at present and can be managed with supplemental oxygen alone. The quickest and easiest method to restore a normal sinus rhythm is synchronized electric cardioversion. If this is unsuccessful or the patient reverts to atrial fibrillation, an antiarrhythmic drug may help convert and stabilize the rhythm. If attempts at cardioversion fail, the patient may be rate controlled with a variety of agents. The calcium channel blockers diltiazem or verapamil are effective at rate control. Both can be given by continuous intravenous infusion. β-blockers also can be used and are ideal after myocardial infarction. The antiarrhythmic amiodarone can slow the heart rate and may help cardiovert the patient back into normal sinus rhythm. Further supportive therapy with nitroglycerin and diuretics also may be used in this situation. Effective pain control, treatment of bronchospasm (with a nonabsorbed anticholinergic, such as ipratropium, that will not stimulate the heart), and reduction of fever are important methods to reduce the cardiac stimulation from catecholamine release.

Case 4. Chronic Congestive Heart Failure from Cardiomyopathy of Coronary Artery Disease

A 55-year-old man with a history of CHF and multiple myocardial infarctions presented with slowly progressive fatigue and shortness of breath over the last week. The patient had his first MI at age 45 years. He initially did well with medical management but at age 53 had a large anterior MI. His course after this MI has been notable for multiple episodes of cardiac failure. After the MI, he was found to have two-vessel coronary disease and a decreased ejection fraction at 20%. He has been managed with an ACE inhibitor and diuretics while he awaits cardiac transplantation. About 3 months ago he was started on carvedilol. The patient was traveling in Italy the last 3 weeks and admits to noncompliance with his low-salt diet. He also ran out of his lisinopril 10 days ago. About 1 week ago he noted some increased dyspnea with exertion and fatigue. The last 3 days he has been sleeping on three to four pillows instead of his usual two, and last night he woke up twice very short of breath. He denies any chest pain but has had some pedal edema.

On exam he was in mild respiratory distress and had a periodic breathing pattern, especially when distracted or resting. Blood pressure was 110/70 mm Hg, heart rate 75 beats/min, and oxygen saturation 95% on 2 L/min nasal cannula. Auscultation of his chest was notable only for a few mild crackles at the bases. His neck veins were elevated to his jaw, there was a large displaced LV apical impulse, and on auscultation a loud S_3 was noted. His legs had 2+ to 3+ pitting edema. Laboratory evaluation was unremarkable, and an ECG showed his usual left bundle branch pattern. A chest radiograph showed cardiomegaly and small bilateral effusions. No pulmonary edema was noted. He was transferred to the critical care unit and while sleeping was noted to desaturate during periods of apnea.

Critical Thinking Questions

- What are the underlying causes for this patient's heart failure exacerbation?
- Why does he desaturate and have apneic episodes during sleep?
- Why doesn't he have pulmonary edema on his chest x-ray?

This patient has decompensated cardiac failure from medical and dietary noncompliance. Conservative therapy with diuretics and restarting of his ACE inhibitor may work; however, an attempt at tailored therapy could also be considered. In this patient a pulmonary artery catheter could be placed to guide therapy. Intravenous diuretics and vasodilators could be used to obtain the lowest filling pressures that provide an adequate $\dot{Q}c$. If needed, an inotrope such as dobutamine could be added. Once hemodynamics are optimized, oral therapy would begin. The presence of periodic breathing is the result of his cardiac failure. An attempt to treat this with noninvasive positive pressure ventilation may help his left ventricular function and overall well-being.

Case 5. Coronary Bypass Surgery

A 68-year-old man with a history of angina underwent coronary bypass surgery for three-vessel disease. When coming off the pump, he experienced hypotension that required high doses of a norepinephrine infusion to stabilize his blood pressure. The patient remained intubated and sedated and was transported to the intensive care unit. He was ventilated with volume ventilation at 6 mL/kg, PEEP 5 cm H_2O, FIO_2 of 1.0, and a rate of 15/min. With this he was hypoxemic with a blood gas of pH 7.46, $PaCO_2$ of 34 mm Hg, and PaO_2 of 50 mm Hg. The pulmonary artery catheter disclosed a right atrial pressure of 14 mm Hg, an RV pressure of 45/14 mm Hg, a pulmonary artery pressure (PAP) of 45/20 mm Hg, and a pulmonary artery occlusion pressure (PAOP) of 8 mm Hg. The $\dot{Q}c$ was normal at 3.8 L/min. A chest radiograph and an ECG were within normal limits. An emergent echocardiogram was notable for a hypocontractile RV with preserved LV function. A patent foramen ovale with right-to-left shunting was noted when air contrast was injected.

Critical Thinking Questions

- Does this patient have right heart failure or left heart failure? What is the difference?
- Is his right atrial pressure normal, too high, or too low?
- What is the significance of the patent foramen ovale with right-to-left shunting?
- What medications can be used to improve his hemodynamics?

This patient has shock from isolated RV dysfunction after cardiopulmonary bypass during cardiac surgery. RV dysfunction after bypass is a well-described complication of cardiac surgery. Several possible etiologies for this dysfunction include air emboli, RV infarction, and stunned myocardium. Air embolism can be fatal and requires prompt treatment with removal of the air or hyperbaric oxygen therapy. The other forms of RV dysfunction after cardiac surgery can reverse if given enough time. The goal is to support the patient with vasoactive drugs until the RV function returns.

In this case the situation is complicated by an intracardiac shunt. The foramen ovale is a hole that exists in utero between the atria. It closes after birth and in most people is fused. A significant portion of the population has a nonfused foramen ovale that remains closed because the left-sided atrial pressure is greater than the right-sided atrial pressure. In this patient, when the pressure increased in the right atrium in association with the decreased compliance of the RV, the foramen ovale opened and shunted blood from the right atrium to the left atrium. This shunted blood is the cause of the refractory hypoxemia.

This patient was stabilized hemodynamically with norepinephrine. The challenge is to reduce the shunt. Increasing PEEP, which generally improves oxygenation in patients with lung disease, may actually be detrimental in this case because it can increase pulmonary vascular resistance and thus increase the fraction of right-to-left shunted blood. Intravenous vasodilators such as nitroprusside and nitroglycerin can lower the PVR but also can lower systemic blood pressure. In addition, these agents will reduce hypoxic vasoconstriction and may potentially worsen hypoxemia. Inhaled nitric oxide is a potent vasodilator with a short half-life. When inhaled, it selectively dilates the pulmonary arteries and improves ventilation-perfusion matching by preferentially dilating the vasculature of ventilated lung units. In this case, a trial of inhaled nitric oxide reduced the shunt and improved RV function by reducing PVR.

If this patient had not responded to inhaled nitric oxide, he could be considered for a trial of extracorporeal membrane oxygenation (ECMO). ECMO uses a large venous catheter to remove deoxygenated blood from the body; the blood is circulated through an external device that oxygenates the blood and removes carbon dioxide, and then it is returned to the body. ECMO can be used in severe cardiac or pulmonary disease as a bridge until those organs recover or until other interventions, such as organ transplantation, can occur.

Key Points

- Cardiac failure is a common occurrence in hospitalized patients and often causes respiratory failure.
- Although there are numerous causes for cardiac failure, it ultimately results from an abnormality of contraction, excessive load, and/or restricted filling.
- Symptoms vary from patient to patient but usually manifest with fatigue and dyspnea on exertion. Often the symptoms occur late in the disease process.
- Treatment for cardiac failure requires a knowledge of its complex pathophysiology.
- The majority of treatments for cardiac failure stabilize the disease and do not reverse the process.
- ACE inhibitors, β-blockers, and diuretics remain the mainstay of therapy in patients with cardiac failure.
- Mechanical ventilation for patients with respiratory failure can be very effective in reversing the abnormalities resulting from pulmonary edema.
- The interactions of the lungs and heart are complex in patients with heart failure, and the use of positive pressure ventilation can often lead to unpredictable results if not used carefully.

References

1. American Heart Association. Forecasting the impact of heart failure in the United States. American Heart Association Policy Statement. November 2014. Available at: http://circheartfailure.ahajournals.org/content/early/2013/04/24/HHF.0b013e318291329a. Accessed November 17, 2014.

2. Hunt SA, Abraham WT, Chin MH, et al. ACC/AHA 2009 focused update incorporated into the 2005 guidelines for the diagnosis and management of chronic heart failure in adults: a report of the American College of Cardiology/American Heart Association Task Force on Practice Guidelines. *Circulation*. 2009;119:e391–e479.
3. Roger V, Lloyd-Jones DM, Benjamin EJ, et al. Heart disease and stroke statistics 2012 update. A report from the American Heart Association Statistics Committee and Stroke Statistics subcommittee. *Circulation*. 2012;125:e20–e220. Erratum in *Circulation*. 2012;125:e1002.
4. Opie LA. *The Heart: Physiology from Cell to Circulation*. Philadelphia: Lippincott Williams & Wilkins; 1998.
5. Guyton AC, Hall JE. *Textbook of Medical Physiology*. 11th ed. Philadelphia: Saunders; 2006:103–245.
6. Ouzounian M. Diastolic heart failure: mechanisms and controversies. *Nat Clin Pract Cardiovasc Med*. 2008;5:375–386.
7. Ashrafian H, Williams L, Frenneaux MP. The pathophysiology of heart failure: a tale of two old paradigms revisited. *Clin Med*. 2008;8:192–197.
8. Monnet X. Cardiopulmonary interactions in patients with heart failure. *Curr Opin Crit Care*. 2007;13:6–11.
9. Pinsky MR. Cardiovascular issues in respiratory care. *Chest*. 2005;128(Suppl 2):592S–597S.
10. New York Heart Association Criteria Committee. *Disease of the Heart and Blood Vessels: Nomenclature for Diagnosis*. Boston: Little, Brown; 1964:114.
11. Achenbach S, Daniel W. Cardiac imaging in the patient with chest pain: coronary CT angiography. *Heart*. 2010;96:1241–1246.
12. Engelmeier RS, O'Connell JB, Walsh R, et al. Improvement in symptoms and exercise tolerance by metoprolol in patients with dilated cardiomyopathy: a double-blind, randomized, placebo-controlled trial. *Circulation*. 1985;72:536–546.
13. Anderson JL, Lutz JR, Gilbert EM, et al. A randomized trial of low-dose β-blockade therapy for idiopathic dilated cardiomyopathy. *Am J Cardiol*. 1985;55:471–475.
14. Krumholz HM. β-blockers for mild to moderate heart failure. *Lancet*. 1999;353:2.
15. Salpeter SR, Ormiston TM, Salpeter EE. Cardioselective β-blockers in patients with reactive airway disease: a meta-analysis. *Ann Intern Med*. 2002;137:715–725.
16. Matera MG, Calzetta L, Cazzola M. *Drugs*. 2013;73:1653–1663.
17. Zannad F, McMurray JJV, Krum H, et al. Eplerenone in patients with systolic heart failure and mild symptoms. *N Engl J Med*. 2011;364:11–21.
18. Dickstein K, Cohen-Solal A, Fillipatos G, et al. ESC guidelines for the diagnosis and treatment of acute and chronic heart failure 2008. *Eur Heart J*. 2008;29:2388–2442. Errata in *Eur Heart J*. 2009;11:110, and 2010;12:416.
19. Boden WE, Gupta V. Reperfusion strategies in acute ST-segment elevation myocardial infarction. *Curr Opin Cardiol*. 2008;23: 613–619.
20. Flaherty JD, Davidson CJ, Faxon DP. Percutaneous coronary intervention for myocardial infarction with left ventricular dysfunction. *Am J Cardiol*. 2008;102:38G–41G.
21. 2013 ACCF/AHA guidelines for the management of ST-elevation myocardial infarction. *J Am Col Cardiol*. 2013;61:485–510.
22. White HD, Chew DP. Acute myocardial infarction. *Lancet*. 2008;372:570–584.
23. Vital FMR, Ladeira MT, Atallah ÁN. Non-invasive positive pressure ventilation (CPAP or bilevel NPPV) for cardiogenic pulmonary oedema. *Cochrane Database Syst Rev*. 2013;5:CD005351.
24. Neto AS, Cardoso SO, Manetta JA, et al. Association between use of lung-protective ventilation with lower tidal volumes and clinical outcomes among patients without acute respiratory distress syndrome: a meta-analysis. *JAMA*. 2012;308:1651–1659.
25. Naughton MT. Common sleep problems in ICU: heart failure and sleep-disordered breathing syndromes. *Crit Care Clin*. 2008;24:565–587.

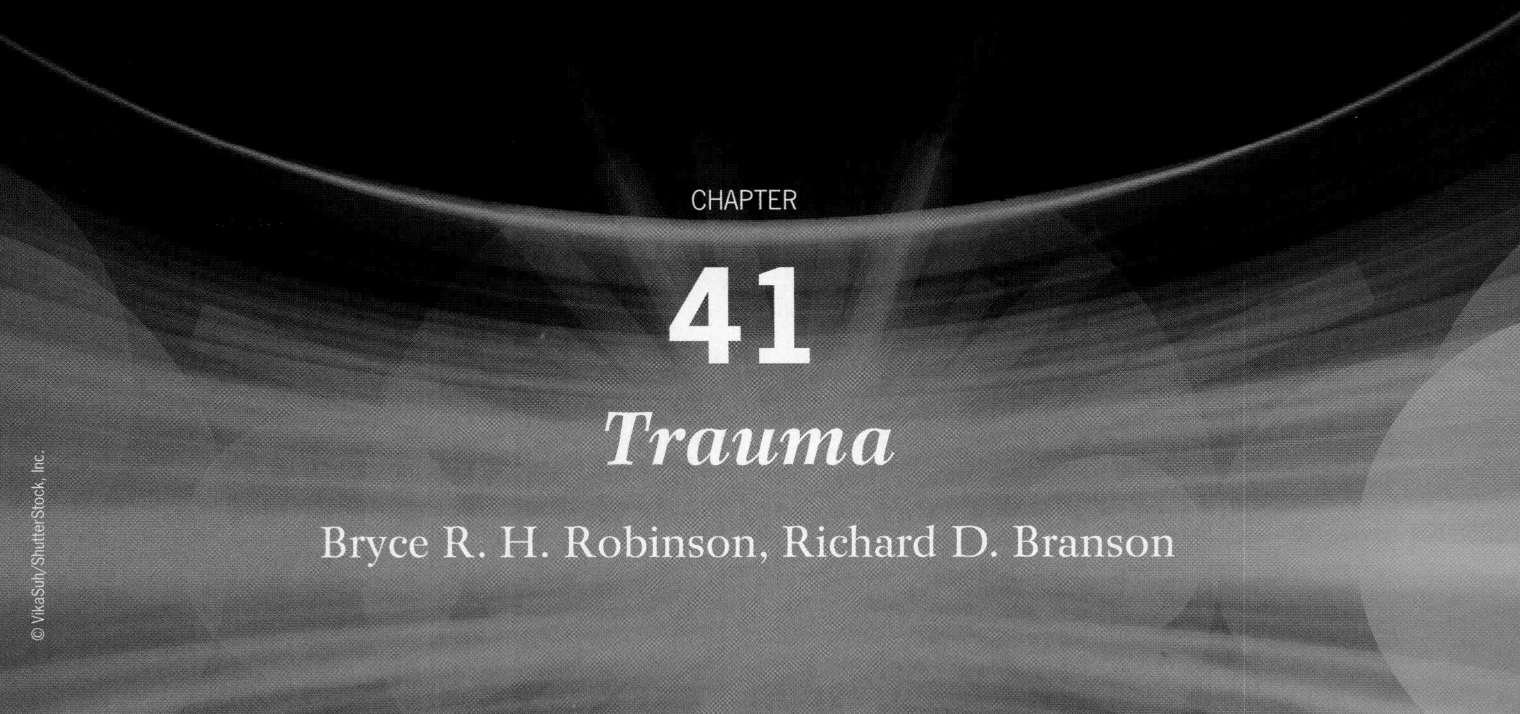

CHAPTER
41
Trauma
Bryce R. H. Robinson, Richard D. Branson

OUTLINE

The Primary and Secondary Surveys
Thoracic Trauma
Airway and Breathing Injuries
Circulation Injuries
Injuries Encountered During the Secondary Survey
Head Trauma
Primary Survey Issues of Head Injury
Secondary Survey Issues of Head Injury
Treatment of Head Injuries

OBJECTIVES

1. Discuss the evaluation of a trauma patient with respect to a primary and secondary survey.
2. List the components of the ABCDE algorithm for assessing the trauma patient.
3. Describe the injuries following trauma that may require respiratory support.
4. Identify common life-threatening injuries encountered during the primary survey.
5. Describe common injuries encountered during the secondary survey.
6. Discuss the importance of pain control.
7. Describe the mechanism of head trauma and traumatic brain injury.
8. Discuss methods to monitor and treat acute traumatic brain injury.

KEY TERMS

Beck's triad
blunt trauma
cardiac tamponade
epidural hematoma
hemothorax
hypovolemic shock
penetrating trauma
pneumothorax
primary survey
pulmonary contusion
secondary survey
subarachnoid (intracerebral) hematoma
subdural hematoma

Introduction

Regardless of the mechanism or anatomic location of injury, the initial evaluation and care of the traumatically injured patient is structured by principles delineated by the advanced trauma life support (ATLS) program of the American College of Surgeons Committee on Trauma.[1] ATLS focuses on the rapid initial assessment and treatment of life-threatening injuries, reevaluation and stabilization of the traumatically injured, and principles for the transfer of these patients to a higher-level care if warranted. Trauma patients die in certain reproducible time frames. A patient without a definitive airway will die of hypoxia more rapidly than a patient with hypovolemic shock. The purpose of this chapter is to familiarize care providers with the evaluation and treatment of injuries to the chest and head.

The Primary and Secondary Surveys

The **primary survey** uses the mnemonic ABCDE for an orderly evaluation and treatment of traumatic injuries based on the rapidity of lethality. *A* is for airway and cervical spine protection, *B* for breathing, *C* for circulation, *D* for deficits, and *E* for exposure (**Figure 41-1**). While the primary survey is occurring, care providers are simultaneously recording vital signs, starting resuscitation, drawing pertinent laboratory specimens, inserting clinically relevant urinary or gastric catheters, obtaining chest and pelvic radiographs, and performing the focused assessment by sonography for trauma (FAST) exam.

A: Airway
B: Breathing
C: Circulation
D: Deficits
E: Exposure

FIGURE 41-1 Primary survey.

The **secondary survey** of the trauma patient is a head-to-toe physical examination that includes a thorough history using the AMPLE mnemonic. AMPLE stands for *a*llergies, current *m*edications used, *p*ast illnesses/*p*regnancy, *l*ast meal, and *e*vents/*e*nvironment related to the traumatic injury. The secondary exam is not performed until the patient is deemed stable by completion of the primary survey and this is confirmed with normal vital signs while resuscitation is under way. After the primary and secondary surveys are complete, patients are triaged for further radiographic evaluation, operative intervention, or inter- or intrahospital transfer or admission.

Thoracic Trauma

Unintentional injuries are responsible for approximately 180,000 deaths and 9 million disabling injuries in the United States each year.[2] This mechanism constitutes the fourth leading cause of death for all Americans and is the leading cause of death for those aged 1 to 44 years.[3,4] Injuries to the chest can be broadly classified as having either a blunt or penetrating mechanism. Twenty-five percent of deaths from **blunt trauma** are the direct result of thoracic injury.[2] For those who survive their initial injuries, blunt thoracic injuries are responsible for 8% of traumatic hospital admissions.[5] Motor vehicle crashes (MVCs) are the dominant cause of blunt force resulting in chest injury.

Penetrating trauma is a common injury pattern endemic to urban trauma centers in the United States. Injuries from stab wounds and handguns result in low-velocity (<1500 ft/s) wounds with injured tissue centered at the trajectory of the object. High-velocity (>1500 ft/s) injuries occur with military assault weapons or hunting rifles. These injuries incur a remarkable amount of tissue damage not only by the trajectory of the missile but also by the simultaneous blast effect, which creates widespread contusion and hemorrhage. High-velocity missiles often are designed to fragment or tumble as they travel, increasing the diameter of the pathway created and resulting in multiple locations of perforation and hemorrhage. Even at the busiest of urban trauma centers, however, penetrating chest injury accounts for only 7% of trauma admissions and 16% of penetrating admissions; these injuries are almost exclusively low-velocity injuries.[6]

Respiratory Recap

Types of Thoracic Trauma

- Blunt
- Penetrating

Airway and Breathing Injuries

Airway injuries detected during the primary survey take precedence over any other injury detected initially due to the temporal nature of their lethality. Initial inspection of the airway includes observing the quality and quantity of air movement at the nose, mouth, and chest. Auscultation of air movement is carried down to the chest onto the lung fields. Inspection of the oropharynx for obstruction occurs rapidly along with the evaluation of the accessory muscles of respiration, specifically, the intercostals and supraclavicular groups.

Laryngotracheal Injuries

Laryngotracheal injuries occurring in the neck or at the thoracic outlet can directly affect the patency of the airway. These injuries occur in both blunt and penetrating mechanisms. Signs and symptoms of presentation include stridor, neck tenderness, hematomas of the neck or upper chest, and subcutaneous emphysema. The evaluation of these injuries requires the use of direct laryngoscopy as well as bronchoscopy. Establishment of a definitive airway is imperative before obstruction occurs, although improperly placed endotracheal airways can worsen an already precarious situation. If such an injury is suspected, operative evaluation and intervention are required.[7]

Obstruction of the airway can occur by a dislocation of the sternoclavicular heads secondary to frontal or lateral blunt impact. Palpation of the sternum with evident posterior dislocation should alert the care team to such an injury. Patients may complain of sternal pain, stridor, and dysphasia due to the direct compression of mediastinal structures. The diagnosis is often confirmed by specific angled radiographs, computed tomography (CT), or both. Closed reduction is the preferred method for correction, although operative open reduction and fixation may be necessary.[8]

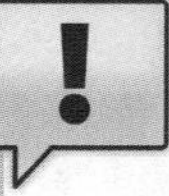

Respiratory Recap

Airway and Breathing Injuries

- Laryngotracheal injuries
- Dislocation of the sternoclavicular heads
- Pneumothorax

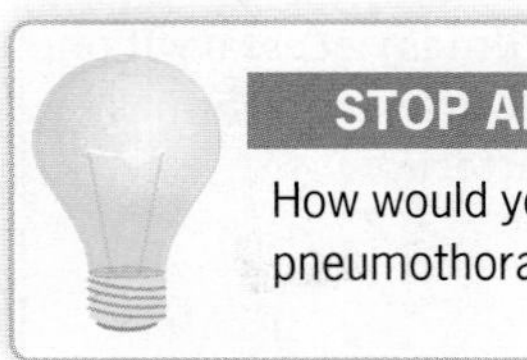

STOP AND THINK

How would you determine if a patient has a pneumothorax?

Pneumothorax

One of the most common and potentially lethal injuries encountered in chest trauma is a **pneumothorax**. It is estimated that 20% of patients who present to a trauma center alive have a pneumothorax,[9] which is the presence of air in the pleural space between the lung and the posterior thoracic wall. Universal signs of pneumothorax are chest pain and respiratory distress. Subcutaneous emphysema found on exam indicates the presence of air escaping from the chest cavity into the subcutaneous tissue from a pneumothorax etiology. The classic yet subtle findings of tracheal deviation and hyperresonance on percussion are difficult and rare to detect in the noisy and busy trauma bay.

Definitive diagnosis is made by chest radiograph, although clinical signs and symptoms can delineate the diagnosis. The rate of missed anterior pneumothoraces on supine anteroposterior chest radiographs is estimated to be between 20% and 35%.[10] Evidence is emerging regarding the utility of detecting pneumothoraces by ultrasound as an adjunct of the FAST exam, although utility may be limited if subcutaneous emphysema is present.[11] Nonetheless, with the increasing rate of CT use for both abdominal and chest imaging, more and more pneumothoraces are being detected. The clinical relevance of these occult pneumothoraces is questionable.

There are three subtypes of pneumothoraces: simple, open, and tension. A simple pneumothorax is one that presents as a collection of air in the pleural space. An open pneumothorax differs in that such an injury is associated with a chest injury that allows air to enter the negatively pressured thoracic cavity. An equalization of pressure between the atmosphere and the chest then occurs. With each inspiration, air is preferentially drawn into the chest via the wound if the diameter of the wound is approximately two-thirds or more greater than that of the trachea. Initial treatment of an open pneumothorax is to place a sterile dressing to the wound with three of four sides taped to the chest. Having one side free allows air to exit the chest during exhalation but prevents air entry into the chest cavity during inspiration by a flap valve mechanism.

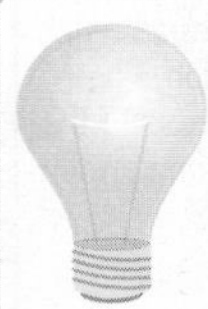

STOP AND THINK

How would you know if there is an air leak in a patient with a chest tube?

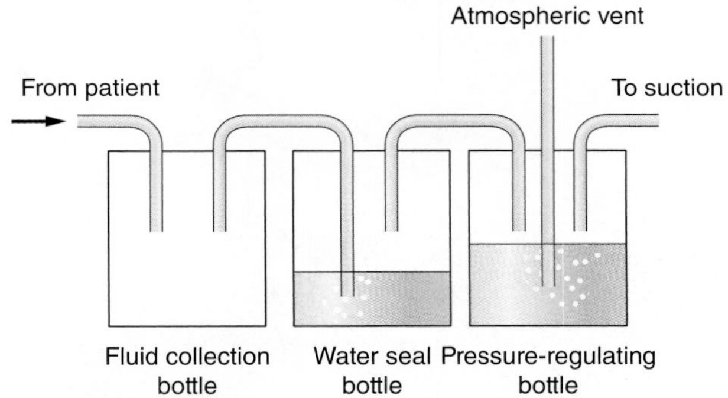

FIGURE 41-2 Schematic of underwater seal showing component parts.

After application of the dressing, a chest tube should be placed away from the wound site. Preferably, a 32-French or larger tube should be placed in the fourth to fifth rib interspace anterior to the midaxillary line. The chest tube is then attached to an underwater seal system, and suction may be applied to prevent air accumulation in the pleural space (**Figure 41-2**).

The most lethal of the subtypes is the tension pneumothorax. A tension pneumothorax occurs via air entering the chest from a lung or chest wall injury but being unable to escape. With enough air entering the cavity through a one-way valve system, pressure accumulates in the chest. This intrathoracic pressure can be higher than the intrinsic venous pressure required to return blood to the heart and may displace the mediastinum. As the pressure builds, less and less blood is able to enter the right heart. This increasing pressure also causes ipsilateral and even contralateral lung parenchymal collapse. Hemodynamic failure and death are imminent unless the pressure is relieved, allowing the return of cardiac preload and pulmonary ventilation and oxygenation.

The diagnosis of tension pneumothorax is made clinically and should not be delayed by waiting for diagnostic imaging. Clinical signs and symptoms include those found for simple pneumothorax, but the presence of tracheal deviation, hyperresonance, and neck vein distention may be more pronounced, although still difficult to detect. Treatment of this breathing emergency starts with immediate chest decompression. This can be accomplished by placing a 14-gauge, 4.5-cm IV catheter needle into the second intercostal space in the midclavicular line on the affected side (**Figure 41-3**). Such decompression is not without drawbacks, in that it is estimated that 30% of trauma patients have a chest wall thickness greater than 5 cm.[12] Definitive treatment often requires the expedient placement of a chest tube or emergent finger decompression to convert a tension to a simple pneumothorax.

Circulation Injuries

After the clearance of potential breathing injuries, the focus shifts to those injuries that can affect the circulatory system. The initial assessment of hemodynamically

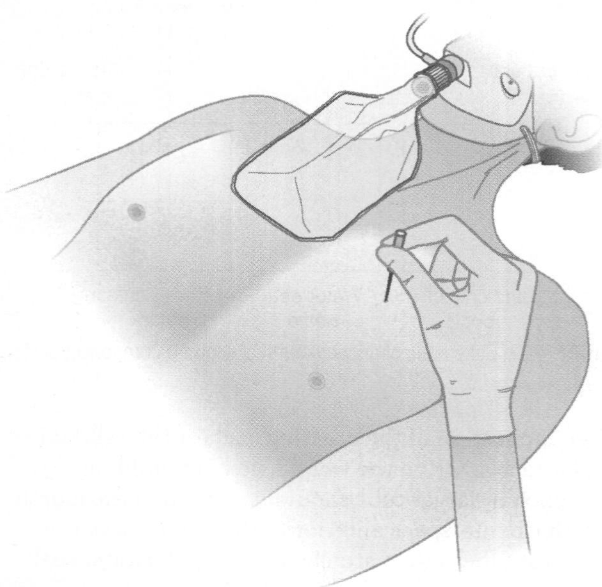

FIGURE 41-3 Chest needle for treating pneumothorax.

unstable patients focuses on the palpation of distal pulses in both the upper and lower extremities. The strength, rate, and rhythm of these pulses need to be evaluated. Objective measurement of vital signs needs to occur. This includes the measurement of heart rate, blood pressure, and respiratory rate. As these parameters are being assessed, a cardiac monitor and pulse oximeter should be attached to the patient. Careful interpretation of the cardiac rhythm is necessary if one suspects blunt thoracic injury, because arrhythmias may occur with such an injury pattern.

Hypovolemic Shock

The diagnosis and treatment of **hypovolemic shock** are the focus at this step in the primary survey. Tissue hypoperfusion from intravascular blood loss (hemorrhagic hypovolemic shock) is the most commonly encountered shock state of injured patients. Signs and symptoms of hemorrhagic hypovolemia include tachycardia, hypotension, and pallor of the skin. Hemorrhage is classified into four categories, using vital signs to aid in the quantification of blood loss (**Table 41-1**). Class I hemorrhage is characterized by a 70-kg patient losing up to 15% of blood volume (<750 mL). Vital signs are often unchanged in a young, healthy—albeit injured—patient with this class of hemorrhage. Class II hemorrhage is characterized by an increase in the heart rate to more than 100 beats per minute for those who have lost 15 to 30% (750–1500 mL) of their volume. Hypotension is the hallmark of class III hemorrhage. These patients have lost 30% to 40% (1500–2000 mL) of their blood volume, affecting their ability to maintain a normal blood pressure. Class IV hemorrhage encompasses patients who have lost more than 40% of their volume (>2000 mL). These patients are in extremis, near the point of death. Those patients who have sustained a thoracic injury and present with a circulatory

TABLE 41-1
Estimated Blood Loss Based on Initial Presentation for a 70-kg Male

	Class I	Class II	Class III	Class IV
Blood loss (mL)	Up to 750	750–1500	1500–2000	>2000
Blood loss (% blood volume)	Up to 15%	15%–30%	30%–40%	>40%
Heart rate	<100	100–120	120–140	>140
Blood pressure	Normal	Normal	Decreased	Decreased
Pulse pressure (mm Hg)	Normal or increased	Decreased	Decreased	Decreased
Respiratory rate	14–20	20–30	30–40	>35
Urine output (mL/h)	>30	20–30	5–15	Negligible
Central nervous system/ mental status	Slightly anxious	Mildly anxious	Anxious, confused	Confused, lethargic
Fluid replacement	Crystalloid	Crystalloid	Crystalloid and blood	Crystalloid and blood

The guidelines in this table are based on the 3-for-1 (3:1) rule, which derives from the empiric observation that most patients in hemorrhagic shock require as much as 300 mL of electrolyte solution for each 100 mL of blood loss. Applied blindly, these guidelines may result in excessive or inadequate fluid administration. For example, a patient with a crush injury to an extremity may have hypotension that is out of proportion to his or her blood loss and may require fluids in excess of the 3:1 guidelines. In contrast, a patient whose ongoing blood loss is being replaced by blood transfusion requires less than 3:1. The use of bolus therapy with careful monitoring of the patient's response may moderate these extremes.

Reproduced from Shock. In: American College of Surgeons Committee on Trauma. *Advanced Trauma Life Support for Doctors: Student Course Manual.* 8th ed. Chicago, IL: American College of Surgeons; 2008:55–71. Reprinted with permission.

deficit detected on the primary survey have by definition fallen into at least class II if they exhibit signs of tachycardia and class III if they are hypotensive.

Controversy surrounds the definition of hypotension. Traditionally, hypotension has been defined as a patient with a systolic blood pressure less than 90 mm Hg. Little evidence supports this rigid physiologic cutoff, however, with recent work demonstrating an inflection of mortality beginning at 110 mm Hg.[13]

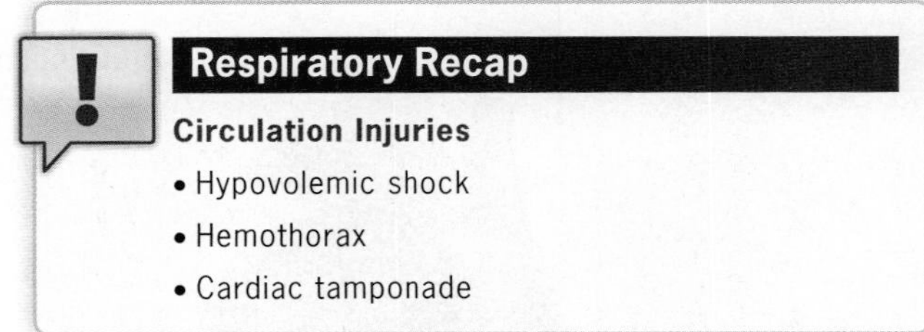

Respiratory Recap

Circulation Injuries

- Hypovolemic shock
- Hemothorax
- Cardiac tamponade

Hemothorax

Massive **hemothorax** is the accumulation of more than 1500 mL of blood in the chest cavity. Such an injury is most commonly caused by a penetrating mechanism, although blunt trauma may be implicated. The classic physical findings of a massive hemothorax are a patient in hemorrhagic shock with decreased breaths sounds and/or dullness to percussion isolated to the affected hemithorax.

The treatment of a massive hemothorax begins with correcting the physiologic derangements associated with hemorrhagic shock. Initial crystalloid resuscitation often occurs in the prehospital environment. This resuscitation continues as the patient is cared for by the evaluating trauma team. A balanced blood product resuscitation of fresh, frozen plasma to packed red blood cells in an effort to mimic whole blood has demonstrated benefit to those individuals requiring a massive transfusion (more than 10 units of blood products in 24 hours).[14–16] Care needs to be taken regarding the amount of resuscitation a patient undergoes. Aggressive fluid resuscitation may be detrimental to the hypotensive patient with penetrating injuries before bleeding is controlled, in that such resuscitation may prevent appropriate clotting at the site of injury and may lead to increased mortality.[17] Furthermore, work in patients with active hemorrhage has implicated relatively small volumes of crystalloid solutions (500-mL aliquots) to be an independent risk factor for the development of acute lung injury.[18]

The management of a massive hemothorax depends on the stability of the patient and the quantification of the hemothorax. In the unstable patient with clinical signs of massive hemothorax, immediate chest cavity decompression is warranted concurrently with ongoing resuscitation. In the hemodynamically stable patient, diagnostic imaging is often performed while the primary and secondary surveys are occurring. Commonly the diagnosis is made by chest radiography, although between 200 and 300 mL of blood needs to be present in the chest for it to be seen on the radiograph. Placing the patient in an upright position will cause the blood to layer in the base of thorax, thus increasing the sensitivity of the radiograph. In the acute setting, this may be the sole imaging from which the diagnosis is made and treatment initiated. This positioning may not be appropriate in those patients in whom a spinal cord injury is suspected. The presence and size of a hemothorax are much more difficult to assess with supine chest radiograph.

Adjuvant methods of imaging are of growing interest in those hemodynamic patients without signs of a massive hemothorax but with evidence of blood within the chest (simple hemothorax). CT is a highly sensitive diagnostic study for the evaluation of chest structures and pathology, although it means both a dramatic increase of cost and radiation exposure as compared with chest radiography.[19] Opponents of the routine use of CT imaging contend that its high sensitivity identifies pathology that is clinically nonsignificant.[20] Such imaging has been demonstrated to be superior over chest radiography in the evaluation of patients with suspected retained hemothorax later in the course of care.[21]

Treatment of both a massive hemothorax and simple hemothorax focuses on the complete evacuation of fluid from the chest cavity. This is first performed by placement of a chest tube into the affected side as described previously. When a massive hemothorax is present, the initial output from the chest tube is dramatic. If more than 1500 mL is immediately evacuated, it is very likely the patient will require emergent thoracotomy, thus necessitating the appropriate surgical consultation. Continued bleeding from the chest (>200 mL per hour for 2 to 4 hours) is traditionally cited as criteria for emergent thoracotomy. Even with these recommended criteria for surgical intervention, the patient's clinical signs and physiology take precedence for determining operative intervention. A patient in hemorrhagic shock, although with output less than the criteria just described, who requires ongoing resuscitation (likely with blood products) is likely experiencing ongoing blood loss and thus will require surgical intervention to control it.

Cardiac Tamponade

Cardiac tamponade is an injury that is most commonly seen after a penetrating injury, although blunt mechanisms have been reported. Cardiac tamponade is defined by the filling of the pericardial sac with blood from the heart, the great vessels, or pericardial vessels. Because the pericardial sac is a fibrous structure with a fixed volume, ever-increasing small amounts of blood that leak into it cause an increase in pressure within this closed space (**Figure 41-4**). This pressure increase directly restricts the activity of the heart and prevents adequate cardiac filling.

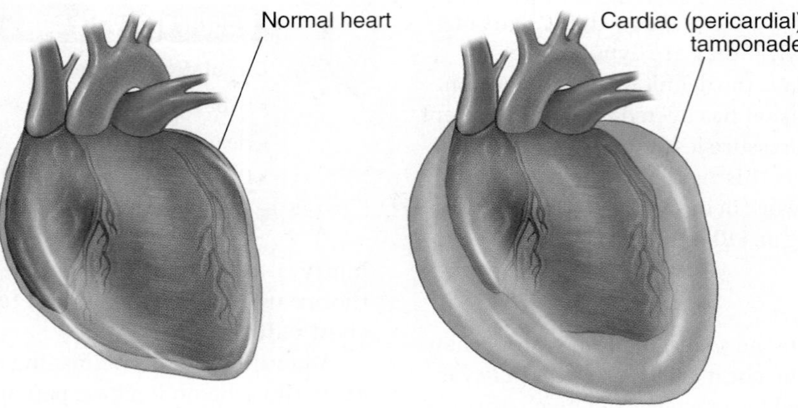

FIGURE 41-4 Cardiac tamponade.

The diagnosis of cardiac tamponade is classically described as **Beck's triad**, which consists of venous pressure elevation (jugular venous distention), a decline in arterial pressure, and muffled heart sounds. In reality, such a triad is difficult to diagnose in a busy and noisy trauma bay. Patients with tamponade present with a spectrum of findings that range from a subtle decrease in blood pressure to hemodynamic collapse with cardiac arrest. A high index of suspicion is required to make a rapid diagnosis. The use of ultrasound has made the detection of pericardial fluid rapid and accurate at the bedside of these patients. The FAST exam allows clinicians to detect blood not only in the pericardial space but also in the abdomen by noninvasive means.[22] Although the precision of such a test is operator dependent, the initial accuracy rate of the FAST exam has been found to be at least 90% from the outset of the experience of the individual clinician.[23]

The treatment of cardiac tamponade begins with volume resuscitation. The goal of intravenous fluids is to increase the central venous pressure to overcome the restrictive pressure created by the accumulated pericardial blood. With an increase in cardiac output created, transient increases in the hemodynamics of the patient are expected. Evacuation of the pericardial blood is necessary for the relief of the tamponade physiology. This is ideally performed in the operating room by a surgical team experienced in repairing injuries to the heart. If surgical intervention is not available, pericardiocentesis using ultrasound is a means to aspirate pericardial blood. This is merely a temporizing measure in that blood may reaccumulate if the cardiac injury is not surgically repaired.

Injuries Encountered During the Secondary Survey

The secondary survey begins after the primary survey is complete and all immediate life-threatening injuries have been addressed. If the patient decompensates hemodynamically during any part of the primary or secondary survey, the clinician must start reevaluating causes using the ordered nature of the primary survey. Injuries described earlier in this chapter may not be detected until the secondary survey based on the temporal nature of their acuity. The secondary survey focuses on an in-depth physical examination of the patient from head to toe. While this exam is occurring, radiographic and laboratory data are collected by members of the team.

If the chest radiograph was not obtained during the primary survey, it should be performed at this time. The anteroposterior chest radiograph is the single most valuable diagnostic study in the evaluation of any patient with chest trauma. Findings on the chest radiograph can suggest the amount of velocity incurred during blunt impact. Multiple broken ribs—specifically, fractures of the first or second ribs—can indicate a high-velocity impact. The chest radiograph may also demonstrate findings to aid in the diagnosis of the eight lethal injuries of the chest, which are tracheobronchial injuries, pneumothorax, hemothorax, pulmonary contusion, blunt cardiac injury, aortic injury, diaphragmatic injury, and esophageal injury. Detection of these injuries during the secondary survey may be subtle as compared with those that present during the primary survey; thus, a high index of suspicion is required for detection.

Pulmonary Contusion

A **pulmonary contusion** is a bruise of the lung parenchyma. The initial trauma, whether direct injury from a blunt impact or contusion injury from a penetrating mechanism, causes the rupture of small blood vessels within the lung or direct injury to lung alveoli. Interstitial edema and intra-alveolar hemorrhage are the end result at the tissue level.[24]

Pulmonary contusion may occur without rib fractures, although the presence of a contusion is almost pathognomonic when a flail segment is present. A flail

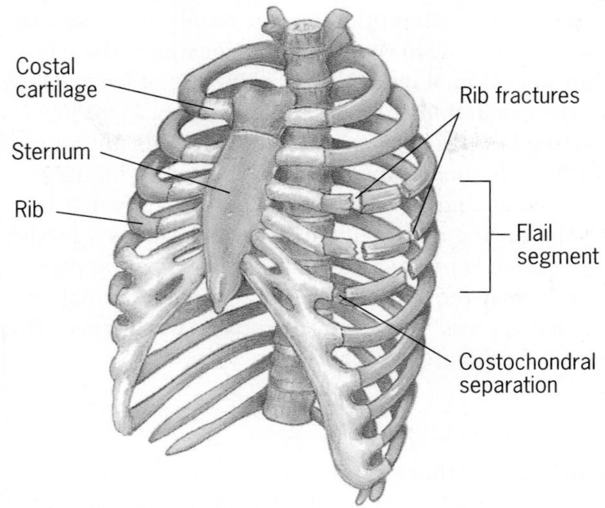

FIGURE 41-5 Flail chest.

chest results from two or more ribs that are fractured in two or more locations, sternal fracture, or costochondral separation (**Figure 41-5**). The term *flail* refers to the paradoxical motion of the affected chest wall segment caused by the lack of structural integrity. During inspiration, the flail segment is drawn into the chest (due to negative intrapleural pressure) while the rest of the thorax expands outward. During exhalation, the opposite occurs, with the flail segment being pushed outward while the rest of the chest retracts. Because the chest wall becomes unstable during impact, the moving segment directly injures the lung parenchyma deep to the thoracic wall.

Pulmonary contusion alters the ventilation-perfusion ($\dot{V}/\dot{Q}$) match and may lead to arterial hypoxia. Patients with significant hypoxia may require intubation rapidly after injury due to the progressive nature of this disease. Pulmonary contusions often develop at 48 hours after injury, with maximal ($\dot{V}/\dot{Q}$) mismatching occurring during this period.[25] Because of the expected progressive nature of significant pulmonary contusions, elective intubation prior to respiratory failure should be considered early in the patient's management.[26] Once the patient's airway is controlled, manipulations of mean airway pressure (e.g., positive end-expiratory pressure, inspiratory-to-expiratory ratio) should be considered to reinflate collapsed pulmonary segments and alveoli to maximize oxygenation. The treatment of contusion is entirely supportive, with resolution occurring at approximately 1 week.

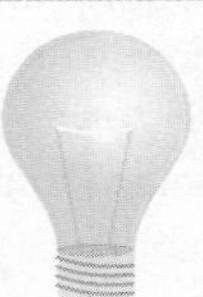

STOP AND THINK

What ventilator settings would you recommend for an intubated patient with flail chest and chest contusion?

Blunt Cardiac Injury

Much like pulmonary contusion is an injury that occurs to lung parenchyma, blunt cardiac injury is trauma to cardiac tissue resulting from a blunt mechanism. Blunt cardiac injury can result in bruising to the heart myocardium, coronary artery injury, chamber rupture, valvular injury, or a combination of these. Cardiac rupture is possible, although it is usually associated with a high transfer of energy such as seen with high-speed MVCs or falls from substantial height.

Patients with blunt cardiac injury present commonly with chest pain. Often these patients have multiple chest wall injuries that can confound this finding. Screening the asymptomatic patient with suspected injury with electrocardiograms (ECGs) and cardiac enzyme levels, the gold standard for myocardial ischemia, remains controversial.[27–29] Symptomatic patients are defined by the finding of hemodynamic instability and dysrhythmias on ECG. These include atrial fibrillation, premature ventricular contractions, sinus tachycardia, bundle-branch block, and ST segment changes. These patients warrant evaluation by echocardiography to determine the presence of pericardial fluid, to quantify the presence of cardiac wall motion abnormality, and to measure cardiac contractility.

Treatment of a blunt cardiac injury follows the same principles described for a penetrating cardiac injury. If pericardial fluid is demonstrated by the initial FAST exam or formal echocardiography, timely drainage of the pericardial space needs to occur, with the possibility that surgical repair of such an injury may be required. In the patient with dysrhythmias or conduction abnormalities found on ECG, supportive care needs to be provided in an intensive care environment with the possibility of concomitant cardiac pharmacology. Nonetheless, these dysrhythmias are often self-limiting, with resolution within 24 to 48 hours.

Aortic Injury

The great majority of injuries to the thoracic aorta have a penetrating mechanism of injury. Unfortunately, these injuries often have a fatal outcome. The identification of an aortic injury by a blunt mechanism often requires a great deal of insight during the secondary survey. The proximal descending aorta is the most common site for injury via a blunt mechanism because of its mobility and susceptibility to shear forces in relation to an otherwise relatively fixed structure.[30] Common types of injuries include a dissection (a tear of the innermost tissue layer of the aorta), a pseudoaneurysm (a full-thickness injury that is contained by surrounding tissue), and rupture, which often is fatal.

The presentation of patients with such an injury pattern is subtle at best during physical examination. Nonspecific clinical signs of a thoracic aorta injury include chest pain, shortness of breath, multiple rib fractures, or a sternal fracture and asymmetric upper extremity blood pressures. Traditional means of diagnosis begin with the chest radiograph. Findings may include a widened mediastinum, loss of the aortopulmonary window, depression of the left main bronchus, blunting of the aortic knob, or deviation of the esophagus or trachea. Abnormalities on chest radiography or a high clinical suspicion dictate the need for further imaging. The historical gold standard for the evaluation of the aorta has been catheter arteriography, although more centers are relying on spiral chest CT because of its speed, accuracy, and noninvasive nature.[31]

When an injury is found, the first step is expedient admission into a critical care environment. The main focus of such an admission is the control of blood pressure via beta blockade to reduce shear forces that are generated by blood flow at the area of injury.[32] Although this treatment is classic teaching for intensivists, the evidence behind such pharmacology is remote and lacks prospective validation. The historical treatment for such injuries has been open surgical repair, whether primary or by replacement of the injured segment by an interposition graft. Endovascular techniques are rapidly becoming favored as an alternative approach secondary to reduced mortality and need for blood transfusions.[33]

Diaphragmatic Injury

Detecting injuries to the diaphragm is often very difficult. The dynamic movement of this structure makes predicting penetrating injuries based on trajectory a guess at best. Penetrating injuries to the diaphragm occur almost three times more frequently than injuries to the diaphragm due to a blunt mechanism.[34] Such penetrating injuries are extremely small, the size of the bullet or the width of a knife, and often are diagnosed and repaired intraoperatively. Blunt trauma often creates large tears secondary to a blow-out effect as force is applied to the external thorax or abdomen. These blunt lacerations are more commonly diagnosed on the left rather than the right because the liver acts to protect or obscure the right hemidiaphragm.

Diaphragmatic injuries are often missed or misinterpreted as normal anatomic variations. If an injury is suspected of the left hemidiaphragm, a nasogastric tube should be placed and a repeat chest radiograph taken. With a nasogastric tube in place, the clinician has an improved ability to determine whether the stomach is within the thoracic cavity. A hemothorax may obscure clear radiographic evaluation of the left diaphragm, and thus a chest tube should be placed before further evaluation. If the diagnosis continues to be unclear, some advocate upper gastrointestinal contrast studies or CT imaging of the chest and abdomen. Unfortunately, there are few specific findings attributable to diaphragmatic injuries, which contributes to a high false-negative rate for these tests.[35]

Operative intervention may be required for the diagnosis to be made in those patients for whom there is a high suspicion of injury. The routine use of laparoscopy for the evaluation of the left hemidiaphragm for penetrating injuries has demonstrated a significant number of otherwise occult injures.[36–38] Penetrating injuries detected during laparoscopy or thoracoscopy may be repaired using minimally invasive techniques if further exploration is not required. Larger or more complex injuries may require a traditional open abdominal or thoracic approach, especially if synthetic mesh is necessary for diaphragmatic closure.

Esophageal Injury

Injuries to the thoracic esophagus are mainly due to gunshot wounds because of the central and deep location of the structure. Penetrating injuries to the esophagus are associated with other central chest injuries (heart, lungs, and great vessels) and thus are associated with a large mortality. Blunt injuries have been reported, although these are suspected to be the result of a blow-out type of mechanism due to force being placed on the chest or abdomen.

Signs and symptoms of an esophageal injury are nonspecific and are often clouded by the patient having multiple severe injuries. A delay in detection of an injury can be catastrophic because of the resultant increase in thoracic contamination, which leads to a higher risk of mediastinitis, sepsis, and death.[39] The evaluation of blunt esophageal injury should be considered in patients with injuries consistent with significant thoracic force. A chest radiograph should be obtained, although accuracy for injury is low. Findings of pneumomediastinum should alert the care team to a possible injury and prompt further evaluation. A high index of suspicion or abnormalities detected on chest radiography should direct the clinician to contrast studies of the esophagus or esophagoscopy, or both. Diagnosed injuries require expedient surgical repair with wide drainage of the contaminated pleural cavity.

Chest Wall Injury

Injuries to the chest often include injuries of the bony thorax, specifically the ribs, clavicles, sternum, and scapulas. Fracture of the upper ribs (ribs 1 and 2), scapula, or sternum requires a great deal of force and thus may give insight into the amount of energy transferred to the chest wall. Such an injury pattern may demand evaluation of the head, spine, lungs, heart, and the great vessels. Fractures of the lower ribs (ribs 10 through 12) may lead to thoracoabdominal injuries, specifically of the spleen and liver.

Although often underappreciated, the sequelae from bone pain of the thorax can be dramatic. The ability of patients to participate in incentive spirometry, clear secretions, ventilate, and oxygenate is compromised by

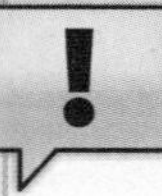

Respiratory Recap

Injuries Found on Secondary Survey

- Pulmonary contusion
- Blunt cardiac injury
- Aortic injury
- Diaphragmatic injury
- Esophageal injury
- Chest wall injury

such pain. In the elderly population, the effects of simple rib fractures can be morbid, likely as a result of the impending consequences of poor pulmonary toilet.[40,41] Splinting of the chest wall may aid in local pain control, although it is contraindicated because of the negative consequences of inadequate pulmonary toilet due to chest wall immobility.

Aggressive pain control should be a primary endpoint for this patient population regardless of whether surgical fixation is warranted. The failure to provide adequate pain control has been associated with hypoventilation, retained secretions, atelectasis, pneumonia, and respiratory failure.[42] Methods of pain medication delivery include parenteral methods (intravenous and intramuscular), enteral means, epidural delivery, and local techniques, including nerve blocks, intrapleural catheters, and extrapleural catheters. These techniques can be controlled by the care team or by the patient. In the latter case, the patient dictates how much pain control is needed by pushing the button of a patient-controlled analgesia (PCA) device.[43] PCA devices prevent periods of breakthrough pain that may delay progress in pulmonary toilet, atelectasis, and cough. PCA devices can have preprogrammed lock-outs for the amount or frequency of medications delivered.

Parenteral narcotics continue to be the standard method by which clinicians treat thoracic pain. Narcotics can be delivered by all of the methods just described. The amount required for pain control is individualized to the patient and thus requires that patients be monitored and evaluated by objective pain measurement tools.[44] Traditionally, approaches focus on the use of short-acting parenteral narcotics for procedural pain or pain control while intubated, with a transition to PCA methods when the patient is able to participate in his or her care. A conversion to longer-acting enteral narcotics often occurs when a diet can be tolerated and more chronic pain medication needs are established. Regardless of whether a narcotic is provided enterally or parenterally, the side effects of confusion, respiratory depression, and cough suppression may occur. A careful balance needs to be achieved between the side effects of narcotic usage and the benefits created by pain-controlled pulmonary care.

The use of regional anesthetics can add a great deal to chest wall pain control while limiting exposure to side effects. Continuous epidural infusions of narcotic and local anesthetics have been successful in controlling chest pain and improving respiratory function. For thoracic trauma patients, it has been demonstrated that epidural delivery of anesthesia may be superior to PCA methods for the control of pain and improvement of pulmonary function.[44] The use of epidural anesthetics has demonstrated an increase in maximum inspiratory and expiratory pressures, vital capacity, and peak expiratory flow. Parenteral narcotics often cause a respiratory depression that leads to a decrease in $Pa{O_2}$ and increase in $Pa{CO_2}$.[45] Epidural analgesia prevents this problem by maintaining normal $Pa{O_2}$ and $Pa{CO_2}$ levels. Epidurals are not without issues, however. Complications at the insertion site, as well as spinal cord injury, have been associated with their use. Epidural analgesia also can cause profound vasodilatory hypotension if fluid management strategies as well as epidural medication infusions are not closely monitored. The use of intercostal catheters with or without medication pumps for the administration of local anesthetic has also been reported, although placement of the catheters requires surgical expertise and the benefits it adds to epidural analgesia are unclear.[46,47]

Head Trauma

Head injuries are commonly encountered by those caring for the traumatically injured. Although most injuries are categorized as minor, it is imperative for the care team to provide timely evaluation and treatment to prevent secondary brain injury in those patients with any signs or symptoms of traumatic brain injury (TBI). Injuries can be the result of either penetrating or blunt mechanisms. Treatment of the patient with a traumatic head injury follows the same orderly steps described previously and outlined by the ATLS guidelines of the American College of Surgeons Committee on Trauma.[48] The focus of the ABCDE and later secondary survey is the identification of a treatable mass lesion, prevention of hypoxia, and avoidance of hypotension to secure adequate cerebral perfusion pressure.

Intracranial Physiology

To understand primary brain injury and to prevent secondary injury, it is important to focus on the unique anatomy and physiology of the head. The brain is enveloped by the arachnoid mater, then by the dura mater, and finally encased by the skull. Because of the nonexpandable nature of the skull, the Monro-Kellie doctrine states that the total volume of the intracranial contents must remain constant. These contents include the brain, cerebrospinal fluid (CSF), and venous blood. If a patient were to have an increase in intracranial blood after a traumatic injury, the resultant volume of

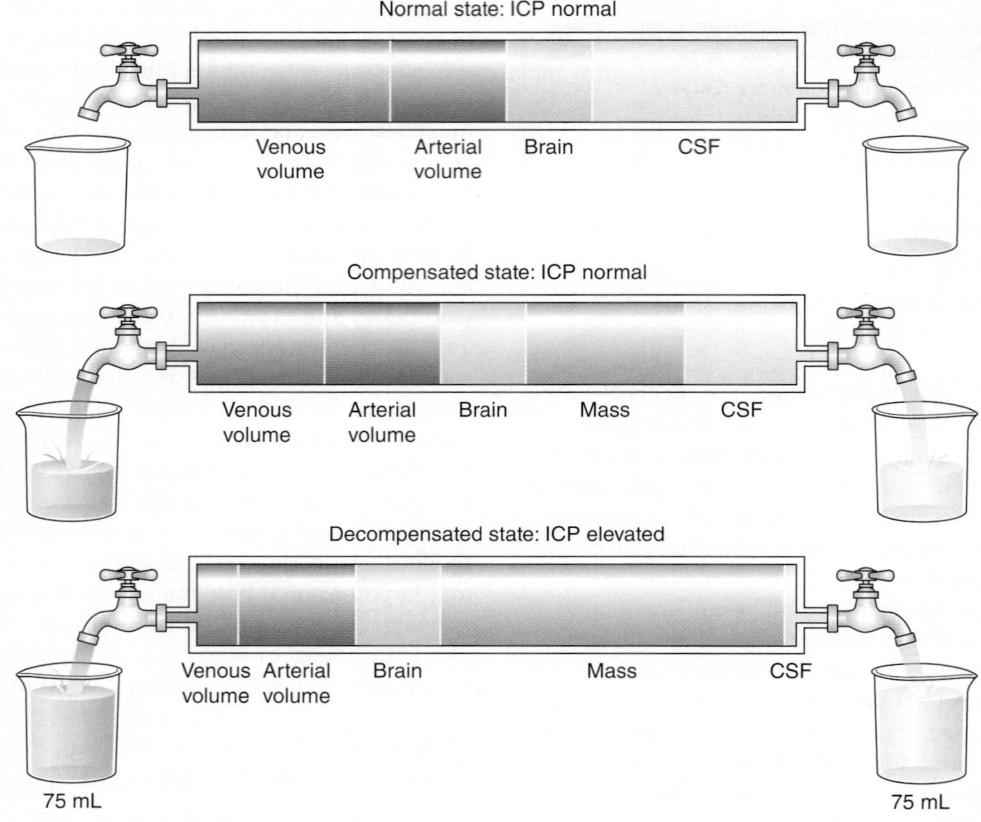

FIGURE 41-6 The Monro-Kellie doctrine.
Reproduced from *Advanced Trauma Life Support.* 8th ed. 2008. With permission of the American College of Surgeons.

CSF and venous blood must exit the skull or intracranial pressure (ICP) will rise (**Figure 41-6**). With both CSF and venous blood being removed by compensatory mechanisms from the intracranial space, ICP will exponentially rise if such a lesion is not externally decompressed.

Blood flow to the brain is directly dependent on the pressure head of the systemic blood pressure but is negated by elevated ICP. When ICP rises, a reflexive increase in mean arterial pressure (MAP) occurs to maintain the appropriate cerebral perfusion pressure (CPP). CPP is defined as the difference between MAP and ICP. The goal of medical and surgical maneuvers is to maintain CPP above 60 mm Hg. This is done by decreasing ICP or increasing MAP, or both. If a normal CPP is unobtainable, cerebral ischemia may result. Normally, the auto-regulation of arterial blood flow to the brain has a dramatic ability to maintain a constant flow over a wide range of systemic pressures. In the injured brain, the autoregulation of flow is decreased, thus making the brain more susceptible to fluctuations of MAP.

Types of Intracranial Lesions

The anatomic layer in which blood is present and whether the lesion is focal or diffusely located define traumatic intracranial lesions. Focal lesions include epidural, subdural, and subarachnoid or intracerebral hematomas. Diffuse injuries are often referred to as *diffuse axonal injuries* or *shear injuries*. Most intracranial lesions are often characterized early in the course of care by obtaining a noncontrasted head CT.

Epidural Hematoma

An **epidural hematoma** is a collection of blood occurring in the potential space between the dura mater and the posterior wall of the skull. These hematomas occur rarely, affecting 0.9% of those with brain injuries and 9% of those in coma.[48] The etiology of such a bleed is the injury of a blood vessel within this space. Blood that accumulates has a biconvex or lenticular shape on head CT because the clot pushes the dura mater away from

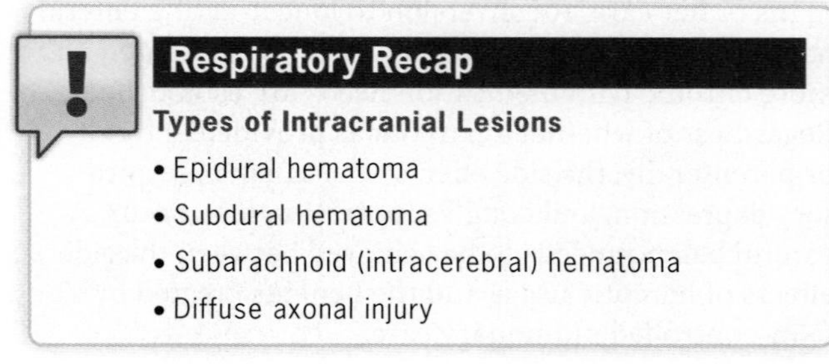

Respiratory Recap

Types of Intracranial Lesions

- Epidural hematoma
- Subdural hematoma
- Subarachnoid (intracerebral) hematoma
- Diffuse axonal injury

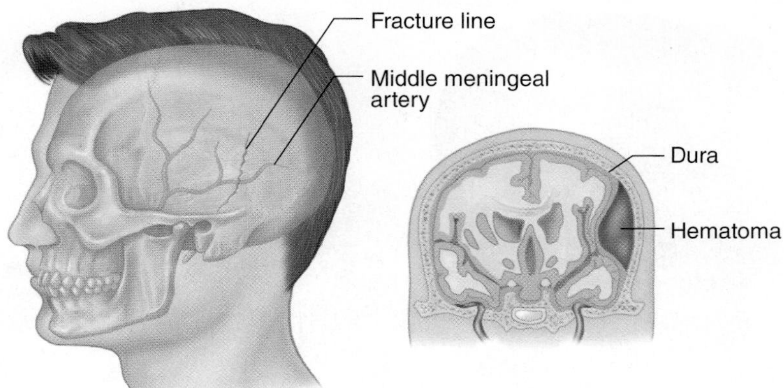

FIGURE 41-7 Epidural hematoma.

the posterior wall of the skull (**Figure 41-7**). Epidural hematomas that accumulate in the temporal or temporoparietal area of the skull often are caused by an injury of the middle meningeal artery.

Subdural Hematoma

A **subdural hematoma** is the result of vascular injury that occurs in the space between the dura mater and the arachnoid mater. Blood that accumulates is often a result of shear injuries of bridging blood vessels originating from the cerebral cortex that travel within this potential space. Subdural hematomas are more common than epidural hematomas in that they occur in approximately 30% of severe brain injuries.[48] The underlying brain injury from a subdural hematoma is often more severe than that from an epidural hematoma. On head CT, subdural hematomas have the appearance of curving to conform to the contours of the brain (**Figure 41-8**).

Subarachnoid Hematoma

Blood that accumulates under the arachnoid mater can have the diffuse appearance common with a **subarachnoid (intracerebral) hematoma** or be a discrete collection as seen with this type of hematoma (**Figure 41-9**). Traumatic subarachnoid hemorrhages have the potential to induce cerebral vasospasm, although the risk is lower than in aneurysmal subarachnoid hemorrhage.[49] Hematomas that occur within the parenchyma may occur in any region of the brain and have the ability to increase in size with time. Often, serial head CT exams are warranted to follow the mass effect of such a bleed.

Diffuse Axonal Injury

Injuries that involve discrete nerve injuries due to shearing forces present during the traumatic event are often referred to as *diffuse axonal injuries*. With multiple nerves being fractured, the potential for pathway injury is present. The spectrum of injury varies from mild concussive symptoms to severe traumatic brain injury. Unfortunately, axonal injury is often difficult to appreciate on head CT and may require magnetic resonance imaging (MRI) for quantification. At present, there are no effective treatments for diffuse axonal injury. The possibility for neuronal healing is present if such nerves are merely injured, not severed, and the exposure to secondary injury is limited.

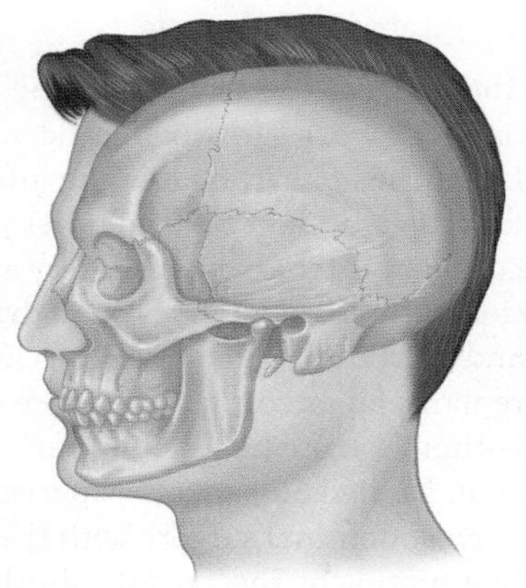

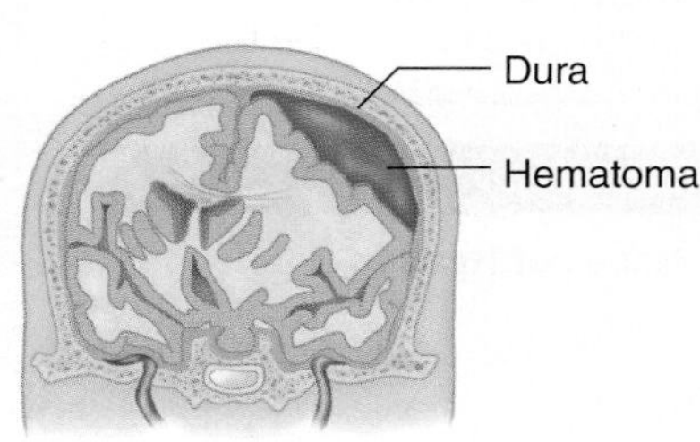

FIGURE 41-8 Subdural hematoma.

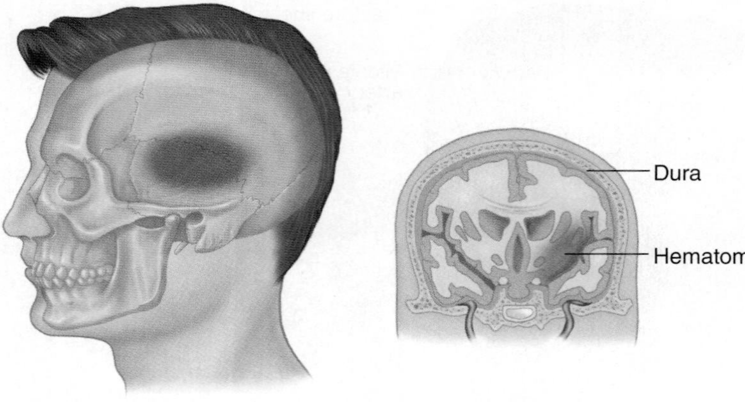

FIGURE 41-9 Subarachnoid (intracerebral) hematoma.

Primary Survey Issues of Head Injury

The primary and secondary survey of a patient with a head injury occurs in the same organized format as it does with any other traumatically injured patient. The effects of brain injury are exacerbated by preventable secondary injury that is encountered and treated during these surveys. It is imperative that the trauma team address these issues rapidly to prevent further neurologic injury.

Hypoxia

The primary survey of the head-injured patient focuses on the prevention of hypoxia. Whether that involves placing a definitive airway or simply providing oxygen to the patient, such interventions need to occur quickly. Those patients who present with severe brain injury may need endotracheal intubation if they are unable to protect their airway or the care team is concerned about the evolution of hypoxia. Pulse oximetry is a useful adjunct in these patients in that a continuous measurement of the blood oxygen saturation is immediately available to all caring for the patient. Hypoxia has been reported to occur in approximately 22% of those with TBI and is an independent predictor of increased morbidity and mortality.[50,51] It appears that even short periods of hypoxia have a significant effect. In one report, an Spo_2 of 90% or less for a median duration of 12 to 20 minutes was found to be an independent predictor of death.[52]

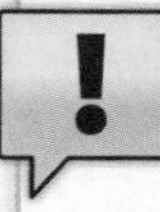

Respiratory Recap

Primary Survey Issues of Head Injury

- Hypoxia
- Hyperventilation
- Hypotension
- Deficits

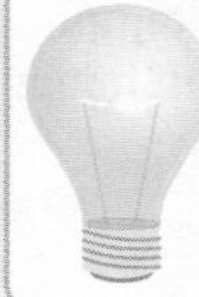

STOP AND THINK

When would you recommend hyperventilation in a patient with head injury?

Hyperventilation

For many years, hyperventilation has been a cornerstone in the care of the patient with severe TBI. Hyperventilating the patient to a $Paco_2$ of less than 25 mm Hg has been demonstrated to rapidly reduce ICP. The mechanism for this reduction is cerebral vasoconstriction, however, with an ultimate reduction of cerebral blood flow.[53] This iatrogenic reduction in cerebral blood flow on top of the innate critical reduction of flow after injury may increase the risk of cerebral ischemia. Cohorts that received prophylactic hyperventilation showed a significantly reduced outcome at 3 and 6 months compared with those who did not receive such treatment.[54] Because of this established risk, the use of prophylactic hyperventilation is not recommended; it should only be used as a temporizing measure for the acute reduction of elevated ICP.[54]

Ventilator Strategies

The impact of intraoperative mechanical ventilation on pulmonary function has been well studied.[55–57] Lellouche et al. evaluated the influence of 10 mL/kg ideal body weight tidal volumes in patients undergoing coronary artery bypass surgery and realized an association with postoperative organ dysfunction, morbidity, and mortality.[57] Nonetheless, a lung protective strategy remains an uncommon practice in subjects with[58] and without[59] acute lung injury during surgery. Severgnini et al. studied 56 patients experiencing 2 hours of open abdominal surgery with the use of a lung protective approach. Their results illustrated that the use of PEEP, recruitment maneuvers, and lower tidal volumes demonstrated improved Clinical Pulmonary Infection Scores, less frequent chest radiograph findings, and enhanced pulmonary function up to 5 days post op.[60] Although these results afford novel options for mitigating postoperative pulmonary complications (PPC), supplementary studies should be performed to reproduce similar results in a larger population. Additionally, Futier et al. related the use of low tidal volumes, PEEP, and recruitment maneuvers during open abdominal surgery with a lower incidence of PPCs, compared to tidal volumes of 10–12 mL/kg and zero PEEP.[61] The patients who were not exposed to a lung protective strategy had a two- to threefold increase in postoperative pneumonia, atelectasis, and re-institution of ventilation. These findings support thorough reconsideration of intraoperative management of mechanical ventilation. PPCs may be avoided with appropriate intraoperative ventilatory management and cost reductions realized by abating complications, and potentially postoperative treatment.

Brueckmann et al. evaluated the prevalence of reintubation subsequent to extubation in the operating room. Their conclusion was consistent with the above findings, and was able to predict reintubation rates in a 1000-patient cohort by combining risk factors and assigning each factor a score. Their 11-point scoring system included the American Society of Anesthesiologists Score ≥3, treatment by a high-risk surgical service, a need for emergent surgical intervention, chronic pulmonary disease, and history of congestive heart failure. Point values of 3, 2, 3, 1, and 2, respectively, were assigned. Of particular note, this system predicts severe PPCs, most remarkably the necessity for reintubation.[62]

Traumatic injury followed by injurious ventilation mimics a two-hit model of organ failure. A lung protective strategy should be considered the standard of care in trauma patients.

Hypotension

The resuscitation of the TBI patient begins immediately in the prehospital setting and continues throughout the patient's evaluation and stay to defend against the deleterious effects of hypotension upon secondary brain injury. Previous work has demonstrated that a single episode of hypotension (<90 mm Hg systolic blood pressure) is associated with an increase in morbidity and a doubling of mortality.[63] The correction of hypotension by fluid resuscitation has been shown to have an impact on beneficial neurologic outcome.[64] Whether resuscitation should occur needs to take into account the CPP of the patient. A systolic blood pressure above 90 mm Hg may not be appropriate if the CPP is compromised. These patients likely would benefit from a closely monitored environment so that alterations in blood pressure can be quickly corrected.

Deficits

The *D* of the primary survey represents evaluating the patient for any neurologic deficits. For a patient who has sustained a traumatic brain injury, calculating the Glasgow Coma Scale (GCS) score is imperative. This scale is an objective clinical measurement of the severity of brain injury. The best GCS score a patient can achieve is 15, whereas the worst is 3. Brain injury is categorized as minor if the score is between 15 and 13, moderate if between 12 and 9, and severe if less than 9. When calculating the GCS score, one uses the highest score response for each of the eye, motor, and verbal components. Accurate scoring is important in that it aids in the prediction of long-term outcome from a variety of injury patterns.

Secondary Survey Issues of Head Injury

The secondary survey exam of a head-injured patient needs to include a thorough neurologic examination. Such an exam needs to be carefully documented so that all others who examine the patient have a clear understanding of the baseline exam. If changes should arise in the neurologic exam, a worsening of the neurologic injury needs to be excluded.

After the secondary survey is complete, an emergency head CT scan is the diagnostic study of choice for all those with moderate or severe brain injury. Controversy exists over the indications for head CT in those with mild brain injury.[65] Regardless, transport of the patient to the CT scanner occurs only after achieving hemodynamic stability. If a change in neurologic exam is encountered during the patient's hospital stay, a repeat head CT is likely indicated.

Treatment of Head Injuries

Medical therapy for the treatment of intracranial injuries focuses on the pharmacologic treatment of elevated ICP. Hyperosmolar agents are the backbone of such therapy. These include mannitol and hypertonic saline. Mannitol acts to lower ICP by creating an osmotic shift of water out of the brain into the intravascular space. Although effective for acutely decreasing ICP, mannitol is a potent diuretic that may exacerbate hypotension. Because of this side effect, the recommended use of mannitol is limited to when signs of transtentorial herniation or progressive neurologic deterioration are present.[66] The use of hypertonic saline to induce an osmotic mobilization similar to mannitol is growing. The use of hypertonic saline as both a bolus agent for treatment of acute ICP and as a continuous infusion for prolonged treatment has been reported, but its long-term efficacy is still unclear.[66]

The surgical treatment of traumatic brain injuries focuses on the rapid decrease of ICP either by open evacuation of the hematoma or by removal of CSF via intraventricular drains. Both of these methods require the expertise of a neurosurgeon in the setting of emergency care. Evidence is emerging that the measurement of brain tissue oxygen levels by an intracranial catheter with the intended goal of manipulating oxygen delivery may have a beneficial effect.[67,68] Nonetheless, placement of these catheters requires neurosurgical support, with values being interpreted by an experienced critical care team.

Key Points

- The mnemonic ABCDE provides for an orderly evaluation and treatment of traumatic injuries.
- The secondary survey of the trauma patient is a head-to-toe physical examination.
- Injuries to the chest can be broadly classified as having either a blunt or penetrating mechanism.
- Traumatic airway and breathing injuries include laryngotracheal injuries, dislocation of the sternoclavicular heads, and pneumothorax.
- There are three subtypes of pneumothoraces: simple, open, and tension.
- Hemorrhage is classified into four categories, using vital signs to aid in the quantification of blood loss.
- Massive hemothorax is accumulation of more than 1500 mL of blood in the chest cavity.
- Treatment of both a massive hemothorax and simple hemothorax focuses on the complete evacuation of fluid from the chest cavity.
- Cardiac tamponade is defined as the filling of the pericardial sac with blood from the heart, the great vessels, or pericardial vessels.
- Lethal injuries of the chest include tracheobronchial injuries, pneumothorax, hemothorax, pulmonary contusion, blunt cardiac injury, aortic injury, diaphragmatic injury, and esophageal injury.
- A flail chest results from two or more ribs that are fractured in two or more locations, sternal fracture, or costochondral separation.
- Pulmonary contusions often develop at 48 hours after injury, with maximal ventilation-perfusion mismatching occurring during this period.
- Although often underappreciated, the sequelae from bone pain of the thorax can be dramatic.
- Traumatic brain injuries can cause epidural hematoma, subdural hematoma, subarachnoid hemorrhage, or diffuse axonal injury.
- Prophylactic hyperventilation is not recommended and should only be used as a temporizing measure for the acute reduction of elevated ICP.
- The correction of hypotension by fluid resuscitation improves neurologic outcome.
- Medical therapy for the treatment of intracranial injuries focuses on pharmacologic treatment of elevated ICP.
- Surgical treatment of traumatic brain injuries focuses on the rapid decrease of ICP.

References

1. American College of Surgeons Committee on Trauma. *Advanced Trauma Life Support for Doctors: Student Manual.* 8th ed. Chicago: American College of Surgeons; 2008.
2. Calhoon JH, Trinkle JK. Pathophysiology of chest trauma. *Chest Surg Clin North Am.* 1997;7:199–211.
3. Centers for Disease Control and Prevention. Injury prevention and control: data and statistics (WISQARS™). Available at: http://www.cdc.gov/ncipc/wisqars/default.htm. Accessed August 21, 2014.
4. MacKenzie EJ, Fowler CJ. Epidemiology. In: Moore EE, Feliciano DV, Mattox KL, eds. *Trauma.* New York: McGraw-Hill; 2004:21–39.
5. Peterson RJ, Tepas JJ, Edwards FH, et al. Pediatric and adult thoracic trauma: age-related impact on presentation and outcome. *Ann Thorac Surg.* 1994;58:14–18.
6. Demetriades D, Velmahos GD. Penetrating injuries of the chest: indications for operation. *Scand J Surg.* 2002;91:41–45.
7. Mathisen DJ, Grillo H. Laryngotracheal trauma. *Ann Thoracic Surg.* 1987;43:254–262.
8. Meyer FN. Upper extremity and hand injuries. In: Moore EE, Feliciano DV, Mattox KL, eds. *Trauma.* New York: McGraw-Hill; 2004:901–937.
9. Di Bartolomeo S, Sanson G, Nardi G, et al. A population based study on pneumothorax in severely traumatized patients. *J Trauma.* 2001;51:677–682.
10. Livingston DH, Hauser CJ. Trauma to the chest wall and lung. In: Moore EE, Feliciano DV, Mattox KL, eds. *Trauma.* New York: McGraw-Hill; 2004:507–538.
11. Kirkpatrick AW, Sirois M, Laupland KB, et al. Hand-held thoracic sonography for detecting post-traumatic pneumothoraces: the Extended Focused Assessment with Sonography for Trauma (EFAST). *J Trauma.* 2004;57:288–295.
12. Marinaro JL, Kenny CV, Smith SR, et al. Needle thoracostomy in trauma patients: what catheter length is adequate? *Acad Emerg Med.* 2003;10:495.
13. Eastridge BJ, Salinas J, McManus JG, et al. Hypotension begins at 110 mm Hg: redefining "hypotension" with data. *J Trauma.* 2007;63:291–299.
14. Borgman MA, Spinella PC, Perkins JG, et al. The ratio of blood products transfused affects mortality in patients receiving massive transfusions at a combat support hospital. *J Trauma.* 2007;63:805–813.
15. Holcomb JB, Wade CE, Michalek JE, et al. Increased plasma and platelet to red blood cell ratios improves outcome in 466 massively transfused civilian trauma patients. *Ann Surg.* 2008;248:447–458.
16. Holcomb JB, del Junco DJ, Fox EE, and the PROMMTT study group. The prospective, observational, multicenter, major trauma transfusion (PROMMTT) study: comparative effectiveness of a time-varying treatment with competing risks. *JAMA Surg.* 2013;148:127–136.
17. Bickell WH, Wall MJ, Pepe PE, et al. Immediate versus delayed fluid resuscitation for hypotensive patients with penetrating torso injuries. *N Engl J Med.* 1994;331:1105–1109.
18. Robinson BR, Cotton BA, Pritts TA, and the PROMMTT study group. Application of the Berlin definition in PROMMTT patients: the impact of resuscitation on the incidence of hypoxemia. *J Trauma Acute Care Surg.* 2013;75(suppl 1):S61–S67.
19. Stafford RE, Linn J, Washington L. Incidence and management of occult hemothoraces. *Am J Surg.* 2006;192:722–726.
20. Kwon A, Sorrells DL, Kurkchubasche AG, et al. Isolated computed tomography diagnosis of pulmonary contusion does not correlate with increased morbidity. *J Pediatr Surg.* 2006;41:78–82.
21. Velmahos GC, Demetriades D, Chan L, et al. Predicting the need for thoracoscopic evacuation of residual hemothorax: chest radiograph is insufficient. *J Trauma.* 1999;46:65–70.

22. Rozycki GS, Feliciano DV, Schmidt JA, et al. The role of ultrasound in patients with possible penetrating cardiac wounds: a prospective multicenter study. *J Trauma*. 1999;46:542–551.
23. McCarter FD, Luchette FA, Molloy M, et al. Institutional and individual learning curves for focused abdominal ultrasound for trauma: cumulative sum analysis. *Ann Surg*. 2000;231:689–700.
24. Fulton RL, Peters ET. Compositional and histologic effects of fluid therapy following pulmonary contusion. *J Trauma*. 1974;14:783–790.
25. Fulton RL, Peters ET. The progressive nature of pulmonary contusion. *Surgery*. 1979;67:499–506.
26. Weiss RL, Brier JA, O'Conner W, et al. The usefulness of transesophageal echocardiography in diagnosing cardiac contusions. *Chest*. 1996;109:73–77.
27. Simon B, Ebert J, Bokhari F, et al; Eastern Association of the Surgery of Trauma. Management of pulmonary contusion and flail chest: an Eastern Association for the Surgery of Trauma practice. *J Trauma Acute Care Surg*. 2012;73(suppl 4):S351–S361.
28. Clancy K, Velopulos C, Bilaniuk JW, et al. Screening for blunt cardiac injury: an Eastern Association for the Surgery of Trauma practice management guideline. *J Trauma Acute Care Surg*. 2012;73 (suppl 4):S301–S306.
29. Bertinchant JP, Polge A, Mohty D, et al. Evaluation of incidence, clinical significance, and prognostic value of circulating cardiac troponin I and T elevation in hemodynamically stable patients with suspected myocardial contusions after blunt chest trauma. *J Trauma*. 2000;48:924–931.
30. Williams JS, Graff JA, Uku JM, et al. Aortic injury in vehicular trauma. *Ann Thorac Surg*. 1994;57:727–730.
31. Demetriades D, Velmahos GC, Scalea TM, et al. Diagnosis and treatment of blunt thoracic aortic injuries: changing perspectives. *J Trauma*. 2008;64:1415–1418.
32. Wheat MW, Palmer RF, Bartley TD, et al. Treatment of dissecting aneurysm of the aorta without surgery. *J Thorac Cardiovasc Surg*. 1965;50:364–373.
33. Demetriades D, Velmahos GC, Scalea TM, et al. Operative repair or endovascular stent graft in blunt traumatic thoracic aortic injuries: results of an American Association for the Surgery of Trauma Multicenter Study. *J Trauma*. 2008;64:561–570.
34. Demetriades D, Murray JA. Traumatic diaphragmatic hernias. In: Fitzgibbons RJ, Greenburg AG, eds. *Nyhus and Condon's Hernia*. Philadelphia: Lippincott Williams & Wilkins; 2002:503–511.
35. Chen JC, Wilson SE. Diaphragmatic injuries: recognition and management in sixty-two patients. *Am Surg*. 1991;57:810–815.
36. Friese RS, Coln CE, Gentilello LM. Laparoscopy is sufficient to exclude occult diaphragm injury after penetrating abdominal trauma. *J Trauma*. 2005;58:789–792.
37. Powell BS, Magnotti LJ, Schroeppel TJ, et al. Diagnostic laparoscopy for the evaluation of occult diaphragmatic injury following penetrating thoracoabdominal trauma. *Injury*. 2008;39:530–534.
38. Scharff JR, Naunheim KS. Traumatic diaphragmatic injuries. *Thorac Surg Clin*. 2007;17:81–85.
39. Abbas G, Schuchert MJ, Pettiford BL, et al. Contemporaneous management of esophageal perforation. *Surgery*. 2009;146:749–755.
40. Bulger EM, Arneson MA, Mock CN, et al. Rib fractures in the elderly. *J Trauma*. 2000;48:1040–1046.
41. Bergeron E, Lavoie A, Clas D, et al. Elderly trauma patients with rib fractures are at greater risk of death and pneumonia. *J Trauma*. 2003;54:478–485.
42. Desai P. Pain management and pulmonary dysfunction. *Crit Care Clin*. 1999;15:151–166.
43. White PE. Use of patient-controlled analgesia for management of acute pain. *JAMA*. 1988;259:243–247.
44. Barr J, Fraser GL, Puntillo K, et al. Clinical practice guidelines for the management of pain, agitation, and delirium in adult patients in the intensive care unit. *Crit Care Med*. 2013;41:263–306.
45. Moon MR, Luchette FA, Gibson SW, et al. Prospective, randomized comparison of epidural versus parenteral opioid analgesia in thoracic trauma. *Ann Surg*. 1999;229:684–691.
46. Haenel JB, Moore FA, Moore EE, et al. Extrapleural bupivacaine for amelioration of multiple rib fracture pain. *J Trauma*. 1995;38:22–27.
47. Allen MS, Halgren L, Nichols FC III, et al. A randomized controlled trial of bupivacaine through intracostal catheters for pain management after thoracotomy. *Ann Thorac Surg*. 2009;88:903–910.
48. Fildes J. Head trauma. In: American College of Surgeons Committee on Trauma. *Advanced Trauma Life Support for Doctors: Student Manual*. 8th ed. Chicago: American College of Surgeons; 2008:131–151.
49. Martin NA, Doberstein C, Zane C, et al. Posttraumatic cerebral arterial spasm: transcranial doppler ultrasound, cerebral blood flow, and angiographic findings. *J Neurosurg*. 1992;77:575–583.
50. Chestnut RM, Marshall LF, Klauber MR, et al. The role of secondary brain injury in determining outcome from severe head injury. *J Trauma*. 1993;34:216–222.
51. Murray GD, Butcher I, McHugh GS, et al. Multivariable prognostic analysis in traumatic brain injury: result from the IMPACT study. *J Neurotrauma*. 2007;24:329–337.
52. Jones PA, Andrews PJD, Midgely S, et al. Measuring the burden of secondary insults in head injured patients during intensive care. *J Neurosurg Anesthesiol*. 1994;6:4–14.
53. Raichle ME, Plum F. Hyperventilation and cerebral blood flow. *Stroke*. 1972;3:566–575.
54. Muizelaar JP, Marmarou A, Ward JD, et al. Adverse effects of prolonged hyperventilation in patients with severe head injury: a randomized clinical trial. *J Neurosurg*. 1991;75:731–739.
55. Fernandez-Perez ER, Sprung J, et al. Intraoperative ventilator settings and acute lung injury after elective surgery: a nested case control study. *Thorax*. 2009;64:121–127.
56. Licker M, Diaper J, Villiger Y, et al. Impact of intraoperative lung-protective interventions in patients undergoing lung cancer surgery. *Crit Care*. 2009;13:R41.
57. Lellouche F, Dionne S, Simard S, et al. High tidal volumes in mechanically ventilated patients increase organ dysfunction after cardiac surgery. *Anesthesiology*. 2012;116:1072–1082.
58. Chaiwat O, Vavilala MS, Philip S, et al. Intraoperative adherence to a low tidal volume ventilation strategy in critically ill patients with preexisting acute lung injury. *J Crit Care*. 2011;26:144–149.
59. Hess DR, Kondili D, Burns E, et al. A 5-year observational study of lung-protective ventilation in the operating room: a single-center experience. *J Crit Care*. 2013;533:e9–e15.
60. Severgnini P, Selmo G, Lanza C, et al. Protective mechanical ventilation during general anesthesia for open abdominal surgery improves postoperative pulmonary function. *Anesthesiology*. 2013;118:1307–1321.
61. Futier E, Constantin JM, Paugam-Burtz C, et al. A trial of intraoperative low-tidal-volume ventilation in abdominal surgery. *N Engl J Med*. 2013;369:428–437.
62. Brueckmann B, Villa-Uribe JL, Bateman BT, et al. Development and validation of a score for prediction of postoperative respiratory complications. *Anesthesiology*. 2013;118:1276–1285.
63. Bratton SL, Chestnut RM, Ghajar J, et al. Guidelines for the management of severe traumatic brain injury. XIV. Hyperventilation. *J Neurotrauma*. 2007;24(suppl 1):S87–S90.
64. Vassar MJ, Fischer RP, O'Brian PE, et al. A multicenter trial for resuscitation of injured patients with 7.5% sodium chloride. The effect of added dextran 70. The Multicenter Group for the Study of Hypertonic Saline in Trauma Patients. *Arch Surg*. 1993;128:1003–1011.
65. Stiell IG, Wells GA, Vandemheen K, et al. The Canadian CT head rule for patients with minor head injury. *Lancet*. 2001;357:1391–1396.
66. Bratton SL, Chestnut RM, Ghajar J, et al. Guidelines for the management of severe traumatic brain injury. II. Hyperosmolar therapy. *J Neurotrauma*. 2007;24(suppl 1):S14–S20.
67. Stiefel MF, Spiotta A, Gracias VH, et al. Reduced mortality rate in patients with severe traumatic brain injury treated with brain tissue oxygen monitoring. *J Neurosurg*. 2005;103:805–811.
68. Narotam PK, Morrison JF, Nathoo N. Brain tissue oxygen monitoring in traumatic brain injury and major trauma: outcome analysis of a brain tissue oxygen-directed therapy. *J Neurosurg*. 2009;111:672–682.

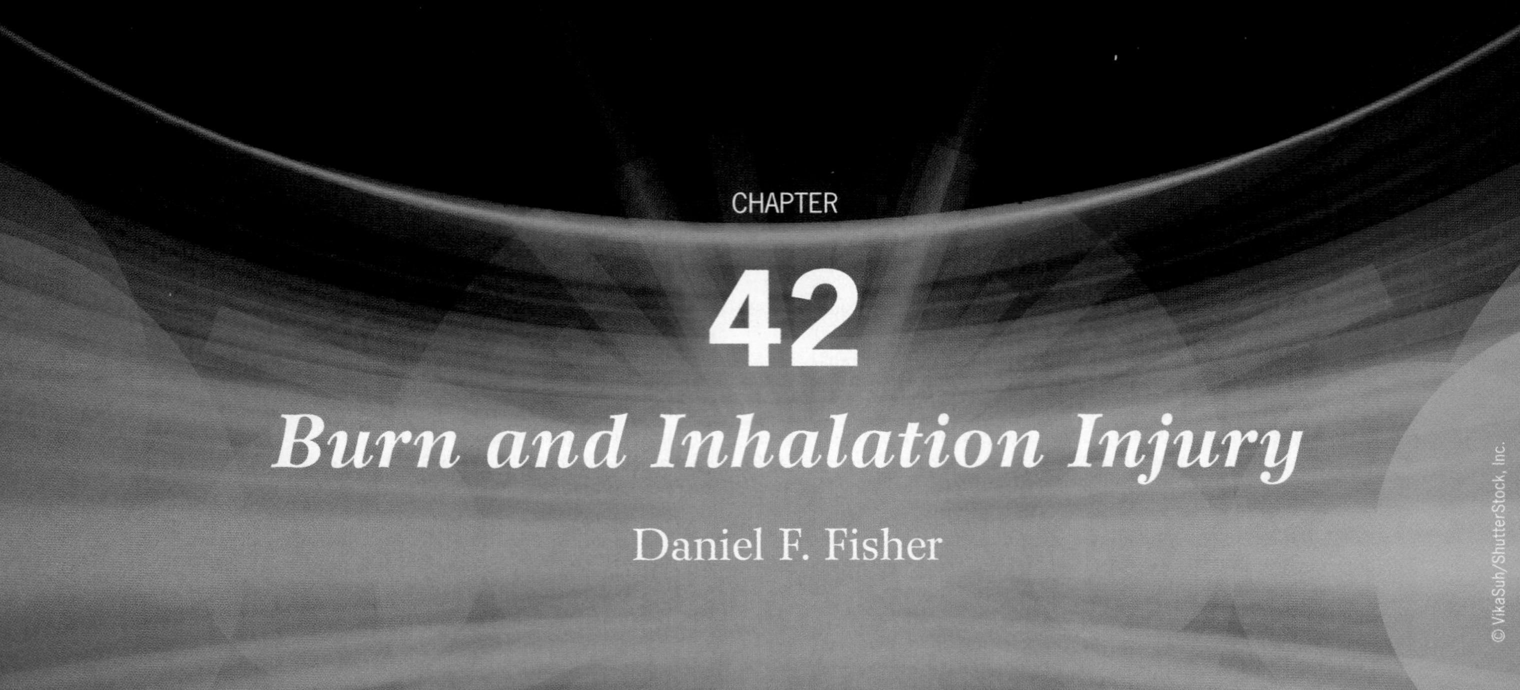

CHAPTER

42
Burn and Inhalation Injury

Daniel F. Fisher

OUTLINE

OBJECTIVES

1. Describe the four phases of burn management.
2. Use the Lund-Browder chart to evaluate the extent of a burn injury.
3. Compare first-, second-, third-, and fourth-degree burns.
4. Discuss issues related to fluid resuscitation of patients with a burn injury.
5. Describe the effect of circumferential burn wounds of the torso on ventilatory function.
6. Discuss issues related to cutaneous heat and water loss in patients with a burn injury.
7. Discuss the physiology of inhalation injury.
8. Describe the diagnosis of inhalation injury.
9. List five predictable events in patients with inhalation injury.
10. Describe the management of upper airway obstruction, bronchospasm, small airway obstruction, pulmonary infection, and respiratory failure in patients with an inhalation injury.
11. Describe the treatment of patients with carboxyhemoglobinemia.

KEY TERMS

allograft
apoptosis
burn shock
carboxyhemoglobin (HbCO)
carboxymyoglobin (MbCO)
CO-oximetry
eschar
escharotomy
fluid resuscitation
full-thickness graft
hyperbaric oxygen (HBO) therapy
inhalation injury
meshing
split-thickness graft
total body surface area (TBSA)
xenograft

Introduction

The term *burn* refers to injuries resulting from the denaturing and destruction of tissue proteins and bone caused by thermal, electrical, or chemical origin. A major burn is defined as an injury involving 20% or more of the **total body surface area (TBSA)**.[1] The quality of life and the outcome for major burn patients have improved dramatically over the past 20 years.[2–4] This change first began with a realization that the natural history of burns can be influenced by prompt surgery; the early removal of **eschar** and rapid biologic closure of the resulting open wounds prevents the otherwise inevitable development of burn wound sepsis. To support a patient with a serious burn injury and associated respiratory failure through the physiologically taxing trial of staged wound closure is not a simple undertaking. Patients who experience a major burn injury have a better outcome when cared for at a specialty burn center staffed with experienced personnel.[5]

Burn Injury

Phases of Burn Care

The function of the skin is to maintain normothermia, protect from infection, and maintain fluid balance within the body. Any injury that damages this organ has an impact on these three factors. Patients with large burns typically have a deep, painful wound that puts them at risk for sepsis and progressive multi-organ dysfunction from the break in skin integrity. Immediate clinical needs must be met, but an organized, overall plan of care must also be created. The initial evaluation of the burn patient should follow the recommendations established by the advanced trauma life support

TABLE 42-1
Four Phases of Burn Care

Phase	Timing	Treatment Objectives
Initial evaluation and resuscitation	First 72 hours	To achieve accurate fluid resuscitation and perform a thorough evaluation
Initial wound excision and biologic closure	Days 1 through 7	To identify and remove all full-thickness wounds and obtain biologic closure
Definitive wound closure	Day 7 through week 6	To replace temporary covers with definitive ones and close small, complex wounds
Rehabilitation, reconstruction, and reintegration	Entire hospitalization and postdischarge.	Initially to maintain range of motion and reduce edema; subsequently to strengthen and prepare patients for return to community

(ATLS) guidelines.[2,6,7] Burn injuries have the potential to distract the caregiver from other injuries; therefore, careful attention needs to be paid to ensure that a complete examination is performed. The patient must be screened for other injuries and comorbid conditions.[1,2,6] This organized plan of care can be described as four phases of care (**Table 42-1**).[8]

Initial Evaluation and Resuscitation of the Burn

The first phase, the initial evaluation and resuscitation, extends from day 1 (day of injury) through day 3. During this phase of care, the crucial events are to determine the size and extent of the injury, as well as provide replacement intravascular volume. Both of these assessments can have a profound effect on the remaining course of the injury. Providing adequate replacement **fluid resuscitation** for the prevention and treatment of **burn shock** has been recognized as the most important factor in treating patients with burn injury.[9–11] Burn shock refers to the multi-organ dysfunction caused by both hypovolemia as well as the systemic release of inflammatory mediators from the wound. Untreated, burn shock is the major cause of morbidity and mortality in the burn patient.[7,12]

Determining the size of the wound with respect to the total surface area of the body has proven to be a daunting task because of variation in practitioner experience as well as inherent calculation errors specific to each method used. The loss of skin integrity provides a conduit for insensible fluid loss through the patient. The rate of fluid lost through the burn wound is predictable based upon previous physiologic observations. The amount of fluid needed to replace the volume lost is a function of burn size, time, and overall body surface area. One of the more common resuscitation formulas is the Parkland Formula, which calculates fluid requirement as:

$$\text{Fluid required} = 4 \text{ mL} \times \%\text{TBSA} \times \text{Weight (kg)}$$

The first half of total fluid is given during the first 8 hours post burn. The remainder is given over the next 16 hours, titrating to urine output.[13,14]

Burned tissue has a dry, leathery appearance and does not easily allow for tissue expansion. If the eschar is circumferential to a limb or the trunk of the body, it can act as a tourniquet, severely restricting blood flow. Circumferential eschar around the thoracic region can make breathing difficult. In this situation, the burn surgeon will cut through the eschar (**escharotomy**) (**Figure 42-1**),

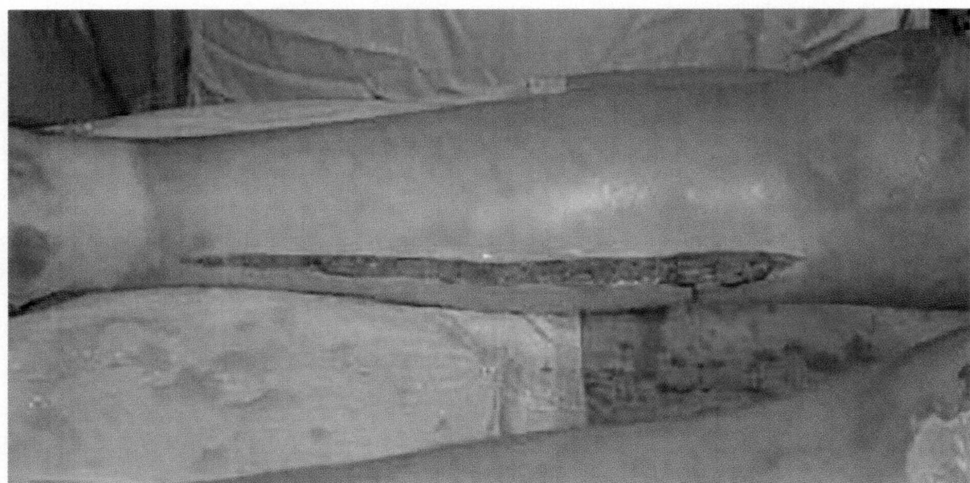

FIGURE 42-1 Escharotomy of the leg with a circumferential deep dermal burn.

Reproduced from Hettiaratchy S, Papini R. Initial management of a major burn: II—assessment and resuscitation. *Brit Med J.* 2004;329:101–103, with permission from BMJ Publishing Group Ltd.

which allows for tissue expansion and ultimately improves perfusion.

Burn Coverage

Wound coverage for burns varies depending upon the severity of the injury. First-degree burns require a dry, sterile dressing while more severe full-thickness second- and third-degree burns may require excision of the damaged tissue and coverage of the area by skin grafting. There are other kinds of dressings as well. Some dressings are impregnated with silver ions (Ag^{++}) because silver has antimicrobial properties; these are applied topically to prevent infection. Other dressing materials are combinations of biologically based and a non-biologic substrate (Alloderm, Biobrane, and Integra). These products have cultured cells from either human or animal (bovine, porcine) origin usually on a silicone backing. These products are used to provide temporary coverage when there is insufficient donor skin available to cover the wound area as well as to prepare the wound bed for subsequent grafting. A common goal for using biologic dressings is to reduce scarring when compared with the non-biologically based dressings.

Types of Grafts

Allografts are skin grafts where the skin being used comes from the patient being treated. The tissue forming the allograft originated from the patient him- or herself and will not pose any rejection of foreign tissue. Sometimes the area needing coverage is larger than the size of the graft; the surgeon will expand the coverage area of the graft by **meshing**. This term refers to passing the graft through a device that creates a matrix of small holes in the tissue, allowing it to be stretched. The holes in the meshed graft help with fluid drainage and decrease hematoma formation, allowing for a healthier graft.

Xenografts refer to skin that is from a donor (usually cadaver). This donated skin is usually stored frozen and only thawed when needed. Another source of xenograft skin is from animals, most typically porcine skin. Regardless of the source of the xenograft, these are temporary coverings that are used to protect the patient from infection and also to prepare the wound bed for healing.

Grafts can be classified as either **split-thickness** or **full-thickness**. Split-thickness grafts have a layer of dermis while full-thickness grafts contain all of the components of the skin: epidermis, dermis, nerve endings, and even hair follicles.[15] Full-thickness grafts are attributed with less scar formation and are thus reserved when function or aesthetics (eyelids, face) are important.[15]

Wound Excision and Biologic Closure

The second phase, initial wound excision and biologic closure, extends from day 1 through day 7. During this phase, the surgery is performed that changes the natural history of the injury. Typically, this period involves a series of staged operations to excise and debride the wound and place temporary covering over the denuded areas. The damaged or dead tissue needs to be removed (escharectomy). Otherwise, it poses an infection risk as well as having an impact on acid–base and electrolytes.

Definitive Wound Closure

The third phase, definitive wound closure, lasts from day 7 through week 6. It involves replacement of temporary wound covers with a definitive cover, as well as closure and acute reconstruction of burns that have a small surface area but are highly complex, such as wounds on the face and hands.

The success of graft healing depends upon the nutritional status of the patient. If patients are not being given adequate nutrition to meet their caloric requirements, they will go into a catabolic state, which has a detrimental impact on graft and donor site healing. If a graft does not adhere to the wound and survive—graft take—then it will need to be treated as a wound with removal of the dead tissue.

Reconstruction, Rehabilitation, and Reintegration

The final stage involves rehabilitation, reconstruction, and reintegration. Although this final stage actually begins during the resuscitation period, it becomes very involved and time consuming toward the end of the acute hospital stay. Because this is an ongoing process, the psychological health of the burn patient is crucial for a successful rehabilitation. Issues that need to be addressed are impaired function, altered body image, and retraining/reconditioning. Still considered investigational, limb (arm, hand), and facial transplantation have been used in the most severe cases where the underlying tissue was destroyed beyond any functionality requiring surgical removal.[16] These procedures are being developed to restore function where a limb has been lost or extreme facial damage has occurred.

Support groups exist for burn survivors. These groups are an important measure in the phase of recovery and rehabilitation as much as surgical intervention. One of these groups, the Phoenix Society for Burn Survivors (http://www.phoenix-society.org) provides peer support for newly burned patients as well as survivors of burn injury. Peer support has been helpful in reintegrating burn survivors into society.

Estimating Burn Size

An extensive cutaneous burn wound has a profound influence on pulmonary function, and accurate evaluation of the wound is important. The process of calculating burn size and depth is the first, crucial step in assessment. This task can prove to be difficult even for an experienced burn surgeon because the burn wound is a dynamic injury and will alter based on both extrinsic and intrinsic factors, such as thrombosis of dermal blood vessels, amount of resultant edema, release of inflammatory mediators, and initial treatment of the wound.[1,15,17,18]

Burns should be evaluated for extent, depth, and circumferential components (**Box 42-1**). It is critical to have an accurate estimate of total body surface area involvement to determine the course and aggressiveness of the resuscitative efforts. Estimation of the involved body surface area involvement in a burn wound is one of the more difficult, yet crucial, tasks to be performed during the assessment of the injury. Various methods to determine body surface area have been developed and introduced over the past 200 years of widely varying complexity. These range from paper templates used to cover the wound, mathematical formulae, estimation based upon the proportion a section of the body is to the total surface area, computer models using digitized photographs, and small measuring devices intended to standardize the measuring area.[19]

The extent of the burn injury is best estimated with a Lund-Browder chart, which is a two-dimensional drawing of both the anterior and posterior surfaces of a generalized body. The Lund-Browder chart accounts for variance in body proportions with growth (**Figure 42-2**). It has recently been noted that most Lund-Browder charts actually total up to 101% because demarcation of the body as described in the original text did not exactly coincide with the drawing and this discrepancy has been carried on throughout the years.[20] Alternative methods for determining burn size are the Wallace Rule of Nines, the palmar method, as well a myriad of computer programs and smartphone applications.[18,21–23] Even with all of the development in this area, there has yet to be a single technique that can be considered as the gold standard.

The Wallace Rule of Nines divides the body into sections representing 9% or multiples thereof to estimate body surface area. This technique is a rapid method of estimating burn surface area and is frequently used by first responders, but the Rule of Nines has a tendency to overestimate the extent of the burn, which has led to excessive fluid resuscitation.[2,9,24,25] The Rule of Nines also does not account for changes in body proportion with age and weight.[26] For example, an infant's head has significantly more surface area in proportion to the body than an adult's head, but they both account for the same area when using this technique.

The palmar method (Rule of Palms) uses only the palmar surface of the patient's hand (without fingers). The assumption for this method is that the palmar surface represents approximately 1% of the body surface area. Realistically, recent data suggest that the palmar area is closer to 0.7% of TBSA.[27] This difference in surface area has a 30% bias.

Most methods used for estimating TBSA make the common assumption of normal body habitus. With morbidly obese patients (BMI >31), the affected BSA is even less. Work has been done to incorporate various body types and shapes into different models using a Lund-Browder type of chart.[26,28,29]

Some of the benefits of these programs are that the computed TBSA involvement is reproducible and can be obtained quickly even by clinicians who may have limited burn experience, and the injury maps can be sent along with the patient when he or she is transferred to a regional burn center. The initial injury thus is also better documented for evaluation by the burn surgeon. Serial measurements can also aid the burn surgeon in observing the progress in wound healing.

BOX 42-1

Evaluation of the Burn Wound

Extent

Lund-Browder chart: An age-specific chart that accounts for changes in body proportions. This is the preferred method used to determine the extent of a burn injury.

Wallace rule of nines: A rough method of estimation that assumes adult body proportions. The head and neck are roughly 9%; the anterior and posterior chest are 9% each; the anterior and posterior abdomen (including buttocks) are 9% each; each upper extremity is 9%; each thigh is 9%; each leg and foot is 9%; and the genitals are 1%.

Palmar surface of the hand: The palmar surface of a person's hand (without the fingers) is approximately 1% of the body surface over all age groups.

Computer Programs/Smartphone applications: These systems are typically based upon either the Lund Browder chart, or the Rule of Nines and calculate involvement based on either photographs or drawings by the user.

Depth

First degree: Red, dry, painful wounds that often are deeper than they appear; sloughing occurs the next day.

Second degree: Red, wet, very painful wounds. Their depth, ability to heal, and propensity to form hypertrophic scars vary immensely.

Third degree: Leathery, dry, insensate, waxy wounds that do not heal.

Fourth degree: Wounds that involve underlying subcutaneous tissue, tendon, or bone.

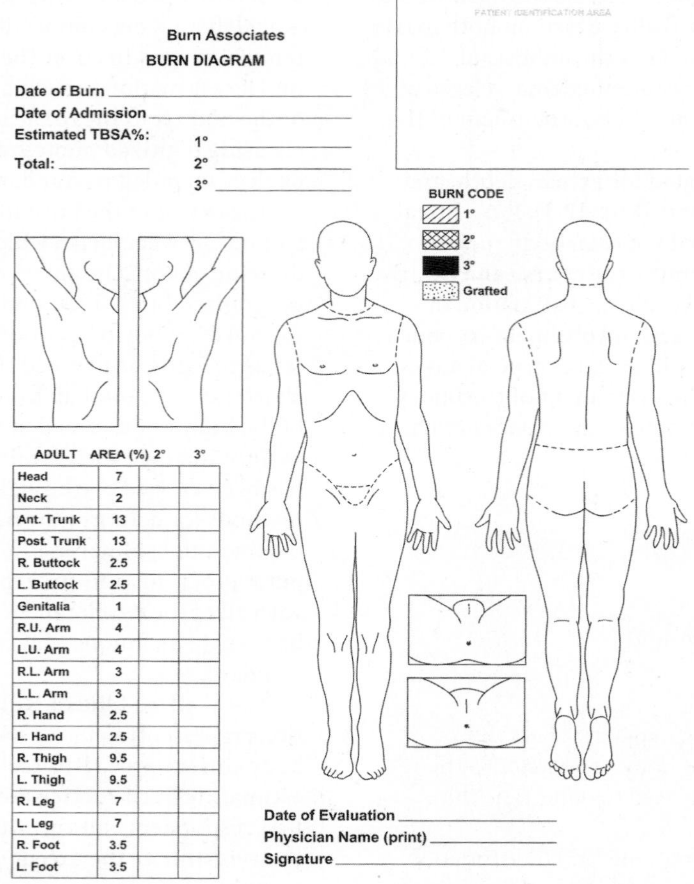

PATIENT IDENTIFICATION AREA

Burn Associates

BURN DIAGRAM

Date of Burn ____________

Date of Admission ____________

Estimated TBSA%: 1° ____________

Total: ________ 2° ____________

3° ____________

BURN CODE

1°

2°

3°

Grafted

ADULT	AREA (%)	2°	3°
Head	7		
Neck	2		
Ant. Trunk	13		
Post. Trunk	13		
R. Buttock	2.5		
L. Buttock	2.5		
Genitalia	1		
R.U. Arm	4		
L.U. Arm	4		
R.L. Arm	3		
L.L. Arm	3		
R. Hand	2.5		
L. Hand	2.5		
R. Thigh	9.5		
L. Thigh	9.5		
R. Leg	7		
L. Leg	7		
R. Foot	3.5		
L. Foot	3.5		

Date of Evaluation ____________

Physician Name (print) ____________

Signature ____________

FIGURE 42-2 Lund-Browder chart for estimating body surface area involvement.

A more direct need for having accurate burn maps is for determining the fluid requirements for the patient based on the severity of the injury. Inaccurate estimates can lead to improper fluid resuscitation.[30] Providing too little fluid during the initial resuscitation can lead to organ system failure. Too much fluid will contribute to systemic edema, which decreases peripheral circulation, leading to collateral tissue injury.[24,25]

Burns are classified as first, second, third, or fourth degree (**Figure 42-3**). In addition, they are classified by the depth of the injury, ranging from superficial to full thickness and finally to deep dermal.[31] It can be difficult for even an experienced examiner to accurately determine the depth of a burn early on. As a general rule, depth usually is underestimated on the initial examination.[17,31,32]

An understanding of the physiologic aberrations that occur with serious burns allows clinicians to provide respiratory care in the burn unit. Successfully resuscitated burn patients manifest a sequence of predictable physiologic changes (**Table 42-2**). These changes can be anticipated, which aids in patient management.

Inhalation Injury

Inhalation injury is a generalized term describing damage to the lungs and upper airway by the inspiration of either superheated gases (temperatures greater than 150° C), steam, or noxious products of incomplete combustion. Inhalation injury also refers to the damage resulting from breathing irritant substances such as chlorine gas, hydrogen sulfide, smoke, or direct aspiration of petrochemicals. Although frequently paired with thermal injury, inhalation injury is more commonly the result from chemical interactions between foreign substances with the lung tissue rather than thermal injury. Despite advances in burn care as well as postinjury resuscitation, inhalation injury remains a critical determinant in burn outcome.[33] Early consequences of inhalation injury include increased alveolar permeability, acute pulmonary edema, and an accumulation of both pro- and anti-inflammatory cytokines that occur with acute respiratory distress syndrome (ARDS).[34,35] Tissue damage resulting from inhalation injury can have an adverse effect on both gas exchange and hemodynamics.[36]

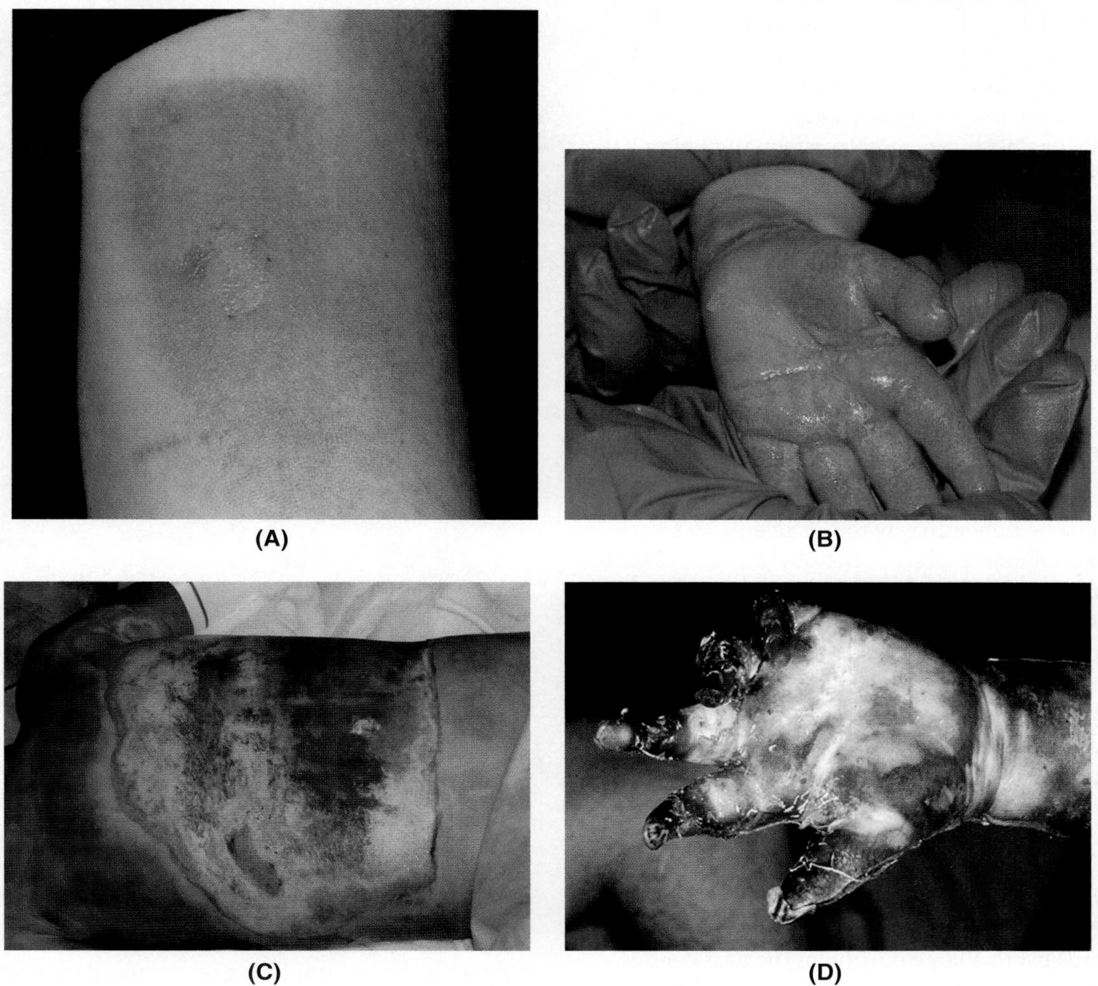

FIGURE 42-3 Various degrees of burn severity. (**A**) First degree. (**B**) Second degree. (**C**) Third degree. (**D**) Fourth degree.

TABLE 42-2
Predictable Physiologic Changes in Burn Patients

Time Frame	Change	Treatment Steps
Resuscitation period (days 0 to 3)	Massive capillary leakage	Fluid resuscitation
Post-resuscitation period (day 3 to 95% definitive wound closure)	Hyperdynamic and catabolic state with high risk of infection	Early wound closure to prevent sepsis (nutritional support is essential)
Recovery period (95% definitive wound closure to 1 year after injury)	Continuing catabolic state and risk of nonwound sepsis	Nutritional support essential; complications anticipated and treated

The severity of inhalation injury varies widely and cannot be predicted during the initial evaluation because of the poor correlation between diagnostic criteria and severity of injury as well as the delayed onset of symptoms. Inhalational injury coupled with thermal injury has a profound effect on mortality: the mortality rate for a person who sustains an inhalation injury with a major burn doubles when compared with the mortality rate predicted based on age and burn size alone.[9]

Inhalational injuries can be divided into the following different phases based on varying pathology and treatment requirements: exudative, degenerative, proliferative, and reparative.[37] It is important to note the surrounding environment and conditions where the injury occurred. Factors to note are whether the exposure took place within an enclosed space, the ventilation of gases in the area, and whether the injury was caused by thermal or chemical exposure as well as the duration of exposure. Although there is no specific treatment for inhalation injury, supportive, lung-protective strategies exist for acute lung injury and can be used in management of the injury. Management involves providing the support required compensating for decrements in gas exchange while the injured endobronchial and alveolar mucosa regenerate.

Smoke inhalation is the most common form of inhalation injury. The components of smoke are determined by the burning material and the availability of oxygen where the fire has taken place. Smoke inhalation injury has been reported to affect anywhere from 5% to 35% of hospitalized burn patients.[9,35,37,38] The concentration of smoke inspired depends on the confines of the space where the fire is occurring as well as the duration of exposure. The larynx is one of the most affected organs in thermal inhalation injury, thus resulting in upper airway dysfunction later in the healing process.[39]

Physiology of Inhalation Injury

An inhalation injury can involve the entire respiratory system, from the upper airway to the alveoli, to a variable and unpredictable degree. The physical and chemical properties, such as water solubility and chemical reactivity, of the inspired irritants are important to understand and may provide insight on how to treat the injury. Water-soluble gases will dissolve into the mucous layer of the upper airway. Gases and other particulates can form concentration gradients throughout the upper and lower airways.[40]

The pathophysiology of inhalational injury with subsequent smoke inhalation can be divided into two subcategories: upper airway involvement and lower airway involvement.[37] The structures of the upper airway, tongue, and oropharynx, including the larynx, act as a heat sink and absorb a large portion of the heat energy, confining the burns to the upper airway. Smoke and the irritating gases that are inspired along with the heated air can trigger bronchospasm and result in inflammation of the lung parenchyma, releasing histamines and cytokines.[36,37] The major airways are denuded of their normal mucosal layer, which impairs the ciliary transport mechanism until resurfacing occurs.[33,41] The smaller airways become obstructed with sloughed endobronchial debris and accumulated secretions (**Figure 42-4**).

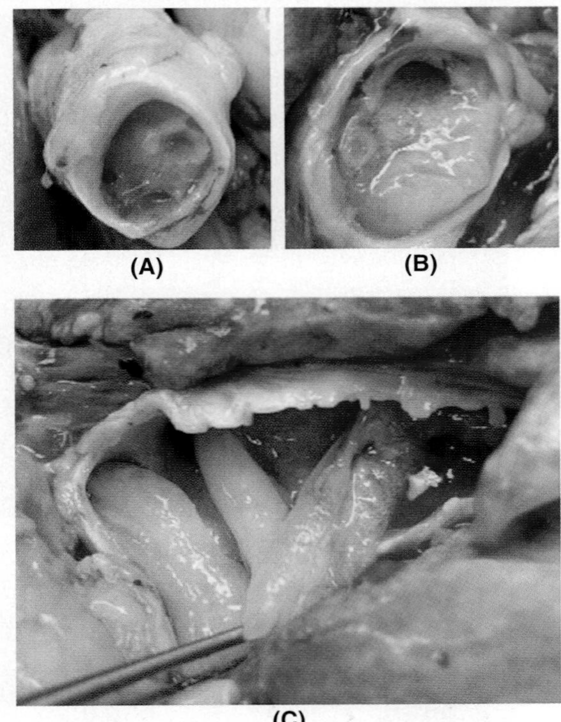

FIGURE 42-4 Macroscopic picture of airway obstructive cast 48 hours after cutaneous burn and smoke inhalation in a sheep. (**A**) Trachea. (**B**) Bronchi. (**C**) Smaller bronchi.

Reproduced from Enkhbaatar P, Cox R, Traber L, et al. Aerosolized anticoagulants ameliorate acute lung.... *Crit Care Med.* 2007;35:2805–2810. Reprinted with permission from Wolters Kluwer Health.

The morbidity of severe burns is increased when accompanied by smoke inhalation because of the stimulation of the inflammatory response and loss of small airway patency.[31] The release of inflammatory mediators contributes to the worsening pulmonary status, ultimately resulting in ARDS. Animal models, specifically ovine, demonstrate that it is this systemic inflammatory response that triggers an increase in cell death (**apoptosis**).[31] Debris from sloughing of the dead cells as well as the hypersecretion of mucous glands contributes to the small airway occlusion. During the initial phase of the injury, superheated gas and liquid burn the upper airway, with resultant mucosal edema and airway obstruction presenting in later stages, which explains why the severity of an inhalational injury can be misleading during the primary evaluation of the patient.

With the mucociliary transport system disrupted, along with the accumulation of cellular debris within the small airways, inhalation injury promotes changes in the lung that favor pneumonia.[42] Pneumonia and tracheobronchitis frequently occur in partially obstructed lung units. The alveolar epithelium is disrupted by toxic products released by the burning of synthetic products, resulting in alveolar flooding.[36–38,43] The clinically important sequelae include loss of airway patency secondary to mucosal edema, bronchospasm, intrapulmonary shunting from small airway occlusion, diminished compliance secondary to alveolar flooding and collapse, pneumonia secondary to loss of ciliary clearance, and respiratory failure secondary to a combination of the previously stated factors.

Diagnosis of Inhalation Injury

Inhalation injury can occur with or without concurrent thermal injury, although it is frequently associated with burns. The process of diagnosing an inhalation injury is difficult in itself because of the lack of a standard definition of what constitutes an inhalation injury, variable inclusion criteria, and the absence of generally accepted and applied methods for quantifying inhalation injury.[44] Diagnosing inhalation injury is difficult because of the pattern of heat distribution along the airway in thermal injury and also chemical reactivity and water solubility of the inspired agent(s).[37] The diagnosis of inhalation injury has traditionally been made by the history and conditions where the burn occurred; enclosed space, elevated HbCO, and soot around the nose and/or mouth as well as bronchoscopic findings.

Numerous proposals have been made to develop an approach to improve the diagnosis and determination of the severity of an inhalation injury.[9,34–36] The abbreviated injury score is one such approach that stratifies the severity of the inhalation injury. Other scoring systems may add a fixed value to the final score if an inhalation injury is present.[45–47] Some patients who have an inhalation injury will present with an initial $Pa{O_2}/F{IO_2}$ that is relatively benign. It is only after the initial resuscitation and the redistribution of fluids within the tissue that there may be a significant change in the $Pa{O_2}/F{IO_2}$. The $Pa{O_2}/F{IO_2}$ does not correlate well with the severity of inhalation injury or outcome.[35] Acute changes could be a reflection of changing lung compliance and airway resistance. It has even been suggested that much of the morbidity/mortality associated with inhalation injury is actually due to ventilator-induced lung injury (VILI).[48]

Inhalation injury should be suspected if there is evidence of carbonaceous material surrounding the nose and mouth, if the fire was in a closed area, and if there is singed skin or nasal hairs. A limited number of tests have been proposed including inflammatory mediators, $Pa{O_2}/F{IO_2}$ and CT scans to aid in the diagnosis of inhalation injury, but they are either inconclusive or not readily available.[34,49,50]

Current methods of diagnosing inhalation injury include history, physical examination, chest radiograph, bronchoscopy, the $Pa{O_2}/F{IO_2}$ and radioisotope scanning (if available). Because there are no specific preemptive therapies for inhalation injury and because current diagnostic measures only loosely predict the degree of subsequent pulmonary dysfunction, diagnostic tests are used only for general evaluation and prognosis. The underlying difficulty with diagnosis is that, much like a cutaneous burn, inhalation injuries evolve over time and involve the entire respiratory system to a variable degree. Another difficulty with diagnosing and grading inhalation injury is the lack of consensus and validated grading systems for inhalation injury.[33] For these reasons, patients at risk for this diagnosis generally are classified as having or not having sustained inhalation injury, with no effort made to quantify the degree of injury.

The circumstances surrounding the burn can provide clues to the burn surgeon as to whether an inhalation injury has occurred. Burns sustained in a closed space or aspiration of hot steam or liquid are pertinent points of the history. Physical findings suggesting the diagnosis include carbonaceous debris in the mouth or sputum, singed nasal hairs, and facial burns. The chest radiograph generally is normal initially, which is consistent with the evolution of these injuries over time.

In addition to bronchoscopy, invasive measures sometimes used include radioisotope scanning and determination of the serum HbCO level. Although logistically more complicated in young children, most clinicians use bronchoscopy as the gold standard for diagnosis of inhalation injury. Bronchoscopic findings include carbonaceous endobronchial debris and mucosal pallor and ulceration (**Figure 42-5**). One study has suggested that inflammatory mediators found in pulmonary secretions can be used to score the extent and severity of the inhalation injury.[51] Two of the findings of this study were surprising: early rise of a specific mediator actually was a positive sign for a positive outcome, and the severity of the injury did not correlate with the level of the cytokines. This system remains to be validated in a large population study.

Two types of radioisotope imaging have been used to diagnose inhalation injury: intravenous administration of technetium-99 or inhalation of xenon-133. Normal lungs rapidly clear both radioisotopes, and asymmetric or delayed clearance is consistent with the diagnosis of inhalation injury, which could indicate an increase

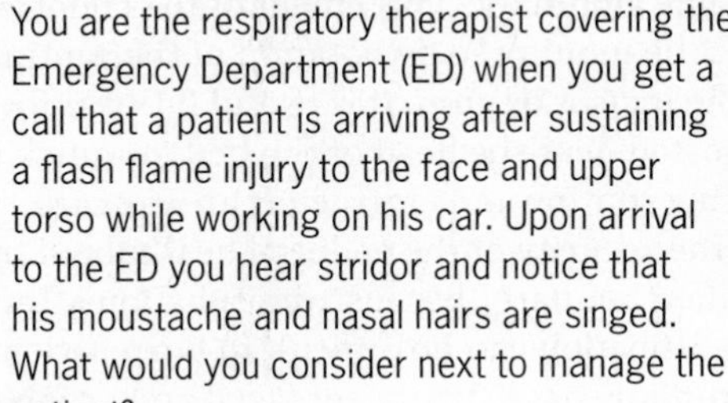

STOP AND THINK

You are the respiratory therapist covering the Emergency Department (ED) when you get a call that a patient is arriving after sustaining a flash flame injury to the face and upper torso while working on his car. Upon arrival to the ED you hear stridor and notice that his moustache and nasal hairs are singed. What would you consider next to manage the patient?

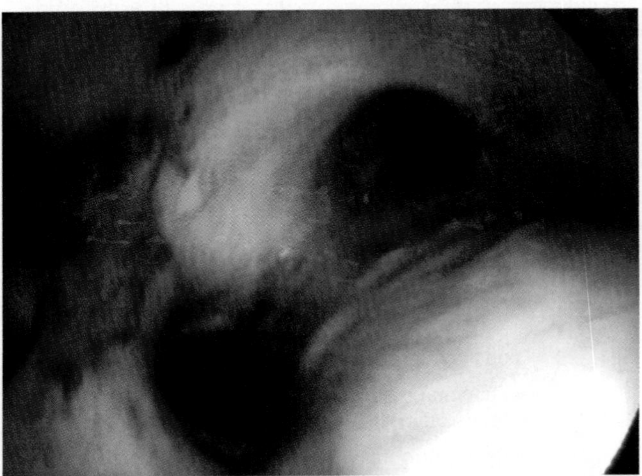

FIGURE 42-5 Bronchoscopic image of airway after sustaining inhalation injury. Note the carbonaceous buildup and inflammation of the airway wall.

in physiologic dead space (V_D). Although physiologically sound, xenon and technetium scanning have not been widely used because of their logistic difficulty and expense.

In small clinical series, tracheobronchial cytologic studies and biopsy have been reported to facilitate the diagnosis of inhalation injury, but these techniques have not been widely used because of logistic difficulties and potential complications. Work continues to identify biologic markers for grading the severity of inhalation injury.[49]

Management of Inhalation Injury

When a diagnosis of inhalation injury is suspected or confirmed, management is supportive only. Treatment of inhalation injury can be broken down into several main categories: ventilator management, pharmacologic treatment to aid pulmonary function using aerosolized medications, early tracheostomy, and using evidence-based medicine to optimize patient outcomes.[35] There are no prophylactic or preemptive therapies for inhalation injury. There is no clear-cut value in using prophylactic antibiotics, and there is evidence to show that such use would promote selection of antibiotic-resistant strains colonizing the airway.[52] Although many patients demonstrate reactive bronchospasm and benefit from early institution of nebulized β_2-agonists, steroids are infrequently required to treat acute bronchospasm. The practice of nebulizing heparin alone or with *N*-acetylcysteine has been studied as a means to prevent or lessen the effects of small airway obstruction resulting from the sloughing of epithelial cells, excessive mucus production, and the formation of fibrin casts in a sheep model.[41,53] This practice has been undertaken by several burn centers, but the supporting evidence is anecdotal and small sample sizes prevent definitive conclusions.[35,38,41,53] It is important, however, to maintain high humidity within the ventilator circuit to prevent a humidity deficit of the airways that results in the desiccation of the secretions of the distal airways. Good pulmonary hygiene is crucial.[54]

Lung-protective strategies should be used in the ventilator management of these patients. The use of a low-tidal-volume (VT) approach similar to the ARDSnet protocol is an acceptable method of managing these patients because it keeps ventilating pressures low, which would otherwise add to the already sustained lung injury.[55,56] Other practices to consider are permissive hypercapnia and prone positioning.[55,57,58]

In patients with inhalation injury, five predictable events occur that have important clinical implications and require intervention: acute upper airway obstruction, bronchospasm, small airway obstruction, infection, and respiratory failure.

Respiratory Recap

Management of Inhalation Injury

- Upper airway obstruction should be bypassed with endotracheal intubation or a tracheostomy; careful attention must be given to the endotracheal tube's position and patency.
- Bronchospasm should be treated with inhaled bronchodilators.
- Adequate humidification of the airway needs to be provided to lessen the chances of secretion desiccation.
- Pulmonary infection should be managed with a focus on organisms identified by sputum culture.
- Respiratory failure is managed with positive end-expiratory pressure and low tidal volumes to avoid alveolar overdistention and subsequent ventilator-induced lung injury.

Acute Upper Airway Obstruction

During inhalation injury, airway obstruction caused by mucosal edema evolves over time (usually within the first 4 to 24 hours after injury) and ideally is anticipated and managed with intubation.[38] Early intubation for airway protection should be considered in the patient with suspected inhalation injury. Intubation attempts of these often difficult airways can be approached in a studied manner if the impending obstruction is anticipated. After resuscitation has occurred, edema of the upper airway can change the anatomic structures from a relatively easy intubation to a difficult airway requiring a well-experienced anesthesiologist or even a surgical airway. Failure to recognize impending airway obstruction can result in serious morbidity and even mortality in burn patients. Clinicians should be alert in cases involving hot liquid aspiration, which can lead to sudden loss of airway patency and late sequelae of upper airway burns.[8,9,35,43,59] The critical importance of initial airway evaluation and proper control cannot be overemphasized, and this need continues throughout the period of intubation.

Oral endotracheal tubes are often used because they are easy to place and are subjectively more comfortable for the patient than nasal endotracheal tubes. Tubes should be secured in a manner that allows room for stabilization and easy adjustment as facial edema changes, but not for gross movement of the airway that might risk unintended extubation. Because the lips are not reliable landmarks, placement of the endotracheal tube must be monitored by notation of the centimeter mark at the incisor or gum. It is useful if this information is posted near the head of the bed for quick reference during routine and emergency airway care.

The security of the endotracheal tube should be verified regularly, because reintubation after accidental extubation can be difficult in burn patients, who commonly have significant facial and oropharyngeal edema. Clinicians who care for these patients should be equipped to deal with sudden airway emergencies and have the appropriate equipment on hand for managing a difficult, unstable airway. Maintenance of endotracheal tubes in burn patients is complicated by shifts in extravascular volume. The method used to secure the tube should facilitate simple loosening and tightening as needed to provide for adjustments coinciding with changes in facial edema. A unique concern with airway securing techniques in burns is for a method that can function in a high relative humidity, heated environment. When facial burns are present, adhesive tape is seldom useful. Cloth ties can be effectively used to secure tubes.[60]

Another aspect of airway care should be maintaining adequate pressure in the cuff of the airway to prevent or at least minimize leakage and aspiration of trapped material from the oropharynx into the lungs. Elevating the head of the bed, if physiologically possible, at a 30-degree supine angle will also help minimize silent aspiration and potential ventilator-associated pneumonia (VAP).[54] By following these interventions, the VAP can be decreased, as this is a population where pulmonary involvements can double the morbidity of the underlying injury.[36,61]

The proper indication and optimum timing for tracheostomy in the burn patient remains the subject of debate. The consensus is that adult burn patients in whom protracted intubation is expected are candidates for tracheostomy, ideally after anterior neck burns have been addressed.

Bronchospasm

Intense bronchospasm from aerosolized irritants is common during the first 24 to 48 hours after injury, especially in young children. This condition is well managed with inhaled β_2-agonists in most patients, although some require low-dose epinephrine infusions or parenteral or inhaled steroids. One option is heliox if the oxygen requirement is minimal. Use of continuous nebulization of high-dose β_2-agonists is another option. Recent evidence, however, has pointed to increased mortality when patients with ARDS are routinely treated with β_2-agonists.[62,63]

Ventilator management strategy for patients with burns and/or inhalation injury is not significantly different from those for any other critically ill patient needing respiratory support. Some points of emphasis specific to burn and inhalation injury patients should be emphasized, such as monitoring airway pressures, lung compliance and resistance, and good pulmonary hygiene techniques.

Thoracic escharotomies may be required to provide adequate chest excursion, allowing the patient to breathe more freely. Until this is done, airway pressures may need to be high in order to overcome the decreased compliance of the chest wall. Techniques used to minimize auto-PEEP, such as using short inspiratory times and high inspiratory flows, as well as attempting to match the auto-PEEP with applied PEEP, often may be necessary, but if air trapping is severe, some degree of carbon dioxide retention is acceptable. Monitoring of plateau airway pressure (Pplat) and mean airway pressure should be performed to assess the patient's gas exchange and transport status.[55,56]

STOP AND THINK

While caring for a mechanically ventilated patient who has sustained 45% TBSA burn, you notice that her oxygenation has been falling over the past few hours and her urine output has decreased. What could be the cause of this and how would you adjust the ventilator?

AGE-SPECIFIC ANGLE

Intense bronchospasm caused by aerosolized irritants is a particular problem in children because of their smaller airways.

Small Airway Obstruction

During the first 24 hours after inhalation injury, airway obstruction is essentially limited to the bronchial airways. Major components of this obstructive material are mucus from extensive glandular secretion, inflammatory cells, fibrin, and exfoliated epithelial cells.[38] As necrotic endobronchial debris sloughs, pulmonary hygiene often becomes increasingly difficult. An aggressive program of pulmonary hygiene, including suctioning and bronchoscopy, is an important component of care. Along with aggressive airway clearance, it is important to provide adequate humidification of inspired gases. Therapeutic bronchoscopy can facilitate clearance of the airways and evaluation of the condition of the airway mucosa. Small endotracheal tubes can suddenly become occluded; staff members should be prepared to respond promptly (**Box 42-2**). Pulmonary hygiene is an essential component of the management of patients with inhalation injury. It is crucial to provide 100% relative humidity to these patients and decrease the potential for creating a humidity deficit that might lead to thickened pulmonary secretions and increase the chances of occluding the endotracheal tube.

The use of mucolytic agents in treating small airway obstruction has been shown not to be as effective as was once believed. The main components of bronchial and small airway casts are fibrin and cellular debris. Use of mucolytic agents has not been shown to be effective in either clinical practice or animal models.[54]

BOX 42-2

Evaluation and Initial Management of Deterioration of the Patient–Ventilator System

A sudden deterioration of the patient–ventilator unit requires immediate assessment for any of four problems: mechanical malfunction, obstruction of the artificial airway, displacement of the endotracheal tube from the trachea or into the main stem bronchus, or pneumothorax.

1. Assess the patient and observe the patient's inspiratory efforts (if any) and compare them with the cycling of the ventilator. Auscultate breath sounds:
   a. If wheezing, provide β_2-agonists.
   b. If coarse, suction the airway.
   c. If the breath sounds are unilaterally decreased, consider a main stem intubation or pneumothorax.
   d. If the breath sounds are absent bilaterally, consider an occluded artificial airway.
2. Observe the monitors.
   a. Is the patient hemodynamically stable?
   b. Check the Spo_2 and provide maximal inspired oxygen. In an emergency, oxygen buys time.
3. Check the ventilator.
   a. Determine which alarms are being triggered. Knowing this is helpful in troubleshooting mechanical problems.
   b. Check the ventilator waveforms; look at the flow–time curve to determine whether the patient is receiving adequate flow or whether the inspiratory time is either too long or too short.
   c. Are the parameters set on the ventilator correct for the patient's needs? If the patient was initially paralyzed and is now able to move and spontaneously trigger the ventilator, it is possible that changes will need to be made.
   d. Is the ventilator functioning as expected? If not, remove the patient from the ventilator, manually ventilate, and exchange with another ventilator.
4. If unable to quickly assess and correct the problem, it may be necessary to disconnect the patient from the ventilator and provide manual breaths with a bag-valve device while troubleshooting the problem. Remember, for patients who require high levels of positive end-expiratory pressure (PEEP), alveolar de-recruitment will occur if the patient is manually ventilated without PEEP.
5. If unable to manually ventilate, the tube may be severely occluded, and extubation followed by mask ventilation may be required.
6. In the event a new airway cannot be passed into the trachea, a surgical airway (cricothyroidotomy, tracheostomy) may be required.

Pulmonary Infection

Pulmonary infection develops in 30% to 50% of patients with an inhalation injury. Pneumonia without the presence of inhalation injury increases the mortality of burn injury up to 40%.[64] It frequently is difficult to distinguish between pneumonia and tracheobronchitis (purulent infection of the denuded tracheobronchial tree), but the difference often has little practical clinical importance. Infection typically occurs toward the end of the first postinjury week; patients with serious inhalation injuries often are seen to deteriorate at this time. A patient with newly purulent sputum, fever, and perhaps diminished gas exchange should be treated with antibiotics, which should be adjusted as necessary after sputum culture information has been obtained. To repeat an important point: the physiology of inhalation injury, which involves injury to endobronchial mucosa with hampered mucociliary clearance, makes good pulmonary hygiene a particularly important component of management.

Respiratory Failure

Respiratory failure is common in individuals with inhalation injury. Respiratory failure among these patients is caused as often by sepsis as by inhalation injury. As in other forms of respiratory failure, the lung volume that can be recruited with mechanical ventilation is limited, and overvigorous attempts to force high pressures into these lungs exacerbate the underlying injury. These patients do well with a volume-targeted, pressure-limited ventilation strategy (**Box 42-3**). If this approach fails, innovative methods of support should be considered, such as extracorporeal membrane oxygenation or inhaled nitric oxide. Prone positioning also has been shown to improve oxygenation. With adequate personnel, the patient can be quickly and safely repositioned

BOX 42-3

Therapeutic Responses to Progressive Respiratory Failure

Address bronchospasm with nebulized β_2-agonist agents.

Address poor chest wall compliance that occurs secondary to overlying eschar with escharotomies.

Ensure ventilator synchrony with adequate opiate and benzodiazepine infusions. Neuromuscular blockade occasionally may be required.

Reset end point of ventilation to a physiologic pH (7.2 or higher). Allow gradual onset of hypercapnia as long as the patient does not have a head injury.

Reset end point of oxygenation to an arterial saturation of at least 88%, typically associated with an arterial oxygen content of 55 mm Hg or higher.

Optimize inflating pressures.

Utilize a lung-protective, low-tidal-volume approach to ventilation. Follow ARDSnet guidelines for adjusting tidal volumes based on ideal body weight for the patient.

Keep plateau pressure (Pplat) below 30 cm H_2O.

Choose optimum positive end-expiratory pressure (PEEP).

Choose optimum mean airway pressure. Lengthen inspiratory time to a target mean airway pressure of 20 to 25 cm H_2O, as long as auto-PEEP is not detectable.

If these measures are inadequate, consider the use of adjuncts such as inhaled nitric oxide or extracorporeal support.

while special attention is given to maintenance of the airway and central lines.[58]

The use of a specific ventilator mode or ventilator often accompanies the discussion of inhalation injury. Some of these modes include high-frequency oscillatory ventilation (HFOV), volume diffusive respiration (VDR), and airway pressure release ventilation (APRV). Each of these ventilation techniques has the common goal of maintaining alveolar recruitment and gas exchange. Both HFOV and VDR require special-purpose ventilators. HFOV has recently been evaluated in several large randomized controlled studies, which have shown either no difference or a negative impact on outcome.[65,66]

VDR is pressure-controlled ventilation with superimposed subtidal oscillations that facilitates clearance of endobronchial debris. Although some data have been encouraging, burn patients with inhalation injury and respiratory failure can be very well managed with any other mode of ventilation with which the center is comfortable, paying particular attention to tidal volume, airway pressure, and aggressive pulmonary hygiene.[9,35,37,64]

Ventilator discontinuation and extubation of burn patients follow the general guidelines applicable to other patients. This patient group has some unique aspects that must be taken into consideration (Box 42-4). Of particular importance is the balance of the pain medication needs of patients with large wounds and donor sites with the need for an alert sensorium for extubation. There is evidence of benefit from combined spontaneous breathing trials along with routine periodic sedation discontinuation in order to assess mental status.[67,68]

Carbon Monoxide Exposure

Many patients injured in structural fires inhale carbon monoxide (CO), and many are obtunded from a combination of CO, anoxia, and hypotension. CO poisoning results in more than 50,000 Emergency Department (ED) visits annually in the United States alone.[69,70] Carbon monoxide is produced from incomplete combustion or combustion in a low-oxygen atmosphere. CO binds avidly to heme-containing enzymes, particularly hemoglobin and the cytochrome proteins, which

BOX 42-4

Important Considerations in Ventilator Discontinuation and Extubation of a Patient with a Burn Injury

Sensorium: The patient must be awake and alert enough to protect the airway.

Airway patency: Upper airway edema must be resolved to the extent that an air leak is audible around the endotracheal tube (with the cuff deflated if the tube is cuffed) at a moderate inflating pressure (20 to 30 cm H_2O).

Muscle strength: Strength must be adequate for ventilation. An indirect measure of this is an unassisted tidal volume of 6 to 10 mL/kg and a maximum inspiratory pressure (PI_{max}) less than −20 cm H_2O.

Compliance: Combined chest wall and lung compliance must be high enough that work of spontaneous breathing is not excessive. Respiratory system compliance should be at least 50 mL/cm H_2O.

Gas exchange: The PaO_2/FIO_2 should be greater than 200 mm Hg.

Spontaneous breathing trial (SBT): The successful completion of an SBT.

inhibits cellular respiration.[21,42,43] CO also binds to myoglobin, forming **carboxymyoglobin (MbCO)**, with heart muscle taking up about three times as much CO as skeletal muscle.[71] The formation of **carboxyhemoglobin (HbCO)** results in an acute physiologic anemia, much like an isovolemic hemodilution. A HbCO concentration of 50% is physiologically similar to an isovolemic hemodilution to 50% of a baseline hemoglobin level. Moreover, CO causes a leftward shift of the oxyhemoglobin dissociation curve, which decreases oxygen release to the tissue. The routine occurrence of unconsciousness at this HbCO level therefore makes it clear that other mechanisms are involved in the pathophysiology of CO injury. It is likely that CO binding to the cytochrome system in the mitochondria, which interferes with oxygen utilization, is more toxic than CO binding to hemoglobin. Many patients with severe CO exposure also have been exposed to cyanide compounds, which are released from burning synthetics. The degree of exposure rarely is such that specific treatment is required.

For unknown reasons, 5% to 25% of patients with serious CO exposure have been reported to develop delayed major neurologic sequelae.[42,43] These patients can be managed with 100% isobaric oxygen or with **hyperbaric oxygen (HBO) therapy**. The half-life of HbCO is about 5 hours breathing 21% oxygen at ambient pressure, about 74 minutes breathing 100% oxygen at ambient pressure (range 26–148 min), and less than 30 minutes breathing 100% oxygen at 3 atm. If serious exposure has occurred and is manifested by overt neurologic impairment or a high HbCO level, HBO is reasonable if it can be safely administered. There is some evidence that neurologic impairment with CO poisoning can be delayed and the effects can be long term.[72,73] With inhalation injury, 100% oxygen should be administered until a safe HbCO level is reached. MbCO has a slower dissociation than HbCO, which can account for a rebound of HbCO several hours after receiving normobaric oxygen.[71]

With inhalation injury the HbCO level should be measured with **CO-oximetry**. In the presence of HbCO, traditional pulse oximetry is unreliable and potentially misleading. Two-wavelength pulse oximetry does not measure HbCO. The pulse oximeter displays high O_2 saturation (Spo_2) despite significant HbCO, misleading the clinician into believing that HbCO is not present. New generation multiple wavelength pulse oximeters allow noninvasive measurement of HbCO. These portable, noninvasive devices can be part of Emergency Medical Services crew equipment providing HbCO measurements closer to the time of exposure. Because HbCO does not affect gas exchange in the lungs, a patient with HbCO who is breathing 100% oxygen may have a very high Pao_2 (more than 400 mm Hg) despite low hemoglobin oxygen saturation as measured by CO-oximetry. The high Pao_2 competes with CO for hemoglobin binding sites, resulting in eventual displacement of CO from the hemoglobin. It is best to use HbCO measurements taken close to the time of exposure. HbCO measurements taken at the hospital can be less because treatment with normobaric oxygen may have already started prior to arrival.[71]

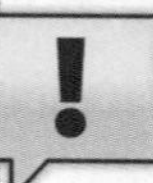

Respiratory Recap

Carboxyhemoglobinemia

- Measure carboxyhemoglobin (HbCO) with CO-oximetry.
- Administer 100% oxygen.
- Consider hyperbaric oxygen therapy, particularly in patients with neurologic depression or delayed neurologic sequelae.

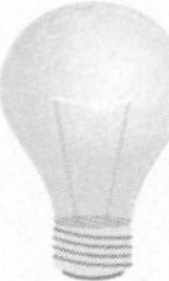

STOP AND THINK

You are working in a hospital that does not have an HBO chamber. A patient presents with CO poisoning. What therapy would you recommend?

HBO has been proposed as a means to improve the prognosis of those who suffer serious CO exposure, but its use remains controversial. On a busy burn service the question of which patient to treat in the hyperbaric chamber commonly arises. Most patients who undergo hyperbaric oxygen therapy are treated in a monoplace hyperbaric chamber (**Figure 42-6**). Treatment regimens

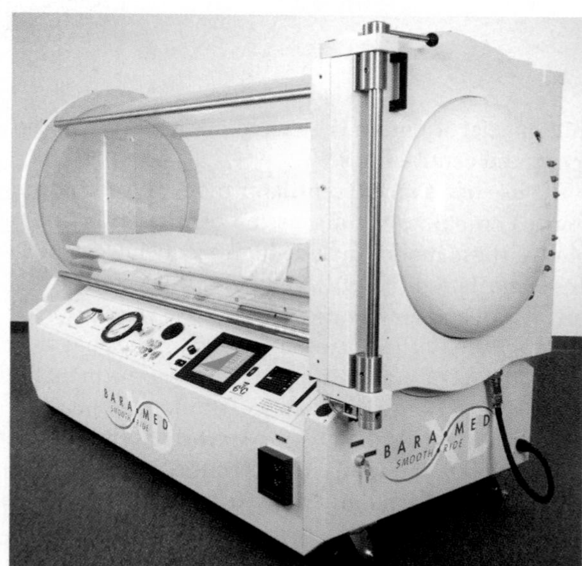

FIGURE 42-6 Monoplace hyperbaric chamber.
Courtesy of ETC BioMedical Systems Group.

vary, but a typical CO poisoning protocol is 3 atm for the first treatment and then 2 atm or 3 atm for subsequent treatments, for 90 minutes, with two 10-minute air breaks to reduce the incidence of oxygen toxicity seizures. Providing HBO to a patient in a monoplace chamber severely limits access to the patient during treatment, so patients in unstable condition are poor candidates. Other relative contraindications are wheezing and air trapping, which increase the risk of pneumothorax, and high fever, which increases the risk of hyperoxia-induced seizures, which are also known as the Paul Bert effect.[74]

If a patient must be mechanically ventilated during HBO, adequate preparation measures before the chamber door is closed can prevent most complications. Prior to the patient's being placed into the chamber, the airway must be well positioned and adequately stabilized because patients who inadvertently awaken during the therapy may attempt self-extubation. For the same reason, patients must be well restrained before HBO regardless of their mental status. The endotracheal tube cuff must be converted from air-filled and refilled with an appropriate volume of sterile water; this conversion prevents collapse of the cuff during the compression phase of the treatment. They must be evaluated for bronchospasm and aggressively treated with bronchodilators just before treatment. Suctioning of both the lower respiratory tract and the oral pharynx is helpful because this cannot be done while the patient is in the hyperbaric chamber. Prophylactic myringotomies are recommended for unconscious or intubated patients to prevent tympanic membrane rupture.

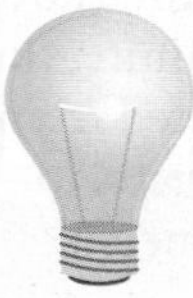

STOP AND THINK

You are caring for a mechanically ventilated patient in HBO. The patient begins to cough, causing the ventilator to pressure limit. The chamber is pressurized to 3 atmospheres absolute and cannot be opened for 2 minutes. What can you do?

Providing mechanical breathing support at hyperbaric pressures can be a technically difficult task. Some considerations that need to be considered are patient and practitioner safety, the type of chamber being utilized (monoplace vs. multiplace), physiologic monitoring needs, as well as sedation requirements. The design of monoplace chambers prevents immediate response in the event of a medical emergency. Multiplace chambers typically have a clinical attendant in the chamber to respond to a crisis.

Ventilators used with monoplace HBO chambers are usually modified versions of a pressure-limited, time-cycled device, although there is a limited choice for commercially available HBO-capable ventilators (**Figure 42-7**).[75,76] A base rate is maintained, but all spontaneous breathing efforts are unassisted. Patients who suddenly awaken during therapy and who cough or inspire vigorously can aspirate oral secretions, leading to an increase in airway pressure and a reduction in tidal volume. These same clinical signs occur with other clinical complications, such as a kinked

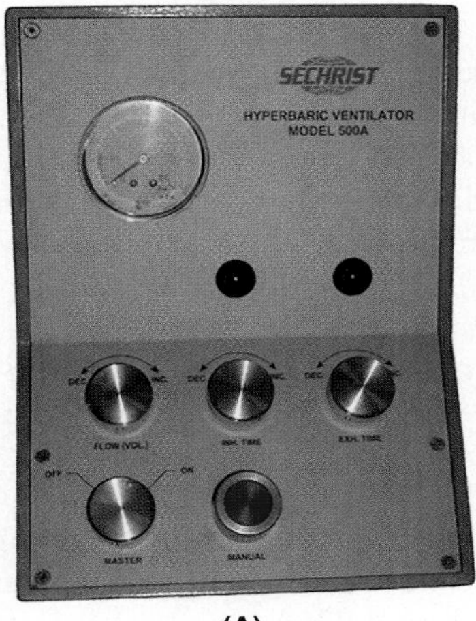

(A)

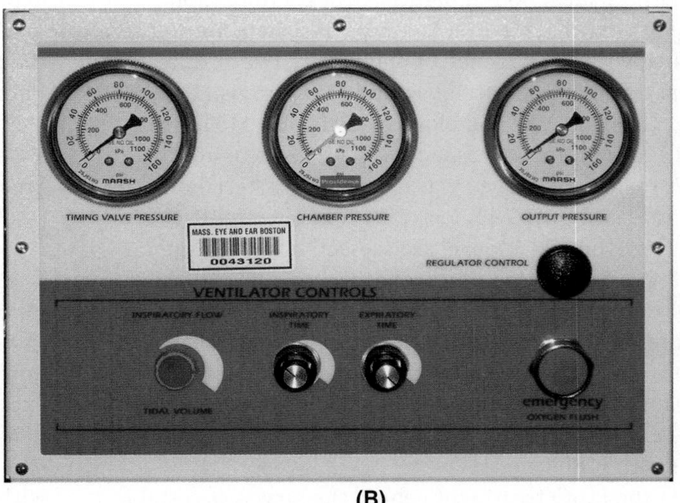

(B)

FIGURE 42-7 Two commercially available hyperbaric-capable ventilators (**A**) Sechrist 500A. (**B**) Providence Global Medical Atlantis.
(**A**) courtesy of Sechrist Industries.

endotracheal tube, main stem intubation, pneumothorax, or bronchospasm. Assessment and ascertaining the cause are difficult because the clinician is isolated from the patient. It may be best, if clinically appropriate, to adequately sedate the patient and avoid spontaneous breathing during the course of treatment.

Hydrogen Cyanide Poisoning

Although carbon monoxide poisoning is the more common condition to treat with inhalation injury, hydrogen cyanide (HCN) poisoning can be present and can result in similar problems with cellular respiration. HCN is produced by the combustion of nitrogen-containing compounds (such as those found in synthetic materials used in furniture) in a low-oxygen atmosphere. Like CO, HCN binds to the cytochrome oxidase system and inhibits cellular metabolism, resulting in tissue and systemic acidosis.[37] The treatments available for HCN poisoning do have risks, and often care may be supportive.[37]

Case Studies

Case 1. Minor Burn with Smoke Inhalation

A 5-foot 10-inch, 47-year-old man was found unconscious on a smoldering mattress with minor burns to the right arm, chest, and thigh. Respirations are shallow and erratic, pulse is 110 beats/min, blood pressure is 140/90 mm Hg, and there is no apparent cyanosis. The patient cannot be aroused and is orally intubated at the scene. He is manually ventilated at an F_{IO_2} of 1.0 and transported to the emergency department.

On admission, the patient is mechanically ventilated with continuous mandatory ventilation, pressure control at 20 cm H_2O, inspiratory time of 1 second, respiratory rate of 12 breaths/min, PEEP of 5 cm H_2O, and F_{IO_2} of 1.0. The tidal volume is approximately 500 mL (≈7 mL/kg ideal body weight). A chest radiograph reveals that the endotracheal tube is 3.5 cm above the carina, with no evidence of pneumothorax or other chest trauma. The patient's pupils are sluggish but reactive. The heart rate and blood pressure are 110 beats/min and 140/90 mm Hg, respectively. The Sp_{O_2} is 100%.

A toxicology screen was drawn. The arterial blood gas values are pH 7.45, Pa_{CO_2} 34 mm Hg, and Pa_{O_2} 360 mm Hg. The HbCO level as assessed by CO-oximetry is 38%. Auscultation of the chest reveals mild diffuse bronchospasm, which resolves with administration of albuterol (six puffs via metered dose inhaler [MDI]). There is no evidence of air trapping or auto-PEEP. Because of the patient's depressed level of consciousness and elevated CO level, the decision is made to treat him with HBO.

At the HBO treatment center, the airway is restabilized, the patient's oropharynx and endotracheal tube are suctioned, and an additional four puffs of albuterol via MDI are delivered. The endotracheal cuff is deflated and refilled with the same volume of sterile water to prevent collapse of the cuff during HBO therapy. Bilateral myringotomies are performed to avoid inadvertent rupture of the eardrums. All intravenous fluids and medications are transferred to specialized infusion pumps designed to operate within the HBO chamber. The patient is connected to a specialized HBO mechanical ventilator at the following settings: V_T 500 mL, respiratory rate 12 breaths/min, F_{IO_2} 1.0, and PEEP 0 cm H_2O. The patient is placed in the HBO monochamber, and the chamber is pressurized to 3 atmospheres absolute. After approximately 15 minutes at this pressure, the V_T becomes erratic, and the peak inspiratory pressure increases by 15 cm H_2O. The patient becomes progressively more awake and attempts to remove the endotracheal tube. Initial attempts to sedate fail, and anesthesia is induced with propofol. The patient is maintained with periodic boluses of propofol for the duration of the treatment, and there are no further complications.

After the HBO treatment, the patient is admitted to the burn intensive care unit, and all sedation is withdrawn. Assessment of ventilatory mechanics and level of consciousness demonstrate intact ventilatory function and responsiveness to commands. The patient is extubated, observed for 12 hours, transferred to a non-ICU floor, and subsequently discharged.

Case 2. Second- and Third-Degree Burns (70% TBSA) with Severe Inhalation Injury

A 5-foot 6-inch, 67-year-old unconscious woman is rescued from a kitchen fire with severe burns over much of her body. Assessment at the scene found significant facial burns and carbonaceous debris in the upper airway. Respiratory rate is 46 breaths/min and labored. The patient is orally intubated, manually ventilated with 100% oxygen, and transported to the emergency department.

On admission the heart rate is 135 beats/min and the blood pressure is 150/100 mm Hg. There is profound wheezing throughout all lung fields. The patient is mechanically ventilated with volume control and a V_T of 475 mL (8 mL/kg IBW), respiratory rate of 16 breaths/min, descending ramp flow pattern, peak inspiratory flow adjusted to provide an inspiratory time of 1 second (≈50 L/min), PEEP 5 cm H_2O, and F_{IO_2} 1. The arterial blood gas values with these settings are as follows: pH 7.35, Pa_{CO_2} 66 mm Hg, and Pa_{O_2} 82 mm Hg. The HbCO level is 27%. Ventilator graphics indicate flow present at end-exhalation and decreased peak expiratory flow. Total PEEP is 17 cm H_2O (12 cm H_2O of auto-PEEP). Pplat is 31 cm H_2O. Albuterol is administered via nebulizer continuously over the next hour with little effect on the total PEEP.

The ventilator is adjusted to address the significant amount of auto-PEEP by increasing the amount of applied PEEP to counterbalance auto-PEEP, and V_T is reduced to 415 mL (7 mL/kg IBW). The inspiratory time is kept at 1 second for synchrony. On reassessment the total PEEP is 6 cm H_2O. Although air trapping is reduced, the diffuse bronchospasm remains refractory to aggressive beta-agonist therapy. HBO therapy is performed due to the risk of barotrauma.

Over the next several days, the patient's arterial blood gas values deteriorate, requiring increases in PEEP to 18 cm H_2O and F_{IO_2} of 0.6 to 1. Air trapping continues to be a problem, and ventilator strategies are modified to include permissive hypercapnia. Bronchoscopy is performed several times to facilitate pulmonary hygiene, and it reveals significant airway injury and edema.

By the fifth day of hospitalization, the patient shows signs of sepsis (increased fever and labile blood pressure) and purulent sputum. Appropriate antibiotic therapy is instituted, and blood pressure is supported with vasopressors. Oxygenation worsens dramatically on day 6 despite various maneuvers to recruit lung volume. Blood pressure becomes progressively unstable and the patient has cardiopulmonary arrest. Cardiopulmonary resuscitation is performed but is unsuccessful.

Key Points

- Respiratory failure is a leading cause of morbidity and mortality in the burn unit.
- An organized plan of care for patients with burn injury has four phases: initial evaluation and resuscitation, initial wound excision and biologic closure, definitive wound closure, and rehabilitation.
- Burn wounds should be evaluated for extent, depth, and circumferential components.
- Adequate fluid resuscitation is vital during the first 24 hours after injury.
- Approximately 20% of burn injury patients suffer inhalation injury.
- Five predictable events occur in patients with inhalation injury: acute upper airway obstruction, bronchospasm, small airway obstruction, infection, and respiratory failure.
- All clinicians who care for burn patients should be prepared to deal with airway emergencies.
- Lung-protective ventilation strategies should be used for patients with inhalation and burn injury.
- Carboxyhemoglobin is treated with 100% oxygen or hyperbaric oxygen therapy, or both.

References

1. Hettiaratchy S, Papini R. Initial management of a major burn: I—overview. *Brit Med J*, 2004;328:1555–1557.
2. Pauldine R, Gibson BR, Gerold KB, Milner SM. Considerations in burn critical care. *Contemporary Critical Care.* 2008;6:1–11.
3. Namias N. Advances in burn care. *Curr Opin Crit Care.* 2007;13:405–410.
4. Meshulam-Derazon S, Nachumovsky S, Ad-El D, et al. Prediction of morbidity and mortality on admission to a burn unit. *Plast Reconstr Surg.* 2006;118:116–120.
5. Sheridan R, Barillo D, Herndon D, et al. Burn specialty teams. *J Burn Care Rehabil.* 2005;26:170–173.
6. Allison K, Porter K. Consensus on the prehospital approach to burns patient management. *Emerg Med.* 2004;21:112–114.
7. Pham TN, Cancio LC, Gibran NS. American Burn Association practice guidelines: burn shock resuscitation. *J Burn Care Res.* 2008;29:257–266.
8. Sheridan RL. Airway management and respiratory care of the burn patient. *Int Anesthesiol Clin.* 2000;38:129–145.
9. Endorf FW, Gamelli RL. Inhalation injury, pulmonary perturbations, and fluid resuscitation. *J Burn Care Res.* 2007;28:80–83.
10. Holm C, Melcer B, Hörbrand F, et al. Intrathoracic blood volume as an end point in resuscitation of the severely burned: an observational study of 24 patients. *J Trauma.* 2000;48:728–734.
11. Klein MB, Hayden D, Elson C, et al. The association between fluid administration and outcome following major burn. *Ann Surg.* 2007;245:622–628.
12. Holm C, Mayr M, Hörbrand F, et al. Reproducibility of transpulmonary thermodilution measurements in patients with burn shock and hypothermia. *J Burn Care Rehabil.* 2005;26:260–265.
13. Mitchell KB, Khalil E, Brennan A, et al. New management strategy for fluid resuscitation: quantifying volume in the first 48 hours after burn injury. *J Burn Care Res.* 2013;34:196–202.
14. Lindford AJ, Lim P, Klass B, et al. Resuscitation tables: a useful tool in calculating pre-burns unit fluid requirements. *Emerg Med J.* 2009;26:245–249.
15. Kagan RJ, Peck MD, Ahrenholz DH, et al. Surgical management of the burn wound and use of skin substitutes: an expert panel white paper. *J Burn Care Res.* 2013;34:e60–e79.
16. Arno A, Barret JP, Harrison RA, Jeschke MG. Face allotransplantation and burns. *J Burn Care Res.* 2012;33:561–576.
17. Hettiaratchy S, Papini R. Initial management of a major burn: II—assessment and resuscitation. *Brit Med J.* 2004;329:101–103.
18. Giretzlehner M, Dirnberger J, Owen R, et al. The determination of total burn surface area: how much difference? *Burns.* 2013;39:1107–1113.
19. Rickard RF, Martin NAJ, Lundy JB. Imprecision in TBSA calculation. *Burns.* 2014;40:172–173.
20. Lundin K, Alsbjørn B. The 101 percent in Lund-Browder charts—a commentary. *Burns* 2013;39:819–820.
21. Prieto MF, Acha B, Gomez-Cia T, et al. A system for 3D representation of burns and calculation of burnt skin area. *Burns.* 2011;37:1233–1240.
22. Godwin ZR, Bockhold JC, Webster L, et al. Development of novel smart device based application for serial wound imaging and management. *Burns.* 2013;39:1395–1402.
23. Lin SY, Chen CC, Mao HF, et al. The development and preliminary validation of the Taiwanese Manual Ability Measure for Burns. *Burns.* 2013;39:1250–1256.
24. Cartotto RC, Innes M, Musgrave MA, et al. How well does the Parkland Formula estimate actual fluid resuscitation volumes? *J Burn Care Rehabil.* 2002;23:258–265.
25. Saffle JR. The phenomenon of "fluid creep" in acute burn resuscitation. *J Burn Care Res.* 2007;28:382–395.
26. Williams RY, Wohlgemuth SD. Does the "Rule of Nines" apply to morbidly obese burn victims? *J Burn Care Res.* 2013;34:447–452.
27. Amirsheybani HR, Crecelius GM, Timothy NH, et al. The natural history of the growth of the hand: hand area as a percentage of body surface area. *Plast Reconstr Surg.* 2001;107:726–733.
28. Williams JF, King BT, Aden JK, et al. Comparison of traditional burn wound mapping with a computerized program. *J Burn Care Res.* 2013;34:e29–e35.
29. Yu CY, Lin CH, Yang YH. Human body surface area database and estimation formula. *Burns.* 2010;36:616–629.
30. Parvizi D, Kamolz LP, Giretzlehner M, et al. The potential impact of wrong TBSA estimations on fluid resuscitation in patients suffering from burns: things to keep in mind. *Burns.* 2014;40:241–245.
31. Papini R. Management of burn injuries of various depths. *Brit Med J.* 2004;329:158–160.

32. Benson A, Dickson WA, Boyce DE. Burns. *Brit Med J.* 2006;332:649–652.
33. Ikonomidis C, Lang F, Radu A, Berger MM. Standardizing the diagnosis of inhalation injury using a descriptive score based on mucosal injury criteria. *Burns.* 2012;38:513–519.
34. Kurzius-Spencer M, Foster K, Littau S, et al. Tracheobronchial markers of lung injury in smoke inhalation victims. *J Burn Care Res.* 2008;29:311–318.
35. Palmieri TL. Inhalation injury: research progress and needs. *J Burn Care Res.* 2007;28:549–554.
36. Brown DL, Archer SB, Greenhalgh DG, et al. Inhalation injury severity scoring system: a quantitative method. *J Burn Care Rehabil.* 1996;17:552–557.
37. Fraser JF, Mullany D, Traber D. Inhalational lung injury in patients with severe thermal burns. *Contemporary Crit Care.* 2007;4:1–12.
38. Cox RA, Mlcak RP, Chinkes DL, et al. Upper airway mucus deposition in lung tissue of burn trauma victims. *Shock.* 2008;29:356–361.
39. Valdez TA, Desai U, Ruhl CM, Nigri PT. Early laryngeal inhalation injury and its correlation with late sequelae. *Laryngoscope.* 2006;116:283–287.
40. Donat N, Weber-Donat G, Bargues L, Tourtier JP. Singular distribution of smoke inhalation injury. *J Trauma.* 2011;70:1013.
41. Enkhbaatar P, Cox RA, Traber LD, et al. Aerosolized anticoagulants ameliorate acute lung injury in sheep after exposure to burn and smoke inhalation. *Crit Care Med.* 2007;35:2805–2810.
42. Edelman DA, Khan N, Kempf K, White MT. Pneumonia after inhalation injury. *J Burn Care Res.* 2007;28:241–246.
43. Smith DD. Acute inhalation injury. *Clin Pulm Med.* 1999;6:224–235.
44. Woodson LC. Diagnosis and grading of inhalation injury. *J Burn Care Res.* 2009;30:143–145.
45. Roberts G, Lloyd M, Parker M, et al. The Baux score is dead. Long live the Baux score: a 27-year retrospective cohort study of mortality at a regional burns service. *J Trauma.* 2012;72:251–256.
46. Andel D, Kamolz L-P, Niedermayr M, et al. Which of the Abbreviated Burn Severity Index variables are having impact on the hospital length of stay? *J Burn Care Res.* 2007;28:163–166.
47. Gomez M, Wong DT, Stewart TE. The FLAMES score accurately predicts mortality risk in burn patients. *J Trauma.* 2008;65: 636–645.
48. Mackie DP. Inhalation injury or mechanical ventilation: which is the true killer in burn patients? *Burns.* 2013;39:1329–1330.
49. Albright JM, Davis CS, Bird MD, et al. The acute pulmonary inflammatory response to the graded severity of smoke inhalation injury. *Crit Care Med.* 2012;40:1113–1121.
50. Jones SW, Zhou H, Ortiz-Pujols et al. Bronchoscopy-derived correlates of lung injury following inhalational injuries: a prospective observational study. *PLoS One* 2013;8:e64250.
51. Neuwalder JM, Sampson C, Breuing KH, Orgill DP. A review of computer-aided body surface area determination. *J Burn Care Rehabil.* 2002;23:55–59.
52. Wahl WL, Taddonio MA, Arbabi S, Hemmila MR. Duration of antibiotic therapy for ventilator-associated pneumonia in burn patients. *J Burn Care Res.* 2009;30:801–806.
53. Holt J, Saffle JR, Morris SE, Cochran A. Use of inhaled heparin/N-acetylcystine in inhalation injury: does it help? *J Burn Care Res.* 2008;29:192–195.
54. Blamoun J. Efficacy of an expanded ventilator bundle for the reduction of ventilator-associated pneumonia in the medical intensive care unit. *Am J Infect Control.* 2009;37:172–175.
55. Anonymous. Ventilation with lower tidal volumes as compared with traditional tidal volumes for acute lung injury and the acute respiratory distress syndrome. *N Engl J Med.* 2000;342:1301–1308.
56. Serpa Neto A, Cardoso S, Manetta J, et al. Association between use of lung-protective ventilation with lower tidal volumes and clinical outcomes among patients without acute respiratory distress syndrome: a meta-analysis. *JAMA.* 2012;308:1651–1659.
57. Galiatsou E. Prone positioning augments recruitment and alveolar overdistension in acute lung injury. *Am J Respir Crit Care.* 2006;174:187–197.
58. Guérin C, Reignier J, Richard J-C, et al. Prone positioning in severe acute respiratory distress syndrome. *N Engl J Med.* 2013;368:2159–2168.
59. Liao W-C, Yeh F-L, Lin J-T, et al. Delayed tracheal stenosis in an inhalation burn patient. *J Trauma.* 2008;64:E37–E40.
60. Lovett PB, Flaxman A, Stürmann KM, Bijur P. The insecure airway: a comparison of knots and commercial devices for securing endotracheal tubes. *BMC Emerg Med.* 2006;6:7.
61. Weireter LJ Jr, Collins JN, Britt RC, et al. Impact of a monitored program of care on incidence of ventilator-associated pneumonia: results of a longterm performance-improvement project. *J Am Coll Surg.* 2009;208:700–705.
62. Anonymous. Randomized, placebo-controlled clinical trial of an aerosolized β_2-agonist for treatment of acute lung injury. *Am J Respir Crit Care Med.* 2011;184:561–568.
63. Gao Smith F, Perkins GD, Gates S, et al. Effect of intravenous beta$_2$-agonist treatment on clinical outcomes in acute respiratory distress syndrome (BALTI-2): a multicentre, randomised controlled trial. *Lancet.* 2012;379:229–235.
64. Freiburg C, Igneri P, Sartorelli K, Rogers F. Effects of differences in percent total body surface area estimation on fluid resuscitation of transferred burn patients. *J Burn Care Res.* 2007;28:42–48.
65. Young D, Lamb SE, Shah S, et al. High-frequency oscillation for acute respiratory distress syndrome. *N Engl J Med.* 2013;368:806–813.
66. Ferguson ND, Cook DJ, Guyatt GH, et al. High-frequency oscillation in early acute respiratory distress syndrome. *N Engl J Med.* 2013;368:795–805.
67. Jackson JC, Girard TD, Gordon SM, et al. Long-term cognitive and psychological outcomes in the awakening and breathing controlled trial. *Am J Respir Crit Care Med.* 2010;182:183–191.
68. Mehta S. Daily Sedation interruption in mechanically ventilated critically ill patients cared for with a sedation protocol. *JAMA.* 2012;308:1985.
69. Hampson NB, Rudd RA, Hauff NM. Increased long-term mortality among survivors of acute carbon monoxide poisoning. *Crit Care Med.* 2009;37:1941–1947.
70. Weaver LK. Carbon monoxide poisoning. *N Engl J Med.* 2009;360:1217–1225.
71. Stoller KP. Hyperbaric oxygen and carbon monoxide poisoning: a critical review. *Neurol Res.* 2007;29:146–155.
72. Weaver LK, Hopkins RO, Chan KJ, et al. Hyperbaric oxygen for acute carbon monoxide poisoning. *N Engl J Med.* 2002; 347:1057–1067.
73. Weaver LK, Valentine KJ, Hopkins RO. Carbon monoxide poisoning. *Am J Respir Crit Care Med.* 2007;176:491–497.
74. Patel DN, Goel A, Agarwal SB, et al. Oxygen toxicity. *J Indian Academy Clin Med.* 2003;4:234–237.
75. Lefebvre J-C, Lyazidi A, Parceiro M, et al. Bench testing of a new hyperbaric chamber ventilator at different atmospheric pressures. *Intensive Care Med.* 2012;38:1400–1404.
76. Weaver LK, Greenway L, Elliott CG. Performance of the Sechrist 500A hyperbaric ventilator in a monoplace hyperbaric chamber. *J Hyperbaric Med.* 1988;3:215–225.

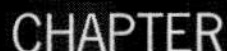

CHAPTER

43

Neuromuscular Dysfunction

Francis C. Cordova, John Mullarkey, Gerard J. Criner

OUTLINE

Overview
Pathophysiology of Neuromuscular Disease on Respiratory Failure
Evaluation of Respiratory Function in Patients with Neuromuscular Disease
Assessment of Respiratory Muscle Function
Upper Motor Neuron Disorders
Lower Motor Neuron Disorders
Disorders of the Peripheral Nerves
Disorders of the Neuromuscular Junction
Inherited Myopathies
Acquired Inflammatory Myopathies
Treatment of Neuromuscular Dysfunction

OBJECTIVES

1. Discuss the effects of neuromuscular disease on respiratory function during wakefulness and sleep.
2. Discuss the relevance of clinical history, physical examination, and pulmonary function testing in the evaluation of respiratory function in patients with suspected neuromuscular disease.
3. Describe the clinical manifestations of neuromuscular disease associated with upper neuron lesions, lower motor neuron lesions, disorders of peripheral nerves, disorders of the neuromuscular junction, and inherited and acquired myopathies.
4. Discuss the treatment of respiratory dysfunction in patients with neuromuscular disease.
5. Describe the role of respiratory muscle training, assisted coughing, glossopharyngeal breathing, mechanical ventilatory support, and diaphragmatic pacing.

KEY TERMS

acid maltase deficiency
amyotrophic lateral sclerosis (ALS)
Becker muscular dystrophy (BMD)
botulism
Cheyne-Stokes breathing
critical illness polyneuromyopathy (CIPNM)
diaphragmatic pacing
Duchenne muscular dystrophy (DMD)
facioscapulohumeral muscular dystrophy (FSHD)
glossopharyngeal breathing
Guillain-Barré syndrome (GBS)
Lambert-Eaton syndrome (LEMS)
limb-girdle muscular dystrophy
maximum expiratory pressure (MEP or PE_{max})
maximum inspiratory pressure (MIP or PI_{max})
mitochondrial myopathy
mouth occlusion pressure ($P_{0.1}$)
multiple sclerosis (MS)
muscular dystrophy
myasthenia gravis (MG)
myotonic dystrophy
Parkinson disease
postpoliomyelitis syndrome
sniff test
stroke
systemic lupus erythematosus (SLE)
tetraplegia
transdiaphragmatic pressure (Pdi)

Introduction

The respiratory system can be divided into two functional parts: the lungs, where gas exchange occurs, and the respiratory muscles and rib cage, which act as a vital pump to enable normal gas exchange. Neuromuscular diseases are a diverse group of neurologic disorders that range from primary muscle diseases that impair all skeletal muscle functions to conditions that selectively involve the diaphragm or the neural control of respiration. The severity of respiratory muscle dysfunction depends on the type of neuromuscular disease, the pattern of respiratory muscle involvement (inspiratory or expiratory muscle), and whether or not effective medical therapies (e.g., plasmapheresis in Guillain-Barré syndrome) are available. The respiratory pump may be impaired at the level of the central nervous system, spinal cord, peripheral nerve, neuromuscular junction, or respiratory muscles. A thorough understanding of the neuroanatomic and pathologic changes brought on by the different neuromuscular disorders is important in the diagnosis and treatment of these diseases. This chapter discusses in detail the etiology, pathophysiology, and treatment of ventilatory dysfunction in the setting of neuromuscular disease.

Overview

Although the list of diseases usually classified under the heading of neuromuscular disorders includes a heterogeneous and pathologically diverse composite of neurologic and muscular diseases (**Table 43-1**), they all commonly lead to a stereotypic clinical course of ineffective cough, recurrent pulmonary infections, and ventilatory insufficiency in advanced disease. Chronic respiratory failure, in association with pulmonary sepsis, is the most common cause of death in these patients.

Some neuromuscular disorders may remain unrecognized by patients and physicians until an intercurrent illness leads to acute respiratory failure. In such cases, neuromuscular dysfunction is only suspected once patients cannot be liberated from mechanical ventilation. In a study involving 293 chronic ventilator-dependent patients, 17% of patients had an underlying neuromuscular disease as the major factor contributing to the development of respiratory failure.[1] Neuromuscular dysfunction frequently contributes to the need for prolonged mechanical ventilation. Overall, the incidence of neuromuscular disease resulting in prolonged mechanical ventilation has been reported to range from 10% to 25% in various ventilator rehabilitation units across the country.[1]

TABLE 43-1
Levels of Pathologic Injury in Neuromuscular Diseases

Level	Disease
Upper Motor Neuron	
Cerebral	Stroke
Spinal cord	Trauma
Lower Motor Neuron	
Anterior horn cells	Poliomyelitis Amyotrophic lateral sclerosis
Peripheral nerves	Phrenic nerve injury Diabetes mellitus Guillain-Barré syndrome Critical illness polyneuropathy
Neuromuscular junction	Myasthenia gravis Lambert-Eaton syndrome Botulism Aminoglycosides
Muscle	Dystrophy Acid maltase deficiency Corticosteroids Acute intensive care myopathy

Pathophysiology of Neuromuscular Disease on Respiratory Function

The changes that occur in ventilation in chronic neuromuscular disorders can best be understood by studying the impact of neuromuscular disease on the respiratory system's different functional components. Neuromuscular diseases can impair the integrity of the respiratory system by affecting its closely interrelated functional parts, such as control of breathing, respiratory muscle function, lung and chest wall mechanics, and upper airway function. In general, the commonly observed changes in the respiratory system found in patients with moderately advanced chronic neuromuscular dysfunction are normal or high central respiratory drive (except in certain diseases that affect the brain stem, such as poliomyelitis); a restrictive ventilatory pattern manifested as a reduction in forced vital capacity and an increase in residual volume; a reduction in respiratory muscle strength; and upper airway dysfunction, which may present as upper airway obstruction, recurrent aspiration pneumonia, and obstructive sleep apnea. All of these pathologic changes may present as subtle signs and symptoms during restful breathing but become magnified during sleep and exercise (**Figure 43-1**).

Control of Breathing

The ventilatory responses to hypoxia and hypercapnia are used to assess the response of the peripheral and central chemoreceptors to chemical stimuli. In normal individuals, the relationship between oxygen saturation and ventilation is linear, such that a fall in oxygen saturation by 1% will trigger an increase of approximately 1 L/min in minute ventilation. A much steeper linear increase in minute ventilation is seen during the hypercapnic breathing test. For every 1 mm Hg rise in $Paco_2$, ventilation increases by 2.5 to 3 L/min. The normally predictable increases in ventilation that occur in response to hypoxia and hypercapnia become disturbed in some neuromuscular disorders.

Patients afflicted with neuromuscular disorders exhibit hypoventilation out of proportion to the severity of the respiratory muscle weakness.[2,3] Definite conclusions cannot be drawn from these early studies, because the ventilatory response to metabolic stress is

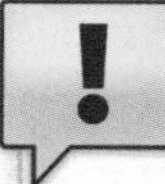

Respiratory Recap

Control of Breathing

- The central respiratory drive in the brain is sensitive to changes in $Paco_2$ and Pao_2.
- The mouth occlusion pressure ($P_{0.1}$) is an accurate measure of the central respiratory drive.
- Respiratory drive is preserved in patients with neuromuscular disease.

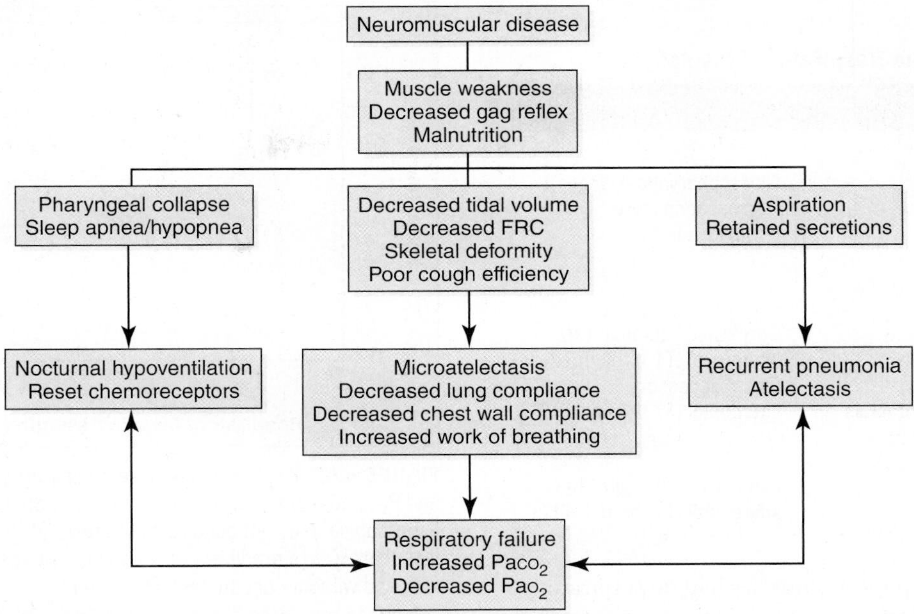

FIGURE 43-1 Pathophysiology of respiratory failure in patients with neuromuscular diseases.

Reproduced from Hill NS, Braman S. 1999. Noninvasive ventilation in neuromuscular disease. In: Cherniack NS, Altose MD, Homma I, eds. *Rehabilitation of the Patient with Respiratory Disease.* New York, NY: McGraw-Hill. (© The McGraw-Hill Companies, Inc.)

not considered a good index of central respiratory drive in the presence of respiratory muscle weakness. The blunted ventilatory responses to hypoxic and hypercapnic challenges observed in patients with chronic neuromuscular disease may be related to inability of the respiratory pump to increase the work of breathing in response to increases in respiratory drive due to respiratory muscle weakness. Alternatively, abnormal chest wall and lung mechanics, a defective afferent input from diseased respiratory muscles, upper airway involvement,[4] and upper motor neuron disorders[5] may all contribute to hypoventilation in selected neuromuscular disorders.

An accurate test of central respiratory drive that is independent of underlying respiratory mechanics is the **mouth occlusion pressure ($P_{0.1}$)**. $P_{0.1}$ refers to the maximum negative mouth pressure generated during the first 100 milliseconds of inspiration measured during complete airway occlusion. Because $P_{0.1}$ is obtained during early inspiration, a small fraction of total inspiratory time, it is not influenced by volitional effort. In addition, because $P_{0.1}$ requires only a fraction of maximum inspiratory muscle strength, it remains valid even in the presence of moderately severe inspiratory muscle weakness.

In contrast to studies that have used ventilation to assess central respiratory drive, $P_{0.1}$ has been found to be normal, or increased, in patients with neuromuscular diseases despite the presence of substantial muscle weakness. Indeed, several studies have shown that despite significant reductions in respiratory muscle strength, $P_{0.1}$ values in patients with Duchenne muscular dystrophy, myotonic dystrophy, and a variety of other neuromuscular diseases are one- to twofold higher than in normal controls.[6] Increases in $P_{0.1}$ were observed in normal human volunteers after severe muscle weakness was induced by curarization.[7] Thus, it appears that central respiratory drive, as measured by $P_{0.1}$, is usually preserved in most patients with underlying neuromuscular diseases.

Respiratory Muscle Function

The respiratory muscles consist of muscles of the upper airway, the diaphragm, chest wall, and abdominal muscles. The respiratory muscles can be further functionally divided into the inspiratory and expiratory muscles. The inspiratory muscles produce rib cage expansion and generate negative intrathoracic pressure, thereby facilitating inspiratory airflow. During rest, exhalation is passive and is driven by the lung and chest wall elastic recoil pressures. Active contraction of the expiratory muscles occurs under conditions in which increased expiratory airflow is required, such as during coughing, exercise, and airway obstruction. **Table 43-2** lists the innervation of the different respiratory muscles and their major functions.

Patients with moderate to severe respiratory muscle weakness due to neuromuscular disease often complain of fatigue, poor sleep quality, and dyspnea, especially on exertion. A significant percentage of these patients may be asymptomatic despite moderate to severe weakness of the inspiratory and expiratory muscles. It has been reported that 27% of patients with moderately advanced neuromuscular disease and severe reduction in both

TABLE 43-2
Innervation of the Respiratory Muscles

Muscle Group	Nerve
Upper airway	
Palate, pharynx	Glossopharyngeal, vagus, spinal accessory
Genioglossus	Hypoglossal
Inspiratory	
Diaphragm	Phrenic
Scalenes	Cervical (C4 through C8)
Parasternal intercostals	Intercostal (T1 through T7)
Sternocleidomastoid	Spinal accessory
Lateral external intercostals	Intercostal (T1 through T12)
Expiratory	
Abdominal	Lumbar (T7 through T11)
Internal intercostals	Intercostal (T1 through T12)

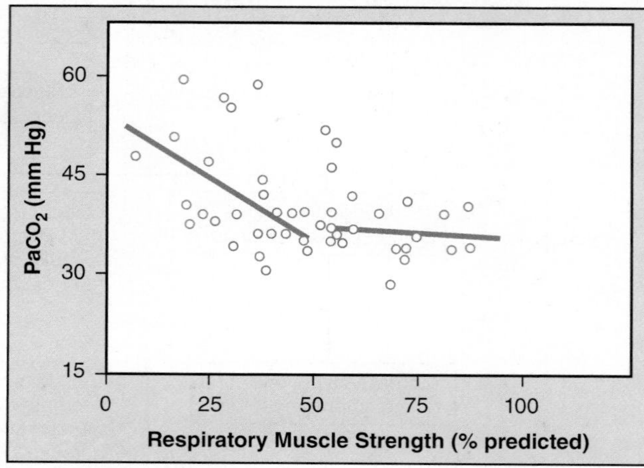

FIGURE 43-2 Relationship between respiratory muscle strength and $Paco_2$ in patients with myopathies. The data suggest that hypercapnia does not occur until the respiratory muscle strength is less than 30% of predicted. Red and blue circles represent patients with and without concomitant lung disease, respectively.

Reproduced from Braun NMT, Arora NS, Rochester DF. Respiratory muscle and pulmonary function in polymyositis and other proximal myopathies. *Thorax*. 1983;38:616–623. © 1983, with permission from BMJ Publishing Group Ltd.

inspiratory and expiratory muscles had no respiratory complaints.[8] Similarly, as many as 50% of patients with severe respiratory muscle weakness due to chronic neuromuscular disease were asymptomatic.[9] It is unclear why there is such a poor correlation between the extent of respiratory muscle weakness and clinical symptoms exhibited by patients. It is possible that the presence of significant respiratory muscle weakness is masked by the inability to achieve significant exercise because of generalized muscle weakness that enforces a sedentary lifestyle. Whatever the case, a substantial number of patients may have significant neuromuscular impairment of the respiratory system that may go initially unnoticed.

The particular type of underlying neuromuscular disorder determines the pattern and severity of respiratory muscle weakness. Some diseases cause global respiratory muscle dysfunction, whereas others cause preferential weakness of the inspiratory or expiratory muscles. Moreover, decreases in inspiratory and expiratory muscle strength may not correlate with general muscle strength assessment. Primary muscle diseases (e.g., polymyositis) may cause more significant impairment of the respiratory muscles compared with the neuropathies. The relationship between inspiratory muscle strength and the onset of ventilatory insufficiency is not linear. Once maximum inspiratory mouth pressure decreases to less than 30% of predicted, hypercapnia ensues (**Figure 43-2**).[10] The clinical course of respiratory muscle dysfunction in different neuromuscular diseases may also be varied. It can be progressive (amyotrophic lateral sclerosis), reversible with therapy (Guillain-Barré syndrome, myasthenia gravis), or improve with time (critical care polyneuropathy).

> **Respiratory Recap**
>
> **Respiratory Muscle Function**
>
> - Isolated or combined inspiratory, expiratory, and bulbar weakness can be seen in neuromuscular diseases.
> - Respiratory muscle weakness can be present in the absence of respiratory muscle weakness.

Lung and Chest Wall Mechanics

Lung volume studies in patients with chronic respiratory muscle weakness often show a restrictive ventilatory pattern with a reduction in total lung capacity (TLC) and forced vital capacity (FVC). There is a moderate decrease in both inspiratory and expiratory reserve volumes. The decrease in FVC is mainly due to respiratory muscle weakness, and its decrease generally parallels the progression of the underlying neuromuscular disease. Because of the sigmoidal shape of the pressure–volume curve, vital capacity is relatively well preserved until respiratory muscle weakness is well advanced (**Figure 43-3**). Indeed, the fall in FVC has been shown to be out of proportion to the reduction in inspiratory muscle strength. A reduction in lung compliance of 40% occurred in 25 patients with moderate to severe neuromuscular disease.[11] Respiratory muscle weakness may also account for a lower vital capacity in these patients. The exact cause or causes of reduced lung compliance in neuromuscular disease patients remain speculative. Several proposed explanations include failed maturation of normal lung tissue in congenital neuromuscular diseases; the presence of micro- or macroatelectasis; an increased alveolar surface tension caused by breathing chronically at low tidal volumes; and an alteration in lung tissue elasticity.

Patients with neuromuscular disease have a rapid, shallow breathing pattern similar to patients with

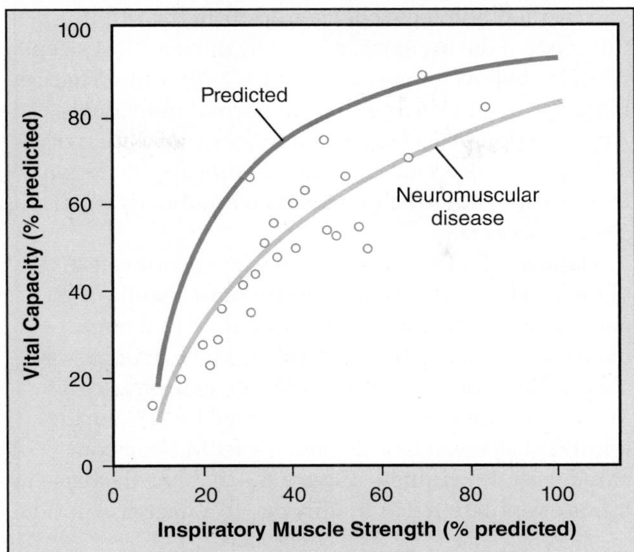

FIGURE 43-3 Relationship between inspiratory muscle strength and vital capacity. The orange line represents the regression line calculated in 25 patients with neuromuscular diseases showing the disproportionate fall in vital capacity for the given degree of inspiratory muscle weakness. The blue line represents the predicted relationship between vital capacity and inspiratory muscle strength.

Modified from De Troyer A, Borensteinm S, Cordier R. Analysis of lung volume restriction in patients with respiratory muscle weakness. *Thorax*. 1980;35:603–610, with permission from BMJ Publishing Group Ltd.

interstitial lung disease. The exact mechanism of this abnormal breathing pattern is unclear but is thought to be secondary to changes in lung and chest wall elastic recoil. Animal studies have demonstrated that breathing at small tidal volumes is associated with reductions in lung compliance and may lead to increased alveolar surface tension. In addition, the lower ventilatory demand induced by a sedentary lifestyle leads to lower lung mechanical stress and over time may result in a reduction in lung tissue elasticity.

Similar to the changes seen in the lungs, a significant reduction in chest wall compliance may occur in patients with chronic neuromuscular disease.[12] The mechanisms of the reduction in chest wall compliance are unclear but may be caused by increased rib cage stiffness due to decreased distensibility of chest wall structures (i.e., tendons, ligaments, costovertebral and costosternal articulations). In patients with type 1 spinal muscular atrophy, the relative preservation of diaphragm strength in the face of marked weakness of the intercostals commonly leads to chest wall deformity characterized by sternal recession and a small bell-shaped chest.

Although a low vital capacity is almost always seen in moderately advanced neuromuscular disease, the changes in functional residual capacity (FRC) and residual volume (RV) are variable and depend on the type, severity, and stage of neuromuscular disease. In general, patients with neuromuscular diseases have moderate reductions in TLC and FRC, with a normal RV.

> **Respiratory Recap**
>
> **Respiratory Mechanics**
>
> - Lung volume shows a restrictive pattern due to reduced chest wall and lung compliance.
> - The breathing pattern is rapid and shallow.
> - The decrease in FVC is relatively attenuated until the respiratory muscle weakness is severe.

Gas Exchange Abnormalities

Hypercapnia and hypoxemia are late findings in patients with neuromuscular disease. Hypercapnia with a relatively normal FVC and static maximum respiratory pressures should raise the possibility of sleep-related breathing disorders (e.g., obstructive sleep apnea, obesity hypoventilation syndrome), the presence of parenchymal lung disease such as chronic obstructive airway disease, or problems with central respiratory drive such as chronic hypoventilation syndrome or hypothyroidism. Even with normal daytime gas exchange parameters, significant hypoxemia and alveolar hypoventilation may occur during sleep, especially during rapid eye movement (REM) sleep, when the activity of the accessory muscles is diminished. In advanced neuromuscular diseases, evidence of alveolar hypoventilation on blood gas examination is likely when the FVC is less than 55% of predicted (**Figure 43-4**) or when the respiratory muscle strength (average of percent predicted inspiratory and expiratory muscle strength) is less than 30% of normal. In addition,

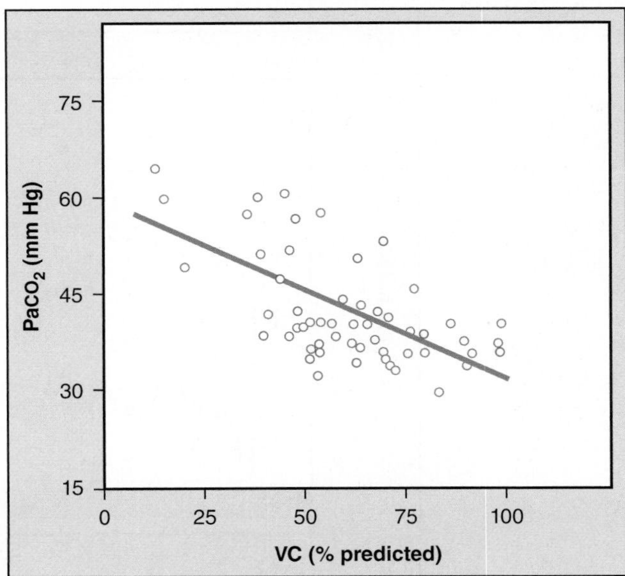

FIGURE 43-4 Relationship between vital capacity and Pa_{CO_2}, showing that hypercapnia occurs when the vital capacity is less than 50% of predicted. Red and blue circles represent patients with and without concomitant lung disease, respectively.

Reproduced from Braun NMT, Arora NS, Rochester DF. Respiratory muscle and pulmonary function in polymyositis and other proximal myopathies. *Thorax*. 1983;38:616–623. © 1983, with permission from BMJ Publishing Group Ltd.

hypercapnia is likely if the FVC is less than 1 L. The onset of hypercapnia in the setting of advanced neuromuscular disease may be abrupt, however, especially in the setting of repeated pulmonary infections. Ventilation-perfusion inequality due to atelectasis is the most common cause of hypoxemia in these patients.

Sleep and Neuromuscular Disease

Sleep-related breathing disorders such as impaired sleep quality and REM-related hypopneas are common in patients with a variety of different neuromuscular diseases. Indeed, significant gas exchange abnormalities may be present and even unsuspected when daytime hypoxemia and hypercapnia are absent. In addition, sleep study usually shows an increased number of awakenings, sleep fragmentation, and disorganization, along with reduced total sleep time.

Several physiologic changes occur in the respiratory system during sleep, especially during REM sleep. Alveolar hypoventilation, causing a 2- to 3-mm Hg rise in $Paco_2$, occurs during sleep in normal individuals. An inhibition of accessory inspiratory muscle activity during REM sleep may lead to a significant reduction in alveolar ventilation in patients with underlying diaphragm weakness.

Hypoventilation during sleep is the major cause of sleep-related oxygen desaturation. In a study of 26 patients with chronic respiratory failure and nocturnal oxygen desaturation (patients with chronic airway obstruction, obesity hypoventilation, neuromuscular disease), minute ventilation decreased by 21% during non-REM sleep and by 39% during REM sleep compared with wakefulness (**Figure 43-5**).[13] The decrease in minute ventilation was mainly due to a decrease in tidal

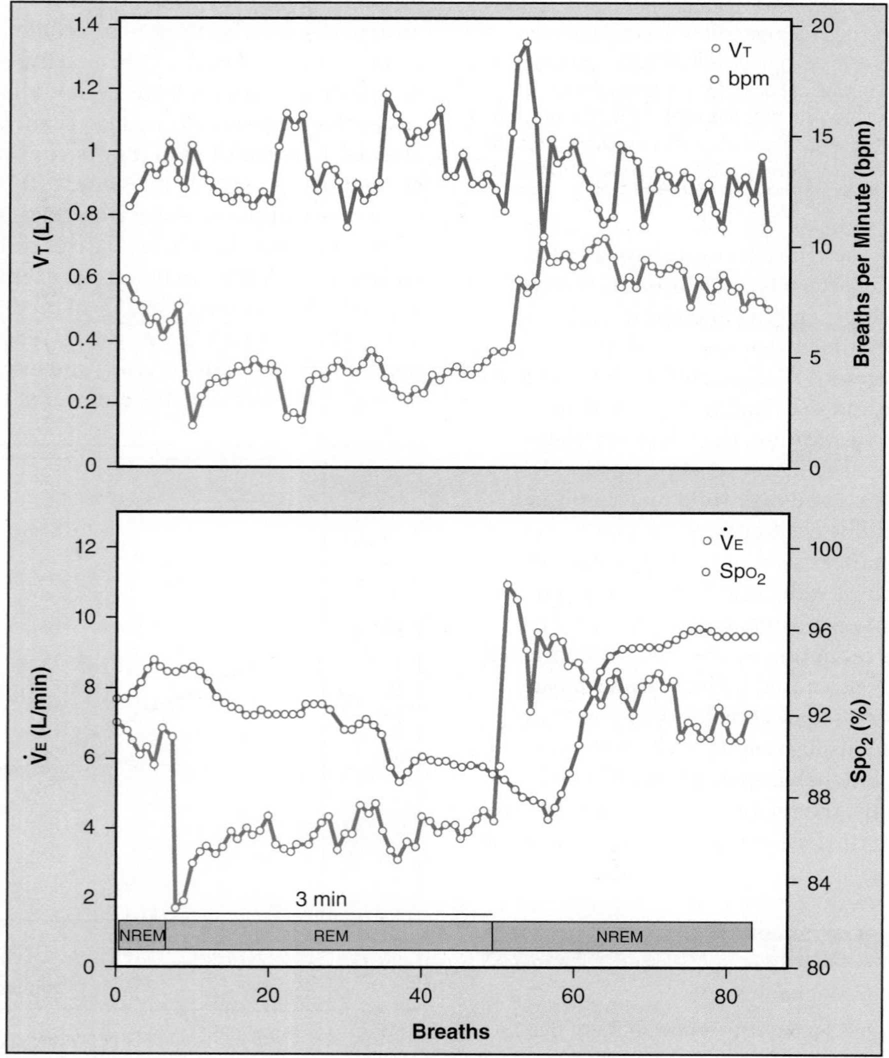

FIGURE 43-5 Both panels show the decrease in tidal volume (VT) and minute ventilation (V̇E) with no change in respiratory rate during transition from nonrapid eye movement (NREM) sleep to rapid eye movement (REM) sleep. Hypoventilation due to decrease in VT during REM sleep appears to be the main reason leading to nocturnal oxygen desaturation in patients with limited pulmonary reserve.

Modified from Becker H, et al. Breathing during sleep in patients with nocturnal desaturation. *Am J Respir Crit Care Med.* 1999;159:112–118. The American Journal of Respiratory and Critical Care Medicine is an official journal of the American Thoracic Society. Reprinted with permission of the American Thoracic Society. Copyright © 2015 American Thoracic Society.

Respiratory Recap

Gas Exchange Abnormalities

- Daytime hypercapnia is likely when FVC is less than 55% or respiratory muscle weakness is less than 30%.
- Hypercapnia is a late sign of respiratory muscle weakness.

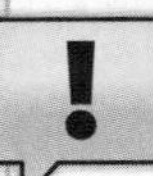

Respiratory Recap

Sleep-Disordered Breathing

- Nocturnal hypoventilation is common and may herald the onset of daytime hypercapnia.
- FVC less than 40% and maximum inspiratory pressure less than 30 cm H_2O predict REM- and non–REM-associated hypoventilation.

volume and was found to be independent of the underlying lung disease. Phasic REM sleep–induced changes in breathing pattern superimposed on the rapid, shallow breathing pattern commonly observed in neuromuscular patients will lead to further increases in dead space ventilation, resulting in more profound degrees of hypoxemia and hypercapnia. In addition to these sleep-induced breathing abnormalities, weakness of the pharyngeal muscles in certain neuromuscular diseases may predispose patients to obstructive sleep apnea and hypopnea due to loss of upper airway tone, especially during REM sleep.

If nocturnal hypoventilation is severe and remains clinically unrecognized, daytime hypercapnia and hypoxemia may ensue even in the absence of severe respiratory muscle dysfunction. Nocturnal gas exchange abnormalities usually precede abnormalities in daytime arterial blood gas results. Indeed, most patients with normal nocturnal gas exchange are unlikely to have abnormal daytime values.

Abnormalities in daytime gas exchange and certain parameters of respiratory mechanics are useful in predicting the subset of patients with neuromuscular disease who are at risk for severe nocturnal oxygen desaturation. In a study of 20 patients with a variety of moderately advanced neuromuscular diseases, it was found that the degree of REM-related oxygen desaturation is directly related to the severity of daytime hypercapnia and hypoxemia.[14] Absolute values for vital capacity, as well as the decrement in vital capacity measured in the supine compared with the seated position, also correlate with the nadir in oxygen saturation measured during REM sleep. The mean decrease in vital capacity measured in the seated compared with supine posture was 21%. In patients with primary myopathies, FVC less than 60% is associated with the development of REM-associated hypopneas. Nocturnal hypopneas occur during REM and non-REM sleep once the vital

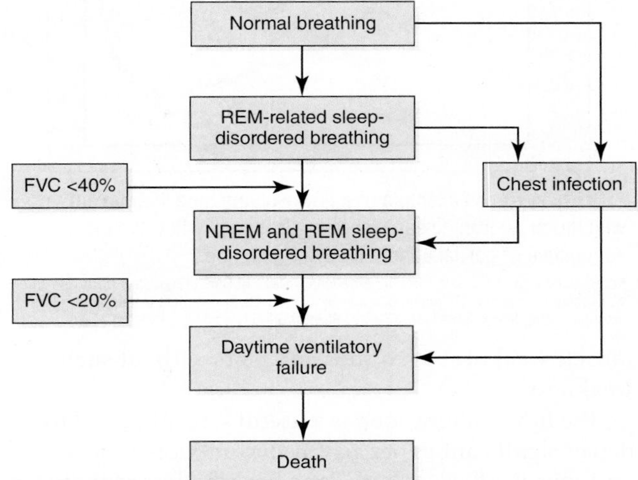

FIGURE 43-6 Respiratory insufficiency in patients with neuromuscular disease is manifested initially as sleep-related breathing disorder during REM sleep and later in NREM sleep. Chronic hypercapnic respiratory failure ensues once forced vital capacity (FVC) is less than 20% of predicted or in the presence of chest infection.

Reproduced from Simonds AK. Recent advances in respiratory care for neuromuscular disease. Chest. 2006;130:1882, with permission from the American College of Chest Physicians.

capacity is less than 40% and the **maximum inspiratory pressure (MIP or PI_{max})** is greater than –30 cm H_2O.[15] **Figure 43-6** shows the evolution of respiratory failure in patients with neuromuscular disease.

Upper Airway Function

Some neuromuscular diseases involve the bulbar muscles and therefore impair upper airway function. Upper airway dysfunction is commonly manifested by repeated pulmonary aspiration, stridor, obstructive sleep apnea, and hypopnea. In patients with chronic neuromuscular disorders, upper airway dysfunction is more common in those who exhibit respiratory

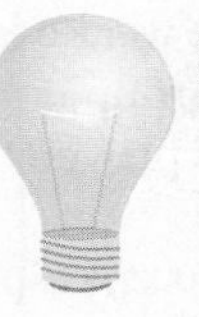

STOP AND THINK

Based on the respiratory pathophysiology of neuromuscular disease, how would you explain to a patient the benefits of nocturnal noninvasive ventilation?

Respiratory Recap

Upper Airway Muscles

- Weakness of the bulbar muscles leads to recurrent aspiration, pneumonia, and upper airway obstruction.
- The flow–volume loop is useful in detecting upper airway obstruction.

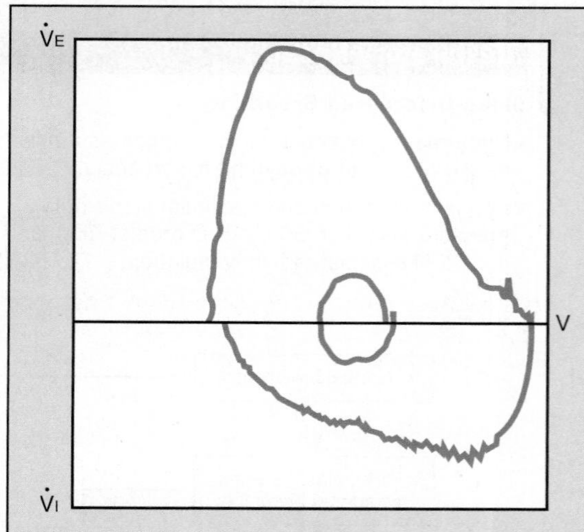

FIGURE 43-7 An example of a flow–volume loop in a patient with motor neuron disease, showing inspiratory flow limitation suggestive of partial upper airway obstruction.

Reproduced with permission from the American College of Chest Physicians from Vincken W, Ellecker G, Cosio M. Detection of upper airway muscle involvement in neuromuscular disorders using flow-volume loop. *Chest*. 1986;90:52–57.

muscle weakness than those patients without such weakness.

The flow–volume loop is a useful screening tool to detect significant upper airway dysfunction. Indeed, an abnormal flow–volume loop has a high sensitivity and specificity in predicting bulbar and upper airway involvement in patients with neuromuscular dysfunction. **Figure 43-7** shows a typical flow–volume loop in a patient with motor neuron disease with bulbar involvement. Sawtoothing of the flow contour can occur in patients with Parkinson disease. In addition, variable extrathoracic obstruction that reverses with drug therapy has been described in patients with myasthenia gravis.[16] Certain features of the flow–volume contour have been shown to correlate with reduced maximum static inspiratory and expiratory mouth pressures: a reduced peak expiratory flow, decreased slope of the ascending limb of the maximum expiratory curve, a drop-off of the forced expiratory flow near residual volume, and a reduction in forced inspiratory flow at 50% of vital capacity (**Figure 43-8**).[17]

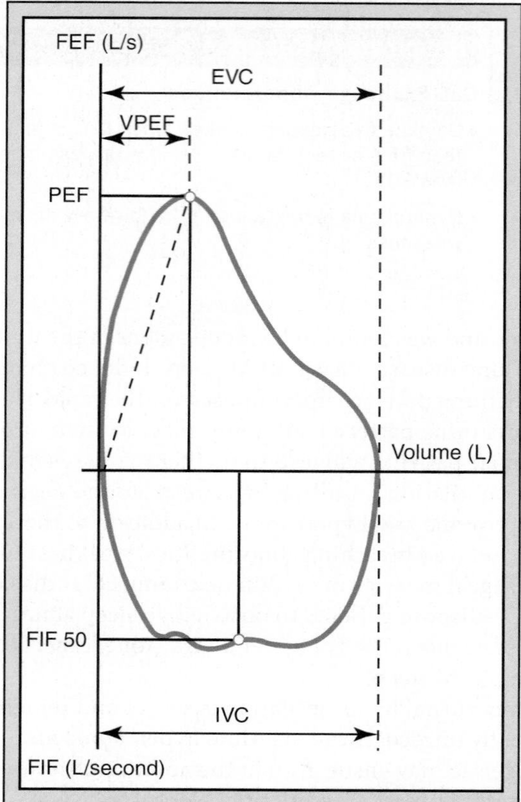

FIGURE 43-8 Analysis of the effort-dependent portion of the flow–volume loop to detect respiratory muscle weakness. These four parameters are (1) peak expiratory flow (PEF); (2) ratio of PEF to the exhaled volume at which PEF was achieved (VPEF); (3) rapid vertical drop of forced expiratory flow (FEF) at residual volume; and (4) forced mid-inspiratory flow. EVC, expired vital capacity; IVC, inspired vital capacity; FIF, forced inspiratory flow.

Reproduced from Vicken W, Ellecker G, Casio M. Flow-volume loop changes reflecting... . *Am J Med*. 1987;83:673–680. © 1987, with permission from Elsevier.

Evaluation of Respiratory Function in Patients with Neuromuscular Disease

Clinical History

The diagnosis of the etiology of muscle weakness may not be readily made on initial clinical evaluation because of the overlapping syndromes among the different neuromuscular diseases. The predominant signs and symptoms of a particular neuromuscular disease depend on the patient's age at the presentation of the clinical symptoms; the acuity, severity, and clinical course of the disease; and the pattern of neuromuscular weakness. Diseases that predominantly affect the pump function of the respiratory system will present as dyspnea, weak cough, and recurrent respiratory tract infections, whereas diseases that primarily affect the limb muscles will present as impaired patient mobility early in the disease evolution. Once respiratory muscles are affected in advanced neuromuscular disease, respiratory failure may occur abruptly due to an intercurrent illness or slowly over months and years, culminating in chronic hypercapnic respiratory failure. In some neuromuscular diseases, however, a typical presentation will help with the correct diagnosis. For example, an acute ascending paralysis of the lower extremities suggests Guillain-Barré syndrome, waxing and waning of neurologic symptoms is commonly seen in multiple sclerosis, and skeletal muscle weakness with repetitive action of a particular muscle group is highly suspicious of myasthenia gravis unless proven otherwise.

In the majority of the neuromuscular diseases, respiratory muscle weakness usually occurs insidiously and is typically associated with weakness of other skeletal muscle groups. Up to 50% of patients with significant respiratory muscle weakness may be asymptomatic until they present with overt respiratory failure.[2] It thus is no surprise that acute respiratory failure has been reported as the initial presentation in patients with motor neuron disease, myasthenia gravis, and adult-onset acid maltase deficiency, and has also been reported with mitochondrial myopathy. Pulmonary physicians and respiratory therapists are involved in the care of these patients when these patients develop either acute respiratory failure or acute or chronic hypercapnic respiratory failure.

In patients who develop acute respiratory failure, the nature of the neuromuscular disease is often not clinically apparent, and the clinical history is often dominated by the symptoms of the precipitating illness that led to respiratory failure. These patients often require early intubation and mechanical ventilation and appropriate treatment of the precipitating intercurrent illness. In most cases, respiratory muscle weakness due to a neuromuscular disease comes to light only after the patient has failed multiple spontaneous breathing trials.

In patients who have chronic stable neuromuscular diseases, such as amyotrophic lateral sclerosis (ALS) or congenital myopathies, progressive respiratory muscle weakness occurs over months and years, eventually leading to chronic progressive hypercapnic respiratory failure. The challenge to both respiratory physicians and therapists is to detect early signs of respiratory muscle weakness before the onset of fulminant respiratory failure and to prevent complications such as aspiration, recurrent respiratory tract infections, and cor pulmonale as well as to preserve remaining lung function. Some studies have shown that early use of noninvasive ventilation may attenuate the decline in respiratory muscle function in certain diseases.[18] The common symptoms of respiratory muscle weakness are dyspnea (especially with activity), inability to clear secretions, and weak cough; frequent respiratory tract infections and choking episodes are often elicited several months before these patients seek medical attention. The presence of chronic headache, lethargy, and somnolence suggests significant daytime and nocturnal hypercapnia. Nocturnal hypercapnia usually heralds the onset of chronic respiratory failure.

Respiratory Recap

Acute Respiratory Failure in Neuromuscular Disease

- Weak cough, inability to clear oral secretions, and failure to liberate from mechanical ventilation should prompt neuromuscular disease workup.

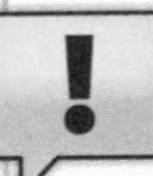

Respiratory Recap

Signs of Respiratory Muscle Weakness

- Subcostal retraction is a sign of diaphragm weakness and heralds impending respiratory failure.
- Tachypnea and use of the respiratory accessory muscles at rest are signs of respiratory muscle weakness.

Physical Examination

A thorough physical examination and a detailed neurologic assessment may reveal a previously undiagnosed neuromuscular disorder. This is particularly true in patients who have mild respiratory muscle weakness but develop acute respiratory failure due to increased ventilatory demand from an acute illness such as an infection. In patients with early or mild neuromuscular weakness, respiratory muscle weakness may not be detected on routine physical examination. Limb muscle weakness is often only recognized after the patient fails multiple liberation attempts. Nevertheless, certain physical examination findings indicate significant respiratory muscle weakness. Tachypnea at rest is very common with the onset of respiratory muscle weakness. As the respiratory muscle weakness progresses, the increase in respiratory rate may be followed by signs of high respiratory workload such as nasal flaring, recruitment of the accessory muscles, and intercostal as well as subcostal retractions. Further progressive weakness of the respiratory muscles will eventually lead to paradoxical inward motion of the rib cage and outward displacement of the abdomen during inspiration. Abnormal paradoxical motion of the rib cage and abdomen may indicate either impending respiratory failure or diaphragm weakness. Indeed, paradoxical inward movement of the abdomen on inspiration that worsens with recumbent position is typically seen in diaphragm weakness.

Arterial Blood Gas Measurements

Abnormalities in arterial blood gas values occur late in patients with severe respiratory muscle weakness and should not be relied on before ventilatory support is initiated. Hypoxemia is commonly the result of

Respiratory Recap

Gas Exchange

- Hypoxemia is caused by retained secretions and atelectasis.
- Hypercarbia is caused by alveolar hypoventilation.

microatelectasis due to ineffective cough and retained secretions causing ventilation-perfusion mismatch or intrapulmonary shunting. More important, alveolar hypoventilation due to respiratory muscle weakness or decreased central respiratory drive may also contribute significantly to hypoxemia. Hypoxemia due mainly to alveolar hypoventilation may be detected by a normal alveolar–arterial Po_2 gradient. Pulse oximetry, which is a measure of arterial oxyhemoglobin saturation, is useful in detecting hypoxemia but is an insensitive indicator of hypoventilation.

Hypercarbia is a late finding in severe respiratory muscle weakness. In fact, hypercarbia does not occur until the respiratory muscle strength is less than 50% of predicted. Careful analysis of the pH and bicarbonate level is helpful in detecting the presence of acute or chronic hypercapnic respiratory failure. Sleep-induced breathing disturbances may also lead to hypercarbia and should be carefully studied in susceptible patients.

Pulmonary Function Tests

Spirometry and lung volume studies are helpful in the initial evaluation as well as in the follow-up of patients with neuromuscular disease. In general, spirometry produces a restrictive pattern characterized by a reduction in FVC and a normal ratio of forced expiratory volume in 1 second to forced vital capacity (FEV_1/FVC). Moreover, there is a decrease in effort-dependent expiratory flow, such as peak expiratory flow, whereas FEV_1 and measurement of mid-expiratory flow rates ($FEF_{25-75\%}$ or FEF_{50}) are often greater than normal predicted values in these patients because of decreased lung compliance resulting in increased lung elastic recoil. Lung volume studies demonstrate a low total lung capacity but a high residual volume due to expiratory muscle weakness. The diffusion capacity is usually normal.

Serial measurement of FVC is helpful in following the progression of respiratory muscle weakness in patients with chronic neuromuscular disease and in the timing of institution of noninvasive positive pressure ventilation. In patients with rapidly progressive respiratory muscle weakness such as seen in Guillain-Barré syndrome, daily measurement of FVC (<10 mL/kg or <1 L) helps in decisions regarding elective airway intubation and mechanical ventilation. Alternatively, FVC can be used as one of the criteria for the initiation of spontaneous breathing trials and liberation from mechanical ventilation.

Respiratory Recap

Spirometry

- FVC is the most important indicator of disease progression and need for ventilator support.

Respiratory Recap

Chest Radiography

- Chest radiograph typically shows small lung volume and basilar atelectasis.

Upper airway dysfunction, commonly seen in chronic neuromuscular diseases, may be detected easily by analyzing the flow–volume loop. For example, an inspiratory plateau of the flow waveform is indicative of extrathoracic upper airway obstruction. In patients with Parkinson disease, instability of the upper airway muscles is reflected in sawtoothing of the contour of the flow–volume loop. An abnormal flow–volume loop in patients with neuromuscular disease is both highly sensitive and specific for predicting bulbar dysfunction in these patients.[4]

Radiographic Assessment

In patients with inspiratory muscle weakness, lung volume appears small on chest radiograph because of an elevated bilateral hemidiaphragm. This radiographic picture can be easily dismissed as a poor inspiratory film. The presence of bilateral basal bandlike atelectasis is suggestive of chronic loss of lung volume due to weak respiratory muscles. Unilateral hemidiaphragm paralysis can be easily recognized on routine chest radiograph as an elevated hemidiaphragm on the one side. The elevation of a hemidiaphragm due to paralysis can be confirmed by performing a **sniff test** under fluoroscopy, which may demonstrate a paradoxical upward movement of the affected hemidiaphragm during a rapid sniff maneuver.

Assessment of Respiratory Muscle Function

Maximum Mouth Pressures

Maximum static respiratory pressures, measured at the airway opening during a voluntary contraction against an occluded airway, are the most sensitive tests to assess respiratory muscle dysfunction in patients with moderately advanced neuromuscular disease even in the absence of symptoms and normal ventilatory function.[8] The extent of respiratory muscle weakness can be quantified by measuring $P_{I_{max}}$ and **maximum expiratory pressure (MEP or $P_{E_{max}}$)** that can be generated by the respiratory muscles. Measurement of static mouth pressures is affected by lung volume. $P_{I_{max}}$ is best when measured near residual volume, when the inspiratory muscles are at their optimum precontraction operating length. In contrast, $P_{E_{max}}$ is greatest when measured near total lung capacity, when the inward recoil of the respiratory system and the ability of the expiratory muscles to generate force are greatest. **Table 43-3** shows normal

TABLE 43-3
Selected Normal Maximum Static Airway Pressure Values in Adults

Study	Sex	$P_{I_{max}}$ (cm H_2O)	$P_{E_{max}}$ (cm H_2O)
Black LF, Hyatt RE. Maximal static respiratory pressures in generalized neuromuscular disease. *Am Rev Respir Dis.* 1971;103:641–649.	Male Female	−124 ± 22 −87 ± 16	233 ± 42 152 ± 27
Braun NMT, Arora NS, Rochester DF. Respiratory muscle and pulmonary function in polymyositis and other proximal myopathies. *Thorax.* 1983;38:616–623.	Male Female	−127 ± 28 −91 ± 25	216 ± 41 138 ± 39
Vincken W, Ghezzo H, Cosio MG. Maximal static respiratory pressures in adults: normal values and their relationship to determinants of respiratory function. *Bull Eur Physiopathol Respir.* 1987;23(5):435–439.	Male Female	−105 ± 25 −71 ± 23	140 ± 38 89 ± 24

$P_{I_{max}}$, maximum inspiratory pressure; $P_{E_{max}}$, maximum expiratory pressure.

values for maximum static inspiratory and expiratory muscle strength in adults. Reported values vary widely in different studies and may be due to differences in the techniques used or to repeated measurements inducing a learning effect.

In chronic neuromuscular disease, $P_{I_{max}}$ and $P_{E_{max}}$ are frequently decreased and range from 37% to 52% of normal.[6] In patients with proximal myopathies, hypercapnic respiratory failure was likely when the average $P_{I_{max}}$ and $P_{E_{max}}$ values were less than 30% of predicted or vital capacity was less than 55% of predicted.[19] A reduction in $P_{I_{max}}$ and $P_{E_{max}}$ may also be seen in patients with only mild generalized nonrespiratory muscle weakness. In a study of 30 patients with stable chronic neuromuscular weakness, up to 30% of patients with relatively preserved general muscle strength had unsuspected severe respiratory muscle weakness (less than 50% predicted).[17] Measurement of $P_{I_{max}}$ and $P_{E_{max}}$ should be routine in the assessment of respiratory status in patients with neuromuscular disease regardless of the severity of the underlying neurologic disease or absence of respiratory symptoms.

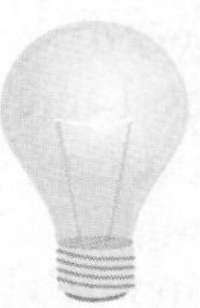

STOP AND THINK

How would you use $P_{I_{max}}$, $P_{E_{max}}$, and FVC to evaluate the respiratory function of a patient with neuromuscular disease?

FVC is also a useful index of global respiratory muscle function. Moreover, it is easy to measure and can be done serially at the bedside to predict impending respiratory failure and the need for ventilatory support. Ventilatory support is often required once FVC is less than 10 to 15 mL/kg or the $P_{I_{max}}$ is greater (i.e., less negative) than −20 to −25 cm H_2O. Mechanical ventilation may be required in select patients above these threshold values in the presence of additional respiratory loads such as occur with pneumonia, atelectasis, or inability to clear secretions. Although measurements of $P_{I_{max}}$, $P_{E_{max}}$, or FVC are useful in quantifying global respiratory muscle strength, they do not distinguish selective weakness of certain respiratory muscle groups.

Maximum Voluntary Ventilation

Maximum voluntary ventilation (MVV) is a commonly performed maneuver in which the subject is asked to breathe in and out as deeply and as fast as he or she can in 15 to 30 seconds. It is a reflection of the global integrity of the respiratory system as a whole. MVV thus decreases with loss of coordination of the respiratory muscles, deformity of the thoracic bellow, neurologic diseases, deconditioning, and ventilatory defects. The MVV is a useful test to assess respiratory muscle endurance. The MVV maneuver is dangerous in patients with myasthenia gravis because it may precipitate acute respiratory failure.

Transdiaphragmatic Pressure Measurement

In contrast to maximum static pressures, which measure global respiratory function, **transdiaphragmatic pressure (Pdi)** specifically measures diaphragm strength. Although transdiaphragmatic pressure measurement is invasive and is not readily available in clinical practice, it may be useful in certain clinical conditions such as phrenic nerve paralysis following cardiac surgery or in cases of idiopathic diaphragm paralysis.

Measurement of diaphragm strength is made by measuring esophageal (Pes) and gastric (Pga) pressures via balloon-tipped catheters placed in the mid-esophagus and in the stomach, respectively. Pdi is then calculated as Pga minus Pes. Several maneuvers with varying degree of difficulty have been used during the measurement of Pdi to obtain maximal voluntary activation of the diaphragm. Pdi obtained during a maximal sniff maneuver (Pdi_{sniff}) is the easiest to perform, whereas Pdi_{max} obtained via a Mueller maneuver combined with active expulsion appears to be the most reproducible and maximal maneuver to measure transdiaphragmatic pressure.[4] Transdiaphragmatic pressure measurement is limited by the need for esophageal and gastric

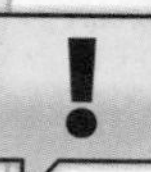

Respiratory Recap

Assessment of Respiratory Muscle Function

- Maximum inspiratory and expiratory pressures, maximum voluntary ventilation, and FVC should be assessed.
- Transdiaphragmatic pressures measure diaphragm muscle strength.
- Serial FVC, PI_{max}, and PE_{max} measurements are useful in predicting impending respiratory failure.

balloon placement, and there is a large variation in measured values (as high as 40%) even in normal individuals. The wide intrasubject variability of Pdi is due to submaximal efforts or activation of the intercostal and accessory muscles, which results in falsely low Pdi values. Direct stimulation of the phrenic nerve (twitch Pdi), by consistently obtaining maximal stimulation of the diaphragm, avoids variability in measured Pdi when only volitional effort is used.

The phrenic nerve is easily stimulated in the neck as it traverses the posterior border of the sternocleidomastoid muscle at the level of the cricoid cartilage. Phrenic nerve stimulation may be performed with either a transcutaneous electrode or a magnetic coil.[20] Care should be taken to ensure supramaximal stimulation as indicated by maximum diaphragm muscle action potential.

A single, unfused twitch contraction of the diaphragm following electrophrenic stimulation is known as Pdi_{twitch}. Pdi_{twitch} is not widely used clinically because of the invasiveness of the procedure and the large coefficient of variation reported in some studies measuring Pdi during volitional efforts. In a study involving 10 patients with diaphragm weakness and 20 normal subjects as controls, there was a large overlap in Pdi_{twitch} between patients with diaphragm weakness (3–27 cm H_2O) and control subjects (9–33 cm H_2O).[21] The Pdi_{twitch} was only consistently decreased when diaphragm weakness was severe. The appropriate role of electrophrenic stimulation in the assessment of respiratory muscle weakness is unclear; currently, it is considered a research tool until further information becomes available.

Upper Motor Neuron Disorders

Stroke

Stroke following an embolic or thrombotic vascular event is one of the major causes of morbidity and mortality in developed countries. Due to the neuroanatomic and functional organization of the brain, different stroke syndromes have a predictable effect on the respiratory system that can be clinically recognized. For example, an acute hemispheric stroke may lead to loss of upper airway function and Cheyne-Stokes breathing, whereas a small stroke in the dorsolateral area of the medulla will lead to sudden death due to respiratory arrest. The pulmonary consequences of the different stroke syndromes include loss of upper airway function, abnormal breathing patterns, decreased diaphragmatic excursion, and loss of automatic or voluntary control of breathing.

Respiratory Recap

Stroke

- Cheyne-Stokes breathing is seen in cortical stroke.
- Swallowing incoordination due to upper airway dysfunction is common.

Upper airway dysfunction resulting in swallowing dyscoordination is a common finding following stroke. This frequently leads to aspiration of oropharyngeal contents, resulting in aspiration pneumonia. Different abnormal breathing patterns may be observed following an acute hemispheric stroke or in rostrocaudal loss of brain stem function, as in brain herniation due to elevated intracerebral pressure. Hemispheric stroke often results in **Cheyne-Stokes breathing**, which is a breathing pattern characteristically described as cyclical hyperpnea and hypopnea often terminating in apnea. Cheyne-Stokes breathing is thought to be due to increased responsiveness to carbon dioxide as a result of interruption of normal cortical inhibition. Brain stem stroke located in the midbrain may lead to central neurogenic hyperventilation, whereas apneustic and ataxic breathing may be seen following injury to the pontomedullary area of the brain stem. After an acute hemispheric stroke, voluntary contraction of the respiratory muscles is reduced on the side of hemiparesis as shown by electromyographic (EMG) activity of the diaphragm and intercostal muscles.

Respiration is under both voluntary and automatic control. The loss of automatic control of respiration (Ondine's curse) occurs following injury to the descending reticulospinal tract in the pons or the nucleus of the vagus, ambiguus, and para-ambiguus. The most common stroke syndrome associated with Ondine's curse is unilateral lateromedullary infarction.[22] A midpontine lesion, which results in the locked-in syndrome, may lead to a loss in the voluntary control of breathing.

Spinal Cord Injury

The degree of respiratory impairment and the need for chronic ventilator support depend on the level and extent of the spinal cord injury. Following traumatic injury to the spinal cord, paresis or paralysis can be easily elicited at or below the level of spinal injury. High cervical cord injury above the origin of the phrenic

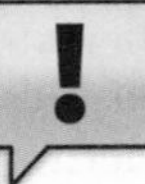

Respiratory Recap

Spinal Cord Injury

- High cervical injury or injury of the phrenic nerve roots (C3 through C5) requires chronic respiratory support.
- Low cervical injury leads to ineffective cough and atelectasis.

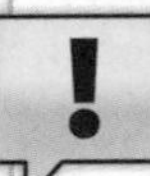

Respiratory Recap

Tetraplegia

- FVC increases in the supine position in patients with tetraplegia because the diaphragm is at its optimal operating length.
- In low cervical injury, training of the clavicular portion of the pectoralis major muscle may improve cough in some patients.

nerve (C1 through C3) leads to paralysis of all the major respiratory muscles except the accessory and bulbar muscles. All patients with high cervical injury invariably require chronic ventilator support. Injury at the level of the phrenic nerve roots (C3 through C5) results in weakness or total paralysis of the diaphragm, requiring continuous ventilatory support. Lower cervical cord injury below the origin of the phrenic nerve (C5 through C6) causes paralysis of the intercostal and abdominal muscles, but because diaphragm function remains intact, the need for long-term ventilator support is obviated. These patients often require ventilatory support in the acute setting. The requirement for chronic ventilatory support thus depends on the level of spinal injury, the ability of the accessory muscles to support ventilation, and the response to strengthening deconditioned muscles.

The effect of the level of spinal cord injury on the mechanical properties of the respiratory system is the same as in patients with chronic neuromuscular disease. Among the changes that may be seen in the respiratory system are a reduction in inspiratory muscle strength to 60% of predicted; a 20% to 30% reduction in both lung and chest wall compliance; and a 50% to 80% reduction in predicted vital capacity, with total lung capacity also moderately reduced.[23] The reduction in lung and chest wall compliance can be observed as early as the first week of injury and usually reaches its nadir by the first month after injury. The reduction in lung compliance may be partly explained by the presence of small lung volumes due to airway closure and atelectasis. On the other hand, the reduction in chest wall compliance is thought to be due to stiffness and ankylosis of the rib cage due to a rapid, shallow breathing pattern and limited chest wall excursion.

In patients with **tetraplegia**, there is a paradoxical increase in FVC measured in the supine compared with the seated position that occurs without a significant increase in total lung capacity. The increase in FVC observed during the supine position is due to cephalad displacement of the end-expiratory position of the diaphragm as a result of gravitational effects on the abdominal visceral organs. The overall effect of these changes is to enable the diaphragm to operate on an optimal portion of its length–tension curve. Alternatively, the increase in FVC in the supine position may be due to a decrease in residual volume because total lung capacity is slightly decreased or unchanged. It has been shown that RV decreases in the supine position by 30% to 38% of seated values in both tetraplegics and paraplegics.[24] The decrease in RV was due to paralysis of the abdominal muscles and the effect of gravity on the abdominal contents. Furthermore, the decrease in RV was not related to an abnormal increase in intrathoracic blood volume as a result of gravitationally induced fluid shifts.[24]

In tetraplegic patients with relatively intact diaphragm function, paradoxical inward motion of the upper rib cage during inspiration occurs due to parasternal and scalene muscle weakness. This abnormal pattern of breathing is even more marked in the supine position than when the subject is seated. In high tetraplegic patients (above C3 through C5), short periods of spontaneous respiration are possible because of contraction of the sternocleidomastoid and trapezius muscles. Analysis of rib cage motion in these patients shows an increase in upper rib cage diameter due to the action of the neck accessory muscles in pulling the sternum cranially and expanding the upper rib cage.

It was previously believed that all of the expiratory muscles were paralyzed in low cervical cord injury. As a result, both cough and other expiratory maneuvers would be passive and solely rely on chest wall elastic recoil. An ineffective cough leads to mucus retention, atelectasis, and pneumonia. Pneumonia is the leading cause of death in this subset of neurologically impaired patients.

EMG activity of the clavicular portion of the pectoralis major is present during voluntary expiration and cough in patients with traumatic low cervical cord injury.[25] Contraction of the clavicular portion of the pectoralis major decreases upper rib cage diameter during cough and could decrease expiratory reserve volume by 60% with the shoulders maintained in abduction. These findings suggest that an active cough can be generated by the clavicular portion of the pectoralis muscles in some tetraplegic patients. Abdominal binding with nonelastic straps to minimize dissipation of intrathoracic forces and training of the clavicular portion of the pectoralis muscle could further improve the effectiveness of cough in tetraplegic patients. Furthermore, 6 weeks of isometric training of the pectoralis muscle increases maximum pectoralis muscle isometric strength and thereby improves cough effectiveness.[26]

Parkinson Disease

Parkinson disease was first described by James Parkinson in 1817 as a symptom complex of cogwheel rigidity, resting tremors, bradykinesia, shuffling gait, and postural instability. The disease affects about 1% of the population older than 50 years and has a disease prevalence of 200 cases per 100,000 individuals. Parkinsonism may be categorized as primary (i.e., idiopathic) or secondary due a variety of causes such as viral encephalitis and drugs. The pathologic findings in primary and secondary parkinsonism are the same and are characterized by the degeneration of pigmented neurons in the substantia nigra, resulting in disruptions of dopaminergic neural pathways.

Ventilatory failure, upper airway obstruction, and aspiration can complicate the clinical course of patients with Parkinson disease. Central alveolar hypoventilation is one of the cardinal features of Parkinsonism associated with Perry syndrome, a rare autosomal dominant parkinsonism. The hypoventilation is thought to be due to neuronal loss in the ventral respiratory group in the ventrolateral medulla, which is critical in the generation of normal respiratory rhythm.[27] Laryngeal somatosensory deficits are common in Parkinson's disease affecting fine motor coordination of the laryngeal muscles and thus speech.[28] Respiratory infection is the most common cause of death in these patients. Both obstructive and restrictive ventilatory patterns have been noted on pulmonary function testing, with about one-third of patients with Parkinson disease having an obstructive ventilatory defect. Both peak inspiratory and expiratory flows are reduced, which may be related to upper airway dysfunction. A concomitant restrictive ventilatory defect appears to be due to weakness and stiffness of the respiratory muscles.

Respiratory muscle dysfunction is common in patients with Parkinson disease.[29] This is usually manifested as either a decrease in respiratory muscle strength or poor coordination, especially when performing repetitive ventilatory tasks similar to what is observed in the limb muscles. Both maximum static inspiratory and expiratory pressures are reduced in Parkinson disease. Poor muscle control, as manifested by difficulty in performing repetitive inspiratory resistive efforts, may be seen even in patients with normal pulmonary function results and respiratory muscle strength. In addition, the performance of this maneuver was associated with a higher oxygen cost of breathing and reduced efficiency of breathing.[30]

Upper airway muscle dysfunction is most likely the cause of the obstructive ventilatory pattern in patients with extrapyramidal disorders. Either regular (type A) or irregular (type B) flow oscillations may be present on the inspiratory and expiratory flow–volume loops (**Figure 43-9**). Oscillations on the flow–volume loop were due to upper airway muscle dyskinesia, which was confirmed by direct endoscopic evaluation. Some patients showed frank intermittent airway closure that caused signs and symptoms of upper airway obstruction. A reduction in FEV_1 should alert the clinician to the possibility of upper airway muscle dysfunction in patients with Parkinsonism. There may be improvement in upper airway obstruction after levodopa

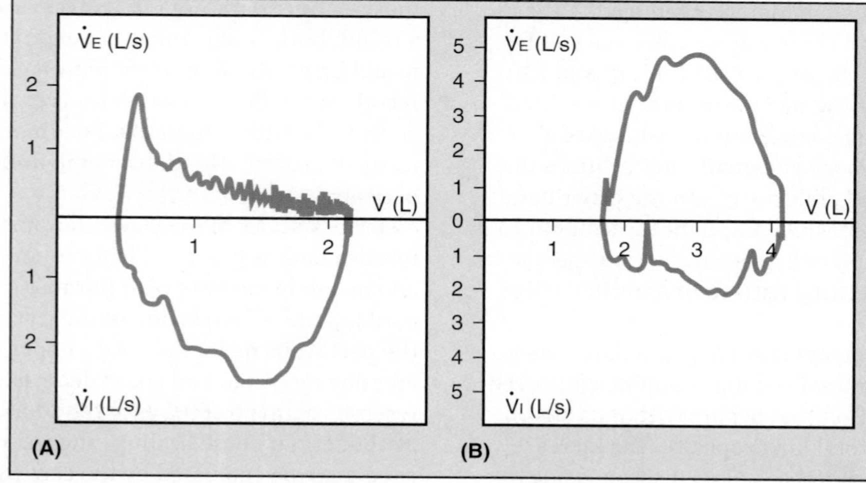

FIGURE 43-9 Two types of abnormal flow–volume loops in patients with extrapyramidal disorders. (**A**) Type A flow–volume loop is characterized by respiratory flutter, a regular consecutive flow deceleration and acceleration representing alternating abduction and adduction of the glottic opening. (**B**) Type B flow–volume loop is characterized by grossly abnormal pattern with abrupt changes in flow indicating intermittent upper airway obstruction due to irregular jerky movements of the glottic structures. V̇E, expiratory flow; V̇I, inspiratory flow.

Reproduced from Vincken WG, et al. Involvement of upper airway muscles in extrapyramidal disorders: a cause of airflow limitation. *N Engl J Med.* 1984;311:438–442. © 1984 Massachusetts Medical Society. Reprinted with permission from Massachusetts Medical Society.

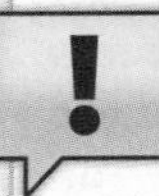

Respiratory Recap

Parkinson Disease

- Respiratory muscle dysfunction either due to weakness or incoordination is common.
- An obstructive ventilatory pattern is often caused by upper airway dysfunction.

therapy in a patient with Parkinson disease.[31] Levodopa therapy may uncommonly induce respiratory dyskinesia, however, which may be managed by decreasing the dose of the medication or using dopamine antagonists.

Patients with Parkinson disease often complain of dyspnea and chronic tachypnea. The abnormal ventilatory pattern discussed earlier improves with levodopa treatment[31] and returns to baseline once therapy is stopped. A modest improvement in FEV_1, FVC, and peak expiratory flow rate has been reported after 1 week of levodopa therapy in 9 of 10 patients with Parkinson disease.[32] Four patients continued to have small, sustained improvements in expiratory flow after 2 weeks of therapy. Patients who did not respond to levodopa therapy did not show an improvement in ventilatory function.

Medications commonly used in the treatment of Parkinson disease can cause pulmonary complications. Levodopa has been reported to cause dyspnea and respiratory distress, presumably due to respiratory muscle dyskinesia. Ergot derivatives such as bromocriptine can cause pleural effusion, pleural thickening, or pulmonary infiltrates.

Multiple Sclerosis

Multiple sclerosis (MS) is a demyelinating disease of the central nervous system clinically characterized by repeated remissions and exacerbations of symptoms. Multiple sclerosis is the most common neurologic disease affecting young adults, with an estimated 350,000 to 400,000 cases in the United States. The exact etiology of the disease remains elusive, although epidemiologic evidence points to both genetic and environmental factors. Classic clinical symptoms include paresthesias, motor weakness, diplopia, blurred vision, bladder incontinence, and ataxia. Symptoms are typically aggravated by an increase in temperature, which causes conduction block in partially demyelinated fibers. The disease may demonstrate remissions and relapses or follow a chronic progressive course. Pathologically, lesions or plaques have a predilection to involve the periventricular white matter of the cerebral hemisphere, the optic nerve, the brain stem, and the cervical spinal cord. Because multiple sclerosis can cause focal lesions anywhere in the central nervous system, different patterns of respiratory impairment can occur. Involvement of the respiratory centers in the medulla can affect either the voluntary or automatic breathing (Ondine's curse) and produce apneustic breathing, paroxysmal hyperventilation, obstructive sleep apnea, or neurogenic pulmonary edema. The three most common patterns of respiratory involvement in multiple sclerosis include respiratory muscle weakness, bulbar dysfunction, and abnormalities in respiratory control.[33]

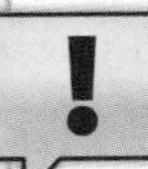

Respiratory Recap

Multiple Sclerosis

- Demyelination of the central nervous system can affect the respiratory center in the medulla and nerve innervation to the bulbar and respiratory muscles.
- Pulmonary impairment depends on the severity of the disease and the functional capacity of the patient.

Acute respiratory failure is rarely encountered in MS but can occur due to severe demyelination of the cervical cord.[34] Diaphragmatic paralysis resulting in respiratory insufficiency has also been reported.[35] More commonly respiratory failure presents insidiously, affecting only those with advanced MS. Even with severe disability and impaired respiratory muscle function, patients with multiple sclerosis seldom complain of dyspnea. The paucity of respiratory complaints may be due to restricted motor activities and greater expiratory than inspiratory muscle weakness. Clinical signs that may be helpful in predicting respiratory muscle involvement are a weak cough and the inability to clear secretions, a limited ability to count on a single exhalation, and the presence of upper extremity weakness.

Expiratory muscles appear to be more frequently involved than the inspiratory muscles in MS patients. FVC, MMV, and PE_{max} are normal in ambulatory MS patients but are severely reduced (39%, 32%, and 36%, respectively) in bedridden patients.[36] Pulmonary dysfunction depends to a large extent on the severity of the disease and the functional capacity of the patient. Those patients who were wheelchair-bound with upper extremity involvement also showed moderate reductions in FVC, MVV, and PE_{max}. In addition, patients with quadriplegia and prominent bulbar muscle involvement were at high risk for acute respiratory failure.

Close respiratory monitoring is required in these patients. Arterial blood gas results are frequently normal even with abnormal respiratory muscle function. Advanced multiple sclerosis is frequently complicated by aspiration, atelectasis, and pneumonia.

Treatment of multiple sclerosis includes adrenocorticotropic hormone (ACTH), high-dose corticosteroids, immunosuppressive agents such as cyclophosphamide and azathioprine, intravenous immunoglobulin therapy, and plasmapheresis. ACTH and prednisone have been shown to hasten the resolution of clinical symptoms in controlled studies.[37] Methylprednisolone 1 g daily for 5 days with or without prednisone taper may be helpful in MS patients with severe respiratory complications. Plasmapheresis has been shown to improve clinical symptoms in patients with severe acute exacerbation and in the relapsing/remitting variety of MS with acute exacerbation.[38] Intravenous immunoglobulin might be beneficial in patients with quadriplegia and respiratory failure following an attack of MS.

Both positive and negative noninvasive pressure ventilation have been successfully used in MS patients with intact bulbar function.[39,40] In the presence of bulbar dysfunction and respiratory failure, tracheotomy and positive pressure ventilation are usually required.

Lower Motor Neuron Disorders

Amyotrophic Lateral Sclerosis

Amyotrophic lateral sclerosis (ALS) is a progressive neurodegenerative disorder of both upper and lower motor neurons leading to a loss of skeletal muscle strength, including respiratory muscles. The incidence of ALS is 1 to 2 cases per 100,000 people. Males are more commonly affected than females, with a ratio of 2:1 involvement. The majority of ALS cases are sporadic (classic ALS), but 5% to 10% of cases are due to an autosomal dominant inheritance (familial ALS). Death is usually due to progressive respiratory failure and repeated respiratory infections. Approximately 80% of ALS patients die within 5 years of initial diagnosis.

The exact etiology of ALS is unknown. A genetic mutation encoding copper-zinc superoxide dismutase, a free oxygen radical scavenger, has been identified in 10% to 15% of familial ALS patients, thus suggesting a susceptibility of the neurons to oxidative stress. Evidence suggests that the motor neurons are susceptible to glutamate-induced neurotoxicity. Glutamate is the principal excitatory brain neurotransmitter. A decreased uptake of glutamate may lead to overstimulation of the glutamate receptors, leading to an increase in intracellular calcium, which then triggers proteolytic enzymes, causing cell membrane injury.

The usual clinical presentation in two-thirds of ALS patients is progressive weakness of the distal extremities, although early involvement of the bulbar muscles occurs in 25% of cases. Acute respiratory failure[41] and nocturnal hypoventilation[42] have been described as initial presentations of ALS. Early involvement of the phrenic nerve neurons within the cervical cord is implicated in this type of presentation.

Although respiratory muscle impairment is usually only evident in advanced stages of the disease, abnormalities in pulmonary function tests are apparent even in patients with mild weakness of the extremities. Serial lung function studies in ALS patients who die show progressive reductions in FVC and MVV, as well as progressive increases in RV compared with patients who survive. In ALS patients who are dyspneic but with relatively preserved pulmonary function tests, $P_{I_{max}}$ and $P_{E_{max}}$ are frequently abnormal.[43] $P_{I_{max}}$ greater (i.e., less negative) than −60 cm H_2O is 100% sensitive for predicting survival of less than 18 months. FVC is the most specific test for predicting survival.

Flow–volume curve shape may identify a subset of patients with greater expiratory muscle weakness. In patients with severe weakness of the expiratory muscles, the flow–volume loop will show a concavity of the maximal expiratory curve, with a sharp drop-off in flow at lower lung volumes. This group of ALS patients exhibits lowers maximal expiratory pressures, smaller vital capacities, and higher residual volumes compared with patients with more normal flow–volume loop contours.[43] Upper airway dysfunction may be detected by oscillations of the flow–volume loop or by direct laryngoscopy. As the disease advances, FVC is reduced and RV is elevated; however, in contrast to other chronic neuromuscular diseases, TLC and FRC are relatively well preserved. These changes are due to earlier involvement of the abdominal muscles with preservation of intercostal and diaphragm function. Weakness of the abdominal muscles causes a reduction in $P_{E_{max}}$ and an increase in RV. In addition, spasticity of the intercostal muscles may attenuate the stiffness of the chest wall, thus preserving lung volumes. Expiratory muscle weakness is often associated with inspiratory muscle weakness. Adequate oxygenation is usually well maintained even with severe deterioration in spirometry. Arterial blood gas monitoring is not useful in early disease. Spirometry, however, is still important in the initial evaluation of patients with ALS because impairment in ventilatory function is frequently underestimated even by experienced examiners.

Phrenic nerve stimulation to assess the diaphragm motor pool has been shown to be an independent predictor of mortality for both spinal- and bulbar-onset ALS patients. The motor response from phrenic nerve stimulation is reported as mean phrenic nerve

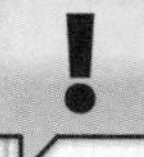

Respiratory Recap

Amyotrophic Lateral Sclerosis

- Progressive weakness of the distal extremities is the most common presentation, but bulbar muscle weakness occurs in one-fourth of patients.
- Serial FVC values and measurements of respiratory muscle strength are useful guides as to when to initiate NIV.
- NIV improves gas exchange and quality of life and decreases mortality.

amplitude and represents the number of excitable motor units in the diaphragm. A small motor unit response following phrenic nerve stimulation suggests impending respiratory failure and warrants full comprehensive respiratory evaluation and need for early ventilatory support.[44,45]

The comprehensive management of ALS patients should include measures to alleviate symptoms, ventilatory support in moderately advanced disease and specific drug therapy to alter the progressive clinical course. Riluzole, an antiglutamate drug, is approved by the Food and Drug Administration (FDA) for treatment of ALS. Riluzole is the only treatment that has been shown to prolong survival in ALS and should be prescribed once a diagnosis of ALS is made.

Despite optimal medical therapy, disease progression invariably occurs, resulting in respiratory insufficiency that requires some form of ventilatory assistance. The onset of respiratory failure often signals a rapid decline in global as well as functional status. The need for mechanical ventilation should be discussed with the patient and family early on to prevent rapid decline in lung function. In a survey of ALS patients, the majority of patients considered mechanical ventilation during the early phase of their disease but eventually declined artificial ventilation as the disease progressed.[46]

In ALS patients who develop respiratory symptoms or have moderate or rapid reductions in lung function, noninvasive forms of ventilation (NIV) should be considered. In patients who can tolerate nasal noninvasive pressure ventilation, the risk of death is decreased by a factor of 3.[18] In one study, 122 patients with ALS were offered NIV once they developed dyspnea or an FVC less than 50% predicted or a fall of more than 15% in FVC in 3 months' follow-up.[47] Those patients who used NIV more than 4 hours per day not only showed a slower decline in lung function but also decreased mortality.

A randomized, controlled trial assessed the effect of NIV versus standard care on survival and quality of life in patients with ALS. Patients were clinically followed every 2 months and were randomly assigned to noninvasive ventilation or standard care when they developed orthopnea with a PI_{max} less than 60% predicted or the presence of hypercarbia. NIV improved survival and quality of life in patients with no bulbar or with moderate bulbar symptoms compared to the best supportive care.[47] In patients with severe bulbar symptoms, NIV improved only the quality of life.

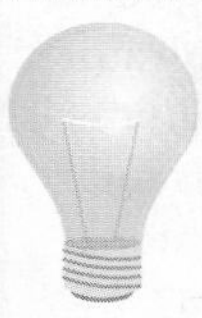

STOP AND THINK

How can a respiratory therapist help in the care of a patient with ALS?

In the intensive care unit (ICU) setting, NIV should be tried first in ALS patients who experience acute or chronic respiratory insufficiency, especially in the absence of significant bulbar symptoms. Patients with significant bulbar symptoms usually cannot tolerate NIV because of difficulty handling oral secretions. Some patients with acute respiratory decompensation may have a partial improvement in respiratory muscle strength after a period of ventilatory assistance.

Diaphragmatic pacing, a technique developed for quadriplegic patients with high cervical cord injury, can be a treatment option for respiratory insufficiency in ALS patients.[48,49] In a pilot study of 16 ALS patients with moderate respiratory muscle weakness (FVC 65%), diaphragmatic pacing increased diaphragm thickness resulting in qualitative improvement in diaphragmatic excursion on maximal voluntary diaphragm excursion, a slower rate of decline in FVC, improvement in the degree of hypercarbia, and improved survival. There was no significant improvement in maximal inspiratory pressures. This was thought to be due to difficulty in performing maximal inspiratory pressures in patients with bulbar involvement.[48] Diaphragmatic pacing is thought to maintain conditioning of the diaphragm and delay the onset of ventilator-dependent respiratory failure. Long-term follow-up showed no safety issues. The FDA has approved the use of diaphragmatic pacing under humanitarian device exemption for orphan diseases.

Poliomyelitis and Postpoliomyelitis

Poliomyelitis was the most common cause of respiratory failure in the early part of the twentieth century, before the advent of the widespread use of the oral polio vaccine. Acute poliomyelitis is now rare in the United States, and recent cases of poliomyelitis are due to exposure to oral polio vaccine and unimmunized individuals. Although most cases of acute polio infections are nonparalytic, as many as 25% of cases are the paralytic form of poliomyelitis that leads to respiratory muscle weakness requiring assisted ventilation. In most cases, respiratory muscle function improves after the acute episode so that assisted ventilation is no longer required. Progressive muscle weakness may occur years later.

Postpoliomyelitis syndrome is recognized as a progressive muscle weakness occurring on average 29 years after recovery from an acute episode of poliomyelitis. Approximately 20% to 60% of poliomyelitis survivors will develop postpoliomyelitis syndrome, with a mean age of onset of 51 years. These patients may complain of dyspnea, exercise intolerance, sleep-related symptoms such as daytime hypersomnolence and morning headaches, and muscle weakness. Muscles that were previously involved are primarily involved in this syndrome, although other muscle groups may also be affected due to previous subclinical involvement.[50]

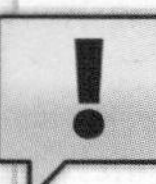

Respiratory Recap

Postpoliomyelitis Syndrome

- Respiratory muscle weakness recurs about 30 years after recovery from acute poliomyelitis.
- Sleep-disordered breathing, both obstructive and central, is common.
- NIV is effective in the reversal of sleep-associated breathing dysfunction.

Several theories have been proposed to explain the pathogenesis of postpoliomyelitis syndrome, including susceptibility to aging of reinnervated motor units, chronic compensatory overuse of damaged muscle fiber, and immune-mediated attack on the abnormal motor units, but the basic pathophysiology appears to be denervation and aberrant reinnervation of motor units.[50–52]

Postpoliomyelitis syndrome often presents insidiously as chronic respiratory failure secondary to respiratory muscle weakness. Serial monitoring of FEV_1, FVC, PI_{max}, and PE_{max} may be helpful in predicting which subset of patients with a prior history of polio develop chronic respiratory failure.[53] The average yearly decline in FVC has been estimated at 18.6 mL/year, or 1.9%. Once the VC is less than 1 L, assisted ventilation is often required. NIV is effective in reversing chronic hypoventilation and its associated symptoms.[54] Nocturnal NIV may also improve respiratory muscle strength and exercise capacity.[55]

Sleep-related breathing disorders are common in patients with postpoliomyelitis syndrome,[56] even in patients who are already on nocturnal ventilatory support. Hypersomnolence was the most common presenting symptom in one review, present in 32 of 35 patients with postpoliomyelitis. The most frequently identified sleep-related breathing disorders were obstructive sleep apnea (19 of 35), hypoventilation (7 of 35), and mixed apnea and hypopnea (9 of 35). Patients with bulbar dysfunction have a greater frequency of sleep apnea compared with those with intact bulbar muscle function. Detailed questioning concerning sleep-related symptoms during initial evaluation helps select those patients with postpoliomyelitis syndrome who may benefit from a formal sleep study evaluation. Even patients who are already on nocturnal assisted ventilation may benefit from a sleep study, especially if they have daytime hypersomnolence, fatigue, and morning headache.

Postpoliomyelitis syndrome may also present as recurrent aspiration due to upper airway muscle weakness and vocal cord paralysis.[57] Asymmetric involvement of the thoracic muscles may lead to kyphoscoliosis and may further compromise respiratory muscle function. Central hypoventilation due to involvement of the brain stem's respiratory center has been reported.[58]

Disorders of the Peripheral Nerves

Phrenic Nerve Injury

Unilateral or bilateral diaphragm paralysis can occur following phrenic nerve injury. Phrenic nerve injury may be seen following cardiac surgery, trauma, mediastinal tumors, pleural space infection, or forceful neck manipulation. Phrenic nerve injury during cardiac surgery is due either to cold exposure or mechanical stretching of the nerve during surgery.[59,60] Diaphragm paralysis may also be seen with motor neuron disease, myelopathies, neuropathies, and myopathies. The majority of cases of diaphragm weakness are idiopathic.

Dyspnea is the main complaint of patients with bilateral diaphragm weakness, especially when lying down, during exertion and when wading in waist-deep water. Cranial displacement of the diaphragm by the abdominal visceral contents in the supine position can further impair the pump function of an already weakened diaphragm. Unexplained severe orthopnea and thoracoabdominal paradoxical breathing, especially in the supine position, thus are clinical clues to the presence of diaphragm dysfunction. Unilateral diaphragm weakness is usually well tolerated by patients even when the FVC and TLC are mildly reduced. In asymptomatic patients, it is often discovered incidentally on chest radiograph as elevated hemidiaphragm. In patients who have significant comorbid conditions such as obesity, parenchymal lung diseases such as COPD or concomitant heart failure, or the presence of weakness of other respiratory muscle groups, unilateral diaphragm paralysis can also result in dyspnea on exertion and limited exercise capacity.

Bilateral diaphragm paralysis usually is identified as a restrictive ventilatory defect on pulmonary function testing. The vital capacity is typically reduced to less than 50% of predicted in the erect posture with further decline in supine vital capacity by 30 to 50%.[61,62] In comparison, the vital capacity is usually >70% in patients with unilateral diaphragm paralysis with less decline in vital capacity in the supine position (10 to 30%).[63] The absence of significant decline in supine vital capacity essentially makes diaphragm dysfunction an unlikely explanation for the patient's dyspnea.

Because the diaphragm is a major respiratory muscle, there is a significant decreased in maximal static inspiratory pressure in bilateral (30% of predicted) and to a lesser extent in unilateral diaphragm paralysis (60%). In isolated diaphragm weakness or paralysis, the maximal expiratory pressure is usually preserved or mildly reduced (70%) due to impaired expiratory muscle function as a consequence of reduced total lung capacity. If both maximum static inspiratory and expiratory pressure are equally decreased, diaphragm weakness is likely due to generalized conditions such as muscular dystrophy involving both inspiratory and expiratory muscles and critical illness myopolyneuropathy.[64]

The chest radiograph typically shows either a unilateral or bilateral elevated hemidiaphragm associated with subsegmental atelectasis. Chest radiograph is a good screening tool for unilateral diaphragm paralysis with good sensitivity (90%) but low specificity (44%).[65] The low specificity is due to parenchymal and pleural diseases such as atelectasis, pulmonary fibrosis, or subpulmonic fluid collections. These may mimic the radiographic picture of diaphragm paralysis, making the diagnosis difficult and frequently delayed.

Fluoroscopy can confirm diaphragmatic weakness or paralysis. The diaphragm is viewed under fluoroscopy while the patient performs a sniff maneuver (sniff test). The rapid increase in intrapleural pressure during the sniff maneuver will cause a paradoxical cephalad movement of the weak hemidiaphragm. Fluoroscopy is not useful in bilateral diaphragm weakness because both hemidiaphragms may descend normally during a sniff maneuver despite profound weakness due to sudden relaxation of the abdominal muscles at the onset of inspiration. The sniff test should be interpreted with caution because paradoxical movement can be seen in up to 6% of normal individuals. The paradoxical movement should be at least 2 cm to increase the specificity of the test.

Ultrasound examination of the diaphragm has been reported to be useful in assessing diaphragm contractile function.[64] This technique has the advantage of being rapid, easy to use, noninvasive, and without radiation exposure. The ultrasound probe is placed in the zone of apposition of the diaphragm with the rib cage to measure change in diaphragm thickness during inspiration. Thickening of the diaphragm during inspiration signifies normal diaphragmatic contractility, and lack of thickening during inspiration is diagnostic of diaphragmatic paralysis. If the thickness of the diaphragm is >2 mm with >20% thickening with inspiration, this essentially rules out clinically significant diaphragmatic paralysis.

Electromyography of the diaphragm can also be used to diagnose diaphragm weakness or paralysis. It is limited by fidelity of the electromyographic signal that may be affected by accuracy of electrode placement, subcutaneous fat, and electromyographic signal from other muscle groups. It is useful in differentiating between neuropathic or myopathic causes of diaphragm dysfunction.

> **Respiratory Recap**
>
> **Phrenic Nerve Injury**
>
> - Injury can lead to unilateral or bilateral diaphragm paralysis.
> - Severe orthopnea and abdominal rib cage paradox are clues to the diagnosis.
> - Chest radiograph shows elevated hemidiaphragm (unilateral) or small lung volume (bilateral).
> - Either fluoroscopy (sniff test) or ultrasound is a useful test to diagnose diaphragm paralysis.

In patients with mild diaphragm weakness, both pulmonary function tests and radiographic examinations may be reported as normal. In this case, measurement of transdiaphragmatic pressure (Pdi), with all of the limitations discussed earlier in mind (i.e., intersubject variability, invasive procedure, and the need for full patient cooperation), is useful in the diagnosis and quantification of diaphragm weakness. If the maximum transdiaphragmatic pressure (Pdi_{sniff} or Pdi_{max}) is greater than 80 cm of water in men and greater than 70 cm of water in women, clinically significant diaphragmatic weakness is ruled out.[62] Total diaphragm paralysis is diagnosed when there is no pressure difference across the two sides of the diaphragm (Pdi) during forceful inspiratory maneuvers against an occluded airway.

Sleep may worsen ventilatory failure in patients with bilateral diaphragm paralysis because of a loss of respiratory accessory muscle activity during REM sleep. Significant nocturnal hypoventilation or daytime hypercapnia was not present in a small study of six patients with isolated bilateral diaphragm paralysis.[61]

Recovery from diaphragm weakness depends on the etiology. In phrenic injury after cardiac surgery, 80% of patients will recover nerve function in 6 months, and 90% will recover in 1 year.[66]

Idiopathic diaphragm paralysis or paralysis due to neuralgic amyotrophy may improve spontaneously. In symptomatic patients with persistent diaphragm paralysis, treatment includes nocturnal or continuous ventilatory support depending on the patient's clinical need. It is recommended to initiate nocturnal ventilatory support in the presence of daytime hypercapnia ($Paco_2$ >45 mm Hg) or the presence of nocturnal hypoxemia (<88% for >5 min) and in progressive neuromuscular weakness with PI_{max} greater (i.e., less negative) than −60 cm H_2O or FVC <50%. Patients with progressive neuromuscular weakness, especially with concomitant oropharyngeal weakness, will eventually need invasive mechanical ventilation.

In symptomatic patients with persistent unilateral diaphragm paralysis with no signs of recovery after 12 to 18 months, plication of the diaphragm may be considered. Plication of the diaphragm is a surgical procedure wherein the diaphragm is made taut by over-sewing of the central tendon and the muscular components of the diaphragm. Plication of the diaphragm may lead to 20% improvement in lung volumes and may ameliorate dyspnea. The improvement in lung volumes is thought to be related to immobilization of the diaphragm resulting in less paradoxical motion. Plication is unlikely to be helpful in bilateral diaphragm paralysis, morbid obesity, and progressive neuromuscular weakness. In patients with high cervical injury and intact phrenic nerve, phrenic nerve pacing in carefully selected patients may provide partial ventilatory support.

Guillain-Barré Syndrome

Guillain-Barré syndrome (GBS) is an acute idiopathic polyneuritis that usually presents as an ascending symmetric paralysis of the lower extremities associated with absent tendon reflexes and autonomic dysfunction. The degree of motor weakness is variable, ranging from mild paresis to complete paralysis. Maximum weakness of the lower extremities occurs within 2 weeks in 50% of cases and in 4 weeks in 80%. Facial (60%), ocular (15%), and oropharyngeal (50%) muscles may be involved. The objective findings of sensory loss are variable, occurring in 40% to 70% of patients. Varying degrees of autonomic dysfunction, such as cardiac arrhythmia, blood pressure lability, gastrointestinal dysfunction, pupillary dysfunction, sweating abnormalities, and urinary retention, can occur in as many as 65% of patients. Involvement of the bulbar and respiratory muscles may lead to swallowing dysfunction, increased risk of aspiration, and respiratory failure.[67,68]

Diagnostic criteria for GBS have been reported.[69] Other variants of GBS (e.g., with asymmetric involvement of the extremities, presence of ataxia, or absence of paresthesia) have also been described. In over 70% of cases, the syndrome is preceded by a history of a recent viral or bacterial infection. The diagnosis of GBS is confirmed by abnormal cerebrospinal fluid (CSF) and nerve conduction studies. The CSF examination characteristically shows an increased protein content with a paucity of cells, commonly referred to as albuminocytologic dissociation. Nerve conduction study typically shows multifocal demyelination.

Although the exact etiology of GBS is unknown, several risk factors have been identified that may precipitate the disease. These risk factors include viral illnesses (e.g., cytomegalovirus, Epstein-Barr virus), *Mycoplasma pneumoniae* infection, influenza vaccination, recent surgery, and malignancy (lymphoma). A strong association between antecedent *Campylobacter jejuni* infection and GBS has also been found in 30% of the patients. The current concept suggests that GBS is a self-limited, reactive autoimmune disease in which an aberrant immune response is directed against bacterial lipopolysaccharides that share similar epitopes with the myelin sheath or Schwann cell basement membrane.

Respiratory failure requiring assisted ventilation occurs in 15% to 30% of cases.[70] Once respiratory muscle dysfunction is evident and requires ICU care, up to 62% of patients will require ventilatory assistance. The average duration of mechanical ventilation in two large series was 50 to 55 days.[71,72] Most patients will require tracheostomy because of the need for prolonged mechanical ventilation and to facilitate pulmonary hygiene, although it has been suggested that tracheostomy be delayed up to 10 days to avoid the procedure in patients who rapidly improve.[68]

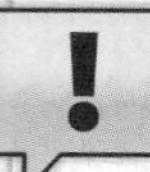

Respiratory Recap

Guillain-Barré Syndrome

- Ascending symmetric paralysis of the lower extremities is a common presentation.
- Acute respiratory failure is a serious complication in one-third of patients.
- Bulbar muscle weakness increases the risk of aspiration and may warrant early intubation.
- Indications for ventilatory support include an FVC less than 12 mL/kg, respiratory distress, inability to handle oral secretions, hypoxemia, and hypercarbia.
- Autonomic dysfunction is common and can cause hemodynamic instability.

A severe reduction in maximum transdiaphragmatic pressures is present during acute ventilatory failure and during recovery from the illness.[71] Among the pulmonary function tests, serial vital capacity measurement is the most useful test in predicting the need for mechanical ventilation. A VC less than 12 to 15 mL/kg is a sign of imminent respiratory failure.[71,72] In patients who developed respiratory failure as a result of Guillain-Barré syndrome, the VC measured serially decreased from a mean of 2.5 L to 0.9 L within 2 weeks. In a study of 81 GBS patients who required mechanical ventilation, the average FVC at the time of intubation was 33% predicted. Other indications for intubation and ventilatory support include respiratory distress, inability to handle oral secretions, hypoxemia (Pa_{O_2} less than 70 mm Hg on room air, or alveolar–arterial P_{O_2} difference of more than 300 mm Hg with F_{IO_2} of 1.0), and hypercapnia. Other predictors of the need for mechanical ventilation include time between onset of disease and hospital admission of less than 7 days, inability to lift the head, presence of bulbar dysfunction, and the presence of anti-GQ1b antibodies.

Neurophysiologic testing is helpful in predicting the need for mechanical ventilation.[70] Of the 154 patients included in this study, patients with the demyelinating form of GBS required mechanical ventilation more

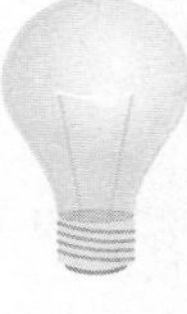

STOP AND THINK

Over 48 hours, the vital capacity of a patient with Guillain-Barré syndrome has progressively decreased to 15% of predicted. What would you recommend regarding the patient's respiratory care needs?

often than patients with axonal or equivocal findings on electrophysiology. The risk of acute respiratory failure was only 2.5% if the proximal/distal compound muscular amplitude potential ratio was greater than 55% and FVC was greater than 80%. It is prudent to initiate early intubation and assisted ventilation to avoid complications that may arise from emergent intubation. Arterial blood gas analysis is used to ensure adequate oxygenation and ventilation. Hypercapnia is a late sign of ventilatory failure. The average Paco_2 at the time of intubation when VC is less than 12 mL/kg was 43 mm Hg in two large series of GBS patients.[70,71]

Upper airway dysfunction due to bulbar involvement may occur in GBS. This may lead to inability to swallow oral secretions, increasing the risk of aspiration. The presence of nasal voice, abnormal gag reflex, dysarthria, and poor mobility of pharyngeal muscles suggests significant bulbar muscle dysfunction. The swallowing mechanism can be roughly assessed at the bedside by asking the patient to drink sips of water and observing for coughing spells. Once significant bulbar dysfunction is observed, early intubation may be necessary to protect the airway even if respiratory muscle strength is still adequate. Delaying intubation might increase the risk of early-onset pneumonia.[68]

Autonomic dysfunction can occur in 65% of patients with GBS. Common manifestations of autonomic dysfunction include labile blood pressure, sinus tachycardia, excessive sweating, urinary retention, and ileus. Autonomic dysfunction is commonly prevalent in patients who require mechanical ventilation and during the progressive and plateau phases of the illness. Particular care should be observed during endotracheal suctioning because it can precipitate tachyarrhythmias and bradyarrhythmias and even asystole from vagal stimulation. Moreover, patients may be overly sensitive to vasoactive medications. Management of severe ileus includes bowel rest and therapeutic trials with erythromycin or neostigmine. The use of promotility agents is contraindicated in patients with dysautonomia.

Aggressive pulmonary toilet is indicated to prevent as well as treat atelectasis. Atelectasis may require repeated bronchoscopy and may decrease the incidence of nosocomial pneumonia. Subcutaneous heparin is preferred for deep venous thrombosis prophylaxis compared with pneumatic boots to avoid prolonged footdrop due to compression of the peroneal nerve. Corticosteroids are not beneficial and may be harmful. Spontaneous breathing trials can be started once VC exceeds 8 to 10 mL/kg, adequate oxygenation can be achieved with an Fio_2 of 0.4 or less, and patients are able to double their minute ventilation.

Immune modulation using either plasma exchange or intravenous immunoglobulin infusion is the mainstay of therapy in GBS. The maximum inspiratory force at the time of successful liberation is more negative than 40 cm H_2O. In multicenter trials, plasmapheresis (250 mL/kg every 2 days for a total of five treatments) using either albumin or fresh frozen plasma as replacement fluid showed short-term benefits in early motor recovery and ambulation, reduced the number of patients who required assisted ventilation, and shortened the duration of mechanical ventilation.[73–75] Immunotherapy should be started within 2 weeks of onset of symptoms or as early as possible. In patients with rapidly deteriorating clinical symptoms, however, plasmapheresis may still offer some benefit even if the duration of the disease is more than 3 weeks. Intravenous immunoglobulin (IVIG) given within 2 weeks of the onset of GBS may be as effective as plasma exchange therapy.[75] In approximately 10% of patients, relapse of neurologic symptoms may follow plasma exchange treatment due to antibody rebound. In such circumstances, additional plasma exchange treatment or IVIG treatment is helpful.

Because IVIG is easier to administer, it is preferred over plasma exchange unless there are specific contraindications to its use, such as low serum immunoglobulin A, presence of uncontrolled hypertension, and a hyperosmolar state. There is no additional benefit conferred by sequential treatment consisting initially of plasmapheresis followed by IVIG when compared with either treatment alone. Corticosteroids alone confer no therapeutic benefit and may slow recovery in GBS; their use is not recommended.[76] The combination of IVIG and intravenous methylprednisolone may hasten recovery, but there has been no documented beneficial effect on long-term outcome.

With the advent of modern ICU care, mortality from Guillain-Barré syndrome dropped from 15% in the 1970s to between 3% and 4% in the 1980s. Common complications are pneumonia, recurrent aspiration, and pulmonary thromboembolic disease. Prognosis for recovery is generally good, but only 15% of patients will have no neurologic residuals. Factors associated with poor prognosis are older age, lower mean compound muscle action potential amplitudes during distal stimulation (less than 20% of normal), need for ventilatory support, and rapid progression to severe weakness in less than 1 week.

Critical Illness Polyneuropathy and Neuromyopathy

Critical illness polyneuromyopathy (CIPNM) presents as flaccid paralysis of both upper and lower extremities and is a common sequela of severe sepsis and multisystem organ failure in both surgical and medical intensive care units. The incidence of CIPNM depends on the severity of illness, the diagnostic criteria used, and the timing of examination from the onset of the critical illness. In prospective studies, 25 to 63% of patients who required mechanical ventilation for at least 7 days developed CIPNM.[77] Patients with sepsis and sepsis syndrome have the highest incidence of CIPNM, approaching 70% to 100%. Axonal polyneuropathy was initially thought to be the main pathologic change in ICU-acquired weakness. EMG and muscle biopsy studies showed that acute myopathy coexists with polyneuropathy, however, and in fact often exists as a separate clinical entity. Four categories of the syndrome are recognized (**Table 43-4**). In a prospective study of 30 patients with critical illness polyneuropathy, biopsy of the quadriceps femoral muscle showed neuropathic changes in 37%, myopathy in 40%, and both neuropathic and myopathic changes in 23% of patients. Muscle necrosis was also present in 30% of the muscle biopsy specimens.[78]

Several risk factors, other than severe sepsis and multisystem organ failure, have been identified in the development of CIPNM. These include prolonged use of corticosteroids and neuromuscular blocking agents, persistent hyperglycemia, hyperosmolality, immobility, use of aminoglycosides, and prolonged mechanical ventilation.[79] Global measures of the severity of critical illness, such as the Acute Physiology, Age, and Chronic Health Evaluation (APACHE) III and the Sequential Organ Failure Assessment Score (SOFA) are also important predictors of the occurrence of CIPNM. Aggressive control of stress-induced hyperglycemia has been reported to decrease the incidence of CIPNM in both surgical and medical ICUs.[80–83] In a prospective, randomized, controlled trial, intensive insulin therapy to maintain normoglycemia (blood glucose levels between 80 and 110 mg/dL) decreased the incidence of critical illness polyneuropathy by 44% compared with conventional insulin therapy (blood glucose level between 180 and 200 mg/dL). The risk of CIPNM was significantly correlated with the mean blood glucose level. In patients who required mechanical ventilatory support for more than 7 days, intensive insulin therapy decreased the duration of mechanical ventilation with an absolute risk reduction of 11.6%. In addition, CIPNM resolved faster in the intensive insulin treatment group compared with the control group, which partially explained the decreased duration of mechanical ventilation.[81] In multivariate analysis, independent predictors of the development of polyneuropathy include conventional insulin treatment and vasopressor support of more than 3 days.

TABLE 43-4
Acute Weakness Syndrome in the Intensive Care Unit

Myopathy	Acute necrotizing myopathy Disuse atrophy
Neuromuscular junction abnormalities	Myasthenia-like syndrome Prolonged neuromuscular blockade
Neuropathy	Critical illness polyneuropathy Acute motor neuropathy
Polyneuromyopathy	Combination of neuropathy and myopathy

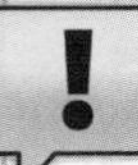

Respiratory Recap

Critical Illness Polyneuromyopathy

- Critical illness polyneuromyopathy is the most common cause of weakness in the ICU.
- Acute ICU myopathy is the most common CIPNM.
- CIPNM is a common cause of failure to liberate from ventilatory support in patients with severe sepsis and multisystem organ failure.
- Quadriparesis in an awake ICU patient following severe sepsis is the usual presentation.
- Control of hyperglycemia can decrease the incidence of CIPNM.

The pathogenesis of CIPNM is not well understood. An exaggerated immune response to severe injury is thought to be the main pathogenic pathway leading to nerve and muscle injury. Both systemic and local inflammatory response mediated by tumor necrosis factor alpha and interleukins 1 and 12 and the recruitment of T helper 1 cells, monocytes, macrophages, and neutrophils lead to endothelial cell injury, increased microvascular permeability, and endoneurial edema resulting in decreased blood flow to the nerve and muscle tissue. The end result of this injury is primary axonal degeneration of the sensory and motor fibers and muscle atrophy with loss of contractile proteins and membrane inexcitability. In animal models, sepsis triggers enhanced muscle protein proteolysis through the ubiquitin-proteasome and calpain system, causing myofibrillar degradation and disruption of the sarcomere. Moreover, animal models of critical illness myopathy reveal altered membrane expression and function of the sodium channels. It has been suggested that critical illness myopathy is not only due to selective myosin loss but also due to muscle fiber membrane electrical inexcitability caused by defective sodium channel regulation.[84,85]

The syndrome is often suspected initially because of failure to liberate from mechanical ventilation as patients recover from their life-threatening illnesses or the presence of new symmetric weakness of both upper and lower extremities. About one-third of these patients have difficulty being liberated from the ventilator, and 70% have evidence of peripheral neuropathy.[86,87] The muscle weakness is most prominent in the lower

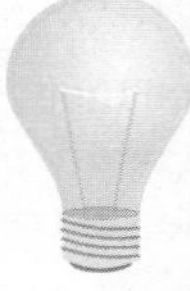

STOP AND THINK

What would you recommend to reduce the risk of critical illness polyneuromyopathy in mechanically ventilated patients?

extremities and is accompanied by muscle wasting and reduced or absent tendon reflexes. Facial muscle weakness, presence of asymmetric weakness of the limbs, or pyramidal signs should prompt further workup to rule out other neurologic causes of weakness. Assessment of peripheral muscle strength can sometimes be difficult in uncooperative patients because of the use of sedative-hypnotic agents or the presence of either delirium or metabolic encephalopathy. Nevertheless, if motor strength assessment is possible, a standardized muscle examination can be used to assess the degree of weakness in individual muscle groups.

The diagnosis of critical care polyneuropathy is supported by nerve conduction and EMG (electroneuromyography, ENMG) studies, which typically show the presence of axonal polyneuropathy with or without the presence of concomitant myopathy. In axonal polyneuropathy, ENMG testing shows a reduction in the amplitude of the compound action potential with normal conduction velocity on motor nerve stimulation, and spontaneous electrical activity on muscle needle recording. This ENMG pattern can be seen in 70% to 100% of ICU patients with severe sepsis and after 5 to 7 days of mechanical ventilation. A myopathic pattern on ENMG is suggested by the presence of a prolonged compound muscle action potential and a short duration and low amplitude of motor unit potentials on voluntary activation. Creatine phosphokinase (CPK) levels are either normal or slightly elevated in CIPNM. Muscle and nerve biopsy can be used to confirm the diagnosis but are not routinely indicated. Muscle biopsy usually shows type II fiber atrophy and occasionally type I atrophy and muscle necrosis. Immunohistochemistry and electron microscopy show a loss of myosin thick filaments. In the right clinical setting, extensive neurologic testing or biopsy of the nerve or muscle is not required to make a confident diagnosis of CIPNM.

The differential diagnosis of muscle weakness in the ICU setting encompasses multiple central nervous system pathologies, including head and spinal cord injury. In acute spinal injury, spinal shock may cause quadriparesis and areflexia mimicking polyneuropathy. Muscle weakness associated with ptosis and bulbar weakness suggests a neuromuscular junction disease such as myasthenia gravis. Axonal variants of Guillain-Barré syndrome are distinguished by the presence of weakness before admission to the ICU, a preceding history of *Campylobacter jejuni* infection, and positive serologic test for anti-GM1 or anti-GD1a antibodies. Prolonged use of neuromuscular blocking agents, especially in the presence of hepatic and renal failure, can lead to persistent neuromuscular blockade due to delayed clearance of the drugs.

Because there is no specific treatment for CIPNM, avoidance of recognized risk factors is important in decreasing the incidence and morbidity and mortality associated with this disease process. Preventive measures include tight blood glucose control, avoidance or minimization of corticosteroids and/or neuromuscular blocking agents, early mobilization and physical therapy, and the institution of a daily interruption of sedation to avoid sedation-related immobilization. Early mobilization in patients on mechanical ventilation improved both short- and long-term functional recovery.[88–90] In a prospective, randomized, blinded trial of physical and occupational therapy implemented at the start of respiratory failure, early mobilization led to improved functional independence at the time of hospital discharge and decreased the duration of mechanical ventilation, decreased delirium, and increased walk distance. Early mobilization is safe even in critically ill patients.[88]

For those patients who survive the acute phase of their injury, CIPNM prolongs the ICU and hospital length of stay, prolongs the duration of mechanical ventilation, and increases mortality. Critical illness neuromyopathy is a predictor of prolonged mechanical ventilation.[91] Clinical recovery of nerve function is often prolonged and is usually associated with residual weakness that causes persistent functional impairment. In a cohort of 100 patients with acute respiratory distress syndrome followed for 1 year, muscle wasting and weakness were the most significant extrapulmonary complications that contributed to persistent functional impairment.[92] The detrimental effect of CIPNM on long-term outcome is best shown by a composite review of 36 studies involving 263 patients. Complete functional recovery occurred in 68% of patients; however, persistent neurologic deficits in the form of absent or reduced deep tendon reflexes, glove and stocking sensory loss, muscle atrophy, painful hyperesthesia, and persistent severe disability due to quadriparesis, quadriplegia, or paraplegia occurred in 28% of patients.[93]

Disorders of the Neuromuscular Junction

Myasthenia Gravis

Myasthenia gravis (MG) is an autoimmune disorder characterized by impaired transmission of neural impulses across the neuromuscular junction due to the destruction of the postsynaptic acetylcholine receptors. It is the most common neuromuscular transmission disorder, with an estimated incidence of 10 to 20 cases per million people and a prevalence of 100 to 200 cases per million. Younger women of childbearing age are affected twice as frequently as men. Thymic tumors are seen in 10% of cases, mostly in older men.

The typical presentation of the myasthenic patient is fluctuating weakness of the involved voluntary muscles that improves with rest or with the administration of anticholinesterase agents (positive Tensilon test) or both. Ocular, facial, and neck muscles are commonly involved. In the generalized form of the disease, variable involvement of bulbar, limb, and respiratory muscles also occurs. Bulbar muscle weakness such as dysarthria, dysphagia, and fatigable chewing is the initial presenting symptom in 15% of cases. Approximately 50% to 60% of patients with the ocular form of the disease progress to generalized weakness involving the oropharyngeal muscles, diaphragm, and other respiratory muscles and limbs within the first 2 years of the onset of symptoms. Respiratory muscle weakness is seen in one-third of patients and may occur in the absence of peripheral muscle weakness. On physical examination, fatigability of the involved muscles can be elicited by asking the patient to do repetitive or sustained muscle activity such as looking upward for several minutes to elicit lid or ocular muscle weakness.

The Tensilon test is a simple test that can be done at the bedside to confirm the diagnosis of myasthenia gravis. Tensilon (edrophonium), a short-acting inhibitor of acetylcholinesterase, can be given intravenously to elicit a transient improvement in muscle weakness. A positive Tensilon test highly suggests myasthenia gravis, but a positive test has also been reported in patients with Lambert-Eaton syndrome, botulism, and ALS. In patients with moderately generalized myasthenia gravis, pulmonary function testing reveals a mild reduction in FVC and a moderate reduction in both inspiratory and expiratory strength, indicating respiratory muscle weakness.

A serologic test may also be used to support the diagnosis of myasthenia gravis. Antibodies to acetylcholine receptors are seen in 80% of patients with generalized myasthenia and 60% of those with ocular myasthenia. The concentration of the acetylcholine receptor antibodies does not correlate with the severity of disease. Acetylcholine receptor antibodies have been found in Lambert-Eaton syndrome and in systemic lupus erythematosus. Studies showed that the presence of anti–muscle specific kinase (anti-MuSK) antibodies identifies a subgroup of patients with myasthenia gravis who have a higher incidence of bulbar weakness (100% vs. 58%) and respiratory failure (46% vs. 7%) compared with seronegative patients.[94] Greater involvement of the respiratory muscles was also reported in patients who tested positive for anti-MuSK.

Electrodiagnostic study is nonspecific for MG but characteristically shows a 10% to 15% decrease in amplitude of the action potential during slow repetitive stimulation in 77% of myasthenic patients. Single-fiber EMG is abnormal in 92% of the patients and is thought to be the most sensitive test, even in patients with a negative serum antibody against acetylcholine receptor or a normal repetitive nerve stimulation test.

Respiratory muscle weakness can occur in the absence of peripheral muscle weakness.[95] Respiratory muscle weakness in MG typically occurs late in the disease process. In patients with moderately generalized MG, performance of pulmonary function tests before the administration of Mestinon reveals mild reduction in FVC and moderate reduction in both maximum static inspiratory (46% of predicted) and expiratory pressures (48% of predicted). There is no evidence of restrictive or obstructive lung disease. Like other chronic neuromuscular diseases, the breathing pattern of patients with MG is rapid and shallow. After Mestinon treatment, FVC, FEV_1, PI_{max}, and PE_{max} show significant improvement, although respiratory muscle strength does not completely normalize. Arterial blood gas examination is unreliable in predicting the severity of respiratory muscle weakness.

Acute respiratory failure usually occurs in the setting of either myasthenic or cholinergic crisis or as the initial presentation of the disease. *Myasthenic crisis* refers to an exacerbation of myasthenia gravis leading to respiratory failure that necessitates the use of mechanical ventilation. This is usually precipitated by discontinuation or decrease in the dosage of anticholinergic medications, surgery (thymectomy), administration of neuromuscular blocking medications (e.g., aminoglycosides, curare-like drugs), or emotional crisis.

Myasthenic crisis can be confirmed by performing Tensilon testing that results in an improvement in muscle strength. Approximately 15% to 20% of patients with myasthenia gravis will experience myasthenic crises, often in the first year of illness. Thymomas are associated with a more fulminant course of MG and are present in one-third of patients who experience myasthenic crises. The initiation of corticosteroid therapy can paradoxically cause a transient increase in muscle weakness during the first and second week of therapy, especially in patients with severe bulbar symptoms and generalized myasthenia gravis.

Cholinergic crisis refers to the worsening of motor weakness due to an excess of anticholinesterase medications, which causes depolarizing blockade at the myoneural junction. This can be diagnosed and

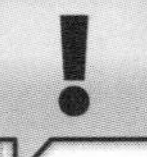

Respiratory Recap

Myasthenia Gravis

- Myasthenia gravis (MG) is an autoimmune disease presenting as fluctuating weakness of ocular, facial, and neck muscles. The muscle weakness improves with anticholinesterase agents.
- In generalized MG, respiratory muscle weakness can lead to acute respiratory failure.
- Both myasthenic crises and cholinergic (due to excess of anticholinesterase medications) crises can lead to acute respiratory failure.
- Surgery can precipitate postoperative respiratory failure.
- Noninvasive ventilation can be helpful in the management of respiratory failure.

differentiated from myasthenic crisis by the presence of muscarinic symptoms such as hypersalivation, sweating, an increase in bronchial secretions, nausea and vomiting, and diarrhea. In addition, these symptoms may worsen with Tensilon testing. Nicotinic symptoms such as fasciculations and cramps are rare. A brittle crisis occurs when the disease is difficult to treat and the patient alternates between myasthenic and cholinergic crises.

Surgery after thymectomy can precipitate acute respiratory failure. In a series of 22 patients, the mean duration of mechanical ventilation was 8 days, with 6 patients (32%) requiring tracheostomy for prolonged mechanical ventilation.[96] Postoperative care of these patients is important because respiratory failure usually occurs within 24 hours of surgery in more than 50% of patients. Serial measurements of VC, PI_{max}, and PE_{max} are helpful in detecting the onset of respiratory failure. It is important to remember that the dosing schedule of anticholinesterase medications will affect the measurement of respiratory parameters. The maximum improvement in respiratory muscle strength occurs about 2 hours after the drug is given and slowly declines before the next dose is given. Consequently, VC, PI_{max}, and PE_{max} should be measured 30 minutes before the next dose of anticholinesterase agents. No single respiratory parameter reliably predicts the need for mechanical ventilation. Once VC is less than 15 mL/kg, PI_{max} is greater (i.e., less negative) than −30 cm H_2O, and PE_{max} is less than 30 cm H_2O, assisted ventilation should be considered.

Other clinical signs of impending acute respiratory failure include signs of upper airway obstruction due to vocal cord paralysis or inability to handle secretions due to severe bulbar involvement. Flow–volume loop analysis may show variable extrathoracic airway obstruction with the characteristic inspiratory plateau in cases of upper airway obstruction. Bilateral basal atelectasis on chest radiograph signifies poor clearance of airway secretions due to a weak cough and is often accompanied by a rapid, shallow breathing pattern. Hypercapnia is a late sign of respiratory muscle fatigue.

Several clinical parameters have been proposed as predictors of postoperative respiratory failure after thymectomy.[97] Severity of disease (Osserman groups 3 and 4), especially with the presence of bulbar symptoms and low VC, appears to be the most important factor in predicting postoperative respiratory failure. In a series of 14 of 122 patients who developed respiratory failure following transsternal thymectomy, independent predictors of postoperative myasthenic crises causing acute respiratory failure included preoperative bulbar symptoms, higher serum levels of acetylcholine receptor antibodies (>100 nmol/L), and intraoperative blood loss.[96]

Sleep-related breathing disturbances may occur in patients with myasthenia gravis. Abnormal sleep study results in MG patients usually reveal mixed central apneas and hypopneas. Patients should be asked about sleep-related symptoms such as daytime hypersomnolence, nocturnal and early morning awakening, and morning headaches. Older patients with moderate obesity and daytime alveolar hypoventilation and restrictive lung defect should undergo sleep study to screen for sleep apnea and nocturnal hypoventilation. The incidence of sleep apnea is higher in patients with a longer duration of MG.

Treatment of MG includes anticholinesterase agents, high-dose corticosteroids, and plasmapheresis in patients who are refractory to steroids and immunosuppressive therapy. Anticholinesterase agents are the first line of treatment. Most patients will improve significantly with this treatment, but only a few patients will regain normal function. Remission can be induced in up to 80% of patients with corticosteroids. Initiation of corticosteroid therapy may cause temporary worsening of muscle weakness, usually on the 6th to 10th day of therapy. Close observation for signs of respiratory insufficiency is advisable. Other immunosuppressive agents (e.g., azathioprine, cyclosporine) are also useful in MG either alone or in combination with steroids.

Thymectomy has been shown, in retrospective study, to improve survival and clinical symptoms even in the absence of thymoma in patients with myasthenia gravis compared with patients who were treated medically.[98] In patients who are younger than 55 years, thymectomy is recommended to prevent malignant transformation of the thymoma. Up to 80% of patients with no thymoma will improve clinically following thymectomy, but the response may be delayed. Because there are no randomized controlled studies documenting the benefit of thymectomy in myasthenia gravis, and given the presence of confounding variables such as age, gender, and severity of myasthenia gravis, the American Academy of Neurology recommends thymectomy in patients with nonthymomatous autoimmune myasthenia gravis only as an option to increase the probability of remission or improvement.

In patients with myasthenic crisis, plasmapheresis and IVIG are effective short-term treatments and help to prepare the symptomatic myasthenia patient for surgery.[99] Improvement in muscle strength is usually apparent in 2 to 3 days, but the improvement does not continue beyond several weeks unless immunosuppressant agents are administered concurrently. Intravenous immunoglobulin given at 1.2 to 2 g/kg over 2 to 5 days has been shown to result in a clinical response comparable with plasmapheresis. However, in a retrospective multicenter study of patients with myasthenic crises, plasmapheresis increased the ability to extubate the patient and improved the patient's functional status at 2 weeks.

Immunosuppressant medications are not appropriate therapy in myasthenic crises because a therapeutic response is often delayed for weeks to months. Corticosteroids have been used in patients who were refractory to plasmapheresis or IVIG; however, steroids may cause a transient worsening of muscle weakness. Corticosteroids and cholinesterase inhibitors are best started several days after a clinical response to plasmapheresis is observed in order to avoid weakness due to corticosteroids and to avoid cholinergic crises.

Acute respiratory failure in patients with myasthenia gravis is usually treated with invasive mechanical ventilation. Noninvasive mechanical ventilation is an alternative ventilatory strategy in patients with severe myasthenic crises with early respiratory failure even in the presence of bulbar symptoms. In a retrospective study of 60 episodes of acute respiratory failure in 52 patients, NIV and invasive mechanical ventilation were the initial method of ventilatory support in 24 and 36 episodes of acute respiratory failure, respectively.[100] In the NIV group, 14 patients (58%) were successfully treated with NIV alone; 10 (52%) eventually required invasive mechanical ventilation. The use of NIV avoids the need for airway intubation, decreases the duration of mechanical ventilation, and decreases both ICU and hospital length of stay. The only predictor of failure of NIV to initially treat respiratory failure in MG was a Pa_{CO_2} of more than 45 mm Hg. NIV thus should be used early in acute respiratory failure, before the onset of hypercapnia. In patients who required invasive ventilatory support, aggressive respiratory management including the use of sighs, positive end-expiratory pressure, frequent suctioning, chest physiotherapy, turning in bed, and the use of antibiotics decreased the prevalence of both atelectasis and bronchopneumonia.

Spontaneous breathing trials can be initiated once an improvement in respiratory status is documented. This includes a PI_{max} less (i.e., more negative) than −20 cm H_2O, PE_{max} greater than 40 cm H_2O, and FVC greater than 10 mL/kg. In a retrospective study of 46 episodes of acute respiratory failure due to myasthenia gravis, extubation failure (defined as the need for reintubation or tracheostomy, or death while on the ventilator) occurred in 44% of cases. Risk factors associated with extubation failures included male sex, history of previous myasthenic crises, atelectasis, and more than 10 days of mechanical ventilation. The FVC, PI_{max}, and PE_{max} were lower in patients who failed extubation but were not statistically different compared with patients who were successfully extubated. Those patients who had lower pH, lower FVC, the presence of atelectasis, and the need for NIV support had a higher risk for reintubation.[101] These data suggest that other factors, such as respiratory muscle fatigue, the presence of bulbar weakness, and the inability to handle upper airway secretions, are not measured by standard weaning parameters and should be considered before attempting extubation.

Lambert-Eaton Syndrome

Lambert-Eaton syndrome (LEMS) is a rare myasthenic-like disorder resulting from a impaired release of acetylcholine from presynaptic terminals. Antibodies against the voltage-gated calcium channel, a large transmembrane protein, interfere with normal calcium flux necessary for the release of acetylcholine into the neuromuscular synapse.[102] The disease is commonly associated with small cell carcinoma of the lung but has also been reported in patients with Hodgkin lymphoma, atypical carcinoid, and malignant thymoma. The prevalence of LEMS in patients with small cell lung cancer is estimated to be 3%.[103] The syndrome can occur throughout the course of the disease but can also serve as a marker of undiagnosed malignancy. In patients without malignancy, LEMS has been associated with autoimmune disorders such as type 1 diabetes mellitus and autoimmune thyroid disorders.

Unlike in myasthenia gravis, limb and girdle muscles are predominantly involved more than ocular and bulbar muscles. Although respiratory failure is infrequent, respiratory muscle weakness is often detected on pulmonary function tests. Acute respiratory failure has been reported as the initial manifestation of LEMS and should be considered as a differential diagnosis in patients with neuromuscular weakness.[104] The diagnosis of LEMS is confirmed by the presence of antibodies against the voltage-gated calcium channel and electrodiagnostic studies.

Botulism

Botulism is a rare disorder caused by toxin produced by *Clostridium botulinum.* Toxin may be ingested via improperly cooked food, wound contamination by the organisms, or absorption of the toxin from the gastrointestinal tract, particularly in infants. There are eight types of toxins, although human disease is caused by types A, B, or E. Botulinum toxin binds with the calcium channel in the presynaptic terminals, impairing neuromuscular transmission of acetylcholine. Gastrointestinal symptoms predominate early in the course of the disease, followed by neurologic impairment including descending paralysis of the neck, trunk, and limb muscles. Weakness of the respiratory muscles requiring ventilatory support is frequent, especially with botulinum type A toxins. Spirometry usually reveals a restrictive ventilatory defect. Recovery from respiratory muscle weakness may take months, requiring prolonged ventilatory support. The average duration of ventilatory support for type A poisoning is 58 days, in contrast to 26 days in type B botulism.[105] Exertional dyspnea and poor exercise tolerance may persist even with normal lung functions.

Inherited Myopathies

Muscular dystrophies refer to a heterogeneous group of progressive, hereditary degenerative skeletal muscle diseases. The respiratory muscles, like any skeletal muscles, become progressively weaker, eventually culminating in respiratory failure and death. In fact, respiratory complications are the most common cause of death in these diseases.

Duchenne and Becker Muscular Dystrophies

Both **Duchenne muscular dystrophy (DMD)** and **Becker muscular dystrophy (BMD)** are progressive myopathies inherited as X-linked recessive traits. Duchenne muscular dystrophy is the most common muscular dystrophy, with an incidence of approximately 1 in 3300 male births and a prevalence rate of 3 per 100,000. Becker muscular dystrophy is less common than DMD and usually has a milder clinical course. Both diseases are caused by mutation of the gene for skeletal protein dystrophin. Dystrophin gene mutations are caused by gene deletions in 65% of patients with DMD and 85% of patients with BMD. The dystrophin protein is thought to stabilize the membrane-bound dystrophin-associated glycoprotein complex and prevent it from degradation. The loss of this associated protein as a result of dystrophin deficiency leads to the degenerative changes that are found in muscular dystrophy. Several potential therapeutic agents targeting the defective gene and its abnormal dystrophin protein are in active clinical trials. Exon skipping agents like eteplirsen and drisapersen are gene product modifiers that act on RNA to correct mutations in the dystrophin gene. Several novel therapeutic agents targeting the downstream effect of the dystrophin gene mutation are in development.[106]

Patients are usually symptomatic early in life, usually at 2 to 3 years of age. Early presenting symptoms are gait disturbances and delayed motor development. Transient improvement may be seen between 3 and 6 years of age (honeymoon period) in DMD, followed by relentless deterioration and becoming wheelchair bound by age 13 years. In contrast, patients with BMD have a milder clinical course and usually do not become wheelchair bound until age 16 years or older. Physical examinations show limb-girdle muscle weakness and pseudohypertrophy of the calf muscles. Muscle weakness is symmetric and selectively affects the proximal and lower limb muscles first before the distal and upper extremity muscle groups. When trying to stand from the floor, affected children often use hand support to push themselves to an upright position (Gower sign). Leg pain is a prominent symptom early in the disease.

Cardiomyopathy is common and becomes clinically significant during the teenage years. In a certain variant of muscular dystrophy called X-linked dilated cardiomyopathy, heart failure occurs early on because the heart muscle is primarily involved. Cognitive impairment in areas of working memory and executive function has been reported. Intestinal hypomotility, presenting as pseudo-obstruction, is a recognized complication in DMD. This gastrointestinal manifestation is thought to be due to smooth muscle degeneration.

The diagnosis is based on myopathic symptoms and signs, markedly increased creatine kinase values, myopathic changes on EMG, and muscle biopsy. A positive family history also is helpful in supporting the diagnosis. The diagnosis is confirmed by a mutation of the dystrophin gene in DNA from peripheral leukocytes or by the absence of or an abnormal dystrophin gene in muscle biopsy. Despite modern respiratory care and better understanding of the abnormal pulmonary mechanics of this disease, survival after the age of 25 is rare. The most common cause of death is progressive respiratory insufficiency and heart failure due to cardiomyopathy.

In Becker muscular dystrophy, the onset of the disease is usually between the ages of 5 and 15 years and in some instances in the third to fourth decades of life. The pattern of muscle weakness is similar to DMD but milder. Cardiac and cognitive impairment is usually uncommon. Gastrointestinal involvement is usually absent. The patients usually remain ambulatory beyond 16 years and into early adulthood and live beyond the age of 30 years. Death as a result of respiratory failure and cardiomyopathy usually occurs between 30 and 60 years of age.

Pulmonary symptoms are often minimal early on despite significant weakness of the respiratory muscles. Serial pulmonary function tests and a few select ancillary procedures such as chest radiography and polysomnography can detect the severity of respiratory muscle weakness and the onset of secondary complications such as scoliosis, abnormal chest wall mechanics, atelectasis due to ineffective cough, and sleep-related breathing disorders. Measurements of FVC, PE_{max},

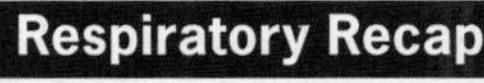

Respiratory Recap

Duchenne Muscular Dystrophy

- DMD is a sex-linked recessive disorder associated with progressive myopathy, culminating in respiratory failure. Becker muscular dystrophy is a milder form of the disease.
- The progression of muscle weakness can be followed by measuring serial vital capacity and maximum mouth pressures.
- Cardiomyopathy is common and can precipitate respiratory failure.
- Development of kyphoscoliosis can contribute to ventilatory pump failure.
- NIV can be used initially, but many patients ultimately require tracheotomy.
- Corticosteroid therapy may improve muscle strength and functional capacity for a few years.

and PI_{max}, when done correctly and in serial fashion, are simple and reproducible tests that are useful in the assessment of respiratory muscle strength. It is important to remember, however, that VC increases with growth during the first decade before it plateaus and progressively decreases and thus may mask early respiratory muscle dysfunction. After age 12 years, VC decreases by about 5% to 6% per year. Maximum inspiratory force is a more useful value during the formative years because it declines gradually despite body growth. Once the initial screening tests show respiratory muscle dysfunction, a more complete battery of pulmonary tests may be needed to further define respiratory muscle endurance, the extent of expiratory muscle weakness, selective weakness of specific respiratory muscle groups, and abnormalities in lung and chest wall mechanics. Once the FVC falls below 1 L, the median survival is 3.1 years, and the 5-year survival is only 8%.[107] An FEV_1 of less than 40% is a sensitive predictor of sleep hypoventilation. Daytime hypercapnia occurs once FEV_1 is less than 20%.[108] Kyphoscoliosis is common and may contribute to a restrictive ventilatory defect.

Maximum voluntary ventilation is useful in detecting respiratory muscle fatigue, but should be avoided in severely weakened patients. Measurement of PE_{max} is important because involvement of the expiratory muscles ($PE_{max} < 60$ cm H_2O) will lead to ineffective cough and inability to handle airway secretions. Because maximum inspiratory pressure measures global inspiratory muscle strength, predominant involvement of the diaphragm muscle may be missed unless transdiaphragmatic pressure is measured using a balloon catheter in the esophagus and the stomach. This procedure is invasive, and many patients may not be able to tolerate it. Alternatively, weakness of the diaphragm can be inferred noninvasively by a greater than 25% decrement in VC from the seated to supine position and by fluoroscopic visualization of diaphragmatic excursion (sniff test). These noninvasive tests are not sensitive enough, however, especially in mild diaphragm weakness.

Although respiratory muscle weakness is progressive, hypercapnia is uncommon in the absence of complicating pulmonary infections. The maintenance of alveolar ventilation in early disease suggests that patients with Duchenne muscular dystrophy have intact diaphragm function until late in the course of the disease. Once hypercapnia sets in, the course is rapidly progressive and prognosis is poor. Mean duration of survival after onset of hypercapnia is about 10 months.[108] Hypoxemia due to ventilation-perfusion inequality is common in moderate to severe disease.

Because ventilation is primarily by the diaphragm in patients with muscular dystrophy, nocturnal hypoventilation may occur especially during REM sleep, when activity of the chest wall and neck muscles is diminished. Indeed, REM-induced hypoventilation has been documented even in patients with normal daytime gas exchange.[109] Sleep-related hypoxemia may contribute to respiratory insufficiency and to the development of cor pulmonale. Hypoxemia is worst during REM sleep when the contribution of the accessory muscles is abolished. Supplemental oxygen may prolong the episode of hypopnea and apnea but does not appear to be clinically significant. NIV has been used successfully in patients with sleep-disordered breathing and DMD.[110,111] In a study of 10 patients with DMD who had pronounced nocturnal oxygen desaturation but normal daytime blood gas values, nocturnal NIV was successfully used to prevent nocturnal oxygen desaturation. Moreover, the progressive decline in lung function appeared to be attenuated with NIV for up to 2 years in follow-up.[112]

Corticosteroids have been shown to improve muscle strength and increase the number of years of effective ambulation as well as preventing decline in VC and PI_{max}. In a randomized, double-blind study, prednisone given at a dose of either 0.75 mg/kg per day or 1.5 mg/kg per day resulted in increased muscle strength and reduced the rate of decline of muscle weakness.[113] Improvement can usually be seen within 10 days of therapy and requires at least 0.75 mg/kg per day of prednisone. Maximal improvement is usually seen at 3 months and is sustained for about 3 years. Side effects associated with prednisone (weight gain, hypertension, behavioral changes, growth retardation, and cataracts) usually necessitate dose reduction of prednisone to 0.35 mg/kg per day.[114]

A synthetic derivative of prednisone, deflazacort, is used in Europe but is currently not available in the United States. Deflazacort may have fewer side effects compared with prednisone, especially regarding weight gain. Clinical studies showed that both deflazacort and prednisone are equally effective in slowing the decline of muscle strength and improving muscle strength and functional performance.[115] A meta-analysis of 15 studies showed that deflazacort improves strength and motor function, but its benefits over prednisone remain unclear.[116] Oxandrolone, a synthetic anabolic steroid, has also been shown to have a beneficial effect comparable with prednisone. In a large randomized controlled trial, oxandrolone significantly improved the mean change in quantitative muscle strength but not the average manual muscle strength when compared with placebo.[117]

Ambulation should be maintained and encouraged as long as possible to retard the development of scoliosis. Surgical correction of severe scoliosis may be helpful in partially correcting the restrictive ventilatory defect, although studies show no significant improvement in respiratory function in patients who undergo spinal fusion surgery. **Table 43-5** presents guidelines for perioperative management of patients with DMD.

TABLE 43-5
Guidelines for Perioperative Management of Patients with Duchenne Muscular Dystrophy

Before Procedure	During Procedure	After Procedure
Consult anesthesiology, pulmonary, cardiology	Succinylcholine should be avoided	Consider extubation to NIV
Measure preoperative FVC, PI_{max}, PE_{max}, PCF, SpO_2; FVC <50%: consider NIV; PCF <270 L/min: consider manual and MIE training	Options for respiratory support include endotracheal intubation, laryngeal mask airway, and NIV	Use supplemental oxygen cautiously Monitor SpO_2 and end-tidal CO_2 Look for hypoventilation, atelectasis, airway secretions
Optimize nutritional status	Consider assisted ventilation if FVC <50%, especially if <30%	Use manually assisted cough and MIE if PE_{max} <60 cm H_2O or PCF <270 L/min
Discuss resuscitation parameters and advance directives, if applicable	Monitor SpO_2 or end-tidal carbon dioxide intraoperatively	Adequate pain control; if sedation and hypoventilation occur, delay extubation for 24 to 48 hours or use NIV Treat constipation and consider prokinetic agents Initiate nutritional support if extubation delayed for more than 24 to 46 hours

NIV, noninvasive ventilation; FVC, forced vital capacity; PI_{max}, maximum inspiratory pressure; PE_{max}, maximum expiratory pressure; PCF, peak cough flow; SpO_2, oxygen saturation measured by pulse oximetry; MIE, mechanical insufflation-exsufflation (cough assist).

NIV and assisted coughing techniques should be initiated before the contemplated procedure if the FVC is less than 50% and the peak cough flow less than 270 L/min.[118] Potential cardiac and gastrointestinal complications should be anticipated and treated appropriately. General physiotherapy is important in preventing contractures.

Patients with chronic neuromuscular disease are at risk for respiratory muscle fatigue because weakened respiratory muscles are working against a high elastic load to maintain the same degree of alveolar ventilation. The effect of respiratory muscle training is variable, however, with some studies reporting substantial improvement whereas other studies show minimal or no significant improvement in respiratory muscle performance.[119] Vigorous respiratory training could be hazardous in patients with advanced disease because it may increase the ventilatory burden on already weakened respiratory muscles. Also, defective nitric oxide release may occur during exercise, potentially causing more muscle injury.[120] Respiratory muscle strength training thus is currently not recommended.[121]

Proper nutrition is important in the maintenance of respiratory muscle function; VC declines as nutritional status deteriorates. In addition, PE_{max} and PI_{max} correlate with body mass in both normal and malnourished persons. High-protein, low-calorie diets aiming to achieve ideal weight may be beneficial.

Nocturnal NIV in patients with DMD has been reported to improve survival and quality of sleep, decrease daytime sleepiness, improve well-being and independence, improve gas exchange, and attenuate the rate of decline of lung function compared with nonventilated control patients.[122–126] Assisted ventilation is required once signs of respiratory insufficiency or symptoms of sleep-related breathing disorders are present. Once VC falls to between 300 to 950 mL, or less than 50% of predicted values, assisted ventilation is often required. Chronic hypercapnic respiratory failure usually develops when the VC is between 500 and 700 mL. Intermittent nasal positive pressure ventilation has been shown to prolong survival and attenuate the decline in VC and MVV in a small controlled study involving patients with advanced DMD. Successful long-term assisted ventilation has been reported in DMD.[125] Intermittent noninvasive ventilation may be used initially for chronic alveolar ventilation, but all patients eventually require positive pressure ventilation via a tracheostomy as the disease advances. Tracheostomy is eventually needed to provide access to the airway secretions in patients who are too weak to cough.

Myotonic Dystrophy

Myotonic dystrophy type 1 (MD type 1) is the most common form of hereditary muscular dystrophy in adults, with an estimated incidence of 1 in 8000. The myotonic dystrophy gene, which is transmitted in an autosomal dominant pattern, is located on the long arm of chromosome 19. The genetic defect in myotonic dystrophy is thought to be due to an amplified trinucleotide CTG repeat that encodes a serine–threonine protein kinase. In normal individuals, the two alleles contain between 5 and 50 copies of the CTG repeat. In patients with MD type 1, there are 50 to 80 copies of the CTG repeat in mildly affected or asymptomatic patients; symptomatic subjects have between 80 and 2000 or more copies. A subset of patients with myotonia and proximal muscle weakness without CTG repeat expansion on chromosome 9 is known; this condition is called myotonic dystrophy type 2, or proximal myotonic myopathy.[127]

Symptoms usually present during adolescence and early adulthood, although the syndrome may be recognized as early as infancy. The cardinal symptoms of myotonic dystrophy are myotonia (delayed relaxation after contraction), weakness and wasting affecting facial muscles and distal limb muscles, frontal balding in males, cataract, cardiomyopathy with conduction block, multiple endocrinopathies (e.g., hyperinsulinism, diabetes, adrenal insufficiency, infertility), hypersomnia, low intelligence, and dementia.

Chronic respiratory failure is common in myotonic dystrophy even in the presence of only mild limb muscle weakness. This is due to the presence of several factors other than respiratory muscle weakness, such as increased respiratory elastance, low central ventilatory drive, and sleep-related breathing disorder, which act in concert to impair lung function. Moreover, myotonia of the respiratory muscles can contribute to an increased work of breathing by increasing the impedance to breathing. Weakness of the expiratory muscles is much more severe compared with the inspiratory muscles in these patients. Weakness of the inspiratory muscles becomes severe once proximal muscle weakness becomes apparent, heralding the onset of alveolar hypoventilation.

Early studies showed a high incidence of hypercapnia and blunted ventilatory response to CO_2, suggesting abnormal central respiratory drive. Subsequent studies have shown that these patients have either a normal or high central ventilatory drive. The abnormal ventilatory response to both hypoxia and hypercarbia has been attributed to respiratory muscle weakness and fatigue. In addition, these patients also may have a chaotic breathing pattern due to impaired afferent input from the respiratory muscles. Daytime hypersomnolence, possibly due to a low central ventilatory drive or sleep apnea, may contribute to the high prevalence of chronic hypercapnia in these patients.

Patients with myotonic dystrophy are particularly susceptible to general anesthesia and respiratory depressants. Avoidance of general anesthesia and muscle relaxants is recommended. If surgery is required, postoperative respiratory monitoring is required. The presence of pharyngeal and laryngeal dysfunction manifesting as nasal speech increases the risks of aspiration. Sleep-related breathing disorders, both central and obstructive sleep apnea, are common in myotonic dystrophy. Nocturnal nasal positive pressure ventilation should be tried once hypercapnia ($Paco_2$ greater than 50 mm Hg) and hypoxemia (Spo_2 <85%) occur.

Acid Maltase Deficiency

Enzymatic defects in the metabolism of carbohydrates (glycogen) lead to an abnormal accumulation of glycogen in the liver, kidney, and cardiac and skeletal muscles. **Acid maltase deficiency** (Pompe disease) is a type II glycogen storage disease that arises because of a deficiency of the lysosomal enzyme responsible for the hydrolysis of both the alpha 1-4 and alpha 1-6 linkages of the glycogen. It is a rare (1 in 40,000 births), inherited, and often fatal disorder that disables the heart and muscles. The disease presents in three clinical forms: infantile, childhood, and adult. In adult-onset disease, the age of onset is usually after age 20 years. The syndrome typically presents with truncal and proximal limb weakness. Respiratory muscle weakness invariably leads to respiratory failure and REM-associated breathing disturbances.

Severe weakness of the diaphragm, out of proportion to limb muscle weakness, may be the predominant clinical manifestation of the disease, which results in respiratory failure.[128] These patients are often misdiagnosed because of the presence of nonspecific symptoms of fatigue, hypersomnolence, morning headaches, and orthopnea. The diagnosis of diaphragm weakness is suspected when paradoxical motion of the abdomen on inspiration is evident, leading to additional neurologic evaluation. Autopsy studies have shown predominant involvement of the proximal respiratory muscles, reflecting predominance of type 1 muscle fibers, which are less efficient in the synthesis and storage of glycogen compared with type 2 muscle fibers. Diagnostic studies reveal elevated serum muscle enzyme levels, myopathic changes on EMG, and vacuoles with glycogen content on muscle biopsy. The diagnosis is confirmed by reduced acid maltase content in muscle and urine assays. Inspiratory muscle training[128,129] and a high-protein diet may be beneficial.[130] Enzyme replacement therapy (alglucosidase alfa) has been shown to decrease heart size; maintain normal heart function; improve muscle function, tone, and strength; and reduce glycogen accumulation.

Facioscapulohumeral Muscular Dystrophy

Facioscapulohumeral muscular dystrophy (FSHD) is an autosomal dominant dystrophy that affects primarily the face and the proximal portion of the upper extremities. The defective gene has been localized to chromosome 4q35. In normal subjects, the number of D4Z4 repeats in chromosome 4q35 ranges from 11 to more than 100. In contrast, most patients with FSHD have 1 to 10 residual repeat units within the subtelomere of chromosome 4q. This forms the basis of the genetic testing, which is positive in 95 to 98% of patients with typical FSHD. It has been hypothesized that deletion of D4Z4 repeat units in chromosome 4q35 leads to overexpression of one or more disease genes.

In the infantile form of FSHD, the disease usually manifests very early in life and is rapidly progressive; patients are usually confined to wheelchairs by the age of 9 to 10 years. In contrast, the classic form of FSHD is slowly progressive, with long periods of disease inactivity. The disease usually affects young adults between the second and third decades of life. The initial manifestations of the disease usually are difficulty in raising the arms above the head and winging of the scapulae. Facial weakness is manifested by the inability to close the eyes, purse the lips, and whistle. In 20% of patients with FSHD, the disease also affects pelvic girdle and trunk muscles, which may impair respiratory function. Spirometry often shows decreased FVC, but facial weakness makes the test unreliable due to poor lip seal.

Limb-Girdle Muscular Dystrophy

Limb-girdle muscular dystrophy is a heterogeneous group of muscle dystrophies that are mainly characterized by weakness of the shoulder and pelvic girdles with sparing of the distal, facial, and extraocular muscles. The mode of inheritance is variable, but the recessive forms are the most common. Similar to other congenital myopathies, symptoms usually become evident during childhood or early adult life. Late-onset disease usually has a benign course. Creatine kinase is usually moderately elevated. EMG shows myopathic changes. Muscle biopsy reveals dystrophic changes with degeneration and regeneration of the muscle fibers, fiber splitting, internal nuclei, fibrosis, and moth-eaten and whorled fibers. Hypercapnic respiratory failure is uncommon even with moderate respiratory muscle weakness. Bilateral paresis of the diaphragm may lead to ventilatory failure. Cardiac involvement is rare.

Mitochondrial Myopathy

Mitochondrial myopathy, one of the manifestations of hereditary mitochondrial disorders, occurs due to a point mutation in mitochondrial DNA (gene mutation at 3250). This group of mitochondrial disorders can also affect other organ systems, particularly the brain. Mitochondrial disorders that manifest polymyopathy as part of the syndrome include myoneural-gastrointestinal encephalopathy; myoclonic epilepsy with ragged red fibers (MERRF); and mitochondrial encephalomyopathy, lactic acidosis, and stroke (MELAS). The disease may present initially in childhood, but onset during adulthood has also been described. The usual clinical manifestations are symmetric proximal muscle weakness that occurs in isolation or in association with central nervous system dysfunction and metabolic derangements. Acute respiratory failure as the initial presentation of the disorder has also been reported.[131] Muscle biopsy is often required to confirm the diagnosis. Modified trichrome stains show marked enlargement of the mitochondria with a reddish tinge, the so-called ragged red fibers. No specific treatment is available. The use of sedative drugs should be avoided.

Acquired Inflammatory Myopathies

Systemic Lupus Erythematosus

Systemic lupus erythematosus (SLE) is an autoimmune disease that can affect almost all organ systems. The pulmonary complications of SLE can be classified as (1) pleuritis and pleural effusions, (2) acute lupus pneumonitis, (3) interstitial lung disease, and (4) respiratory muscle weakness.

Respiratory muscle weakness and diaphragm muscle dysfunction may occur without significant limb weakness. It is estimated that up to 25% of patients with SLE have significant diaphragm weakness even in the absence of generalized myopathy. The diaphragm weakness can be apparent on the chest radiograph, which shows bilateral diaphragm elevation, called by Hoffbrand and Beck the "shrinking lung syndrome."[132]

Steroid Myopathy

Unlike the acute myopathy encountered in the ICU setting, steroid myopathy results from the prolonged use of corticosteroids (as short as 2 weeks of therapy). Myopathy can occur with any glucocorticosteroid preparation but is unusual in patients treated with less than 10 mg/day of prednisone or its equivalent. Myopathy induced by glucocorticoids is largely due to their direct catabolic effects and interference with insulin-like growth factor-1 signaling, which leads to increased myocyte apoptosis. It usually manifests subacutely as proximal limb and girdle muscle weakness. Affected patients thus have difficulty combing their hair, reaching overhead for an object, and climbing stairs. Muscle enzyme levels are usually normal. EMG is either normal or reveals only slight myopathic changes. Muscle biopsy usually shows loss of type IIa muscle fibers with no evidence of inflammation or fiber necrosis. There is a poor correlation between the total dose of steroids given and the severity of muscle weakness. A gradual improvement in muscle strength is usually observed with discontinuation or significant reduction in corticosteroid dosage.

Treatment of Neuromuscular Dysfunction

The proper care of these complicated patients often requires a multidisciplinary team of healthcare workers consisting of pulmonary specialists, respiratory therapists, pulmonary trained nurses, physiatrists, physical therapists, nutritionists, social workers, and clinical psychologists. Depending on the acuity of care required in an individual case, patients can be initially treated in

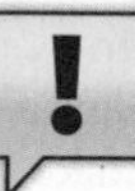

Respiratory Recap

Treatment of Neuromuscular Dysfunction

- Respiratory muscle training may be helpful.
- Assisted coughing techniques are useful in clearance of airway secretions.
- Glossopharyngeal breathing (frog breathing) allows short periods of spontaneous ventilation in ventilator-dependent patients.
- Noninvasive ventilation includes positive and negative pressure devices, rocking beds, and pneumobelts.
- Diaphragmatic pacing is an option in ventilator-dependent patients with high cervical cord injury.

an ICU setting until the resolution of their acute illness and then transferred to a respiratory rehabilitation unit specializing in the care of these patients. Frequent family interaction with the healthcare team is beneficial to facilitate the transition of care from the hospital to home. It is helpful to admit patients with stable chronic respiratory failure to a noninvasive respiratory rehabilitation unit for a few days to familiarize them with the different types of noninvasive ventilator support available in a relaxed and supportive environment.

The goals of therapy in the treatment of patients with chronic neuromuscular diseases are similar to those for other groups of patients with chronic lung disease: to maintain lung function and to restore independent and functional lifestyle for as long as possible. Clearly, some patients with advanced disease will not be able to achieve these goals. Nevertheless, a rapid decline in lung function may be avoided by following judicious pulmonary rehabilitation techniques such as the use of respiratory aid devices to facilitate clearance of airway secretions, early use of noninvasive ventilation to augment alveolar ventilation, especially during periods of acute decline, and the timely treatment of respiratory infections with appropriate antibiotics. Maintenance of proper nutrition is of utmost importance. Both obesity and undernutrition can further contribute to respiratory muscle dysfunction. The decreased chest wall compliance observed in obese patients will lead to an increased work of breathing and may induce respiratory muscle fatigue in already weakened respiratory muscles. On the other hand, under-nutrition has also been shown to decrease respiratory muscle strength in a variety of chronic lung diseases.

Respiratory Muscle Training

Respiratory muscle training improves strength and ventilatory endurance in normal subjects and in patients with pulmonary diseases. The clinical benefits of regular exercise training aim specifically toward increasing ventilatory capacity and facilitating the clearance of airway secretions in patients with chronic neuromuscular diseases. Uncontrolled studies performed in patients with muscular dystrophy have shown that inspiratory muscle training may improve respiratory muscle endurance and strength.[133,134] In a prospective, controlled trial of 19 patients with DMD, 9 patients who received respiratory muscle training 30 minutes a day, 5 days a week, for 2 months showed no significant improvements in VC or in PI_{max} and PE_{max} values at the end of the 2-month training period compared with baseline; however, both increased inspiratory and expiratory times during loaded breathing suggested an improvement in respiratory muscle endurance. In contrast, studies looking at the effect of inspiratory resistive training in tetraplegic patients showed an improvement in inspiratory muscle strength and endurance after 6 to 16 weeks of exercise.[135,136] Furthermore, 6 weeks of pectoralis muscle isometric training significantly increased expiratory reserve volume in C6 through C8 tetraplegic patients. The increase in expiratory reserve volume in these patients may have improved effective cough and diminished the incidence of lower respiratory tract infections.

Concerns have been raised about the potential detrimental effects of respiratory muscle training in patients with advanced neuromuscular weakness. Breathing through resistive loads may potentially lead to muscle fiber damage and fatigue already weakened respiratory muscles. Moreover, no study has correlated any improvement in respiratory mechanics with an improvement in clinical outcome. The beneficial effect of respiratory muscle training thus remains unresolved.

Assisted Coughing

Effective mucus clearance depends on the mucociliary escalator and cough. Cough is usually the limiting function in patients with a neuromuscular dysfunction. This may result from ineffectiveness in phase 1, phase 2, or both phases, depending on the pathology. A weakness of inspiratory muscles such as the diaphragm will limit inspiratory volume. A weakness in abdominal muscles will limit the effect of compressing gas in the lungs. When the peak cough flow is less than 160 L/min (**Figure 43-10**), the patient needs assistance in clearing secretions. Modalities that assist the patient with an ineffective cough include hyperinflation, quad cough, insufflator/exsufflator cough assist, and mechanical aspiration.

Spontaneous cough efforts can be improved in patients with weak inspiratory muscle strength using manual or mechanical insufflation. Manual hyperinflation can be administered using a resuscitator bag with a one-way valve and mouthpiece (**Figure 43-11**). A series of breath-stacking maneuvers is applied until the lungs are maximally insufflated. Mechanical insufflation can also be administered mechanically using volume

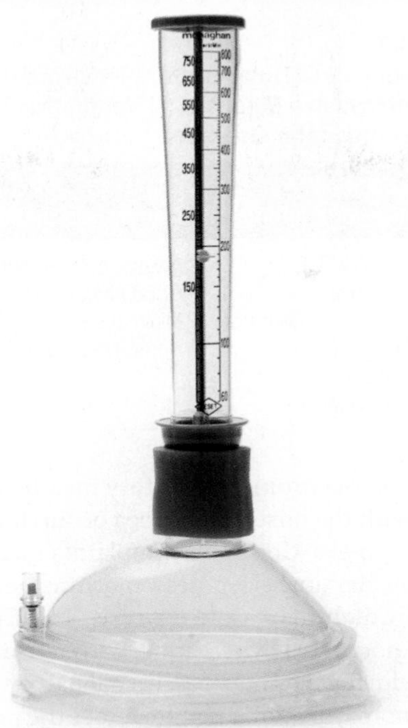

FIGURE 43-10 Peak cough flow meter with an air-cushion face mask.

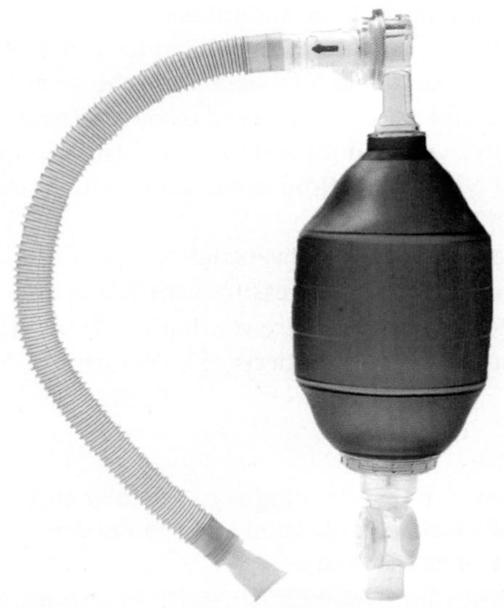

FIGURE 43-11 Resuscitator bag, one-way valve, flexible tube, and mouthpiece for manual hyperinflation.

control ventilation with a mouthpiece. The stored elastic recoil energy of the lungs may produce a peak cough flow sufficient to clear secretions.

The cough assist (insufflator/exsufflator) inflates the lungs with a positive pressure and then produces a negative pressure to create a peak cough flow great enough to clear secretions. Positive and negative pressures between 10 and 60 cm H_2O are selected according to patient tolerance and the effectiveness of the treatments. Inhalation and exhalation times of 1 to 3 seconds and a pause of 0 to 5 seconds may be selected. The ability of the patient to tolerate the settings and the effectiveness of the therapy will dictate the best settings. Most patients will need an oronasal mask as the patient interface if they cannot tighten their lips on a mouthpiece. If a mouthpiece is used, a nose clip will also be necessary. The cough assist can also be attached to a tracheostomy tube.

The quad cough is used to strengthen the patient's cough efforts. The clinician places the thumb of each hand below the xiphoid process, with all fingers placed below the ribs. The patient takes a deep inhalation and coughs on exhalation. The clinician pushes in and up as the patient coughs. Quad cough can be combined with hyperinflation or the cough assist (insufflator/exsufflator).

If the patient has excessive airway secretions, airway clearance therapies such as postural drainage, high-frequency chest wall compression, positive expiratory pressure (PEP), and oscillatory PEP can be used. The effectiveness of these therapies is often limited for patients with neuromuscular dysfunction. Inhaled bronchodilators have limited value in patients with neuromuscular disease unless the patient also has pulmonary disease such as asthma. Tracheal suction is useful in some patients with a tracheostomy tube, but nasotracheal suction is not usually indicated. In patients with bulbar disease and poor swallowing function, oral suction is helpful.

Glossopharyngeal Breathing

Glossopharyngeal breathing, also known as frog breathing, is a technique involving the use of oropharyngeal muscles to inject air into the trachea and thus augment ventilation to provide short periods of spontaneous ventilation, improve effective cough, and increase the volume of the voice. With this technique, the patient gulps in air by lowering and raising the tongue against the palate in a piston-like fashion, thereby injecting air into the trachea. With practice, patients may be able to gulp in 50 to 150 mL of air every half second. With six to eight successive gulps, a tidal volume of approximately 500 to 600 mL may be achieved and sustained for several hours, thus liberating the patient from ventilatory support. Although some patients have difficulty in learning and mastering the technique, patients with spinal cord injuries, postpolio syndrome, and other neuromuscular diseases have successfully used this technique.

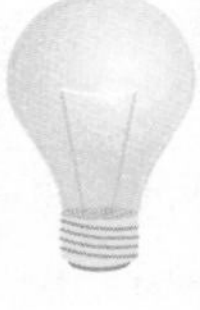

STOP AND THINK

You are asked to assist in the care of a patient with neuromuscular disease who is having difficulty clearing airway secretions. What would you recommend?

Mechanical Ventilation

Although ventilatory insufficiency leading to chronic respiratory failure is a common sequela of progressive neuromuscular diseases, acute respiratory failure is commonly seen after aspiration pneumonia, lower respiratory tract infections, or other acute illnesses that place an additional burden on already compromised ventilatory reserve. Pneumonia is the most common cause of increased morbidity and mortality in patients with advanced chronic neuromuscular disease. Once impending respiratory failure is recognized, mechanical ventilation should be used early to support spontaneous breathing until the acute precipitating event is identified and treated. **Table 43-6** lists the indications for mechanical ventilation.

In patients who present with severe dyspnea, acute hypercapnia with respiratory acidosis, moderate to severe hypoxemia, and hemodynamic instability, translaryngeal intubation and mechanical ventilation are often necessary and are preferred over noninvasive mechanical ventilation. In some clinical situations, NIV may be used to augment minute ventilation in patients who present with acute hypercapnic respiratory failure who remain alert and cooperative, with intact upper airway function and minimal airway secretions. **Table 43-7** compares invasive ventilation and NIV.

In patients who present with chronic respiratory failure or acute or chronic respiratory failure due to progression of their underlying neuromuscular disorder, NIV has been effective in reversing hypercapnia and hypoxemia and is the treatment of choice because of patient comfort, effectiveness, and portability. Moreover, NIV has been shown to decrease the incidence of pneumonia and reduce hospitalization rates in a survey of 654 patients with neuromuscular diseases with up to 20 years of follow-up.[137] In this group of patients, the manifestation of chronic respiratory insufficiency may be subtle, with the onset of dyspnea occurring gradually over days to weeks. Common complaints include lethargy, fatigue, daytime sleepiness, morning headache, and occasionally nightmares and enuresis. These patients often have nocturnal hypercapnia with normal arterial gas values during daytime. Nocturnal oximetry or polysomnogram may be indicated to detect the presence of nocturnal oxygen desaturation and hypercapnia, which may contribute to daytime symptoms. The presence of nocturnal hypoventilation usually leads to chronic hypercapnia and progressive symptoms of respiratory failure within 2 years. In a randomized controlled trial of 26 patients with nocturnal hypercapnia and daytime normocapnia, nocturnal NIV decreased the severity of hypercapnia and improved arterial oxygen saturation. In patients who were randomized to the control group, 9 of 10 required NIV for daytime hypercapnia after a mean follow-up of 8.3 months.

Noninvasive mechanical ventilation can be divided into noninvasive positive pressure ventilation and noninvasive negative pressure ventilation. **Table 43-8** lists the benefits and limitations of both forms of NIV.

TABLE 43-7
Comparisons of Clinical Factors Favoring Invasive Versus Noninvasive Mechanical Ventilation in Patients with Neuromuscular Disease

Invasive Ventilation (Endotracheal Intubation)	Noninvasive Ventilation
Copious secretions Poor airway control Inability to tolerate or failure of noninvasive ventilation Impaired cognition Unstable hemodynamics	Awake, cooperative patient Good airway control Minimal secretions Hemodynamic stability

TABLE 43-6
Indications for Mechanical Ventilation in Patients with Neuromuscular Disorders

Disorder	Indications
Acute respiratory failure	Severe dyspnea Marked accessory muscle use Inability to handle secretions Unstable hemodynamic status Hypoxemia refractory to supplemental O_2 Acute respiratory acidosis
Chronic respiratory failure	
Nocturnal hypoventilation	Morning headache Lethargy Nightmares Enuresis
Nocturnal oxygen desaturation	Spo_2 <88% despite supplemental O_2
Cor pulmonale	Due to hypoventilation with $Paco_2$ >45 mm Hg, pH <7.32

TABLE 43-8
Advantages and Disadvantages of Positive and Negative Pressure Ventilation Used in Patients with Neuromuscular Disease

Type	Advantages	Disadvantages
Negative pressure ventilators (tank, pulmowrap, cuirass)	Dependable Airway cannulation not required Minimal hemodynamic effect Maintenance of speech	Cumbersome Predispose to obstructive apnea Limit nursing care Controlled ventilation
Positive pressure by mask or mouthpiece	Avoids upper airway obstruction Pressure preset, compensates leak Patient-initiated machine breaths	Aerophagia Pressure sores Leaks Problems with interface

Noninvasive positive pressure ventilation is preferred over negative pressure ventilation because of ease of use, portability, and maintenance of upper airway patency during sleep. In addition, noninvasive positive pressure provides better maintenance of alveolar ventilation and airway stability during sleep. Different types of masks may be used (e.g., nasal, oronasal, full face mask) depending on patient comfort and preference. In patients with significant mouth air leaks, the use of a chin strap or changing to an oronasal or total face mask will often solve the problem.[138,139] In chronic NIV use, facial ulcers may rarely develop due to contact pressure from a particular mask interface. In this situation, using two different mask interfaces and rotating their use may promote healing of the facial ulcers and prevent recurrence. Alternatively, mouthpiece interfaces—either a generic mouthpiece with a plastic lip seal or one custom fitted by orthodontics—have been used to administer continuous ventilatory support in some patients.[140]

A wide variety of positive pressure ventilators may be used to deliver NIV. In the intensive care setting, use of a standard ICU ventilator allows either continuous mandatory ventilation or pressure support mode. Some features that are available in standard ventilators that are useful in the acute care setting are the ability to monitor respiratory pattern and to supply supplemental oxygen. In patients with stable chronic respiratory failure, portable bilevel ventilators are widely used.

The initial ventilator settings should be low and slowly increased to achieve an increase in tidal volume of 30% to 50% and/or a decrease in $Paco_2$ of 5 to 10 mm Hg. The expiratory airway pressure during present bilevel ventilation is usually set at 4 cm H_2O or greater to minimize rebreathing, increase functional residual capacity, or counterbalance auto-PEEP. Supplemental oxygen can be titrated into the circuit of the bilevel ventilator.

The duration of ventilatory assistance depends on the severity of respiratory failure and patient tolerance. In the acute setting, ventilatory assistance of 20 hours or more may be needed. In the chronic setting, patients use NIV during the daytime for a few hours followed by nocturnal use of 6 to 8 hours once they become accustomed to the NIV settings. A Cochrane review that included eight randomized or quasi-randomized controlled studies on the efficacy of nocturnal mechanical ventilation for chronic hypoventilation in patients with neuromuscular and chest wall disorders concluded that NIV resulted in short-term improvement of symptoms of chronic hypoventilation, daytime hypercapnia, and nocturnal mean oxygen saturation compared with no ventilation. In three studies in which a 1-year mortality rate was reported, the estimated risk of death following nocturnal ventilation was significantly reduced. The survival advantage of NIV was shown only in patients with ALS.[141]

Negative pressure ventilators intermittently apply subatmospheric pressures to the thorax and abdomen to increase transpulmonary pressure and inflate the lungs. The efficacy of negative pressure ventilation is determined by thoracic and abdominal compliance and the surface area over which the negative pressure is applied. Tank ventilators are the most efficient form of negative pressure ventilation because of the amount of body surface area covered compared with cuirass ventilators, which cover only the upper torso. Tank ventilators are reliable, but they are seldom used today because they are large, cumbersome, have the potential to induce claustrophobia, and interfere with nursing care. Chest cuirass ventilators are more portable than tank ventilators but must be used in the recumbent position to be effective. A limitation to all forms of negative pressure ventilators is that they may induce obstructive sleep apnea due to upper airway collapse during a mechanically delivered breath.

In patients with mild to moderate ventilatory failure, rocking beds and pneumobelts may be used, depending on patient preference, comfort, and the amount of ventilatory support required by the individual patient. These devices act as abdominal displacement devices that augment diaphragmatic motion by displacing abdominal viscera against gravity. The rocking bed consists of a mattress on a motorized platform that rocks in an arc of 40 degrees with the patient recumbent. As the bed moves with the head dependent, gravity induces the abdominal contents and diaphragm to move cranially, assisting exhalation. In the next cycle, as the bed tilts upward, gravity acts to move the diaphragm and abdominal contents in a caudad direction, assisting inspiration. The bed rocks between 12 and 24 times per minute and may be adjusted to optimize patient comfort so as to achieve the desired minute ventilation. The pneumobelt is an inflatable bladder that is worn over the anterior abdomen and is connected to a positive ventilator that intermittently inflates it. With the patient seated upright, bladder inflation increases intra-abdominal pressure, forcing the diaphragm cephalad and thereby inducing active exhalation. When the bladder deflates, gravity moves the abdominal contents and diaphragm caudally, thereby facilitating passive inspiration.

Both devices are limited by their constraint on patients and posture and the amount of ventilatory assistance they provide. The rocking bed is bulky and stationary. Similarly, the pneumobelt requires that the patient use it in the upright posture, and some patients complain of pain and discomfort when high bladder inflation pressures are required to sufficiently augment ventilation.

With the increasing popularity of NIV, several studies have showed impressive improvements in daytime gas exchange even though NIV was given only at night or intermittently throughout the 24-hour period. At the end of 3 months of NIV, the Pa_{O_2} increased by approximately 15 mm Hg while Pa_{CO_2} decreased by approximately 14 mm Hg.[142,143] Moreover, patients had a significant improvement in their symptoms and functional capacity. The exact mechanisms responsible for the improvement of daytime gas exchange in patients with neuromuscular diseases using chronic intermittent noninvasive ventilation are unknown. Some of the proposed mechanisms are that (1) intermittent ventilatory assistance rests already fatigued respiratory muscles; (2) the Pa_{CO_2} central threshold is reset by preventing nocturnal alveolar hypoventilation; (3) ventilation-perfusion matching is improved; and (4) the higher lung volume achieved during assisted ventilation improves lung and chest wall compliance, which decreases the work of breathing.

Diaphragmatic Pacing

Diaphragmatic pacing consists of a radio frequency transmitter and an antenna that discharge signals to a receiver to transmit electrical impulses to an electrode placed over the phrenic nerve or directly on the diaphragm in some cases. Both the electrodes and receiver are surgically implanted. Electrode implantation around the phrenic nerves can be divided via a cervical and thoracic approach; however, the thoracic approach is preferred to ensure stimulation of all phrenic nerve roots while avoiding the brachial plexus. The subcutaneous receiver is usually placed in the lower anterolateral rib cage to allow it to be superficial but in an area where soft tissue movement is limited.

Patients who appear to benefit most from this technology are ventilator-dependent patients following high cervical cord injury. The central nervous system injury must be above the second or third cervical level, above the origin of the phrenic nerve root. Approximately one-third of patients with this type of injury may be suitable for this type of treatment. Potential candidates for diaphragmatic pacing include patients with complete upper cervical injuries leading to apnea, those with some type of central sleep apnea such as congenital central alveolar hypoventilation syndrome, and those with brain stem tumors or infarction. In addition, candidates should have normal cognitive function, complete respiratory muscle paralysis without recovery for 3 months, and viable phrenic nerves. Contraindications to diaphragmatic pacing include failure of the diaphragm to contract with percutaneous stimulation of the phrenic nerves, coma, and severe primary pulmonary disease.

A period of diaphragm conditioning is necessary in patients who have had no diaphragm function for more than 6 months. Successful implantation and conditioning of the diaphragm allow the patients to be independent from ventilator support for prolonged periods of time and enable them to regain speech and olfaction.

In retrospective studies of patients with ventilatory failure due to high spinal cord injury, brain stem injury, and congenital central alveolar hypoventilation, long-term diaphragm pacing full time was well tolerated in carefully selected patients.[144–147] In a study of 50 adult patients with high spinal cord injuries, direct diaphragm stimulation by a device inserted via laparoscopic technique was successful in liberating the patients from the ventilator for at least 4 hours each day in 96% of cases. Diaphragmatic pacing is safe in tetraplegic patients with prior cardiac pacemaker. In a long-term follow-up of 20 tetraplegic patients who have both diaphragmatic pacing and cardiac pacemakers, there was no immediate or long term interaction between the two devices.[148] For patients with ALS, diaphragmatic pacing delayed the need for mechanical ventilation for up to 2 years. The widespread use of diaphragmatic pacing is limited by its high cost, the potential for sudden failure of the hardware, the development of upper airway obstruction, and the induction of diaphragm fatigue.

Key Points

- Neuromuscular diseases impair the pump function of the respiratory muscles, leading to chronic respiratory failure or failure to liberate from mechanical ventilation.
- Severe respiratory muscle weakness may occur in the absence of clinical symptoms.
- Measurements of static respiratory muscle strength and vital capacity help predict impending respiratory failure.
- Sleep-related breathing disorders and nocturnal oxygen desaturation may occur and often precede changes in daytime gas exchange abnormalities.
- A strong clinical suspicion is often required for the proper diagnosis and treatment of neuromuscular diseases.
- Upper motor neuron lesions include stroke, spinal cord injury, Parkinson disease, and multiple sclerosis.
- Lower motor neuron lesions include amyotrophic lateral sclerosis, poliomyelitis, and postpoliomyelitis muscular dystrophy.
- Disorders of peripheral nerves include phrenic nerve injury, Guillain-Barré syndrome, and critical illness polyneuropathy.
- Disorders of the neuromuscular junction include myasthenia gravis, Lambert-Eaton syndrome, and botulism.
- Inherited myopathies include Duchenne muscular dystrophy, Becker muscular dystrophy, myotonic dystrophy, acid maltase deficiency, facioscapulohumeral muscular dystrophy, limb-girdle muscular dystrophy, and mitochondrial myopathy.
- Acquired inflammatory myopathies include systemic lupus erythematosus, acute ICU steroid myopathy, and chronic steroid myopathy.

- NIV is the preferred mode of ventilatory assistance in patients with respiratory insufficiency who have intact bulbar function.

References

1. Votto J, Brancifort J, Scalise P, et al. COPD and other diseases in chronically ventilated patients in a prolonged respiratory care unit. *Chest.* 1998;113:86–90.
2. Johnson DC, Kazemi H. Central control of ventilation in neuromuscular disease. *Clin Chest Med.* 1994;15:607–617.
3. Spinelli A, Marconi G, Gorini M, et al. Control of breathing in patients with myasthenia gravis. *Am Rev Respir Dis.* 1992;145:1359–1366.
4. Vincken W, Ellecker G, Cosio M. Detection of upper airway muscle involvement in neuromuscular disorders using flow-volume loop. *Chest.* 1986;90:52–57.
5. Mier-Jedrzejowicz A, Green M. Respiratory muscle weakness associated with cerebellar atrophy. *Am Rev Respir Dis.* 1988;137:673–677.
6. Baydur A. Respiratory muscle strength and control of ventilation in patients with neuromuscular disease. *Chest.* 1991;99:330–338.
7. Holle R, Shoene R, Pavlin E. Effect of respiratory muscle weakness in $P_{0.01}$ induced by partial curarization. *J Appl Physiol.* 1984;57:1150–1157.
8. Demedts M, Beckers J, Rochette F, Bulcke J. Pulmonary function in moderate neuromuscular disease without respiratory complaints. *Eur J Respir Dis.* 1982;63:62–67.
9. Vincken W, Elleker MG, Cosio M. Determinants of respiratory muscle weakness in stable neuromuscular disorders. *Am J Med.* 1987;82:53–58.
10. Toussaint M, Steens M, Soudon P. Lung function accurately predicts hypercapnia in patients with Duchenne muscular dystrophy. *Chest.* 2007;131:368–375.
11. De Troyer A, Borenstein S, Cordier R. Analysis of lung volume restriction in patients with respiratory muscle weakness. *Thorax.* 1980;35:603–610.
12. Estenne M, Heilporn A, Delhez L, et al. Chest wall stiffness in patients with chronic respiratory muscle weakness. *Am Rev Respir Dis.* 1983;128:1002–1007.
13. Becker H, Piper A, Flynn W, et al. Breathing during sleep in patients with nocturnal desaturation. *Am J Respir Crit Care Med.* 1999;159:112–118.
14. Bye PTP, Ellis ER, Issa FG, et al. Respiratory failure and sleep in neuromuscular disease. *Thorax.* 1990;45:241–247.
15. Ragette R, Mellies U, Schwake C, et al. Patterns and predictors of sleep disordered breathing in primary myopathies. *Thorax.* 2002;57:724–728.
16. Schmidt-Nowara W, Marder E, Feil P. Respiratory failure in myasthenia gravis due to vocal cord paralysis. *Arch Neurol.* 1984;41:567–568.
17. Vincken W, Elleker MG, Cosio MG. Flow-volume loop changes reflecting respiratory muscle weakness in chronic neuromuscular changes. *Am J Med.* 1987;83:673–680.
18. Aboussouan L, Khan S, Meeker D, et al. Effect of noninvasive positive pressure ventilation on survival in amyotrophic lateral sclerosis. *Ann Intern Med.* 1997;6:450–453.
19. Braun NMT, Arora NS, Rochester DF. Respiratory muscle and pulmonary function in polymyositis and other proximal myopathies. *Thorax.* 1983;38:616–623.
20. Laporta D, Grassino A. Assessment of transdiaphragmatic pressure in humans. *J Appl Physiol.* 1996;58:1469–1476.
21. Mier A, Brophy C, Moxham J, Green M. Twitch pressures in the assessment of diaphragm weakness. *Thorax.* 1989;44:990–996.
22. Vingerhoets F, Bogousslavsky J. Respiratory dysfunction in stroke. *Clin Chest Med.* 1994;15:729–737.
23. Scanlon PD, Loring SH, Pichurko BM, et al. Respiratory mechanics in acute quadriplegia. *Am Rev Respir Dis.* 1989;139:615–620.
24. Estenne M, De Troyer A. Mechanism of the postural dependence of vital capacity in tetraplegic subjects. *Am Rev Respir Dis.* 1987;135:367–371.
25. De Troyer A, Estenne M, Heilporn A. Mechanism of active expiration in tetraplegic subjects. *N Engl J Med.* 1986;314:740–744.
26. Estenne M, Knoop C, Vanvaerenbergh J, et al. The effect of pectoralis muscle training in tetraplegic subjects. *Am Rev Respir Dis.* 1989;139:1218–1222.
27. Aji BM, Medley G, O ' Driscoll K, et al. Perry syndrome: a disorder to consider in the differential diagnosis of Parkinsonism. *J Neuro Sci.* 2013;330:117–118.
28. Hammer MJ, Barlow SM. Laryngeal somatosensory deficits in Parkinson's disease: implications for speech respiratory and phonatory control. *Exp Brain Res.* 2010;201:401–409.
29. Bogaard JM, Hovestadt A, Meerwaldt J, et al. Maximal expiratory and inspiratory flow-volume curves in Parkinson's disease. *Am Rev Respir Dis.* 1989;139:610–614.
30. Estenne M, Hubert M, De Troyer A. Respiratory muscle involvement in Parkinson's disease. *N Engl J Med.* 1984;311:1516–1517.
31. Vincken WG, Darauay CM, Cosio MG. Reversibility of upper airway obstruction after levodopa therapy in Parkinson's disease. *Chest.* 1989;96:210–212.
32. Mehta AD, Wright WB, Kirby BJ. Ventilatory function in Parkinson's disease. *BMJ.* 1978;1:1456–1457.
33. Carter JL, Noseworthy JH. Ventilatory dysfunction in multiple sclerosis. *Clin Chest Med.* 1994;15:693–703.
34. Kuwahira I, Kondo T, Ohta Y, et al. Acute respiratory failure in multiple sclerosis. *Chest.* 1990;97:246–248.
35. Balbierz J, Ellenberg M, Honet J. Complete hemidiaphragmatic paralysis in a patient with multiple sclerosis. *Am J Phys Med Rehabil.* 1988;67:161.
36. Smeltzer S, Utell M, Rudick R, et al. Respiratory function in multiple sclerosis. *Arch Neurol.* 1988;45:1245–1249.
37. Carter JL, Rodriquez M. Immunosuppressive treatment of multiple sclerosis. *Mayo Clin Proc.* 1984;64:664–669.
38. Weiner HL, Dau PC, Khatri BO, et al. Double-blind study of true vs. sham plasma exchange in patients treated with immunosuppression for acute attacks of multiple sclerosis. *Neurology.* 1989;39:1143–1149.
39. Bach J, Alba A, Saporito L. Intermittent positive pressure ventilation via the mouth as an alternative to tracheostomy for 257 ventilator users. *Chest.* 1993;103:174–182.
40. Splaingard M, Frates R, Jefferson L, et al. Home negative pressure ventilation: report of 20 years of experience in patients with neuromuscular disease. *Arch Phys Med Rehabil.* 1985;66:239–243.
41. Fromm GB, Wisdom PJ, Block AJ. Amyotrophic lateral sclerosis presenting with respiratory failure. *Chest.* 1977;71:612–614.
42. Carre PC, Didier AP, Tiberge YM, et al. Amyotrophic lateral sclerosis presenting with sleep hypopnea syndrome. *Chest.* 1988;93:1309–1312.
43. Kreitzer SM, Saunders NA, Tyler HR, Ingram RH. Respiratory muscle function in amytrophic lateral sclerosis. *Am Rev Respir Dis.* 1978;117:437–447.
44. Singh D, Verma R, Garg R, Singh MK. Assessment of respiratory function by spirometry and phrenic nerve studies of amyotrophic lateral sclerosis. *J Neurol Sci.* 2011;76–81.
45. Pinto S, Pinto A, de Carvalho M. Phrenic nerve studies predict survival in amyotrophic lateral sclerosis. *Clin Neurophysiol.* 2012;123:2452–2459.
46. Silverstein M, Stocking C, Antel J. Amyotrophic lateral sclerosis and life-sustaining therapy: patients' desires for information, participation in decision making, and life-sustaining therapy. *Mayo Clin Proc.* 1991;66:906–913.
47. Bourke SC, Tomlinson M, Williams TL, et al. Effects of noninvasive ventilation on survival and quality of life in patients with amyotrophic lateral sclerosis: a randomized controlled trial. *Lancet Neurol.* 2006;5;140–147.
48. Onders RP, Elmo M, Kaplan C, et al. Final analysis of the pilot trial of diaphragm pacing in amyotrophic lateral sclerosis with long

term follow-up: diaphragm pacing positively affects diaphragm respiration. *Am J Surg*. 2014;207:393–397.

49. Schmiesing CA, Lee J, Morton JM, Brock-Utne JG. Laparoscopic diaphragmatic pacer placement—a potential new treatment for ALS patients: a brief description of the device and anesthetic issues. *J Clin Anesth*. 2010;22:549–552.
50. Dalakas MC, Elder G, Hallett M, et al. A long term follow-up study of patients with post-poliomyelitis neuromuscular symptoms. *N Engl J Med*. 1986;314:959–963.
51. Cashman N, Maselli R, Wollman R, et al. Late denervation in patients with antecedent paralytic poliomyelitis. *N Engl J Med*. 1981;317:7–12.
52. Perry J, Barnes G, Gronley J. The postpolio syndrome: an overuse phenomenon. *Clin Orthop Related Res*. 1988;223:145–162.
53. Deans E, Ross J, Road JD, et al. Pulmonary function in individuals with a history of poliomyelitis. *Chest*. 1991;100:118–123.
54. Bach JR, Alba AS, Bohatiuk G, et al. Mouth intermittent positive pressure ventilation in the management of postpolio respiratory insufficiency. *Chest*. 1987;91:859–864.
55. Curran FJ, Colbert AP. Ventilator management in Duchenne muscular dystrophy and post-myelitis syndrome: a twelve years' experience. *Arch Phys Med Rehabil*. 1989;70:180–185.
56. Hsu A, Staats B. "Postpolio" sequelae and sleep-related disordered breathing. *Mayo Clin Proc*. 1998;73:216–224.
57. Canon S, Ritter FN. Vocal cord paralysis after post-myelitis syndrome. *Laryngoscope*. 1987;97:981–983.
58. Solliday N, Gaensler E, Schwaber J, Parker T. Impaired central chemoreceptor function and chronic hypoventilation many years following poliomyelitis. *Respiration*. 1974;31:177–192.
59. Large B, Heywood LJ, Flower CD, et al. Incidence and aetiology of a raised hemidiaphragm after cardiopulmonary bypass. *Thorax*. 1985;40:444–447.
60. Markand ON, Moorthy SS, Mahomed Y, King RD, Brown JW. Postoperative phrenic nerve palsy in patients with open-heart surgery. *Thorax*. 1985;35:603–610.
61. Chan CK, Loke J, Virgulto JA, et al. Bilateral diaphragmatic paralysis: clinical spectrum, prognosis, and diagnostic approach. *Arch Phys Med Rehabil*. 1988;69:976–979.
62. Mier-Jedrzejowicz A, Brophy C, Moxham J, Green M. Assessment of diaphragm weakness. *Am Rev Respir Dis*. 1988;137:877–883.
63. Laroche CM, Carroll N, Moxham J, Green M. Clinical significance of severe isolated diaphragm weakness. *Am Rev Respir Dis*. 1988;138:862–866.
64. McCool D, Tzelepis GE. Dysfunction of the diaphragm. *N Engl J Med*. 2012;366:932–942.
65. Chetta A, Rehman AK, Moxham J, et al. Chest radiography cannot predict diaphragm function. *Respir Med*. 2005;99:39–44.
66. DeVita MA, Robinson LR, Rehder J, et al. Incidence and natural history of phrenic nerve neuropathy occurring during open heart surgery. *Chest*. 1993;103:850–856.
67. Ropper AH. The Guillain-Barré syndrome. *N Engl J Med*. 1992;326:1130–1136.
68. Yuki N, Hartung H. Guillain-Barré syndrome. *N Engl J Med*. 2012;366:2294–2304.
69. Asbury A, Cornblath D. Assessment of current diagnostic criteria for Guillain-Barré syndrome. *Ann Neurol*. 1990;27(suppl 1):S21–S24.
70. Gracey DR, McMihan JC, Divertie MB, Howard FM. Respiratory failure in Guillain-Barré syndrome. *Mayo Clin Proc*. 1982;57:742–746.
71. Orlikowski D, Sharshar T, Porcher R, Annane D, Raphael JC, Clair B. Prognosis and risk factors of early onset pneumonia in ventilated patients with Guillain-Barré syndrome. *Intensive Care Med*. 2006;32:1962–1969.
72. Borel CO, Tilford C, Nichols DG, Hanley DF, Traystman RJ. Diaphragmatic performance during recovery from acute ventilatory failure in Guillain-Barré syndrome and myasthenia gravis. *Chest*. 1991;99:444–451.
73. Guillain-Barré Syndrome Study Group. Plasmapheresis and acute Guillain-Barré syndrome. *Neurology*. 1985;35:1096–1104.
74. French Cooperative Group on Plasma Exchange in Guillain-Barré Syndrome. Efficiency of plasma exchange in Guillain-Barré syndrome: role of replacement fluids. *Ann Neurol*. 1987;22:753–761.
75. van der Meche FGA, Schmitz PIM, The Dutch Guillain-Barré Study Group. A randomized trial comparing intravenous immune globulin and plasma exchange in Guillain-Barré syndrome. *N Engl J Med*. 1992;326:1123–1129.
76. Hughes RAC, Swan AC, van Koningsveld R, van Doorn P. Corticosteroids for Guillain-Barré syndrome. *Cochrane Database Syst Rev*. 2007;(4):16625544.
77. Leijten F, De Weerd A, Poortvliet D, et al. Critical illness polyneuropathy in multiple organ dysfunction syndrome and weaning from the ventilator. *Intensive Care Med*. 1996;22:856–861.
78. De Letter MA, van Doorn PA, Savelkoul HF, et al. Critical illness polyneuropathy and myopathy (CIPNM): evidence for local immune activation by cytokine-expression in the muscle tissue. *J Neuroimmunol*. 2000;106:206–213.
79. Bednarik J, Vondracek P, Dusek L, et al. Risk factors for critical illness polyneuropathy. *J Neurol*. 2005;252:343–351.
80. Van den Berghe G, Schoonheydt K, Becx P, et al. Insulin therapy protects the central and peripheral nervous system of intensive care patients. *Neurology*. 2005;64:1348–1353.
81. Van den Berghe G, Wouters P, Weekers F, et al. Intensive insulin therapy in the critically ill patient. *N Engl J Med*. 2001;345:1359–1367.
82. Van de Berghe G, Wilmer A, Hermans G, et al. Intensive insulin therapy in the medical ICU. *N Engl J Med*. 2006;354:449–461.
83. Hermans G, Wilmer A, Meerseman W, et al. Impact of intensive insulin therapy on neuromuscular complication and ventilator dependency in the medical intensive care unit. *Am J Respir Crit Care Med*. 2007;175:480–489.
84. Allen DC, Arunnachalam R, Mills KR. Critical illness myopathy: further evidence from muscle-fiber excitability studies of an acquired channelopathy. *Muscle Nerve*. 2008;37:14–22.
85. Witt N, Zochodne D, Bolton C. Peripheral nerve function in sepsis and multiple organ failure. *Chest*. 1991;199:176–184.
86. Garnacho-Montero J, Amaya-Villar R, Garcia-Garmendia JL, et al. Effect of critical illness polyneuropathy on the withdrawal from mechanical ventilation and the length of stay in septic patients. *Crit Care Med*. 2005;33:349–354.
87. De Jonghe B, Bastuji-Garin S, Sharshar T, et al. Does ICU acquired paresis lengthen weaning from mechanical ventilation? *Intensive Care Med*. 2004;30:1117–1121.
88. Schweickert WD, Pohlman MC, Pohlman AS, et al. Early physical and occupational therapy in mechanically ventilated, critically ill patients; a randomized, controlled trial. *Lancet*. 2009;373:1874–1882.
89. Morris PE, Griffen L, Berry M, et al. Receiving early mobilization during an intensive care unit admission is a predictor of improved outcomes in acute respiratory failure. *Am J Med Sci*. 2011;341:373–377.
90. Morris PE, Goad A, Thompson C et al. Early intensive care unit mobility therapy in the treatment of acute respiratory failure. *Crit Care Med*. 2008;36:2238–2243.
91. Kress JP, Hall JB. ICU-Acquired weakness and recovery from critical illness. *N Engl J Med*. 2014;370:1626–1635.
92. Herridge MS, Cheung AM, Tansey CM, et al. One-year outcomes in survivors of the acute respiratory distress syndrome. *N Engl J Med*. 2003;348:683–693.
93. Latronico N, Peli E, Botteri M. Critical illness myopathy and neuropathy. *Curr Opin Crit Care*. 2005;11:126–132.
94. Sanders DB, El Salem K, Massey JM, et al. Clinical aspects of MuSK antibody positive seronegative MG. *Neurology*. 2003;60:1978–1980.
95. Dushay KM, Zibrak JD, Jensen WA. Myasthenia gravis presenting as isolated respiratory failure. *Chest*. 1990;97:232–234.
96. Watanabe A, Watanabe T, Obama T, et al. Prognostic factors for myasthenic crises after transsternal thymectomy in patients with myasthenia gravis. *J Thorac Cardiovasc Surg*. 2004;127:868–876.

97. Juel VC. Myasthenia gravis: management of myasthenic crises and perioperative care. *Semin Neurol.* 2004;24:75–81.
98. Gronseth GS, Barohn RJ. Practice parameter: thymectomy for autoimmune myasthenia gravis (an evidence-based review). Report of the quality standards subcommittee of the American Academy of Neurology. *Neurology.* 2000;55:7–15.
99. Qureshi AI, Choudhry MA, Akbar MS, et al. Plasma exchange versus intravenous immunoglobulin treatment in myasthenic crises. *Neurology.* 1999;52:629–632.
100. Seneviratne J, Mandrekar J, Wijdicks EFM, Rabinstein AA. Noninvasive ventilation in myasthenic crisis. *Arch Neurol.* 2008;65:54–58.
101. Seneviratne J, Mandrekar J, Wijdicks FM, Rabinstein AA. Predictors of extubation in myasthenic crisis. *Arch Neurol.* 2008;65:929–933.
102. Lang B, Pinto A, Giovanini F, et al. Pathogenic autoantibodies in the Lambert-Eaton myasthenic syndrome. *Ann N Y Acad Sci.* 2003;998:187.
103. Elrington GM, Murray NM, Spiro SG, Newsom-Davis J. Neurological paraneoplastic syndromes in patients with small cell lung cancer. A prospective survey of 150 patients. *J Neurol Neurosurg Psychiatry.* 1991;54:764.
104. Nicolle MW, Stewart DJ, Remtulla H, et al. Lambert-Eaton myasthenic syndrome presenting with severe respiratory failure. *Muscle Nerve.* 1996;19:1328–1333.
105. Hughes JM, Blumenthal JR, Merson MH, et al. Clinical features of type A and type B food-borne botulism. *Ann Intern Med.* 1981;95:442–445.
106. Ruegg UT. Pharmacological prospect in the treatment of Duchenne muscular dystrophy. *Curr Opin Neurol.* 2013;26:577–584.
107. Phillips MF, Quinlivan RC, Edwards RH, Calverley PM. Changes in spirometry over time as prognostic marker in patients with Duchenne muscular dystrophy. *Am J Respir Crit Care Med.* 2001;164:2191–2194.
108. Begin P, Mathieu J, Almirall J, Grassino A. Relationship between chronic hypercapnia and inspiratory-muscle weakness in myotonic dystrophy. *Am J Respir Crit Care Med.* 1997;156:133–139.
109. Hukins CA, Hillman DR. Daytime predictors of sleep hypoventilation in Duchenne muscular dystrophy. *Am J Respir Crit Care Med.* 2000;161:166–170.
110. Fanfulla F, Berardinelli A, Gaultieri G, Zoia M. The efficacy of noninvasive mechanical ventilation on nocturnal hypoxemia in Duchenne's muscular dystrophy. *Monaldi Arch Chest.* 1998;53:9–13.
111. Guilleminault C, Philip P, Robinson A. Sleep and neuromuscular disease: bilevel positive airway pressure by nasal mask as a treatment for sleep disordered breathing in patients with neuromuscular disease. *J Neurol Neurosurg Psychiatry.* 1998;65:225–232.
112. Vianello A, Bevilacqua M, Salvador V, et al. Long-term nasal intermittent positive pressure ventilation in advanced Duchenne's muscular dystrophy. *Chest.* 1994;105:445–449.
113. Mendell JR, Moxley RT, Griggs RC, et al. Randomized, double-blind six months trial of prednisone in Duchenne's muscular dystrophy. *N Engl J Med.* 1989;320:1592–1597.
114. Backman E, Henriksson KG. Low-dose prednisolone treatment in Duchenne and Becker muscular dystrophy. *Neuromuscul Disord.* 1995;5:233–241.
115. Bonifati MD, Ruzza G, Bonometto P, et al. A multicenter, double-blind, randomized trial of deflazacort versus prednisone in Duchenne muscular dystrophy. *Muscle Nerve.* 2000;23:1344–1347.
116. Campbell C, Jacob P. Deflazacort for the treatment of Duchenne dystrophy: a systematic review (abstract). *BMC Neurol.* 2003;3:7.
117. Fenichel GM, Florence JM, Pestronk A, et al. A randomized efficacy and safety trial of oxandrolone in the treatment of Duchenne dystrophy. *Neurology.* 2001;56:1075–1079.
118. Birnkrant DJ, Panitch HB, Benditt JO, et al. American College of Chest Physicians statement on the respiratory and related management of patients with Duchenne muscular dystrophy undergoing anesthesia and sedation. *Chest.* 2007;132:1977–1986.
119. Wanke T, Toifl K, Merkle M, et al. Inspiratory muscle training in patients with Duchenne muscular dystrophy. *Chest.* 1994;105: 475–482.
120. Sander M, Chavoshan B, Harris S, et al. Functional muscle ischemia in neuronal nitric oxide synthase-deficient skeletal muscle of children with Duchenne muscular dystrophy. *Proc Natl Acad Sci USA.* 2000;97:13818–13823.
121. ATS Consensus Statement. Respiratory care of patients with Duchenne muscular dystrophy. *Am J Respir Crit Care Med.* 2004;170:456–465.
122. Annane D, Orlikowski D, Chevret S, et al. Nocturnal mechanical ventilation for chronic hypoventilation in patients with neuromuscular and chest wall disorders. *Cochrane Database Syst Rev.* 2007;(4):CD001941.
123. Ward S, Chatwin M, Heather S, Simonds AK. Randomized controlled trial of non-invasive ventilation (NIV) for nocturnal hypoventilation in neuromuscular and chest wall disease patients with daytime normocapnia. *Thorax.* 2005;60:1019–1024.
124. Simonds AK, Muntoni F, Heather S, Fielding S. Impact of nasal ventilation on survival in hypercapnic Duchenne muscular dystrophy. *Thorax.* 1998;53:949–952.
125. Baydur A, Layne E, Aral H, et al. Long term non-invasive ventilation in the community for patients with musculoskeletal disorders: 46 years of experience and review. *Thorax.* 2000;55:411.
126. Barbe F, Quera-Salva MA, de Lattre J, et al. Long-term effects of nasal intermittent positive-pressure ventilation on pulmonary function and sleep architecture in patients with neuromuscular diseases. *Chest.* 1996;110:1179–1183.
127. Thornton CA, Griggs RC, Moxley RT 3rd. Myotonic dystrophy with no trinucleotide repeat expansion. *Ann Neurol.* 1994;35:269–272.
128. Sivak E, Ahmad M, Hanson M, Mitsumoto H. Respiratory insufficiency in adult-onset acid maltase deficiency. *South Med J.* 1987;80:205–208.
129. Martin R, Sufit R, Ringel S, et al. Respiratory muscle improvement by muscle training in adult-onset acid maltase deficiency. *Muscle Nerve.* 1983;6:201–203.
130. Margolis ML, Hill AR. Acid maltase deficiency in an adult: evidence for improvement in respiratory function with high-protein dietary therapy. *Am Rev Respir Dis.* 1986;134:328–331.
131. Lynn DJ, Woda RP, Mendell JR. Respiratory dysfunction in muscular dystrophy and other myopathies. *Clin Chest Med.* 1994;15: 661–674.
132. Hoffbrand B, Beck E. "Unexplained" dypnea and shrinking lungs in systemic lupus erythematosus. *Br Med J.* 1965;1:1273–1277.
133. DiMarco A, Kelling J, DiMarco M, et al. The effects of inspiratory resistive training on respiratory muscle function in patients with muscular dystrophy. *Muscle Nerve.* 1985;8:284–290.
134. Martin A, Stern L, Yeates J, et al. Respiratory muscle training in Duchenne dystrophy. *Med Child Neurol.* 1986;8:284–290.
135. Gross D, Ladd H, Riley E, Macklem P, Grassino A. The effect of training on strength and endurance of the diaphragm in quadriplegia. *Am J Med.* 1980;68:27–35.
136. Huldtgren A, Fugl-Myers A, Jonasson E, Bake B. Ventilatory dysfunction and respiratory rehabilitation in post-traumatic quadriplegia. *Eur J Respir Dis.* 1980;61:347–356.
137. Bach JR, Rajaraman R, Ballanger F, et al. Neuromuscular ventilatory insufficiency: effect of home mechanical ventilator use vs oxygen therapy on pneumonia and hospitalization rates. *Am J Phys Med Rehabil.* 1998;77:8–19.
138. Criner G, Travaline J, Brennan K, Kreimer D. Efficacy of a new full face mask for noninvasive positive pressure ventilation. *Chest.* 1994;106:1109–1115.
139. Roy B, Cordova F, Travaline J, et al. Full face mask for noninvasive positive pressure ventilation in patients with acute respiratory failure. *J Am Osteopath Assoc.* 2007;107:148–156.
140. Bach J, Alba A, Saporito L. Intermittent positive pressure ventilation via the mouth as an alternative to tracheostomy for 257 ventilator users. *Chest.* 1993;103:174–182.
141. Annane D, Orlikowski D, Chevret S, et al. Nocturnal mechanical ventilation for chronic hypoventilation in patients with neuromuscular and chest wall disorders. *Cochrane Database Syst Rev.* 2007;4: CD001941.

142. Gay P, Patel A, Viggiano R, et al. Nocturnal nasal ventilation for treatment of patients with hypercapneic respiratory failure. *Mayo Clin Proc.* 1991;144:1234–1239.
143. Heckmatt J, Loh L, Dubowitz V. Nighttime nasal ventilation in neuromuscular disease. *Lancet.* 1990;335:579–581.
144. Elefteriades JA, Hogan JF, Handler A, Loke JS. Long-term follow-up of bilateral pacing of the diaphragm in quadriplegia. *N Engl J Med.* 1992;326:1433–1434.
145. Elefteriades JA, Quin JA, Hogan JF, et al. Long term follow-up of pacing of the conditioned diaphragm in quadriplegia. *Pacing Clin Electrophysiol.* 2002;25:897–906.
146. Garrido-Garcia H, Mazaira Alvarez J, Martin Escribano P, et al. Treatment of chronic ventilatory failure using a diaphragmatic pacemaker. *Spinal Cord.* 1998;36:310–314.
147. Onders RP, Khansarinia S, Weiser T, et al. Multicenter analysis of diaphragm pacing in tetraplegic with cardiac pacemakers: positive implications for ventilator weaning in intensive care unit. *Surgery.* 2010;148:893–898.
148. Onders RP, Elmo M, Khansarinia S, et al. Complete worldwide operative experience in laparoscopic diaphragm pacing: results and differences in spinal cord injured patients and amyotrophic lateral sclerosis patients. *Surg Endosc.* 2009;23:1433–1440.

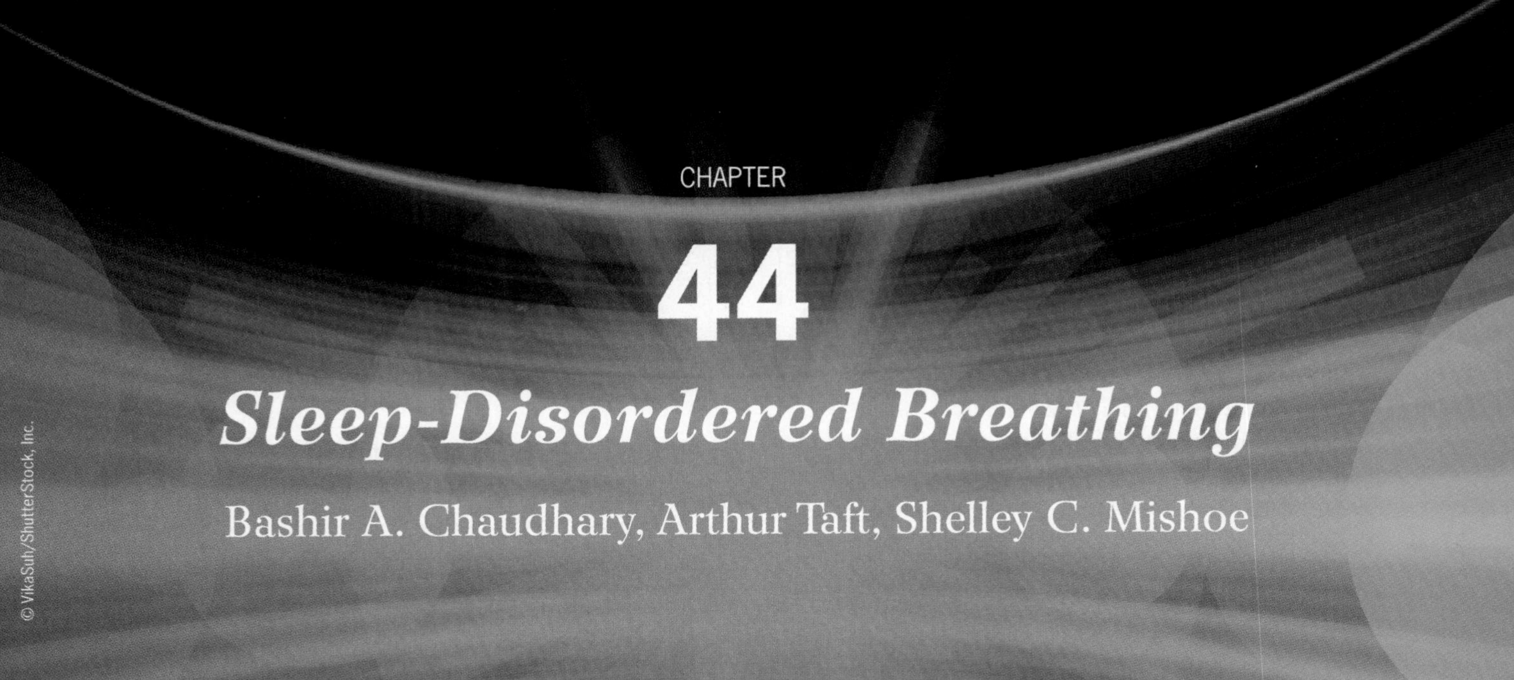

CHAPTER
44
Sleep-Disordered Breathing
Bashir A. Chaudhary, Arthur Taft, Shelley C. Mishoe

OUTLINE

OBJECTIVES

1. Define obstructive sleep apnea.
2. Compare obstructive sleep apnea (OSA), central sleep apnea, and mixed apnea.
3. Discuss the prevalence and pathogenesis of OSA.
4. Describe the clinical features of OSA.
5. Describe the systemic effects of OSA.
6. Compare the advantages and disadvantages of various treatment strategies for OSA.
7. Define central sleep apnea (CSA).
8. Describe the conditions that encompass CSA including idiopathic CSA (ICSA), Cheyne-Stokes breathing, high altitude–induced periodic breathing, narcotic-induced central apnea, and obesity hypoventilation syndrome (OHS).
9. Describe the features and treatments for restless legs syndrome.

KEY TERMS

apnea
arousals
central apnea
Cheyne-Stokes breathing
complex sleep apnea syndrome
continuous positive airway pressure (CPAP)
hypersomnolence
hypopnea
mixed apnea
obesity hypoventilation syndrome (OHS)
obstructive apnea
oral appliance
polysomnography
restless legs syndrome (RLS)
sleep apnea
uvulopalatopharyngoplasty (UPPP)

Introduction

Sleep is an essential biological function that serves many purposes from regulation of metabolism and the immune system to memory consolidation. Recent research at the molecular level suggests that sleep's basic purpose it to clear the brain of toxic metabolic by-products.[1] Without adequate sleep, health is jeopardized due to safety risks from unexpectedly falling asleep and physiologic effects on the body that can lead to serious complications affecting the cardiac, pulmonary, psychological, sexual, endocrine, central nervous, renal, vascular, and ophthalmic systems.

This chapter describes the most common sleep disorders including obstructive sleep apnea, central sleep apnea, upper airway resistance syndrome, high altitude periodic apnea, obesity hypoventilation syndrome, and restless leg syndrome. This chapter describes central and obstructive sleep apneas from prevalence and pathogenesis to effect on the different systems of the body. Obstructive sleep apnea is characterized by continued chest and abdominal efforts to breath during periods of airflow cessation. Central apnea is characterized by cessation of both the effort to breathe and airflow. Mixed apnea has characteristics of both types of apnea: central in the beginning and obstructive at the end. Upper airway resistance syndrome (UARS) is a milder sleep-related breathing problem In UARS, the sleep study does not show apneas, but there is an increase in the number of arousals related to increased respiratory effort. This chapter includes discussion of the advantages and disadvantages of various treatment strategies and how treatment can improve health and prolong a person's life.

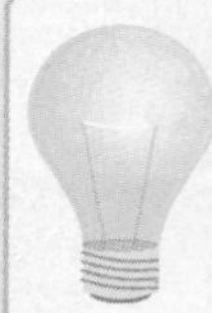

STOP AND THINK

Why should respiratory therapists be knowledgeable of sleep-disordered breathing?

Descriptions and Common Terms

Symptoms suggestive of sleep apnea were well described in Charles Dickens's novel *The Pickwick Papers*. In 1906, William Osler in his book *The Principles and Practice of Medicine* referred to obese patients with uncontrollable sleepiness as *Pickwickians*, "like the fat boy Joe in *Pickwick Papers*." The recognition of episodic cessation of breathing during sleep in drowsy patients heralded the modern era of sleep medicine. **Sleep apnea** is a chronic disorder characterized by daytime **hypersomnolence**, snoring, disrupted sleep, hypoxemia, and repeated episodes of **hypopnea** or **apnea**, or both, during sleep.[2] **Table 44-1** lists some of the common terms used for describing sleep-related breathing problems.

During the past 35 years, much has been published about various aspects of sleep apnea. Two longitudinal studies have provided a wealth of information about the long-term effects of sleep apnea. The Wisconsin Sleep Cohort Study is an epidemiologic study of sleep apnea and other sleep problems, based on a random sample of 1522 Wisconsin state employees that began in 1989.[3] In 1994 the National Heart, Lung and Blood Institute initiated the Sleep Heart Health Study as a multicenter prospective cohort study to assess the contribution of sleep apnea to hypertension and cardiovascular disease.[4]

Types of Sleep-Disordered Breathing

Three types of sleep apnea are recognized: obstructive apnea, central apnea, and mixed apnea.[2] During normal sleep, chest and abdominal movements are in synchrony and airflow is normal (**Figure 44-1**). **Obstructive apnea** is characterized by continued chest and abdominal efforts to breathe during periods of airflow cessation (**Figure 44-2**). When the obstruction is not complete and airflow does not cease, but diminishes to 30% or less of average, these episodes are known as *hypopneas* (**Figure 44-3**). **Central apnea** is characterized by cessation of both the effort to breathe and airflow (**Figure 44-4**). **Mixed apnea** has characteristics of both types of apnea: central in the beginning and obstructive at the end (**Figure 44-5**). Mixed apnea often is combined with obstructive apnea, since the pathogenesis and clinical manifestations are similar. The usual description of sleep apnea refers to patients with obstructive sleep apnea (OSA).

TABLE 44-1
Definitions for Describing Sleep-Related Breathing Problems

Term	Definition
Apnea	Cessation of airflow for at least 10 seconds
Obstructive apnea	Continuation of chest and abdominal effort during apnea
Central apnea	Cessation of both airflow and the respiratory effort
Mixed apnea	Both central and obstructive apnea characteristics
Hypopnea	Reduction of airflow by 30% with oxygen desaturation of at least 4%
Apnea index	Number of apneas per hour of sleep
Hypopnea index	Number of hypopneas per hour of sleep
Apnea-hypopnea index (AHI)	Number of apneas and hypopneas per hour of sleep
Respiratory disturbance index	Apneas, hypopneas, and respiratory arousals per hour of sleep
RERA index	Number of respiratory effort–related arousals per hour of sleep

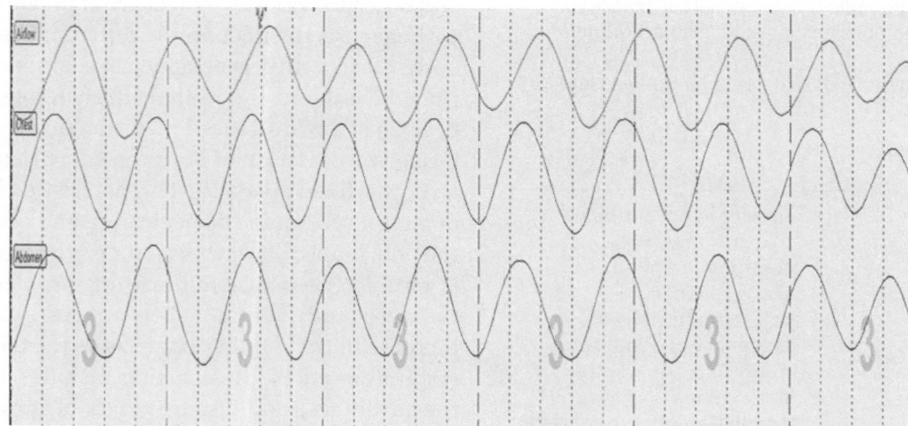

FIGURE 44-1 Normal breathing pattern. Upper tracing: airflow. Middle tracing: chest movements. Lower tracing: abdominal movements.

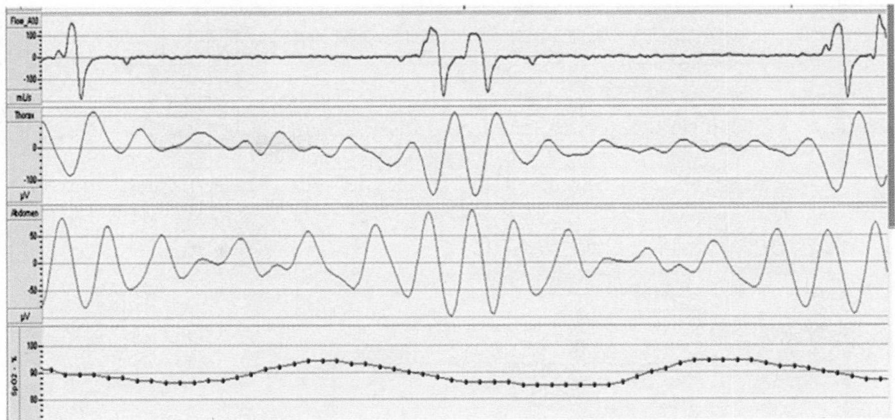

FIGURE 44-2 Obstructive apnea. First tracing: airflow. Second tracing: chest movements. Third tracing: abdominal movement. Fourth tracing: oxygen saturation.

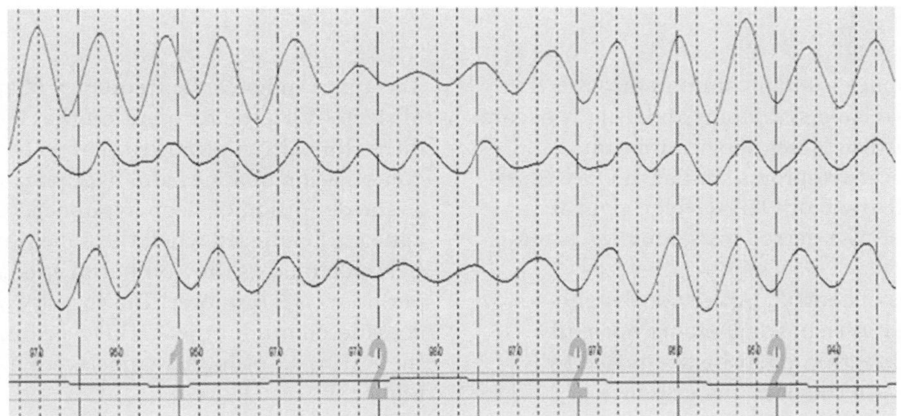

FIGURE 44-3 Hypopnea. First tracing: airflow. Second tracing: chest movements. Third tracing: abdominal movements. Fourth tracing: oxygen saturation.

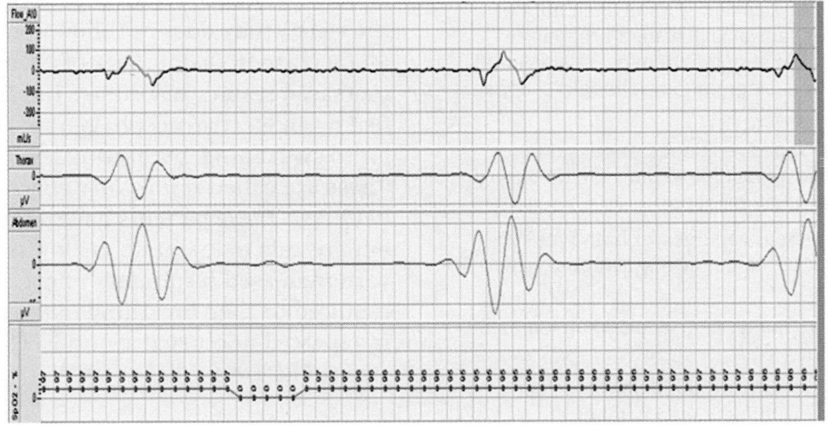

FIGURE 44-4 Central sleep apneas. First tracing: airflow. Second tracing: chest movements. Third tracing: abdominal movement. Forth tracing: oxygen saturation.

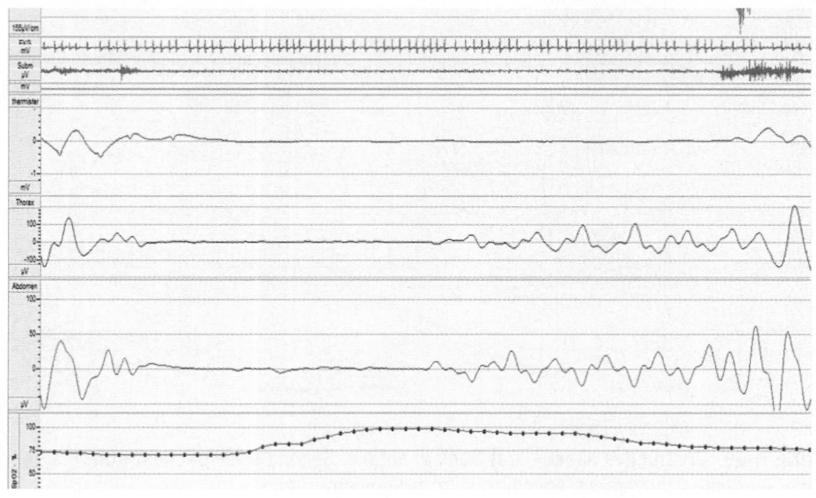

FIGURE 44-5 Mixed apneas. First tracing: airflow. Second tracing: chest movements. Third tracing: abdominal movements. Fourth tracing: oxygen saturation.

Central sleep apnea is an uncommon disorder that causes mild sleep-related symptoms and usually occurs in patients with cardiac or neurologic problems.[5] Patients have clinical symptoms similar to OSA. Some patients who are treated for OSA develop central apneas during therapy, referred to as **complex sleep apnea syndrome**.

When episodes of central, mixed, or obstructive apnea are greater than what occurs normally, sleep-disordered breathing may be diagnosed by **polysomnography**. In the past, the presence of 30 apneas during a 6- to 8-hour polysomnogram and/or an apnea index of 5 was used to define sleep apnea.[2]

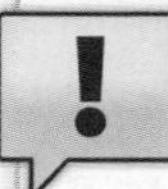

Respiratory Recap

Types of Sleep-Disordered Breathing

- *Obstructive sleep apnea*: greater than normal episodes of absent or diminished breathing, but continued chest and abdominal movements during sleep, causing pathophysiologic changes while awake.
- *Central sleep apnea*: episodes of cessation of airflow and chest/abdominal movements during sleep, greater than expected.
- *Mixed sleep apnea*: episodes of both types of apnea, central in the beginning and obstructive at the end.
- *Complex sleep apnea*: central sleep apnea as a result of treating OSA.
- *Upper airway resistance breathing*: a milder sleep disorder with increased number of respiratory effort–related arousals due to increased upper airway resistance, but with normal number of apneas and hypopneas.

The apnea index is the frequency of apneas per hour of sleep. With the recognition that hypopnea can produce clinical symptoms similar to those of apneas, a combination of apnea and hypopnea was suggested as the definition of sleep hypopnea.[6] Currently, sleep apnea is diagnosed when the apnea-hypopnea index (AHI, defined as the number of apneas plus hypopneas per hour) is 5 or more.[2] The severity of sleep apnea is considered mild if the AHI is 5 or higher, moderate if the AHI is 15 or higher, and severe if the AHI is 30 or higher.[7]

The presence of daytime hypercapnia and hypoxemia defines hypercapnic and hypoxemic respiratory failure. Sleepy obese patients with respiratory failure were diagnosed as having Pickwickian syndrome before it was known that the underlying cause for their symptoms was the sleep-disordered breathing.

A milder sleep-related breathing problem is upper airway resistance syndrome (UARS). In UARS, the sleep study does not show apneas, but there is an increase in the number of **arousals** related to increased respiratory effort. The arousals are identified by an electroencephalogram (EEG) pattern similar to awakening, but lasting less than 15 seconds. These are called *respiratory effort–related arousals* (RERAs). These patients have upper airway narrowing but are able to maintain airflow in the normal range with increased respiratory effort. The increased effort required to keep breathing in the normal range results in repeated nocturnal arousals. Consequently, the symptoms are similar to OSA.

Prevalence

Sleep apnea is a very common disorder. The Wisconsin Sleep Cohort Study has provided valuable information

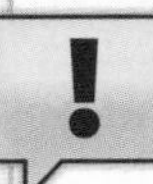

Respiratory Recap

Prevalence of Sleep Apnea

- People older than 65 years are three times more likely to develop sleep apnea than middle-aged persons.
- The risk of sleep apnea is two to four times higher among family members of sleep apnea patients regardless of age, weight, or gender.

about risk factors and the prevalence of sleep apnea in a community population.[3,8] Using the criteria of an AHI of more than 5 and the presence of daytime sleepiness revealed a prevalence of 2% in women and 4% in men. The prevalence is about 17% (24% in men and 9% in women) if sleep apnea is defined by solely an AHI of more than 5. It is estimated that about 6% of the general population has moderate sleep apnea (defined as an AHI of 15 or above). The prevalence of sleep apnea increases with age and obesity. People older than 65 years are about three times more likely to have sleep apnea compared with middle-aged persons.

Most patients clinically diagnosed to have sleep apnea are obese. There is progressive increase in the prevalence of sleep apnea with increasing severity of obesity. A person with a body mass index (BMI) of 30 kg/m^2 has more than a 30% chance of having sleep apnea. A BMI of 40 kg/m^2 increases the chance of having sleep apnea to 50%.[9] Neck circumference is a better predictor for the presence of sleep apnea than BMI. A neck circumference of 16 inches in women and 17 inches in men suggests the high likelihood of sleep apnea, requiring further testing to confirm it.

About one-third of patients with hypertension have sleep apnea. The prevalence is more than 50% in patients with hypothyroidism and acromegaly. Persons with anatomic upper airway abnormalities have a high prevalence of the disease. The prevalence of sleep apnea in many Asian populations is similar to that in the United States, even though obesity is uncommon among Asians.[10] This may be related to craniofacial characteristics of Asian populations.

There is a two to four times higher risk of sleep apnea among the family members of sleep apnea patients, independent of the effects of obesity, gender, and age. The risk of sleep apnea increases with the number of affected family members. **Table 44-2** shows some of the common risk factors for the presence of sleep apnea.

TABLE 44-2
Common Risk Factors Associated with Sleep Apnea

Obesity	Most patients are obese (body mass index >30 kg/m^2)
Age	Progressive increase in incidence with age
Gender	Twice as common in men
Snoring	Almost all sleep apnea patients snore
Sleepiness	Very common in sleep apnea
Alcohol use	Increases the number of apneas
Hypertension	Three times more common in hypertensive patients
Congestive heart failure (CHF)	Over half of CHF patients have sleep apnea
Stroke	Over two-thirds of acute stroke patients have sleep apnea
Hypothyroidism, acromegaly	High incidence of sleep apnea
Medications	Sedatives and narcotics increase the number of apneas
Upper airway abnormalities	Higher incidence in persons with upper airway narrowing
Family history	Two to four times higher risk among family members regardless of other factors such as obesity, age, or gender

Screening for Sleep-Disordered Breathing

Many screening questionnaires have been developed to clinically identify patients who have sleepiness and might have sleep apnea. These questionnaires are based on patient reported symptoms, demographics, physical examination, and the presence of comorbid conditions.

Sleepiness is usually assessed by the Epworth Sleepiness Scale (ESS), in which the patient is asked to rate the likelihood of falling asleep from 0 (no chance of dozing off) to 3 (high chance of dozing off) in eight situations (sitting and reading, watching TV, sitting inactive in a public place, as a passenger in a car for an hour, lying down in the afternoon, sitting and talking to someone, sitting quietly after lunch, and in a car while stopped in traffic).[11–13] An ESS score of 10 or more is suggestive of significant daytime sleepiness.[11] Objective assessment of daytime sleepiness can be obtained by the Multiple Sleep Latency Test (MSLT), in which a patient is given an opportunity to nap for 20 minutes.[13]

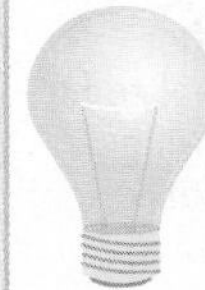

STOP AND THINK

You are caring for a patient with a BMI of 35 kg/m^2. How would you screen this patient for OSA?

This is repeated every 2 hours four more times. The time it takes to fall asleep during these five naps is calculated. The mean sleep latency in the general population is more than 8 minutes. In patients with sleepiness, the mean sleep latency is less than 8 minutes. This test, however, is not needed for routine care of sleep apnea patients.

Many screening questionnaires have been developed to clinically identify patients who might have sleep apnea.[14,15] The most commonly used tool to screen for possible obstructive sleep apnea is the STOP-BANG questionnaire.[16] Scoring is based on yes or no answers for 8 questions: presence of ***s***noring, ***t***iredness, ***o***bserved apneas, elevated blood ***p***ressure, ***b***ody mass index ≥35 kg/m^2, ***a***ge above 50 years, ***n***eck size ≥40 cm, and male ***g***ender. Three or more "yes" answers are suggestive of increased risk for having sleep apnea. Higher scores not only increase the likelihood of the presence of sleep apnea but also the likelihood that the sleep apnea is going to be severe. For example, its use in sleep clinics show that a STOP-BANG score of 8 suggests the probability of having severe sleep apnea in more than 80% of patients.[17] Based on the screening results, a complete sleep study may be performed to confirm a diagnosis.

The Epworth Sleepiness Scale and the STOP-BANG Questionnaire are useful screening tools that can uncover potential sleep disorders that require further testing using polysomnography for a complete sleep study.

Obstructive Sleep Apnea

Pathogenesis

Hypopnea and apnea result from the narrowing and occlusion of the upper airway.[18,19] The upper airway from the back of the nasal septum to the epiglottis has minimal bony support and can collapse easily. Normally this region is maintained open by a balance of the forces that tend to dilate and the forces that tend to narrow this area. Forces that tend to dilate this area include the tonic and phasic activity of the genioglossus (tongue) and upper airway muscles. The tonic activity is present throughout the respiratory cycle, and the phasic activity is present during inspiration. Conversely, inspiration creates negative pressure inside the airway. The negative pressure inside a collapsible tube can reduce the size of the tube. Increased inspiratory effort opens the intrathoracic airway but reduces the luminal area of the upper airway. This effect is similar to sucking though a collapsible straw. The harder one sucks at the straw, the narrower the lumen of the straw becomes. Airflow linearly decreases as the pressure in the upper airway becomes negative. When the negative pressure exceeds a critical pressure (e.g., –10 cm H_2O in normal persons), airway occlusion occurs.

During sleep, as the tone of the pharyngeal dilator muscles decreases, the soft palate and the tongue move backward, causing narrowing of the oropharynx. Maximum narrowing occurs during rapid eye movement (REM) sleep, when the muscle tone is further reduced, and also in the supine posture, where gravity has the greatest effect. Occasional apnea and hypopnea thus can occur during REM sleep and in supine posture, even in normal individuals. The site of occlusion is variable and may occur at multiple sites, but most commonly occurs at the velopharynx and in the retroglossal area. The velopharynx consists of the velum (soft palate), the lateral pharyngeal walls (side walls of the throat and the posterior pharyngeal wall), and the back wall of the throat. The velum rests against the back of the tongue during normal nasal breathing. During inhalation, air can flow through the nose and pharynx to the lungs without obstruction. Velopharyngeal closure occurs during speech, swallowing, gagging, vomiting, sucking, blowing, and whistling. Velopharyngeal closure during sleep is a major contributing cause of obstructive sleep apnea.

Four interdependent factors that play a role in upper airway occlusion during sleep are narrowing of the pharyngeal cavity, decreased activity of the pharyngeal dilator muscles, increased respiratory effort (i.e., more negative intraluminal pressure), and increased compliance (collapsibility) of the pharyngeal airway. When there is fat in the neck and tongue, it causes enlargement of the tongue with narrowing of the upper airway. Many abnormalities that can cause narrowing of the upper airway have been identified (**Table 44-3**).

Respiratory Recap

Pathogenesis of Obstructive Sleep Apnea

- The pathogenesis of OSA is related to upper airway anatomy characteristics, pharyngeal tone during sleep, airway pressure changes during inspiration, and inspiratory efforts associated with airway narrowing or occlusion.

TABLE 44-3
Common Upper Airway Abnormalities Associated with Obstructive Sleep Apnea

Nose	Enlarged turbinates, deviated septum, polyps, nasal valve dysfunction
Nasopharynx	Enlarged adenoids, tumors, pharyngeal flap
Oropharynx	Enlargement of uvula and soft palate, tonsillar hypertrophy, tumor, macroglossia
Larynx	Vocal cord paralysis, epiglottic edema
Jaw	Micrognathia, retrognathia

Alcohol and sedatives reduce upper airway muscle activity, predisposing patients to apnea.[20] These substances result in narrowing of the airway from the decreased muscle tone. This leads to reduced airflow, causing an increased respiratory effort to try to restore the airflow. Narrowing above the site of occlusion (i.e., upstream resistance) causes more negative intraluminal pressure, leading to even more narrowing. A vicious cycle, therefore, occurs in which the harder the patient tries to breathe, the more the airways become obstructed. Deposition of fat makes the upper airway more compliant. That is, a small increase in negative pressure can pull the upper airway muscles together. Thus, in obese patients with sleep apnea, occlusion occurs with less negative pressure and, at times, even with positive airway pressure.

Clinical Features

Apneas cause hypoxemia and hypercapnia, which are terminated by arousals. Most of the clinical manifestations of sleep apnea result from repeated arousals and hypoxemia. Snoring, daytime hypersomnolence, and disturbed sleep are the usual reasons patients seek medical attention. Many times, patients are unaware of their problems and are brought for evaluation because their spouses are bothered by the snoring and disturbed sleep. **Box 44-1** lists the usual symptoms associated with OSA. A wide spectrum of clinical manifestations exists, ranging from mild nocturnal snoring and daytime tiredness to acute or chronic hypoxemic and hypercapnic respiratory failure (**Table 44-4**).

Snoring is the most common symptom among patients with OSA. It is usually loud enough to be heard from outside the room. The loudness of snoring is a predictor of the severity of sleep apnea. The snoring may be continuous, but usually it has an intermittent pattern. Snoring is caused by the oscillation of pharyngeal soft tissues. Snoring is common in the general population, and it is estimated that about 48% of men and 34% of women snore habitually.[21] Snoring is present in almost all patients seen in sleep clinics. Occasionally a patient with sleep apnea may deny snoring, but either he or she is sleeping alone or the bed partner does not corroborate the denial. The snoring is often described as being similar to the noise coming from a freight train. Loud snoring disturbs the bed partner's sleep and frequently leads to sleeping in separate beds or rooms.

Hypersomnolence during the daytime is one of the main reasons for seeking evaluation. Falling asleep during periods of relative inactivity, such as watching television, driving, and attending meetings, is common. In advanced cases, the patient may fall asleep even when engaged in an activity (e.g., talking, walking, and eating). Many patients seen in sleep clinics complain of daytime tiredness and general decreased performance. In sleep studies performed in the general population, regardless of the presence of symptoms, sleepiness is present in only about 50% of the subjects who are diagnosed to have sleep apnea.[22] Sleepiness is also uncommon in sleep apnea patients with congestive heart failure. Some patients complain of daytime tiredness instead of sleepiness. "I am tired of being tired" is a common complaint. Both repeated nocturnal awakenings (i.e., sleep fragmentation) and hypoxemia have been implicated as the cause of daytime somnolence, but sleep fragmentation appears to be the main determinant.[11]

Other symptoms are common with OSA. The sleep pattern of patients with OSA is characterized by frequent tossing and turning. Patients wake up repeatedly from their sleep because of choking, shortness of breath, dry mouth, or for no apparent reason. Some patients' primary complaint may be the inability to have a good night sleep. Nocturnal sweating, probably related to increased breathing effort, is common. Hallucinations may occur because of awakening from REM sleep. Patients do not feel fresh when they wake up in the morning. Morning headaches, personality changes, and decreased hearing acuity are common.

BOX 44-1

Symptoms of Sleep Apnea

Daytime Symptoms

Sleepiness
Nonrefreshing sleep
Morning headaches
Intellectual dysfunction
Personality changes

Nighttime Symptoms

Snoring
Apneic, choking, gasping awakenings
Restless sleep
Nocturia
Dry mouth
Drooling
Diaphoresis
Erectile dysfunction

Complications of Obstructive Sleep Apnea

Blood gas abnormalities, repeated arousals, and increased negative intrathoracic pressure are the main

TABLE 44-4
Clinical Spectrum of Sleep Apnea

	Snoring	Arousals	Somnolence	Hypoxemia	Hypercarbia	AHI*
Normal	–	–	–	–	–	–
Snorers	+	+–	–	–	–	+–
UARS†	++	+	+–	–	–	<5
Mild sleep apnea	+++	++	+	+–	–	>5
Moderate sleep apnea	++++	+++	++	+	–	>15
Severe sleep apnea	++++	++++	+++	+++	+–	>30
Sleep apnea with respiratory failure	++++	++++	++++	++++	+	>30

*AHI, apnea-hypopnea index

†UARS, upper airway resistance syndrome

mechanisms responsible for a myriad of complications occurring in severe sleep apnea patients. Many biochemical abnormalities have been identified that may be playing a role in the pathogenesis of these complications. Hypoxemia occurs with apneic episodes and, with increasing severity of the disease, may become sustained and occur during the daytime. Hypoxemia appears to be the main determinant of most sleep apnea–related complications.

Hypoxemia causes tissue ischemia, induces pulmonary artery constriction leading to pulmonary hypertension, and causes increased sympathetic discharge (catecholamines). Long-standing pulmonary hypertension may result in right-sided heart failure, or cor pulmonale. Transient hypercapnia also occurs with apneas and can become sustained and chronic. If left untreated, this can lead to chronic respiratory failure. Repeated arousals from sleep lead to higher catecholamine release during the night. Increased respiratory effort needed to overcome upper airway narrowing causes increased negative pressure in the chest cavity. This increased negative intrathoracic pressure affects the heart in two ways. It makes it easier for blood to come back to the right side of the heart but makes it more difficult for the left heart to pump blood into the aorta. Because of the increased negative pressure around it (i.e., the heart is being pulled to the outside), the heart has to work harder (produce more positive pressure) to pump the blood out. This increased cardiac workload may lead to left-sided heart failure.

Patients with OSA have increased blood levels of C-reactive protein (CRP), a marker of inflammation.[23] An elevated CRP level causes blunting of endothelium-dependent vasodilation and correlates with increased risk of developing cardiovascular disease. Similarly, levels of fibrinogen, tumor necrosis factor-α (TNF-α), interleukin-6 (IL-6), homocysteine, and other biomarkers are increased,[24] causing increased cardiovascular disease. Leptin is a protein secreted by fat cells and is thought to be an appetite suppressant. Serum leptin levels are high in patients with OSA, suggesting there is resistance to this protein.[25] Increased leptin levels are linked to cardiovascular disease.[26] Circulating nitric oxide level is decreased with OSA, and the level improves with therapy.[27]

Almost all parts of the body are affected by the presence of sleep apnea. Complications are common and become more frequent as the severity of disease increases. Some of the common complications of OSA are discussed in the following subsections according to their effects on various systems of the body.

Central Nervous System

Cognitive dysfunction and sleepiness are common in patients with OSA. Neuropsychological measures of overall performance are moderately impaired, and cognitive abilities have an inverse correlation with oxygen desaturation and apnea. Patients may have problems related to attention, concentration, memory, and vigilance. Some patients become irritable and have difficulty with social interaction. Sleepiness at work is associated with reduced efficiency. Sleepiness in patients who operate heavy equipment or drive for work, such as long-haul truck drivers and bus drivers, may be particularly hazardous. The rate of automobile accidents in patients with sleep apnea is about three times higher than in the general population. The rate of auto accidents goes down as patients are successfully treated.[28] Most children with lack of adequate sleep resist sleepiness and are restless during the day. These patients may be labeled as having attention deficit hyperactivity disorder (ADHD). Children and adults with ADHD who snore need to be evaluated for possible sleep apnea.[29]

Cardiovascular

Sleep apnea has been implicated in many cardiovascular abnormalities.[30] Cardiac arrhythmias and both right and left ventricular dysfunction ultimately leading to congestive heart failure can occur in patients with OSA. The heart rate slows during an apneic episode and speeds up when the apnea is terminated. Nocturnal bradycardia (30 to 50 beats per minute) during apneic episodes, followed by tachycardia (90 to 120 beats per minute) at the resolution of apnea is the most common pattern of arrhythmias.[31] Other cardiac arrhythmias are seen in about 20% of patients undergoing polysomnography. These arrhythmias occur more frequently in patients with hypoxemia and include premature atrial and ventricular contractions, atrial and ventricular tachycardia, sinus pauses, and heart block. The incidence of OSA in patients with atrial fibrillation is high, and the recurrence rate of fibrillation after cardioversion remains high if the OSA remains untreated.[32] Both right and left ventricular hypertrophy and congestive cardiac failure can develop secondary to OSA. Additionally, the incidence of both central and obstructive sleep apnea is very common in patients with congestive heart failure.[33]

Hypertension occurs in about 50% of patients with sleep apnea; conversely, the prevalence of sleep apnea in the hypertensive population is estimated to be about 30%. There is a progressive increase in the prevalence of hypertension with the severity of sleep apnea, but even mild sleep apnea is associated with an increased prevalence of hypertension.[34] The prevalence of hypertension is about two to three times higher in sleepy patients compared with nonsleepy patients.[22] Almost all male patients and two-thirds of female patients with refractory hypertension (defined as continued elevation of blood pressure in spite of taking three or more antihypertensive medications) have OSA.[35] The likelihood of developing hypertension over time progressively increases with the severity of OSA. Although both hypertension and sleep apnea occur more commonly in middle-aged obese men, sleep apnea is an independent risk factor for hypertension. Successful therapy for sleep apnea may lead to improvement in hypertension.

Patients with OSA have an increased incidence of angina, myocardial infarction, and congestive heart failure.[31] Like hypertension, smoking, and obesity, OSA is considered an independent risk factor for myocardial infarction. The prevalence of OSA is higher in patients with cardiovascular disorders than in the general population.

There is a strong association between sleep apnea and cerebral vascular accidents.[6] Patients with OSA are about two to three times more likely to develop stroke compared with controls. Because OSA is a risk factor for hypertension, which is one of the strongest risk factors for stroke, it is not surprising that the risk of stroke is increased. It appears, however, that the risk of stroke in patients with sleep apnea is higher even in the absence of hypertension. The prevalence of OSA in patients with stroke is very high. More than two-thirds of patients admitted with acute stroke have sleep apnea.[6]

Pulmonary

Pulmonary hypertension during apneic episodes is common. In patients with severe hypoxemia, extremely high levels of pulmonary hypertension may be observed.[36] Sustained pulmonary hypertension during the day is found in about 20% of patients with OSA, primarily in those with hypoxemia and hypercapnia during the day and severe oxygen desaturation during the night.[37] Occasionally, acute pulmonary edema may be the presenting feature of the disease in patients with severe sleep apnea.[36] A paradoxical shift of the interventricular septum can occur because of increased right ventricular pressure.

Endocrine

The prevalence of type 2 diabetes is higher in patients with OSA; conversely, the prevalence of OSA is higher in patients with type 2 diabetes.[38] Although obesity is a common risk factor for both diseases, OSA is an independent risk factor for the development of insulin resistance. There is improvement in insulin resistance with **continuous positive airway pressure (CPAP)** therapy in patients with OSA and diabetes.[38]

Renal

Proteinuria is known to commonly occur in obese patients, but it appears that sleep apnea may be a stronger determinant of its frequency and severity.[39] Proteinuria may be significant enough to be in the nephrotic range and is usually reversible with adequate therapy for sleep apnea.[40] Proteinuria usually occurs in patients with severe sleep apnea and appears to be related to the degree of hypoxemia.[41,42]

Gastrointestinal

Gastroesophageal reflux symptoms are present in more than 50% of patients with OSA. Patients with reflux disease have a higher prevalence of snoring and sleep apnea. The paradoxical breathing pattern (chest and abdomen moving in opposite directions) during apneic episodes predisposes the development of reflux. Increased negative intrathoracic pressure during an apneic episode encourages the movement of gastric acid into the esophagus. At the same time, abdominal pressure is increased due to the inward movement of the abdominal muscles causing the same effect. Therapy with CPAP leads to improvement in reflux symptoms.[43]

Ophthalmic

Several associations between OSA and various eye-related problems have been suggested. Optic disk swelling, teardrop retinal hemorrhages, normotensive glaucoma, ischemic optic neuropathy, and increased intracranial pressure associated with disc edema (pseudo tumor cerebri) have all been reported in patients with OSA.[44]

Psychiatric

Sleep disturbances are frequently seen in patients with depression. Depression is common in patients with sleep apnea. Patients with depression and hypertension have a high prevalence of sleep apnea. CPAP therapy results in improvement in symptoms of depression in many patients with sleep apnea and depression.[45]

Sexual

Erectile dysfunction is common in patients with severe OSA, particularly in patients with hypoxemia. CPAP therapy is associated with improvement in erectile dysfunction.[46]

Diagnosis of Obstructive Sleep Apnea

Many clinical findings, such as degree of obesity, neck circumference, snoring, nocturnal choking, hypertension, age, sleepiness during driving, and the presence of upper airway abnormalities, have been identified as predictors of the presence of OSA. A flow–volume loop usually shows the presence of upper airway obstruction or a sawtooth pattern, or both.[47] Holter monitoring can reveal characteristic arrhythmias present predominantly during sleep. None of these, however, is strong enough to obviate the need for polysomnography for a definite diagnosis.

Nocturnal pulse oximetry showing repeated episodes of oxygen desaturation is strongly suggestive of sleep apnea.[48] In many countries an oxygen desaturation of 4% is considered equivalent to an apneic episode. Instead of using the AHI, an oxygen desaturation index (ODI) is reported. In most patients with sleep apnea and hypoxemia there is a high correlation between the AHI and ODI. Hypoxemia may not be present in patients with mild sleep apnea, however.

Overnight polysomnography, with recording of the electroencephalogram, electro-oculogram, electromyogram, electrocardiogram, oronasal airflow, chest and abdominal movements, and oxygen saturation, remains the standard diagnostic test for sleep apnea. Polysomnography reveals the frequency, type, and duration of apnea and hypopnea; the presence of cardiac arrhythmias; and the quality and quantity of sleep. In addition, the presence of repeated arousals and episodes of nocturnal myoclonus that can produce hypersomnolence can be identified. The American Academy of Sleep Medicine has published guidelines for scoring of sleep and sleep-related breathing problems.[49]

Usually single-night polysomnography is a sufficiently sensitive test to exclude clinically significant sleep apnea. Sometimes, however, the first polysomnogram may be falsely negative. Factors that may cause a false-negative polysomnogram include a technically poor study, an inadequate amount of sleep, reduced REM sleep, sleeping in a lateral posture, recent weight loss, or recent therapy for suspected sleep apnea.

Respiratory Recap

Complications of Sleep-Disordered Breathing

- Sleep-disordered breathing causes a variety of serious complications affecting the cardiac, pulmonary, psychological, sexual, endocrine, central nervous, renal, vascular, and ophthalmic systems.
- Cognitive dysfunction and sleepiness are common in patients with OSA. The rate of automobile accidents in patients with sleep apnea is about three times higher than in the general population. There may also be problems related to attention, concentration, memory, and vigilance.

Treatment of Obstructive Sleep Apnea

Tracheostomy was considered the standard treatment for very sick patients with OSA during the 1970s. Currently, most patients, including those with acute or chronic respiratory failure, can be adequately treated with CPAP therapy. **Oral appliances** also are considered first-line therapy for mild sleep apnea. Surgical therapy can be used if there are significant correctable anatomic abnormalities. Other helpful strategies include weight loss, sleeping in nonsupine posture, and avoiding aggravating factors such as alcohol, smoking, sedatives, and narcotics. Treatment of diseases contributing to sleep apnea, such as hypothyroidism, can also improve sleep apnea symptoms.

Weight Loss

Fat deposition in neck and pharyngeal tissue contributes to the anatomic and physiologic narrowing of the upper airway. Weight loss is quite effective in reducing the number of apneas and improving nocturnal oxygen desaturation and the quality of sleep. Generally, for every 1% decrease in weight there is a 3% decrease in the apnea-hypopnea index.[50,51] Usually, about a 10% to 20% weight loss is needed for a significant effect on clinical symptoms to be seen. In some patients, however, even a modest amount of weight loss may have a significant effect on the severity of sleep apnea. Regular follow-up with dietary counseling and nutritional consultation is helpful. Weight reduction surgery or medications can also be considered in patients with significant weight-related problems.

Posture

Sleeping on the back is associated with the highest number of apneas and hypopneas. Sleeping on the side improves apnea and hypopnea and, in some patients, may totally control the problem.[52] Sleeping with a tennis ball sewn in the back of the shirt or a lateral wedge pillow can help reduce time spent sleeping on the back. Most spouses are aware of this improvement and use elbow therapy to make sure the patient sleeps on the side. Sleeping with the head and upper body elevated to 30 to 60 degrees has been effective in decreasing the severity of sleep apnea.[53]

Positive Airway Pressure Therapy

Positive airway pressure (PAP) for treating OSA was first described in 1981[54] and has become the most commonly used therapy for sleep apnea.[55,56] Positive airway pressure acts as a pneumatic splint in the upper airway counteracting the negative inspiratory pressure and preventing airway collapse (**Figure 44-6**). There is a progressive increase in the upper airway size with increasing positive airway pressure. It is now considered the first-line therapy for sleep apnea and can be successfully used in most patients.

PAP can be applied using many techniques. The most common method is to apply preselected constant pressure during sleep from an airflow generator (machine). Because the same pressure level is maintained during both inspiration and expiration, it is called continuous positive airway pressure (CPAP) therapy. Many patients are uncomfortable during exhalation when they breathe against the airflow, which is still coming in at the same pressure level. The normal respiratory pattern is altered during CPAP therapy, with exhalation becoming active. Most CPAP machines provide pressures ranging from 4 to 20 cm H_2O. The most commonly used CPAP pressure range for treating OSA is between 8 and 10 cm H_2O.

Bilevel machines provide two pressure levels: higher pressure during inspiration and a lower pressure during exhalation. The pressure difference is usually about 4 cm H_2O. Because of the lowered expiratory pressure during bilevel therapy, exhalation may be less uncomfortable than with CPAP. It was anticipated that the compliance would be better with bilevel machines than with CPAP. Compliance, however, does not seem to be better with bilevel machines.[56] Bilevel machines are most commonly used when the pressure level during expiration is high (mostly above 15 cm H_2O), to the point that the patient cannot tolerate CPAP therapy. Bilevel machines are more expensive than CPAP machines.

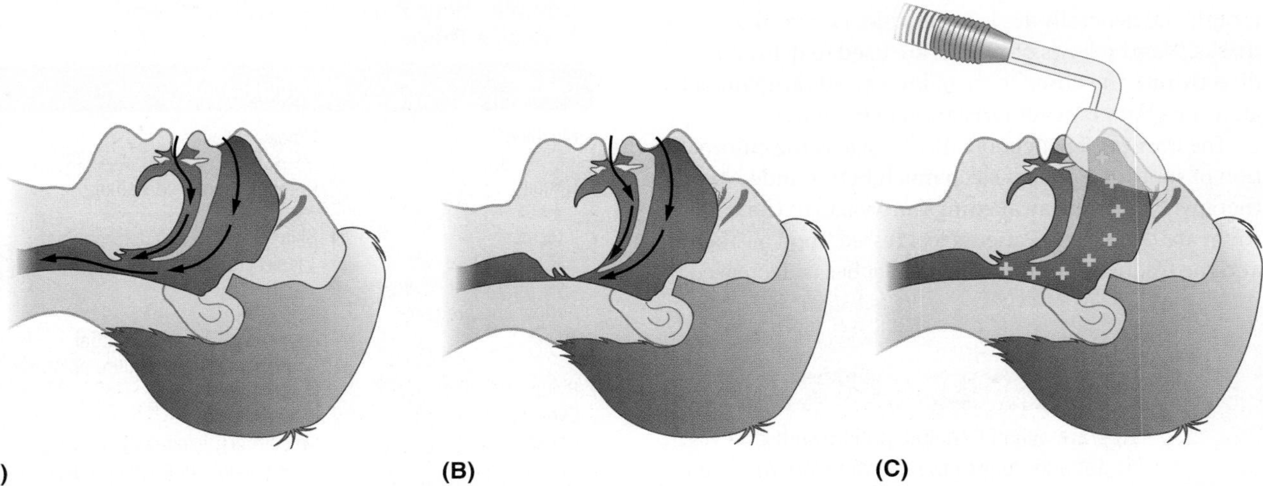

FIGURE 44-6 (**A**) Normal upper airway. (**B**) Upper airway obstruction. (**C**) Upper airway obstruction relieved with the addition of continuous positive airway pressure (CPAP) circuit for acute respiratory failure.

Adapted from Branson RD. Spontaneous breathing systems: IMV and CPAP. In: Branson RD, Hess DR, Chatburn RL, eds. *Respiratory Care Equipment*. 2nd ed. JB Lippincott; 1999.

Autotitrating PAP machines detect airway narrowing and progressively adjust the pressure until airflow becomes normal again. They are being used for the diagnosis and therapy of obstructive sleep apnea and to predict the pressure needed for CPAP therapy.[57] The mean pressure with autotitrating machines is lower than with CPAP machines because the pressure goes to the maximum only when needed. These machines have not been shown to improve compliance with CPAP therapy. They have the potential to decrease the need for CPAP titration studies. One drawback with autotitrating machines is that these machines can overcompensate if there is leakage around the mask or if the mouth is open. This overcompensation can unnecessarily increase the airway pressure, which has the potential to cause even more air leakage and can also disturb sleep. Conversely, the patient may be undertreated because of the time delay in reaching the optimal pressure needed to correct apneas. Because one of the mechanisms in some autotitrating machines is the detection of reduced inspiratory airflow, these machines may not be able to treat patients with central apneas. Also, they may not be able to treat patients with OSA who develop central apnea during CPAP therapy (complex sleep apnea). Autotitrating CPAP machines are more expensive than conventional CPAP machines.

A useful feature of CPAP machines is a ramp, in which the pressure starts at a low level and gradually increases to the prescribed level. A ramp helps some patients better tolerate this therapy. The newer CPAP machines have the capability of reducing pressure (expiratory pressure relief and C-Flex modes) briefly by 1 to 4 cm H_2O at the beginning of exhalation, which may improve patient comfort and compliance.

Many different interfaces are available for CPAP. Oronasal masks are big and cover both nose and mouth. These masks are useful for patients who keep their mouth open during PAP therapy. Nasal masks are smaller and cover only the nose. Oral masks deliver air through the mouth and generally are less well tolerated than other masks. Nasal pillows or prongs are used to deliver air directly into the nose. These pillows avoid skin-contact abrasions but may cause irritation of the nares.

The immediate effect of CPAP usage is the elimination of snoring. Spouses sleep much better and love this therapy! Nighttime awakenings and visits to the bathroom are decreased. Patients feel rested upon awakening, and the frequency of morning headaches is decreased.

STOP AND THINK

You are asked to help a patient with OSA who is not adherent to the use of CPAP. What can you do to help?

Daytime sleepiness and tiredness are reduced or eliminated in a significant number of patients. Improvement in sleep-related complications (driving, functioning at work) is noted. There is improvement in cognitive functions. Long-term CPAP usage is associated with improvement in most of the complications of sleep apnea.[55–57]

The side effects of PAP therapy are caused either by the interface or the air pressure and flow (**Table 44-5**). Newer PAP machines produce only a minimal humming noise. The main reason for noise at the face is the leakage of air because of poor fit or movement of the mask. Some patients may get entangled with the circuit. Fitting the mask too tightly can lead to skin irritation and skin abrasions at the contact site. The nasal bridge is the usual site of skin and bony erosion. Many patients complain of nasal or oral dryness, nasal congestion, sneezing, and even nosebleeds. The use of heated humidity reduces symptoms in most patients.[58] Chinstraps can help in keeping the mouth closed, thereby reducing oral dryness in patients who keep their mouth open during PAP therapy. Using intranasal ipratropium can help rhinorrhea. Pressures in the lower range are well tolerated; however, at higher pressures, some patients experience hyperinflation. In such patients, the CPAP apparatus can be modified to give lower pressure during exhalation. Swallowing air (aerophagy) may be associated with CPAP use and can be reduced by using lower pressure. Pneumothorax is potentially a serious complication but occurs rarely in the usual pressure range used for sleep apnea. Pneumocephaly is also rare and is related to air leakage from the nose to the cranium.

The major reason for the failure of PAP therapy is lack of adherence to the treatment plan. Most new PAP

TABLE 44-5
Complications Related to Positive Airway Pressure Therapy

Cause	Complication
Machine	Noise
Circuit	Entanglement, rebreathing
Interface	Skin abrasions, claustrophobia, leaks, rebreathing
Airflow and pressure	
Nose	Dryness on nose and throat, rhinorrhea, congestion, epistaxis
Sinus	Discomfort
Eyes	Conjunctivitis
Chest	Discomfort, expiratory difficulty, hyperinflation, pneumothorax
Gastrointestinal system	Aerophagy
Central nervous system	Pneumocephalus

machines have the capability to provide hourly, nightly, and long-term data about when the machine is turned on and the actual usage of the machine. Because the beneficial effect of PAP therapy is directly proportional to the amount of time it is used, all-night usage should be encouraged. Arbitrarily, a patient is considered compliant if his or her PAP machine usage is a minimum of 4 hours per night on 70% of the nights under consideration. Patient adherence during the first month predicts long-term usage. Adherence is better in patients with severe symptoms and in better-educated individuals. A higher pressure level does not reduce patient adherence, as is sometimes assumed. Patient adherence to therapy can be improved by positive reinforcement and treatment of PAP-related side effects (e.g., uncomfortable mask, oronasal dryness). Unfortunately, only about 55% of patients use CPAP therapy regularly, which is an adherence rate similar to the intake rate of oral medications for other medical diseases.

The Centers for Medicare and Medicaid Services has recommended AHI-based criteria for CPAP therapy. Reimbursement for CPAP is approved if the patient has an AHI of 15 or above (moderate and severe sleep apnea). Reimbursement is also approved for patients with an AHI greater than or equal to 5 and less than or equal to 14 (mild sleep apnea) who have at least one of the following: (1) symptoms of excessive daytime sleepiness; (2) impaired cognition, mood disorders, or insomnia; or (3) cardiovascular disease such as hypertension, ischemic heart disease, or history of stroke.

Oral Appliances

Oral appliances are used to enlarge the oropharynx by either advancing the mandible or keeping the tongue in a forward position.[59,60] Mandibular repositioning appliances (MRAs) cause forward and downward movement of the mandible when attached to one or both dental arches. Tongue-retaining devices (TRDs) keep the tongue in the anterior position by creating negative pressure in a plastic bulb, a flange that fits between the lips and the teeth. Oral appliances increase the airway space in both the retropalatal and retroglossal areas. Both types of devices also increase upper airway muscle tone, thereby making it easier for the airway to remain open. Previously, these appliances required dental impressions, bite registration, and fabrication by a dental laboratory. Newer appliances, however, are available in prefabricated thermolabile forms that can be molded in the office or at home.

Oral appliances are generally used in patients who present with snoring, upper airway resistance syndrome, or mild sleep apnea that does not respond to conservative therapy. These appliances can also be used in patients who have moderate or severe sleep apnea and cannot use CPAP therapy. Oral appliances are not considered the first-line therapy for severe sleep apnea.

Oral appliances are effective in reducing the severity of symptoms and various objective measures used to express the severity of sleep apnea. There is significant improvement in the intensity and frequency of snoring in most patients. Reduction in daytime sleepiness occurs in most patients. Apnea and hypopnea are improved, and the rate of improvement depends on how the improvement is defined.[61] The success rate is about 65% if the most liberal definition of improvement (i.e., 50% reduction in AHI) is used. The success rates are 52% and 42% if AHI reductions down to 10 or 5 are used, respectively. About one-half of patients continue to have significant apneas, and about 10% may have worsening of AHI with these appliances. The four main predictors of successful therapy with oral appliances are lower severity of OSA, lower body mass index, more severe OSA when the patient sleeps on his or her back compared with his or her side, and the amount of mandibular or tongue advancement by the appliance.[62] Improvement is least in obese patients with severe OSA, particularly those who do not have significant improvement in apneas in the nonsupine posture. The usual protrusion of mandible necessary to improve OSA varies between 5 and 10 mm. Improvement is seen in only one-third of patients if the protrusion is 50% of the maximum, but increases with more protrusion.

The compliance rate with oral appliances is high, and about three-fourths of patients use their appliance regularly. Compliance rate falls somewhat over time because of side effects and lack of efficacy. Overall compliance rates are similar to CPAP in various crossover studies.

Some oral discomfort occurs, but most patients tolerate these appliances well. Common side effects include mouth dryness, excessive salivation, tooth discomfort, occlusive change, and jaw pain. Side effects may improve with continued use. In addition, long-term use may result in a mild reduction in overbite or overjet and minor movements of teeth. In some patients bite changes persist after cessation of therapy.

Currently, oral appliances and CPAP are considered the first lines of therapy for mild sleep apnea. The patient acceptance rate is high, and many patients prefer these appliances compared with CPAP therapy. The reduction in apneas and hypopneas and oxygen desaturation is less than with CPAP therapy, but the improvement in symptoms is similar. The improvement in apneas and hypopneas is better with oral appliances than with surgical therapy.[62]

Edentulous patients are unable to use MRAs but may be able to use TRDs. Patients should have at least six teeth in each dental arch to be able to hold an MRA, and they should be able to open the mouth and protrude the mandible forward. Significant temporomandibular joint problems and severe bruxism are contraindications for oral appliance therapy.

Surgery

Tracheostomy is very effective in eliminating apnea and reversing the consequences of apnea; however, complications commonly occur. Most patients are reluctant to have it done; consequently, tracheostomy is rarely performed for OSA. Although many surgical procedures can be undertaken to correct anatomic abnormalities and to open the upper airway (**Box 44-2**), **uvulopalatopharyngoplasty (UPPP)** remains the most common surgical procedure.[63,64]

Upper airway obstruction in sleep apnea usually occurs at the retropalatal and/or retroglossal area. UPPP enlarges the posterior pharynx by removing the uvula, tonsils, and excessive tissue from the lateral pharyngeal wall and pharyngopalatal arch. Following surgery, symptomatic improvement may be reported by up to 90% of patients. Objective improvement (50% reduction in apneas) occurs in about two-thirds of patients, and cure (reduction of apneas to the normal range) is seen in less than half. Unfortunately, many patients have recurrence of symptoms of OSA after initial improvement. Some patients have worsening of apneas and hypopneas after surgery. Many modifications of UPPP, including laser-assisted uvuloplasty (LAUP) and radio frequency ablation, have not been any more successful.

The efficacy of UPPP is highest in patients with mild to moderate sleep apnea. Patients with severe OSA and particularly those who have excessive body weight are not helped much by this procedure. The failure of UPPP is probably related to the multiplicity of causes of OSA and multiple sites of airway obstruction. Multiple modalities, including computed tomography of the upper airway, cephalometric analysis, pharyngeal pressure measurements, the Mueller maneuver, and direct visualization by nasoendoscope, have been used to predict the site of airway obstruction and the success of UPPP, but none of the techniques has been consistently beneficial.

Many other surgical procedures have been used for enlarging the upper airway. The overall success rate with additional procedures has been reported by some centers to be better than UPPP alone. Correction of deviated nasal septum and resection of enlarged turbinates and nasal polyps can enlarge the nasal passage. The tongue (genioglossus muscle) is attached to the inner side of the mandible at the geniotubercle. Pulling the geniotubercle forward to attach it to the front part of the mandible (mandibular osteotomy) can put tension on the tongue, preventing it from falling back to the pharynx. Moving the lower jaw forward alone or with the upper jaw (mandibular or maxillomandibular osteotomy) can increase the space at the base of the tongue. Partial resection of the center part of the tongue (midline glossectomy) has been tried in a few patients.

Surgical procedures are associated with pain, bleeding, infection, and even deaths. Persistent side effects related to UPPP surgery occur in about half of the patients and include difficulty swallowing, globus sensation, and voice changes.[64] Because of complications and the low success rate, surgical therapy is usually considered when patients do not want to use CPAP or oral appliances. If there are significant anatomic abnormalities causing airway obstruction, such as enlarged tonsils, adenoids, or deviated nasal septum, surgical therapy may be considered as the primary therapy.

BOX 44-2

Surgical Therapies for Sleep Apnea Syndromes

Uvulopalatopharyngoplasty (UPPP)
Genioglossal advancement
Partial glossectomy
Hyoid bone advancement
Maxillomandibular advancement
Tracheostomy
Combinations

Pharmacologic Therapy

Many pharmacologic agents have been tried, but none has been consistently effective. Drugs have the potential to improve apneas by many different mechanisms. Because apneas occur more frequently during REM sleep, reduction of this sleep stage by medications may be beneficial. Most antidepressant agents significantly reduce REM sleep time. In those patients with mild sleep apnea who have the majority of their apneic episodes occurring in REM sleep, a trial of a nonsedating tricyclic antidepressant (e.g., protriptyline) or selective serotonin reuptake inhibitor (SSRI) such as fluoxetine can be undertaken to see if improvement occurs in apneas and oxygen desaturation. These antidepressants also reduce upper airway narrowing by increasing the upper airway muscle tone. Medroxyprogesterone stimulates ventilation and was initially shown to have some beneficial effect, but subsequent studies have shown no improvement in apneas. Because of the limited clinical benefit and the potential for many side effects, drug therapy is not considered as a standard therapy for OSA.

Oxygen therapy can improve nocturnal oxygen desaturation as well as the frequency of apnea. However, a high concentration of inspired oxygen therapy may prolong apneic episodes and should be avoided. In patients who present with acute respiratory failure, oxygen therapy is used in conjunction with CPAP and diuretic therapy. Long-term oxygen therapy usually is reserved for patients who remain hypoxemic despite other forms of therapy.

Treatment of diseases that cause upper airway narrowing and apnea may be beneficial. Treatment of nasal allergies and the use of nasal steroids, decongestants, and antihistamines may improve nasal breathing in patients with rhinitis.[65] About 10% of patients with snoring and apneas can benefit from nasal vasoconstrictors. Apneas commonly occur in patients with hypothyroidism and acromegaly. Hypothyroidism causes narrowing of the upper airways and reduced ventilatory drive. The possibility of hypothyroidism should be considered during evaluation of patients with sleep apnea. Drug therapy of these disorders is associated with an improvement of apneas and nocturnal oxygen desaturation. Successful therapy of these disorders may reduce the need for long-term CPAP.

Some patients remain significantly sleepy in spite of adequate therapy of sleep apnea. The reason for the residual sleepiness is not clear. It has been suggested that it may be related to hypoxemia damage to wake-promoting regions of the brain.[66] Wakefulness-promoting medications such as modafinil may be considered in patients who continue to remain sleepy.[67] This medication improves daytime alertness; however, there is a potential risk that the patient may reduce the usage of CPAP therapy. The patient needs to be informed that this medication does not reduce apneas or apnea-related hypoxemia.

Mechanical Devices

In selected patients, nasopharyngeal tubes that can keep the upper airway open have been used successfully.[68,69] The control of apnea and hypopnea is less than with CPAP therapy, and the quality of sleep remains poor. Nasopharyngeal tubes are not well tolerated and have limited clinical utility.

Both external and internal dilators have been tried to treat patients with OSA.[68–70] There is improvement in snoring intensity, and some reduction in apneas, although patients continue to have oxygen desaturation and poor quality of sleep. Nasal dilators can be tried to reduce snoring but are not recommended as therapy of moderate and severe sleep apnea.

Mortality Associated with Obstructive Sleep Apnea

Many studies have shown increased cardiovascular mortality in untreated sleep apnea patients, but the mortality rates have not been consistent. Mortality rate variability seems to be related to multiple factors, including the severity of disease, age, obesity, hypertension, medical illnesses, and therapy. Most studies show increased mortality in moderate to severe OSA, whereas the role of mild sleep apnea is not clear. Increased mortality rates have been shown in both clinical and community populations with sleep apnea. A study of a community population (the Wisconsin Sleep Cohort) with 18 years of follow-up showed that after adjustments for age, sex, and body mass index, all-cause mortality was 3.8 times higher in patients with severe OSA compared with those with no sleep-disordered breathing.[70] In the same study, the cardiovascular mortality in severe OSA was 5.2 times compared with normal subjects. Other studies have shown annual mortality rates of 2% to 4% but have also emphasized the contribution of associated risk factors.

Sleep apnea causes increased highway and industrial accidents.[28,71] Increased mortality may occur in the perioperative period from anesthesia and medications. Successful therapy of sleep apnea is associated with reduction in mortality. Cardiovascular events such as angina and myocardial infarction and the death rates in patients with severe OSA who are treated with CPAP therapy are similar to controls, however.[72]

Central Sleep Apnea

Central sleep apnea (CSA) is diagnosed when there is simultaneous cessation of airflow and ventilatory effort. Because of apneas, fragmentation of sleep with nocturnal awakening occurs resulting in daytime sleepiness. There is considerable overlap in both clinical symptoms and polysomnographic findings between OSA and CSA patients. If more than 50% of the apneas are scored as

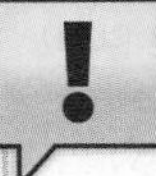

Respiratory Recap

Treatment of Obstructive Sleep Apnea

- There are many types of treatments, including mechanical, surgical, and pharmacologic approaches.
- The mechanical approach using positive airway pressure is one of the most common and effective treatments for OSA.
- Only about 55% of patients use the PAP device every night during sleep.

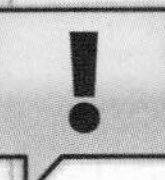

Respiratory Recap

Mortality Associated with Obstructive Sleep Apnea

- Untreated OSA can result in serious complications and even death.
- Proper diagnosis and patient adherence to required treatments are imperative. The respiratory therapist plays an important role in the diagnosis, treatment, education, and management of the patient.

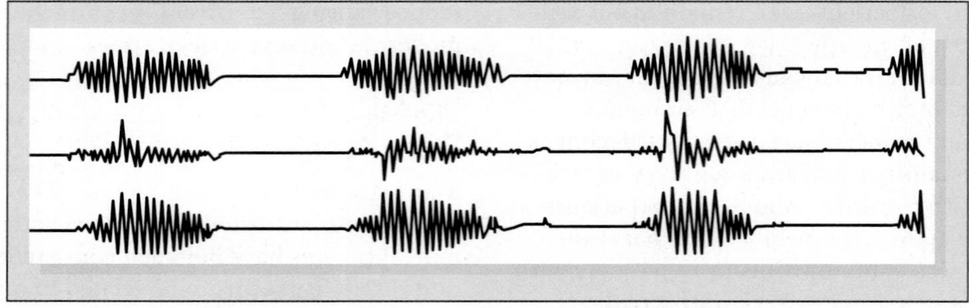

FIGURE 44-7 Cheyne-Stokes breathing. Upper: oronasal airflow. Middle: chest movements. Lower: abdominal movements.

central then CSA is considered the primary diagnosis.[49] Patients with central sleep apnea are usually not obese and have milder sleep related symptoms. Snoring and daytime sleepiness are less common. Many patients complain about insomnia and restless sleep. Nocturnal hypoxemia is less severe compared to persons with OSA. In most cases of CSA there is increased ventilatory response to CO_2.

CSA encompasses several clinical conditions including idiopathic CSA (ICSA), **Cheyne-Stokes breathing**, high altitude–induced periodic breathing, narcotic-induced central apnea, and **obesity hypoventilation syndrome (OHS)**.[73,74] Rarely, central sleep apnea may occur without any known cause and is called primary or idiopathic central sleep apnea. Both central and obstructive apneas may occur with acute administration of opioids. In long-term users of methadone, morphine, and hydrocodone CSA may be seen in up to 50% of patients.

Cheyne-Stokes Breathing

Cheyne-Stokes breathing, also known as periodic breathing, is characterized by prolonged periods of waxing and waning of ventilation separated by central apneas or hypopneas (**Figure 44-7**). This is usually seen in male subjects who are more than 60 years of age. It is rarely seen in female subjects. This pattern of breathing is seen in 25% to 40% of patients who have congestive heart failure and in about 10% of patients with stroke.

Central apneas in Cheyne-Stokes breathing occur because $Paco_2$ drops below the apneic threshold. Carbon dioxide is the primary stimulus for respiration. When $Paco_2$ levels decrease by a few mm Hg from baseline (usually 3–6 mm Hg), breathing comes to a standstill. The $Paco_2$ level at which the subjects stop breathing is called apneic threshold. During central apneas in congestive heart failure there is rise in blood CO_2 during the apneic episode. When that blood gets to the brain it stimulates an increase in breathing and CO_2 is lowered in pulmonary blood. Because circulatory time is prolonged, it takes a while for the lowered $Paco_2$ to reach the brain and decrease ventilation. The respiratory center response thus lags behind the changes in blood CO_2 and blood CO_2 changes are exaggerated, resulting in periods of hyperventilation and apnea. On polysomnogram, the apnea-ventilation cycle duration reflects the circulation time for blood from lungs to chemoreceptors. Cheyne-Stokes breathing pattern typically occurs during transition from wakefulness to sleep, mostly in stage 1 and 2, and rarely in stage 3 and REM sleep.

Treatment of Cheyne-Stokes breathing is mainly directed toward improving cardiac function.[74] Nocturnal oxygen therapy reduces the frequency of apneas and improves daytime symptoms. Some medications including theophylline and hypnotics have been shown to be helpful. CPAP therapy improves both the frequency of apneas and cardiac functions.

High Altitude Periodic Breathing

High altitude periodic breathing is characterized by cyclical periods of central apnea and hyperpnea with cycle length of 12 to 34 seconds. This pattern of breathing is seen in almost everybody at altitudes higher than 7600 meters and in some even at altitudes lower than 5000 meters. In high altitude, hypoxemia also becomes a factor in driving respiration. Individuals will hyperventilate due to hypoxemia that can drive CO_2 levels below the apneic threshold resulting in periods of apnea.

Obesity Hypoventilation Syndrome

Obesity hypoventilation syndrome is defined as a combination of obesity (body mass index ≥30 kg/m^2) and arterial hypercapnia ($Paco_2$ ≥45 mm Hg) during wakefulness. Hypercapnia worsens during sleep, particularly during REM sleep. Both obstructive and central apneas can be seen in these patients.

The patient with OHS who first presents for evaluation of a sleep complaint is clinically almost indistinguishable from the typical obese, snoring, sleepy patient with sleep apnea. If blood gases are not drawn it can be missed that a patient has OHS. It is only on careful analysis of the sleep study that hypoventilation will be suspected. The OHS sleep study will show a prolonged, rather than intermittent, desaturation pattern.

In the past, arterial blood gases were routinely drawn on all patients presenting for evaluation of sleep disorders. The present practice is to rely on noninvasive oximetry, however, and hypercapnia can remain unrecognized. Elevated serum bicarbonate on the venous blood is often the only hint that an arterial $Paco_2$ needs to be sampled. Although the oxygen saturation while awake may be low in patients with hypercapnia, it is often only modestly reduced until sleep. Noninvasive measurement of hypercapnia by end-tidal CO_2 has proven difficult and inconsistent for technical and clinical reasons, which is why obtaining a blood gas for assessment of $Paco_2$ is recommended in any patient presenting with an elevated venous bicarbonate level and/or associated chronic obstructive pulmonary disease (COPD) or predisposition to respiratory depression (e.g., medication such as opiods).[75]

Restless Legs Syndrome

Restless legs syndrome (RLS) is a sensorimotor disorder characterized by irresistible urges to move the legs accompanied by uncomfortable symptoms in legs that are difficult to describe. RLS causes paresthesias (abnormal sensations) or dysesthesias (unpleasant abnormal sensations), with sensations varying in severity from uncomfortable to irritating to painful. Some descriptions of these symptoms include: ants are crawling under my skin; soda is running in my veins; there is creepy crawly feeling. These symptoms usually occur during periods of rest and reclining. Though the symptoms may be present all day, they get worse in the evenings. The most distinctive or unusual aspect of the condition is that lying down and trying to relax activates the symptoms. Most people with RLS have difficulty falling asleep and staying asleep.

Prevalence

Approximately 10% of the U.S. population may have RLS. Several studies have shown that moderate to severe RLS affects approximately 2% to 3% of adults (more than 5 million individuals). Childhood RLS is estimated to affect almost 1 million school-age children, with one-third having moderate to severe symptoms.[75] RLS occurs in both men and women, although the incidence is about twice as high in women. It may begin at any age and the cause is not known, but may be genetic. Many individuals who are severely affected are middle-aged or older, and the symptoms typically become more frequent and last longer with age.

About 80% of the patients with RLS symptoms have periodic leg movement during sleep (PLMS).[76] The PLMS is frequently associated with arousals causing both insomnia and daytime sleepiness. PLMS is characterized by involuntary leg twitching or jerking movements during sleep that typically occur every 15 to 40 seconds, sometimes throughout the night. The symptoms cause repeated awakening and severely disrupted sleep. Although many individuals with RLS also develop PLMS, most people with PLMS do not experience RLS. PLMS may be a variant of RLS and thus respond to similar treatments.

Considerable evidence suggests that RLS is related to a dysfunction in the brain's basal ganglia circuits that use the neurotransmitter dopamine, which is needed to produce smooth, purposeful muscle activity and movement. Disruption of these pathways frequently results in involuntary movements. Individuals with Parkinson disease, another disorder of the basal ganglia's dopamine pathways, often have RLS as well.

Treatment of RLS

Movements such as walking or stretching often relieve symptoms. Consequently, people with RLS will often pace or frequently move their legs. Finding and treating an associated medical condition, such as peripheral neuropathy or diabetes, can sometimes control RLS symptoms. Certain lifestyle changes and activities that may reduce mild to moderate symptoms include: decreased use of caffeine, alcohol, and tobacco; supplements to correct deficiencies in iron, folate, and magnesium; a regular sleep pattern; moderate exercise; and massage of the legs, a hot bath, and heating pad or ice pack.

Medications are usually helpful, but no single medication effectively manages RLS for all individuals. Trials of different drugs may be necessary. In addition, medications taken regularly may lose their effect over time or even worsen symptoms, making it necessary to change medications periodically. Common drugs prescribed to treat RLS include *dopaminergic agents*, which are drugs that increase dopamine that are used to treat Parkinson disease. These agents at bedtime are the initial treatment of choice. Ropinirole, pramipexole, and rotigotine are FDA approved to treat moderate to severe RLS. These drugs are generally well tolerated but can cause nausea, dizziness, or other side effects. Good short-term results of treatment with levodopa plus carbidopa have been reported. With chronic use, a person may begin to experience symptoms earlier in the evening than in the afternoon until finally the symptoms are present around the clock.

Gabapentin enacarbil can also be prescribed to treat moderate to severe RLS. It metabolizes in the body to become gabapentin. Other medications may be prescribed off-label (not specifically designed to treat RLS) to relieve some of the symptoms. These include benzodiazepines, opioids, and anticonvulsants. Side effects of these medications can actually cause sleep apnea and should be considered alternative options under careful supervision.

Left untreated, the condition can cause exhaustion, daytime fatigue, and depression. Many people with RLS report that their job, personal relations, and activities of daily living are strongly affected as a result of their sleep deprivation and inability to concentrate.

Key Points

- Sleep apnea is common and is associated with significant complications and even death in patients who remain untreated.
- Persons who exhibit symptoms suggestive of sleep apnea should see a sleep specialist who can perform polysomnography, leading to the appropriate diagnosis and treatment.
- The most common type of sleep-disordered breathing is obstructive sleep apnea (OSA).
- Central sleep apnea (CSA) encompasses several clinical conditions including idiopathic CSA (ICSA), Cheyne-Stokes breathing, high altitude–induced periodic breathing, narcotic-induced central apnea, and obesity hypoventilation syndrome (OHS).
- Rarely, central sleep apnea may occur without any known cause and is called primary or idiopathic central sleep apnea.
- Restless legs syndrome (RLS) is a sensorimotor disorder characterized by an irresistible desire to move legs accompanied by uncomfortable symptoms in legs that can occur throughout the day but is most common in the evening.
- Respiratory therapists should have an understanding of the basics of polysomnography and sleep-disordered breathing because they may frequently be in contact with persons who have undiagnosed sleep apnea.
- Several different treatment modalities are available to alleviate the symptoms and reverse most of the complications associated with this disease.
- Respiratory therapists have an important role in the diagnosis, treatment, and management of sleep-disordered breathing.
- Patient education is a key component of patient adherence to treatment of OSA.
- Successful therapy of sleep-disordered breathing can significantly improve quality of life.

References

1. Lulu Xie, Hongyi Kang, Qiwu Xu, et al. Sleep drives metabolite clearance from the adult brain. *Science*. 2013;342:373–377.
2. Guilleminault C, Tilkian A, Dement WC. The sleep apnea syndromes. *Annu Rev Med*. 1976;27:465–484.
3. Young T, Palta M, Dempsey J, et al. The occurrence of sleep-disordered breathing among middle-aged adults. *N Engl J Med*. 1993;328:1230–1235.
4. Gottlieb, DJ. The Sleep Heart Health Study: a progress report. *Curr Opin Pulm Med*. 2008;14:537–542.
5. Yumino D, Bradley TD. Central sleep apnea and Cheyne-Stokes respiration. *Proc Am Thorac Soc*. 2008;5:226–236.
6. Yaggi HK, Concato J, Kernan W, et al. Obstructive sleep apnea as a risk factor for stroke and death. *N Engl J Med*. 2005;353:2034–2041.
7. Epstein LJ, Kristo D, Strollo PJ, et al. Clinical guideline for the evaluation, management and long-term care of obstructive sleep apnea in adults. *J Clin Sleep Med*. 2009;5:263–276.
8. Young T, Skatrud J, Peppard PE. Risk factors for obstructive sleep apnea in adults. *JAMA*. 2004;29:2013–2016.
9. Resta O, Foschino-Barbaro MP, Legari G, et al. Sleep related breathing disorders, loud snoring and excessive daytime sleepiness in obese subjects. *Int J Obes Relat Metab Disord*. 2001;25:669–675.
10. Lam B, Lam DC, Ip MS. Obstructive sleep apnoea in Asia. *Int J Tuberc Lung Dis*. 2007;11:2–11.
11. Johns MW. Daytime sleepiness, snoring, and obstructive sleep apnea. The Epworth Sleepiness Scale. *Chest*. 1993;103:30–36.
12. Johns MW. A new method for measuring daytime sleepiness: the Epworth Sleepiness Scale. *Sleep*. 1991;14:540–545.
13. Littner MR, Kushida C, Wise M, et al. Practice parameters for clinical use of the multiple sleep latency test and the maintenance of wakefulness test. *Sleep*. 2005;28:113–121.
14. Abrishami A, Khajehdehi A, Chung F. A systematic review of screening questionnaires for obstructive sleep apnea. *Can J Anaesth*. 2010;57:423–438.
15. Ramachandran, CK, Josephs, LA. A meta-analysis of clinical screening tests for obstructive sleep apnea. *Anesthesiology*. 2009;110:928–939.
16. Chung F, Subramanyam R, Liao P, et al. High STOP-BANG score indicates a high probability of obstructive sleep apnoea. *Br J Anaesth*. 2012;108:768–775.
17. Farney RJ, Walker BS, Farney RM, Snow GL, Walker JM. The STOP-BANG equivalent model and prediction of severity of obstructive sleep apnea: relation to polysomnographic measurements of the apnea/hyponea index. *J Clin Sleep Med*. 2011;7:459–465.
18. White DP. Pathogenesis of obstructive and central sleep apnea. *Am J Respir Crit Care Med*. 2005;172:1363–1370.
19. Ryan CM, Bradley TD. Pathogenesis of obstructive sleep apnea. *J Appl Physiol*. 2005;99:2440–2450.
20. Peppard PE, Austin D, Brown RL. Association of alcohol consumption and sleep disordered breathing in men and women. *J Clin Sleep Med*. 2007;3:265–270.
21. Kapur VK, Resnick HE, Gottlieb DJ. Sleep disordered breathing and hypertension: does self-reported sleepiness modify the association? *Sleep*. 2008;31:1127–1132.
22. Arzt M, Young T, Finn L, et al. Sleepiness and sleep in patients with both systolic heart failure and obstructive sleep apnea. *Arch Intern Med*. 2006;166:1716–1722.
23. Lui MM, Lam JC, Mak HK, et al. C-reactive protein is associated with obstructive sleep apnea independent of visceral obesity. *Chest*. 2009;135:950–956.
24. Bravo Mde L, Serpero LD, Barcelo A, et al. Inflammatory proteins in patients with obstructive sleep apnea with and without daytime sleepiness. *Sleep Breath*. 2007;11:177–185.
25. Kapsimalis F, Varouchakis G, Manousaki A, et al. Association of sleep apnea severity and obesity with insulin resistance, C-reactive protein, and leptin levels in male patients with obstructive sleep apnea. *Lung*. 2008;186:209–217.
26. Schafer H, Pauleit D, Sudhop T, et al. Body fat distribution, serum leptin, and cardiovascular risk factors in men with obstructive sleep apnea. *Chest*. 2002;122:829–839.
27. Atkeson A, Yeh SY, Malhotra A, Jelic S. Endothelial function in obstructive sleep apnea. *Prog Cardiovasc Dis*. 2009;51:351–362.

28. Ellen RL, Marshall SC, Palayew M, et al. Systematic review of motor vehicle crash risk in persons with sleep apnea. *J Clin Sleep Med.* 2006;2:193–200.
29. Naseem S, Chaudhary B, Collop N. Attention deficit hyperactivity disorder in adults and obstructive sleep apnea. *Chest.* 2001;119:294–296.
30. Parish JM, Somers VK. Obstructive sleep apnea and cardiovascular disease. *Mayo Clin Proc.* 2004;79:1036–1047.
31. Guilleminault C, Connolly SJ, Winkle RA. Cardiac arrhythmia and conduction disturbances during sleep in 400 patients with sleep apnea syndrome. *Am J Cardiol.* 1983;52:490–494.
32. Caples SM, Somers VK. Sleep-disordered breathing and atrial fibrillation. *Prog Cardiovasc Dis.* 2009;51:411–415.
33. MacDonald M, Fang J, Pittman SD, et al. The current prevalence of sleep disordered breathing in congestive heart failure patients treated with beta-blockers. *J Clin Sleep Med.* 2008;4:38–42.
34. Nieto FJ, Young TB, Lind BK, et al. Association of sleep disordered breathing, sleep apnea and hypertension in a large community based study. Sleep Heart Health Study. *JAMA.* 2000;283: 1829–1836.
35. Logan AG, Perlikowski SM, Mente A, et al. High prevalence of unrecognized sleep apnea in drug-resistant hypertension. *J Hypertens.* 2001;19:2271–2277.
36. Chaudhary BA, Nadimi M, Chaudhary TK, Speir WA. Pulmonary edema due to obstructive sleep apnea. *South Med J.* 1984;77:499–501.
37. Atwood CW Jr, McCrory D, Garcia JG, et al. Pulmonary artery hypertension and sleep disordered breathing. *Chest.* 2004;126:72s–77s.
38. Tasali E, Mokhlesi B, Van Cauter E. Obstructive sleep apnea and type 2 diabetes: interacting epidemics. *Chest.* 2008;133:496–506.
39. Chaudhary BA, Sklar AH, Chaudhary TK, et al. Sleep apnea, proteinuria, and nephrotic syndrome. *Sleep.* 1988;11:69–74.
40. Sklar AH, Chaudhary BA. Reversible proteinuria in obstructive sleep apnea syndrome. *Arch Intern Med.* 1988;148:87–89.
41. Chaudhary BA, Rehman O, Brown T. Proteinuria in patients with sleep apnea. *J Fam Pract.* 1995;40:139–141.
42. Faulx MD, Storfer-Isser A, Kirchner HL, et al. Obstructive sleep apnea is associated with increased urinary albumin excretion. *Sleep.* 2007;30:923–929.
43. Green BT, Broughton WA, O'Conner JB. Marked improvement in nocturnal gastroesophageal reflux in a large cohort of patients with obstructive sleep apnea treated with continuous positive airway pressure. *Ann Intern Med.* 2003;163:41–45.
44. Marcus DM, Lynn J, Miller JJ, et al. Sleep disorders: a risk factor for pseudotumor cerebri. *J Neuroophthalmol.* 2001;21:121–123.
45. Schwartz DJ, Karatinos G. For individuals with obstructive sleep apnea, institution of CPAP therapy is associated with an amelioration of symptoms of depression which is sustained long term. *J Clin Sleep Med.* 2007;3:631–635.
46. Goncalves MA, Guilleminault C, Ramos E, et al. Erectile dysfunction, obstructive sleep apnea syndrome and nasal CPAP treatment. *Sleep Med.* 2005;6:333–339.
47. Dennison FH, Taft AA, Chaudhary BA. Noise or upper airway disorder? *Respir Care.* 1993;38:202–206.
48. Zou D, Grote L, Peker Y, et al. Validation of a portable monitoring device for sleep apnea diagnosis in a population based cohort using synchronized home polysomnography. *Sleep.* 2006;29:367–374.
49. Iber C, Ancoili-Israel S, Chesson A, Quan SF, for the American Academy of Sleep Medicine. *The AASM Manual for the Scoring of Sleep and Associated Events: Rules, Terminology and Technical Specifications.* Westchester, IL: American Academy of Sleep Medicine; 2007.
50. Veasey SC, Guilleminault C, Strohl KP, et al. Medical therapy for obstructive sleep apnea: a review by the Medical Therapy for Obstructive Sleep Apnea Task Force of the Standards of Practice Committee of the American Academy of Sleep Medicine. *Sleep.* 2006;29:1036–1044.
51. Young T, Peppard PE, Taheri S. Excess weight and sleep-disordered breathing. *J Appl Physiol.* 2005;99:1592–1599.
52. Chaudhary BA, Chaudhary T, Kolbeck RC, et al. Therapeutic effect of posture in sleep apnea. *South Med J.* 1986;79:1061–1063.
53. Neil AM, Angus SM, Sajklov D, McEvoy RD. Effects of sleep posture on upper airway stability in patients with obstructive sleep apnea. *Am J Respir Care Med.* 1997;155:199–204.
54. Kakkar RK, Berry RB. Positive airway pressure treatment for obstructive sleep apnea. *Chest.* 2007;132:1057–1072.
55. Kushida CA, Littner MR, Hirshkowitz M, et al. Practice parameters for the use of continuous and bilevel positive airway pressure devices to treat adult patients with sleep-related breathing disorders. *Sleep.* 2006;29:375–380.
56. Morgenthaler TI, Aurora RN, Brown T, et al. Practice parameters for the use of autotitrating continuous positive airway pressure devices for titrating pressures and treating adult patients with obstructive sleep apnea syndrome: an update for 2007. *Sleep.* 2008;31:141–147.
57. Fitzgerald MP, Mulligan M, Parthasarathy S. Nocturic frequency is related to severity of obstructive sleep apnea, improves with continuous positive airways treatment. *Am J Obstet Gynecol.* 2006;194:1399–1403.
58. Neill AM, Wai HS, Bannan SP, et al. Humidified nasal continuous positive airway pressure in obstructive sleep apnoea. *Eur Respir J.* 2003;22:258–262.
59. Ferguson KA, Cartwright R, Rogers R, et al. Oral appliances for snoring and obstructive sleep apnea: a review. *Sleep.* 2006; 29;244–262.
60. Kushida CA, Morgenthaler TI, Littner MR, et al. Practice parameters for the treatment of snoring and obstructive sleep apnea with oral appliances: an update for 2005. *Sleep.* 2006;29:240–243.
61. Hoekema A, Doff MHJ, de Bont LGM, et al. Predictors of obstructive sleep apnea-hypopnea treatment outcome. *J Dent Res.* 2007;86:1181–1186.
62. Walker-Engstrom ML, Tegelberg A, Wilhelmsson B, Ringqvist I. 4-year follow-up of treatment with dental appliance or uvulopalatopharyngoplasty in patients with obstructive sleep apnea: a randomized study. *Chest.* 2002;121:739–746.
63. Fujita S, Conway W, Zorick F, Roth T. Surgical correction of anatomic abnormalities in obstructive sleep apnea syndrome: uvulopalatopharyngoplasty. *Otolaryngol Head Neck Surg.* 1981;89:923–934.
64. Franklin KA, Anttila H, Axelsson S, et al. Effects and side-effects of surgery for snoring and obstructive sleep apnea—a systematic review. *Sleep.* 2009;32:27–36.
65. Kiely JL, Nolan P, McNicholas WT. Intranasal corticosteroid therapy for obstructive sleep apnea in patients with co-existing rhinitis. *Thorax.* 2004;59:50–55.
66. Zhan G, Serrano F, Fenik P, et al. NADPH oxidase mediates hypersomnolence and brain oxidative injury in a murine model of sleep apnea. *Am J Respir Crit Care Med.* 2005;172:921–929.
67. Santamaria J, Iranzo A, Ma Montserrat J, de Pablo J. Persistent sleepiness in CPAP treated obstructive sleep apnea patients: evaluation and treatment. *Sleep Med Rev.* 2007;11:195–207.
68. Schonhofer B, Franklin KA, Brunig H, et al. Effect of nasal-valve dilation on obstructive sleep apnea. *Chest.* 2000;118:587–590.
69. Ellegard E. Mechanical nasal alar dilators. *Rhinology.* 2006; 44:239–348.
70. Yong T, Finn L, Peppard PE, et al. Sleep-disordered breathing and mortality: eighteen-year follow-up of the Wisconsin Sleep Cohort. *Sleep.* 2008;31:1071–1078.
71. Ulfberg J, Carter N, Edling C. Sleep-disordered breathing and occupational accidents. *Scand J Work Environ Health.* 2000;26:237–242.
72. Marin JM, Carrizo SJ, Vicente E, Agusti AG. Long-term cardiovascular outcomes in men with obstructive sleep apnoea-hypopnoea with or without treatment with continuous positive airway pressure: an observational study. *Lancet.* 2005;365:1046–1053.

73. Aurora RN, Chowdhuri S, Ramar K, et al. The treatment of central sleep apnea syndromes in adults: practice parameters with an evidence-based literature review and meta-analyses. *Sleep.* 2012;35:17–40.
74. Campbell AJ. Ferrier K. Neill AM. Effect of oxygen versus adaptive pressure support servo-ventilation in patients with central sleep apnoea-Cheyne Stokes respiration and congestive heart failure. *Intern Med J.* 2012;42:1130–1136.
75. Berger KI, Goldring RM, Rapoport DM. Obesity hypoventilation syndrome. *Semin Respir Crit Care Med.* 2009;30:253–261.
76. Rye DB. Trotti LM. Restless legs syndrome and periodic leg movements of sleep. *Neurol Clin.* 2012;30:1137–1166.

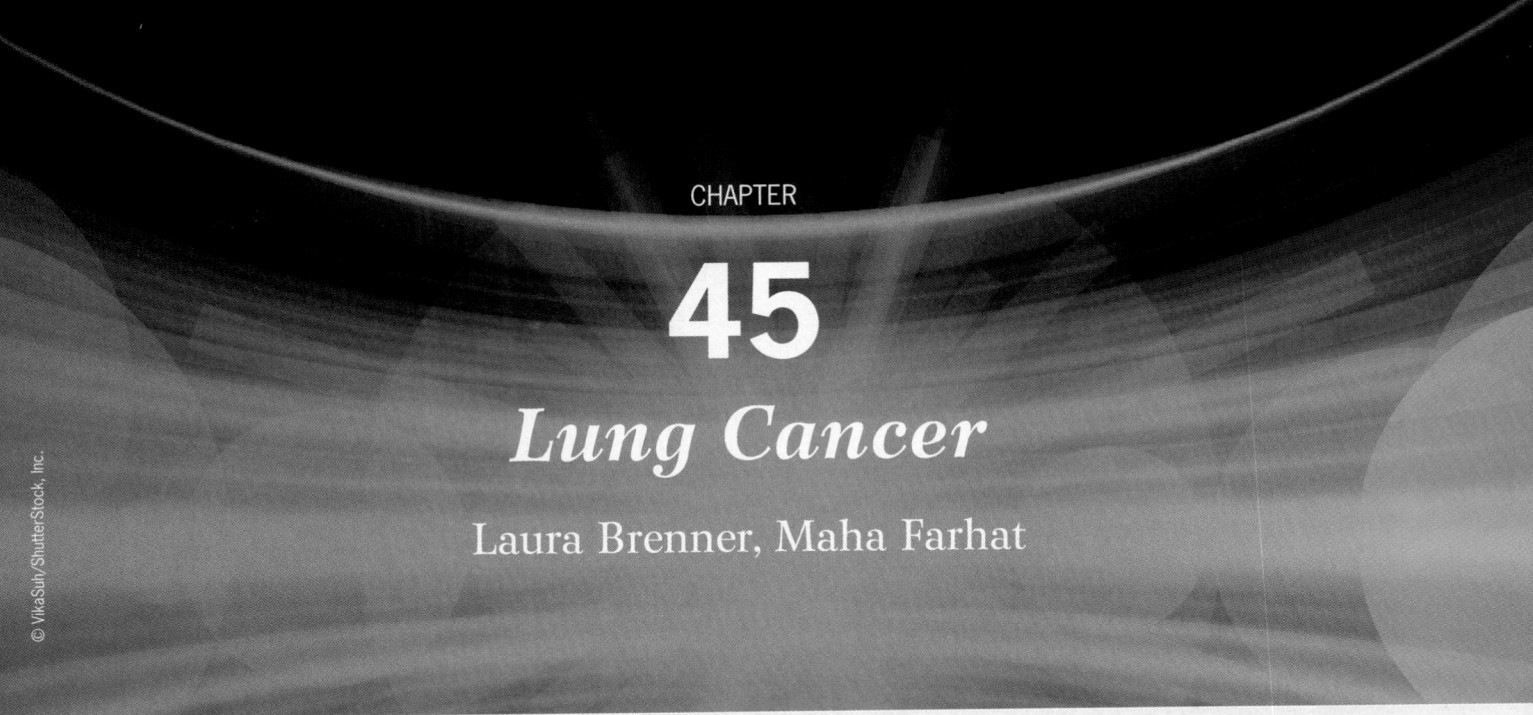

OUTLINE

OBJECTIVES

1. Discuss the magnitude of the worldwide problem of bronchogenic cancer.
2. Classify the different types of lung cancer.
3. Explain the importance of cigarette smoking as a risk factor for lung cancer.
4. Describe the approach to staging of small cell and non-small-cell lung cancer.
5. List the different treatment options for lung cancer and the associated prognoses.
6. Discuss possible future advances in the screening, diagnosis, and treatment of lung cancer.

KEY TERMS

adenocarcinoma
adjuvant therapy
benign
bronchogenic carcinoma
chemotherapy
malignant
mediastinoscopy
metastasis
neoadjuvant therapy
non-small-cell lung cancer (NSCLC)
radiotherapy
small cell lung cancer (SCLC)
solitary pulmonary nodule (SPN)
squamous cell carcinoma
transbronchial needle aspiration (TBNA)
tumor suppressor gene

Introduction

Bronchogenic cancer is a common disease with major health implications. Each year, approximately 228,000 patients are diagnosed with primary carcinoma of the lung in the United States,[1] and 83% die within 5 years. Lung cancer causes as many as 1.4 million deaths annually worldwide,[2] and it currently is the leading cause of death from cancer in adults. Although it is largely preventable, lung cancer kills more people than breast cancer, colon cancer, and prostate cancer combined.[3] Despite extensive research, the mortality rate for lung cancer has not improved substantially over the past several decades. The U.S. cost of treatment is estimated to be $12.2 billion a year.[4] This makes lung cancer one of the most expensive cancers to treat in the country. As the frequency of smoking has decreased, the incidence of lung carcinoma in men has declined, and in the past 10 years the incidence in women has finally started to decline as well, albeit at a lower rate. This fact, in addition to new guidelines on screening and diagnosis, stereotactic radiotherapy, and new targeted therapies, offers some basis for optimism. However, the persistently dismal prognosis of patients with lung cancer in developed countries and the continued rising incidence of disease among both women and men in developing countries show that this disease remains a substantial cause for concern.

Classification

Lung tumors can be classified as primary or secondary, **benign** or **malignant**, endobronchial or parenchymal. **Box 45-1** presents the World Health Organization's histologic classification of lung and pleural tumors.

BOX 45-1

World Health Organization's Histologic Classification of Lung and Pleural Tumors

Tumors of the Lung

Malignant Epithelial Tumors

- Squamous cell carcinoma
  - Papillary
  - Clear cell
  - Small cell
  - Basaloid
- Small cell carcinoma
  - Combined small cell carcinoma
- Adenocarcinoma
- Adenocarcinoma, mixed subtype
- Acinar adenocarcinoma
- Papillary adenocarcinoma
- Bronchoalveolar carcinoma
  - Nonmucinous
  - Mucinous
  - Mixed mucinous and nonmucinous or indeterminate
- Solid adenocarcinoma with mucin
  - Fetal adenocarcinoma
  - Mucinous ("colloid") carcinoma
  - Mucinous cystadenocarcinoma
  - Signet ring adenocarcinoma
  - Clear cell adenocarcinoma
- Large cell carcinoma
  - Large cell neuroendocrine carcinoma
  - Combined large cell neuroendocrine carcinoma
  - Basaloid carcinoma
  - Lymphoepithelioma-like carcinoma
  - Clear cell carcinoma
  - Large cell carcinoma with rhabdoid phenotype
- Adenosquamous carcinoma
- Sarcomatoid carcinoma
  - Pleomorphic carcinoma
  - Spindle cell carcinoma
  - Giant cell carcinoma
  - Carcinosarcoma
  - Pulmonary blastoma
- Carcinoid tumor
  - Typical carcinoid
  - Atypical carcinoid
- Salivary gland tumors
  - Mucoepidermoid carcinoma
  - Adenoid cystic carcinoma
  - Epithelial-myoepithelial carcinoma
- Preinvasive lesions
  - Squamous carcinoma in situ
  - Atypical adenomatous hyperplasia
  - Diffuse idiopathic pulmonary neuroendocrine cell hyperplasia

Benign Epithelial Tumors

- Papillomas
  - Squamous cell papilloma
    - Exophytic
    - Inverted
  - Glandular papilloma
  - Mixed squamous cell and glandular papilloma
- Adenomas
  - Alveolar adenoma
  - Papillary adenoma
  - Adenomas of salivary gland type
    - Mucous gland adenoma
    - Pleomorphic adenoma
    - Others
- Mucinous cystadenoma

Mesenchymal Tumors

- Epithelioid hemangioendothelioma
- Angiosarcoma
- Pleuropulmonary blastoma
- Chondroma
- Congenital peribronchial myofibroblastic tumor
- Diffuse pulmonary lymphangiomatosis
- Inflammatory myofibroblastic tumor
- Lymphangioleiomyomatosis
- Synovial sarcoma
  - Monophasic
  - Biphasic
- Pulmonary artery sarcoma
- Pulmonary vein sarcoma

Lymphoproliferative Tumors

- Marginal zone B-cell lymphoma of the MALT type
- Diffuse large B-cell lymphoma
- Lymphomatoid granulomatosis
- Langerhans cell histiocytosis

Miscellaneous Tumors

- Hamartoma
- Sclerosing hemangioma
- Clear cell tumor
- Germ cell tumors
  - Teratoma, mature
  - Immature
  - Other germ cell tumors
- Intrapulmonary thymoma
- Melanoma

Metastatic Tumors

Tumors of the Pleura

Mesothelial Tumors

Diffuse malignant mesothelioma
- Epithelioid mesothelioma
- Sarcomatoid mesothelioma
- Desmoplastic mesothelioma
- Biphasic mesothelioma

Localized malignant mesothelioma

Other tumors of mesothelial origin
- Well-differentiated papillary mesothelioma
- Adenomatoid tumor

Lymphoproliferative Disorders

Primary effusion lymphoma

Pyothorax-associated lymphoma

Mesenchymal Tumors

Epithelioid hemangioendothelioma
- Angiosarcoma

Synovial sarcoma
- Monophasic
- Biphasic

Solitary fibrous tumor

Calcifying tumor of the pleura

Desmoplastic round cell tumor

Reproduced from Travis WD, Brambilla E, Muller-Hermelink HK, Harris CC. *Pathology and Genetics of Tumours of the Lung, Pleural, Thymus and Heart.* World Health Organization Classification of Tumours. Lyon, France: IARC Press; 2004.

Epithelial tumors of the lung, or **bronchogenic carcinomas**, are by far the most common type of primary pulmonary tumor (other histologies constitute well under 1%). Bronchogenic carcinomas are classified as **small cell lung cancer (SCLC)** or **non-small-cell lung cancer (NSCLC)**. NSCLC includes **squamous cell carcinoma**, marked by histologic evidence of keratinization; **adenocarcinoma**, marked by glandular organization and mucus secretion; and large cell undifferentiated cancer, a diagnosis of exclusion when there is no evidence of either squamous or glandular differentiation with light microscopy. Advances in electron microscopy and immunohistochemistry have led to an expansion of the original classification, providing subtypes of NSCLC. These subtypes do not have a major influence on management of the disease, although some differences in presentation and pattern of spread have been noted. As more is learned about the genetic underpinnings of cancers, and as drugs are developed targeting specific mutations, the histologic classifications of tumors are being superseded by genetic identification methods for diagnosis and treatment.[5]

Over the past 30 to 40 years, the relative incidence of adenocarcinomas has increased. Adenocarcinomas are the most common subtype of bronchogenic carcinoma and are by far the most common type in lifetime nonsmokers. They have a slightly greater propensity for early distant spread, especially to the brain, compared with squamous cell tumors. These tumors most often are peripherally located in the lung and include bronchoalveolar carcinoma, a subtype with unique behavior. The reason for the increased risk of adenocarcinoma is unclear but may be related to changes in smoking behavior (depth of inspiration, type of filter, nitrosamine content). Squamous cell tumor incidence superseded that of adenocarcinoma in men in the mid-1990s. Squamous cell tumors arise from the proximal respiratory epithelium and can form large central masses, often with associated necrosis. Large cell tumors are the least common type of NSCLC. Similar to adenocarcinomas, they are most often peripheral, but they may be necrotic (more similar to squamous cell tumors).

SCLC differs from NSCLC in its cell of origin and its aggressiveness. Although tumors with mixed histology have led to the idea of a pluripotent stem cell origin for all bronchogenic cancers, small cell cancers appear to be derived from the neuroendocrine cells of the airway, the so-called enterochromaffin or amine precursor uptake and decarboxylation (APUD) cells. SCLC is highly associated with tobacco smoking, especially heavy smoking, and accounts for 15% to 25% of all bronchogenic carcinomas.[6] Overall the relative incidence of SCLC has been declining and has mirrored that of squamous cell carcinoma. The name derives from the histologic appearance of the tumors, which are seen as small, round, blue cells with hematoxylin-eosin staining. These tumor cells are about twice as big as lymphocytes and have a high mitotic rate and metastatic potential. Small cell tumors have a rapid doubling time,

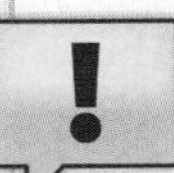

Respiratory Recap

Lung Cancer Classification
- Primary or secondary
- Benign or malignant
- Endobronchial or parenchymal

Respiratory Recap

Types of Bronchogenic Carcinoma
- Small cell lung cancer
- Non-small-cell lung cancer

and early distant spread is the rule. Although small cell cancers are sensitive to chemotherapy and radiotherapy, the survival rate is dismal. This is partly because SCLC frequently presents in an advanced stage.

Epidemiology

There were 228,190 new cases of lung cancer in the United States in 2013 (13.7% of all new cancer cases).[1] Incidence peaked in the mid-1980s in men, and around the year 2000 in women. These trends have followed the peak and decline in cigarette smoking in the United States; worldwide, however, the rate of cigarette smoking has dramatically increased in the past two decades.[7] At the current rate the worldwide incidence of lung cancer is expected to continue to increase and may reach a staggering level. Although traditionally considered a disease of men, lung cancer increasingly is seen in women, who account for 44% of new cases.[1] These gender-specific trends are largely explained by smoking behaviors. The increase in tobacco use among girls and young women makes these data a matter of particular concern.[8]

TABLE 45-1
Relative Risk of Lung Cancer

Patient History	Risk Ratio*
Never smoked; no significant industrial contact	1
Cigarette smoker	
½ pack/day	15
½ to 1 pack/day	17
1 to 2 packs/day	42
More than 2 packs/day	64
Cigar smoker†	3
Pipe smoker†	8
Former smoker	2–10
Nonsmoking woman exposed to secondhand smoke	1.4–1.9
Asbestos worker	
Nonsmoker	5
Cigarette smoker	92
Uranium miner	
Nonsmoker	7
Cigarette smoker	38
Relatives of lung cancer patients	
Nonsmoker	4
Cigarette smoker	14

*The risk ratio is the relative risk of an individual developing lung cancer compared with the risk faced by a comparable individual without the listed exposure.

†Although cigarette smoking carries the greatest risk of lung cancer, the differences among tobacco products are small when adjusted to similar amounts of tobacco consumption.

Reproduced from Murray JF, Nadel JA. *Textbook of Respiratory Medicine*. 2nd ed. Philadelphia: WB Saunders; 1994. Reprinted with permission.

Risk Factors and Etiology

The major risk factor for lung cancer is cigarette smoking (**Table 45-1**). Lung cancer thus differs from most other cancers in that it is largely preventable. The relative risk of developing lung cancer is 10 to 30 times higher for smokers than for lifelong nonsmokers. For a heavy smoker, the lifetime risk of developing lung cancer may be as high as 30% and is proportional to the total quantity and duration of cigarette use. The link between lung cancer and cigarette smoke is based not only on population level correlations and associations but also through a direct causal link demonstrated by the induction of damage to specific loci of a **tumor suppressor gene** (*p53*, seen in roughly 60% of lung cancers) by benzopyrene, a chemical in tobacco smoke.[9] Moreover, proto-oncogenes can produce proteins that regulate cell growth and differentiation. For example, mutations of the *ras* proto-oncogenes have been identified in as many as one-third of patients with NSCLC, with *K-ras* mutations commonly identified in adenocarcinomas in smokers.[10] Other carcinogens present in industrial pollutants can act similarly to tobacco smoke carcinogens and induce initial genetic abnormalities that lead to epithelial cell proliferation. The genetic abnormalities seen vary among different carcinoma histologies and between smokers and nonsmokers and hold promise in devising new methods for the early detection and therapy of lung carcinoma.[11] In summary, tobacco exposure causes more than 70% of lung cancer deaths worldwide, and thus primary prevention, through limiting tobacco exposure, is the only cost-effective and sustainable means to reduce the burden of lung cancer.[12]

Environmental tobacco smoke (ETS), also known as secondhand smoke, has important health effects as well. Although the amount of exposure is clearly less than in smokers, the onset of exposure generally occurs at a younger age. Although it varies across studies, the relative risk of lung cancer increases above that of lifelong nonsmokers in a dose-dependent fashion and is on the order of 1.2 to 1.3 times that in nonsmokers. The recognition of the significance of ETS has led to public health policies to reduce smoking and exposure in public spaces.

Risk factors unrelated to tobacco use that have also been proven to increase the risk for lung cancer development include exposure to chromium, asbestos,

Respiratory Recap

Primary Risk Factor for Lung Cancer

- The major risk factor for lung cancer is cigarette smoking.

bis(chloromethyl) ether, ionizing radiation, nickel, mustard gas, arsenic, radon, and polycyclic aromatic hydrocarbons (**Box 45-2**). Risk factors may act in concert to increase the risk of lung cancer substantially—for example, smoking in a patient with asbestosis. Low-level exposure to asbestos (e.g., nonoccupational exposure) without the development of asbestosis does not significantly change the risk of lung cancer.[13]

Genetic and dietary factors also may increase the risk of lung cancer.[14] First-degree relatives of patients with lung cancer have a twofold to threefold higher risk. It was initially believed that females were at increased risk of lung cancer at all levels of tobacco use, but further epidemiologic evidence has brought this hypothesis into question.[15] In addition, numerous recent studies suggest that certain benign diffuse parenchymal lung diseases (e.g., scleroderma, sarcoidosis, idiopathic pulmonary fibrosis, emphysema) may increase the relative risk of developing lung cancer.[16,17]

Infection with the human immunodeficiency virus (HIV) may influence the development and progression of lung cancer and other non-AIDS–defining malignancies. This has been particularly notable since the advent of highly active antiretroviral therapy (HAART) and the dramatic reduction in the rate of AIDS-defining illnesses, including malignancies, and the prolongation of life expectancy for patients with HIV infection. The reasons behind this increased risk are not clear, but it is postulated that the prolonged survival on HAART with only partial recovery of the immune system can account for this observation.[18]

BOX 45-2

Occupational Carcinogens for Lung Cancer

Proven Carcinogens

Passive/environmental tobacco smoke
Metals (e.g., arsenic, chromium, iron oxide, nickel)
Asbestos
Industrial (bis[chloromethyl]ether)
Radon gas
Mustard gas
Polycyclic aromatic hydrocarbons
Ionizing radiation
Formaldehyde
Aristolochic

Suspected Carcinogens

Air pollution
Acrylonitrile
Beryllium
Vinyl chloride
Silica
Wood dust
History of tuberculosis

Information from Murray JF, Nadel JA. *Textbook of Respiratory Medicine*. 2nd ed. Philadelphia: WB Saunders, 1994; and Hanley ME, Welsh CH. *Current Diagnosis and Treatment in Pulmonary Medicine*. New York: McGraw-Hill; 2003.

Screening

Prior studies including the Mayo Lung Project and the Prostate, Lung, Colorectal and Ovarian (PLCO) Cancer Screening Trial demonstrated that screening using chest x-ray with or without sputum cytology does not result in lives saved from lung cancer.[19,20] The National Lung Cancer Screening Trial (NLST) screened more than 53,000 high-risk individuals using low-dose helical chest CT or chest x-ray.[21] This study showed a reduction of mortality in the population of CT-screened patients with 320 high-risk subjects screened to save one life from lung cancer. The Danish randomized Lung Cancer CT Screening Trial (DLCST) compared low dose CT scan for screening versus no screening in a smaller number of subjects (4104) and demonstrated no difference in mortality between the groups.[22] Several other randomized CT-screening trials are currently under way in Europe, the results of which are yet to be released.[23] These results remain debated. Several professional societies are now advocating for CT screening of patients who meet the NLST criteria: (1) age 55 to 74 years, (2) 30 or more pack-years of cigarette smoking history, (3) former smokers within the previous 15 years, or (4) have no history of lung cancer. This screening practice has not yet been widely adopted as there are several concerns with implementation including the following: (1) the morbidity and expense associated with false-positive CT scan results (i.e., scan that identifies suspicious lesions that turn out to be benign after biopsy or other investigations are performed), (2) the overdiagnosis of small or non-aggressive cancers that may never result in patient morbidity or mortality, (3) excess radiation exposure with annual CT scanning, (4) the high predicted cost and resources needed for CT scanning interpretation and follow-up of the estimated 7 million Americans that meet the entry criteria for the NLST. Recommendations around screening for lung cancer are expected to continue to evolve as clinical centers gain experience with this practice and as additional clinical trial data become available.

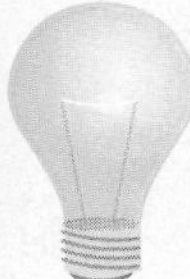

STOP AND THINK

When would you recommend a screening CT for a patient?

Presentation

Bronchogenic cancers may be found incidentally, through active screening, or because of local or systemic symptoms.[24] Because the outcome for individuals with symptomatic lung cancer is dismal, prevention and screening have been emphasized. Roughly 90% of patients found to have lung cancer are symptomatic at presentation.

Symptoms of lung cancer are of three types: symptoms related to the primary lesion, those related to distal spread or **metastasis**, and those related to paraneoplastic phenomena. Symptoms related to the primary lesion, such as cough, are common at presentation (**Table 45-2**). Along with dyspnea and hemoptysis, cough often is thought to indicate a central tumor. Persistent pneumonic infiltrates or recurrent same-segment pneumonias should suggest an obstructing airway lesion. Similarly, a unifocal wheeze on physical examination may be a diagnostic clue to an obstructing airway lesion.

Dyspnea that occurs as a direct result of lung cancer may be caused by airway obstruction with atelectasis, postobstructive pneumonitis, lymphangitic spread of the tumor, or a compressive malignant pericardial or pleural effusion. Local invasion of the phrenic nerve or the diaphragm may contribute to dyspnea related to diaphragmatic dysfunction.

TABLE 45-2
Initial Symptoms of Bronchogenic Carcinoma*

Symptom	Occurrence (%)
Cough	21
Hemoptysis	21
Chest pain	16
Dyspnea	12
Extrathoracic pain	6
Anorexia and weight loss	5
Cervical mass	5
Fatigue	3
Superior vena caval obstruction	3
Hoarseness	3
Central nervous system symptoms	3
Shoulder pain	2
Clubbing of the fingers	1

*Patients were seen at University of Texas MD Anderson Cancer Center, Houston, Texas.

Reproduced from Murray JF, Nadel JA. *Textbook of Respiratory Medicine*. 2nd ed. Philadelphia: WB Saunders; 1994. Reprinted with permission.

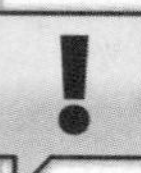

Respiratory Recap

Presentation of Lung Cancer

- Dyspnea
- Hemoptysis
- Chest pain
- Dysphagia
- Clubbing of the fingers
- Endocrine syndromes
- Neurologic syndromes
- Signs of metastases

Hemoptysis is a common symptom in patients with lung cancer, to some extent reflecting concurrent chronic bronchitis. Although lung cancer is in the differential diagnosis of massive hemoptysis because in rare cases tumors may erode into hilar vessels, low-volume but recurrent hemoptysis is most characteristic of bleeding tumors. Typically a high-resolution computed tomographic (CT) scan of the chest is performed to help identify suspicious lesions, direct bronchoscopy, and define common benign etiologies such as bronchiectasis.[25]

Substantial chest pain in lung cancer patients usually represents extension of a peripheral mass to the pleura or the chest wall. Pancoast syndrome is chest wall and spinal nerve root/sympathetic chain invasion by an apical bronchogenic tumor, the so-called superior sulcus tumor.[26] The syndrome consists of pain in the shoulder and medial scapula, an ulnar distribution of radicular pain or muscle atrophy (or both), and Horner syndrome (unilateral ptosis, miosis, anhydrosis, and enophthalmos). Superior sulcus tumors are most commonly squamous cell carcinomas.

Local spread of proximal tumors or lymph node masses may also cause dysphagia related to esophageal compression, hoarseness related to recurrent laryngeal nerve involvement, chylothorax secondary to thoracic duct compromise, or superior vena caval (SVC) syndrome related to central venous obstruction. Although the differential diagnosis is wide, the most common cause of the SVC syndrome is intraluminal thrombosis related to extrinsic compression by bronchogenic cancer, usually SCLC. Patients with SVC syndrome have symptoms and signs of upper body venous congestion, such as headache or flushing, plethora, and a prominent upper body pattern of venous collaterals. Although controversy exists as to whether SVC syndrome is a true emergency, chemoradiotherapy in SCLC promptly resolves the syndrome.[27] Commonly these patients also require anticoagulation.

Lesions in the lung that represent the spread of a primary lung cancer consist of secondary nodules, lymphangitic spread, and tumor emboli. Tumor emboli, increasingly recognized as a syndrome, may result in subacute or acute dyspnea, disseminated intravascular coagulation, and obstructive shock. The diagnosis may be made by cytologic analysis of a wedged sample obtained by pulmonary artery (PA) catheter. This is rarely performed because of concern for the morbidity associated with PA catheter placement. Lymphangitic spread, which causes dry cough, weight loss, and progressive dyspnea, may manifest as asymmetric pulmonary edema on the chest radiograph. In the appropriate clinical context, the presence of Kerley B lines on the chest radiograph is suggestive of this diagnosis (especially if unilateral) and is highly characteristic on high-resolution CT if they are seen as thickened, beaded, intralobular septae. The diagnosis also is made with high sensitivity and specificity by transbronchial biopsy.

Spread of the tumor itself can result in a variety of manifestations, depending on the mechanism.[28] Extrathoracic symptoms may be related to hematogenous spread of the cancer itself. Common sites include the central nervous system (CNS), bone (axial more often than appendicular skeleton), liver, and adrenal glands. CNS and bone lesions are exceedingly important, because they may lead to substantial pain and disability and often are amenable to palliation, usually through radiotherapy. Liver and adrenal metastases, however, are often asymptomatic and may be suspected because of an infiltrative picture of elevated liver enzyme levels or may be found on a CT scan of the chest or abdomen.

The paraneoplastic manifestations of bronchogenic carcinoma are those that are unrelated to the mechanical effects of primary or metastatic tumor. These paraneoplastic syndromes may occur in at least 10% of lung cancer patients (**Table 45-3** and **Box 45-3**). Several specific syndromes deserve mention. Weight loss is a common feature of lung cancer and is thought to be a paraneoplastic syndrome associated with enhanced inflammatory cytokine production, which results in anorexia and hypermetabolism. The debility associated with weight loss is an important negative prognostic factor.[29]

Clubbing of the fingers, which is caused by an increase in subungual soft tissue with associated straightening of the nail bed (Lovibond angle), is an important, albeit nonspecific, finding in lung cancer. Other causes of clubbing include chronic pulmonary infections (bronchiectasis, lung abscess, or empyema), restrictive lung diseases (idiopathic pulmonary fibrosis, pulmonary alveolar phospholipoproteinosis), cyanotic congenital heart disease, infective endocarditis, inflammatory bowel disease, and alcoholic cirrhosis.[30] Both clubbing and the related hypertrophic pulmonary osteoarthropathy (HPO), a symmetric, painful syndrome involving the long bones, are less commonly seen in SCLC than NSCLC. Both signs may disappear with successful tumor therapy. One interesting

TABLE 45-3
Endocrine and Hematologic Syndromes Associated with Lung Tumors

Syndrome	Tumor	Proteins/Cytokines Involved
Hypercalcemia of malignancy	Non-small cell	Parathyroid hormone–related peptide, parathormone
Hyponatremia of malignancy	Small cell Non-small cell	Antidiuretic hormone (arginine vasopressin) Atrial natriuretic peptide
Ectopic ACTH syndrome	Small cell Carcinoid	Adrenocorticotropic hormone Corticotropin-releasing hormone
Acromegaly	Carcinoid, small cell	Growth hormone–releasing hormone
Granulocytosis	Non-small cell	C-CSF, GM-CSF, IL-6
Thrombocytosis	Non-small cell, small cell	IL-6
Thromboembolism	Non-small cell, small cell	Unknown

ACTH, adrenocorticotropic hormone; C-CSF, granulocyte colony-stimulating factor; GM-CSF, granulocyte-macrophage colony-stimulating factor; IL-6, interleukin 6.

BOX 45-3

Lung Cancer Paraneoplastic Syndromes

Cachexia (e.g., anorexia, weight loss, weakness)
Fever
Hypertension
Endocrinologic: hypercalcemia, hyponatremia, Cushing syndrome, gynecomastia, acromegaly, hypoglycemia
Neurologic: Lambert-Eaton myasthenic syndrome, peripheral neuropathy, cerebellar degeneration, limbic encephalitis, encephalomyelitis
Musculoskeletal: clubbing, hypertrophic pulmonary osteoarthropathy, dermatomyositis, polymyositis
Hematologic: anemia, autoimmune hemolytic anemia, leukocytosis/thrombocytosis, vasculitis, noninfectious thrombotic endocarditis, idiopathic thrombocytopenic purpura

Reproduced from Hanley ME, Welsh CH. *Current Diagnosis and Treatment in Pulmonary Medicine.* New York: McGraw-Hill; 2003. Reprinted with permission.

association has been made between unilateral facial pain and HPO in a small number of patients with lung cancer. Both syndromes have been postulated to result from afferent vagal nerve compression from an intrathoracic tumor.

Endocrine syndromes are another relatively common feature of lung cancer, especially SCLC. The syndrome of inappropriate antidiuretic hormone secretion (SIADH, manifesting with hyponatremia) and ectopic Cushing syndrome (manifesting with weakness, glucose intolerance, and hypokalemia related to an excess of adrenocorticotropin hormone) may be found in patients with established malignancy or may be the first clue to a previously occult tumor. Hypercalcemia, seen most often with squamous cell carcinoma, presents with malaise, dehydration, and gastrointestinal and neurologic abnormalities. Differentiating paraneoplastic hypercalcemia from metastatic bone hypercalcemia that occurs secondary to osseous metastases (through identification of excess parathyroid hormone–related peptide) may be important in the determination of therapy. Hypercalcemia is a very poor prognostic factor in patients with bronchogenic carcinoma.[31]

Neurologic syndromes are recognized as rare (3% to 5% of SCLC) but devastating paraneoplastic manifestations of lung cancer. In general these syndromes result from the aberrant production of antibodies against neural antigens expressed by the tumor and that are present in normal neuronal tissues.[32] A notable example is the antibody ANNA-1 (anti-Hu), associated with SCLC, with a variety of clinical manifestations. In addition to cerebellar ataxia and a sensory neuropathy, ANNA-1 can lead to alterations in gastric motility, manifesting with nausea, anorexia, and weight loss. Although SCLC often is localized to the chest at the time of diagnosis, the overall survival rate is still dismal. Although some authors report slower tumor growth in patients with ANNA-1, the prognosis remains poor because of associated weight loss, malnutrition, and immobility from gait ataxia.[29–32]

Solitary Pulmonary Nodule

A **solitary pulmonary nodule (SPN)**, a lesion seen on the chest radiograph, is completely surrounded by lung parenchyma, without other radiographic abnormalities such as pleural effusion or adenopathy. An arbitrary size cutoff of 3 cm distinguishes SPN from pulmonary masses, which generally are malignant. SPNs, or *coin lesions,* usually are asymptomatic and generally are found on routine radiographs. In adults, an SPN is considered malignant until proven otherwise, but a number of alternative etiologies are included in the differential diagnosis (**Box 45-4** and **Table 45-4**).[33]

Diagnostic algorithms and advances in imaging have focused on differentiation of benign lesions from malignant ones. This distinction is important because

BOX 45-4

Causes of Solitary Pulmonary Nodules

Malignant Nodules

- Bronchogenic carcinoma
  - Adenocarcinoma
  - Squamous cell carcinoma
  - Small cell carcinoma
- Metastatic lesions
  - Breast
  - Head and neck
  - Melanoma
  - Colon
  - Kidney
  - Sarcoma
  - Germ cell tumor
  - Others
- Pulmonary carcinoid

Benign Nodules

- Infectious granuloma
  - Histoplasmosis
  - Coccidioidomycosis
  - Tuberculosis
  - Atypical mycobacteria
  - Cryptococcosis
  - Blastomycosis
- Other infections
  - Bacterial abscess
  - *Dirofilaria immitis*
  - *Echinococcus* cyst
  - Ascariasis
  - *Pneumocystis carinii*
  - Aspergilloma
- Benign neoplasms
  - Hamartoma
  - Lipoma
  - Fibroma
- Vascular
  - Arteriovenous malformation
  - Pulmonary varix
- Developmental
  - Bronchogenic cyst
- Inflammatory
  - Wegener granulomatosis
  - Rheumatoid nodule
- Other
  - Amyloidoma
  - Rounded atelectasis
  - Intrapulmonary lymph nodes
  - Hematoma
  - Pulmonary infarct
  - Pseudotumor (loculated fluid)
- Mucoid impaction

TABLE 45-4
Clinical and Radiologic Criteria in the Differentiation of Benign and Malignant Solitary Pulmonary Nodules

Criteria	Benign Nodule	Malignant Nodule
Clinical		
Age	Under 35 years of age; exception is hamartoma	Over 35 years of age
Symptoms	Absent	Present
Past history and functional inquiry	Geographic area with high incidence of granulomata; exposure to tuberculosis; nonsmoker	Diagnosis of primary lesion elsewhere; smoker; exposure to carcinogens
Radiographic		
Size	Small (<5 mm diameter are 1% malignant)	Large (>2 cm diameter are 80% malignant)
Location	No predilection except for tuberculosis (upper lobes)	Predominantly upper lobes except for lung metastases
Contour	Margins smooth	Margins spiculated
Calcification	Almost pathognomonic of a benign lesion if laminated, diffuse, or central	Rare, may be eccentric (engulfed granuloma)
Satellite lesions	More common	Less common
Serial studies showing no change over 2 years	Almost diagnostic of benign lesion	Most unlikely (one exception is small nodules of bronchoalveolar carcinoma)
Doubling time	<30 or >490 days	Between these extremes
Computed Tomography		
Calcification	Diffuse or central	Absent or eccentric
Fat	Virtually diagnostic of hamartoma	Absent
Bubblelike lucencies	Uncommon	Common in adenocarcinomas
Enhancement with intravenous contrast material	<15 Hounsfield units (HU)	>25 HU

an SPN is the most curable presentation of bronchogenic carcinoma. The 5-year survival rate for resected T1N0M0 lesions ranges from 60% to 80%.[34] In addition, nonsurgical identification of a benign lesion may eliminate the need for thoracotomy or thoracoscopy. There is greater ability of computed tomography to identify benign lesions.[35] The local frequency of malignant SPN depends to a large extent on the likelihood of obtaining chest radiographs in young people, the population's age distribution, the smoking prevalence, and the prevalence of infectious granulomatous disease, such as endemic fungi and tuberculosis. The differential diagnosis of an SPN also includes metastatic nodules, adenomas and other benign tumors, hamartomas, embolic phenomena, and nodules associated with rheumatologic lesions.[36]

Historical risk factors for a malignant cause of an SPN are age over 35 years, exposure to tobacco or another known lung carcinogen, and previous malignancy (or metastatic disease). Radiographic signs of malignancy include larger size (more than 2 cm in diameter) and a spiculated border (**Figure 45-1**, **Figure 45-2**, and **Figure 45-3**). Most important, when comparison of current radiographs with previous ones shows growth of the nodule, with a volumetric doubling time of 20 to 400 days, malignancy is likely. Signs of benignity include stable lesions (i.e., no growth over a 2-year period) and calcification. Although not 100%

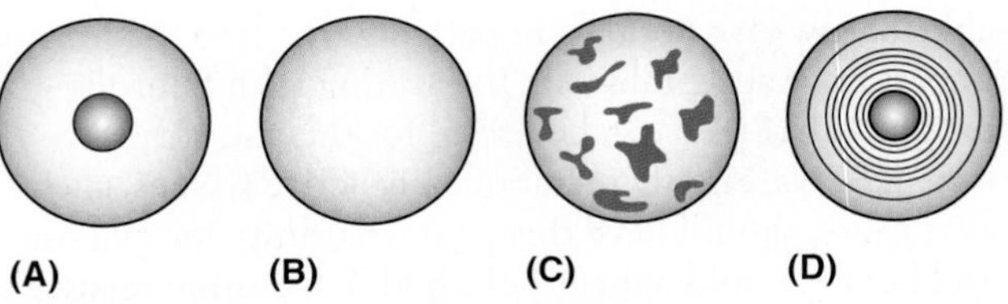

FIGURE 45-1 Patterns of benign calcification. Schematic representation of different patterns of benign calcification. (**A**) Target. (**B**) Diffuse. (**C**) Popcorn. (**D**) Lamellated calcification.

Redrawn with permission from Stark P. Computed tomographic and positron emission tomographic scanning of pulmonary nodules. In: UpToDate, Basow DS, ed. UpToDate: Waltham, MA; 2010. Copyright © 2010 UpToDate, Inc. For more information visit www.uptodate.com.

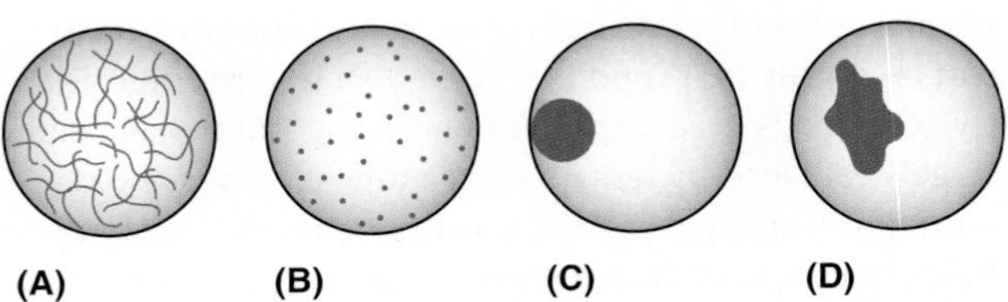

FIGURE 45-2 Patterns of malignant calcification. Schematic representation of different patterns of malignant calcification. (**A**) Reticular. (**B**) Psammomatous (punctate). (**C**) Eccentric. (**D**) Amorphous calcification.

Redrawn with permission from Stark P. Computed tomographic and positron emission tomographic scanning of pulmonary nodules. In: UpToDate, Basow DS, ed. UpToDate: Waltham, MA; 2010. Copyright © 2010 UpToDate, Inc. For more information visit www.uptodate.com.

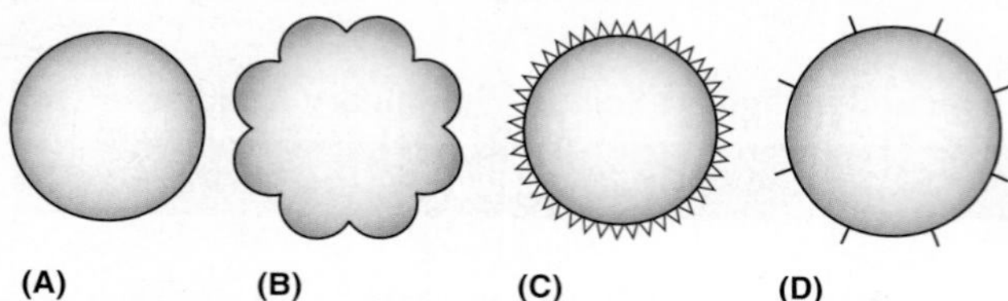

FIGURE 45-3 Margin of pulmonary nodules. Schematic representation of different patterns of the margin of pulmonary nodules. (**A**) Smooth. (**B**) Scalloped. (**C**) Corona radiata. (**D**) Spiculated.

Redrawn with permission from Stark P. Computed tomographic and positron emission tomographic scanning of pulmonary nodules. In: UpToDate, Basow DS, ed. UpToDate: Waltham, MA; 2010. Copyright © 2010 UpToDate, Inc. For more information visit www.uptodate.com.

specific, a high calcium content of nodules correlates with benign diagnoses, and certain patterns (popcorn, laminated, diffuse, and central calcification) are very suggestive of benignity. On the other hand, peripheral eccentric calcification is thought to be compatible with a diagnosis of malignancy.

Possible approaches to clinically indeterminate nodules include serial follow-up, transthoracic or bronchoscopic lung biopsy, contrast CT scanning, and positron emission tomography (PET) scanning. The choice of approach depends on the pretest probability of a diagnosis of malignancy, local practice patterns, and the patient's values (i.e., the individual's comfort or discomfort in observing a lesion with a low likelihood of malignancy). In general, serial follow-up is acceptable for low-risk nodules in patients who find diagnostic uncertainty acceptable. PET scanning with fluorodeoxyglucose (FDG) can be useful for the risk stratification of SPNs. Highly metabolically active tissues, such as tumors, should have the greatest affinity for glucose and hence should appear hot on PET scanning relative to normal tissue or benign nodules. PET scanning is usually used concomitantly with CT scan for anatomic correlation. The current mainstay of PET-CT scanning is for staging of known malignancies and for follow-up after treatment. Additionally, it can accurately characterize lesions larger than 7 to 15 mm as benign or malignant. The resolution of PET scanning deteriorates significantly for lesions smaller than 1 cm. The specificity of PET scanning is on the order of 70% to 90%, because other lesions with infection or inflammation can be highly PET avid. For high-risk lesions, definitive diagnosis is required. Open thoracotomy has been largely replaced by less invasive video-assisted thoracoscopic surgery (VATS) techniques. The accuracy of bronchoscopic or transthoracic needle techniques used to diagnose SPN varies widely based on the size of the lesion, its position in the chest, local practice patterns, and the practitioner's skill.[37]

Transthoracic needle aspiration (TTNA) is carried out under imaging guidance, commonly CT, but occasionally fluoroscopy or ultrasound. Overall the diagnostic yield is between 80% and 90%; however, the false-negative rate has been reported to be as high as 29%, especially for smaller lesions (<2 cm diameter). The indications for TTNA include tissue sampling in a patient with a presumed benign lesion, the establishment of a diagnosis in patients who are high risk for VATS or surgery, and when there is a concern that the pulmonary nodule is a metastatic nonpulmonary tumor. Electromagnetic navigation (EMN) bronchoscopy and radial endobronchial ultrasound (R-EBUS)-guided lung biopsy are emerging technologies for the diagnosis of both central and peripheral tumors with a diagnostic yield of about 70%. These techniques have the advantage of lower rate of pneumothorax as compared with TTNA.[38] Otherwise, VATS or surgical resection remains the standard of care for patients with SPN and a medium to high probability of malignancy.

Diagnosis

The diagnosis of bronchogenic cancer may be based on symptoms, the results of asymptomatic screening, or an incidental radiographic abnormality. Induced sputum can sometimes be useful to reach a diagnosis in patients with a central lung mass on the chest radiograph. Sputum can be pooled over 24 hours, which increases the diagnostic yield of this study; overall, however, the yield is limited with a sensitivity of about 66%.[35,38]

The diagnostic approach is similar to that for SPNs. In addition, bronchoscopy with EBUS and **transbronchial needle aspiration (TBNA)** can be helpful in the workup of central and mediastinal lesions. While mediastinoscopy is still considered the surgical gold standard, the improved yield of bronchoscopy when guided by EBUS and its decreased invasiveness has made it increasingly popular. This fact, combined with the high sensitivity of EBUS in combination with PET-CT, may make EBUS the future in lung cancer staging.[39,40]

Mediastinoscopy can be used for individuals with mediastinal lymphadenopathy (**Figure 45-4**). This technique is useful for diagnostic purposes if TBNA fails and for staging once the diagnosis of NSCLC has been established.

Occasionally the diagnosis of metastatic bronchogenic cancer can be made on the basis of a biopsy of a remote lesion (e.g., cervical node, adrenal gland). In addition, pleural fluid may be sampled, and pleural

Respiratory Recap

Diagnosis of Lung Cancer

- Sputum tests
- Bronchoscopy
- Mediastinoscopy
- Biopsy

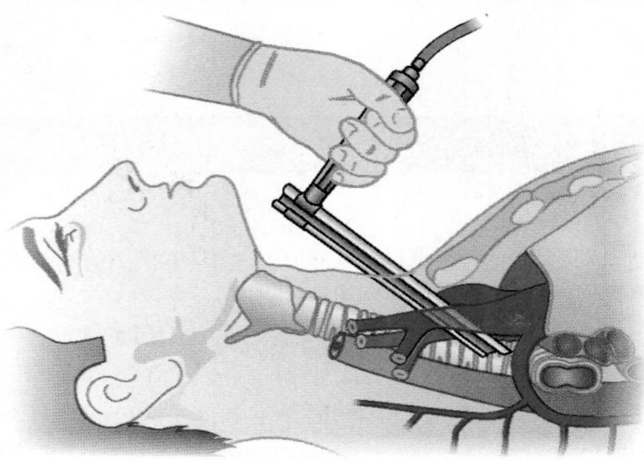

FIGURE 45-4 Mediastinoscope in place demonstrating the superior mediastinal plane.

Adapted from Fishman AP. *Fishman's Pulmonary Diseases and Disorders*. 3rd ed. McGraw Hill; 1998.

biopsy can be performed for the diagnosis of malignant effusion. The advantage of pleural fluid sampling is that it can provide both diagnostic and staging information because the presence of a malignant effusion implies a lesion and that disease is effectively metastatic with the stage being IV.

Workup and Staging

Once the diagnosis has been established, staging of disease is the next step. Knowledge of the staging system can help determine the necessary workup. **Table 45-5** and **Table 45-6** reflect the 2009 NSCLC staging classification advocated by the International Association for the Study of Lung Cancer (IASLC). **Table 45-7** illustrates survival according to the stage of lung cancer. The TNM system is of most use for early-stage disease (stage I), when the disease is amenable to resection and adjuvant chemotherapy.

The tests required after a diagnosis of lung cancer are controversial. A careful history and physical examination should be followed by tests of blood chemistry (serum calcium, alkaline phosphatase, aspartate aminotransferase, alanine aminotransferase, and lactate dehydrogenase levels, and a complete blood count) and CT scanning of the entire chest, extending caudally to the level of the adrenal glands. Additional tests that may be useful are CT or magnetic resonance imaging (MRI) scans of the head and a bone scan. The yield on these tests for metastasis is low if the patient has no symptoms; however, they are not generally indicated in such patients.[41]

With SCLC, some advocate complete staging, including a head MRI, bone scan, and unilateral or bilateral bone marrow biopsies; others perform a sequential, symptom-based workup. In patients with clinical limited stage SCLC, PET imaging is recommended for staging. If a PET is obtained, the bone scan may be omitted. With NSCLC, mediastinoscopy versus EBUS is recommended to assess the extent of mediastinal node involvement because PET and/or CT scanning can be misleading (false positives and false negatives) in the mediastinum.[42]

For patients who may be candidates for surgery, pulmonary function testing is useful to determine the patient's ability to undergo such a procedure. Ideally, a postoperative forced expiratory volume in 1 second (FEV_1) of 800 mL or 40% of predicted should be sought. This value, however, is based largely on empiric data. In borderline cases a quantitative ventilation-perfusion scan can help estimate the amount of resection a patient can physiologically tolerate. Exercise testing also may help predict morbidity associated with thoracotomy; for example, patients with maximum oxygen consumption under 10 mL/kg do poorly. On the other hand, if patients' predicted FEV_1 is less than 40% predicted, they can still safely undergo surgery if their exercise capacity is high. Improvements in surgical and anesthetic techniques and the reemergence of lung volume reduction surgery (LVRS) have helped lower the threshold for surgical resection of NSCLC.[43]

Treatment

Treatment options include surgery, **radiotherapy**, and **chemotherapy**. Newer options, although not the mainstays of treatment, include immunotherapy, brachytherapy, gene therapy, bronchoscopic treatments, and photodynamic therapy (PDT).[44] Because the individual chemotherapeutic agents and combinations of agents tend to change frequently, the underlying therapeutic principles in the treatment of lung cancer are emphasized here.

Small Cell Lung Cancer

Because of the aggressive nature of these tumors, most patients with SCLC who seek medical treatment have extensive disease at the time of diagnosis. Without treatment, patients with limited SCLC survive an average of 12 weeks; for extensive disease, survival is only 5 weeks. In addition to moderate improvements in survival to 15–20 and 8–13 weeks for limited and extensive disease respectively, combination chemotherapy in some cases can lead to substantial improvements in the patient's quality of life.[45]

Chemotherapeutic agents have long been known to affect SCLC tumors in patients with both limited (90%

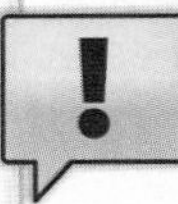

Respiratory Recap

Treatment of Lung Cancer

- Surgery
- Radiotherapy
- Chemotherapy

TABLE 45-5
Tumor Node Metastisis (TNM) Descriptors

Descriptors	Definitions	Subgroups*
T	Primary tumor	
T0	No primary tumor	
T1	Tumor ≤ 3 cm† surrounded by lung or visceral pleura, not more proximal than the lobar bronchus	
T1a	Tumor ≤ 2 cm†	T1a
T1b	Tumor > 2 but ≤ 3 cm†	T1b
T2	Tumor > 3 but ≤ 7 cm† or tumor with any of the following:‡ Invades visceral pleura, involves main bronchus ≥ 2 cm distal to the carina, atelectasis/obstructive pneumonia extending to hilum but not involving the entire lung	
T2a	Tumor > 3 but ≤ 5 cm†	T2a
T2b	Tumor > 5 but ≤ 7 cm†	T2b
T3	Tumor > 7 cm;	$T3_{>7}$
	or directly invading chest wall, diaphragm, phrenic nerve, mediastinal pleura, or parietal pericardium;	$T3_{Inv}$
	or tumor in the main bronchus < 2 cm distal to the carina;§	$T3_{Centr}$
	or atelectasis/obstructive pneumonitis of entire lung;	$T3_{Centr}$
	or separate tumor nodules in the same lobe	$T3_{Satell}$
T4	Tumor of any size with invasion of heart, great vessels, trachea, recurrent laryngeal nerve, esophagus, vertebral body, or carina;	$T4_{Inv}$
	or separate tumor nodules in a different ipsilateral lobe	$T4_{Ipsi\ Nod}$
N	**Regional lymph nodes**	
N0	No regional node metastasis	
N1	Metastasis in ipsilateral peribronchial and/or perihilar lymph nodes and intrapulmonary nodes, including involvement by direct extension	
N2	Metastasis in ipsilateral mediastinal and/or subcarinal lymph nodes	
N3	Metastasis in contralateral mediastinal, contralateral hilar, ipsilateral or contralateral scalene, or supraclavicular lymph nodes	
M	**Distant metastasis**	
M0	No distant metastasis	
M1a	Separate tumor nodules in a contralateral lobe;	$M1a_{contr\ Nod}$
	or tumor with pleural nodules or malignant pleural dissemination‖	$M1a_{P1\ Dissem}$
M1b	Distant metastasis	M1b
Special situations		
TX, NX, MX	T, N, or M status not able to be assessed	
Tis	Focus of *in situ* cancer	Tis
T1§	Superficial spreading tumor of any size but confined to the wall of the trachea or mainstem bronchus	$T1_{ss}$

*These subgroup labels are not defined in the IASLC publications[7–10] but are added here to facilitate a clear discussion.

†In the greatest dimension.

‡T2 tumors with these features are classified as T2a if ≤ 5 cm.

§The uncommon superficial spreading tumor in central airways is classified as T1.

‖Pleural effusions are excluded that are cytologically negative, nonbloody, transudative, and clinically judged not to be due to cancer.

Reproduced with permission from the American College of Chest Physicians from Detterbeck FC, Postmus PE, Tanoue LT. The stage classification of lung cancer: diagnosis and management of lung cancer, 3rd ed: American College of Chest Physicians evidence-based clinical practice guidelines. *Chest.* 2013;143:e191S–210S.

TABLE 45-6
Tumor Node Metastasis (TNM Elements) Included in Stage Groups

Stage Groups	Descriptors T	N	M	% of All Patients*
Ia	T1a,b	N0	M0	15
Ib	T2a	N0	M0	13
IIa	T1a,b	N1	M0	2
	T2a	N1	M0	4
	T2b	N0	M0	4
IIb	T2b	N1	M0	2
	T3	N0	M0	14
IIIa	T1-3	N2	M0	20
	T3	N1	M0	6
	T4	N0,1	M0	2
IIIb	T4	N2	M0	1
	T1-4	N3	M0	3
IV	T_{Any}	N_{Any}	M1a,b	14

*Percentage of patients in IASLC database according to best stage (rounded to nearest integer).

Reproduced with permission from the American College of Chest Physicians from Detterbeck FC, Postmus PE, Tanoue LT. The stage classification of lung cancer: diagnosis and management of lung cancer, 3rd ed: American College of Chest Physicians evidence-based clinical practice guidelines. *Chest.* 2013;143:e191S–210S.

TABLE 45-7
Overall Survival by Clinical and Pathologic Stage

	Deaths/N	Median Survival Time (in months)	5-Year Survival (%)
Clinical Stage			
cIa	443/831	60	50
cIb	750/1284	43	43
cIIa	318/483	34	36
cIIb	1652/2248	18	25
cIIIa	2528/3175	14	19
cIIIb	676/758	10	7
cIV	2627/2757	6	2
Pathologic Stage			
pIa	1168/3666	119	73
pIb	1450/3100	81	58
pIIa	1485/2579	49	46
pIIb	1502/2252	31	36
pIIIa	2896/3792	22	24
pIIIb	263/297	13	9
pIV	224/266	17	13

Adapted from Goldstraw P, Crowley J, Chansky K, et al. The IASLC Lung Cancer Staging Project: proposals for the revision of the TNM stage groups in the forthcoming (seventh) edition of the TNM classification of malignant tumours. *J Thorac Oncol.* 2007;2:706–714.

of patients) and extensive disease (70% of patients). Despite the sensitivity of these tumors to chemotherapeutic agents, relapse is very common. There has been no substantial improvement in survival of this disease over the past 20 to 30 years. Commonly used agents include etoposide, platinum agents (e.g., cisplatinum, carboplatin), ifosfamide, vincristine, irinotecan, paclitaxel, and anthracyclines. In general, the platinum-based regimens are considered superior to non-platinum-based regimens, and cisplatin plus etoposide or irinotecan are the most frequently used combinations based on their clinical activity and toxicity profile. In general, adding additional agents and using higher doses can lead to a higher response rate, but the regimens with the higher number of agents have a higher rate of toxicity.[46,47]

Patients with limited-stage SCLC treated with chemotherapy alone commonly develop local tumor progression. Studies have shown that the addition of thoracic radiotherapy reduces intrathoracic recurrence and provides a small but significant improvement in survival. Early administration of radiotherapy is superior to late radiation, especially in patients who are receiving etoposide and cisplatin chemotherapy. Delivering the radiotherapy in more intense but briefer doses (accelerated hyperfractionation) is superior to daily dosing. Furthermore, concurrent chemoradiotherapy is considered superior to sequential chemotherapy and radiotherapy in terms of survival. There may be some increased toxicity with the concurrent administration of chemoradiotherapy. In patients who do not tolerate it, radiation can be delayed until chemotherapy is completed. Radiation therapy also can be used for treatment of metastatic disease. Radiotherapy has been shown to improve mortality in the treatment of patients with limited-stage SCLC. Another role for radiation in SCLC is in prophylactic cranial irradiation (PCI). Brain metastases are common in SCLC, even in patients who appear to have responded to systemic therapy; this may be because of poor penetration of chemotherapy through the blood–brain barrier. PCI is indicated in patients with limited or extensive disease who achieve a partial or complete response to initial therapy.

Traditionally, surgery was not considered useful for SCLC because of the disease's systemic nature at the time of diagnosis. Immediate surgery, however, should be considered for individuals who have biopsy-proven T1N0M0 tumors, but only after node negativity has been confirmed by bronchoscopy or mediastinoscopy. Surgical resection may also improve survival after induction chemotherapy in highly selected patients with early disease. Currently no prospective data are available to inform definitive recommendations. Adjuvant chemotherapy as well as prophylactic cranial irradiation is recommended in patients who undergo surgery. If the surgical margins are positive or there is nodal disease, patients should also receive adjuvant radiotherapy.[41,43]

Non-Small-Cell Lung Cancer

Several principles are important in the approach to treatment of patients with NSCLC. First, surgical resection is used much more commonly in NSCLC than in SCLC, particularly for early-stage disease. Second, the probability of achieving cure in early-stage NSCLC is quite good (5-year survival after surgery for stage I disease is 47%). Third, in multiple stages of the disease, there is an increasingly recognized role for multimodality therapy (i.e., **neoadjuvant therapy** and **adjuvant therapy** [chemotherapy and radiotherapy] followed by surgical resection). Adjuvant therapy is given in addition to the primary therapy (i.e., chemotherapy in addition to surgery). Neoadjuvant therapy is therapy (usually chemotherapy) given before the main treatment (usually surgery).

For early-stage NSCLC, surgical resection is the treatment of choice, with excellent long-term survival reported in several series (63% to 85% stage IA 5-year survival).[48] Most deaths that occur are caused by recurrent disease. Currently the recommendation for patients with stage I and II is for lobectomy rather than sublobar resection. There are ongoing studies in combined sublobar resection and adjuvant therapy. If patients cannot tolerate lobar resection because of reduced pulmonary function, sublobar resection is recommended over nonsurgical therapy. Another option for patients with borderline medical fitness for surgery is stereotactic body radiotherapy. Adjuvant chemotherapy is not recommended after resection of stage IA,B tumors as there is no survival advantage. In stage IIA,B after complete resection, postoperative platinum-based therapy is recommended. With patients who have N2 disease, postoperative radiation therapy may be beneficial, and prospective trials addressing this are ongoing. Further, molecular profiling of tumors may be predictive of chemotherapeutic response, which would allow *a priori* prediction of which patients would benefit from additional or more aggressive therapy.[49,50]

The treatment of locally advanced NSCLC with multimodality therapies has become increasingly popular. Curative intent remains the standard of care of patients with stage III disease. Surgery remains the standard of care for patients without N2 (mediastinal lymphadenopathy) disease. Formerly, patients with stage IIIA and nonbulky N2 burden were considered surgical candidates; however, it has become more recognized that cure is difficult to achieve even with surgery in this patient population, and combination chemoradiotherapy is now considered the standard of care.[51] For stage III disease, neoadjuvant chemotherapy has been studied and is a controversial topic. Overall it offers no survival advantage when compared with postoperative (adjuvant) chemotherapy, although it may be used in cases of superior sulcus (Pancoast) tumors (in addition to preoperative radiation) or in cases of T4 disease with mediastinal invasion with curative intent to facilitate surgery.[52,53] Adjuvant chemotherapy offers a survival advantage after resection of stage III disease and is considered the standard of care.[54,55] Postoperative radiation therapy has been studied to reduce the risk of local recurrence. Although it was associated with a survival advantage in patients with N2 disease in a subset analysis, overall there does not seem to be a large survival advantage to postoperative radiotherapy because survival seems to be limited more frequently by distant metastases than by local recurrence.[56] Concurrent chemoradiation is considered the standard of care for nonresectable stage III NSCLC. Chemotherapy is usually with a platinum-based regimen.[57]

There are emerging opportunities for personalized treatment in lung cancer care, based on the ability to detect gene targets that drive cancer growth and the availability of effective therapeutic agents that target these genetic pathways. The targets known so far in NSCLC are *EGFR* (epidermal growth factor receptor) mutations and the fusion gene *ELM4-Alk* (echinoderm microtubule-associated protein-like 4 and anaplastic lymphoma kinase). The *EGFR* small molecule inhibitor gefitinib is now recommended as a frontline agent for patients with advanced NSCLC who have any clinical predictors or molecular predictors of response. Crizotinib is a small molecule tyrosine kinase inhibitor that is specific for *cMET*, *ALK*, and *ROS-1*. Crizotinib has been shown to slow down progression of disease. Cetuximab, a monoclonal antibody that inhibits *EGFR*, has been shown to have a small benefit in patients who express the *EGFR* by immunohistochemistry without carrying an activating mutation.[58] Other molecular agents such as bevacizumab (antivascular endothelial growth factor) are recommended in combination with standard chemotherapy. Bevacizumab increases the risk of bleeding and is contraindicated in patients with brain metastases and with hemoptysis.

Lung cancer, especially stage IV, is associated with high mortality and morbidity rates and can be associated with a significant amount of suffering. Palliative care is a subspecialty of medicine aimed at treating patients' symptoms as the focus of their care. It is aimed at providing support in a holistic manner to patients and their families. The Early Intervention with Palliative Care (EIPC) trial randomized patients with newly diagnosed NSCLC to receive either palliative care in conjunction with usual treatment or usual treatment alone. The patients assigned to receive conjunctive palliative care had a better quality of life (QOL), less aggressive end of life care, and a longer median survival. Other studies have shown a high

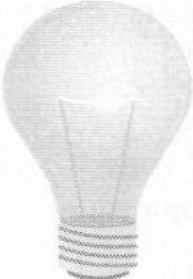

STOP AND THINK

You are caring for a patient with SCLC. What is the main difference between treatment of SCLC and NSCLC?

psychological burden in patients with advanced stage diseases. Patients with poor QOL at baseline were more likely to have worse outcomes than patients with higher QOL. Patients with high symptoms burden, or stage IV cancer, should have usual care combined with palliative care treatment early in their course.[59,60]

Complications of Therapy

The complications of the individual chemotherapeutic drugs are beyond the scope of this chapter.[61] Roughly 1% of treatment-associated mortality is a result of chemotherapy itself. Several important general points can be made, as follows:

- In the week or two after chemotherapy, neutropenia can occur and greatly increases the risk of superimposed bacterial and opportunistic fungal pneumonias and sepsis. Growth factors can be used to prevent neutropenia in a susceptible or previously afflicted patient.
- Mucositis, which represents acute toxicity of the highly active lining cells of the gastrointestinal tract, leads to substantial discomfort and can increase infectious sequelae as a result of an increased risk of aspiration and altered gastrointestinal permeability.
- Various chemotherapeutic agents have acute or chronic pulmonary sequelae, which complicate the distinction between tumor spread or recurrence, infection, and drug toxicity; early invasive diagnostic attempts often are warranted in these cases. Fortunately the chemotherapeutic agents typically used for lung cancers do not, for the most part, have major pulmonary toxicities.
- Platinum-based chemotherapeutic drugs are commonly used in lung cancer and are frequently associated with renal failure and with neurologic toxicity, specifically peripheral neuropathy. This side effect can range from asymptomatic to nuisance to severe and disabling; therefore, it must be considered and discussed with patients undergoing chemotherapy.
- The tyrosine kinase inhibitors mentioned above are overall well tolerated. Rash and diarrhea are the most common side effects. Bevacizumab is associated with hemorrhage, poor surgical wound healing, and gastrointestinal perforation as less common but serious side effects.

Radiation damage to the lung parenchyma remains the limiting factor in chest radiotherapy. The complications of radiation therapy may be characterized as acute or chronic. The incidence of acute radiation pneumonitis is higher for patients receiving larger daily or cumulative doses and those receiving radiation to a larger amount of tissue. In addition, certain chemotherapeutic drugs used in lung cancer regimens, such as doxorubicin and vincristine, are radiosensitizers and can increase radiation-induced injury. Acute pneumonitis occurs within the first 6 months of therapy (mean is approximately 1 to 3 months) and is manifested by cough and dyspnea. It typically but not exclusively is confined to the radiation port, and the histopathology may be consistent with a lymphocytic alveolitis or diffuse alveolar damage. In addition, a nonspecific reaction, cryptogenic organizing pneumonia (COP) can occur in the lung in response to radiation injury. Corticosteroid therapy usually is given for acute pulmonary radiation toxicity, although human data are sparse.

Chronic complications of radiotherapy include injury to lung and mediastinal structures. Lung fibrosis can be seen 6 months after discontinuation of radiotherapy and manifests with progressive dyspnea and restrictive pulmonary function tests. Mediastinal radiotherapy has been associated with a number of complications, including mediastinal fibrosis, constrictive pericarditis, restrictive cardiomyopathy, accelerated coronary artery disease, and valvular fibrosis.[62]

With thoracotomy, mortality rates as low as 1% are now reported, a considerable improvement compared with 30 to 40 years ago. Smoking cessation at least 2 months before surgery has been associated with an improved outcome in elective coronary artery bypass patients. These data are generally extrapolated to thoracotomy patients as well.[63] Other preoperative measures, such as exercise, good nutrition, pulmonary rehabilitation, and deep breathing regimens, may facilitate smooth the perioperative course. Meticulous attention must be paid to postsurgical pulmonary toilet to prevent and treat respiratory complications of atelectasis, lobar collapse, and pneumonia. Care after discharge from the hospital, through transitional care units and visiting nurses, is crucial in many cases. Late complications, such as postthoracotomy pain syndromes, which occur in as many as 50% of patients, are somewhat underappreciated.

Prognosis

The prognosis for lung cancer is still quite poor; the 5-year survival rate is only 14%. The following are some useful prognostic variables:

- *Tumor stage, including size.* In addition to the tumor's stage, its size appears to linearly predict survival, with increasing mortality associated with larger size.
- *Weight loss.* As with many diseases and other cancers, weight loss is an important prognostic indicator. The poor outcome associated with patients with lung cancer who lose weight has prompted some to aggressively place percutaneous gastrostomy feeding tubes. Thus, even when oral intake is poor, caloric requirements can be met. Appetite stimulants such as megestrol acetate can help increase body weight. Minimal outcome data support these approaches, however. Other systemic symptoms similarly predict a poor outcome.

- *Performance status*. The Karnofsky Performance Scale (**Table 45-8**) provides a quantitative measure of patient performance as a percentage of normal activities. As with many tumors, a lung cancer patient with good performance status has a much better outcome.
- *Histologic subtype*. In NSCLC, a few studies have suggested a superior outcome for squamous cell carcinoma compared with adenocarcinoma. Several other studies, however, have not shown important differences in survival or recurrence risk. The histologic subtype, therefore, is probably not a major prognostic factor in NSCLC. Subtyping of adenocarcinomas may be useful, because bronchoalveolar cell carcinoma may have an improved outcome compared with other adenocarcinomas.
- *Tumor differentiation*. Variable results have been published in different papers regarding the importance of this factor. Although some data suggest a worse outcome for patients with undifferentiated cancers, other studies report no important differences in survival on this basis.
- *Vascular or lymphatic invasion*. A resected tumor that demonstrates invasiveness may warrant more aggressive treatment than one that does not.
- *Molecular markers*. Molecular markers, such as *K-ras* mutations, have not yet had a major impact on prognostication or prediction of relapse, although early data from gene expression profiling are promising.[64] Tumor expression of the *EGFR* mutation or the *ALK* rearrangement predicts response to targeted agents as mentioned above.
- *Male gender*. Disease in men is associated with a worse outcome than disease in women.

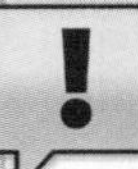

Respiratory Recap

Prognosis for Lung Cancer

- The 5-year survival rate for lung cancer is only 14%.

Prevention

The most important cause of cancer death in North America is preventable. Primary prevention of lung cancer requires smoking cessation, avoidance of exposures, and early detection. Evidence clearly suggests a decline in the risk of lung cancer among former smokers compared with current smokers. Although statistics vary, the lung cancer risk falls by 5 years after smoking cessation and continues to decline thereafter. These individuals probably do not completely return to the baseline risk seen in those who have never smoked.

In the case of lung cancer, smoking cessation is the best defense. Achieving this requires the establishment of policies to restrict access to tobacco products through taxation and regulation, in addition to education campaigns and banning of smoking in public areas among other interventions.[65] From a health provider perspective it is important to encourage and to

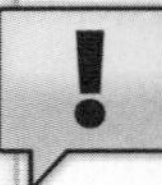

Respiratory Recap

Lung Cancer Prevention

- Smoking cessation
- Screening
- Interventions to prevent disease progression

TABLE 45-8
Karnofsky Performance Scale

Definition	Percentage	Criteria
Able to carry on normal activity and to work; no special care needed	100	Normal; no complaints; no evidence of disease
	90	Able to carry on normal activity; minor signs or symptoms of disease
	80	Normal activity with effort; some signs or symptoms of disease
Unable to work; able to live at home and care for most personal needs; varying amount of assistance needed	70	Cares for self; unable to carry on normal activity or do active work
	60	Requires occasional assistance but is able to care for most needs
	50	Requires considerable assistance and frequent medical care
Unable to care for self; requires equivalent of institutional or hospital care; rapid progression of disease possible	40	Disabled; requires special care and assistance
	30	Severely disabled; hospitalization indicated, although death may not be imminent
	20	Very sick; hospitalization necessary; active supportive treatment required
	10	Moribund; fatal processes progressing rapidly

facilitate the cessation of tobacco use in 1:1 encounters. The modest success of tobacco control programs in North America should not distract health professionals from the huge problem of an estimated 1.1 billion smokers worldwide. For example, estimates suggest that 66% of all young men in China currently are smokers.[66] Primary prevention must target the problem on both a global and an individual level. Emphasis is placed on the need for repeated discussions with smokers and planned follow-up. Several attempts by patients and healthcare providers often are required to successfully overcome this addiction. Group or family therapy may be useful for some smokers. Smoking cessation programs are cost-effective, particularly if they use personnel who are not physicians.[67]

Recent data support the usefulness of nicotine replacement therapies to facilitate smoking cessation. Bupropion (150 mg given orally twice a day) has been shown to facilitate withdrawal from nicotine. Only 23.1% of participants in one study were tobacco free at 1 year, compared with 12.4% in the placebo group.[68,69] The combination of nicotine replacement and bupropion may have a higher probability of success. Varenicline (a nicotinic receptor partial agonist) is another first-line agent to help patients quit smoking. Compared with bupropion, it was found to be more efficacious. Uncertainty exists about the role of e-cigarettes in tobacco control despite its increasing popular use and requires further investigation.[70]

Some limited data suggested a benefit of certain dietary supplements, especially antioxidants, in preventing lung and other cancers in high-risk groups. Randomized controlled trials of vitamin A and beta-carotene have yielded disappointing results, disproving any efficacy in primary prevention of disease.[71,72] There remains some evidence of a protective role for vitamins C and E. As it stands, however, the data are insufficient to recommend their use routinely in clinical practice.[73]

Future Directions

Worldwide smoking trends dictate that bronchogenic carcinoma will continue to be a major health problem in the foreseeable future. Current epidemiologic statistics likely will be eclipsed. Although advances in imaging, chemotherapy radiotherapy, and genetics may produce some incremental benefit, prevention is the only secure answer. Primary prevention, through political and financial pressure on tobacco companies, would help limit the supply of tobacco and related products. Worldwide education programs through mass media could help limit the demand. Secondary prevention through screening for early detection of lung cancer is likely to gain momentum for high-risk individuals. Immune-related therapies and the personalization of treatment through the detection of biomarkers predicting response are anticipated to be the way of the future.[74]

Case Studies

Case 1. Lung Cancer Screening

A 45-year-old man who smoked two packs a day for 20 years but who quit 2 years ago consults his physician. A friend of the patient recently has been diagnosed with lung cancer, and the patient is concerned that he might develop the same condition. He otherwise is healthy and has no diagnosed lung disease. The review of systems is negative for weight loss, chest pain, and hemoptysis. The patient is taking no medications, and his family history also is negative for cancer. The patient works in an office and has never been exposed to any dusts, fumes, or toxic chemicals. His physical examination is normal.

This individual, although asymptomatic, is clearly at risk of developing lung cancer, given his 40 pack year history of smoking. He has no additional risk factors from other exposures, from his family history, or from chronic obstructive pulmonary disease. He has no active symptoms or signs suggestive of lung cancer. This frequently is the case until the cancer becomes quite advanced, however. By the time a patient develops symptomatic lung cancer, the prognosis is quite poor because of the advanced disease. The emphasis thus has been placed on attempts at early diagnosis, before the onset of symptoms and signs.

Until recently, trials of screening for lung cancer in populations at risk have been largely unsuccessful. Sputum cytology and chest radiography have yielded some benefit in terms of increased detection of early-stage tumors but have had no substantial impact on patient outcome. Using spiral CT scanning has provided encouraging data in this field and has been shown to reduce mortality in high-risk patients. These scans can be performed quickly, with minimal radiation exposure, and at relatively low cost. False-positive results (e.g., identification of benign lesions that would not otherwise have been detected) could limit the utility of this technique.

Case 2. Early-Stage Lung Cancer

A 63-year-old woman seeks medical attention after an abnormality is noted on a chest radiograph. She is a former smoker of 38 pack years who quit smoking 5 years ago. She otherwise is quite healthy and has no active medical problems. Her exposure history, social history, and family history are unremarkable, as is her physical examination. The chest radiograph shows a 2-cm peripheral lesion in the right upper lobe. No other abnormalities are seen on the film, specifically, no pleural effusion, no bony invasion, and no evidence of mediastinaladenopathy.

A transthoracic needle aspirate tests positive for squamous cell carcinoma. A CT scan of the chest to the level of the adrenal glands reveals no abnormalities apart from the 2-cm lesion. A complete blood count and serum calcium and liver enzyme values were all within normal limits. Mediastinoscopy revealed no evidence of adenopathy. Pulmonary function testing revealed an FEV_1 of 2.2 L (70% predicted). Because of the absence of symptoms, a bone scan and a CT scan of the head were not performed.

This patient has T1N0M0 disease, which represents stage IA non-small-cell lung cancer. The treatment of choice is surgical resection. The patient's pulmonary function tests are quite good and should easily allow resection of a single lobe. There is no proven role for postoperative chemotherapy or radiotherapy in this setting. The 5-year survival rate for this type of patient after resection is 70%. If this patient had a larger tumor (3 cm or more) and the presentation was otherwise identical, the clinical stage would be stage IB. Survival for this stage is lower, at about 58%. For this stage there are emerging data that postoperative chemotherapy may improve survival.

Case 3. Metastatic Lung Cancer

A 72-year-old man sees his physician because of new onset of headaches. The patient currently smokes and has smoked two packs of cigarettes a day for the past 40 years. His past medical history is remarkable for two myocardial infarctions. His medications include daily aspirin, atenolol, and captopril (all for his heart). His family history and social history are unremarkable. His physical examination is remarkable for marked gait instability and asymmetric deep tendon reflexes, which are consistent with a pathologic condition in the central nervous system.

His chest radiograph reveals a 5-cm mass in the right mid-lung zone with enlargement of the mediastinum, which is consistent with substantial adenopathy in the paratracheal region and the aorticopulmonary window. A right-sided pleural effusion also is present. A CT scan of the head reveals three intracranial lesions, a finding consistent with metastatic disease. A diagnostic thoracentesis yields a positive result for adenocarcinoma of the lung.

This patient has metastatic non-small-cell lung cancer. The staging would be T2N3M1. The T2 status is based on the 5-cm size of the tumor, whereas the N3 status is based on the radiographic evidence of contralateral mediastinaladenopathy. The metastatic lesion is evident from the pleural effusion and head CT scan. For diagnostic certitude, drainage of the pleural effusion should be performed; this will likely both confirm the diagnosis and stage the patient as stage IV.

The therapeutic goal in this situation should be palliation. The patient sought attention for his headaches, and cranial irradiation could be performed to control these symptoms. Because the patient has several intracranial metastases, surgical resection of these lesions is not recommended. Most would advocate offering chemoradiotherapy for palliative purposes. This decision is based on discussion with the patient and his family regarding his wishes. Although treatment would not offer a cure, there are data that suggest that survival is improved with chemoradiotherapy if a patient has a good performance status. However, the median survival still is likely to be less than 1 year.

Key Points

- Lung cancer is common and can be preventable.
- A tissue-based diagnosis generally is required. This can be obtained by analysis of sputum or pleural fluid or of bronchoscopic, surgical, or needle biopsy specimens.
- Lung cancer generally is classified as small cell or non-small-cell cancer.
- Small cell lung cancer generally is treated with chemotherapy or radiotherapy or both but rarely with surgery.
- Surgical resection is the preferred treatment for early-stage non-small-cell lung cancer.
- Chemotherapy and radiotherapy in nonresectable non-small-cell lung cancer in patients with a good performance status is the standard of care.
- For patients with advanced disease and a poor performance status, supportive care and palliation remain the only options available.
- Prevention and early diagnosis are future areas of emphasis in lung cancer.

References

1. Howlader N, Noone AM, Krapcho M, et al. *SEER Cancer Statistics Review, 1975–2010*. National Cancer Institute. Bethesda, Md. Available at: http://seer.cancer.gov/csr/1975_2010/, based on November 2012 SEER data submission, posted to the SEER website, April 2013.
2. World Health Organization. Global cancer rates could increase by 50% to 15 million by 2020. Available at: http://www.iarc.fr/en/media-centre/pr/2013/pdfs/pr223_E.pdf. Accessed August 28, 2014.
3. Centers for Disease Control and Prevention. *Lung cancer trends*. Available at: http://www.cdc.gov/cancer/lung/statistics/trends.htm. Accessed August 28, 2014.
4. Mariotto AB, Yabroff KR, Shao Y, et al. Projections of the cost of cancer care in the United States: 2010–2020. *J Natl Cancer Inst*. 2011;103:117–128.
5. Reck M, Heigener DF, Mok T, et al. Management of non-small-cell lung cancer: recent developments. *Lancet*. 2013; 382:709–719.
6. Osann K, Lowery J, Schell M. Small cell lung cancer in women: risk associated with smoking, prior respiratory disease, and occupation. *Lung Cancer*. 2000;28:1–10.
7. Molina JR, Yang P, Cassivi SD, et al. Non-small cell lung cancer: epidemiology, risk factors, treatment and survivorship. *Mayo Clin Proc*. 2008;83:584–594.
8. Christiani DC. Smoking and the molecular epidemiology of lung cancer. *Clin Chest Med*. 2000;21:87–93.
9. Molina JR, Yang P, Cassivi SD, et al. Non-small cell lung cancer: epidemiology, risk factors, treatment and survivorship. *Mayo Clin Proc*. 2008;83:584–594.
10. Nana-Sinkam SP, Powell CA. Molecular biology of lung cancer. In Diagnosis and management of lung cancer, 3rd ed: American College of Chest Physicians evidence-based clinical practice guidelines. *Chest*. 2013;143(5 suppl):e30S–e39S.
11. Reck M, Heigener DF, Mok T, et al. Management of non-small-cell lung cancer: recent developments. *Lancet*. 2013;382:709–719.

12. Lung cancer: a global scourge. *Lancet*. 2013;382:659.
13. Alberg AJ, Brock MV, Ford JG, et al. Epidemiology of lung cancer. In Diagnosis and management of lung cancer, 3rd ed: American College of Chest Physicians evidence-based clinical practice guidelines. *Chest*. 2013;143(5 suppl):e1S–e29S.
14. Du Y, Zhou BS, Wu JM. Lifestyle factors and human lung cancer: an overview of recent advances. *Int J Oncol*. 1998;13:471–479.
15. Jemal A, Travis WD, Tarone RE, et al. Lung cancer rates convergence in young men and women in the United States: analysis by birth cohort and histologic type. *Int J Cancer*. 2003;105: 101–107.
16. Hubbard R, Venn A, Lewis S, et al. Lung cancer and cryptogenic fibrosing alveolitis: a population-based cohort study. *Am J Respir Crit Care Med*. 2000;161:5–8.
17. Yamasawa H, Ishii Y, Kitamura S. Concurrence of sarcoidosis and lung cancer: a report of four cases. *Respiration*. 2000;67:90–93.
18. Bedimo R. Non-AIDS-defining malignancies among HIV-infected patients in the highly active antiretroviral therapy era. *Curr HIV/AIDS Rep*. 2008;5:140–149.
19. Marcus PM, Bergstrahl EJ, Fagerstrom RM, et al. Lung cancer mortality in the Mayo Lung Project: impact of extended follow-up. *J Natl Can Inst*. 2000;92:1308–1316.
20. Oken MM, Hocking WG, Kvale PA, et al. Screening by chest radiograph and lung cancer mortality: the Prostate, Lung, Colorectal, and Ovarian (PLCO) randomized trial. *JAMA*. 2011;306:1865–1873.
21. Aberle DR, Adams AM, Berg CD, et al. Reduced lung-cancer mortality with low-dose computed tomographic screening. *N Engl J Med*. 2011;365:395-409.
22. Saghir Z, Dirksen A, Ashraf H, et al. CT screening for lung cancer brings forward early disease. The randomised Danish Lung Cancer Screening Trial: status after five annual screening rounds with low-dose CT. *Thorax*. 2012;67:296–301.
23. Ru Zhao Y, Xie X, de Koning HJ, et al. NELSON lung cancer screening study. *Cancer Imaging*. 2011;11(suppl 1A):S79–S84.
24. Patel A, Peters S. Clinical manifestations of lung cancer. *Mayo Clin Proc*. 1993;68:273–277.
25. Crapo JD, et al., eds. *Baum's Textbook of Pulmonary Disease*. 7th ed. Philadelphia: Lippincott Williams & Wilkins; 2004.
26. Arcasoy SM, Jett J. Superior pulmonary sulcus tumors and Pancoast's syndrome. *N Engl J Med*. 1997;337:1370–1376.
27. Yano S, Shimada K. Changes in superior vena cava pulsed Doppler flow patterns: possible indicator of improvement of superior vena cava syndrome due to lung cancer. *J Ultrasound Med*. 1997;16: 707–710.
28. Kashitani N, Eda R, Masayoshi T, et al. Lobar extent of pulmonary lymphangitic carcinomatosis: Tl-201 chloride and Tc-99m MIBI scintigraphic findings. *Clin Nucl Med*. 1996;21:726–729.
29. Patel A, Davila D, Peters S. Paraneoplastic syndromes associated with lung cancer. *Mayo Clin Proc*. 1993;68:278–287.
30. Sridhar K, Lobo C, Altman RD. Digital clubbing and lung cancer. *Chest*. 1998;114:1535–1537.
31. Strewler GJ. The physiology of parathyroid hormone-related protein. *N Engl J Med*. 2000;342:177–185.
32. Rossato M, Zabeo E, Burei M, et al. Lung cancer and paraneoplastic neurologic syndromes. Case report and review of the literature. *Clin Lung Cancer*. 2013;14:301–309.
33. Kagan A, Steckel R, Braun R. Asymptomatic peripheral lung nodule. *AJR Am J Roentgenol*. 1980;135:417–420.
34. Detterbeck FC, Boffa DJ, Tanoue LT, Wilson LD. The new lung cancer staging system. *Chest*. 2009;136:260–271.
35. Gould MK, Donington J, Lynch WR, et al. Evaluation of individuals with pulmonary nodules: when is it lung cancer? Diagnosis and management of lung cancer, 3rd ed: American College of Chest Physicians evidence-based clinical practice guidelines. *Chest*. 2013;143(5 suppl):e93S–e120S.
36. Rubins JB, Rubins HB. Temporal trends in the prevalence of malignancy in solitary pulmonary lesions. *Chest*. 1996;109:100–103.
37. Sagel S, Ferguson T, Forrest JV, et al. Percutaneous transthoracic aspiration needle biopsy. *Ann Thorac Surg*. 1978;26:399–405.
38. Rivera MP, Mehta AC, Wahidi MM. Establishing the diagnosis of lung cancer: Diagnosis and management of lung cancer, 3rd ed: American College of Chest Physicians evidence-based clinical practice guidelines. *Chest*. 2013;143(5 suppl):e142S– e165S.
39. Preciado M, Duvall A, Koop SH. Mediastinoscopy: a review of 450 cases. *Laryngoscope*. 1973;83:1300–1310.
40. Herth FJ, Rabe KF, Gasparini S, Annema JT. Transbronchial and transoesophageal (ultrasound-guided) needle aspirations for the analysis of mediastinal lesions. *Eur Respir J* 2006;28:1264–1275.
41. Lau CL, Harpole D. Noninvasive clinical staging modalities for lung cancer. *Semin Surg Oncol*. 2000;18:116–123.
42. Tasci E, Tezel C, Orki A, et al. The role of integrated positron emission tomography and computed tomography in the assessment of nodal spread in cases with non-small cell lung cancer. *Interact Cardiovasc Thorac Surg*. 2010;10:200–203.
43. Lefrak S, Yusen R, Trulock EP, et al. Recent advances in surgery for emphysema. *Annu Rev Med*. 1997;48:387–398.
44. Sutedja G, Postmus P. Bronchoscopic treatment of lung tumors. *Lung Cancer*. 1994;11:1–17.
45. van Meerbeeck JP, Fennell DA, De Ruysscher DK. Small cell lung cancer. *Lancet*. 2011;378:1741–1755.
46. Pujol JL, Carestia L, Daures JP. Is there a case for cisplatin in the treatment of small-cell lung cancer? A meta-analysis of randomized trials of a cisplatin-containing regimen versus a regimen without this alkylating agent. *Br J Cancer*. 2000;83:8–15.
47. Reck M, Heigener DF, Mok T, et al. Management of non-small-cell lung cancer: recent developments. *Lancet*. 2013;382:709–719.
48. Reif M, Socinski M, Rivera MP. Evidence-based medicine in the treatment of non-small cell lung cancer. *Clin Chest Med*. 2000;21:107–120.
49. El-Sherif A, Gooding WE, Santos R, et al. Outcomes of sublobar resection versus lobectomy for stage I non-small cell lung cancer: a 13-year analysis. *Ann Thorac Surg*. 2006;82:408–415.
50. Rowell NP, Williams CJ. Radical radiotherapy for stage I/II non-small cell lung cancer in patients not sufficiently fit for or declining surgery (medically inoperable): a systematic review. *Thorax*. 2001;56:628–638.
51. Albain KS, Swann RS, Rusch VW, et al. Radiotherapy plus chemotherapy with or without surgical resection for stage III non-small-cell lung cancer: a phase III randomised controlled trial. *Lancet*. 2009;374:379–386.
52. Bradbury PA, Shepherd FA. Chemotherapy and surgery for operable NSCLC. *Lancet*. 2007;369:1903–1904.
53. Attar S, Krasna M, Sonnett JR, et al. Superior sulcus (Pancoast) tumor: experience with 105 patients. *Ann Thorac Surg*. 1998;66: 193–198.
54. National Comprehensive Cancer Network. *NCCN Guidelines®*. Available at: www.nccn.org/professionals/physician_gls/f_guidelines.asp. Accessed August 28, 2014.
55. Pisters KM, Evans WK, Azzoli CG, et al. Cancer Care Ontario and American Society of Clinical Oncology adjuvant chemotherapy and adjuvant radiation therapy for stages I-IIIA resectable non small-cell lung cancer guideline. *J Clin Oncol*. 2007;25: 5506–5518.
56. Lally BE, Zelterman D, Colasanto JM, et al. Postoperative radiotherapy for stage II or III non-small-cell lung cancer using the Surveillance, Epidemiology, and End Results database. *J Clin Oncol*. 2006;24:2998–3006.
57. Douillard JY, Rosell R, De Lena M, et al. Adjuvant vinorelbine plus cisplatin versus observation in patients with completely resected stage IB-IIIA non-small-cell lung cancer (Adjuvant Navelbine International Trialist Association [ANITA]): a randomised controlled trial. *Lancet Oncol*. 2006;7:719–727.
58. Azzoli CG, Baker S Jr, Temin S, et al. American Society of Clinical Oncology clinical practice guideline update on chemotherapy for stage IV non-small-cell lung cancer. *J Clin Oncol*. 2009;27: 6251–6299.
59. Bakitas M, Lyons KD, Hegel MT, et al. Effects of a palliative care intervention on clinical outcomes in patients with advanced cancer:

the Project ENABLE II randomized controlled Trial. *JAMA*. 2009; 302:741–749.

60. Temel JS, Freer JA, Muzikansky A, et al. Early palliative care for patient with metastatic non-small-cell lung cancer. *N Engl J Med*. 2010;363:733–742.
61. Byhardt R, Scott C, Sause WT, et al. Response, toxicity, failure patterns, and survival in five Radiation Therapy Oncology Group (RTOG) trials of sequential and/or concurrent chemotherapy and radiotherapy for locally advanced non-small cell carcinoma of the lung. *Int J Radiat Oncol Biol Phys*. 1998;42:469–478.
62. Monson J, Stark P, Reilly JJ, et al. Clinical radiation pneumonitis and radiographic changes after thoracic radiation therapy for lung carcinoma. *Cancer*. 1998;82:842–850.
63. Warner MA, Offord K, Warner ME, et al. Role of preoperative cessation of smoking and other factors in postoperative pulmonary complications: a blinded prospective study of coronary artery bypass patients. *Mayo Clin Proc*. 1989;64:609–616.
64. Rom W, Hay JG, Lee TC, et al. Molecular and genetic aspects of lung cancer. *Am J Respir Crit Care Med*. 2000;161:1355–1367.
65. Lung cancer: a global scourge. *Lancet*. 2013;382:659. Abstract.
66. Zhang H, Cai B. The impact of tobacco on lung health in China. *Respirology*. 2003;8:17–21.
67. Croghan I, Offord K, Patten CA, et al. Cost-effectiveness of the AHCPR guidelines for smoking. *JAMA*. 1998;279:836–837.
68. Hurt R, Sachs D, Glover ED, et al. A comparison of sustained-release bupropion and placebo for smoking cessation. *N Engl J Med*. 1997;337:1195–1202.
69. Gonzales D, Rennard SI, Nides M, et al. Varenicline, an a4b2 nicotinic acetylcholine receptor partial agonist, vs sustained-release bupropion and placebo for smoking cessation: a randomized controlled trial. *JAMA*. 2006;296:47–55.
70. Bullen C, Howe C, Laugesen M, et al. Electronic cigarettes for smoking cessation: a randomised controlled trial. *Lancet*. 2013;382: 1629–1637.
71. The Alpha-Tocopherol Beta Carotene Cancer Prevention Study Group. The effect of vitamin E and beta carotene on the incidence of lung cancer and other cancers in male smokers. *N Engl J Med*. 1994;330:1029–1035.
72. Ruano-Ravina A, Figueiras A, et al. Antioxidant vitamins and risk of lung cancer. *Curr Pharm Des*. 2006;2:599–613.
73. Omenn G, Goodman G, Thornquist MD, et al. Effects of a combination of β-carotene and vitamin A on lung cancer and cardiovascular disease. *N Engl J Med*. 1996;334:1150–1155.
74. Reck M, Heigener DF, Mok T, et al. Management of non-small cell lung cancer: recent developments. *Lancet*. 2013;382:709–719.

CHAPTER

46

Neonatal and Pediatric Respiratory Disorders

Sherry L. Barnhart

OUTLINE

Apnea of Prematurity
Respiratory Distress Syndrome
Bronchopulmonary Dysplasia and Chronic Lung Disease
Transient Tachypnea of the Newborn
Pneumonia in the Neonate
Meconium Aspiration Syndrome
Persistent Pulmonary Hypertension of the Newborn
Congenital Diaphragmatic Hernia
Congenital Pulmonary Anomalies
Air Leak Syndrome
Retinopathy of Prematurity
Bronchiolitis
Laryngotracheobronchitis
Epiglottitis

OBJECTIVES

1. List the factors that may predispose an infant or child to pulmonary disease.
2. Explain the pathophysiology of pulmonary diseases affecting the newborn and child.
3. Identify the signs and symptoms of pulmonary diseases affecting the newborn and child.
4. Discuss diagnosis of pulmonary diseases affecting the newborn and child.
5. Recognize the radiographic appearance of various diseases of the newborn and child.
6. Integrate the history, physical examination, laboratory, and radiographic findings that are used in the diagnosis of diseases of the infant and child.
7. Discuss treatment options for pediatric pulmonary disease.
8. Explain the significance of monitoring oxygen at preductal and postductal sites.
9. Discuss the impact that hypoxia in a neonate has on the pulmonary vasculature.
10. Describe the development of retinopathy of prematurity.
11. Define apnea of prematurity and periodic breathing.
12. Differentiate between pulmonary agenesis, pulmonary aplasia, and pulmonary hypoplasia.
13. Compare laryngotracheobronchitis and epiglottitis.

KEY TERMS

air leak syndrome
apnea of prematurity
bronchiolitis
bronchogenic cyst
bronchopulmonary dysplasia (BPD)
chronic lung disease (CLD)
congenital diaphragmatic hernia (CDH)
congenital pulmonary airway malformation (CPAM)
epiglottitis
laryngotracheobronchitis (LTB)
meconium aspiration syndrome (MAS)
persistent pulmonary hypertension of the newborn (PPHN)
pulmonary agenesis
pulmonary aplasia
pulmonary hypoplasia
pulmonary sequestration
respiratory distress syndrome (RDS)
retinopathy of prematurity (ROP)
transient tachypnea of the newborn (TTN)

Introduction

Respiratory illness is the most common cause of infant and childhood morbidity in developed countries. There are many disorders that result in respiratory distress and place an infant or child at high risk of cardiopulmonary failure. Respiratory disease may begin early in life, even in utero, and remain a challenging problem that affects the infant's survival and quality of life. The causes are many. In utero abnormalities, such as congenital diaphragmatic hernia, can inhibit lung development. Maternal factors, such as medication or illicit drug use, often cause severe respiratory depression. Events at birth will affect the infant's respiratory status, as is found with transient tachypnea of the newborn and meconium aspiration syndrome. Premature birth with lungs that are unable to adequately support gas exchange may result in apnea and respiratory distress syndrome. Ironically, therapy for respiratory disorders can actually lead to more disease, which is what occurs with chronic lung disease, air leaks, and retinopathy of prematurity.

As for the child, acute respiratory tract infections may be mild or life threatening. Infections resulting in bronchiolitis, laryngotracheobronchitis, and epiglottitis are often causes for emergency department and hospital admissions. Although we have witnessed significant advances in the medical management of infants and children, the fact remains that all of the factors just described continue to have an impact on neonatal and pediatric respiratory care.

Apnea of Prematurity

The successful progression from fetal to neonatal life is dependent on complex physiologic changes that include moving from fetal respiratory activity to normal spontaneous breathing. When an infant is born premature, the immaturity of the central respiratory control center interrupts this normal transition and often leads to apnea. The standard definition of **apnea of prematurity** is the cessation of breathing for at least 20 seconds or for shorter periods if the apnea is followed by bradycardia, oxygen desaturation, cyanosis, or pallor.[1] Apnea of prematurity is different from the periodic breathing common to premature as well as some full-term infants. Periodic breathing is a respiratory pattern characterized by periodic pauses of breathing lasting between 5 and 10 seconds and then followed by regular breathing. It has no pathologic significance, does not result in bradycardia or cyanosis, and spontaneously resolves without the need for intervention.

Apnea of prematurity affects at least 85% of infants born at less than 34 weeks' gestation and 50% of infants of less than 1500 grams birth weight.[2] It is the most common cause of apnea in neonates, with peak incidence usually occurring between 2 and 7 days' postnatal age.

Pathophysiology and Etiology

Apnea of prematurity is largely due to immaturity of the medullary brain stem center that regulates breathing. This immaturity leads to impaired responses to hypoxia and hypercapnia and an exaggerated inhibitory response to stimulation of airway receptors.

Apnea is traditionally classified as obstructive, central, or mixed, depending on the presence or absence of upper airway obstruction. No airflow, chest wall motion, or inspiratory efforts occur in central apnea. In obstructive apnea, inspiratory efforts and chest wall motion persist, but airflow is absent. Mixed apnea, the most common type associated with apnea of prematurity, has components of both central and obstructive apnea: inspiratory efforts with airway obstruction preceding or following central apnea.

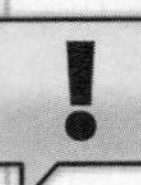

Respiratory Recap

Apnea of Prematurity

- Cessation of breathing for at least 20 seconds
- Caused by immaturity of the brain stem
- Treated with respiratory stimulants, oxygen, CPAP, and mechanical ventilation
- Home apnea monitor may be used

Clinical Manifestations

In premature infants who are breathing spontaneously with no assistance, apnea usually occurs on the first or second day of life. If lung disease exists or the infant is receiving any form of mechanical ventilation, including noninvasive ventilation (NIV) or continuous positive airway pressure (CPAP), apnea may be delayed or not present until the infant no longer needs ventilator assistance. Bradycardia, hypotension, cyanosis, pallor, and oxygen desaturation typically accompany the apneic episodes. Apnea of prematurity has usually resolved by 37 weeks' postconceptional age but may persist beyond term, especially in infants delivered at 24 to 28 weeks' gestation.[3] If apnea presents immediately after birth, first presents in a premature infant that is older than 2 weeks, or reoccurs after a 1- to 2-week period without apnea, it may signify an underlying pathophysiologic condition. Immediate investigation of possible causes is always warranted.

Diagnosis

A diagnosis of apnea of prematurity is made after other disorders have been considered and excluded. Several studies are routinely used to confirm the diagnosis. Laboratory studies performed when infection is suspected include a complete blood count, blood and spinal fluid cultures, and urinalysis. Electrolyte levels and glucose levels are tests useful in diagnosing a metabolic process. Chest radiographs and electrocardiograms (ECGs) are routine, whereas echocardiograms are obtained if symptoms are suggestive of cardiac disease. Imaging studies of the head and neck may be obtained if obstructive apnea is suspected. A swallow study or abdominal ultrasound is used to detect gastrointestinal problems.

Management

Clinical management includes cardiorespiratory monitoring and tactile stimulation. When apnea lasts for only a few seconds, stimulating the infant by patting

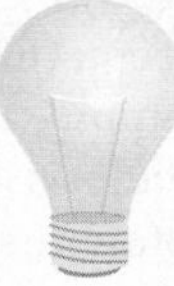

STOP AND THINK

A neonate born at 28 weeks' gestation has received caffeine for 12 days. He is ready for discharge home. Bradycardia and apnea spells that resolve on their own are noted during feedings. Should an impedance (apnea) monitor be ordered for home use or should discharge be delayed until there are no further events?

the infant or flicking the feet is usually the only intervention needed. Pharmacologic treatment with methylxanthines, most often caffeine or theophylline, has been used since the 1970s to stimulate respirations, thereby reducing the frequency of apnea and need for mechanical ventilation. Caffeine is preferred over theophylline because it has a longer half-life that allows for once-daily dosing, a larger gap between therapeutic and toxic levels, and fewer side effects.[4]

Depending on the frequency and severity of the apneic episodes, oxygen therapy, NIV, CPAP, and intubation with assisted ventilation may be required. When apnea results in oxygen desaturation, oxygen is administered and manual ventilation applied if the apnea is prolonged. High-flow nasal cannula, NIV, or CPAP is initiated when the apneic events continue or become more frequent in spite of methylxanthine therapy. If apnea with oxygen desaturation, bradycardia, or both continues, intubation and mechanical ventilation may be indicated.[5] **Box 46-1** contains a suggested treatment protocol for apnea of prematurity. Although the time interval is not clearly established, methylxanthine therapy is discontinued when there have been no significant events for 7 to 14 days. The infant is discharged without methylxanthine treatment if no further events occur.

In some infants the apnea will reoccur, and medication is restarted. If the infant continues to need methylxanthines at discharge, an impedance monitor (apnea monitor) is provided for use at home. This monitor stores data and documents apneic, bradycardic, and tachycardic events. Parents and other caregivers receive training in cardiopulmonary resuscitation as well as observation and stimulation techniques. They also are instructed on monitor use, including how to apply monitor leads and correctly respond to alarms. The monitor can be safely discontinued after the infant has had no true and significant apneic and bradycardic events for 1 to 2 months after discharge home.[6] **Box 46-2** lists the indications for apnea monitoring at home.

BOX 46–1

Protocol for Treating Apnea of Prematurity

1. Monitor with cardiorespiratory monitor and pulse oximeter.
2. Provide tactile stimulation and reposition head and neck.
3. Administer oxygen for bradycardia or oxygen desaturation.
4. Begin methylxanthine therapy (caffeine preferred).
5. Apply high-flow nasal cannula or nasal continuous positive airway pressure.
6. Intubate and begin mechanical ventilation.

BOX 46-2

Indications for Home Apnea Monitoring in Infants

Methylxanthine treatment at home
Bradycardia with methylxanthine use
GERD with apnea
Documented ALTE
Risk of central apnea
Twin or sibling with SIDS-related death*

*The American Academy of Pediatrics does not recommend home apnea monitoring to prevent SIDS.

GERD, gastroesophageal reflux disease; ALTE, apparent life-threatening event; SIDS, sudden infant death syndrome.

Complications and Outcome

Apnea that leads to hypoxemia and bradycardia increases the risk of cerebral injury; however, treatment with caffeine decreases this risk.[7] Apnea due to prematurity is usually resolved by 44 weeks' conceptional age. Studies indicate that it does not cause an infant to be at a higher risk for sudden infant death syndrome (SIDS).[8]

Respiratory Distress Syndrome

Infants born before the 37th week of gestation are considered premature. The consequences of a premature birth are complex, with the earliest recognized complication being **respiratory distress syndrome (RDS)**. Previously referred to as hyaline membrane disease, RDS is the most common cause of respiratory distress in the premature infant and occurs most often in infants born at less than 28 weeks' gestation. RDS rarely occurs in term infants.[9]

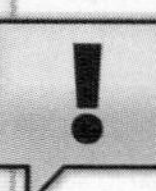

Respiratory Recap

Respiratory Distress Syndrome

- Complication of prematurity.
- Biochemical tests of amniotic fluid can be used to evaluate lung maturity.
- Treatment includes oxygen, surfactant replacement, CPAP, mechanical ventilation, and supportive therapy.

Pathophysiology and Etiology

Box 46-3 lists factors that may predispose an infant to RDS. The risk of RDS may decrease if the mother has pregnancy-induced hypertension, prolonged rupture of membranes, or a history of narcotic addiction. It is believed that the stress of these situations helps the lungs to mature. Antenatal corticosteroid therapy to mothers with preterm labor accelerates maturation of the neonate's lung and significantly reduces the incidence of RDS and mortality.

High surface tension and a lack of pulmonary surfactant in the lungs are responsible for the development of RDS in premature infants. Surfactant is a complex mixture of phospholipids and proteins that is produced by type II pneumocytes and stored in the lamellar bodies. Synthesis begins near 20 weeks of gestation and continues with accelerated production around 36 weeks. As surfactant spreads along the alveolar air–liquid interface, surface tension is decreased and lower pressures are required to keep alveoli inflated. In the premature infant, immature type II alveolar cells produce less surfactant, causing alveoli to collapse.[10] The result is decreased compliance, reduced functional residual capacity (FRC), diffuse atelectasis, and increased airway resistance and dead space.[11] Well-perfused but poorly ventilated areas result in ventilation-perfusion mismatch with hypoxia and right-to-left shunting of blood.

BOX 46-3

Risk Factors Associated with Respiratory Distress Syndrome

Male infant
Hypothermia
Premature birth
Maternal diabetes
Perinatal asphyxia
Multifetal pregnancy
Family history of respiratory distress syndrome
Cesarean delivery without labor

Because of the weak respiratory muscles and overly compliant chest that are characteristic of the premature neonate, work of breathing increases as lung compliance is reduced. Hypercarbia and respiratory acidosis quickly develop as the diaphragm and intercostal muscles fatigue. Prolonged hypoxemia leads to vasoconstriction of pulmonary arteries, decreased pulmonary blood flow, and direct damage to the respiratory epithelium, allowing plasma to leak into the alveoli, where hyaline membranes are formed, hence the term hyaline membrane disease.[12,13]

Clinical Manifestations

RDS is suspected in the premature infant who develops respiratory distress at or shortly after delivery. Tachypnea with respiratory rates of 60 breaths per minute or greater is often the initial symptom. Other hallmark clinical signs are nasal flaring, subcostal and intercostal retractions, and expiratory grunting. Grunting occurs as air is forced through the partially closed glottis in an attempt to increase the FRC. As the work of breathing continues, grunting becomes ineffective, and the alveoli collapse. Cyanosis and hypoxia are common, and breath sounds are diminished. Upon examination the infant may be inactive and have edema and decreased perfusion in peripheral extremities. Oxygen requirements and apnea often increase after birth, and within 48 hours the infant has rapidly progressed to respiratory failure with hypercarbia and respiratory acidosis. Extremely premature neonates with severe atelectasis and loss of compliance may have lungs so stiff that they are apneic before they leave the delivery room.

Diagnosis

Clinical features and risk factors aid in the diagnosis, which is confirmed with physical findings, chest radiographs, and lab values consistent with RDS. A detailed history is also critical in the differential diagnosis. Details should include gestational age and maternal history. Age is important because RDS typically occurs in premature infants, unlike term infants affected by transient tachypnea or postterm infants with meconium aspiration syndrome. Information concerning labor and delivery is vital and should include fetal heart tracings, color and amount of amniotic fluid, method of delivery, and maternal temperature. Pneumonia due to β-hemolytic *Streptococcus* has been associated with rupture of membranes occurring more than 24 hours prior to delivery. Transient tachypnea of the newborn usually occurs in term infants following cesarean delivery without maternal labor.

Although the chest radiograph may not be typical in the first few hours after birth, RDS is characterized by a large thymus, markedly decreased lung expansion, atelectasis, and a diffuse symmetric reticulogranular

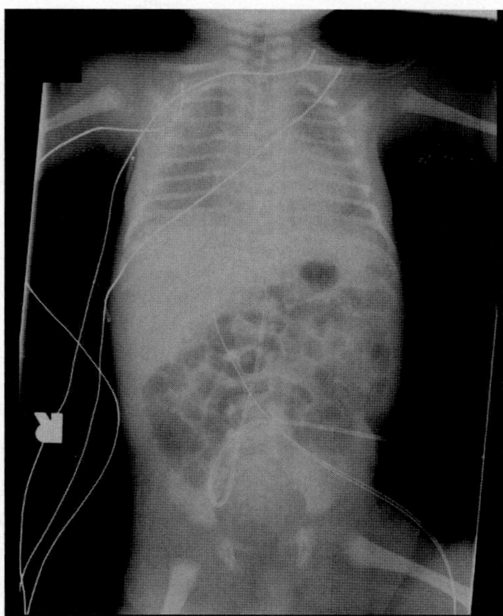

FIGURE 46-1 Chest radiograph of a preterm infant presenting with a bilateral diffuse fine granular (ground glass) appearance and reduced lung expansion, typical of respiratory distress syndrome.
Courtesy of Chetan Chandulal Shah, MBBS, DMRD, MBA, Arkansas Children's Hospital.

(ground glass) appearance that extends to the periphery of the lungs. With severe disease, the chest radiograph may progress to complete whiteout that is difficult to distinguish from pneumonia (**Figure 46-1**).

Biochemical tests of lung maturity began in 1971 with the introduction of the lecithin-to-sphingomyelin (L/S) ratio. Lecithin and sphingomyelin are both phospholipids found in the amniotic fluid. Lecithin levels increase as the lung matures and begins producing surfactant, whereas the amount of sphingomyelin remains fairly constant. A calculated L/S ratio of 2 or more is considered an accurate indication that sufficient surfactant is being produced and the risk of RDS is low. The assessment of amniotic fluid for phosphatidylglycerol, first reported in 1976, was the next biochemical test developed to determine fetal lung maturity. The presence of phosphatidylglycerol is associated with a low risk for RDS. Recent studies, however, have shown that it is gestational age and not the presence of a mature fetal lung index that correlates most highly with improved neonatal outcomes. Although widely used at one time, these and other biochemical tests, including the foam stability index (also known as the shake test) and the lamellar body count, may have passed the point of being clinically useful.[14,15]

Management

When there is a high risk of delivery occurring between 23 and 34 weeks' gestation, mothers are given tocolytics to delay delivery and then receive corticosteroids 24 to 48 hours before delivery. This has been shown to accelerate fetal lung maturation and surfactant production, thereby decreasing the incidence of RDS as well as intraventricular hemorrhage and neonatal mortality.[16]

Maintaining an airway with adequate oxygenation is vital in the management of RDS. Depending on the infant's clinical presentation, initial oxygen therapy is delivered using blow-by oxygen, a hood, or resuscitation bag and mask. In very low birth weight infants, attempts are made to maintain the fraction of inspired oxygen (FIO_2) to keep the oxygen saturation as measured by pulse oximetry (SpO_2) between 85% and 92% or the PaO_2 at 50 to 80 mm Hg. Nasal CPAP should be considered when there is increasing respiratory distress and the heart rate is greater than 100 beats/minute. In some institutions, heated and humidified high-flow nasal cannulas with flows greater than 2 L/min are used in place of nasal CPAP.[17] The high-flow therapy may prevent the need for intubation and mechanical ventilation, or it may be used to facilitate extubation.[18,19]

Before the use of exogenous surfactant therapy, RDS was associated with significant morbidity and mortality. Following its introduction in the 1980s, surfactant replacement therapy for RDS has proven to be undoubtedly one of the greatest advances in neonatal care.[20] Today it is a standard of care for the infant with RDS; early administration is associated with a significant reduction in mortality, duration of mechanical ventilation, and incidence of air leaks.[21]

Two approaches have emerged in surfactant replacement therapy: prophylactic and rescue treatment. In an attempt to replace surfactant before the development of severe RDS, prophylactic treatment consists of surfactant administration in the delivery room. It is given within 10 to 30 minutes following intubation and radiographic confirmation of RDS features. Studies have concluded that prophylactic surfactant replacement is associated with a lower incidence and severity of RDS and pulmonary air leaks.[22] One disadvantage to this approach is that some infants who might manage perfectly well on CPAP are unnecessarily treated with intubation and ventilation, increasing the risk of bronchopulmonary dysplasia. This is avoided with rescue treatment, in which surfactant is administered within the first 12 hours after birth and only to those infants who have a diagnosis of RDS and are requiring mechanical ventilation. Early rescue surfactant replacement is defined as administering surfactant within 1 to 2 hours of birth, whereas late rescue replacement is administration 2 or more hours after birth.[23] A criticism of rescue therapy is that the delay in surfactant replacement could result in progression of RDS.

Two types of surfactant preparations are available to treat RDS. The natural surfactants are derived from animal sources, including minced lung extracts from cows or pigs or surfactant extracted after lavage of cow lungs. The latest synthetic surfactants contain biologically active peptides or whole proteins that mimic the human surfactant protein.[24,25]

Prior to surfactant replacement, the infant must be intubated and the endotracheal tube placement confirmed with a chest radiograph. If needed, the infant is suctioned prior to instillation of surfactant. Suctioning is then avoided for at least 2 hours after surfactant administration unless airway compromise develops. A bolus, portion of small aliquots, or infusion of surfactant is administered inline through an adapter port on the proximal end of the endotracheal tube. Currently there is insufficient evidence to recommend the optimal method of delivery, number of doses, or body position.[23] Although data are limited on their effectiveness, alternatives to intratracheal administration include nebulized surfactant, delivery with a laryngeal mask, and using laryngoscopy to guide a thin intratracheal catheter; all of these eliminate the need for intubation.[26–28] To reduce the need for prolonged pressure ventilation and the risk of developing bronchopulmonary dysplasia, some institutions provide intubation and ventilation primarily for surfactant administration and then quickly extubate to nasal CPAP.[29]

Lung compliance can change rapidly following surfactant replacement and often necessitates adjusting ventilator and FIO_2 settings. Close monitoring of ventilator waveforms, transcutaneous CO_2 levels, blood gas values, and SpO_2 is essential in determining safe and effective settings. To reduce the risk of hyperoxia and pulmonary air leaks, the FIO_2 is weaned and tidal volumes or peak inspiratory pressures are reduced empirically within a few minutes following administration.

With the clinical goal of maintaining FRC, CPAP applied to the stiff lungs of the infant with RDS results in improved lung compliance, alveolar inflation, and oxygenation, which in turn decrease intrapulmonary shunting and work of breathing. CPAP is indicated when the FIO_2 required is greater than 0.30 and the infant continues to have respiratory distress or whenever the required FIO_2 is greater than 0.40, regardless of the presence of respiratory distress. Nasal CPAP may be applied shortly after birth in an attempt to avoid the need for mechanical ventilation with prolonged intubation and thereby prevent ventilator-induced lung injury that may lead to chronic lung disease. Administering pressures of 4 to 7 cm H_2O are usually adequate; however, pressures up to 10 cm H_2O may be necessary to improve alveolar recruitment in the infant with severely noncompliant lungs. It is believed that pressures greater than 10 cm H_2O provide no significant benefit and may in fact increase the risk of gastric insufflation. Extremely premature infants weighing less than 1000 g with a gestational age less than 28 weeks are typically intubated and begun on ventilator support immediately after delivery so they can receive preventive surfactant.[30]

CPAP may also be applied following mechanical ventilation. Extubation to CPAP stabilizes the airways and may decrease the risk of respiratory failure and need for reintubation. When the FIO_2 is weaned to less than 0.40, CPAP pressures can be decreased by increments of 1 cm H_2O until 4 cm H_2O is reached. At that point CPAP is discontinued and the infant provided oxygen therapy with a low-flow nasal cannula or oxygen hood.[31] Heated, humidified high-flow nasal cannula appears to have a similar effect to nasal CPAP when it is applied early for respiratory distress or when applied immediately postextubation.[18,19]

For some infants, CPAP or high-flow nasal cannula alone cannot adequately support ventilation, especially in very low birth weight infants (<1000 g) or the extremely premature neonate with a gestational age of less than 26 weeks. Intubation and mechanical ventilation are indicated if the infant has an FIO_2 requirement greater than 0.40, more frequent or prolonged episodes of apnea, or hypercarbia and acidosis in spite of increased levels of CPAP or cannula flow. Mechanical ventilation that optimizes lung volume while limiting hyperexpansion is vital to protecting the fragile neonatal lung. Using volume-targeted ventilation has been shown to reduce the duration of mechanical ventilation and the incidence of chronic lung disease, intraventricular hemorrhage, pneumothorax, and episodes of hypocarbia.[32–35] Initial ventilation settings typically include a tidal volume of 4 to 6 mL/kg, a rate of 30 to 60 breaths per minute, a positive end-expiratory pressure (PEEP) of 4 to 5 cm H_2O, and an inspiratory time between 0.25 and 0.35 second.[36] The FIO_2 is adjusted to keep the appropriate SpO_2 levels (see oxygen therapy values). When initiating pressure-limited ventilation, peak inspiratory pressures of 15 to 25 cm H_2O are usually required to maintain a tidal volume of 4 to 6 mL/kg.

If respiratory failure persists, high-frequency ventilation is implemented using high-frequency oscillatory ventilation (HFOV), high-frequency jet ventilation (HFJV), or high-frequency flow-interrupter (HFI). Studies report that infants treated with HFOV have a lower mortality rate and significantly reduced development of air leak syndrome, display fewer signs of bronchopulmonary dysplasia, and require fewer days of mechanical ventilation and lower oxygen

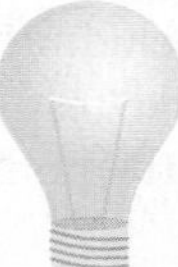

STOP AND THINK

A neonate weighing 690 grams is born at 25 weeks' gestation to a mother whose pregnancy was complicated by preterm labor. Upon delivery the neonate has peripheral cyanosis and is limp and tachypneic with irregular respirations and a heart rate of 60 beats per minute. What procedures should be performed to manage the respiratory distress while minimizing lung injury?

concentrations. There is no clear evidence that choosing HFOV as the initial primary mode of ventilation or as rescue ventilation following conventional ventilation is more beneficial, except that there may be a small reduction in chronic lung disease when using HFOV. There is support of the use of HFOV over conventional ventilation in conjunction with nitric oxide therapy to treat PPHN.[37,38] Inhaled nitric oxide may be used to treat PPHN, but it is not administered to treat RDS alone.

To prevent hypothermia, which increases oxygen consumption, the infant is placed in a neutral thermal environment using either an incubator or a radiant warmer. Although maintaining minimal stimulation is vital, it is necessary to constantly monitor the heart rate, respiratory rate, and Spo_2 and to obtain lab tests. Perfusion and blood pressure are monitored, and blood or volume expanders may be required. An echocardiogram is performed to diagnose a patent ductus arteriosus (PDA) and to determine the presence of pulmonary hypertension and congenital heart defects. Because it is difficult to distinguish between RDS and pneumonia at birth, infants receive empiric antibiotic therapy. Blood cultures are obtained, and antibiotics are discontinued after 2 to 4 days if cultures remain negative.

Complications and Outcomes

Beginning in the 1980s, there has been a significant improvement in the prognosis for RDS, with survival to as low as 23 weeks' gestational age. This is believed to be a result of the administration of antenatal steroids to mothers with preterm labor, surfactant replacement, and volume-targeted ventilation techniques. With adequate treatment, RDS usually resolves within 4 to 5 days in infants with a gestational age of more than 30 weeks. However, the more premature the infant, the greater the probability of requiring ventilator support for several weeks.

Acute complications of RDS, especially in infants who receive mechanical ventilation, include pneumothorax and pulmonary interstitial emphysema (PIE), intraventricular hemorrhage, necrotizing enterocolitis, PDA, and sepsis. With the increased survival of extremely premature infants, a higher incidence of long-term complications is expected. Persistent RDS involving prolonged intubation and mechanical ventilation has a high incidence of chronic lung disease, retinopathy of prematurity, and neurologic impairment with learning disabilities. RDS also increases the incidence of wheezing, asthma, respiratory infection, and pulmonary function test abnormalities.[23,39]

Bronchopulmonary Dysplasia and Chronic Lung Disease

Bronchopulmonary dysplasia (BPD), the chronic lung disease of prematurity, is the most common complication associated with premature birth. Use of antenatal corticosteroids, surfactant replacement, improved nutrition, and advances in ventilation strategies have markedly improved the survival rates of infants born before 28 weeks' gestation with birth weights of less than 1 kg.[40,41] With more births and the dramatic decrease in mortality rates of extremely low birth weight infants, however, the prevalence of long-term complications of prematurity has actually increased.[42,43] The incidence of BPD increases with decreasing gestational age and birth weight. It is characterized by respiratory failure, the need for supplemental oxygen and mechanical ventilation, and a progressive deterioration of lung function that results in chronic lung injury.

When BPD was first described in 1967, mechanical ventilation of premature neonates was just beginning and infants with birth weights less than 1 kg rarely survived.[44] At that time BPD was considered a syndrome of severe lung injury in preterm infants with RDS who received high levels of supplemental oxygen and prolonged mechanical ventilation using high airway pressures. This classic BPD occurred in relatively larger preterm infants and was based on progressive chest radiographic changes that typically revealed areas of increased density, fibrosis, and marked hyperinflation and emphysema. Exposure of the premature lung to mechanical ventilation and oxygen was considered the major factor in its development.

As practices and outcomes have changed, this severe form of BPD, characterized by diffuse lung disease and injury to the immature lung, has become less common and a new BPD has emerged in very low birth weight infants who often have received antenatal steroid therapy and surfactant replacement.[45] Instead of the diffuse progressive lung injury that characterized BPD before surfactant use, the chronic lung disease seen today is predominantly disrupted alveolar development and abnormal pulmonary vascular growth.[46] These preterm infants may or may not have RDS, and their initial respiratory course is often mild, needing little or no ventilatory support. When required, oxygen is administered at low concentrations and ventilation is supported using low tidal volumes to avoid volutrauma and hypocarbia. Typically triggered by infections and a PDA, increased oxygen requirement and mechanical ventilation usually occur in the second or third week of life. As lung function progressively deteriorates, the need for mechanical ventilation and supplemental oxygen is prolonged. Chest radiographs revealing hazy lungs, cystic emphysema, and more uniform inflation characterize this form of BPD.

BPD is best described as chronic lung disease in the premature infant who requires prolonged mechanical ventilation and high oxygen concentrations to treat RDS and continues to be oxygen dependent at 28 postnatal days.[47] Although sometimes used interchangeably with BPD, **chronic lung disease (CLD)** can be defined as the milder new form of BPD and is simply based on a continued oxygen requirement at 36 weeks' gestational age.[48] It refers to the very low birth weight preterm infant with chronic lung disease who initially responded favorably to surfactant replacement and may or may not have a history of RDS.

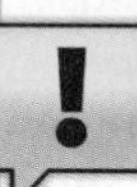

Respiratory Recap

Chronic Lung Disease

- Occurs in premature infants with progressive deterioration of lung function.
- A milder form of bronchopulmonary dysplasia based on continued oxygen therapy at 36 weeks' gestation.
- Causes are multifactorial and include ventilator- and oxygen-induced injury.
- Treatment includes oxygen, mechanical ventilation, corticosteroids, and bronchodilators.

Pathophysiology and Etiology

BPD is no longer believed to be predominantly a ventilator- and oxygen-induced injury but instead is multifactorial and includes inflammation, inadequate nutrition and fetal growth, infection, high oxygen levels that increase free radical exposure, mechanical ventilation with volutrauma, and genetic factors.[49] **Box 46-4** lists risk factors responsible for the development of BPD.

Lung inflammation is a major contributor to BPD and may actually begin prior to birth. It often continues after delivery if the infant requires mechanical ventilatory support or supplemental oxygen. Limited fetal growth has been attributed to failure of the placenta to provide adequate oxygenation and nutrition, which can in turn interfere with alveolar and pulmonary artery development.[50] Any process that limits fetal growth has the ability to continue to adversely affect lung growth after birth, making the lung more vulnerable to injury.

With supplemental oxygen, the lungs are exposed to toxic free radicals, ions that disrupt chemical bonds. Excessive free radical exposure further damages cell membranes and the already-injured pulmonary tissues. Because of inadequate concentrations of antioxidant enzymes, preterm infants are poorly equipped to handle free radicals and are more susceptible to oxygen exposure injury.

The surfactant-deficient fetal lung is easily injured, with injury very likely occurring during resuscitation. Ventilating with lower tidal volumes minimizes the injury but may not prevent hypercarbia. As positive pressure ventilation inflates and stretches the lung, the walls and alveolar septa are damaged, triggering an inflammatory response.[45]

Prenatal infection is believed to be a risk factor for the development of BPD. The lungs of infants born before 30 weeks' gestation may be exposed to inflammation as a result of chorioamnionitis. *Ureaplasma urealyticum* and *Mycoplasma* are the most frequent contaminant organisms in amniotic fluid, and it is believed that the ascending intrauterine infection can inflame the infant lungs within hours.[51]

BOX 46-4

Risk Factors in the Development of Bronchopulmonary Dysplasia

Prematurity
Preeclampsia
Postnatal hyperoxia
Aspiration syndromes
Postnatal pneumonia and/or sepsis
Patent ductus arteriosus (PDA)
Intrauterine growth restriction
Genetic variants in surfactant proteins
Mechanical ventilation with volutrauma
Prenatal infection (chorioamnionitis) and inflammation

Clinical Manifestations and Diagnosis

Physical examination of the infant with BPD reveals tachypnea, tachycardia, wheezing, crackles, noisy breathing, and retractions. The infant is usually fussy and may be difficult to feed due to the increased work of breathing. The ECG and echocardiogram may reveal right ventricular hypertrophy and pulmonary hypertension. Chest radiographs vary widely, depending on the degree of lung injury. Typically there is a gradual progression from minimal findings to a picture of hyaline membranes with decreased lung volumes, areas of atelectasis and hyperexpansion, fine or coarse interstitial opacities, and a bubbly appearance with irregular dense areas (**Figure 46-2**). There is typically a medical history of prematurity, mechanical ventilation, and supplemental oxygen therapy. The diagnosis of BPD is based on clinical manifestations and radiographic changes.

Management

Management goals are to maintain adequate oxygenation and ventilation, reduce inflammation, improve lung function, relieve symptoms, promote optimal lung growth, and prevent further lung injury.

Supplemental oxygen is essential in maintaining adequate oxygenation and preventing right ventricular hypertrophy (RVH), which often accompanies BPD. It is provided by nasal cannula or through mechanical ventilation and is weaned to maintain an Spo_2 of 92%

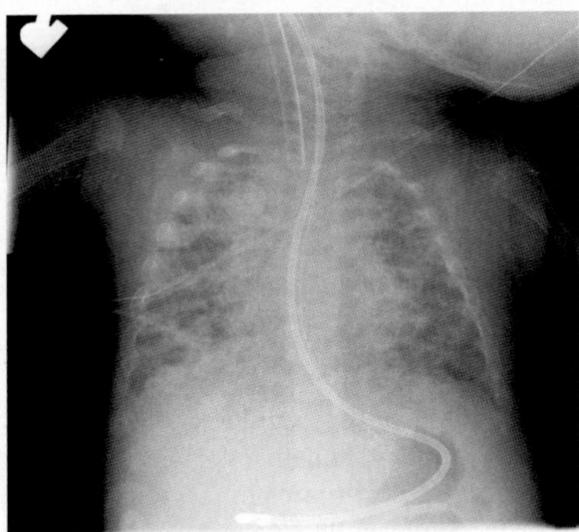

FIGURE 46-2 Chest radiograph of an infant with bronchopulmonary dysplasia showing areas of hyperaeration and reticular opacities with small cystic radiolucencies, giving a coarse, bubbly appearance.
Courtesy of Chetan Chandulal Shah, MBBS, DMRD, MBA, Arkansas Children's Hospital.

to 94%. When RVH is present oxygen is maintained at saturations greater than 97%. Because RVH resolves gradually, many infants continue oxygen use at home following discharge. Although the use of nasal CPAP to avoid intubation and pressure ventilation is a strategy to reduce the risk of BPD, there remain infants who cannot be adequately oxygenated or ventilated with CPAP alone.[52,53] These infants often have moderate to severe BPD. Weaning from ventilation may be difficult and result in chronic ventilator dependence.

Inflammation is considered to be one of the main contributors to the pathogenesis of BPD. This led to treatment with systemic corticosteroids, primarily dexamethasone, which yielded several short-term benefits. Data indicate that the adverse effects of systemic corticosteroids outweigh the short-term benefits. These adverse effects include hyperglycemia, hypertension, infection, cerebral palsy, poor weight gain and brain growth, gastrointestinal bleeding and perforation, and hypertrophic obstructive cardiomyopathy.[54] In view of these data, the American Academy of Pediatrics strongly discourages the routine use of systemic corticosteroids.[55] Inhaled corticosteroids, however, have been used and offer promise in reducing inflammation without the adverse effects of systemic administration. Currently clinical trials are evaluating the use of low-dose hydrocortisone therapy and also intratracheal delivery of budesonide during surfactant replacement administration.[56,57]

It is believed that premature infants have enough bronchial smooth muscle to constrict, so it would appear logical to provide β-agonist therapy; however, this remains controversial. Use has not been proven to reduce F_{IO_2} requirements, number of days with mechanical ventilation, or mortality, and may actually cause $\dot{V}/\dot{Q}$ mismatch in some infants.[58] Administration may only be effective against acute bronchospasm, and routine use for prevention of BPD is not advised.

Multiple efforts should be made to prevent further illness. Doses of palivizumab given monthly between November and March have been shown to reduce hospital admissions for respiratory syncytial virus (RSV) and also to reduce hospital stays.[59] In the early fall, the influenza vaccine is given to those infants who are 6 months of age and older; siblings, parents, and caregivers are highly encouraged to also be vaccinated. Environmental control is essential in minimizing the risk of illness. Parents are advised to avoid day-care settings, large crowds, and people with respiratory infections; schedule elective medical procedures outside the viral season; eliminate exposure to tobacco smoke, dander-producing pets, and kerosene- or wood-burning stoves; wash hands frequently; and use liquid hand sanitizer prior to touching the infant.

BPD is a disease that must be outgrown, with clinical recovery and lung repair dependent on growth. Airways become larger and alveolarization continues up to 5 years of age. For this reason, optimal nutrition is essential. Unfortunately, the infant with BPD often experiences gastroesophageal reflux and oral aversion that lead to feeding intolerance. Hypoxemia, infections, and fluid or caloric restriction can also lead to growth failure, necessitating complex therapy in the home for several months or years. In addition to feeding supplies, respiratory equipment required by this technology-dependent child may include a home oxygen system, mechanical ventilator and humidifier, pulse oximeter, end-tidal CO_2 monitor, apnea monitor, and airway clearance devices. Parents and caregivers often require extensive education on how to care for their child and ongoing psychosocial support to help deal with the transition to home.

Pulmonary hypertension is increasingly associated with significant morbidity and mortality in infants with BPD.[60] Selective pulmonary vasodilator therapy is used to decrease pulmonary vascular resistance. Delivered directly to the pulmonary vasculature, inhaled nitric oxide (NO) with its rapid onset of action remains the first line of therapy. Dosage typically begins at 20 ppm with doses subsequently decreased. Treatment with prostacyclin promotes pulmonary vasodilation; however, caution must be used as it may result in systemic hypotension. Although currently used off-label, pulmonary vasodilators, such as sildenafil and bosentan, may reduce pulmonary arterial pressure and improve oxygenation.[61]

Complications and Outcome

The majority of infants with BPD will survive; however, they are at considerable risk for numerous pulmonary, cardiac, and neurologic impairments. Nearly 50% of these infants continue to wheeze or have asthma, and lung function tests are consistently abnormal in school-aged children with a history of BPD.[62] Most infants can be weaned off oxygen by age 2 years, but hospitalization rates remain high, with up to 50% of infants with BPD requiring readmission in the first year of life. Recurrent episodes of hypoxemia place these infants at risk of persistent RVH or pulmonary hypertension that may progress to heart failure if left untreated. Infants with BPD are at greater risk of cerebral palsy and have greater impairment of fine and gross motor skills, language, and academic delay. Growth failure is common and is likely due to frequent respiratory exacerbations, an elevated resting metabolic rate, feeding problems, fluid restriction, chronic oxygen desaturation during sleep, and aggressive weaning from oxygen.[62]

Adolescents and adults with a history of BPD are often smaller, but their growth is usually still within normal range. Lung function continues to be compromised and includes diminished airflow, obstructive lung disease, and reactive airways. Cough and wheeze are more common, and there is an increased risk of hospitalization for respiratory illness.[63,64] Future strategies for the prevention or treatment of BPD are on the horizon. Stem cell–based therapies are showing promise in their potential for preventing and repairing neonatal lung inflammation and injury.[65] Clinical trials with aerosolized surfactant, bubble CPAP, and neurally adjusted ventilator assist (NAVA) for noninvasive ventilation are also underway.[26,66,67]

Transient Tachypnea of the Newborn

In 1966, Mary Ellen Avery and her associates were the first to use the term **transient tachypnea of the newborn (TTN)** to describe those infants who shortly after birth present with rapid respirations that usually resolve within 24 to 48 hours.[68] Also known as transient RDS, type II RDS, wet lungs, and retained fetal lung liquid syndrome, TTN is a self-limiting disorder that most often affects term or near-term infants. TTN is considered the most common cause of neonatal respiratory distress, affecting approximately 11 in every 1000 births.[69]

Pathophysiology and Etiology

At term gestation, the fetal lung is filled with approximately 20 mL/kg fluid. This fluid is equivalent to the FRC of the newborn lung and is what distends the airways and alveoli. Rapid removal of this fluid is vital for a smooth transition from placental to pulmonary gas exchange.[70]

Production of lung fluid begins to decrease 2 to 3 days prior to labor. During labor, fluid is reduced through lymphatic drainage and pulmonary epithelial cell adsorption. Fluid is also removed with the thoracic squeeze that occurs during labor contractions.

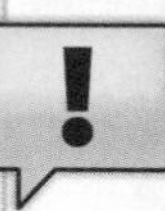

Respiratory Recap

Transient Tachypnea of the Newborn

- A self-limiting disorder of term and near-term infants
- Respiratory rates of 60 to 100 breaths/min common
- Treatment: oxygen therapy

Fetal lung fluid is usually completely cleared within 24 hours after birth. When absorption of the fluid is delayed and fluid accumulates in fetal lung tissue, the resulting bronchiolar collapse causes air trapping and decreased lung compliance, resulting in TTN.[71]

TTN is particularly common in infants of mothers with a history of failure to progress in labor resulting in cesarean delivery. Other risk factors include male sex, maternal diabetes, maternal sedation, perinatal asphyxia, and macrosomia.[72] Maternal asthma also appears to increase the risk of TTN.[73]

Clinical Manifestations

Immediately after or within 2 hours of birth, the infant with TTN presents with respiratory rates of 60 to 100 breaths/minute. Along with tachypnea, the clinical presentation can include grunting, intercostal retractions, cyanosis, and nasal flaring, with symptoms lasting for a few hours to days. Air trapping and hyperinflation may result in a barrel-shaped chest with the liver and spleen more palpable. Breath sounds are usually clear, and blood gas analysis may reveal a respiratory acidosis with mild to moderate hypoxemia.

Diagnosis

The diagnosis is based on history, clinical and radiologic findings, and laboratory data. Because of the tachypnea, $Paco_2$ is usually normal; however, if they begin to rise, the infant should be monitored closely for respiratory fatigue and failure. Should the infant's respiratory status worsen, blood gas analysis and chest radiographs are repeated to rule out complications or another diagnosis.

Chest radiography is the standard for diagnosis of TTN. It often reveals fluid in the interlobar fissures and perihilar streaking with alveolar edema presenting as fluffy, parenchymal infiltrates. There are no areas of consolidation, and the lungs may be hyperinflated, with widening of intercostal spaces and flattened diaphragms. Within 72 hours the findings are usually unremarkable except for perihilar markings, which may remain for up to 7 days (**Figure 46-3**).[74]

Other diagnoses to consider include RDS, meconium aspiration syndrome, pneumonia, PPHN, pneumothorax, pneumomediastinum, birth asphyxia, and congenital heart disease. Because it is often a diagnosis of

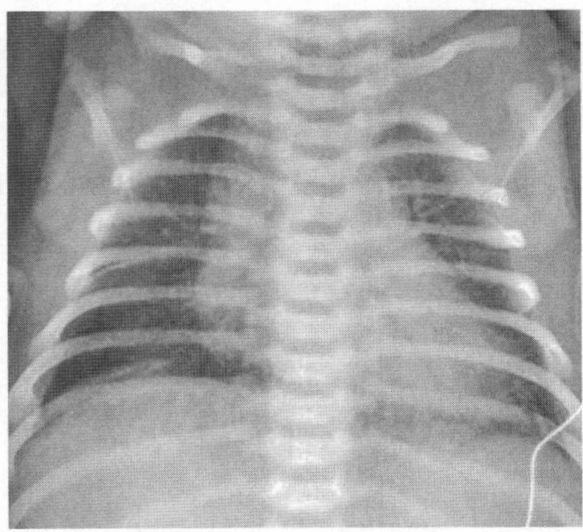

FIGURE 46-3 Transient tachypnea of the newborn is shown in this radiograph by flattened diaphragms, mild cardiomegaly, bulging intercostal spaces, and streaky perihilar markings.
Courtesy of Chetan Chandulal Shah, MBBS, DMRD, MBA, Arkansas Children's Hospital.

exclusion, some infants may not be given a definitive diagnosis of TTN until the tachypnea has resolved.

Management

Because TTN is self-limited, treatment is directed at maintaining oxygenation and ventilation. Oxygen by nasal cannula at 1 to 2 L/min or by hood at FIO_2 levels less than 0.50 is usually sufficient; however, nasal CPAP may be indicated if the oxygen requirement increases. Although rare, a worsening clinical picture may require intubation and mechanical ventilation and be cause for concern that TTN is not the diagnosis. Ventilator settings at a rate of 20 with a tidal volume of 4 to 6 mL/kg and PEEP of 4 to 5 cm H_2O are usually adequate. Continuous monitoring of the SpO_2, respiratory rate, and heart rate is essential. Because it is initially difficult to rule out pneumonia, empiric antibiotics are given for the first 24 to 48 hours until blood cultures are negative. Recent studies, however, are suggesting that empiric use may not be warranted.[75,76] While waiting for the respiratory rate to improve enough to allow oral feeds, the infant is supported by intravenous fluids or gavage feedings. Supportive care also includes maintaining a neutral thermal environment with minimal stimulation. Although not common practice, corticosteroids may be given to the mother 48 hours before an elective cesarean section when the gestational age is greater than 36 weeks.

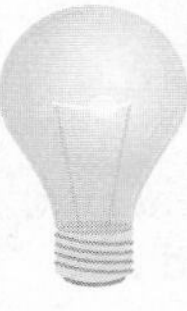

STOP AND THINK

A full-term infant is delivered by cesarean section. Respiratory distress develops within 15 minutes following delivery. TTN is suspected. What other diagnoses should be considered, and what can be done to aid in the diagnosis?

Complications and Outcome

Tachypnea due to TTN usually resolves within 72 hours of birth. Although air leaks may occur, few potential complications exist, and the prognosis is good.[77] Reports have associated TTN with the later development of childhood asthma, especially among male infants.[78]

Pneumonia in the Neonate

The neonate is highly susceptible to infection, and when compared with the term infant has at least a tenfold increase in the incidence of pneumonia. The World Health Organization estimates that 25% of neonatal deaths globally are caused by severe infections, with about one-third due to pneumonia.[79] Pneumonia in neonates is classified according to age at onset. Early-onset pneumonia presents at or within hours of birth through day 6 of life, while late-onset pneumonia occurs after 7 days of age.

Pathophysiology and Etiology

Pneumonia can occur at any gestational age and does not have an increased risk associated with sex, race, or ethnic group; however, premature infants are affected more often than term newborns. Immature mucociliary clearance, small conducting airways, and compromised host defense mechanisms render the fetus and neonate especially susceptible to infection. Invading microorganisms or foreign material that obstructs airways and increases airway resistance, mucus secretion, and inflammatory cells causes the pathologic findings in neonatal pneumonia. In addition there are cell necrosis, damaged alveolocapillary epithelium, and disrupted alveolar capillary membrane permeability. The result is loss of surfactant activity, air trapping, atelectasis, consolidation, decreased lung compliance, and intrapulmonary shunting.

Neonatal pneumonia is divided into three categories: congenital, intrapartum, and postnatal. Congenital pneumonia is transplacentally acquired and is established before birth. The infant presents at birth or shortly after with clinical signs of pneumonia. In congenital pneumonia, infection from the mother is transmitted to the fetus in utero. This occurs when infection crosses the placenta or with intrauterine aspiration of amniotic fluid. Intrapartum pneumonia is acquired when the infant passes through the birth canal and aspirates infected maternal fluids, contaminated meconium, or blood. Symptoms usually occur a few hours after birth. Postnatal pneumonia originates after delivery. Infection is often acquired through invasive therapies, such as intravenous catheter insertion and intubation, or by aspiration of enteral feeds. Infection may also be transmitted through bacteria on the hands of hospital staff or parents.

Bacterial organisms are the most likely cause of neonatal pneumonia, with group B β-hemolytic

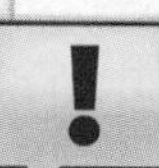

Respiratory Recap

Pneumonia

- Can occur at any gestational age.
- Congenital, intrapartum, and postnatal forms.
- Treatment is aimed at eradicating the infection and providing supportive care.

Streptococcus (GBS) the cause of about 25% of cases of neonatal pneumonia, especially in the premature infant. GBS can also cause meningitis and sepsis. Also common among very low birth weight infants is infection with *Escherichia coli*. Other bacterial pathogens responsible for pneumonia include *Listeria monocytogenes, Streptococcus pneumoniae, Haemophilus influenzae, Klebsiella*, and *Staphylococcus aureus*. Common viral causes include herpes simplex virus, enterovirus, and adenovirus. Congenital infection with cytomegalovirus and *Toxoplasma gondii* often presents within 24 hours of birth, whereas *Chlamydia* infection tends to develop several weeks later.

Clinical Manifestations

Fetal distress and tachycardia may present prior to delivery. Infected infants may present with respiratory distress immediately after birth, or symptoms may develop several hours later, usually within 8 to 10 hours. The initial signs of distress are similar to other respiratory disorders and include persistent tachycardia (respiratory rates greater than 60 breaths/min), grunting, use of accessory muscles, nasal flaring, and marked retractions. Airway secretions may be increased, and the skin and nails may be discolored or stained with meconium or blood. Other physical findings include abdominal distention, jaundice, cyanosis, and poor perfusion with low blood pressure. Early signs of infection can also include hypoglycemia or hyperglycemia, fever or hypothermia, poor feeding, irritability, lethargy, and seizures.

Diagnosis

Box 46-5 lists radiographic findings associated with neonatal pneumonia. A chest radiograph with bilateral patchy alveolar densities is a common finding. Diffuse infiltrates resembling the ground glass pattern of RDS may be present, making it difficult to determine in the premature infant whether the findings are RDS or pneumonia. It may also be difficult to differentiate between pneumonia and meconium aspiration syndrome in term infants (**Figure 46-4**).[80]

Maternal history, chest radiographs, and clinical presentation can assist in the differential diagnosis of neonatal pneumonia (**Box 46-6**). Definitive diagnosis, however, is made with cultures identifying the infecting organism. Cultures of blood, urine, endotracheal and gastric aspirates, and cerebrospinal fluid should be performed when pneumonia is suspected. Results of cultures will facilitate the diagnosis of pneumonia and provide information necessary to determine what antibiotic should be used.

BOX 46-5

Radiographic Findings Associated with Neonatal Pneumonia

Cardiomegaly
Pneumatoceles
Pleural effusion
Air bronchograms
Pneumomediastinum
Thickened minor fissure
Bilateral patchy densities
Pulmonary interstitial emphysema
Diffuse granular pattern (ground glass)

BOX 46-6

Differential Diagnosis in Neonatal Pneumonia

Air leak syndrome
Respiratory distress syndrome
Meconium aspiration syndrome
Transient tachypnea of the newborn

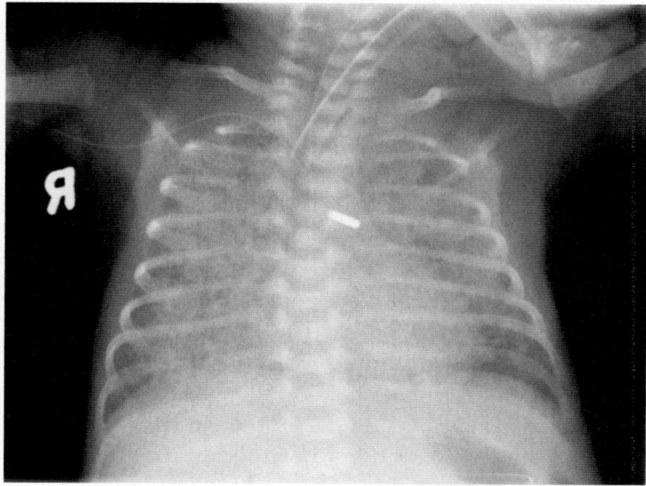

FIGURE 46-4 *Klebsiella* pneumonia in a neonate shows coarse and patchy opacity of the lung field and what appears to be some free air at the bases.
Courtesy of Chetan Chandulal Shah, MBBS, DMRD, MBA, Arkansas Children's Hospital.

Management

Treatment of neonatal pneumonia is aimed at eradicating the infection and providing respiratory support to maintain adequate oxygenation and ventilation. Antibiotic or antiviral therapy is essential. Delays in treatment for infections, especially those caused by GBS, have potentially devastating consequences. Neonates with signs highly suggestive of sepsis therefore should be thoroughly evaluated. This includes a complete blood count, blood cultures, and a lumbar puncture if the infant is stable enough to undergo the procedure.[81] Antibiotics are given to neonates with a clinical presentation or risk factors for pneumonia even though diagnosis is not confirmed. Intravenous ampicillin and gentamicin are recommended for initial empiric antibiotic therapy. Other agents may be used once the causative organism is identified.[82]

Oxygen therapy is provided using a nasal cannula, oxygen hood, or nasal CPAP. If oxygen requirements increase or respiratory failure is imminent, then endotracheal intubation and mechanical ventilation are indicated. Oxygenation and ventilation may be so compromised that the infant may require extracorporeal membrane oxygenation (ECMO). Screening for GBS and intrapartum antibiotic therapy are recommended in mothers with risk factors for early-onset GBS pneumonia. This preventive strategy that screens and identifies mothers who are GBS carriers has significantly reduced the number of reported cases.[83] **Box 46-7** lists maternal risk factors for GBS infection.

Complications and Outcome

The clinical course of neonatal pneumonia depends strongly on the causative organism. Circulatory collapse, respiratory failure, and death within 24 hours of birth are most often associated with GBS and *Listeria monocytogenes*. Complications include pleural effusion, air leaks, septic shock, pulmonary hypertension, hypoperfusion, BPD, and long-term ventilator dependency.

BOX 46-7

Maternal Risk Factors for Group B *Streptococcus* Pneumonia

Amniocentesis
Premature labor
Intrapartum fever
Pelvic examinations
Birth canal colonization
Intrauterine catheter placement
Premature rupture of membranes (longer than 18 hours before delivery)

Meconium Aspiration Syndrome

Meconium is a viscous, dark green-black substance that as a normal event in gastrointestinal maturation constitutes the first intestinal discharge from a newborn infant. Passage usually occurs within 48 hours after birth but can also occur in utero, especially in term or postterm infants. Mixed with amniotic fluid, it is a sterile mixture of water, mucus, ingested lanugo hair, bile, and digestive enzymes, all toxic to the infant's lungs. Meconium passage in utero is associated with hypoxia, fetal distress, abnormal fetal heart tracings, fetal acidosis, and low Apgar scores.[84]

Meconium aspiration syndrome (MAS) occurs when the infant aspirates stained amniotic fluid prior to, during, or immediately after birth. Approximately 5% of infants born through meconium-stained fluid will develop MAS, with 30% to 50% of the affected infants requiring intubation and mechanical ventilation. The incidence of MAS may be decreasing and is thought to be due to changes in obstetric practice that have resulted in a reduction in postterm deliveries.[85,86]

Pathophysiology and Etiology

Aspiration of meconium is no longer considered purely a postnatal event that may be prevented by suctioning the airway immediately following delivery. Instead, it is now believed that the most severe cases occur prior to delivery with the first breath an intrauterine gasp in which aspiration is induced by hypoxia and acidosis. Although meconium is sterile, within hours of aspiration it induces an inflammatory response that causes alveolar and parenchymal edema and a chemical pneumonitis. Protein leakage into alveoli inactivates surfactant and results in atelectasis and decreased lung compliance. The effect on surfactant is dose dependent: the more meconium present, the worse the effect. Aspiration of meconium may cause complete airway obstruction with regional atelectasis and $\dot{V}/\dot{Q}$ mismatch. Occurring more often is partial airway obstruction, in which the airways expand with air during inspiration but then collapse around meconium during expiration, trapping the air. This is commonly referred to as a *ball-valve effect*. The trapped air causes hyperinflation and may result in a pneumothorax, pneumomediastinum, or pneumopericardium. Pulmonary air leaks often develop during resuscitation of the infant with MAS. The lungs respond to the hypoxemia with thickening of the pulmonary vessels and pulmonary vasoconstriction, both of which may contribute to the PPHN that is often associated with MAS.[87] **Box 46-8** lists perinatal risk factors associated with MAS. Postterm delivery seems to be the greatest risk factor.

BOX 46-8

Perinatal Risk Factors Associated with Meconium Aspiration Syndrome

Preeclampsia
Fetal distress
Fetal hypoxia
Oligohydramnios
Chorioamnionitis
Maternal diabetes
Postterm delivery
Maternal tobacco use
Placental insufficiency
Maternal hypertension
Gestational age greater than 40 weeks
Abnormal fetal heart tracings
Meconium-stained amniotic fluid
Maternal drug abuse, especially cocaine
Meconium remaining in the airway prior to the first breath
Positive pressure ventilation before clearing the airway of meconium

Clinical Manifestations

The infant with MAS is usually born at term or postterm and has a history of delivery through meconium-stained amniotic fluid. The fingernails, skin, and umbilical cord may have yellow-green staining. The postmature infant will have long fingernails and peeling skin with a wrinkled appearance. Meconium staining may be visible in the oropharynx, larynx, and trachea. Meconium pigment can be absorbed by the lung and excreted in urine, making the urine green. Some infants will have only mild symptoms, which may represent a smaller amount of aspirated meconium. Other infants will present with marked distress, including high oxygen requirements and respiratory failure requiring intubation and mechanical ventilation. The more pronounced symptoms may be due to a thicker or larger amount aspirated into the lungs. Symptoms include severe respiratory distress with tachypnea, grunting, nasal flaring, retractions, and cyanosis. With marked hyperinflation the infant may present with a barrel chest. Onset of respiratory distress may occur immediately after birth or several hours later. Breath sounds may be diminished, with rales and sometimes rhonchi. Results of arterial blood gas analysis will indicate hypoxemia and metabolic acidosis. Depending on the degree of distress, analysis may reveal hypercapnia and a mixed respiratory and metabolic acidosis. Mild symptoms will result in normal $Pa{CO_2}$ levels or hypocarbia if tachypnea is present.

Diagnosis

Chest radiographs vary depending on the degree of disease, with the severity of findings not predictive of the severity of illness. A contradictory combination of areas of hyperexpansion with areas of collapse is typical of MAS. Patchy and linear fluffy infiltrates are common, with diffuse, white areas indicative of atelectasis. Radiographs typically progress from atelectasis to widespread patchy opacification, hyperinflation, and atelectasis (**Figure 46-5** and **Figure 46-6**).

A diagnosis of MAS is suspected when an infant presents with respiratory distress after delivery through meconium-stained amniotic fluid. Diagnosis is confirmed by a chest radiograph with hyperinflation, variable areas of atelectasis, and flattened diaphragms.

Management

Since the 1970s, the standard practice to prevent MAS in infants delivered through meconium-stained amniotic fluid has been to provide oropharyngeal and nasopharyngeal suctioning before the infant's shoulders are delivered. Unfortunately, intrapartum suctioning may cause vagal stimulation, postnatal fetal depression, and bradycardia. The efficacy of this procedure was debated after evidence suggested that meconium is aspirated in utero and not at the time of delivery.[88,89] Routine suctioning before delivery of the shoulders is no longer advised, and delivery is not delayed. Instead, the infant is evaluated immediately following delivery. If meconium is present and the infant has bradycardia with depressed respirations and muscle tone, then the trachea should be intubated

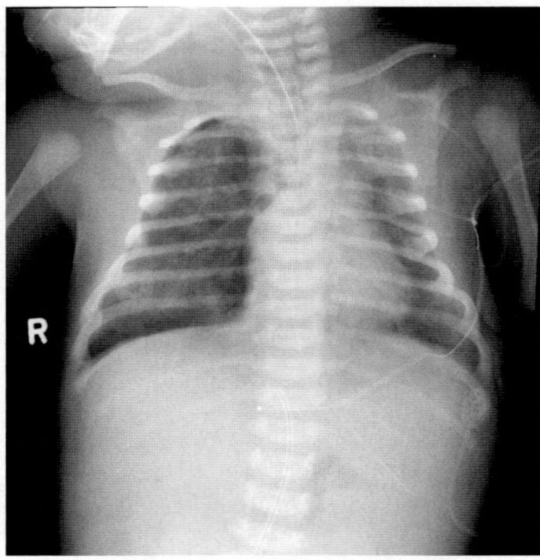

FIGURE 46-5 Chest radiograph of meconium aspiration syndrome with lung hyperexpansion, patches of atelectasis, and infiltrates that are more severe on the right.

Courtesy of Chetan Chandulal Shah, MBBS, DMRD, MBA, Arkansas Children's Hospital.

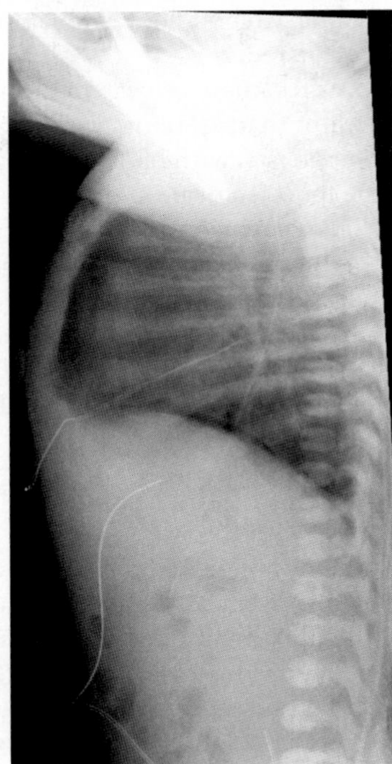

FIGURE 46-6 Lateral chest radiograph of an infant with meconium aspiration syndrome and lung hyperinflation.
Courtesy of Chetan Chandulal Shah, MBBS, DMRD, MBA, Arkansas Children's Hospital.

and meconium suctioned from beneath the glottis. If the infant has a heart rate greater than 100 beats per minute, a strong respiratory rate, and good muscle tone, then selective intubation and tracheal suctioning is contraindicated.[90]

Oxygen administration is critical to the infant with MAS and should be provided at the first sign of respiratory distress. Once the diagnosis of MAS is established, the infant is maintained at a preductal Spo_2 greater than 95%. In some infants oxygen is the only therapy required. High-flow nasal cannula or nasal CPAP is considered if oxygen requirements exceed an FIO_2 of 0.4 to 0.5 and $Paco_2$ is stable. The infant in marked respiratory distress will require intubation and mechanical ventilation, often needing high FIO_2 and ventilator settings to maintain adequate gas exchange. With chronic hypoxia, pulmonary vasoconstriction and increased pulmonary resistance often lead to the development of PPHN. PPHN is confirmed with echocardiography and treated with oxygen, nitric oxide, and continued mechanical ventilation.

Inhaled nitric oxide is approved for use as a pulmonary vasodilator. High-frequency ventilation is used if conventional ventilation fails to meet the infant's respiratory requirements or if air leaks occur. When all other therapies have been exhausted, then ECMO is considered. The infant with MAS is easily agitated, which causes right-to-left shunting, hypoxia, and acidosis. Supportive care includes maintaining

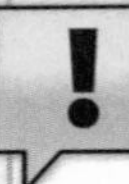

Respiratory Recap

Meconium Aspiration Syndrome

- Occurs when the infant aspirates meconium-stained amniotic fluid.
- Usually occurs in infants born at term or postterm.
- Treatment includes suctioning, oxygen therapy, mechanical ventilation, inhaled nitric oxide, extracorporeal membrane oxygenation, and surfactant replacement.

an optimal thermal environment with minimal stimulation.

Using the rationale that aspiration of meconium in the lungs causes surfactant to be altered or inactivated, surfactant replacement therapy has been used in infants with respiratory failure due to MAS. Studies suggest that lung lavage with diluted surfactant or through bolus therapy may be beneficial.[91] Airway lavage consists of instilling a small volume of dilute surfactant into the infant's airway and then suctioning the airway. This removes meconium debris, but leaves behind surfactant.[92] Bolus therapy is analogous to surfactant replacement in infants with RDS. Recently in an attempt to reduce the meconium-induced inflammation, the glucocorticoid budesonide has been added into the surfactant preparation.[93,94] Further studies are needed to determine the effectiveness of treatment, compare lavage with bolus therapy, and evaluate the benefit of a combined surfactant/anti-inflammatory drug approach.[95,96]

Complications and Outcomes

The clinical course of MAS is quite variable, with mild cases resolving within 2 to 4 days. Infants with severe aspiration requiring mechanical ventilation, nitric oxide therapy, or ECMO have a more guarded recovery, however. Air leak syndromes further complicate the clinical course and often result in less favorable outcomes. Infants may have an increased incidence of infections during the first year of life. Unfortunately, those who have required more intensive therapy are at risk of developing BPD.[97] Infants who have developed severe parenchymal disease and PPHN have a mortality rate as high as 20%. Mortality risk factors include first-born infants, shock, air leaks, PPHN, renal failure, and resuscitation outside the hospital.[98]

Infants who had prenatal or postnatal hypoxia and acidosis are at increased risk of long-term neurologic deficits that include seizures, cerebral palsy, central nervous system damage, and mental retardation.[99] Despite advances in treatment and early diagnosis, term infants with MAS continue to represent a high-risk population with significant morbidity.[100]

Persistent Pulmonary Hypertension of the Newborn

For postnatal survival, a dramatic cardiopulmonary transition must occur. Within minutes after birth, the lungs must fill with air and the pulmonary vasculature resistance (PVR) must fall. When this decrease in vascular tone does not occur, pulmonary blood flow is shunted to the systemic circulation. The resulting arterial hypoxemia, cyanosis, and severe respiratory distress are referred to as **persistent pulmonary hypertension of the newborn (PPHN)**. This syndrome has also been described as pulmonary vasospasm, neonatal pulmonary hypertension, persistent transitional circulation, and persistent fetal circulation. Recent estimates are that severe PPHN occurs in 2 per 1000 live births, with mortality at 20%.[101] Although it may present without underlying pulmonary disease, it most often complicates the clinical course of infants with neonatal cardiorespiratory disorders, with approximately half of those having MAS.

Pathophysiology

Prior to birth, pulmonary hypertension is a natural state, with the placenta serving as the gas exchange organ. Pulmonary vessels are constricted and pulmonary vascular resistance is high. This causes blood to be shunted through the foramen ovale and ductus arteriosus with only a small percentage of right ventricle blood flowing to the pulmonary circulation. When the umbilical cord is cut, the function of gas exchange is transferred from the placenta to the lungs and from fetal to neonatal circulation. Loss of the placenta elevates systemic vascular resistance and increases left atrium and ventricle pressures, leading to functional closure of the foramen ovale. As the lungs expand with the first breath, mechanically compressed pulmonary vessels are physically pulled open, carbon dioxide tension drops, and oxygen tension increases, constricting the ductus arteriosus and ultimately dilating pulmonary vessels and reducing PVR. The greatest decline in resistance occurs within 24 hours of birth and continues for the next 2 weeks. The elevated systemic vascular resistance now directs blood to the low-resistance pulmonary circulation, leading to an eight- to tenfold increase in pulmonary blood flow. Transition from fetal circulation has occurred.[102]

In PPHN the PVR remains elevated after birth and is equal to or greater than systemic vascular resistance. Fetal circulation persists, with blood continuing to flow through the foramen ovale and PDA. A right-to-left shunt develops, causing pulmonary perfusion to be inadequate. Arterial oxygen tension drops, and the infant experiences significant and possibly refractory hypoxemia, cyanosis, and respiratory distress. When the heart must work harder to pump blood through this highly resistant vascular bed, the risk of right heart dilatation and failure is high.[102]

> **Respiratory Recap**
>
> **Persistent Pulmonary Hypertension of the Newborn**
>
> - Occurs when fetal circulation persists after birth.
> - Echocardiography used to make the diagnosis.
> - Treatment includes oxygen, mechanical ventilation, inhaled nitric oxide, extracorporeal membrane oxygenation, and supportive therapy.

Etiology

Although the specific abnormality is unknown, three underlying etiologies are most often associated with PPHN. The most common etiology is hypoxia associated with parenchymal lung disease (e.g., RDS, MAS, pneumonia). The second cause, often referred to as idiopathic PPHN, is associated with infants who have no evidence of lung disease and is most likely due to a structurally abnormal pulmonary vascular bed occurring secondary to chronic fetal stress. Intrauterine closure of the ductus arteriosus is also a form of idiopathic PPHN. Repeated closure may occur during the third trimester if the mother ingests nonsteroidal anti-inflammatory drugs (NSAIDs), such as ibuprofen and naproxen, or high doses of the prostaglandin inhibitor aspirin. After determining that selective serotonin reuptake inhibitor (SSRI) antidepressants also have this effect, the Food and Drug Administration (FDA) ordered that a warning be placed on SSRI labels stating that ingestion after the 20th week of pregnancy could increase the chance of PPHN. The third abnormality is underdeveloped pulmonary vasculature, as seen in pulmonary hypoplasia, congenital diaphragmatic hernia, and oligohydramnios syndrome.[103,104] **Box 46-9** lists both prenatal and antenatal conditions that may predispose an infant to PPHN.[105]

Clinical Manifestations

Although PPHN may affect premature infants, it is most noted in term or postterm infants within 12 hours of birth. Early signs include cyanosis, tachypnea, and respiratory distress. The infant may have a gradual onset of distress with grunting, nasal flaring, tachycardia, and retractions that progressively worsen within 12 to 24 hours following birth. Depending on the etiology, however, the infant may present at birth in severe distress with low Apgar scores, poor perfusion, and shock. Work of breathing may not be severe unless there is coincidental parenchymal lung disease. Typically, cyanosis and hypoxemia respond poorly to supplemental oxygen. The infant often experiences oxygen desaturation with any form of stimulation, such as feeds, diaper changes,

BOX 46-9

Conditions That Predispose an Infant to Persistent Pulmonary Hypertension of the Newborn

Prenatal Conditions

Fetal hypoxia
Maternal asthma
Maternal obesity
Maternal diabetes
Poor prenatal care
Cesarean delivery
Maternal use of SSRI
Maternal use of NSAID
Abnormal fetal heart rate
Term or near-term gestation
Maternal tobacco smoke exposure
Maternal use of prostaglandin inhibitors

Antenatal Conditions

Sepsis
Pneumonia
Hypothermia
Polycythemia
Pneumothorax
Hypoglycemia
Birth asphyxia
Myocardial failure
Low Apgar score
Pulmonary hypoplasia
Large for gestational age
Respiratory distress at birth
Meconium aspiration syndrome
Transient tachypnea of the newborn

SSRI, selective serotonin reuptake inhibitor; NSAID, nonsteroidal anti-inflammatory drug.

noise, and suctioning. The worst cases require intubation and mechanical ventilation shortly after birth.[106]

Diagnosis

Diagnosis of PPHN is usually based on the clinical features. It should be suspected in the term infant who is in respiratory distress with cyanosis and who has a history that includes risk factors of PPHN. There should be an even higher index of suspicion when an infant presents with hypoxemia that is refractory to oxygen therapy and lung recruitment strategies, especially if there is a history of fetal hypoxia, birth asphyxia, or delivery through meconium-stained amniotic fluid.

The chest radiograph of an infant with idiopathic PPHN is typically clear with decreased vascular markings and a slightly enlarged heart. When PPHN is a result of an underlying lung disease, the radiograph will demonstrate abnormalities typical of that disorder. Scattered pulmonary parenchymal densities may be mild compared with the level of hypoxia.

Because the clinical presentation of PPHN mimics that of congenital heart defects, two-dimensional echocardiography is essential for diagnosing PPHN and excluding cyanotic heart disease. Findings characteristic of PPHN include right-to-left shunting across the foramen ovale or ductus arteriosus or both, right-to-left atrial septum deviation, right atrial enlargement, and tricuspid regurgitation. Diagnosis is confirmed by demonstrating right-to-left shunting at the ductal or atrial level and absence of a structural heart defect. The echocardiogram is also useful in assessing myocardial function, the severity of PPHN, and response to treatment. In the past, cardiac catheterization was used to monitor pulmonary artery pressures to diagnose PPHN; however, that is no longer needed and is not recommended.[107]

Diagnosis may also be established by comparing preductal and postductal Spo_2. By placing a pulse oximeter probe on a preductal extremity (right hand) and a second probe on a postductal extremity (right or left foot), the Spo_2 can be obtained simultaneously. The left hand should not be used as a site because it may be preductal or postductal. A preductal Spo_2 that is higher than the postductal Spo_2 occurs when deoxygenated blood flows from the pulmonary circulation into the descending aorta by way of a PDA. Because the majority of right-to-left shunting in PPHN occurs through the ductus arteriosus, postductal Spo_2 is lower than preductal Spo_2. Preductal Spo_2 higher than postductal Spo_2 indicates a right-to-left shunt. If there is little to no difference when the Spo_2 are compared, then ductal shunting is not present. When using Pao_2 values for comparison, blood is drawn from an upper extremity artery (preductal) and compared with that from the umbilical artery catheter. A difference greater than 15 mm Hg indicates ductal shunting. Oxygen values obtained through transcutaneous monitoring may also be compared by placing a probe on the infant's right upper chest (preductal) and a lower extremity (postductal). The hyperoxia test may be considered to diagnose PPHN if two-dimensional echocardiography is not available, but it cannot be definitive because some congenital heart defects will produce results similar to PPHN.[108]

Management

Treatment of PPHN is aimed at maintaining adequate oxygenation, lowering PVR, reversing right-to-left shunting, improving systemic blood pressure, correcting acidosis and hypercarbia, and minimizing complications. Continuous monitoring of blood pressure, oxygenation, and perfusion is essential.

To minimize hypoxia-induced pulmonary vascular constriction, treatment should always begin with oxygen administration and adjustments made to maintain adequate oxygenation.[109] Improvement in alveolar oxygenation reduces pulmonary vasoconstriction and improves pulmonary blood flow, factors that are especially important in infants with underlying parenchymal lung disease. Preductal and postductal Spo_2 should be continuously monitored. It is important to know whether the ductus arteriosus has remained open because shunting blood through it allows the right ventricle to decompress. This reduces the work of the ventricle, ultimately preventing right heart failure. An indication that the ductus is constricted or closed is preductal desaturation in an otherwise stable infant. Confirmation by echocardiography would necessitate a trial of prostaglandin therapy to maintain a PDA. Mild PPHN can be managed by nasal cannula; however, when hypoxia persists despite maximal administration of oxygen, then intubation with mechanical ventilation is indicated.

The goal of mechanical ventilation is to improve oxygenation using optimal lung volumes that minimize the risk of volutrauma lung injury while targeting an Spo_2 greater than 97% and $Paco_2$ levels of 35 to 50 mm Hg. Because hyperventilation with hypocapnia is a known risk factor for hearing impairment in PPHN survivors, the $Paco_2$ levels should not be lower than 35 mm Hg.[107] Lung recruitment strategies are dependent on the basis of underlying parenchymal lung disease. Treatment of idiopathic PPHN usually does not require pressures or volumes as high as those needed for ventilation of the infant with pneumonia or MAS. Infants with significant airspace disease or lung hypoplasia often require lung recruitment strategies attainable only through HFOV. Newborns with PPHN generally require sedation to achieve adequate mechanical ventilation. Although muscle paralysis can be used, adverse circulatory effects often occur, leading to overdistension of some areas of the lung and alveolar collapse in others.[110]

HFOV is used as rescue therapy for infants who are not improving or are showing signs of deterioration with conventional ventilation as well as infants who have developed air leaks. Response to HFOV depends on the underlying disease pathophysiology. HFOV has been shown in numerous studies to greatly improve the outcome in treatment of PPHN and to improve the response to inhaled nitric oxide in infants with severe lung disease.[111] The infant without significant lung disease may have a better response to inhaled nitric oxide when used with conventional mechanical ventilation than with HFOV.

Inhaled nitric oxide has proven to be a potent vasodilator with specific relaxation of pulmonary vasculature. In general the starting dose for treatment of PPHN is 20 ppm, which is then slowly lowered according to response and stability. It is increasingly recognized that adequate lung inflation is needed to optimize delivery of nitric oxide within the lungs. Some infants with PPHN either do not respond to therapy or have only transient improvements in oxygenation. This tends to occur most often in infants with abnormalities of vascular development, especially those with congenital diaphragmatic hernia. Although inhaled nitric oxide has been shown to reduce the need for ECMO support, there is no proof that it reduces length of hospital stay, the risk of neurodevelopmental impairment, or mortality.[112,113] Approximately 30% of infants fail to respond to inhaled nitric oxide, and others experience rebound pulmonary hypertension when nitric oxide is discontinued.[114]

Advances in the understanding of vasoactive mediators have led to the use of other pulmonary vasodilators. Sildenafil is a phosphodiesterase inhibitor that selectively reduces PVR and produces vasodilation. In 2005, the FDA approved the use of sildenafil in adults with pulmonary hypertension, which led to studies testing its effect in the treatment of PPHN. Numerous case reports and controlled studies have since continued to demonstrate improved oxygenation and lower mortality with no clinically important side effects.[115] Despite its controversial beginnings, sildenafil remains a valuable option for the treatment of PPHN and may be considered as first-line treatment when initiation of inhaled NO, ECMO, or HFV must be delayed.[115,116] Bosentan, an oral dual endothelin-1 receptor, has been successful in the treatment of severe cases of PPHN.[117] More studies are needed to evaluate potential adverse outcomes in this patient population.

ECMO support remains an effective rescue method and is considered in infants with PPHN who fail to maintain adequate oxygenation or systemic arterial pressure or who fail to wean from support with HFOV. By itself ECMO is purely supportive, allowing time for the lungs and pulmonary vasculature to recover. The usual criteria for ECMO use are a pH less than 7.15, oxygenation index (OI) greater than 40, and failure to respond to all available treatment.[118] There are some cases in which it may be considered earlier.

It is essential to maintain a neutral thermal environment to reduce oxygen consumption.[108] Myocardial function is often poor, requiring volume replacement and inotropic agents to maintain systemic vascular resistance and improve cardiac output. Infants with PPHN are particularly vulnerable to medical procedures that involve handling and respond with a decrease in oxygenation. A minimum stimulation protocol dictates that infants be handled only when medically necessary. **Box 46-10** lists intervention strategies to facilitate minimal stimulation. Studies have proven that when a neonatal intensive care unit is altered for minimal light, noise, infant handling, and staff activity,

BOX 46-10

Intervention Strategies for Minimal Stimulation

Place a sign at the bed announcing minimal stimulation.
Minimize frequency of baths.
Minimize positioning of the infant.
Suction only when absolutely necessary.
Decrease visual/auditory stimulation:

- Keep lights turned down low.
- Discourage loud talking at the bedside.
- Open incubator portholes quietly.
- Place phones away from beds.
- Place covers on incubators.
- Set equipment alarms at safest low level.
- Reduce fluid condensation in ventilator tubing.
- Carry out medical rounds away from bedside.
- Cluster activities.

there is a decrease in infant mean diastolic pressure and mean arterial pressure.[119]

Complications and Outcome

PPHN may last anywhere from 36 hours to several weeks after birth. There is no question that it contributes significantly to morbidity and mortality, regardless of the infant's gestational age. The use of inhaled nitric oxide and ECMO has led to a reduction in mortality rates, which were as much as 50% prior to the use of ECMO. Although ECMO support has improved overall survival to approximately 80%, the survival rate varies. Survival is highest in individuals with reversible parenchymal lung disease. Survival rates are as low as 50% in infants with congenital diaphragmatic hernia and as high as 90% in infants with MAS.[110,118]

Despite advances in treatment and the remarkable decrease in mortality, survivors of PPHN remain at substantial risk for long-term disability. Complications are often a result of treatment; however, birth asphyxia and perinatal hypoxia are largely responsible for the neurodevelopmental impairments. Survivors of PPHN have an increased incidence of sensorineural hearing loss, motor disability, behavioral problems that include hyperactivity and conduct disorders, and reactive airway disease.

Congenital Diaphragmatic Hernia

Congenital diaphragmatic hernia (CDH) is an anomaly that occurs in about 1 in 2500 live births. It is a developmental abnormality in which the infant's diaphragm allows abdominal organs to protrude into the thoracic cavity during a period when bronchi and pulmonary arteries are undergoing branching. CDH is not just a hole in the diaphragm but a malformation with a complex pathophysiology that results in pulmonary hypoplasia and PPHN.

Pathophysiology and Etiology

Diaphragm development is still not completely understood but is believed to require the fusion of embryonic structures during the 8th to 10th weeks of gestation. Improper fusion prevents the diaphragm from completely closing and allows abdominal organs, most often the stomach and small intestine, to migrate into the chest cavity. Herniation of abdominal contents during gestation impedes normal development of the lung on the herniated side, resulting in hypoplasia. Although not as severe, hypoplasia can also occur on the unaffected side, possibly due to the mediastinal shift to that side. **Pulmonary hypoplasia** is characterized by a permanent reduction in the number of airways, fewer alveoli, and a small pulmonary artery and pulmonary vascular bed. Pulmonary hypoplasia causes inadequate gas exchange and contributes to the hypercarbia that is present. The reduced number of arterial branches in the pulmonary vascular bed, abnormal muscular hypertrophy, and thickening of the arterial walls increase vasoconstriction and PVR.[120] The size of the defect varies, ranging from very small to complete agenesis of the diaphragm.

There are three basic types of hernias. The most common is the posterolateral Bochdalek hernia, representing approximately 90% of all hernias. These hernias are usually on the left side. It is thought that the left side is affected most because the liver may block herniation through the right side. With a left-sided hernia, there is herniation of the small and large intestine, stomach, and possibly liver into the thoracic cavity. The anterior Morgagni hernia represents less than 5% of all cases, with 90% occurring on the right side. These infants are often asymptomatic. Usually only the liver and a portion of the bowel herniate on the right side. Bilateral hernia is rare and nearly always fatal. Hiatal hernia and diaphragmatic eventration are rare types of CDH.[11,121,122]

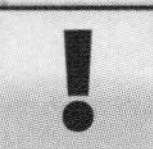

Respiratory Recap

Congenital Diaphragmatic Hernia

- Abnormality in which the infant's diaphragm allows the abdominal organs to protrude into the thorax.
- Treatment includes delivery room stabilization, mechanical ventilation, inhaled nitric oxide, extracorporeal membrane oxygenation, surgery, and supportive therapy.

Clinical Manifestations

Within the first minutes or hours after birth, infants with CDH will typically develop severe respiratory distress and cyanosis that is unresponsive to supplemental oxygen. It is common for the infant to fail to respond to resuscitation immediately following delivery. The majority of infants who present with severe distress have left-sided hernias. Breath sounds are decreased or absent on the affected side, and chest movement is asymmetric secondary to the hypoplasia. Bowel sounds may be audible in the thorax on the affected side, and heart sounds are shifted to the unaffected side. As a result of abdominal organs in the chest cavity, the infant usually presents at birth with a scaphoid abdomen and possibly a barrel-shaped chest. The most severely affected infants will develop PPHN, and the hypoplastic lung places them at high risk of developing a pneumothorax on the unaffected side.

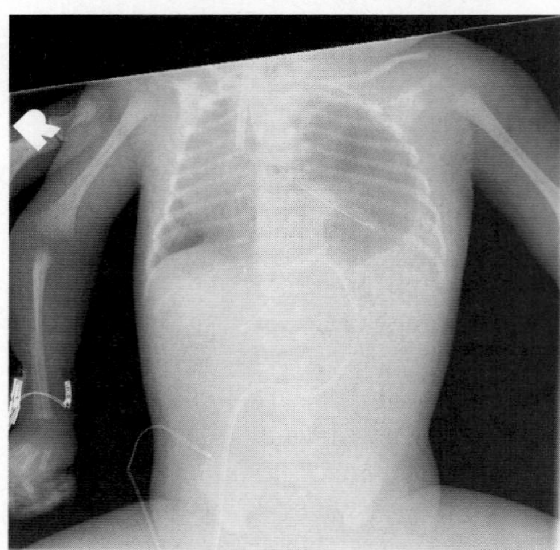

FIGURE 46-7 Chest radiograph of an infant with a left congenital diaphragmatic hernia showing herniation of bowel into the left hemithorax.

Courtesy of Chetan Chandulal Shah, MBBS, DMRD, MBA, Arkansas Children's Hospital.

Diagnosis

Most cases of CDH are diagnosed prenatally on routine ultrasound scans or scans obtained following the discovery of polyhydramnios in the mother. Previously undiagnosed cases still occur, presenting at or very soon after birth depending on the severity of the hernia. By 15 weeks of gestation, prenatal diagnosis is possible using ultrasonography. CDH is confirmed when abdominal contents are visualized in the chest and there is a mediastinal shift away from the affected side. Defects on the right side are more difficult to diagnose and can be missed if the stomach is not in the thorax at the time of the scan. Gallbladder visualized in the chest is indicative of a right-sided hernia. The extent of pulmonary hypoplasia cannot be predicted with an ultrasound, however. A prenatal diagnosis is no indication for cesarean section delivery. Fetal hydrops may be noted as well as polyhydramnios, which tends to have a poorer prognosis. Low levels of maternal serum alpha fetoprotein have been associated with CDH and other defects. This is not considered a definitive test for CDH but calls for more investigation. Following delivery, diagnosis is confirmed by a chest radiograph that reveals air-filled loops of intestine in the thoracic cavity on the affected side with the mediastinum shifted to the unaffected side. The affected lung may be hypoinflated or hypoplastic (**Figures 46-7 to 46-10**).

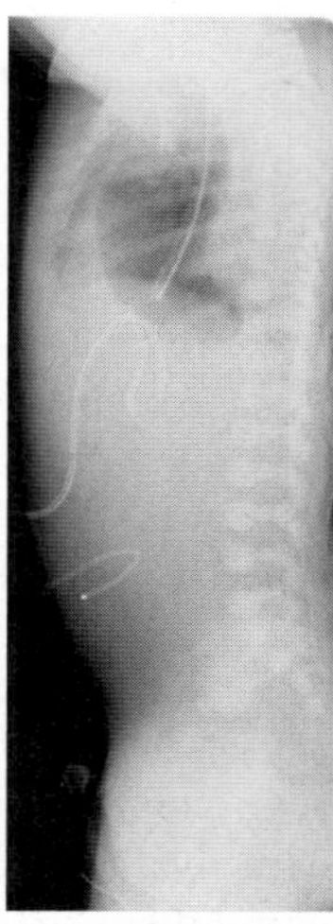

FIGURE 46-8 Lateral view of a left congenital diaphragmatic hernia.

Courtesy of Chetan Chandulal Shah, MBBS, DMRD, MBA, Arkansas Children's Hospital.

Management

Stabilization following delivery is critical. The infant is intubated immediately to avoid bag-mask ventilation and prevent stomach and bowel distention. Mechanical ventilation is implemented, and an orogastric or nasogastric tube using low continuous suction is inserted to decompress the stomach and avoid further lung compression.[123] Because air leak in either lung is highly possible, the infant is observed closely for signs of a pneumothorax, and a chest tube is immediately inserted if necessary. Care includes continuous monitoring of blood pressure and preductal and postductal Spo_2. It is important to monitor preductal Spo_2 because it reflects cerebral oxygenation. Successful delivery room resuscitation focuses on the avoidance of high airway pressures and an acceptable preductal Spo_2 that is greater than 85%.

Although there is no single specific best strategy for mechanical ventilation of infants with CDH, mortality risk is reduced when ventilation is approached with the goals of lung protection, improved oxygenation, and decreased PVR. Gentle ventilation with strategies that avoid high peak pressures is recommended in an attempt to lower the risk of air leaks.[124,125] Although controversy still exists

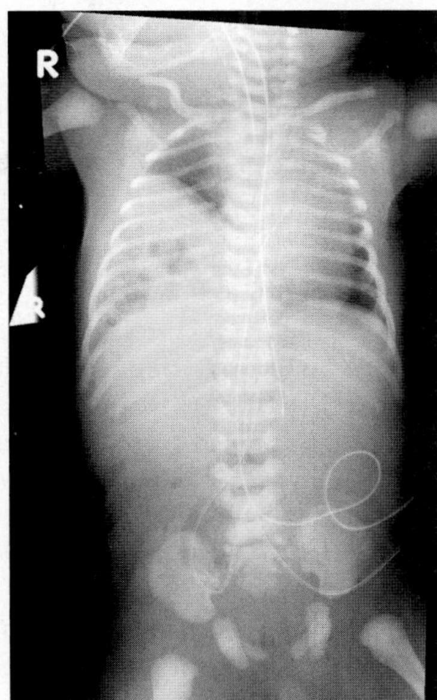

FIGURE 46-9 Chest radiograph of an infant with a right congenital diaphragmatic hernia. Gas-filled loops of bowel are in the right hemithorax, and there is a mediastinal shift to the left compressing the left lung.

Courtesy of Chetan Chandulal Shah, MBBS, DMRD, MBA, Arkansas Children's Hospital.

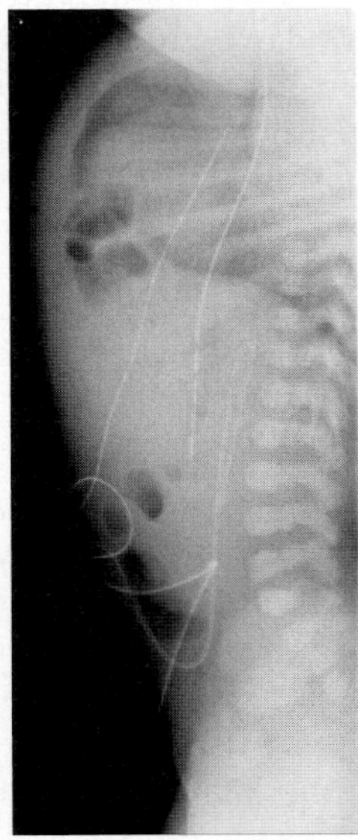

FIGURE 46-10 Lateral view of a right congenital diaphragmatic hernia showing bowel loops in the anterior mediastinum.

Courtesy of Chetan Chandulal Shah, MBBS, DMRD, MBA, Arkansas Children's Hospital.

concerning the appropriate target for the $Paco_2$ level, more centers are using permissive hypercarbia to allow for ventilation at lower pressures and shorter inspiratory times.[126] HFOV is recommended when conventional ventilation is unable to prevent hypoxemia or hypercarbia. For many years treatment of CDH with HFOV was considered a rescue mode to be used only when hyperventilation with conventional ventilation had failed. Some recommend HFOV as an early intervention strategy to avoid barotrauma.[127]

Nitric oxide has proven to be a powerful vasodilator and effective in reducing PVR and dilating the pulmonary vascular bed. Infants with CDH who present with PPHN, significant hypoxia, acidosis, and right ventricular failure may benefit from inhaled nitric oxide. Trials using inhaled nitric oxide in infants with PPHN have included infants with CDH; unfortunately, the latter was the group that responded least well, with no impact on survival or the use of ECMO.[128]

Despite the use of nitric oxide, some infants with CDH will progress to refractory pulmonary hypertension. Using the same selection criteria as PPHN, ECMO should be considered when pH is less than 7.15, OI is greater than 40, preductal Spo_2 is less than 85%, and all other support has been exhausted. The purpose of ECMO in the treatment of CDH is to serve as a lung-protective strategy during the preoperative period.[118,129]

Deferred surgery after stabilization with gentle ventilation and reversal of pulmonary hypertension remains the cornerstone of management. In the past, surgery was believed to be critical to reducing the hernia and allowing expansion of the unaffected lung. Understanding that CDH is not just a surgical disease and that the problems of pulmonary hypoplasia and PPHN are largely responsible for outcome has led to a delayed surgical approach. Removing abdominal contents from the chest cavity is no longer emergent; instead, time is allowed for respiratory and hemodynamic stabilization. Survival rates have been reported to be as high as 81% when the management of CDH includes delayed surgical repair, early postnatal HFOV, and selective referral for ECMO. Survival rates are favorable and respiratory morbidity just as low when treating isolated CDH with early HFOV and delayed surgery but excluding ECMO.[130,131]

It is critical that infants with CDH receive continuous monitoring. This includes preductal and postductal Spo_2 monitoring with pulse oximetry and transcutaneous CO_2 monitoring to avoid hyperventilation. A central venous line is placed for monitoring and fluid infusion and an umbilical arterial line is placed for pressure monitoring and arterial blood gas analysis. Umbilical venous lines are needed for fluid resuscitation and fluid maintenance, although the umbilical venous line may be difficult to insert if there is liver herniation. In an effort to minimize the effects of PPHN, minimal-stimulation protocols should be in place and routine sedation and analgesia used.

Complications and Outcome

Infants with CDH are at considerable risk for long-term complications. The majority of these are due to pulmonary hypoplasia, respiratory failure, and

BOX 46-11

Complications Associated with Congenital Diaphragmatic Hernia

Scoliosis
Hypotonia
Hearing loss
Oral aversion
Failure to thrive
Cortical atrophy
Ventriculomegaly
Chest asymmetry
Chronic lung disease
Patch-related infections
Reactive airway disease
Gastroesophageal reflux
Small airway obstruction
Limited pulmonary reserve
Intraventricular hemorrhage
Pectus, most often excavatum
Learning and attention problems
Recurrent pulmonary hypertension
Lifelong limited exercise tolerance

PPHN and have very little to do with surgical repair of the defect. **Box 46-11** lists complications associated with CDH.[132]

Morbidity and mortality are largely dependent on three factors: the size of the defect and herniation, the degree of lung hypoplasia, and the severity of PPHN. Predictors of postnatal outcome prior to delivery are difficult, but extent of the herniation may be a reliable predictor. Simply stated, the more abdominal contents involved in the herniation, the poorer the prognosis. Occurrence of a left-sided CDH has a good prognosis if there is no herniation of the liver. Unfortunately, when liver herniation is present, survival rate is less than 50%. Nearly all infants with a right-sided defect will present with a portion of the liver in the chest cavity. Prognosis is worse if more than 50% of the liver is in the chest.[133,134]

Congenital Pulmonary Anomalies

In addition to CDH, there is a spectrum of rare congenital lung malformations that vary widely in their presentation and severity. They are a result of an insult during fetal lung development. Anomalies of the lung can range from small cystic masses to complete absence of the lung and bronchus.

Pulmonary Hypoplasia

In 1955, Boyden classified three degrees of lung maldevelopment: hypoplasia, aplasia, and agenesis.[135] With pulmonary hypoplasia there is normal pulmonary tissue but a decrease in the number of airway generations, lung cells, alveoli, and in some cases corresponding pulmonary arterioles. The result is a smaller lung that weighs less than normal. Involvement can range from simple involvement of an isolated lobe to bilateral hypoplasia of the lungs. Occurring in about 1 per 1000 live births, it is the most commonly encountered anomaly of underdeveloped lung parenchyma. It may present as primary (idiopathic) hypoplasia, which is rare, or as secondary hypoplasia in association with other anomalies that most often include CDH.[136]

Clinical presentation varies depending on the degree of lung involvement and presence of associated abnormalities but may include asymmetric chest wall movement and reduced breath sounds on the affected side. The infant may present at birth with severe respiratory distress or remain asymptomatic for months to years and be diagnosed incidentally.[136]

Diagnosis often requires a high index of clinical suspicion. Chest radiographic findings vary but can include reduced or absent lung volume with the heart and trachea displaced, a mediastinal shift, and hyperinflation of the contralateral lung. A chest CT scan or MRI may be required to better establish the defect and differentiate it from other conditions. Treatment, when required, is directed at supporting oxygenation and ventilation and controlling recurrent respiratory infections. Morbidity and mortality rates are directly related to the degree of hypoplasia, the health of the normal lung, and the presence of comorbidities.[137]

Pulmonary Aplasia

Occurring much less often than hypoplasia, **pulmonary aplasia** is the presence of a rudimentary bronchus coming off of the trachea with incomplete development of lung tissue. The carina and bronchus are present but the bronchial trunk is seen as a stump and lung tissue and pulmonary vessels are absent.[135] As with pulmonary hypoplasia, infants may remain asymptomatic or present within hours of birth with respiratory distress. Diagnosis may be confirmed with noninvasive radiographic imaging, typically revealing an opaque hemithorax suggestive of massive atelectasis, tracheal and mediastinal shift, rib crowding, and hyperinflation of the unaffected lung. Treatment is required only if the patient is symptomatic. If lower respiratory tract infections become chronic, surgical removal of the bronchial stump may be an option. As there is a high incidence of associated malformations, prognosis depends upon the functional integrity of the normal lung and the severity of other anomalies.[138]

Pulmonary Agenesis

Pulmonary agenesis refers to the complete absence of the lung and its associated bronchus and pulmonary vessels.[135] There is no pleural cavity on the affected side and no carina or bronchial stump. The incidence is approximately 1 in 15,000 live births. It can be bilateral, where the trachea ends in a cul-de-sac, or unilateral, in which the trachea essentially becomes the bronchus. Bilateral pulmonary agenesis is extremely rare and incompatible with life; most infants die in utero or within the first hour after birth. Unilateral agenesis, especially when it involves the right side, is associated with cardiovascular, gastrointestinal, skeletal, facial, and renal anomalies.[139]

Although some infants will remain asymptomatic, especially in the absence of associated anomalies, most cases present with some degree of respiratory distress or increased oxygen requirement. Affected infants tend to have recurrent respiratory infections that may lead to pneumonia and respiratory failure.

Pulmonary agenesis is difficult to diagnose with a prenatal ultrasound because many anomalies can have a similar appearance. Instead fetal magnetic resonance imaging is a more useful tool in clarifying a diagnosis. Massive atelectasis, crowded ribs, and tracheal deviation with a cardiomediastinal shift seen on a chest radiograph should be the first clue suggesting possible lung agenesis. In less symptomatic infants the diagnosis may be delayed even into adulthood when a routine chest radiograph or chest CT is obtained for some other complaint. High-resolution CT of the chest is considered the most definitive tool in diagnosing pulmonary agenesis and is needed to confirm absence of the bronchus, lung tissue, and branches of the pulmonary artery (**Figure 46-11**). Prognosis is better when the normal lung remains healthy and free from disease processes, such as atelectasis or infection. The poorer prognosis with right-sided agenesis is thought to be due to its greater association with other congenital malformations. Prognosis of unilateral agenesis overall has improved, however, as fetal MRI has made antenatal diagnosis more definitive.[140]

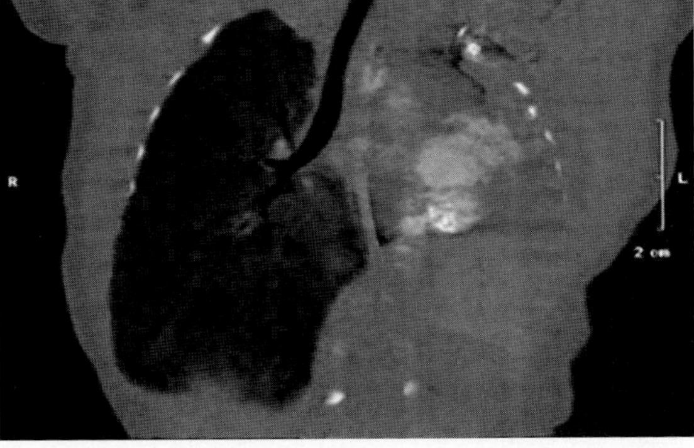

FIGURE 46-11 CT of the chest of an infant with unilateral pulmonary agenesis. The trachea continues as the right bronchus and there is no evidence of a left bronchus or lung tissue on the left.

Congenital Pulmonary Airway Malformation

Congenital pulmonary airway malformation (CPAM) is a rare developmental anomaly of the lower respiratory tract that was previously known as congenital cystic adenomatoid malformation. The malformations are cysts or lesions of varying size and cellular composition and are connected to the tracheobronchial tree. They contain mostly elements from tracheal, bronchial, bronchiolar, or alveolar tissue. Although they can arise in any lobe, they are usually limited to only one lobe and are nearly always unilateral. Size can range from a maximum diameter of 0.5 cm to large enough to comprise an entire lobe or several lobes. The most common cysts range from 2 to 10 cm in diameter. According to population registries CPAM occurs in 1 per 8300 to 35,000 live births.[141]

Clinical presentation of affected infants is variable. Symptoms are most often dependent on the size of the cyst and the extent of air trapping and lung involvement. Infants with small cysts are asymptomatic or may present months or years later with respiratory infection. Large cysts may compress the lung in utero resulting in pulmonary hypoplasia of the contralateral lung, mediastinal shift, fetal hydrops, and severe respiratory distress that progresses to respiratory failure. The most common complication of CPAM is recurrent respiratory infections. There is also significant risk of developing the malignancy pleuropulmonary blastoma, which is also associated with spontaneous pneumothorax.

Diagnosis of CPAM is made through radiographic imaging. Fetal MRI can provide a prenatal diagnosis while a chest radiograph or CT scan of the chest is diagnostic after birth. The differential diagnosis of CPAM includes pulmonary sequestration, CDH, bronchogenic cyst, congenital lobar emphysema, and pulmonary interstitial emphysema.

Treatment is dependent upon the symptoms and the type and size of lesion present. For asymptomatic infants, surgical resection of the lesions at 3 to 6 months of age is recommended in an effort to prevent infection or malignancy. An alternative to surgery is surveillance with serial chest CT scans; however, surveillance is not an option when the lesions are the type that can rapidly develop into solid blastomas. Surgical resection is recommended in symptomatic infants. With a fetal diagnosis of CPAM with hydrops, options for treatment are maternal steroid administration, cyst aspiration, and open fetal resection, which is considered strongly in cases of large CPAMs or when hydrops

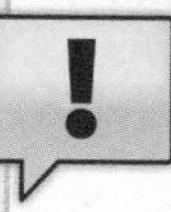

Respiratory Recap

Congenital Pulmonary Anomalies

- Timeline of insult in relation to fetal lung development determines type and severity of anomaly.
- Early diagnosis possible with fetal ultrasound, CT, and MRI imaging.
- Prognosis depends largely on presence of associated congenital malformations and health of the normally developed lung.

develops before 32 weeks' gestation. The type of CPAM and its association with other anomalies largely determines the prognosis. In some cases surgical resection is curative with an excellent prognosis. Infants with CPAM and severe hypoplasia of the contralateral lung often develop pulmonary hypertension, and the prognosis is not as favorable.[142]

Bronchogenic Cyst

A **bronchogenic cyst** is a rare congenital malformation that buds off from the primitive esophagus and tracheobronchial tree. They are usually 2 to 10 cm, single, thin-walled cysts filled with fluid or mucus. Located most often in the middle of the mediastinum around the carina, they are usually not connected to the tracheobronchial tree. Bronchogenic cysts occur in 1 in 42,000 to 1 in 68,000 births.[143]

Infants are rarely symptomatic unless the cyst is large enough to compress the airways, esophagus, or heart, which would result in severe respiratory distress with wheezing and stridor, hemoptysis, or dysphagia. If the cyst becomes infected it enlarges rapidly, and symptoms include fever, chest pain, cough, respiratory distress, and wheezing. Diagnosis is best obtained through a chest radiograph or CT scan. A chest radiograph can usually detect larger cysts or lung masses and tracheal deviation and compression, but is limited in differentiating masses from fluid. CT of the chest or an MRI can both provide a more accurate diagnosis but are challenged in differentiating lymph nodes and other solid lesions. As is the case with CPAM, a fetal MRI is a vital diagnostic tool to determine a cyst is present and if it is severely compressing normal lung tissue or the heart, which can result in pulmonary hypoplasia or hydrops with fetal death. A cyst should be aspirated if it is large enough to cause an in utero mediastinal shift or pneumothorax.[144] Care must be taken during air travel transport where cystic lesions have been known to expand up to 30% and cause significant compression of the airways, lungs, and heart.

Treatment choice is controversial with some advocating surgical resection only if symptoms are present, while others encourage preventive excision of all cysts because of the strong potential for infection, pulmonary compression, and malignancy. Surgery may include a thoracotomy or the minimally invasive video-assisted thoracoscopic surgery (VATS) with cyst excision. Intrapulmonary bronchogenic cysts may require a wedge resection, segmental resection, or lobectomy depending upon the size and location. Cysts can also be treated with transbronchial or percutaneous aspiration under CT guidance. In the case of small cysts, the infant may not undergo surgery but instead be followed with serial MRI or CT scans.[145]

Pulmonary Sequestration

Representing approximately 6% of all congenital malformations, **pulmonary sequestration** is a cystic or solid mass of abnormal lung tissue that is not connected to the tracheobronchial tree but appears within a lobe (intrapulmonary) or next to the lung (extrapulmonary). Over 75% of all sequestrations are intrapulmonary and are most often located in the left lower lobe. These sequestrations tend to present in late childhood or adulthood as recurrent lung infections. Enclosed in its own pleural sac, an extrapulmonary sequestration nearly always occurs on the left side and is four times more likely to be found in males than females. It is usually located between the left lower lobe and the diaphragm, however on rare occasions it has occurred in the mediastinum and pericardium. An extrapulmonary sequestration usually presents as respiratory distress, cyanosis, and signs of sepsis in neonates and children less than one year of age.[146]

A chest radiograph will show an opacity or cystic spaces. Chest CT scans are helpful in determining if the sequestration is intrapulmonary or extrapulmonary. A fetal ultrasound may detect an extrapulmonary sequestration as early as 16 weeks' gestational age. When detected in utero the fetus is monitored closely, and the majority of infants are treated after birth.[147] Because there is a high volume of blood flowing through the sequestration, there is the risk of heart failure and treatment is surgical resection of the sequestration. This can usually be done without removing normal lung tissue, although an intrapulmonary sequestration may require resection of a lung segment or the entire lobe. Unless recurrent respiratory infections occur, most infants do well following surgery and have normal lung function.

Air Leak Syndrome

Pulmonary **air leak syndrome** comprises a group of clinically recognizable disorders that are characterized by the escape of air into tissue in which air is not normally present. These disorders include pulmonary interstitial emphysema, pneumothorax, pneumomediastinum, and pneumopericardium. Less common forms are subcutaneous emphysema and pneumoperitoneum.

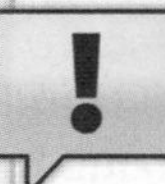

Respiratory Recap

Air Leak Syndrome

- Includes pulmonary interstitial emphysema, pneumothorax, pneumomediastinum, and pneumopericardium
- Transillumination used to make immediate diagnosis of pneumothorax

The incidence is greatest in premature infants who have existing lung disease. Term infants are also affected, especially those who had long periods of rupture of membranes prior to delivery or long durations of labor.[148] Although occurrence can be spontaneous, it is most often a complication of positive pressure mechanical ventilation. The decline in the incidence of air leak syndrome in newborns is believed to be due to surfactant replacement therapy and changes in ventilator management strategies. The use of shorter inspiratory times, lower peak inspiratory pressures, permissive hypercapnia, and the early introduction of CPAP are also believed to contribute to this decline.[149]

The common cause of the disorders comprising air leak syndrome is overdistention due to air trapping or uneven distribution of gas. As the volume in the lung exceeds its physiologic limit, tissue in the alveoli or terminal airspaces rupture and air leaks are created. The resulting disorders depend on where the free air is located. Clinical presentation is specific, and intervention varies for each condition. In every case definitive diagnosis is made with a chest radiograph.

Pneumothorax

Pneumothorax is the most common air leak and occurs most often in neonates. It refers to the presence of air in the pleural cavity between the visceral and parietal pleura. Air from ruptured alveoli moves toward the hilum, where blebs form and then dissect into the pleural space to develop a pneumothorax. With sufficient accumulation of air, a tension pneumothorax develops and the loss of intrapleural negative pressure causes lung collapse. Gas exchange is impaired as air accumulates and pressure increases, shifting mediastinal structures and compressing the uninvolved lung. Compression of the vena cava results in a decrease in venous return and consequently a decreased cardiac output that can emergently progress to hypotension, shock, and death. Risk factors for a pneumothorax include RDS, mechanical ventilation, MAS, pulmonary hypoplasia, and other air leak conditions. Although the majority of infants who develop a pneumothorax are receiving mechanical ventilation, healthy term infants can spontaneously develop a pneumothorax immediately after birth.

A pneumothorax should always be suspected if there is sudden deterioration in an infant's respiratory status, especially if the infant is receiving mechanical ventilation. Distress is often accompanied by nasal flaring, cyanosis, grunting, severe retractions, hypercarbia, and hypoxia. An infant may be asymptomatic or have only mild tachypnea, retractions, and grunting, however. Heart sounds are shifted and breath sounds are diminished on the affected side, although it may be difficult to appreciate breath sounds because they are so widely transmitted in the neonate's small thorax.[150]

In an emergent situation, transillumination of the chest is used for an immediate diagnosis. With lights lowered around the immediate area of the infant's bed, a fiberoptic light probe is held firmly against the infant's skin, about halfway down the chest and in line with the axilla. The side of the chest with the air leak transmits a bright light, whereas the lung is solid tissue and does not illuminate. Confirmation of a diagnosis of pneumothorax is provided with chest radiography, both anteroposterior (AP) and lateral views. Transillumination does not take the place of a chest radiograph. The affected lung will typically have increased lucency and decreased lung markings, with the free air appearing dark on the radiograph. As the leak increases, the affected lung is hyperinflated, with a flattened diaphragm and widened intercostal spaces (**Figures 46-12 and Figures 46-13**).

A small pneumothorax usually resolves spontaneously without need for intervention. In an effort to resolve it more quickly, oxygen at an F_{IO_2} of 1.0 may be administered with a nasal cannula to an infant with increased work of breathing. This treatment should be carefully considered and closely monitored in the preterm infant who is at risk of retinopathy of prematurity. Needle aspiration or thoracentesis is indicated if the pneumothorax is large, symptomatic, or under tension. If the infant has a tension pneumothorax and is

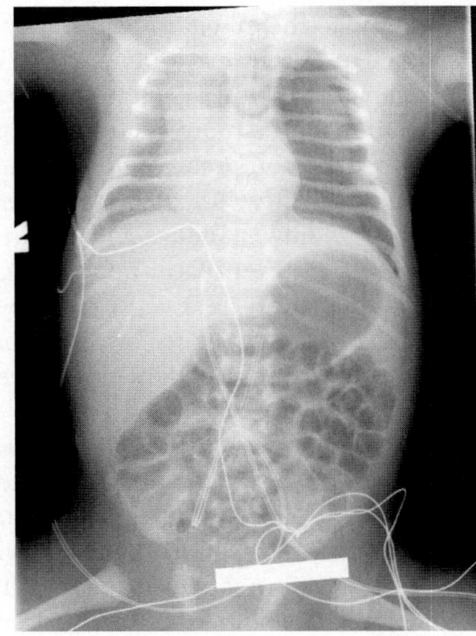

FIGURE 46-12 Chest radiograph showing large left pneumothorax.
Courtesy of Chetan Chandulal Shah, MBBS, DMRD, MBA, Arkansas Children's Hospital.

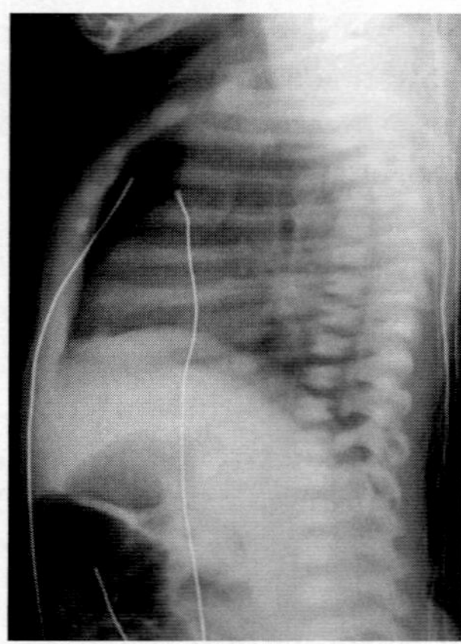

FIGURE 46-13 Lateral chest radiograph of a pneumothorax.
Courtesy of Chetan Chandulal Shah, MBBS, DMRD, MBA, Arkansas Children's Hospital.

receiving mechanical ventilation, chest tube placement will be needed.[151] When the air leak is large, most of the gas will exit the lung through the bronchopleural fistula and not participate in gas exchange. With deteriorating blood gases and decreased oxygenation, HFV is often the only means to provide adequate ventilation and oxygenation.

Pulmonary Interstitial Emphysema

Pulmonary interstitial emphysema (PIE) begins with an air leak from the alveoli or terminal bronchioles that spreads into the pulmonary interstitium and perivascular tissues of the lungs. The air may form subpleural blebs that can rupture into the pleural space, resulting in a pneumothorax. Air does not rupture through the pleura. This development occurs usually, although not exclusively, in association with mechanical ventilation. If the resulting PIE affects only one lung, there is a mediastinal shift that compresses the normal adjacent lung. The extent of PIE is variable. It may involve one or both lungs and may have a diffuse or localized pattern within each lung. The more widespread the air leak, the more acute the respiratory distress. As trapped air compresses the pulmonary circulation, areas of healthy lung become atelectatic and pulmonary blood flow is reduced. The degree of air trapping and required ventilator pressures can decrease venous return and right ventricular outflow, increase PVR, and markedly reduce oxygenation. PIE that lasts longer than 1 week is referred to as persistent pulmonary interstitial emphysema.[152]

PIE often presents as hypotension and a slow, progressive deterioration of arterial blood gas values with increasing oxygen and ventilatory support requirements. In some cases the infant presents first with a pneumothorax, and PIE is not appreciated until after the collapsed lung is reexpanded. PIE is more common in infants of lower gestational age, typically occurring during the first week of life in preterm infants requiring mechanical ventilation or who have received late surfactant replacement therapy. Other conditions associated with PIE include MAS, aspiration of amniotic fluid or blood, low Apgar scores, resuscitation at birth, main stem intubation, and infection.

Diagnosis is based on chest radiography that typically demonstrates tubular or small bubblelike radiolucencies. They may be focal or diffuse, unilateral or bilateral, and may be described as "salt and pepper." When PIE is confined to one lung, there is hyperinflation with a mediastinal shift that compresses the contralateral lung. When this occurs, the compressed lung will look small and opaque. The heart looks smaller as intrathoracic pressure increases. If PIE involves both lungs, the mediastinum and cardiac silhouette will appear narrowed. The radiograph may look similar to that seen with BPD or may be confused with aspiration pneumonia, pulmonary edema, and air bronchograms similar to those seen with RDS (**Figure 46-14**).[153]

Treatment is mainly supportive, with HFOV or minimal volume ventilation being the most successful interventions.[154] Lateral decubitus positioning is an easy and effective treatment for PIE if one lung is significantly more affected than the other. The infant is placed in the lateral decubitus position, lying on the side with the more severe PIE. This will help compress the lung, thereby decreasing leakage and possibly improving ventilation to the other lung.[155] Selective intubation and ventilation has been somewhat successful in treating infants with severe PIE who have failed conservative treatment. Intubation of the main bronchus and ventilation of the lung on the unaffected side decompresses the hyperinflated lung tissue in the affected lung, protecting it from high ventilator pressures and allowing time for the emphysema to regress. Once the air leak has stopped, which usually takes 24 to 48 hours, the endotracheal tube is pulled back and ventilation is provided again to both lungs. PIE may resolve over 1 or 2 days or it may persist on radiography for weeks, progressing into other air leak conditions.[156] A 3-day course of dexamethasone has been reported to provide significant

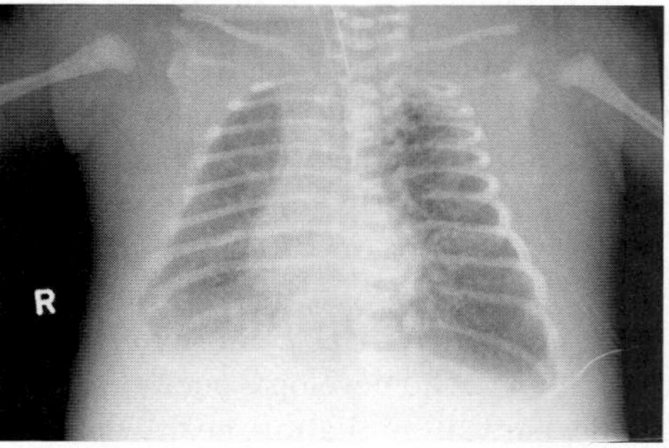

FIGURE 46-14 Chest radiograph of an infant with pulmonary interstitial emphysema on the left and granular appearance of the right lung consistent with respiratory distress syndrome.
Courtesy of Chetan Chandulal Shah, MBBS, DMRD, MBA, Arkansas Children's Hospital.

clinical improvement in the treatment of PIE, possibly due to reduced airway obstruction, edema, and inflammation.[157] A lobectomy in which the hyperinflated lobe is removed is rare but may be indicated in the infant who fails all other medical interventions.

Very low birth weight infants with PIE have a high risk of mortality and significant complications, including CLD and intraventricular hemorrhage. There is also an increased occurrence of other air leaks, especially pneumothoraces and pneumomediastinum.

Pneumomediastinum

A pneumomediastinum occurs when ruptured alveolar air breaks through the visceral pleura into the connective tissue spaces of the mediastinum, neck, and scalp. Unlike a pneumothorax, the visceral pleura and parietal pleura remain in contact and the lungs remain inflated. The causes of pneumomediastinum are essentially the same as those for a pneumothorax. Known predisposing factors are lung diseases including pneumonia and MAS, mechanical ventilation, and other conditions of air leak syndrome; however, many infants develop a pneumomediastinum for no apparent reason.

Most cases of pneumomediastinum are completely asymptomatic. A preterm infant may experience mild to moderate respiratory distress with tachypnea and cyanosis and may also present with an increased AP diameter of the chest. Often preceded by PIE, pneumomediastinum should be suspected when heart sounds are distant or muffled during a routine newborn exam.

A chest radiograph with mediastinal air extending down and outlining the heart is diagnostic for pneumomediastinum. The thymus is often seen to be elevated, giving the appearance of a sail or angel wings. This is referred to as the thymic sail sign or spinnaker sign. In some cases pneumomediastinum is more obvious on the lateral view than on the AP view. A lateral decubitus film will rule out a pneumothorax if the AP film is unclear. Pneumomediastinum and pneumothorax can coexist, and some infants will be affected by both at the same time.[158]

A pneumomediastinum usually resolves spontaneously, and treatment is rarely required; however, the infant must be observed for other air leaks, especially a pneumothorax. HFOV may be indicated if the condition is severe or accompanied by other air leak conditions. Mortality and morbidity are generally attributed to underlying disease states.

Pneumopericardium

Pneumopericardium is a rare but potentially life-threatening form of air leak syndrome in which air is in the pericardial sac. It is the least common form of air leak syndrome and is almost exclusively preceded by other forms of air leak, most often PIE or a pneumothorax. It rarely occurs in an infant who is not requiring assisted ventilation. Although not well understood, it is believed that pneumopericardium is caused by air tracking along vascular sheaths, ending with dissection into the pericardium.

Clinical presentation of pneumopericardium varies from asymptomatic to life-threatening cardiac tamponade. An abrupt onset of tachycardia followed by severe cyanosis, hypotension, and bradycardia with distant heart sounds is the typical presentation of hemodynamic compromise due to cardiac tamponade. The first sign of pneumopericardium is often hypotension or a decreased pulse pressure.

Diagnosis is suspected when the infant experiences sudden clinical deterioration with acute circulatory collapse. It is confirmed with a chest radiograph or the return of air on pericardiocentesis. Pneumopericardium has the most classic radiograph of all the air leaks: the characteristic halo sign. Thin streaks of air may outline the left ventricle and right atrium or completely surround the heart with a radiolucent halo if there is a large amount of free air. Pneumomediastinum and pneumopericardium are not mutually exclusive and can occur together. Radiographs suggestive of both diagnoses should not be disregarded.

Treatment for pneumopericardium depends on the presence of cardiac tamponade and aortic blood pressure monitoring. Cardiac tamponade with a stable blood pressure requires minimal intervention. Symptomatic infants with a fall in aortic blood pressure should be treated emergently with pericardiocentesis and surgical insertion of a pericardial drain. The prognosis is dire and outcome fatal unless emergency treatment with pericardiocentesis is available.[159]

Retinopathy of Prematurity

Retinopathy of prematurity (ROP) is a complex disease that affects growth of the blood vessels needed to support the retina. Full-term infants have fully developed retinas and are not susceptible to ROP. It primarily affects premature infants with birth weights less than 1500 g. The severity is related to gestational age: the more premature the infant, the more severe the disease. Today ROP is the second most common cause of childhood visual impairment and blindness in premature infants. Of the approximately 28,000 infants who are born in the United States weighing less than 1250 g, about 14,000 to 16,000 have some degree of ROP, with 400 to 600 of these infants legally blind.[160] The incidence is greater in Caucasian infants than African-American infants, and boys are more vulnerable than girls.

ROP was first described in 1942 and referred to as retrolental fibroplasia (RLF). Not coincidently, this was shortly after Julius Hess developed the infant oxygen unit, an incubator that had a small porthole used for continuous oxygen administration.[161] In the decade that followed, thousands of children became blind. This was

Respiratory Recap

Retinopathy of Prematurity

- Affects growth of blood vessels needed to support the retina.
- Prevention is the best treatment: restrict oxygen therapy, use steroid therapy, reduce exposure to light, provide adequate nutrition.

a direct result of abnormal blood vessel growth causing scarring and detachment of the retina. In 1951, Kate Campbell determined that there was a link between using oxygen and the development of this disease. Her suggestion was to avoid using oxygen except for treatment of cyanosis.[162] One year later strict guidelines were created to maintain oxygen concentrations at less than 40%.[163] As oxygen administration was controlled, this epidemic of blindness came to an end. In fact, in 1965 the incidence of RLF in the United States was only 4%, compared with 50% in 1950.[164] In the 1970s and 1980s, however, an increase in the survival rate of very low birth weight infants brought with it an increase in ROP. Today, with advanced technology and surfactant replacement therapy, the survival rates for infants with extremely low gestational ages and birth weights have markedly improved, placing these infants at the highest risk for ROP.

Pathophysiology

The function of the retina is to form images. Vessels that will support the retina begin to grow from the optic disk into the retina at approximately 16 weeks' gestation. Complete formation of the capillary bed occurs by 40 to 44 weeks' gestation. Once complete the vessels are no longer susceptible to injury.[165] When an infant is born prematurely, the retinal blood vessels have not had adequate time to mature, and normal vascular growth is terminated. These fragile retinal vessels are extremely vulnerable to injury.

The development of ROP begins when exposure to oxygen causes the delicate retinal vessels to constrict. Perfusion to the retina is interrupted, and capillary cells are destroyed. As the infant matures, the vessels grow, but unfortunately growth is excessive and abnormal. The result is hemorrhage, scar tissue formation, and retinal detachment with functional or complete blindness.

The most significant risk factors for ROP are extreme premature birth, low birth weight, and supplemental oxygen therapy. Genetic factors may contribute to ROP, which may be why it occurs in some premature infants who have not received oxygen therapy.[166] A number of other risk factors have been identified and include acidosis, intraventricular hemorrhage, *Candida* sepsis, mechanical ventilation, and twin pregnancy.[167]

Clinical Manifestations and Diagnosis

The progression of ROP is sequential; therefore, timely screening and treatment is necessary to reduce the risk of blindness.[168] To minimize the risk of retinal detachment and traumatic eye exams, the American Academy of Pediatrics (AAP) developed a policy statement that suggests a schedule be developed for timing eye examinations. This schedule is based on gestational and postnatal age.[169] The AAP's recommendation is to screen any infant with a birth weight of less than 1500 grams or gestational age of 32 weeks or less, or infants with an unstable clinical course who are believed to be at high risk for ROP. Retinal screening examinations are performed by a pediatric ophthalmologist and are done 4 to 6 weeks after birth, with repeat exams every 1 to 2 weeks. There is no need for a second exam if the initial examination shows that the retina in each eye is fully vascularized.

Because changes in the blood vessels cannot be visualized with the naked eye, the ophthalmologist uses a binocular with special lens for evaluation. Topical anesthetic eye drops are instilled 30 minutes prior to the examination. The infant is swaddled during the exam. The exam may cause reflex bradycardia, hypertension, and apnea; therefore, the infant should be relatively stable before an exam is performed.

An international classification of ROP was established in 1984.[170] It is based on the location, stage, and extent of the disease. Location and extent of the disease are described using zones.

Management

ROP is easiest to treat when it is caught early. Prevention remains the best treatment option. Possible preventive measures are restriction of oxygen therapy, use of steroid therapy, reduced exposure of the retina to light, and nutritional factors.[171] Current treatment begins with close monitoring of Spo_2 levels. Although the ideal pulse oximetry range is debatable, most nurseries have policies in place that recommend a normal Spo_2 range of 85% to 95%. Administration of vitamin E may help prevent ROP, along with covering the infant's eyes. This is accomplished by keeping nursery lights low and by placing a mask over the infant's eyes or placing a blanket on top of the incubator.

Usually infants with stages 1, 2, and 3 spontaneously resolve and surgical treatment is not needed. Two forms of surgery are available to stop the progression of ROP. Cryosurgery requires an incision into the conjunctiva. It consists of applying an extremely cold probe to the infant's eye and freezing hypoxic areas of the retina. This prevents the spread of abnormal vessels but has a high risk of visual complications, including retinal scarring and detachment. Laser photocoagulation is the newest surgical treatment. This technique involves applying a laser directly to the retina. It condenses protein material in the eye and destroys any abnormal blood vessels. This treatment has less risk of tissue damage and only requires a topical anesthetic. Complications include scarring, intraocular hemorrhage, corneal haze, burns of the iris, and possibly cataracts. Most infants completely recover following treatment.[168,172]

Complications and Outcomes

Fortunately, ROP is of variable severity, and most infants recover with no lasting visual problems. It is impossible to accurately predict the outcomes, however. Some infants will progress to retinal scar formation or retinal detachment resulting in blindness. Strabismus, glaucoma, astigmatism, nystagmus, and amblyopia may also occur. Early screening and treatment for ROP along with surgical repair have improved long-term outcomes. In spite of limiting oxygen exposure, ROP remains a common problem in infants who weigh less than 1251 grams.[173]

Bronchiolitis

Bronchiolitis, defined as inflammation of the bronchioles, is an acute infectious disease that often occurs in epidemics. Although bronchiolitis may occur at any age, it usually affects children under the age of 24 months, with a peak incidence in infants 3 to 6 months old. It may be more prevalent in urban areas and occurs more frequently in males than females. Typically bronchiolitis is seasonal, appearing more frequently between November and April, and remains one of the most common reasons for an infant to be hospitalized during winter and early spring.[174]

Pathophysiology

Bronchiolitis begins with a viral infection in the upper respiratory tract and can spread to the terminal bronchiolar cells within 1 to 3 days. Pathologic changes begin 18 to 24 hours following the infection. The virus initiates an inflammatory response causing increased mucus production with bronchiolar and ciliated epithelial cell necrosis. The developing edema, airway debris, and sloughed epithelium cause partial or total obstruction to airflow. Airway narrowing during expiration produces a decrease in airflow along with air trapping that may lead to complete obstruction and atelectasis. Hypoxia is a result of $\dot{V}/\dot{Q}$ mismatch, and work of breathing is increased due to a decrease in lung compliance. The epithelial cells begin recovery after 3 to 4 days; however, it may take 2 or more weeks for cilia to regenerate.[175]

Etiology

Respiratory syncytial virus (RSV) is the most common cause of bronchiolitis and may be responsible for 50% to 80% of all cases.[176] Less frequently identified viruses include adenovirus, influenza A and B, parainfluenza viruses, human metapneumovirus, rhinovirus, and measles virus. Some bacteria have been associated with bronchiolitis, including *Mycoplasma pneumoniae* and *Chlamydia pneumoniae*. RSV is so common that it is estimated that by the time infants are 12 months old, more than half of them have been exposed to the virus. Unfortunately, RSV is extremely contagious and is transmitted from person to person by inhaling airborne droplets of infected secretions or by direct contact with objects contaminated with respiratory secretions. These droplets can survive for several hours on contaminated objects, including bed rails and the hands of caregivers.

Box 46-12 lists risk factors that increase the likelihood that a child will develop bronchiolitis. Children at high risk of developing severe, life-threatening RSV infection include those with underlying cardiopulmonary disease, including congenital heart disease and BPD, infants younger than 6 weeks, and infants with congenital or acquired immunodeficiency. Multiple infections, such as RSV and metapneumovirus, also tend to result in more severe cases.[177]

Clinical Manifestations

RSV infection in older children and adults causes generally mild symptoms similar to the common cold. The bronchioles of an infant are much narrower than those of an adult, causing infants with RSV infection to present with more severe respiratory distress.

Bronchiolitis follows a variable course characterized by wheezing, tachypnea, and hypoxia. Clinical presentation typically begins with nasal congestion and rhinorrhea followed by mild coughing, and possibly a low-grade fever. The child may also have conjunctivitis or otitis media. Apnea may be the presenting feature of bronchiolitis, especially in younger infants with a history of premature birth. Over a period of 2 to 3 days,

BOX 46-12

Risk Factors for Development of Bronchiolitis

- Day-care attendance
- Younger than 6 months
- Exposure to wood smoke
- Exposure to cigarette smoke
- Never having been breastfed
- Having siblings who attend school
- Exposure to traffic-related air pollutants
- Exposure to an adult or child with a cold
- Premature birth (before 37 weeks' gestation)

Respiratory Recap

Bronchiolitis

- Greatest incidence is in infants aged 3 to 6 months.
- Respiratory syncytial virus is the most common cause.
- Treatment includes nasotracheal suctioning, hydration, and oxygen.
- Bronchodilator therapy is controversial.

tachypnea develops with respiratory rates of up to 100 breaths/min in infants and 60 breaths/min in the older child. Audible wheezing with a prolonged expiratory phase is common, and fine inspiratory crackles are heard on auscultation. Dyspnea develops and symptoms progress to tachycardia, marked intercostal retractions, nasal flaring, grunting, and head bobbing with the use of accessory muscles. The infant may be irritable and appear anxious and toxic. Fever and tachypnea increase insensible fluid loss, while respiratory distress makes it difficult for an infant to take a bottle. This, along with a decreased appetite, can quickly lead to dehydration. The liver and spleen may be palpable from hyperinflation of the lungs and depression of the diaphragm. Persistent hypoxia and increased work of breathing lead to fatigue, more shallow respirations, and eventually respiratory failure.

Severe disease most often develops in toxic-appearing infants who are younger than 3 months and have an Spo_2 of less than 95% on room air. Infants with respiratory rates greater than 70 breaths/min, apneic episodes, or chest radiographs with atelectasis are also at higher risk of developing acute respiratory distress.

Diagnosis

Bronchiolitis is diagnosed and the severity of the disease assessed on the basis of history and physical examination of the child. Although the clinical syndrome of bronchiolitis is well recognized, diagnosis can be supported by additional tests. Because hypoxemia is common, Spo_2 is monitored; no further testing is warranted when Spo_2 is normal. RSV rapid antigen testing is done using a nasal swab, and although it is diagnostic for RSV it is not generally necessary for disease management.

Laboratory tests and radiographs are not routinely recommended but may be useful in ruling out other disorders in children with complicating or worsening symptoms.[178] Although the white blood cell count is usually within normal limits, a complete blood count may be ordered if bacterial illness is suspected. If chest radiographs are indicated they should include AP and lateral views. Bronchiolitis typically presents

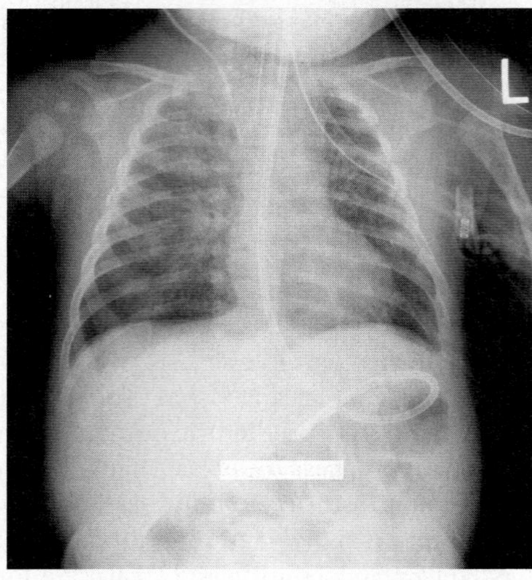

FIGURE 46-15 Chest radiograph with bilateral hyperinflation and widespread pulmonary infiltrates in an infant with bronchiolitis.
Courtesy of Chetan Chandulal Shah, MBBS, DMRD, MBA, Arkansas Children's Hospital.

as hyperinflation with flattened diaphragms, air bronchograms, peribronchial cuffing, and prominent hilar markings. Atelectasis and patchy infiltrates may be present as well as pneumonia (**Figure 46-15**).

When the child presents with atypical symptoms, additional tests are warranted and may reveal evidence of other diagnoses, including bronchitis, pneumonia, and congenital heart disease. Gastroesophageal reflux or dysphagia with aspiration of gastric contents may also present with a clinical picture similar to bronchiolitis. Foreign body aspiration should be considered when there is a history of sudden-onset wheezing without symptoms of upper respiratory tract infection. Asthma may present similarly but is much more likely to occur in a child who is older than 18 months. Vascular rings, tracheomalacia, and other anatomic airway abnormalities should be included in the differential diagnosis.

Management

In the majority of cases, bronchiolitis can be successfully treated in the outpatient setting. Indications for hospitalization include hypoxemia, tachypnea with respiratory rates greater than 60 breaths/min, retractions at rest, apnea, poor oral intake, and children with underlying cardiopulmonary disease or immunodeficiency. Many institutions use pathways or guidelines to standardize the management of bronchiolitis. There is mounting evidence that the use of pathways is associated with a decrease in unwarranted treatment, use of antibiotics, and hospital length of stays.[179] Because of the highly contagious nature of the virus, early efforts should be made to isolate infants confirmed to have RSV infection or who present with a clinical picture suggestive of bronchiolitis.

Nasopharyngeal suctioning is an effective component of the care of infants with bronchiolitis and should be used to clear nasal secretions. Saline drops may be instilled in the nose prior to suctioning. Parents and other caregivers must be proficient in bulb suctioning techniques to use at home and be educated on proper hand sanitation.

With oxygenation and hydration the primary goals, treatment is largely supportive and usually requires only fluids, oxygen, and suctioning of secretions. The risk of dehydration makes it essential that fluid intake and urine output be monitored. Frequent small feeds and IV fluid administration are used to maintain adequate hydration if the child's respiratory rate is greater than 80 breaths/min or the child has respiratory distress or oxygen desaturation during feedings.

Although not routinely recommended, supplemental oxygen is administered with a nasal cannula or oxygen hood if the Spo_2 of a previously healthy infant is persistently below 92%. Ventilation is assessed by monitoring the Pco_2 of arterial, capillary, or venous blood. A Pco_2 greater than 55 mm Hg is an indication for high-flow nasal cannula or mechanical ventilation.[180] Recurrent apnea requires intubation with mechanical ventilation. Oxygen may be discontinued when the Spo_2 is at or above 92%, the infant has adequate oral intake, and respiratory distress is at a minimum. Weaning oxygen in premature infants or infants with cardiopulmonary disease must be closely monitored.

Bronchodilator use would seem to be the logical choice for treatment of wheezing; however, it continues to be controversial in the management of bronchiolitis. Recent guidelines from the AAP recommend that bronchodilators not be used routinely. A carefully monitored trial is an option, with use continued only if there is evidence of clinical improvement.[178] Chest physiotherapy is not recommended because no benefit has been documented and it may actually increase respiratory distress and irritability. Because bronchiolitis is viral in nature, antibiotics are ineffective and should not be administered unless there is evidence of concomitant bacterial infection (e.g., otitis media, pneumonia). Because clinical trials have reported that there is no benefit in using corticosteroids to treat bronchiolitis, routine use is not recommended.[181] There is evidence that nebulized hypertonic saline (3%) results in clinically significant reductions in hospital stay and is a safe and effective treatment for viral bronchiolitis.[182]

When first approved for use in the United States in 1986, the antiviral agent ribavirin was administered by continuous aerosol for 18 hours a day for 3 to 6 days.[183] Multiple studies since that time have criticized its application, concluding that there is marginal benefit from this expensive drug that requires a complicated aerosol delivery system and has the potential of teratogenic risks for pregnant caregivers. Present recommendations are that it not be used.[178] As of this date there is no RSV vaccine available for bronchiolitis. Since its introduction in 1998, however, the humanized monoclonal antibody palivizumab (Synagis) has been shown to help protect high-risk infants from RSV infection and limit severity of the illness. The recommended dosage of palivizumab is 15 mg/kg body weight administered by a single intramuscular injection in five monthly doses during RSV season, usually beginning in November.[184] Recommendations made by the AAP currently limit its use to infants and children who are at high risk of developing severe disease from RSV. **Box 46-13** lists those who may benefit from palivizumab prophylaxis. Discharge is considered when the child is stable without supplemental oxygen, the respiratory rate is within normal range, and oral intake is adequate to maintain hydration.

BOX 46-13

Indications for Palivizumab Prophylaxis

- Infants born at 32 weeks' gestation or earlier
- Infants born between 32 and 35 weeks' gestation with at least two risk factors*
- Infants and children younger than 24 months with chronic lung disease
- Infants and children younger than 24 months with congenital heart disease

*Risk factors: day-care attendance, school-aged sibling, exposure to environmental air pollutants, congenital airway abnormalities, severe neuromuscular disease, acquired immunodeficiency.

Complications and Outcome

Complications of bronchiolitis are most severe in high-risk infants and children. Apnea often occurs in young infants or those with previous episodes of apnea. Severe respiratory distress may lead to respiratory failure and require intubation and mechanical ventilation. Although uncommon, a secondary bacterial pneumonia may occur. Although the association is controversial, there is some indication that infants hospitalized with bronchiolitis have increased risk for recurrent wheezing and development of early childhood asthma. Whether

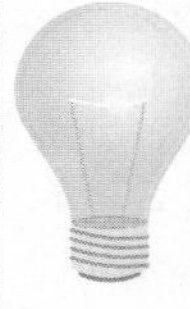

STOP AND THINK

A 3-month-old previously healthy infant is admitted to the hospital with nasal congestion, bilateral wheezing and crackles, a respiratory rate of 70 breaths/minute, and an Spo_2 of 92%. What tests should be obtained and what results would be expected to confirm a diagnosis of bronchiolitis?

these children have an inherited asthma tendency that makes them more prone to bronchiolitis or whether bronchiolitis triggers asthma is uncertain.[185,186]

Most infants, regardless of the severity of illness, recover in 3 to 5 days. Wheezing, cough, and disruption in feeding and sleeping patterns often continue for 2 to 4 weeks. Although rare, death occurs most often in infants younger than 6 months and depends largely on comorbidities. The mortality rate is less than 1%, with this rate decreasing with increasing birth weight.

Laryngotracheobronchitis

Acute respiratory tract infections are common in the pediatric patient and are the number one reason for children under the age of 4 years to be hospitalized. Upper airway infections can be particularly severe because of the anatomy of the child's airway. Unlike an adult, whose glottis is the narrowest part of the airway, a child's narrowest airway segment is the subglottis. The subglottic area is cone-shaped, with the cricoid ring being the narrowest area. Because it is completely surrounded by the cricoid cartilage and loose connective tissue, a small amount of inflammation and edema of this subglottic tissue can result in significant airway obstruction.

Laryngotracheobronchitis (LTB), also referred to as croup, is the most common cause of infectious upper airway obstruction in children between the ages of 6 months and 3 years. It rarely occurs in children younger than 1 year or older than 6 years and is more prevalent in males than females.[187] About 15% of affected children have a family history of LTB. It is epidemic by nature and occurs most often between early fall and late spring. The vast majority of children with LTB are not hospitalized.

Pathophysiology and Etiology

This disorder is termed laryngotracheobronchitis because it is characterized by diffuse inflammation that affects the airway from the larynx to the bronchus. It involves edema of the subglottic area and exudate in the airway, resulting in varying degrees of airway narrowing. It is usually due to a viral invasion, particularly parainfluenzae types 1 and 2. Although not as common, a number of other viruses have been reported, including influenza type A and B, adenovirus, rhinovirus, enterovirus, respiratory syncytial virus, herpes simplex type 1, measles, and varicella. A disruption in the laminar airflow through the constricted or partially obstructed airway during inspiration produces the characteristic harsh, brassy sound of stridor.

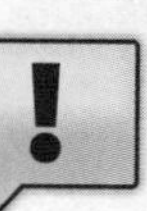

Respiratory Recap

Laryngotracheobronchitis

- Most common cause of infectious upper airway obstruction in children between the ages of 6 months and 3 years.
- Treatment includes corticosteroids, racemic epinephrine, oxygen, heliox, and, in rare cases, intubation.

Clinical Manifestations

The spectrum of disease severity is broad with LTB. The child typically presents with a several-day history of upper respiratory–type symptoms that include a low-grade fever, rhinorrhea, sore throat, and mild cough.[188] Over the next 2 to 3 days, the symptoms progress to hoarseness and the barking-seal cough that is characteristic of LTB. The cough often begins abruptly in the middle of the night and may occur in spasms. Stridor is heard mainly on inspiration, typically occurring when the child is irritated or crying. With more significant airway narrowing, it becomes audible even when the child is resting quietly and during both inspiration and expiration, which is referred to as biphasic stridor. Physical examination usually reveals an apprehensive-appearing child with mild fever, tachypnea, tachycardia, suprasternal and substernal retractions, head bobbing, and breath sounds that are mostly clear.

Diagnosis

The diagnosis of viral LTB is most often based on the characteristic clinical presentation. It does not require radiography in children with typical histories and mild symptoms that respond effectively to treatment. Lateral neck films typically reveal a normal epiglottis and supraglottic structures, an overdistended hypopharynx, and haziness within the subglottis with subglottic narrowing greater on inspiration. These films help confirm the diagnosis of LTB while ruling out other disorders, including epiglottitis, hemangioma, and congenital abnormalities such as a tracheal web or vascular ring. The AP view of the neck will demonstrate narrowing immediately below the vocal cords with the usual squared-shoulder appearance of the subglottic area replaced with airway narrowing referred to as a steeple sign or pencil-point sign (**Figure 46-16**). The absence of abnormalities, however, does not rule out the diagnosis of LTB, because radiographs may be normal in as many as 50% of children with LTB and diagnosis is made from history and clinical presentation alone (**Figure 46-17**).[189]

Management

For the majority of children, LTB is self-limiting and only supportive care is needed. Despite the lack of strong scientific evidence, there is anecdotal support for treating LTB at home with humidification using a humidifier or vaporizer at the bedside or sitting with

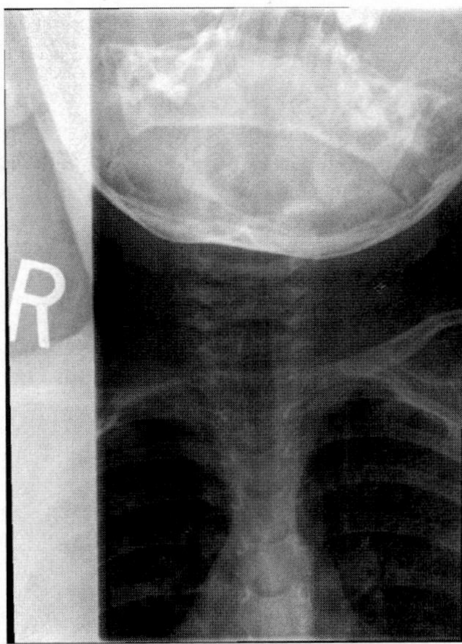

FIGURE 46-16 Chest radiograph of a child with laryngotracheobronchitis shows the pencil-point or steeple sign.
Courtesy of Chetan Chandulal Shah, MBBS, DMRD, MBA, Arkansas Children's Hospital.

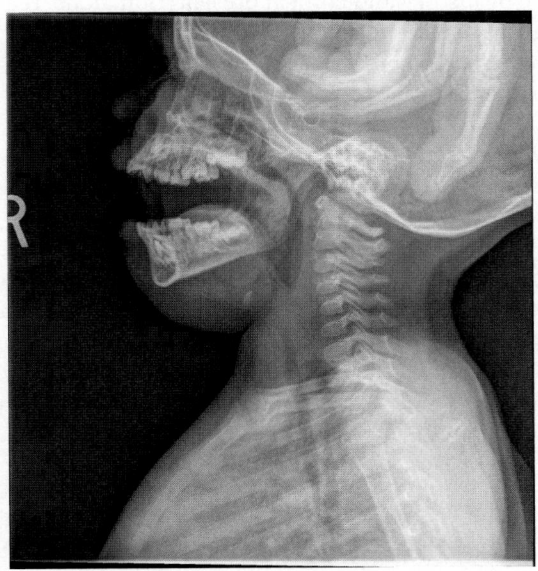

FIGURE 46-17 Lateral neck radiograph of a child with laryngotracheobronchitis shows a hypopharynx that is overdistended and subglottic haziness.
Courtesy of Chetan Chandulal Shah, MBBS, DMRD, MBA, Arkansas Children's Hospital.

the child in the bathroom with the door closed and a hot shower running. Although the benefit of such treatment may only be a placebo to make parents feel like they are helping their child, it is still used. It is not without risks, however, which may include scalding, unnecessary discomfort, and anxiety that worsens symptoms.[190]

Management of LTB has undergone dramatic changes, including the use of corticosteroids in both outpatient and inpatient settings. It is believed that the potent vasoconstrictive and anti-inflammatory properties of corticosteroids reduce mucosal edema and the inflammatory reaction. Use has been shown not only to reduce symptoms and the need for hospital admission but also to reduce the need for and duration of intubation. Oral dexamethasone has been shown to provide quick relief with many children responding to a single dose. Aerosolized budesonide is another option that can be given alternatively to children unable to tolerate oral dexamethasone.[189]

Available in the United States since 1971, racemic epinephrine has a vasoconstrictive α-adrenergic effect on the vasculature mucosa that rapidly reduces upper airway edema. Upon presentation in the emergency department, children typically receive aerosolized racemic epinephrine by face mask with a handheld nebulizer using a 2.25% solution diluted in normal saline. The amount of medication used is dependent on the child's response. Recommended dosage is 0.05 mL/kg/dose of a 2.25% solution diluted in 2.5 mL normal saline with a maximum recommended dose of 0.5 mL. Nebulized L-epinephrine is as effective as racemic epinephrine.[191] The recommended dose is 0.5 mL/kg/dose of a 1:1000 solution in 2.5 mL of normal saline, with a maximum recommended dose of 5 mL. With either form the effect is generally short lived, usually lasting only 2 hours. For some children a single dose is all that is required for relief, however, and they can be discharged home if symptom-free for at least 3 hours following the treatment.

For the child who has poor to no response to treatment in the emergency department, hospitalization is advised. Corticosteroid therapy is continued, and nebulized epinephrine treatments are continued, given as often as every 30 minutes. Respiratory rate is the simplest predictor of hypoxemia in the child with LTB. To prevent the anxiety and crying that often trigger stridor and retractions, noninvasive monitoring with pulse oximetry is preferred over blood gas testing. Supplemental oxygen is provided only if the child's Spo_2 is less than 92%. Because LTB is usually caused by a virus, antibiotics are not indicated unless the child has cultures suggestive of a bacterial infection. Although heliox has shown benefit as a useful alternative to intubation, it has not been shown to be more effective than inhaled racemic epinephrine in the management of LTB.[192]

On rare occasions a child will fail medical intervention and require endotracheal intubation. Because of the subglottic edema and narrowed airway, intubation should be with an endotracheal tube that is at least 1 mm smaller than the normal estimate. As airway edema and inflammation are resolved, an air leak will develop around the endotracheal tube, and extubation attempts are usually successful at that time. Close monitoring for the return of stridor and respiratory distress is necessary in the first 12 hours following extubation.

Complications and Outcome

Complications that develop from LTB are rare but can include dehydration as a result of tachypnea and increased respiratory distress or secondary infections of otitis media and pneumonia. LTB usually resolves within 72 hours of onset, although some cases last up to 7 days, with complete uncomplicated resolution. Some children have repeat episodes of LTB. Only 5% to 10% of LTB patients are hospitalized, with approximately only 2% of that group requiring intubation. Subglottic stenosis in the child with LTB is uncommon but is a possible complication if intubation is prolonged.[193]

Epiglottitis

The life-threatening bacterial infection known as **epiglottitis** is a true airway emergency. It was first described in 1878 and given the name epiglottitis, although today we appreciate that it is an infection that affects the supraglottic structures. These include the epiglottis, aryepiglottic folds, arytenoid soft tissue, and occasionally the uvula. It tends to occur in children aged 2 to 6 years, although cases have been reported in which the child is younger than 1 year, and may present at no particular season.

Pathophysiology and Etiology

Epiglottitis is purely a supraglottic lesion in which swelling pushes the epiglottis posteriorly and edema produces partial or complete airway obstruction. There is ballooning of the hypopharynx, thickened aryepiglottic folds, and circumferential narrowing of the subglottic portion of the trachea during inspiration. *Haemophilus influenzae* type b (Hib) is the most common causative organism; however, pneumococcus, group A β-hemolytic *Streptococcus pneumoniae*, *Klebsiella*, and viruses such as herpes simplex 1 and parainfluenzae have also been implicated.[187]

Clinical Manifestations

Clinical findings include the classic four Ds of epiglottitis: drooling, dysphagia, dysphonia, and dyspnea. History is common for an abrupt onset of sore throat with refusal to eat, high fever (>38° C), irritability, and a muffled-sounding voice. The child is toxic appearing and drooling. In contrast to laryngotracheobronchitis, the respiratory pattern of the child with epiglottitis is one of very deliberate slow breaths with large tidal volumes. This is an effort to reduce turbulent airflow and airway resistance. Suprasternal and substernal retractions are evident, with nasal flaring and cyanosis if obstruction is severe. Typical presentation is in the tripod position: sitting upright supported by both hands and leaning forward with the neck extended in a sniffing position in an attempt to keep the airway open. Inspiratory stridor is heard but may diminish as airway obstruction worsens.

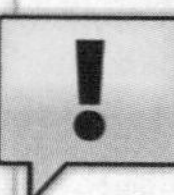

Respiratory Recap

Epiglottitis

- Epiglottitis is a life-threatening bacterial infection.
- Common findings include drooling, dysphagia, dysphonia, and dyspnea.
- Many cases respond to antibiotics and oxygen.
- If epiglottitis is severe and intubation is indicated, it should be performed in the operating room.

Diagnosis

Manipulation of the epiglottis with a tongue depressor, radiographs, and blood gas analysis are painful and anxiety-provoking procedures that greatly increase the risk of complete airway obstruction. For that reason they should be avoided if at all possible and diagnosis made by history and clinical presentation alone. If a diagnosis is in question, however, lateral neck films are valuable in confirming the diagnosis and ruling out other disorders, including LTB, foreign body aspiration, and retropharyngeal abscess. Patient age, clinical presentation, and radiographic findings can contribute to differentiation from LTB.[194] **Table 46-1** lists those factors that assist in the differential diagnosis. The radiograph will typically reveal an enlarged epiglottis, described as the thumb sign, and a distended hypopharynx. It should be noted that if neck radiographs are performed, the child should never be left alone and must remain in an upright position during the study because the supine position may result in total airway obstruction.

Management

The overriding goal in treating the child with epiglottitis is to obtain and maintain a secure airway. Many patients will respond to intravenous antibiotics and supplemental oxygen and not require intubation but must be closely monitored in an intensive care setting.[195] If epiglottitis is severe and emergency intubation is indicated, it should be performed in an operating suite where an emergent tracheostomy can be performed if needed. After the patient is anesthetized, fiberoptic-assisted intubation is performed and airway specimens obtained for culture and sensitivity. As with LTB, intubation of the swollen airway will require an endotracheal tube that is one size smaller than that estimated for age and weight. Extubation should be attempted only after an air leak is noted and there is evidence of clinical improvement. A nasotracheal tube is preferred because it is more stable and better able to keep secured. If the child will need to be transported

TABLE 46-1
Clinical Differentiation of Epiglottitis and Laryngotracheobronchitis

	Epiglottitis	Laryngotracheobronchitis
Age	2 to 6 years	6 months to 3 years
Gender	No prevalence	More prevalent in males
Onset	Sudden, within 4 to 8 hours	2- to 4-day history of cold symptoms
Seasons	All	Fall through spring
Fever	High	Low-grade
Respiratory rate	Bradypnea with deliberate, large tidal volumes	Late-onset tachypnea
Heart rate	Early-onset tachycardia	Late-onset tachycardia
Retractions	Severe	Mild to severe
Stridor	Inspiratory	Inspiratory and expiratory
Cough	Minimal	Barking seal
Voice	Muffled	Hoarse
Drooling	Yes	No
Dysphagia	Yes	No
Position	Supine worsens stridor	No effect on stridor
Appearance	Toxic, acutely ill	Irritable, restless
Radiograph	Lateral neck view: thumb sign	Anteroposterior view: steeple sign

to another facility, the airway must be secured and the child should be sedated to prevent anxiety that can worsen airway compromise.[188]

Complications and Outcome

With a quick response to antibiotic therapy and corticosteroid administration, intubation is usually required for no more than 48 hours. Nearly half of all patients with epiglottitis will develop another infection, most often pneumonia and otitis media. Bacteremia can also lead to cellulitis and meningitis. Accidental extubation increases the risk of airway complications. Mortality rate can be as high as 10% when there is airway obstruction without intubation, in contrast to only 1% when intubation is performed. Introduction of the Hib vaccine in 1985 has led to a marked decrease in the number of cases of epiglottitis, with 41 cases reported per 100,000 children in 1987 compared with 1.3 cases per 100,000 children in 1997.[196]

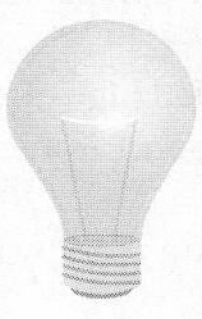

STOP AND THINK

A 2-year-old child presents to the emergency department with stridor, marked suprasternal and substernal retractions, and a temperature of 102° F (39° C). Parents state that he has had nasal congestion for over 24 hours and is more restless than normal. What treatment should be provided at this time, and what tests should be performed to confirm a diagnosis?

Key Points

- Apnea of prematurity is due to immaturity of the brain stem.
- Apnea of prematurity is treated with respiratory stimulants, oxygen, CPAP, and mechanical ventilation.
- Home apnea monitoring may be used with apnea of prematurity.
- Respiratory distress syndrome is a complication of prematurity.
- Biochemical tests of amniotic fluid can be used to evaluate lung maturity.
- Treatment of respiratory distress syndrome includes oxygen, surfactant replacement, CPAP, mechanical ventilation, and supportive therapy.
- A milder form of bronchopulmonary dysplasia, chronic lung disease is based on continued oxygen therapy at 36 weeks' gestation.
- Chronic lung disease occurs in premature infants with progressive deterioration of lung function.
- Causes of chronic lung disease in newborns are multifactorial and include ventilator- and oxygen-induced injury.
- Treatment of chronic lung disease in newborns includes oxygen, mechanical ventilation, corticosteroids, and bronchodilators.
- Transient tachypnea of the newborn is a self-limiting disorder of term and near-term infants.
- Pneumonia can occur at any gestational age and includes congenital, intrapartum, and postnatal forms.
- Treatment of neonatal pneumonia is aimed at eradicating the infection, along with supportive care.
- Meconium aspiration syndrome occurs when the infant aspirates stained amniotic fluid.
- Meconium aspiration syndrome usually occurs in infants born at term or postterm.
- Treatment of meconium aspiration syndrome includes suctioning, oxygen therapy, mechanical ventilation, inhaled nitric oxide, extracorporeal membrane oxygenation, and surfactant replacement.

- Persistent pulmonary hypertension of the newborn occurs when fetal circulation persists after birth.
- Echocardiography is used to make the diagnosis of persistent pulmonary hypertension of the newborn.
- Treatment of persistent pulmonary hypertension of the newborn includes oxygen, mechanical ventilation, inhaled nitric oxide, extracorporeal membrane oxygenation, and supportive therapy.
- Congenital diaphragmatic hernia is an abnormality in which the infant's diaphragm allows the abdominal organs to protrude into the thorax.
- Treatment of congenital diaphragmatic hernia includes delivery room stabilization, mechanical ventilation, inhaled nitric oxide, extracorporeal membrane oxygenation, surgery, and supportive therapy.
- The type and severity of a congenital pulmonary anomaly depend upon the time during fetal lung development that an insult occurred resulting in the malformation.
- Early diagnosis of congenital pulmonary anomalies using fetal ultrasound, CT, and MRI imaging has improved prognosis, which depends largely on the presence of associated congenital malformations and health of the normally developed lung.
- Air leak syndrome in the newborn includes pulmonary interstitial emphysema, pneumothorax, pneumomediastinum, and pneumopericardium.
- Transillumination is used to make an immediate diagnosis of pneumothorax.
- Retinopathy of prematurity affects growth of blood vessels needed to support the retina.
- Prevention is the best treatment for retinopathy of prematurity and includes restriction of oxygen therapy, steroid therapy, reduced exposure to light, and adequate nutrition.
- The greatest incidence of bronchiolitis occurs in infants aged 3 to 6 months.
- Respiratory syncytial virus is the most common cause of bronchiolitis.
- Treatment of bronchiolitis includes nasotracheal suctioning, hydration, and oxygen.
- Bronchodilator therapy for the treatment of bronchiolitis is controversial.
- Laryngotracheobronchitis (LTB) is the most common cause of infectious upper airway obstruction in children between the ages of 6 months and 3 years.
- Treatment of LTB includes corticosteroids, racemic epinephrine, oxygen, heliox, and, in rare cases, intubation.
- Epiglottitis is a life-threatening bacterial infection.
- Common findings in epiglottitis include drooling, dysphagia, dysphonia, and dyspnea.
- Many cases of epiglottitis respond to antibiotics and oxygen.
- If epiglottitis is severe and intubation is indicated, it should be performed in the operating room.

Figures 46-1 to 46-10 and 46-12 to 46-17 are courtesy of Chetan Chandulal Shah, MBBS, DMRD, MBA, Arkansas Children's Hospital.

References

1. Finer NN, Higgins R, Kattwinkel J, et al. Summary proceedings from the apnea-of-prematurity group. *Pediatrics.* 2006;117(suppl 1): S47–S51.
2. Barrington K, Finer N. The natural history of the appearance of apnea of prematurity. *Pediatr Res.* 1991;29:372–375.
3. Eichenwald E, Aina A, Stark AR. Apnea frequently persists beyond term gestation in infants delivered at 24 to 28 weeks. *Pediatrics.* 1997;100:354–359.
4. Schmidt B. Methylxanthine therapy in premature infants: sound practice, disaster, or fruitless byway? *J Pediatr.* 1999;135:526–528.
5. American Academy of Pediatrics, Committee on Fetus and Newborn. Apnea, sudden infant death syndrome, and home monitoring. *Pediatrics.* 2003;111:914–917.
6. Sychowski SP, Dodd E, Thomas P, et al. Home apnea monitor use in preterm infants discharged from newborn intensive care units. *J Pediatr.* 2001;139:245–248.
7. Schmidt B, Roberts RS, Davis P, et al. Long-term effects of caffeine therapy for apnea of prematurity. *N Engl J Med.* 2007;357:1893–1902.
8. Hoffman HJ, Damus K, Hillman L, et al. Risk factors for SIDS. Results of the National Institute of Child Health and Human Development SIDS Cooperative Epidemiological Study. *Ann N Y Acad Sci.* 1988;533:13–30.
9. Hintz SR, Van Meurs KP, Perritt R, et al. Neurodevelopmental outcomes of premature infants with severe respiratory failure enrolled in a randomized controlled trial of inhaled nitric oxide. *J Pediatr.* 2007;151:e1–e3.
10. Ghodrat M. Lung surfactants. *Am J Health Syst Pharm.* 2006;63:1504–1521.
11. Rodriguez RJ. Management of respiratory distress syndrome: an update. *Respir Care.* 2003;48:279–287.
12. Pickerd N, Kotecha S. Pathophysiology of RDS. *J Paediatr Child Health.* 2009;19:153–157.
13. Cole FS. Defects in surfactant synthesis: clinical implications. *Pediatr Clin North Am.* 2006;53:911–927.
14. McGinnis KT, Brown JA, Morrison JC. Changing patterns of fetal lung maturity testing. *J Perinatol.* 2008;28:20–23.
15. Yarbrough ML, Grenache DG, Gronowski AM. Fetal lung maturity testing: the end of an era. *Biomark Med.* 2014;8:509–515.
16. NIH Consensus Development Panel. Effect of corticosteroids for fetal maturation on perinatal outcomes. *JAMA.* 1995;274:413–417.
17. Haq I, Gopalakaje S, Fenton AC, et al. The evidence for high flow nasal cannula devices in infants. *Paediatr Respir Rev.* 2014;15:124–134.
18. Kugelman A, Riskin A, Said W, et al. A randomized pilot study comparing heated humidified high-flow nasal cannulae with NIPPV for RDS. *Pediatr Pulmonol.* 2014:March 12. Doi; 10.1002/ppul.23022. (Epub ahead of print).
19. Yoder BA, Stoddard RA, Li M, et al. Heated, humidified high-flow nasal cannula versus nasal CPAP for respiratory support in neonates. *Pediatrics.* 2013;131:e1482–e1490.
20. Fujiwara T, Maeta H, Chida S, et al. Artificial surfactant therapy in hyaline-membrane disease. *Lancet.* 1980;1:55–59.
21. Ramanathan R. Choosing a right surfactant for respiratory distress syndrome treatment. *Neonatology.* 2009;95:1–5.
22. Rojas-Reyes MX, Morley CJ. Prophylactic versus selective use of surfactant in preventing morbidity and mortality in preterm infants. *Cochrane Database Syst Rev.* 2012;3:CD000510.
23. Polin RA, Carlo WA, American Academy of Pediatrics, Committee on Fetus and Newborn. Surfactant replacement therapy for

preterm and term neonates with respiratory distress. *Pediatrics.* 2014;133:156–163.

24. Proquitte H, Dushe T, Hammer H, et al. Observational study to compare the clinical efficacy of the natural surfactants Alveofact and Curosurf in the treatment of respiratory distress syndrome in premature infants. *Respir Med.* 2007;101:169–176.
25. Moya F. Synthetic surfactants: where are we? Evidence from randomized, controlled clinical trials. *J Perinatol.* 2009;29(suppl 2): S23–S28.
26. Abdel-Latif ME, Osborn DA. Nebulised surfactant in preterm infants with or at risk of respiratory distress syndrome. *Cochrane Database Syst Rev.* 2012;10:CD008310.
27. Attridge JT, Stewart C, Stukenborg GJ, et al. Administration of rescue surfactant by laryngeal mask airway: lessons from a pilot trial. *Am J Perinatol.* 2013;30:201–206.
28. Martinelli S, Gatelli I, Proto A. Surfactant administration during spontaneous breathing via a thin endotracheal catheter. *Acta Biomed.* 2013;84(suppl 1):22–24.
29. Pfister RH, Soll RF. Initial respiratory support of preterm infants: the role of CPAP, the INSURE method, and noninvasive ventilation. *Clin Perinatol.* 2012;39:459–481.
30. Morley CJ, Davis PG, Doyle LW, et al. Nasal CPAP or intubation at birth of very preterm infants. *N Engl J Med.* 2008;358:700–708.
31. DiBlasi RM. Nasal continuous positive airway pressure (CPAP) for the respiratory care of the newborn infant. *Respir Care.* 2009;54:1209–1235.
32. Chowdhury O, Patel DS, Hannam S, et al. Randomised trial of volume-targeted ventilation versus pressure-limited ventilation in acute respiratory failure in prematurely born infants. *Neonatology.* 2013;104:290–294.
33. Shah S, Kaul A. Volume targeted ventilation and arterial carbon dioxide in extremely preterm infants. *J Neonatal Perinatal Med.* 2013;6:339–344.
34. Guven S, Bozdag S, Saner H, et al. Early neonatal outcomes of volume guaranteed ventilation in preterm infants with respiratory distress syndrome. *J Matern Fetal Neonatal Med.* 2013;26:39–401.
35. Peng W, Zhu H, Shi H, et al. Volume-targeted ventilation is more suitable than pressure-limited ventilation for preterm infants: a systematic review and meta-analysis. *Arch Dis Child Fetal Neonatal Ed.* 2014;99:F158–F165.
36. Morley CJ. Volume-limited and volume-targeted ventilation. *Clin Perinatol.* 2012;39:513–523.
37. Lampland AL, Mammel MC. The role of high-frequency ventilation in neonates: evidence-based recommendations. *Clin Perinatol.* 2007;34:129–144.
38. Henderson-Smart DJ, Cools F, Bhuta T, et al. Elective high frequency oscillatory ventilation versus conventional ventilation for acute pulmonary dysfunction in preterm infants. *Cochrane Database Syst Rev.* 2007;3:CD000104.
39. Kovisto M, Marttila R, Saarela T, et al. Wheezing illness and re-hospitalization in the first two years of life after neonatal respiratory distress syndrome. *J Pediatr.* 2005;147:486–492.
40. Carlo WA, McDonald SA, Fanaroff AA, et al. Association of antenatal corticosteroids with mortality and neurodevelopmental outcomes among infants born at 22 to 25 weeks' gestation. *JAMA.* 2011;306:2348–2358.
41. Baraldi E, Filippone M. Chronic lung disease after premature birth. *N Engl J Med.* 2007;357:1946–1955.
42. Thomas W, Speer CP. Prevention and treatment of bronchopulmonary dysplasia: current status and future prospects. *J Perinatol.* 2007;27(suppl 1):S26–S32.
43. Henderson-Smart DJ, Hutchinson JL, Donoghue DA, et al. Prenatal predictors of chronic lung disease in very preterm infants. *Arch Dis Child Fetal Neonatal Ed.* 2006;91:F40–F45.
44. Northway WH, Rosan RC, Porter DY. Pulmonary disease following respiratory therapy of hyaline membrane disease: bronchopulmonary dysplasia. *N Engl J Med.* 1967;276:357–368.
45. Jobe AH. The new bronchopulmonary dysplasia: an arrest of lung development. *Pediatr Res.* 1999;46:641–643.
46. Coalson JJ. Pathology of new bronchopulmonary dysplasia. *Semin Neonatol.* 2003;8:73–81.
47. Truog WE. Chronic lung disease and randomized interventional trials: status in 2005. *Neoreviews.* 2005;6:e278.
48. Lal MK, Manktelow BN, Draper ES, et al. Chronic lung disease of prematurity and intrauterine growth retardation: a population based study. *Pediatrics.* 2003;111:483–488.
49. Peterson SW. Understanding the sequence of pulmonary injury in the extremely low birth weight, surfactant-deficient infant. *Neonatal Netw.* 2009;28:221–229.
50. Neerhof MG, Thaete LG. The fetal response to chronic placental insufficiency. *Semin Perinatol.* 2008;32:201–205.
51. Been JV, Rours IG, Kornelisse RF, et al. Histologic chorioamnionitis, fetal involvement, and antenatal steroids: effects on neonatal outcome in preterm infants. *Am J Obstet Gynecol.* 2009; 201:e581–e588.
52. Bhandari V. The potential of non-invasive ventilation to decrease BPD. *Semin Perinatol.* 2013;37:108–114.
53. Vendettuoli V, Bellu R, Zanini R, et al. Changes in ventilator strategies and outcomes in preterm infants. *Arch Dis Chld Fetal Neonatal Ed.* 2014;99:F321–F324.
54. Halliday HL, Ehrenkranz RA, Doyle LW. Moderately early (7–14 days) postnatal corticosteroids for preventing chronic lung disease in preterm infants. *Cochrane Database Syst Rev.* 2003:CD001144.
55. Watterberg KL. Policy statement—postnatal corticosteroids to prevent or treat bronchopulmonary dysplasia. *Pediatrics.* 2010;126:800–808.
56. National Institutes of Health. PREMILOC trial to prevent bronchopulmonary dysplasia in very preterm neonates. ClinicalTrials.gov. Identifier: NCT00623740. Available at: http://clinicaltrials.gov/show/NCT00623740. Accessed September 19, 2014.
57. Yeh TF, Lin HC, Chang CH, et al. Early intratracheal instillation of budesonide using surfactant as a vehicle to prevent chronic lung disease in preterm infants: a pilot study. *Pediatrics.* 2008;121:e1310–e1318.
58. Deakins KM. Bronchopulmonary dysplasia. *Respir Care.* 2009;54:1252–1262.
59. Impact-RSV Study Group. Palivizumab, a humanized respiratory syncytial virus monoclonal antibody, reduces hospitalization from respiratory syncytial virus infection in high-risk infants. *Pediatrics.* 1998;102:531–537.
60. Baker CD, Abman SH, Mourani PM. Pulmonary hypertension in preterm infants with bronchopulmonary dysplasia. *Pediatr Allergy Immunol Pulmonol.* 2014;27:8–16.
61. Papoff P, Cerasaro C, Caresta E, et al. Current strategies for treating infants with severe bronchopulmonary dysplasia. *J Matern Fetal Neonatal Med.* 2012;25(suppl 3):15–20.
62. Broughton S, Thomas MR, Marston L, et al. Very prematurely born infants wheezing at followup: lung function and risk factors. *Arch Dis Child.* 2007;92:776–780.
63. Doyle L, Faber B, Callanan C, et al. Bronchopulmonary dysplasia in very low birth weight subjects and lung function in adolescence. *Pediatrics.* 2006;118:108–113.
64. Walter E, Ehlenbach W, Hotchkin D, et al. Low birth weight and respiratory disease in adulthood. *Am J Respir Crit Care Med.* 2009;180:176–180.
65. Strueby L, Thebaud B. Advances in bronchopulmonary dysplasia. *Expert Rev Respir Med.* 2014;8:327–338.
66. Claure N, Bello JA, Jain D. Strategies to reduce mechanical ventilation and bronchopulmonary dysplasia in preterm infants. *Respir Care.* 2013;58:1257.
67. Brown MK, DiBlasi RM. Mechanical ventilation of the premature neonate. *Respir Care.* 2011;56:1298–1313.
68. Avery ME, Gatewood DB, Brumley G. Transient tachypnea of the newborn: possible delayed resorption of fluid at birth. *Am J Dis Child.* 1966;111:380–385.
69. Guglani L, Lakshminrusimha S, Ryan R. Transient tachypnea of the newborn. *Pediatr Rev.* 2008;29:e59–e65.

70. Barker PM, Olver RE. Invited review: clearance of lung liquid during the perinatal period. *J Appl Physiol.* 2002;93:1542–1548.
71. Jain L, Eaton DC. Physiology of fetal lung fluid clearance and the effect of labor. *Semin Perinatol.* 2006;30:34–43.
72. Riskin A, Abend-Weinger M, Riskin-Mashiah S, et al. Cesarean section, gestational age, and transient tachypnea of the newborn: timing is the key. *Am J Perinatol.* 2005;22:377–382.
73. Demissie K, Marcella SW, Breckenbridge MB, et al. Maternal asthma and transient tachypnea of the newborn. *Pediatrics.* 1998;102:84–90.
74. Jain L, Dudell GG. Respiratory transition in infants delivered by cesarean section. *Semin Perinatol.* 2006;30:296–304.
75. Weintraub AS, Cadet CT, Perez R, et al. Antibiotic use in newborns with transient tachypnea of the newborn. *Neonatology.* 2013;103:235–240.
76. Salama H, Abughalwa M, Taha S, et al. Transient tachypnea of the newborn: is empiric antimicrobial therapy needed? *J Neonatal Perinatal Med.* 2013;6:237–241.
77. Al Tawil K, Abu-Ekteish FM, Tamimi O, et al. Symptomatic spontaneous pneumothorax in term newborn infants. *Pediatr Pulmonol.* 2004;37:443–446.
78. Birnkrant DJ, Picone C, Markowitz W, et al. Association of transient tachypnea of the newborn and childhood asthma. *Pediatr Pulmonol.* 2006;41:978–984.
79. The United Nations Children's Fund/World Health Organization. *Pneumonia: The Forgotten Killer of Children.* 2006. Available at: http://www.unicef.org/publications/files/Pneumonia_The_Forgotten_Killer_of_Children.pdf. Accessed September 19, 2014.
80. Haney PJ, Bohlman M, Sun CC. Radiographic findings in neonatal pneumonia. *Am J Roentgenol.* 1984;143:23–26.
81. Committee on Infectious Diseases and Committee on Fetus and Newborn. Recommendations for the prevention of perinatal group b streptococcal (GBS) disease. *Pediatrics.* 2011;128:1–6.
82. Schrag S, Gorwitz R, Fultz-Butts K, et al. Prevention of perinatal group B streptococcal disease. *Morb Mortal Wkly Rep.* 2002;51:1–22.
83. Oh W. Early onset neonatal group B streptococcal sepsis. *Am J Perinatol.* 2013;30:143–147.
84. Velaphi S, Vidyasagar D. Intrapartum and postdelivery management of infants born to mothers with meconium-stained amniotic fluid: evidence-based recommendations. *Clin Perinatol.* 2006;33:29–42.
85. Walsh MC, Fanaroff JM. Meconium stained fluid: approach to the mother and the baby. *Clin Perinatol.* 2007;34:653–665.
86. Yoder BA, Kirsch EA, Barth WH, et al. Changing obstetric practices associated with decreasing incidence of meconium aspiration syndrome. *Obstet Gynecol.* 2002;99:731–739.
87. Gelfand SL, Fanaroff JM, Walsh MC. Controversies in the treatment of meconium aspiration syndrome. *Clin Perinatol.* 2004;31:445–452.
88. Vain NE, Szyld EG, Prudent LM, et al. Oropharyngeal and nasopharyngeal suctioning of meconium-stained neonates before delivery of their shoulders: multicenter, randomized controlled trial. *Lancet.* 2004;364:597–602.
89. Wiswell TE, Gannon CM, Jacob J, et al. Delivery room management of the apparently vigorous meconium-stained neonate: results of the multicenter, international collaborative trial. *Pediatrics.* 2000;105:1–7.
90. ACOG Committee on Obstetric Practice. ACOG Committee Opinion No. 379. Management of delivery of a newborn with meconium-stained amniotic fluid. *Obstet Gynecol.* 2007;110:739.
91. Choi HJ, Hahn S, Lee J, et al. Surfactant lavage therapy for meconium aspiration syndrome: a systematic review and meta-analysis. *Neonatology.* 2012;101:183–191.
92. Kinsella JP. Meconium aspiration syndrome. Is surfactant lavage the answer? *Am J Respir Crit Care Med.* 2003;168:413–414.
93. Mokra D, Mokry J, Tonhajzerova I. Anti-inflammatory treatment of meconium aspiration syndrome: benefits and risks. *Respir Physiol Neurobiol.* 2013:187;52–57.
94. Mikolka P, Mokra D, Kopincova J, et al. Budesonide added to modified porcine surfactant Curosurf may additionally improve the lung functions in meconium aspiration syndrome. *Physiol Res.* 2013;62(suppl 1):S191–S200.
95. Mokra D, Calkovska A. How to overcome surfactant dysfunction in meconium aspiration syndrome? *Respir Physiol Neurobiol.* 2013;187:58–63.
96. Hahn S, Choi HJ, Soll R, et al. Lung lavage for meconium aspiration syndrome in newborn infants. *Cochrane Database Syst Rev.* 2013;4:CD003486.
97. Hamutcu R, Nield TA, Garg M, et al. Long-term pulmonary sequelae in children who were treated with extracorporeal membrane oxygenation for neonatal respiratory failure. *Pediatrics.* 2004;114:1292–1296.
98. Lin HC, Su BH, Lin TW, et al. Risk factors of mortality in meconium aspiration syndrome: review of 314 cases. *Acta Paediatr Taiwan.* 2004;45:30–34.
99. Beligere N, Rao R. Neurodevelopmental outcome of infants with meconium aspiration syndrome: report of a study and literature review. *J Perinatol.* 2008;28(suppl 3):S93–S101.
100. Singh BS, Clark RH, Powers RJ. Meconium aspiration syndrome remains a significant problem in the NICU: outcomes and treatment patterns in term neonates admitted for intensive care during a ten-year period. *J Perinatol.* 2009;29:497–503.
101. Nair J, Lakshminrusimha S. Update on PPHN: mechanisms and treatment. *Semin Perinatol.* 2014;38:78–91.
102. Dakshinamurti S. Pathophysiologic mechanisms of persistent pulmonary hypertension of the newborn. *Paediatr Pulmonol* 2005;39:492–503.
103. Hernandez-Diaz S, Van Marter LJ, Werler MM, et al. Risk factors for persistent pulmonary hypertension of the newborn. *Pediatrics.* 2007;120:e272–e282.
104. Ostrea EM, Villanueva-Uy ET, Natarajan G, et al. Persistent pulmonary hypertension of the newborn: pathogenesis, etiology, and management. *Paediatr Drugs.* 2006;8:179–188.
105. Delaney C, Cornfield DN. Risk factors for persistent pulmonary hypertension of the newborn. *Pulm Circ.* 2012;2:15–20.
106. Jaillard S, Houfflin-Debarge V, Storme L. Higher risk of persistent pulmonary hypertension of the newborn after cesarean. *J Perinat Med.* 2003;31:538–539.
107. Teng RJ, Wu TJ. Persistent pulmonary hypertension of the newborn. *J Formos Med Assoc.* 2013;112:177–184.
108. Puthiyachirakkal M, Mhanna MJ. Pathophysiology, management, and outcome of persistent pulmonary hypertension of the newborn: a clinical review. *Front Pediatr.* 2013;1:23.
109. Sasidharan P. An approach to diagnosis and management of cyanosis and tachypnea in term infants. *Pediatr Clin North Am.* 2004;51:999–1021.
110. Konduri GG, Kim UO. Advances in the diagnosis and management of persistent pulmonary hypertension of the newborn. *Pediatr Clin North Am.* 2009;56:579–600.
111. Boden G, Bennett C. The management of persistent pulmonary hypertension of the newborn. *Curr Paediatr.* 2004;14:290–297.
112. American Academy of Pediatrics, Committee on Fetus and Newborn. Use of inhaled nitric oxide. *Pediatrics.* 2000;106:344–345.
113. Steinhorn RH. Nitric oxide and beyond: new insights and therapies for pulmonary hypertension. *J Perinatol.* 2008;28(suppl 3):S67–S71.
114. Shah PS, Ohlsson A. Sildenafil for pulmonary hypertension in neonates. *Cochrane Database Syst Rev.* 2011;8:CD005494.
115. Yaseen H, Darwich M, Hamdy H. Is sildenafil an effective therapy in the management of persistent pulmonary hypertension? *J Clin Neonatol.* 2012;1:171–175.
116. Samiee-Zafarghandy S, Smith PB, van den Anker JN. Safety of sildenafil in infants. *Pediatr Crit Care Med.* 2014;15:362–368.
117. Mohammed WA, Ismail M. A randomized, double-blind, placebo-controlled, prospective study of bosentan for the treatment of persistent pulmonary hypertension of the newborn. *J Perinatol.* 2012;32:608–613.
118. Betit P, Craig N. Extracorporeal membrane oxygenation for neonatal respiratory failure. *Respir Care.* 2009;54:1244–1251.

119. Slevin M, Farrington N, Duffy G, et al. Altering the NICU and measuring the infants' responses. *Acta Paediatrica.* 2007;89:577–581.
120. Clugston RD, Greer JJ. Diaphragm development and congenital diaphragmatic hernia. *Semin Pediatr Surg.* 2007;16:94–100.
121. Rottier R, Tibboel D. Fetal lung and diaphragm development in congenital diaphragmatic hernia. *Semin Perinatol.* 2005;29:86–93.
122. Al-Salem AH, Zamakhshary M, Al Mohaidly M, et al. Congenital Morgagni's hernia: a national multicenter study. *J Pediatr Surg.* 2014;49:503–507.
123. Bohn D. Congenital diaphragmatic hernia. *Am J Respir Crit Care Med.* 2002;166:911–915.
124. Chess PR. The effect of gentle ventilation on survival in congenital diaphragmatic hernia. *Pediatrics.* 2004;113:917.
125. Logan J, Cotten CM, Goldberg RN, et al. Mechanical ventilation strategies in the management of congenital diaphragmatic hernia. *Semin Pediatr Surg.* 2007;16:115–125.
126. Garcia A, Stolar CJ. Congenital diaphragmatic hernia and protective ventilation strategies in pediatric surgery. *Surg Clin North Am.* 2012;92:659–668.
127. Van den Hout L, Tibboel D, Vijfhuize S, et al. The VICI-trial: high frequency oscillation versus conventional mechanical ventilation in newborns with congenital diaphragmatic hernia: an international multicenter randomized controlled trial. *BMC Pediatr.* 2011;11:98.
128. Finer NN, Barrington KJ. Nitric oxide for respiratory failure in infants born at or near term. *Cochrane Database Syst Rev.* 2001;4:CD000399.
129. Bryner BS, West BT, Hirschl RB, et al. Congenital diaphragmatic hernia requiring extracorporeal membrane oxygenation: does timing of repair matter? *J Pediatr Surg.* 2009;44:1165–1171.
130. Datin-Dorriere V, Walter-Nicolet E, Rousseau V, et al. Experience in the management of eighty-two newborns with congenital diaphragmatic hernia treated with high-frequency oscillatory ventilation and delayed surgery without the use of extracorporeal membrane oxygenation. *J Intensive Care Med.* 2008;23:128–135.
131. Bosenberg AT, Brown RA. Management of congenital diaphragmatic hernia. *Curr Opin Anaesthesiol.* 2008;21:323–331.
132. Badillo A, Gingalewski C. Congenital diaphragmatic hernia: treatment and outcomes. *Semin Perinatol.* 2014;38:92–96.
133. Gucciardo L, Deprest J, Done E, et al. Prediction of outcome in isolated congenital diaphragmatic hernia and its consequences for fetal therapy. *Best Pract Res Clin Obstet Gynaecol.* 2008;22:123–138.
134. Chiu PP, Sauer C, Mihailovic A. The price of success in the management of congenital diaphragmatic hernia: is improved survival accompanied by an increase in long-term morbidity? *J Pediatr Surg.* 2006;41:888–892.
135. Boyden EA. Developmental anomalies of the lungs. *Am J Surg.* 1955;89:79–89.
136. Abrams ME, Ackerman VL, Engle WA. Primary unilateral pulmonary hypoplasia: neonate through early childhood—case report, radiographic diagnosis and review of the literature. *J Perinatol.* 2004;24:667–670.
137. Hsu JS, Lee YS, Lin CH, et al. Primary congenital pulmonary hypoplasia of a neonate. *J Chin Med Assoc.* 2012;75:87–90.
138. Fitoz S, Ucar T, Erden A, et al. DiGeorge syndrome associated with left lung aplasia. *Br J Radiol.* 2001;74:764–766.
139. Khurram MS, Rao SP, Vamshipriya A. Pulmonary agenesis: a case report with review of literature. *Qatar Med J.* 2013;2013:38–40.
140. Russell BC, Whitecar P, Nitsche JF. Isolated unilateral pulmonary agenesis and other fetal thoracic anomalies. *Obstet Gynecol Surv.* 2014;69:335–345.
141. Shanti CM, Klein MD. Cystic lung disease. *Semin Pediatr Surg.* 2008;17:2–8.
142. Azizkhan RG, Crombleholme TM. Congenital cystic lung disease: contemporary antenatal and postnatal management. *Pediatr Surg Int.* 2008;24:643–657.
143. Sanli A, Onen A, Ceylan E, et al. A case of a bronchogenic cyst in a rare location. *Ann Thorac Surg.* 2004;77:1093–1094.
144. Levine D, Jennings R, Barnewolt C, et al. Progressive fetal bronchial obstruction caused by a bronchogenic cyst diagnosed using prenatal MR imaging. *AJR. Am J Roentgenol.* 2001;176:49–52.
145. Shah DS, Lala R, Rajegowda B, et al. Bronchogenic cyst and its progress in a premature infant. *J Perinatol.* 1999;19:150–152.
146. Corbett HJ, Humphrey GM. Pulmonary sequestration. *Paediatr Respir Rev.* 2004;5:59–68.
147. Paterson A. Imaging evaluation of congenital lung abnormalities in infants and children. *Radiol Clin North Am.* 2005;43:303–323.
148. Mirosh MD, Hayes B, Payton N. 187 risk factors associated with respiratory distress in term neonates with and without air leak. *Pediatr Res.* 2004;56:496.
149. Carlo WA. Permissive hypercapnia and permissive hypoxemia in neonates. *J Perinatol.* 2007;27(suppl 1):S64–S70.
150. Watkinson M, Tiron I. Events before the diagnosis of a pneumothorax. *Arch Dis Child Fetal Neonatal Ed.* 2001;85:F201–F203.
151. Litmanovitz I, Carlo W. Expectant management of pneumothorax in ventilated neonates. *Pediatrics.* 2008;122:e975–e979.
152. Phatak RS, Pairaudeau CF, Smith CJ, et al. Heliox with inhaled nitric oxide: a novel strategy for severe localized interstitial pulmonary emphysema in preterm neonatal ventilation. *Respir Care.* 2008;53:1731–1738.
153. Jabra AA, Fishman EK, Shehata BM, Perlman EJ. Localized persistent pulmonary interstitial emphysema: CT findings with radiographic-pathologic correlation. *Am J Roentgenol.* 1997;169:1381–1384.
154. Clark RH, Gerstman DR, Null DM, et al. Pulmonary interstitial emphysema treated by high frequency oscillatory ventilation. *Crit Care Med.* 1986;14:926–930.
155. Schwartz AN, Graham CB. Neonatal tension pulmonary interstitial emphysema in bronchopulmonary dysplasia: treatment with lateral decubitus positioning. *Radiology.* 1986;16:351–354.
156. Chalek LF, Kaiser JR, Arrington RW. Resolution of pulmonary interstitial emphysema following selective left main stem intubation in a premature newborn: an old procedure revisited. *Paediatr Anesth.* 2007;17:183–186.
157. Fitzgerald D, Willis D, Usher R. Dexamethasone for pulmonary interstitial emphysema in preterm infants. *Biol Neonate.* 1998;73:34–39.
158. Bejvan SM, Godwin JD. Pneumomediastinum: old signs and new signs. *Am J Roentgenol.* 1996;166:1041–1048.
159. Carey BE. Neonatal air leaks: pneumothorax, pneumomediastinum, pulmonary interstitial emphysema, pneumopericardium. *Neonatal Netw.* 1999;18:81–84.
160. National Eye Institute. Retinopathy of prematurity. Available at: http://www.nei.nih.gov/health/rop/. Accessed September 19, 2014.
161. Terry TL. Extreme prematurity and fibroplastic overgrowth of persistent vascular sheath behind each crystalline lens. Preliminary report. *Am J Ophthalmol.* 1942;25:203–204.
162. Campbell K. Intensive oxygen therapy as a possible cause for retrolental fibroplasia: a clinical approach. *Med J Austr.* 1951;2:48–50.
163. Patz A, Hoeck L, DeLaCruz E. Studies on the effect of high oxygen administration in retrolental fibroplasia: nursery observations. *Am J Ophthalmol.* 1952;35:1248–1253.
164. Wheatley CM, Dickinson JL, Mackey DA, et al. Retinopathy of prematurity: recent advances in our understanding. *Arch Dis Child Fetal Neonatal Ed.* 2002;87:F78–F82.
165. Forrester JV, Dick AD, McMenamin PG, et al. Embryology and early development of the eye and adnexa. In: Forrester JV, Dick AD, McMenamin PG, et al., eds. *The Eye: Basic Sciences in Practice.* Philadelphia: Elsevier; 2002:99–113.
166. Holmstrom G, van Wijngaarden P, Coster DJ, et al. Genetic susceptibility to retinopathy of prematurity: the evidence from clinical and experimental animal studies. *Br J Ophthalmol.* 2007;91:1704–1708.
167. Karna P, Muttineni J, Angell L, et al. Retinopathy of prematurity and risk factors: a prospective cohort study. *BMC Pediatr.* 2007;26:371–378.
168. Harrell SN, Brandon DH. Retinopathy of prematurity: the disease process, classifications, screening, treatment, and outcomes. *Neonatal Netw.* 2007;26:371–378.

169. Section on Ophthalmology, American Academy of Pediatrics; American Academy of Ophthalmology; American Association for Pediatric Ophthalmology and Strabismus. Screening examination of premature infants for retinopathy of prematurity. *Pediatrics.* 2006;572–576.
170. International Committee for the Classification of Retinopathy of Prematurity. The international classification of retinopathy of prematurity revisited. *Arch Ophthalmol.* 2005;123:991–999.
171. DiBiasie A. Evidence-based review of retinopathy of prematurity prevention in VLBW and ELBW infants. *Neonatal Netw.* 2006;25:393–403.
172. Quiram PA, Capone A Jr. Current understanding and management of retinopathy of prematurity. *Curr Opin Ophthalmol.* 2007;18:228–234.
173. Good WV, Hardy RJ, Dobson V, et al. The incidence and course of retinopathy of prematurity: findings from the early treatment for retinopathy of prematurity study. *Pediatrics.* 2005;116:15–23.
174. Mullins JA, Lamonte AC, Bresee JS, et al. Substantial variability in community respiratory syncytial virus season timing. *Pediatr Infect Dis J.* 2003;22:857–862.
175. Hall CB. Respiratory syncytial virus and parainfluenza virus. *N Engl J Med.* 2001;344:1917–1928.
176. Zorc JJ, Hall CB. Bronchiolitis: recent evidence on diagnosis and management. *Pediatrics.* 2010;125:342–349.
177. Karr CJ, Demers PA, Koehoorn MW, et al. Influence of ambient air pollutant sources on clinical encounters for infant bronchiolitis. *Am J Respir Crit Care Med.* 2009;180:995–1001.
178. American Academy of Pediatrics, Subcommittee on Diagnosis and Management of Bronchiolitis. Clinical practice guidelines: diagnosis and management of bronchiolitis. *Pediatrics.* 2006;118:1774–1793.
179. Mittal V, Darnell C, Walsh B, et al. Inpatient bronchiolitis guideline implementation and resource utilization. *Pediatrics.* 2014;133:e730–e737.
180. Milesi C, Baleine J, Matecki S, et al. Is treatment with a high flow nasal cannula effective in acute viral bronchiolitis? A physiologic study. *Intensive Care Med.* 2013;39:1088–1094.
181. Davison C, Ventre KM, Luchetti M, et al. Efficacy of interventions for bronchiolitis in critically ill infants: a systematic review and meta-analysis. *Pediatr Crit Care Med.* 2004;5:482–489.
182. Kuzik BA, Al Quadhi SA, Kent S, et al. Nebulized hypertonic saline in the treatment of viral bronchiolitis. *J Pediatr.* 2007;151:266–270.
183. Taber LH, Knight V, Gilbert BE, et al. Ribavirin aerosol treatment of bronchiolitis associated with respiratory syncytial virus infection in infants. *Pediatrics.* 1983;72:613–618.
184. Committee on Infectious Diseases and Bronchiolitis Guidelines Committee. Updated guidance for Palivizumab prophylaxis among infants and young children at increased risk of hospitalization for respiratory syncytial virus infection. *Pediatrics.* 2014;134:415–420.
185. Stein RT. Early-life viral bronchiolitis in the causal pathway of childhood asthma: is the evidence there yet? *Am J Respir Crit Care Med.* 2008;178:1097–1098.
186. Jartti T, Makela MJ, Vanto T, et al. The link between bronchiolitis and asthma. *Infect Dis Clin North Am.* 2005;19:667–689.
187. Sobol SE, Zapata S. Epiglottitis and croup. *Otolaryngol Clin North Am.* 2008;41:551–566.
188. Rotta AT, Wiryawan B. Respiratory emergencies in children. *Respir Care.* 2003;48:248–260.
189. Petrocheilou A, Tanou K, Kalampouka E, et al. Viral croup: diagnosis and a treatment algorithm. *Pediatr Pulmonol.* 2014;49:421–429.
190. Lavine E. Scolnik D. Lack of efficacy of humidification in the treatment of croup: why do physicians persist in using an unproven modality? *CJEM.* 2001;3:209–212.
191. Bjornson C, Russell KF, Vandermeer B, et al. Nebulized epinephrine for croup in children. *Cochrane Database Syst Rev.* 2011;CD006619.
192. Myers TR. Use of heliox in children. *Respir Care.* 2006;51:619–631.
193. Custer JR. Croup and related disorders. *Pediatr Rev.* 1993;14:19–29.
194. Tibbals J, Watson T. Symptoms and signs differentiating croup and epiglottitis. *J Paediatr Child Health.* 2011;47:77–82.
195. Glynn F, Fenton JE. Diagnosis and management of supraglottitis (epiglottitis). *Curr Infect Dis Rep.* 2008;10:200–204.
196. Centers for Disease Control and Prevention. Progress toward eliminating Haemophilus influenza type b disease among infants and children – United States, 1977-1997. *Morbid Mortal Wkly Rep.* 1998;47:993–998.

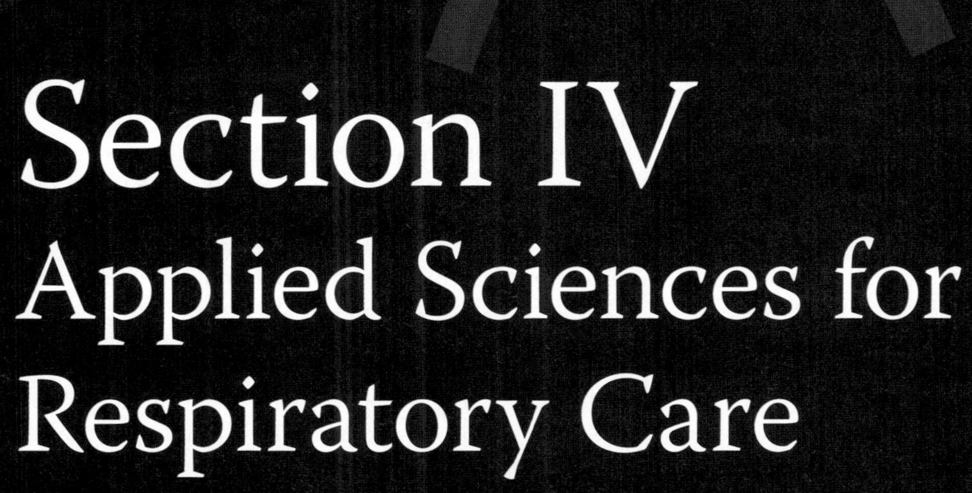

Section IV
Applied Sciences for Respiratory Care

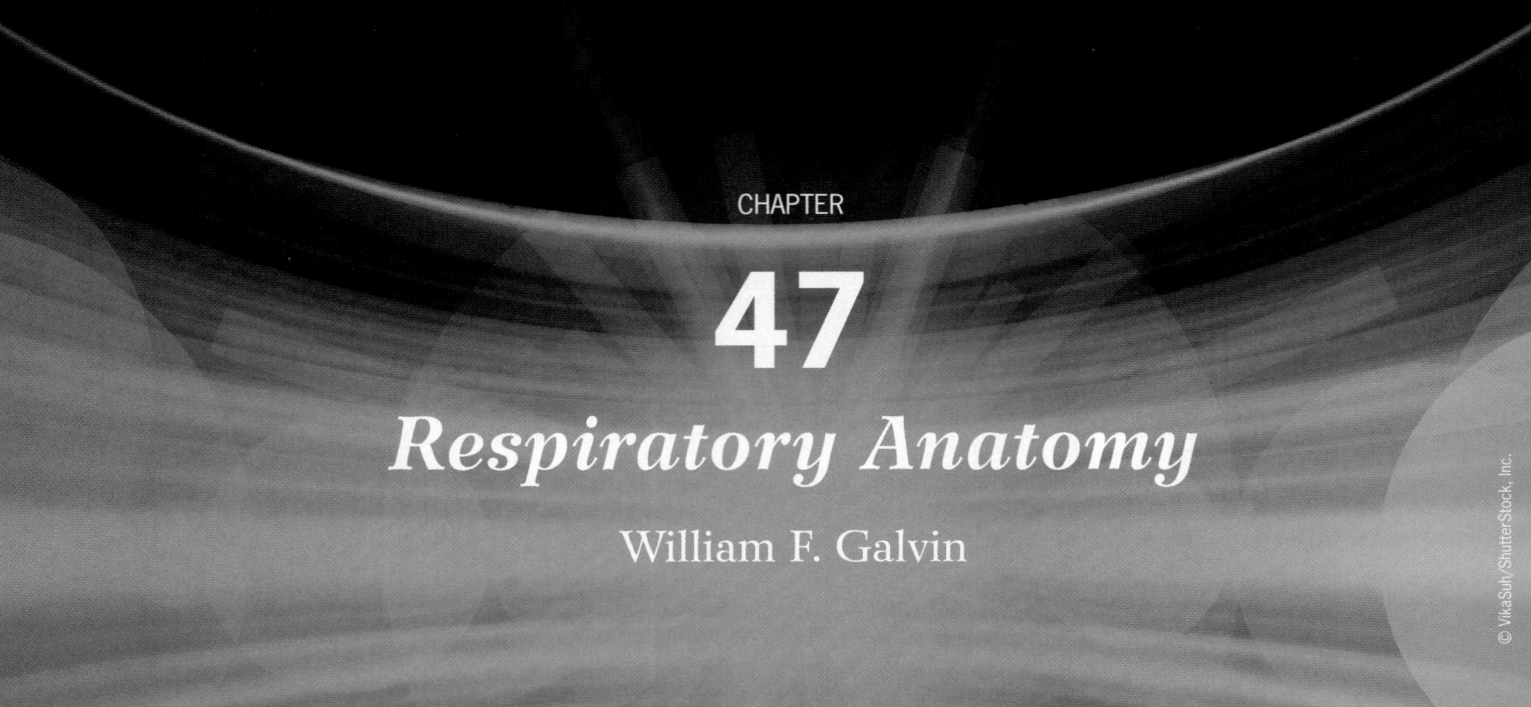

OUTLINE

Growth and Development of the Respiratory System
Gross Anatomy of the Respiratory System
Anatomy of the Thorax
Microanatomy of the Respiratory System

OBJECTIVES

1. Explain the purpose of the respiratory system.
2. List and briefly explain the five stages of fetal development.
3. Describe key changes in the transition from prenatal to postnatal development.
4. Describe the gross anatomy of the respiratory system.
5. Describe the anatomy of the upper airway.
6. Describe the anatomy of the lower airway.
7. Discuss the relationship between the bony elements of the thorax.
8. Identify and explain the roles of the diaphragm, accessory inspiratory muscles, and abdominal muscles.
9. Describe the visceral pleura, parietal pleura, and pleural space.
10. Describe the microanatomy of the respiratory system.
11. Describe the mucociliary apparatus.
12. Describe the smooth muscle function of the airways.
13. Compare macrophages and dendritic cells found in the respiratory system.
14. Compare alveolar type I and type II cells.
15. Describe the interstitial space in the lungs.

KEY TERMS

abdominal muscle
accessory muscle
acinus
alveolar stage
alveolus
bronchus
canalicular stage
carina
channels of Lambert
concha
dendritic cell
diaphragm
embryonic stage
epiglottis
glottis or glottic opening
hilum
laryngopharynx
larynx
lobe
macrophage
mast cell
mediastinum
mucociliary apparatus
nasopharynx
oropharynx
parietal pleura
pericardium
phrenic nerve
pleural space
pores of Kohn
pseudoglandular stage
saccular stage
segment
senescence
thorax
trachea
type I cell
type II cell
visceral pleura
work of breathing

Introduction

A thorough understanding of the growth and development of the human lung is fundamental and indispensable to the respiratory therapist. It is virtually impossible to gain an appreciation of the physiology of the lung and the pathophysiology of respiratory diseases without first knowing the anatomy of the respiratory system. One must first know the parts (anatomy) and their function (physiology) before understanding abnormalities associated with respiratory diseases (pathophysiology).

The respiratory system is a gas exchanger as well as a gas distributor. Gas exchange is respiration and respiration comprises five distinct processes: ventilation, perfusion, diffusion, external respiration, and internal respiration. Ventilation is the movement of air from the atmosphere to the lung. Perfusion entails the movement (or circulation) of blood through the cardiovascular system. Diffusion is the movement of gases (oxygen and carbon dioxide) from a relatively high pressure to a low pressure across the alveolocapillary membrane. External respiration is gas exchange at the interface of the **alveoli** and the blood, and internal respiration is gas exchange at the interface of the blood and the tissues.

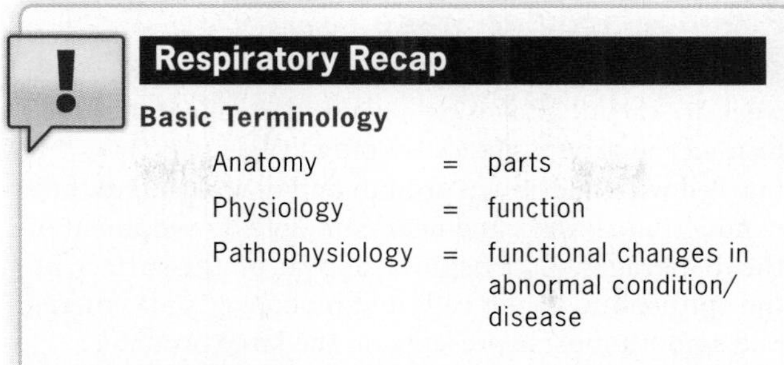

Respiratory Recap

Basic Terminology

Anatomy	=	parts
Physiology	=	function
Pathophysiology	=	functional changes in abnormal condition/ disease

Gas exchange occurs exclusively at the **acinus** or alveolar level, the functioning portion of the lung located at the very end of the respiratory tract.

Gas distribution represents the other major purpose and entails gas traversing the pathways of the upper airway as well as the conducting airways of the lower respiratory tract. Identifying the components of the respiratory system and understanding their function are essential concepts to understand. This chapter focuses on the individual components and the normal development of the respiratory system. It provides a general overview of this growth and development from the earliest stage of conception, a fetus, to the fully functioning stage of adult. In addition, it addresses the gross anatomy and microanatomy of the lung as well as the anatomy of the thorax.

Growth and Development of the Respiratory System

The growth and development of the respiratory system is a remarkable event evolving from embryo, to fetus, to neonate, to infant, to child, to adolescent, through adulthood, and finally to the elderly state of **senescence** when function begins to diminish and eventually declines to death. This evolution begins at conception with the fertilization of a single cell that grows and develops progressively and proportionately into a fully functioning organ. It transitions from the microscopic to the macroscopic, entailing a single bud at the beginning of the embryonic stage, to a developing infant consisting of some 50 million alveoli, to a fully developed adult with a surface area of approximately 70 m^2 and 300 million alveoli. Degeneration begins later in life during senescence (old age) and continues until death. The life stages of development are noted in **Table 47-1**.

TABLE 47-1
Life Stages of Development

Life Stage	Period
Embryo	Conception to end of eighth week of gestation
Fetus	Week nine of gestation to birth
Neonate	Birth to end of week 4
Infant	End of week 4 to 1 year
Child	1 year to puberty
Adolescent	Puberty to adulthood
Adult	Approximately 18 years to old age
Senescence	Old age to death

Respiratory Recap

Key Respiratory Concepts

Ventilation	=	movement of air from atmosphere to the lung
Perfusion	=	movement or circulation of blood
Diffusion	=	movement of gas across the alveolocapillary membrane
Respiration	=	gas exchange
External respiration	=	gas exchange between alveoli and blood
Internal respiration	=	gas exchange between blood and tissues

Prenatal Development

The prenatal period begins with fertilization and ends with birth. The time spent in prenatal development is called gestation, and gestation entails growth (increase in size and number of newly formed cells) as well as development (continuous process of change from one life phase to another). Prenatal development is often expressed in terms of lung stages, gestational age, and developmental events. **Table 47-2** represents the five stages of lung development as well as the corresponding gestational age and significant developmental events. **Figure 47-1** provides a visual illustration of these significant events.

Embryonic Stage

The first period of lung development exists for approximately 2 months and is called the **embryonic stage**. It entails primitive development of the lung. It begins at approximately 21 days after conception with the formation of a lung bud that emerges from the foregut, an out-pouching of the pharynx. The lung bud elongates forming the trachea and two bronchial buds that go on to become the mainstem bronchi. The pharynx evolves to become the esophagus, and the mainstem bronchi

TABLE 47-2
Stages of Lung Development, Approximate Gestational Age, and Significant Developmental Events

Stage	Gestational Age	Significant Developmental Events
Embryonic	4–6 weeks	Development of proximal airways (trachea and major bronchi, early formation of segmental bronchi)
Pseudoglandular	6–16 weeks	Development of conducting airways (smooth muscle, cilia, mucous glands, goblet cells, and respiratory bronchioles)
Canalicular	17–26 weeks	Development of vascular bed and framework of respiratory acini
Saccular	27–36 weeks	Development of gas exchange units (presence of surfactant and early development of alveoli)
Alveolar	36–beyond birth	Rapid alveolar development (increase in size and number)

evolve to form lobar bronchi and finally remnants of segmental bronchi. Simultaneously, three germ layers evolve and give rise to eventual formation of respiratory epithelium, pulmonary interstitium, smooth muscle, blood vessels, and cartilage. **Figure 47-2** illustrates lung development from week 4 through week 8.

Pseudoglandular Stage

Starting around the sixth week and extending through week 16, the lung takes on a glandular appearance termed the **pseudoglandular stage.** This stage is marked with continued growth and development of the conducting airways and near complete development of the diaphragm. Cilia begin to appear on the surface of the epithelium, goblet cells and mucous glands emerge, and smooth muscle presents on the large bronchi. Survival at this stage of development is highly unlikely.

Canalicular Stage

The **canalicular stage** represents the third stage of lung development and extends from approximately week 17 through week 26. It is so named because of the connotation to canals or channels, signifying the formation of capillary network around the air passages. Additionally, this stage reflects the appearance of type I and type II alveolar cells giving rise to development of the alveolo-capillary membrane as well as the production of surfactant. This is quite significant as limited gas exchange becomes possible and thus a prematurely born fetus is capable of extrauterine survival at this stage if provided intensive and advanced medical care.

Saccular Stage

The fourth stage of lung development is the **saccular stage**. The hallmark of this stage is a marked increase in the potential gas-exchanging surface area of the lung. It is so named because the terminal structures of the airways develop into saccules, which eventually become alveoli.

Alveolar Stage

The final stage of lung development is called the **alveolar stage.** It is marked by significant alveolar maturation and proliferation. The estimated number of alveoli ranges from 20 to 150 million with an average of approximately 50 million at birth. This number will reach its peak at about 300 million by age 8, which

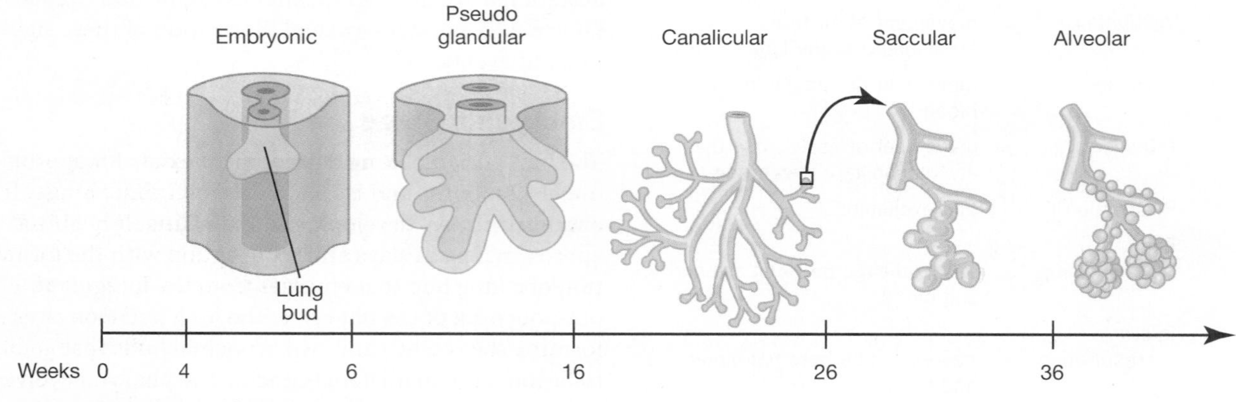

FIGURE 47-1 Stages of development.

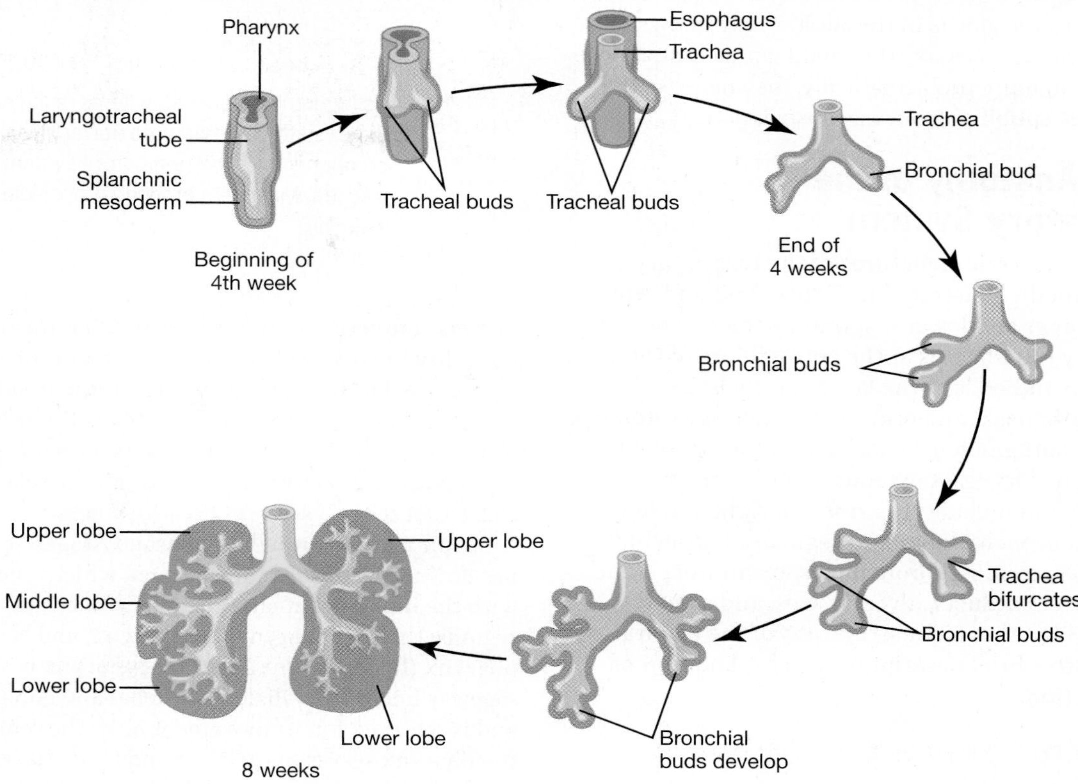

FIGURE 47-2 Lung development, week 4 through week 8.

is when alveolar development is considered complete. While completely developed, the fluid-filled nature of the lung precludes its ability to function in a gas-exchanging capacity.

Postnatal Lung Development

While the postnatal period theoretically extends from birth until death, this section highlights the significant developmental events that occur at the time of birth as well as the major differences between infants/children and adults. Subsequent sections of this chapter address the gross anatomy and microanatomy of the adult lungs and adult thorax.

Prior to the first breath, the infant lung is fluid-filled. Throughout gestation, fluid maintains lung expansion and facilitates pulmonary growth. This fluid is constantly replenished at a rate of approximately 250 to 300 mL per day and continuously flows to the oropharynx where it is swallowed or expelled into the amniotic fluid. While the body applies various mechanisms to reduce and clear lung fluid at the time of birth, an infant's first breath must be deep and forceful; an exceedingly high transpulmonary pressure gradient is required to open and replace the remaining lung fluid. This pressure gradient varies; however, reports estimate that approximately 40 to 80 cm H_2O pressure and a volume of approximately 40 mL are needed to overcome the surface tension of the alveoli and the viscosity of the remaining lung fluid. Subsequent breaths require a lower transpulmonary pressure as more and more alveoli remain inflated after each successive breath. In the normal term infant, fluid removal to the interstitial space is complete within several breaths, although it may take several hours to remove excess fluid from the interstitial space by means of the capillaries and lymphatics.

> **Respiratory Recap**
>
> **Five Stages of Lung Development**
>
> - Embryonic
> - Pseudoglanduar
> - Canalicular
> - Saccular
> - Alveolar

In addition to the replacement of fluid with air within the lung of the newborn, other anatomic differences exist between the infant/child and the adult. The head and the upper airway of the infant are significantly different compared to the adult. The infant' s head is larger and heavier relative to the size of its body, the nasal passages are proportionately smaller than that of the adult, and the tongue much larger relative to the size of the oral cavity. The infant's jaw is much rounder, the larynx positioned higher in the neck, and the cricoid ring is the narrowest portion of the upper airway compared to the glottis in the adult. Many of these anatomic variations make the infant a preferential nose breather but, more problematically, they increase the infant's susceptibility to airway obstruction.

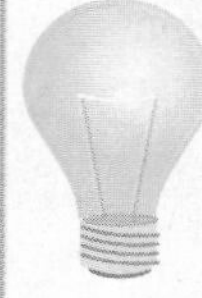

STOP AND THINK

Using common everyday items, such as a dime, a straw, or a coffee stirrer, illustrate the components of the respiratory system: the trachea, mainstem bronchi, bronchioles, and alveoli.

Gross Anatomy of the Respiratory System

The gross anatomic structures of the respiratory system are broadly illustrated in **Figure 47-3** and represent the upper and lower respiratory tracts. The upper respiratory tract begins at the entry points of the nose and mouth and ends at the larynx. It includes the nose, mouth, nasal and oral cavities, pharynx, tongue, epiglottis, soft and hard palates, and the larynx. The lower respiratory tract extends from the trachea to the alveoli and includes the trachea, right and left main stem bronchi, lobar and segmental bronchi, bronchioles, terminal bronchioles, respiratory bronchioles, alveolar ducts, alveolar sacs, and alveoli. **Table 47-3** list the major structures of the respiratory system with a brief description and explanation of their function.

Upper Respiratory Tract

The air conditioning and filtering goals of the upper airway begin the moment air enters the upper respiratory tract (**Figure 47-4**). Primary entry is through two external openings in the nose called nostrils or external nares. The nostrils open into the nasal cavity, which is comprised of bone and cartilage. Mucus-coated epithelial membranes line the cavities and this mucus-secreting epithelium is called the respiratory mucosa. The nasal **conchae**, also known as turbinates, are bony ridges that laterally project into the nasal cavity. The main function of this area is to filter, warm, and humidify the inspired air. The frontal and sphenoid sinuses are located above (superior to the nasal cavity) while the hard and soft palate lie below (inferior to the nasal cavity). Within the cavity, sensory neurons allow smell (via the olfactory nerve) and initiate reflexes that cause sneezes or a sense of breathlessness.

As air travels through the nasal passages, it continues downward toward the pharynx, which combines with the inner ear canals. The pharynx has three regions: the nasopharynx, oropharynx, and laryngopharynx (hypopharynx). The **nasopharynx** is a passageway lined with ciliated epithelial and goblet cells and is reserved for air movement only; the remainder of the pharynx serves to carry air and food. The **oropharynx** is distal to the mouth and is lined with stratified squamous epithelium that is continuous with the oral cavity. Tonsils are two masses in the back of the throat. Adenoids are a single pharyngeal tonsil located high in the throat behind the nose and the roof of the mouth (soft palate) and are not visible through the mouth. The uvula is the visible projection of the middle of the soft palate—easily seen in an open mouth. Enlargement of these structures may impede breathing, especially during sleep. The **laryngopharynx** is the most inferior

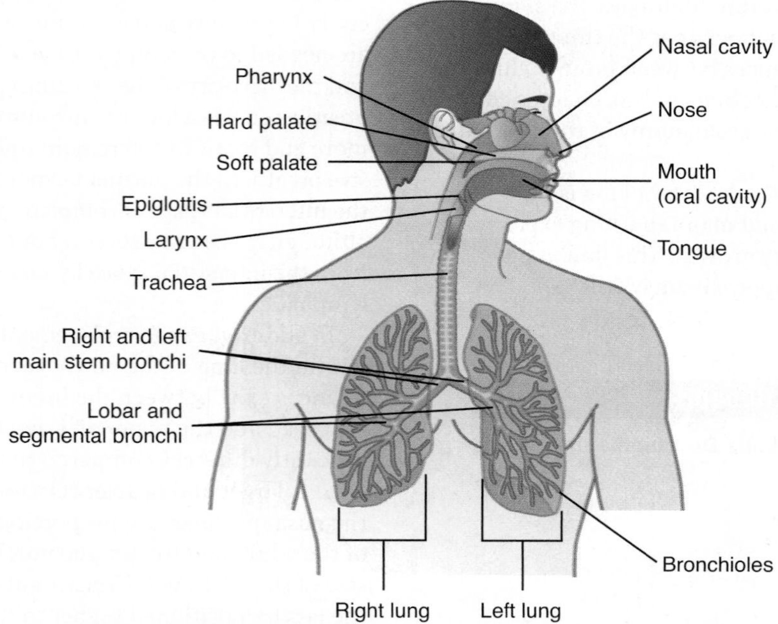

FIGURE 47-3 Anatomy of the respiratory system. Highlights of upper respiratory tract, lower respiratory tract, and alveolar sacs.

TABLE 47-3
Major Components of the Respiratory System

Component	Description	Function
Nose	Centered above the mouth as well as inside and below the space between the eyes	Contains the nostrils, which provide entrances to the nasal cavity
Nasal cavity	Hollow space behind the nose	Transports air to the pharynx; it filters, warms, and moistens air
Oral cavity	The mouth cavity, containing the teeth, tongue, salivary glands, etc.	Allows passage of air and food; transports air to the pharynx as well as warming and moistening it; aids in the production of vocal sounds
Paranasal sinuses	Hollow spaces in certain skull bones	Serve as resonant chambers; they also help to reduce the weight of the skull
Pharynx	A chamber located behind the nasal cavity, oral cavity, and larynx; also known as the throat	Transports air to the larynx
Epiglottis	Flap-like cartilaginous structure at the back of the tongue, near the entrance to the trachea	Covers the opening to the trachea when swallowing occurs
Larynx	Enlargement at top of trachea; commonly known as the voice box; it houses the vocal cords	Produces sounds; transports air to the trachea; helps to filter, warm, and moisten incoming air
Trachea	Tubular structure in the neck through which air passes	Warms, filters, and moistens air; transports air to the lungs
Bronchial tree (including bronchi and bronchioles)	Tubes that branch outward, connecting the trachea to the alveoli	Conducts air from trachea to alveoli, with a mucous lining that filters incoming air
Lungs	A pair of organs in the chest that are responsible for providing oxygen to the blood and for exhaling carbon dioxide waste	Contain air passages, alveoli (the area where oxygen and carbon dioxide exchange occurs), blood vessels, connective tissues, lymphatic vessels, and nerves of the lower respiratory tract

portion of the pharynx. In the pharynx, the air and food passages coincide below the oral cavity. Air is directed to the larynx by the negative thoracic pressure generated primarily by the diaphragm, and food is directed posterior into the esophagus by a complex coordination of muscles during swallowing. The **epiglottis**, a valve-like structure, can close the entry to the larynx, preventing aspiration of food particles.

The **larynx** is a cartilaginous structure that serves as the passageway for air between the pharynx and trachea.

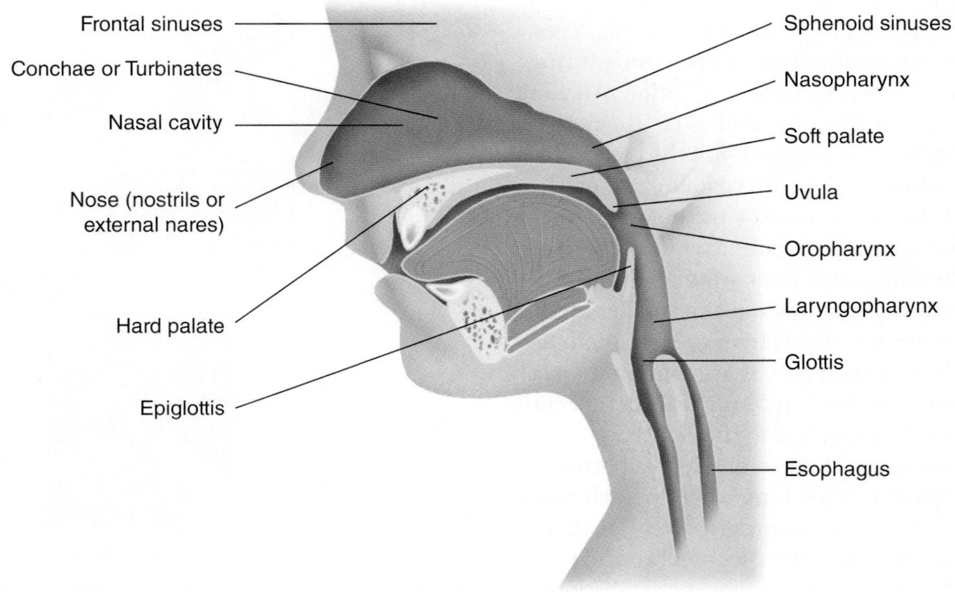

FIGURE 47-4 Anatomy of the upper respiratory tract.

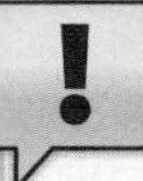

Respiratory Recap

Major Components of the Upper Respiratory Tract

- Nasal cavity
- Oral cavity
- Pharynx (nasal, oral, laryngeal)
- Larynx

The hyoid bone is seated above the larynx. The epiglottis is the uppermost cartilage of the larynx. The largest cartilage of the larynx is the thyroid cartilage, which protrudes more prominently in men (the Adam's apple). The only complete ring cartilage around the airway is the cricoid cartilage, which is located below the thyroid cartilage. The cricothyroid membrane (between the two cartilages) can be opened in an emergency to obtain access to the lower airways. Small cartilage pairs—the corniculates and arytenoids—complete the posterior larynx. The vocal cords are mucosal folds supported by elastic ligaments, and the opening between the cords is called the **glottis or glottic opening**. The glottis is a triangular slit, and when food or liquid is swallowed, the glottis closes to prevent food or liquid from entering the trachea. When air moves through the vocal cords, they can be vibrated to create sounds.

Lower Respiratory Tract

Major structures of the lower respiratory tract include the trachea, mainstem bronchi, bronchioles, and alveoli. The **trachea**, commonly called the windpipe, is a large hollow tube that bifurcates at the carina into the two primary **bronchi**. The trachea marks the beginning of the conducting system and because it resembles an inverted tree is often referred to as the tracheobronchial tree. The trachea measures 10 to 13 cm in length. It is protected and supported by 16 to 20 C-shaped pieces of cartilage, which keep the trachea open even during the negative thoracic pressures of inspiration. An adult trachea is about 2.0 to 2.5 cm in diameter. The mucosa that lines the trachea and a majority of the tracheobronchial tree is pseudostratified ciliated columnar epithelium. Smoking is known to destroy the cilia that line the airways. The trachea bifurcates asymmetrically at a point in the division called the **carina**, with the right main stem bronchus branching out at a smaller angle (20 to 30 degrees from vertical) than the left (45 to 55 degrees). Therefore, foreign bodies are aspirated mainly into the right bronchus, and endotracheal suction catheters will commonly advance into the right lung.

The main bronchi continue to divide in a pattern known as dichotomous branching whereby each consecutive airway splits into two progressively smaller airways giving rise to lobar, then segmental, and then to approximately 40 subsegmental bronchi. The lobar bronchi correspond with the five lobes of the lung

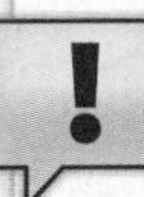

Respiratory Recap

Major Components of the Lower Respiratory Tract

- Trachea
- Mainstem bronchi
- Bronchioles
- Alveoli

and the segmental bronchi to the 18 segments of the lung. The airways continue to divide as they penetrate deeper into the lung where hundreds of smaller bronchi branch into thousands of bronchioles. Up until this point, the airways have been supported by cartilage. The bronchioles, however, which are less than 1 mm in diameter, do not contain any cartilage. They retain their patency and avoid collapse during exhalation by adhering to the retractile forces of the lung's elastic parenchymal tissue. The bronchioles continue to divide and branch into still smaller airways called terminal bronchioles. Terminal bronchioles number approximately 30,000 to 40,000 and have a diameter of approximately 0.65 mm. They represent the last component of the conducting airway, the conducting zone.

The respiratory bronchioles, the alveolar ducts, alveolar sacs, and the alveoli constitute the 16th to the 23rd generation of airway branching and the end of the lower respiratory tract. They are often called the acinus or respiratory zone (**Figure 47-5**). Surrounding the acinus is a rich capillary network where gas exchange occurs. **Figure 47-6** illustrates the conducting zone (trachea to respiratory bronchioles) as well as the respiratory zone (respiratory bronchioles to alveoli). **Table 47-4** provides

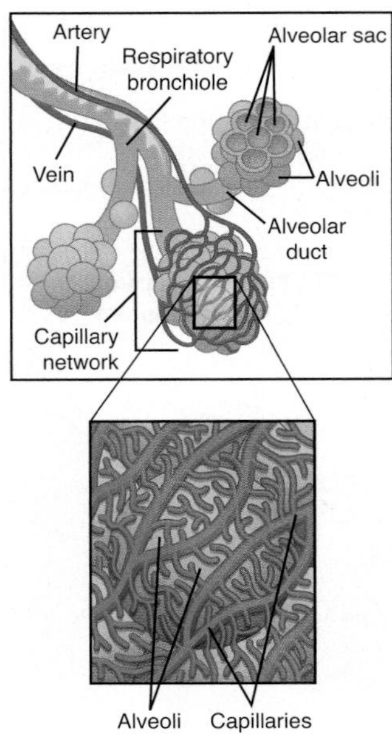

FIGURE 47-5 Acinus: terminal bronchioles, alveolar ducts, alveolar sacs, and alveoli.

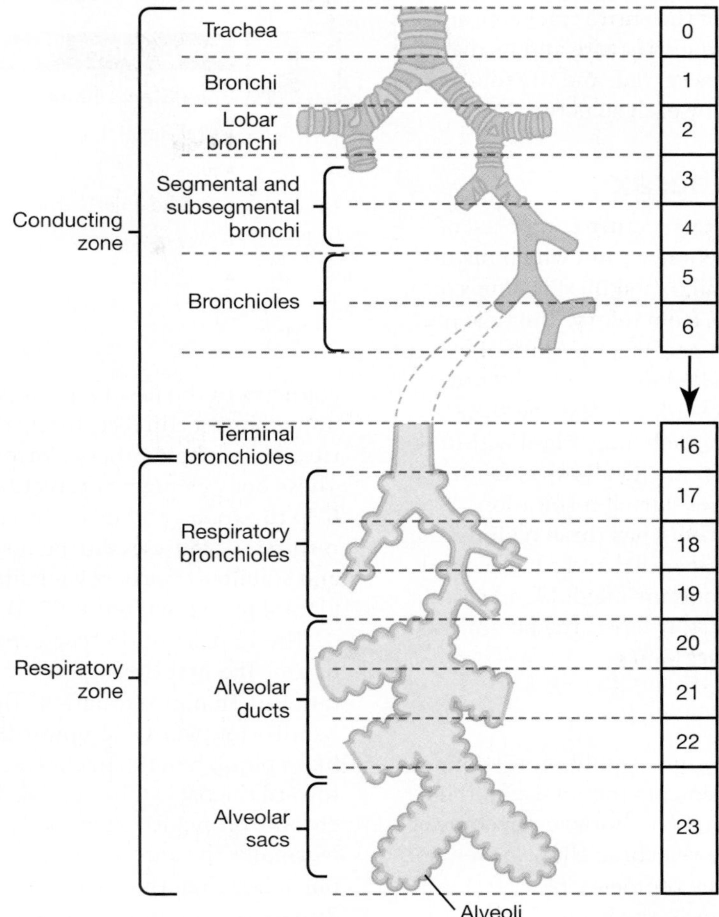

FIGURE 47-6 Airways of the conducting zone and the respiratory zone.
Reproduced from Hicks G. *Cardiopulmonary Anatomy and Physiology*. 4th ed. St. Louis: Mosby; 1999:687.

TABLE 47-4
Structural Characteristics of Tracheobronchial Tree

Structure	Generation	Number of Generations	Diameter	Area(s) Served	Cross-sectional Area
Trachea	0	1	2.5 cm	Both lungs	5.0 cm^2
Main stem bronchi	1	2	11–19 mm	Individual lungs	3.2 cm^2
Lobar bronchi	2	5	4.5–13.5 mm	Lobes	2.7 cm^2
Segmental bronchi	3	18	4.5–6.5 mm	Segments	3.2 cm^2
Small bronchi	4–10	~40–1020	Varies	Secondary lobules	Varies
Bronchioles	11	~2 thousand	Varies	Pulmonary acinus	Varies
Terminal bronchioles	14	~16–32 thousand	0.65 mm	Pulmonary acinus	116 cm^2
Respiratory bronchioles	16	65–260 thousand	Varies	Pulmonary acinus	Varies
Alveolar ducts	19	524 thousand–8.8 M	0.40 mm	Pulmonary acinus	1.71 m^2
Alveoli	24	300 M	0.25–0.30 mm	Pulmonary acinus	70 m^2

Modified from Lumb A. *Nunn's Applied Respiratory Physiology*, 7th ed., 2011, Elsevier.

structural characteristics of the entire tracheobronchial tree to include each anatomic structure and its diameter, the generation and area served, and the total cross-sectional area represented by each structure.

Anatomy of the Thorax

The **thorax** contains an infrastructure composed of the chest wall and the vertebrae within which major organs reside. The chest wall (i.e., skin, ribs, intercostal muscles) protects the lungs from injury. Thoracic muscles such as the **diaphragm** perform the work of breathing. A serous membrane called the **parietal pleura** adheres firmly to the chest wall, whereas the **visceral pleura** covers the surface of each lung. Fluid within the pleural cavity prevents friction and allows smooth sliding between the two surfaces during respiration.

The thorax or thoracic cavity has three regions: the mediastinum, a right pleural cavity, and a left pleural cavity. The **mediastinum** contains major blood vessels, the esophagus, and the heart, whereas the pleural cavities contain the lungs (**Figure 47-7**).

Bony Thorax

The bony elements provide support and protection for the heart and lungs. The elements that make up the thorax include the sternum, ribs, thoracic vertebrae, clavicles, and scapulae. The vertebrae allow movement, rotation, and elevation of the thoracic ribs. The sternum, which anchors the ribs to the front of the chest wall, is subdivided into three parts: the manubrium, the body, and the xiphoid process. The manubrium connects to the first two ribs, and the body of the sternum connects directly to the third through seventh ribs. The xiphoid process forms the tip of the sternum. These bony elements protect the contents of the thorax, help to expand and relax the chest via contraction of respiratory muscles during inspiration and expiration, and stabilize the chest wall during changes in intrapleural pressure (**Figure 47-8**).

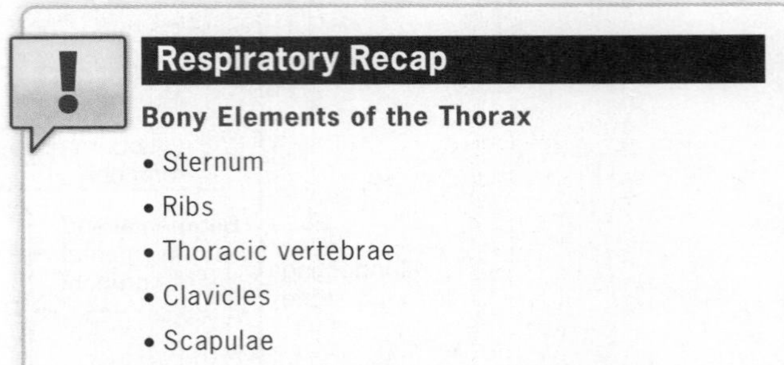

Respiratory Recap

Bony Elements of the Thorax

- Sternum
- Ribs
- Thoracic vertebrae
- Clavicles
- Scapulae

The 12 pairs of ribs correspond to their vertebrae of origin. The first through seventh ribs play an important function in ventilation. These ribs lift like bucket handles (outward and upward), while the sternum rises like a pump handle. In contrast, the lower ribs rotate toward the back. Obstructive lung disorders such as chronic bronchitis or emphysema limit the expansion. Normally, the anterior-to-posterior (AP) diameter is much less than the chest width, but with obstructive disease, air trapping expands the lungs and increases the AP diameter of the chest, forming the so-called barrel chest.

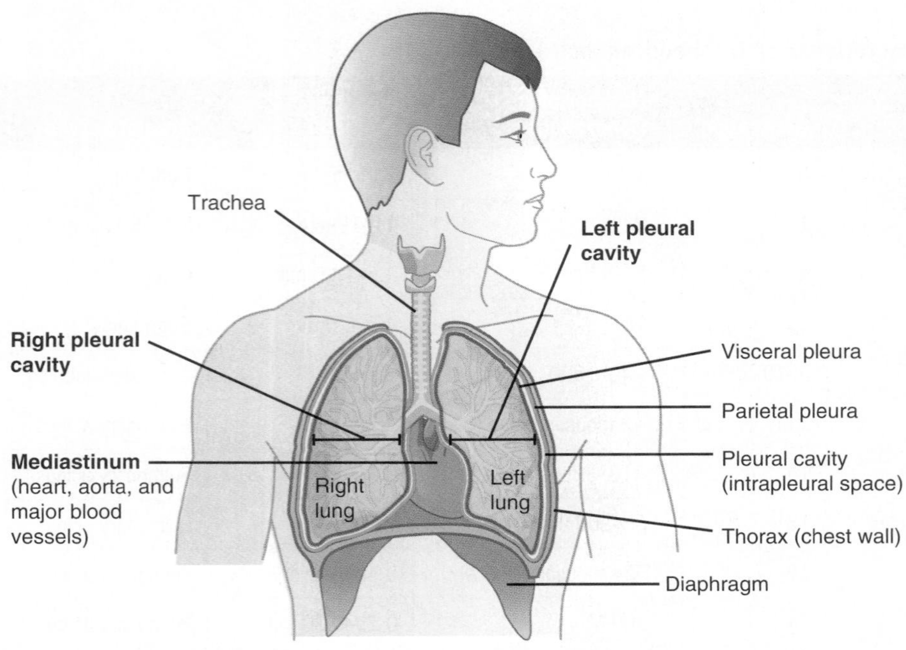

FIGURE 47-7 Thorax: mediastinum and right and left pleural cavity.

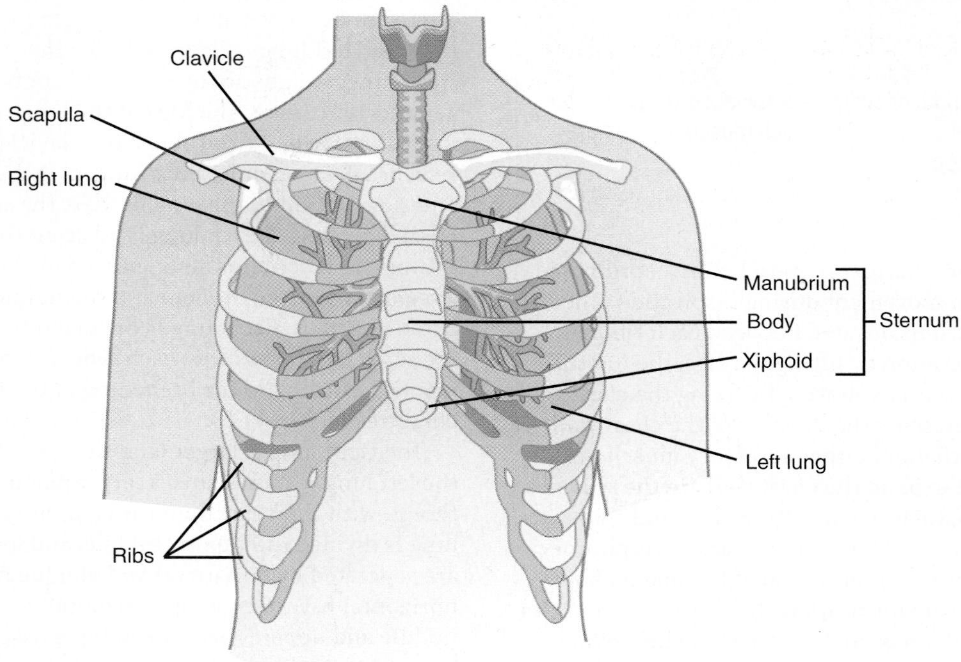

FIGURE 47-8 Bony structures of thorax in relation to lungs.

Respiratory Muscles

The muscles of respiration are divided into primary and accessory, with the accessory further divided into accessory muscles of inspiration and accessory muscles of expiration. The major muscle of respiration is the diaphragm. It is a large muscle that provides the primary force for the **work of breathing**. It is normally dome-shaped and attaches to the large vertebrae, the ribs, and the xiphoid process. Fibers of the diaphragm connect to a broad connective sheet called the *central tendon*. During inspiration, the diaphragm contracts and becomes flat, causing lung expansion. During exhalation, the elastic recoil of the lungs and relaxation of the diaphragm allow the lungs to return to their end-expiratory volume and position.

During normal tidal breathing, the diaphragm moves approximately 1.5 cm. At high levels of stress and movement with increasing work of breathing, the diaphragm can move up to 6 to 10 cm with each breath. When diaphragmatic contraction draws the central tendon down, flattening the diaphragm, intrathoracic pressure is decreased, creating a pressure differential with atmospheric pressure. Due to how it attaches to the ribs, it creates a zone of apposition, which causes outward movement of the thorax during inspiration.

The diaphragm receives its major nerve supply from the **phrenic nerve** that exits the cervical region at C3–C5. A hiccup is a reflex spasm of the diaphragm caused by an irritation of the phrenic nerve. Cervical fractures between C1 and C5 are likely to affect the phrenic nerve and disrupt or impair the ability to breathe.

The accessory muscles of inspiration are the scalene, sternocleidomastoid, pectoralis major, trapezius, and external intercostal muscles. The accessory muscles of expiration are the internal intercostal, rectus abdominus, external abdominis oblique, internal abdominus oblique, and transverse abdominus muscles. Various muscles contracting in synchrony maintain the elasticity and ease of lung movement. Contraction of a coordinated set of muscles of respiration moves air into the lungs, leading to inspiration. Although exhalation is typically passive, thoracic muscles can fix the chest, and **abdominal muscles** can contract to force air out of the lungs, most dramatically in coughing or sneezing.

During exercise, **accessory muscles** can be recruited on inspiration and expiration to increase the

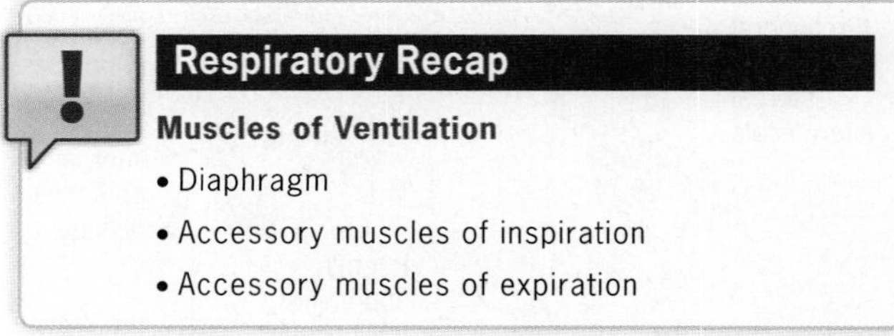

Respiratory Recap

Muscles of Ventilation

- Diaphragm
- Accessory muscles of inspiration
- Accessory muscles of expiration

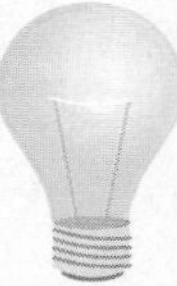

STOP AND THINK

If a patient sustains a spinal cord injury at the level of C3 or C6, which muscle groups are affected?

respiratory effort. Accessory muscles are coordinated with diaphragm movement during inspiration. The external intercostals, located between each rib pair, assist with inspiration by lifting the ribs; the internal intercostals aid with expiration by fixing the chest wall. **Figure 47-9** represents the muscles of the chest wall involved in ventilation. Other accessory muscles of inspiration that expand the chest wall are the scalenes, sternocleidomastoids, pectoralis majors, and trapezius. A way to evaluate whether subjects are in respiratory distress is to observe a retraction at the notch above the clavicles during inspiration. The accessory muscles of expiration (which is normally passive) help exhalation if resistance to expiration is significant or demands on ventilation greatly increase, as with exercise. These muscles include the rectus abdominis, external abdominis oblique, internal abdominis oblique, transversus abdominis, and internal intercostal muscles. Consequently, active exhalation can be observed if contraction of the abdomen is apparent. In patients with severe obstructive disease with increased work of breathing, both inspiratory and expiratory accessory muscles are often active.

Lungs

The lungs are cone shaped, with a broad and concave base surrounded by the thoracic ribs and diaphragm.

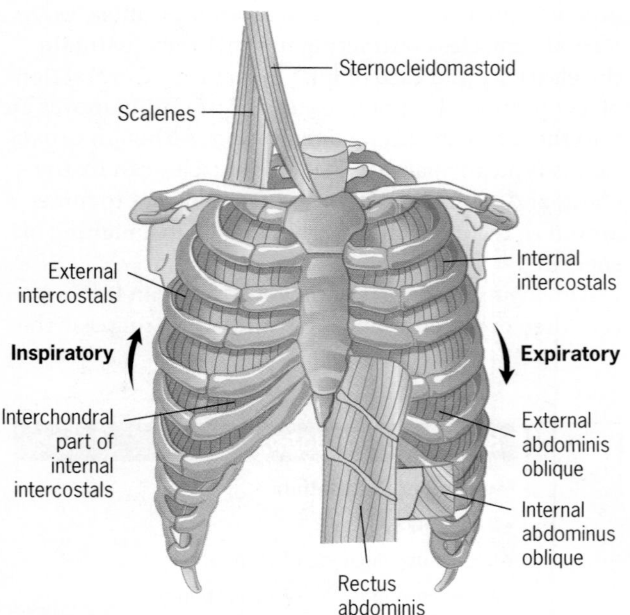

FIGURE 47-9 Muscles of the chest wall involved in ventilation.

There are five **lobes** and 18 lung **segments** between the right and left lungs (**Figure 47-10**). The average pair of adult lungs weighs about 800 g and contains about 90% gas and 10% tissue. The tops of the lungs are called the *apices* and extend from above the clavicle to the first vertebra. During quiet breathing, at end-expiration, the anterior portion of the lung borders the sixth rib. The medial portion of each lung is adjacent to the mediastinum and contains an opening called the **hilum**—a region where the bronchi and the pulmonary vessels enter the lungs. Each lung is divided into lobes, which are separated by fissures; each lobe is divided into segments according to the branching of the tracheobronchial tree (**Table 47-5**).

The right lung is larger (and therefore heavier) than the left lung, which shares a larger portion of its hemithorax with the heart than the right lung. The right lung is divided into upper, middle, and lower lobes that are separated by horizontal and oblique fissures. The horizontal fissure extends horizontally, separating the middle and upper lobes. The oblique fissure separates the middle and lower lobes. The left lung is divided into two lobes (upper and lower) separated by an oblique fissure. Knowledge of lobe and segment anatomy is required of bronchoscopists and those assisting in the procedures.

The lungs consist of two major anatomic divisions: the airways and the parenchyma (the functional part of an organ). Within the lung parenchyma, adults have approximately 300 million alveoli. Each alveolus is between 200 and 300 microns in diameter. Small pulmonary capillaries that provide perfusion to the alveoli cover about 85% to 90% of the alveolar surface area. The alveolar sacs originate from a single terminal bronchiole referred to as a *primary lobule*. There are about 130,000 primary lobules in the lung, each containing 2000 alveoli. Capillary blood and alveolar gas are separated by vascular endothelium, interstitial space, and alveolar epithelium. Gas exchange occurs via diffusion across the alveolocapillary membrane encompassing the alveolar sacs (**Figure 47-11**).

The alveolar epithelium is composed of two principal cell types: type I and type II cells. **Type I cells** are the structural squamous pneumocytes that cover 90% to 95% of the alveolar surface. They are the major sites of alveolar gas exchange. Their thickness ranges from 0.1 to 0.5 microns. **Type II cells** cover the remaining 5% to 10% of the alveolar surface. Small and cuboidal in shape, they are the primary source of surfactant production. Surfactant helps to inflate the alveoli and

Respiratory Recap

Anatomy of the Lungs

- Airways and alveoli
- Lobes and segments

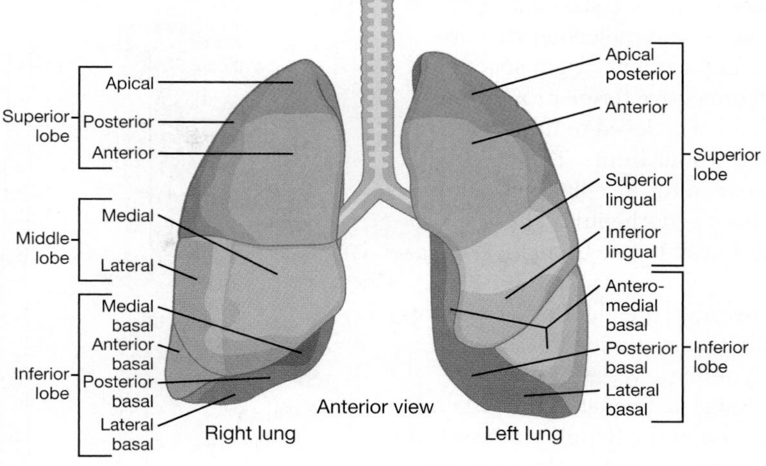

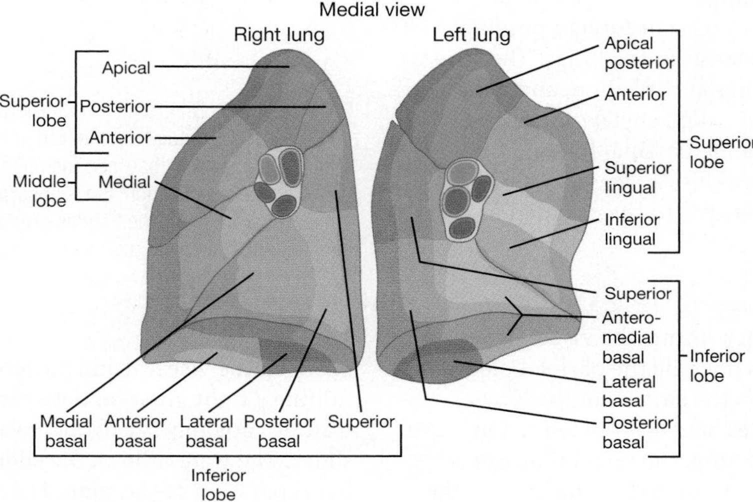

FIGURE 47-10 Lobes and segments of the lungs.

TABLE 47-5
Lobes and Segments of the Lungs

Lung	Lobe	Segments
Right	Upper	Apical Anterior Posterior
	Middle	Lateral Medial
	Lower	Superior Anterior basal Posterior basal Lateral basal Medial basal
Left	Upper	Apical posterior Anterior Superior lingular Inferior lingular
	Lower	Superior Anterior medial basal Lateral basal Posterior basal

prevent collapse by reducing the surface tension of the air–fluid interface within the alveoli.

Adjacent alveoli communicate through connections called the **pores of Kohn** and **channels of Lambert**. Alveolar macrophages, or type III cells, play a defensive role by removing bacteria from the acini or lung units.

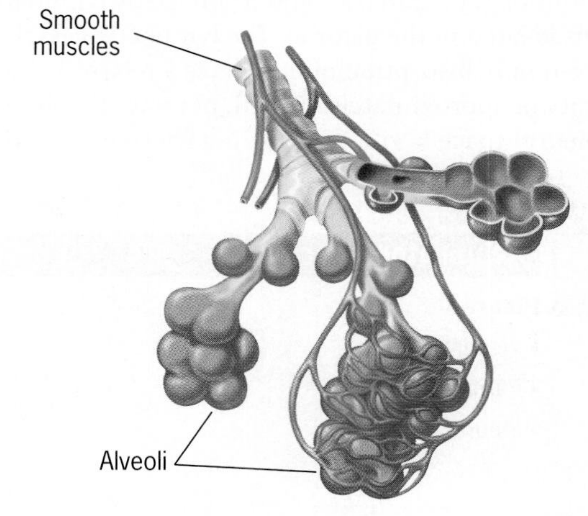

FIGURE 47-11 Gas exchange at the alveolocapillary membrane.

The interstitium (the space between cells) contains a gel-like substance made up of acid molecules that are contained in two major compartments: tight space and loose space. Collagen (a connective tissue protein) surrounds the interstitium and is believed to limit the alveolar distention beyond hazardous limits. Tight space is the area in the alveoli between the alveolar epithelium and the pulmonary capillary endothelium. Loose space surrounds the bronchioles, respiratory bronchi, alveolar ducts, and alveolar sacs.

The lungs and their covering, the pleura, also are well endowed with lymphatic circulation and lymph nodes. The open-ended lymphatic vessels are found superficially around the lungs just beneath the visceral pleura. The primary function of the lymphatic vessels is to remove excess fluid and protein molecules that leak from the capillaries. Lymphatic drainage also allows lungs to defend against bacteria or foreign products and helps achieve homeostasis in the lungs. The lymphatic vessels exit the lungs at the hilum, and lymph (i.e., a clear or milky fluid called chyle) drains away from the lung toward the mediastinal lymph nodes. The mediastinal nodes are the storage sites for lymph fluid, which eventually returns to the circulation via the thoracic duct.

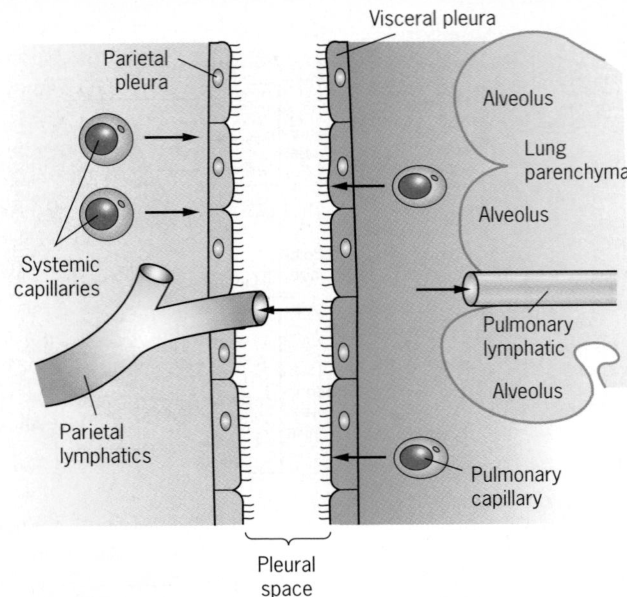

FIGURE 47-12 Diagram of the structures making up the pleurae and the pleural space. The pleurae are lined with mesothelial cells containing microvilli that face the pleural space. The arrows denote the direction for filtration and reabsorption of pleural fluid. This fluid emanates from capillaries and is predominantly reabsorbed by the lymphatics.

Pleurae

Each lung is covered with a lining, the visceral pleura, whereas the chest wall is lined by the parietal pleura. The visceral pleura covers the surface of the lungs, extending into the fissures between the lobes. On the medial surface of the lung, the visceral pleura is reflected onto the mediastinum to become part of the parietal pleura. The pleurae thus isolate the right and left lungs from the heart, which sits within its own container, the **pericardium**. Ciliated mesothelial cells line both pleurae.

Between the two pleurae is the **pleural space** (**Figure 47-12**), a cavity containing a small amount of thin fluid (<20 mL) that has a low protein concentration. Regulation of the fluid volume within the pleural space involves balancing of leakage from systemic and pulmonary capillaries and drainage by lymphatic vessels located in the pleurae. The lymphatic vessels involved in reabsorption of fluid have a relatively high capacity of approximately 700 mL per day. The fluid in the pleural space is vital in allowing frictionless sliding between the visceral and parietal pleurae and maintaining a tight junction between the lungs and chest wall. An analogy is a drop of water between two glass slides. The water allows the slides to be moved slightly, but separation of the slides is difficult. In addition, the opposing mechanical forces between the lungs and chest wall—the lungs tending to collapse and the chest wall tending to expand—helps ensure a negative pressure (below atmospheric pressure) within the pleural space. Intrapleural pressure was first measured through placement of a catheter within the pleural space. Intrapleural pressure is currently estimated through measurement of the pressure in the lower esophagus using an esophageal balloon.

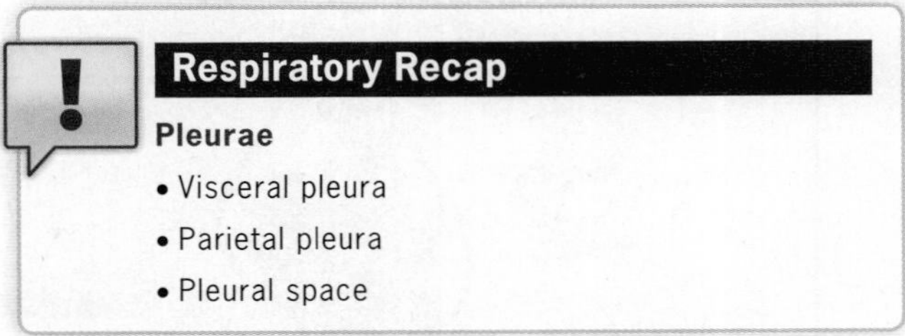

Respiratory Recap

Pleurae

- Visceral pleura
- Parietal pleura
- Pleural space

Innervation of the visceral pleura is by the vagus nerve, whereas intercostal and phrenic nerves supply the parietal pleura. Importantly, irritation of the visceral pleura does not result in pain sensation because it has no nerves of general sensation, whereas the parietal pleura is extremely sensitive to irritation. Severe pain that may be referred to the root of the neck and over the shoulder occurs in pleurisy as sensed in the parietal pleura.

The mediastinum is the area between the two pleural sacs and is divided into superior and inferior as well as anterior, middle, and posterior regions. All structures within the thorax other than the lungs and pleurae are located in the mediastinum. The superior mediastinum contains the thymus, great vessels associated with the heart, esophagus, trachea, and thoracic duct, and numerous nerves, including the vagus and esophageal plexus. Within the other regions are located the heart (within the pericardium), main bronchi, great vessels, phrenic nerves, and portions of the thymus and esophagus.

Microanatomy of the Respiratory System

As previously noted, the main function of the lung is to provide adequate gas exchange. The following sections describe the microanatomy of the respiratory system as it relates to maintaining a balanced ventilation-perfusion relationship while providing normal mucus transport to remove debris and particles from the airways.

Mucociliary Clearance

As air moves in and out of the lungs, gas exchange in the alveoli maintains adequate homeostasis in the body. While a normal tidal volume is approximately 400 to 500 mL, ventilation of between 12,000 and 24,000 liters of air per day can expose the lungs to damaging agents, including pollutants, viruses and bacteria, and organic agents such as antigens. Responses to foreign body inhalation can lead to respiratory compromise. The body reacts to these exposures by coughing, sneezing, bronchoconstriction, and increasing mucus production to expel or avoid damaging effects from these inhaled agents.

The primary defense mechanism within the conducting airways is the pseudostratified ciliated columnar epithelium that lines the airways and serves as an escalator of mucus from the lungs (**Figure 47-13**). Goblet cells secrete mucus, which catches the inhaled debris. The trachea contains both ciliated and nonciliated epithelial cells as the proportion of ciliated cells increases down the bronchi. Immediately bathing the epithelial cells is a watery fluid (sol) where the cilia beat, on top of which sits a mucous (gel) layer. In the bronchioles are also cuboidal cells and secretory Clara cells. Under the ciliated cell bed is a layer of fibroblasts, nerves, lymphatics, and smooth muscle cells extending from the nose to the bronchioles. The ratio of ciliated cells to goblet cells is about 4:1. Each ciliated cell contains about 200 to 250 cilia, with each cilium in the trachea having a length of about 6 microns and a diameter of about 2 microns. Ciliary beat frequency is between 1000 and 1500 per minute, with faster rates in larger airways. Boluses of mucus that move in a rhythmical fashion upward will lead to expulsion from the airway to be, most often, swallowed.

It is important for the **mucociliary apparatus** to maintain a fluid homeostasis. Dehydration prevents the ability of patients to adequately produce secretions. The volume of expelled tracheobronchial secretions in a normal subject has been estimated to be between 10 and 100 mL/day. The viscosity of mucosal secretions is mainly attributed to mucoglycoproteins.

Many factors and conditions adversely affect mucociliary transport and clearance. Among them are smoking and diseases such as cystic fibrosis, COPD, and asthma. Additionally, general and specific medications can impede the function of the mucociliary apparatus and stimulate the production of secretions. Among this list are narcotics, ethyl alcohol, atropine, acetylsalicylic acid (aspirin), β-adrenergic antagonists, and inhaled and intravenous anesthetics, to name but a few.

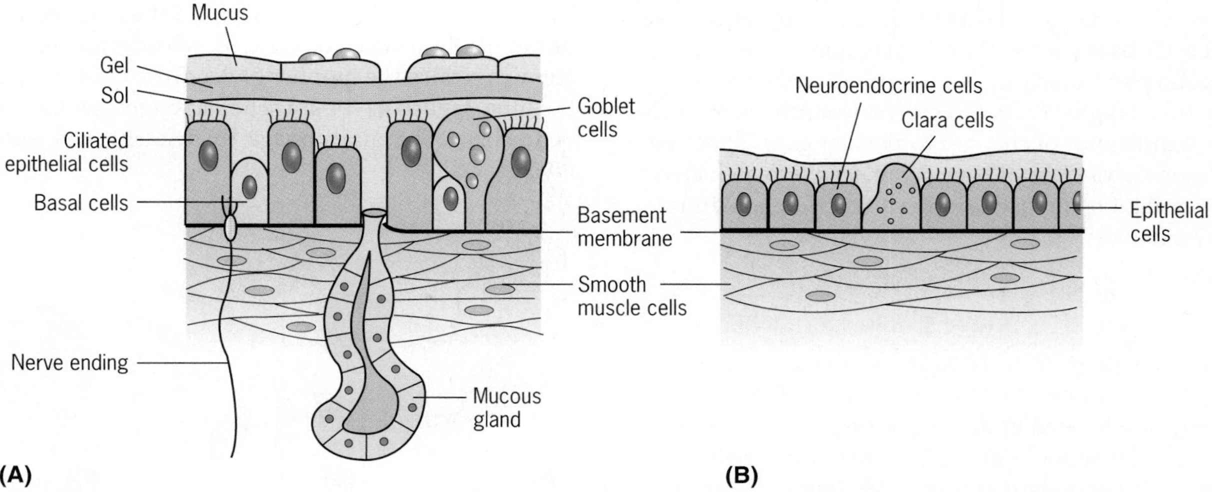

FIGURE 47-13 Cells that contribute to the mucociliary clearance apparatus in (**A**) large and (**B**) small airways. Basal cells are thought to be stem or progenitor cells that give rise to epithelial and goblet cells when the epithelium is damaged.

Respiratory Recap

Mucociliary Apparatus

- Contains mucous layer
- Contains cilia that move the mucous layer

The paranasal sinuses (air cavities in the maxillae, frontal sphenoid, and ethmoid bones) are lined with ciliated epithelium. When infections occur, mucus often drains from these sinuses into the nasal cavities. This postnasal drip can cause local irritation at the level of the larynx and is one of the common causes of a chronic cough.

Airway and Vascular Smooth Muscle

Both the airways and pulmonary vasculature are lined with smooth muscle cells. Smooth muscle control is involuntary. When smooth muscles contract, the cells become shorter and wider. When stimulated, airways, pulmonary vasculature, mast cells, and epithelial cells can alter smooth muscle tone.

Smooth muscle within the pulmonary vasculature, especially the pulmonary artery bed, is scarcer than that found in systemic arteries. Moreover, vascular tone in the pulmonary vessels is low, as are pressure and resistance compared with the systemic circulation. Smooth muscles direct blood flow within the lung parenchyma by changing the caliber of pulmonary vessels. Factors that influence smooth muscle tone thus affect regional lung perfusion.

Chemicals that affect vascular tone are produced locally or metabolized by endothelial cells, nerves, and mast cells, or by other organs. Nerve endings within the pulmonary vasculature can release acetylcholine and norepinephrine. Finally, mast cells produce histamine and leukotrienes. Pulmonary vascular tone is potently affected by changes in surrounding gas concentrations and acid–base status. Thus, hypercapnia, a decrease in pH, and particularly hypoxia cause vascular vasoconstriction. Hypoxia acts directly on smooth muscle cells. The significance of changes in alveolar gases affecting pulmonary vasomotor tone is the need to match alveolar ventilation and perfusion and therefore maximize gas exchange.

Mast Cell, Macrophages, and Dendritic Cells

Mast cells range from 10 to 20 μm in diameter and may be oval or more irregularly shaped. They frequently are located in the respiratory mucosal surfaces and alveolar septa. A major feature of mast cells is the presence of abundant granules. Mediators released from mast cell granules are one of three classes: (1) granule-associated mediators, such as histamine and serotonin; (2) membrane-derived lipid mediators, such as leukotrienes; and (3) cytokines. In individuals with asthma, mast cell numbers in bronchial and alveolar tissue are elevated, as are protease and histamine levels in bronchoalveolar lavage fluid. Stabilization of mast cell membranes and administration of drugs that counter the production or activity of these mediators help prevent the symptoms manifested during an asthma attack.

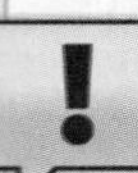

Respiratory Recap

Mast Cells, Macrophages, and Dendritic Cells

- Mast cells: cells that release mediators
- Macrophages: phagocytic cells
- Dendrites: antigen-presenting cells

Two types of cells derived from bone marrow stem cells that reside in different parts of the lung are macrophages and dendritic cells. **Macrophages** have three functions: phagocytosis, antigen presentation, and cytokine production. Macrophages engulf and digest bacteria, viruses, or other foreign material (phagocytosis). Antigen presentation is the transfer and display of antigen shapes to other immune system cells that can launch an antibody response. Macrophages also produce cytokines, the most significant being interleukine-1 (IL-1) and tumor necrosis factor (TNF).

Dendritic cells are mobile cells with irregular shapes and long processes. Normally they are found in small numbers within the airway epithelium and lung parenchyma. Their major function in the lung is as antigen-presenting cells. When exposed to antigens, dendritic cells phagocytose antigens and process them, migrate to lung-draining lymph nodes, and present the antigens to T lymphocytes, thus activating T lymphocytes. If an individual is chronically exposed to inhaled irritants, the number of dendritic cells within the lung increases dramatically. Inhaled or systemically administered steroids reduce the number of dendritic cells within the lung. **Figure 47-14** is a schematic representation of an (a) alveolar macrophage, (b) dendritic cell, and (c) mast cell.

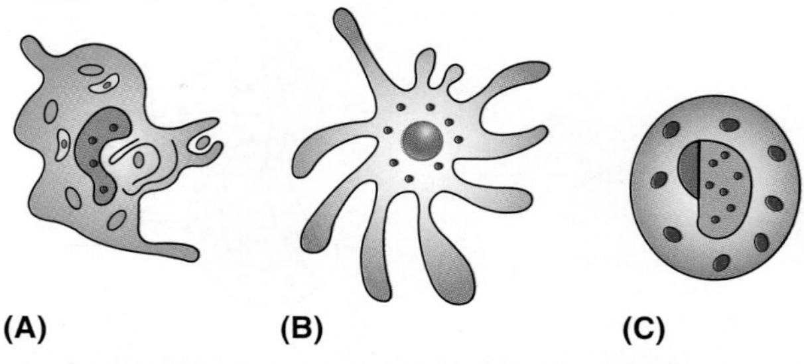

FIGURE 47-14 A schematic representation of an (**A**) alveolar macrophage, (**B**) dendritic cell, and (**C**) mast cell.

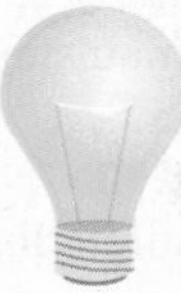

STOP AND THINK

Identify specific diseases that adversely affect the function of the mucociliary apparatus. Explain the mechanism by which this occurs.

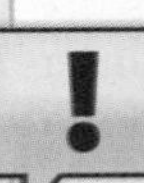

Respiratory Recap

Alveolar Cells

- Type I – cover greatest surface area
- Type II – produce surfactant

Alveolar Cells

The most distal functional units of the lungs arising from bronchioles are the air sacs known as alveoli. There are millions of alveoli in each lung. The alveolocapillary division outlines two alveolar epithelial cells (type I and type II), a basement membrane, an interstitial space, and endothelial cells that make up the pulmonary capillaries that contain red blood cells (**Figure 47-15**).

Alveolar type I pneumocytes are the smallest, most abundant cells covering the alveoli. Type I pneumocytes are extremely flat and cover about 95% of the alveolar surface. Type I cells have a mean thickness of approximately 0.1 to 0.5 µm. Gases move easily across these cells' walls. Type I cells are sensitive to injury, including high levels of O_2, bacteria, bleomycin, cyclophosphamide, and particulates.

Alveolar type II cells, or granular pneumocytes, are cube shaped and cover only 5% of the alveolar surface. They are located predominantly in corners of alveolar sacs and form tight junctions with type I cells, which helps impede the movement of excess fluid into the alveolar spaces. Type II cells exhibit a number of functions, including the production of surfactant, differentiation into type I cells when the latter have been damaged, and transport of sodium and water toward the endothelial cells and blood to help minimize fluid accumulation in the alveolar space.

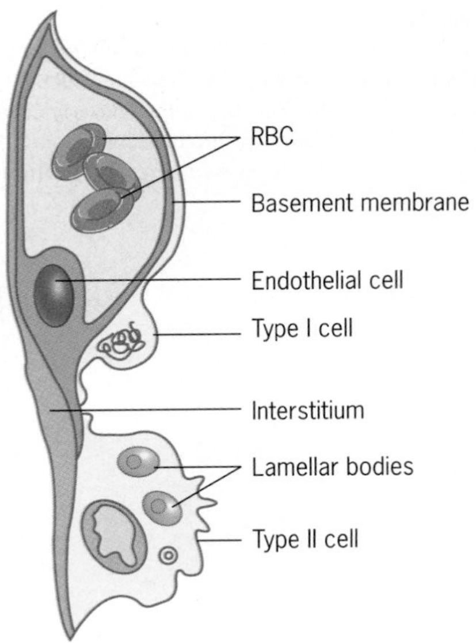

FIGURE 47-15 A schematic representation of the alveolocapillary complex showing the structural relationships between type I and type II cells and endothelial cells that make up the pulmonary capillaries. RBC, red blood cells (within the pulmonary capillary).

Type II cells are larger and more irregularly shaped than type I cells. The surfactants produced by type II cells contain lipoproteins that coat the inner surface of the alveoli and lower the surface tension at end-expiration, preventing alveolar collapse. Pulmonary surfactant is composed of 90% phospholipids and 10% protein. The primary surface tension–lowering chemical in the pulmonary surfactant is phospholipid dipalmitoyl phosphatidylcholine (DPPC). DPPC contains hydrophobic (water-insoluble) and hydrophilic (water-soluble) substances. The average surface tension of the alveolus varies from 5 to 15 dynes/cm (small) to about 50 dynes/cm (large or fully distended alveolus). As the radius gets smaller, surface tension decreases. As the radius grows larger, surface tension increases. As the alveolar area decreases, the surfactant molecules are crowded together and begin to repel one another.

Absence of pulmonary surfactant can cause collapse of the alveoli, resulting in atelectasis. Pulmonary complications are often seen when there is a reduction in surfactant. Conditions associated with a deficiency in surfactant or type II cell instability include neonatal respiratory distress syndrome, congenital surfactant deficiency, and pulmonary alveolar proteinosis.

The following safety factors within the alveolocapillary complex help prevent fluid accumulation within the alveoli:

- Tight junctions that exist between alveolar cells
- Transport of water from the alveolar spaces into the pulmonary vessels as hydrostatic pressure within the pulmonary vasculature is low
- Surfactant and its associated proteins, which help repel water
- An active defense system within the alveolar sacs that helps prevent injury to alveolar membranes, thus maintaining their structural integrity
- An extensive lymphatic system within the lung that helps drain fluid that accumulates within the interstitial space.

Interstitial Space

The pulmonary interstitium is the space between the alveolar epithelial and the endothelial cells lining the vasculature. The interstitium serves as mechanical support, containing various cell types associated with the maintenance of fluid balance in the lung. The interstitium is a continuum that pervades the entire lung, from the visceral pleura to the hilum, where it is connected to the mediastinum. Cells within the interstitium include fibroblasts, myofibroblasts, smooth muscle cells, pericytes, lymphatic endothelial cells, and inflammatory/immune cells such as lymphocytes, mast cells, and macrophages. Structural components that form the matrix within the interstitium include collagens, elastic fibers, proteoglycans, and fibronectin.

In pulmonary interstitial lung disease there is a marked increase in the number of cells that reside in the interstitium, with an increase in its thickness. These components consist of elastin and collagen fibers, fibronectin, proteoglycans, and constituents of the epithelial and endothelial basement membranes. The scaffolding that forms the alveolar walls and septa consists primarily of collagen and elastin fibers. Collagen represents 15% to 20% of lung dry weight. Elastin fibers form a three-dimensional network that contributes to the elastic recoil characteristics of the lung. Although normally the adult lung features very little elastin turnover, the presence of elastases or a deficiency of alpha-1 antitrypsin can lead to considerable lung damage.

Key Points

- The primary functions of the respiratory system are gas distribution and gas exchange.
- The five stages of fetal lung development are embryonic, pseudoglandular, canalicular, saccular, and alveolar.
- Postnatal development entails significant anatomic differences between the infant/child and the adult.
- Key structures in the upper airway of the respiratory system consist of the nose, nasopharynx, oropharynx, laryngopharynx, and larynx.
- Key structures in the lower airway of the respiratory system consist of the trachea, mainstem bronchi, bronchioles, and alveoli.
- The lungs consist of the airways and alveoli.
- The bony thorax consists of the sternum, ribs, thoracic vertebrae, clavicles, and scapulae.
- The respiratory muscles are the diaphragm, accessory muscles of inspiration, and accessory muscles of expiration.
- The visceral pleurae surround the lungs, the parietal pleurae line the chest wall, and the pleural space is between the visceral and parietal pleurae.
- The mucociliary apparatus clears inhaled agents from the lower respiratory tract.
- Important cells in the lower respiratory tract include mast cells, macrophages, and dendritic cells.
- The alveolus is composed of type I and type II cells.
- The interstitial space is located between the alveolar epithelia and the vascular endothelia.

Suggested Reading

Beachey W. *Respiratory Care Anatomy and Physiology: Foundations for Practice*. 3rd ed. St. Louis: Mosby; 2012.

Des Jardins T. *Cardiopulmonary Anatomy and Physiology: Essentials for Respiratory Care*. 6th ed. Clifton Park, NY: Delmar; 2013.

Hicks G. *Cardiopulmonary Anatomy and Physiology*. Philadelphia: WB Saunders; 2000.

Huether S, McCrane K. *Understanding Pathophysiology*. 4th ed. St. Louis: Mosby; 2004.

Loengenbaker S. *Understanding Human Anatomy and Physiology*. 6th ed. New York: McGraw Hill; 2008.

Moini J. *Anatomy and Physiology for Health Professionals*. Burlington, MA: Jones & Bartlett Learning; 2012.

Scanlon V, Sander T. *Essentials of Anatomy and Physiology*. 5th ed. Philadelphia: FA Davis; 2007.

Shier D, Butler JL, Lewis R. *Hole's Essentials of Human Anatomy and Physiology*. 9th ed. New York: McGraw Hill; 2006.

Standring S. *Gray's Anatomy: The Anatomical Basis of Clinical Practice*. 40th ed. New York: Elsevier Churchill Livingstone; 2008.

Thibodeau T, Patton K. *Anatomy and Physiology*. 4th ed. St. Louis: CV Mosby, 1999.

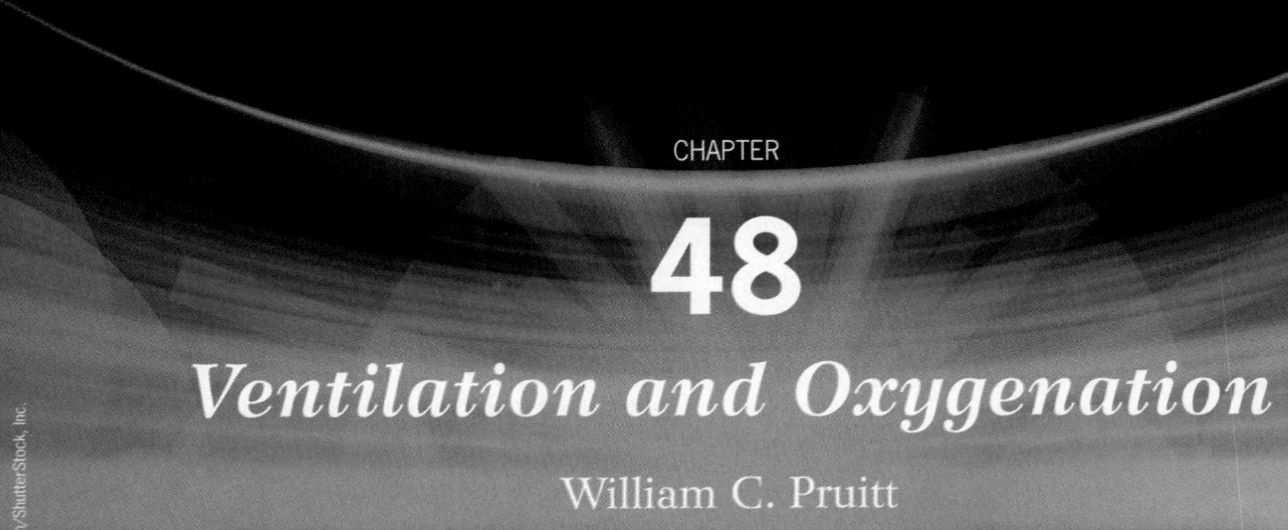

CHAPTER

48

Ventilation and Oxygenation

William C. Pruitt

OUTLINE

OBJECTIVES

1. Discuss the physiology of gas exchange.
2. Calculate alveolar Po_2.
3. Describe oxygen uptake from the lungs.
4. Describe oxygen and carbon dioxide transport between the lungs and tissues.
5. Compare the distribution of ventilation and blood flow within the lungs.
6. Discuss the importance of the ventilation-perfusion ratio.
7. Compare the oxyhemoglobin dissociation curve and the carbon dioxide dissociation curve.
8. Distinguish between hypoxemia and hypoxia.
9. Describe the relationships among $Paco_2$, carbon dioxide production, and alveolar ventilation.
10. List causes of hypoxemia, hypoxia, and hypercapnia.

KEY TERMS

Bohr effect
dead space
fetal hemoglobin (Hb F)
Fick equation
Fick's law
Haldane effect
hemoglobin
hypercapnia
hypoxemia
hypoxia
methemoglobin
oxyhemoglobin dissociation curve (ODC)
partial pressure of the alveolar CO_2 (P_{ACO_2})
shunt
ventilation-perfusion ratio ($\dot{V}/\dot{Q}$)

Introduction

The primary function of the lungs is ventilation and proving a suitable place for gas exchange to occur. Ventilation is the movement of gas in and out of the lungs; this movement allows oxygen (O_2) to enter the body and carbon dioxide to be removed. The body must have O_2 coming through the lungs and into the circulatory system and then delivered to the tissues in a constant supply to allow for normal metabolism. O_2 is an essential element for life, and insufficient O_2 (**hypoxia**) results in damage to the cells in the major organs (heart, brain, etc.). This damage may be reversible or permanent, depending on the injury, and if hypoxia continues eventually the damage becomes extensive, organs fail, and death occurs. Carbon dioxide (CO_2) is a waste product of metabolism and it has to be removed from the body; a build-up of CO_2 causes a decrease in pH (acidosis). If the pH, is too low, organ systems begin to malfunction. If acidosis is too severe, death can occur. On the other hand, having too much CO_2 removed from the body (hyperventilation) will increase pH, causing an alkalosis. A severe alkalosis can also bring organ system failure and death. This chapter will discuss the physiology of ventilation—how gas moves into and out of the lungs—and oxygenation—how O_2 is moved from the ambient air into the tissues.

Ventilation

The mechanics of gas movement in and out of the body through the process of ventilation and the neurologic guidance and drive to breathe are described elsewhere in the text. Ambient air (room air) includes two primary gases: O_2, which makes up 21%, and nitrogen (N_2), which makes up about 78%. The remaining 1% is made up of mixed gases (argon, carbon dioxide, neon, methane, etc., in descending order of concentration). Air, and O_2 in particular, moves from outside the body into the lungs and eventually to the blood through two mechanisms: bulk flow and diffusion.

During inspiration, bulk flow of gas moves into the nose and mouth as a result of negative pressure, which is generated in the thoracic cavity by the diaphragm and other muscles of ventilation. Expiration is normally a passive event brought about by the relaxation of the muscles of inspiration and by the normal recoil of the lung tissue. During quiet breathing, there is about 400 mL to 500 mL of gas moving in and out of the body. Normal tidal volume (V_T) is determined by gender and height.

Dead Space Ventilation

From its entrance to the upper airway at the mouth and nose, gas moves through the opening in the glottis into the lower airway, through the trachea and bronchi, and into the terminal bronchioles, respiratory bronchioles, alveolar ducts, and alveoli. The region of the airways from the mouth and nose to the terminal bronchioles, the conducting airways, is called anatomic dead space ($V_{D_{anat}}$). The volume of the anatomic dead space for an adult male is about 150 mL (about a third of the normal tidal volume). Movement of gas into and out of this region is called dead space ventilation. The term **dead space** is used because this volume of gas moves in and out of the lungs without taking part in gas exchange. This is also called wasted ventilation. O_2 moves out of the alveoli into the blood, and CO_2 moves out of the blood into the alveoli. The movement of gas in and out of the gas exchange part of the lungs (alveoli) is called alveolar ventilation. Alveolar ventilation makes up about 350 mL of the 500 mL V_T. Assuming a breath rate or frequency of about 12 times per minute, the minute ventilation (that is, expired volume unit per minute of time, $\dot{V}_E$) is 6000 mL/min or 6 L/min.[1] V_T and $\dot{V}_E$ are typically measured from exhaled gas.

$$V_T = V_A + V_D$$

$$500 \text{ mL} = 350 \text{ mL} + 150 \text{ mL}$$

$$\dot{V}_E = V_T \times f = 500 \text{ mL} \times 12 \text{ breaths/min} = 6 \text{ L/min}$$

where V_A is alveolar volume, V_D is dead space volume, and f is frequency (respiratory rate).

With loss of blood flow to alveoli, gas exchange will not occur even though ventilation of that area continues. This results in an increase of dead space ventilation, and this abnormal condition is called alveolar dead space ($V_{D_{alv}}$). Total dead space ventilation, also called physiologic dead space (V_D), is the sum of the anatomic dead space ($V_{D_{anat}}$) plus the $V_{D_{alv}}$.

$$V_D = V_{D_{anat}} + V_{D_{alv}}$$

Alveolar Ventilation

Alveolar ventilation ($\dot{V}_A$) is the amount of air that moves in and out of the alveoli, and this is the air that is involved with the bloodstream in what is called gas exchange. O_2 moves from the alveolus into the blood, and CO_2 moves out of the blood into the alveoli. Not all of the $\dot{V}_E$ is involved with gas exchange; dead space ventilation ($\dot{V}_D$) is not a part of this process.[2]

$$\dot{V}_A = \dot{V}_E - \dot{V}_D$$

These concepts are important because ventilation of the lungs is what brings O_2 to the alveoli and what takes CO_2 out of the body. If minute ventilation increases (hyperventilation), it has a direct impact on removal of CO_2 from the lungs and the CO_2 levels in the blood will drop. Conversely, if $\dot{V}_E$ decreases (hypoventilation), less CO_2 is removed and CO_2 blood levels rise.

Physiologic Mechanisms of Hypercapnia

A common mechanism for **hypercapnia** (high Pa_{CO_2}) is alveolar hypoventilation. Pa_{CO_2} is inversely related to alveolar ventilation ($\dot{V}_A$). Because $\dot{V}_A$ is the difference between $\dot{V}_E$ and $\dot{V}_D$, hypercapnia can be caused by a decrease in $\dot{V}_E$ or an increase in $\dot{V}_D$. The dead space fraction (V_D/V_T) can be calculated from the Bohr equation:

$$V_D/V_T = (Pa_{CO_2} - P\bar{E}_{CO_2}) / Pa_{CO_2}$$

where $P\bar{E}_{CO_2}$ is the partial pressure of mixed exhaled CO_2. If Pa_{CO_2} is 40 mm Hg and $P\bar{E}_{CO_2}$ is 27 mm Hg, the V_D/V_T ratio is 0.33. The Bohr equation requires measurement of $P\bar{E}_{CO_2}$ in exhaled gas. The relationship between V_D/V_T, Pa_{CO_2}, and $\dot{V}_E$ is shown in **Figure 48-1**.

Physiologic dead space consists of the anatomic dead space and abnormally high $\dot{V}/\dot{Q}$ (underperfused) units in the gas exchange regions (alveolar dead space). CO_2 exchange between gas and blood does not occur in anatomic dead space. Its volume varies little in disease but does increase with V_T because airways dilate slightly with inspiration. In practice, measurement of anatomic dead space is not necessary because its size can be predicted (anatomic dead space = 1 mL per pound ideal body weight). In patients receiving positive pressure ventilation, the volume of $V_{D_{anat}}$ may be increased because of mechanical bronchodilation. Tubing in the

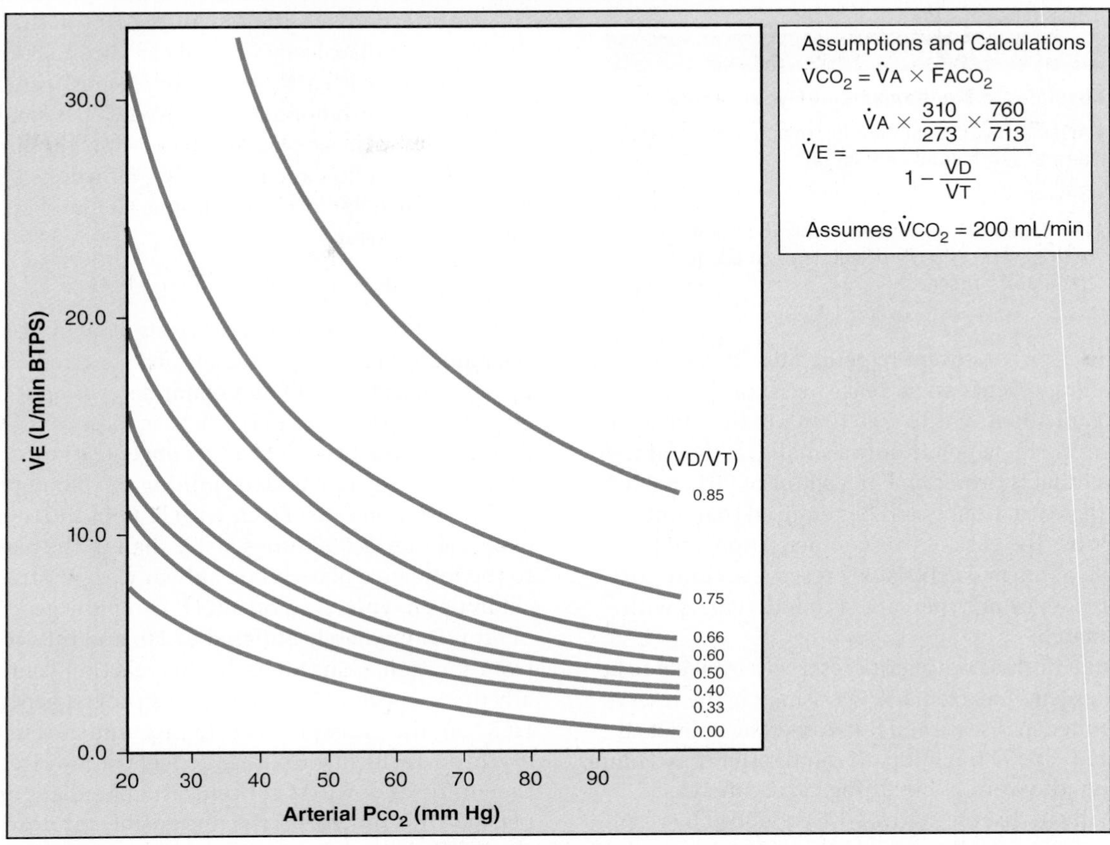

FIGURE 48-1 An isopleth nomogram used to estimate VD/VT from minute ventilation ($\dot{V}E$) and arterial P_{CO_2}.
Adapted from Baum GL, et al. *Textbook of Pulmonary Diseases.* 6th ed. Lippincott Williams & Wilkins; 1998.

ventilator circuit between the Y-adaptor and the artificial airway also increases dead space (mechanical dead space). An artificial airway (endotracheal tube or tracheostomy tube) decreases VD_{anat}.

Pa_{CO_2} is determined by the relationship between tissue CO_2 production ($\dot{V}CO_2$) and $\dot{V}A$.

$$Pa_{CO_2} = (0.863 \times \dot{V}CO_2)/\dot{V}A$$

The factor 0.863 is used to convert standard conditions to body conditions and to account for measurement of $\dot{V}CO_2$ in mL/min and $\dot{V}A$ in L/min. When $\dot{V}CO_2$ and $\dot{V}A$ are measured in the same units and at body conditions, 0.863 is replaced with barometric pressure (e.g., 760 mm Hg) in the equation.

High $\dot{V}/\dot{Q}$ units (increased VD_{alv}) are less efficient in CO_2 exchange than units with normal $\dot{V}/\dot{Q}$; that is, more ventilation is required to produce a change in Pa_{CO_2}. In the sitting position, VD/VT is about 0.3 and varies little with age. It can increase to 0.6 or more in lung disease characterized by increased number of high $\dot{V}/\dot{Q}$ units, such as emphysema, shock, and pulmonary embolism. During exercise, VD/VT normally decreases to below 0.2, primarily because of an increase in VT.[3] In disease, VD/VT may not decrease, and in severe cases it may increase with exercise.[4]

Although CO_2 exchange is affected by severe $\dot{V}/\dot{Q}$ mismatch, it usually does not cause hypercapnia. As $\dot{V}/\dot{Q}$ falls, partial pressure of carbon dioxide (P_{CO_2}) in the low $\dot{V}/\dot{Q}$ areas of the lung rises, reaching the value of the mixed venous P_{CO_2} at a $\dot{V}/\dot{Q}$ of 0. The resulting increase in P_{CO_2} is small (changing from 40 to 47 mm Hg), but CO_2 content increases due to the steep slope of the CO_2 dissociation curve. Elimination of CO_2 retained in the blood due to high $\dot{V}/\dot{Q}$ usually is accomplished by an increased ventilation in alveoli with better blood flow, which means total ventilation must increase to maintain a normal Pa_{CO_2}. The increase in ventilation occurs rapidly because of the sensitivity of central chemoreceptors to altered levels of Pa_{CO_2}.

The ventilatory work required for this compensation is usually small, as can be illustrated by the following extreme example. If half the cardiac output goes to alveoli that are not ventilated, there is no CO_2 removed from the blood in the unventilated area (50% shunt). As a result the remaining alveoli would need to double

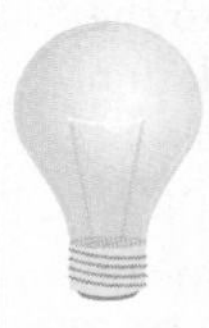

STOP AND THINK

You are caring for a mechanically ventilated patient with a Pa_{CO_2} of 70 mm Hg. What are the potential physiologic causes for the hypercapnia and how would you determine which is most likely?

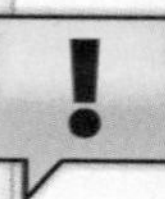

Respiratory Recap

Physiologic Mechanisms of Hypercapnia

- Alveolar hypoventilation (increased dead space, decreased minute ventilation)
- Severe $\dot{V}/\dot{Q}$ mismatch
- Increased CO_2 production (only in patients with severe $\dot{V}/\dot{Q}$ abnormalities and borderline ventilatory reserve

their ventilation to prevent hypercapnia. This increased ventilation represents an increase over normal resting ventilation of about 25% to 30% to maintain a P_{CO_2} of about 40 mm Hg, which is only a small fraction of the normal ventilatory reserve. For a shunt of 90%, a 200% increase in ventilation would be required to maintain normal P_{CO_2}. The ease of this compensation and the magnitude of normal ventilatory reserve account for the low incidence of hypercapnia in individuals with $\dot{V}/\dot{Q}$ mismatch.

Although normal ventilatory reserve is unlikely to be exceeded except in extreme $\dot{V}/\dot{Q}$ mismatch, the reserve may be limited in disease and if stressed, the individual with limited reserve might tip over into respiratory failure. In addition, the work of breathing can be increased substantially in disease states. CO_2 produced by respiratory muscles may place an additional burden on the lungs when increases in ventilation require high levels of muscular work. A decreased ventilatory reserve combined with a high work of breathing and severe $\dot{V}/\dot{Q}$ mismatch thus can lead to significant hypercapnia.

Occasionally an increase in CO_2 production (e.g., overfeeding, fever, sepsis) may cause hypercapnia in patients with severe $\dot{V}/\dot{Q}$ abnormalities and borderline ventilatory reserve. This is most likely in patients in whom the $\dot{V}_A$ is fixed, as occurs in the paralyzed mechanically ventilated patient.

Carbon Dioxide Transport

CO_2 is produced as a by-product of metabolism, and diffuses from the tissues into the blood. The heart circulates the blood from the tissues to the alveolar capillaries, where CO_2 diffuses into the alveoli and is eliminated by ventilation. These gas transport mechanisms use the physical processes of diffusion (gas movement between lungs and blood and between tissues and blood), dissolution (the gases dissolve as they move into the body's tissues), chemical reactions (between O_2 or CO_2 and **hemoglobin**), and bulk gas and blood movement (ventilation and blood flow).

About 90% of the CO_2 that enters the blood diffuses into the red blood cells, where it undergoes one of three chemical reactions: (1) it remains as dissolved CO_2, (2) it combines with hemoglobin (Hb) to form carbaminohemoglobin, or (3) it combines with water to form carbonic acid (H_2CO_3), which dissociates into H^+ and HCO_3^- (bicarbonate). The remaining 10% of the CO_2 in the plasma is dissolved CO_2 and carbamino compounds after reacting with NH_2 groups of plasma proteins.

Although the amount of dissolved CO_2 is small, it is in equilibrium with the plasma Pa_{CO_2}, which in turn determines the direction and rate of CO_2 diffusion at body tissue and alveolar levels. In plasma, CO_2 undergoes the following reaction:

$$CO_2 + H_2O \rightarrow H_2CO_3 \rightarrow HCO_3^- + H^+$$

The rate of this reaction is relatively slow in plasma, and the amount of H_2CO_3 in the plasma is extremely small. Even so, plasma H_2CO_3 is a major determinant of blood H^+ concentration (i.e., pH). Because dissolved CO_2 determines the plasma H_2CO_3 concentration, dissolved CO_2 plays a key role in determining the blood pH.

The reaction rate of CO_2 with H_2O in the erythrocyte is about 13,000 times faster than in the plasma due to the influence of carbonic anhydrase, an intracellular catalytic enzyme. As a result, H^+ is rapidly generated, but it is immediately buffered by Hb and thus removed from solution. Consequently, this reaction continually draws more CO_2 into the erythrocyte, generating HCO_3^- in the process. As HCO_3^- accumulates in the erythrocyte, its intracellular concentration rises. HCO_3^- then diffuses down its concentration gradient into the plasma. This mechanism is responsible for nearly all of the HCO_3^- in the plasma.

Before Hb buffers H^+, its negative charges are exactly balanced by the positive ions inside the erythrocyte. As it buffers H^+, the net negative charge is reduced, but this reduction is exactly matched by newly generated HCO_3^-, and intracellular electroneutrality is maintained. However, when negatively charged HCO_3^- ions diffuse out of the erythrocyte, an electropositive environment develops inside the erythrocyte. In response, Cl^-, the most abundant anion in the plasma, diffuses into the erythrocyte (the so-called *chloride shift*), which maintains intracellular electrical neutrality.

At the alveolus, CO_2 carried in the Hb is released to diffuse out of the red blood cell into the plasma. Dissolved CO_2 also moves into the plasma. The CO_2 carried as HCO_3^- combines with H^+ to form carbonic acid, which then dissociates into CO_2 and H_2O. Note that the arrows in the formula below go both ways and recall the effect of carbonic anhydrase.

$$CO_2 + H_2O \leftrightarrow H_2CO_3 \leftrightarrow HCO_3^- + H^+$$

(Carbonic anhydrase)

The CO_2 diffuses into the plasma, and then into the alveolus, where it is removed by alveolar ventilation.

Carbon Dioxide Dissociation Curve

The CO_2 Hb dissociation curve is essentially linear over the physiologic range of Pa_{CO_2} (**Figure 48-2**). This means a change in alveolar ventilation is much more effective in changing arterial CO_2 content than O_2

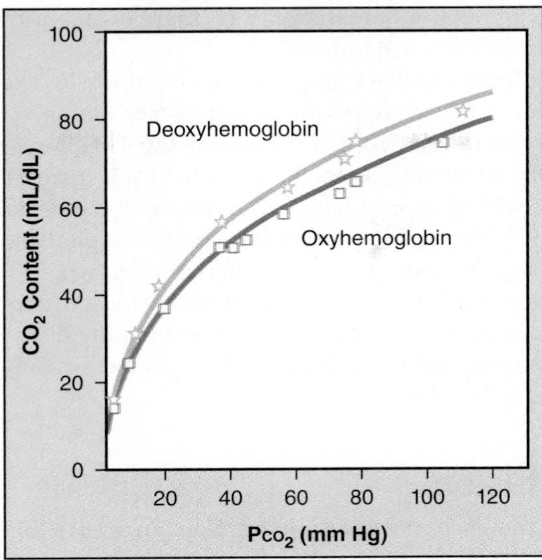

FIGURE 48-2 Carbon dioxide curve of blood that shows the relationship between CO_2 content and PCO_2.

Modified from Baum GL, et al. *Textbook of Pulmonary Diseases*. 7th ed. Lippincott Williams & Wilkins; 2003.

content. For example, a doubling of the alveolar ventilation in healthy lungs reduces the blood CO_2 content in half but changes arterial O_2 content very little because Hb is already nearly 100% saturated with O_2 during normal ventilation. The steepness of the CO_2 Hb dissociation curve also permits continued excretion of CO_2 even in the presence of significant mismatching of pulmonary ventilation and blood flow. This explains why CO_2 retention is seen only in patients with severe ventilation-perfusion mismatch.

The Hb molecule simultaneously carries O_2 and CO_2, but not at the same binding sites. O_2 combines with the molecule's heme groups, whereas CO_2 combines with the amino groups of the α- and β-polypeptide chains. The presence of O_2 on the heme portions of Hb hinders the combination of amino groups with CO_2 (i.e., it hinders formation of carbaminohemoglobin). The affinity of Hb for CO_2 thus is greater when it is not combined with O_2 (**Haldane effect**). Conversely, carbaminohemoglobin has a decreased affinity for O_2 (Bohr effect). Oxygenated blood, therefore, carries less CO_2 for a given $PaCO_2$ than deoxygenated blood.

The Alveolar Gas Equation

The inspired PO_2 (PIO_2) in ambient air is calculated from the barometric pressure (PB) and the fraction of O_2 in the inspired gas (FIO_2).

$$PIO_2 = FIO_2 \times PB$$

At sea level, PB is 760 mm Hg and FIO_2 is 0.21.

$$PIO_2 = 0.21 \times 760 \text{ mm Hg} = 160 \text{ mm Hg}$$

At an elevation greater than sea level, PB decreases and PIO_2 decreases (**Table 48-1**). The barometric pressure

TABLE 48-1
Barometric Pressure, Ambient PO_2, and Alveolar PO_2 at Different Altitudes

Altitude (Feet)	PB (mm Hg)	Ambient PO_2 (mm Hg)	Alveolar PO_2 (mm Hg)
0	760	159	109
3000	682	143	103
5000	630	132	92
8000	564	118	78
10,000	523	110	70
12,000	483	101	61
15,000	412	90	50
18,000	379	80	40
20,000	349	73	33
30,000	226	47	7

PB, barometric pressure; PO_2 = partial pressure of oxygen.

in Denver, Colorado, is 630 mm Hg and the PIO_2 is thus 132 mm Hg. FIO_2 also affects PIO_2. For example, changing the FIO_2 to 0.60 with the PB at 760 mm Hg causes the PIO_2 to increase to 456 mm Hg.

As the inspired gas passes through the upper airway, humidification occurs such that the gas becomes fully (100%) saturated with water vapor. The partial pressure of water vapor P_{H_2O}) is 47 mm Hg at normal body temperature. PB thus is adjusted for P_{H_2O} to calculate PIO_2.

$$PIO_2 = FIO_2 \times (PB - P_{H_2O})$$

$$PIO_2 = 0.21 \times (760 \text{ mm Hg} - 47 \text{ mm Hg}) = 150 \text{ mm Hg}$$

When the inspired gas reaches the alveoli, PO_2 is reduced further due to the loss of O_2 to the surrounding pulmonary capillaries. If the amount of O_2 diffusing out of the alveoli into the capillary blood were exactly equal to the amount of CO_2 diffusing from the capillary blood into the alveoli, the partial pressure of alveolar O_2 would be calculated by subtracting the **partial pressure of the alveolar CO_2 ($PACO_2$)** from the PIO_2 as calculated above. O_2, however, diffuses out of the alveoli at a greater rate than CO_2 diffuses into the alveoli. At rest, capillary blood removes about 250 mL/min of O_2 from the alveoli while replacing it with only about 200 mL/min of CO_2. The ratio of alveolar CO_2 excretion from the blood to O_2 uptake into the blood is called the respiratory exchange ratio (R) and has a value of about 0.8; R = (200 mL/min)/(250 mL/min) = 0.8. This uneven exchange has the ultimate effect of amplifying the effect of $PaCO_2$ on PAO_2. This amplification is calculated by the following factor in the alveolar gas

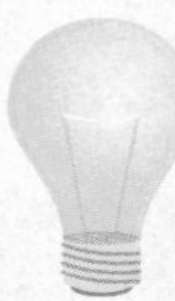

STOP AND THINK

Why will hypercapnia have a greater effect on Pa_{O_2} in Salt Lake City than in New York City?

equation: $F_{IO_2} + (1 - F_{IO_2})/R$. The P_{AO_2} is thus calculated using the alveolar gas equation:

$$P_{AO_2} = F_{IO_2} \times (P_B - P_{H_2O}) - \{Pa_{CO_2} \times [F_{IO_2} + (1 - Pa_{CO_2})/R]\}$$

The simplified alveolar gas equation for computing P_{AO_2} is shown below. R is replaced by the value 0.8.

$$P_{AO_2} = F_{IO_2} \times (P_B - P_{H_2O}) - Pa_{CO_2}/R$$

$$P_{AO_2} = 0.21 \times (760 \text{ mm Hg} - 47 \text{ mm Hg}) - 40 \text{ mm Hg}/0.8 = 100 \text{ mm Hg}$$

The following is a summary of the various partial pressures of O_2 as it moves from the atmosphere to the alveoli and into the blood using normal barometric pressure and breathing an F_{IO_2} of 0.21 (**Figure 48-3**).

P_{IO_2} = 160 mm Hg in the atmosphere just before the air has entered the mouth and nose
P_{IO_2} = 150 mm Hg once the inspired O_2 has been fully saturated with water vapor
P_{AO_2} = 100 mm Hg in the alveoli
Pa_{O_2} = 95 mm Hg (measured from an arterial blood gas)

Barometric pressure decreases with altitude. In Denver, Colorado, where the elevation is 5280 feet above sea level, the normal barometric pressure is 630 mm Hg, as mentioned above. The P_{IO_2}, P_{AO_2}, and Pa_{O_2} values thus are lower than at sea level. When commercial airplanes fly long distances at high altitudes (often at 30,000 feet), the cabin is pressurized to the equivalent of about 8000-foot elevation, a pressure of 564 mm Hg, to prevent severe hypoxemia.[5]

Patients who have lung disease often have low Pa_{O_2} (**hypoxemia**). Based on the alveolar gas equation, the P_{AO_2} can be increased by increasing the F_{IO_2}, increasing the P_B, or decreasing the Pa_{CO_2}. The F_{IO_2} is increased by providing supplemental O_2, something that is done every day for millions of patients in the hospital and at home. Increasing the P_B to increase the P_{AO_2} is uncommon but can be accomplished using a hyperbaric chamber.[6] For patients with severe lung disease and hypercapnia, reducing the Pa_{CO_2} can effectively increase the P_{AO_2}.

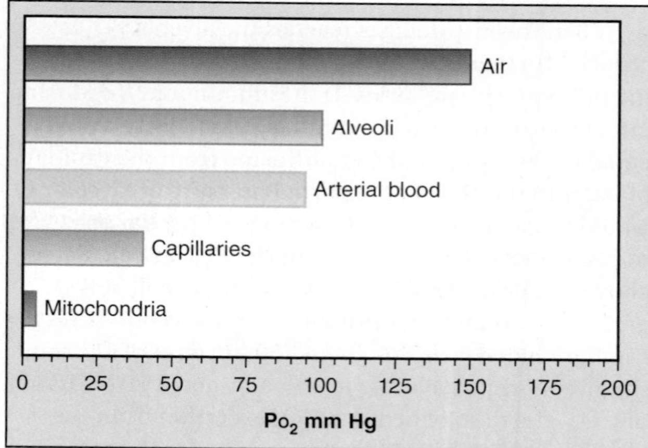

FIGURE 48-3 The oxygen gradient from the alveolar space to the mitochondria. Note the stepwise decrement in P_{O_2} from 100 mm Hg in the alveolar space to values of a few mm Hg at the mitochondria, where most of the oxygen is consumed.

Adapted from Baum GL, et al. *Textbook of Pulmonary Diseases*. 6th ed. Lippincott Williams & Wilkins; 1998.

Diffusion

Diffusion occurs by gas moving from an area of high concentration (high partial pressure) to an area of low concentration (low partial pressure).

Fick's Law

The rate of diffusion of gases from the alveolus into the capillary (called the alveolocapillary or A-C membrane) is affected by several factors, which are given in Fick's Law for Diffusion. **Fick's law** states that the amount of gas that moves across the A-C membrane is directly proportional to the surface area of the membrane, the diffusion coefficient (a measure of diffusivity unique for each gas in the mixture), and the pressure gradient from one side of the membrane to the other. The volume of gas moving across the A-C membrane is inversely proportional to the thickness of the membrane. Fick's Law of Diffusion (also known as the **Fick equation**) is as follows:[7]

$$Vgas = \frac{A}{T} \times D \times (P_1 - P_2)$$

where Vgas is the volume of gas diffusing across the A-C membrane (measured in mL/min); A is the surface area of the A-C membrane that is available for diffusion; D is the diffusion coefficient of the particular gas; $P_1 - P_2$ is the pressure gradient across the A-C membrane (high pressure – low pressure); and T is the thickness of the A-C membrane. The P_{AO_2} is P_1 in Fick's law and P_2 is P_{O_2} in the pulmonary capillary. A decrease in P_{AO_2} thus will decrease the rate of diffusion.

Diffusion can be altered by changes in the volume of blood in the pulmonary capillaries. For example, increasing the pulmonary artery pressure when left atrial pressure is low can increase the perfusion pressure of the pulmonary circulation. This increases diffusion because the higher perfusion pressure recruits and distends pulmonary capillaries, and hence increases the volume of blood in the pulmonary capillaries. The increase in diffusion during exercise and with changes from the upright to the supine position also can be explained by capillary dilation and recruitment, resulting in an increase in blood volume in the pulmonary capillary bed.

A reduction in alveolar surface area, as occurs with emphysema or lung resection, results in a decrease in diffusing capacity. An increased thickness of the A-C membrane, as occurs with pulmonary fibrosis, also results in decreased diffusing capacity. Abnormalities that increase the thickness or surface area of the A-C membrane rarely result in hypoxemia at rest. During exercise, however, blood flow velocity associated with these abnormalities may prevent equilibration of Po_2 between alveolar gas and capillary blood during the short transit through the lung, causing hypoxemia. Exercise, therefore, can unmask diffusion defects that are not apparent at rest. A falling Pao_2 with exercise indicates that diffusion defect may be a contributing factor for hypoxemia.

Ventilation-Perfusion

Disruption of either ventilation or perfusion can change the volume of gas diffusing across the A-C membrane. This relationship is the **ventilation-perfusion ratio ($\dot{V}/\dot{Q}$)**. The normal $\dot{V}/\dot{Q}$ ratio is 0.8. If the perfusion is reduced relative to ventilation, $\dot{V}/\dot{Q}$ will increase. This can happen if an area of the lung's blood supply is reduced due to pulmonary embolus. An increase in $\dot{V}/\dot{Q}$ results in physiologic dead space and in particular, an increase in alveolar dead space (in a complete loss of blood flow $\dot{V}/\dot{Q}$ will be infinity, or ∞). On the other hand, if ventilation is reduced relative to perfusion, $\dot{V}/\dot{Q}$ will decrease. For example, this happens with bronchospasm or airway secretions. If the alveolus is collapsed, fluid filled, or consolidated, this creates a condition called a **shunt**; $\dot{V}/\dot{Q}$ is 0.

Exchange of O_2 and CO_2 occur in the more than 300,000,000 alveoli. There are more than 100,000 functional units, which correspond to acini supplied with ventilation by respiratory bronchioles.[8,9] Overall gas exchange is determined by the relative contributions of these functional units, determined by the distribution of ventilation and perfusion throughout the lungs. Inadequate ventilation relative to perfusion (low $\dot{V}/\dot{Q}$ and shunt) reduces O_2 uptake by the lungs and thus results in hypoxemia. On the other hand, excessive ventilation relative to perfusion (high $\dot{V}/\dot{Q}$ and dead space) hinders the lungs' ability to eliminate CO_2 and may cause hypercapnia, especially in individuals with limited ability to increase ventilation.

> **Respiratory Recap**
>
> **Ventilation-Perfusion Ratio**
>
> - Ideal: 1.0
> - Normal: 0.8
> - Shunt: 0
> - Dead space: infinity

$\dot{V}/\dot{Q}$ Mismatch

With aging, $\dot{V}/\dot{Q}$ decreases. As much as 10% of the total blood flow may go to lung units with $\dot{V}/\dot{Q}$ values of less than 0.1, but still no shunt is detected. The increased regions with low $\dot{V}/\dot{Q}$ adequately explain the decreased Pao_2 and increased alveolar-arterial O_2 difference with aging. The cause of such age-related $\dot{V}/\dot{Q}$ mismatch often is attributed to degenerative processes in the small airways, which occurs with aging.

In patients with chronic obstructive pulmonary disease (COPD) characterized by emphysema, large amounts of ventilation go to lung units with extremely high $\dot{V}/\dot{Q}$.[10] The increased numbers of high $\dot{V}/\dot{Q}$ regions results in dead space and hypercapnia. The presence of coexisting low $\dot{V}/\dot{Q}$ regions results in mild hypoxemia responsive to O_2 therapy.

Abnormal $\dot{V}/\dot{Q}$ distributions produce hypoxemia (low blood O_2 levels), but not necessarily hypercapnia. Even though a low $\dot{V}/\dot{Q}$ interferes with the efficiency of CO_2 elimination, it is often associated with a normal or even low $Paco_2$. The reason is that the regulatory chemoreceptors increase the ventilatory drive in response to a rising $Paco_2$. This increases ventilation and subsequently the $Paco_2$ will remain normal to low. A significant portion of the increased ventilation is inefficient with respect to CO_2 elimination because it goes to lung units with high $\dot{V}/\dot{Q}$, however. This regional hyperventilation lowers the $Paco_2$ of these units, balancing out the high $Paco_2$ of the units with low $\dot{V}/\dot{Q}$. Depending on the severity of $\dot{V}/\dot{Q}$ mismatch (i.e., the relative numbers of high $\dot{V}/\dot{Q}$ and low $\dot{V}/\dot{Q}$ units), a hypoxemic patient therefore can have low, normal, or high arterial CO_2. $\dot{V}/\dot{Q}$ mismatch is the primary mechanism for hypercapnia seen in severe COPD patients. These patients require an increased ventilation to achieve a given Pao_2 or $Paco_2$ and thus incur an increased work of breathing.

The P_{AO_2} is an important factor in regulating the distribution of $\dot{V}/\dot{Q}$ within the lung. Hypoxemia causes pulmonary vasoconstriction, called hypoxic pulmonary vasoconstriction. This increases resistance to blood flow in hypoxic (underventilated or low $\dot{V}/\dot{Q}$) regions of the lungs. Hypoxic pulmonary vasoconstriction tends to restore the $\dot{V}/\dot{Q}$ matching of the regions by reducing blood flow to underventilated units and redistributing it to normally ventilated lung units. In a localized disease like pneumonia, this is a helpful mechanism to maintain a proper $\dot{V}/\dot{Q}$. Generalized hypoxic pulmonary vasoconstriction occurring over a long period of time, however, as in severe COPD, can cause increased work on the right heart and lead to cor pulmonale.[11] People living in high altitudes, who are chronically exposed to low ambient O_2 concentrations, will have hypoxemic vasoconstriction.[12]

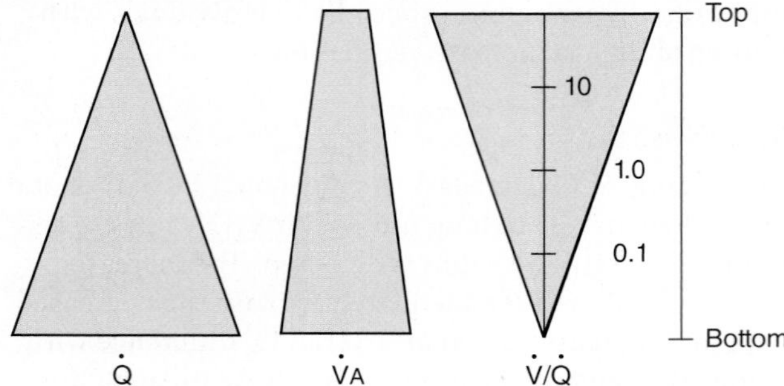

FIGURE 48-4 Ventilation-perfusion matching showing the relative distribution of perfusion ($\dot{Q}$), ventilation ($\dot{V}$), and the ratio ($\dot{V}/\dot{Q}$) throughout the lungs of an upright individual breathing at functional residual capacity. Top denotes alveoli and capillaries in the hilar regions of the lung, and bottom denotes these structures at the base of the lung.

Hydrostatic factors and lung volume influence $\dot{V}/\dot{Q}$ in an upright individual (**Figure 48-4**). At the top of the lungs, alveolar pressure is greater than pulmonary vascular pressure, resulting in no blood flow (dead space), called *West zone 1*. At the bottom of the lungs, pulmonary vascular pressure is greater than alveolar pressure, called *West zone 3*. In *West zone 2*, between zones 1 and 3, blood flow is determined by the difference between pulmonary vascular pressure and alveolar pressure. Blood flow at the top of the lung is less than that at the bottom. The distribution of ventilation and blood flow in the lungs is such that $\dot{V}/\dot{Q}$, and thus PO_2, is higher at the top of the lungs and lower at the bottom of the lungs. This explains, in part, the small difference between PAO_2 and PaO_2 in normal individuals.

Assessment of Oxygenation

The simplest approach to assessment of oxygenation is to measure PaO_2. The advantage of this measurement is its simplicity. Normal values of PaO_2 decrease with age. The definition of hypoxemia in adults depends on the age of the individual and the altitude (**Table 48-2**). In general, a low PaO_2 while breathing room air at rest indicates the presence of $\dot{V}/\dot{Q}$ mismatch, shunt, or alveolar hypoventilation.

The alveolar-arterial PO_2 difference, or $P(A - a)O_2$, is calculated as the difference between the PAO_2 and the PaO_2. The $P(A - a)O_2$ is more sensitive and specific than the PaO_2 alone as an indicator of $\dot{V}/\dot{Q}$ abnormalities. The $P(A - a)O_2$ in healthy adults breathing room air increases with age. As a general rule, the $P(A - a)O_2$ for an individual should be no more than half the chronologic age and no more than 25 mm Hg while breathing room air.[13,14] The upper normal limit of the $P(A - a)O_2$ for a 30-year-old person is thus 15 mm Hg, whereas the upper normal limit of $P(A - a)O_2$ for a 60-year-old individual is 25 mm Hg while breathing room air. The $P(A - a)O_2$ in normal adults is the result of the combination of mild $\dot{V}/\dot{Q}$ mismatch and a small anatomic right-to-left shunt. At sea level, none of the $P(A - a)O_2$ in normal individuals is caused by diffusion limitation, even during heavy exercise. Diffusion disequilibrium may contribute to an increased $P(A - a)O_2$ during exercise and at high altitudes.[15]

The $P(A - a)O_2$ increases with increasing PAO_2. In lungs with severe non-uniform $\dot{V}/\dot{Q}$ distribution, the $P(A - a)O_2$ reaches a maximum at FIO_2 of about 0.6 to 0.7 and then decreases at higher FIO_2. The decline in the $P(A - a)O_2$ at higher FIO_2 is caused by more uniform rises in PAO_2, which overcome the nonuniform distribution of $\dot{V}/\dot{Q}$ ratios. This nonlinear relationship between the $P(A - a)O_2$ and FIO_2 makes reference $P(A - a)O_2$ values obtained with supplemental O_2 difficult to use in critically ill patients, whose FIO_2 values vary frequently.

The PaO_2/FIO_2 is a simple, bedside index of O_2 exchange when $\dot{V}/\dot{Q}$ mismatch is the primary cause of hypoxemia. A normal PaO_2/FIO_2 is about 450 if using 95 mm Hg for the PaO_2 and 0.21 for the FIO_2. This ratio loses reliability when hypoventilation contributes to hypoxemia, however. The PaO_2/PAO_2 is another easily calculated index of oxygenation. It has advantages and disadvantages similar to those of the PaO_2/FIO_2. In addition, the PaO_2/PAO_2 can be misleading if $P\bar{v}O_2$ fluctuates. For example, when cardiac output decreases, the $P\bar{v}O_2$ falls because the tissues have more time to extract O_2 from the blood. $P\bar{v}O_2$ decreases PaO_2, resulting in lower PaO_2/PAO_2, but the decrease is not because of worsening gas exchange in the lungs but because of low cardiac output. The PaO_2/FIO_2 is also affected by $PaCO_2$ (e.g., hypoventilation increases $PaCO_2$, which will drop the PAO_2 and the PaO_2).

TABLE 48-2
Acceptable PaO_2 Ranges for Adults in Supine Position at Sea Level*

Age (y)	30	40	50	60	70	80	90
PaO_2 (mm Hg)	>90	>85	>80	>75	>70	>65	>60

PaO_2 = partial pressure of oxygen, arterial.

*Values are calculated with the equation of Sorbini CA, Grassi V, Solinas E, Muiesan G. Arterial oxygen tension in relation to age in healthy subjects. *Respiration*. 1968;25(1):3–13.

Shunt

Hypoxemia due to the presence of right-to-left shunt can be differentiated from that caused by low $\dot{V}/\dot{Q}$ by breathing 100% O_2 and obtaining blood for gas analysis. While the individual breathes pure O_2, lung units with low $\dot{V}/\dot{Q}$ ratios increase their PAO_2 maximally with

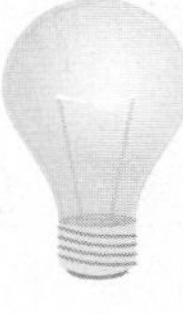

STOP AND THINK

Your patient has a PaO_2 of 80 mm Hg breathing 60% O_2. How can shunt be differentiated from $\dot{V}/\dot{Q}$ mismatch? Why might this information be important?

elevation of the P_{IO_2} but areas with shunt do not. The amount of the shunt can be calculated:

$$\dot{Q}_S/\dot{Q}_T = (Cc'o_2 - Cao_2)/(Cc'o_2 - C\bar{v}o_2)$$

where $\dot{Q}_S$ is the shunt (expressed as a fraction of cardiac output), $\dot{Q}_T$ is cardiac output, $Cc'o_2$ is end-capillary O_2 content from the non-shunt alveoli, Cao_2 is arterial O_2 content, and $C\bar{v}o_2$ is mixed venous O_2 content.

Breathing 100% O_2 increases the Pao_2 to greater than 600 mm Hg in normal adults. If Pao_2 only rises to 250 mm Hg during 100% O_2 breathing, the shunt is about 25% of the cardiac output. This procedure does not determine the location of a shunt, which may be intracardiac (e.g., ventricular septal defect) or intrapulmonary (e.g., atelectasis caused by a mucous plug that occludes a lung segment), but the calculation can help the clinician focus the differential diagnosis for causes of hypoxemia that develop predominantly by shunt mechanisms. Furthermore, because Pao_2 shows little response to variations in F_{IO_2} at shunt fractions that exceed 25%, the clinician may be encouraged to avoid administration of high F_{IO_2} and reduce the risk of O_2 toxicity. The shunt calculation frequently overestimates the true shunt, however, because alveoli with very low $\dot{V}/\dot{Q}$ (< 0.1) may collapse completely during O_2 breathing (due to absorption atelectasis, also called nitrogen washout atelectasis).

Physiologic Mechanisms of Hypoxemia

Hypoxemia is an abnormal condition of having low O_2 level in the blood (low Pao_2). Hypoventilation decreases the Pao_2 and increases the $Paco_2$. If $\dot{V}/\dot{Q}$ distribution is normal, no alveolar-arterial Pao_2 difference is present for either O_2 or CO_2. Although hypoxemia caused by hypoventilation can be corrected with supplemental O_2, the primary treatment should be directed toward support of alveolar ventilation.

$\dot{V}/\dot{Q}$ mismatch (low $\dot{V}/\dot{Q}$ units) is the most common cause of hypoxemia (**Figure 48-5**). **Figure 48-6** illustrates how $\dot{V}/\dot{Q}$ mismatch can cause hypoxemia with a two-compartment lung model. High $\dot{V}/\dot{Q}$ units do not cause hypoxemia because the blood perfusing these units is well oxygenated. Hypoxemia associated with asthma, COPD, and interstitial lung disease is mostly caused by $\dot{V}/\dot{Q}$ mismatch. Hypoxemia caused by $\dot{V}/\dot{Q}$ mismatch usually responds to supplemental O_2.

When blood passes through the pulmonary circulation without going past functional alveoli, it returns to the left heart as unoxygenated blood. This is called a right-to-left shunt. The effects of a right-to-left shunt on gas exchange are shown schematically in **Figure 48-7**. In this example, 33% of the total blood flow (2.0 L/min) is shunt, bypassing the normal path around the alveoli. Although gas exchange in units A and B is unimpaired (these units have normal $\dot{V}/\dot{Q}$), the net result from the mixture of blood from these two units and the shunt pathway is a reduction of Pao_2 and an increased A-a gradient. This effect on Pao_2 is similar to that caused by $\dot{V}/\dot{Q}$ mismatch.

Because of the absence of ventilation in the shunt pathway, hypoxemia resulting from right-to-left shunt cannot be corrected via breathing of 100% O_2. Thus breathing 100% O_2 allows $\dot{V}/\dot{Q}$ mismatch to be differentiated from shunt as the cause of hypoxemia. Classic examples of right-to-left shunt include atelectasis, arteriovenous malformation caused by hereditary hemorrhagic telangiectasia (Osler-Weber-Rendu disease), liver cirrhosis, and congenital heart diseases (Eisenmenger syndrome, tetralogy of Fallot).

A reduction in diffusion (also called a diffusion defect or impaired diffusion) may be a cause of hypoxemia under certain circumstances. In healthy individuals resting at sea level, O_2 equilibrates quickly between the blood and gas phases in the alveolar region of the lung, and diffusion limitation does not occur. During exercise at higher altitudes (greater than 10,000 feet), the $P(A - a)O_2$ may increase because of diffusion

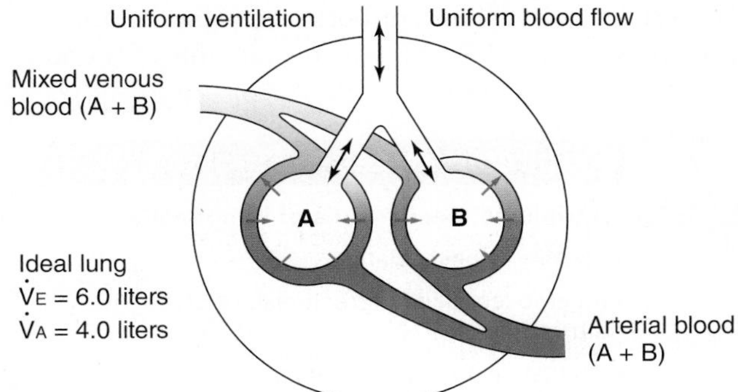

	A	B	(A + B)
Alveolar ventilation (L/min)	2.0	2.0	4.0
Pulmonary blood flow (L/min)	2.5	2.5	5.0
Ventilation/perfusion distribution	0.8	0.8	0.8
Mixed venous Po_2 (mm Hg)	40.0	40.0	40.0
Mixed venous O_2 saturation (%)	75.0	75.0	75.0
Alveolar Po_2 (mm Hg)	101.0	101.0	101.0
Arterial Po_2 (mm Hg)	101.0	101.0	101.0
Arterial O_2 saturation (%)	97.5	97.5	97.5

FIGURE 48-5 Ventilation-perfusion relationships of an ideal lung (**A**) and a healthy lung (**B**) are illustrated with a two-compartment model. Note that the ventilation-perfusion maldistribution is responsible for an alveolar-arterial Po_2 difference of about 4.4 mm Hg; the remainder of the normal Po_2 difference is caused by anatomic shunts (ignored in this illustration).

Adapted from Forster RE, et al., eds. *The Normal Lung: Physiological Basis of Pulmonary Function Tests*. 3rd ed. Year-Book; 1986.

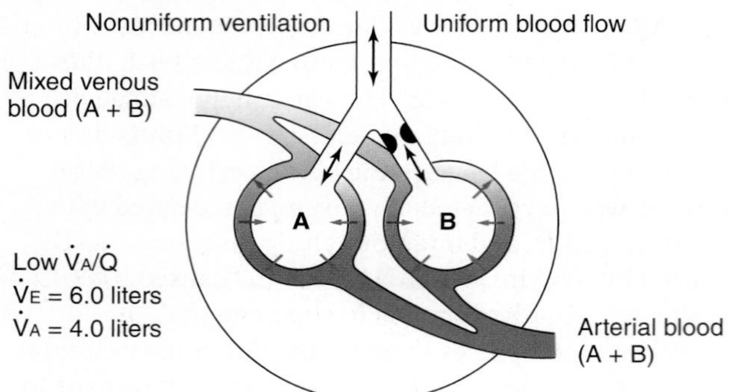

	A	B	(A + B)
Alveolar ventilation (L/min)	3.2	0.8	4.0
Pulmonary blood flow (L/min)	2.5	2.5	5.0
Ventilation/perfusion distribution	1.3	0.3	0.8
Mixed venous Po_2 (mm Hg)	40.0	40.0	40.0
Mixed venous O_2 saturation (%)	75.0	75.0	75.0
Alveolar Po_2 (mm Hg)	116.0	66.0	106.0
Arterial Po_2 (mm Hg)	116.0	66.0	84.0
Arterial O_2 saturation (%)	98.2	91.7	95.0

FIGURE 48-6 Effects of nonuniform distribution of ventilation with uniform blood flow on gas exchange in a two-compartment lung model. If the total ventilation remains at 4 L/min, but unit A receives four times as much ventilation as unit B (3.2 L/min versus 0.8 L/min) and the distribution of perfusion is uniform (2.5 L/min for each unit), the $\dot{V}/\dot{Q}$ ratio for unit A becomes 1.3, whereas that for unit B is 0.3. Oxygen tension and saturation must decrease in blood, leaving unit B with low $\dot{V}/\dot{Q}$; oxygen saturation must rise in blood, leaving unit A with high $\dot{V}/\dot{Q}$. Because of the sigmoid shape of the oxyhemoglobin equilibrium curve, high Po_2 in the blood leaving high-$\dot{V}/\dot{Q}$ unit A is not sufficient to compensate for the low Po_2 contributed by low-$\dot{V}/\dot{Q}$ unit B. The final Po_2 in the pulmonary venous blood, which is derived from blood flow–weighted average of oxygen content, decreases. The arterial blood then would have a Po_2 of 84 mm Hg instead of 100 mm Hg, as in the healthy lung.

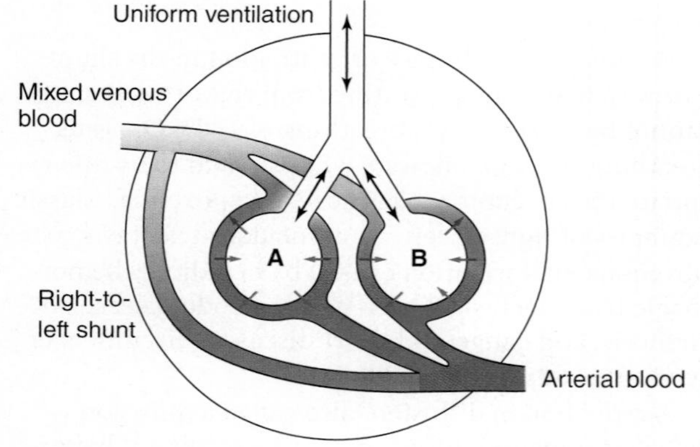

	A + B	Shunt	(A + B + shunt)
Alveolar ventilation (L/min)	4.8	0.0	4.8
Pulmonary blood flow (L/min)	4.0	2.0	6.0
Ventilation/perfusion distribution	1.2	0.0	0.8
Mixed venous Po_2 (mm Hg)	40.0	40.0	40.0
Mixed venous O_2 saturation (%)	75.0	75.0	75.0
Mixed venous Pco_2 (mm Hg)	46.0	46.0	46.0
Alveolar Po_2 (mm Hg)	114.0	—	114.0
Arterial Po_2 (mm Hg)	114.0	40.0	59.0
Arterial O_2 saturation (%)	98.2	75.0	90.5
Arterial Pco_2 (mm Hg)	36.0	46.0	39.0
$P(A - a)O_2$ difference (mm Hg)	0.0	—	55.0

FIGURE 48-7 Effects of right-to-left shunt on gas exchange in a two-compartment lung model.
Adapted from Baum GL, et al. *Textbook of Pulmonary Diseases*. 6th ed. Lippincott Williams & Wilkins; 1998.

impairment. There is a low barometric pressure at high altitude, so exercise-induced diffusion abnormality is a result of the combined effects of a lower ambient Po_2, which decreases the diffusion gradient, and an increase in the rate of blood flow, which shortens the capillary transit time. In individuals with severe lung diseases who exercise, diffusion impairment also can be an important determinant of hypoxemia because the pulmonary capillary blood volume is decreased, further exacerbating the effect of short capillary transit time during exercise. Similar to $\dot{V}/\dot{Q}$ mismatch, hypoxemia caused by diffusion impairment can be corrected by breathing 100% O_2.

Low mixed venous O_2 content ($C\bar{v}o_2$) may also contribute to hypoxemia. The O_2 content of pulmonary artery (mixed venous) blood usually has little effect on Pao_2 in individuals with normal lungs. In the presence of abnormal lungs with a substantial amount of either $\dot{V}/\dot{Q}$ abnormalities, however, or a large right-to-left shunt, or both, the O_2 content in the mixed venous blood has a considerable effect on

Respiratory Recap

Physiologic Mechanisms of Hypoxemia

- Alveolar hypoventilation
- Right-to-left shunt (intracardiac or intrapulmonary)
- Ventilation-perfusion mismatch
- Diffusion defect
- Low mixed venous O_2 content
- Low Pio_2 (e.g., at altitude)

Pa_{O_2} because the abnormal lung is unable to fully oxygenate the blood when it traverses the pulmonary circulation. For a given $\dot{V}/\dot{Q}$ mismatch, the lower the mixed venous O_2 content, the lower the Pa_{O_2}. This mechanism of hypoxemia is particularly important in critically ill individuals with serious cardiopulmonary diseases. The response to supplemental O_2 depends on the relative contributions of $\dot{V}/\dot{Q}$ mismatch and right-to-left shunt to hypoxemia if $C\bar{v}_{O_2}$ remains the same. Correcting low $C\bar{v}_{O_2}$ (e.g., by increasing cardiac output) can significantly increase Pa_{O_2}. Tissue hypoxia may occur when hypoxemia is present and may also be caused by other issues.

Oxygen Transport

The O_2 pathway begins in the atmosphere, where P_{O_2} is about 160 mm Hg at sea level, and ends at the mitochondria, where P_{O_2} is only a few millimeters of mercury. The only blood–air interface is the alveolar-capillary membrane. O_2 and CO_2 exchange therefore occurs only in the alveoli and nowhere else in the lungs (the thickness of the airways blocks the diffusion of the gases). Alveolar ventilation is the only portion of the minute ventilation that affects arterial blood gases. O_2 is taken up by the approximately 300 million alveoli, each of which is about 300 μm in diameter. The huge alveolar surface area (approximately 75 m^2) and the thin alveolar-capillary membrane (<0.5 μm thick) provide an extremely efficient mechanism for O_2 movement from alveolus to capillary.

Deoxygenated blood travels to the heart and is pumped forward by the right ventricle into the pulmonary artery and the pulmonary circulation. As the pulmonary circulation reaches the alveoli, gas exchange occurs (CO_2 exits the blood and O_2 enters). Pulmonary capillary blood leaving the alveoli contains the same P_{O_2} as alveolar gas. The Pa_{O_2} is slightly lower than $P_{A_{O_2}}$, however, because local matching of ventilation and perfusion in normal lungs is imperfect. In addition, a small amount of unoxygenated blood is added to pulmonary capillary blood through anatomic shunts connecting the venous bronchial circulation to the pulmonary venous blood. Oxygenated blood travels from the lungs back to the heart and is pumped out of the heart by the left ventricle into the aorta and the systemic circulation. The arterial blood travels to the systemic capillaries, where O_2 diffuses into the tissue cells to support aerobic metabolism. The bulk of molecular O_2 (about 90%) is consumed in the cellular mitochondria.

When alveolar O_2 diffuses into the pulmonary capillaries, it binds with Hb in the erythrocytes. Each erythrocyte traverses the pulmonary capillary in about 0.75 s (pulmonary capillary transit time) (**Figure 48-8**). Within the first third of this brief transit time (0.25 s), the partial pressure of the O_2 in the alveoli and capillary bed reaches equilibrium and Hb approaches full O_2 saturation (measured as Hb saturation). At the same time, CO_2 diffuses into the alveoli and is removed by ventilation. Transportation of the blood gases is carried out by the heart and circulation of the blood. Normal cardiac output is 5 L/min. A decrease in cardiac output will decrease the supply of O_2 to the tissues.

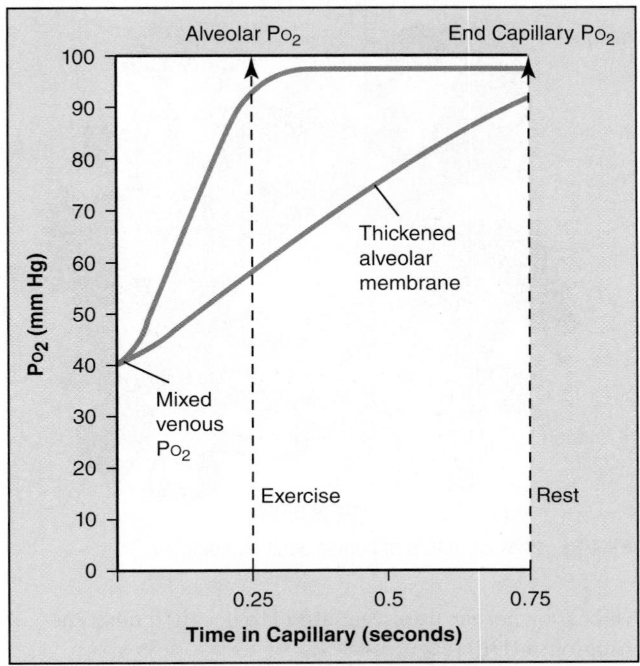

FIGURE 48-8 Typical time courses for the change in P_{O_2} in the pulmonary capillary. Note that it takes an average of 0.75 second for each erythrocyte to traverse the pulmonary microcirculation. In healthy lungs the hemoglobin becomes virtually completely oxygenated within 0.25 second. In abnormal lungs with significant $\dot{V}/\dot{Q}$ mismatch and thickened alveolocapillary membrane, the hemoglobin at end capillary may not be fully saturated. This effect is further accentuated by exercise, which shortens the capillary transit time.

Modified from Baum GL, et al. *Textbook of Pulmonary Diseases*. 7th ed. Lippincott Williams & Wilkins; 2003.

The Oxyhemoglobin Dissociation Curve

Once O_2 diffuses into the pulmonary capillaries, it binds rapidly to Hb. O_2 does not oxidize hemoglobin. Rather, it oxygenates Hb in a reversible process. Each Hb molecule can bind with four O_2 molecules. Hb is the major protein of erythrocytes, which allows it to transport molecular O_2 from the lungs to the tissues and CO_2 from the tissues to the lungs. Because Hb exists inside the red blood cell, high concentrations can be carried without affecting the blood's oncotic pressure. Human Hb has four polypeptide chains that make up the globin part (two α-polypeptides and two β-polypeptides), and each of the four has a heme group that contains iron. The iron in the heme group is where O_2 molecules attach reversibly to the Hb molecule. Combined with O_2, Hb is called oxyhemoglobin

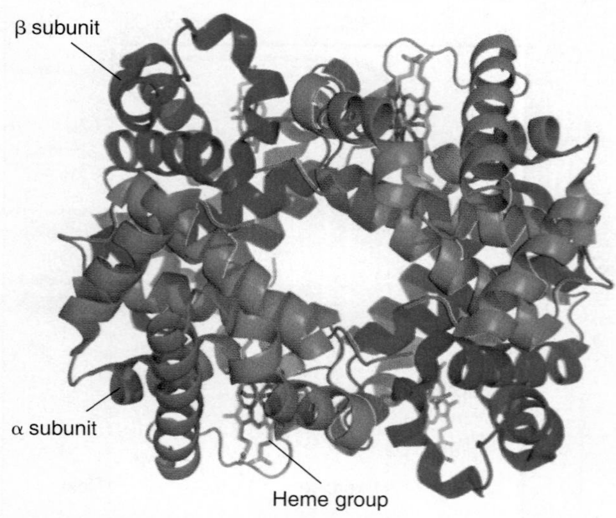

FIGURE 48-9 Structure of human adult hemoglobin.

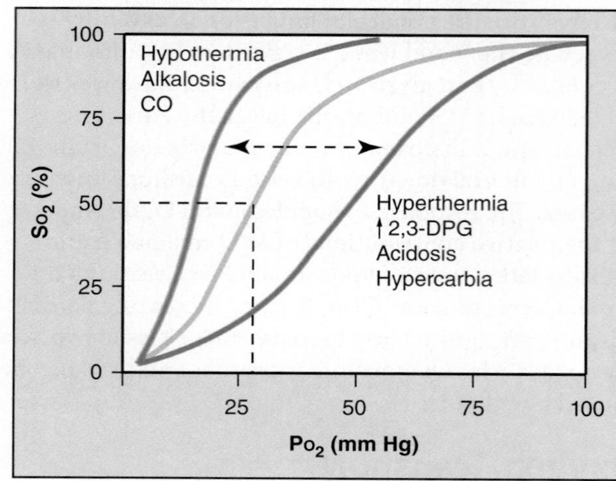

FIGURE 48-10 Oxyhemoglobin dissociation curve. The normal P_{50} value is indicated by the dashed lines. The changes in position of the curve associated with various effector molecules are indicated by the dashed arrows.

Modified from Baum GL, et al. *Textbook of Pulmonary Diseases*. 7th ed. Philadelphia: Lippincott Williams & Wilkins; 2003.

(HbO_2), whereas unoxygenated Hb is called deoxyhemoglobin (Hb) (**Figure 48-9**).

The Hb molecule takes up and releases O_2 molecules in a process known as cooperative binding. As O_2 molecules successively bind with Hb, the Hb molecule physically changes its shape, which increases its affinity for the next O_2 molecule. Similarly, the release of the first O_2 molecule facilitates the release of each remaining molecule. The change in the shape of the Hb molecule that occurs with loading or unloading O_2 molecules causes it to reflect and absorb light differently when it is oxygenated than when it is deoxygenated. This phenomenon is responsible for the bright red color of oxygenated Hb in arterial blood and the deep purple color of deoxygenated Hb in venous blood. This difference in light absorption and reflection makes it possible to measure the amount of oxygenated Hb present in a blood sample through a process known as spectrophotometry, or as it is clinically known, oximetry. The cooperative binding phenomenon is responsible for the sigmoid shape of the **oxyhemoglobin dissociation curve (ODC)** (**Figure 48-10**). The curve is plotted with HbO_2 saturation (Sao_2) as a function of Po_2. As Po_2 increases, the more O_2 binds to Hb. When the Po_2 is low, Hb picks up very little O_2, the curve is flattened, and Hb saturation is very low. As Po_2 increases, Hb binds with O_2 much more quickly and the slope of the curve rises rapidly. As Po_2 reaches about 70 mm Hg, the curve flattens and O_2 saturation becomes high, approaching 100%.

The ODC relates to the attraction between Hb and O_2. This is described as the affinity of Hb for O_2. When affinity is increased, the attraction between Hb and O_2 is high and O_2 binds quickly and easily to the Hb receptor sites. Decreased affinity allows O_2 to release easily from Hb. The position of the ODC changes due to the influence of many factors. Its position is expressed by the P_{50}, or the Po_2 that corresponds with 50% O_2 saturation. The normal P_{50} for human Hb is approximately 27 mm Hg. When the ODC shifts to the left, the Hb affinity for O_2 increases and is reflected in a lower value for P_{50}. When the ODC shifts to the right the Hb affinity for O_2 decreases and is reflected in a higher value for P_{50}.

The position of the ODC is influenced primarily by four factors; pH, temperature, Pco_2, and 2,3-DPG. When there is an increase in temperature, Pco_2, or 2,3-DPG, or a decrease in pH (acidemia), the ODC shifts to the right (**Table 48-3**). When there is a decrease in temperature, Pco_2, or 2,3-DPG, or an increase in

TABLE 48-3
Effect of Various Factors on the Affinity of Hemoglobin to Oxygen and P_{50}

Factors	Changes	O_2 Affinity	P_{50}
pH	↑ (Alkalemia)	↑	↓
	↓ (Acidemia)	↓	↑
2,3-DPG	↑	↓	↑
	↓	↑	↓
Temperature	↑	↓	↑
	↓	↑	↓
Pco_2	↑	↓	↑
	↓	↑	↓
CO	↑	↑	↓
Methemoglobin	↑	↑	↓
Fetal hemoglobin	↑	↑	↓

P_{50}, Po_2 that corresponds with 50% O_2 saturation; 2,3-DPG, 2,3-diphosphoglycerate; Pco_2, partial pressure of carbon dioxide; CO, carbon monoxide.

pH (alkalemia), the ODC shifts to the left. 2,3-DPG is produced in the erythrocytes during glycolysis. An increase in 2,3-DPG facilitates release of O_2 by shifting the ODC to the right. Through this important mechanism, erythrocytes defend against tissue hypoxia after vigorous exercise, after ascent to high altitude, and in numerous diseases associated with reduction in O_2 availability (such as anemia, right-to-left shunt, congestive heart failure, and the chronic hypoxemia of chronic obstructive pulmonary disease). Low levels of 2,3-DPG with corresponding increases in O_2 affinity have been observed in individuals with hypophosphatemia and septic shock. Low levels of 2,3-DPG are also found in stored blood used for transfusions.

The shifts in the ODC help the uptake of O_2 in the lungs and the unloading of O_2 at the tissue. At the tissue, the ODC is shifted to the right due to the relatively higher level of CO_2. Hb affinity for O_2 is decreased and O_2 releases easily from the Hb to diffuse into the tissues for use by the mitochondria. CO_2 diffusion into the blood at the tissue level decreases Hb affinity for O_2, thus enhancing the release of O_2 to the tissues. This is called the **Bohr effect**. At the same time, O_2 dissociates from the Hb molecule and diffuses out of the blood into the tissues. The release of O_2 enhances Hb's ability to carry CO_2. This is called the Haldane effect. It should be appreciated that the Haldane and Bohr effects are mutually enhancing. As O_2 diffuses into the tissue cells, it dissociates from the Hb, enhancing its ability to carry CO_2 (Haldane effect). At the same time, CO_2 diffusion into the blood at the tissue level decreases Hb affinity for O_2 (Bohr effect), enhancing the release of O_2 to the tissues.

In the lungs, CO_2 diffuses out of the blood, into the alveoli, and is then exhaled. As the blood level of CO_2 falls, this shifts the ODC to the left and Hb affinity for O_2 is increased. This shift enhances the uptake of O_2 by Hb. With fever, body temperature is increased and the ODC shifts to the right (linked to a decrease in Hb affinity for O_2). The opposite is true for a person who is hypothermic (low body temperature), which occurs with exposure to cold water or prolonged exposure to cold temperatures outside.

> **Respiratory Recap**
>
> **Oxyhemoglobin Dissociation Curve**
>
> - The sigmoid curve describes the relationship between O_2 saturation and Po_2
> - A shift to the left causes an increased affinity of Hb for O_2
> - A shift to the right causes a decreased affinity of Hb for O_2
> - Numerous physiologic conditions affect the position of the curve

O_2 Content in the Blood

The Cao_2 is a measurement of the O_2 carrying capacity of the blood, but it may not give a good measurement of O_2 delivery, which is dependent on both Cao_2 and the circulation. O_2 is carried in the blood in two forms: (1) as dissolved O_2 in the plasma and (2) combined with Hb. One gram of Hb can combine with a maximum of 1.34 mL O_2, whereas the dissolved O_2 depends on the Pao_2. For each 1 mm Hg Pao_2, 0.003 mL O_2 will dissolve in 100 mL of plasma. Note that Hb concentration is expressed in g/100 mL. To calculate the Cao_2 the following formula is used:

$$Cao_2 = ([Hb] \times 1.34 \times Sao_2) + (Pao_2 \times 0.003)$$

Assuming that the Hb is 15 g/100 mL, the Pao_2 is 100 mm Hg and the Sao_2 is 97%, the Cao_2 will be about 20 mL/100 mL.

Hb carries the majority of the O_2 in the blood; this is reflected in the first part of the formula ([Hb] × 1.34 × Sao_2). The dissolved O_2 transported in the blood is reflected in the last part of the formula (100 mm Hg × 0.003 mL/100 mL), which is 0.3 mL/100 mL. So Hb carries about 98% of the blood's O_2 content and the dissolved portion is only 2%. The Cao_2 is very steady and relatively unchanging from the time blood leaves the left ventricle and into the aorta until the blood reaches the capillary beds at the tissues. At this point Hb releases O_2 for use by the tissues.

The Cao_2 demonstrates that Hb is the primary carrier for O_2. If a person has anemia, the capacity for carrying O_2 to the tissues is greatly reduced. If the Hb drops to 8 g/dL with a Pao_2 of 100 mm Hg and the Sao_2 is 97%, the Cao_2 will drop to 10.7 mL/100 mL. This demonstrates that although the Pao_2 and the Sao_2 are normal, when anemia is present, the delivery of O_2 to the tissues will be poor. Methemoglobin, fetal hemoglobin, and carbon monoxide (CO) poisoning will also decrease delivery of O_2 to the tissues by increasing Hb affinity for O_2 and interfering with the release of O_2 when the blood delivers the Hb to the capillary bed.

Methemoglobin occurs when the normal state of iron in the Hb (the ferrous state) is changed to an abnormal ferric state. When this happens, the iron molecule is not able to bind with O_2. Methemoglobin is formed when the ferrous (Fe^{+2}) iron center of the heme molecule is oxidized to the ferric state (Fe^{+3}). Normal red blood cells contain less than 1% methemoglobin. Levels of methemoglobin may be elevated if too much nitrate or nitrite is ingested or administered (found in sodium nitrite, amyl nitrite, nitroglycerin, nitroprusside, silver nitrate, inhaled nitric oxide). Methemoglobin may also occur due to an inherited abnormality (hemoglobin M disorder). **Box 48-1** lists clinical conditions associated with increased methemoglobin formation.

Fetal hemoglobin (Hb F) occurs naturally in the fetus. Fetal Hb has higher affinity for O_2 than adult

BOX 48-1

Conditions Associated with Methemoglobinemia

Hereditary

M hemoglobins
Cytochrome b_5 reductase deficiency

Acquired

Nitrites and nitrates: sodium nitrite, amyl nitrite, nitroglycerin, nitroprusside, silver nitrate, inhaled nitric oxide
Aniline dyes: aminobenzenes, nitrobenzene
Acetanilid and phenacetin
Sulfonamides, sulfasalazine
Other: lidocaine, chlorate, phenazopyridine, ferrous sulfate, quinones

Hb (Hb A). The ODC is naturally shifted to the left in the fetus, and the Hb F allows for rapid and vigorous O_2 uptake from the placenta. Most of the Hb F is gone by 6 months of age and is naturally replaced by Hb A.

CO poisoning occurs when a person breathes gases from an incomplete combustion of a carbon-based material. Examples include fire in an enclosed space, the exhaust from a car, a space heater that burns fuel, or a gas-powered electrical generator. Hb affinity for CO is about 200 times more than for O_2.[16] So when CO is present, Hb will bind to it very aggressively. At the same time, CO increases Hb affinity for O_2 and shifts the ODC to the left. This interferes with the release of O_2 at the tissue level.

O_2 Delivery and O_2 Consumption

Arterial blood carries the O_2 to the capillary beds in the tissues where O_2 is released from Hb to be used for cellular metabolism. But only a portion of the O_2 is released. Blood that returns from the tissues to the right side of the heart (venous blood) still carries a fair amount of O_2. The difference between the arterial blood and the venous blood reflects O_2 used by the tissues is called O_2 consumption. A blood sample taken from the pulmonary artery provides a measurement of the residual O_2 left in the blood just before the blood picks up the incoming supply of O_2. The pulmonary artery sample of blood is called a mixed venous sample because the blood from all parts of the body has been thoroughly mixed by the time it reaches the pulmonary arteries. If blood was taken from one of the larger accessible veins like the subclavian veins in the upper anterior chest, the O_2 levels reflect the O_2 demand from the region drained by those veins (namely, the chest, neck, and head). These measurements of O_2 may be different compared to blood coming back to the heart through the femoral veins found in the legs. The mixed venous oxyhemoglobin saturation ($S\bar{v}O_2$) and the mixed venous PO_2 ($P\bar{v}O_2$) are normally 75% and 40 mm Hg, respectively.

The mixed venous O_2 content ($C\bar{v}O_2$) is calculated in the same fashion as the CaO_2 but using the mixed venous measurements for the saturation and partial pressure of O_2. To calculate the $C\bar{v}O_2$ the following formula is used:

$$C\bar{v}O_2 = ([Hb] \times 1.34 \times S\bar{v}O_2) + P\bar{v}O_2 \times 0.003)$$

Assuming that the Hb is 15 g/dL, the $P\bar{v}O_2$ is 40 mm Hg, and the $S\bar{v}O_2$ is 75%, the $C\bar{v}O_2$ will be about 15 mL/100 mL. The portion carried by the Hb is 15.1 mL/100 mL and the dissolved portion is 0.12 mL/100 mL.

Normal cardiac output ($\dot{Q}c$) is 5 L/min. O_2 delivery to the tissue (DO_2) is calculated as:

$$DO_2 = CaO_2 \times \dot{Q}c$$

In a normal adult at sea level and at rest, DO_2 is approximately 1000 mL/min with a Hb concentration of 15 g/100 mL, 97.5% SaO_2, and a $\dot{Q}c$ of 5 L/min). Without Hb (i.e., if the only O_2 being carried in the blood was dissolved O_2 in plasma), one would need a $\dot{Q}c$ of at least 80,000 mL/min to support the normal resting O_2 consumption of about 250 mL/min in adult humans. The most efficient way to increase O_2 to the peripheral tissues is by increasing Hb (the major carrier for O_2) or by increasing $\dot{Q}c$ (**Figure 48-11**).

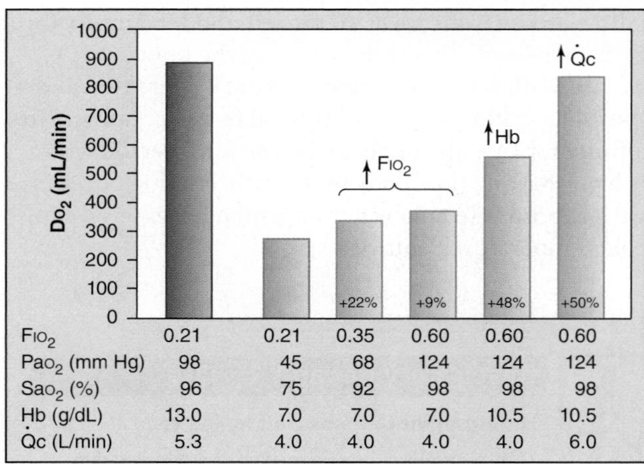

FIO_2	0.21	0.21	0.35	0.60	0.60	0.60
PaO_2 (mm Hg)	98	45	68	124	124	124
SaO_2 (%)	96	75	92	98	98	98
Hb (g/dL)	13.0	7.0	7.0	7.0	10.5	10.5
$\dot{Q}c$ (L/min)	5.3	4.0	4.0	4.0	4.0	6.0

FIGURE 48-11 Relative effects of changes in PaO_2, hemoglobin, and $\dot{Q}c$ on oxygen delivery (DO_2) in a critically ill patient. DO_2 in a normal 75-kg subject at rest is shown in the purple bar, and DO_2 in a patient with hypoxemia, anemia, and reduced $\dot{Q}c$ is shown in the blue bar. The red bars show the effect of sequential interventions on DO_2. The numbers in each bar represent the calculated increase in DO_2 compared with the preceding value.

Reproduced from Huang Y-C. Monitoring oxygen delivery in the critically ill. *Chest.* 2005;125:554–560.

O_2 consumption ($\dot{V}O_2$), the amount of O_2 used by the tissues per minute, can be calculated:

$$\dot{V}O_2 = (CaO_2 - C\bar{v}O_2) \times \dot{Q}c$$

For CaO_2 of 20 mL/100 mL, 15 mL/100 mL for $C\bar{v}O_2$, and 5/min for $\dot{Q}c$, the $\dot{V}O_2$ is about 250 mL/min. (Note: the units for oxygen content are mL/100 mL, so it is necessary to multiply by 10 to convert to L.)

Under normal resting conditions, therefore, the tissues extract about 25% of O_2 delivered to them. The O_2 extraction fraction can increase under conditions such as exercise (increased tissue O_2 demand), congestive heart failure (decreased $\dot{Q}c$ and DO_2), and severe anemia (reduced CaO_2), leading to a lower $C\bar{v}O_2$. Conversely, the O_2 extraction fraction decreases in disease states that greatly increase $\dot{Q}c$ (e.g., sepsis), leading to a higher $C\bar{v}O_2$. Brain tissue and cardiac muscle extract a much higher percentage of the O_2 delivered to them than do other organs. For this reason, the brain and heart are highly susceptible to O_2 deprivation caused by lack of blood flow (ischemia) and low CaO_2 (hypoxemia).

Tissue Hypoxia

Hypoxemia is the abnormal condition of low O_2 levels in the blood. Tissue hypoxia is the condition of low O_2 levels in the tissues. Hypoxemia is one of the causes of hypoxia but there are several other causes as well. Hypoxia brings about complex disturbances of cellular function, primarily because of inadequate production of high-energy phosphate compounds such as ATP during aerobic metabolism of glucose. When the O_2 supply to the tissues is insufficient, glucose is metabolized anaerobically to pyruvate and lactate. Organs that use large amounts of O_2, such as the brain and heart, are more susceptible to hypoxia. When PaO_2 is reduced acutely (hypoxemia), symptoms and signs of cerebral hypoxia (such as impaired judgment, motor incoordination, or altered mental status) and cardiac hypoxia (such as myocardial ischemia or arrhythmias) tend to manifest first. When hypoxia becomes more severe and prolonged, the respiratory centers of the brain stem are affected, and death usually occurs as a result of respiratory failure. Although tissue hypoxia may be associated with a variety of clinical conditions, it is generally divided into five categories (**Table 48-4**).

TABLE 48-4
Mechanisms of Tissue Hypoxia

Mechanism	Examples	Response to Oxygen
Hypoxemic	Lung diseases, high altitude	Good in most cases (except in right-to-left shunt)
Anemic	Severe anemia, carbon monoxide poisoning, methemoglobinemia	Generally ineffective in pure anemia; high FIO_2 effective in CO poisoning
Stagnant	Cardiac failure, hypovolemia, peripheral vascular diseases, cardiac arrest	Poor
Affinity	Alkalosis, carbon monoxide poisoning	Ineffective for alkalosis; high FIO_2 effective in CO poisoning
Histotoxic	Cyanide poisoning	Poor

FIO_2, fraction inspired oxygen; CO, carbon monoxide.

Hypoxemic hypoxia results from an inadequate amount of O_2 in the blood (reduced PaO_2) caused by either lung diseases or decreased O_2 in the inspired air (such as being at high altitude). Supplemental O_2 corrects tissue hypoxia by raising the PaO_2 in most cases, except right-to-left shunt.

Anemic hypoxia results from a reduction in blood O_2 content, which may be caused by severe anemia or the presence of dyshemoglobin states (such as CO poisoning, which forms carboxyhemoglobin or increases in methemoglobin). In individuals with severe anemia, PaO_2 is normal but the absolute amount of O_2 transported per unit volume of blood is diminished. Because the Hb is well saturated with O_2, supplemental O_2 provides little benefit in augmenting O_2 delivery to the tissues unless the PaO_2 is raised into the hyperbaric range. CO poisoning decreases the O_2-binding capacity of Hb by this means. CO molecules bind to the Hb and form carboxyhemoglobin (HbCO). This prevents the Hb from binding with O_2. Also, HbCO shifts the oxyhemoglobin dissociation curve to the left, impairing the unloading of O_2 at the peripheral tissues. Supplemental O_2 is useful in treating CO poisoning because it displaces CO from Hb and decreases the half-life of carboxyhemoglobin and CO in the tissues. This effect is greatly facilitated by hyperbaric O_2 therapy, which can bring about a huge increase in the dissolved O_2 in the blood.

Stagnant hypoxia is a result of poor tissue perfusion, as may be seen in cases of severe cardiac failure, hypovolemic shock, cardiac arrest, and peripheral vascular diseases. The amount of O_2 delivered to the tissues each minute is reduced in these conditions due to low cardiac output or poor tissue perfusion. Poor perfusion may increase tissue edema, increasing the distance through which O_2 has to travel before it reaches the cells. This further increases tissue hypoxia. Supplemental O_2 usually is not helpful unless tissue perfusion can be restored.

Affinity hypoxia occurs when the Hb does not release O_2 to the tissues. This occurs with a left shift of the ODC, such as with alkalosis. CO poisoning leads to both anemic hypoxia and affinity hypoxia, because it causes a left shift of the ODC.

Respiratory Recap

Mechanisms of Tissue Hypoxia

- Hypoxemic hypoxia
- Anemic hypoxia (including carboxyhemoglobin, methemoglobinemia)
- Stagnant hypoxia (e.g., venous stasis)
- Affinity hypoxia
- Histotoxic hypoxia (e.g., cyanide poisoning)

Histotoxic hypoxia is an inability to use O_2 at the cellular level, as with cyanide or sulfide poisoning. These chemical poisons produce cellular hypoxia by inhibiting electron-transfer function by cytochrome oxidase so that O_2 cannot be reduced to water. Because O_2 delivered to the tissues by the blood is not used, the venous blood tends to have a high Pao_2. Supplemental O_2 has little benefit unless the underlying toxic process is reversed.

Mixed Venous O_2

Mixed venous Po_2 ($P\bar{v}o_2$) is the Po_2 in blood of the pulmonary artery. It is a measurement that reflects the O_2 concentration of the pooled venous blood returning from the body to the heart. Both $P\bar{v}o_2$ and $S\bar{v}o_2$ are important in the assessment of Do_2 and $\dot{V}o_2$. $S\bar{v}o_2$ should be measured in blood drawn from the distal port of the pulmonary artery catheter, which represents the true mixture of venous blood from the upper body via the superior vena cava (SVC), the lower body via the inferior vena cava (IVC), and the heart via the coronary sinuses. The measured values of $P\bar{v}o_2$ and $S\bar{v}o_2$ are considered the gold standard for assessing venous O_2 levels. A blood sample from a peripheral vein should not be used for this purpose.

At rest, the normal $P\bar{v}o_2$ is 35 to 45 mm Hg and $S\bar{v}o_2$ is 65% to 75%. A $P\bar{v}o_2$ below 35 mm Hg in a critically ill individual suggests that O_2 extraction is increased and that tissues may be hypoxic. A normal or a higher-than-normal value, however, does not always mean that the tissues have adequate oxygenation. For example, in sepsis, blood may bypass tissues through the peripheral arterial-venous shunting. Less O_2, therefore, is extracted by the tissues, leading to higher-than-normal $P\bar{v}o_2$, but tissue oxygenation is impaired. In the individual with cyanide poisoning, O_2 delivered to the tissues cannot be used because the cytochrome oxidase of the respiratory transport chain is inhibited. $P\bar{v}o_2$ increases despite severe tissue hypoxia in the absence of impaired O_2 utilization (e.g., cyanide poisoning and sepsis). $P\bar{v}o_2$ and $S\bar{v}o_2$ are directly related to cardiac output. When cardiac output and thus O_2 decrease, the tissues respond by extracting more O_2 from the blood to maintain tissue oxygenation, causing $P\bar{v}o_2$ and $S\bar{v}o_2$ to fall.

Because of the declining use of pulmonary artery catheters, many clinicians now measure O_2 saturation in blood withdrawn from a central venous catheter ($Scvo_2$). Because of its easy accessibility, $Scvo_2$ has been used to guide medical therapy, for example, in assessing the adequacy of fluid resuscitation in septic shock.[17] It is important to remember that this measurement, although frequently called mixed venous measurement, in fact only assesses the SVC venous saturation. $Scvo_2$ does not include venous saturation from coronary sinuses. $Scvo_2$ also may vary depending on the location of the tip of the central venous catheter. The measurement may vary if the tip is in the superior vena cava (SVC), inferior vena cava (IVC), or the junction. Although $S\bar{v}o_2$ and $Scvo_2$ follow a parallel course in normal individuals, their relationship in critically ill patients is variable.[18] In one study, the differences between $S\bar{v}o_2$ and $Scvo_2$ ranged from −8% to 16.5%.[19] But in a more recent study, if the placement of the tip of the catheter is placed in the right atrium, the gap between the $Scvo_2$ and the $S\bar{v}o_2$ is greatly reduced. A measurement of the $Scvo_2$ taken with the tip 15 cm away from the opening into the right atrium was 8% higher than the $S\bar{v}o_2$ while the measurement taken in the right atrium showed a +1% error when compared to the $S\bar{v}o_2$.[20]

Key Points

- Physiologic mechanisms of hypoxemia include $\dot{V}/\dot{Q}$ mismatch, shunt, hypoventilation, diffusion defect, and, in patients with critical illnesses, low mixed venous Po_2.
- The shifts in the oxyhemoglobin dissociation curve help the uptake of O_2 in the lungs and the unloading of O_2 at the tissue level.
- Causes of tissue hypoxia include hypoxemic hypoxia, anemic hypoxia, stagnant hypoxia, affinity hypoxia, and histotoxic hypoxia.
- Physiologic mechanisms of hypercapnia include hypoventilation, severe $\dot{V}/\dot{Q}$ mismatch, and, in patients with borderline lung function, increased CO_2 production.
- Oxygenation and ventilation operate under a variety of rules, laws, and physiologic systems.
- Ventilation and oxygenation are regulated in an interdependent fashion involving the cardiopulmonary, cardiovascular, musculoskeletal, neurologic, and renal systems.
- Respiratory therapists must understand the physiology of ventilation and oxygenation to be effective in practice.

References

1. Alveolar ventilation. In: Levitzky M. *Pulmonary Physiology*. 8th ed. New York: McGraw-Hill; 2013.
2. Ventilation. In: West J. *Respiratory Physiology: The Essentials*. 9th ed. Baltimore: Lippincott Williams & Wilkins; 2012.

3. Murray J. *The Normal Lung*. Philadelphia: WB Saunders; 1986.
4. Jones N. Determinants of breathing patterns in exercise. In: Whipp B, Wasserman K, eds. *Exercise: Pulmonary Physiology and Pathophysiology*. New York: Marcel Dekker; 1991.
5. Luks AM. Do lung disease patients need supplemental oxygen at high altitude? *High Alt Med Biol.* 2009;10:321–327.
6. Danesh-Sani SA, Shariati-Sarabi Z, Feiz MR. Comprehensive review of hyperbaric oxygen therapy. *J Craniofacial Surg.* 23:e483–e491.
7. Gas diffusion. In: Beachy W. *Respiratory Care Anatomy and Physiology: Foundations for Clinical Practice*. 3rd ed. St. Louis: Mosby; 2013.
8. Hedenstierna G, Hammond M, Mathieu-Costello O, Wagner PD. Functional lung unit in the pig. *Respir Physiol.* 2000;120: 139–149.
9. Young I, Mazzone RW, Wagner PD. Identification of functional lung unit in the dog by graded vascular embolization. *J Appl Physiol.* 1980;49:132–141.
10. Kent BD. Mitchell PD. McNicholas WT. Hypoxemia in patients with COPD: cause, effects, and disease progression. *Inter J Chron Obstruct Pulmon Dis*. 2011;6:199–208.
11. Weitzenblum E. Chaouat A. Cor pulmonale. *Chronic Resp Dis.* 2009;6:177–185.
12. Cruz JC, Hartley LH, Vogel JA. Effect of altitude relocations upon $AaDo_2$ at rest and during exercise. *J Appl Physiol.* 1975;39:469–474.
13. Mellemgaard K. The alveolar-arterial oxygen difference: its size and components in normal man. *Acta Physiol Scand.* 1966;67:10–20.
14. Sorbini CA, Grassi V, Solinas E, Muiesan G. Arterial oxygen tension in relation to age in healthy subjects. *Respiration*. 1968;25:3–13.
15. Gale GE, Torre-Bueno JR, Moon RE, Saltzman HA, Wagner PD. Ventilation-perfusion inequality in normal humans during exercise at sea level and simulated altitude. *J Appl Physiol.* 1985;58:978–988.
16. Centers for Disease Control and Prevention (CDC). *Carbon Monoxide*. In: Workplace Safety & Health Topics. Available at: http://www.cdc .gov/niosh/topics/co-comp/. Accessed Aug. 31, 2014.
17. Rivers E, Nguyen B, Havstad S, et al. Early goal-directed therapy in the treatment of severe sepsis and septic shock. *N Engl J Med.* 2001;345:1368–1377.
18. Reinhart K, Kuhn HJ, Hartog C, Bredle DL. Continuous central venous and pulmonary artery oxygen saturation monitoring in the critically ill. *Intensive Care Med.* 2004;30:1572–1578.
19. Varpula M, Karlsson S, Ruokonen E, Pettila V. Mixed venous-oxygen saturation cannot be estimated by central venous oxygen saturation in septic shock. *Intensive Care Med*. 2006;32:1336–1343.
20. Kopterides P, Bonovas S, Mavrou I, Kostadima E, Zakynthinos E, Armaganidis A. Venous oxygen saturation and lactate gradient from superior vena cava to pulmonary artery in patients with septic shock. *Shock* 2009;31:561–567.

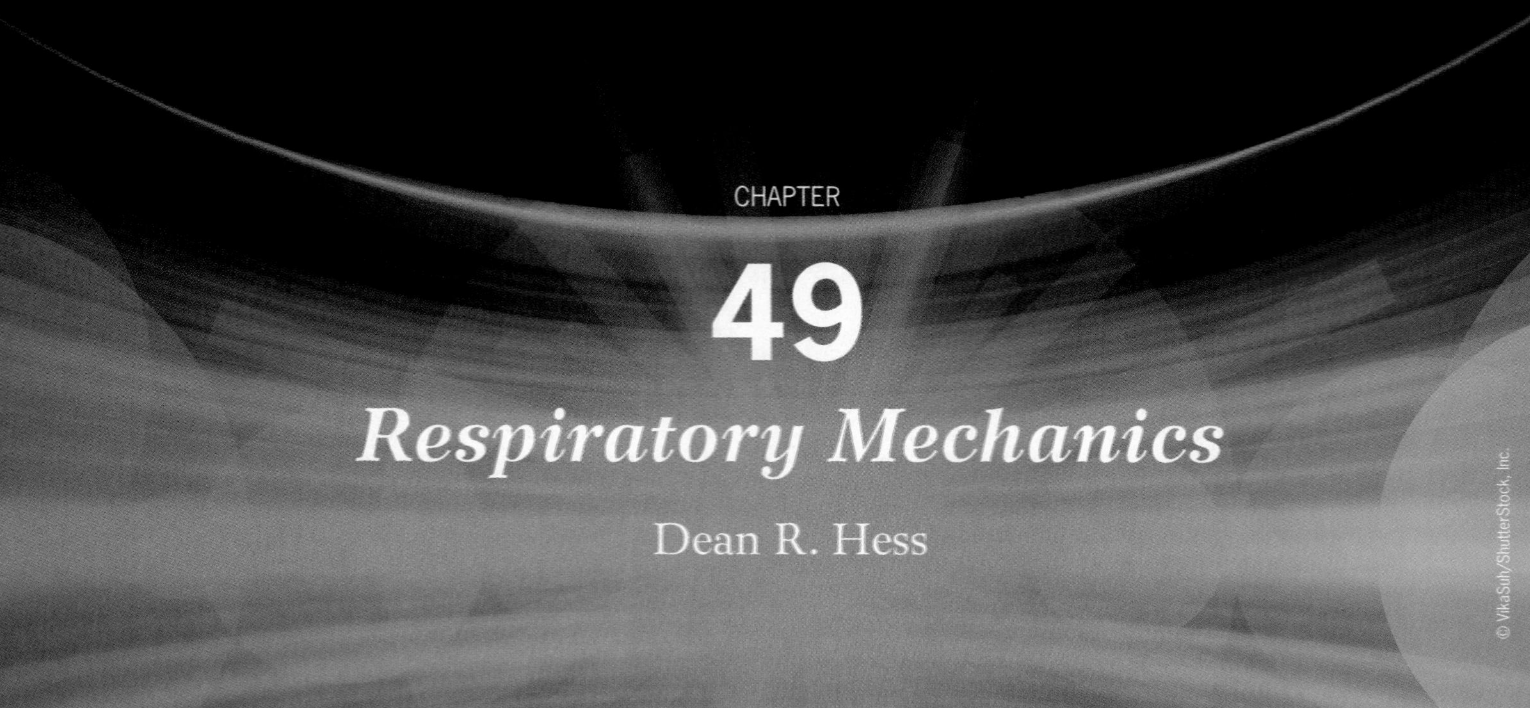

CHAPTER

49 Respiratory Mechanics

Dean R. Hess

OUTLINE

Airways Resistance
Compliance
Pleural Pressure Gradient
The Chest Wall
Respiratory Mechanics During Mechanical Ventilation

OBJECTIVES

1. Define resistance and compliance.
2. Explain why small airways normally contribute little to overall airways resistance.
3. List physiologic factors that increase airways resistance.
4. Describe the concept of flow limitation.
5. Compare lung compliance, chest wall compliance, and respiratory system compliance.
6. Describe the normal pleural pressure gradient.
7. Draw a normal pressure–volume curve for the lungs, chest wall, and respiratory system.
8. Calculate respiratory system compliance and airways resistance for a mechanically ventilated patient.
9. Explain how esophageal pressure can be used to estimate pleural pressure.
10. Use stress and strain to describe ventilator-induced lung injury.
11. Explain how compliance, stress index, pressure–volume curve, and esophageal pressure can be used to titrate PEEP.
12. Discuss the measurement of end-expiratory lung volume during mechanical ventilation.
13. Define work of breathing, pressure-time product, and tension–time index.

KEY WORDS

airways resistance
chest wall compliance
equal pressure point
esophageal pressure (P_{ES})
flow limitation
lung compliance
pressure-time product (PTP)
pressure–volume curve
respiratory mechanics
respiratory system compliance
strain
stress
stress index
tension–time index (TTI)
work of breathing (WOB)

Introduction

Respiratory mechanics relates to the forces needed to move the lungs and the chest wall.[1] These forces overcome resistance and compliance during inspiration. Expiration is passive; elastic recoil pressure and airways resistance determine expiratory flow. **Respiratory mechanics** refers to the expression of lung function through measures of pressure and flow. From these measurements, a variety of derived indices can be determined such as volume, compliance, resistance, and work of breathing.

The most important muscle of inspiration is the diaphragm (**Figure 49-1**). When it contracts, the abdominal contents are forced downward, the vertical dimension of the chest wall is increased, and the rib margins are lifted outward. The external intercostal muscles connect adjacent ribs, and when they contract, the ribs are pulled upward and forward to increase the lateral and the anteroposterior diameters of the thorax. Accessory muscles of inspiration include the scalene muscles, which elevate the first two ribs, and the sternomastoids, which raise the sternum. During exercise and hyperventilation, expiratory muscles become active. The most important muscles of expiration are the rectus abdominis, internal and external oblique muscles, the transversus abdominis, and the internal intercostal muscles.

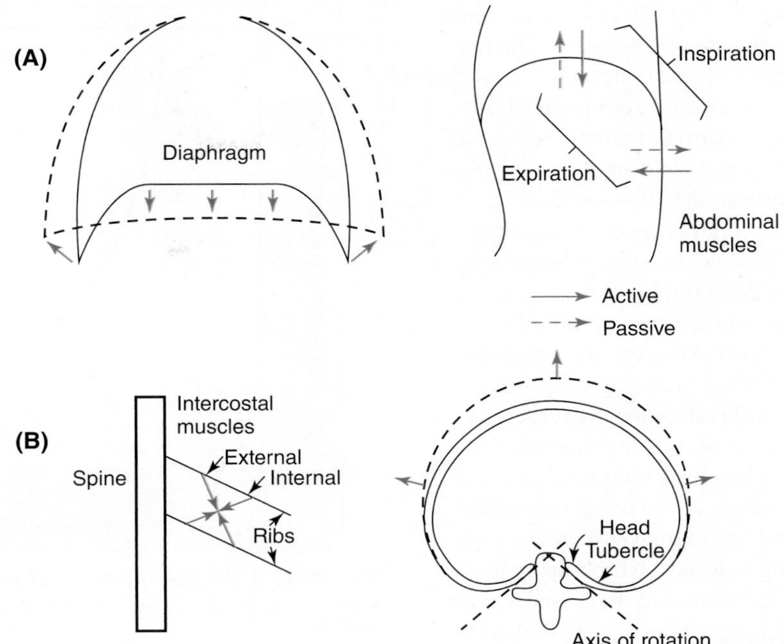

FIGURE 49-1 (**A**) On inspiration, the dome-shaped diaphragm contracts, the abdominal contents are forced down and forward, and the rib cage is widened. Both increase the volume of the thorax. On forced expiration, the abdominal muscles contract and push the diaphragm up. (**B**) When the external intercostal muscles contract, the ribs are pulled upward and forward, and they rotate on an axis joining the tubercle and the head of a rib. As a result, both the lateral and anteroposterior diameters of the thorax increase. The internal intercostals have the opposite action.

Reproduced from West JB. *Respiratory Physiology: The Essentials*. Lippincott (Wolters Kluwer Health); 2011.

In this chapter, the physiology of resistance and compliance of the respiratory system is discussed. After that, the physiology of respiratory mechanics during mechanical ventilation is discussed in detail.

Airways Resistance

At end-expiration, intrapleural pressure is −5 cm H_2O due to the elastic recoil of the lungs. Because there is no flow, alveolar pressure is the same as proximal airway pressure (0 cm H_2O relative to atmospheric pressure). The alveolar pressure decreases to establish the driving pressure necessary for gas to flow into the lungs (**Figure 49-2**). Flow and **airways resistance** determines the magnitude of the pressure needed. In normal individuals, the alveolar pressure required is about 1 cm H_2O. But in patients with obstructive lung disease, however, the alveolar pressure required for flow is greater.

Alveolar pressure decreases during inspiration due to a decrease in intrapleural pressure. The decrease in intrapleural pressure during inspiration is determined by the elastic properties of the lung parenchyma and airways resistance. During expiration, intrapleural pressure is less negative than expected due to airways resistance. Alveolar pressure is positive during expiratory flow, and intrapleural pressure becomes positive with forced expiration, such as a cough.

Moving from the trachea toward the alveoli, the branching of airways becomes more numerous and

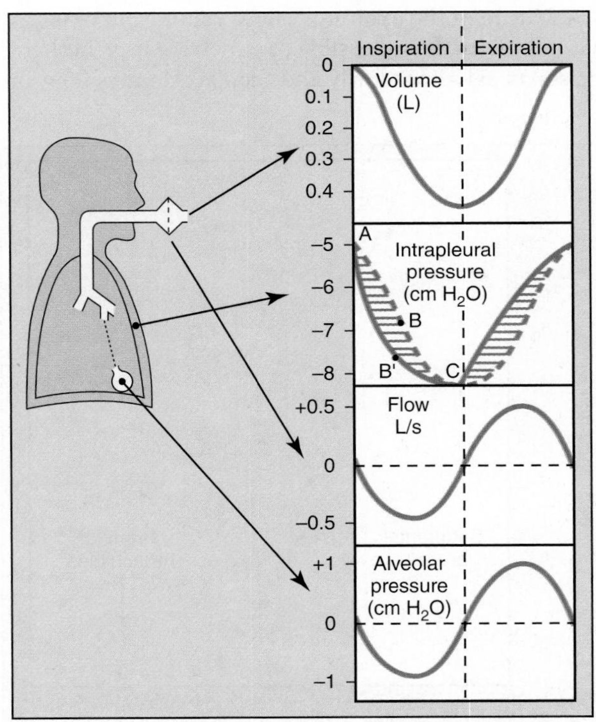

FIGURE 49-2 Pressures during the breathing cycle. If there was no airway resistance, alveolar pressure would remain at zero, and intrapleural pressure would follow the broken line ABC, which is determined by the elastic recoil of the lung. The fall in alveolar pressure is responsible for the hatched portion of intrapleural pressure.

Reproduced from West JB. *Respiratory Physiology: The Essentials*. Lippincott (Wolters Kluwer Health); 2011.

airways become narrower (**Figure 49-3**). Airways resistance, however, is less in the smaller airways. The reason is that the large number of small airways is parallel, such that their total cross-sectional area is very large. That the peripheral airways contribute little resistance is important in the development of lung diseases such as chronic obstructive pulmonary disease (COPD). Because there are so many small airways, they must be significantly affected by disease before the patient becomes symptomatic or detected by spirometry.

Lung volume is an important determinant of airways resistance (**Figure 49-4**). Airways are supported by the radial traction of the surrounding lung. Thus, airway radius increases, and resistance decreases, as the lungs expand. Airway resistance increases as lung volume decreases. At very low lung volumes, small airways in the dependent regions of the lungs may close completely. Patients who have increased airways resistance breathe at high lung volumes, which decreases airways resistance. Clinical causes of increased airways resistance includes bronchospasm (e.g., asthma) and increased airway secretions (e.g., cystic fibrosis). Gas density and viscosity also affects resistance to flow. Changes in density have a greater effect than changes in viscosity because gas flow in medium-sized airways, the major site of resistance in normal lungs, is turbulent (density dependent), whereas flow in small airways is laminar (viscosity dependent).

A feature of the expiratory flow-volume curve is that it is virtually impossible to penetrate it. Whether one starts exhaling slowly and then accelerates flow, or makes a less forceful expiration, the descending portion of the flow-volume curve takes nearly the same path. Flow thus is independent of effort—greater effort has a limited effect on expiratory flow. This is illustrated in **Figure 49-5**. If the flow and intrapleural pressures are

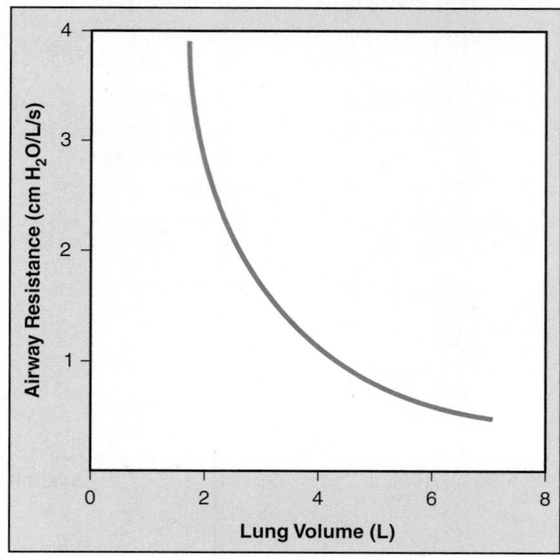

FIGURE 49-4 Variation of airway resistance with lung volume.
Reproduced from West JB. *Respiratory Physiology: The Essentials*. Lippincott (Wolters Kluwer Health); 2011.

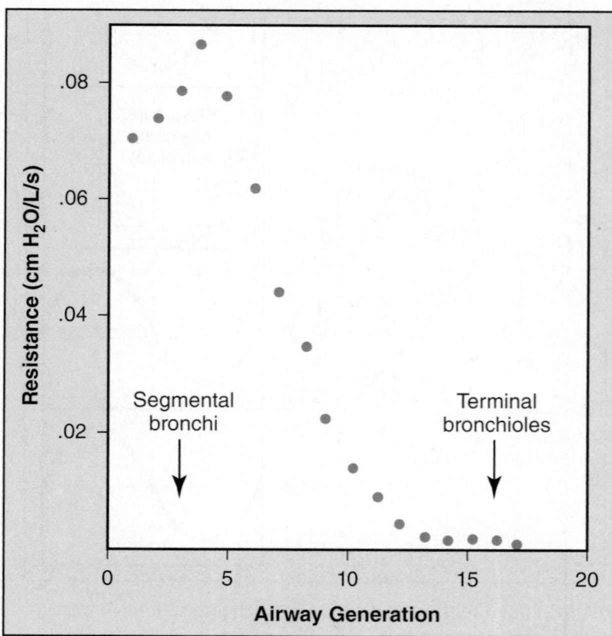

FIGURE 49-3 Location of the chief site of airways resistance. Note that the intermediate-sized bronchi contribute most of the resistance and that relatively little is located in the very small airways.
Reproduced from West JB. *Respiratory Physiology: The Essentials*. Lippincott (Wolters Kluwer Health); 2011.

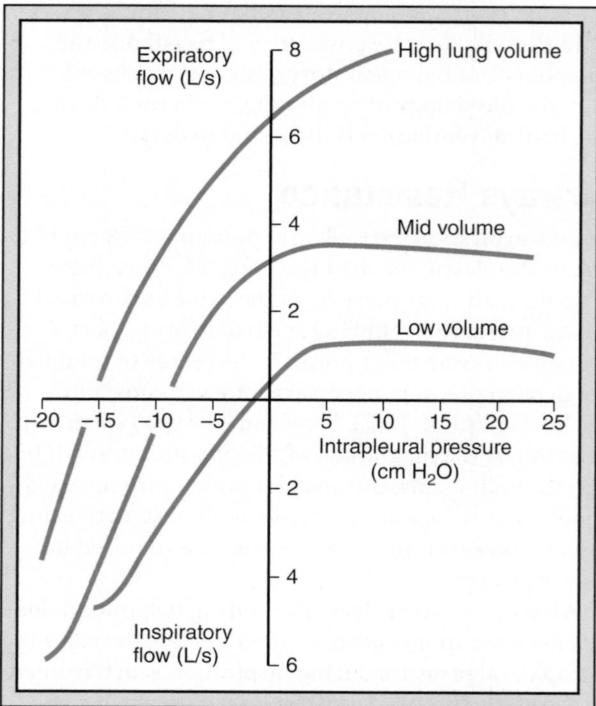

FIGURE 49-5 Isovolume pressure-flow curves drawn for three lung volumes. Each of these was obtained from a series of forced expirations and inspirations. Note that at the high lung volume, a rise in intrapleural pressure (obtained by increasing expiratory effort) results in a greater expiratory flow. At mid and low volumes, however, flow becomes independent.
Reproduced from West JB. *Respiratory Physiology: The Essentials*. Lippincott (Wolters Kluwer Health); 2011.

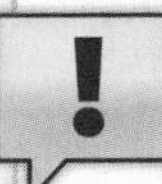

Respiratory Recap

Airways Resistance

- The peripheral airways normally offer little overall resistance because their total cross section is large.
- Lung volume is an important determinant of airways resistance.
- Clinical causes of an increase in airways resistance include bronchospasm and increased airway secretions.
- Flow limitation is the result of airway compression by intrathoracic pressure.

plotted at the same lung volume for each breath, isovolume pressure-flow curves are obtained. At high lung volumes, the expiratory flow increases with effort until a plateau in flow is reached and cannot be increased with further increases in intrapleural pressure.

Flow limitation is the result of airway compression by intrathoracic pressure (**Figure 49-6**). The pressure outside the airways is intrapleural pressure. At end-expiration, airway pressure is zero due to no flow. Because intrapleural pressure is –5 cm H_2O, there is a pressure of 5 cm H_2O holding the airway open. During the inspiratory phase, both intrapleural and alveolar pressure decrease, and there is a net positive distending pressure holding the airway open. At the onset of forced expiration, alveolar pressure is the sum of intrapleural pressure and elastic recoil pressure. Airway compression occurs due to the positive intrapleural pressure. The effective driving pressure, therefore, is elastic recoil pressure because intrapleural pressure compresses alveoli and airways equally.

This is a Starling resistor mechanism. If intrapleural pressure is raised by increased expiratory muscle effort, the effective driving pressure is unaltered because the difference between alveolar pressure and intrapleural pressure is determined by lung volume. In this way, flow is independent of effort. Maximal flow decreases with lung volume because elastic recoil pressure decreases, and also because airway radius decreases. It also follows that flow is independent of the resistance of the airways downstream of the point of collapse, which is called the **equal pressure point**. As expiration proceeds, the equal pressure point moves more distal in the lungs due to loss of elastic recoil pressure and increased airways resistance.

Flow limitation can be made worse in disease by moving the equal pressure point more distal. An increase in resistance of the peripheral airways magnifies the pressure drop along the airway (e.g., bronchospasm, secretions). Low lung volume reduces the driving pressure due to less elastic recoil pressure. Elastic recoil pressure is also reduced with parenchymal destruction, such as occurs in emphysema. With parenchymal destruction, radial traction on the airways is reduced and they are more easily compressed. If the equal pressure point causes dependent airways to collapse, there can be a precipitous decrease in expiratory flow, as observed on the expiratory flow-volume curve of patients with severe COPD.

When the lungs and chest wall move, pressure is required to overcome the viscous forces within the tissues as they slide over each other. Tissue resistance, however, is only about 20% of the total resistance in young normal subjects. Total resistance is called pulmonary resistance to distinguish it from airway resistance.

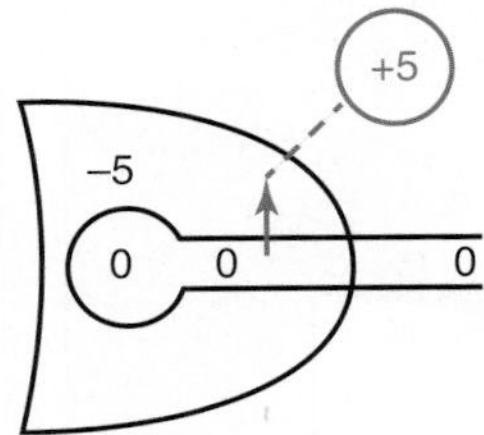

Preinspiration

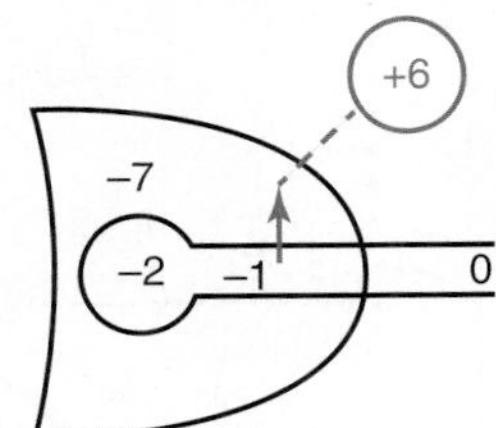

During inspiration

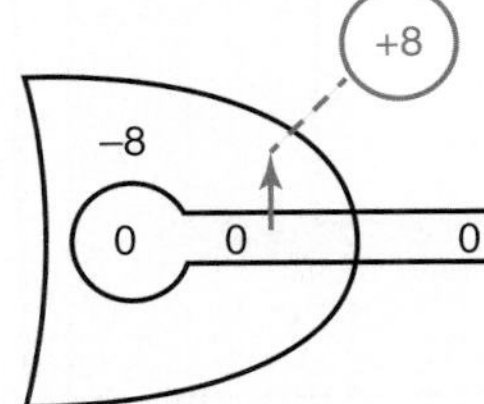

End-inspiration

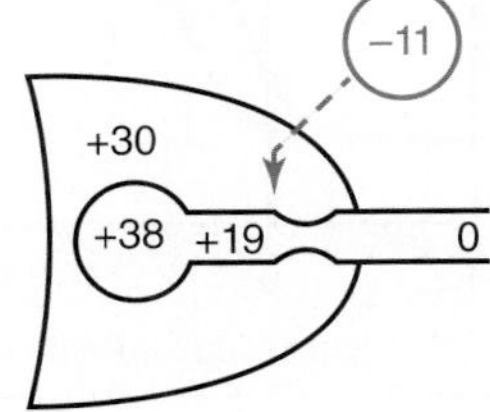

Forced expiration

FIGURE 49-6 Scheme showing why airways are compressed during forced expiration. Note that the pressure difference across the airway is holding it open, except during a forced expiration.

Reproduced from West JB. *Respiratory Physiology: The Essentials*. Lippincott (Wolters Kluwer Health); 2011.

Compliance

Imagine that the lungs are placed inside a rigid container, with the trachea open to atmosphere, and then the pressure within the container is decreased in a stepwise manner (**Figure 49-7**). As the pressure is decreased, the corresponding volume in the lungs is recorded. In this way, the **pressure-volume curve** of the lungs is recorded. In humans, the decrease in pressure is caused by an increase in volume of the chest wall due to respiratory muscle contraction. In Figure 49-7, it can

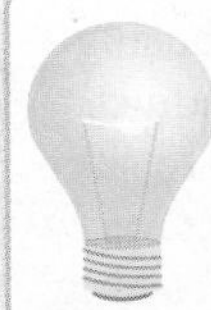

STOP AND THINK

For a mechanically ventilated patient, why does it require proportionately more pressure to ventilate at excessive levels of PEEP than at an appropriate level of PEEP?

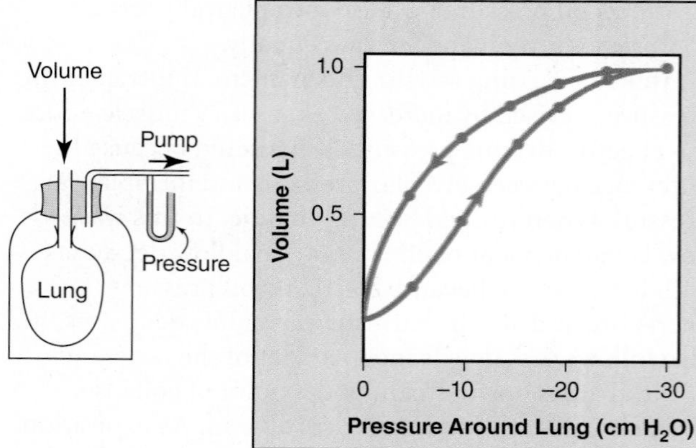

FIGURE 49-7 Measurement of the pressure-volume curve of excised lung. The lung is held at each pressure for a few seconds while its volume is measured. The curve is nonlinear and becomes flatter at high expanding pressures. Note that the inflation and deflation curves are not the same; this is called hysteresis.

Reproduced from West JB. *Respiratory Physiology: The Essentials*. Lippincott (Wolters Kluwer Health); 2011.

be seen that the pressure-volume curves are different for inflation and deflation, which is known as hysteresis. The lung volume at any pressure during deflation is larger than during inflation. Also, the lungs without any distending pressure contain some gas because small airways close, trapping gas in the alveoli. Airway closure occurs at higher lung volumes with increasing age and with disease such as COPD. The difference in pressure between the inside and the outside of the lungs is called *transpulmonary pressure*.

Compliance is the slope of the pressure-volume curve, or the volume change per unit pressure change. In the normal range of distending pressure of −5 to −10 cm H_2O, the lungs are very compliant. At high expanding pressures and high lung volumes, the lungs are stiffer, and compliance is smaller. Compliance can be decreased with pulmonary fibrosis, pulmonary edema, and atelectasis. An increased compliance occurs with COPD due to parenchymal destruction and loss of elastic tissue (emphysema). Compliance also increases in the normal aging lungs (senile emphysema). **Lung compliance** depends on size and therefore the compliance per unit volume of lung (specific compliance) is calculated to assess the intrinsic elastic properties of lung tissue.

The pressure surrounding the lungs is subatmospheric because of the elastic recoil of the lungs. The elastic behavior of the lungs is due to elastic tissue (elastin and collagen) in the lung parenchyma. Another important factor in the pressure-volume behavior of the lungs is the surface tension of the liquid film lining the alveoli. The pressure generated due to surface tension can be predicted using the Law of Laplace: pressure $\propto$ (surface tension/radius).

Surface tension is decreased in the lungs due to surfactant produced by type II alveolar cells. Surfactant lowers the surface tension in alveoli and increases lung compliance. Surfactant also promotes alveolar stability. Due to surface tension and the Law of LaPlace, there would be a tendency for small alveoli to collapse into larger ones (the smaller the radius, the larger the pressure). As the radius of the alveolus decreases, however, surfactant molecules come closer together, surface tension is reduced, and the pressure does not increase as one would expect in the absence of surfactant. In the absence of surfactant, lung compliance is reduced and atelectasis results. If the blood flow to a region of lung is absent as the result of an embolus, surfactant in that region is depleted and atelectasis occurs. Because surfactant is formed late in fetal life, babies born prematurely without adequate amounts of surfactant develop severe respiratory distress.

Another mechanism that contributes to alveolar stability is interdependence. Alveoli are supported by one another. Due to alveolar interdependence, any tendency for one group of alveoli to reduce its volume is opposed by surrounding alveoli. For example, if a group of alveoli has a tendency to collapse, large expanding forces will be developed because the surrounding parenchyma is expanded.

Pleural Pressure Gradient

Due to the weight of the lungs, the intrapleural pressure is more negative at the top of the lungs than the bottom of the lungs. Alveoli at the bottom and at the top of the lungs thus are subjected to different distending pressures (**Figure 49-8**). The lungs are easier to inflate at low volumes than at high volumes, where they become stiffer.

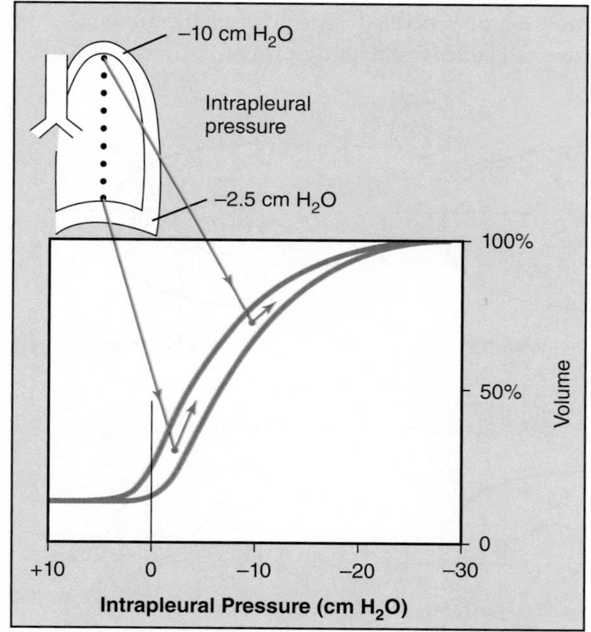

FIGURE 49-8 Explanation of the regional differences of ventilation down the lung. Because of the weight of the lung, the intrapleural pressure is less negative at the base than at the apex. As a consequence, the basal lung is relatively compressed in its resting state but expands more on inspiration than the apex.

Reproduced from West JB. *Respiratory Physiology: The Essentials*. Lippincott (Wolters Kluwer Health); 2011.

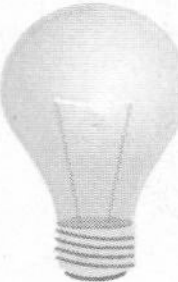

STOP AND THINK

How would you position a patient with unilateral atelectasis to take advantage of the pleural pressure gradient?

Because the expanding pressure at the base of the lung is small, alveoli in this region have a small resting volume. But because they are located on a steep part of the pressure-volume curve, they expand well on inspiration. On the other hand, alveoli at the apex of the lungs have a large expanding pressure, a larger resting volume, and smaller change in volume during inspiration.

Although the bases of the lungs are relatively poorly expanded compared with the apex, they are better ventilated. The same occurs in dependent lung regions in the supine and lateral positions. At low lung volumes, intrapleural pressure is less negative because elastic recoil forces are smaller. The pleural pressure gradient is still present because of the weight of the lungs, however. Now the intrapleural pressure at the bases exceeds atmospheric pressure (**Figure 49-9**). In this circumstance, ventilation is not possible until the intrapleural pressure falls below atmospheric pressure. In this case, the apex of the lungs is on a favorable part of the pressure-volume curve and ventilates well. It is important to note, however, that the compressed region at the bases of the lungs is not airless because airway closure occurs.

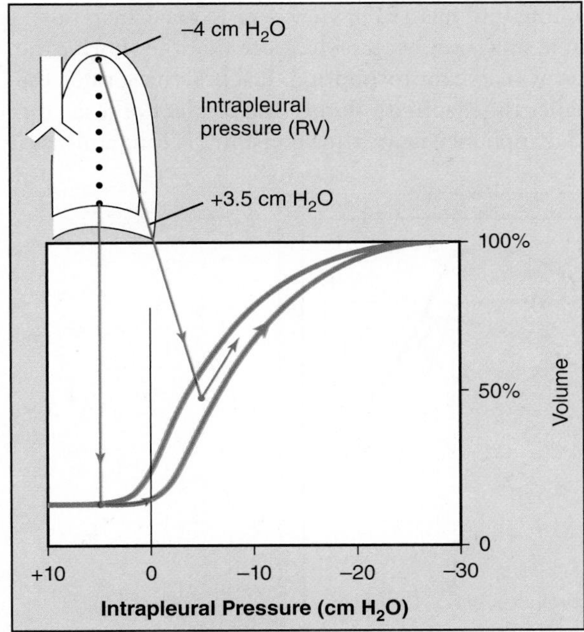

FIGURE 49-9 Situation at very low lung volumes. Now intrapleural pressures are less negative, and the pressure at the base actually exceeds airway (atmospheric) pressure. As a consequence, airway closure occurs in this region, and no gas enters with small inspirations.

Reproduced from West JB. *Respiratory Physiology: The Essentials*. Lippincott (Wolters Kluwer Health); 2011.

The Chest Wall

At equilibrium, the chest wall is pulled inward while the lung is pulled outward, thus producing the normal subatmospheric intrapleural pressure. When air is introduced into the intrapleural space, as with a pneumothorax, the lung collapses inward and the chest wall expands outward. The pressure-volume curve for the lungs and the chest wall is shown in **Figure 49-10**. At functional residual capacity (FRC), the elastic recoil of the lungs is balanced by the outward expansion of the chest wall. At volumes above FRC, the relaxation pressure is positive, and at volumes below FRC, the relaxation pressure is negative. In Figure 49-10, note that at zero pressure the lungs are at their minimal volume, which is below RV. At FRC, the relaxation pressure of the chest wall is negative. It is not until volume is increased to about 75% of the vital capacity that the relaxation pressure of the chest wall is atmospheric. At any volume, the relaxation pressure of the respiratory system (lungs plus chest wall) is the sum of the pressures for the lungs and the chest wall measured separately.

The total compliance of the lung and chest wall (**respiratory system compliance**) is the sum of the reciprocals of the lung and chest wall compliances measured separately:

$$1/Crs = 1/C_L + 1/Ccw$$

Normal lung compliance is 200 mL/cm H_2O and normal **chest wall compliance** is also 200 mL/cm H_2O. Normal respiratory system compliance, therefore, is 100 mL/cm H_2O. Because elastance is the inverse of compliance, this relationship can be rewritten as:

$$Ers = E_L + Ecw$$

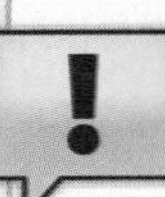

Respiratory Recap

Compliance

- Compliance is the slope of the pressure-volume curve: volume change per pressure change.
- The lungs are less compliant at high lung volumes.
- Compliance is decreased with pulmonary fibrosis, pulmonary edema, and atelectasis.
- An increased compliance occurs with COPD and aging.
- The elastic behavior of the lungs is due to elastic tissue and surface tension.
- Interdependence contributes to alveolar stability.
- The intrapleural pressure is more negative at the top of the lungs than at the bottom of the lungs.
- At functional residual capacity, elastic recoil of the lungs is balanced by chest wall expansion.

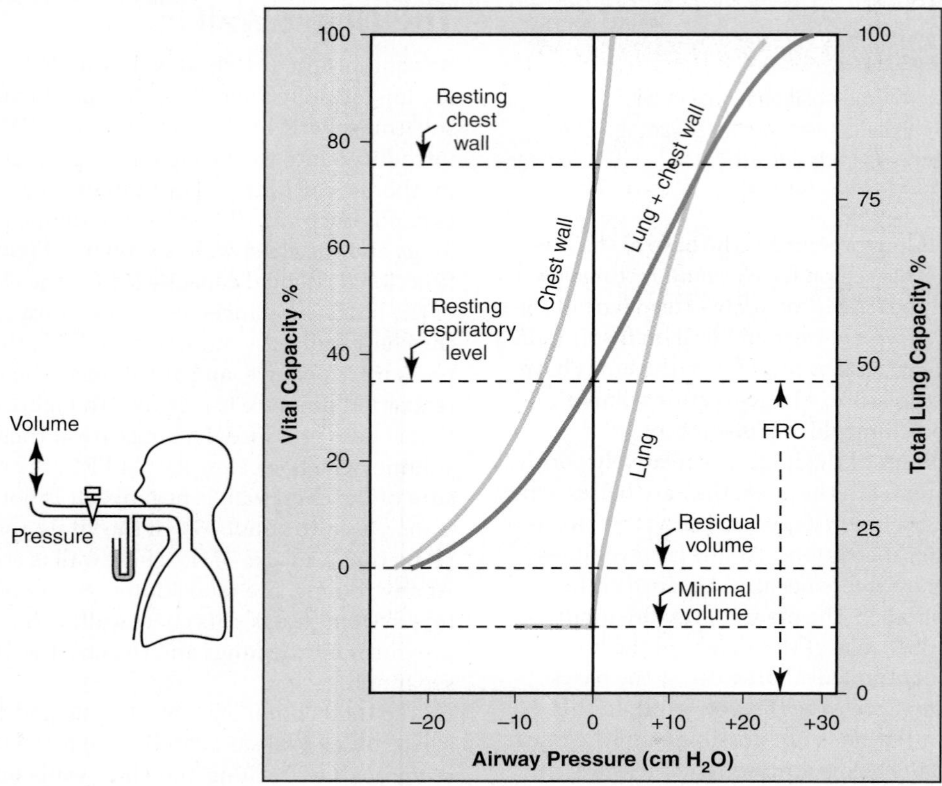

FIGURE 49-10 Relaxation pressure-volume curve of the lung and chest wall. The subject inspires (or expires) to a certain volume from the spirometer, the tap is closed, and the subject then relaxes his respiratory muscles. The curve for lung + chest wall can be explained by the addition of the individual lung and chest wall curves.

Reproduced from West JB. *Respiratory Physiology: The Essentials*. Lippincott (Wolters Kluwer Health); 2011.

Causes of Uneven Ventilation

The ventilation of an individual lung unit depends on the compliance of the alveoli and the resistance of the airway leading to the alveoli (**Figure 49-11**). For a lung unit with normal resistance and compliance, volume change is large and rapid. If a lung unit has a low compliance, its change in volume is rapid but small. If a lung unit has a high airway resistance, inspiration is slow and incomplete. Note that the shorter the time available for inspiration (fast breathing rate), the smaller the inspired volume. The product of resistance and compliance is the time constant. A lung unit with

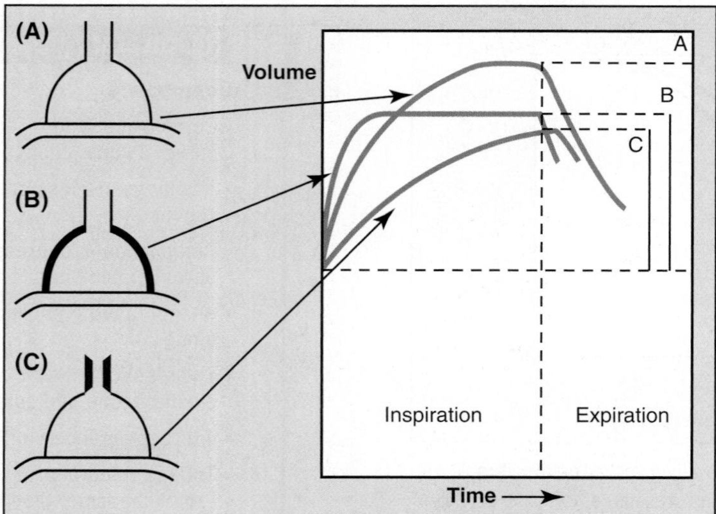

FIGURE 49-11 Effects of decreased compliance (**B**) and increased airways resistance (**C**) on ventilation of lung units compared with normal (**A**). In both instances, the inspired volume is abnormally low.

Reproduced from West JB. *Respiratory Physiology: The Essentials*. Lippincott (Wolters Kluwer Health); 2011.

a low compliance has a fast time constant, whereas a lung unit with a high airways resistance has a slow time constant.

Respiratory Mechanics During Mechanical Ventilation

All current-generation positive pressure ventilators provide monitoring of pulmonary mechanics and graphics in real time at the bedside. When interpreting these measurements, it is important to remember that bedside monitoring of mechanics and graphics during positive pressure ventilation depicts the lungs as a single compartment and assumes a linear response over the range of tidal volume. Respiratory mechanics is useful to evaluate lung function, to assess response to therapy, and to optimize mechanical ventilator support.[2–4]

Equation of Motion

Airway pressure is predicted mathematically by the equation of motion:

$$\text{Pvent} + \text{Pmus} = \text{V}_\text{T}/\text{C} + \text{R} \times \dot{\text{V}} + \text{PEEP} + \text{PEEPi} + \text{inertance}$$

where Pvent is the proximal airway pressure applied by the ventilator, Pmus is the pressure generated by the patient's inspiratory muscles, V_T is tidal volume, C is respiratory system compliance, R is airways resistance, $\dot{V}$ is inspiratory flow, PEEP is the positive end-expiratory pressure set on the ventilator, and PEEPi is intrinsic PEEP (auto-PEEP). The inertance variable, representing the effect of inertia, is assumed to be low and thus disregarded.

R and C can be obtained by fitting the equation of motion to P, V, and $\dot{V}$ with a multiple linear regression analysis, called linear least squares fitting.[4] This is incorporated into the software of some ventilators, allowing display of R, C, and auto-PEEP. The least squares fitting method assumes that Pmus is zero and is thus less valid if the patient is actively breathing.

Alveolar Pressure

During volume control, alveolar pressure (Palv) at any time during inspiration is determined by the volume delivered and respiratory system compliance:

$$\text{Palv} = \text{V}/\text{C} + \text{PEEP}$$

For pressure control, Palv at any time after the initiation of inspiration is:

$$\text{Palv} = \Delta\text{P} \times (1 - e^{-t/\tau}) + \text{PEEP}$$

where ΔP is the pressure applied to the airway above PEEP, e is the base of the natural logarithm, t is the elapsed time after initiation of the inspiratory phase, and τ is the time constant.

Alveolar pressure is estimated with an end-inspiratory hold maneuver. Plateau pressure (Pplat) is measured during mechanical ventilation by applying an end-inspiratory breath hold for 0.5 to 2 seconds, during which time pressure equilibrates so that the pressure measured at the proximal airway approximates alveolar pressure.

Pplat is determined by V_T, respiratory system compliance, and PEEP during full ventilatory support: $\text{Pplat} = V_T/C + \text{PEEP}$. A high Pplat indicates risk of alveolar overdistension; it should ideally be kept ≤30 cm H_2O,[5] and lower is better.[6,7]

Incomplete emptying of the lungs occurs if the expiratory phase is terminated prematurely. The pressure produced by this trapped gas is called auto-PEEP, intrinsic PEEP, or occult PEEP. Auto-PEEP increases end-expiratory lung volume and thus causes dynamic hyperinflation.[8,9] Auto-PEEP is measured by applying an end-expiratory pause for 0.5 to 2 seconds. The pressure measured at the end of this maneuver in excess of the PEEP set on the ventilator is defined as auto-PEEP. For a valid measurement, the patient must be relaxed and breathing in synchrony with the ventilator, as active breathing invalidates the measurement. The end-expiratory pause method can underestimate auto-PEEP when some airways close during expiration, as may occur during ventilation of the lungs of patients with severe asthma (**Figure 49-12**). In spontaneously breathing patients, measurement of esophageal pressure can be used to determine auto-PEEP (**Figure 49-13**).

Auto-PEEP is a function of ventilator settings (tidal volume and expiratory time) and lung function (airways resistance and lung compliance):

$$\text{auto-PEEP} = \text{V}_\text{T}/[\text{C} \times (e^{\text{Kx} \times \text{T}_\text{E}} - 1)]$$

where Kx is the inverse of the expiratory time constant (1/τ) and T_E is the expiratory time. Note that auto-PEEP is increased with increased resistance and compliance, increased respiratory rate or increased inspiratory time (both decrease expiratory time), and increased tidal volume. Clinically, auto-PEEP is reduced by decreasing

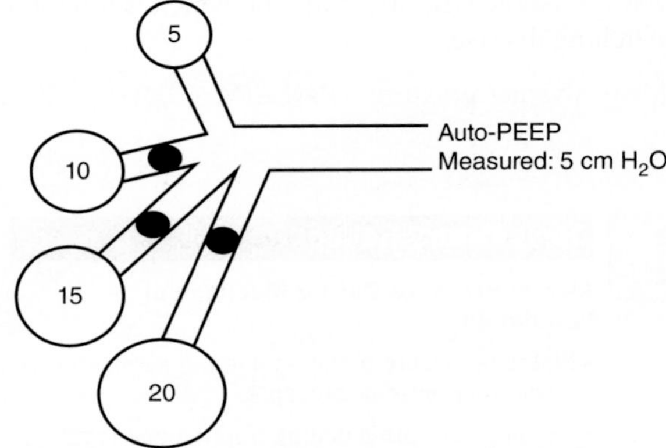

FIGURE 49-12 As illustrated here, the measured auto-PEEP can be considerably less than the auto-PEEP in some lung regions if airways collapse during expiration.

Reproduced from Hess DR. Respiratory mechanics in mechanically ventilated patients. *Respir Care.* 2014;59:1773–1794.

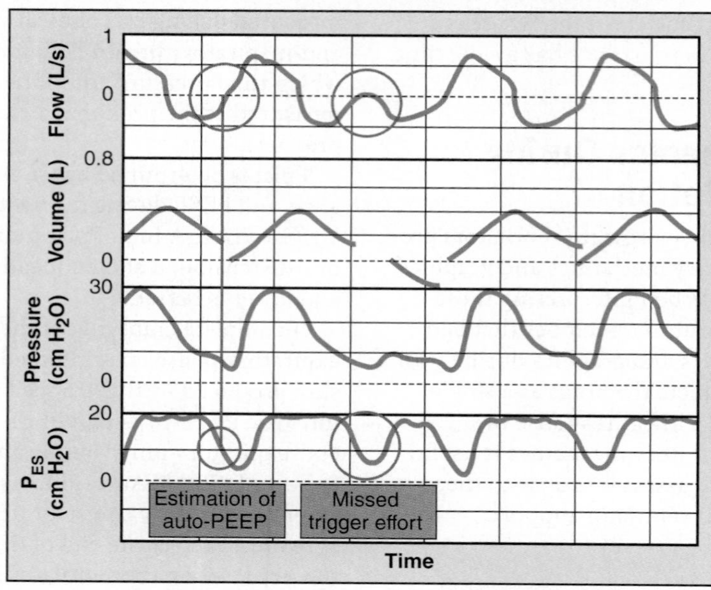

FIGURE 49-13 Auto-PEEP. Note the amount of effort required to trigger the ventilator, represented by the amount of decrease in esophageal pressure required for triggering. Also note the presence of an inspiratory effort that does not trigger the ventilator.

minute ventilation (rate or tidal volume), increasing expiratory time (decreasing rate or inspiratory time), or decreasing airways resistance (e.g., bronchodilator administration and clearing secretions).

Mean airway pressure ($\bar{P}aw$) is determined by peak inspiratory pressure (PIP), the fraction of time devoted to the inspiratory phase (T_I/T_{TOT}), and PEEP. For constant flow volume ventilation, in which the airway pressure waveform is triangular, mean airway pressure can be calculated as:

$$\bar{P}aw = 0.5 \times (PIP - PEEP) \times (T_I/T_{TOT}) + PEEP$$

During pressure ventilation, in which the airway pressure waveform is rectangular, $\bar{P}aw$ can be estimated as:

$$\bar{P}aw = (PIP - PEEP) \times (T_I/T_{TOT}) + PEEP$$

The mean alveolar pressure may be different than $\bar{P}aw$ if the inspiratory airways resistance (R_I) and expiratory airways resistance (R_E) are different, which is often the case in lung disease:

$$\text{Mean alveolar pressure} = \bar{P}aw + (\dot{V}_E/60) \times (R_E - R_I)$$

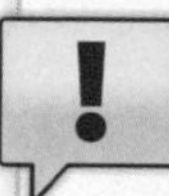

Respiratory Recap

Airway Pressure During Mechanical Ventilation

- Plateau pressure (Pplat) is used to estimate end-inspiratory alveolar pressure.
- The pressure produced by trapped gas is called auto-PEEP.
- Mean airway pressure ($\bar{P}aw$) is determined by peak inspiratory pressure (PIP), the fraction of time devoted to the Ti/Ttot, and PEEP.

Esophageal Pressure

The traditional approach to assess pleural pressure (Ppl) is the use of an esophageal balloon,[10–13] which consists of a thin catheter with multiple small holes in the distal 5 to 7 cm of its length. A 10-cm long balloon is placed over the distal end of the catheter to prevent the holes in the catheter from being occluded by esophageal tissue and secretions, and the balloon is inflated with a small amount of air (0.5 mL). The proximal end of the catheter is attached to a pressure transducer.

The catheter is inserted orally or nasally to about 35 to 40 cm from the airway opening. Correct positioning of the esophageal balloon is necessary to ensure accurate **esophageal pressure (P_{ES})** measurements. After the balloon is inflated and the pressure is measured, the esophageal pressure waveform should be compared to the airway pressure waveform. If they appear similar in pressure and shape, the catheter is likely in the trachea and should be removed. If the catheter is in the esophagus, cardiac oscillations should be visible on the esophageal pressure waveform, indicating that the balloon is positioned in the lower third of the esophagus directly behind the heart (**Figure 49-14**). Some clinicians use a technique in which the catheter is intentionally inserted into the stomach, air is added to the balloon,

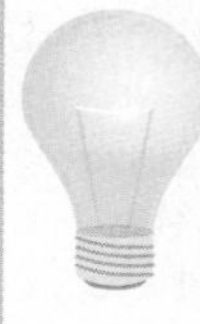

STOP AND THINK

In a paralyzed mechanically ventilated patient, would you expect esophageal pressure to move in the positive direction or the negative direction when the lungs are inflated with a tidal volume?

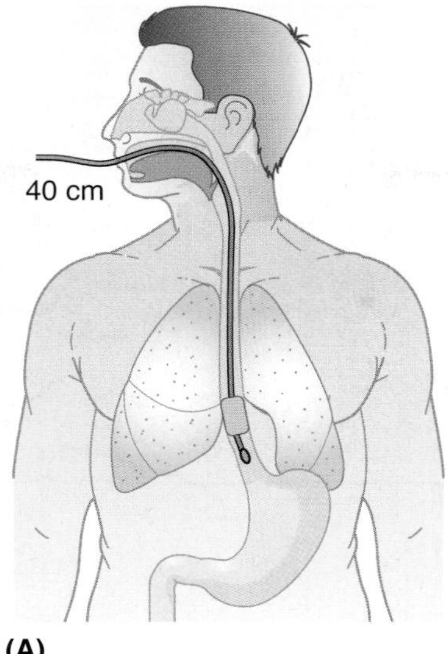

(A)

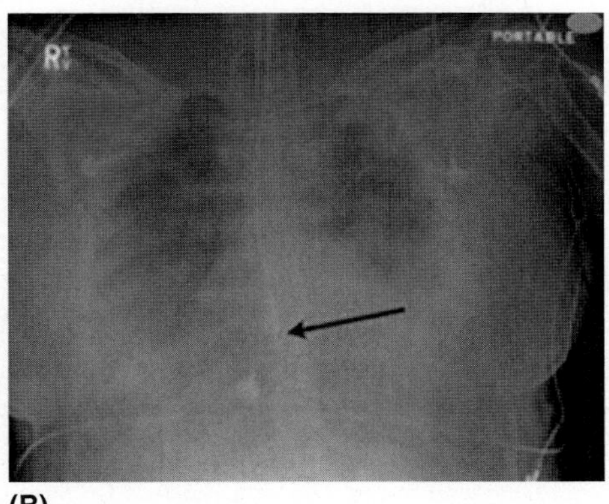

(B)

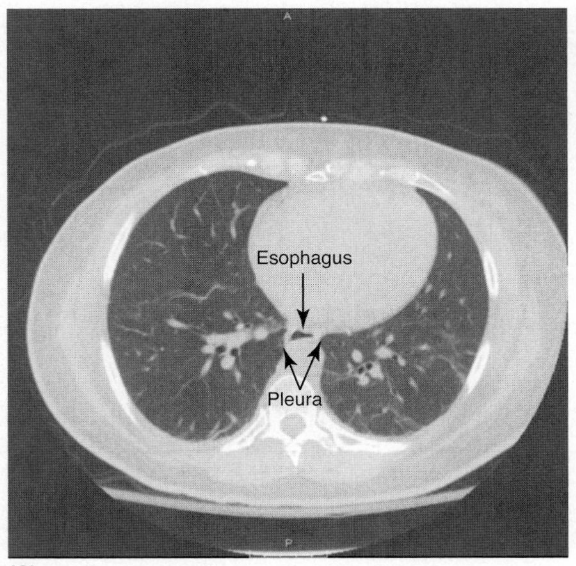

(C)

FIGURE 49-14 (**A**) Correct positioning of the esophageal balloon, about 40 cm from the lips. (**B**) Chest radiograph showing correct balloon placement. (**C**) Note that the esophagus borders the pleural space in the mid-thorax.

(**A–B**) reproduced from Piraino T, Cook DJ. Optimal PEEP guided by esophageal balloon manometry. *Respir Care.* 2011;56:510–513; (**C**) reproduced from Hess DR. Respiratory mechanics in mechanically ventilated patients. *Respir Care.* 2014;59:1773–1794.

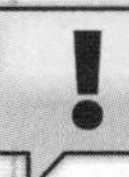

Respiratory Recap

Esophageal Pressure

- Pleural pressure (Ppl) is estimated by use of an esophageal balloon.
- Transpulmonary pressure (P_L) is the difference between pressure measured at the mouth and esophageal (pleural) pressure.
- During no flow, transpulmonary pressure becomes the alveolar distending pressure.
- A stiff chest wall increases esophageal (pleural) pressure during mechanical ventilation.
- The ventilator should be set to avoid a negative transpulmonary pressure during expiration (contributing to cyclical alveolar opening and closing injury) and to avoid excessive transpulmonary pressure at end-inspiration (alveolar overdistention).

and then the catheter is withdrawn until cardiac oscillations are observed.

The classic technique used to validate the balloon's position requires the patient to perform static Valsalva and Mueller maneuvers with the glottis open. In patients unable to cooperate, P_{ES} and airway pressure are assessed during a gentle push on the abdomen with the airway occluded using the expiratory pause on the ventilator. When changes in P_{ES} are equal to airway pressure, it is assumed that transmission of Ppl to P_{ES} is unimpeded and P_{ES} accurately reflects Ppl. There are potential sources of error in the use of P_{ES} to estimate Ppl.[13,14] P_{ES} estimates Ppl mid-thorax, and Ppl is more negative in the nondependent thorax and more positive in the dependent thorax. The weight of the heart can bias the P_{ES} by as much as 5 cm H_2O.

Transpulmonary pressure (P_L) is the difference between pressure measured at the mouth and esophageal (pleural) pressure. During no flow (inspiratory or expiratory pause maneuvers), P_L becomes the alveolar distending pressure. The ventilator should be set to avoid a negative P_L during expiration (contributing to cyclical opening and closing injury) and to avoid excessive P_L at end-inspiration (overdistention). Chest wall effects can increase pleural pressure and, if pleural pressure is high relative to alveolar pressure, there may be potential for alveolar collapse. In that case it is desirable to set PEEP greater than pleural pressure. The use of an esophageal balloon to assess intrapleural pressure has been advocated to allow more precise setting of PEEP (**Figure 49-15** and **Figure 49-16**).[15]

Intra-Abdominal Pressure

Interactions between the abdominal compartment and the thoracic compartment are important

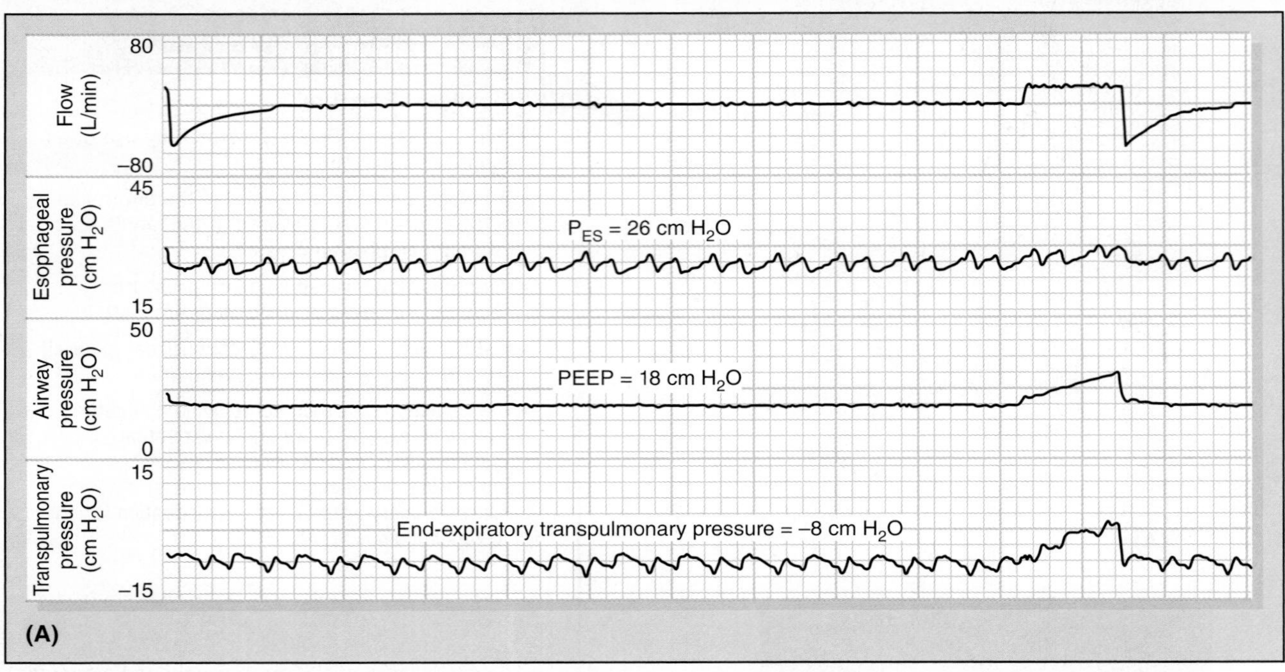

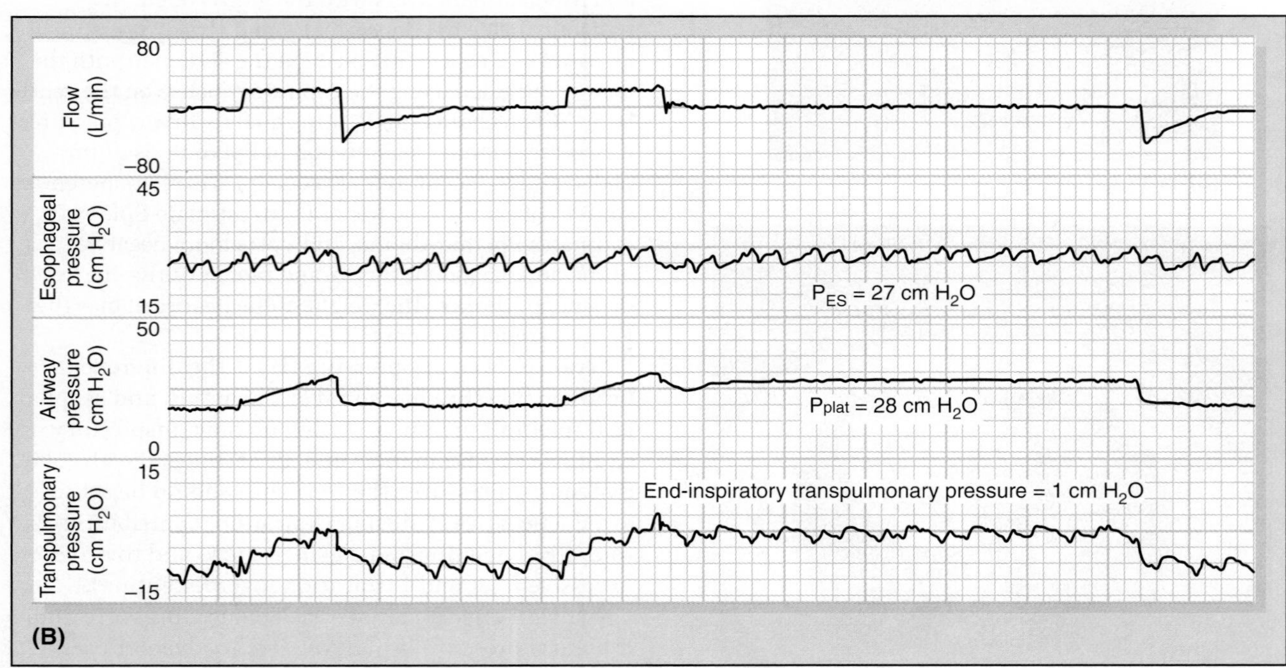

FIGURE 49-15 Esophageal pressure, airway pressure, and transpulmonary pressure with PEEP set at 18 cm H_2O. (**A**) During expiratory pause. (**B**) During inspiratory pause. (**C**) As shown in the cartoon, there is a net collapsing pressure on the lungs, heart, and central circulation at end-expiration. At the mid-thoracic level (position of the esophageal balloon), the end-inspiratory transpulmonary pressure is slightly positive.

(**A–C**) reproduced from Hess DR. Respiratory mechanics in mechanically ventilated patients. *Respir Care.* 2014;59:1773–1794.

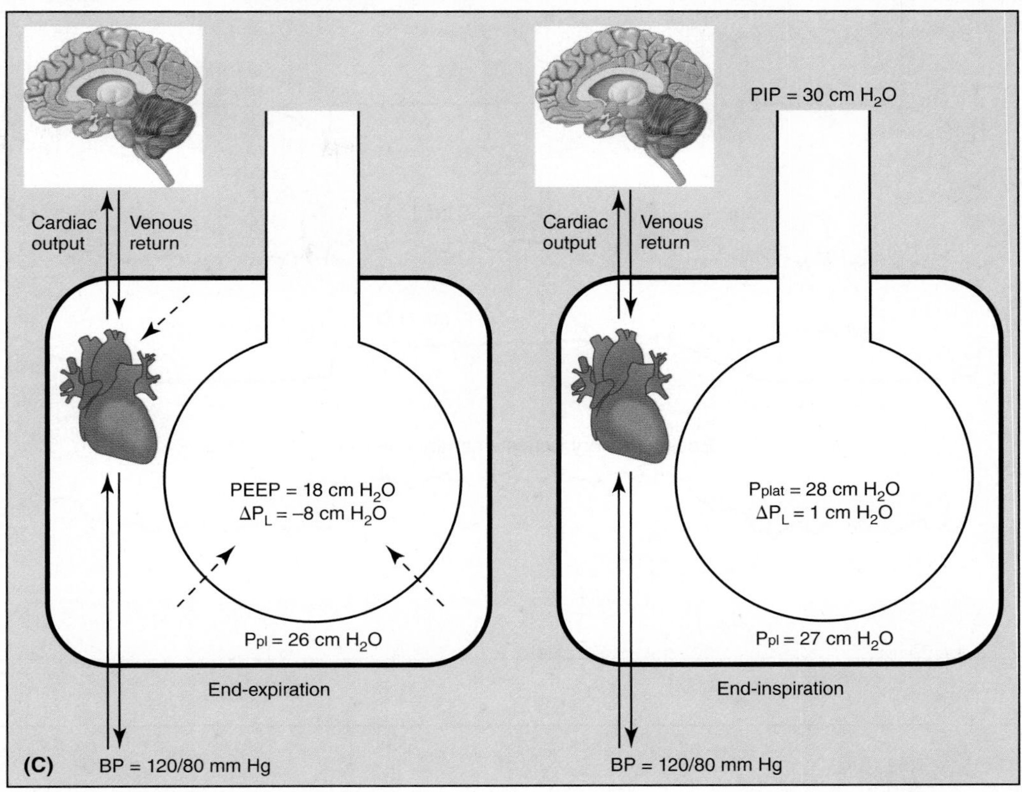

FIGURE 49-15 *(Continued)*

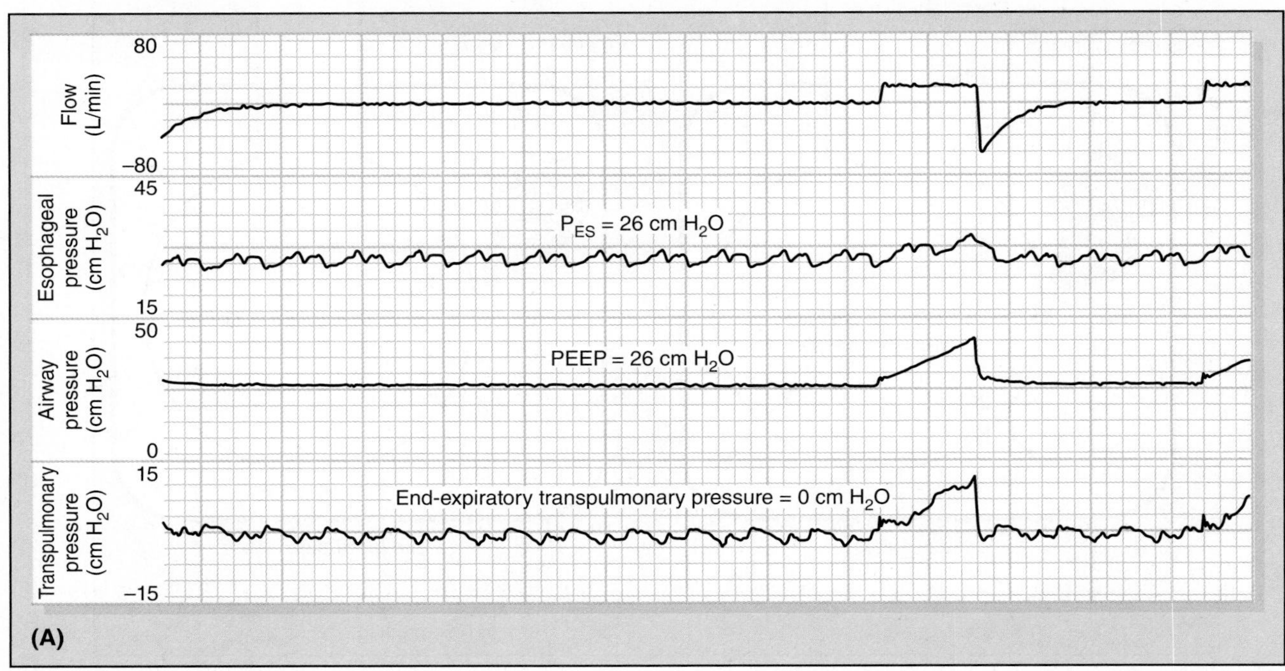

FIGURE 49-16 Esophageal pressure, airway pressure, and transpulmonary pressure with PEEP set at 26 cm H_2O (same patient as Figure 49-15). (**A**) During expiratory pause. (**B**) During inspiratory pause. (**C**) As shown in the cartoon, the PEEP is counter-balancing the esophageal pressure (pleural pressure). Note that the same pressure is exerted on the heart and central circulation at end-expiration. At the mid-thoracic level (position of the esophageal balloon), the end-inspiratory transpulmonary pressure is 10 cm H_2O, which is likely safe, despite that the Pplat is 40 cm H_2O. Note that blood pressure (BP) is not affected because there is no increase in pleural pressure with the addition of PEEP.
(**A–C**) reproduced from Hess DR. Respiratory mechanics in mechanically ventilated patients. *Respir Care.* 2014;59:1773–1794.

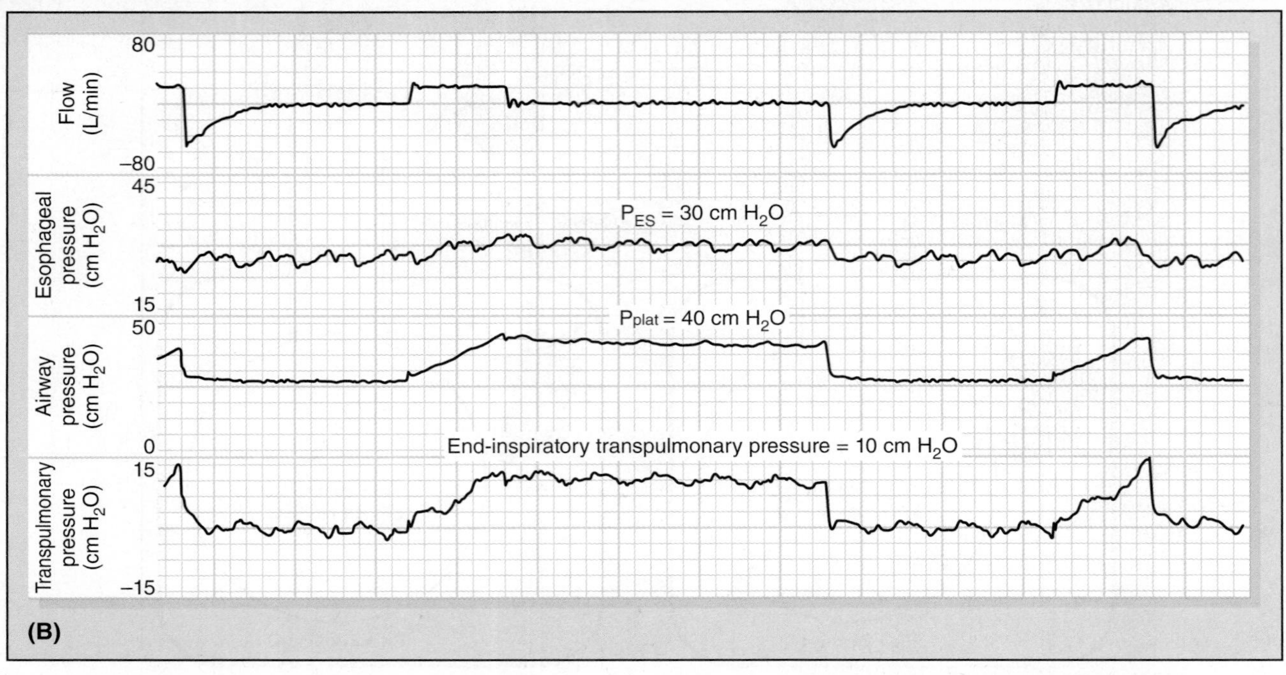

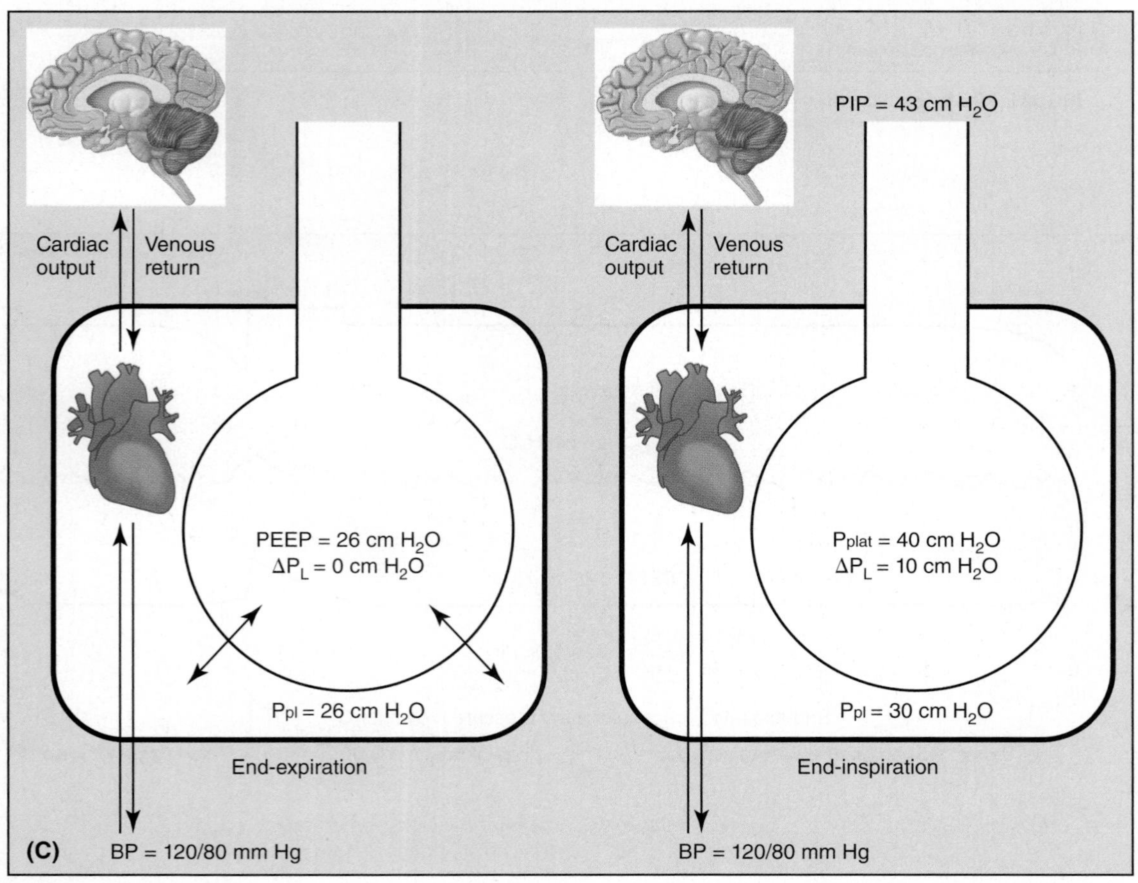

FIGURE 49-16 *(Continued)*

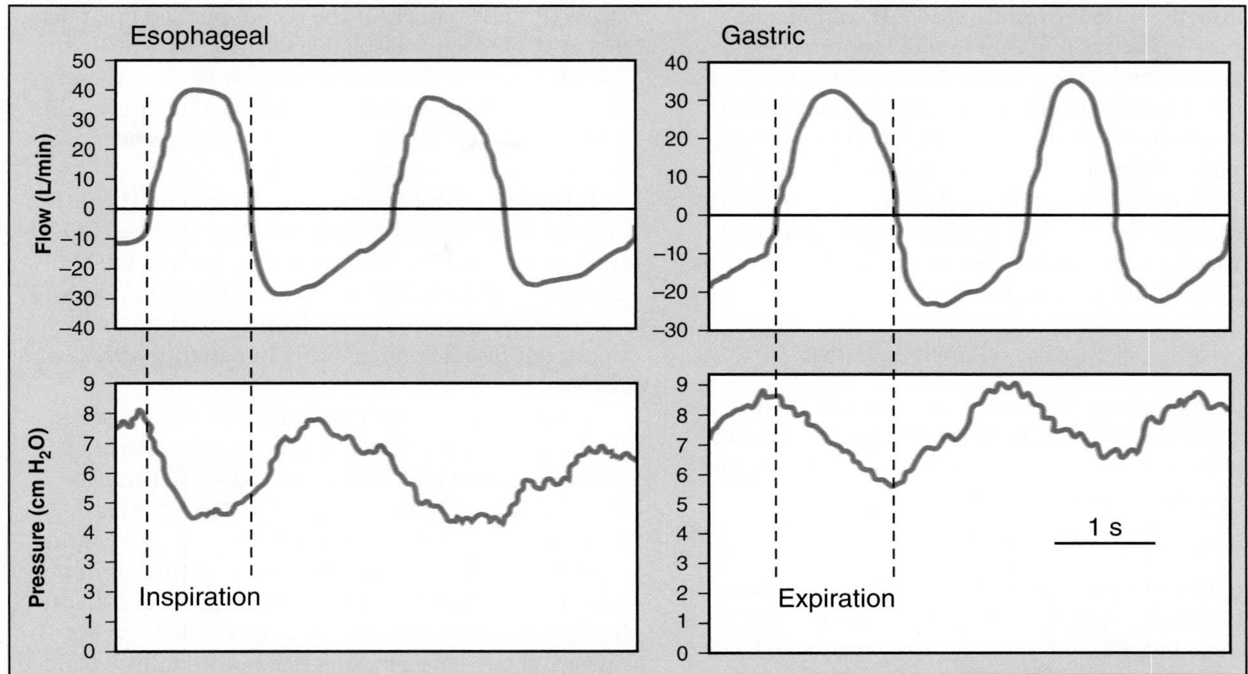

FIGURE 49-17 Esophageal (left) and gastric (right) pressures. Positive flow represents inspiration, and negative flow represents expiration. Both esophageal and gastric pressures decrease during inspiration, consistent with diaphragmatic paralysis.

Reproduced from Lecamwasam HS, Hess D, Brown R, Kwolek CJ, Bigatello LM. Diaphragmatic paralysis after endovascular stent grafting of a thoracoabdominal aortic aneurysm. *Anesthesiology.* 2005;102:690–692.

considerations in the critically ill patient, as the diaphragm links these compartments.[16] If the diaphragm is allowed to freely shift upward into the thorax with increased abdominal pressure, lung volume will be reduced. If lung volume is restored with PEEP, the increased abdominal pressure will result in an increase in intrathoracic pressure. On average, half of the pressure in the intra-abdominal compartment (range 25% to 80%) has been noted to be present in the intrathoracic space. This wide range in transmitted pressure is likely related to the amount of PEEP that has been applied to restore lung volume.

Intra-abdominal pressure (IAP) is the steady-state pressure in the abdominal cavity. Normal IAP is 5 mm Hg, and it increases during inspiration with diaphragm contraction. Bladder pressure is most commonly used for intermittent IAP measurement. The bladder is a passive structure, transmitting IAP after infusion of saline volumes between 50 and 100 mL.

Transdiaphragmatic Pressure

Normally during spontaneous inspiration, the pleural pressure decreases and the intra-abdominal pressure increases. Transdiaphragmatic pressure (P_{di}) represents the pressure across the diaphragm; the difference between P_{AB} and pleural pressure (Ppl):

$$P_{di} = P_{AB} - Ppl$$

P_{AB} is measured from a catheter in the stomach (gastric pressure) and Ppl is measured as P_{ES}. Abdominal

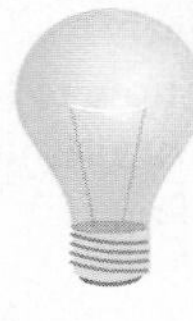

STOP AND THINK

How would you use compliance, stress index, esophageal pressure, and/or pressure-volume curve to determine the best level of PEEP for a patient with ARDS?

paradox is a clinical sign of diaphragm paralysis. In the circumstance, both esophageal and gastric pressures have a negative deflection during inspiration, suggestive of diaphragmatic paralysis (**Figure 49-17**).[17]

Stress Index

The **stress index** is used to assess the shape of the pressure-time curve during constant-flow volume control (**Figure 49-18**).[18] A linear increase in pressure (constant compliance, stress index = 1) suggests adequate alveolar

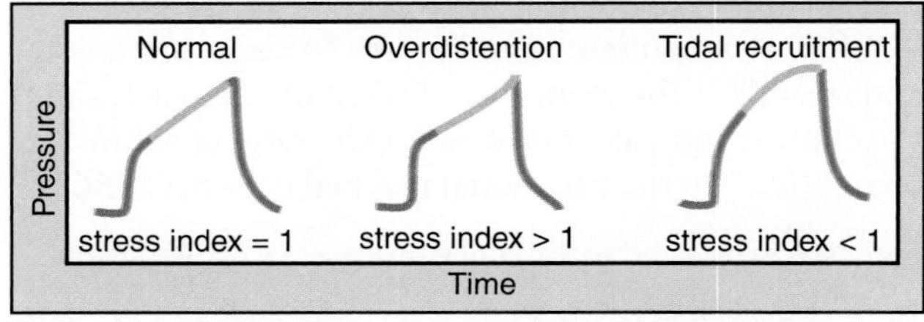

FIGURE 49-18 Normal stress index (left), stress index with overdistention (center), and stress index with tidal recruitment (right).

Reproduced from Hess DR. Respiratory mechanics in mechanically ventilated patients. *Respir Care.* 2014;59:1773–1794.

recruitment without overdistention. If compliance is worsening as the lungs are inflated (progressive decrease in compliance, upward concavity, stress index > 1), this suggests overdistention and the recommendation is to decrease the PEEP, the VT, or both. If the compliance is improving as the lungs are inflated (progressive increase in compliance, downward concavity, stress index < 1), this suggests tidal recruitment and potential for additional recruitment, and thus a recommendation to increase PEEP.

Flow

During volume control, the inspiratory flow is that which is set on the ventilator. During passive pressure control, flow is the pressure applied to the airway, airways resistance, and τ:

$$\dot{V} = (\Delta P/R) \times e^{-t/\tau}$$

where ΔP is the pressure applied to the airway above PEEP, R is resistance, C is compliance, t is the elapsed time after initiation of the inspiratory phase, and e is the base of the natural logarithm.

Expiratory flow is normally passive and is determined by alveolar driving pressure (Palv), R, the elapsed time since initiation of expiration, and τ:

$$\dot{V} = -(Palv/R) \times e^{-t/\tau}$$

Note that, by convention, expiratory flow is negative and inspiratory flow is positive. End-expiratory flow is present if airways resistance is high and expiratory time is not sufficient, which indicates the presence of air trapping (auto-PEEP).

Stress and Strain

Stress is a force applied to an area, such as pressure applied to the lung parenchyma. Force applied at an angle generates shear stress. **Strain** is the physical deformation or change in shape of a structure, such as an alveolus, caused by stress. Elasticity is the reversible deformability of the alveolus generated by a stress, but allows the alveolus to return to its original shape. A stress that stretches the lungs may not seem to permanently change the size or shape of the lung, but it may affect lung integrity. The lungs are elastic structures that respond in an elastic manner to stress and strain.

Esophageal pressure can be used to assess stress and strain.[19,20] The clinical equivalent of stress is P_L, and the clinical equivalent of strain is the ratio of volume change (ΔV) to the functional residual capacity (FRC):

$$P_L \text{ (stress)} = \text{specific lung elastance} \times \Delta V/FRC \text{ (strain)}$$

ΔV is the change in lung volume above resting FRC with the addition of PEEP and VT. Specific lung elastance is constant at 13.5 cm H_2O. A harmful threshold of strain is more than 2; therefore, the harmful threshold of stress (P_L) is 27 cm H_2O. The recommended Pplat below 30 cm H_2O is thus reasonable for most patients with ARDS. A higher Pplat, however, may be safe when P_L is reduced due to an increase in pleural pressure. This makes a case for measurement of esophageal pressure in a patient with a stiff chest wall.

It is also possible to measure strain and then calculate stress, if the end-expiratory lung volume (EELV) is measured as FRC. However, strain is the lung volume above resting FRC without PEEP. EELV, thus, is measured without PEEP to determine strain, which might not be safe, particularly in patients with severe ARDS.

This concept is illustrated in **Figure 49-19**. When the PEEP is set at 26 cm H_2O, the end-inspiratory P_L (stress) is 10 cm H_2O and strain is 0.74. In this case, stress at 10 cm H_2O and strain at 0.74 are both safe, despite that the Pplat is 40 cm H_2O.

Stress will be concentrated in the setting of inhomogeneity within the lungs where regions of collapse border regions of ventilation. This is called a stress raiser.[20] If two adjacent lung regions are fully expanded at 30 cm H_2O and if one of the two regions loses elasticity (i.e., consolidation or collapse), the applied force concentrates in the other, thereby increasing its strain and stress. If the volume ratio of the two regions goes from 10/10 (both regions distended) to 10/1 (one region distended and the other collapsed), the stress of the open regions increases from 30 cm H_2O to 130 cm H_2O. In an inhomogeneous lung, therefore, as usually is the case in a mechanically ventilated patient, the presence of these areas of stress raisers might create dangerous regional P_L despite that the Pplat is acceptable.

End-Expiratory Lung Volume

Calculation of end-expiratory lung volume (EELV) is based on a step-change in FIO_2 and the assumption that N_2 is the balance gas.[21,22] Baseline determinations are made of $\dot{V}O_2$, $\dot{V}CO_2$, and end-tidal N_2 ($FETN_2$). It is assumed that $\dot{V}O_2$ and $\dot{V}CO_2$ remain constant throughout the measurement. A step-change in FIO_2 then occurs and the EELV is calculated as:

$$EELV = \Delta VN_2/\Delta FETN_2$$

where $FETN_2$ is the last recorded value following the step change in FIO_2. The breath-to-breath changes are calculated over approximately 20 breaths:

$$EELV = \frac{\sum_{time} \Delta VN_2}{\text{baseline } FETN_2 - \text{last } FETN_2}$$

The use of EELV during PEEP titration would seem attractive. However, a PEEP-induced increase in EELV might be the result of recruitment or it might be the result of overdistention of already open alveoli. EELV by itself thus might not be useful to assess PEEP response.

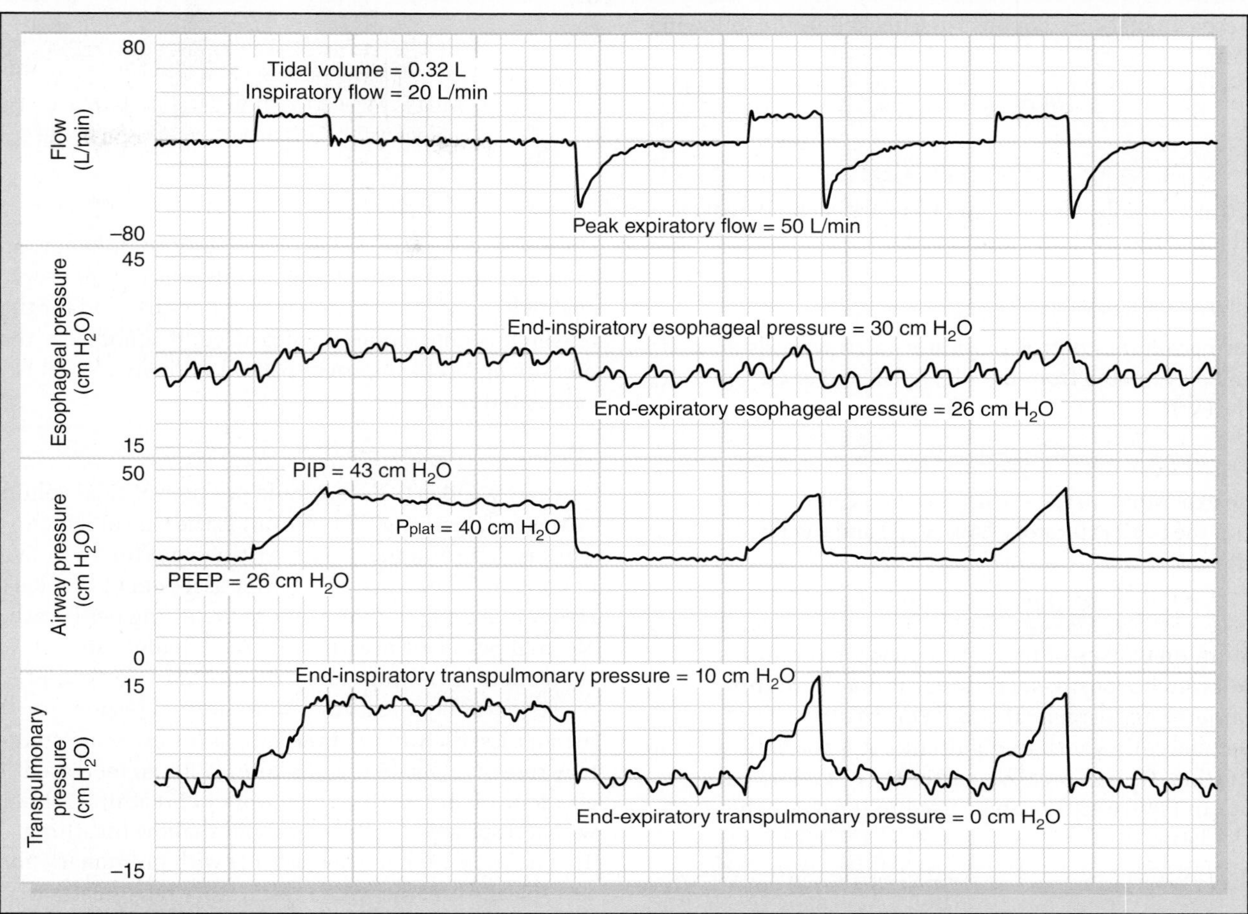

FIGURE 49-19 Flow, esophageal pressure, airway pressure, and transpulmonary pressure can be used to calculate respiratory system compliance, chest wall compliance, lung compliance, inspiratory airway resistance, and expiratory airway resistance. See text for details.

Reproduced from Hess DR. Respiratory mechanics in mechanically ventilated patients. *Respir Care.* 2014;59:1773–1794.

Respiratory System Compliance

Respiratory system compliance (Crs) is calculated as the tidal volume divided by the pressure required:

$$Crs = \Delta V/\Delta P = V_T/(Pplat - PEEP)$$

Acceptable Crs is 50 to 100 mL/cm H_2O in mechanically ventilated patients. It is determined by the compliance of the lungs and chest wall. Crs has been used to determine the optimal level of PEEP in patients with ARDS; the highest level of Crs corresponds to best PEEP.

Chest Wall Compliance

To calculate chest wall compliance (Ccw), changes in esophageal pressure (pleural pressure) are used during passive inflation:

$$Ccw = \Delta V/\Delta P = V_T/\Delta P_{ES}$$

The patient data in Figure 49-19 can be used to calculate Ccw:

$$Ccw = 320\ mL/4\ cm\ H_2O = 80\ mL/cm\ H_2O$$

Ccw is normally 200 mL/cm H_2O and is decreased due to morbid obesity, abdominal hypertension, chest wall edema, chest wall burns, and thoracic deformities (e.g., kyphoscoliosis). Ccw is also decreased with an increase in muscle tone (e.g., a patient who is asynchronous with the ventilator). Ccw is increased with flail chest and paralysis.

Lung Compliance

To calculate lung compliance (CL), the change in transpulmonary pressure when the lungs are inflated is used:

$$C_L = \Delta V/\Delta P = V_T/\Delta P_L$$

Normal CL is 200 mL/cm H_2O. Lung compliance is decreased with ARDS, cardiogenic pulmonary edema, pneumothorax, consolidation, atelectasis, pulmonary fibrosis, pneumonectomy, mainstem intubation, and overdistention. Lung compliance is increased with emphysema.

The patient data in Figure 49-19 can be used to illustrate these calculations:

$$Crs = 320\ mL/(40\ cm\ H_2O - 26\ cm\ H_2O) = 23\ mL/cm\ H_2O$$

$$Ccw = 320\ mL/4\ cm\ H_2O = 80\ mL/cm\ H_2O$$

$$C_L = 320\ mL/10\ cm\ H_2O = 32\ mL/cm\ H_2O$$

These calculations can be crosschecked in the following manner:

$$1/Crs = 1/Ccw + 1/C_L$$

$$1/23 \approx 1/80 + 1/32$$

In this example, Crs, CL, and Ccw are each decreased, but CL is the most compromised.

Airways Resistance

During volume control, inspiratory airways resistance (R_I) can be estimated from the PIP, Pplat, and end-inspiratory flow ($\dot{V}_I$):

$$R_I = (PIP - Pplat)/\dot{V}_I$$

The expiratory airways resistance (R_E) can be estimated from the peak expiratory flow ($\dot{V}_{EXP}$) and the Pplat – PEEP difference:

$$R_E = (Pplat - PEEP)/\dot{V}_{EXP}$$

Common causes of increased airways resistance are bronchospasm, secretions, and a small inner diameter endotracheal tube. For intubated and mechanically ventilated patients, R_I should be <10 cm H_2O/L/s. R_E is typically greater than R_I. The patient data in Figure 49-19 can be used to illustrate these calculations:

$$R_I = (43\ cm\ H_2O - 40\ cm\ H_2O)/0.33\ L/s = 9\ cm\ H_2O/L/s$$

$$R_E = (40\ cm\ H_2O - 26\ cm\ H_2O)/0.83\ L/s = 17\ cm\ H_2O/L/s$$

Work of Breathing

The Campbell diagram (**Figure 49-20**) includes the effects of Ccw, CL, and R on the **work of breathing (WOB)**. Note that WOB is increased with decreased chest wall compliance, decreased lung compliance, or increased airways resistance. WOB requires an esophageal balloon to properly quantify pressure, and for that reason it is not frequently measured. It is not clear that measuring WOB improves patient outcome. WOB is calculated from the $\dot{V}_I$ and the P:

$$WOB = \int P \times \dot{V}dt$$

Normal WOB is 0.3 – 0.7 joule per liter of tidal volume. Power-of-breathing (WOB/min) is the rate at which work is done as a measure over time, not for an individual breath.[19] This may be a better assessment of respiratory muscle load than work of breathing per breath. Normal power-of-breathing is 4 to 8 joule/min.

Work of breathing can be divided into elastic and resistive work of breathing. With normal respiratory mechanics, the work of breathing is lowest at a respiratory rate of about 15 breaths/min. With an increased elastic work of breathing, the work of breathing is lowest with a respiratory pattern or rapid shallow breathing. This helps to explain why patients with pulmonary fibrosis typically breathe with a respiratory rate greater than normal. With an increased resistive work of breathing, such as a patient with COPD, the work of breathing is lowest with a lower respiratory rate (**Figure 49-21**).

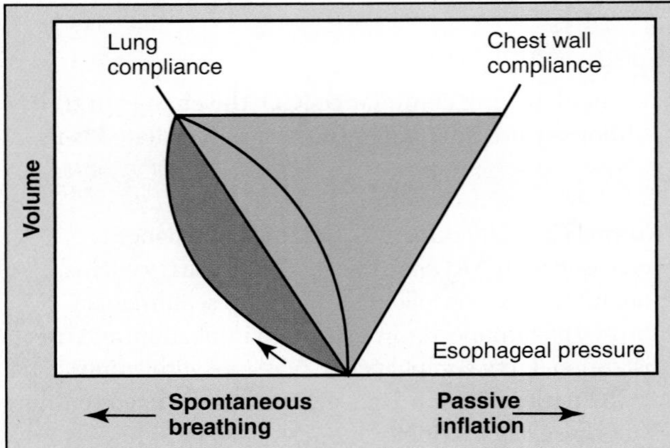

FIGURE 49-20 Campbell diagram as used to calculate work of breathing. The green area represents elastic work of breathing and the blue area represents resistive work of breathing. The total shaded area represents the total work of breathing.

Reproduced from Hess DR. Respiratory mechanics in mechanically ventilated patients. *Respir Care*. 2014;59:1773–1794.

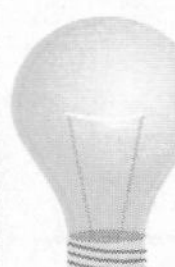

STOP AND THINK

What is the work of breathing in which a patient with COPD makes an effort that does not trigger?

Pressure-Volume Curves

Pressure-volume (PV) curves are displayed with volume as a function of pressure;[23–25] the slope of the PV curve is respiratory system compliance. The most common methods used to measure PV curves during mechanical ventilation are the use of a super syringe, inflation with a constant slow flow (<10 L/min), and the Pplat at various inflation volumes. Correct interpretation of the PV curve during non-constant-flow ventilation (e.g., pressure-control), and with higher inspiratory flows, is problematic.

An approach for setting PEEP is based on inflection points determined from the PV curve (**Figure 49-22**). The lower inflection point is thought to represent the pressure at which a large number of alveoli are recruited, and the upper inflection point is thought to indicate overdistention. Recruitment, however, is likely to occur along the entire inflation PV curve and the upper inflection point might represent the end of recruitment rather than overdistention.

A number of issues preclude the routine use of PV curves to set the ventilator in patients with ARDS. Measurement of the PV curve requires sedation, and often paralysis, to correctly make the measurement.

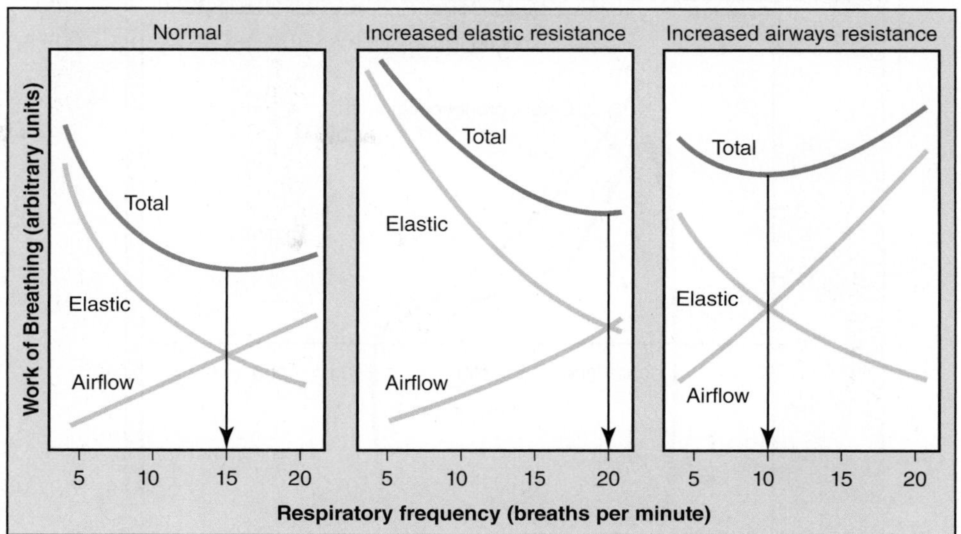

FIGURE 49-21 Effect of respiratory mechanics on work of breathing.
Reproduced from Hess DR. Respiratory mechanics in mechanically ventilated patients. *Respir Care.* 2014;59:1773–1794.

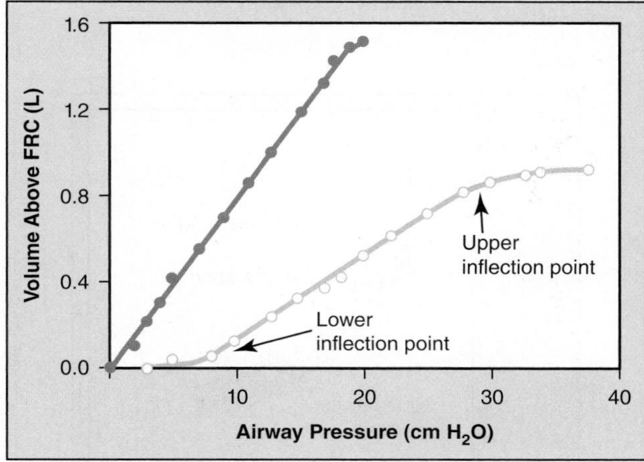

FIGURE 49-22 Pressure-volume curve for normal lungs (solid circles) and ARDS (open circles). Note the presence of a lower and upper inflection point on the pressure-volume curve for ARDS.

Precise identification inflection points may require mathematical curve fitting to precisely identify the inflection points. Although the inflation limb of the PV curve is most commonly measured, the deflation limb may be more useful for setting PEEP. Chest wall mechanics potentially affect the shape of the PV curve, necessitating esophageal pressure measurement to separate lung from chest wall effects. The PV curve, as with most measures of respiratory mechanics, treats the lungs as a single compartment, disregarding the inhomogeneity of the lungs of patients with ARDS that are heterogeneous.

Flow-Volume Loops

Flow-volume loops are displayed with flow as a function of volume. Some systems display expiratory flow

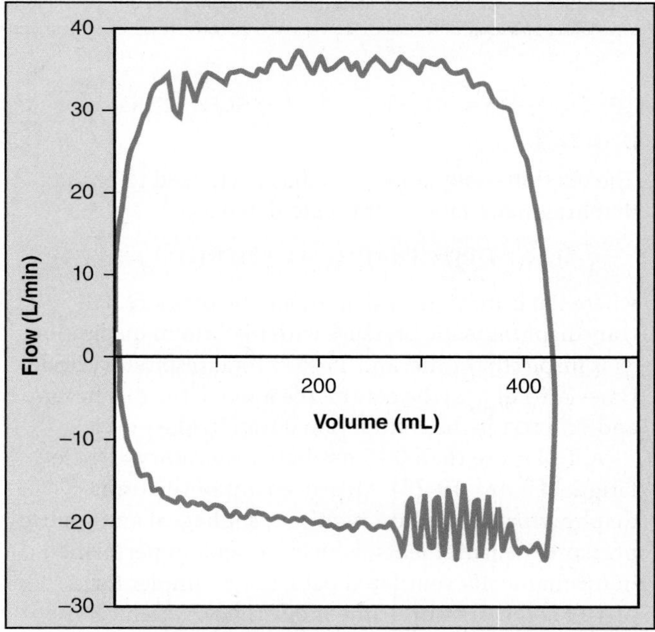

FIGURE 49-23 Sawtooth pattern on flow-volume curve representing secretions in the airway.

in the positive position, whereas other systems display expiratory flow in the negative position. Analysis of the flow-volume loop may be helpful for identifying reduced expiratory flow, flow limitation during expiration, the presence of secretions in the airway (**Figure 49-23**), and bronchodilator response (**Figure 49-24**). The flow-volume curve can provide an indication of excessive secretions more reliably than clinical examination, with the presence of excessive secretions in the airways producing a sawtooth pattern on both the inspiratory and expiratory flow-volume curves.

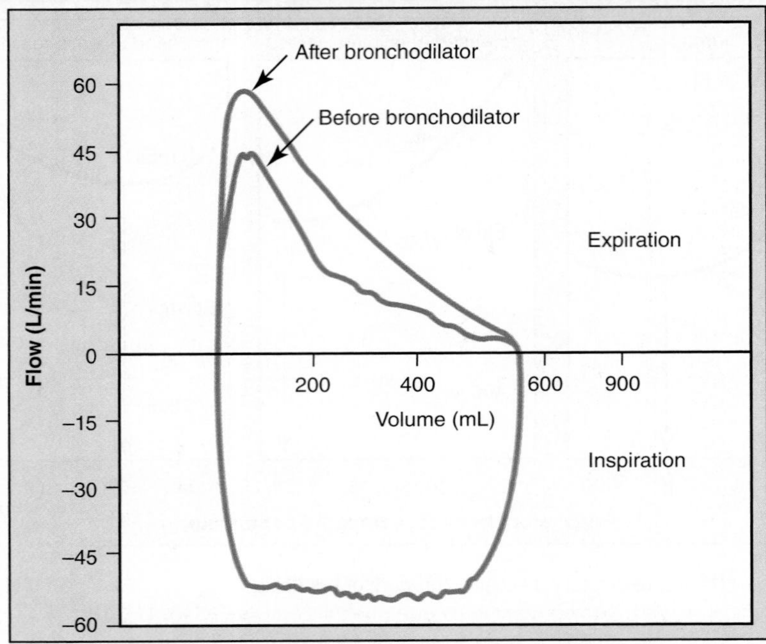

FIGURE 49-24 Flow–volume loops showing a response to bronchodilator administration. The expiratory limb of the curve is concave in patients with expiratory flow limitation. Administration of a bronchodilator aerosol leads to improvement in expiratory flow.
Reproduced from MacIntyre NM, Branson RD. *Mechanical Ventilation*. Philadelphia: WB Saunders; 2001:17.

Tension–Time Index and Pressure-Time Product

The **tension–time index (TTI)** has been used to predict diaphragmatic fatigue; it is calculated as:

$$TTI = (Pdi/Pdi_{max}) \times (T_I/T_{TOT})$$

where Pdi is mean transdiaphragmatic pressure, Pdi_{max} is transdiaphragmatic pressure with maximum inspiration, T_I is inspiratory time, and T_{TOT} is total respiratory cycle time. Pdi/Pdi_{max} is the contractile force of the diaphragm, and T_I/T_{TOT} is the contraction duration (duty cycle).

A TTI more than 0.15 predicts respiratory muscle fatigue (**Figure 49-25**). Measurement of the transdiaphragmatic pressure requires esophageal and gastric pressure measurements, which are seldom performed in mechanically ventilated patients. A simpler form of TTI is the pressure-time index (PTI), which can be determined more readily with equipment available in the intensive care unit. It is calculated as:

$$PTI = (P_{breath}/P_{I_{max}}) \times (T_I/T_{TOT})$$

where P_{breath} is the pressure required to generate a spontaneous breath. The P_{breath} can be determined with esophageal balloon measurements during a short trial of spontaneous breathing. $P_{I_{max}}$ is the maximum pressure that can be generated against an occluded airway.

The **pressure-time product (PTP)** accounts for energy expenditures during the dynamic and isometric phases of respiration.[26] WOB does not account for the isometric phase of respiration because there is no volume change. For example, energy is expended to overcome the threshold load of auto-PEEP, but technically this is not work because there is no volume moved into the lungs. Different patients thus might have the same WOB, but the respiratory efficiency (WOB/$\dot{V}O_2$ of respiratory muscles) could be quite different. The PTP is measured as the time integral of the difference between the esophageal pressure tracing and the recoil pressure of the chest wall (**Figure 49-26**). The traditional measurement of PTP may fail to account for the energy needed for active expiration, which has led to the determination of upper bound PTP and lower bound PTP to enable calculations of PTP throughout the respiratory cycle so that total energy expenditure can be approximated.

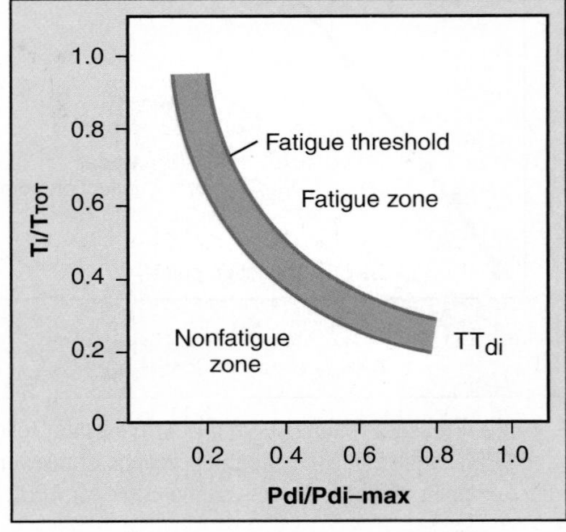

FIGURE 49-25 Tension–time index; note that the fatigue threshold is a tension–time index of about 0.15 to 0.18.
Reproduced from Grassino A, Macklem PT. Respiratory muscle fatigue and ventilatory failure. *Ann Rev Med.* 1984;35:625–647. Reprinted with permission.

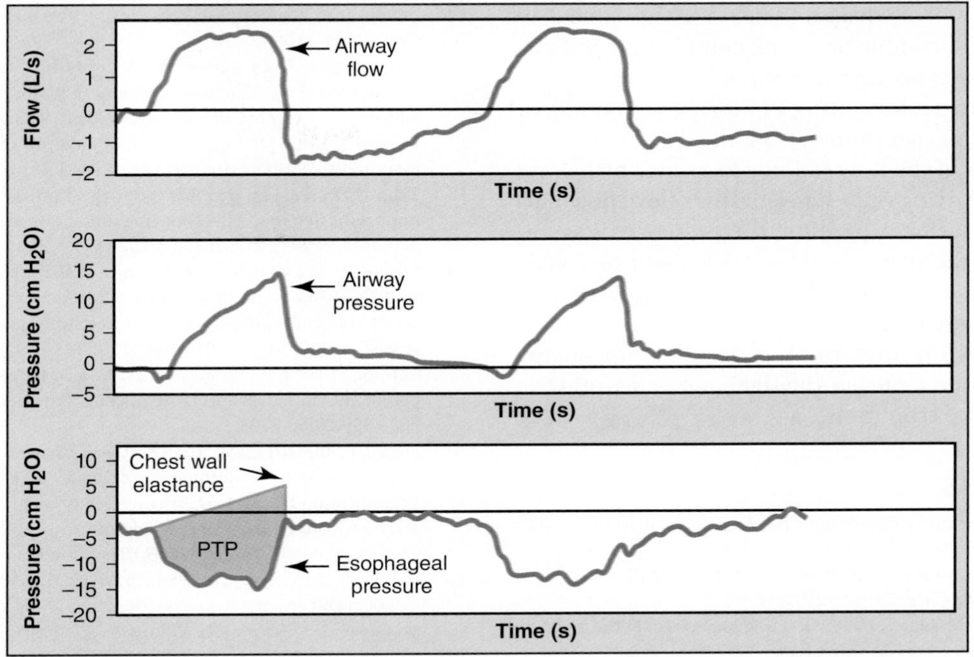

FIGURE 49-26 An illustration of the determination of pressure-time product (PTP); the shaded area is PTP.
Reproduced from Hess DR. Respiratory mechanics in mechanically ventilated patients. *Respir Care.* 2014;59:1773–1794.

Key Points

- Respiratory mechanics relates to the forces needed to move the lungs and the chest wall.
- The most important muscle of inspiration is the diaphragm.
- Alveolar pressure decreases during inspiration due to a decrease in intrapleural pressure.
- Airways resistance is less in the smaller airways because the large numbers of small airways are in parallel, such that their total cross-sectional area is very large.
- Lung volume is an important determinant of airways resistance.
- Flow limitation is the result of airway compression by intrathoracic pressure.
- Compliance is the slope of the pressure-volume curve, or the volume change per unit pressure change.
- Surfactant lowers the surface tension in alveoli and increases lung compliance.
- Due to alveolar interdependence, any tendency for one group of alveoli to reduce its relative volume is opposed by surrounding alveoli.
- The chest wall is pulled inward while the lung is pulled outward, thus producing the normal subatmospheric intrapleural pressure.
- The ventilation of an individual lung unit depends on the compliance of the alveolus and the resistance of the airway leading to that alveolus.
- Airway pressure is predicted mathematically by the equation of motion.
- Plateau pressure is determined by tidal volume, respiratory system compliance, and PEEP during full ventilatory support.
- The pressure produced by this trapped gas is called auto-PEEP, intrinsic PEEP, or occult PEEP.
- Mean airway pressure is determined by peak inspiratory pressure, the fraction of time devoted to the inspiratory phase, and PEEP.
- The traditional approach to assess pleural pressure is the use of an esophageal balloon.
- Transpulmonary pressure is the difference between pressure measured at the mouth and pleural pressure.
- The use of an esophageal balloon to assess intrapleural pressure can be used to set PEEP relative to the collapsing effect of the chest wall.
- Intra-abdominal pressure is the steady-state pressure in the abdominal cavity.
- The stress index is used to assess the shape of the pressure-time curve during constant-flow volume control.
- Stress is a force applied to an area, such as pressure applied to the lung parenchyma.
- Force applied at an angle generates shear stress.
- Strain is the physical deformation or change in shape of a structure, such as an alveolus, caused by stress.
- Calculation of end-expiratory lung volume (EELV) is based on a step-change in F_{IO_2} and the assumption that N_2 is the balance gas.

- The Campbell diagram includes the effects of chest wall compliance, lung compliance, and airways resistance on the work of breathing.
- An approach for setting PEEP is based on inflection points determined from the PV curve.
- Analysis of the flow-volume loop may be helpful for identifying reduced expiratory flow, flow limitation during expiration, the presence of secretions in the airway, and bronchodilator response.
- The tension–time index is used to predict diaphragmatic fatigue.
- The pressure-time product accounts for energy expenditures during the dynamic and isometric phases of respiration.

References

1. West JB. *Respiratory Physiology: The Essentials.* Baltimore, MD: Lippincott (Wolters Kluwer Health); 2011.
2. Hess DR. Respiratory mechanics in mechanically ventilated patients. *Respir Care.* 2014;59:1773–1794.
3. Lucangelo U, Bernabe F, Blanch L. Lung mechanics at the bedside: make it simple. *Curr Opin Crit Care.* 2007;13:64–72.
4. Lucangelo U, Bernabe F, Blanch L. Respiratory mechanics derived from signals in the ventilator circuit. *Respir Care.* 2005;50:55–67.
5. Ventilation with lower tidal volumes as compared with traditional tidal volumes for acute lung injury and the acute respiratory distress syndrome. The Acute Respiratory Distress Syndrome Network. *N Engl J Med.* 2000;342:1301–1308.
6. Terragni PP, Filippini C, Slutsky AS, et al. Accuracy of plateau pressure and stress index to identify injurious ventilation in patients with acute respiratory distress syndrome. *Anesthesiology.* 2013;119:880–889.
7. Terragni PP, Rosboch G, Tealdi A, et al. Tidal hyperinflation during low tidal volume ventilation in acute respiratory distress syndrome. *Am J Respir Crit Care Med.* 2007;175:160–166.
8. Marini JJ. Dynamic hyperinflation and auto-positive end-expiratory pressure: lessons learned over 30 years. *Am J Respir Crit Care Med.* 2011;184:756–762.
9. Blanch L, Bernabe F, Lucangelo U. Measurement of air trapping, intrinsic positive end-expiratory pressure, and dynamic hyperinflation in mechanically ventilated patients. *Respir Care.* 2005;50:110–124.
10. Benditt JO. Esophageal and gastric pressure measurements. *Respir Care.* 2005;50:68–77.
11. Akoumianaki E, Maggiore SM, Valenza F, et al. The application of esophageal pressure measurement in patients with respiratory failure. *Am J Respir Crit Care Med.* 2014;189:520–531.
12. Piraino T, Cook DJ. Optimal PEEP guided by esophageal balloon manometry. *Respir Care.* 2011;56:510–513.
13. Talmor DS, Fessler HE. Are esophageal pressure measurements important in clinical decision-making in mechanically ventilated patients? *Respir Care.* 2010;55:162–174.
14. Loring SH, O'Donnell CR, Behazin N, et al. Esophageal pressures in acute lung injury: do they represent artifact or useful information about transpulmonary pressure, chest wall mechanics, and lung stress? *J Appl Physiol.* 2010;108:515–522.
15. Talmor D, Sarge T, Malhotra A, et al. Mechanical ventilation guided by esophageal pressure in acute lung injury. *N Engl J Med.* 2008;359:2095–2104.
16. Hess DR, Bigatello LM. The chest wall in acute lung injury/acute respiratory distress syndrome. *Curr Opin Crit Care.* 2008;14:94–102.
17. Lecamwasam HS, Hess D, Brown R, et al. Diaphragmatic paralysis after endovascular stent grafting of a thoracoabdominal aortic aneurysm. *Anesthesiology* 2005;102:690–692.
18. Grasso S, Stripoli T, De Michele M, et al. ARDSnet ventilatory protocol and alveolar hyperinflation: role of positive end-expiratory pressure. *Am J Respir Crit Care Med.* 2007;176:761–767.
19. Chiumello D, Carlesso E, Cadringher P, et al. Lung stress and strain during mechanical ventilation for acute respiratory distress syndrome. *Am J Respir Crit Care Med.* 2008;178:346–355.
20. Gattinoni L, Carlesso E, Caironi P. Stress and strain within the lung. *Curr Opin Crit Care.* 2012;18:42–47.
21. Branson RD, Johannigman JA. Innovations in mechanical ventilation. *Respir Care.* 2009;54:933–947.
22. Owens RL, Stigler WS, Hess DR. Do newer monitors of exhaled gases, mechanics, and esophageal pressure add value? *Clin Chest Med.* 2008;29:297–312.
23. Harris RS. Pressure-volume curves of the respiratory system. *Respir Care.* 2005;50:78–99.
24. Blanch L, Lopez-Aguilar J, Villagra A. Bedside evaluation of pressure-volume curves in patients with acute respiratory distress syndrome. *Curr Opin Crit Care.* 2007;13:332–337.
25. Albaiceta GM, Blanch L, Lucangelo U. Static pressure-volume curves of the respiratory system: were they just a passing fad? *Curr Opin Crit Care.* 2008;14:80–86.
26. Grinnan DC, Truwit JD. Clinical review: respiratory mechanics in spontaneous and assisted ventilation. *Crit Care* 2005;9:472–484.

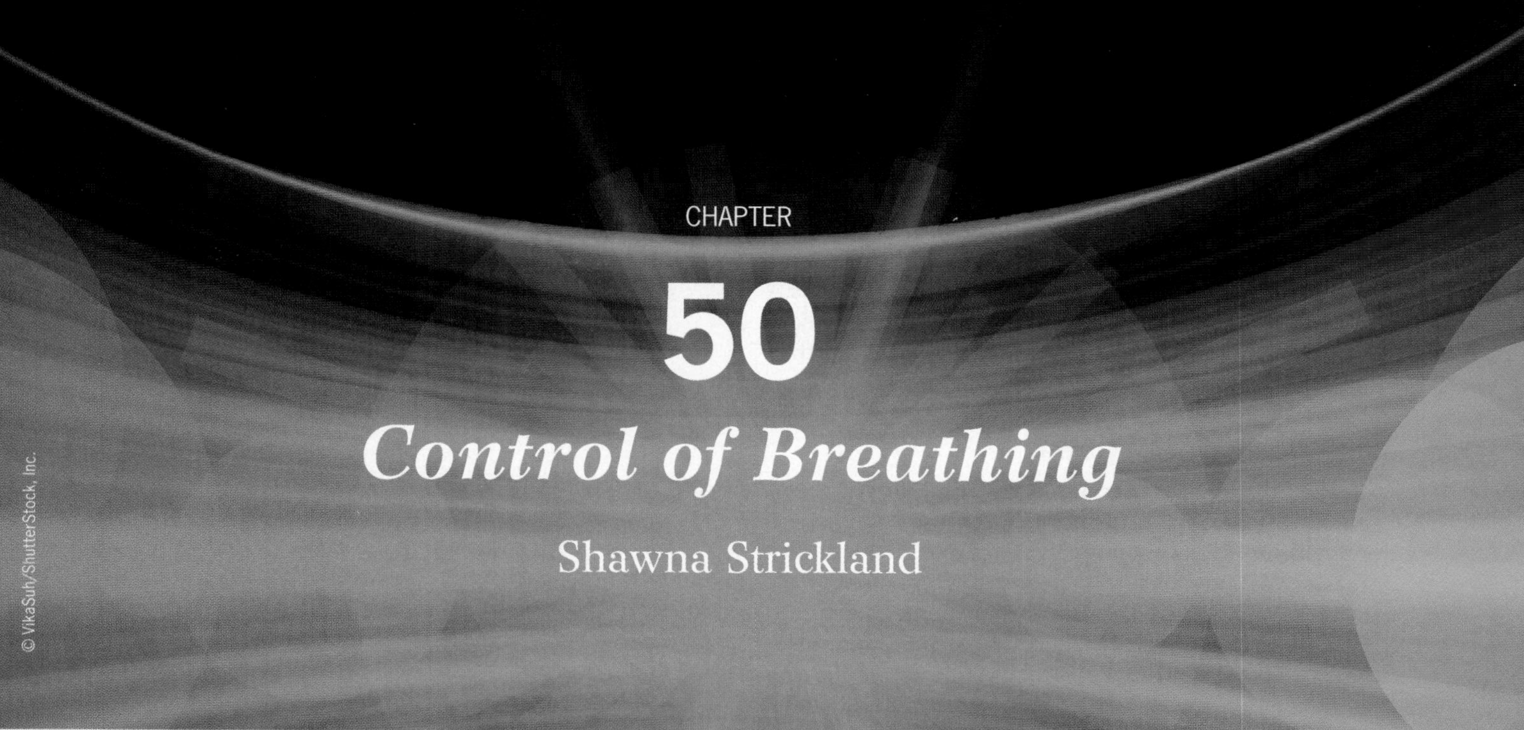

OUTLINE

Control of Breathing
Effects of Acid–Base Disorders
High Altitude and Control of Breathing
Hypoxic Drive
Opioid Drugs and Respiratory Drive
Abnormal Breathing Patterns
Respiratory Drive and Exercise
Assessing Respiratory Drive

OBJECTIVES

1. Identify the location of the structures that regulate breathing.
2. Describe the role of the medulla in regulating breathing.
3. Describe the role of the pons in regulating breathing.
4. Identify the respiratory reflexes and describe their effect on the control of breathing.
5. Describe innervation of the lungs.
6. Identify the location, purpose, and mechanisms of stimulation of the central and peripheral chemoreceptors.
7. Describe the medullary adjustment that occurs in the presence of respiratory and metabolic acid–base disorders.
8. Identify the various factors that stimulate or depress ventilation.
9. Identify acute and chronic effects of high altitude on ventilation.
10. Describe the effects of hypercapnia on cerebral circulation.
11. Identify two mechanisms by which supplemental O_2 administration might result in hypercapnia in patients with carbon dioxide–retaining diseases.
12. Describe the characteristics of abnormal breathing patterns.
13. Explain how respiratory drive is assessed.

KEY TERMS

afferent impulse
aortic body
apnea
apneustic breathing
apneustic center
ataxic breathing
Biot breathing
bradypnea
carotid body
central chemoreceptor
Cheyne-Stokes breathing
compensated respiratory alkalosis
deflation reflex
dorsal respiratory group (DRG)
dyspnea
efferent impulse
eupnea
Head paradoxical reflex
Hering-Breuer reflex
hyperpnea
hypopnea
hypoxic drive theory
juxtacapillary receptor
Kussmaul breathing
medulla oblongata
$P_{0.1}$
peripheral chemoreceptor
peripheral proprioceptor
pneumotaxic center
pons
ventral respiratory group (VRG)

Introduction

To completely understand cardiopulmonary disorders, the respiratory therapist must understand how breathing is controlled. Understanding how physiologic changes affect the control of breathing provides the key elements to identifying appropriate therapeutic interventions. This chapter discusses the anatomy and function of control of breathing as well as identifies factors that alter breathing patterns.

Control of Breathing

While gas exchange occurs within the lungs, the control of breathing originates in the central nervous system. There are two regulatory mechanisms for breathing: automatic (involuntary) control and conscious (voluntary) control. The control of breathing is regulated by the **medulla oblongata**, located at the base of the spinal cord, and the **pons**, located just above the medulla oblongata in the spinal cord (**Figure 50-1**).

Role of the Medulla Oblongata

The medulla oblongata contains the respiratory control center, which controls the normal, rhythmic pattern of breathing. This center receives impulses from other areas of the body, such as the cerebral cortex, the pons, the upper airway reflexes, the phrenic nerve, peripheral chemoreceptors, and central chemoreceptors. Impulses that are carried toward a central organ, such as the medulla oblongata, are called **afferent impulses**. These impulses are interpreted within the respiratory control center, and then **efferent impulses** are created and transmitted. Efferent impulses are those created within the central nervous system (CNS) and then sent to other areas of the body.

Located within the medulla oblongata are two major areas of respiratory-related neurons: the **dorsal respiratory group (DRG)** and the **ventral respiratory group (VRG)** (Figure 50-1). Neurons in these groups send different types of efferent impulses to specific areas to assist in the control of breathing.

> **Respiratory Recap**
>
> **Control of Breathing Regulation**
> - Medulla oblongata
> - Pons

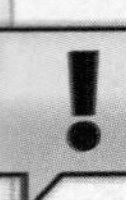

> **Respiratory Recap**
>
> **Medulla Oblongata**
> - The respiratory control center that receives impulses from the cerebral cortex, pons, upper airway reflexes, peripheral chemoreceptors, and carotid chemoreceptors
> - It houses two areas of respiratory-related neurons, the dorsal respiratory group (DRG) and the ventral respiratory group (VRG)

The DRG is located along the lateral walls within the medulla oblongata referred to as the nucleus tractus solitarius (NTS) (see Figure 50-1). The DRG is the initial processing center for afferent impulses from the vagus (X) and glossopharyngeal (IX) nerves. These afferent impulses modify the basic breathing pattern by stimulating inspiration. The DRG is also the place of origin of efferent impulses to the phrenic nerve, which in turn stimulates diaphragmatic movement, and to external intercostal motor nerves. The DRG is the primary controller of the depth and rate of inspiration. Inspiration is normally a ramp signal that increases in force gradually for approximately 2 seconds followed by a cessation of inspiration for approximately 3 seconds. This gradual increase results in a progressively stronger contraction of inspiratory muscles and a gradual increase in lung inflation. In stressed breathing or breathing during exercise, peripheral receptors and reflexes send afferent impulses that alter the ramp signal. This steeper signal results in lung inflation that is more rapid than during normal breathing.

The VRG is located in the medulla in two separate nuclei, which are anterior and lateral to each DRG, and contain inspiratory and expiratory neurons

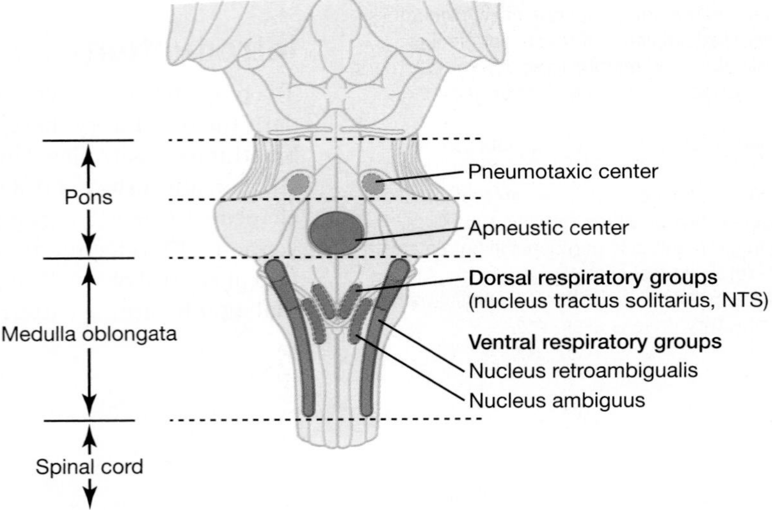

FIGURE 50-1 Major components of the brain stem.

(Figure 50-1). These neurons are located in the nucleus ambiguus and the nucleus retroambigualis. The nucleus ambiguus contains inspiratory neurons that send efferent impulses to innervate laryngeal and pharyngeal muscles. The nucleus retroambigualis contains both inspiratory and expiratory neurons. The inspiratory neurons send efferent impulses to the diaphragm and external intercostal muscles via the phrenic and intercostal nerves, respectively. The expiratory neurons send efferent impulses to the internal intercostal and abdominal muscles. It is important to remember that the afferent impulses are processed in the DRG, and the VRG is inactive during normal breathing. The inspiratory efferent impulses are sent from the VRG during stressed breathing and during exercise.

Role of the Pons

The pons, located above the medulla oblongata, houses two centers that contain afferent respiratory neurons: the **pneumotaxic center** and the **apneustic center** (Figure 50-1). The pons modifies the output, or the efferent impulses, from the medulla oblongata. Sometimes called the pontine centers, the pneumotaxic and apneustic centers can cause alterations in respiratory rate and tidal volume depending on location of injury to the spinal cord.

The pneumotaxic center is located in the upper pons (see Figure 50-1). It receives afferent impulses from the vagus nerve that help fine-tune the respiratory rhythm and blocks stimulation of the DRG and VRG from the apneustic center. The result is control of the stopping point of the inspiratory ramp signal created by the DRG. Specifically, the impulses inhibit the apneustic center and shorten the inspiratory phase of respiration. A strong signal from the impulse results in a shorter inspiratory time and a faster respiratory rate, which results in lower tidal volumes. Conversely, a weak signal from the impulse results in a longer inspiratory time and lower respiratory rate, which results in higher tidal volumes. If the pneumotaxic center is destroyed, the apneustic center controls the respiratory pattern.

The apneustic center is located in the lower pons (see Figure 50-1). It stimulates the inspiratory neurons of the DRG and the VRG. Normally, the pneumotaxic center inhibits this signal. If the pneumotaxic center is destroyed, the afferent impulses from the apneustic center prevent the inspiratory ramp signal from shutting off. The result is a prolonged inspiration with a shortened expiratory time. This respiratory pattern is called **apneustic breathing** (**Figure 50-2**). Some causes of apneustic breathing include cerebral edema, acute poliomyelitis, and medications that cause CNS depression. If both the pneumotaxic center and the apneustic center are destroyed, the respiratory pattern is rapid and irregular.

> **Respiratory Recap**
>
> **Two Centers in the Pons Contain Afferent Respiratory Neurons**
>
> - Pneumotaxic center
> - Apneustic center

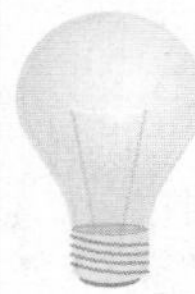

> **STOP AND THINK**
>
> A patient with severe cerebral edema has a respiratory pattern characterized by a prolonged inspiratory phase. What is the cause of this pattern?

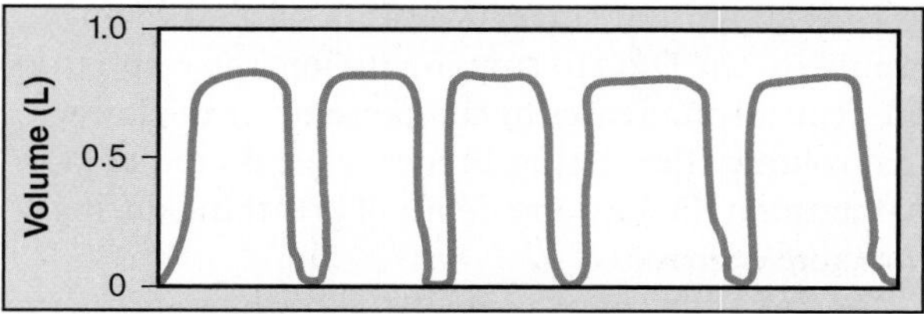

FIGURE 50-2 Apneustic breathing.

Respiratory Reflexes

The DRG receives afferent impulses from multiple areas of the body. The respiratory reflexes send these afferent impulses to manage the rate and depth of breathing in various situations. Different reflexes stimulate different responses in unique situations.

Reflexes of the upper airway are located in the nose, the nasopharynx, the larynx, and the trachea. When stimulated, each sends an afferent impulse to the DRG to produce a specific response. Potential responses from the upper airway reflexes are provided in **Table 50-1**.

TABLE 50-1
Location of Upper Airway Reflexes and Potential Stimulant Responses

Location	Potential response
Nose	• Forceful exhalation (sneeze) • Apnea • Bradycardia
Nasopharynx	• Sniff • Aspiration reflex • Rapid inhalation
Larynx	• Apnea • Slow, deep breathing • Bronchoconstriction • Cough • Hypertension
Trachea	• Cough • Hypertension • Bronchoconstriction

The receptors, called pulmonary stretch receptors, involved in the **Hering-Breuer reflex** are located in the walls of the bronchi and the bronchioles. These receptors are stimulated when the lung inflates and the transpulmonary pressure rises. When the lung inflates and the transpulmonary pressure rises, the receptors send an afferent impulse to the DRG to stop inhalation. In adults, this typically occurs when the tidal volume exceeds 800 to 1000 mL. As a result of the afferent impulse to the DRG to stop inhalation, the respiratory rate typically increases to compensate for the lower tidal volume. The Hering-Breuer reflex is credited for maintaining the rate and depth of breathing during moderate exercise.

The **deflation reflex** is mediated by the vagus nerve. This means that the vagus nerve carries the afferent impulse to the DRG in the medulla oblongata. This reflex causes the respiratory rate to increase during a time of lung collapse. For example, when a patient suffers a pneumothorax, the tidal volume drops significantly. This reflex signals the DRG to increase the respiratory rate to compensate for the lower tidal volume and maintain the minute ventilation. The resulting respiratory pattern is called **hyperpnea**.

The irritant receptors are vagal sensory fibers located in the epithelium of the nose, pharynx, trachea, and bronchi. They produce a vasovagal response, meaning that they stimulate afferent impulses from both sensory and motor neurons. These receptors can adjust their firing rate very rapidly in the event of a stimulus. Causes such as an inspired irritant (e.g., histamine), inhaled particulate matter, and anaphylaxis can result in coughing, sneezing, tachypnea, glottis narrowing, bradycardia, bronchoconstriction, and hyperpnea. Respiratory therapists must be aware that common hospital procedures such as bronchoscopy, tracheal suctioning, and intubation may stimulate this response as well.

Juxtacapillary receptors, also called C-fibers, are located in the lung parenchyma near the capillary walls. Because the receptors are located near the capillary wall, they are stimulated by conditions that affect the capillaries such as alveolar inflammation, pulmonary vascular congestion, and edema. This stimulation may result in rapid shallow breathing, dyspnea, expiratory narrowing of the glottis (i.e., grunting), and bradycardia.

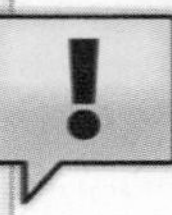

Respiratory Recap

Hering-Breuer Reflex

- Primarily stretch receptors
- Stimulated when the lung inflates and transpulmonary pressure rises
- Sends impulses to DRG to stop inhalation

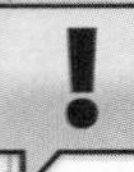

Respiratory Recap

Respiratory Reflexes

- Upper airway reflexes
- Hering-Breuer reflex
- Deflation reflex
- Irritant reflex
- Juxtacapillary receptors
- Head paradoxical reflex
- Peripheral proprioceptors

The **Head paradoxical reflex** is not completely understood, but the basic mechanism of action is a vagal block of the Hering-Breuer reflex. This means that when the lung is overinflated, the stimulus allows the lung to continue to inflate and does not stop the inflation. This may help maintain an increased tidal volume during exercise. It is also suspected that this reflex is responsible for the baby's first breath after delivery.

These receptors, stimulated with movement and pain, are found in muscles, tendons, and joints. When the **peripheral proprioceptors** are stimulated, afferent impulses to the medulla oblongata cause an increase in respiratory activity. This breathing pattern is called hyperpnea. Interventions such as moving limbs, applying cold water, and causing mild pain can stimulate breathing in the patient suffering from respiratory depression. One example of this phenomenon can be found in the neonatal unit. A premature infant experiencing spells of apnea can be stimulated to breathe by rubbing the back or tapping the soles of the feet.

Innervation of the Lungs

Breathing occurs when there are changes within intrapulmonary pressure. During breathing, the diaphragm contracts, changing the muscle from its resting dome shape to a flat, taut muscle. In addition, the muscles of the chest wall are stimulated to contract, which causes the rib cage to move up and out. The resultant negative pressure created within the lung causes a pressure gradient with the atmospheric pressure, and air is drawn into the lungs. Exhalation relies on the passive recoil of the diaphragm and rib cage returning to their natural positions, which then causes a pressure in the lungs higher than that of atmospheric pressure, and air flows out of the lungs.

The diaphragm receives efferent impulses from the phrenic nerve, which is located near the C3-C5 segment of the spinal cord. The external intercostal muscle receives efferent impulses from external intercostal nerves, located near the T1-T12 segment of the spinal cord. These nerves receive impulses from the DRG that stimulate motor activity, resulting in the constriction of muscle fibers and inspiration. When the signal ceases, the muscle fibers relax and the structures return to their natural shape, which results in exhalation.

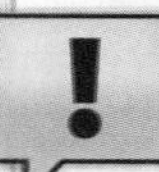

Respiratory Recap

Innervation of Lungs

- Diaphragm receives efferent impulses from phrenic nerve
- External intercostal muscle receives efferent impulses from external intercostal nerves

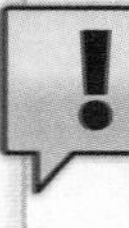

Respiratory Recap

Peripheral Chemoreceptors

- Carotid bodies located in bifurcation of common carotid artery and innervated by glossopharyngeal nerve
- Aortic bodies located in aortic arch and innervated by vagus nerve

Central and Peripheral Chemoreceptors

Specific breathing patterns are activated based on information received from several different monitoring systems throughout the body. Chemoreceptors are nerve cells that are sensitive to changes within the blood chemistries. They lie outside the central nervous system and control breathing patterns based on the information they receive from the different monitoring systems. The chemoreceptors that affect the control of breathing are the **peripheral chemoreceptors** and the **central chemoreceptors**.

Peripheral Chemoreceptors

Two groups of peripheral chemoreceptors have been identified as primary contributors to the control of breathing (**Figure 50-3**). The **carotid bodies** are located in the bifurcation of the common carotid artery and are innervated by the glossopharyngeal nerve. The **aortic bodies** are located in the aortic arch and are innervated by the vagus nerve. These cells have direct contact with blood, and the cell membranes are permeable to H^+ ion concentration and $Paco_2$. Both the carotid bodies and the aortic bodies are stimulated by a decreased Pao_2, a decreased pH, and an increased $Paco_2$. In the presence of hypoxia and acidemia, a synergistic effect is noted.

The peripheral chemoreceptors are not directly stimulated by the Pao_2, but by the amount of dissolved O_2. Like all cells, the peripheral chemoreceptors need O_2 to survive. When the O_2 supply is not enough for the cells' metabolic needs, they are stimulated. The peripheral chemoreceptors' response to the stimulation is an increase in ventilation. This usually occurs when the Pao_2 reaches 60 mm Hg (corresponding Spo_2 90%). At that point, the chemoreceptors are stimulated to send an afferent impulse to the DRG in an effort to increase ventilation. Note that Pao_2 does not stimulate the peripheral chemoreceptors until the Pao_2 level reaches

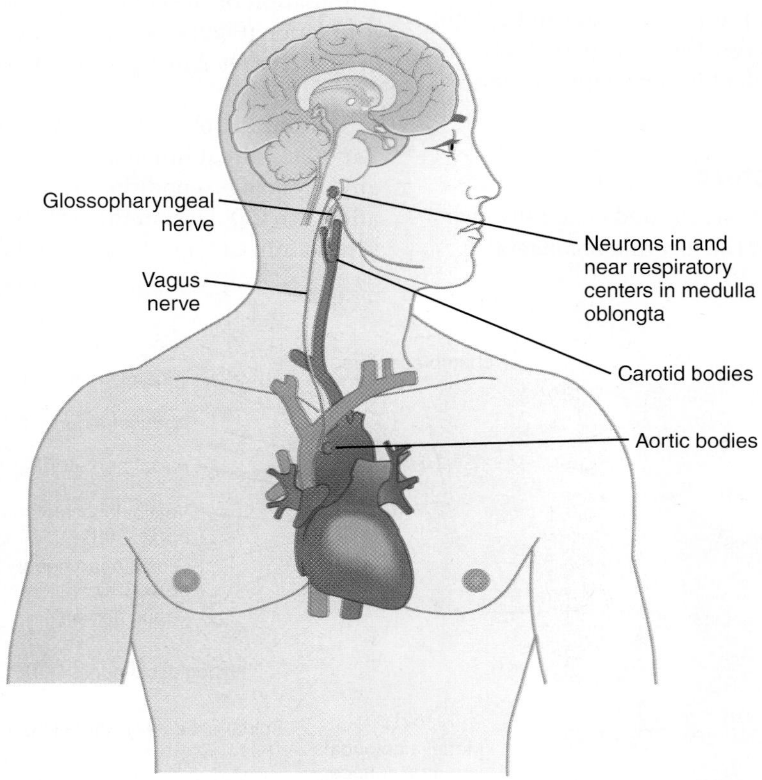

FIGURE 50-3 Peripheral chemoreceptors contributing to control of breathing: the carotid and aortic bodies.

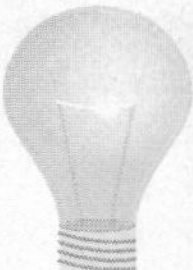

STOP AND THINK

What causes you to hyperventilate at high altitude?

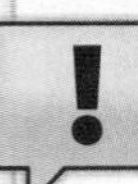

Respiratory Recap

Central Chemoreceptors

- Are located bilaterally on the ventrolateral surface of the medulla oblongata
- Changes in $Paco_2$ affect CSF and ultimately stimulate the central chemoreceptors to affect minute ventilation

60 mm Hg. This means that, in normal circumstances, O_2 does not play a role in the control of breathing.

Low Pao_2, not O_2 content (Cao_2), stimulates the peripheral chemoreceptors. Therefore, conditions where the Pao_2 remains normal but the Cao_2 is dangerously low will not stimulate an increased ventilatory pattern based on O_2 stimulus alone. Examples include chronic anemia, carbon monoxide poisoning, and methemoglobinemia.

The peripheral chemoreceptors are also sensitive to Pao_2 and H^+ ion concentration. Remember that $Paco_2$ changes result in H^+ ion (pH) changes. If the $Paco_2$ increases, therefore the H^+ ion concentration increases and stimulates the peripheral chemoreceptors. The peripheral chemoreceptors thus are stimulated directly by the change in H^+ ion concentration and indirectly by the change in $Paco_2$. The peripheral chemoreceptors are stimulated more by an increase in H^+ ion concentrations and less by a decrease in H^+ ion concentrations. If the peripheral chemoreceptors are stimulated by an increase in H^+ ion concentration (decreased pH), the result is an increase in respiratory rate and an increase in tidal volume. If the peripheral chemoreceptors are stimulated by a decrease in H^+ ion concentration, the result is a slight decrease in respiratory rate and a slight decrease in tidal volume. Over time, the peripheral chemoreceptors learn to adapt to the changing body acid–base balance.

Central Chemoreceptors

The central chemoreceptors are located bilaterally near the ventrolateral surface of the medulla oblongata (**Figure 50-4**). These groups of cells are in contact with the cerebral spinal fluid (CSF) and arterial blood. Between the arterial blood and the CSF lies a thin membrane called the blood-brain barrier (BBB). This barrier protects the CSF from various substances within the arterial blood. The only substance that easily diffuses from the arterial blood through the blood-brain barrier into the CSF is CO_2. HCO_3 and H^+ ions do not readily diffuse across the blood-brain barrier.

Changes in $Paco_2$ result in changes in the diffusion of CO_2 across the blood-brain barrier. For example, an increased $Paco_2$ results in an increased CO_2 in the CSF. CO_2 in the CSF hydrolyzes and releases H^+ ions. The increased amount of H^+ ions decreases the pH in the CSF, which stimulates the central chemoreceptors to increase ventilation. Conversely, a decreased $Paco_2$ results in a decreased level of CO_2 in the CSF. Lower CO_2 in the CSF results in fewer H^+ ions from the hydrolysis process. The decreased amount of H^+ ions increases the pH in the CSF, which decreases stimulation of the central chemoreceptors to decrease ventilation (**Figure 50-5**). In general, alveolar ventilation ($\dot{V}_A$) increases 2 to 3 L/min for every 1 mm Hg rise in $Paco_2$.

Various factors affect the CO_2 levels in the CSF. The $Paco_2$ is a direct influence on the CO_2 in the CSF, so any physiologic condition that affects the $Paco_2$ will affect the CO_2 level in the CSF. Alterations in alveolar ventilation, CO_2 production, and CO_2 content of venous

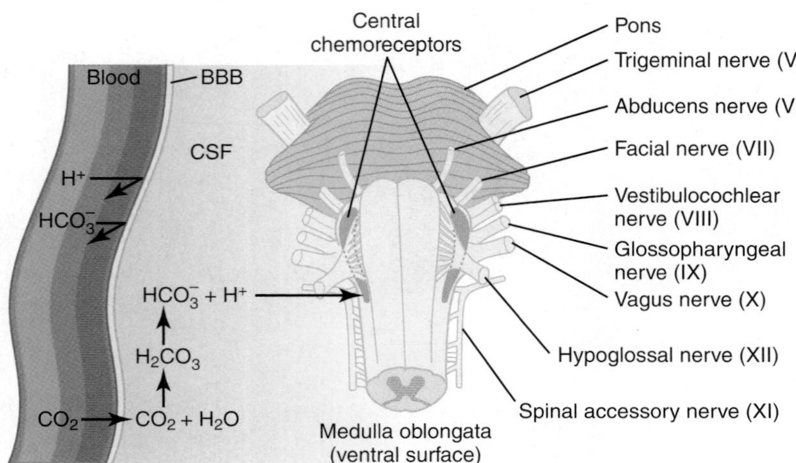

FIGURE 50-4 Central chemoreceptors.

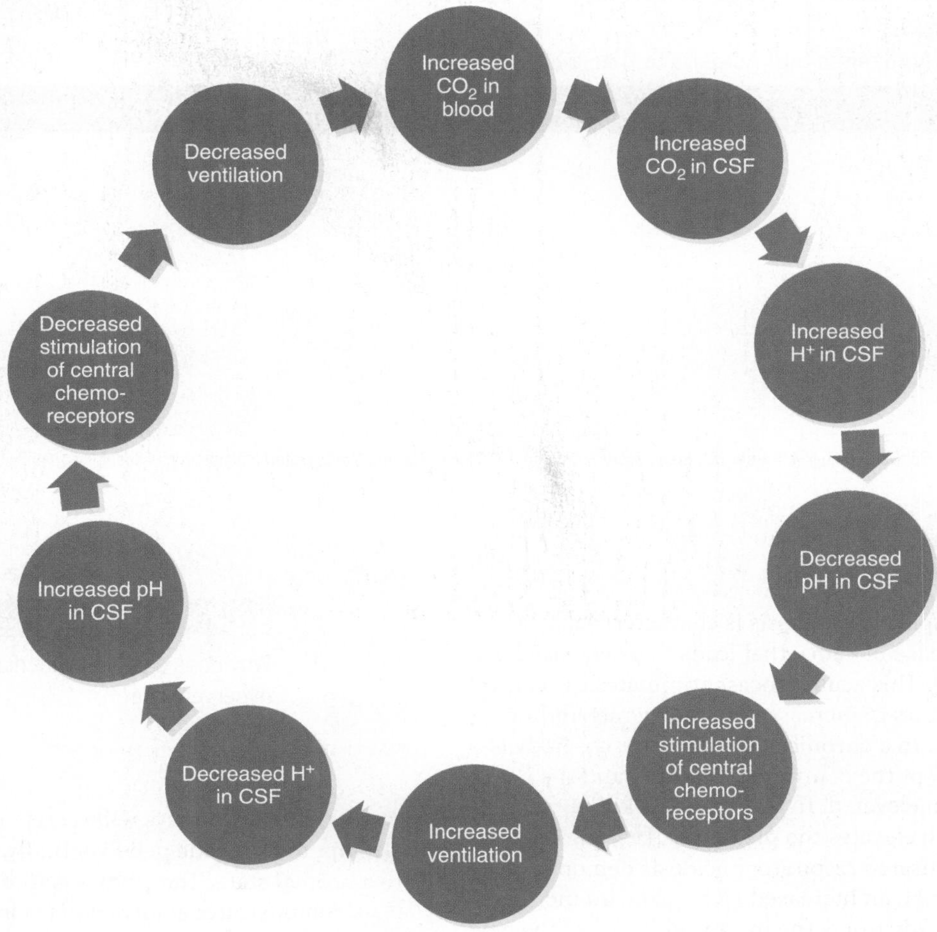

FIGURE 50-5 Central chemoreceptor stimulation cycle.

blood are contributors. Also, the volume of cerebral blood flow can affect the CO_2 levels in the CSF.

Cortical Effects

Behavioral and subjective respiratory control mechanisms in the cerebral cortex are responsible for the wakefulness drive to breathe. This volitional control of breathing allows voluntary hyperventilation and breath holding. It might also be responsible for the hyperventilation that occurs with anxiety.

Factors That Affect Control of Breathing

The control of breathing is affected by many factors. Some factors result in a decreased (depressed) drive to breathe while others result in an increased (stimulated) drive to breathe (**Table 50-2**).

TABLE 50-2
Factors That Stimulate and Depress Drive to Breathe

Factors That Stimulate	Factors That Depress
Hypercapnia	Hypocapnia
Acidosis	Alkalosis
Hypoxemia	Drugs: narcotics, propofol, barbiturates
Pain	
Sepsis	
Anxiety	
Drugs: aspirin, xanthine, progesterone, doxapram	

Effects of Acid–Base Disorders

Acute acid–base disorders produce short-term effects based on the level of Pa_{O_2}, Pa_{CO_2}, and pH. When the acid–base balance is disrupted for long periods of time, however, the body compensates and the responses from the DRG and VRG are slightly altered. Acid–base disorders that occur for a prolonged (chronic) period of time are called compensated. The effects of acid–base disorders on respiratory drive are summarized in **Table 50-3**.

TABLE 50-3
Effects of Hypoxemia and Acid–Base Disorders on Respiratory Drive

Stimulus	Peripheral Chemoreceptors	Central Chemoreceptors	Response of the Controller
Hypoxemia			
Acute	↑↑	↓	↑
Chronic	↑↑↑	0	↑↑↑
Hypercapnia			
Acute	↑↑	↑↑↑	↑↑↑↑↑
Chronic	↑	↑↑	↑↑↑
Mild metabolic acidosis			
Acute	↑↑	↓	↑
Chronic	↑	0	↑

Reproduced from Schwartzstein RM, Parker MJ. *Respiratory Physiology: A Clinical Approach (Integrated Physiology)*. Philadelphia: Lippincott Williams & Wilkins; 2005.

Respiratory Acidosis

An acute respiratory acidosis is characterized by a sudden increase in $Paco_2$ that leads to a decreased pH (higher $[H^+]$). This acute process stimulates the central chemoreceptors to increase respiratory rate and/or tidal volume. In a chronic state, however, the body is unable to adapt the control of breathing and the $Paco_2$ levels remain elevated. In this case, the kidney retains HCO_3^-, which elevates the pH (lower $[H^+]$) toward normal. Compensated respiratory acidosis demonstrates a normalized pH, an increased HCO_3^-, and an increased $Paco_2$. The body resets the increased $Paco_2$ as the new baseline level. This leads to a decrease in the central chemoreceptors' ability to control breathing and a decreased sensitivity to changes in $Paco_2$. In disease processes with a prolonged hypercapnic state, such as severe COPD, O_2 may play the primary role in control of breathing.

Metabolic Acidosis

An acute metabolic acidosis is characterized by a decreased HCO_3^- and decreased pH. Remember that HCO_3^- and pH have a direct relationship as well as the fact that neither can cross the blood-brain barrier. Instead, the low pH in the plasma stimulates the peripheral chemoreceptors to increase ventilation. The $Paco_2$—which does cross the blood-brain barrier—decreases and increases the CSF pH. Over time, this adjustment decreases respiratory drive.

Respiratory Alkalosis

An acute respiratory alkalosis is characterized by a decreased $Paco_2$, which increases the pH. This acute process is precipitated by some conditions that cause the patient to hyperventilate. This stimulates the central chemoreceptors to decrease either the respiratory rate or the tidal volume. If the condition that causes the hyperventilation continues, the lower $Paco_2$ will persist.

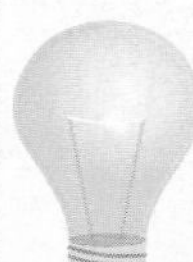

STOP AND THINK

Why does a patient with diabetic ketoacidosis hyperventilate?

As a result, the kidneys will secrete more HCO_3^- in an attempt to lower the pH. Eventually, the pH will return to a normal state. The **compensated respiratory alkalosis** demonstrates a normal pH, a low HCO_3^-, and a low $Paco_2$. Again, the chemoreceptor sensitivity to $Paco_2$ is reset to the new baseline level, which is lower than normal.

Compensated Metabolic Alkalosis

An acute metabolic alkalosis is characterized by an increased HCO_3^- and increased pH. Plasma pH stimulates the peripheral chemoreceptors. The peripheral chemoreceptors interpret the high pH to mean that there is also a low $Paco_2$. In response, the peripheral chemoreceptors send a stimulus to decrease ventilation. As a result, the $Paco_2$ increases and decreases the pH. Over time, this ventilatory adjustment corrects the pH. The compensated metabolic alkalosis demonstrates a normal pH, a higher than normal $Paco_2$, and a high HCO_3. The chemoreceptor sensitivity is reset to the new baseline $Paco_2$ level. Because an elevated $Paco_2$ is a strong drive to breathe, compensation for metabolic acidosis might not occur.

High Altitude and Control of Breathing

The partial pressure of inspired O_2 (PIO_2) is lower at higher altitudes. Note the differences in barometric pressure (PB) and PAO_2 for a patient breathing room air (FIO_2 of 0.21) at various elevations (**Table 50-4**).

TABLE 50-4
Effects of Altitude

Altitude (meters)	Altitude (feet)	Point of Reference	PB (mm Hg)	PAO_2 (mm Hg)
Sea level	Sea level	Dallas, TX	760	149
1524	5,000	Denver, CO	632	122
3048	10,000	Breckenridge, CO	523	100
4572	15,000	Mount Hubbard, AK	429	80
6096	20,000	Mount McKinley, AK	349	63

FIO_2 is 0.21.

Acute Effects

Persons who rapidly ascend to high altitudes are susceptible to high altitude illness, defined as cerebral and pulmonary syndromes that can develop in persons shortly after ascent to high altitude.[1] Preventative measures for high altitude illness include ascending at a slow rate, spending a night at an intermediate altitude before ascending to the final altitude, and avoiding overexertion. High altitude illnesses include acute mountain sickness (AMS), high altitude cerebral edema (HACE), and high altitude pulmonary edema (HAPE). All have the same risk factors:

- Rate of ascent
- Prior history of high altitude illness
- Resident below 900 m (2952 feet)
- Exertion

Persons at all levels of physical fitness may be susceptible to high altitude illness.[1,2] The incidence of AMS among visitors to moderate altitudes in the United States is approximately 25%, but the incidence of HACE and HAPE are much lower (0.1% to 4.0%).[2,3]

AMS occurs when a person rapidly ascends to an altitude over 2500 m (8202 feet). The proposed pathophysiology of AMS is inability to compensate for the sudden hypoxemia at the higher altitude. The peripheral chemoreceptors sense the drop in PaO_2 and send an afferent impulse to the DRG to trigger increased ventilation in an effort to increase the amount of O_2 available to the tissues. The cardinal symptom of AMS is headache; others include gastrointestinal symptoms such as nausea, vomiting, and anorexia; insomnia; dizziness; fatigue; and sleep disturbance. Though some cases have been noted to occur within an hour of ascent, most persons with AMS develop symptoms between 6 to 10 hours after ascent to an altitude over 2500 m (8202 ft). With early diagnosis, descending to a lower altitude and controlling symptoms with analgesics and antiemetics are used to treat AMS. Moderate AMS may require the administration of low-flow O_2 (1 to 2 L/min) or the application of hyperbaric O_2 in addition to treatment of symptoms. Failure to recognize and treat AMS early may result in the development of HACE.[1–3]

High altitude cerebral edema is considered end-stage disease for AMS. With HACE, the patient demonstrates ataxia (lack of muscle coordination), altered consciousness, or both. HACE progresses over a period of hours or days. Though the pathophysiology of AMS and HACE is not completely known, the suspected path of the disease begins with hypoxia resulting from the lower PIO_2. If the body is unable to compensate and maintain tissue oxygenation, hypoxemia leads to increased cerebral blood flow, increased cerebral blood volume, and increased permeability of the blood-brain barrier. These lead to brain swelling and the inadequate buffering of the CSF. At this point, the patient demonstrates hypoventilation, impaired gas exchange, fluid retention, and increased intracranial pressure (ICP). The cause of death in HACE is brain herniation. Treatment of HACE includes immediate descent to lower altitude, application of O_2 or hyperbaric O_2 therapy, and dexamethasone to reduce inflammation.[1–3]

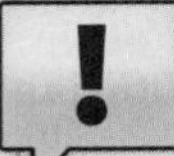

Respiratory Recap

Acute Mountain Sickness

- Occurs at an altitude of over 8202 feet (2500 meters)
- Headache is a cardinal sign
- If detected early can be easily treated with rapid descent, analgesics, and antiemetics

Respiratory Recap

High Altitude Cerebral Edema (HACE)

- Is considered end stage of acute mountain sickness (AMS)
- Results in ataxia (lack of muscle coordination)
- Death is due to brain herniation

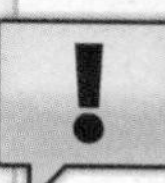

Respiratory Recap

High Altitude Pulmonary Edema (HAPE)

- Manifests 2 to 4 days following ascension to 8202 feet (2500 meters)
- Presents with dyspnea on exertion and decreased exercise tolerance at higher altitude
- Treatment entails immediate descent to lower altitude, application of O_2 or hyperbaric O_2 therapy, and dexamethasone to reduce inflammation

Unlike HACE, high altitude pulmonary edema (HAPE) is a disease process independent from AMS, though a significant percentage of those with HAPE also have AMS (50%).[1] HAPE begins to manifest between days 2 and 4 following ascension to an elevation of 2500 m (8202 ft) or higher. Preliminary symptoms are nondefinitive and include dyspnea on exertion and a decreased exercise tolerance at the higher altitude. Soon after, the patient develops a dry cough. As the disease progresses, symptoms such as pink or blood-tinged sputum, respiratory distress, tachycardia, tachypnea, orthopnea, frank hemoptysis, and fever develop. Breath sounds reveal crackles and the electrocardiogram reveals sinus tachycardia with a right bundle branch block. Arterial blood gases reveal severe hypoxemia and respiratory alkalosis.[1,2]

The exact pathophysiology of HAPE is not completely understood. However, it is believed that the body is unable to compensate for the initial hypoxia that occurs with the lower P_{IO_2} and that results in a noncardiogenic pulmonary edema with pulmonary hypertension. The pulmonary hypertension results from uneven pulmonary vasoconstriction due to hypoxemia. This may lead to overperfusion of capillaries, endothelial stress, and capillary leakage. Treatment for HAPE includes immediate descent to lower altitude, O_2 therapy, continuous positive airway pressure, hyperbaric O_2 therapy, and dexamethasone.[1,2] Of the three high altitude illnesses, HAPE accounts for the greatest number of deaths.[2]

Chronic Effects

Approximately 140 million people live in high altitudes.[2] Persons who reside at altitudes over 2500 m (8202 feet) develop various physiologic responses.

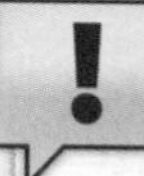

Respiratory Recap

Chronic Effects of High Altitude

- Hyperventilation is normal response to lower P_{aO_2}
- Healthy persons demonstrate pulmonary hypertension, right ventricular hypertrophy, and increased amount of smooth muscle cells in distal pulmonary arteries

Hyperventilation is a normal response to the lower P_{IO_2} found in the higher altitude. Healthy persons in these locations demonstrate pulmonary hypertension, right ventricular hypertrophy, and an increased amount of smooth muscle cells in the distal pulmonary arteries.[4] Persons who are unable to compensate tend to hypoventilate and experience greater hypoxemia, resulting in chronic mountain sickness (CMS). The reported prevalence ranges from 8% to 28%. Men are more likely to develop CMS, and the risk of CMS increases with age, smoking, and pollution. CMS is characterized by an increased hemoglobin (≥21 g/dL in males; ≥19 g/dL in females), severe hypoxemia, severe pulmonary hypertension, cor pulmonale, and congestive heart failure. Symptoms recede when the patient is transferred to a lower altitude but return upon ascension to higher altitude.[4,5]

Hypoxic Drive

Chronic respiratory illnesses, such as COPD and cystic fibrosis, may lead to alteration in baseline blood chemistries. These patients, called "CO_2 retainers," develop compensated respiratory acidosis. This new baseline changes the chemoreceptors' sensitivity to P_{aCO_2}. As a result, P_{aO_2}, which is usually not a major influence on control of breathing, is now the primary stimulus. Significant changes to P_{aO_2} may result in significant changes in control of breathing.

The **hypoxic drive theory** emerged in the 1950s and 1960s. The premise of this theory is that high levels of P_{aO_2}, resulting from supplemental O_2, increase the P_{aO_2} and cause the O_2 chemoreceptors to decrease ventilation. This response causes the P_{aO_2} to rise.[6–8]

The increased P_{aO_2} from supplemental O_2 administration is only one aspect of this hypoventilation phenomenon. Patients with chronic respiratory disease have pulmonary vasoconstriction from the persistent hypoxic state. When the delivery of supplemental O_2 increases P_{aO_2}, the pulmonary vasculature responds with vasodilation. This causes increased perfusion to underventilated alveoli, increasing the capillary P_{CO_2} and the P_{aCO_2}. Another factor contributing to an increase in P_{aCO_2} with oxygen administration is the Haldane effect.[7,8] According to the Haldane effect, CO_2 is released from hemoglobin with an increase in oxygen saturation, thus causing the P_{aCO_2} to increase. Patients with chronic respiratory disease may have poor outcomes from both hyperoxemia (S_{pO_2} >96%) and hypoxemia (S_{pO_2} <88%). Titrated O_2 therapy to patients with chronic respiratory disease with appropriate monitoring is a vital component to successful disease management.

Opioid Drugs and Respiratory Drive

Opioid drugs such as morphine are a mainstay for pain relief. They are also used during mechanical ventilation not only for pain control but to promote patient-ventilator synchrony. Opioid receptors are abundant in the respiratory center, and thus an important consequence of opioid administration is respiratory depression.[9] In the case of the mechanically ventilated patient, this might be an intended effect in the presence of asynchrony, but it becomes an unintended effect when attempting to liberate the patient from the ventilator.

The most opioid effect on breathing is rhythm generation. At lower opioid doses, changes in the respiratory rate (**bradypnea**) occur. Higher opioid doses cause reduction in tidal volume. Respiratory depression secondary to opioid (narcotic) administration is an important cause of postoperative morbidity. These patients should be monitored closely, including the use of pulse oximetry and capnography. Narcotic drug overdose is a cause of admission to the hospital. Such patients require mechanical ventilation until the drug is cleared or reversed with naloxone.

Anesthetic drugs other than opioids can also produce respiratory depression. Propofol and barbiturates are respiratory depressants. Although the respiratory depressant effects of ethanol and benzodiazepines are mild, the concurrent use of these drugs with opioids is often present in drug addicts with fatal opioid overdose. Similarly, in the postoperative period, the residual effects of anesthetic agents and sedative premedication can further exacerbate the opioid-mediated depression of breathing.[9]

Abnormal Breathing Patterns

A normal adult human breathes approximately 12 to 20 breaths/minute. The breathing pattern is regular and rhythmic. This breathing pattern is called **eupnea.**

When the only change in the breathing pattern is an increased rate, the breathing pattern is called *tachypnea*. The regularity and rhythm are consistent, but the respiratory rate is increased to over 20 breaths/min. Causes of tachypnea include fever, infection, pain, fear, and anxiety. The breathing pattern is called bradypnea when the only change in the breathing pattern is a decreased rate. The regularity and rhythm are consistent, but the respiratory rate is less than 10 breaths/minute. Causes of bradypnea include electrolyte imbalance, alkalosis, and pharmacologic depressants.

At times, the breathing pattern changes only in the tidal volume. The rate, rhythm, and regularity of the pattern are normal but the person is inhaling tidal volumes greater than normal. This breathing pattern is called hyperpnea. Causes of hyperpnea include ketoacidosis, head injury, and hyperventilation syndrome. Conversely, when the only deviation from eupnea is a lower than normal tidal volume, the breathing pattern is called **hypopnea**. Causes of hypopnea include head trauma, narcotic suppression, and cerebral hypoxia. Persons with sleep apnea may also display several episodes of hypopnea during sleep due to defects of the nasal passages, obesity, or weakened respiratory muscles. **Kussmaul breathing** is characterized by a rapid respiratory rate and a higher than normal tidal volume. This breathing pattern is associated with severe diabetic ketoacidosis.

Cheyne-Stokes breathing is characterized by gradual increases in respiratory rate and tidal volume, followed by gradual decreases in respiratory rate and tidal volume, followed by a period of cessation of breathing (apnea). After the period of apnea, the cycle begins again. This breathing pattern is associated with severe cardiovascular disease (specifically those with low cardiac output) and severe traumatic brain injuries, including stroke and tumors.

A breathing pattern with irregular tidal volumes and respiratory rates is called **ataxic breathing**. Periods of apnea may be interspersed as well. This breathing pattern is typically caused by damage to the medulla oblongata, either by trauma or stroke. The presence of this breathing pattern indicates impending respiratory failure. **Biot breathing** is characterized by short bursts of rapid respiratory rates and high tidal volumes followed by 10 to 30 seconds of apnea. Note that the respirations are uniformly deep and relatively regular. This breathing pattern is associated with severe brain stem injury and meningitis. Apneustic breathing is characterized by deep respirations and a prolonged inspiratory phase followed by a short expiratory phase. Apneustic breathing is associated with injury to the pons.

Apnea is the complete cessation of respiratory effort. Without intervention, death will occur within a few minutes of onset. Apnea can be caused by an obstructive defect or can be mediated by the central nervous system.

Orthopnea is the term used to describe a situation in which the patient is most able to breathe comfortably in the upright position. The patient experiences shortness of breath when lying flat. Conditions in which patients might experience orthopnea include pulmonary edema, sleep apnea, and various chronic respiratory diseases.

Dyspnea is the medical term used to describe shortness of breath. Dyspnea may occur due to heavy exercise or exertion or from a multitude of medical conditions.

Respiratory Drive and Exercise

Ventilation increases during exercise in three phases: the neurologic phase, the metabolic phase, and the compensatory phase.[10] The initial increase in ventilation at the onset of exercise is too quick to be explained by changes in metabolism or other factors. It is possible that this first phase is partly a learned response (neurologic phase). As exercise continues, ventilation increases linearly with the increase in O_2 consumption and CO_2 production that results from the increased physical activity (metabolic phase). Pao_2 and $Paco_2$ are normal during this phase of exercise. When the anaerobic threshold is reached, lactic acid is produced. This lowers the pH of the blood, which stimulates the peripheral and central chemoreceptors (compensatory phase).

Assessing Respiratory Drive

Because the Pao_2 can usually be reduced a lot without evoking a ventilatory response (**Figure 50-6**), hypoxia is generally not used as a test of respiratory drive. The ventilatory response to CO_2 is normally measured by inhaling CO_2 (e.g., 7% CO_2 with 93% O_2) or rebreathing so that the inspired Pco_2 increases gradually.[11] As can be seen in **Figure 50-7**, minute ventilation increases by 2 to 3 L/min for each 1 mm Hg rise in . There is considerable variation between subjects, making it difficult to apply normal values. The ventilatory response to CO_2 is reduced by sleep; increasing age; genetic, racial, and personality factors; narcotics and barbiturates; and increased work of breathing. Trained athletes and divers have a low CO_2 sensitivity.

Measuring inspiratory pressure during a brief period of inspiratory airway occlusion can assess respiratory drive.[11] The patient breathes through a mouthpiece. A shutter is closed during exhalation, with the patient unaware, so that the first part of the next inspiration is occluded, and the shutter is opened after 0.5 second. The pressure measured during the first 0.1 s (**$P_{0.1}$**) against the closed shutter is a measure of respiratory center output. It is relatively unaffected by the mechanical properties of the respiratory system. This method can be used to study the respiratory sensitivity to CO_2, O_2, and other variables. Some mechanical ventilators allow the measurement of $P_{0.1}$, and this might be useful when considering liberation from the ventilator. Either a very low or a very high $P_{0.1}$ is associated with failure of liberation from the ventilator.

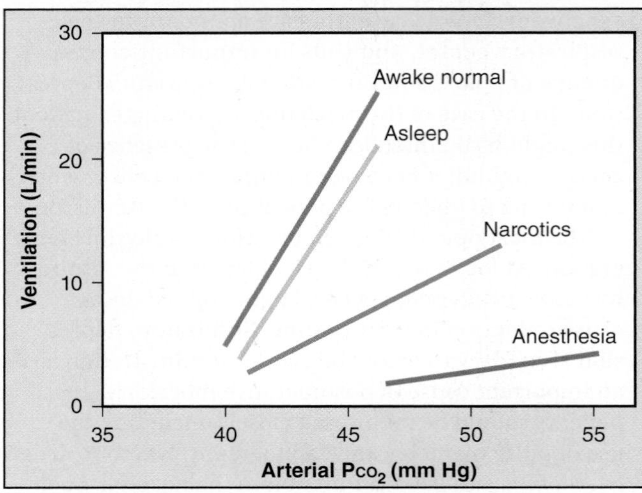

FIGURE 50-7 The ventilatory response to hypercapnia. The ventilatory response to hypercapnia is linear in nature. The normal range of the response is an increase of 2 to 5 L/min in ventilation for each 1 mm Hg increase in $Paco_2$. When a patient is asleep, the curve is shifted to the right. When a patient is under the effects of anesthesia or narcotics, both of which inhibit the response of the controller, the curves are shifted to the right, and the slope is diminished.

Reproduced from Schwartzstein RM, Parker MJ. *Respiratory Physiology: A Clinical Approach.* Philadelphia: Lippincott Williams & Wilkins; 2005.

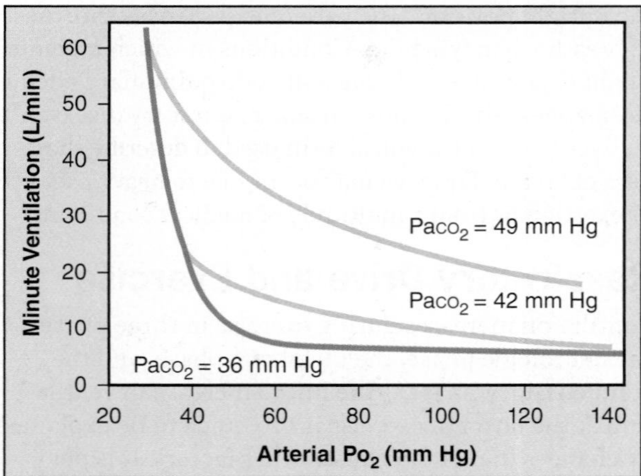

FIGURE 50-6 Ventilatory response to hypoxemia. Minute ventilation is plotted as a function of Pao_2. Note that ventilation changes little as Pao_2 decreases from supranormal levels through the normal range. As Pao_2 decreases below 60 mm Hg, ventilation starts to increase, and the rate of increase becomes marked when Pao_2 is below 40 mm Hg. The same degree of hypoxemia, when combined with acute hypercapnia, produces even more marked increases in ventilation.

Adapted from Leff A, Schumacker P. *Respiratory Physiology: Basics and Applications*. 1st ed. Philadelphia: WB Saunders; 1993:114. As shown in Schwartzstein RM, Parker MJ. *Respiratory Physiology: A Clinical Approach*. Philadelphia: Lippincott Williams & Wilkins; 2005.

Key Points

- Control of breathing is regulated by the medulla oblongata and the pons.
- The two major areas of respiratory control in the medulla oblongata are the dorsal respiratory group (DRG) and the ventral respiratory group (VRG).
- The pons modifies the output from the medulla oblongata.
- Respiratory reflexes send signals to manage the rate and depth of breathing based on stimulus received.
- Chemoreceptors modify the control of breathing based on input from various bodily monitoring systems.
- DRG and VRG control of breathing are altered by compensated (chronic) acid–base disorders.
- The control of breathing may not adapt to either acute or chronic exposure to high altitude (lower PAO_2) and may have significant negative effects.
- A hyperventilation mechanical ventilation strategy may not be optimal in managing the patient with traumatic brain injury.
- Titrated O_2 delivery to chronic respiratory disease patients with appropriate monitoring is a vital component to successful disease management.
- $P_{0.1}$ is a measure of respiratory drive.

References

1. Hacket PH, Roach RC. High-altitude illness. *N Engl J Med.* 2001;345: 107–114.
2. Basnyat B, Murdoch DR. High-altitude illness. *Lancet.* 2003;361: 1967–1974.
3. Honigman B, Theis MK, Koziol-McLain J, et al. Acute mountain sickness in a general tourist population at moderate altitudes. *Ann Intern Med.* 1993;118:587–592.
4. Penaloza D, Arias-Stella J. The heart and pulmonary circulation at high altitudes: healthy highlanders and chronic mountain sickness. *Circulation.* 2007;115:1132–1146.
5. Leon-Velarde F, Maggiorini M, Reeves JT, et al. Consensus statement on chronic and subacute high altitude diseases. *High Altitude Med Biol.* 2005;6:147–157.
6. Branson RD, Johannigman JA. Pre-hospital oxygen therapy. *Respir Care.* 2013;58:86–94.
7. New A. Oxygen: kill or cure? Prehospital hyperoxia in the COPD patient. *Emerg Med J.* 2006;23:144–146.
8. Robinson TD, Freiberg DB, Regnis JA, Young IH. The role of hypoventilation and ventilation-perfusion redistribution in oxygen-induced hypercapnia during acute exacerbations of chronic obstructive pulmonary disease. *Am J Respir Crit Care Med.* 2000;161:1524–1529.
9. Pattinson KTS. Opioids and the control of respiration. *Br J Anaesth.* 2008;100:747–758.
10. Schwartzstein RM, Parker MJ. *Respiratory Physiology: A Clinical Approach (Integrated Physiology).* Philadelphia: Lippincott Williams & Wilkins; 2005.
11. West JB. *Respiratory Physiology: The Essentials.* Philadelphia: Lippincott Williams & Wilkins; 2011.

CHAPTER

51

Cardiovascular, Renal, and Neural Anatomy and Physiology

Georgianna Sergakis, Crystal Dunlevy, Sarah Varekojis

OUTLINE

Cardiovascular Anatomy and Physiology
Renal Anatomy and Physiology
Neural Anatomy and Physiology

OBJECTIVES

1. Describe the gross and functional anatomy of the heart and circulatory system.
2. Describe the structure and function of the heart chambers and valves.
3. Trace blood flow through the heart.
4. Describe the components and conduction system of the heart.
5. Name the waves and intervals of the ECG and indicate what each represents.
6. Describe the timing and events of the cardiac cycle.
7. Explain the various factors regulating stroke volume and heart rate.
8. Explain the importance of renal function to the regulation of serum pH.
9. Describe the location and structure of the kidney.
10. Explain the processes of glomerular filtration, tubular reabsorption, and tubular secretion performed by the nephron.
11. Differentiate the central nervous system from the peripheral nervous system.
12. Describe the major divisions of the human brain.
13. Describe the major functions of the cerebrum and spinal cord.
14. Describe the structure of neurons, dendrites, and axons.
15. Describe the role of neurotransmitters in the peripheral nervous system and the autonomic nervous system.
16. Identify the difference between sensory and motor neurons.
17. Differentiate between the sympathetic and parasympathetic divisions of the autonomic nervous system.

KEY TERMS

acetylcholine
afferent neuron
aorta
aortic valve
artery
atrioventricular (AV) node
autonomic nervous system
axon
baroreceptor
brain stem
bundle of His
cerebellum
cerebral cortex
cerebral hemisphere
cerebrum
chordae tendinae
collecting duct
contractility
coronary sinus
corpus callosum
dendrite
diastole
endocardium
epicardium
glomerular capsule
glomerular filtration rate (GFR)
glomerulus
hypothalamus
inferior vena cava
left atrioventricular (bicuspid) valve
loop of Henle
mediastinum
medulla
meninges
midbrain
mitral valve (bicuspid valve)
myocardial infarction
myocardial ischemia
myocardium
nephron
neuron
papillary muscle
parasympathetic system
pericardium
pons
preload
pulmonary artery
pulmonary semilunar valve
pulmonary trunk
pulmonary vein
Purkinje fiber
renal corpuscle
renal pelvis
renal tubule
right atrioventricular (tricuspid) valve
right atrium
sinoatrial (SA) node
somatic nervous system
spinal cord
stroke volume
superior vena cava
sympathetic system
synapse
systole
thalamus
ureter
urethra
urinary bladder
vein

Introduction

Knowledge of the functional anatomy and physiology of the cardiovascular, renal, and neural systems is essential for understanding the extent and course of cardiopulmonary disorders. The anatomic and physiologic details of these systems provide the basis for monitoring changing pathology and response to treatment. This chapter discusses the basic anatomy and physiologic principles related to the cardiovascular, renal, and neural systems.

Cardiovascular Anatomy and Physiology

The Heart

The cardiovascular system, which includes the heart and an extensive network of blood vessels, provides the force and the transport system essential to maintain homeostasis, or a state of equilibrium in the body. The central organ of this system is the heart. The heart (**Figure 51-1**) is located in the **mediastinum**, intermediate to the lungs, posterior to the sternum, anterior to the vertebral column, and rests on the superior surface of the diaphragm. The heart is hollow, cone-shaped, and varies in size. The average human heart is 9 centimeters wide by 14 centimeters long and weighs between 250 and 350 grams. The base of the heart, which is the upper portion, lies beneath the second rib. The apex, or the blunt, pointed end, extends distally to the fifth intercostal space at the mid-clavicular line.

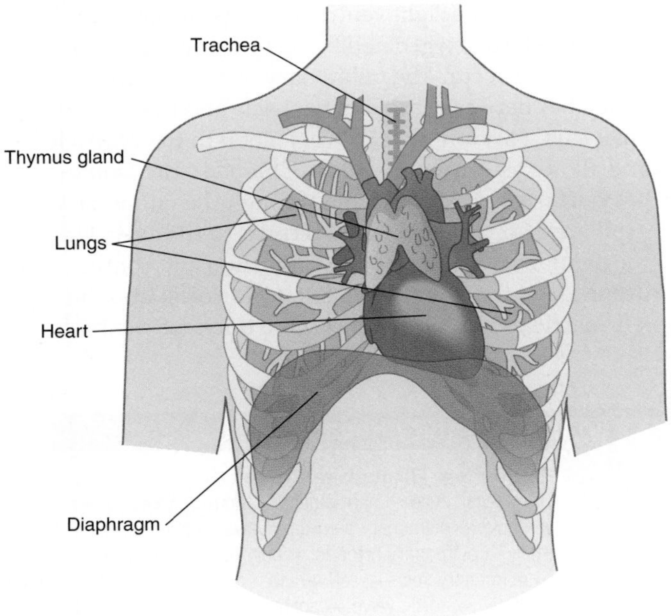

FIGURE 51-1 The heart.

Surrounding the heart is the **pericardium** (**Figure 51-2**), a serous membrane that has an inner (visceral) layer, a fibrous outer (parietal) layer, and an area between (the pericardial space). A small volume of serous fluid between these layers (approximately 5 mL) reduces friction between the pericardial membranes as the heart moves within the pericardial sac. Pericarditis, or pericardial inflammation, results in the heart rubbing against this sac and causing a sound heard by stethoscope called the pericardial friction rub. The area usually filled with a small amount of serous fluid may become overly filled with inflammatory fluid. This is known as a pericardial effusion, which causes a condition known as cardiac tamponade, where the overfilled sac puts pressure on the beating heart, reducing its pumping ability. The condition can be resolved through pericardiocentesis, when a physician drains the area with a needle and syringe.

The heart wall is composed of three layers: the epicardium, myocardium, and endocardium (**Figure 51-3**). The **epicardium**, a thin membrane, covers the outside of the heart. The innermost lining of the heart is the **endocardium**, composed of a single layer of endothelial cells. The endocardium contains specialized cardiac muscle fibers, called **Purkinje fibers**, important for electrical conduction. Finally, the **myocardium** consists

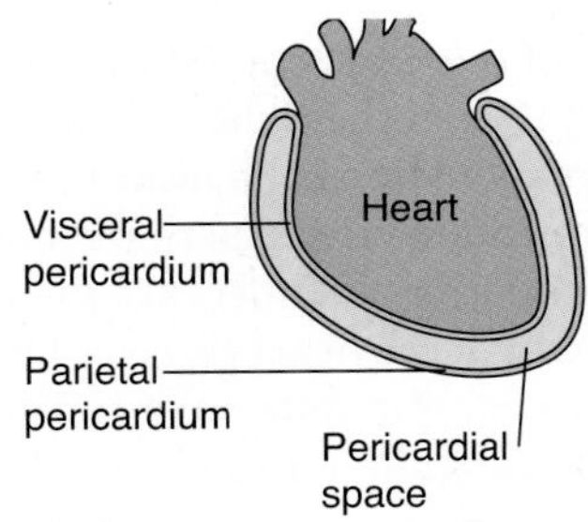

FIGURE 51-2 The pericardium.

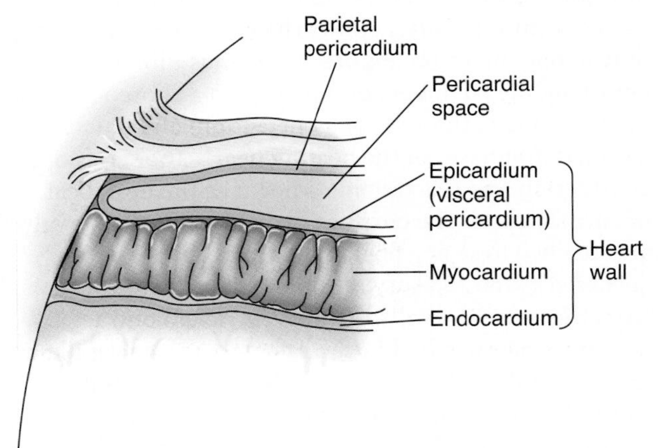

FIGURE 51-3 The heart wall.

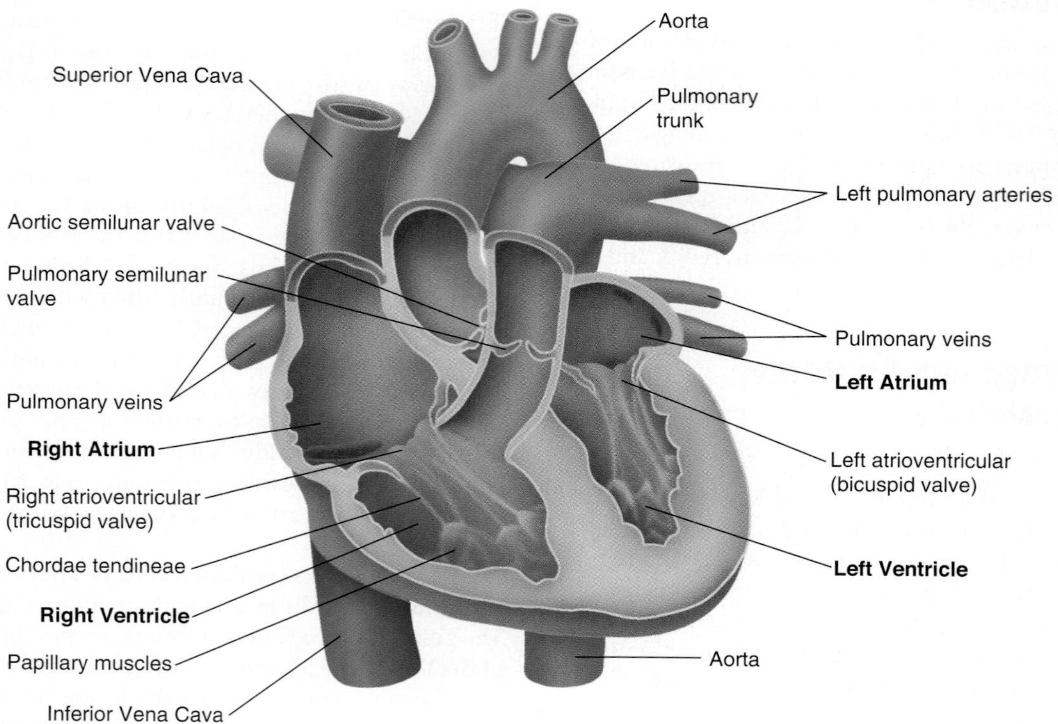

FIGURE 51-4 Heart chambers and related structures.

of cardiac muscle, functioning as the primary pump action of the heart.

The inside of the heart consists of four chambers (**Figure 51-4**); two on the right and two on the left which are separated by a solid, wall-like structure known as the septum. The superior chambers are the atria, and the inferior chambers are the ventricles. The **right atrium** of the heart receives blood from two large veins, the **inferior vena cava** and **superior vena cava**. The **coronary sinus** also collects blood originating from the heart's myocardium and drains it into the right atrium. The **right atrioventricular (tricuspid) valve** and **left atrioventricular (bicuspid) valve** separate the atria and ventricles, which ensure one-way blood flow toward the ventricles. Strategic placement of the valves within the heart allows the movement of blood only in one direction (**Figure 51-5**), thus filling and emptying the chambers of the heart in a choreographed manner during the **systole** (contraction) and **diastole** (relaxation) phases of the beating heart. The series of contraction and relaxation is known as the heartbeat, or cardiac cycle. The cusps of each atrioventricular valve are attached to strong fibers called **chordae tendinae**, anchored by the **papillary muscles** that project inward from the ventricle walls. As the ventricles contract, compressing the blood in their chambers, the papillary muscles pull on the chordae tendinae and prevent the valves from everting back into the atria, effectively closing the valves. **Table 51-1** lists the heart valves, their location, and action.

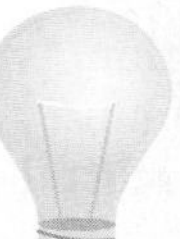

STOP AND THINK

What are the only locations in the body that deoxygenated blood travels in arteries and oxygenated blood is carried in veins?

The wall of the right ventricle assists the heart in pumping the deoxygenated blood to the lungs for gas exchange to occur. The **pulmonary semilunar valve**, which lies between the right ventricle and the **pulmonary trunk**, prevents backflow of blood to the ventricle and allows forward movement of blood to the **pulmonary arteries**. After traveling through the pulmonary capillaries, oxygenated blood returns to the heart via the **pulmonary veins** into the left atrium and continues through the **mitral valve (bicuspid valve)** into the left ventricle. The contraction of the thick, left ventricle

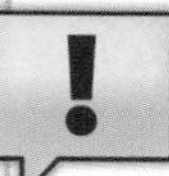

Respiratory Recap

Blood Flow Through the Heart

From vena cavae → right atrium → tricuspid valve → right ventricle → pulmonary semilunar valve → pulmonary trunk → pulmonary arteries → pulmonary capillaries → pulmonary veins → left atrium → mitral valve → left ventricle → aortic valve → aorta → systemic capillaries → vena cavae

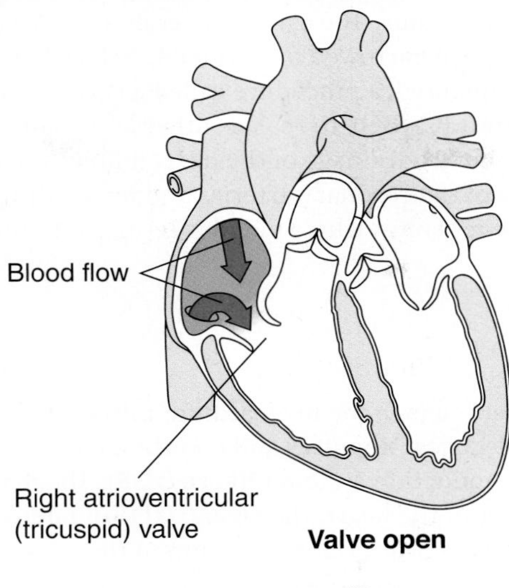

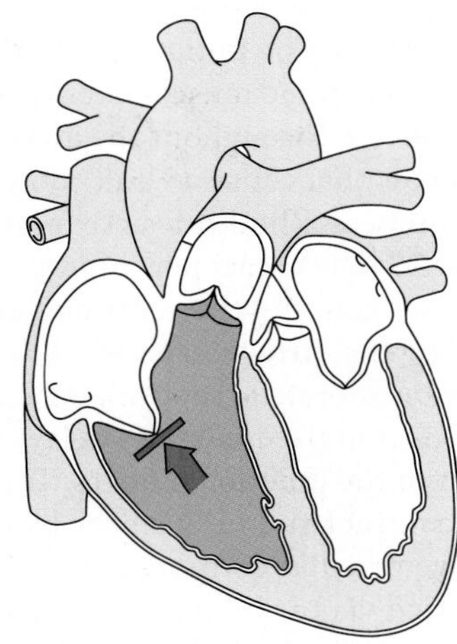

FIGURE 51-5 Opening and closing of valves.

TABLE 51-1
Heart Valves

Heart Valve	Location	Action
Tricuspid valve	Between right atrium and right ventricle	During ventricular contraction, it prevents blood from moving from the right ventricle into the right atrium
Pulmonary valve	At entrance to pulmonary trunk	During ventricular relaxation, it prevents blood from moving from the pulmonary trunk into the right ventricle
Mitral valve	Between left atrium and left ventricle	During ventricular contraction, it prevents blood from moving from the left ventricle into the left atrium
Aortic valve	At entrance to aorta	During ventricular relaxation, it prevents blood from moving from the aorta into the left ventricle

generates pressures of approximately 120 mm Hg, which drives blood through the **aortic valve** and into the **aorta**, forcing the blood into the systemic circulation at a pressure of about 120/80 mm Hg. Valves can leak (regurgitate) or can narrow (stenosis) from disease; in either case, pressures will increase in the preceding chambers and vessels. A faulty valve (commonly the mitral valve) can be surgically replaced by a cow or pig valve (treated to prevent rejection), mechanical valve, or cryopreserved cadaverous human valve.

The major function of the heart is to generate pressure that will propel blood through the lungs and systemic circulation. Blood travels through several pathways or circuits. The right ventricle supplies the pulmonary circuit and the left ventricle supplies the systemic circuit (**Figure 51-6**). The pulmonary circuit is unique because it is the only place in the body that the arteries carry deoxygenated blood and the veins carry oxygenated blood. Elsewhere in the body, it is exactly the opposite.

The blood supply to the heart, the coronary circuit or coronary circulation (**Figure 51-7**), arises from the ascending aorta. The right coronary artery passes anteriorly over the heart until it reaches the inferior surface, where it connects with the terminal branch of the left coronary artery. Major branches of the right coronary artery include the artery to the sinoatrial (SA) node, the intraventricular artery supplying both the septum and the rest of the electrical conduction system of the heart. The left main coronary artery branches into the left anterior descending and circumflex arteries. The former supplies blood to the walls of both ventricles and the interventricular septum. A branch of the left descending artery forms the diagonal artery that supplies blood to the left ventricular wall. The circumflex artery, a continuation of the left coronary artery, follows the surface of the heart to its inferior portion. Blockage of the coronary circulation can be serious and/or fatal. Stress or increased physical demand can cause the coronary arteries to spasm. These spasms result in decreased blood delivery to the myocardium and may cause the individual to experience angina pectoris, or thoracic pain. Prolonged blockage of the coronary arteries is much more serious and can lead to **myocardial infarction**, also known as a heart attack. About 35% of all deaths in the United States are attributed to coronary artery disease. Occlusions or strictures of the coronary arteries are extremely dangerous; therefore, they are promptly treated with stents, vessel-widening balloons, and transplanted vessels to route blood

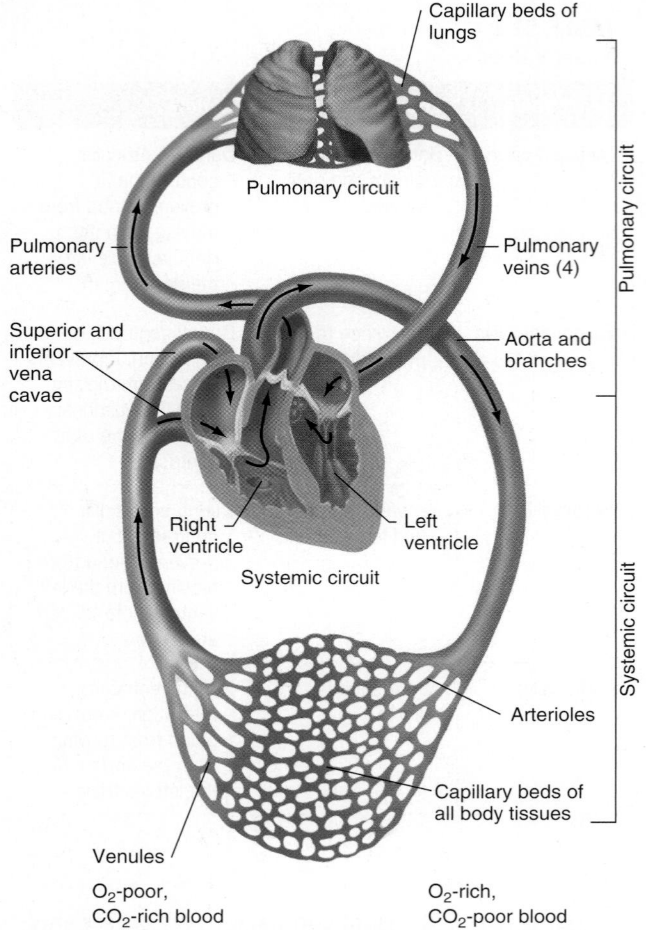

FIGURE 51-6 Blood pathway—pulmonary and systemic circuit.

around the lesions. The carotid arteries are bypassed when they are narrowed or occluded. Arterial grafts can be implanted, a procedure called a coronary artery bypass graft (CABG), to replace other large damaged vessels. Venous drainage of the heart follows the major branches of the coronary arteries and finally drains into the coronary sinus, where blood is returned to the right atrium.

Intrinsic Conduction

Specialized cells in the myocardium initiate and distribute electrical impulses and coordinate the intrinsic cardiac conduction system (**Figure 51-8**). The major pacemaker of the heart, the **sinoatrial (SA) node**, is located just beneath the epicardium in the upper right atrium. As the pacemaker, the SA node generates rhythmic activity by initiating impulses that cause coordinated cardiac muscle fiber contraction. A conduction system throughout the atria distributes electrical signals that cause a weak contraction of the two atrial chambers. Rhythmic activity in a normal adult occurs at 70 to 80 beats per minute.

Impulses travel to the ventricles after they are received by the **atrioventricular (AV) node**, located in the inferior interatrial septum, beneath the endocardium. This impulse is slightly delayed due to the small diameter of the junctional fibers. This allows for the atria to contract and fully empty blood to the ventricles prior to ventricular contraction. The cardiac impulse is then carried via the **bundle of His** down the right and

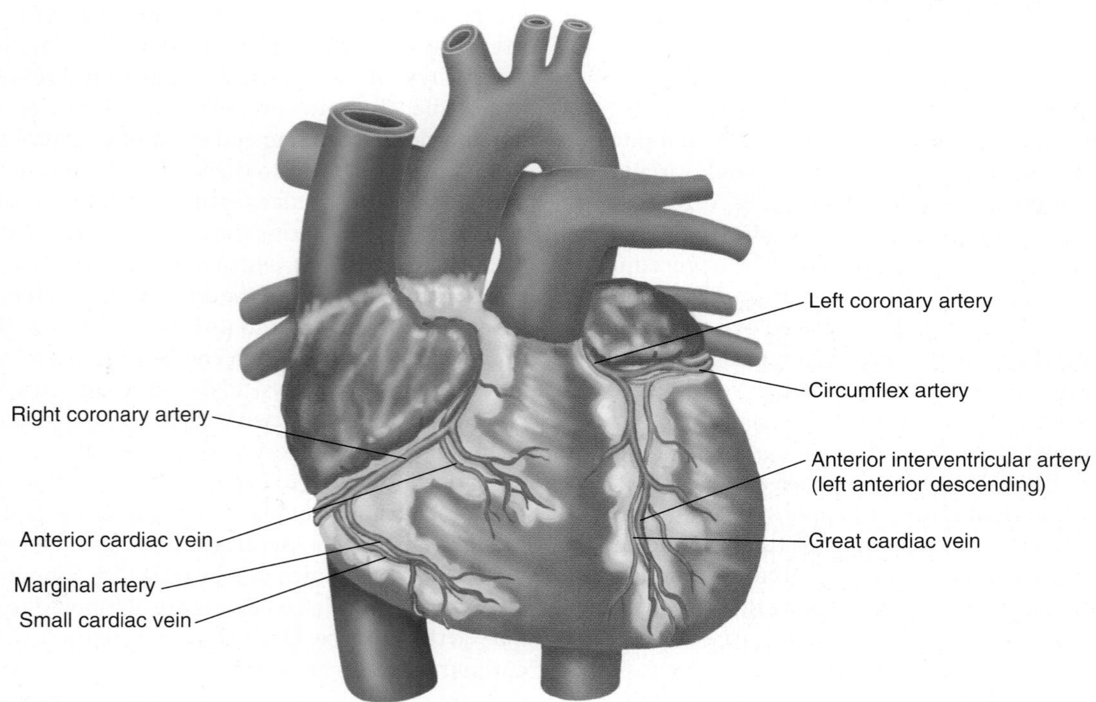

FIGURE 51-7 Coronary circulation.

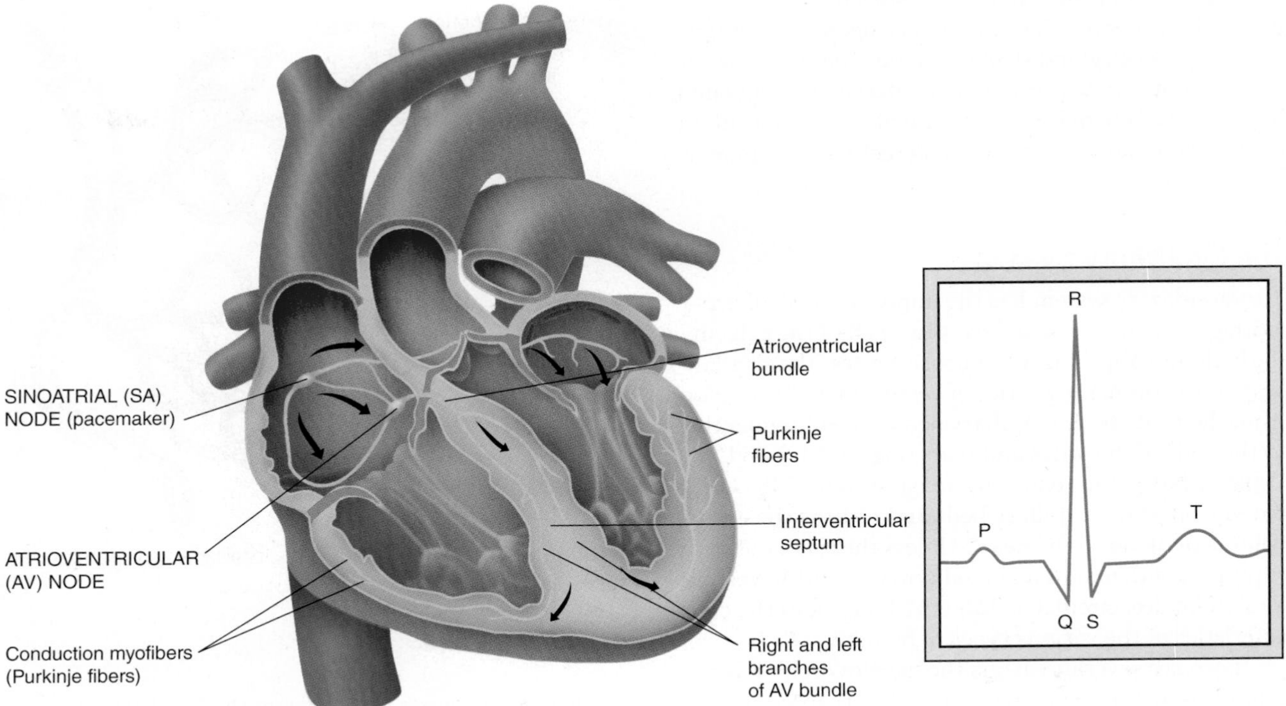

FIGURE 51-8 Conduction system of heart.

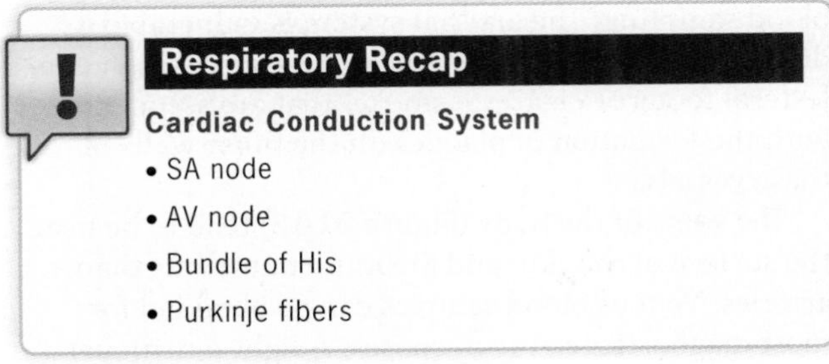

Respiratory Recap

Cardiac Conduction System

- SA node
- AV node
- Bundle of His
- Purkinje fibers

left bundle branches along Purkinje fibers that innervate both ventricular myocardia. When the ventricles contract via this pathway, they contract simultaneously in a twisting motion, efficiently forcing blood into both the aorta and pulmonary trunk.

An electrocardiogram (ECG) records the electrical changes in the myocardium during the cardiac cycle. Nodes connected to wires are placed on the skin and connected to an ECG machine. The nodes translate the electrical changes of the heart to an ECG tracing.

Each electrical impulse produces a characteristic recordable wave (deflection) on the ECG. The first movement recorded in the cardiac cycle is the P wave, which corresponds to depolarization of the atrial fibers leading to atrial contraction. As the impulse reaches the thicker ventricular walls, a greater electrical change, or depolarization, called the QRS complex, results. The T wave results from ventricular repolarization. Atrial repolarization is not visible in this pattern because the atrial fibers repolarize at the same time that the ventricular fibers are depolarizing.

The ECG is examined closely and the patterns are used to assess the patient. Impulses traveling via irregular pathways are, typically, inefficient (e.g., premature ventricular contractions). Another example of the diagnostic value of the ECG is the elevation of the S-T segment, or length between the S and T wave, which is characteristic of a totally blocked coronary artery. Complete blockage leads to oxygen deprivation, or **myocardial ischemia**, which can eventually lead to cell death. Cardiac markers, such as troponin, as well as potassium and calcium levels are also examined closely to assess possible heart conditions.

Extrinsic Conduction

The extrinsic innervation of the heart is supplied by the autonomic nervous system. The sympathetic supply is from the upper thoracic segments of the spinal cord, through the sympathetic trunk. These nerve fibers join the cardiac plexus beneath the arch of the aorta and innervate the SA and AV nodes, the myocardium, and the coronary arteries. Stimulation of the sympathetic nervous system increases both the rate and force of the heartbeat. To increase contraction force and rate, nerve impulses stimulate sympathetic fibers reaching the nodes and heart structures, causing the release of norepinephrine. Parasympathetic innervation is supplied by the vagus nerve. Stimulation of the parasympathetic nervous system results in an opposite effect of the sympathetic nervous system, that is, decrease in heart rate, contractility, and stroke volume. The responses of sympathetic and parasympathetic nerves are regulated by **baroreceptor** reflexes in the cardiac control center of the brain. Baroreceptors also detect changes in blood pressure.

The Circulatory System

The circulatory system has the important task of providing nutrients, ions, and oxygen to all of the cells in the body and disposing of metabolic wastes. The arterial system is a branching series of vessels that carries blood from the heart to the capillary beds and subsequently to the cells of the lungs and body (**Figure 51-9** and **Figure 51-10**). The venous drainage system collects the blood from those capillary beds and returns the entire volume of blood to the heart. Unless there is a cut or rupture in either system, blood remains within vessels and, therefore, circulates. **Table 51-2** provides the characteristics of the various types of blood vessels.

There are several reasons the cardiovascular system is important. Primarily, an uninterrupted flow of oxygen must be supplied to the tissues of the body. The cardiovascular system is susceptible to injuries and diseases that can be rapidly fatal. Also, in care settings, access to arteries and veins allows healthcare providers to monitor cardiovascular pressures, obtain blood specimens for analysis, and administer medications rapidly into veins.

Arteries of the body (**Figure 51-11**) tend to be deeper, but arterial blood pressure can be felt or palpated on the skin surface if circulation is adequate. Normal arterial pressure is relatively uniform at about 120/80 mm Hg throughout the arterial system. The major arteries—the aorta, subclavian, and abdominal aorta—are deep. Palpation is usually possible at several sites, such as the radial, brachial, dorsalis pedis, carotid, and femoral arteries. Blood pressure is measured, most often, with a sphygmomanometer from the brachial artery. Catheters can be inserted into the radial, brachial, or femoral arteries to monitor arterial pressure and allow sampling of arterial blood for blood gas analysis. The radial artery is the usual site for intermittent arterial blood sampling. The arterial system is vulnerable to disease as a result of consuming substances (high cholesterol foods or cigarette smoke) that are associated with the formation of plaques on the inner walls of these vessels.

The **veins** of the body (**Figure 51-12**) tend to be near the surface of the skin and are more numerous than arteries. Venous blood samples can be obtained for most diagnostic testing purposes. A light tourniquet on the upper arm will cause veins to become prominent, including the easily accessible antecubital vein. An intravenous catheter can usually be placed in the

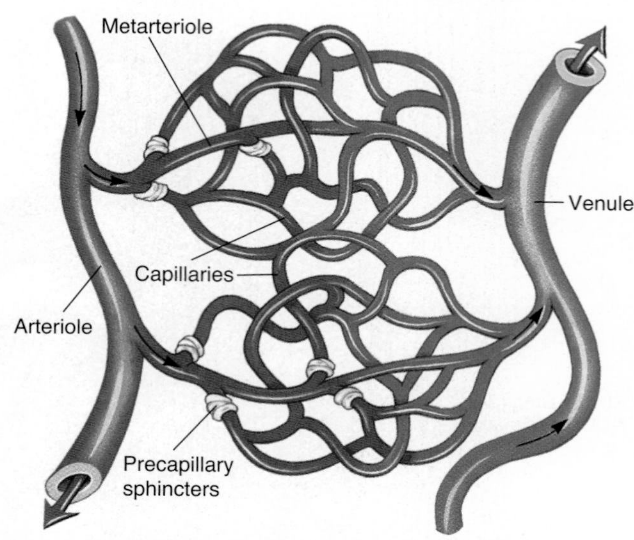

FIGURE 51-10 Network of arterioles, capillaries, and venules.

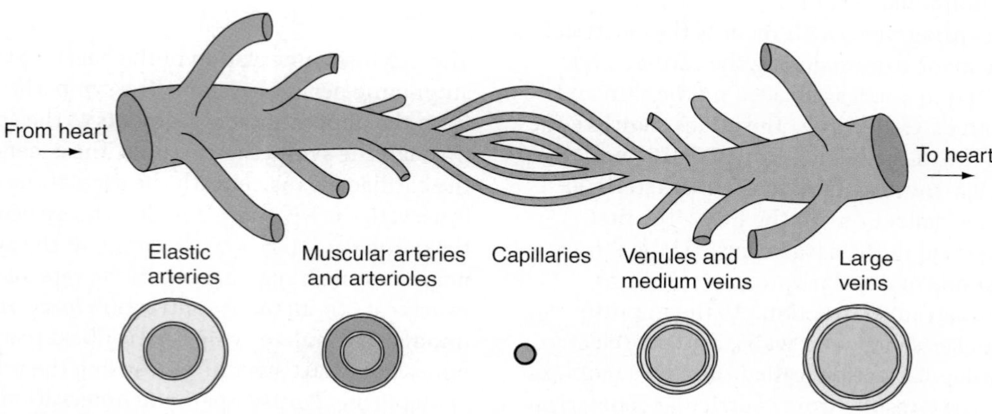

FIGURE 51-9 Composition and diameter of various blood vessel walls.

TABLE 51-2
Characteristics of Various Types of Blood Vessels

Type of Vessel	Vessel Wall	Actions
Artery	Three-layer thick wall	Carries relatively high pressure blood from the heart to the arterioles
Arteriole	Three-layer thin wall	Helps control blood flow from arteries to capillaries by vasoconstricting or vasodilating
Capillary	One layer of squamous epithelium	Has a membrane allowing nutrients, gases, and waste to be exchanged between blood and tissue fluid
Venule	Thinner wall than arterioles, less smooth muscle and connective tissue	Connects capillaries to veins
Vein	Thinner wall than arteries but similar layers	Carries relatively low pressure blood from venules to the heart; valves prevent blood backflow; veins serve as blood reservoirs

forearm to ensure continual access for medication delivery. When venous access is required in patients with unreliable circulation, a central venous catheter is placed via the internal jugular, subclavian, or femoral veins. Thrombi that form in the venous system present the risk of breaking free and becoming emboli, which may lodge in the lungs. Medications are available to prevent thrombi formation and to actively dissolve the clots. Large thrombi can be trapped by an implanted vascular umbrella or physically extracted if necessary.

The vessels have characteristics that relate to their role within the circuitry; that is, they have an anatomic structure to withstand pressures, avoid leaks, and control distribution of flow and contain valves to send blood in the right direction. The vessels have layers: a basement membrane is innermost, followed by the tunica intima, tunica media, and tunica adventitia (**Figure 51-13**). Arteries are thicker and flexible to withstand the higher pressures required for blood flow to and through major organs. Veins are thinner and they serve as more passive conduits for returning blood to the heart. The driving pressures within the arteries are not adequate both to deliver blood to the capillary beds and to push the blood back to the heart, however. Many veins (primarily in the legs) thus have one-way valves aimed toward the heart to prevent backflow. Muscular contraction in the lower extremities helps move blood back to the heart. Stagnant blood tends to clot and form thrombi—a risk that is greatest in the legs. The tunica media of the arteries is larger and is composed of elastic fibers and longitudinal muscles. The control of these muscles is autonomic; that is, sympathetic and parasympathetic nerves control the tone of the longitudinal muscles in the arterial walls. Medications with specific autonomic effects (i.e., sympathomimetic) can be administered to control blood pressure.

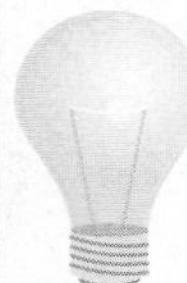

STOP AND THINK

What is the cardiac output of an individual with a normal resting heart rate (75 beats/min) and normal stroke volume (70 mL/beat)?

The circulating blood volume is only about 10% to 15% of the 40 liters of fluid in the body. The remaining fluid is intracellular or in the interstitial space between the cells. The output generated by each heartbeat is measured in terms of cardiac output and stroke volume. Cardiac output ($\dot{Q}c$) is the amount of blood discharged by each ventricle in one minute; it is the product of the heart rate and stroke volume. **Stroke volume** is the volume of blood generated by one ventricle with each beat. Generally, the stroke volume is the result of the overall force of the ventricular contraction.

Average adult blood volume is approximately 5 L (75 mL/kg for men and 65 mL/kg for women). In the example, you can see that the entire blood supply passes through each side of the heart in one minute. $\dot{Q}c$ varies with SV and HR. When the heart beats faster, or stroke volume increases, or both occur, the $\dot{Q}c$ increases. Cardiac reserve is the difference between resting and maximal $\dot{Q}c$. During exercise, $\dot{Q}c$ can increase markedly (typically 4 to 5 times resting $\dot{Q}c$) to as much as 25 L/min as the additional output (with its oxygen) is sent to the working muscles. Trained athletes can have a cardiac reserve of up to seven times resting $\dot{Q}c$ (35 L/min). Blood flow is not circulated evenly throughout the body, however; in fact, there is an elaborate control system for routing blood to organs and tissues that require more oxygen or nutrients according to varying needs. Normally, blood flow proportionally favors the brain and kidneys. More discussion of cardiac output and hemodynamic monitoring are located elsewhere in this text.

A circulatory model for blood movement within the body is used to help understand the mechanisms of cardiac performance, blood pressure control (or blood delivery to the capillary beds), and venous drainage. Basically, the heart is the pump that ejects blood with a certain force, or **contractility**. The strength of the heart's contractility can be increased by medications.

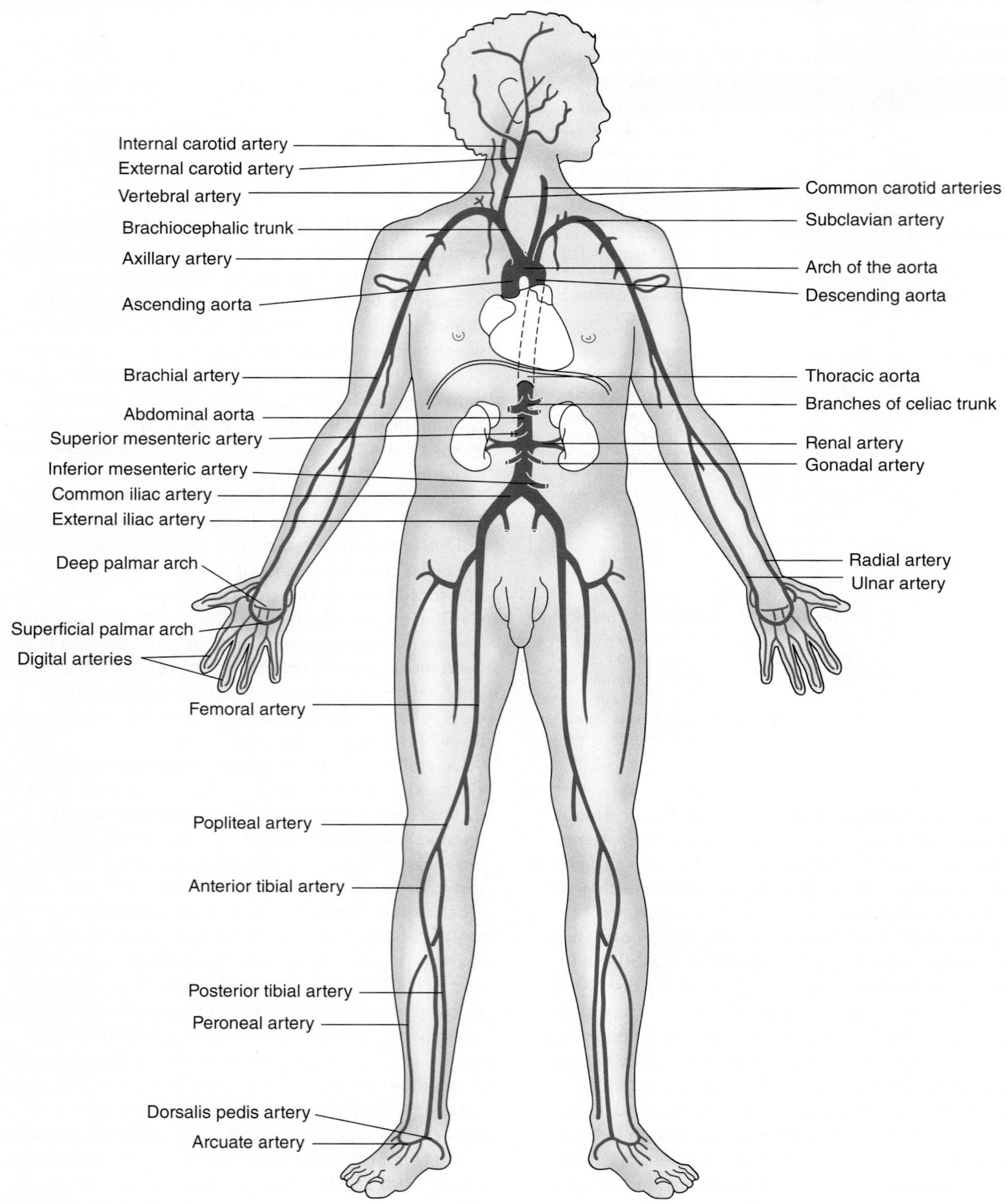

FIGURE 51-11 Arteries.

Cardiac performance can be described (and affected) in terms of contractility, afterload, and preload. The heart pump must be primed with enough blood to function properly. The end-diastolic volume, or amount of blood available for ejection by the ventricle during diastole, is called the **preload.** Preload, which controls stroke volume, can be controlled by fluid administration, fluid restriction, or fluid withdrawal, as illustrated by the use of diuretics. In a normal heart, an increase in preload will result in increased stroke volume.

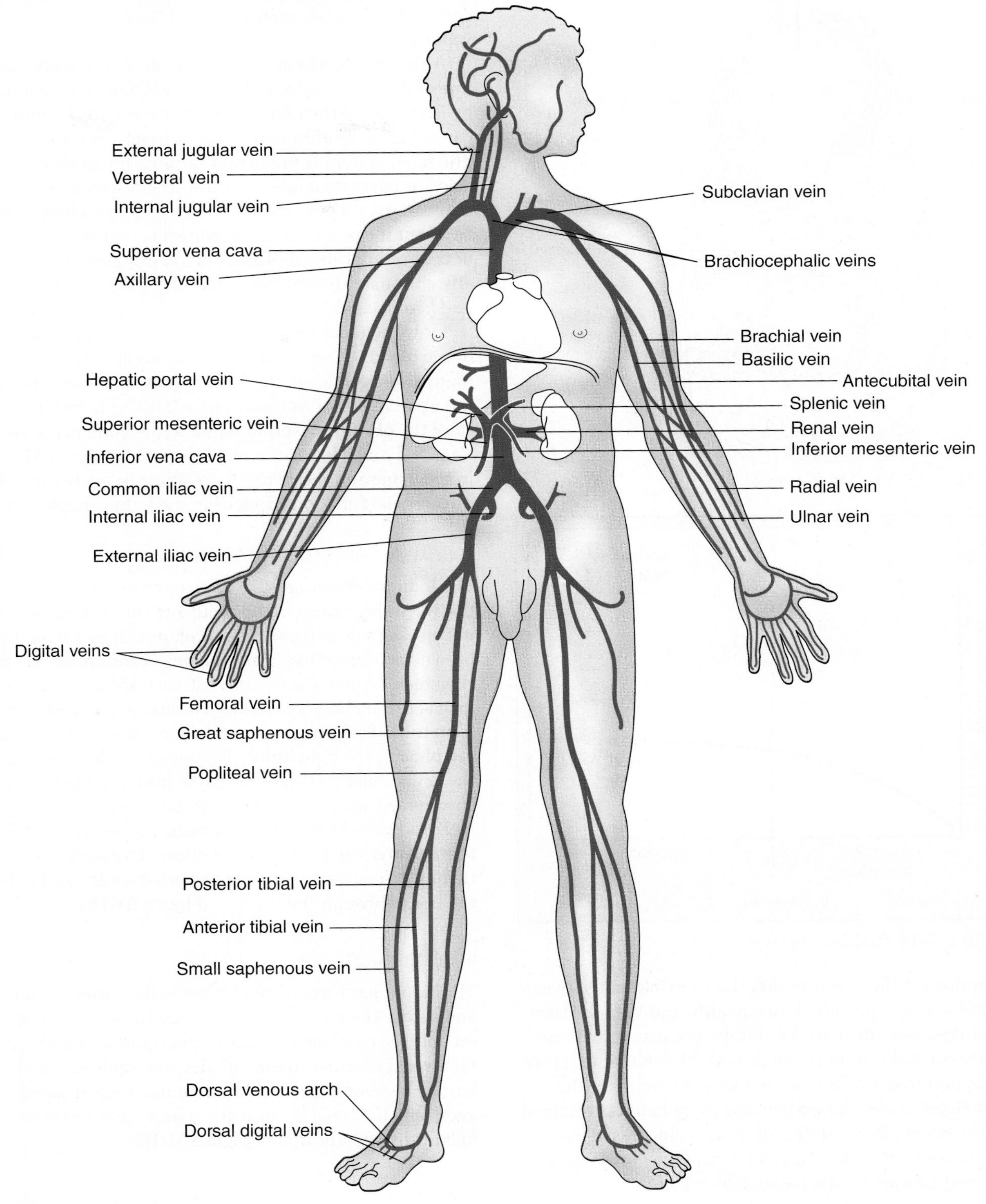

FIGURE 51-12 Veins.

The relationship between blood volume and cardiac performance is graphically displayed by the Frank-Starling curve (**Figure 51-14**). This curve demonstrates that the stroke volume of the heart increases as preload increases. As you can see from the illustration, in the failing heart (such as in congestive heart failure) this can lead to congestion. The arterial blood flow creates a backpressure exerted on the aortic and pulmonary valves. End-systolic volume is the volume of blood remaining in the ventricle after contraction (systole).

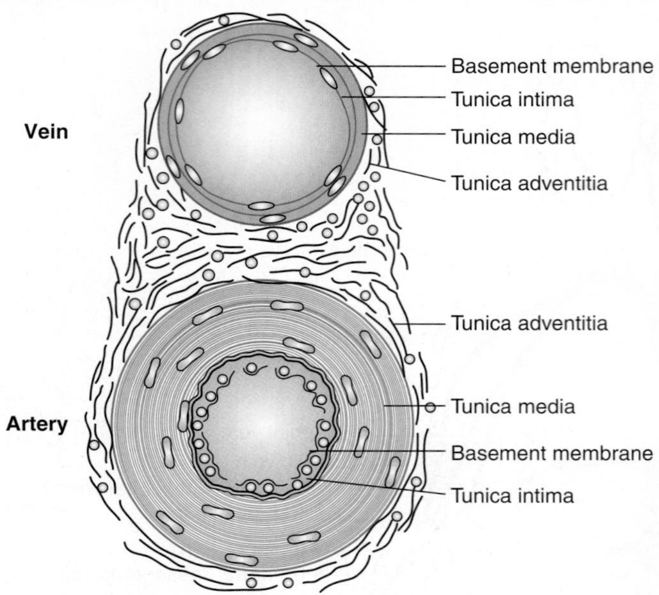

FIGURE 51-13 Structure of a vessel.

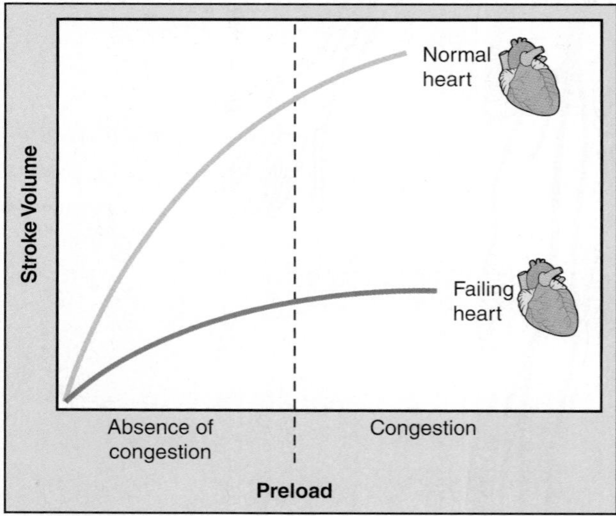

FIGURE 51-14 Frank-Starling curve.

Afterload is the pressure that the ventricles must overcome to eject this blood. In a healthy individual, afterload does not affect stroke volume because it remains fairly constant. In individuals with high blood pressure, or hypertension, afterload reduces the ability of the ventricles to eject blood because more blood is retained in the heart after systole. Afterload is increased by medications or stiffened arteries and may be decreased by medications or disease such as sepsis.

Renal Anatomy and Physiology

In order to have a good understanding of acid–base balance, it is essential for the respiratory therapist (RT) to understand the structure and function of the renal system. The kidneys play a vital role in homeostasis. They are responsible for regulation of blood volume and its chemical composition as well as maintaining the correct balance between acids and bases and between water and salts.

Although the chemical buffer system (the body's first line of defense) reacts within seconds to a change in pH by inactivating the excess acids or bases, this system cannot actually eliminate acids or bases from the body. The renal system is important because it can eliminate acids or bases through the urine. The respiratory system can get rid of carbonic acid (H_2CO_3) by eliminating CO_2, but it cannot excrete other acids that are the products of cellular metabolism. The renal system can actually eliminate these other acids (phosphoric, uric, lactic, and ketone acids).

Only the renal system can regulate alkaline balance in the blood. When extracellular fluids are acidic (too many hydrogen ions), the renal system eliminates H^+ in the urine and retains bicarbonate (HCO_3^-) in order to raise the pH. On the other hand, if the blood pH is alkalotic (too much base), the renal system eliminates HCO_3^- in the urine and retains H^+ in an effort to lower the pH. This crucial function happens in the kidney nephrons.

External Anatomy of the Kidney

The kidneys are situated in a retroperitoneal position (between the posterior body wall and the peritoneal cavity) on each side of the vertebral column. They are reddish-brown and shaped like beans (kidney beans are named for this shape). About the size of a fist, each kidney is 12 cm long (4 to 5 inches), 3 cm wide (a little over an inch), and 3 cm thick. Each weighs about 5 ounces (the size of a small cell phone). The right kidney is situated a little lower than the left because it is underneath the liver. Each kidney is surrounded and protected by a fibrous capsule.

Blood vessels, lymphatic vessels, nerves, and the **ureter** enter the kidney at the hilum. Urine moves through the ureters into the **urinary bladder** and exits the body through the **urethra** (**Figure 51-15**).

Internal Anatomy

The kidney has three distinct regions: the cortex, medulla, and pelvis. The renal cortex is the outermost, superficial section; the renal medulla is the innermost area and contains renal pyramids (renal tubules and capillaries are located here, which gives the pyramids a striped appearance); and the **renal pelvis** collects urine that will leave the kidney through the ureter (**Figure 51-16**).

Nephron

The functional units of the kidneys are the **nephrons**, and each kidney has approximately one million nephrons. The nephron is made up of a **renal corpuscle** (**glomerulus** and **glomerular capsule**) and a **renal tubule.** On the proximal end of the renal tubule is the glomerular capsule or Bowman's capsule. The glomerular capsule completely surrounds the glomerulus like a baseball glove surrounds a ball.

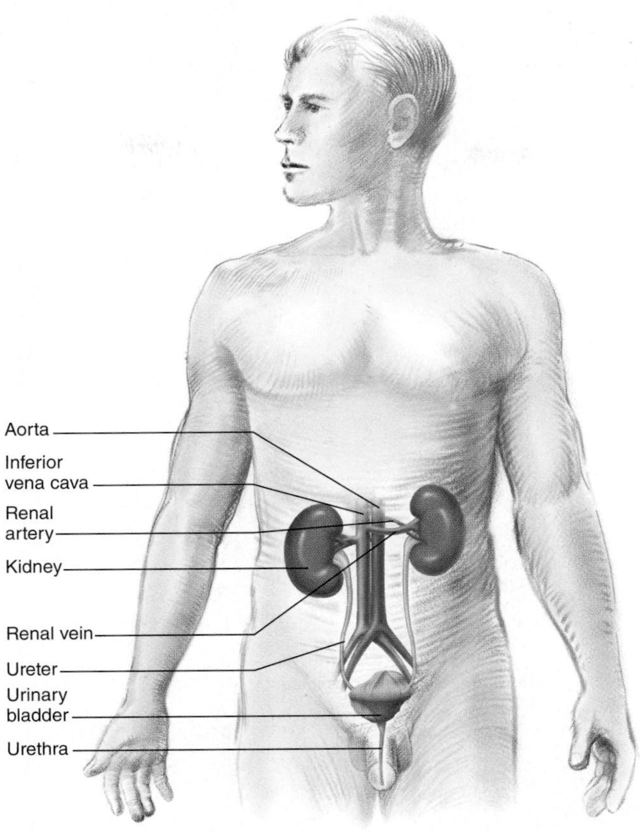

FIGURE 51-15 The kidney.

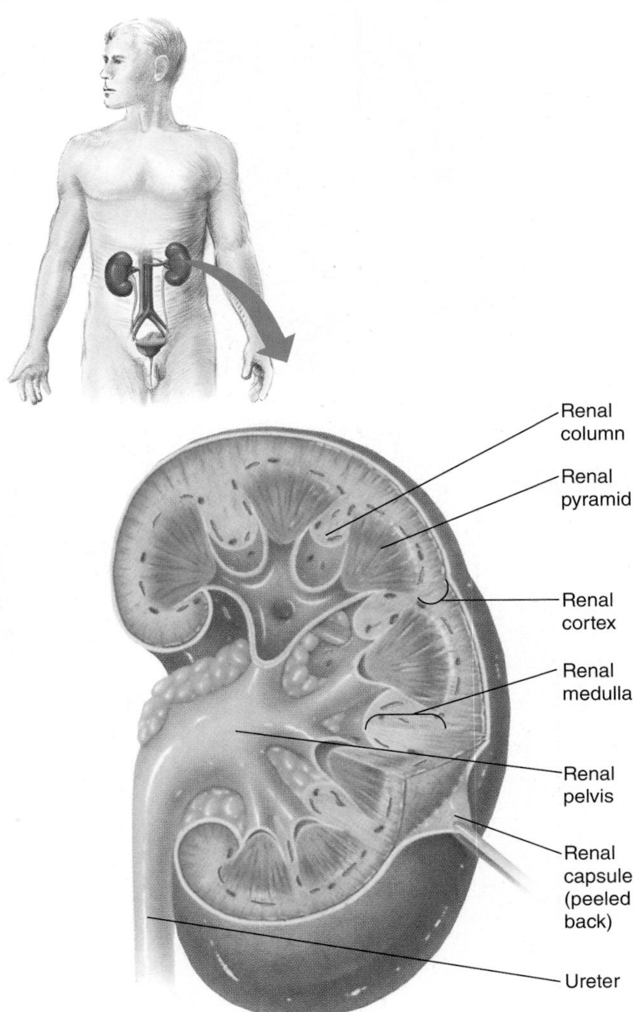

FIGURE 51-16 Gross anatomy of the kidney.

The renal tubule has three main parts, each named for its shape and distance from the renal corpuscle: proximal convoluted tubule, **loop of Henle** (it has a descending segment/limb and an ascending limb), and distal convoluted tubule (**Figure 51-17**). The renal tubules empty into **collecting ducts**, with each duct collecting filtrate from many nephrons, eventually emptying into the renal pelvis.

Blood Supply

Renal arteries supply the kidney with blood, branching many times before reaching the nephron. Afferent arterioles lead to the glomerular capillaries and, subsequently, the efferent arterioles. Glomerular capillaries are very porous, which allows fluid to move easily from the blood into the glomerular capsule. Efferent arterioles branch into interconnected capillary networks called peritubular capillaries, which surround the renal tubules (**Figure 51-18**).

Physiology of the Kidney

Nearly 200 liters of blood are filtered every day by the kidneys, the majority of which is reabsorbed (normal urine output is only 1 to 2 L/day). The kidneys utilize a considerable amount of oxygen, approximately 20% to 25% of all the oxygen used by the body at rest. The majority of filtration occurs within the nephron, which is the

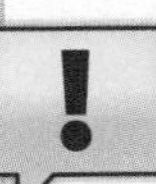

Respiratory Recap

Renal Structure

- Paired kidneys are located retroperitoneally, on each side of the vertebral column.
- Urine flow: formed in kidney → ureter → urinary bladder → urethra → elimination
- Filtrate flow: glomerular capillaries → glomerular capsule → proximal convoluted tubule → loop of Henle (descending, then ascending limb) → distal convoluted tubule → collecting duct → renal pelvis (urine)
- Blood flow: descending aorta → renal arteries → afferent arterioles → glomerular capillaries → efferent arterioles → peritubular capillaries → venules → renal veins → inferior vena cava (IVC)

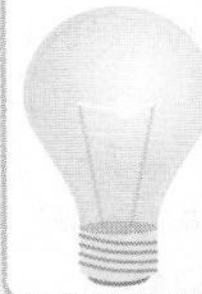

STOP AND THINK

What happens if the majority of urine was not reabsorbed?

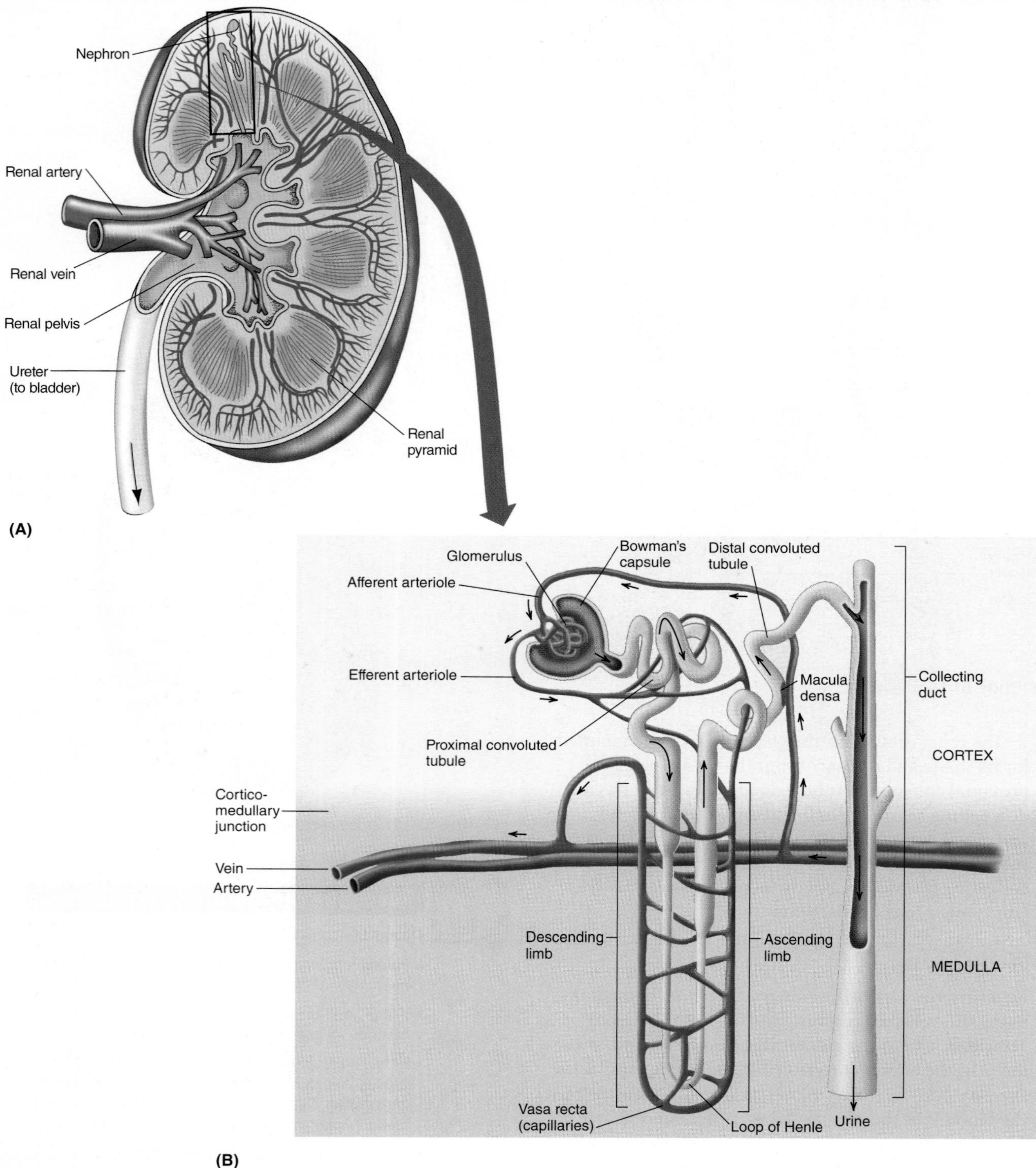

FIGURE 51-17 (**A**) Main branches of renal artery and vein. (**B**) Structure of the nephron.

functional unit of the kidney. The nephron performs three key functions: glomerular filtration, tubular reabsorption, and tubular secretion.

Glomerular Filtration

Glomerular filtrate is mostly water—it has the same composition as blood plasma, except for large plasma protein molecules. Glomerular filtration is the process of turning that filtrate into urine. The process is passive; hydrostatic pressure forces the filtrate (fluids and solutes) through a filtration membrane (glomerulus). The glomerulus is a much more efficient filter than other capillary beds because its membrane has a large surface area that is much more permeable to water and solutes,

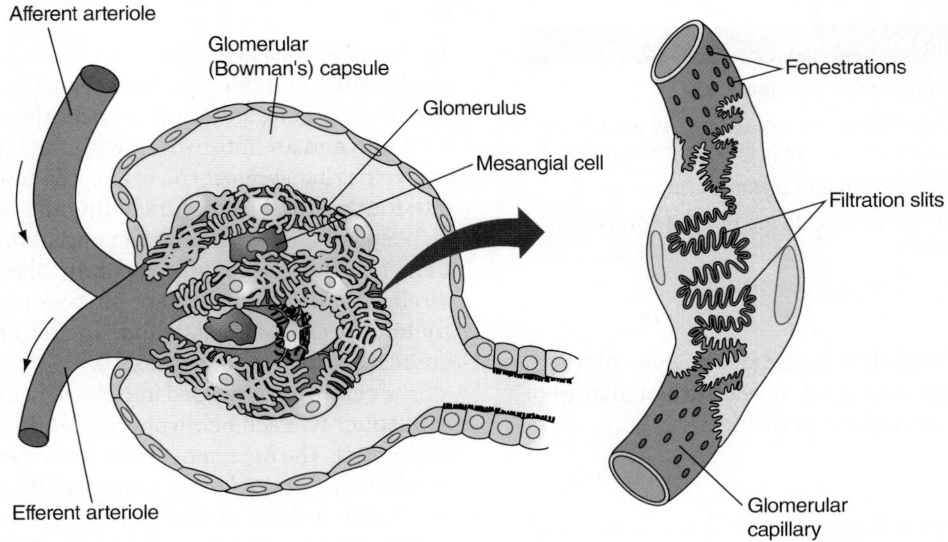

FIGURE 51-18 Structure of the renal corpuscle.

and glomerular blood pressure is much higher than in other capillary beds. This results in a much higher net filtration pressure (NFP). Larger molecules like plasma proteins, which are greater than 5 nm, generally do not enter the tubule. Molecules smaller than 3 nm, like water, glucose, amino acids, and nitrogenous wastes, pass easily from the blood into the glomerular capsule.

The **glomerular filtration rate (GFR)** is the volume of filtrate formed each minute by the collective glomeruli. Recall that the kidneys have about 2 million nephrons between them, and each nephron has a glomerulus; this means there are 2 million glomeruli contributing to the GFR. Normal GFR in adults is approximately 120 to 125 mL/min and is directly proportional to NFP. GFR may decrease if the body needs to conserve fluids (dehydration) or increase if the body has excessive fluids (heart failure).

The kidneys need a relatively constant GFR in order to function and maintain homeostasis. GFR is regulated both locally/intrinsically within the kidney and extrinsically by maintaining systemic blood pressure via the nervous and endocrine systems. When there are extreme changes in blood pressure (mean arterial pressure <80 mm Hg or >180 mm Hg), extrinsic mechanisms exert greater control than intrinsic mechanisms.

Tubular Reabsorption

If our bodies did not reabsorb most of the contents of the renal tubules, our plasma would be drained away as urine in about half an hour! Tubular reabsorption is the process of reclaiming plasma. It begins as soon as the filtrate enters the proximal tubules. Normally, almost all nutrients (glucose, amino acids, and vitamins) are completely reabsorbed. Water, small proteins, cations (Na^+, K^+, Mg^{++}, Ca^{++}), and anions (Cl^- and HCO_3^-) are also reabsorbed in the renal tubules. Water reabsorption follows sodium reabsorption; if more sodium is reabsorbed in the renal tubule, more water will also be reabsorbed, and vice versa. The proximal tubule is the primary site for reabsorption of HCO_3^-.

By the time the filtrate reaches the distal convoluted tubule, only about 25% of the water and 10% of the NaCl remain. Most reabsorption from this point on depends on what the body needs and is regulated by hormones. If necessary almost all of the water and Na^+ can be reabsorbed.

Tubular Secretion

Tubular secretion is the process of clearing waste and unwanted substances from the plasma (certain drugs and metabolites, urea, uric acid). Substances like H^+, K^+, NH_4^+ (ammonium), creatinine, and certain organic acids are either produced in the renal tubule and secreted or move into the filtrate through the peritubular capillaries. The urine that is excreted contains both secreted and filtered substances.

Tubular secretion is also important for the control of blood pH. The distal tubules are involved in secreting acids. The main urinary buffers used for acid excretion are phosphate and ammonia. When serum pH decreases to the acidic end of its homeostatic range (<7.35), the renal tubule cells actively secrete more H^+ into the filtrate and retain more HCO_3^-. The result is an increase in serum pH due to the excess H^+ eliminated in the urine and retention of HCO_3^-. On the other hand,

STOP AND THINK

Your patient has a pH is 7.31. How will the renal system respond?

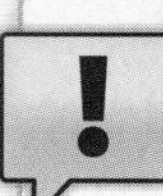

Respiratory Recap

Renal (Nephron) Function

- Glomerular filtration: large particles are filtered out, small particles pass into the renal tubule
- Tubular reabsorption: plasma is regained
- Tubular secretion: rids the body of toxins and metabolites

when serum pH increases to the alkaline end of its homeostatic range (>7.45), Cl^- is reabsorbed instead of HCO_3^-, which is eliminated in the urine.

Urine

Urine is about 95% water and is the final product of glomerular filtration and tubular reabsorption and secretion. Urine passes from the collecting ducts to the renal pelvis to the ureter. Each ureter is about 30 cm long and runs parallel to the vertebral column. The ureters descend from each kidney to the urinary bladder, where urine remains until it is forced through the urethra and out of the body through the process of micturition (urination).

Neural Anatomy and Physiology

There are many reasons for RTs needing to possess knowledge of the nervous system, the first and foremost of which is to understand the control and process of spontaneous breathing. It is also necessary to understand diseases and disorders the RTs will encounter, including neuromuscular diseases, spinal cord injuries, and central sleep apnea, to name a few. Respiratory therapists also frequently administer a variety of medications. Knowledge of the nervous system is essential to understanding the mechanism of action, effects, and side effects of many of these classes of drugs, which can include bronchodilators, neuromuscular blocking agents, sedatives, anesthetics, and analgesics. In addition, modes and methods of providing mechanical ventilation are continuously evolving, becoming more and more sophisticated and better coordinated with patients' spontaneous breathing efforts. Respiratory therapists must use knowledge of the nervous system to understand and correctly apply these advances in mechanical ventilation.

The nervous system is divided into two parts, the central nervous system (CNS) and the peripheral nervous system (PNS). The CNS includes the brain and spinal cord. The PNS includes nerves that connect the brain and spinal cord to muscles, glands, and sense organs in the body. This section will focus on those structures and functions of both the CNS and PNS that are important to respiratory therapists.

Brain

The brain is encased in the skull and is floating in cerebrospinal fluid (CSF). The **meninges** are connective tissue membranes that connect the subdivisions of the brain and are interwoven with the major arteries and veins that support the brain. The brain is divided into four main divisions, including the cerebrum, the diencephalon (thalamus and hypothalamus), the brain stem, and the cerebellum. The brain also includes four cerebral ventricles. These are interconnected cavities containing cerebrospinal fluid. The four divisions of the brain are shown in **Figure 51-19**.

The **cerebrum** is divided into the right and left **cerebral hemispheres**. Each hemisphere contains several layers of material. The outermost layer is the **cerebral cortex**, consisting of gray matter composed of mostly cell bodies. The inner layer of white matter is composed of mostly myelinated nerve fiber tracts. While the right and left hemispheres are largely separated, the **corpus callosum** is a massive bundle of nerves that connects the two (**Figure 51-20**). Each hemisphere is divided into four main lobes by sulci or fissures (similar to lung fissures), including the frontal, parietal, occipital, and temporal lobes (**Figure 51-21**).

The cerebral cortex is the most complex integrating area of the nervous system, serving to coordinate sensory and motor functions and to manage higher mental functions like memory and reasoning. The

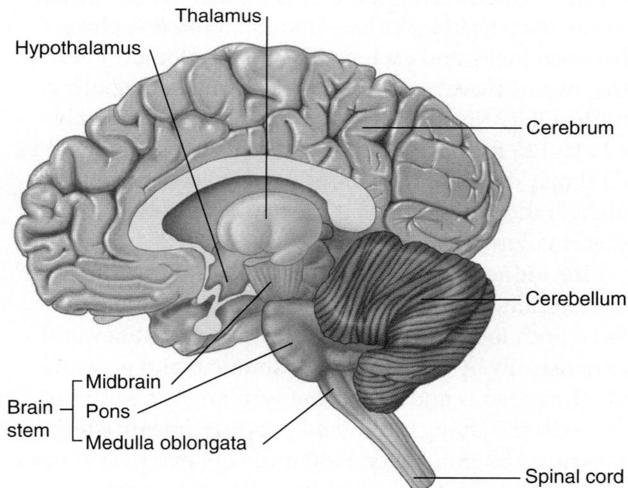

FIGURE 51-19 Structures of the brain.

Respiratory Recap

Four Divisions of the Brain

- Cerebrum
- Diencephalon (thalamus and hypothalamus)
- Brain stem
- Cerebellum

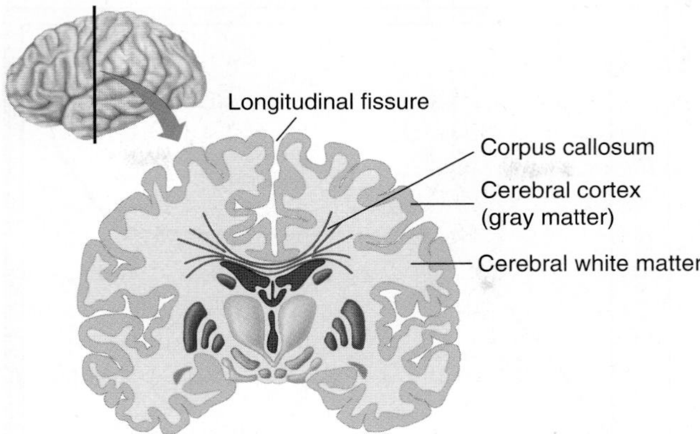

FIGURE 51-20 Coronal section through cerebrum.

cerebral cortex is composed of many nerve fibers that bring information into the cerebrum to be processed into meaningful perceptions, carry information out of the cerebrum to control systems that govern skeletal muscle movement, and connect different areas of the cerebrum.

The diencephalon forms the central core of the forebrain and is connected to the midbrain, the uppermost portion of the brain stem. Nerve fibers enter the cerebral cortex through the diencephalon, carrying information about specific events in the environment. Its two main parts, the **thalamus** and the **hypothalamus**, aid in processing sensory information. Specifically, the thalamus serves as a relay station for nerve impulses and as an integration center for inputs to the cerebral cortex, and it is the entry point for nerve fibers into the cerebral cortex. The hypothalamus is the master command center for endocrine coordination and for homeostatic regulation of the body. It is largely responsible for the functions necessary to preserve the individual, like eating and drinking.

The **brain stem** is composed of the **midbrain, pons**, and **medulla**. The midbrain is responsible for the regulation of hearing and vision, the pons is responsible for the maintenance of regular breathing, and the medulla is responsible for regulating coughing, sneezing, swallowing, and vomiting. All nerve fibers relaying signals between the forebrain, cerebellum, and spinal cord go through the brain stem, and it is responsible for the regulation of visceral activities like breathing and heart rate. These functions are coordinated through the reticular formation. It is a collection of nerve fibers running through the core of the brain stem. The reticular formation is essential for life, as it receives and integrates input from all areas of the CNS and is involved in cardiovascular and respiratory control as well as motor function, regulation of sleep and wakefulness, and focusing attention. In addition, the brain stem processes information for 10 of the 12 pairs of cranial nerves. These are peripheral nerves that connect directly to the brain and innervate muscles, glands, and sensory receptors of the head, the thoracic, and the abdominal cavities.

The **cerebellum** is located dorsal to the pons. It too is covered by an outer layer of cells, called the cerebellar cortex, and has an inner layer of nerve cell clusters. The cerebellum is important for coordinating movement, posture, and balance, but it does not initiate voluntary movement. In order to accomplish these functions, it receives input from muscles and joints, skin, eyes and ears, and other parts of the brain involved in the control of movement. The major parts of the brain and their structures and functions are further explained in **Table 51-3**.

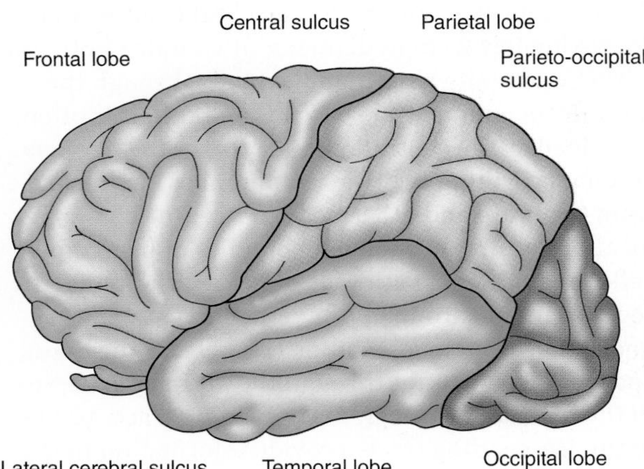

FIGURE 51-21 Lobes of the cerebrum.

Intracranial Pressures and Cerebral Perfusion Pressure

Because the skull is rigid and thus intracranial volume increases result in an increase in intracranial pressure (ICP). The relationship between intracranial volume and intracranial pressure is described by the cerebral compliance curve (**Figure 51-22**). Although small increases in intracranial volume are tolerated without an increase in ICP, larger increases in volume result in large increases in ICP. An increase in ICP thus decreases cerebral blood flow, resulting in cerebral hypoxia. With large increases in ICP, the swelling brain herniates through the tentorium, resulting in compression of the brain stem.

Cerebral perfusion pressure (CPP) is defined as the difference between mean arterial pressure (MAP) and ICP:

$$CPP = MAP - ICP$$

Normally, ICP is <10 mm Hg and MAP is about 90 mm Hg, resulting in a normal CPP >80 mm Hg. The target CPP is >60 mm Hg. Treatments that decrease MAP (e.g., positive pressure ventilation, diuresis, vasodilator therapy) decrease CPP, whereas treatments that decrease ICP (hyperventilation, mannitol) increase CPP. A normal physiologic response to an acute increase in ICP is hypertension with bradycardia, which is called the Cushing response. Mechanical

TABLE 51-3
Key Functions of Four Major Parts of the Brain

Structure	Function
Cerebrum	Provides higher brain functions Interprets sensory impulses and initiates voluntary muscular movements Stores information that makes up memory and utilizes it to reason Controls intelligence and personality
Diencephalon	Thalamus is the central relay station for sensory impulses except smell Produces awareness of sensations such as pain, touch, and temperature Hypothalamus maintains homeostasis by regulating visceral, nervous, and endocrine activities (heart rate, arterial blood pressure, temperature, water and electrolyte balance, hunger and body weight, movement control, glandular secretions, control of pituitary, and sleep patterns)
Brain stem	Midbrain is made up of gray matter Pons relays impulses to and from other brain parts and the PNS, including regular breathing Medulla oblongata is made up of white matter. Other nuclei inside it control coughing, sneezing, swallowing, and vomiting
Cerebellum	Communicates with the CNS Is a reflex center controlling body position, posture, skeletal muscle movements, muscle tone, and equilibrium

ventilation can increase ICP and decrease CPP because of the increased intrathoracic pressure associated with mechanical ventilation. PEEP has the potential of decreasing MAP and venous return. A decrease in venous return increases ICP and a decrease in MAP decreases CPP.

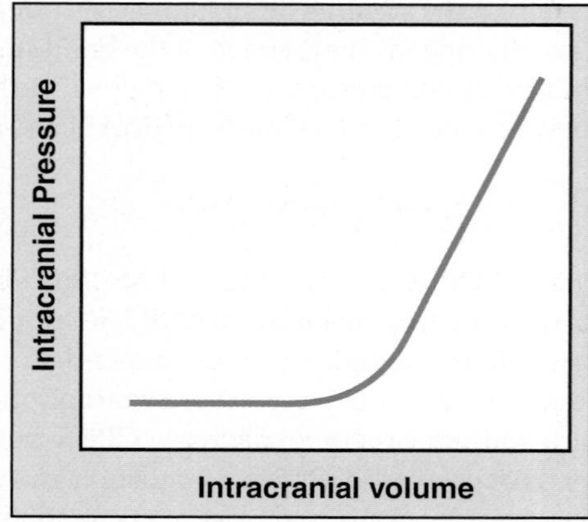

FIGURE 51-22 Relationship between intracranial pressure and intracranial volume.

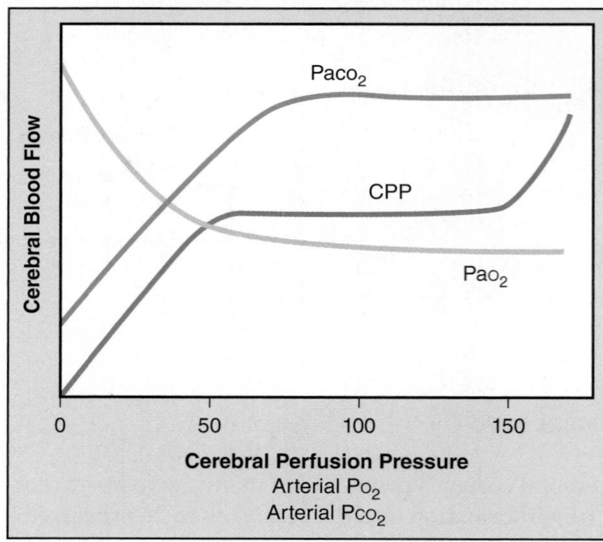

FIGURE 51-23 Relationship between cerebral blood flow, cerebral perfusion pressure, Pao_2, and $Paco_2$.

An increase in $Paco_2$ and a decrease in Pao_2 result in increases in ICP (**Figure 51-23**). $Paco_2$ has an indirect effect on cerebral vascular tone due to the effect of Pco_2 on pH. The change in pH affects the tone of cerebral blood vessels and thus cerebral blood volume and intracranial pressure. A decrease in pH (increased $Paco_2$) causes cerebral vascular dilatation and an increase in ICP. An increase in pH (decreased $Paco_2$) causes a decrease in ICP. With hyperventilation, the brain quickly equilibrates to changes in $Paco_2$ and a new steady state is established. Within 4 to 6 hours of the onset of hyperventilation, the pH normalizes. Although iatrogenic hyperventilation is not recommended in the management of ICP, permissive hypercapnia may be associated with unacceptable elevations in ICP.

Spinal Cord

The **spinal cord** is the other component of the CNS and serves as the link between the CNS and the PNS. It is located within the vertebral column and is approximately 2 cm in diameter. It contains both gray matter and white matter and extends through the foramen magnum at the base of the skull. It is often described as the central relay station in the nervous system, providing two-way communication to and from the brain and other body parts. This communication occurs through long bundles of nerve fibers called major nerve pathways or tracts. The spinal cord receives input through peripheral nerves from the body and through descending tracts from the brain, and it projects output through the peripheral nerves to the body and through the ascending tracts to the brain. Descending tracts provide information to the muscles and glands in the body, including motor commands that arise from the higher centers in the brain

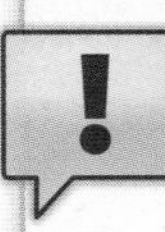

Respiratory Recap

Functions of the Spinal Cord

- Transmit output from the brain
- Relay input to the brain

that descend through the spinal cord along motor pathways. Ascending tracts provide information and input to the brain, including sensory signals that originate in sensory receptors in the body and limbs and are transmitted through the spinal cord to the brain along ascending sensory pathways. The peripheral nerves that connect the CNS and the PNS include the 12 pairs of cranial nerves mentioned earlier and the 31 pairs of spinal nerves that arise from the spinal cord segments named for the level of the vertebral column where they exit: cervical, thoracic, lumbar, sacral, and coccygeal (**Figure 51-24**).

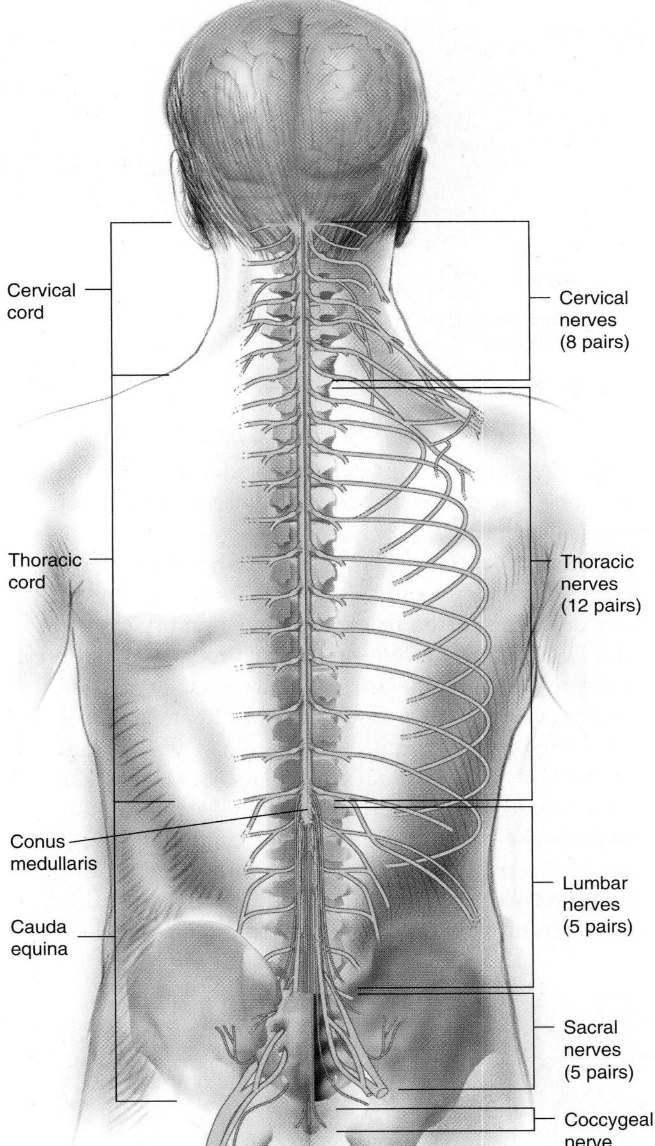

FIGURE 51-24 The spinal cord.

Peripheral Nervous System

An individual nerve cell is called a **neuron**, serving as both the structural and the functional unit of the nervous system. Neurons generate electric signals that move from cell to cell. These electrical signals trigger the release of chemical messengers called neurotransmitters that communicate with other cells both inside and outside the nervous system. All neurons have a similar structure but vary in size and in shape. Neurons contain a cell body and long extensions called processes that connect neurons to each other and transmit input and output for the neuron. There are two types of processes: **dendrites** and **axons**. Dendrites are branching outgrowths of the cell body that increase a cell's capacity to receive signals from other neurons. Axons are often referred to as nerve fibers. They are long processes that extend from the cell body. Bundles of axons constitute nerves. Functionally, they carry output from the neuron to the target cell. Electrical signals are generated at the connection of the axon to the cell body. These electrical signals are transmitted through the length of the axon. At the end, the axon terminal releases neurotransmitters that diffuse across the extracellular gap to the receiving neuron (**Figure 51-25**). Many axons are covered by myelin, which consist of modified plasma membrane, to speed conduction and conserve energy. This myelin gives axons a distinctive white color. Axons and other supporting cells thus are referred to as the white matter in the nervous system, and the cell bodies, dendrites, and additional supporting cells are referred to as the gray matter in the nervous system.

The junction between two communicating neurons is called a **synapse**. There are two types of synapses, electrical and chemical. Electrical synapses are only found in cardiac and smooth muscles. In these synapses, the electrical activity of one neuron directly influences the electrical activity of another neuron. Chemical synapses are much more common, and the majority of synapses in the body are chemical. In these synapses, communication of the electrical signals occurs through neurotransmitters that bind with specific protein receptors on the membrane of the receiving neuron. The neurotransmitters either excite, by triggering a nerve impulse, or inhibit, by decreasing the chance a nerve impulse will trigger the receiving cell (**Figure 51-26**). There are over 50 different neurotransmitters in the body. Several of the most common include **acetylcholine**, which plays a role in the control of skeletal muscle,

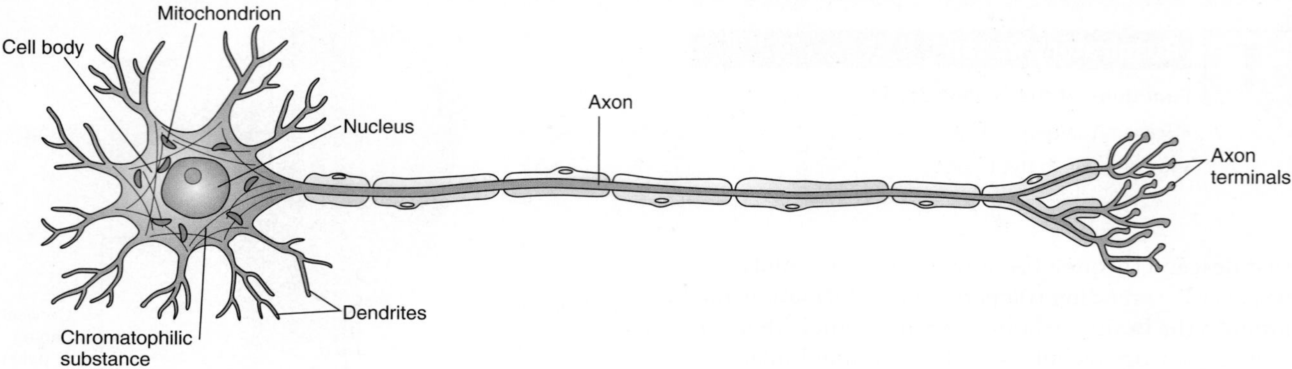

FIGURE 51-25 A typical neuron.

dopamine and norepinephrine, which control a person's sense of well-being, and serotonin, which causes sleepiness.

There are two types or classes of neurons that connect the body and the CNS. **Afferent neurons** convey information from the tissue and organs into the CNS, while efferent neurons convey information from the CNS to effectors, such as muscles, glands, and other cells in the body. Sensory fibers are afferent—they convey input from the sensory receptors in the body to the spinal cord. Sensory receptors, at ends of peripheral neurons, create electrical signals in response to various physical or chemical changes in the internal and external environment, including temperature, light, sound, and O_2 levels. Motor fibers are efferent; they convey output from the spinal cord to voluntary skeletal and striated muscles (including the diaphragm) and involuntary smooth muscles and cardiac muscles (**Figure 51-27**). As mentioned above, the cranial and spinal nerves connect the CNS and the PNS. Spinal nerves contain both afferent and efferent fibers, while some cranial nerves contain only afferent fibers.

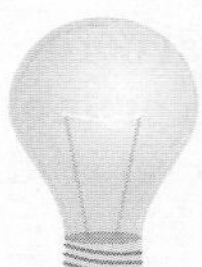

STOP AND THINK

What effect would a fracture between C1 and C5 have on a patient's ability to breathe?

Within the PNS, motor functions are controlled by either the **somatic nervous system** or the **autonomic nervous system**. The somatic nervous system regulates consciously controlled skeletal muscles, and

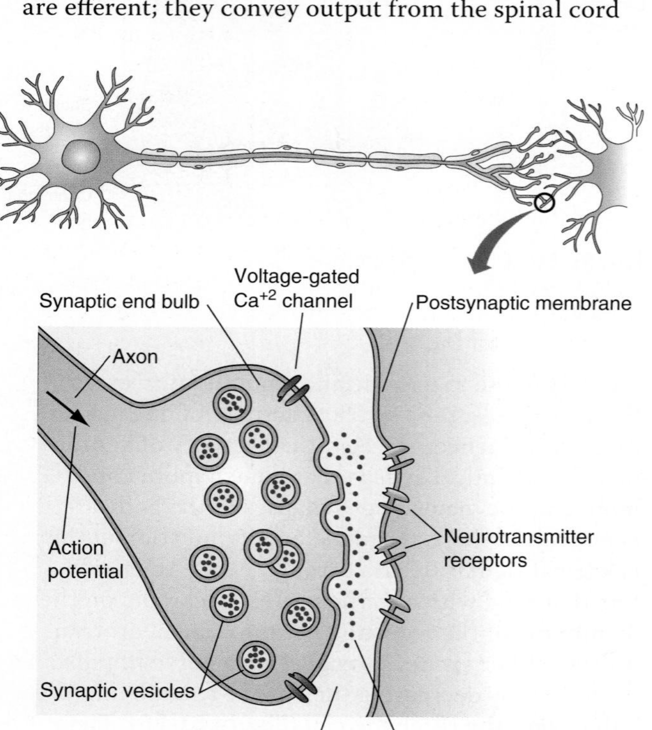

FIGURE 51-26 Chemical synapse.

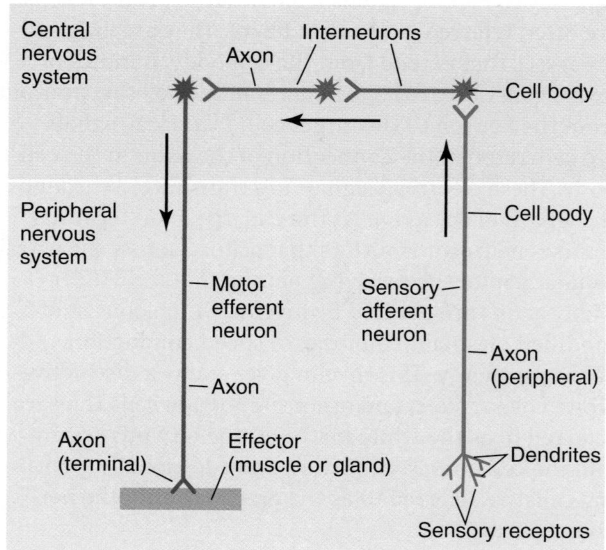

FIGURE 51-27 Classification of neurons by function and structure.

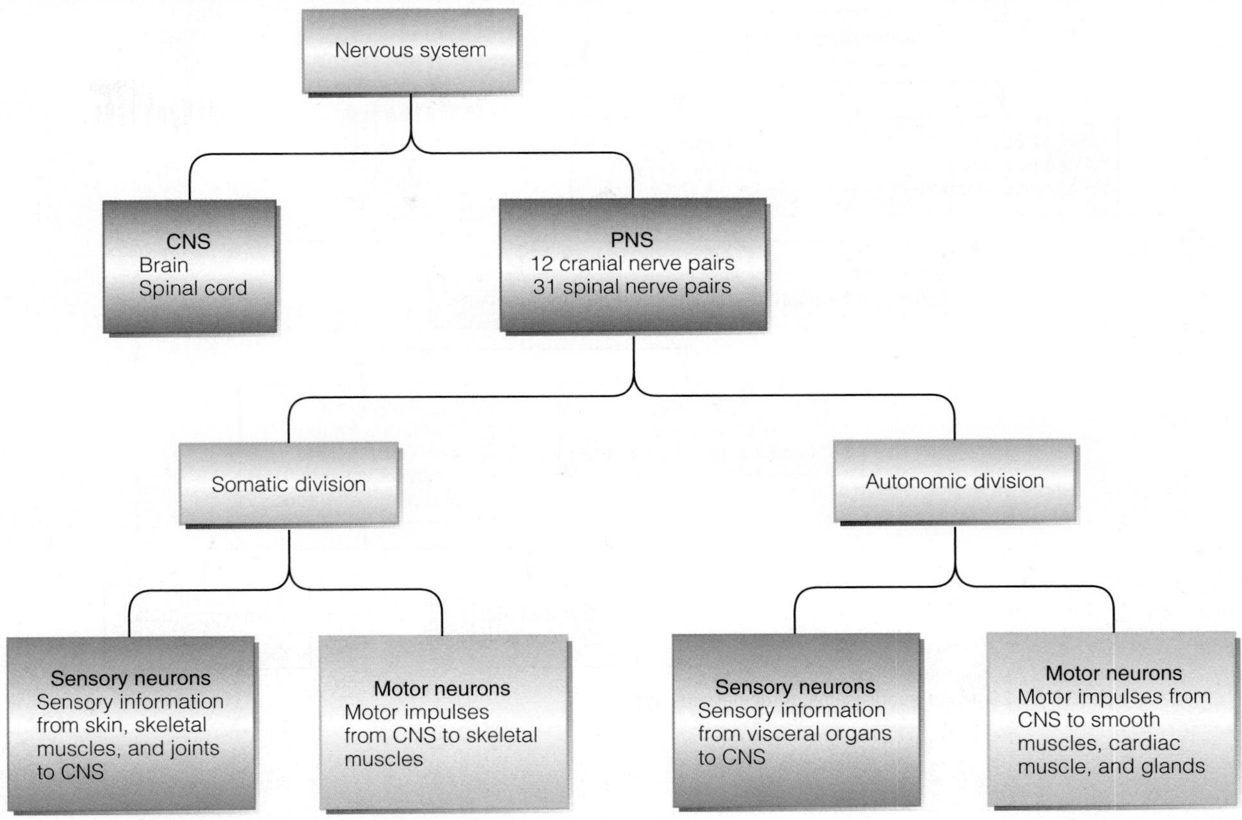

FIGURE 51-28 Motor pathways of somatic and autonomic nervous system.

the autonomic nervous system regulates involuntary controlled effectors like cardiac muscle, smooth muscle, and various glands. The cranial nerves—arising from the cerebrum and brain stem—and the spinal nerves—arising from the spinal cord—are included in the somatic nervous system and connect to the skeletal muscles. The diaphragm is a skeletal muscle and is voluntarily or consciously controlled by the somatic nervous system. Nerve fibers from the third, fourth, and fifth cervical nerves are combined into the right and left phrenic nerves, conducting motor impulses to the diaphragm. The autonomic nervous system functions autonomously, independently, and without conscious effort. Stimulation of autonomic nerve pathways in the medulla oblongata stimulates muscles and glands to control cardiac, vasomotor, and respiratory activities, all of which are necessary to maintain homeostasis (**Figure 51-28**).

The autonomic nervous system is further subdivided into the **sympathetic** and the **parasympathetic systems**. The sympathetic system regulates what is commonly referred to as the fight-or-flight response, preparing the body for stressful or emergency situations, including increasing heart rate and respiratory rate. In contrast, the parasympathetic system regulates the rest-and-digest response, returning the body to normal after activation of the sympathetic response and leading to a decreased heart rate and respiratory rate. These represent the final subdivisions of the nervous system (**Figure 51-29**).

Some of the neurons within the autonomic nervous system secrete acetylcholine and are called cholinergic fibers. Other neurons secrete norepinephrine and are called adrenergic fibers. The heart responds to cholinergic stimulation by decreasing heart rate and to adrenergic stimulation by increasing heart rate. The bronchioles in the lung respond to cholinergic stimulation by constricting and to adrenergic stimulation by dilating. Additional effects on other organs by both cholinergic stimulation and adrenergic stimulation are listed in **Table 51-4**.

> **Respiratory Recap**
>
> **Common Neurotransmitters in the Autonomic Nervous System**
>
> - Acetylcholine
> - Norepinephrine

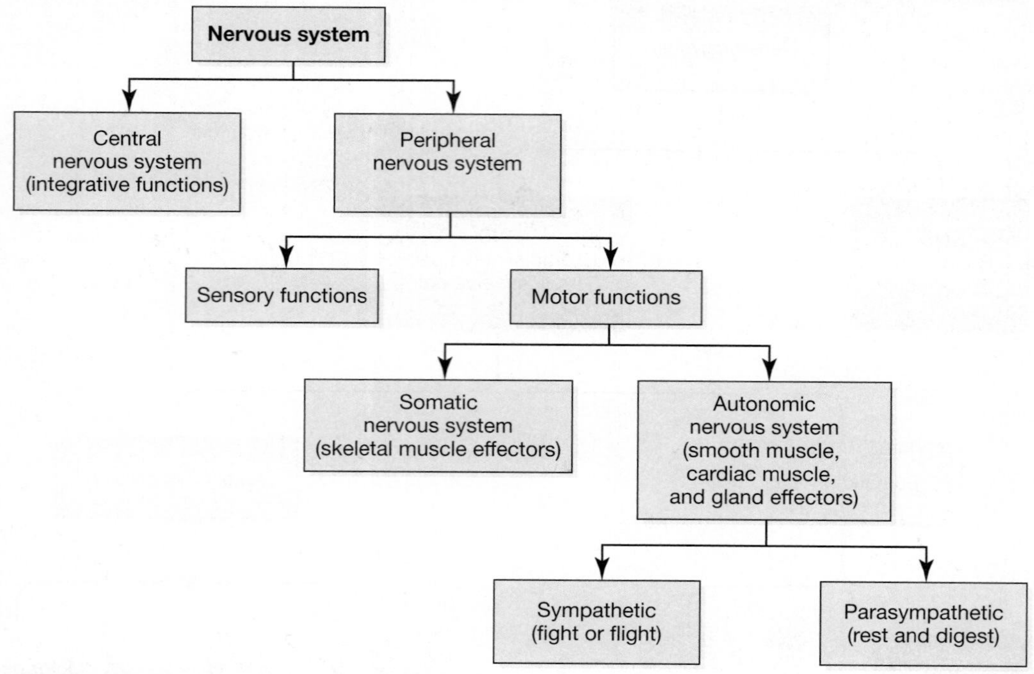

FIGURE 51-29 Major subdivisions of the nervous system.

TABLE 51-4
Adrenergic and Cholinergic Effects on Select Organs/Body Parts (Effectors)

Effector	Response to Adrenergic Stimulation	Response to Cholinergic Stimulation
Pupils	Dilation	Constriction
Heart rate	Increasing	Decreasing
Lung bronchioles	Dilation	Constriction
Distribution of blood	Increasing skeletal muscle blood, decreasing digestive organ blood	Increasing digestive organ blood, decreasing skeletal muscle blood
Salivary glands	Decreasing secretion	Increasing secretion
Tear glands	No action	Secretion

Key Points

- The primary function of the heart is to generate pressure to propel blood through the lungs and the systemic circulation.
- The gross anatomy of the cardiovascular system includes the heart muscle, valves and chambers, arteries, veins, capillaries, coronary circulation, and the conduction system.
- The major pacemaker of the heart is the SA node.
- The cardiac conduction system entails the SA node, AV node, bundle of His, and the Purkinje fibers.
- The circulating volume of blood in the body is 5 liters in an adult.
- The kidneys' primary function is regulation of blood volume and its chemical composition and maintaining the correct balance between acids and bases and between water and salts.
- The functional unit of the kidney is the nephron.
- Glomerular filtration is the process of turning filtrate into urine.
- Tubular reabsorption is the process of reclaiming plasma.
- Tubular secretion is the process of clearing waste and unwanted substances from the plasma.
- The nervous system is divided into the CNS and PNS.
- The four divisions of the brain are the cerebrum, diencephalon, brain stem, and cerebellum.
- The brain stem is composed of the midbrain, pons, and medulla.
- The spinal cord provides two-way communication between the brain and other body parts.
- Afferent neurons convey information from the tissues and organs to the CNS.
- Efferent neurons convey information from the CNS to effectors: muscles, glands, and cells in the body.
- The sympathetic nervous system is referred to as the fight-or-flight response.
- The parasympathetic system regulates rest-and-digest.

Suggested Reading

Des Jardins T. *Cardiopulmonary Anatomy and Physiology: Essentials for Respiratory Care*. 5th ed. Clifton Park, NY: Delmar; 2008.

Huether S, McCrane K. *Understanding Pathophysiology*. 4th ed. St. Louis: Mosby; 2004.

Loengenbaker S. *Understanding Human Anatomy and Physiology*. 6th ed. New York: McGraw-Hill; 2008.

Marieb EN, Hoehn KN. *Human Anatomy & Physiology*. 9th ed. San Francisco: Pearson; 2012.

Moini J. *Anatomy and Physiology for Health Professionals*. Burlington, MA: Jones & Bartlett; 2012.

Netter FH. *Atlas of Human Anatomy*. 2nd ed. East Hanover, NJ: Novartis; 1997.

Saladin KS. *Anatomy & Physiology: The Unity of Form and Function*. 6th ed. New York: McGraw-Hill; 2011.

Scanlon V, Sander T. *Essentials of Anatomy and Physiology*. 5th ed. Philadelphia: FA Davis; 2007.

Shier D, Butler JL, Lewis R. *Hole's Essentials of Human Anatomy and Physiology*. 9th ed. New York: McGraw-Hill; 2006.

Standring S. *Gray's Anatomy: The Anatomical Basis of Clinical Practice*. 40th ed. New York: Elsevier Churchill Livingstone; 2008.

Widmaier EP, Raff H, Strang KT. *Vander's Human Physiology; the Mechanisms of Body Function*. 11th ed. New York: McGraw-Hill; 2008.

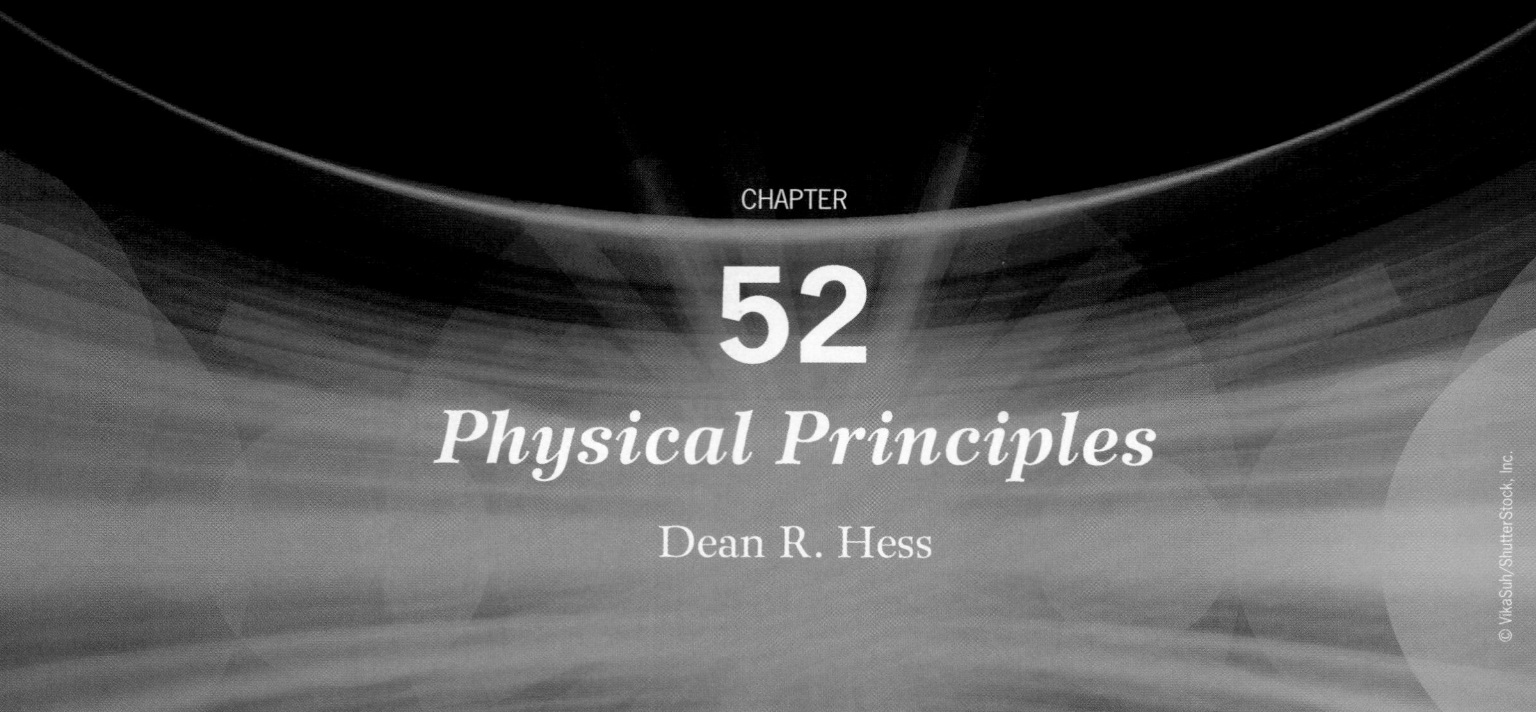

OUTLINE

OBJECTIVES

1. Identify the physical principles that are most important to respiratory physiology and respiratory care.
2. Explain the behaviors of fluids at various pressures, volumes, temperatures, and flows.
3. Describe units of measurement and states of matter.
4. Discuss physical principles affecting force, stress, pressure, and work.
5. Describe surface tension and its relationship to lung function.
6. Discuss Boyle's, Charles's, and Gay-Lussac's laws and the ideal gas law, and explain how changes in pressure, temperature, and volume affect the behavior of gases.
7. Describe applications of physical principles to monitoring, measurement, and assessment of the lung.

KEY TERMS

Bernoulli principle
Boyle's law
Charles's law
compliance
Dalton's law
density (ρ)
elastance
Fick's law
flow
force
Gay-Lussac's law of combining volumes
Gay-Lussac's law of pressure and temperature
Graham's law
gravity
Hagen-Poiseuille equation
humidity deficit
hydrostatic pressure
ideal gas law
joule (J)
laminar flow
mass
Ohm's law
pascal
percentage of body humidity (%BH)
pressure
resistance
Reynolds number
strain
stress
surface tension
Système International d'Unités (SI system)
temperature
turbulent flow
velocity
Venturi principle
viscosity
work

Introduction

Respiratory therapists must understand the physical principles important to respiratory physiology and the practice of respiratory care, particularly the behavior of gases and liquids under varying conditions of pressure, temperature, and flow. Physical forces have primary effects on gas movement, ventilation of the lungs, and blood flow. Some of the equations and relationships presented in this chapter simplify the physics and physiology, but a simplified approach provides insight into the usefulness of these important concepts.

Basic Physics

Molecules and States of Matter

Atoms, molecules, and compounds are the building blocks of all matter. The periodic table displays all known atoms, the elemental units of matter. Molecules are composed of two or more atoms. A molecule may be a pure element, in which the atoms are the same, or a compound of different atoms. Molecular oxygen (O_2) is composed of two atoms of the same element (oxygen), whereas carbon dioxide (CO_2) is a compound, a molecule with different atoms, made up of one carbon atom and two oxygen atoms.

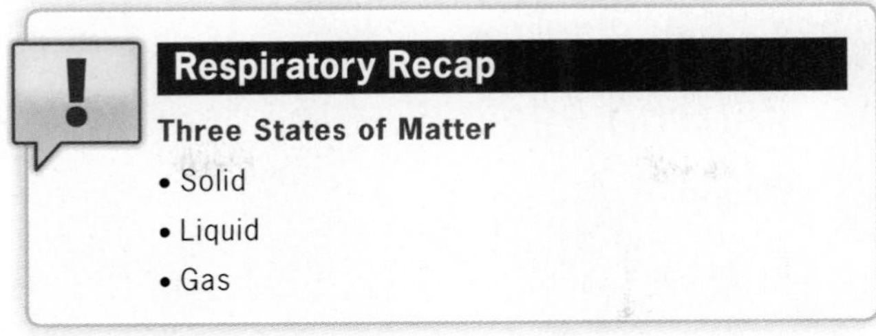

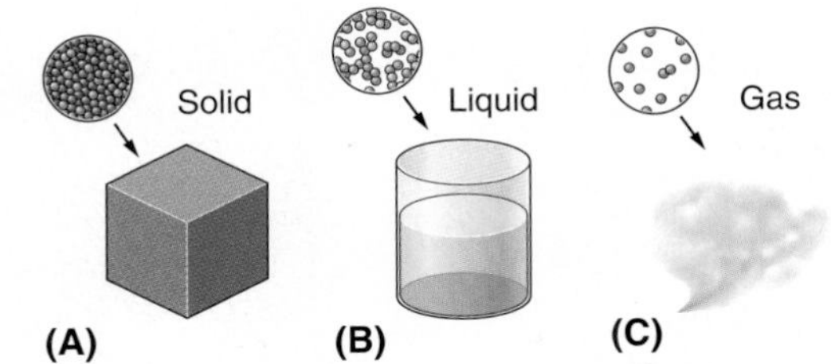

FIGURE 52-1 Simplified models of the three states of matter. (**A**) Solid. (**B**) Liquid. (**C**) Gas.

Molecular theory describes three states of matter: solid, liquid, and gas. The amount of kinetic energy present and interactions among molecules determine the physical state that molecules assume. For example, water can exist as a solid, liquid, or gas (**Figure 52-1**). A solid is a condensed structure in which strong intermolecular bonds determine a definite shape and volume. Solids do not move and are difficult to compress. A liquid, which is composed of molecules that move freely, has a definite volume without definite shape. Liquids are denser than gases. Like solids, liquids are difficult to compress. The intermolecular bonds of a gas, on the other hand, are weak. A gas is compressible and completely fills an enclosed space. Both gases and liquids are considered fluids, that is, substances that can flow.

All three states of matter have a characteristic elasticity, or reversible deformability. An ideal gas may be considered perfectly elastic: when the molecules collide with the wall of a vessel or with each other, no energy is lost. Gases in the real world are not quite ideal, but for our purposes they are close enough to ideal to be analyzed as if they were.

Units of Measurement

A common system of measurement is important to establish clear, consistent communication. Unfortunately, several units of measure are used in respiratory physiology. The **Système International d'Unités (SI system)** is an international system of measurement that is universally accepted but not always used. SI units are preferred, particularly in scientific and healthcare settings; however, for some measures both SI and clinical units are used. In the SI system the **pascal** (Pa; 1 newton/m^2) is the primary unit of pressure (**Table 52-1**); for ease of calculation, the kilopascal (kPa; 1000 Pa) is commonly used because the pascal is too small in the physiologic range. In the clinical setting, however, the more common units of measurement for pressure are cm H_2O for gases and mm Hg for liquids. **Table 52-2** shows these conversions.

Familiarity with the symbols used in respiratory physiology is essential to understand common terminology. The symbols of respiratory physiology have particular meanings and may be modified by characters placed above the symbol and by superscripts or subscripts. A dot over a symbol indicates the rate of change (i.e., distance over time or velocity), whereas two dots indicate the change in the rate of change (i.e., change in velocity over time, acceleration). For example, V indicates volume, and $\dot{V}$ is flow or change in volume over time. A bar over a symbol indicates a mean quantity, such as mean airway pressure ($\overline{P}aw$). **Table 52-3** lists commonly used symbols.

Mass, Force, Stress, Pressure, and Work

Mass is the amount of a substance, determined by the number and type of molecules. The molecular mass of a substance is a number of moles (mol) of a substance, and 1 mole is Avogadro's number (6.023×10^{23}) of atoms or molecules of that substance.

Force is a mechanical energy applied to a body. In mathematic terms, force is the product of mass times acceleration. *Weight* describes the force due to the acceleration of **gravity** acting on a mass (**Equation 52-1**). The acceleration of gravity is approximately 9.8 m/s^2. **Density (ρ)** is mass per unit volume, or m/V. The product

TABLE 52-1
International System (SI) Base and Derived Units

SI Base Units			SI Derived Units			
Measurement	**Unit**	**Abbreviation**	**Measurement**	**Unit**	**Abbreviation**	**Derivation**
Length	Meter	m	Force	Newton	N	$kg \times m \times s^{-2}$
Mass	Kilogram	kg	Pressure	Pascal	Pa	$N \times m^{-2}$
Time	Second	s	Work	Joule	J	N × m (L × kPa)
Temperature	Kelvin	K	Frequency	Hertz	Hz	s^{-1}

TABLE 52-2
Common Conversions in Units of Measurement

Measurement	Unit of Measure	Conversions*
Pressure	1 kilopascal (kPa)	7.5 mm Hg 10.2 cm H_2O 0.00987 atm 10^4 dyne × cm^{-2}
	1 millimeter of mercury (mm Hg)	1 torr 0.133 kPa 1.36 cm H_2O 1.33 × 10^3 dyne × cm^{-2}
	1 atmosphere	101.3 kPa 760 mm Hg 1033 cm H_2O 10 m seawater
Work	1 joule	0.239 calories 1 L × kPa
Power	1 watt	1 J × s^{-1}

*Atmospheres (atm) and millimeters of mercury (mm Hg) are not International System (SI) units, but they are in common use.

EQUATION 52-1

Weight

$$F = m \times a$$

$$\text{Weight} = m \times g$$

$$\text{Weight} = \rho \times V \times g$$

where:

F = Force

m = Mass

a = Acceleration

ρ = Density (mass/volume)

V = Volume

g = Acceleration of gravity

TABLE 52-3
Symbols and Modifiers Commonly Used in Respiratory Physiology

Symbol	Meaning	Modifier*	Meaning
V	Volume of gas	T	Tidal
$\dot{V}$	Flow of gas	A	Alveolar
Q	Volume of liquid	a	Arterial
$\dot{Q}$	Blood flow, perfusion	v	Venous
S	Saturation	atm	Atmospheric
F	Fraction	rc	Rib cage
P	Pressure	cw	Chest wall
T	Temperature	pl	Pleural
C	Compliance	es	Esophageal
E	Elastance		
R	Resistance		
T	Time		
f	Frequency (rate)		

*A modifier usually is expressed as a subscript or suffix.

of density, volume, and the acceleration of gravity also is weight.

Stress is a force applied to an area. Force applied at an angle generates shear stress. **Pressure** (force per unit area) is the same concept applied to fluids, including gases (**Equation 52-2**). Examples include the pressure

EQUATION 52-2

Pressure and Force

$$F = P \times A$$

$$P = F/A$$

where:

F = Force

P = Pressure

A = Area

of the atmosphere (barometric pressure) and the pressure measured at the airway during a respiratory cycle. Force is the product of pressure and area.

Strain is the physical deformation or change in shape of a structure or substance caused by stress. Elasticity is the *reversible* deformability that can be generated by stress, yet allows the structure or substance to return to its original shape. A gas is highly elastic, which means that its volume can be compressed relatively easily. Other fluids, such as liquids, are less elastic and behave as if incompressible. **Viscosity** is the resistance to movement between adjacent fluid molecules. Solids lack elasticity compared with gases or liquids. A stress applied to solid materials can alter the strength or soundness of a substance without changing its apparent shape.

A force causing displacement of matter does **work**. For gases, a force can be measured as pressure, and the displacement is the volume change to the lungs. Using SI units, work is expressed in newton meters (N × m) or **joules (J)** or joules per liter.

Pressure is transmitted without reduction throughout any enclosed static fluid, an observation known as *Pascal's law*. In terms of molecular theory, the collisions of molecules with one another and the wall of their containing vessel generate pressure. If conditions are at equilibrium, pressure is constant throughout the fluid if the pressure caused by the weight of the fluid is neglected. The weight of a fluid generates static fluid pressure (**hydrostatic pressure**) due to the force of gravity, which varies according to the density and depth within the fluid container. This static fluid pressure is important in liquids but negligible for gases (**Equation 52-3**). As shown in **Figure 52-2**, the height of the fluid and its density

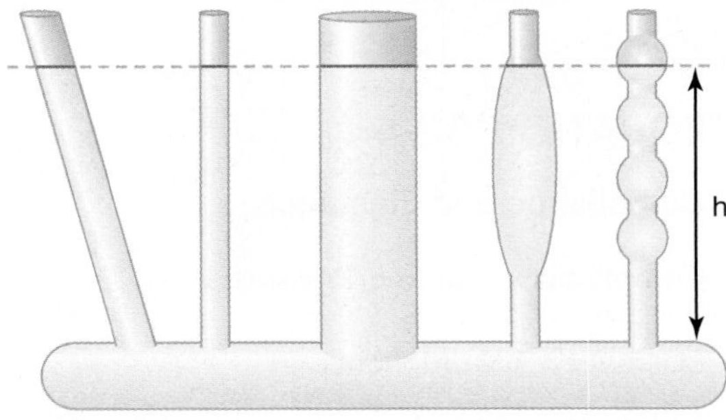

FIGURE 52-2 Pascal's law. Liquid pressure depends only on the height (h) of the vessel and not on the vessel's shape or the total volume of liquid.

determine the fluid pressure. The shape of the container does not affect pressure.

Because pressure is force applied to an area, if pressure is equal throughout an enclosed fluid, the force exerted on a larger area of a container must be greater than the force at a smaller area, known as the *hydraulic press principle*. Given two syringes of different diameters, the syringe with the larger diameter can generate greater force than the syringe with the smaller diameter. Because work is the product of force and distance, the distance the syringe with the smaller diameter (less force) moves is greater than the distance that the larger-diameter syringe moves. If equal force is applied simultaneously to syringes of different diameters, a greater pressure will be generated in the syringe of lesser cross-sectional area.

Atmospheric (barometric) pressure is an example of static fluid pressure. Atmospheric pressure is the pressure generated by the weight of atmospheric gas above the barometer at any particular altitude. As elevation increases, atmospheric pressure decreases. The decrease in atmospheric pressure at a higher altitude is due to a shorter column of atmospheric gas. At a fixed altitude, comparatively minor changes in barometric pressure such as those witnessed in low- and high-pressure systems can cause major differences in weather.

The volume change to sphere-like structures such as alveoli caused by a pressure change is the **compliance**, or stiffness, of the sphere (**Equation 52-4**). A balloon that is difficult to inflate is an example of a low-compliance sphere. The compliance of the respiratory system is a composite of two compliances—lung compliance and chest wall compliance—like springs pulling in opposite directions. The reciprocal of respiratory system compliance is the sum of the reciprocals of lung and chest wall compliance (refer to Equation 52-4). **Elastance** (pressure per unit volume) is the reciprocal of compliance; therefore, respiratory system elastance is the sum of the lung elastance and chest wall elastance.

EQUATION 52-3

Hydrostatic Pressure

$$P = h \times \rho \times g$$

where:

P = Pressure

h = Height

ρ = Density

g = Acceleration of gravity

EQUATION 52-4

Compliance and Elastance

Compliance = Volume/Pressure

Elastance = 1/Compliance

$1/C_{RS} = 1/C_{CW} + 1/C_{L}$

where:

C_{RS} = Total respiratory system compliance

C_{CW} = Chest wall compliance

C_{L} = Lung compliance

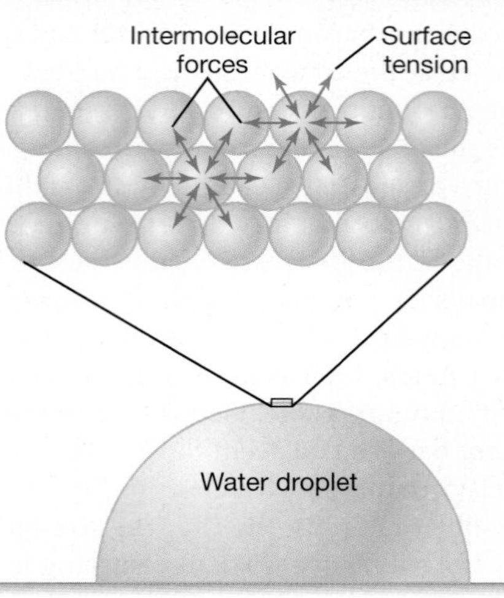

FIGURE 52-3 The force of surface tension in a drop of liquid. Cohesive force (arrows) attracts molecules inside the drop to one another. Cohesion can pull the outermost molecules inward only, creating a centrally directed force that tends to contract the liquid into a sphere.

Wall Tension and Surface Tension

Although Pascal's law states that pressure is equal throughout a containing structure (ignoring hydrostatic pressure), the wall tension varies. Laplace's law describes the tension of the wall of a sphere or cylinder (**Equation 52-5**). Wall tension increases with radius. A smaller structure generates a greater inward pressure, resulting in a tendency to collapse due to surface tension.

Surface tension describes the property of a liquid that tends to reduce the surface of a liquid toward a minimum, pulling the surface molecules inward. This causes water to bead up on a surface rather than spread out. Surface tension is the force acting at the boundary surface between two regions, such as the boundary between liquid and the adjoining air (**Figure 52-3**). The force generated across the wall of a structure is a combination of wall and surface tension.

Surfactant reduces surface tension. Soap is a common example of a surfactant. In the lungs, surfactant reduces the pressure required to expand an alveolus. Surfactant also reduces the pressure differences between alveoli of different diameters. Without surfactant, smaller alveoli would empty into larger ones because of the greater surface tension in the smaller alveoli (**Figure 52-4**). Surfactant is necessary for normal

EQUATION 52-5

Laplace's Law for a Sphere

$T = (P \times r)/2$

$P = (2T)/r$

where:

T = Tension

P = Pressure

r = Radius

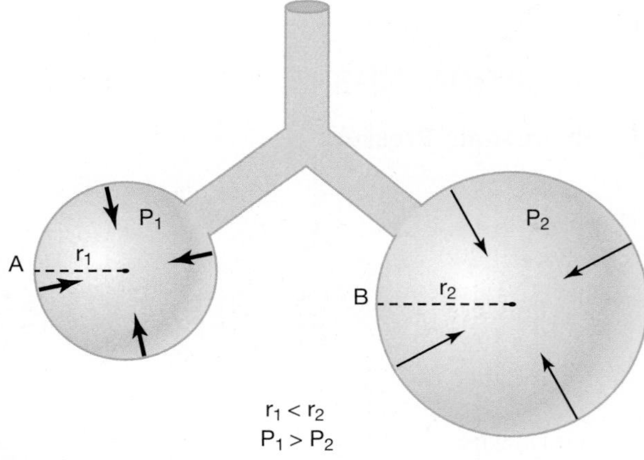

FIGURE 52-4 Relationship described by Laplace's law. Bubble A (**left**), which has the smaller radius, has the greater inward or deflating pressure and is more prone to collapse than is bubble B (**right**). Because the two bubbles are connected, bubble A would tend to deflate and empty into bubble B. Conversely, because of bubble A's greater surface tension, it would be harder to inflate than bubble B.

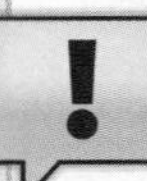

Respiratory Recap

Surface Tension and Surfactant

- Surface tension tends to reduce the surface of a liquid to a minimum.
- Surfactant reduces surface tension.

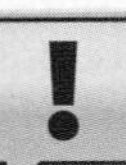

Respiratory Recap

Temperature Scales

- Fahrenheit (F)
- Celsius (C)
- Kelvin (absolute) (K)

lung function because it reduces the work of breathing (by reducing the surface tension) and allows alveoli or lung regions of various sizes to remain open, allowing the equalization of volumes and pressures between regions.

Temperature

Temperature describes the amount of heat, or thermal energy, present in a system. Three temperature scales are in common use. The Fahrenheit and Celsius scales are used in health care and are calibrated in reference to the freezing and boiling points of water—distinct points of reference (**Table 52-4**). The Fahrenheit scale divides the temperature range between freezing and boiling into 180 gradations, or degrees, whereas the Celsius scale uses 100 gradations. In scientific settings, the scales are referenced to 0° or absolute zero (without minus degrees) and are the Kelvin scale, which uses Celsius units, and the Rankin scale, which uses Fahrenheit units. The Rankin scale is rarely used.

The formula for converting Celsius to Fahrenheit takes into consideration the difference in zero points (32°) and the ratio of the two degree sizes because Celsius degrees are 1.8 times larger than Fahrenheit degrees (**Equation 52-6**).

EQUATION 52-6

Celsius and Fahrenheit Temperature Conversions

Conversion from Celsius to Fahrenheit

$$\text{Fahrenheit} = 32 + (\text{Celsius degrees} \times 9/5)$$

Conversion from Fahrenheit to Celsius

$$\text{Celsius} = (\text{Fahrenheit degrees} - 32) \times 5/9$$

Thermodynamics and Heat Exchange

Thermodynamics describes changes in the thermal state of a system by adding or removing energy, such as when changes in pressure, volume, or temperature alter the state of the substance. When a change of state requires the addition of energy, the process is called *endothermic*. An *exothermic* process gives off energy. **Table 52-5** lists common endothermic and exothermic processes as the states of matter change between gas, liquid, and solid states. Substances usually condense into liquids before becoming solids.

Gas Laws

Solids and liquids follow the same basic principles but do not exhibit the perfectly elastic intermolecular behavior of an ideal gas. Theoretical, or ideal, gases

TABLE 52-4
Temperature Scales

	Fahrenheit (° F)	Celsius (° C)	Kelvin (K)
Absolute zero	−460	−273	0
Oxygen boils	−297	−183	90
Water freezes	32	0	273
Normal body temperature	98.6	37	310
Water boils	212	100	373

TABLE 52-5
Changes in the State of Matter

Type of Change	Conversion	Example
Exothermic Change (Energy Given Up)		
Condensation Freezing	Gas to liquid or solid Liquid to solid	Water condensing on a cold glass Ice forming
Endothermic Change (Energy Added)		
Sublimation Melting Evaporation	Solid to gas Solid to liquid Liquid to gas	Dry ice Ice melting Water boiling

obey gas laws and behave precisely the same at all temperatures and pressures. Real gases act ideal but are not ideal under all conditions; however, under the relatively low pressure and temperature conditions encountered in respiratory physiology, their behavior can be predicted quite well by ideal gas laws.

The **ideal gas law** defines a relationship between pressure, volume, temperature, and the number of molecules of a gas (**Equation 52-7**). Pressure and volume are inversely related, whereas temperature is directly proportional to volume or pressure (**Figure 52-5**):

$$PV = nRT$$

The term n in the ideal gas law accounts for the number of gas molecules present. The universal gas constant, R, expresses the force (or work) required to move a quantity of ideal gas. This has a value of 8.1314 joules × degrees Kelvin^{-1} × moles^{-1}. If one or more quantities change, the others must change to compensate and keep the equation in balance. In particular, if the amount and makeup of a gas stay constant, then the quantity PV/T must remain constant, although these three quantities may each change within their fixed relationship.

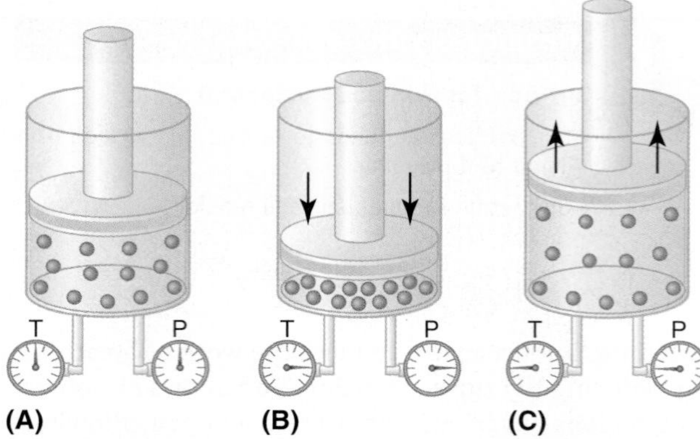

FIGURE 52-5 (**A**) A mass of gas in the resting state exerts a given pressure at a given temperature in a cylinder. (**B**) As the piston compresses the gas, the molecules are crowded closer together, and the increased energy of molecular collisions increases both the temperature and the pressure. (**C**) Conversely, as the gas expands, molecular interaction diminishes and the temperature and pressure fall.

EQUATION 52-7

Ideal (Combined) Gas Law

$$(P_1 \times V_1)/T_1 = (P_2 \times V_2)/T_2$$

where:

P = Pressure

V = Volume

T = Absolute temperature

$$PV = nRT$$

where:

P = Pressure

V = Volume

n = Number of moles

R = Gas constant

T = Absolute temperature

Gay-Lussac's law of combining volumes states that volumes of gases combine chemically in volumetric proportions that are small whole numbers (**Equation 52-8**). This observation confirms that under equivalent conditions, equal volumes of ideal gases contain an equal number of molecules. Under standard conditions of 0° C and barometric pressure of 1 atmosphere (1 atm), 1 mol of an ideal gas has a volume of 22.4 L.

Boyle's law states that pressure is inversely proportional to volume (**Equation 52-9**); therefore, the product of pressure and volume is expressed as a constant, k. Boyle's law predicts the relationship of a volume of gas to a pressure change. If the volume of a gas is halved, pressure will double, given a constant mass and

EQUATION 52-8

Gay-Lussac's Law of Combining Volumes

$$V = k \times n$$

$$V_1/n_1 = V_2/n_2$$

where:

V = Volume

k = Constant

n = Number of moles

EQUATION 52-9

Boyle's Law

$$P \times V = k$$

$$P_1 \times V_1 = P_2 \times V_2$$

where:

P = Pressure

V = Volume

k = Constant

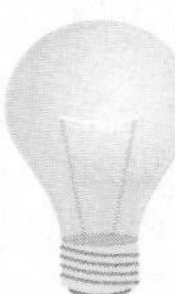

STOP AND THINK

Why are divers instructed to exhale during ascent?

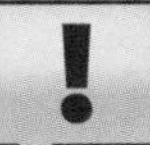

Respiratory Recap

Gas Laws

- Gay-Lussac's law of combining volumes
- Boyle's law
- Charles's law
- Gay-Lussac's law of pressure and temperature
- Ideal (combined) gas law

temperature. A pressure change important in pulmonary function testing is the change in lung pressure while attempting to pant against a blocked airway. This application of Boyle's law allows a calculation of lung volume in body plethysmography studies.

Charles's law predicts the effect of temperature on a fixed amount of dry gas. At constant pressure, gas expands proportionally to changes in absolute temperature (**Equation 52-10**). A constant multiplied by temperature predicts volume; for example, an ideal gas expands 37.5% when heated from 0° C to 100° C. For this reason, a volume of inhaled gas at room temperature expands when inhaled into a 37° C body. When exhaled, the volume will remain proportionally larger according to its temperature; pulmonary function testing systems account for this warming effect.

Gay-Lussac's law of pressure and temperature (**Equation 52-11**) describes the direct relationship between pressure and temperature given a fixed mass and volume of gas. If the absolute temperature of a fixed gas volume is increased, then the pressure will be increased proportionally. The pressure in an oxygen tank will change directly with changes in temperature.

Gases can deviate slightly from ideal gas behavior even under commonly encountered conditions. For example, ideal gases assume purely elastic collisions between molecules. Non-ideal gases require quantitative modifications of the classic gas laws to describe their behavior. For example, under standard conditions, the volume of 1 mole of carbon dioxide is 22.2 L rather than 22.4 L. Factors that describe attraction or repulsion between

EQUATION 52-10

Charles's Law

$$V = k \times T$$

$$V_1/T_1 = V_2/T_2$$

where:

V = Volume

k = Constant

T = Absolute temperature

EQUATION 52-11

Gay-Lussac's Law of Pressure and Temperature

$$P = k \times T$$

$$P_1/T_1 = P_2/T_2$$

where:

P = Pressure

k = Constant

T = Absolute temperature

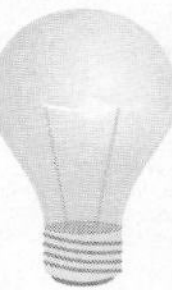

STOP AND THINK

The gas flowing from a high-pressure oxygen cylinder often feels cool. Why is that?

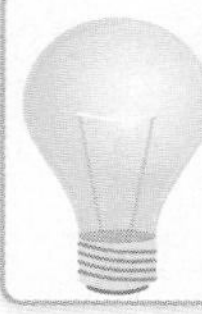

STOP AND THINK

Why are airplanes pressurized?

molecules (e.g., Van der Waals forces) attempt to predict these differences from ideal behavior.

Gas Mixtures and Partial Pressures

Dalton's law of partial pressures describes the behavior of physical mixtures of gases and vapors. In these mixtures, each separate gas acts according to the ideal gas law as if it were alone. The partial pressure of each particular gas is equal to its fraction times the total atmospheric pressure. Oxygen accounts for approximately 21% of atmospheric air, a percentage that can be expressed as the fraction of 0.21. At 1 atm (760 mm Hg), the partial pressure of oxygen is therefore 159.6 mm Hg (**Equation 52-12**). Nitrogen, which accounts for approximately 78% of air, has a partial pressure that can be similarly calculated to be 592.8 mm Hg at 1 atm.

Physical combinations of gases mix uniformly. Gases are continuously in motion, are at equilibrium, and are evenly distributed in any particular confined space. The same fractions of oxygen and nitrogen are present in Death Valley (86 m below sea level) as on Mount Everest (elevation 8850 m), although their partial pressures vary greatly.

EQUATION 52-12

Dalton's Law

Pressure of Oxygen at 1 Atmosphere

$$P_{IO_2} = F_{IO_2} \times Patm$$

$$P_{IO_2} = 0.21 \times 760 \text{ mm Hg} = 160 \text{ mm Hg}$$

Pressure of Nitrogen at 1 Atmosphere

$$P_{IN_2} = F_{IN_2} \times Patm$$

$$P_{IN_2} = 0.78 \times 760 = 593 \text{ mm Hg}$$

P_{IO_2} = Partial pressure of inspired oxygen

F_{IO_2} = Fraction of oxygen in inspired gas

Patm = Atmospheric pressure

P_{IN_2} = Partial pressure of inspired nitrogen

F_{IN_2} = Fraction of nitrogen in inspired gas

Humidity, Water Vapor, and Evaporation

Most gases encountered in physiologic conditions are combinations of various dry gases, but they also contain water vapor (gas), which combines with the other gases according to Dalton's law of partial pressures. Water is particularly important as a vapor under conditions encountered in respiratory care.

Evaporation and Condensation

A water surface emits molecules of vapor continuously by evaporation. As vapor molecules hit the surface of a liquid, some are absorbed into the liquid by condensation. The net change due to evaporation or condensation depends on which is greater—the rate of condensation or the rate of evaporation. Because energy is needed to change state from liquid to gas, evaporation is a cooling process. Above 100° C at atmospheric pressure, water is largely a vapor. Below 0° C, water is a solid. Between those temperatures, where humans generally live, there is a saturation pressure (or partial pressure of water) at any given temperature at which water will condense (**Figure 52-6**). Temperature defines a limit to the maximum amount of water vapor that can be contained in air at that temperature.

Humidity can be quantified by partial pressure of water (P_{H_2O}), absolute humidity, or relative humidity. *Absolute humidity* (**Equation 52-13**) is the amount of water vapor in the air or the mass of water present in a volume of gas, usually measured in milligrams per liter. Humidity is most often expressed as *relative humidity*, or the total water content in a gas, such as air, compared with the capacity for water content at that temperature. A sample of gas having a relative humidity of 50% at 20° C has a vapor pressure of 8.75 mm Hg (0.5 × 17.5 mm Hg). At the usual body temperature of 37° C, 50% relative

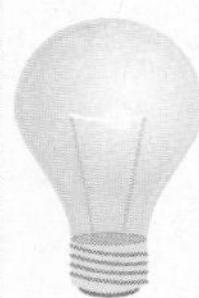

STOP AND THINK

Why is an unheated humidifier cool to the touch?

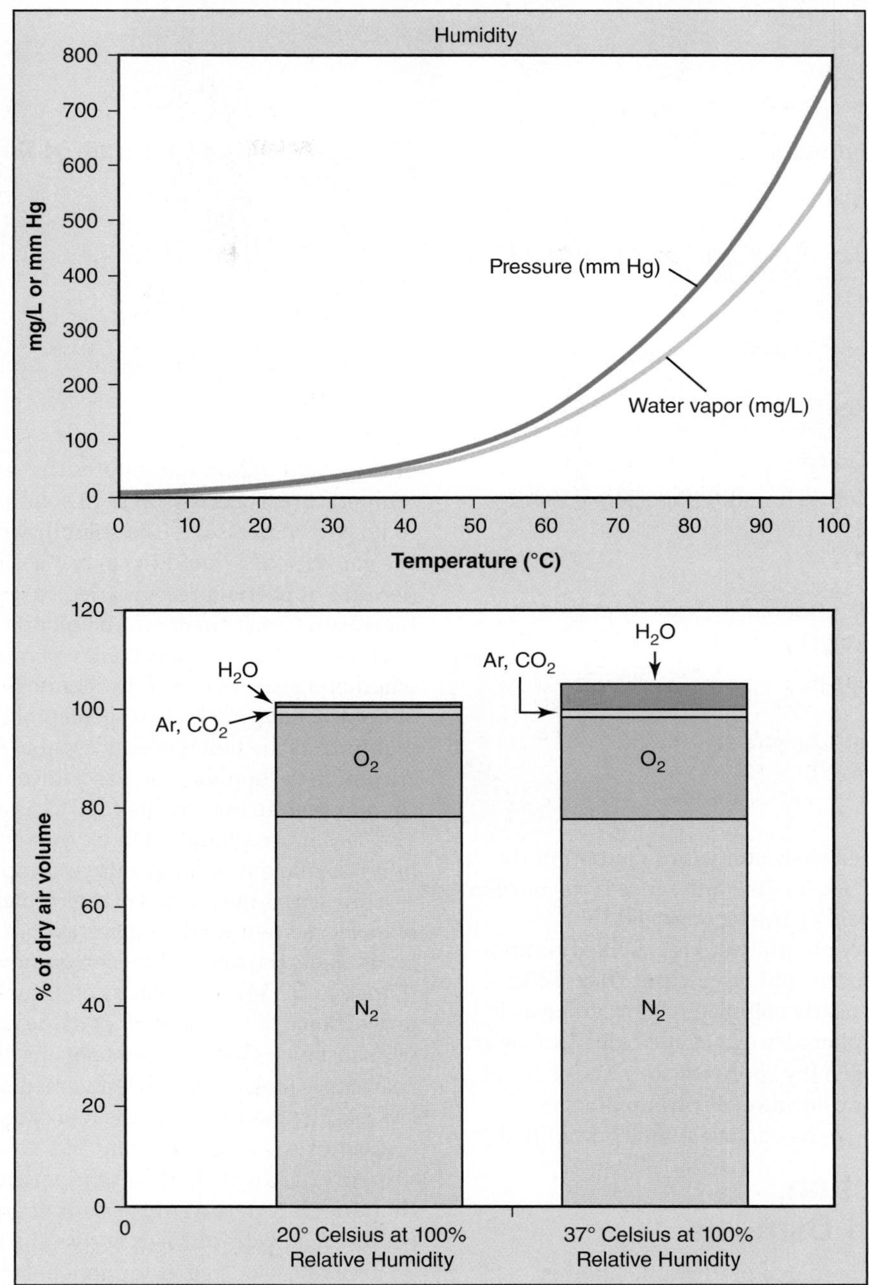

FIGURE 52-6 Absolute humidity and water vapor pressure as a function of temperature.

humidity has a water vapor pressure of 23.5 mm Hg, or one-half the maximum of 47 mm Hg.

If temperature is decreased and vapor pressure (and absolute humidity) remains the same, condensation occurs. As temperature decreases along a ventilator circuit as gases move away from the heated humidifier, condensation occurs. Adding heated wires to the circuitry can prevent or reduce this condensation.

When conditions such as pressure and temperature are constant, a vapor can be analyzed in the same manner as any gaseous substance. At 1 atm, fully humidified or saturated air at body temperature has a P_{H_2O} of 47 mm Hg. Other gases account for the remainder of the 760 mm Hg, or 713 mm Hg. Respiratory therapists have used an additional measure of humidity—**percentage of body humidity (%BH)**—as an assessment of humidity deficit. The %BH is the ratio of actual water vapor content to the water vapor capacity in a saturated gas at 37° C. The water content (absolute humidity) of fully saturated gas at body temperature is 43.8 mg/L. A **humidity deficit** occurs whenever inspired gas is not fully saturated at body temperature, requiring the body to add water to inspired gases to achieve full saturation. Humidity deficit is determined by calculating

EQUATION 52-13

Calculating Humidity

Absolute Humidity

$$\text{Absolute humidity} = (16.42 - 0.73 \times T) + 0.04 \times T^2$$

where:

T = temperature (Celsius)

Relative Humidity

% Relative humidity =
(Absolute humidity/Humidity capacity) × 100%

Humidity Deficit

Humidity deficit = Content − Capacity at 37° C = Content − 43.8 mg/L

Body Humidity (BH)

%BH = (Content/Capacity) × 100% = (Content/43.8 mg/L) × 100

the difference between the water vapor content of the inspired gas and 43.8 mg/L. This difference is the burden on the airway to humidify the inspired gas.

Unconditioned (dry or ambient) air is a fixed composition of oxygen, nitrogen, and other gases (**Box 52-1**). Inhaled air becomes nearly completely humidified as it passes through the upper airway. Exhaled air has a lower concentration of oxygen (by approximately 5%, or about 16%), a significant concentration of carbon dioxide of approximately 5% and exhaled air remains humidified.

Gases in Solution, Diffusion, and Osmosis

Gases dissolve in a liquid in a predictable manner according to Henry's law and the solubility coefficient

BOX 52-1

Composition of Unconditioned Dry Air

Nitrogen: 78.08%
Oxygen: 20.95%
Carbon dioxide: 0.03%
Argon: 0.93%
Trace gases: 0.01%

Water vapor at 20° C and 50% relative humidity accounts for 1.1% of air volume.

EQUATION 52-14

Graham's Law for Rate of Diffusion of Gases

$$\frac{\text{Rate}_A}{\text{Rate}_B} = \sqrt{\frac{\text{MW}_B}{\text{MW}_A}}$$

where:

MW = molecular weight

of the liquid. *Henry's law* states that at a constant temperature, a gas dissolves in solution in proportion to its partial pressure. The solubility coefficient, or the capacity of a liquid to carry a gas (mass dissolved per unit of partial pressure) decreases as temperature increases. Constituents in the blood affect the solubility coefficient. For example, Henry's law does not predict whether a gas will combine chemically with a constituent of the fluid, such as oxygen combining with hemoglobin, and the blood is very capable of carrying CO_2. Although carbon dioxide has a lower partial pressure than oxygen in air and blood, CO_2 is approximately 19 times more soluble than oxygen due to its high solubility coefficient or large carrying capacity in blood.

Diffusion is the process of intermingling and movement of molecules as a result of their random motion. **Graham's law** predicts the rate of diffusion or movement of a gas (**Equation 52-14**). The velocity of diffusion is inversely proportional to the square root of the molecular weight of a substance; therefore, lighter gases diffuse faster than heavier gas molecules. In a liquid medium, both Graham's law and Henry's law affect the rate of diffusion of gases.

Osmosis is the movement of a solvent by diffusion, primarily, through a semipermeable membrane that does not permit movement of larger solute molecules. A solvent diffuses across the membrane from an area of lesser to greater concentration. **Fick's law** (**Equation 52-15**) relates the factors that affect the transmembrane transfer of solute during osmosis. The total diffusion rate of a gas across a barrier (such as the alveolar membrane in the lung) is directly proportional to the cross-sectional area available for diffusion (lung size), to the difference in concentration gradients of the diffusing gases, and to the perpendicular distance of that cross-sectional area (thickness of the alveolocapillary membrane).

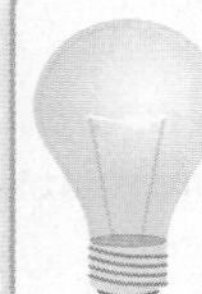

STOP AND THINK

Why does the Po_2 decrease in a blood gas syringe placed into an ice water bath?

EQUATION 52-15

Fick's Law

$$V_{gas} = \frac{A}{T} \times D_{gas}(P_1 - P_2)$$

where:

V_{gas} = Volume of gas diffusing across a membrane

A = Surface area for diffusion

T = Thickness of the membrane

$(P_1 - P_2)$ = Pressure gradient

D_{gas} = Diffusibility of the gas (solubility coefficient/density)

$$Do_2 = \frac{0.023}{\sqrt{32 / 22.4}} = 0.0192$$

$$Dco_2 = \frac{0.51}{\sqrt{44 / 22.4}} = 0.364$$

The diffusibility of carbon dioxide (Dco_2) is 19 times greater than that of oxygen (Do_2).

EQUATION 52-16

Gas Conversion Formulas

$$V_{BTPS} = V_{ATPS} \times \frac{Patm - P_{H_2O}(T)}{Patm - P_{H_2O}(37)} \times \frac{273 + 37}{273 + T}$$

$$V_{STPD} = V_{ATPS} \times \frac{Patm}{Patm\ (standard)} \times \frac{273}{273 + T}$$

$$V_{BTPS} = V_{STPD} \times \frac{Patm\ (standard)}{Patm - P_{H_2O}(T)} \times \frac{310}{273}$$

$$V_{STPD} = V_{ATPS} \times \frac{273}{273 + T} \times \frac{Patm\ (standard)}{Patm - P_{H_2O}(T)}$$

where:

V_{BTPS} = Volume at body temperature and pressure, saturated

V_{ATPS} = Volume at atmospheric temperature and pressure, saturated

Patm = Atmospheric pressure

P_{H_2O} = Partial pressure of water

T = Temperature

V_{STPD} = Volume at standard temperature and pressure, dry

V_{ATPD} = Volume at atmospheric temperature and pressure, dry

Patm (standard) = Standard pressure

Conversion of Gas Volumes

Pressure, temperature, and humidity have important effects on gas volume. Several sets of conditions are commonly encountered in respiratory therapy because of the conditions under which certain gases are stored (dry) or measured (body temperature, humidified). These are (1) standard temperature and pressure, dry (STPD); (2) body temperature and pressure, saturated (BTPS); (3) atmospheric temperature and pressure, dry (ATPD); and (4) atmospheric temperature and pressure, saturated (ATPS) (**Table 52-6**). Gas is transformed from ATPD to BTPS on inspiration, causing volume changes due to warming and humidifying. Similarly, although gas may be collected and measured under BTPS conditions, measurement of gas exchange (such as oxygen consumption) usually is reported at STPD, or 1 atm and 0° C. **Equation 52-16** shows conversions between

TABLE 52-6
Common Sets of Conditions Affecting Gas Volume

Condition	Description	Temperature (° C)	Atmospheres (atm)	Relative Humidity (%)
STPD	Standard temperature and pressure, dry	0	1 (760 mm Hg)	0
BTPS	Body temperature and pressure, saturated	37	1	100
ATPD	Atmospheric temperature and pressure, dry	Ambient (<25)	Ambient	0
ATPS	Atmospheric temperature and pressure, saturated	Ambient (<25)	Ambient	100

conditions of BTPS, STPD, and ATPD. Although tables and conversions are readily available, the basis of these equations must be understood, and some conversion factors should be committed to memory.

A frequently needed conversion is between STPD and BTPS. The *gas constant* (which is different from the universal gas constant) is used to convert between the standard temperature and pressure of 1 atm and 0° C and body temperature and pressure of 37° C and 1 atm (**Equation 52-17**). This conversion is important in the calculation of dead space from measurements of carbon dioxide production and minute ventilation. Production of CO_2 is measured in STPD, whereas minute ventilation is directly measured in BTPS.

EQUATION 52-17

Gas Constant

$$(760-47) \div \left(\frac{273}{310} \times \frac{713}{760}\right) = 863$$

$$\text{mm Hg} - \text{mm Hg} \div \left(\frac{°K}{°K} \times \frac{\text{mmHg}}{\text{mmHg}}\right)$$

This constant is the standard partial pressure of dry gas (partial pressure of vapor pressure subtracted from standard atmospheric pressure) divided by the ratio of standard temperature and body temperature in Kelvin (273 and 310 degrees, respectively) multiplied by the ratio of the partial pressure of humidified gas at body temperature to dry gas at 1 atmosphere (760 mm Hg). It is used to express moles of carbon dioxide (CO_2) production in terms of volumes measured at standard temperature and pressure, dry (STPD). Units of temperature cancel.

Expressing Pa_{CO_2} in mm Hg and CO_2 production in mL/min, the gas constant is 0.863:

$$Pa_{CO_2} = \frac{\dot{V}_{CO_2} \times 0.863}{\left(1 - \frac{V_D}{V_T}\right) \times \dot{V}_E}$$

where:

Pa_{CO_2} = Partial pressure of arterial carbon dioxide

$\dot{V}_{CO_2}$ = Carbon dioxide production

V_D = Dead space

V_T = Tidal volume

$\dot{V}_E$ = Minute ventilation

Conservation of Energy

When analyzing a system, one can assume that the total energy of that system is constant. Energy may change forms, but the total amount of energy must remain the same. There are many types of energy, but for the purposes of respiratory care, important types include the following:

- Potential (e.g., a ball on a shelf)
- Kinetic (e.g., a moving ball)

Subtypes of energy are:

- Thermal (e.g., kinetic energy of molecules in hot water)
- Chemical (e.g., potential energy of molecules in unburned fuel)
- Pressure (e.g., potential energy of molecules in a fluid, especially a compressible gas)

When a ball falls off a shelf, its potential energy (a product of its mass and height) is converted to kinetic energy (a function of its mass and velocity), but the same total energy must exist. If chemical energy in the form of fuel is released by burning (oxidization) and heats a pot of cold water, the temperature of the water will increase, or convert to thermal energy. The temperature of the water, or thermal energy, is actually a manifestation of the kinetic energy of the water molecules. The total energy of the system remains the same, with less chemical energy and greater thermal energy. Some of the thermal energy will undoubtedly be lost to increasing the temperature (kinetic energy) of the surrounding air.

Fluid Flow

Flow is the movement of a specified volume of fluid (gas or liquid) in a particular period of time. Both liquids and gases can flow. Gas flow through tubes is a key physical phenomenon in respiratory physiology, whether in reference to the flow of air into and from the lungs or the flow of gas through a ventilator circuit. Flow is central to other areas of physiology as well, such as blood flow through vessels. Flow can be determined mathematically by dividing volume change by time. That is, the rate of volume change determines the rate of flow. Volume can be calculated by multiplying a constant flow rate by time.

Principle of Continuity

If any liquid flows through a rigid pipe, the mass of fluid entering a tube must equal the mass leaving the tube. This concept is the principle of continuity (**Equation 52-18** and **Figure 52-7**). Considering geometry alone, during flow conditions any thin segment of fluid moves a particular distance in a set time. This movement of fluid over a time period is flow **velocity**. The product of velocity and the area of the tube define the volume of fluid moving over

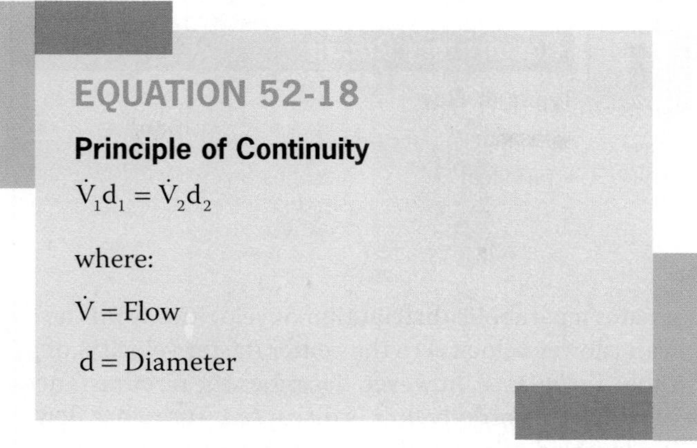

EQUATION 52-18

Principle of Continuity

$$\dot{V}_1 d_1 = \dot{V}_2 d_2$$

where:

$\dot{V}$ = Flow

d = Diameter

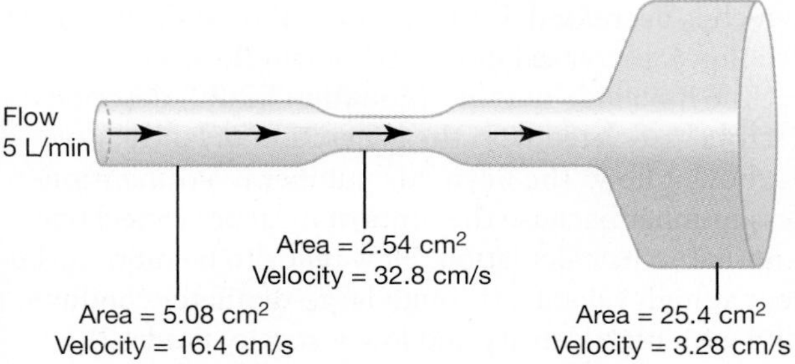

FIGURE 52-7 Principle of continuity. Note that fluid velocity is related inversely to the cross-sectional area.

time. If the diameter (hence, area) of a section of tube increases, the velocity decreases through that segment because the same mass entering must equal the mass exiting the tube. Diameter and velocity therefore are inversely related.

Bernoulli and Venturi Principles

The **Bernoulli principle** generally describes the pressure in a fluid as the velocity changes. The Bernoulli principle explains the lift caused by airplane wings. More specific to respiratory care, if a fluid flowing into a tube reaches a section where the diameter is reduced or constricted, the velocity must increase according to the law of continuity. In the high-velocity section, pressure will be reduced. This occurs because energy must be conserved. In the large-diameter section, velocity is lower, so most of the energy is associated with the pressure. When the diameter is reduced and velocity increases, kinetic energy increases. Because the total energy must remain the same, the pressure energy must decrease as velocity increases. If the diameter of the tubing returns to its original size, the reverse energy shift occurs: kinetic energy will exchange again for pressure energy, and the pressure will return to its original value. This is ideally, but not strictly, true because fluids have viscosity and there is some loss of energy due to viscous friction between the tubing and the fluid and within the fluid itself. But for gas flows (with low viscosity), this analysis is approximately correct.

This phenomenon is particularly important in respiratory care. For instance, in a constricted airway, the reduced pressure will cause a narrow airway to collapse even further. Similarly, vessels tend to collapse with increased blood flow in constricted or partially occluded vessels. The Bernoulli principle is used in some nonrespiratory fields of flow measurement because simple pressure measurements at two diameter points in a tube can estimate a reading of flow; however, these types of devices are not often seen in respiratory care applications.

The **Venturi principle** is an application of the Bernoulli principle and the law of continuity that explains the entrainment of fluids through an open port in a tube. A common misconception is that air entrainment oxygen delivery masks (so-called Venturi masks) operate according to the Bernoulli principle. This is not correct, because such masks operate by entraining a flow of gas through an orifice. The system is open, and, therefore, regions of different diameters will not attain the pressure changes expected from the Bernoulli principle effect. These devices use the converging funnel half of the Venturi tube, increasing the velocity of flow as the same amount of gas moves through a reduced diameter. The higher-velocity gas traveling through the narrowed tube interacts with stagnant ambient air. Molecules of gas exiting the jet collide with molecules in the surrounding air and drag them along, entraining air molecules into the forward flow of gas. The pressure drop across a narrowed section that allows entrainment can be restored if the postsection angle of divergence is less than 15 degrees.

Viscosity

All real fluids, both gases and liquids, have the property of viscosity, which is not accounted for by the Bernoulli principle. The Bernoulli principle assumes that fluids have zero viscosity. Viscosity can be described as the internal friction of a fluid and is independent of the density of a fluid. Molecules of a liquid flowing through a tube collide with the walls and reduce the overall velocity of the liquid. For gas movement, viscosity increases with temperature because the frequency of collisions between molecules is greater at higher temperatures. Viscosity in liquids, however, is increased at lower temperatures. For a viscous fluid such as molasses or oil, viscosity is highly dependent on temperature.

Viscosity most frequently refers to dynamic, or molecular, viscosity. A fluid in motion may be viewed as a set of thin parallel layers that move past each other. Dynamic viscosity is the stickiness between the layers. If a constant force pushes against an upper layer while the lower one is fixed, the upper layer moves with a flow velocity. The required force to achieve a velocity depends on the area of the layer, the viscosity, and the distance between layers (**Equation 52-19**). Measurement of viscosity using SI units is in

EQUATION 52-19

Force and Viscosity

$F = \eta vA/z$

$\eta = Fz/vA$

where:

F = Force

η = Viscosity

v = Velocity

A = Area

z = Distance between plates

pascal-seconds, a unit without a specific name. The poise (dyne × second × cm^2) is a non-SI unit for viscosity that remains in frequent use. Poise is approximately one-tenth the unnamed SI unit. Typically, a gas is less viscous than a liquid. Air is approximately 50 times less viscous than water.

Laminar and Turbulent Flow

Flow of any fluid can be characterized as laminar or turbulent. **Laminar flow** is the orderly flow of a fluid through a straight tube as a series of concentric cylinders slide over one another (**Figure 52-8**). Laminar flow creates a parabolic distribution of velocities from the wall (slower velocity) to the center (faster velocity) of a tube. *Turbulence*, however, describes the circumstances in which this orderly flow is disrupted. **Turbulent flow** is a jumbled mixture of velocities across the section of tube. Friction also has a prominent effect on flow, which is decreased during laminar flow and, conversely, friction is increased during turbulent flow.

Respiratory Recap

Types of Flow

- Laminar
- Turbulent

The **Reynolds number** (**Equation 52-20**) describes factors associated with the generation of laminar or turbulent flow. The Reynolds number is a dimensionless number because the units of measure cancel one another in its calculation. Flow tends to be more turbulent at high velocity, through large-diameter conduits, and with high-density and low-viscosity fluids. The equation shows that density and viscosity are independent factors affecting turbulence. Whereas viscosity is inversely related to the Reynolds number, the fluid density, velocity, and conduit radius are directly related. On a qualitative basis, Reynolds numbers describe a ratio of inertial forces to viscous forces. A fluid with significant inertia (the tendency to continue in the direction of movement) is more likely to be turbulent. A low Reynolds number (under 2000) in smooth tubes with a length substantially longer than the diameter indicates laminar flow, whereas a high number (more than 3000) indicates turbulent flow.

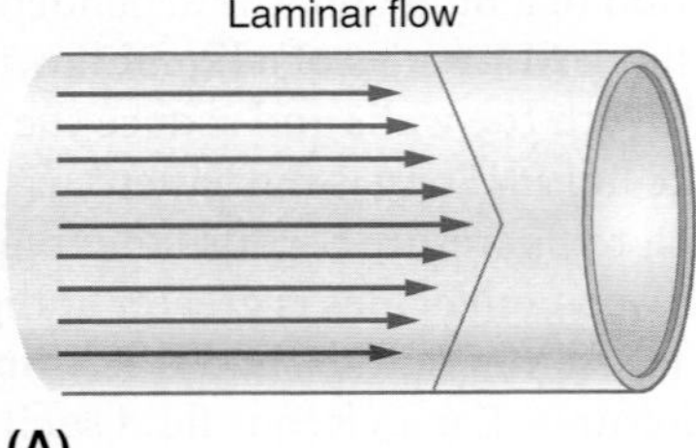

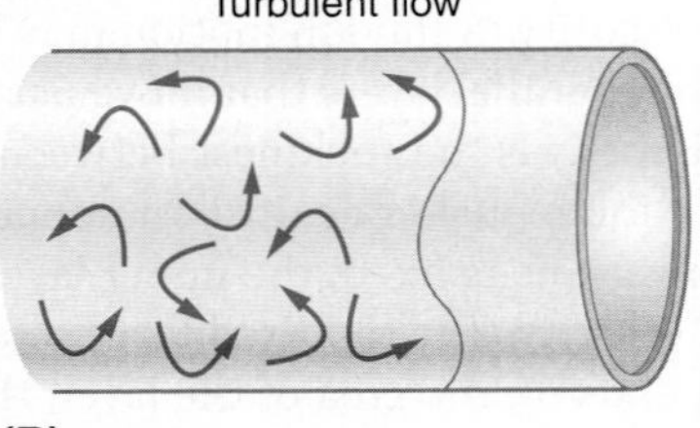

FIGURE 52-8 (**A**) Laminar flow. (**B**) Turbulent flow.

EQUATION 52-20

Reynolds Number

$Re = \text{Inertial forces/Viscous forces} = vr\rho/\eta$

where:

Re = Reynolds number

v = Velocity

r = Radius

ρ = Density

η = Viscosity

Hagen-Poiseuille Equation

If a viscous fluid is flowing without turbulence through a tube (i.e., is laminar), the layer of fluid next to the wall of the tube (the boundary layer) has low velocity due to friction, whereas the layer at the center of the tube has the maximum velocity. The different flow rates create fronts with parabolic configurations. Because of viscosity, analysis beyond the principle of continuity and the Bernoulli principle must be applied. The force required to push flow through a tube is the product of the pressure difference and the area of the tube.

After several mathematic transformations, the **Hagen-Poiseuille equation** can be derived (**Equation 52-21**). A most relevant factor is that flow or pressure drop is related to the fourth power of the radius. Flow is inversely related to the viscosity of the fluid and the length of the tube through which the fluid passes and directly related to the pressure gradient. If these variables remain constant, the pressure gradient over the length of the tubular structure is directly proportional to flow. Most importantly, differential pressure pneumotachographs within ventilators use this principle to measure flow.

The relationship between pressure and a tube's radius is very important in respiratory care. A change in the inside diameter of a tracheal tube from 6 mm to 5 mm increases the pressure drop across the tube by a factor of 2 if constant flow is maintained. Endotracheal tube size can have a dramatic effect on work of breathing.

In contrast to laminar flow, turbulent flow varies directly with the square of flow rate and carries a term for friction, implying greater resistance at equivalent flows. Density rather than viscosity is a more prominent fluid characteristic. These differences explain the use and possible effectiveness of ventilating with helium–oxygen mixtures when the upper airways are narrowed. Although the viscosities of helium, oxygen, and air are not markedly different, helium is much less dense. **Equation 52-22** describes the effects of density when flow is turbulent. Flow velocity is greater in the upper airway and trachea than in the more numerous small airways, as explained by the principle of continuity. The total area of the smaller airways is greater; thus, velocity is less.

Flow, Resistance, and Pressure

An analysis of flow/pressure and resistance relationships assumes linear relationships without the loss of thermal energy or effects of turbulence. This analysis allows application of easily measured quantities, such as resistance, to other circular systems of single or connected circuits in which measurements may be more technically difficult. The more general expression of **Ohm's law** involving electrons flowing in electrical circuits describes the relationships among voltage, current, and resistance (**Equation 52-23**).

In physiologic terms, voltage correlates with pressure differences, current with flow rate, and electrical

EQUATION 52-21

Hagen-Poiseuille Equation

$$\dot{V} = \frac{\Delta P r^4}{8 \eta l}$$

where:

$\dot{V}$ = Flow

ΔP = Pressure gradient

r = Radius

η = Viscosity

l = Length

EQUATION 52-22

Laminar and Turbulent Flow

Laminar Flow

$$\Delta P = \frac{8 \eta l \dot{V}}{r^4}$$

Turbulent Flow

$$\Delta P = \frac{\rho l \dot{V}^2}{4 \pi r^5}$$

where:

ΔP = Pressure gradient

η = Viscosity

l = Length

r = Radius

$\dot{V}$ = Flow

ρ = Density

EQUATION 52-23

Ohm's Law

$$V = I \times R$$

Current

$$I = \frac{V}{R}$$

Resistance

$$R = \frac{V}{I}$$

where:

V = Voltage

R = Resistance

I = Current

For fluid flow, this becomes:

$$\Delta P = \dot{V} \times R$$

Flow

$$\dot{V} = \frac{\Delta P}{R}$$

Resistance

$$R = \frac{\Delta P}{\dot{V}}$$

where:

ΔP = Pressure gradient

R = Resistance

$\dot{V}$ = Flow

resistance with airflow resistance. Ohm's law gives a general expression for **resistance**, the ratio of pressure gradient to flow.

Application of Physical Principles to Measurement and Physiology

Principles of Measurement

Any measurement device will convert a physical entity into a number or signal. Even a water column manometer converts a pressure existing somewhere in a system of interest into a column of water height that can be measured. Electronic transducers are in common use for the purposes of measurement. Important considerations in the ability of measurement devices to record physical signals faithfully include: linearity, the proportional output of a system including hysteresis (i.e., a difference between responses to increasing and decreasing pressure), drift, or the long-term shift in the system output in response to a constant signal, and dynamic response, or distortion of the signal caused by the way the physical signal reaches the transducer.

An analog meter or gauge measures by a physical continuous scale, such as a spring (mechanical) or voltage range (electronic). Passing the signal into a suitable circuit allows simple manipulation of the signal (e.g., integration, differentiation). A digital meter, on the other hand, measures the signal of interest not continuously but at regular, discrete intervals. Digital analysis of a signal permits a more flexible and complicated analysis but must sample the signal at a sufficiently rapid frequency to reproduce it faithfully.

Noise is unwanted effects detected by the recording system. Noise may be intrinsic, such as oscillations or physical movements occurring in a catheter system attached to a pressure manometer, or extrinsic, such as electrical interference occurring between a transducer and an amplifier. A goal is to maximize the signal-to-noise ratio.

Calibration refers to the process by which the output of a measurement system is adjusted to a known input. Calibration may be passive, in which the output is compared with a static input signal (such as a particular set pressure) or dynamic, which compares the system output with a forcing function or probe in which a varying signal is used for calibration.

Common Methods of Measuring Flow in Respiratory Care

Devices that measure flow are capable of faster responses to changes than are devices that directly measure volume. This limitation in frequency response, or ability to faithfully reflect changes in volume over short periods, has restricted the use of volumetric spirometers. Most volume measurement devices in wide use today therefore measure flow and calculate volume by integration.

The following device types are found in mechanical ventilators, spirometers for measurements of pulmonary function, and other specialty devices.

Pneumotachometer

A device that actually measures a pressure difference between two sides of a resistance element. As flow increases, the pressure drop across the element also increases due to viscous forces. If the flow is laminar (nonturbulent), the change in pressure versus flow is nearly linear (i.e., a doubling in flow results in a doubling of pressure). An element can be inserted to laminarize the flow, such as a screen, filter paper, or an array of smaller-diameter tubes, also known as a laminar flow element.

Fixed Orifice Meter

A variant on the pneumotachometer uses a fixed orifice that is not linear because the flow is generally turbulent. This is a simple device that is resistant to fouling with secretions or humidity but requires more sophisticated software to calculate the actual flow. Generally, the total resistance at the highest flow rate will be higher than that measured by a linear pneumotachometer.

Thermal Meter

As flow increases, so does convective heat transfer (think of wind chill). Devices heat an element electrically and measure the power required to maintain a particular temperature. Hence, some method of measuring the temperature of the heated element is also required. One common thermal meter is a hot-wire anemometer.

Ultrasonic Meter

This type of meter operates similar to sonar or radar by measuring the speed of sound as affected by flow toward and away from an ultrasonic signal. The difference represents the gas velocity.

Rotating Vane Anemometer (Wright Respirometer)

This uses a rotating vane set in a tube with oblique slots through which air enters. This device is not linear at low flows because gas can enter the tube before the vanes rotate.

The most straightforward method of flow measurement is direct, timed collection of volume (e.g., of blood or gas); however, this method cannot be applied to a closed system. Any measurement applied must add minimal resistance and generate a signal that is linear over the range of expected flows. Devices used to measure the flow of some liquids include electromagnetic flow meters, which rely on a conductor moving through a magnetic field; ultrasonic flow meters, in which frequency changes of reflected sound waves are measured (the Doppler frequency shift principle); radioactivity counting devices; and direct volume measurement, in which a volume change is directly measured when outflow is occluded for a set period. All these methods have been used to determine blood flow, but the underlying principles do not apply (electromagnetic, ultrasound techniques) or are impractical (plethysmography) to measure airflow.

Key Points

- Molecular theory describes physical entities and their response to physical forces by describing atoms and molecules and the interactions between them.
- Pascal's law describes the way in which pressure is transmitted without reduction throughout any enclosed static fluid; this law is the basis for manometric measurements.
- Laplace's law describes the tension of the wall of a sphere or cylinder (wall tension) and is useful for understanding pressures in an alveolus.
- Surface tension describes the property of liquid that tends to reduce the surface of a liquid toward a minimum, pulling the surface molecules inward.
- The ideal gas law states that pressure and volume are inversely related, whereas temperature is directly proportional to volume or pressure.
- Common conditions for reporting of gas volumes are STPD, BTPS, ATPD, and ATPS.
- A humidity deficit occurs whenever inspired gas is not fully saturated at body temperature.
- Graham's law predicts the rate of diffusion of a gas as inversely proportional to the gram molecular weight of the gas.
- Fick's law describes the transfer of a solute by diffusion.
- The Bernoulli principle describes the pressure drop when fluid passes through a constriction in a rigid tube.
- The Venturi principle states that a pressure drop across an obstruction can be restored provided the angle of divergence is less than 15 degrees.
- The Hagen-Poiseuille equation states that flow is related to the fourth power of the radius, the viscosity of the fluid, the length of the tube, and the pressure gradient.
- The Reynolds number is a dimensionless number used to describe laminar or turbulent flow.
- Ohm's law describes the relationship among pressure, flow, and resistance.

CHAPTER

53

Chemistry for Respiratory Care

Carl F. Haas, Allan G. Andrews, Andrew J. Weirauch

OUTLINE

Basic Chemistry
Inorganic Molecules
Organic Molecules
Fluid Balance
Metabolic Pathways

OBJECTIVES

1. Describe the structure of the atom.
2. Compare ionic, covalent, and hydrogen bonds.
3. Describe synthesis, decomposition, and exchange reactions.
4. List factors that affect the solubility of solutions.
5. Compare methods used to state concentrations of solutions.
6. List colligative properties of solutions.
7. Compare organic and inorganic compounds.
8. Describe the physical and chemical properties of water, oxygen, carbon dioxide, and electrolytes.
9. Describe the chemical properties of acids, bases, buffers, and salts.
10. Discuss the biologic importance of carbohydrates, lipids, proteins, nucleic acids, vitamins, hormones, cytokines, and enzymes.
11. Explain the biologic basis of fluid balance.
12. Describe the energy-producing metabolic pathways.

KEY TERMS

acid
adenosine triphosphate (ATP)
adsorption
allele
amino acid
anabolism
anion
atom
atomic mass unit (amu)
atomic number
atomic weight
base
boiling point
buffer
carbohydrate
catabolism
cation
cholesterol
chromosome
citric acid (Krebs) cycle
colligative property
colloid
compound
concentrated
covalent bond
crenation
cytokine
deoxyribonucleic acid (DNA)
dilute
eicosanoid
electrolyte
electron
electron transport system
element
enzyme
freezing point
genotype
glucose
glycolysis
heat of vaporization
hemolysis
Henderson-Hasselbalch equation
hormone
hydrogen bond
hydrophilic
hydrophobic
hypertonic
hypotonic
ionic bond
ion
isotonic
isotope
lipid
mass number
matter
milliequivalent
molar solution
mole
neutron
nucleic acid
osmosis
osmotic pressure
oxidative phosphorylation
peptide
percent solution
periodic table
pH
phenotype
phospholipid
polar
precipitate
protein
proton
ribonucleic acid (RNA)
saturated
saturated fatty acid
semipermeable membrane
single-nucleotide polymorphism (SNP)
solute
solution
solvent
specific heat
steroid
suspension
triglyceride
unsaturated fatty acid
valence electron
vapor pressure
vitamin

Introduction

Chemistry is the science of the composition, structure, properties, and reactions of matter. An understanding of basic chemistry is essential to the practice of respiratory care. This chapter covers basic chemistry, the chemistry of inorganic and organic molecules, fluid balance, and metabolic pathways.

Basic Chemistry

Matter

Anything that occupies space and has mass is **matter**. Matter is classified as an element or a compound. An **element** cannot be broken down into two or more substances; it is a pure substance containing only one type of atom. Although oxygen is a good example of an element, most living materials are not composed of pure elements but rather are a combination of elements. When two or more elements join to form a chemical combination, the result is a **compound**. Three important examples of compounds in the human body are water (H_2O), in which two hydrogen atoms combine with one oxygen atom; carbon dioxide (CO_2), in which one carbon atom combines with two oxygen atoms; and glucose ($C_6H_{12}O_6$), in which six carbon atoms combine with twelve hydrogen and six oxygen atoms.

The **atom** often is called the building block of the universe. It is the smallest portion of an element that retains all the properties of the element. Each atom is composed of a small, heavy, core-like nucleus with particles surrounding it at relatively great distances.

Three fundamental particles that make up the atom are the proton, the neutron, and the electron. **Protons** have a positive electrical charge (+1) and are located in the nucleus. **Neutrons** have no net electrical charge and are also located in the nucleus. **Electrons** have a negative electrical charge (–1) and are located outside the nucleus (**Figure 53-1**). This gives the atomic nucleus a positive charge and the surrounding electron cloud a negative charge.

The number of protons in the nucleus defines the element and is known as the **atomic number**. Because all atoms are electrically neutral, the number of electrons is the same as the number of protons. The sum of the protons and neutrons determines the atom's **mass number**. The naturally occurring sodium atom has an atomic number of 11 and a mass number of 23, indicating 11 protons and electrons and 12 neutrons. The relative weight of an atom is its **atomic weight**, a term often used interchangeably with *mass number*. The carbon atom, which has a mass number of 12 (carbon-12), has been assigned the weight of 12 **atomic mass units (amu)**, to which all other atoms are referenced.

Each element has a unique atomic number, suggesting a specific and unchanging number of protons in the nucleus, but not necessarily the same mass number. **Isotopes** are atoms with nuclei that have the same number of protons (atomic number) but a different number of neutrons (mass number). All elements have isotopes. Oxygen has three isotopes, each having eight protons and eight electrons but 8, 9, or 10 neutrons (99.8% of atmospheric oxygen is composed of oxygen-16, 0.04% is oxygen-17, and 0.16% is oxygen-18). Isotopes of the same element have the same basic chemical properties because they have the same number of electrons and protons, but they have different physical properties because they differ in the number of neutrons. Most isotopes are stable and do not break up, particularly the lighter elements. Isotopes of some of the heavier unstable elements give off radiation when they break up and are referred to as being *radioactive*.

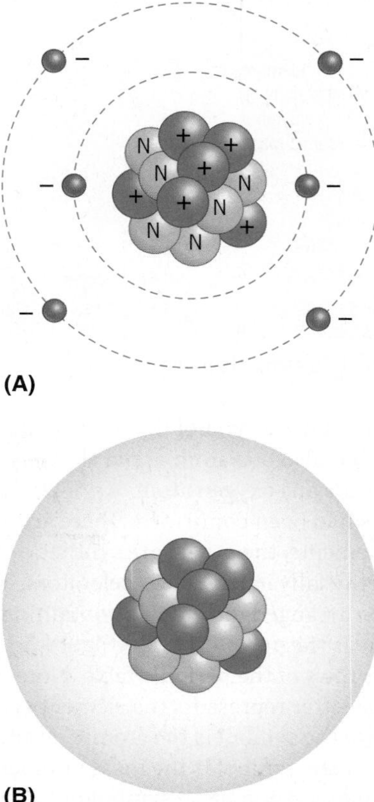

FIGURE 53-1 Model of the atom. (**A**) The nucleus contains protons (+1 change) and neutrons (0 charge). Electrons (–1 charge) occupy the outer regions, which are called electron shells. This figure represents the carbon atom, which has six protons and six neutrons in the nucleus and six electrons orbiting the nucleus. Two electrons are in the first electron shell, and the remaining four are in the outer shell. (**B**) The outer shells can be thought of collectively as an electron cloud.

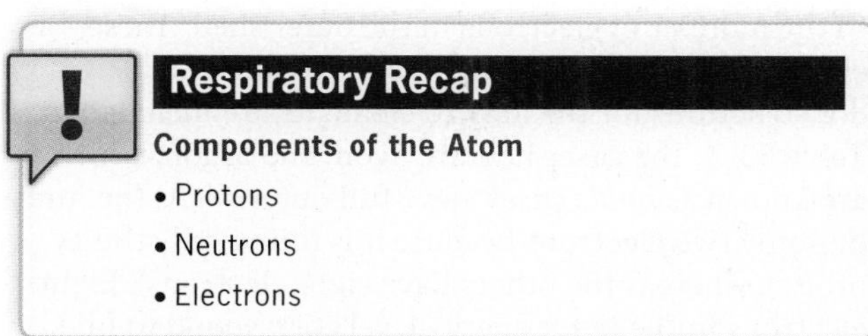

Respiratory Recap
Components of the Atom
• Protons
• Neutrons
• Electrons

Element	hydrogen
Atomic number	1
Symbol	H
Atomic mass	1.01

Metals
Metalloids
Nonmetals

1 IA	2 IIA	3 IIIB	4 IVB	5 VB	6 VIB	7 VIIB	8 VIII	9 VIII	10 VIII	11 IB	12 IIB	13 IIIA	14 IVA	15 VA	16 VIA	17 VIIA	18 VIIIA
																	helium 2 He 4.00
lithium 3 Li 6.94	beryllium 4 Be 9.01											boron 5 B 10.81	carbon 6 C 12.01	nitrogen 7 N 14.01	oxygen 8 O 16.00	fluorine 9 F 19.00	neon 10 Ne 20.18
sodium 11 Na 22.99	magnesium 12 Mg 24.31											aluminum 13 Al 26.98	silicon 14 Si 28.09	phosphorus 15 P 30.97	sulfur 16 S 32.07	chlorine 17 Cl 35.45	argon 18 Ar 39.95
potassium 19 K 39.10	calcium 20 Ca 40.08	scandium 21 Sc 44.96	titanium 22 Ti 47.88	vanadium 23 V 50.94	chromium 24 Cr 52.00	manganese 25 Mn 54.94	iron 26 Fe 55.85	cobalt 27 Co 58.93	nickel 28 Ni 58.69	copper 29 Cu 63.55	zinc 30 Zn 65.39	gallium 31 Ga 69.72	germanium 32 Ge 72.61	arsenic 33 As 74.92	selenium 34 Se 78.96	bromine 35 Br 79.90	krypton 36 Kr 83.80

FIGURE 53-2 The first 36 elements of the periodic table of the elements.

Each element has a symbol that represents not only the element but also one atom of the element. The symbol O stands for one oxygen atom. As of 2014, 117 chemical elements had been confirmed. There are 94 naturally occurring elements; the others are synthetic elements produced artificially in particle accelerators. These elements can be arranged into a table containing seven rows, known as the **periodic table. Figure 53-2** shows the first four rows of the periodic table. Note in each box that the large letter represents the element symbol, the number above the symbol is the atomic number, and the number below the symbol is the mass number.

For example, carbon has a symbol of C, an atomic number of 6, and a mass number of 12.01. Elements in a vertical column belong to the same *group.* They have similar chemical properties because they have the same number of electrons in their outer shell. For example, each element in column IA has one electron in its outer shell, whereas elements in column VIIA have seven electrons. Elements in a horizontal row belong to the same *period.* It is interesting that 21 of the first 36 elements on the periodic table are found in the body. **Table 53-1** lists elements that are important to the functioning of the human body.

Electrons are arranged in a definite order in the atom. They occupy various principal energy levels, or *shells,* which can be thought of as a volume occupied by an electron cloud. Each level can hold a maximum number of electrons, which is defined by the formula $2n^2$, where n is the number of energy levels or orbits from the nucleus. The first level can hold 2 electrons; the second, 8; the third, 18, and so on. Each element in a given period (row) in the periodic table has the same number of energy levels, or orbitals. For example, the elements in the first row have one orbital for their electrons, the elements in the second row each have two energy levels, and so on. Currently the maximum number of orbitals or shells is seven.

Each energy level has sublevels, called *subshells.* As the energy level increases, so does the number of subshells. The atoms of known elements have four types of subshells, labeled *s, p, d,* and *f.* In excited atoms, electrons may occur in subshells labeled *g, h, i,* and so on, but further detail is beyond the scope of this discussion.

The number of subshells is equal to the shell (energy level) number. The first energy level has one subshell, the *s* subshell, which contains two electrons (one pair). The second energy level has two subshells: an *s* subshell (2*s*) containing two electrons, and a *p* subshell (2*p*) that has six electrons (three pairs). The third energy level has an *s* subshell (3*s*) with two electrons, a *p* subshell (3*p*) with six electrons, and a *d* subshell (3*d*), which holds 10 electrons (five pairs). The fourth energy level has the *s, p, d* subshells and an *f* subshell, which can hold 14 electrons (seven pairs). Electrons fill shells in an orderly manner: first the orbital 1*s*; then 2*s*; then 2*p* and 3*s*; then 3*p* and 4*s*; then 3*d*, 4*p*, and 5*s*; then 4*d*, 5*p*, and 6*s*; then 4*f*, 5*d*, 6*p*, and 7*s*; followed by 5*f*, 6*d*, and 7*p*. Overlapping of shells begins with the transition from shell 3 to shell 4.

The number of electrons in the various energy levels of an element can be represented by a notation referred to as the *electron configuration.* For example, the electron configuration for the element sodium (Na, atomic number 11) is $1s^22s^22p^63s^1$. This representation indicates that the 1*s* subshell has two electrons, the 2*s* subshell has two electrons, the 2*p* subshell has six electrons, and the 3*s* (outermost) subshell has one electron. **Table 53-2** shows the electron configuration for the first 20 elements.

Chemical Bonding

The outermost electron shell is most important to determine an element's chemical properties, because these orbitals are involved in the formation of chemical bonds and in chemical reactions. An electron dot structure, known as a *Lewis dot structure,* often is used to represent the structure of an atom. The nucleus and all the filled energy levels are represented by the element's symbol; the symbol is surrounded by dots equal to the number of electrons in the outer shell. These electrons are known as **valance electrons.** The Lewis dot structures for the first 20 elements are included in Table 53-2. The gases helium, neon, and argon, which are known as *noble gases,* have full outer shells (helium has only two electrons because it is filling only the 1*s* orbital, whereas the others have eight electrons). Eight electrons in the outer energy level correspond to filled

TABLE 53-1
Important Elements Found in the Body

Element	Symbol	Atomic Number	Percentage of Body Weight	Function or Importance
Major Elements				
Oxygen	O	8	65.0	Cellular respiration; a component of water and organic compounds
Carbon	C	6	18.5	Backbone of organic molecules
Hydrogen	H	1	9.5	Component of water and most organic molecules; necessary for energy transfer and respiration
Nitrogen	N	7	3.3	Component of all proteins and nucleic acids
Calcium	Ca	20	1.5	Component of bones and teeth; necessary for certain enzymes, nerve and muscle function, hormonal action, cellular motility, and blood clotting
Phosphorus	P	15	1.0	Main component of nucleic acids; required for bones and teeth; important in energy transfer and for phospholipids and some proteins
Potassium	K	19	0.4	Main positive intracellular ion; important in muscle and nerve function
Sulfur	S	16	0.3	Component of most proteins and some organic compounds
Sodium	Na	11	0.2	Important positive ion surrounding cells; important in muscle and nerve function and in fluid balance
Chlorine	Cl	17	0.2	Important negative ion surrounding cells
Magnesium	Mg	12	0.1	Component of many energy-transferring enzymes
Trace Elements				
Silicon	Si	14	<0.1	Helps form connective tissue and bone
Iron	Fe	26	<0.1	Critical component of blood hemoglobin and many enzymes
Manganese	Mn	25	<0.1	Requirement for many enzymes
Fluorine	F	9	<0.1	Requirement for bones and teeth; inhibitor of certain enzymes
Chromium	Cr	24	<0.1	Relationship to action of insulin
Copper	Cu	29	<0.1	Requirement for many enzymes, for the synthesis of hemoglobin, and for normal bone formation
Boron	B	5	<0.1	Aids in the use of Ca, P, and Mg
Cobalt	Co	27	<0.1	Assistance to vitamin B_{12} in blood clot production
Zinc	Zn	30	<0.1	Requirement for many enzymes; related to action of insulin; essential for normal growth and reproduction
Selenium	Se	34	<0.1	Close relationship to action of vitamin E
Molybdenum	Mo	42	<0.1	Key component of many enzymes
Iodine	I	53	<0.1	Component of thyroid hormone

TABLE 53-2
Electron Representations of the First 20 Elements

Element	Atomic Number	Electron Configuration	Lewis Dot Structure
H	1	$1s^1$	H·
He	2	$1s^2$	He:
Li	3	$1s^22s^1$	Li·
Be	4	$1s^22s^2$	Be:
B	5	$1s^22s^22p^1$	B̈·
C	6	$1s^22s^22p^2$	C̣̈·
N	7	$1s^22s^22p^3$	:Ṇ̇·
O	8	$1s^22s^22p^4$	:Ọ̈·
F	9	$1s^22s^22p^5$	:F̤̈·
Ne	10	$1s^22s^22p^6$	:N̤̈e:
Na	11	$1s^22s^22p^63s^1$	Na·
Mg	12	$1s^22s^22p^63s^2$	Mg:
Al	13	$1s^22s^22p^63s^23p^1$	Äl·
Si	14	$1s^22s^22p^63s^23p^2$	S̈ịi·
P	15	$1s^22s^22p^63s^23p^3$	·P̣̈·
S	16	$1s^22s^22p^63s^23p^4$	:S̈ị·
Cl	17	$1s^22s^22p^63s^23p^5$	:C̤̈l·
Ar	18	$1s^22s^22p^63s^23p^6$	:Ä̤r:
K	19	$1s^22s^22p^63s^23p^64s^1$	K·
Ca	20	$1s^22s^22p^63s^23p^64s^2$	Ca:

H, hydrogen; He, helium; Li, lithium; Be, beryllium; B, boron; C, carbon; N, nitrogen; O, oxygen; F, fluorine; Ne, neon; Na, sodium; Mg, magnesium; Al, aluminum; Si, silicon; P, phosphorus; S, sulfur; Cl, chlorine; Ar, argon; K, potassium; Ca, calcium.

s and *p* orbitals, which lead to great stability. This tendency to fill the *s* and *p* levels is known as the *octet rule.* Elements with the same number of valance electrons are in the same column in the periodic table. They belong to the same group or family and have similar chemical properties. Such elements tend to form similar compounds and often substitute for each other.

Atoms bond in such a way that each atom participating in the chemical bond either acquires a completed outer shell and attains the configuration of the closest noble gas to satisfy the octet rule or obtains at least a spin pair of electrons in the outer shell. Stable configurations are achieved by the transfer of electrons (**ionic bond**) or by the sharing of electrons (**covalent bond**). Elements with only one, two, or three valence electrons tend to give them up, thereby becoming positive **ions**. Positively charged ions are known as **cations**. Sodium (Na) loses its one valance electron and takes on a +1 charge (11 protons and 10 electrons); aluminum (Al) loses its three valance electrons and takes on a +3 charge (13 protons and 10 electrons) (**Equation 53-1**). Elements with six or seven valance electrons tend to gain electrons to reach stability. Chlorine (Cl), which has seven valance electrons, gains one electron to fill its outer shell, thereby taking on a –1 charge and becoming a negative ion. Similarly, sulfur (S) takes on two electrons to fill its outer shell and becomes an ion with a –2 charge. Negatively charged ions are known as **anions**.

Ions of opposite charge are attracted to each other. When a sodium atom (Na) combines with a chlorine atom (Cl) to form a sodium chloride molecule (NaCl), the sodium atom loses (or donates) an electron, and the

EQUATION 53-1

Cations and Anions

Cations

$Na - 1e \rightarrow Na^{+}$

$Al - 3e \rightarrow Al^{+3}$

Anions

$Cl + 1e \rightarrow Cl^{-}$

$S + 2e \rightarrow S^{-2}$

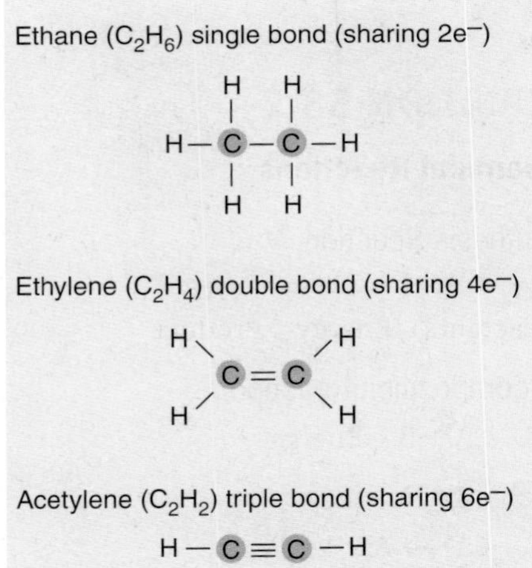

FIGURE 53-3 Formation of carbon–carbon single, double, and triple bonds.

chlorine atom gains (or accepts) the electron. In the process a positive sodium cation (Na^+) and a negative chloride (Cl^-) anion are formed. The two opposite-charged ions are held together by electrostatic attraction of their opposite charges to form a sodium chloride molecule:

$$Na^+ + Cl^- \rightarrow NaCl$$

Compounds having ionic bonds, called *ionic compounds*, share some characteristics, such as high melting and boiling points and the ability to conduct electricity in the gaseous or liquid state. Ions are very important in the chemistry of the body, especially as electrolytes and minerals.

Another type of bonding involves the sharing of one or more pairs of electrons to achieve a stable electron configuration. When each of the two bonding atoms shares one of its valance electrons, the bond is referred to as a *covalent bond*. When one of the atoms shares two of its valance electrons with another atom, the bond is called a *dative bond*. Once formed, both covalent and dative bonds produce a shared pair of electrons and therefore have identical structures. The molecular orbital theory is used to describe the sharing of electrons and the overlap of atomic orbitals. When the atomic orbital of one atom overlaps with the atomic orbital of another atom, two new molecular orbitals are formed that encompass both nuclei. Each molecular orbital can hold one spin pair of electrons, which is the property of the whole molecule, not just the atoms forming the bond. This molecular arrangement is more stable than a combination in which each nucleus retains its own electrons.

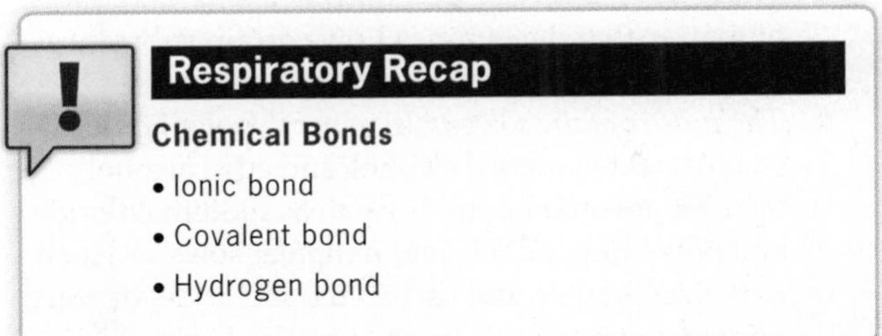

Respiratory Recap
Chemical Bonds
• Ionic bond
• Covalent bond
• Hydrogen bond

Atoms often share more than one pair of electrons. When one, two, or three pairs of electrons are shared, the covalent bonds formed are called *single* (–), *double* (=), or *triple* (≡) bonds, respectively. The carbon atom has four valence electrons that can be shared to form covalent bonds (**Figure 53-3**). It uses all three types of covalent bonds when bonding with another carbon atom, often with the remaining valence electrons single bonded with hydrogen atoms.

The covalent bond is particularly important in physiology because the major elements of the body (carbon, oxygen, hydrogen, and nitrogen) almost always share electrons to form bonds. Carbon, nitrogen, and oxygen form covalent bonds using atomic orbitals of the second principal energy level (elements in the second row on the periodic table). Table 53-2 shows that oxygen (atomic number 8) has six valence electrons and that the two unpaired electrons in the 2*p* subshell are available to form covalent bonds. Oxygen exists naturally as a diatomic molecule (O_2), which uses a double covalent bond to form. When two oxygen atoms unite to form molecular oxygen, each oxygen atom shares its two unpaired 2*p* electrons.

In addition to covalent and ionic bonds, which form molecules, a third type of bond can exist within or between biologically important molecules. The **hydrogen bond** is a weak bond and requires much less energy to break than a covalent or ionic bond. It forms as the result of unequal charge distribution on a molecule rather than from sharing or transfer of electrons. This type of molecule is called a **polar** molecule. Water is a polar molecule; although it is electrically neutral, it has a partial positive charge on the hydrogen side and a partial negative charge on the oxygen side. Hydrogen bonds weakly attach the negative (oxygen) side of one water molecule with the positive (hydrogen) side of an adjacent water molecule. This ability of water to form hydrogen bonds

EQUATION 53-2

Chemical Reactions

Synthesis Reaction

$$\underset{\text{Reactants}}{A + B} \xrightarrow[\text{Energy}]{} \underset{\text{Product}}{AB}$$

Decomposition Reaction

$$AB \rightarrow A + B + \text{Energy}$$

Exchange Reaction

$$AB + CD \rightarrow AD + CB$$

$$H \cdot \text{Lactate} + NaHCO_3 \rightarrow Na \cdot \text{Lactate} + H_2CO_3$$

makes water an ideal medium for the chemistry of life. Hydrogen bonds also help maintain the three-dimensional structure of proteins and nucleic acids.

Chemical Reactions

Chemical reactions involve the formation or breaking of chemical bonds between atoms and molecules. The three basic types of chemical reactions are synthesis reactions, decomposition reactions, and exchange reactions (**Equation 53-2**). *Synthesis reactions* combine two or more substances (reactants) to form a different, more complex substance (product). Energy is required for this reaction to occur and the new product to be formed.

Decomposition reactions break down complex substances into two or more simpler substances. During this reaction chemical bonds are broken, and energy is released. The energy can be released in the form of heat energy, or it can be captured and stored for future use. An example of a decomposition reaction is the breakdown of a complex nutrient in a cell to release energy for other cellular functions. The products of such reactions are ultimately waste products. Synthesis and decomposition reactions are opposites: synthesis forms chemical bonds and builds up, whereas decomposition undoes bonds and breaks down. Often the two opposite processes are coupled in such a way that the energy released through decomposition is used to drive a synthesis reaction.

Respiratory Recap

Chemical Reactions

- Synthesis reaction
- Decomposition reaction
- Exchange reaction

An *exchange reaction* allows two reactants to exchange components and to form two new products. Exchange reactions break down two compounds and synthesize two new compounds. An example of such a reaction in the blood is the reaction of lactic acid with sodium bicarbonate to form sodium lactate and carbonic acid.

Liquid Mixtures

Most chemical reactions in the body take place in a liquid environment. Water is the primary liquid in the body, making up about 45% to 80% of the human body. Every cellular process takes place in a watery environment, and water is essential to the processes of digestion, circulation, elimination, and regulation of body temperature. Water allows substances and particles to get into a liquid form as one of three types: a solution, a suspension, or a colloid.

A **solution** is a homogeneous mixture of two or more substances, meaning that the substances mix evenly and occupy the entire volume of the solution in equal proportions. A liquid solution consists of two parts: the **solute**, which is the solid, liquid, or gaseous material being dissolved, and the **solvent**, which is the liquid material into which the solute is dissolved. Water is the most common solvent in the body. Common nonbody solvents are alcohol, which forms the basis of medicinal tinctures, and ether, which dissolves fats and oils.

Solutions have several common characteristics: they have a variable concentration; they are transparent; they are homogeneous; they do not settle; they may be separated by physical means; and they can pass through filter paper. When a salt crystal is dropped into a glass of water and stirred, the crystal dissolves and the solution remains clear. The same thing occurs when sugar is mixed with water. If more salt or sugar (solute) is mixed into the water (solvent), the solution becomes more concentrated but remains clear. If the solution is poured into a funnel with filter paper, the solute particles pass though, indicating that solute particles in a solution are very small. If the glass is left undisturbed for a time, the solute particles do not settle out provided evaporation does not occur. Should the solvent evaporate, the solute particles would be left behind.

The degree to which solute particles can dissolve into a solvent is referred to as the *solubility of the solution.* A high solubility indicates that the solvent allows many solute particles to be dissolved. The following factors affect solubility.

- *The nature of the solute*: A physical characteristic of matter that determines how certain substances dissolve in a solvent.
- *The nature of the solvent*: In general, polar liquids (such as water, methyl alcohol, and ethyl alcohol) dissolve polar compounds (such as sodium chloride and potassium iodide), and nonpolar solvents (such as benzene, ether, and carbon tetrachloride) dissolve nonpolar compounds (such as oils and waxes).

- *Temperature*: Most solids become more soluble as temperature increases (i.e., the solubility of solids is directly related to temperature), although sodium chloride shows little change; gases become less soluble as temperature increases (the solubility of gases is inversely related to temperature).
- *Pressure*: The solubility of a gas is directly related to pressure, although pressure has little effect on solid or liquid solutes.
- *Surface area*: Although the actual solubility is not changed, the rate of dissolution is directly related to surface area, which explains the rationale for a powder solute.
- *Agitation*: Stirring a solution brings solute particles in contact with fresh solvent more quickly, which increases the rate of dissolution but not the actual solubility.

The relative concentration, or strength, of a solution is classified as dilute or concentrate. **Dilute** means that the solution contains a small amount of solute. As more solute is added, the solution becomes more **concentrated**. No specific point exists at which dilute becomes concentrated; these are relative terms, used only in a comparative sense, and do not provide a specific quantitative meaning. The term **saturated** means that the maximum amount of solute is dissolved for given conditions. If conditions such as temperature or pressure change, the maximum amount of solute that a given volume of solvent can dissolve also changes. An unsaturated solution contains fewer solute particles than it maximally could under normal conditions. A supersaturated solution contains more solute particles than it normally does under specific conditions. Such a solution is formed by the addition of solute as a mixture is heated, until the solution is saturated. On slow cooling, if the solution is not disturbed, excess solute remains in solution. Such a solution is very unstable, and any physical disturbance causes the excess solute to crystallize and form a solid, or **precipitate**, at the bottom of the container.

The terms related to saturation are relative and do not indicate the quantity of solute in solution. In hospitals, chemical laboratories, and industry it is important to be specific; therefore, more precise terms must be used. A **molar solution** is defined as a solution that contains 1 mole (mol) of solute per liter of solution. One **mole** of a substance is equal to its gram molecular weight, which has 6.02×10^{23} atoms (Avogadro's number). Carbon-12 has an atomic weight of 12 amu; therefore, the gram molecular weight of carbon-12 is 12 g. One mole of carbon-12 weighs 12 g. When 1 mole of an element combines with 1 mole of another element, the result is 1 mole of a new molecule or substance. For example, a mole of potassium chloride (KCl) contains 1 mole of potassium (K) atoms and 1 mole of chlorine (Cl) atoms, or 6.02×10^{23} KCl molecules. Therefore, the weight of KCl (74.4 g) is the sum of the gram molecular weights of K (39 g) and Cl (35.4 g).

EQUATION 53-3

Calculation of Moles

Number of moles = Number of grams / Gram molecular weight

Example: Given the gram molecular weight of carbon is 12 g, calculate the number of moles in 8 grams of carbon.

12 g carbon / mol = 8 g carbon / x moles

12 g (x) = 8 g

x = 0.67 mol

The concept of molarity is commonly used in chemistry to quantify solute in solutions. It reflects the number of moles of a solute per volume of solvent:

Molarity (M) = Number of moles (mol) / Liter (L)

Given the weight (grams) and the gram molecular weight of a solute, it is possible to determine the number of moles (**Equation 53-3**) and therefore the molarity of a solution (**Equation 53-4**).

In clinical situations, a **percent solution** is used more often. *Percent* implies parts per hundred, so *percent solution* specifies the number of parts of solute

EQUATION 53-4

Calculation of Molarity

Example: Calculate the molarity of a 150 mL solution containing 10 g of NaCl.

Step 1: Determine the weight of 1 mol of NaCl. (Given the gram molecular weight of sodium is 23 g and that of chloride is 35 g.)

1 mol NaCl = 23 g + 35 g = 58 g

Step 2: Determine the number of moles of NaCl in 10 g.

1 mol / 58 g = x mol / 10 g

58 g (x mol) = 10 g

x = 0.172 mol

Step 3: Convert 150 mL to L

150 mL (1 L / 1000 mL) = 0.15 L

Step 4: Determine the molarity.

M = 0.172 mol NaCl / 0.15 L = 1.15 M

EQUATION 53-5

Weight/Weight Percent Solutions

w/w% =

(Grams of solute × 100%) / (Grams of solute + Grams of solvent)

Example: Calculate the percent solution containing 2.5 g of sugar in 47.5 g of water. Because both the solute and solvent are expressed as weights, the weight/weight percent method is used.

w/w% =

(2.5 g sugar × 100%) / (2.5 g sugar + 47.5 g H_2O) = 5% (w/w%)

present per 100 parts of solution. Dilute concentrations are sometimes given as parts per million (ppm), such as the dose of inhaled nitric oxide. The three commonly used percent measurements are weight/weight percent, weight/volume percent, and volume/volume percent.

The weight/weight percent method (w/w%) describes the relative weight of the solute (in grams) compared with the total weight of the solution (**Equation 53-5**). The weight/volume percent method (w/v%) describes the weight of the solute with the relative volume of solution (in milliliters) and is commonly used in clinical situations and in pharmacology (**Equation 53-6**).

EQUATION 53-6

Weight/Volume Percent Solutions

w/v% =

(Grams of solute / mL of solution) × 100%

Example: What percent solution is the bronchodilator albuterol if its concentration is 2.5 mg/0.5 mL? Because the solute is expressed as a weight and the solvent as a volume, the weight/volume percent method is used.

w/v% = (2.5 mg / 0.5 mL) × 100%

= 500 mg/mL

Then convert to grams:

= (500 mg/mL) × (1 g/1000 mg) × 100%

= 5% (w/v%)

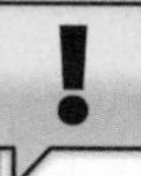

Respiratory Recap

Concentration of a Solution

- Molar
- Percent
- Weight/weight
- Weight/volume
- Volume/volume
- Ratio
- Normal

The volume/volume percent method (v/v%) describes the volume of solute compared with the total volume of solution and is commonly used with liquid solutes (such as in expressions of the alcohol content of beer or wine) (**Equation 53-7**).

Simple ratios are sometimes used to describe the concentration of certain drugs. A ratio of 1:100 indicates that 1 g of solute is dissolved in 100 mL of solvent (**Equation 53-8**). In clinical medicine it often is necessary to prepare a weaker solution from a stronger (stock) solution. This usually is done by the addition of water or 0.9% NaCl to the stock solution (**Equation 53-9**).

Gram equivalent weight is the mass of a substance that will supply or react with one mole of hydrogen ions (H^+) in an acid–base reaction. The gram equivalent weight of a compound can be calculated by dividing the gram molecular weight by the number of positive or negative electrical charges that result from the dissolution of the compound. The normality of a solution is the number of gram equivalent weights in a liter of solution. A 1 normal (N) solution contains 1-gram equivalent weight in 1 L of solution.

The properties of a pure solvent are different from those of a solution. The term **colligative properties** refer to the properties of solutions that depend on the

EQUATION 53-7

Volume/Volume Percent Solutions

v/v% = (mL of solute / mL of solution) × 100%

Example: A 0.75 L bottle of wine contains 60 mL of ethanol. What is the percentage (v/v%) of ethanol in this aqueous solution? Because both the solute and solvent are expressed as volumes, the volume/volume percent method is used.

v/v% = (60 mL / 750 mL) × 100%

= 8% (v/v%)

EQUATION 53-8

Ratio Concentrations

Example: How much solute (active drug) of epinephrine is contained in 0.5 mL of a 1:200 solution?
Step 1: Determine the concentration of a 1:200 solution.

$$1{:}200 = 1\ \text{g} / 200\ \text{mL} = 1000\ \text{mg} / 200\ \text{mL} = 5\ \text{mg/mL}$$

Step 2: Calculate the amount of solute.

$$0.5\ \text{mL epinephrine}\ (5\ \text{mg}/1\ \text{mL}) = 2.5\ \text{mg solute}$$

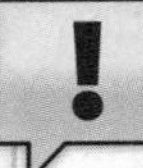

Respiratory Recap

Colligative Properties of Solutions

- Depress vapor pressure
- Depress freezing point
- Elevate boiling point
- Elevate osmotic pressure

number of solute particles dissolved and not on chemical properties. Such properties include vapor pressure, boiling point, freezing point, and osmotic pressure. When a solute is added to a solvent, the solute dilutes the solvent and displaces some of the solvent particles at the surface of the solution. This displacement allows fewer solvent particles to escape in the form of gas particles, thereby reducing the **vapor pressure** of the solution. As a result of the lower vapor pressure, a higher temperature is required to raise the vapor pressure to atmospheric pressure. The solute particles in effect raise the **boiling point** of the solution compared with a pure solvent. For every mole of solute particles added per kilogram of water (1 kg of water has a volume of 1 L), the boiling point is raised 0.52° C. Solute particles also reduce the likelihood that water will enter the solid state and freeze, effectively reducing the **freezing point** of the solution. This is why salt is added to water when pasta is boiled (to raise the boiling point) and why salt is added to ice on sidewalks or antifreeze is added to radiators (to reduce the freezing point).

Another colligative property of solutions involves osmosis. **Osmosis** is the process by which water molecules are transferred through a semipermeable membrane. A **semipermeable membrane** allows water but no other molecules to pass through it. Osmosis is very important in the maintenance of water balance between intracellular and extracellular fluid. It involves the movement of water from an area of high concentration of water to an area of low concentration in an attempt to make the concentrations equal. As an example, **Figure 53-4** shows the effect of the placement of equal volumes of 20% NaCl and 40% NaCl in a U-tube container, with the two sides separated by

EQUATION 53-9

Dilution of Stock Solutions

$$V_1 \times C_1 = V_2 \times C_2$$

where V_1 and V_2 are the initial and final volumes, and C_1 and C_2 are the initial and final concentrations, respectively.
Example: Prepare 5 mL of a 10% solution, given a 20% stock solution. Given C_1 (20%), C_2 (10%), and V_2 (5 mL), solve for V_1 (x mL of stock solution).

$$x\ \text{mL stock solution} \times 20\% = 5\ \text{mL} \times 10\%$$

$$20x = 50\ \text{mL}$$

$$x = 2.5\ \text{mL}$$

To prepare the solution, take 2.5 mL of the 20% stock solution and add 2.5 mL of water to dilute it to a final 5 mL 10% solution.

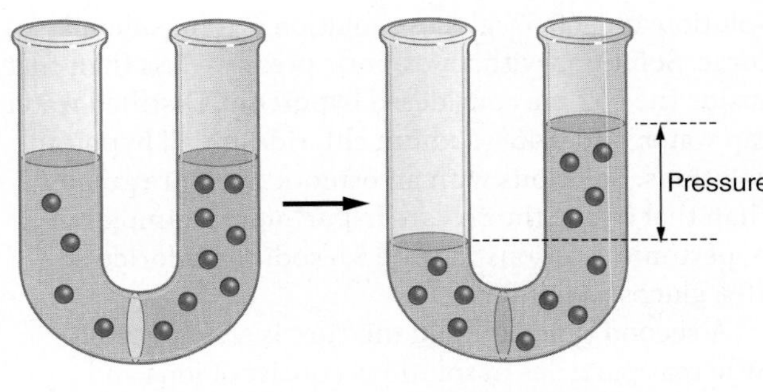

FIGURE 53-4 Osmotic pressure. (**A**) A U-shaped tube divided by a semipermeable membrane has a 20% sodium chloride (NaCl) solution on the left side of the membrane and an equal volume of 40% NaCl solution on the right side. As time passes, water moves from the area of the high-solvent (water) and the low-solute (NaCl) concentration (left side) to the area of low-solvent and high-solute concentration (right side). (**B**) Because the membrane allows movement only of the solvent and not of the solute, the volume on the right side increases. The difference in the height of the water column creates back pressure, which helps stop the flow of water.

a semipermeable membrane. Because the concentration of NaCl is higher on the right, the concentration of water must be lower on that side. Water therefore moves from an area of high water concentration (the left side) to an area of low concentration (the right side). This net movement of water results in both sides of the membrane having equal concentrations of solution, but because the membrane did not allow solute particles to pass through, the volume of fluid on the right is now much greater than on the left. The increased volume raises the height of the column of fluid, which exerts a pressure. External pressure (hydrostatic) can be applied to the right side of the column to push the higher column down and make the sides equal again. The externally applied pressure that would just stop the flow of solvent through the membrane is called the **osmotic pressure**. The osmotic pressure of pure water is always zero, whereas the osmotic pressure of a solution is directly related to the number of solute particles in solution. The greater the concentration of the solution, the greater the osmotic pressure the solution exerts.

Cells in the body can be harmed if the concentrations of solutes in the body fluids are not carefully maintained. If the concentration of water outside a red blood cell is less than that inside the cell (i.e., the osmotic pressure is higher outside the cell), water leaves the cell, causing it to shrivel, a process called **crenation**. In the reverse situation, when the water concentration is higher outside the cell (i.e., the osmotic pressure is lower outside the cell), water passes into the cell and may burst it, a process called **hemolysis**.

When intravenous fluids are administered, the composition of the fluid must be carefully considered. Solutions with an osmotic pressure equal to that found inside the cell are **isotonic**. A 0.9% sodium chloride solution and a 5.5% glucose solution are considered isotonic. Solutions with an osmotic pressure less than that inside the cell are considered **hypotonic**. Distilled water, tap water, and 0.45% sodium chloride are all hypotonic solutions. Solutions with an osmotic pressure greater than that inside the cell are **hypertonic**. Examples of hypertonic solutions include 5% sodium chloride and 10% glucose solutions.

A second type of liquid mixture is a **suspension**. Whereas particles in solutions consist of ions and molecules, particles in suspensions consist of large clumps of molecules. Properties of suspensions include the following: they consist of an insoluble substance dispersed in a liquid; they are heterogeneous (not the same throughout); they are not clear; they settle out over time; and they do not pass through filter paper or membranes. Certain medications are dispensed as suspensions, such as milk of magnesia. Water often is the suspending medium, although oils can also be used, as is the case with certain antibiotics. An aerosol is an example of a liquid suspended in a gas.

A third type of liquid mixture, a **colloid**, consists of tiny particles suspended in a liquid. Although similar to suspensions, colloids have entirely different properties. Colloids do not settle; they can pass through filter paper but not through membranes; they adsorb (hold) particles on their surface; they have electrical charges, owing to the adsorption of charged particles (ions); and they exhibit the Tyndall effect and Brownian movement. **Table 53-3** compares the properties of colloids, solutions, and suspensions.

The particles in a colloid are larger than those in a solution (<1 nm) but smaller than those in a suspension (>100 nm); colloid particles therefore are small enough to pass though filter paper but too large to pass through a membrane. Colloids have a vast surface area because they consist of so many tiny particles. The property of adsorption is due to this tremendous surface area. **Adsorption** is defined as the ability to hold substances to a surface. Most colloids have selective adsorption, or the ability to adsorb only certain substances. Colloidal charcoal adsorbs large amounts of gas. Coconut charcoal selectively adsorbs poisonous gas but not ordinary gas, which is why it is used in gas masks. Colloids can selectively adsorb ions and take on an electrical charge. If a colloidal mixture consists of like charges, the particles repel each other and have minimal likelihood of coming together to form larger particles that would settle. On the other hand, if colloids of opposite charges come in contact, they attract each other and settle out. When the poison bichloride of mercury ($HgCl_2$) is swallowed, it forms a positive colloid in the stomach. Drinking egg white, a negative colloid, is the antidote. These two opposite-charged colloids neutralize each other and coagulate in the stomach. The coagulant must be pumped out of the stomach before the egg

TABLE 53-3
Comparison of the Properties of Solutions, Suspensions, and Colloids

	Size	Passes Through Filter Paper	Passes Through Membranes	Settles	Adsorbs	Charged
Solution	<1 nm	Yes	Yes	No	No	No
Suspension	>100 nm	No	No	Yes	No	No
Colloid	1–100 nm	Yes	No	No	Yes	Yes

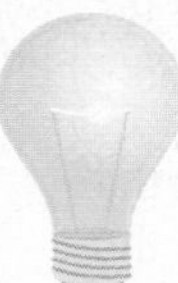

STOP AND THINK

Why does hypertonic saline assist with induced sputum?

white is digested, which would expose the body to the poison again.

When a beam of light is passed through a colloid, the beam reflects off the colloidal particles and scatters. Such a beam passes directly through a solution without scattering because the particles are so small. This phenomenon, referred to as the *Tyndall effect*, is used as a way to distinguish between colloids and solutions. Colloids also exhibit a haphazard, irregular motion, known as *Brownian movement*, that never ceases. This movement is thought to be due to constant bombardment of the colloid particles by the molecules of the suspending medium, which are in continuous, random motion.

Colloidal dispersions can be **hydrophilic** (water attracting) or **hydrophobic** (water repelling). Systems in which a strong attraction exists between the colloidal particles and water (hydrophilic systems) are called *gels*. Gels, such as gelatin, are semisolid or semirigid and do not flow easily. When little attraction exists between the colloid and water (hydrophobic systems), the system is referred to as a *sol*. Such dispersion in air is called an *aerosol*; when it is in water, it is called a *hydrosol*. When a gel is heated, it turns into a sol, which returns to a gel on cooling. Protoplasm has the ability to change from gel to sol and vice versa.

Several clinical applications use the concept by which solutions and colloids are passed through membranes. Dialysis involves the separation of solute particles from colloid particles with a semipermeable membrane. Peritoneal dialysis involves bathing of the gut with a solution, after which water-soluble waste particles are allowed to pass through the semipermeable intestinal wall. Hemodialysis involves passing blood by a semipermeable membrane, where soluble waste products are removed and the blood cells and plasma proteins retained. Antitoxins are prepared by placement of an impure material inside a membrane suspended in running water. The soluble impurities are washed out, leaving the pure antitoxin. Low-sodium milk is produced by a similar method.

Inorganic Molecules

The compounds that make up living organisms can be divided into two broad categories: organic compounds and inorganic compounds. Organic compounds generally are composed of molecules containing carbon–carbon (C—C) or carbon–hydrogen (C—H) covalent bonds. Inorganic compounds do not have any C—C or C—H bonds, although several inorganic compounds do contain carbon. Organic compounds usually are larger and more complex than inorganic compounds. The human body contains both types of compounds. As shown in Table 53-1, the body is made up of 23 important elements. Eleven are considered major elements, and the remaining 12 are referred to as *trace elements*. More than 96% of body weight is made up of oxygen, carbon, hydrogen, and nitrogen; oxygen alone is responsible for 65% of the body's weight. The most abundant molecule in the body is water (H_2O).

Water

The importance of water in the human body is evidenced by the fact that the body can stay alive for several weeks without food but only a few days without water. Water is essential for existence. Water accounts for 45% to 80% of the total weight of the human body and is essential for proper digestion, circulation, elimination, and regulation of body temperature. Every activity in each cell in the body takes place in a watery environment.

Pure water is colorless, odorless, and tasteless. Many physical constants are based on water as a reference. The freezing point (0° C or 32° F) and the boiling point (100° C or 212° F) of water at 1 atmosphere of pressure are the standard reference points for the measurement of temperature. The calorie is defined as the amount of heat required to change the temperature of 1 g of water 1° C. The metric standard of weight, the gram, is equal to the weight of 1 mL of water at 4° C (its maximum density). The concept of specific gravity is based on water and is defined as the weight of a substance compared with the weight of an equal volume of water.

The atomic structure of water results from the combination of two covalent bonds between a single oxygen atom and two hydrogen atoms. The water molecule is not arranged in a straight line (such as HOH) but rather in a nonlinear manner, with the angle between the hydrogen atoms being approximately 105 degrees (**Figure 53-5**). The shared electrons between the hydrogen and oxygen are attracted to the oxygen more than the hydrogen, which results in a slight negative charge at the oxygen end of the molecule and a slight positive charge at the hydrogen end. This polar nature of water is what makes it such an effective solvent. As a polar solvent, water has a tendency to ionize substances in solution. This allows large compounds to be broken into smaller, more reactive particles (ions), getting them ready for chemical reactions to occur.

Water also has several chemical properties worth noting (**Equation 53-10**). When an electric current is passed through water, it undergoes electrolysis and forms hydrogen gas (H_2) and oxygen gas (O_2). Water is extremely stable; when it boils and turns into a gas (steam), it does not decompose, even at extreme temperatures (≈0.3% decomposition at 1600° C). When

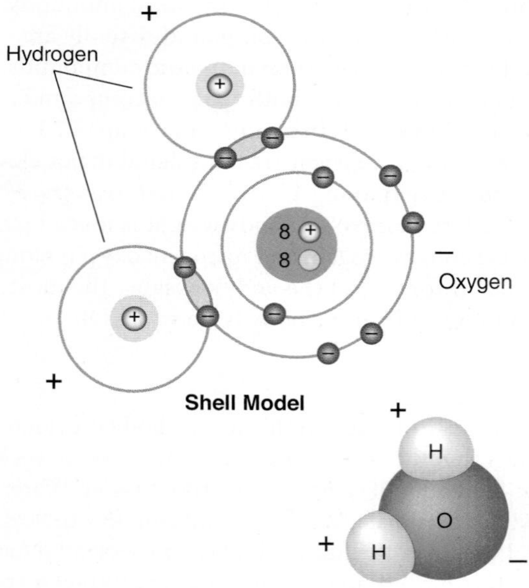

FIGURE 53-5 Structure of the water molecule.

water reacts with a metal oxide (metals are found on the left side of the periodic table), it forms a compound known as a *base*. When water reacts with a nonmetal (nonmetals are found on the right side of the periodic table), it forms a compound known as an *acid*. When water reacts with active metals, such as sodium or potassium, a vigorous reaction occurs and hydrogen gas is formed.

EQUATION 53-10

Reactions of Water

Electrolysis (with the symbol ↑ *indicating* a gas):

$$2\,H_2O \xrightarrow[\text{Electric current}]{} 2\,H_2\uparrow + O_2\uparrow$$

Reaction with metal oxide to produce a base:

$$CaO + H_2O \rightarrow Ca(OH)_2$$

Calcium oxide (metal oxide) → Calcium hydroxide (base)

Reaction with nonmetals to produce an acid:

$$CO_2 + H_2O \rightarrow H_2CO_3$$

Carbon dioxide (nonmetal) → Carbonic acid (acid)

Reaction with metals:

$$2\,Na + 2\,H_2O \rightarrow 2\,NaOH + H_2\uparrow$$

Sodium → Sodium hydroxide

Water plays a crucial role in the transport of many essential materials in the body. For example, by dissolving oxygen and food substances in the blood, water enables these materials to enter and leave the blood capillaries in the lungs and digestive organs and eventually to enter cells in every area of the body. Water then transports waste products from the place where they are produced to the excretory organs, where they are eventually eliminated.

Water's ability to absorb and give up heat slowly gives it a major role in another unique and important bodily function—maintaining a relatively constant temperature. Chemists refer to water's ability to lose and gain large amounts of heat with little change in temperature as its high **specific heat**. Because the body has a large water content, it can resist sudden changes in temperature. For example, it can transport the heat produced by muscle contraction during exercise to the surface of the body to be evaporated, with little change in core temperature.

Another important physical property of water is its high **heat of vaporization**; this refers to the fact that a significant amount of heat must be absorbed to change water from a liquid to a gas (specifically, 540 calories per gram). The energy is used to break the hydrogen bonds holding adjacent water molecules together in the liquid state. When water is placed on the skin, the heat required to make it evaporate comes from the skin. In this manner the skin loses heat and is cooled. In a similar manner, the skin is cooled by the evaporation of perspiration.

Oxygen and Carbon Dioxide

Oxygen and carbon dioxide are inorganic substances that play an important role in cellular respiration (**Figure 53-6**). Oxygen is required to complete the decomposition reactions required for the release of energy from nutrients burned by the cells. Carbon dioxide is a waste product of these same decomposition reactions and is important to acid–base homeostasis of the body.

Electrolytes

Electrolytes constitute another large group of inorganic compounds. They include acids, bases, and salts. **Electrolytes** are substances that break down, or dissociate, in solution to form ions. Positively charged ions are called *cations* and negatively charged ions are called *anions*. In solution, electrolytes are capable of carrying an electrical current.

The unit of measurement for electrolytes is the number of milliequivalents per liter of solution (mEq/L). **Milliequivalents** measure the number of ionic charges or electrovalent bonds in a solution and therefore are an

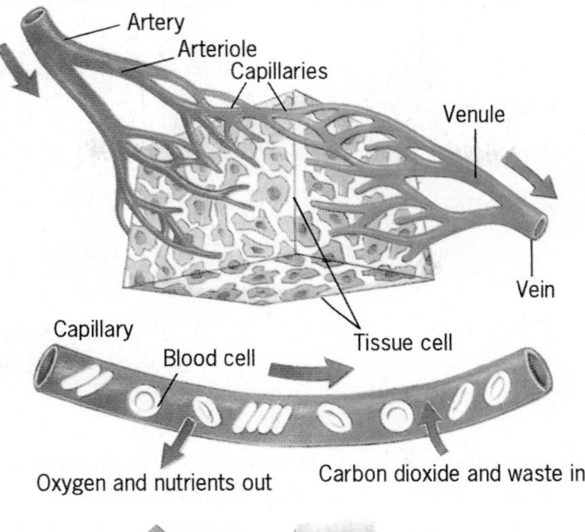

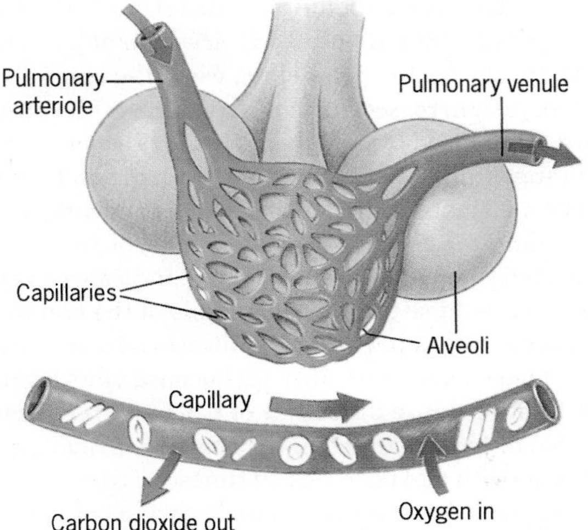

FIGURE 53-6 Transport of carbon dioxide (CO_2) and oxygen (O_2) at the (**A**) tissue and (**B**) lung levels. Note that the process of CO_2 uptake and O_2 release at the tissue level is reversed at the lung level (O_2 uptake and CO_2 release).

accurate measure of the chemical combining power, or reactivity, of the electrolyte solution. The number of milliequivalents can be determined from the weight of the ion in 100 mL of the solution (mg%) (**Equation 53-11**).

Acids, Bases, and Buffers

An **acid** is a compound that donates, or yields, a hydrogen ion (H^+) in an aqueous solution. Acid solutions have a sour taste. Citric acid gives a sour taste to lemons and grapefruits, acetic acid gives a sour taste to vinegar, and lactic acid makes milk taste sour. Because a hydrogen ion is the result of the hydrogen atom losing its only electron, it becomes a single proton, because it has no neutron in its nucleus. Actually, an aqueous hydrogen ion, H^+ (aq), is not a bare proton but rather a proton chemically bonded to water as H_3O^+ (aq). According to the Brönsted-Lowry theory, an acid is the species that donates a proton in a transfer reaction. An acid, then, can also be thought of as a substance that donates protons.

EQUATION 53-11

Calculation of mEq/L

mEq/L = (mg/100 mL × 10 [the conversion factor for 100 mL to L] × valence) / Atomic weight

Example: Convert 16 mg% of potassium to mEq/L, given potassium's atomic weight = 39 and valence = 1.

$$\text{mEq/L} = (16 \times 10 \times 1) / 39 = 160 / 39 = 4.1$$

Some common acids are hydrochloric acid (HCl), sulfuric acid (H_2SO_4), nitric acid (HNO_3), carbonic acid (H_2CO_3), phosphoric acid (H_3PO_4), and acetic acid (CH_3CO_2H). Acids yield ions when placed in water (**Equation 53-12**). Strong acids (such as HCl, HNO_3, and H_2SO_4) almost completely ionize in solution to form H^+ ions, whereas weak acids (such as H_2CO_3) dissociate very little and therefore produce few excess H^+ ions. Acids react with metal oxides and hydroxides to form water and a salt.

The water molecule dissociates continually in a reversible reaction to form hydrogen ions and hydroxide ions (OH^-):

$$H_2O \leftrightarrow H^+ + OH^-$$

EQUATION 53-12

Acid Reactions

Reactions in Water

Acids with a single ionizable hydrogen ionize into one cation and one anion:

$$HCl \rightarrow H^+ + Cl^-$$

$$HNO_3 \rightarrow H^+ + NO_3^-$$

Acids with multiple ionizable hydrogen atoms donate their protons in stages:

Stage 1: $H_2SO_4 \rightarrow H^+ + HSO_4^-$

Stage 2: $HSO_4^- \rightarrow H^+ + SO_4^{-2}$

that can be combined and represented as:

$$H_2SO_4 \rightarrow 2\,H^+ + SO_4^{-2}$$

Reactions with Metal Oxides and Hydroxides to Form Water and a Salt

$$H_2SO_4 + 2\,NaOH \rightarrow 2\,H_2O + Na_2SO_4$$

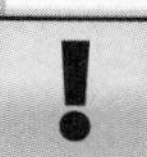

Respiratory Recap

Acids and Bases

- *Acid*: donates hydrogen ions
- *Base*: accepts hydrogen ions
- *Buffer*: minimizes change in the hydrogen ion concentration
- *Salt*: produced by a reaction between an acid and a base

The single unpaired valence electron makes hydrogen unstable, and by losing or donating the electron, it becomes more stable. This is why the dissociation of water occurs. Rather than share its electron with oxygen, hydrogen would just as soon give up its electron to OH to maintain stability. In pure water the balance between the two ions is equal, but when an acid, such as HCl, dissociates into H^+ and Cl^-, it shifts the H^+/OH^- balance in favor of H^+ ions, increasing the acidity level.

A **base** is a solution that yields a hydroxide ion (OH^-) in an aqueous solution. The base, or alkaline compound, shifts the H^+/OH^- balance in favor of OH^-, as shown in the ionization reaction of sodium hydroxide (**Equation 53-13**). A base can also be thought of as the substance that accepts the proton in a transfer reaction. With this definition the bicarbonate ion (HCO_3^-) also is a base because it can accept a proton. Basic solutions feel slippery and soapy and have a bitter, biting taste. A strong base has a high hydroxide concentration and is corrosive to tissues because of its ability to react with proteins and fats.

The concentration, or strength, of an acid or base is expressed as pH. The **pH** indicates the hydrogen ion concentration $[H^+]$ in a solution and is mathematically defined as the negative logarithm of the hydrogen ion concentration:

$$pH = -\log[H^+]$$

EQUATION 53-13

Chemical Reactions Involving Bases

The ionization reaction of sodium hydroxide to yield OH^-:

$$NaOH \rightarrow Na^+ + OH^-$$

Reactions that accept a proton:

$$\underset{\text{Base}}{HCO_3^-} + \underset{\text{Proton}}{H^+} \rightarrow H_2CO_3$$

EQUATION 53-14

The pH of a Solution

$pH = -\log [H^+]$

A solution with a $[H^+]$ of 10^{-7} mol / L has a pH of 7:

$pH = -\log [H^+] = -\log 10^{-7} = -(-7) = 7$

Because a logarithm is an exponent, the logarithm (log) of 100, or 10^2, is 2, and log 10^{-4} is -4 (10^{-4} is 0.0001). Therefore, a solution with a $[H^+]$ of 10^{-7} mol/L has a pH of 7 (**Equation 53-14**). The sum of $[H^+]$ and $[OH^-]$ is always 10^{-14}; therefore, when the concentration of one increases, the concentration of the other must be reduced by an equal amount. The values for pH range from 0 to 14. For example, a pH of 0 indicates a $[H^+]$ mol/L of 10^0 mol/L (or 1 mol/L) and a $[OH^-]$ of 10^{-14} mol/L. A pH of 14 indicates a $[H^+]$ of 10^{-14} mol/L and a $[OH^-]$ of 10^0 mol/L. A pH of 7 indicates a neutral solution, because the concentrations of the two ions are the same, 10^{-7}. A pH above 7 indicates a base, whereas a pH below 7 indicates an acid. Because of its logarithmic relationship, a difference of 1 pH unit represents a 10-fold difference in strength. This means that an acid solution with a pH of 5.5 is 10 times as strong as one with a pH of 6.5 and that a base with a pH of 9.0 is 10 times as strong as one with a pH of 8.0.

Buffers maintain a relative constant pH when a strong acid or a strong base is added. Blood is an effective buffer. For the bicarbonate buffer system, the degree to which the pH changes depends on the ratio of base bicarbonate to carbonic acid. A ratio of 20:1 produces a pH of 7.4. This is mathematically expressed by the **Henderson-Hasselbalch equation**, which includes the ionization constant for carbonic acid:

$$pH = 6.1 + \log\frac{[HCO_3^-]}{(P_{CO_2} \times 0.03)}$$

The ratio of HCO_3^- to H_2CO_3 for a pH of 7.4 is 20:1. If the ratio goes up by means of an elevation in bicarbonate or a reduction in the partial pressure of carbon

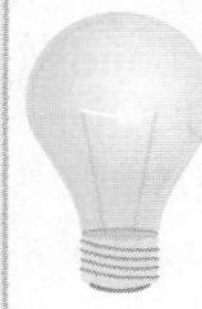

STOP AND THINK

How will the body respond to an increased level of P_{CO_2} in the blood?

EQUATION 53-15

Chemical Reactions Involving Salts

Neutralization reaction:

$HCl + NaOH \rightarrow NaCl + H_2O$

Acid Base Salt Water

Salts in solution yield a positive and negative ion:

$NaCl \rightarrow Na^+ + Cl^-$

$K_2SO_4 \rightarrow 2\ K^+ + SO_4^{-2}$

dioxide (Pco_2), the pH increases, or becomes more basic or alkaline. Either a reduction in the bicarbonate or an increase in Pco_2 causes the pH to decrease and become more acidic.

Salts

When an acid and a base react, the result is a salt. When the result is a salt and water, the reaction is known as a *neutralization reaction* (**Equation 53-15**). Although acids (H^+) and bases (OH^-) all have an ion in common, salts do not. Salts in solution yield a positive and negative ion. Many of the major and trace minerals listed in Table 53-1 are derived from inorganic salt sources, which are common in many body fluids and specialized tissue such as bone. Often, these elements can exert a full physiologic effect only when present as an ion in solution. **Table 53-4** lists some common inorganic salts.

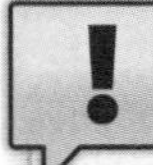

Respiratory Recap

Biologically Important Organic Molecules

- Carbohydrates
- Lipids
- Proteins
- Nucleic acids
- Vitamins
- Hormones
- Enzymes

Organic Molecules

Organic chemistry is the chemistry of carbon compounds. Carbon compounds have a separate category because although there are tens of thousands of known inorganic compounds, there are millions of known organic compounds. Some important organic compounds in the body are carbohydrates, lipids, proteins, nucleic acids, vitamins, hormones, and enzymes. Other common materials that contain organic compounds include drugs, wool, silk, cotton, linen, nylon, rayon, Dacron, perfumes, dyes, flavors, soaps, detergents, plastics, gasoline, and oils.

Organic compounds are different from inorganic compounds in many ways. **Table 53-5** lists some of the most important differences. One of the unique characteristics of carbon is its ability to bond other carbon atoms to itself to form very large, complex molecules. The carbon atoms may form continuous or branched chains, creating substances known as *aliphatic compounds*. Carbon atoms also can form in the shape of a ring. If the ring is formed of all carbon atoms, the compound is called a *cyclic* or *aromatic compound*; if

TABLE 53-4
Common Inorganic Salts in the Body

Salt	Chemical Formula	Electrolyte Combination	Medicinal Use
Sodium chloride	$NaCl$	$Na^+ + Cl^-$	Replacement therapy, irrigation, diluent
Calcium chloride	$CaCl_2$	$Ca^{+2} + 2\ Cl^-$	Reduction in blood clotting time
Sodium bicarbonate	$NaHCO_3$	$Na^+ + HCO_3^-$	Antacid, buffering agent
Potassium chloride	KCl	$K^+ + Cl^-$	Potassium replacement therapy
Sodium sulfate	Na_2SO_4	$2\ Na^+ + SO_4^{-2}$	Cathartic agent
Calcium carbonate	$CaCO_3$	$Ca^{+2} + CO_3^{-2}$	Antacid
Calcium phosphate	$Ca_3(PO_4)_2$	$3\ Ca^{+2} + 2\ PO_4^{-3}$	Replacement therapy
Magnesium sulfate	$MgSO_4$	$Mg^{+2} + SO_4^{-2}$	Cathartic agent, anticonvulsant, laxative
Potassium iodide	KI	$K^+ + I^-$	Expectorant, antitussive

TABLE 53-5
Comparison of Common Characteristics of Most Organic and Inorganic Compounds

Organic Compounds	Inorganic Compounds
Complex structure	Simpler structure
Flammability	Nonflammability
Low melting point	High melting point
Low boiling point	High boiling point
Solubility in nonpolar liquids	Insolubility in nonpolar liquids
Insolubility in water	Solubility in water
Covalent bonds	Ionic bonds
Reactions usually formed between molecules	Reactions usually formed between ions
Generally many atoms	Usually relatively few atoms

another element, such as nitrogen, is substituted for one of the carbon atoms in the ring, the compound is called a *heterocyclic compound*.

Because the carbon atom has four valence electrons and needs four more to reach a full shell of eight electrons, carbon can form up to four covalent bonds. This requirement can be satisfied by its bonding to four separate atoms by use of four single bonds; to three atoms by use of two single bonds and one double bond; or to two atoms by use of one triple bond and one single bond (**Figure 53-7**). The three atoms most commonly bound with carbon are hydrogen, which needs one electron to fill its outer shell and can form only one bond; oxygen, which forms two bonds; and nitrogen, which forms three bonds. With this brief overview, let us move on to the four major groups of organic substances most important in the human body: carbohydrates, proteins, lipids, and nucleic acids.

Carbohydrates

All **carbohydrate** molecules contain the elements carbon, hydrogen, and oxygen; the word *carbohydrate* literally means "carbon and water." The carbon atoms

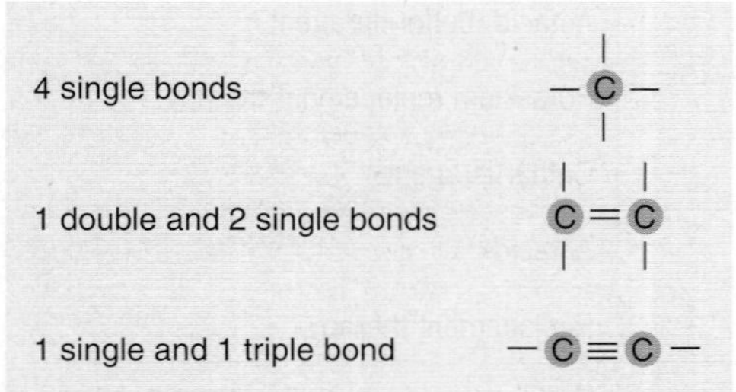

FIGURE 53-7 Covalent bonds formed by carbon. Each dash represents a pair of shared electrons.

are linked to form chains of varying lengths. Sugars and starches are carbohydrates and the primary sources of chemical energy required by each cell in the body. Carbohydrates are divided into four groups based on the length of the carbon chain: monosaccharides (simple sugars), disaccharides (double sugars), oligosaccharides (few sugars), and polysaccharides (complex sugars).

The basic unit of the carbohydrate molecule is the monosaccharide. **Glucose** (dextrose), the most important monosaccharide, is a six-carbon sugar with the formula $C_6H_{12}O_6$. Because it is a six-carbon molecule, it is referred to as a *hexose* (*hexa* means six). Glucose is present in a straight chain in the dry state but forms a cyclic compound when in solution. Glucose is the primary source of energy for the cells. Fructose and galactose are other important hexoses. Some monosaccharides consist of five-carbon atoms and are referred to as *pentoses*. Two important pentoses are ribose and deoxyribose, which are integral to the formation of the nucleic acids ribonucleic acid (RNA) and deoxyribonucleic acid (DNA).

Disaccharides are composed of two simple sugars bonded together through a synthesis reaction that involves the removal of water. Examples of disaccharides include sucrose (table sugar from cane or beet sugar), maltose (grain sugar), and lactose (milk sugar). Each consists of two linked monosaccharides. The combining of glucose and fructose forms sucrose. After they are eaten, these important dietary disaccharides are broken down into monosaccharides so that the cells can utilize them.

Oligosaccharides are made up of 3 to 20 monosaccharides linked together. They are often bound to proteins on the outer surface of cell membranes as a self-antigen. Having self-antigens on our own cells allows the immune system to recognize antigens that are nonself.

Polysaccharides are made up of many chemically linked monosaccharides. Glycogen is the body's most important polysaccharide. It sometimes is referred to as *animal starch*. Because it has a molecular weight of several million atomic mass units, it is considered a macromolecule. When excess glucose is present in the blood, it is converted to glycogen by the liver and stored in liver and muscle cells for later use.

Proteins

Proteins are very large molecules composed of carbon, hydrogen, oxygen, and nitrogen. The molecular weight of a protein reaches several million atomic mass units. The basic protein unit or building block is the **amino acid**. Proteins are composed of 20 such amino acids, and nearly all 20 are present in every protein. Of the 20, only 8 are considered *essential amino acids* because they cannot be produced by the body and must be included in the diet (**Box 53-1**). The remaining 12 are known as *nonessential amino acids* because they can be produced from other amino acids or from simple organic molecules readily available to the body cells.

BOX 53-1

Essential Amino Acids

Histidine
Isoleucine
Leucine
Methionine
Phenylalanine
Theonine
Tryptophan
Valine

The basic structure of an amino acid consists of a carbon atom (called the α-carbon) to which are bonded an amino group (NH_2), a carboxyl group (COOH), a hydrogen atom, and a side chain (**Figure 53-8**). The side chain is a group of elements denoted by the letter R. It is the side chain that constitutes the unique and identifying characteristic of an amino acid.

To link amino acids, the OH from the carboxyl group of one amino acid and the H from the amine group of another amino acid split off to form water plus a new compound called a **peptide**. A long chain of peptides is called a *polypeptide*, and the compound is finally considered a protein when the chain reaches about 50 amino acids or more in length.

The shape of a protein molecule determines its function, and there are two main classes of proteins: fibrous and globular. Fibrous proteins are long linear chains of amino acids that are usually water insoluble. Examples of fibrous proteins are collagen (in skin) and keratin (in hair). Globular proteins are usually soluble in water and are highly folded, spherical in shape. Examples of globular proteins include hormones, hemoglobin, antibodies, and enzymes. Proteins can also bind with other organic compounds to form mixed molecules, such as a glycoprotein (sugar with a protein) or a lipoprotein (a lipid and a protein).

Lipids

A **lipid** is an organic biomolecule that is soluble in nonpolar organic solvents, such as ether, alcohol, or benzene.

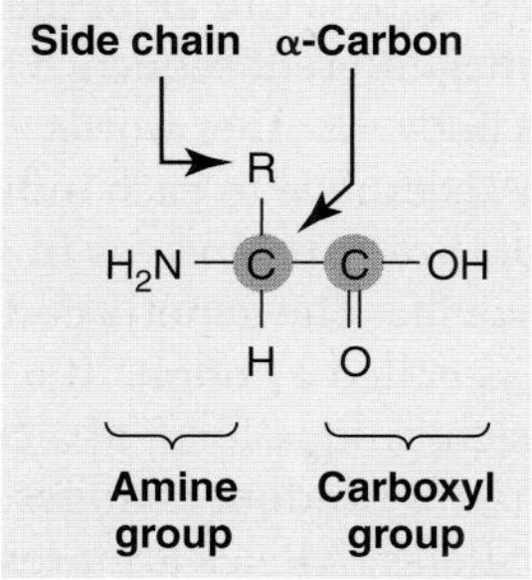

Side chain α-Carbon
R
H_2N—C—C—OH
H O
Amine group
Carboxyl group

FIGURE 53-8 Basic structure of an amino acid.

Lipids are not soluble in water. Lipids are composed primarily of carbon, hydrogen, and oxygen, although nitrogen and phosphorus are also used. The proportion of oxygen is much lower in lipids than it is in carbohydrates. The different lipid categories include triglycerides (fats), phospholipids, steroids, and eicosanoids.

Lipids have critically important biologic functions. They provide energy (they yield more energy per unit of weight than carbohydrates or proteins); structure (phospholipids and cholesterol are required components of cell membranes); essential nutrients in the form of vitamins (fat-soluble vitamins include vitamins A, D, E, and K); protection (fat surrounds and protects organs); insulation (skin fat minimizes heat loss; fatty tissue, or myelin, covers nerve cells and electrically insulates them); and regulation (steroid hormones such as estrogen, testosterone, and eicosanoids regulate many physiologic processes).

Triglycerides are the most abundant lipids and function as the body's most concentrated source of energy. Fats and oils are both triglycerides; fats are solid at room temperature (e.g., butter, lard), and oils are liquid (e.g., corn oil, olive oil). The basic building blocks of the triglyceride are a glycerol molecule and three fatty acids. The glycerol unit is the same for all triglycerides; the specific type of fatty acid determines the identity and chemical nature of the fat.

Naturally occurring fats have long fatty acid chains, consisting of an even number of carbons that range from 12 to 24 carbons long. A **saturated fatty acid** is one in which all available bonds of the hydrocarbon chain are filled with hydrogen atoms. The chain has all single carbon–carbon bonds. **Unsaturated fatty acids** have one or more double carbon–carbon bond in their hydrocarbon chain because not all of the chain carbon atoms are saturated with hydrogen atoms. The degree of saturation determines the physical and chemical properties of fatty acids. Fats become more oily and liquid as the number of unsaturated double bonds increases. Double bonds cause the chain to bend or kink, thereby keeping the molecules from fitting closely together. For example, animal fats such as lard are saturated, whereas vegetable oils are not.

Phospholipids are similar to triglycerides in structure but do not store energy. Instead of three fatty acids attached to a glycerol, one of the fatty acid chains is replaced by a chemical structure containing phosphorus and nitrogen. The shape of the phospholipid molecule resembles a head with two tails: the head is the phosphorus and nitrogen group, and the tails are the two fatty acids. The head is hydrophilic (attracts water), whereas the tails are hydrophobic (repel water). This unique property allows the phospholipid molecule to bridge or join two different chemical environments—for example, a water environment on one side and a lipid environment on the other. Phospholipids are a primary component of cell membranes, pulmonary surfactant (a surface tension–reducing agent in the lungs), and myelin.

Steroids are an important lipid group. They are widely distributed throughout the body and are involved in many important structural and functional roles. **Cholesterol** is a steroid lipid that combines with phospholipids in the cell membrane to help stabilize the membrane's bilayer structure. The body also uses cholesterol as a starting point for making steroid hormones such as estrogen, testosterone, and cortisol and for bile salts used in digestion.

Eicosanoids are signaling molecules made by oxidation of three different 20-carbon essential fatty acids (EFA): eicosapentaenoic acid (EPA), arachidonic acid (AA), and dihomo-gamma-linolenic acid (DGLA). Eicosanoids are not stored within cells but are synthesized as required. Some of the most complex pathways in the human body depend on eicosanoids. The four families of eicosanoids are prostaglandins (PG), prostacyclins (PGI_2), thromboxanes (TX), and leukotrienes (LT).

Prostaglandins are lipids composed of a 20-carbon unsaturated fatty acid that has a 5-carbon ring. They are often referred to as *tissue hormones*. Sixteen types of prostaglandins have been classified into nine broad categories, labeled PGA through PGI. Prostaglandins are produced by cell membranes in almost every body tissue. They are formed and released in response to specific stimuli. Once released, they have a very local effect and are then inactivated. Prostaglandins help regulate blood pressure and the secretion of digestive juices, enhance the immune system and inflammatory response, play an important role in blood clotting, and help regulate the effects of several hormones. The use of prostaglandin and prostaglandin inhibitor drugs is gaining attention for the treatment of conditions ranging from relief of menstrual cramps to treatment of asthma, high blood pressure, and ulcers. Because prostaglandins have a short half-life, their effect is felt primarily locally or within the cell of origin. **Table 53-6** summarizes some of the physiologic actions of prostaglandins.

Prostacyclin also has a short half-life. Prostacyclin is an inhibitor of platelet aggregation and a potent vasodilator. *Thromboxanes* have an effect opposite to that of prostacyclin. They facilitate platelet aggregation and have a contractive effect on a variety of smooth muscle. *Leukotrienes* play an important role in asthma and allergic reactions and sustain inflammatory reactions. As multifunctional mediators, leukotrienes probably play a role in other diseases. The role of leukotrienes in cardiovascular and neuropsychiatric illnesses is actively being investigated.

TABLE 53-6
Physiologic Actions of Prostaglandins

Constriction or dilation in vascular and bronchial smooth muscle cells	Sensitize spinal neurons to pain
Aggregation or disaggregation of platelets	Decrease intraocular pressure
Regulate inflammatory mediation	Regulate calcium movement
Control hormone regulation	Control cell growth
Regulate gastric acid secretion	Stimulate release of insulin from pancreas

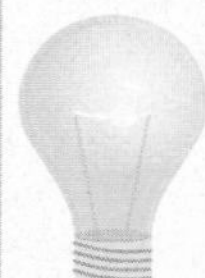

STOP AND THINK

What happens when someone takes an inhaled corticosteroid to treat a respiratory disease?

Nucleic Acids

The two principal forms of **nucleic acid** are **deoxyribonucleic acid (DNA)** and **ribonucleic acid (RNA)**. The basic building blocks of nucleic acids are nucleotides. Just as proteins are made from chains of amino acids, nucleic acids are made from chains of nucleotides. Each nucleotide consists of a phosphate group, a five-carbon sugar, and a nitrogenous base. The sugar component in DNA is deoxyribose, whereas ribose is used in RNA. The five nitrogenous bases are uracil (U), thymine (T), cytosine (C), guanine (G), and adenosine (A). Both DNA and RNA use the bases cytosine, guanine, and adenosine; DNA also uses thymine, and RNA also uses uracil.

DNA molecules are the largest molecules in the body. They are composed of two long polynucleotide chains that run parallel to each other (**Figure 53-9**). The sugar–phosphate part of the molecule faces toward the outside, and its bases point inward, toward the bases of the other chain. Each base in one chain is joined to a base in the other chain by hydrogen bonds, forming a base pair. DNA base pairs always consist of A with T and G with C. The double chains coil around each other to form a double helix. The DNA molecule looks like a twisted ladder, with the rails of the ladder being the sugar–phosphate backbone of the nucleotide chain and the rungs of the ladder the base pairs connected by hydrogen bonds.

Although a DNA molecule contains only two types of base pairs (A-T and G-C), millions of them are present in each DNA molecule. The millions of base pairs occur in the same sequence in all of the DNA molecules in the body but in a different sequence in the DNA of another person's body. In other words, the base pair sequence in DNA is unique to each individual.

A sequence of three nucleotides in a strand of DNA or RNA provides the genetic code for a specific amino acid and is called a codon. The codons make up a *gene*, and each unique form of a gene is called an **allele**. Mutations are random changes in genes and can create new alleles. Alleles are present in pairs, one on each of a **chromosome** pair. Human somatic

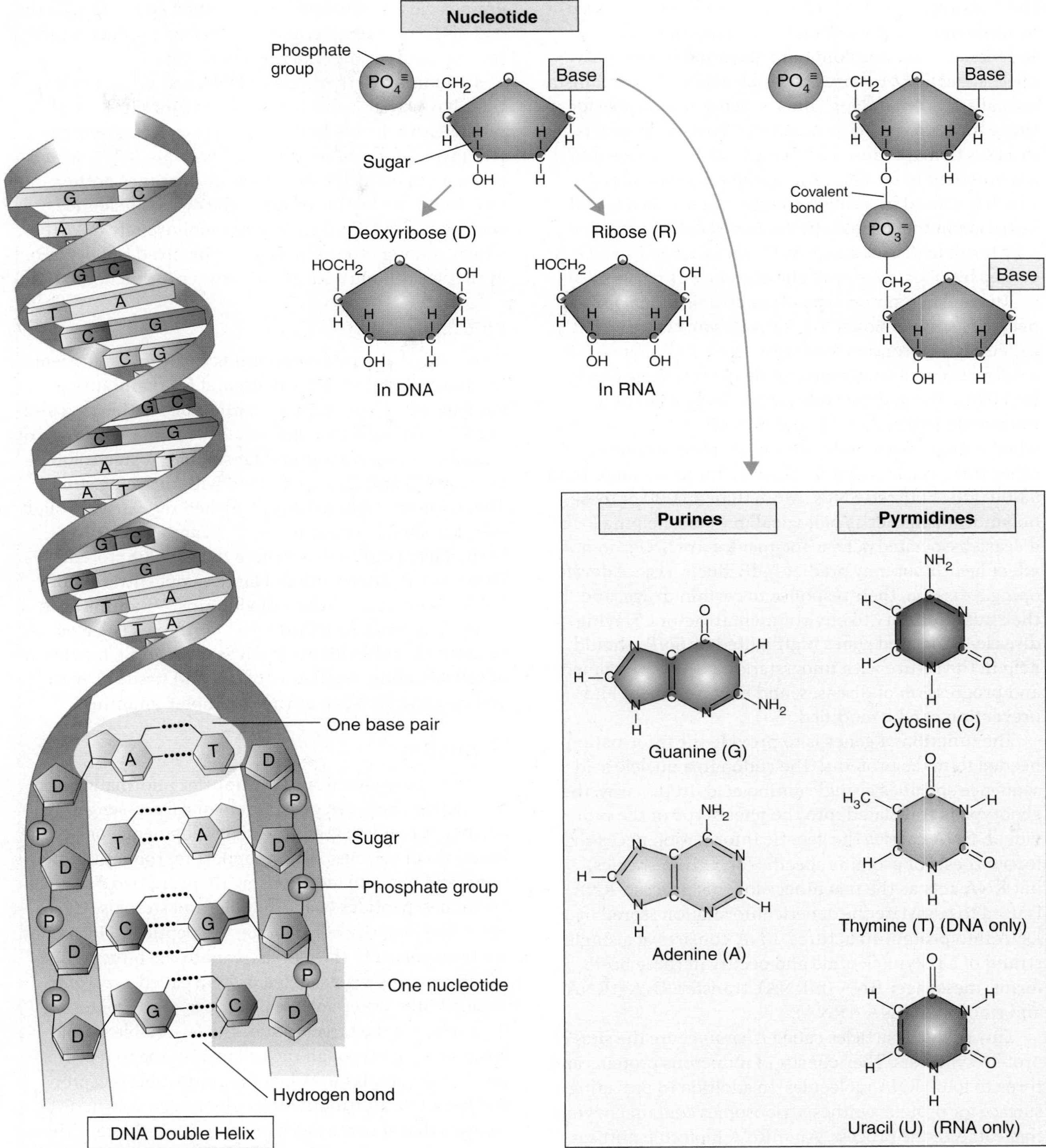

FIGURE 53-9 Structure of the DNA molecule.

cells (body cells) are diploid, having two sets of 23 chromosomes (46 total), one from the mother and one from the father. Gametes, or reproductive cells, are haploid and have one set of chromosomes. One of the 23 pairs of chromosomes determines sex, and diseases transmitted on this pair of chromosomes are called *sex-linked*. Examples include hemophilia and Duchenne muscular dystrophy. The other 22 pairs of chromosomes are called *autosomal*.

Homozygous refers to having identical alleles for a single trait, whereas *heterozygous* refers to having two different alleles for a single trait. If one allele overrides the instructions from another, it is called the *dominant allele*, and the allele that is overridden is called the *recessive allele*. For a recessive trait to be expressed, its allele must be present on both chains of DNA. Individuals with one dominant allele and one recessive allele are called *carriers*. The visible traits of an organism are called its **phenotype**, and the genes responsible for those traits are called its **genotype**. Genetic disorders are diseases that are caused by a single allele of a gene and are inherited in families. An example is cystic fibrosis, which is caused by a single recessive gene called CFTR. Variation in the normal chromosomal content of a cell may result in diseases such as Down syndrome, which is caused by an extra copy of chromosome 21 (trisomy 21).

The most common type of genetic variation among people is **single nucleotide polymorphisms**, frequently called **SNPs** (pronounced *snips*). Each SNP represents a difference in a single nucleotide (the building blocks for DNA). The genetic code is specified by the four nucleotide letters A, C, T, and G. SNP variation occurs when a single nucleotide, such as A, replaces one of the other three nucleotides: C, G, or T. There are more than 5,000,000 validated SNPs. More than 40,000 of these polymorphisms act as biological markers, helping locate disease-associated genes. The majority of SNPs do not affect health but may predict individuals' risk of developing a disease, their response to certain drugs, and their susceptibility to environmental factors. Having disease-associated genes highlighted by SNPs should help in the future with understanding the development and progression of diseases, and how treatment and prevention can be modified.

The function of genes is to provide the information needed to make proteins. The codon in a nucleic acid sequence specifies a single amino acid. In this way, the genotype is translated into the phenotype of the individual. DNA carries the genetic information necessary for synthesis of proteins specific for a given species, but RNA acts as the machinery for this process. RNA is used to translate the genetic information stored in DNA into protein structures. RNA consists of a single strand of a polynucleotide and occurs in three basic forms: messenger RNA (mRNA), transfer RNA (tRNA), and ribosomal RNA (rRNA).

Tiny cellular particles called *ribosomes* are the sites of protein synthesis. They consist of numerous proteins and three to four rRNA molecules. In addition to providing a surface for protein synthesis, ribosomes contain enzymes that catalyze the process. An mRNA molecule diffuses about the cell and attaches itself to a ribosome, where it acts as a pattern for protein synthesis. A sequence of three base pairs in a mRNA molecule acts as the code for a particular amino acid. This sequence is called a *codon*, and each codon represents one of the 20 different amino acids. The attached mRNA codons provide the sequence of amino acids for a protein that will be synthesized. A tRNA molecule then bonds to a particular amino acid and carries it to a ribosome. It attaches itself to a mRNA codon through base pairing. Once the sequence of amino acids is complete, a termination codon signals the end of the polypeptide, and the finished product, a protein, is released from the ribosome.

In addition to their role in DNA and RNA, nucleotides have other important biologic functions. Most notable is their role in the production of high-energy triphosphate, or **adenosine triphosphate (ATP)**, which is the main molecule used to store energy. Another important nucleotide group is the cyclic nucleotides, such as cyclic 3′5′-adenosine monophosphate (cAMP), which, among other functions, is involved in relaxation of the smooth muscles of the airways (bronchodilation).

Vitamins

Vitamins are organic compounds required as nutrients in minute amounts for growth and for maintaining good health. Most vitamins cannot be synthesized and must be obtained through diet. There are two classes of vitamins: water soluble and fat soluble. Water-soluble vitamins (B and C) are excreted without being stored. This requires them to be replenished regularly through diet. Fat-soluble vitamins (A, D, E, and K) dissolve in the fats of our bodies, where they can be stored. Diseases can arise from too large a concentration of vitamins or from a deficit of vitamins. Vitamins have many functions, functioning as hormones (such as vitamin D), antioxidants (such as vitamin E), mediators of cell signaling, regulators of cell and tissue growth, and coenzymes (such as the B complex vitamins).

Hormones

Hormones are chemicals that transfer information and instructions between cells. As chemical messengers, hormones regulate growth and development, control the functions of various tissues, support reproductive functions, and regulate metabolism. There are two classes of hormones: peptides (water soluble) and steroids (fat soluble). The majority of hormones are peptides. Hormones are transported in the bloodstream to the target tissue, which contains a specialized protein called a *receptor*. Typically, the water-soluble peptide uses a receptor on the surface of the target tissue. The fat-soluble steroid hormones pass through the cell membrane to receptors in the cytoplasm. When the compatible receptor and hormone bind, both molecules undergo structural changes that activate mechanisms within the cell. These mechanisms produce the desired effect dictated by the hormone. Hormonal effects are complex. Some hormones change the permeability of the cell membrane. Others can alter enzyme activity, and some hormones stimulate the release of other hormones.

Cytokines

Cytokines are substances that carry signals between cells and thus have an effect on other cells. They encompass a large and diverse family of polypeptide regulators that are produced widely throughout the body. Cytokines are classified as lymphokines, interleukins (IL), and chemokines. Hormones circulate in nanomolar concentrations, whereas some cytokines circulate in picomolar concentrations that can increase up to 1000-fold during trauma or infection. The widespread distribution of cellular sources for cytokines is another feature that differentiates cytokines from hormones. Virtually all nucleated cells (especially endothelial cells, epithelial cells, and macrophages) produce IL-1, IL-6, and tumor necrosis factor-α (TNF-α). In contrast, classic hormones, such as insulin, are secreted from discrete glands (e.g., the pancreas). In recent years, it has been shown that lung injury, such as may occur with ventilator-induced lung injury, can result in increased release of cytokines from the lungs. The cytokines released from the lungs can induce downstream organ failures.

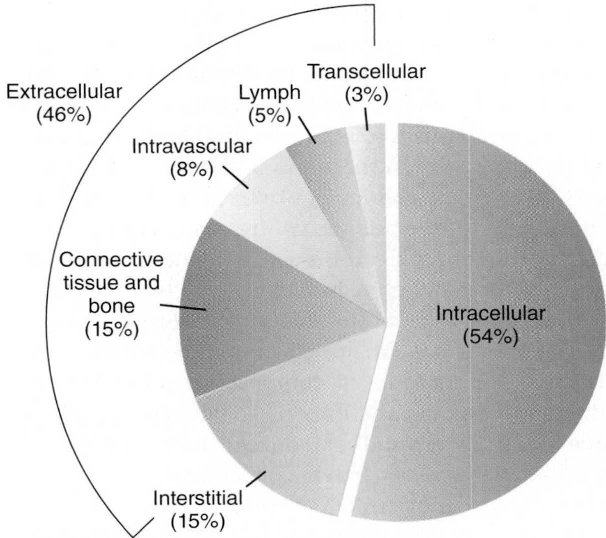

FIGURE 53-10 Fluid compartments of the body.

Enzymes

Enzymes are proteins secreted by cells that act to speed up (catalyze) chemical changes in other substances while they remain unchanged in the process. Most enzymes are globular proteins. Enzymes work by temporarily binding to one or more reactants, thus decreasing the amount of activation energy needed for reactions and increasing the rate of the reaction. The activity of enzymes is affected by temperature, pH, the concentration of the reactant, and inhibitors such as drugs and poisons. Enzymes have a wide variety of functions, including signal transduction and cell regulation, muscle contraction, acting as ion pumps involved in active transport and creating metabolic pathways.

Fluid Balance

The human body is composed primarily of water. The weight of a newborn infant is 75% to 80% water; that of a woman, 45% to 50%; and that of a man, 55% to 60%. These percentages vary depending on gender, age, and weight. People with a higher fat content have lower water content per kilogram of body weight. Women have relatively less total water content than men primarily because of their higher percentage of fat.

Water in the body is functionally distributed between two major areas: the intracellular compartment and the extracellular compartment. Intracellular fluid is a solvent in the cells that facilitates intracellular chemical reactions. Extracellular fluid serves the dual roles of providing a relatively constant environment for cells and transporting substances to and from the cell. Approximately 54% of the body's water is intracellular and 46% is extracellular (**Figure 53-10**). The extracellular fluid compartment is composed of five areas: the interstitial compartment, which accounts for the fluid outside or between the cells (15% of total body water); the intravascular (plasma) compartment, which accounts for the fluid in the heart and blood vessels (8%); dense connective tissue, cartilage, and bone (15%); lymph (5%); and the transcellular compartment, which includes the fluid in the salivary glands, thyroid gland, gonads, mucous membranes of the respiratory and gastrointestinal tracts, kidneys, liver, pancreas, cerebrospinal fluid, joint fluid, and the fluid in the spaces of the eyes (3%). The interstitial and intravascular compartments are the extracellular areas most involved with fluid balance.

The normal daily water intake is 2400 to 2500 mL, which is offset by an equal amount of fluid output. Fluid is taken in primarily through daily food (≈700 mL) and drink (≈1500 mL), but some also comes from body metabolism (≈200 mL a day). In the oxidation of food, about 14 mL of water is produced for every 100 kcal of energy released. The type of energy substrate oxidized determines the volume of water produced: 100 g of carbohydrate produces 55 g of water; 100 g of fat produces 107 g of water; and 100 g of protein produces 41 g of water.

Fluid loss occurs as a sensible loss through the kidneys as urine (≈1400 mL/day) and through the gastrointestinal tract as feces (≈200 mL/day) or as an insensible loss through the skin as perspiration (≈450 mL/day) or from the lungs as expired water vapor (≈350 mL/day). The volume of insensible loss is higher with vigorous muscular exercise; with an increased respiratory rate; in a hot, dry environment; with a fever; or with severe skin burns.

The various compartments are separated by semipermeable membranes that allow certain fluids and solutes to move freely between them. The movement of water between compartments is maintained by a dynamic equilibrium among five interdependent factors: intake and output, osmotic and hydrostatic pressure, hormones, electrolyte concentration, and the cardiovascular system.

An important concept in fluid balance is that the amount of fluid taken in must equal the amount of fluid leaving the body. If this does not occur, the fluid level in the various compartments must change. The body's primary mechanism to maintain total body fluid volume is adjustment in the amount of fluid leaving the body through the volume of urine excreted. Although it is difficult for the body to control the amount a person eats or drinks, it can influence the desire to do so through thirst and hunger.

The composition of the solutions in the different compartments has a major effect on fluid balance. The principal difference in the composition of the intracellular, intravascular, and interstitial fluids is the difference in the protein and salt concentrations. As shown in **Table 53-7**, the electrolyte concentration of the extracellular compartments is very similar, with the major cation being sodium and the major anions being chlorine and bicarbonate. The intravascular compartment has a much higher protein concentration than the interstitial compartment, thereby generating an osmotic pressure that helps keep fluid in the vascular space and out of the interstitial space. Extracellular and intracellular fluids are more unlike chemically than they are similar. The primary intracellular cation is potassium, and the major anion is phosphate; the protein content is highest in the cells.

One important mechanism used to control extracellular fluid (ECF) volume is the electrolyte concentration, particularly sodium. The phrase, "Where sodium goes, water soon follows" can aid in remembering this concept. The arterial blood pressure declines when the ECF and blood volume are reduced from lack of fluid intake. This stimulates pressure receptors (baroreceptors) in the hypothalamus and thorax to stimulate the adrenal cortex to increase secretion of the hormone aldosterone. Aldosterone increases resorption of sodium in the kidney tubule, which leads to an increase in kidney tubule resorption of water and a reduction in urine volume. The reduced urine volume increases the ECF volume and steers it back toward a normal balance.

Stimulation of the hypothalamus also triggers the pituitary gland to secrete antidiuretic hormone (ADH). ADH functions to reduce the amount of water excreted by promoting resorption of water into the circulation at the renal tubules. The pituitary gland can also trigger secretion of ADH after receiving a signal from the baroreceptors in the aortic bodies that the blood pressure is low.

Two factors working together determine urine volume: the kidney glomerular filtration rate and the rate of water resorption by the renal tubules. Except under abnormal conditions, the filtration rate is fairly constant and is not a major factor in urine excretion. The rate of tubular resorption, on the other hand, fluctuates considerably. During the course of a single day, the kidneys filter 190 L of water and reabsorb 189 L. As already

TABLE 53-7
Electrolyte Concentrations of Body Fluids

Electrolyte	Intravascular Concentration (mEq/L)	Interstitial Concentration (mEq/L)	Intracellular Concentration (mEq/L)
Cations			
Sodium (Na^+)	142	145	10
Potassium (K^+)	4	4	158
Magnesium (Mg^{+2})	3	2	35
Calcium (Ca^{+2})	5	3	2
Total	154	154	205
Anions			
Chloride (Cl^-)	103	115	2
Bicarbonate (HCO_3^-)	27	30	8
Phosphate (PO_4^{-3})	2	2	140
Sulfate (SO_4^{-2})	1	1	—
Protein ($Prot^-$)	16	1	55
Organic acids	5	5	—
Total	154	154	205

EQUATION 53-16

Starling's Law

Starling's law is expressed as

$$Q_f = K_1 (Pch - Pih) - K_2 (Pco - Pio)$$

where:

Q_f = Effective filtration pressure between blood and interstitial fluid, which determines the bulk or net outward flow of fluid from the capillaries
Pch = Capillary hydrostatic pressure
Pih = Interstitial hydrostatic pressure
Pco = Capillary osmotic pressure
Pio = Interstitial osmotic pressure
K_1 = Capillary permeability coefficient for fluids and electrolytes
K_2 = Capillary permeability coefficient for proteins

discussed, the amounts of the hormones secreted by the pituitary gland (e.g., ADH) and the adrenal cortex (aldosterone) regulate water resorption.

Another important mechanism that regulates the water and electrolyte levels in the extracellular fluid is the pressure gradient. According to the physical laws governing filtration and osmosis, hydrostatic pressure tends to push fluid out of its compartment, whereas osmotic pressure tends to pull water into its compartment. English physiologist Ernest Starling proposed a mechanism that controls movement across capillary membranes (**Equation 53-16**).

Because the intravascular compartment contains a larger number of proteins than the interstitial compartment (refer to Table 53-7), a larger osmotic pressure is generated in the vascular space. At the arterial end of tissue capillaries, normal values for the various pressures are as follows: capillary hydrostatic pressure (Pch), 35 mm Hg; capillary osmotic pressure (Pco), 24 mm Hg; interstitial fluid hydrostatic pressure (Pih), 2 mm Hg; and interstitial osmotic pressure (Pio), 0 mm Hg (**Figure 53-11**). The net filtration pressure at the arterial end of the capillaries therefore is as follows:

$$(35 - 2) - (24 - 0) = 33 - 24 = 9 \text{ mm Hg}$$

This suggests that a net positive pressure of 9 mm Hg tends to push fluids from the vascular space at the arterial end of the capillaries.

At the venous end of the tissue capillaries, normal pressures are as follows: Pch, 15 mm Hg; Pco, 25 mm Hg; Pih, 1 mm Hg; and Pio, 3 mm Hg. The net filtration pressure of the venous end of the capillaries is as follows:

$$(15 - 1) - (25 - 3) = 14 - 22 = -8 \text{ mm Hg}$$

This suggests that a net negative pressure of 8 mm Hg tends to pull fluids in toward the vascular space at the venous end of the capillaries. As blood flows through the capillary tissue bed, the tendency is for fluid to be pushed out into the interstitial space at the arterial end (net outward pressure of 9 mm Hg) and pulled back into the capillaries from the interstitial space at the venous end (−8 mm Hg). Interstitial fluid that is not pulled back into the capillaries is drained via the lymphatic system.

Of the three main body compartmental fluids, interstitial fluid varies the most. Plasma volume usually fluctuates only slightly and briefly. If an abnormally large amount of fluid shifts to the interstitial (and eventually to the intercellular) tissue space, the condition is known as *edema*. Edema can be caused by any of the factors governing the movement of fluids between the vascular and interstitial compartments, including (1) retention of electrolytes (especially sodium) in the extracellular fluid as a result of increased aldosterone secretion or after serious renal disease; (2) an increase in capillary

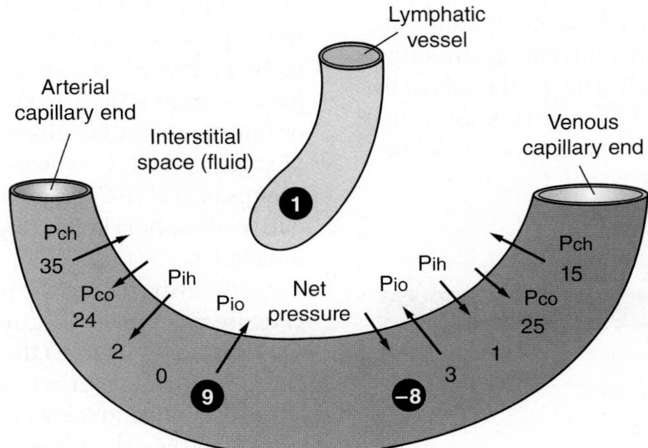

FIGURE 53-11 Starling's law governs the movement of fluids between the capillary and interstitial compartments based on hydrostatic (capillary [Pch] and interstitial [Pih]) and osmotic (capillary [Pco] and interstitial [Pio]) pressure differences.

hydrostatic pressure, as is seen in congestive heart failure caused by left ventricular failure; and (3) a decrease in plasma proteins because of a low overall protein concentration, such as that caused by poor nutrition (reflected in a low serum albumin level) or because of increased capillary permeability, such as that caused by infection, burns, or shock. Increased capillary permeability allows protein molecules to leak out of the vascular space into the interstitial space, where they exert an osmotic pressure and pull fluid toward that area.

Metabolic Pathways

Food is broken down into nutrients that are used by the body to promote growth, maintenance, and repair. The six classes of nutrients are carbohydrate, fat, protein, vitamins, minerals, and water.

The word *metabolism* is derived from the Greek word *meta*, meaning "change." Metabolism involves the processes by which these nutrients are used after they are ingested, digested, absorbed, and circulated to the cells of the body. It uses them in two ways: as an energy source to drive vital functions (carbohydrates, fat, and protein are the energy nutrients) or as the ingredients to make complex chemical compounds. Before nutrients can be used, catabolism must occur. **Catabolism** involves reactions in which large molecules are broken down to smaller ones that can be used by the cells, where they undergo many chemical changes. The process by which the nutrients are used to build more complex biomolecules is **anabolism**.

Catabolism is a decomposition process involving the oxidation of nutrient molecules. It releases energy (exergonic metabolism) in two forms: as heat or as chemical energy. Heat energy helps maintain the homeostasis of body temperature, but it cannot be used as a form of energy by the cells. Chemical energy, on the other hand, can be used by the cells, but it must first be transferred to high-energy bonds of ATP molecules. These bonds break more easily than other types of chemical bonds and therefore give up their energy more readily. ATP is one of the crucial compounds of the biologic world because it supplies energy directly to the energy-using reactions of all cells in all kinds of living organisms, from one-celled plants to trillion-celled human beings. The end products of catabolism include such molecules as lactic acid, ethanol, CO_2, urea, ammonia, and water.

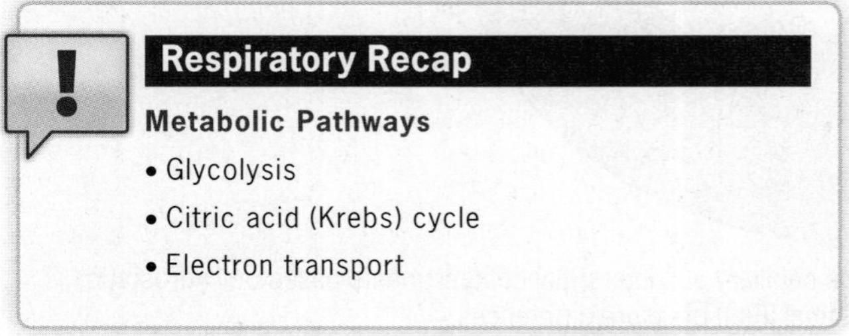

Respiratory Recap

Metabolic Pathways

- Glycolysis
- Citric acid (Krebs) cycle
- Electron transport

Anabolism is a synthesis process that assembles precursor molecules, such as amino acids, sugars, fatty acids, and nitrogenous bases, into cell macromolecules such as proteins, polysaccharides, lipids, and nucleic acids. This process requires energy (endergonic metabolism), which is supplied by the ATP generated during catabolism.

These two metabolic processes occur simultaneously in the cell in that some of the energy released and the products produced during catabolism are immediately used in the process of anabolism. The cell manages the conflicting demands of concomitant catabolism and anabolism in two ways. First, the cell maintains a tight and separate regulation of both processes through the use of literally hundreds of enzymatic reactions organized into discrete pathways. Second, the metabolic pathways are localized in different cellular compartments. For example, the enzymes responsible for fatty acid biosynthesis are found in the cytosol, whereas the fatty acid oxidation process takes place in the mitochondria.

The pathways of catabolism converge to a few end products, and the process consists of three stages (**Figure 53-12**). Stage 1 involves the breakdown of protein, polysaccharide, and lipid macromolecules into their respective building blocks. Proteins give up their 20 component amino acids; polysaccharides break down to carbohydrate units that are ultimately converted to glucose; and lipids produce glycerol and fatty acids. The cells prefer glucose as their primary energy fuel and therefore catabolize most of the carbohydrates absorbed and anabolize a relatively small portion of it. Fats and proteins are catabolized only when the amount of glucose entering cells is inadequate for their energy needs.

Stage 2 converts the products from stage 1 into an even more limited set of simpler metabolic by-products. Fatty acids break down into two-carbon units of acetyl coenzyme A (acetyl-CoA). Glucose and the glycerol from lipids generate the three-carbon α-keto acid pyruvic acid (pyruvate), which breaks down into acetyl-CoA in the presence of oxygen (aerobic metabolism) or to lactic acid when oxygen is absent (anaerobic metabolism). Amino acids give rise to pyruvate, acetyl-CoA, or intermediates fed directly into the citric acid cycle of stage 3. Stage 3 involves the combustion of the acetyl groups of acetyl-CoA by the citric acid cycle and oxidative phosphorylation to yield CO_2, water, and ATP molecules.

Carbohydrates are the primary source of energy. Glucose metabolism begins with the breakdown of a six-carbon glucose chain ($C_6H_{12}O_6$) to two three-carbon pyruvate (pyruvic acid) molecules by means of a process called **glycolysis**. Glycolysis takes place in the cytosol of the cell. It is an anaerobic process in that it does not use oxygen and as such is the only process that provides cells with energy when the oxygen supply is

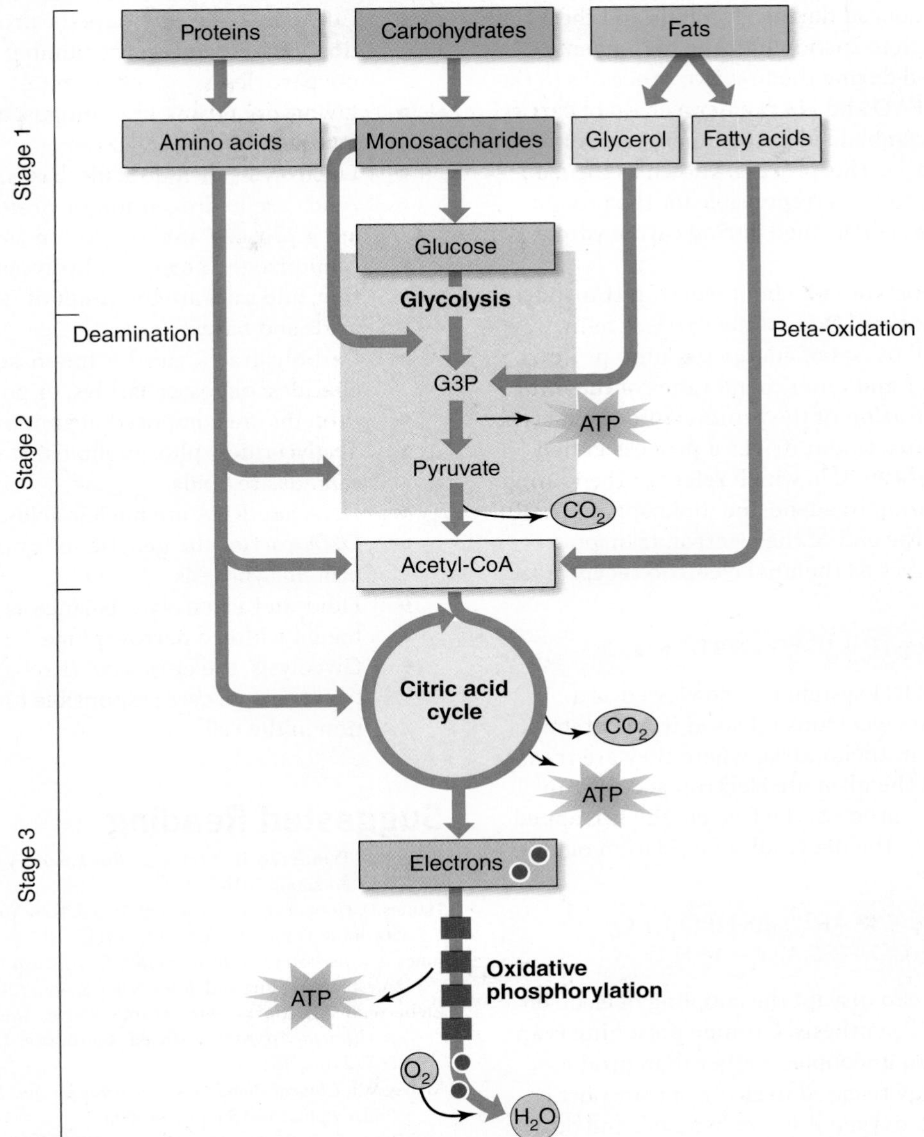

FIGURE 53-12 Three stages of catabolism.

inadequate or even absent. Glycolysis releases about 5% of the energy stored in the glucose molecule, releasing some energy as heat and the rest as energy transferred to ATP molecules and to reduced nicotinamide adenine dinucleotide (NAD) molecules (NADH). For every glucose molecule undergoing glycolysis, a net of two ATP molecules is formed. Although only a small amount of energy is released during glycolysis, it is an essential process because it prepares glucose for the second step in catabolism, namely, the citric acid cycle.

The **citric acid (Krebs) cycle** converts two pyruvic acid molecules into six CO_2 molecules and six water molecules. The citric acid cycle takes place in the presence of oxygen in the mitochondria of the cell. Before pyruvic acid molecules enter the mitochondria, they combine with coenzyme A to split off CO_2 and a pair of high-energy electrons to form acetyl-CoA. Coenzyme A then detaches from acetyl-CoA, leaving a two-carbon acetyl group to enter the citric acid cycle. The citric acid cycle consists of a series of eight reactions, the first of which is the formation of citric acid from the combination of the two-carbon acetyl group with the four-carbon oxaloacetic acid (which was formed as a product in the eighth step of the cycle). Citric acid is also known as *tricarboxylic acid (TCA)*, and the citric acid cycle therefore is also known as the *TCA cycle*; it is also called the *Krebs cycle* because Sir Hans Krebs deciphered the cyclic nature of pyruvate oxidation, earning the 1935 Nobel Prize for his work on this metabolic pathway. In addition to eight acids, the citric acid cycle produces CO_2, a small amount of ATP, a small amount of reduced flavin adenine dinucleotide (FAD), and a large amount of reduced NAD (NADH).

The energy produced during glycolysis and the TCA cycle is not enough to sustain life. The high-energy electrons removed during the first two processes in the form of reduced FAD and NAD enter a chain of carrier molecules that is embedded in the inner membrane of the mitochondria. This process, known as the **electron transport system**, is responsible for the production of 90% of the ATP formed during carbohydrate catabolism.

The most important fact about electron transport is that as electrons move down the carrier chain, they release small bursts of energy to pump protons between the inner and outer membranes of the mitochondria. The diffusion of the protons into the matrix in the inner compartment drives a process called **oxidative phosphorylation**, which refers to the joining of a phosphate group to adenosine diphosphate (ADP) to form ATP. At the end of the electron transport chain, oxygen serves as the final electron receptor to form water:

$$NADH + H^+ + \tfrac{1}{2}O_2 \rightarrow NAD^+ + H_2O$$

The NAD^+-NADH system can be viewed as a shuttle that carries electrons released from catabolic substrates to the mitochondria, where they are transferred to oxygen, the ultimate electron acceptor in catabolism. In the process, the free energy is trapped in ATP molecules. The net result of oxidation of glucose is as follows:

$$\text{Glucose} + 38\ ADP + 38\ HPO_4^{-2} + O_2 \rightarrow 6\ CO_2 + 38\ ATP + 44\ H_2O$$

Certain drugs can disrupt the coupling of electron transport and ATP synthesis. Cyanide poisoning is an example of such an uncoupler. Rather than producing ATP, the energy released in electron transport is dissipated as heat, oxygen is not consumed, and death eventually occurs.

Key Points

- Atoms consist of protons, neutrons, and electrons.
- Atoms join to produce ionic, covalent, and hydrogen bonds.
- Chemical reactions involve the forming or breaking of chemical bonds.
- The degree to which solute particles dissolve into a solvent is called *solubility*.
- The concentration of a solution can be stated as moles, percent, ratio, or mEq/L.
- Colligative properties are the properties of a solution that depend on the number of dissolved solute particles.
- Living organisms are composed of organic and inorganic compounds.
- Electrolytes include acids, bases, and salts.
- Acids are hydrogen ion or proton donors, bases are hydrogen ion or proton acceptors, buffers minimize the change in hydrogen ion concentration, and salts are the result of reactions between acids and bases.
- Carbohydrates can be monosaccharides, disaccharides, oligosaccharides, or polysaccharides.
- Proteins are composed of amino acids.
- Triglycerides, phospholipids, steroids, and eicosanoids are lipids.
- DNA and RNA are nucleic acids.
- DNA carries the genetic information (genes) for protein synthesis.
- Fluid and electrolyte balance is normally maintained within a narrow range.
- Glycolysis, the citric acid (Krebs) cycle, and electron transport are responsible for energy production in the cell.

Suggested Reading

Berg JM, Tymoczko JL, Stryer L. *Biochemistry*. 7th ed. New York: WH Freeman; 2010.

Hames D, Hooper N. *Biochemistry*. 4th ed. New York: Garland Science, Taylor & Francis Group, LLC; 2011.

Jones A. *Chemistry: An Introduction for Medical and Health Sciences*. West Sussex, England: John Wiley & Sons; 2005.

Lieberman M, Marks AD. *Mark's Basic Medical Biochemistry: A Clinical Approach*. 4th ed. Baltimore: Lippincott Williams & Wilkins; 2012.

Malley WJ. *Clinical Blood Gases: Assessment and Intervention*. 2nd ed. Philadelphia: WB Saunders; 2005.

McMurry J, Ballantine D, Hoeger C. *Fundamentals of General, Organic, and Biological Chemistry*. 7th ed. Glenview, IL: Pearson Education Inc; 2012.

Mooney S. Bioinformatics approaches and resources for single nucleotide polymorphism functional analysis. *Brief Bioinform*. 2008;6:44–56.

Murry RM, Rodwell VW. *Harper's Illustrated Biochemistry*. 29th ed. New York: Lange Medical Books/McGraw-Hill; 2012.

Nelson DL, Cox MM. *Lehniger Principles of Biochemistry*. 6th ed. New York: WH Freeman; 2012.

Raymond KW. *General, Organic, and Biological Chemistry: An Integrated Approach*. 4nd ed. Hoboken, NJ: John Wiley & Sons; 2014.

Sackheim GI, Lehman DD. *Chemistry for the Health Sciences*. 8th ed. Upper Saddle River, NJ: Prentice Hall; 1998.

Scanlon VC, Sanders T. *Essentials of Anatomy and Physiology*. 6th ed. Philadelphia: FA Davis; 2010.

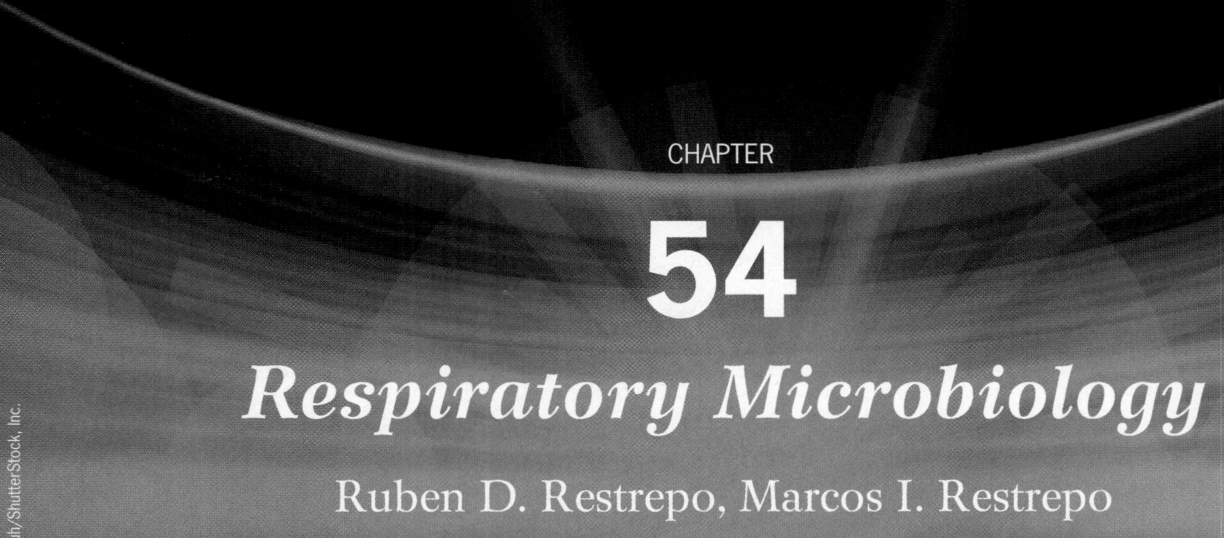

CHAPTER

54
Respiratory Microbiology

Ruben D. Restrepo, Marcos I. Restrepo

OUTLINE

OBJECTIVES

1. Identify the major microorganisms causing respiratory infections.
2. Compare bacteria, viruses, fungi, and parasites.
3. List the most common pathogens infecting the upper airway and lower respiratory tract.
4. Compare the techniques of sputum induction, bronchoscopy, and bronchoalveolar lavage.
5. Describe microbiology techniques to identify pathogens.
6. Discuss the mechanisms of antibiotic resistance.

KEY TERMS

acid-fast bacillus (AFB)
aerobe
anaerobe
antibiotic resistance
antigen detection
bacillus
bacterium
biofilm
bronchoalveolar lavage (BAL)
bronchoscopy
coccus
culture
fungus
gram-negative bacterium
gram-positive bacterium
Mantoux test
microbiology
multiresistant
mutation
normal flora
parasite
purified protein derivative (PPD)
spirochete
sputum induction
transtracheal aspiration (TTA)
virologic study
virus

Introduction

The respiratory therapist encounters patients with upper and lower airway infections every day. The pathogens responsible for these common illnesses are diverse, representing essentially the entire spectrum of **microbiology**, from bacteria to viruses, fungi, and occasionally parasites.

Bacteria

Bacteria are a large group of unicellular microorganisms first observed by Antonie van Leeuwenhoek in 1676.[1] Their name derives from the Greek word *baktērion*, which means "small staff."

Bacterial Microbiology

Bacteria typically measure between 0.5 and 5 μm in diameter. *Mycoplasma*, however, a very important bacterium in respiratory infections, only measures 0.3 μm. The human body contains approximately 10 times more bacterial cells than human cells. Most of these bacteria reside on the skin and in the gastrointestinal tract. Bacteria are classified as prokaryotes. Unlike the larger eukaryotes and other animal cells that contain a fully differentiated nucleus, prokaryotic bacterial deoxyribonucleic acid (DNA) forms only in a single, circular chromosome (a nucleoid) that is not bound by a membrane. Like animals and plants, bacteria use ribosomes to translate ribonucleic acid (RNA) into protein products. Bacteria (excluding the mycobacteria) are surrounded by both a cell membrane and a rigid cell wall. Eukaryotes lack a cell wall. **Figure 54-1** shows a schematic diagram of a typical bacterium.

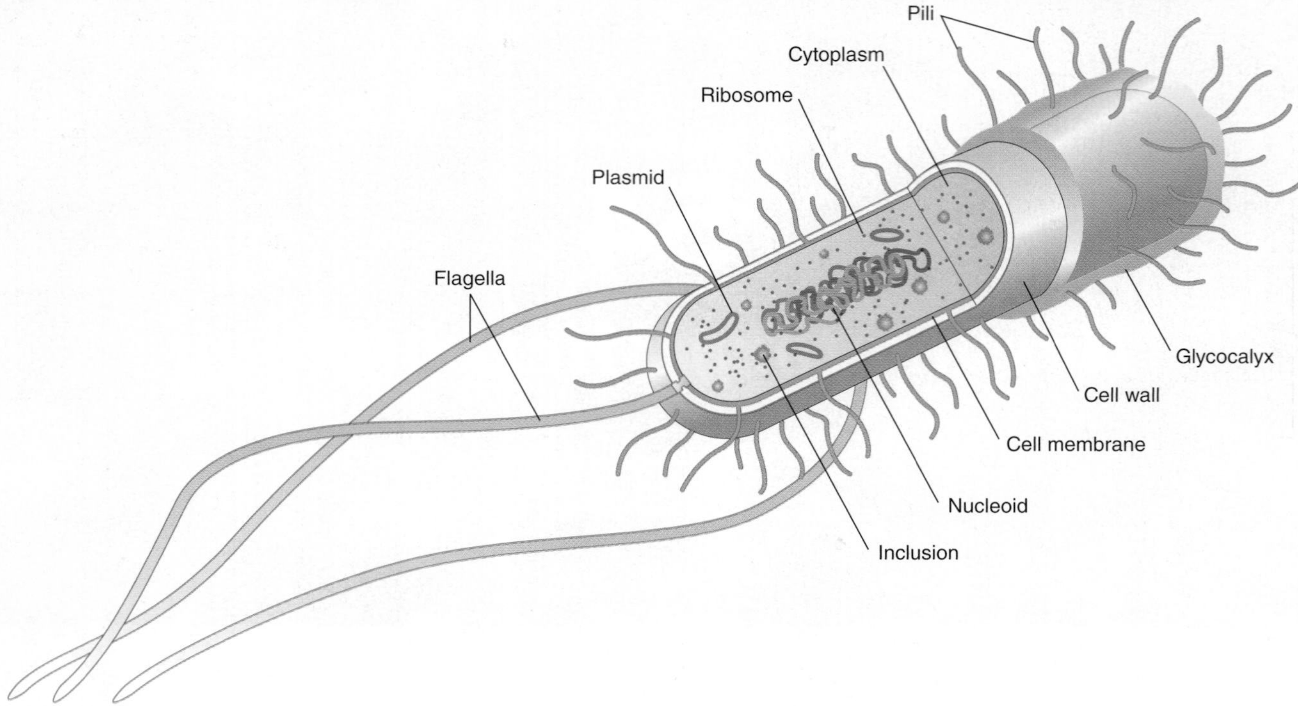

FIGURE 54-1 A typical bacterium.

Bacteria are free-living organisms that vary in their survival requirements. Oxygen is a variable of particular clinical importance. An **aerobe** requires oxygen for survival, an **anaerobe** requires the absence of oxygen, and a *facultative anaerobe* has limited oxygen tolerance. Bacteria are ubiquitous but are found preferentially in certain sites. For example, anaerobes such as *Clostridium* are found in soil, where oxygen concentrations are lower, explaining why soil-contaminated wounds are more prone to tetanus infection and gas gangrene (*C tetani* and *C perfringens*, respectively; both are anaerobes). Because *Pseudomonas aeruginosa* commonly colonizes the leaves of plants, live flowers are frequently banned from ventilator and burn units.

Bacteria display a wide variety of morphologies, as seen in **Figure 54-2**. Most bacterial species are either spherical (**cocci**) or rod-shaped (**bacilli**). Some are comma shaped (vibrio), spiral shaped (spirilla), or coiled (**spirochetes**). These different shapes can influence the ability of bacteria to acquire nutrients, swim through liquids, attach to surfaces, and escape predators. Some bacteria also associate in characteristic patterns: *Streptococcus* forms pairs or chains, *Staphylococcus* forms clusters like grapes, and *Neisseria* forms pairs. These typical morphologic features help clinicians in the rapid recognition of infections when samples are analyzed under the microscope.

Bacterial cell walls, which are essential for their survival, are made of peptidoglycan. Penicillin kills bacteria by inhibiting synthesis of peptidoglycan. According to the reaction of the cell wall to the Gram stain, bacteria can be classified as gram positive and gram negative. **Gram-positive bacteria** retain the crystal violet dye when washed in a decolorizing solution, whereas **gram-negative bacteria** do not retain the crystal violet dye in the Gram staining protocol. A safranin counterstain that is added after the crystal violet is washed out is responsible for coloring all gram-negative bacteria pink or red (**Figure 54-3**).

Gram-positive bacteria have a thick cell wall, whereas gram-negative bacteria have a thin cell wall with a few layers of peptidoglycan surrounded by a lipid membrane. This difference in coloration is one of the most important criteria used to classify bacteria and to

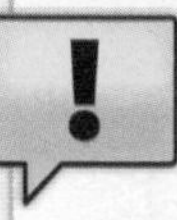

Respiratory Recap

Bacterial Shape Classification

- Cocci: round
- Bacilli: rod
- Spirochetes: spirals

Respiratory Recap

Bacterial Reaction to Gram Staining

- *Gram-positive bacteria*: peptidoglycan in cell wall; stains violet
- *Gram-negative bacteria*: no violet stain; pink appearance due to safranin counterstain

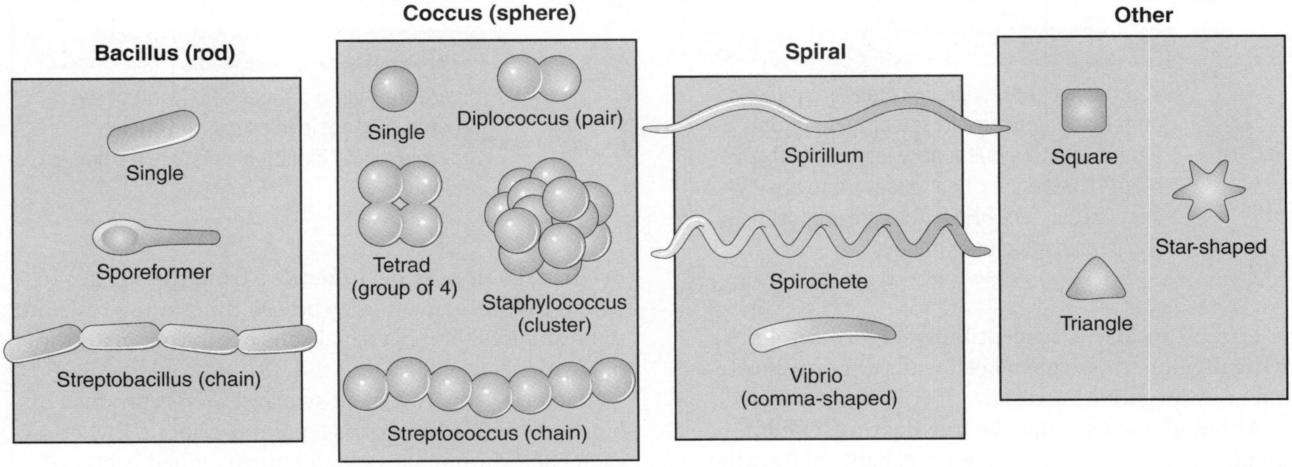

Bacillus (rod)

Single

Sporeformer

Streptobacillus (chain)

Coccus (sphere)

Single

Diplococcus (pair)

Tetrad (group of 4)

Staphylococcus (cluster)

Streptococcus (chain)

Spiral

Spirillum

Spirochete

Vibrio (comma-shaped)

Other

Square

Star-shaped

Triangle

(A)

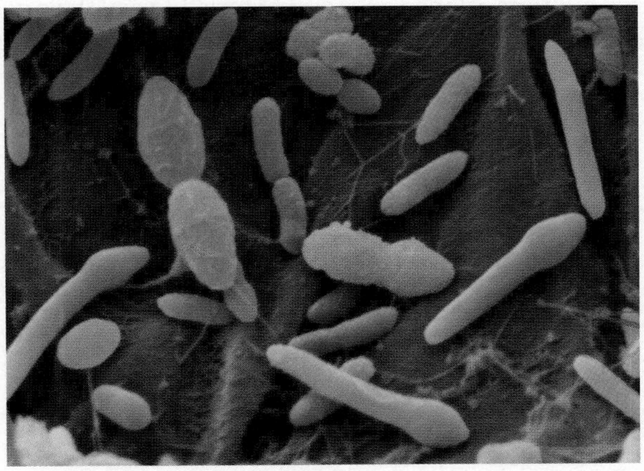

(B)

FIGURE 54-2 Basic bacterial shapes (**A**) and (**B**).

(**B**) © Medical-on-Line/Alamy Images.

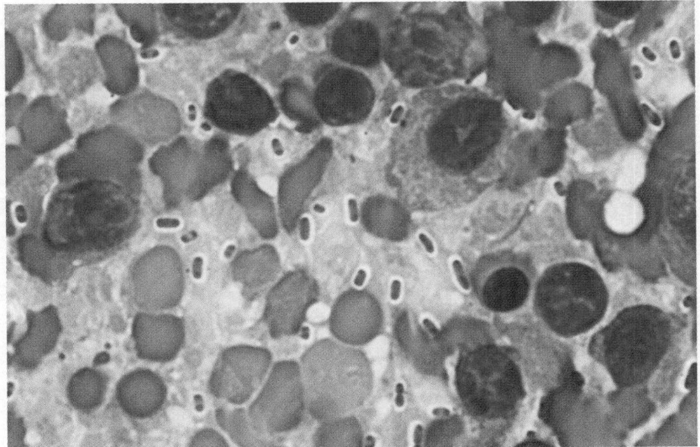

FIGURE 54-3 Electron micrograph of gram-negative bacilli (*Klebsiella pneumoniae*).

© CNRI/Science Source.

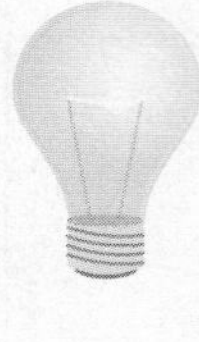

STOP AND THINK

You receive a preliminary report from the lab on the sputum sample you obtained from a patient with a pulmonary infection, which reads, "presence of abundant gram-positive cocci in clusters." How does this report help you in managing your patient?

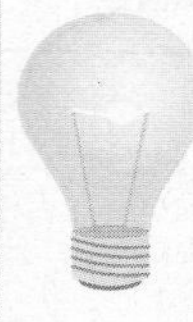

STOP AND THINK

You are treating a patient who is intubated and receiving positive pressure ventilation. What role would biofilm play in this particular situation?

determine antibiotic susceptibility. **Figure 54-4** schematically illustrates typical cell walls of gram-positive and gram-negative bacteria.

Although bacteria may be free floating (exhibiting planktonic behavior), they are capable of forming complex and stable aggregate communities, also known as bacterial mats or **biofilms**. These biofilms attach to any surface, liquid or solid. Once formed, biofilms may be virtually impossible to remove from the surface to which they attach and may be 100 times more resistant to antibiotics than bacterial cells exhibiting planktonic behavior.

Bacteria grow to a fixed size and then reproduce by binary fission, a form of asexual reproduction whereby each bacterium makes two identical cloned bacterial cells. Because this process is asexual, the ability of bacteria to vary their genetic traits is limited. Given an environment that provides unlimited nutrients, binary

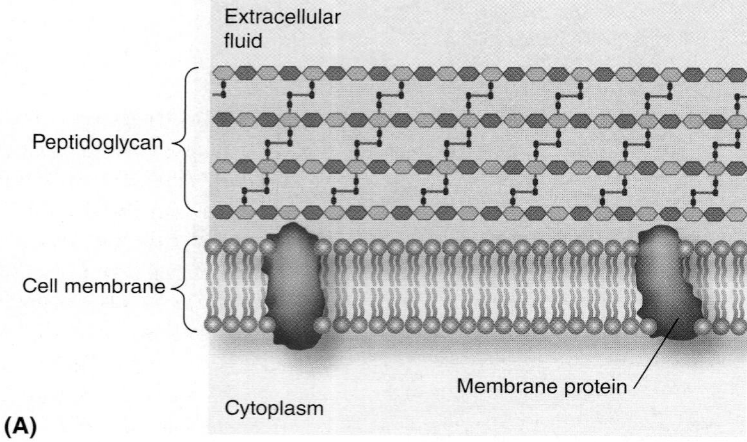

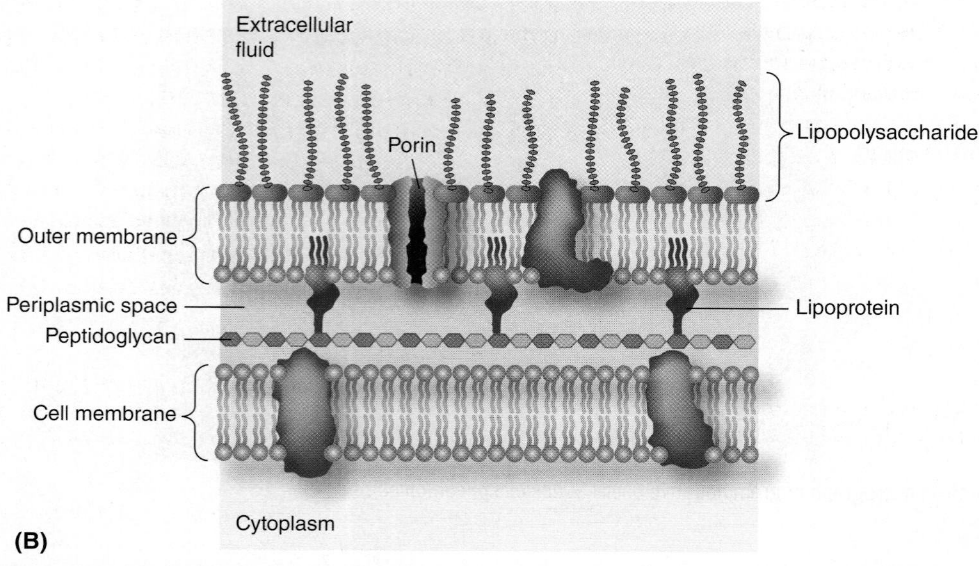

FIGURE 54-4 Gram-positive and gram-negative bacteria. (**A**) A gram-positive bacterium has a thick layer of peptidoglycan. (**B**) A gram-negative bacterium has a thin peptidoglycan layer and an outer membrane.

fission produces rapid bacterial growth. Because the number of bacteria doubles with each division, the pattern of growth is exponential (logarithmic). Each bacterium has a characteristic doubling time under ideal conditions. Although it can be as fast as 9.8 minutes (for *Pseudomonas natriensis*),[2] it typically ranges from 20 minutes (for *Escherichia coli*) to 24 hours (for *Mycobacterium tuberculosis*). For example, under ideal conditions, a single *E coli* bacterium can yield over 50 million bacteria in 8 hours. At this pace, the bacterial growth would fill a patient's room within 24 hours.

Because nutrients are limited in natural environments, bacteria cannot continue to reproduce at these fast rates and need to adapt to a low-nutrient environment by three different growth stages:

1. *Lag phase:* Period of slow growth when cells are adapting to the new environment.
2. *Log (logarithmic) phase:* Rapid exponential growth. Nutrients are metabolized at maximum speed until depleted.
3. *Stationary phase:* Nutrients are locally depleted, and waste products accumulate, growth rate slows, and the population reaches a steady state. The cells consume nonessential cellular proteins.

If conditions continue to deteriorate, bacterial counts begin to decline to low levels. This phase occurs in abscesses or as a consequence of immune system activity.

Gene transfer between bacterial cells is important in understanding antibiotic resistance. It occurs in three ways: mutation, conjugation, and transduction. **Mutation**, or transformation, is a genetic alteration that can result from the uptake of foreign DNA. This genetic material is added to or replaces part of a bacterium's DNA. Although some mutations are repaired and most produce nonfunctional genes, an occasional fortuitous mutation occurs, producing an improved gene. This altered gene then is passed on as the bacterium divides. If the new gene imparts a survival advantage, bacteria carrying it may come to predominate over normal, wild type bacteria. In bacterial *conjugation*, the DNA is transferred through direct cell contact, a process also known as horizontal gene transfer. *Transduction* involves the integration of a virus that infects bacteria (a bacteriophage), introducing foreign DNA into the chromosome. When viruses are released, they carry this DNA to newly infected bacteria.

TABLE 54-1
Common Disease-Causing Toxins

Toxin	Producer	Effect
Toxic shock	*Staphylococcus aureus*	Causes fever, rash, shock, tissue necrosis
Diphtheria	*Corynebacterium diphtheriae*	Inhibits protein synthesis, causing cell death
Erythrogenic	*Streptococcus pyogenes*	Causes scarlet fever rash
Tetanus	*Clostridium tetani*	Inhibits release of the neurotransmitter glycine, causing muscle spasm and rigidity
Botulism	*Clostridium botulinum*	Blocks release of the neurotransmitter acetylcholine, causing paralysis and flaccidity
Enterotoxin	*Escherichia coli*	Stimulates adenylate cyclase, increasing fluid secretion into the gut and causing diarrhea

Bacteria cause disease through three major mechanisms: toxin formation, direct damage, and inflammatory response. In addition to the endotoxin contained in the cell walls of gram-negative bacteria, many bacteria secrete exotoxins. These toxins are the primary virulence factor capable of damaging the plasma membrane of eukaryotic cells, inhibiting their protein synthesis or altering cellular proteins without killing the intoxicated cell. **Table 54-1** lists some important examples of toxins. Some bacterial infections do not require direct invasion of the bacteria into tissue or even the presence of viable bacteria. Particularly in foodborne illnesses, preformed toxins may be ingested even when all bacteria have been killed during brief cooking. Cooking or sterilization must produce high enough temperatures for sufficient duration to break down toxins as well as kill bacteria.

Although some bacterial illnesses are due solely to toxins, most bacteria cause direct damage by invading the host tissue and depleting its nutrients. More important, many bacteria produce substances that cause damage to adjacent tissues, facilitating bacterial spread. Examples include the collagenase and hyaluronidase

Respiratory Recap

Bacterial Growth

- Lag phase
- Log phase
- Stationary phase

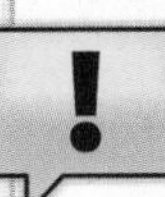

Respiratory Recap

Mechanisms of Bacterial Disease

- Toxin formation by bacteria
- Direct local tissue damage from bacteria
- Damage as a result of the immune response (pyogenic or granulomatous)

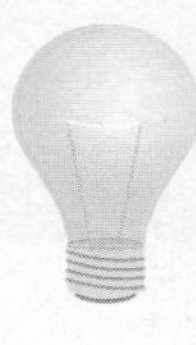

STOP AND THINK

One of your patients has been diagnosed with a pulmonary abscess. Why, despite intense antimicrobial therapy, might this patient's infection not resolve?

produced by *Streptococcus pyogenes*, which digest components of the intercellular matrix. *Staphylococcus aureus* produces coagulase, which forms a fibrin clot around the site of infection, protecting *S aureus* from immune attack. New strains of methicillin-resistant *S aureus* (MRSA) acquired in the community produce the Panton-Valentine leukocidin toxin, which is associated with tissue necrosis, abscess formation, and a high mortality.[3,4]

Immune responses to bacterial invasion are responsible for clinical manifestations that include fever, hypotension, muscle aches, malaise, loss of appetite, confusion, and temporary liver and heart dysfunction. Immune cells also cause local tissue damage in their attempt to directly kill bacteria as often seen in pyogenic or granulomatous patterns. With the pyogenic pattern the predominant immune cells are neutrophils. Intense activity kills bacteria and host cells, producing a collection of neutrophils and dead tissue called *pus*. A cavity called an *abscess* may form where tissue has been destroyed. Because immune cells tend to travel along tissue surfaces, bacteria may survive within the center of an abscess unless it is drained. Some bacteria, of which *Mycobacterium tuberculosis* is the archetype, stimulate the formation of granulomas, which are collections of macrophages arranged in a palisade, or wall, around a focus of infection. The macrophages are surrounded by T lymphocytes, a formation that tends to wall off the infection, preventing its spread. Organisms then are phagocytized (ingested) by the macrophages. The interior of a granuloma may become filled with dead cells, forming a cheesy substance that gives these granulomas the name *caseating necrotizing granulomas*.

Many areas of the body normally contain bacteria, known as the **normal flora**, that do not usually cause disease at that site. However, when normal flora from one site contaminates another site, serious illness may result. **Table 54-2** lists the normal flora of several important sites.

TABLE 54-2
Normal Human Flora by Body Site

Site	Normal Flora
Pharynx and upper gastrointestinal tract	*Moraxella catarrhalis*; *Staphylococcus epidermidis* and *S aureus*; α-hemolytic streptococci; viridans group streptococci; *Streptococcus pneumoniae*; *Peptostreptococcus*, *Lactobacillus*, and *Fusobacterium* species; *Actinomyces israelii*; *Haemophilus influenzae* and *parainfluenzae*; *Corynebacterium* species; *Neisseria meningitidis*, *Bacteroides* species, and other anaerobes; and *Candida* (yeast) species
Colon	*Enterococcus* species; *Escherichia coli*; *Pseudomonas*, *Bacteroides*, and *Clostridium* species and other gram-negative bacilli and anaerobes; also *Candida* (yeast) species; organisms known as coliforms or enteric bacteria because of their location in the colon
Skin	*Staphylococcus epidermidis* and *S aureus*; streptococci; *Corynebacterium* species; *Clostridium perfringens*; *Propionibacterium aenes*; *Candida* (yeast) species
Lower respiratory tract	Essentially sterile; possibility of colonization when illness or structural lung disease compromises immune function

Common Bacteria Associated with Respiratory Disease

Streptococcus pneumoniae

Streptococcus pneumoniae, or pneumococcus, is a gram-positive, α-hemolytic (turns blood agar green) facultative anaerobe. It is also known as *Diplococcus pneumoniae* because of its characteristic appearance in gram-stained sputum (**Figure 54-5**). *S pneumoniae*'s polysaccharide capsule is variably resistant to phagocytosis, which determines its virulence, prevalence, and extent of drug resistance. This bacterium is normally found in the nasopharynx of 20% to 40% of healthy children and 5% to 10% of healthy adults. Its count may be higher in environments where people are in close proximity to each other for long periods of time, however, such as day-care centers and hospitals. Although *S pneumoniae* causes respiratory infections such as pneumonia, acute sinusitis, and otitis media, it is also

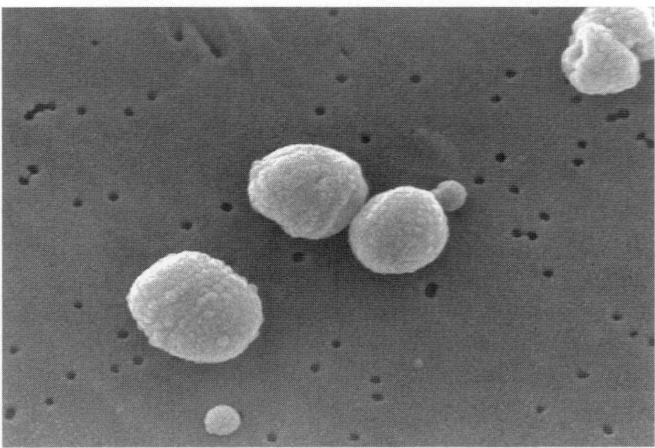

FIGURE 54-5 Electron micrograph of *Streptococcus pneumoniae* showing its characteristic appearance in pairs.
Courtesy of Janice Haney Carr/CDC.

responsible for causing endocarditis, pericarditis, osteomyelitis, and bacteremia. *S pneumoniae* is the most common cause of bacterial meningitis in children and adults. It spreads to the bloodstream from the site of original infection.

A heptavalent pneumococcal conjugate vaccine (PCV-7) is recommended for all children aged 2 to 23 months and for at-risk children aged 24 to 59 months. Immunization with the PCV is suggested for those at highest risk of infection, including those 65 years or older.

Staphylococcus aureus

Staphylococcus aureus is a spherical gram-positive coccus, a facultative anaerobe bacterium that appears as grapelike clusters under the microscope (**Figure 54-6**). It forms round, golden (*aureus* in Latin) colonies when grown on blood agar. *S aureus* is primarily coagulase positive; therefore, it causes clot formation. Some strains of *S aureus* carry the Panton-Valentine leukocidin (PVL) toxin, which is responsible for increased virulence and resistance to antibiotics. This toxin is associated with severe necrotizing pneumonia in children. Nearly 25% to 30% of otherwise healthy people carry *S aureus* on the skin or in the nose. *S aureus* can cause a range of illnesses, from minor skin infections to life-threatening diseases such as pneumonia, meningitis, osteomyelitis, endocarditis, toxic shock syndrome (TSS), and septicemia. It is one of the four most common causes of nosocomial infections and is responsible for most postsurgical wound infections.

Nosocomial and healthcare-associated *S aureus* bacteremia are more likely to be caused by methicillin-resistant *Staphylococcus aureus* (MRSA). MRSA is a strain of *S aureus* resistant to a large group of antibiotics called the β-lactams, which include the penicillins and the cephalosporins. Patients with open wounds, invasive devices, and weakened immune systems are at greater risk for infection by MRSA than the general public. Patients with community-associated MRSA (CA-MRSA) pneumonia may require hospitalization or admission to the intensive care unit (ICU). MRSA is easily transferred from patient to patient if hospital isolation protocols are not rigorously followed. Either linezolid or vancomycin can be used for the treatment of MRSA pneumonia.[5]

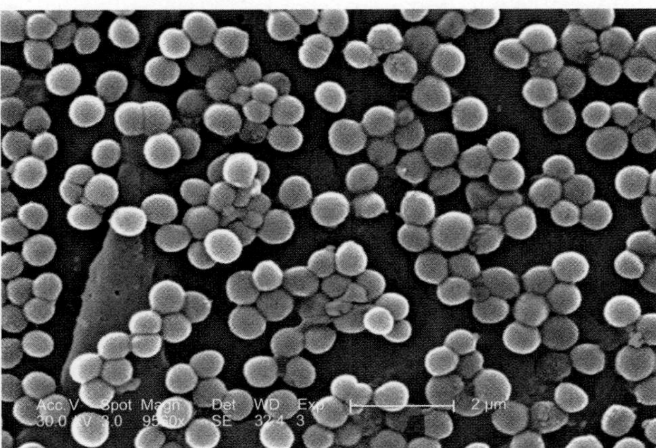

FIGURE 54-6 Electron micrograph depicting numerous grapelike clusters of *Staphylococcus aureus*.
Courtesy of Janice Haney Carr/Jeff Hageman, M.H.S./CDC.

Haemophilus influenzae

Haemophilus influenzae is a nonmotile, gram-negative coccobacillus with two defined strains: encapsulated and nonencapsulated (**Figure 54-7**). There are six types of *H influenzae:* a, b, c, d, e, and f. The encapsulated type b (Hib) is seen in conditions such as epiglottitis. Similar to *S aureus*, the capsule makes *H influenzae* resistant to phagocytosis. Most strains of *H influenzae*

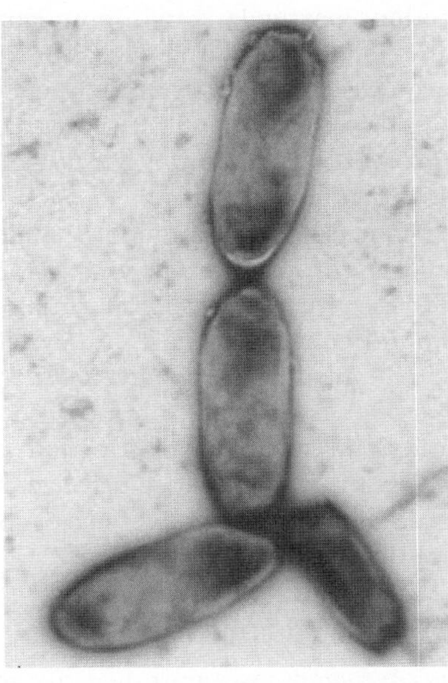

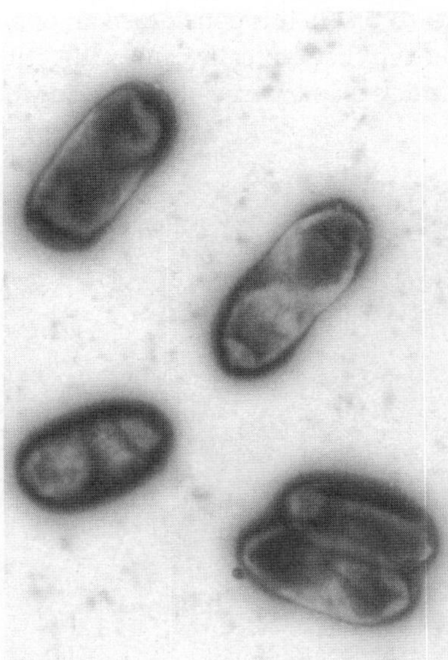

FIGURE 54-7 Electron micrographs of *Haemophilus influenzae*.
Courtesy of Wadsworth Center, NYS Department of Health.

are opportunistic bacteria. Since 1990, the routine use of the Hib conjugate vaccine has dramatically reduced the rate of severe meningitis and pneumonia in young children. Non–b type *H influenzae* cause otitis media, sinusitis, conjunctivitis, and pneumonia. Due to increase proportion of strains that produce β-lactamase, either a combination of amoxicillin and clavulanic acid, trimethoprim-sulfamethoxazole, or second- and third-generation cephalosporins can be considered.

Klebsiella pneumoniae

Klebsiella pneumoniae is a gram-negative, nonmotile, encapsulated, facultative anaerobic bacillus (**Figure 54-8**). It causes some of the most common gram-negative infections seen worldwide. *K pneumoniae* is commonly associated with hospital-acquired urinary tract and wound infections, particularly in immunocompromised and malnourished individuals. It causes bacterial pneumonia, typically as a result of aspiration in alcoholics, and is a common opportunistic pathogen for patients with chronic obstructive pulmonary disease (COPD) and diabetes. Pneumonia caused by *K pneumoniae* is associated with necrotic, inflammatory, and hemorrhagic changes in the lung parenchyma that produce the characteristic red currant jelly sputum.

K pneumoniae contains a β-lactamase that confers a resistance to ampicillin. Although *Klebsiella* bacteria remain largely susceptible to aminoglycosides and cephalosporins, the emergence of infections due to multidrug-resistant gram-negative pathogens in the ICU has resulted in a more frequent use of colistin, a polymyxin antibiotic.

Pseudomonas aeruginosa

Pseudomonas aeruginosa is a gram-negative aerobic bacillus (**Figure 54-9**). It is considered an opportunistic human pathogen that typically causes infection of the respiratory tract, urinary tract, burns, and wounds, as well as causing other blood infections. It is the most common cause of infections in burned patients and the most common pathogen found in invasive medical devices such as catheters. *P aeruginosa* can cause community-acquired pneumonia, healthcare-associated pneumonia, and ventilator-associated pneumonia. Patients with cystic fibrosis are frequently predisposed to respiratory infections caused by *P aeruginosa*.

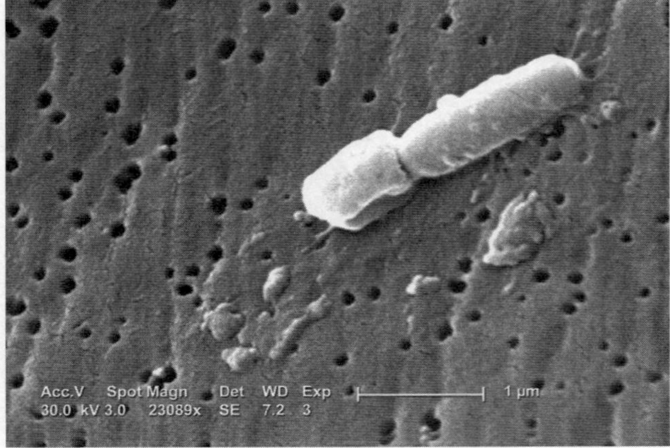

FIGURE 54-8 Electron micrograph of *Klebsiella pneumoniae*.
Courtesy of Janice Haney Carr/CDC.

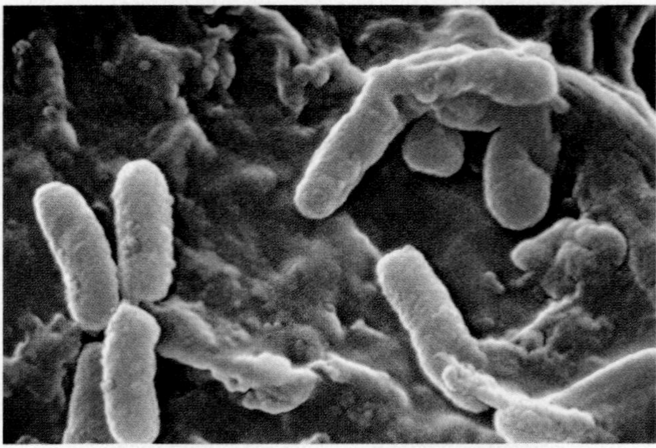

FIGURE 54-9 Electron micrograph of *Pseudomonas aeruginosa*.
Courtesy of Janice Haney Carr/CDC.

Laboratory sensitivity studies rather than empiric antibiotic therapy should guide treatment of *P aeruginosa* infections. Some of the antibiotics considered active against *P aeruginosa* are aminoglycosides (gentamicin, amikacin, and tobramycin) or quinolones (ciprofloxacin and levofloxacin but *not* moxifloxacin) in combination with cephalosporins (ceftazidime and cefepime but *not* cefuroxime, ceftriaxone, or cefotaxime), ureidopenicillins (piperacillin or ticarcillin. *P aeruginosa* is intrinsically resistant to all other penicillins), carbapenems (meropenem, imipenem, and doripenem but *not* ertapenem), polymyxins (polymyxin B and colistin), and monobactams (aztreonam).

Acinetobacter baumannii

Acinetobacter baumannii is a gram-negative aerobic bacillus similar in appearance to *H influenzae* on the Gram stain (**Figure 54-10**). *A baumannii* is associated with opportunistic infections and enters the body through catheters, endotracheal tubes, and open wounds. It has emerged as a very important pathogen among wounded soldiers. *A baumannii* commonly colonizes irrigation solutions and intravenous fluids. Healthcare workers can become carriers of *Acinetobacter* and be responsible for hospital-acquired infections. Prolonged hospitalization or antibiotic therapy is known to predispose to *Acinetobacter* colonization. *Acinetobacter* pneumonias usually occur as a consequence of colonized respiratory support equipment or fluids. Bacteremia may be associated with mortality rates as high as 75%. *A baumannii* is a multidrug-resistant bacillus sensitive to relatively few

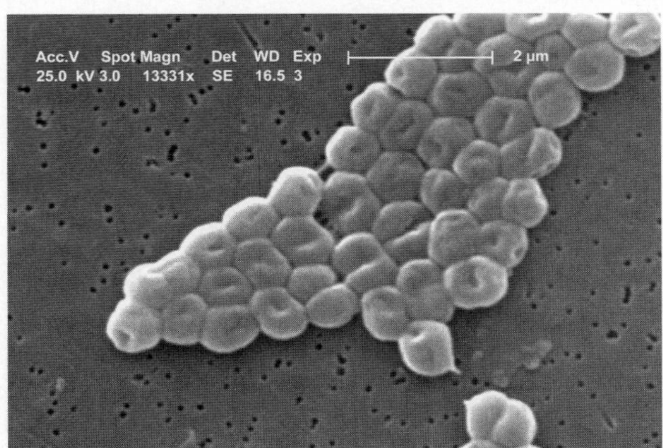

FIGURE 54-10 Electron micrograph of a highly magnified cluster of gram-negative, nonmotile *Acinetobacter baumannii* bacteria.
Courtesy of Janice Haney Carr/CDC.

antibiotics. A combination of sulbactam and ampicillin is recommended for a mild-to-severe infection, while carbapenems and polymyxins are recommended for multidrug-resistant strains.[6,7]

Chlamydophila pneumoniae

Chlamydophila (formerly *Chlamydia*) *pneumoniae*, *Mycoplasma pneumoniae*, and *Legionella pneumophila* are known as atypical bacteria because they do not appear in standard culture and staining techniques. *C pneumoniae* is an obligate intracellular gram-negative bacterium that belongs to the genus *Chlamydia* (**Figure 54-11**). *C pneumoniae* is an airborne organism. Chlamydiae commonly cause pharyngitis, bronchitis, and atypical pneumonia. There is increasing evidence to support an association between atypical bacterial infection—particularly with *C pneumoniae* and *M pneumoniae*—and stable asthma and asthma exacerbations.[8] The clinical presentation of *C pneumoniae* infection is indistinguishable from other causes of pneumonia and includes dry cough, fever, and dyspnea. Doxycycline has been considered the treatment of choice for *C pneumoniae* pneumonia, except in children younger than 9 years of age and in pregnant women. Several other medications used to treat patients with *C pneumoniae* infection include tetracyclines, macrolides, and fluoroquinolones. Telithromycin is the first antibiotic in a new class called ketolides approved for *C pneumoniae* pneumonia by the U.S. Food and Drug Administration (FDA).

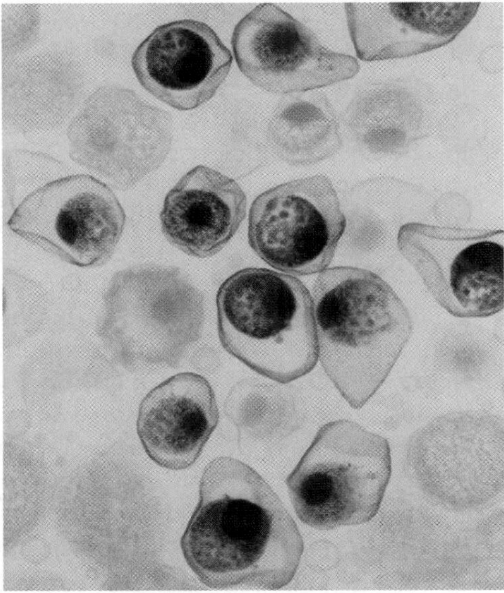

FIGURE 54-11 Electron micrograph of chlamydial particles (pear-shaped cells) of *Chlamydophila pneumoniae*.
© Phototake/Alamy Images.

Mycoplasma pneumoniae

Mycoplasma bacteria are the smallest free-living organisms, with diameters as small as 0.3 µm, similar to large viruses (**Figure 54-12**). These bacteria lack a cell wall. Without a cell wall, they are unaffected by many common antibiotics such as penicillin or other β-lactam antibiotics that target cell wall synthesis. Several species are pathogenic in humans, including *Mycoplasma pneumoniae*, which is the most common cause of atypical pneumonia and among the most common causes of pneumonia in children and young adults.[9] *M pneumoniae* is spread through respiratory droplet transmission, causing pharyngitis, bronchitis, and pneumonia. The atypical pneumonia caused by *M pneumoniae* is characterized by its relatively slow progression of symptoms, lack of sputum production, and a positive blood test for cold hemagglutinins in 50% to 70% of patients

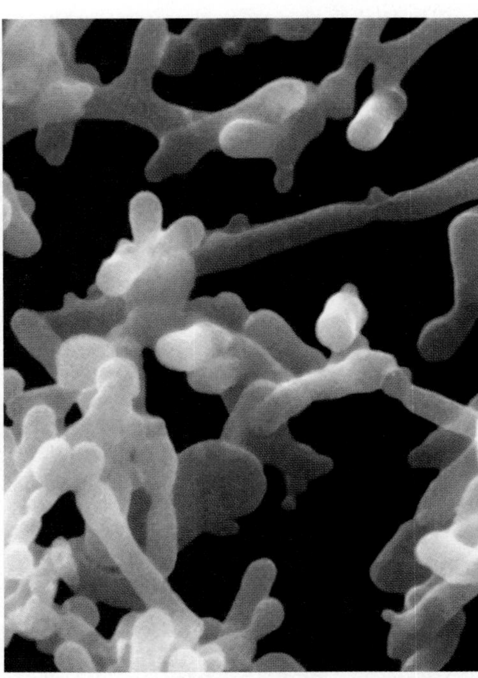

FIGURE 54-12 Electron micrograph showing *Mycoplasma pneumoniae*.
© Michael Gabridge/Visuals Unlimited, Inc.

after 10 days of infection. The most sensitive and rapid test to diagnose *M pneumoniae* infection in children is a combination of oropharyngeal polymerase chain reaction (PCR) and IgM enzyme immunoassay. Second-generation macrolide antibiotics, doxycycline, and fluoroquinolones are effective antimicrobials against infections caused by *Mycoplasma* species.[10]

Legionella pneumophila

Legionella pneumophila is a flagellated, noncapsulated, aerobic gram-negative bacillus that produces β-lactamase (**Figure 54-13**). *L pneumophila* is the etiologic agent of legionellosis or Legionnaire disease. *Legionella* is transmitted via inhalation of mist droplets containing the bacteria. *Legionella* earned its name after an outbreak of illness among people at a convention of the American Legion in Philadelphia in 1976. Legionnaire disease is a form of pneumonia that often goes undiagnosed and is difficult to distinguish from other types of pneumonia. It is typically not harmful except in elderly individuals or those with an immunocompromised system. On the other hand, hospital-acquired *Legionella* pneumonia carries a mortality rate as high as 28%. Current therapy for Legionnaire disease includes quinolones and newer macrolides such as azithromycin, clarithromycin, and roxithromycin.[11]

Rickettsiae

Like chlamydiae, rickettsiae are small bacteria that are obligate intracellular organisms. Rickettsiae are maintained within a mammalian reservoir (humans in the case of *Rickettsia prowazekii*). Rickettsiae are transmitted to humans indirectly, however, through the bite of specific arthropods (lice, mites, fleas, or ticks) that have previously encountered an infected mammal (**Figure 54-14**). The agent causing Q fever, originally named *Rickettsia burnetii* but recently renamed *Coxiella burnetii*, is an exception to this pattern. *C burnetii* is spread by aerosol emitted directly from cats, dogs, sheep, cattle, and goats.

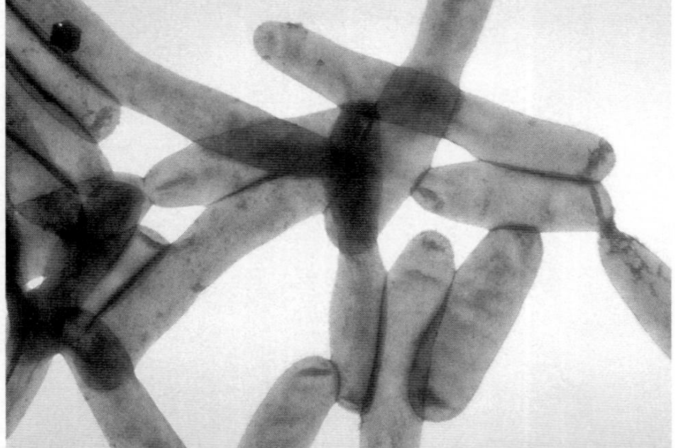

FIGURE 54-13 Electron micrograph of *Legionella pneumophila*.
Courtesy of CDC.

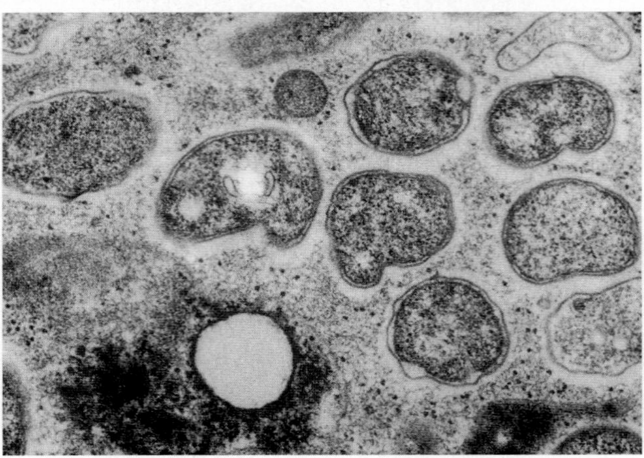

FIGURE 54-14 Electron micrograph of *Rickettsia prowazekii* inside host cells.

Aerosolization from the surface of the placenta is particularly effective, so attendance at an animal birth is a risk factor for infection.

Rickettsial diseases manifest as fever, severe headache, and influenza symptoms. Rickettsial diseases with important pulmonary manifestations include Q fever (*C burnetii*), epidemic typhus (*R prowazekii*), endemic typhus (*Rickettsia typhi*), and scrub typhus (*Rickettsia tsutsugamushi*). Cell culture is possible but not commonly used. Diagnosis is based on serology, that is, the detection of a specific antibody response to the organism. Serology may not show positive results for up to 2 weeks after infection. The majority of *Rickettsia* bacteria are susceptible to antibiotics of the tetracycline group.

Mycobacteria

Mycobacteria are rod-shaped bacteria distinguished by an unusual staining pattern in response to the Ziehl-Nielsen stain. Because mycobacteria's cell walls retain red carbolfuchsin stain despite rinsing with hydrochloric acid, they are called **acid-fast bacilli (AFB)**. The cell wall is neither truly gram negative nor positive, and it is resistant to a number of antibiotics, such as penicillin, that work by destroying bacterial cell walls.[12]

Mycobacterium tuberculosis (MTB) causes most cases of tuberculosis (**Figure 54-15**). Nontuberculous mycobacteria (NTM) are a large group of mycobacteria that includes *Mycobacterium avium-intracellulare* (MAI) and *Mycobacterium intracellulare*—together called *Mycobacterium avium* complex (MAC)—*Mycobacterium gordonae, Mycobacterium kansasii, Mycobacterium fortuitum, Mycobacterium chelonae,* and *Mycobacterium abscessus*; the last three are also known as rapid growers. Mycobacteria causing primarily nonpulmonary disease include *Mycobacterium marinum, Mycobacterium leprae, Mycobacterium bovis* (used to produce bacille Calmette-Guérin [BCG] vaccine for tuberculosis), and *Mycobacterium scrofulaceum*. Mycobacteria are slow-growing obligate aerobes

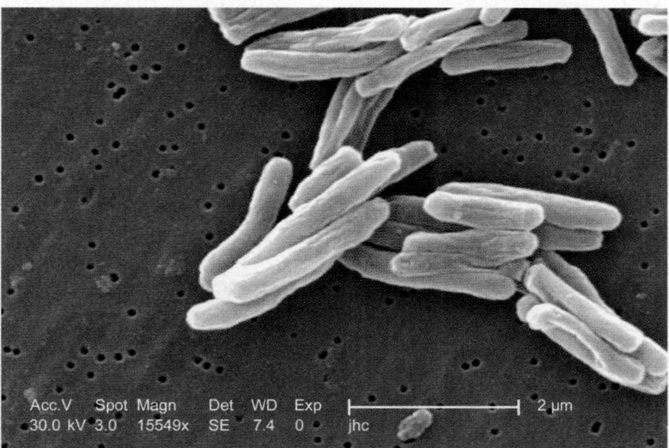

FIGURE 54-15 Electron micrograph depicting numerous clusters of *Mycobacterium tuberculosis*.
Courtesy of Janice Haney Carr/CDC.

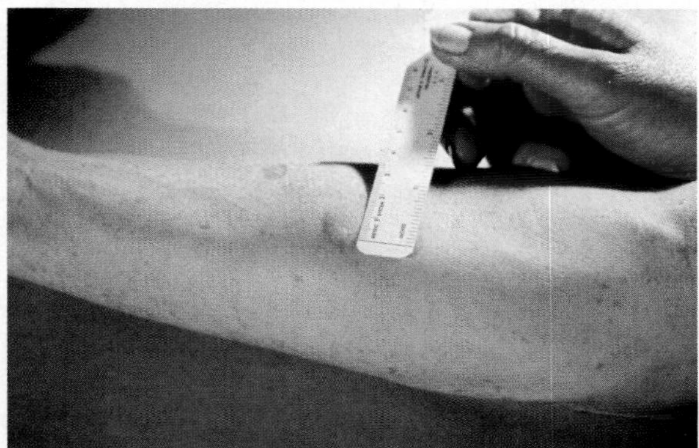

FIGURE 54-16 A 48-hour purified protein derivative (Mantoux or tuberculin) test being measured.
Courtesy of CDC.

that cause a slowly progressive, wasting disease over months to years.

Tuberculosis (TB) is spread through the air when people who have the disease cough, sneeze, or spit. One-third of the world's population has been infected with *M tuberculosis*; however, most of these infections remain asymptomatic or latent. New infections occur at a rate of one per second. Despite the fall in the number of cases of TB worldwide, an estimated 8.6 million people developed TB and 1.3 million died from the disease in 2012. TB is the leading killer of people with HIV.[13] Typical symptoms of tuberculosis include fever, night sweats, chronic cough with blood-tinged sputum, and weight loss. The presence of these symptoms should merit respiratory isolation until further laboratory tests confirm or rule out the presence of tuberculosis. Chest radiography, the tuberculin skin test, blood tests, and microscopic examination and microbiological culture of bodily fluids are the most commonly used diagnostic tools. Immunofluorescence has largely replaced actual acid-fast staining for AFB. This technique uses antibodies that bind specifically to mycobacteria and are joined to a molecule that fluoresces under ultraviolet light. The presence of fluorescence is evaluated microscopically. Like staining, this technique is limited by the very small numbers of organisms present in most cases of active disease. Therefore these techniques, although rapid, are insensitive. Additionally, neither test distinguishes MTB from other species of mycobacteria. Mycobacterial culture remains essential to reliably detect the presence of mycobacteria, identify the species, and determine the pattern of susceptibility to antibiotics. The major drawback to mycobacterial culture is the slow growth rate of mycobacteria; even with newer, rapid-growth techniques, results may take longer than 1 week.

Placement of **purified protein derivative (PPD)** subcutaneously, called the **Mantoux test** or tuberculin skin test, detects the presence of an immune response to mycobacteria by eliciting a delayed-type hypersensitivity response. This response manifests as induration of the injection site within 72 hours (**Figure 54-16**). A positive test is defined as an induration of 5 to 15 mm in diameter, depending on the population group (**Table 54-3**), representing exposure to mycobacteria at some time in the past, but not necessarily infection. Once converted to a positive PPD status, most patients remain positive indefinitely.

TABLE 54-3
Criteria for Purified Protein Derivative (PPD) Test Positivity

Threshold for Positive Test (Diameter of Induration at 48 to 72 Hours)	Group
5 mm	Recent TB exposure, chest radiograph suggestive of TB, immunocompromised because of disease (e.g., HIV infection) or drugs (e.g., corticosteroids)
10 mm	High-prevalence groups: born in a country with high prevalence of TB; poor access to health care; persons who live or spend time in certain facilities (e.g., nursing homes, prisons, shelters); persons who inject drugs High-risk groups: children younger than 4 years; close contact with infectious TB; chest radiograph suggestive of old TB; PPD conversion to positive in the past 2 years; certain medical conditions (diabetes, silicosis, prolonged therapy with corticosteroids, immunosuppressive therapy, leukemia, Hodgkin disease, head and neck cancers, severe kidney disease, malnutrition)
15 mm	General population

TB, tuberculosis; HIV, human immunodeficiency virus.

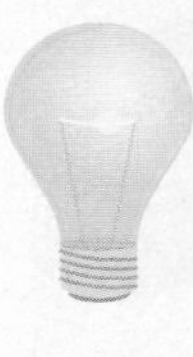

STOP AND THINK

A patient on the ward has a history of fever, night sweats, chronic cough with blood-tinged sputum, and weight loss. The PPD was negative. Should the patient be placed in respiratory isolation?

Some patients fail to demonstrate an immune response even after exposure and are termed *anergic*. The BCG vaccine rarely produces an induration greater than 15 mm into adulthood, so Mantoux tests can be useful in this population and should be read as if no prior BCG vaccination had been applied. The Mantoux test should not be applied to patients who have received BCG vaccine recently or to patients known to be PPD positive, because a vigorous immune response may produce tissue damage at the test site. A positive Mantoux test may be produced by exposure to any *Mycobacterium* species.

In the past few years, drug-resistant strains of MTB leading to multidrug-resistant TB (MDR TB) and extensively drug-resistant TB (XDR TB) have emerged, carrying a high mortality, especially in developing countries.[14] Drug-resistant tuberculosis is transmitted in the same way as regular TB. Multidrug-resistant TB is typically resistant to at least two first-line drugs (isoniazid [INH] and rifampin [RFP]) used to treat all persons with TB. Extensively drug-resistant TB is a relatively rare disease defined as TB resistant to INH and RFP plus resistant to any fluoroquinolone and at least one of three injectable second-line drugs (i.e., amikacin, kanamycin, or capreomycin). Healthcare providers can help prevent MDR-TB by quickly diagnosing cases, following recommended treatment guidelines, monitoring patients' response to treatment, and making sure therapy is completed. Healthcare providers should avoid exposure to patients who have TB in closed or crowded places and should consult infection control or occupational health experts to determine environmental procedures for preventing exposure to TB. The Xpert MTB/RIF is an automated, cartridge-based nucleic amplification assay (NAA) for the simultaneous detection of TB and rifampicin resistance directly from sputum in less than 2 hours.[15] This test looks at the genetic sequence of the organism to identify mutations in the genome of MDR-TB. The Centers for Disease Control and Prevention (CDC) has published updated guidelines for the use of NAA in the diagnosis of tuberculosis.

Viruses

With the exception of prions, **viruses** are the smallest and simplest class of pathogens. They are about 100 times smaller than bacteria, ranging in size from 0.02 to 0.3 μm. Viruses consist of genetic material, either RNA or DNA, surrounded by a protein coat called a *capsid*. Some viruses also are surrounded by a lipoprotein membrane called an *envelope* (**Figure 54-17**).

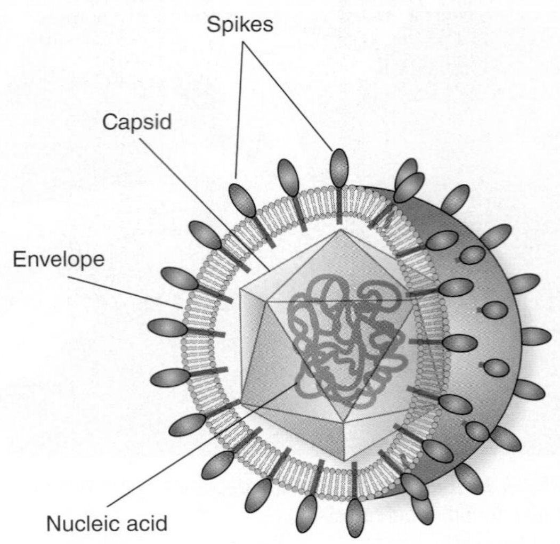

FIGURE 54-17 Diagrammatic view of a virus depicting its parts.

Viruses are infectious agents that are unable to grow or reproduce outside a host cell. After gaining entry into a host, viruses attach themselves selectively to certain host cells; for example, rhinovirus infects the upper airway mucosa, whereas human immunodeficiency virus (HIV) has a predilection for CD41 lymphocytes. This specificity is imparted by different proteins embedded in the outer surface of the capsid or, in enveloped viruses, by glycoproteins embedded in the envelope. These proteins or glycoproteins bind to specific cell surface receptors, and the virus then is taken up into the host cell and sheds its capsid or envelope to expose its genetic material, a process known as *uncoating*. Whereas replication of most DNA viruses takes place in the cell's nucleus, RNA viruses replicate in the cytoplasm. A reverse transcribing virus is any virus that forms DNA from an RNA template. The Baltimore classification places viruses into one of seven groups depending on a combination of their nucleic acid (DNA or RNA), strandedness (single stranded or double stranded), genome type, and method of replication.

Viruses themselves are metabolically inactive, but once inside a cell they use the host cell metabolism to replicate. The mechanism of viral replication varies, depending on the type of virus, but its goal is always to produce messenger RNA (mRNA), from which viral proteins are translated by the host cell. Most positive-polarity RNA viruses simply use their genome directly as mRNA, whereas negative-polarity RNA viruses carry their own RNA-dependent RNA polymerase to transcribe their genome into positive-polarity mRNA. Some RNA viruses—the retroviruses, of which the best known is HIV—first transcribe their RNA into DNA (**Figure 54-18**).

Because eukaryotic cells lack the reverse transcriptase necessary for DNA production from RNA, the retroviruses must carry a copy of their own reverse transcriptase. The resulting viral DNA then is transcribed by the host cell's RNA polymerase to produce mRNA. The genome of DNA viruses is transcribed directly into

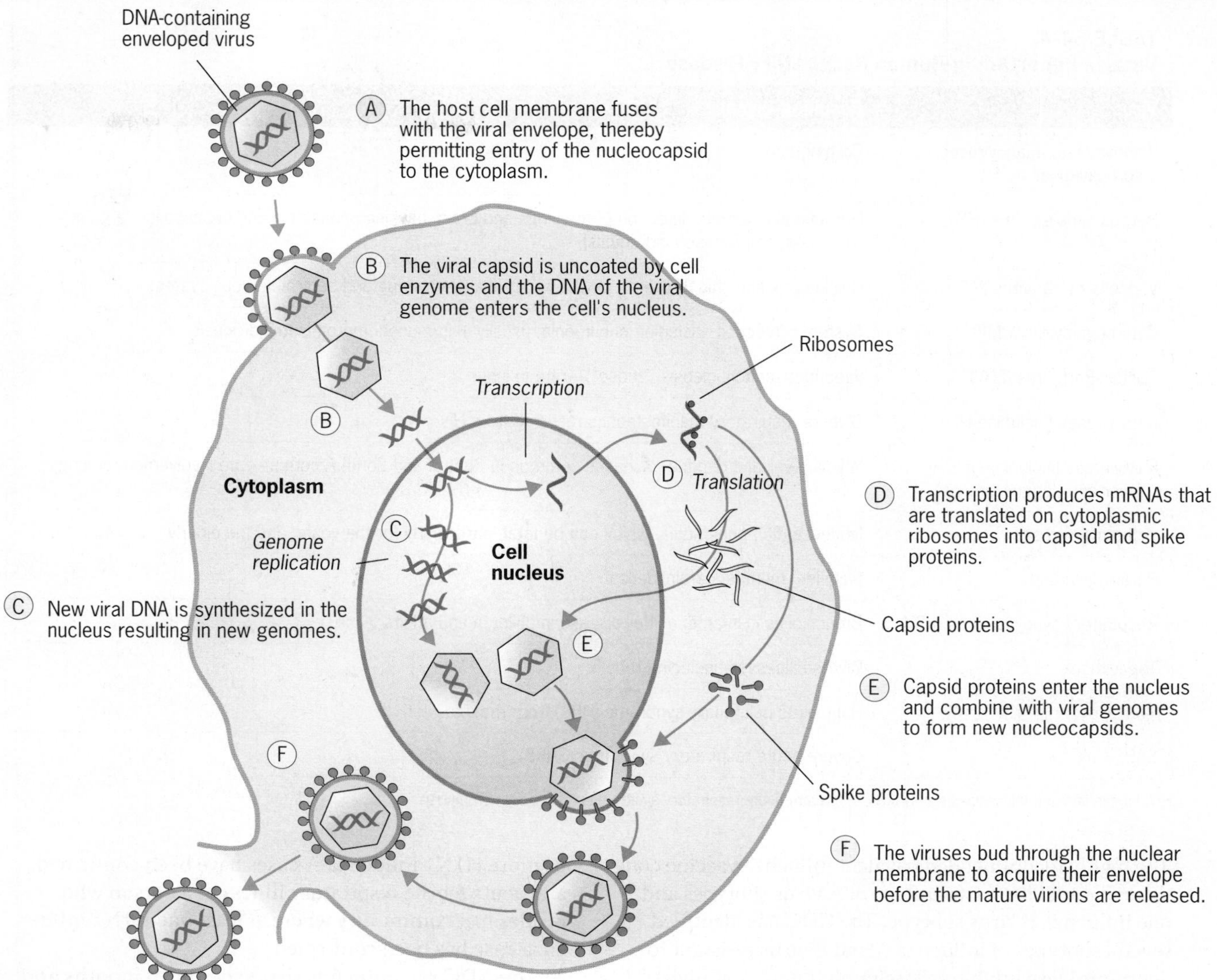

FIGURE 54-18 Process of viral replication from viral attachment to the cell to release of viral particles to infect the other cells.

mRNA by the host cell RNA polymerase. Regardless of the mechanism used, the host cell eventually fills with newly synthesized virions—sometimes clustered together as a recognizable inclusion body—and then ruptures, releasing the virus into the environment.

It is believed that viruses produce clinical disease by causing host cell rupture and death; by causing host cell dysfunction, including fusion with other cells to produce multinucleate giant cells; by malignant transformation; and by stimulating the body's cellular host defenses against infection. Although local disease is mediated by cell dysfunction and death, the final mechanism (stimulation of cellular host defenses) is responsible for many systemic symptoms associated with viral infection, including fever, malaise, loss of appetite, and increased mucus production. Because viruses use the host cell to reproduce and then reside within it, they are difficult to eliminate without killing the host cell. Despite their limitations, vaccinations and antiviral drugs continue to be the most effective therapies against viral infections.

Because a large number of virus species exist, they are usually considered in groups; **Table 54-4** lists some of the more important viral respiratory pathogens. Respiratory syncytial virus (RSV), rhinovirus, influenza virus, and the severe acute respiratory syndrome–associated coronavirus (SARS-CoV) cause respiratory infections that affect the practice of respiratory care around the world due to their widespread epidemiologic and clinical impact. RSV is the most common cause of bronchiolitis and pneumonia in children younger than 1 year.[16] A very contagious disease, RSV infection is spread as a result of direct or indirect contact with nasal or oral secretions from infected persons. There seems to be an association between asthma diagnosed at early school age and severe viral infections caused by RSV and group C human rhinoviruses.[17,18]

Influenza virus is responsible for seasonal flu epidemics that result in the deaths of hundreds of thousands annually. In severe cases, influenza causes life-threatening pneumonia, particularly in young children and the elderly.

TABLE 54-4
Viruses Important in Human Respiratory Disease

Virus	Resulting Disease
Rhinoviruses, adenoviruses, coronaviruses	Common cold
Herpes simplex virus (HSV)	Herpetic skin lesions; infection of the lungs and brain, causing pneumonia and encephalitis (e.g., in immunocompromised individuals)
Varicella-zoster virus (VZV)	Chickenpox and shingles, both of which may involve the lung and central nervous system
Cytomegalovirus (CMV)	Systemic infection, including pneumonia, usually in immunocompromised individuals
Epstein-Barr virus (EBV)	Infectious mononucleosis ("mono")—rare in lungs
Retroviruses (including HIV)	Diverse respiratory manifestations resulting from HIV
Flaviviruses (including yellow fever and dengue viruses)	Yellow fever and dengue, diseases common in Central and South America—rare involvement of lungs
Orthomyxoviruses	Influenza (flu); pneumonia, which can be fatal, particularly for the young and the elderly
Paramyxoviruses	Measles, mumps, parainfluenza
Respiratory syncytial virus (RSV)	Bronchiolitis in infants; milder disease in children and adults
Togaviruses	Diverse illnesses, including rubella
Hantavirus	Hantavirus pulmonary syndrome (HPS) from rodents
SARS-CoV	Severe acute respiratory syndrome (SARS)

HIV, human immunodeficiency virus; SARS-CoV, severe acute respiratory syndrome–associated coronavirus.

The highly recommended trivalent influenza vaccine contains material from two influenza A virus subtypes and one influenza B virus subtype. The CDC has identified several subtypes of influenza A and B virus resistant to neuraminidase inhibitors (oseltamivir and zanamivir).[19]

The H1N1 virus that emerged in 2009 caused the first global pandemic in more than 40 years and resulted in substantial hospitalizations and deaths due to respiratory failure. H1N1 Influenza, also known as swine flu, is a highly contagious respiratory disease in pigs caused by one of several swine influenza A viruses. The main swine influenza viruses circulating in U.S. pigs in recent years are the swine triple reassortant (tr) H1N1 influenza virus, the trH3N2 virus, and the trH1N2 virus. Although transmission of swine influenza viruses to humans is uncommon, it can be transmitted to humans via contact with infected pigs or environments contaminated with swine influenza viruses. Manifestations of H1N1 influenza are similar to those of seasonal influenza. Patients present with symptoms of acute respiratory illness, plus at least two of the following symptoms: fever, cough, sore throat, body aches, headache, and chills. The CDC criteria for suspected H1N1 influenza include an onset of acute febrile respiratory illness within 7 days of close contact with a person who has a confirmed case of H1N1 influenza A virus infection, onset of acute febrile respiratory illness within 7 days of travel to a community (within the United States or internationally) where one or more H1N1 influenza A cases have been confirmed, and acute febrile respiratory illness in a person who resides in a community where at least one H1N1 influenza case has been confirmed.

The CDC recommends that everyone 6 months and older get a flu vaccine since it does protect against an H3N2 virus, an influenza B virus, and the 2009 H1N1 virus. Although treatment is largely supportive, high-dose oseltamivir may hasten viral clearance in patients with severe infection even more than 48 hours after illness onset.[20]

Severe acute respiratory syndrome (SARS) is a respiratory disease caused by the SARS-CoV that reached almost a pandemic state between late 2002 and early 2003, when the infection spread over 37 countries around the world with a mortality rate of nearly 10%. There have not been any known cases of SARS reported anywhere in the world since 2004.[21] Other than isolation and supportive measures, no therapy has been found to be effective against SARS-CoV infection. Although it is considered a rare viral infection today, its legacy has been much stricter infection control policies to protect the public, healthcare workers, and patients around the world.

Outbreaks caused by Ebola virus in 2014 have brought special attention to potentially fatal viral infections. Ebola disease is a severe zoonotic filovirus infection caused by five species: *Zaire* ebolavirus, *Sudan* ebolavirus, *Taï Forest* ebolavirus, *Bundibugyo* ebolavirus, and

Reston ebolavirus. The *Zaire* ebolavirus is responsible for the 2014 epidemic in West Africa, considered the largest outbreak since the virus was discovered in 1976. Human-to-human transmission occurs by close contact with body fluids of infected patients. There is no evidence of airborne transmission, and respiratory failure is unusual except for the most severe disease. Outside endemic areas, Ebola infection is rare and usually carried by travelers from affected areas. Although the incubation period is usually 5 to 9 days, it can range between 1 and 21 days in the majority of patients. Clinical diagnosis is challenging due to its nonspecific presentation. Fever, fatigue, loss of appetite, vomiting, diarrhea, headache, abdominal pain, and unexplained bleeding have been the most common clinical manifestations in the 2014 outbreak. Human infection carries a fatality rate that ranges from 30% to 90%. The use of personal protective equipment is fundamental in preventing the spread of the virus among healthcare workers.

Fungi

Fungi differ from the other organisms in that they are eukaryotic and thus share many features with human cells. This homology makes difficult the development of antifungal therapy that is nontoxic to humans. Fungal structure differs in the following two important ways from human cells: (1) the fungal cell membrane contains ergosterol and zymosterol instead of cholesterol, and (2) fungi have a rigid cell wall composed of chitin (unlike the peptidoglycan cell wall of bacteria). Fungi occur in two forms. The majority of species grow as multicellular filaments called *hyphae*, forming a mycelium; some fungal species also grow as single cells or yeasts (**Figure 54-19**). Although individual yeasts are approximately 4 μm each, mycelia can be quite large, covering up to 1500 acres, and are claimed to be the world's largest organisms.[22] Some fungi are dimorphic, existing as molds in soil but forming yeasts at human body temperatures. All fungi reproduce by spore formation, which may occur either sexually or asexually, depending on the species.

With the exception of *Candida*, which is part of the normal human flora, fungi are found naturally in soil, bird feces, and other decaying material. Therefore, they often produce disease after an individual has been exposed to dust, rotting wood, or dried bird droppings. Skin infection can be caused by direct contact, as in cases of tinea pedis (athlete's foot).

Because inhalation is a significant route for transmitting fungal infection, the lungs are second only to the skin as the major site of fungal infection. The clinical manifestations of fungal disease, known as mycosis, depend on the number of organisms introduced into the lungs (the inoculum) and mechanisms such as direct tissue damage (*Aspergillus*, *Mucor*, and *Rhizopus* species), inflammatory response (*Candida albicans*), and allergy. In cases of prolonged infection or colonization, an immune response may develop. An excellent example is allergic bronchopulmonary aspergillosis (ABPA). In

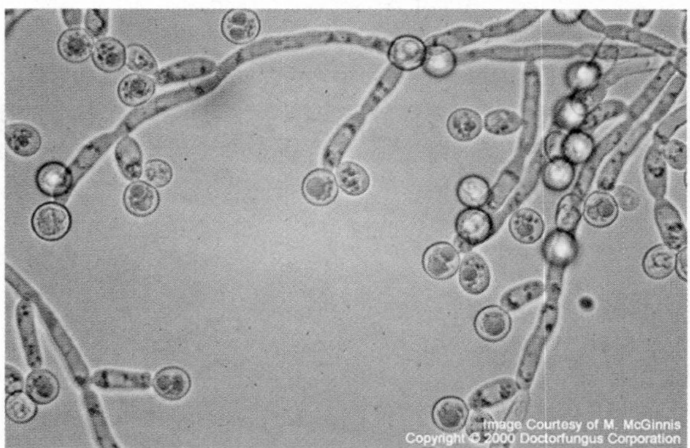

FIGURE 54-19 Electron micrograph of *Candida* showing clusters of budding yeast cells and branching pseudohyphae.
Courtesy of www.doctorfungus.org © 2007.

this condition, pulmonary colonization with *Aspergillus* leads to chronic fevers, cough, and pulmonary infiltrates that represent a delayed-type hypersensitivity reaction (allergy) and not a direct effect of the *Aspergillus*. Because the *Aspergillus* cannot be eradicated, treatment requires immune suppression such as steroids and itraconazole. **Table 54-5** lists important fungal respiratory pathogens in normal hosts, whereas **Table 54-6** lists mycoses known as *opportunistic* because they generally occur in response to lowered host immune activity.

Fungi may be cultured by special techniques but grow more slowly than bacteria. Diagnosis can be made either by cytology or microscopic observation after treatment with potassium hydroxide (KOH), which dissolves most tissue but leaves the chitinous fungal wall intact. Serology is often useful, but its utility is limited in endemic areas, where the majority of healthy individuals may be seropositive. Latex agglutination is frequently used as a rapid detection test for cryptococci in cerebrospinal fluid.

Pneumocystis jiroveci

Pneumocystis jiroveci was previously known as and is still often referred to as *Pneumocystis carinii*. Little was known about *Pneumocystis jiroveci* before the era of the acquired immunodeficiency syndrome (AIDS), and it has only recently been classified as a fungus, based on genetic studies. *P jiroveci* is dimorphic, existing as trophozoites and cysts (**Figure 54-20**).

Pneumocystis carinii pneumonia (PCP) was a common opportunistic infection during the first decade of AIDS and remains an important complication, although its incidence has dropped since the institution of trimethoprim-sulfamethoxazole (TMP-SMX) or aerosolized pentamidine prophylactic therapy. PCP caused by *P jiroveci* is common among people with weakened immune systems, such as patients on medium- to high-dose long-term corticosteroids, those receiving transplants, premature or severely malnourished children, the elderly, and especially AIDS patients, in whom it is most commonly observed today.[23] The risk of PCP increases when CD4 levels are less than 200 cells/μL. Symptoms of PCP

TABLE 54-5
Important Fungal Respiratory Pathogens in Normal Hosts

Organism	Disease	Comments
Coccidioides immitis, Coccidioides posadii	Coccidioidomycosis	Commonly found in the arid regions of the southwest United States (Arizona, central California, and Texas). It causes valley fever, bilateral pneumonia, and may later form thin-walled pulmonary cavities.
Histoplasma capsulatum	Histoplasmosis	Commonly found along the Mississippi and Ohio River valleys. A high, inhaled *Histoplasma* inoculum may cause acute fever and pneumonia. Some patients develop disseminated infection, often causing skin lesions. In rare cases, fibrosis of the mediastinum may result. Most residents of endemic areas have had asymptomatic infection, causing elevated antibody titers, and often one or more calcified granulomas are visible on chest radiographs.
Blastomyces dermatitidis	Blastomycosis	Commonly found in the central United States. The disease varies from mild fever and pulmonary infiltrates to severe illness, nodular pulmonary infiltrates, and dissemination.
Paracoccidioides brasiliensis	Paracoccidioidomycosis	Occurring in Central America, this clinical disease is similar to mild coccidioidomycosis.

include fever, nonproductive cough, dyspnea on exertion, night sweats, and weight loss. The disease causes marked thickening of the alveolar septa and alveoli, leading to significant hypoxia. A hallmark of PCP is that the patient's degree of hypoxia often is greater than expected based on the chest radiographic findings. A Pa_{O_2} of less than 70 mm Hg is an indication for systemic corticosteroids, which have significantly reduced mortality.[24] Pathologic identification of the organism in induced sputum or bronchial washings obtained by bronchoscopy via coloration by toluidine blue or immunofluorescence assay will show characteristic cysts. *Pneumocystis* infection can also be diagnosed by immunofluorescent or histochemical staining of the specimen. Molecular analysis of PCR products, comparing DNA samples, is one of the most recent diagnostic tools.

The most commonly used medication is trimethoprim-sulfamethoxazole. Alternative medications include pentamidine, trimetrexate, dapsone, atovaquone, primaquine, and clindamycin. Treatment is usually for a period of about 21 days.

Parasites

A **parasite** is defined as a plant or animal that lives with or on another, deriving benefit from the association but having a detrimental effect on the host. Those that live inside the host are called *endoparasites*, and those that live on the host's surface are called *ectoparasites*. Essentially any pathogen can be considered a parasite by this definition, but in practical usage the term *parasite* is usually limited to protozoa and helminths (worms). Parasites are an important cause of disease in developing countries but are rare pulmonary pathogens in developed countries and thus will be discussed in this chapter only briefly. Examples of pulmonary parasites include

TABLE 54-6
Opportunistic Fungal Respiratory Pathogens

Organism	Disease	Comments
Candida albicans	Candidiasis (thrush, esophagitis, intertrigo)	Organism is commonly found in infants and the elderly and also in HIV-infected and critically ill patients. Thrush also may be precipitated by inhaled steroid deposition in the mouth. True candidal pneumonia is rare.
Aspergillus species	Aspergillosis	Disease causes otitis externa in normal hosts; may infect skin, sinuses, or lung of immunocompromised individuals and can disseminate, with extremely high mortality. Preexisting lung cavities from tuberculosis or emphysema are particularly prone to infection, with formation of a "fungus ball" inside.
Cryptococcus neoformans	Cryptococcosis	Organism is found in kitten feces and causes pneumonia and meningitis.
Mucor and *Rhizopus* species	Mucormycosis	Organism can infect the sinuses, lungs, or gut, forming a black eschar. Treatment is difficult, often requiring surgical debridement.

HIV, human immunodeficiency virus.

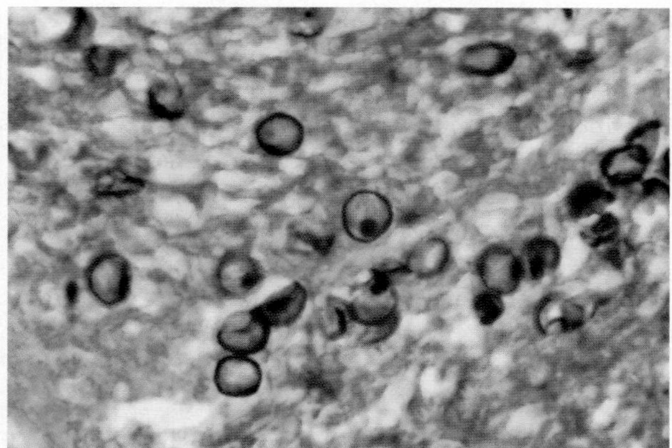

FIGURE 54-20 Methenamine silver stain showing cysts of *Pneumocystis jiroveci* in AIDS.
Courtesy of Dr. Edwin P. Ewing, Jr./CDC.

Entamoeba histolytica (amebiasis), *Paragonimus westermani* (paragonimiasis), and *Echinococcus multilocularis/Echinococcus granulosus* (echinococcosis: hydatid cysts). *Plasmodium falciparum* (malaria) may cause pulmonary manifestations in 3% to 10% of individuals.

The single-celled protozoa usually cause pulmonary disease through abscess formation or stimulation of a vigorous inflammatory response in the lungs. The multicellular helminths frequently produce focal lesions in the lungs—cysts or larvae—and usually are easily visible on chest radiographs. Manifestations are most frequently malaise, fever, cough, and dyspnea. Chest pain may be present, and eosinophilia is a frequent occurrence.

Common Respiratory Infections

Upper Respiratory Tract Infections

Otitis and Sinusitis

The nasopharynx is surrounded by several airspaces in the skull that drain into it via channels. These airspaces include the middle ear, which drains into the posterior nasopharynx via the eustachian tube, along with the frontal, sphenoid, and maxillary sinuses, which drain into the nasopharynx through ostia located above the superior turbinate and under the middle turbinate. In addition, two collections of small air cells are present in the skull: the ethmoid air cells above the nose and the mastoid cells behind the ears. Because the drainage passages to the middle ear and sinuses are vulnerable to obstruction by mucosal swelling, thick secretions, or mechanical obstruction by tubes or nasal polyps, these spaces can become essentially closed spaces, prone to infection. Anatomic differences in the child's eustachian tube predispose it to obstruction, explaining the higher incidence of otitis media in children.

The organisms that cause upper respiratory tract infections (URTIs) may be acquired by inhalation of infected aerosol drops, as with *S pneumoniae* and viruses. Infection frequently represents an overgrowth of local flora after normal drainage of the airspace is compromised, however, explaining why sinusitis frequently follows a viral URTI that has caused mucosal edema. The most common organisms causing otitis and sinusitis therefore reflect the normal flora of the nasopharynx to a great extent. In decreasing order of frequency, they are *S pneumoniae, S aureus, H influenzae,* and *Moraxella catarrhalis.*

Pharyngitis, Parapharyngeal Abscess, Epiglottitis, and Tracheitis or Tracheobronchitis (Croup)

The trachea and posterior pharynx are also frequent sites of infection. Infections in these regions are primarily acquired via aerosol spread. Examples include group A β-hemolytic streptococci (*S pyogenes*) and *C diphtheriae.* Infection of the pharynx rarely causes respiratory complications, although the thick gray peel of necrotic mucosa generated in cases of diphtheria can cause airway obstruction. Infection of the trachea can be more severe, especially in infants, in whom even minor mucosal swelling can significantly narrow the airway. Croup, the viral tracheobronchitis that causes stridor and brassy cough in infants, can produce respiratory failure in severe cases. Infection and swelling of the epiglottis (acute epiglottitis) can rapidly produce severe airway compromise in young children and represents a true emergency because acute airway obstruction may occur. If the infection spreads to the soft tissues around the pharynx and trachea (parapharyngeal abscess), local swelling can compress the airway. Alternatively, the deep tissue planes of the neck may facilitate the rapid spread of infection down into the mediastinum (Ludwig's angina).

Lower Respiratory Tract Infections

The lungs may become infected by two major routes: aspiration of secretions and inhalation of infected aerosols. Infection also may be carried to the lung by the bloodstream (hematogenous spread). Up to 98% of the cardiac

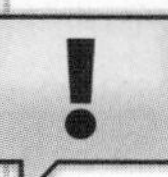

Respiratory Recap

Upper Respiratory Pathogens

- *Streptococcus pneumoniae*
- *Haemophilus influenzae*
- *Moraxella catarrhalis*

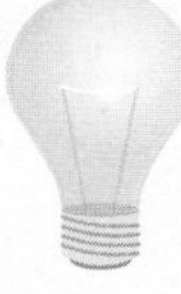

STOP AND THINK

One of your pediatric patients with severe stridor has been diagnosed with epiglottitis. What should be the priority in the management of this patient?

output flows through the pulmonary capillary bed, which is the first filter encountered by organisms or objects returning to the heart from the body via the venous system of the body. Nevertheless, hematogenous infection is much less common than aspiration or inhalation.

Lower respiratory infections are thought to originate from the person's own flora, which gain access to the lung by aspiration of secretions, usually from the pharynx and upper digestive tract. Organisms from the upper digestive tract find their way to the pharynx via gastroesophageal reflux, which occurs nearly universally in healthy individuals. Once organisms are present in the pharynx, they are readily aspirated into the lower respiratory tract. Up to 45% of healthy individuals aspirate small amounts of secretions (microaspiration). Weakened hospitalized patients, spending long periods of time flat and often with nasogastric tubes traversing the pharynx, experience an even greater incidence of aspiration. Intubated, mechanically ventilated patients are believed to universally aspirate.

The aspirated organisms generally represent the normal flora, but illness and extensive exposure to antibiotics may modify the flora substantially, as is particularly evident in the increasing role of gram-negative organisms in healthcare-associated pneumonia.

Risk factors that increase pharyngeal colonization with potentially pathogenic gram-negative bacteria are as follows: depressed level of consciousness (e.g., alcoholism, coma, hypotension), compromised immune function (e.g., acidosis, alcoholism, azotemia, diabetes mellitus, leukocytosis, leukopenia), anatomic alteration of the respiratory system (e.g., nasogastric or endotracheal tubes, preexisting pulmonary disease), exposure to antibiotics, and extreme age (either very young or very old).

Aerosol spread is another common route of lower respiratory infection. Coughing and sneezing project large quantities of aerosol a surprising distance, but even quiet breathing produces aerosol capable of spreading infection. In the case of fungi, large numbers of organisms may be present in the general environment. Aerosol transmission can occur in the hospital, although isolation of patients with pneumonia is not a common practice. An important exception is tuberculosis, which requires immediate respiratory (aerosol) isolation as soon as a reasonable suspicion of the disease is present.

> **Respiratory Recap**
>
> **Mechanisms of Infection**
>
> - Overgrowth of normal flora
> - Aspiration of oral and gastric flora
> - Aerosol inhalation
> - Hematogenous spread
> - Direct contact (rare except during instrumentation)

Direct contact rarely causes pneumonia but is believed to be a common mode by which bacteria are spread between patients and caregivers. These bacteria often include antibiotic-resistant and unusual organisms, such as MRSA and vancomycin-resistant enterococcus (VRE). Once spread to a new individual, these bacteria frequently reside in the nasopharynx, skin, and digestive tract, where they displace normal flora. From these locations, they infect the lower respiratory tract, providing a reason why hand washing is an effective and essential technique used to limit the spread of infectious agents in the healthcare setting. Direct contact does become an important mechanism of infection when instrumentation is introduced into the lower respiratory tract.

The cause of lower respiratory tract infections (LRTIs) varies with age and setting. Community-acquired pneumonia (CAP) originates outside a healthcare setting and must be distinguished from nosocomial pneumonia and ventilator-associated pneumonia (VAP). Nosocomial pneumonia (defined as pneumonia diagnosed more than 48 hours after hospital admission) is hospital acquired, whereas VAP is a subset of nosocomial pneumonia occurring in patients who are mechanically ventilated for more than 48 hours.[25] **Box 54-1** lists the microorganisms commonly responsible for all types of pneumonia.

A term recently added to the literature is *healthcare-associated pneumonia* (HCAP), which is caused by the pathogens often seen in nosocomial pneumonia. Risk factors for HCAP are residence in nursing homes or long-term care facilities; recent hospitalization for more than 2 days in the previous 3 months; infusion therapy; hemodialysis; and having contact with family members with MDR pathogens.

Anaerobes are as important in nosocomial pneumonia and VAP as they are in community-acquired pneumonia. Identifying the causative organisms in nosocomial pneumonia, and especially VAP, may be difficult because of the high rate of lower respiratory tract colonization. Pathogen identification is important in order to define susceptibility and determine and quickly initiate the most appropriate antimicrobial therapy.

Sampling Methods

Respiratory therapists are often responsible for obtaining respiratory specimens for different diagnostic studies. Adequate sampling using methods such as bronchoscopy, tracheal aspiration, and nonbronchoscopic bronchoalveolar lavage is critical to the diagnosis and management of respiratory infections.

Sputum Induction

When a patient is unable to produce sputum for analysis, the sample can be obtained as an endotracheal

BOX 54-1

Etiologic Agents of Community-Acquired, Hospital-Acquired (HAP), Healthcare-Associated (HCAP), Ventilator-Associated (VAP), and Nosocomial Pneumonias

Community-Acquired Pneumonia

Streptococcus pneumoniae
Mycoplasma pneumoniae
Viruses
Chlamydophila pneumoniae
Haemophilus influenzae
Legionella species
Staphylococcus aureus
Mycobacterium tuberculosis
Fungi (*Histoplasma, Coccidioides, Blastomyces* species)
Gram-negative bacilli, nonpseudomonal (*Klebsiella*, enteric species)
Pseudomonas species
Gram-negative bacilli, nonpseudomonal

Nosocomial (HAP/HCAP/VAP) Pneumonia

Not multidrug resistant
- *S pneumoniae*
- *H influenzae*
- Gram-negative rods

Multidrug resistant
- *S aureus* (MRSA)
- *P aeruginosa*

Extended-spectrum β-lactamases (ESBLs)
Acinetobacter species

aspirate or after inhalation of nebulized 3% saline. The hypertonic saline increases the tonicity of the fluid layer lining the airways, both drawing fluid into these secretions and stimulating an irritant cough response. In the patient who is able to produce sputum spontaneously, induction does not improve sensitivity. Care must be taken during **sputum induction** in a patient with suspected contagious illness, especially tuberculosis, to prevent transmission of the disease to the respiratory therapist and other healthcare providers. Because some patients may experience severe bronchospasm after a sputum induction, a bronchodilator must be at hand to relieve induced bronchospasm.[26]

Acceptable Sputum Specimens

The collection of sputum specimens from which microbiologic diagnoses can be made is quite difficult, accounting for the low percentage of pneumonias identified by sputum alone (less than half). Three criteria must be met to obtain a useful sputum specimen. First, the specimen must be collected in a sterile container and handled with sterile technique. Second, the specimen must be transported to the laboratory promptly. Some respiratory pathogens are very sensitive to bacterial overgrowth, which may occur if the sputum remains unprocessed for long periods of time. Finally, the sample must be screened to verify that it is in fact sputum from the lower respiratory tract and not saliva, which is accomplished by counting the number of squamous epithelial cells per microscopic low-power field (lpf). Because these cells originate from the oropharynx, a large number of them (>25/lpf) indicate a specimen that is unacceptably contaminated with oral secretions. Sputum with fewer than 25 squamous epithelial cells and more than 10 polymorphonuclear leukocytes per low-power field is considered a good specimen.

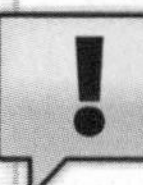

Respiratory Recap

Acceptable Sputum Specimens

- Less than 25 squamous cells per low-power field
- More than 10 polymorphonuclear leukocytes per low-power field

Bronchoscopy

Fiberoptic **bronchoscopy** is a powerful technique that enables the collection of many sample types from the lower airways. The working channel is generally contaminated with upper airway secretions, so simple suctioned specimens yield unreliable cultures. This problem has been addressed with the protected specimen brush (PSB), also called the protected brush catheter (PBC). A sterile brush is passed through the working channel into the bronchus. The brush is advanced from the catheter and worked back and forth to collect secretions and cells before it is withdrawn into the protective sheath and retrieved for culture. The reported sensitivity of PSB varies from 47% to 54%, with specificity of 87% to 100%.[27,28]

Another common technique used to diagnose pneumonia is **bronchoalveolar lavage (BAL)**. The bronchoscope is positioned as far distally as possible in the airway leading to the site of interest. Aliquots of 20 to 50 mL of sterile saline, usually 100 mL, are introduced via the working channel. This saline migrates distally, mixing with secretions, and each aliquot then is suctioned back and collected in a sterile trap. Bronchoalveolar lavage is a sensitive technique and is used to detect organisms that are not reliably isolated from sputum, including nontuberculous mycobacteria, cytomegalovirus, and *Pneumocystis* species, for which sensitivities may be more than 90%, with near-100% specificity. When used to diagnose acute nosocomial pneumonia, BAL has been reported to produce a sensitivity between 55% and 91% and a specificity between 63% and 100%.[29–33]

Regardless of the technique used for specimen collection, quantitative culture is superior to qualitative culture techniques because of its increased ability to distinguish contaminants from true infection.

Biopsy of the lung parenchyma is useful for diagnosis of pneumonia, especially fungal and granulomatous infections, and is accomplished bronchoscopically by tearing of small pieces of tissue (approximately 1 mm) from the lung parenchyma with small grasping biopsy forceps that are placed through the working channel. For bacterial pneumonia, transbronchial biopsy (TBB) has a reported sensitivity of 57% and specificity of 100%.[34] Because the technique appears to offer little advantage over PSB and BAL and carries a much higher risk of hemorrhage and pneumothorax, TBB is not often used to diagnose acute pneumonia.

Transtracheal Aspiration

Transtracheal aspiration (TTA) is a sputum-collection technique designed to bypass the upper airway, with its potential contaminants. The method begins with a careful skin preparation of the anterior neck, followed by the insertion of a sterile needle directly into the trachea through the cricothyroid membrane. Proper position is ensured by aspiration of air from the needle, and tracheal secretions are aspirated. The obvious disadvantage of this procedure is its invasive nature, which explains why it is no longer used in clinical practice.

Nonbronchoscopic Bronchoalveolar Lavage

Bronchoalveolar lavage can be performed with a blind, nonbronchoscopic technique in mechanically ventilated patients. With this technique a catheter is advanced through the endotracheal tube until resistance is felt in the distal airways of the (usually) right lower lobe, usually at a distance of 50 to 60 cm. Aliquots of sterile saline are instilled and suctioned. In studies in the same patients, the reported sensitivities of nonbronchoscopic BAL (NB-BAL) and traditional bronchoscopic BAL (B-BAL) were 73% and 93%, respectively; specificities were 96% and 100%, respectively.[27] Although B-BAL is superior to NB-BAL, the nonbronchoscopic technique is useful because of its ease of performance and substantially lower cost. It is also a method that can be available at all times without the need of a bronchoscopist. Respiratory therapists can be trained to perform this procedure.

Pleural Fluid Analysis

The presence of significant pleural fluid usually demands sampling and analysis of the fluid to determine its nature, unless a cause is readily apparent. Pleural fluid analysis may address two principal issues. First, the measurement of fluid characteristics, such as cell type, pH, protein, amylase, lactate dehydrogenase, and others, may provide clues to the effusion's cause. For example, demonstration of increased adenosine deaminase in the fluid, a predominance of lymphocytes in the white blood cell differential, and a paucity of mesothelial cells (which make up the pleural surface and are usually found in abundance) all suggest tuberculosis as a potential cause.

A second issue is frequently addressed when a pleural effusion is adjacent to an area of pneumonia. These parapneumonic effusions are at risk for becoming secondarily infected from the pneumonia. When pus is present, this is known as *empyema*. If organisms are cultured from the normally sterile pleural space, this technique usually identifies the cause of the pneumonia. Parapneumonic effusions also tend to be highly proteinaceous, prone to developing loculations and forming peels around the adjacent lung, permanently limiting its expansion. For this reason, parapneumonic effusions are most frequently drained completely at the time of sampling.

Microbiology Techniques

Once a good respiratory specimen is obtained, different diagnostic techniques allow identification of the pathogen. These techniques include cultures and virologic antigen identification.

Sputum Culture

After Gram stains are used on the specimen, the sputum or tracheal aspirate is cultured. A microbiological **culture** is one of the primary methods to diagnose bacterial infection. It is a method in which microorganisms are allowed to reproduce in a predetermined culture media under controlled laboratory conditions. To distinguish contamination from colonization and from active infection, the number of colony-forming units (CFUs) per milliliter is counted from the culture; this is called a *quantitative culture*. Colony-forming units measure viable bacterial cells and therefore the microbiologic load that correlates with the magnitude of the infection. After pathogens are isolated, the in vitro testing of bacterial cultures with antibiotics is performed to determine the bacteria's susceptibility to specific antibiotic therapy. Specimens containing more than 10 epithelial cells per low-power field are considered inappropriate for culture and are rejected. Typically, only one sputum specimen per patient is cultured per day. A preliminary report is given in 24 hours, but the final report takes between 48 and 72 hours.

Respiratory Tract Culture

Evaluation of sputum cultures does not examine for *Legionella pneumoniae*, *Chlamydophila pneumoniae*, or *Mycoplasma pneumoniae*, since these pathogens require specialized testing. Adequate samples for culture, excluding sputum, can be obtained from bronchoalveolar lavage, bronchial wash, lung aspirates, sinus aspirates, and quantitative bronchoalveolar lavage. Specimens from nasal passages may be cultured to determine the presence of MRSA or *Neisseria meningitidis* carrier status. A preliminary report is typically available in 24 hours and the final report in 72 hours.

Virologic Studies

Culture

Respiratory specimens for **virologic studies** such as culture include nasopharyngeal washes or aspirates, sputum, bronchial wash, BAL, and lung tissue. Viruses are grown in cell culture, where they produce recognizable cytopathic changes, a process that can take up to 2 weeks. A rapid shell vial culture technique is used to obtain a diagnosis of cytomegalovirus (CMV) infection within 48 hours and is frequently performed on respiratory secretions and bronchoscopy specimens. Certain viruses, especially CMV and Epstein-Barr virus, produce characteristic microscopically visible inclusion bodies in infected cells. Virus culture tests for the presence of RSV, influenza A and B, adenovirus, and parainfluenza.

Viral Antigen Detection

Detection of the influenza A and B antigen is possible through optical immunoassay of nasal specimens. However, the test should not be part of therapeutic decision making because of the insufficient negative predictive value of the test. A result is available in 30 to 60 minutes. RSV **antigen detection** also requires the use of an optical immunoassay and direct fluorescent antibody.[35] Specimens of choice are nasopharyngeal aspirates and washes.

Antimicrobial Therapy

Antimicrobials are often prescribed for patients admitted to the hospital. While some patients are on antibiotics that cover only a few organisms (narrow spectrum), others receive antibiotics that cover multiple organisms (broad spectrum). For the respiratory therapist, the most important antibiotics are those used to treat community-acquired pneumonia or hospital-acquired pneumonia in the intensive care unit. **Table 54-7** summarizes the common classes of antimicrobials, their spectra of action, and common side effects.

Antimicrobial Resistance

Antibiotic resistance is the ability of bacteria and fungi to withstand the effects of antibiotics that would normally kill them or limit their growth. The widespread and increased use of antimicrobials in humans, animals, and agriculture has resulted in many microorganisms developing resistance to these powerful drugs. Antibiotic resistance is a growing concern worldwide and has become a major problem, especially in environments that are constantly exposed to antibiotics, such as hospitals, where resistant bacterial strains can become a dominant part of the endogenous flora.[36]

Microorganisms adapt to their environment and change to ensure their survival. Antibiotic resistance is a complex process of adaptation that evolves as the result of mutation, gene transfer, and selective process. With each replication, genetic mutations may help an individual microorganism survive exposure to an antibiotic. Once such a resistant gene is generated, microorganisms can transfer or acquire this new genetic material via plasmid exchange. In the presence of an antibiotic, bacteria are killed unless they carry resistance genes. These survivors then become the dominant type throughout the microbial population. When a microorganism possesses several resistance genes, it is called **multiresistant**, or a *superbug*.

The most important mechanism of resistance to penicillins and cephalosporins is the production of β-lactamases, which digest the β-lactam ring structure of these antibiotics. The most important mechanisms of resistance to aminoglycosides and chloramphenicol are the production of various inactivating enzymes.

The activity of antibiotics may be improved by modification of their targets, which usually involves a change in the chromosomal genes of the microorganism. The second-most-important mechanism of resistance to penicillins and cephalosporins is modification of the penicillin-binding proteins in the bacterial cell membrane to which the drugs attach. Resistance to aminoglycosides, macrolides, sulfonamides, fluoroquinolones, and rifampin is imparted by mutations in the bacterial ribosomes or enzymes that make up the targets of these antibiotics.

Resistance to aminoglycosides, tetracyclines, and isoniazid results from decreased permeability of the cell wall and membrane to the antibiotic, reducing the antibiotic levels inside the bacterium. Antibiotics also may be actively transported from the bacteria by an enzymatic pump, which is usually plasmid encoded. Resistance to tetracyclines and sulfonamides is also accomplished by active transport of the antibiotic from the bacteria.

Gram-negative ventilator-associated pneumonia in critically ill patients is associated with substantial morbidity, longer ICU stays, prolonged mechanical ventilation, and higher mortality. Aerosolized aminoglycosides may play a valuable role as adjunct therapy in selected patients with multidrug-resistant gram-negative organisms.[37–39]

TABLE 54-7
Common Antimicrobials, Mechanisms, Spectra of Activity, and Toxicities

Class	Examples	Spectrum of Activity	Toxicity
Antibacterials			
Penicillins	Generally in combinations (i.e., amoxicillin-clavulanic acid, ampicillin-sulbactam, ticarcillin-clavulanic acid, piperacillin-tazobactam)	G+, G–, and anaerobic activities increasing with successive generations	Hypersensitivity (fever and rash)
Cephalosporins	First generation: cefazolin, cephalexin Second generation: cefuroxime, cefaclor, cefotetan Third generation: ceftriaxone, cefotaxime, ceftazidime Fourth generation: cefepime Other: ceftaroline	Same as penicillins; third and fourth generations used against *Pseudomonas aeruginosa*	Rare cytopenias
Carbapenems	Imipenem, meropenem, ertapenem, doripenem	Broad G+, G–, anaerobic coverage	Seizure, phlebitis (meropenem, doripenem)
Monobactams	Aztreonam	G–	Similar to penicillins, except nephrotoxicity
Aminoglycosides	Gentamicin, tobramycin, amikacin	G– rods	Nephrotoxicity, ototoxicity, rare paralysis; levels require monitoring
Tetracyclines	Tetracycline, doxycycline, minocycline	G+, atypicals	Tooth and bone defects, phototoxicity, GI intolerance, benign intracranial hypertension, mild hepatitis
Sulfonamides	Trimethoprim/sulfamethoxazole (TMP/SMX)	G+, G–, *Pneumocystis jiroveci, Nocardia* species	Hypersensitivity, possible trigger of hemolysis in G6PD deficiency
Fluoroquinolones	Ciprofloxacin, levofloxacin, moxifloxacin, norfloxacin, clinafloxacin, gemifloxacin	G–, G+, atypical, TB/NTM	GI intolerance, CNS, arrhythmias, drug–drug interactions. Not administered in children, except those with cystic fibrosis
Macrolides	Erythromycin, clarithromycin, azithromycin, roxithromycin, dirithromycin	G+, some G–; good atypical coverage, including *Legionella* species; TB/NTM	GI intolerance and arrhythmias
Others	Vancomycin	G+, including MRSA; *Enterococcus faecalis* species	Hypotension and rash with infusion, ototoxicity, nephrotoxicity, hematological disturbances
	Metronidazole	Anaerobes, parasites	Ethanol intolerance, seizures, peripheral neuropathy
	Chloramphenicol	G+, many G–, anaerobes, rickettsiae	Aplastic anemia
	Clindamycin	G+ and anaerobes	*Clostridium difficile* colitis or diarrhea
	Linezolid	G+, including MRSA	Diarrhea, headache, nausea, thrombocytopenia
	Daptomycin	G+ only, but no effect in pulmonary processes	Gastrointestinal adverse effects, headache, rash
	Tigecycline	G+, G–, anaerobes, MRSA and multidrug-resistant *Acinetobacter baumannii*	Diarrhea, nausea, vomiting
Antifungals			
Imidazoles	Miconazole, ketoconazole, clotrimazole, econazole	*Aspergillus, Blastomyces,* and *Histoplasma* species, onychomycosis	Hepatotoxicity
Triazoles	Fluconazole, itraconazole, ravuconazole, posaconazole, voriconazole	Yeasts, molds, and dimorphic fungi	Hypertension, hypokalemia, edema, headache, and alterations in mental status are seldom observed; hepatotoxicity is rare

(*continued*)

TABLE 54-7
Common Antimicrobials, Mechanisms, Spectra of Activity, and Toxicities (*Continued*)

Class	Examples	Spectrum of Activity	Toxicity
Antifungals			
Polyenes	Amphotericin, natamycin, candicin, nystatin	Preferred for severe infections; nystatin for *Candida* infection only	Fever, rigors, hypotension with infusion, nephrotoxicity, hypersensitivity, hepatotoxicity, cytopenias
Allylamines	Terbinafine, amorolfine, naftifine, butenafine	Dermatomycoses (tinea pedis)	Headache, rash, GI upset
Echinocandins	Anidulafungin, caspofungin, micafungin	*Candida* species, *Aspergillus*, *Blastomyces*, *Histoplasma*	
Antivirals			
	Acyclovir, famciclovir, valacyclovir	HSV, VZV, CMV	Headache, nausea
	Amantadine, rimantadine	Influenza A	Reversible neurotoxicity
	Ganciclovir, valacyclovir, famciclovir	CMV	Cytopenias, impaired male fertility
	Foscarnet	HSV, VZV, CMV, EBV	Nephrotoxicity in most patients, electrolyte abnormalities, seizures, anemia
	Ribavirin	RSV	Clogging of ventilator valves, bronchospasm, rash, hemolytic anemia
	Oseltamivir	Treatment and prevention of influenza A and B virus	Nausea, vomiting, diarrhea, abdominal pain, and headache
	Zanamivir (inhalation)	Treatment and prophylaxis of influenza A and B virus	Bronchospasm, psychiatric problems
	Peramivir	Hospitalized patients with known or suspected H1N1 influenza	Diarrhea, nausea, vomiting, leukopenia
Antituberculous			
	Rifampin, rifabutin	G+, G–, MTB, NTM	Flulike syndrome, hepatotoxicity
	Isoniazid (INH)	MTB	Hepatotoxicity, neurotoxicity, hypersensitivity
	Ethambutol (EMB)	MTB, NTM	Optic neuritis, peripheral neuropathy
	Pyrazinamide (PZA)	MTB	Hepatotoxicity, hyperuricemia
	Streptomycin	MTB, G–, NTM	Hypersensitivity, ototoxicity, neurotoxicity

G+, gram-positive bacteria; G–, gram-negative bacteria; GI, gastrointestinal; TB, tuberculosis; NTM, nontuberculous mycobacteria; G6PD, glucose-6-phosphate dehydrogenase; MRSA, methicillin-resistant *Staphylococcus aureus*; HSV, herpes simplex virus; VZV, varicella-zoster virus; CMV, cytomegalovirus; EBV, Epstein-Barr virus; RSV, respiratory syncytial virus; MTB, *Mycobacterium* tuberculosis.

Key Points

- Respiratory infections are caused most frequently by typical and atypical bacteria and by viruses. Some species of rickettsiae, mycobacteria, and fungi also are commonly encountered.
- Bacteria are classified by three major characteristics: oxygen requirement, Gram staining, and shape.
- Normal flora bacteria are generally present in certain areas of the body but are major causes of respiratory infection when they overgrow in the upper airway or are introduced to the normally near-sterile lower airways.
- The modes of infection and the most common respiratory pathogens vary significantly, depending on an individual's age and setting.
- Among normal adults the major pathogens of upper airway infection are *Streptococcus pneumoniae*, *Haemophilus influenzae*, and *Moraxella catarrhalis*. The most common community-acquired lower respiratory pathogens are *S pneumoniae*, viruses, and *H influenzae*. *Mycoplasma pneumoniae*, *Chlamydophila pneumoniae*, and assorted gram-negative bacteria are also common.
- Aspiration represents the major route of pulmonary infection, especially among hospitalized patients.
- A wide variety of respiratory care equipment has been implicated in the spread of infection.
- Viruses are responsible for a variety of seasonal respiratory infections, are highly contagious, and require strict adherence to infection control policies.
- Induced sputum is frequently useful for diagnostic purposes, but some infections are much more reliably diagnosed with bronchoscopy or nonbronchoscopic bronchoalveolar lavage.
- Selection of an adequate sampling method and obtaining an acceptable sputum specimen are

critical elements for the diagnosis and management of respiratory infections.

- A large number of antibiotics are available to treat respiratory infections, each with toxicities that must be considered. Use of nebulized antibiotics can reduce toxicity.
- Antibiotic resistance is now a common phenomenon and has necessitated use of multiple antibiotics for some infections, such as tuberculosis and *Pseudomonas* pneumonia.

References

1. Porter JR. Anthony van Leeuwenhoek: tercentenary of his discovery of bacteria. *Bacteriol Rev.* 1976;40:260–269.
2. Eagon R. *Pseudomonas natrienses*, a marine bacterium with generation time of less than 10 minutes. *J Bacteriol.* 1962;83:736–737.
3. Shallcross LJ, Fragaszy E, Johnson AM, Hayward AC. The role of the Panton-Valentine leucocidin toxin in staphylococcal disease: a systematic review and meta-analysis. *Lancet Infect Dis.* 2013;13:43–54.
4. Catena V, Baiocchi M, Lentini P, et al. Necrotizing pneumonia caused by Panton-Valentine leukocidin-producing methicillin-susceptible *Staphylococcus aureus* (MSSA). *Infez Med.* 2012;20:205–210.
5. Wunderink RG. How important is methicillin-resistant *Staphylococcus aureus* as a cause of community-acquired pneumonia and what is best antimicrobial therapy? *Infect Dis Clin North Am.* 2013;27:177–188.
6. Michalopoulos A, Falagas ME. Treatment of *Acinetobacter* infections. *Expert Opin Pharmacother.* 2010;11:779–788.
7. Wisplinghoff H, Paulus T, Lugenheim M, et al. Nosocomial bloodstream infections due to *Acinetobacter baumannii*, *Acinetobacter pittii* and *Acinetobacter nosocomialis* in the United States. *J Infect.* 2012;64:282–290.
8. Metz G, Kraft M. Effects of atypical infections with *Mycoplasma* and *Chlamydia* on asthma. *Immunol Allergy Clin North Am.* 2010;30:575–585.
9. Wang K, Gill P, Perera R, et al. Clinical symptoms and signs for the diagnosis of *Mycoplasma pneumoniae* in children and adolescents with community-acquired pneumonia. *Cochrane Database Syst Rev.* 2012;10:CD009175.
10. Mulholland S, Gavranich JB, Gillies MB, Chang AB. Antibiotics for community-acquired lower respiratory tract infections secondary to *Mycoplasma pneumoniae* in children. *Cochrane Database Syst Rev.* 2012;9:CD004875.
11. Carratalà J, Garcia-Vidal C. An update on *Legionella*. *Curr Opin Infect Dis.* 2010;23:152–157.
12. Parish T, Brown A, eds. *Mycobacterium: Genomics and Molecular Biology*. Norfolk, England: Caister Academic Press; 2009.
13. World Health Organization. *Global tuberculosis report 2013*. Available at: http://www.who.int/tb/publications/global_report/en/. Accessed September 8, 2014.
14. Dooley KE, Obuku EA, Durakovic N, et al: Efficacy Subgroup, RESIST-TB. World Health Organization group 5 drugs for the treatment of drug-resistant tuberculosis: unclear efficacy or untapped potential? *J Infect Dis.* 2013;207:1352–1358.
15. Walusimbi S, Bwanga F, De Costa A, et al. Meta-analysis to compare the accuracy of GeneXpert, MODS and the WHO 2007 algorithm for diagnosis of smear-negative pulmonary tuberculosis. *BMC Infect Dis.* 2013;13:507.
16. Centers for Disease Control and Prevention. Respiratory Syncytial Virus Infection (RSV). Available at: http://www.cdc.gov/rsv/. Accessed September 8, 2014.
17. Szabo SM, Levy AR, Gooch KL, et al. Elevated risk of asthma after hospitalization for respiratory syncytial virus infection in infancy. *Paediatr Respir Rev.* 2013;13(Suppl 2):S9–S15.
18. Proud D. Role of rhinovirus infections in asthma. *Asian Pac J Allergy Immunol.* 2011;29:201–208.
19. Centers for Disease Control and Prevention. *FluView: 2013–2014 influenza season week 3 ending January 18, 2014*. Available at: http://www.cdc.gov/flu/weekly. Accessed January 27, 2014.
20. Centers for Disease Control and Prevention. *Interim Guidance on Specimen Collection and Processing for Patients with Suspected Swine Influenza A (H1N1) Virus Infection*. Available at http://www.cdc.gov/flu/swineflu/index.htm. Accessed September 8, 2014.
21. Centers for Disease Control and Prevention. *Severe Acute Respiratory Syndrome (SARS)*. Available at: http://www.cdc.gov/sars/. Accessed September 8, 2014.
22. Carrier R, ed. *Guinness Book of World Records*. New York: Bantam Books; 1999:236.
23. Miller RF, Huang L, Walzer PD. Pneumocystis pneumonia associated with human immunodeficiency virus. *Clin Chest Med.* 2013;34:229–241.
24. Consensus statement on the use of corticosteroids as adjunctive therapy for pneumocystis pneumonia in the acquired immunodeficiency syndrome. The National Institutes of Health–University of California Expert Panel for Corticosteroids as Adjunctive Therapy for Pneumocystis Pneumonia. *N Engl J Med.* 1990;323:1500–1504.
25. Guidelines for the management of adults with hospital-acquired, ventilator-associated, and healthcare-associated pneumonia. *Am J Respir Crit Care Med.* 2005;171:388–450.
26. Paggiaro PL, Chanez P, Holz O, et al. Sputum induction. *Eur Respir J.* 2002;37(Suppl):3S–8S.
27. Hussain SM, Abubaker J, Ali M, et al. Comparison of quantitative bronchoscopic lavage cultures (B-BAL) with blind NG tube lavage (N-BAL) cultures in the diagnosis of ventilator associated pneumonia (VAP). *J Coll Physicians Surg Pak.* 2009;19:245–248.
28. Ramirez P, Valencia M, Torres A. Bronchoalveolar lavage to diagnose respiratory infections. *Semin Respir Crit Care Med.* 2007;28:525–533.
29. Fagon JY. Diagnosis and treatment of ventilator-associated pneumonia: fiberoptic bronchoscopy with bronchoalveolar lavage is essential. *Semin Respir Crit Care Med.* 2006;27:34–44.
30. Goldberg AE, Malhotra AK, Riaz OJ, et al. Predictive value of broncho-alveolar lavage fluid Gram's stain in the diagnosis of ventilator-associated pneumonia: a prospective study. *J Trauma.* 2008;65:871–876.
31. Leo A, Galindo-Galindo J, Folch E, et al. Comparison of bronchoscopic bronchoalveolar lavage vs blind lavage with a modified nasogastric tube in the etiologic diagnosis of ventilator-associated pneumonia. *Med Intensiva.* 2008;32:115–120.
32. Clec'h C, Jauréguy F, Hamza L, et al. Agreement between quantitative cultures of postintubation tracheal aspiration and plugged telescoping catheter, protected specimen brush, or BAL for the diagnosis of nosocomial pneumonia. *Chest.* 2006;130:956–961.
33. Kirtland SH, Corley DE, Winterbauer RH. The diagnosis of ventilator-associated pneumonia: a comparison of histologic, microbiologic and clinical criteria. *Chest.* 1997;112:445–457.
34. Rao VK, Ritter J, Kollef MH. Utility of transbronchial biopsy in patients with acute respiratory failure: a postmortem study. *Chest.* 1998;114:549–555.
35. Prendergast C, Papenburg J. Rapid antigen-based testing for respiratory syncytial virus: moving diagnostics from bench to bedside? *Future Microbiol.* 2013;8:435–444.
36. Lusti-Narasimhan M, Pessoa-Silva CL, Temmerman M. Moving forward in tackling antimicrobial resistance: WHO actions. *Sex Transm Infect.* 2013;89(Suppl 4):iv57–iv59.
37. Mohr AM, Sifri ZC, Horng HS, et al. Use of aerosolized aminoglycosides in the treatment of gram-negative ventilator-associated pneumonia. *Surg Infect (Larchmont).* 2007;8:349–357.
38. Dhand R. The role of aerosolized antimicrobials in the treatment of ventilator-associated pneumonia. *Respir Care.* 2007;52:866–884.
39. Michalopoulos A, Fotakis D, Virtzili S, et al. Aerosolized colistin as adjunctive treatment of ventilator-associated pneumonia due to multidrug-resistant gram-negative bacteria: a prospective study. *Respir Med.* 2008;102:407–412.

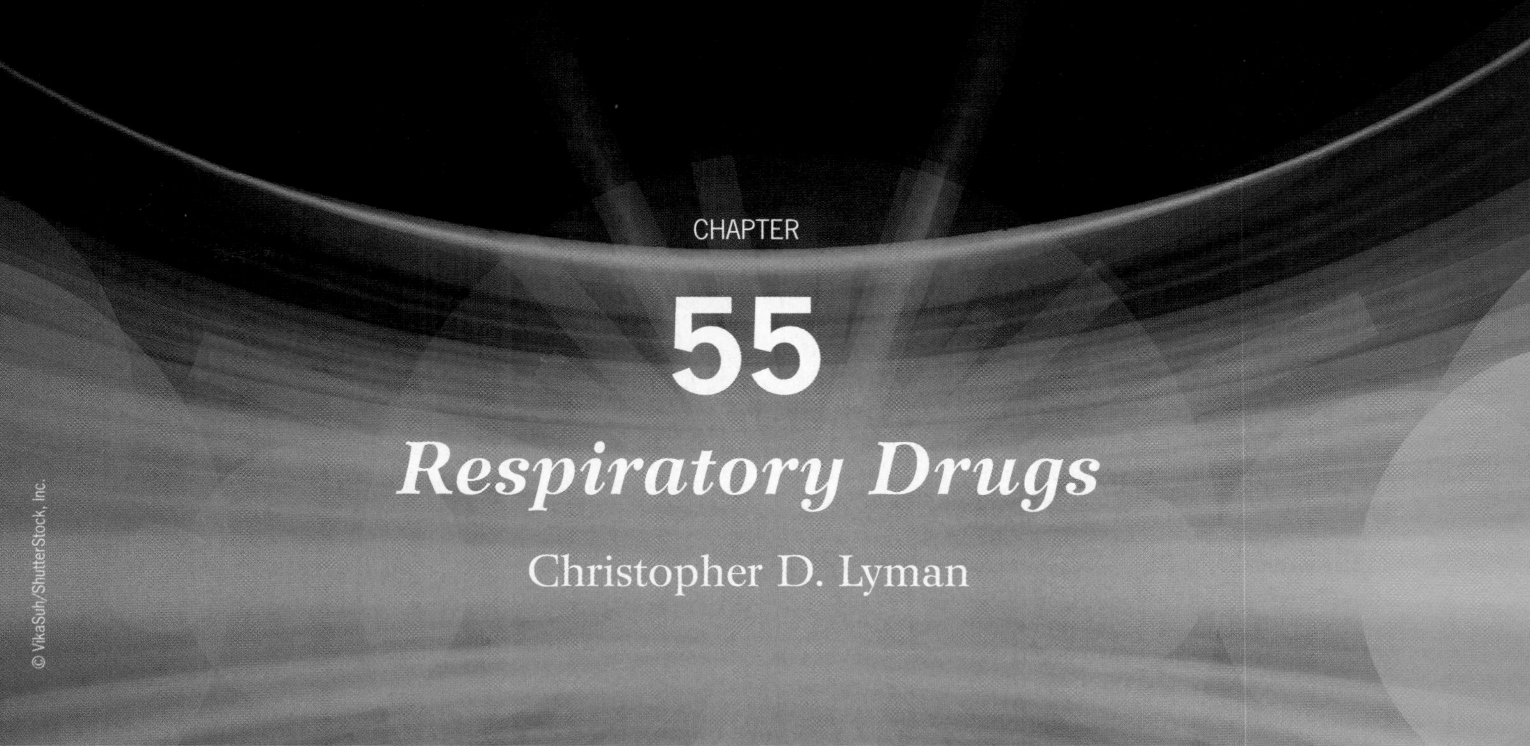

OUTLINE

OBJECTIVES

1. Discuss the concepts of pharmacokinetics and pharmacodynamics as they relate to drug response and disposition in the body.
2. Discuss the need for different routes of administration of medications and advantages to different routes.
3. Describe the different agents used in the management of airway diseases with attention to the mechanism of actions and modification realized to the pathophysiology of these diseases.
4. Discuss adjunct medication introduced via aerosol to maximize penetration to lung tissue.
5. Discuss the pharmacology of agents used in the management of respiratory secretions.
6. Discuss the pharmacology of agents used to establish an airway through intubation and the agents used to optimize management of patients on mechanical ventilators.
7. Describe the pharmacology of agents used for the treatment of pulmonary arterial hypertension and the targeted disease pathways of the different agents.

KEY TERMS

albuterol
anticholinergic
antihistamine
anti-immunoglobulin E
antimicrobial
bambuterol
benzodiazepine
corticosteroid
formoterol
ipratropium
leukotriene modifier
long-acting β_2-agonist (LABA)
mast cell stabilizer
methylxanthine
neuromuscular blocking agent
opiate
pharmacodynamics
pharmacokinetics
salmeterol
sedative
short-acting β_2-agonist (SABA)
theophylline
tiotropium

Introduction

Respiratory illnesses affect millions by impacting the quality of life and interfering with their health. Advances to pharmacotherapy of many respiratory illnesses over the past decade have improved quality of life and survival. Pharmacotherapy options have expanded and changes to routes of delivery have allowed for improved side effect profiles. This chapter discusses options for drug delivery, summarizes the classes of agents used in respiratory illness, and provides a review of agents that offer synergistic or additive benefits when used together.

Pharmacokinetics, Pharmacodynamics, and Drug Delivery

Many pharmacologic options that act on the respiratory system are available for parenteral, oral, or inhaled therapy. The advantages and disadvantages relate to the patient's response and the side effect profiles of agents. **Pharmacokinetics** of drugs refers to how the body acts on drugs, specifically absorption, distribution, metabolism, and elimination. **Pharmacodynamics** refers to the clinical response of the body to a drug.[1]

Absorption concerns with a drug are related to the bioavailability of these agents after administration into the systemic circulation. *Bioavailability* is a pharmacokinetic term that refers to the amount of a drug available to the systemic circulation as compared to the intravenous route. The intravenous (IV) parenteral route is the standard for which all other routes of administration are compared for characterizing the bioavailability. An IV dose of a drug is said to be 100% bioavailable as the complete dose reaches the systemic circulation because it is injected directly into the blood. Barriers to absorption are the size and charge of a drug molecule, its water solubility or lipid solubility, and its abilities to cross membranes.

Parenteral routes, such as the intramuscular and subcutaneous routes of administration, often approach equivalent systemic concentrations to the intravenous route with absorption from tissues near complete. There is a delay in the drug reaching systemic concentrations during the time the drug is absorbed from the tissue into the blood, however. Although the bioavailability is close to 100%, the onset of action therefore is slower than with the intravenous route and the degree of response may be less, although the duration of response may be prolonged. Oral administration of drugs exposes a drug to the gastrointestinal system and first pass metabolism through the liver. First-pass metabolism will decrease bioavailability. Some drugs have limited oral bioavailability and need to be administered via other routes for clinical effect. Understanding oral bioavailability is important to dosing of medications. When administered via the inhaled route, through a nebulizer or inhalers, oral bioavailability can be observed due to poor administration technique and may result in side effects.

Bioavailability is also affected by the distribution and metabolism characteristics of a drug molecule. Distribution is related to the protein or other binding characteristics of the drug and the ability of the drug molecule to pass across membranes into tissues. Highly lipophilic drugs will easily cross membranes and may have prolonged time in tissues as compared with the blood.

Metabolism refers to the conversion of a drug when acted upon by enzymes found in the tissues, primarily the liver, blood, kidney, and lungs. Most enzymes convert drugs to inactive forms (metabolites), but some metabolites can have similar effects as the parent drug, referred to as active metabolites. Most drugs undergo first-order kinetics, for which drug concentration is independent of the rate of metabolism of the drug. But for some drugs, such as theophylline, the enzymes involved in metabolism can become saturated. The metabolism will switch from first-order kinetics to zero-order kinetics (*saturation kinetics*) where the rate of metabolism is dependent on the blood concentration. This will put a patient at risk of toxicity as the ability to metabolize higher concentrations of drug is impaired. Small increases in dose can cause large increases in blood concentrations, resulting in side effects without gain in efficacy. Fortunately, the list of medications undergoing zero-order kinetics is limited. Most drugs follow first-order kinetic metabolism.

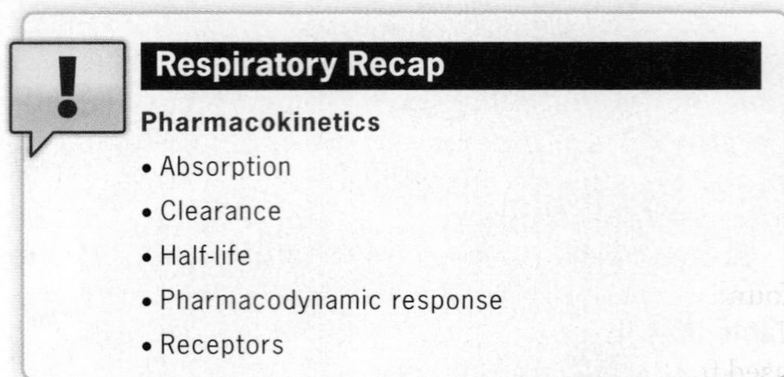
Respiratory Recap

Pharmacokinetics

- Absorption
- Clearance
- Half-life
- Pharmacodynamic response
- Receptors

Elimination is the pharmacokinetic term that refers to the method by which the body removes the drug from systemic circulation. Many organs are associated with some degree of drug elimination; however, the kidney and liver are the major organs of elimination and the lungs, saliva, and sweat are minor routes of elimination. The degree to which the lungs participate in drug elimination of most drugs is poorly quantified. The elimination of drugs via the kidney is quantified based on renal function. Creatinine clearance (CrCl) is a calculation that allows for estimating the efficiency of renal elimination; an alternative is the estimated glomerular filtration rate (eGFR). The liver participates in drug elimination through enzymatic degradation to metabolites. In addition, plasma enzymes can act to metabolize drugs. Metabolism often results in more water-soluble forms so that elimination via the kidney or packaging into bile can then be accomplished.

Characterizing the time a drug stays in the blood is referred to as the *serum elimination half-life* ($t_{½}$). The elimination half-life is the time it takes for the concentration in the blood to reach half of its original concentration. Half-life can be affected by age, disease states, renal and liver function, genetics, drug interactions, and other patient factors. Half-life tells us about time in the blood but does not tell us about time in tissues or the interaction with receptors. It is helpful to understand $t_{½}$ because the time to a steady blood level (*steady state*) and the time needed for near complete elimination from the body will be guided by $t_{½}$, which allows for prediction of maximal response (*efficacy*) and elimination (*loss of efficacy*). Although this is helpful, for many drugs, the response of a drug is determined by its time in the target tissue and the response of the receptor, a term referred to as pharmacodynamics.

The response to a dose of a drug is referred to as the *pharmacodynamic response*.[2] The pharmacodynamic response is due to the drug binding to the receptor in target tissues. All patients will not have the same response to a similar dose. Interpatient variability in response will dictate the dose required for the desired effect. For any individual patient, during a disease flare, the pharmacodynamic response can differ from when a patient is at his or her baseline, requiring higher and more frequent dosing.

Receptors of interest in respiratory diseases can be found on the surface or within the cell membrane.[2] **Table 55-1** lists some of the receptors targeted by drugs used in the treatment of respiratory diseases. Receptors are binding targets for drugs. Affinity for the receptor describes the degree to which a drug will attach to the receptor and disassociate from the receptor. Some drugs will tightly bind to a receptor and stay bound for prolonged periods, producing a prolonged duration of response, while others have weaker binding properties and a shorter duration of response. It is not enough to bind to a receptor, however, to produce an effect. The intrinsic activation of the receptor is required. Drugs that activate a receptor are called *agonists*. Drugs that bind to the receptor but do not activate the receptor are called *antagonists*.

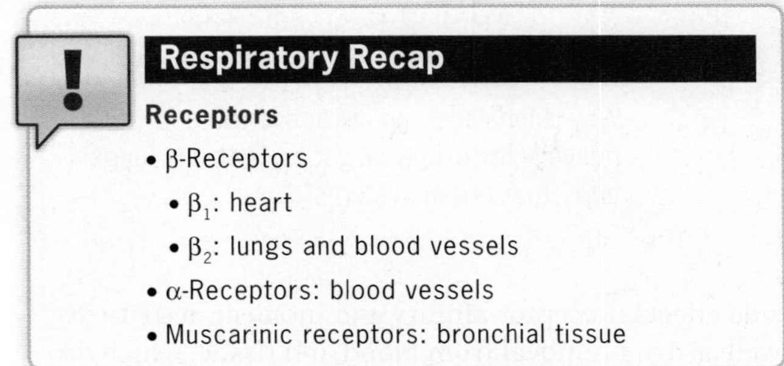

Respiratory Recap

Receptors

- β-Receptors
  - β_1: heart
  - β_2: lungs and blood vessels
- α-Receptors: blood vessels
- Muscarinic receptors: bronchial tissue

Duration of response can vary and will dictate re-dosing. If the duration is prolonged, the desired response may allow for a patient to extend the interval and minimize the need for medication. Patients may benefit from fewer side effects. More frequent and higher dosing will expose the patient to higher blood and tissue concentration, increasing the potential for

TABLE 55-1
Receptors Affecting Respiratory Function

Receptor	Type	Respiratory Effects	Heart and Vascular Effects	Other Effects
α_1	Adrenergic	Bronchoconstriction	Vasoconstriction	Bladder contraction, glycogenolysis, potassium release by the cells, platelet aggregation
α_2	Adrenergic		Vasoconstriction	
β_1	Adrenergic		Increased heart rate (chronotropy) and pumping force (inotropy)	
β_2	Adrenergic	Bronchodilation, increased edema clearance	Vasodilation	Sphincter relaxation, glycogenolysis, tremor
H_1	Histamine	Bronchoconstriction; increases secretions and airway edema by direct stimulation and by increasing vascular permeability		
H_2	Histamine	Possible bronchodilation (minimal)		Primary effects on gastric acid secretion
H_3	Histamine	Bronchoconstriction		
M_1	Cholinergic			
M_2	Cholinergic			
M_3	Cholinergic	Enhanced mucus production, bronchoconstriction		
ET_A	Endothelin		Vasoconstriction, smooth muscle proliferation	CNS- decreased blood flow; seizures (?)
ET_B	Endothelin		Vasoconstriction, smooth muscle proliferation	CNS- decreased blood flow; seizures (?)

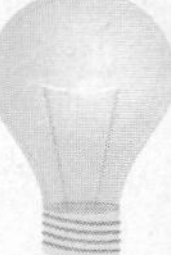

STOP AND THINK

Why is inhalation an attractive route for drug delivery for drugs targeting both the lungs and other organ systems?

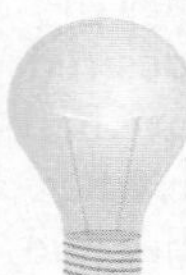

STOP AND THINK

A patient with asthma asks, "What are the side effects of steroids?" How would you respond?

side effects. Receptor affinity and intrinsic activity as well as drug removal from blood and tissue, which are dependent on distribution and elimination characteristics, all play roles in duration of response.

Potency of a drug refers to the amount of drug necessary to elicit a response in target tissue. Two drugs may differ in potency if one drug can have a similar response at lower dose. The extent of the response may be similar at equivalent doses. The drug requiring a smaller dose is said to be more potent. This is suggested to be due to the drug's ability to bind and activate the receptor at lower concentrations.

In lung diseases, the aerosolized inhaled route of administration allows drug delivery directly to the tissue affected by the disease process. Systemic exposure is limited and absorption is thought to be minimal. Aerosol inhalation bypasses the gastrointestinal system and minimizes or eliminates first pass metabolism through the liver. There remains some oral systemic absorption via this route due to deposition of the dose into the oral cavity that then is swallowed. Dose exposure is less, however, as the majority of the dose is delivered directly into the lung when proper medication administration techniques are utilized. Aerosol inhalation is the preferred method for many pharmacologic agents used in respiratory illness due to direct administration to the affected organ and target tissues. This allows for rapid onset of action, smaller doses resulting in equal clinical effect relevant to oral or intravenous administration, and fewer side effects secondary to limited systemic bioavailability. Corticosteroids and β-sympathomimetic agents can be administered via the inhalation route, as oral agents, or parenterally. Certain bronchodilator medications, such as **tiotropium** and **ipratropium**, are only available for administration via inhalation due to a lack of oral bioavailability.

Transcutaneous administration is an alternative route that uses the skin as a reservoir for drug deposition and slowly releases drug from a patch, cream, or ointment. This route has not been exploited for administration of agents used in respiratory illness to date.

Systemic Corticosteroids

The effects of **corticosteroids** are numerous and widespread. The major biologically active corticosteroid in humans is cortisol, while aldosterone is the major biologically active mineralocorticoid. Modification of the structure of cortisol has led to increases in the ratio of anti-inflammatory to sodium-retaining potency (mineralocorticoid effects). This has allowed for the development of many compounds with excellent anti-inflammatory properties but little effect on the body's handling of electrolytes and water. In addition, pharmacokinetic properties have been modified and agents with oral activity, intravenous activity, topical activity, and inhaled activity have resulted.

Corticosteroids act by controlling the rate of synthesis of proteins by reacting with receptor proteins in the cytoplasm of sensitive cells.[3] The steroid-receptor complex is modified and moves into the nucleus where its effect is to modify transcription of specific genes. For most genes, transcription is enhanced as manifested by increased amounts of specific mRNA. Corticosteroids, however, can decrease transcription in other genes, as demonstrated by the gene that codes for adrenocorticotropic hormone (ACTH) production, the endogenous stimulator of cortisol synthesis.[3]

Corticosteroids influence carbohydrate, protein, and lipid metabolism, electrolyte and water balance, and the function of many organ systems (cardiovascular, skeletal muscle, central nervous system, and blood elements) and tissues. Administration of corticosteroids promotes an increase in production of glucose from proteins and promotes glycogen production for storage in the liver.[3] Prolonged high-dose corticosteroids lead to an exaggeration of these changes, producing a diabetes-like state, with elevated plasma glucose concentrations and resistance to insulin. In addition, a redistribution of body fat occurs with deposition of fat in the back of the neck (buffalo hump), subclavicular area, and face (moon face), and a loss of fat from the extremities. Synthetic corticosteroids often have mineralocorticoid properties similar to aldosterone. Mineralocorticoid effects result due to the action on the distal tubules and collecting ducts of the kidney to enhance reabsorption of sodium (Na^+) and promote urinary excretion of potassium (K^+) and hydrogen ions (H^+).[3] This creates a positive Na^+ balance in the plasma, hypokalemia, and alkalosis. Cortisol and systemically administered corticosteroids are less effective than aldosterone in causing Na^+ retention and K^+ excretion. Hypokalemia therefore is usually modest as is the water retention accompanying the Na^+ retention.

Corticosteroid-induced hypertension is in part due to water retention but is also associated with increased plasma renin activity. Corticosteroids administered at high doses tend to cause muscle wasting of skeletal muscle, the mechanism of which is not known. This steroid myopathy is responsible for weakness and fatigue and can complicate attempts to extubate patients from mechanical ventilation. Central nervous system effects of systemic corticosteroids include changes in mood and sleep. Most patients respond with elevation in mood characterized by euphoria, increased energy, and increased motor activity. Insomnia and restlessness are described. A smaller but significant percentage of patients will exhibit psychotic symptoms. Corticosteroids have been associated with delirium in the critically ill.[3]

Systemic corticosteroid effects on formed blood elements have been used for therapeutic benefit. Administration of corticosteroids will decrease the number of lymphocytes, monocytes, eosinophils, and basophils. In contrast, an increase in leukocytes is seen due to demargination from the vascular walls, increased rate of entrance into the blood from the marrow, and diminished rate of removal from the circulation. T lymphocytes are decreased to a greater degree than B lymphocytes. The response of lymphocytes to mitogens is altered actions of anti-inflammation and immunosuppression. A major indication for corticosteroids is suppression of the development of manifestations of inflammation, which is only a palliative effect as the underlying cause remains. Undesirable immune reactions are often the target of therapy, from those of humoral immunity, such as urticaria, to cellular immunity seen in rejection of transplanted organs.[4]

Corticosteroids endow the body with the capacity to resist many types of noxious stimuli and environmental changes. Administration of corticosteroids for the suppression of inflammation and its consequences has made these agents of great clinical value. Corticosteroids interfere with the early and late phases of the inflammatory process.[3] During the early phase, they decrease edema, fibrin deposition, capillary dilation, leukocyte migration, and phagocytic activity. Also suppressed are the later manifestations of proliferation of capillaries and fibroblasts and the deposition of collagen. This anti-inflammatory activity may suppress progression of the disease process and interfere with a physician's diagnosis. Infections are of concern when treatment with corticosteroids is initiated due to their ability to mask symptoms. The ability of corticosteroids to inhibit the recruitment of leukocytes and monocytes/macrophages is important because it results in a decrease in chemotactic substances and factors important to mediating capillary permeability, vasodilation, and contraction of various nonvascular smooth muscles.[5]

Systemic exposure may be limited with the ability to deliver the dose via nebulizer or metered dose inhaler, yet efficacy is still retained. This has become the preferred route of administration for chronic treatment of COPD or asthma as it retains efficacy while sparing systemic side effects of corticosteroid treatment.[6] Actions useful in treating asthma include increasing the number of β_2-receptors and improving receptor responsiveness, reducing mucus production and hypersecretion, reducing bronchial hyperresponsiveness (BHR), and preventing and reversing airway remodeling. Adverse effects of systemic corticosteroids are of concern with long-term administration or frequent short-burst therapy. Of particular concern are hypothalamus-pituitary-adrenal suppression, growth retardation, osteoporosis, electrolyte and water disturbances, hypertension, and impaired wound healing.[3] As corticosteroids affect the nucleus and membrane receptors of most cells, the adverse effect profile of these agents is extensive. **Table 55-2** lists the potencies of the most frequently used systemic corticosteroids.

Systemic corticosteroids are indicated in all patients with acute severe asthma not responding to inhaled β_2-agonist administration. Intravenous therapy offers no advantage over oral administration. Usually, this is continued until discharge from the hospital.[7] Tapering therapy is generally unnecessary if inhaled therapy is continued following discharge. Forced expiratory volume in the first second of expiration (FEV_1) improvement is

TABLE 55-2
Comparative Systemic Steroid Potencies of Selected Agents

Name	Glucocorticoid Potency	Mineralocorticoid Potency	Duration of Action (half-life in hours)
Cortisol (hydrocortisone)	1	1	8
Prednisone	3.5–5	0.8	16–36
Prednisolone	4	0.8	16–36
Methylprednisolone	5–7.5	0.5	18–40
Dexamethasone	25–80	0	36–54
Fludrocortisone acetate	15	200	24
Aldosterone	0.3	200–1000	–

usually 50% after 48 hours of treatment and 80% after 6 days of therapy. Maintaining systemic therapy for 10 to 14 days may be unnecessary. For patients not admitted to the hospital, 3 to 5 days of systemic corticosteroid therapy is usually sufficient. Infants and young children respond to short-term administration of prednisone for 3 to 10 days. It is recommended that a full dose of corticosteroid be continued until FEV_1 reaches 80% of predicted or personal best.[7,8]

Systemic corticosteroids reduce the treatment failure rates, show a more rapid improvement in FEV_1, and reduce hospital stay as compared to placebo when used for acute exacerbations of COPD. The optimal dose has not been defined as studies have used both intravenous and oral therapy at various doses. Duration of therapy appears to be a 9-day to 14-day treatment course, as longer duration has not been shown to be more beneficial. If therapy is continued for more than 2 weeks, a tapering regimen should be employed to avoid hypothalamus-pituitary-adrenal axis suppression. Adverse effects include hyperglycemia, insomnia, and hallucinations at higher doses.

Systemic corticosteroids have been used for other respiratory illnesses involving immune response. Interstitial lung disease (ILD) has been shown to respond to systemic corticosteroids administration. Idiopathic pulmonary fibrosis has been shown to have some response to prednisone at 1 mg/kg/day for 3 to 6 months than when tapered off over 4 to 6 months.[9] Side effects may necessitate alternative agents for immunosuppression. ILD from sarcoidosis or collagen vascular disease has also been shown to respond to systemic corticosteroids.

Inhaled Corticosteroids

The principal advantage of inhaled corticosteroids (ICS) is their high topical potency to reduce inflammation in the lung and their low systemic activity. The ICSs have anti-inflammatory potencies 1000-fold greater than endogenous cortisol. A number of inhaled agents are now available for inhalation therapy (**Table 55-3** and **Table 55-4**). The anti-inflammatory differences between agents can differ by four- to sixfold, but this can be overcome by giving equipotent microgram doses of each drug. The aerosol dose delivered of each drug has great variability depending on patient technique and delivery device. There are some differences in pharmacokinetic properties that will determine frequency of dosing. Dose response curves for the different agents are relatively flat due to the fact that the measures used to determine efficacy (lung function, BHR, symptoms, as-needed short-acting β_2-agonist use) are downstream events from the anti-inflammatory activity.[5]

Pharmacokinetic differences between agents produce differences in the topical-systemic effect ratio (therapeutic index). Pharmacokinetic properties that enhance improved topical selectivity (efficacy) include long residence time in the lung, poor oral bioavailability, and rapid systemic clearance.[6] Owing to their high lipophilicity, systemic clearance of the ICS is very rapid, approaching the rate of liver blood flow. ICSs differ in oral bioavailability, however, although they all undergo significant first-pass metabolism.[6] The ICSs produce dose-dependent systemic effects from a combination of increased oral absorption and increased fraction absorbed from the lung tissue. Essentially every drug that reaches the lungs is absorbed systemically. Oral bioavailability can be altered by using a spacer device to prevent oral mucosal deposition as approximately 80% of the dose will be contained in the spacer.[6]

Most ICSs can be dosed twice daily for patients with moderate disease. Twice daily dosing may allow for fewer local side effects. There does not appear to be any specific pharmacologic or pharmacokinetic aspect of the ICSs that allow for once daily dosing. More severe patients require multiple daily dosing. The inflammatory response of asthma has been shown to inhibit steroid-receptor binding. This provides strong theoretical evidence for initially beginning patients on higher, more frequent doses and then tapering down once control has been achieved. The National Asthma Education and Prevention Program (NAEPP) recommends this approach.

Response to ICSs will often be delayed, with most patients seeing improvement within the first 1 to 2 weeks of therapy and maximal response within 4 to 8 weeks. Improvement in baseline FEV_1 and PFTs usually shows maximal response within 3 to 6 weeks, and improvement in BHR may require 2 to 3 weeks. Maximal response is seen in 1 to 3 months but may continue to improve over 1 year. There is large variability in response with up to 10% of patients not seeing any improvement. Whether nonresponders show no improvement in exacerbations is not well understood. Nonresponders will show decreases in sensitivity to exercise and partial improvement to antigen challenge. These two effects are likely due to a reduction in mucosal mast cells.[5]

Local adverse effects of ICSs include oropharyngeal candidiasis and dysphonia that are dose-dependent. Dysphonia is thought to be due to local myopathy of the vocal chords due to the corticosteroid.[6] A spacer or valved holding chamber can minimize oropharyngeal deposition and decrease the frequency and severity of local side effects. Systemic side effects can be seen with all ICS agents when used at high doses. Long-term side effects of concern include growth suppression in children, osteoporosis, cataracts, and adrenal suppression and crisis. Of these, only growth suppression occurs in low to medium doses. Growth suppression is transient during the first 6 months to 1 year of therapy, and then growth velocity will return to normal. The effect is small and not cumulative. Attainment of predicted adult height is expected.[10] The effect of ICSs on HPA

TABLE 55-3
Clinically Comparable Doses of Inhaled Corticosteroids

Drug	Comparative Daily Dosages (μg)					
	Low		Medium		High	
	Child*	Adult	Child	Adult	Child	Adult
Beclomethasone dipropionate						
HFA-pMDI	80–160	80–240	>160–320	>240–480	>320	>480
Budesonide						
DPI	180–400	200–600	>400–800	>600–1200	>800	>1200
Nebules	500	UK	1000	UK	2000	UK
Ciclesonide†						
HFA-pMDI	80–160	160–320	>160–320	>320–640	>320	>640
Flunisolide						
HFA-pMDI	160	320	320	>320–640	≥640	>640
Fluticasone propionate						
HFA-pMDI	88–176	88–264	>176–352	264–440	>352	>440
DPI	100–200	100–300	>200–400	300–500	>400	>500
Mometasone furoate‡						
DPI	110	220	220–440	440	>440	>440

DPI, dry powder inhaler; HFA-pMDI, hydrofluoroalkane-propelled pressurized metered dose inhaler; UK, unknown.
*Child age is 5–11 years
†Beclomethasone dipropionate and ciclesonide are prodrugs that are activated in the lung to their active metabolites beclomethasone 17-monopropionate and desciclesonide, respectively
‡Mometasone furoate studied in a different receptor system. Value estimated from relative values of beclomethasone dipropionate, triamcinolone acetonide, and fluticasone propionate in that system
Reproduced from Kelly HW. Comparison of Inhaled Corticosteroids: An Update. *Annals of Pharmacotherapy.* 2009;43:519–527. Reprinted by Permission of SAGE Publications.

TABLE 55-4
Pharmacodynamic/Pharmacokinetic Properties of Inhaled Corticosteroids

Drug	Receptor Binding Affinity	Lung Delivery (%)	Protein Binding (%)	Oral Bioavailability (%)	Systemic Clearance (L/h)	Distribution Volume (L)	Half-Life (h)	
							IV	Inhaled
Beclomethasone dipropionate/ 17-monopropionate	0.4/13.5	50–60	87	20/40	150/120	20/424	0.5/2.7	UK/2.7
Budesonide	9.4	15–30	88	11	84	280	2.8	2.0
Ciclesonide/ desciclesonide	0.12/12.0	50	99/99	<1/<1	152/228	207/897	0.36/3.4	0.5/4.8
Flunisolide	1.8	68	80	20	58	96	1.6	1.6
Fluticasone propionate	18	20	90	≤1	66	318–859	7.8	14.4
Mometasone furoate	23	11	99	<1	53	152	5.0	UK

Reproduced from Kelly HW. Comparison of Inhaled Corticosteroids: An Update. *Annals of Pharmacotherapy.* 2009;43:519–527. Reprinted by Permission of SAGE Publications.

axis suppression and bone mineralization is not clinically significant except at high doses.

In the latter 1990s, several large international trials failed to demonstrate any long-term benefit from ICSs in modifying the long-term decline in lung function that is characteristic of COPD.[11] In patients with more advanced disease (usually classified as an FEV_1 <50% predicted) there is evidence that the number of exacerbations per year and the rate of deterioration in health status can be reduced by inhaled corticosteroids in COPD. Evidence from four large prospective 3-year studies showed no effect of inhaled corticosteroids on rate of change of FEV_1 in any severity of COPD.[12] Combining long-acting inhaled β-agonists and inhaled corticosteroids in one inhaler seemed a convenient way of delivering treatment. The initial trial data showed a significant additional effect on pulmonary function and a reduction in symptoms in those who received combination therapies compared with those receiving its components. The largest effects in terms of exacerbations and health status were found in patients with an FEV_1 <50% predicted, where combining treatment was clearly better than either component drug used by itself.[13]

Beta-Adrenoceptor Agonists

β-receptors of the adrenergic nervous system are targets of the endogenous catecholamines, norepinephrine and epinephrine. The three subtypes of β-receptors, β_1, β_2, and β_3 are found in many tissues. Activation of β-adrenergic receptors leads to relaxation of smooth muscle in the lung and dilation and opening of the airways. β-adrenergic receptors are coupled to a stimulatory G protein of adenylyl cyclase. This enzyme produces the second messenger cyclic adenosine monophosphate (cAMP). In the lung, cAMP decreases calcium concentrations within cells and activates protein kinase A.[14] Both of these changes inactivate myosin light chain kinase and activate myosin light chain phosphatase. In addition, β_2-agonists open large conductance calcium-activated potassium channels and thereby tend to hyperpolarize airway smooth muscle cells. The combination of decreased intracellular calcium, increased membrane potassium conductance, and decreased myosin light chain kinase activity leads to smooth muscle relaxation and bronchodilation.[14]

The β-agonists drugs used in respiratory illnesses are designed for selectivity for the β_2-specific receptors. These receptors are abundant in the smooth muscle of the bronchioles. Other tissues also have β_2-receptors, however. These include the smooth muscle of the arteries and uterus, adipose tissue, pancreas, liver, and GI tract. Specificity to β_2-receptors can be lost when doses are increased, causing β_1-receptor stimulation that may lead to unwanted side effects, specifically stimulation of cardiac β_1-receptors that cause tachycardia and a concern for angina.

Short-Acting β_2-Agonists

The **short-acting β_2-agonists (SABA)** are the most effective bronchodilating agents and the treatment of choice for the management of severe bronchoconstriction and severe acute asthma.[15,16] Aerosolized β_2-agonists have demonstrated equal to greater efficacy over systemic β_2-agonists and have a safer side effect profile. Systemic adverse effects include tachycardia and dysrhythmias, hypokalemia, and hyperglycemia. Nebulized β_2-agonists can be delivered safely to children younger than 2 years old.[15] For patients with severe obstruction and respiratory failure, aerosolized or nebulized β_2-agonists can be given to patients on ventilators via the circuit.[17] For severe obstruction frequent nebulization or continuous nebulization has been shown to have greater benefit at improving FEV_1 and peak expiratory flow (PEF) and reduces length of hospitalization when compared to equivalent doses delivered at 1-hour intervals.[16] Continuous nebulization should be considered when there is suboptimal response following three nebulized treatments of short-acting β_2-agonists 20 minutes apart. [18]

The doses of inhaled β_2-agonists used for severe bronchoconstriction have been derived empirically and the dose response will vary with degree of bronchospasm. During acute exacerbations of asthma, the dose necessary for relief may vary 5- to 10-fold over the dose needed in chronic stable asthma.[16] The degree of inflammatory response to the inciting event may also play a role in the response to typical doses. The safety profile via inhalation provides for the clinician and patient to use much higher doses than if systemic administration was required. This ability to increase the dose supports the efficacy of these agents in acute bronchospasm. Excessive cardiac stimulation, palpitations, hyperglycemia, and tremor are evident when higher doses are used. Drug interactions are infrequent.

Coordination of inhalation technique for pressurized metered dose inhalers (pMDI) requires education. Delivery of the drug into the lungs can be compromised with poor technique. Dry powders have been formulated with delivery devices intended to improve drug delivery to the lungs. For nebulized β_2-agonists, administration with other bronchodilators for an additive effect is a frequent practice.[19]

Albuterol is the prototype drug representative in the class of β_2-agonist agents. Albuterol is available as pMDI nebulizer solution, and as an oral agent in both tablet and liquid form. Nebulizer doses are 2.5 to 5 mg per dose, administered every 20 minutes during exacerbations and then every 1 to 4 hours as needed upon evidence of response. The pMDI delivers 90 μg/dose and are usually 4 to 8 puffs every 30 minutes, and then 2 to 4 puffs every 4 hours as needed. In patients with severe distress, nebulization may be preferred, as the pMDI requires coordination of inhalation that may be difficult for patients in severe distress.[15] Also of concern

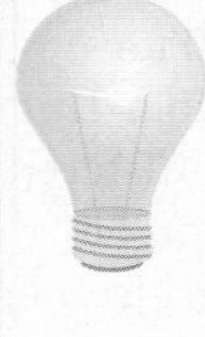

STOP AND THINK

You are caring for a patient with a COPD exacerbation in the emergency department. He has a heart rate of 120 beats/min but also needs an inhaled bronchodilator. What options are available?

is the high cost associated with the HFA formulations of inhalers.

Racemic albuterol is a mixture of the dextro rotatory (S) and levo rotatory isomer (R). Only the l-isomer (R-albuterol) contributes to albuterol's bronchodilatory effects. Levalbuterol contains only the l-isomer and is likely to be twice as potent allowing for one-half the dose. In the absence of the r-isomer, at the lower dose, the side effect profile is improved, specifically focusing on less tachycardia associated with equivalent doses.[20] The clinical data supporting this claim have been challenged. During exacerbations, higher doses of levalbuterol caused tachyarrhythmias similar to those seen with racemic albuterol.[20–22] Superiority of the l-isomer over the racemic mixture is unproven.

The oral route of administration of short-acting β_2-agonists is mostly used in children for ease of administration when nebulization is not an option. Pediatric dosing for children ages 2 to 6 years old is 0.1 to 0.2 mg/kg three times daily, not to exceed 12 mg/day (divided doses). For children ages 6 to 12 years, a 2 mg/dose three to four times daily, maximum not to exceed 24 mg/day (divided doses) is recommended. For children 12 years and older to adults, the recommendation is 2 to 4 mg/dose three to four times daily, not to exceed 32 mg/day (divided doses). An extended release tablet is available as a 4 mg tablet and is administered every 12 hours. Elderly adults may be more sensitive to the side effects of oral therapy, and dosage recommendations are 2 mg three to four times daily with a maximum 8 mg dose three to four times daily.[15]

Long-Acting β_2-Agonists

Long-acting β_2-agonists (LABA) are selective for β_2-receptors. Currently three agents are available in the United States: **salmeterol, formoterol,** and **bambuterol**. A fourth ultra-long-acting β_2-receptor agonist, indacaterol, was recently approved. LABAs are used for moderate to persistent asthma, nocturnal asthma, and chronic obstructive pulmonary disease (COPD). The duration of action is extended, approximately 12 hours for salmeterol and formoterol. Formoterol has an onset of action similar to albuterol and retains the prolonged duration of effect. Bambuterol is only available as an oral formulation. Salmeterol and formoterol are preferred over short-acting β_2-agonists in the treatment of moderate to persistent asthma as chronic therapy. Three other agents have recently been approved for COPD—indacaterol, vilanterol, and olodaterol—and these are ultra-long acting, allowing for once daily administration. LABAs are not intended as first-line agents in the treatment of moderate to persistent asthma but rather as add-ons to inhaled corticosteroids. LABAs are not intended to replace short-acting β_2-agonists for rescue therapy, so patients need to be counseled to continue use of their short-acting β_2-agonist.[16] LABAs are available singularly or as fixed-dose combination therapy with inhaled corticosteroids. Combination therapy in asthma provides greater control than increasing the dose of the inhaled corticosteroid alone.[22–24] LABAs, like short-acting β_2-agonists, are devoid of anti-inflammatory properties and should not be used alone in chronic asthma.

Since their introduction, concern has existed that use of LABAs provides an increased risk of asthma exacerbations and asthma-related deaths. Initially, the risk was believed to be due to inappropriate initial therapy of acute exacerbations.[25,26] The SMART study was halted owing to poor enrollment and an increased risk of asthma-related deaths in African American patients receiving salmeterol.[27] This result may be due to greater severity of asthma in this population or undertreatment with inhaled corticosteroids, although it is difficult to discern. Tolerance is produced with chronic administration of LABAs.[27] Responsiveness to short-acting β_2-agonists is slightly decreased but can be overcome by increasing the dose of the short-acting β_2-agonists.[28] Evidence for LABAs reducing exacerbation rates in pediatrics is still ongoing.

In COPD, combination LABA and ICS have been approved for several fixed-dose products. Initial evidence with the combination salmeterol/fluticasone and formoterol/budesonide has demonstrated improved clinical outcomes such as FEV_1, health status, and frequency of exacerbations as compared to inhaled corticosteroids or long-acting bronchodilators alone.[29,30] These combination inhalers provide more convenience for patients and decrease the total number of inhalations needed daily. Long-acting β_2-agonists should not be used for quick relief of symptoms or on an as needed basis. The U.S. Food and Drug Administration (FDA) approved the ultra-long-acting β_2-agonist indacaterol as a monotherapy for COPD in 2011. Clinical trials comparing this agent to placebo showed improvement in lung function at 5 minutes that was maintained throughout the 24-hour dosing period. This effect held for the 12 weeks of the study.[31] The need for rescue therapy with inhaled short-acting β_2-agonists and inhaled anticholinergic agents was reduced. Additionally, patients reported improved health-related quality of life. In 2013, the FDA approved the combination ultra-short-acting β_2-agonist/inhaled corticosteroid, vilanterol/fluticasone furoate, for COPD. Approval of once daily administration of three fixed-dose vilanterol/fluticasone combinations showed improved FEV_1 for all combinations as compared to placebo through 24 weeks of therapy. As with LABAs, ultra-long-acting agents should not be used for quick relief of symptoms or on an as needed basis.

Epinephrine

The endogenous hormone epinephrine has activity at alpha-receptors (α) and β-receptors of the adrenergic nervous system.[14] Primary use in respiratory diseases is for anaphylaxis when administered via the intramuscular or subcutaneous route. The bronchodilator benefits of epinephrine support the use in status asthmaticus as an intravenous infusion, but this has been shown to be no better than continuous nebulization of a short-acting β_2-agonist. The α-effects provide vasoconstriction of the periphery and lungs, decreasing capillary leakage. The β-effects are nonspecific for receptor subtypes and stimulate β_1-receptors to promote heart rate and contractility and the β_2-receptors to promote bronchodilation.[14] Epinephrine is available as an injectable formulation (1:1000 injectable solution = 1 mg/mL) and is given as an intramuscular injection into the deltoid. Adult dosing (and patients weighing >30 kg) is 0.3 mg to 0.5 mg and may be repeated in 15 to 20 minutes if needed. Pediatric dosing (patients weighing 15 to 30 kg) is 0.15 mg as an IM injection and may be repeated if needed.[32] Epinephrine is available as an auto-injector for ease of administration in patients with a significant allergy history or history of anaphylaxis. Epinephrine has an absence of oral bioavailability, making this route unacceptable. The use in asthma exacerbations and status asthmaticus has fallen out of favor, as there is no proven advantage of systemic administration over aerosolized β_2-agonists. Guidelines still include this as an option.

Aerosolized epinephrine is used for laryngeal obstruction following extubation causing inspiratory narrowing signaled by the onset of stridor. The cause is believed to be airway swelling. Aerosolized epinephrine may relieve the airway swelling so as to prevent reintubation. If the patient is not *in extremis*, aerosolized epinephrine using 2.5 mL of epinephrine 1:1000 for injection (l-isomer) is an appropriate intervention. This dose may be diluted with normal saline or administered as straight drug via nebulizer. A racemic solution of epinephrine, which contains equal amounts of the l-isomer and d-isomer, is commercially available as a 2.25% solution for inhalation, but the standard l-isomer is equally effective. Dosing of the racemic mixture is 0.5 mL diluted with normal saline to a volume of 3 mL and administered via nebulizer. This has been proven effective in children, and the practice is carried to adults despite it being unproven in this population. The effect of epinephrine on α-receptors causes vasoconstriction of the mucosal vessels that is aimed at reducing airway swelling.

Respiratory Recap

Medications for Respiratory Disease

- Corticosteroids
- β-Agonists
- Anticholinergics
- Methylxanthines
- Magnesium
- Leukotriene modifiers
- Mast cell stabilizers
- Anti-IgA
- Antimicrobials
- Secretion modifiers

Anticholinergic Agents

The parasympathetic nervous system plays a major role in regulating the tone of smooth muscles lining the respiratory airways.[11] Drugs that inhibit the actions of the neurotransmitter acetylcholine at muscarinic receptors for acetylcholine in the periphery are referred to as **anticholinergic** agents. The two types of receptors for acetylcholine are nicotinic and muscarinic receptors. Muscarinic receptors are of interest in respiratory medicine as they are found on exocrine glands and smooth muscle of the larger airways.[33] A diverse set of stimuli results in reflex increases in parasympathetic activity that result in bronchoconstriction.[11] The submucosal glands are also innervated by parasympathetic neurons. Although older anticholinergic agents were utilized for bronchodilation, they were largely supplanted by the introduction of epinephrine and **methylxanthines** until the introduction of ipratropium.[11] Ipratropium and other anticholinergic bronchodilators are effective against stimulants to bronchoconstriction such as methacholine but only partially antagonize the effects of histamine and bradykinin on bronchial reflexes.[33] These indirect actions on inflammatory mediators of bronchoconstriction released during asthmatic attacks form the basis of their use in asthma and other reversible airway diseases.

Ipratropium and tiotropium are two agents currently approved and available for inhalation administration.[34,35] Ipratropium exhibits broncholytic action by reducing cholinergic influence on the bronchial musculature. It blocks muscarinic acetylcholine receptors without specificity for subtypes and therefore promotes the degradation of cyclic guanosine monophosphate (cGMP), resulting in a decreased intracellular concentration of cGMP.[33,34] Most likely due to actions of cGMP on intracellular calcium, this results in decreased contractility of smooth muscle in the lung, inhibiting bronchoconstriction and mucus secretion. It is a nonselective muscarinic antagonist and does not diffuse into the blood, which prevents systemic side effects. Combination with β-adrenergic agonists increases the dilating effect on the bronchi.

Inhibiting the secretion of mucous membranes in the upper and lower respiratory system will thicken secretions. Concern for the mucociliary clearance with systemic anticholinergics as well as other systemic side effects makes them unattractive. Inhaled ipratropium does not decrease mucociliary clearance, however,[11] but it can cause headache and irritation of the throat in some patients. If ipratropium is inhaled, side effects resembling those of other anticholinergics are minimal. Dry mouth and sedation have been reported. Also, other effects such as skin flushing, tachycardia, acute angle-closure glaucoma, nausea, palpitations, and headache have been observed. Urinary retention has been reported in patients receiving doses by nebulizer. As a result, caution may be warranted, especially in men with prostatic hypertrophy.[36]

Ipratropium is used for reversible airway disease as adjunctive therapy to short-acting β_2-agonists. It is available as a pMDI and nebulizer solution. The combination product albuterol and ipratropium is available in both formulations. These agents can be administered together for acute asthma exacerbations. The recommendation is to dose every 6 hours. Much like albuterol, more frequent dosing is often employed in severe bronchospastic disease due to its safety profile.[11]

Combination agents are often employed in COPD. The benefits are often seen during disease progression and worsening of symptoms. Combining agents with differing mechanisms of action allows for the lowest possible dose to minimize side effects than with individual agents used alone. In COPD, the combination of either long-acting β_2-agonists or short-acting β_2-agonists with ipratropium improves both symptomatic relief and pulmonary function.

Tiotropium is a long-acting agent not used for acute exacerbations of reversible airway disease. Approved for use in COPD patients, it has a prolonged duration at the receptor that allows for once daily administration.[35] Tiotropium does not display selectivity for specific muscarinic receptors. When topically applied, it acts mainly on M_3 muscarinic receptors located on smooth muscle cells and submucosal glands.[37] This leads to a reduction in smooth muscle contraction and mucus secretion and thus produces a bronchodilatory effect. Currently available formulations require use of a dry powder inhaler. It is not available for nebulization or as a pMDI. Tiotropium has been shown more effective than either salmeterol or ipratropium alone to decrease exacerbations and hospitalization in moderate to severe COPD.[35]

Methylxanthines

Caffeine and **theophylline** are plant-derived methylxanthines that were studied for medicinal purposes in the early 1900s. The diverse pharmacologic actions of methylxanthines have found many therapeutic uses and have been available for six decades. Theophylline and the salt of theophylline, aminophylline, have been employed extensively to relax bronchial smooth muscle in the treatment of asthma and to relieve dyspnea in the treatment of chronic obstructive pulmonary disease. With the advent of short-acting and long-acting β_2-agonists and anticholinergics, theophylline has largely fallen out of favor in the treatment of asthma and COPD. At higher doses, caffeine has similar effects to theophylline and can be used in the treatment of asthma but offers no advantage over theophylline. Regular use of theophylline has not been shown to either a beneficial or detrimental effect on the progression of COPD. When added to the treatment plan of a patient with COPD maintained on a β-agonist and anticholinergic agents, it provides added benefit. This supports the hypothesis that there is a synergistic bronchodilator effect.

Methylxanthines have several pharmacological properties of therapeutic interest. They relax smooth muscle, notably bronchial muscle, stimulate the central nervous system, stimulate cardiac muscle, and act on the kidney to produce diuresis. Theophylline competitively inhibits phosphodiesterase, the enzyme that degrades cAMP. Increased concentrations of cAMP may mediate the observed bronchodilation. Other proposed mechanisms of action include inhibition of the release of intracellular calcium and competitive antagonism of the bronchoconstrictor adenosine.[38] Chronic theophylline has been shown to improve lung function, including vital capacity, FEV_1, minute ventilation, and gas exchange. Subjectively, COPD patients report reduced dyspnea, improved exercise tolerance, and improved respiratory drive.

Therapeutic serum ranges for the efficacy and toxicity of theophylline have been identified. The recognized therapeutic concentration of theophylline in the plasma for bronchodilation was reported as between 5 and 20 μg/mL.[39] Serum concentrations between 5 and 12 μg/mL have been recognized as being a safer therapeutic range with the hope of avoiding toxicities. Theophylline concentrations are dependent on clinical factors as well as many drug interactions. Methylxanthines are substrates for many cytochrome p450 liver enzymes and, therefore, the list of drugs that interact with it is extensive. The upper range between 12 and 20 μg/mL is associated with some toxicity. Effects on the CNS and on the cardiovascular system can be particularly problematic as serum levels are elevated outside of therapeutic ranges.[40,41]

Methylxanthines stimulate the medullary respiratory centers in the brain stem, resulting in increased sensitivity to stimulatory effects of elevated levels of CO_2 increasing respiratory minute volume. At therapeutic levels, CNS stimulation can cause nervousness, anxiety, tremors, and insomnia. At higher levels, in excess of 25 μg/mL, concern for seizure activity has been reported. Nausea and vomiting are also associated with CNS effects seen within the upper therapeutic range for theophylline and suggest serum levels approaching toxic ranges. The central nervous system stimulatory effects of methylxanthines have been used in the treatment of prolonged apnea sometimes seen in preterm infants. In addition, stimulation of respiratory drive in COPD may be advantageous for oxygen exchange.[38]

Cardiovascular effects of theophylline include modest increases in heart rate seen in therapeutic ranges. Improvement in contractile force and decreases in preload have been described, but these effects are reported no to be long-lasting and are of little clinical benefit. Sinus tachycardia can be common in patients initiated on theophylline. Tachyarrhythmias can be problematic in patients with a history of atrial rhythm disturbances and may necessitate discontinuation.[38,40]

Benefits to skeletal muscle function are also described. At therapeutic concentrations, both caffeine and theophylline improve diaphragmatic contractility and reduce diaphragmatic fatigue in normal human subjects and in patients with COPD.[38] These effects contribute to the decreased sensation of breathlessness in patients with COPD. Some adverse effects related to effects on skeletal muscle that are more common in the elderly include gastric reflux and ulcer aggravation, difficulty urinating in elderly males with prostatism, and tremor.

Pharmacokinetics parameters are variable depending on age, liver function, cardiac function, lung disease, and smoking history. Neonates and children younger than 3 months old will eliminate about 50% of the drug unchanged in the urine, whereas for children older than age 3 months to adults, less than 10% is found unchanged in the urine.[42] Absorption and time to peak concentration are dosage form dependent. Dosage formulations have been modified to promote avoidance of higher peak serum concentrations and allow for once or twice daily dosing to promote compliance. Serum half-life is highly variable dependent on factors mentioned above as well as drug interactions.[41,42]

Theophylline is available as an intravenous formulation, as immediate-release syrup and tablets, and as sustained-release tablet and capsule formulations. These all have different pharmacokinetic characteristics requiring deliberation if switching from one formulation to another.[40] The role of theophylline in COPD is as maintenance therapy in nonacutely ill patients. Despite being available as an intravenous formulation, therefore, the acute use of intravenous theophylline for exacerbations of COPD is no longer supported. Monitoring of theophylline for toxicities is important. Monitor heart rate, CNS effects, respiratory rate, and arterial blood gases. Serum concentrations should be monitored prior to making dose increases especially in the presence of signs and symptoms of toxicity. Drug and disease interactions should be considered and serum monitoring performed when identified.

Magnesium

Intravenous magnesium has been used for asthma exacerbations for many years, as magnesium has been shown to have moderate bronchodilator properties similar to theophylline. Its use in patients presenting to the emergency department is controversial. Magnesium is known to be a relaxant of smooth muscle. When given intravenously, the adverse effect profile includes hypotension, facial flushing, sweating, loss of deep tendon reflexes, and respiratory depression. Its use as a bronchodilator has largely fallen out of favor.

Leukotriene Modifiers

Leukotrienes are released during the inflammatory process in response to certain antigens. *Leukotrienes* are substances that induce numerous biological effects, including augmentation of neutrophil and eosinophil migration, neutrophil and monocyte aggregation, leukocyte adhesion, increased capillary permeability, and smooth muscle contraction.[43,44] These effects contribute to inflammation, edema, mucus secretion, and bronchoconstriction in the airways of asthmatic patients. LTB4, a chemoattractant for neutrophils and eosinophils, and cysteinyl leukotrienes (LTC4, LTD4, LTE4) can be measured in a number of biological fluids, including bronchoalveolar lavage fluid, blood, urine, and sputum from patients with asthma, causing bronchoconstriction, increased mucous production, and inflammation.[44]

The **leukotriene modifiers**—zafirlukast, montelukast, and zileuton—are mediator-specific therapy for the treatment of asthma and allergic rhinitis. Two clinically distinct cysteinyl leukotriene antagonists, zafirlukast and montelukast, are synthetic peptides that inhibit the binding of three leukotrienes (LTC4, LTD4, and LTE4) responsible for smooth muscle constriction and hyperresponsiveness after contact with an allergen challenge, including exercise. Zileuton is a 5-lipoxygenase inhibitor. It affects 5-lipoxygenase pathway activation by limiting the production of LTA4, LTB4, LTC4, and the derivatives of cysteinyl leukotriene, LTD4 and LTE4, which are potent vasoconstrictors.[43]

Leukotriene modifiers appear to have a beneficial role in the treatment of both asthma and allergic rhinitis and are currently recommended as alternative therapy to inhaled corticosteroids or in combination depending on severity of symptoms.[45] The use of leukotrienes as monotherapy for asthma has demonstrated an improvement in pulmonary function tests (FEV_1 and PEF), decreased nocturnal awakenings and β-agonist use, and improved asthma symptoms.[46] Leukotriene modifiers are an alternative medication for use in children with mild persistent asthma, especially those unable to comply with inhaled steroids.[47] Leukotriene modifiers are also considered to be an additional medication for the step-up approach, or combination therapy, recommended by the National Asthma Education Prevention Program (NAEPP) for moderate and severe persistent asthma not controlled with inhaled corticosteroids alone.[48] There is some evidence that patients with aspirin-sensitive asthma do well with leukotriene modifiers. Antileukotrienes also have modest efficacy in allergic rhinitis.

In a systematic review comparing the use of inhaled glucocorticoids with leukotriene antagonists as monotherapy in the treatment of asthma, Ducharme concluded that leukotriene antagonists are less effective than inhaled glucocorticoids when used as a single agent in the treatment of asthma.[49] Gonyeau and Partisano, in their review of leukotriene antagonists as a treatment for seasonal allergic rhinitis, also concluded that leukotriene antagonists appear to have a primary role, not as a single treatment agent but as an adjunct to intranasal corticosteroids.[50] Montelukast has been approved as monotherapy for allergic rhinitis by the FDA.

Zafirlukast and montelukast have distinctions. Zafirlukast should be taken on an empty stomach as food reduces the mean bioavailability by about 40%. Montelukast can be taken with or without food. Zafirlukast has significant drug interactions with warfarin, resulting in prolonged prothrombin times, and with theophylline, elevating theophylline serum levels. Montelukast is free of these drug interactions and with many other medications that potentially interact with zafirlukast. Zafirlukast has FDA approval for use in asthma for children older than 7 years. Montelukast has FDA approval for asthma in children 1 year old and older and for perennial allergic rhinitis in those ages 6 months and older.

Zafirlukast is recommended for twice daily dosing. Once daily dosing is recommended for montelukast, with evening administration to reduce the frequent nocturnal and early morning symptoms of asthma and allergic rhinitis. The most frequently reported side effect is headache, occurring in almost 20% of treated individuals. Other side effects were reported in fewer than 5% of individuals and included abdominal pain, cough, increased liver function tests (LFTs), diarrhea, and rash. An idiosyncratic syndrome similar to the Churg-Strauss syndrome, with marked circulating eosinophilia, heart failure, and associated eosinophilic vasculitis, was reported in a small number of patients treated with zafirlukast and montelukast. The majority of these patients received high-dose oral or inhaled corticosteroids and the leukotriene modifier allowed for dose reduction, which may have unmasked this underlying condition. Whatever the cause, the incidence is fewer than 1 in 15,000 to 20,000 patient-years of treatment.[51] The Churg-Strauss syndrome has not been reported in children and the drug has been very well tolerated.

Zileuton is indicated for children 12 years of age and older for the treatment of chronic asthma. The recommended dose is 600 mg four times a day for the immediate-release preparation and two 600-mg tablets of the extended-release preparation twice daily. Zileuton should be taken on an empty stomach. Zileuton is contraindicated for children with liver disease or elevated LFTs and allergy to zileuton. The most serious side effect is elevated liver enzymes, so LFTs should be monitored on a regular basis. Headache is a side effect experienced by 25% of patients taking zileuton. Additional reported side effects include unspecified pain, dyspepsia, nausea, and abdominal pain. Patients taking theophylline, warfarin, and propranolol should be monitored closely and have their medications adjusted accordingly.[52]

Mast Cell Stabilizers

Cromolyn sodium and necromil sodium are pharmacologically similar **mast cell stabilizers**. Mast cells are found in many types of tissues and are similar to basophils, possessing granules containing histamine and heparin. Both cells release histamine upon binding with immunoglobulin E (IgE). Mast cells are present in most tissues, characteristically surrounding blood vessels and nerves, and are especially prominent near the boundaries between the outside world and the internal milieu, such as the skin, mucosa of the lungs, and digestive tract as well as the mouth, conjunctiva, and nose.[53]

Mast cell–stabilizing drugs (sodium cromolyn, nedocromil) block a calcium channel essential for pulmonary mast cell degranulation, stabilizing the cell and preventing release of histamine and related mediators. When activated, mast cells release the content of their granules, histamine and other autacoids. Histamine dilates postcapillary venules, activates the endothelium, and increases blood vessel permeability. This leads to local edema (swelling), warmth, redness, and the attraction of other inflammatory cells to the site of release. Cromolyn sodium and nedocromil inhibit neurally mediated bronchoconstriction through c-fiber sensory nerve stimulation in the airway, although both agents are devoid of bronchodilating activity. They have been shown to markedly reduce the production of leukotrienes. Mast cell stabilizers inhibit the early and late phase response to allergens.[53]

In 2010, the FDA announced that seven agents available for the treatment of asthma would be discontinued in the United States and Canada to come in line with legislation regarding propellants in pMDI and their negative effects on Earth's ozone layer. Both cromolyn and nedocromil inhalation production were discontinued, but these agents remain available in Europe. The use of these agents in the treatment of asthma as a controller has largely been replaced by leukotriene modifiers.[5] Mast cell stabilizers are no more or less effective than leukotriene modifiers or theophylline for persistent asthma.[5] Cromolyn in the form of a nasal spray is available for symptoms associated with seasonal and perennial allergic rhinitis.[54]

Anti-IgE Therapy

Immunoglobulin E (IgE) plays a central role in the pathogenesis of allergic diseases, including asthma, making this immunologic pathway an attractive target for therapeutic agents. Most asthmatic patients have elevated circulating IgE concentrations when levels are adjusted for age. The bridging of IgE molecules on mast cells and basophils by protein allergens results in the activation of these cells. Activation leads to release of preformed mediators such as histamine and increased synthesis of lipid mediators such as prostaglandins and cysteinyl leukotrienes, which in turn result in bronchoconstriction and plasma exudation. IgE thus plays a central role in the mechanism of immediate bronchoconstriction in allergic asthmatic patients after inhalation of allergen.[55]

Omalizumab is an IgG monoclonal antibody that inhibits IgE binding (i.e., **anti-immunoglobulin E**) to high-affinity IgE receptors on mast cells and basophils. Omalizumab is approved for the treatment of asthma that is not well controlled on high-dose ICS. Omalizumab requires subcutaneous administration. Patient weight and pretreatment serum IgE levels determine dose. IgE levels remain elevated up to 1 year following therapy and therefore cannot be used as a dosage guide. The drug is slowly absorbed from subcutaneous tissues and peaks between 3 and 14 days, with an elimination half-life of 17 to 22 days. Serum IgE levels return to baseline in about 3 weeks. It is indicated for patients who require oral corticosteroids or are on high-dose ICS with continued symptoms and high IgE levels.[56]

Omalizumab has a black box for anaphylaxis, including delayed-onset anaphylaxis following administration that usually occurs within 2 hours of administration but can be seen up to 24 hours and in some cases more than 1 year after initiation of regular therapy. Malignant neoplasms have been reported with use. Upper respiratory infections, sinusitis, pharyngitis, and viral infections have occurred in excess of 10% of patients during clinical trials.

Antimicrobial Therapy Via Nebulization

Some **antimicrobials** are formulated for nebulization and use in treatment of chronic infections or in patients with known colonization, such as that seen in patients with cystic fibrosis. Oropharyngeal colonization with gram-negative organisms is thought to be the precursor of pneumonia in patients with cystic fibrosis, patients with non–cystic fibrosis bronchiectasis, patients with chronic lung conditions, and in ventilator-supported patients. Once established in the oropharynx, organisms gain entry to the lower respiratory tract by several mechanisms, including gross aspiration of oropharyngeal secretions, microaspiration around the low-pressure cuff of the endotracheal tube, or along the artificial airway via biofilm colonization. Antimicrobial therapy can be pursued with two goals in mind: long-term therapy to prevent infection in the patient with colonization and treatment of active infection.

Aerosolized delivery of antimicrobial agents for management of pulmonary infections provides high local drug concentrations while minimizing systemic exposure. Knowledge on the pulmonary pharmacokinetics, efficacy, and safety of antimicrobial agents administered by this route is insufficient. Only a few drug products for treatment or prevention of infection are specifically formulated for this route of administration. No consensus regarding the safety, efficacy, and means with which to use aerosolized antimicrobials exists.

Two key concepts related to the direct delivery of antimicrobial agents to the respiratory tract are the characteristics of the aerosolized particles and the methods of aerosol delivery. The physical properties of antimicrobial formulations can have significant effects on drug delivery as well as patient tolerability. A primary determinant of deposition into the small airways and alveoli is the mean mass aerodynamic diameter (MMAD) of the aerosol particles. The MMAD is the average size of particles generated by a drug–nebulizer combination. Particles <1 μm are likely to be eliminated during exhalation, whereas particles >5 μm are deposited into the oropharynx and swallowed. Hence, the target of 1–5 μm is optimal for aerosol drug delivery. Given the fact that MMAD differs for each drug–nebulizer combination, these data are frequently unavailable for aerosolized antimicrobial therapies.[57]

Evidence supporting the use of nebulized antimicrobials for treatment of pulmonary infections differs depending on indication. Antibiotics administered by means of nebulization should not be routinely used for treatment of exacerbations in patients with cystic fibrosis, non–cystic fibrosis bronchiectasis, and community-acquired pneumonia. In regards to hospital-acquired pneumonia, which includes hospital ventilator-associated pneumonia (HAP), because of a lack of treatment options, adding aerosolized antibiotics to systemic antibiotics may be considered in the following situations: treatment of patients who are nonresponsive to systemic antibiotics or have recurrent HAP or treatment of patients with multiple-drug-resistant HAP. For isolates that are sensitive to aminoglycosides and colistin, using an aminoglycoside may be preferred because of fewer adverse events.

Evidence supporting the use of nebulized antimicrobials for prophylaxis of pulmonary infections in cystic fibrosis differs for agents. Nebulized tobramycin has strong evidence to support its use in patients with chronic *P aeruginosa* infection and moderate-to-severe lung disease, to improve lung function and reduce acute exacerbations, and is recommended for use in patients with early *P aeruginosa* lower airway colonization to prevent chronic infection and in patients who have colonization with *P aeruginosa* and are asymptomatic or have mild lung disease, to reduce exacerbations and antibiotic use.[57,58]

Aztreonam, a monobactam antibacterial, is approved for the indication to improve respiratory symptoms in cystic fibrosis patients with *P aeruginosa*. Inhaled colistin should not be used routinely for chronic suppression in patients with cystic fibrosis who have colonization with *P aeruginosa* (level B-II). There is insufficient evidence to support use of nebulized antibiotics other than tobramycin for chronic suppression of *Pseudomonas* species in patients with cystic fibrosis.[57]

The clinical impact of nebulized antibiotics, including tobramycin, on the prevention of non–cystic fibrosis bronchiectasis, particularly with regard to decreased hospitalizations and improvement in quality of life, has not been adequately demonstrated. A subset of patients may benefit, but the routine use of aerosolized antimicrobial agents for the prevention of exacerbations in patients with non–cystic fibrosis bronchiectasis is not recommended. Similarly, studies evaluating the role of aerosolized antibiotics in the prevention of HAP are inconclusive and the routine use of aerosolized antibiotics for prevention of HAP, including ventilator-associated pneumonia, is not recommended.[57,58]

Tobramycin

Tobramycin interferes with bacterial protein synthesis by binding 30S and 50S ribosomal subunits, resulting in defective bacterial cell membranes. Tobramycin is indicated for patients colonized with *Pseudomonas aeruginosa*. The nebulizer solution is available as a 300 mg solution (60 mg/mL) and the usual dose is 300 mg twice daily for 28 days followed by 28 days off.[60] It is also available as a dry powder inhaler (Podhaler; four capsules twice daily for 28 days). Tobramycin is a polar molecule that does not readily cross epithelial membranes. Following administration, tobramycin remains concentrated primarily in the airways. Bioavailability varies with nebulizer performance and airway pathology. Sputum concentrations have little correlation with serum concentrations. The average serum concentration of tobramycin 1 hour after inhalation of a single 300 mg dose was 0.95 μg/mL. There was no appreciable accumulation with continued therapy. After 20 weeks of therapy, the average serum tobramycin concentration 1 hour after dosing was 1.05 μg/mL. The elimination half-life of tobramycin from serum is approximately 2 hours after IV administration, and assuming tobramycin absorbed following inhalation behaves similarly to tobramycin following IV administration, systemically absorbed tobramycin is eliminated principally by glomerular filtration. Unabsorbed tobramycin is probably eliminated primarily in expectorated sputum. Bronchospasm can occur with inhalation of tobramycin. Renal toxicity and hearing loss have not been described with the use of inhaled tobramycin, but ringing of the ears and hoarseness have been described in patients.[60]

Colistimethate

Colistimethate is hydrolyzed to colistin and a toxic metabolite after mixture with a diluent. Colistin acts as a cationic detergent, which damages bacterial cytoplasmic membrane causing leakage of intracellular substances and cell death. Colistimethate has an unlabeled/investigational use via nebulization for the prevention of *P aeruginosa* respiratory tract infections in immunocompromised patients and as adjunct therapy in patients with cystic fibrosis and other seriously or chronically ill patients. The drug is only available as a parenteral formulation (150 mg vials). The dose via nebulizer is 75 to 150 mg dissolved to a final volume of 3 to 4 mL and administered twice daily.[61]

A concern with the use of inhaled colistimethate is the loss of efficacy for the intravenous formulation with continued aerosolized administration due to the development of resistance. Inhaled colistimethate can be associated with serious adverse effects; however, these are rare. Severe bronchospasm has been reported during administration. Potential nephrotoxicity has been reported in two of eight treated patients in one small clinical trial. Compared with tobramycin, colistimethate appears to have a higher rate and more severe presentation of pulmonary adverse events. It is important that the medication be compounded immediately before use to avoid potentially fatal pulmonary toxicity. The product should be used within 24 hours of mixing.[61,62]

Aztreonam

Aerosolized aztreonam exhibits activity against gram-negative aerobic pathogens, including *P aeruginosa*, by binding penicillin-binding proteins, leading to inhibition of bacterial cell wall synthesis and death. Aerosolized aztreonam is available as a nebulizer kit, which includes the nebulizer apparatus, drug, and diluent. Aerosolized aztreonam is dosed as 75 mg administered three times daily. Sputum aztreonam concentrations are variable between patients and show no accumulation with continued use. Serum concentrations are minimal as compared with intravenous administration, suggesting very little systemic absorption. Common side effects include cough, nasal congestion, wheezing, sore throat, fever, chest discomfort, stomach area (abdominal) pain, and vomiting. Bronchospasm has been described during administration. Severe adverse effects such as rash, swelling of the face, and throat tightness warrant discontinuation.[63]

β-lactams Antibiotics

Aerosolized β-lactams antibiotics (amoxicillin, carbenicillin, ceftazidime, and cefotaxime) were well tolerated in clinical trials. Conclusions on safety and tolerability cannot be ascertained, however, due to the small sample sizes that were primarily case series. Of importance, imipenem should not be aerosolized because of its questionable solubility and delivery to the lungs.[57]

Amphotericin B

Fungal infections are a major cause of morbidity and mortality in immunocompromised patients. Nebulized amphotericin B has been advocated for the prophylaxis of invasive aspergillosis in immunocompromised patients and in lung transplant patients, although these studies are limited by small population size. A recent study suggested that administration of nebulized liposomal amphotericin B as infrequently as every 2 weeks may be adequate to prevent aspergillosis. Amphotericin B binds to ergosterol, altering cell membrane permeability in susceptible fungi, causing leakage of cell components and death. In lung transplant patients, nebulized amphotericin deoxycholate demonstrated preferential deposition in the allografted lung and a greater accumulation in the distal zones of the bronchial tree. Dosage in clinical trials has varied depending on which of the four formulations was studied. All have been shown to achieve concentrations in excess of that needed for prophylaxis. Absorption into the blood is minimal as shown by serum concentrations as compared with intravenous administration. As with other anti-infectives, adverse effects associated with aerosolized amphotericin B are mostly pulmonary, including cough, chest tightness, and decline in pulmonary function tests. Tongue numbness, taste disturbances, nausea, and vomiting are other adverse effects.[59]

Pentamidine

Aerosolized pentamidine is a relatively well-tolerated alternative to oral agents for primary and secondary prophylaxis of *Pneumocystis jiroveci* pneumonia (PJP) in appropriate patients with HIV infection (level A-I) or patients with immunosuppressive conditions, such as recent hematopoietic stem cell transplant recipients. The mechanism of action is not well characterized, but there is some evidence that it may involve mitochondrial function. It interferes with RNA/DNA, phospholipids and protein synthesis through inhibition of phosphorylation in protozoa. Aerosolized pentamidine is indicated for prophylaxis but not for treatment of PJP.[57] Acute PJP can develop despite aerosolized pentamidine therapy, as excess failure compared to sulfamethoxazole/trimethoprim has been demonstrated. Pentamidine is dosed 300 mg usually once every 4 weeks. Pentamidine comes as a solution to be delivered via a Respigard nebulizer over 30 to 45 minutes. Pentamidine may induce bronchospasm.[64] Other side effects include light-headedness, fatigue, dizziness, fever, throat irritation, and conjunctivitis. Use precautions to minimize exposure to healthcare personnel due to Pregnancy Category C warnings. Despite this warning, pentamidine may be used in pregnant patients if they are unable to tolerate other options.

Ribavirin

Ribavirin is an antiviral agent for inhalation. It is only administered through a small-particle aerosol generator (SPAG). The recommendation is to administer continuous aerosolization for 6 to 8 hours per day for 3 to 7 days. Use of ribavirin has been shown to reduce ventilator and hospital days but has not been proven to be cost-effective because of its high price. Its effects on mortality, respiratory deterioration, and long-term pulmonary function are not clear.[65]

Secretion Modifiers

Acetylcysteine

Acetylcysteine (n-acetyl L-cysteine, NAC) is an adjunctive mucolytic therapy used for abnormal or viscid mucus secretions in patients with acute and chronic bronchopulmonary diseases. Such conditions include COPD, tuberculosis, bronchiectasis, pulmonary fibrosis, amyloidosis, and cystic fibrosis. It is also used postoperatively, as a diagnostic aid, and in tracheotomy care.[66] NAC exerts mucolytic action through its free sulfhydryl group that opens up the disulfide bonds in mucoproteins, thus lowering mucus viscosity. The inhalation solution is available as a 10% solution or a 20% solution. The 20% solution requires further dilution with normal saline. In adults, 3 to 4 mL of the 10% solution is administered 3 or 4 times daily. The onset of action is 5 to 10 minutes and duration is >1 hour. Patients should receive an aerosolized bronchodilator prior to administration. Though infrequent, bronchospasm has been reported to occur unpredictably in some patients and has caused this agent to largely fall out of favor. Other adverse effects for inhalational formulations of acetylcysteine include nausea, vomiting, stomatitis, fever, rhinorrhea, drowsiness, clamminess, and chest tightness.[55] Most important, the benefit of NAC to promote airway clearance is unproven.

Dornase Alfa

Dornase alfa is a recombinant human deoxyribonuclease used in the management of patients with cystic fibrosis (CF) to reduce the frequency of respiratory infections and to improve pulmonary function when used in conjunction with standard therapies. The presence of abundant, purulent airway secretions composed of highly polymerized DNA is the hallmark of CF. The source of this DNA is the nuclei of degenerating neutrophils found in infected lung tissue of patients with CF.[58,67] Dornase alfa selectively cleaves DNA, reducing mucus viscosity, improving airflow, and potentially decreasing the risk of infection. More importantly, dornase alfa may help to decrease the incidence or lengthen the time between respiratory exacerbations and improve quality of life and indirectly the cost of care in patients with mild to moderate CF.[58] Enzyme activity is evident within 15 minutes of aerosolization, but the duration of effect rapidly declines. Dornase alfa for nebulization is available as 1 mg/mL to 2.5 mL preservative-free solution and the drug should be stored in the refrigerator prior to administration. It is approved for use in ages >3 months to adults in a dose of 2.5 mg once daily. Some patients will benefit from twice-daily administration. Cough is the most frequent adverse effect seen in up to 45% of patients. Fever, pharyngitis, rhinitis, and dyspnea are frequent in patients with an FEV_1 <40%. Other less frequent adverse effects are chest pain, rash, voice alteration, and dyspepsia.

Antihistamines

Antihistamines are competitive antagonists to histamine at the H1 receptors, binding without activating them. They may alter components of the inflammatory response such as histamine release, generation of adhesion molecules, and the influx of inflammatory cells. Antihistamines have anticholinergic properties that are responsible for the drying effect, reducing nasal, salivary, and lacrimal gland hypersecretion. Drowsiness is usually the chief complaint of patients who take antihistamines. The anticholinergic effects can cause dry mouth, difficulty in urination, and constipation. The elderly may have a predisposition to these side effects. Antihistamines are most effective when taken in anticipation of exposure to an allergen.[43]

Anticholinergic Agents

Anticholinergic agents block the effects of acetylcholine at parasympathetic sites in smooth muscle, salivary glands, and the CNS. Anticholinergic agents are used to inhibit salivation and excessive secretions of the respiratory tract preoperatively and as adjunctive therapy to control airway secretions in respiratory illness. The side effect profiles of these agents when used for drying secretions have limited the use. In respiratory illness, difficulty in mobilizing secretions may predispose to infection. Glycopyrrolate, scopolamine, and atropine are the most common agents used. Glycopyrrolate and atropine are available as both oral and parenteral formulations. In addition to dry mouth, difficulty in urination, and constipation, cardiovascular effects of tachycardia and other arrhythmias can be of concern. CNS adverse effects include confusion, dizziness, drowsiness, and nervousness. Seizures have been described with toxic concentrations.[33]

Neuromuscular Blocking Agents

The first task in managing acutely unstable patients is to secure an airway through intubation. This is achieved through rapid sequence intubation (RSI) using **sedative** agents and paralytic agents. The choice of pharmacologic agents for sedation during intubation will depend on the pharmacokinetic and pharmacodynamic characteristics of the different agents and concomitant clinical conditions. RSI incorporates a rapid-acting sedative administered almost simultaneously with a paralytic agent. The patient is rendered unconscious and flaccid to allow for optimal conditions for placement of the endotracheal tube.[68]

The action of acetylcholine is elicited when two molecules bind to the nicotinic receptor, causing an end-plate potential in the muscle. This action potential causes local excitation and propagation of the impulse throughout the muscle, ultimately causing muscle contraction.[69] Neuromuscular blockers (NMBs) are used for rapid sequence intubation (RSI) and to facilitate mechanical ventilation and prevent uncontrolled muscle contractions and patient interference with ventilator strategies (**Table 55-5**). The latter use is employed when this goal cannot be achieved with adequate sedation.

Succinylcholine, a depolarizing **neuromuscular blocking agent**, acts to depolarize the membrane and open sodium channels. Because succinylcholine is fairly resistant to acetylcholinesterase and not metabolized locally at the neuromuscular junction, it persists longer than acetylcholine and results in longer depolarization and a brief initial period of fasciculation. This is followed by a block in neurotransmission and the onset of flaccid

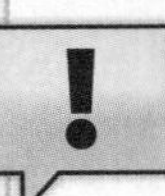

Respiratory Recap

Drugs Used for Airway Management

- Neuromuscular blocking agents
- Induction agents
- Benzodiazepines
- Opiates
- Ketamine
- Propofol
- Dexmedetomidine

TABLE 55-5
Pharmacokinetics of Neuromuscular Blockers

Agent	Structure	Onset (min)	Duration (min)	Half-life (min)
Succinylcholine	Acetylcholine-like	1–1.5	5–10	Unknown
Mivacurium	Benzylisoquinolinium	2–4	12–18	2
Atracurium	Benzylisoquinolinium	2–4	30–40	20
Cisatracurium	Benzylisoquinolinium	2–5	30–70	20–30
Vecuronium	Steroid-based	2–4	20–60	60–130
Rocuronium	Steroid-based	1–2	30–67	80–100
Metocurine	Benzylisoquinolinium	1–4	35–90	280
Pancuronium	Steroid-based	4–6	120–180	110–140
Doxacurium	Benzylisoquinolinium	4–6	90–120	100 (+/–154)
Pipecuronium	Steroid-based	2–4	0–100	137 (+/–168)

Reproduced from McManus MC. Neuromuscular blockers in surgery and intensive care, part 2. *Am J Health-Syst Pharm.* 2001;58:2381–2399.

paralysis, both of which are secondary to the inability of acetylcholine to initiate a propagating action potential on an already depolarized end plate.[70]

Succinylcholine is used for RSI due to its quick onset of action and short duration of effect. Recommended doses are 1 to 1.5 mg/kg as an IV push to produce complete muscle relaxation in 30 to 60 seconds with a duration that lasts 4 to 5 minutes. Succinylcholine is degraded by butyrylcholinesterase, a plasma cholinesterase. This hydrolysis by butyrylcholinesterase is much slower than that of acetylcholine by acetylcholinesterase.[70] Declines in renal and hepatic function do not necessitate dose reductions. Acid–base disorders may predispose to potentiating or antagonizing the effects of succinylcholine. Succinylcholine should be used with caution in patients with a personal or familial history of malignant hyperthermia, a life-threatening complication.

Other adverse effects include bradycardia mediated through increased vagal tone. The risk increases if a second dose is necessary. Ventricular fibrillation has also been reported. Due to the depolarization of the muscle, increases in serum potassium can occur acutely by as much as 0.5 to 1.0 mmol/dL. It should be used with caution in patients at risk of hyperkalemia, such as those in the acute phase of injury from major burns, multiple trauma, or extensive denervation of skeletal muscle. Succinylcholine can increase intragastric pressure, increasing the risk of vomiting and aspiration during intubation. Histamine release has been described with succinylcholine and can stimulate bronchospasm. Succinylcholine has the potential for many drug interactions.[69]

Nondepolarizing NMBs, or competitive NMBs, combine with the nicotinic receptors and block the action of acetylcholine. They reduce the frequency of channel-opening events but do not affect the magnitude of conductance or the duration of opening of a single channel. Neuromuscular blocking agents are used in a large but highly variable proportion of patients with ARDS. Current guidelines indicate that neuromuscular blocking agents are appropriate for facilitating mechanical ventilation when sedation alone is inadequate, most notably in patients with severe gas-exchange impairments.[71]

There are multiple nondepolarizing NMBs available with rapid onset of action that make them suitable for rapid sequence intubation. They differ from succinylcholine in mechanism of action, duration of effect, metabolism and elimination, and side effect profiles. For patients being intubated, a rapid onset makes the agent most suitable and duration is less important as patients' respiratory function will be managed by mechanical ventilation. The drugs' elimination profile may be the most important feature in choice of agent. Rocuronium has an onset of action that is two to three times faster than vecuronium but with a similar duration of action. Cisatracurium and atracurium are eliminated by ester hydrolysis and Hofmann elimination in the plasma and are good choices for patients with multiple-organ dysfunction syndrome. Doxacurium and pipecuronium have a long duration of action, which renders these agents less useful to facilitate intubation.[69]

For management of mechanical ventilation, prolonged infusions of NMBs have been used. The nondepolarizing agents are distinguished by the elimination profile to avoid accumulation and prolonged muscle paralysis when the agents are stopped. As mentioned, cisatracurium and atracurium are eliminated by ester hydrolysis and Hofmann elimination. These agents are metabolized to an active but potentially toxic metabolite, laudanosine. In patients with renal failure, prolonged use of atracurium has been associated with rare reports of seizure activity. Vecuronium and rocuronium have bimodal elimination via renal and biliary routes of elimination. Most of the other agents are less suitable for continuous infusion due to a longer half-life, resulting in prolonged duration of paralysis when discontinued.[70]

A concern with prolonged paralysis is a disuse atrophy or muscle weakness ascribed to the adversely affected functions of peripheral nerves, neuromuscular junctions, and skeletal muscles in the critically ill that may interfere with the ability to wean from the ventilator. An acute necrotizing myopathy has been associated with NMB use. The pathophysiology is not well known. Critical illness myopathy is strongly associated with sepsis and multiple-organ dysfunction syndrome, in which muscle is injured directly by toxins. Acute necrotizing myopathy may relate to the pathology induced by the combined use of corticosteroids and NMBs. Most clinicians will make strong efforts to discontinue NMBs as soon as possible through maximizing sedation to achieve ventilator synchrony.[69,70]

Sedatives

Etomidate

Etomidate is an ultra-short-acting nonbarbiturate sedative-hypnotic agent that is frequently used for RSI. Etomidate acts directly on the gamma amino butyric acid (GABA) receptor complex, blocking neuroexcitation and producing anesthesia. It has no analgesic properties. When given as an intravenous push over 30 to 60 seconds, etomidate has a rapid onset within 30 to 60 seconds, a peak effect in 1 minute, and a short duration of action of 3 to 5 minutes. Etomidate dosing is weight based; recommended doses are 0.2 to 0.6 mg/kg. Etomidate is metabolized in the liver and by plasma esterases.[72,73]

Etomidate inhibits 11-β-hydroxylase, an enzyme important in adrenal steroid production. Induction doses block the stress-induced increase in adrenal cortisol production for 4 to 6 hours and up to 24 hours in the elderly and debilitated patients.[73] Etomidate is associated with hemodynamic stability, making it attractive for use in hypotensive patients or those with intracranial pathology, when hypotension must be avoided. The drug has little effect on airway resistance and may be used in patients with bronchospasm. Etomidate decreases cerebral metabolic oxygen demand while preserving cerebral perfusion pressure. Aside from the adrenal effects, etomidate has exhibited some regional cerebral excitation and myoclonus misidentified as seizure activity. Concomitant use of paralytic agents makes these effects of no clinical significance. In patients with sepsis, some clinicians recommend the use of corticosteroids for 24 hours after a dose of etomidate.[74] Etomidate should not be used as an infusion or in repeated bolus doses for maintenance of sedation after intubation.

Benzodiazepines

Benzodiazepines act on receptors for drugs found on the GABA receptor complex, causing sedation and amnesia. Midazolam is a water-soluble benzodiazepine most often used for RSI. Midazolam provides anticonvulsant effects, making it effective in patients with status epilepticus. It possesses no analgesic, antidepressant, or antipsychotic properties. The induction dose of 0.1 to 0.3 mg/kg is given as an intravenous push. Midazolam has a rapid onset of action in 1 to 3 minutes with duration of 15 to 30 minutes, but onset and duration can be variable, particularly in elderly and debilitated patients. Midazolam is extensively metabolized via the hepatic cytochrome p4503A4. The half-life is 1 to 4 hours and midazolam has an active metabolite that is renally eliminated. Midazolam causes a modest drop in mean arterial blood pressure of 10% to 25% and should be avoided for RSI in hypotensive patients or those with shock.[75]

Midazolam can be used as an infusion for long-term sedation. Safe and effective doses of 0.05 mg/kg to 0.4 mg/kg per hour IV have been used in intubated critically ill patients, including neonates and children. Dosing should be titrated to an endpoint of adequate sedation, preferably using a sedation scale. Tachyphylaxis and tolerance have been described with long-term use. Midazolam has an active metabolite that accumulates in patients with renal failure, so daily assessment of dosage should be undertaken to prevent overaccumulation.[76]

Benzodiazepines have been associated with paradoxical reactions, including hyperactive and combative behavior, particularly in adolescent/pediatric or psychiatric patients. More recently, drugs with primary actions on GABA receptors have been reported to be associated with the development of delirium. Studies have shown that the benzodiazepines, including midazolam and lorazepam, are more often associated with the development of delirium than propofol or dexmedetomnidine.[77] This remains a controversial area, but strategies to reduce benzodiazepine use do support intermittent dosing and frequent awakening to avoid accumulations and allow for improved evaluation.

Lorazepam and diazepam can be used for long-term sedation following intubation but are not recommended for RSI. Both require propylene glycol as a diluent, and there are reports of propylene glycol toxicity associated with long-term infusions or frequently scheduled, high-dose intermittent IV push doses. In addition, lorazepam has a much longer half-life than midazolam. Diazepam has active metabolites that can accumulate and contribute to oversedation.

Opioids

Opioids (morphine, hydromorphone, fentanyl, remifentanyl) remain important for analgesic therapy in critically ill patients. This class of agents provides sedative properties and facilitates mechanical ventilation due to potent respiratory depressant effects. All opioids depress respiratory drive in a dose-dependent manner and this effect increases when given in combination with benzodiazepines. Although advantageous for ventilator synchrony, respiratory depression can be problematic if accumulation occurs during the period leading up to extubation.[78]

Opiates exhibit their effect by stimulating the mu, delta, and kappa receptors, which are widely distributed in the brain and spinal cord and throughout peripheral tissues. Opioids are divided into three primary classes based on structure: (1) morphine-like agents (including morphine and hydromorphone); (2) meperidine-like agents (e.g., meperidine, fentanyl, remifentanil, alfentanil, and sufentanil); and (3) diphenylheptanes (including methadone). The use of meperidine should be avoided due to its low potency, propensity to cause nausea and vomiting, and metabolism to normeperidine, which can accumulate in renal insufficiency and cascade into neuroexcitatory effects, including seizures. Methadone has effects at NMDA receptors and may be useful for patients who develop opioid tolerance or neuropathic pain.[79]

Remifentanil, alfentanil, and sufentanil are derivatives of fentanyl with some pharmacokinetic differences. For alfentanil, neonates and infants will differ in elimination half-life. All these agents have rapid onset, short duration of clinical effect, and are less often associated with accumulation and prolonged respiratory depression. When compared with fentanyl in single-dose studies, they may allow for quicker time to extubation.[80] In the ICU with continuous infusion, however, this benefit is not often clinically relevant due to spontaneous awakening trials and spontaneous breathing trials. The cost of these fentanyl derivatives can be prohibitive when used as long-term continuous infusions for ventilator synchrony.

Morphine, hydromorphone (dilaudid), and fentanyl are the most commonly used opioid in the management of pain in the ICU. Pharmacokinetic information on opioids comes primarily from single-dose studies or from intermittent dose studies. The half-life and the duration of response are not reliable for analgesic efficacy or effects on ventilator drive. Information relative to continuous infusions is mostly lacking. Individual pharmacodynamic response is most relative to doses needed for ventilator synchrony. Intravenous infusions are preferred in critically ill ventilated patients. Daily awakening trials and spontaneous breathing trials have become practice to assist in the assessment of readiness for extubation and to assist in identifying patients for whom accumulation of opioids may be occurring.

Fentanyl has an almost immediate onset of action as compared with morphine and hydromorphone, which take about 5 minutes. Most patients will receive a bolus dose and then be started on a continuous infusion. Histamine release is not associated with fentanyl bolus dosing, which is a concern when bolus doses of morphine and hydromorphone are administered. Because histamine release can cause hypotension, fentanyl is often preferred in patients with labile blood pressure. Dose ranges and half-life of opioids can be wide, often requiring bolus doses to achieve sedation and ventilator synchrony as the continuous infusion is titrated to effect (**Table 55-6**).

TABLE 55-6
Infusion Rates for Opioids in Critical Care

Drug	Half-life (min)	Dose (μg/kg/h)	Onset (min)
Morphine	100–180	50–100	5–10
Fentanyl	185	1–5	<1
Remifentanil	3–20	30–60	<1
Hydromorphone	120–180	7–15	5–10
Alfentanil	90 (adults)	30–60	<1
Sufentanil	160–210	0.3–1	<1

Based on references 78, 79.

Following metabolism in the liver, opioids are eliminated renally. Morphine is metabolized via glucuronidation to an inactive (morphine-3-gluconidate) and active metabolite (morphine-6-glucuronidate) with significant analgesic activity. The morphine-6-glucuronidate metabolite can accumulate in renal failure. Fentanyl does not have active metabolites, but the parent compound may accumulate in renal failure. Hydromorphone is also metabolized to hydromorphone-3-glucuronidate that is inactive. Hydromorphone will not accumulate in renal failure and may be preferred over fentanyl for this reason. Fentanyl has a high extraction ratio by the liver. Concerns for accumulation in patients with liver failure need consideration. Fentanyl is a substrate of cyp3A4 and has the potential to interact with inhibitors of this liver enzyme.[79]

Tolerance is a concern in patients who are exposed to opioids for prolonged periods of time. Continuous infusions may need to be increased in patients requiring prolonged sedation with opioids. Increased pain and other factors interfere with assessment of tolerance. Adverse effects are dose related. Nonintubated patients often complain of nausea and vomiting. Fentanyl given in larger bolus doses has been associated with muscle rigidity and spasm. Hypotension in patients with hemodynamic instability is seen as opioids affect sympathetic tone. Volume-depleted patients may be at higher risk. As previously mentioned, morphine is associated with histamine release, which produces more hypotension, urticaria, flushing, bronchospasm, and itching. QTc prolongation is associated with methadone.

Gastric motility and ileus are common with opioid use. Bowel regimens are recommended for prevention using prokinetic agents and stimulant laxatives. Methylnaltrexone, an opioid antagonist with peripheral effects, only is approved for use in patients with opioid-induced constipation. Oral naloxone, an IV antagonist for reversal of respiratory depression, has been used for constipation but is not recommended due to concerns for reversing the central analgesic and sedative opioid effects as well as limited studies on efficacy for constipation. Opioid-induced urinary retention is rarely seen.

Ketamine

Ketamine is characterized as a unique dissociative anesthetic agent that provides analgesia, amnestic effects, and sedation. It produces a cataleptic-like state in which patients feel disassociated from their surrounding environment. Ketamine acts on a number of receptors in the central nervous system.[81] The action of ketamine on the NMDA receptor of the GABA receptor complex causes neuroinhibition and anesthesia. By stimulating the catecholamine receptors, it causes a release of catecholamines and increases heart rate, contractility, mean arterial pressure, and cerebral blood flow. It excites opioid receptors, producing analgesia. Ketamine also reduces production of vascular nitric oxide, thereby diminishing vasodilatory effects and inhibiting nicotinic acetylcholine receptors.

Given intravenously in doses of 1 to 2 mg/kg, ketamine has a time to effect of 45 to 60 seconds and duration of action of 10 to 20 minutes. Ketamine is a substrate for the liver cytochrome enzymes CYP2B6, 2C9, and 3A4. The drug has active metabolites with one-third to one-fifth less activity. Ketamine can be given orally, but this route is not used for RSI.

Ketamine preserves respiratory drive, allowing for awake intubations in patients who are topically anesthetized but not paralyzed due to concerns about a difficult airway. The sympathetic stimulation caused by ketamine provides hemodynamic stability, making it an attractive agent for hypotensive and hemodynamically unstable patients. This catecholamine effect theoretically provides bronchodilatory effects and ketamine may be preferred in asthmatics for this reason. A reemergence phenomenon, in which patients experience disturbing dreams, has been described with ketamine-induced anesthesia. This has limited the use of the drug for procedural sedation or elective anesthesia in adult patients. Treatment with a benzodiazepine is reported to reduce emergence phenomenon.[81] Ketamine's effects to increase cerebral blood flow may be beneficial in patients with a neurologic injury. However, this is controversial because of reports of ketamine increasing intracerebral pressure secondary to sympathetic stimulation.[81]

Propofol

Propofol is a highly lipid-soluble alkyl-phenolic compound with intravenous general anesthetic properties. It is unrelated to any of the currently used barbiturates, opioids, benzodiazepines, and other intravenous agents. Propofol has been proposed to have several mechanisms of action. It acts at the GABA-A receptor, thereby slowing the channel-closing time, and also may serve as a sodium channel blocker. The endocannabinoid system has also been reported to contribute to its anesthetic action. Propofol causes prominent reduction in the brain's information integration capacity. Sedation occurs through direct suppression of brain activity, while amnesia appears to result from interference with long-term memory creation.[75,82]

Induction doses of 1.5 to 3 mg/kg IV can be used, with a time to effect of approximately 15 to 45 seconds and duration of action of 3 to 10 minutes. Propofol is highly protein bound. Propofol has a large volume of distribution and may accumulate in adipose tissue. The elimination half-life is biphasic, initially 40 minutes, then a terminal half-life of 4 to 7 hours due to redistribution to fat and other tissues. With continued infusion (>10 days), the terminal half-life can be up to 1 to 3 days. The duration of effect is much shorter than its half-life. Propofol is primarily metabolized in the liver through conjugation and excreted in the urine as inactive metabolites. Dosage must be individualized based on total body weight and titrated to clinical effect.

Propofol reduces airways resistance and can be a useful induction agent for patients with bronchospasm undergoing RSI. Because of its neuroinhibitory effects, propofol is a good induction agent for patients with intracranial pathology, provided they are hemodynamically stable. A decrease in mean arterial pressure caused by propofol can reduce cerebral perfusion pressure, thereby exacerbating a neurologic injury. Propofol suppresses sympathetic activity, has negative inotropic effects, and causes peripheral vasodilation and reductions in mean arterial pressures. Propofol does not provide analgesia.[82]

Propofol has respiratory depression effects, which limits its use as a sedative agent in nonintubated patients. Propofol is also used to sedate individuals receiving mechanical ventilation who are not undergoing surgery, such as those in the ICU. Doses for ICU sedation are 0.3 mg/kg/h to 3 mg/kg/h, but higher doses may be needed. Due to its high lipophilicity, actual body weight should be considered when initiating dosing. In critically ill patients, propofol has been found to be superior to lorazepam in effectiveness for sedation. The predictable onset and offset of sedation allows for keeping a patient at a desired sedation level and daily awakening and spontaneous breathing trials to assess if patients are ready for extubation.

Long-term infusions for sedation have been associated with adverse events. Elevation in triglycerides is an expected side effect with high-dose and long-term infusion due to the lipid vehicle (10% fat emulsion). It should be used with caution in patients with preexisting pancreatitis. Propofol-related infusion syndrome is a rare but serious side effect with a high mortality.

This syndrome is characterized by dysrhythmias (bradycardia or tachycardia), heart failure, hyperkalemia, lipemia, metabolic acidosis, and rhabdomyolysis or myoglobulinuria with subsequent renal failure. Risk factors have been identified, including doses >5 mg/kg/h, poor oxygen delivery, sepsis, and cerebral injury. The onset can be rapid, occurring within 4 days of initiation of therapy.[83]

Dexmedetomidine

Dexmedetomidine, a selective α_2-adrenergic agonist, is used for sedation in critical care. The sedative and anesthetic properties are thought to be due to activation of G proteins by α_{2a}-adrenoceptors in the brain stem, resulting in inhibition of norepinephrine release. Peripheral α_{2b}-receptors are activated at high doses or with rapid IV administration. Dexmedetomidine's pharmacokinetic and pharmacodynamic characteristics preclude its use for rapid sequence intubation as the onset of effect is delayed after IV administration, occurring 5 to 10 minutes after a bolus infusion.

Intravenous infusion of dexmedetomidine is commonly initiated with a 1 µg/kg loading dose, administered over 10 minutes, followed by a maintenance infusion of 0.2 to 1.0 µg/kg/h. There may be great individual variability in the hemodynamic effects (especially on heart rate and blood pressure) as well as the sedative effects of this drug. The dose is adjusted to achieve desired sedation levels. As mentioned, onset following a bolus loading dose is 5 to 10 minutes. The loading dose may not be needed for ICU sedation when transitioning from another agent and may be responsible for the higher incidence of bradycardia seen in clinical trials as compared to other sedative agents. Peak effect is seen in 5 to 30 minutes and titration of dose can be made every 20 to 30 minutes. The duration of effect is variable and dose dependent. The elimination half-life is approximately 6 minutes with a terminal half-life of about 2 hours. The duration of effect when infusions are discontinued can vary depending on the dose and are usually 60 to 20 minutes. Dexmedetomidine is metabolized via hepatic N-glucuronidation and N-methylation as well as through CYP2A6 enzymes. Metabolites are inactive and renally eliminated.[84,85]

Dexmedetomidine is primarily used in ICU patients for continuous sedation of intubated and nonintubated patients. It is relatively unusual in its ability to provide sedation without causing respiratory depression. Limiting its usefulness is the caution that concerns around bolus doses exist due to peripheral α_2-receptor stimulation with resulting hypotension and bradycardia. Dexmedetomidine appears to shorten mechanical ventilation compared with midazolam but not compared with propofol. Time to extubation is reduced compared with both midazolam and propofol.

Dexmedetomidine enhances patients' ability to communicate pain to the nursing staff, possibly contributing to the earlier extubation. Accordingly, dexmedetomidine may provide clinically relevant benefits compared with standard sedation, even when measures to reduce the risks of oversedation are implemented. The better arousability and ability to communicate pain should allow more appropriate use of opioids and facilitate earlier mobilization and functional recovery. Delirium may be less frequently observed with dexmedetomidine as compared with lorazepam and midazolam.[77]

Dexmedetomidine should be used with caution in patients with heart block or severe ventricular dysfunction, hypovolemia, chronic hypertension and in the elderly. Transient hypertension has been observed in association with the bolus dose administration and is associated with the initial peripheral vasoconstriction effects of dexmedetomidine. When withdrawn abruptly in patients who have received it for more than 24 hours, withdrawal symptoms similar to clonidine withdrawal may result, such as hypertension, nervousness, agitation, and headache.[86]

Agents for the Treatment of Pulmonary Arterial Hypertension

Pulmonary arterial hypertension (PAH) is a disease of the small pulmonary arteries characterized by vascular cell proliferation, aberrant remodeling, and thrombosis in situ. The syndrome results from restricted flow through the pulmonary arterial circulation, resulting in increased pulmonary vascular resistance and leading to right heart failure. Improved understanding of the disease pathways has led to therapeutic strategies with targeted drug therapy. Three targets of drug therapy are described below. The World Health Organization has five classifications for pulmonary hypertension. Group I PAH patients have been shown to respond to drug therapies targeting these pathways.[87,88]

Prostacyclin and thromboxane A_2 have been implicated due to an imbalance in these two prostanoids. Prostacyclin is a potent vasodilator, inhibits platelet activation, and has antiproliferative properties. Thromboxane A_2 is a potent vasoconstrictor and promotes proliferation and platelet activation. In PAH there is a shift toward thromboxane A_2, favoring thrombosis, proliferation, and vasoconstriction. Prostacyclin synthase is decreased in the small and medium-sized pulmonary arteries.[87]

Endothelin-1 (ET-1) is a potent vasoconstrictor and stimulates pulmonary artery smooth muscle cell proliferation. Plasma levels of ET-1 are elevated in PAH. In addition, clearance of ET-1 in the pulmonary vasculature is reduced.[87]

Nitric oxide (NO) is a vasodilator and inhibitor of platelet activation and vascular smooth muscle cell

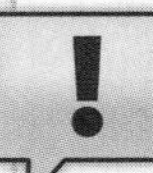

Respiratory Recap

Agents for the Treatment of Pulmonary Arterial Hypertension

- Inhaled nitric oxide
- Prostaglandins (epoprostenol, trepostinil, and iloprost)
- Endothelin (ET) receptor antagonists (bosentan, ambrisentan, macitentan)
- Phosphodiesterase-5 (PDE5) inhibitors (sildenafil, tadalafil)

proliferation. Nitric oxide synthase (NOS) is responsible for NO synthesis and one of the isoenzymes of NOS is decreased in endothelial cells of patients with PAH. Effects of NO are mediated by cyclic 3′,5′-guanosine monophosphate (cGMP) that is rapidly inactivated by the isoenzyme phosphodiesterase-5 (PDE-5) that is found in large amounts in the lung.[87] Dosages of 5 to 80 parts per million usually are targeted. Toxicities are few but include methemoglobinemia.

Prostaglandins (Epoprostenol, Treprostinil, and Iloprost)

Epoprostenol is administered via intravenous continuous infusion. This agent requires patients to learn techniques for sterile preparation and operation of ambulatory infusion pumps. IV epoprostenol is usually started in the hospital at a dose of 2 ng/kg/min and slowly titrated up based on symptoms of PAH and side effects. During initiation of therapy, the dose is titrated to the highest tolerated dose and then reduced by 2 ng/kg/min for continued therapy. Common side effects are headache, jaw pain, flushing, nausea, skin rash, and musculoskeletal pain. Dosing is highly individualized. Tachyphylaxis is seen, requiring most patients to need dose adjustment to higher doses with continued therapy.

Epoprostenol is rapidly hydrolyzed subject to enzymatic degradation. The half-life is approximately 6 minutes. Epoprostenol is unstable when stored or kept at room temperature for prolonged times. The specific brand should be referenced for stability data. Patients require teaching on proper care. Use is limited to patients seen at centers with considerable experience and appropriate follow-up. Infusion interruptions can be life threatening due to increases in pulmonary pressures resulting in pulmonary edema and symptoms of right heart failure. Infections to central catheters are of major concern.[88] Patients and clinicians caring for PAH patients managed with epoprostenol should be familiar with signs and symptoms of drug toxicity and loss of efficacy.

Treprostinil is a stable prostanoid with an elimination half-life of about 4.5 hours. Treprostinil can be administered as a subcutaneous or intravenous infusion. The dose of treprostinil as compared to epoprostenol for comparable effects will usually result in more than twice the dose. Intravenous treprostinil has a side effect profile similar to epoprostenol. The longer half-life allows for short interruptions in therapy without major concern for decompensation. Issues with stability and administration are similar to epoprostenol as well as infection concerns.[88]

Treprostinil is available as a nebulized solution delivered via a specialized nebulizer system. Immediate access to a backup inhalation device is essential to prevent treatment interruptions. The dose is 18 μg (delivered as 3 inhalations) every 4 hours for 4 doses daily. If tolerated, the dose can be increased by 3 inhalations at every 1- or 2-week interval. The maximum dose is 54 μg four times daily.[88]

Iloprost is prostacyclin I-2 delivered by an aerosol device six to nine times daily while the patient is awake. The dose is initiated at 2.5 μg and increased as tolerated to 5 μg/dose for a maximum of 45 μg daily. Long-term benefits in terms of improved outcomes are conflicting. Side effects include cough, headache, jaw pain, and flushing.[89]

Endothelin Receptor Antagonists (Bosentan, Ambrisentan, and Macitentan)

Bosentan was the first endothelin (ET) antagonist introduced for the treatment of PAH. Endothelin binds to ET_A and ET_B receptors and acts to help regulate vascular tone in the pulmonary vasculature. Bosentan blocks ET receptors on vascular endothelium and smooth muscle, preventing the vasoconstriction and proliferation stimulated by these receptors. ET may be overexpressed in PAH.[87,90]

Bosentan is a dual ET_A/ET_B receptor antagonist and is available as 62.5 mg and 125 mg tablets. The usual adult dose is 62.5 mg twice daily for 4 weeks and then increased to 125 mg twice daily. The bosentan dose may need to be reduced due to liver toxicity. Bosentan has an unlabeled indication in children ages 12 years or younger and the dose is weight based. Ambrisentan is a once-daily oral ET receptor antagonist with a 4000-fold selectivity for the ET_A receptor over the ET_B receptor. Ambrisentan does not appear to have the risk of hepatotoxicity seen with bosentan.[91] Macitentan is a newer agent recently approved by the FDA with 50-fold selectivity for ET_A receptors over ET_B receptors and a slow dissociation from receptors. Like ambrisentan, hepatotoxicity does not appear to be a problem.

Side effects common to the ET receptor antagonists include low red blood cell count (anemia), common cold-like symptoms (nasopharyngitis), sore throat, bronchitis, headache, flu, and urinary tract infection. These agents are all Pregnancy Category X and carry a REMS program associated with their dispensing.

Drug interactions are common as these agents are substrates for the cyp3A4 and cyp2C19 isoenzymes. In addition, interactions with p-glycoproteins have been described.

Phosphodiesterase-5 Inhibitors (Sildenafil, Tadalafil)

Phosphodiesterase-5 (PDE5) inhibitors work via the NO pathway. The release of NO from the endothelium stimulates an increase in intracellular cGMP, resulting in vasodilation. PDE5 is the predominant isoenzyme in the pulmonary vasculature responsible for the degradation of cGMP. Inhibition of PDE5 prolongs the effects of this vasodilating cyclic nucleotide.[92]

Sildenafil has an onset of action of approximately 30 minutes and duration of about 4 hours. Sildenafil is a major substrate for cyp3A4 and cyp2C9 as well as undergoing N-demethylation to an active metabolite in the liver. The elimination half-life is 4 hours and is prolonged in the elderly and in patients with severe renal failure and reduced clearance of the active metabolite. Due to the multiple enzymatic pathways, many drugs can interact with sildenafil.[92]

Sildenafil is dosed three times daily and was the first PDE5 inhibitor approved for PAH. Sildenafil can be initiated with 20 mg and quickly titrated to the maximum tolerated dose, with the usual maximum being 80 mg three times daily. Sildenafil has been shown to increase the 6-minute walk test, reduce pulmonary artery pressures, and improve symptoms of PAH. The major dose-limiting side effect is hypotension. Another side effect is epistaxis.

Tadalafil is a long-acting PDE5 antagonist. It has an onset of action of 1 hour, similar to sildenafil. The peak effect on pulmonary vasculature is seen in 75 to 120 minutes and the duration of effect can last for 36 hours. The elimination half-life is 15 to 17.5 hours, longer in patients not receiving bosentan. Tadalafil is metabolized via cyp3A4 to inactive metabolites and is primarily eliminated via feces (61%), with 36% found in urine as the metabolite.[92]

Tadalafil starting doses in patients with a creatinine clearance of >31 mL/min is 20 mg daily and may be increased to 40 mg dosed once daily based on tolerability. For patients with a creatinine clearance less than 30 mL/min, tadalafil should be avoided due to increased exposure and limited clinical experience. Tadalafil will interact with inhibitors and inducers of the cyp3A4 enzyme. Potential for drug interactions should be identified with initiation of therapy or as agents are added to the regimen. Common side effects are headache, flushing dyspepsia, nausea, and myalgia. Epistaxis has been reported in fewer than 2% of patients in clinical trials.

Combination therapy with two or more targeted therapies for PAH is common practice. Targeting additional pathogenic pathways or augmenting a parallel pathway may result in improved symptom management and disease control. Most new agents are studied in patients maintained on a background treatment. Research is needed to determine optimal combination therapies. Some limiting factors may include side effects, drug interactions, and cost justification for perceived benefit.[88]

Key Points

- ▶ Routes for administering medications include inhalation, oral, and parenteral.
- ▶ The inhalational route treats the lungs directly, incurring fewer systemic effects.
- ▶ Pharmacokinetics describes how the body handles a drug as influenced by absorption, bioavailability, distribution, volume of distribution, clearance, and half-life.
- ▶ Pharmacodynamics describes the effect of a medication on the body as determined by potency and receptor sites.
- ▶ Categories of therapeutic agents to treat the lungs include β-agonists, anticholinergics, corticosteroids, methylxanthines, magnesium, leukotriene inhibitors, anti-IgE, antimicrobials, and secretion modifiers.
- ▶ Drugs used in airway and ventilator management include neuromuscular blocking agents, induction agents, benzodiazepines, opiates, propofol, ketamine, and dexmedetomidine.
- ▶ Drugs used in the treatment of pulmonary arterial hypertension include inhaled nitric oxide, prostaglandins, endothelin receptor antagonists, and phosphodiesterase-5 inhibitors.

References

1. Wilkinson GR. Pharmacokinetics: the dynamics of drug absorption, distribution, and elimination. In: *Goodman and Gilman's the Pharmacological Basis of Therapeutics*. 10th ed. New York: McGraw-Hill; 2001.
2. Ross EM. Pharmacodynamics: mechanisms of drug action and the relationship between drug concentration and effect. In: *Goodman and Gilman's the Pharmacological Basis of Therapeutics*. 10th ed. New York: McGraw-Hill; 2001.
3. Schimmer BP, Parker KL. Adrenocorticoptropic steroids and their synthetic analogs; inhibitors of the synthesis and actions of adrenocortical hormones. In: *Goodman and Gilman's the Pharmacological Basis of Therapeutics*. 10th ed. New York: McGraw-Hill; 2001.
4. McKay LI, Cidlowski JA. Physiologic and pharmacologic effects of corticosteroids. In: *Holland-Frei Cancer Medicine*. 6th ed. Hamilton (ON): BC Decker; 2003.
5. Kelly HW, Sorkness CA. Asthma. In: DiPiro JT, ed. *Pharmacotherapy: A Pathophysiologic Approach*. 6th ed. New York: McGraw-Hill; 2005.
6. Kelly HW. Comparison of inhaled corticosteroids: an update. *Ann Pharmacother.* 2009;43:519–527.
7. Global Initiative for Asthma (GINA). *Global Strategy for Asthma Management and Prevention, Global Initiative for Asthma*. 2014. Available at: http://www.ginasthma.org/documents/4. Accessed September 24, 2014.
8. McFadden ER Jr. Acute severe asthma. *Am J Respir Crit Care Med.* 2003;168:740–759.
9. Raghu G, Collard HR, Egan JJ, et al., for the ATS/ERS/JRS/ALAT Committee on Idiopathic Pulmonary Fibrosis. An official ATS/

ERS/JRS/ALAT statement: idiopathic pulmonary fibrosis: evidence based guidelines for diagnosis and management. *Am J Respir Crit Care Med.* 2011;183:788–824.

10. Zhang L, Prietsch SOM. Inhaled corticosteroids in children with persistent asthma: dose-response effects on growth. *Cochrane Database Syst Rev.* 2012;CD009878.
11. Bourdet SV, Williams DM. Obstructive pulmonary disease. In: DiPiro JT, ed. *Pharmacotherapy: A Pathophysiologic Approach.* 6th ed. New York: McGraw-Hill; 2005.
12. Decramer M, Janssens W, Miravitlles M. Chronic obstructive pulmonary disease. *Lancet.* 2012;379:1341–1351.
13. Shafazand S. ACP Journal Club. Review: inhaled medications vary substantively in their effects on mortality in COPD. *Ann Intern Med.* 2013;158:JC2.
14. Hoffman BB. Catecholamines, sympathetic drugs, and adrenergic receptor antagonists. In: *Goodman and Gilman's the Pharmacological Basis of Therapeutics.* 10th ed. New York: McGraw-Hill; 2001.
15. Albuterol sulfate (Inhalation, Oral). DRUGDEX Evaluation, *Micromedex 2.0.* (retrieved May 2014). Available at: http://www.micromedexsolutions.com/micromedex2/librarian. Accessed October 11, 2014.
16. Boulet L. Long- versus short-acting β_2-agonists. *Drugs.* 2012;47:207–222.
17. Dhand R. Inhalation therapy with metered-dose inhalers and dry powder inhalers in mechanically ventilated patients. *Respir Care.* 2005;50:1331–1344.
18. Camargo CA Jr, Spooner CH, Rowe BH. Continuous versus intermittent beta-agonists for acute asthma. *Cochrane Database Syst Rev.* 2003;4:CD001115.
19. Burchett DK, Darko W, Zahra J, et al. Mixing and compatibility guide for commonly used aerosolized medications. *Am J Health-Syst Pharm.* 2010;67:227–230.
20. Bio LL, Willey VJ, Poon CY. Comparison of levalbuterol and racemic albuterol based on cardiac adverse effects in children. *J Pediatr Pharmacol Ther.* 2011;16:191–198.
21. Levalbuterol. DRUGDEX Evaluation, *Micromedex 2.0.* (retrieved May 2014). Available at: http://www.micromedexsolutions.com/micromedex2/librarian. Accessed October 11, 2014.
22. Op't Holt TB. Inhaled beta agonists. *Respir Care.* 2007;52:820–832.
23. Ni Chroinin M, Greenstone IR, Ducharne FM. Addition of inhaled long-acting beta2-agonists to inhaled steroids as first line therapy for persistent asthma in steroid-naïve adults. *Cochrane Database Syst Rev.* 2008;3:CD005307.
24. Nelson SH, Weiss ST, Bleecker ER, et al. The Salmeterol Multicenter Asthma Research Trial: a comparison of usual pharmacotherapy for asthma or usual pharmacotherapy plus salmeterol. *Chest.* 2006;129:15–26.
25. Oppenheimer J, Nelson HS. Safety of long-acting beta-agonists in asthma: a review. *Curr Opin Pulm Med.* 2008;14:646–649.
26. Patela M, Shirtcliffea P, Beasleya R. The b-2 agonist debate: is there still a problem? *Curr Opin Allergy Clin Immunol.* 2013;13:58–62.
27. Currie GP, Lee DK, Lipworth BJ. Long-acting beta2-agonists in asthma: not so SMART? *Drug Saf.* 2006;29:647–656.
28. Nishikawa M, Mak JCW, Barnes PJ. Effect of short- and long-acting beta-adrenoceptor agonists on pulmonary beta-adrenoceptor expression in human lung. *Eur J Pharmacol.* 1996;318:123–129.
29. Rossi A, Khirani S, Cazzola M. Long-acting β_2-agonists (LABA) in chronic obstructive pulmonary disease: efficacy and safety. *Int J Chron Obstruct Pulmon Dis.* 2008;3:521–529.
30. Rodriguez-Roisin R. COPD exacerbations: management. *Thorax.* 2006;61:535–544.
31. Cazzola M, Bardaro F, Stirpe E. The role of indacaterol for chronic obstructive pulmonary disease (COPD). *J Thorac Dis.* 2013;5:559–566.
32. Epinephrine. DRUGDEX Evaluation, *Micromedex 2.0.* (retrieved May 2014). Available at: http://www.micromedexsolutions.com/micromedex2/librarian. Accessed October 11, 2014.
33. Brown JH, Taylor P. Muscarinic receptor agonists and antagonists. In: *Goodman and Gilman's the Pharmacological Basis of Therapeutics.* 10th ed. New York: McGraw-Hill; 2001.
34. Wellington K. Ipratropium bromide HFA. *Treat Respir Med.* 2005;4:215–220.
35. Barr RG, Bourbeau J, Camargo CA, Ram FS. Tiotropium: for stable chronic obstructive pulmonary disease: a meta-analysis. *Thorax.* 2006;61:854–862.
36. Ipratropium. DRUGDEX Evaluation, *Micromedex 2.0.* (retrieved May 2014). Available at: http://www.micromedexsolutions.com/micromedex2/librarian. Accessed October 11, 2014.
37. Tiotropium. DRUGDEX Evaluation, *Micromedex 2.0.* (retrieved May 2014). Available at: http://www.micromedexsolutions.com/micromedex2/librarian. Accessed October 11, 2014.
38. Undem BJ, Lichtenstein LM. Drugs used in the treatment of asthma. In: *Goodman and Gilman's the Pharmacological Basis of Therapeutics.* 10th ed. New York: McGraw-Hill; 2001.
39. Barnes PJ. Theophylline for COPD. *Thorax.* 2006;61:742–744.
40. Theophylline. DRUGDEX Evaluation, *Micromedex 2.0.* (retrieved May 2014). Available at: http://www.micromedexsolutions.com/micromedex2/librarian. Accessed October 11, 2014.
41. Barnes PJ. Theophylline in chronic obstructive pulmonary disease. *Proc Amer Thor Soc.* 2005;2:334–339.
42. Simons E. Guidelines for the use of theophylline in children with asthma *CMAJ.* 1985;132:1011–1012.
43. Brown NJ, Roberts LJ. Histamine, Bradykinins and their antagonists. In: *Goodman and Gilman's the Pharmacological Basis of Therapeutics.* 10th ed. New York: McGraw-Hill; 2001.
44. Aharony D. Pharmacology of leukotriene receptor antagonists. *Am J Respir Crit Care Med.* 1998;157(6 Pt. 1):S214–S219.
45. Banasak NC, Meadows-Oliver M. Leukotrienes: their role in the treatment of asthma and seasonal allergic rhinitis. *Pediat Nurs.* 2005;31:35–38.
46. Virchow JA, Bachert C. Efficacy and safety of montelukast in adults with asthma and allergic rhinitis. *Respir Med.* 2006;100:1952–1959.
47. Doherty GM. Is montelukast effective and well tolerated in the management of asthma in young children? Part A: evidence-based answer and summary. *Paediatr Child Health.* 2007;12:307–308.
48. Joos S, Miksch A, Szecsenyi J, et al. Montelukast as add-on therapy to inhaled corticosteroids in the treatment of mild to moderate asthma: a systematic review. *Thorax.* 2008;63:453–462.
49. Ducharme FM, Schwartz Z, Kakuma R. Addition of anti-leukotriene agents to inhaled corticosteroids for chronic asthma. *Cochrane Database Syst Rev.* 2004;2:CD003133.
50. Gonyeau MJ, Partisano A. A review of leukotriene inhibitors in the treatment of allergic rhinitis. *Formulary.* 2003;38:368–378.
51. Bibby S, Healy B, Steele R, at al. Association between leukotriene receptor antagonist therapy and Churg-Strauss syndrome: an analysis of the FDA AERS database. *Thorax.* 2010;65:132–138.
52. Zileuton. DRUGDEX Evaluation, *Micromedex 2.0.* (retrieved May 2014). Available at: http://www.micromedexsolutions.com/micromedex2/librarian. Accessed October 11, 2014.
53. Miyatake A, Fujita M, Nagasaka Y, et al. The new role of disodium cromoglycate in the treatment of adults with bronchial asthma. *Allergol Int.* 2007;56:231–239.
54. Cromolyn sodium. DRUGDEX Evaluation, *Micromedex 2.0.* (retrieved May 2014). Available at: http://www.micromedexsolutions.com/micromedex2/librarian. Accessed October 11, 2014.
55. D'Amato G. Role of anti-IgE monoclonal antibody (omalizumab) in the treatment of bronchial asthma and allergic respiratory diseases. *Eur J Pharmacol.* 2006;533:302–307.
56. Hendeles L, Sorkness CA. Anti-immunoglobulin E therapy with omalizumab for asthma. *Ann Pharmacotherapy.* 2007;41:1397–1410.
57. Le J, Ashley ED, Neubauser MM, et al. Consensus summary of aerosolized antimicrobial agents: application of guideline criteria: insights from the society of infectious disease pharmacists. *Pharmacotherapy.* 2010;30:562–584.
58. Milavetz G, Smith JJ. Cystic fibrosis. In: DiPiro JT, ed. *Pharmacotherapy: A Pathophysiologic Approach.* 6th ed. New York: McGraw-Hill; 2005.
59. Chuchalin A, Csiszér E, Gyurkovics K, et al. A formulation of aerosolized tobramycin (Bramitob) in the treatment of patients with cystic

fibrosis and *Pseudomonas aeruginosa:* a double-blind, placebo-controlled, multicenter study. *Pediatric Drugs.* 2007;9(Suppl 1):21–31.

60. Tobi (Tobramycin Inhalation Solution) Package Insert. New York: Novartis Pharmaceutical Corporation. Available at: https://www.pharma.us.novartis.com/product/pi/pdf/tobi.pdf. Accessed September 29, 2014.
61. Conway SP. Nebulized antibiotic therapy: the evidence. *Chronic Respir Dis.* 2005;2:35–41.
62. Shirk MB, Donahue KR, Shirvani J. Unlabeled uses of nebulized medications. *Am J Health Syst Pharm.* 2006;63:1704–1716.
63. Cayston (Aztreonam for inhalation solution) Product Monograph. Gilead Sciences, Inc. Available at: https://www.cayston.com/. Accessed September 29, 2014.
64. Pentamidine isethionate (Inhalation, Injection). DRUGDEX Evaluation, *Micromedex 2.0.* (retrieved May 2014). Available at: http://www.micromedexsolutions.com/micromedex2/librarian. Accessed October 11, 2014.
65. Ventre K, Randolph A. Ribavirin for respiratory syncytial virus infection of the lower respiratory tract in infants and young children. *Cochrane Database Syst Rev.* 2007;1:CD000181.
66. Acetylcysteine (Inhalation, Intravenous, Oral). DRUGDEX Evaluation, *Micromedex® 2.0.* (retrieved May 2014). Available at: http://www.micromedexsolutions.com/micromedex2/librarian. Accessed October 11, 2014.
67. Jones, AP, Wallis C. Dornase alfa for cystic fibrosis. *Cochrane Database Syst Rev.* 2010;17:CD001127.
68. McManus MC. Neuromuscular blockers in surgery and intensive care, part 1. *Am J Health-Syst Pharm.* 2001;58:2287–2399.
69. Taylor P. Agents acting at the neuromuscular junction and autonomic ganglia. In: *Goodman and Gilman's the Pharmacological Basis of Therapeutics.* 10th ed. New York: McGraw-Hill; 2001.
70. McManus MC. Neuromuscular blockers in surgery and intensive care, part 2. *Am J Health-Syst Pharm.* 2001;58:2381–2399.
71. Papazian L, Forel JM, Gacoiun A, et al. Neuromuscular blockers in early acute respiratory distress syndrome. *N Engl J Med.* 2010;363:1107–1116.
72. Yeung JK, Zed PJ. A review of etomidate for rapid sequence intubation in the emergency department. *CJEM.* 2002;4:194–198.
73. de la Grandville B, Arroyo D, Walder B. Etomidate for critically ill patients. Con: do you really want to weaken the frail? *Eur J Anaesthesiol.* 2012;29:511–514.
74. Chan CM, Mitchell AL, Shorr AF. Etomidate is associated with mortality and adrenal insufficiency in sepsis: a meta-analysis. *Crit Care Med.* 2012;40:2945–2953.
75. Gommers D, Bakker J. Medications for analgesia and sedation in the intensive care unit: an overview. *Crit Care.* 2008;12(Suppl 3):S4.
76. Panharipande P, Shintani A, Peterson J, et al. Lorazepam is an independent risk factor for transitioning to delirium in intensive care unit patient. *Anesthesiology.* 2006;104:21–26.
77. Reardon DP, Anger KE, Adams CD, Szumita PM. Role of dexmedetomidine in adults in the intensive care unit: an update. *Am J Health-Syst Pharm.* 2013;70:767–777.
78. Smith HS. The metabolism of opioid agents and the clinical impact of their active metabolites. *Clin J Pain.* 2011;27:824–838.
79. Devlin JW, Roberts R. Pharmacology of commonly used analgesics and sedatives in the ICU: benzodiazepines, propofol and opioids. *Crit Care Clin.* 2009;25:431–439.
80. Ahonen J, Olkkolal KT, Hynynen M, et al. Comparison of alfentanil, fentanyl and sufentanil for total intravenous anaesthesia with propofol in patients undergoing coronary artery bypass surgery. *Br J Anaesth.* 2000;85:533–540.
81. Craven R. Ketamine. *Anaesthesia.* 2007;62(Suppl 1):48–53.
82. Lundstrom S, Twycross R, Mihalyom M, Wilcock A. Propofol. *J Pain Symptom Manage.* 2010;40:466–470.
83. Kam PC, Cardone D. Propofol infusion syndrome. *Anaesthesia.* 2007;62:690–701.
84. Hoy SM, Keating GM. Dexmedetomidine. A review of its use in sedation of mechanically ventilated patients in the intensive care setting and procedural sedation. *Drugs.* 2011;71:1481–1501.
85. Gerlach AT, Murphy CV, Dasta JF. An updated focused review of dexmedetomidine in adults. *Ann Pharmacother.* 2009;43:2064–2074.
86. Dexmedetomidine. DRUGDEX® Evaluation, *Micromedex 2.0.* (retrieved May 2014). Available at: http://www.micromedexsolutions.com/micromedex2/librarian. Accessed October 11, 2014.
87. McLaughlin VV, Archer SL, Badesch DB, et al. ACCF/AHA 2009 Expert consensus document on pulmonary hypertension. *J Am Coll Cardiol.* 2009;53:1573–1619.
88. Taichman DB, Ornelas J, Chung L, et al. Pharmacological therapy for pulmonary arterial hypertension in adults: CHEST Guideline. *Chest.* 2014;146:449–475.
89. Iloprost. DRUGDEX Evaluation, *Micromedex 2.0.* (retrieved May 2014). Available at: http://www.micromedexsolutions.com/micromedex2/librarian. Accessed October 11, 2014.
90. Channick RN, Simonneau G, Sitbon O, et al. Effects of the dual endothelin-receptor antagonist bosentan in patients with pulmonary hypertension: a randomized placebo-controlled study. *Lancet.* 2001;358:1119–1123.
91. Galié N, Badesch D, Oudiz R, et al. Ambrisentan therapy for pulmonary arterial hypertension. *J Am Coll Cardiol.* 2005;46:529–535.
92. Buckley MS, Staib RL, Wicks LM, Feldman JP. Phosphodiesterase-5 inhibitors in management of pulmonary hypertension: safety, tolerability, and efficacy *Drug, Healthcare and Patient Safety.* 2010;2:151–161.

Section V
The Respiratory Care Profession

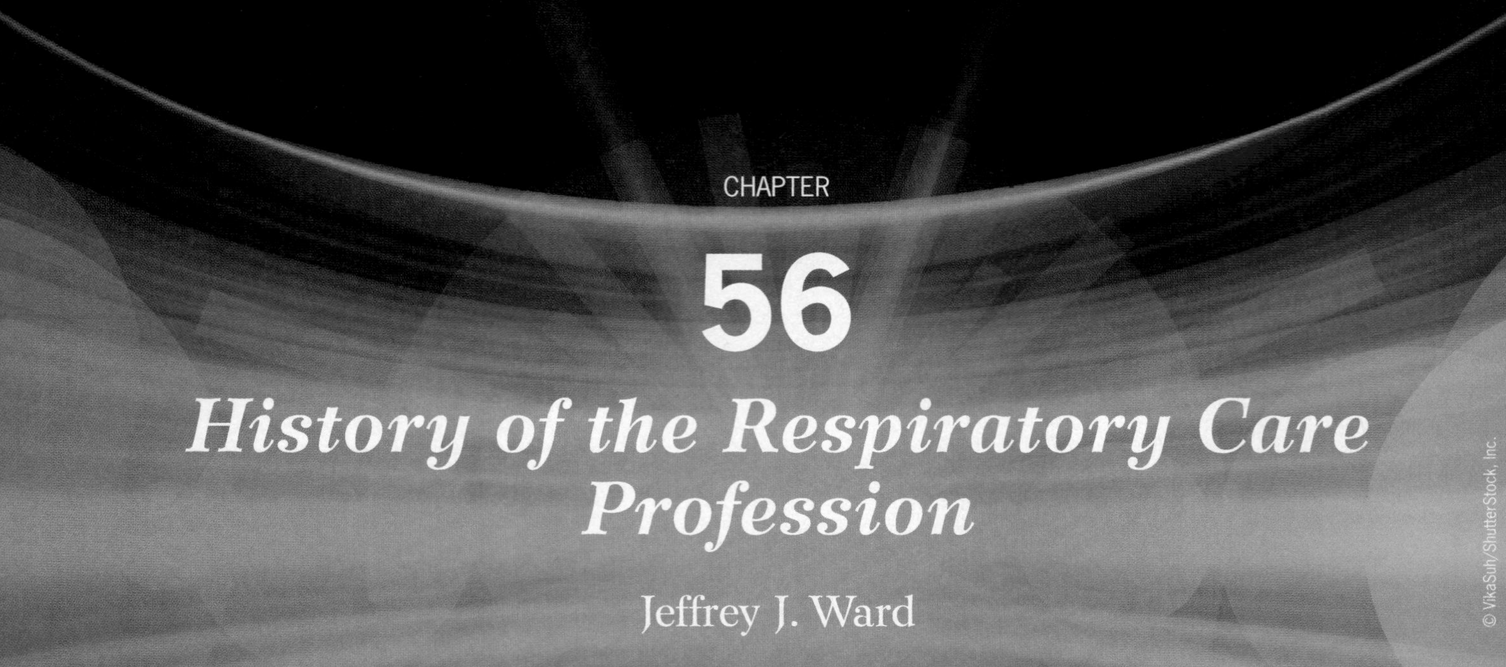

CHAPTER
56
History of the Respiratory Care Profession
Jeffrey J. Ward
© VikaSuh/ShutterStock, Inc.

OUTLINE

Historical Events and Key Advances in Medical-Related Sciences
Historical Events That Signaled the Evolution of Respiratory Care
Milestones in the Organizations Within the Respiratory Care Profession: Beginning Years
Respiratory Care's Continuing Evolution: Contemporary and Future Changes

OBJECTIVES

1. Identify early philosophers, scientists, inventors, and physicians whose discoveries were important to the evolution of Western medicine.
2. Note key events and pioneers in the areas of medical gases, aerosol medications, airway care, resuscitation, and mechanical ventilation.
3. Recognize advances in medicine that were the result of lessons learned in military conflicts.
4. Trace the evolution of the professional, credentialing, and educational organizations involved in the infrastructure of the respiratory care profession.
5. Identify current major trends that are likely to shape the future of respiratory care.

KEY TERMS (NAMES)

Albert H. Andrews
Alvan Barach
Andreas Vesalius
Antoine Lavoisier
Archie Brain
Åsmund Laerdal
Chevalier Jackson
Forrest Bird
Galen
H. Fred Helmholz Jr.
Hippocrates
John Emerson
John Haldane
John Hutchinson
John Severinghaus
Joseph Priestley
Karl Albert Hasselbalch
Lawrence Henderson
Leland Clark
Linus Pauling
Louis Pasteur
Peter Safar
Philip Drinker
René T. H. Laennec
Thomas Beddoes
Thomas Petty
V. Ray Bennett
Virginia Apgar
William Harvey

Introduction

A historical review provides beginning respiratory care practitioners with a perspective on the evolution of both clinical practice and the related professional organizations. We are all travelers in history. An understanding of the past may allow an explanation for the present and also can provide insight into what lies ahead. This chapter notes major events and trends that became important milestones. Behind these milestones are personal contributions. It would be impossible to note them all. Respiratory care is a relatively young field; a few of the pioneers are still with us! Although the focus of this chapter is on respiratory care practice as it developed in North America, international connections will be placed in context. Events that occurred following World War II are highlighted. More comprehensive coverage is available both in books and on the Internet.[1–6]

Historical Events and Key Advances in Medical-Related Sciences

Respiratory care has its roots in a diverse history that includes the unraveling of key scientific concepts in chemistry, physics, biology, and pharmacology. A long list of pioneers allowed concurrent development of impressive technology, a medical infrastructure, and insights into the ethics, art, and science of clinical practice. **Table 56-1** summarizes major historical contributors to the background and clinical science related to respiratory care.

TABLE 56-1
Major Contributors to Medical Sciences and Respiratory Clinical Medicine

Contributor	Country; Birth and Death Dates	Contribution
Ancient Period		
Hippocrates	Greece; 460–370 BC	Early guidelines for medical profession; importance of observation and diagnostic logic
King Pandukabhaya	Sri Lanka; 437–367 BC	Founded first institutions specifically dedicated to the care of the sick (other than religious temples)
Aristotle	Greece; 384–322 BC	Animal experiments; observed suffocation
Early Renaissance		
Leonardo da Vinci	Italy; 1578–1657	Human dissection; inflation of lungs caused by subatmospheric intrapleural pressures
Andreas Vesalius	Belgium; 1514–1564	Experiments with respiration in animals; early resuscitation
William Harvey	England; 1578–1657	Elucidated arterial and venous systemic and pulmonary circulations
Antonie van Leeuwenhoek	Netherlands; 1632–1723	Development of microscope lenses and discovery of single-cell organisms
Isaac Newton	England; 1643–1727	Mathematics and physics, especially motion and gravitation
18th Century		
Daniel Bernoulli	Holland and Switzerland; 1700–1782	Aerodynamics and hydrodynamics
Joseph Black	Scotland; 1728–1799	Discovery of carbon dioxide
Carl Scheele	Sweden; 1742–1786	Manufacture and discovery of oxygen
Joseph Priestley	England; 1733–1804	Discovery of oxygen
Antoine Lavoisier	France; 1743–1794	Discovery of role of oxygen and carbon dioxide in metabolism
Thomas Beddoes	England; 1760–1808	Clinical use of supplemental oxygen
Jacques Alexandre César Charles	France; 1746–1823	Gas law
René Laennec	France; 1781–1826	Invention of the stethoscope
Joseph Louis Gay-Lussac	France; 1778–1850	Gas law
Edward Jenner	England; 1749–1832	Microbiology; smallpox vaccination
19th Century		
John Dalton	England; 1766–1844	Gas pressure and atomic theory
William Henry	England; 1775–1836	Absorption of gases in fluids
Thomas Graham	Scotland; 1805–1869	Diffusion of gases through membranes
Louis Pasteur	France; 1822–1895	Bacteriology; germ theory
Robert Koch	Germany; 1843 1910	Bacteriology; discovery of cause of tuberculosis
Eduard Pfluger	Germany; 1829–1910	Oxygen consumption; respiratory quotient
Christian Bohr	Denmark; 1856–1911	Oxyhemoglobin dissociation curve
Adolf Fick	Germany; 1828–1901	Cardiac output measurement; contact lenses
Florence Nightingale	England; 1820–1910	Nursing care, hygiene, and sterile technique; medical statistics
Clara Barton	United States; 1821–1912	Battlefield evacuation; distribution of medical resources; American Red Cross
William Roentgen	Germany; 1845–1923	Discovered the x-ray
20th Century		
Karl Albert Hasselbalch	Denmark; 1874–1962	Blood oxygen physiology and acid–base chemistry
John Scott Haldane	England; 1880–1936	Hemoglobin oxygen physiology; regulation of breathing; gas therapy devices
Lawrence J. Henderson	United States; 1878–1942	Blood oxygen physiology and acid–base chemistry
Willem Einthoven	Holland; 1860–1927	Cardiac electrophysiology; invented the electrocardiogram
Ernest Henry Starling	England; 1866–1927	Cardiac muscle physiology; Frank-Starling law
Otto Frank	Germany; 1865–1944	Isotonic contractile behavior of cardiac muscle
Gerhard Domagk	Germany; 1895–1964	Antimicrobials; sulfanilamide
Alexander Fleming	Scotland; 1881–1956	Discovered penicillin
Selman Waksman	Russia, United States; 1888–1973	Antituberculosis use of streptomycin
Edward Kendall and Philip Hench	United States; 1886–1972 and 1896–1965	Isolated the corticosteroid cortisone
Carl Gottfried von Linde	Germany; 1842–1934	Manufacture of oxygen by fractional distillation
Alvan Barach	United States; 1895–1977	Oxygen and helium–oxygen therapy; constant positive pressure breathing (CPPB)
Linus Pauling	United States; 1901–1994	Chemistry and molecular biology; oxygen analysis using paramagnetic qualities
Chevalier Jackson	United States; 1865–1958	Endoscopy; tracheal intubation and tracheotomy
Leland C. Clark Jr.	United States; 1918–2005	Membrane oxygen electrochemical analysis
Philip Drinker	United States; 1894–1972	Coinventor of the iron lung
John H. Emerson	United States; 1907–1997	Inventor of iron lung and early volume-controlled mechanical ventilator
Forrest M. Bird	United States; 1921–	Aviation medicine; inventor of Bird Mark-7 and Baby Bird ventilators
Virginia Apgar	United States; 1909–1974	Developed the Apgar score for assessment of newborn infants
Willam Ganz	United States; 1919–2009	Cardiologist & codeveloper of balloon-tip pulmonary artery catheter
John Severinghaus	United States; 1922–	Membrane pH and carbon dioxide electrochemical analysis
Harold James C. (Jeremy) Swan	Ireland; United States; 1922–2005	Cardiologist & codeveloper of balloon-tip pulmonary artery catheter
Peter Safar	Austria and United States; 1924–2003	Modern CPR procedures; EMT training, intensive care units and critical care education
Mary Ellen Avery	United States; 1927–2009	Furthered understanding of perinatal lung pathophysiology
Thomas Petty	United States; 1932–2011	Pulmonologist & coauthored landmark work on ARDS, PEEP, and long-term oxygen therapy
Takuo Aoyagi	Japan; 1936–	Reported findings leading to development of pulse oximeter

Ancient Times

The earliest records of practical medicine are from ancient Egypt and Mesopotamia, dating before 3000 BC. Their medicine was highly advanced for the time and included simple surgery, setting of bones, and an extensive pharmacy. Medical texts specified a rational, stepwise approach to diagnosis and treatments. These beliefs were synergistic with mysticism and religion. Egyptians developed a theory of channels that carried air, water, and blood to the body.

By 2000 BC the ancient Chinese had developed a part-philosophic and part-physiologic concept of breathing. They believed that what was breathed from the air was transmitted to the soul. They developed rituals for taking a pulse. They also practiced moxibustion, burning substances on the skin. Medicines included herbal teas, such as ephedra (ma huang, from the plant *Ephedra sinica*) for asthma and hay fever. The ancient Indian pharmacopeia had even more extensive antiasthma drugs, including ginger. The Bible's Old Testament records the story of the prophet Elisha's resuscitating a Shunammite child by relieving a tracheal obstruction (II Kings 4:34).[2–6] In early history, the East and Middle East were well ahead of the West in medical sciences and practice. About 430 BC the Sinhalese royalty (modern-day Sri Lanka) appeared to be the first governance to provide dedicated institutions for their sick.

A key part of Western medicine's scientific heritage began with the Greeks, who felt such knowledge had both altruistic and practical value. Pythagoras (580–489 BC) defined life's four elements as being earth, fire, water, and air. **Hippocrates** of Cos II (460–370 BC; **Figure 56-1**) is considered the father of medicine.

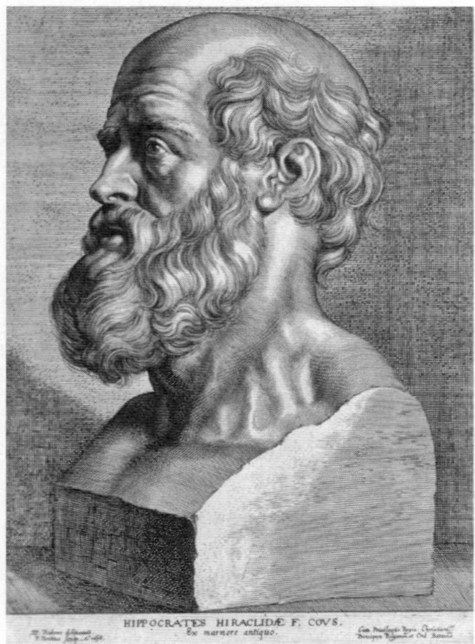

FIGURE 56-1 Hippocrates of Cos II, the father of Western medicine (ca. 460–370 BC).
Courtesy National Library of Medicine.

He established medicine as a separate discipline, aligned with philosophy and science and incorporating professional attributes that continue today. He believed that diseases were not punishments from the Gods but rather were disorders of essential humors. This promoted a lucid approach of careful examination and identification of physical signs. For example, Hippocrates is given credit for the first description of digital clubbing (Hippocratic fingers), an important diagnostic sign in chronic suppurative lung disease, lung cancer, and cyanotic heart diseases. Aristotle (384–322 BC) is likely to have recorded the first respiratory physiology experiment after observing that animals died when kept in air-tight chambers. He believed the heart to be the source of the body's heat and nervous center. Erasistratus (304–250 BC), a Greek anatomist who worked in the school of anatomy in Alexandria, Egypt, believed respiration involved the lungs passing air into the left ventricle and then to the body using air-filled arteries.

Galen of Pergamum (AD 130–199), a prominent Roman physician, probably was the most accomplished medical researcher of the Roman period. His theories dominated Western medicine for over a millennium. He believed blood carried "pneuma" from inspired air via a pulmonary and then via an arterial circulation. By dissection of animals and observation of gladiators' injuries, he demonstrated that nervous control originated in the brain and spinal cord. The Romans established the importance of physicians on the battlefield. The Romans also established the value of public health measures to prevent and control epidemics.[2–6]

The Middle Ages

Little scientific or medical investigation was done in Europe after Galen. During the early Middle Ages (AD 400–500), the collapse of the Roman Empire and invasion by Germanic tribes threatened both written records and civilized infrastructure. The survival of some medical texts from Rome, Greece, and Persia is credited to monastic communities in Ireland, France, and Italy that preserved and transcribed original documents.[7] The works of ancient Greek and Moslem scientists and philosophers were reintroduced into the Western world. These works provided new intellectual material for European scholars.

The first hospital incorporated into an organized component for clinical education of physicians was the Academy of Gudishapur (Persia) in late AD 400. In Europe, though, medical care was mostly limited to some monasteries. These monasteries incorporated almshouses for the poor, infirmaries, leprosaria, and hospices open to both clergy and lay populations. The term *hospital* is derived from the Latin *hospes*, which is also the root for the English words *hospitality*, *hostel*, and *hotel*.

A series of more than nine major Crusades occurred from 1092 through the 13th century. Although undertaken with Christian religious purpose, there was significant brutality and intolerance of both Moslem and other minorities. Over the course of 200 years, some 2 million Europeans died in the Middle East Crusades. There was some benefit, however, since much knowledge in areas such as science, medicine, and architecture was transferred from the Islamic to the Western world during the Crusade era. There also was a resurgence of commerce in the 1300s. By the 14th century, the Crusades had decreased the centralized power of the papacy, which kindled the foundation of modern nation-states in Europe.

Populations became more concentrated in cities, and problems with public health became significant. A series of pandemic plagues occurred, which began in Asia and reached Europe during the mid and late 14th century, where it was known as the Black Death (bubonic plague). It is estimated that one-fourth of the European population (20 million) died. Initially the disease was blamed on comets or scapegoats such as lepers or Jews. The actual cause of the plague was the bacteria *Yersinia pestis*, which inhabited the intestines of fleas. The impact of the plague was most significant in killing off old-school physicians, thereby allowing those with new ideas regarding medicine to establish a practice.

The Renaissance: The 14th to 17th Centuries

The period beginning in the late 14th century and spanning to the 17th century reflected a general revival of learning based on classical sources and widespread educational reform, which included the arts and sciences. Men such as Leonardo da Vinci (1452–1519) took up human dissection to better understand human physiology. He was the first to report that subatmospheric pressures were required to inflate mammalian lungs. In 1543, **Andreas Vesalius** (1514–1564) published his masterful anatomy text, *De Humani Corporis Fabrica* ("On the Artistry of the Human Body"), which dispelled many of Galen's premises (**Figure 56-2**). The record shows that Vesalius performed a thoracotomy on a live pig. He then documented pneumothorax, subsequent ventricular fibrillation, and recovery after ventilation via a primitive tracheostomy tube.

Educational reform was not without setbacks due to the Western Roman Catholic Church, which suppressed scientific theories and practices (such as autopsy and dissection) that it saw as heresy. Spanish anatomist Michael Servetus (1509–1563) was burned at the stake after his revolutionary anatomy text stated that blood in the pulmonary circulation, once it mixed with air from the lungs, returned to the left heart. It was another 75 years (1628) before English physician

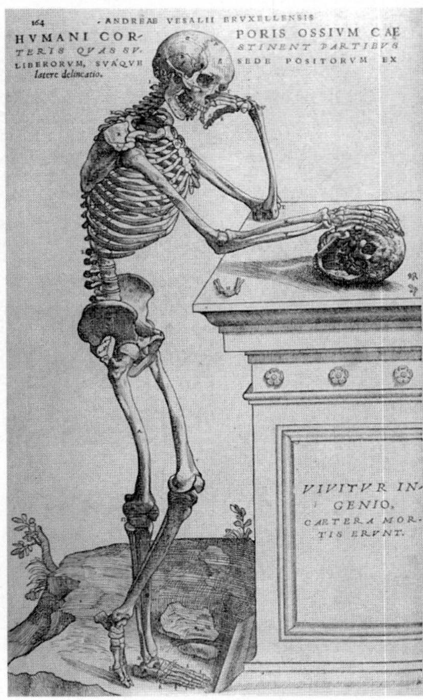

FIGURE 56-2 Illustration from Vesalius's De Humani Corporis Fabrica, 1543.
Courtesy National Library of Medicine.

William Harvey (1578–1657) correctly described details of the arterial and venous circulations.[2–6]

Advances in understanding the primary and physical sciences continued throughout Europe during the 17th century. In Italy, Evangelista Torricelli (1608–1647; **Figure 56-3**) and associates made the first barometer by 1643. In France, Blaise Pascal (1623–1662) documented the relationship between barometric pressure and altitude. Irish theologian, alchemist, and gentleman scientist Robert Boyle (1627–1691; **Figure 56-4**) is regarded as one of the founders of modern chemistry. He received credit for espousing the inverse relationship between gas volumes and pressure, a hypothesis that was originally formulated by Henry Power in 1661. A multitalented assistant of Boyle, Robert Hooke (1635–1703), played important roles in the scientific revolution. He built vacuum pumps for Boyle's experiments as well as telescopes and microscopes. Hooke is known principally for his law of elasticity but is also acknowledged as a father of microscopy. It is believed that Hooke coined the word *cell* to describe the basic unit of biological life.

In the Netherlands, cloth merchant Antonie van Leeuwenhoek (1632–1723) was intrigued after reading Robert Hooke's book on microscopes in the mid-1600s. Van Leeuwenhoek's skill in glass making and lens grinding allowed him to improve on the early microscope. His revolutionary findings about single-celled organisms were published in 1673. This period in history would not be complete without mentioning the

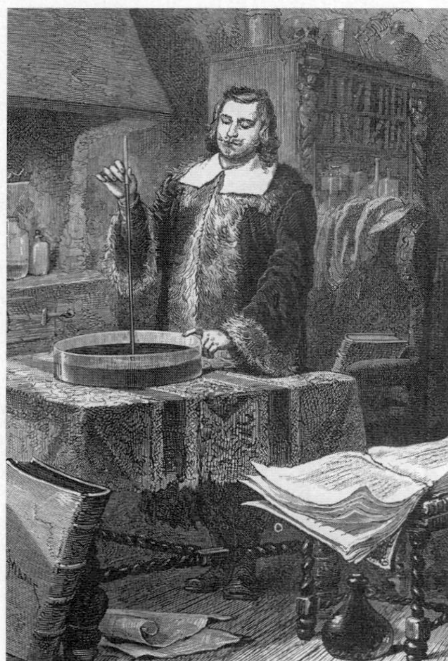

FIGURE 56-3 Evangelista Torricelli with his mercury barometer (circa 1640).

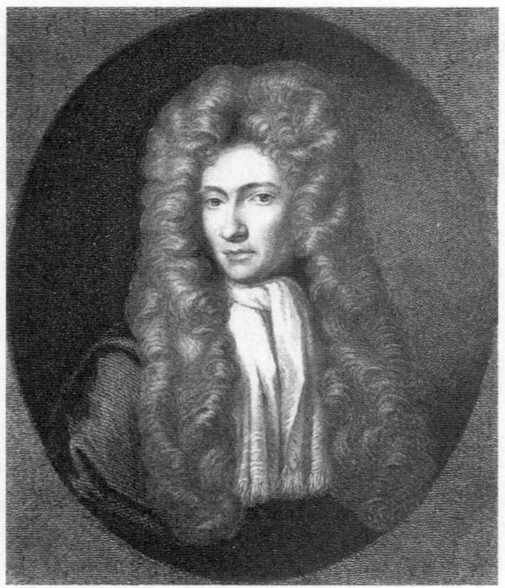

FIGURE 56-4 Robert Boyle, Irish chemist, physicist, and inventor, best known for the formulation of Boyle's law.

major contribution of Sir Isaac Newton (1643–1727). His work in mathematics, physics, the mechanics of motion, and gravitation as well as light and optics suggests that he was one of the most influential scientists in human history.

The 18th Century

During the 1700s, advances continued in the understanding of physical and chemical sciences. Daniel Bernoulli (1700–1782), a Dutch-Swiss mathematician, studied mechanics, especially fluid and gas hydrodynamics. Bernoulli's principle was critical in the area of aerodynamics. In addition, his statistical-epidemiologic work was notable in his 1766 analysis of smallpox morbidity and mortality data to demonstrate the efficacy of vaccination. This was prior to Edward Jenner's 1796 findings.

The identification of respiratory gases that occurred during this period provided valuable insight into scientific competition, publication, and communication. Priority for discovery of a respiratory gas implies both preparation and identification. But it also involves communication of the work (oral or written) to other scientists and publication in either a book or journal. This sequence remains true today. Scotsman Joseph Black (1728–1799) is credited with the discovery of carbon dioxide (which he called "fixed air") by heating limestone in 1754. This discovery, however, was reported previously by Flemish chemist Baptiste van Helmont (1580–1644). He was the first to understand that there are distinct gases within atmospheric air and reported that carbon dioxide ("gas sylvestre") was given off by burning charcoal, which he believed was the same gas as produced during fermentation.

For some time, English theologian-scientist and politician **Joseph Priestley** (1733–1804) was credited with the discovery of oxygen ("dephlogisticated air"). These findings were communicated in September of 1774, but he later confessed that he had no clear comprehension of oxygen. Priestley published his findings in November 1775. He believed this work would defend German scientist George Stahl's phlogiston theory and disprove the new chemical revolution of atomic theory. The former believed that combustible substances consumed phlogiston, which had negative mass when burned. Rejection of atomic theory eventually left Priestley isolated within the scientific community.

Swedish apothecary Carl Scheele (1742–1786) appears to have generated oxygen ("fire air") by heating magnesium oxide with sulfuric acid in June of 1771, three years ahead of Priestley. He communicated these findings by letter to **Antoine Lavoisier** in October 1774 and later in his book *Air and Fire* in August 1777. Of interest is that Scheele also discovered the element molybdenum and a method to mass-produce phosphorus. He likely died prematurely due to exposure to mercury from heating mercuric oxides.[8]

In France, a third scientist, Antoine Lavoisier (1743–1794; **Figure 56-5**) capitalized on the work of Scheele and Priestley. He too has strong claims to the discovery of the gas that he termed "oxygen" (Greek *oxys* = sharp [acid] + *genes* = begetter), a description of which he published in May 1775. Lavoisier dispelled

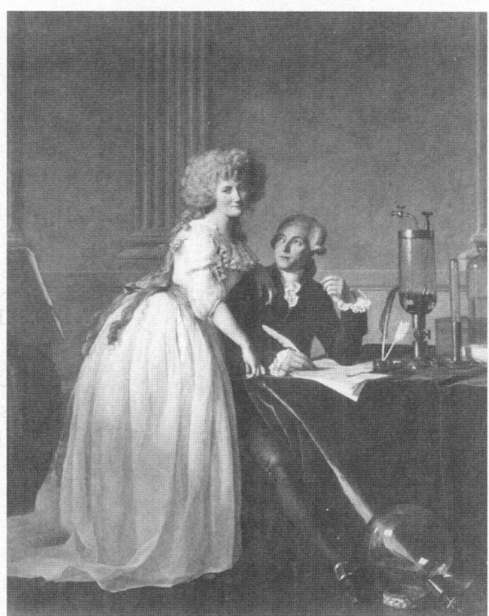

FIGURE 56-5 Marie and Antoine Lavoisier.
Courtesy National Library of Medicine.

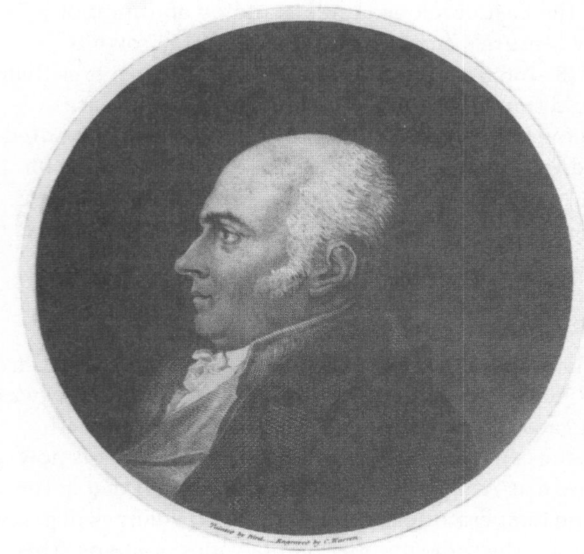

FIGURE 56-6 Thomas Beddoes (1760–1808), father of respiratory therapy.
Courtesy National Library of Medicine.

the phlogiston theory. His research included some of the first quantitative chemical analyses supporting the law of conservation of mass, which he was the first to state. His later work confirmed that the body consumed oxygen, that carbon dioxide and water vapor were primary components of exhalation, and that nitrogen was essentially unchanged in the breathing process. Unfortunately, knowledge that his laboratory was supported by the French royalty resulted in his death by guillotine in the prime of his career.

In summary, Scheele probably has priority for actual chemical manufacture of oxygen. As for written communication of the discovery, Priestley and Scheele seem to have equal priority. The criterion of earliest publication by the individual scientist of his own work would give Priestley an edge. However, the criteria of earliest publication by other than the original investigator and a true understanding of the discovery's physiologic significance would give Lavoisier the credit.[8] Similar issues relate to Charles's law of gases. This was first published in 1808 by Joseph Louis Gay-Lussac (1778–1850), but he referenced an earlier unpublished work by fellow Frenchman Jacques Alexandre César Charles (1746–1823) around 1787.

Thomas Beddoes (1760–1808; **Figure 56-6**) deserves special mention for his scholarly contribution and for being the first clinician to implement therapeutic use of medical gases as well as nitrous oxide. In 1784, his multilingual skills were employed as he translated Scheele's *Chemical Essays* from German to English. He then reviewed Priestley's work and visited Lavoisier. He may be considered the father of respiratory therapy because he applied and investigated the "medical powers of factitious airs and gases." He solicited funds from a wide circle of intellectual friends. He gained technical support to generate gases from the inventor James Watt. In 1798 a Pneumatic Institute was established at Clifton, overlooking Bristol, England.[9] The facility was a spa-like environment incorporating a dispensary (clinic), hospital, and laboratory (**Figure 56-7**). The latter was supervised by Sir Humphrey Davy (1778–1829), who used oxygen and nitrous oxide to treat a number of conditions, including dyspnea, asthma, scrofulous infections, and congestive heart failure. Unfortunately the pneumatic component was overshadowed by demand for general care due to a typhus epidemic in 1800; the Institute was largely abandoned by 1801.

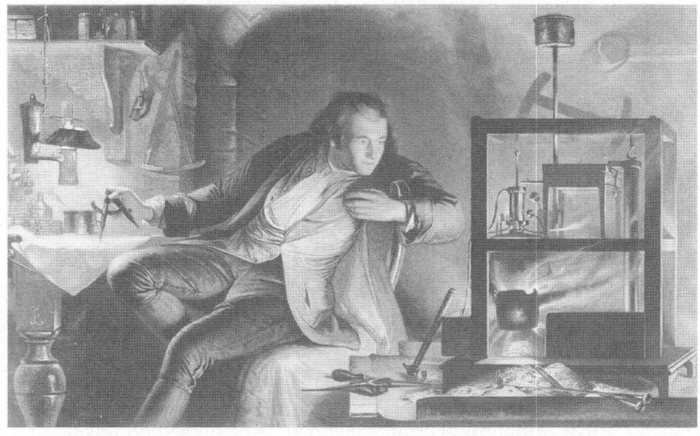

FIGURE 56-7 The Pneumatic Institute's early apparatus to generate medical gases, invented by James Watt.

The East developed understanding of immunology centuries before Italian Fracastoro Girolamo (1478–1563) proposed that tiny particles or spores that could transmit infection caused epidemic diseases. Fellow Italian Agostino Bassi (1773–1856) is often credited with having stated the germ theory of disease for the first time, based on his observations. Englishman Edward Jenner (1749–1832) published his findings on smallpox vaccination in 1789.

The 19th Century

Italian savant Lorenzo Romano Amedeo Carlo Avogadro di Quaregna e di Cerreto (1776–1856; **Figure 56-8**) was educated in law but then dedicated himself to mathematics and physics. In 1811 he proposed what is now known as Avogadro's hypothesis. He stated that at the same temperature and pressure, equal volumes of gases contain the same number of molecules or atoms. This was a radical statement at the time and was not widely accepted for 50 years. Avogadro developed this hypothesis after Joseph Louis Gay-Lussac had published his law in 1808 on volumes and combining gases. Of interest is that Avogadro had not resolved the question of whether molecules were made up of atoms.[2–6] John Dalton (1766–1844), an English chemist and meteorologist, is best known for his pioneering work in the development of modern atomic theory. In 1803 Dalton published his work on his principles of gas partial pressures, which constitute Dalton's law. Fellow English chemist William Henry (1775–1836) quantified the absorption of gases by water at different temperatures and under different pressures. This later became known as Henry's law.

Closely related to concepts about the physics of gases was the understanding of factors that govern diffusion through membranes. This was quantitated first by the Scotsman Thomas Graham (1805–1869) in 1831. Heinrich Gustav Magnus (1802–1870) was a German-born chemist and physicist who studied under Gay-Lussac in Paris. Between the 1830s and 1860s he is credited with extending the understanding of vapor pressures of water, electrolysis, the conduction of heat in gases, and the thermal effects produced by condensation. He is credited with the first quantitative analysis of arterial and venous O_2 and CO_2 content.

Advances in science likely promoted initial acceptance of the metric system in 1875 in an international treaty known as the Convention du Mètre. The idea of a metric system has been attributed to John Wilkins, first secretary of the Royal Society of London in 1668. French abbot and scientist Gabriel Mouton proposed a decimal system of linear measurement based on the circumference of the earth in 1670. He then suggested a system of subunits, dividing successively by factors of 10 into the centuria, decuria, virga, virgula, decima, centesima, and millesima.

Paris became a center of modern medicine in the first half of the 19th century. Based on recent understanding of physics and chemistry, its institutions used a scientific approach based on experiment and observation. French physicians who provided clinical-related advances included Jean-Nicolas Corvisart, who assessed heart disease by tapping on the chest, and **René T. H. Laennec** (1781–1826; **Figure 56-9**), inventor of the stethoscope (a 2-cm by 25-cm hollow wooden

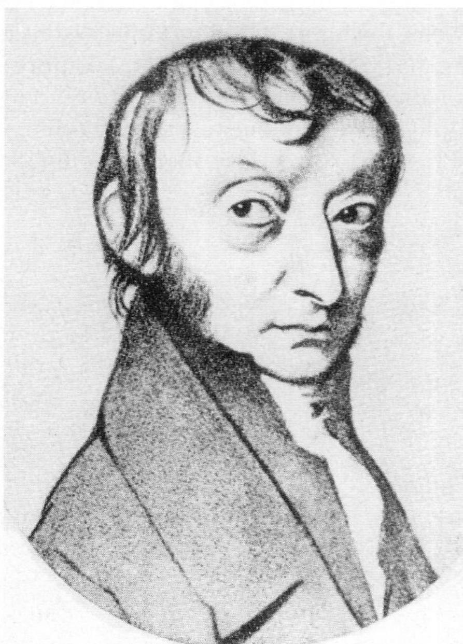

FIGURE 56-8 Amedeo Avogadro, who in 1811 published *Essay on Determining the Relative Masses of the Elementary Molecules of Bodies and the Proportions by Which They Enter These Combinations.*
© National Bureau of Standards Archives, courtesy AIP Emilio Segre Visual Archives.

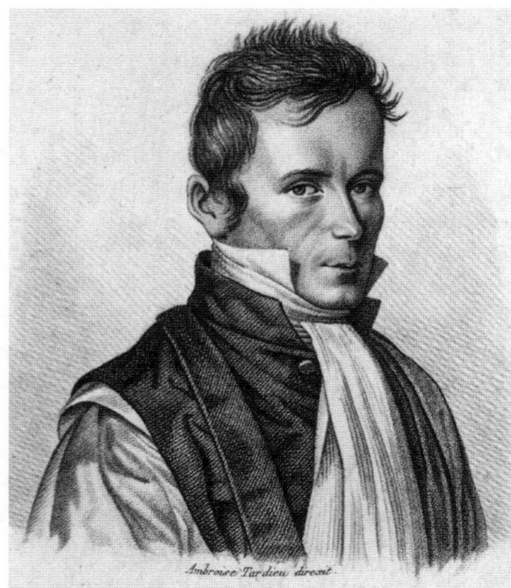

FIGURE 56-9 René Laennec, who developed the science of auscultation and is credited with inventing the stethoscope (Greek *stethos*, meaning "chest," and *skopos*, meaning "to look at").
Courtesy National Library of Medicine.

tube) in 1819. There is conjecture as to whether his skill as a flutist, his interest in preventing the embarrassment of direct ear-to-chest contact with the opposite sex, or his desire to distance himself from patients' body odor and lice prompted this invention. French chemist Charles Fredrick Gerhardt was the first to prepare acetylsalicylic acid in 1853, which was patented under the name Aspirin in 1899.

The sciences of microbiology/bacteriology and immunology also advanced rapidly toward the middle of the 19th century. French chemist and microbiologist **Louis Pasteur** (1822–1895) continued work on germ theory and bacteriology. He conducted experiments in the mid-1800s that clearly validated the concepts of spoilage of beer, wine, and milk. By 1862 he and Claude Bernard showed that treating fluids with heat could kill bacteria. This process became known as pasteurization. Pasteur's immunology work, initially done on chicken cholera, led to a patent for his vaccination against anthrax in 1870. German Heinrich Hermann Robert Koch also studied cholera and anthrax. His most important contribution was the discovery of *Mycobacterium tuberculosis* in 1882, for which he was awarded a Nobel Prize in 1905. Both he and Pasteur are regarded as the fathers of germ theory and bacteriology.

In England, surgeon **John Hutchinson** (1811–1861) developed a spirometer to measure the effect of disease on lung volumes. He coined the term *vital capacity*. In 1846 he published results of vital capacities of over 2000 subjects (at autopsy and live patients). He found decreased volumes in those with tuberculosis or heart failure and in coal miners.[10]

By the mid-1800s education in medicine was promoted by French and German universities. Religion no longer dominated the curriculum, and education became increasingly more accessible for all students. The German approach became an international model because a university could support both basic sciences as well as clinical medicine. German scientists are credited with development of the laryngoscope, ophthalmoscope, and cystoscope. William Roentgen discovered x-rays in 1895. German physiologist Eduard Pfluger (1829–1910) noted that oxygen consumption in tissues was proportional to their needs and devised the term *respiratory quotient*. By 1885 his laboratory also revealed that hypoxemia and hypercarbia both stimulated ventilation. Miescher-Rusch showed that carbon dioxide was the more potent stimulator.[11]

Danish physician-physiologist Christian Bohr (1856–1911; **Figure 56-10**) constructed the oxyhemoglobin-hemoglobin dissociation curve in 1886 and in 1891 characterized dead space. German physiologist and biophysicist Adolf Eugene Fick (1828–1901; **Figure 56-11**) made contributions in gas diffusion and described the direct method for measuring cardiac output in 1870. He also is credited with inventing contact lenses. About 1860, Bunsen and Kirchhoff invented the spectroscope. Later, Georg Gabriel Stokes realized that hemoglobin's absorption of oxygen changed its color. The first effort to monitor human blood oxygenation was reported by Karl von Vierordt (1818–1854), a German physiologist in 1874. He noted that red light diminished when tissues became ischemic.

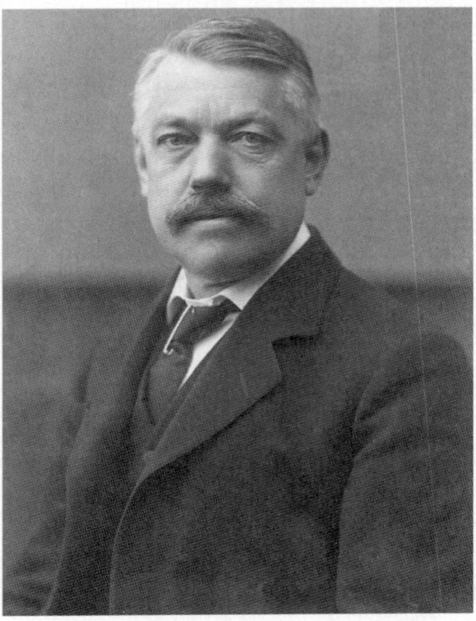

FIGURE 56-10 Danish physician Christian Bohr was educated at the University of Leipzig, Germany, and is credited with describing physiologic relationships involving oxygen–hemoglobin dissociation and dead space ventilation.
Courtesy of the Niels Bohr Archive, Copenhagen.

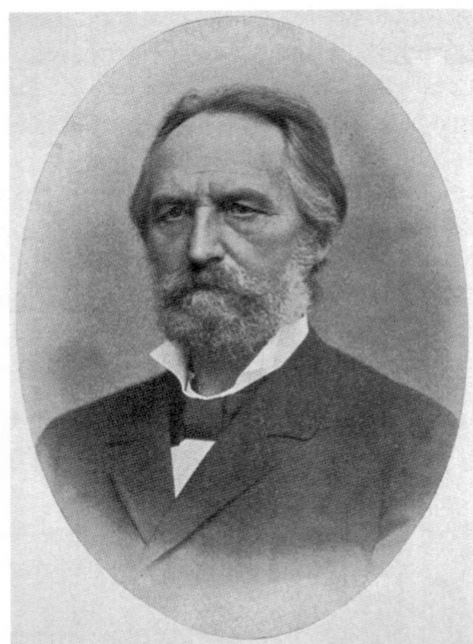

FIGURE 56-11 Adolf Fick, a German physiologist, is credited with the invention of contact lenses as well as an explanation of the diffusion of gases across a membrane and a method for determining cardiac output.
Courtesy National Library of Medicine.

Warfare during the 19th century provided some positive benefit to medicine in spite of its human and economic devastation. Napoleon realized the importance of medical care. His army physicians began the practice of triage. Advances in surgery, including limb amputation, elevated the competency of battlefield surgeons, who returned to civilian practice after the Napoleonic wars (1803–1815). Newspaper correspondents during the Crimean War (1853–1856) reported the scandalous treatment of soldiers in British field hospitals. Deaths due to typhus, typhoid, cholera, and dysentery were 10 times as frequent as those from battlefield wounds. This prompted the advancement of nursing care of the wounded by Florence Nightingale (1820–1910; **Figure 56-12**). Her introduction of clean and sterile techniques and emphasis on the importance of diet and activity reduced death rates from 42% to 2%. She also had skills in mathematics and statistics, using pie charts to document causes of mortality and the effects of sanitation practices.[12]

The American Civil War (1861–1865) provided a similar grisly lesson for the American public and its physicians. Recently, a review of 1850–1880 census records has increased the previously estimated total death count (both Union and Confederate) by 20% to approximately 752,000.[13] That translates to the loss of 1 in 10 men of military age or 2.4% of the U.S. population at that time. Only some soldiers pinned their name on paper notes inside uniforms or scratched identification on the back of belt buckles; sketchy or lost casualty records (especially Confederate) and burial sites left most soldiers unidentified. The upper bounds of actual deaths may have been as high as 850,000.

Advances in military technology such as heavy artillery and the rifled barreled gun exceeded battle tactics left over from the Revolutionary War. Many soldiers were left wounded to die on the battlefield; approximately 80% died from lack of sanitary conditions or epidemics of smallpox and measles as there was no immunization. Death statistics do not include the huge toll on widows, orphans, and the 500,000 men who survived but with disabling physical or psychological wounds. The financial impact was estimated to be over $10 billion in 1860 dollars. Like all wars, medical lessons learned did somewhat offset some of the cost. The importance of identification (dog tags), military records, immunization, sanitation, and hygiene for troops was realized. Union physician Jonathan Letterman developed a more modern system to care for mass casualties, including an ambulance core, first aid stations, field hospitals, and pavilion-style general hospitals. Battlefield physicians realized the need for metal combat helmets, immediate care of wounds and performing major operative procedures within 24 hours, and the importance of nurses. Besides the technical experience gained by physicians, many lessons set the stage for improved management in World Wars I and II. Mortality from battle wounds decreased from the Civil War's 13.3% to 4.5% in World War II.[14]

Women's roles in medicine advanced slowly in the United States. Elizabeth Blackwell became the first woman to earn a medical degree in 1849 but was banned from practice in most hospitals. As nurses were introduced to the hospital, Blackwell trained nurses for the Union. The requirements of the Civil War did allow Dr. Mary Edwards Walker (1832–1919) to become the first woman U.S. Army surgeon. She received the Medal of Honor for her service. Clara Barton (1821–1912; **Figure 56-13**) served as a nurse on Union Civil War ambulances behind enemy lines. She was also an organizer to improve distribution of medical supplies.

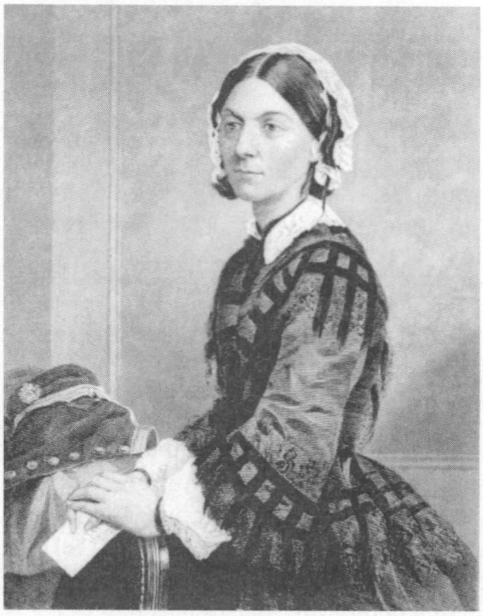

FIGURE 56-12 Florence Nightingale was a pioneering nurse who reduced the mortality of British soldiers in the Crimean War. She also was an early medical statistician.
Courtesy National Library of Medicine.

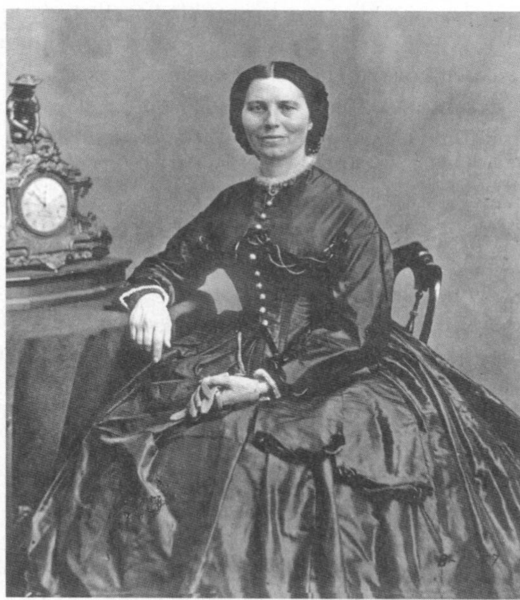

FIGURE 56-13 Clara Barton served as a nurse in the American Civil War and was instrumental in establishing the American Red Cross.
Courtesy National Library of Medicine.

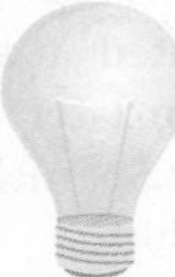

STOP AND THINK

What advances in medical care and preventing military casualties did the American Civil War promote?

Barton became involved in the International Red Cross movement. By 1873, she helped establish the American Red Cross, which had a scope broader than war crises.

Anesthesia was available at the time of the Civil War in the form of chloroform, and analgesia in the form of opium or morphine. In 1842, American medical student William Clark used diethyl ether during a tooth extraction for its anesthetic properties. A country physician in Georgia, Dr. Crawford Long, also used it during a surgical operation in that same year. William Thomas Green Morton in Boston conducted the first public demonstration of ether for surgery in 1846. This provided the documentation that established anesthesia internationally. In that same year Morton used the anesthetic gas nitrous oxide for a dental extraction. Forty-seven years earlier, Thomas Beddoes's chemist associate Humphrey Davy had used nitrous oxide for recreational purposes in 1799.[15]

Evolution of Respiratory Care in the 20th and 21st Centuries

The 20th century ushered in a wave of advancements. Medical practice was affected by international contributions in the fields of human physiology, pathophysiology, and technology. In the area of cardiopulmonary physiology, Christian Bohr, **Karl Albert Hasselbalch** (1874–1962), Joseph Barcroft (1882–1947), and August Krogh (1874–1949) made major contributions. Edward Pfluger and Krogh developed a bubble method that involved equilibration of small gas bubbles with large volumes of blood followed by analysis of gas tensions in the bubbles. Important research was conducted by John Gillies Priestley (1880–1941), Yandell Henderson (1873–1944), and **John Scott Haldane** (1980–1936; **Figure 56-14**). In 1898, Haldane created his gas analysis apparatus to measure oxygen content in blood. He also worked on regulation of breathing. Haldane discovered the effect of oxygen on hemoglobin dissociation of CO_2 (the Haldane effect). His interests included study of respiration under both hypobaric and hyperbaric conditions. The former resulted in a U.S. expedition to Colorado in 1911, where he conducted high-altitude research on Pikes Peak. His interest in mining disasters in the United Kingdom promoted study of carbon monoxide, hydrogen sulfide, and dust (silica) exposure.[16]

In the United States, physiologist-biochemist **Lawrence J. Henderson** (1878–1942; **Figure 56-15**), while working at Harvard, calculated the oxygen dissociation constants for oxygenated and reduced hemoglobin. He also calculated the law of mass action for the CO_2/bicarbonate buffer system. Wilhelm Ostwald first measured the concentration of hydrogen ions in 1896 using a platinum electrode in solutions saturated with hydrogen gas. He discovered that the potential generated by the platinum electrode was a logarithmic function of the strength of the acid. The Ostwald platinum electrode was later modified and used by Karl Albert Hasselbalch in 1912 to measure blood acidity. In 1916, Hasselbalch converted Henderson's 1908 equation to logarithmic form, which is now known as the Henderson-Hasselbalch equation. In 1920, August Krogh was awarded the Nobel Prize in Physiology or

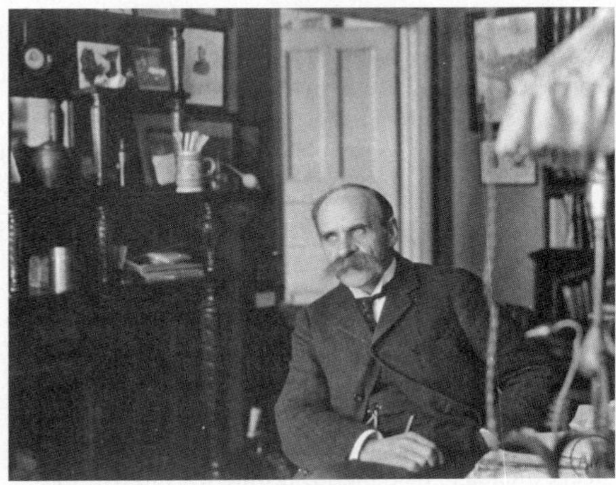

FIGURE 56-14 John Scott Haldane was a Scottish physiologist and biochemist whose work included research on respiration at extremes of pressure, exposure to toxic gases, and hemoglobin's interaction with oxygen and carbon dioxide, as well as the development of gas masks and oxygen delivery systems.
Courtesy National Library of Medicine.

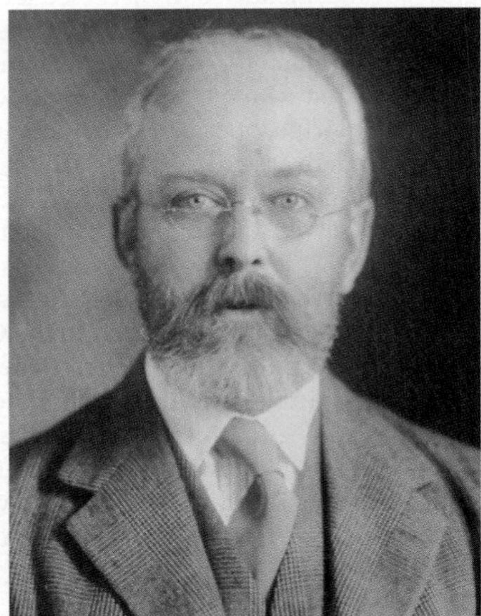

FIGURE 56-15 Lawrence J. Henderson investigated acid–base regulation, finding that acid–base balance is regulated by buffer systems of the blood (hemoglobin), in complex coordination with respiration, and the kidneys.
Courtesy of Harvard University Archives, HUP Henderson, L.J. (2)

Medicine for the discovery of the mechanism of capillary blood flow regulation in skeletal muscle. Wallace O. Fenn (1893–1917) contributed primary research in understanding the mechanics of breathing and became the founder of the *Journal of Applied Physiology*. He and Herman Rahn devised a diagram for displaying alveolar gas information.[17]

Cardiac physiology also experienced a rapid evolution. Dutch physician Willem Einthoven (1860–1927; **Figure 56-16**) invented the electrocardiogram in 1903 as well as methods for understanding rhythm disturbances. For that work, he received the Nobel Prize for Medicine in 1924. German physiologist Otto Frank (1865–1944) studied the isotonic contractile behavior of heart muscle. His collaboration with Englishman Ernest Henry Starling (1866–1927) resulted in the Frank-Starling law of the heart, which was first presented in 1915.

The first global war, World War I (1914–1918) resulted in the death of over 37 million military personnel and civilians. Like the American Civil War, technological advancements led to increased lethality in weaponry. Tanks, machine guns, and long-distance artillery replaced antiquated cavalry and cannons. One of the most feared weapons was chemical warfare with toxic gases (chlorine, phosgene, and mustard gas) released from cylinders or artillery shells. Haldane's physiology work prompted development of masks for gas attacks and to deliver supplemental oxygen to treat survivors.[16]

World War I provided yet another horrific lesson for both surgeons and internists. Compared to the Civil War there was less mortality due to nonbattlefield problems; only one-third of military deaths were due to disease. Some advances in microbiology included use of tetanus antitoxin to prevent or treat gangrenous infections. Gunshot wounds were treated with Dakin's solution (sodium hypochlorite). The Spanish influenza pandemic followed the end of hostilities in 1918. Influenza A virus, which probably originated at the Fort Riley, Kansas, U.S. Army training camp, later evolved to a more virulent strain in France. The Spanish flu resulted in the death of approximately 680,000 Americans and 22 million to 40 million people worldwide. This was 2% to 5% of the world population at that time. The virus elicited a storm of macrophage-derived chemokines and cytokines, which resulted in the lungs becoming infiltrated by inflammatory cells, causing severe pulmonary hemorrhage.[18]

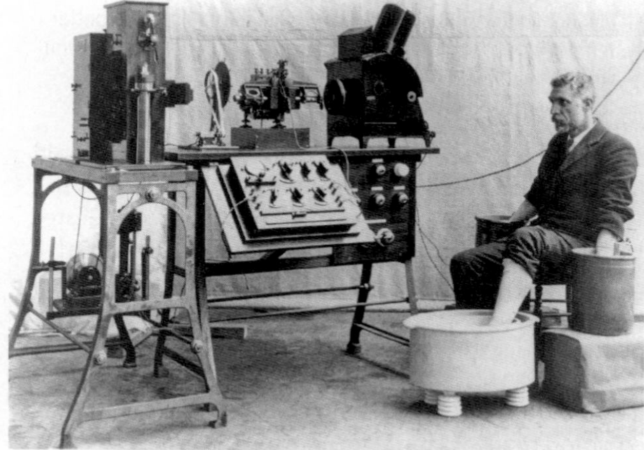

FIGURE 56-16 Willem Einthoven invented the electrocardiogram and methods to evaluate cardiac electrophysiologic disturbances.

By 1921 the cause of diabetes had been discovered. A research team in Toronto, Canada, led by Dr. Fredrick Banting, isolated insulin. The antibiotic era began as German chemist Gerhard Domagk (1895–1964) discovered the antimicrobial properties of an industrial dye that was converted to sulfanilamide in the body. He received the Nobel Prize for Medicine in 1939 for his work. He was forced by the Nazi regime to refuse the prize and was arrested by the Gestapo.

While serving in World War I, Scottish physician-pharmacist Alexander Fleming (1881–1956) saw the devastation of septicemia and the limited value of antiseptics. The lack of cleanliness in his lab's sinks led to the accidental discovery of penicillin. He shared the Nobel Prize for Medicine with Howard Florey and Ernst Chain in 1945 for the discovery of penicillin. Biochemist and microbiologist Selman Waksman (1888–1973) immigrated to the United States from Russia in 1910 to work at Rutgers University, where he isolated the antituberculosis agent streptomycin in 1944. Mayo Clinic chemists Edward Kendall and Philip Hench isolated the steroid hormone cortisone, for which they later received the Nobel Prize for Medicine in 1950.[19] This allowed the treatment of Addison disease and rheumatologic disorders.

Historical Events That Signaled the Evolution of Respiratory Care

Clinical Oxygen Therapy

Earlier in this chapter, the work of Thomas Beddoes during the late 1700s was noted. He applied the chemical discovery of Scheele, Priestley, and Lavoisier to patients. The first oxygen devices began appearing as modified anesthetic masks made of oiled canvas, velveteen leather, mouth pipes, and cheek pieces (**Figure 56-17**). Fresh oxygen was manufactured on location using electrolysis in local apothecaries. By 1868, copper cylinders were developed to store and transport oxygen.[20]

Only gradually did the medical community embrace oxygen therapy, after significant strides were made in understanding the physiology of oxygen transport by Bohr, Krogh, Haldane, and Barcroft (**Figure 56-18**).[19,20] The first reports of potentially toxic effects of sustained breathing of oxygen at high concentrations also began

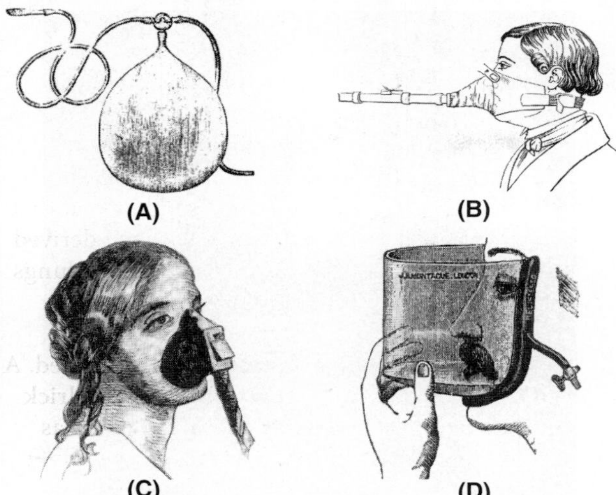

FIGURE 56-17 (**A**) Oxygen (mouthpiece) inhaler after design of Beddoes and Watt (circa 1796). (**B**) Oxygen face-piece mask of canvas and oiled silk (circa 1847). (**C**) Lead mask covered with leather and velveteen (circa 1847). (**D**) Open face-tent originally used for nitrous oxide (circa 1899).

Reproduced with permission from Leigh JM. The evolution of the oxygen therapy apparatus. *Anaesthesia*. 1974;25:210.

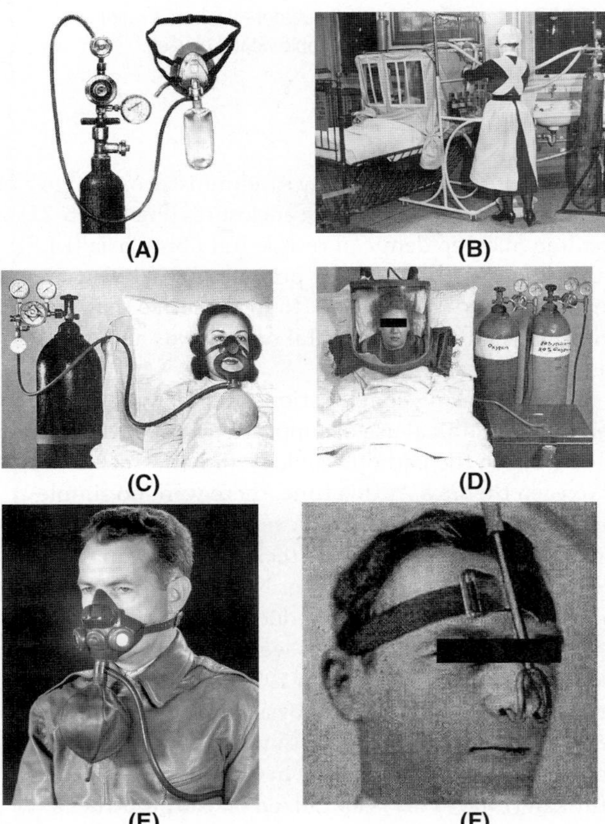

FIGURE 56-18 (**A**) Haldane's reservoir oxygen mask (circa 1919). (**B**) Apparatus for supplying patients with oxygen (circa 1950). (**C**) Barach's mix-o-mask. (**D**) Barach's heliox constant positive airway pressure device. (**E**) World War II aviator with BLB mask. (**F**) Metallic nasal cannula.

(**A**) Reproduced from Leigh JM. The evolution of the oxygen therapy apparatus. *Anaesthesia*. 1974;25:210, with permission; (**B**) © William Vanderson/Fox Photos/Getty Images, Creative; (**C**) courtesy of Aerospace Medical Association; (**D**) reproduced from Barach. Principles and Practices of Inhalation Therapy. J.B. Lippincott; 1944. Reprinted with permission from Wolters Kluwer Health; (**E**) reproduced with permission of Mayo Foundation for Medical Education and Research. All rights reserved; (**F**) reproduced from Barach. Principles and Practices of Inhalation Therapy. J.B. Lippincott; 1944. Reprinted with permission from Wolters Kluwer Health.

to appear in the literature. Sir Arbutot Lane introduced the nasal catheter using simple rubber tubing in 1907. He first used these nasal catheters for sick children and adult victims of World War I gas poisoning. Haldane's previously mentioned oxygen mask consisted of a 2-liter reservoir bag to extend the performance of the catheter to treat soldiers with pulmonary edema caused by chlorine gas inhalation inducing chemical pneumonitis (refer to Figure 56-18A). Haldane and Barcroft exposed themselves to subambient (15%) oxygen in experimental chambers to simulate hypoxia, in addition to their work at altitude.

Oxygen enclosures for clinical use appeared in England and Canada around 1910. Carl Gottfried von Linde (1842–1934) was a German engineer who invented technologies for refrigeration, which facilitated cooling for gas separation by fractional distillation. There had been much demand for CO_2 in European breweries. He was successful in generating oxygen in 1895, and the process was quickly commercialized. A U.S. patent was granted in 1903, and the Linde Air Products Company was formed by 1907. By 1926, U.S. physician and oxygen therapy proponent Dr. **Alvan Barach** (1895–1977; **Figure 56-19**) saw to the development of closed-system oxygen tents, which removed CO_2 with calcium chloride and used chunk ice for cooling (refer to Figure 56-18B).

American inventors Thomas Midgley and Charles Kettering developed Freon for refrigeration in 1928; oxygen tents soon took advantage of that technology (**Figure 56-20**). Barach and Haldane both developed types of meter masks with diluting valves to allow specific entrainment of room air (refer to Figure 56-18C).[21] Barach also conducted trials with spontaneously breathing patients using helium–oxygen mixtures (heliox) as well as heliox with constant positive airway pressure (CPAP) hoods in 1934 (refer to Figure 56-18D).[22,23]

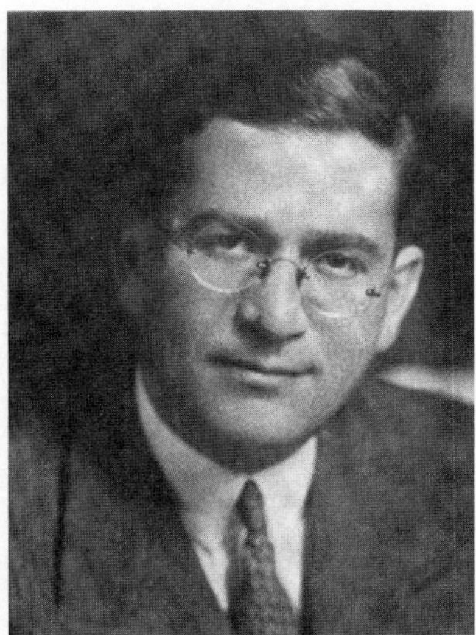

FIGURE 56-19 Dr. Alvan Barach (1895–1977).

© Archives & Special Collections, Columbia University Health Sciences Library.

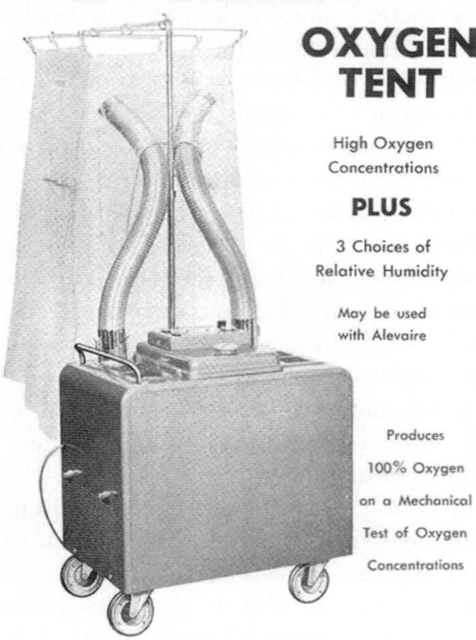

FIGURE 56-20 Electrically powered refrigerated oxygen tent (circa 1956).
Courtesy of John Bunn, a Graham-Field Brand.

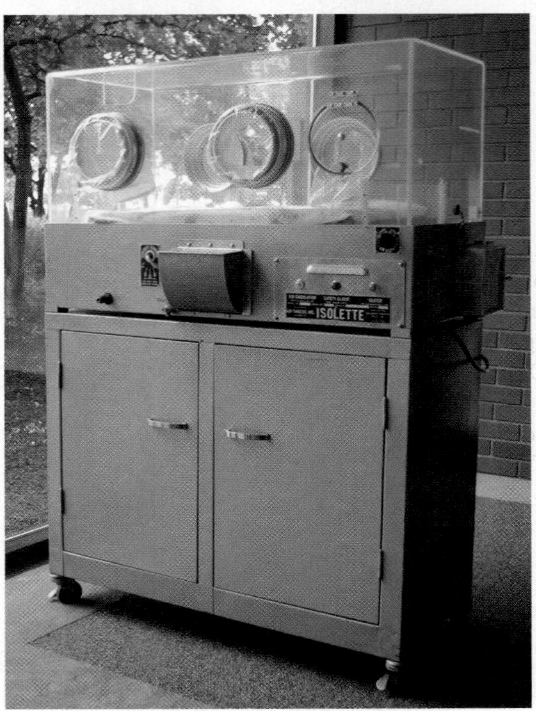

FIGURE 56-21 Infant warmer-incubators (Isolette brand) were fitted with adaptors to provide supplemental oxygen.
Courtesy of Draeger Medical Systems, Inc.

World War II (1939–1945) was the deadliest military conflict in history. Estimates range from 60 million to more than 85 million deaths, which was 2.5% to 3.5% of the world population at the time. It saw a significant increase in civilian casualties due to famine, war-related disease, ethnic genocide, and use of aircraft as a weapon of war for strategic bombing. World War II sped the development of mass-produced penicillin that saved thousands of Allied soldiers from infections and subsequently introduced antibiotics into civilian medical practice.

The need for military aircraft to fly both at greater altitudes to avoid antiaircraft artillery and at higher speeds prompted further study of oxygen physiology at low barometric conditions as well as effect of gravity, that is, g-force, on the cardiovascular system. A group of physicians (William Boothby, W. Randolph Lovelace, and Arthur Bulbulian) with the Mayo Clinic's Aero Medical Unit developed a partially valved reservoir mask capable of providing 80% to 100% oxygen in 1938. Later they termed this the BLB mask, which was made commercially available by Ohio Chemical (refer to Figure 56-18E). The Mayo Aero Medical Unit was also instrumental in creating the G-suit, which allowed external compression of a pilot's legs and abdomen to prevent hypotension-induced blackouts during acceleration in higher performance fighter aircraft. Metal cannulas became available as an alternative to the nasal catheter (refer to Figure 56-18F).

In the late 1940s, the ability to administer oxygen to premature infants in warming enclosures (**Figure 56-21**) resulted in an epidemic of retrolental fibroplasia (RLF), later named retinopathy of prematurity (ROP). Theodore Terry was the first to hypothesize that indiscriminate use of supplemental oxygen was a potential cause.[24]

Both increasing complications and increased demand for clinical use of supplemental oxygen escalated work in the pathophysiology and new technology of oxygen therapy. At this time, there were no simple methods to measure oxygen levels in inspired gas or blood. Efforts to provide this technology began with Heinrich Danneel and Walther Nernst, who determined the electrochemical reduction of oxygen in 1897. Polarographic characteristics were accidently discovered by Jaroslav Heyrovsky in 1922 using platinum cathodes. In 1935, German physiologist Kurt Kramer (1906–1985) used photocells to measure oxygen saturations using an in vivo cuvette in dogs. American Glen Millikan (1906–1947) capitalized on Karl Matthes's (1905–1962) work by using two hemoglobin absorption wavelengths for his external ear oximeter. **Linus Pauling** (1901–1994) exploited the characteristic that increased oxygen enhanced a magnetic field. The Arnold Beckman Company developed the D-2 oxygen analyzer in 1945 in collaboration with Pauling.

By this time demand for gas supplies and knowledgeable personnel to support physicians and nurses

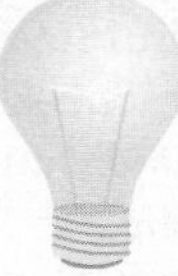

STOP AND THINK

How does learning the history of blood gas analysis contribute to your understanding of modern blood gas analysis?

in a 24-hour-per-day service heralded the beginning of organized inhalation therapy departments. In 1942, Francis Roughton and Per Scholander modified Krogh's oxygen testing method to measure carbon monoxide (CO) using a syringe with a calibrated capillary for equilibration so that only a small amount of blood was needed. Richard Riley adapted this syringe method later for measuring PO_2 in the blood, and it became known as the *Riley bubble method*. The Riley bubble method was widely used, primarily as a research tool to study ventilation-perfusion relationships in the lung. In 1954, **Leland C. Clark Jr.** (1918–2005) was credited with developing the first membrane oxygen electrode that was not poisoned by blood proteins.[25]

By the mid-1960s, commercially available arterial blood gas (ABG) electrodes developed by Clark and **John Severinghaus** (1922) allowed analyses of PaO_2, $PaCO_2$, and pH. Their operation often became incorporated within the clinical services of respiratory therapy departments. Arterial blood collection and interpretation skills were one more skill set added to the growing list of job functions. Millikan's ear oximeter was made clinically available by 1974, and by the early 1980s ABG-type electrodes had been miniaturized so they could be applied transcutaneously. In 1974, Japanese bioengineer Takuo Aoyagi published an abstract of his serendipitous discovery of pulse oximetry. His discovery occurred while working on an ear probe densitometer for recording dye dilution curves for cardiac output.[26] The pulse oximeter has become a standard device for monitoring patient oxygenation in emergency departments, operating rooms, intensive care units, and hospital floors.

The goal of improving titration of oxygen levels to patients, especially those with chronic obstructive pulmonary disease (COPD), led E. J. Moran Campbell to develop the Venturi mask in 1960. It was similar in function to Barach's meter mask and provided high-flow controlled FIO_2 to meet the inspiratory demands of tachypneic patients while minimizing the risk of induced carbon dioxide retention.[27] Reliable air–oxygen blenders became commercially available by the mid-1970s and were quickly put into use in nurseries and intensive care units. They were also incorporated into mechanical ventilators. The oxygen concentrator and portable liquid systems also became available by the mid-1970s. Conserving devices such as reservoir masks or cannulas, demand pulse units, and transtracheal catheters were developed in response to a growing demand for out-of-hospital oxygen therapy. The benefit of that approach was made clear in 1980 as the Nocturnal Oxygen Therapy Trial (NOTT) group published its findings. These investigators showed a positive mortality benefit when oxygen was continuously used for hypoxic patients with COPD.[28]

By the 1990s oxygen therapy had evolved to require significant skills in assessing patients' medical requirements, recommending care, and evaluating its effects. Therapist-driven protocols (TDPs) were now required to better define the science and patient applications. It was not surprising that oxygen therapy became the subject of one of the first in a series of clinical practice guidelines (CPGs) developed by the American Association for Respiratory Care.[29,30]

Medicated Aerosols

For the purposes of reviewing the history of clinical aerosols, the concept should also include use of mists, fogs, vapors, or fumes. The practice of inhaling sulfuric vapors from the slopes of Mt. Vesuvius was mentioned by Galen (AD 130–201). The practice of inhaling burning medicinal substances from smoking pipes goes back thousands of years. The leaves and roots of *Datura ferrox* were used to treat asthma. Jimsonweed (*Datura stramonium*) was also used for its added psychotropic effect. Commercially produced antiasthma cigarettes (e.g., Asmador) were available until 1992, when they were withdrawn because of the potential for abuse. Home therapy also included flame-heated vaporizers to administer a range of inhalable liquid medications (**Figure 56-22**).

In 1912, adrenaline to treat asthma was made available and delivered with perfume-type squeeze-ball atomizers. By 1940, more sophisticated pneumatic nebulizers evolved from work by Lucien Dautrebande and others, which improved these devices with baffling designs.

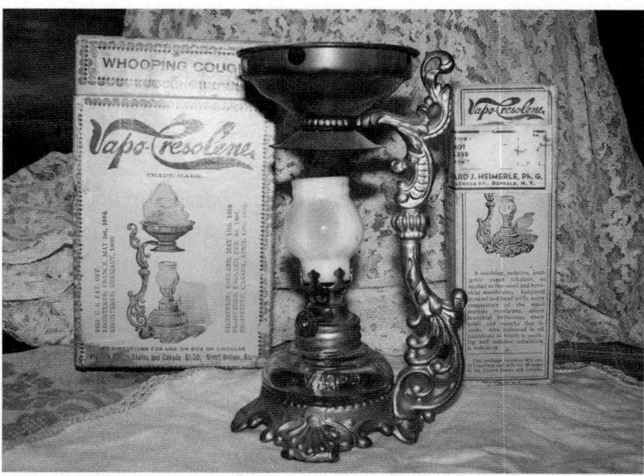

FIGURE 56-22 Vaporizers were commonly used for home therapy. An alcohol- or kerosene-lamp burner heated liquid medication in a chamber to be vaporized into a room or inhaled directly.
Courtesy of Susanna Connelly Holstein, www.grannysu.blogspot.com.

High-velocity jet-type nebulizers were applied via self-inflating bags, intermittent positive pressure breathing (IPPB) devices, and volume-controlled mechanical ventilators, for both humidification and medication delivery. The most commonly used β-agonist in 1940 was isoproterenol (Isuprel), which became appreciated for its robust bronchodilation. It also was known for its tendency to produce tachycardia. Ultrasonic nebulizers became available in 1949, first used as room humidifiers. Later physicians added medications and directed aerosol output to patients with masks.[31]

Pharmacologic research provided medications that targeted specific airway receptors. The first introduced was Bronkosol, which was available by 1951. A proliferation of more β-specific agonists, anticholinergics, and corticosteroid medications subsequently occurred. Chlorofluorocarbon (CFC)-powered metered dose inhalers (MDIs) were developed in 1956 and became the most commonly used devices because of their low cost, simplicity, and ability for self-administration. Dry powder inhaler (DPI) use began in the United States with delivery of cromolyn sodium via the Spinhaler in 1973. Concerns about the environmental effects of CFCs on Earth's ozone layer resulted in international cooperation to discontinue the use of CFC propellants, including those in MDIs, by 2009. Other propellants have since been introduced. Use of MDIs and DPIs has increased, especially for nonacute care application.

Antimicrobial agents have been administered by pneumatic nebulizers for many years. Evidence for their efficacy occurred in the treatment of cystic fibrosis patients with *Pneumocystis carinii* infections. That patient group was also treated with rhDNase aerosols to diminish the viscosity of pulmonary secretions.[31] Aerosol therapy has continued to advance in terms of new devices using technologies such as porous mesh and medications such as insulin.[32]

Airway Management and Resuscitation

Tracheotomy is an ancient medical procedure. Its use was first recorded in Hindi and Egyptian literature from about 3600 to 2000 BC. Homerus of Byzantium wrote that Alexander the Great performed the procedure with a sword to treat an ailing soldier in about 1000 BC. Hippocrates campaigned against the tracheotomy because of serious and frequent complications from vascular damage as well as unsterile instruments. In 1542 Andreas Vesalius performed a tracheotomy on a pig on which he had previously performed a thoracotomy, using a reed for the tracheostomy tube. Once ventilation was applied, he observed its recovery from (presumed) ventricular fibrillation following a pneumothorax. The procedure was first named tracheotomy in 1718. Until the early 1900s, it was largely regarded as a last-ditch effort or considered only in emergency situations.

German surgeon Fredrich Trendelenburg reportedly did the first tracheal intubation for anesthesia in 1869. He introduced the tube through a temporary tracheostomy. In 1878, the Scottish surgeon William MacEwan reported the first elective oral intubation. During World War I, Drs. Ivan Magill and Robert Macintosh advanced the procedure for direct tracheal intubation. American laryngologist **Chevalier Jackson** (1865–1958; **Figure 56-23**) is credited with inventing the first anesthetic laryngoscope in 1913. Magill, Miller, and Macintosh then developed modifications to the instrument. Jackson largely invented the science of endoscopy of the upper airway and esophagus by refining procedures to reduce complications and improve physician training. A model of metallic tracheostomy tube still bears his name. Subsequent advances included blind nasal intubation, described by Magill in 1930, and catheters for secretion removal, described by F. J. Murphy in 1941.[33] The polio pandemic renewed interest in tracheostomy. With the dwindling availability of the costly iron lung, tracheostomy allowed positive pressure ventilation. This was often applied by simple hand-powered bag-valve systems.

The modern techniques of resuscitation were developed from the late 1940s to the 1960s. Impetus came from successful experience with mobile army surgical hospital (MASH) units developed in 1945 and deployed during the Korean War (1950–1953). A system was developed for medics to treat at the point of injury,

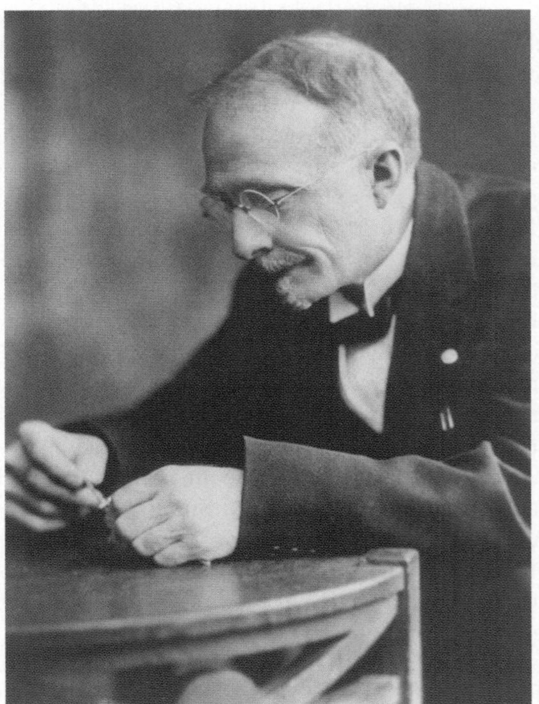

FIGURE 56-23 Dr. Chevalier Jackson was a pioneer in laryngoscopy, bronchoscopy, and endoscopy. He refined the procedures for tracheotomy and endotracheal intubation.
Courtesy of Thomas Jefferson University, Archives & Special Collections.

then transport first to battalion aid stations for stabilizing surgery, and finally route soldiers to a MASH where they had 97% chance of survival. Watchers of the popular MASH TV series may recall surgeon Hawkeye Pierce performing open-heart cardiac massage in several episodes. That procedure was first done in 1901 for anesthesia-induced arrest in the operating room (OR), but in 1958 William Kouwenhoven documented the effectiveness of closed-chest cardiac massage.[33] Successful open-chest defibrillation was first performed by Claude Beck in 1947, and by 1956 Paul Zoll had documented it to work if applied externally. In 1958, **Peter Safar** (1924–2003; **Figure 56-24**) and colleagues published their work on mouth-to-mouth resuscitation compared with the older Silvester arm-lift technique.[34] Airway management procedures, manual or mechanical ventilation, and closed-chest circulation methods were integrated and advocated by Safar's landmark publication in 1961, and the first national cardiopulmonary resuscitation (CPR) guidelines were published.[35–37]

Modern CPR became an international standard of practice necessary for hospital personnel, not just emergency squads. Resuscitation tools were initially only used by rescue teams (outside the hospital). Special procedures such as intubation or mechanical ventilation were not performed outside the operating or recovery room. Safar collaborated with **Åsmund Laerdal** to have a Norwegian card and toy manufacturer produce the Resusi Anne manikin to allow simulator training for medical personnel and the lay public. Advances in the science of and effective instrumentation for cardiac defibrillation with direct current closely followed.[38] Safar and others recognized the need for specialized resuscitation equipment and skills in critical care to be made rapidly available to any hospitalized patient. He developed both the first intensive care unit and intensivist physician-training program in the United States. He also was active in early medical disaster planning.[39]

Direct oral endotracheal intubation became an essential skill and the advanced airway of choice following bag-mask ventilation. More frequent and larger numbers of intubated patients resulted in significant complications from high-pressure cuffs. Improved design and plastic compounds quickly reduced the occurrence of this complication.

Dr. **Archie Brain** developed the laryngeal mask airway in the mid-1980s. He also developed the Mallampati system for identifying potentially difficult intubation candidates.[40,41] These concepts were incorporated into the American Society of Anesthesiology's first publication of a difficult airway algorithm in 1993.[42] In 1985, equipment and procedures for the percutaneous dilatational tracheostomy, a variant of the standard surgical tracheotomy, were developed that could be performed in an intensive care setting.[43]

Operation Iraqi Freedom was the last military campaign by the United States that used the MASH. New approaches employed in Iraq and Afghanistan included better body armor, updated frontline kits to treat hemorrhage and pneumothorax, and combat surgical hospitals (CSH). The severely injured could then immediately be sent in flying-ICUs to comprehensive military hospitals in Germany with respiratory therapists as part of those medical flight teams. Soldiers finally were transported to U.S. hospitals for definitive and rehabilitative care.

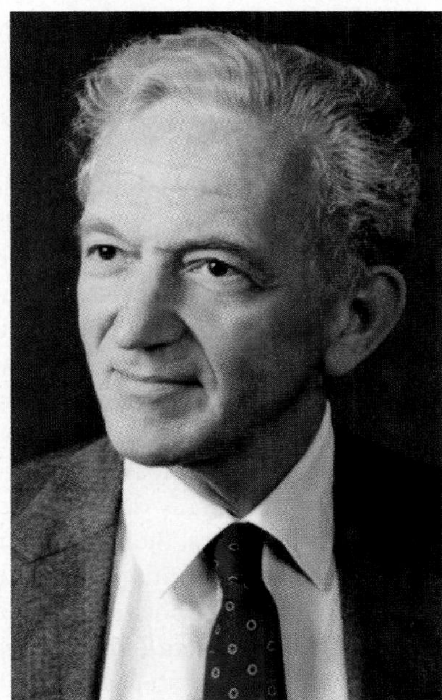

FIGURE 56-24 Dr. Peter Safar is recognized as the father of CPR for his research, promotion, and teaching of both cardiopulmonary resuscitation and intensive care practice.

Courtesy of the Safar Center for Resuscitation Research, University of Pittsburgh.

Mechanical Ventilation

A complete historical review of mechanical ventilation is beyond the scope of this chapter.[43–45] Mechanical ventilating devices that were more than fireplace bellows began appearing in the mid-1800s. Most early devices, such as the Woillez 1876 Spirophone (**Figure 56-25**), followed a physiologic approach, using a body-enclosing chamber and bellows to create subatmospheric pressure. The head was allowed to protrude. A sealing membrane around the neck allowed pressure to be applied only to the chest. The problems of providing

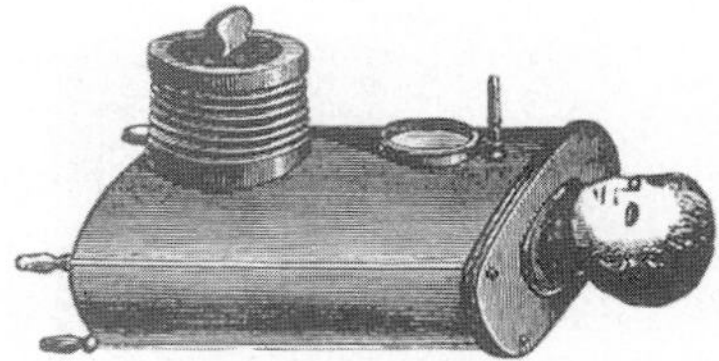

FIGURE 56-25 Woillez's Spirophone negative pressure ventilator (circa 1876).

This article was published in Morch ET. History of mechanical ventilation. In: Kirby RR, Banner MJ, Downs JB, eds. *Clinical Applications of Ventilatory Support.* Copyright Elsevier (Churchill Livingstone) 1990.

and maintaining an artificial airway were avoided. Because problems of patient access prevented using such devices for any surgical application, German surgeon Ernst Sauerbruch developed a negative pressure-operating chamber in 1904.

The difficulty of transporting negative pressure devices prompted early development of positive pressure resuscitators for use by rescue squads. The operating room and the ambulance became the early incubators for positive pressure ventilator development. The Fell-O'Dwyer apparatus (circa 1888; **Figure 56-26**) combined a metallic laryngeal tube and a foot-operated bellows. In 1907, German inventor Heinrich Dräger patented his Pulmotor (**Figure 56-27**). Henry Janeway constructed an anesthesia machine capable of automatic ventilation by 1910.[44,45]

The poliomyelitis pandemic signaled both the heyday of the iron lung and its demise. A variable pattern of polio events occurred in America and Europe (**Figure 56-28**). An early epidemic in New York in 1916 prompted **Philip Drinker**, Charles McKhann, and Louis Shaw to develop the first iron lung at Harvard in Boston by 1928 (refer to Figure 56-28B). It became the most widely used iron lung, costing $1500 (the price of a modest home in those days). In 1932, **John H. Emerson** constructed his version, which had an optional transparent dome to provide positive pressure ventilation while the device was opened for patient care (refer to Figure 56-28A).[46]

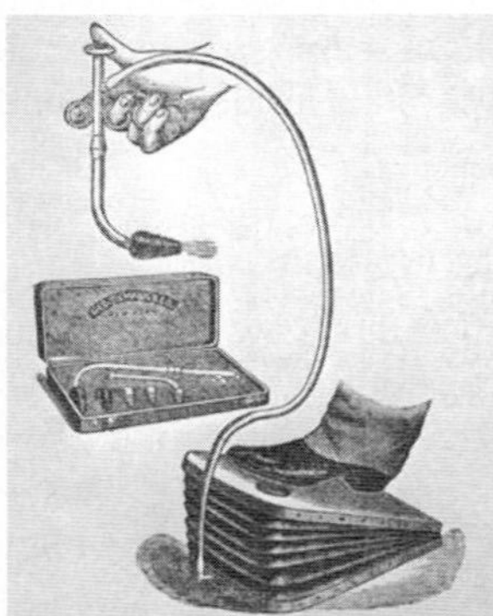

FIGURE 56-26 Fell-O'Dwyer bellows and endotracheal intubating device (circa 1888).

This article was published in Morch ET. History of mechanical ventilation. In: Kirby RR, Banner MJ, Downs JB, eds. *Clinical Applications of Ventilatory Support*. Copyright Elsevier (Churchill Livingstone) 1990.

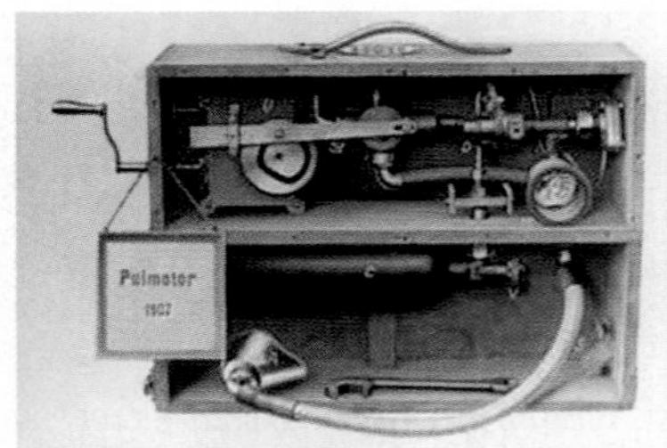

FIGURE 56-27 Drager Pulmotor (circa 1907).

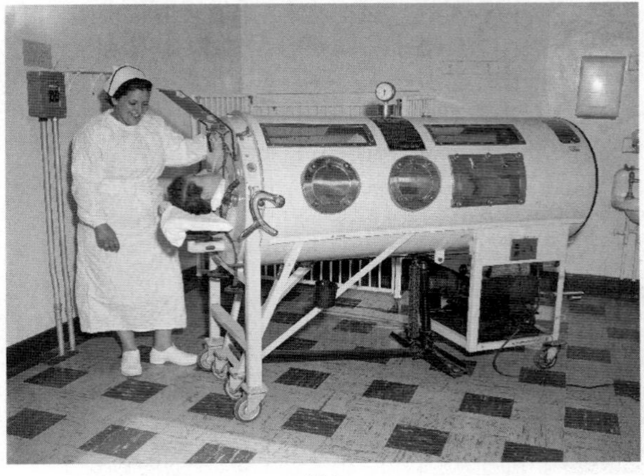

(A)

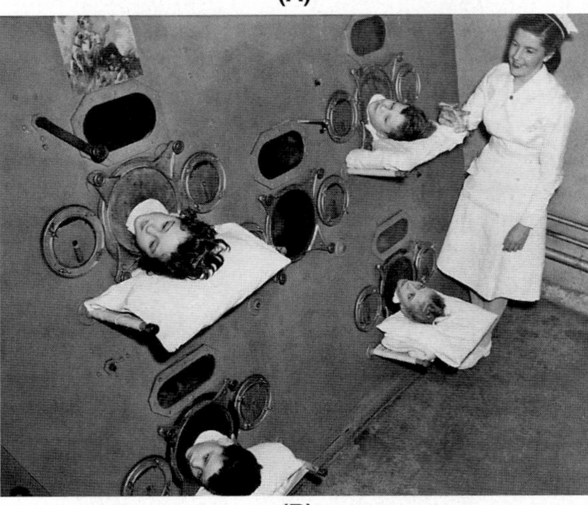

(B)

FIGURE 56-28 (**A**) Emerson iron lung. (**B**) A nurse at Children's Hospital in Boston, Massachusetts, in 1938 shown tending to young polio patients lying in a four-place iron lung room, which was developed by Philip Drinker. Their bodies were contained inside the room; falling then rising pressure allowed their lungs to inhale and exhale, respectively.

(**A**) Courtesy of CDC; (**B**) courtesy of Boston Children's Hospital Archives, Boston, Massachusetts.

Significant numbers of polio patients developed respiratory muscle paralysis with or without bulbar involvement. Many urban hospitals were faced with caring for long-term patients. Facilities such as Rancho Los Amigos Rehabilitation Center were established (**Figure 56-29**). The Scandinavian countries were hit hard by polio in the early 1950s. The main hospital serving Copenhagen, Denmark, which previously had only three negative pressure devices, was faced with ventilating up to 70 patients daily during the summer of 1952. Physicians such as Drs. Bjorn Ibsen and H. C. Lassen were pioneers in abandoning the iron lung in place of anesthesia methods of positive pressure ventilation with artificial airways (cuffed tracheostomy). Lassen's simple device incorporated a humidifier, a canister of soda lime for CO_2 absorption, and valves for administration of 50% oxygen from a high-pressure gas cylinder (**Figure 56-30**). A rubber bag allowed manual ventilation by personnel such as medical students.[47]

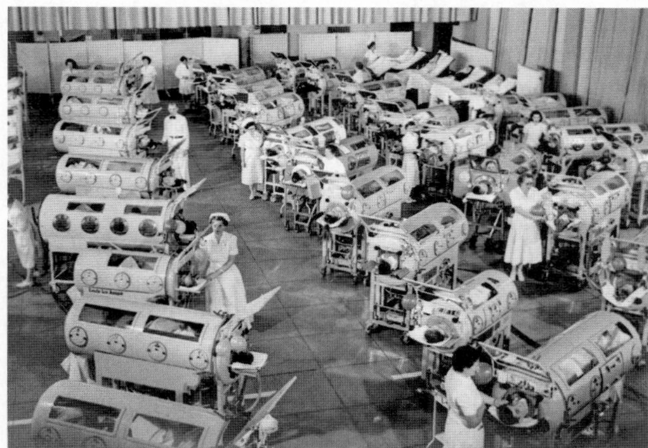

FIGURE 56-29 Polio ward at Rancho Los Amigos Rehabilitation Center, California (circa 1952). Various-sized Drinker iron lungs can be seen. The angled plates above patients' heads contained a mirror to allow patients to observe their surroundings.
Courtesy of Rancho Los Amigos National Rehabilitation Center/LADHS.

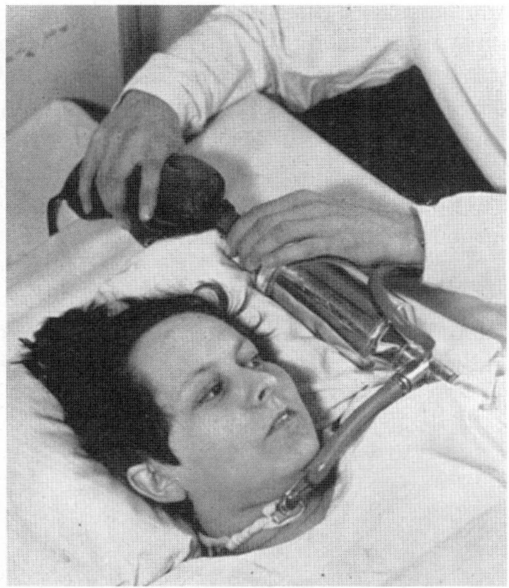

FIGURE 56-30 H. C. Lassen's manual positive pressure ventilation was used for polio patients in Copenhagen, Denmark, when negative pressure became unavailable.
Reproduced from Elsevier, reprinted from *Management of Life Threatening Poliomyelitis*, Lassen, © 1956 Livingstone.

The experience with long-term ventilators for polio patients underscored the importance of preventing pulmonary complications, largely pneumonia. Secretion clearance in the form of suctioning, frequent turning, and postural drainage was used to prevent pneumonia.

Skin care and frequent turning helped prevent pressure ulcers. In Europe and America, automated ventilators were developed rapidly. Besides interest in their use in long-term care, there was increasing interest in their use in the operating room. Positive pressure ventilation was also used for prophylactic postoperative care following thoracic and cardiac surgery.[46]

During the German occupation of Denmark in 1942, Dr. Ernst Trier Mørch developed a piston device using scavenged sewer pipe for the cylinder. After World War II, he immigrated to the United States, where Mueller, Inc., manufactured his refined designs in Chicago by 1953. The Mørch III (**Figure 56-31**) maintained his original rotary piston design, fitting under the bed in a polio ward. It also was adapted for use in the ICU. In Denmark, Dr. C. Bang developed a ventilator that used a solenoid valve that cycled to interrupt minute volume gas flow to provide a tidal volume.[48,49] Around this same time, the Swedish Engstrom ventilator was developed for application in either the operating room or respiratory unit. In Germany, the Dräger Company developed the Poliomat in 1951 and the Spiromat by 1958. British anesthesiologists adept at mechanical tinkering came up with a range of devices in the early 1950s, including the Beaver, Blease, Radcliffe, and Clevedon ventilators. The polio experience also allowed physiologic research to help guide selection of ventilatory parameters. The Radford nomogram provided a scientific basis for estimating initial selection of tidal volume and rate. Edward P. Radford predicted tidal volumes in the 7 to 8 mL/kg range for polio patients who typically had normal lung mechanics.[50]

In contrast to the Europeans, who used a mechanical approach with pistons or concertina bags, Americans initially favored positive pressure using pressure valves often spawned from World War II military applications (**Figure 56-32**). **V. Ray Bennett's** (Figure 56-32A) Ben X-2 flow-sensing valve had been used to deliver oxygen

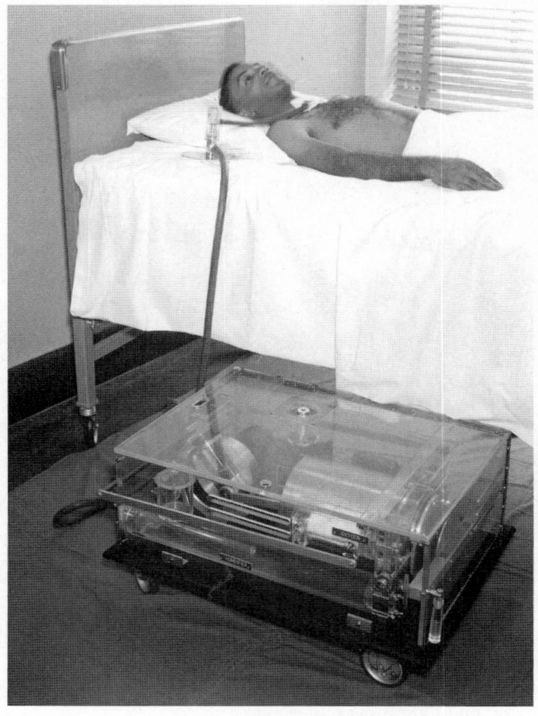

FIGURE 56-31 Mørch III piston ventilator (circa 1953).
Courtesy of Sys Trier Morch.

in unpressurized aircraft. He incorporated the valve into the TV-2P assister and BA-2 anesthesia machine in 1948. **Dr. Forrest Bird** (Figure 56-32B) introduced the clinical magnetic respirator in 1951. With the addition of automatic cycling mechanisms, the Bird Mark 7 and the Mark 4 anesthesia version were available in 1956 and 1959, respectively. The Bennett PR-1 and PR-2 were in large-scale production after 1961. The Bird and Bennett positive pressure ventilators were often the first post–iron lung ventilators in newly formed inhalation therapy departments in the United States.

The importance of volume-controlled ventilation became a dominant theme about the same time that intensive care units were undergoing their rapid growth phase in the 1960s. J. H. Emerson (**Figure 56-33**) took the lead in 1964 with the manufacture of his rotary piston volume- and time-controlled 3-PV ventilator. A fleet of American ICU workhorses soon followed, including the Puritan Bennett MA-1 (1967), Ohio 560 (1968), Ohio/Monaghan 225 (1972), and Bourns Bear I (1975). By the mid- to late 1960s arterial blood gas electrodes had become available in most hospitals. This technology provided the ability to monitor both ventilation and oxygenation. Anesthesiologists developed a new awareness of the hypoxemia-causing effects of intraoperative atelectasis, which was initially treated by increasing tidal volume to 10 to 15 mL/kg. Unfortunately, that approach was indiscriminately transferred from the OR to the ICU for all patients, including those with diseased or injured lungs.[51,52] The Vietnam War provided further insight into critical care medicine. Drs. David Ashbaugh, **Thomas Petty** (**Figure 56-34**), and Boyd Bigelow published their landmark paper on acute respiratory distress syndrome (ARDS) in 1967, and the use of positive end-expiratory pressure (PEEP) soon followed.[53–55]

In perinatal and pediatric medicine, **Dr. Virginia Apgar** (1909–1974; **Figure 56-35**) developed her scoring system for newborns in 1956. In the 1970s, research on fetal lambs elucidated the cause of respiratory distress syndrome in infants. Soon CPAP systems were

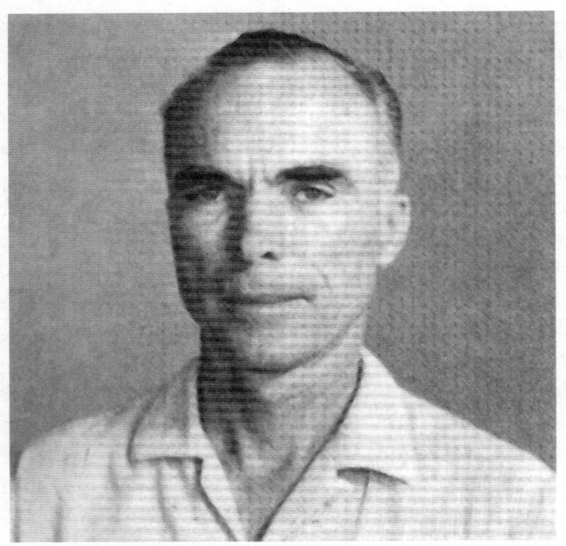

(A)

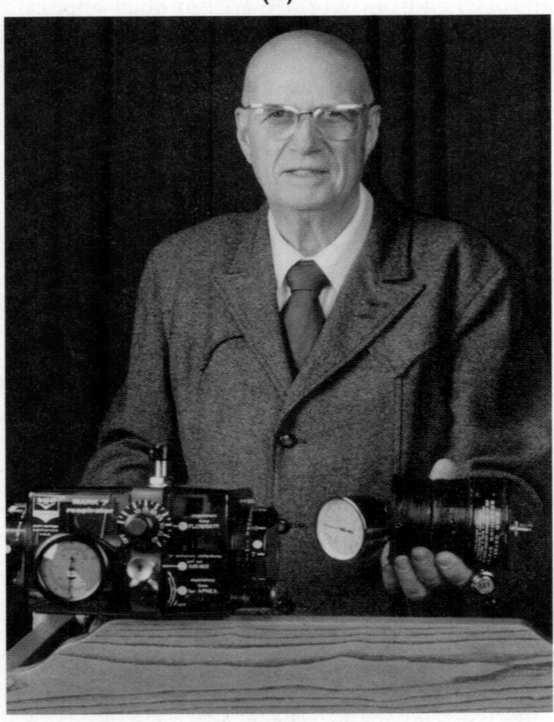

(B)

FIGURE 56-32 (**A**) V. Ray Bennett, developer of the flow-sensitive valve used on early Puritan-Bennett assistors and anesthesia machines. (**B**) Dr. Forrest Bird, shown holding his original magnetic device (right) and a Bird Mark 7 (left).

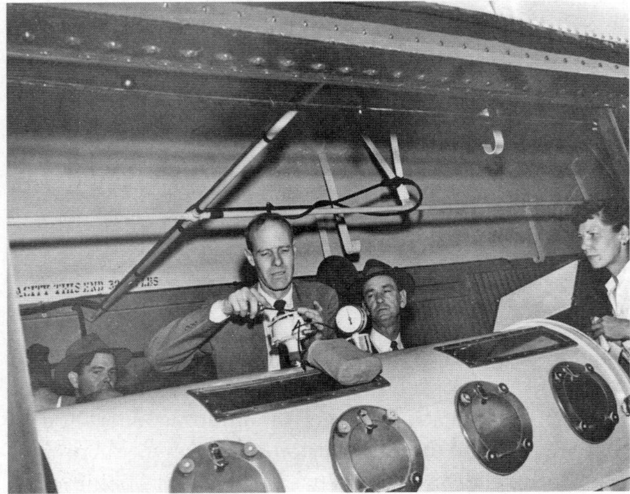

FIGURE 56-33 J. H. (Jack) Emerson was a notable inventor of mechanical ventilators. He is shown working on his version of the iron lung (circa 1932), which was less costly and lighter weight than the Drinker. He also invented an early positive pressure piston-driven (3-PV) ventilator in 1964 that became one of the early workhorses. He later modified that device for IMV in the 1970s.

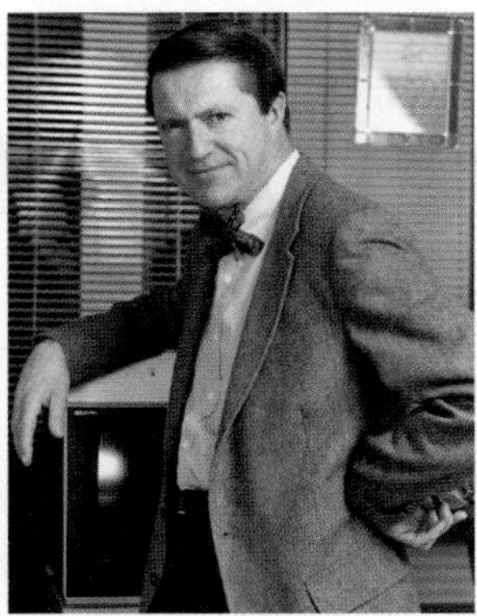

FIGURE 56-34 Dr. Thomas Petty, pulmonologist who coauthored the initial publications on acute respiratory distress syndrome, positive end-expiratory pressure, and the benefits of long-term oxygen therapy.
Courtesy of Louise Nett.

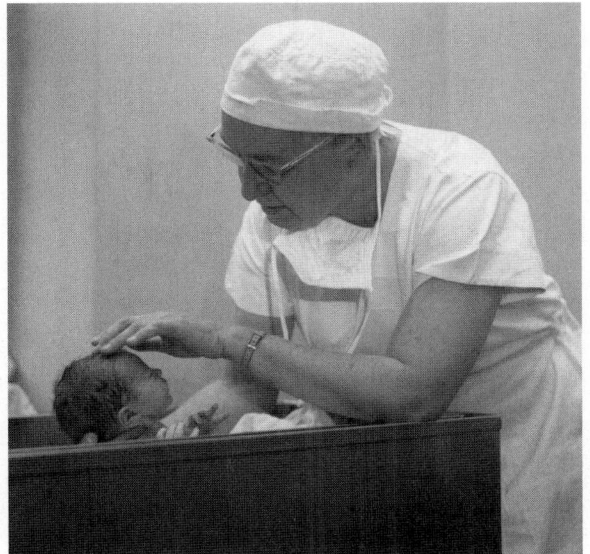

FIGURE 56-35 Dr. Virginia Apgar developed a newborn infant scoring system based on physical assessment to aid in guiding care in the delivery room.
© Archives & Special Collections, Columbia University Health Sciences Library; photograph by Elizabeth Wilcox.

promoted by Gregory.[55] Exogenous surfactant therapy followed. Ventilators specifically designed for infants began to appear. In 1964, Bourns Inc. developed a linear piston-driven infant volume ventilator, the LS104-150. However, intermittent mandatory ventilation with PEEP/CPAP, developed by Kirby, evolved to be the standard of practice. Kirby collaborated with Bird in the development of the Baby Bird in 1971.[56] Similar ventilators, such as the Bourns PB-200, Bear Cub, and Sechrist IV-100B, became familiar sights in neonatal ICUs, along with respiratory therapists with specialized skills.

Adult and perinatal/pediatric mechanical ventilators have evolved steadily (**Table 56-2**). Technology advancements, first in printed circuits and later in microprocessors, have allowed manufacturers to usher in new operational characteristics (modes), improved breathing valve response, and enhanced monitoring and alarm capabilities. The 1960s classification system devised by Mushin was updated by respiratory therapist Robert Chatburn.[57] In contrast to the many modes of ventilation, there have been few changes that have translated into decreased morbidity and mortality.

In the mid-1980s, the use of noninvasive ventilation (NIV) for patients with either acute exacerbations of COPD or neurologic respiratory failure was proposed.[58] Over time, NIV modes have become the standards of practice. In addition, improved diagnosis of sleep-disordered breathing resulted in a phenomenal increase in the use of nasal CPAP for obstructive sleep apnea (OSA) and of NIV for patients with a central component. Advances in mask design, CPAP generators, and ventilators to meet those needs have rapidly occurred in the past few years.[58,59] Alternative ventilator modes, such as airway pressure release ventilation (APRV), first appeared in 1987.[60] Ventilator manufacturers have aggressively marketed newer modes. Dual-control models permit switching from pressure or volume control. Weaning modes include auto mode, proportional assist ventilation, adaptive support ventilation, and automatic tube compensation.[61]

Animal studies and a multicenter human study by the Acute Respiratory Distress Syndrome Network (ARDSnet) resulted in a major rethinking of tidal volume size during mechanical ventilation.[62,63] Reducing the tidal volume from 12 mL/kg to 6 mL/kg can provide lung-protection and reduce mortality. Use of high-frequency modes such as high-frequency oscillatory ventilation (HFO) has seen greater acceptance for use with premature infants.[64] Its use for adults with ARDS has not demonstrated significant outcome differences. Adjuncts such as prone positioning and the use of inhaled nitric oxide have shown some benefit to improve oxygenation in ARDS patients. Research continues to better identify which patients might benefit most.[65]

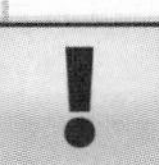

Respiratory Recap

Historical Developments in Respiratory Care

- Clinical medical gas therapy
- Pulmonary diagnostics: spirometry and lung volume measurement
- Medicated aerosol therapy
- Modalities to prevent atelectasis and pulmonary secretion retention
- Airway management: intubation and tracheostomy care
- Patient–mechanical ventilator management
- Critical care monitoring
- Cardiopulmonary rehabilitation
- Case management for asthma, COPD, and cystic fibrosis

TABLE 56-2
Adult and Infant Ventilator Development

Year Introduced	Brand/Model	Year Introduced	Brand/Model
1907	Dräger Pulmotor	1984	Sechrist Adult 2200B
1948	Bennett TV-2P	1985	Bear Medical Bear 5
1951	Engstrom 150	1985	Ohmeda CPU
1953	Dräger Poliomat	1986	Hamilton Veolar
1953	Thompson portable	1986	Bird 6400 ST
1954	Morch III	1986	Infrasonics Infant Star
1956	Bird MK-7	1988	Bear Medical Bear 3
1956	Emerson Assistor	1988	Hamilton Amadeus
1958	Dräger Spiromat	1988	Bird 8400 ST
1961	Bennett PR-1	1988	Respironics S/T D-30
1963	Air Shields 1000	1989	Bunnell Life Pulse
1964	Emerson Post-op 3-PV	1989	PPG Irisa/Drager Evita
1964	Bourns LS104-150	1989	Infrasonics Adult Star
1967	Puritan-Bennett MA-1	1991	Siemens Servo 300
1968	Ohio 560	1993	Bear Medical Bear 1000
1968	Engstrom ER 300	1993	Dräger Evita
1970	Veriflow CV 2000	1996	Respironics Vision
1970	Hamilton Standard PAD-1	1997	Dräger Evita 2 Dura
1971	Siemens 900	1998	Hamilton Galileo
1972	Monaghan 225 fluidic	1998	Puritan Bennett 840 & 740
1972	Baby Bird	2001	Siemens Servo-i (now Maquet)[i]
1972	Bird IMV	2001	Respironics Esprit
1973	Chemtron Gill 1	2001	Viasys/Cardinal Health Vela
1974	Emerson 3-MV	2001	Dräger Savina
1974	Searle VVA	2001	Newport Medical e500
1974	Ohio 560 fluidic	2001	Pulmonetics LTV 1000
1975	Bourns Bear I	2002	Viasys/Cardinal Health Avea
1976	Forreger 210	2003	Dräger Evita XL
1978	Puritan Bennett MA-2 & MA-2+2	2005	GE Datex-Ohmeda Engström Carestation
1980	Engstrom Erica	2006	Hamilton Medical Raphael
1980	Respironics BiPAP	2007	Hamilton Medical G-5
1982	Siemens 900C	2010	Phillips Healthcare V-60 & V-200
1982	Bear Medical Bear 2	2013	Maquet Servo-U
1983	Biomed IC-5 Microprocessor	2014	Coviden-Puritan Bennett 980
1984	Puritan Bennett 7200		

Milestones in the Organizations Within the Respiratory Care Profession: Beginning Years

In 1943, Chicago-based otolaryngologist **Albert H. Andrews** (**Figure 56-36**) wrote a monograph entitled *Manual of Oxygen Therapy Techniques* in which he proposed that formal hospital departments of inhalation therapy should be established. Inhalation therapy departments would function under the medical direction of a knowledgeable staff physician. Pulmonologist Edwin R. Levine and anesthesiologist Max Sadov (Figure 56-36) joined Andrews to teach every 2 weeks for a 9-month period. They realized the importance of both scientific background and a well-organized inhalation therapy hospital department. Early oxygen technicians were employed through central supply or the orderly staff. Their job was to ensure that oxygen cylinders with functioning regulators and flow meters were available on demand for the bedside care of postsurgical patients who needed masks or oxygen tents.

A core group formed, consisting of Chicago-based oxygen technicians, from Michael Reese and Alexian Brothers Hospitals, and nurse anesthesia students from area schools. The founders organized the Inhalational Therapy Association (ITA) on July 13, 1946, at the University of Chicago Hospital. It became apparent that much work was needed to gain financial support and to devise a systematic approach for developing an infrastructure for a national organization, an educational system, and a method for awarding a credential. On April 5, 1947, articles of incorporation for chartering this nonprofit organization were filed with the Illinois secretary of state. The mission statement, which suggested fostering a cooperative relationship with physicians and the need to advance the art and science of inhalation therapy through education, is summarized:

- To promote higher standards in methods and the professional advancement of members of the association
- To create mutual understanding and cooperation among the technicians, physicians, and all others working in the interest of individual or public health
- To advance the knowledge of inhalation therapy through institutes, lectures, and other means under the sponsorship of physicians
- To grant certificates of qualification to individuals who have completed educational requirements

There were 59 charter members, including pharmacists, nurse anesthetists, nurses, inhalation therapy department managers, an attorney, a member of the oxygen medical industry, and nine physicians. George A. Kneeland served as chairman. Brother Roland Maher, a nurse anesthetist, served as assistant chairman (**Figure 56-37**). Drs. Andrews, Levine, and Sadov served as medical advisors for the next 9 years.[1,66]

In 1948, the fledgling group changed its name to the Inhalation Therapy Association. To act on its mission statement, a quarterly newsletter entitled the *ITA Bulletin* was published from 1950 to mid-1954 and sent

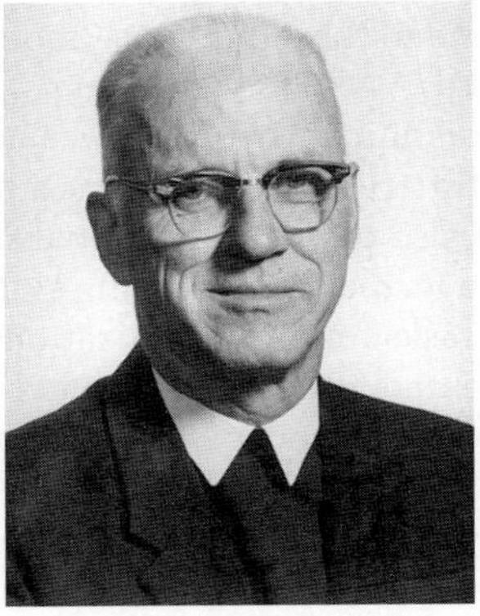

FIGURE 56-37 Brother Roland Maher was the second president of the Inhalational Therapy Association (ITA). He worked at Alexian Brothers Hospital in Chicago. He served as president from 1949 to 1951 and from 1953 to 1954.

Courtesy of the American Association for Respiratory Care.

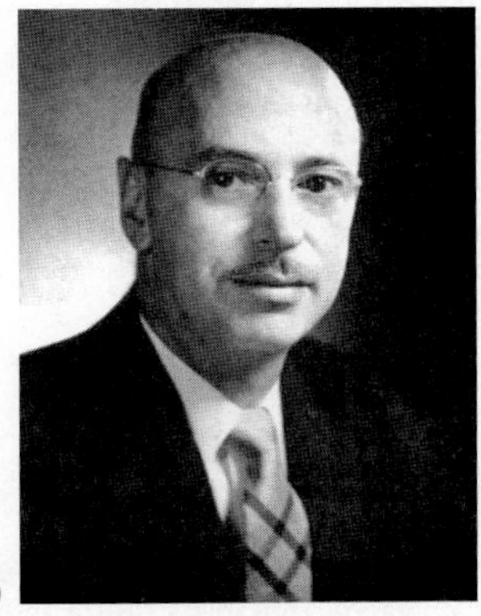

(A)

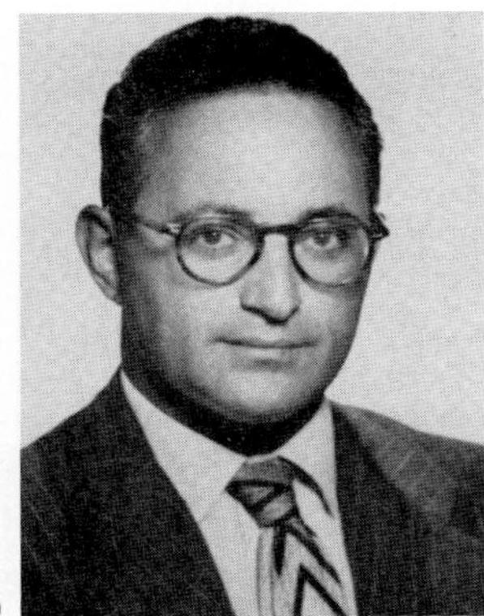

(B)

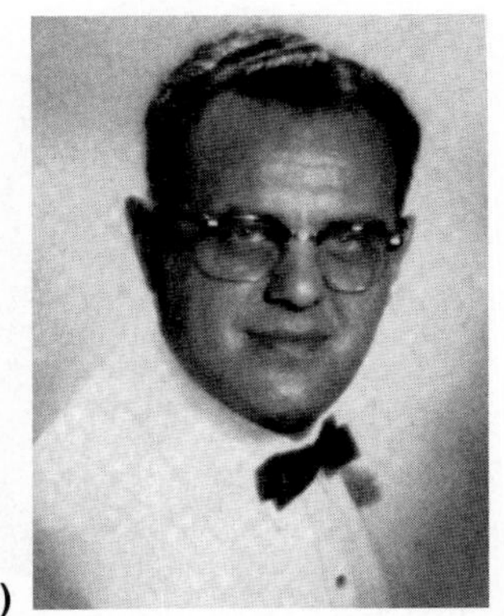

(C)

FIGURE 56-36 (**A**) Dr. Albert Andrews Jr., (**B**) Dr. Edwin Levine, and (**C**) Dr. Max Sadov were physicians in the Chicago metropolitan area who promoted education for those who provided oxygen therapy.

(**A, B, C**) Reproduced from *Inhalation Therapy.* 1956;1:19. Reprinted with permission from Respiratory Care and the American Association for Respiratory Care.

to 1500 U.S. hospitals free of charge. Also in 1950, the ITA began sponsoring a series of lectures and workshops. The first glimpse of credentialing was the awarding of 31 certificates to those who had attended 16 of the workshops. In the following year, a more formal 5-day workshop was cosponsored with the American College of Chest Physicians (ACCP).

In 1954 membership grew to over 200 members, representing 14 states. The national scope was reflected in a name change to the American Association of Inhalation Therapists (AAIT). Because of the increasing need for administrative management, in 1956 the association's president, Sister Mary Borromea, OSF, CRNA, hired a public relations firm to manage the association's business affairs. Albert Carrière (**Figure 56-38**), a principal in the firm, was named the first executive director of the AAIT and served until 1967. The profession established a code of ethics in 1958. To broaden the base of governance, in 1966 the AAIT established its House of Delegates. In 1972 the association changed its name to the American Association for Respiratory Therapy (AART) to better reflect changing medical practice, which had come to include pulmonary and cardiovascular diagnostics. In 1982, the professional association changed its name to the American Association for Respiratory Care (AARC).

The initial mission of the AAIT was not only to establish an infrastructure to serve as a professional association but also to provide national standards for education and a formal credentialing system. These were daunting tasks for one organization, however, and also held a potential for conflicts of interest. This set the stage for two other independent organizations to assist the AAIT as part of an educational system and credentialing board. Education took a step forward when Drs. Alvan Barach, Edwin Emma, and Vincent Collins published formalized minimum standards for training programs in 1950. They received support from the Committee on Public Health Relations of the New York Academy of Medicine. In the document, they specified a curriculum and conditions of training. They noted that in most medical schools, inhalation therapy was rarely part of the curriculum.[67]

The first hospital-based training programs were in place by 1960, as it became apparent that a formal system for school accreditation was necesary. The Board of Schools (BOS) was formed under the American Medical Association (AMA) Council on Medical Education and Hospitals (CMEH) in 1963. The board was composed of two members from each of the sponsoring physician organizations (the ACCP and the American Society of Anesthesiologists [ASA]) and three representatives from the AAIT. In early 1964, the first survey teams began evaluating training programs. Over the years the accreditation group has evolved; currently, that function is the mission of the Commission for Accreditation of Respiratory Care (CoARC).

By November 1960, the credentialing portion of the tripartite system was formalized. A core group of three ITA members along with three physicians formed the American Registry of Inhalation Therapists (ARIT). The initial plan was for a written exam and a set of two oral exams. The group's exam standards were purposely quite rigorous because of the modest educational requirements compared with other allied health professions. The rigor was also attributed to the significant responsibility a respiratory therapist has for a patient's life. The first executive group consisted of Dr. Albert Andrews, president; Dr. Duncan Holiday, vice president; Sr. Mary Yvonne Jenn (**Figure 56-39**), registrar; and Jim Whitacre, secretary. Twelve candidates passed the first pilot exam in 1960. Because the ARIT was not legally incorporated until January 1961, the first group of 28 registered respiratory therapists (RRT) was awarded their credentials after a second session of examinations in April of that year. Like the AIT, the ARIT has had a series of name changes. In 1975 it became the National Board for Respiratory Therapy (NBRT), and in 1983 it took its current title as the National Board for Respiratory Care (NBRC).

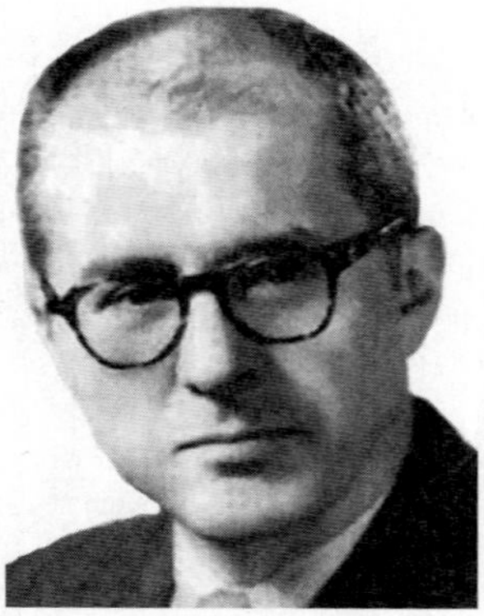

FIGURE 56-38 Albert Carrière, first executive director of the AAIT (from 1955 to 1966).

Reproduced from *Inhalation Therapy.* 1960;5:19. Reprinted with permission from RESPIRATORY CARE and the American Association for Respiratory Care.

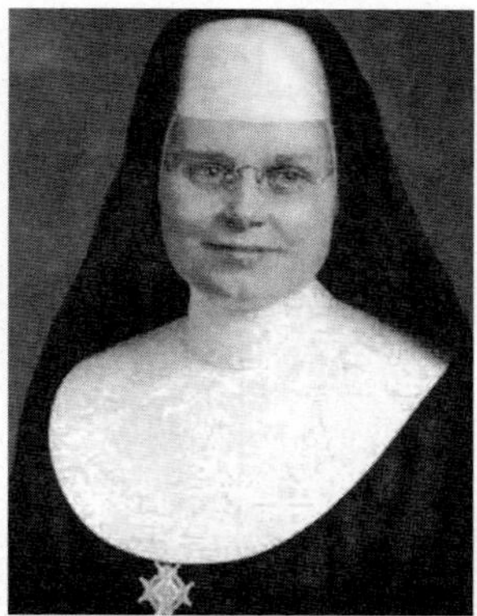

FIGURE 56-39 Sister Mary Yvonne Jenn, BS, RN, first registrar of the American Registry of Inhalation Therapists (ARIT) and registered therapist number 1.

Reproduced from *Inhalation Therapy.* 1956;1:17. Reprinted with permission from RESPIRATORY CARE and the American Association for Respiratory Care.

Professional Publications

Since the early days of the quarterly *ITA Bulletin* (1950–1954), the professional association has supported publications for its members to stay informed of association news. Its news magazine, *AARC Times*, began in 1978. Its peer-reviewed scientific journal, *Inhalation Therapy*, published its first issue in February 1956 (**Figure 56-40**). It featured original research, special articles, journal symposia proceedings, case reports, and teaching cases. The first volunteer editor was James Whitacre, MS, RRT (refer to Figure 56-40A), who served until 1966 when Allan Saposnick, MS, RRT followed him as editor. As the scientific nature of the profession began to mature, the role of the journal became more important and the role of editor more demanding. In 1971 the journal was renamed RESPIRATORY CARE. Philip Kittredge became the first full-time staff therapist editor (Figure 56-40B). In 1998 Dr. David Pierson became the first physician editor.

Table 56-3 records the journal's editors and their years of service. The journal is a major international publication that is focused on respiratory care. Its special proceedings and consensus conferences publish the work of world-class experts in specific content areas. These have tremendous value to the entire field of cardiopulmonary medicine. In 2000, the journal was included in *Index Medicus*. This recognition validated the steadily increasing level of scholarship and quality of scientific research within the respiratory care profession. It also documented that respiratory therapy professionals clearly understood that professional journalism is an attribute of a medical professional. The journal has also increased the submission of original research from a broader base of practitioners through its sponsorship of Open Forum abstract presentations at the annual AARC International Congress.

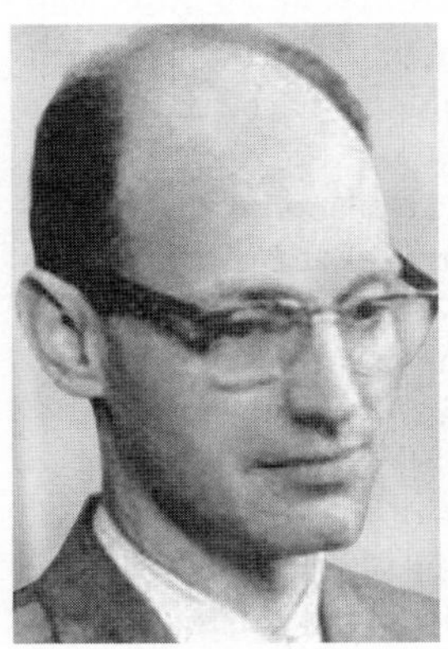

(A)

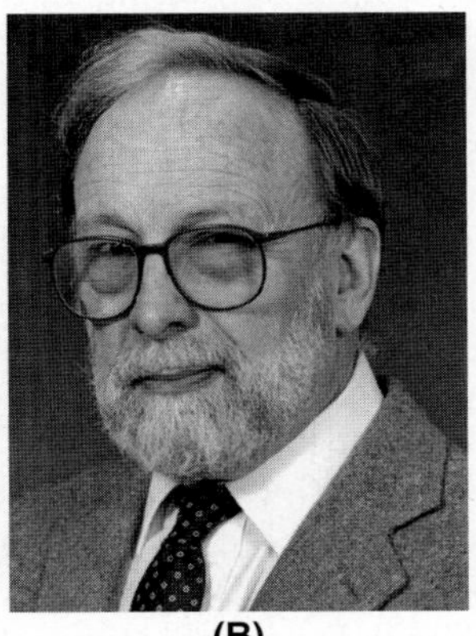

(B)

FIGURE 56-40 (**A**) James F. Whitacre, MS, RRT, first secretary of the American Registry of Inhalation Therapists (ARIT) and first editor of *Inhalation Therapy: Journal of the American Association of Inhalation Therapists*. (**B**) Phil Kittredge, BA, RRT, second editor of RESPIRATORY CARE (1968–1986). He coedited with Pat Brougher, BA, RRT, from 1987 to 1989.

(**A, B**) Reproduced from *Inhalation Therapy*. 1964;9:15. Reprinted with permission from RESPIRATORY CARE and the American Association for Respiratory Care.

TABLE 56-3
Editors of the AARC Scientific Journal *Respiratory Care*

Years	Editor(s)
1956–1966	James F. Whitacre, MS, RRT
1967–1968	Alan Saposnick, MS, RRT
1969–1986	Philip Kittredge, BA, RRT
1987–1989	Philip Kittredge, BA, RRT, and Pat Brougher, BA, RRT
1990–1997	Pat Brougher, BA, RRT
1998–2007	David J. Pierson, MD
2008–	Dean R. Hess, PhD, RRT

History of the Credentialing Organization and State Licensure

Credentialing is a generic term that refers to recognition of individuals who have attained a specified level of competency in an occupation. The two major forms of credentialing are by voluntary national certification/registry and by state licensure. The NBRC is the nationally recognized, voluntary credentialing body in respiratory care. Through its examination systems, therapists demonstrate competency. Each state legislature, or state medical board, typically determines laws that define the right to practice, provide title recognition, or require registration/listing of practitioners. At present, Puerto Rico and all U.S. states except Alaska have licensure/registration provisions. In addition to documentation of successful completion and graduation from an accredited respiratory care program, state licensure (in most states) is based on completion of the certified respiratory therapist (CRT) credentialing exam administered by the National Board for Respiratory Care. The registered respiratory therapist (RRT) credential requires completion of a second written exam, as well as a clinical simulation exam.

The history of the profession's two-tiered CRT and RRT system is the source of some controversy and continued discussion. In the 1960s, the leadership of the AARC (then the AAIT) and NBRC (then the ARIT) originally envisioned one registry credential, to be provided via the latter organization. In 1968, however, AAIT president John R. Julius appointed Louise H. Julius to head a committee to undertake the process of both educating and granting a credential for certified inhalation therapy technicians (CITT). It appears there was pressure within the AAIT membership to have some recognition for those who were not able to complete the more rigorous registry exams. It was thought that this could help maintain employment, by having a credential (for the future) if pending state licensure acts were enacted. By the fall of 1969, the AAIT had established a Technician Certification Board (TCB) and established a training process and programs. It administered its first pilot exam to 100 practitioners. This concept was not originally supported by the ARIT.[1]

After significant deliberations, in 1972 the AARC (then the ARRT) transferred the TCB credentialing role to the ARIT. By 1975 the latter began administering its version of the CITT exam. During this time, the U.S. Department of Health, Education, and Welfare conducted a survey of the profession of respiratory therapy.[68] Not surprising, the study found significant overlap in the tasks performed by those with technician and therapist credentials. By 1978 a national job analysis by the NBRC (then NBRT) found a similar employment pattern. With support from the AART, the NBRC agreed to develop an initial written examination that would reflect the tasks and competency level required of all candidates for entry to practice. Successful completion would allow certification. After a 6-month interval, completion of a second set of exams (written and clinical simulation) would allow the registry credential for the advanced practitioner graduates of therapist-level programs. This hierarchical certified-to-registered system was put into place in 1983.

Over the next 20 years, as most states implemented licensure systems, completion of the entry-level (CRT) examination became the criterion. But over that same time period, as job responsibilities became more complex, there has been a gradual decline in the employment demand for CRTs. Currently there are no longer technician-only training programs. Therefore, a decision made in 1968 has resulted in a two-tiered system becoming embedded into the licensure process, even though it was not originally intended by the profession's original leaders in credentialing.[1]

Beginning in 2015, one exam is administered, in contrast to graduates having to take two separate multiple-choice exams for both the entry-level and registered therapist credentials. The level of passing score determines whether the examinee receives only the CRT credential or also qualifies to take the clinical simulation examination to complete the second phase of the registry credential.

In addition to the CRT and RRT credentials, the NBRC currently provides specialty board exams in pulmonary function diagnostics, perinatal/pediatrics, sleep diagnostics, and adult critical care. **Table 56-4** summarizes all NBRC examinations and credentials attained upon successful completion.

TABLE 56-4
National Board for Respiratory Care Examinations

Examinations	Credentials
Primary Examinations	
Therapist multiple choice examination & clinical simulation	Certified respiratory therapist (CRT) Registered respiratory therapist (RRT)
Specialty Examinations	
Entry-level pulmonary function	Certified pulmonary function technologist (CPFT)
Advanced pulmonary function	Registered pulmonary function technologist (RPFT)
Neonatal/pediatric respiratory care	Certified neonatal/pediatric specialist (CRT-NPS) or registered neonatal/pediatric specialist (RRT-NPS)
Sleep disorders	Certified respiratory therapist–sleep disorders specialist (CRT-SDS) or registered respiratory therapist–sleep disorders specialist (RRT-SDS)
Adult critical care	Adult critical care specialist (RRT-ACCS)

History of Respiratory Care Education and Program Accreditation

The Board of Schools (BOS) was charged with reviewing applications for new training programs and conducting site visits to grant approval status. The original members of the BOS were four therapists and three physicians. At that time, schools were primarily based in hospitals. By the 1960s, reports from the National Advisory Health Council, National Advisory Commission on Health Manpower predicted increasing service roles for allied health personnel as well as the need for educators for training programs. In 1963 the BOS was incorporated and placed within the AMA's Council on Medical Education (AMA CME), which served as overseer of accreditation. By 1969 that group approved a minimum program length of 18 months of training. In that same year the BOS was disbanded because of resistance to orienting programs with academic institutions, problems with funding site visits, and continued concerns about the quality of the school accreditation process. Its replacement, the Joint Review Committee for Respiratory Therapy Education (JRCRTE) was incorporated in 1970 and approved by the AMA CME for its role as the national program accreditation agency for respiratory care programs. The first chairman was **H. Fred Helmholz Jr.**, MD (**Figure 56-41**), a representative of the ACCP. He was an experienced cardiopulmonary physiologist, having worked in the Mayo Aero Medical Unit during World War II. During this time, all programs were required to be sponsored by a formally accredited academic institution.

In 1971, the Study of Accreditation of Selected Health Education Programs (SASHEP) was published, which was highly critical of the inconsistency and methods for insuring quality of training programs. A national third-party accreditor with more uniform

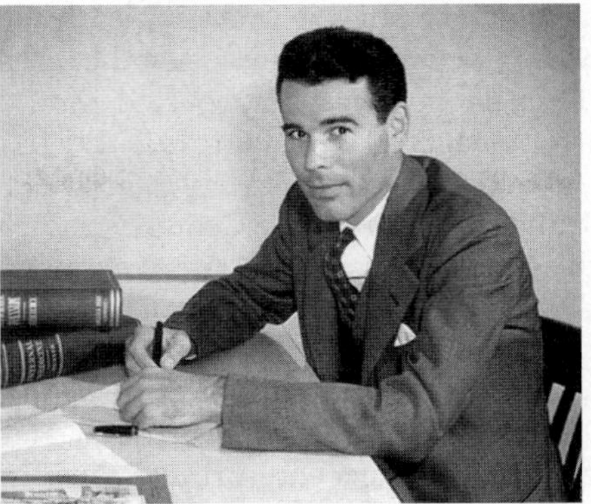

FIGURE 56-41 Dr. H. F. Helmholz Jr. (circa 1942), first chairman of the Joint Review Committee for Respiratory Therapy Education, 1970 to 1976.
Courtesy of the American Association for Respiratory Care.

process was recommended, and in 1977 the AMA CME withdrew and the Committee on Health Education Accreditation (CAHEA) was established under the U.S. Office of Education.

JRCRTE became one of the 25 other allied education review committees under the umbrella accreditor, CAHEA. Upon the retirement of Dr. Helmholz in 1976, the office was moved from Rochester, Minnesota, to the Dallas, Texas, area. Over the years, the process of accreditation has continued to evolve. In 1986, the JRCRTE became the first allied health programmatic accrediting committee to support a focus on outcomes of education. This shift focused on board exam performance rather than the training process. The Essentials and Guidelines have gone through multiple updates to reflect the escalating demands of education and clinical practice experiences.

Following recommendations by a Pew Commission Report, the CAHEA accreditation system was restructured into the Commission on Accreditation of Allied Health Education Programs (CAAHEP) in 1994. In 1994, the AARC experienced difficulties with JRCRTE in the matter of accreditation and withdrew its sponsorship. It temporarily set up a separate Respiratory Care Accreditation Board (RCAB). The concerns were resolved by 1996, and as a result the JRCRTE was renamed the Commission on Accreditation for Respiratory Care (CoARC). In an effort to provide broader and more responsive accreditation service to programs, CoARC withdrew from CAAHEP in 2009 and established itself as an independent accrediting agency under the Council for Higher Education Accreditation (CHEA). Besides members at large and the lay public, other sponsor and representative organizations of CoARC include the AARC, ASA, ATS, ACCP, Association of Schools of Allied Health Professions (ASAHP), and National Network of Health Career Programs in Two-Year Colleges (NN2).

Respiratory care educators have maintained a pragmatic approach in terms of teaching strategies,

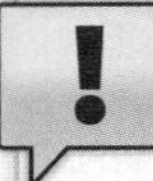

Respiratory Recap

Achievements of the Beginning Years of the Respiratory Care Profession

- Circulation of the foundational documents
- Creation of the professional organization
- Establishment of a professional scientific journal
- Development of the credentialing organization
- Establishment of a system for accreditation of respiratory educational programs

blending classroom, laboratory, and clinical practicums. They have been challenged to adapt curriculum as the scope of practice, responsibilities, and technology continued to escalate, however. Recognizing the need to plan for future change, during 1992 and 1993 the AARC sponsored two educational consensus conferences and supported research on the future scope of the practice and education of therapists.[69,70] The first conference documented those practice demands and the difficulty in providing entry-level education in less than an associate degree's 2-year time frame. The second conference's recommendations resulted in the AARC, JRCRTE, and NBRC all agreeing to set the associate degree as the minimum academic entry level in 2002. This resulted in the decline and eventual closure of training programs at the CRT-only level.

Respiratory Care's Continuing Evolution: Contemporary and Future Changes

This chapter has chronicled the history of respiratory care prior to the establishment of the profession as well as the past 60 years since it officially began in 1947. The original AIT mission statement of caring for patients and supporting the art and science of respiratory care has not changed. However, the technology, scope of practice, and level of responsibility of today's respiratory care practitioners hardly resemble that of the original respiratory therapists who were oxygen orderlies. It is difficult to imagine practicing respiratory care without medical gas supplies, sterile techniques, full-ranging pharmaceuticals, microprocessor-based mechanical ventilators, and Internet communication.

Throughout this period, the demand for therapists exceeded the supply, and the pressure to meet workforce needs may have maintained the lower-division academic degree as compared with other health professions. Respiratory care has evolved from conducting limited, task-based technical functions in 1947 to performing an array of services requiring more complex cognitive abilities and patient management skills in the 21st century. In the early 1990s the AARC sponsored two conferences where the Delphi method was used to summarize experts' forecasts for the profession and steps to realize future projections.[69,70] In 2008, the AARC sponsored a similar process based on a three-part series of conferences with key stakeholder experts to again project how the education and credentialing systems can prepare to meet the evolving roles of the respiratory therapist.[71] Data presented at the first conference documented that respiratory therapists have and will likely become more involved in public health, end-of-life and palliative care, smoking cessation, home care, and sleep diagnostics. Because of increasing pressures to reduce medical costs, responsibility for outpatient case management will likely become a major new role for therapists for patients with asthma, COPD, cystic fibrosis, lung cancer, and pulmonary interstitial fibrosis as well as cardiovascular diseases. Therapists are, and will continue to be, more involved in providing patient education and in coordinating care in cost-effective approaches and multiple settings.

To meet these future needs, educational programs will likely respond by expanding both didactic curricula and clinical practicums beyond the traditional settings. These new responsibilities require additional professional competencies. The roles of both outpatient case manager and respiratory consultant to interdisciplinary hospital teams demand higher levels of communication, assessment abilities, and integrative critical thinking skills to operate within protocols and best-practice consensus guidelines. Besides applying a scientific approach, therapist recommendations need to be individualized based on economic and humanistic (ethical and moral) dimensions.[71–73] Department managers will also need therapists who are multicompetent—bedside caregivers who have added abilities to assist in management tasks, patient and staff development and education, and research. These trends may be reflected in the increasing number of baccalaureate degree programs, which grew from 7 in 1970 to approximately 60 in 2013. There also is more interest in developing postgraduate residency programs, following models of physician and pharmacy education.[74]

In the United States, medical education took a huge step forward with the Carnegie Foundation–commissioned Flexner report.[75] After studying every school in the United States, Abraham Flexner found several different approaches (apprenticeship, proprietary, and university) and vastly different curricula (e.g., scientific, homeopathic, botanical, physiomedical, spiritual). His study revealed some good schools, but also many deplorable schools with incompetent faculty, dismal laboratories, and haphazard clinical experiences, all of which contributed to ill-prepared graduates.

A lack of a scientific approach, without much research-based science, was notable in the early days of inhalation therapy education and practice in spite of school standards and early textbooks on inhalation/respiratory therapy by Drs. Alvan Barach, Peter Safar, and Donald Egan.[76–78] This was clearly identified in 1974 by the first Conference on the Scientific Basis of Respiratory Therapy, supported jointly by the then-National Heart and Lung Institute (NHLI) and the American Thoracic Society (ATS), held at Temple University Conference Center at Sugarloaf in Philadelphia.[79] Prominent scientists nationwide reviewed available evidence (or lack of evidence) for oxygen therapy, aerosol therapy, physical therapy, and IPPB therapy. IPPB therapy, a major clinical task of the 1960s and early 1970s, was scrutinized, and the evidence suggested a vast enterprise of abuse in spite of good science that showed no value of IPPB for conditions such as emphysema.[80] The lesson was clear: the scientific method, not tradition, needed to be applied to respiratory care practice. Physicians and therapists needed to assess patients and perform only justified care with identifiable, measureable outcomes and individualized needs.

This premise was clearly promoted in 1988 in Respiratory Care.[81] By 1992 the term *evidence-based medicine (EBM)* began to appear in the literature.[82] Exponential explosions of medical science, technology, and improved information management have all promoted use of EBM resources. EBM is often defined as a set of principles and methods for conscientious, explicit, and judicious use of mathematical estimates of the risk of benefit and harm, derived from high-quality research on population samples. The purpose is to promote informed clinical decision making both for population-base management and individual patients.[82–85]

In addition, there has been a heightened concern for patient safety and growing demand by the public and governmental agencies for medical accountability. A 1999 report by the Institute of Medicine's (IOM) Quality of Health Care in America Committee, *To Err Is Human: Building a Safer Health System*, revealed a disturbing statistic: between 44,000 and 98,000 patients were dying annually in U.S. hospitals due to preventable medical errors.[86] That report and a 2001 follow-up publication, *Crossing the Quality Chasm: A New Health System for the 21st Century* by (IOM), also reviewed the financial cost of errors; some faults were identified, including overly complex, cumbersome, and uncoordinated systems.[87] That report identified potential aims and set goals for error reduction, and system redesign rules were based on approaches using knowledge that already existed.[87]

An approach to reduce human error has supported increasing use of simulation-based medical education as both a teaching strategy as well as a tool for competency evaluation. Although the military and aviation industries used this approach effectively, medicine embraced this tactic only recently.[88] Because medical care is increasingly being delivered by teams, aviation's flight crew-resource management is increasingly applied through simulation to enhance performance and safety of critical care teams.[89] The evidence of the positive impact of simulation-based medical education has been documented.[90,91] Current standards from the Accreditation Council for Graduate Medical Education (ACGME) have mandated that simulation training be embedded as part of residency training curricula.[92] The U.S. Department of Health and Human Services (HHS) Agency for Healthcare Research and Quality (AHRQ) has developed a comprehensive set of evidence-based training resources for hospitals, clinicians, and professional educators in order to foster safe practice for both individuals and teams. The latter is in the form of comprehensive resources with strategies and tools to enhance team performance and patient safety; they are called TeamStepps.[93]

Mortality data have been studied in an effort to objectively identify major external modifiable (nongenetic) factors that result in death in the United States. For the past 30 years, analysis has revealed several factors that cause fatal diseases related to lifestyle patterns. Smoking remains the leading cause of years lost due to premature mortality and is the major modifiable root problem of the four most common causes of death: (1) heart disease, (2) cancer, (3) stroke, and (4) chronic lower respiratory disease (e.g., COPD). Both lung cancer and COPD are increasing in absolute numbers but declining in age-standardized rates. Early mortality is also related to increasing prevalence of obesity and diabetes due to poor diet and physical inactivity.[94–96] Analysis from 1990 to 2010 has shown that with a huge increase in expenditure of the United states gross domestic product (GDP), life expectancy has increased from 75.2 to 78.2 years.[97] The number of years spent living with disabling health problems has increased from 9.4 to 10.1 years. Despite spending 17.9% of its gross domestic product (GDP) on health care, the highest health expense per capita in high-income countries, the United States ranks 26th in healthy life expectency.[97]

The largest contributors of years living with disabilities are mental and musculoskeletal disorders, which tend to receive less attention and research funding than disorders with less of a burden. Mediocre health outcomes in the United States have been blamed on lack of universal health coverage, inefficiency, and marked disparity across geographic, socioeconomic groups, and race and ethnicity groups. Problems have been compounded by lack of political initiatives on tobacco control and the physical environment.[97]

The clinical practice of respiratory care has also evolved to better identify best evidence, focus on patient safety, and improve value of diagnostics and outcome of therapeutics. This theme began by using committees of therapist and physician experts to systematically review the literature on specific respiratory care practices. The goal was to assist clinicians by making current information readily available so resources for delivering the best care could be disseminated nationally and internationally. In 1991, the AARC began publication of *Clinical Practice Guidelines* (CPGs) in its scientific journal, Respiratory Care. Over 50 types of respiratory care practices have been reviewed and are available on the Respiratory Care website (www.rcjournal.com). More recently, they have been categorized as reference-based expert panel guidelines and evidence-based CPGs.[98] Most CPGs provide citations within an outline formatted text based on indications; contraindications, hazards/complications, limitations; monitoring; and assessment of outcome. Many CPGs provide a final recommendation based on the strength or grade of quality of the current evidence.[99]

Similar approaches have been used by major medical groups and/or professional organizations to guide best practice. In addition to literature-based and/or expert consensus, many have further identified *critical pathways,* also known as care maps or critical paths. They use an algorithm decision-making format to recommend optimal use and sequence/timing of assessment/tests and to guide interventions based on outcomes at various points in the process.[100–106] **Table 56-5** provides examples of both guidelines and critical pathways from other groups involved in respiratory patient care.

In addition to national or international acceptance of clinical pathways, there has been an evolution of *therapist-driven protocols (TDPs)* within medical institutions. The goal of protocol-based care is to enhance patient safety but also increase flexibility for respiratory therapy and nursing staff. Algorithm-like decision plans initiate, modify, or discontinue therapy without detailed physician direction or written orders.

TABLE 56-5
Examples of Consensus/Expert Guidelines and Critical Pathways

- Management of the Difficult Airway [American Society for Anesthesiology (ASA)][100]
- National Asthma Education and Prevention Program. *Expert Panel Report 3: Guidelines for the Diagnosis and Management of Asthma.* [National Institutes of Health, Heart, Lung, and Blood Institute][101]
- Global Strategy for Diagnosis, Management and Prevention of COPD. [Global Initiative for Chronic Obstructive Lung Disease (GOLD)][102]
- 2010 American Heart Association Guidelines for Cardiopulmonary Resuscitation and Emergency Cardiovascular Care Science [American Heart Association (AHA)][103]
- Recommendations for End-of-Life Care in the Intensive Care Unit: A Consensus Statement. [American College of Critical Care (ACCM)][104]
- Clinical Guideline for the Evaluation, Management and Long-term Care of Obstructive Sleep Apnea in Adults. [American Academy of Sleep Medicine (AASM)][105]
- Standardization of Lung Function Testing: General Considerations for Lung Function Testing [American Thoracic Society & European Respiratory Society (ATS/ERS)][106]

TDPs are based on accepted practice but require approval and acceptance by an institution's medical staff. Typically there are predetermined situations in which the protocol specifies that physicians be consulted. Clinical research has documented that expeditious use of TDPs can result in both improved resource utilization and improved quality of care. Areas studied have included weaning from mechanical ventilation, medicated aerosol therapy, and oxygen therapy.[107–112]

The United States' healthcare system is positioned for dramatic changes. The *Affordable Care Act (ACA)* was signed into law in 2010.[113] The hope is to improve access to care for almost 50 million people in the United States (15.7% of the population) who have been uninsured.[114] That population tends to have below average health, is less successful in managing chronic conditions, and tends not to seek medical care when sick or injured. Consequently, lack of insurance has been implicated in annual deaths of approximately 50,000.[114] The cost of caring for the uninsured is either absorbed as charity care or passed on to the insured through higher premiums or to taxpayers through higher taxes. The uninsured tend to see the emergency room as their only safety net.

The *Emergency Medical Treatment and Active Labor Act (EMTALA)*, enacted in 1986, required hospital emergency rooms to treat patients regardless of their ability to pay. But no direct payment mechanism was provided to accompany the law. Indirect payment and reimbursement by federal or state programs have been inadequate; approximately half of all care goes uncompensated. Billing uninsured patients directly as fee-for-service has resulted in overcharging, bankruptcy, and lawsuits. Another aspect of the ACA is to increase accountability and quality by reducing reimbursement to hospitals if patients require readmission within 30 days after discharge. The *Centers for Medicare & Medicaid Services (CMS)* monitor hospitals over a 3-year period for excessive readmission for conditions including acute myocardial infarction, congestive heart failure, and pneumonia.[115]

Similar to surveillance of readmission by Medicare agencies, the *Centers for Disease Control's National Healthcare Safety Network (NHSN)* has implemented an updated reporting system to better follow ventilator-associated events (VAE) of adult patients. This system was initially put in place because of the high risk for complications such as ventilator-associated pneumonia (VAP). Additional problems of sepsis, ARDS, and pulmonary thromboembolism also are now followed; they, too, result in increased cost, extended ICU admission, and poor health outcomes, including death. A more qualitative analysis in the updated version is hoped to improve objectivity of surveillance, since benchmarking of quality in this area is difficult.[116,117]

Just as the governmental agencies have reviewed the evolving changes in medicine, respiratory care's professional groups have continued to assess the capacity to provide a workforce in terms of adequate numbers and preparedness for advancing levels of technology and clinical skills. In 2003, educators within the AARC identified concerns in the difficulty in preparing graduates to meet the increasingly technical tasks and clinical responsibilities within the 2-year associate-degree format. Many of those schools had reached or exceeded length or credit limit of state community college requirements. Although some existing programs had already expanded to a 4-year degree, the report recommended that future programs for entry level be transitioned to the baccalaureate degree, and master's programs should also be made more available.[118]

As the AARC was celebrating its 60th anniversary in 2007, it responded to that concern by initiating a formal process similar to the Carnegie Foundation's Flexner study of U.S. medical schools. In the early 20th century, American medical education was in a state of disarray. Flexner's review transformed mostly mediocre college programs and charlatan-like proprietary apprenticeships into a high-quality scientific-based system. The escalating demand for well-prepared respiratory therapists in the early 1970s paralleled the birth of the U.S. community college system that became the most common training format. Until 2002, respiratory therapy education programs continued to include a mixed bag of 18-month certificate and associate-degree programs that were limited to awarding the certified respiratory therapist; at that time all nonassociate degree CRT-only programs were eliminated. In 2013, the minimum academic level for attaining the therapist credential remains the associate degree.

Three *2015 and Beyond Conferences* were conducted in 2008, 2009, and 2010. Invited participants included representatives from government, education, clinical practice, licensure, credentialing groups, and medical-oriented consumer groups. As previously noted, the first conference identified the expected changes in health care, the medical workforce, and respiratory care. A pending perfect storm was predicted with problems in increasing costs; increased complexity of medical care, technology, and informatics; greater demand for quality; and shortages of all types of healthcare providers.[71] Trends identified a shift from episodic care of acute problems to a greater need for prevention and management of chronic diseases. It was believed that, because of the foundations in physiology, pathophysiology, and applied technology, respiratory therapists could be in a unique position to accept future responsibilities if some additional competencies could be assured.[71]

The second 2015 and Beyond Conference focused on need for expanding competencies. Clinical and education experts reviewed current and future knowledge, skills, and behaviors needed by the graduate respiratory therapists to best maintain and match projected future demands. These included medical and technical knowledge, clinical skills, use of computers, and critical thinking as well as abilities to effectively communicate and interact with teams as they served in both critical care and case management settings.[119] In addition, therapists must be able to evaluate research for application to EBM; have problem-solving skills, the ability to implement protocol-based care, leadership capabilities; and assume roles in multidisciplinary teams. The latter point was underscored as the Affordable Care Act's Section 3506, which encourages greater use of shared decision making in health care.[120] The latter functions are supported by recommendations found in the IOM's report *Crossing the Quality Chasm* and AHRQ's Team STEPPs training resources.[86,93] A 2009 survey of accredited respiratory care programs identified that a majority of baccalaureate programs had imbedded curricula in EBM, research, as well as subclinical specialization.[121]

The third 2015 and Beyond Conference tackled the difficult problem of identifying what changes and approaches would be needed to upgrade both the current workforce and the education and credentialing infrastructure. More advanced education and skills, identified in conferences one and two, would need to be incorporated into school curricula, and both board exams and licensure systems revised.[122] This is a complex issue because of ramifications to the current educational system, program accreditation system, credentialing agency as well as individual state medical licensing boards.

The 2015 third conference attendees reached majority agreement that future demands for career entry will exceed the educational and clinical capability of the traditional 2-year associate degree format. They recommended that additional support and resources be provided to allow the current workforce increased access to baccalaureate and graduate level education. This would include courses and clinical opportunities in areas of subspecialization such as perinatal pediatrics, diagnostics, case management, and critical care.[122]

Other allied health professions have also been faced with challenges as the time needed to teach entry-level professional skills and clinical responsibilities began to exceed constraints imposed by credit limits of academic degrees. Many college or university programs moved to higher degrees as advisory boards responded to needs of local or regional employers. Some professional associations or program accreditation agencies have collaborated on comprehensive approaches to change by mandating new educational requirements. Often this has been done over an extended time with support to transition existing programs or placing a moratorium on starting any new programs under former guidelines. There has been much debate in both respiratory care and nursing on the outcome or value added by requiring longer programs or more advanced degrees for career entry. The Physician Assistant Education Association required all programs to be at the masters level by 2014. Physical therapy, pharmacy, and nurse anesthesia are moving to clinical doctorate degrees.[123,124] Some professions have chosen to require that students complete clinical internships/residencies or fellowships similar to the physician training models.

Like respiratory care, nursing continues to have multiple education levels for professional entry: diploma, associate degree (ADN), and baccalaureate degree (BSN). Approximately 20% complete diploma programs; 45% complete ADN programs; and 34% of nurses complete BSN or higher degrees. Because of the variations in training programs and hospital practice, it is very difficult to document outcome differences between ADN and BSN practitioners. Like respiratory care, nursing does differentiate competency levels versus education and training skills at entry level.[125]

In 2010, an Institute of Medicine (IOM) report cited a need for increased numbers of entry BSN graduates based on similar factors noted in the 2015 and Beyond Conferences; the IOM also recommended a system with more seamless academic and career transition be implemented.[126] Nursing does have well-defined career ladders for advanced practice registered nurses (APRNs) that link education with specific credentials and licensure. These include master's or doctoral degrees with associated examinations for certified nurse midwife (CNM), nurse practitioner (NP), clinical nurse specialist (CNS), and certified registered nurse anesthetist (CRNA). NPs constitute 63% of APRNs.[127] Like nursing, respiratory care remains a profession with significant patient care responsibility levels that for years has hesitated in moving its professional entry education level to the baccalaureate entry level.[122,128] Currently, 56 (8%) of the approximately 435 respiratory care programs in the United States award a baccalaureate degree and four at the master's level. The respiratory care profession does have specialized credentialing exams, but they are not interconnected in an organized way with advanced levels of education in a defined career ladder system.[118]

The 2015 and Beyond Conference identified evidence to guide the profession into the 21st century. Clearly there is a need for better coordination and collaboration between the education, credentialing, and state licensure. To properly evolve, the current educational system will require resources to support access and assist current associate degree graduates and staff

STOP AND THINK

How do you anticipate that the education level and practice of respiratory therapists will evolve in the next 50 years?

therapists to move up both the educational and better organized career ladders. The reimbursement systems (both through hospitals, private insurers, and government) must then appropriately reward competency based on advanced skills and services. The final 2015 Conference recommendations were then sent to the AARC Board of Directors for approval and implementation with its collaborative organizations CoARC and NBRC.[122] Evidence for change has thoughtfully been provided to both nursing and respiratory care by independent groups whose primary interest is in providing high-quality care to patients.[122,126] Unfortunately, history has shown that decisions are influenced by scientific discoveries, governmental policy, political events, personalities, and leadership that may distract from the primary mission of their professions.

The Vision/Mission Statement of the AARC is:

> The American Association for Respiratory Care (AARC) will continue to be the leading national and international professional association for respiratory care. The AARC will encourage and promote professional excellence, advance the science and practice of respiratory care, and serve as an advocate for patients, their families, the public, the profession and the respiratory therapist.[129]

In 1947 the profession of respiratory therapists in the United States started from a handful of oxygen orderlies conducting specific tasks with strict physician direction. In 2009 over 145,000 clinicians were performing diagnostic and therapeutic tasks using protocols and serving as team consultants in the United States.[130] There is also a growing representation in other countries. In 1963, the first group of 28 registered therapists received the registered therapist credential. As of 2013, there were 224,340 registered and 133,875 certified respiratory therapists credentialed by the NBRC, and this number is projected to grow by over 20% in 2020.[131] Informal hospital conferences have evolved into over 435 accredited respiratory therapy educational programs at colleges and universities. The profession's growth reflects both the demand for a wider array of diagnostic and therapeutic services and attraction for entering clinicians who are interested in both challenging technical and interpersonal responsibilities. **Table 56-6** summarizes future changes and challenges identified by the 2015 and Beyond Conferences and related events.

A quote from medical historian Henry Sigerist should set the theme for those who have read this chapter and either have practiced or are about the enter the profession of respiratory care.

> Medical history teaches us where we came from, where we stand in medicine at the present time, and what direction we are marching. It's the compass that guides us into the future. If our plan is not to be hap-hazard but to follow a well-laid plan, we need the guidance of history, and it is not by accident that all great medical leaders were fully aware of historical studies.[132]

TABLE 56-6
Future Changes and Challenges Facing Respiratory Care Professions

Expected Changes
• Increasing age and burden of chronic cardiac and respiratory diseases • Shortages of all types of healthcare providers • Increased accountability for patient safety • Greater impact of government-related involvement in health care including reimbursement keyed to: safety, outcome performance such as readmission following hospital discharge • Increased use of healthcare information management systems
Future Competencies
• Increasing complexity of respiratory care technology • Need for incorporating protocols and communication skills to serve as leaders within teams (both acute care and disease management) • Greater need for ability to evaluate new evidence and application to new clinical practice
Transitions for Education, Credentialing, and Career Ladders
• Demand for advanced preparation at professional entry will increase need for baccalaureate degree • Need for better structuring of career ladders with education to document competencies at professional entry and for postgraduate education for advanced practices and/or specialization. • Providing credentials and licenses that parallel educational preparation and competency documentation • Increased use of medical simulation for training and competency assessment • Enhanced use of online educational technology to provide initial and continuing education

Key Points

- Key scientists helped establish the foundation for respiratory care modalities and treatments.
- A variety of discoveries in math, science, and engineering contributed to the development of respiratory care as an allied health profession.
- Several key individuals, organizations, and events led to the establishment of respiratory care as an allied health profession.
- Throughout history and up to the current time, many organizations have promoted, supported, sponsored, and funded the respiratory care profession.
- The goals of each supporting organization ultimately improve the scope, practice, education, credentials, quality, and professional growth of respiratory care, which ultimately benefits society through health and wellness.
- The AARC and related professional organizations enhance the entire respiratory care profession, with far-reaching effects beyond each organization's membership.

- The increasing complexity of respiratory care science has been documented, including increasing acute and chronic health problems of an aging population, which supports increasing professional education levels to provide expanded competencies to provide high-quality patient care into the future.
- Knowing the history of the profession serves as a guide and compass, pointing individuals and organizations into the future.

References

1. Smith GA, ed. *Respiratory Care: Evolution of a Profession*. Lenexa, KS: Applied Measurement Professionals; 1989.
2. Loudon I, ed. *Western Medicine: An Illustrated History*. New York: Oxford University Press; 1997.
3. Magner LN. *A History of Medicine*. 2nd ed. New York: Informa Healthcare; 2005.
4. Bynum WF. *The History of Medicine: A Very Short Introduction*. New York: Oxford University Press; 2008.
5. National Institutes of Health. *History of Medicine*. Available at: http://www.nlm.nih.gov/hmd. Accessed September 28, 2014.
6. Perkins JF. Historical development of respiratory physiology. In: Fenn WO, Rahn H, eds. *Handbook of Physiology: Respiration*. Washington, DC: American Physiological Society; 1964: 1–58.
7. Cahill T. *How the Irish Saved Civilization*. New York: Doubleday; 1996.
8. Cassebaum H, Schufle JA. Scheele's priority for the discovery of oxygen. *J Chem Ed*. 1975;52:442–444.
9. Gottlieb LS. Thomas Beddoes, MD, and the pneumatic institution at Clifton, 1798–1801. *Ann Intern Med*. 1965;63:530–533.
10. Petty TL. John Hutchinson's mysterious machine revisited. *Chest*. 2002;121(5 Suppl):219S–223S.
11. Colice GL. Historical perspective on the development of mechanical ventilation. In: Tobin MJ, ed. *Principles and Practice of Mechanical Ventilation*. New York: McGraw-Hill; 1994.
12. Miracle VA. The life and impact of Florence Nightingale. *Dimens Crit Care Nurs*. 2008;27:21–23.
13. Hacker JD. A census-based count of the Civil War dead. *Civil War History*. 2011;57:307–348.
14. Blaisdell FW. Medical advances during the Civil War. *Arch Surg*. 1988;123:1045–1050.
15. Bergman NA. *The Genesis of Surgical Anesthesia*. Park Ridge, IL: Wood Library–Museum of Anesthesiology; 1998.
16. Haldane JS. *Respiration*. New Haven, CT: Yale University Press; 1922.
17. Helmholz HF. Professional champions (1900–1940). In: Smith GA, ed. *Respiratory Care: Evolution of a Profession*. Lexena, KS: Applied Measurement Professionals; 1989.
18. Kobasa D, Takada A, Shinya K, et al. Enhanced virulence of influenza A viruses with the haemagglutinin of the 1918 pandemic virus. *Nature*. 2004;431:703–707.
19. Perkins JF. Historical development of respiratory physiology. In: Fen WO, Rahn H, eds. *Handbook of Physiology*. Vol. 3. Washington, DC: American Physiological Society; 1964.
20. Leigh JM. The evolution of the oxygen therapy apparatus. *Anaesthesia*. 1974;29:462–485.
21. Barach AL. Symposium: inhalation therapy historical background. *Anesthesiology*. 1962;23:407–421.
22. Barach AL. Use of helium as a new therapeutic gas. *Proc Soc Exp Biol Med*. 1934;32:462–464.
23. Barach AL. The therapeutic use of helium. *JAMA*. 1936;107:1273.
24. Terry TL. Extreme prematurity and fibroblastic overgrowth of persistent vascular sheath behind each crystalline lens. *Am J Opthalmol*. 1942;25:203–204.
25. Severinghaus JW, Astrum PB. History of blood gas analysis: IV. Leland Clark's oxygen electrode. *J Clin Monit*. 1986;2:125–139.
26. Severinghaus JW, Honda Y. History of blood gas analysis: VII. Pulse oximetry. *J Clin Monit*. 1987;3:135–138.
27. Campbell EJM. A method of controlled oxygen administration which reduces the risk of CO_2 retention. *Lancet*. 1960;276:12–14.
28. Nocturnal Oxygen Therapy Trial Group. Continuous and nocturnal oxygen therapy in hypoxic chronic obstructive lung disease: a clinical trial. *Ann Intern Med*. 1980;93:931–932.
29. AARC clinical practice guideline: oxygen therapy in the acute care hospital. *Respir Care*. 1991;36:1410–1413.
30. AARC clinical practice guideline: oxygen therapy in the home or extended care facility. *Respir Care*. 1992;37:918–922.
31. Dessanges JF. A history of nebulization. *J Aerosol Med*. 2001;14:65–71.
32. Dhand R. Nebulizers that use a vibrating mesh or plate with multiple apertures to generate aerosols. 2002;47:1406–1416.
33. Stoller JK. History of intubation, tracheostomy and airway appliances. *Respir Care*. 1999;44:595–603.
34. Safar P, Escarraga LA, Elam JO. A comparison of the mouth-to-mouth and mouth-to-airway methods of artificial respiration with the chest pressure arm-lift methods. *N Engl J Med*. 1958;258:671–677.
35. Kouwenhoven WB, Jude JR, Knickerbocker GG. Closed-chest cardiac massage. *JAMA*. 1960;173:1064–1067.
36. Safar P, Brown T, Holtey W, Wider R. Ventilation and circulation with closed-chest massage in man. *JAMA*. 1961;176:574–576.
37. Ad Hoc Committee on Cardiopulmonary Resuscitation of the Division of Medical Sciences, National Academy of Sciences–National Research Council. Cardiopulmonary resuscitation. *JAMA*. 1966;198:138–145.
38. Lown B, Neuman J, Amarasingham R, Berkovits BV. Comparison of alternating current with direct current electroshock across the closed chest. *Am J Cardiol*. 1962;10:223–233.
39. Hilberman M. Evolution of intensive care units. *Crit Care Med*. 1975;3:159–165.
40. Brain AIJ. The laryngeal mask: a new concept in airway management. *Br J Anaesthesia*. 1983;56:801–806.
41. Mallampati SR, Gatt SP, Gugino LD, et al. A clinical sign to predict difficult tracheal intubation: a prospective study. *Can Anaesth Soc J*. 1985;32:429–434.
42. ASA Task Force on Management of the Difficult Airway. Practice guidelines for management of the difficult airway. *Anesthesiology*. 1993;78:597–602.
43. Ciaglia P, Firsching R, Syniec C. Elective percutaneous dilational tracheostomy. A new simple bedside procedure; preliminary report. *Chest*. 1985;87:715–719.
44. Mørch ET. History of mechanical ventilation. In: Kirby RR, Banner MJ, Downs JB, eds. *Clinical Applications of Ventilatory Support*. New York: Churchill Livingstone; 1990.
45. Mushin WW, Rendel-Baker L, Thompson PW, Mapleson WW. *Automatic Ventilation of the Lungs*. 3rd ed. London, UK: Blackwell Scientific; 1980.
46. Colice G. Historical background. In: Tobin MJ, ed. *Principles and Practice of Mechanical Ventilation*. New York: McGraw-Hill; 2002.
47. Lassen HCA. A preliminary report on the 1952 epidemic of poliomyelitis in Copenhagen—with special reference to the treatment of acute respiratory insufficiency. *Lancet*. 1953;1:37–41.
48. Rosenberg H, Axelrod JK. Ernst Trier Mørch: inventor, medical pioneer, heroic freedom fighter. *Anesth Analg*. 2000;90:218–221.
49. Avery EE, Mørch ET, Benson DW. Critically crushed chests, a new method of treatment with continuous mechanical hyperventilation to produce alkalotic apnea and internal pneumatic stabilization. *J Thoracic Surg*. 1956;32:291–309.
50. Radford EP. Ventilation standards for use in artificial respiration. *J Appl Physiol*. 1956;7:451–460.
51. Hedley-Whyte J, Pontoppidan H, Morris MJ. The response of patients with respiratory failure and cardiopulmonary disease to different levels of constant volume ventilation. *J Clin Invest*. 1966;45:1543–1564.

52. Bendixen HH, Hedley-Whyte J, Laver MB. Impaired oxygenation in surgical patients during general anesthesia with controlled ventilation. *N Engl J Med*. 1963;269:991–997.
53. Asbaugh DG, Bigelow DB, Petty TL. Acute respiratory distress in adults. *Lancet*. 1967;1:319–323.
54. Asbaugh DG, Petty TL, Bigelow DB, et al. Continuous positive pressure breathing in adult respiratory distress syndrome. *J Thorac Cardiovasc Surg*. 1969;57:31–41.
55. Gregory GA, Kitterman JA, Phibbs RH. Treatment of the idiopathic respiratory distress syndrome with continuous positive airway pressure. *N Engl J Med*. 1971;284:1333–1340.
56. Kirby R, Robison E, Schulz J, de Lemos R. Continuous-flow ventilation as an alternative to assisted or controlled ventilation in infants. *Anesth Analg*. 1972;51:871–875.
57. Chatburn R. Classification of ventilator modes: update and proposal for implementation. *Respir Care*. 2007;52:301–323.
58. Meduri GU, Conoscenti CC, Menashe P, Nair S. Noninvasive face mask ventilation in patients with acute respiratory failure. *Chest*. 1989;95:865–870.
59. Quon BS, Gan WQ, Sin DD. Contemporary management of acute exacerbations of COPD: a systematic review and meta-analysis. *Chest*. 2008;133:756–766.
60. Downs JB, Stock MC. Airway pressure release ventilation: a new concept in ventilatory care. *Chest*. 1987;15:459–461.
61. Branson RD, Johnnigman JA. What is the evidence base for the newer ventilation modes? *Respir Care*. 2004;49:742–760.
62. Dreyfus D, Saumon G. Ventilator-induced lung injury. Lessons from experimental studies. *Am J Respir Crit Care Med*. 1998;157:294–323.
63. The Acute Respiratory Distress Syndrome Network. Ventilation with lower tidal volumes as compared with traditional tidal volumes for acute lung injury and the acute respiratory distress syndrome. *N Engl J Med*. 2000;342:1301–1308.
64. The HIFI Study Group. High-frequency oscillatory ventilation compared with conventional mechanical ventilation in the treatment of respiratory failure in preterm infants. *N Engl J Med*. 1989;320:88–93.
65. Marini JJ, Gattinoni L. Propagation prevention: a complementary mechanism for "lung protective" ventilation in acute respiratory distress syndrome. *Crit Care Med*. 2008;36:3252–3258.
66. Andrews AH Jr. *Manual of Oxygen Therapy Techniques*. Chicago: Year-Book; 1947.
67. Barach AL, Collins V, Emma E. Minimum standards for inhalation therapy. *JAMA*. 1950;144:25.
68. American Association for Respiratory Care (AARC). *Delineation of Roles and Functions of Respiratory Therapy Personnel. Final Report for Division of Allied Health Manpower, Bureau of Health Manpower Education, National Institutes of Health, Department of Health Education and Welfare (US)*. Dallas: AARC; 1973.
69. American Association for Respiratory Care. *Year 2001: Delineating the Education Direction for the Future Respiratory Care Practitioner*. Dallas: AARC; 1992.
70. American Association for Respiratory Care. *Year 2001: An Action Agenda*. Dallas: AARC; 1993.
71. Kacmarek RM, Durbin CG, Barnes TA, et al. Creating a vision for respiratory care in 2015 and beyond. *Respir Care*. 2009;54:375–389.
72. Mishoe SC, MacIntyre NR. Expanding professional roles for respiratory care practitioners. *Respir Care*. 1997;42:71–85.
73. Mishoe SC. Educating respiratory care professionals: an emphasis on critical thinking. *Respir Care*. 2002;47:568–569.
74. AARC CoBGRTE Steering Committee. Development of baccalaureate and graduate degrees in respiratory care. *Respir Care Educ Ann*. 2003;12:29–39.
75. Flexner A. *Medical Education in the United States and Canada*. New York: Carnegie Foundation for the Advancement of Teaching; 1910.
76. Barach AL. *Inhalation Therapy*. Philadelphia: JB Lippincott; 1944.
77. Safar P, ed. *Respiratory Therapy*. Philadelphia: F.A. Davis; 1965.
78. Egan DF. *Fundamentals of Inhalation Therapy*. St. Louis: Mosby; 1969.
79. Pierce AK, Saltzman HA. Conference on the scientific basis of respiratory therapy. *Am Rev Respir Dis*. 1974;110:1–3.
80. Fowler WS, Helmholz HF, Miller RD. Treatment of pulmonary emphysema with aerosolized bronchodilator drugs and intermittent positive pressure breathing therapy. *Proc Staff Mayo Clin*. 1953;28:743.
81. Pierson DJ. Respiratory care as a science. *Respir Care*. 1988;33:27.
82. Guyatt G, Cairns J, Churchill D, et al. Evidence-based medicine. A new approach to teaching the practice of medicine. *JAMA*. 1992;268:2420–2425.
83. Sackett DL, Rosenberg WM, Gray JA, Haynes RB, Richardson WS. Evidence based medicine: what it is and what it isn't. *BMJ*. 1996;312:71–72.
84. Greenhalgh T. *How to Read a Paper: The Basics of Evidence-Based Medicine*. 4th ed. Hoboken, NJ: Wiley-Blackwell Inc.; 2010.
85. Taylor R, Reeves B, Ewings P, et al. A systematic review of the critical appraisal skills training for clinicians. *Med Ed*. 2000;34: 120–125.
86. Kohn LT, Corrigan JM, Donaldson MD, eds. Committee on Quality of Health Care in America, Institute of Medicine. *To Err Is Human: Building a Safer Health System*. Washington, DC: The National Academies Press; 2000.
87. National Research Council. *Crossing the Quality Chasm: A New Health System for the 21st Century*. Washington, DC: The National Academies Press; 2001.
88. Bradley P. The history of simulation in medical education and possible future directions. *Med Ed*. 2006;40:254–262.
89. Gaba DM. The future vision of simulation in health care. *Qual Saf Health Care*. 2004;13:2–10.
90. McGaghie WC, Issenberg SB, Petrussa ER, Scalese TJ. A critical review of simulation-based medical education research: 2003–2009. *Med Ed*. 2010;44:50–63.
91. McGaghie WC, Issenberg BS, Cohen ER, et al. Does simulation-based medical education with deliberate practice yield better results than traditional clinical education? A meta-analytic comparative review of the evidence. *Acad Med*. 2011;86:706–711.
92. Accreditation Council for Graduate Medical Education. *ACGME Internal Medicine Program Requirements*. 2011. Available at: http://www.acgme.org. Accessed September 9, 2014.
93. Agency for Healthcare Research and Quality. TeamSTEPPS®: Strategies and Tools to Enhance Performance and Patient Safety. Available at: http://www.ahrq.gov/professionals/education/curriculum-tools/teamstepps/index.html. Accessed September 9, 2014.
94. McGinnes JM, Foege WH. Actual causes of death in the United States. *JAMA*. 1993;270:2207–2212.
95. Mokdad AH, Marks JS, Stroup DF, Gerberding JL. Actual causes of death in the United Sates. *JAMA*. 2000;291:1238–1245.
96. Xu J, Kochanek KD, Murphy SL, Tejada-Vera B. Deaths: final data for 2007. *Natl Vital Stat Rep*. 2010;58:1–117. Available at: http://www.cdc.gov/nchs/products/nvsr.htm#vol58. Accessed September 28, 2014.
97. Murray JL and US Burden of Disease Collaborators. The state of US health, 1990–2010 Burden of disease, injuries and risk factors. *JAMA*. 2013;310:591–608.
98. *Respiratory Care*. Clinical practice guidelines. Available at: http://www.rcjournal.com/cpgs. Accessed September 29, 2014.
99. Restrepo RD. AARC clinical practice guidelines: from "reference-based" to "evidence-based." *Respir Care*. 2010;56:787–788.
100. Apfelbaum JL and Committee on Standards and Practice Parameters. Practice guidelines for the management of the difficult airway—an updated report by the American Society of Anesthesiologists Task Force on Management of the Difficult Airway. *Anesthesiology*. 2013;118:251–270.
101. National Asthma Education and Prevention Program. *Expert Panel Report 3: Guidelines for the Diagnosis and Management of Asthma*. Bethesda, MD: National Institutes of Health—Heart, Lung, and Blood Institute; 2007.

102. American Heart Association guidelines for cardiopulmonary resuscitation and emergency cardiovascular care. Part 1 executive summary. *Circulation.* 2013;122(Suppl 3):S640–S656.
103. Global Strategy for diagnosis, management and prevention of COPD. Updated February 2013. Global Initiative for Chronic Obstructive Lung Disease (GOLD). Available at: http://www.goldcopd.org/Guidelines/guidelines-resources.html. Accessed September 28, 2014.
104. Truog RD, Campbell ML, Curtis JR, et al. Recommendations for end-of-life care in the intensive care unit: a consensus statement by the American College of Critical Care Medicine. *Crit Care Med.* 2008;36:953–963.
105. Epstein LJ and Adult Obstructive Sleep Apnea Task Force. Clinical guideline for the evaluation, management and long-term care of obstructive sleep apnea in adults. *J Clin Sleep Med.* 2009;5:263–276.
106. Miller MR, Crapo R, Hankinson J, et al. ATS/ERS Standardization of lung function testing: general considerations for lung function testing. *Eur Respir J.* 2005;26:153–161.
107. Ely EW, Bennett PA, Boston DL, et al. Large scale implementation of a respiratory therapist-driven protocol for ventilator weaning. *Am J Respir Crit Care Med.* 1999;159:439–446.
108. Haas C, Loik PS. Ventilator discontinuation protocols. *Respir Care.* 2012;57:1649–1662.
109. Svircevic V, Nierich AP, Moons KG, et al. Fast-track anesthesia and cardiac surgery: a retrospective cohort study of 7989 patients. *Anesth Analg.* 2009;108:727–733.
110. Muehling BM, Halter GL, Schelzig H, et al. Reduction of postoperative pulmonary complications after lung surgery using a fast track clinical pathway. *Eur J Cardio-Thorac.* 2008;34:174–180.
111. Kallam A, Meyerink K, Modrykamien AM. Physician-ordered aerosol therapy versus respiratory therapist-driven aerosol protocol: the effect on resource utilization. *Respir Care.* 2013;58:431–437.
112. Christman SL, Volsko TA. Evaluation of an oxygen protocol in long-term care. *Respir Care.* 2006;51:1424–1431.
113. U.S. Department of Health & Human Services. The Affordable Care Act. Available at: http://www.hhs.gov/healthcare/rights/index.html. Accessed September 28, 2014.
114. Wilper AP, Woolhandler S, Lasser KE, et al. Health insurance and mortality in the US. *Am J Pub Health.* 2009;99:2289–2295.
115. Brock J, Mitchell J, Irby K, et al. Care Transitions Project Team. Association between quality improvement for care transitions in communities and rehospitalizations among Medicare beneficiaries. *JAMA.* 2013;309:381–391.
116. Centers for Disease Control and Prevention. National Healthcare Safety Network. *Surveillance for Ventilator-Associated Events.* Available at: http://www.cdc.gov/nhsn/acute-care-hospital/vae/. Accessed September 28, 2014.
117. Klompas M. Complications of mechanical ventilation—the CDC's new surveillance paradigm. *N Engl J Med.* 2013;368:1472–1475.
118. Barnes TA, Black CP, Douce FH, et al. AARC CoBGRTE Steering Committee. Development of baccalaureate and graduate degrees in respiratory care. *Respir Care Educ Ann.* 2003;12:29–39.
119. Barnes TA, Gale DD, Kacmarek RM, Kageler WV. Competencies needed by graduate respiratory therapists in 2015 and beyond. *Respir Care.* 2010;56:601–616.
120. Lee EO, Emanuel EJ. Shared decision making to improve care and reduce costs. *N Engl J Med.* 2013;368:6–8.
121. Barnes TA, Ward JJ. Survey and analysis of baccalaureate and graduate respiratory therapy education programs. *Respir Care Ed Ann.* 2010;19:1–12.
122. Barnes TA, Kacmarek RM, Morris MJ, et al. Transitioning the respiratory therapy workforce for 2015 and beyond. *Respir Care.* 2011;56:681–690.
123. Jones PE. Physician assistant education in the United States. *Acad Med.* 2007;82:882–887.
124. Hoslin VH, Cook PA, Ballweg R, et al. Value added: graduate-level education in physician assistant programs. *J Physician Assist Educ.* 2006;17:16–30.
125. Aiken LH, Clarke SP, Cheung RB, et al. Education levels of hospital nurses and surgical patient mortality. *JAMA.* 2003;290:1617–1623.
126. Institute of Medicine. *The Future of Nursing: Leading Change, Advancing Health.* Available at: http://iom.edu/Reports/2010/The-Future-of-Nursing-Leading-Change-Advancing-Health.aspx. Accessed September 28, 2014.
127. American Nurses Association. Registered nurses in the US: nursing by the numbers. Available at: http://nursingworld.org/Content/NNW-Archive/NationalNursesWeek/MediaKit/NursingbytheNumbers.pdf. Accessed September 28, 2014.
128. Hader R. Education matters: does higher learning yield higher income? *Nursing Management.* 2011;42:22–27.
129. American Association for Respiratory Care. We Have a Vision. Mission Statement. Available at: https://www.aarc.org/headlines/vision.asp. Accessed September 28, 2014.
130. Dubbs W. *2009 AARC Manpower Study.* Irving, TX: American Association for Respiratory Care (AARC); 2009.
131. Lockard CB, Wolf M. Occupational employment projections to 2020. *Monthly Labor Review.* 2012;135:84–108.
132. Marti-Ibanez F, ed. *Henry E. Sigerist on the History of Medicine.* New York: MD Publications; 1960.

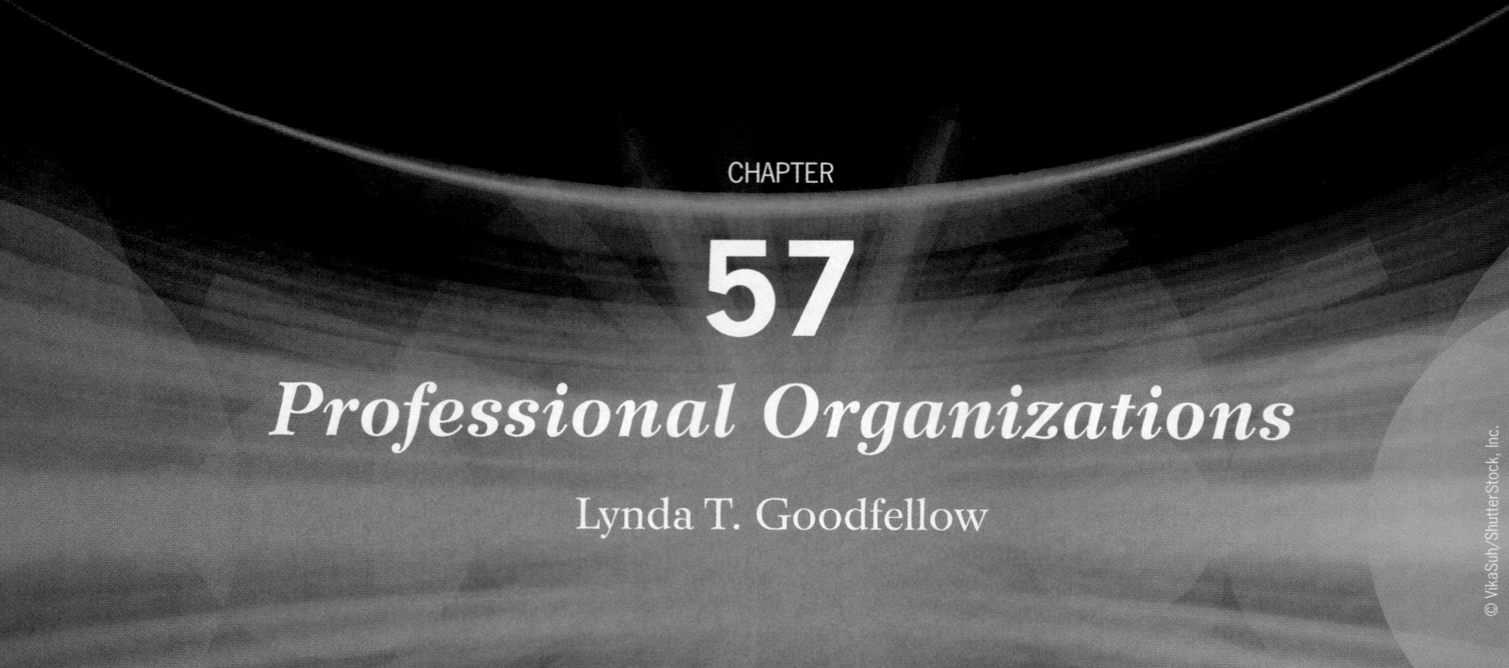

CHAPTER

57 Professional Organizations

Lynda T. Goodfellow

OUTLINE

American Association for Respiratory Care
American Respiratory Care Foundation
National Board for Respiratory Care
Commission on Accreditation for Respiratory Care
National Association for Medical Direction of Respiratory Care
American College of Chest Physicians
American Thoracic Society
American Society of Anesthesiologists
Society of Critical Care Medicine
The Joint Commission
National Asthma Educator Certification Board
Association of Asthma Educators
American Academy of Sleep Medicine
Board of Registered Polysomnographic Technologists

OBJECTIVES

1. Describe the organization and function of the American Association for Respiratory Care.
2. Describe the roles of the National Board for Respiratory Care and the Commission on Accreditation for Respiratory Care.
3. Describe the way in which medical professional organizations contribute to the respiratory care profession.
4. Discuss the accreditation, credentialing, and medical direction aspects of the respiratory care profession.
5. Identify the primary medical sponsoring and representative organizations of the respiratory care profession.
6. Discuss the physician organizations that contribute to the art and science of the respiratory care profession.
7. Describe the various credentialing examinations available for respiratory therapists.
8. Discuss the role of the Joint Commission regarding patient safety in healthcare organizations.
9. Identify the role that each professional must play in the future growth of the respiratory care profession.

KEY TERMS

AARC Times
accreditation
American Academy of Sleep Medicine (AASM)
American Association for Respiratory Care (AARC)
American Respiratory Care Foundation (ARCF)
Association of Asthma Educators (AAE)
Board of Medical Advisors (BOMA)
Board of Registered Polysomnographic Technologists (BRPT)
certification
Commission on Accreditation for Respiratory Care (CoARC)
credentialing
credential
House of Delegates (HOD)
licensure
National Association for Medical Direction of Respiratory Care (NAMDRC)
National Asthma Educator Certification Board (NAECB)
National Board for Respiratory Care (NBRC)
President's Council
RESPIRATORY CARE
specialty section
The Joint Commission (TJC)

Introduction

This chapter describes the role of professional organizations in the respiratory care profession, identifying each organization (**Table 57-1**) and discussing its importance to the profession's principles and practice. The primary professional organization for respiratory care is the **American Association for Respiratory Care (AARC)**. The AARC and related organizations contribute to the scientific basis, governance, stature, and growth of respiratory care. Many of the organizations described in this chapter have been involved with the respiratory care profession since its inception, either in the current form or via a former name or function. Respiratory

TABLE 57-1
Common Acronyms in Respiratory Care Related to Professional Organizations

Acronym	Organization or Credential
AARC	American Association for Respiratory Care
AAE	Association of Asthma Educators
AASM	American Academy of Sleep Medicine
ASME	Asthma Self-Management Education
AE-C	Certified Asthma Educator
BOMA	Board of Medical Advisors
BRPT	Board of Registered Polysomnographic Technologists
BOD	(AARC) Board of Directors
CoARC	Commission on Accreditation for Respiratory Care
HOD	(AARC) House of Delegates
NBRC	National Board for Respiratory Care
NAECB	National Asthma Educator Certification Board
NAMDRC	National Association for Medical Direction of Respiratory Care
ACCP	American College of Chest Physicians
AAP	American Academy of Pediatrics
AAAAI	American Academy of Allergy, Asthma, and Immunology
ACAAI	American College of Allergy, Asthma, and Immunology
ATS	American Thoracic Society
ALA	American Lung Association
RCP	Respiratory Care Practioner
ASA	American Society of Anesthesiologists
RPSGT	Registered Polysomnographic Technologist
SCCM	Society of Critical Care Medicine

care would not be as valued a member of the healthcare team without the contributions of such organizations.

American Association for Respiratory Care

The AARC is the national association that represents the respiratory care profession to communities of interest. The AARC also addresses larger societal changes to advocate and enhance the professionalism of respiratory therapists. A profession is described by its advancing science, technology, and practice; continuing education; active participation of its members; credentials; leadership; research; and innovation. The AARC was organized in 1946 as the Inhalation Therapy Association (ITA). As the profession progressed, the name changed and the organization evolved into the professional entity it is today.

The art and science of respiratory care are supported by the publications of the AARC, which include **Respiratory Care**, **AARC Times**, Education Annual, and others published by specialty sections. The editorial board for the scientific journal, Respiratory Care, comprises researchers who are also respiratory therapists or physicians. The AARC has various standing and special committees to support the profession.

Funding for operations of the AARC is derived from member dues, advertising, and revenues from educational programs and conventions throughout the year. The AARC has a membership of over 52,000, with approximately 42,000 active members as of September 2013. The AARC also offers student, associate, life, and honorary memberships. The AARC has consistently provided some of the highest member benefits found in the health professions while maintaining nearly the lowest dues of all national healthcare organizations. The AARC has 10 specialty sections that support major subsets of therapists, including management, education, perinatal/pediatrics, adult critical care, home care, subacute care, transport, diagnostics, sleep, and continuing care and rehabilitation. Many AARC members belong to different specialty sections based both on their work activities and on their professional interests.

The AARC will continue to be the leading national and international professional association for respiratory care. The AARC encourages and promotes professional excellence, advances the science and practice of respiratory care, and serves as an advocate for patients, their families, the public, the professions, and the respiratory therapist.[1] The AARC comprises several governance and advisory bodies, including the Board of Directors, House of Delegates, Board of Medical Advisors, and executive office, located in Irving, Texas.[2]

Board of Directors

The executive government of the AARC is composed of the Board of Directors (BOD) made up of no more

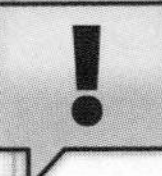

Respiratory Recap

Description of a Profession

- Advancing science and technology
- Evolving practice, scope, credentialing, and accreditation
- Advanced degrees and continuing education
- Active participation by members
- Leadership, research, and innovation

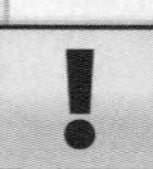

Respiratory Recap

Governance of the AARC

- The Board of Directors is the governing body of the AARC, with fiduciary responsibility for the professional organization and its members.

than 18 Active AARC Members, with at least 5 officers and 12 directors-at-large and section chairs serving as directors from each specialty section with a minimum of 1000 active members of the association. The officers consist of the president, immediate past president, vice president for internal affairs, vice president for external affairs, secretary-treasurer, and, in alternate years, president-elect.[2] So long as the number of section chairs serving as directors is at least six, the number of at-large directors is equal to the number of section chairs serving as directors. If the number of section chairs serving as directors is fewer than six, the number of at-large directors is increased to ensure a minimum of 12 director seats on the Board of Directors. The significance of the section chairpersons is magnified by their inclusion as BODs (provided that section has more than 1000 members), which allows growth of the AARC through the potential inclusion of new associations and specialties that relate to the profession. The specialty section chairpersons serve a dual role as both section chairs and BOD directors.

In general, the AARC term of office is 3 years. Up to one-third of the at-large directors are elected each year, and the term of office for all directors begins following the annual business meeting. The immediate past speaker of the House of Delegates (HOD), chair of the President's Council, and current chairperson of the Board of Medical Advisors serve 1-year terms as non-voting members of the BOD.[1]

The current executive director of the AARC serves as an advisor to the BOD, reporting to the current AARC president. In addition, the incoming AARC president appoints a parliamentarian to the BOD to help with parliamentary procedures for BOD activities before, during, and between board meetings. The BOD meets three times per year, usually during April, directly after the AARC Summer Forum and directly preceding the AARC International Congress in the fall. The BOD and HOD meet simultaneously during the summer and fall meetings, facilitating communications, costs, and actions required by bylaws that govern activities of the budget, nominations, and joint members of various BOD and HOD committees. The seven standing committees that include bylaws, elections, executive, finance, judicial, program, and strategic planning assist the BOD in fulfilling their fiduciary governance role.

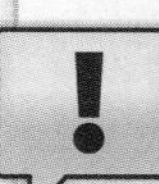

Respiratory Recap

AARC Standing Committees

- Bylaws
- Elections
- Executive
- Finance
- Judicial
- Program
- Strategic planning

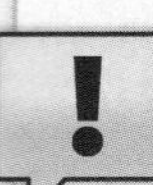

Respiratory Recap

House of Delegates

- Each chartered affiliate of the HOD elects active members of the AARC (from their respective affiliates) to represent the membership of the professional association.

House of Delegates

The **House of Delegates (HOD)** is a representative body for the chartered affiliate societies to contribute to the growth, existence, governance, and future of the respiratory care profession. The general membership can bring wishes and concerns to the national organization through local representatives in the HOD. The HOD further serves as a communication bridge, reporting activities, data, information, and needs to the AARC chartered affiliates and members. Its structure, organization, and function are similar to the United States Congress. The HOD is an advisor to the BOD. The HOD helps govern the AARC through approval of bylaws, budgets, nominations, and audits and through consideration of resolutions and motions forwarded to the BOD for consideration.[1] Any AARC member can bring issues to his or her state delegation, which in turn broaches the issue in a resolution or motion for consideration by the entire HOD.

The HOD is composed of one to three members from each chartered affiliate and meets preceding the annual business meeting of the association and at such other times as called by its speaker or by the majority vote of the House of Delegates.[2] Currently, 50 delegations represent 48 states. A two-state delegation comprises Vermont and New Hampshire. One state-and-district combination is composed of Maryland and the District of Columbia. The territory of Puerto Rico has its own delegation. The HOD elects officers, including the speaker-elect, speaker, immediate past speaker, treasurer/secretary. The speaker appoints the parliamentarian for a 1-year term. As with the BOD, HOD officers also serve 1-year terms, with the exception of the 3-year term as speaker-elect, speaker, and past speaker.

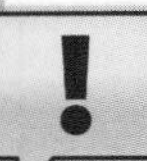

Respiratory Recap

Medical Societies Composing the Board of Medical Advisors

- American Society of Anesthesiologists (ASA)
- American College of Chest Physicians (ACCP)
- American Thoracic Society (ATS)
- Society for Critical Care Medicine (SCCM)
- American Academy of Pediatrics (AAP)
- American College of Allergy, Asthma, and Immunology (ACAAI)
- National Association for Medical Directors of Respiratory Care (NAMDRC)

Board of Medical Advisors

The **Board of Medical Advisors (BOMA)** consists of professional medical societies that provide significant input to the art and science of the profession of respiratory care. The current societies include the American Society of Anesthesiologists (ASA), the American College of Chest Physicians (ACCP), the American Thoracic Society (ATS), the American Academy of Pediatrics (AAP), the American College of Allergy, Asthma, and Immunology (ACAAI), the National Association for Medical Directors of Respiratory Care (NAMDRC), and the Society of Critical Care Medicine (SCCM). BOMA consists of no less than 12 individual members nominated from each society, who serve staggered terms.[2] The BOMA chairperson is designated in a rotation so that each society has a representative serve as chair.

Specialty Sections

AARC **specialty sections** consist of members with special interests in specific areas of respiratory practice. Like AARC membership, specialty section membership is voluntary. Members of a section pay special dues over and above their annual AARC dues. Each section has a chairperson, chair-elect, and various committee chairpersons and committee members. Many AARC professionals are members of multiple specialty sections.

The specialty sections usually meet during the Summer Forum and the International Respiratory Care Congress. The sections may introduce recommendations directly to the BOD through their liaison, and the board takes action on such reports during meetings. The AARC vice president for internal affairs serves as the liaison between the specialty sections and the BOD. In response to the fast pace of healthcare policy and practice changes, specialty sections are popular and play a broadened role in governing the AARC.

Roundtables have also formed as special interest groups to allow sharing of ideas and information with other members who have an interest in specific niches within the profession. Examples of roundtables include asthma disease management, disaster response, and tobacco-free lifestyle. Roundtable discussions as well as other electronic discussions are through AARC Connect, the social media venue.

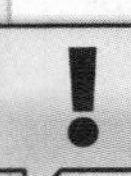

Respiratory Recap

AARC Specialty Sections

- Management
- Education
- Adult acute care
- Perinatal/pediatrics
- Long-term care
- Home care
- Diagnostics
- Continuing care and rehabilitation
- Transport
- Sleep

President's Council

The **President's Council** was formed in 1971. The council is composed of past presidents of the AARC who have been elected to membership by the council. The President's Council serves as an advisory body to the Board of Directors and performs other duties assigned by the Board of Directors.[2] This council has significant experience and wisdom gained through its members' experiences as elected officials of the AARC. The chair of the President's Council is elected by the members to serve a 1-year term and presides at meetings of the council. The chair also serves as a nonvoting member of the AARC Board of Directors.

Executive Office

The executive office is composed of those individuals employed on behalf of the AARC. The BOD, HOD, and BOMA are composed of professional volunteers who meet membership requirements and work on behalf of the profession. Members of the executive office are hired to focus on the daily activities of the AARC. The executive offices are located in Irving, Texas.

The AARC executive office has an executive director who reports to the president of the AARC. In addition,

Respiratory Recap

President's Council

- The President's Council comprises past presidents of the AARC who advise the current Board of Directors and perform other duties as assigned by the BOD.

associate executive directors and staff members support the membership and educational functions of the AARC. The AARC has an in-depth website (http://www.aarc.org). Users can access membership and respiratory care information, special articles, and announcements at the website. Members can visit a special members-only section of the website for specific information and services.

The AARC in 2015 and Beyond

The profession has been involved in a strategic planning process since 2009 by directing activities designed to chart a path for the future by identifying the clinical and nonclinical skills, attributes, and characteristics of the respiratory therapist for 2015 and beyond. The planning process has involved projecting the future role of the profession based on the expected needs of the public, patients, profession, and the evolving healthcare system. This process occurred through a series of three conferences organized by the AARC with its many allied professional partners so that organizational and functional changes were planned for and implemented as appropriate.[3–5]

The first conference considered the changes in the profession that are needed to reflect the transformations in health care, science, technology, education, and communications.[3] The second conference created a list of competencies that graduate respiratory therapists need to become proficient at to meet the evolving challenges.[4] This list includes diagnostics, disease management, evidence-based practice and protocols, patient assessment, and leadership. The third conference mapped the needed changes to education and clinical practice so that the profession is capable of transitioning to 2015 and beyond.[5]

The recommendations of the last conference have created much discussion on several fronts such as the BS degree as entry into practice, requiring the RRT for licensure, and the appropriate timeline needed for change. Since 2012, the AARC BOD has accepted the direction and competencies of the first two conferences. A task force was established to provide further direction to the AARC from the third conference and several initiatives were established to develop mechanisms for implementation of the recommendations. Specifically, the task force was established to review entry and practice competency mechanisms; validate standards for simulation competency models; explore consortia and cooperative AS to BS program models; and validate career ladder models for advanced competencies and education. Consequently, the AARC continuously examines its structure, organization, and operations while assessing its relationships to its members, current practices, and communities of interest. Updates regarding 2015 and Beyond can be found on the AARC home page (www.aarc.org).

American Respiratory Care Foundation

The **American Respiratory Care Foundation (ARCF)** is a not-for-profit organization formed to support research, education, and charitable activities. ARCF activities include the funding of clinical and economic research, granting educational recognition awards, supporting educational activities, granting literary awards, and supporting scholarly publications. The ARCF is committed to health promotion, disease prevention, and improving the quality of the environment. The ARCF also educates the public about respiratory health and assists in the training and continuing education of healthcare providers.

National Board for Respiratory Care

The **National Board for Respiratory Care (NBRC)** is a voluntary health-certifying board founded in 1960 for the evaluation of the professional competence of respiratory therapists.[6] The organization first was named the American Registry of Inhalation Therapists (ARIT) to reflect the designation of the profession at that time. The primary purpose of the NBRC and its board of trustees is to provide high-quality voluntary credentialing examinations for respiratory therapists.

The NBRC has established standards for the **credentialing** of practitioners who work under medical direction and cooperates with accrediting agencies to support respiratory therapy education. The NBRC supports the ethical and educational standards of respiratory care. The NBRC also publishes an electronic newsletter called *NBRC Horizons* as well as a directory of credentialed individuals.

By September 2013, the NBRC had issued more than 350,000 professional credentials to more than 209,000 individuals and currently tests nearly 40,000 candidates per year.[6] The NBRC has established itself as a credible credentialing organization. Its respiratory therapy examinations are used as the standard for **licensure** or **certification** in the 49 states that currently regulate the profession. The national offices of the NBRC have been located in the greater Kansas City area since 1974, when the ARIT and the technician certification board of the AARC merged to form a single, independent credentialing organization. The offices are currently located in Olathe, Kansas.

Respiratory Recap

National Board for Respiratory Care

- The NBRC is the national credentialing organization for respiratory therapists.

The NBRC is accredited by the National Commission for Certifying Agencies (NCCA) and is a member of the National Organization for Competency Assurance (NOCA). The NBRC is sponsored by the AARC, ACCP, ASA, and ATS. Each sponsoring organization appoints members who serve on the 31-member NBRC board of trustees. The three physician groups and the National Society for Pulmonary Technology appoint 5 members each, and the AARC appoints 10 members and a public member.

The NBRC uses periodic assessments of the practice of respiratory care through direct profiles of current practice provided by active practitioners. The board's credentialing examinations are consistent with the federal government's Uniform Guidelines on Employee Selection Procedures. The credentialing examinations are also consistent with the American Psychological Association's standards for job-relatedness, validity, and criterion-referenced passing points. The clinical simulation examination was one of the first credentialing examinations of its kind in the United States. All credentialing examinations are developed, prepared, and administered through Applied Measurement Professionals, Inc. (AMP), a wholly owned subsidiary of the NBRC. All NBRC examinations are administered by computer.

Examinations

All NBRC examinations have a common education requirement that includes graduation from a program recognized by the Commission on Accreditation for Respiratory Care. **Table 57-2** provides an overview of the different professional **credentials** awarded by the NBRC.

NBRC examinations are graded with a minimum pass level (MPL) preestablished by the examination committee using a modified Angoff procedure. This accepted psychometric procedure uses the judgments of content experts to determine the number of correct answers required to achieve a passing score for the examination.[7] Canadian Registered Respiratory Therapists (RRTs) may be admitted as candidates for the certification examination (certified respiratory therapists) and seek reciprocity for their credential in the United States by successful completion of the clinical simulation section of the registry examination. NBRC credentialing examinations have specific admittance criteria for applicants, which may be reviewed through applications available from the NBRC website at http://www.nbrc.org. Examinations are administered in over 43 countries around the world through AMP. From 1960 to 2013, over 386,200 NBRC credentials have been earned by practitioners.[8]

The NBRC also offers examinations for respiratory care practitioners in Spanish. The Latin American Board for Proficiency Certification in Respiratory Therapy partners with the NBRC to offer credentialing exams. Registrants can attempt the Professional Certification in Respiratory Therapy exam, which is recognized by members of the Latin American Board. Other countries are in the initial stages of creating their own versions of respiratory therapy proficiency examinations with the assistance of the NBRC.

TABLE 57-2
National Board for Respiratory Care (NBRC) Respiratory Care Credentials

Credential	Acronym
Adult Critical Care Specialty	ACCS
Registered Respiratory Therapist	RRT
Certified Respiratory Therapist	CRT
Registered Pulmonary Function Technologist	RPFT
Certified Pulmonary Function Technologist	CPFT
Perinatal/Pediatric Respiratory Care Specialist	RRT-NPS or CRT-NPS
Sleep Disorders Specialist	RRT-SDS or CRT-SDS

Certified Respiratory Therapist

The Certified Respiratory Therapist (CRT) examination is the entry-level credential for practice in respiratory care. Candidates for the CRT exam must be 18 years of age and graduates of an accredited associate's degree program in respiratory therapy. In the recent past, graduate respiratory therapists needed to successfully complete the CRT exam before attempting any portion of the registry exam. In January 2015, however, the CRT exam was no longer offered and was replaced with a new exam with an established CRT cut score. Competence exhibited at the CRT level is the primary credential used for licensure by state licensure boards that regulate respiratory care practice, but the Ohio Board of Respiratory Therapy moved to the RRT credential for state licensure on January 1, 2015.[9]

Registered Respiratory Therapist

The Registry Examination System was developed to objectively measure essential knowledge, skills, and abilities required of advanced respiratory therapists. The RRT examination contains two parts, the written registry exam (WRRT) and the Clinical Simulation Examination (CSE), which may be taken on the same day or at separate times. The WRRT uses a multiple-choice question format. The clinical simulation exam presents layered clinical problems that can be solved successfully in many ways. On the written registry examination, the graduate therapist demonstrates a sufficient factual database of information. The clinical simulation examination focuses on the graduate's ability to critically think and to assess patient data in clinical practice components. Candidates for the RRT exam must possess the CRT credential and have satisfied other degree or semester-hour requirements. By 2013, 133,174 practitioners had earned the RRT credential.[8]

Major changes to the RRT exam were established, beginning January 2015. The WRRT is renamed the Therapist Multiple Choice (TMC) Examination. Candidates are no longer required to take the CRT exam in order to attempt the TMC. As of January 2015, the exam includes 140 total questions of which 20 questions are used for test-validation purposes. The exam is scored with two cut scores: a lower score to signify passage of the CRT and a higher score associated with eligibility to take the CSE. Admission criteria for the TMC are 18 years of age, an AS degree from a CoARC accredited program, graduated on or before November 11, 2009, from a CAAHEP program, or a Canadian RRT. Compared to the CRT Examination, the TMC Examination will reflect fewer items in recall and application and more items in the analysis domain.[10]

The CSE format also changed in January 2015. The number of patient cases to complete increased from 10 to 20 cases. Candidates can see a sum of positive and negative scores by type of problem (for instance, adult COPD, pediatric, neonatal) and by data gathering and decision making.[10]

Certified Pulmonary Function Technologist

The Certified Pulmonary Function Technologist (CPFT) examination is an entry-level certification exam for pulmonary function technologists. It is designed to validate core competencies in pulmonary function testing, data analysis, equipment, and instrumentation. Candidates must be 18 years old, have an associate's degree from an approved program, or be a CRT or RRT. Another way to attain eligibility is to complete 62 semester hours of college credit, including college credit–level courses in biology, chemistry, and mathematics. A minimum of 6 months of clinical experience in the field of pulmonary function technology under the direction of a medical director of a pulmonary function laboratory is also required prior to applying for the examination.[7] By 2013, 12,824 had earned the CPFT credential.[8]

Registered Pulmonary Function Technologist

The Registered Pulmonary Function Technologist (RPFT) examination is for advanced practice credentialing in pulmonary function technology. The areas of core competency are the same as for the CPFT exam but at a higher level of practice. Candidates must meet the common eligibility requirements and must possess the CPFT credential to write this exam. By 2013, 4315 had earned the RPFT credential.[8]

Perinatal/Pediatric Respiratory Care Specialist

The perinatal/pediatric specialty certification examination recognizes advanced practice in perinatal, neonatal, and pediatric respiratory care. The successful candidate must demonstrate advanced practice knowledge desirable by employers seeking to hire individuals to perform primary duties. The exam validates competency in core areas of clinical data, equipment, and therapeutic procedures. Candidates must meet the common eligibility requirements and hold the RRT or the CRT credential, plus 1 year of clinical experience in perinatal/pediatric respiratory care after attaining NBRC certification. By 2013, 11,687 had earned the NPS-CRT or the NPS-RRT credential.[8]

Sleep Disorders Specialist

The specialty certification for sleep disorders recognizes respiratory therapists performing sleep disorders testing and therapeutic interventions. The successful candidate must demonstrate advanced practice knowledge desirable by employers seeking to hire individuals to perform sleep-testing duties. Admission eligibility includes being a CRT or RRT who has graduated from an accredited respiratory therapy program including a sleep add-on track or who has achieved the CRT credential plus 6 months of full-time clinical experience or the RRT credential plus 3 months of full-time clinical experience. Required clinical experience for this specialty credential must be in a sleep diagnostics and treatment setting under medical supervision. The examination covers five major content areas: pretesting, sleep disorders testing, study analysis, administrative functions, and treatment plan. Candidates are given 4 hours to complete this examination and should expect to find polysomnography tracings based on old and new recording guidelines in the examination. By 2013, 242 had earned the CRT-SDS or RRT-SDS credential.[8]

Adult Critical Care Specialist

The Adult Critical Care Specialty Examination program is designed specifically for a respiratory therapist with the RRT credential and experience in the field of adult critical care. Eligible candidates have already demonstrated advanced knowledge in the field of respiratory care; therefore, this examination focuses on competencies unique to therapists practicing in an adult critical care setting and not basic competencies of general respiratory care. By 2013, 305 had earned the ACCS credential.[8]

Commission on Accreditation for Respiratory Care

Accreditation is a status that provides assurance to prospective students, their families, and the general public that an institution (or a program) meets minimum requirements (i.e., Accreditation Standards) and that there are reasonable grounds to believe the institution (or program) will continue to meet those standards in the future.[11] The **Commission on Accreditation for Respiratory Care (CoARC)**, founded in 1954, is located in Bedford, Texas. CoARC primarily accredits first professional respiratory care degree programs at the associate, baccalaureate, and master's degree levels in the United States and internationally. The CoARC also accredits professional respiratory care degree programs offering certificates in polysomnography. CoARC's mission is to serve the public by promoting high-quality respiratory care education through accreditation services. The composition of CoARC includes board members at-large and from each collaborating and representative organization, including the AARC, ACCP, ASA, ATS, the Association of Schools of Allied Health Professions (ASAHP), and the National Network of Health Career Programs in Two-Year Colleges (NN2). CoARC receives no financial support from the collaborating or representative organizations.

The Committee on Accreditation preceded CoARC for Respiratory Care, which made recommendations to the Commission on Accreditation of Allied Health Education Programs (CAAHEP). The CoARC board of directors made a decision in 2008 to proceed with the option of leaving the CAAHEP and becoming a free-standing **accreditation** agency of respiratory therapy education programs. The Commission on Accreditation for Respiratory Care became a free-standing accreditation agency of respiratory therapy education programs on November 12, 2009, and received Council of Higher Education Accreditation (CHEA) recognition in September 2012.

CoARC evaluates the accreditation findings of respiratory care programs and makes all accreditation decisions. Accreditation is voluntary, but failure to submit to the accreditation process may be construed as a program's failure to meet the standards and expectations set forth for all allied health education programs. Furthermore, the NBRC requires graduation from an accredited educational program for eligibility for its credentialing examinations. As of December 2012, there were 382 programs that educated AS graduates, 42 programs that graduate BS graduates, and 3 programs that offer the master's degree as entry into the profession.[12] More information about CoARC may be found at www.coarc.com.

> **Respiratory Recap**
>
> **Commission on Accreditation for Respiratory Care**
>
> - CoARC is the national accreditation body for respiratory care education programs.

Accreditation Process

Respiratory care educational programs prepare for the critical CoARC on-site survey visit by following the commission's manual of policies and procedures detailing the expectations for accreditation of a program.[13] The standards by which CoARC measures programs include sponsorship, outcome orientation, resources, student disclosure, instructional planning, and program evaluation. Each critical area has objective standards of expectation established through careful scrutiny of successful high-quality programs. The manuals, policies, procedures, and written information provided by the prospective program for the accreditation decision process are confidential. The confidentiality requirement protects the hard work of each program's educators in their preparation for accreditation. CoARC uses periodic written reviews, reports, and evaluations with an on-site visit by a team of accreditation experts to determine the worthiness of an applicant program for accreditation.[14]

The on-site review process ensures that policies and procedures submitted before an on-site visit reflect the reality of the educational experience at any prospective school. In addition, the accreditation and review process provides a measurable benchmark by which all such programs can be compared. The on-site evaluation team is composed of two individuals, such as one physician and one respiratory therapist, both of whom have completed a site-visitor training program. Either member may serve as the team captain during the site visit. The assignment process for CoARC site-visit teams ensures that any on-site visit team members do not have any potential or real conflicts of interests. Avoidance of potential or actual conflicts of interest ensures objectivity.

CoARC publishes on-site team behavioral expectations so that the program directors are aware of the expectations of on-site accreditation visitors. The policies and procedures create a formal matrix that guides the on-site team in its objective consideration of the quality of a prospective program. The accreditation process allows outsiders, prospective students, and government educational oversight groups an objective measure of a program's accomplishments and the quality of respiratory care education.

The on-site survey team provides its written findings to the referee for the program's accreditation process, and a final written report is provided to the program. The assigned program referee provides a report following the site visit with proposed accreditation recommendations. The analytic report of CoARC findings indicates any potential or actual violations of the accreditation standards. The prospective program also provides written evaluation feedback about the on-site survey team, which provides CoARC with information about the objectivity, knowledge, and demeanor of its on-site team members. A flowchart of the accreditation process is found on the CoARC website at www.coarc.com/14.html.

National Association for Medical Direction of Respiratory Care

The **National Association for Medical Direction of Respiratory Care (NAMDRC)** has existed for over 30 years. The mission of NAMDRC is to educate its members and address regulatory, legislative, and payment issues that relate to the delivery of health care to patients with respiratory disorders.[15] NAMDRC's national offices are located in Vienna, Virginia. Currently, NAMDRC's members comprise the medical directors at more than 2000 hospitals. Medical direction of respiratory care departments has been described in many states and through the Joint Commission as most appropriate for those physicians with special training and background in respiratory disease and management. NAMDRC members therefore provide respiratory care medical direction consistent with the guidelines of most oversight agencies.

Most frequently, medical direction for respiratory care has stemmed from pulmonary medicine physicians as well as anesthesiologists and a small percentage of individuals in other medical specialties, including sleep specialists. NAMDRC seeks to provide support across a full range of cardiopulmonary services, including respiratory care, critical care, ventilator management, cardiopulmonary rehabilitation, pulmonary physiology assessment, respiratory home healthcare services, hyperbaric oxygen therapy, and sleep disorders. More extensive information about NAMDRC may be obtained through its publications or its website at www.namdrc.org.

Publications

NAMDRC prints several publications, including *Washington Watchline*, the *Presidential Update*, the *Clinical and Management Quarterly Newsletter*, *Understanding Oxygen Therapy*, and the *Medical Director's Handbook*. The *Washington Watchline* is a monthly publication that keeps NAMDRC membership current on legislative and reimbursement issues associated with pulmonary care.

NAMDRC also publishes and distributes position and policy statements in the *Medical Director's Handbook*. Examples of pertinent position statements for respiratory care include "The Delivery of Hospital Respiratory Care and Duties" and "Responsibilities of the Medical Director of Respiratory Care Services and Pulmonary Function Laboratories." In many cases, related organizations use these position statements when certain issues require a respected physician perspective. For example, the AARC may use the position statement entitled "The Delivery of Hospital Respiratory Care" as a basis for the promotion of the respiratory therapist as the best provider of high-quality respiratory care. The related professional organization may have members in multiple roles, such as NAMDRC or BOMA members or representatives of a sponsoring organization.

STOP AND THINK

What are the similarities and differences among professional, credentialing, and accreditation organizations? What is the importance of each type of organization?

American College of Chest Physicians

The American College of Chest Physicians (ACCP) provides resources for the worldwide improvement of cardiopulmonary health and critical care. Its primary mission is to promote prevention and treatment of diseases of the chest through membership, leadership, education, research, communication, and government relations. Communication occurs through publication of *Chest: The Cardiopulmonary and Critical Care Journal*, clinical practice guidelines, and consensus statements. Philanthropy is achieved via the Chest Foundation. The ACCP, established in 1935, is located in Northbrook, Illinois. Up-to-date information about its conferences, new initiatives, and current publications is available at www.chestnet.org.

Membership

Membership includes more than 19,000 physicians and other professionals in this unique multidisciplinary society dedicated to the advancement of research, teaching, and clinical practice of cardiopulmonary medicine, surgery, and critical care. The designation Fellow College of Chest Physicians (FCCP) indicates recognition as a specialist in the field.[16]

Allied health professionals who provide direct patient care, department supervision at a hospital, or practice administration or who engage in clinical, academic, or research activities are eligible for ACCP membership as allied members. The ACCP

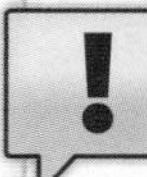

Respiratory Recap

Physician Organizations That Provide Resources for Respiratory Therapists and Offer Membership as Affiliate Members

- American College of Chest Physicians
- American Thoracic Society
- American Society for Anesthesiologists
- American Academy for Sleep Medicine

also grants the FCCP designation to nonphysicians, specialists, and scientists with distinguished accomplishments in cardiopulmonary research, teaching, and clinical practice.

Educational Offerings

The ACCP offers and sponsors a large array of educational materials through meetings, video, audiotapes, compact discs, hands-on workshops, and online self-study. The ACCP is accredited for physician continuing medical education, holding large seminars or meetings and cosponsoring educational meetings with professional organizations such as the AARC. The Health and Science Policy Committee of the ACCP is a leading resource for the assessment of the science and development of clinical policy in cardiopulmonary medicine and critical care. Its mission is to oversee and monitor significant developments in the scientific and clinical arenas of cardiopulmonary health and critical care, to transfer research findings to clinical practice, and to provide scientific conferences. A major goal of the scientific conferences is to discuss research initiatives for future research activities.

Relationship with Respiratory Care

The ACCP assists the AARC, NBRC, and CoARC, providing board members to these organizations. The ACCP also provides leadership for the AARC by naming ACCP members to BOMA.

American Thoracic Society

The American Thoracic Society (ATS) was founded in 1905 by a small group of physicians desiring to improve the care of tuberculosis patients. The ATS was originally formed as the American Sanatorium Association. Later, it was renamed the American Trudeau Society in 1938, which became the ATS in 1960. Today, it is an international professional and scientific society focusing on respiratory and critical care medicine. Currently the society has over 15,000 members. The primary mission of the ATS is the prevention and treatment of respiratory disease. Through education, research, and patient care, the ATS works to decrease morbidity and mortality associated with respiratory disease.[17]

The ATS has a long history of cooperation and advocacy through the American Lung Association (ALA), for which the ATS serves as the medical section. The ALA mission is to promote lung health and prevent lung disease. In the past decade, the ATS has become more active in critical care medicine and in the prevention, control, and treatment of diseases such as pneumonia, tuberculosis, and human immunodeficiency virus (HIV) infection. Recently, the ALA and ATS severed their organizational ties. More information about the ATS may be obtained at www.thoracic.org.

Research

The ATS promotes research through discovery of new knowledge related to respiratory and critical care medicine in health and disease. The ATS accomplishes this through assistance to the ALA in peer review process and interaction with agencies and organizations that fund new research. In addition, the ATS helps in the creation of new research funds through philanthropic organizations.

Education

Educational initiatives at the ATS promote the dissemination of new scientific information. ATS education encourages high standards for training, education, research, and clinical practice and facilitates rapid transfer of new scientific information to practice. The ATS also synthesizes new information for the public through the ALA.

The ATS publishes the *American Journal of Respiratory and Critical Care Medicine*, the *American Journal of Respiratory Cell and Molecular Biology*, and *Proceedings of the American Thoracic Society*. Each is highly respected and used worldwide by pulmonary and critical care practitioners.

Patient Care

Patient care initiatives include promotion of the highest standards for quality in health care, establishment of partnerships between pulmonary and critical care medicine, and evaluation of the relationship between cost and quality in the delivery of health care.

Advocacy

The ATS encourages growth in programs and methods that provide high-quality care. In addition, the ATS advises and promotes cooperation by and between governmental and nongovernmental agencies for matters of common interest. For example, the ATS sponsors the AARC, which includes activities in BOMA, NBRC, and CoARC.

American Society of Anesthesiologists

The ASA is an educational, research, and scientific association of physicians organized in 1905 to raise and maintain the standards of anesthesiology and improve patient care. Contact with respiratory care usually involves postsurgical care, most prominently in the area of critical care.[18] The anesthesiologist maintains analgesia and life functions during the surgical procedures in the operating suite. After surgery, the anesthesiologist maintains contact with the patient's care team to ensure a comfortable and stable recovery after surgery.

Members of ASA must be doctors of medicine who are licensed practitioners and have successfully completed a training program approved by the Accreditation Council for Graduate Medical Education (ACGME). Members may also be doctors of osteopathy who have successfully completed training approved by the American Osteopathic Association (AOA). By 2013, more than 50,000 practitioners were ASA members.[19] The ASA is currently located in Park Ridge, Illinois, a suburb of Chicago. More information is available at www.asahq.org.

Relationship with Respiratory Care

The ASA is currently a sponsoring or collaborating member of the AARC, NBRC, and CoARC. Through clinical expertise, provision of members to BOMA for AARC, and other support mechanisms, the ASA contributes to the practice and science of respiratory care. The ASA supports AARC activities and professional issues, developing position statements and clinical practice guidelines to denote the need for respiratory therapy personnel in all areas of clinical practice. The anesthesiologist is the perioperative physician who provides medical care to the patient throughout his or her surgical experience.

True to this definition, the anesthesiologist may order preoperative testing, including arterial blood gases and pulmonary function studies, to determine the current health status of the patient. In addition, the anesthesiologist may order respiratory care procedures to help promote a higher level of lung function in preparation for surgery. The chances of a healthy patient suffering an intraoperative death attributable to anesthesia is less than 1 in 200,000 when an anesthesiologist is involved in patient care.[19]

Mission

The ASA supports the world's largest educational program for anesthesiology practice and science. The annual meeting of ASA provides up-to-date research, science, and continuing education to its members. The ASA sponsors the self-education and evaluation (SEE) program and publishes its own monthly peer-reviewed journal, *Anesthesiology.*

Governmental Affairs

The ASA's Office of Governmental Affairs (OGA), located in Washington, D.C., monitors legislative activities and regulations at the state and federal levels to ensure the continuance of high-quality care in all areas of health care. Examples include Medicare and Medicaid. The ASA works closely with others groups, such as the AMA and AARC, on clinical practice issues of regulation that may influence anesthesiology and respiratory care.

Governance

The ASA's governance structure is similar to that of the AARC. The ASA has a House of Delegates distributed by geographic region that meets at the ASA annual meeting. Officers, past presidents, the editor in chief of *Anesthesiology,* and chairs of sections for education and residency all contribute to the practice, governance, and direction of anesthesiology.

Society of Critical Care Medicine

The Society of Critical Care Medicine (SCCM), formed in 1970, is the youngest organization related to the practice of respiratory care. The SCCM was formed to further a multidisciplinary and multiprofessional approach to the care of the critically ill patient. The society boasts more than 16,000 members in over 100 countries by 2013.[20] The SCCM's membership is evidence of its multiprofessional approach. Members include intensivists, nurses, respiratory therapists, pharmacists, pharmacologists, scientists, researchers, bioengineers, critical care industry executives, and other interested allied health professionals.

The use of a multidisciplinary approach to research and patient care promotes a continuum of care. This continuum begins at the moment of injury or illness and proceeds through full recovery. Critical care may be practiced at the site of an accident or in the perioperative setting. Most activity involving the respiratory therapist occurs in the emergency and intensive care areas, however. More information may be found at www.sccm.org.

Journals and Relationship with Respiratory Care

The SCCM publishes *Critical Care Medicine,* a monthly journal dedicated to the science and treatment of critically ill patients. As a multidisciplinary organization, SCCM is engaged in respiratory care in ways similar to previously described medical groups and professional organizations. The SCCM is directly involved in the AARC through BOMA and as a BOD member during its rotation as BOMA chair. SCCM sponsors AARC, NBRC, and CoARC, providing a valuable multiprofessional perspective to advances in care and regulatory issues affecting respiratory care.

The Joint Commission

The Joint Commission (TJC) is the nation's predominant standards setting and accrediting body in health care. This organization changed its name in 2007 from the Joint Commission on Accreditation of Health Care Organizations to The Joint Commission. The central office is located in Oakbrook Terrace, Illinois, with a satellite office in Washington, D.C. The Joint Commission is an independent, not-for-profit organization.

Since 1951, TJC has maintained state-of-the-art standards that focus on improving the quality and safety of care provided by healthcare organizations.

TJC evaluates and accredits more than 20,000 healthcare organizations and programs in the United States. Joint Commission certification is recognized nationwide as a symbol of quality that reflects an organization's commitment to meeting certain performance standards.[21] To earn and maintain certification, an organization must undergo an on-site survey by a Joint Commission survey team at least every 3 years.

TJC also awards disease-specific care certification to health plans, disease management service companies, hospitals, and other care delivery settings that provide disease management and chronic care services. TJC also has a healthcare staffing services certification program. It is developing a certification program for transplant centers and healthcare services.

Mission

The mission of TJC is to continuously improve health care for the public, in collaboration with other stakeholders, by evaluating healthcare organizations and inspiring them to excel in providing safe and effective care of the highest quality and value.[21] Programs accredited by TJC include not only hospitals but also home care, laboratory services, assisted living, long-term care, and office-based surgery. Requirements and survey guides are provided for all these program-specific certifications on the Commission's website at www.jointcommission.org.

Relationship to Respiratory Care

Respiratory therapists are directly involved with Joint Commission surveyors when their facility or program is under review. Technical directors of respiratory care services are responsible for the core performance measures of patient care related to respiratory care in the hospital or home care setting. The AARC also appoints members to TJC to provide input and influence professional and technical advisory committees (PTACs). The Joint Commission PTACs are designed to assist in important matters pertaining to its accreditation programs. Periodically, TJC seeks input from respiratory therapists to comment on proposed standards. The use of medication management in acute care settings is an example of how respiratory therapists have added value to this organization.

National Asthma Educator Certification Board

The **National Asthma Educator Certification Board (NAECB)** was established in 2000 as a result of over 50 stakeholder groups coming together to discuss the need for an asthma certification exam. The mission of the NAECB is to promote optimal asthma management and quality of life among individuals with asthma, their families, and communities by advancing excellence in asthma education through the Certified Asthma Educator (AE-C) process.[22] The 17-member board represents the multiple disciplines involved in asthma education, including allergy/immunology, behavioral science, emergency medicine, nursing, patient advocacy, environmental health, health education, medicine, pediatrics, pharmacy, public health, pulmonary medicine, and respiratory therapy.

Certified Asthma Educator

A Certified Asthma Educator (AE-C) is an expert in teaching, educating, and counseling individuals with asthma and their families in the knowledge and skills necessary to minimize the impact of asthma on their quality of life.[23] The AE-C possesses comprehensive, current knowledge of asthma pathophysiology and management, including developmental theories, cultural dimensions, the impact of chronic illness, and principles of teaching and learning. Respiratory therapists make ideal asthma educators because they are very knowledgeable on the optimal use of medications and delivery devices. Respiratory therapists are particularly good at explaining technical concepts to individuals in language each can understand.

Other roles and duties of the AE-C include assessments of individuals and families to identify strengths and resources as well as negative psychological factors, the social and economic impact of asthma, educational needs, and barriers to optimal health care and self-management.[23] The educator works with an individual with asthma, his or her family, and other healthcare professionals to develop, implement, monitor, and revise an asthma action plan customized to the individual's needs, environment, disease severity, and lifestyle to optimize the individual's self-management skills.

AE-C Examination

The NAECB administers the AE-C exam in a manner similar to the process used by the NBRC, through Applied Measurement Professionals. Registrants can apply for the exam if they meet eligibility requirements, which include being a licensed or credentialed healthcare professional. **Box 57-1** lists the healthcare professions eligible for the AE-C. Individuals who are not licensed but who have provided professional asthma education and counseling with a minimum of 1000 hours experience in these activities also can register to take the exam.

The examination is based on seven major content areas. Content areas are outlined in detail in the candidate handbook, including the exam matrix. As of October 2, 2013, there were 4030 individuals certified, with a national pass rate of 68.1%. Recertification is by examination or by a new continuing education process[23] that includes obtaining 35 clock hours in areas pertaining to asthma education. Recertification is required every 5 years. Information regarding the AE-C exam,

BOX 57-1

Healthcare Professionals Eligible for the AE-C Examination

Physicians (MD, DO)
Physician assistants (PA-C)
Nurse practitioners (NP)
Nurses (RN, LPN)
Respiratory therapists (RRT, CRT)
Pulmonary function technologists (CPFT, RPFT)
Pharmacists (RPh)
Social workers (LSW, MDW, LMSW)
Health educators (CHES)
Physical therapists (PT)
Occupational therapists (OT)

recertification, and the NAECB can be found at www.naecb.org.

Association of Asthma Educators

The **Association of Asthma Educators (AAE)** is an interdisciplinary professional organization with the goal of raising the competency of individuals who educate patients and families affected by asthma.[24] Formed in 1998, the majority of AAE members are asthma educators who do not have prescribing privileges. One of the AAE's primary goals is to be the leading resource for asthma educators to help improve health outcomes for individuals and families affected by asthma. An annual conference is held each year. The AAE also offers an online review course to prepare participants to take the AE-C exam. Other programs available are listed on the organization's website at www.asthmaeducators.org. Membership is open to all licensed healthcare professionals. Associate and student memberships are also available.

American Academy of Sleep Medicine

Established in 1975 as the Association of Sleep Disorders Centers, the **American Academy of Sleep Medicine (AASM)** is the only professional society that is dedicated exclusively to the medical subspecialty of sleep medicine. The AASM sets standards and promotes excellence in health care, education, and research. The AASM serves its members and advances the field of sleep health care by setting the clinical standards for sleep medicine; advocating for the recognition, diagnosis, and treatment of sleep disorders; educating professionals to provide optimal sleep health care; and fostering the development and application of scientific knowledge.[25]

Publications

The journal *Sleep* is a publication of the Associated Professional Sleep Societies, LLC, which is a joint venture of the AASM and the Sleep Research Society. *Sleep* was the first journal published that was dedicated exclusively to sleep. As the official publication of the AASM, the *Journal of Clinical Sleep Medicine* publishes applied sleep science of clinical trials, clinical reviews, case series and reports, and commentaries and debates. It also publishes reports, news, and updates from the AASM.[25]

Membership

The AASM membership consists of more than 12,000 physicians, researchers, and other healthcare professionals. These members specialize in studying, diagnosing, and treating disorders of sleep and daytime alertness such as insomnia, narcolepsy, and obstructive sleep apnea. Respiratory therapists are eligible to join for affiliate membership if they have special training in sleep disorders. Special training includes sleep technologists or sleep center managers who are active in the clinical or research aspects of sleep medicine.

Board of Registered Polysomnographic Technologists

The **Board of Registered Polysomnographic Technologists (BRPT)** based in McLean, Virginia, is an independent, nonprofit certification board that sets professional and ethical standards for polysomnographic technologists. Established in 1978 to benefit the developing field of polysomnographic technology and set credentialing standards for technologists, the BRPT developed the registry examination for polysomnographic technology (RPSGT). The BRPT also maintains and administers the RPSGT exam. There are more than 19,000 registered polysomnographic technologists.

Examinations

The RPSGT credential indicates that the technologist has a level of experience and competence aligned with an international standard. Since March 2013, there have been a number of changes to the eligibility pathway to becoming a RPSGT.[26] For example, a

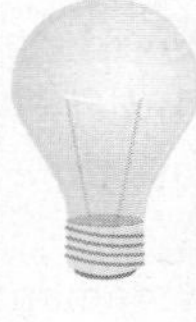

STOP AND THINK

How do professional, credentialing, and accreditation organizations benefit the principles and practice of respiratory care? What role should you have in these organizations and why is your involvement important?

few options include completing an 18-month polysomnographic (PSG) experience through on-the-job training, or obtaining 6 months of PSG experience (credentialed health professionals only), or graduating from a CAAHEP-accredited or CoARC-accredited polysomnographic technology program, to name a few. In March 2010 the BRPT launched the Certified Polysomnographic Technician (CPSGT) certificate-level exam, intended specifically for individuals new to a career in sleep. The CPSGT certificate is time-limited; certificate holders must earn the RPSGT credential within 3 years or lose the CPSGT designation.[27]

Key Points

- Many organizations sponsor and support the respiratory care profession.
- Certain organizations have very specific and limited missions, whereas others are more diverse in purpose and mission.
- The goals of each supporting organization ultimately improve the scope, practice, education, credentials, quality, and professional growth of respiratory care.
- The AARC provides various forms of education and educational opportunities through meetings, publications, grants, awards, fellowships, activities, and services for its members to facilitate continued growth of the profession.
- Although some supporting organizations are restricted to physician membership, many are not, providing numerous opportunities for participation by respiratory therapists.
- The AARC and related professional organizations enhance the entire respiratory care profession, with far-reaching effects beyond each organization's membership.
- Membership in the AARC should be considered an integral part of a respiratory care professional's identity.

References

1. American Association for Respiratory Care. *In the News. We Have a Vision*. Available at: http://www.aarc.org/headlines/vision/asp. Accessed September 9, 2014.
2. American Association for Respiratory Care. *AARC Bylaws*. Irving, TX: AARC; 2007.
3. Kacmarek RM, Durbin CG, Barnes TA, et al. Creating a vision for respiratory care and beyond. *Respir Care*. 2009;54:375–389.
4. Barnes TA, Gale DG, Kacmarek RM, Kageler WV. Competencies needed by graduate respiratory therapists in 2015 and beyond. *Respir Care*. 2010;55:601–616.
5. Barnes TA, Kacmarek RM, Kageler WV, Morris MJ. Transitioning the respiratory care workforce for 2015 and beyond. *Respir Care*. 2011;56:681–690.
6. National Board for Respiratory Care. *About the National Board for Respiratory Care*. Available at: http://www.nbrc.org/Pages/about.aspx. Accessed September 9, 2014.
7. National Board for Respiratory Care. *Candidate Handbook and Application*. Olathe, KS: National Board for Respiratory Care; 2013.
8. Ohio Board of Respiratory Therapy. 761-5-01 Waiver of licensing requirements pursuant to division (B) of section 4761.04 of the Revised Code. Available at: http://codes.ohio.gov/oac/4761-5-01. Accessed September 9, 2014.
9. National Board for Respiratory Care. Credentialing for the profession. *NBRC Horizons*. 2013;39:11.
10. National Board for Respiratory Care. *The Jimmy A Young Memorial Lecture: Unveiling the New Therapist Multiple Choice Examination*. Available at: http://www.nbrc.org/Documents/2013%20Jimmy%20A.%20Young%20Memorial%20Lecture.pdf. Accessed on September 9, 2014.
11. Commission on Accreditation of Respiratory Care. Available at: http://www.coarc.com. Accessed on September 9, 2014.
12. Commission on Accreditation of Respiratory Care. *2012 Report on Accreditation in Respiratory Care Education*. Available at: http://www.coarc.com/29.html. Accessed September 9, 2014.
13. Commission on Accreditation of Respiratory Care. *CoARC Accreditation Policies and Procedures*. Available at: http://www.coarc.com/31.html. Accessed September 9, 2014.
14. Commission on Accreditation of Respiratory Care. *Accreditation Process Flow Chart*. In: *Overview of the Accreditation Process*. Available at: http://www.coarc.com/14.html. Accessed September 9, 2014.
15. National Association for Medical Direction of Respiratory Care. *What is NAMDRC?* Available at: http://www.namdrc.org. Accessed September 9, 2014.
16. American College of Chest Physicians. *Membership Opportunities*. Available at: http://www.chestnet.org/Get-Involved/ACCP-Membership/Membership-Opportunities. Accessed on September 9, 2014.
17. American Thoracic Society. *ATS at a Glance*. Available at: http://www.thoracic.org/about/ats-at-a-glance.php. Accessed on September 9, 2014.
18. American Society for Anesthesiology. *About ASA: Advancing the Practice and Securing the Future*. Available at: http://www.asahq.org/For-the-Public-and-Media/About-ASA.aspx. Accessed September 9, 2014.
19. American Society for Anesthesiology. *Anesthesia Fast Facts*. Available at: http://www.asahq.org/For-the-Public-and-Media/Press-Room/Anesthesia-Fast-Facts.aspx. Accessed on September 9, 2014.
20. Society for Critical Care Medicine. *Critical Care Statistics*. Available at: http://www.sccm.org/Communications/Pages/CriticalCareStats.aspx. Accessed on September 9, 2014.
21. The Joint Commission. *Facts about the Joint Commission*. Available at: http://www.jointcommission.org/facts_about_the_joint_commission/. Accessed September 9, 2014.
22. National Asthma Education Certification Board. Home page. Available at: http://www.naecb.org. Accessed September 9, 2014.
23. National Asthma Education Certification Board. *Recertification by Education as a Certified Asthma Educator (AE-C®)*. Available at: http://naecb.com/pdf/NAECBBookletEMAIL.pdf. Accessed September 9, 2014.
24. Association of Asthma Educators. Welcome to AAE! Available at: http://www.asthmaeducators.org. Accessed September 9, 2014.
25. American Academy of Sleep Medicine. Home page. Available at: http://www.aasmnet.org. Accessed September 9, 2014.
26. Board of Registered Polysomnographic Technologists. *RPSGT: Eligibility*. Available at: http://www.brpt.org/default.asp?contentID=34. Accessed September 9, 2014.
27. Board of Registered Polysomnographic Technologists. *The RPSGT and CPSGT Credentials*. Available at: http://www.brpt.org/default.asp?contentID=22. Accessed September 9, 2014.

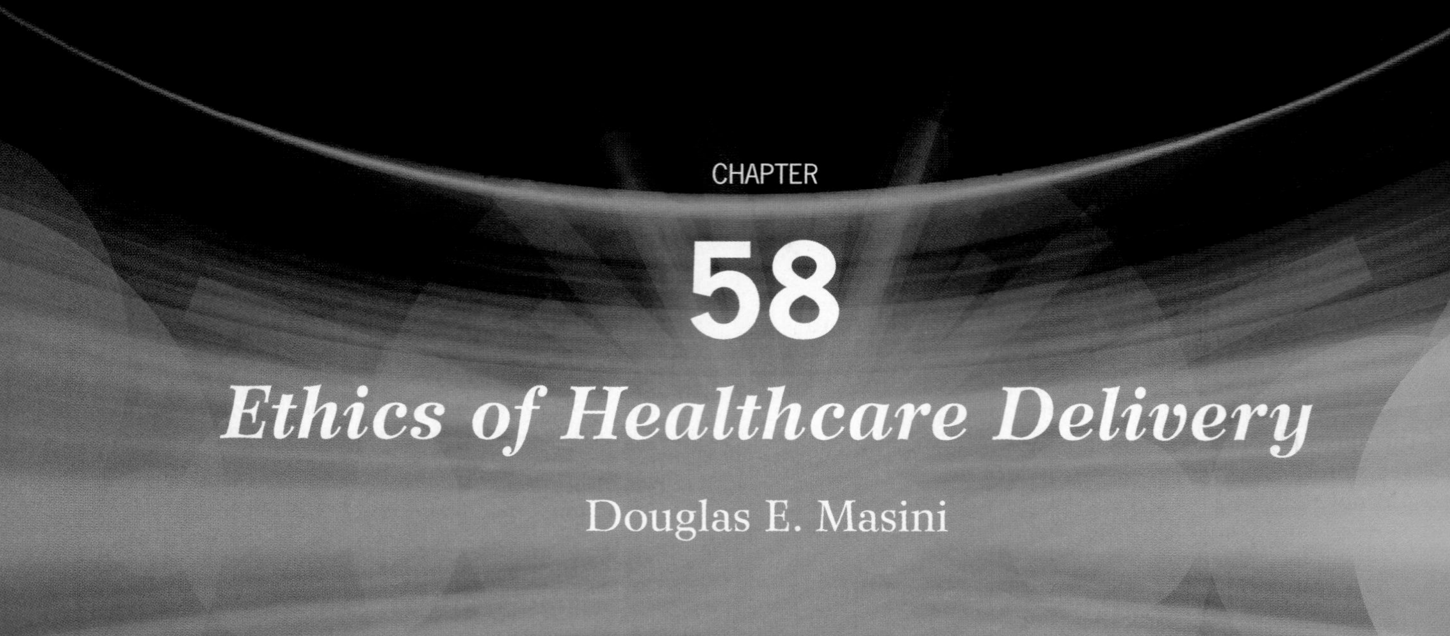

OUTLINE

Definition of Ethics
Foundations of Ethical Thinking
Ethical Versus Legal Behavior
Ethical Theories
Ethical Principles
Role of Professional Organizations in Ethics
Ethics Committees
Case Studies

OBJECTIVES

1. Define ethics.
2. Describe methods by which an ethical orientation is formed.
3. Distinguish between ethical and legal behavior.
4. Describe an ethical dilemma.
5. State the role of ethics in the delivery of effective respiratory care.
6. Define common ethical theories.
7. Define seven contemporary ethical principles.
8. Describe the way the analysis method is used to solve ethical dilemmas.
9. Describe three common ethical dilemmas associated with the delivery of respiratory care.
10. Describe key components of the American Association for Respiratory Care's statement of ethics and professional conduct.
11. Discuss the role of ethics committees and the respiratory therapist.
12. List components of the Patient Care Partnership.
13. Discuss the way technology has increased the incidence of confidentiality violations.
14. List ways in which managed care has affected basic ethical principles.

KEY TERMS

AARC Code of Ethics
advance directive
analysis method
autonomy
beneficence
bias
capacity
confidentiality
deontological theory
Durable Medical Power of Attorney
ethics
ethics or optimum care committee
fidelity
justice
living will
moral philosophy
nonmaleficence
Patient Care Partnership
personal belief system
personal value system
prejudice
proxy
surrogate
teleological theory
veracity

Introduction

Increasingly, respiratory therapy literature has called for respiratory therapists to take on new roles and have new levels of autonomy and independence in decision making, especially in the context of respiratory care protocols. The new student and the seasoned therapist must recognize that such a paradigm shift requires not only experience and technical training but enhanced communication skills to promote their knowledge of professional ethics and ethical considerations in the delivery of respiratory care. In other words, we have to walk the walk and talk the talk when we discuss the ethical practice of respiratory therapy with other caregivers.

Every working day, the respiratory therapist is faced with ethical dilemmas and new questions that have to be answered. For example, how can respiratory therapists continue to provide quality patient care while departmental staffing is undergoing a reduction in force? How can respiratory therapists maintain patient confidentiality in the information age? Is there a place for the respiratory therapist on the community ethics or optimal care committee? What roles do respiratory

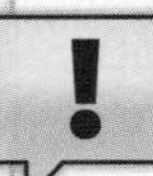

Respiratory Recap

Ethics

- Ethical principles have long been a part of medical practice, dating back to the time of Hippocrates.
- Ethics is a decision-making process, and in that process societies and individuals made a decision regarding what was right or wrong.

therapists play in assisting families with the difficult decision to use life support equipment or agree to "do-not-resuscitate" orders for their loved ones? Should advanced and expensive monitoring, use of intravascular lines, and heroic mechanical ventilation be used in every critical care situation?

These ethical questions and more confront both students and clinicians every day. Ethical discussions and decisions are never easy. With ethical questions in particular, answers are rarely black or white and often lie within gray zones. Ethical decisions depend on the specific value systems and decisions of the individuals involved.

Although discussions about medical ethics have increased in recent years, the topic is not a new one. Medical ethics have been discussed since the days of ancient Greece. The Hippocratic Oath, established in the fourth century BC, outlined ethical guidelines and behaviors for physicians, who vowed "to keep their patients from harm and injustice."[1]

The Oath contained other provisions that addressed confidentiality for patients and the role of the physician. These and other ethical issues in patient care have transcended time, but society continues to reestablish, refine, and then redefine its code of ethics for health care. In this chapter, the respiratory therapist learns how to model and communicate the ethical practice of respiratory care.

Definition of Ethics

The American Medical Association (AMA) stated that the term "ethical" is used in opinions of the AMA's Council on Ethical and Judicial Affairs to refer to matters involving (1) moral principles or practices and (2) matters of social policy involving issues of morality in the practice of medicine. The term "unethical" is used to refer to professional conduct which fails to conform to these moral standards or policies."[2] The study of ethics is not specifically the determination of right or wrong answers but the study of the ways in which individuals come to the judgment that their decision is right or wrong; ethics is the study of the decision-making pathway one takes in determining what she or he believes is right or wrong.

Two important variables worthy of discussion when we talk about personal or clinical decision making are bias and prejudice. **Bias** is defined as "A preference or an inclination, especially one that inhibits impartial judgment" or "an unfair act or policy stemming from prejudice."[3] **Prejudice** can be defined as "... [a] judgment formed before due examination and consideration of the facts—a premature or hasty judgment."[4] Both bias and prejudice inform clinical decision making, and the student and seasoned clinicians both must confront their own bias and prejudices prior to making that decision. Conflict-of-interest statements, signed by the speaker or presenter, are now standardized as documentation that a speaker has reflected upon his or her professional relationships and influences and considered his or her bias or prejudice prior to presentation of information to a larger audience. For example, one must identify specific conflict-of-interest relationships to include remuneration, travel expenses, or honorariums that one has received from vendors, manufacturers, or pharmaceutical companies. This relationship has the potential to skew a presentation, which in turn could bias or prejudice the opinions or decision made by an individual respiratory therapist.

No individual is born knowing what is right or wrong. **Ethics** are based in part on values individuals develop as they mature both professionally and personally. Often these values are influenced by gender, geographic location, social and economic standards, religious convictions, family members, ethnicity, prejudice, bias, political beliefs, education, life experience, and culture.

Foundations of Ethical Thinking

Personal Belief System

As individuals experience life and are educated in the morals and mores of our society, they develop a set of personal beliefs. These beliefs are not necessarily right or wrong and are certainly not objective. Yet they are deeply ingrained in an individual's thoughts and their decision-making processes.

Attitudinal Orientation

Attitudinal orientation is the outward expression of an individual's **personal belief system**. It is what a person says and how that person behaves and is based on what the individual believes. Attitudes have a large effect on behavior; this is most evident when an individual is confronted with an ethical dilemma.

Personal Value System

The **personal value system** is formed when the decision is made to continue to believe and express a conviction even when a person or event challenges it. For example, having a particular belief about the death penalty is easy, as is expression of this belief when no opposition exists. Maintaining a belief and defending it to others becomes more difficult in the face of opposition,

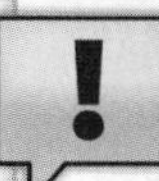

Respiratory Recap

Personal Value Systems

- Personal beliefs include the mores and morals of our society.
- Attitudinal orientation is the outward expression of a personal belief system.
- The personal value system is formed when beliefs become convictions.
- An individual's moral philosophy can be viewed as a behavioral code.

however, especially if a person's bias or prejudice is without evidence or merit. When an individual is willing to maintain a belief in the face of opposition, that belief becomes a conviction. When the individual integrates convictions into a personal value system and maintains them in the face of opposition, they become personal principles. This progression is an important step in the formation of an individual's ethical orientation because personal principles influence that individual's ethical orientation and decision making.

Moral Philosophy

An individual's **moral philosophy** can be viewed as a behavioral code. Morals define what individuals will or will not do in a given situation, and moral philosophy is based on the individual's previously adopted personal principles. Ethics can be viewed as a work in progress, and ethical principles often reflect the current society. As a society evolves and changes, so will its ethical beliefs; two timely examples include abortion and the death penalty. Changes in the way society views these issues are reflected in newer laws governing these practices.

Ethical Versus Legal Behavior

Ethical Orientation

A discussion of ethical behavior is difficult without at least an allusion to legal behavior. Legal behavior in this sense simply means abiding by the law. Sometimes the line between the ethical and the legal is fine; sometimes that line disappears and the behaviors merge; other times the gap between the two widens. A given behavior can be described as both ethical and legal, and it often has the same foundation. Ethical and legal behaviors differ primarily in the individual freedom allowed for decision making. For example, an individual may be free to adhere to a given ethical code but required to abide by the legal code under the threat of punishment by law.

Legal Standards

Ideally, behavior would always be both ethical and legal. In reality, however, that standard is not always met. Several reasons exist for the discrepancy between the legal and the ethical, the primary reason being that neither ethical behavior nor legal requirements are static standards. Ethical and legal standards of behavior change as society grows and changes.

In recent history abortion is a classic example that demonstrates the way major societal issues influence both ethical and legal standards. Before 1973, when the Supreme Court's *Roe v. Wade* decision was handed down, abortion was clearly illegal. Needless to say, the Supreme Court did not decide in a vacuum on that day to legalize abortion. Instead, the argument had grown over the previous decades that all abortions should not be illegal. It may not have been stated as such, but this view marked a gradual change in society's ethical orientation. Although not every American citizen agreed that abortion should be legalized, at the time of the Supreme Court decision, society's ethical orientation had shifted so significantly that the Court's interpretation was inevitable. Some legal scholars might argue that the Court simply interpreted the Constitution and the ruling had nothing to do with society's ethical orientation. However, constitutional interpretation is usually related to society's ethical orientation. Take, for example, the Supreme Court's decisions on the death penalty and slavery. The range of legal decisions handed down by courts, whether deemed positive or negative, reflect society's orientation at these times in history.

A major ethical and legal shift in the area of death and dying is pending. The right to die appears to have gained a growing acceptance from an ethical standpoint. Customary in these kinds of shifts is for legal standards to lag behind ethical development. For example, Jack Kevorkian, a Michigan pathologist, was found legally responsible for the death of one of his patients. Close examination of the opinions surrounding his work reveals a subtle shift from a view that his work is ethically wrong to one of a right to die. This shift in ethical viewpoints in the United States toward euthanasia is primarily evident in the nonscientific literature.[5] In 1997, however, Oregon introduced legislation to legalize the "Death with Dignity" act for physician-assisted

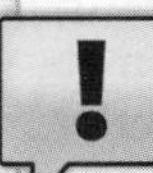

Respiratory Recap

Ethical Versus Legal Behavior

- Legal behavior simply means abiding by the law, whereas ethical behavior involves personal beliefs, attitudinal orientation, and moral philosophy.
- Legal and ethical behaviors are not static.
- Ideally, behavior would always be both ethical and legal.
- A major pending shift in ethical and legal behavior is presently happening in death and dying.

suicide, and 22 other states have proposed similar legislation. Respiratory therapists practicing today and in the future will no doubt confront the ramifications of this legislation in their daily practice.[6,7]

The preceding discussion on legal standards and ethical orientation may appear unrelated to ethics for the respiratory therapist. It is, however, important in helping respiratory therapists to understand the dynamics of ethical dilemmas. Ethical dilemmas are not static issues that remain constant but change as society changes. The most important point for the therapist to learn is how to deal with ethical dilemmas in situational settings.

The respiratory therapist may encounter many ethical dilemmas, ranging from dramatic life support and end-of-life issues to the basic staffing and level of care issues prevalent in today's managed care environment. In fact, most dilemmas the average therapist faces are the less dramatic ones. That these dilemmas are less dramatic does not make them less important.

Ethical Theories

Two main theories are used to describe the decision-making process an individual undertakes in deriving an ethical conclusion to a dilemma. Teleological and deontological theories guide ethical decision making. In addition to these two major ethical theories, the analysis method is used, which combines teleological and deontological theory, recognizing that most ethical decisions require systematic analysis.

Teleological Theory

Teleological theory is based on consequences. The right or wrong of an action is based on the outcomes or consequences of predicted outcomes. The most common type of consequential theory is known as utilitarianism, in which an individual chooses the act that brings about the best outcome. To determine the best outcome the individual must follow a system of steps, during which the problem first is described, all solutions then are listed, and the solutions finally are compared with the good each can provide. The correct answer is the most useful solution and becomes the best outcome. For example, enough money is available for either a heart transplant for one patient or vaccines for hundreds of infants. Using the teleological theory, the consequences of helping hundreds would be better than helping one patient. The best outcome therefore would be to use the money to buy the vaccines. Patient triage is another example of utilitarianism. In today's fast-paced respiratory care department, triage skills are critical when, simply put, the right person must give the right therapy to the right patient at the right time.

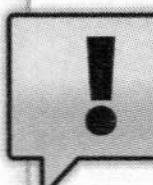

Respiratory Recap

Teleological Theory

- Teleological theory is consequential theory, based on consequences.
- The most common type of consequential theory is known as utilitarianism.
- Utilitarianism looks for the best outcome.

STOP AND THINK

Discuss an example that demonstrates a clinical issue that may be legally valid but presents ethical dilemmas. Discuss another clinical issue that may be ethically valid but presents legal ramifications. Provide evidence to support decision making.

Deontological Theory

Deontological theory is based on duty and states that an act is either right or wrong based on its intrinsic character rather than on its consequences. Although deontological theory is concerned with doing the best thing, it also tries to do the right thing. The philosophical works of Immanuel Kant, as well as many religions, identify with this theory. The steps involved in the deontological theory are much more complicated than those in teleological theory and are outlined in **Figure 58-1**.

Analysis Method

One other theory used in ethics is the **analysis method**, which combines key components from teleological and

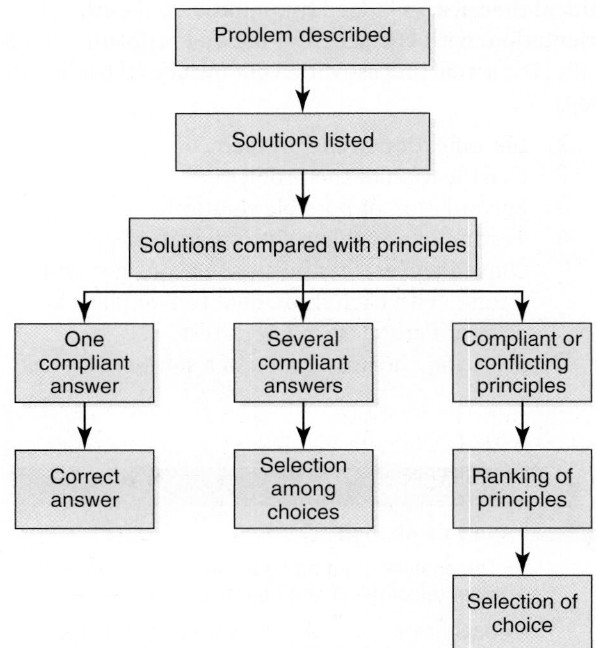

FIGURE 58-1 Deontological theory of reasoning.

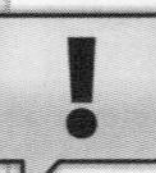

Respiratory Recap

Deontological Theory

- Deontological theory is an ethical theory based on duty.
- An act is either right or wrong based on its intrinsic character (duty) rather than on its consequences.
- The philosophical works of Immanuel Kant as well as many religions identify with this theory.

deontological theories. It recognizes that in the final analysis, most ethical decisions are made by a systematic analytic process devised by the individual.[8]

Fletcher and coworkers established a Case Method of Moral Problem solving, using clinical pragmatism in the spirit of John Dewey's pragmatic philosophy. In their method they suggested: (1) assessment, (2) moral diagnosis, (3) goal setting, and (4) evaluation. The Case Method of Moral Problem solving asked many incisive questions; it evaluates patient medical condition, relevant contextual factors, patient capacity for decision making, patient preferences, needs of the patient as a person, preferences of family or **surrogate** decision makers, interests other than and potentially competing with the patient's, and issues of power or conflict in the interactions of the key actors in the case that need to be addressed. This method asks, "Have the parties had the opportunity to be heard, and have all institutional factors contributing to problems posed by the case been addressed?"[9]

Analysis methodology became increasingly popular in the 21st century. Most ethical dilemmas were solved with analysis method, which combines the best of the ethical theories, as judged by an individual's ethical orientation, with critical-thinking and problem-solving skills. The actual process varied but includes the following steps:

1. Identification of the problem.
2. Clarification of the problem.
3. Formulation of possible solutions.
4. Testing of possible solutions against consequences, feasibility, sense of right and wrong, with each individual free to place a different emphasis on each test.
5. Selection and application of a solution.

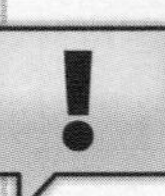

Respiratory Recap

Analysis Method

- The analysis method combines key components from teleological and deontological theories.
- Healthcare professionals resolve most ethical dilemmas using the analysis method.

Ethical Principles

Using ethical theories, society has developed several principles or standards of behavior to help determine right or wrong actions. These principles change over time as societies change. Eight ethical principles considered important in contemporary medicine are (1) beneficence, (2) capacity, (3) nonmaleficence, (4) veracity, (5) autonomy, (6) confidentiality, (7) justice, and (8) role fidelity.

Beneficence

Beneficence means charity or mercy. This principle imposes on the clinician the responsibility to seek good for the patient under all circumstances. The healthcare professional should do only what will benefit the patient.

Healthcare professionals enter their professions with the genuine desire to help patients and receive intrinsic rewards by helping and caring for those who need their expertise. Beneficence has long played a role in the delivery of health care. Hippocrates wrote, "I will apply dietetic measures for the benefit of the sick according to my ability and judgment."[1] This desire to provide care to benefit patients has been a continuing principle. Healthcare and professional organizations recognize the need for continued education to foster growth and competence in health care.

Determining what is good is a difficulty encountered with beneficence. If beneficence means the seeking of good for the patient, who will decide what is good? Will the patient make the determination or the healthcare worker? Just as individuals have different values, so will patients have different opinions as to what will benefit them the most.

Beneficence is becoming increasingly more difficult to determine in today's advanced technological world. For example, the technology now exists to prolong lives that would have been lost just two decades ago. At the same time remains the question of whether this technology should be used to save every life. An individual with terminal cancer could be kept alive for months on life support. Should technology be used in this case? Would it benefit the patient? Is it good for the patient? Is it good for the family? Who decides?

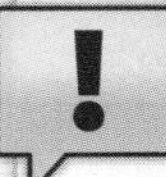

Respiratory Recap

Beneficence

- Beneficence imposes the responsibility to seek good for the patient under all circumstances.
- Determining what is good can be difficult.
- Beneficence is becoming increasingly more difficult to determine in today's advanced technological world.

Patients Who Refuse Intubation and Ventilation

Advance directives communicate a patient's wishes to their physician and caregivers. They may be modified to assert a patient's wishes, what they want done and what they do not want done. In particular, an advance directive can specify whether patients do not wish to have an artificial airway placed, such as the do-not-intubate (DNI) order. Authors examined the use of noninvasive ventilation (NIV) in patients who did not wish to be intubated. In some patients who have declined or are reluctant to undergo intubation, NIV was used to lessen dyspnea, preserve patient autonomy, and permit verbal communication with loved ones. This indication is controversial, however, and may in theory prolong the dying process and lead to inappropriate utilization of scarce resources.[10] Mehta and Hill suggest that the use of NIV for patients who are not to receive invasive ventilation is justifiable if the patient understands that NIV is being used as a form of life support, and there is the potential for reversal of the acute process.[10]

In European respiratory intermediate and high dependency care units, the most common end-of-life practices were withholding treatment, the use of noninvasive mechanical ventilation as a ceiling therapy, and provision of DNR/DNI.[11] Nava et al concluded that patients, when competent, and their families together with nurses were most often involved in reaching these key decisions.[11]

When determining the overall value of NIV at the end of life, physicians should ask patients if they meant that they do not wish to be intubated, if they do not want the discomfort of an endotracheal intubation or a mechanical ventilator, or if they mean that they do not want any intervention and are prepared to die.[12] When patients say they do not want to be intubated, they may simply mean that they do not wish to be subjected to the discomfort of an endotracheal tube or mechanical ventilator but might be willing to receive NIV.[12] The most critical issues with regard to NIV for DNI and comfort measures only (CMO) patients are patient and family education and informed consent. The respiratory therapist must ask, "Have the risks and potential benefits of NIV been clearly discussed, and would the patient agree to accept the risks?" Data from patients with terminal cancer suggest that patient-important factors were retaining control over their end-of-life care decisions and having adequate time to prepare for their death. If control over care decisions is assured, NIV may be able to reverse acute respiratory failure that is not necessarily a life-terminating event and improve patient comfort and sustain life until the patient can put his or her affairs in order.[13]

Capacity

Capacity is the deduction of one or more principal caregivers, based upon the best evidence available, that the patient is capable of making a sound decision to accept or to withhold care. "The capable patient has a duty implied within the context of shared decision making...to articulate as clearly as possible what motivates a decision to refuse (or accept) treatment."[9] Such a decision may be motivated by coherent personal reasons, religious beliefs, social or political ideology, or emotions. Treatment refusals by capable patients are valid when the elements of informed consent have been satisfied with the patient demonstrating (1) understanding of his/her medical condition, (2) understanding of the consequences of his/her decision, and (3) voluntariness.[9]

Some have described competency testing, an indicator of capacity, to include "Evidencing a choice—a very low-level test, most respectful of autonomy, looking only for consent or denial; reasonable outcome of choice; choice based upon rational reasons; ability to understand; and actual understanding, the highest test. In cases where there is doubt as to the patient being capable, psychiatric or neurologic consultants would be a valued asset in the case."[14] The establishment of capacity may be clouded by the severity of injury, blood loss or shock, medications, cardiopulmonary or neurologic decompensation, or pressures from family members, caregivers, or others who are directly or indirectly involved, influencing the patient in question. Recognizing such influences and evaluating the perceived impact on capacity are important roles for the caregiving team.

Nonmaleficence

Nonmaleficence is the principle that requires therapists to avoid or refrain from harm. It is often viewed as the opposite of beneficence. This principle is outlined in the Hippocratic Oath with the words "I will keep them from harm and injustice."[1] Violations of this principle are the basis for most lawsuits.

As with beneficence, nonmaleficence can be seen as a double-edged sword. Often the benefits or beneficence of a treatment is accompanied by undesirable side effects that could cause harm, known as the principle of double effects. A common example of this dilemma is the use of narcotics to relieve pain. Although use of narcotics may relieve a patient's pain (beneficence), the patient also may suffer respiratory depression or addiction (nonmaleficence).

Respiratory Recap

Nonmaleficence

- Nonmaleficence is the principle that requires clinicians to avoid or refrain from harm.
- The principle of double effects occurs when the benefit (or beneficence) of a treatment is accompanied by undesirable side effects that could cause harm.

Clinicians use these guiding elements to deal with the principle of double effects:[15]

1. The action taken must be good or at least morally neutral.
2. The good must not follow as a consequence of the secondary harmful effects.
3. The harm must never be intended but tolerated as casually connected with the good intended.
4. The good must outweigh the harm.

Veracity

Veracity means truth. This principle implies that the clinician should tell the patient the truth at all times and is based on the belief that health care is best served in a relationship of trust in which the clinician and the patient are both bound by truth.

Veracity has not always been the norm in medical practice. A few decades ago, doctors made decisions about what their patients should or should not be told about their conditions. In a 1961 study, 90% of the 219 physicians surveyed stated that they would not disclose a diagnosis of cancer to a patient, believing that the patient would not be able to handle the news or would give up. A similar study was done 20 years later with 264 physicians surveyed; 97% stated that they would disclose a diagnosis of cancer.[16] Research has also demonstrated that patient attitudes concerning veracity have changed in recent years. Patients are more knowledgeable about medical treatments and more active in the decision-making process involving their health care and they expect that healthcare providers will be truthful with them.

Truth in medicine serves several purposes. By telling patients the truth about their medical condition, an important bond is created between the public and the medical community. Without trust, many patients would not seek medical attention or they would make uninformed decisions about their condition. The absence of veracity, however, can result in legal action. Before undergoing procedures or participating in research studies, health professionals must give patients adequate information about the procedure or the research. Patients must then have an opportunity to ask questions and understand the risks involved, before they accept or decline.

Although the medical community realizes the importance of veracity, it also recognizes that in certain instances a physician not telling the patient the truth is equally important. Benevolent deception is the view that the physician can withhold information from a patient for that patient's own good. For instance, telling the patient the truth can result in psychologic or physiologic harm in certain situations; other times patients may not wish to know everything about their medical conditions. Some patients do not want elaboration of all the possible side effects or risks involved in a procedure and may rely on the principle that ignorance is bliss.

In some cultures, life is present in the body as long as the heart beats. Asian cultures, for example, may not regard the truth as we know it to be as important as it is in the American culture. Family members with this type of cultural background may ask that information such as a terminal condition be kept from the patient. This situation requires patience, tact, and respect for cultural differences, and the healthcare professional must work closely with the family to establish the best course for the patient, including how to obtain the required informed consent.

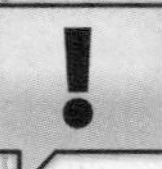

Respiratory Recap

Veracity

- This principle states that the clinician should tell the patient the truth at all times.
- Benevolent deception is the view that the clinician can lie to a patient for that patient's own good.
- Veracity has not always been the norm in medical practice.

Autonomy

Autonomy is the right and the ability to govern one's self. In medical terms, it allows patients to make decisions about the medical treatment they will receive and decide which treatments they do not wish to receive. In the past, physicians took a more paternalistic role in the delivery of care, making the treatment choices for their patients, and were rarely questioned. Patients viewed doctors as the experts who would take care of them.

With recent advancements in medical science and telecommunications, patients have become more aware of treatment options and more vocal about making decisions regarding their health. Additionally, involving patients and families in care decisions and delivery is the new norm in the United States to ensure patient safety, quality, and outcomes. The Patient Care Partnership and informed consent are the results of this changing view of autonomy.

The Patient Care Partnership

The American Hospital Association established the **Patient Care Partnership** in 2003 to outline the rights and responsibilities patients have regarding their medical care (**Box 58-1**). The Partnership was previously called the Patient's Bill of Rights. Provisions of the Patient Care Partnership state that the patient has the right to know about all aspects of their care, to include their diagnosis, who is treating them, potential outcomes, financial issues, and that the patient may refuse treatment to the extent permitted by law. The patient should

Box 58-1

The Patient Care Partnership

The Patient Care Partnership replaced the American Hospital Association's (AHA) Patient's Bill of Rights in 2003.[17]

Introduction

Effective health care requires collaboration between patients and physicians and other healthcare professionals. Open and honest communication, respect for personal and professional values, and sensitivity to differences are integral to optimal patient care. As the setting for the provision of health services, hospitals must provide a foundation for understanding and respecting the rights and responsibilities of patients, their families, physicians, and other caregivers. Hospitals must ensure a healthcare ethic that respects the role of patients in decision making about treatment choices and other aspects of their care. Hospitals must be sensitive to cultural, racial, linguistic, religious, age, gender, and other differences as well as the needs of persons with disabilities.

The American Hospital Association presented the Patient Care Partnership with the expectation that it will contribute to more effective patient care and be supported by the hospital on behalf of the institution, its medical staff, employees, and patients. The American Hospital Association encouraged healthcare institutions to tailor this partnership to their patient community by translating and/or simplifying the language of this patient care partnership as necessary to ensure that patients and their families understood their rights and responsibilities.

Patient Care Partnership: What to expect during your hospital stay

(Excerpted from the AHA's patient brochure.)*

High quality hospital care

Hospital care, when needed, is provided with skill, compassion, and respect. You have the right to know the identity of doctors, nurses, and others involved in your care, and you have the right to know when they are students, residents or other trainees.

A clean and safe environment

The hospital works hard to keep a patient safe. Special policies and procedures are aimed at preventing mistakes and keep you free from abuse and neglect. If anything unexpected and significant happens during your hospital stay, you will be told what happened, and any resulting changes in your care will be discussed with you.

Involvement in your care

You and your doctor often make decisions about your care before you go to the hospital. Other times, especially in emergencies, those decisions are made during your hospital stay. When decision-making takes place, it should include:

Discussing your medical condition and information about medically appropriate treatment choices

To make informed decisions with your doctor, you need to understand:

The benefits and risks of each treatment,

Whether your treatment is experimental or part of a research study,

What you can reasonably expect from your treatment and any long-term effects it might have on your quality of life,

What you and your family will need to do after you leave the hospital,

The financial consequences of using uncovered services or out of network providers.

Please tell your caregivers if you need more information about treatment choices.

Discussing your treatment plan

When you enter the hospital you sign a general consent to treatment. In some cases, such as surgery or experimental treatment, you may be asked to confirm in writing that you understand what is planned and agree to it. This process protects your right to consent to or refuse a treatment. Your doctor will explain the medical consequences of refusing recommended treatment. It also protects your right to decide if you want to participate in research study.

*These rights can be exercised on the patient's behalf by a designated surrogate or proxy decision maker if the patient lacks decision making capacity, is legally incompetent, or is a minor. Courtesy of the American Hospital Association. T*he Patient Care Partnership*. Chicago: American Hospital Association; 2003.

(*continues*)

Box 58-1 *(continued)*

Getting information from you

Your caregivers need complete and correct information about your health and coverage so that they can make good decisions about your care. That includes:

Past illnesses, surgeries or hospital stays.

Past allergic reactions.

Any medicines or dietary supplements (such as vitamins and herbs) that you are taking.

Any network or admission requirements under your health plan.

Understanding your healthcare goals and values

You may have healthcare goals and values or spiritual beliefs that are important to your well-being. They will be taken into account as much as possible throughout your hospital stay.

Make sure your doctor, your family and your care team know your wishes.

Understanding who should make decisions when you cannot

If you have signed a healthcare power of attorney stating who should speak for you if you become unable to make healthcare decisions for yourself, or a "living will" or "advance directive" that states your wishes about end-of-life-care, give copies to your doctor, your family and your care team. If you or your family need help making difficult decisions, counselors, chaplains and others are available to help.

Protection of your privacy

We respect the confidentiality of your relationship with your doctor and other caregivers, and the sensitive information about your health and health care that are part of that relationship. State and federal laws and hospital operating policies protect the privacy of your medical information.

You will receive a Notice of Privacy Practices that describes the ways that we use, disclose and safeguard patient information and that explains how you can obtain a copy of information from our records about your care.

Preparing you and your family for when you leave the hospital

Your doctor works with hospital staff and professionals in your community. You and your family also plays an important role in your care. The success of your treatment often depends on your efforts to follow medication, diet and therapy plans. Your family may need to help care for you at home. You can expect us to help you identify sources of follow-up care and to let you know if your hospital has a financial interest in any referrals. As long as you agree that we can share information about your care with them, we will coordinate our activities with your caregivers outside the hospital. You can also expect to receive information and, where possible, training about the self-care you will need when you go home.

Help with your bill and filing insurance claims

Our staff will file claims for you with health care insurers or other programs such as Medicare and Medicaid. They also will help your doctor with needed documentation. Hospital bills and insurance coverage is often confusing. If you have questions about your bill, contact our business office. If you need help understanding your insurance coverage or health plan, start with your insurance company or health benefits manager. If you do not have health coverage, we will try to help you and your family receive financial help or make other arrangements. We need your help with collecting needed information and other requirements to obtain coverage or assistance.

Discussion

The collaborative nature of health care requires patients or their families/surrogates to participate in their care. The effectiveness of care and patient satisfaction with the course of treatment depend, in part, on the patient fulfilling certain responsibilities. Patients are responsible for providing information about past illnesses, hospitalizations, medications, and other matters related to health status. To participate effectively in decision making, patients must be encouraged to take responsibility for requesting additional information or clarification about their health status or treatment when they do not fully understand information and instructions.

Patients are also responsible for ensuring that the healthcare institution has a copy of their written advance directive if they have one. Patients are responsible for informing their physicians and other caregivers if they anticipate problems in following prescribed treatment. Patients should also be aware of the hospital's obligation to be reasonably efficient and equitable in providing care to other patients and the community. The hospital's rules and regulations are designed to help the hospital meet this obligation. Patients and their families are responsible for making reasonable accommodations to the needs of the hospital, other patients, medical staff, and hospital employees.

Patients are responsible for providing necessary information for insurance claims and for working with the hospital to make payment arrangements, when necessary. A person's health depends on much more than health-care services. Patients are responsible for recognizing the impact of their lifestyle on their personal health.

Conclusion

Hospitals have many functions to perform, including the enhancement of health status, health promotion, and the prevention and treatment of injury and disease; the immediate and ongoing care and rehabilitation of patients; the education of health professionals, patients, and the community; and research. All these activities must be conducted with an overriding concern for the values and dignity of patients.

Courtesy American Hospital Association. *The Patient Care Partnership*. Chicago: American Hosptial Association; 2003.

also be informed of the medical consequences of their actions if they accept or refuse treatment.[17]

Informed Consent

Informed consent includes disclosure, understanding, voluntarism, competence, and permission. Before undergoing or refusing treatments, a patient must be provided with all of this information. The Patient Care Partnership has a provision dealing specifically with informed consent, in which the patient has the right to receive information necessary to give consent. The patient also has the right to know about significant medical alternatives and the names of the individuals responsible for the treatment and/or procedure.[17]

Refusal of Treatment

The patient has the right to refuse treatment or go against medical authority in any situation. The caregiver should attempt to evaluate the patient's capacity at the time of refusal, document same, and attempt to assess the patient's understanding of the nature of his/her condition and the consequences of various options. The patient should have the mental capacity, or competency, to process the information required to make these decisions, which must be within the law.

Increasingly, caregivers are considering their right to refuse to participate in medical procedures or treatments that go against their ethical or religious values. Controversial topics—including the gathering and use of stem cells, the morality of late term abortion, and assisted suicide—are frequently discussed in the medical and popular literature. While several states have looked at such legislation, only three (Oregon, Washington, and Vermont) have a statute in place, the Death with Dignity statute, allowing a patient at the point of medical futility to take a prescribed lethal dose of medication. Caregivers in Oregon may be concerned about their legal status if they are involved in caring for a patient who chooses to end their own life. In Oregon, the Death with Dignity statute states, in part, that "Except as provided in ORS 127.890.1, No person shall be subject to civil or criminal liability or professional disciplinary action for participating in good faith compliance with ORS 127.800 to 127.897. This includes being present when a qualified patient takes the prescribed medication to end his or her life in a humane and dignified manner."[18] Many caregivers may not feel comfortable about caring for patients who have made decisions about assisted suicide, chemical contraception, or abortion, and some clinicians will have misgivings about participating in practices that violate their own ethical, moral, or spiritual beliefs.

Statutes called "conscience clauses" or Protection of Rights of Conscience legislation[19] exist to protect individuals engaged in medical and allied health practice. Respiratory therapists and other clinicians are not bound to participate in acts they believe are outside of their moral or religious beliefs. An example of such a statute in Florida stated that "...refusal to participate in termination of a pregnancy or to refuse to participate in contraception, provision of supplies for contraception for religious or medical reasons will not be held liable for such refusal, nor will the refusal be the basis for disciplinary or other recriminatory action."[20] It should be noted that the Federal Health Care Provider Conscience Protection Statutes[21] allow a clinician to file a complaint through Health and Human Services (HHS) if "...you believe you have suffered discrimination on the basis of your objection to, participation in, or refusal to participate in, specific medical procedures, including abortion and sterilization, and related training and research activities; or if you believe that you have been coerced into performing procedures that you find religiously or morally objectionable."[21] Individuals concerned about Rights of Conscience laws in their state should consult their state respiratory care board, their Medical Practice Act, and read the statutes concerning Rights of Conscience in their state.

Advance Directives

An **advance directive** is one or more documents that are generally designed by knowledgeable case managers, social workers, legal entities, or healthcare agencies. Ideally, advance directives communicate a person's foresight and planning and document their thoughts, ideas, and wishes concerning what they want done in the event they are unable to verbally or otherwise direct their medical treatment, resuscitation, nutritional support, or other specifics related to their health and welfare.

People should discuss the content of advance directives with their spouse, children, family members, and a legal advisor if desired. Likewise, a person should speak with his or her primary healthcare provider about the content of their advance directive, as this communicates his or her wishes to those who would be speaking for them, interpreting their documents, consulting, or being physically present when the person is in an extreme or incapacitated state. A well-designed advance directive gives clear instructions that detail many health-related issues and includes the most current forms, such as those published by several state attorneys general, incorporate a living will, pain-management directives, acceptance or rejection of nutritional support and hydration, healthcare **proxy**, do-not-intubate/do-not-resusitate (DNI/DNR) or comfort measures only (CMO) forms, into the published state-sponsored advance directive document (**Appendices 58-1** through **58-5**). As previously discussed, patients may also be advised to discuss and note their preferences on other forms of technology, such as whether NIV should or should not be used to prolong life.

Patients' perception of their pain is a critical facet of providing comfort at the end of life. An example is one family member who discussed the improved comfort of her husband, an anesthesiologist, after working with a palliative care team's respiratory therapist who recommended nebulized morphine sulfate by aerosol inhalation.[22] Moneymaker suggested that a patient may include a set of orders in their advance directive that specify CMO when the following are noted by the patient: a cure or prolongation of life is no longer a reachable goal, and comfort is the priority, when the expected quality of the rest of life is at a level that is not acceptable, and when the durable Power of Attorney for Health Care indicates comfort is a priority in this situation.[23] When the patient is in pain, the alleviation of pain becomes an important goal regardless of the patient's stage of life. The Joint Commission has encouraged patients to discuss pain management goals with the healthcare team using the acronym *Speak Up*. The framework of the Speak Up program urges patients to:

- Speak up if you have questions or concerns, and if you don't understand, ask again. It's your body and you have a right to know.
- Pay attention to the care you are receiving. Make sure you're getting the right treatments by the right healthcare professionals. Don't assume anything.
- Educate yourself about your diagnosis, the medical tests you are undergoing, and your treatment plan.
- Ask a trusted family member or friend to be your advocate.
- Know what medications you take and why you take them. Medication errors are the most common healthcare errors.
- Use a hospital, clinic, surgery center, or other type of healthcare organization that has undergone a rigorous on-site evaluation against established state-of-the-art quality and safety standards, such as that provided by the Joint Commission.
- Participate in all decisions about your treatment. You are the center of the healthcare team.[24]

A frequently discussed advance directive is a DNR order. Advance directives do not routinely include a DNR order, and a patient can have a DNR order without other advance directives. Generally, a patient would speak with their family and physician to have a DNR inserted into the medical record. The order would clearly state that if their heart stops beating or they stop breathing, they would not receive cardiopulmonary resuscitation, no effort to institute an airway, no assisted breathing, and no chest compressions (formerly called external cardiac massage). Advance directives may specify "Do-Not-Intubate," "No Tracheostomy," or other types of limited resuscitation. It is important to clarify exactly what the patient wants done, however, and not confuse the staff regarding the patient's true code status. Unusual practices or variations in resuscitation status, such as the "Show Code" or "Slow Code," are widely discussed in the literature and strongly discouraged.[25,26]

Advance directive documents do not come in a one-size-fits-all format, and even the best advance directive document needs to be customized for the individual patient and reviewed carefully, as the value of resuscitation or medical intervention may change as a person grows older or acquires a new diagnosis. The **living will** is a document that details the types of medical treatments and life-prolonging measures that you do or do not want performed if you are incapacitated. A surrogate decision maker, or **durable medical power of attorney**, requires a legal document allowing someone to serve as your decision maker, or *medical proxy*, in the event you are incapable of making a decision. It is critical to note that any and all facets of the advance directive can be modified or terminated if there is a change in the health of the patient. And, after full recovery, the durable medical power of attorney can be relinquished. Likewise, advance directives enabling a durable medical power of attorney do not restrict or involve matters of ownership of property or finance.

Regardless of the sophistication of the family and the level of advance directive preparation, decision making at the end of life is difficult for all parties, including healthcare providers. A physician recounted the experience of acknowledging his mother's desire to discontinue intravenous antibiotics and supporting her wish to expedite her death by stopping all hydration and nutrition.[27] Investigators studied nurses who worked with hospice patients who had decided to expedite

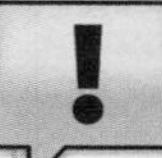

Respiratory Recap

Autonomy

- Autonomy is the ability and right to govern oneself.
- The Patient Care Partnership outlined the rights and responsibilities of patients regarding their medical care.
- For a patient to refuse treatment that individual must understand the nature of the condition and the consequences of various options.
- Advance directives, living wills, and medical power of attorney specify which treatments patients desire.

their death by stopping food and fluids. These nurses reported that they believed the quality of the process of dying for most patients was good, and the authors suggested that caregivers evaluate the standards of care and policies when caring for these special types of patients.[28]

Advance directives grew from efforts by the courts and government to resolve ethical dilemmas. In 1990 the U.S. Supreme Court, in an attempt to determine whether a patient has a right to refuse medical treatment, handed down a decision in *Cruzan v. Director Missouri Dept. of Health*, a landmark decision that recognized a competent patient's right to refuse medical treatment.[29] Although the decision clarified the rights of competent patients, it raised many questions about informed consent, which is based on the ethical principle of autonomy. An opposing ethical principle no longer considered valid is the principle of paternalism, which stems from the word *parent* and assumes that an individual with more knowledge, in this case the healthcare professional, is more capable of making decisions for the patient.

As a result of the Court's decision and the autonomy-paternalism conflict related to informed consent, Congress passed the Patient Self-Determination Act, effective December 1991.[30] The Act requires healthcare facilities receiving Medicaid or Medicare reimbursement to inform patients of their right to refuse treatment and of the availability of advance directives. Because these facilities depend financially on Medicaid and Medicare reimbursement, all states immediately passed statutes recognizing advance directives.

Confidentiality

Confidentiality ensures that the information entrusted to healthcare professionals in the line of duty is not revealed to others except when necessary to carry out their duties. This principle has a long past and is included in the Hippocratic Oath, which states: "What I may see or hear in the course of treatment…I will keep to myself holding such things shameful to be spoken aloud."[1] The principle of confidentiality remains one of the most cherished medical ethical principles, and the Patient's Care Partnership guarantees confidentiality by stating that "We respect the confidentiality of your relationship with your doctor and other caregivers, and the sensitive information about your health and health care that are part of that relationship."[13]

Respiratory Recap

Confidentiality

- Confidentiality ensures that the information entrusted to healthcare professionals in the line of duty is not revealed to others except when necessary to carry out such duties.
- Maintaining confidentiality is important because it contributes to the trust patients need in the medical community.
- Confidentiality has become more difficult to maintain due to technologic advances.

Need

Maintaining confidentiality is important because it contributes to necessary trust in the practice of medicine. Patients often reveal personal or embarrassing information in the course of receiving medical treatment. If this information is not guarded, they lose this trust and may not provide healthcare professionals with the information they need to be properly diagnosed and treated. Many laws have been passed to protect patient confidentiality, including the Privacy Act of 1974, Conditions of Participation for Hospitals in Medicare and Medicaid Programs, Conditions of Participation for Long Term Care Facilities, and the Uniform Health Care Information Act.

Violations of Confidentiality

Confidentiality is the most violated of the ethical principles. As the medical system has expanded in recent years, so has the number of individuals with access to medical records. Estimations are that more than 75 individuals see a medical chart during a patient's hospital stay.[15] Confidentiality has become more difficult to maintain due to technologic advances; although fax machines, cellular phones, and computers have made healthcare jobs easier, they also have helped decrease patient confidentiality.[31] For example, celebrity medical records have been viewed by unauthorized personnel, videos and pictures of accident victims have been taken using cell phone cameras, patient records have been faxed accidentally to restaurants, and conversations concerning patients have been overheard in elevators and nursing station phones. This has become even more problematic with social media, where it is tempting to place photographs or confidential information in a Facebook or Twitter post.

Computers offer even faster and more dangerous access to medical records. Databases can be accumulated containing information gathered legitimately by businesses. For example, drug companies may enter prescription purchases into a billing database. If an insurance company obtains these records, they could screen potential clients for high-risk conditions and deny them coverage.

Breaking Confidentiality

Although respect for confidentiality is an important tenet, at times healthcare professionals must break confidentiality. In such situations the clinician must balance the need to protect others from foreseeable harm with the need to protect confidentiality. For example, if a patient threatens to harm someone, the healthcare worker has a responsibility to warn the individual potentially in danger.

An example of this is the case of *Tarasoff v. Regents of the University of California*.[32,33] In this case a psychologist had reason to believe that one of his patients would kill a woman whose name was Tatiana Tarasoff. The psychologist had the campus police arrest his patient, but the police later released the man when he assured them he would not contact Tarasoff. Neither the campus police nor the psychologist warned Tarasoff of the potential danger to her, and the man in question later killed Tarasoff. The woman's family brought a lawsuit against the University of California, resulting in an important decision in which the courts ruled that healthcare providers have a duty to warn individuals of foreseeable danger.

Breaking confidentiality is often necessary when the public's welfare may be jeopardized. Many states have laws requiring certain diseases, such as tuberculosis or sexually transmitted diseases, to be reported to public health agencies so that others who might have been exposed to the disease are informed and can receive the necessary treatment. Most states have laws requiring healthcare workers who suspect child or elder abuse to file confidential reports. In such cases a concern exists for the public's welfare, so confidentiality may be violated. Most state licensure boards and hospital codes of ethics provide guidance for practitioners who observe what they believe is an ethical violation or potentially dangerous situation; this issue is covered in most human resource departmental orientations.

> **Respiratory Recap**
>
> **Confidentiality**
>
> - When confidentiality is broken, one must balance the need to protect others from foreseeable harm with the need to protect confidentiality.
> - Confidentiality may be broken when a concern exists for the public's welfare.

Justice

Justice is the principle that deals with fairness and equity in the distribution of scarce resources, such as time, services, equipment, and money. Although this concept may seem simple, in reality it is one of the most difficult principles to implement, creating numerous questions. For example, which criteria should be used to decide who receives life-saving organ transplants? Should a person's lifestyle (for instance, being overweight, smoking, or drinking) be considered? Researchers have suggested that a patient's lifestyle choices, particularly smoking, should be considered prior to the prescription of home oxygen therapy after actively smoking patients were identified and advised of the dangers but later housemates and neighbors died in oxygen accelerated house fires. The danger to patients and others from an oxygen accelerated fire should be considered and inform a physician's decision to prescribe or withhold domiciliary oxygen for active smokers.[34–37]

Theories

How should limited healthcare resources be distributed? Several theories deal with this question, with the egalitarian theory stating that all individuals should have equal access to goods and services. This theory, however, does not always translate into reality, For instance, healthcare availability in rural areas of the country is not the same as availability in metropolitan areas.

Other theories approach the question from different angles. The utilitarian theory of justice states that the distribution of resources should be such that it achieves the greatest good for the greatest number of individuals. The libertarian theory emphasizes the personal rights to society and economic liberty. Another theory

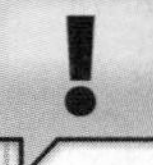

> **Respiratory Recap**
>
> **Justice**
>
> - Justice is the principle that deals with fairness and equity in the distribution of scarce resources, such as time, services, equipment, and money.
> - The egalitarian theory of justice states that all individuals should have equal access to goods and services.
> - The utilitarian theory of justice states that the distribution of resources should be such that it achieves the greatest good for the greatest number of individuals.
> - The maximin theory of justice states that the individual most needing the resources is helped, even if others are not helped.

is the maximin view of justice.[38] Using this theory the individual maximizes the minimum, even if doing so does not maximize the total amount of good done. In other words the individual needing the resources is helped the most, even if others are not helped. Another way to look at this theory is that the maximum amount of health care goes to a minimum number of patients (that is, the most critical).

With healthcare resources stretched these days, decisions about who gets the resources are never easy. This question has created robust discussions in Congress, public rallies, and at the supper table in homes nationwide. Distribution of health care can be seen in changes in payment structures for Medicare and insurance companies, which have influenced the country's healthcare system. The distribution of justice affects all levels of health care and remains one of the more problematic ethical principles facing healthcare professionals today.

Managed Care and Justice

The implementation of managed care has changed the distribution of medical resources. Managed care uses a variety of techniques that influence the clinical behavior of healthcare providers and patients. These techniques, including utilization of restraints and preapproval criteria, often integrate the payment and delivery of health care and are used with the overall goal of cost efficiency.

To keep costs down, managed care reduces resources such as time spent with patients, medications, tests, and treatments and offers incentives to physicians who are cost effective. Many physicians receive bonuses if they stay within the guidelines of the managed care provider. Those who are not cost efficient may be penalized with reduced income or receive peer pressure from superiors to become more cost efficient.

The distribution of healthcare resources often is debated, but managed care has fueled this controversy as efforts to contain the rising cost of health care compete with its fair distribution. Companies and policies, instead of healthcare professionals, often dictate the decisions as to how resources are distributed. As managed care continues to expand, healthcare professionals will continue to face more ethical dilemmas, particularly those dealing with justice.

Fidelity to Patients

Fidelity implies an obligation or faithfulness to duty. Each member of the healthcare team has a role with specific tasks and responsibilities or a scope of practice, which is usually set by tradition and/or the state legislature that regulates healthcare practice. Each clinician has a duty to practice within this role (role fidelity). Keeping within the scope of practice is considered in the best interests of the patient. The American Association for Respiratory Care (AARC) has made this preference clear in its statement on ethics, as shown in **Box 58-2**.[39] Respiratory therapists should perform only those procedures or functions in which they are individually competent and that are within the scope of accepted and responsible practice. The nature of this role is one in which a relationship is established between the healthcare provider and the patient and in which the patient expects truth and the loyalty of the provider. Patients place trust in their providers to perform their duties to the best of their abilities and refrain from duties not in their expertise.

Fidelity to Colleagues

Role **fidelity** exists among colleagues, with an obligation of loyalty to coworkers and the profession. At times, this loyalty may interfere with loyalty to the patient, and loyalty to colleagues does have exceptions. For example, most state license boards and professional organizations have ethical codes that require members to report incompetent or dishonest practices or impaired colleagues. In such cases, loyalty to the patient would outweigh loyalty to colleagues. The AARC states in its position statement that the respiratory therapist "shall refuse to conceal illegal, unethical or incompetent acts of others."[39]

Conflicts with Fidelity

Role fidelity creates a number of problems. In many cases, roles that once were clearly established by tradition

Respiratory Recap

Managed Care and Justice

- Managed care uses techniques that influence the clinical behavior of healthcare providers and patients.
- To meet efficiency goals, managed care companies offer incentives to physicians who control costs.
- As managed care grows, so will the ethical dilemmas associated with justice.

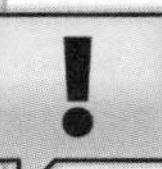

Respiratory Recap

Role Fidelity

- Fidelity implies an obligation or faithfulness to duty.
- Each clinician has a duty to practice within this role.
- Problems with role fidelity occur more often today because of changes in traditional roles, conflicts of interest, and referrals.

BOX 58-2

AARC Statement of Ethics and Professional Conduct

In the conduct of professional activities the respiratory therapist is bound by certain ethical and professional principles and demonstrate the following:

1. Demonstrate behavior that reflects integrity, supports objectivity, and fosters trust in the profession and its professionals.
2. Actively maintain and continually improve their professional competence and represent it accurately.
3. Perform only those procedures or functions in which they are individually competent and that are within the scope of accepted and responsible practice.
4. Respect and protect the legal and personal rights of patients they treat, including the right to informed consent and refusal of treatment.
5. Divulge no confidential information regarding any patient or family unless disclosure is required for responsible performance of duty or is required by law.
6. Provide care without discrimination on any basis, with respect for the rights and dignity of all individuals.
7. Promote disease prevention and wellness.
8. Refuse to participate in illegal or unethical acts and refuse to conceal illegal, unethical, or incompetent acts of others.
9. Follow sound scientific procedures and ethical principles in research.
10. Comply with state or federal laws governing and related to their practice.
11. Avoid any form of conduct that creates a conflict of interest and follow the principles of ethical business behavior.
12. Promote the positive evolution of the profession and health care in general through improvement of the access, efficacy, and cost of patient care.
13. Refrain from indiscriminate and unnecessary use of resources, both economic and natural, in practice.

Reproduced from American Association for Respiratory Care. *AARC Statement of Ethics and Professional Conduct.* Effective December 1994; revised December 2007 and July 2009. Available at: http://www.aarc.org/resources/position_statements/ethics.html. Reprinted with permission.

are now changing. Managed care and a desire for cost efficiency have created overlapping jobs. Various professionals now perform tasks that were once assigned to one particular profession, creating conflicts with role fidelity.

Other practices, such as joint ventures and referrals, have added to the fidelity question. Joint ventures involve physicians who have investments in healthcare services to which they may refer their patients (for example, a physician who owns a radiology center and refers all of his patients to that facility for radiographs). Referrals also create problems with role fidelity. For instance, a therapist refers or recommends a home health company or equipment company to a patient and then collects a finder's fee from that company. To deal with this problem the AARC issued a statement regarding the ethical performance of therapists and prohibiting this type of conduct. In some states, self-referral and finder's fees are illegal, resulting in legal violations in addition to ethical misconduct.

Role of Professional Organizations in Ethics

Need for Professional Ethics

Professional medical organizations recognize the need for guidelines in helping their members maintain high ethical standards. The respiratory care profession, although still new compared with other professions, has established a code of ethics for its members. New professions must establish themselves as entities that embrace guidelines and standards and are willing to set

Respiratory Recap

Professional Organizations' Role in Ethics

- Professional medical organizations recognize the need for guidelines in helping their members maintain high ethical standards.
- The AARC code tends to the legal and professional growth needs of the profession.

direction and provide some degree of self-governance for their members. Along the same lines, new professionals must establish themselves as responsible clinicians who adhere to guidelines and standards. Important characteristics of a professional include the abilities to operate with integrity and demonstrate self-governance and direction.

AARC Code of Ethics

The **AARC Code of Ethics** and professional conduct[39] has evolved through several revisions over the life of the respiratory therapy profession. In its present form (see Box 58-2), it closely resembles the ethical theories and principles discussed in this chapter and embraces the major legal concerns that all professionals face today in the performance of their professional duties. The following discussion analyzes each of the code's discrete components:

Item 1: Demonstrate behavior that reflects integrity, supports objectivity, and fosters trust in the profession and its professionals.

Item 1 of the statement addresses the need for integrity, objectivity, trust, and role fidelity for respiratory care professionals. These traits can be incorporated into the principle of veracity, or truth. By fostering integrity, healthcare professionals demonstrate that in performing their duties, they adhere to unimpaired standards of care that are free of flaws. Fidelity is upheld as long as clinicians work within their professional competence.

A common trait is that all professionals adhere to a community standard of care. *Community* in this case may refer to both the profession and a physical community, as in a state or region of the country. Adherence to a community standard of care can be extremely important when clinicians are required to defend themselves in legal actions. Objectivity in the delivery of care ensures that the clinician does not discriminate on any basis—ethnicity, gender, or type of disease. The objective clinician simply delivers the best care possible to whoever needs it. Public trust in the professional is essential both to establish and maintain professional status and to maximize adherence to the service and directions of the professional.

Item 2: Actively maintain and continually improve their professional competence and represent it accurately.

Item 3: Perform only those procedures or functions in which they are individually competent and that are within the scope of accepted and responsible practice.

Items 2 and 3 reflect the need for research and continuing education, along with the requirement for professionals to self-govern themselves by acknowledging their own limitations. These items also address fidelity in reflecting the need for continuing education because the therapist's scope of practice will grow. Therapists must continue to enhance their education by learning about new procedures, treatments, and equipment. With continual learning beneficence and nonmaleficence are served; therapists will be better able to treat their patients and provide them with the best care while avoiding unnecessary therapy or harm.

Item 4: Respect and protect the legal and personal rights of patients they treat, including the right to informed consent and refusal of treatment.

Item 4 of the AARC statement emphasizes the need for informed consent, which relates to autonomy, the patient's right to decide care. This item respects the patient's right to make decisions regarding care, including the right to refuse treatments.

Item 5: Divulge no confidential information regarding any patient or family unless disclosure is required for responsible performance of duty or is required by law.

Item 5 refers to one of the oldest and best-established ethical principles, confidentiality, a mainstay of healthcare delivery. The respiratory therapist has a duty to uphold the confidentiality of information shared in the course of treatment unless the information is required to perform the job or disclosure is required by law.

Item 6: Provide care without discrimination on any basis, with respect for the rights and dignity of all individuals.

Item 6 refers to the principles of justice and autonomy. The distribution of healthcare resources should be provided without discrimination. At the same time, respiratory therapists must respect the autonomy and dignity of the patient.

Item 7: Promote disease prevention and wellness.

Item 7 supports the principles of role fidelity, justice, beneficence, and nonmaleficence. Role fidelity is addressed by the need for respiratory therapists to educate the public about disease prevention and wellness. Because therapists are the allied health experts, their involvement in the cardiopulmonary aspect of health is vital. By educating individuals about disease prevention and wellness, the public may become healthier, thus lowering the demand for respiratory resources. Justice can be served by provision of these services to those who need them. Through education, clinicians can provide good to their patients and prevent harm, serving beneficence and nonmaleficence.

Item 8: Refuse to participate in illegal or unethical acts and refuse to conceal illegal, unethical, or incompetent acts of others.

Item 11: Avoid any form of conduct that creates a conflict of interest and follow the principles of ethical business behavior.

Items 8 and 11 discuss the importance of fidelity and veracity. With fidelity, patients expect loyalty from their therapists, a trait evident in competent, ethical respiratory therapists. Therapists also have a duty to the profession to identify members of the profession who are not maintaining competency and ethical behavior, thus enforcing nonmaleficence.

In addition, sound research includes veracity. Research subjects must be informed of the risks of any research and have the opportunity to ask questions and receive truthful answers. Individuals have the right to refuse to participate in research studies without any adverse effects or discontinuance of their health care.

Item 9: Follow sound scientific research procedures and ethical principles in research.

Item 10: Comply with state or federal laws governing and related to their practice.

Items 9 and 10 again deal with fidelity. State and federal laws dictate the scope of practice, and respiratory therapists should be familiar with these laws, particularly state laws that usually define the scope of care. Item 9 also addresses the need for ethical research, which has led to many breakthrough discoveries and enhanced beneficence. Ethical standards must be maintained so that patients can benefit from research, not be harmed by it.

Item 12: Promote the positive evolution of the profession and health care in general through improvement of the access, efficacy, and cost of patient care.

Item 13: Refrain from indiscriminate and unnecessary use of resources, both economic and natural, in practice.

Items 12 and 13 deal with justice. The current distribution of resources in the United States is imperfect and unequal. To deal with this problem the AARC has stated that every respiratory therapist has a duty to try to improve the principle of justice.[38] Respiratory therapists should be aware of the distribution of healthcare resources and constantly seek measures to improve their delivery and access. They should be conscious of the cost of the care provided and seek cost-efficient, effective ways to deliver care.

Ethics Committees

In 1991, the Joint Commission on Accreditation of Healthcare Organizations (JCAHO), now the Joint Commission (TJC), adopted guidelines requiring each accredited organization to establish a mechanism to consider ethical issues in patient care and education for healthcare professionals. Most facilities responded by establishing ethics committees, sometimes called **ethics or optimum care committees**, the composition, duties, and activities of which vary widely from institution to institution. A typical committee is composed of approximately 12 members ranging from medical staff, administration, and various service departments. A member of the clergy also may serve on the ethics committee, along with a medical ethicist, often an ethics professor or researcher, and representatives of the community. Townsend noted that "Toleration of and receptivity to divergent viewpoints, important for cultural diversity and understanding, can also serve to win the trust of various constituencies."[40] The knowledge and insight of the respiratory therapist into advanced resuscitation, life support, and weaning procedures, particularly terminal weaning,[41] would be critical and useful resources to any ethics or optimum care committee.

Committees may develop policies and procedures, sponsor educational activities, and serve as clearinghouses for the distribution of information on ethical issues. The committee may consider specific ethical dilemmas, but when ethics committees become involved in patient care, their only goal is to issue a recommendation. Further research on the outcomes and effectiveness of ethics committees is recommended, as ethics committees are now being strongly recommended or required by accreditation agencies such as the TJC.

Adherence to ethical standards improves patient outcomes, decreases the likelihood that a facility will encounter accountability problems, and assures patients that they can trust their healthcare system. Given the current state of healthcare accountability, more important than ever is that healthcare providers, including respiratory therapists, take every precaution possible to ensure that the services they provide meet the highest ethical standards.

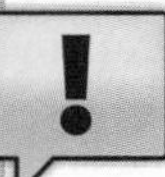

Respiratory Recap

Ethics Committees

- Ethics committees were formed to consider ethical issues in patient care and education for the healthcare professional.
- Committees may develop policies and procedures, sponsor educational activities, and serve as clearinghouses for the distribution of information on ethical issues.

Case Studies

Case 1. Two Lives Inseparable

Anne was the daughter of the respiratory therapy department director, D., a seasoned registered respiratory therapist who had moved to the region in 1990. Anne was a beautiful young lady who was stricken with systemic lupus erythematosis (SLE) in 1993. Within 3 years of diagnosis, Anne quickly developed lupus cerebritis, pericardial and pleural effusions, renal failure, and a commitment to hemodialysis. Anne survived multiple critical care admissions, mechanical ventilation, exploratory craniotomy, *C. difficile* colitis, and long-term anticonvulsant therapy. Anne's serum complement and immune system were delicate, with no detectable immunoglobulin (Ig) A and declining levels of IgM and IgG. Despite the many volunteers from a long list of family, friends, and the extended donor community, her immune system problems complicated the search for a compatible donor. Anne remained on circulating (CCPD) and ambulatory (CAPD) peritoneal dialysis for four and one-half years. Anne and her family discussed and documented what she wanted done at the time of her death, funeral and burial arrangements, disposition of her estate, and in particular the care of her beloved cats. At 17 years of age, Anne, a deeply spiritual young lady, made peace with her God and decided that if she continued on dialysis therapy and ceased to breathe on her own, or her heart stopped, she declined to be intubated or resuscitated. D. and family agonized over the dilemma of honoring Anne's wishes for a do-not-resuscitate (DNR) advance directive. Having worked for many years in critical care, D. knew that patient outcomes in end-stage renal disease differed, especially in young patients, and that Anne's compliance with regimen made her an excellent transplant candidate once a donor was located. How could D., his wife, and son stand by and not aggressively resuscitate and care for this precious daughter?

Anne's desire to work with empirical and experimental therapy for the sequelae of lupus led her to participate in research protocols requiring chemotherapy, and despite the resulting nausea and side effects, she was a highly compliant patient. In the late hours of August 7, 1998, Anne received a call from the regional organ transplant coordinator, noting that she had a near perfect match with a 3-year-old donor, and it was time to go to the hospital and receive her transplant. The transplantation was a success and after many challenges, Anne initiated contact through the regional donor organization, making contact with the donor family. Since 1998, the two families have enjoyed a warm friendship and regular visits. Anne is married, teaches school, and has had no issues with renal function since 1998. All of the modern miracles of medicine came together to bring this story to a happy ending. The joy of receiving the transplant is tempered by the reality of the situation, however, and the death of the 3-year-old has weighed heavily on everyone involved. Her father keeps a photo of the child donor on his desk, never forgetting the courage of her parents in making the decision to donate their child's organs and their child's role in uniting these families, two lives made inseparable by the gift of organ donation.

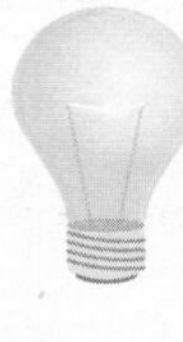

STOP AND THINK

How does Anne's story demonstrate that the advance directive can be modified or terminated if there is a change in the health of the patient? What is shown in this case about durable medical power of attorney? What does this case illustrate about advance directives enabling a durable medical power of attorney?

Case 2. A Fifty for Your Trouble

You are a student in clinical training, based in a large metropolitan hospital. You have been on the floor for 3 weeks and previously cared twice for an older gentleman with chronic obstructive lung disease named Mr. Duills. Today, after you administered medicated aerosol treatment to Mr. Duills, you are washing your hands and your clinical instructor has just stepped out of the room to answer a page. Mr. Duills's wife approaches you and puts a fifty dollar bill in your pocket, stating, "I know you students have a tough time financially, and my husband just wanted to say 'Thank you' for the excellent care you have been giving him. Let's just keep this our little secret."

Accepting money for performing duties that will be documented and billed by the hospital will compromise your future as a therapist. A caregiver should gently but firmly tell Mrs. Duills that accepting gifts or money is strictly forbidden, because accepting this gift creates a conflict of interest. The AARC suggests that respiratory therapists avoid any conflict of interest, and if you accepted a gift of money from a patient, that would also be a breach of the principles of ethical business behavior.[38] You are duty bound to reveal anything outside the ordinary that occurs while under the instructor's supervision, because a student's role fidelity requires that you do not conceal information from the instructor.

Case 3. A Double-Edged Sword

Casey is a respiratory therapist working in a regional burn center. One of her patients has second-degree burns on his lower extremities and is in considerable pain. He is crying and thrashing about in his bed, begging Casey, "Please give me something for the pain!" Casey is concerned that the patient will pull out his intravenous (IV) line and hurt himself if he doesn't stop

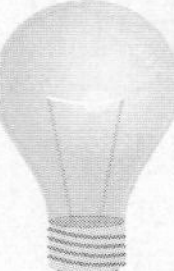

STOP AND THINK

How would you handle a situation where a patient offered you money?

thrashing. The intern on call orders more morphine, but Casey is concerned that the additional morphine could depress the patient's respiratory drive.

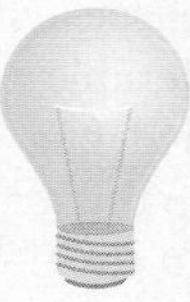

STOP AND THINK

Should the additional morphine be given to Casey? Does pain relief outweigh the possibility of respiratory depression?

Case 4. To Intubate or Not to Intubate

Mrs. Ray is 68 years old and has a history of chronic obstructive pulmonary disease (COPD), congestive heart failure (CHF), and renal disease. She has been admitted to the hospital numerous times in the past 3 years, and the respiratory therapy staff members know her well. On previous admissions, she stated to several respiratory therapy staff members that she never wanted to be intubated or placed on mechanical ventilation.

Mrs. Ray's current admission is for pneumonia. The respiratory therapist assigned to give Mrs. Ray her nebulizer treatments receives a stat page; on arrival in the patient's room, the therapist finds Mrs. Ray's daughter and physician in a discussion outside. Mrs. Ray is unresponsive and in impending respiratory failure. The physician explains that the antibiotics have not had time to treat Mrs. Ray's pneumonia and that without mechanical ventilation, the woman will suffer respiratory failure and likely die.

The physician says that they must decide whether to intubate Mrs. Ray. The daughter insists, "I want everything done for my mother! Put her on the breathing machine!" The physician agrees with the daughter and asks the respiratory therapist to intubate and ventilate the woman per the respiratory care protocol. The therapist informs the physician of Mrs. Ray's previous requests regarding intubation and mechanical ventilation, but the physician angrily states, "Mrs. Ray doesn't have an advance directive. It is the daughter's decision to make. We can treat the pneumonia and then probably extubate her."

This case involves several ethical principles, including autonomy, beneficence, and nonmaleficence. The respiratory therapist, knowing that Mrs. Ray previously requested not to be intubated or placed on mechanical ventilation, may think that Mrs. Ray's autonomy is being compromised with intubation. Although the patient did not formally put her wishes in writing, she made her wishes well known to the respiratory staff members. Whether the patient fully understood the nature of her condition and the consequences of this decision are not known. These two criteria are required for a patient to make an autonomous decision to refuse therapy. If she understood that her medical condition could at some point in time require intubation with mechanical ventilation and that refusing this therapy could result in her death, then she made a conscious decision invoking her autonomy. She had the right to make this decision for herself.

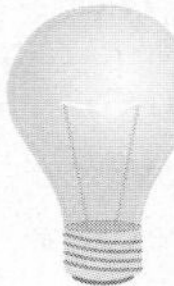

STOP AND THINK

In Case 4, should Mrs. Ray be intubated and placed on mechanical ventilation? Which ethical principles are involved? What decision-making processes are the respiratory therapist and physician each using to make their judgments?

The physician's decision to intubate could be based on the principle of beneficence, which involves the performance of procedures and treatments to benefit the patient. The assumption may be made that Mrs. Ray did not inform the physician of her past decision to refuse intubation and mechanical ventilation. The physician believes the pneumonia can be treated and that Mrs. Ray will be extubated. By performing these procedures, the physician thinks that in the long run, the patient will benefit and that beneficence must be upheld in this matter. From this viewpoint, not treating Mrs. Ray would result in nonmaleficence or harm.

The physician is guided by a consequential, or teleological, theory and is basing the decision to intubate on the possible consequences or outcomes of the actions. If the patient is not placed on mechanical ventilation, the physician believes she will die. If she is placed on mechanical ventilation and treated for her pneumonia, the physician believes that recovery and subsequent extubation are likely. According to the physician's beliefs the consequences or likely outcomes of this situation should direct the decision making. Based on this reasoning, the physician has sufficient reason to intubate.

The respiratory therapist is guided by the principle of duty, or deontology, in the decision to inform the doctor of Mrs. Ray's wishes. The therapist believes in a duty to the patient to abide by previously stated wishes and that the patient's autonomous decision should be upheld, despite her daughter's wishes. Because the therapist appears to have known Mrs. Ray and has discussed intubation with her in the past, the respiratory therapist may be aware of possible psychological or financial impacts on Mrs. Ray if her autonomy is not upheld. By refusing to uphold the patient's autonomous decision regarding life support, the therapist

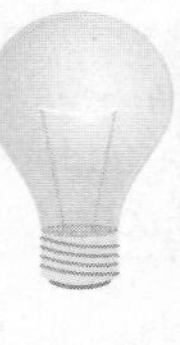

STOP AND THINK

How would a deontological view determine Bill and Lisa's decision in Case 5? How would a teleological view determine their decision? What ethical principles were violated in this case? What ethical principles could be violated based on their decision?

may believe that the principle of nonmaleficence is being violated and that intubating her against the patient's wishes would harm her. This situation is not uncommon in today's medical practice. The absence of advance directives and poor communication among family members and attending physicians often lead to ethical dilemmas in which all parties involved in the patient's care must balance the beneficence of an action with its nonmaleficence.

Case 5. Nosey Therapists

Bill and Lisa are respiratory therapists working in a hospital. They have discovered that they can uncover personal information about their coworkers by using the hospital computer. They already have learned that two of their coworkers are living together and that one of these individuals has a history of psychological problems. In addition, they have discovered that the husband of another coworker, Joan, recently tested positive for human immunodeficiency virus (HIV) and they are concerned that Joan, who frequently draws arterial blood gases on patients, may be HIV positive and could be a risk to the patients if standard aseptic techniques were compromised. They wonder whether they should inform their boss.

In this case, two employees have learned to use the computer for some dangerous snooping. In the process they have most likely not only violated hospital policy regarding computer access but also violated patient confidentiality. They have learned that one of their coworkers has been exposed to HIV, are concerned about patient risk, and are making some assumptions regarding that coworker, including the assumption that their boss does not know about her husband's positive HIV test. This may not be true. They also are assuming that Joan has tested HIV positive, which also may not be true. Furthermore, none of these matters involve them because they are not supervisors, and neither has a right or need to know the information in question. From a deontological viewpoint, Bill and Lisa could argue they should inform their boss of their discovery. They believe that patients are at risk for harm and that they have a duty to protect their patients. Informing their supervisor could protect Joan's patients from potential harm.

A teleological view of this scenario involves listing of all of the consequences. Bill and Lisa believe that if they

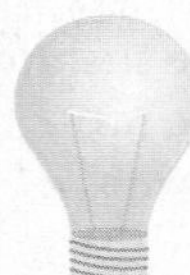

STOP AND THINK

What should the therapist do in Case 6? How would you respond in this situation?

do not tell their boss, Joan could be placing her patients at risk. They could tell their boss but would most likely have to admit how they gained this information, which would place them both at risk for punishment. Bill and Lisa would have to decide which consequence would have the best outcome.

Case 6. You Can Tell Mom

A patient has been admitted to the hospital with an acute myocardial infarction (MI). The respiratory therapist on duty receives a phone call from his mother, who works with the patient's wife. The therapist's mother asks him to ensure that the physicians are telling the patient's wife the full story. She also wants her son to fill her in on the details.

Case 7. Who Gets the Therapy?

John is a respiratory therapy supervisor at a large metropolitan hospital. When he arrives to start his shift, the departing supervisor notifies him that two members on his shift have called in sick for the night and that replacements for both are unavailable. The hospital is extremely busy that night, with each staff member already taking a full load of patients, and performance of all of the respiratory therapy procedures needed is impossible. John must decide how to distribute the available resources.

Policy states that patients who are either in the intensive care unit (ICU) or on mechanical ventilation receive priority over those receiving general floor therapies. John knows that several ventilator patients are stable and have not been weaned in several weeks. Several patients with asthma cannot afford to be without therapy. He also knows that the nurses in the ICU are educated in respiratory therapy procedures and in a better position to help with treatments than the nurses in the general nursing units.

John has several choices. He could decide that all patients will receive one less treatment during this shift. For instance, a patient who was scheduled to receive three jet nebulizer treatments would receive only two treatments. He also could decide that several

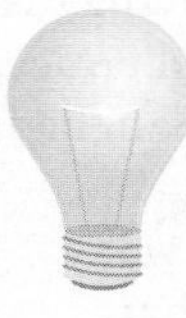

STOP AND THINK

In Case 7, what should John do? What ethical principles come into consideration as John makes his decision on how to divide his time in the care of the patients assigned to his care?

patients will not receive any therapy so that the others who need their treatments the most will receive therapy as ordered. Furthermore, he could assign all the procedures and allow his staff members to decide who receives the therapy.

In making his decision, John may choose to look at issues from several viewpoints. If he decides to reduce the therapy received by all patients, he would be taking an egalitarian position. This theory states all individuals should have equal access to goods and services. In this case, he could argue that all patients would be treated fairly in that they all would receive reduced services.

John may choose to assume a maxmin position of justice. This theory states that justice would be served if the therapists maximized the minimum. In other words, John and the staff would provide therapy to those who need it most. John would not deliver therapy to some patients but instead would concentrate his resources on those with the greatest need.

A respiratory care policy addresses the way in which care should be delivered during a shortage of staff members, stating that respiratory care should be prioritized to treat patients in the ICU first. John does not think this policy fairly distributes the resources, however. If John were to approach the problem with a utilitarian theory, he would look at the consequences of all the possible alternatives and decide on the choice that maximizes the total amount of good done, regardless of who benefits. Because John believes the patients with asthma have the greatest need for respiratory care, he could utilize the utilitarian theory to support his decision to perform the treatments on the asthmatic patients instead of the stable, ventilated ICU patients. According to John's values, the patients with asthma would receive the greatest good from the treatments and thus would receive therapy.

By making a decision in opposition to hospital policy, John places his values above those of the hospital. By violating policy as a supervisor, he sets a poor example for his staff members. Failure to follow policies can result in detrimental actions not only to the individual disregarding the policy but also to the hospital. The hospital could face legal action if policies are not followed and patients suffer ill consequences. John will have to deal with any consequences that occur as a result of his actions. If he believes the policy is incorrect, he should address this issue with his superiors.

Case 8. A Couple of Beers

After a busy evening shift, respiratory therapist Tony is glad when Sam arrives to relieve him. While giving his report, Tony smells alcohol on Sam's breath and notices that Sam's speech is slurred. Tony knows that Sam had mentioned he was going to watch the football game at a bar with some friends before coming in to work the night shift. Tony suspects that Sam might have had some alcohol and might not be in shape to work.

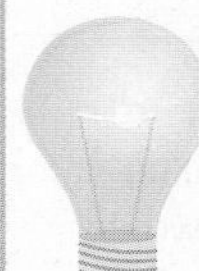

STOP AND THINK

What would you do if a coworker shows up for work under the influence of drugs or alcohol?

He decides to question him about his suspicion. Sam admits, "I had a couple of beers. It's no big deal." Tony asks him whether he is competent to do his job, and Sam replies, "Be a friend. Don't make so much out of this. Don't worry; I can do my job."

Tony is torn between fidelity to his patients and fidelity to his coworker. He can allow his colleague to maintain his autonomy and do nothing. Tony is not convinced his colleague has the capacity to make that decision, however, because he believes Sam is impaired by alcohol.

Tony believes that his patients could be at risk if Sam is allowed to care for them. Following this line of thinking, he believes that fidelity to his patients and nonmaleficence take precedence. The respiratory therapy code of ethics also states he has a duty to the profession to report incompetence among fellow members. Tony thus would do best to report the incident to his supervisor immediately so that managerial decisions about staffing for the shift can be made.

Key Points

- Ethics is the study of the ways individuals and societies make judgments regarding right and wrong.
- Many factors affect decisions about right and wrong, including culture, religion, morals, societal mores, prejudice, and bias.
- Two main theories, teleological and deontological, are used to describe the decision-making process an individual undertakes in making an ethical decision.
- Seven important ethical principles help guide health care: beneficence, capacity, nonmaleficence, veracity, autonomy, confidentiality, justice, and role fidelity.
- Beneficence is the principle that imposes on the healthcare professional the responsibility to seek good for the patient.
- Capacity is the measureable capability of a patient to make an informed decision that accepts, changes, or withholds therapy, treatment, or medical care.
- Nonmaleficence is the principle by which the healthcare professional refrains from harming the patient.
- Veracity requires the healthcare professional to tell the patient the truth.
- Confidentiality ensures that information revealed to the healthcare professional is not revealed to others except when necessary to perform duties or when silence may result in harm to an individual or the public.

- Justice deals with the fair and equitable distribution of healthcare resources.
- Role fidelity refers to one's faithfulness to duty.
- The Patient Care Partnership defines what a patient can expect prior to and during a hospital admission.
- Professional organizations such as the AARC recognize the need to establish guidelines for professional ethical behavior.
- The AARC Code of Ethics describes ethical behaviors for respiratory therapists that guide professional practice.
- Hospitals have established ethics or optimum care committees to deal with ethical issues in patient care and educate healthcare professionals.
- Each respiratory therapist has a duty and responsibility to provide quality health care guided by legal and ethical principles.

References

1. Hippocrates. The Oath. In: *Jones, W.H.S., translator. Hippocrates* (the Loeb Classic Library). Vol. 1. Cambridge, MA: Harvard University Press; 1923:299–301.
2. American Medical Association. *Opinion 1.01*. Available at: http://www.ama-assn.org/ama/pub/physician-resources/medical-ethics/code-medical-ethics/opinion101.page? Accessed September 11, 2014.
3. Bias, defined in *The American Heritage Dictionary of the English Language*. 4th ed. Boston: Houghton Mifflin Company; 2006.
4. Allport GW. *The Nature of Prejudice*. Reading, MA: Perseus Publishing; 1979.
5. Evans RW. The physician-assisted-killing fallacy. *Life Adv.* May/June 1999;13(6).
6. Sullivan AD, Hedberg K, Fleming K. Legalized physician-assisted suicide in Oregon—the second year. *N Engl J Med.* 2000;342;598–604.
7. Oregon.gov. *Death with Dignity Act. Records and Report Data on the Act.* Available at: http://www.oregon.gov/DHS/ph/pas/. Accessed September 11, 2014.
8. Carroll C. Ethical theories and methods. In: Carroll C. *Legal Issues and Ethical Dilemmas in Respiratory Care*. Philadelphia: FA Davis; 1996:68–74.
9. Fletcher JC, Lombardo PA, Marshall MF, Miller FG. *Introduction to Clinical Ethics.* 3rd ed. Hagerstown, MD: University Publishing Group; 2005:30–31, 71–81.
10. Mehta S, Hill NS. Noninvasive ventilation. *Am J Respir Crit Care Med.* 2001;163:540–577.
11. Nava S, Sturani C, Hartl S, et al. End-of-life decision-making in respiratory intermediate care units: a European survey. *Eur Respir J.* 2007;30:156–164.
12. Levy M, Tanios MA, Nelson D, et al. Outcomes of patients with do-not-intubate orders treated with noninvasive ventilation. *Crit Care Med.* 2004;32:2002–2007.
13. Kacmarek RM. Should noninvasive ventilation be used with the Do-Not-Intubate patient? *Respir Care.* 2009;54:223–229.
14. Roth LH, Meisel A, Lidz CW. Tests of competency to consent to treatment. *Am J Psychiatry.* 1977;134:279–284.
15. Edge RS, Groves JR. *Basic Principles of Healthcare Ethics—A Guide for Clinical Practice.* Albany, NY: Delmar; 1994:38.
16. Hebert PC, Hoffmaster B, Glass KC, et al. Bioethics for clinicians: truth telling. *CMAJ.* 1997;156:225–228.
17. American Hospital Association. *Patient Care Partnership*. Available at: http://www.aha.org/aha/issues/Communicating-With-Patients/pt-care-partnership.html. Accessed September 11, 2014.
18. *Oregon Revised Statutes*. (Death With Dignity Act) 127.885 s.4.01. Immunities; basis for prohibiting health care provider from participation; notification; permissible sanctions. Available at: http://public.health.oregon.gov/ProviderPartnerResources/EvaluationResearch/DeathwithDignityAct/Pages/ors.aspx. Accessed September 11, 2014.
19. *Protection of Conscience Laws. United States. Federal Laws and Regulations.* Available at: http://www.consciencelaws.org/law/laws/usa.aspx. Accessed September 11, 2014.
20. *The 2011 Florida Statutes.* Title XXIX Public Health, Chapter 381. Public Health General Provisions. 381.0051. Family planning. Available at: http://www.leg.state.fl.us/statutes/index.cfm?mode=View%20Statutes&SubMenu=1&App_mode=Display_Statute&Search_String=family+planning&URL=0300-0399/0381/Sections/0381.0051.html. Accessed September 11, 2014.
21. Federal Health Care Conscience Protection Statutes. http://www.hhs.gov/ocr/civilrights/understanding/ConscienceProtect/index.html. Accessed September 18, 2014.
22. Miller KL. Pain management from the other side of the mountain. *Am Soc Anesthesiol Newsletter*. 1997;61.
23. Moneymaker KM. Comfort measures only. *J Palliat Med.* 2005;8:688.
24. Powers K. *Joint Commission Urges Patients to Speak Up About Pain.* Joint Commission News Release. September 16, 2008.
25. Gazelle, G. The slow code: should anyone rush to its defense? *N Engl J Med.* 1998;338:467–469.
26. The Legal Information Institute, Cornell University. *Cruzan v. Director, Missouri Department of Health (88-1503), 497 U.S. 261 (1990).* Available at: http://www.law.cornell.edu/supct/html/88-1503.ZS.html. Accessed September 11, 2014.
27. Eddy D. A conversation with my mother. *JAMA.* 1994;272:179–181.
28. Ganzini L, Goy ER, Miller LL, et al. Nurses' experiences with hospice patients who refuse food and fluids to hasten death. *N Engl J Med.* 2003;349:359–365.
29. *Cruzan v. Director Missouri Dept. of Health.* US Supreme Court. 88-1503; 1990.
30. Logue BJ. *Last Rights: Death Control and the Elderly in America.* New York: Macmillan; 1993.
31. Dodek DY, Dodek A. From Hippocrates to facsimile: protecting patient confidentiality is more difficult and more important than ever. *CMAJ.* 1997;156:847–852.
32. *Tarasoff v. Regents of the University of California.* 529 P2d 553,118 Cal Rpt 129; 1974.
33. *Tarasoff v. Regents of the University of California.* Reargued 17 Cal3d 425,551 P2d 334,131 Cal Rptr 333; 1976.
34. Lacasse Y, LaForge J, Maltais F. Got a match? Home oxygen therapy in current smokers (editorial). *Thorax.* 2006;61:374–375.
35. U.S. Veteran's Administration National Ethics Teleconference. *Home Oxygen for Patients Who Smoke: Prescription vs. Proscription.* Teleconference minutes of October 23, 2001. Available at: http://www.ethics.va.gov/ETHICS/docs/net/NET_Topic_20011023_Home_Oxygen_For_Smokers.doc. Accessed September 11, 2014.
36. McDonald CF, Crockett AJ, Young I. Adult domiciliary oxygen therapy. Position Statement of the Thoracic Society of Australia and New Zealand. *Med J Aust.* 2005;182:621–626.
37. Lambert AEC. Adult domiciliary oxygen therapy: a patient's perspective. *Med J Aust.* 2005;183:472–473.
38. Rawls J. *A Theory of Justice.* Cambridge, MA: Harvard University Press; 1999.
39. American Association for Respiratory Care (AARC). *Position Statement. Ethics and Professional Conduct.* (December 1994, updated July 2000). Available at: http://www.aarc.org/media_center/position_statements/ethics.html. Accessed September 11, 2014.
40. Townsend T. Health care ethics committees. In: Roberts LW, Dyer AR, eds. *Ethics in Mental Health Care.* Arlington, VA: American Psychiatric Publishing, Inc; 2004:295–311.
41. Keene S, Samples DA, Masini DE, Byington R. Ethical concerns that arise from terminal weaning procedures of a ventilator dependent patient—a respiratory therapist's perspective. *Internet Journal of Law, Healthcare and Ethics.* 2007;4(2).

APPENDIX 58-1

GENERAL INSTRUCTIONS: Use this Durable Health Care Power of Attorney form if you want to select a person to make future health care decisions for you so that if you become too ill or cannot make those decisions for yourself the person you choose and trust can make medical decisions for you. Talk to your family, friends, and others you trust about your choices. Also, it is a good idea to talk with professionals such as your doctor, clergyperson and a lawyer before you sign this form.

Be sure you understand the importance of this document. If you decide this is the form you want to use, complete the form. **Do not sign this form until** your witness or a Notary Public is present to witness the signing. There are further instructions for you about signing this form on page three.

1. Information about me: (I am called the "Principal")

My Name: ____________ My Age: ____________
My Address: ____________ My Date of Birth: ____________
My Telephone: ____________

2. Selection of my health care representative and alternate: (Also called an "agent" or "surrogate")

I choose the following person to act as my representative to make health care decisions for me:

Name: ____________ Home Telephone: ____________
Street Address: ____________ Work Telephone: ____________
City, State, Zip: ____________ Cell Telephone: ____________

I choose the following person to act as an alternate representative to make health care decisions for me if my first representative is unavailable, unwilling, or unable to make decisions for me:

Name: ____________ Home Telephone: ____________
Street Address: ____________ Work Telephone: ____________
City, State, Zip: ____________ Cell Telephone: ____________

3. What I AUTHORIZE if I am unable to make medical care decisions for myself:

I authorize my health care representative to make health care decisions for me when I cannot make or communicate my own health care decisions due to mental or physical illness, injury, disability, or incapacity. I want my representative to make all such decisions for me except those decisions that I have expressly stated in Part 4 below that I do not authorize him/her to make. If I am able to communicate in any manner, my representative should discuss my health care options with me. My representative should explain to me any choices he or she made if I am able to understand. This appointment is effective unless and until it is revoked by me or by an order of a court.

The types of health care decisions I authorize to be made on my behalf include but are not limited to the following:

- To consent or to refuse medical care, including diagnostic, surgical, or therapeutic procedures;
- To authorize the physicians, nurses, therapists, and other health care providers of his/her choice to provide care for me, and to obligate my resources or my estate to pay reasonable compensation for these services;
- To approve or deny my admittance to health care institutions, nursing homes, assisted living facilities, or other facilities or programs. By signing this form I understand that I allow my representative to make decisions about my mental health care except that generally speaking he or she cannot have me admitted to a structured treatment setting with 24-hour-a-day supervision and an intensive treatment program – called a "level one" behavioral health facility – using just this form;

Developed by the Office of Arizona Attorney General Updated December 3, 2007
TERRY GODDARD (All documents completed before December 3, 2007 are still valid)
www.azag.gov 1 DURABLE HEALTH CARE POWER OF ATTORNEY

- To have access to and control over my medical records and to have the authority to discuss those records with health care providers.

4. DECISIONS I EXPRESSLY DO NOT AUTHORIZE my Representative to make for me:

I do not want my representative to make the following health care decisions for me (describe or write in "not applicable"):

____
____
____
____
____

5. My specific desires about autopsy:

NOTE: Under Arizona law, an autopsy is not required unless the county medical examiner, the county attorney, or a superior court judge orders it to be performed. See the General Information document for more information about this topic. Initial or put a check mark by one of the following choices.

____ Upon my death I DO NOT consent to (want) an autopsy.
____ Upon my death I DO consent to (want) an autopsy.
____ My representative may give or refuse consent for an autopsy.

6. My specific desires about organ donation: ("anatomical gift")

NOTE: Under Arizona law, you may donate all or part of your body. If you do not make a choice, your representative or family can make the decision when you die. You may indicate which organs or tissues you want to donate and where you want them donated. Initial or put a check mark by A or B below. If you select B, continue with your choices.

____ **A.** I DO NOT WANT to make an organ or tissue donation, and I do not want this donation authorized on my behalf by my representative or my family.
____ **B.** I DO WANT to make an organ or tissue donation when I die. Here are my directions:

1. What organs/tissues I choose to donate: (Select a or b below)
____ **a.** Any needed parts or organs.
____ **b.** These parts or organs:
1.) ____________
2.) ____________
3.) ____________

2. What purposes I donate organs/tissues for: (Select a, b, or c below)
____ **a.** Any legally authorized purpose (transplantation, therapy, medical and dental evaluation and research, and/or advancement of medical and dental science).
____ **b.** Transplant or therapeutic purposes only.
____ **c.** Other: ____________

3. What organization or person I want my parts or organs to go to:
____ **a.** I have already signed a written agreement or donor card regarding organ and tissue donation with the following individual or institution: (Name) ____________
____ **b.** I would like my tissues or organs to go to the following individual or institution: (Name) ____________
____ **c.** I authorize my representative to make this decision.

Developed by the Office of Arizona Attorney General Updated December 3, 2007
TERRY GODDARD (All documents completed before December 3, 2007 are still valid)
www.azag.gov 2 DURABLE HEALTH CARE POWER OF ATTORNEY

7. Funeral and Burial Disposition: (Optional)

My agent has authority to carry out all matters relating to my funeral and burial disposition wishes in accordance with this power of attorney, which is effective upon my death. My wishes are reflected below:

Initial or put a check mark by those choices you wish to select.
____ Upon my death, I direct my body to be buried. (As opposed to cremated)
____ Upon my death, I direct my body to be buried in ____________. (Optional directive)
____ Upon my death, I direct my body to be cremated.
____ Upon my death, I direct my body to be cremated with my ashes to be ____________. (Optional directive)
____ My agent will make all funeral and burial disposition decisions. (Optional directive)

8. About a Living Will:

NOTE: If you have a Living Will and a Durable Health Care Power of Attorney, **you must attach** the Living Will to this form. A Living Will form is available on the Attorney General (AG) web site. Initial or put a check mark by box A or B.

____ **A.** I have SIGNED AND ATTACHED a completed Living Will in addition to this Durable Health Care Power of Attorney to state decisions I have made about end of life health care if I am unable to communicate or make my own decisions at that time.
____ **B.** I have NOT SIGNED a Living Will.

9. About a Prehospital Medical Care Directive or Do Not Resuscitate Directive:

NOTE: A form for the Prehospital Medical Care Directive or Do Not Resuscitate Directive is available on the AG Web site. Initial or put a check mark by box A or B.

____ **A.** I and my doctor or health care provider HAVE SIGNED a Prehospital Medical Care Directive or Do Not Resuscitate Directive on paper with ORANGE background in the event that 911 or Emergency Medical Technicians or hospital emergency personnel are called and my heart or breathing has stopped.
____ **B.** I have NOT SIGNED a Prehospital Medical Care Directive or Do Not Resuscitate Directive.

HIPAA WAIVER OF CONFIDENTIALITY FOR MY AGENT/REPRESENTATIVE

____ **(Initial)** I intend for my agent to be treated as I would be with respect to my rights regarding the use and disclosure of my individually identifiable health information or other medical records. This release authority applies to any information governed by the Health Insurance Portability and Accountability Act of 1996 (aka HIPAA), 42 USC 1320d and 45 CFR 160-164.

SIGNATURE OR VERIFICATION

A. I am signing this Durable Health Care Power of Attorney as follows:

My Signature: ____________ Date: ____________

B. I am physically unable to sign this document, so a witness is verifying my desires as follows:

Witness Verification: I believe that this Durable Health Care Power of Attorney accurately expresses the wishes communicated to me by the principal of this document. He/she intends to adopt this Durable Health Care Power of Attorney at this time. He/she is physically unable to sign or mark this document at this time, and I verify that he/she directly indicated to me that the Durable Health Care Power of Attorney expresses his/her wishes and that he/she intends to adopt the Durable Health Care Power of Attorney at this time.

Developed by the Office of Arizona Attorney General Updated December 3, 2007
TERRY GODDARD (All documents completed before December 3, 2007 are still valid)
www.azag.gov 3 DURABLE HEALTH CARE POWER OF ATTORNEY

Witness Name (printed): ____________
Signature: ____________ Date: ____________

SIGNATURE OF WITNESS OR NOTARY PUBLIC:

NOTE: At least one adult witness OR a Notary Public must witness the signing of this document and then sign it. The witness or Notary Public CANNOT be anyone who is: (a) under the age of 18; (b) related to you by blood, adoption, or marriage; (c) entitled to any part of your estate; (d) appointed as your representative; or (e) involved in providing your health care at the time this form is signed.

A. Witness: I certify that I witnessed the signing of this document by the Principal. The person who signed this Durable Health Care Power of Attorney appeared to be of sound mind and under no pressure to make specific choices or sign the document. I understand the requirements of being a witness and I confirm the following:

- I am not currently designated to make medical decisions for this person.
- I am not directly involved in administering health care to this person.
- I am not entitled to any portion of this person's estate upon his or her death under a will or by operation of law.
- I am not related to this person by blood, marriage or adoption.

Witness Name (printed): ____________
Signature: ____________ Date: ____________
Address: ____________

Notary Public (NOTE: If a witness signs your form, you DO NOT need a notary to sign):

STATE OF ARIZONA) ss
COUNTY OF ____________)

The undersigned, being a Notary Public certified in Arizona, declares that the person making this Durable Health Care Power of Attorney has dated and signed or marked it in my presence and appears to me to be of sound mind and free from duress. I further declare I am not related to the person signing above by blood, marriage or adoption, or a person designated to make medical decisions on his/her behalf. I am not directly involved in providing health care to the person signing. I am not entitled to any part of his/her estate under a will now existing or by operation of law. In the event the person acknowledging this Durable Health Care Power of Attorney is physically unable to sign or mark this document, I verify that he/she directly indicated to me that this Durable Health Care Power of Attorney expresses his/her wishes and that he/she intends to adopt the Durable Health Care Power of Attorney at this time.

WITNESS MY HAND AND SEAL this ___ day of ____________, 20___.
Notary Public ____________ My Commission Expires: ____________

OPTIONAL:
STATEMENT THAT YOU HAVE DISCUSSED YOUR HEALTH CARE CHOICES FOR THE FUTURE WITH YOUR PHYSICIAN

NOTE: Before deciding what health care you want for yourself, you may wish to ask your physician questions regarding treatment alternatives. This statement from your physician is not required by Arizona law. If you do speak with your physician, it is a good idea to have him or her complete this section. Ask your doctor to keep a copy of this form with your medical records.

Developed by the Office of Arizona Attorney General Updated December 3, 2007
TERRY GODDARD (All documents completed before December 3, 2007 are still valid)
www.azag.gov 4 DURABLE HEALTH CARE POWER OF ATTORNEY

On this date I reviewed this document with the Principal and discussed any questions regarding the probable medical consequences of the treatment choices provided above. I agree to comply with the provisions of this directive, and I will comply with the health care decisions made by the representative unless a decision violates my conscience. In such case I will promptly disclose my unwillingness to comply and will transfer or try to transfer patient care to another provider who is willing to act in accordance with the representative's direction.

Doctor Name (printed): ____________
Signature: ____________ Date: ____________
Address: ____________

FIGURE 58A-1 Developed by the Office of Arizona Attorney General, Terry Goddard. www.azag.gov

Appendix 58-1 *(continued)*

Instructions: Competent adults and emancipated minors may give advance instructions using this form or any form of their own choosing. To be legally binding, the Advance Care Plan must be signed and either witnessed or notarized.

I, ______________________, hereby give these advance instructions on how I want to be treated by my doctors and other health care providers when I can no longer make those treatment decisions myself.

Agent: I want the following person to make health care decisions for me:

Name: ______________ Phone #: __________ Relation: ______________
Address: ______________________________

Alternate Agent: If the person named above is unable or unwilling to make health care decisions for me, I appoint as alternate:

Name: ______________ Phone #: __________ Relation: ______________
Address: ______________________________

Quality of Life:

I want my doctors to help me maintain an acceptable quality of life including adequate pain management. A quality of life that is unacceptable to me means when I have any of the following conditions **(you can check as many of these items as you want):**

- ☐ **Permanent Unconscious Condition:** I become totally unaware of people or surroundings with little chance of ever waking up from the coma.
- ☐ **Permanent Confusion:** I become unable to remember, understand or make decisions. I do not recognize loved ones or cannot have a clear conversation with them.
- ☐ **Dependent in all Activities of Daily Living:** I am no longer able to talk clearly or move by myself. I depend on others for feeding, bathing, dressing and walking. Rehabilitation or any other restorative treatment will not help.
- ☐ **End-Stage Illnesses:** I have an illness that has reached its final stages in spite of full treatment. Examples: Widespread cancer that does not respond anymore to treatment; chronic and/or damaged heart and lungs, where oxygen needed most of the time and activities are limited due to the feeling of suffocation.

Treatment:

If my quality of life becomes unacceptable to me and my condition is irreversible (that is, it will not improve), I direct that medically appropriate treatment be provided as follows. **Checking "yes" means I WANT the treatment. Checking "no" means I DO NOT want the treatment.**

☐ ☐ Yes No	**CPR (Cardiopulmonary Resuscitation):** To make the heart beat again and restore breathing after it has stopped. Usually this involves electric shock, chest compressions, and breathing assistance.
☐ ☐ Yes No	**Life Support / Other Artificial Support:** Continuous use of breathing machine, IV fluids, medications, and other equipment that helps the lungs, heart, kidneys and other organs to continue to work.
☐ ☐ Yes No	**Treatment of New Conditions:** Use of surgery, blood transfusions, or antibiotics that will deal with a new condition but will not help the main illness.
☐ ☐ Yes No	**Tube feeding/IV fluids:** Use of tubes to deliver food and water to patient's stomach or use of IV fluids into a vein which would include artificially delivered nutrition and hydration.

PLEASE SIGN ON PAGE 2 — Page 1 of 2

Other instructions, such as burial arrangements, hospice care, etc.: ______________________

(Attach additional pages if necessary)

Organ donation (optional): Upon my death, I wish to make the following anatomical gift (please mark one):
☐ Any organ/tissue ☐ My entire body ☐ Only the following organs/tissues: ______________

SIGNATURE

Your signature should either be witnessed by two competent adults or notarized. If witnessed, neither witness should be the person you appointed as your agent, and at least one of the witnesses should be someone who is not related to you or entitled to any part of your estate.

Signature: ______________________ (Patient) DATE: ______________

Witnesses:

1. I am a competent adult who is not named as the agent. I witnessed the patient's signature on this form. ______________ Signature of witness number 1
2. I am a competent adult who is not named as the agent. I am not related to the patient by blood, marriage, or adoption and I would not be entitled to any portion of the patient's estate upon his or her death under any existing will or codicil or by operation of law. I witnessed the patient's signature on this form. ______________ Signature of witness number 2

This document may be notarized instead of witnessed:

STATE OF TENNESSEE
COUNTY OF ______________

I am a Notary Public in and for the State and County named above. The person who signed this instrument is personally known to me (or proved to me on the basis of satisfactory evidence) to be the person who signed as the "patient". The patient personally appeared before me and signed above or acknowledged the signature above as his or her own. I declare under penalty of perjury that the patient appears to be of sound mind and under no duress, fraud, or undue influence.

My commission expires: ______________ ______________ Signature of Notary Public

WHAT TO DO WITH THIS ADVANCE DIRECTIVE

- Provide a copy to your physician(s)
- Keep a copy in your personal files where it is accessible to others
- Tell your closest relatives and friends what is in the document
- Provide a copy to the person(s) you named as your health care agent

Approved by Tennessee Department of Health, Board for Licensing Health Care Facilities, February 3, 2005
Acknowledgement to Project GRACE for inspiring the development of this form.

Page 2 of 2

FIGURE 58A-2 Approved by the Tennessee Department of Health, Board for Licensing Health Care Facilities, February 3, 2005. Acknowledgment to Project GRACE for inspiring the development of this form.

I, ______________________, give my agent named below permission to make health care decisions for me if I cannot make decisions for myself, including any health care decision that I could have made for myself if able. If my agent is unavailable or is unable or unwilling to serve, the alternate named below will take the agent's place.

Agent:	Alternate:
Name	Name
Address	Address
City State Zip Code	City State Zip Code
( ) Area Code Home Phone Number	( ) Area Code Home Phone Number
( ) Area Code Work Phone Number	( ) Area Code Work Phone Number
( ) Area Code Mobile Phone Number	( ) Area Code Mobile Phone Number
Patient's name (please print or type) Date	Signature of patient (must be at least 18 or emancipated minor)

To be legally valid, **either** block A **or** block B must be properly completed and signed.

Block A Witnesses (2 witnesses required)

1. I am a competent adult who is not named above. I witnessed the patient's signature on this form. ______________ Signature of witness number 1
2. I am a competent adult who is not named above. I am not related to the patient by blood, marriage, or adoption and I would not be entitled to any portion of the patient's estate upon his or her death under any existing will or codicil or by operation of law. I witnessed the patient's signature on this form. ______________ Signature of witness number 2

Block B Notarization

STATE OF TENNESSEE
COUNTY OF ______________

I am a Notary Public in and for the State and County named above. The person who signed this instrument is personally known to me (or proved to me on the basis of satisfactory evidence) to be the person whose name is shown above as the "patient." The patient personally appeared before me and signed above or acknowledged the signature above as his or her own. I declare under penalty of perjury that the patient appears to be of sound mind and under no duress, fraud, or undue influence.

My commission expires: ______________ ______________ Signature of Notary Public

Approved by Tennessee Department of Health, Board for Licensing Health Care Facilities, February 3, 2005

FIGURE 58A-3 Approved by the Tennessee Department of Health, Board for Licensing Health Care Facilities, February 3, 2005.

I, ______________________ (**Designated Physician**) made the decision to appoint ______________________ (**Name of Surrogate**) as surrogate for ______________________ (**Name of Patient**).

Surrogate Contact Information: Home: ______________
Work: ______________
Cell Phone: ______________

Reasons for Appointment (check all that apply):

- ___ Knows patient's wishes
- ___ Knows patient's best interest
- ___ Had regular contact with patient
- ___ Available and willing to serve
- ___ Demonstrates care and concern
- ___ Visits patient regularly during illness
- ___ Engages in face-to-face contact with caregiver
- ___ Participates in decision making process

______________ **Physician Signature** ______________ **Date/Time**

If designated physician is to act as surrogate, one of the following signatures must be obtained:

______________ **Ethics Committee Representative Date** or ______________ **Concurring Second Physician Date**

Any individuals in disagreement? Yes ___ No ___
If yes, please explain ______________________

ACCEPTANCE OF SURROGATE SELECTION

I accept the appointment as surrogate for ______________________ (**Patient**)
and understand I have the authority to make all medical decisions.

______________ **Signature of Surrogate** ______________ **Date/Time**

Approved by Tennessee Department of Health, Board for Licensing Health Care Facilities, May 3, 2005

FIGURE 58A-4 Approved by the Tennessee Department of Health, Board for Licensing Health Care Facilities, February 3, 2005.

(continues)

Appendix 58-1 (*continued*)

COPY OF FORM SHALL ACCOMPANY PATIENT WHEN TRANSFERRED OR DISCHARGED

Physician Orders
for Scope of Treatment (POST)

This is a Physician Order Sheet based on the medical conditions and wishes of the person identified at right ("patient"). Any section not completed indicates full treatment for that section. When need occurs, first follow these orders, then contact physician.

Patient's Last Name
First Name/Middle Initial
Date of Birth

Section	
Section A *Check One Box Only*	**CARDIOPULMONARY RESUSCITATION (CPR): Patient has no pulse and/or is not breathing.** ☐ **Resuscitate (CPR)** ☐ **Do Not Attempt Resuscitate (DNR/no CPR)** When not in cardiopulmonary arrest, follow orders in **B, C,** and **D.**
Section B *Check One Box Only*	**MEDICAL INTERVENTIONS. Patient has pulse and/or is breathing.** ☐ **Comfort Measures** Treat with dignity and respect. Keep clean, warm, and dry. Use medication by any route, positioning, wound care and other measures to relieve pain and suffering. Use oxygen, suction and manual treatment of airway obstruction as needed for comfort. **Do not transfer to hospital for life-sustaining treatment. Transfer only if comfort needs cannot be met in current location.** ☐ **Limited Additional Interventions** Includes care described above. Use medical treatment, IV fluids and cardiac monitoring as indicated. Do not use intubation, advanced airway interventions, or mechanical ventilation. **Transfer to hospital if indicated. Avoid intensive care.** ☐ **Full Treatment.** Includes care above. Use intubation, advanced airway interventions mechanical ventilation, and cardioversion as indicated. **Transfer to hospital if indicated. Include intensive care.** *Other Instructions:* ______
Section C *Check One Box Only*	**ANTIBIOTICS – Treatment for new medical conditions:** ☐ **No Antibiotics** ☐ **Antibiotics** *Other Instructions:* ______
Section D *Check One Box Only in Each Column*	**MEDICALLY ADMINISTERED FLUIDS AND NUTRITION.** Oral fluids and nutrition must be offered if medically feasible. ☐ **No IV fluids** (provide other measures to assure comfort) ☐ **No feeding tube** ☐ **IV fluids for a defined trial period** ☐ **Feeding tube for a defined trial period** ☐ **IV fluids long-term if indicated** ☐ **Feeding tube long-term** *Other Instructions:* ______
Section E *Must be Completed*	**Discussed with:** ☐ Patient/Resident ☐ Health care agent ☐ Court-appointed guardian ☐ Health care surrogate ☐ Parent of minor ☐ Other: ______ (Specify) **The Basis for These Orders Is:** (Must be completed) ☐ Patient's preferences ☐ Patient's best interest (patient lacks capacity or preferences unknown) ☐ Medical indications ☐ (Other) ______ **Physician Name** (Print) | **Physician Phone Number** | **Office Use Only** **Physician Signature** (Mandatory) | **Date**

COPY OF FORM SHALL ACCOMPANY PATIENT WHEN TRANSFERRED OR DISCHARGED

HIPAA PERMITS DISCLOSURE OF POST TO OTHER HEALTH CARE PROFESSIONALS AS NECESSARY

Signature of Patient, Parent of Minor, or Guardian/Health Care Representative

Significant thought has been given to life-sustaining treatment. Preferences have been expressed to a physician and/or health care professional(s). This document reflects those treatment preferences.

(If signed by surrogate, preferences expressed must reflect patient's wishes as best understood by surrogate.)

Signature	Name (print)	Relationship (write "self" if patient)

Contact Information

Surrogate	Relationship	Phone Number	
Health Care Professional Preparing Form	Preparer Title	Phone Number	Date Prepared

Directions for Health Care Professionals

Completing POST

Must be completed by a health care professional based on patient preferences, patient best interest, and medical indications.

POST must be signed by a physician to be valid. Verbal orders are acceptable with follow-up signature by physician in accordance with facility/community policy.

Photocopies/faxes of signed POST forms are legal and valid.

Using POST

Any incomplete section of POST implies full treatment for that section.

No defibrillator (including AEDs) should be used on a person who has chosen "Do Not Attempt Resuscitation".

Oral fluids and nutrition must always be offered if medically feasible.

When comfort cannot be achieved in the current setting, the person, including someone with "Comfort Measures Only", should be transferred to a setting able to provide comfort (e.g., treatment of a hip fracture).

IV medication to enhance comfort may be appropriate for a person who has chosen "Comfort Measures Only".

Treatment of dehydration is a measure which prolongs life. A person who desires IV fluids should indicate "Limited Interventions" or "Full Treatment".

A person with capacity, or the surrogate of a person without capacity, can request alternative treatment.

Reviewing POST

This POST should be reviewed if:

(1) The patient is transferred from one care setting or care level to another, or
(2) There is a substantial change in the patient's health status, or
(3) The patient's treatment preferences change.

Draw line through sections A through E and write "VOID" in large letters if POST is replaced or becomes invalid.

Approved by Tennessee Department of Health, Board for Licensing Health Care Facilities, February 3, 2005

COPY OF FORM SHALL ACCOMPANY PATIENT WHEN TRANSFERRED OR DISCHARGED.

DO NOT ALTER THIS FORM !

FIGURE 58A-5 Approved by the Tennessee Department of Health, Board for Licensing Health Care Facilities, February 3, 2005.

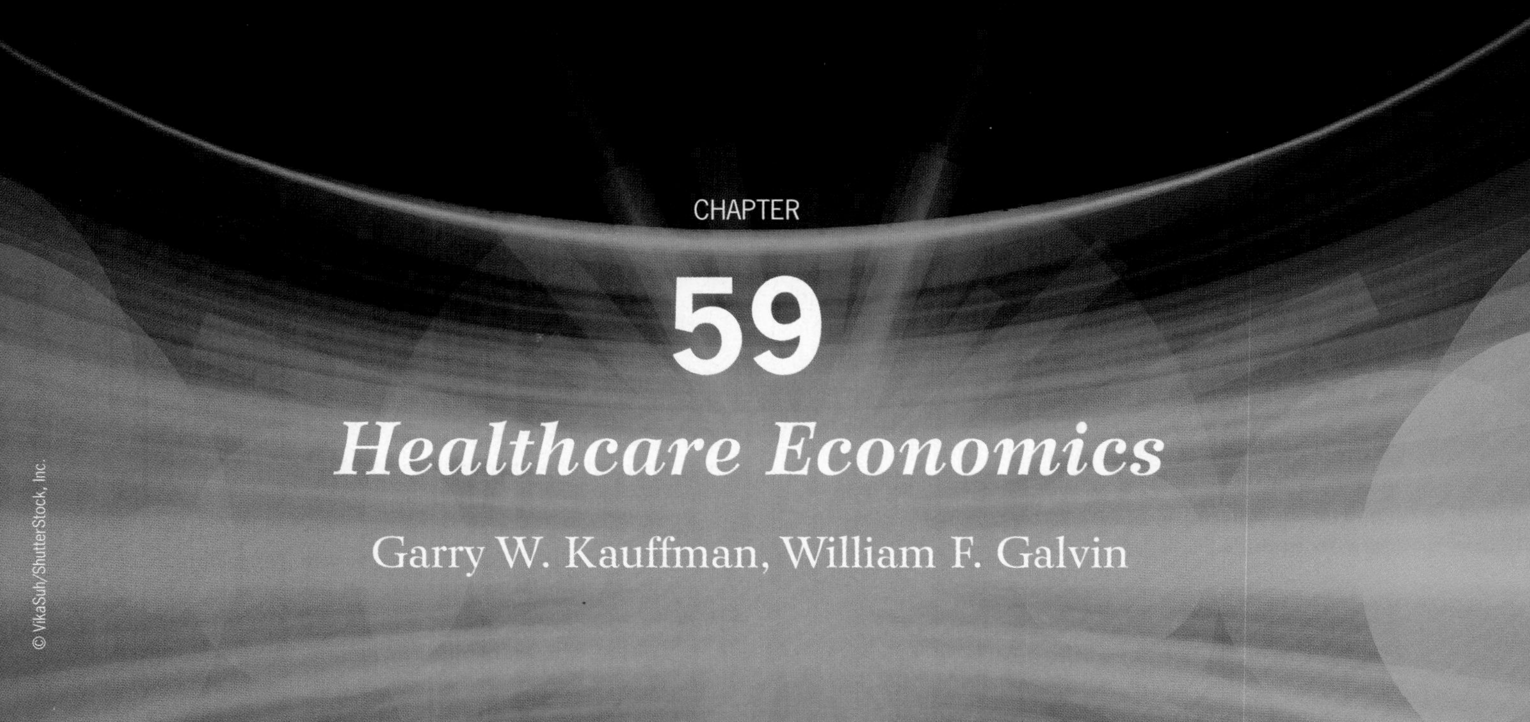

OUTLINE

Basic Healthcare Functions
Stakeholders in the U.S. Healthcare System
The Respiratory Therapist's Role in Balancing Cost and Care
Forces Influencing Healthcare Costs
A Brief History and Overview of Financing Health Care
The Era of Managed Care
Reimbursement Methodologies
The Future of Healthcare Funding
Respiratory Therapist Documenting and Demonstrating Value

OBJECTIVES

1. Explain four major functions of the healthcare system.
2. Identify and explain the role of the major stakeholders in healthcare delivery.
3. Discuss forces influencing healthcare change and costs.
4. Describe general healthcare payment systems.
5. Explain the history and evolution of managed care.
6. Explain the types of managed care organizations.
7. Describe prominent reimbursement methodologies.
8. Discuss the future of healthcare financing.
9. Discuss role of respiratory therapist in documenting and demonstrating value.

KEY TERMS

all-patient refined diagnosis-related group (APR-DRG)
bundled charges
capitation
case mix
Centers for Medicare and Medicaid Services (CMS)
copayment
diagnosis-related group (DRG)
evidence-based medicine (EBM)
exclusive provider organization (EPO)
fee-for-service system
health maintenance organization (HMO)
indemnity insurance plan
insurance
managed care organization (MCO)
Medicaid
Medicare
minimum data set (MDS)
pay for performance (P4P)
point-of-service plan (POS)
preferred provider organization (PPO)
prospective payment system (PPS)
resource-based relative value scale (RBRVS)
resource intensity
retrospective payment system (RPS)
risk of mortality
severity of illness
skilled nursing facility (SNF)
third-party payer

Introduction

The economic climate of the U.S. healthcare system is extremely volatile and unpredictable. Numerous forces—both complementary and opposing—are at play within the private and public sectors attempting to shape it to better understand and gain control of what many believe are unwarranted and unnecessary escalating healthcare costs. While the healthcare system is constantly evolving and undergoing change, the way in which it reimburses has a profound impact on its delivery of services and practice patterns. Reimbursement and economic considerations are central issues for healthcare executives. In fact, some would say that the U.S. healthcare system is driven primarily by economics rather than **evidence-based medicine (EBM)**. The astute respiratory therapist (RT) must recognize the paramount importance placed on healthcare financing. Converting care and services into financial returns to the provider has become critical to survival of the healthcare organization. Current economic pressures are not likely to change in the foreseeable future, at least until such time that federal and state governmental leadership are convinced that health care is delivering on the investment.

Respiratory therapy schools and departments have historically not taught students and practitioners to understand the critical importance of healthcare financing and the underlying economic principles guiding the healthcare system. This chapter identifies and discusses the basic functions of health care, provides an overview of the forces driving the system, identifies and explains the role of the major stakeholders, provides a basic and simplified view of the history and various forms of reimbursement, and explains the role and function of the RT within this system. The theme of the chapter is that the RT can no longer limit his or her involvement to simply the provision of quality care. Today's healthcare environment demands that respiratory therapists (RTs) be a valued-added member of the healthcare team and are savvy with regard to healthcare economics.

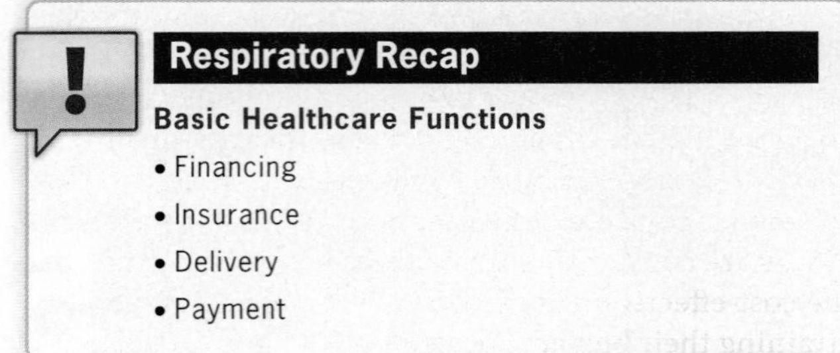

Respiratory Recap

Basic Healthcare Functions

- Financing
- Insurance
- Delivery
- Payment

Basic Healthcare Functions

The four major functions of the healthcare system in the United States are financing, insurance, delivery, and payment.[1] **Table 59-1** depicts the four major functions, their roles, and the group or organization that is associated with each.

The first major function in health care is *financing*, which involves the purchase of insurance and serves as the means to pay for healthcare services consumed by the patient or client. Historically, employers, including governmental and private industry, offered free or discounted health care as a fringe benefit to attract and retain employees. The federal, state, and local government also can provide it.

Strictly speaking, the **insurance** function entails protection of the patient, client, or consumer against catastrophic risk. *Insurance* also refers to the administration of the customer's benefits package and is provided by an insurance company or managed care organization (MCO) that serves as an intermediary between the purchaser and the recipient or consumer. Interestingly, providers (especially hospitals) are increasingly contracting directly with employers to provide healthcare services and, by doing so, are bypassing the middleman. Of recent note were announcements that several large employers will be directly contracting with only a few healthcare providers. For example, Wal-Mart announced that it would be the first retailer to offer a national program that covers heart, spine, and transplant procedures for its employees. Essentially, when any of the 1.1 million employees and dependents enroll in the company's health plan and need those procedures, Wal-Mart will direct them to six "centers of excellence" around the nation, including the Cleveland Clinic and Mayo Clinic, at no additional cost.[2]

Healthcare *delivery*, the third major function, involves the provision of services by the physician or other healthcare provider to the patient or consumer. *Delivery* also can refer to the hospital, skilled nursing home, clinic, or home care company. The RT is closely involved in this function.

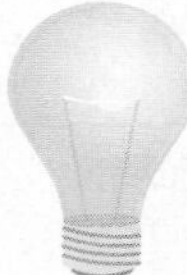

STOP AND THINK

Why should the RT develop an understanding of healthcare economics?

TABLE 59-1
Four Major Functions of Health Care

Function	Role	Affected Group or Organization
Financing	Purchase of health insurance	Private sources: employers, individuals Public sources: federal, state, and local governments
Insurance	Protection against risk	Commercial insurance companies: Aetna US Healthcare, Met Life, Prudential, others Blue Cross/Blue Shield
Delivery	Provision of services	Short-term acute care hospitals, long-term acute care hospitals, acute and chronic rehabilitation services, skilled nursing facilities, clinics, physicians, physician-extenders, home health agencies, durable medical equipment companies, pharmacies, urgent care centers, and retail health clinics
Payment	Determination of reimbursement methodology and disbursement of funds	Commercial insurance companies Blue Cross/Blue Shield Third-party claims processors

Perhaps the most complex function of the system is *payment*, which increasingly defines how services are delivered. The RT must understand that payment deals specifically with reimbursement and disbursement of funds. It is an infinitely complicated process that undergoes continuous change and ceaseless revision. Payers are constantly searching for ways to optimize the cost-effectiveness of care delivery in pursuit of attaining their business goals. It is critically important for the RTs to understand the goals and objectives of each segment in order to align and market their value.

The sources of these funds for disbursement are employers; the federal, state, and local governments; fraternal organizations; MCOs; and self-pay. These disbursements take the form of premiums or entitlement payments. The insurance company is the intermediary providing payment to the provider orchestrated by a claim submitted by the consumer. The provider or patient submits the claim to the intermediary, which processes it according to a previously defined and agreed-upon contract. The RT should recognize that the U.S. healthcare system is exceedingly complex. While the primary goal is to deliver healthcare services, it is clear that opportunity exists to move from a fragmented and disease-focused system to one that fosters wellness and preventative services for the consumer.

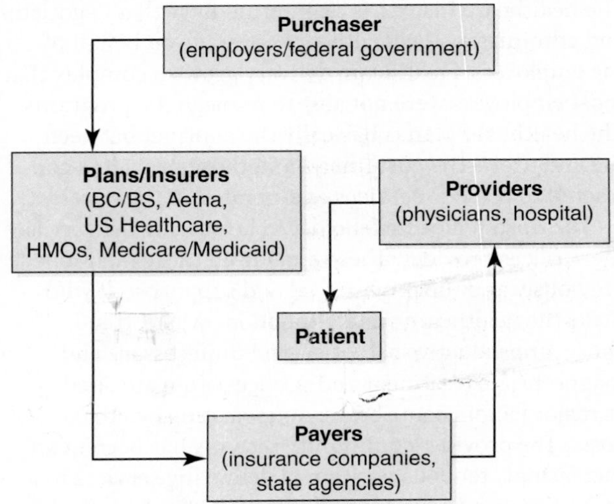

FIGURE 59-1 Stakeholders in healthcare reimbursement.

Stakeholders in the U.S. Healthcare System

Providing and delivering healthcare services involve several stakeholders. Historically, three major stakeholders existed: the patient (primary payer), the provider (secondary payer), and the insurer (**third-party payer**). Over the years the system has become increasingly more complicated and complex, particularly with the rise of new delivery models. Today we acknowledge the roles and functions of the following five significant stakeholders in the U.S. healthcare system: purchasers, plans, providers, payers, and patients (**Figure 59-1**).

At times the role and function of each stakeholder overlaps, often clouding the lines of responsibilities. Purchasers are generally employers or the federal, state, or local governments and presently subsidize much of the cost of health care. Employers purchase healthcare packages and typically offer several options as a means to best meet the needs of each customer. The government funds health care in the form of entitlement and shared assistance programs. Employers began providing this benefit early in the 20th century as a means to provide a tangible benefit to their employees' compensation packages, both to attract as well as retain employees. Medical coverage was viewed as a way to safeguard both the employee and the company from catastrophic healthcare losses. In addition, it was viewed as a way to add a benefit without having to incur a more direct expense in the form of salary increases. The federal government entered healthcare reimbursement by instituting Medicare and Medicaid in 1965 to assist the elderly and the poor. In addition to programs serving the elderly and the poor, other programs were initiated to assist those with special needs (e.g., Childrens' Health Insurance Program). While beyond the scope of this chapter, RTs are encouraged to explore these specialty programs with regard to how we may become engaged not only to provide high-quality care but to do so in a cost-effective and patient-centric manner. In recent years, purchasers have become increasingly concerned with the dramatic increases in overall costs and attendant financial risk. Program costs have soared and thus employers are interested in better managing the programs and controlling the costs while at the same time providing a tangible benefit to their employees.

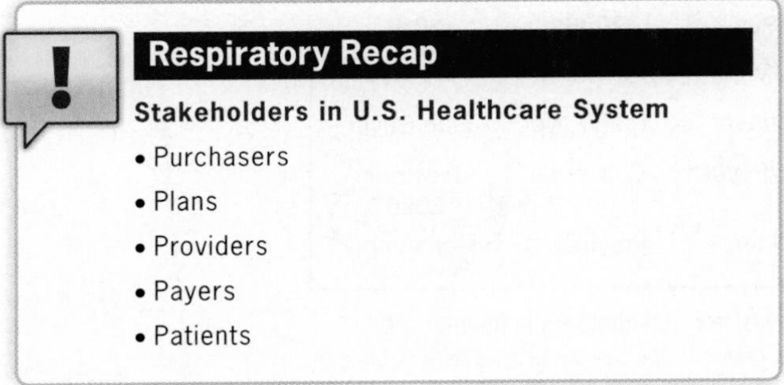

Respiratory Recap

Stakeholders in U.S. Healthcare System

- Purchasers
- Plans
- Providers
- Payers
- Patients

The organizations or groups that provide healthcare plans to purchasers make up the second group of stakeholders, generally insurance companies, insurers, or plans. The insurer or plan is either the public or private sector and is represented by the federal/state government or commercial insurers. Examples of the larger and more prominent healthcare insurers include Blue Cross/Blue Shield, Aetna, US Healthcare, and Kaiser Permanente, among many other smaller organizations.

The healthcare insurer is an intermediary that negotiates and administers the healthcare coverage on behalf of the employers. Healthcare delivery grew so complex that most employers were not able to manage the programs. The healthcare plan is basically the contract between the end user—the customer—and those providers contracted to provide services enumerated in the contract.

The third major stakeholder in healthcare delivery is the services provider. These include all those mentioned previously and the professional and support staff who make the healthcare system function. Waste, fraud, abuse, unproductive activities, and unnecessary and inappropriate treatment and services often are cited as major factors contributing to escalating healthcare costs. The provider community recently has been in an increasingly tenuous position of delivering services in a more cost-conscious manner. These cost reductions have involved employees, facilities, equipment, supplies, and services.

The fourth stakeholder is the payer, that is, the group or organization that processes the claim and disburses the funds. The payer is either the insurer or a third party that administers the process. The health plan or insurer performs the insurance function, whereas the payer provides payment or disbursement. The payer also is known as the *third-party administrator* (*TPA*).

The final stakeholder is the ultimate recipient of care—the patient—who is typically referred to as the healthcare consumer. Most healthcare consumers have historically assumed a passive role and one that expected and assumed the delivery of high-quality care. The cost of this care was not preeminent in the minds of consumers. Their passivity stemmed from their historically employer-provided healthcare coverage that shielded the true cost of health care from them. This consumer passivity is changing as a result of a shift in financial obligations to the consumer. Employers are simply unable to sustain the added expense and burden of escalating healthcare premiums and still compete in a global economy. The escalating healthcare premiums are negatively impacting budgets, reducing company profitability, and, in some instances, leading to dissolution of the business. Consequently, employers have begun to shift some of these expenses to employees in the form of higher copayments, higher deductibles, increased limits for out-of-pocket expenses, and constraining of healthcare services. Consumers are becoming increasingly more responsible for managing their health care.

All five stakeholders attempt to limit their financial risk. **Figure 59-2** depicts a theoretic view of the amount of risk incurred by the major stakeholders during various time periods. While speculative, it appears the evolving healthcare system is increasingly exposing the provider network to more financial risk. Insurers are attempting to manage risk by placing increasing pressure on providers to increase productivity, reduce staffing, improve patient satisfaction, eliminate inefficiency, and decrease inappropriate utilization. Providers are being challenged to demonstrate that the delivery of services, which are predicated on a scientific basis that substantiates the services, are provided. In short, gone are the days where "Doing More with More" was the mantra for much of the modern healthcare system's existence. With the dramatic focus on cost-containment, this has been replaced by "Do Less with Less." For RTs, this is a phenomenal opportunity to demonstrate the value of their services in terms of clinical outcomes, patient/family satisfaction, and cost-effectiveness.

As a result, the consumer is pulled into the equation and required to more actively participate by changing copayments, increased deductibles, or reduced services. In some scenarios, health service rationing has been enacted with a reward-and-punishment system implemented to acknowledge and reward healthy lifestyle behaviors and practices and, concomitantly, to financially punish unhealthy behaviors and practices. For example, significantly reduced premiums, copayments, or deductibles can be provided to consumers who choose not to smoke or who engage in healthy lifestyle behaviors that include regular exercise, annual vaccinations or immunization, and preventive health checkups. Participating in regular exercise by joining a gym or health club can translate into reimbursement for a portion of the health club membership fee. Conversely, higher premiums are being applied to those employees who choose to continue unhealthy behaviors and practices. While this consumer-centric model is still in its infancy, there are some signs that engaging people to be more active in their healthcare delivery system may be working.

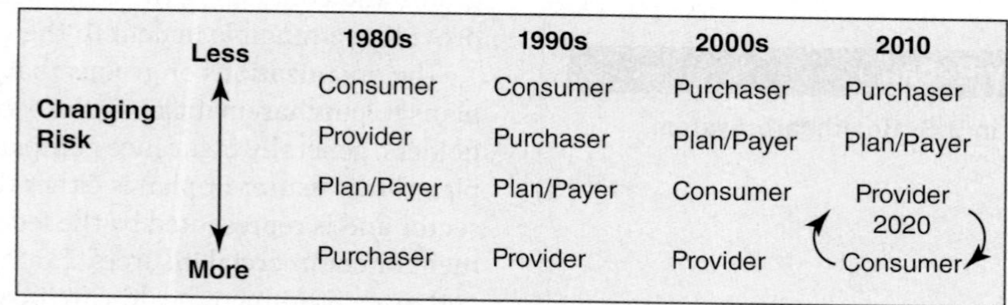

FIGURE 59-2 Theoretic view of risk incurred by major stakeholders in health care.

Information from U.S. Department of Health and Human Services, Centers for Medicare and Medicaid Services, Office of Information Services.

The Respiratory Therapist's Role in Balancing Cost and Care

Most RTs enter the healthcare profession primarily to care for patients, and most services are delivered in the acute care venue. Most RTs' primary function is as bedside clinicians and, as such, as the nonphysician experts in cardiorespiratory care and care management. Although little has changed with regard to this primary purpose, the system in which it occurs has changed significantly. The system is beginning to question the need and efficacy of care as well as whom the most appropriate provider of each service should be. Additionally, pressure is increasing to address the burgeoning increase in healthcare costs that is seen to be negatively impacting the U.S. economy and its citizens. **Figure 59-3** provides a graphic display of the exponential growth of healthcare expenditures and selected healthcare indicators, namely, total healthcare expenditures, average expenditure per person, and healthcare expenditure as a percentage of gross domestic product.[3]

Health care is becoming too costly. Cost containment is rising in prominence and is a critical concern to all stakeholders, including the RT. The RT must learn the business of health care, develop a better understanding of financial considerations associated with the patient care decisions, and learn to create a value proposition in the evolving healthcare system.

Forces Influencing Healthcare Costs

A number of forces drive the changes seen in health care.[1,4,5] Each will be discussed with a brief commentary on the implications to the RT.

Increase in Cost Without Increase in Quality

Numerous studies within the United States as well as comparing our health status to that of other nations have repeatedly documented that the increasing cost of health care has not generated a concomitant improvement in overall health. In fact, despite the fact that the United States spends a greater percentage of its economy on health care and has markedly higher per person expenditures, little can be shown when clinical outcomes are compared to those of other nations, including some third world countries. **Figure 59-4** illustrates this point by comparing U.S. statistics with

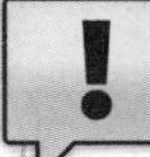

Respiratory Recap

Forces Driving Health Care

- Increase in cost without increase in quality
- Technology
- Aging population
- Fragmentation of the industry
- Excess capacity
- Unnecessary care and defensive medicine
- Growth of underinsured and uninsured
- Consumerism

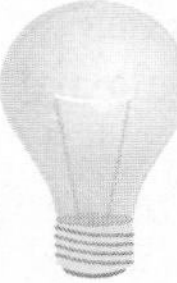

STOP AND THINK

Healthcare spending in the United States is estimated to be 2½ times that of the average country in the Organisation for Economic Co-operation and Development (OECD). Comment on the model of health care practiced in some of these OECD countries and, more importantly, identify reasons/factors behind the higher cost in the United States.

Year	Total Expenditures (in billions)	Expenditures per Person (in thousands)	As a Percentage of GDP
1960	27.4	0.147	5.2
1970	74.9	0.356	7.2
1980	255.8	1.110	9.2
1990	724.3	2.854	12.5
2000	1,377.2	4.878	13.8
2010	2,600.0	8.417	17.9
2013	2,915	9,216	18.0
2014	3,093.2 (projected)	9,697 (projected)	18.3 (projected)
2020	4,416.2 (projected)	13,142 (projected)	19.2 (projected)

FIGURE 59-3 Healthcare expenditures and selected healthcare indicators. Total healthcare expenditures, average expenditure per person, and healthcare expenditure as a percentage of gross domestic product.

Information from Centers for Medicare and Medicaid Services. Available at: http://www.cms.gov/Research-Statistics-Data-and-Systems/Statistics-Trends-and-Reports/NationalHealthExpendData/NationalHealthAccountsProjected.html.

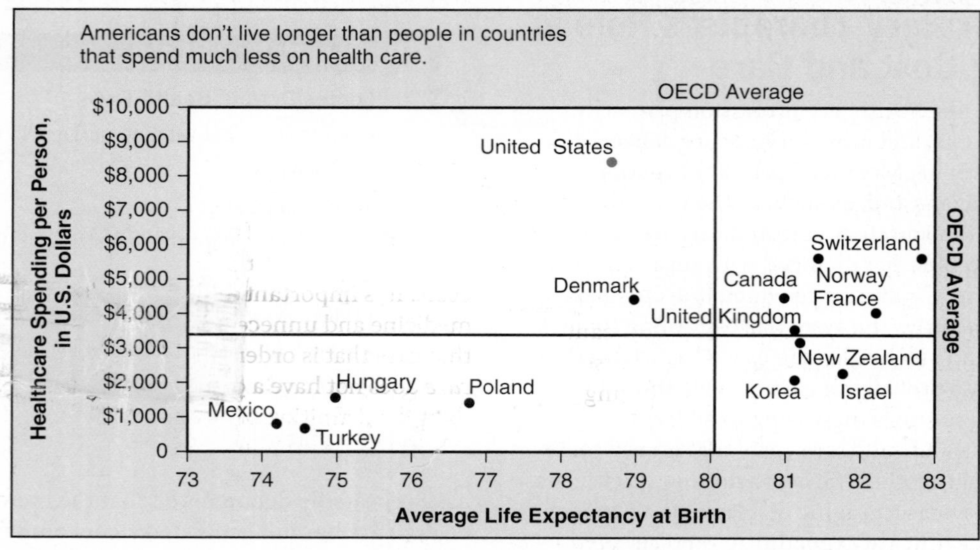

FIGURE 59-4 Comparison of healthcare spending per person between the United States and selected OECD countries and average life expectancy at birth.

Reproduced from The Huffington Post, information from OECD Health Data 2013.

select countries in the Organisation for Economic Co-operation and Development (OECD) in terms of average life expectancy at birth and healthcare spending per person in U.S. dollars. The proportion of the U.S. economy consumed by healthcare services has more than tripled in the past three decades, an alarming increase.

In 2011, the most recent year in which most of the countries reported data, the United States spent 17.9% of its gross domestic product (GDP) on health care; the projection for 2014 is 18.3%. This is concerning since no other country tracked by the OECD reported more than 11.9%.[6] On a positive note, the growth in U.S. healthcare costs, after a peak in 2002, has actually decreased each year through 2011, and the myriad of change forces appear, at least at this time, to be slowing the rate of increase.[7] But more troubling than the cost increase is the fact that the increased financial resources dedicated to health care have not resulted in an improvement in infant mortality, diabetes, chronic pulmonary disease, and a host of other conditions. One example of the so-called cost–quality chasm is that the U.S. infant mortality compared to other nations has worsened for several decades. As of 2010, the United States ranked only 26th compared to other nations.[8]

The implication for RTs is that the value of service in terms of quality, customer service, and cost must be documented. Services that provide a documented improvement should be utilized, while those that cannot document improvement should be eliminated.

Technology

Traditionally, hospital administrators focus on technology associated with electronic medical records, imaging, and operation of the medical laboratory. Sophisticated and essential capital equipment employed by RTs, such as mechanical ventilators, are closely monitored for their high costs. Therapeutic and diagnostic technologies utilized by RT departments continue to take an increasingly larger percentage of capital expenditures, however, and are subjected to increased scrutiny for virtually every organization.

The implication for the RTs is that for each new technology under consideration, the impact of that technology must be documented. Historically, this mandate with new technology that purported to improve care was not done. RTs must demonstrate the impact of technology, which can include decreasing patients' length of stay, reducing time on the ventilator, reducing readmissions, and/or decreasing the cost of services, to name but a few factors affecting the budget.

Aging Population

The American population continues to grow increasingly older and at a rate greater than the general population. RTs are encountering both older sick and older healthy senior citizens. Unlike the generations preceding them, the new generations of older adults are increasingly dying secondary to chronic disease rather than from acute disease. Clearly, this population will consume a disproportionately greater amount of healthcare services and concomitantly more of the healthcare dollar.

For RTs, the services provided to maintain the health of senior citizens should increase in value in the eyes of all stakeholders, particularly in light of the changing reimbursement methodology. Pulmonary rehabilitation and RT services provided in subacute and home environments, which are currently not widely accepted as value-added by many stakeholders, will be recognized, if appropriately provided and documented, for high quality as well as decreased cost.

Fragmentation of the Industry

Despite recent attempts by the federal government to assist in coordination of services between providers, there remains little coordination between different care venues. The chest radiograph taken in the physician's office is duplicated in the urgent care center and is duplicated again in the hospital emergency department. Reimbursement methodology has been a significant driver of these practices, but changes in reimbursement, notably bundling of services, will be driving drastic changes in these practices.

One of the newest care delivery models, Integrated Practice Units (IPUs), appears to be making a change in patient outcomes as it is designed to improve the coordination of patient care across the continuum. IPUs have demonstrated better quality (i.e., improved patient clinical outcomes) and lower costs with several patient conditions.[9] While still in its infancy, this is a model with which RTs should become familiar, particularly with regard to how they can integrate respiratory care services within this care continuum to demonstrate value in terms of patient outcomes, patient/family satisfaction, and cost-effectiveness.

One way to increase value and partner with physician colleagues is to identify physician practices that provide pulmonary function testing and offer to create a hub and spoke arrangement whereby the RT assumes responsibility for testing within the hospital and also for managing these services within the physician offices. There are quality control concerns with such disseminated testing, and the RT is perfectly positioned to assist in improving quality, decreasing cost, and improving patient and customer satisfaction.

Excess Capacity

The American Hospital Association (AHA) reports annually on a variety of hospital performance indicators. These show a continued decrease in inpatient bed utilization and occupancy. Even if hospitals are able to shutter beds and proportionately decrease the staffing, services, and support for these closed wings, their overhead does not decrease proportionately. This is one of the driving factors in hospital affiliations, mergers, and acquisitions. A second major source of excess capacity was cited previously with regard to the duplication of services between providers.

The RT needs to examine the possibility of utilizing some of these closed wings or near vacant hospitals to judiciously expand current diagnostic and rehabilitative services with the goals of increasing capacity and customer satisfaction. While some hospitals have been forced to create sleep labs in hotels, such services can be returned to the hospital, which would decrease operational costs. With the renewed understanding of the value of pulmonary rehabilitation, hospitals that eliminated their rehabilitation programs and shuttered their space are now able to reinstitute this value-added service.

Unnecessary Care and Defensive Medicine

Defensive medicine has been reported by numerous sources to be a contributor to driving up healthcare costs. It is important to distinguish between defensive medicine and unnecessary care. *Defensive medicine* is that care that is ordered to avoid litigation. *Unnecessary care* does not have a clinical justification but may be seen to fit the definition of "it doesn't hurt and might help."

The RT needs to utilize clinical practice guidelines, appropriateness filters, and patient-focused clinical protocols. The RT must be able to document the appropriateness of the care, measure the patient response to the services, and report the value of the services rendered.

Growth of Underinsured and Uninsured

As noted previously, the United States continues to witness a sustained growth in the number of Americans who are either uninsured or underinsured. RTs may see this in patients who don't fill their discharge prescriptions after discharge from the hospital. The result is that patients either do not receive the prescribed care they need or they succumb to poor health status and utilize inappropriate resources, such as the emergency department rather than a family physician. This will clearly add to the overall cost of healthcare delivery.

RTs need to identify their patients, particularly those at highest risk, and deliver the services in a manner that the patients will accept. This may mean providing pulmonary function services in a health clinic, moving an asthma education program to a local inner city school or church, or transitioning some of the respiratory therapy staff to perform home visits. While innovative in nature and absent documented outcomes, continuing to repeat what has been done in the past and expecting improvement cannot continue.

Consumerism

Perhaps more significant than any issue is the expanding role of consumerism in the process of redesigning, delivering, measuring, and reporting the value of healthcare services. Concomitantly, a shift in the financial burden of health care from acute care to chronic disease has occurred. While genetics and other innovations hold promise in the future, RTs are witnessing a burgeoning demand for our limited health services as a result of self-inflicted health problems, including heart disease, diabetes, COPD, obesity, and others. While the problems are understood and RTs have provided both education and support to those individuals with self-inflicted diseases, there is no significant progress.

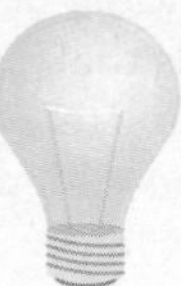

STOP AND THINK

Which of the forces driving health care do you view as most significant? Why? Are there others? Explain.

Summary of Forces Influencing Healthcare Costs

In summarizing the forces influencing healthcare costs, there is little question that Americans are concerned about issues such as the right to health, broader access, lower costs, and measurable outcomes. Also evident is that the entire institution of medicine is being demystified. The consumer movement, patient advocacy, the proliferation of support groups, and the Internet have brought about a more intelligent and informed public that is questioning medical practices and the costs of services. The existing healthcare model in this country is still based on treatment rather than prevention. Americans have not completely bought into the concept of practicing healthy lifestyle behaviors. A representative example of this comes from the Public Health Service that estimates the cost per smoker for smoking cessation interventions to be $165.59. Yet a projected 25% of Americans continue to smoke, at an estimated expenditure of $193 billion annually ($97 billion in lost productivity and $96 billion in healthcare expenditures).[10] A redefined focus on health promotion and disease prevention would add considerably to healthcare cost reductions.

The RT must document and communicate the value of services in such a manner that the general public, payers, and federal/state leaders will support and provide funding. Critical and insightful questions exist that include: how do healthcare services impact the practice of respiratory care? What can the individual RT do to aid his/her director, department, or institution? How can one add value in terms of quality, service, and cost? In short, these questions need to be asked and answered in an affirming manner.

A Brief History and Overview of Financing Health Care

Payment for healthcare services in the form of reimbursement is crucial to the survival of any healthcare institution, facility, or provider. There are limited instances of self-pay, out-of-pocket, or direct pay in which the patient deals directly with the provider. The more common practice entails a third-party, such as an insurance company, the government, or MCO. Reimbursement models and methodologies are constantly evolving, and hybridization is blurring the distinction between models that were in the past exclusive. Nonetheless, an attempt to simplify and eliminate some of the complexity is provided in the sections to follow. One of the most complex of systems, healthcare finance, is addressed in terms of three general payment systems: the **retrospective payment system (RPS)**, the **prospective payment system (PPS)**, and **capitation**.

Retrospective Payment

Traditional Health Insurance

The origins of American health insurance are rooted in the historical inability of individuals and their families to sustain expenses incurred by extensive medical care. Medical care, in the form of extended hospital stays as well as repeated office visits to the family physician, was unaffordable to most individuals. Community hospitals and family doctors recognized that some means to finance health care was required to prevent the inevitable consequences of unpaid medical bills, personal destitution, catastrophic bankruptcy, and ultimate economic disaster for the patient, physician, hospital, and ultimately the U.S. economy. Out of this concern grew the concept of health insurance, whereby individuals pooled funds and distributed the risk of illness among a larger group. Thus grew the concepts of shared risk and shared losses.

The beginning of modern private health insurance was in 1929 when a group of teachers made a contract with Baylor Hospital in Dallas, Texas, to provide coverage against certain hospital expenses. This event was considered the birth of the first Blue Cross plan.[11] Blue Cross and Blue Shield plans, considered service plans, historically reimbursed providers for the total costs of covered benefits. This system is in contrast to an **indemnity insurance plan**, a commercial plan that provided a benefit only if and when a medical event occurred. Indemnity plans provided payment of a fixed sum for a covered benefit.

Around this period, employers were equally concerned with the health and well-being of their workers. World War II was under way, and businesses such as the railroad, steel, aluminum, and shipbuilding industries needed assurance that the workforce could maintain productivity and sustain the war effort. Coupled with this desire to sustain a consistent, dependable, and healthy workforce was the desire to optimize company profits and provide additional employee incentives and rewards, the latter being especially true after the war as employers wanted to provide their employees with additional but small fringe benefits and yet avoid the costly burden of salary increases. Providing healthcare coverage was the perfect solution, and this benefit enhancement became a reality endorsed and sanctioned by hospitals, physicians, and employers.

Respiratory Recap

Three General Payment Systems

- Retrospective payment system (RPS)
- Prospective payment system (PPS)
- Capitation

Government Involvement

In 1965, the federal government entered the healthcare reimbursement scene with the U.S. Congress legislating and amending the Social Security Act of 1935 and establishing the Medicare (Title XVIII) and Medicaid (Title XIX) entitlement programs. **Medicare** provides health insurance for the elderly, whereas **Medicaid** helps states pay for the healthcare of the poor and certain other groups, such as the elderly, infants and children, and the blind and other people with disabilities. In 1973, additional legislation extended Medicare coverage to other groups, including persons with disabilities and end-stage renal disease requiring dialysis or kidney transplant.

The Medicare program consisted of Parts A and B. Medicare Part A is considered hospital coverage, and Part B is considered supplemental outpatient coverage. Part A pays the institutional provider for inpatient hospital care, care in a **skilled nursing facility (SNF)**, home health services, and hospice services provided to enrolled recipients. Part A covers all inpatient hospital care, including semiprivate room, meals, regular nursing services, operating and recovery room costs, intensive care, drugs, laboratory tests, x-rays, and all other medically necessary services and supplies. It does not cover physician fees, however, because it was designed solely as hospital insurance. **Box 59-1** addresses the

BOX 59-1

Medicare Part A: Financing, Eligibility, Coverage, and Benefits

Financing

Mandatory employer and employee payroll taxes are collected under Social Security paid by all working individuals, including the self-employed.

Eligibility

The benefits usually are provided automatically to persons 65 years of age or older, most people who are disabled for at least 24 months, and those who have end-stage renal disease.

Coverage

Hospital inpatient services, care in a skilled nursing facility (SNF), home health visits, and hospice care are covered.

Premiums*

No premium is required if the individual or spouse has worked for at least 10 years in Social Security/Medicare-covered employment. Other eligible individuals can purchase coverage. Medicare Part B premiums are based on income.

Deductibles/Copayments*

A cost-sharing deductible is assessed per benefit period. No copayments are required for the first 60 days of hospitalization, with a copayment for days 61 through 150. No copayments are assessed for skilled nursing for the first 20 days, with a copayment schedule for days 21 through 100. No copayments are required for home health visits, whereas small copayments are assessed for medications through hospice care.

Benefits

The benefit period is defined as the period beginning when the beneficiary first enters the hospital and ending when the beneficiary has been out of the hospital or other facility for 60 concurrent days. Benefit periods cannot exceed 90 days of inpatient hospital care, but the number of benefit periods is unlimited. If the 90 days of inpatient hospital care are exhausted, the beneficiary can draw from a nonrenewable "lifetime reserve" of up to 60 additional days. Skilled nursing care pays up to 100 days only if it follows within 30 days of a hospitalization of 3 or more days and is certified as medically necessary. Home care through a home health agency is covered when a beneficiary is homebound and requires intermittent or part-time skilled nursing or rehabilitation care. No limits exist for time or visits for home health care. Hospice services to the terminally ill with life expectancy of 6 months or less also are covered.

* Premium, deductible, and copayment information current as of April 2010. Values are subject to change.

Information from Centers for Medicare & Medicaid Services. Available at: http://www.cms.gov/Medicare/Medicare-General-Information/MedicareGenInfo/index.html.

specifics of Part A as they pertain to eligibility, the benefit period, coverage, copayments, SNFs, and hospice services.

Medicare Part B is a voluntary, supplemental insurance program that covers services not provided under Part A. Part B pays for covered physician services, such as diagnostic tests, medical and surgical services, approved ambulatory services, drugs that cannot be self-administered, home health, durable medical equipment, and outpatient services. **Box 59-2** addresses the specifics of Part B as they pertain to cost sharing, deductibles, and coverage of home medical and home respiratory equipment. **Box 59-3** details the specific Part B coverage requirements for home respiratory equipment that a patient must meet for Medicare reimbursement.

In 2005 Medicare initiated **pay for performance (P4P)** with the intent of encouraging increased quality in health care for the recipients of Medicare. This initiative crossed all venues of care, from inpatient hospital care to physician offices. Initially, this was done with demonstration projects that encouraged participation from healthcare providers by giving increased payment for top performance, as measured with defined clinical outcomes. Eventually, acceptance of evidence-based care led to improvements such as preventing community-acquired pneumonia via strict attention to the type of antibiotics used and their timely delivery. As P4P has evolved, there are now payment penalties for patient care that does not follow scientific evidence or for a health provider who does not perform to a set level.

Medicaid provides medical assistance for certain individuals and families with low incomes and resources. It is a jointly funded cooperative venture between the federal and state governments to assist states in the provision of adequate medical care to eligible needy persons. Within broad national guidelines set by the federal government, each state establishes its

BOX 59-2

Medicare Part B: Financing, Eligibility, Coverage, and Benefits

Financing

The voluntary program is financed by general tax revenues and requires individual premium contributions.

Eligibility

All resident citizens over 65 years of age, even those who are not entitled to Part A services, and disabled beneficiaries entitled to Part A are eligible.

Coverage

Part B coverage is optional. Coverage of home medical equipment requires that the item be used in the home, medically useful, able to stand up to repeated use, and reasonable and necessary for the treatment of illness or injury or the improvement of function. (Equipment that satisfies these criteria is considered durable medical equipment [DME].) To be reimbursed, the supplier must have a physician's order for the items and in some cases a certificate of medical necessity (CMN).

Premiums

Beneficiaries must pay a monthly premium, which in most cases is automatically deducted from the Social Security payment.

Deductibles

An annual deductible and a coinsurance payment of 20% of most allowable charges are assessed.

Benefits

Covered physician services include (excluding routine physical exams) emergency department services, outpatient surgery, diagnostic tests, and laboratory services; outpatient physical, occupational, and speech therapy; outpatient mental health services; ambulance; renal dialysis; blood transfusion and blood components; medical equipment and supplies; rural health clinic services; and some limited preventive services (e.g., Pap smears, mammography, and influenza shots).

Information from Centers for Medicare & Medicaid Services (CMS). Available at: http://www.cms.gov/Medicare/Medicare-General-Information/MedicareGenInfo/Part-B.html.

BOX 59-3

Medicare Part B: Coverage of Home Respiratory Equipment

Medicare has set specific eligibility and qualifying requirements for all durable medical equipment (DME) used in the home. That a physician prescribes a certain item is no guarantee that Medicare will pay for it. The majority of private insurers and many managed care organizations also follow the Medicare guidelines in determining eligibility and reimbursement.

Oxygen

Medicare pays a flat monthly amount for oxygen, the same whether provided from cylinders, a concentrator, or a liquid source and regardless of the liter flow. While the details are beyond the scope of this chapter, the rental fee is all-inclusive, covering the oxygen, equipment, most disposable supplies, and all services, such as delivery, maintenance, and repair, with some exceptions.

In addition, Medicare has no required standards of service specific to providers of oxygen therapy. The supplier is not required to be accredited, perform any type of initial instruction or ongoing follow-up, or employ RTs. Suppliers who do provide these services are reimbursed at the same level as those who do not.

Medicare has created specific criteria for the patient to "qualify" to receive home oxygen. While beyond the scope of this chapter, it is important for the RT to fully understand these criteria in order to support the provision of high-quality care via the most appropriate equipment for the patient's condition, mobility, and physical layout of the home environment. The company providing the oxygen cannot do the testing, which must be performed by an objective third party, such as an independent laboratory, a hospital, or a physician.

Continuous Positive Airway Pressure (CPAP)

CPAP is covered if the patient has obstructive sleep apnea that has been documented during studies done in a sleep laboratory and demonstrates at least 30 episodes of apnea, each lasting a minimum of 10 seconds, during 6 to 7 hours of recorded sleep. Bilevel devices also qualify for reimbursement for treatment of obstructive sleep apnea but only if the patient meets all of the previous criteria and CPAP has been tried without appropriate patient response.

Noninvasive Ventilation and Respiratory Assistive Devices

Since 1999 these devices have been covered for chronic obstructive pulmonary disease (COPD), restrictive thoracic disorders, central sleep apnea, and obstructive sleep apnea when specific qualifying awake ABGs, nocturnal oximetry, and certain other criteria are met.

Ventilators

Ventilators, either positive- or negative-pressure types, are covered if the patient has a diagnosis of neuromuscular disease, thoracic restrictive disease, or chronic respiratory failure due to COPD.

Suction Machine

A device for nasal, oral, or tracheal suctioning is covered only if the patient has difficulty raising and clearing secretions secondary to cancer or surgery of the throat, dysfunction of the swallowing muscles, unconsciousness or obtundent state, or tracheostomy.

Information from Centers for Medicare & Medicaid Services. Available at: http://www.cms.gov/medicare-coverage-database/details/ncd-details.aspx?NCDId=169&ncdver=1&DocID=240.2&SearchType=Advanced&bc=IAAAABAAAAAA&.

own eligibility standards; determines the type, amounts, duration, and scope of services; sets the rate of payment for services; and administers its own program. Medicaid thus varies considerably from state to state.

Medicare and Medicaid have been heralded as perhaps one of the most massive and sweeping social welfare initiatives undertaken by the federal government. These programs have targeted large segments of the population and have been tasked with successfully improving the health and quality of life of millions of seniors, people with disabilities, and the poor and indigent of society. **Table 59-2** reflects Medicare data for selected years, and **Table 59-3** represents Medicaid data for selected years.

TABLE 59-2
Medicare Data for Selected Years

Year	Beneficiaries (Millions)	Expenditures (Billions)
1970	20.5	$7.7
1980	28.5	$37.5
1990	34.3	$111.5
2000	39.7	$224.8
2010	47.7	$522.0
2012	50.7	$574.2

Information from Boards of Trustees, Federal Hospital Insurance, and Federal Supplementary Medical Insurance Trust Funds. *2013 Annual Report*. Available at: http://www.cms.gov/ReportsTrustFunds/downloads/tr2013.pdf.

TABLE 59-3
Medicaid Data for Selected Years

Year	Beneficiaries (Millions)	Expenditures (Billions)
1970	17.6	$5.3
1980	21.6	$26.1
1990	25.3	$75.3
2000	42.8	$200.5
2010	66.4	$397.7

Information from Boards of Trustees, Federal Hospital Insurance, and Federal Supplementary Medical Insurance Trust Funds. *2011 Annual Report*. Available at: http://www.cms.gov/ReportsTrustFunds/downloads/tr2011.pdf.

Prospective Payment

The prospective payment system (PPS) arose because of increasing pressure from employers and the federal government to curtail spiraling healthcare costs. Initiated in 1983, it involves reimbursement that establishes fixed and preestablished payment for the actual primary reason for admission. The rates are determined annually by the plan administrator, who is the federal government (under the direction of the **Centers for Medicare and Medicaid Services [CMS]**, previously known as the Health Care Financing Administration [HCFA]) or commercial insurance carriers such as Blue Cross or Aetna US Healthcare. A multiyear phase-in of the PPS for hospital reimbursement through Medicare began in 1983.

Physician reimbursement under the PPS is based on a methodology known as the **resource-based relative value scale (RBRVS)**. A relative value scale is a reimbursement methodology developed by a Harvard research team that assigned values to physician services based on the resource costs of providing those services.[12] The RBRVS was implemented in 1992 by HCFA as a fee schedule for physicians who participate in Medicare Part B. It is based on a national fee schedule and replaces the previous payment method outlining "usual, customary, and reasonable charges." The RBRVS assigns a relative value to each current procedural terminology (CPT) code. The relative value units are based on the time, skill, and **resource intensity** it takes to provide a service and the actual reimbursement is derived from a complex formula. Relative values were designed with the objective of narrowing the gap between the incomes of specialists and generalists.[1]

Capitation

Capitation is a prepaid, fixed amount negotiated in advance by the payer or plan and the provider. It involves payment for each eligible person for a particular time period regardless of the care or services provided and also is known as the *per-member, per-month* (*PMPM*) system, which represents or reflects the amount paid by each participating member each month enrolled in the plan. Managed care programs for primary care providers commonly use capitation, but specialists (e.g., pulmonologists) are still more likely to be paid under a negotiated fee schedule.

The Era of Managed Care

Managed care is actually a generic term for a payment system alternative to traditional insurance plans, such as fee-for-service or indemnity plans. The concept of managed care is considered similar to managed costs, but a distinction should be made between the techniques of care and costs management versus the organization that performs those functions. Managing care or costs may involve a variety of interventions, such as health promotion, disease prevention, wellness, disease management, patient education, and utilization control, to name a few. Managed care organizations are the organizations that can implement these strategies but mainly are responsible for delivering and financing health services. In other words, managed care organizations are more than just the claims payers; they actively manage the delivery of the care.

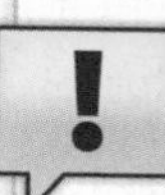

Respiratory Recap

Types of Managed Care

- Health maintenance organization (HMO)
- Preferred provider organization (PPO)
- Exclusive provider organization (EPO)
- Point-of-service plan (POS)

TABLE 59-4
Breakdown of Enrollment by Plan Type, 2008 and 2014

Plan Type	Percentage 2008	Percentage 2014
Managed Care		
Health maintenance organization (HMO)	20	13
Preferred provider organization (PPO)	58	58
Point-of-service plan (POS)	12	8
Nonmanaged Care		
High-deductible health plan	8	20
Conventional/indemnity	2	<1

Information from The Henry J. Kaiser Family Foundation and Health Research and Educational Trust. *2014 Employer Health Benefits Survey.* Available at: http://ehbs.kff.org.

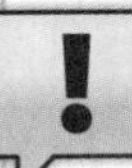

Respiratory Recap

General Characteristics of an HMO

- Emphasis on preventive services
- Provision of a complete range of services for a fixed fee
- Requirement that all care be provided by participating providers
- Adherence of services to established standards of quality

A **managed care organization (MCO)** is an integrated network of doctors, hospitals, and other healthcare providers that delivers health services to an insured population. Over the past two decades, managed care has become the predominant form of health care in most parts of the United States. More than 70 million Americans have enrolled in health maintenance organizations (HMOs), and almost 90 million have been part of preferred provider organizations (PPOs).[13] Overall enrollment numbers in HMOs peaked in 2001 and are declining with increases occurring in the high-deductible health plans. Managed care, however, generally remains a dominant type of healthcare coverage (**Table 59-4**).

The four different types of MCOs are HMOs, PPOs, exclusive provider organizations (EPOs), and point-of-service plans (POSs). These are discussed individually in the following sections.

Health Maintenance Organizations

Unknown to most who believe that HMOs are a new methodology, managed care models have existed for more than a century. The first cited example of an MCO was the Western Clinic in Tacoma, Washington. This was a prepaid group practice created in 1910 to provide a broad range of medical services to lumber mill owners and their employees. These eligible individuals were provided services for a premium payment of a mere 50 cents per member per month. A number of additional examples can be cited, including the rural workers' cooperative in Elk City, Oklahoma; the Kaiser Foundation Health Plan of Southern California; the Group Health Association of Washington, D.C.; the Health Insurance Plan of Greater New York; and the Group Health Cooperative of Puget Sound.

Despite the insurgence of this new system, managed care plans developed relatively slowly. President Nixon believed that this model could provide better control of the healthcare delivery system, however, and championed the managed care model. In 1973, President Nixon signed into law the federal HMO Act, which reflected concern with the fee-for-service system that rewarded healthcare providers for increased volume of services. Little in the way of checks and balances was in place under the fee-for-service system, and the incentives encouraged overuse. The HMO movement in the 1970s is considered the brainchild of Dr. Paul Ellwood, who spearheaded the effort. Because of Ellwood's expertise, President Nixon asked him to devise ways to curtail the spiraling healthcare costs in Medicare.

The **health maintenance organization (HMO)** model of health care is uniquely different from the traditional model. Rather than just pay for care when the individual is ill, HMOs promote and reimburse services to maintain health—thus the term *health maintenance*—placing considerable emphasis on preventive services encouraging wellness and healthy lifestyle practices. It also provides a wide array of services for a fixed fee per month, use of which is coordinated and managed by the HMO. This type of managed care is an attempt to address the fragmentation of basic healthcare delivery functions alluded to previously. Under the HMO model, the subscriber must secure all services from providers participating in the plan or pay a higher amount for using a nonparticipating provider, with some exceptions permitted for extenuating circumstances. Finally, services are provided and monitored according to established standards of quality.[1]

HMOs have four general models: the staff model, group model, network model, and independent practice association (IPA) model. Their distinction from one another is based on the way the organization relates to its participating physicians.

The staff model entails the provision of physician services through a salaried staff of physicians employed by the HMO. Physicians in this model work exclusively for the HMO and provide care to its enrollees only. The HMO exercises considerable control over the physician practice, and thus physician performance and practice are typically subject to a greater degree of oversight to ensure compliance with standards of practice and care. In the staff model the HMO assumes the financial risk, as opposed to the physician.

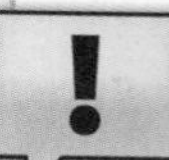

Respiratory Recap

General Types of HMOs

- Staff model
- Group model
- Network model
- Independent practice association (IPA) model

In the group model the HMO contracts with a multispecialty group practice. The physicians are not employees of the HMO but rather employees of the group. This model is seen to provide more choice to the consumer when compared with the staff model.

The network model entails the HMO contracting with more than one physician group. The model is more attractive to the enrollee because the larger number of physicians involved in the network provides greater choice.

The IPA model is unique in that the association serves as an intermediary, between the HMO and physicians, handling the logistics of arranging physician services. The IPA is paid a capitated amount, reimburses the physicians based on a methodology determined by both parties, and assumes some of the risk. The IPA's degree of control over physician practices varies widely, but enrollee choice is typically enhanced.

Preferred Provider Organizations

Preferred provider organizations (PPOs) date back to the late 1970s. PPOs differ from traditional HMOs in that services are provided on a discounted fee-for-service basis. In contrast to HMOs' employment of a capitated model, PPOs use a discounted fee-for-service system. Additionally, enrollees are required to use a particular group of physicians, hospitals, and other providers that the PPO has preselected. Enrollees are free to choose physicians or hospitals outside the system, but nonpreferred providers constitute additional charges. PPOs thus encourage enrollees, via financial impact to use their preferred providers, to abide by the PPO's guidelines.

Point-of-Service Plans

Point-of-service plans (POSs) entered the market in the late 1980s and are a hybrid of HMOs and PPOs. They represent features of both organizations, attempting to provide the tight utilization controls of the HMO and the ability to choose a nonparticipating provider at the point (time) at which service is received, thus the phrase *point of service*. The POS addresses the unpopular feature of limited choice that is seen by consumers to be overly restrictive.

Exclusive Provider Organizations

Exclusive provider organizations (EPOs) are designed to provide the greatest degree of control of service utilization and the associated costs. Enrollees are required to use the physician, hospital, and other providers stipulated in the plan, with certain exemptions to all for accessing services while on vacation, and so forth. While it would appear that these models are distinct, the evolution of managed care is increasingly blurring these once clear distinctions.

A new entry into this market is a novel variation of the traditional POS delivery system. This model is a direct contract between the employer and the healthcare provider. The most visible example of this was the announcement by Wal-Mart and Lowe's to create a preferred provider network for their employees to receive care at Cleveland Clinic and Mayo Clinic for heart and spine surgeries.[14] The employee would have no out-of-pocket costs and the arrangement would include coverage of all medical costs, travel, food, and lodging. Not long after this announcement, these two national companies expanded this model to four other hospitals/systems for hip and knee replacements, again with no cost to the employee. The selection process focused on quality outcomes and rates were subsequently negotiated. While this model is considered experimental, it is gaining popularity throughout the insurance and healthcare provider communities.

Reimbursement Methodologies

Reimbursement and its methodologies involve payment for healthcare delivery. Intermediaries or third-party payers generally perform this function and are responsible for determining the method and amount of reimbursement as well as the actual disbursement of funds. Examples of intermediaries are the federal government, MCOs, and insurance companies.

Box 59-4 lists a number of models for reimbursing hospitals. The four most popular hospital reimbursement methodologies by HMOs are fee schedule (or fee for service), per diem, diagnosis-related groups (DRGs), and capitation.[15] The more popular physician methodologies are fee-for-service systems and capitation.

BOX 59-4

Models for Reimbursing Hospitals

- Fee-for-service
- Per diem
- Diagnosis-related groups (DRGs)
- Capitation

Respiratory Recap

Popular Types of Physician Reimbursement

- Fee for service
- Capitation

Fee for Service

The **fee-for-service system** is a reimbursement methodology in which the provider establishes the fee for each distinct service. Billing is based on an itemized account of each service provided. For example, the pulmonologist could submit a claim for a physical examination, chest radiograph, and pulmonary function test in which each service would constitute a separate charge to be submitted for reimbursement.

Initially, the insurer paid fee-for-service reimbursement after care was delivered (retrospectively), without any restrictions or limitations. Insurers transitioned to a usual, customary, and reasonable charge methodology, however, which limited the fee to a standard determined through regional or statewide surveys. If the provider-determined charge exceeded the usual, customary, and reasonable amount, either the patient or the contracted provider was responsible for the difference. Some managed care plans, notably PPOs, adopted a discounted fee-for-service methodology. The main drawback to this method is that providers are still rewarded for providing additional services, with less incentive to be cost-conscious.

Cost Plus or Charge Minus

In another methodology, rates are preestablished on a cost-plus or charge-minus basis. The cost-plus method was used by the federal government in its Medicare and Medicaid programs to establish inpatient rates for hospitals, nursing homes, and home health care. The institution was required to submit a cost report to the third-party payer detailing the total costs that facility incurred. This methodology was tied directly to costs of providing services, number of services provided, and length of stay. Historical data were utilized to determine the amount to be paid in future years. As with the fee-for-service methodology, cost plus also presented an incentive for providers to increase service utilization and no incentive for cost containment.

Prospective Reimbursement

The PPS was introduced by the federal government in 1983 under Part A of its Medicare program as a means of curtailing spiraling healthcare costs. Reimbursement was fixed at a preestablished amount in advance of the services rendered, still set annually by the CMS. Prospective payment was applied to SNFs in 1998, and provisions were made to implement this system for hospital outpatient services and home health agencies through the Balanced Budget Act of 1997.

Diagnosis-Related Groups

The **diagnosis-related groups (DRG)** system is based on a classification of patients into over 500 groupings with reimbursement tied to resource utilization. DRGs establish a rate based on bundled services for a principal diagnosis established at the time of admission that the physician determined to be the cause of the admission.

This system provides an incentive for providers to utilize only those services—in type and amount—that will be most effective in treating the patient. Each DRG assumes that all patients with the same diagnosis require the same level of clinical services. Differences in DRG reimbursement are provided for the following extenuating circumstances, including variations in regional wage index, location of institution, existence of residency programs, and disproportionate indigent care, among other variables that were created to make the payment system more fair between healthcare providers. Additionally, extensive lengths of stay (LOS) and costs for extraordinary circumstances, classified as outliers, allow for higher payment rates. While the increased LOS and increased payment for certain extenuating circumstances were initially felt to be a method to consistently obtain higher reimbursement, providers should not utilize these as a means of working around the DRG system.

The DRG system, based on total inpatient stay, is in direct contrast to the per diem methodology, which is based on a daily charge. The DRG methodology is an attempt to shift financial risk to the hospital (provider). If the hospital provides the service for less than the predetermined DRG reimbursement rate, a profit is generated for that case. If the hospital's costs exceed the predetermined allotment, the facility incurs a financial loss. **Table 59-5** lists examples of common respiratory-related DRGs.

All-Patient Refined Diagnosis-Related Groups

Originally, DRGs were created based upon the intensity of care and the resources consumed to care for a patient with a principal diagnosis. Over time, the need arose to refine the system to more accurately describe the patient's condition. In particular, a refined patient classification system was needed for the following:

- Comparison of hospitals across a wide range of resource and outcome measures
- Evaluation of differences in inpatient mortality rates
- Implementation and support of critical pathways
- Identification of continuous quality improvement projects

TABLE 59-5
Common Respiratory-Related DRGs

DRG Code	Description
190	Chronic obstructive pulmonary disease
181	Pulmonary infections and inflammations, age >17 with comorbid condition
202	Bronchitis and asthma, age 0 to 17
207	Respiratory system diagnosis with ventilator support
189	Pulmonary edema and respiratory failure
180	Respiratory neoplasms
011	Tracheostomy for face, mouth, and neck diagnosis
184	Major chest trauma with comorbid condition
176	Pulmonary embolism
945	Rehabilitation
194	Simple pneumonia and pleurisy, age >17 without comorbid condition
313	Chest pain
007	Lung transplantation

Data from Centers for Medicare and Medicaid Services. *List of Diagnosis Related Groups (DRGS), Fiscal Year 2008*. Available at: https://www.cms.gov/Research-Statistics-Data-and-Systems/Statistics-Trends-and-Reports/MedicareFeeforSvcPartsAB/downloads/DRGdesc08.pdf.

- Serving as the basis of internal management and planning systems
- Serving as the management of capitated payment arrangements

To meet these changing needs, the system needed to incorporate additional information regarding the **severity of illness** and the **risk of mortality** while maintaining a measurement for resource intensity.

All-patient refined diagnosis-related groups (APR-DRGs) were created and include four multiple subclasses to each original DRG to address the severity of illness and the risk of mortality. This requires more specific documentation in the medical record for each patient, including details about the illness and possible complications of the patient. The four subclasses represent minor, moderate, major, or extreme severity of illness and risk of mortality.[16]

Resource-Based Relative Value Scale

The RBRVS, mentioned previously, is an initiative to reimburse physicians according to services provided. It replaces the fee-for-service methodology and was intended to narrow what was seen as an inappropriate disparity in reimbursement between specialists and general practitioners. In reality, it simply reimburses the provider predicated on the intensity of services rendered. The scale is based on the time, skill, and intensity of the services provided. The RBRVS, developed by the federal government under the Medicare fee schedule (MFS), is composed of more than 7000 covered services. To compute the physician's payment, the relative value unit is adjusted for geographic area and then multiplied by a conversion factor, a monetary amount set annually by the federal government.

Bundled Charges

Bundled charges describe a type of packaged pricing, a form of reimbursement in which a number of related services are grouped together and provided for one fee. An example of a bundled charge would be the provision of pulmonary rehabilitation. Rather than charge separately for each component, all the services falling under this service, such as education and training in pursed-lip breathing, chest physiotherapy, and pulmonary hygiene, are packaged or bundled together and a single price charged.

Managed Care Approaches

Managed care approaches consist of the HMO, PPO, POS, and EPO methodologies. The HMO plan provides or arranges for a comprehensive array of services through a defined network of providers for a monthly fee. Members are required to stay within the network of physicians, outpatient providers, and hospitals. Coverage restrictions apply to services provided outside the network, except in certain emergencies or when specific approval is provided in advance of care. The HMO receives a monthly premium in advance for each member, who then has unlimited use of most of the health plan's services, provided that the services are considered medically necessary. Each member usually pays a specified fee for each physician visit, prescription, or other service stipulated in the plan, referred to as a **copayment**, or *copay*.

Figure 59-5 depicts the relative level of patient choice and provider control (particularly of costs) for a variety of plans.[15] As one moves from one end of the continuum to another, one adds greater degrees of control and accountability and responsibility and greater or lesser degrees of cost and quality. The more restrictive plans are on the right-hand side of the continuum. These offer fewer choices and greater restrictions but yield lower costs. The managed care approaches are variations of a common theme, all focusing on cost containment.

Case Mix

Case mix refers to the overall intensity of conditions requiring medical and nursing intervention. It involves extensive assessment of the patient's condition, followed by a determination of specific services or

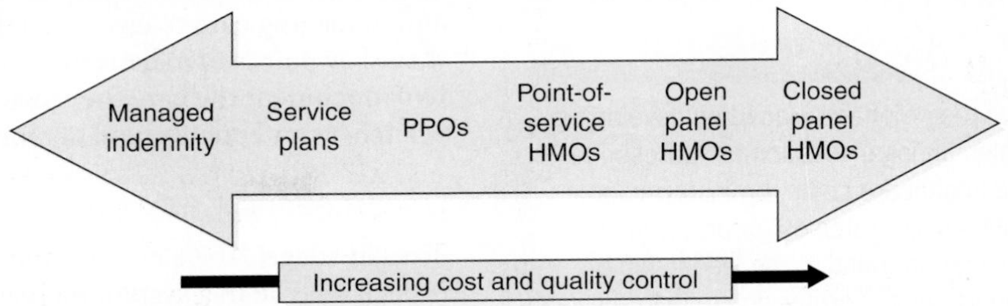

FIGURE 59-5 Continuum of cost control in U.S. health care.

procedures considered necessary or essential to effectively manage the patient. The case mix approach is used extensively in SNFs and is driven by the **minimum data set (MDS)**, which consists of a core of screening elements that are assessed for each patient admitted to the facility. These elements focus on patient care; function, health, and mental status; and treatment.

The Future of Healthcare Funding

There are numerous factors spurring renewed interest in an overhaul of the U.S. healthcare system. In 2010 President Obama signed into law the Patient Protection and Affordable Care Act (PPACA). The issues that drove this initiative are beyond the scope of this chapter; however, the following issues bear particular meaning and criticality to the future of respiratory care services and practice:

- Rising cost of health care, particularly without concomitant increase in quality outcomes (e.g., mortality, morbidity, life span)
- Improving overall community health, reducing health disparities, protecting households from impoverishment secondary to medical expenses, and providing services that respect the dignity of persons
- Burgeoning costs of health care that are driving employers to reduce or in some cases eliminate health insurance coverage for their employees
- Existence of a healthcare system where approximately 49 million Americans are disenfranchised and without health insurance, creating a situation where health needs have been ignored and/or this segment of the population is forced to use inappropriate services, such as emergency departments.

There are three key provisions within the PPACA[17] that most directly impact the practice of respiratory care, namely: hospital readmissions, value-based purchasing, and innovation center.

Hospital Readmissions

The readmissions program, begun in federal fiscal year (FY) 2013, reduces payments to hospitals that have excess readmissions within 30 days after discharge. The first year penalty was 1% and this increases to 3% by FY15. The initial three diagnoses being monitored were acute myocardial infarction, congestive heart failure, and pneumonia. COPD has just been approved for inclusion in FY15. RTs should review their hospital's performance on the CMS website (www.hospitalcompare.hhs.gov).

Value-Based Purchasing

The Value-Based Purchasing (VBP) program began rewarding hospitals for high-quality and safe care effective October 1, 2012. These payments are based upon comparisons within like groups of hospitals (patient volumes are not included) and how well a hospital improves relative to a baseline period. Presently, PPACA is only applied to short-term acute care hospitals; however, the plan is to extend this to skilled nursing facilities, home health agencies, and physicians. This program is of particular interest to RTs because it is consistent with the AARC's movement to convince federal leadership to allow RTs to practice under the general direction of a physician and also extend their role to other care settings.

Innovation Center

While numerous pilots are in operation, three demonstration programs are worthy of brief description so that the RT can appreciate the opportunities provided for our professions as well as other health professionals.

- *Community-Based Care Transitions Program* This new CMS office was created by PPACA and designed to test new models for effective health-care delivery. For those innovative models that are deemed successful in terms of improving health and lowering cost, improved payment is funded. The Community-Based Care Transitions Program (CCTP) involves hospitals with high readmission rates partnering with community-based organizations that provide care transition services (e.g., hospital to SNF/home). There are already signs that this program, while in its infancy, is being successfully managed in several sites. For the RT, this program should provide another opportunity

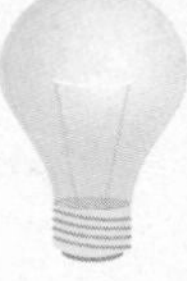

STOP AND THINK

In light of the emphasis placed on developing and implementing innovation to address the spiraling healthcare costs, brainstorm some methodologies, strategies, or programs that you could recommend to the leadership of your department or profession to help alleviate or curtail these spiraling costs.

to demonstrate the value of our services as we transition pulmonary-compromised patients from the hospital to their next site of care.

- *Accountable Care Organizations*
  Accountable care organizations (ACOs) are groups of hospitals, physicians, postacute providers, and others who voluntarily agree to collaborate and provide coordinated high-quality care to Medicare patients. The goal is to ensure that patients receive the right care at the right time at the right place. This program should decrease or eliminate duplicative services, reduce medical errors, and improve medication reconciliation across providers—all of which are well known to increase the cost of care, reduce quality of care, and increase readmissions.
- *Patient-Centered Medical Home (PCMH)*
  The patient-centered medical home (PCMH) model is designed to make advanced primary practices, also known as medical homes, readily available to all persons and particularly those with chronic conditions. Physicians serve as the team leader and engage other professions and systems in a team approach with the patient at the center of all activities. The goals are to improve the delivery of quality health care and improve the overall health of each individual. CMS is funding this model by reimbursing the physician on a monthly basis for high-resource-consuming individuals with chronic conditions. While still early in evaluation, the program is growing steadily and there is clearly a value-added role for RTs to contribute.

Discussion on innovative programs and strategies continues at the federal and state levels and the respiratory therapy community must keep abreast of changes and proactively plan and retroactively respond to such changes as they impact the delivery of services and the roles and responsibilities of RTs.

Respiratory Therapist Documenting and Demonstrating Value

So what does the changing face of healthcare economics mean for RTs? In short, reasoning supports the theory that managed care will continue to evolve and dominate the market. In order to better control escalating costs and managing care to ensure quality, RTs must address three key points to effectively contribute to such a system: document the care they provide, ensure its appropriateness and quality, and demonstrate value.

Documenting Care: Charting

The old adage, "If it's not charted, it wasn't done," rings especially true in a system increasingly focused on cost reduction. RTs must recognize that payers are focused on cost control and are increasingly investigating whether provided services are done according to evidence-based medicine or at least best practices. Therefore, therapists must document every procedure and service, including the rationale for services selected and the patient response to those services, so that the medical coder can capture the appropriate information.

Three Rights

Ensuring appropriateness of care can be represented by adherence to the three rights of healthcare delivery: provision of the right care, in the right setting, by the right provider.

RTs must recognize that they are rewarded for appropriate care, not merely by providing what the physician ordered. Under former reimbursement methodologies, overuse of services was actually rewarded in that respiratory therapy departments were revenue generators. An increase in services meant increased revenue for the institution. In today's system, which is heavily based on capitation, DRGs, and per diems, institutions are paid on a fixed-income structure, effectively eliminating the incentives or rewards to provide additional services. To be clear, the goal is not to provide less care. Rather, the goal is to provide care that will result in desired outcomes.

Conversely, although underuse may at first glance appear to result in a profit for an institution (i.e., given that the DRG payment is made without regard to service utilization), constraining appropriate care will result in lower quality care, including increasing the length of stay, increased readmissions, and, ultimately, perhaps increasing the overall costs of care.

In addition to providing the right care, RTs must understand the importance of providing care in the right setting. Critical care areas represent the most expensive settings in which to provide inpatient healthcare services. The estimated daily charge for one day of admission to an intensive care unit (ICU) is approximately two to five times greater than the charge for a non-ICU ward. The number, intensity, and critical nature of services in an ICU are more costly and labor intensive. RTs must recognize this and make every effort to assist in decision making regarding the transfer of patients to less costly and less intensive settings. In contrast to critical care costs, general medical-surgical wards are one-half to one-third of the cost; skilled nursing facilities less than half of the cost of a typical medical-surgical ward; and home care is but a fraction of these costs. In addition to cost, it has been confirmed that patients prefer the comfort and familiarity of the home over the hospital environment. Clearly, compelling evidence suggests that the home, when feasible, is the most desirable and cost-effective environment for the provision of healthcare services. In short, the RT, as a key member of the healthcare team, should make every effort to assist the team to provide services in the most appropriate care venue.

Equally important is that the healthcare provider possesses the appropriate skill, training, and education to effectively care for the patient, satisfying professional credentialing standards and matching education and skill set. A highly compensated provider, who routinely performs skills that should be delegated to another, is neither economical nor cost-effective. This concept has been central in the development of the profession in that RTs are physician extenders, trained and competency tested to properly perform a wealth of services formerly provided by physician and others.

Demonstrating Value

Much has been written about the future role of the RT, with potential roles including clinician, diagnostician, patient advocate, technical expert, consultant, counselor, case manager, and educator. Convincing and growing evidence suggests that RTs are best suited for these value-added roles, both because of their training and competency testing and because RTs utilize critical thinking skills.

Demonstrating value, central to the success of any professional, can occur clinically at the bedside; diagnostically in the pulmonary function laboratory; in consultation with the physician, nurse, or other healthcare provider; in counseling and education as a patient advocate and educator; and in the role of case manager who efficiently and effectively transitions the patient through the healthcare system. Physicians, nurses, other healthcare professionals and especially patients have heralded RTs as significant contributors to quality care, and therapists must continue to function on the basis of evidence-based medicine when it exists, or at least via best practice protocols, algorithms, and guidelines. The future for RTs will be bright as long as high-quality services are provided, outcomes of our services are documented, and our value-added role is communicated to all stakeholders.

Key Points

- ▶ The four major functions of the healthcare system in the United States are financing, insurance, delivery, and payment.
- ▶ Managed care is an attempt to integrate and coordinate the various functions of health care and create a system that functions effectively and efficiently.
- ▶ The key players in the healthcare system are the patients, purchasers, plans, payers, and providers.
- ▶ The drivers of health care include increase in cost without increase in quality, technology, aging population, excess capacity, unnecessary care, defensive medicine, growth of underinsured and uninsured, and consumerism.
- ▶ The retrospective payment system uses a per diem methodology for inpatient hospital reimbursement and a fee-for-service system and "usual, customary, and reasonable" fee schedule for physician services.
- ▶ Employer-based insurance continues to be the dominant model among most consumers, but this is changing dramatically and the future of employer-based insurance is not as clear as it was just a few years ago.
- ▶ Government, both federal and state, is a major player in healthcare reimbursement through its programs of Medicare and Medicaid.
- ▶ Diagnosis-related groups (DRGs) are an attempt to curtail escalating costs with a fixed reimbursement rate based on a predetermined formula for inpatient hospital admissions.
- ▶ The all-patient refined DRG (APR-DRG) was added to the reimbursement mix to address the severity of illness and the risk of mortality.
- ▶ The resource-based relative value scale (RBRVS) has replaced the "usual, customary, and reasonable" fee payment methodology and is used to pay physicians under Medicare Part B.
- ▶ The capitated system entails a per-member, per-month payment methodology.
- ▶ The four major types of managed care are the health maintenance organization, preferred provider organization, point-of-service plans, and exclusive provider organizations.
- ▶ Managed care emphasizes prevention, provides a complete range of services for a fixed fee, requires participants to use designated providers, and adheres to established standards of quality.
- ▶ The more popular methodologies used in healthcare reimbursement are fee for service, cost plus or charge minus, prospective payment, DRGs, resource-based relative value scales, bundled charges, multiple managed care approaches, and case mix.
- ▶ The successful RT of the future must document care, ensure appropriateness and quality, and demonstrate value.

References

1. Shi L, Singh DA. *Delivering Health Care in America: A Systems Approach.* 5th ed. Sudbury, MA: Jones & Bartlett Learning; 2011.
2. Diamond D. *How Wal-Mart May Have Just Changed the Game on Health Care.* 2012. Available at: http://www.californiahealthline.org/road-to-reform/2012/how-wal-mart-may-have-just-changed-the-game-on-health-care. Accessed January 9, 2015.

3. Centers for Medicare and Medicaid Services. *National Health Expenditure Data*. Available at: http://www.cms.gov/NationalHealthExpendData/02_NationalHealthAccountsHistorical.asp. Accessed September 16, 2014.
4. Kacmarek R, Durbin CG, Barnes TA, et al. Creating a vision for respiratory care in 2015 and beyond. *Respir Care*. 2009;54:375–389.
5. Sultz HA, Young KM. *Health Care USA: Understanding Its Organization and Delivery*. 8th ed. Burlington, MA: Jones & Bartlett Learning; 2014.
6. Organisation for Economic Co-operation and Development (OECD). *Health Policies and Data*. Available at: http://www.oecd.org/health/healthdata. Accessed September 16, 2014.
7. *Washington Post. Wonkblog*. Yearly Archives. Available at: http://www.washingtonpost.com/blogs/wonkblog/wp/2013. Accessed September 16, 2014.
8. National Center for Health Statistics. *Health, United States, 2013: With Special Feature on Prescription Drugs*. Hyattsville, MD. 2014. Available at: http://www.cdc.gov/nchs/data/hus/2012/016.pdf. Accessed October 8, 2014.
9. Porter ME, Lee TH. The strategy that will fix health care. *Harvard Business Review*. 2013;91:50–70.
10. Centers for Disease Control and Prevention. *Smoking and Tobacco Use: Fast Facts*. Available at: http://www.cdc.gov/tobacco/data_statistics/fact_sheets/fast_facts/index.htm. Accessed September 16, 2014.
11. Williams SJ, Torrens PR. *Introduction to Health Services*. 5th ed. Albany, NY: Delmar; 1999.
12. Kimball AM, Miller EK. *Making Sense of Managed Care*. Vol. 1. San Francisco: Jossey-Bass; 1997.
13. National Conference of State Legislatures. *Managed Care, Market Reports and the States* (updated February 2011; new material added June 2013). Available at: http://www.ncsl.org/research/health/managed-care-and-the-states.aspx. Accessed September 16, 2014.
14. Modern Healthcare. *Wal-Mart, Lowe's to offer leg up on knee and hip work—at certain systems*. Available at: http://www.modernhealthcare.com/article/201310081/NEWS/310089966. Accessed September 16, 2014.
15. Kongstvedt P. *Essentials of Managed Health Care*. 6th ed. Burlington, MA: Jones & Bartlett Learning; 2013.
16. Averill RF, Goldfield N, Hughes JS, et al. *All Patient Refined Diagnosis Related Groups (APR-DRGs): Methodology Overview*. Version 20.0. Wallingford, CT, and Murray, UT: 3M Health Information Systems; 2003. Document GRP–041.
17. U.S. Department of Health and Human Services (DHHS). *About the Law (Affordable Care Act)*. Available at: http://www.hhs.gov/healthcare/rights/law/index.html. Accessed September 16, 2014.

CHAPTER

60

Respiratory Care Research and Evidence-Based Practice

Dean R. Hess

OUTLINE

Research Design
Statistical Issues
Study Types
What Is Evidence-Based Respiratory Care?
Hierarchy of Evidence
Evidence for a Diagnostic Test
Evidence for a Therapy
Meta-Analysis
Finding the Evidence
Narrative Reviews and Systematic Reviews
Clinical Practice Guidelines

OBJECTIVES

1. Describe and explain the purposes of study design factors.
2. Emphasize key points about statistics used in research.
3. Describe the types of medical study reports.
4. Define evidence-based medicine.
5. List the hierarchy of evidence.
6. Use the tools of evidence-based medicine to evaluate the evidence for a diagnostic test and for a therapy.
7. Describe the details of a forest plot resulting from a meta-analysis.
8. Use techniques to identify the best evidence.
9. Compare narrative and systematic reviews.
10. Use the recommendations of clinical practice guidelines.

KEY TERMS

Bland-Altman plot
blinding
case control study
case report
case series
clinical practice guideline (CPG)
cohort study
correlation coefficient
cross-sectional study
crossover study
descriptive statistics
evidence-based medicine
forest plot
incidence
inferential statistics
informed consent
institutional review board (IRB)
interventional study
Kaplan-Meier plot
likelihood ratio (LR)
matching
meta-analysis
N-of-1 randomized controlled trial
observational study
prevalence
prospective studies
randomization
randomized controlled trial (RCT)
receiver operating characteristic curve
regression analysis
retrospective study
sensitivity
specificity
standard deviation (SD)
survey
systematic review
type I error
type II error

Introduction

Advancements in the profession of respiratory care have been driven by supportive research. Uniquely, respiratory care has developed in parallel with advancements in pulmonary medicine, critical care, and technical devices. To critically assess the investigations reported in journals, a framework for evaluating their relevancy includes knowledge of design factors, basic statistics issues, and study types.

One of the important movements affecting healthcare practice in the 21st century is the emergence of **evidence-based medicine**.[1,2] Respiratory care practice demands evidence for the accuracy of diagnostic tests, as well as the efficacy and safety of treatments. The principles of evidence-based medicine provide the tools to incorporate the best evidence into everyday respiratory care practice. Research evidence has a short doubling time—perhaps 10 years or less. Thus, it can be a challenge for clinicians to stay abreast of the newest research findings. The evolving research evidence

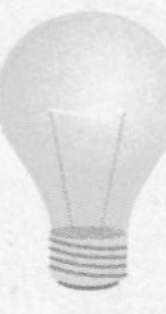

STOP AND THINK

Why is it important that respiratory therapists understand the basic principles of research design?

replaces currently accepted diagnostic tests and treatments with new ones that are more powerful, more accurate, more efficacious, and safer. The availability of evidence is not sufficient, however. It is increasingly recognized that the translation of evidence into practice is often slow. This chapter reviews the core elements of research and the principles of evidence-based medicine as it applies to respiratory care practice.

Research Design

The research process is shown in **Table 60-1**. The language of research is described in the sections that follow.

Controls

Study participants who do not receive the new treatment but receive instead the usual treatment, a placebo, or a sham treatment are the controls. A new treatment will be judged effective if it performs better in the treatment group than in the control group. Controls are studied in the same manner as the treatment group to guard against the investigators fooling themselves (or the public) into believing a new therapy is effective when nontherapy might be similar or safer or less costly.

Matching

Subjects in the control group must be similar to those in the treatment group. **Matching** may be necessary to prevent factors other than the treatment from confounding or confusing the study results. For example, controls should not enter a study sicker than the treatment group members, or the results may favor the treatment group for that reason. A common method of matching illness severity in critical care studies is to enroll patients with similar illness severity into the treatment and control groups. The APACHE (Acute Physiology and Chronic Health Evaluation) scoring system is used to quantify illness severity by assigning severity points to 12 routine physiologic measurements. If treatment and control groups are well matched in APACHE scores, then differences between groups in results (positive, negative, or no difference) should be due to the treatment.

TABLE 60-1
The Research Process

Generate an idea
Determine the research team; establish authorship
Solicit help from statistician and others as needed
Determine conflicts of interest: industry involvement
Develop a study question
State the null hypothesis
Search the literature
Design the experiment
Write the protocol
Obtain permission: Institutional Review Committee/Ethics Committee, department leadership, clinical trials registry
Obtain funding
Collect data
Analyze data: statistician
Reject or concede hypothesis
Write paper
Incorporate the findings into practice
Perform another study

Randomization

To achieve a balance (similar patients, similar status) between treatment and control group members and to avoid investigator bias, a **randomization** process is used after enrollment to assign the patient to either the treatment or control group of a study. This process can be completed by a simple coin flip or, preferably, by randomization software that is readily available via the Internet. Randomization seems simple, but it is potentially complex. Bias can be suspected when groups are not well matched if a truly random process for assigning treatment is not guaranteed.

Blinding or Masking

Whenever possible, investigators and participants should be unaware of the treatment being delivered (i.e., be blinded). If investigators or participants know who is receiving treatment, they might be able to affect the study outcome, even subconsciously, in a preferred direction. This tendency to alter a study is well known, and **blinding** can prevent this possible influence on the results. When both investigators and participants are blinded, the study is said to be *double blinded*. When the participants alone are unaware of their treatment status, the study is *single blinded*. For example, in medication studies, a new drug and the placebo are dispensed in coded bottles containing tablets that are identical in appearance and taste. Both the investigators and participants are unaware of, or blinded to, the real drug bottle and tablets. An independent investigator

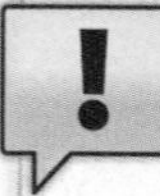

Respiratory Recap

Design Factors for Avoiding Potential Investigator Biases

- Controls
- Matching
- Randomization
- Blinding
- Crossover

decodes the bottles after the results are collected. Drug studies are frequently double blinded, whereas treatment studies usually cannot easily blind the investigators; however, the participants can often be blinded. A sham or fake treatment, like a placebo, can be administered to blind the study participants. Patients and investigators are usually unblinded or unmasked after the study is completed.

Crossover

As a method of matching controls to study patients and designing a more efficient study by reducing the number of subjects, the same patient can be assigned to both the treatment and control groups if the patient can cross over between therapies during the study. In a **crossover study**, the age, gender, disease state, and entire patient history are, of course, identical for both study limbs. The sequencing of the treatment-to-control or control-to-treatment crossover can be randomized or alternated, or, if possible, the participant can cross over back to the original therapy (double crossover) to avoid a sequencing effect.

Observational Versus Interventional

An **observational study** does not change current practice but simply observes activities or results. Observational studies can be useful to report problems or to provide indices for quality assurance monitoring (e.g., timeliness of therapy or compliance with orders). Chart reviews are observational. Privacy rights must be considered even when reviewing charts or observing activities. External observations or reviews cannot be reported (without consent) if the person's identity might be determined by the report. In an observational study in which investigators were hidden, higher hand washing rates were observed for respiratory therapists than physicians or nurses.[3]

An **interventional study** involves a change in care with approval by the patient or relative via informed consent. Studies of major questions such as setting a safe tidal volume or a best PEEP require carefully planned interventions that are administered under tightly controlled conditions.

Prospective and Retrospective

Prospective studies are conducted going forward, whereas **retrospective studies** look back at records to analyze what has already happened (**Figure 60-1**).

> **Respiratory Recap**
>
> **Classification of Studies**
> - Observational or interventional
> - Retrospective or prospective

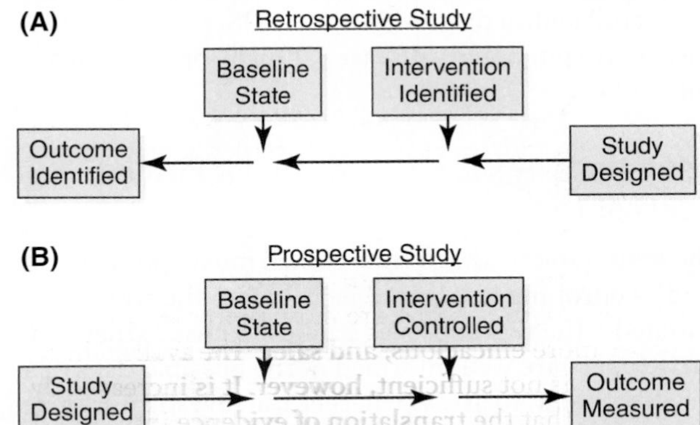

FIGURE 60-1 (**A**) Retrospective studies look back at records to analyze what has already happened. (**B**) Prospective studies are conducted going forward.

> **STOP AND THINK**
>
> Why is a prospective study design always better than a retrospective design?

Retrospective data are susceptible to choosing the best data available and ignoring contrary data. Retrospective studies can also become fishing expeditions—looking for a discovery. There are no real controls in retrospective studies, but an attempt to match a control group to a cases group can be performed. The biggest issue with a retrospective study is that the investigator has no control over the quality of data collection or recording. Missing data can be another big issue with retrospective studies. There are lessons to be learned from retrospective analyses, but prospective studies are preferred because a carefully designed study can avoid most sources of investigator bias. Interventional studies are prospective. Quality assurance projects are often retrospective reviews from the medical records (chart review).

Inclusion and Exclusion Criteria

Before candidates can be entered into or excluded from a study, clearly defined enrollment criteria must be decided upon—the inclusion criteria and exclusion criteria. In addition, conditions should be stated that would withdraw a patient from a study. Enrollment will typically require that patients are restricted to an age range (e.g., older than 16 years), an illness severity level

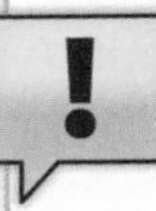

> **Respiratory Recap**
>
> **Incidence Versus Prevalence**
>
> *Incidence* is the number of new cases and usually refers to acute diseases.
>
> *Prevalence* is the number of people who currently have the disease and is a measure of chronic disease.

(e.g., ventilated), a diagnosis (e.g., ARDS, sepsis, chronic obstructive pulmonary disease [COPD]), or a combination of these.

Institutional Review Boards and Informed Consent

The **institutional review board (IRB)** must approve studies enrolling human subjects before the study is initiated.[4] The IRB approves studies to ensure that participants are well informed of the possible risks of a new treatment, to assess whether the investigators are capable of conducting the study, and to judge whether the study has a reasonable probability of answering the study question. The IRB approves the **informed consent** form that must be signed by the patient, relative, or guardian to approve the participant's entry into the treatment or control group. Retrospective studies and surveys also require IRB approval if there is a risk of revealing a patient's identity by the reporting of results. Most studies require IRB approval.

Clinical Trial Registration

A clinical trials registry is an official platform and catalog for registering a clinical trial. ClinicalTrials.gov, run by the United States National Library of Medicine (NLM), was the first online registry for clinical trials and is the largest and most widely used today. The goal of a clinical trials registry is to provide increased transparency and access to clinical trials made available to the public. Clinical trials registries are searchable (for example, trials can be searchable by disease/indication, drug, location). Those sponsoring the study, most often by the investigators, are responsible to register trials. It is now considered unethical if the study is not registered and most journals will not publish clinical trials that are not registered. The requirement to register clinical trials should address the issue of publication bias. Investigators tend not to publish negative studies. Thus, these studies will not be found in a PubMed search but should be found by searching the clinical trials registry.

Measurements

The measured variables of prime interest in a study will, preferably, be common parameters (e.g., mortality, ventilator-free days, Pa_{O_2}, infection rates) with known degrees of accuracy and variability. The measurements must be part of an analysis plan that will be used to answer the study question. This plan also estimates a minimum number of participants (the sample size determination) required to obtain statistically significant results.

Incidence and Prevalence

Incidence is the number of new cases of a disease contracted or diagnosed in a given time period, usually a year. **Prevalence** is the number of individuals in a given population who have the disease or condition at a given time. The importance of these terms becomes relevant in studies of acute and chronic diseases. For example, approximately 40,000 deaths are caused by influenza each year in the United States.[5] Although millions may be contracting flu each year (the cases), the incidence of death due to the flu—the case fatality ratio—is the important metric for evaluating the severity of the influenza season each year. For chronic disease management, the prevalence rate measures the continuing burden of that disease on the healthcare system. For example, there are an estimated 13 million COPD patients in the United States, a prevalence associated with cigarette smoking that explains why COPD is the fourth leading cause of death.[6] Incidence and prevalence studies fall within the field of epidemiology, the branch of medicine involved with the transmission and control of diseases.

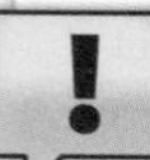

Respiratory Recap

Requirements for Conducting a Study

- Inclusion and exclusion criteria
- Approval from an IRB
- Clinical trials registration
- Measurements
- Contingencies for dealing with missing values

Missing Values and Dropouts

Even the best-designed studies conducted by meticulous investigators have problems with missing values or dropouts or both, because complete acquisition of clean data in any study is unusual. Fortunately, if there is no particular pattern to the missing values, they can be disregarded; if a pattern exists, statistical adjustments can be made to account for this problem. Studies over time (longitudinal studies) will frequently have missing data due to patients lost to follow-up.

A dropout rate can be a positive finding. For example, liberation from ventilator support is a success, as displayed in **Figure 60-2**.[7] The plot in this figure shows that the use of a therapist-driven liberation protocol reduces ventilator hours when compared with the usual nonprotocol liberation method. This type of graph, a **Kaplan-Meier plot**, is most often used to analyze survival rates in mortality studies. The Kaplan-Meier curves in **Figure 60-3** display mortality caused by lung cancer according to high or low depressive coping. The overall low survival rates in lung cancer have been strongly associated with cigarette smoking, and the coping behavior connection with survival may result from differing physical conditions rather than a beneficial psychological makeup such as high depressive coping.

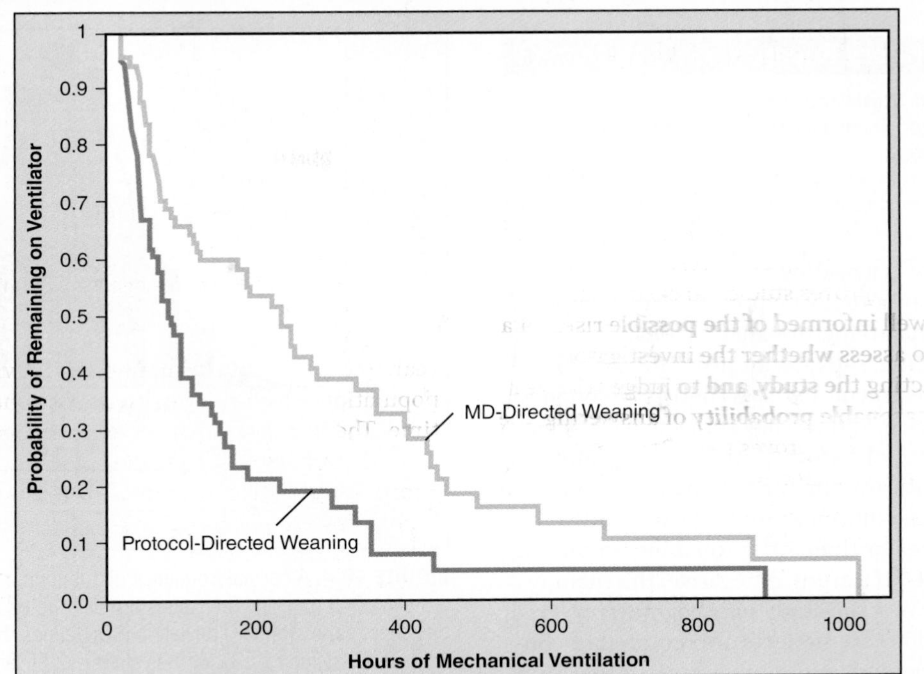

FIGURE 60-2 Kaplan-Meier analysis of the duration of mechanical ventilation after adjustment for the severity of illness at baseline (as measured by the APACHE II score), age, sex, race, location of the intensive care unit, and duration of intubation before enrollment. Mechanical ventilation was discontinued more rapidly in the therapist-driven protocol group than in the control group.

Reproduced from Ely EW, Baker AM, Dunagan DP, et al. Effect on the duration of mechanical ventilation of identifying patients capable of breathing spontaneously. *N Engl J Med.* 1996;335:1864–1869. © 1996 Massachusetts Medical Society. Reprinted with permission from Massachusetts Medical Society.

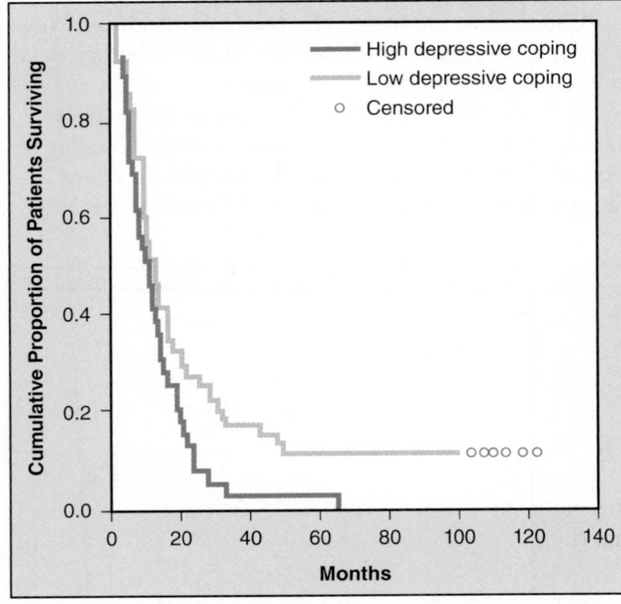

FIGURE 60-3 Kaplan-Meier survival curves showing probability of mortality over a 10-year follow-up period in lung cancer patients with high and low levels of depressive coping.

Reproduced from Faller H, Bülzebruck H. Coping and survival in lung cancer: a 10-year follow-up. *Am J Psychiatry.* 2002;159:2105–2107. Reprinted with permission from the American Journal of Psychiatry. © 2002 American Psychiatric Association.

Statistical Issues

Statistics can be complex, but knowledge of statistics is essential to thoroughly evaluate the merit of research reports. Although there is no substitute for learning statistics in an organized program of study, the following are pointers that can aid in interpreting the statistical methods used in a study.

Descriptive statistics, such as means with standard deviations of obtained variables, are often presented to provide an overview of the measurements from the study. Figures such as histograms, line graphs, scatter plots, and tables will display the data more clearly than descriptions within the narrative of the text. Statistics used to answer the study questions (i.e., to reject the hypotheses) are known as **inferential statistics**, which require significance testing. Equipoise should be observed when the study question or hypothesis is written. The purpose of research is to "determine whether" and not to "prove that."

A statistically significant result *infers* that the results can be applied to other settings (i.e., beyond the study itself). There are two important types of statistical errors (type I and type II errors) that can be committed when drawing conclusions from significance testing. The primary goal of statistics is to provide data to argue that a study has identified a truth that can be applied to other settings, but statistics can also lie. A **type I error** occurs when a conclusion appears to be true but may actually be false. To avoid this possibility, P (probability) values are calculated to assess whether the probability of making this type of error is less than 5% ($P < .05$). Whereas this criterion does not guarantee that the inference is true, the likelihood of making a type I error is low if this criterion is met.

Respiratory Recap

Types of Statistical Errors

Type I error: There appears to be an effect, but, in fact, there is none.

Type II error: There appears to be no effect, but in fact an effect exists but has not been detected.

A **type II error** is a finding that appears to show no effect when it may actually be present. An example of a type II error is the premature analysis of an incomplete study that is finding, thus far, an insignificant effect of the drug or treatment. Perhaps there is a tendency toward significance, and too few subjects have been studied. The *power* of a study is its ability to detect a statistically significant difference between groups using some standard assumptions. Studies are usually powered to have a greater than 80% probability of finding significant results. If a study is negative, the therapy may be ineffective *or* the study may be underpowered (type II error) and more subjects are required to confirm an effect—possibly more subjects than the study can afford to enroll.

Measurements in a study can be continuous variables, such as Pao_2, plateau pressure, cardiac output, or FEV_1. Continuous variables can be normally distributed (i.e., evenly on both sides of the mean) or skewed toward lower values (e.g., oximetry) or toward positive values (e.g., Pao_2 for patients receiving oxygen). Categorical variables place outcomes into one or more categories such as yes or no, dead or alive, male or female, presence or absence of dyspnea or cyanosis. Variables can also be ordinal, which have an order or ranking according to an accepted scale system, such as the Borg score or APACHE score. Parametric data are continuous and normally distributed. Nonparametric data are ordinal or continuous, but not normally distributed (i.e., skewed).

Many variables will follow a normal distribution, that is, they are graphically characterized by a bell-shaped curve. **Figure 60-4** shows a normal distribution of $Paco_2$ data from a large number of patients. Values from a normal distribution of $Paco_2$ values have an average, or *mean*, of 40 mm Hg, displayed by the peak in the center. The dispersion of values about the mean is quantified by the **standard deviation (SD)**, where ±1 SD encompasses 68% of the values, ±2 SD encompasses 95% of the values, and ±3 SD encompasses 99% of the values. The *median* is defined as the mid-value where half the values are above and half are below that median. The *mode* is the most frequent value; categorical and ordinal data are often described by modes. The mean, median, and mode are the same value in a normal distribution but differ when the data are skewed (i.e., there is a tail in the positive or negative direction).

Depending on a variable's distribution, either the mean, median, or mode may best characterize the data. When data are parametric, the mean and SD are used. For nonparametric data, median and interquartile range are used. The interquartile range is the spread of the data between the 25th and 75th percentile. For categorical data, the fraction (or percentage) and 95% confidence interval are reported.

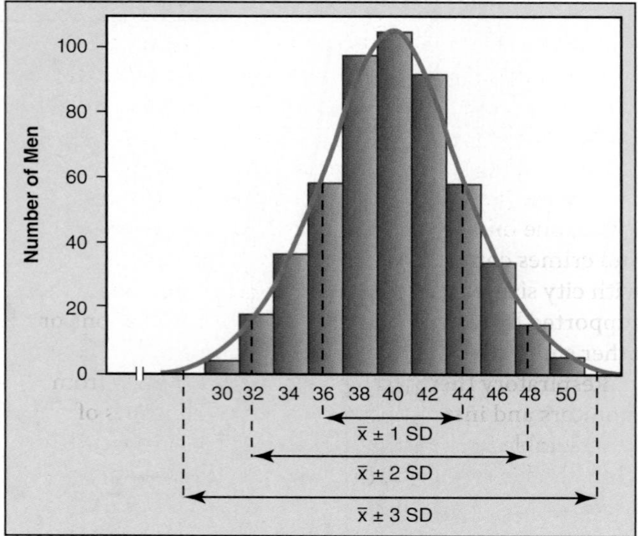

FIGURE 60-4 A normal frequency distribution of $Paco_2$ values about a mean of 40 mm Hg. The values are distributed about the mean in a bell shape. The standard deviation (SD) defines the width of the bell, with ±1 SD including 68% of the values, ±2 SD encompassing 95%, and ±3 SD encompassing 99% of the values.

Associations are frequently the major findings from a study. **Correlation coefficients** indicate whether associations exist (+1 = positive or direct, −1 = negative or indirect, 0 = no relationship). A **regression analysis** can definitively quantify the strength of the association or associations. For example, age and FEV_1 are negatively correlated, but **Figure 60-5** shows that FEV_1

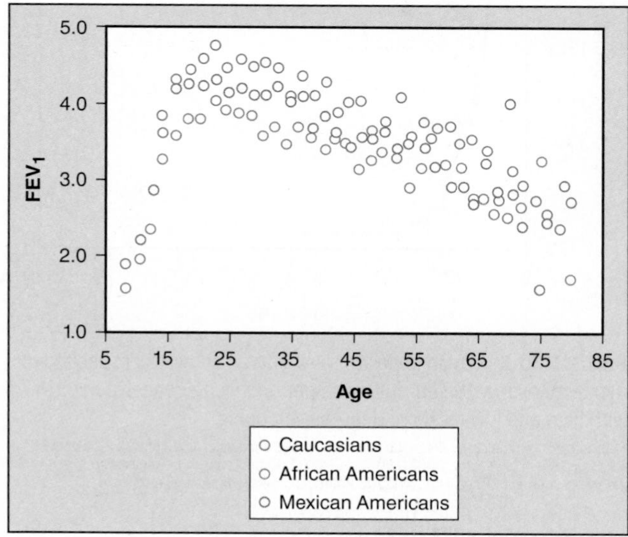

FIGURE 60-5 The association or regression of FEV_1 (*y* axis) with age (*x* axis) for men.

declines about 20 to 25 mL for every year that we age. The measurement and interpretation of associations often require a statistician's assistance. Unfortunately, associations can be deceptive and may not tell us about causality. The classic example is the direct association between the number of churches in a city and the city's crime rate. Instead of concluding that churches cause crime, one must consider that the number of churches and crimes committed in a city are both associated with city size. Reports of associations should be further supported by reasonable causes for the associations or other supportive data, or both.

Respiratory therapists rely on measurements from monitors and instruments, and their accuracy is of considerable interest. A new measurement instrument or method is frequently compared to the current gold standard instrument to assess its potential usefulness. A **Bland-Altman plot** is often used to display the values obtained by each method, easily illustrating the average differences (bias) and the variability (standard deviation of the differences) between the new and old instruments. In **Figure 60-6**, Bland-Altman plots display comparisons between CO_2 readings from arterial blood ($Paco_2$) and readings from a transcutaneous CO_2 monitor and an end-tidal CO_2 monitor.[8] The bias or average difference between the $Paco_2$ and transcutaneous values was +5.6 mm Hg, whereas the mean end-tidal CO_2 difference was −14 mm Hg. Variability of the differences was 3.4 mm Hg and 7.4 mm Hg, respectively. Note that the transcutaneous sensor overestimates $Paco_2$, whereas the end-tidal adapter underestimates $Paco_2$.

Be wary of multiple comparisons. As studies become more complex, several variables are frequently tested to detect any possible significant effects between the variables of interest. When a number of comparisons are made there is an increased risk of discovering chance relationships that may not be real. Statistical testing can be adjusted or changed to reduce this possibility. For example, if 20 factors are studied to assess the potential for ventilator liberation, one factor can be expected to be positive *due to chance* if the common criterion of $P < .05$ is used to define significance. Lowering the P value by a factor related to the number of comparisons will reduce the risk of this error.

Simple calculations of mean and standard deviation can be readily performed by available spreadsheets, as can the creation of figures. Meaningful inferential statistics must be calculated with the use of statistical packages such as SAS, SPSS, or R. Increasingly, a statistician is becoming a critical member of the investigative team, and the statistician deserves co-authorship on most study reports. When reading the results of a study, it is important to question whether the proper statistical tests were used. For example, if a parametric statistical test was used for nonparametric data, the results may be misleading. **Table 60-2** shows the proper statistical test for the type of data that are analyzed.[9]

The statistical findings with inferences often define the importance of a study. Ultimately, the importance of a study may not depend on the statistics but on the clinical relevance of the findings. Although an effect measured in a study may be statistically significant, it may have minor clinical importance. In contrast, a small but statistically significant reduction in mortality can justify approval of a major new cardiovascular drug. Therefore, a reader must judge a study's relevance after considering the author's discussion and the overall relevance of the study for improving patient care.

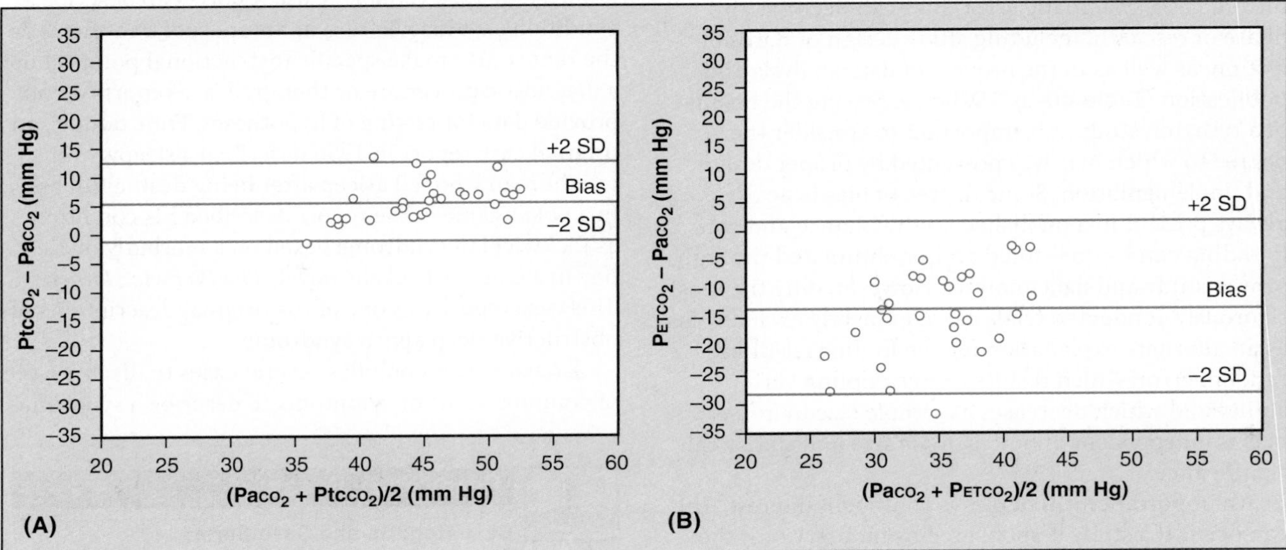

FIGURE 60-6 Bland-Altman plots of comparisons between $Paco_2$ and Pco_2 measured by a transcutaneous CO_2 capnometer (**A**) and an end-tidal CO_2 capnometer (**B**). The transcutaneous sensor overestimates $Paco_2$, whereas the end-tidal adapter underestimates $Paco_2$.

Reproduced from Stein N, et al. An evaluation of a transcutaneous and an end-tidal capnometer for noninvasive monitoring of spontaneously breathing patients. *Respir Care*. 2006;51:1162–1166. Reprinted with permission.

TABLE 60-2
Appropriate Statistical Test Determined by the Type of Data

Unpaired groups (parallel and independent groups)					
Parametric		**Nonparametric**		**Categorical**	
2 groups	**>2 groups**	**2 groups**	**>2 groups**	**2 groups**	**>2 groups**
Unpaired t-test	Analysis of variance	Mann-Whitney or Wilcoxon	Kruskall-Wallis	Chi-square or Fisher Exact Test	Chi-square
Paired groups					
Parametric		**Nonparametric**		**Categorical**	
2 groups	**>2 groups**	**2 groups**	**>2 groups**		
Paired t-test	Repeated measures analysis of variance	Wilcoxon signed-rank test	Friedman's analysis of variance	McNamar's test	Cochran's Q test
Association between variables					
Both Variables Parametric		**Nonparametric**		**Categorical**	
Pearson's product moment correlation coefficient		Spearman's or Kendall's rank correlation coefficient		Relative risk, risk ratio, odds ratio, logistic regression	
Agreement between assessment techniques					
Continuous Data			**Categorical Data**		
Intraclass correlation coefficient or Bland-Altman plot			Cohen's kappa		

Information from Nayak BK, Hazra A. How to choose the right statistical test? *Indian J Ophthalmol.* 2011;59:85–86.

Bias

Bias is anything that prevents unprejudiced consideration of a question. Bias occurs in research when selecting or encouraging one outcome over others introduces a systematic error. Bias can occur at any phase of research, including study design or data collection, as well as in the process of data analysis and publication (**Table 60-3**).[10] When assessing the results of a research study, it is important to consider the degree to which bias was prevented by proper design and implementation. Some degree of bias is nearly always present in a published study. Chance and confounding can be quantified and/or eliminated through proper study and data analysis. However, only the most rigorously conducted trials can completely exclude bias as an alternate explanation for the findings. Unlike random error, which results from sampling variability and which decreases as sample size increases, bias is independent of both sample size and statistical significance.

An important form of bias is conflict of interest. This can occur if a study is sponsored by industry or if the investigators have a financial relationship with a company. It is important that all potential conflicts of interest are disclosed when the study is published.

Study Types

Case Reports and Case Series

A detailed description of an unusual, interesting case is known as a **case report.**[11] Case reports can describe a condition that may be rare or an unusual treatment, or the report may make specific instructional points about a diagnostic procedure or therapy. Case reports do not provide data for testing of hypotheses. For example, an original case report in 1956 described a sleepy, overweight man who fell asleep after being dealt a full house in a poker game.[12] The report described his condition as Pickwickian syndrome based on a morbidly obese boy in a Charles Dickens novel, *The Pickwick Papers.* This case report was one of the original descriptions of obstructive sleep apnea syndrome.

A **case series** compiles several cases to discuss a set of common signs or symptoms to describe a syndrome

Respiratory Recap

Case Reports and Case Series

Case reports and case series are effective ways of reporting unusual observations or unique treatments or emphasizing instructional points.

TABLE 60-3
Common Types of Bias That Can Be Introduced into a Study

Type of Bias	How to Avoid
Pre-Study Bias	
Flawed study design	Clearly define risk and outcome, preferably with objective or validated methods. Standardize and blind data collection.
Selection bias	Select patients using rigorous criteria to avoid confounding results. Subjects should be selected from the same population. Well-designed prospective studies help to avoid selection bias.
Channeling bias	Assign subjects to study cohorts using rigorous criteria. Allocation should be concealed so that the investigator does not know to which group the subject will be assigned until enrollment.
Conflict of interest	Investigators should not have a relationship with any company that could benefit from the study's results.
Bias During the Study	
Interviewer bias	Blind interviewer to exposure status. Standardize data collection tool.
Chronology bias	Use prospective study design. Avoid use of historical controls, as this can lead to confounding due to practice changes over time that affect outcomes unrelated to study design.
Recall bias	Use objective questions. Conduct prospective studies; retrospective studies can be confounded by poor recall of the subject and missing data.
Transfer bias	Carefully design plan to account for subjects lost to follow-up. Perform intent-to-treat analysis.
Exposure misclassification	Clearly define exposure *a priori* and avoid using proxies of exposure.
Outcome misclassification	Use objective diagnostic studies or validated measures. Avoid surrogate endpoints.
Performance bias	Be certain that investigators and subjects perform interventions correctly. This can be an issue in respiratory care due to poor procedure performance by subjects or investigators (for example, using an inhaler incorrectly).
Bias After Trial	
Citation bias (publication bias)	Register trial and check trial registries for similar unpublished or in-progress trials prior to publication. Publish results even if the trial is negative.
Confounding	Known confounders can be controlled with study design (case control design or randomization) or during data analysis (regression). Unknown confounders can be controlled only with randomization.

Reproduced from Pannucci CJ, Wilkins EG. Identifying and avoiding bias in research. *Plast Reconstr Surg*. 2010;126:619–625.

or to further characterize cases or a treatment. The expectation is that reports of cases or a case series will lead to studies that further clarify the disease, syndrome, or its treatment. Twelve severe lung injury cases were described by Petty in *The Lancet* in 1970.[13] The common features of these patients led to an acceptance of the adult respiratory distress syndrome as a disease entity. In another example, an investigator observed a notch in the expiratory flow limb of a ventilator waveform. A bronchoscopy was performed that found a partially occlusive unilateral mucous plug, and further examination of the waveform identified distinct graphic signs that indicated the presence of the partial occlusion (**Figure 60-7**). A detailed case report was published to alert clinicians of these waveform signs as indicators of large unilateral mucous plugging.[14]

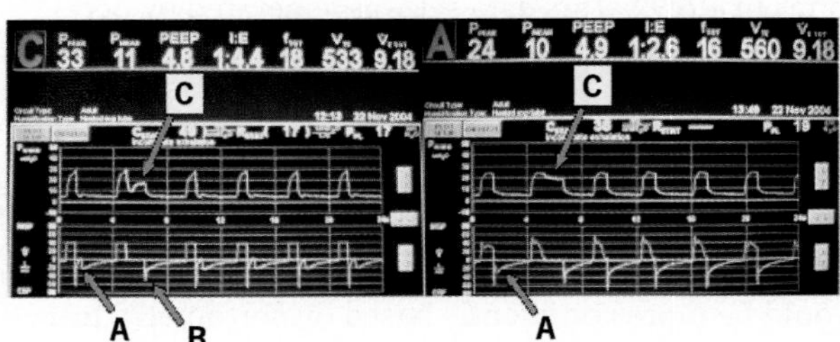

FIGURE 60-7 Airway pressure and flow tracings recorded before and after bronchoscopy. Arrow A in the prebronchoscopy panel indicates a flow stutter step that attenuates after clearance of plugs after bronchoscopy. Arrow B shows a normal exponential flow decay after a pause prior to bronchoscopy. The C arrows display an unusual rising plateau pressure before bronchoscopy when plugs are present that resolves to a normal plateau pressure display after plug clearance postbronchoscopy.

Reproduced from Zamanian M, Marini JJ. Pressure-flow signatures of central-airway mucus plugging. *Crit Care Med*. 2006;34:223–226. Reprinted with permission from Wolters Kluwer Health.

Case Control Studies

Case control studies, which are often retrospective, involve the accumulation of a number of disease cases that must meet a specific case definition to be compared with controls. The goal is to find a cause for—or important associations with—the cases. Controls are found from a reasonable source such as medical records, interviews, or patients receiving similar care. Controls do not have the case condition, but they should be compared to the cases by available factors that might be associated with becoming a case: age, gender, location, related medical history, potential exposures, and so on. The factors for the cases that the controls do not have are the associations with becoming a case (such as what was eaten or not eaten at a particular event). The associations will characterize the risk factors for becoming a case, but they may not reveal the actual cause or causes. Pathology, microbiology, or biochemical pathway studies are often required to determine causality. Case control studies can involve exhaustive medical record reviews.

Cross-Sectional Studies

Studies of a sampling from the population at a given point in time are **cross-sectional studies** because they cut across the population. Cross-sectional data are generated by surveying or calculating parameters from existing data sets to determine a case rate (prevalence) or by measuring current values for a specific test or polling opinions. For example, the percentage of the United States population who smoked cigarettes in 2009 was 21%, as determined by cross-sectional data from surveys,[15] compared with a 42% rate in 1961. The drop in smoking rates over time helps to explain the recent stabilization in COPD prevalence and lung cancer incidence rates.

Spirometry standards, or normal predicted values according to age, gender, and height, are based on a large cross-sectional study of persons with normal lungs in 1999.[16] This data set was generated by performing spirometry using a standardized technique on 16,000 normal individuals. From this study (HANES III), mean values and regression equations for FEV_1, FEV_6, and vital capacity were determined to become the basis for predicting normal spirometric values (according to one's age, height, and gender). Predicted values would be more confidently based on spirometry testing from the same people as they age throughout their lives—a cohort study.

Cohort Studies

Cohort studies attempt to answer important questions about the cause, treatment, progression, or prevention of a disease. These studies enroll large numbers of participants (the cohort) and follow them over years, even decades. The research team will test, treat, or monitor the cohort with the goal of detecting insights into disease progression and the effects of treatment as the participants get older. Cohort studies require a continual effort to track participants. Follow-up is often difficult, and dropouts can be a serious problem. The Scandinavian countries are known for conducting meticulous cohort studies. The Framingham heart studies have followed individuals in Framingham, Massachusetts (the cohort), over decades to identify factors associated with many diseases, particularly coronary heart disease.[17] The Framingham data have documented the important role of primary care such as cholesterol reduction and blood pressure control in the reduction of cardiovascular disease. In a study of COPD in the Framingham cohort, investigators reported that smoking increases the rate of lung function decline and that quitting smoking has a beneficial effect at any age but that the benefit is more pronounced in earlier quitters.[18] Although these results seem logical, this type of solid evidence continues to emphasize and confirm the detrimental effects of smoking.

Animal Studies

The use of animals in medical research is controversial, but nearly all significant advancements in medicine have been made possible through discoveries from animal studies. There are strict regulations in the United States governing the use of animals in research to guarantee their humane treatment, including the avoidance of pain or discomfort. Investigators who conduct animal research are monitored by an Animal Care and Use Committee that is directed by *The Guide for the Care and Use of Laboratory Animals*.[19]

To study lung disease, several animal models have been developed to simulate the human diseased state. Models of ARDS can be caused by oleic acid infusion, high airway pressures or ventilator-induced lung injury, saline lavage to wash out surfactant, or instillation of bacteria to cause a severe pneumonia. The procedures are often 4 to 12 hours in duration and are designed to study pressing critical care questions. Generally, the animals studied most frequently in research are small animals such as mice and rats, while swine or sheep often serve as models for the human cardiopulmonary system. Limiting factors to large animal studies are the short-term nature of the studies and minor anatomic differences from humans; generally, however, their cardiopulmonary physiology is similar to humans.

Equipment Evaluations

The innovation of industry continues to develop machines and instruments for use in the treatment, monitoring, and diagnosis of illnesses. Devices that are similar to a previously tested device (the predicate device) do not require additional testing and can be marketed as is. But as technology progresses, newly

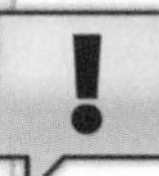

Respiratory Recap

Equipment Evaluations

- Equipment that is similar to previous devices can be marketed as is and does not require additional studies.
- New devices are studied by comparing their measures to gold standard measurements from established devices.

introduced instruments must be compared in some manner to a standard measurement. If an equipment evaluation study of a new instrument provides comparable values to the standard device or if the instrument is more accurate, more efficient, less expensive, or safer, the instrument will be adopted. Although some comparisons can be made easily in the laboratory, convincing comparisons should be made in the clinical setting to fairly assess the safety and accuracy of the instrument. New techniques and machines are often tested, initially, under normal conditions, but their reliability must be determined under abnormal or challenging conditions to learn limitations to their use.

Surveys

Surveys use questionnaires or a set of questions sometimes called an *instrument* to obtain results. A survey goal may be to determine opinions, practice patterns, or purchasing intentions. Surveys or polling can be carefully conducted to be more accurate by using small samples that are highly representative of the target group. Surveys are not interventional. In a survey of clinicians involved with the ARDSnet studies, the investigators attempted to determine barriers to implementing a lung-protective ventilatory strategy. Lung-protective strategies include reduced tidal volume (V_T) settings to reduce pressure exposure. The potentials for tachypnea, discomfort, hypoxemia, and acidosis were important concerns or barriers to implementing a lung-protective or lower-V_T ventilator strategy.[20]

Randomized Controlled Trials

The **randomized controlled trial (RCT)** (**Figure 60-8**) is the most important type of study of medical interventions in clinical care. Proposed changes in care must undergo the scrutiny of RCTs to investigate a change in treatment or a new treatment in the clinical setting through comparison with the current (or usual)

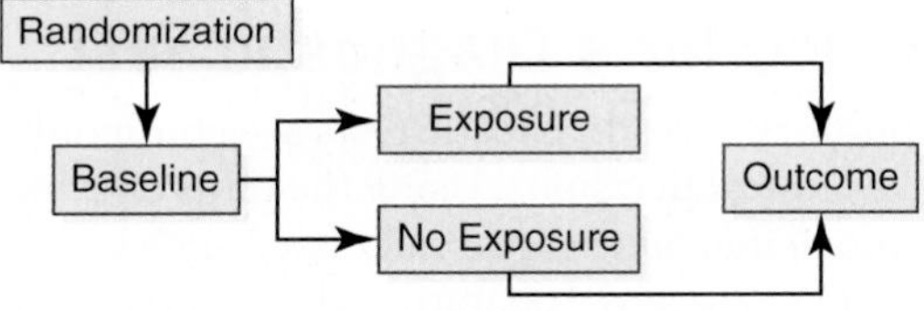

FIGURE 60-8 Design of a randomized controlled trial.

Respiratory Recap

Randomized Controlled Trials

RCTs are the primary means of testing the safety and effectiveness of new medications or therapies.

therapy. Most RCTs are lengthy (1 to 3 years) and expensive, and are often investigations of new treatments. An RCT is interventional, prospective, randomized, and blinded (if possible), and the treatment group will, it is hoped, match with the control group at baseline. In the FDA clearance process of new medications, phases of an investigational drug are formalized (in phases I through III) to examine a drug's safety, effectiveness, and applicability to human use.

RCTs conducted within the ARDSnet collaboration of hospitals have produced important discoveries in the treatment of ARDS. This consortium is a disciplined group of investigative teams that have recruited ARDS patients into RCTs to study tidal volume settings, PEEP, fluid resuscitation, and methylprednisolone, ketoconazole, and lisofylline use.[21] The first decisive RCT study of 887 ARDS patients found that high V_T compared with low V_T (12 vs. 6 mL/kg) was associated with increased mortality.[22] In another RCT, 550 patients tested the use of high versus low PEEP and found no difference in mortality between the PEEP settings.[3]

What Is Evidence-Based Respiratory Care?

Evidence-based respiratory care is the integration of individual clinical expertise with the best available research evidence from systematic research and a patient's values and expectations.[1,2] The best evidence is not static but rather changes when better evidence becomes available. Evidence-based medicine does not devalue clinical skills and clinical judgment. To the contrary, evidence-based medicine demands a high level of clinical skill and judgment. The practice of evidence-based medicine requires us to apply the evidence to the right patient, at the right time, in the right place, at the right dose, and using the right resources. We need to recognize the correct patient diagnosis before applying the evidence to the care of the patient. For example, the best evidence for management of asthma may not apply to a patient with chronic obstructive pulmonary disease (COPD).

Research evidence comes from real clinical research among intact patients. Animal studies do not trump patient studies. That is not to say that animal studies are not important to test proof of concept or to explore physiologic mechanisms. However, care must always be taken when extrapolating animal studies to patient care. The findings of properly conducted studies in a relevant patient population should never be discarded in favor of the findings from an animal study. No number of animal studies can outweigh the findings of even a single well-done human study.

Patient values and expectations are an important part of evidence-based medicine. For example, there is a compelling body of high-level research evidence supporting the use of noninvasive ventilation (NIV) in patients with an exacerbation of COPD. The patient with COPD exacerbation may choose not to accept NIV. Another example relates to the choice of an aerosol delivery device. The evidence shows that similar outcomes result from the use of a nebulizer and a pressurized metered dose inhaler (pMDI) with valved holding chamber. A patient may reject the use of the MDI in favor of the nebulizer. Although this may contradict the bias of the clinician, the patient's choice should be respected; moreover, the nebulizer may result in better compliance if it better meets the expectations of the patient.

Evidence-based respiratory care is not cookbook medicine or cost-cutting care. The best evidence needs extrapolation to the patient's unique pathophysiology and values. With the implementation of evidence-based medicine, costs may increase, decrease, or remain unchanged.

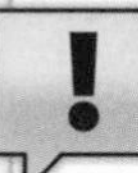

Respiratory Recap

Evidence-Based Medicine

- Evidence-based medicine is the integration of individual clinical expertise with the best available research evidence from systematic research and a patient's values and expectations.
- A hierarchy of evidence can be used to assess the strength upon which clinical decisions are made.

Hierarchy of Evidence

A hierarchy of evidence can be used to assess the strength upon which clinical decisions are made (**Box 60-1**).[23] Respiratory therapists should seek the highest available evidence from this hierarchy. Evidence always exists, but sometimes it may be weak. The best available evidence may be the unsystematic observation of a single clinician or a generalization from physiologic studies.

Note that randomization is an important attribute of higher levels of evidence. The highest level of evidence is an **N-of-1 randomized controlled trial** (RCT). In the N-of-1 RCT, an individual patient undertakes pairs of treatment periods in which the patient receives a target treatment in one period of each pair and a placebo or alternative in the other. The order of the target treatment and the control is randomized, and quantitative ratings are made for each treatment. The N-of-1 RCT continues until both the patient and clinician conclude that there is, or is not, benefit from the intervention. For example, imagine that a decision is made to try flutter therapy for a patient with cystic fibrosis. The clinician and patient agree that a clinically useful outcome measure is sputum production. A 12-week trial is designed. For 1 week, the only sputum clearance technique used is huff coughing. For a second week, flutter therapy in addition to huff coughing is used. For a third week, sham therapy is used. The order of treatments is randomized (the patient flips a coin), and the sequence is repeated four times. Each day, the sputum produced during the therapy session is weighed. A diary is also kept in which events such as chest infections are logged. At the end of 12 weeks, the results are analyzed (this may include statistical analysis), reviewed together by the clinician and patient, and a collaborative decision is made regarding the benefit of the therapy. In this manner, an objective decision is made regarding the benefits of this therapy for this individual patient.

There are some therapies for which there has not been a randomized trial, and one might argue that a randomized trial is either unethical or unnecessary. For example, it is unlikely that a randomized trial will ever be conducted to study the survival benefit of mechanical ventilation in patients with apnea, transfusion for massive blood loss, or antibiotics for bacterial pneumonia. In such cases, the benefit of therapy is overwhelmingly obvious and a randomized controlled trial is unnecessary. In respiratory care, some therapies are unproven. In other words, the evidence to support their use is weak. Because a therapy is unproven does not mean that it is wrong, but it also does not mean that it is right.

BOX 60-1

Hierarchy of Evidence

N-of-1 randomized trial
Meta-analysis of randomized trials
Single randomized controlled trial
Systematic reviews of observational studies
Single observational study
Physiologic studies
Unsystematic clinical observations

Evidence for a Diagnostic Test

In respiratory care, diagnostic tests are commonly used to make clinical decisions. Using the tools of evidence-based medicine, metrics are calculated such as sensitivity, specificity, receiver operating characteristic curves, and likelihood ratios (**Figure 60-9**).

		Reference Standard	
		Positive	Negative
Test Result	Positive	a	b
	Negative	c	d

True Positive = a
True Negative = d
False Positive = b
False Negative = c
Sensitivity = a/(a + c)
Specificity = d/(b + d)
Likelihood Ratio for Positive Test (LR+) = sensitivity/(1 – specificity)
Likelihood Ratio for Negative Test (LR–) = (1 – sensitivity)/specificity
Positive Predictive Value (PPV) = a/(a + b)
Negative Predictive Value (NPV) = d/(c + d)
Diagnostic Accuracy = (a + d)/(a + b + c + d)

(A)

		Extubation	
		Successful	Unsuccessful
RSBI	<100	32	12
	>100	1	19

True Positive = 32
True Negative = 19
False Positive = 12
False Negative = 1
Sensitivity = 32/(32 + 1) = 97%
Specificity = 19/(12 + 19) = 61%
Likelihood Ratio for Positive Test (LR+) = 0.97/(1 – 0.61) = 2.49
Likelihood Ratio for Negative Test (LR–) = (1 – 0.97)/0.61 = 0.05
Positive Predictive Value (PPV) = 32/(32 + 12) = 0.73
Negative Predictive Value (NPV) = 19/(1 + 19) = 0.95
Diagnostic Accuracy = 51/64 = 0.80

(B)

FIGURE 60-9 (**A**) Statistical tests commonly used to assess a diagnostic test. (**B**) Comparison of the results of a diagnostic test (ratio of rate to tidal volume) with the results of a reference standard (successful spontaneous breathing trial), assuming that a ratio less than 100 indicates successful extubation. RSBI, rapid shallow breathing index.

(A, B) Information from Yang KL, Tobin MJ. A prospective study of indexes predicting the outcome of trials of weaning from mechanical ventilation. *N Engl J Med.* 1991;324:1445.

Sensitivity and Specificity

Sensitivity is the proportion of patients who have a disorder and are correctly identified by the test. **Specificity** is the proportion of patients who are free of a disorder and are correctly identified by the test.

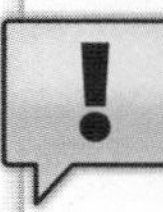

Respiratory Recap

Evidence for a Diagnostic Test

- Sensitivity and specificity
- Likelihood ratio
- Receiver operating characteristic curve

Likelihood Ratio

Likelihood ratio (LR) is used for assessing the value of performing a diagnostic test.

An LR of 1 indicates that the posttest probability is exactly the same as the pretest probability. Thus, diagnostic tests with an LR of 1 are not helpful.

An LR greater than 1 increases the probability that the target condition is present, and an LR less than 1 decreases the probability that the target condition is present.

An LR greater than 10 or less than 0.1 generates large and conclusive changes in the probability of a given diagnosis.

An LR in the range of 5 to 10 or 0.1 to 0.2 generates moderate and usually useful shifts in pretest to posttest probability.

An LR in the range of 2 to 5 or 0.5 to 0.2 generates small, but sometimes important, changes in pretest probability.

An LR in the range of 1 to 2 or 0.5 to 1.0 alters the probability of a given condition to a small and rarely important degree.

The rapid shallow breathing index (RSBI) can be used to illustrate the use of these statistical metrics.[24] Meade et al. suggest an LR of 1.58 and 0.22 for positive and negative predictions, respectively.[25] An LR of this magnitude generates a small change in pretest probability. A nomogram can be used to derive posttest probabilities from the pretest probability and the likelihood ratio. Imagine an intubated 30-year-old patient following multiple trauma. In your clinical experience, 80% of similar patients extubate successfully following resolution of the chest trauma (the pretest probability of successful extubation is 80%). Suppose that the patient's RSBI is 85 (test is positive for extubation). As shown in **Figure 60-10**, the likelihood ratio produces a posttest probability of successful extubation that differs little from the pretest probability. If the RSBI is 120 (test is negative for extubation), however, the posttest probability of successful extubation does change the pretest probability.

Imagine an 85-year-old patient with resolving COPD exacerbation. In your experience, only 20% of similar patients extubate successfully following resolution of the COPD exacerbation (the pretest probability of successful extubation is 20%). Suppose that this patient's RSBI is 85. As shown in Figure 60-10, using the likelihood ratio produces a posttest probability of successful extubation that increases the pretest probability, but not by a lot. However, if the RSBI is 120, the posttest probability of successful extubation is extremely low.

Receiver Operating Characteristic Curve

The **receiver operating characteristic curve** is a figure showing the power of a diagnostic test. It plots the true-positive rate (sensitivity) on the vertical axis and the false-positive rate (specificity) on the horizontal axis for different cut points, thus dividing a positive from a negative test. For a perfect test, the area under the curve is 1. For a test that performs no better than chance, the area under the curve is 0.5. In **Figure 60-11**, note that the modest area under the curve (0.7) demonstrates that the RSBI has no more than modest accuracy in predicting extubation readiness.

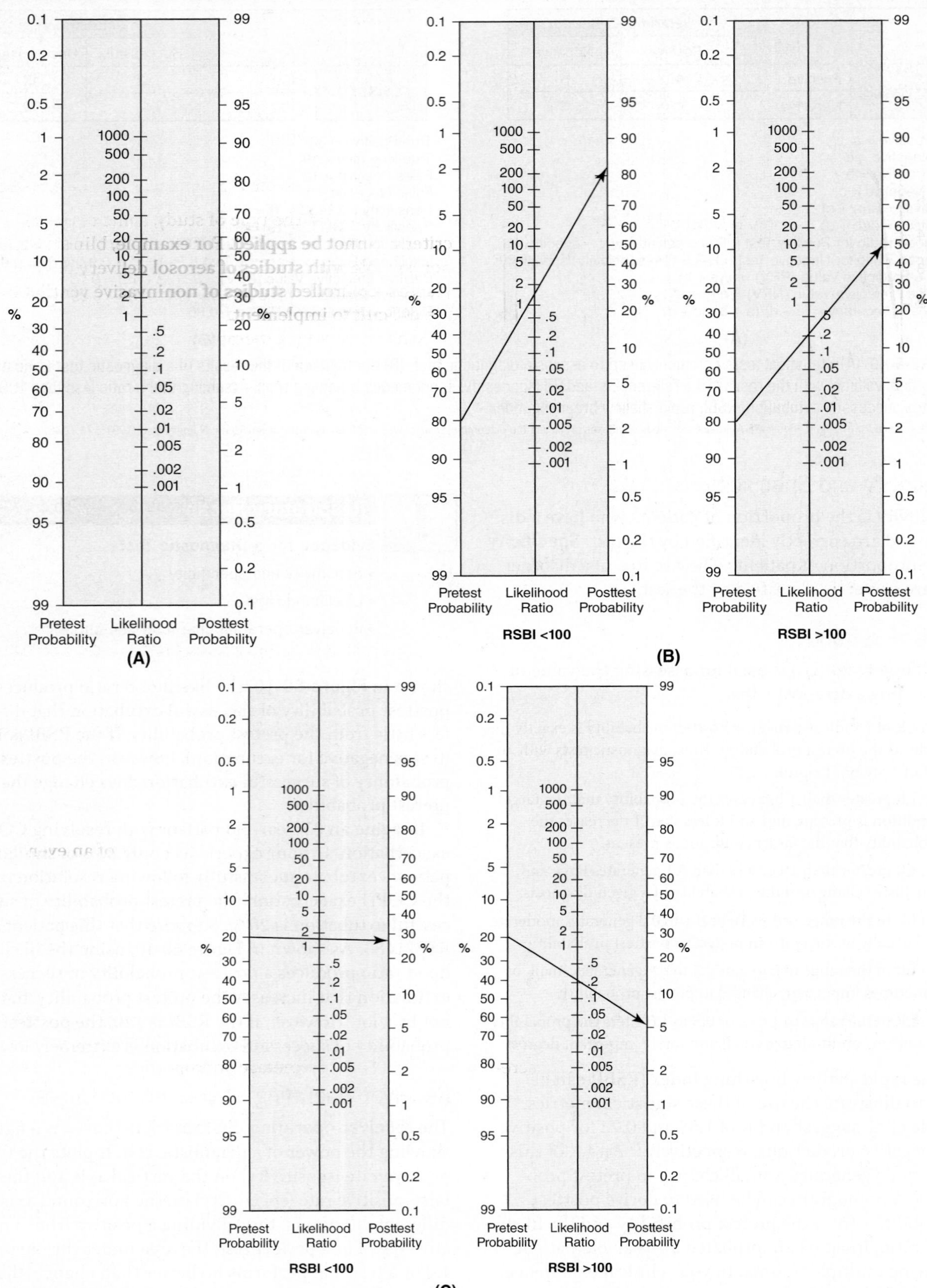

FIGURE 60-10 **(A)** A nomogram to determine posttest probability from pretest probability and likelihood ratio. **(B)** Patient recovering from acute respiratory distress syndrome (ARDS) with 80% pretest probability of weaning. The solid line represents the likelihood ratio. **(C)** Patient recovering from chronic obstructive pulmonary disease (COPD) with 20% pretest probability of weaning. The solid line represents the likelihood ratio. RSBI, rapid shallow breathing index.

(A, B, C) Information from Meade M, Guyatt G, Cook D, et al. Predicting success in weaning from mechanical ventilation. *Chest.* 2001;120:400S–424S.

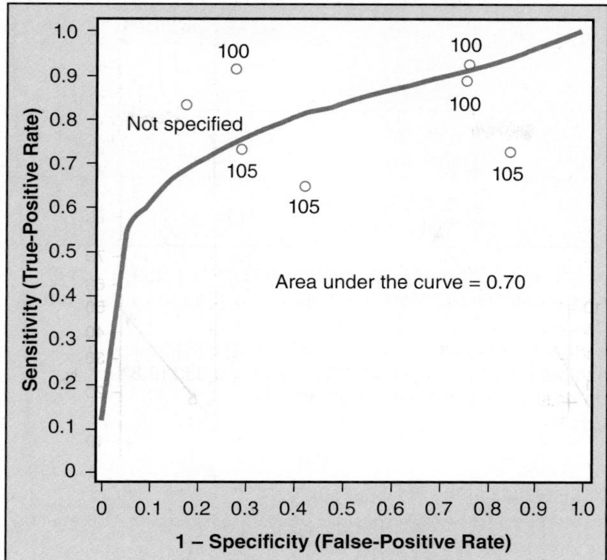

FIGURE 60-11 Summary receiver operating characteristic curve for the rapid shallow breathing index (RSBI) predicting successful extubation. The numbers in the figure represent the RSBI cut points from the various studies.

Reproduced from Meade M, et al. Predicting success in weaning from mechanical ventilation. *Chest.* 2001;120:400S–424S, with permission from the American College of Chest Physicians.

Evidence for a Therapy

High-level studies are prospective, randomized, blinded, placebo controlled, concealed allocation, and of parallel design and assess patient-important outcomes.

- *Prospective study:* Prospective investigation of the factors that might cause a disorder in which a cohort of individuals who do not have evidence of an outcome of interest but who are exposed to the putative cause are compared with a concurrent cohort who are also free of the outcome but not exposed to the putative cause. Both cohorts are then followed to compare the incidence of the outcome of interest.
- *Randomization:* Allocation of individuals to groups by chance, usually done with the aid of tables of random numbers. This differs from systematic allocation (e.g., even and odd days of the month) or allocation at the convenience or discretion of the investigator.
- *Blind (or blinded or masked):* The participant of interest is unaware of whether patients have been assigned to the experimental or control group. Patients, clinicians, those monitoring outcomes, assessors of outcomes, data analysts, and those writing the paper can all be blinded.
- *Placebo:* An intervention without biologically active attributes.
- *Concealment:* Randomization is concealed if the person who is making the decision about enrolling a patient is unaware of whether the next patient enrolled will be entered in the treatment or control group.
- *Parallel design:* With a parallel study design, subjects are randomly assigned to the treatment or control group, an intervention is applied, and the outcome is identified for each subject. This is different from a crossover study, in which subjects receive both the treatment and control intervention.

Depending on the type of study, some of these criteria cannot be applied. For example, blinding is not possible with studies of aerosol delivery devices. Placebo-controlled studies of noninvasive ventilation are difficult to implement.

When assessing a therapy, it is important to evaluate a patient-important outcome. Clinicians are often interested in physiologic outcomes such as an improvement in arterial blood gas results. Patients, on the other hand, are more interested in outcomes such as survival. There are a number of examples in which an improvement in physiologic outcomes does not correlate with patient-important outcomes. For patients with acute respiratory distress syndrome (ARDS), inhaled nitric oxide improves Pa_{O_2}, but not mortality.[26,27] High tidal volumes in patients with ARDS improve the Pa_{O_2}, but mortality is lower for small tidal volumes.[22]

Using the tools of evidence-based medicine, metrics such as event rate, relative risk, relative risk reduction, absolute risk reduction, number needed to treat, and odds ratio can be calculated.

- *Event rate:* The proportion of patients in a group in whom an event is observed. *Control event rate* and *experimental event rate* refer to this metric in control and experimental groups of patients, respectively.
- *Relative risk:* The ratio of the risk of an event among an experimental group to the risk among the control group. A relative risk less than 1 means benefit, a relative risk greater than 1 means harm, and a relative risk equal to 1 means the intervention has no effect.
- *Relative risk reduction:* An estimate of the proportion of baseline risk that is removed by the therapy.
- *Absolute risk reduction:* The difference in the absolute risk (percentage or proportion of patients with an outcome) in the exposed (experimental event rate) versus the unexposed (control event rate) group.
- *Number needed to treat:* The number of patients who need to be treated to prevent one bad outcome.
- *Odds ratio*: The ratio of the odds of an event in an exposed group to the odds of the same event in a group that is not exposed.
- *Survival curve:* Survival analysis involves the modeling of time to event data. In this context, death or failure is considered an event in the survival analysis literature. Survival analysis asks questions such as "What is the fraction of a population that

		Outcome	
		Present	Absent
Treatment	Present	a	b
	Absent	c	d

Control Event Rate (CER) = c/(c + d)
Experimental Event Rate (EER) = a/(a + b)
Relative Risk (RR) = EER/CER = [a/(a + b)] / [c/(c + d)]
Relative Risk Reduction (RRR) = 1 – RR
Absolute Risk Reduction (ARR) = c/(c + d) – a/(a + b)
Number Needed to Treat (NNT) = 1/ARR
Odds Ratio (OR) = (a × d) / (c × b)

(A)

		Outcome	
		Death at 28 days	Alive at 28 days
Treatment	6 mL/kg tidal volume	134	298
	12 mL/kg tidal volume	171	259

Control Group Mortality (12 mL/kg) = 171/(171 + 259) = 0.398
Experimental Group Mortality (6 mL/kg) = 134/(134 + 298) = 0.31
Relative Risk (RR) = 0.31/0.398 = 0.787
Relative Risk Reduction = 1 – 0.787 = 0.213 (21.3%)
Absolute Risk Reduction = 0.398 – 0.31 = 0.088 (8.8%)
Number Needed to Treat = 1/0.088 = 11
Odds Ratio = (134 × 259) / (171 × 298) = 0.68

(B)

FIGURE 60-12 (**A**) Statistical tests commonly used to assess a therapy. (**B**) The results of the ARDSnet study.

Information from the Acute Respiratory Distress Syndrome Network. Ventilation with lower tidal volumes as compared with traditional tidal volumes for acute lung injury and the acute respiratory distress syndrome. *N Engl J Med.* 2000;342:1301–1308.

will survive past a certain time?" In medicine, a typical application might involve grouping patients into categories and then determining whether one group dies more quickly than the other.

- *Confidence interval:* The range of values within which it is probable that the true value lies for the whole population of patients from which the study patients were selected. The confidence interval is affected by sample size and effect size (i.e., the difference in outcomes between the intervention and control groups divided by some measure of variability, typically the standard deviation). A larger sample size narrows the range of the confidence interval, increasing the precision of the study results. A larger sample size also decreases the risk of a type II (beta) error, in which the study fails to detect an important difference. High-level studies conduct a power analysis as part of the study design so that an appropriate sample size can be determined *a priori*.

The Acute Respiratory Distress Syndrome Network (ARDSnet) study can be used as an example (**Figure 60-12**).[22] In this study, 861 patients with ARDS were randomly assigned to be mechanically ventilated with a tidal volume of 12 mL/kg or 6 mL/kg. The primary outcome was mortality. Mortality for the control group (12 mL/kg tidal volume) was 39.8%, and mortality for the experimental group (6 mL/kg tidal volume) was 31%. The relative risk of mortality was lower for the 6 mL/kg group (0.787), with a relative risk reduction of 0.213 compared with the 12 mL/kg group. The absolute risk reduction for mortality was 8.8%, resulting in a number needed to treat of 11 patients. In other words, for every 11 mechanically ventilated patients with ARDS who received a tidal volume of 6 mL/kg (rather than 12 mL/kg), one additional life will be saved. The survival curves from this study are shown in **Figure 60-13**.

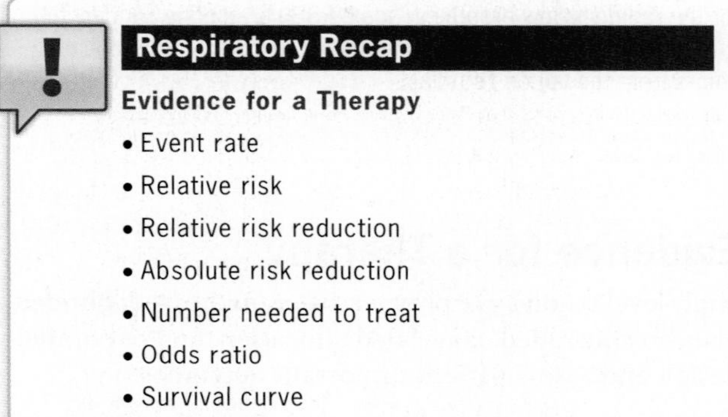

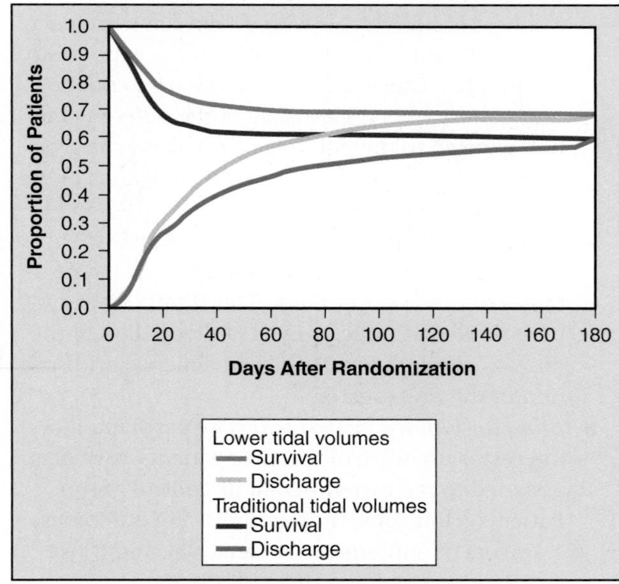

FIGURE 60-13 Probability of survival and of being discharged home and breathing without assistance during the first 180 days after randomization in patients with acute lung injury and the acute respiratory distress syndrome.

Reproduced from the Acute Respiratory Distress Syndrome Network. *N Engl J Med.* 2000;342:1301–1308. © 2000 Massachusetts Medical Society. Reprinted with permission from Massachusetts Medical Society.

Meta-Analysis

Clinical trials related to respiratory care are often expensive, and it may be difficult to recruit an adequate sample size to avoid a beta error. A **meta-analysis** uses statistical methods to combine the results of several studies into a single pooled metric. Meta-analysis is a statistical approach that combines the results of several independent studies. As with any study design, the question asked will influence the design and the method of meta-analysis. Because it is usually based on a literature review, the meta-analysis is observational rather than experimental in nature. The person conducting the meta-analysis has limited control over the availability of the data reported in individual studies. The studies included in the meta-analysis should be comparable, but the degree of comparability is subjective and determined by the person conducting the meta-analysis. Included studies should be identified from a comprehensive review of the literature, and unpublished data should ideally be included to reduce the risk of publication bias. Ideally, the meta-analysis will be conducted from the discrete data from the included studies, but more commonly it is conducted using summary data published in the individual studies.

One type of meta-analysis is a study-level meta-analysis, in which the summary outcomes of the individual studies are pooled. Alternatively, the meta-analysis can be an individual subject meta-analysis, where individual subject data are pooled across studies. An individual subject meta-analysis is more powerful and allows subgroup comparisons. A study-level meta-analysis found that treatment with higher versus lower levels of PEEP was not associated with improved hospital survival (**Figure 60-14**).[28] However, in an individual subject meta-analysis, higher levels of PEEP were associated with improved survival among the subgroup of patients with moderate and severe ARDS.[29]

The results of a meta-analysis are often displayed as a **forest plot** (see Figure 60-14). The name refers to the forest of lines produced. Forest plots are commonly presented with two columns. The left-hand column lists the names of the studies, commonly in chronological order from the top downward. The right-hand column is a plot of the measure of effect for each of these studies, often represented by a square, incorporating confidence intervals represented by horizontal lines. The graph often is plotted on a logarithmic scale when using ratio-based effect measures so that the confidence intervals are symmetrical about the means from each study. The size of each square is proportional to the study's weight in the meta-analysis. The overall measure of effect is commonly plotted as a diamond, the lateral points of which indicate confidence intervals for this estimate. A vertical line representing no effect is also plotted. If the confidence intervals for individual studies overlap with this line, it demonstrates that their effect sizes do not differ from no effect.

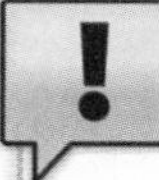

Respiratory Recap

Meta-Analysis

- Uses statistical methods to combine the results of several studies.
- Results are often displayed as a forest plot.

Finding the Evidence

Finding the evidence begins with a question.[30,31] There are two types of questions: background questions and foreground questions.[23] Background questions are those that might be answered by referring to a textbook or performing a basic Internet search. Examples include the following:

1. How many lobes are in the right lower lobe?
2. What are normal blood gas values for a newborn?
3. How does a noninvasive ventilator work?

Foreground questions are asked by more seasoned clinicians and require the ability to find the evidence, assess its validity, and determine whether it applies to

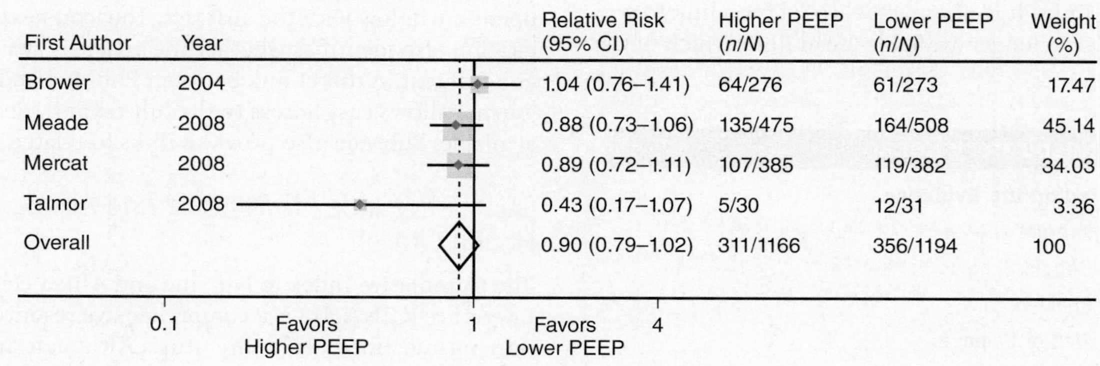

First Author
Year
Relative Risk (95% CI)
Higher PEEP (n/N)
Lower PEEP (n/N)
Weight (%)
Brower 2004 1.04 (0.76–1.41) 64/276 61/273 17.47
Meade 2008 0.88 (0.73–1.06) 135/475 164/508 45.14
Mercat 2008 0.89 (0.72–1.11) 107/385 119/382 34.03
Talmor 2008 0.43 (0.17–1.07) 5/30 12/31 3.36
Overall 0.90 (0.79–1.02) 311/1166 356/1194 100
0.1
Favors Higher PEEP
1
Favors Lower PEEP
4

FIGURE 60-14 Results of a study level meta-analysis comparing higher versus lower levels of PEEP in patients with ARDS.

Reproduced from Dasenbrook EC, Needham DM, Brower RG, Fan E. Higher PEEP in patients with acute lung injury: a systematic review and meta-analysis. *Respir Care.* 2011;56:568–575.

the unique patients seen by the clinician. Examples of foreground questions are as follows:

1. What is the current role of inhaled steroid therapy in patients with COPD?
2. How should positive end-expiratory pressure be set when ventilating a patient with ARDS?
3. Should NIV be used in patients with hypoxemic respiratory failure?

Internet Search

The Internet is a confederation of networks around the world that allows computers connected to the Internet to communicate with other computers across the Internet. Browsers such as Internet Explorer and Safari access documents called Web pages that are linked to each other via hyperlinks.

A common method to find information is a basic Web search. Many search engines are available free of charge, and the choice of one over the other is based on personal preference. A commonly used search engine is Google (www.google.com). Because Google returns only Web pages that contain all the words in the query, refining or narrowing the search is done by adding more words to the search terms. The result is a smaller subset of the pages found by Google for the original broad query. It is important to choose key words carefully.

- Try the obvious words first. For information on noninvasive positive pressure ventilation, enter "noninvasive ventilation" rather than "mechanical ventilation."
- Use words that are likely to appear on a website with the information you want. "BiPAP" gets more specific results than "equipment for noninvasive ventilation."
- Choose key words that are as specific as possible. "Noninvasive positive pressure ventilation" gets more relevant results than "positive pressure ventilation."

Conducting a Web search is a quick way to find lots of information. In fact, the amount of information obtained can be overwhelming and involve a considerable amount of time filtering through Web pages and hypertext links. It is not unusual to follow a link to a page that is no longer available (dead link). Much of the information that is found may be irrelevant. Moreover, the validity of information may be suspect. Information posted on the Web may be outdated or incorrect; it is almost never subjected to peer review.

> **Respiratory Recap**
>
> **Finding the Evidence**
>
> - Internet search
> - Google Scholar
> - PubMed
> - Web of Science
> - Ovid
> - Journal websites

Google Scholar

Google Scholar (http://scholar.google.com) is a freely accessible Web search engine that indexes the full text of scholarly literature across an array of publishing formats and disciplines. Scholarly searches appear using the references from full-text journal articles, technical reports, preprints, theses, books, and other documents that are deemed to be scholarly.

PubMed

PubMed (www.pubmed.gov) provides access to citations to medical journals dating to the mid-1960s and includes links to many sites that provide full-text articles and other related resources. To search PubMed, enter search terms in the site's query box (**Figure 60-15**). The search rules are straightforward:

- Enter one or more search terms.
- Enter author names in the format "Hess DR" (initials are optional).
- Enter journal titles in full or using abbreviations.

A search strategy helps identify the information needed. First, identify the key concepts and search those terms. Then consider alternative terms and search those. It may then be useful to refine the search to dates, study groups, and other limits as appropriate. The Boolean operators "AND," "OR," and "NOT" can be used to refine the search. There is no right or wrong way to do a search. Search strategies differ according to personal choice, and efficient searching requires practice and a systematic approach.

Note that PubMed provides some suggestions for additional searches to the right of the screen. This can be helpful to refine your search. Using the Limits feature of PubMed, one can limit the search to citations in English. Using the Advanced feature, one can search for papers in a specific journal. Clicking on the citation opens a window with the abstract. The icon next to the citation also identifies whether the article is available as a full text. A direct link between PubMed and the journal allows easy access to the full-text article if it is available. PubMed also provides links to related papers.

Cumulative Index to Nursing and Allied Health Literature

The Cumulative Index to Nursing and Allied Health Literature (CINAHL) is a comprehensive resource for nursing and allied health literature. Although there is considerable overlap between PubMed and CINAHL, there are a number of nursing and allied health journals listed in CINAHL that are not found in PubMed.

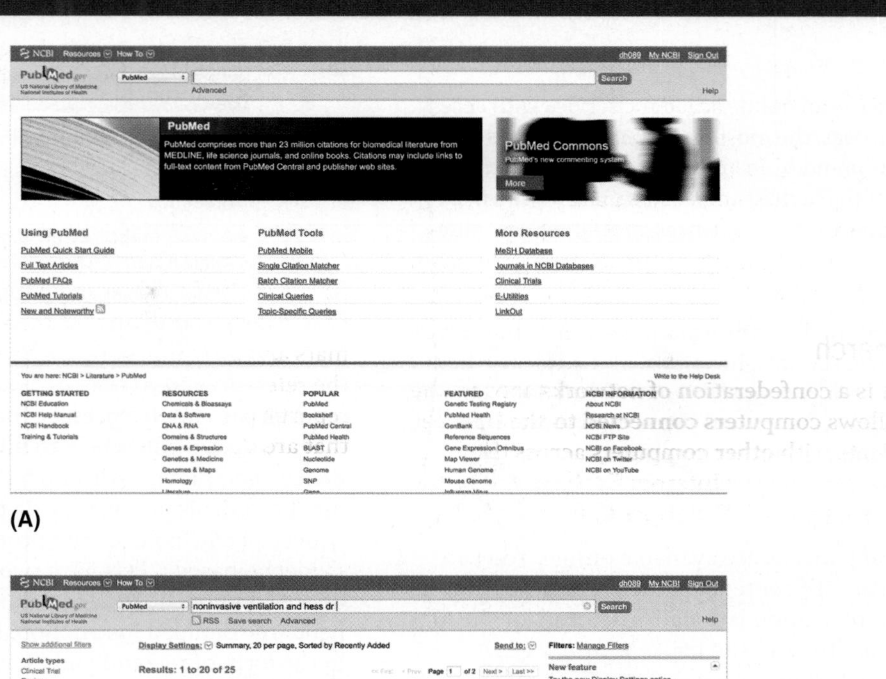

(A)

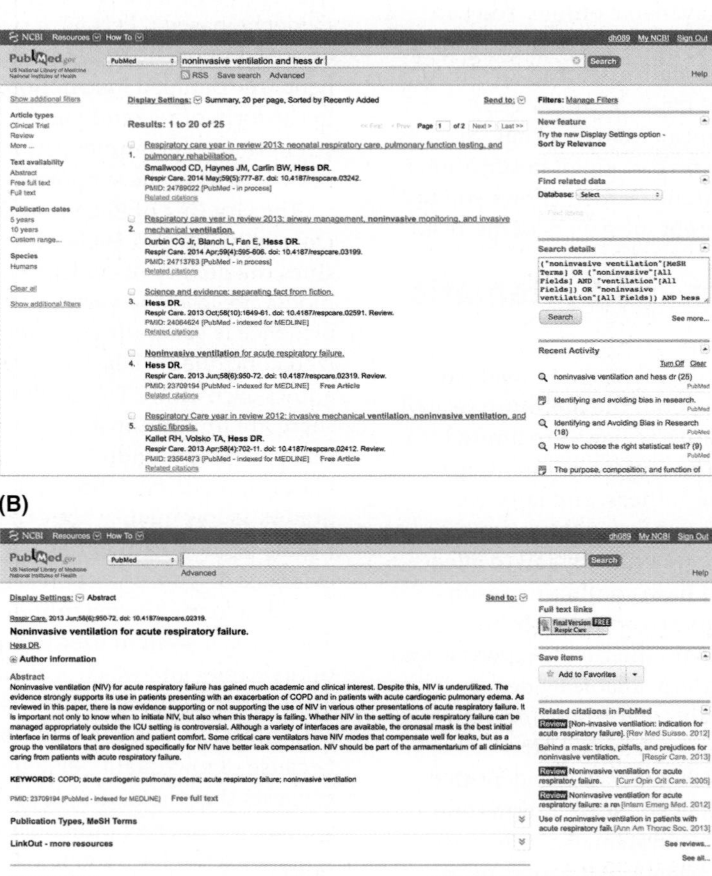

(B)

(C)

FIGURE 60-15 (**A**) The PubMed home page. (**B**) The results of a PubMed search. (**C**) When a citation is clicked, note the "Related citations" links on the side of the window.

Courtesy National Library of Medicine.

Web of Science

Web of Science is an online academic service with access to seven databases, the most important of which is the Science Citation Index. Its multidisciplinary content covers over 10,000 of the highest-impact journals worldwide. It covers the sciences, social sciences, arts, and humanities.

Ovid

Ovid provides medical information services to individuals in medical schools, hospitals, and academic institutions. Ovid offers content in more than 3000 ebooks, more than 1200 peer-reviewed journals, and more than 100 bibliographic and full-text databases.

Journal Websites

Most medical journals are available online. You can access the journal's content via the journal website, although a subscription is usually required for the most recent content. The website for *Respiratory Care* (www.rcjournal.com) is typical. Many journal websites provide the opportunity to receive email notifications of the journal's table of contents, which allows you to survey the most recent content for papers of interest.

Narrative Reviews and Systematic Reviews

Review papers are commonly published in medical journals and summarize in detail the literature related to a subject matter.[32] Narrative reviews are limited by incomplete searches of the literature, intentional or unintentional bias by the authors, and failure to account for the quality of individual publications. Additionally, narrative reviews typically fail to effectively deal with studies that have conflicting results. Narrative reviews by experts are notoriously biased because experts tend to rely on their own expertise and experience rather than on the available evidence.

A **systematic review** is different from a narrative review in purpose and process. A systematic review details the methods by which papers were identified in the literature. This includes the search terms and the search engines utilized. A systematic review uses predetermined criteria for selection of papers to be included in the review. Explicit methods for appraising the literature are used to evaluate the quality and validity of individual studies. Many systematic reviews include a quantitative review of the literature in the form of a meta-analysis. The Cochrane Collaboration (www.cochrane.org) is a good source of high-level systematic reviews and meta-analyses.

Clinical Practice Guidelines

Clinical practice guidelines (CPGs) are systematically developed statements to help clinicians deliver appropriate care in specific clinical circumstances.[33] Well-designed CPGs help to fill the gap between evidence and practice. Although the CPGs are not treatment protocols per se, they do provide a context within which specific policies and protocols can be developed. Evidence-based CPGs have two components: the evidence component and the detailed instructional component. The detailed instructional component is expressed in the form of recommendations. Furthermore, the strength of a recommendation is given a grade based on the strength of the supporting evidence.

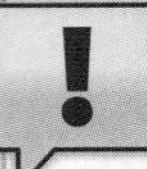

Respiratory Recap

Reviews and Clinical Practice Guidelines

- Narrative reviews are often incomplete and biased.
- A systematic review uses explicit methods to search and appraise the literature.
- Clinical practice guidelines provide recommendations for care.

The Grading of Recommendations Assessment, Development, and Evaluation (GRADE) system classifies the quality of evidence using four levels: high, moderate, low, and very low.[34,35] The highest-quality evidence is generally considered to arise from randomized controlled trials. However, the GRADE system allows even an RCT to be downgraded in strength if there are important study limitations (e.g., inconsistency of results, indirectness of evidence, reporting bias, imprecision). Observational studies are usually graded as low quality but can be upgraded if the magnitude of the treatment effect is very large, if there is evidence of a dose–response relationship, or if all biases would increase the magnitude of a treatment effect. The GRADE system uses two grades of recommendations, strong and weak. A strong recommendation is given when desirable effects clearly outweigh undesirable effects. When the trade-offs are less certain, either because of low-quality evidence or because evidence suggests that the desirable and undesirable effects are similar, a weak recommendation is given. Many professional societies have adopted GRADE for writing clinical practice guidelines.

A number of CPGs have been published by the American Association for Respiratory Care and can be found at www.rcjournal.com. The National Guideline Clearinghouse (www.guideline.gov) is a comprehensive database of evidence-based CPGs and related documents produced by the U.S. Department of Health and Human Services Agency for Healthcare Research and Quality. Several sources can be searched for evidence-based systematic reviews and clinical practice guidelines. PubMed can be searched using the limits of "meta-analysis" or "practice guideline."

Key Points

- A study design is a plan for conducting the study that avoids bias and attempts to answer the study question or questions.
- Statistics are necessary to describe and display results and to show that the study's conclusions apply elsewhere.
- Studies are reported in a range of formats that reflect the design features and the overall importance of the findings.
- Evidence-based respiratory care is the integration of individual clinical expertise with the best available research evidence from systematic research and a patient's values and expectations.
- A hierarchy of evidence can be used to assess the strength upon which clinical decisions are made.
- To evaluate a diagnostic test, metrics such as sensitivity, specificity, receiver operating characteristic curves, and likelihood ratios are calculated.
- High-level studies are prospective, randomized, blinded, placebo controlled, concealed allocation, and of parallel design and assess patient-important outcomes.
- When assessing a therapy, it is important to evaluate a patient-important outcome.
- To evaluate a therapy, metrics such as event rate, relative risk, relative risk reduction, absolute risk reduction, number needed to treat, and odds ratio can be calculated.
- A meta-analysis uses statistical methods to combine the results of several studies into a single pooled metric.
- A number of electronic search strategies can be used to find the best evidence.
- A systematic review details the methods by which papers were identified in the literature, uses predetermined criteria for selection of papers to be included in the review, and uses explicit methods for appraising the literature based on the quality and validity of individual studies.
- Clinical practice guidelines are systematically developed statements to help clinicians deliver appropriate care in specific clinical circumstances.

References

1. Hess DR. What is evidence-based medicine and why should I care? *Respir Care.* 2004:730–741.
2. Hess DR. Science and evidence: separating fact from fiction. *Respir Care.* 2013;58:1649–1661.
3. Donowitz LG. Handwashing technique in a pediatric intensive care unit. *Am J Dis Child.* 1987;141:683–685.
4. Enfield KB, Truwit JD. The purpose, composition, and function of an institutional review board: balancing priorities. *Respir Care.* 2008;53:1330–1336.
5. Dushoff J, Plotkin JB, Viboud C, et al. Mortality due to influenza in the United States—an annualized regression approach using multiple-cause mortality data. *Am J Epidemiol.* 2006;163: 181–187.
6. Halbert RJ, Isonaka S, George D, et al. Interpreting COPD prevalence estimates: what is the true burden of disease? *Chest.* 2003;123:1684–1692.
7. Ely EW, Baker AM, Dunagan DP, et al. Effect on the duration of mechanical ventilation of identifying patients capable of breathing spontaneously. *N Engl J Med.* 1996;335:1864–1869.
8. Stein N, Matz H, Schneeweiss A, et al. An evaluation of a transcutaneous and an end-tidal capnometer for noninvasive monitoring of spontaneously breathing patients. *Respir Care.* 2006;51:1162–1166.
9. Nayak BK, Hazra A. How to choose the right statistical test? *Indian J Ophthalmol.* 2011;59:85–86.
10. Pannucci CJ, Wilkins EG. Identifying and avoiding bias in research. *Plast Reconstr Surg.* 2010;126:619–625.
11. Pierson DJ. How to read a case report (or teaching case of the month). *Respir Care.* 2009;54:1372–1378.
12. Bickelmann AG, Burwell CS, Robin ED, et al. Extreme obesity associated with alveolar hypoventilation: a Pickwickian syndrome. *Am J Med.* 1956;21:811–818.
13. Petty TL, Ashbaugh DG. The adult respiratory distress syndrome. Clinical features, factors influencing prognosis and principles of management. *Chest.* 1971;60:233–239.
14. Zamanian M, Marini JJ. Pressure-flow signatures of central-airway mucus plugging. Case report. *Crit Care Med.* 2006;34: 223–226.
15. U.S. Department of Health and Human Services, Centers for Disease Control and Prevention, National Center for Health Statistics. *Health, United States, 2008.* Available at: http://www.cdc.gov/nchs/data/hus/hus08.pdf#063. Accessed September 29, 2014.
16. Hankinson JL, Odencrantz JR, Fedan KB. Spirometric reference values from a sample of the general U.S. population. *Am J Respir Crit Care Med.* 1999;159:179–187.
17. Preis SR, Hwang SJ, Coady S, et al. Trends in all-cause and cardiovascular disease mortality among women and men with and without diabetes mellitus in the Framingham Heart Study, 1950 to 2005. *Circulation.* 2009;119:1728–1735.
18. Kohansal R, Martinez-Camblor P, Agusti A, et al. The natural history of chronic airflow obstruction revisited: an analysis of the Framingham offspring cohort. *Am J Respir Crit Care Med.* 2009;180:3–10.
19. Institute of Laboratory Animal Resources. *Guide for the Care and Use of Laboratory Animals.* Washington, DC: National Academies Press; 1996.
20. Rubenfeld GD, Cooper C, Carter G, et al. Barriers to providing lung-protective ventilation to patients with acute lung injury. *Crit Care Med.* 2004;32:1289–1293.
21. Kallet RH. What is the legacy of the National Institutes of Health Acute Respiratory Distress Syndrome Network? *Respir Care.* 2009;54:912–924.
22. The Acute Respiratory Distress Syndrome Network. Ventilation with lower tidal volumes as compared with traditional tidal volumes for acute lung injury and the acute respiratory distress syndrome. *N Engl J Med.* 2000;342:1301–1308.
23. Guyatt G, Drummond R, Meade M, Cook D. *Users' Guides to the Medical Literature: Essentials of Evidence-Based Clinical Practice.* 2nd ed. New York: McGraw-Hill; 2008.
24. Yang KL, Tobin MJ. A prospective study of indexes predicting the outcome of trials of weaning from mechanical ventilation. *N Engl J Med.* 1991;324:1445–1450.
25. Meade M, Guyatt G, Cook D, et al. Predicting success in weaning from mechanical ventilation. *Chest.* 2001;120:400S–424S.
26. Adhikari NK, Burns KE, Friedrich JO, et al. Effect of nitric oxide on oxygenation and mortality in acute lung injury: systematic review and meta-analysis. *BMJ.* 2007;334:779.
27. Adhikari NKJ, Dellinger RP, Lundin S, et al. Inhaled nitric oxide does not reduce mortality in patients with acute respiratory distress syndrome regardless of severity: systematic review and meta-analysis. *Crit Care Med.* 2014;42:404–412.

28. Dasenbrook EC, Needham DM, Brower RG, Fan E. Higher PEEP in patients with acute lung injury: a systematic review and meta-analysis. *Respir Care*. 2011;56:568–575.
29. Briel M, Meade M, Mercat A, et al. Higher vs lower positive end-expiratory pressure in patients with acute lung injury and acute respiratory distress syndrome: systematic review and meta-analysis. *JAMA*. 2010;303:865–873.
30. Hess DR. Information retrieval in respiratory care: tips to locate what you need to know. *Respir Care*. 2004;49:389–400.
31. Chatburn RL. How to find the best evidence. *Respir Care*. 2009;54:1360–1365.
32. Callcut RA, Branson RD. How to read a review paper. *Respir Care*. 2009;54:1379–1385.
33. Hess DR. Evidence-based clinical practice guidelines: where's the evidence and what do I do with it? *Respir Care*. 2003;48: 838–839.
34. Guyatt GH, Oxman AD, Vist GE, et al. GRADE: an emerging consensus on rating quality of evidence and strength of recommendations. *BMJ*. 2008;336:924–926.
35. Restrepo RD. AARC clinical practice guidelines: from "reference-based" to "evidence-based." *Respir Care*. 2010;55:787–788.

Glossary

A

a wave On the central venous pressure tracing, the wave created by the increased atrial pressure during right atrial contraction. It correlates with the P wave on an electrocardiogram.

AARC Code of Ethics The professional policy document of the American Association for Respiratory Care that describes ethical behaviors for respiratory therapists that should guide professional practice.

AARC Times The premier news and feature magazine of the respiratory care profession, which includes management tips, educational articles, human interest features, how-to articles, profiles of leaders in the profession, reports on current government trends, and job opportunities nationwide.

abdominal muscles Muscles in addition to those directly involved in respiration that nevertheless aid in expiration, including the rectus abdominis, external and internal oblique muscles, and the transversus abdominis muscles, which depress the lower ribs, increase intra-abdominal pressure, and flex the thoracic spine.

absorption The incorporation of a substance in one state into another substance in a different state, such as a liquid being absorbed by a solid or a gas being absorbed by a liquid.

accessory muscles Muscles outside the principal respiratory muscles that nevertheless affect inspiration, including the pectoralis minor and major (innervated by C5 through C8 and T1), the serratus anterior (innervated by C5 through C7), and the erector spinae, which all help raise the ribs, push the sternum forward and upward, and straighten the concavity of the thoracic spine.

accreditation A voluntary process intended to help establish and maintain the standards and expectations for all allied health education programs. Although accreditation is voluntary, the National Board for Respiratory Care requires graduation from an accredited educational program for eligibility for its credentialing examinations for individual professionals.

acetylcholine The neurotransmitter that stimulates skeletal muscle to contract.

acid A compound that donates or yields a hydrogen ion (H^+) in an aqueous solution.

acid-fast bacilli (AFB) Bacteria in which the cell wall, because of the presence of waxes such as mycolic acid, retains a red carbolfuchsin stain despite rinsing with hydrochloric acid. Acid-fast bacteria are considered neither gram positive nor gram negative.

acid maltase deficiency Type II glycogen storage disease that arises because of a deficiency of the lysosomal enzyme responsible for the hydrolysis of glycogen.

acidosis A pathologic condition resulting from the accumulation of acid or depletion of alkaline reserve (bicarbonate) in the blood and tissues; it is characterized by a low blood pH.

acinus A small, sac-like structure that serves as the gas-exchanging portion of the lung.

acoustic technology Noninvasive and continuous monitoring of the respiration rate using an adhesive sensor with an integrated acoustic transducer applied to the patient's neck.

activated partial thromboplastin time (aPTT) A direct way of evaluating overall coagulation status; used to assess the intrinsic clotting pathway, especially the early stages involving factors XII, XI, IX, and VIII. This measurement is often used to monitor patients on heparin therapy.

active cycle of breathing A breathing maneuver that combines breathing control, thoracic expansion control, and forced expiration technique.

active error An error that occurs at the point of contact between a human and some aspect of a larger system (e.g., a human–machine interface). Such errors are generally readily apparent (e.g., pushing an incorrect button, ignoring a warning light) and almost always involve someone at the front line.

active humidifier A humidification device in which energy (heat) is used to add water to the inspired gas.

acute respiratory distress syndrome (ARDS) A respiratory disorder characterized by the abrupt onset of respiratory distress. It is associated with severe hypoxemia and diffuse pulmonary opacities on chest radiograph that are not caused by congestive heart failure or volume overload; Pa_{O_2}/F_{IO_2} <300 mm Hg.

adaptive pressure control A volume feedback mechanism for pressure-controlled or pressure-supported breaths. The desired tidal volume is set, and the ventilator adjusts the inspiratory pressure to deliver the minimal target tidal volume.

adaptive support ventilation (ASV) A mode of ventilation in which the ventilator automatically selects tidal volume and frequency on the basis of the respiratory system mechanics and target minute ventilation.

adenocarcinoma Any one of a large group of malignant epithelial cell tumors.

adenosine triphosphate (ATP) A high-energy triphosphate that is the main molecule used to store energy; it supplies energy directly to the energy-using reactions of all cells in all kinds of living organisms.

adjuvant therapy A substance, especially a drug, added to a prescription to assist in the action of the main ingredient; also, an additional treatment or therapy.

adsorption The ability to hold substances to a surface.

advance directive A document to be used on a patient's behalf, in the absence of competency, specifying which treatments the patient does or does not want in such a case and sometimes, in some states, specifying a surrogate to make decisions in the event that the patient cannot. See also *durable medical power of attorney*.

advanced cardiovascular life support (ACLS) Treatment implemented after a patient experiences cardiac arrest. It includes (1) maintaining the airway with equipment and advanced techniques, (2) monitoring the electrocardiogram and recognizing dysrhythmias, (3) using conventional defibrillators, and (4) administering supplemental oxygen and drugs via parenteral or endotracheal routes.

aerobe A free-living organism that requires oxygen for its survival.

aerosol A suspension of solid or liquid particles in a gas.

affective domain The area of learning involved in appreciation, interests, and attitudes. This domain describes the way people react emotionally and their ability to feel another person's pain or joy.

afferent impulses Impulses that are carried toward a central organ.

afferent neuron A neuron that conveys information from tissues and organs into the central nervous system.

afterload Resistance in the circulation against which the ventricle must eject blood during contraction; the load that opposes myocardial shortening.

air bronchogram A radiographic abnormality in the image of the bronchi that occurs when the alveolar airspaces become filled with fluid, causing increased contrast between the air-filled bronchi and the adjacent fluid-filled lung parenchyma, rendering the bronchi lucent and projecting them as branching tubular air-filled structures.

air-entrainment mask An oxygen delivery device in which air is entrained proportional to oxygen flow for a fixed oxygen concentration delivered to the patient.

air leak syndrome The movement of gas from the lungs into spaces where it is not normally present; includes pneumothorax, pneumomediastinum, pneumopericardium, pneumoperitoneum, pulmonary interstitial emphysema, and subcutaneous emphysema.

air-oxygen blender A mechanical device designed to proportion air and oxygen to a specific concentration.

air-to-oxygen mix ratio The proportion of oxygen and air required to produce a specific oxygen concentration.

air trapping A condition in the lungs in which air is not exhaled because of decreased lung elasticity and increased expiratory airway resistance; it is accompanied by hyperinflation.

airborne precautions Actions taken to prevent the transmission of infectious agents over a long distance when those pathogens are suspended in the air.

airway cuff An inflatable balloon that surrounds the endotracheal tube (or tracheostomy tube) near its distal end to seal the airway for mechanical ventilation and to minimize aspiration.

airway hyperresponsiveness A marker associated with asthma that is responsive to both specific and nonspecific factors (such as environment, exercise, allergens, and viral infections), whereby the airways constrict too easily and frequently.

airway inflammation A condition that exacerbates asthmatic reactions through the release of mediators, including mast cells, eosinophils, macrophages, epithelial cells, and T lymphocytes, resulting in recurrent exacerbations that manifest as wheezing, progressive shortness of breath, chest tightness, and coughing; may be classified as acute, subacute, or chronic.

airway pressure release ventilation (APRV) A mode of ventilation that is time cycled and pressure controlled. An active exhalation valve allows the patient to breathe spontaneously throughout the ventilator-imposed pressures. This mode is often used with a long inspiratory:expiratory timing pattern.

airway stent An endobronchial device designed to maintain the patency of the airway in the presence of central airways obstruction due to benign or malignant causes.

airways resistance (Raw) Pressure difference developed per unit flow as gas flows into or out of the lungs; normally, it is less than 2.4 cm H_2O/L/s at 0.5 L/s. Measurements of Raw can complement other tests evaluating airway responsiveness to bronchial provocation or bronchodilation.

alarm fatigue A decrease in attentiveness and sensitivity to the daily cacophony of bells, beeps, and tones from medical devices that overwhelms medical personnel with information and desensitizes them to the alarms themselves.

albuterol A β_2-agonist medication used as a treatment for asthma, COPD, and other obstructive lung diseases.

alkalosis A pathologic condition resulting from the accumulation of base or loss of acid without a comparable loss of base in the body fluids; it is characterized by a high blood pH.

all-patient refined diagnosis-related groups (APR-DRGs) An enhancement of the original diagnosis-related groups (DRGs), designed to apply to a population broader than that of Medicare beneficiaries; it includes four subclasses to each original DRG to address the severity of illness and the risk of mortality.

allele Either of a pair or alternative forms of a gene.

Allen test A test performed before radial arterial puncture or cannulation to ascertain whether there is adequate ulnar artery perfusion to the hand.

allergen Common triggering mechanism for asthmatic reactions; can be indoor factors (e.g., mold, animal dander, cleaning chemicals, cockroach antigen, dust mites) or outdoor factors (e.g., noxious fumes, grass, tree pollens).

allograft A skin graft in which the skin being used comes from the patient being treated, a technique that eliminates the rise of rejection of foreign tissue.

alpha$_1$-antitrypsin (AAT) deficiency A condition in which the liver does not produce sufficient amounts of α_1-antitrypsin, a plasma protein that inhibits trypsin and other proteolytic enzymes; deficiency is associated with the development of emphysema.

alveolar stage The final stage of lung development, generally considered to last from birth to 8 years of age.

alveoli Small sacs through which gas exchange takes place between alveolar gas and capillary blood; composed of type I and type II cells.

American Academy of Sleep Medicine (AASM) A professional society dedicated exclusively to the medical subspecialty of sleep medicine that sets standards; it promotes excellence in health care, education, and research.

American Association for Respiratory Care (AARC) The primary professional organization for respiratory care. The AARC and related organizations contribute to the scientific basis, governance, stature, and future growth of respiratory care; assist chartered affiliates in their efforts to pursue meaningful, nonrestrictive licensure; and promote the sequential functions of higher education—namely, research, archiving, and dissemination of knowledge.

American Respiratory Care Foundation (ARCF) A trusteeship that administers awards, education recognition, fellowships, and grants as well as provides financial support of the consensus and special proceedings conferences of the American Association for Respiratory Care.

American Standard Safety System (ASSS) A system for categorizing the connections on compressed air cylinders that uses a combination of the following factors specific for each gas or gas combination contained in the cylinder: diameter of the outlet, number of threads per inch, whether the outlet has right-handed or left-handed threads, whether the threads are external or internal, and the shape of the mating nipple on the corresponding regulator.

amino acid The basic building block of proteins. Its structure consists of a carbon atom (the alpha carbon) to which are bonded an amino group (NH_2), a carboxyl group (COOH), a hydrogen atom, and a side chain that constitutes the unique and identifying characteristic of the amino acid.

amplifier Any device that changes (usually increases) the amplitude of a signal. An amplifier multiplies an input signal with a constant, which is usually in the range of 2 to 1000. The amplification factor is referred to as gain and can be expressed as V_{out}/V_{in}.

amyotrophic lateral sclerosis (ALS) A progressive neurodegenerative disorder of both upper and lower motor neurons leading to a loss of skeletal muscle strength, including the respiratory muscles.

anabolism The synthesis process that assembles precursor molecules, such as amino acids, sugars, fatty acids, and nitrogenous bases, into cell macromolecules, such as proteins, polysaccharides, lipids, and nucleic acids.

anaerobe A free-living organism that requires an absence of oxygen. Anaerobes are thought to be a minor cause of community-acquired pneumonia but are becoming increasingly important in nosocomial pneumonia and ventilator-associated pneumonia.

analysis method An ethics theory that combines key components from the teleological and deontological theories, asserting that in the final analysis, most ethical decisions are made by a systematic analytic process devised by the individual.

Andrews, Albert H. A Chicago-based otolaryngologist who promoted education in inhalation therapy.

angina A choking, crushing, painful feeling most often associated with cardiac pain caused by hypoxia of the myocardium.

anion A negatively charged ion that is attracted to the positive electrode (anode) in electrolysis; a negatively charged atom, molecule, or radical.

anion gap (AG) The difference between the concentrations of serum cations and anions such that the anion gap = $([Na^+] + [K^+]) - ([HCO_3^-] + [Cl^-])$. If the anion gap exceeds 12 mmol/L, excessive unmeasured anions are likely present. Because its concentration is normally low, $[K^+]$ is often omitted from this calculation.

anteroposterior (AP) projection A chest radiographic view in which the x-ray beam passes through the chest from the front to the back.

anthropometry Study of human body measurements and components, including measurement of height, weight, body mass index, midarm muscle circumference, skinfold thicknesses, and skeletal breadths.

antibiotic A chemical substance capable of inhibiting the growth of, or killing, certain microorganisms but generally nontoxic enough to be used chemotherapeutically in the treatment of infectious diseases.

antibiotic resistance The ability of bacteria and fungi to withstand the effects of antibiotics that would normally kill them or limit their growth.

anticholinergic agent Any agent that blocks the parasympathetic nerves. Such drugs are often used as bronchodilators, delivered by inhalation (e.g., ipratropium bromide for chronic obstructive pulmonary disease). They decrease both bronchial and upper airway secretions. Such agents act through the blockade of acetylcholine receptors, which results in the inhibition of the transmission of parasympathetic nerve impulses; they function by competing with the neurotransmitter acetylcholine for its receptor sites at synaptic junctions.

anticoagulant Any substance that in vivo or in vitro suppresses, delays, or nullifies the coagulation of blood.

anticoagulation Use of an agent that prevents or delays coagulation of the blood.

antigen detection Technique that is applied to sputum, serum, urine, and body fluid samples to help in the rapid identification of pathogens that may be difficult to culture or pathogens scarcely growing due to prior antibiotic treatment. It is most valuable in the diagnosis of difficult-to-culture organisms such as *Mycoplasma pneumoniae, Legionella pneumophila, Chlamydophila pneumoniae,* and viral pneumonias.

antihistamine A drug or substance capable of reducing the physiologic and pharmacologic effects of histamine, including a wide variety of drugs that block histamine receptors.

anti-immunoglobulin E An antibody class used as a pharmacologic therapy to treat respiratory disease.

antimicrobial An agent that kills microorganisms or inhibits their growth.

antisepsis The use of chemical agents (antiseptics) to inhibit microbial growth.

aorta The largest artery in the body; it arises in the left ventricle of the heart and splits into the common iliac arteries that go to the legs.

aortic bodies Peripheral chemoreceptors located in the aortic arch that are innervated by the vagus nerve; they contribute to the control of breathing.

aortic valve A valve located at the base of the aorta; it has three cusps, and opens to allow blood to leave the left ventricle during contraction.

Apgar, Virginia Developer of a newborn infant scoring system based on physical assessment.

Apgar score A system used to assess the heart rate, respiratory effort, muscle tone, reflex irritability, and color in newborns.

apical lordotic A chest radiographic view that provides a good view of the lung apex, lingula, and right middle lobe.

apnea Cessation of airflow (*a*: absence; *pnea*: breathing).

apnea of prematurity Category or type of cessation of airflow in a premature infant's breathing. Its resolution may be determined more by the maturation of the respiratory control center than by an underlying disease process. Prevalence is higher at lower gestational ages and may be the result of an immature respiratory control system. This apnea is manifested by frequent periodic breathing, a decreased ventilatory response to CO_2, and a depression of respiration produced by hypoxemia.

apneustic breathing A prolonged inspiration with a shortened expiratory time; it may be caused by cerebral edema, acute poliomyelitis, and medications that cause central nervous system depression.

apneustic center The portion of the lower pons that stimulates the inspiratory neurons of the dorsal and ventral respiratory groups.

apoptosis Programmed cell death.

ARDS Network (ARDSnet) A clinical research network developed by the National Heart, Lung, and Blood Institute of the National Institutes of Health to accelerate the development of successful management strategies for acute respiratory distress syndrome.

arousal index A value derived from the data gathered during a polysomnogram: the number of arousals divided by the total sleep time, expressed in arousals per hour, which normally should be less than 15.

arousals Sudden changes from sleep to wakefulness or from a deeper stage of nonrapid eye movement sleep to a lighter stage, characterized by an abrupt shift in electroencephalographic frequency.

arterial blood gas (ABG) A blood component whose primary measurements (Po_2, Pco_2, and pH) provide important information about oxygenation, ventilation, and acid–base status.

arterial blood pressure One of the four vital signs. Monitoring techniques range from intermittent manual determinations using sphygmomanometry to use of automated noninvasive devices or an indwelling arterial catheter providing continuous measurement and waveform graphics.

artery An elastic vessel able to carry blood away from the heart under high pressure.

artificial nose A passive humidifier, also known as a heat and moisture exchanger (HME), that captures exhaled heat and moisture and transfers part of that heat and humidity to the next inspired breath. It can include condensers, hygroscopic condensers, and hygrophobic condensers.

aspiration pneumonia A respiratory inflammation and infection caused by inhalation of bacteria-rich oropharyngeal or gastric secretions.

assisted breath A breath during which all or part of inspiratory (or expiratory) flow is generated by the ventilator doing work for the patient.

Association of Asthma Educators (AAE) A professional society that promotes asthma education as an integral component of a comprehensive asthma program to raise the competence of healthcare professionals who educate individuals and families affected by asthma and to raise the standard of care and quality of asthma education delivered to those with asthma.

asthma A chronic inflammatory disorder of the airways in which many cells and cellular elements play a role—in particular, mast cells, eosinophils, T lymphocytes, macrophages, neutrophils, and epithelial cells. It causes recurrent episodes of wheezing, breathlessness, chest tightness, and coughing, particularly at night or in the early morning.

asthma education program A plan implemented by the clinician to ensure patient and caregiver compliance, which seeks to minimize exacerbations and healthcare costs by providing maximum understanding of current asthma treatment and management.

asthma trigger Any mechanism that can cause an asthmatic reaction, including allergens, pollution, food and drug additives, and viral agents.

ataxic breathing A breathing pattern characterized by irregular tidal volumes and respiratory rates; periods of apnea may be interspersed as well.

atelectasis Incomplete expansion of the lung or collapse of previously expanded lung tissue, a common noninfectious pulmonary complication that occurs after surgery. It may be due to many factors, including small, monotonous tidal volumes and inadequate lung distending forces, airway obstruction with gas absorption, and reduction in surfactant levels.

atom The smallest portion of an element that retains all the properties of the element.

atomic mass unit (amu) The unit for expressing masses of atoms or molecules.

atomic number The number of protons contained inside the nucleus of an atom, determining the actual element.

atomic weight The relative weight of an atom; often used interchangeably with the term "mass number."

atrioventricular (AV) node A specialized mass of cardiac muscle fibers in the interatrial septum of the heart; it transmits cardiac impulses from the sinoatrial node to the atrioventricular bundle.

atypical organism A strain of unusual type; examples include *Legionella* species, *Mycoplasma pneumoniae, Chlamydia psittaci, Chlamydophila pneumoniae*, and *Coxiella burnetii*.

atypical pneumonia Pneumonia caused by any strain of unusual type that is characterized by a flulike disease with prodromal symptoms, dry cough, myalgia, malaise, rhinorrhea, and moderate fever. The usual pathogens in atypical pneumonia include *Mycoplasma pneumoniae, Chlamydia psittaci, Coxiella burnetii, Chlamydophila pneumoniae*, and respiratory viruses.

auscultation The most commonly used physical assessment technique; it involves listening to sounds produced by the body with the aid of a stethoscope placed on the bare skin.

autogenic drainage A technique that aims to achieve the highest possible airflow in the different generations of bronchi to move secretions.

automated external defibrillator (AED) A portable device capable of diagnosing life-threatening cardiac arrhythmias and using electrical therapy to reestablish an effective rhythm.

automatic resuscitator A device designed to replace the need for manual ventilation.

autonomic nervous system The part of the nervous system that handles involuntary effectors such as the heart, certain glands, and smooth muscle in blood vessels.

autonomy The right and ability to govern oneself, particularly in regard to medical treatment and personal and financial care.

auto-PEEP End-expiratory alveolar pressure that is greater than the pressure at the proximal airway, which results from high airways resistance and a short expiratory time.

auto-positive airway pressure (APAP) A feature on some devices that deliver continuous positive airway pressure through which they actively monitor one or more airway variables during sleep and respond to upper airway changes by automatically adjusting the pressure.

axon An extension from a neuron that sends out electrochemical messages.

B

baby boomers The generation born between 1946 and 1964.

bacillus A rod-shaped bacterium. Plural: bacilli.

backup ventilator A secondary ventilator that performs two functions: it facilitates patient mobility and can be used in the event the primary ventilator fails. In situations in which patients need ventilator support most or all of the hours of the day at home, the primary ventilator is usually provided at the bedside, and a backup ventilator is often mounted on the patient's wheelchair.

bacteremia The presence of bacteria in the blood, as determined from blood cultures.

bacteria A large group of unicellular, prokaryote microorganisms.

bactericidal Pertaining to a method of killing bacteria.

bag technique A procedure used to minimize the likelihood of cross-contamination as a clinician travels from house to house. The bag technique requires the clinician to remove all needed care supplies from the bag with clean hands and to clean all used items prior to returning them to the bag.

bambuterol A long-acting β_2 agonist.

Barach, Alvan (1895–1977) A U.S. physician who developed the closed-system oxygen tent. Also did early work on breathing of helium-oxygen (heliox) gas mixtures.

baroreceptor A sensory nerve terminal that is stimulated by changes in pressure.

barrel chest A chest configuration in which the diameter of the individual's anteroposterior chest is equal to the lateral diameter.

basal metabolic rate (BMR) The amount of energy required to maintain the most basic bodily functions, expressed as kilocalories per day. The BMR has a fixed relationship with gender, weight, height, and age.

base A compound that yields a hydroxide ion (OH^-) in an aqueous solution.

basic life support (BLS) A primary patient assessment and treatment procedure that is performed to stabilize the emergency patient. It includes preliminary actions such as assessing unresponsiveness and conducting the primary ABCD survey.

Becker muscular dystrophy (BMD) An X-linked recessive inherited disorder characterized by slowly progressive muscle weakness; it affects males.

Beck's triad The three classic symptoms or signs of cardiac tamponade: hypotension, distended neck veins, and distant heart sounds.

Beddoes, Thomas (1760–1808) The first clinician to make therapeutic use of medical gases as well as nitrous oxide; the father of respiratory therapy.

Beer-Lambert law Law defining the relationship between the concentration of a substance and the amount of light (I) transmitted through it: $I_{out} = I_{in}\ e^{-A}$ and $A = L \times C \times \varepsilon$, where L is the optical path length, C is the concentration of the substance, and ε is the absorption of the particular wavelength used.

behavior modification The use of basic learning techniques, such as conditioning, biofeedback, reinforcement, and aversion therapy, to alter human behavior.

behavioral contracting Teaching technique creating a higher level of learner accountability and responsibility and calling on one's own integrity and autonomy.

beneficence Charity or mercy toward a patient. This principle imposes on the practitioner the responsibility to seek good for the patient under all circumstances.

benign Noncancerous.

Bennett, V. Ray Developer of the flow-sensitive valve used on early Puritan-Bennett assistors and anesthesia machines.

benzodiazepine Any of a class of drugs that possess sedative, hypnotic, anxiolytic, anticonvulsant, muscle relaxant, and amnesic actions, which may be useful in critically ill, mechanically ventilated patients.

Bernoulli principle The first law of fluid dynamics, used in 1738 by David Bernoulli to describe the relationship of fluid flow through a tube and, therefore, to explain the pressure drop that occurs when fluid passes through a constriction in a rigid tube by showing how potential energy, kinetic energy, and pressure energy interact.

bias A preference or an inclination that inhibits impartial judgment. Bias may result in an unfair act or policy stemming from prejudice.

bicarbonate buffer system A system influenced by the independent and direct effect of P_{CO_2} on $[HCO_3^-]$. It is made up of two components—hydration of CO_2 into carbonic acid (HCO_3^-) and the dissociation of carbonic acid into HCO_3^- and hydrogen ion.

bilirubinemia Increased level of bilirubin in the blood.

biofilm A complex aggregation of microorganisms that adhere to one another or to a surface, or both.

biomarker A substance (e.g., hormone, protein, and cytokine) produced by the body, which is indicative of a certain condition (e.g., cancer, infections).

Biot respirations (Biot breathing) A pattern of breathing symptomatic of elevated intracranial pressure and meningitis; it is characterized by a short burst of uniform, deep respirations followed by a period of apnea lasting 10 to 30 seconds.

Bird, Forrest A pioneer in aviation medicine who invented the clinical magnetic respirator, and subsequently ventilators offering automatic cycling and anesthesia options.

bite block A device that is placed between the teeth to prevent the patient from biting an orotracheal airway or the tongue or lips, thereby causing bleeding and trauma to the mouth. This device is also used during bronchoscopy.

bland aerosol therapy A humidification therapy that uses inspired gas consisting of water, saline solution, or other substances without important pharmacologic action. It is used primarily to humidify, liquefy, or otherwise change the character of thick secretions.

Bland-Altman plot A method of displaying the level of agreement between two measurement methods.

blinding A research technique for ensuring that the investigators or the participants in a study, or both, are as unaware as possible of the treatment being investigated to avoid any tendency to prefer a specific outcome (bias).

blood urea nitrogen (BUN) The most common nonprotein nitrogenous compound in the blood; its measurement is used to assess renal function in the adult. Normal values for BUN are between 7 and 21 mg/dL.

blunt trauma Any traumatic injury that occurs due to a force that does not penetrate the body of the patient. Common mechanisms of blunt trauma include motor vehicle crashes, falls, and being struck by an automobile.

blunted costophrenic angle A finding on chest x-ray consistent with pleural effusion.

Board of Medical Advisors (BOMA) One of several governance and advisory entities of the American Association for Respiratory Care (AARC); it consists of four AARC sponsoring professional medical societies that provide significant input concerning the art and science of the profession of respiratory care.

Board of Registered Polysomnographic Technologists (BRPT) An independent, nonprofit certification board that oversees a program of competency-based testing for sleep technicians and technologists.

body plethysmography A diagnostic tool that is used to achieve measurements of airways resistance (Raw), airway conductance (Gaw), and static lung volumes, based on Boyle's law. In practice, the patient is placed inside a fixed-volume, air-sealed body box in which the effects of excursion of the chest wall can be measured by small pressure changes in the box and airway.

Bohr effect The relationship between hydrogen ion concentration and hemoglobin affinity for oxygen. An increase in hydrogen ion concentration decreases the affinity of hemoglobin for oxygen.

boiling point The temperature required to raise the vapor pressure of a solution to atmospheric pressure.

botulism A rare disorder caused by toxin produced by *Clostridium botulinum*, often ingested via improperly cooked food, wound contamination by the organisms, or absorption of the toxin from the gastrointestinal tract, particularly in infants. Gastrointestinal symptoms predominate initially, followed by neurologic impairment.

Bourdon gauge flow meter A flow control device with a fixed outlet orifice that allows for adjustment of inlet pressure.

Boyle's law The observation credited to Robert Boyle, early in the 18th century, that predicts the relation of a volume of a fixed mass of gas to a pressure change; when temperature is held constant, volume is inversely related to pressure.

brachytherapy Radiotherapy treatment that involves applying an ionizing radiation source near the body area being treated; in respiratory treatment, this usually entails the endobronchial placement of encapsulated radionuclide in close proximity to an endobronchial malignancy.

bradypnea Slow respiratory rate.

Brain, Archie The developer of the laryngeal mask and the Mallampati system for identifying potentially difficult intubation candidates.

brain natriuretic peptide (BNP) A polypeptide secreted by the ventricles of the heart in response to excessive stretching of heart muscle cells; also known as B-type natriuretic peptide.

brain stem The portion of the brain that regulates visceral activities such as breathing and heart rate.

brain tissue PO_2 ($PbtO_2$) A measurement of the partial pressure of oxygen obtained via an electrode placed into the brain tissue; it is most commonly used in patients with traumatic brain injury.

breath A positive change in airway flow (inspiration) paired with a negative change in airway flow (expiration), associated with ventilation of the lungs. This definition allows the superimposition of, for example, a spontaneous breath on a mandatory breath, or vice versa. The flows are paired by size, not necessarily by timing.

breathing retraining A component of pulmonary rehabilitation, consisting of pursed-lip breathing and diaphragmatic breathing.

bronchi Larger air passages of the lungs.

bronchial artery embolization (BAE) A method used to occlude or restrict blood flow within the bronchial artery; the therapy of choice when bleeding is from the bronchiectatic airways.

bronchial breath sounds Auscultation sounds normally heard over the trachea, at the manubrium anteriorly and between the scapulae posteriorly. When such sounds are heard over the periphery of the lungs, they suggest consolidation of lung tissue.

bronchial challenge testing Use of either methacholine or histamine to measure responsiveness to general stimuli, usually administered in a pulmonary function laboratory and followed (usually within 15 minutes) with a short-acting β_2-agonist that results in a 12% to 15% increase in a patient's forced expiratory volume in 1 second (FEV_1).

bronchiolitis Inflammation of the bronchioles caused by infection.

bronchiolitis obliterans with organizing pneumonia (BOOP) An acute interstitial lung disease that appears to be a response of the lung to a variety of injuries affecting the smaller airways and alveoli as a unit, including infections, exposures to toxic gases, radiation therapy, drug toxicity, eosinophilic pneumonia, Wegener granulomatosis, and hypersensitivity pneumonitis.

bronchoalveolar lavage (BAL) A procedure for collecting an alveolar specimen by use of a bronchoscope or other hollow tube through which saline is instilled into distal bronchi and then withdrawn; also used to describe the specimen thus obtained.

bronchogenic carcinoma A malignant lung tumor that originates in the bronchi.

bronchogenic cyst A cyst occurring as a mass usually near the carina in the mediastinum; it results from abnormal budding from the bronchopulmonary foregut during the fourth through sixth weeks of gestation.

bronchophony An auscultation sound typically heard with consolidation of lung tissue, meaning that the normally aerated tissue has been filled with fluid, mucus, pus, or cellular debris. In bronchophony, the patient's repetition of "99" becomes easily audible, as opposed to its normal muffling.

bronchopulmonary dysplasia (BPD) A chronic iatrogenic lung disease caused by oxygen toxicity and barotrauma resulting from positive pressure ventilation. Its incidence is greater in premature infants, perhaps related to the increased requirement for oxygen therapy and mechanical ventilation in this patient population.

bronchoscopic brushing A technique in which a brush is introduced into the airway via a bronchoscope to collect cells or microorganisms for diagnostic purposes.

bronchoscopic washing A technique designed to sample the airway, rather than the alveolar space, particularly in cytologic sampling when a patient has an exophytic lesion obstructing a lobar or segmental orifice.

bronchoscopy Examination using a bronchoscope that enables inspection of the interior of the tracheobronchial tree and related diagnostic and therapeutic maneuvers, including taking specimens for culture, biopsy, and removal of foreign bodies.

bronchovesicular Referring to breath sounds heard over the junction between the bronchi and the alveoli.

bubble echocardiogram A technique that uses agitated saline injected into the venous circulation to detect the presence of an intracardiac shunt.

bubble humidifier A system in which dry gas is directed toward the bottom of a water-filled reservoir, where the stream of gas is broken into bubbles that gain humidity as they rise through the water.

buffer A substance that maintains a relatively constant pH level when strong acids or strong bases are added to it.

bullae Airspace enlargements greater than 1 cm; they can progressively enlarge and compress adjacent lung tissue, impairing respiratory function.

bullectomy Removal of giant bullae (airspace enlargements that occupy one-third of a hemithorax), which represent a reversible cause of pulmonary decompensation, particularly in patients with emphysema.

bundle of His The bundle of cardiac muscle fibers that begins at the atrioventricular node and passes through the right atrioventricular fibrous ring to the membranous part of the interventricular septum. It conducts the electrical impulse that regulates the heartbeat from the right atrium to the ventricles.

bundled charges A single comprehensive group of related charges. Payments for bundled charges have become the norm in recent years, and unbundled services are investigated closely by the Health Care Financing Administration and other payers for evidence of fraud.

burn shock Multi-organ dysfunction caused by hypovolemia as well as the systemic release of inflammatory mediators from a burn wound.

C

CABD sequence The primary patient assessment and treatment steps to be taken in emergency or resuscitation situations, including circulation, airway, breathing, and defibrillation, focusing on basic CPR and defibrillation.

canalicular stage The third stage of lung development, generally considered to last from week 17 to week 26 of gestation.

cannulation Introduction of a tube into a blood vessel, duct, or body cavity that remains in place for a period of time as part of medical care.

capacity The measurable capability of a patient to make an informed decision that accepts, changes, or withholds therapy, treatment, or medical care.

capillary blood gas Samples taken from the cutaneous layer of the skin in a highly vascularized area that is warmed before sampling to estimate pH and P_{CO_2} in infants or other individuals; it is used when arterial blood gas analysis is indicated, but arterial access is difficult.

capitation A prepaid and fixed amount that is negotiated in advance by the payer or plan and the provider; it involves payment for each person for a particular period of time regardless of the care or services provided.

capnogram Assessment of gas levels at the proximal airway that plots CO_2 on the vertical axis and time or volume on the horizontal axis.

capnography A noninvasive technique that measures CO_2 levels in inspired and expired gas; the results are displayed in the form of a capnogram.

capnometry Numeric display of CO_2 measurements taken from the proximal airway.

carbogen An oxygen–carbon dioxide mixture, usually consisting of 90% O_2 and 10% CO_2 or 95% O_2 and 5% CO_2.

carbohydrate An organic compound containing the elements carbon, hydrogen, and oxygen.

carbon dioxide CO_2; a colorless, transparent, odorless to pungent, and tasteless or slightly acid-tasting gas.

carbon dioxide production (CO_2) The amount of CO_2 produced by the tissues and excreted by the lungs each minute; normally about 200 mL/min in adults.

carbonic acid (H_2CO_3) The product of the hydration of carbon dioxide that ionizes to H^+ and bicarbonate; carbonic acid then forms bicarbonate.

carboxyhemoglobin (HbCO) A compound produced by exposing hemoglobin to carbon monoxide; carbon monoxide is usually inhaled into the lungs and subsequently becomes bound to hemoglobin in the blood, blocking the sites for oxygen transport.

carboxymyoglobin (MbCO) A compound formed by binding of carbon dioxide to myoglobin.

cardiac arrest Cessation of cardiac mechanical activity, as confirmed by the absence of signs of circulation.

cardiac arrhythmia A condition in which the heartbeat may be too fast or too slow, and may be regular or irregular.

cardiac catheterization An invasive means to quantify valvular stenosis and regurgitation and assess coronary artery blood flow.

cardiac enzymes A group of enzymes that are released from myocardial tissue and appear in the serum during myocardial injury (usually ischemia).

cardiac failure A complex clinical syndrome that can result from any structural or functional cardiac disorder that impairs the ventricle from filling with or ejecting blood.

cardiac output ($\dot{Q}c$) The volume of blood expelled by the heart's ventricles, equal to the amount of blood ejected at each beat multiplied by the heart rate (in beats per minute).

cardiac tamponade A life-threatening complication of penetrating wounds to the heart, most often characterized by Beck's triad (distention of neck veins, muffled heart sounds, and hypotension) and often by elevated central venous pressure; it involves compression of the heart by fluid or blood within the pericardial space. The increase in pressure generated by an increase in fluid volume may prevent blood return to the heart.

cardiomyocytes Muscle cells that make up the heart.

cardiomyopathy Any disease that affects the heart's structure and function.

cardiopulmonary exercise testing (CPET) A relatively noninvasive test that measures respiratory gas exchange (oxygen uptake and carbon dioxide output, minute ventilation, and anaerobic threshold), electrocardiography, blood pressure, and pulse oximetry during maximal exercise tolerance.

cardiopulmonary resuscitation (CPR) A formalized approach to maintain blood flow in an individual who has experienced a sudden cessation of heartbeat or respiration; the goal is to delay or prevent death caused by lack of the oxygen needed to support cellular function.

care management An umbrella term referring to the coordination of patient interventions, encompassing many loosely related terms: component management, demand management, case management, and disease management.

carina Bifurcation of the trachea into right and left main stem bronchi.

carotid bodies Peripheral chemoreceptors located in the bifurcation of the common carotid artery that are innervated by the glossopharyngeal nerve; they contribute to the control of breathing.

case control study A research study that involves, initially, the accumulation of a number of cases, which are then matched as much as possible with those that do not have the condition; both the cases and the noncases (controls) can then be studied for differences that may account for why the cases contracted the disease.

case management A collaborative process that assesses, plans, implements, coordinates, monitors, and evaluates the options and services required to meet an individual's health needs, using communication and available resources to promote quality, cost, and effective outcomes.

case mix A relatively new form of reimbursement that refers to the overall intensity of conditions requiring medical and nursing intervention. It involves extensive assessment of the patient's condition, followed by a determination of specific services or procedures considered necessary or essential to manage the patient effectively.

case report A detailed, observational report of an unusual, interesting case. Case reports are observational and can be reported easily. The disease described in the case may be rare, the treatment may be unusual, or there may be specific instructional points.

case series Several case reports presented over time.

catabolism The process of releasing chemical energy from food molecules in a decomposition process involving the oxidation of nutrient molecules. Energy is released (exergonic metabolism) in two forms: as heat or as chemical energy.

cation A positively charged ion; one of the most common serum electrolytes.

cell-mediated immunity The primary component of the immune system, which relies on lymphocytes; it is adversely affected by protein-calorie malnutrition.

Centers for Medicare and Medicaid Services (CMS) The branch of the U.S. Department of Health and Human Services that administers the Medicare and Medicaid programs; previously known as the Health Care Financing Administration.

central apnea Loss of diaphragmatic and other respiratory muscle function, resulting in the cessation of respiratory effort and stemming from the central nervous system.

central chemoreceptors Nerve cells sensitive to changes in the blood chemistry that are located bilaterally near the ventrolateral surface of the medulla oblongata.

central venous pressure (CVP) Pressure measured in the superior vena cava or right atrium, which is used to estimate intravascular volume status.

cepacia syndrome A rapid clinical decline characterized by fever and frank sepsis at some point after initial infection by *Burkholderia cepacia*. The precise pathogen and host factor(s) that trigger this dramatic decompensation are unknown.

cerebellum The structure in the brain responsible for coordinating movement, posture, and balance.

cerebral cortex The thin layer of gray matter making up the outer portion of the cerebrum.

cerebral hemisphere Either of the left and right divisions of the cerebrum.

cerebrum The largest part of the brain, which is responsible for many nervous system functions.

certification Verification from a professional organization that a person is able to competently complete a job or task, usually involving the passing of an examination.

channel A medium through which a message is transmitted to its intended audience, such as print media or broadcast (electronic) media.

channels of Lambert Anatomic connections between alveoli and adjacent terminal bronchioles that allow collateral ventilation (along with the pores of Kohn).

Charles's law The principle that predicts the effect of temperature on a fixed amount of dry gas, such that, at constant pressure, gas expands proportionally to changes in temperature. This law describes, at least at a qualitative level, the effect of kinetic energy on volume; when pressure is held constant, volume and temperature vary directly.

chemical agent Any chemical power, active principle, or substance that can produce an effect in the body by interacting with various body substances.

chemotherapy Treatment of cancer, infections, and other diseases with chemical agents.

chest compressions The rhythmic application of pressure on the lower half of the sternum to facilitate blood flow by compressing the heart during CPR.

chest physiotherapy (CPT) A technique used to help remove mucus and fluid from the lungs. Conventional CPT consists of postural drainage, percussion, and vibration.

chest radiograph An image produced by x-ray beams passing through the thorax.

chest wall compliance The elastic properties of the chest wall; normally 200 mL/cm H_2O.

Cheyne-Stokes breathing A repeating pattern of breathing in which the rate and depth of breathing increase to a peak, followed by a decrease in the rate and depth of breathing, followed by a period of apnea.

cholesterol A steroid lipid that combines with phospholipids in the cell membrane to help stabilize its bilayer structure; it is also used by the body as a starting point in making steroid hormones such as estrogen, testosterone, and cortisol.

chordae tendinae Strong fibers originating from the papillary muscles that attach to the cusps of the cardiac valve.

chromosome A strand of DNA in the cell nucleus that carries the genes.

chronic bronchitis A type of chronic obstructive pulmonary disease defined by the presence of cough and sputum production for three or more months in two successive years in patients who do not have other causes of cough.

chronic care model (CCM) A model identifying the essential elements of a healthcare system that encourage high-quality chronic disease care—namely, the community, the health system, self-management support, delivery system design, decision support, and clinical information systems.

chronic lung disease (CLD) Any lung disease that progressively damages lung tissue and airways over a period of years, ultimately resulting in a depletion of ventilatory reserves; a chronic condition referring to the very low birth weight preterm infant who initially responded favorably to surfactant replacement and who may or may not have a history of RDS, but has a continued oxygen requirement at 36 weeks' gestational age.

chronic obstructive pulmonary disease (COPD) A progressive, irreversible condition characterized by dyspnea and airflow obstruction, and sometimes including chronic cough.

citric acid (Krebs) cycle The aerobic process in stage 3 catabolism that converts two pyruvic acid molecules into six carbon dioxide molecules and six water molecules; it takes place within the mitochondria of the cell.

clarification A questioning or interviewing technique that attempts to correct ambiguity and clear up the meaning of confusing communication.

Clark, Leland C., Jr. The inventor of the first membrane oxygen electrode that was not poisoned by blood proteins.

Clark electrode A Po_2 electrode, consisting of a platinum cathode and a silver anode immersed in a dilute, buffered potassium chloride solution; it measures Po_2 using the principle of polarography.

cleaning Removal of visible soil from surfaces of equipment.

client education The use of the educational process for individuals who are partners in the health education effort.

Clinical Laboratory Improvement Amendment (CLIA) U.S. federal law regulating general aspects of laboratory quality control.

clinical practice guideline (CPG) A statement intended to assist clinicians with selecting the appropriate healthcare options for specific clinical circumstances. CPGs are often developed by professional associations.

clinical respiratory services A term used by some accrediting agencies to describe the hands-on services provided by a respiratory therapist, usually within the patient's home—for example, administering nebulizer medications, managing a ventilator, or performing pulmonary function tests.

closed-ended question A questioning technique that limits respondents to a limited number of responses or to a simple *yes* or *no*.

clubbing Enlargement of the distal phalanges, particularly the fingers.

CO-oximetry A means of measuring carboxyhemoglobin; also the standard technique used to measure hemoglobin oxygen saturation and methemoglobin.

coccus A spherical bacterium. Plural: cocci.

cognitive domain The area of learning involved in knowledge, comprehension, and critical thinking.

cohort study A research study that attempts to definitively answer an important question about the cause, treatment, or prevention of disease by enrolling a large number of participants and following them over time so that the study participants are measured, tested, or treated and followed up for years.

collagen vascular disease Any of a group of diseases that can present with interstitial lung disease, including progressive systemic sclerosis, systemic lupus erythematosus, polymyositis and dermatomyositis, Sjögren syndrome, and mixed connective tissue disease. The clinical presentation and histopathologic features are comparable to those of idiopathic pulmonary fibrosis, with additional features of lymphoid hyperplasia, cellular interstitial pneumonitis, lymphoid interstitial pneumonitis, diffuse alveolar damage, and bronchiolitis obliterans with organizing pneumonitis.

collecting duct One of a series of small tubes inside the kidneys that empty into the renal pelvis.

colligative property A property of a solution that depends on the number of solute particles dissolved, not on the solution's chemical properties.

colloid A liquid mixture that consists of tiny particles suspended in a liquid.

Commission on Accreditation for Respiratory Care (CoARC) A constituency group that makes the final accreditation decisions for respiratory therapy educational programs.

community-acquired pneumonia (CAP) Pneumonia acquired outside the hospital.

compensated respiratory alkalosis A type of respiratory alkalosis characterized by a normal pH, a low HCO_3^-, and a low Pa_{O_2}.

complex sleep apnea syndrome Sleep apnea that displays both obstructive and central characteristics.

compliance A lung characteristic that, with resistance, serves as a determinant in the mechanics of airflow in and out of the lungs; the ratio of volume change and pressure change.

component management A method of controlling healthcare costs that focuses on limiting the use of resources or services such as therapeutic procedures, diagnostic tests, medications, or hospital lengths of stay.

compound A substance formed by the reaction of two or more chemical elements.

compound question When more than one question is combined in what seems to be a single question. It generally results in confusion and a response to only the last portion of the question.

Compressed Gas Association (CGA) An industry technical trade organization that has developed numerous safety standards for cylinders, fittings, and connections on compressed gas cylinders.

compressed gas system Oxygen stored in a high-pressure cylinder, usually at 2000 to 3000 pounds per square inch. Flow of gas to the patient is regulated through a pressure-reducing valve combined with a flow metering device.

compressible volume The volume of gas that remains compressed in the ventilator circuit and, therefore, is not delivered to the patient.

computed tomographic angiography (CTA) A technique used to examine the pulmonary arteries to detect pulmonary embolism.

computed tomography (CT) A radiographic technique that produces a film representing detailed cross sections of tissue using an array of detectors in a variety of angles and a collimated beam of x-rays that rotates in a continuous 360-degree motion around the patient to create cross-sectional images.

concentrated A solution that contains a large amount of solute relative to the amount that could potentially dissolve.

conchae Three curled bony plates or turbinates that project downward from the walls of the nasal cavity and greatly enlarge the surface area of the nose, move mucus toward the nasopharynx, and warm and humidify incoming air.

confidentiality The legally protected right afforded to (and duty required of) specifically designated healthcare professionals not to disclose information discerned or communicated during consultation with a patient, except in cases of suspected abuse, commission of a crime, or threat of harm to self or others.

confrontation In a therapeutic context, the process by which a therapist provides direct, reality-oriented feedback to a client regarding the client's own thoughts, feelings, or behavior.

congenital diaphragmatic hernia (CDH) A condition associated with a left posterolateral diaphragmatic defect and the failure of the pleuroperitoneal canal to close early in gestation (5th to 10th weeks of fetal life), resulting in compression of the developing lung by abdominal organs.

congenital pulmonary airway malformation (CPAM) Abnormal developmental branching of the lung resulting in cysts of varying sizes that are connected to the tracheobronchial tree involving one or multiple lobes. Large cysts can compress the esophagus, mediastinum, and inferior vena cava.

consumer education The use of the educational process by an individual or group of individuals who are independent decision makers.

contact precautions Actions taken to prevent transmission of infectious agents that are spread by direct or indirect contact with a patient or the patient's environment.

continuous-flow oxygen (CFO) The traditional method of oxygen delivery in which oxygen is metered to the patient continuously via a delivery system. The amount of oxygen a patient receives is determined by the flow and the inspiratory time.

continuous mandatory ventilation (CMV) A system for delivering a set tidal volume (or pressure) and a minimum respiratory rate, in which the patient can trigger additional breaths above the minimal rate, but the set volume or pressure is constant at the preset level. Also called assist/control (A/C).

continuous positive airway pressure (CPAP) A ventilation method by which a constant pressure greater than atmospheric pressure is applied to the airway through the respiratory cycle.

continuous spontaneous ventilation (CSV) A breath sequence in which all breaths are spontaneous.

contractility A feature of muscle tissue, especially cardiac muscle, that allows it to contract by shortening sarcomeres.

control system A design feature in a mechanical ventilator that generates the signals that operate the ventilator's output valve and exhalation manifold.

controller medication Any of a number of pharmacologic interventions whose goal is to maintain normal (or near normal) lung function, including inhaled corticosteroids, nonsteroidal anti-inflammatory agents, long-acting β-agonists, methylxanthines, and leukotriene modifiers.

copayment A limited fee paid by enrollees of managed care organizations for each physician visit, prescription, or other service stipulated in the plan.

cor pulmonale Hypertrophy and dilatation of the right ventricle; right heart failure.

coronary angiography Direct imaging of the coronary arteries using cardiac catheterization and subsequent injection of contrast dye. This technique can identify atherosclerotic lesions as well as coronary anomalies, areas of spasm, and acute thrombi.

coronary artery bypass surgery A surgical procedure that can improve myocardial function by reducing ischemia after restoration of normal blood flow. An area of obstruction in a coronary artery is bypassed.

coronary sinus An enlarged vein joining the cardiac veins; it empties into the right atrium.

corpus callosum A deep bridge of nerve fibers connecting the brain hemispheres.

correlation coefficient A statistical parameter used to measure the strength of the relationship between two variables.

corticosteroid Any of a major class of anti-inflammatory drugs that generally produce two types of effect: (1) the glucocorticoid effect, which reduces inflammation, increases blood glucose, and generally induces a catabolic state; and (2) the mineralocorticoid effect, which is active primarily at the kidney, promoting sodium conservation.

cough etiquette The procedure whereby one covers the nose and mouth when coughing/sneezing, uses tissues to contain respiratory secretions and disposes of those tissues in the nearest receptacle after use, and performs hand hygiene after having contact with respiratory secretions or contaminated objects.

covalent bond A stable atomic configuration formed when each of the two bonding atoms shares one of its valance electrons.

crackles Fine, high-pitched, discontinuous sounds heard during auscultation of the lungs.

C-reactive protein (CRP) A protein found in the blood, the levels of which rise in response to inflammation.

creatinine A substance formed from creatine metabolism that may be measured in blood and urine and serves as an indicator of kidney function. Creatinine levels are a function of skeletal muscle breakdown, and most creatinine is filtered in the glomeruli with little reabsorption.

credentialing The formal identification of professionals who meet predetermined standards of professional skill or competence; it can include both licensure and certification.

credentials An attestation of qualification, competence, or authority issued to an individual by a third party with relevant or assumed competence. Examples of credentials include diplomas, academic degrees, certifications, security clearances, and powers of attorney.

crenation The process in which water leaves a cell, causing it to shrivel, as a result of greater osmotic pressure outside that cell.

cricothyrotomy An incision into the larynx between the cricoid and thyroid cartilages, usually done emergently when no other airway access is available.

critical care ventilator A full-featured ventilator designed for use with critically ill patients in respiratory failure.

critical illness polyneuromyopathy (CIPNM) A disease affecting several areas of the peripheral nervous system at once. Diagnosis is confirmed by electromyographic studies, which show primary axonal polyneuropathy rather than demyelination, as suggested by the reduction in the amplitude of the compound action potential without significant prolongation of the conduction latency period. This condition may be caused by hyperglycemia that leads to nerve ischemia by endovascular shunting or nerve toxins generated from multiple organ failure.

crossover study A research study in which each patient is randomized to either a treatment group or a control group and, after measurements are made, each patient is then restudied in the other group (control or treatment).

cross-sectional study A research study based on sampling from the population at a given point in time.

cuirass A body ventilator consisting of a lightweight rigid dome that fits over the anterior chest wall and connects to a negative pressure generator; also called a chest shell or turtle shell.

culture In context of microbiology, a method of multiplying microorganisms by letting them reproduce in predetermined culture media under controlled laboratory conditions.

culture of safety A commitment to safety that permeates all levels of an organization, from frontline personnel to executive management.

cyanosis A bluish hue to the skin that suggests hemoglobin is poorly saturated with oxygen.

cycle The signal that ends the inspiratory phase of breathing.

cystic fibrosis (CF) A disorder that is inherited in an autosomal recessive pattern and that affects the exocrine glands, resulting in abnormally thick secretions of mucus.

cystic fibrosis–related diabetes (CFRD) A type of diabetes associated with cystic fibrosis and characterized by insidious onset, failure to gain or maintain weight despite nutritional intervention, poor growth, or an unexplained chronic decline in pulmonary function.

cystic fibrosis transmembrane conductance regulator (CFTR) The gene responsible for cystic fibrosis.

cytokine A small protein that is secreted by cells and carries signals between cells.

D

Dalton's law The principle of partial pressures that describes the behavior of physical mixtures of gases and vapors such that each separate gas acts as predicted by the combined gas law, as if it were present alone. In such a mixture, the partial pressure of each particular gas is proportional to the fractional concentration of that gas and equal to the product of fraction concentration and total atmospheric pressure.

dead space The volume of gas that moves in and out of the lungs without taking part in gas exchange; wasted ventilation.

decannulation The removal of a tracheostomy tube.

decoding The process by which information (words, symbols, actions, pictures, numbers, or gestures) is interpreted back into the thought, feeling, or attitude communicated from the source.

deep sulcus sign The distinctive radiographic appearance of a pneumothorax in patients in the supine position; it appears as free air in the pleural space rising to the highest portion of the thorax, usually the anterior costophrenic sulcus, and projecting over the upper abdomen and diaphragm.

deep vein thrombosis (DVT) Blood clotting in the legs and pelvis, which usually occurs as a result of venostasis. It is common in surgical patients and with other causes of immobility, damage to the endothelial wall of the blood vessels, and hypercoagulability states.

defibrillation Use of an electrical current passed through the heart to eliminate the chaotic asynchronous activity of ventricular fibrillation by depolarizing cardiac cells and repolarizing them in a uniform manner with resumption of coordinated cardiac contraction. This therapy is indicated for ventricular fibrillation, pulseless ventricular tachycardia, and asystole (with the possibility that the rhythm is actually fine ventricular fibrillation).

deflation reflex Signaling of the dorsal respiratory group via an afferent impulse, which causes the respiratory rate to increase during a time of lung collapse.

delta wave Electroencephalographic activity with a frequency less than 4 Hz. Conventionally, in sleep stage scoring, the minimum criteria for scoring delta waves are 75-μV (peak-to-peak) amplitude and 0.5-second duration (2 Hz).

demand delivery device A system of oxygen delivery that responds to the patient's inspiratory effort and cycles off upon receiving the expiratory signal. Some demand systems (hybrid units) provide a higher flow of oxygen initially, then return to a set base flow during the inspiratory cycle.

demand management Any organized effort or program designed to guide healthcare consumers into the most appropriate level of healthcare service by involving them in their own care.

dendrite An extension from a neuron that receives electrochemical messages.

dendritic cells Mobile cells with irregular shapes and long processes.

density (ρ) Mass per unit volume.

deontological theory An ethical theory based on duty, asserting that an act is either right or wrong based on its intrinsic character rather than its consequences.

deoxyribonucleic acid (DNA) A nucleic acid in which the sugar component is deoxyribose. The largest molecule in the body, it is composed of two long polynucleotide chains running parallel to each other. DNA carries the genetic information necessary for synthesis of proteins specific for a given species.

Department of Transportation (DOT) U.S. government agency that regulates cylinder manufacture and the testing and the transporting of hazardous materials, including compressed gases and cryogenic liquids.

descriptive statistics Data or raw information obtained from conducting a study whose results are often presented more clearly and efficiently in tables, graphs, or figures.

diabetic ketoacidosis A buildup of ketones in the blood due to the breakdown of stored fats for energy; a potentially life-threatening complication in patients with diabetes mellitus.

diagnosis-related group (DRG) A system developed for Medicare as part of the prospective payment system that utilizes a predetermined rate per case or type of discharge.

diagnostic bronchoscopy A procedure involving the direct observation of the airways using a bronchoscope to elucidate the cause of a pulmonary abnormality.

dialogue Purposeful, reciprocal, and close or intimate expression between participants; two-way communication.

Diameter Index Safety System (DISS) One of three indexed safety systems for medical gas distribution station outlets. In this system, a female nut and nipple are manually tightened onto the outlet until contact is made with the plunger, moving it forward until it seats on the stem, thereby allowing gas to flow from the piping system.

diaphragm The membranous muscle that separates the abdomen and thorax and serves as a major inspiratory muscle.

diaphragmatic pacing Use of a radio-frequency transmitter and an antenna that discharges signals to a surgically implanted receiver to transmit electrical impulses to a surgically implanted electrode placed over the phrenic nerve to ensure stimulation of all phrenic nerve roots.

diastole In the cardiac cycle, a period of relaxation during which venous blood returns to the heart.

diastolic Pertaining to the diastole; the nadir of a blood pressure measurement.

diastolic dysfunction Impaired ventricular filling, recognized increasingly as a cause of congestive heart failure symptoms; failure of the cardiac muscle to relax normally.

diet-induced thermogenesis An increase in metabolic rate of 10% to 15% that occurs after eating as a result of the energy cost of digesting and storing nutrients.

diffusing capacity The number of milliliters of gas that transfer from the lungs across the alveolocapillary membrane into the bloodstream each minute, for each 1 mm Hg difference in the pressure across the membrane.

diffusion defect A deficiency in the ability of gases to cross the alveolocapillary membrane.

dilute A description of the relative concentration or strength of a solution indicating that it contains a small amount of solute.

disaster management plan A predetermined plan for responding to disaster.

disease management An approach to patient care that emphasizes coordinated, comprehensive care along the continuum of disease and across healthcare delivery systems.

disinfection A process that eliminates all pathogenic microorganisms except bacterial spores.

distal intestinal obstruction syndrome (DIOS) Blockage of the intestines by thickened stool, which occurs in individuals with cystic fibrosis.

documentation Recording or charting individual patient education, including the date and time of the intervention, the subject matter or content addressed, the method of instruction, and the response of the learner or the results of the learning.

dorsal respiratory group (DRG) A group of respiratory-related neurons located along the lateral walls within the medulla oblongata; it serves as the initial processing center for afferent impulses from the vagus (X) and glossopharyngeal (IX) nerves.

Drinker, Philip A co-developer of the iron lung, which was used for patients with poliomyelitis in the 20th century.

droplet precautions Actions taken to prevent transmission of pathogens spread through close respiratory or mucous membrane contact with respiratory secretions.

dry powder inhaler (DPI) A device that creates aerosols by drawing air through a dose of powdered medication. DPIs produce aerosols in which most of the drug particles are in the respirable range.

Duchenne muscular dystrophy (DMD) A hereditary familial muscle disease transmitted via an X-linked recessive gene, although about one-third of cases may be caused by spontaneous mutation. Early presenting symptoms are gait disturbances and delayed motor development, as well as limb-girdle muscle weakness and pseudohypertrophy of the calf muscles.

durable medical equipment (DME) company A company that provides products to aid in the care of the patient at home, including, but not limited to, mobility aids (wheelchairs, walkers, electric or semi-electric hospital beds), respiratory equipment (apnea monitors, bilevel and continuous positive airway pressure devices, home oxygen therapy, mechanical ventilators), enteral products (pumps and enteral formula), and wound and skin care products (lymphedema pumps, special seating and mattresses). Also called home medical equipment (HME) company.

durable medical power of attorney A document that names an individual or agent who can make decisions specifically related to health care for another individual.

dynamic airway compression A condition occurring as a result of decreased lung elasticity and leading to increased expiratory airway resistance, which ultimately results in air trapping and hyperinflation.

dynamic hyperinflation An increase in lung volume secondary to air trapping.

dyspnea Shortness of breath or breathlessness; the distressing feeling of inability to breathe or great effort required to breathe.

E

echocardiography A diagnostic and assessment tool that uses ultrasound to examine the heart structures and function by transmission of high-frequency ultrasound waves through the chest and calibration of the velocity of sound waves in the medium under examination; a noninvasive form of cardiac imaging used extensively to diagnose a variety of valvular and myocardial diseases.

ECMO circuit The combination of a large-bore cannula placed into a patient's central vein that drains blood from the patient, an artificial gas exchanger that oxygenates the blood, and a cannula that returns the oxygenated/ventilated blood to the patient as part of corporeal membrane oxygenation.

EEG rhythms A means of categorizing electroencephalographic waves based on their frequency (i.e., cycles per second); examples include alpha, beta, delta, and theta rhythms.

efferent impulses Impulses created within the central nervous system that are sent to other areas of the body.

egophony An auscultation sound typically heard with consolidation of lung tissue, meaning that the normally aerated tissue has been filled with fluid, mucus, pus, or cellular debris. In egophony, the verbalized *e* sounds like *a*.

eicosanoid A naturally occurring substance derived from one of the 20-carbon polyunsaturated fatty acids. Eicosanoids include the prostaglandins, thromboxanes, leukotrienes, and epoxyeicosatrienoic acids and function as hormones.

ejection fraction (EF) The percentage of blood pumped from the ventricle during a single cardiac contraction. The normal left ventricular ejection fraction is greater than 50%.

elastance The ratio of pressure change to volume change (i.e., the reciprocal of compliance).

elastic load A component of the patient–ventilator interaction, describing the elastance of the respiratory system (lungs and chest wall) and volume of flow as a function of time.

elastic recoil The tendency of a structure to return to its resting position after it is stretched.

electrical impedance tomography (EIT) A thoracic imaging technique in which conductivity is inferred from surface electrical measurements.

electrically powered portable ventilator A portable ventilator that requires a battery or external power source for operation; a pneumatic gas source may not be required.

electrocardiography (ECG) A test that evaluates the electrical activity of the heart.

electroencephalogram (EEG) Recording through the scalp of electrical potentials (activity) from the brain and the changes in those potentials.

electrolyte Any substance containing free ions that make the substance electrically conductive.

electromyogram (EMG) Recording of electrical activity from the muscular system.

electron A particle with a negative charge (−1) located outside the nucleus of an atom.

electron transport system Movement of high-energy electrons (removed during glycolysis and the tricarboxylic acid cycle in the form of reduced flavin adenine dinucleotide and nicotinamide adenine dinucleotide) down a chain of carrier molecules embedded in the inner membrane of the mitochondria, resulting in the production of some 90% of the adenosine triphosphate formed during carbohydrate catabolism.

electronic health record (EHR) An individual patient's medical record in digital format. Electronic health record systems coordinate the storage and retrieval of individual records with the aid of computers. See also *electronic medical record (EMR)*.

electronic medical record (EMR) A medical record in digital format. In health informatics, an EMR is considered by some to be one of several types of electronic health records (EHRs), but in general usage *EMR* and *EHR* are synonymous.

electronic signature A unique code or password that verifies the individual making the entry and creates an individual signature on the record, then stores it on magnetic, optical, or some other computer storage media. This is a legally recognized electronic means of signing that indicates that a person adopts the contents of an electronic message.

electrooculogram (EOG) Recording of voltage changes resulting from shifts in position of the eyeball, made possible by the fact that each globe has a positive (anterior) dipole and a negative (posterior) dipole. Sleep recordings use surface electrodes placed near the eyes to record the movement of the eyeballs. Rapid eye movements in sleep indicate a stage of sleep (usually REM sleep).

element A pure chemical substance consisting of one type of atom, distinguished by its atomic number.

embryonic stage The first stage of lung development, generally considered to last from 26 days after conception to the end of the fifth week of gestation.

emergency plan A plan developed by the home care therapist, the patient, and the patient's family that includes an analysis of the most likely emergencies the patient and family may experience, based on the patient's medical needs, the home environment, and the geographical area in which the patient lives.

Emerson, John H. The inventor of the iron lung and several types of volume-controlled ventilators.

emotional filter A perspective that assists in determining what someone is feeling.

emphysema A type of chronic obstructive pulmonary disease occurring in patients who experience damage to the lung parenchyma; it results in histopathologic evidence of alveolar wall destruction without fibrosis and physiologic evidence of decreased lung elastic recoil, resulting in bullae that eventually enlarge and compress adjacent lung tissue, impairing respiratory function.

empyema Infection of the pleural space.

EMS portable ventilator A ventilator used in patient transport, typically in emergency care delivered by emergency medical services (EMS) personnel via ambulance.

encoding The process by which information (words, symbols, actions, pictures, numbers, or gestures) is interpreted into the thought, feeling, or attitude communicated from the source.

end-tidal PCO_2 The partial pressure of carbon dioxide at end-exhalation; symbolized as P_{ETCO_2}.

endobronchial biopsy A method for sampling endoscopically visible exophytic central tumors or mucosal ulceration, irregularity, or infiltration.

endocardium The inner layer of the heart wall.

endotracheal intubation Establishment of an artificial airway by placing a tube through the mouth or nose, through the glottis, and into the trachea.

endotracheal tube A large-bore tube inserted through the mouth or nose and into the trachea.

enteral nutrition Provision of nutrients through the gastrointestinal tract when the patient is unable to chew or swallow.

enzyme A protein that is produced by cells and acts as a catalyst in specific biochemical reactions.

eosinophilic granuloma A rare, predominantly pulmonary disorder that occurs almost exclusively in smokers or ex-smokers between 10 and 40 years old; it is likely an inflammatory response by Langerhans cells to a component of tobacco smoke.

epicardium The outer layer of the heart wall.

epidemic Incidence of new cases of a disease, in a given human population and during a given period, that substantially exceeds what is expected.

epidural hematoma A traumatic brain injury resulting in the accumulation of blood between the skull and the outer covering of the brain (dura mater).

epiglottis The cartilaginous structure overhanging the entrance to the larynx that serves to prevent food or foreign material from entering the larynx and trachea while a person is swallowing.

epiglottitis Rapidly progressing inflammation of the epiglottis and surrounding tissue that can result in severe airway obstruction.

equal pressure point The point in the airway where the pressure outside (pleural pressure) equals the pressure inside; the result is flow limitation.

equation of motion A mathematical model of patient–ventilator interaction: $Pvent + Pmus = EV + R\dot{V}$, where Pvent is inspiratory pressure generated by the ventilator, Pmus is the inspiratory pressure generated by the respiratory muscles, E is the elastance of the respiratory system, V is volume, R is respiratory system resistance, and $\dot{V}$ is flow.

equipment management service The provision of durable medical equipment, usually to the patient's home, to aid in the patient's home care. These services include helping the patient and family select the proper equipment for the patient's needs, ensuring the adequacy of the home environment for the intended equipment, delivering and setting up the equipment, training the patient and family on how to safely and properly use the equipment, and performing the appropriate maintenance of the equipment.

equipment surveillance A quality assurance program in which cultures of equipment are processed to ensure that high-level disinfection or sterilization is effective.

eschar A scab or dry crust that develops after trauma, such as a thermal or chemical burn, infection, or excoriating skin disease.

escharotomy Surgical incision into necrotic tissue resulting from a severe burn to prevent edema from generating sufficient interstitial pressure to impair capillary filling, thereby causing ischemia.

esophageal pressure (P_{ES}) The pressure measured by a balloon-tipped catheter in the esophagus; it is used as a proxy for pleural pressure.

ethics Matters involving (1) moral principles or practices and (2) matters of social policy involving issues of morality in the practice of medicine. *Unethical* is used to refer to professional conduct that fails to conform to these moral standards or policies.

ethics committee A committee consisting of physicians, administrators, service department members, clergy, a medical ethicist, and community members, who are brought together to consider divergent viewpoints related to the ethical issues in patient care. When involved in patient care, its goal is to issue a recommendation. Also called an optimum care committee.

eupnea The normal breathing pattern, which is regular and rhythmic, at 12 to 20 breaths/minute.

evaluation In a patient education context, monitoring of the ongoing process of teaching effectiveness, the teaching process, and the learner's response.

evidence-based medicine (EBM) An approach to incorporate the best current evidence based on scientific methods, which is then integrated in the decision-making process along with the needs of an individual patient to achieve the best outcome of medical treatment; medical practices that have been thoroughly evaluated by peer-reviewed journals and have been deemed safe and effective by the scientific community.

exacerbation Sudden worsening of respiratory symptoms accompanied by deteriorating lung function. Most often, patients will present with increased dyspnea, cough, and changes in the quality or quantity of sputum.

exclusive provider organization (EPO) A managed care model in which choice is completely eliminated and enrollees must seek care from the physician and the hospital stipulated in the plan; the most affordable but most restrictive of the managed care models.

exercise assessment An assessment that performs two functions: (1) it quantitates the level of disability and provides information for setting initial exercise loads and program expectations, and (2) it provides insight into the various cardiorespiratory factors that are involved in functional disabilities.

exercise capacity The ability to perform behaviors such as activities of daily living.

exercise-induced asthma (EIA) A form of asthma characterized by transient airway obstruction, typically occurring 5 to 15 minutes after strenuous exertion.

exercise training One of the key components of pulmonary rehabilitation, in which the patient's exercise capability and functional status are improved.

exertional dyspnea Shortness of breath that occurs during exercise.

exhaled nitric oxide (eNO) Measurement of the concentration of nitric oxide in the exhaled breath to assess inflammation in patients with asthma.

expiratory positive airway pressure (EPAP) Pressure applied to the airway during the expiratory phase with ventilators designed for noninvasive ventilation; synonymous with positive end-expiratory pressure (PEEP).

extracellular fluid Fluid found outside the cells.

extracorporeal life support (ECLS) The use of venoarterial and venovenous approaches to remove CO_2 and add O_2 to blood; also called extracorporeal membrane oxygenation (ECMO).

Extracorporeal Life Support Organization (ELSO) An industry organization that has published guidelines for initiating extracorporeal membrane oxygenation.

extracorporeal membrane oxygenation (ECMO) A method of gas exchange in which a large-bore cannula drains blood from the patient, the blood is pumped through an oxygenator, and the oxygenated/ventilated blood is returned to the patient.

extraglottic airway An artificial airway that bypasses the upper airway soft tissue. With this device, a mask forms a seal around the glottic aperture, and the tip of the device engages the proximal esophageal sphincter posterior to the cricoid cartilage. Also called a supraglottic airway.

extubation The process of removing an endotracheal tube.

exudative A classification of fluid based on laboratory findings suggesting an inflammatory or malignant etiology.

F

face shield Apparatus used to provide emergency exhaled-gas ventilation.

facilitation A technique whereby words, postures, or actions encourage more detail; the process or act of assisting or making easier the progress or improvement of something.

facioscapulohumeral muscular dystrophy (FSHD) An autosomal dominant, slow-progressing dystrophy that affects primarily the face and the proximal portion of the upper extremities.

fee-for-service system A payment model in which services are unbundled and paid for separately, and in which healthcare providers are paid for each service (e.g., an office visit, test, or procedure).

feedback Helpful information or criticism that is given to someone to say what can be done to make improvements.

fetal hemoglobin (HbF) Hemoglobin F; it has higher affinity for O_2 than adult hemoglobin (hemoglobin A), which can be attributed to the replacement of β-chains in hemoglobin A by γ-chains.

fiberoptic plethysmography A measurement of how much rib cage or abdominal displacements stretch an elastic belt; the changes in light transmission through the fibers of the belt indicate respiratory motion.

Fick equation A mathematical equation describing the relationship between cardiac output, oxygen consumption, and the difference between the arterial and mixed venous oxygen contents.

Fick's law A description of transfer by diffusion, demonstrating that the diffusion rate across a barrier is directly proportional to the cross-sectional area available for diffusion and the difference in concentration gradient per unit distance perpendicular to that cross section.

fidelity The principle dealing with one's faithfulness to duty.

flail chest Multiple rib fractures on one side of the chest or two or more rib fractures in two or more places, resulting from sternal fracture or costochondral separation. The term "flail" refers to the paradoxic motion of the chest resulting from loss of chest wall stability.

flexible fiberoptic bronchoscope A bronchoscope constructed with a fiberoptic light conduit, which allows for visualization of the airways through the bronchoscope.

flow The movement of a specified volume of fluid (gas or liquid) in a specific period of time.

flow-inflating bag A manual resuscitator that requires a continuous flow from an external gas source; pressure is determined by the flow and the pressure release valve.

flow limitation A Starling resistor effect, in which greater expiratory effort does not produce greater flow as the result of airway compression.

flow restrictor An orifice that allows a specific flow of gas to pass through a flow control device, provided the inlet pressure is a constant 50 psig.

flow triggering An alternative to pressure triggering in mechanical ventilation, in which the ventilator responds to a change in flow rather than a pressure drop.

fluid resuscitation Intravascular fluid administration to treat shock.

Food and Drug Administration (FDA) The agency of the U.S. Department of Health and Human Services that enforces regulations and standards concerning drugs.

force Mechanical energy applied to a body.

forced expiratory technique (FET) A breathing maneuver that consists of one or two forced expirations or huffs, combined with a period of controlled breathing.

forced vital capacity (FVC) A test of pulmonary function that measures the maximal volume of gas that can be expelled forcibly after full inspiration.

foreign body obstruction (FBO) Presence of any object lodged in any part of the airway, interfering with the individual's ability to breathe and causing sudden choking.

forest plot A graphical display designed to illustrate the relative strength of treatment effects in multiple quantitative scientific studies addressing the same question.

formoterol A long-acting β_2-adrenoceptor agonist medication.

fractional distillation of liquefied air The process by which the two major components of air (oxygen and nitrogen) are produced in bulk commercial quantities.

frailty The state of being weak in health or body (especially from old age).

freezing point The temperature at which a liquid will enter the solid state and freeze (0° C or 32° F at 1 atmosphere of pressure for water).

full-thickness graft A skin graft that contains all of the components of the skin: epidermis, dermis, nerve endings, and hair follicles.

fungal pneumonia Respiratory infection caused by fungi and including the following: histoplasmosis, blastomycosis, coccidioidomycosis, cryptococcosis, aspergillosis, and *Candida* respiratory infection.

fungi A large group of eukaryotic organisms that includes microorganisms such as yeasts and molds, as well as the more familiar mushrooms.

G

Galen (AD 130–199) A prominent Roman physician, who was probably the most accomplished medical researcher of the Roman period.

Gay-Lussac's law of combining volumes The principle that volumes of gases combine chemically in volumetric proportions that are small whole numbers.

Gay-Lussac's law of pressure and temperature A description of the direct relationship between pressure and temperature given a fixed mass and volume of gas.

genotype The genetic makeup of an organism.

geometric standard deviation (GSD) A measure of the magnitude of variation in particle size distribution. A monodisperse aerosol, in which all particles are basically the same size, has a GSD less than 1.2, whereas a heterodisperse aerosol, with a wider range of particle sizes, has a GSD higher than 1.2.

geriatrics A specialty that focuses on health care of the elderly.

gerontology The study of the social, psychological, and biological aspects of aging.

glomerular capsule Also known as the Bowman's capsule, the structure that encloses the glomerulus.

glomerular filtration rate (GFR) The volume of glomerular filtrate formed each minute in the nephrons of both kidneys.

glomerulus The collection of capillaries located within the glomerular capsule at the proximal end of the renal tubule.

glossopharyngeal breathing A technique involving the use of oropharyngeal muscles to inject air into the trachea, thereby augmenting ventilation to provide short periods of spontaneous ventilation, improve effective cough, and increase the volume of the voice; also known as frog breathing.

glottis (glottic opening) The opening in the larynx where the vocal cords reside that separates the upper and lower airways.

glucose A six-carbon sugar with the formula of $C_6H_{12}O_6$, which is found in fruits and other foods; the primary source of energy for cells.

glycolysis An anaerobic process necessary for glucose metabolism that begins with the breakdown of a 6-carbon glucose chain ($C_6H_{12}O_6$) into two 3-carbon pyruvate (pyruvic acid) molecules in the cytosol of the cell; it prepares glucose for the second step in catabolism, the citric acid cycle.

go-bag A carefully prepared bag that includes the equipment and supplies a patient may need when away from home (such as a resuscitation bag, a metered dose inhaler adapter, a list of important phone numbers, a copy of the prescribed ventilator settings, and a flashlight). It is helpful if this bag is kept always stocked and ready so that crucial items are not forgotten should a last-minute excursion occur.

Graham's law The principle predicting the rate of diffusion of a gas to be inversely proportional to the square root of its density.

gram-negative bacteria Bacteria that have a cell wall composed of a thin layer of peptidoglycan covered by an outer membrane of lipoprotein and lipopolysaccharide and that lose the stain or are decolorized by alcohol in Gram staining. Examples include *Haemophilus influenzae, Moraxella catarrhalis, Pseudomonas aeruginosa, Klebsiella* species, *Escherichia coli, Enterobacter* species, *Serratia* species, *Acinetobacter* species, and *Proteus mirabilis.*

gram-positive bacteria Bacteria whose cell walls are composed of a thick layer of peptidoglycan with attached teichoic acids and that retain the stain or resist decolorization by alcohol in Gram staining. Examples include *Streptococcus pneumoniae, Staphylococcus aureus*, and *Enterococcus* species.

gravitational sedimentation Deposition of aerosol particles due to gravity.

gravity The force of attraction between all masses in the universe.

ground circuit detector An inexpensive device that, when plugged into an electrical outlet, identifies whether the electrical outlet is properly grounded.

ground glass appearance A hazy increased attenuation of the lungs, with preservation of bronchial and vascular margins.

grunting A sound heard in newborns with respiratory distress. It occurs when the glottis closes as the body attempts to maintain lung volume.

Guillain-Barré syndrome (GBS) An acute idiopathic polyneuritis usually presenting as an ascending symmetric paralysis associated with absent tendon reflexes.

gum elastic bougie An endotracheal tube introducer that assists with intubation; it is generally used in case of a difficult intubation.

H

Hagen-Poiseuille equation An equation relating flow to the fourth power of the radius, directly and inversely related to the viscosity of the fluid and the length of the tube through which the fluid passes, and directly related to the pressure gradient. If these variables are kept constant, the pressure gradient over the length of the tubular structure in question is directly proportional to flow.

Haldane, John A Scottish physiologist and biochemist who discovered the effect of oxygen on hemoglobin dissociation of carbon dioxide (the Haldane effect) and conducted important research in regulation of breathing. He also contributed to development of gas masks and oxygen masks in World War I.

Haldane effect The influence of O_2 on the CO_2 dissociation curve; it ensures that the CO_2 content of deoxygenated blood is greater than the CO_2 content of oxygenated blood at any P_{CO_2}.

Hampton hump A wedge-shaped peripheral infiltrate that may be seen after a pulmonary embolus occludes distal vessels in the pulmonary arterial tree.

hand hygiene Hand washing with soap and water for 15 to 20 seconds or using alcohol-based gels, foams, or rubs that do not require water.

handoff A transfer of responsibility for a patient from one caregiver to another. The goal of a handoff is to provide timely, accurate information about a patient's care plan, treatment, current condition, and any recent or anticipated changes.

Harvey, William (1578–1657) An English physician who correctly described the arterial and venous circulations.

Hasselbalch, Karl Albert (1874–1962) Developer of an equation that measures blood acidity.

Head paradoxical reflex A vagal block of the Hering-Breuer reflex, which allows the overinflated lung to continue to inflate; the process helps maintain an increased tidal volume during exercise.

health belief model A theory focusing on prevention of disease and asserting that taking action depends on one's perception of four issues: one's level of susceptibility to the condition, the severity of the consequences that might result from contracting the condition, the potential benefits of the health action in preventing or reducing susceptibility, and the barriers or costs related to starting or continuing the proposed behavior.

Health Insurance Portability and Accountability Act (HIPAA) A federal law that establishes the rights, protections, and other standards of care for working people with preexisting medical conditions.

health maintenance organization (HMO) An organization that provides or arranges managed care for health insurance, self-funded healthcare benefit plans, individuals, and other entities in the United States and acts as a liaison with healthcare providers (e.g., hospitals, physicians) on a prepaid basis.

health promotion An individual's voluntary adoption of a wellness model and choice to gain an awareness or knowledge of healthy lifestyle practices, incorporate such practices into the daily routine, and ultimately reach a higher level of well-being and wellness.

healthcare-associated infection (HAI) An infection associated with the delivery of health care in any setting.

healthcare utilization The use of health-related resources such as drugs, medical devices, and hospitalization.

heart rate The number of heart beats in 1 minute.

heat of vaporization The amount of heat required to convert a liquid into a gas at constant temperature and pressure.

heliox A gaseous mixture of helium and oxygen; it is used clinically because of its low density.

helium An inert gas with a lower density than either air or O_2.

helium dilution One of the most commonly used methods of measuring functional residual capacity.

helmet An interface for noninvasive ventilation or continuous positive airway pressure that fits over the entire head of the patient.

Helmholz, H. Fred, Jr. The first chairman of the Joint Review Committee for Respiratory Therapy Education.

hematocrit The proportion of whole blood that is composed of red blood cells.

hemoglobin An iron-containing globular protein consisting of two pairs of polypeptides; its primary function is the transport of oxygen from the lungs to the tissues.

hemolysis The process where water passes through a cell, bursting it, such as occurs when the water concentration is higher outside the cell.

hemothorax Blood trapped in the pleural space, causing a space-occupying lesion. The source of blood is typically from fractured ribs lacerating the intercostal blood vessels or lacerating the lung.

Henderson, Lawrence A U.S. physiologist and biochemist whose research into acid–base regulation elucidated the role of the carbon dioxide/bicarbonate buffer system in the blood.

Henderson-Hasselbalch equation An equation showing that the pH of a buffer is determined by the ratio of the concentration of base to the concentration of weak acid.

heparin A drug used to prevent further clot formation.

hepatojugular reflux Inappropriate elevation of a usually normal jugular venous pressure when the abdomen is compressed for 1 minute over the liver.

Hering-Breuer reflex Stimulation of pulmonary stretch receptors when the lung inflates and the transpulmonary pressure rises, which sends an afferent impulse to the dorsal ventral group to stop inhalation; this process maintains the rate and depth of breathing during moderate exercise.

hertz (Hz) Unit of measure for wave frequency; equal to 1 cycle per second.

high-flow/fixed-performance device An oxygen delivery device that provides a premixed oxygen concentration at a flow that meets or exceeds a patient's inspiratory demand.

high-flow nasal cannula A delivery device in which humidified oxygen in excess of 6 L/min is delivered to the nares via well-fitted nasal prongs.

high-frequency chest wall compression (HFCWC) An airway clearance technique that uses a vest to compress the chest externally with short, rapid expiratory flow pulses; it relies on chest wall elastic recoil to return the lungs to their functional residual capacity.

high-frequency chest wall oscillation (HFCWO) An airway clearance technique that uses a chest cuirass to generate biphasic changes in transrespiratory pressure difference.

high-frequency flow interrupter ventilation (HFFIV) One of four general types of high-frequency ventilation; it delivers inspiratory flow to the patient in short bursts via a rotating ball valve or microprocessor-controlled solenoid valve, producing breath rates of 2 to 22 Hz (1 Hz = 60 breaths/min). With this therapy, both the inspiratory and expiratory phases are active.

high-frequency jet ventilation (HFJV) One of four general types of high-frequency ventilation; it delivers short pulses of gas directly into the trachea through a narrow-bore cannula or jet injector.

high-frequency oscillatory ventilation (HFOV) One of four general types of high-frequency ventilation; essentially an airway vibrator, usually using piston pumps or a vibrating diaphragm that operates at frequencies ranging from 3 to 15 Hz. Both inspiratory and expiratory phases are active with this therapy.

high-frequency positive pressure ventilation (HFPPV) Conventional positive pressure ventilation at high breath rates (>150 breaths/min) and small tidal volumes, with a short inspiratory time to facilitate the increased respiratory rate. With this therapy, exhalation is passive.

high-frequency ventilation (HFV) A mode of mechanical ventilation used in neonatal and pediatric critical care. It features positive pressure ventilation at rates greater than 150 breaths/min and tidal volumes approximating the anatomic dead space, with an ability to deliver an adequate minute volume with a lower airway pressure. HFV is often used when conventional mechanical ventilation has failed.

high-reliability organization (HRO) An organization or system that operates in hazardous conditions but has fewer than its fair share of adverse events. The features of high-reliability organizations include a preoccupation with failure; a commitment to resilience; sensitivity to operations; and a culture of safety, in which individuals feel comfortable drawing attention to potential hazards or actual failures without fear of censure from management.

hilum The depression in the lung where the vessels and nerves enter.

Hippocrates (460–370 BC) The father of Western medicine.

home medical equipment (HME) company A company that provides products to aid in the care of the patient at home, including, but not limited to, mobility aids (wheelchairs, walkers, electric or semi-electric hospital beds), respiratory equipment (apnea monitors, bilevel and continuous positive airway pressure devices, home oxygen therapy, mechanical ventilators), enteral products (pumps and enteral formula), and wound and skin care products (lymphedema pumps, special seating and mattresses). Also called durable medical equipment (DME) company.

home respiratory care Those prescribed respiratory care services provided in a patient's personal residence; they may include patient assessment and monitoring, as well as diagnostic and therapeutic modalities and providing education regarding respiratory equipment, disease management, and health-promoting behaviors for the patient and the family caregiver(s).

honeycomb appearance The presence of cystic airspaces with thick fibrous walls lined by bronchiolar epithelium.

hormone A chemical substance produced in the body that controls and regulates the activity of certain cells or organs.

hospital-acquired pneumonia (HAP) Pneumonia that develops after hospital admission, excluding any infection that is incubating at the time of admission.

Hounsfield units (HU) A measurement system used in computed tomography to indicate density, in which air is given a value of −1000 and water is given a value of 0, causing most soft tissues to have values ranging from −100 to 100 and bone to range from 600 to over 2000.

House of Delegates (HOD) One of several governance and advisory entities of the American Association for Respiratory Care.

huff coughing A forced expiratory technique that is performed by sharply exhaling from high- to mid-lung volumes through an open glottis; it is used for patients who are unable to generate an effective cough.

human immunodeficiency virus (HIV) A retrovirus that causes acquired immune deficiency syndrome (AIDS) by infecting helper T cells of the immune system.

humidity deficit A condition in which inspired gas is not fully saturated at body temperature, requiring the body to add water to inspired gases to achieve full saturation.

humidity therapy A respiratory therapy that delivers water vapor or aerosol.

Hutchinson, John (1811–1861) The developer of the spirometer to measure the effect of disease on lung volumes.

hybrid stent An airway stent composed of a nitinol frame and a silicone or polyurethane sheath.

hydrogen bond The connection that holds adjacent water molecules together in a liquid state; it requires a significant amount of heat to be absorbed to change water from a liquid to a gas.

hydrophilic Water-loving; describes molecules that tend to be attracted to, and mix well with, water molecules.

hydrophobic Water-hating; describes molecules that tend to be repelled by, and to repel, water molecules.

hydrostatic pressure Static water pressure, generated by the water's weight and varying on the basis of the density of the fluid and its height, reflecting the force of gravity; with other fluids, this pressure is called manometric pressure.

hydrostatic testing A process that measures the expansion characteristic of a compressed air cylinder when it is exposed to internal pressures two-thirds greater than normal. The test is performed by totally suspending the cylinder in a tank of water and then pumping water into the cylinder.

hyperbaric oxygen (HBO) therapy A treatment modality in which a patient breathes 100% oxygen intermittently while the pressure of the treatment chamber is increased to a point higher than sea-level pressure.

hypercalcemia An increased serum level of calcium; it is characterized by anorexia, vomiting, polyuria, mental confusion, obtundation, and death.

hypercapnia Excess carbon dioxide in the blood; it can be caused by hypoventilation, increased dead space, and increased CO_2 production.

hypercarbia Elevation of $Paco_2$ to more than 40 mm Hg.

hyperchloremia An increased serum level of chloride.

hyperinflation A lung condition in which air is not easily exhaled, resulting from decreased lung elasticity and subsequent increased expiratory airways resistance and air trapping as a result of dynamic airway compression.

hyperkalemia An increased serum level of potassium; it can produce hyporeflexia and muscle weakness. Paralysis can occur in severe cases, but death because of cardiac arrhythmias usually takes place before this occurs.

hypermagnesemia An increased serum level of magnesium.

hypernatremia An increased serum level of sodium.

hyperosmolar An osmolar concentration of the body fluids that is abnormally increased.

hyperoxia A term to describe increased oxygen in the body.

hyperphosphatemia An increased serum level of phosphorus.

hyperpnea Rapid, deep, labored breathing.

hyperresonant A loud, low-pitched, long sound produced using percussion technique. This sound is often heard over an emphysematous lung.

hypersomnolence A condition characterized by excessive sleepiness.

hypertonic A property of a solution with an osmotic pressure greater than that within the cell.

hyperventilation Rapid, deep, labored breathing resulting in a lowered $Paco_2$.

hypocalcemia A decreased level of calcium in the blood.

hypochloremia A decreased level of chloride in the blood.

hypokalemia A decreased level of potassium in the blood.

hypomagnesemia A decreased level of magnesium in the blood.

hyponatremia A decreased level of sodium in the blood, which creates a significant shift in the relationship between the intracellular and extracellular fluid compartments.

hypophosphatemia A decreased level of phosphorus in the blood, primarily caused by decreased absorption, intracellular shifts, or increased excretion.

hypopnea Shallow respiration (*hypo*: less; *pnea*: breathing).

hypothalamus The command center for homeostatic regulation of the body.

hypothermia A core temperature of 95° F (35° C) or less.

hypotonic A property of a solution with an osmotic pressure less than that within the cell.

hypoventilation Reduction in the amount of breathing, which causes an increase in $Paco_2$.

hypovolemic shock Hypotension with end-organ dysfunction caused by intravascular volume loss; most commonly due to hemorrhage in a traumatically injured patient.

hypoxemia A deficiency in blood oxygenation. Hypoxemia in adults is usually defined as a Pao_2 of less than 80 mm Hg at sea level.

hypoxemic drive A secondary ventilatory drive that triggers increased minute ventilation when Pao_2 is less than 60 mm Hg.

hypoxic drive theory The theory that high levels of Pao_2, resulting from supplemental O_2, increase the Pao_2 and cause the O_2 chemoreceptors to decrease ventilation; this response causes the $Paco_2$ to rise.

hypoxia A broad term to describe diminished oxygen to body tissues.

hypoxic pulmonary vasoconstriction Narrowing of the lumen in a pulmonary blood vessel because of low oxygen level.

I

ideal gas law PV = nRT; that is, the product of pressure (P) and volume (V) is equal to the product of the number of molecules of gas (n), absolute temperature (T), and a gas constant (R).

idiopathic pulmonary arterial hypertension (IPAH) Pulmonary hypertension of unknown origin.

idiopathic pulmonary fibrosis (IPF) This is an interstitial lung disease of unknown pathogenesis but that likely reflects an aberrant host response to injury of the alveolar epithelium and endothelium or a protracted response to the same.

illness/wellness continuum A perspective in patient education in which health is viewed both from a traditional perspective and from a wellness perspective.

impedance pneumography A method for measuring respiratory rate and excursion in which two electrodes are placed on the chest wall and a high-frequency, low-ampere AC current is then passed between the electrodes.

impedance threshold valve (ITV) An airway adjunct for resuscitation that produces a small vacuum in the chest during the recoil phase of chest compression, thereby improving venous return.

implementation In a patient education context, putting the teaching plan into action; a dynamic, didactic encounter between the teacher and the learner.

immunosenescence Aging of the immune system.

incentive spirometry (IS) A technique designed to mimic natural sighing or yawning maneuvers; also referred to as sustained maximal inspiration.

incidence How often a disease or condition is contracted or diagnosed in a time period.

incident report An occurrence report filed for an untoward incident in a healthcare system, such as administration of an incorrect medication; also called a safety report.

indemnity insurance plan A type of commercial insurance plan that provides a benefit only if and when a medical event occurs. Indemnity plans provide payment of a fixed sum for a covered benefit.

indirect calorimetry A technique for measuring energy requirements, based on the primary measurement of oxygen consumption and carbon dioxide production.

infection control Policies and procedures to minimize the risk of spreading infections.

inferential statistics Statistical methods to allow inference to other settings; often involves the reporting of a P-value.

inferior vena cava Along with the superior vena cava, one of the two largest veins in the body; it is formed by the joining of the common iliac veins.

inferior vena cava (IVC) filter A vascular filter that is implanted into the inferior vena cava to prevent fatal pulmonary emboli.

informed consent The right of the patient to receive all pertinent information before undergoing or refusing treatment; it includes the components of disclosure, understanding, voluntary nature, competence, and permission giving.

inhalation injury Sequela of aspiration of superheated gases, steam, or noxious products of incomplete combustion, generating adverse effects on both gas exchange and hemodynamics.

inspection An examination technique that ranges from casual observation to visual scrutiny of the patient.

inspiratory positive airway pressure (IPAP) The level of pressure specified on ventilators designed to provide noninvasive positive pressure ventilation.

institutional review board (IRB) A facility-specific group that officially approves proposed studies, ensures the safety of participants for a new treatment, and verifies that informed consent forms are signed by the patient, nearest relative, or guardian to approve the treatment or control.

insurance A guarantee against loss or harm; the act, system, or business of insuring one's person against loss or harm; the equitable transfer of the risk of a loss from one entity to another in exchange for payment. This form of risk management is primarily used to hedge against the risk of illness.

integrated care A concept bringing together inputs, delivery, management, and organization of services related to diagnosis, treatment, care, rehabilitation, and health promotion; an organizational process of coordination that seeks to achieve seamless and continuous care, tailored to the patient's needs, and based on a holistic view of the patient.

intensive program A pulmonary rehabilitation program that generally provides two to five sessions per week for periods of 4 to 12 weeks.

intermittent asthma The least severe category of asthma. It is characterized by symptoms of coughing or wheezing fewer than two times per week with asymptomatic or normal peak expiratory flow (PEF) values between brief exacerbations; nocturnal symptoms of coughing, wheezing, or breathlessness fewer than two times per month; and measured FEV_1 or PEF that is consistently more than 80% of predicted, while maintaining less than 20% variability in PEF routinely.

intermittent-flow device A device that gives oxygen intermittently only during the inspiratory cycle.

intermittent-flow oxygen Oxygen delivery that is provided based on the patient's inspiratory effort and turns off during exhalation, eliminating oxygen waste associated with continuous flow during exhalation.

intermittent mandatory ventilation (IMV) A mode of breath delivery or ventilation in which a mandatory breath rate is set and the patient determines the tidal volume and rate of the spontaneous breaths between the mandatory breaths.

intermittent positive pressure breathing (IPPB) Episodic mechanical ventilation for the primary purpose of providing short-duration hyperinflation therapy. It is usually administered with pneumatically driven, pressure-triggered, and pressure-cycled ventilators.

international 10-20 system A system developed in 1958 to standardize the placement of electrodes for electroencephalogram (EEG) recording. The system is termed 10-20 because electrodes are placed either at 10% or 20% of the total distance between two skull landmarks. This system allows for comparison of electrical activity from different areas of the brain and serial comparison of follow-up EEGs in a single patient.

interstitial lung disease (ILD) Any of the approximately 200 distinct diseases in which the pulmonary interstitium is altered by inflammation or fibrosis, or both.

interventional study A research study that modifies care.

intra-aortic balloon pump (IABP) A catheter-based balloon that is inserted into the descending aorta just below the aortic arch and inflated during diastole, causing increased coronary blood flow, and deflated during systole, causing decreased afterload.

intracellular fluid Fluid inside cell membranes that contains dissolved solutes essential to electrolytic balance and healthy metabolism.

intrapulmonary percussive ventilation (IPV) A form of airway clearance therapy that uses a pneumatic device called a Percussionator. The patient breathes through the mouthpiece, which delivers high-flow mini-bursts of air, along with an aerosolized medication, at rates of more than 200 cycles/minute.

intrinsic positive end-expiratory pressure End-expiratory alveolar pressure that is greater than the pressure at the proximal airway, which results from high airways resistance and a short expiratory time. Also called auto-PEEP.

ion An electrically charged atom or group of atoms.

ionic bond A stable atomic configuration accomplished by transferring electrons.

I-PASS A mnemonic developed as a handoff that acts as a checklist for information to include in the handoff. **I**: Illness severity; **P**: Patient summary (the standard clinical summary); **A**: Action list for the next team; **S**: Situation awareness/contingency plans; **S**: Synthesis—a chance for a read-back of the information by the provider being briefed.

ipratropium An anticholinergic medication.

iron lung An airtight ventilator that consists of a metal tank enclosing the entire body, except the head; the prototype negative pressure ventilator.

ischemia A decrease in oxygenated blood in a body part or organ.

isothermic saturation boundary (ISB) The point at which inspired gas is fully saturated at body temperature (44 mg/L at 37° C), approximately 5 cm below the carina at the level of the third-generation airways.

isotonic A property of a solution that occurs when the osmotic pressure is equal to that found within cells.

isotope Any of a group of atoms whose nuclei have the same number of protons (atomic number) but a different number of neutrons (mass number).

J

Jackson, Chevalier (1865–1958) An American laryngologist credited with inventing the first anesthetic laryngoscope.

jaundice A yellowish skin color arising from an elevated serum bilirubin level.

jet nebulizer An aerosol-producing device that uses a jet of compressed gas that passes through a restricted orifice, creating a low-pressure area near the tip of a narrow tube; fluid is drawn from the device's reservoir and sheared or shattered into droplets by the airstream.

The Joint Commission (TJC) A private-sector, not-for-profit organization in the United States that operates accreditation programs for a fee to subscriber hospitals and other healthcare organizations. Formerly known as the Joint Commission on Accreditation of Healthcare Organizations.

joule (J) A unit of energy in the meter-kilogram-second system equivalent to the product pressure and volume, or equivalent to 107 erg or 1 watt/second.

justice The principle dealing with fairness and equity in the distribution of scarce healthcare resources, such as time, services, equipment, and money.

juxtacapillary receptors C-fibers. Their stimulation by conditions that affect the capillaries (e.g., alveolar inflammation, pulmonary vascular congestion, or edema) may result in rapid shallow breathing, dyspnea, expiratory narrowing of the glottis, and bradycardia.

K

K complexes A sharp, negative, high-voltage electroencephalographic wave, followed by a slower, positive component. K complexes occur spontaneously during nonrapid eye movement sleep, beginning in (and defining) stage 2.

Kaplan-Meier plot A graphical display of the survival rate over time.

Kerley B lines Short lines that appear perpendicular to the pleural surface on a chest radiograph; they are associated with congestive heart failure.

kinesics Messages created through body motion.

Kussmaul breathing Hyperventilation that occurs as a compensatory mechanism in metabolic acidosis.

kyphosis Forward curvature of the spine.

L

lactate An anion of lactic acid most commonly formed in ischemic cells as a consequence of anaerobic glycolysis; it is frequently used as an indicator of the severity of shock.

lactate threshold The point where lactate (lactic acid) begins to accumulate in the bloodstream; also known as the anaerobic threshold.

Laennec, René (1781–1826) The French developer of the science of auscultation who invented the stethoscope.

Laerdal, Åsmund With Peter Safar, the developer of a manikin to allow simulator training for medical personnel and the lay public.

Lambert-Eaton syndrome (LEMS) A rare myasthenic-like disorder resulting from a reduction of transmitter release from presynaptic terminals. It is commonly associated with small cell carcinoma of the lung; limb and girdle muscles predominantly are involved.

laminar flow A pattern of flow in which concentric layers of fluid flow parallel to the tube wall at linear velocities that increase toward the center; a smooth, uninterrupted flow.

large-volume nebulizer An aerosol-producing device designed to deliver enough humidified inspired gases to provide adequate flow to meet patient inspiratory flow rates.

laryngeal mask airway (LMA) A supraglottic airway that consists of a tube with a mask and an inflatable cuff that is inserted into the pharynx. It may be used for both routine management of the airway during general anesthesia and as an emergency airway adjunct in the difficult airway.

laryngopharynx The inferior portion of the pharynx, which contains openings into the larynx and esophagus.

laryngoscope An instrument used to visualize the larynx.

laryngotracheobronchitis (LTB) Acute inflammation of the larynx, trachea, and bronchi marked by swelling of the tissues.

larynx The musculocartilaginous structure behind the tongue and hyoid bone that acts as a sphincter to protect the entrance to the trachea; it functions secondarily as the voice box.

latent error A human error that is likely to be made due to systems or routines developed in such a way that humans are disposed to making these errors.

lateral decubitus A chest radiographic view in which the patient is lying on the side.

Lavoisier, Antoine (1743–1794) A French scientist who stated the law of conservation of mass.

leading question A question that is phrased in such a way that a predetermined or expected response is inevitable.

lecithin-to-sphingomyelin (LS) ratio A test performed on amniotic fluid to determine lung maturity. When the LS ratio is more than 2:1, the lungs are considered mature.

left atrioventricular (bicuspid) valve A valve on the left side of the heart, between the left atrium and the left ventricle.

leukocyte A white blood cell.

leukocytosis Elevated white cell count; it is often a sign of significant infection but also can be associated with elevated glucocorticoids (e.g., stress reaction, steroid administration) and a number of hematologic malignancies.

leukopenia Decreased white cell count; it often indicates the presence of overwhelming infection.

leukotriene modifier A member of the most recent class of asthma medications, which are available in oral tablet or chewable (montelukast) form. These agents are beneficial as add-on therapy in patients with moderate to severe asthma.

licensure Government permission to legally practice or work in a profession, obtained by demonstrating a certain level of knowledge involving a high level of skill. Such licenses are usually issued to regulate some activity that is deemed to be dangerous or a threat to the person or the public; they often require accredited training and examinations.

life expectancy The average number of years an individual is expected to live, either from birth or in terms of the number of years remaining at any given age.

life span The typical length of time a species is expected to live.

likelihood ratio (LR) A statistic used for assessing the value of performing a diagnostic test. A likelihood ratio greater than 1 indicates the test result is associated with the disease; a likelihood ratio less than 1 indicates that the result is associated with absence of the disease.

limb-girdle muscular dystrophy A heterogeneous group of muscle dystrophies characterized primarily by weakness of the shoulder and pelvic girdles, with sparing of the facial muscles.

lipid An organic biomolecule that is soluble in nonpolar organic solvents, such as ether, alcohol, or benzene, but is not soluble in water. It is composed primarily, but not exclusively, of carbon, hydrogen, and oxygen.

liquid oxygen (LOX) storage system A superinsulated container, commonly called a dewar, that eliminates heat transfer to the contents of the container. A LOX system keeps the liquid oxygen at −298° F.

living will A document that details the types of medical treatments and life-prolonging measures that an individual does or does not want performed if he or she were to be incapacitated.

lobes The major divisions within each lung. The right lung has three lobes and the left lung two lobes. The lobes are further subdivided into bronchopulmonary segments that correspond to the distribution of a specific bronchus.

locus of control Attitude toward one's responsibility for one's own behavior. Persons with an internal locus of control believe they can control their own destiny; those with an external locus of control believe that their lives are controlled by forces outside themselves.

long-acting β_2-agonist (LABA) A β_2-agonist medication taken routinely to control and prevent bronchoconstriction. These agents are not intended for fast relief; they take longer to begin working, but relieve airway constriction for up to 12 hours.

long-acting muscarinic antagonist (LAMA) An anticholinergic medication that is taken routinely to control and prevent bronchoconstriction. Such agents are not intended for fast relief; they take longer to begin working, but relieve airway constriction for up to 24 hours. Tiotropium is the most commonly prescribed long-acting anticholinergic drug in COPD.

long-term acute care hospital (LTACH) A hospital or facility that specializes in treating patients who require extended hospitalization. Such a facility provides rehabilitation for patients who are too sick to be in a nursing home but not sick enough to be in a traditional hospital.

long-term oxygen therapy (LTOT) Administration of oxygen for at least 20 hours/day; a life-prolonging therapy for hypoxemic patients with chronic obstructive pulmonary disease.

longevity Length or duration of life.

loop of Henle The long U-shaped section of the renal tubule between the proximal convoluted tubule and the distal convoluted tubule; it includes a descending limb and an ascending limb.

lordosis Backward curvature of the spine.

low-flow/variable-performance device An oxygen delivery device that provides supplemental oxygen at a concentration that varies because the delivered oxygen is mixed with variable amounts of inhaled room air.

lung compliance The elastic properties of the lungs; normally 200 mL/cm H_2O.

lung injury score A measure that incorporates the level of positive end-expiratory pressure, the PaO_2/FIO_2 ratio, a chest radiograph score, and lung compliance into a summary score that can be used to describe the severity of acute lung injury.

lung-protective ventilator strategy A ventilatory technique in which the target tidal volume is 6 mL/kg of predicted body weight, the plateau pressure is kept below 30 cm H_2O, and positive end-expiratory pressure is applied to maintain alveolar recruitment.

lung capacity A combination of two or more lung volumes: vital capacity, inspiratory capacity, functional residual capacity, or total lung capacity.

lung transplantation Transfer of a pulmonary organ system from a donor to a recipient; it is recognized as an accepted therapy for end-stage cystic fibrosis lung disease.

lung volume A measure of the size of the lungs: tidal volume, inspiratory reserve volume, expiratory reserve volume, or residual volume.

lung-volume reduction A procedure that removes 20% to 30% of the lung tissue most severely affected by emphysema, encouraging the remaining lung to gain recoil elasticity and improve lung, chest wall, and diaphragmatic mechanics in addition to right ventricular performance. Also called lung-volume reduction surgery.

lung-volume reduction surgery (LVRS) A procedure that removes 20% to 30% of the lung tissue most severely affected by emphysema, encouraging the remaining lung to gain recoil elasticity and improve lung, chest wall, and diaphragmatic mechanics in addition to right ventricular performance.

M

Macklin effect The dissection of air into the mediastinum, which creates vertical linear streaks on the chest radiograph.

macrophages Cell type derived from blood monocytes or through local proliferation that resides in many locations in the lung; they are associated with defense of the lung against inhaled agents and with phagocytosis of particulates and debris.

magnetic resonance imaging (MRI) Imaging that takes advantage of nuclear magnetic resonance.

maintenance program A medically supervised facility- or home-based pulmonary rehabilitation program for patients with pulmonary disease who reside locally.

malignant Tending to become worse and to cause death; a malignant cancer is anaplastic, invasive, and metastatic.

managed care organization (MCO) A system of financing and delivery of health care that is intended to reduce the cost of providing health benefits and to improve the quality of care.

mandatory breath A breath for which the start or end of inspiration (or both) is determined by the ventilator, independent of the patient.

Mantoux test Placement of purified protein derivative (PPD) subcutaneously to detect the presence of an immune response to mycobacteria by eliciting a delayed-type hypersensitivity response.

manual resuscitator A bag-valve device consisting of a self-inflating bag, an air-intake valve, a nonrebreathing valve, an oxygen inlet nipple, and an oxygen reservoir to aid in resuscitation and breathing.

mass The amount of a substance determined by the number and type of molecules.

mass casualty respiratory failure (MCRF) An event resulting in patients requiring mechanical ventilation in excess of the space available to care for them and the devices available to provide ventilatory support.

mass median aerodynamic diameter (MMAD) A measurement that expresses the geometric size of the particles of an aerosol. For medical use, aerosol generators should produce respirable particles with an MMAD range of 1 to 5 μm.

mass number The sum of the protons and neutrons inside the nucleus of an atom; often used interchangeably with the term "atomic weight."

mass spectrometer An instrument capable of measuring all respiratory gases, including respiratory and anesthetic gases, breath by breath.

mast cell A cell that produces histamine and leukotrienes, both of which constrict airway smooth muscles. The two types of mast cells are classified according to their neutral protease composition (chymase and/or tryptase).

mast cell stabilizer A type of medication used to treat respiratory disease.

matching A research evaluation parameter of a study that asserts that the controls must be similar to the treatment group in as many respects as are feasible to avoid other factors confounding (confusing) the results.

matter Any substance that has mass and occupies space.

maximum expiratory pressure (MEP or PE_{max}) After a full inhalation, the pressure generated by forced exhalation against an occluded airway.

maximum inspiratory pressure (MIP or PI_{max}) After a full exhalation, the pressure generated by forced inhalation against an occluded airway.

mean airway pressure ($\bar{P}aw$) Average pressure, relative to atmospheric pressure, within the airway during one complete respiratory cycle. It is directly related to the inspiratory time, respiratory rate, peak inspiratory pressure, and positive end-expiratory pressure.

mechanical insufflation–exsufflation A technique in which a device inflates the lungs with positive pressure followed by negative pressure to simulate a cough; also called cough assist.

mechanical ventilation Use of a device to help patients breathe, by assisting with the inhalation of oxygen into the lungs and the exhalation of carbon dioxide.

meconium aspiration syndrome (MAS) A condition that develops when the fetus or newborn inhales meconium. The most common cause of severe hypoxemic respiratory failure, it can block the air passages and cause failure of the lungs to expand or other pulmonary dysfunction such as pneumonia or emphysema.

meconium ileus Obstruction of the small intestine in the newborn resulting from an impaction of thick, dry, cohesive meconium, usually occurring at or near the ileocecal valve. Meconium is a thick, dark green material that collects in the intestines of the full-term fetus and forms the first stools of a newborn; it consists of a mixture of intestinal gland secretions, some amniotic fluid, and intrauterine debris, such as bile pigments, fatty acids, epithelial cells, mucus, lanugo, and blood.

mediastinal shift Movement of the tissues and organs that constitute the mediastinum (heart, great vessels, trachea, and esophagus) to one side of the chest cavity.

mediastinoscopy Examination of the mediastinum using an endoscope with light and lenses inserted through an incision in the suprasternum.

mediastinum The area between the lungs; the mediastinum contains the heart and its vessels, the esophagus, trachea, phrenic and cardiac nerves, thoracic duct, thymus, and lymph nodes of the central chest.

Medicaid A healthcare insurance program funded jointly by the federal and state governments that pays for medical services for the elderly, disabled, poor, and dependent children.

medical gas cylinders Containers used to store medical gas. They range from small, lightweight units containing a few cubic feet of gas to large cylinders with capacities of several hundred cubic feet. U.S. Department of Transportation regulations specify that high-pressure medical gas cylinders be made of seamless construction from high-quality steel, chromium–molybdenum alloy, or aluminum.

medical record A collection of documentation of patient assessments, problem identification, care plans, treatments, and outcomes, typically including discharge summaries, progress notes, physician orders, laboratory results, and flow sheets, as well as additional media, which may include online reports, photographs, videotapes, films, and audio recordings.

Medicare The federal government's healthcare insurance program for the elderly, the disabled, and persons with certain diseases, such as end-stage renal disease.

medication reconciliation The process of avoiding inadvertent inconsistencies across transitions in care by reviewing the patient's complete medication regimen at the time of admission, transfer, and discharge and comparing it with the regimen being considered for the new setting of care.

medium The means of transmitting information between a sender and a receiver.

medulla oblongata A structure in the brain stem that contains the respiratory control center; it is responsible for regulating breathing, coughing, sneezing, swallowing, and vomiting.

meninges Layered membranes that protect the brain and spinal cord.

mesh nebulizer An aerosol-generating device that forces a solution through a mesh to generate particles.

meshing The process of passing a skin graft through a device that creates a matrix of small holes in the tissue, allowing it to be stretched.

message The information, facts, data, ideas, thoughts, feeling, or attitude conveyed during communication.

meta-analysis A statistical process that combines the results of several studies that address a set of related research hypotheses.

metabolic acidosis A decrease in pH associated with a loss of buffer (HCO_3^-).

metabolic alkalosis An increase in pH associated with an increase in buffer (HCO_3^-).

metabolic cart A device used to perform indirect calorimetry.

metabolic equivalent (MET) A physiological concept expressing the energy cost of physical activity as a multiple of resting oxygen consumption.

metallic stent An airway stent constructed of a lattice of nitinol, a metallic alloy with excellent shape memory. The nitinol allows the stent to be deployed in a contracted state but then self-expand to return to its originally constructed size.

metastasis The process by which tumor cells spread to distant parts of the body.

methemoglobin The form of hemoglobin that is produced when the iron in heme is oxidized from Fe^{+2} to Fe^{+3}.

methylxanthine An agent that serves as a smooth muscle relaxant and cardiac muscle and CNS stimulant. Clinically, methylxanthine is employed as a bronchodilator, though it is declining in popularity for long-term care.

microbiology The branch of biology that studies microorganisms and their effects on other living organisms.

midbrain The structure in the brain stem that is responsible for regulation of hearing and vision.

mild persistent asthma Category of asthma characterized by symptoms of coughing or wheezing more than two times per week but less than once per day, with symptoms that affect normal daily activities of living or normal nighttime sleep patterns; nocturnal symptoms of coughing, wheezing, or breathlessness more than two times per month; and measured FEV_1 or peak expiratory flow (PEF) that is consistently more than 80% of predicted or personal best, while maintaining approximately 20% to 30% variability in PEF rates.

milliequivalent One-thousandth of a gram equivalent of a chemical element, an ion, a radical, or a compound.

minibronchoalveolar lavage (mini-BAL) A nonbronchoscopic method of performing a small-volume bronchoalveolar lavage for quantitative culture; the results are used to guide antibiotic therapy prescribed for patients suspected of having ventilator-associated pneumonia.

minimum data set (MDS) Part of the U.S. federally mandated process for clinical assessment of all residents in Medicare- or Medicaid-certified nursing homes. This process provides a comprehensive assessment of each resident's functional capabilities and helps nursing home staff identify health problems.

mitochondrial myopathy One of the manifestations of hereditary mitochondrial disorders, occurring as a result of a point mutation in mitochondrial DNA. It can also affect other organ systems, particularly the brain.

mitral valve (bicuspid valve) A valve that lies between the left atrium and left ventricle, and prevents blood from flowing back into the left atrium from the ventricle.

mixed apnea A combination of central and obstructive apnea.

mode A preset pattern of interaction between the ventilator and the patient.

moderate persistent asthma Category of asthma characterized by symptoms of coughing or wheezing on a near-daily basis, with exacerbations experienced more than two times per week, and often persisting for multiple days. It manifests with symptoms that routinely interfere with normal daily activities of living or normal nighttime sleep patterns; nocturnal symptoms of coughing, wheezing, or breathlessness more than one time per week; and measured FEV_1 or peak expiratory flow (PEF) that is routinely 60% to 80% of predicted or personal best, while consistently maintaining more than 30% variability in PEF rates.

molar solution A solution containing one mole of solute per liter of solution.

mole A quantity of a substance equal to its gram molecular weight, which contains 6.02×10^{23} atoms (Avogadro's number).

moral philosophy An individual's behavioral code, defining behavior in a given situation, based on personal principles the individual has previously adopted.

motivation The patient's interest in changing an undesirable behavior associated with his or her condition.

motivational interviewing (MI) A directive, client-centered counseling style for eliciting behavior change that focuses on helping clients explore and resolve ambivalence.

mouth occlusion pressure ($P_{0.1}$) A test of the central respiratory drive that is independent of underlying respiratory mechanics. The maximum negative mouth pressure generated during the first 100 milliseconds (0.1 second) of inspiration is measured during complete airway occlusion.

mucociliary apparatus A mechanism that clears inhaled agents from the lower respiratory tract.

mucokinetic agent A drug that is intended to reduce mucus viscosity and assist with the mobilization of airway secretions.

multiple sclerosis (MS) A demyelinating disease of the central nervous system characterized clinically by repeated remissions and exacerbations of symptoms, including paresthesias, motor weakness, diplopia, blurred vision, bladder incontinence, and ataxia.

multiresistant The state of possessing resistance to multiple drugs (especially antibiotics).

murmur An extra-cardiac sound heard in conjunction with S_1 and S_2.

muscular dystrophy A heterogeneous group of progressive, hereditary degenerative skeletal muscle diseases in which the respiratory muscles, like any skeletal muscle, become progressively weaker, eventually culminating in respiratory failure and death. Respiratory complications are the most common cause of death in these diseases.

mutation An event that changes the genetic structure of a living organism.

myasthenia gravis (MG) An autoimmune disorder characterized by impaired transmission of neural impulses across the neuromuscular junction resulting from the destruction of the postsynaptic acetylcholine receptors.

myocardial infarction Prolonged blockage of the coronary arteries; also known as heart attack.

myocardial ischemia A condition of inadequate blood flow in the coronary arteries that supply the heart muscle; it often results in angina.

myocardial perfusion imaging An imaging technique that involves intravenous injection of a radionuclide agent, which accumulates in the myocardium in proportion to regional myocardial perfusion.

myocardium The thick middle layer of the heart wall.

myotonic dystrophy A chronic, slowly progressing, inherited disease characterized by wasting of the muscles (muscular dystrophy), cataracts, heart conduction defects, endocrine changes, and myotonia.

N

N-of-1 randomized controlled trial An approach to treatment in which patients undergo pairs of treatment periods during which they receive a target treatment in one period and a placebo or alternative in the other period.

nasal continuous positive airway pressure (NCPAP) Therapeutic support for potential low lung volumes and associated hypoxemia (particularly in infants); also commonly used in the treatment of obstructive sleep apnea.

nasal high flow (NHF) A therapy that delivers high flows of blended, heated, and humidified oxygen through a specially designed nasal cannula.

nasal mask An interface for noninvasive ventilation or continuous positive airway pressure that fits over the nose of the patient.

nasal oxygen cannula A low-flow variable performance delivery device consisting of nasal prongs that are loosely placed in the nares.

nasal pillows An interface for noninvasive ventilation or continuous positive airway pressure featuring prongs that fit into the nose of the patient.

nasopharyngeal airway An airway device that is inserted into the nose and directed along the floor of the nose parallel to the hard palate; it represents an alternative to the oropharyngeal airway.

nasopharynx The uppermost region of the throat or pharynx, located behind the nasal cavity and extending from the posterior nares to the level of the soft palate.

nasotracheal intubation An intubation technique in which the tube is passed through the nasal passage.

nasotracheal suctioning A maneuver used to remove secretions from the lower respiratory tract.

National Association for Medical Direction of Respiratory Care (NAMDRC) A national organization of physicians whose mission is to educate its members and address regulatory, legislative, and payment issues that relate to the delivery of healthcare services to patients with respiratory disorders.

National Asthma Education and Prevention Program (NAEPP) An expert panel of the National Institutes of Health that focuses specifically on the needs of, and programs affecting, individuals with asthma.

National Asthma Educator Certification Board (NAECB) The organization that oversees the voluntary testing program used to assess qualified health professionals' knowledge in asthma education.

National Board for Respiratory Care (NBRC) A voluntary health certifying board founded in 1960 for the purpose of evaluating the professional competence of respiratory therapists by providing high-quality voluntary credentialing examinations for respiratory care and pulmonary function technology.

National Patient Safety Goals A series of specific actions that accredited organizations are required to take to prevent medical errors such as miscommunication among caregivers, unsafe use of infusion pumps, and medication errors.

near-infrared spectroscopy (NIRS) A technique for noninvasive monitoring of peripheral tissue oxygenation.

nebulizer A device that produces an aerosol, or suspension, of particles in gas.

negative pressure ventilation Use of a ventilator that applies less than ambient pressure to the external chest wall.

neoadjuvant therapy A cancer treatment, such as chemotherapy or radiation, that usually precedes another phase of treatment.

nephron The functional unit of the kidneys, which consists of the renal corpuscles and renal tubules.

neurally adjusted ventilatory assist (NAVA) A mode of ventilation that is triggered, limited, and cycled by the electrical activity of the diaphragm (diaphragmatic EMG).

neuromuscular blocking agent A chemical substance that interferes locally with the transmission or reception of impulses from motor nerves to skeletal muscles.

neuron A nerve cell.

neutral thermal environment An environment that provides adequate warmth and humidity to minimize insensible heat and water loss for premature and newborn infants. It can be achieved with use of an incubator for a premature, sick, or low-birth-weight infant.

neutron A particle with no mass but a net charge, found inside the nucleus of an atom.

new oral anticoagulant An anticoagulant agent that is administered by mouth.

nitric oxide (NO) A colorless gas that is naturally synthesized in human tissue and plays an important role in vascular smooth muscle relaxation, inhibition of platelet aggregation, neurotransmission, and immune regulation.

nitrogen A gas that makes up approximately 80% of the earth's atmosphere.

nitrogen balance Study involving a 24-hour urine collection and calculation of the difference between nitrogen intake and excretion; it helps determine protein requirements and assess changes in visceral protein store status over time.

nitrogen washout A method for measuring functional residual capacity.

nitrogen washout atelectasis Alveolar collapse due to replacement of nitrogen with oxygen.

nocturnal asthma A marker for uncontrolled or more severe asthma; it indicates a decrease in lung function of patients who are sleeping.

nodular appearance Multiple round opacifications on the chest radiograph.

noninvasive open ventilation (NIOV) A battery-operated, portable ventilator and nasal pillows interface that is intended for use as a home-based ventilation system.

noninvasive positive pressure ventilation Mechanical ventilation provided without an artificial airway.

noninvasive ventilation (NIV) A form of mechanical ventilation that does not involve an endotracheal tube or tracheostomy tube.

nonmaleficence The principle by which the healthcare practitioner refrains from harming the patient.

nonprotected bronchial brush An instrument used for cytologic sampling of proximal airways and central tumors under direct vision as well as peripheral lesions under fluoroscopic guidance. A catheter with a brush (open or enclosed in a sheath) at its distal end is introduced through the working channel of the bronchoscope for sampling of proximal airways or central tumors.

nonrapid eye movement (NREM) sleep Phases of sleep during which there is an absence of rapid eye movement. NREM sleep is subdivided into three stages: N1, N2, and N3. Stages N1 and N2 represent superficial sleep, whereas stage N3 represents deep sleep.

nonrebreathing mask An oxygen mask with a one-way valve between the bag and the mask and another one-way valve over one or both mask ports; this arrangement causes all of the patient's exhaled volume to be directed out of the mask through the mask ports. The valve positioned between the mask and the bag prevents exhaled gases from entering the bag.

non-small-cell lung cancer (NSCLC) A major category of histologic types of lung carcinomas, including adenocarcinoma of the lung, large cell carcinoma, and squamous cell carcinoma. This type of lung cancer is characterized histologically by keratinization or glandular differentiation and has no features of small cell lung cancer on histology; it is believed to arise from bronchial epithelial cells.

nontuberculous mycobacterial infection (NTM) Noninfectious mycobacterial microorganisms found in soil and water.

nonverbal communication The process of conveying meaning in the form of non-word-oriented messages.

nonverbal cue A form of communication without words. Cues include messages created through body motion, the use and interpretation of space, the use of sounds, and touch.

normal flora Bacteria that normally exist in a particular area of the healthy body and do not usually cause disease at that site.

nosocomial Pertaining to an infection that is acquired in a hospital or nursing home.

nosocomial pneumonia Pneumonia occurring in hospitalized patients.

nucleic acid An organic molecule, principally occurring as either deoxyribonucleic acid or ribonucleic acid, that is made from chains of nucleotide, each of which consists of a phosphate group, a five-carbon sugar, and a nitrogenous base.

O

obesity hypoventilation syndrome A combination of obesity (body mass index ≥30 kg/m^2) and arterial hypercapnia ($Paco_2$ ≥45 mm Hg) during wakefulness.

observational study A study design that draws inferences about the possible effect of a treatment on subjects, where the assignment of subjects into a treatment group versus a control group is outside the control of the investigator.

obstructive apnea Reduction in airflow to less than 90% of baseline despite persistent respiratory effort.

obstructive lung disease Disease characterized by a reduced lumen of the airways within the lungs.

Ohm's law The principle describing properties of electric systems, assuming linear relations between a pressure, resistance, and flow term, without loss of thermal energy, or turbulence. This law may be applied to easily measured quantities, such as electric resistance, and to other circular systems of single or connected circuits in which measurement may be more technically difficult.

oncotic pressure The osmotic pressure of a colloid in solution, such as exists with a higher concentration of protein in the plasma on one side of a cell membrane than in the neighboring interstitial fluid.

opacifications Areas on a chest radiograph that block the passage of x-ray energy and, therefore, appear white.

open-ended question A questioning technique that generally involves short probes followed by periods of silence in which the recipient of the communication is permitted to develop a more in-depth and personal response; almost always begins with *what*, *why*, or *how*.

opiate A natural or synthetic derivative of morphine, derived from the opium poppy, which stimulates opiate receptors in the brain and spinal cord to decrease the sensation of pain. Opiates also act as potent sedatives, respiratory depressants, and cough suppressants.

optimum care committee A committee consisting of physicians, administrators, service department members, clergy, a medical ethicist, and community members, who are brought together to consider divergent viewpoints related to the ethical issues in patient care. When involved in patient care, its goal is to issue a recommendation. Also called an ethics committee.

oral appliance A dental device for clinical use; it can be characterized primarily as either a tongue-retaining device or a mandibular-advancing device.

oronasal mask An interface for noninvasive ventilation or continuous positive airway pressure that fits over the nose and mouth of the patient.

oropharyngeal airway An artificial airway with a relatively rigid structure that is designed to be inserted into the mouth between the lips and teeth and extend from the lips to the pharynx, following the natural curvature of the tongue, without entering the larynx or esophagus.

oropharynx One of the three components of the throat or pharynx, extending behind the mouth from the soft palate to the hyoid bone; it contains the palatine and lingual tonsils.

orotracheal intubation Establishment of an artificial airway by placing a tube through the mouth into the trachea.

orthopnea Breathlessness, especially when an individual is recumbent.

orthostatic hypotension A decrease in blood pressure that occurs when changing from a reclining position to an upright position.

osmosis The process of transferring water molecules through a semipermeable membrane; it involves the movement of water from an area of high concentration to an area of low concentration in an attempt to make the concentrations equal.

osmotic pressure Externally applied hydrostatic pressure that stops the flow of a solvent through a membrane.

oxidative phosphorylation Joining of a phosphate group to adenosine diphosphate to form adenosine triphosphate during catabolism.

oximeter A spectrophotometer that uses specific wavelengths in the oxyhemoglobin spectrum to measure hemoglobin oxygen saturation in the blood.

oximetry Determination of the hemoglobin oxygen saturation of arterial blood using an oximeter.

oxygen analyzer A device used to measure the concentration of oxygen administered to patients.

oxygen concentrator A device designed to produce a low flow (typically, 0.5 to 5.0 L/min) of high-purity oxygen (90% to 95%) from room air by either molecular adsorption of nitrogen or filtration of air through a membrane; it is the most widely used source of oxygen in the home and in extended care facilities.

oxygen-conserving device (OCD) A device that supplies a flow of oxygen only when it is needed, on demand at the initiation of inspiration. The conserver is placed between the oxygen supply and the delivery device, which can be a nasal catheter, a nasal cannula, or a transtracheal catheter.

oxygen consumption (O_2) The rate of O_2 uptake by the body, measured by analyzing inspired and expired O_2; it is approximately 250 mL/min in the adult under resting conditions.

oxygen delivery (DO_2) The rate of O_2 transport to the peripheral tissues; it is determined by the cardiac output and arterial O_2 content. Also referred to as O_2 availability or O_2 transport.

oxygen extraction The difference between the amount of oxygen delivered to the tissues and the amount of oxygen remaining when the blood leaves the tissues.

oxygen hood A clear rigid plastic device that can be placed over an infant's head for oxygen administration.

oxygen-induced hypoventilation Reduced ventilation that results from the administration of high concentrations of oxygen.

oxygen pulse A physiological term for oxygen uptake per heartbeat at rest.

oxygen tent A device used for both oxygen administration and for high humidity therapy; it is rarely used in modern practice.

oxygen toxicity A pathologic response of the body and its tissues to long-term exposure to high partial pressures of oxygen.

oxygenation index (OI) A measure calculated from mean airway pressure FIO_2 and PaO_2 and used to estimate the severity of hypoxemia.

oxygenator In an extracorporeal membrane oxygenation system, the device that provides the artificial gas exchange; it is external to the patient.

oxyhemoglobin Hemoglobin that is bound to oxygen.

oxyhemoglobin dissociation curve (ODC) The nonlinear in vivo relationship between PO and O_2 saturation; commonly called the oxyhemoglobin dissociation curve.

P

$PaCO_2$ The partial pressure of carbon dioxide in the blood.

PaO_2 The partial pressure of oxygen in the blood.

PaO_2/FIO_2 A number calculated by dividing PaO_2 by FIO_2 and used to estimate the severity of hypoxemic respiratory failure.

pack years Measure of a patient's smoking exposure; one pack per day for 1 year equals 1 pack year.

pallor Diminished skin color accompanying anemia or, in case of severe peripheral vasoconstriction, accompanying shock.

palpation The examiner's use of his or her hands to feel for body movement, lumps, masses, and skin characteristics.

papillary muscle A muscle that contracts as the heart's ventricles contract, pulling on the chordae tendinae to prevent the cusps from swinging back into the atrium.

paradoxical respiration Flail chest movement, which is characterized by chest wall movement outward on expiration and inward on inspiration.

paralinguistics The use of sound in the communication process.

parasites Plants or animals that live with or on another organism, deriving benefit from the association but having a detrimental effect on the host.

parasympathetic system The part of the nervous system that decreases heart and breathing rates; it is responsible for the "rest-and-digest" response.

parenteral nutrition Administration of nutrients by a route other than the alimentary canal.

parietal pleura A serous membrane of mesothelial cells and connective tissue that lines the chest wall, covers the diaphragm, and extends over the structures of the mediastinum.

Parkinson disease A neurologic disorder characterized by hypokinesia, tremor, and muscular rigidity.

paroxysmal nocturnal dyspnea Sudden shortness of breath that occurs several hours after a patient lies down; it suggests the presence of cardiac dysfunction.

partial rebreathing mask A simple oxygen mask equipped with a reservoir bag. The oxygen supply tube is positioned between the mask and the reservoir bag, and the oxygen flow is set at a rate sufficient to keep the bag at least partially inflated throughout inspiration.

partial thromboplastin time (PTT) Clotting time in anticoagulation therapy; ideally, it is 2 to 2.5 times the control value.

pascal Under the SI system, the primary unit of pressure; that is, 1 N/m^2. For ease of calculation, the kilopascal (kPa) is commonly used so that 1 standard atmosphere (at sea level) is approximately 101 kPa.

passive humidifier A humidifying device that uses exhaled heat and moisture to humidify the inspired gas; also called a heat and moisture exchanger.

passover humidifier A humidifying device that directs gas over the surface of a body of water; an example is a passover wick humidifier.

Pasteur, Louis (1822–1895) A French chemist and microbiologist whose immunology work led to an anthrax vaccine; the developer, with Claude Bernard, of the pasteurization process.

pasteurization A process for killing or reducing the number of pathogens and organisms other than bacterial spores.

pathway One of the main tools used to manage quality in health care concerning the standardization of care processes. Such processes are designed to provide the greatest efficiency of care with the greatest quality. Also referred to as clinical pathway, critical pathway, care pathway, integrated care pathway, or care map.

Patient Care Partnership A definition established by the American Hospital Association in 2003 that outlines the rights and responsibilities patients have regarding their medical care; previously called the Patient Bill of Rights.

patient-controlled analgesia (PCA) A method of pain control in which the patient can self-administer intravascular pain medication. The computerized device administers doses and includes a lockout interval to automatically inactivate the system if a patient tries to increase the amount of drug used within a predetermined time period.

patient education The use of the educational process for individuals, their families, and other significant persons when they are dependent upon the healthcare system for diagnosis, treatment, or rehabilitation.

patient–ventilator asynchrony A condition in which there is a mismatch between how the patient is breathing and how the ventilator is delivering breaths.

Pauling, Linus (1901–1994) A U.S. scientist who exploited the characteristic that increased oxygen enhances a magnetic field to develop the D-2 oxygen analyzer.

pay for performance (P4P) A concept to reward (pay) physicians based on the quality of care provided to patients instead of the current concept of paying based on the volume of care.

peak flow meter A monitoring device for the management of asthma, which is used to measure peak expiratory flow.

peak inspiratory pressure (PIP) The highest pressure measured at the proximal airway during positive pressure ventilation.

pectus carinatum A condition in which the chest bows out at the sternum, similar to a pigeon's chest.

pectus excavatum A condition in which the sternum is depressed and deviated somewhat like a funnel.

penetrating trauma A mechanism of traumatic injury in which the body of the patient is incised. Common forms of penetrating injuries are stab wounds and gunshot wounds.

penumbra effect A condition that can occur during the application of pulse oximetry in which the sensor is not correctly positioned. This effect causes incorrect readings when the sensor is not symmetrically placed, causing one wavelength to be overused in the calculations of saturation.

peptide A compound created when amino acids are linked together, with the OH from the carboxyl group of one amino acid and the H from the amine group of another amino acid splitting off.

percent solution Concentration measure of a solute, usually expressed in units of mass or volume in ratios such as weight/weight, weight/volume, and volume/volume; commonly used in clinical situations.

percentage of body humidity (%BH) In clinical practice, a measure of humidity to assess humidity deficit.

percussion An examination technique in which the examiner places a finger firmly against a body part and then strikes that finger with a fingertip from the other hand. The sounds produced may suggest the presence of either normal or abnormal tissue.

percussion therapy The technique of rapidly clapping, cupping, or striking the external thorax directly over the lung segment being drained, with either cupped hands or a mechanical device.

percutaneous coronary intervention (PCI) The use of balloon angioplasty or placement of stents in occluded or stenotic coronary arteries to improve flow through affected arteries.

perfusion index (PI) A value derived from the photoelectric plethysmographic signal of a pulse oximeter and calculated as the ratio of the pulsatile component (arterial compartment) and the nonpulsatile component (other tissues—venous blood, bone, connective tissue) of the light reaching the device's detector.

pericardium A membranous structure that encloses the heart and proximal ends of the large blood vessels; it consists of several different layers.

periodic limb movements (PLMs) of sleep A condition characterized by pathologic repetitive myoclonic contractions, which can result in frequent arousals or awakenings and can cause daytime symptoms such as excessive daytime sleepiness.

periodic table A tabular arrangement of the chemical elements according to atomic number.

perioperative program A pulmonary rehabilitation program designed to optimize a patient's functional status prior to surgery.

peripheral chemoreceptors Nerve cells sensitive to changes in the blood chemistry that are found outside the brain.

peripheral proprioceptors Nerve receptors that sense the relative positioning and activity of the various body parts in relation to one another.

permissive hypercapnia High $Paco_2$ resulting from protective ventilation strategies.

persistent pulmonary hypertension of the newborn (PPHN) A clinical syndrome characterized by a sustained elevation of pulmonary vascular resistance after birth, resulting in hypoxemia and right-to-left extrapulmonary shunting of blood.

personal belief system A set of personal beliefs that an individual develops based on life experience. These beliefs are not necessarily right or wrong and are certainly not objective, but they are deeply ingrained in an individual's thoughts and decision-making processes.

personal protective equipment (PPE) Protective clothing (gowns), gloves, goggles, or other garments or devices used alone or in combination to protect mucous membranes, airways, skin, and clothing from coming in contact with infectious agents.

personal value system A value system that is formed when a decision is made to continue to believe and express a conviction even when a person or event challenges it.

Petty, Thomas A coauthor of an influential paper on acute respiratory distress syndrome, which led to development of positive end-expiratory pressure as a therapy. Also contributed to the understanding of the value of long-term oxygen therapy and pulmonary rehabilitation.

pH An indicator of the hydrogen ion concentration $[H^+]$ in a solution; mathematically defined as the negative logarithm of the hydrogen ion concentration.

pharmacodynamics A drug's action in the body, both at a molecular level and in terms of its overall clinical effect.

pharmacokinetics A drug's movement in the body through the processes of absorption, distribution, and elimination.

phenotype The observable physical or biochemical characteristics of an organism, as determined by both genetic makeup and environmental influences.

phospholipid A lipid similar to triglyceride except that instead of three fatty acids attached to a glycerol, one of the fatty acid chains is replaced by a chemical structure containing phosphorus and nitrogen. Phospholipids are primary components of cell membranes and of pulmonary surfactant.

phrenic nerve Nerves that exit the third through fifth cervical vertebrae and provide motor innervation to the diaphragm.

piezoelectric plethysmography A measurement of how much rib cage or abdominal displacements stretch an elastic belt; the plethysmography apparatus utilizes a piezoelectric buckle, which encloses a sensor that generates a voltage in response to stretch passed through the ends of the belts, thereby measuring respiratory motion.

Pin Index Safety System (PISS) One of three indexing safety systems for medical gases. It uses a specific combination of two holes in the post valve just below the gas outlet for each gas or gas mixture; any regulator or device intended to connect to the valve will have pins that correspond to the holes, allowing a proper connection.

planning In a patient education context, setting learning goals, objectives, and learning outcomes.

plateau pressure (Pplat) End-inspiratory alveolar pressure attained during mechanical ventilation. It should be kept below 30 cm H_2O in conjunction with an overall lung-protective ventilation strategy.

platelet A blood cell critical to clot formation after vascular injury; produced in the bone marrow.

platypnea Difficulty breathing that is experienced whenever the individual is not lying flat.

plethora Fullness of blood vessels at the skin surface, often occurring with vasodilation or hypercapnia.

plethysmographic variability index (PVI) A measure of the dynamic changes in the perfusion index (PI) that occur during the respiratory cycle. Used during pulse oximetry, it provides information about changes in the balance between intrathoracic pressure and intravascular fluid volume.

pleural effusion A collection of an abnormal volume of fluid in the pleural space in the thoracic cavity.

pleural friction rub A continuous grating sound heard with auscultation of the lungs, resembling two pieces of leather or two hands being rubbed together; this sound occurs when pleurae are inflamed or when fluid accumulates in the pleural cavity.

pleural space The space between the visceral and parietal layers of the pleurae.

pleurodesis Obliteration of the pleural space produced by inflammation in the visceral and parietal pleural surfaces, resulting in symphysis of the pleural surfaces.

pneumatically powered portable ventilator A portable ventilator that requires a compressed gas source for its operation; an electrical power source is not required.

pneumobelt An unconventional ventilation device that consists of an inflatable rubber bladder held over the abdomen by an adjustable corset; it assists with diaphragmatic motion by causing piston-like motions of the abdominal viscera.

pneumonia Any of several subgroups of respiratory infections that are characterized by the inflammation and consolidation of lung tissue caused by infectious agents.

pneumotaxic center The portion of the upper pons that receives afferent impulses from the vagus nerve that help fine-tune the respiratory rhythm and blocks stimulation of the dorsal and ventral respiratory groups from the apneustic center.

pneumothorax Air in the pleural space that can cause collapse of the lung.

point-of-care testing (POCT) Diagnostic testing at or near the site of patient care.

point-of-service plan (POS) A type of health insurance plan that represents a hybrid of the health maintenance organization (HMO) and preferred provider organization (PPO) plans. Point-of-service plans attempt to provide the tight utilization controls of the HMO coupled with the ability to choose a nonparticipating provider at the point (time) of receiving the service.

polar Type of molecule that forms as the result of unequal charge distribution on a molecule, rather than the sharing or transfer of electrons.

polysomnogram A comprehensive recording made in a sleep diagnostics lab; it includes all multichannel respiratory recording variables, plus electroencephalographic, electrooculographic, and electromyographic measurements made during sleep, for the diagnosis of sleep-disordered breathing.

polysomnography A sleep study that produces a polysomnogram.

pons The structure in the brain stem that is responsible for maintenance of regular breathing.

pores of Kohn Openings between the alveoli that allow collateral ventilation between adjacent alveoli.

portable oxygen concentrator (POC) An oxygen system that includes a power source (battery), which allows for mobility of the oxygen concentrator. Most POCs are small enough to be moved by the patient and usually weigh less than 20 pounds.

positive end-expiratory pressure (PEEP) The baseline pressure applied during exhalation with mechanical ventilation.

positive expiratory pressure (PEP) An airway clearance technique in which the patient exhales against a fixed-orifice flow resistor to aid in the movement of secretions into the larger airways.

positron emission tomography (PET) An imaging modality used for assessing thoracic pathology, in particular for tumor imaging. It provides physiologic and metabolic information and focuses on the biochemical properties of cells.

posteroanterior (PA) projection A chest radiographic view in which the x-ray beam passes through the chest from the back to the front.

postpoliomyelitis syndrome Progressive muscle weakness occurring, on average, 29 years after recovery from an episode of acute poliomyelitis.

postural drainage (PD) Use of positioning and gravity to drain secretions from areas of the bronchi and lungs into the trachea.

PRECEDE-PROCEED model A model widely used in the health promotion movement, focusing on factors external to the individual that shape healthcare behavior. The acronym PRECEDE stands for predisposing, reinforcing, and enabling constructs in education/environmental diagnosis and evaluation; the acronym PROCEED stands for policy, regulatory, and organizational constructs in educational and environmental development.

precipitate To crystallize within a solute.

precordium Part of the front chest wall that overlays the heart and epigastrium.

preferred provider organization (PPO) An organization in which member physicians, pharmacists, and hospitals offer their health services to subscriber patients on a discounted fee-for-service basis.

prejudice A judgment formed before due examination and consideration of the facts; a premature or hasty judgment. Both bias and prejudice inform clinical decision making, and both the student and the seasoned practitioner must confront their own biases and prejudices prior to making decisions.

preload Distending pressure within the ventricle during diastole.

President's Council An ex-officio group of the American Association for Respiratory Care (AARC) Board of Directors, consisting of past presidents of the AARC.

pressure Force per unit area.

pressure amplitude A means of manipulating the P_{CO_2} level during high-frequency oscillatory ventilation. Increasing the amplitude increases displacement of the bellows, thereby increasing tidal volume delivery. An increased pressure amplitude at the airway opening results in a lower Pa_{CO_2}.

pressure control (PC) Breath type in which airway pressure is set and remains constant with changes in resistance and compliance.

pressure support (PS) Breath type in which patient effort is augmented by a clinician-determined level of pressure during inspiration; no rate is set.

pressure-time product (PTP) The time integral of the difference between the esophageal pressure tracing and the recoil pressure of the chest wall; it accounts for energy expenditures during the dynamic and isometric phases of respiration.

pressure triggering A form of triggering in which the ventilator detects a pressure drop at the proximal airway as the inspiratory effort of the patient and initiates the inspiratory phase.

pressure–volume curve A plot of pressure and increasing or decreasing lung volume; the shape of the curve is determined by the elastic properties of the system. The upper and lower inflection points can be used to set PEEP on the ventilator and to avoid overdistention.

pressurized metered dose inhaler (pMDI) The most commonly prescribed method of aerosol delivery; it is used to administer bronchodilators, anticholinergics, anti-inflammatory agents, and steroids. The device consists of a pressurized canister containing a drug in the form of a micronized powder or solution that is suspended with a mixture of propellants, surfactant, preservatives, flavoring agents, and dispersal agents.

prevalence How many persons have a given disease or condition in a location at a given time.

prevention Measures taken to avoid the development of disease, as opposed to treating disease.

Priestley, Joseph (1733–1804) An English theologian-scientist and politician who discovered oxygen.

primary apnea A period of rapid breathing followed by a period of gasping or no breathing; it may be observed in stressed neonates.

primary ARDS Acute lung injury caused by direct injury to the lungs, such as pneumonia, aspiration of gastric contents, inhalation of toxic gases, or pulmonary contusion.

primary survey The initial evaluation of life-threatening injuries of the trauma patient using the mnemonic ABCDE: airway and cervical spine protection, breathing, circulation, deficits, and exposure.

procalcitonin A precursor of the hormone calcitonin that is involved with calcium homeostasis and is produced by the C cells of the thyroid gland. It has also has been proposed as a marker of infection in critically ill patients.

procedural sedation Use of sedative medications by properly trained healthcare providers to enhance relaxation while maintaining adequate spontaneous respiratory efforts by the patient during an invasive procedure.

programmed instruction A learning method and materials that allow the patient to learn at his or her own pace and that require little time on the part of the respiratory therapy patient educator.

prone position Position in which the patient is lying face-downward. Changing patients with acute respiratory distress syndrome from a supine to a prone position may result in a significant improvement in oxygenation; prone positioning may also improve secretion clearance from the lungs.

proportional assist ventilation (PAV) A positive feedback control that provides ventilatory support in proportion to neural output of the respiratory center; the ventilator calculates the pressure required from the equation of motion.

prospective payment system (PPS) A payment mechanism for reimbursing hospitals for inpatient healthcare services in which a predetermined rate is set for treatment of specific illnesses.

prospective study A research study that is designed and then conducted to avoid bias.

prostacyclin A pulmonary vasodilator that is the most effective therapy available for patients with primary pulmonary hypertension.

protected bronchial brush An instrument used for collecting microbiologic samples to ensure that the bacteria collected represent lower-tract pathogens and not upper airway contaminants. The brush is enclosed within two telescoping catheters, the outer of which protects the catheter tip from contamination as it is advanced through the bronchoscope and proximal airways.

protein A large molecule composed of carbon, hydrogen, oxygen, and nitrogen; it forms when a chain of peptides reaches about 100 amino acids or more in length.

protein-calorie malnutrition (PCM) Nutritional deficit affecting all muscle fiber types, but impairing fast-twitch fibers most profoundly, and resulting in decreased contractile strength. The primary component of the immune system adversely affected by protein-calorie malnutrition is cell-mediated immunity.

prothrombin time (PT) A test for coagulation defects, which is used to evaluate the extrinsic pathway, depending on the levels of factors V, VII, X, and eventually I and II.

protocol A written plan specifying the procedure to be followed in giving a particular examination, in conducting research, or in providing care for a certain condition.

proton A particle with a positive charge (+1) located inside the nucleus of an atom.

proxemics The use and interpretation of space in the communication process.

proxy A person, specified by the patient in a legal document, who will make decisions for the patient in the event he or she is incapable of making a decision.

pseudoglandular stage The second stage of lung development, generally considered to last from week 17 to week 26 of gestation.

pseudohypoxemia Factitious hypoxemia; a condition in which the $Pa{O_2}$ within a blood gas sample decreases rapidly in the presence of extreme leukocytosis; the result is a measured $Pa{O_2}$ much lower than the $Pa{O_2}$ in the patient.

psychomotor domain The area of learning involved in physical movement, coordination, and use of motor skills. It entails a person's ability to perform a task or procedure.

pulmonary agenesis Developmental malformation during the fourth week of gestation characterized by complete absence of the bronchus, bronchial tree, alveolar parenchyma, and pulmonary and bronchial vasculature. It is most often unilateral but can involve both lungs, which is incompatible with life.

pulmonary alveolar proteinosis (PAP) An interstitial lung disease characterized by filling of alveolar spaces with a lipoproteinaceous exudate and interstitial fibrosis; it usually presents with dyspnea and cough.

pulmonary angiography Radiographic examination of the blood vessels of the lungs after injection of an opaque contrast medium into the pulmonary circulation.

pulmonary aplasia A congenital abnormality that develops during the fourth week of gestation in which the lung and pulmonary artery are absent but there is a rudimentary bronchus coming off the trachea.

pulmonary arterial hypertension (PAH) An increase in blood pressure in the pulmonary arterial vasculature.

pulmonary artery A blood vessel that supplies blood to the lungs.

pulmonary artery (PA) catheter A Swan-Ganz catheter, which is inserted into the pulmonary artery and provides pressure measurements, cardiac output determinations, and mixed venous blood analysis.

pulmonary artery pressure Blood pressure within the pulmonary artery; a reflection of pulmonary vascular resistance and left heart failure.

pulmonary artery wedge pressure (PAWP) A measure that provides an estimate of left atrial (LA) and left ventricular end-diastolic or filling pressure (LVDEP).

pulmonary contusion A bruise in the lung that is usually the primary culprit in gas exchange abnormalities following chest trauma. Blood and edema collect at the site of lung injury, causing decreased focal air exchange.

pulmonary edema Accumulation of excess fluid in the interstitial and alveolar spaces in the lung.

pulmonary embolism (PE) Blockage of a pulmonary artery by foreign matter, such as fat, air, tumor tissue, or a thrombus. It is characterized by dyspnea, sudden chest pain, shock, and cyanosis.

pulmonary function tests (PFTs) Breathing tests that are used to detect restrictive or obstructive patterns, the gas transfer abnormalities that accompany some restrictive and some obstructive lung diseases, and respiratory muscle weakness.

pulmonary hypertension (PH) Abnormally high pressure within the pulmonary circulation.

pulmonary hypoplasia A congenital anomaly in which there is a decrease in the number or size of airways, alveoli, alveolar cells, and pulmonary vessels, resulting in a small lung. This condition may be primary or secondary to intrauterine conditions that limit fetal lung growth and may involve one or both lungs.

pulmonary rehabilitation Any of a variety of outpatient programs that provide opportunities to restore patients to the highest possible level of independence and functioning in the community. Such programs typically include exercise training, education for patients and their families, instruction in use of inhalers and airway clearance, and psychological support.

pulmonary semilunar valve A valve located at the base of the pulmonary trunk; it has three cusps and allows blood to leave the right ventricle while preventing backflow into the ventricular chamber.

pulmonary sequestration A result of abnormal fetal development of the lung bud; the formation of a cystic or solid piece of lung tissue, most often within a lung segment or next to the lung usually near the diaphragm. It is treated by surgical resection to prevent excessive blood flow through the lesion.

pulmonary trunk A vessel that arises from the right ventricle of the heart, extends upward, and divides into the right and left pulmonary arteries that convey deoxygenated blood to the lungs.

pulmonary vascular resistance (PVR) Resistance in the pulmonary vascular bed against which the right ventricle must eject blood.

pulmonary vein A blood vessel that carries oxygenated blood from the lungs to the left atrium of the heart.

pulse contour waveform analysis A method of measuring stroke volume and cardiac output through analysis of the contour of the arterial pressure waveform; this technology uses the principle that area under the arterial pressure curve correlates with stroke volume.

pulse flow Flow from an oxygen delivery system that is triggered by the patient's inspiratory effort but is terminated based on a timing mechanism, either electronic or pneumatic. Pulse flow systems usually deliver a set bolus of oxygen at a specific flow rate.

pulse oximetry A technique that measures oxyhemoglobin saturation noninvasively in arterial blood; it rapidly detects changes in arterial oxygen saturation.

pulse pressure variation (PPV) The variation of pulse pressure over the respiratory cycle (particularly during positive pressure ventilation), used to assess fluid responsiveness.

pumpless extracorporeal lung assist (PECLA) A type of extracorporeal membrane oxygenation system that relies on an oxygenator attached to the patient's arterial and venous systems; it uses the patient's own arterial pressure as the driving force for blood flow through the pump.

purified protein derivative (PPD) A dried form of tuberculin that is injected subcutaneously during a Mantoux test to detect past or present infections with tubercle bacilli by eliciting a delayed-type hypersensitivity response.

Purkinje fiber One of the branches of the atrioventricular bundle that spread and enlarge, located near the papillary muscles; these fibers continue to the heart's apex and cause the ventricular walls to contract in a twisting motion.

Q

quick-relief medication Any of a group of primarily short-acting agonists used to combat acute exacerbations of bronchoconstriction or provide quick, complete resolution of airflow obstruction and its accompanying symptoms of cough, wheezing, and chest tightness. This category includes short-acting β_2-agonists and anticholinergics.

R

radiodensity The ability of an object to block x-ray energy, determined by its composition and thickness.

radiolucent Pertaining to body tissues that are penetrated by x-rays, such that they produce black areas on the chest radiograph.

radionuclide angiocardiography A noninvasive technique for evaluating left ventricular function, which uses intravenous injection of a radioisotope (most commonly technetium-99m) and imaging via a gamma-ray scintillation camera to detect the isotope's signal within the left ventricle.

radiopaque Pertaining to body tissues that cannot be penetrated by x-rays, such that they produce white areas on the chest radiograph.

radiotherapy Primary treatment of an intrathoracic tumor or metastatic disease, involving the use of x-rays or gamma rays to slow or stop the proliferation of malignant cells.

Raman spectroscopy A method used to measure the concentration of CO_2 in the inspired and expired gas.

randomization The process of avoiding bias by ensuring random assignments of, for example, subjects to either a treatment group or a control group.

randomized controlled trial (RCT) The primary study method for testing the effectiveness of a medical treatment. Patients are randomized to receive either a treatment or usual care, with their outcomes then being compared to evaluate the effect of the treatment.

rapid eye movement (REM) sleep The phase of the sleep cycle marked by the presence of rapid eye movements on electrooculography.

rapid response team A group of clinicians with critical care expertise who quickly respond to the patient's bedside in the event that the patient develops a life-threatening condition.

Rating of Perceived Exertion (Modified Borg Scale) A numeric scale for assessing dyspnea, whose values range from 0 (representing no dyspnea) to 10 (maximal dyspnea).

receiver operating characteristic curve A graphical plot of the sensitivity, or true positives, versus (1 – specificity), or false positives.

refeeding syndrome The metabolic and clinical disturbances that occur after the reinstitution of nutrition to patients who are malnourished or starved.

regression analysis A statistical method of evaluating the relationship of independent variables to dependent variables.

remote alarm A device that transmits the sound of a ventilator alarm to another (remote) location. Depending on the ventilator and the type of remote alarm, the remote alarm may be physically connected to the ventilator via a long cable, or it may transmit the sound from the ventilator wirelessly to the remote alarm.

renal corpuscle The glomerulus and glomerular capsule.

renal pelvis The funnel-shaped extension of the ureter's upper end, where urine is collected.

renal tubule Part of the nephron, where fluid is secreted and reabsorbed, resulting in the formation of urine.

resistance Ratio of pressure to flow; a lung characteristic that, with compliance, serves as a determinant in the mechanics of airflow in and out of the lungs.

resistive load A component of the patient–ventilator interaction, describing the resistance of the respiratory system (lungs and chest wall) and volume of flow as a function of time.

resonant A quality of sound produced in percussion that is loud, low, and long, such as may be heard over normal lung tissue.

resource-based relative value scale (RBRVS) A reimbursement methodology that assigns values to physician services based on the resource costs (time, skill, and resource intensity) of providing those services. It is based on a national fee schedule and replaces the previous payment method outlining usual, customary, and reasonable charges.

resource intensity The relative volume and types of diagnostic, therapeutic, and bed services used in the management of a particular illness.

Respimat Soft Mist Inhaler A device that delivers a metered dose of medication as a fine mist without the use of a propellant or external power source.

respiratory acidosis A decrease in pH associated with an elevated Pa_{CO_2}.

respiratory alkalosis An increase in pH associated with a decreased Pa_{CO_2}.

respiratory arrest Cessation of breathing.

respiratory bronchiolitis A rare lung disorder that occurs exclusively in cigarette smokers. It is characterized by intracytoplasmic golden-brown, granular pigment within alveolar macrophages in respiratory and terminal bronchioles.

RESPIRATORY CARE The official science journal of the American Association for Respiratory Care, which is published monthly and indexed in PubMed.

respiratory dialysis A low-flow extracorporeal carbon dioxide removal system that uses a double-lumen catheter to remove the patient's blood, pass the blood through a gas exchanger, and return it to the patient.

respiratory distress syndrome (RDS) Condition of a newborn characterized by dyspnea with cyanosis; the most common cause for hypoxemic respiratory failure in premature neonates.

respiratory effort–related arousal A sequence of breaths lasting 10 seconds, which is characterized by increasing respiratory effort leading to an arousal from sleep, when the sequence of breaths does not meet the criteria for apnea or hypopnea.

respiratory exchange ratio (RER) Ratio of CO_2 to O_2 (CO_2/O_2). During steady-state exercise at moderate to low levels of exertion, the RER reflects the respiratory quotient, which is the ratio of CO_2 to O_2 in the mitochondria.

respiratory inductance plethysmography (RIP) A method for indirectly measuring tidal volume, in which sensors use a circuit of coiled wire woven into an elastic band and excited by an AC current. Inductance results from alternating electrical currents that create magnetic fields around themselves; those changing magnetic fields alter other electrical currents that they encounter.

respiratory mechanics The forces needed to move the lungs and the chest wall; an expression of lung function through measures of pressure and flow.

respiratory quotient The ratio of carbon dioxide produced to oxygen consumed in the stoichiometric oxidation of a particular substrate.

respiratory system compliance The elastic properties of the respiratory systems (lungs with chest wall); normally 100 mL/cm H_2O.

resting energy expenditure (REE) Energy requirements, either estimated by prediction equations or measured by calorimetry.

restless legs syndrome (RLS) A sensorimotor disorder characterized by irresistible desire to move the legs accompanied by uncomfortable, irritating, or painful symptoms in the legs that can occur throughout the day but that are most common in the evening.

restrictive lung disease An abnormality detected by spirometry that is characterized by reduced lung volumes.

retinopathy of prematurity (ROP) Formation of fibrous tissue behind the lens of the eye, caused by excessive oxygen administration to premature infants. It produces blindness in its worst form. Also called retrolental fibroplasia.

retrospective payment system (RPS) A system of reimbursement based on costs actually incurred.

retrospective study A study that looks back at records to determine what has been done.

Reynolds number A dimensionless number that describes factors associated with the generation of laminar or turbulent flow, such that units of measurement cancel each other when consistent units are used; describes a ratio of inertial forces to viscous forces.

rhonchus A deep, rumbling respiratory sound that is more pronounced in auscultation on expiration and is usually continuous; it is caused by air passing through a partially obstructed airway.

ribonucleic acid (RNA) A nucleic acid in which the sugar component is ribose; it acts as the machinery for the protein synthesis process by translating the genetic information stored in DNA into protein structures.

right atrioventricular (tricuspid) valve A valve on the right dorsal side of the heart, between the right atrium and the right ventricle.

right atrium One of the four chambers of the heart. It receives deoxygenated blood from the superior and inferior vena cavae, the coronary sinus, and the anterior and cardiac veins, and pumps the blood into the right ventricle through the tricuspid valve.

rigid bronchoscope A metal tube introduced into the central airways for diagnostic and therapeutic purposes.

risk of mortality The likelihood of dying.

robust process improvement (RPI) Methods and tools to improve safety and quality of health care; examples include Lean, Sigma Six, and change management processes, among others.

rocking bed An unconventional ventilation device whose action has been compared to a piston in a cylinder. As the patient's head moves down, the diaphragm slides cephalad, assisting with exhalation. In the foot-down position, the diaphragm slides caudad, assisting with inhalation.

root-cause analysis (RCA) A structured process for identifying the causal or contributing factors underlying adverse events or other critical incidents.

S

saccular stage The fourth stage of lung development, generally considered to last from week 26 of gestation to birth.

Safar, Peter (1924–2003) Author of an influential study of mouth-to-mouth resuscitation versus the Silvester arm-lift technique, which led to the development of cardiopulmonary resuscitation guidelines.

safe harbor An environment in which individuals are able to report errors or near misses without fear of reprimand or punishment.

salmeterol A long-acting β_2-adrenoceptor agonist medication.

Sanz electrode A modern pH electrode.

sarcoidosis An interstitial lung disease (ILD) in which multiple organ systems usually have noncaseating granulomas; the most prevalent ILD of unknown etiology.

sarcopenia Age-related loss of muscle mass, which starts to develop somewhere between ages 40 and 60 for both sexes.

saturated The strength of a solution indicating that it contains the maximum amount of a given dissolved solute for the given conditions.

saturated fatty acid A naturally occurring fatty acid that has all available bonds of its hydrocarbon chain filled with hydrogen atoms so that the chain contains all single carbon–carbon bonds.

sclerosing agent A chemical introduced into the pleural space to cause pleurodesis.

scoliosis Lateral curvature of the spine.

secondary apnea An irregular breathing pattern in neonates that follows primary apnea, requiring positive pressure ventilation.

secondary ARDS Acute lung injury caused by indirect injury to the lungs, such as sepsis and multiple trauma.

secondary survey The portion of the history and physical examination of the trauma patient that follows the identification and treatment of life-threatening injuries of the primary survey (ABCDE). It includes a head-to-toe physical examination and a thorough history delineating allergies, current medications used, past illnesses and pregnancies, last meal, and events or environment related to the traumatic injury.

sedative A drug taken for its calming or sleep-inducing effect.

segments Subdivisions within each lobe of the lung; each segment corresponds to the distribution of a specific bronchus.

self-inflating bag A manual resuscitator that inflates automatically and does not require an external gas source to provide positive pressure.

self-instructional Pertaining to a learning technique in which a learner (with others or alone) works without the direct control of a teacher.

semipermeable membrane A structure that separates the body's various compartments from one another and allows certain fluids and solutes to move freely between them.

senescence The state of being old or the process of aging.

sensitivity In the context of data analysis, the proportion of actual positives that are correctly identified as such.

sentinel event An adverse event in which death or serious harm to a patient has occurred; usually an event that is not expected or acceptable—for example, an accidental patient–ventilator disconnect.

serum electrolyte A substance found in the blood that dissociates into ions when melted or dissolved and is able to conduct an electric current. The most common serum electrolytes are the cations Na^+, K^+, Ca^{+2}, and Mg^{+2} and the anions HCO_3^-, Cl^-, PO_4^-, and SO_4^-.

severe persistent asthma Highest level of the four classes of asthma severity. It manifests with symptoms of coughing or wheezing almost continually with frequent exacerbations often persisting for multiple days or sometimes weeks; symptoms that limit normal daily activities of living or normal nighttime sleep patterns, with nocturnal symptoms of coughing, wheezing, or breathlessness almost every night and measured FEV_1 or peak expiratory flow (PEF) that is routinely less than 60% of predicted or personal best, while consistently maintaining more than 30% variability in PEF rates.

Severinghaus, John The co-developer of arterial blood gas electrodes.

Severinghaus electrode A modern PCO_2 electrode that represents a modification of the electrode developed by Stowe in the early 1950s.

severity of illness The extent of physiologic decompensation or organ system loss of function.

short-acting β_2-agonist (SABA) The most effective bronchodilator and the treatment of choice for severe bronchoconstriction. These rescue medicines are used for quick relief of asthma symptoms.

shunt Any cardiac or pulmonary condition in which blood passes from the right side of the heart to the left side of the heart without participating in gas exchange.

silhouette sign A radiologic sign, usually taking the form of an obliterated border, that helps to localize a radiographic opacity. For example, if the contiguous lung becomes opacified from any cause, the normal contrast between these structures is lost and the border between them is obliterated, producing the silhouette sign.

silicone stent An airway stent constructed of a silicone sleeve that is introduced into the central airways via a rigid bronchoscope.

simple oxygen mask A low-flow, variable-performance oxygen delivery device.

single-breath nitrogen test A test of ventilation distribution.

single-nucleotide polymorphism (SNP) A difference in a single nucleotide within DNA.

sinoatrial (SA) node A small mass of specialized tissue located just beneath the epicardium in the right atrium; it initiates impulses through the myocardium to stimulate contraction of cardiac muscle fibers.

situation, background, assessment, recommendation (SBAR) A technique that provides a framework for communication between members of the healthcare team about a patient's condition.

skilled nursing facility (SNF) An institution or part of an institution that fulfills the criteria for accreditation outlined by the sections of the Social Security Act that determine the basis for Medicaid and Medicare reimbursement for skilled nursing care.

sleep apnea A sleep disorder in which a person temporarily does not maintain airflow through the nose and mouth, resulting in periodic absence of breathing.

sleep apnea hypopnea syndrome (SAHS) A sleep disorder that affects the individual's breathing for short periods of time during sleep.

sleep efficiency A sleep study scoring category that measures the amount of time a patient is asleep per electroencephalographic criterion divided by the total recording time.

sleep latency A sleep study scoring category that measures the time from when lights are turned off to when the patient falls asleep.

sleep spindles A burst of brain activity visible on an EEG that occurs during stage 2 sleep.

sleep stages The phases of sleep that are based on the frequencies recorded during an electroencephalogram.

small cell lung cancer (SCLC) A type of lung cancer characterized histologically by the presence of small cells that appear blue on hematoxylin and eosin staining; it is believed to arise from bronchial neuroendocrine cells.

smoking cessation A structured program to assist individuals to quit smoking.

sniff test A test performed under fluoroscopy to confirm the elevation of a hemidiaphragm resulting from paralysis. An affected individual will demonstrate paradoxical upward movement of the affected hemidiaphragm when the patient sniffs rapidly.

solitary pulmonary nodule (SPN) A lesion, seen on a chest radiograph, that is completely surrounded by lung parenchyma, without other radiographic abnormalities such as pleural effusion or adenopathy.

solute A solid, liquid, or gaseous material that is being dissolved.

solution A homogeneous mixture of two or more substances, meaning that the substances mix evenly and occupy the entire volume in equal proportions.

solvent The liquid material into which a solute is dissolved.

somatic nervous system The part of the nervous system that handles consciously controlled motor functions, including skeletal muscle movements.

spacer A simple open-ended tube or bag that, with sufficiently large device volume, provides space for the pressurized metered dose inhaler plume to expand by allowing the propellant to evaporate.

speaking valve A device that enables a patient with a tracheostomy to communicate verbally.

specialty sections The nine divisions within the American Association for Respiratory Care (AARC) that support various major subsets of therapists.

specific heat The amount of heat per unit mass required to raise the temperature by one degree Celsius.

specificity In the context of data analysis, the proportion of actual negatives that are correctly identified.

spectrophotometry A method of identifying substances by their absorption (also called extinction) of specific wavelengths in the electromagnetic spectrum.

spinal cord A thin column of nerves leading from the brain to the vertebral canal.

spirochete A spiral-shaped bacterium.

spirometer A device used to measure lung volumes and flows; it is most commonly used for the forced vital capacity maneuver.

spirometry Breathing tests used to measure the forced vital capacity, forced inspiratory vital capacity, slow vital capacity, and maximal voluntary ventilation.

split-thickness graft A skin graft that consists of a layer of dermis, but not the other components of skin.

spontaneous breath A breath determined by the patient independent of any ventilator settings for inspiratory time and expiratory time.

spontaneous breathing trial (SBT) A process in which the patient is removed from ventilatory support and allowed to breathe spontaneously; the goal is to identify readiness for extubation.

sputum Gram stain and culture Culture of a sputum sample, followed by application of a test that stains microorganisms with crystal violet dye, followed by an iodine solution, decolorizing, and then counterstaining with safranin. The retention of either the violet color of the stain or the pink color of the counterstain serves as a primary means of identifying and classifying bacteria by revealing details of the cell wall structure; gram-positive microorganisms stain blue and gram-negative microorganisms stain pink.

sputum induction A method of facilitating the coughing up of material from the lungs, often through the administration of bland aerosols. Induced sputum contains a higher proportion of viable cells than does spontaneously produced sputum.

squamous cell carcinoma A slow-growing malignant tumor consisting of scaly or platelike epithelium.

standard deviation (SD) A measure of the dispersion of data about the mean.

standard precautions A group of infection prevention practices that apply to all patients regardless of suspected or confirmed infection status in any setting where healthcare services are provided.

Starling's law of cardiac function The longer the initial sarcomere length, the greater the force generated with contraction.

steatorrhea Greater than normal amounts of fat in the feces, characterized by frothy, floating fecal matter with a foul odor. It is seen in cystic fibrosis, celiac disease, some malabsorption syndromes, and any condition in which fats are malabsorbed by the small intestine.

sterilization Equipment-processing modality that involves the complete killing of all organisms; it requires adequate heat and time. This process destroys or eliminates all forms of microbial life.

steroid Any member of an important lipid group that is widely distributed throughout the body and involved in many important structural and functional roles.

strain Physical deformation or change in shape of a structure or substance, usually caused by stress; in the lungs, the increase in volume above resting lung volume.

stress Force applied to an area; in the lungs, the transpulmonary pressure.

stress index The shape of the pressure–time curve during constant-flow volume control; used to assess overdistention and tidal alveolar recruitment.

stress response to critical illness The wide fluctuation in metabolic rate that occurs in critically ill patients.

stress test A functional study of the coronary circulation in which a stressor is used to induce an imbalance between the coronary blood supply and myocardial demand; a means to detect the ischemic response.

stridor A crowing inspiratory sound, commonly caused by inflammation and edema of the larynx, such as may occur postextubation or with croup.

stroke Cerebrovascular accident; a sudden brain abnormality characterized by occlusion by an embolus, thrombus, or cerebrovascular hemorrhage, resulting in ischemia of the brain tissues normally perfused by the damaged vessels.

stroke volume The absolute volume of blood ejected during a single contraction of a ventricle; in adults, it is usually about 70 mL.

strong ion difference (SID) Net negative or positive charge exerted by strong ions. The underlying principle is similar to that of the anion gap, but the SID has the advantage of functioning as an independent variable in acid–base regulation.

subarachnoid (intracerebral) hematoma A traumatic brain injury characterized by the accumulation of blood in the space between the arachnoid mater and the pia mater that attaches directly to the brain. Subarachnoid hematomas often are caused by the traumatic rupture of brain aneurysms or direct bleeding from brain parenchyma.

subdural hematoma A traumatic brain injury that results in accumulation of blood in the space between the arachnoid mater and the dura mater. It is often caused by the shearing of bridging veins that run in this potential space.

suction catheter A flexible tube used to aspirate secretions.

superior vena cava Along with the inferior vena cava, one of the two largest veins in the body; the superior vena cava is formed by the joining of the brachiocephalic veins.

surface tension A property of a liquid that tends to reduce the surface of the liquid to a minimum.

surfactant A surface-active agent, such as soap or detergent, that is dissolved in water to decrease its surface tension or the tension between the water and another liquid.

surrogate An individual appointed by a patient, in a legal document such as an advance directive, living will, or durable medical power of attorney, to make decisions for that patient in the event that the patient cannot do so.

survey A means of collecting quantitative information about a population, usually via questionnaire.

suspension A liquid mixture in which the particles consist of large clumps of molecules. Its properties include the following: consisting of an insoluble substance dispersed in a liquid, being heterogeneous, not being clear, settling out over time, not passing through filter paper, and not passing through membranes.

sweat test A method of assessing sodium and chloride excretion from the sweat glands; often the first test done in the diagnosis of cystic fibrosis.

sweep gas In an extracorporeal membrane oxygenation system, the oxygen/air mixture that is passed through the oxygenator to provide gas exchange.

sympathetic system The part of the nervous system that increases heart and breathing rates; it is responsible for the "fight-or-flight" response.

synapse A functional connection where neurons communicate with other cells.

synchronization window During mechanical ventilation, a short period, at the end of a preset expiratory time or at the end of a preset inspiratory time, during which a patient signal may be used to synchronize the beginning or ending of inspiration to the patient's actions.

synchronized intermittent mandatory ventilation (SIMV) A mode of breath delivery or ventilation in which a mandatory breath rate is set and the patient determines the tidal volume and rate of the spontaneous breaths between the mandatory breaths, which are synchronized with the patient's spontaneous efforts.

systematic review A literature review focused on a single question that tries to identify, appraise, select, and synthesize all high-quality research evidence relevant to that question.

Système International d'Unités (SI system) An internationally agreed system of units in wide, but not universal use; the generally preferred system in scientific and healthcare settings.

systemic lupus erythematosus (SLE) An autoimmune disease that can affect almost all organ systems. Complications are classified as pleuritis and pleural effusions, acute lupus pneumonitis, interstitial lung disease, and respiratory muscle weakness.

systemic vascular resistance (SVR) The resistance against which the left ventricle must force its stroke volume with each beat.

systole In the cardiac cycle, a period of contraction during which the heart pumps blood into the pulmonary and systemic circulation.

systolic Pertaining to the systole; the peak of a blood pressure measurement.

systolic dysfunction Inability of the heart to pump because of direct impairment in the force of contraction or in the frequency of contractions (as in arrhythmias).

T

tachypnea Increased respiratory rate.

tactile fremitus Palpation of vibrations of the chest wall as a patient speaks.

teaching moment Any opportunity to impart critical and meaningful information to a captive audience.

team resource management The use of team members' various skills and characteristics to optimal effect, while minimizing the risk of human error.

teleological theory An ethical theory that guides decision making regarding the right or wrong qualities of an action based on the consequences of predicted outcomes.

temperature The amount of heat, or thermal energy, present in a system.

tension-time index (TTI) A measurement used to predict respiratory muscle fatigue.

tetraplegia Paralysis of all four limbs; quadriplegia.

thalamus A relay station for nerve impulses; the entry point for nerve fibers into the cerebral cortex.

theophylline A plant-derived methylxanthine.

therapeutic bronchoscopy A bronchoscopic procedure aimed at relieving central airways obstruction.

thermistor A thermometer that can measure extremely small changes in temperature.

thermocouple An apparatus that detects bidirectional airflow at the nose and mouth by sensing the temperature difference between inspired room air and exhaled air that has been warmed to body temperature; an active sensor used to measure temperature.

thermodilution A method of measuring cardiac output by injecting a cold or cool indicator and sampling with a thermistor.

third-party payer An insurer; one of the five major stakeholders in the provision and delivery of healthcare services.

thoracentesis Removal of pleural fluid from the chest cavity using a needle or small catheter.

thorax The lungs, pleura, respiratory muscles, and skeletal elements, including the sternum, ribs, thoracic vertebrae, the clavicles, and scapulae. Within the thorax, the mediastinum contains major blood vessels, the esophagus, and the heart enveloped within the pericardial sac.

Thorpe tube flow meter A flow control device that provides an accurate display of flow, provided it remains in a vertical position and the inlet pressure is constant. Unlike flow restrictors and Bourdon gauges, pressure-compensated Thorpe tube flow meters display the actual outlet flow in the face of downstream resistance.

thrombolytic therapy Use of drugs such as tissue plasminogen activator, urokinase, or streptokinase to dissolve an arterial clot.

timed walk test A test focused on functional performance that generally involves having a patient walk over a measured course for a set duration of time (for example, 6 or 12 minutes).

tiotropium A long-acting anticholinergic agent.

tissue plasminogen activator (TPA) A thrombolytic agent used to help dissolve clots.

tonometry The measurement of exact gas tensions in whole, fresh blood. Because of the unique O_2-binding characteristics of hemoglobin and the complex viscosity characteristics of normal fresh blood, whole blood must be carefully tonometered so that exact gas tensions can be prepared for analysis by a blood gas instrument.

total body surface area (TBSA) The area of involvement in thermal injury represented as a percentage of the whole body.

total enteral nutrition (TEN) Nutrition administration via direct access to the gastrointestinal tract, bypassing the mouth and throat in a patient who cannot eat but who has adequate gastric motility and emptying.

total face mask An interface for noninvasive ventilation or continuous positive airway pressure that fits over the entire face of the patient.

total lung capacity The volume of gas in the lungs at the end of a maximal inspiration and the total volume of air in the lungs seen on most chest radiographs and lung computed tomography scans.

total parenteral nutrition (TPN) Administration of a nutritionally adequate hypertonic solution that can meet the needs of a patient who cannot eat by mouth.

trachea The tubelike segment of the respiratory tract located between the larynx and the carina.

tracheostomy tube A hollow, curved tube of metal, rubber, or plastic that is surgically inserted into the trachea to relieve a breathing obstruction.

transbronchial biopsy (TBB) A procedure that collects samples of lung tissue for histopathologic review.

transbronchial needle aspiration (TBNA) An innovative bronchoscopic diagnostic technique used for staging mediastinal lymph nodes in suspected bronchogenic lung cancer, diagnosing submucosally infiltrating or extrinsically compressing tumors, approaching endobronchial tumors with necrotic or friable outer layers, and, increasingly, diagnosing peripheral nodules.

transcutaneous monitoring A means of respiratory monitoring of blood gases through electrodes applied to the skin.

transdiaphragmatic pressure (Pdi) A specific measure of diaphragm strength; made by measuring esophageal (P_{ES}) and gastric (Pga) pressures via balloon-tipped catheters placed in the midesophagus and the stomach, respectively. Pdi is then calculated by subtraction of P_{ES} from Pga (Pdi = Pga − P_{ES}).

transesophageal echocardiography (TEE) A diagnostic test in which a small ultrasound transducer is passed posterior to the heart via the esophagus, allowing close investigation of valvular heart disease because of the proximity of the transesophageal probe to the heart and the absence of intervening anatomic barriers such as the thoracic ribs. It includes all aspects of transthoracic imaging, including two-dimensional, Doppler, and color Doppler techniques.

transient tachypnea of the newborn (TTN) A self-limiting disorder that presents in term or near-term infants shortly after birth and is characterized by rapid respirations; it usually resolves within 24 to 48 hours.

transillumination A technique used to identify a suspected pneumothorax in the neonate. A fiberoptic light source is placed on the chest wall in a darkened room. A large pneumothorax will glow, or seem very pink and illuminated, in comparison with the other areas of the chest.

transtracheal aspiration (TTA) A sputum-collection technique designed to bypass the upper airway. After skin preparation of the anterior neck, a sterile needle is inserted directly into the trachea through the cricothyroid membrane and tracheal secretions are aspirated.

transtracheal oxygen Passing oxygen directly into the trachea. A transtracheal catheter passes from the skin of the lower neck through a tract that ends directly in the trachea. Oxygen is usually delivered at a lower flow rate because the upper airway dead space is bypassed.

transtracheal oxygen catheter A small-diameter Teflon catheter that is surgically inserted into the trachea between the second and third tracheal rings, connected to a small flange, and held in place by an adjustable chain. Oxygen supply tubing is connected directly to the catheter and delivers oxygen into the midtrachea.

transudative A classification of pleural fluid based on laboratory findings suggestive of a hydrostatic cause of pleural fluid accumulation.

trigger The signal that begins the inspiratory phase of respiration.

trigger window A period of time comprising the entire respiratory time minus a short refractory period required to reduce the risk of triggering a breath before exhalation is complete.

triglyceride The most abundant type of lipid, which functions as the body's most concentrated source of energy; its basic building blocks are a glycerol molecule and three fatty acids.

troponin A complex of three regulatory proteins that is integral to muscle contraction in skeletal and cardiac muscle, but not smooth muscle; it is useful as a diagnostic marker for various heart disorders.

tube compensation (TC) A mode of mechanical ventilation that overcomes the flow-resistive work of breathing imposed by an artificial airway; it measures the resistance of the artificial airway and applies a pressure proportional to that resistance.

tube exchanger A flexible tube used to maintain a pathway to the trachea, thereby permitting one endotracheal tube to be replaced with another.

tuberculosis (TB) An infection that arises by inhalation of *Mycobacterium tuberculum* organisms from infected, coughing individuals and manifesting with malaise, fever, or no symptoms.

tumor suppressor gene A genetic unit that is able to reverse the effect of a specific kind of mutation in certain tumors.

turbulent flow A mixture of fluid velocities in which friction has a particularly prominent effect (as opposed to laminar flow) and varies directly with the square of the flow rate; the term for friction implies greater resistance may occur at equivalent flows.

tympanic The quality of a loud, drum-like, high-pitched sound typically heard over a gastric bubble during percussion examination.

type I cells Alveolar epithelial cells that form part of the alveolocapillary complex and cover a large portion (90%) of the alveolar surface, facilitating the movement of gases across this surface.

type I error Occurs when a conclusion appears to be true but may actually be false. To avoid this possibility, *P* (probability) values are calculated to assess whether the probability of making this type of error is less than 5% ($P < .05$).

type II cells Alveolar cells that produce surfactant and surfactant-associated proteins.

type II error Occurs when a finding appears to show no effect when an effect may actually be present.

typical pneumonia Any of several pneumonias usually caused by pneumococci, but also by *Haemophilus influenzae*, *Enterobacteriaceae*, and *Staphylococcus aureus*. It is characterized by abrupt onset of chills, high fever, pleuritic chest pain, and cough productive of rusty or purulent sputum. Physical signs of consolidation such as bronchial breath sounds and inspiratory crackles are present; lobar or segmental consolidation is seen on the chest radiograph, and leukocytosis is present.

U

ultrasonic nebulizer A device that uses a piezoelectric crystal, vibrating at a high frequency, to convert electricity to sound waves, thereby creating standing waves in the liquid immediately above the transducer, disrupting the liquid surface, and forming a geyser of aerosolized droplets.

Universal Protocol A protocol developed to prevent wrong-site, wrong-procedure, and/or wrong-person surgery. The three principal components are conducting a preprocedure verification process, marking the procedure site, and performing a time-out before the procedure.

unmeasured anions Anionic proteins and other substances in serum that are not measured in routine serum electrolyte determinations but whose presence can be suspected by calculating the anion gap.

unsaturated fatty acid A naturally occurring fatty acid that has one or more double carbon–carbon bonds in its hydrocarbon chain because not all of the chain carbon atoms are saturated with hydrogen atoms.

ureter One of a pair of tubes that carry urine from the kidney to the bladder.

urethra The canal running from the bladder to the outside of the body, through which urine is eliminated.

urinary bladder The membranous sac that serves as a reservoir for urine, which it receives through the ureters and eliminates through the urethra.

uvulopalatopharyngoplasty (UPPP) The oldest and most commonly performed surgery to treat obstructive sleep apnea.

V

v wave On the central venous pressure tracing, the wave that arises from the pressure produced when the blood filling the right atrium comes up against a closed tricuspid valve. It occurs as the T wave is ending on an electrocardiogram.

valence electron An electron in the outer shell of an atom.

valved holding chamber A device used with a pressurized metered dose inhaler that consists of a spacer with a one-way valve to prevent loss of the dose.

valvular heart disease Any valvular lesion or abnormality that can be differentiated hemodynamically into two types, although a combination of both may exist: (1) stenotic lesions due to a decreased valve orifice size or impaired valve opening or (2) regurgitant lesions due to impairment of valve closure.

valvular regurgitation A condition in which a proportion of the ventricular stroke volume moves retrograde through the valve.

valvular stenosis Narrowing of a heart valve.

vapor pressure A colligative property of a solution that depends on the number of solute particles dissolved and not on chemical properties. For example, a solute added to a solvent dilutes it, displacing the solution surface's solvent particles and allowing fewer solvent particles to escape in the form of gas, thereby reducing the vapor pressure.

vehicle transmission A form of indirect contact transmission that involves transfer of an infectious agent through a contaminated intermediate object.

vein A blood vessel that carries blood back to the atria; veins are less elastic than arteries.

velocity A property of flow that determines diffusion and that is inversely proportional to the square root of the molecular weight of a substance; equivalent to the kinetic energy of a fluid.

venoarterial (VA) ECMO An extracorporeal membrane oxygenation method that returns blood to the arterial system.

venous return Filling of the heart with blood from the venous circulation.

venovenous (VV) ECMO An extracorporeal membrane oxygenation method that returns blood to the venous system.

ventilation-perfusion ($\dot{V}/\dot{Q}$) mismatch A mismatch in the amount of air and the amount of blood reaching the alveoli.

ventilation-perfusion ratio ($\dot{V}/\dot{Q}$) The relationship between alveolar ventilation and blood flow past the alveolus. Ideally, this ratio is 1; normally, it is 0.8. A decrease in this ratio results in shunt-like physiology; an increase results in dead space–like physiology.

ventilator A device designed to do all or part of the work required to ventilate or move gas into and out of the lungs.

ventilator-associated event (VAE) A term that groups all the conditions that result in a significant and sustained deterioration in oxygenation, defined as a greater than 0.2 increase in the daily minimum F_{IO_2} or an increase of at least 3 cm H_2O in the daily minimum PEEP to maintain oxygenation. It entails both infectious and noninfectious conditions. VAEs are categorized into three tiers: Tier 1—ventilator-associated condition (VAC); Tier 2—infection-related ventilator-associated complication (IVAC); and Tier 3—probable or possible ventilator-associated pneumonia (VAP).

ventilator-associated pneumonia (VAP) A new or progressive and persistent radiographic abnormality developing in a patient on mechanical ventilation, who also demonstrates one or more systemic signs (fever, leukopenia or leukocytosis, or altered mental status in those older than 70 years of age) and selected pulmonary criteria (e.g., change in respiratory secretions, new onset of cough, dyspnea, crackles, bronchial breath sounds, or worsening oxygenation).

ventilator-induced lung injury (VILI) Damage to the lungs sustained during mechanical ventilation and caused by any of several factors, including alveolar overdistention and cyclical opening of an alveolus during inhalation and closure during exhalation.

ventilator pattern The possible breathing sequences with a mechanical ventilator, based on two control variables (volume control and pressure control) and three breath sequences (continuous mandatory ventilation, intermittent mandatory ventilation, and continuous spontaneous ventilation).

ventilatory equivalent The relationship between minute ventilation and oxygen consumption or carbon dioxide production.

ventral respiratory group A group of respiratory-related neurons located in the medulla oblongata that include inspiratory and expiratory neurons. The inspiratory neurons send efferent impulses to the diaphragm and external intercostal muscles; the expiratory neurons send efferent impulses to the internal intercostal and abdominal muscles.

ventricular interdependence Interaction between the left ventricle (LV) and the right ventricle (RV) both in systole and diastole through alterations in systemic and pulmonary venous return, LV and RV dimensional changes, and functional changes.

ventriculography Radiographic examination of a ventricle of the heart after injection of a radiopaque contrast medium.

Venturi principle A physical rule stating that a pressure drop across an obstruction can be restored provided that the angle of divergence is less than 15 degrees.

veracity The principle by which the healthcare practitioner tells the patient the truth.

verbal expression In communication, the use of language, jargon, choice of words or questions, voice tone and quality, and feedback.

Vesalius, Andreas (1514–1564) A Renaissance-era researcher and author of a well-known anatomy text.

vesicular breath sounds Low-pitched, low-intensity sounds heard over healthy lung issue.

vibration therapy A maneuver used as part of airway clearance that assists patients in mobilizing secretions from the lower respiratory tract.

video laryngoscope A device that provides a digitally produced, real-time view of the larynx without having to directly view this structure through the patient's open mouth. The image is displayed on a screen and can prove useful in difficult airway situations.

videobronchoscope A bronchoscope that includes a charge-coupled device that forms an image on a video monitor during its use.

viral pneumonia An uncommon but often severe pneumonia caused by any of the following viruses: influenza, parainfluenza, respiratory syncytial virus, cytomegalovirus, adenovirus, measles, varicella zoster, herpes simplex, Epstein-Barr, and hantavirus.

virologic study A method designed to determine the presence of and identify viruses.

viruses Small infectious agents that replicate only within cells of living organisms.

visceral pleura The inner layer of the pleura adjacent to the external lung tissue.

viscosity Force applied to interaction between adjacent fluid molecules; also, the internal friction of a fluid, which is independent of the density of that fluid.

vital capacity The maximum volume of gas that can be exhaled from the lungs after a maximal inspiration or maximum volume inhaled from a point of maximal exhalation.

vitamin Any of a group of organic substances essential in small quantities to normal metabolism.

volume control (VC) Breath type in which the ventilator controls the inspiratory flow and tidal volume; the tidal volume in this mode is delivered regardless of resistance or compliance.

voxels Volume elements that make up a computed tomography slice image.

W

weaning parameters Measurements made to determine when liberation from the ventilator might be possible.

wellness A multidimensional state of being describing the existence of positive health in an individual as exemplified by quality of life and a sense of well-being.

Westermark sign Decreased vascularity in one lung causing a unilateral increase in radiographic lucency; it suggests the presence of a large pulmonary embolus.

wheezes A form of rhonchus characterized by either a high-pitched musical-quality sound or a low-pitched snoring-type sound. It is caused by high-velocity airflow through a narrowed airway.

whispered pectoriloquy A voice sound heard during auscultation of the lungs. With lung consolidation, whispered sounds are louder than are heard in nonconsolidated lungs.

Wood units A simplified measurement of vascular resistance that uses pressures instead of more complicated units. For example, pulmonary vascular resistance is measured by subtracting the pulmonary capillary wedge pressure from the mean pulmonary arterial pressure and dividing by the cardiac output in liters per minute.

work The amount of energy transferred by a force acting through a distance; for work of breathing, the amount of pressure required to deliver a volume of gas into the lungs.

work of breathing (WOB) A measurement of the amount of pressure required to inflate the lungs; normal value is 0.3 to 0.7 joule per liter of tidal volume.

work rate The rate at which work is performed or energy is converted from one form to another.

X

xenograft A skin graft in which the skin being used comes from a donor (usually a cadaver). This technique brings the rise of rejection of foreign tissue.

Index

Note: The letter *f* indicates a figure on the page. The letter *t* indicates a table.

B

C

D

E

F

G

H

J

P

S

T

U

V